Rubin's
Pathology

MECHANISMS OF HUMAN DISEASE

Eighth Edition

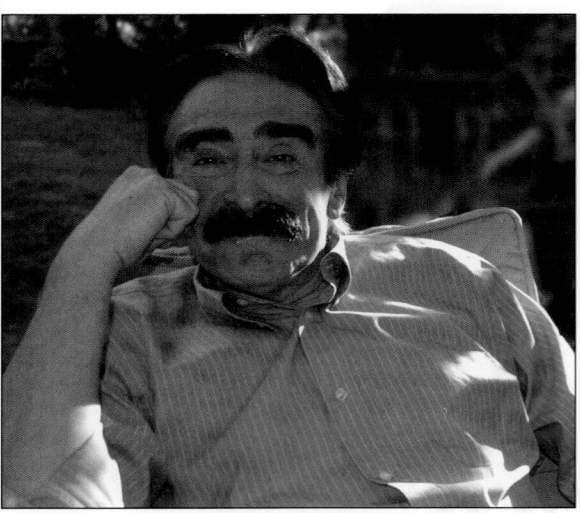

Editor
David S. Strayer, MD, PhD
Professor
Department of Pathology, Anatomy and Cell Biology
Sidney Kimmel Cancer Center
Thomas Jefferson University
Philadelphia, Pennsylvania

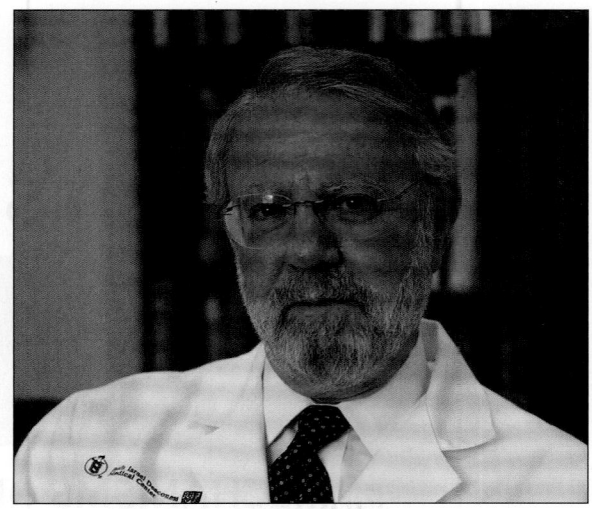

Editor
Jeffrey E. Saffitz, MD, PhD
Mallinckrodt Professor of Medicine
Harvard Medical School
Chairman, Department of Pathology
Beth Israel Deaconess Medical Center
Boston, Massachusetts

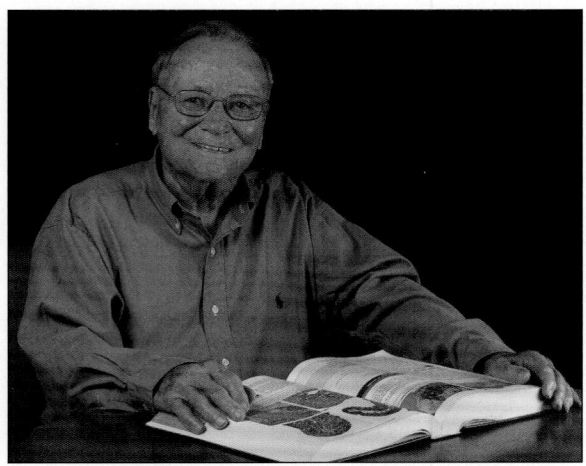

Founder and Consulting Editor
Emanuel Rubin, MD
Distinguished Professor of Pathology, Anatomy and Cell Biology
Sidney Kimmel Medical College of Thomas Jefferson University
Philadelphia, Pennsylvania

Rubin's
Pathology
MECHANISMS OF HUMAN DISEASE
Eighth Edition

EDITORS

David S. Strayer, MD, PhD

Professor
Department of Pathology, Anatomy and Cell Biology
Sidney Kimmel Cancer Center
Thomas Jefferson University
Philadelphia, Pennsylvania

Jeffrey E. Saffitz, MD, PhD

Mallinckrodt Professor of Medicine
Harvard Medical School
Chairman, Department of Pathology
Beth Israel Deaconess Medical Center
Boston, Massachusetts

FOUNDER AND CONSULTING EDITOR

Emanuel Rubin, MD

Distinguished Professor of Pathology, Anatomy and Cell Biology
Sidney Kimmel Medical College of Thomas Jefferson University
Philadelphia, Pennsylvania

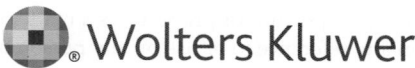

Philadelphia • Baltimore • New York • London
Buenos Aires • Hong Kong • Sydney • Tokyo

Acquisitions Editor: Crystal Taylor
Product Development Editor: Andrea Vosburgh
Editorial Coordinator: Kerry McShane
Marketing Manager: Jason Oberacker
Production Project Manager: Bridgett Dougherty
Design Coordinator: Holly McLaughlin
Art Director: Jennifer Clements
Manufacturing Coordinator: Margie Orzech
Prepress Vendor: Aptara, Inc.

8th edition

Library of Congress Cataloging-in-Publication Data available upon request.
978-1-4963-8614-4

Library of Congress Control Number: 2019908240

shop.lww.com

CCS0919

We dedicate this edition of *Rubin's Pathology* to our families, who patiently put up with our long hours, and provided encouragement, emotional sustenance, and endless devotion in the face of our work on this volume; to our colleagues and residents whose constant challenging and curiosity helped inform our efforts and focus them on the needs of today's and tomorrow's medical students and professionals; to our chapter authors, who worked hard to rewrite and revise this text, and whose selfless efforts make this book what it is; and to students everywhere, in the hopes that they, their careers and, ultimately, their patients may benefit from this volume's contents.

On a personal note, this 8th edition is also dedicated to the loving memory of Marlene Strayer, PhD. I (DS), who have made a career of putting words on paper (or computer screen)—find myself at a loss; I am unable to express how much her love, wit, and understanding were the cornerstone of my life, family, and career, and how they made my involvement with this textbook possible. Everything about her was beautiful and loving. Even as her death and suffering from terrible disease leaves me and my family diminished, I cherish every moment we spent together and try to take inspiration from her courage, warmth, and kindness.

Contributors

Ronnie M. Abraham, MD
Dermatopathologist
Western Diagnostic Services Laboratory
Santa Barbara, California

Michael F. Allard, BSc, MD, FRCPC
Professor and Head of Pathology and Laboratory Medicine
University of British Columbia
Cardiovascular Pathologist
Pathology and Laboratory Medicine
St. Paul's Hospital
Vancouver, British Columbia, Canada

Jeffrey P. Baliff, MD
Clinical Assistant Professor
Department of Pathology, Anatomy and Cell Biology
Sidney Kimmel Medical College of Thomas Jefferson University
Philadelphia, Pennsylvania

Leomar Y. Ballester, MD, PhD
Assistant Professor
Pathology and Laboratory Medicine
University of Texas Health Science Center at Houston
Houston, Texas

Mary Beth Beasley, MD
Professor of Pathology
Mount Sinai Medical Center
New York, New York

John L. Berk, MD
Assistant Director
Amyloidosis Center/Department of Medicine
Boston University School of Medicine
Associate Professor of Medicine
Department of Medicine
Boston Medical Center
Boston, Massachusetts

Parul Bhargava, MD
Professor
Department of Laboratory Medicine
Medical Director, Clinical Laboratories at
    Moffitt-Long
University of California, San Francisco
San Francisco, California

Thomas W. Bouldin, MD
Professor
Department of Pathology and Laboratory Medicine
University of North Carolina at Chapel Hill
Attending Pathologist
University of North Carolina Hospitals
Chapel Hill, North Carolina

Christine R. Bryke, MD
Instructor
Department of Pathology
Harvard Medical School
Medical Director
Cytogenetics Laboratory
Department of Pathology
Beth Israel Deaconess Medical Center
Boston, Massachusetts

Diane L. Carlson, MD
Affiliate Associate Professor
Department of Pathology
Florida Atlantic University College of Medicine
Boca Raton, Florida
Director
Breast and Head and Neck Pathology
Cleveland Clinic Florida
Weston, Florida

Emily Y. Chu, MD, PhD
Assistant Professor
Dermatology, Pathology, and Laboratory Medicine
Perelman School of Medicine, University of Pennsylvania
Hospital of the University of Pennsylvania
Philadelphia, Pennsylvania

Philip L. Cohen, MD
Professor Emeritus
Department of Medicine, Section of Rheumatology
Lewis Katz School of Medicine at Temple University
Philadelphia, Pennsylvania

Myron I. Cybulsky, MD
Professor
Department of Laboratory Medicine and Pathology
University of Toronto
Staff Pathologist
Laboratory Medicine Program
University Health Network
Toronto, Ontario, Canada

Jeffrey M. Davidson, PhD
Professor
Department of Pathology, Microbiology and Immunology
Vanderbilt University Medical Center
Nashville, Tennessee

Elizabeth G. Demicco, MD, PhD
Associate Professor
Department of Laboratory Medicine and Pathobiology
University of Toronto
Staff Pathologist
Department of Pathology and Laboratory Medicine
Mount Sinai Hospital
Toronto, Ontario, Canada

Luisa A. DiPietro, DDS, PhD
Professor
Periodontics Department
University of Illinois at Chicago
Chicago, Illinois

David E. Elder, MD, ChB, FRCPA
Professor of Pathology and Laboratory Medicine
Hospital of the University of Pennsylvania
Philadelphia, Pennsylvania

Alina Dulau Florea, MD
Hematopathologist
Staff Physician
Department of Laboratory Medicine
Clinical Center
National Institutes of Health
Bethesda, Maryland

Gregory N. Fuller, MD, PhD
Professor and Chief Neuropathologist
Department of Pathology
The University of Texas MD Anderson Cancer Center
Houston, Texas

Joaquín J. García, MD
Associate Professor
Mayo Clinic School of Medicine
Vice Chair, Anatomic Pathology
Department of Laboratory Medicine and Pathology
Mayo Clinic
Rochester, Minnesota

Roberto A. Garcia, MD
Associate Attending Pathologist
Pathology and Laboratory Medicine
Hospital for Special Surgery
New York, New York

Jonathan N. Glickman, MD, PhD
Associate Professor
Department of Pathology
Harvard Medical School
Director of Surgical Pathology
Beth Israel Deaconess Medical Center
Boston, Massachusetts

Krzysztof Glomski, MD, PhD
Resident
Department of Pathology
Massachusetts General Hospital
Boston, Massachusetts

J. Clay Goodman, MD, FAAN
Professor
Departments of Pathology and Laboratory Medicine, and
    Neurology
Baylor College of Medicine
Houston, Texas

Avrum I. Gotlieb, MDCM, FRCPC
Professor
Department of Laboratory Medicine and
    Pathobiology
University of Toronto
Toronto, Ontario, Canada

Jennifer L. Hammers, DO
Cyril H. Wecht and Pathology Associates
Pittsburgh, Pennsylvania

Kim HooKim, MD
Assistant Professor
Department of Pathology, Anatomy and
    Cell Biology
Thomas Jefferson University
Philadelphia, Pennsylvania

S. David Hudnall, MD
Professor
Department of Pathology and Laboratory Medicine
Yale University School of Medicine
Attending Hematopathologist
Department of Pathology and Laboratory Medicine
Yale New Haven Hospital
New Haven, Connecticut

J. Charles Jennette, MD
Kenneth M. Brinkhous Distinguished Professor and Chair
Department of Pathology and Laboratory Medicine
School of Medicine
Chief of Pathology and Laboratory Medicine Services
UNC Hospitals
Executive Director, UNC Nephropathology Division
University of North Carolina at Chapel Hill
Chapel Hill, North Carolina

Sergio A. Jimenez, MD
Professor and Co-Director
Jefferson Institute of Molecular Medicine
Director, Connective Tissue Diseases Section
Associate Director, Joan and Joel Rosenbloom Center for
    Fibrotic Diseases,
Director, Scleroderma Center
Thomas Jefferson University
Philadelphia, Pennsylvania

Lawrence C. Kenyon, MD, PhD
Associate Professor
Department of Pathology, Anatomy and Cell Biology
Thomas Jefferson University
Surgical Pathologist and Neuropathologist
Department of Pathology
Thomas Jefferson University Hospital
Philadelphia, Pennsylvania

Michael J. Klein, MD
Professor
Pathology and Laboratory Medicine
Weill Cornell School of Medicine
Pathologist in Chief Emeritus
Pathology and Laboratory Medicine
Hospital for Special Surgery
New York, New York

David S. Klimstra, MD
Professor
Pathology and Laboratory Medicine
Weill Cornell Medical College
Attending Pathologist and Chairman
Department of Pathology
Memorial Sloan Kettering Cancer Center
New York, New York

David Benner Lombard, MD, PhD
Associate Professor
Department of Pathology and Institute of Gerontology
Attending Pathologist
Department of Pathology
University of Michigan
Ann Arbor, Michigan

Scott B. Lovitch, MD, PhD
Instructor
Department of Pathology
Harvard Medical School
Associate Pathologist
Department of Pathology
Brigham and Women's Hospital
Boston, Massachusetts

Peter A. McCue, MD
Professor
Department of Pathology
Thomas Jefferson University
Philadelphia, Pennsylvania

Bruce Maxwell McManus, MD, PhD
Professor
Department of Pathology and Laboratory Medicine
University of British Columbia
Chief Executive Officer
PROOF Centre of Excellence
St. Paul's Hospital
Vancouver, British Columbia, Canada

Anna Marie Mulligan, MB BCh, MSc, FRCPath (UK)
Associate Professor
Department of Laboratory Medicine and Pathobiology
University of Toronto
Staff Pathologist
Laboratory Medicine Program
University Health Network
Toronto, Ontario, Canada

George L. Mutter, MD
Professor of Pathology
Department of Pathology
Harvard Medical School
Pathologist
Division of Women's and Perinatal Pathology
Brigham and Women's Hospital
Boston, Massachusetts

Vania Nosé, MD, PhD
Professor
Department of Pathology
Harvard Medical School
Associate Chief, Anatomic and Molecular Pathology
Department of Pathology
Massachusetts General Hospital
Boston, Massachusetts

Frances P. O'Malley, MB, FRCPC
Professor Emerita
Department of Laboratory Medicine and Pathobiology
University of Toronto
Consulting Pathologist
Department of Laboratory Medicine
Humber River Hospital
Toronto, Ontario, Canada

Jaime Prat, MD, PhD, FRCPath
Professor of Pathology
Department of Pathology
Autonomous University of Barcelona Medical School
Senior Consultant
Department of Pathology
Hospital de la Santa Creu i Sant Pau
Barcelona, Spain

Gordana Raca, MD, PhD
Associate Professor of Pathology, USC Keck School of Medicine
Director of Clinical Cytogenomics, Center for Personalized
    Medicine
Department of Pathology and Laboratory Medicine
    Children's Hospital Los Angeles
Los Angeles, California

Daniel Remick, MD
Chair and Professor
Department of Pathology and Laboratory Medicine
Boston University School of Medicine
Chief
Pathology and Laboratory Medicine
Boston Medical Center
Boston, Massachusetts

Emanuel Rubin, MD
Professor and Chair Emeritus
Department of Pathology, Anatomy and Cell Biology
Sidney Kimmel Medical College of Thomas Jefferson University
Philadelphia, Pennsylvania

Jeffrey E. Saffitz, MD, PhD
Mallinckrodt Professor of Pathology
Department of Pathology
Harvard Medical School
Pathologist-in-Chief
Department of Pathology
Beth Israel Deaconess Medical Center
Boston, Massachusetts

Barbara A. Sampson, MD, PhD
Chief Medical Examiner
Office of Chief Medical Examiner
Chairman and Professor
Forensic Medicine
NYU Langone Medical Center
New York, New York

Vaishali Sanchorawala, MD
Director
Amyloidosis Center
Boston University School of Medicine
Professor
Department of Medicine
Boston Medical Center
Boston, Massachusetts

Alan Lewis Schiller, MD
Founding Chair and Professor
Department of Pathology
Nova Southeastern University
Fort Lauderdale, Florida
Director—Pathology Residency
Department of Pathology
Kendall Regional Medical Center
Miami, Florida
Professor and Chair Emeritus of Pathology
Icahn School of Medicine at Mount Sinai
New York, New York

David A. Schwartz, MD, MS Hyg, FCAP
Clinical Professor
Department of Pathology
Medical College of Georgia
Augusta University
Augusta, Georgia

Gregory C. Sephel, PhD
Associate Professor
Department of Pathology, Microbiology and Immunology
Vanderbilt University School of Medicine
Director, Clinical Pathology
Department of Pathology and Laboratory Medicine
Veterans Affairs Tennessee Valley Healthcare System
Nashville, Tennessee

Harsharan Kaur Singh, MD
Professor of Pathology and Laboratory Medicine
Director, Electron Microscopy Services, UNC Health Care
Associate Director, Division of Nephropathology
Department of Pathology and Laboratory Medicine
The University of North Carolina at Chapel Hill
Chapel Hill, North Carolina

Elias S. Siraj, MD, Dr Med
Professor and Chief
Endocrinology and Metabolic Disorders
Eastern Virginia Medical School
Norfolk, Virginia

Edward Benjamin Stelow, MD
Professor
Department of Pathology
University of Virginia
Charlottesville, Virginia

Isaac Ely Stillman, MD
Associate Professor
Department of Pathology
Harvard Medical School
Director, Renal Pathology Service
Department of Pathology
Beth Israel Deaconess Medical Center
Boston, Massachusetts

David S. Strayer, MD, PhD
Professor
Department of Pathology, Anatomy and Cell Biology
Sidney Kimmel Cancer Center
Thomas Jefferson University
Philadelphia, Pennsylvania

Arief Antonius Suriawinata, MD
Professor
Department of Pathology and Laboratory Medicine
Geisel School of Medicine at Dartmouth
Hanover, New Hampshire
Section Chief of Anatomic Pathology
Department of Pathology and Laboratory Medicine
Dartmouth-Hitchcock Medical Center
Lebanon, New Hampshire

Nasreen A. Syed, MD
Clinical Professor
Departments of Ophthalmology and Pathology
Director
F.C. Blodi Eye Pathology Laboratory
Department of Ophthalmology and Visual Sciences
University of Iowa
Iowa City, Iowa

Swan N. Thung, MD
Professor
Department of Pathology
Icahn School of Medicine at Mount Sinai
Director of Liver Pathology Division
Department of Pathology
Mount Sinai Medical Center
New York, New York

William D. Travis, MD
Professor of Pathology
Department of Pathology
Weill Medical College of Cornell University
Attending Thoracic Pathologist
Department of Pathology
Memorial Sloan Kettering Cancer Center
New York, New York

Jeffrey S. Warren, MD
Aldred S. Warthin Endowed Professor
Department of Pathology
University of Michigan
Director, Clinical Immunology
Department of Pathology
Michigan Medicine
Ann Arbor, Michigan

Olga K. Weinberg, MD
Assistant Professor
Department of Pathology
Harvard Medical School
Director of Hematopathology and Flow Cytometry Lab
Department of Pathology
Boston Children's Hospital
Boston, Massachusetts

Kevin Jon Williams, MD
Professor of Medicine and Chief, Section of Endocrinology,
    Diabetes, and Metabolism
Department of Medicine
Lewis Katz School of Medicine at Temple University
Philadelphia, Pennsylvania
Visiting Professor
Department of Molecular and Clinical Medicine
Sahlgrenska Academy of the University of Gothenburg
Gothenburg, Sweden

Bobby Yanagawa, MD, PhD, FRCSC
Assistant Professor
Department of Medicine
University of Toronto
Surgeon
Division of Cardiac Surgery
St. Michael's Hospital
Toronto, Ontario, Canada

Preface

A little over 100 years ago, in 1910, Abraham Flexner published a report assessing medical education in America. He found it wanting. Severely. Many medical schools had failed to base their instruction on the sound scientific principles that underlie medicine. Many were proprietary, run to enrich a small number of people, rather than to teach medicine. Student preparation for the profession of medicine was poor, owing to inadequate scientific instruction, insufficient experience with patient care, and other shortcomings. Within a short time, about 1/3 of US medical colleges closed. Medical licensure examinations became the norm. A remarkable era of scientific discovery followed and continues, providing medicine with the intellectual underpinnings that have made a massive impact on human health, conquered or diminished societal impact of many diseases, and advanced our understanding of both normal and abnormal human conditions.

Our appreciation of chemistry and biochemistry, cell and molecular biology, physiology and pathophysiology, population and environmental sciences, pathology and microbiology, genetics and genomics, and so much else has mushroomed. This growth of knowledge and understanding has made possible hitherto unimagined therapies that turned once inexorably fatal illnesses into routine matters that are addressed cavalierly in everyday medical practice.

It has led to vaccines that have eliminated—or all but eliminated—scourges that killed and destroyed the lives of untold millions in the past. Work on preventing diseases will hopefully continue—and continue to build on—their path to basic scientific discovery and development, despite those segments of society that loudly distort, disparage, and downplay much of the science that has prevented so much suffering and saved so many lives.

In medical education, this continuing explosive growth of our understanding of human health and disease, has begun to seem formidable and overwhelming. Thus, it has become fashionable to take the scientific foundations of medicine for granted, and to look at the science that has made so much possible and to dismiss it as dry, arcane, and of only peripheral relevance to modern day-to-day patient care. This urge in teaching medicine to treat basic medical sciences like geology or astrophysics—serious subjects, to be sure, but too distant from the business of seeing patients to merit significant attention—comes at a time when there is more than ever to know. These trends concern us.

They also come at considerable cost. Established diseases are increasingly better understood and new ones arise. Therapeutics relies increasingly on meshing basic biochemistry, pathophysiology, genetics, and molecular biology, and is becoming ever more precise and sophisticated in targeting specific steps and mediators of disease. This progressively greater reliance on the foundation provided by basic medical sciences requires medical practitioners to understand in greater—not less—depth the nature of the diseases they treat and the scientific principles that they apply in treating them.

It may be tempting to dismiss investing energy in understanding disease pathogenesis and mechanisms of therapeutics to an annoying, fusty professorial insistence on memorizing minutiae. But each patient is an individual. If one is diagnosing and treating people who are ill, one should have a good idea of what one is doing and why, rather than—as is a current trend—following formulaic scripts designed by someone else for generic patients. (Understanding what you're doing is, of course, a good idea under any circumstances—and especially when treating patients.) Only then can a physician understand symptoms and clinical presentations. Only then can appropriate treatments be brought to bear. Only then will consequences of those treatments make sense, to be looked for, evaluated, and addressed appropriately. At a time when it is estimated that roughly a quarter million deaths in the United States annually result directly from unanticipated effects of increasingly sophisticated medical interventions, it cannot possibly be more important for doctors to understand the pathogenesis of the diseases that afflict their patients, how therapies are supposed to achieve beneficial results, and what the ramifications—good and untoward—of those therapies are.

This is a textbook of Pathology. As physicians, our adversary is disease. In order to help developing physicians, we hope to nourish their understanding of what they are up against, believing that professional strength and effectiveness reside in that understanding. We focus here, as the subtitle indicates, on mechanisms of human disease. Our goal is to help future internists, pediatricians, surgeons, and others prepare for their specialties by acquainting them with their opponents and how they behave: how diseases develop and how they affect patients. We provide a foundation on which future clinicians of all specialties can build.

Pathology is well positioned for this task, since, as a clinical specialty, it basically aims to tell stories. Pathology is not just a compilation of burdensome, isolated facts, or hazy and nameless pathways to be memorized and promptly forgotten. It is the drama of inevitable human frailty and mortality that affects each of us, presented as concepts and principles to understand and apply. It is not only about disease, but also about what people do to each other. Hence, the importance of our discussions of environmental and forensic pathology.

Although it may be easily overlooked amid the time and financial pressures of modern medical practice, each patient's medical history is a tale, beginning with the array of social, environmental, familial, and other influences that bear on a person's life and health, and then continuing to the current illness and its course. Like the string around a package, Pathology tries to make sense out of these elements—to link them so as to turn a patient's presentation and course into an intelligible narrative.

In this vein, we try to give students of medicine the background they need to prepare them to diagnose and treat patients—choosing to present here what is basically important for all doctors, and to put aside topics best left to more specialized publications. Still, what there is to understand remains overwhelming. We therefore have tried to focus on what students of medicine *must* know in order to become good doctors, to prepare for a lifetime of professional learning and to understand how advances in medical sciences will affect their patients. Appreciating what a good doctor must understand, as well as students' limited time and energy, we have tried to avoid being comprehensive, preferring instead to be useful.

Our approach is integrative. Many processes and diseases affect multiple organ systems, and are best understood as such. It does not suffice, for example, only to describe aging as a series of separate effects on cells in culture, or on the brain or cardiovascular system. As we can attest from personal experience, aging—apart from the dubious wisdom that some people believe accompanies it—affects almost everything a person does, and what he or she can and cannot do. Its effects on one organ system are linked inextricably to its effects on others.

Accordingly, we include a section on systemic processes—aging, autoimmune diseases, sepsis and pregnancy, as well as amyloidosis and obesity, diabetes and their consequences—that affect whole human beings, beyond isolated effects on kidneys, lungs, or joints. These integrated discussions should help to present, and to understand, these processes and their effects on health. Organ-specific chapters still cover respective manifestations of these processes.

Traditional, printed textbooks are being supplanted by texts on portable devices. Medical school courses prepare their own syllabi. Online information and other resources are abundantly available (if not always reliable). Many faculty feel their time and energy are more profitably invested seeing patients, doing research, administering. Some students may feel that the key to navigating medicine is to plow through quick recall question-and-answer compendia endlessly, rather than developing understanding by reading systematic discussions (like this).

Here, experts from around the world present a thorough but digestible understanding of how diseases occur and, we hope, stimulate excitement for medical advances yet to come. Medical knowledge is always in flux. This new edition is quite different from its predecessors. Many chapters have been rewritten or extensively revised. Timely topics, like climate change, have been added. New authors in 16 chapters join the outstanding contributors whose continuing efforts have been so valuable, and exemplify this goal. The dedicated and selfless work of all these authors is the backbone of this textbook. We cannot thank them enough.

We emphasize what is understood, but also note the limits of our current knowledge. Hopefully, inquisitive minds will find here a door to further exploration, and students and colleagues will share the excitement of discovery that we have been privileged to experience in our education and careers.

Rubin's Pathology has always been characterized by its stylistic consistency and readability, its strikingly visual presentation, its effective application of mechanistic drawings and color to its portrayal of disease mechanisms, and its focus on currency and clinical relevance in all material presented. Included instructional ancillaries are designed to help students learn, and to help teachers teach. The editors and authors are determined to achieve these goals, and believe that medical education can best be provided in this format.

David S. Strayer, MD, PhD
Philadelphia, 2019

Jeffrey E. Saffitz, MD, PhD
Boston, 2019

Acknowledgments

Many dedicated people, too numerous to list, provided insight that made this 8th edition of *Rubin's Pathology* possible. The editors would like especially to thank the managing and editorial staff at Wolters Kluwer, and in particular Crystal Taylor, Nancy Dickson, and Andrea Vosburgh, whose encouragement and support throughout all phases of this endeavor have both touched us personally and also been a key to the successful publication of this text and its ancillaries.

The editors also acknowledge contributions made by our colleagues who participated in writing previous editions and those who offered suggestions and ideas for the current edition.

Stuart A. Aaronson
Mohammad Alomari
Adam Bagg
Karoly Balogh
Sue Bartow
Douglas P. Bennett
Marluce Bibbo
Hugh Bonner
Patrick J. Buckley
Lindas A. Cannizzaro
Stephen W. Chensue
Daniel H. Connor
Jeffrey Cossman
John E. Craighead
Mary Cunnane
Ivan Damjanov
Giulia DeFalco
Hormuz Ehya
Joseph C. Fantone
John L. Farber
Kevin Furlong
Antonio Giordano
Barry J. Goldstein
Leana A. Guerin
Stanley R. Hamiliton

Terrence J. Harrist
Philip N. Hawkins
Arthur P. Hays
Steven K. Herrine
Kendra Iskander
Serge Jabbour
Robert B. Jennings
Kent J. Johnson
Anthony A. Killeen
Robert Kisilevsky
Gordan K. Klintworth
William D. Kocher
Robert J. Kurman
Ernest A. Lack
Shauying Li
Amber Liu
Antonio Martinez-Hernandez
Steven McKenzie
Wolfgang J. Mergner
Maria J. Merino
Marc Micozzi
Frank Mitros
Hedwig S. Murphy
George L. Mutter
Victor J. Navarro

Adebeye O. Osunkoya
Juan Palazzo
Stephen Peiper
Robert O. Peterson
Roger J. Pomerantz
Martha Quezado
Timothy R. Quinn
Stanley J. Robboy
Raphael Rubin
Brian Schapiro
Roland Schwarting
Stephen M. Schwartz
Benjamin H. Spargo
Charles Steenbergen, Jr.
Craig A. Storm
Steven L. Teitelbaum
Ann D. Thor
John Q. Trojanowski
Benjamin F. Trump
Ricardo Valdez
Jianzhou Wang
Beverly Y. Wang
Bruce M. Wenig
Mary Zutter

Contents

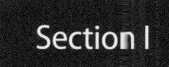

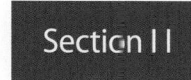

Section II — Pathogenesis of Systemic Conditions

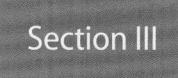

Section III — Diseases of Individual Organ Systems

Mechanisms of Disease

David S. Strayer, Jeffrey E. Saffitz

To understand disease, one must begin by studying how cells are injured, and the consequences of cell injury. One then progresses to how tissues are injured and the consequences of that injury, etc. This study begins by recognizing that cells sustain themselves in a hostile environment: they must generate energy and so have to maintain a structural and functional barrier between themselves and their surroundings. Maintaining that barrier's structural and functional integrity requires endless vigilance. The **plasma membrane** does this by:

■ keeping a constant internal ionic composition against very large chemical gradients between interior and exterior compartments.
■ selectively admitting some molecules while excluding or extruding others.
■ providing a structural envelope to contain the cell's informational, synthetic, and catabolic constituents.

■ housing signal transduction molecules that communicate with each other and link the cell's external and internal milieus.

Cells have to adapt to fluctuating environmental conditions, like changes in temperature, solute concentrations, oxygen supply, noxious agents, etc. The evolution of multicellular organisms eased the precarious lot of individual cells by establishing controlled extracellular environments, in which temperature, ionic content, availability of oxygen and nutrients, and so on, remain relatively constant. It also permitted the luxury of cell differentiation for such diverse functions as energy storage (glycogen in hepatocytes, lipids in adipocytes), communication (neurons), contractile activity (heart muscle), protein synthesis for export (pancreas, endocrine cells), absorption (intestine) and defenses from foreign invaders (immune system).

Notwithstanding such adaptations, changes in an organism's internal and external environments strain the tranquility of its constituent cells. *Patterns of response to such stresses constitute the cellular basis of disease.* If an insult exceeds a cell's adaptive capacity, that cell dies. A cell exposed to persistent sublethal injury has limited available responses, expression of which we interpret as cell injury. *Thus, pathology begins with injury to cells and organs and the consequences of such injuries.*

REVERSIBLE CELL AND TISSUE INJURY

To deal with shifts in environmental conditions, cells have ion channels that open or close. Cells detoxify harmful chemicals. They store energy as fat or glycogen which may be mobilized when needed. Their catabolic processes allow them to segregate internal particulate materials. When environmental changes exceed a cell's capacity to maintain homeostasis, we recognize acute cell injury. If the stress is removed in time, or if the cell can withstand the assault, the damage is reversible and complete structural and functional integrity is restored. Thus, when circulation to the heart is interrupted for under 30 minutes, restored blood supply allows repair of structural damage and recovery of function. Cells can also be exposed to persistent sublethal stress, as in skin that is repeatedly irritated mechanically or bronchial mucosa exposed to tobacco smoke. In that setting, cells have time to adapt to nonlethal injury in several ways, each of which has a morphologic counterpart.

On the other hand, a severe insult may cause irreversible injury and cell death. The "point of no return," at which reversible injury becomes irreversible, is not known.

Hydropic Swelling Is a Reversible Increase in Cell Volume

In hydropic swelling, increased cellular water content causes the cell to swell and the cytoplasm to become enlarged and pale. The nucleus remains normally situated (Fig. 1-1). Hydropic swelling reflects acute, reversible cell injury, caused by diverse stimuli, such as chemical and biologic toxins, viral or bacterial infections, ischemia, or excessive heat or cold.

In hydropic swelling, the number of organelles remains constant, but they appear to be dispersed in a larger volume. The excess fluid accumulates mainly in endoplasmic reticulum (ER) cisternae. These are conspicuously dilated, presumably because ionic shifts bring water into this compartment (Fig. 1-2).

Hydropic swelling occurs when the cell cannot control ionic concentrations in the cytoplasm, which in turn leads to impaired cellular volume regulation. This dysregulation, particularly for sodium, involves three components: (1) the plasma membrane, (2) the plasma membrane sodium (Na^+) pump, and (3) adenosine triphosphate (ATP). An intact plasma membrane prevents gradient-driven ion flows: especially Na^+ flow from the extracellular fluid into the cell, and potassium (K^+) flow out of the cell. The barrier to sodium is imperfect and its relative leakiness permits some passive entry of sodium into the cell. To compensate for this intrusion, the energy-dependent, plasma membrane

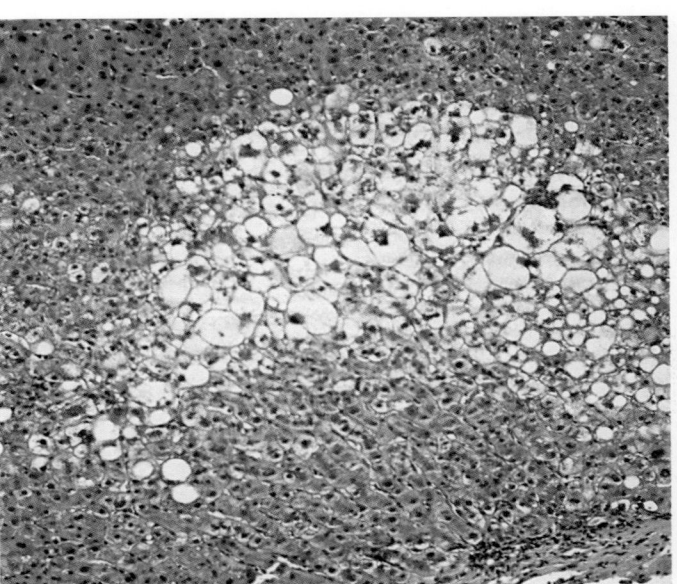

FIGURE 1-1. Hydropic swelling. The liver from a patient with toxic hepatic injury shows severe hydropic swelling in the centrilobular zone. In affected hepatocytes, the cytoplasm is distended by excess fluid and the nuclei remain centrally situated.

sodium pump (Na^+/K^+-ATPase), which is fueled by ATP, extrudes sodium from the cell. Noxious agents may interfere with this membrane-regulated process by (1) increasing plasma membrane permeability to Na^+, to a point that exceeds the pump's ability to expel the ion; (2) damaging the pump directly; or (3) depriving the pump of its fuel by interfering with ATP synthesis. In any event, if Na^+ accumulates within the cell, intracellular water must also increase, in order to maintain isosmotic conditions. The cell then swells.

Subcellular Changes in Reversibly Injured Cells

- **Endoplasmic reticulum (ER):** In hydropic swelling, ER cisternae become distended by fluid (Fig. 1-2B). Membrane-bound polysomes may disaggregate and detach from the surface of the rough ER (Fig. 1-2C).
- **Mitochondria:** In some forms of acute injury, particularly ischemia (poor oxygen delivery by the blood; see below), mitochondria swell (Fig. 1-2D). This is due to dissipation of the mitochondrial energy gradient (membrane potential), which impairs volume control. These effects are fully reversible on recovery.
- **Plasma membrane:** Blebs of plasma membrane—focal extrusions of the cytoplasm—are occasionally noted. They can detach from the membrane into the external environment without impairing cell viability.
- **Nucleus:** Reversible injury to the nucleus manifests mainly as segregation of fibrillar and granular nucleolar constituents. Sometimes, the granular component is diminished, leaving only a fibrillar core.

These changes in cell organelles (Fig. 1-3) impair cell functions (e.g., they reduce protein synthesis, impair energy production). *Once the stress that caused the reversible injury has dissipated, by definition, the cell returns to its normal state.*

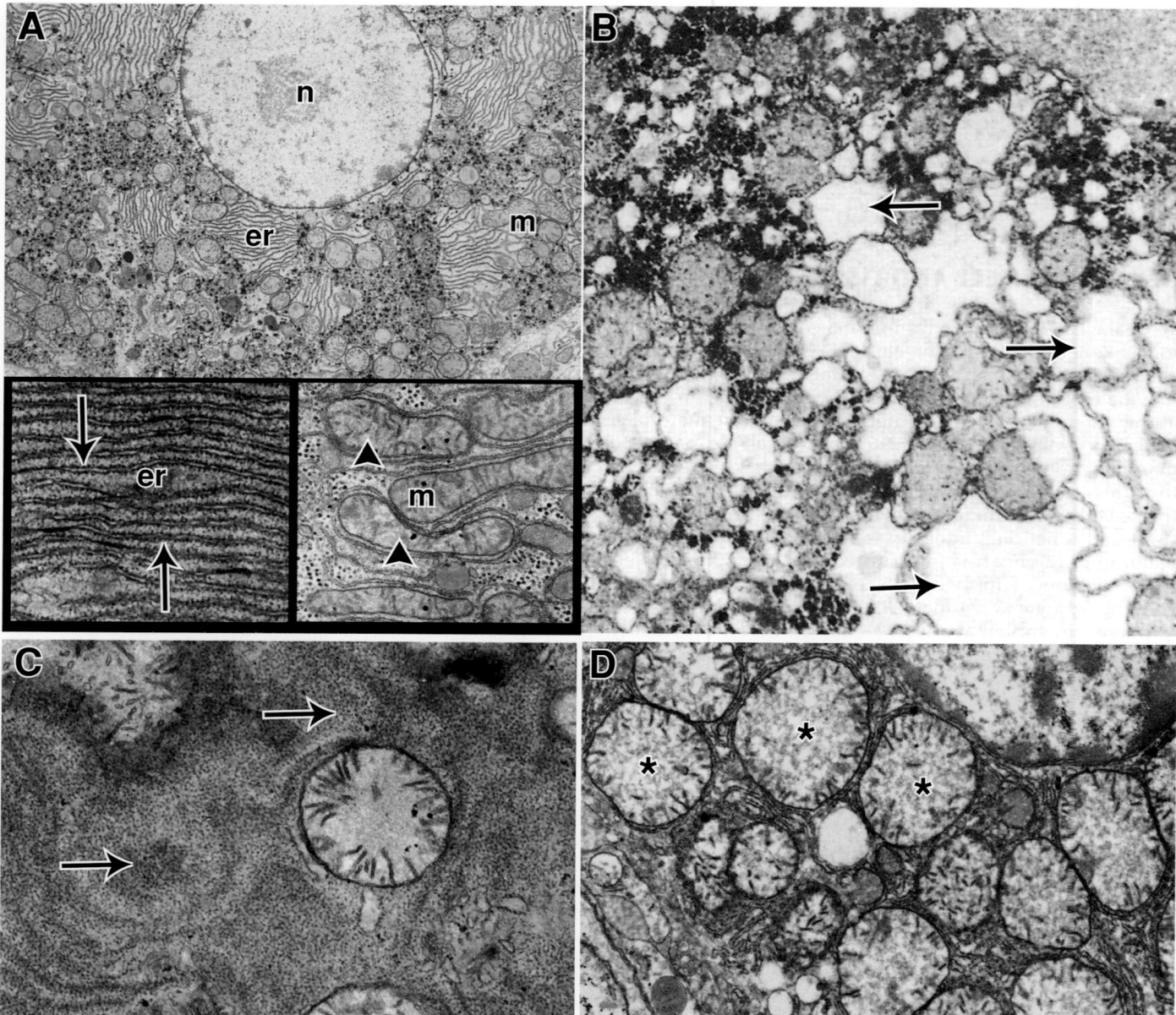

FIGURE 1-2. Subcellular changes in reversible cellular injury. A. Electron micrograph of a normal hepatocyte shows tightly organized, parallel arrays of rough endoplasmic reticulum (*arrows,* left inset) and normal mitochondria (*arrowheads, right inset*). *n* = nucleus; *m* = mitochondria; *er* = endoplasmic reticulum. **B.** In hydropic swelling, ER cisternae are dilated by excess fluid (*arrows*). **C.** Disaggregation of membrane-bound ribosomes in acute, reversible liver injury, with ribosomes detached from the ER membranes and accumulating free in the cytosol *(arrow)* (compare with inset in **A**, above). **D.** Mitochondria swell in acute ischemic injury, with decreased matrix density and less prominent cristae (*; compare with **A**, right inset).

Oxygen Deprivation May Cause Cell Injury

If blood flow to a tissue is interrupted or diminished, affected cells lack adequate oxygen for normal function. In this situation, called *ischemia,* the cells cannot make ATP by aerobic metabolism. Instead, they generate ATP inefficiently anaerobically. Ischemia triggers a series of chemical and pH imbalances, accompanied by increases in injurious free radical species (see below). Cells may recover from damage due to short periods of ischemia if circulation is restored. However, long periods of ischemia lead to irreversible cell injury and death. The mechanisms of cell damage are discussed below.

Intracellular Storage Is Retention of Materials Within Cells

Such substances may be normal or abnormal, endogenous or exogenous, harmful or innocuous.

- **Nutrients,** such as fat, glycogen, vitamins and minerals, are stored for later use.
- **Degraded phospholipids,** from membrane turnover, are engulfed in lysosomes and may be recycled.
- **Substances that are not metabolized** accumulate in cells. These include (1) endogenous substrates that are not further processed because a key enzyme is missing (hereditary

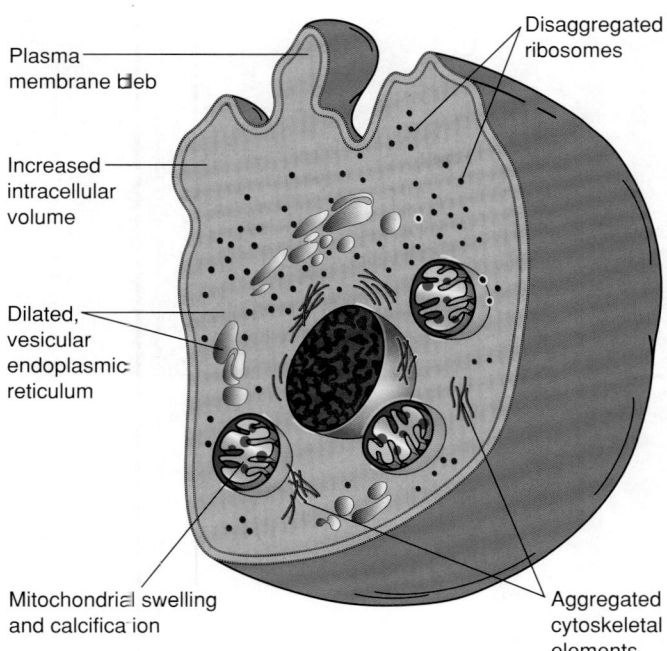

Plasma membrane bleb

Increased intracellular volume

Dilated, vesicular endoplasmic reticulum

Mitochondrial swelling and calcification

Disaggregated ribosomes

Aggregated cytoskeletal elements

FIGURE 1-3. How reversible cell injury affects cells.

storage diseases), (2) insoluble endogenous pigments (e.g., lipofuscin, melanin), (3) aggregates of normal or abnormal proteins, and (4) foreign particulates, such as inhaled silica or carbon.

- **Overload of normal body constituents,** including iron, copper and cholesterol, may injure cells.
- **Abnormal forms of proteins** may be toxic if they are retained within cells (e.g., Lewy bodies in Parkinson disease and mutant α_1-antitrypsin; see below).

Fat

Unlike unicellular organisms, mammals eat only periodically, and can survive prolonged fasting because they store nutrients for later use in specialized cells—fat in adipocytes and glycogen in the liver, heart, and muscle.

Abnormal fat accumulation is most conspicuous in the liver (Fig. 1-4A; see Chapter 20). Hepatocytes normally contain some fat, because they take up free fatty acids released from adipose tissue and convert them to triglycerides. The liver secretes most such newly synthesized triglycerides as lipoproteins. However, in some disease states, like diabetes or alcohol-related altered intrahepatic lipid metabolism, there is increased free fatty acid delivery to the liver, and triglycerides accumulate in hepatocytes. Fatty liver is visualized as cytoplasmic lipid globules. Other organs, including the heart, kidney, and skeletal muscle, also store fat. *Fat storage is always reversible. There is no evidence that excess cytoplasmic fat* **per se** *impairs cell function.*

Glycogen

Glycogen is a long-chain polymer of glucose, formed and largely stored mostly in the liver and, to a lesser extent, in muscle. When energy is needed, glycogen is converted to

glucose stepwise by a series of enzymes, any of which may be inactivated by mutation. Whatever the specific enzyme deficiency, the result is a glycogen storage disease (see Chapter 6). These inherited disorders affect the liver, heart, and skeletal muscle and range from mild and asymptomatic conditions to inexorably progressive and fatal diseases (see Chapters 11, 20, 31).

Blood glucose levels normally regulate intracellular glycogen storage. Hyperglycemic states, like poorly controlled diabetes, may cause increased glycogen stores, where hepatocytes and renal proximal tubule epithelial cells are swollen by glycogen.

Inherited Lysosomal Storage Diseases

Catabolism of certain complex lipids and mucopolysaccharides (glycosaminoglycans) requires multiple enzymatic steps, which take place in lysosomes. If an enzyme for one of those steps is inactive, incompletely degraded lipids accumulate in lysosomes, for example, cerebrosides (Gaucher disease), gangliosides (Tay–Sachs disease), or products of mucopolysaccharide catabolism (Hurler and Hunter syndromes). These disorders are all progressive, but they vary in severity from asymptomatic organomegaly to rapidly fatal brain disease (see Chapters 6 [general principles], 30, 32 [organ-specific manifestations]).

Cholesterol

Cholesterol is a double-edged sword for the human body. On the one hand, it is a key component of all plasma membranes and a precursor in steroidogenesis. On the other hand, its storage in excess is associated with atherosclerosis and cardiovascular disease, the leading cause of death in the Western world (see Chapter 16).

Briefly, the initial lesion of atherosclerosis (fatty streak) reflects accumulation of cholesterol and cholesterol esters in macrophages within the arterial intima. As the disease progresses, smooth muscle cells also store cholesterol. Advanced lesions of atherosclerosis are characterized by extracellular deposition of cholesterol (Fig. 1-4).

In some disorders characterized by very high blood levels of cholesterol (e.g., familial hypercholesterolemia), macrophages store cholesterol. Clusters of these cells may be grossly visible in subcutaneous tissues as **xanthomas** (Fig. 1-4).

Lipofuscin

Lipofuscin is a golden-brown mixture of lipids and proteins. Some call it, "wear and tear" pigment. It reflects ongoing accretion of indigestible peroxidized unsaturated lipids and oxidized, cross-linked proteins. The usual disposal mechanisms (see Autophagy, below) may be unable to rid the cell of these aggregates, which simply continue to accrue. Lipofuscin accumulates mainly in postmitotic cells (e.g., neurons, cardiac myocytes) or in cells that cycle infrequently (e.g., hepatocytes) (Fig. 1-4) and increases with age. In fact, fisheries measure lipofuscin in optic neurons to estimate age in lobsters and other crustaceans. It may be more conspicuous in conditions associated with atrophy of an organ.

It was once considered to be benign, but increasing evidence suggests that lipofuscin may be both a result and a

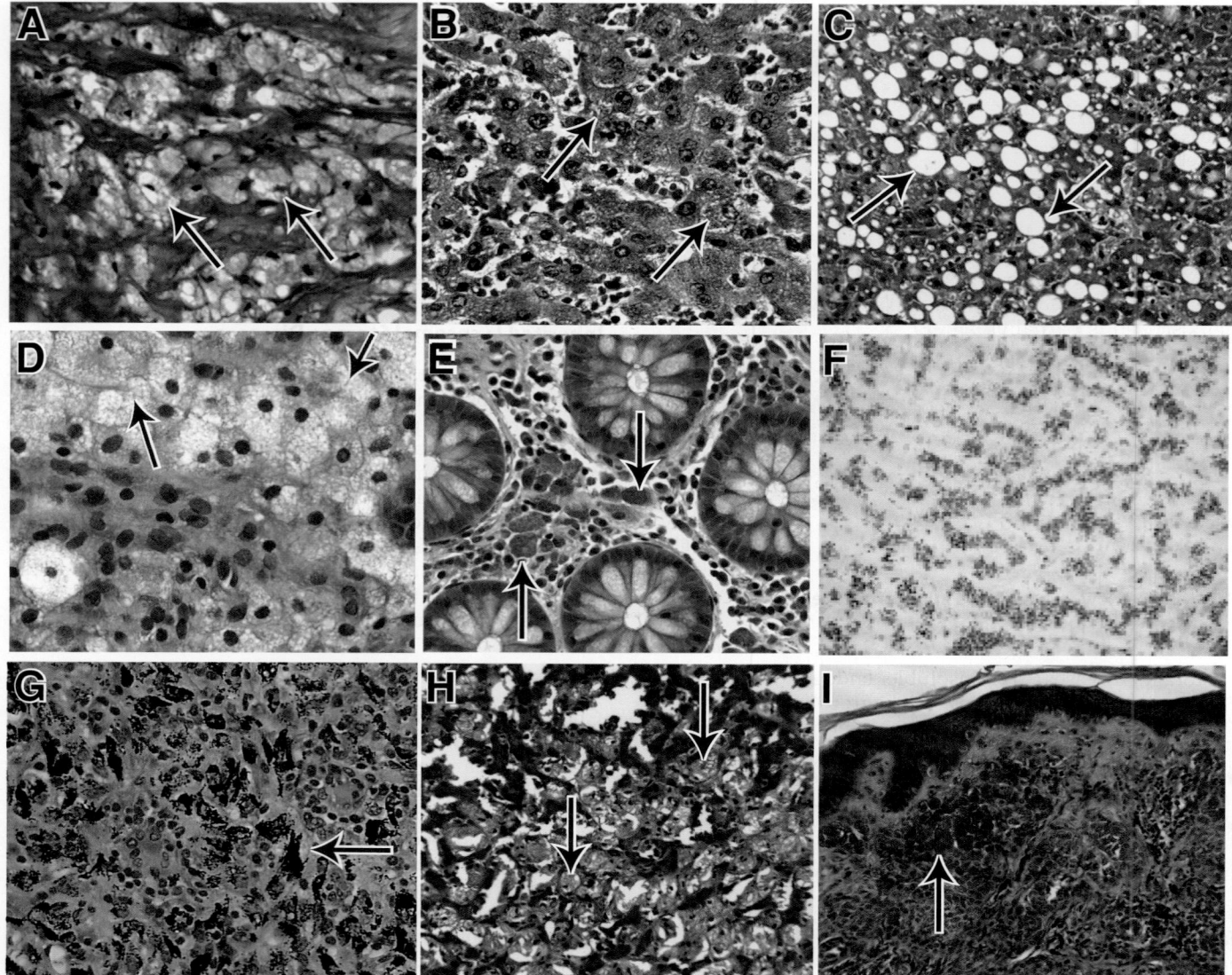

FIGURE 1-4. Abnormal intracellular storage. A. Abnormal cholesterol accumulation (*arrows*) in an atherosclerotic plaque. **B.** Lipofuscin in the liver of an elderly man (*arrows*) as golden cytoplasmic granules. **C.** Triglyceride accumulation in hepatocytes in a diabetic patient (*arrows*). **D.** Lipid stored in macrophages (*arrows*) in a cutaneous xanthoma. **E.** Melanosis coli. Pigment from plant-derived laxatives stored in colonic macrophages (*arrows*). **F.** Iron storage, highlighted by Prussian blue stain of the liver, in hereditary hemochromatosis. **G.** Carbon pigment storage in a mediastinal lymph node. Macrophages migrated to the lymph node, carrying inhaled black anthracotic (carbon) pigment that was originally deposited in the lungs. **H.** Abnormal glucocerebroside storage in hepatic macrophages (Kupffer cells, *arrows*) due to deficiency of glucocerebrosidase in Gaucher disease. **I.** Melanin (*arrow*) stored in cells of an intradermal nevus.

cause of increasing oxidant stress in cells. It may impair proteasomal and lysosomal degradation of senescent or poorly functioning organelles, and so facilitate cellular oxidant injury. Inefficient or malfunctioning mitochondria may accumulate, make more reactive oxygen species (ROS) and continue the cycle.

Melanin

Melanin is an insoluble, brown-black pigment found in epidermal cells, in the eye and elsewhere (Fig. 1-4). Melanocytes make melanin by polymerizing tyrosine oxidation products in intracellular organelles called melanosomes. In the skin, melanocytes "feed" melanin granules to other cells,

according to genetic determinants or environmental stimuli. Because it absorbs ultraviolet light, melanin protects from the harmful effects of sun exposure. In white people, exposure to sunlight increases melanin production (tanning). The amount of melanin in the skin determines skin color among the various races. Benign (nevi) and malignant (melanomas) tumors of melanocytes also produce melanin (see Chapters 28, 33). Hereditary inability to manufacture melanin is **albinism**.

Exogenous Pigments

Anthracosis is storage of carbon particles in the lung and regional lymph nodes (Fig. 1-4). Virtually, all city dwellers inhale particulates of organic carbon that are generated by burning of fossil fuels. Alveolar macrophages phagocytose these particles and transport the indigestible material to hilar and other lymph nodes, where it remains indefinitely. Grossly, anthracotic lungs may be striking, but the condition is innocuous.

Iron and Other Metals

Iron
About 25% of the body's iron is stored intracellularly, bound to the proteins, **ferritin** and **hemosiderin**. Ferritin is ubiquitous, and most abundant in the liver and bone marrow. Hemosiderin is partially denatured ferritin that aggregates easily and appears microscopically as yellow-brown cytoplasmic granules, mainly in the spleen, bone marrow, and Kupffer cells of the liver.

Total body iron may increase with increased need, as when the intestine absorbs more in some anemias, or if a patient receives repeated blood transfusions. If the body takes in more iron than it needs, the excess accumulates intracellularly as ferritin and hemosiderin. In **hemosiderosis**, greatly increased total stored iron accumulates in, for example, skin, pancreas, heart, kidneys, and endocrine organs. By definition, intracellular iron accumulation in hemosiderosis does not injure cells.

Excessive iron storage in some organs may increase the risk of cancer. For example, metal polishers with pulmonary siderosis tended to develop lung cancer more often.

Hereditary hemochromatosis (HH) occurs when there are mutations in the genes that regulate iron absorption and storage. It leads to extreme iron overload causes organ damage, mainly in the heart, liver, testes, and pancreas (Fig. 1-4). Tissue injury in HH most likely reflects iron-generated oxidative stress (see below), and is associated with increased risk of liver cancer (see Chapter 20).

Other Metals
Excess accumulation of several metals is dangerous. Lead, particularly in children, causes mental retardation and anemia (see Chapter 8). In Wilson disease (Chapter 20), copper accumulates in the liver and brain and damages those organs.

Cellular Adaptation to Ongoing Stresses

Persistent stress often requires that a cell adapt or die. The major adaptive responses are atrophy, hypertrophy, hyperplasia, metaplasia, dysplasia, and intracellular storage. Sometimes, tumor development (neoplasia) may follow adaptive responses.

The following sections describe mechanisms that mediate adaptive changes in cell and tissue mass and function, and how they manifest morphologically. At the core of these processes is cells' machinery for translating environmental changes into appropriate adaptive responses. Such plasticity is important in clinical medicine because it is often these adjustments, and their occasionally maladaptive consequences, that determine the course and outcome of many diseases.

Thus, one begins to study cellular adaptation to persistent environmental challenges by examining how cells change their composition: the ubiquitin system, proteasomal degradation, proteostasis, and autophagy.

SAFEGUARDING THE INTEGRITY OF CELLULAR CONSTITUENTS AND PROCESSES

Forces, both internal and external, constantly stress cells and cell constituents. Proteins need to fold correctly as they are produced and processed, and continually as they participate in cellular activities. If not, they will be non-functional, aggregate and interfere with cell homeostasis. Some proteins mediate tasks that are time-limited, such as driving cell division or expression of certain genes. Cells must eliminate them once their jobs are complete. Oxidative and other injuries to proteins and organelles may render them inefficient, ineffective or harmful, and so necessitate their removal. Pathogens may produce alien gene products, which cells must destroy and present to the immune system, in order to protect the organism from these invaders.

A complex meshwork of intracellular apparatus protects cells from all these stressors. The major players in this process are:

1. **proteasomes**, which execute ubiquitin (Ub)-dependent and Ub-independent protein degradation
2. large families of molecular **chaperones**, which guide protein folding and, if correct folding is impossible, escort recalcitrant proteins to their destruction
3. **autophagy**, in which lysosomes handle degradative activities that proteasomes cannot

These are not separate systems. Rather, they interrelate and intertwine extensively. When they go awry—whether by increased or decreased activity—diseases ensue. Because of their ubiquity and their importance for protecting cells, proteasomes, chaperones, and autophagy are often impaired in acquired diseases. These systems are tantalizing targets for developmental therapeutics, as well as for destructive manipulation by diverse pathogens.

Conjugation to Ubiquitin May Trigger Protein Degradation

Ubiquitin (Ub) is an evolutionarily conserved 76-amino acid protein that is critical to intracellular protein trafficking. It links to proteins, mostly via its seven lysine groups, and directs them to the diverse intracellular compartments, including to proteasomes, where partial or total protein degradation occurs. The fate of ubiquitinated proteins depends on the number of Ub molecules conjugated, the nature of the Ub linkage, the specific protein itself and, undoubtedly, other factors yet to be identified. While there are no hard and fast rules, several useful generalizations help to understand how this system works, as long as one accepts that each individual situation may be different.

The Different Types of Ubiquitination and Their Consequences

Proteins may be monoubiquitinated, polyubiquitinated in chains of Ub moieties or multiply monoubiquitinated. To

types of ubiquitin modifications

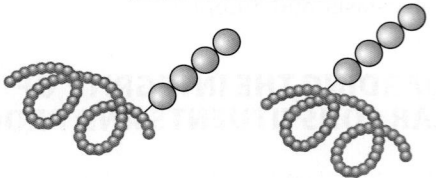

Polyubiquitination at different sites

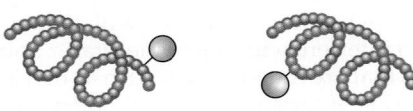

Monoubiquitination at different sites

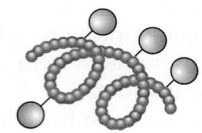

Multiple monoubiquitination

FIGURE 1-5. The diversity of ubiquitination. The several lysines of the Ub (ubiquitin) molecule can be used either to form poly-Ub chains or for mono- or oligoubiquitination. Ubiquitination of different lysine residues (represented here by *K*) imparts different functions to the target protein.

make things yet more complicated, the consequences of Ub conjugation to proteins reflect which Ub lysine (K) moiety is involved and the complexity of the Ub chains so formed. These different structures are illustrated in Figure 1-5. Among the diverse results of protein ubiquitination are:

- DNA damage response and DNA repair
- endocytosis
- proteasomal degradation
- autophagic destruction
- transcriptional regulation
- intracellular signaling
- protein trafficking, that is, directing proteins to one or another intracellular site
- regulating catalytic activities

Four Catalytic Functions Mediate Protein Ubiquitination

First, a *Ub-activating enzyme (E1)* binds and activates Ub (Ub*), and transfers it to one of dozens of *Ub-conjugating enzymes (E2)*. One of about 800 known *E3 Ub ligases* then conjugates the Ub* to the target protein (Fig. 1-6). One should note at this point that the importance of E3 Ub ligases as a class of enzymes cannot be overestimated: they determine the existence or destruction of specific proteins and so regulate a great many cellular processes. These steps occur generally whenever proteins are ubiquitinated. If a protein is in store for a poly-Ub chain, a fourth (somewhat controversial) type of enzyme (E4) conjugates Ub moieties to each other, by binding one or another lysine moiety to the C-terminus of the previous Ub molecule. The nature of this linkage determines to a degree a protein's fate. Thus, generally, a string of

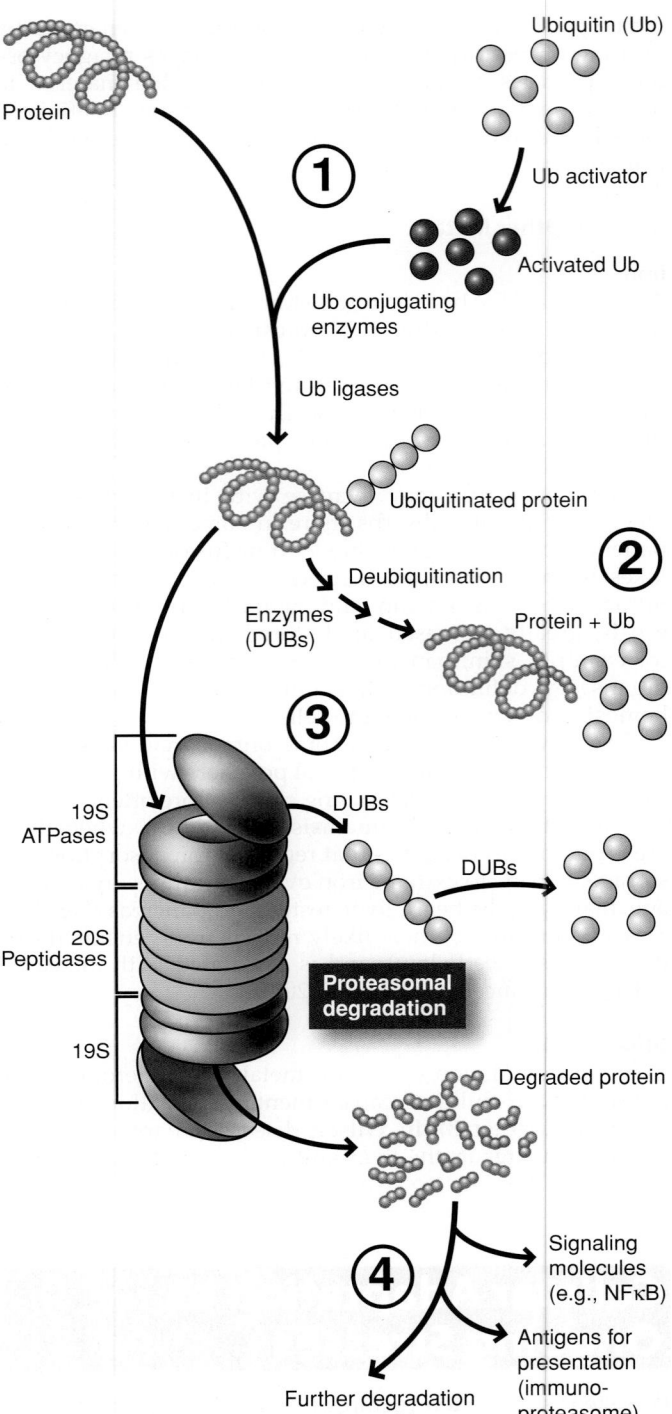

FIGURE 1-6. Ubiquitin–proteasome pathways. Ub (ubiquitin) targets proteins for specific elimination in proteasomes. **1.** Ub is activated by E1 ubiquitin-activating enzyme, after which it is transferred to an E2 ubiquitin-conjugating enzyme. The E2–Ub complex interacts with an E3 ubiquitin ligase to bind a particular protein. The process may be repeated multiple times to append a chain of Ub moieties. There follows a choice: **2.** These complexes may be deubiquitinated by deubiquitinating enzymes (DUBs). **3.** If degradation is to proceed, 26S proteasomes recognize the poly-Ub-conjugated protein via their 19S subunit and degrade it into oligopeptides. In the process, Ub moieties are returned to the cell pool of Ub monomers by DUBs. **4.** After release from the proteasome, partially degraded proteins may follow alternative fates.

four K48-linked Ub's is most efficient for targeting proteins for proteasomal degradation. (This is not absolute, however, as proteasomes may degrade proteins with four K63-linked Ub's, monoubiquitinated or even nonubiquitinated proteins, depending on the specific protein.)

Anything that can be done, can also be undone. About 100 known *deubiquitinating enzymes (DUBs)* can remove Ub moieties or pare poly-Ub chains. DUBs therefore may reverse the effects of ubiquitination on such processes as protein degradation, cell cycle regulation, gene expression, signaling, and DNA repair.

Proteasomes Catalyze Protein Degradation

Proteasomes are the cell's main apparatus for eliminating individual proteins. These come in several flavors, each of which appears to play a different and specific role. In general, the various types of proteasomes share basic features:

1. a 20S cylindrically shaped central proteolytic core of stacked subunits (β_{1-7}), different members of which cleave proteins via different enzymatic activities (caspase-like, chymotrypsin-like, trypsin-like);
2. an antechamber composed of α (α_{1-7}) and β particles controls access to the proteolytic core
3. complex heteromeric *regulatory particles*, which may attach to one or both ends of the core and are the gatekeepers.

The 26S Proteasome

These are the cell's executioners for (usually) ubiquitinated proteins, especially K48-linked polyubiquitinated proteins. They have 19S regulatory particles at one or both ends of the catalytic chamber. These regulators recognize Ub, contain DUB activity to excise the poly-Ub chains for recycling, bind proteins targeted for degradation, and have the ATPase activity needed to open the gates to the proteins' doom.

These proteasomes are present constitutively, and serve several key functions. They:

1. destroy proteins that are in native conformation, that the cell uses transiently and then must be eliminated (like proteins that drive cell division).
2. exercise quality control over ribosomal mRNA translation, so that protein products of defective RNAs are ubiquitinated near ribosomes, and targeted for removal.
3. are the destination for proteins that, upon completing ribosomal synthesis, are not—or cannot be—folded correctly by chaperones (see below). *Chaperones* and *co-chaperones* work with E3 ligases (e.g., CHIP) to ubiquitinate such proteins and direct them to proteasomes.
4. protect the cell from suffocating in its own secretory waste. Chaperones conduct cell membrane proteins, or proteins to be secreted, to the ER secretory pathway. There, they are folded, cleaved, activated, etc., as necessary. If they cannot be rendered useful this way, the *ER-associated protein degradation system (ERAD)* oversees their ubiquitination, retrograde transport back to the cytosol and removal by proteasomes.

Immunoproteasomes (20S)

Stress-related protein modifications (e.g., due to heavy metals, heat, oxygen radicals; see below) can alter protein folding, exposing hydrophobic moieties that are normally hidden. This impairs protein function and causes them to aggregate. The job of protecting cells from such damaged proteins belongs to 20S *immunoproteasomes*.

Stress-related increases in the inflammation- and infection-associated moieties IFNγ, TNFα, lipopolysaccharide, and *advanced glycation end products* (AGEs; see Chapter 13) cause the constitutive 26S proteasome to disassemble and upregulate a different cap, the **11S regulator**. Stress-induced catalysts (iβ_1, iβ_2, iβ_5) replace their respective catalytic units of constitutive proteasomes (26S, above) and combine with 11S regulators and remnants of 26S proteasomes to make immunoproteasomes. These 20S proteasomes assemble rapidly, under the management of iβ_5, and are quickly ready to handle damaged proteins. They remain intact briefly, and disassemble when the job is done, usually 3 to 24 hours.

Unlike 26S proteasomes, immunoproteasomes do not process ubiquitinated proteins. The mediators that induce them and the circumstances under which they are generated suggest that they play a role in antigen processing for immune recognition. In addition, there is felt to be a connection between immunoproteasomal response to oxidative modification of nuclear proteins and stress-activated DNA repair mediated by **poly-ADP-ribose polymerases (PARPs)**.

Other Proteasomes

There are additional regulatory caps, which most likely mediate specific protein degradative processes. Mixed-type, or hybrid, proteasomes also exist, bearing one regulatory cap at one end of their structures, and another at the other. Further, a specific β_5 catalytic subunit, called β_5t, is present only in the thymus and is part of a *thymoproteasome*, which appears to play a role in selecting specific cytotoxic (CD8+) T lymphocytes.

The UPS Regulates Key Cellular Processes

Examples of this are many. Among the best understood is the role of the UPS in gene expression. **Nuclear factor-κB (NFκB)** is an important transcription factor that is activated in two different ways by the UPS. The active form of NFκB is a heterodimer, composed of two different protein subunits. Inactive precursor forms of the two NFκB subunits are ubiquitinated and cleaved to their active forms in proteasomes. *This is an example of incomplete protein degradation by the UPS.* Also, the inhibitor of NFκB, called **IκB**, is degraded following ubiquitination. This step releases active NFκB, which drives expression of genes that promote cell survival. Proteasome inhibition permits the IκB–NFκB complex to persist, and so decreases NFκB-induced transcriptional activation. In cancer cells, which depend in part on NFκB-induced survival functions, inhibiting proteasome function may cause tumor cell death, and so is a target for pharmaceutical manipulation.

Proteasomal Activities Are Subject to Regulation at Multiple Levels

Cells control proteasome function in many ways. Thus, shuttling factors may deliver candidate proteins for degradation to proteasomes. DUBs may act as the appeals court of last resort, and can stay or abrogate proteins' death sentences.

Transcriptional regulation determines which, and how many, proteasomes are made. *Nrf* genes, about which we shall read more later, are key players in responses to oxidative stress, including regulating proteasomal constituents that participate in stress responses. Post-translational changes of many kinds, similarly, may up- or downregulate proteasome activity.

Some Pathogens Manipulate the UPS

Some pathogens can subvert Ub/DUB pathways at multiple points. Certain bacterial proteins, called effectors, resemble E3 Ub ligases and activate ubiquitination, allowing exquisite exploitation of host cells to facilitate invasion and pathogenicity. Other bacteria (e.g., *Salmonella typhimurium, Chlamydia trachomatis*) and viruses (e.g., herpes simplex) encode proteins that act as DUBs, suggesting that interfering with ubiquitination gives these pathogens a selective advantage. Viral control of cell membrane proteins may protect infected cells from immune destruction, so that HIV-1 Vpu protein causes CD4 degradation via a mechanism resembling ERAD. Cytomegalovirus (CMV) does something similar with MHC-1, and prions are reportedly able to block protein entry into proteasomes.

Some modifications of proteins may protect them from ubiquitination. For example, DNA damage leads to p53 phosphorylation (see Chapter 5), which protects it from Ub-mediated degradation.

There are several proteins that resemble Ub but are structurally and functionally distinct from it, and that subserve somewhat different functions. Such proteins (e.g., SUMO and NEDD8) may participate in forming some E3 complexes. Their polymeric chains may direct protein localization and diverse protein activities.

CLINICAL FEATURES: Ubiquitination and Deubiquitination are Key to Many Diseases: Ubiquitination and specific protein elimination are critical to cellular adaptation to stress and injury. Changes in UPS functionality, both up and down, are central to many diseases. Not surprisingly, diseases characterized by abnormal protein accumulation often entail impaired UPS function. Thus, some hereditary forms of Parkinson disease reflect mutations in *Parkin*, a ubiquitin ligase: undegraded Parkin accumulates as Lewy bodies (see Chapter 32). In some other neurodegenerative diseases, such as Alzheimer and Huntington diseases and inherited forms of amyotrophic lateral sclerosis, mutant proteins accumulate and cause neuron dysfunction and death. Similar pathologic protein accumulation may cause apoptosis of cardiac myocytes in ischemia/reperfusion injury and pressure overload. Therapies for diseases of impaired UPS function may aim to activate the UPS by inhibiting processes, such as are noted above, that restrict proteasome activity.

The opposite phenomenon, that is, excessive UPS activity, leads to sarcopenia during aging and in patients with advanced malignancies. In certain cancers, proteasomal activity increases, often targeting tumor suppressor proteins for elimination. Thus, human papillomavirus strains associated with human cervical cancer (see Chapters 5, 24) produce E6 protein. E6 inactivates p53 tumor suppressor by facilitating association between a Ub ligase with p53 and, in so doing, accelerating p53 degradation.

Along these lines, inhibiting proteasomal activity is an important pharmacologic tool in treating several different types of disease. Some malignancies that are characterized by excessive protein secretion, such as plasma cell myeloma (see Chapter 26), are treated effectively with proteasome inhibitors, causing cells to suffocate in their own protein products. Some immunologically mediated diseases, which feature increased inflammatory and immune responses, are susceptible to proteasome inhibition. For example, activated T lymphocytes are more susceptible to the inhibitory effects of proteasome inhibition than are resting T cells, so that proteasome inhibition may alleviate diseases caused by excessive T-cell–mediated immunity (e.g., graft vs. host disease) without compromising defenses against pathogens.

Heat Shock Proteins Are the Guardians of the Cell's Proteome

Every cell must synthesize proteins, fold them into proper three-dimensional configurations, deliver them to places they should go, oversee association(s) with other molecules that activate or inactivate them as needed and then repair their structures when proteins suffer the slings and arrows of outrageous fortune (i.e., internal and external stresses).

If cells cannot prevent proteins from misfolding, they try to prevent misfolded proteins from forming disruptive and toxic aggregates. Should they fail at that task, they then try to pry proteins away from those masses and to refold them properly. If a cell fails at these tasks, or when a protein has outlived its usefulness, the cell may tag it for destruction.

This constellation of cellular functions is *proteostasis*. Every organism must be able to establish and maintain proteostasis in order to survive. Several families of *heat shock proteins (HSPs)* mediate these functions. Convention groups these HSPs into the following basic families: small HSPs (sHSPs, e.g., HSP27), HSP40s (also called J-proteins), HSP60s, HSP70s, HSP90s, and HSP100s. Different HSPs mediate different functions, but they collectively preserve a cell's viability in the face of internal and external forces that damage proteins, change their structures, or impair their function. HSPs have diverse structures and functions, many being specific to particular client proteins. Some HSPs are produced constitutively. Others are induced by various stresses, such as heat, oxidants, ischemia, heavy metals, starvation, infections, inflammation, irradiation, etc. The importance of these proteins and the functions they mediate is exemplified by the fact that in nonstressed cells, HSP70 may constitute as much as 3% of total cellular protein. Stress conditions may amplify this percentage.

HSP Functions

HSPs are *molecular chaperones*: like teachers at a high-school dance, they supervise and guide other proteins to assume proper postures and behaviors. To do this, HSPs may act individually or in concert with each other, with helpers of various kinds, which may be called co-chaperones and bridge proteins of several kinds.

HSPs and proteostasis promote cell survival. *These mechanisms do not discriminate between normal and abnormal cells. If a cell is normal, its survival benefits the organism. However, if a cell is malignant, or if it harbors a virus infection, its* *survival may jeopardize the whole organism's survival* (see below and Chapter 5).

The Menace of Misfolded Proteins

Misfolded proteins with exposed hydrophobic residues (see below) potentially jeopardize cell functionality and viability. Protein surface nonpolar moieties tend to associate with other similar structures, forming aggregates. Small may be soluble or insoluble, but either way, they endanger cell viability.

Soluble aggregates are extremely damaging. They may form pores in membranes or puncture them. If the plasma membrane is involved, cytosol constituents may leak out. If a mitochondrial membrane is damaged, leakage of intramitochondrial species may lead to apoptosis (see below).

Soluble aggregates may encourage delinquent tendencies in normally folded proteins and cause them to become misfolded. Or, they may coalesce with other soluble aggregates to form larger, insoluble aggregates. These latter may disrupt cytoskeleton and intracellular transport, magnify oxidant injury, and interfere with protein repair and replacement. Large insoluble protein aggregates are important in the pathogenesis of many neurodegenerative diseases (see Chapter 32). Perhaps counterintuitively, such large insoluble aggregates are actually less cytotoxic than their smaller, soluble cousins.

Helping Newly Synthesized Proteins to Fold Correctly

When a ribosome synthesizes a protein, the mRNA template only specifies the proper amino acid sequence, not the protein's architecture (i.e., its tertiary structure). HSP70, sometimes in concert with HSP40s, awaits the nascent protein strand as it exits the ribosome (Fig. 1-7). This complex may stabilize the emerging protein until it is completely synthesized, so as to assure proper alignment, the final touches to which may be provided by HSP90 or other HSPs (e.g., HSP60). Alternatively, HSP70 may hold the protein in an unfolded or partially folded state in order to facilitate its transport to a noncytoplasmic subcellular destination (see below).

HSP70 (which, in the context of protein synthesis, is sometimes called constitutive HSP70, or HSC70) has other important functions in this regard. When protein synthesis is proceeding in a setting of cellular stress, HSP70 rushes to put out the fire—that is, HSP70s focus on restoring order when cellular stresses (oxidative, heat, chemical, etc.) cause protein misfolding. Translation at the ribosome stops until the stress passes and the HSP70/HSP40 complex can return to assist.

Refolding Proteins That Assume Improper Configurations After Their Synthesis

Proteins, once folded into a particular structure, are not static. The may assume multiple geometries over their lifetimes. If, in the course of this process, a protein winds up in

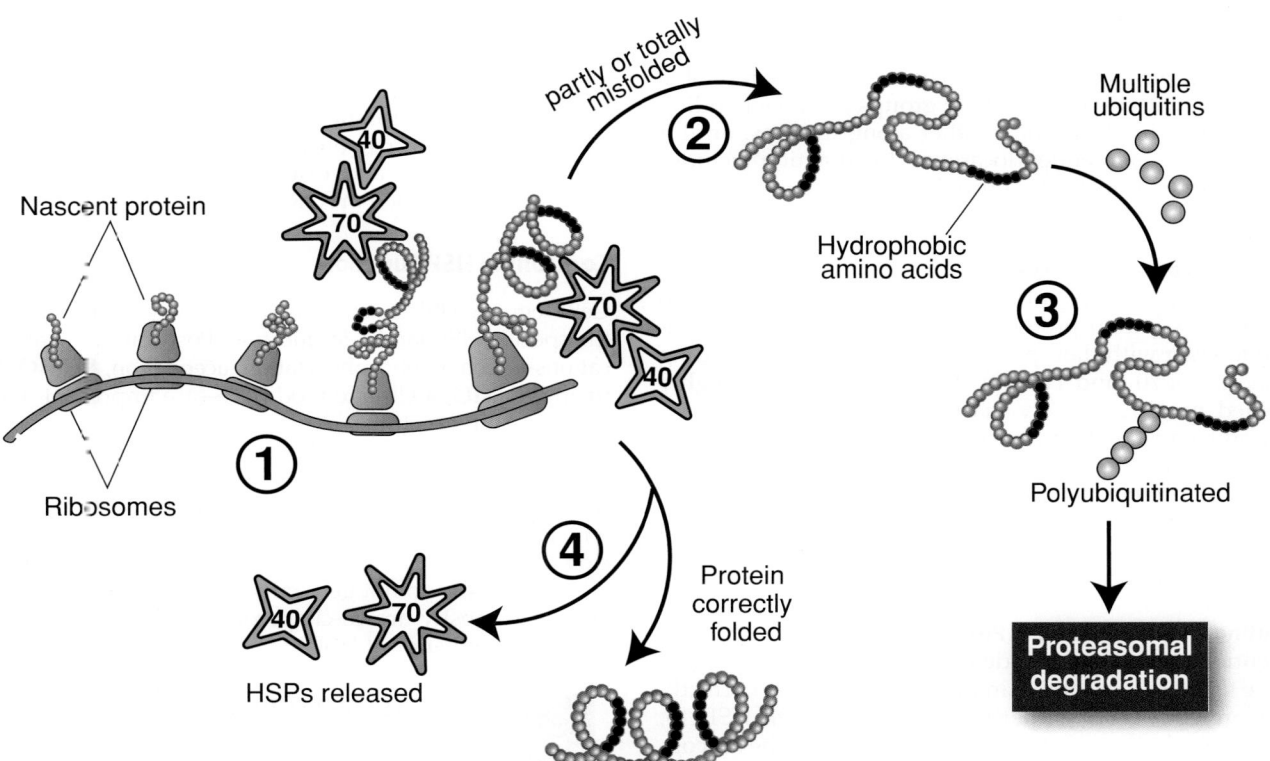

FIGURE 1-7. Role of HSPs in assuring proper folding of proteins during translation. 1. In normal (nonstressed) settings, HSP70 (and, often, HSP40) situate themselves at ribosomes, as they translate mRNAs into polypeptide chains. The black moieties represent hydrophobic amino acids, which are most appropriately nestled within the core of the protein's tertiary structure and not exposed to the surface. **2.** If the chain is incorrectly folded, and cannot be corrected by the chaperones, it becomes part of the ubiquitin-proteasomal system. **3.** The incorrigibly misfolded protein is polyubiquitinated, and degraded by proteasomes. **4.** HSP70 (often with the assistance of HSP40) assures that proteins assume their correct configuration. Correctly folded proteins are then chaperoned from the ribosomes that produce them to their ultimate cellular destination.

an improper configuration after being buffeted by intra- and extracellular forces, interior hydrophobic stretches may be exposed at the protein's external surface, and there face the protein's hydrophilic milieu. HSP40s, sHSPs, and HSP70s recognize those acquired misfoldings. In the presence of an accessory protein called Hip, HSP40 then activates HSP70 conversation of ATP to ADP and the folding of the new protein begins. The folding process is often completed when a representative of a third HSP family, HSP90, joins the fray. This newcomer is also accompanied by an accessory protein, aptly named Hop, and the protein folding process is completed. The product is a new peptide, correctly folded.

In times of stress, sHSPs may bind misfolded proteins and hold them in a folding-ready state until the stress passes and the sHSPs may then deliver the bound proteins to larger HSP complexes for refolding. This helps to decrease protein aggregate formation. Should aggregates form despite sHSP binding, the presence of the sHSP facilitates aggregate dissolution once the stress has waned.

If Proteins Do Not Fold Correctly

Recalcitrant proteins may be too stubbornly misfolded to be amenable to even the most persuasive HSPs. To deal with such malingering, some HSPs associate with proteases that digest target proteins into peptides that can later be further broken down into recyclable amino acids. Alternatively, protein obduracy may lead directly to proteasomal or other cellular degradation.

Shepherding Proteins to Their Appropriate Destinations

HSPs usher properly folded proteins to their proper sites of action. Simple as this process may seem, it may resemble a relay race, with several HSPs or groups of HSPs handing the client protein off to one another along the way, until it finally reaches its intended location. This function includes transmembrane transport, and delivering proteins to (e.g.) secretory vesicles or subcellular organelles.

Positioning Proteins for Success

An important function of HSPs, especially HSP90, is to assure that its bound protein targets are in proper orientation to interact with their partners or ligands. In the folding sequence, HSP70 (and HSP60) (Fig. 1-8) recognizes highly misfolded proteins, mostly via exposed hydrophobic residues, and wrestles them back into shape so they do not aggregate. With the help of Hop (see below) HSP70 then hands select proteins to HSP90, which optimizes their structures to facilitate their functions, be it enzymatic activity (e.g., Cdk4; see Chapter 5), ligand binding (e.g., glucocorticoid receptor), or other downstream functions.

Preventing and Disassembling Protein Aggregates

As mentioned above, misfolded proteins tend to aggregate because they are less soluble in the cytosol than are correctly folded proteins. HSP70s, perhaps in concert with HSP110, may help break down some of these aggregates. They recognize a protein's exposed hydrophobic residues, disentangle and unfold it, and then try to reorient it. If they fail in doing that, they may direct the pertinacious molecule to the cell's degradative apparatus.

Inhibiting Apoptosis

Some HSPs play a key role in maintaining cell survival, above and beyond preventing accumulation of toxic protein aggregates, etc., as outlined above. HSPs bind and block several proteins that trigger programmed cell death (PCD) (which is discussed below). HSP pro-survival actions include the following:

- inhibiting mitochondrial release of cytochrome *c* and **SMAC/Diablo**
- preventing Bax from entering mitochondria
- inhibiting apoptosis protease activating factor (**Apaf-1**)
- blocking **procaspases-3** and -9 from conversion to their active, apoptosis-triggering forms, caspases-3 and 9
- preventing signaling via certain cell death–related receptors (FasR, TNFα)

Other Known HSP Activities

The HSP system plays an important role in tumor development and dissemination (see Chapter 5). Some of these HSP activities reflect their cytoprotective nature, but more complex HSP roles also come into play.

Several HSPs (HSP70, HSP90, HSP27) may be secreted and/or insert into cell membranes. How HSPs work in these settings is under study. They may have both pro- and anti-inflammatory activities, wound healing and, at least in some settings, appear to play a major role in immune regulation. This type of cellular protection shelters tumor cells or cells that carry intracellular pathogens (e.g., viruses) from immune recognition and elimination.

Controlling HSP Levels

From the foregoing discussion, it is clear that HSPs represent one of the key mechanisms by which cells assure their survival in sometimes hostile and changing environments. A transcription factor, **heat shock factor-1** (**HSF-1**), induces HSP expression in response to heat or other environmental stresses. mTOR (see above) also activates HSF-1, so HSPs are more abundant when mTOR is active.

Controlling HSP Function

Cells regulate HSP functions in diverse ways, which depend on the specific HSP family in question. Post-translational modifications—such as phosphorylation, acetylation, **SUMOylation** (using **SUMO**, a Ub-like modifier)—are important determinants of HSP function.

However, the best understood determinants of chaperone function are co-chaperones. These proteins include Hip, which helps activate HSP70 in the presence of HSP40, Hop, which facilitates target protein (or, in the parlance of HSP aficionados, "client") transfer from HSP70 to HSP90 and many others. HSP40s do not generally act as independent chaperones, but mostly are co-chaperones for HSP70. Aha1 is an important activator of HSP90.

 CLINICAL FEATURES: Proper or improper functioning of HSPs and the protein folding system are central to many human diseases, including some that may not meet the eye. These include:

- Neurodegenerative diseases. In this setting, neuronal dysfunction and death may involve accumulations of insoluble protein aggregates, such as Alzheimer disease, some forms of amyotrophic lateral sclerosis, Parkinson disease (see Chapter 32).

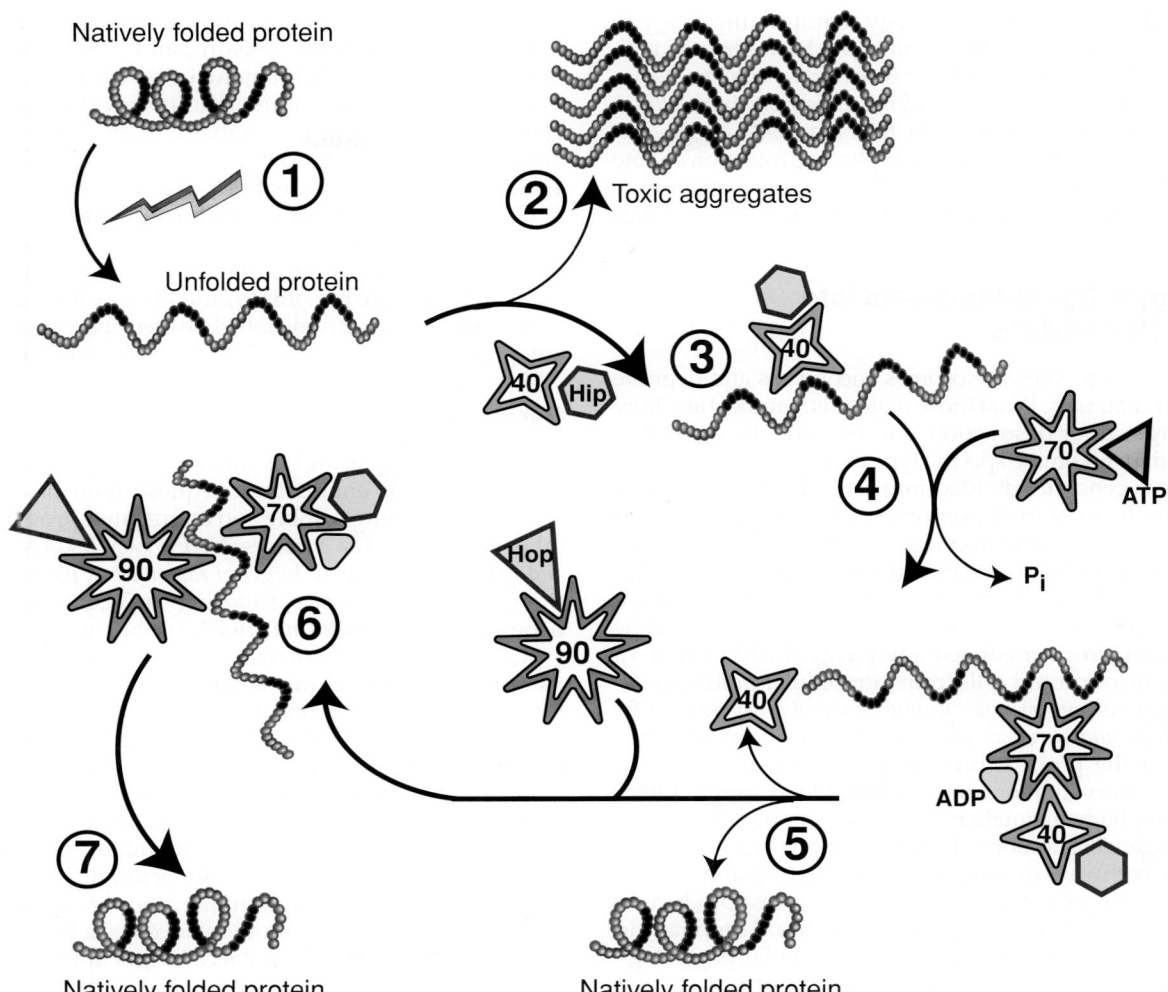

FIGURE 1-8. Role of HSPs in proteostasis. 1. A protein in its correct configuration is subject to many stresses and toxic stimuli, which may cause it to unfold, exposing normally hidden hydrophobic amino acids (*black*). **2.** If the now incorrectly folded protein cannot be corrected by the chaperones, it may cluster with other, similarly misfolded proteins, to form insoluble intracellular aggregates, which are potentially toxic and interfere with cell function. **3.** Alternatively, the now misfolded protein is recognized with HSP40, which joins with the linker protein, Hip. **4.** The HSP40-Hip complexed to the incorrectly folded protein then binds to HSP70. As a result of this association, HSP70-bound ATP is hydrolyzed to ADP, thus activating HSP70. **5.** This complex may be sufficient to wrestle the mischievous protein back to its proper conformation, in which case the several components dissociate. **6.** However, additional help may be needed. The cavalry arrives, in the form of HSP90, which, with a linker protein, Hop, may be sufficient persuasive that the protein finally resumes its correct structure.

- Cancers. Rapid proliferation of malignant cells usually begins with mutant proteins and generates more mutant proteins. Chapter 5 has more detail, but suffice it to say here that misfolded non-native (mutant) proteins would aggregate and be toxic to cancer cells, were it not for the soothing ministrations of HSPs, particularly HSP90, which protect cancer cells from such calamity.
- Infections. Like cancer cells, viruses replicate rapidly. In so doing they generate many misfolded and mutant viral proteins which normally would be toxic for infected cells. That toxicity for infected cells would curtail viral infectious cycles and short-circuit infections. HSPs help assure proper folding of viral proteins (including mutant proteins) and allow infection to proceed.

- Genetic diseases. In some inherited diseases (e.g., cystic fibrosis; see Chapter 6) HSP90 does not fold the mutant protein (cystic fibrosis transmembrane conductance regulator, or CFTR) and prevents from reaching the cell membrane, leaving cells without a chloride channel. Pharmacologic inhibition of HSP90 may allow that mutant CFTR protein to reach the cell membrane, where it may function as a chloride channel.

AUTOPHAGY

Autophagy (Greek: "auto," *self;* "phagy," *eating*) *is a highly conserved process that helps cells respond to stress.* When cellular stress sensors are activated, autophagy recognizes intracellular targets and delivers them to lysosomes for digestion and removal. Normal cell physiology requires autophagy to work smoothly so that cells can navigate between survival, death, and adaptation. *Autophagy is central to cellular adaptation to diverse circumstances. It defends cells from intracellular and foreign enemies—sometimes to the organism's benefit, but sometimes to its detriment.* When autophagy protections wane or go awry, consequences to the cell and the organism may be catastrophic, in the forms of organ degeneration, malignant tumors, and other diseases.

Autophagy Is Tightly Integrated Into the Cell's Homeostasis

In all forms of autophagy, lysosomes encompass and degrade intracellular materials. What those materials (cargoes) are, how they are targeted for destruction, and the route they travel to lysosomes depend on the specific type of autophagy involved. Autophagy is generally divided into several categories. **Macroautophagy** handles bulk portions of cytoplasm. Both macroautophagy and **microautophagy** target damaged cellular organelles, aggregated proteins, and other potentially injurious materials. In addition, some defective proteins require interaction with molecular chaperones to enter the autophagic system via **chaperone-mediated autophagy** (**CMA**) (Fig. 1-9). **Xenophagy** helps protect cells from intracellular pathogens.

Autophagy systems operate continuously and are obligatory for cell homeostasis and survival. Bulk autophagy, the most primitive form of the process, protects cells when nutrients are lacking, as in starvation or compromised blood supply. Other forms of autophagy maintain homeostasis among cellular proteins and organelles in normal settings and in times of stress. Autophagic pathways are ongoing physiologic quality control mechanisms that protect from, for example, excess production of ROS by inefficient or damaged mitochondria. Autophagy in its various forms is thus essential for basal cellular physiology and for adaptation to adversity, in such settings as:

- Starvation
- Ischemia
- Recycling nutrients from cellular organelles and macromolecules
- Clearance of misfolded or damaged proteins and organelles
- Antigen presentation
- Inflammation
- Protection from tumorigenesis
- Protection from neurodegeneration

Autophagy is a multistep process, which entails autosome initiation, growth, maturation, movement, fusion with lysosomes and, finally, up- and downregulation. These steps require that the cell activate many components—and inactivate many others—and then assemble several multicomponent complexes to act in concert. Autophagy is immensely complex, involving multiple members of several large families of proteins—ATGs, TRIMs, SECs, EXOs, CULLINs, and others—some of which are discussed below. The *Dramatis Personae* of autophagy is enormous, and the cast of characters and their roles are beyond the scope of this discussion.

Autophagy Walks a Tightrope Between Activation and Suppression, Fine Tuning Constantly

Dire consequences await if it is too active or not active enough (see below). The following sections illustrate

mechanisms of autophagy, how they relate to other systems, how they maintain health, and their (beneficial and not-so-beneficial) involvement in disease. Since cell survival requires continuous maintenance of intracellular components, impaired autophagy in any form may cause abnormal proteins and defective organelles to accumulate. The result may be cell death or disease.

The pathways of autophagy (above) all lead to one common end: lysosomal destruction of targeted cargoes. However, these processes differ in (1) regulation, (2) types of cargo, (3) how doomed targets are recognized, and (4) how they are delivered to lysosomes. Fine distinctions between the various forms of autophagy may be fuzzy, and some overlap probably exists.

Macroautophagy

Macroautophagy is the best understood of the several forms of autophagy. It entails bulk sequestration of cytoplasmic contents, including soluble and aggregated proteins and cellular organelles. *The enzymes AMPK (AMP kinase, see below) and mTOR (mammalian target of rapamycin), play central—and antagonistic—roles in macroautophagy.* mTOR is part of a multicomponent complex (**mTORC1**, see below).

Cells express autophagy proteins constitutively, so autophagy is poised for action at a moment's notice, via post-translational modifications of existing molecules—like phosphorylation and ubiquitination—rather than transcription. In the resting (well-fed) state, autophagy is ready, but quiescent. A number of factors restrain the process. External to the cell, growth factors such as insulin and IGF-I increase with nutrient abundance. They maintain inhibitory pathways by receptor-mediated **Akt** activation. In turn, Akt activates mTORC1, which inhibits autophagy (Fig. 1-10). (In reality, the process is far more nuanced, see below.)

In a setting of stress (like starvation), cellular sensors detect scarcity of amino acids. Endocrine and paracrine growth factor production declines. The intracellular AMP/ATP ratio increases, which activates AMPK. This enzyme (about which more will be said below) does several things. It activates **TSC1** (see Chapter 5), which inhibits mTORC1, and sets the process in motion. mTORC1 normally binds and inhibits ULK1. Activated TSC1 frees ULK1 from its inhibitory binding by mTORC1, allowing ULK1 to activate Beclin-1, so autophagic complexes may assemble and begin to act. AMPK also phosphorylates and activates ULK1, and helps assemble critical multicomponent autophagy execution complexes.

Then, bulk cytoplasm, containing cytoplasmic organelles and including proteins, lipids, and other constituents, is partially sequestered by a membrane (the **phagophore**). The latter fuses at its ends to enclose a structure, the **autophagosome**. Autophagosome membranes may derive from several cytoplasmic sources, including the outer mitochondrial membrane, ER, plasma membrane, or Golgi apparatus. The autophagosome then fuses with lysosomes, whose enzymes reduce autophagosome contents to small molecules for reutilization by the cell (Fig. 1-9).

Identifying Targets in Macroautophagy

Starvation-related autophagy is mostly nonselective for soluble cytoplasmic constituents and organelles, although even in this setting, recycling of cell contents is not totally random. Macroautophagy also handles damaged cytoplasmic organelles and aggregated proteins, for both of which specific recognition is needed.

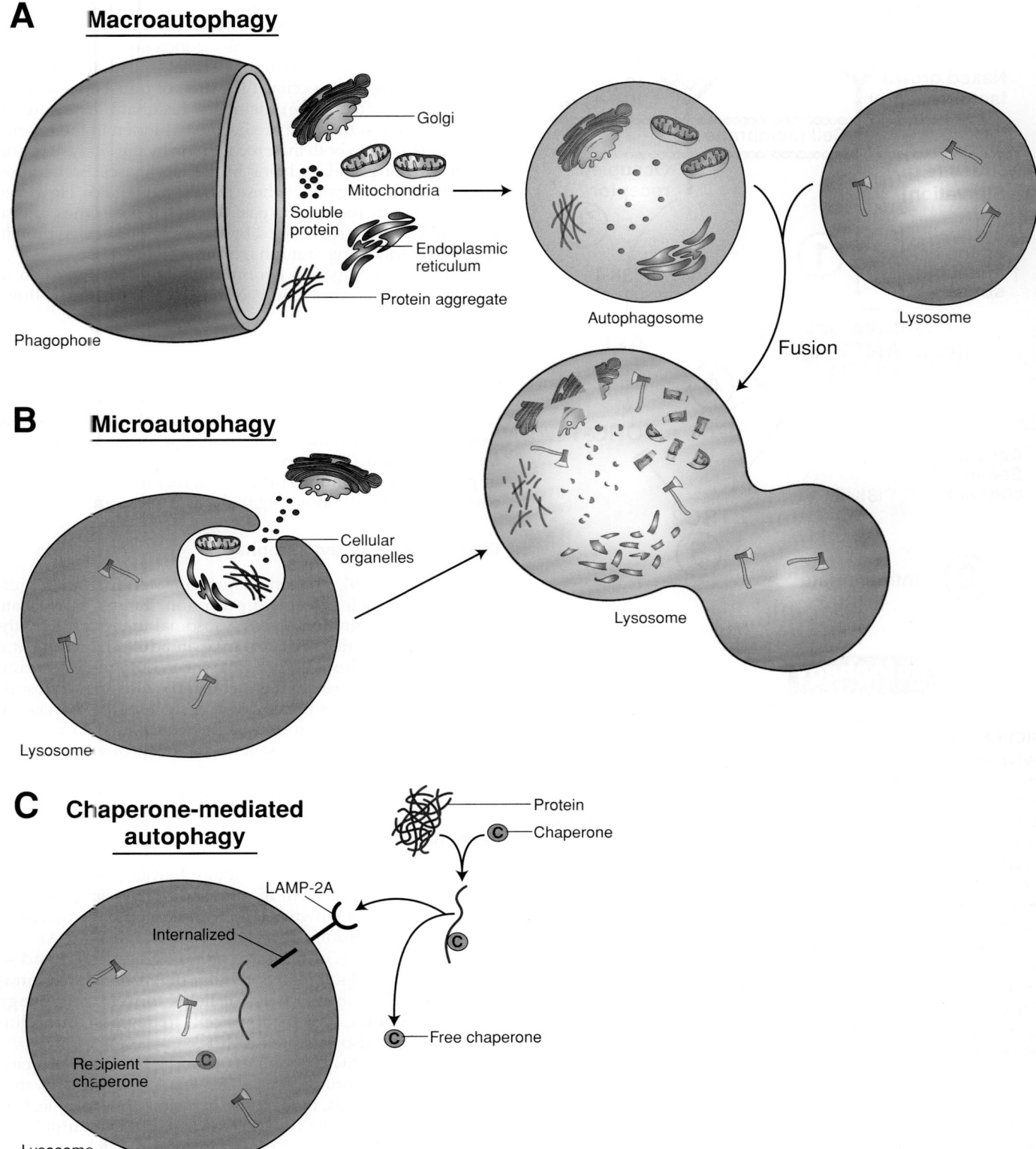

FIGURE 1-9. Types of autophagy. A. Macroautophagy. Cytoplasmic organelles are partially sequestered by an open membrane, the phagophore. Upon closure by fusion, the phagophore becomes an autophagosome, which then delivers its contents to a lysosome. Lysosomal enzymes degrade the contents to small molecules for reutilization. **B. Microautophagy.** Cytosolic cargoes are engulfed by invagination of the lysosomal membrane. The contents are then degraded by lysosomal enzymes. **C. Chaperone-mediated autophagy.** Proteins conjugated to chaperones (e.g., Hsc70) are recognized by lysosomal receptor proteins (LAMP-2A) and translocated to the lysosomal interior, where they are received by a second chaperone and then degraded. The original, extralysosomal chaperone survives to work further.

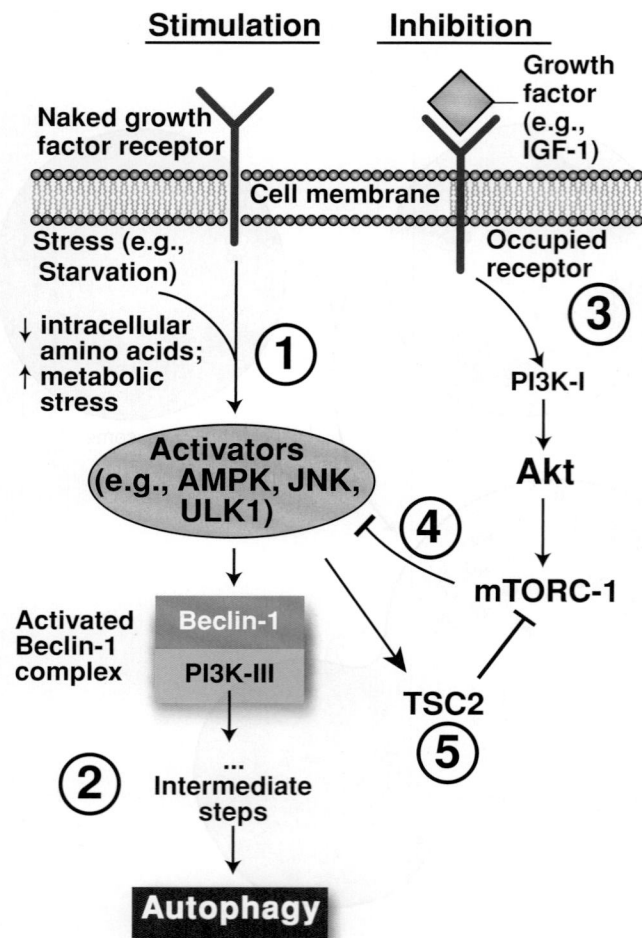

FIGURE 1-10. Factors contributing to triggering and inhibiting autophagy. Stimulation (left). **1.** In the setting of starvation or other initiators of autophagy, lack of growth factors leads to depletion of nutrients and metabolic stress. A consortium of upstream molecules is triggered. **2.** As a result, an autophagy-activating complex containing Beclin-1 and class III phosphatidylinositol-3-kinase (PI3K-III) is formed. This complex triggers autophagy, from the phagophore to the fusion of the phagosome with the lysosome. **3.** Inhibition (right).Autophagy is inhibited when nutrients or other stimuli elicit growth factors (e.g., insulin-like growth factor-I [IGF-I], insulin), which bind to their cell membrane receptors. This process activates class I PI3K (PI3K-I), which produces phosphatidylinositol-tris-phosphate (PIP3). **4.** PIP3 then recruits Akt to the cell membrane, where it is activated and in turn stimulates the mTOR-related complex, mTORC1. The latter directly blocks the autophagy cascade, including Beclin-1, to prevent autophagy. **5.** AMPK activates the tuberous sclerosis tumor suppressor complex, TSC2, which inhibits mTORC1.

In that case, target identification depends on the nature of the problem. For example, a damaged, inefficient, mitochondrion that generates too much reactive oxygen from dysfunctional electron transport suffers altered membrane potential. A cytosol protein, Nix, then binds the outer mitochondrial membrane. This complex recruits a protein, **Parkin** (for its likely involvement in Parkinson disease), which in turn binds to several members of a series of Ub-like (**UBL**) recognition proteins, called autophagy-related proteins, or **ATGs**. A bridge protein, **p62**, recognizes these UBLs and

attaches the damaged mitochondrion to the interior of the developing phagophore (Fig. 1-11).

Protein aggregates are usually concretions of misfolded proteins and are handled by a parallel, but different, pathway. Misfolding may occur at the time of translation or from acquired (e.g., oxidative) damage. Resultant exposure of hydrophobic residues that are normally hidden in the interior of proteins leads to both their recognition by the Ub system and attachment of poly-Ub chains by E3 Ub ligases. Sometimes, Atgs are also conjugated to these protein aggregates. However, these masses are too large to pass through proteasomes, and so Ubs and UBLs are recognized by the same p62 bridge protein and incorporated into autophagosomes (Fig. 1-11).

Macroautophagy is a continuously vigilant guardian of protein quality control, and is central to maintaining cellular integrity.

Microautophagy

Microautophagy (Fig. 1-9) is a process by which cytosolic cargoes are directly engulfed by invagination of lysosomal membranes, then transferred into the interior of lysosomes for degradation. This process is largely constitutive and is important for continuous turnover of membranes and organelles and for maintaining organelle size and composition.

Chaperone-Mediated Autophagy

In CMA (Fig. 1-9), chaperone proteins conduct all targets selectively to their lysosomal execution. Targets translocate via receptor recognition across lysosomal membranes, without phagosome intermediates. Like an adult chaperone at a teenage dance, who is responsible for maintaining decorum in conduct and for removing incorrigible violators, cytosolic molecular chaperones preside over correct folding of nascent proteins and destruction of misfolded or damaged proteins via CMA. There is a modest level of constitutive CMA, but this pathway can be further activated when the cell is stressed (e.g., starvation, oxidant stress, toxic exposures, etc.).

Xenophagy

Xenophagy is a selective autophagy that targets intracellular pathogens. It is a form of macroautophagy, triggered by several different pathways. Intracellular pathogen sensors may activate immunity-related GTPase M (**IRGM**). Among these, **TRAF6** (an E3 Ub-ligase) ubiquitinates IRGM and so activates it. IRGM stimulates cellular defenses against intracellular invaders in two ways: it helps form an autophagy initiation complex, which allows cells to degrade intracellular invaders. It also activates AMPK.

A parallel pathway revolves around a family of proteins called tripartite motif proteins (**TRIMs**). TRIMs are activated by type II interferons, in response invasion, for example, free noncellular DNA. Like IRGM, TRIMs help form autophagy initiation complexes. Type I interferons, separately, may stabilize Beclin-1.

The role of xenophagy in protecting from viral and other (e.g., mycobacterial) invaders is discussed below.

Crosstalk Among Degradative Pathways

Some branches of the autophagic pathway are regulated by sequential enzymatic activation of Ub and UBLs, the latter

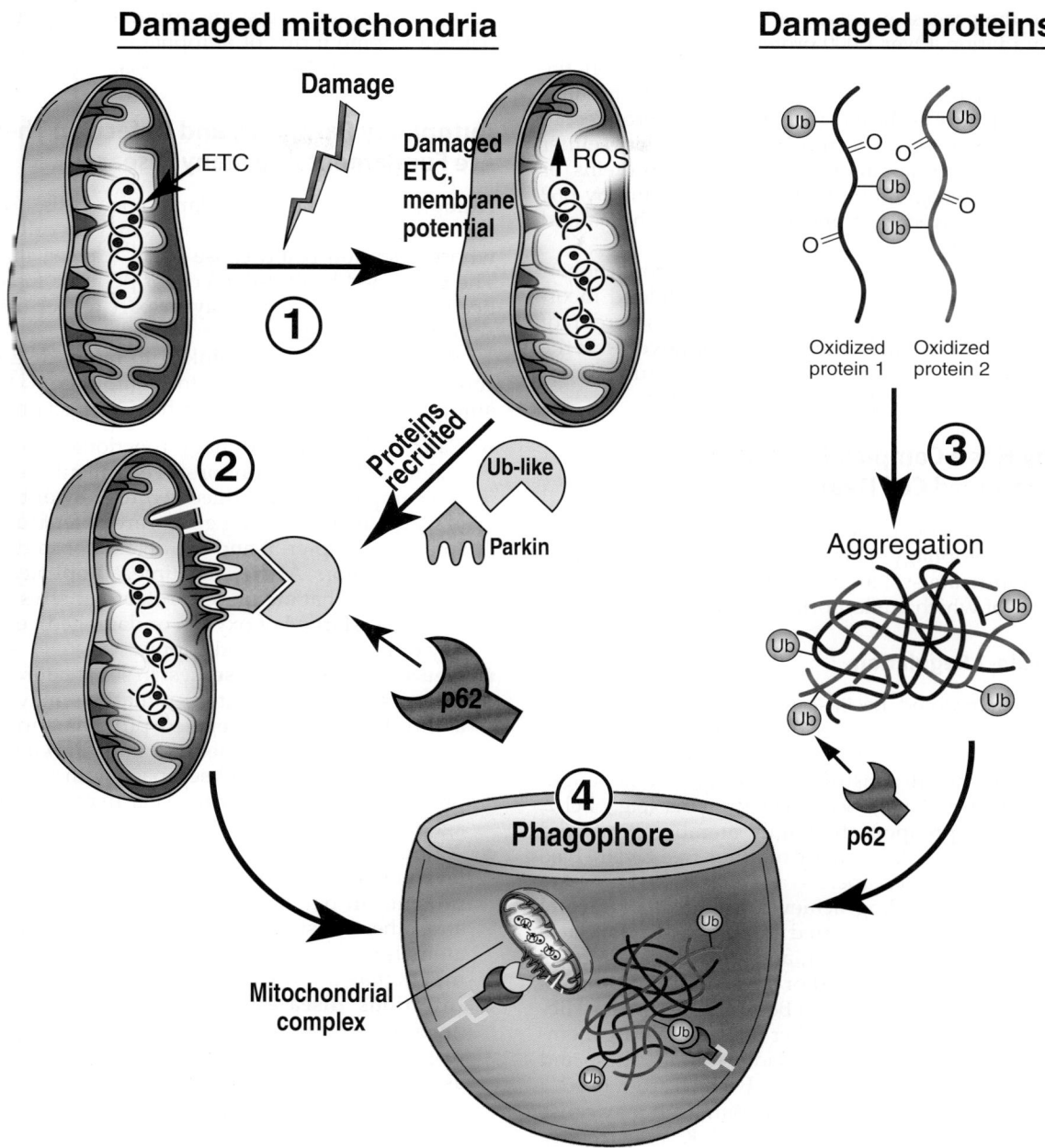

FIGURE 1-11. Role of autophagy in handling damaged cellular organelles and protein aggregates. 1. Damaged cellular organelles (left): Damage (here) to mitochondria disrupts electron transport and dissipates the electrochemical gradient across the mitochondrial membrane. Increased ROS both cause and result from oxidative damage. **2.** This leads to recruitment of cytosolic proteins, Parkin and a Ubiquitin-like protein (Ub-like, or UBL). The complex of fragmented mitochondria–Parkin–UBL binds to p62. **3.** Proteins that have sustained oxidative damage are conjugated to Ub or a UBL and form aggregates, which are then bound by p62. **4.** The p62-bound complexes with damaged mitochondria or aggregated proteins are recognized by a specific receptor in the phagophore, leading to autophagy. *ETC* = electron transport chain; *ROS* = reactive oxygen species; *Ub* = ubiquitin; *UBL* = Ub-like protein.

resembling the activation cascade of the UPS (see above). Short-lived proteins are generally specifically digested by the UPS, whereas autophagy tends to remove longer-lived proteins selectively. This division of labor is not rigid: if one system is compromised, the other may compensate, at least in part. The UPS cannot handle protein aggregates or large cytoplasmic structures, like organelles or endocytosed foreign matter (e.g., bacteria). These two systems thus complement each other. There are also molecular interactions among the different types of autophagy, so if one pathway is impaired, another may compensate.

Both autophagy and the UPS operate continuously, and impairment of either may have harmful consequences. Although autophagy can act as a bulk recycling mechanism for nutrients in times of starvation, both systems may be remarkably selective. This specificity reflects the participation of many molecules in the process of selective identification of materials for degradation. Over 1,000 proteins confer on the UPS precision in target selection. Autophagy depends on the diversity of the Ub system, as well as additional families of proteins, such as TRIMs and the parallel Atg proteins, to maintain a broad scope and accuracy. As noted above, either Ub or Atg protein conjugation to aggregated proteins or organelles allows recognition of a targeted structure by p62 linker protein, followed by transport to phagophores and autophagic degradation.

Why is selectivity important? A significant proportion of newly synthesized proteins are translated or folded incorrectly. Oxidative damage further increases a cell's burden of defective proteins. Such molecules must be removed, lest the cell accumulate large, insoluble aggregates that cause abnormal protein–protein interactions or other mischief.

Autophagy Has a Complex Relationship With Programmed Cell Death

In general, signals and species that mediate apoptosis (see below) inhibit autophagy. This, however, is an oversimplification of an intricate system of checks and balances, a few characteristics of which are important to understand.

PCD and Beclin-1 Regulation

If autophagy is to proceed, Beclin-1 must be free and available. The protein has a BH3 domain (see below), just like many pro- and antiapoptotic proteins of the Bcl-2 family of apoptosis-controlling proteins. In unstressed settings, some antiapoptotic (i.e., pro-survival) Bcl-2–like proteins (e.g., Bcl-2, Mcl-1) and even a proapoptotic family member, Bim, bind and inactivate Beclin-1. Autophagy requires free Beclin-1, so the cell must arrange its escape.

Stress-activated signaling achieves this goal in several ways. JNK1, a starvation-activated kinase, phosphorylates Bcl-2, forcing it to release Beclin-1, and allowing autophagy to proceed. Other stress-activated or stress-induced proteins may interpose themselves between Bcl-2 and Beclin-1, to liberate the latter. Among these are other BH3-containing members of the Bcl-2 clan, for example, Bad or Puma. These and other proteins (e.g., HMGB-1) displace Beclin-1 from Bcl-2.

Independently of these interactions, Bim itself may cause Beclin-1 sequestration. Stress-activated JNK may relieve Beclin-1's bondage by phosphorylating Bim. In addition, caspases, which signal apoptosis (see below), cleave and inactivate Beclin-1.

Other Cross-Talk Between Autophagy and PCD

P53 may up- and downregulate autophagy, depending on circumstances. It inhibits AMPK, and so impedes autophagy signaling. On the other hand, it upregulates PUMA, an antiapoptotic Bcl-2 family member, which directly promotes mitophagy.

Caspases and their relatives, calpains, may cleave key proteins that are required for autophagy, including Atg proteins and other proteins that stimulate autophagy (e.g., Ambra1). Inactivating these autophagy promoting proteins has the effect of facilitating apoptosis.

This type of behavior, however, is a two-way street: just as apoptosis-related proteins may impair autophagy, autophagy-related proteins may block apoptosis signaling.

Thus, Atg5 inhibits signaling through the extrinsic apoptotic pathway. Some forms of autophagy signaling also degrade caspases, thereby blocking apoptosis.

Autophagy Pathways, and Defects in Them, Are Fundamental to Many Diseases

Autophagy maintains cellular homeostasis during starvation and removes obsolete or damaged cell constituents, whose retention could cause harm (cancer, infection, etc.). The presumed healthful effects of periodic fasting, as practiced by many cultures, may in part reflect the fact that it activates autophagy.

Because autophagy is linked to many diseases, there is considerable focus on ways to manipulate it. For example, autophagy and defective autophagy impact on

- **Cancer:** Because autophagy functions to protect cellular viability, its role in tumor development and progression is a complex double-edged sword. Key autophagy genes (e.g., Beclin-1, some Atg genes) are potent tumor suppressors (see Chapter 5) and are deleted or mutated in many human tumors. At the same time, autophagy also protects cancer cells that are under proteotoxic stress, deprived of nutrients, starved of oxygen or damaged because of therapy or insufficient blood supply.
- **Neurodegenerative diseases:** In some neurodegenerative diseases (e.g., Huntington) mutations may impair cells' ability to remove aggregated proteins and/or defective mitochondria. In Alzheimer and Parkinson diseases, autophagy may fail to keep pace with the rate at which protein aggregates accrue. This may be due in part to age-related decreases in Beclin-1 synthesis.
- **Aging:** Macroautophagy and CMA decline with age, as do levels of Beclin-1, ATGs, and certain lysosomal membrane proteins. In parallel, aggregates of unprocessed proteins and other substances accumulate. Experimental data in animals suggest that facilitating autophagy by inhibiting mTOR may improve longevity.
- **Infectious diseases:** Autophagy is an important host defense mechanism against pathogens. Xenophagy is responsible for eliminating many pathogen species, such as intracellular parasites, several types of viruses, including HIV-1 and bacteria such as *Shigella, Streptococcus,* and *Mycobacterium tuberculosis.* Not surprisingly, many pathogens have evolved ways to evade or subvert this process. Some viruses, for example, encode Bcl-2–like proteins that bind Beclin-1. *M. tuberculosis* and *Shigella flexneri* interfere with phagosome–lysosome fusion, so they may survive and replicate unmolested. Conversely, some viruses, particularly RNA viruses such as poliovirus and hepatitis C virus, benefit from increased autophagy; autophagic vesicles serve as membrane scaffolds for their replication.
- **Inflammatory bowel disease:** Mutations in two autophagy-related genes are associated with increased risk of Crohn disease. Both genes normally facilitate xenophagy. Mutations in them that impair bacterial clearance tend to increase production of pro-inflammatory molecules.
- **Pulmonary diseases:** Both increased and decreased autophagy may contribute to smoking-related respiratory illnesses. Increased autophagy activity characterizes some cases of chronic obstructive pulmonary disease (COPD; see Chapter 18). On the other hand, alveolar macrophages from chronic smokers reportedly show lower than normal

autophagy, and clearance of mutant protein aggregates in airway epithelial cells reportedly contributes to the pathogenesis of cystic fibrosis.

- **Cardiovascular diseases:** Mutations in autophagy proteins may cause certain inherited cardiomyopathies. Impaired autophagy may contribute to cardiac injury and dysfunction in settings of ischemia/reperfusion, as well as heart failure.

Diverse Chemical and Physical Triggers Cause Atrophy and Hypertrophy

Atrophy is decreased cell or organ size. It may both cause and result from altered function. *Hypertrophy is its converse: increased cell or organ size.* Usually, hypertrophy entails increased functional capacity.

Normal Homeostasis Determines Cell and Tissue Mass

A cell's size reflects its equilibrium between anabolic and catabolic forces. Many cell types can undergo atrophy and hypertrophy, but most studies focus on skeletal muscle, which is the paradigm of these mechanisms. Myocytes can adapt to increased functional demand by increasing synthesis of muscle proteins and downregulating their degradation. Conversely, muscle atrophy (wasting) may have many causes and leads to reduced synthesis and increased degradation of contractile proteins. Within a cell, the signaling pathways that control hypertrophy and atrophy are closely interconnected.

Atrophy

Atrophy may result from disuse of skeletal muscle or loss of hormonal signals after menopause. It may also allow a cell to accommodate changes in its environment, while remaining viable. Atrophy may also be harmful, as in some chronic diseases and biologic aging (see below).

Atrophy of an organ differs from cellular atrophy. Reduced organ size may be caused by reversible cell shrinkage or by irreversible loss of cells. Thus, when a broken leg is casted, lack of physical activity may cause that limb's muscle cells to lose volume as adaptation to their disuse. When the case is removed, myocytes are used again, and resume their usual size and function. On the other hand, brain atrophy in Alzheimer disease[1] reflects extensive cell loss; the organ's size cannot be restored (Fig. 1-12). Atrophy occurs under a variety of conditions as outlined in Table 1-1.

Hypertrophy

When trophic signals or functional demands increase, cells adapt to satisfy these changes. Larger cells (hypertrophy) and, in some cases, increased cell number (hyperplasia; see above), result. In several organs (e.g., heart, skeletal

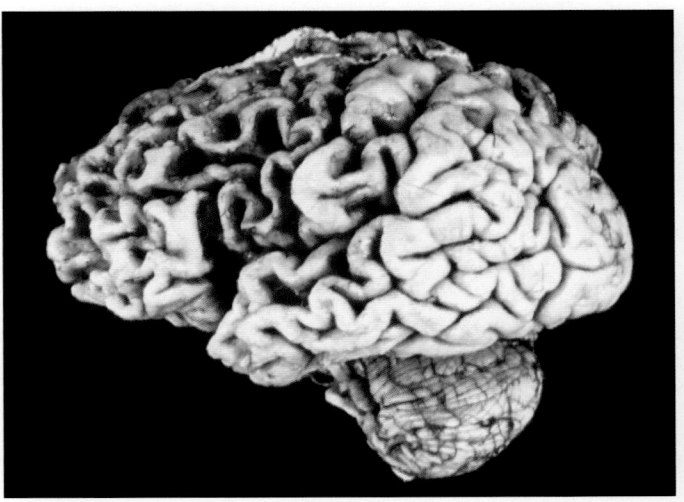

FIGURE 1-12. Atrophy of the brain. Marked atrophy of the frontal lobe is characterized by thinned gyri and widened sulci. (From Okazaki H, Scheithauer BW. *Atlas of Neuropathology*. New York: Gower Medical Publishing; 1988. By permission of the author.)

muscle), such adaptive responses are achieved mainly by increased cell size, which leads to increased organ mass (Fig. 1-13). In other organs (e.g., kidney), cell numbers and size may both increase.

TABLE 1-1 REACTIVE OXYGEN SPECIES (ROS)	
Molecule	**Attributes**
Hydrogen peroxide (H_2O_2)	Forms free radicals via Fe^{2+}-catalyzed Fenton reaction Diffuses widely within the cell
Superoxide anion (O_2^-)	Generated by leaks in the electron transport chain and some cytosolic reactions Produces other ROS Does not readily diffuse far from its origin
Hydroxyl radical (OH•)	Generated from H_2O_2 by Fe^{2+}-catalyzed Fenton reaction The intracellular radical most responsible for attack on macromolecules
Peroxynitrite (ONOO•)	Formed from the reaction of nitric oxide (NO) with O_2^- Damages macromolecules
Lipid peroxide radicals (RCOO•)	Organic radicals produced during lipid peroxidation
Hypochlorous acid (HOCl)	Produced by macrophages and neutrophils during respiratory burst that accompanies phagocytosis Dissociates to yield hypochlorite radical (OCl^-)

Fe^{2+} = ferrous iron.

---

[1]A note about eponymous diseases (i.e., diseases named after people). In common usage, such diseases are cited as possessives (e.g., Alzheimer's disease, Crohn's disease), but medical convention prefers that they to be identified *without the possessive proper noun* ("Classification and nomenclature of morphological defects", *Lancet* 1975;1:513). Like many other journals and texts, we honor this convention.

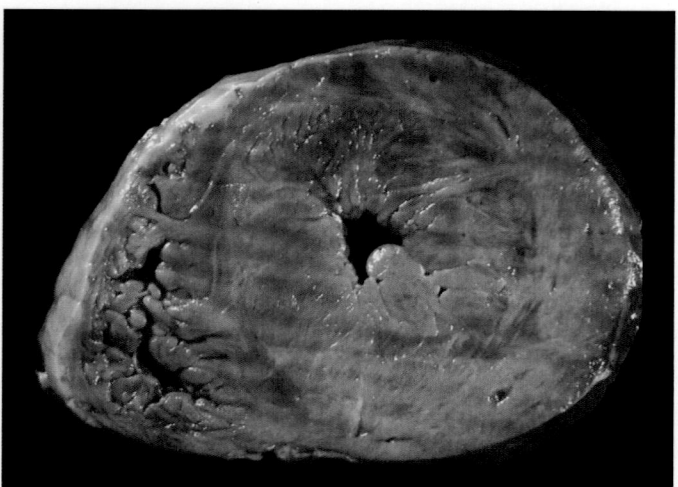

FIGURE 1-13. Myocardial hypertrophy. Cross-section of the heart of a patient with long-standing hypertension shows pronounced, concentric left ventricular hypertrophy.

Conditions That Cause Atrophy Are Often Inverses of Those That Stimulate Hypertrophy

Conditions Leading to Atrophy

Reduced Functional Demand
Atrophy commonly follows reduced functional demand. For example, after a motor nerve is injured, muscles it serves lose mass, and strength correspondingly diminishes.

Impaired Oxygen Supply
Ischemia *is interference with blood supply to tissues.* It causes oxygen deprivation. If cells survive, they may be atrophic and functionally impaired. For example, cells in poorly perfused areas at the margins of ischemic necrosis due to vascular occlusion (**infarcts,** see below) in the heart, kidneys, etc., may become atrophic.

Insufficient Nutrients
Starvation or malnutrition leads to wasting (decreased mass) of skeletal muscle and adipose tissue. Microscopically, this appears as cell atrophy. Decreased cell (e.g., myocytes, adipocytes) size results.

Interruption of Trophic Signals
Many cells depend on hormonal or other stimulatory signals. If these signals wane or vanish (e.g., endocrine ablation, or muscle denervation [Fig. 1-14]), cells dependent on those stimuli will atrophy. Injury to the anterior pituitary (e.g., Sheehan syndrome; see Chapter 14) may lead to deficiency of its many hormones, causing thyroid, adrenal cortical, etc., atrophy.

Atrophy due to altered hormone levels may be physiologic: the endometrium atrophies when estrogen levels decrease after menopause (Fig. 1-15), as does the breast after lactation is completed. Even some cancer cells may atrophy after hormonal deprivation. Androgen-dependent prostatic cancers and estrogen-responsive breast cancers may regress after treatment with hormone antagonists.

Increased Pressure
Prolonged pressure in inappropriate locations may cause atrophy. Sustained bed rest can put continued, localized

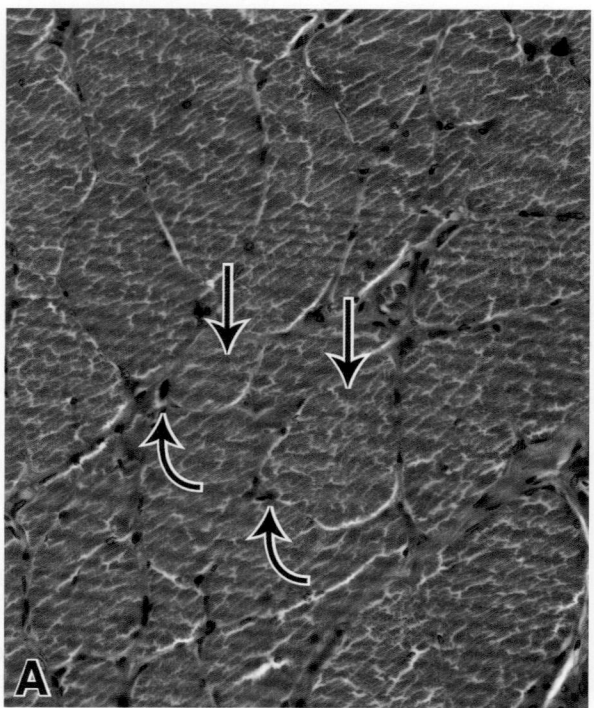
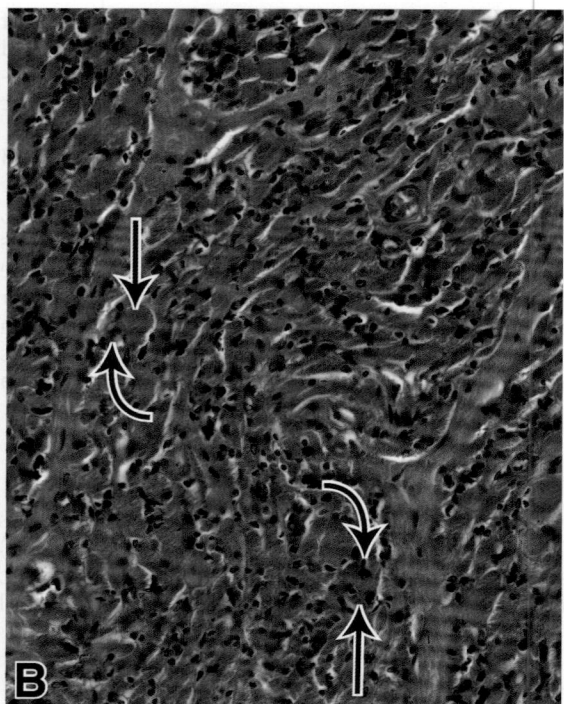

FIGURE 1-14. Loss of cell volume following loss of trophic signal. Muscle from a patient who experienced traumatic muscle denervation. **A.** Normal muscle from the patient, showing large muscle bundles (*straight arrows*) with inconspicuous peripheral nuclei (*curved arrows*). **B.** Area of denervated muscle, showing loss of myocyte protein (*straight arrows*), with comparative increase in prominence of myocyte nuclei (*curved arrows*).

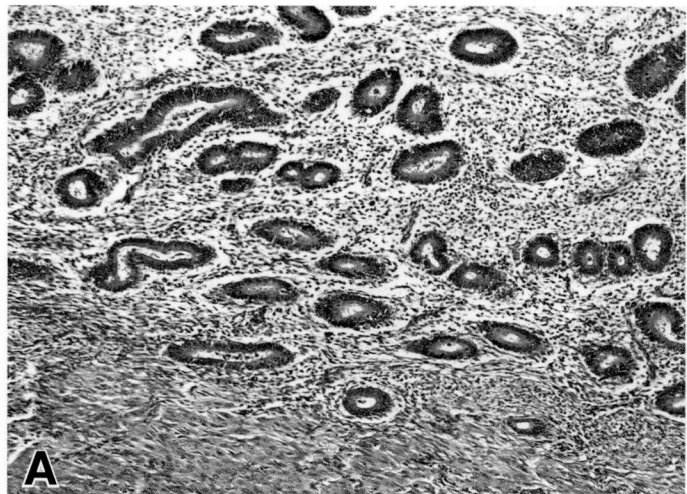
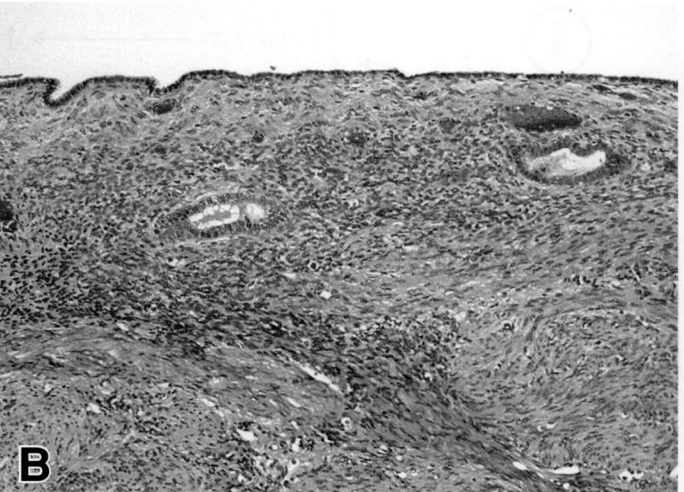

FIGURE 1-15. Atrophy of the endometrium. A. A section of the normal uterus from a woman of reproductive age reveals a thick endometrium composed of proliferative glands in an abundant stroma. **B.** The endometrium of a 75-year-old woman (shown at the same magnification) is thin and contains only a few atrophic and cystic glands.

pressure on the skin and cause it to atrophy, leading to decubitus ulcers (bed sores). Hepatocytes in the center of liver lobules atrophy when poor hepatic venous return due to congestive heart failure increases intrasinusoidal pressure.

Aging

One hallmark of aging (see Chapter 10) is decreased size and/or number of neurons, cardiac myocytes, and skeletal muscle cells (called **sarcopenia**). All these organs decrease in size, leading to weakness, debility, and accelerated death.

Chronic Disease

People afflicted with chronic inflammatory or wasting diseases (see below) often show atrophy of many tissues. Tissue loss exceeds what can be attributed to decreased caloric intake, and reflects alterations in cytokines and other mediators (see below).

Conditions Leading to Hypertrophy

Situations associated with increased cell and organ mass are often converse of those that lead to atrophy. Greater functional demand or increased trophic signaling (see below) elicits adaptive increases in cell or organ size. Unfortunately for many of us, although starvation may cause both muscle and fat to atrophy, excess nutrient intake increases only fat.

Increased Functional Demand

The classical example of demand-driven adaptation and tissue hypertrophy is skeletal muscle in athletes, which is familiar to us all.

Human skeletal muscle contains slow-twitch (type I) and fast-twitch (type II) fibers. Each responds to different types of increased functional demand, and responds differently. Differences between them include different types of myosin and vastly different metabolisms—in particular mitochondrial numbers and activities, and responsiveness to demand. A marathon runner undergoing endurance training with light loads will increase highly oxidatively effective type I fibers. Muscle mass remains constant (see below). Type I

fibers depend principally on aerobic metabolism, mediated by mitochondria. Thus, endurance training increases mitochondrial aerobic activity by type I fibers, dynamically augmenting mitochondrial numbers and oxygen consumption (Fig. 1-16).

Endurance training entails adaptive increases in mitochondrial activity, requiring more mitochondria, quality control surveillance to remove those mitochondria damaged by increased oxidative activity and, as we shall see, increased vascularity and so improved oxygen delivery. Low-resistance exercise activates both AMPK (see above) and the MAP kinase pathway (p38MAPK). These both increase the amount and activation levels of the key effector, **Pgc-1α** (Fig. 1-17).

PGC-1α upregulates mitochondrial DNA and mitochondrial fusion via a cascade involving **nuclear respiratory factors** (Nrfs), which, in turn, upregulate **transcription factor of activated mitochondria (TFAM)**. TFAM stimulates mitochondrial biogenesis and fusion, which foster metabolic adaptation to exercise.

As in many settings of rapid adaptation to changed circumstances, healthy new organelles are produced and damaged ones must be removed. A parallel mechanism identifies damaged mitochondria and eliminates them by autophagy (**mitophagy**, see above).

The nature of tissues' adaptations to increased functional demand also depends on the magnitude of the demand. Above, we illustrated adaptive responses to repetitive exercise with low loads. However, weightlifters impose different types of adaptive needs on their muscles. In response to high load stresses, type II fibers hypertrophy. Responses to repeated need to handle high loads are more complex than those described above, and are illustrated in Figure 1-18. The forces that drive muscle hypertrophy in this setting reorganize cellular metabolism, to favor anaerobic glycolysis over oxidative phosphorylation.

Increased Trophic Signals

Cells and organs, like thyroid or breast, that respond to hormones and other physical and soluble mediators (estrogens

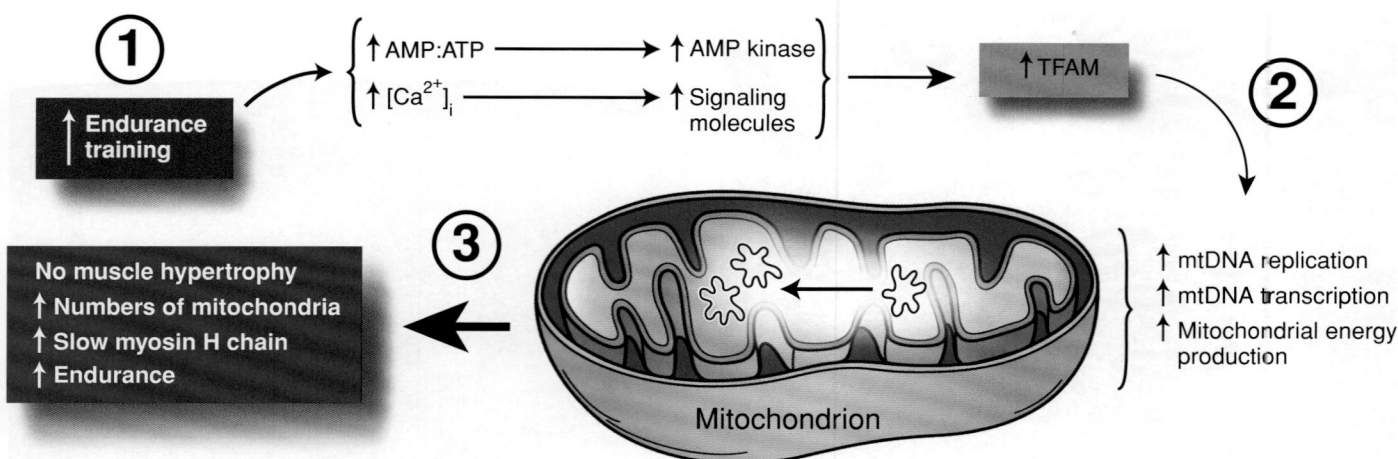

FIGURE 1-16. Mechanisms involved in muscle hypertrophy: Endurance training. 1. Muscle strengthening for endurance entails repeated or prolonged exercise with small loads and raises the adenosine monophosphate-to-adenosine triphosphate (AMP:ATP) ratio, stimulating AMP kinase activity. Such training also increases cytosolic calcium concentration ($[Ca^{2+}]_i$), which triggers a number of cellular signaling intermediates. **2.** Consequent peroxisome activation triggers TFAM (transcription factor–activating mitochondrial transcription), which in turn leads to both replication and transcription of mitochondrial DNA. **3.** The consequence is augmentation of muscle content of slow myosin H chains, increased numbers of mitochondria, and improved endurance without muscle cell hypertrophy.

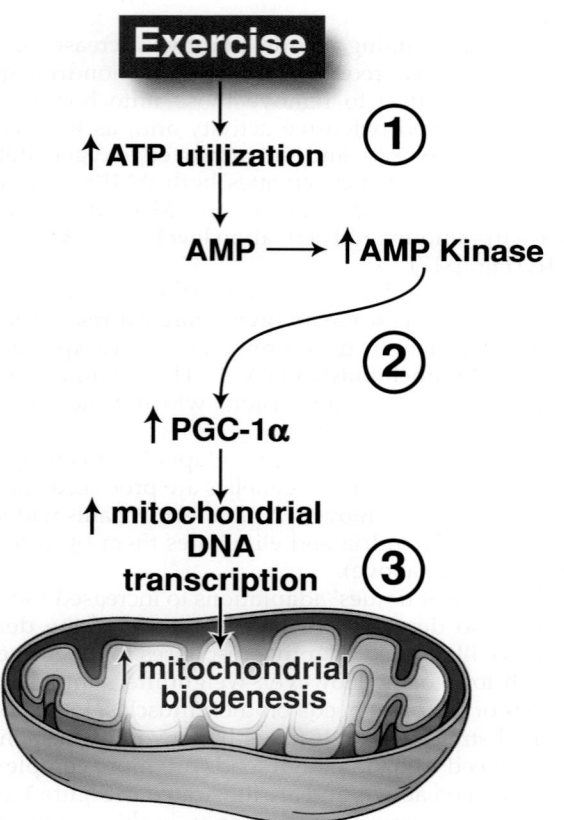

FIGURE 1-17. Akt-independent muscle hypertrophy. 1. Exercise requires adenosine triphosphate (ATP), which is then converted to adenosine monophosphate (AMP), in turn stimulating AMP kinase. **2.** AMP kinase activates PGC-1a (a transcription factor coactivator that upregulates energy production), leading to increased transcription of mitochondrial DNA. **3.** The final result is an increased number of mitochondria.

and progestins) may undergo hypertrophy when those hormones increase.

Atrophy and Hypertrophy Are Active Results of Checks and Balances Among Extracellular Stimuli and Interwoven Intracellular Mediators

CLINICAL FEATURES: Why study the mechanisms of atrophy and hypertrophy? They are much more than abstract details of little practical importance to anyone in real life (save, perhaps, sports trainers, or researchers). Quite the contrary, loss of muscle mass as a consequence of starvation or disease (**cachexia**) is a major medical problem affecting patients with cancer, congestive heart failure, COPD, AIDS, and many other chronic illnesses. **Sarcopenia**, which is muscle loss during advanced (or advancing) years, affects a large percentage of the elderly. Both have significant medical and human consequences. Cachexia impairs responsiveness to therapy, decreases resilience, and may cause and accelerate death, regardless of the status of the patient's underlying disease. Sarcopenia restricts individuals' mobility, limits their self-sufficiency, leads to loss of independence, and greatly increases the cost of care.

These processes can be slowed or even prevented by attention to approaches that lead to muscle hypertrophy. The signaling mechanisms that underlie atrophy and hypertrophy are related, as described below. Not only do some pathways stimulate or facilitate one, there are also pathways that seem mainly to inhibit the other. The clinical and societal impact of atrophy and hypertrophy makes them subjects of intense diagnostic and therapeutic study. Atrophy and hypertrophy represent quintessential cellular responses to changes in their environment. They

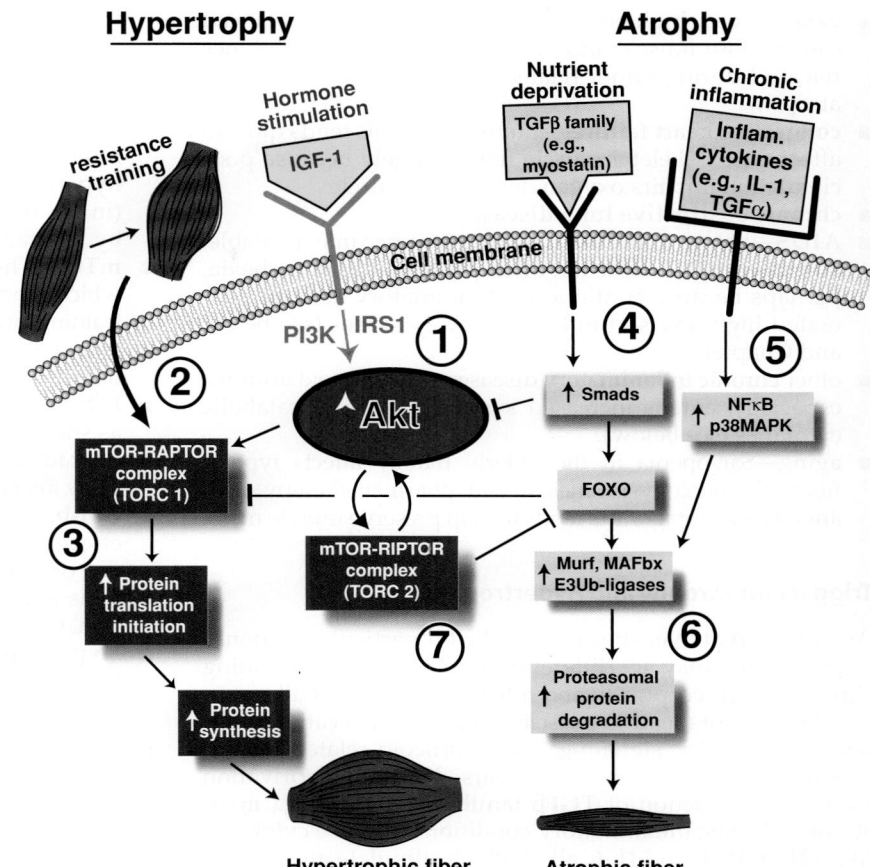

FIGURE 1-18. **Interrelationship between muscle atrophy and hypertrophy: Centrality of Akt to both atrophy and hypertrophy. 1.** In resistance-induced hypertrophy, binding of insulin-like growth factor-I (IGF-I) to its receptor stimulates Akt activity, which leads to **2**, activation of the mTOR complex and consequent increases in protein synthesis. **3.** Conversely, in atrophy, transforming growth factor-b (TGF-b) binding by its receptor triggers Smad activity, which in turn inhibits Akt. **4.** Smads also stimulate a transcription factor (FOXO). FOXO is also inhibited by the Akt-activated mTOR complex, TORC2. Blocking of FOXO relieves its inhibition of the mTORC complex, TORC1, thereby leading to greater protein production during hypertrophy. **5.** Concurrently, FOXO increases protein degradation, which is characteristic of atrophy.

are best understood—in fact, can only be understood—in the context of protein degradation and autophagy (see above).

Stimuli Leading to Cellular Hypertrophy

Puberty

The surge in androgens and growth hormone (GH) during puberty, especially in boys, leads to greater bone and muscle mass. GH stimulates IGF-1 production, which (see below) is a major stimulant for hypertrophy-related signaling and inhibition of atrophy. Beyond puberty, *physiologic* stimuli (as opposed to pharmacologic manipulation) for muscle hypertrophy do not clearly reflect increased IGF-1 or other hormones or cytokines.

Increased Demand Leading to Increased Cell and Tissue Mass

Early in the process, cells accelerate degradation of selected proteins (see proteasomes, above) that do not contribute to the need for hypertrophy. This occurs even as cells make more of proteins that promote hypertrophy. Thus, some genes are expressed more, some less. Some proteins accumulate or become activated, while others are reduced.

Factors Stimulating Hypertrophy

Signals that elicit hypertrophic responses vary depending on cell type and circumstances. Consequences of such signaling vary from cell type to cell type, and reflect each cell's context.

Further, as we shall see, some signals promote hypertrophy by interfering with atrophy, while other signals stimulate hypertrophy directly.

Prototypically, type II skeletal muscle fibers and cardiac muscle respond to increased demand by hypertrophy. Repeated use for high resistance tasks leads to cellular hypertrophy.

Hypertrophy is not simply cells accumulating mass. It is accumulation of the right cell mass, with simultaneous elimination of cell constituents that do not contribute to the task at hand. Factors that participate in this process include:

- physical forces—for example, weight load (resistance)
- growth factors—physiologically (e.g., during childhood or puberty) and adaptively to environmental changes
- neuroendocrine stimulation—for example, the β-adrenergic system
- ion channels—for example, Ca^{2+} fluxes across membranes
- other mediators—such as oligopeptides or small molecules
- angiogenesis—to supply cells' increased needs for oxygen, glucose, and other nutrients
- antagonists

Factors Favoring Atrophy

Atrophy is an active process, like hypertrophy, reflecting selective synthesis and degradation of cellular constituents. Unlike hypertrophy, atrophy tends to predominate in the setting of certain systemic conditions or diseases. Among these are:

- **cancer**—very high percentages of patients with advanced cancers lose muscle and adipose tissue mass. Cytokines released during tumor-related lipolysis stimulate muscle atrophy.
- **congestive heart failure**—interestingly, this tends most to affect type I skeletal muscle fibers, largely because poor circulation impairs oxygen delivery to muscle
- **chronic obstructive lung disease**
- **AIDS**—before antiretroviral treatment became available, advanced HIV-1 infection often presented with cachexia, perhaps because continuous inflammatory activity generated high levels of inflammatory cytokines (see below and Chapter 2).
- other **chronic inflammatory diseases**—rheumatoid arthritis, especially, entails increased systemic levels of catabolic cytokines (see below).
- **aging**—Sarcopenia in the elderly mainly affects type II fibers. Its etiology is unclear, but pharmacotherapy with angiotensin antagonists tends to help preserve muscle mass.

Triggers for Atrophy and Hypertrophy

As indicated above, stimuli that elicit a particular response in one setting may act differently in others. Some initiating stimuli reflect receptor-ligand interactions, but not all.

Many factors lead to muscle atrophy. Denervation interferes with trophic signaling. Glucocorticoid-related muscle wasting has been known for years. Nutrient deprivation increases production of **TGFβ** family cytokines (e.g., **myostatin**). Chronic inflammatory conditions increase cytokines like **TNFα**, **IL-1**, and **IL-6**, all of which stimulate atrophy.

Some hormones, such as androgens and IGF-1, may cause muscle hypertrophy during early years and especially puberty, but not later in life. Otherwise, physiologic levels of these mediators appear to play little role in stimulating hypertrophy directly.

Resistance training induces muscular hypertrophy via as yet unclear triggers. Some evidence suggests that membrane phospholipid products and, perhaps, G protein–coupled receptors, may initiate downstream hypertrophy-generating signals, but this remains conjectural. There are data suggesting that β-adrenergic stimulation may be important in hypertension-related cardiac myocyte hypertrophy (see Chapter 17).

Mechanisms leading to atrophy and hypertrophy are intertwined. In many cases, settings favoring one or the other do not directly stimulate one process, so much as they inhibit the other. The outcome, then, depends on the nature of the balance (Fig. 1-18).

Hypertrophy reflects a net increase in protein production and a net decrease in protein degradation. In atrophy, the net balance is opposite: less protein is made than is degraded. In hypertrophy, every step of the process increases protein production, from transcription of specific genes, through more effective mRNA translation because ribosomes increase both in number and efficiency. In atrophy, protein degradation increases because of increased ubiquitination and proteasomal degradation of specific proteins (including those that stimulate protein synthesis) and increased autophagic activity.

Several species and steps appear to be central to the outcome of this minuet between atrophy and hypertrophy:

- **IGF-1 and anabolic cytokines.** In childhood, these are critical to muscle and bone growth. Thereafter, they appear less to stimulate hypertrophy than to facilitate

it and to inhibit atrophy. IRS-1 is activated when IGF-1 binds its receptor, and is a key signaling intermediate in IGF-1-activated cell functions.
- **Akt** (also called protein kinase B, or PKB). Like IGF-1, Akt in adults mainly inhibits atrophy, for example, by inhibiting FOXO (see below), rather than directly eliciting hypertrophy. It may, however, magnify increased mTOR (in the TORC1 complex, below) activity that is stimulated by resistance training.
- **mTOR.** This protein participates in two complexes, TORC1, which is activated via unknown intermediates by resistance training, and which leads to hypertrophy; and TORC2, activation of which is even less well understood and which participates in an autocrine stimulatory loop with Akt.
- **FOXO.** This family of transcription factors is activated, as shown, by several pathways. FOXOs stimulate protein degradation by increasing production of E3-Ub ligases. They also inhibit TORC1.
- **Cbl-b.** This E3-Ub ligase has many activities and biologic effects. In the context of this discussion, it complexes with one or more members of the Cullin family of scaffold proteins to polyubiquitinate IRS-1 and target it for degradation. Cbl-b thus inhibits hypertrophy.
- **Hypertrophy antagonists.** Some molecules impede hypertrophy, or promote its nemesis, atrophy.

Ancillary processes that contribute to atrophy and hypertrophy include:

- **Survival signaling.** Stimulating hypertrophy entails inhibiting cell death. Key intermediates in the cascade, such as Akt and PI3K, inhibit PCD (see below).
- **Extracellular matrix (ECM).** In some situations, hypertrophy involves changes in a cell's environment, such as remodeling ECM.
- **Recruitment of satellite cells.** Skeletal muscle hypertrophy includes recruiting perimuscular satellite cells. These may generate additional myocytes and may also fuse with myocyte syncytia to provide additional nuclei, supporting the enlarging muscle's expanded proteosynthetic needs.
- **Apoptosis** (see below). Actomyosin is specifically degraded by Ub-related pathways that are activated as part of atrophic responses. Proteasomal actomyosin degradation is greatly enhanced by prior actomyosin cleavage by caspase-3 or calpain. Both of these enzymes also participate in apoptosis (see below).
- **Energy utilization.** Muscle cells selectively decrease free fatty acid (as opposed to glucose) utilization as an energy source in adapting to unloading.

The factors that are involved are variably well—or poorly—understood, and are summarized in Figure 1-19.

5'-AMP–Activated Kinase Is Central to Cellular Adaptive Responses

AMPK, as earlier parts of this chapter indicate, is a key player in many different types of cellular adaptive responses. Its principal antagonist in almost all of these activities is mTOR, in its complex, mTORC1, and the signaling pathways that activate mTOR.

AMPK Activation and Inactivation

In large part, AMPK activation reflects a cell's, and so also the body's, energy status: decreased ATP and increased AMP

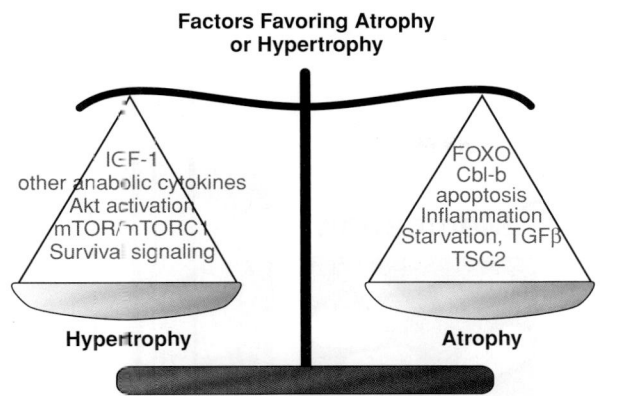

Factors Favoring Atrophy
or Hypertrophy

IGF-1
other anabolic cytokines
Akt activation
mTOR/mTORC1
Survival signaling

FOXO
Cbl-b
apoptosis
Inflammation
Starvation, TGFβ
TSC2

Hypertrophy   Atrophy

FIGURE 1-19. Balance between forces favoring atrophy and hypertrophy.

indicates energy depletion. High levels of AMP or ADP phosphorylate and so turn on AMPK. Increased ROS, if cells have adequate antioxidant capacity, may do the same. The tumor suppressor enzyme, LKB1, is an important AMPK activator (see below). Several pharmacologic agents, particularly salicylates and metformin, increase AMPK activity (see below) (Fig. 1-20A).

High levels of ATP, indicating abundant energy stores, inhibit AMPK. Other inhibitory pathways involve insulin-activated AKT signaling, inflammation, and molecules (e.g., diacylglycerol [DAG]) that reflect high blood glucose or lipid levels. Adipogenesis, which reflects overnutrition and entails increased fatty acid synthase (FAS), increases inflammation by activating toll-like receptor-4 (TLR4; see Chapter 2) and stimulating insulin resistance (see Chapter 13). AMPK activity also tends to be less vigorous as people age (Fig. 1-20B).

How AMPK Acts

In general, AMPK increases autophagy, improves cellular resistance to oxidant injury, improves insulin sensitivity, lowers blood lipid levels and circulating glucose. It achieves the latter by increasing cellular glucose uptake, while inhibiting gluconeogenesis. It strongly affects lipid metabolism—decreasing FAS and so fatty acid synthesis, while upregulating fatty acid uptake and β-oxidation via fatty acid oxidase (FAO)—decrease oxidant generation. Stimulating mitophagy and enhancing mitochondriogenesis also decrease oxidant exposure by removing dysfunctional mitochondria, which generate excess ROS, and replacing them with more efficient ones. AMPK also downregulates HMG-CoA reductase, the rate limiting step in cholesterol biosynthesis. These combined effects increase NADPH and lower the NADP/NADPH ratio. To conserve energy, AMPK decreases overall protein synthesis, but maintains production of those proteins necessary for cell survival.

It also downregulates inflammation by several routes, including decreasing fatty acid synthesis and inhibiting the proinflammatory factor, NFκB (Fig. 1-21). AMPK's anti-inflammatory activity also reflects the fact that it switches metabolism from glycolysis to mitochondrial oxidation, the latter favoring anti-inflammatory activity (e.g., in macrophages), while the former favors proinflammatory activity.

Implications of AMPK Activity

AMPK functions in several ways to maintain health and longevity.

■ It improves insulin sensitivity, while reducing insulin resistance. In so doing, it helps protect from type II diabetes, a disease that largely reflects insulin resistance (see Chapter 13).

■ It reduces inflammation and so oxidant stress, which protects both from inflammatory tissue injury and related accumulated DNA alterations. In the process, it decreases the likelihood of tumor development. Once a tumor has become established, however, the enzyme's role may protect the tumor from some therapies (see Chapter 5).

Postmitotic Cells May Turn Over

Historically, neurons, cardiac myocytes, and skeletal muscle cells were considered to be incapable of mitosis and essentially static throughout their life span. This view was generally interpreted to imply that such cells cannot be replaced, and therefore that their respective tissues cannot respond to cell loss or increased demand by adding cells. This conclusion is now considered only partially correct.

The Concept of Postmitotic Cells and Terminal Differentiation

Neurons and cardiac myocytes may not undergo mitosis, but committed progenitor cells in the brain and heart can proliferate and differentiate in response to cell loss and injury or, in the case of striated muscle, increased functional demand. Thus, there is a natural, albeit low, rate of cell loss and replacement among cells that were once considered irreplaceable. If the kinetics of such replacement favor cell loss, organ atrophy results, as in the heart, muscle, and brain of the very aged. If progenitor cell activity predominates (e.g., in the skeletal muscle), hypertrophy may result.

MORPHOLOGY OF REACTIONS TO PERSISTENT STRESSES

Hyperplasia Is Increased Cell Numbers in an Organ or Tissue

Stimuli that induce hyperplasia and mechanisms by which they act vary greatly among different tissues and cell types. A stress that causes one tissue to undergo hyperplasia may not do so in another, or may do so by different mechanisms. When so stimulated, a tissue's cells divide so that one or more of its cell populations increase in number (**hypercellular**). The stimulated cells may already be cycling or may come from resting progenitors. Hypercellularity has diverse causes, such as increased endocrine stimulation, greater functional demand, or chronic injury. **Hypertrophy** (increased organ and/or cell size; see below) may occur simultaneously with hyperplasia.

Hormonal Stimulation

Changes in hormone concentrations can cause responsive cells to proliferate, reflecting physiologic, developmental,

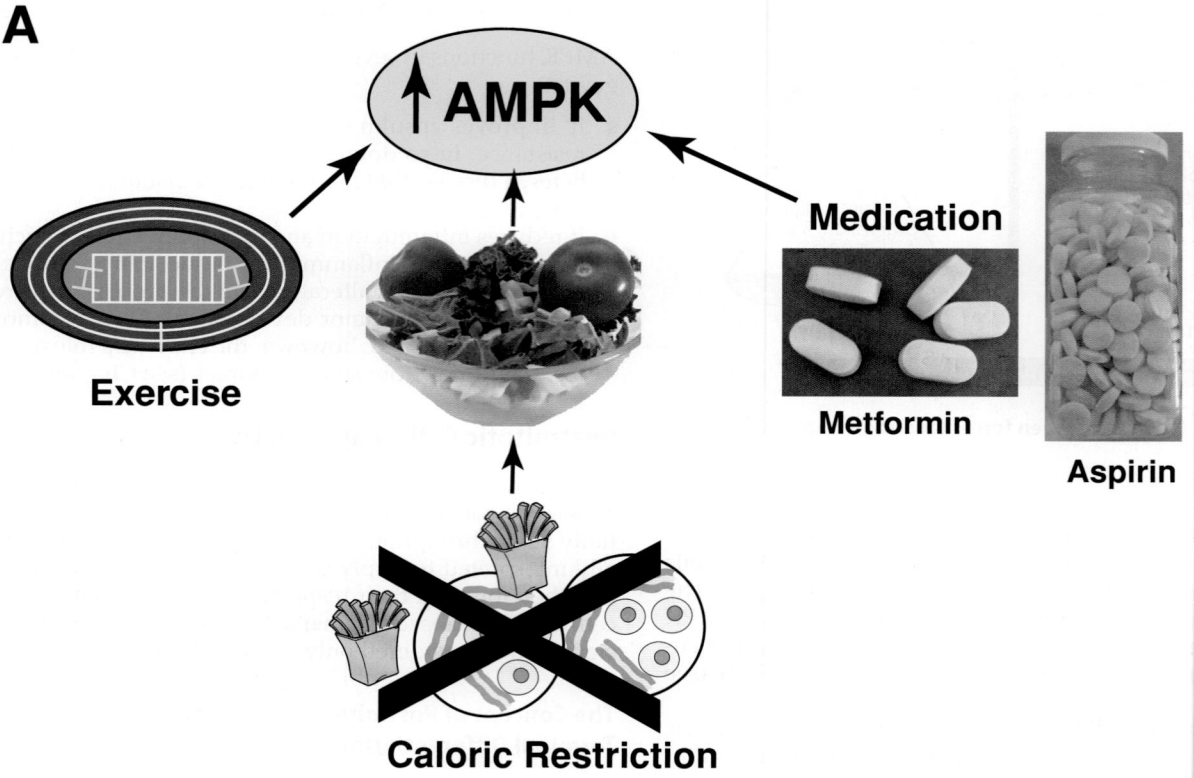

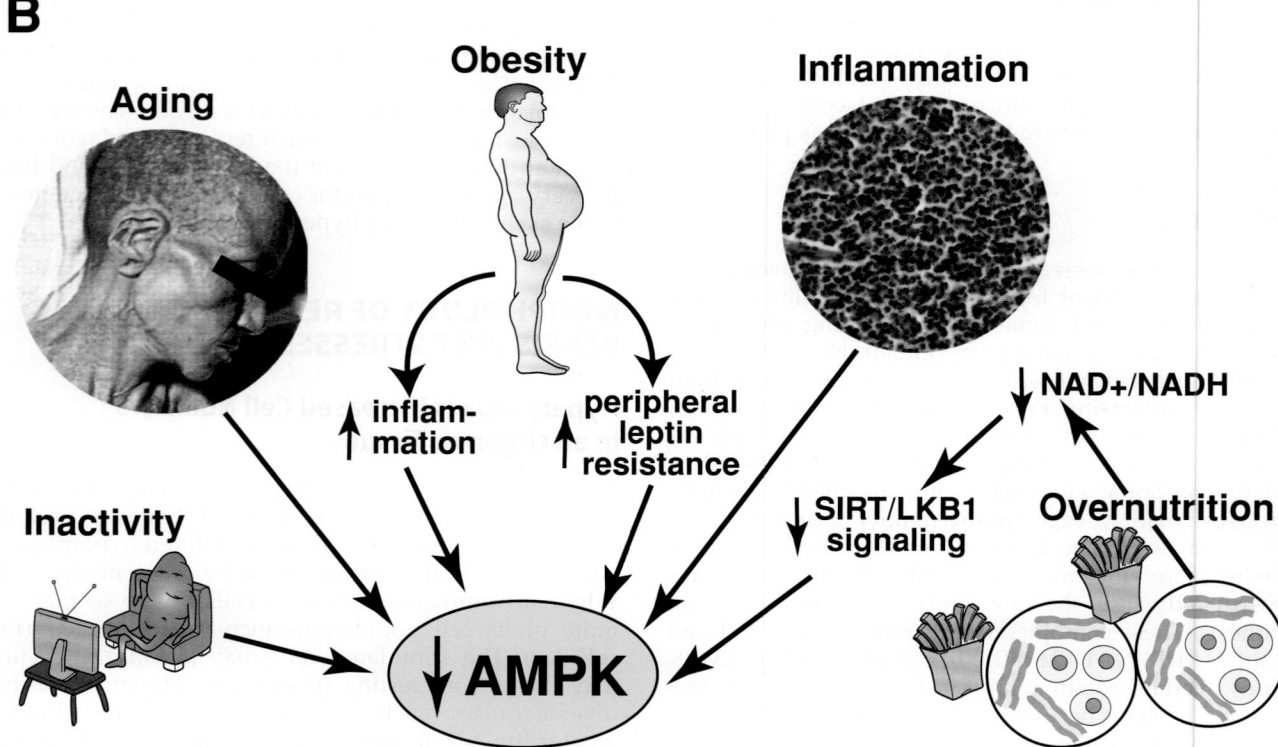

FIGURE 1-20. Factors relating to AMPK activation and downregulation. A. Factors activating AMPK. **B.** Factors leading to AMPK downregulation.

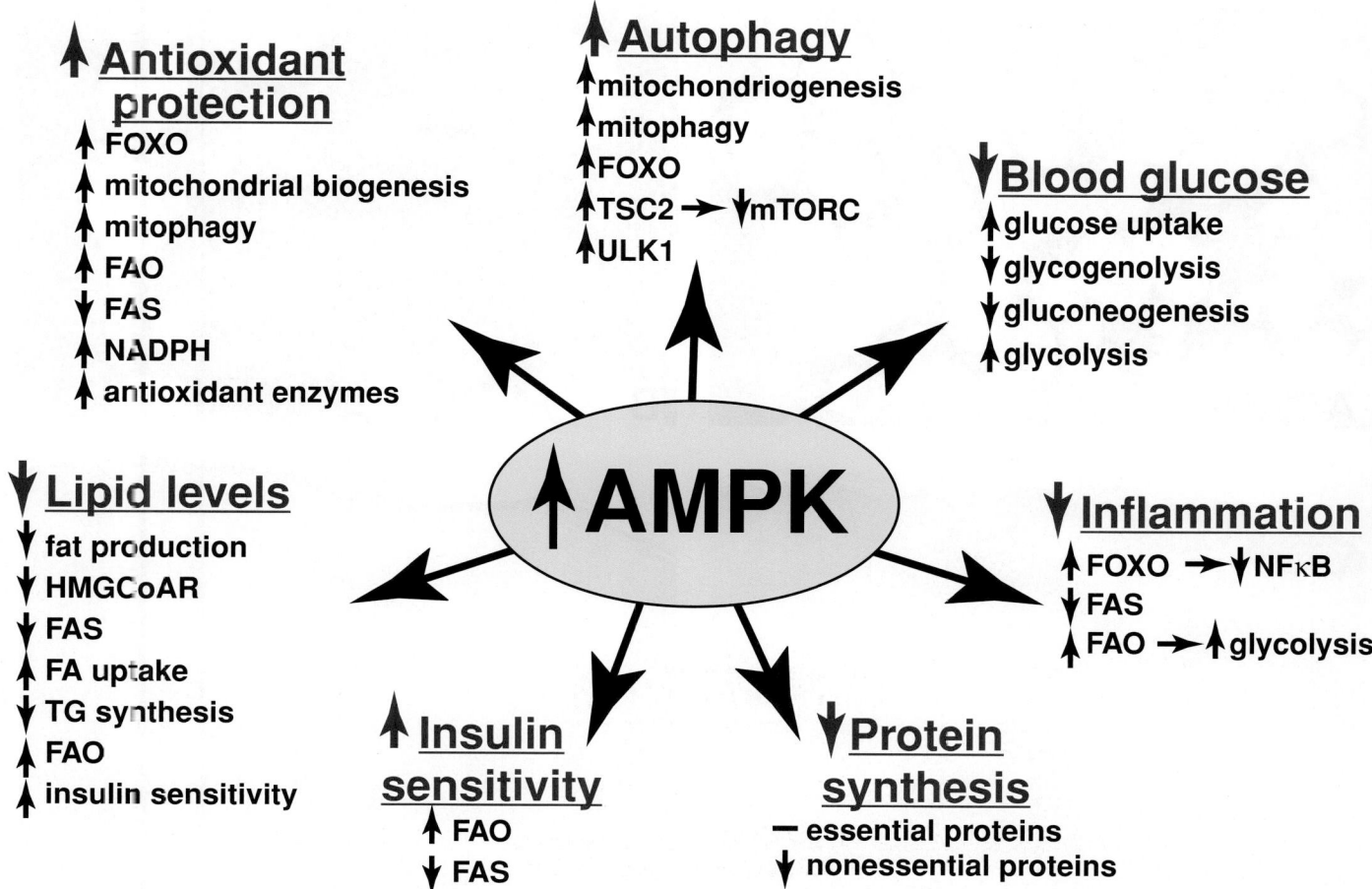

FIGURE 1-21. Consequences of AMPK activation and the mechanisms and mediators by which they act.

pathologic, or pharmacologic effects. For example, estrogens normally increase at puberty or early in the menstrual cycle, uterine epithelial and stromal cells respond by proliferating. Exogenous estrogen has the same effect (e.g., in postmenopausal women). Breast enlargement in males, **gynecomastia** may occur in men with excess estrogens (e.g., due to estrogen therapy for prostate cancer or poor detoxification of circulating estrogens by a diseased liver). Excess or ectopic hormone production may be a tumor's first presenting symptom (e.g., erythropoietin secretion by renal tumors stimulating bone marrow erythroid hyperplasia).

Increased Functional Demand

Increased physiologic requirements may result in hyperplasia. For example, low ambient oxygen tension at high altitudes elicits compensatory erythroid hyperplasia in the bone marrow and increased blood erythrocytes (secondary polycythemia) (Fig. 1-22). Red blood cell numbers increase to compensate for the decreased oxygen carried per erythrocyte. Hematocrit normalizes on return to sea level.

Bacterial infections may stimulate the bone marrow to produce and release more neutrophils than normal (myeloid hyperplasia). Immune responses to many antigens may lead to lymphoid hyperplasia (e.g., enlarged tonsils and swollen lymph nodes in streptococcal pharyngitis). Altered calcium metabolism in chronic renal failure may lead to parathyroid hyperplasia, in an attempt to maintain blood calcium levels.

Chronic Injury

Persistent injury may result in hyperplasia. Long-standing or repeated irritation, or chronic physical or chemical injury, may lead to protective hyperplasia of affected areas. Calluses, or epidermal hyperplasia, protects the skin from persistent rubbing. Chronic irritation in the urinary bladder may lead to chronic inflammation and epithelial hyperplasia.

Not all injurious stimuli that elicit hyperplasia are adaptive. Thus, psoriasis reflects ongoing uncomfortable epidermal proliferation, without apparent cause (Fig. 1-22).

Hyperplasia thus may reflect adaptive or nonadaptive cellular and molecular mechanisms that lead to increased mitotic activity, and may entail altered control of cell proliferation. In this vein, every mitosis carries a finite risk of mutation, which in turn may lead to autonomous cellular proliferation, that is, neoplasia (see Chapter 5).

Metaplasia Is Conversion of One Differentiated Cell Type to Another

Since some epithelial types are more resistant than others to some insults, metaplasia is usually an adaptive response to persistent injury. Tissues thus assume a phenotype that best protects them from the stressor. Most often, squamous epithelium replaces chronically irritated, or stressed, glandular epithelium. Squamous metaplasia in the bronchial lining of a

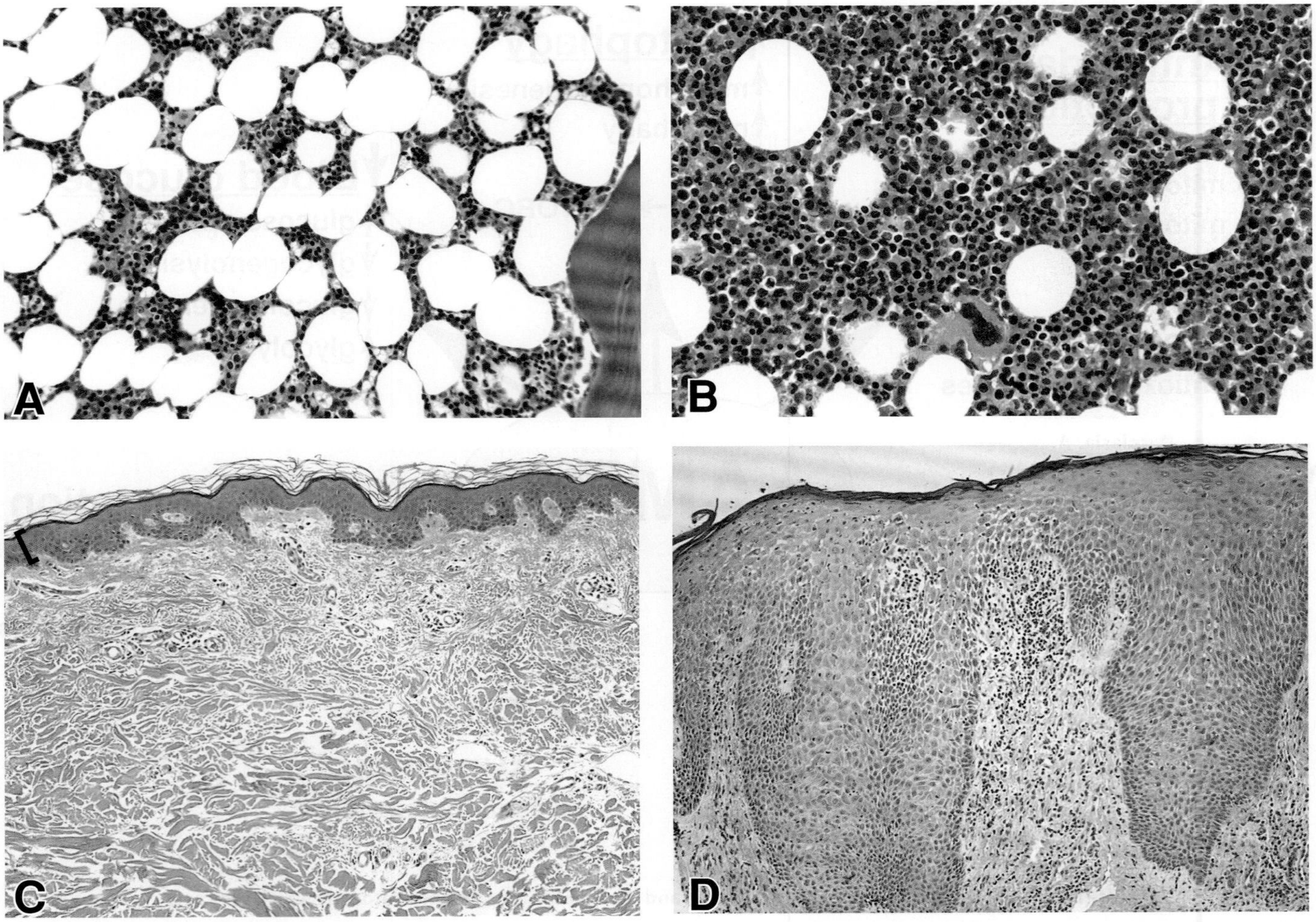

FIGURE 1-22. Hyperplasia. A. Normal adult bone marrow. Normocellular marrow with normal ratio of fat to hematopoietic cells. **B. Bone marrow hyperplasia**, with increased cellularity relative to fat. **C. Normal epidermis.** Epidermal thickness is modest (*bracket*) compared to the dermis (below). **D. Epidermal hyperplasia** in psoriasis, at the same magnification as in **C**. Thickened epidermis due to increased numbers of squamous cells.

long-term smoker is an example. Similarly, chronic infection in the endocervix may lead columnar epithelium to become squamous (Fig. 1-23). It is not clear whether metaplasia reflects altered differentiation of maturing cells or altered commitment of tissue stem cells to one lineage rather than another.

The process can go in both directions. If highly acidic gastric contents chronically reflux into the lower esophagus, intestinal-type glandular epithelium may replace the normal squamous epithelium (**Barrett esophagus**). This adaptation protects the esophagus from injury by gastric acid and pepsin, to which glandular mucosa is more resistant. Similarly, when the bladder is chronically inflamed, its transitional epithelium may undergo metaplasia to glandular epithelium (cystitis glandularis).

One glandular epithelium may also replace another. In chronic gastritis, chronic inflammation causes small intestinal type cells to replace atrophic stomach glands.

Metaplasia may be adaptive or protective, but it is not necessarily innocuous. Thus, although squamous metaplasia may protect a bronchus from tobacco smoke, it also limits mucus production and impairs ciliary clearance.

Metaplasia is usually fully reversible if the noxious stimulus is removed. Thus, when one stops smoking,

bronchial squamous metaplasia eventually returns to its prior columnar phenotype. However, as indicated above, continued irritant-stimulated epithelial proliferation may cause cancers. Lung, stomach, bladder, and other malignancies often arise in such areas.

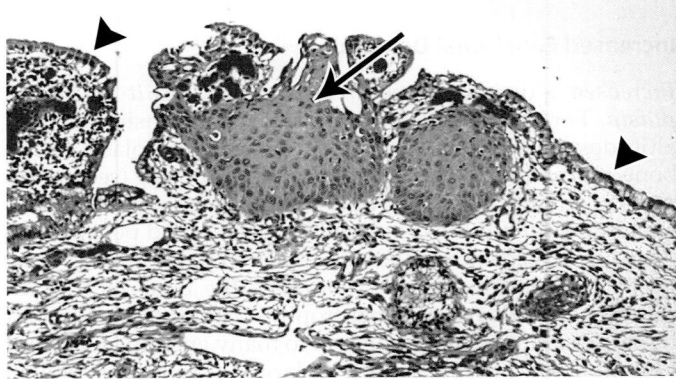

FIGURE 1-23. Squamous metaplasia. A section of endocervix shows the normal columnar epithelium at both margins (*arrowheads*) and a focus of squamous metaplasia in the center (*arrow*).

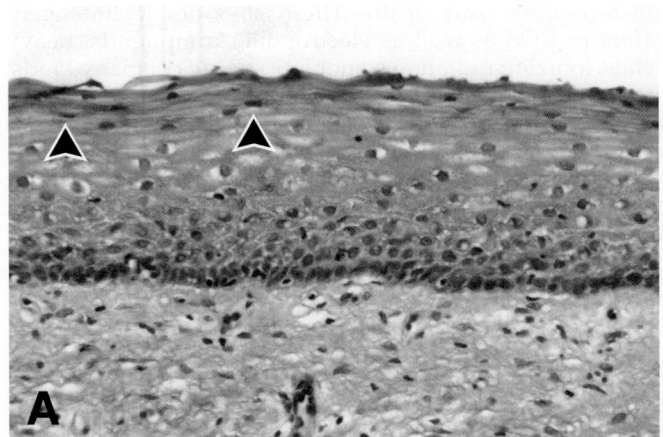
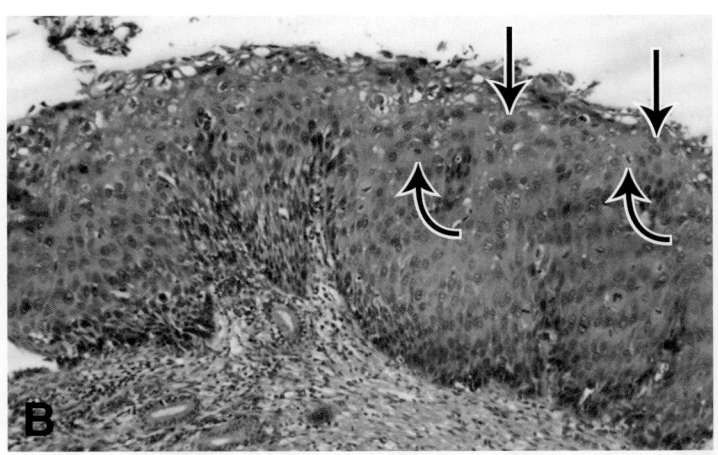

FIGURE 1-24. Dysplasia. A. Nondysplastic cervical epithelium. Normal cervix shows no mitotic activity above the most basal layers, but rather shows epithelial maturation, with flattening of the cells and progressive diminution of nuclei (*arrowheads*). **B.** At the same magnification, dysplastic epithelium of the uterine cervix lacks normal polarity, and individual cells show hyperchromatic nuclei and a greater than normal nucleus-to-cytoplasm ratio. Compare, for example, the size and hyperchromaticity of nuclei in the dysplastic cells (*straight arrows*) with the characteristics of normal counterparts at comparable height in the normal cervix. In contrast to normal cervix, cellular arrangement in dysplastic epithelium is disorderly, largely lacking appropriate histologic maturation, from the basal layers to the surface. Mitotic figures far above the basal layers (*curved arrows*) are common.

Dysplasia Is Disordered Cellular Growth and Maturation

Epithelial cells and their nuclei normally show uniform size and shape, and mature in an orderly pattern. For example, squamous epithelium progresses from plump basal cells that may undergo mitosis, through progressively less mitotically active cells with more cytoplasm and relatively smaller nuclei, eventually to flat superficial cells. This orderliness is disturbed in dysplasia. Dysplastic cells vary in size and shape. Mitoses occur distant from the basal layer. Nuclei enlarge, and are irregular and hyperchromatic. Normal, orderly maturation becomes disorderly (Fig. 1-24). *Dysplasia is the morphologic manifestation of disturbed growth and maturation.*

Dysplasia may occur in all epithelia: in epidermal keratinocytes in actinic keratosis (caused by sunlight), in a chronically inflamed colonic columnar mucosa in ulcerative colitis, in papilloma virus (HPV)-infected uterine cervix. It may affect areas of metaplasia, as in a smoker's bronchial lining or in metaplastic glandular epithelium in a patient with Barrett esophagus (see Chapter 19).

Like metaplasia, dysplasia is a kind of response to persistent injury and will usually regress when the stressor ceases: if a person stops smoking or if the immune system eliminates HPV-infected cells from the cervix. However, dysplasias share many cytologic features with frank cancer, and the line between the two may be fuzzy. Severe cervical dysplasia and in situ cervical cancer are very similar. *Dysplasia is preneoplastic: it is a precursor morphologic phenotype in cancer development* (see Chapter 5), and is part of morphologic progression of intraepithelial neoplasia in several organs (e.g., cervix, prostate, bladder). Severe dysplasia is considered an indication for aggressive preventive therapy to cure the underlying cause, eliminate a noxious agent, or surgically remove the abnormal tissue.

Like cancer (see Chapter 5), dysplasia results from cumulative sequential mutations in proliferating cells. DNA replication is imperfect, and every mitosis may lead to mutations. If one cell's particular mutation confers a growth or survival advantage, progeny of that original mutant cell will have a

survival advantage over their neighbors, and will tend to predominate. Those cells' more rapid proliferation helps their progeny to develop still additional mutations. As such mutations accumulate, they help free affected cells from normal regulatory constraints. Unlike cancer cells, dysplastic cells are not entirely autonomous. With intervention, the tissue may still revert to normal.

Persistent Stresses or Injuries May Manifest as Extracellular Accumulations

Tissue Calcification

Calcification is, of course, part of normal bone maturation. However, after cell injury, calcium enters dead or dying cells because such cells lose the ability to maintain a steep calcium gradient (see below). Such intracellular calcium accumulation only appears as inclusions within mitochondria.

In "dystrophic" calcification, macroscopic calcium salts deposit in injured tissues. Calcium leaves blood and interstitial fluids and deposits extracellularly in injured tissues. Cellular fatty acids are released from membranes when cells die, bind calcium, and cause it to precipitate. Dystrophic calcification is often grossly apparent visibly, and its feel varies from gritty, sand-like grains to firm, rock-hard material. Small tissue calcifications may reflect cell death because of rapid turnover in breast tumors or in the brains of infants who developed certain infections in utero.

Dystrophic calcification may have no functional ramifications, as in lungs or lymph nodes with tuberculosis. However, calcification may impair a structure's flexibility, and so limit its function. Thus, a calcified mitral or aortic valve (Fig. 1-25), it may limit blood flow or be unable to open completely during the cardiac cycle. Calcified atherosclerotic coronary arteries may compromise oxygen delivery to the heart. Underlying mechanisms are obscure, but molecules that drive physiologic bone calcium deposition (e.g., osteopontin, osteonectin, osteocalcin) may also lead to dystrophic calcification.

Unlike dystrophic calcification, which begins with cell injury, "metastatic" calcification reflects deranged calcium

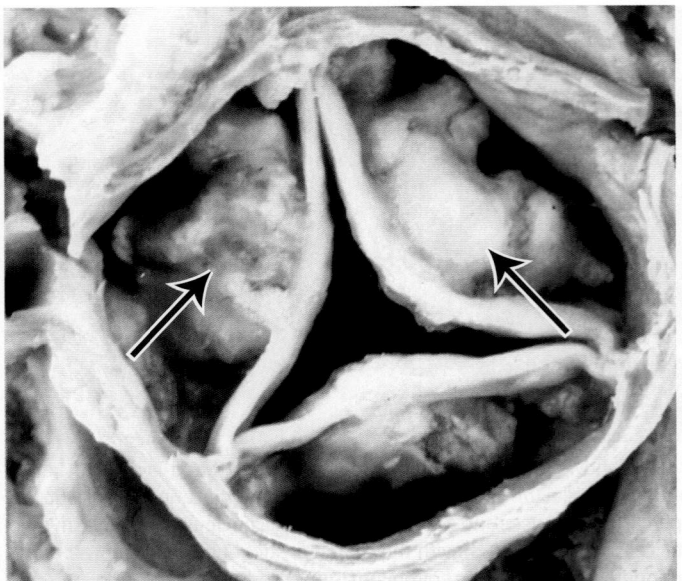

FIGURE 1-25. Calcific aortic stenosis. Deposits of solid calcium salts (*arrows*) are seen in the cusps and the free margins of the thickened aortic valve, viewed from above.

metabolism and hypercalcemia. Almost any disorder that increases blood calcium (e.g., chronic renal failure, vitamin D intoxication, primary hyperparathyroidism) can cause calcification in such inappropriate places as pulmonary alveolar septa, renal tubules, and blood vessels.

Calcium-containing stones may form because local fluids may become supersaturated with calcium, which can precipitate when nidi of organic material are present, for example, in the biliary tract, renal pelvis, or urinary bladder, as another type of pathologic calcification. Those who have suffered the agony of biliary or renal colic can attest to the unpleasant consequences of this type of calcification.

Hyaline

The term "hyaline" is an anachronism. Classically, authors used it to describe any homogeneous eosinophilic material seen on routine tissue staining. It encompassed diverse and unrelated lesions, like arteriolosclerosis, protein accumulations in alcoholic livers, material deposited along alveolar lining in respiratory distress syndrome were designated **"hyaline."** Such lesions have nothing in common. Alcoholic hyaline contains cytoskeletal filaments; hyaline in renal arterioles derives from basement membranes; and hyaline membranes in the lung consist of plasma proteins that deposit in alveoli. The term, though etiologically useless, persists as a morphologic descriptor.

OXIDANTS, OXIDATIVE INJURY, AND PROTECTION FROM OXIDANT-RELATED INJURY

Oxidative Stress Causes Cell and Tissue Injury and Triggers Adaptive Responses

Stressors, both internal and external, may cause oxidant-related damage, leading to cellular dysfunction, malignant transformation, and death. These stressors include generators of ROS as well as electrophilic compounds: heavy metals, ionizing radiation, xenobiotics, drugs of many kinds, infectious agents, and endogenously generated reactive species derived from the cell's own metabolism and organisms' responses to injury and disease. In this sense, oxygen is a blessing and a curse. Without it, life is impossible, but some of its partially reduced derivatives can react with, and damage, virtually any molecule they contact.

Reactive Oxygen Species

ROS cause cell and tissue injury in many settings. Mitochondria use molecular oxygen (O_2) as a terminal electron acceptor, reducing it to H_2O, and harnessing the resulting electrochemical potential across the inner mitochondrial membrane.

O_2 becomes H_2O by accepting four electrons. Three intermediate, partially reduced, species represent transfers of one to three electrons (Fig. 1-26). These are O_2^-, superoxide (one electron); H_2O_2, hydrogen peroxide (two electrons); and OH•,

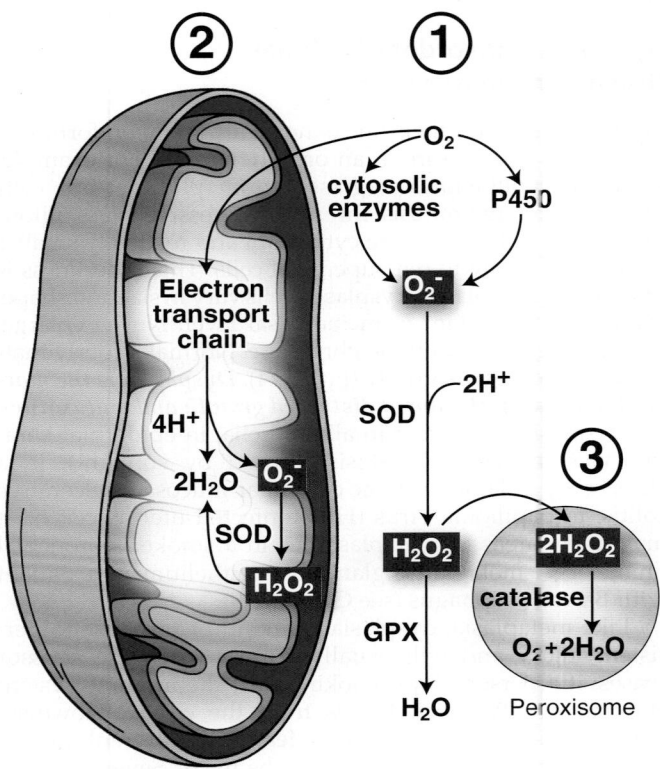

FIGURE 1-26. Mechanisms by which reactive oxygen radicals are generated from molecular oxygen and then detoxified by cellular enzymes. Circulating oxygen delivered to the cell may follow one of three paths: **1.** Molecular O_2 is converted to O_2^- in the cytosol. O_2^- is reduced to H_2O_2 by cytosolic superoxide dismutase (Cu/Zn SOD), and finally to water. **2.** O_2 enters the mitochondria, where inefficiencies in electron transport result in conversion of O_2 to O_2^-. This superoxide is rendered less reactive by further reduction to H_2O_2, via mitochondrial SOD (MnSOD). This H_2O_2 is then converted to H2O by GPX. **3.** Cytosolic H_2O_2 enters peroxisomes where it is detoxified to H_2O by catalase. *CoQ* = coenzyme Q; *GPX* = glutathione peroxidase; *H*[+] = hydrogen ion; *H_2O* = water; *H_2O_2* = hydrogen peroxide; *O_2* = oxygen; *O_2^-* = superoxide; *SOD* = superoxide dismutase.

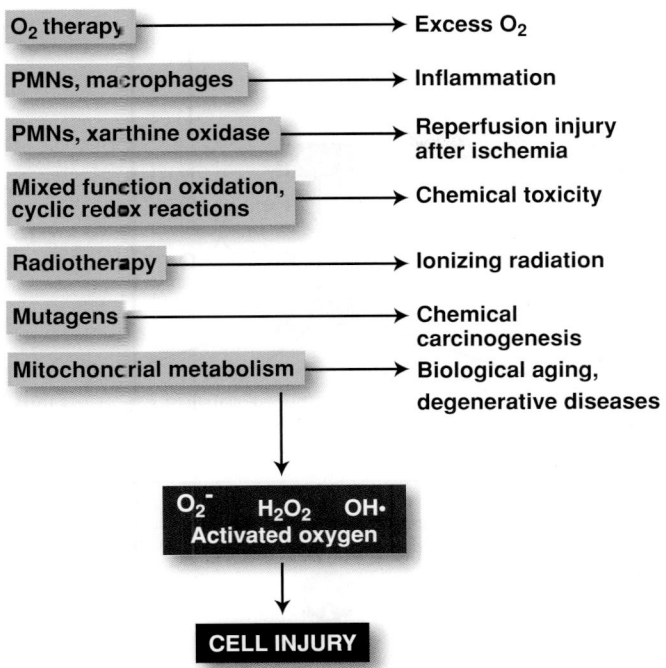

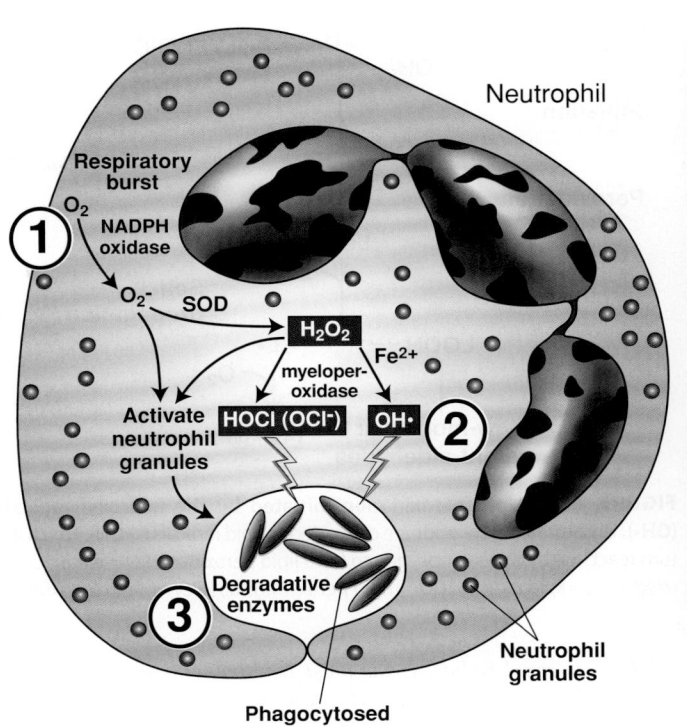

FIGURE 1-27. Exposure to oxidizing agents, and types of resulting cell injury. H_2O_2 = hydrogen peroxide; O_2 = oxygen; O_2^- = superoxide; $OH\bullet$ = hydroxyl radical; *PMNs* = polymorphonuclear neutrophils.

FIGURE 1-28. Generation of reactive oxygen species in neutrophils as a result of phagocytosis of bacteria. 1. The respiratory burst in neutrophils begins with reduction of O_2 to O_2^- by NADPH oxidase. In turn, O_2^- is converted to H_2O_2 by SOD. **2.** Reactive oxygen species (ROS) (HOCl, OH•) are produced from H_2O_2 by myeloperoxidase. Concurrently, O_2^- and H_2O_2 activate neutrophil granules to release degradative enzymes. **3.** Bacteria are engulfed by neutrophils, where they are destroyed by ROS and degradative enzymes. *Fe²⁺* = ferrous iron; H_2O_2 = hydrogen peroxide; *HOCl* = hypochlorous acid; *NADPH* = reduced nicotinamide adenine dinucleotide phosphate; *OCl⁻* = hypochlorite radical; *OH•* = hydroxyl radical; *SOD* = superoxide dismutase.

the hydroxyl radical (three electrons). These ROS normally come from several sources, including inefficiencies in mitochondrial electron transport and mixed-function oxygenases (P450). ROS are also important cellular signaling intermediates. The major forms of ROS are listed in Table 1-1. Excessive ROS may derive from many stimuli or exposures, and can both cause and aggravate many disorders (Fig. 1-27).

Superoxide

Superoxide anion (O_2^-) may come from several sources. Leaks in mitochondrial electron transport reflect the promiscuity of coenzyme Q (CoQ) and other imperfections in the electron transport chain (ETC), which allow electron transfer to O_2 to produce O_2^-. Phagocytic inflammatory cells entail activation of a plasma membrane oxidase that produces O_2^-, which is then converted to H_2O_2 and eventually to other ROS (Fig. 1-28). These ROS are key effectors of cellular defenses that destroy phagocytosed material, like microbial pathogens, dead cells, etc. (see Chapter 2). ROS also are important intracellular signaling intermediates in pathways that mediate many critical functions, such as release of proteolytic and other degradative enzymes, that help to destroy bacteria and other foreign materials.

Hydrogen Peroxide

O_2^- anions are converted by superoxide dismutases (SODs) to hydrogen peroxide, H_2O_2. Oxidases in cytoplasmic peroxisomes may also produce peroxide directly (Fig. 1-26). By itself, H_2O_2 is not particularly injurious, and is largely metabolized to H_2O by catalase. However, when peroxide is present in excess, it may be converted to the very destructive and highly reactive hydroxyl radical, OH•. Neutrophil

myeloperoxidase may transform H_2O_2 to another potent radical, hypochlorite (OCl⁻), which is lethal for microorganisms and, if released extracellularly, can kill cells.

Most cells have efficient mechanisms for removing H_2O_2. Two different enzymes reduce H_2O_2 to water: (1) catalase within peroxisomes and (2) glutathione peroxidase (GPX) in the cytosol and mitochondria (Fig. 1-26). GPX uses reduced glutathione (GSH) as a cofactor in a reaction yielding oxidized glutathione (GSSG). Because H_2O_2 is membrane permeable, it affects oxidant balance in many cellular compartments, not only in mitochondria that produce it.

Hydroxyl Radical

Hydroxyl radicals (OH•) are formed by (1) radiolysis of water (caused, e.g., by ionizing radiation), (2) H_2O_2 reaction with ferrous iron (Fe^{2+}) or cuprous copper (Cu^{1+}) in the Fenton reaction:

$$Fe^{2+} + H_2O_2 \rightarrow Fe^{3+} + OH^- + OH\bullet$$

and (3) conversion of O_2^- with H_2O_2, which is called the Haber–Weiss reaction:

$$O_2^- + H^+ + H_2O_2 \rightarrow O_2 + H_2O + OH\bullet$$

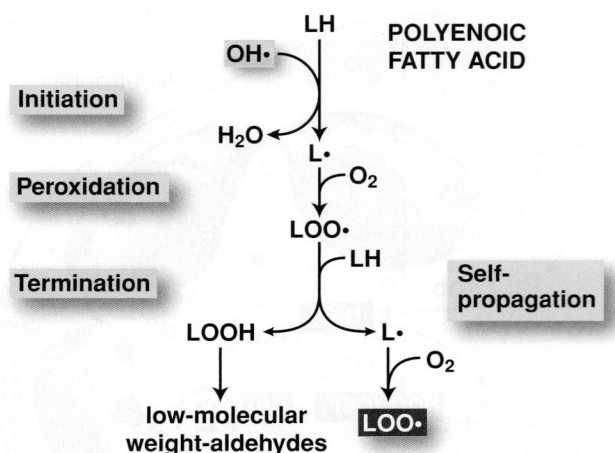

FIGURE 1-29. Lipid peroxidation initiated by the hydroxyl radical (OH·). Unsaturated fatty acids are converted to lipid radicals by OH·, which in turn reacts with molecular oxygen to form lipid peroxides. H_2O = water; O_2 = oxygen; $L·$ = lipid radical; $LOO·$ = lipid peroxy radical; $LOOH$ = lipid peroxide.

The hydroxyl radical is the most reactive, and so destructive, ROS, and there are several mechanisms by which it can damage macromolecules.

Iron and other cations often participate actively in oxidative damage to cells (see below) by virtue of the Fenton reaction. In several cell types, H_2O_2 stimulates iron uptake and so increases hydroxyl radical production.

- **Lipid peroxidation:** Hydroxyl radicals remove a hydrogen atom from unsaturated fatty acids in membrane phospholipids, a process that forms a free lipid radical (Fig. 1-29). The lipid radical then reacts with molecular oxygen to generate a lipid peroxide radical. Lipid peroxides then act as initiators, removing a hydrogen atom from a second unsaturated fatty acid, to create a lipid peroxide and a new lipid radical, initiating a chain reaction. Lipid peroxides are unstable and break down into smaller molecules. Destruction of unsaturated fatty acids in phospholipids impairs membrane integrity.
- **Protein interactions:** Hydroxyl radicals may also attack proteins. Sulfur- and nitrogen-containing amino acids, cysteine, methionine, arginine, histidine, and proline, are especially vulnerable to attack by OH•. Oxidative damage causes proteins to fragment and undergo cross-linking, aggregation, and eventually degradation (see below).
- **Sugars:** OH• can attack sugars and other carbohydrates to generate reactive intermediates that may, in turn, modify proteins to form harmful products, called AGEs.
- **DNA damage:** Hydroxyl radicals can attack DNA, causing strand breaks, modifying bases, and cross-linking DNA strands. Genomic integrity can usually be restored by the various DNA repair pathways. However, if oxidative damage to DNA is too extensive, permanent DNA mutations or cell death may result.

Figure 1-30 summarizes the mechanisms of cell injury by ROS.

Nitric Oxide and Peroxynitrite

Nitric oxide (NO) is a reactive nitrogen molecule found in many cells. Its half-life is measured in seconds. NO is the

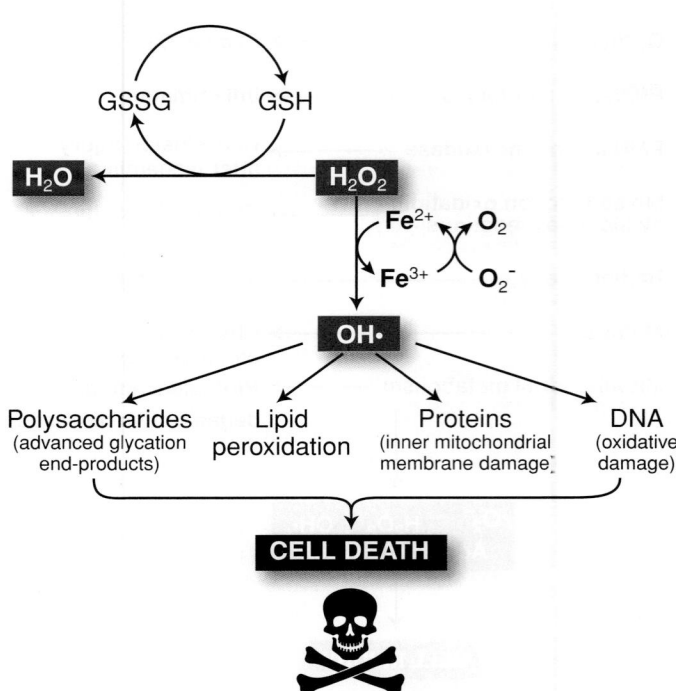

FIGURE 1-30. Mechanisms of cell injury by activated oxygen species. Fe^{2+} = ferrous iron; Fe^{3+} = ferric iron; GSH = glutathione; $GSSG$ = oxidized glutathione; H_2O_2 = hydrogen peroxide; O_2 = oxygen; O_2^- = superoxide anion; $OH•$ = hydroxyl radical.

product of nitric oxide synthase (NOS), a ubiquitous enzyme that comes in two flavors: inducible NOS (iNOS) and constitutive NOSs, which are found in several tissues. NO participates in cellular signaling, and may be harmful or protective to cells, depending on the circumstances. As a free radical, it reacts with many molecular targets, and so may activate or inhibit diverse cell functions.

When NO and oxygen interact, other free radicals result. These secondary radicals may nitrosate amines or modify other available groups, such as sulfurs on some amino acids. NO can also react with superoxide to generate another free radical, peroxynitrite (ONOO⁻):

$$NO• + O_2^- \rightarrow ONOO^-$$

Peroxynitrite attacks many important cellular molecules, including lipids, proteins, and DNA. Its actions may be beneficial or harmful, again, depending on the context.

Miscellaneous ROS

Other ROS, particularly singlet oxygen (O•) and carbonyl radical (CO_3^-•), may play important roles in oxidative stress.

The Effectiveness of Cellular Defenses May Determine the Outcome of ROS-Mediated Injury

Cells carry strong protection against damage mediated by electrophilic and ROS-mediated injury, including detoxifying enzymes and exogenous free radical scavengers. These defenses are diverse, and include the Nrf2 signaling system as the most potent generator of self-protective antioxidants, many additional enzymes, and reduced GSH as the most abundant and effective antioxidant substance.

Detoxifying Enzymes

Some key enzymes that convert ROS to less reactive molecules are the following:

- **SODs** are a small family of cytosolic, nuclear, and extracellular enzymes that defend against O_2^- by converting it to H_2O_2 and O_2 ($2O_2^- + 2H^+O_2 + H_2O_2$).
- **Catalase**, mainly located in peroxisomes, is one of two enzymes that complete the detoxification process by converting H_2O_2 to water ($2H_2O_2 \rightarrow 2H_2O + O_2$).
- **GPX** (see above) catalyzes H_2O_2 and lipid peroxide reduction in mitochondria and the cytosol ($H_2O_2 + 2GSH \rightarrow 2H_2O + GSSG$).
- **NQO1** is a cytosolic enzyme that belongs to the NAD(P)H dehydrogenase family. It reduces quinones, which generate ROS, to hydroquinones.
- **Heme Oxygenase** helps form biliverdin from heme, and generates carbon monoxide (CO) in the process. CO downregulates lipid peroxidation and upregulates anti-inflammatory cytokines, such as IL-10 (see Chapters 2, 4).
- **Peroxiredoxins** reduce H_2O_2 to water, and then use **thioredoxins** to regenerate their enzymatically active, reducing form.

Scavengers of ROS

- **Vitamin E (α-tocopherol)** is a terminal electron acceptor that aborts free radical chain reactions. As it is fat soluble, α-tocopherol protects membranes from lipid peroxidation.
- **Vitamin C (ascorbate)** is water soluble and reacts directly with O_2, OH•, and some lipid peroxidation products. It also helps regenerate the reduced form of vitamin E.
- **Retinoids,** the precursors of vitamin A, are lipid soluble and interrupt the chain reactions that propagate antioxidant species generation.
- **NO•** may scavenge ROS, mainly by chelating iron and combining with other free radicals.

Reduced Glutathione

Most oxidants are electrophiles (electron acceptors), and so antioxidants are characteristically nucleophilic (electron donors). The most abundant endogenous antioxidant is GSH. In the presence of GPX, two molecules of GSH give up two electrons to form the oxidized dimer, GSSG. GSH is then regenerated by the action of GSH reductase. Cells may also disencumber themselves of the oxidized form, and so reestablish oxidant balance, by exporting GSSG into the extracellular fluid.

Nrf2 and Nrf2 Signaling

The most potent single activator of nucleophilic defenses (including antioxidant defenses) is Nrf2 signaling. Nrf2 is a transcription factor, which mediates transcription of genes (see below) whose promoters contain antioxidant response elements (AREs).

Under unstressed conditions, Nrf2 is bound (and inactive) in the cytosol in a complex with a protein called **Keach1** and a CULLIN family E3 Ub ligase (see above). This complex shuttles Nrf2 to proteasomes, where it is degraded (Fig. 1-31).

Disentangling Nrf2 from this fate requires participation by a series of intermediates. Among these is p53, which senses stress and induces transcription of a family of intermediates, **Sestrins**, which liberate Nrf2 and activate a series

TABLE 1-2

EXAMPLES OF ANTIOXIDANT PROTEINS RESPONSIVE TO NRF2-UPREGULATION

General Function	Enzyme Name
Thioredoxin family	Peroxiredoxins
	Thioredoxin
Hydrolyzing, oxidizing, and reducing foreign chemicals	Aldehyde dehydrogenases
	Cytochrome p450s
	Epoxide hydrolase
	NADPH-quinone oxidoreductase (NQO1)
Conjugating foreign chemicals	Glutathione S-transferases (GST)
	UDP glucuronosyl transferases
Glutathione-related	Glutaredoxin
	Glutathione peroxidases
Carbohydrates and related	Glucose-6-phosphate dehydrogenase (G6PD)
	Isocitrate dehydrogenase
	Transaldolase
	Transketolase
Lipids and related	Acetyl CoA thioesterases
	Acetyl CoA oxidases
	Lipases
	Phospholipases
Iron-related	Ferritins
	Heme Oxygenase

of downstream effectors. Once Sestrins disentangle Nrf2 from Keach1, p62 (see above) mediates Keach1 degradation by autophagy. Sestrins also activate AMPK and inhibit mTORC1.

Free Nrf2 travels to the nucleus, where it turns on production of members of many families of antioxidant enzymes (Table 1-2).

Oxidant Sensors

Cells have a complex system of damage and oxidant sensors. These include the ubiquitous cellular guardian, p53 (see below and Chapter 5), among whose many functions is to sense and transduce DNA and other damage-related signaling, as well as a series of oxidant sensors. The latter include multiple protein tyrosine phosphatases and kinases. Tyrosine phosphatases dephosphorylate proteins, and all have unique structures with active site cysteines that render them sensitive to H_2O_2-mediated oxidation to one or another acid moiety. This inactivates tyrosine phosphatases. Since tyrosine phosphatases counteract tyrosine kinase-related signaling, when oxidants inactivate tyrosine phosphatases, tyrosine kinase activity is increased.

Furthermore, some protein kinases also function as oxidant sensors. Key signaling protein kinases, such as MAP kinases, which are usually activated by upstream kinases, are sensitive to, and may also be activated by, ROS.

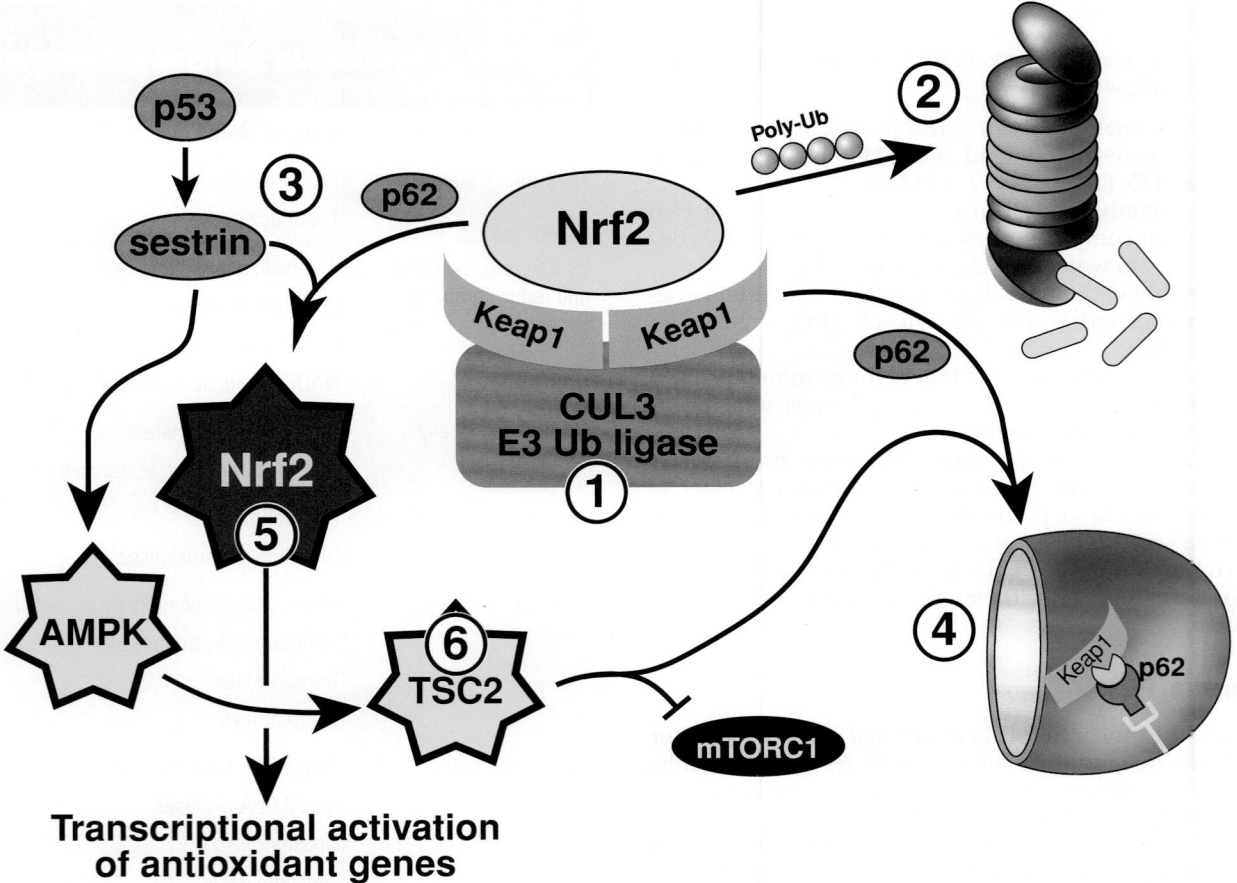

FIGURE 1-31. Nrf2: Steady state and activation. 1. Under unstressed circumstances, Nrf2 is sequestered in the cytosol, bound to a complex containing Keap1 and a CULLIN E3-ubiquitin ligase. **2.** This leads to rapid degradation of Nrf2, via proteasomes. **3.** When stress sensors are activated, p53 drives production of sestrin. This, together with p62, abstracts Nrf2 from its complex, and activates it. **4.** Simultaneously, p62 mediates autophagic Keap1 degradation. **5.** Nrf2 translocates to the nucleus, where it activates transcription of antioxidant genes. **6.** In parallel, sestrin activates AMPK, which in turn inactivates TSC2. This leads to mTORC1 inactivation. The presence of p62, plus mTORC1 inactivation, contribute to autophagic Keap1 digestion.

Activation of these pathways triggers signaling by MAPK, and activates transcription factors AP-1 and NFκB, as well as Nrf2 (Fig. 1-32). The result is increased antioxidant production.

Extracellular Oxidants and Antioxidants

Many intracellular processes generate ROS that diffuse or are transported outside cells, where they then may act as precursors of further oxidants. Such molecules include H_2O_2, lipid hydroperoxides, halogenated species such as hypochlorous acid (HOCl) derived from myeloperoxidase and related enzymes, as well as other compounds. Extracellular molecules that act as antioxidants include albumin, GSH, ascorbate (vitamin C), a-tocopherol (vitamin E), and an extracellular form of SOD.

Although the consequences of oxidative stress in the ECM are not well understood, matrix proteins such as collagen, elastin, fibronectin, and laminin are damaged. Nonprotein ECM constituents (glycosaminoglycans, chondroitin sulfate, hyaluronan, etc.) may also be altered. Damage to these ECM molecules may lead to functional impairments in skin, bone, and cartilage. Basement membranes throughout the body are also affected, particularly in the kidney and lungs.

p53 May Enhance or Inhibit Oxidative Damage

p53 is a versatile actor that plays diverse roles in the drama of cell survival and death. On the one hand, p53 helps to prevent and repair DNA damage, thereby rescuing cells from injury caused by many endogenous and exogenous insults. On the other hand, if DNA damage is irreparable, p53 activates cell death programs (see below). In addition to these activities, p53 orchestrates cellular metabolic activity in response to levels of oxidative stress.

Under normal conditions with low oxidant stress and normal levels of metabolic activity, this protein maintains expression of many antioxidant genes, thus promoting cell survival. In the face of severe oxidant stress, p53 performs an about-face and activates a different suite of target genes that impair oxidant defenses, allow cellular damage to accumulate and culminate in cell death. In addition to these effects on gene transcription, p53 directs metabolic pathways that reinforce its transcriptional activity.

Chaperonopathies

Defects in molecular chaperones contribute to several disorders, called "chaperonopathies." These diseases are

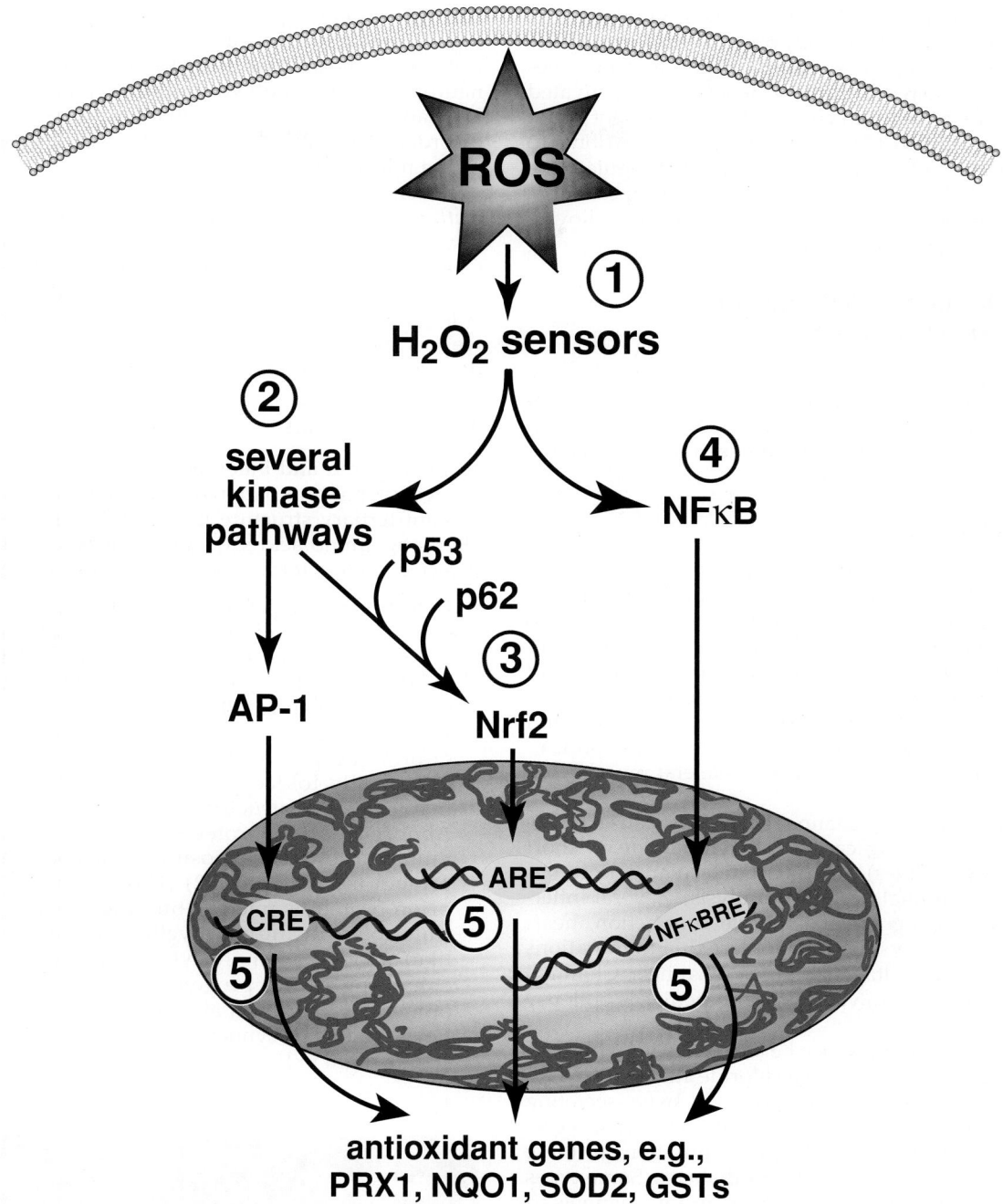

FIGURE 1-32. Activating expression of antioxidant genes. 1. In a setting of oxidant stress, endogenous peroxide sensors detect H_2O_2. **2.** This leads to activation of several different cytosolic kinase pathways, leading to activation of AP-1 transcription factor, and **3.** activating Nrf2. **4.** In parallel, NFκB is released from its inhibitor, IκB. **5.** These transcription factors bind their cognate response elements: CRE (cAMP response element, for AP-1), ARE (antioxidant response element for Nrf2) and NFκBRE (for NFκB), upregulating transcription of many antioxidant species, of which the ones are but a small number.

characterized by defects, excesses, or mistakes in chaperone proteins.

Genetic chaperonopathies mainly reflect inherited germline mutations in one or another of the molecular chaperones, and are implicated in developmental disorders, neuropathies, dilated cardiomyopathies, and polycystic liver and kidney diseases. A mutation in a chaperone cofactor causes a form of X-linked retinitis pigmentosa. Hereditary spastic paraplegia is related to a mutation in HSP60, a mitochondrial chaperone. If von Hippel–Lindau protein (VHL) is mutated, it may bind its chaperone poorly, leading to its being misfolded and inactive as a tumor suppressor. Affected people develop tumors of the adrenal, kidney, and brain. Moreover, mutant chaperone genes are responsible for certain types of cancer.

Acquired chaperonopathies arise for several reasons. Impairment of stress responses may result in inadequate amounts of chaperone proteins. By contrast, high levels of substrate (misfolded or degraded) proteins may exceed the capacity of the chaperone system. Chaperone molecules may also be sequestered in protein deposits or inactivated by exogenous toxins (e.g., an enzyme from a virulent strain of *E. coli* cleaves HSP70). Chaperones may also contribute to tumorigenesis through effects on proteins that regulate the cell cycle and cell death (see below). Acquired chaperonopathies are also implicated in biologic aging and in cardiovascular and neurodegenerative diseases.

Mutations May Impair Cell Function Without Causing Cell Death

Mutations in genes that encode a variety of proteins may lead to a wide array of clinical syndromes, but they do not necessarily cause affected cells to die. Such mutations help to provide pathogenetic links among seemingly unrelated diseases.

Channelopathies

Channelopathies are inherited or acquired disorders of ion channels. Ion channels are transmembrane pore-forming proteins that allow ions, such as Na^+, K^+, Ca^{2+}, and Cl^-, to enter or exit cells. Such ion traffic is critical for control of heartbeat, muscle contraction and relaxation, regulation of insulin secretion in pancreatic β cells, and many other functions. For example, activation and inactivation of Na^+ and K^+ channels determine neuronal action potentials, and Ca^{2+} channels are important in cardiac and skeletal muscle contraction and relaxation.

Mutations in many ion channel genes may cause a variety of diseases, including cardiac arrhythmias (e.g., short and long QT syndromes) and neuromuscular syndromes (e.g., myotonias, familial periodic paralysis). Several inherited disorders affecting skeletal muscle contraction, heart rhythm, and nervous system function are due to mutations in genes that encode voltage-gated Na^+ channels. Channelopathies may also be involved in certain pediatric epilepsy syndromes.

Nonexcitable tissues may also be affected. Cystic fibrosis, which is caused by a mutation in a chloride channel (**CFTR**), is a channelopathy affecting mucus- and sweat-secreting cells of several organs. In pancreatic β cells, ATP-sensitive K^+ channels regulate insulin secretion, and mutations in these channel genes lead to certain forms of diabetes. Some types of retinitis pigmentosa reflect mutations in ion channels. It deserves mention that mutations in gap junctions, channels that provide direct communication between cells, are also associated with a variety of inherited diseases.

Channelopathies may entail gains (epilepsy, myotonia) or losses (weakness) of ion channel function. Different mutations involving the same ion channel may cause different disorders. For instance, distinct mutations in a single skeletal muscle Na^+ channel can lead to either hyperkalemic or hypokalemic periodic paralysis. Sometimes, mutations in different genes may give rise to the same phenotype, so that mutations in different skeletal muscle Na^+ channels can cause hyperkalemic periodic paralysis.

Not all channelopathies are inherited: acquired channelopathies facilitate the evolution of some cancers (see Chapter 5) and autoimmune neurologic conditions. Autoantibodies (see Chapter 4) may cause disorders of both ligand-gated ion channels (receptors) and voltage-gated ones. Thus, autoantibodies versus nicotinic acetylcholine receptors, which control ion channels, cause myasthenia gravis and autoimmune neuropathy. Autoantibodies against voltage-gated Ca^{2+} and K^+ channels are also responsible for diverse neuromuscular disorders. Ion channels that affect cell cycle progression may play a role in tumor development.

Channelopathies are not merely esoteric diseases, but often are matters of life and death. Up to 20% of sudden unexplained deaths and 10% of sudden infant death syndrome (SIDS; see Chapter 6) reflect cardiac arrhythmias associated with mutations in the Na^+ channel responsible for long-QT syndrome. A large majority of patients with mucolipidosis type IV, as well as those with autosomal dominant polycystic kidney disease, have mutations in cell membrane Ca^{2+} channels.

Abnormal Proteins

Many acquired and inherited diseases are characterized by intracellular accumulation of abnormal proteins. A protein's deviant tertiary structure may result from a mutation that alters the amino acid sequence or may reflect an acquired defect in protein folding. The following are a few examples:

- **In α_1-antitrypsin deficiency**, mutations in the α_1-antitrypsin gene cause liver cells to produce an insoluble protein that is not exported, as it should be. It accumulates in hepatocytes (Fig. 1-33), injures them and eventually causes cirrhosis (see Chapter 19).
- **Prion diseases** are neurodegenerative disorders (spongiform encephalopathies) caused by accumulation of abnormally folded prion proteins. The protein's normal α-helical structure becomes a β-pleated sheet. Abnormal prion proteins may result from inherited mutations or from exposure to the aberrant form of the protein (see Chapter 32). The function of the normal prion protein is unclear, but data suggest several possible roles, including myelination, antioxidant (SOD-like) activity, T-lymphocyte–dendritic cell interactions, enhancing neural progenitor proliferation and development of long-term memory.
- **Lewy bodies** (α-synuclein) occur in neurons of the substantia nigra in Parkinson disease (see Chapter 32).

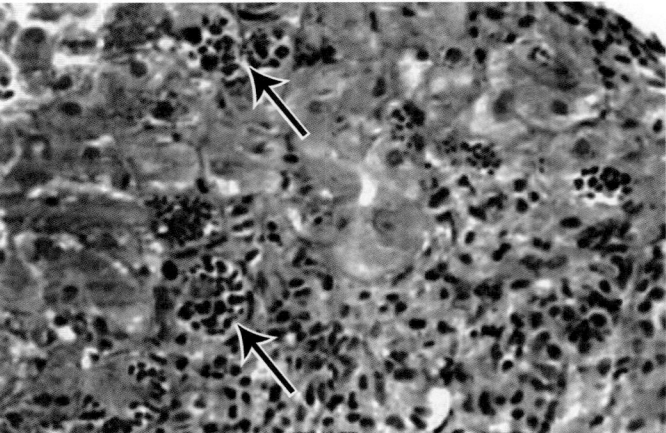

FIGURE 1-33. Storage of abnormal, mutant α_1-antitrypsin in the liver. Periodic acid–Schiff (PAS) stain after diastase treatment to remove glycogen highlights the aggregates of α_1-antitrypsin protein (*arrows*).

- **Neurofibrillary tangles** (tau protein) characterize cortical neurons in Alzheimer disease (see Chapter 32).
- **Mallory bodies** (intermediate filaments) are hepatocellular inclusions in alcoholic liver injury (see Chapter 20).

MOLECULAR PATHOGENESIS: As discussed above, when ribosomes translate messenger RNA (mRNA), they make a linear chain of amino acids without a defined three-dimensional structure. Curiously, it is energetically more favorable for cells to produce many foldings, even abnormal ones, and then edit the protein repertoire than to construct only a single correct conformation. As a result, protein misfolding is intrinsic to cellular protein production, and occurs all the time. However, there is an escape valve: evolution favors energy conservation, and so dictates that a substantial proportion of newly made proteins are rogues unsuitable for the company of civilized cells. Several outcomes are possible:

- The primary sequence is correct and the protein folds properly into the appropriate functional conformation.
- The primary sequence may be correct but the protein does not fold correctly, due to random energetic fluctuations.
- A mutant protein (one with an incorrect amino acid sequence) folds incorrectly.
- A conformationally correct protein may become unfolded or misfolded due to an unfavorable environment (e.g., altered pH, high ionic strength, oxidation, etc.). A malfunction of protein quality control or system overload may prevent the cell from correcting the problem. Misfolded proteins then accumulate as amorphous aggregates or fibrils and may cause cell injury by (1) decreasing a necessary activity (**loss of function**) or (2) a harmful increase in a cellular activity that alters a delicate balance of forces within the cell (**gain of function**).
- **Loss of function:** Some mutations prevent crucial proteins from folding correctly. These, then, do not function properly or cannot localize at the correct site. Thus, abnormal cystic fibrosis proteins are misfolded chloride ion channels, which are then degraded. As they do not reach their intended destination at the cell membrane, the resulting defect in Cl⁻ transport produces the disease. Other examples of loss of function include mutations of the low-density lipoprotein (LDL) receptor in certain types of hypercholesterolemia and mutations of a copper-transporting ATPase in Wilson disease.
- **Formation of toxic protein aggregates:** Defects in protein structure may be acquired as well as genetic. Impaired antioxidant defenses, particularly in non-dividing cells, may fail to prevent protein oxidation, which in turn alters protein tertiary structure, exposing interior hydrophobic amino acids that are normally hidden. If oxidative stress is mild to moderate, 20S proteasomes recognize these exposed hydrophobic moieties and degrade the proteins. However, when oxidative stress is excessive, a combination of hydrophobic and ionic bonds causes these proteins aggregate (Fig. 1-34). Resulting, often disordered, aggregates are insoluble and tend to sequester Fe²⁺ ions. The trapped Fe²⁺ helps generate additional ROS (see above), further increasing aggregate size. Disordered aggregates

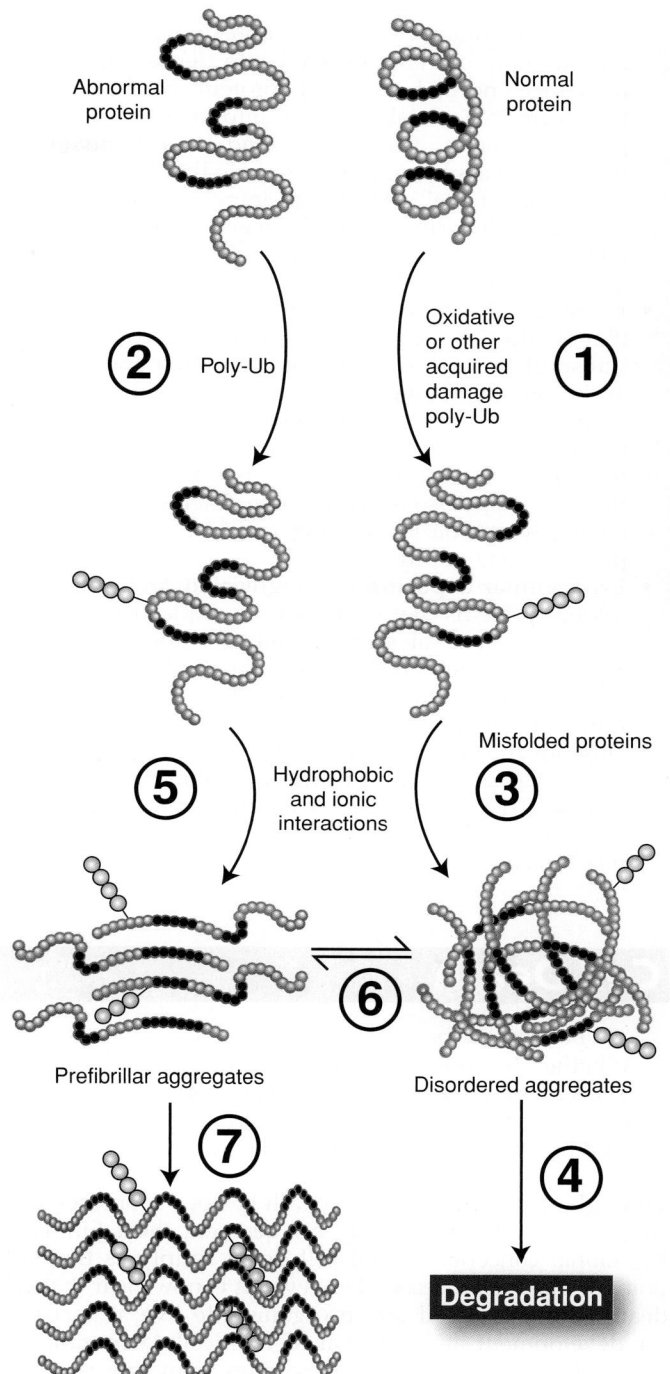

FIGURE 1-34. Formation of toxic protein aggregates. 1. Normal proteins can become damaged by exposure to reactive oxygen species and other stresses. **2.** Nonnative proteins may result from genetic mutations or translational errors. In any event, the resulting abnormal proteins may become misfolded, with hydrophobic moieties (*black*) that are normally internal to the protein appearing on the surface. The proteins are then poly-ubiquitinated, after which two paths are open. **3.** Some of the misfolded proteins may become disordered aggregates, which can be degraded (**4**). Alternatively (**5**), the normal α-helical structure may be transformed into less soluble forms, consisting, to a variable extent, of β-pleated sheets (prefibrillar aggregates). The latter may exist to some extent (**6**) in equilibrium with disordered aggregates or they may evolve irreversibly into insoluble amyloid fibrils (**7**). *Ub* = ubiquitin.

may be degraded (e.g., by autophagy; see above) or may become partially ordered into denser structures in which normal α-helical protein conformations transform to a variable degree into insoluble fibrillar β-pleated sheets. These latter tend to accumulate as indigestible agglomerations. Any Ub bound to them is lost, depleting cellular Ub and impairing proteostasis in general. By virtue of their both generating toxic ROS and inhibiting proteasomal degradation, these aggregates may lead to cell death.

- **Retention of secretory proteins:** Many cellular proteins that are destined to be secreted must fold correctly for transport through cellular compartments and release at the cell membrane. Mutations in genes that encode such proteins (e.g., α$_1$-antitrypsin) lead to cell injury because misfolded proteins accumulate massively within the cell. Failure to secrete this antiprotease into the circulation also leads to unregulated proteolysis of connective tissue in the lung and loss of pulmonary parenchyma (emphysema).

- **Extracellular deposition of aggregated proteins:** Misfolded proteins tend to assume β-pleated conformations instead of random coils or α-helices. These abnormal proteins often form insoluble aggregates, which may be deposited extracellularly. Such accumulations often assume the forms of various types of amyloid and produce cell injury in systemic amyloidosis (see Chapter 15) and a variety of neurodegenerative diseases (see Chapter 32). Accumulation of β-amyloid protein in Alzheimer disease may occur by this type of mechanism.

Cell Death

"To be or not to be—that is the question
Whether 'tis nobler in the mind to suffer
The slings and arrows of outrageous fortune
Or to take arms against a sea of troubles
And by opposing end them. To die …" (*Hamlet, III:i*)

Throughout recorded history, death has been considered as tragic, especially when youth has been cut short. Similarly, traditional concepts viewed cell death simply as the endpoint of disease processes. However, it is now clear that cell death is often needed for an organism to live; it is crucial for development and survival of multicellular organisms. Just as the grim reaper himself assumes many guises, so cell death takes diverse forms. Sometimes it represents the consequences of nonphysiologic and unregulated injury, but in others, complex intracellular molecular pathways respond to external and internal triggers to cause the cell's demise. Such PCD oversees the size and diversity of many tissue compartments by eliminating obsolescent cells, as in the gastrointestinal tract, skin, and hematopoietic system. Not all such mechanisms eliminate only older, senescent cells; in some cases, young upstarts, like autoreactive lymphocyte clones, may be targeted for destruction.

In addition to unplanned murder of cells by external violence, which is called **necrosis**, there are diverse suicide programs: apoptosis, autophagic cell death, necroptosis, NETosis, and so forth. To further complicate matters, many

of these pathways interconnect, so that clear-cut distinctions are not always possible. Outcomes of such overlapping mechanisms are usually parallel, but on occasion they are opposite and may fulfill adaptive or maladaptive functions. For example, while autophagy may impede malignant transformation, it also protects malignant cells from the effects of chemotherapy (see Chapter 5). In its many forms, PCD is integral to many disease processes.

The multiplicity and connectivity of the various networks are confusing and challenge the student to understand how processes whose consequences seem so different can be tightly linked. The field of cell death is evolving rapidly, and the following discussion is necessarily limited to those issues about which there is a consensus and that are important for an appreciation of disease development.

Understanding cell death is not simply an academic exercise; manipulation of cell viability is currently a major area of research. For example, if we understand the biochemistry of ischemic death of cardiac myocytes, which is responsible for the leading cause of death in the Western world, we may be able to prolong myocyte survival after a coronary occlusion until circulation is restored.

Once upon a time, all cell death was called necrosis. Now, we know better. Three main avenues leading to cell death have been delineated: necrosis, apoptosis, and autophagy. Other, more specialized forms of cell death are also described (see below). Necrosis was defined as an unplanned form of cell death caused by a hostile environment to which a cell could not adapt effectively. It was thus seen as a passive process in which the cell was a victim of injury over which it had no control. By contrast, apoptosis is a form of cellular suicide in which the cell participates actively in its own demise. Individual cells activate their own signaling systems to sacrifice themselves for the preservation of the organism. Autophagy (see above) is also an active signaling process that is elicited when a stressful environment requires autodigestion of a portion of the cell's macromolecular constituents. Since the principal pathways of cell death may overlap, it is important to understand how the processes manifest morphologically.

MORPHOLOGY OF CELL DEATH

Necrosis Is Reflected in Geographic Areas of Cell Death

Necrosis occurs when hostile external forces overwhelm cells' adaptive abilities. Diverse insults can cause necrotic cell death, which typically affects geographically localized groups of cells. The response to this process is usually acute inflammation, which itself may generate further cell injury (see Chapter 2). Stimuli that initiate pathways leading to necrosis are highly variable, and produce diverse and recognizable histologic and cytologic patterns.

Coagulative Necrosis

Coagulative necrosis describes specific light microscopic appearances of dead or dying cells (Fig. 1-35). Shortly after a cell dies, its outline is maintained. When stained with the usual combination of hematoxylin and eosin, the cytoplasm of necrotic cells is more deeply eosinophilic (i.e., more intensely red) than usual. This occurs because of rapid degradation of cytoplasmic RNA which, like nuclear DNA,

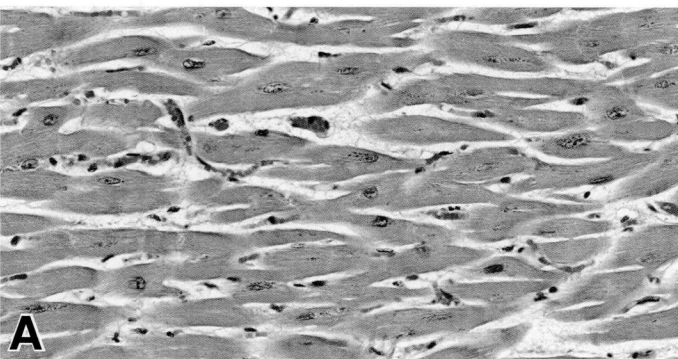
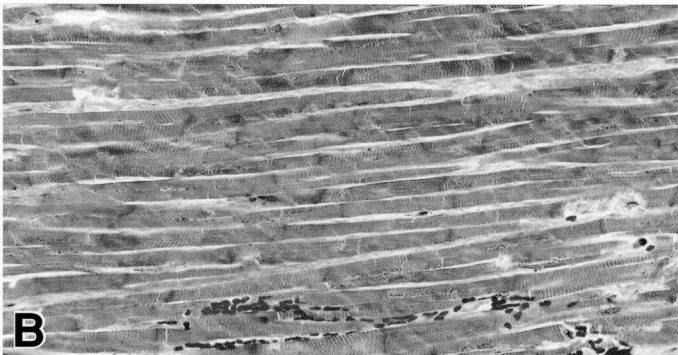

FIGURE 1-35. Coagulative necrosis. A. Normal heart. All myocytes are nucleated, and striations are clear. The cytoplasm has a slightly bluish tinge due to binding of the blue dye hematoxylin by RNA. **B. Myocardial infarction.** The heart from a patient following acute myocardial infarction. The necrotic cells are deeply eosinophilic and most have lost their nuclei. The more eosinophilic appearance is due to rapid degradation of cytoplasmic RNA.

binds the blue dye hematoxylin. The loss of such cytoplasmic staining produces the characteristic "eosinophilia" of acute coagulative necrosis. Nuclear chromatin is initially clumped, and then redistributes along the nuclear membrane. Three morphologic changes follow:

- **Pyknosis:** The nucleus becomes smaller and stains deeply basophilic as chromatin clumping continues.
- **Karyorrhexis:** The pyknotic nucleus breaks up into many smaller fragments scattered about the cytoplasm.
- **Karyolysis:** The pyknotic nucleus may be extruded from the cell or it may progressively lose chromatin staining.

Early ultrastructural changes in dying or dead cells reflect extensions of alterations associated with reversible cell injury (Fig. 1-2). In addition to nuclear changes described above, dead cells have dilated ER, disaggregated ribosomes, swollen and calcified mitochondria, aggregated cytoskeletal elements, and plasma membrane blebs and/or discontinuities.

After a variable time, depending on the tissue and circumstances, the lytic activity of intracellular and extracellular enzymes causes the cell to disintegrate. This is particularly the case when necrotic cells have elicited an acute inflammatory response.

The appearance of necrotic tissue has traditionally been described as **coagulative necrosis** because it resembles the coagulation of proteins that occurs upon heating. This term, while based on obsolete concepts, remains useful as a morphologic descriptor.

Liquefactive Necrosis

When the rate at which necrotic cells dissolve greatly exceeds the rate of repair, the resulting appearance is termed **liquefactive necrosis**. Polymorphonuclear leukocytes of the acute inflammatory reaction (see Chapter 2) contain potent hydrolases capable of digesting dead cells. A sharply localized collection of these acute inflammatory cells, generally in response to bacterial infection, produces rapid cell death and tissue dissolution. The result is often an **abscess** (Fig. 1-36), a cavity formed by liquefactive necrosis in a solid tissue. In time, the abscess is walled off by a fibrous capsule that contains its contents.

Coagulative necrosis in the brain may occur after cerebral artery occlusion and is often followed by rapid dissolution—liquefactive necrosis—of the dead tissue by a mechanism

that cannot be attributed to acute inflammation. It is not clear why coagulative necrosis in the brain and not elsewhere is followed by the disappearance of necrotic cells, but the abundant lysosomal enzymes, or different hydrolases specific to cells of the CNS, may be responsible. Liquefactive necrosis of large areas of the CNS can lead to an actual cavity or cyst that persists for the lifetime of the person.

Fat Necrosis

Fat necrosis specifically affects adipose tissue and most commonly results from pancreatitis or trauma (Fig. 1-37). The unique feature determining this type of necrosis is the presence of triglycerides in adipose tissue. In the peripancreatic fat, for example, the process begins when digestive enzymes that are normally found only in the pancreatic duct and small intestine lumen are released from injured pancreatic acinar cells and ducts into extracellular spaces. Upon extracellular activation, these enzymes digest both the pancreas itself and surrounding tissues, including adipocytes.

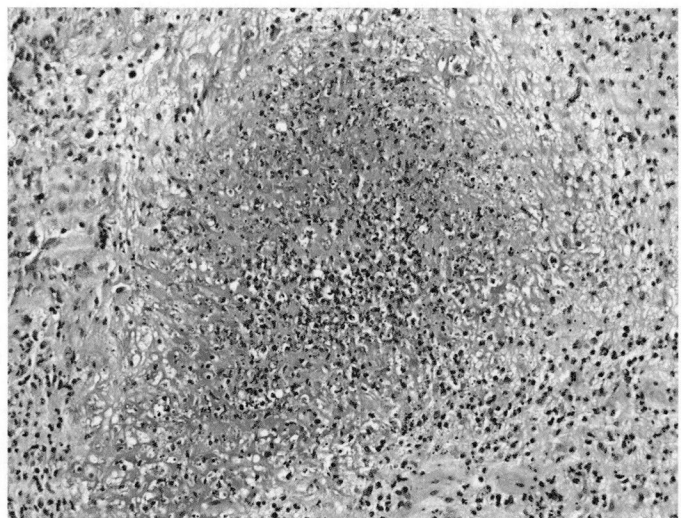

FIGURE 1-36. Liquefactive necrosis in an abscess of the skin. The abscess cavity composed of amorphous eosinophilic material in the center of the image is filled with polymorphonuclear leukocytes.

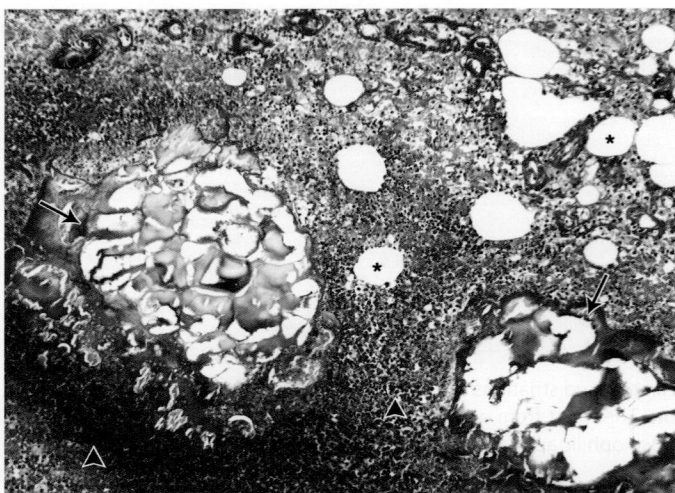

FIGURE 1-37. Fat necrosis. Peripancreatic adipose tissue from a patient with acute pancreatitis shows fatty acids precipitated as calcium soaps, which appear as amorphous, basophilic deposits (*arrows*). These intermingle with extensive acute inflammation (*arrowheads*) and remnants of adipocytes (*).

1. Phospholipases and proteases attack plasma membranes of adipocytes, releasing intracellular triglycerides.
2. Pancreatic lipase hydrolyzes the triglycerides in adipocytes, which produces free fatty acids.
3. Free fatty acids bind Ca^{2+} and precipitate as soaps. These appear as amorphous, basophilic deposits at the edges of irregular islands of necrotic adipocytes.

Grossly, fat necrosis appears as an irregular, chalky white area embedded in otherwise normal adipose tissue. In the case of traumatic fat necrosis, triglycerides and lipases are released from the injured adipocytes. In the breast, fat necrosis due to trauma is common and may mimic a tumor, particularly if calcification has occurred.

Caseous Necrosis

Caseous necrosis is characteristic of tuberculosis but occurs, less often, in other settings. The lesions of tuberculosis are

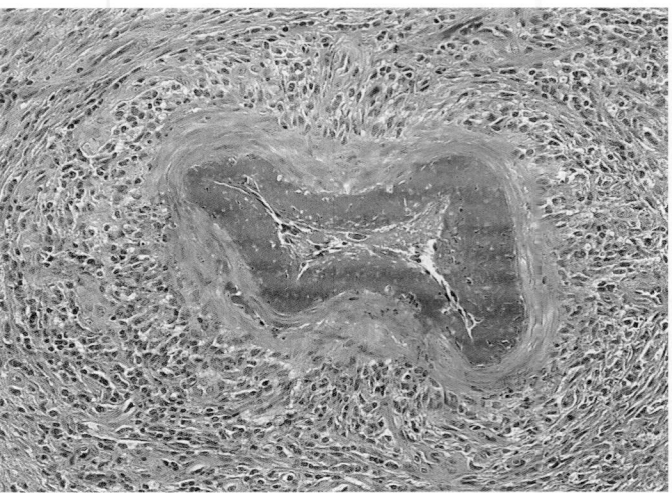

FIGURE 1-39. Fibrinoid necrosis. An inflamed muscular artery in a patient with systemic arteritis shows a sharply demarcated, homogeneous, deeply eosinophilic zone of necrosis.

granulomas or tubercles (Fig. 1-38). In the center of such granulomas, the accumulated mononuclear cells that mediate a chronic inflammatory reaction to the offending mycobacteria are killed. Unlike coagulative necrosis, dead cells in granulomas lose their cellular outlines. They do not disappear by lysis, however, as in liquefactive necrosis, but rather persist indefinitely as amorphous, coarsely granular, eosinophilic debris. Grossly, this material is grayish white, soft, and friable. It resembles clumpy cheese, hence the name **caseous necrosis**. This distinctive type of necrosis is generally attributed to the toxic effects of mycobacterial cell walls, which contain complex waxes (peptidoglycolipids) that exert potent biologic effects. In fact, granuloma formation may really be orchestrated by mycobacteria, to facilitate the organism's survival in the face of host immune responsiveness.

Fibrinoid Necrosis

Fibrinoid necrosis occurs in injured blood vessels, where insudation and accumulation of plasma proteins cause the vessel wall to stain intensely with eosin (Fig. 1-39). The term

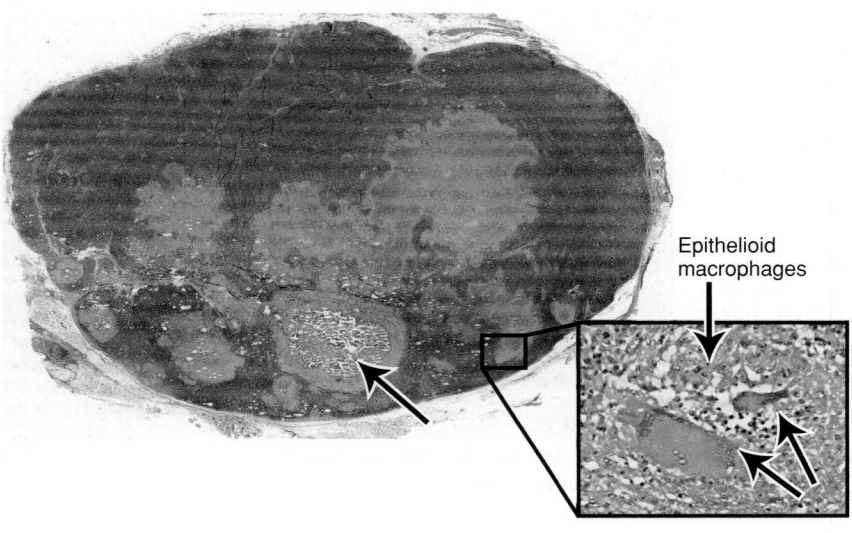

Epithelioid macrophages

FIGURE 1-38. Caseous necrosis in a tuberculous lymph node. Hilar lymph node from a patient with active tuberculosis. Irregular pink areas of caseous necrosis (*arrow*) are evident against a background of lymphocytes. **Inset:** Granulomas on the periphery of necrotic areas show epithelioid macrophages and multinucleated giant (Langhans) cells (*arrows*).

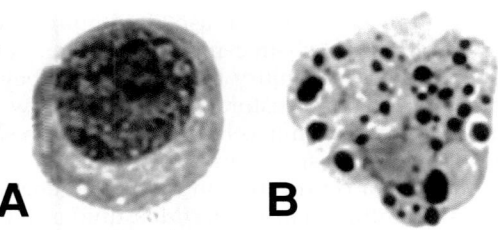

FIGURE 1-40. Apoptosis. A viable cell (**A**) contrasts with an apoptotic cell (**B**) in which the nucleus has undergone condensation and fragmentation but within an intact cell membrane.

is a misnomer, however, as the eosinophilia of the accumulated plasma proteins obscures the underlying alterations in the blood vessel, making it difficult, if not impossible, to determine whether there truly is necrosis in the vascular wall.

Apoptosis Produces Individual Cell Death Amidst Viable Cells

Morphology of Apoptosis

Apoptosis is a pattern of cell death that is triggered by a variety of extracellular and intracellular stimuli and is carried to its conclusion by organized cellular signaling cascades. Apoptotic cells are recognized by nuclear fragmentation and pyknosis, generally against a background of viable cells. Unlike necrosis, which characteristically involves larger geographic areas of cell death, apoptosis occurs in single cells or small groups of cells. In this process: (1) nuclei condense and fragment, (2) cytoplasmic organelles segregate into distinct regions, (3) blebs form in the plasma membrane, and (4) cells fragment into membrane-bound structures, which often lack nuclei (Fig. 1-40).

Removal of Apoptotic Cells Prevents Exposure of Viable Tissues to Toxic Molecules

The process by which dead cells (either from apoptosis or necrosis) are removed is called **efferocytosis** (from Greek meaning to "carry the dead to the grave"). In the normal

adult human body, more than one million cells undergo apoptotic cell death every second. Their removal must, therefore, be carefully regulated and orchestrated. Both professional phagocytes (e.g., macrophages) and cells (epithelial cells and fibroblasts) adjacent to dead cells participate in efferocytosis. It is of paramount importance that dead cells be distinguished from viable cells in the removal process. This is ensured by multiple regulatory mechanisms. Dead or dying cells release chemoattractant "find me" signals that recruit phagocytes to sites of cell death. They also express opsonin-like bridging molecules that help link phagocytes to their targets. Specific "eat me" signals, such as phosphatidyl serine or calreticulin, which normally reside within the inner phospholipid layer of the cell membrane, become exteriorized. Their appearance on the surface of dead or dying cells activates engulfment receptors on phagocytes. Counterbalancing "don't eat me" signals, which are expressed ubiquitously by viable cells, are rapidly downregulated during apoptosis.

Once the self-destructive process of apoptosis has propelled a cell to DNA fragmentation and cytoskeletal dissolution, the final remnant, the ***apoptotic body***, remains. These are illustrated in Figures 1-40 and 1-41. Apoptotic bodies are phagocytosed by tissue macrophages before membrane integrity breaks down, thus preventing exposure of neighboring viable cells to injurious agents such as oxidants, proteases, and caspases, and also avoiding an inflammatory reaction. This is unlike necrotic cell death, which tends to elicit acute inflammatory responses.

Defective efferocytosis has been implicated in many diseases including cystic fibrosis, bronchiectasis, and atherosclerosis.

Cells May Participate Actively in Their Own Death

There is increasing agreement that the various forms of cell death are not strictly separate, but rather share molecular effectors and signaling pathways. They may also exhibit overlapping morphologic features. Cell processes incriminated in one may be co-conspirators with the others, and a particular cell's death may involve combinations of two, or more, of these mechanisms. For the sake of clarity, mechanisms of cell death by necrosis, apoptosis, and autophagy

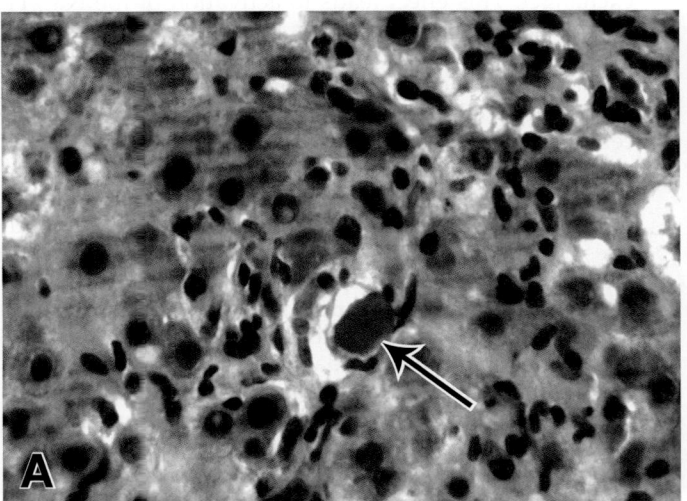
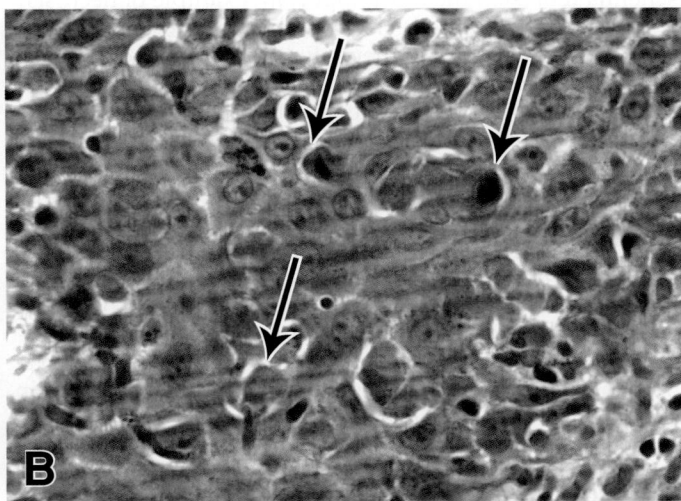

FIGURE 1-41. Apoptosis in the liver in viral hepatitis (**A**) and in the skin in erythema multiforme (**B**). Apoptotic cells are indicated by *arrows*.

are presented separately, but it is important to understand that all of these processes involve signaling, borrow from one another and collaborate with each other.

NECROSIS

Necrosis Refers to "Unprogrammed" Death of Cells and Tissues

Necrotic cell death is caused by external types of injury. It typically follows ischemia/reperfusion injury, but may also result from physical trauma leading to disruption of cells, thermal effects (burns or frostbite), toxins or pathogens such as virus and bacteria. By contrast to apoptotic cell death, necrotic cells release enzymes and other injurious mediators that typically elicit an inflammatory response and may harm viable neighboring cells. While necrosis has traditionally been considered to be "unregulated," we now recognize a regulated form, necroptosis, which resembles necrosis morphologically but shares some signaling mechanisms with apoptotic cell death. Necroptosis is considered later in this chapter as a specialized form of cell death. Here, we focus on classical necrosis in response to ischemia and reperfusion.

Ischemia Injures Cells During Both Deprivation and Restoration of Oxygen Supply

Ischemia is interruption of blood flow, the result of which may be myocardial infarction or stroke. Cessation of blood flow interrupts delivery of O_2 and key nutrients, such as glucose, to cells and prevents removal of metabolic byproducts such as CO_2. Rapid loss of ATP impairs energy-dependent ionic pumps and exchangers, leading to intracellular acidosis, loss of glycogen stores, accumulation of injurious metabolites, and progressive mitochondrial injury. Ischemia promotes ROS generation, which is greatly magnified during reperfusion of acutely ischemic tissues.

Ischemic Cell Death

Myocardial infarction and stroke, together the most common cause of mortality in the Western world, are both due to ischemic cell death. Thus, cellular injury and death due to ischemia represent the most important example of necrosis.

Living cells maintain electrochemical gradients relative to their external environment. Extracellular levels of Na^+ and Ca^{2+} are normally orders of magnitude more than intracellular concentrations. The opposite holds for K^+. Resting membrane potential (i.e., the voltage difference between the inside of a cell and its external environment) ranges from -5 to -10 mV for erythrocytes to -70 to -90 mV for electrically excitable cells such as neurons and muscle cells. Maintenance of such gradients depends on a plethora of ion channels, pumps, transporters, and exchangers, along with an intact plasma membrane and a considerable amount of energy (ATP). Compartments within cells (e.g., sarcoplasmic reticulum and mitochondria) also maintain specific electrochemical gradients with a similar dependency on ion-selective protein assemblies, intact organelle membranes and, of course, ATP. Acute ischemia causes ATP levels to plummet with dissipation of normal gradients, rapid onset of intracellular acidosis, and production of injurious metabolites such as ROS and lysophospholipids. If the ischemic episode is brief, normal ionic equilibrium can be re-established without tissue damage. With prolonged ischemic injury, however, cell membranes sustain sufficient injury to push the cell beyond the "point of no return" and restoration of blood flow will not save the cell. Thus, ischemic cell injury and death share the same pathophysiologic spectrum.

Calcium plays a central role in the pathogenesis of cell death. Ca^{2+} concentration in extracellular fluid is in the millimolar range (10^{-3} M), but cytosol Ca^{2+} concentration ($[Ca^{2+}]_i$) is 1/10,000 of that—that is, about 10^{-7} M. Furthermore, resting membrane potentials of normal ventricular myocytes are approximately -90 mV (i.e., the interior of the cell has a negative charge compared with the exterior). As a result, there is a large electrical and concentration gradient for Ca^{2+}. Many crucial cell functions are regulated by tiny fluctuations in $[Ca^{2+}]_i$. **Massive influx of Ca^{2+} through a damaged plasma membrane is thus key to ischemic cell damage** and may ensure loss of viability. This is the mechanism for "contraction band" necrosis in the heart (see Chapter 17).

Cell death by necrosis varies according to the cause, organ, and cell type. The best-studied and most clinically important example is ischemic necrosis of cardiac myocytes. Mechanisms underlying the death of these cells are in part unique, but basically are comparable to those in other organs. Some of these events may occur simultaneously; others may be sequential (Fig. 1-42):

1. **Interruption of blood supply decreases delivery of O_2 and energy nutrients (glucose and fatty acids).** For most cells, but especially for cardiac myocytes and neurons, which do not store much energy and have high energy expenditures, this combined insult is formidable.

2. **Anaerobic glycolysis leads to overproduction of lactate and decreased intracellular pH.** Decreased O_2 during myocardial ischemia blocks ATP production and inhibits mitochondrial oxidation of pyruvate. Instead of entering the citric acid cycle, pyruvate is reduced to lactate in the cytosol, a process called **anaerobic glycolysis**. Lactate accumulation lowers cytosol pH (acidification), thus initiating a spiral of events that propels the cell downward toward disaster.

3. **Distortion of the activities of pumps in the plasma membrane skews the cell's ionic balance.** Na^+ accumulates because lack of ATP impairs the Na^+/K^+ ion exchanger. This effect leads to activation of the Na^+/H^+ ion exchanger. This pump is normally quiescent, but when intracellular acidosis threatens, it pumps H^+ out of the cell in (one-for-one) exchange for Na^+ to maintain proper intracellular pH. The resulting increase in intracellular sodium activates the Na^+/Ca^{2+} ion exchanger, which increases calcium entry. Ordinarily, excess intracellular Ca^{2+} is extruded by an ATP-dependent calcium pump, but with ATP in very short supply, Ca^{2+} accumulates in the cell.

4. **Activation of phospholipase A_2 (PLA$_2$) and proteases disrupts plasma membrane and cytoskeleton.** Elevated $[Ca^{2+}]_i$ in an ischemic cell activates PLA$_2$, leading to membrane phospholipid degradation and consequent release of free fatty acids and lysophospholipids. The latter act as detergents that solubilize cell membranes. They also exert deleterious effects on various ion channels and pumps, further impairing ionic homeostasis. Both fatty acids and lysophospholipids are potent mediators of inflammation, which may further injure the already compromised cell.

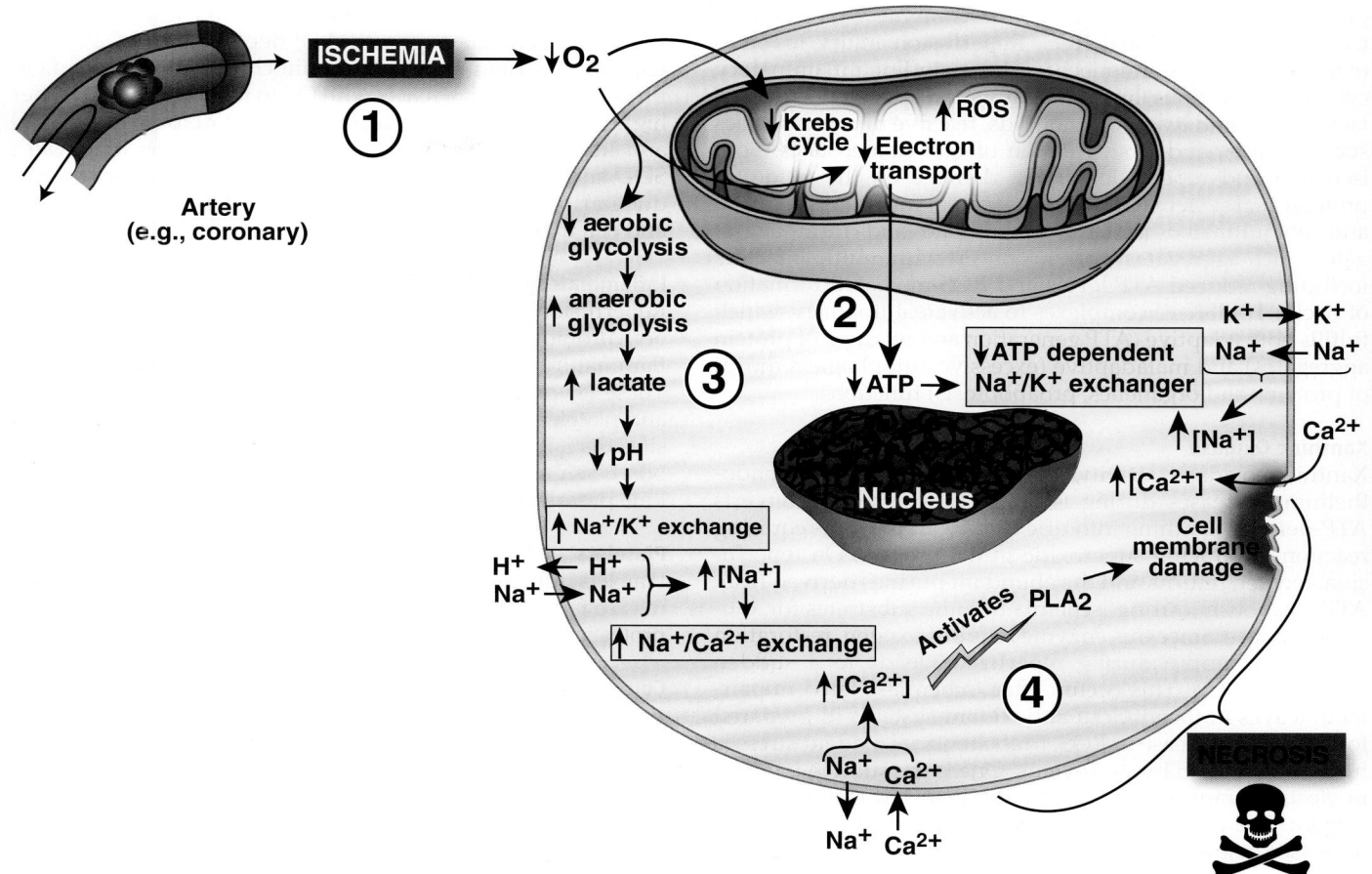

FIGURE 1-42. Mechanisms by which ischemia leads to cellular death by necrosis. 1. Loss of oxygen due to vascular occlusion impairs mitochondrial function, resulting in decreased energy (adenosine triphosphate [ATP]) production by aerobic processes. **2.** Decreased ATP impairs ATP-dependent ion pumps and exchangers. **3.** The loss of aerobic processes causes anaerobic glycolysis to predominate, with consequent intracellular acidosis, eventually leading to increased cytosolic [Ca^{2+}]. **4.** Ca^{2+}-dependent phospholipases are then activated, causing loss of cell membrane integrity and necrosis.

5. Calcium also activates proteases that attack the cytoskeleton and its attachments to the cell membrane. As connections between cytoskeletal proteins and the plasma membrane are disrupted, membrane blebs form, causing the cell's shape to change. The combination of electrolyte imbalance and increased cell membrane permeability makes the cell swell, often a morphologic prelude to its dissolution.

6. **Lack of O_2 impairs mitochondrial electron transport, decreasing ATP and increasing ROS.** Normally, 1% to 3% of oxygen entering mitochondria is converted to ROS, because of inefficiencies in the ETC. During ischemia, more ROS are generated because of damage to ROS detoxification mechanisms and impaired processing of reactive oxygen intermediates. ROS cause peroxidation of cardiolipin, a membrane phospholipid unique to mitochondria and sensitive to oxidative damage because of its high content of unsaturated fatty acids. This attack impairs the ETC and decreases its ability to produce ATP.

7. **Mitochondrial damage promotes cytochrome c (Cyt c) release into the cytosol.** In normal cells, the mitochondrial permeability transition pore (MPTP; see below) opens and closes sporadically. Ischemic injury to mitochondria causes sustained opening of the MPTP. Resulting loss of Cyt c from the ETC further diminishes ATP

synthesis and may also trigger apoptotic cell death (see below).

8. **The cell dies.** When a cell can no longer maintain itself as a metabolic unit, it dies. The line between reversible and irreversible cell injury (i.e., the "point of no return") is not precisely defined.

Reperfusion Injury

Restoration of blood flow after a period of ischemia is **reperfusion**. Although beneficial in salvaging viable, reversibly injured cells, reperfusion can itself cause damage by "**reperfusion injury**." Such injury most often occurs in settings of organ ischemia, such as spontaneous or therapeutic reperfusion in acute myocardial infarction, but also in other situations (e.g., organ transplantation).

Reperfusion injury reflects the interplay of transient ischemia and its consequent tissue damage with exposure of damaged tissue to the oxygen that arrives when blood flow is re-established (reperfusion). The extent to which reperfusion kills injured cells that otherwise might have been salvaged by mitigating interventions is significant. In the heart, it may account for up to half of the final size of myocardial infarcts. Initially, ischemic cellular damage leads to generation of free radical species (see above). Reperfusion then provides abundant molecular O_2 to combine with free radicals to form additional ROS. Reperfusion injury involves many other factors and mechanisms including inflammatory cytokines, injurious lipid mediators like platelet-activating factor (PAF) and lysophospholipids, reactive nitrogen species such as NO•, and dysregulation of Ca^{2+} homeostasis. Both ischemia and reperfusion inflict damage on the ubiquitin proteasomal system (UPS)—proteasomal function is reduced and ubiquitinated proteins accumulate and form aggregates. Such aggregates work in concert with multiple factors including reduced ATP levels and ROS-mediated formation of Beclin-1/PI3K-III complexes to activate autophagy, which fulfills both adaptive (ATP generation and removal of protein aggregates) and maladaptive (excessive autophagic removal of proteins and organelles, proapoptosis) functions.

Xanthine Oxidase

Xanthine oxidase activity, particularly in vascular endothelium, increases during ischemia. The enzyme converts ATP-derived xanthine into uric acid in an oxygen-requiring reaction, producing superoxide in the process. On reperfusion, oxygen returns and the abundant purines derived from ATP catabolism during ischemia become substrates for xanthine oxidase. Since this enzyme requires oxygen, restoration of oxygen supply during reperfusion leads to a sudden increase in ROS. This occurs after ischemia-related impairment leaves mitochondrial antioxidant systems ill-prepared for the rapid increase in ROS. Mitochondrial oxidant stress is further magnified by two events. One is the sudden increase in electron transport, driven by the renewed availability of oxygen. The other is changes in pH and calcium concentrations (see below).

The Role of Neutrophils

Neutrophils are an additional source of ROS during reperfusion. Reperfusion prompts endothelial cells to move preformed P-selectin to the cell surface, increasing neutrophil binding to the intercellular adhesion molecule-1 (ICAM-1) at the endothelial cell membrane (see Chapter 2). Neutrophils release large quantities of ROS and hydrolytic enzymes, both of which further injure the previously ischemic cells.

Ion Fluxes During Reperfusion

Ischemia-altered cell ion transporter activities become even more deranged with reperfusion. When blood flow is re-established, cellular pH is suddenly rectified. Ca^{2+} overload, which began during ischemia, is then exacerbated by reversal of the Na^+/Ca^{2+} exchanger. Increased $[Ca^{2+}]_i$ activates Ca^{2+}-dependent proteases to generate more ROS. It also acts in concert with increased mitochondrial ROS to open the MPTP dissipating the mitochondrial membrane potential and triggering mitochondria-related cell death programs (see below).

The Role of Nitric Oxide (NO•) and Nitric Oxide Synthase (NOS)

NO is generated from arginine by constitutive and inducible NOSs. NO exerts powerful protective effects, dilating microvasculature by relaxing smooth muscle, inhibiting platelet aggregation, and decreasing leukocyte adhesion to endothelial cells. It also decreases transferrin-mediated iron uptake, limiting the amount of iron available to generate OH• from other ROS. These activities largely reflect the ability of NO to decrease $[Ca^{2+}]_i$ by both extruding it from the cell and sequestering it in intracellular stores.

NO and NOS are double-edged swords, however. In the setting of ischemia-triggered ATP depletion and Ca^{2+} overload and nutrient deprivation, mitochondrial NOS tends to produce NO• which reacts with O_2^- to form $ONOO^-$, another highly reactive species. Normally, O_2^- is detoxified by SOD and little $ONOO^-$ is produced, but reperfusion inactivates SOD and provides abundant O_2^-, which together favor production of $ONOO^-$. ONOO promotes DNA strand breaks and cell membrane lipid peroxidation.

Inflammatory Cytokines

Reperfusion injury is complicated by cytokine release, which both promotes inflammation and modulates its severity. Proinflammatory cytokines such as TNFα, IL-1, and IL-6 are keys. These (1) promote vasoconstriction, (2) stimulate neutrophil and platelet adherence to endothelium, and (3) have effects at sites distant from the ischemic insult itself. They also activate NFκB signaling pathways, which stimulates additional cytokine production and activates proapoptotic cascades.

Platelets

Platelets adhere to the microvasculature of injured tissue and release factors that play a role in both tissue damage and cytoprotection. These include cytokines, TGFβ, serotonin, and NO•.

Complement

Activation of the complement system (see Chapter 2) during reperfusion leads to deposition of membrane attack complexes and elaboration of chemotactic agents and proinflammatory cytokines. The net result is recruitment and adhesion of neutrophils.

Summary of Ischemia and Reperfusion Injury

We can put reperfusion injury in perspective by emphasizing that there are three different degrees of cell injury, depending on the duration of the ischemia:

- After short periods of ischemia, reperfusion (and, thus, resupply of oxygen) totally restores a cell's structural and functional integrity. Cell injury in this case is completely reversible.
- With longer periods of ischemia, reperfusion leads to cell deterioration and death: lethal cell injury occurs during reperfusion. In this setting, interventions to counteract specific mechanisms of reperfusion injury may salvage vulnerable cells and limit infarct size.
- Lethal cell injury may develop during the period of ischemia itself, in which case reperfusion need not be a factor. A longer period of ischemia is required to produce this third type of cell injury.

Processes involved in reperfusion injury are summarized in Table 1-3.

Ischemic Preconditioning

Prolonged ischemia may cause cell death before adaptive mechanisms come into play, but repeated transient episodes of ischemia, each one of which is insufficient to cause irreversible injury, may stimulate adaptive responses referred to as **ischemic preconditioning**. This can occur, for example, in the heart of a patient who experiences repetitive bouts of angina pectoris without actual myocardial infarction. Such "preconditioning" activates protective mechanisms that limit the amount of necrosis that follows a subsequent, more prolonged, episode of ischemia. Exactly how ischemic

TABLE 1-3
CELL INJURY MECHANISMS ACTIVE IN REPERFUSION INJURY

Formation of reactive oxygen species

Generated by xanthine oxidase

Produced by neutrophils

Made by mitochondria

Altered ionic composition

Rapid pH normalization following period at acidic pH

Increased [Na⁺]

Increased [Ca²⁺]

Abnormalities of nitric oxide metabolism

Decreased endothelial cell NOS with subsequent vasoconstriction, increased platelet aggregation and neutrophil recruitment

ONOO generation

Altered vascular function and inflammation

Vasoconstriction and inhibition of vasodilatation

Increase in proinflammatory cytokines

High cell membrane levels of adhesion molecules

Clumping of platelets

Migration of neutrophils

Complement

Cell death

Opening of MPTP

Activation of apoptosis

Activation of autophagy

MPTP = mitochondrial permeability transition pore; NOS = nitric oxide synthase; ONOO = peroxynitrite.

preconditioning affords protection is complex—more than 100 different signaling molecules and mechanisms have been implicated in experimental studies. Among the most important chemical mediators and signaling cascades are the reperfusion injury salvage kinase (RISK) pathway involving activation of Akt and its downstream targets such as ERK and GSK3β which exert cardioprotective effects, and the survival activating factor enhancement (SAFE) pathway involving TNFα and its receptor-mediated activation of STAT3 which promotes expression of cardioprotective proteins. Another key player is hypoxia-inducible factor-1α (HIF-1α; see Chapter 5), the master regulator of transcriptional responses to low O_2 tension. HIF-1α activates genes whose protein products limit ROS production, Ca^{2+} accumulation, and ATP depletion. As a result, HIF-1α tends to protect against mitochondrial injury, DNA damage and oxidative stress, and so improves chances of survival in response to a subsequent episode of ischemia.

PROGRAMMED CELL DEATH

PCD covers processes that are lethal to individual cells and are regulated by preexisting signaling pathways. First noted

170 years ago and thought to represent a passive form of cell death, various forms of PCD entail activation of cellular signaling cascades.

PCD is part of the balance between cellular life and death, determining whether a cell dies when it is no longer useful or if its survival harm the organism. Without PCD to limit the size of bodily compartments, an estimated two tons of bone marrow and lymph nodes and 16 km (10 miles) of intestines would have accumulated by age 80. To balance the rate of new cell production, *more than one million cells per second undergo PCD* in a normal human body. In adults, this mainly entails removal of aged and senescent cells. PCD is also a self-defense mechanism: cells infected with pathogens or carrying genomic alterations are destroyed.

Classification of PCD

Diverse mechanisms eventuate in PCD. This term originally was synonymous with apoptosis, but we now recognize *multiple interrelated pathways of PCD, activated under various conditions and settings.* These are:

- **Apoptosis** is a highly conserved cell death program that depends on a family of cysteine proteases (caspases) as crucial signaling intermediates and executioners. Among the various forms of PCD, it is the most studied and best understood (see below).
- **Necroptosis** is a type of cell death in which cells can execute necrosis in a programmed fashion. It occurs, for example, in the setting of viral infection in which cells undergo "suicide" via caspase-independent pathways in the presence of viral caspase inhibitors. Necroptosis also occurs in noninfectious inflammatory settings such as Crohn disease, myocardial infarction, and pancreatitis.
- **Pyroptosis** is related to necroptosis. It occurs in response to infection with intracellular pathogens such as bacteria or viruses. Recognizing the presence of intracellular "foreign danger signals," immune cells respond by producing proinflammatory cytokines which, along with other mechanisms, cause the infected cells to swell and burst. Unlike apoptosis, pyroptotic cell death involves plasma membrane rupture, releasing damage-associated molecular pattern (DAMP) molecules into the extracellular space. DAMPs recruit additional immune cells to help clear the infection. For example, macrophages infected with *Salmonella* undergo pyroptosis caused by recognition of the bacteria protein flagellin.
- **Anoikis** is a form of PCD in anchorage-dependent cells that become detached from the ECM. Metastatic tumor cells are especially adept at evading this type of cell death (see Chapter 5).
- **Entosis** is another response to loss of attachment to the ECM, in which a living detached cell invades the cytoplasm of another cell. First described in cancer, entotic tumor cells may grow within invaded cells and cannibalize their nutrients.
- **NETosis** is a form of PCD that involves neutrophil extracellular traps (NETs), extracellular fibrous networks composed mainly of DNA and proteins released by neutrophils which bind pathogens and aid in their elimination. As a first line of defense against invading pathogens, NETosis by neutrophils not only immobilizes pathogens, but also aids incoming neutrophils in killing pathogens while minimizing damage to host cells. NETosis also facilitates tumor growth and spread (see Chapter 5).

Detailed discussion of all these processes is beyond the scope of this chapter, and this rapidly evolving field remains incompletely understood. Here, we focus on the highlights of the major pathways: apoptosis, autophagy, and necroptosis. Other, more restricted, forms of PCD are addressed briefly. For the sake of clarity, we use the term "apoptosis" for PCD involving specific caspase signaling pathways (see below). "Necroptosis" describes cell death resembling necrosis, but utilizing programmed signaling pathways.

Apoptosis Relies on Caspase Cascades

Once apoptosis begins, it is irreversible, and so is, highly regulated. There are two major pathways: the **intrinsic pathway** (also called the mitochondrial pathway) is a suicide program activated in a cell that is undergoing stress; in the **extrinsic pathway**, a cell kills itself in response to signals sent by other cells. Both pathways induce cell death by first activating "initiator" caspases to enter the death program and then activating "executioner" caspases that "carry out the sentence" by degrading proteins indiscriminately. Apoptosis plays fundamental roles in normal development and physiology, and defects in apoptosis are implicated in many diseases.

Apoptosis in Development and Physiology

During embryogenesis, many evolutionary relics sequentially appear, then regress. Some aortic arches do not persist. The pronephros and mesonephros regress in favor of the metanephros. Structures required by only one sex disappear in embryos of the other sex. Thus, Müllerian ducts, progenitors of the uterus, disappear in males, and Wolffian ducts, which form part of the male genital tract, vanish in females. In some organs, such as the brain and ovaries, cells are overproduced, then culled by apoptosis. Apoptosis also causes interdigital webs to disappear, yielding discrete fingers and toes. Likewise, apoptosis converts solid primordia to hollow tubes (e.g., GI tract), produces a four-chamber heart, and sculpts other bodily structures. On an individual cellular basis, apoptosis eliminates autoreactive lymphocyte clones (see Chapter 4).

Physiologic apoptosis mainly affects progeny of stem cells that are constantly dividing (e.g., stem cells of the hematopoietic system, gastrointestinal mucosa, and epidermis). Apoptosis of mature cells in these organs protects those compartments from overpopulation. Thus, normal organ size and architecture are maintained (Fig. 1-43).

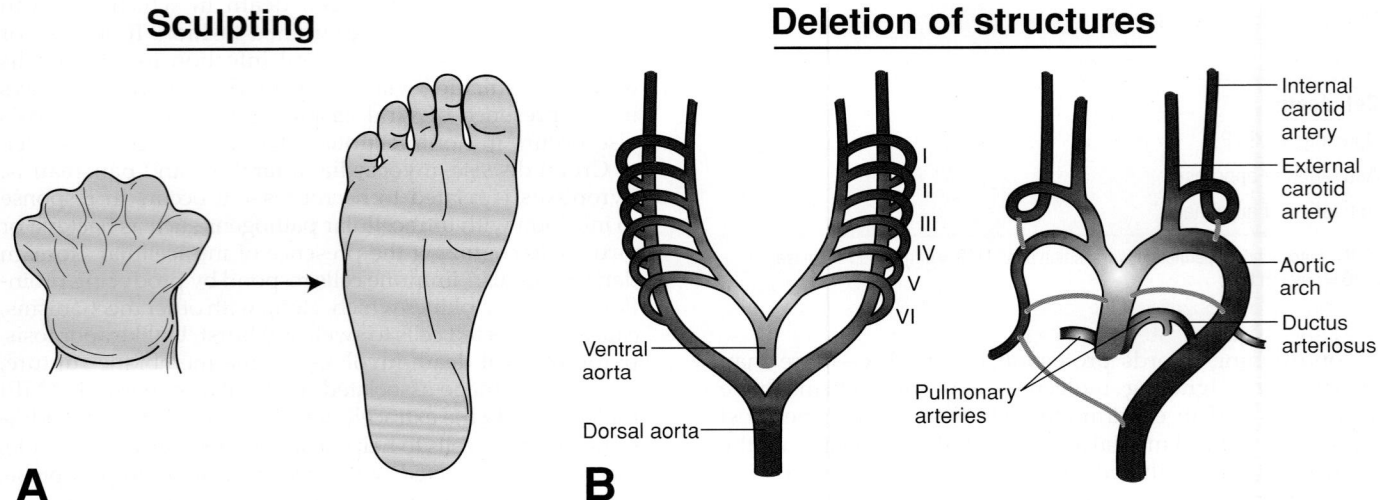
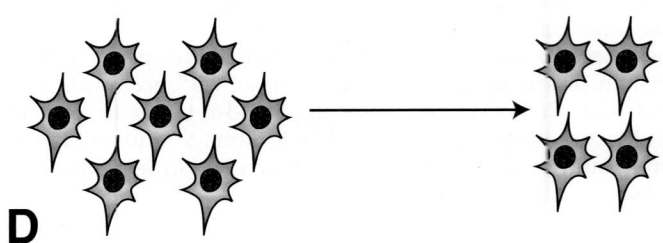

FIGURE 1-43. Activities of apoptosis during embryonic development. A. Sculpting. Apoptosis eliminates interdigital tissue. **B. Aortic arches.** Multiple embryonic aortic arches (**left**), which are evolutionary relics, are eliminated and transformed by apoptosis into the eventual adult circulatory system (**right**). **C. Dangerous cells.** Autoreactive lymphocytes and other errant cells are eliminated by apoptosis. **D. Population control.** Excessive numbers of diverse cell types, such as central nervous system neurons, are pruned by apoptosis.

Apoptosis Eliminates Obsolescent Cells

Cell turnover is essential to maintaining the size and function of many organs. For example, as new cells are continuously supplied to circulate in the blood, older and less functional ones must be eliminated to maintain normal numbers of cells. Pathologic accumulation of polymorphonuclear leukocytes in chronic myeloid leukemia (see Chapters 5, 26) results from a mutation that inhibits apoptosis and so allows these cells to persist. In the small intestine mucosa, cells migrate from the deep crypts to villous tips, where they undergo apoptosis and are sloughed into the lumen.

Apoptosis also maintains cellular balance in organs that respond to hormones and other trophic stimuli, as in regression of lactational breast hyperplasia when a woman stops nursing. Later in life, postmenopausal endometrial atrophy follows loss of hormonal support.

An interesting facet of apoptosis is its impact on gametogenesis. Adult men produce about 1,000 new spermatozoa per second, most of which undergo apoptosis because of intrinsic defects or external damage. Excessive apoptosis among spermatozoa contributes to some forms of male infertility. Similarly, in females, apoptosis eventually eliminates 99% of neonatal ovarian oocytes.

Apoptosis Deletes Mutant Cells

The wellbeing of an organism requires that cells that have accumulated genetic defects during their lifespans be eliminated. There is a finite, albeit low, error rate in DNA replication, reflecting imperfect fidelity of DNA polymerases. Environmental stresses such as ultraviolet (UV) light, ionizing radiation, and DNA-binding chemicals may also alter DNA structure. There are several means, the most important of which probably involve p53, by which cells recognize genomic abnormalities and "assess" whether or not they can be repaired. If DNA damage is too severe to be repaired, a cascade of events leads to apoptosis. This process protects organisms from the consequences of a nonfunctional cell or one that cannot control its own proliferation (e.g., a cancer cell). Perversely (and quiet effectively!), cancer cells often evolve mechanisms to circumvent apoptosis that might otherwise eliminate them (see Chapter 5).

Apoptosis Defends From Disseminated Infection

When a cell "detects" nonchromosomal DNA replication, as in viral infection, it tends to initiate apoptosis. By destroying infected cells, the body limits viral spread. Viruses have evolved mechanisms to manipulate apoptosis. Many viruses carry genes whose products inhibit apoptosis. Some such viral proteins bind and inactivate key cellular triggers for apoptosis (e.g., p53). Others may interfere with apoptosis signaling pathways.

MECHANISMS OF APOPTOSIS

Apoptosis Comprises Several Signaling Pathways

Different subtypes of PCD are mediated by complex interrelated signaling pathways. Here, we focus on the major pathways involved in apoptosis. As mentioned above, these are, broadly, the *intrinsic pathway* activated in cells under stress, and the *extrinsic pathway* which responds to signals from other cells. These pathways may be initiated by diverse external injurious agents such as invading pathogens, toxins, or ionizing radiation, all of which activate inflammatory cascades. They may also be stimulated by endogenous molecules such as p53, in response to stress-related and/or genetic changes. The ER may elicit apoptosis in which calcium signaling plays a central role.

These categories are not rigid, but rather are paradigms of varied signaling mechanisms. The different routes to apoptosis intersect and overlap.

A family of cysteine proteases, **caspases**, is central to apoptosis. Sequential activation of these enzymes, which entails conversion from proenzyme forms to catalytically effective enzymes, is central to apoptotic pathways. Some 14 caspases are now known, of which about half are important participants in apoptotic signaling. Others function in mediating pyroptosis in response to intracellular pathogens.

These various pathways may start differently and signal via different caspases. However, just as all roads lead to Rome, these diverse paths all generally lead to apoptosis via "executioner" enzymes: caspases-3, -6, and -7.

Cell Membrane Receptor–Ligand Interactions Trigger Extrinsic Apoptosis

TNFα, a soluble cytokine, triggers apoptosis by binding its receptor (TNFR). Similarly, caspase signaling is activated when Fas receptor (Fas) binds its ligand (FasL), at the plasma membrane of certain cells, such as cytotoxic effector lymphocytes.

Transmembrane cell surface receptors, TNFR and Fas, become activated upon binding their ligands. Specific amino acid sequences in the cytoplasmic tails of these receptors, "death domains," act as docking sites for corresponding death domains of other proteins (Fig. 1-44). After binding to ligand-activated receptors, docking proteins stimulate downstream signaling, especially procaspases-8 and -10, which are converted to their operational forms, caspases-8 and -10. In turn, these caspases activate downstream caspases in the apoptosis pathway.

The ultimate caspases in this process are "effector," or "executioner," caspases-3, -6, and -7. Caspase-3 is the most commonly activated effector caspase. It stimulates enzymes that cause nuclear fragmentation (e.g., caspase-activated DNase [CAD], which degrades chromosomal DNA). Caspase-3 also destabilizes the cytoskeleton as the cell begins to fragment into apoptotic bodies.

Notably, TNFR activation by TNFα may also stimulate the antiapoptotic protein NFκB, a transcription factor that directs production of proteins that inhibit apoptosis (NFκB serves many purposes, including as a master regulator of immune responses to infections, see below, in the discussion of necroptosis).

The extrinsic (death receptor) apoptosis pathway intersects the intrinsic (mitochondrial) pathway via caspase-8, which cleaves a cytoplasmic protein, Bid (Fig. 1-45). Truncated Bid (tBid) translocates to mitochondria, where it activates apoptosis through a separate signaling mechanism (see below). As detailed in a later section, caspase-8 also inhibits necroptosis.

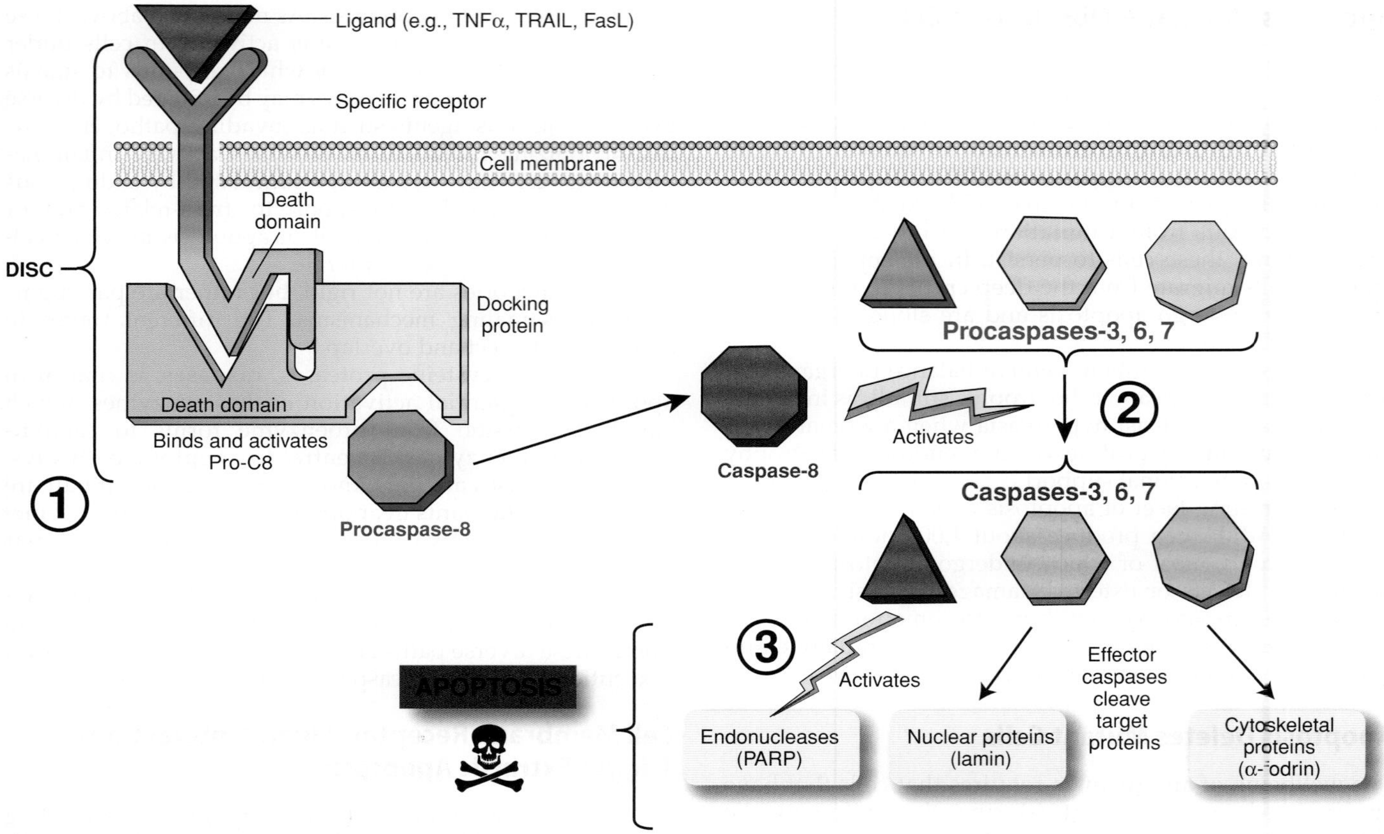

FIGURE 1-44. Extrinsic pathway of apoptosis. Ligand–receptor interactions that lead to caspase activation. **1.** Diverse extrinsic injury-related ligands bind their respective cell membrane receptors. These ligand interactions stimulate the cytoplasmic tails of these receptors bind the "death domains" of docking proteins, to form a death-inducing signaling complex (DISC). In turn, these proteins activate procaspase-8. **2.** The conversion of procaspase-8 to activated caspase-8 then converts procaspases-3, -6 and -7 to their respective active forms. **3.** Caspases-3, -6 and -7, especially caspase-3, are executioners that cleave target proteins, thereby initiating an irreversible process that culminates in cell death by apoptosis. *TNF* = tumor necrosis factor; *TNFR* = tumor necrosis factor receptor; *PARP* = poly-ADP-ribosylpolymerase.

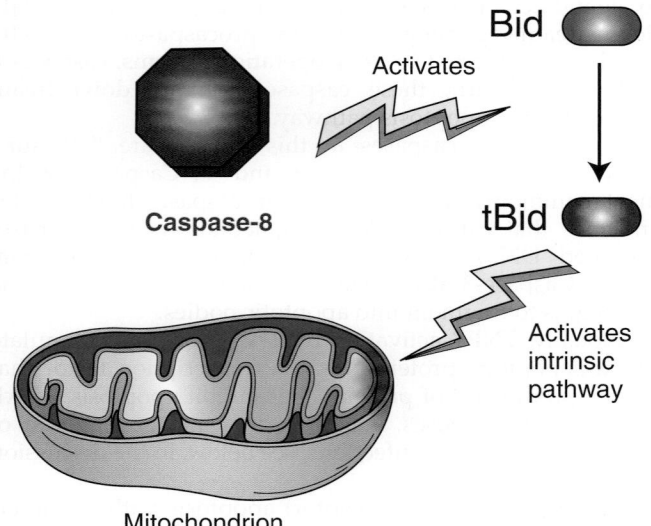

FIGURE 1-45. Intersection of the extrinsic and intrinsic pathways of apoptosis. Caspase-8, activated by, for example, a receptor–ligand interaction such as in Figure 1-40, may in turn cleave cytosolic Bid to yield a truncated derivative, tBid. In turn, tBid translocates to mitochondria, thereby activating the intrinsic (mitochondrial) pathway of apoptosis.

Diverse Intracellular Stimuli Activate the Mitochondrial Intrinsic Pathway of Apoptosis

From the perspective of cell survival and adaptation, mitochondria are akin to Dr. Jekyll and Mr. Hyde. On the one hand, in their Dr. Jekyll persona, they generate the energy needed to sustain the cell and participate in carbohydrate and fatty acid metabolism. On the other hand, as Mr. Hyde, they can trigger cell death. Indeed, cell death caused by cessation of aerobic respiration by mitochondria involves activation of several apoptotic pathways.

Key protein mediators of apoptosis affect mitochondria in multiple ways. Current understanding of this route of apoptosis involves two sequential series of events. The specific order of events is not completely understood, and some steps presented below may occur simultaneously or in a different sequence.

Mitochondrial Matrix and Inner Membrane Pathways

The composition of the mitochondrial matrix, within these organelles, is determined to a large extent by the impermeability of the inner mitochondrial membrane. This barrier is traversed by the MPTP, which is normally closed. The MPTP is a protein but its structure is poorly understood. Its formation in the inner mitochondrial membrane is stimulated by various pathologic conditions and its opening increases mitochondrial membrane permeability to small (<1,500 Daltons) molecules. Various factors including high levels of Ca^{2+}, NO, and ROS induce MPTP opening. Under normal basal conditions, there is an electrochemical potential ($\Delta\psi_m$) across the inner membrane, with the organelle's interior charged negatively relative to the exterior. MPTP opening dissipates $\Delta\psi_m$, which contributes to destruction of the ETC, markedly impairing ATP generation. Several molecules that are attached to the inner membrane play key roles as the apoptotic drama unfolds. These molecules may become released and gain access to the cytosol via the **mitochondrial apoptosis-induced channel** (MAC) which is formed on the outer mitochondrial membrane in response to various apoptotic signals. These molecules include **Cyt c** (a member of the ETC) and second mitochondrial-derived activator of caspases (**SMACs**) which are released into the cytosol when the MPTP opens. Once released, Cyt c binds **Apaf-1** and ATP, which then binds an inactive form of **caspase-9**, which normally resides in the cytosol. This creates a protein complex (the **apoptosome**, described further below) that converts procaspase-9 to its active form, which then activates the executioner enzymes including caspase-3. SMACs released into the cytosol reinforce the proapoptotic signals by binding to and inactivating normal cytosolic proteins that inhibit apoptosis (so called **IAPs**).

Thus, SMACs neutralize antiapoptotic factors and so allow apoptosis to proceed. Another inner mitochondrial membrane protein released when the MPTP opens is **apoptosis-inducing factor (AIF)**. Once released, AIF acts as a caspase-independent death effector. It enters the nucleus, where it mediates chromatin condensation and DNA fragmentation. To summarize, the key events involving mitochondrial matrix and inner membrane pathways are:

If mitochondria accumulate Ca^{2+} or generate excessive ROS, or if $D\psi_m$ or mitochondrial pH decrease, the MPTP opens (Fig. 1-46).

1. MPTP opening allows water, protons (H^+), and salts into the mitochondrial matrix.
2. Influx of H^+, water, and solutes collapses $\Delta\psi_m$. Resulting loss of membrane potential impairs mitochondrial ATP production.
3. Water entry causes mitochondria to swell. Outer mitochondrial membrane permeability increases, either due to its rupture or to opening of outer membrane pores.
4. Release of inner membrane constituents (Cyt c, SMACs, AIF, etc.) into the cytosol activates the next phase of apoptotic signaling.

The Outer Membrane Components

The normal constituents of the outer mitochondrial membrane include proapoptotic and antiapoptotic proteins of the Bcl-2 family. At least 25 known genes belong to this family. Bcl-2 proteins are all composed of hydrophobic α-helix cores surrounded by amphipathic domains. Some have transmembrane domains that help localize them in the outer mitochondrial membrane. They all share one or more of four characteristic Bcl-2 homology (BH) domains (BH1–BH4) which are critical determinants of their pro- versus anti-apoptotic properties.

The Bcl-2 Family Is the Cell's Life/Death Switch

Bcl-2 family members are grouped into three subfamilies, depending on the number of BH domains (Fig. 1-47).

1. Antiapoptotic (i.e., prosurvival) members all contain BH1 and BH2 domains. Some also have an N-terminal BH4 domain (which may also be seen in proapoptotic members). Antiapoptotic family members include Bcl-2, Bcl-xL, Mcl-1, and others.
2. Proapoptotic (antisurvival) members all contain BH3 domains which are necessary for dimerization with other Bcl-2 family members and activation of cell death pathways. They belong to two groups:
   a. One group contains three BH domains (Fig. 1-47). Bak and Bax are the key members of this group. A third member, Bok, is less well understood. Bak is mainly a mitochondrial protein. Bax is largely cytoplasmic.
   b. A larger group of proapoptotic proteins, BH3-only proteins, carry a single BH3 domain. These include Bim, Bid, Bik, Bad, and others. Different BH3-only proteins can elicit apoptosis by inactivating prosurvival functions of Bcl-2 family members or by directly stimulating death-inducing properties of Bax and Bak.

Mechanisms That Control the Intrinsic Pathway

The Normal Mitochondrion
Among other proteins, Cyt c, SMACs, and AIF are attached to the inner mitochondrial membrane, facing the intermembranous space. Opposite these, and attached to the outer membrane, are complexes of Bax and/or Bak bound to antiapoptotic Bcl-2 family members. In this peaceful equilibrium, Bcl-2 (Bcl-xL, Mcl-1, etc.) inhibits proapoptotic functions of Bax/Bak. The mitochondrial default setting is prosurvival.

Triggering the Intrinsic Pathway of Apoptosis via the Bcl-2 Family of Proteins
Many intracellular *agents provocateurs*, often involving stress or injury, act via BH3-only family members. Such actions may include increasing concentrations of some BH3-only proteins (e.g., by activating transcription), altering their conformations from quiescent to active, modifying enzymes and so forth. The now-active BH3-only molecules may interpose themselves into Bcl-2 (Bcl-xL, etc.) complexes with Bak and Bax, causing these complexes to dissociate, and so liberate Bax and Bak to form channels in the outer mitochondrial membrane. These channels—**mitochondrial apoptosis-induced channels (MACs)**—allow release of toxic mitochondrial proteins (Cyt c, SMACs, etc.) into the cytosol (Fig. 1-48). Free Bax can also be activated directly by BH3-only proteins to form MACs.

Apoptosis Activated by p53

Cells are continually perched on a precipice between life and death. p53, a tetrameric transcription factor that controls expression of dozens of genes, is pivotal to the outcome of that balancing act. Its multiple functions include activating DNA repair proteins and cell cycle arrest when DNA has been damaged, actions designed to promote cell survival. However, if DNA damage is extensive and beyond repair, p53 can initiate apoptosis. Here, we focus on the role of p53 in cell death. (p53 is discussed in greater detail in Chapter 5.)

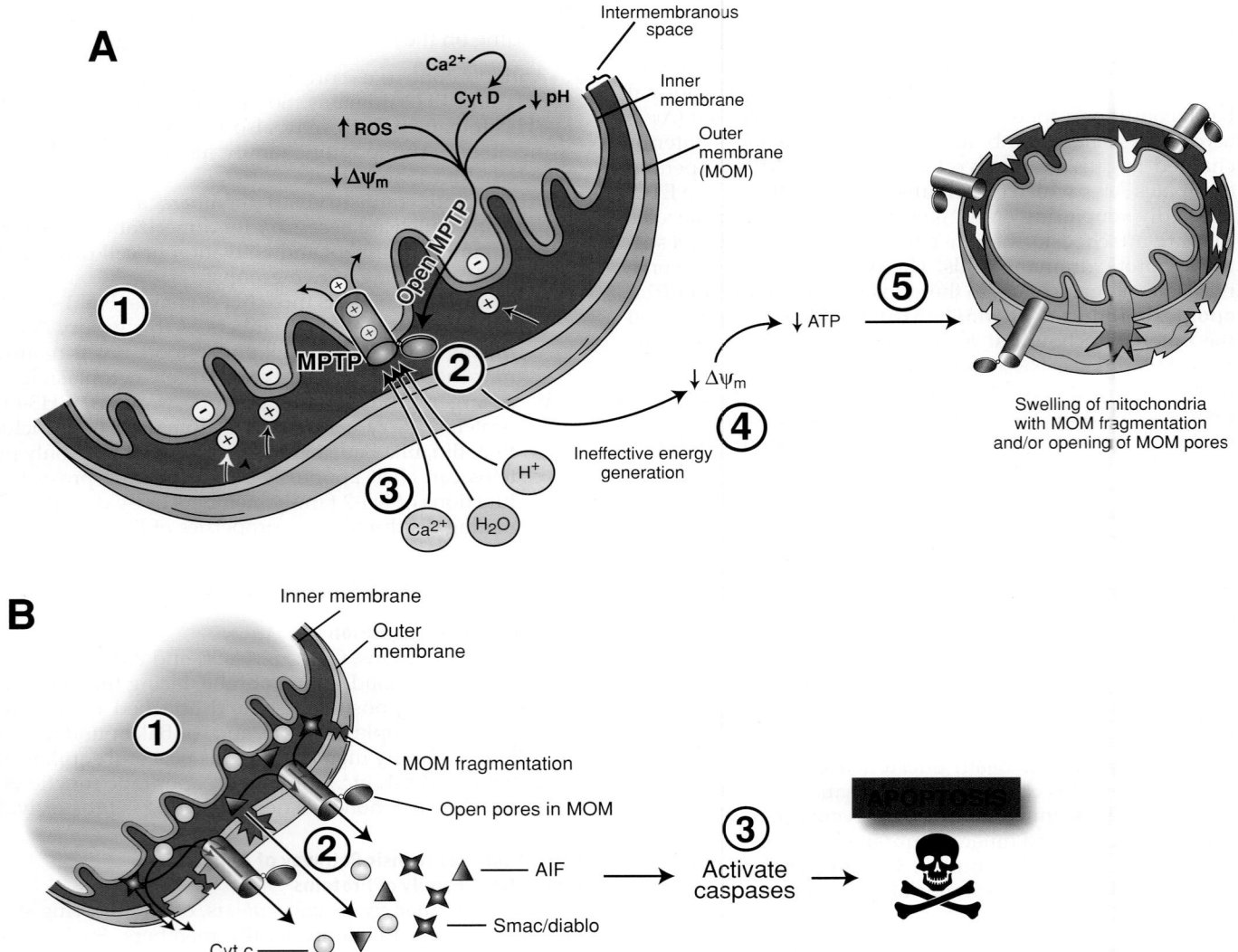

FIGURE 1-46. The intrinsic pathway of apoptosis. A. Causes and consequences of mitochondrial permeability transition pore (MPTP) activation. 1. A variety of stresses occurring within (i.e., intrinsic to) the cell affect mitochondria via multiple mechanisms including altered mitochondrial membrane potential ($\Delta\psi_m$), increased reactive oxygen species (ROS) and Ca^{2+}, and decreased pH differential. **2.** As a result, the MPTP opens. **3.** The high colloid oncotic pressure of the mitochondrial matrix drives an influx of water and accompanying solutes through the MPTP into the mitochondrial matrix. Concomitant cation influx neutralizes the cross-membrane $\Delta\psi_m$ and pH differential. **4.** This disrupts energy production, which further impairs the mitochondrion's ability to rectify the imbalance. **5.** Water influx leads to swelling of the organelle and fragmentation of the mitochondrial outer membrane (MOM). **B. The MOM in the intrinsic pathway of apoptosis. 1.** Molecules—SMACs, cytochrome c (Cyt c), apoptosis-inducing factor (AIF)—that are attached to the inner membrane, or are free within the intermembranous space, become detached. **2.** They then exit through outer membrane pores or holes and **3.** activate cytosolic effectors of apoptosis.

Homeostasis of p53

Normally, p53 is present in very small amounts owing to its rapid turnover. It is mostly in the cytosol, where it is bound mainly to Mdm2, an E3 Ub ligase. Mdm2 promotes p53 degradation via polyubiquitination. Even so constrained, p53 can foster cell health and effective responses to stress.

When a cell is injured or its equilibrium is disturbed, p53 undergoes diverse molecular modifications. These include phosphorylation, monoubiquitination at multiple sites (i.e., adding single Ub moieties at several points on p53 protein, rather than polymeric Ub chains at a single site, see above) and others. These alterations release p53 from Mdm2. So liberated, p53 evades

proteasomal degradation and accumulates. It also targets it to the mitochondria or nucleus, depending on the specific molecular modification (Fig. 1-49).

Apoptosis-Related Activities of p53

Within the nucleus, p53 is both a transcriptional activator and a repressor, depending on the target gene. It activates transcription of many proapoptotic proteins, such as Bad, Bax, NOXA (a proapoptotic Bcl-2 family member), and PUMA (p53 upregulated modulator of apoptosis) which binds and neutralizes antiapoptotic Bcl-2 family members. Simultaneously, nuclear localization of p53 represses transcription of such prosurvival proteins as Bcl-2, Bcl-xL, and Mcl-1.

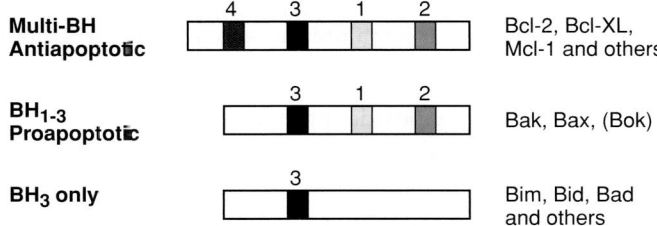

Multi-BH Antiapoptotic	4 3 1 2		Bcl-2, Bcl-XL, Mcl-1 and others
BH$_{1-3}$ Proapoptotic	3 1 2		Bak, Bax, (Bok)
BH$_3$ only	3		Bim, Bid, Bad and others

FIGURE 1-47. Bcl-2 family of apoptosis-related proteins. These proteins are divided into three groups, differentiated by structure and function. This division reflects the numbers of Bcl-2 homology (BH) domains in the protein. The presence of the BH4 domain characterizes the antiapoptotic family members. By contrast, proapoptotic Bcl-2 family members lack the BH4 domain and may have BH1-3 or only BH3. The latter are referred to as BH3-only proteins.

Cytosolic p53 may directly activate Bax, whereupon Bax relocates to mitochondria to cause apoptosis via release of mitochondrial proteins (see above). Mitochondria-targeted (i.e., [poly-monoubiquitinated] p53 acts as a functional BH3-only protein. In this mode, it disrupts complexes between Bak and its inhibitor, Mcl-1, and tips mitochondrial Bcl-2 family equilibrium to favor apoptosis.

p53 has many other functions, which are addressed more fully in Chapter 5.

Ca^{2+} Release From the ER May Elicit Apoptosis

Normally, Ca^{2+} concentration ([Ca^{2+}]) in the extracellular fluid is about 10,000× cytosolic Ca^{2+} concentration ([Ca^{2+}]$_i$). Ligand-induced and other changes in [Ca^{2+}]$_i$ are central to many biologic processes such as excitation–contraction coupling, hormone secretion, and immune activation. However, excessive changes in [Ca^{2+}]$_i$ may induce apoptosis. The ER stores considerable ionized calcium, which may be released in response to various stimuli (stress response). Excessive and, especially, prolonged ER Ca^{2+} release lead to apoptosis.

The juxtaposition of the ER and mitochondria is key to this process. Ca^{2+} released by the ER may be taken up by mitochondria, especially where the two organelles are in close proximity. Mitochondrial Ca^{2+} uptake is mediated by the mitochondrial calcium uniporter which has a very low affinity for calcium. Thus, cytosolic levels must be relatively high (i.e., pathologic) for there to be significant transport into mitochondria. When that happens, the MPTP opens, releasing Cyt c, SMACs, and AIF, activating downstream apoptosis pathways.

Sustained Ca^{2+} release from ER stores also promotes release of caspase-12. This protein, which is normally bound to the ER membrane, becomes activated upon its release. Activated caspase-12 activates caspase-9 in the apoptosome (see below), thus triggering executioner caspases (mainly caspase-3).

Metabolic Factors in the Mitochondrial Apoptosis Pathway

Just as mitochondrial function is fundamental to cell survival, its loss can contribute to the mitochondrial mechanism of apoptosis. Thus:

- Because Cyt c, AIF, and other mitochondrial proteins released into the cytosol are also integral to the ETC, their loss impairs mitochondrial ATP generation. The cell's

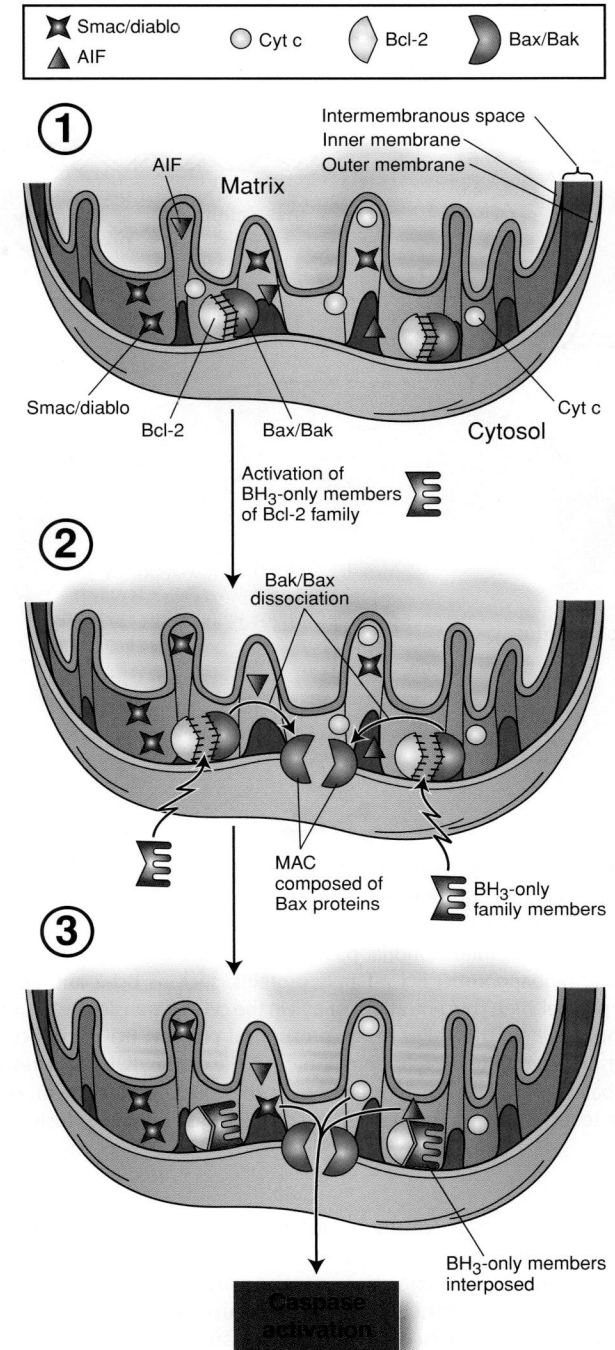

FIGURE 1-48. Formation of pores in the outer mitochondrial membrane during activation of the intrinsic pathway of apoptosis. 1. At equilibrium, Cyt c, SMACs, and apoptosis-inducing factor (AIF) either are attached to the mitochondrial inner membrane or float within the intermembranous space. The complex composed of oligomeric Bak/Bax with antiapoptotic Bcl-2 family cousins resides at the outer membrane. **2.** When BH3-only members of the Bcl-2 clan are activated, they interpose themselves between their prosurvival relatives and Bak/Bax, thereby freeing Bak/Bax proteins. The latter then form a pore (MAC) in the outer mitochondrial membrane. **3.** Proapoptotic proteins Cyt c, SMACs, AIF, and others exit from the mitochondrion via the MAC pore. Once in the cytosol, these proteins facilitate activation of the caspase cascade and so cause apoptosis. *Cyt c* = cytochrome C; *MAC* = mitochondrial apoptosis-induced channel.

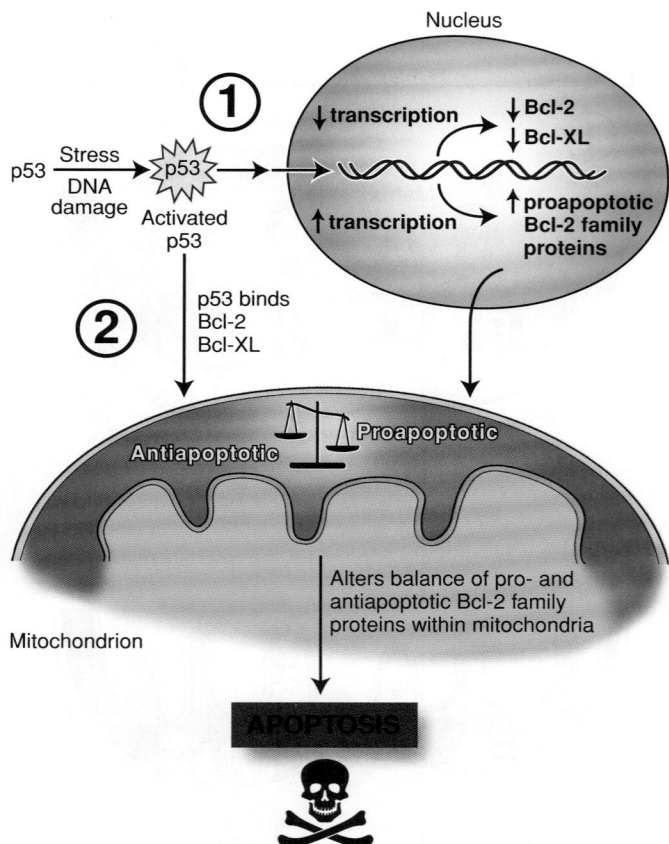

FIGURE 1-49. Activation of p53 and apoptosis. When p53 is activated (e.g., by DNA damage), it translocates to the nucleus. **1.** If DNA damage is irreparable, p53 promotes transcription of proapoptotic proteins, which then migrate to mitochondria. p53 also decreases transcription of pro-survival (antiapoptotic) Bcl-2 family proteins, such as Bcl-2 and Bcl-xL. **2.** In parallel, high concentrations of p53 in the cytosol translocate to mitochondria, where they bind to the prosurvival proteins Bcl-2 and Bcl-xL, releasing their bound proapoptotic partners (e.g., Bax/Bak). As a result, the balance of Bcl-2 family members at the mitochondrial membrane shifts to favor proapoptotic forces, and the cell undergoes apoptosis.

ability to repair injury is consequently suboptimal. If the causative insult is limited or transient, remaining functional mitochondria may compensate for the temporary loss of energy generation and sustain repair.

- Bax alters mitochondrial metabolism, directly and indirectly, to increase generation and decrease detoxification of ROS. This, in turn magnifies mitochondrial injury. ROS increase release of Cyt c and other proteins.
- Caspase-3 directly impairs parts of the ETC.
- Antioxidant defenses are weakened, because of both p53-directed decreases in antioxidant enzymes and the defects in electron transport that increase ROS generation.
- Imbalances in Ca^{2+} metabolism affect mitochondria. Physiologic increases in $[Ca^{2+}]$ (e.g., in excitable cells like neurons and myocytes) are transient, coinciding with stimulated and tightly regulated release from the ER. While this leads to brief MPTP opening, it does not impair cell viability. However, if Ca^{2+} influx into mitochondria is prolonged, increased mitochondrial ROS and other factors can lead to sustained, fatal MPTP opening.

- p53 may promote mitochondrial respiration, which, when electron transport is impaired (see above), generates more ROS. Harmful consequences of this may be further exacerbated by p53-related transcriptional repression of SOD, which decreases antioxidant protection.

It should be noted that ATP, even depleted by the events mentioned above, is required for apoptosome activity (see below). Thus, if MPTP opening is prolonged and ATP supply is exhausted, a cell may undergo necrotic, rather than apoptotic, death.

Proteins Released From Mitochondria Lead to Apoptosis via Several Pathways

As noted above, permeabilization of the outer mitochondrial membrane causes several mitochondrial molecules—Cyt c, SMACs, AIF, and others—to exit into the cytosol. Once in the cytosol, Cyt c binds cytosolic **Apaf-1** and procaspase-9 to form the **apoptosome**. This structure releases activated caspase-9, which then cleaves procaspases-3, -6, and -7, resulting in cell death (Fig. 1-50, left side).

Caspases-3, -7, and -9 may be inactivated by a family of E3 Ub ligases, called **inhibitors of apoptosis (IAPs)**. SMACs, and other similar proteins, bind IAPs and relieve caspases from IAP-mediated inhibition, thereby allowing them to execute the cell (Fig. 1-50, right side).

In addition, AIF and other proteins that are released from mitochondria through MACs can initiate apoptosis directly. They do so by activating destructive enzymes including **CAD** that cause nuclear condensation and DNA fragmentation, thus generating a *caspase-independent form of PCD.*

Complex Pathways Regulate Apoptosis and Cell Survival

The multiple specific mechanisms that give rise to and prevent apoptosis are themselves regulated by many other cellular pathways. For example, the Ub–proteasome system can target proapoptotic proteins, like caspases, for degradation. Ubiquitination, in turn, is controlled by DUBs and other modulators (see above). The balance between apoptosis and cell survival is thus influenced by the interplay between inducers and inhibitors of apoptosis, HSPs, protein kinases that may alter caspases or other enzymatic activities, and a host of other factors. Recent studies have implicated microRNAs (miRs) in regulating intracellular levels of many key proteins in apoptosis, mainly to protect viable cells from untoward activation of cell death pathways. For example, miR-125b suppresses expression of proapoptotic Bak. Bcl-xL and Mcl-1, both antiapoptotic Bcl-2 family members, are suppressed by miR-491 and miR-133a. Other microRNAs downregulate expression of caspase-3 and thereby attenuate apoptosis. *Thus, whether a cell lives or dies is therefore not determined solely by unique apoptosis-related mechanisms, but rather by a complex array of pathways whose functions converge on that single point.*

Some survival signals are transduced through receptors linked to PI3K. By antagonizing apoptosis, PI3K enhances cell viability. A prototypical receptor that signals via PI3K is insulin-like growth factor-I receptor (IGF-IR). Paradoxically, PI3K is also activated by TNFR binding TNFα. Thus, the same cell membrane receptor that induces apoptosis in some settings may initiate survival signaling in other situations.

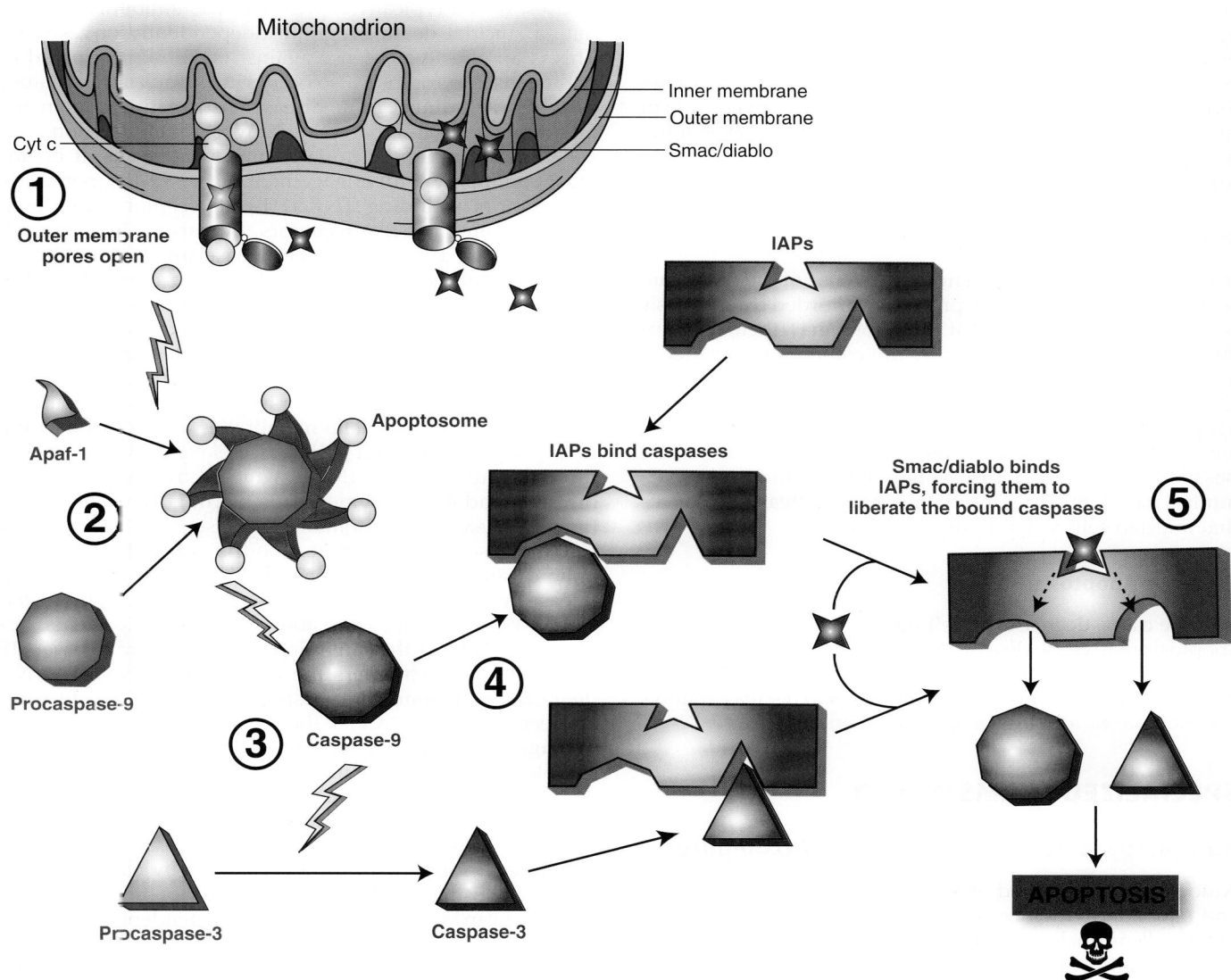

FIGURE 1-50. Opening of the mitochondrial outer membrane, leading to Apaf-1 activation, thereby triggering the apoptotic cascade.
1. Upon triggering by proapoptotic stimuli, pores in the outer membrane open and release proapoptotic proteins. **2.** Cyt c activates multiple molecules of Apaf-1 and both together recruit procaspase-9 to form a structure called the apoptosome, in which the procaspase is activated to caspase-9. Two sets of events may then occur to caspase-9. **3.** It may activate the effector caspases, particularly caspase-3. **4.** As well, IAPs may bind and sequester active forms of several caspases, including caspase-3 and -9. In so doing, IAPs impede apoptosis. **5.** However, SMACs and other mitochondrial proteins that are released when apoptosis is triggered may bind IAPs, causing them to release their bound caspases. The latter then cause the cell to undergo apoptosis. *Apaf-1* = apoptosis-activating factor; *Cyt c* = cytochrome c; *IAP* = inhibitor of apoptosis.

PI3K exerts antiapoptotic effects through intracellular mediators, which favor survival by activating Akt (see above). Akt inactivates several important proapoptotic proteins (e.g., Bad). More importantly, it activates NFκB, thus driving expression of prosurvival proteins (Bcl-xL, A1).

Cell survival and PCD are thus part of an intricate and highly complex balance, like a symphony orchestra. Each member of the symphony has many parts to play and the outcome depends on how all the members harmonize. However, unlike a symphony, the cell does not have a conductor or a score by which to direct its music, but rather a balance between proapoptotic and prosurvival influences.

Other Functions of Caspases

The caspase family has many functions unrelated to apoptosis. Caspases participate in (1) inflammation and immunity, (2) cell proliferation and differentiation in embryonic and extraembryonic life, (3) remodeling of cellular structures and projections, (4) mitogenesis, and (5) many other processes.

Apoptosis Is Central to Many Disease Processes

When regulation of apoptosis goes awry, there is the devil to pay. Apoptosis is vital for correct progression of embryologic development, eliminating self-reactive B- and T-lymphocyte clones and many other normal functions. Thus, defective apoptosis has been implicated in autoimmune diseases. Similarly, apoptosis guards against uncontrolled cell proliferation due to mutations in DNA. It is not surprising, therefore, that dysregulated apoptosis likely plays a major role in cancer (see Chapter 5). For example, overexpression of antiapoptotic Bcl-2 has been identified in some highly aggressive forms of lymphoma.

Insufficient Apoptosis

If a major protein that mediates the defense of the organism, such as p53, is mutated, the protection afforded by apoptosis is compromised. Subsequent mutations may then accumulate unhindered. Such pathways are commonly considered to be important in tumor development and progression (see Chapter 5). As another example, some viruses can block apoptosis, allowing them to replicate with less interference, and to disseminate more widely than would otherwise be possible. Oncogenic viruses often inhibit apoptosis (e.g., human papillomavirus inactivates p53), increasing chances that infected cells will progress to cancer.

Excessive Apoptosis

In some cases, decreases in cell numbers due to "excessive" apoptosis may cause disease. For example, in some neurodegenerative diseases intracellular proteins accumulate within neurons and trigger apoptosis. This leads to decreased numbers of neurons and loss of specific functions.

SPECIALIZED FORMS OF PCD

Autophagy in PCD: Is It a Killer or an Accomplice?

Autophagy is described above. It helps cells survive stress and injury, but whether, or how, it functions independently to kill cells is unclear. Experimental inhibition of autophagy prevents cell death induced by a variety of agents. At the same time, recent studies suggest that autophagy in dying cells might serve prosurvival functions. Thus, it is currently unclear whether, or to what extent, autophagy is responsible for cell death independently of other forms of PCD.

Necroptosis Is a Form of PCD Morphologically Indistinguishable From Necrosis

As discussed above, cellular morphology in necrosis involves cell swelling, plasma membrane fragmentation, and nuclear pyknosis, followed by an inflammatory response. In apoptosis, plasma membranes bleb and nuclei fragment without inflammation. There is, however, a "programmed" form of necrosis—**necroptosis**—in which cells undergo signaled or "suicidal" necrotic cell death. Under physiologic circumstances, necroptosis participates in development, particularly at the bone growth plate. It is also active normally in some adult tissues such as deep intestinal crypts. If physiologic apoptosis is unavailable to cells, cell death may default to necroptosis pathways. In this context, necroptosis may be an important mechanism of PCD in cancer cells in which apoptotic pathways are blocked.

Necroptosis is also closely related to targeting of pathogens by the immune system. For example, cells infected with viruses, which typically express caspase inhibitors, can initiate a suicidal death program independently of caspases. This is an effective defense against unrestrained spread of pathogens. Necroptosis also occurs in various inflammatory diseases including Crohn disease, pancreatitis and in the inflammatory phase that follows myocardial infarction.

Necroptosis can be initiated in several ways. It begins most commonly with engagement of the TNF superfamily of receptors including TNFr1, T-cell receptors, interferon receptors, and Toll-like receptors, by various ligands such as Fas ligand (FasL) or TNFα. These interactions recruit **TNF receptor-associated death domain protein (TRADD)** which, in turn, binds the receptor-interacting proteins, **RIP1** and **RIP3**, which form a microfilament-like complex called the **necrosome**. The necrosome activates the proapoptotic protein MLKL which initiates necrotic cell death by inserting into the lipid bilayers of the plasma membrane and intracellular organelle membranes and compromising their integrity (Fig. 1-51). RIP3 also elevates $[Ca^{2+}]_i$, in part through activation of CaMKII, which activates calpain and other degradative enzymes. This disrupts lysosome membranes, releasing lysosomal hydrolases into the cytosol. Calpain also damages mitochondria, precipitating metabolic dysfunction with impaired ATP generation and iron release, with consequent increased ROS (via Fenton and Haber–Weiss reactions, see above), damaging proteins, lipids, and DNA. At the same time, mitochondria release AIF (see above), which enters the nucleus and activates DNA degradation. Bioenergetic crisis with morphologic features of necrosis ensues. Cells then release molecules (called **damage-associated molecular patterns**, or **DAMPS**; see Chapter 2) that provoke inflammation.

There seems to be considerable interplay between apoptosis and necroptosis pathways. For example, caspase-8, which initiates apoptosis by activating executioner enzymes, can prevent formation of the necrosome by cleaving RIP1. By an opposing mechanism, inhibition of necroptosis by caspase-8 can be bypassed through independent interactions that sequester caspase-8 into a nonfunctional heterodimer with the antiapoptotic protein **cFLIP**. Decisions to follow apoptosis or necroptosis pathways thus depend on multiple fine control mechanisms.

Anoikis Is Activated by Loss of Cell Attachments

Anoikis (Greek: "homelessness") is a variety of apoptosis that occurs when anchorage-dependent cells, mainly epithelial cells, become detached from their native ECM. Proper cell binding to ECM helps determine whether that cell is in its appointed location. The significance of anoikis is that it efficiently deletes cells that have been displaced from their proper residence, preventing wandering cells or cell clusters from developing colonies at distant or improper ECM sites. It thus inhibits cancer metastases (see Chapter 5).

Anoikis utilizes intrinsic or extrinsic classical apoptotic pathways, both of which are upregulated when a cell becomes detached (Fig. 1-52). If a cell loses contact with its normal ECM, like one that is pushed off the tip of an intestinal villus by proliferating cells deeper in the crypts, loss of integrin-mediated survival signaling triggers anoikis. Similarly, if a detached cancer cell makes contact with inappropriate ECM components, anoikis may be activated. Nevertheless, errant tumor cells can evade anoikis (see Chapter 5).

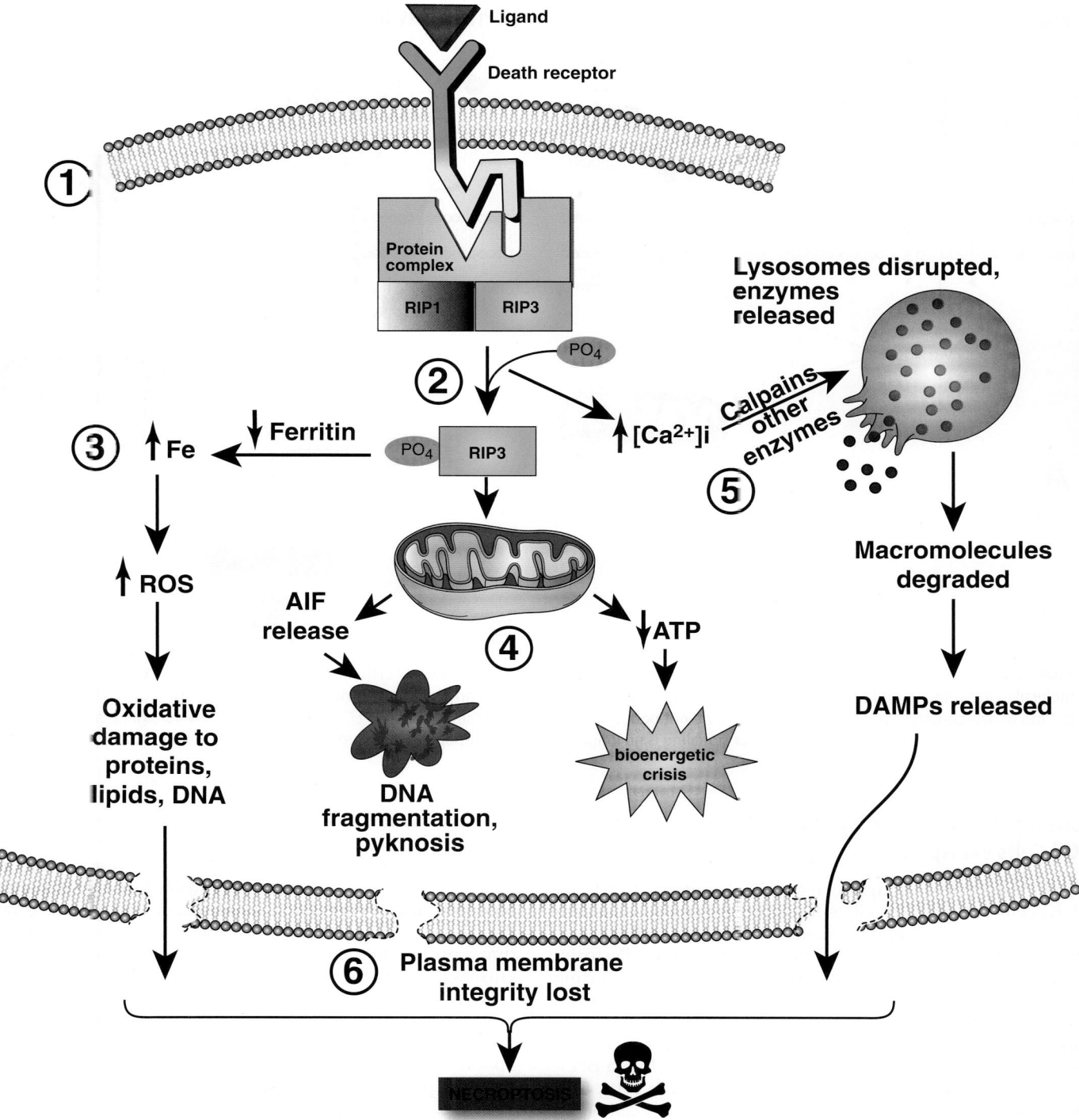

FIGURE 1-51. Pathways leading to necroptosis. 1. Binding of a ligand to a death receptor results in formation of a protein complex that binds RIPs. **2.** As a result, RIP3 becomes phosphorylated, which leads to necroptosis by several paths. **3.** Phosphorylated RIP3 increases free iron and so increases reactive oxygen species (ROS). **4.** Damage to mitochondria leads to apoptosis-inducing factor (AIF) release and also impairs adenosine triphosphate (ATP) production. **5.** Also, increased [Ca²⁺] leads to activation of Ca²⁺-dependent degradative enzymes including phospholipases, which disrupt lysosomes and release lysosomal enzymes that degrade cellular macromolecules. **6.** The final steps in each of these pathways consist of necroptosis: AIF triggers DNase activity and leads to nuclear pyknosis; loss of ATP precipitates a bioenergetic crisis; and plasma membrane damage due to oxidative disruption of membrane lipids produces holes in the cell membrane and leads to release of macromolecular breakdown products that stimulate inflammation (DAMPS). *DAMPs* = damage-associated molecular products; *RIP* = receptor-interacting protein.

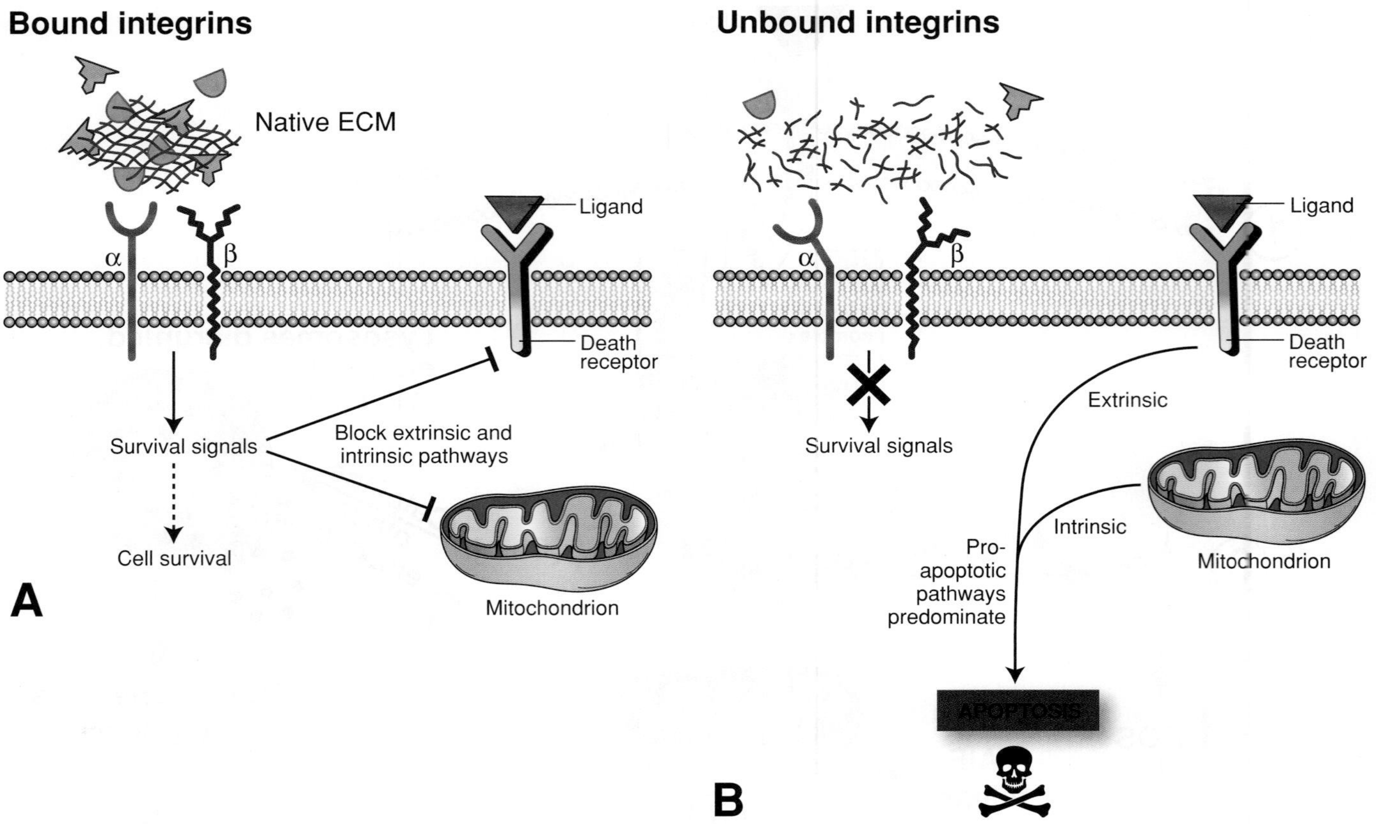

Bound integrins

Unbound integrins

FIGURE 1-52. Mechanisms of anoikis. A. Normal. Under normal circumstances, epithelial cells are bound to their native ECM by transmembrane molecules, including α- and β-integrins. These molecules activate survival signals and block both intrinsic and extrinsic apoptotic signaling pathways. **B. Loss of attachment.** When the cell's integrins are not bound, or not bound by the appropriate ECM moieties, their survival signals are eliminated. Then, activation of apoptosis by death receptor signaling is no longer blocked, and apoptosis may proceed. *ECM* = extracellular matrix.

Granzymes Released by Cytotoxic Lymphocytes Kill Cells via Apoptosis

When cytotoxic T lymphocytes (CTLs) and natural killer (NK) cells recognize a cell as foreign, they attack it via activating caspase signaling. These lymphocytes release two major molecular species: perforin and granzymes. Perforin, as its name suggests, punches a hole in a target cell's plasma membrane, making a conduit through which proteins from the lymphocyte enter. Granzymes are a family of multifunctional serine proteases, among which the best understood is granzyme B. This protease activates cytosolic Bid, a BH3-only protein, by cleaving it to tBid (Fig. 1-53). In turn, tBid increases mitochondrial release of Cyt c and other cell death effector proteins. It also converts several procaspases (notably procaspase-3) to active caspases.

Granzyme A is also released by NK cells and CTLs into target cells. Granzymes A and B together induce cell death by caspase-independent mechanisms. They activate the DNA nicking enzyme, CAD (see above), which degrades genomic DNA (Fig. 1-53).

Pyroptosis Contributes to Innate Immune Defenses

Pyroptosis is a form of PCD that occurs in the setting of intense inflammatory responses, typically associated with infection with intracellular pathogens. Many infectious agents, particularly viruses, but also bacteria and others, stimulate inflammatory reactions by interacting with members of a group of cell membrane receptors called **pattern recognition receptors** (see Chapters 2, 4). Once it recognizes the presence of an invading pathogen, an infected cell produces proinflammatory cytokines and activates other mechanisms that ultimately cause it to swell and burst.

Pyroptosis relies on caspase-1. Although caspase-1 is a cysteine protease involved in PCD, it is independent of apoptotic signaling, and its activation does not bring about apoptosis (Fig. 1-54). Instead, caspase-1 is a proinflammatory protease produced by a structure called an **inflammasome**. This structure is formed when intracellular pathogen molecules, **pathogen-associated molecular patterns** or **PAMPs**, bind to intracellular **NOD-like receptors (NLRs)**. This stimulates expression of inflammatory cytokines and activates caspase-1 (Fig. 1-54). Once activated, caspase-1 cleaves select cellular molecules, including enzymes that are important for glycolysis, thereby depleting cellular energy. It also produces ion-permeable plasma pores, allowing influx of water and solutes to provoke cell swelling and then death. Furthermore, by activating a number of proinflammatory cytokines, the dead cell elicits inflammation.

In addition to its host-protective role in encounters with nefarious pathogens, pyroptosis has been implicated in the pathogenesis of metabolic syndrome, obesity, and the

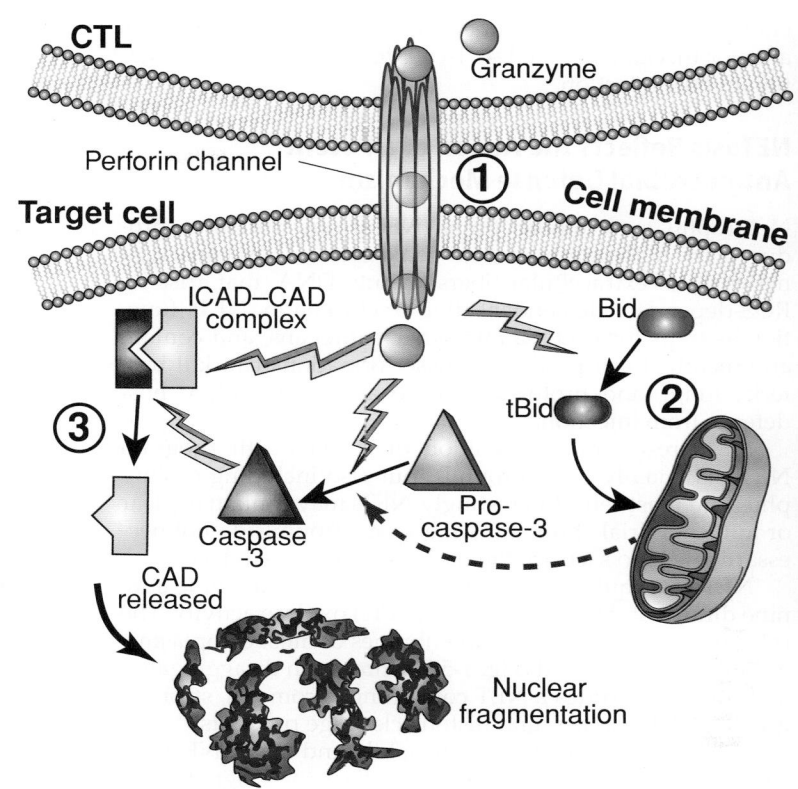

FIGURE 1-53. Cell death caused by CTLs. 1. Granzyme and perforin are made mainly by CTLs and natural killer (NK) cells. Once a CTL binds its cellular victim, perforin molecules combine to create an intercellular channel through which granzymes enters the target cell. **2.** Granzymes cleave cytoplasmic Bid to its active form, tBid, which translocates into mitochondria and triggers the intrinsic pathway of apoptosis. It also activates procaspase-3 to caspase-3, via which apoptosis may proceed. **3.** Granzymes may also disrupt the complex between CAD and its inhibitor, ICAD. This effect releases the DNase (CAD) to elicit a caspase-independent form of apoptosis. The CAD–ICAD complex may also be cleaved by caspase-3. *CAD* = caspase-activated DNase; *CTL* = cytotoxic T lymphocyte; *ICAD* = inhibitor of CAD.

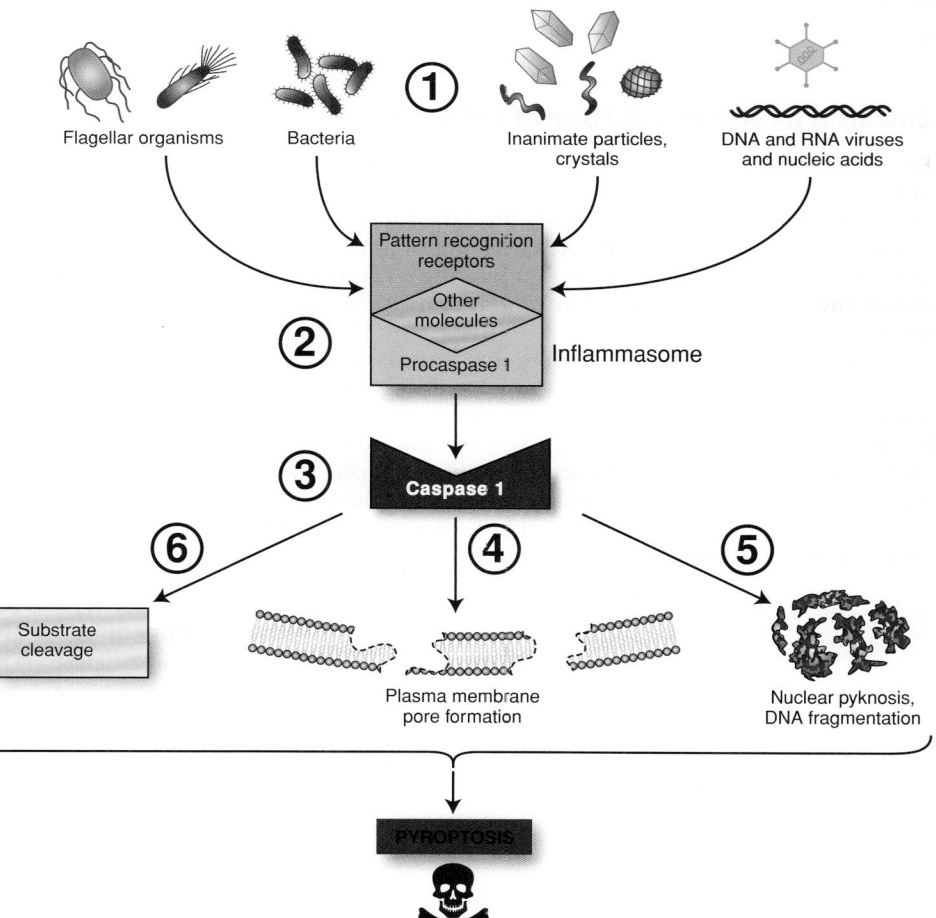

FIGURE 1-54. Pyroptosis. 1. The cell is exposed to injurious agents, both infectious and irritative (e.g., mineral crystals). **2.** Complexes called inflammasomes recognize these exogenous agents via diverse pattern recognition receptors. Inflammasomes contain procaspase-1. **3.** When inflammasome-linked receptors are activated, procaspase-1 is converted to its active form, caspase-1, which has several consequences. **4.** Caspase-1 forms pores in the plasma membrane, allowing intracellular components to leak out of the dying cell. **5.** At the same time, the nucleus is damaged, and **(6)** important intracellular substrates, including cytoskeletal proteins, chaperones, glycolytic proteins, and caspase-7, are cleaved. **7.** All these effects contribute to pyroptotic cell death.

etiology of type 2 diabetes mellitus (see Chapter 13). It also is a major mechanism of CD4+ T-cell depletion and inflammation in HIV infection.

NETosis Reflects the Action of a Potent Antimicrobial Defense Mechanism

Neutrophil extracellular traps (NETs) are structures produced by polymorphonuclear leukocytes. They consist of networks of extracellular fibers, mainly DNA, that arise by ROS-dependent de-condensation of chromatin. NETs function as traps for bacteria and other pathogens, and contain antimicrobial cell products. These formations can kill bacteria, fungi, and protozoa, and so are an important host defense from infection.

NETs result from activation of a cell death program **NETosis**, mainly in neutrophils, but also including eosinophils and mast cells. Interestingly, NETs may contain nuclear or mitochondrial chromatin, and so neutrophils do not necessarily need to sacrifice themselves to generate NETs.

NETosis requires both autophagy and nicotinamide adenine dinucleotide phosphate (NADPH) oxidase activity. The cell's nuclear envelope and membranes of most cytoplasmic granules are destroyed (Fig. 1-55). Chromatin disaggregates, and the cell extrudes a NET containing chromatin, strongly microbicidal histones, and histone cleavage products.

Unlike apoptotic cells, neutrophils and other NETosis-susceptible cells do not present the "eat me" signals (cell membrane phosphatidyl serine; see above) characteristic of apoptosis. Lacking such signals, NETotic cells are not preemptively removed by macrophages and can stimulate inflammatory responses.

Entosis Is a Cell-Eat-Cell Form of Cell Death

Entosis is a type of cellular cannibalism in which cells that are not professional phagocytes engulf nearby living cells. Aggressor cells may engulf cells of either the same or other lineages. For example, hepatocytes may ingest and destroy autoreactive T lymphocytes, thus inhibiting experimental autoimmune liver disease. More often, entosis occurs in tumors.

Vacuoles containing cells undergoing entosis may fuse with lysosomes, in which case target cells usually die, although death is not an inevitable outcome. The cannibalized cell, or parts thereof, may survive the process. Its nuclear material may become part of the aggressor cell, leading to multinucleate cells, polyploidy, or aneuploidy. Some engulfed cells escape their captors and re-emerge unscathed. Mechanisms governing entosis are largely obscure.

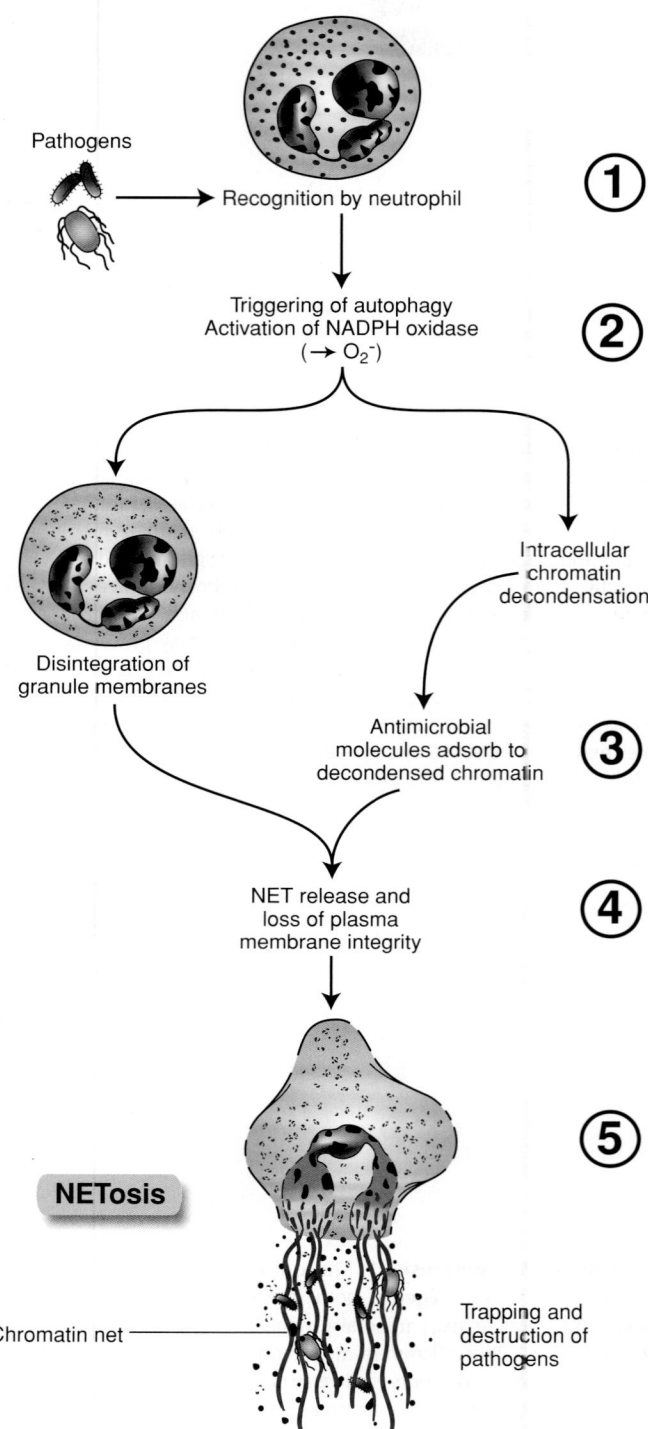

FIGURE 1-55. NETosis. 1. Neutrophils recognize pathogens, after which **(2)** autophagy and NADPH oxidase are activated, the latter yielding reactive oxygen species (ROS). **3.** As a result, intracellular chromatin becomes dispersed and membranes of cytoplasmic granules disintegrate. **4.** NETotic activity leads to release of neutrophil chromatin traps containing antimicrobial cellular products. **5.** These traps then catch and destroy pathogens.

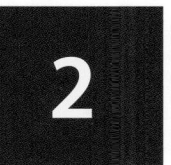

2 Inflammation

Scott B. Lovitch

Inflammation as a Concept: Overview and Historical Perspective

Inflammation is the systemic and local tissue response to injury. Fundamentally, it is a *protective* response optimized to eliminate the cause of cell injury, plus the cells and tissues that died from the original insult. The goal is to restore injured tissues to physical integrity and, ideally, normal function. There are many potential injurious stimuli, but the body responds to all of them in a similar manner: the vascular changes and recruited cells and mediators degrade and sterilize the zone of injury, and set events in motion that will eventually heal and reconstitute those sites.

The word "inflammation" is derived from the Latin verb *inflammare*—literally, "to set afire"—in reference to the heat and redness of tissue that are among its characteristic features. The cardinal features of inflammation, first described by the Roman encyclopedist Aulus Celsus in the first century AD, can be recalled using the Latin mnemonic *calor, dolor, rubor, et tumor*—heat, pain, redness, and swelling, respectively. A fifth cardinal feature, *functio laesa* (loss of function), was added by Rudolf Virchow, the father of modern pathology, in the 19th century.

The main pathways in acute inflammation involve three elements (Fig. 2-1):

- **Vascular** response: locally increased blood flow and increased vascular permeability
- **Cellular** response: recruitment and activation of a specific population of innate immune cells—polymorphonuclear leukocytes (PMN's, poly's, neutrophils, etc.)
- **Effector** cascades: activating pathways, for example, eicosanoids, and including circulating proteins largely synthesized by the liver—like complement and coagulation factors.

These pathways directly trigger the cardinal features of inflammation described by Celsus: *calor* (heat) from increased blood flow (and therefore heat dissipation); *rubor* (redness) from increased blood flow and dilated blood vessels; *tumor* (swelling) from increased vascular permeability causing fluid leakage into surrounding tissue; and *dolor* (pain) from release of inflammatory mediators.

While its cardinal features have been known for centuries, the molecular and cellular mechanisms of acute inflammation have only been elucidated over the last several decades. Many essential drugs in the modern pharmacopeia, including aspirin, corticosteroids, and nonsteroidal anti-inflammatory drugs (NSAIDs), work by targeting acute inflammation, its mediators, and its consequences.

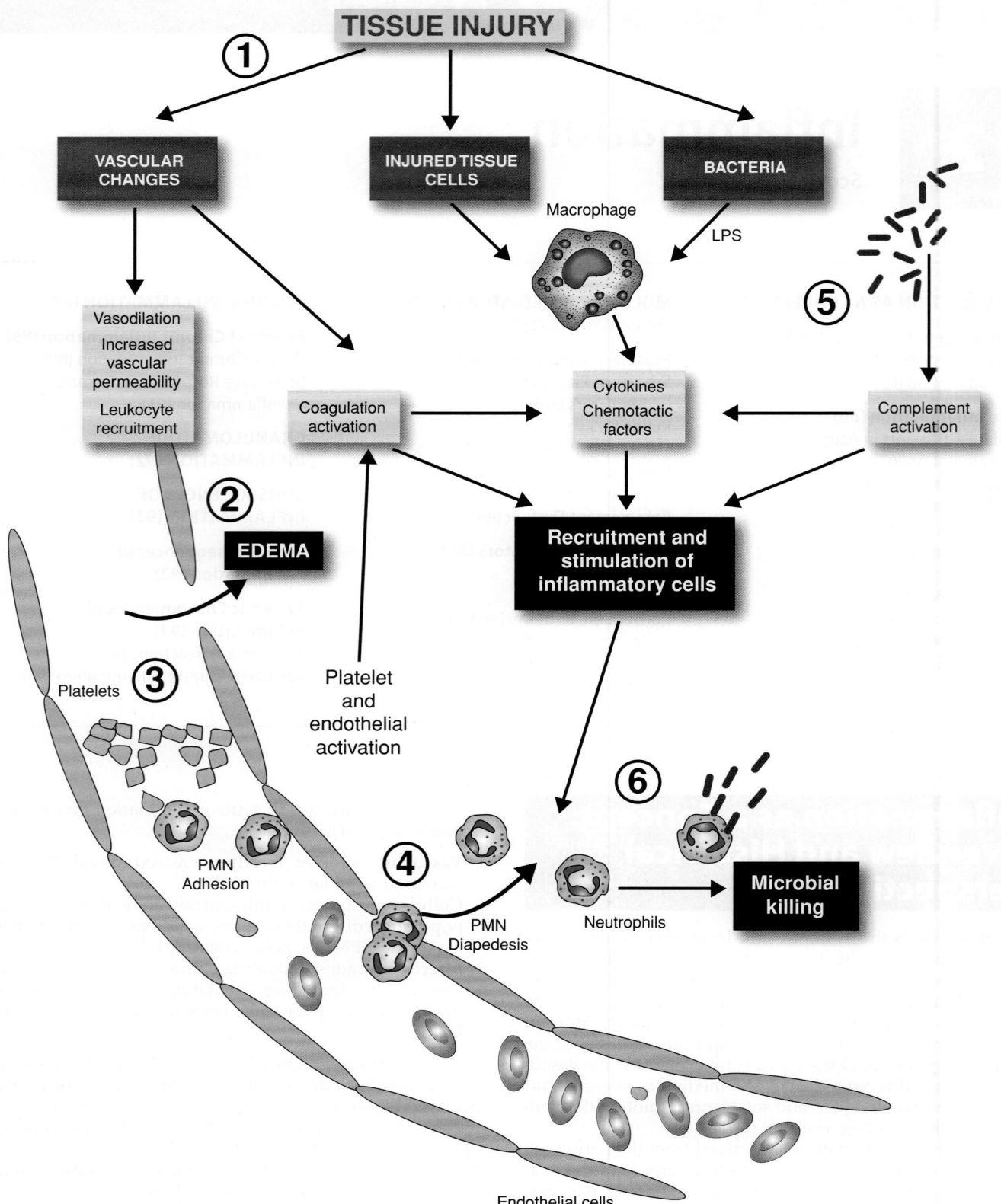

FIGURE 2-1. The inflammatory response to injury. *1.* Tissue injury results in immediate and prolonged vascular changes. Chemical mediators and damaged tissue cells stimulate vasodilation and vascular injury, leading to (*2*) leakage of fluid into tissues (edema). *3.* Platelets are activated to initiate clot formation and hemostasis and to increase vascular permeability via histamine release. *4.* Vascular endothelial cells contribute to clot formation, anchor circulating neutrophils via their upregulated adhesion molecules, and retract to allow increased vascular permeability to plasma and to inflammatory cells. At the same time, microbes (*red rods*) (*5*) initiate activation of the complement cascade, which, along with soluble mediators from macrophages, (*6*) recruits neutrophils to the site of tissue injury. Neutrophils and macrophages eliminate microbes and remove damaged tissue so that repair can begin. *PMN* = polymorphonuclear leukocyte.

Furthermore, while inflammation helps resolve infections and clear debris from injury and make wound healing possible, it may also cause tissue injury and disease in its own right. Dysregulated or overexuberant inflammation in many common diseases, including cancer and cardiovascular disease, is increasingly also a target for therapy.

CHRONOLOGY OF INFLAMMATION

The character of inflammatory responses to tissue injury depends on several factors, including the nature of the offending agent, duration of the insult, extent of damage, and the site of injury and its specific microenvironment. However, the process generally follows a reproducible sequence of events (Fig. 2-1):

- **Initiation:** Soluble mediators are activated and inflammatory cells are recruited to the area. Molecules released from invading agents, damaged cells and extracellular matrix rapidly trigger a sequence of **vascular** changes increasing nearby blood vessel permeability to plasma, causing rapid flooding of injured tissues with fluid, coagulation factors, cytokines, chemokines, platelets and inflammatory cells, particularly neutrophils (Fig. 2-2). These changes are characteristic of **acute inflammation.**
- **Amplification:** Depending on the extent of injury and activation of mediators like kinins and complement, more leukocytes and macrophages are recruited to the area.
- **Destruction:** Eliminating damaging agents brings the process under control. Enzymatic digestion and phagocytosis reduce or remove foreign material or infectious organisms. Simultaneously, damaged tissue components are also removed and debris is cleared.
- **Termination:** Intrinsic anti-inflammatory mechanisms limit tissue damage and allow for tissue healing and

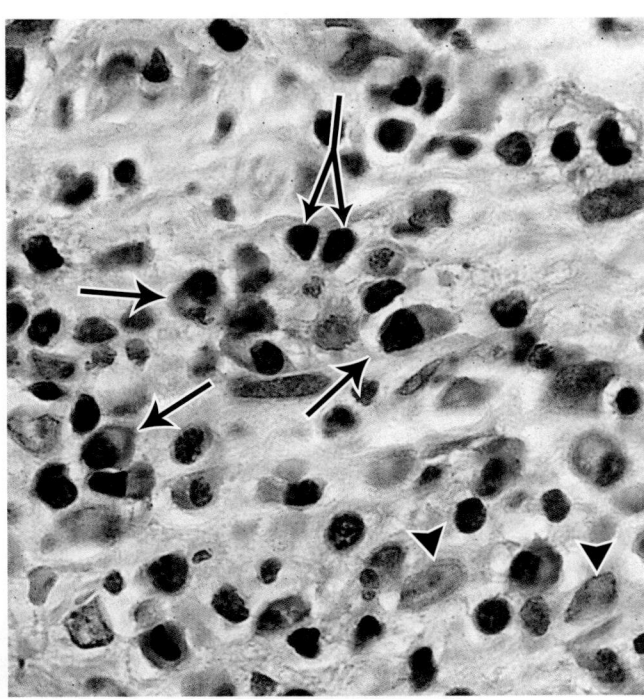

FIGURE 2-3. Chronic inflammation. Lymphocytes (*double-headed arrow*), plasma cells (*arrows*) and a few macrophages (*arrowheads*) are present.

repair (see **Chapter 3**). Depending on the nature of the injury and specific inflammatory and repair responses, the tissue returns to normal function (regeneration) or a scar develops in place of normal tissue (fibrosis).

Intrinsic mechanisms terminate the inflammatory process; prevent further influx of fluid, mediators and inflammatory cells and limit damage to normal cells and tissues.

If acute inflammation fails to resolve the insult, or an infectious agent persists, inflammation may continue, and **chronic inflammation** can supervene. Unlike acute inflammation, chronic inflammation entails infiltration by mononuclear cells (lymphocytes, macrophages and plasma cells) and deposition of extracellular matrix (fibrosis) (Fig. 2-3). Acute and chronic inflammation may also coexist. Chronic inflammation can cause scarring and loss of function, and is the basis for many degenerative diseases.

Each Cellular Component of Inflammation Has Specific Roles

The cast of cellular characters in inflammation includes neutrophils, the key cells of acute inflammation, as well as T and B lymphocytes, monocytes, macrophages, eosinophils, mast cells and basophils. These cells' functions overlap and change as inflammation evolves (Fig. 2-4). Inflammatory and resident tissue cells interact continuously during inflammation.

Neutrophils

These cells, also called polymorphonuclear leukocytes or PMNs, are the *sine qua non* of acute inflammation; as a general rule, if you see an inflammatory infiltrate consisting mainly of neutrophils, you are looking at an acute

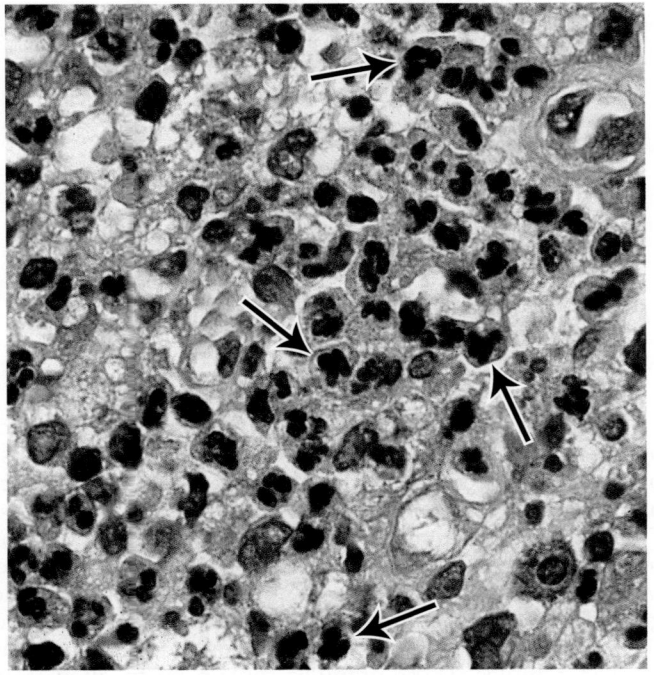

FIGURE 2-2. Acute inflammation. Densely packed polymorphonuclear leukocytes (PMNs) with multilobed nuclei (*arrows*).

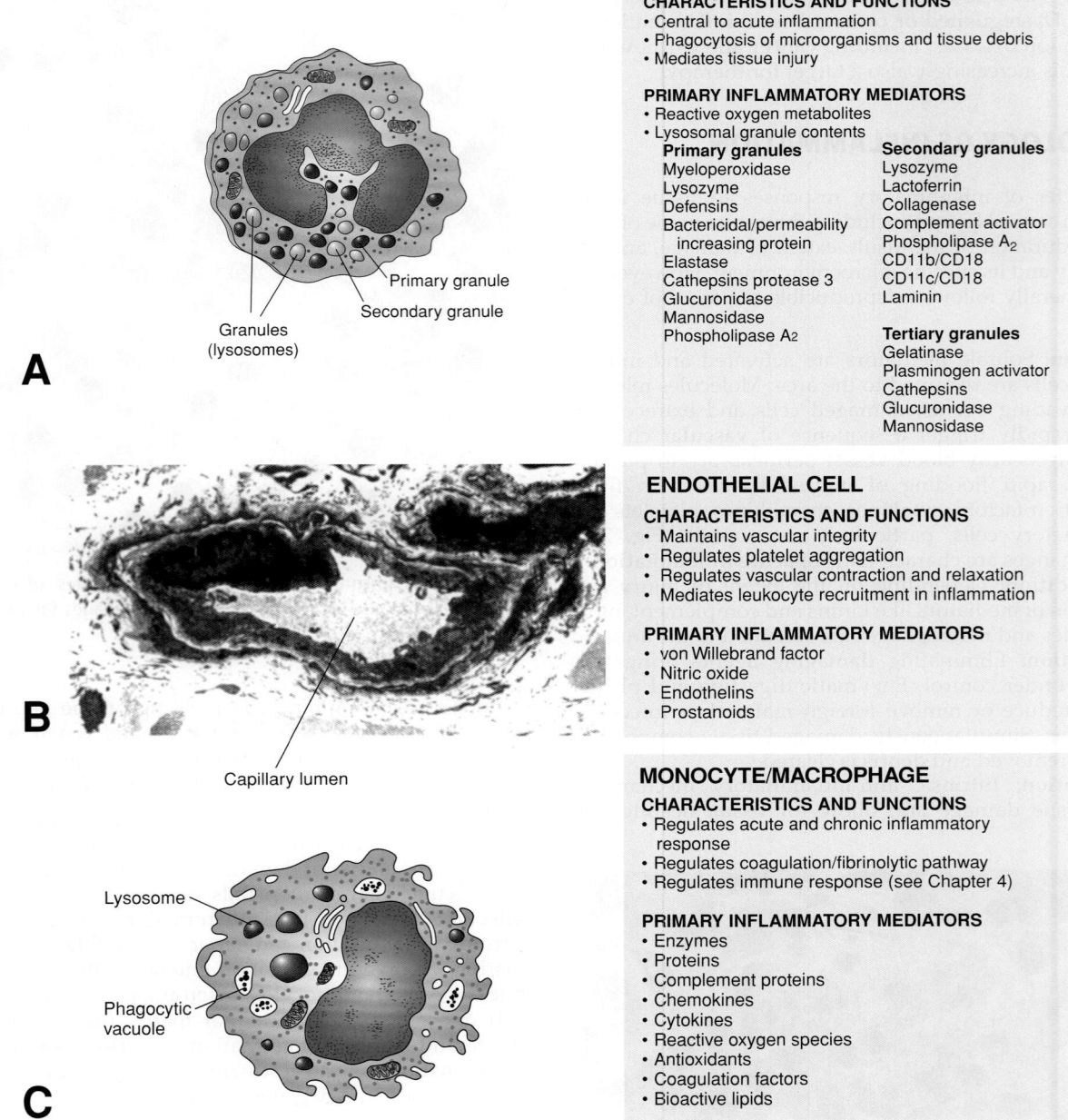

POLYMORPHONUCLEAR LEUKOCYTE

CHARACTERISTICS AND FUNCTIONS
• Central to acute inflammation
• Phagocytosis of microorganisms and tissue debris
• Mediates tissue injury

PRIMARY INFLAMMATORY MEDIATORS
• Reactive oxygen metabolites
• Lysosomal granule contents

Primary granules	**Secondary granules**
Myeloperoxidase	Lysozyme
Lysozyme	Lactoferrin
Defensins	Collagenase
Bactericidal/permeability	Complement activator
increasing protein	Phospholipase A₂
Elastase	CD11b/CD18
Cathepsins protease 3	CD11c/CD18
Glucuronidase	Laminin
Mannosidase	
Phospholipase A₂	**Tertiary granules**
	Gelatinase
	Plasminogen activator
	Cathepsins
	Glucuronidase
	Mannosidase

ENDOTHELIAL CELL

CHARACTERISTICS AND FUNCTIONS
• Maintains vascular integrity
• Regulates platelet aggregation
• Regulates vascular contraction and relaxation
• Mediates leukocyte recruitment in inflammation

PRIMARY INFLAMMATORY MEDIATORS
• von Willebrand factor
• Nitric oxide
• Endothelins
• Prostanoids

MONOCYTE/MACROPHAGE

CHARACTERISTICS AND FUNCTIONS
• Regulates acute and chronic inflammatory response
• Regulates coagulation/fibrinolytic pathway
• Regulates immune response (see Chapter 4)

PRIMARY INFLAMMATORY MEDIATORS
• Enzymes
• Proteins
• Complement proteins
• Chemokines
• Cytokines
• Reactive oxygen species
• Antioxidants
• Coagulation factors
• Bioactive lipids

FIGURE 2-4. Cells of inflammation: morphology and function. A. Neutrophil. **B.** Endothelial cell. **C.** Monocyte/macrophage.

inflammatory process. Neutrophils are typically 12 to 15 micrometers (μm, or microns) in diameter (comparable to other granulocytes, e.g., eosinophils and basophils), and have a multilobed nucleus—three lobes are most common, but neutrophils with two or four lobes are frequently seen. Their cytoplasm contains fine granules that do not stain well in conventional preparations (hence "neutrophil," reflecting the "neutral" staining qualities of these granules). Neutrophils are stored in bone marrow, circulate in the blood and accumulate rapidly at sites of injury or infection (Figs. 2-4A and 2-5). They are short-lived cells, with a circulating half-life of about 10 hours.

Neutrophils express many cell-surface receptors, that recognize **pathogen-associated molecular patterns (PAMPs)** produced by infectious agents and **danger-associated molecular patterns (DAMPs)** released by injured and dead cells. They also have receptors for Fc portions of IgG and IgM; complement components C5a, C3b and iC3b; arachidonic acid (AA) metabolites; chemokines; and cytokines. Chemotactic gradients of ligands for these receptors recruit neutrophils to sites of injury, where they release the contents of their intracellular granules. Those granules contain potent mediators that sterilize and degrade injured tissue, and phagocytose invading microscopes and dead tissue. They then undergo

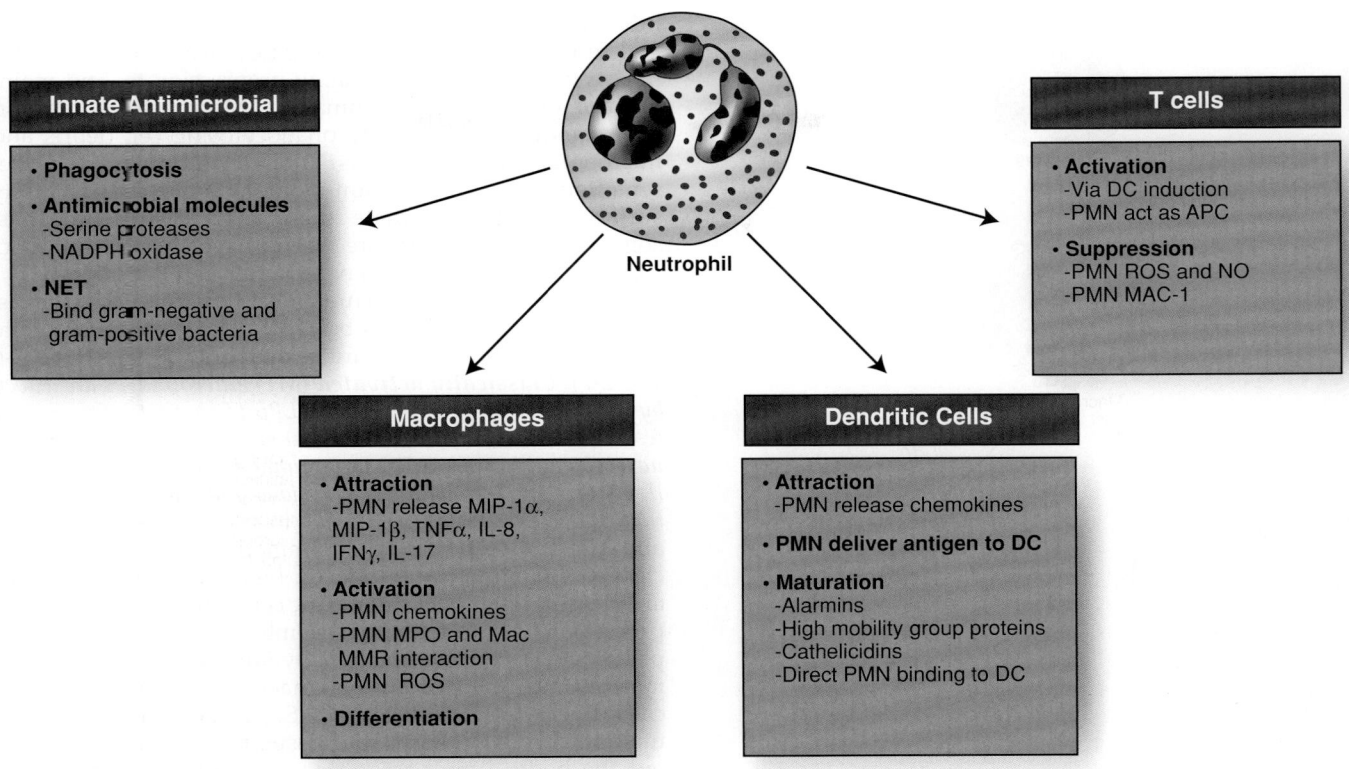

Innate Antimicrobial

- **Phagocytosis**
- **Antimicrobial molecules**
  - -Serine proteases
  - -NADPH oxidase
- **NET**
  - -Bind gram-negative and gram-positive bacteria

Neutrophil

T cells

- **Activation**
  - -Via DC induction
  - -PMN act as APC
- **Suppression**
  - -PMN ROS and NO
  - -PMN MAC-1

Macrophages

- **Attraction**
  - -PMN release MIP-1α, MIP-1β, TNFα, IL-8, IFNγ, IL-17
- **Activation**
  - -PMN chemokines
  - -PMN MPO and Mac MMR interaction
  - -PMN ROS
- **Differentiation**

Dendritic Cells

- **Attraction**
  - -PMN release chemokines
- **PMN deliver antigen to DC**
- **Maturation**
  - -Alarmins
  - -High mobility group proteins
  - -Cathelicidins
  - -Direct PMN binding to DC

FIGURE 2-5. Effector functions of neutrophils.

apoptosis, largely during the resolution phase of acute inflammation. Neutrophil apoptosis both limits the extent of tissue injury caused by neutrophil activity and helps to sterilize tissue via release of **neutrophil extracellular traps (NETs)** which ensnare and kill pathogens (NETosis; see Chapter 1). In addition to their microbicidal and proinflammatory properties, neutrophils regulate dendritic cell, T cell and macrophage functions. They also help trigger subsequent chronic inflammation, through mediators they release and products that dead and dying cells leave behind in their wake.

Endothelial Cells

Endothelial cells line blood vessels, creating a functional barrier between the intravascular and extravascular spaces. They produce antiplatelet and antithrombotic agents that maintain blood vessel patency and secrete vasodilators and vasoconstrictors that regulate vascular tone (see Chapter 16). Injury to a vessel wall interrupts the endothelial barrier and exposes local procoagulant signals (Fig. 2-4B). Endothelial cells are gatekeepers in inflammatory cell recruitment; they may promote or inhibit tissue perfusion and inflammatory cell influx. Inflammatory agents such as **bradykinin** and **histamine, endotoxins** and cytokines induce endothelial cells to display adhesion molecules that anchor and activate leukocytes, causing them to present major histocompatibility complex (MHC, see Chapter 4) class I and II molecules, and generate key vasoactive and inflammatory mediators. These mediators include:

- **Nitric Oxide (NO):** NO is a low–molecular-weight vasodilator that inhibits platelet aggregation, regulates vascular

tone by stimulating smooth muscle relaxation and reacts with ROS to create highly active free radicals (see above).
- **Endothelins:** Endothelins-1, -2, and -3 are low–molecular-weight peptides that are potent vasoconstrictor and pressor agents. They induce prolonged vasoconstriction of vascular smooth muscle.
- **AA–derived factors:** Oxygen radicals generated by the hydroperoxidase activity of cyclooxygenase, and prostanoids, for example, TXA2 and PGH2, induce smooth muscle contraction, while the biologic opponent of TXA2, PGI2, inhibits platelet aggregation and causes vasodilation.
- **Cytokines:** IL-1, IL-6, TNFα and other inflammatory cytokines are generated by activated endothelial cells.
- **Anticoagulants:** Heparin-like molecules and thrombomodulin inactivate the coagulation cascade (see Chapters 16, 26).
- **Fibrinolytic factors: Tissue-type plasminogen activator (t-PA)** promotes fibrinolysis.
- **Prothrombotic agents:** von Willebrand factor facilitates platelet adhesion, and tissue factor activates the extrinsic clotting cascade.

Monocytes/Macrophages

Circulating monocytes (Fig. 2-4C) are bone marrow–derived cells with a single lobed, or kidney-shaped, nucleus. They may exit the circulation to migrate into tissues, to become resident macrophages that accumulate at sites of acute inflammation. Macrophages clear pathogens, cell debris, and apoptotic cells. Monocytes/macrophages produce potent

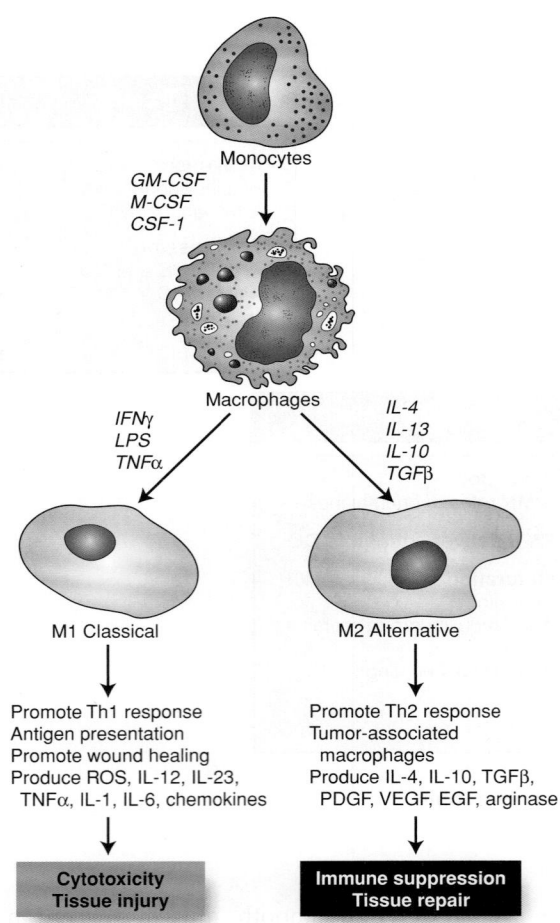

FIGURE 2-6. Macrophage activation states.

inflammatory mediators, influencing initiation, progression, and resolution of acute inflammatory responses. They also have a central role in regulating progression to, and maintenance of, chronic inflammation. Macrophages respond to inflammatory stimuli by phagocytosing cell debris and microorganisms, chemotaxis, antigen processing, and presentation and secreting immunomodulatory factors. Many surface receptors mediate these macrophage functions; some immune receptors are macrophage specific, but macrophages share others with neutrophils and lymphocytes.

There are basically two functional types of macrophages, although in practice it can be difficult to distinguish them, as their expression of cell surface markers overlaps (Figs. 2-6 and 2-7). *Classically activated (M1) macrophages are driven by interferon-γ (IFNγ), TNFα and LPS to support inflammatory responses and release ROS and immune defense cytokines. Alternatively activated (M2) macrophages respond to IL-4 and IL-13 to help clear parasitic infections and suppress inflammation.* Macrophages also respond to cytokines such as IL-10 and TGFβ to help resolve inflammation or switch acute to chronic inflammatory responses. Like PMNs, macrophages are phagocytes and, like dendritic cells, are crucial in antigen processing and presentation. Members of this mononuclear phagocyte system are functionally diverse and include bone marrow macrophages, alveolar macrophages (lung), Kupffer cells (liver), microglial cells (CNS), Langerhans cells (skin), mesangial cells (kidney), and tissue macrophages throughout the body. Tumor-associated macrophages (TAMs) can recognize and lyse tumor cells.

Dendritic Cells

Dendritic cells derive from bone marrow progenitors, circulate in the blood as immature precursors, then settle widely in tissues, where they differentiate. They are highly efficient

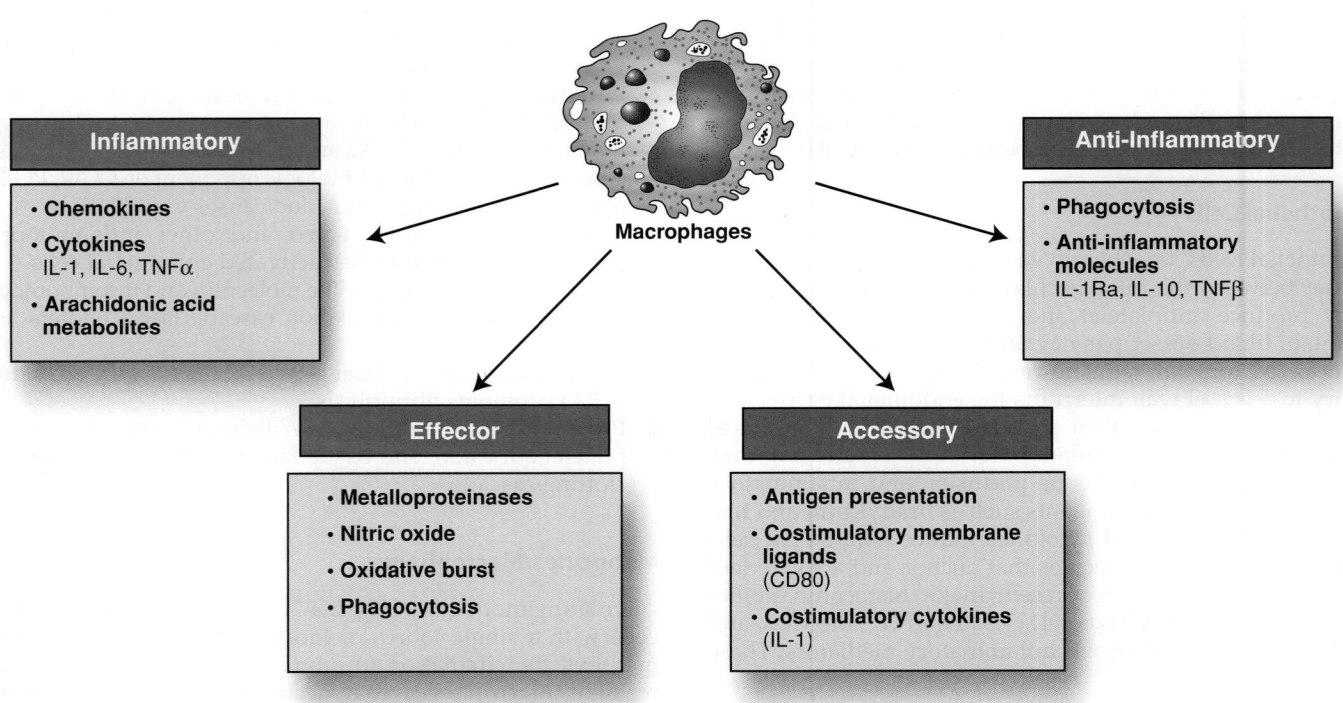

FIGURE 2-7. Effector functions of macrophages.

antigen-presenting cells, and are the primary cell type that stimulates naive T cells to initiate adaptive immune responses. Antigens bind MHC class II on dendritic cells. These then present antigens to lymphocytes and activate them (see **Chapter 4**).

Mast Cells and Basophils

Basophils (Fig. 2-8A) are the least common leukocyte in the blood. They can migrate into tissue to participate in immunologic responses. Functionally similar mast cells are long-lived and reside in all supporting tissues in connective tissues, on lung and gut mucosal surfaces, in the dermis and in the microvasculature. Both mast cells and basophils have cell surface receptors for **IgE**. Antigens, physical agonists (cold, trauma) or cationic proteins may stimulate IgE-sensitized mast cells or basophils to release inflammatory mediators that the cells store in dense cytoplasmic granules. These granules contain acid mucopolysaccharides (including heparin), serine proteases, chemotactic mediators for neutrophils and eosinophils, and histamine. Histamine binds specific H1 receptors in the vascular wall, inducing endothelial cell contraction, gap formation and edema, and so stimulates increased vascular permeability (which can be blocked pharmacologically by H1-receptor antagonists [antihistamines]). Stimulated mast cells and basophils also release leukotrienes (products of AA metabolism) and cytokines such as TNFα and IL-4.

Eosinophils

Eosinophils (Fig. 2-8B) circulate in blood and are recruited to tissues similarly to PMNs. They often accumulate during IgE-mediated reactions, such as allergy and asthma. Eosinophils express IgA receptors and have large granules containing eosinophil major basic protein (MBP), both of which are involved in defense against parasites (see Chapter 4). Their granules also contain **leukotrienes**, **platelet-activating factor (PAF)**, acid phosphatase, and peroxidase.

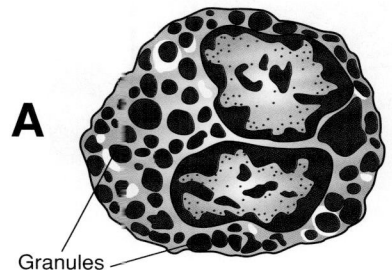

MAST CELL (BASOPHIL)

CHARACTERISTICS AND FUNCTIONS
- Binds IgE molecules
- Contains electron-dense granules

PRIMARY INFLAMMATORY MEDIATORS
- Histamine
- Leukotrienes (LTC, LTD, LTE)
- Platelet-activating factor
- Eosinophil chemotactic factors
- Cytokines (e.g., TNFα IL-4)

A — Granules

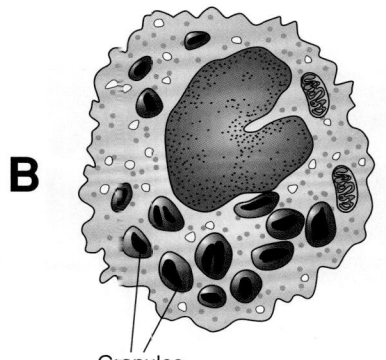

EOSINOPHIL

CHARACTERISTICS AND FUNCTIONS
- Associated with:
  - Allergic reactions
  - Parasite-associated inflammatory reactions
  - Chronic inflammation
- Modulates mast cell–mediated reactions

PRIMARY INFLAMMATORY MEDIATORS
- Reactive oxygen metabolites
- Lysosomal granule enzymes (primary crystalloid granules)
  - Major basic protein
  - Eosinophil cationic protein
  - Eosinophil peroxidase
  - Acid phosphatase
  - β-glucuronidase
  - Arylsulfatase B
  - Histaminase
- Phospholipase D
- Prostaglandins of E series
- Cytokines

B — Granules

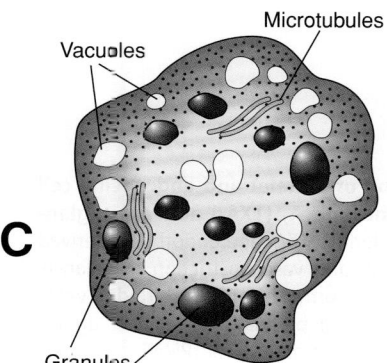

PLATELET

CHARACTERISTICS AND FUNCTIONS
- Thrombosis; promotes clot formation
- Regulates permeability
- Regulates proliferative response of mesenchymal cells

PRIMARY INFLAMMATORY MEDIATORS
- Dense granules
  - Serotonin
  - Ca^{2+}
  - ADP
- α-Granules
  - Cationic proteins
  - Fibrinogen and coagulation proteins
  - Platelet-derived growth factor (PDGF)
- Lysosomes
  - Acid hydrolases
- Thromboxane A_2

C — Vacuoles, Microtubules, Granules

FIGURE 2-8. **More cells of inflammation: morphology and function. A.** Mast cell/basophil. **B.** Eosinophil. **C.** Platelet. *ADP* = adenosine diphosphate.

Platelets

Platelets (Fig. 2-8C) are essential for initiating and regulating clotting (see **Chapter 26**). Platelets are small (1 to 2 μm in diameter) and lack nuclei. They have three types of inclusions: (1) dense granules, rich in serotonin, histamine, calcium, and ADP; (2) α-granules, containing fibrinogen, coagulation proteins, platelet-derived growth factor (PDGF) and other peptides and proteins; and (3) lysosomes, which sequester acid hydrolases. In addition to their role in hemostasis, platelets produce inflammatory mediators—potent vasoactive substances and growth factors that modulate mesenchymal cell proliferation. Platelets adhere, aggregate, and degranulate when they contact fibrillar collagen (e.g., after vascular injury that exposes interstitial matrix proteins)

or thrombin (after coagulation is activated) (Fig. 2-9). Degranulation releases serotonin (5-hydroxytryptamine), which, like histamine, directly increases vascular permeability. In addition, the platelet AA metabolite thromboxane A2 (TXA2) plays a key role in the second wave of platelet aggregation and mediates smooth muscle constriction. On activation, platelets, like phagocytic cells, secrete cationic proteins that neutralize the negative charges on endothelium and increase permeability.

ACUTE INFLAMMATION

Acute inflammation represents a tissue's first response after most forms of injury. It is of relatively short duration,

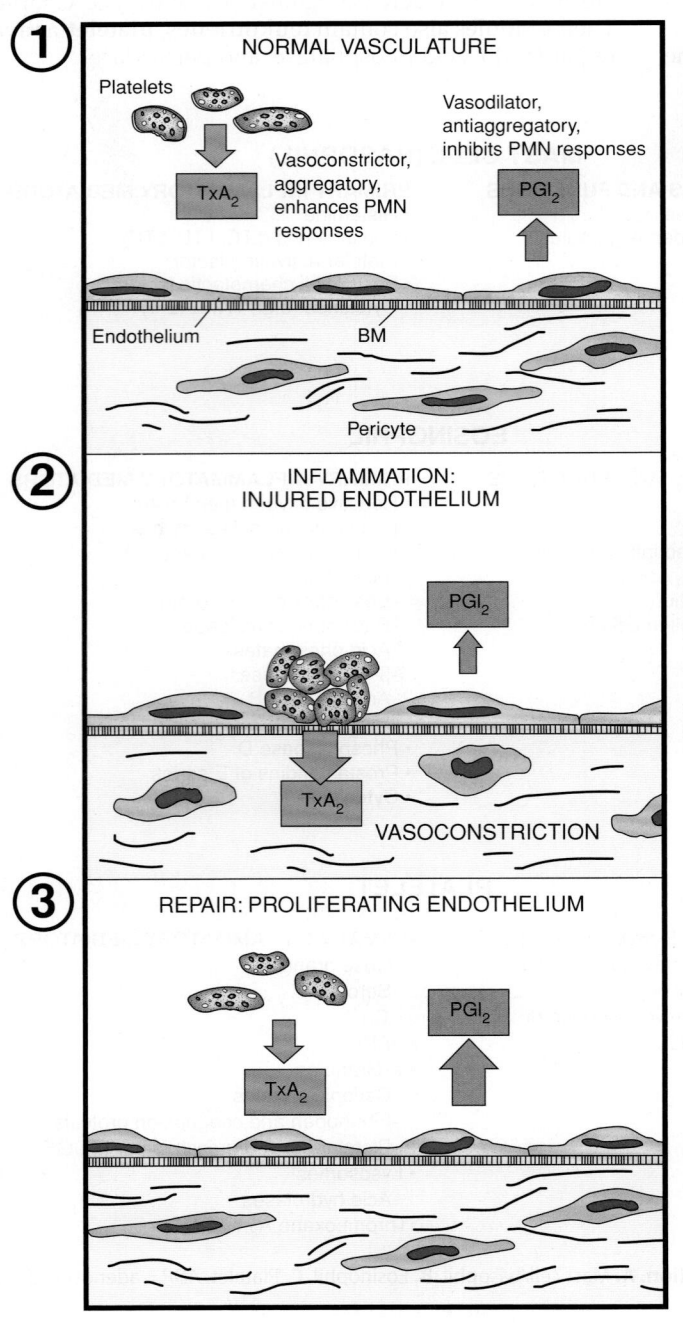

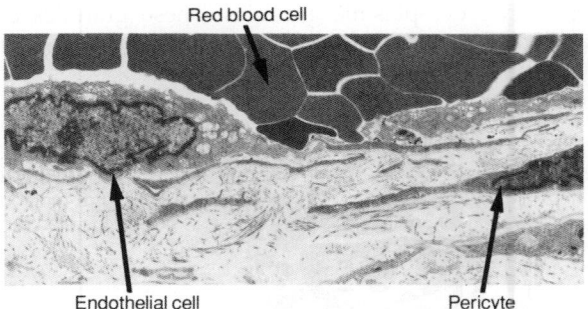

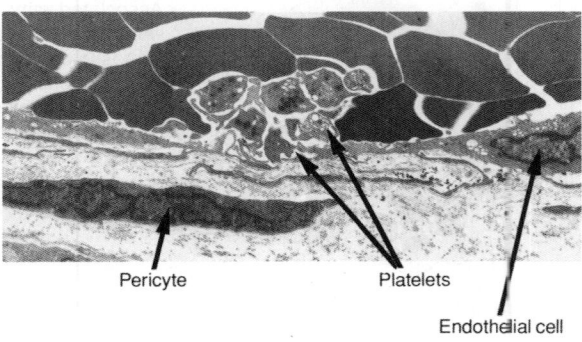

FIGURE 2-9. Regulation of platelet and endothelial cell interactions by thromboxane A₂ (TXA₂) and prostaglandin I₂ (PGI₂). 1. Platelet-derived TXA₂ and endothelial-derived PGI₂ maintain vasodilation and vasoconstriction in balance. **2.** During inflammation, the normal balance is shifted to vasoconstriction, increased vascular permeability, platelet aggregation, and polymorphonuclear neutrophil (PMN) responses. **3.** During repair, the prostaglandin effects predominate, inhibiting PMN responses and promoting normal blood flow. *BM* = basement membrane.

lasting from minutes to days (hence the name). It is the immediate and early response to injury, designed to deliver leukocytes to sites of injury and set them in motion. A *fluid and plasma protein exudate* accumulates, accompanied by an infiltrate mainly of neutrophils (Figs. 2-1 and 2-2). Once there, leukocytes clear any pathogenic organisms present in the tissue and begin removing dead (necrotic) or damaged tissues.

Acute Inflammation Results From an Interplay of Circulating and Resident Cells, Soluble Factors, and Supporting Tissues

Participants include circulating blood cells, cells that reside in vascular walls—particularly endothelial cells and underlying smooth muscle cells that regulate vascular tone—as well as plasma proteins and surrounding connective tissue cells, including macrophages, lymphocytes, mast cells, and fibroblasts.

Acute inflammation has two major components, visible grossly and microscopically:

- **Vascular changes**: alterations in diameter and in permeability of the vessel wall, increases blood flow (vasodilation) and efflux of plasma proteins from the circulation.
- **Cellular events**: emigration of leukocytes from the circulation to the site of injury (cellular recruitment and activation).

These changes are driven by many **molecular mediators**, both soluble and cell associated; the most important of these will be discussed below.

The major events of acute inflammation occur in waves, with vascular events occurring predominantly within the first 6 hours after injury, and influx of neutrophils peaking at 12 hours and persisting for about 24 hours. The initial influx of monocytes, signaling the transition to chronic inflammation, starts at about 48 hours postinjury; by 96 hours, the infiltrate should be mostly mononuclear.

Vascular changes and cellular recruitment cause three of the five classic local signs of acute inflammation: heat (calor), redness (rubor), and swelling (tumor). The two additional cardinal features of acute inflammation, pain (dolor) and loss of function (functio laesis), reflect soluble mediators and leukocyte-mediated tissue damage.

Vascular Changes in Acute Inflammation Begin Shortly After Injury

Once triggered, these changes develop at variable rates, depending on the tissue site and the nature and severity of the injury. They reflect the "triple response" first described by Sir Thomas Lewis in 1924. In those experiments, a dull red line developed at the site of mild trauma to skin, followed by a flare (red halo) and then a wheal (swelling). Lewis postulated that a vasoactive mediator caused vasodilation and increased vascular permeability at the site of injury.

- **As the immediate response to injury or insult, blood vessels rapidly and transiently (within seconds) constrict, and then dilate**. Vasodilation, which occurs under the influence of NO, histamine, and other soluble agents, allows increased blood flow and expansion of the capillary bed; this causes the redness (**erythema**) and warmth associated with acute inflammation.

- **Increased vascular permeability allows fluid and plasma components to accumulate in affected tissues**. Endothelial cells are connected to each other by tight junctions and separated from surrounding tissues by a limiting basement membrane (Fig. 2-10A). Endothelium normally functions as a permeability barrier: it regulates and limits fluid movement between intravascular and extravascular spaces. **Disruption of this barrier function is a hallmark of acute inflammation**. Shortly after tissue injury, inflammatory mediators produced at the site of injury directly increase permeability of capillaries and postcapillary venules. Vascular leakage reflects endothelial cell contraction and retraction, and alterations in transcytosis. Endothelial cells are also damaged, either directly, or indirectly by leukocytes. Disruption of the permeability barrier causes leakage of fluid (**edema**) and cells into the extravascular space (Fig. 2-10B,C).

- **Soluble mediators (e.g., kinins, complement) stimulate intravascular platelets and inflammatory cells**. These molecules bind receptors on vascular endothelial and smooth muscle cells, causing vasoconstriction or vasodilation. Arteriolar vasodilation increases blood flow and exacerbates fluid leakage into tissue, while vasoconstriction of postcapillary venules increases capillary bed hydrostatic pressure, further stimulating edema. Activated complement components further increase vascular permeability and contribute to edema (Fig. 2-11).

- **Neutrophils are recruited to the injured site**. As fluid leaks into the extravascular space, effectively concentrating erythrocytes and leukocytes, blood viscosity increases and circulation slows (**vascular stasis**). This appears microscopically as many dilated, congested small vessels. As stasis develops, leukocytes (particularly neutrophils) begin to settle out of flowing blood and accumulate along endothelial surfaces (**margination**), where they can adhere to receptors expressed by endothelial cells, and eventually squeeze between the endothelial cells and migrate into the tissue, a process called **diapedesis**. Chemotactic factors then recruit leukocytes into the injured tissue. Once in tissues, leukocytes start attacking invading pathogens so that damaged components can be removed, and tissue repair can start. Neutrophils also secrete additional mediators, which may enhance or inhibit inflammation. The specific receptor-ligand interactions mediating this process are discussed below.

Inflammation and Edema

Under conditions of physiologic homeostasis, fluid continually leaks from the intravascular compartment into the extravascular space. Lymphatics clear this fluid and return it to the circulation. Fluid interchange between vascular and extravascular compartments reflects a balance of forces that draw fluid into vascular spaces or out into tissues (see **Chapter 7**). **Hydrostatic pressure,** from blood flow and plasma volume, forces fluid out of the vasculature. This pressure is countered by **osmotic pressure** generated by electrolyte gradients between plasma and tissue, and **oncotic** pressure generated by plasma proteins (particularly albumin), which are generally too large to cross the endothelium and therefore remain intravascular.

Vascular changes in acute inflammation disturb this balance of forces, producing edema. Increased blood flow

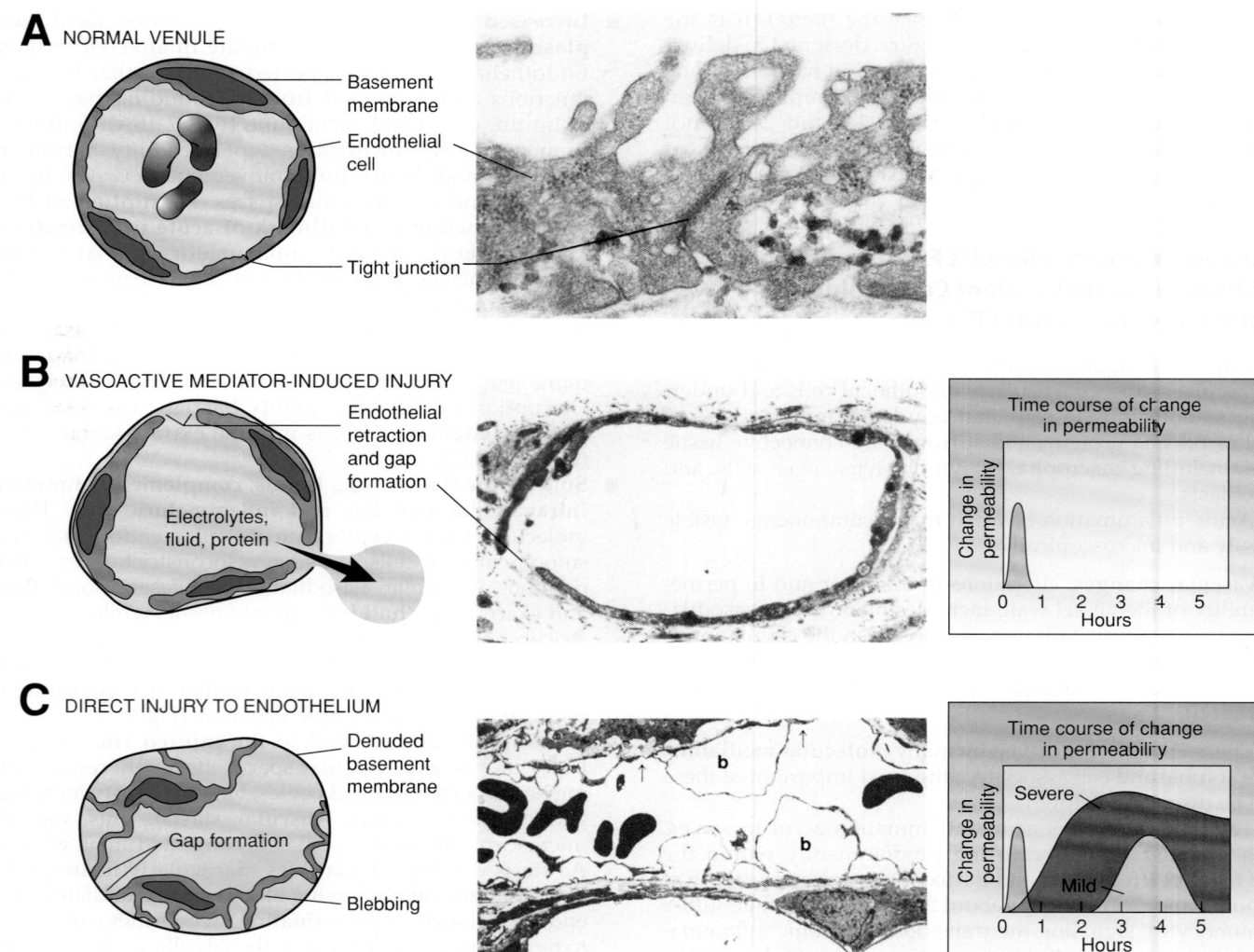

FIGURE 2-10. Responses of the microvasculature to injury. A. The wall of the normal venule is sealed by tight junctions between adjacent endothelial cells. **B.** During mild vasoactive mediator-induced injury, the endothelial cells separate and permit the passage of the fluid constituents of the blood. **C.** With severe direct injury, the endothelial cells form blebs (*b*) and separate from the underlying basement membrane. Areas of denuded basement membrane (*arrows*) allow a prolonged escape of fluid elements from the microvasculature.

and increased hydrostatic pressure work with increased vascular permeability (see above) and endothelial injury to move fluid from the intravascular to the extravascular space. Initially, this fluid is essentially a **transudate**: an ultra-filtrate of blood plasma. However, as vascular permeability increases and cells begin to migrate through the endothe-lium, the fluid that accumulates in tissues becomes an **exu-date**, rich in proteins and cells. Transudatives and exudates can be distinguished by their specific gravity—a specific gravity under 1.015 indicates low protein content, and is characteristic of transudates, while exudates have specific gravity >1.015. Specific measurements of proteins in fluid, compared to plasma, also help make this distinction.

Many clinical conditions cause transudative or exuda-tive fluid accumulation. For example, obstruction of venous outflow (thrombosis) or decreased right ventricular function (congestive heart failure) increases vascular back pressure, and so hydrostatic pressure (see **Chapter 7**). Decreased plasma albumin, whether via renal loss or decreased hepatic synthesis, reduces plasma oncotic pressure. Any abnormality

of sodium or water retention alters osmotic pressure and the balance of fluid forces. Finally, lymphedema may occur if lymphatic drainage is impaired (e.g., after surgery, radiation, or tumor or infection).

Several key terms describe edema and its consequences:

- **Effusions** are accumulations of excess fluid in body cavi-ties (e.g., peritoneal or pleural space).
- **Serous** exudates (or effusions) are characterized by scant cellular response and a yellow, straw-like color.
- **Serosanguineous** fluids are serous exudates, or effusions, containing red blood cells. These have a reddish tinge.
- **Fibrinous** exudates contain large amounts of fibrin, due to clotting system activation. When a fibrinous exudate occurs on a serosal surface, such as the pleura or pericar-dium, it is "fibrinous pleuritis" or "fibrinous pericarditis."
- **Purulent** exudates contain prominent cellular compo-nents, and are often associated with pyogenic infections, in which neutrophils predominate.
- **Suppurative inflammation** is a purulent exudate with sig-nificant liquefactive necrosis (see **Chapter 1**); that is, pus.

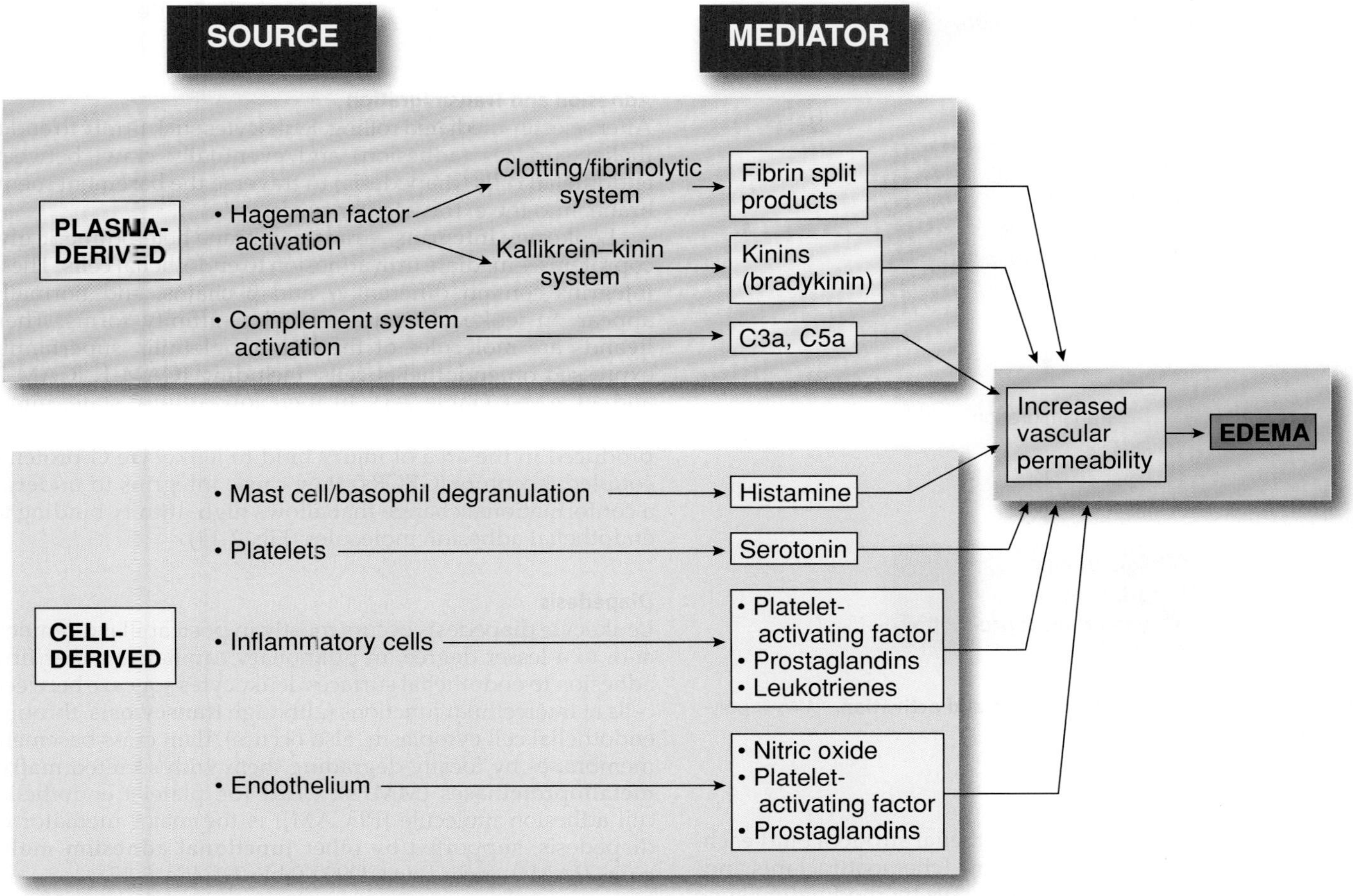

SOURCE / MEDIATOR

PLASMA-DERIVED

- Hageman factor activation → Clotting/fibrinolytic system → Fibrin split products
- Hageman factor activation → Kallikrein–kinin system → Kinins (bradykinin)
- Complement system activation → C3a, C5a

CELL-DERIVED

- Mast cell/basophil degranulation → Histamine
- Platelets → Serotonin
- Inflammatory cells → • Platelet-activating factor • Prostaglandins • Leukotrienes
- Endothelium → • Nitric oxide • Platelet-activating factor • Prostaglandins

→ Increased vascular permeability → **EDEMA**

FIGURE 2-11. nflammatory mediators of increased vascular permeability. Plasma and cell-derived products generate potent vasoactive mediators.

Leukocytes, Especially Neutrophils, Accumulate in Affected Tissues

Swift recruitment requires a response orchestrated by chemoattractants that induce directed cell migration; lipid mediators, eicosanoids, serum proteins (complement products C3a, C5a, and cytokines), and chemokines function sequentially for optimal responses (Fig. 2-12). Diverse inflammatory stimuli, including proinflammatory cytokines, bacterial endotoxins, and viral proteins, stimulate endothelial cells, causing loss of barrier function and recruiting leukocytes. Leukocytes adhere to activated endothelium and are themselves activated in the process. They then flatten and migrate from the vascular space, through the vessel wall and into surrounding tissue. Once in extravascular tissues, PMNs ingest foreign material, microbes, and debris (Fig. 2-13).

Leukocyte Recruitment

Leukocytes (mainly neutrophils) exit the vascular lumen into the extravascular space in three phases: (1) *margination and rolling*; (2) *adhesion* and transmigration between endothelial cells; and (3) *migration* in interstitial tissues toward a chemotactic stimulus (Figs. 2-14 and 2-15). Rolling, adhesion, and transmigration begin when complementary adhesion

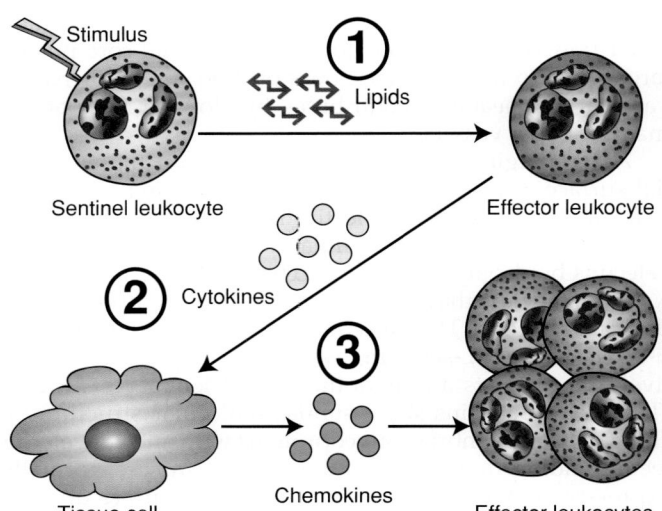

FIGURE 2-12. A schema of orchestrated initiation of inflammatory responses. *1*. Lipid mediators (eicosanoids) are released from activated cells, resulting in early recruitment of inflammatory cells from bone marrow into the vascular system. *2*. Proinflammatory cytokines activate resident tissue cells, which in turn (*3*) release chemokines to amplify inflammatory cell recruitment.

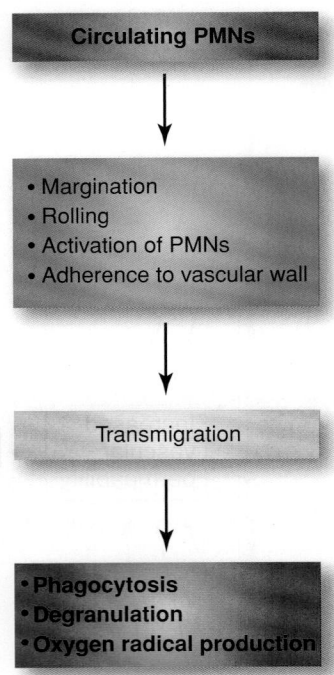

FIGURE 2-13. Leukocyte recruitment and activation. *PMNs* = poly-morphonuclear neutrophils.

molecules on leukocytes and endothelial surfaces bind each other (Fig. 2-16). Chemical mediators (chemoattractants and certain cytokines) affect these processes by modulating surface expression or avidity of these adhesion molecules.

Margination and Rolling

In *margination* leukocytes accumulate at the periphery of vessels. This occurs through a combination of flow changes occurring at the level of capillaries to postcapillary venules: faster flow of erythrocytes down vessels' axial core pushes larger cells to the periphery. Loss of fluid due to increased vascular permeability contributes by slowing flow at the margins of the vessels.

After margination, leukocytes tumble on the endothelial surface, transiently sticking along the way; this *rolling* is facilitated by **selectins**, lectin-like molecules (hence the name) that express extracellular sugar-binding domains. Selectins bind sialylated oligosaccharides (e.g., sialyl-Lewis X on leukocytes) that decorate mucin-like glycoproteins on their target cells. The selectin family includes **P-selectin, E-selectin**, and **L-selectin**, which are expressed respectively on platelets and endothelial and leukocyte surfaces (Table 2-1). Selectins share similar molecular structures: a chain of transmembrane glycoproteins with an extracellular lectin-binding domain. Endothelial selectins are normally expressed only at low levels or not at all, but are upregulated upon stimulation by specific mediators. This allows a degree of specificity of binding restricted to sites where there is ongoing injury. Thus, in nonactivated endothelial cells, P-selectin occurs mainly in intracellular **Weibel–Palade bodies**, but within minutes of exposure to mediators like histamine or thrombin, P-selectin redistributes to the cell surface. Some selectins (e.g., E-selectin) are also

transcriptionally upregulated by inflammatory mediators such as IL-1 or TNFα.

Adhesion and Transmigration

After selectin-mediated rolling, leukocytes stick firmly to endothelial surfaces (adhesion) and eventually crawl between endothelial cells (diapedesis) to traverse the basement membrane, into the extravascular space.

Leukocyte **integrins**—transmembrane heterodimeric glycoproteins—mediate firm adhesion to endothelial cells. These integrins contain different α and β chains, and normally appear on leukocyte surfaces in low-affinity forms. Their ligands are molecules of the immunoglobulin superfamily expressed on endothelial cells, including ICAM-1, ICAM-2, and VCAM-1 (Table 2-1). In their low-affinity state, integrins bind those ligands poorly. However, when chemokines produced in the area of injury bind to leukocyte G-protein–coupled receptors (GPCRs) they cause integrins to undergo a conformational change that allows high-affinity binding to endothelial adhesion molecules (Fig. 2-14).

Diapedesis

Leukocyte diapedesis occurs mostly in postcapillary venules, and, to a lesser degree, in pulmonary capillaries. After firm adhesion to endothelial surfaces, leukocytes squeeze between cells at intercellular junctions (although **transcytosis**, through endothelial cell cytoplasm, also occurs), then cross basement membranes by focally degrading them with secreted **matrix metalloproteinases (MMPs)**. CD31 (or, platelet endothelial cell adhesion molecule [PECAM]) is the major mediator of diapedesis, supported by other **junctional adhesion molecules (JAMs)**, including CD99 (Table 2-1, Fig. 2-17).

Chemotaxis and Activation

After exiting the blood, leukocytes migrate toward sites of injury along a chemical gradient (**chemotaxis**, Fig. 2-14). Both exogenous and endogenous substances can be chemotactic for leukocytes, including: (1) soluble bacterial products, particularly peptides with N-formyl-methionine termini; (2) components of the complement system, particularly C5a (see below); (3) products of the lipoxygenase pathway of AA metabolism, particularly **leukotriene B4 (LTB4)** (see below); and (4) cytokines, especially of the chemokine family (e.g., IL-8). In addition to stimulating locomotion, chemotactic factors activate leukocytes to: (1) induce degranulation and secretion of lysosomal enzymes; (2) generate an oxidative burst; (3) produce AA metabolites via DAG- and calcium-induced activation of phospholipase A2 (PLA2); and (4) modulate leukocyte adhesion molecules.

Neutrophils, monocytes, eosinophils and various types of lymphocytes use different—but overlapping—molecules for rolling and adhesion. The type of recruited leukocyte thus reflects the nature of the inciting stimulus and the age of the inflammatory site. In most forms of acute inflammation, neutrophils predominate for the first 6 to 24 hours, then are replaced by monocytes in the next 24 to 48 hours (Fig. 2-3). This pattern is best explained by the sequential expression of different adhesion molecules and chemotactic factors at different phases of an inflammatory response. In addition, neutrophils are rather short lived, undergoing apoptosis within 10 to 12 hours or so after exiting the blood stream, while monocytes survive substantially longer and may persist for extremely long periods as tissue macrophages.

ENDOTHELIAL CELLS

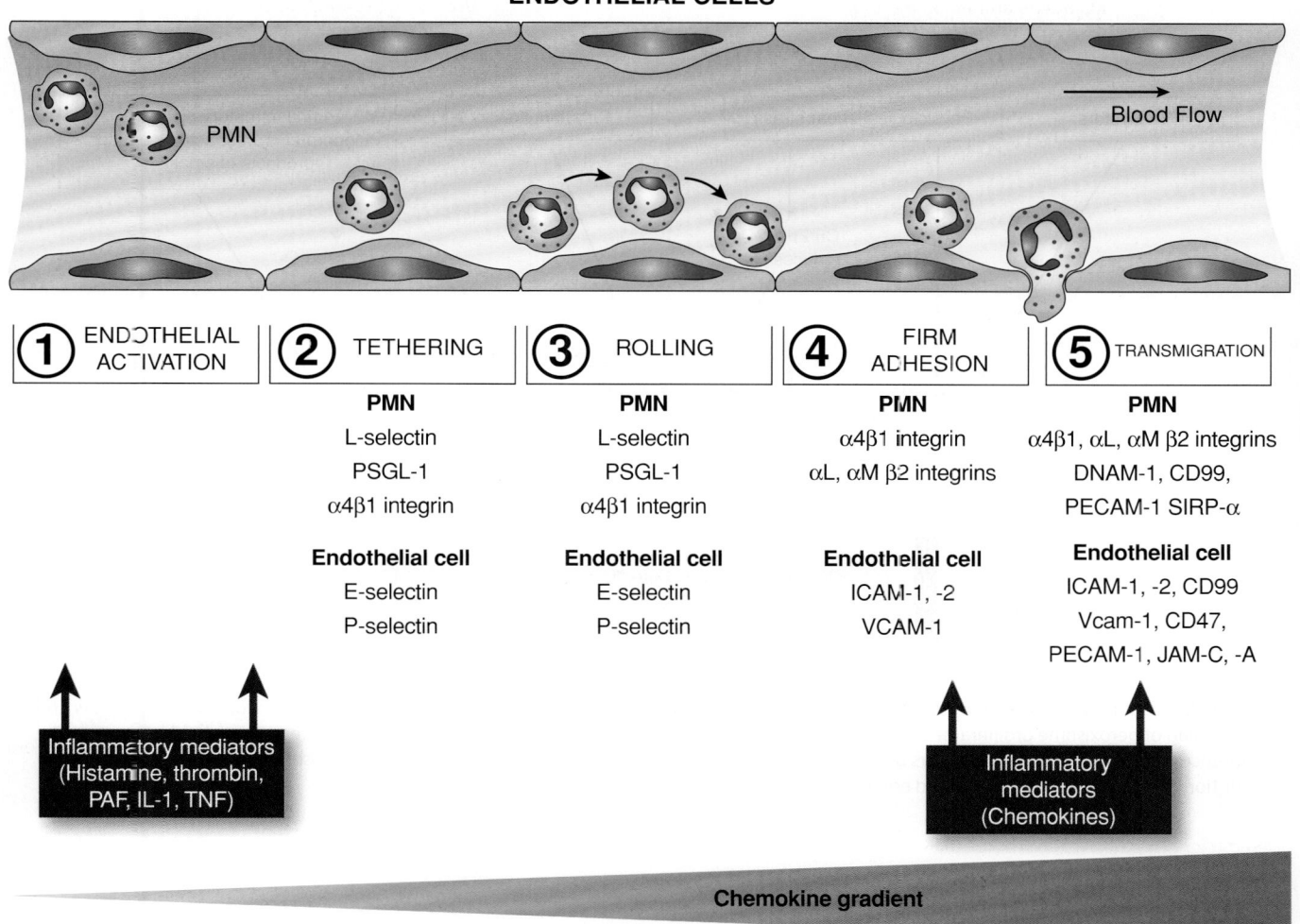

FIGURE 2-14. Neutrophil adhesion and extravasation. *1*. Inflammatory mediators activate endothelial cells to increase expression of adhesion molecules. Sialyl-Lewis X on neutrophil P-selectin glycoprotein-1 (PSGL-1) and E-selectin ligand (ESL-1) binds to P- and E-selectins to facilitate (*2*) tethering and (*3*) rolling of neutrophils. Increased integrins on activated neutrophils bind to intercellular adhesion molecule-1 (ICAM-1) on endothelial cells to form (*4*) a firm attachment. *5*. Endothelial cell attachments to one another are released and neutrophils then pass between separated cells to enter the tissue. *EC* = endothelial cell; *IL* = interleukin; *PAF* = platelet-activating factor; *PMN* = polymorphonuclear neutrophil; *TNF* = tumor necrosis factor.

Leukocyte Effector Functions Begin With Phagocytosis

Monocytes, tissue macrophages, dendritic cells, and neutrophils recognize, internalize, and digest foreign material, microorganisms, or cellular debris by **phagocytosis**. This term, first used over a century ago by Elie Metchnikoff, entails ingestion by eukaryotic cells of large (usually >0.5 μm) insoluble particles and microorganisms. The complex process involves a sequence of four distinct but interrelated steps.

Recognition and Attachment

Phagocytosis starts when specific receptors on phagocytic cell surfaces recognize their targets (Fig. 2-18). Microbes express **PAMPs**. *These are motifs unique to the microbes in question, and do not occur in the human body. They are important, indispensable structural or functional molecules and so are obligatory for microbial function.* The cells that mediate innate immunity (neutrophils, monocytes/macrophages) exploit this by binding the motifs with a standard array of **pattern recognition receptors (PRRs)**. Recognition and attachment of leukocytes to most microorganisms is also facilitated by serum **opsonins**, which bind specific molecules on microbial surfaces and facilitate their binding with specific opsonin receptors on leukocytes. The most important opsonins are immunoglobulin G (IgG) (specifically its Fc region; see **Chapter 4**), C3b fragment of complement and plasma carbohydrate-binding lectins that bind microbial cell wall sugar groups. IgG binding a target often triggers activation of the complement cascade, which causes C3b fragments to deposit on the targeted particle. However, many stimuli (e.g., microbial surfaces) can directly activate complement independently of IgG. Leukocyte receptors that mediate these interactions include the Fc receptor (FcR) for IgG, complement receptors 1, 2, and 3 (CR 1, 2, and 3) for complement fragments and specific receptors for circulating lectin-like molecules.

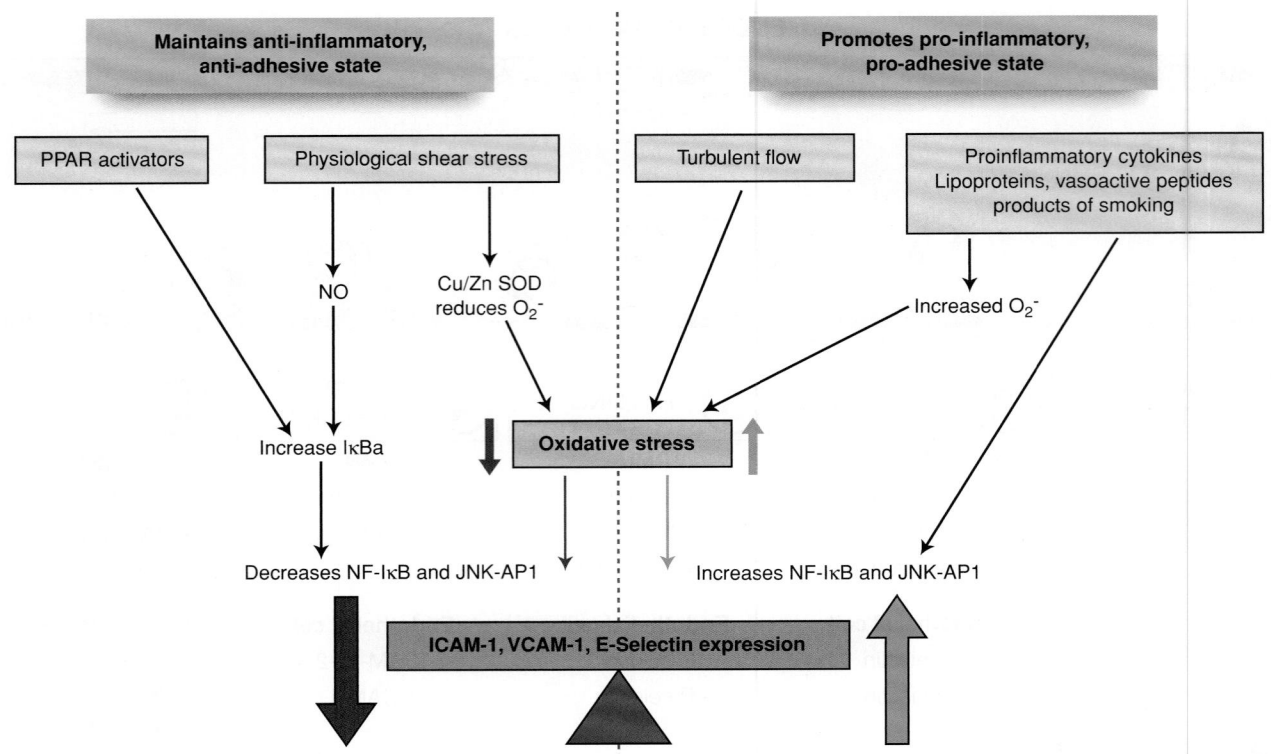

FIGURE 2-15. Balance of pro- and antiadhesive forces in vascular endothelial cells. Under physiologic conditions of vascular flow and expression of peroxisome proliferator-activated receptors (PPARs), oxidative stress and adhesion molecule expression are held in check. In the presence of proinflammatory mediators and turbulent flow or oscillatory shear stress, oxidative stress increases, followed by increased transcription of proinflammatory genes and enhanced expression of adhesion molecules.

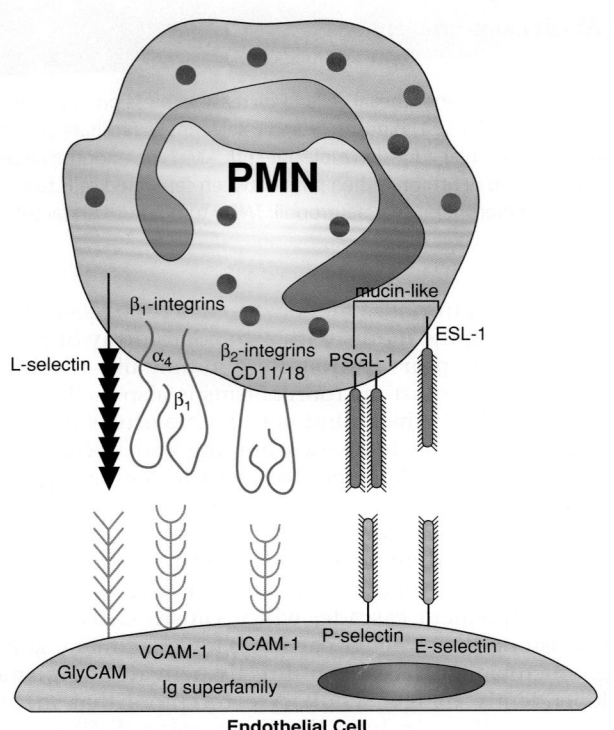

FIGURE 2-16. Leukocyte and endothelial cell adhesion molecules.
GlyCAM = glycan-bearing cell adhesion molecule; *ICAM-1* = intercellular adhesion molecule-1; *VCAM* = vascular cell adhesion molecule.

TABLE 2-1
MAJOR ADHESION MOLECULE PAIRS IN ACUTE INFLAMMATION

Endothelial Molecule	Leukocyte Molecule	Function
P-selectin	Sialyl-Lewis–X modified proteins	Rolling (neutrophils, monocytes, lymphocytes)
GlyCAM-1	L-selectin	Rolling (neutrophils, monocytes)
E-selectin	Sialyl-Lewis–X modified proteins	Rolling (neutrophils, monocytes, T lymphocytes)
VCAM-1	VLA-4 integrin	Adhesion (eosinophils, monocytes, lymphocytes)
ICAM-1	CD11/CD18 integrins (LFA-1, Mac-1)	Adhesion, arrest, transmigration (neutrophils, monocytes, lymphocytes)
CD31 (PECAM-1)	CD31 (PECAM-1)	Arrest, transmigration (neutrophils, monocytes, lymphocytes)

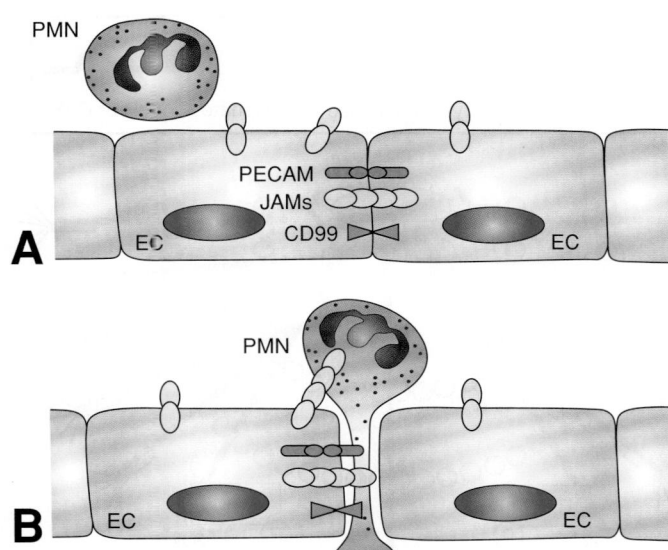

FIGURE 2-17. Endothelial cell junctional molecules participate in leukocyte recruitment. A. Junctional molecules contribute to cell–cell adhesion and maintenance of endothelial barrier function. **B.** These same molecules regulate paracellular transmigration of leukocytes. *PMN* = polymorphonuclear neutrophil; *EC* = endothelial cell; *PECAM* = platelet endothelial cell adhesion molecule, CD31; *JAMs* = junctional adhesion molecules.

Many devious pathogens have evolved ways to evade phagocytosis by leukocytes. Polysaccharide capsules, protein A, protein M, or peptidoglycans around bacteria can prevent complement deposition or antigen recognition and receptor binding.

Signaling

Clumping of opsonins at bacterial surfaces causes phagocyte plasma membrane Fcγ receptors to cluster. Subsequent phosphorylation of the cytosolic (γ) domain of **immunoreceptor tyrosine-based activation motifs (ITAMs)** triggers intracellular signaling via tyrosine kinases that associate with the Fcγ receptor (Fig. 2-19).

Internalization and Engulfment

Then, pseudopods from the cell extend around the object, eventually forming a phagocytic vacuole. IgG binding to FcR activates cellular actin assembly directly under the phagocytosed target, with polymerized actin filaments pushing the plasma membrane forward. The plasma membrane then remodels to increase surface area and surround the foreign material. The resulting phagocytic cup engulfs the foreign agent. The membrane then "zippers" to enclose it in a vacuole—the phagosome (Fig. 2-18).

Digestion

The phagosome containing the foreign material fuses with cytoplasmic lysosomes to form a **phagolysosome**, into which lysosomal enzymes are released. Acid pH in the phagolysosome activates these hydrolytic enzymes, which then degrade the phagocytosed material. Ever sneaky, some microorganisms have evolved mechanisms to survive, by preventing lysosomal degranulation or inhibiting neutrophil enzymes.

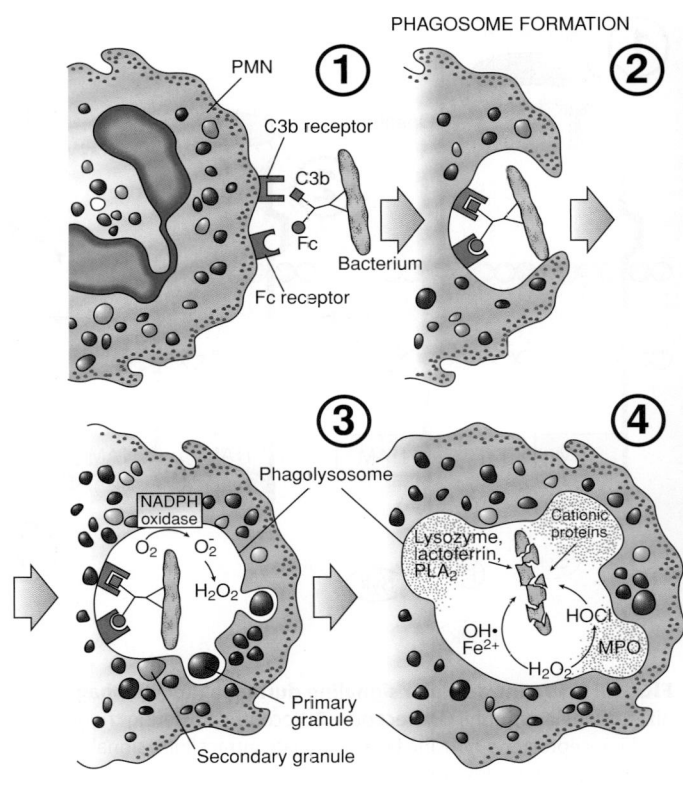

- Degranulation and NADPH oxidase activation
- Bacterial killing and digestion

FIGURE 2-18. Mechanisms of neutrophil bacterial phagocytosis and cell killing. 1. Opsonins such as C3b coat the surface of microbes, allowing recognition by the neutrophil C3b receptor. **2.** Receptor clustering triggers intracellular signaling and actin assembly within the neutrophil. Pseudopods form around the microbe to enclose it within a phagosome. **3.** Lysosomal granules fuse with the phagosome to form a phagolysosome, into which the lysosomal enzymes and oxygen radicals are released to (**4**) kill and degrade the microbe. Fe^{2+} = ferrous iron; $HOCl$ = hypochlorous acid; MPO = myeloperoxidase; PLA_2 = phospholipase A_2; PMN = polymorphonuclear neutrophil.

ROS Are Neutrophils' Main Microbe Killers

Phagocytosis stimulates an **oxidative burst**, with a sudden increase in oxygen consumption, glycogen catabolism (glycogenolysis), increased glucose oxidation and production of reactive oxygen metabolites (ROS) (Fig. 2-18; see **Chapter 1**). These include, but are not limited to:

- *Superoxide anion (O_2^-)*: In neutrophil cell membranes, phagocytosis activates an **NADPH oxidase**, a multicomponent electron transport complex that reduces molecular oxygen to O_2^-. Prior exposure of cells to a chemotactic stimulus or bacterial lipopolysaccharide (LPS) enhances NADPH oxidase activation. NADPH oxidase increases oxygen consumption and stimulates the hexose monophosphate shunt. Together, these cell responses are known as the **respiratory burst**.
- *Hydrogen peroxide (H_2O_2)*: O_2^- is rapidly converted to H_2O_2 at the cell surface and in phagolysosomes, either spontaneously or superoxide dismutase (SOD). Amounts of hydrogen peroxide produced are generally insufficient to kill most

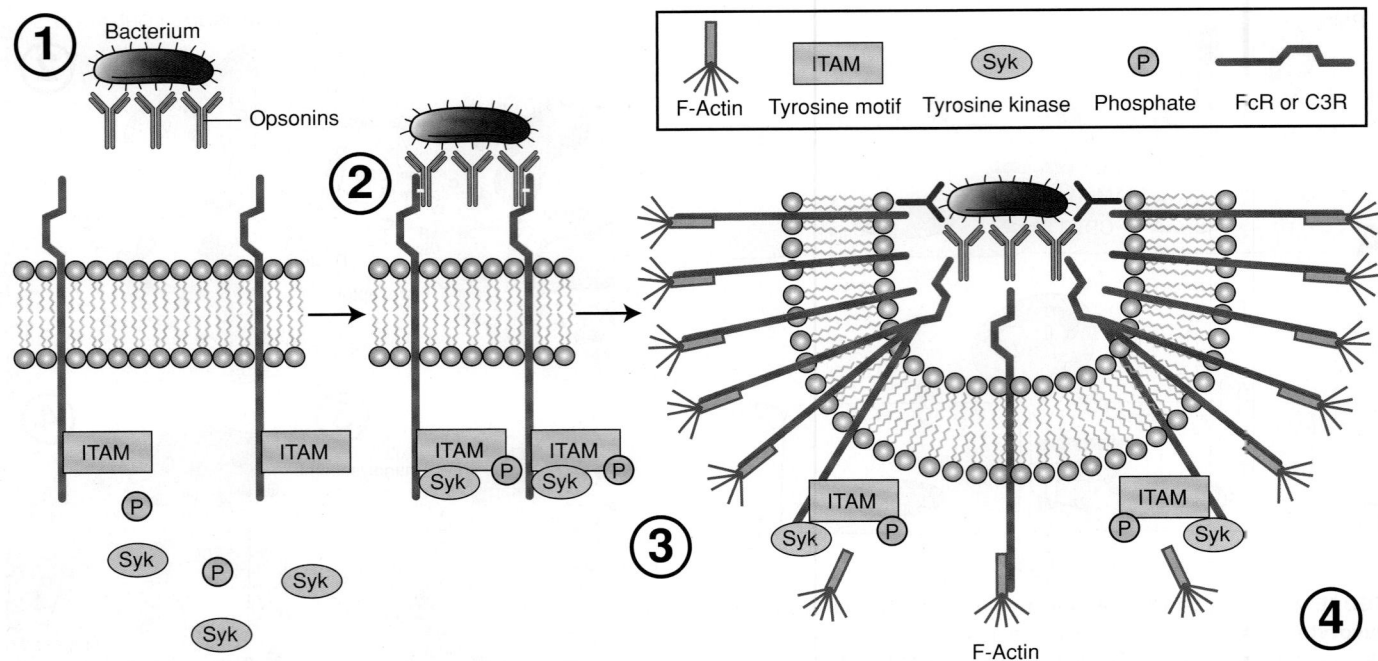

FIGURE 2-19. Intracellular signaling during leukocyte phagocytosis. 1. Opsonins coating the surface of microbes or foreign material are recognized by the neutrophil C3b receptor. **2**. Receptor clustering triggers (**3**) phosphorylation of immunoreceptor tyrosine-based activation motifs (ITAMs) on the receptor, and tyrosine kinases initiate intracellular signaling. **4**. Polymerized actin filament aggregates beneath the plasma membrane to form a pseudopod to enclose the foreign agent.

bacteria effectively (although superoxide and hydroxyl radicals may be sufficient to do so). However, H_2O_2 is stable and is a source for generating additional reactive oxidants.

- *Hypochlorous acid (HOCl•):* Neutrophil lysosomes (called azurophilic granules) contain the enzyme **myeloperoxidase (MPO)**. In the presence of a halide anion such as Cl^-, MPO converts H_2O_2 to HOCl• (hypochlorous radical). HOCl• is a powerful oxidant and antimicrobial agent (NaOCl is the active ingredient in chlorine bleach) that kills bacteria by halogenation, or by protein and lipid peroxidation. It also helps activate neutrophil-derived collagenase and gelatinase, both of which are secreted as latent enzymes, and inactivates α_1-antitrypsin.
- *Hydroxyl radical (OH•):* Reduction of H_2O_2 via the Haber–Weiss reaction forms the highly reactive OH• radical. This occurs slowly at physiologic pH, but if ferrous iron (Fe^{2+}) is present, the Fenton reaction rapidly converts H_2O_2 to OH•, which is a powerful bactericidal agent. Further reduction of OH• yields H_2O (see **Chapter 1**).
- *Nitric oxide (NO•):* Phagocytes and endothelial cells produce NO• and its derivatives, which have many physiologic and nonphysiologic effects. NO• and other free radicals interact with one another to balance their cytotoxic and cytoprotective effects. NO• reacts with oxygen radicals to form toxic molecules such as peroxynitrite and S-nitrosothiols, or it can scavenge O_2^-, thus reducing the amount of toxic radicals.

Besides neutrophils, monocytes, macrophages, and eosinophils also make oxygen radicals, depending on their state of activation and the stimulus to which they are exposed. ROS made by these cells contributes to their bactericidal and fungicidal activity, and to their ability to kill certain parasites. The importance of oxygen-dependent bacterial killing is

exemplified in chronic granulomatous disease of childhood, a hereditary deficiency of NADPH oxidase. Affected patients fail to produce O_2^- and H_2O_2 during phagocytosis, and so are prone to recurrent infections, especially with gram-positive cocci. Patients with a related genetic deficiency in MPO cannot make HOCl• and are excessively susceptible to *Candida* fungal infections (Table 2-2).

TABLE 2-2	
CONGENITAL DISEASES OF DEFECTIVE PHAGOCYTIC CELL FUNCTION	
Disease	**Defect**
Leukocyte adhesion deficiency (LAD)	LAD-1 (defective β_2-integrin expression or function [CD11/CD18])
	LAD-2 (defective fucosylation, selectin binding)
Hyper-IgE-recurrent infection (Job) syndrome	Poor chemotaxis
Chediak–Higashi syndrome	Defective lysosomal granules, poor chemotaxis
Neutrophil-specific granule deficiency	Absent neutrophil granules
Chronic granulomatous disease	Deficient NADPH oxidase, with absent H_2O_2 production
Myeloperoxidase deficiency	Deficient HOCl production

H_2O_2 = hydrogen peroxide; HOCl = hypochlorous acid; Ig = immunoglobulin; NADPH = nicotinamide adenine dinucleotide phosphate.

NADPH oxidase is only active after its cytosolic subunit translocates to the phagolysosome membrane; thus, the reactive end products are generated only within that compartment. After the oxidative burst, H_2O_2 is eventually broken down to water and O_2 by catalase, and the other ROS are also degraded. **Lysosomal acid hydrolases** then digest the dead microorganisms.

Leukocytes Can Also Kill Microorganisms by Nonoxidative Mechanisms

Even without an oxidative burst, other constituents of the leukocyte granules can kill bacteria and other infectious agents, predominantly via bactericidal proteins in cytoplasmic granules, for example, lysosomal acid hydrolases and specialized noncatalytic proteins unique to inflammatory cells.

- *Lysosomal hydrolases:* Primary and secondary PMN granules and lysosomes of mononuclear phagocytes contain hydrolases—sulfatases, phosphatases, and other enzymes—that can digest polysaccharides and DNA.
- *Bactericidal/permeability-increasing protein (BPI):* This cationic protein in PMN primary granules can kill many gram-negative bacteria but is not toxic to gram-positive bacteria or eukaryotic cells. BPI inserts into bacterial envelope outer membranes and increases their permeability. Activation of certain phospholipases and enzymes then degrades bacterial peptidylglycans.
- *Defensins:* Primary granules of PMNs and lysosomes of some mononuclear phagocytes contain these cationic proteins, which kill many gram-positive and gram-negative bacteria, fungi, and some enveloped viruses. Some also kill host cells. Defensins are chemotactic for phagocytes, immature dendritic cells, and lymphocytes and so help mobilize and amplify antimicrobial immunity.

- *Lactoferrin:* Lactoferrin is an iron-binding glycoprotein in neutrophil secondary granules and in most body secretory fluids. It chelates iron and so competes with bacteria for iron. It may help generate OH• for oxidative killing of bacteria.
- *Lysozyme:* This bactericidal enzyme is found in many tissues and body fluids, in primary and secondary granules of PMNs and in lysosomes of mononuclear phagocytes. Peptidoglycans of gram-positive bacterial cell walls are sensitive to degradation by lysozyme; gram-negative bacteria are usually resistant to it.
- *Eosinophil bactericidal proteins:* Eosinophils have several granule-bound cationic proteins, the most important of which are MBP and eosinophilic cationic protein. Both are potent killers of many parasites, though not bacteria. MBP accounts for half of the total protein of eosinophil granules.

Molecular Mediators of Acute Inflammation

PLASMA-DERIVED MEDIATORS

Cell- and plasma-derived mediators work in concert to activate cells by binding specific receptors, activating cells, recruiting cells to sites of injury, and stimulating release of additional soluble mediators (Fig. 2-20). These mediators are inherently short lived or are inhibited by intrinsic

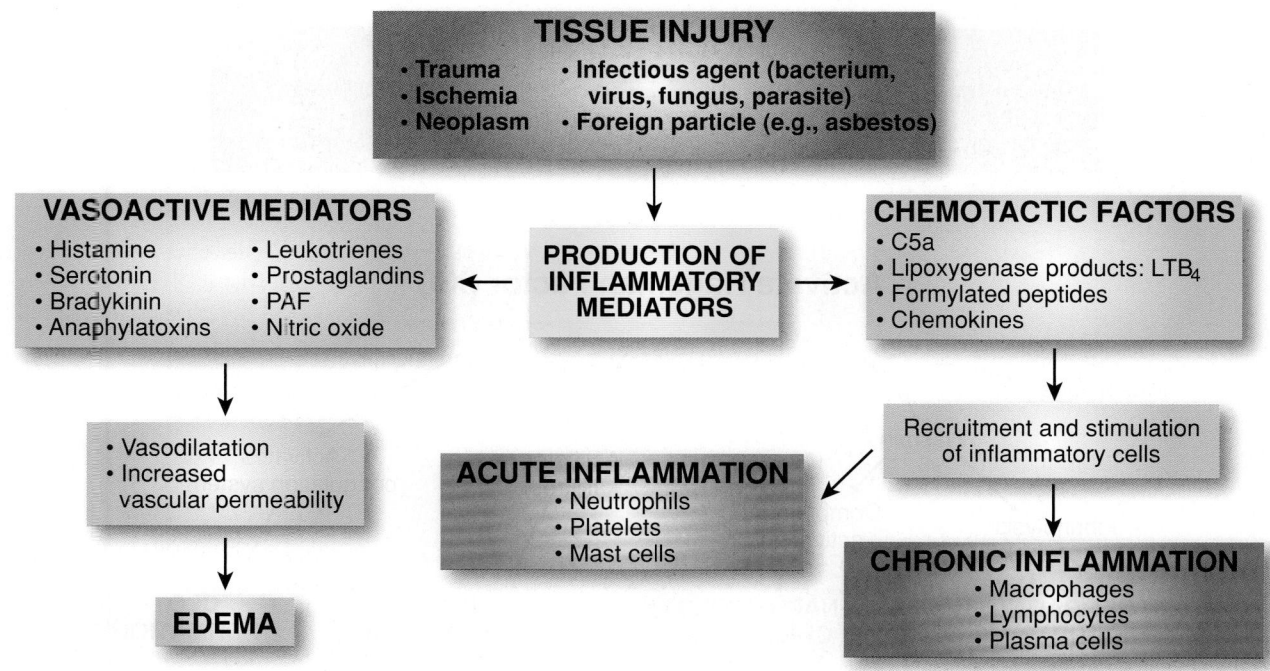

FIGURE 2-20. Mediators of the inflammatory response. Tissue injury stimulates the production of inflammatory mediators in plasma and released into the circulation. Additional factors are generated by tissue cells and inflammatory cells. These vasoactive and chemotactic mediators promote edema and recruit inflammatory cells to the site of injury. *PMNs* = polymorphonuclear leukocytes.

mechanisms, effectively turning off the response and allowing the process to resolve. Thus, these are important "on" and "off" control mechanisms of inflammation. While specific mediator types will be discussed below, there are several important conceptual principles governing their function:

- *Mediators may be produced locally by cells at the site of inflammation or circulate in the plasma (typically synthesized by the liver).* Plasma-derived mediators include the complement, kinin and coagulation cascades; these circulate as inactive precursors that must undergo proteolytic cleavage to become biologically active. Cell-derived mediators are normally stored in intracellular granules that are secreted upon activation (e.g., histamine in mast cells), or are synthesized *de novo* in response to a stimulus (e.g., prostaglandins, leukotrienes).
- *Most mediators act by binding to specific receptors on target cells.* However, some have direct enzymatic and/or toxic activities (e.g., lysosomal proteases or ROS).
- *Mediators can stimulate target cells to release secondary effector molecules.* These secondary mediators may have activities similar to their initial effector molecules, amplifying a particular response. Or they may oppose those initial stimulators, as a counter-regulatory mechanism.
- *Mediators may have only one, a few or many targets,* causing widely differing outcomes, depending on which cell type they affect.
- *Mediator function is generally tightly regulated.* Most mediators are potent and can potentially be harmful. Fortunately, most mediators quickly decay once activated and released from the cell (e.g., **AA** metabolites), are inactivated by enzymes (e.g., kininase inactivates bradykinin), are eliminated (e.g., antioxidants scavenge ROS), or are inhibited (complement inhibitory proteins).

Plasma-Derived Inflammatory Mediators Belong to Three Major Systems: Coagulation, Kinins, and Complement

Plasma contains the elements of these three major enzyme cascades, each composed of a series of proteases. Sequential activation of proteases results in release of important chemical mediators (Fig. 2-21). The coagulation cascade is discussed in **Chapters 16 and 26**; the kinin and complement systems are presented here.

All three cascades are mechanistically linked by initial activation of Hageman factor (Factor XII of the coagulation cascade). This protein is synthesized by the liver and circulates in an inactive form until it encounters collagen, basement membrane, or activated platelets (as at a site of endothelial injury). Assisted by a high–molecular-weight kininogen (HMWK) cofactor, factor XII then changes conformation (becoming activated factor XIIa), exposing an active serine center that can cleave a number of protein substrates, and triggers activation of other plasma proteases, including:

- *Conversion of plasminogen to plasmin:* Plasmin generated by activated Hageman factor induces clot dissolution (fibrinolysis). Products of fibrin degradation (fibrin-split products) increase vascular permeability in the skin and lung. Plasmin also cleaves complement components, to generate biologically active products, including anaphylatoxins, C3a, and C5a.
- *Conversion of prekallikrein to kallikrein:* Plasma kallikrein, also generated by activated factor XII, cleaves HMWK to several vasoactive low–molecular weight peptides, collectively called kinins.
- *Activation of the alternative complement pathway.*
- *Activation of the coagulation system* (see **Chapters 16, 26**).

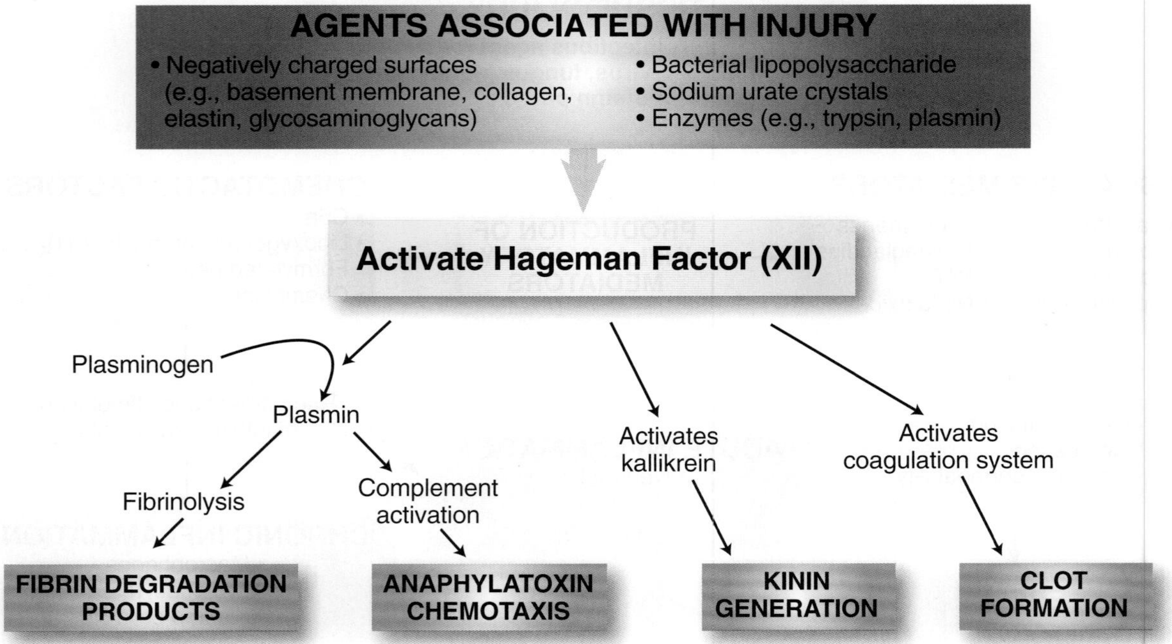

FIGURE 2-21. Hageman factor activation and inflammatory mediator production. Hageman factor activation is a key event leading to conversion of plasminogen to plasmin, resulting in generation of fibrin split products and active complement products. Activation of kallikrein produces kinins and activation of the coagulation system results in clot formation.

Kinins Amplify Inflammatory Responses

Kinins are potent inflammatory agents formed in plasma and tissue when kallikrein proteases cleave kininogens, specific plasma glycoproteins. Factor XIIa causes release of **bradykinin** from its circulating precursor, HMWK. Bradykinin and related peptides regulate multiple physiologic processes, including blood pressure, smooth muscle contraction and relaxation, plasma extravasation, cell migration, inflammatory cell activation and inflammatory-mediated pain responses. The immediate effects of kinins are mediated by B1 and B2 receptors. The former are induced by inflammatory mediators and selectively activated by bradykinin metabolites. B2 receptors are expressed constitutively and widely. Kinins act quickly and then are rapidly inactivated by kininases.

Perhaps the most significant function of kinins is that they amplify inflammatory responses by stimulating local tissue cells and inflammatory cells to generate additional mediators, such as prostanoids, cytokines (e.g., TNFα and interleukins), NO, and tachykinins.

Three Separate Pathways Can Activate Complement to Form the Membrane Attack Complex

The complement system is a group of proteins found in plasma and on cell surfaces. Its main function is defense against infections. First identified as a heat-labile serum factor that kills bacteria and "complements" antibodies, there are over 30 complement proteins, including plasma enzymes, regulatory proteins, and cell lysis proteins. They are mainly made in the liver and are activated in sequence. Their physiologic activities include: (1) defense against pyogenic bacterial infection by opsonization, chemotaxis, activating leukocytes, and lysing bacteria and cells; (2) bridging innate and adaptive immunity to defend against microbial agents by augmenting antibody responses and enhancing immune memory; and (3) eliminating immune products and products of inflammatory injury by removing immune complexes and apoptotic cells.

Some complement components, **anaphylatoxins**, are vasoactive mediators. Others fix opsonins to cell surfaces. Still others lyse cells by generating a lytic **membrane attack complex** (MAC) made of C5b-9. Proteins that activate complement are themselves activated by three convergent routes: the classical, mannose-binding lectin (MBL), and alternative pathways.

The Classical Complement Pathway

Activators of the classical pathway include antigen–antibody (Ag–Ab) complexes, products of bacteria and viruses, proteases, urate crystals, apoptotic cells and polyanions (polynucleotides). Complement proteins C1 through C9 are numbered in their historical order of discovery. Ag–Ab complexes activate C1, triggering a cascade that leads to formation of the MAC (Fig. 2-22):

1. *Antibodies bound to antigens on bacterial cell surfaces bind the C1 complex,* which contains C1q and two molecules each of C1r and C1s. The complexed antibodies activate C1q, which in turn activates C1r and C1s.
2. *C1s cleaves C4, which binds the bacterial surface,* then cleaves C2. Resulting split molecules form the C4b2a enzyme complex, also called **C3 convertase**, which binds the bacterial surface covalently, anchoring the complement

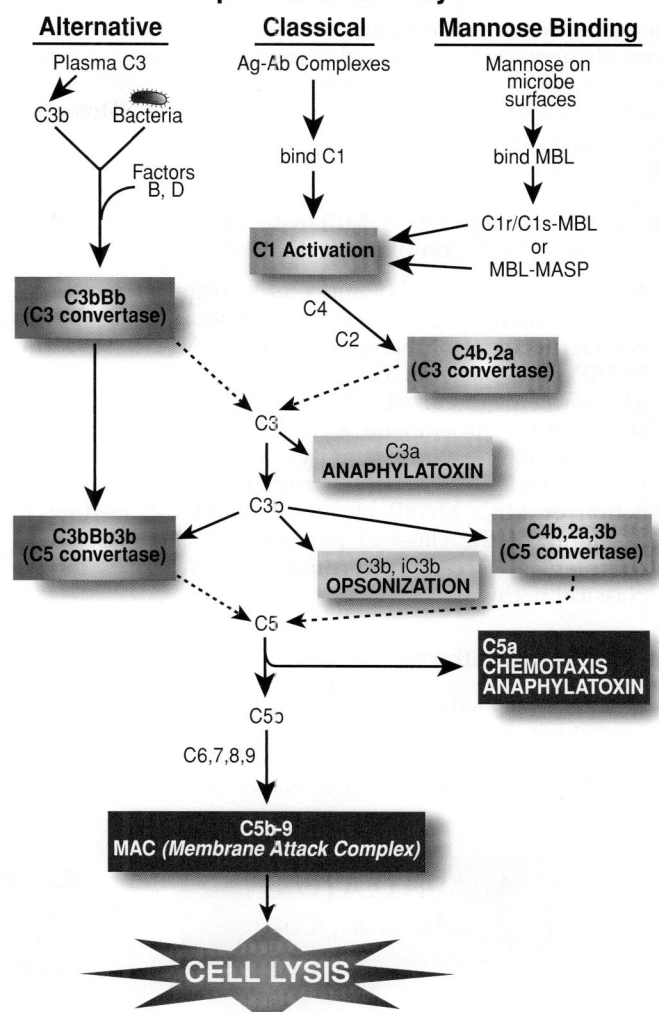

Complement Pathways

FIGURE 2-22. Complement activation. The alternative, classical, and mannose-binding pathways lead to generation of the complement cascade of inflammatory mediators and to cell lysis by the membrane attack complex (MAC). *MBL* = mannose-binding lectin; *MBL-MASP* = MBL-associated serine protease.

system at specific tissue sites. If a covalent bond is not formed, the complex is inactivated, thus aborting the cascade in normal host cells or tissues.
3. *C3 convertase cleaves C3 into C3a and C3b. This is a critical step.* C3a is released as an anaphylatoxin. C3b reacts with cell proteins to localize, or "fix," on the cell surface. C3b and its degradation products, especially iC3b, on the surface of pathogens enhance phagocytosis. This process of coating a pathogen with a molecule that enhances phagocytosis is opsonization; the molecule that does this is an **opsonin**.
4. *The complex of C4b, C2a, and C3b (called C5 convertase) cleaves C5 into C5a and C5b.* C5a also is an anaphylatoxin, and C5b acts as the nidus for subsequent sequential binding of C6, C7, and C8 to form the MAC.
5. *The MAC assembles on target cells.* The MAC directly inserts into plasma membranes as C7 binds the lipid bilayer via hydrophobic interactions. The result is a cylindrical transmembrane channel through the plasma membrane, leading to cell lysis.

The Mannose-Binding Pathway

The mannose- or lectin-binding complement pathway shares some elements with the classical pathway. It begins when microbes with terminal mannose groups bind **MBL**, in the family of calcium-dependent lectins (**collectins**). This multifunctional acute phase protein resembles IgM in binding many oligosaccharides, IgG in recognizing phagocytic receptors and C1q in interacting with C1r–C1s. It also interacts with a serine protease, MBL-associated serine protease (MASP), to activate complement (Fig. 2-22):

1. MBL interacts with C1r and C1s to trigger C1 esterase activity. Alternatively, and preferentially, MBL complexes with a precursor of the serine protease, MASP. MBL and MASP bind bacterial cell surface mannose groups on glycoproteins or carbohydrates. Once MBL binds a substrate, MASP proenzyme is cleaved into two chains and expresses a C1-esterase activity.
2. C1-esterase activity, either from C1r/C1s–MBL interaction or MBL–MASP, cleaves C4 and C2, leading to assembly of the classical pathway C3 convertase. The complement cascade then continues as described for the classical pathway.

The Alternative Pathway

This pathway is activated by products of microorganisms, like endotoxin (from bacterial surfaces), zymosan (yeast cell walls), polysaccharides, cobra venom factor, viruses, tumor cells and foreign materials. Alternative pathway members

are "factors," followed by a letter. Activation of this pathway proceeds as follows (Fig. 2-22):

1. A small amount of C3 in plasma cleaves to C3a and C3b. This C3b binds covalently proteins and carbohydrates on microbial cell surfaces. It binds factors B and D to form alternative pathway C3 convertase, C3bBb, which is stabilized by properdin.
2. C3 convertase generates more C3b and C3a. Binding of a second C3b molecule to C3 convertase converts it to a C5 convertase, C3bBb3b.
3. As in the classical pathway, cleavage of C5 by C5 convertase generates C5b and C5a and leads to assembly of the MAC.

Complement Components Have Diverse Proinflammatory Activities

The endpoint of complement activation is MAC formation and cell lysis. However, in addition to catalyzing the next step in the cascade, cleavage products generated at each step play supporting roles as key inflammatory mediators (Fig. 2-23):

- *Anaphylatoxins (C3a, C4a, C5a):* These proinflammatory molecules mediate smooth muscle contraction and increase vascular permeability.
- *Opsonins (C3b, iC3b):* In bacterial opsonization, a specific molecule (e.g., IgG or C3b) binds the surface of a bacterium. The process enhances phagocytosis by allowing receptors on phagocyte cell membranes (e.g., FcR or C3b

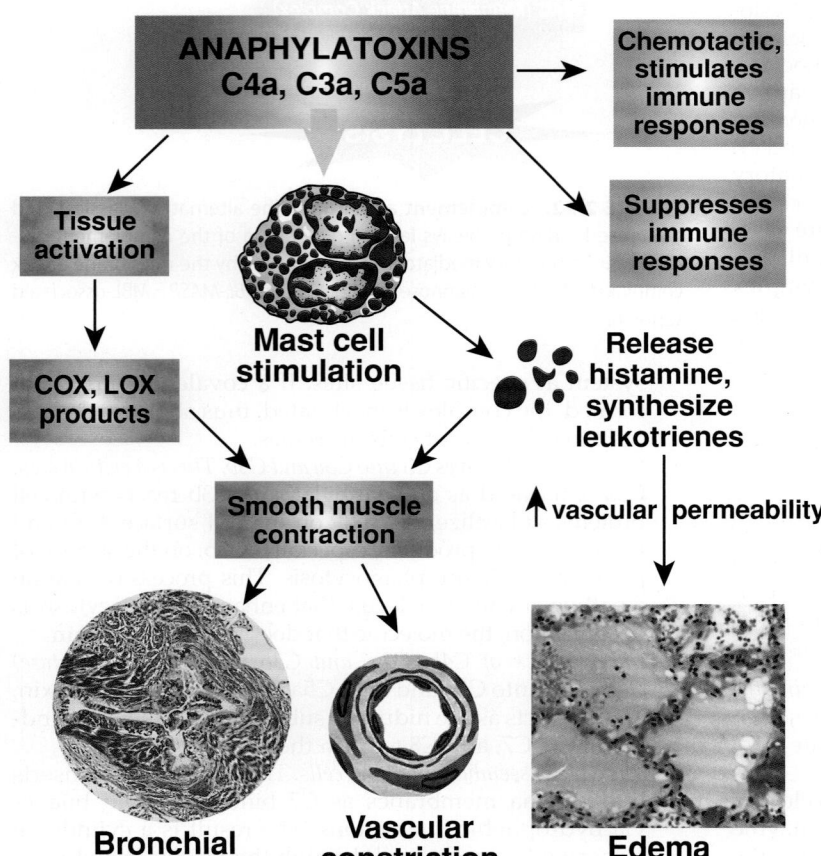

FIGURE 2-23. Biologic activity of the anaphylatoxins. Complement activation products, generated during activation of the complement cascade, regulate vascular permeability, cell recruitment, and smooth muscle contraction.

receptor) to recognize and bind the opsonized bacterium. Viruses, parasites, and transformed cells also activate complement similarly, which leads to their inactivation or death.

- *Proinflammatory molecules (MAC, C5a):* These chemotactic factors also activate leukocytes and tissue cells to generate oxidants and cytokines, and induce mast cell and basophil degranulation.
- *Lysis (MAC):* C5b binds C6 and C7, and subsequently C8 to the target cell; C9 polymerization is catalyzed to lyse the cell membrane.

Regulating the Complement System

Proteins in serum and on cell surfaces tightly regulate complement activation, to protect the host from indiscriminate injury. Four major mechanisms mediate this effect:

- *Spontaneous decay:* C4b2a and C3bBb and their cleavage products, C3b and C4b, decrease by decay.
- *Proteolytic inactivation:* Plasma inhibitors include **factor I** (which inhibits C3b and C4b) and serum **carboxypeptidase N (SCPN)**. SCPN removes a carboxyl terminal arginine from anaphylatoxins C4a, C3a, and C5a, thereby markedly decreasing their biologic activities.
- *Binding active components:* C1 esterase inhibitor (C1 INA) binds C1r and C1s to form an irreversibly inactive complex. Other binding proteins in the plasma include factor H– and C4b-binding protein. These complex with C3b and C4b, respectively, increasing their susceptibility to proteolytic cleavage by factor I.
- *Cell membrane–associated molecules:* **Decay-accelerating factor (DAF)** and **protectin (CD59, membrane cofactor protein)** are cell membrane—bound proteins. DAF breaks down alternative pathway C3 convertase; CD59 binds membrane-associated C4b and C3b, promotes inactivation by factor I, and prevents MAC formation.

Complement Dysfunction May Cause Tissue Injury and Disease

When mechanisms regulating this equilibrium malfunction, or are lacking because of mutation, resulting imbalances in complement activity can cause tissue injury. Uncontrolled systemic complement activation may occur in sepsis (see **Chapter 19**), playing a central role in the development of septic shock. Clinical situations in which complement dysfunction plays a pathogenic role include:

- *Immune complex-mediated disease.* Immune (Ag–Ab) complexes form on bacterial surfaces and associate with C1q, activating the classical pathway. Complement then promotes physiologic clearance of circulating immune complexes. However, if these complexes are made continuously and in excess (e.g., in chronic immune responses), relentless activation consumes and depletes complement. Complement inefficiency, whether due to complement depletion, deficient complement binding or defects in complement activation, results in immune deposition and inflammation, which in turn may manifest as autoimmunity.
- *Infectious Disease.* Complement is a key defense against infection. If the system functions poorly, the person is overly susceptible to infection. Defects in antibody production, complement proteins or phagocyte function

increase susceptibility to pyogenic infections with organisms such as *Haemophilus influenzae* and pneumococcus, while deficiencies in MAC formation predispose to infections with meningococci, and deficiency of complement MBL may result in recurrent infections in young children. Interestingly, many pathogens have evolved mechanisms to evade complement. Thick capsules protect some bacteria from complement-mediated lysis, and bacterial enzymes can inhibit the effects of complement components, especially C5a. Bacteria can also increase catabolism of components, such as C3b, thus reducing formation of C3 convertase. Viruses, on the other hand, may use cell-bound components and receptors to facilitate their infectivity. *Mycobacterium tuberculosis*, Epstein–Barr virus, measles virus, picornaviruses, HIV, and flaviviruses use complement components like a Trojan horse, to infect inflammatory or epithelial cells.

- *Inflammation and Necrosis.* Complement amplifies inflammatory responses. Anaphylatoxins C5a and C3a activate leukocytes, and C5a and MAC stimulate endothelial cells, thus generating excess ROS and cytokines that injure tissues (see **Chapter 1**). Nonviable or damaged tissues cannot regulate complement normally.
- *Complement Deficiencies.* The importance of an intact and appropriately regulated complement system is underscored by the consequences of acquired or congenital deficiencies of specific complement components or regulatory proteins (Table 2-3).

The most common congenital defect is C2 deficiency, inherited as an autosomal codominant trait. Acquired deficiencies of early complement components occur in patients with some autoimmune diseases, especially those associated with circulating immune complexes. These include certain forms of membranous glomerulonephritis and systemic lupus erythematosus (SLE). Deficiencies in early components of complement (e.g., C1q, C1r, C1s, C4) are strongly associated with susceptibility to SLE. Patients lacking the middle (C3, C5) components are prone to recurrent pyogenic infections, membranoproliferative glomerulonephritis, and rashes. Those who lack terminal complement components (C6, C7, C8) are vulnerable to *Neisseria* infections.

TABLE 2-3

HEREDITARY COMPLEMENT DEFICIENCIES

Complement Deficiency	Clinical Association
C3b, iC3b, C5, MBL	Pyogenic bacterial infections Membranoproliferative glomerulonephritis
C3, properdin, MAC proteins	Neisserial infection
C1 inhibitor	Hereditary angioedema
CD59	Hemolysis, thrombosis
C1q, C1r and C1s, C4, C2	Systemic lupus erythematosus
Factor H and factor I	Hemolytic–uremic syndrome Membranoproliferative glomerulonephritis

MAC = membrane attack complex; MBL = mannose-binding lectin.

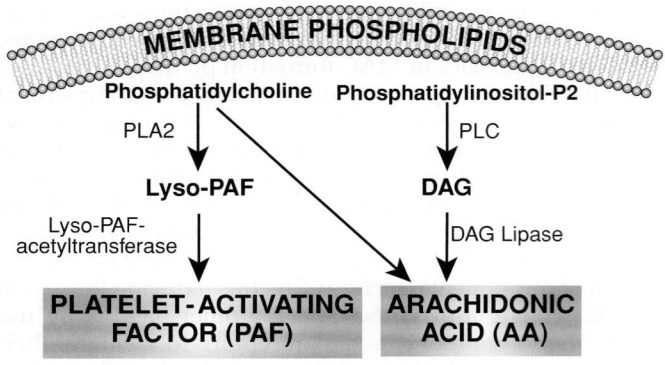

FIGURE 2-24. Cell membrane–derived mediators. Platelet-activating factor (PAF) is derived from choline-containing glycerophospholipids in the membrane. Arachidonic acid derives from phosphatidylinositol phosphates and from phosphatidyl choline.

Component-specific disease susceptibilities underscore how individual complement components protecting from specific pathogens. Congenital defects in proteins that regulate the complement system (e.g., C1 inhibitor, SCPN) lead to chronic complement activation. Lack of C1 inhibitor is associated with hereditary angioedema.

Cell-Derived Inflammatory Mediators

Platelets, basophils, PMNs, endothelial cells, monocyte/macrophages, mast cells, and injured tissue itself all can generate vasoactive and inflammatory mediators. These molecules may: reflect metabolism of membrane phospholipids (eicosanoids, PAF); be preformed and stored in cytoplasmic granules (histamine, serotonin, lysosomal hydrolases); or indicate altered production of normal vascular regulators (e.g., NO, neurokinins).

Lipid Mediators: Arachidonic Acid Metabolites and Platelet-Activating Factor

Phospholipids and fatty acid derivatives released from plasma membranes are metabolized into mediators and homeostatic regulators by inflammatory cells and injured tissues (Fig. 2-24). As part of a complex regulatory network, **prostanoids, leukotrienes,** and **lipoxins,** all AA derivatives, both promote and inhibit inflammation (Table 2-4). The net impact of AA metabolites, also known as **eicosanoids**, depends on levels and profiles of prostanoid production, both of which change during an inflammatory response.

Arachidonate Metabolites: Prostanoids, Leukotrienes and Lipoxins

Depending on the specific inflammatory cell and type of stimulus, activated cells generate AA by one of two routes. In one pathway, AA is liberated from the glycerol of cell membrane phospholipids (particularly, phosphatidylcholine) by stimulus-induced **PLA2** activation. **Phospholipase C (PLC)** can also generate AA by cleaving phosphatidylinositol phosphates (PIPs, see **Chapter 1**) to diacylglycerol (DAG) and inositol phosphates; DAG lipase then extracts AA from DAG (Fig. 2-24). AA is further metabolized by either: (1) **cyclooxygenation**, to produce **prostaglandins and thromboxanes**; or (2) **lipoxygenation**, to **leukotrienes and lipoxins** (Fig. 2-25).

TABLE 2-4	
BIOLOGIC ACTIVITIES OF ARACHIDONIC ACID METABOLITES	
Metabolite	**Biologic Activity**
PGE$_2$, PDG$_2$	Induce vasodilation, bronchodilation; inhibit inflammatory cell function
PGI$_2$	Induces vasodilation, bronchodilation; inhibits inflammatory cell function
PGF$_{2a}$	Induces vasodilation, bronchoconstriction
TXA$_2$	Induces vasoconstriction, bronchoconstriction; enhances inflammatory cell functions (esp. platelets)
LTB$_4$	Chemotactic for phagocytic cells; stimulates phagocytic cell adherence; enhances microvascular permeability
LTC$_4$, LTD$_4$, LTE$_4$	Induce smooth muscle contraction; constrict pulmonary airways; increase microvascular permeability

PG… = prostaglandin; LT… = leukotriene; TXA$_2$ = thromboxane A$_2$.

PROSTANOIDS: AA is further metabolized by **cyclooxygenases 1 and 2 (COX-1, COX-2)** to generate **prostanoids**, which include the prostaglandins and **TXA2** (Fig. 2-25). COX-1 is constitutively expressed by most cells and increases upon cell activation. It is a key enzyme in synthesizing *prostaglandins*, which in turn: (1) protect gut mucosa; (2) regulate water/electrolyte balance; (3) stimulate platelet aggregation to maintain normal hemostasis; and (4) maintain resistance to thrombosis on vascular endothelial cell surfaces. COX-2 expression is generally low or undetectable but increases substantially with stimulation to yield metabolites that are important in inducing pain and inflammation. Early inflammatory prostanoid responses are COX-1-dependent. As inflammation proceeds, COX-2 takes over as the major source of prostanoids.

Both COX isoforms generate **prostaglandin H2 (PGH2)**, from which **prostacyclin** (PGI2), PGD2, PGE2, PGF2α, and **TXA2 (thromboxane)** derive. How much and which prostaglandins are produced during inflammation depends in part on the cells present and their state of activation. Thus, mast cells make mostly PGD2; macrophages generate PGE2 and TXA2; platelets are the major source of TXA2; and endothelial cells secrete PGI2.

Prostanoids trigger many intracellular-signaling pathways in immune and resident tissue cells by binding G-protein–coupled cell surface receptors. Repertoires of prostanoid receptors on various immune cells differ, so these cells' functional responses may vary according to the prostanoids present.

LEUKOTRIENES: Alternatively, AA may be metabolized by **5-lipoxygenase (5-LO)**, the main AA-metabolizing enzyme in neutrophils. 5-LO synthesizes **5-hydroperoxye-icosatetraenoic acid (5-HpETE)** and **leukotriene A4 (LTA4)** from AA; LTA4 is a precursor for other leukotrienes. In neutrophils and some macrophage populations, LTA4 is metabolized to **LTB4**, a potent chemotactic agent for neutrophils, monocytes, and macrophages. In other cells, especially mast

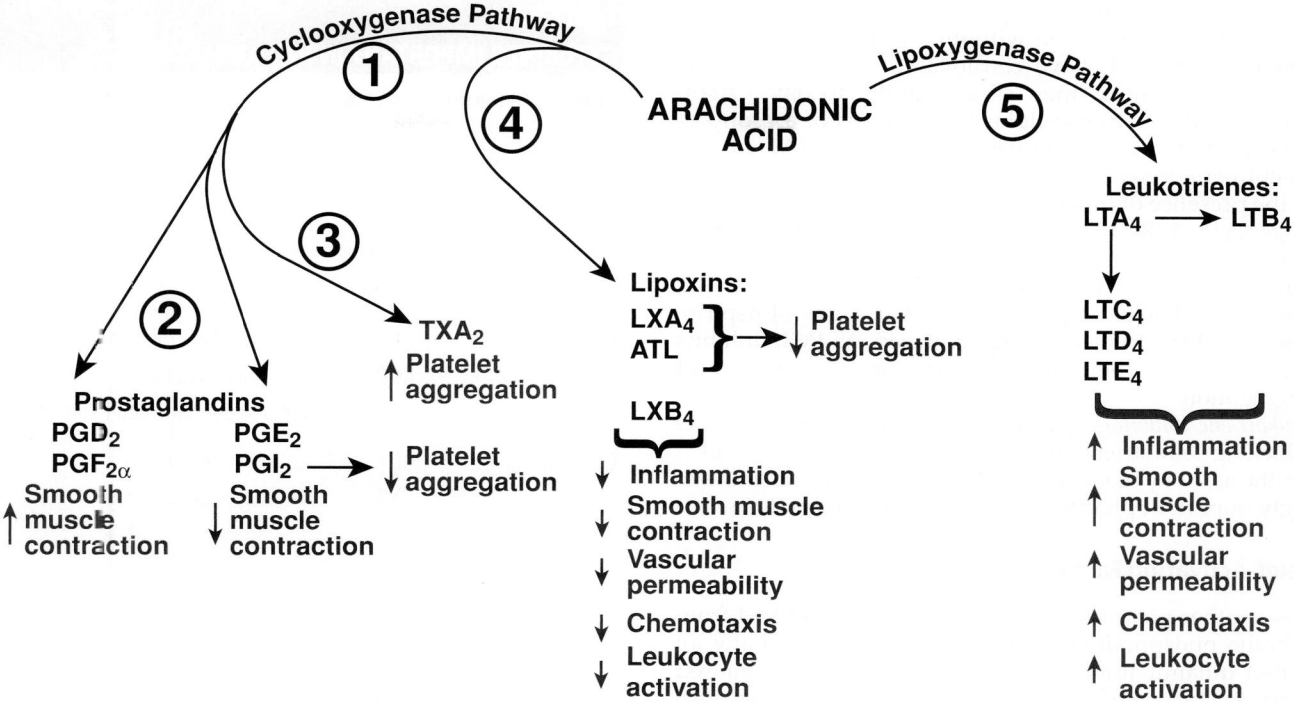

FIGURE 2-25. Major biologically active arachidonic acid (AA) metabolites. Species and activities that tend to promote inflammation are shown in red; those that tend to inhibit it are shown in blue. Two major types of enzymes activate AA: cyclooxygenase (COX) and lipoxygenase (LOX). *1.* COX-1 and COX-2, the major isoforms, produce multiple metabolites. *2.* Prostaglandins, the major ones being shown here, either mediate or antagonize smooth muscle contraction (bronchoconstriction, vasoconstriction). PGI_2 is, in addition, a crucial endogenous inhibitor of platelet aggregation. *3.* Thromboxane A_2 is a platelet substance that strongly stimulates platelet aggregation. *4.* Lipoxins derive from AA or from 15S-HETE (hydroxyleicosatetraneoic acid). The major lipoxins, shown, strongly inhibit inflammatory responses. LXA_4 and ATL (aspirin-triggered lipoxin) both strongly inhibit platelet aggregation. *5.* The lipoxygenase pathway generates leukotrienes, as shown, LTA_4 being the precursor for the other major members of this class of proinflammatory mediators. Although not all members of each group possess all the activities shown, the general characteristics of the groups are indicated. Aspirin, depending on dose, and other NSAIDs, inhibit COX-1 and COX-2. For simplicity, intermediate metabolites are not shown.

cells, basophils, and macrophages, LTA4 is converted to LTC4 and then to LTD4 and LTE4. These three leukotrienes stimulate smooth muscle contraction, enhance vascular permeability, and are responsible for many of the clinical symptoms associated with allergic-type reactions. Thus, they play a pivotal role in the development of asthma.

LIPOXINS: Lipoxins, the third class of AA products, are made in vascular lumens by cell–cell interactions (Fig. 2-25). They are anti-inflammatory, trihydroxytetraene-containing eicosanoids, generated during inflammation, atherosclerosis, and thrombosis. Several cell types synthesize lipoxins from leukotrienes. LTA4, released by activated leukocytes, is available for transcellular enzymatic conversion by nearby cells. When platelets adhere to neutrophils, LTA4 from neutrophils is converted by platelet 12-lipoxygenase to **lipoxin A4 and B4 (LXA4, LXB4)**. To make LXA4 or LXB4, platelets require the intermediate LTA, from adjacent neutrophils. Monocytes, eosinophils, and airway epithelial cells generate 15S-hydroxyeicosatetraenoic acid (15S-HETE), which is taken up by neutrophils and converted to lipoxins via 5-LOX. Activation of this pathway also inhibits leukotriene biosynthesis, thus regulating the process.

Lipoxins are generally anti-inflammatory: LXA4 causes vasodilation and antagonizes LTC4-stimulated vasoconstriction. Other activities inhibit neutrophil chemotaxis and adhesion while stimulating monocyte adhesion. An inverse relationship between lipoxin and leukotriene formation suggests that lipoxins may be endogenous counterweights to leukotriene actions.

Clinical Significance of AA Metabolites

The central role of eicosanoids in inflammatory processes is emphasized by the clinical utility of agents that block their synthesis:

- *Corticosteroids* induce synthesis of an inhibitor of PLA2 and block AA release by inflammatory cells. They are widely used to suppress tissue destruction associated with many inflammatory diseases, including allergic responses, rheumatoid arthritis and SLE. However, prolonged corticosteroid use can increase risk of infection and can damage connective tissue.
- *Aspirin and other NSAIDs* inhibit COX, blocking prostanoid—but not leukotriene or lipoxin—synthesis. Aspirin irreversibly acetylates and alters COX activity; other NSAIDs (e.g., ibuprofen, naproxen) reversibly block COX activity. In either case, the result is upstream inhibition of COX activity, and thus of downstream prostaglandin synthesis; hence their efficacy in treating pain and fever. Aspirin and NSAIDs inhibit both COX-1 and COX-2 and so reduce inflammation by blocking prostaglandin synthesis. They also predispose to gastric

ulceration. (Selective COX-2 inhibitors, which theoretically block inflammation without affecting the epithelial benefits of COX-1, have cardiovascular adverse effects which have limited their clinical utility to date.) Aspirin also initiates transcellular biosynthesis of a group of lipoxins termed "aspirin-triggered lipoxins (ATLs)," or 15-epimeric-lipoxins (15-epi-LXs). Aspirin administered in the presence of inflammatory mediators, causes COX-1 to generate 15R-HETE, which activated neutrophils convert to 15-epi-LXs, both of which are anti-inflammatory.

- Low-dose aspirin inhibits COX-1 and so blocks TXA2, impeding platelet aggregation. Higher doses of aspirin, however, tend to block PGI2 synthesis. As PGI2 inhibits TXA2, these higher aspirin doses may restore platelet aggregation.
- *Leukotriene inhibitors*, which act either by inhibiting 5-LO (blocking leukotriene and lipoxin—but not prostanoid—synthesis) or by blocking leukotriene receptors, are increasingly important pharmacologically in treating asthma.

Platelet-Activating Factor

PAF is another potent inflammatory mediator derived from membrane phospholipids. It is synthesized by virtually all activated inflammatory cells, endothelial cells, and injured tissue cells. During inflammatory and allergic responses, PAF comes from cell membrane choline-containing glycerophospholipids, by PLA2 catalytic action, followed by acetylation (Fig. 2-24). PAF has many functions. It favors inflammation by enhancing leukocyte adhesion, chemotaxis, leukocyte degranulation, and the oxidative burst; it also stimulates synthesis of other mediators, particularly eicosanoids. (As its name suggests, PAF also induces platelet aggregation, but this is not its main function.) In addition, it is a powerful vasodilator and augments microvascular permeability at sites of tissue injury. In this regard, it is 100 to 10,000 × more potent than histamine. Like most comparably strong inflammatory mediators, it is tightly regulated: **PAF-acetylhydrolase**, circulates in plasma, hydrolyzes PAF, and limits its function.

CELL-DERIVED PROTEIN MEDIATORS

Cytokines Are Low–Molecular-Weight Proteins Secreted by Activated Cells

They are produced at sites of tissue injury, and act via specific receptors on target cells. Cytokines regulate inflammatory responses from initial changes in vascular permeability to resolution and restoration of tissue integrity.

Many different cytokines, including interleukins, growth factors, colony-stimulating factors, interferons and chemokines, are produced at sites of inflammation (Table 2-5). Cytokines may act in one of several modes: *autocrine*, affecting the cells that make them; *paracrine*, affecting neighboring cells; and *endocrine*, acting via the bloodstream on distant cells (Fig. 2-26). Most cells produce cytokines, but differ in cytokine repertoires. Many cells make multiple cytokines, with both **pleiotropic effects** (affecting different cells differently) and **redundant effects** (multiple cytokines with similar activities).

Cytokine production is generally triggered when PAMPs and/or DAMPs bind receptors on inflammatory cells. In particular, **LPS**, a gram-negative bacterial outer membrane

TABLE 2-5
CYTOKINES IMPORTANT IN INFLAMMATION

Class of Cytokine	Species	Inflammation-Related Actions
Interleukins	IL-1	Inflammatory cell activation
	IL-6	
	IL-8	
	IL-10	
	IL-13	
Growth Factors	GM-CSF	Stimulate macrophage population
	M-CSF	Bactericidal activity
		NK and dendritic cell function
Chemokines	CC	Leukocyte chemotaxis
	CXC	Leukocyte activation
	XC	
	CX3C	
Interferons	IFNα	Antiviral
	IFNβ	Leukocyte activation
	IFNγ	
Proinflammatory cytokines	TNFα	Fever
		Anorexia
		Shock
		Cytotoxicity
		Cytokine induction
		Activation of endothelial and tissue cells

GM-CSF = granulocyte-monocyte colony-stimulating factor; IL = interleukin; NK = natural killer; IFN = interferon; TNF = tumor necrosis factor.

component, is a potent activator of macrophages, endothelial cells and leukocytes (Fig. 2-27). When LPS binds its receptor, it activates macrophages to synthesize TNFα, IL-1, IL-6, IL-8, IL-12, and others. These then modulate endothelial cell–leukocyte adhesion (TNFα), leukocyte recruitment (IL-8), acute phase responses (IL-6, IL-1), and immune function (IL-1, IL-6, IL-12).

Cytokine secretion is self-limited and tightly regulated. Excessive or inappropriate cytokine production can cause significant harm. For example, many cases of **sepsis** reflect unbalanced cytokine production (see **Chapter 12**).

IL-1 and TNFα

IL-1 and **TNFα** made by macrophages and other cells, are central to developing and amplifying inflammatory responses. These cytokines activate endothelial cells to express adhesion molecules and then release cytokines, chemokines, and ROS. TNFα causes priming and aggregation of neutrophils. IL-1 and TNFα also trigger fever by acting on the hypothalamic thermoregulatory center (via local prostaglandin production), and stimulate muscle catabolism, shifts in protein synthesis, and altered hemodynamics (Fig. 2-27). **IL-6** stimulates hepatic synthesis of plasma proteins, including

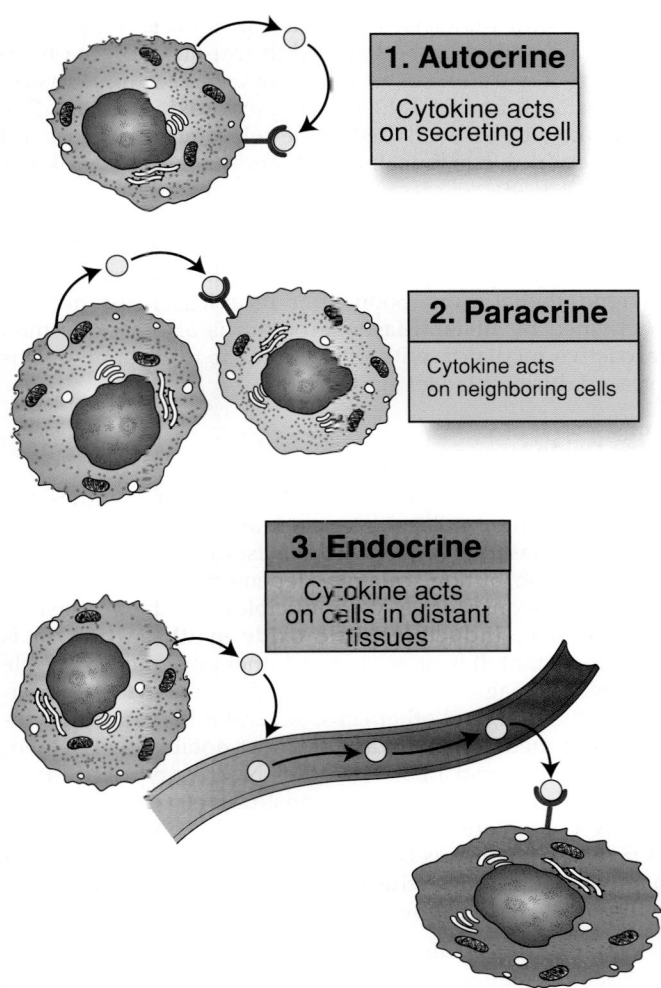

FIGURE 2-26. Types of cytokine signaling. *1.* Autocrine signaling occurs when secreted products act through receptors on the secreting cell. *2.* Paracrine signaling occurs when secreted products act on nearby cells. *3.* In endocrine signaling, products are carried in the vascular system to act on distant cells.

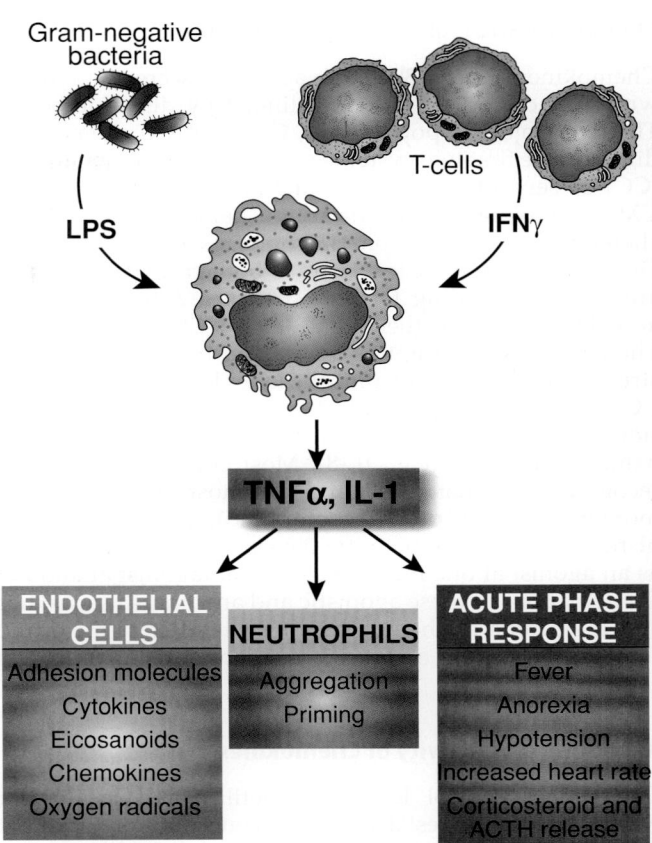

FIGURE 2-27. Central role of interleukin (IL)-1 and tumor necrosis factor (TNF)-α in inflammation. Lipopolysaccharide (LPS) and interferon-γ (IFN-γ) activate macrophages to release inflammatory cytokines, principally IL-1 and TNF-α, responsible for directing local and systemic inflammatory responses. *ACTH* = adrenocorticotrophic hormone.

fibrinogen, and also acts on the hypothalamus to induce fever. Together, these three cytokines (IL-1, IL-6, TNFα) are the **endogenous pyrogens** (pyro = fever), and are among the most important mediators of the systemic effects of acute inflammation (**acute-phase reactions,** see below).

Interferon-γ

IFNγ, another potent stimulus for macrophage activation and cytokine production, is produced by a subset of T lymphocytes as part of the immune response (see Chapter 4). It is also synthesized by natural killer (NK) cells in the primary host response to intracellular pathogens (e.g., *Listeria monocytogenes*) and certain viruses. NK cells migrate to tissues at sites of injury where, when exposed to IL-12 and TNF-α, they produce IFNγ. Thus, there is an amplification pathway by which activated tissue macrophages produce TNFα and IL-12, stimulating IFNγ production by NK cells, with subsequent activation of additional macrophages. IFNγ is one of the most important mediators of chronic inflammation.

Chemokines Are Small Cytokines That Act as Leukocyte Chemoattractants and Activators

Concentration gradients of chemokines are sensed by inflammatory cells, usually via binding GPCRs on the surface of a sensing cell. Unique combinations of chemokines recruit particular cell populations (e.g., neutrophils vs. eosinophils vs. lymphocytes) to sites of injury. In addition, chemokines can stimulate hematopoietic precursor cells, and recruit and activate mesenchymal cells, for example, fibroblasts, smooth muscle cells. Like other cytokines, chemokines are *redundant* (many different ones have the same effect) and *pleiotropic* (they often bind several different receptors, with different outcomes).

Inflammatory Chemokines and Homing Chemokines

Inflammatory chemokines are elicited by bacterial toxins and inflammatory cytokines (especially IL-1, TNFα, IFNγ), by many tissue cells, and by leukocytes themselves. They recruit leukocytes during host inflammatory responses. **Homing chemokines** are constitutively expressed, but upregulated in disease. They direct trafficking and homing of lymphocytes and dendritic cells to lymphoid tissues during an immune response (see **Chapter 4**).

Chemokine Structure and Nomenclature

Chemokines are 70–130 amino acid-long secretory proteins with four conserved cysteines linked by disulfide bonds. The two major subpopulations, CXC and CC chemokines, differ by the first two cysteines' positioning: either adjacent (CC) or separated by one amino acid (CXC). In general, CXC chemokines act primarily on neutrophils, while CC chemokines act mainly on macrophages and lymphocytes. Of course, there are exceptions to both rules. Chemokines are named according to their structure, followed by "L" and the number of their gene (e.g., CCL1, CXCL1, etc.). Their chemokine receptors are named by the number and structure of their ligand, plus the letter R (for receptor) (e.g., CCR1, CXCR1, etc.). To add to, or perhaps dispel, confusion, many chemokines and their receptors have common names still in use (e.g., IL-8). Most chemokine receptors recognize more than one ligand, and most chemokines bind more than one receptor. Receptor binding may trigger agonistic or antagonistic activity: the same chemokine may act as an agonist at one receptor and an antagonist at another. Combinations of these agonistic and antagonistic activities, and the profile of chemokines at a site, dictate the attraction and activation of specific resident and inflammatory cell types.

Anchoring and Activity of Chemokines

Chemokines control leukocyte motility and localization within tissues by establishing a concentration gradient. Some chemokines establish gradients as soluble peptides. *Others bind extracellular matrix* thus maintaining chemotactic gradients needed for directed migration of recruited cells and allowing high concentrations of chemokines to persist at sites of tissue injury. Specific membrane receptors on migrating leukocytes recognize matrix-bound chemokines and associated adhesion molecules, causing cells to move along chemotactic gradients to a site of injury. Cell responses to matrix-bound chemoattractants is called **haptotaxis**. During this migration, a cell extends a pseudopod toward increasing chemokine concentrations. At the leading front of the pseudopod, marked changes in levels of intracellular calcium correspond to assembly and contraction of cytoskeleton proteins. This pulls the rest of the cell along the chemical gradient. Chemokines are also displayed on cytokine-activated vascular endothelial cells.

Chemokines—especially IL-8—are not the only regulators of chemotaxis of inflammatory cells, or even the most important. Neutrophil chemotaxis responds to C5a from complement; bacterial and mitochondrial products, particularly low–molecular-weight N-formylated peptides; and prostanoids, especially LTB4.

Chemokines participate in many acute and chronic diseases, particularly when tissue inflammation is involved. Examples include rheumatoid arthritis, ulcerative colitis, Crohn disease, chronic bronchitis, asthma, autoimmune diseases, and vascular diseases, including atherosclerosis.

Vasoactive Amines

Vasoactive amines like **histamine** and **serotonin** (5-hydroxytryptamine) play important roles in acute inflammation. Histamine is widely distributed in tissues, particularly in mast cells adjacent to vessels, and in circulating basophils and platelets. Preformed histamine is stored in mast cell granules, to be released in response to: (1) physical injury like trauma or heat; (2) immune reactions involving mast cell-bound IgE; (3) anaphylotoxins (C3a, C5a); (4) leukocyte-derived histamine-releasing proteins; (5) neuropeptides (e.g., substance P); and (6) certain cytokines (e.g., IL-1, IL-8).

In humans, histamine causes arteriolar dilation and orchestrates the immediate phase of increased vascular permeability, inducing venular endothelial contraction and interendothelial gaps. Soon after its release, histamine is inactivated by **histaminase**. Serotonin is also a preformed vasoactive mediator, with effects similar to histamine. It is released during platelet aggregation.

Nitric Oxide

NO is a short-lived, soluble, free radical gas synthesized from L-arginine, molecular oxygen and NADPH by **nitric oxide synthase (NOS)**. The three isoforms of NOS vary in tissue distribution, calcium dependence and modes of expression (constitutive vs. inducible). In the context of inflammation, **inducible nitric oxide synthase (iNOS)** is most important. It is present in endothelium, smooth muscle cells, macrophages, hepatocytes, cardiac myocytes, respiratory epithelium, and other cells. Several inflammatory cytokines and mediators activate it—most notably IL-1, TNFα, IFNγ, and bacterial LPS. The other NOS isotypes are neuronal NOS (nNOS), which is constitutively expressed (its activity is regulated by intracellular Ca^{++}), and endothelial NOS (eNOS), which is constitutively synthesized but found mainly (though not exclusively) in endothelium. NO plays multiple roles in inflammation:

- When produced by endothelium (generally via eNOS), it activates guanylyl cyclase in vascular smooth muscle, increasing cGMP and ultimately relaxing smooth muscle (vasodilation). This is the basis for using cardiac nitrates (e.g., nitroglycerin) to treat acute myocardial ischemia. They increase NO generation and increase venous return to the heart.
- Antagonism of all stages of platelet activation (adhesion, aggregation, and degranulation)
- Reduction of leukocyte recruitment at inflammatory sites.
- Acting as a microbicidal agent in activated macrophages; NO can be converted to the highly reactive and cytotoxic peroxynitrite (ONOO–, see **Chapter 1**), particularly in the presence of superoxidase.

Lysosomal Constituents

Neutrophil and monocyte lysosomal granules carry multiple mediators of acute inflammation. These may be released after cell death, by leakage during formation of phagocytic vacuoles or by "frustrated phagocytosis"—attempted phagocytosis of large, nondigestible surfaces. While acid proteases have acidic pH optima and are generally active only in phagolysosomes, **neutral proteases**—like elastase, collagenase, and cathepsin—are active in the extracellular matrix and can injure tissue by degrading elastin, collagen, and other matrix proteins. Neutral proteases can also cleave C3 and C5, generating C3a and C5a anaphylatoxins, and can catalyze generation of active kinins (e.g., bradykinin) from their kininogen precursors.

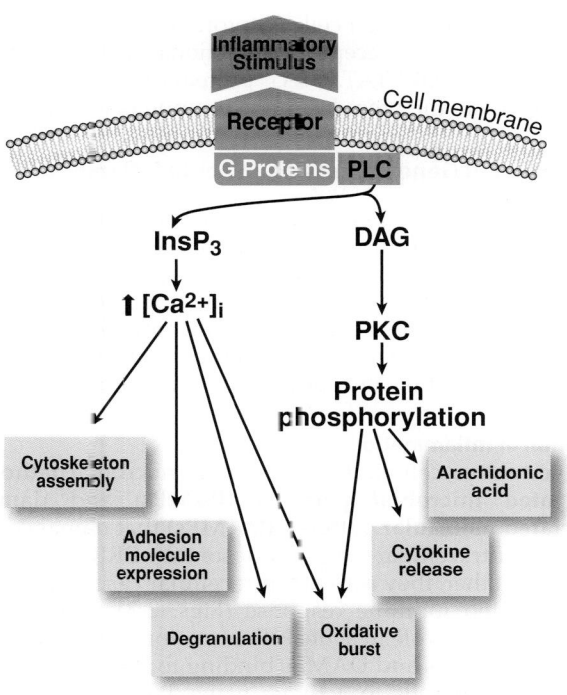

FIGURE 2-28. G-protein–mediated intracellular signal transduction pathway common to many inflammatory stimuli.

Unchecked Acute Inflammation Can Cause Tissue Injury and Death

However, genetic and biochemical regulation mitigates "bystander" such effects of acute inflammation, and allows resolution and repair. Many factors downregulate and modulate acute inflammatory responses. They include soluble pro- or anti-inflammatory mediators, positive- and negative-feedback intracellular signaling pathways and regulated gene expression.

The process by which diverse stimuli lead to functional inflammatory responses is **stimulus–response coupling**. Stimuli include microbial products and the many plasma- or cell-derived inflammatory mediators described in this chapter. Although intracellular-signaling pathways are complex and vary with cell type and stimulus, soluble mediator share common intracellular pathways that activate inflammatory cells: GPCR, TNF receptor (TNFR) and JAK-STAT pathways (Figs. 2-28 to 2-30, respectively).

Soluble Mediators

Plasma- and cell-derived proinflammatory mediators can amplify tissue responses in positive feedback loops. Complement, proinflammatory cytokines and, in some cases, immune complexes activate signal transduction pathways that control expression of proinflammatory mediators, including TNFα, IL-1, chemokines, and adhesion molecules. Secreted cytokines then propagate responses by activating other cell types via these and similar pathways.

The inflammatory response is also regulated to limit these cascades, and to protect tissues from damage (negative feedback). Inducible cytokines, including IL-4, IL-10, and IL-12, block NFκB activation by stabilizing its inhibitor, Iκb, thus reducing the response (Fig. 2-29). Protease inhibitors,

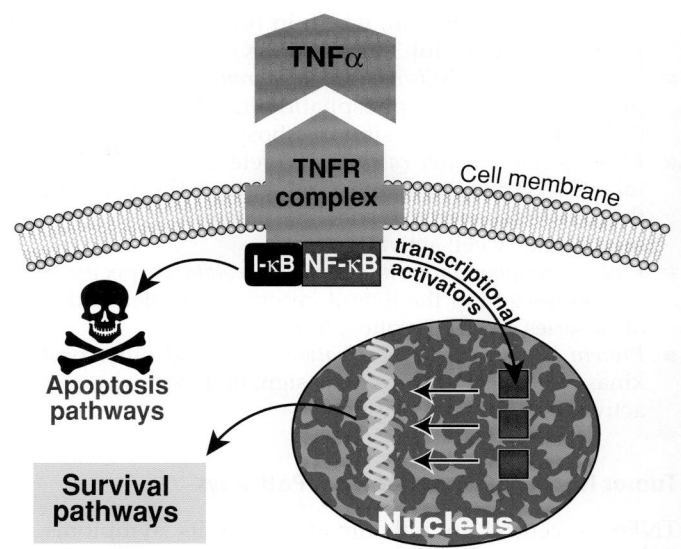

FIGURE 2-29. Tumor necrosis factor (TNF) receptor–mediated intracellular signal transduction pathway.

for example, secreted leukocyte protease inhibitor (SLPI); matrix metalloprotease (MMP) inhibitors (e.g., tissue inhibitor of MMPs [TIMPs]); antioxidant enzymes (e.g., SOD); lipoxins; glucocorticoids and phosphatases; and transcriptional regulatory factors, like suppressor of cytokine signaling (SOC)—all inhibit activation of proinflammatory factors, oxidants, and signaling pathways.

G-Protein–Coupled Receptor Pathways

Many chemokines, hormones, neurotransmitters, and other mediators signal via GPCRs (Fig. 2-28). GPCRs activate diverse downstream intracellular-signaling pathways (covered in more detail in **Chapter 1**), but common activities include:

- *Ligand–receptor binding:* When a stimulatory factor binds a specific cell membrane receptor, the resulting ligand–receptor complex triggers exchange of GDP for GTP. This

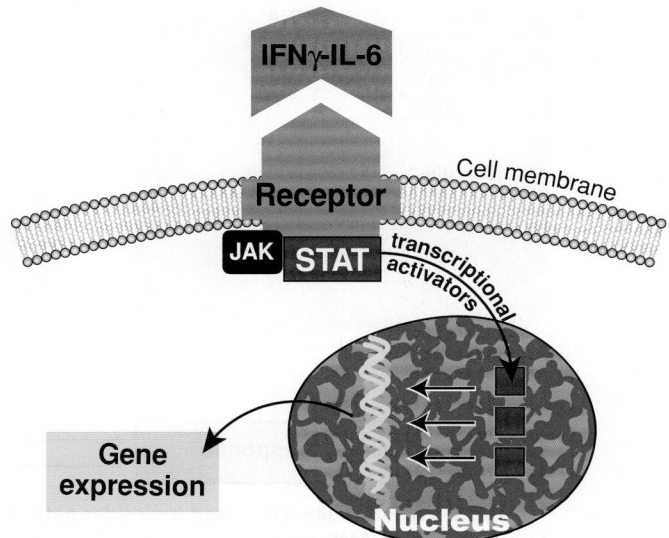

FIGURE 2-30. JAK-STAT–mediated intracellular transduction pathway. *IFN* = interferon; *IL* = interleukin.

activates the G protein, which in turn, activate PLC and phosphatidylinositol-3-kinase (PI3K).

- *Phospholipid metabolism of cell membranes:* PLC hydrolyzes plasma membrane phosphatidylinositol bisphosphate (PIP2) to DAG and inositol trisphosphate (IP3).
- *Elevated cytosolic free calcium:* IP3 releases stored intracellular Ca^{2+}. Acting with influx of Ca^{2+} from the extracellular fluid, IP3 increases cytosolic free calcium, a key event in inflammatory cell activation.
- *Protein phosphorylation and dephosphorylation:* Specific tyrosine kinases bind the ligand–receptor complex and initiate a series of protein phosphorylations.
- *Protein kinase C (PKC) activation:* PKC and other protein kinases activate intracellular-signaling pathways, often activating gene transcription.

Tumor Necrosis Factor Receptor Pathways

TNFα is central to inflammation and its symptoms. It induces tumor cell apoptosis and regulates immune functions (Fig. 2-29). TNFα and related proteins bind receptors to form a multiprotein-signaling complex at the cell membrane. This complex can activate: (1) caspases to trigger apoptosis (see **Chapter 1**); (2) inhibitors of apoptosis; or (3) NFκB transcription factor, causing it to dissociate from its inhibitor, IκB, and then translocate to the nucleus, where NFκB can activate transcription. This NFκB pathway is critical to regulating TNF-mediated events during inflammation.

JAK-STAT Pathway

This pathway provides a direct route from extracellular polypeptides (e.g., growth factors) or cytokines (e.g., interferons or interleukins) through cell receptors to gene promoters in the nucleus. Ligand–receptor interactions elicit transcription complexes of JAK-STAT. STAT proteins translocate to the nucleus, where they regulate gene promoters (Fig. 2-30).

Regulation of Gene Expression in Acute Inflammation

Regulated gene expression is essential to controlling acute inflammation. It occurs in multiple phases, including when inflammation starts (*initiation*) (often triggered by microbial products); when proinflammatory mediator *genes are activated*; *reprogramming* to silence acute proinflammatory genes and activate anti-inflammatory mediators; and *gene silencing* to terminate inflammation and allow tissue to recover its integrity.

Initiation of Inflammation

As noted above, cellular **PRRs** recognize microbial **pathogen-associated microbial patterns (PAMPs)** and **damage-associated molecular patterns (DAMPs)** that damaged cells release. (Intracellular—e.g., endosomal—PRRs also bind these.) Together, they activate intracellular cascades to drive a coordinated immune response (Figs. 2-31 and 2-32). In addition to their role in acute inflammation, gene expression driven by PAMPs and DAMPs binding to PRRs primes antigen-presenting cells to activate naive T cells, functionally linking innate and adaptive immunity (Fig. 2-32). Four families of PRRs are found on inflammatory and immune cells: (1) toll-like receptors (TLRs); (2) nucleotide oligomerization domain leucine-rich repeat proteins (NOD-like receptors [NLRs]); (3) cytoplasmic caspase activation and recruitment domain helicases; and (4) C-type lectin receptors.

- **TLRs** are a major class of PRRs on immune, inflammatory, and tissue cells, including macrophages, endothelial

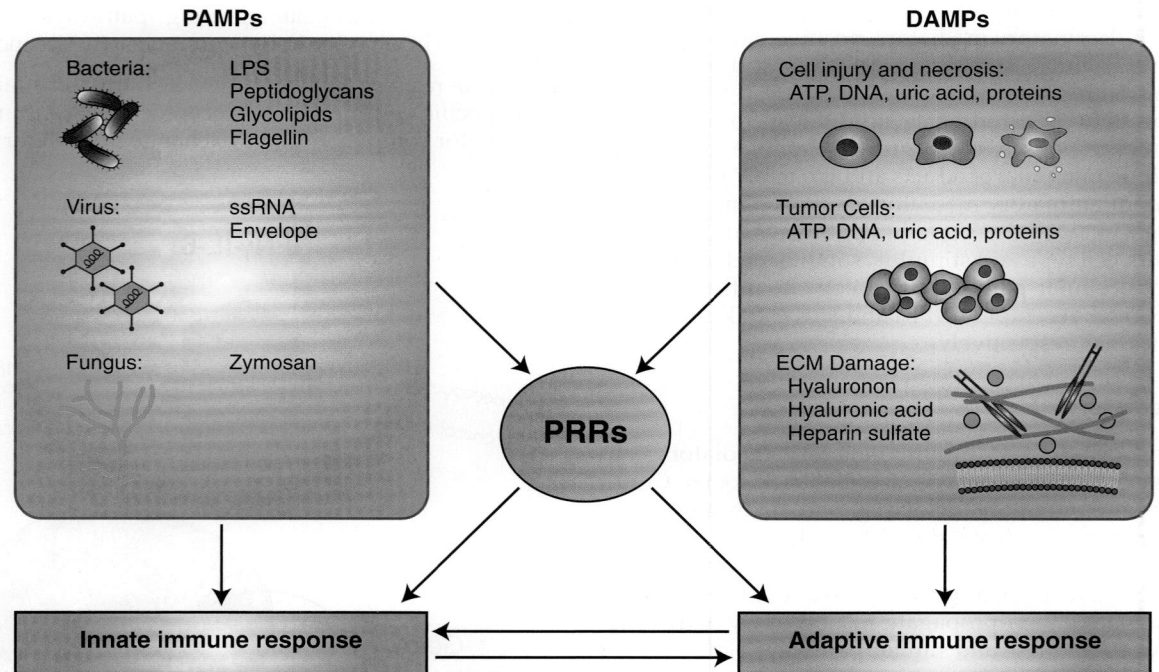

FIGURE 2-31. Pathogen-associated molecular pattern molecules (PAMPs) and damage-associated molecular pattern molecules (DAMPs) initiate adaptive and innate immune responses. Microbes release PAMPs. Damaged cells and tissue release DAMPs. Binding to receptors belonging to the family of pattern recognition receptors (PRRs) mediates innate and adaptive immune responses.

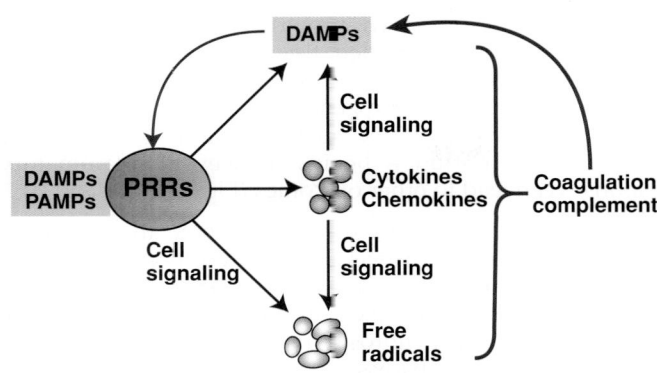

FIGURE 2-32. Damage-associated molecular pattern molecules (DAMPs) and pathogen-associated molecular pattern molecules (PAMPs) drive the multifaceted inflammatory response. Interaction of PAMPs and DAMPs with pattern recognition receptors (PRRs) initiates cell signaling, leading to enhanced activation of inflammatory mediators. These inflammatory signals can lead to further release of DAMPs and maintenance of the inflammatory response.

cells, and epithelial cells (Table 2-6). TLRs on the cell surface recognize bacterial cell wall components and viruses. Genetic polymorphisms of TLRs relate to specific cellular responses. Thus, specific TLRs recognize lipid and carbohydrates on gram-positive bacteria, fungi, LPS of gram-negative bacteria, and viral RNA. TLR engagement activates intracellular defenses against microbial organisms, and may also activate cytokine cascades.

■ **NLRs**. NLRs are *intracellular* soluble proteins that form large molecular complexes, **inflammasomes**, involved in proteolytic activation of proinflammatory cytokines.

■ **Cytoplasmic caspase activation and recruitment domain helicases**. This large family includes receptors (e.g., retinoic acid inducible gene-1 [RIG-1]-like receptors) of macrophages, dendritic cells, and fibroblasts. These cytoplasmic RNA helicases survey for microbes and recognize viral RNA in the cytosol.

■ **C-type lectin receptors.** Glycosylated proteins have pathogen recognition functions, in addition to participating in cell adhesion. Mainly expressed on macrophages and dendritic cells, these receptors recognize fungal pathogens and modulate innate immunity. Members include mannose receptor, **dendritic cell–specific ICAM-3–grabbing nonintegrin (DC-SIGN),** dectins-1 and -2, and collectins. When pathogens bind these receptors on epithelial and endothelial cells, additional DAMPs are released. This stimulates inflammatory cells and amplifies activation of coagulation and complement cascades. These, in turn, positively feed back to drive production of inflammatory mediators (i.e., cytokine, chemokines, DAMPs) (Fig. 2-32).

Gene Activation

The main function of PRRs is to activate three major signaling pathways: (1) the **NFκB** pathway; (2) the **mitogen-activated protein kinase/activator protein-1 (MAPK/AP-1)** pathway; and (3) **the interferon regulatory factor (IRF)** pathway. Activation of NFκB and MAPK/AP-1 induces proinflammatory cytokines, while IRFs activate type 1 IFNs and proinflammatory mediators. Via these pathways, microbial recognition activates transcription of mediators of acute inflammation, especially inflammatory cytokines.

TABLE 2-6
PATHOGEN RECOGNITION RECEPTORS

Toll-like Receptor	Cell Expression	Pathogen-Associated Molecule(s) Recognized
TLR1	Macrophages Neutrophils	Lipid and carbohydrates from gram-positive bacteria
TLR2	Macrophages Basophils Neutrophils	Lipid and carbohydrates from gram-positive bacteria Fungal organisms
TLR3	Macrophages	Nucleic acid and derivatives Double-stranded RNA (viral DNA)
TLR4	Macrophages Basophils Neutrophils	LPS from gram-negative bacteria
TLR5	Macrophages Neutrophils	Bacterial flagellin
TLR6	Macrophages Neutrophils	Lipid and carbohydrates from gram-positive bacteria
TLR7	Macrophages Neutrophils	Nucleic acid and derivatives (viral DNA)
TLR8	Macrophages Neutrophils	Nucleic acid and derivatives (viral DNA)
TLR9	Macrophages Neutrophils	Nucleic acid and derivatives Bacterial DNA containing unmethylated CpG motifs
TLR10	Macrophages Neutrophils	Ligand unknown
TLR11 (pseudogene)	Macrophages Neutrophils	Bacterial profilin

LPS = lipopolysaccharide.

Negative Regulators of Acute Inflammation

Acute inflammation resolves when inflammation eliminates the initial stimulus and inflammatory cells undergo apoptosis. Proinflammatory mediator production wanes and anti-inflammatory mediators brake the process. Proper healing can proceed when damaged tissue and debris are removed. The process varies, however, genetics and the patient's sex and age determine response to injury, extent of healing and, especially, progression to chronic inflammatory disease. Negative regulators of inflammation include:

■ **Gene silencing and reprogramming:** These processes: (1) silence acute proinflammatory genes (e.g., TNFα, IL-1β); (2) increase anti-inflammatory gene expression; and (3) allow the process to start to resolve. Simultaneously, expression of anti-inflammatory factors, like IL-1 receptor antagonist (IL-1RA), TNFα receptors, IL-6 and IL-10, increases.

- **Cytokines:** Several interleukins (IL-6, IL-10, IL-11, IL-12, IL-13) limit inflammation by reducing TNFα production, possibly by preserving IκB, thus blocking cell activation and release of inflammatory mediators.
- **Protease inhibitors:** Secretory leukocyte proteinase inhibitor (SLPI) and TIMP-2 reduce responses of several cell types, including macrophages and endothelial cells, and limit connective tissue damage.
- **Lipoxins:** Lipoxins and aspirin-triggered lipoxins are anti-inflammatory lipid mediators that block leukotriene biosynthesis.
- **Glucocorticoids:** Hypothalamic–pituitary–adrenal axis stimulation increases release of immunosuppressive glucocorticoids. They suppress proinflammatory genes transcriptionally and posttranscriptionally.
- **Kininases:** Kininases in plasma and blood degrade the potent proinflammatory mediator bradykinin.
- **Phosphatases:** As kinases activate inflammatory signaling by phosphorylating proteins, their opposites, phosphatases, decrease inflammatory signaling by rapidly dephosphorylating those proteins.
- **TGFβ:** Apoptotic cells, particularly PMNs, upregulate TGFβ, which suppresses proinflammatory cytokines and chemokines, switches AA–derived mediators to favor production of lipoxin and resolvin (resolution phase interaction products; ω-3 unsaturated fatty acid), causes recognition and clearance of apoptotic cells and debris by macrophages and stimulates anti-inflammatory cytokines and fibrosis.

The Outcome of Acute Inflammation Depends on a Balance Between Cell Recruitment, Division, Emigration, and Death

Optimally, when inflammation recedes, normal tissue architecture and physiologic function are restored. If a tissue is to return to normal, inflammation must be reversed: the stimulus to injury removed, proinflammatory signals extinguished, cellular influx ended, tissue fluid balance restored, debris removed, vascular function restored, epithelial barriers repaired and ECM regenerated. As signals for acute inflammation wane, PMN apoptosis limits the immune response and resolution begins. However, inflammatory responses can lead to other outcomes (Fig. 2-33):

- **Scar:** Although the body may eliminate the offending agent if a tissue is irreversibly injured, normal architecture is often replaced by a scar (see **Chapter 3**).
- **Abscess:** If inflammatory cells blockade an area of acute inflammation with fibrosis, PMN products destroy the tissue, leaving an abscess.
- **Lymphangitis/Lymphadenitis:** Localized acute and chronic inflammation may cause secondary inflammation of lymphatic channels (lymphangitis) and lymph nodes (lymphadenitis). Inflamed lymphatic channels appear as red streaks, and lymph nodes are enlarged and painful. Affected nodes show follicular hyperplasia and abundant mononuclear phagocytes in sinuses (sinus histiocytosis).
- **Persistent inflammation:** Inflammation may persist if the offending agent persists or resolution is incomplete. A prolonged acute response, with continued neutrophil influx and tissue destruction—or, more often, chronic inflammation—result.

Chronic Inflammation

If acute inflammation does not resolve an infection or other injury, **chronic inflammation** supervenes. Then, inflammatory cells persist, the stroma becomes hyperplastic and tissue destruction and scarring may cause organ dysfunction. Acute and chronic inflammation are ends of a dynamic continuum with overlapping morphologies: (1) inflammation

Outcomes of Acute Inflammation

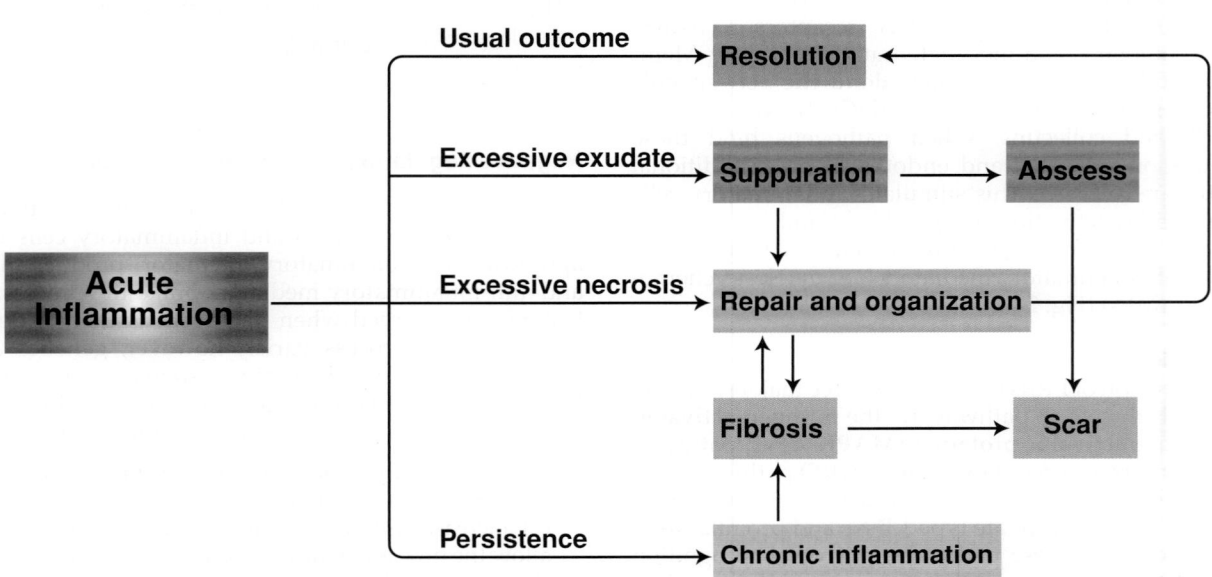

FIGURE 2-33. Outcomes of acute inflammation.

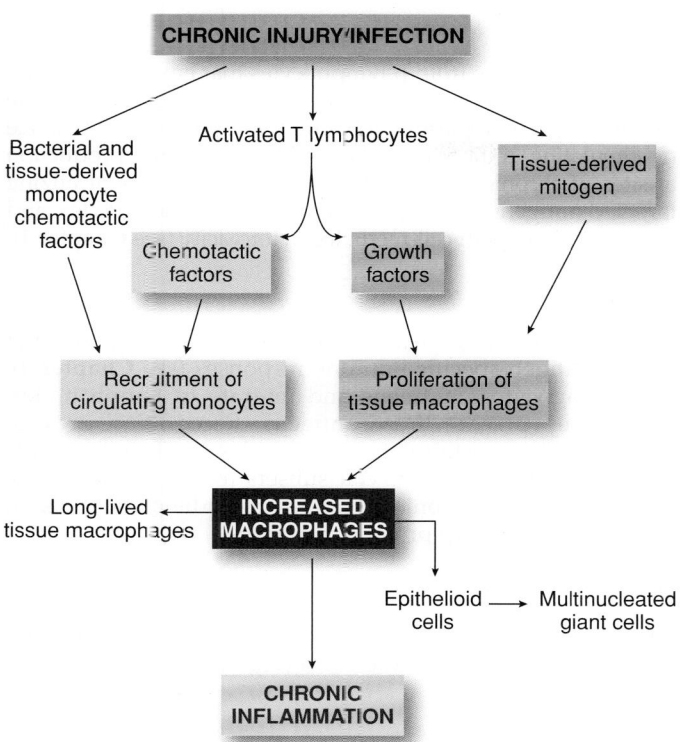

FIGURE 2-34. Accumulation of macrophages is central to development of chronic inflammation.

featuring continued recruitment of chronic inflammatory cells is followed by; (2) tissue injury due to prolonged inflammation; and (3) an often disordered attempt to restore tissue integrity. Macrophages are key determinants of the outcome (Fig. 2-34). Unresolved chronic inflammation may cause ongoing disability, as in chronic lung disease, rheumatoid arthritis, ulcerative colitis, granulomatous diseases, autoimmune diseases, and chronic dermatitis.

THE EVENTS OF CHRONIC INFLAMMATION

Chronic inflammatory triggers resemble those of acute inflammation:

- **Specific activators**, microbial products or injury, initiate the response.
- **Chemical mediators direct recruitment, activation and interaction of inflammatory cells.** Activation of coagulation and complement generates small peptides that prolong inflammatory responses. Cytokines, specifically IL-6 and RANTES, regulate a switch in chemokines, so mononuclear cells are directed to the site. Other cytokines (e.g., IFNγ) then promote macrophage proliferation and activation.
- **Inflammatory cells migrate in from the blood.** Interactions between lymphocytes, macrophages, dendritic cells, and fibroblasts generate antigen-specific responses. Macrophages have a central, controlling role. They produce inflammatory mediators that activate other macrophages, lymphocytes, and tissue fibroblasts (Fig. 2-34) either promoting resolution or perpetuating injury.
- **DAMPs and PAMPs drive multifaceted inflammatory responses** Interaction of PAMPs, DAMPs, and PRRs increases activation of inflammatory mediators. This can cause more damage, thus more DAMPs, and perpetuate the inflammation, even after the inciting event has passed (Fig. 2-32).
- **Stromal cell activation and ECM remodeling** both affect cellular immune responses. Variable fibrosis may result, depending on the extent of tissue injury and the persistence of injury and inflammation.

Chronic inflammation is not synonymous with chronic infection. It does not even require infection, but may follow an acute inflammatory or immune response to a foreign antigen. Signals that lead to extended responses include:

- **Bacteria, viruses, and parasites:** These provide signals to support persistent inflammatory responses, which may act to isolate the invader from the host.
- **Apoptosis**: Apoptotic PMNs induce an anti-inflammatory reaction, but defective recognition or responses to their remnants may lead to chronic inflammation.
- **Defective gene silencing:** Delayed or persistent expression of late proinflammatory genes helps perpetuate inflammatory environments. Then, a gene silencing phase does not occur, cytokine onslaught persists and pathologic inflammation develops.
- **Trauma:** Extensive tissue damage releases mediators that prolong the inflammatory environment.
- **Cancer:** Tumors recruit chronic inflammatory cells, especially macrophages and T-cells to support their growth (see **Chapter 5**).
- **Immune factors:** In many autoimmune diseases, for example, rheumatoid arthritis, chronic thyroiditis, and primary biliary cirrhosis, chronic inflammatory responses occur in affected tissues (see **Chapter 4**). Persistent injury in affected organs may reflect ongoing immune-mediated inflammation.

Chronic Inflammatory Cells Come From the Circulation and Affected Tissues

The blood contributes macrophages, lymphocytes, plasma cells, dendritic cells, and eosinophils, while affected tissues provide fibroblasts and endothelial cells. *The key chronic inflammatory cells are mononuclear cells, particularly monocytes/macrophages and lymphocytes.*

Monocytes/Macrophages

Activated macrophages and their cytokines are central to chronic inflammation and to prolonging responses that lead to it. Tissue macrophages are stimulated and proliferate as circulating monocytes arrive and differentiate into tissue macrophages (Fig. 2-34). Urged by the microenvironment, resident tissue macrophages become either classically activated M1 macrophages or alternatively activated M2 macrophages (Figs. 2-6 and 2-7). Macrophages produce inflammatory and immunologic mediators, and regulate reactions leading to chronic inflammation. They also regulate lymphocyte responses to antigens and secrete other mediators that modulate fibroblast and endothelial cell proliferation and activities.

Within different tissues, resident macrophages differ in their armamentaria of enzymes and responses to local inflammatory signals. Granules of circulating monocytes contain serine proteinases, like those in PMNs. Blood monocytes synthesize additional enzymes, especially MMPs. When monocytes enter tissue and differentiate into macrophages, they acquire the ability to make additional MMPs and cysteine proteinases, but no longer produce serine proteinases. The activities of these degradative enzymes are central to tissue destruction in chronic inflammation. For example, in emphysema, resident macrophages generate proteinases, particularly MMPs with elastolytic activity, which destroy alveolar walls and recruit blood monocytes into the lung. Other macrophage products include oxygen metabolites, chemotactic factors, cytokines and growth factors (Fig. 2-4C).

Lymphocytes

naïve lymphocytes home to secondary lymphoid organs, where they encounter antigen-presenting cells and become antigen-specific lymphocytes. Plasma cells and T-cells exit secondary lymphoid organs to circulate in the blood, from which they are recruited to peripheral tissues. T cells regulate macrophage activation and recruitment by secreting specific mediators (lymphokines), modulate antibody production and cell-mediated cytotoxicity and maintain immune memory (Fig. 2-35A). NK and other lymphocyte subtypes help eliminate viruses and bacteria.

Plasma Cells

Plasma cells derive from B lymphocytes that have encountered antigen and differentiated into antibody-secreting cells. They are rich in rough endoplasmic reticulum and are the main source of circulating antibodies (Fig. 2-35B). Antibody production at sites of chronic inflammation is important for neutralizing targeted antigens, clearing foreign antigens and particles, and antibody-dependent cell-mediated cytotoxicity (see **Chapter 4**).

Dendritic Cells

Dendritic cells are professional antigen-presenting cells that trigger antigen-specific immune responses (see **Chapter 4**). They phagocytose antigens and migrate to lymph nodes, where they present those antigens. Recognition of antigen and other costimulatory molecules by T cells results in recruitment of specific cell subsets to the inflammatory process. During chronic inflammation, dendritic cells in inflamed tissues help prolong responses.

Fibroblasts

Fibroblasts are long-lived, ubiquitous cells, that mainly produce components of the ECM (Fig. 2-35C). They are the

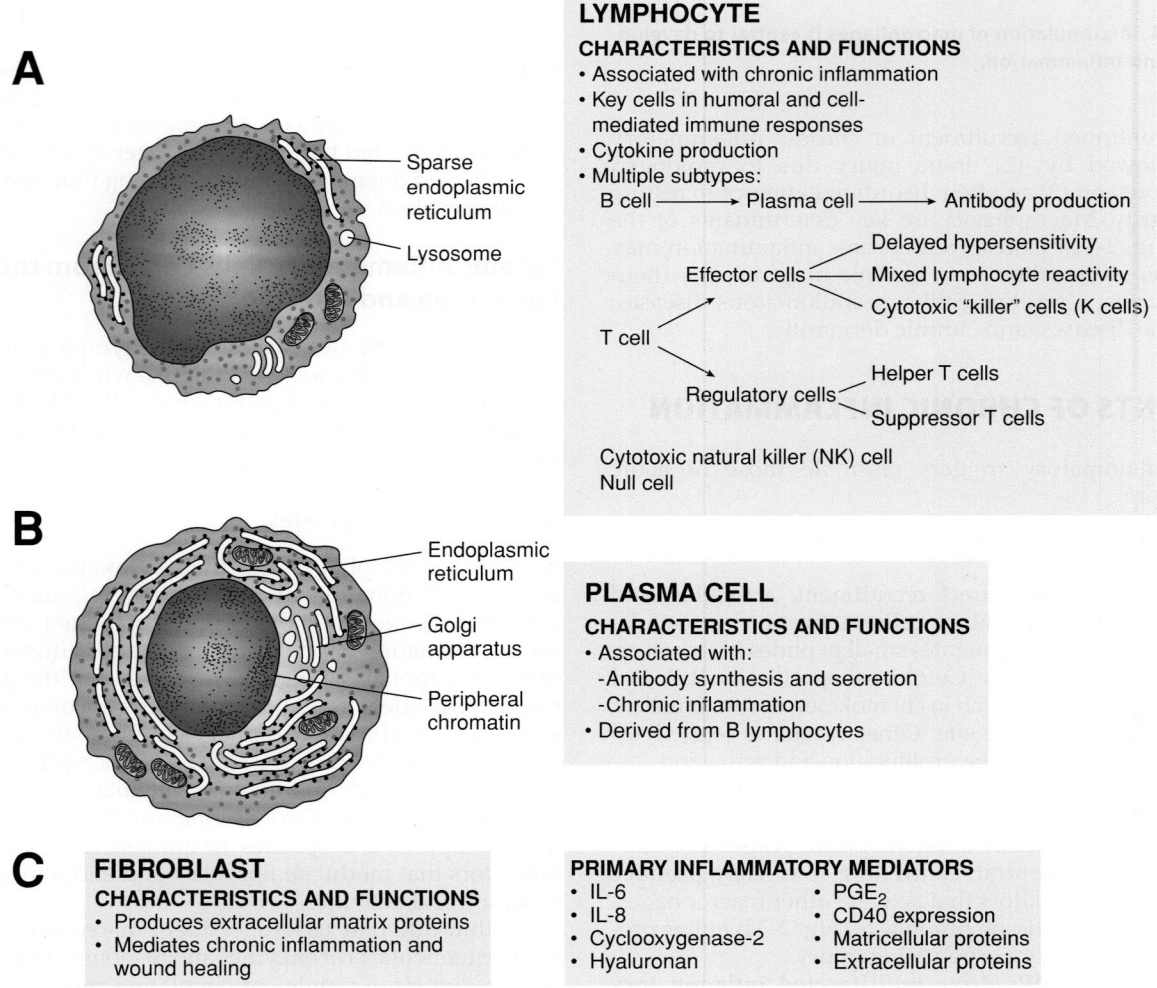

FIGURE 2-35. More cells of inflammation: morphology and function. A. Lymphocyte. **B.** Plasma cell. **C.** Fibroblast.

tissue construction crew, rebuilding the ECM scaffolding upon which tissue can be reestablished. They also differentiate into other connective tissue cells (e.g., chondrocytes, adipocytes, osteocytes, smooth muscle cells). Fibroblasts not only respond to immune signals that induce their proliferation and activation, but also actively abet immune responses. They interact with inflammatory cells, particularly lymphocytes, via surface molecules and receptors on both cells. For example, when CD40 on fibroblasts binds its ligand on lymphocytes, both cells are activated. Activated fibroblasts produce cytokines, chemokines, and prostanoids, creating a tissue microenvironment that further regulates inflammatory cell behavior in damaged tissues. This process results in resolution and subsequent wound healing or chronic persistent inflammation (see **Chapter 3**).

Acute Inflammatory Cells

Neutrophils, although characteristically acute inflammatory cells, may also participate in chronic inflammation if there is ongoing infection and tissue damage. Eosinophils are particularly prominent in allergic reactions and parasitic infestations.

Reparative Responses in Chronic Inflammation Include Granulation Tissue and Fibrosis

Repair processes initiated as part of inflammation can restore normal architecture and function. However, if inflammation is prolonged or exaggerated, repair may be ineffective, alter tissue architecture, and impair tissue function (Fig. 2-33). Thus:

- Ongoing proliferation of epithelial cells can cause metaplasia (see **Chapter 1**). Goblet cell metaplasia, for example, occurs in smokers' airways.
- Fibroblast proliferation and activation increase ECM, which now occupies space previously devoted to tissue cells. Organ function may thus be impacted.
- ECM may be altered. Matrix degradation and production change the normal mix of extracellular proteins. Altered ECM (e.g., fibronectin) can be a chemoattractant for inflammatory cells and alter cellular scaffolding.

Persistent tissue injury in chronic inflammation contributes to the pathogenesis of several diseases, including emphysema, rheumatoid arthritis, some immune complex diseases, gout, hepatic cirrhosis, and pulmonary fibrosis. Phagocytic cell adherence, escape of ROS, and release of lysosomal enzymes all increase cytotoxicity and tissue degradation. Proteinase activity is elevated in chronic wounds, creating a proteolytic environment that prevents healing. Many of these diseases can be treated with drugs that broadly inhibit lymphocyte and macrophage activity (immunosuppressive agents), or that block specific cytokines involved in chronic inflammation.

Granulomatous Inflammation

Granulomatous inflammation develops when phagocytosis is persistently stimulated. This may occur in several settings including:

- The presence of inherently indigestible material (i.e., a foreign body present in tissue)

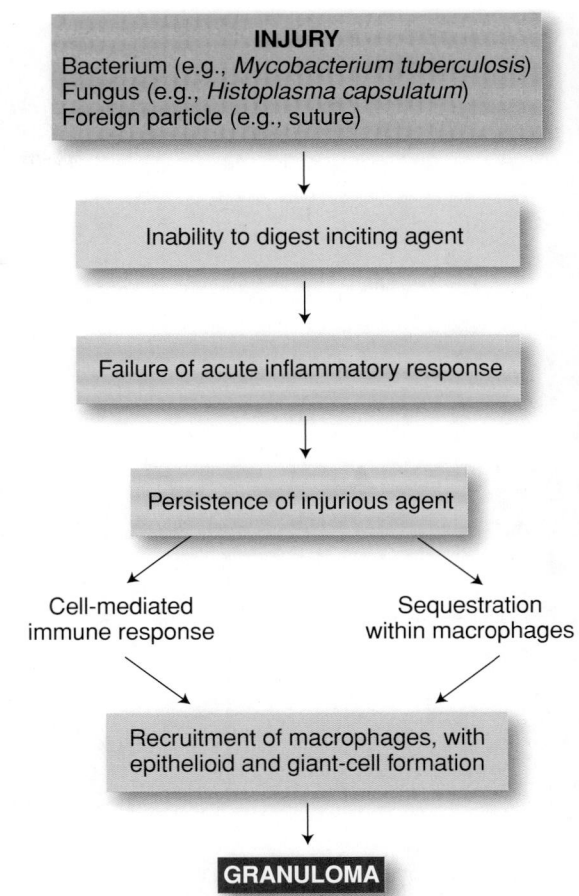

FIGURE 2-36. **Mechanism of granuloma formation.**

- Persistent infection
- Chronic stimulation of macrophages due to persistent cytokine production in autoimmune disease

These represent potential dangers, because they can lead to a vicious cycle of:

1. Phagocytosis
2. Failure of digestion
3. Phagocytic cell death
4. Release of undigested provoking agents, and
5. Rephagocytosis by newly recruited cells

Granuloma formation (Fig. 2-36) is a protective response that occurs in this setting, and may be seen in chronic infection (e.g., some fungi, tuberculosis) and in the presence of foreign material (e.g., silk suture, asbestos). It isolates a persistent offending agent, preventing it from disseminating and restricting inflammation, thus protecting the host. (Evidence suggests that some pathogens, e.g., *M. tuberculosis*, stimulate granuloma formation, which protects them from elimination by host cells.) Some autoimmune diseases are also associated with granulomas (e.g., Crohn disease, sarcoidosis).

The main cells of granulomatous inflammation are epithelioid macrophages, which have abundant pinkish cytoplasm and so vaguely resemble squamous cells, and lymphocytes (Fig. 2-37). Nodular collections of macrophages accumulate at the site of an indigestible phagocytic stimulus (Fig. 2-37A). "Frustrated" macrophages also fuse

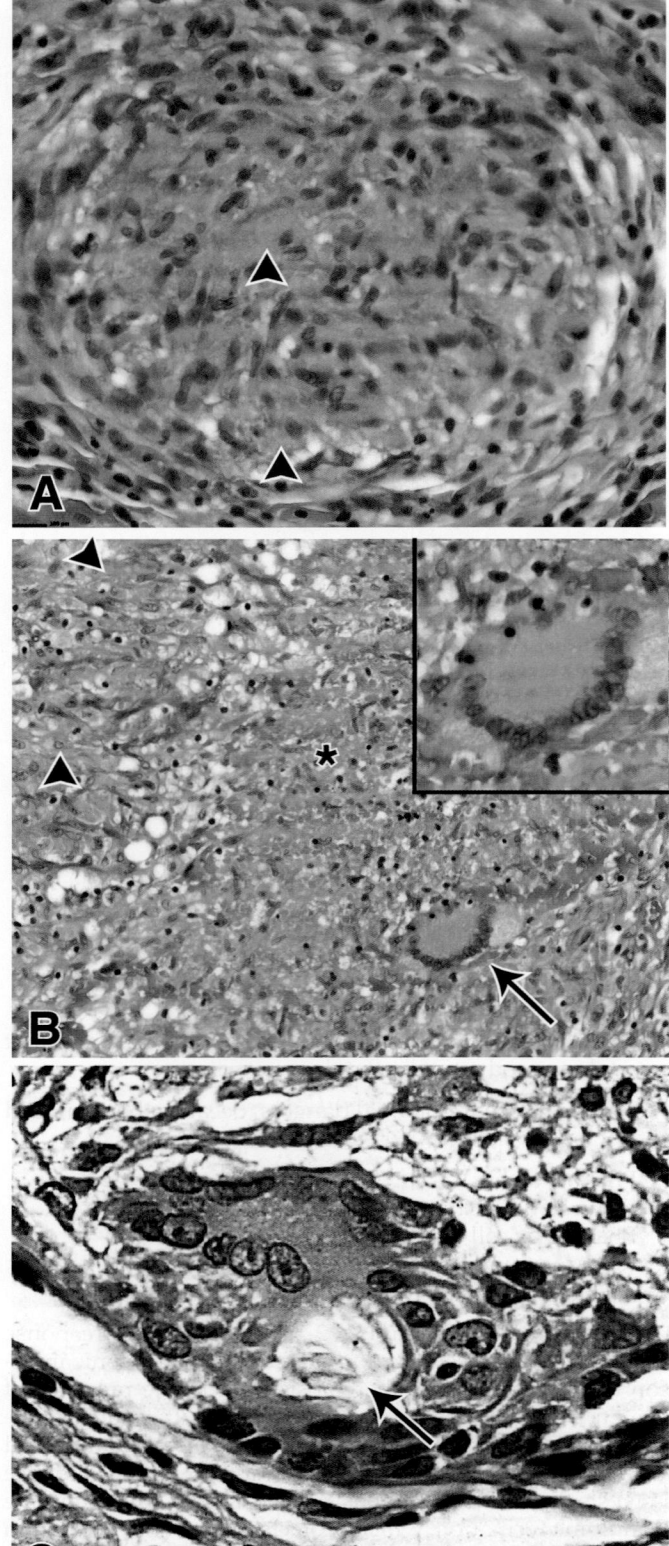

their cytoplasm to become syncytial multinucleated **giant cells**, of which there are several types. When their multiple nuclei are arrayed around the cell's periphery in a horseshoe pattern, the cell is called a *Langhans giant cell* (Fig. 2-37B); if a foreign agent (e.g., silica) or other indigestible material persists in the cytoplasm of a multinucleated giant cell, the multiple nuclei tend to disperse throughout the cytoplasm; this is a *foreign body giant cell* (Fig. 2-37C). In addition to macrophages, granulomas contain CD4+ T lymphocytes; these are recruited to the site of inflammation by cytokines produced by activated macrophages and giant cells, and form a concentric ring or "collar" around the central core of macrophages, giant cells and sometimes, necrotic debris. Several T-cell cytokines stimulate macrophage function (e.g., IFNγ), while others inhibit macrophage activation (e.g., IL-4, IL-10). Thus, lymphocytes are vital for regulating development and resolution of inflammatory responses.

Granulomas are further subdivided according to whether they show necrosis. Some infectious agents, such as *M. tuberculosis*, ultimately kill the macrophages that phagocytose them and destroy nearby tissue, to produce **necrotizing granulomas**, with centers filled with amorphous mixtures of debris and dead microorganisms and cells. When the initiating stimulus is not lethal to macrophages and local tissues, as in sarcoidosis, **nonnecrotizing granulomas** result. Centers these granulomas contain viable epithelioid macrophages and giant cells.

The outcome of granulomatous reactions depends on the immunogenicity and toxicity of the inciting agent. Cell-mediated immune responses may modify granulomatous reactions by recruiting and activating more macrophages and lymphocytes. Under the influence of T-cell cytokines, like IL-13 and TGFβ, granulomas may burn out and become fibrotic nodules.

Consequences of Inflammation

Effective inflammatory responses will:

1. Limit the area of injury
2. Clear the inciting pathologic agent and damaged tissue; and
3. Restore tissue integrity (and, if possible, tissue function).

However, unchecked or inappropriate inflammation can damage the site of initial injury, and lead to potentially severe or even fatal systemic consequences.

LOCAL CONSEQUENCES OF INFLAMMATION

As described above, significant local consequences of inflammation include edema (which may cause significant morbidity and even mortality if it occurs in a confined space, such as within the brain) and abscess formation. In addition, local consequences of acute inflammation include:

■ **Fibrinous exudate**. Occasionally, fibrin deposition dominates acute inflammation. When this occurs on a serosal surface, for example, the pericardium, *fibrinous pericarditis* occurs. If sufficiently severe, this may compromise

FIGURE 2-37. Types of granulomas. A. Granuloma with many pale epithelioid cells (e.g., *arrowheads*). **B.** Necrotizing granuloma with central necrosis (*), peripheral epithelioid cells (*arrowheads*) and Langhans giant cell with multiple nuclei arrayed peripherally and abundant cytoplasm (*arrow* and *inset*). **C.** Foreign body giant cell with scattered nuclei randomly arranged in the cytoplasm and foreign material (*arrow*) in the center.

cardiac function. Similarly, *fibrinous pleuritis* entails fibrinous pleural exudation, and may compromise lung function.
- **Ulceration.** Injury to epithelial structures due to neutrophils and the mediators they release (plus ROS and NO), can denude the epithelium and expose the underlying connective tissue. This is **ulceration.** As the underlying connective tissue is vascular, significant bleeding can result, and can be severe if an ulcer erodes into a large blood vessel in the subepithelial connective tissue.
- **Keloid formation.** Fibrosis may continue after the physical continuity of the injured tissue is restored, and may create collagenous masses—**keloids** or **hypertrophic scars** (see **Chapter 3**).

SYSTEMIC CONSEQUENCES OF INFLAMMATION

Acute Phase Reactions

Symptomatically, these manifest as fever, malaise, somnolence and anorexia (reduced appetite)—that is, the general features of feeling ill. In tissues, acute phase reactions include degradation of skeletal muscle proteins, hypotension, hepatic synthesis of complement and coagulation factors and altered circulating white blood cell (WBC) pools. As discussed above, **IL-1, IL-6,** and **TNFα** are the most important culprits. The overall increase in circulating plasma proteins in acute-phase responses increases the **erythrocyte sedimentation rate (ESR)**—the rate at which cells in uncentrifuged, anticoagulated blood settle by gravity (measured in mm/hr). Though qualitative and nonspecific, ESR is clinically useful as an indicator of systemic inflammation.

- **Leukocytosis** (increased WBC count) is common in inflammatory reactions, especially those caused by bacterial infections. WBC counts (normally 4,000 to 10,000 cells/μL) typically increases to 15,000 to 20,000 cells/μL, and exceptionally may reach 25,000 to 50,000 cells/μL, which is sometimes called a *leukemoid reaction,* mimicking chronic myeloid leukemia (see **Chapter 26**). During infectious stress, IL-1 and TNFα may cause the bone marrow to release immature neutrophil precursors. This increases total WBC count, and is called a "left-shift." Prolonged infection also induces compensatory proliferation of WBC precursors in the bone marrow, due to IL-1- and TNFα-driven production of colony-stimulating factors. Increased WBC counts in most bacterial infections are relatively selective for neutrophils (neutrophilia). In parasitic infections and allergies, eosinophils may be increased (eosinophilia), and certain viruses may increase circulating lymphocytes (lymphocytosis).
- **Leukopenia** is an absolute decrease in circulating WBCs. Although leukocytosis is far more common with infections, patients who are malnourished or who have chronic debilitating diseases like disseminated cancer may respond to infection with leukopenia, rather than leukocytosis. Leukopenia may also occur in typhoid fever, and certain viral and rickettsial infections.
- **Fever** is a classical clinical hallmark of inflammation. As discussed above, molecules that induce fever—

pyrogens—may be endogenous (most importantly IL-1, IL-6, and TNFα) or exogenous, including bacterial and viral products. IL-1 stimulates prostaglandin synthesis in hypothalamic thermoregulatory centers, thus altering the "thermostat" that controls body temperature. This is the basis for the antipyretic effect of cyclooxygenase inhibitors (e.g., aspirin). TNFα and IL-6 also increase body temperature by acting directly on the hypothalamus. Chills (sensations of cold), rigors (profound chills with shivering and piloerection), and sweats (to allow heat dissipation) may occur with fever.
- **Pain** associated with inflammation is mostly a neural response, initiated in injured tissues by specific *nociceptors,* high-threshold receptors for thermal, chemical, and mechanical stimuli. Most chemical mediators of inflammation discussed in this chapter activate peripheral nociceptors directly or indirectly. **Kinins,** especially bradykinin, formed after tissue trauma and during inflammation, activate primary sensory neurons to transmit pain signals. Cytokines, particularly TNFα and IL-1, -6, and -8, increase sensitivity to pain caused by mechanical and thermal stimuli. Prostaglandins and growth factors may directly activate nociceptors but act mostly by enhancing nociceptor sensitivity, which may cause people to perceive pain, even with normally innocuous stimuli.
- **Disseminated intravascular coagulation (DIC)** occurs when coagulation pathway activation leads to widespread microthrombi, consuming clotting components and so predisposing to bleeding. This occurs most often with endothelial injury so extensive that coagulation is activated systemically, overwhelming local regulatory mechanisms (see **Chapters 12 and 26**). This may occur in systemic infection (sepsis) or severe trauma.
- **Shock.** The most dangerous systemic consequence of inflammation occurs if tissue injury is massive, or if infection invades the blood (sepsis, **Chapter 12**). Then, large quantities of cytokines, especially TNFα, overwhelm local regulatory mechanisms and enter the systemic circulation where they cause generalized vasodilation and increase vascular permeability, thus reducing effective intravascular volume. This causes cardiac output to drop, and may lower blood pressure to the point that critical organs and tissues receive inadequate perfusion. Multiorgan system failure and death may result.

The **hypothalamic–pituitary–adrenal axis** is central to many of the systemic effects of inflammation, particularly fever. Notably, since inflammation triggers adrenal cortical release of anti-inflammatory glucocorticoids, loss of adrenal function can magnify the severity of inflammation.

Persistent Chronic Inflammation

Several chronic infectious diseases are associated with eventual tumor development. For example, schistosomiasis in the urinary bladder leads to squamous carcinoma of that organ. Pulmonary tuberculosis is associated with adenocarcinoma of the lung. Inflammation that is not specifically linked to infection may also be a risk factor for cancer; for example, patients with reflux esophagitis or ulcerative colitis have increased risk for adenocarcinomas in those organs. Chronic inflammation promotes malignant transformation by several mechanisms (see **Chapter 5**):

- **Increased cell proliferation:** Chronically increased mitotic activity raises the chance that a transforming mutation may occur in proliferating cells.
- **Oxygen and NO• metabolites:** Inflammatory metabolites, for example, nitrosamines, may damage DNA (see **Chapter 5**).

- **Chronic immune activation:** The cytokine milieu of chronic antigen exposure suppresses cell-mediated immunity, and so antitumor immune surveillance.
- **Angiogenesis:** Inflammation stimulates angiogenesis, which may also facilitate and sustain tumor growth.
- **Inhibition of apoptosis:** Chronic inflammation suppresses apoptosis. Combined with increased cell division, decreased apoptosis favors survival and expansion of mutant cell clones.

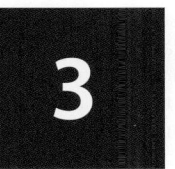

3 Repair, Regeneration, and Fibrosis

Jeffrey M. Davidson, Luisa A. DiPietro, Gregory C. Sephel

INTRODUCTION

From scarring to regeneration, damaged tissues heal in ways that ensure the organism's immediate survival. Observations regarding wound repair (healing) date to physicians in ancient Egypt and battle surgeons in classical Greece. Clotting of blood to prevent exsanguination was recognized as the first necessary event in wound healing. With the advent of the microscope, studies of infected wounds led to the discovery that inflammatory cells are primary actors in the repair process. The importance of antisepsis to wound healing is now taken for granted. However, from the 2nd-century Greco-Roman physician Galen until Pasteur and Lister at the end of the 19th century, the presence of pus at a wound site was praised and even referred to as "laudable pus." In 1876, British physician Joseph Lister was invited to serve as president of the Surgical Section of the International Medical Congress in Philadelphia. Five years later, President Garfield died after being shot by an assassin, succumbing not to damage from the bullet but several months later to pus and sepsis, the result of tissue probing by doctors leery of the germ theory and antiseptic methods. The importance of extracellular matrix (ECM), specifically collagen, in tissue integrity and wound healing was first recognized through study of scurvy, a disease that claimed the lives of millions (see Chapter 8). In 1747, Dr. James Lind, a surgeon in England's Royal Navy, conducted what is thought to be the first controlled clinical trial. Aboard the HMS Salisbury, he separated scurvy-ridden sailors into six treatment groups and observed that sailors given oranges and lemons derived the greatest benefit by preventing the reopening of wounds and loss of teeth. In 1907, the role of vitamin C began to be clarified when Norwegians Axel Holst and Theodor Frølich discovered that guinea pigs, like humans, were unable to synthesize vitamin C (ascorbic acid). Ascorbate was eventually found necessary for the action of prolyl hydroxylase, an enzyme required for proper posttranslational folding and stabilization of the collagen triple helix,

a fundamental process in establishing tissue integrity and building a strong scar.

While thoughts of regeneration evoke visions of flatworms and starfish, human liver regeneration was the basis of the Greek myth of Prometheus, whose liver regenerated daily. Modern concepts of regeneration and cell differentiation progressed in the latter half of the 20th century. In the 1950s, Sir John Gurdon determined that transplanting somatic cell nuclei into a *Xenopus* egg could form a normal adult organism; his work presaged current technologies that have yielded clonal propagation of several mammalian species and generation of inducible pluripotent stem cells (iPSC) from many tissues. Current studies on epigenetic control of gene expression, stem and progenitor cell biology, and directed control of differentiation patterns in cells are rapidly advancing the fields of regenerative healing and tissue engineering.

Wound healing encompasses diverse cell types, matrix proteins, growth factors, and soluble signals (e.g., cytokines) that collectively regulate and modulate the repair process. Nearly every stage in this process is redundantly controlled, and there are few rate-limiting factors except uncontrolled infection, blood coagulation, and availability of oxygenated blood and nutrients. ECM (see below) is central to both repair and regeneration. Matrix deposition and composition are fundamental to tissue repair and fibrosis, and to maintaining undifferentiated stem and progenitor cell populations, so as to promote regeneration and repair. In adults, *successful healing maintains tissue function and repairs tissue barriers, preventing blood loss and infection, but it is usually accomplished through excessive collagen deposition or scarring (fibrosis).* Better understanding of growth factors, ECM, and inflammatory and stem cell biology improves healing, and opens avenues to restoring injured tissues to their pre-existing architecture and of engineering replacement tissues.

Successful repair relies on a crucial balance between the *yin* of tissue formation and the *yang* of tissue remodeling. *Regeneration is favored when matrix composition and tissue architecture are fully restored.* Thus, wounds that do not heal may reflect excess proteinase activity, reduced signaling, decreased matrix accumulation, or altered matrix assembly. Conversely, fibrosis and scarring may result from inadequate proteinase activity or increased matrix production. Although new collagen formation during repair is essential for restoring strength at the healing site, fibrosis is a major complication of diseases that involve chronic injury.

THE BASIC PROCESSES OF HEALING

Many of the basic cellular and molecular participants required for wound healing also contribute to other processes of dynamic tissue change, such as morphogenesis and tumor growth. Key mechanisms required for wound healing, once hemostasis is achieved, are:

- **Cellular migration**
- **Inflammation**
- **ECM organization and remodeling**
- **Cell proliferation**

Cell Migration Initiates Repair

Cells That Migrate to the Wound

Several factors activate local cells and cause cells to migrate into a wound. There are changes in the local mechanical environment. The injury causes **mast cells and platelets** to secrete preformed stores of mediators, and stimulates them to make others. Preformed mediators include cytokines, chemoattractants, proteases, and proinflammatory chemicals that influence vascular tone and permeability, degrade damaged tissue, and initiate repair.

Collagen that is exposed at sites of endothelial damage activates platelets, which then aggregate. Together with fibrin clot formation, this limits blood loss. Activated platelets release **platelet-derived growth factor (PDGF)** and other molecules that facilitate adhesion, coagulation, vasoconstriction, cell proliferation, and clot resorption. Mast cells are bone marrow–derived cells that reside in connective tissue near small blood vessels. They recognize and respond to foreign antigens by releasing the contents of their granules, which contain high concentrations of vasoactive amines like histamine and serotonin, and chemoattractant molecules. Many of these modulate capillary function. **Resident macrophages,** tissue-fixed mesenchymal cells, and epithelial cells also contribute mediators that stimulate early responses to injury. The cellularity of wound sites increases rapidly and transiently via cell proliferation and cell recruitment (Fig. 3-1). *Cell types characteristic of skin wounds are:*

- **Leukocytes** arrive quickly at the wound site early. They adhere to activated endothelium, exit the circulation, and migrate rapidly into tissue by forming small focal adhesions with matrix molecules (fibrin, fibronectin, collagen). A family of small peptide chemoattractants **(chemokines)** mediates both restricted and broad recruitment of particular leukocyte subtypes (see Chapter 2). Several leukocyte subtypes are critical to healing:
  - **Neutrophils** from the circulation and bone marrow can invade the wound site within minutes. They degrade and destroy nonviable tissue and infectious organisms

by ingesting foreign substances, releasing their granular contents, and generating reactive oxygen species (ROS). Neutrophils are short lived, and soon undergo apoptosis, whereupon macrophages ingest and remove them. Dying neutrophils release dense nets of nuclear DNA (see Chapter 1) that trap bacteria.

- **Macrophages** reside in tissues, and additional macrophages are recruited from **monocytes** that are available in large numbers from the circulation, bone marrow, and spleen. Monocyte recruitment begins shortly after neutrophils enter a wound, but the newly differentiated macrophages spend much more time in wounds. They phagocytose debris and apoptotic neutrophils. By releasing cytokines, chemoattractants, and eventually, growth factors, they also orchestrate the inflammatory cascade and development of granulation tissue. Wound macrophages include a continuum of phenotypes. In early wounds, macrophages promote inflammation by releasing proinflammatory mediators. In later stages of repair, most macrophages adopt a healing phenotype, and produce growth factors that stimulate cell proliferation, protein synthesis, and active restoration of new tissue. Macrophages are essential for tissue repair: defects in macrophage function impair wound healing in many conditions, such as diabetes.

- **Mast cells** are resident tissue cells that respond to injury and other stimuli by quickly releasing mediators that promote inflammation. Because they degranulate quickly and completely, mast cells often appear only as ghosts in early wounds. With time, bone marrow progenitors replenish mast cell numbers. Mast cells release many mediators that influence tissue repair. After injury, resident mast cells quickly release vasoactive amines and lipid mediators that cause capillaries to dilate and become more permeable, causing tissue edema. Mast cells release multiple proinflammatory cytokines/chemokines. They also secrete a variety of factors that promote tissue growth, including epithelial growth and angiogenesis. The ability of mast cells to promote fibrotic growth involves the production of multiple mediators that promote fibrosis, such as **tryptase, chymase, transforming growth factor-β₁ (TGFβ₁),** and other factors. The presence of large numbers of mast cells is linked to eventual scar formation.

- **Dendritic cells (DCs)** are resident antigen-presenting cells that regulate innate and adaptive immunity. They can proliferate in some tissues, such as skin, are also recruited from bone marrow or derive from closely related macrophages.

- **Dendritic epidermal T cells (DETCs)** are the major population of T cells in the skin. They exhibit an invariant surface receptor, and promote tissue homeostasis and repair in skin. Injured keratinocytes communicate with DETCs, which in turn produce growth factors that stimulate repair. In contrast to DETCs, **antigen-specific CD4⁺ and CD8⁺ T cells,** although present in skin wounds, do not appear to play critical roles in normal healing. In skin fibrotic diseases, such as scleroderma, T-cell subsets appear to have multiple roles (see Chapter 28).

- **Fibroblasts, myofibroblasts, pericytes, and smooth muscle cells** are a spectrum of mesenchymal cells that are recruited locally and are also populated from progenitors in bone marrow. They migrate and propagate via

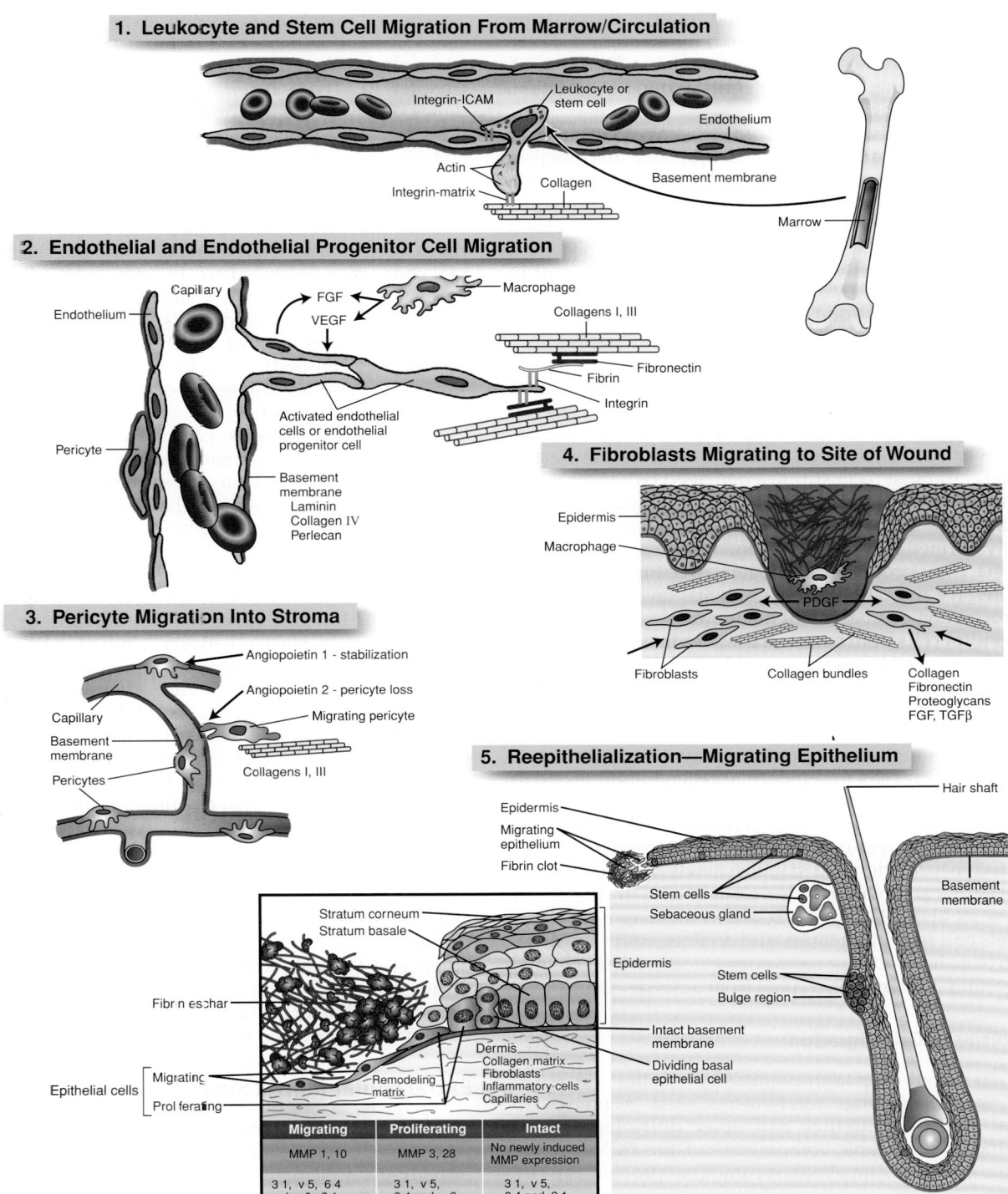

FIGURE 3-1. Resident and migrating cells initiate repair and regeneration. 1. After cytokine activation of capillary endothelium, leukocytes and bone marrow–derived circulating stem cells attach to, and migrate between, capillary endothelial cells; penetrate the basement membrane; and enter the interstitial matrix in response to chemotactic signals. **2.** Under the influence of locally released angiogenic factors, capillary endothelial cells lose their connection with the basement membrane and extend through the provisional matrix to form new capillaries. Pericytes and basement membranes are required to stabilize new and existing capillary structures. **3.** Pericytes detach from capillary endothelial cells and their basement membranes to migrate into the matrix. **4.** Under the influence of growth factors such as platelet-derived growth factor (PDGF), fibroblasts become bipolar and migrate through the matrix to the site of injury where transforming growth factor-β (TGFβ) can cause differentiation into smooth muscle actin–containing myofibroblasts. These then become bipolar and migrate through the matrix to the site of injury. **5.** During reepithelialization, groups of basal keratinocytes at the wound edge release from underlying basement membrane, take on a migratory behavior, and penetrate between the fibrin eschar (if present) and the granulation tissue that generates wound dermis. Migrating cells switch to a different display of integrin matrix receptors that recognize provisional matrix and stromal collagen (type I) and to different metalloproteinases that favor migration and matrix remodeling. *FGF* = fibroblast growth factor; *VEGF* = vascular endothelial growth factor.

signals from growth factors and matrix degradation products, populating a skin wound by day 3 or 4. These cells mediate synthesis of connective tissue (fibroplasia), tissue remodeling, vascular integrity, wound contraction, and wound strength.

- **Endothelial cells** sprout from existing postcapillary venules and also arise from circulating bone marrow progenitors. Nascent capillaries form in response to growth factors and are visible in wound granulation tissue, together with fibroblasts, beyond day 3. Vascularization is critical for gas exchange, nutrient delivery, and influx of inflammatory cells. Capillary growth is exuberant in healing wounds, with vascular density exceeding that of normal tissue manyfold. Most newly formed capillaries eventually regress, as tissue remodels and returns to a more normal architecture.
- **Epidermal cells** move across the surface of a skin wound (Fig. 3-1.5). If the wound is superficial, epithelial cells can migrate quickly and restore epithelial barrier function. However, epithelialization is slower if the migrating epithelial cells must reconstitute a damaged basement membrane. In open wounds, keratinocytes migrate between a desiccated fibrin clot (see below) and pre-existing or newly formed stromal collagen, which is coated with plasma glycoproteins, fibrinogen, and fibronectin. The progressive migration of the epithelial layer depends on the formation of a basement membrane.
- **Progenitor cells** from bone marrow, dermis, and epidermis provide renewable sources of epidermal and dermal cells that can migrate, proliferate, and differentiate. Marrow-derived, multipotential progenitors of fibroblasts and endothelium are recruited to sites of injury (Fig. 3-1.1) as well, although they appear to play a temporary role in repair. Stem cells for epidermal regeneration reside in both the bulge region of the hair follicle and the interfollicular epidermis (Fig. 3-1.4). Perivascular mesenchymal cells can also be recruited to wound sites to aid in connective tissue formation and stabilize newly formed capillaries. Dermal progenitors, also associated with the lower hair shaft and follicular bulb, aid in forming new blood vessels and new epithelium, and regenerating skin structures (e.g., hair follicles, sebaceous glands). Mesenchymal progenitor cells may also come from adipose tissue.

Mechanisms of Cell Migration

Activation of cell migration requires two critical processes during wound healing: receptor-mediated responses to chemical signals (**cytokines** and other diffusible chemokines) and the insoluble components of the ECM. At the inception of injury, ameboid locomotion propels rapidly migrating leukocytes via wave-like membrane extensions, or **lamellipodia.** Slower-moving cells, like fibroblasts, extend narrower, finger-like membrane protrusions called **filopodia.** Chemical gradients of growth factors and chemokines bind and activate specific cell surface receptors, and influence cell polarization and membrane extensions in response to chemokine concentration gradients. Intracellular **actin fibrils** polymerize and form a network at the membrane's leading edge, propelling lamellipodia and filopodia forward, with traction achieved by engaging extracellular substrates. Actin-related proteins modulate actin assembly and control regional cell rigidity by rapidly assembling, stabilizing, and destabilizing actin networks.

The cell membrane's leading edge impinges upon adjacent ECM and adheres to it through allosterically activated, transmembrane adhesion receptors, called **integrins** (see Chapter 2). These heterodimers show significant redundancy; many of the 24 known vertebrate integrin combinations recognize the same matrix components (e.g., collagen, laminin, fibronectin) with varying affinity. The relative proportions of different integrins and their state of activation allow distinction of basement membrane, provisional, and stromal matrices. Focal contacts develop when the integrin extracellular domain adheres to the provisional or stromal connective tissue matrix. In vitro, focal adhesions form under the cell body, while smaller focal contacts form at the leading edges of migrating cells. The focal contact anchors actin stress fibers, against which myosins pull to extend or contract the cell body. As cells move forward, older adhesions at the rear are weakened or destabilized, allowing the trailing edge to retract.

Hundreds of proteins participate in forming adhesion plaques. Cytoplasmic domains of integrins trigger a protein cascade that anchors actin stress fibers. The Rho family of GTPases (Rho, Rac, Cdc42; see Chapter 5) is molecular switches that interact with surface receptors to regulate matrix assembly, generate focal adhesions, and organize the actin cytoskeleton.

Integrins transmit intracellular signals that also regulate cellular survival, proliferation, and differentiation (see Chapter 5). Integrin functions are affected by additional matrix receptors, such as collagen-binding discoidin domain receptors (DDRs), tetraspanins, and other cell activators (e.g., growth factors, chemokines). These molecules allosterically alter the binding avidity of integrins' extracellular domains by signaling via activation of integrin cytoplasmic tails (inside-out signaling). Thus, cytokines also influence organization and tension in matrix and tissue.

Integrin binding is also essential for many growth factor receptor signaling processes. Growth factors and integrins share several common signaling pathways, but integrins are unique in their ability to organize and anchor cytoskeleton. The interplay between cell–cell and cell–matrix connections also regulates cytoskeletal connections, and determines the shape and differentiation of epithelial, endothelial, and other cells. These same cytoskeletal connections are changed during epithelial-to-mesenchymal transitions (EMTs; see Chapter 5) that occur as epithelial cells migrate across a wound surface, during wound surface reepithelialization.

Extracellular Matrix Sustains the Repair Process

We discuss ECM in some detail, as it is critical for repair and regeneration. ECM defines the mechanical environment by providing key elements of scar tissue and contributing to the stem cell niche. Three types of ECM participate in organizing and defining the physical properties and function of tissue:

- **Basement membrane**
- **Provisional matrix**
- **Connective tissue (interstitial matrix or stroma)**

Basement Membrane

Basement membrane, or **basal lamina,** is a thin, well-defined layer of specialized ECM that separates the cells that make it from subjacent connective tissue (Fig. 3-2). This biologic boundary is important in development, healing, regeneration, and neoplasia. It provides key signals for cell differentiation,

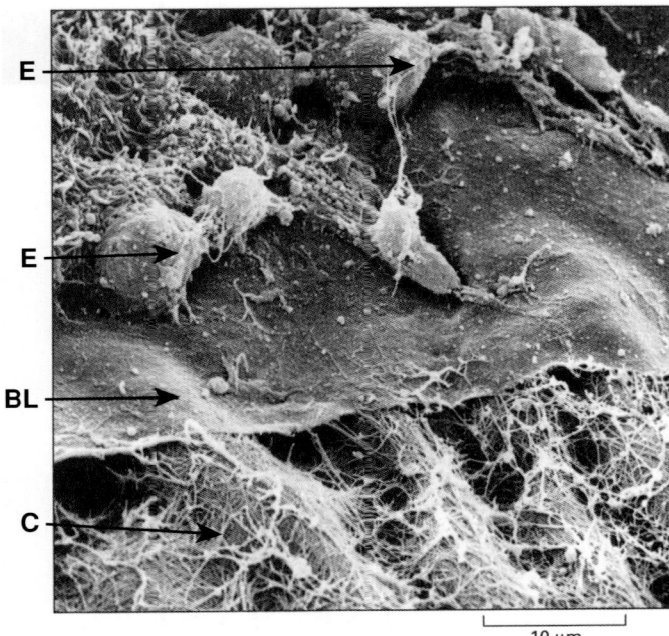

FIGURE 3-2. Scanning electron micrographs of basement membrane. The basement membrane (*BL* = basal lamina) separates chick embryo corneal epithelial cells (*E*) from underlying stromal connective tissue with collagen fibrils (*C*).

defines polarity, and contributes to tissue organization. Basement membranes are thin laminae that react with periodic acid–Schiff (PAS) stain, reflecting high glycoprotein content. Different basement membranes underlie each type of epithelium, surround epithelial ducts and tubules of skin and organs, form around adipocytes, over smooth and skeletal muscle cells and peripheral nerve Schwann cells, around capillary endothelium, and enveloping pericytes.

- Basement membranes are made from a unique set of ECM molecules, including isoforms of collagen IV, isoforms of the glycoprotein laminin, entactin/nidogen, and perlecan, a heparan sulfate proteoglycan (Table 3-1). These components self-assemble into a sandwich-like, planar structure with a covalently cross-linked type IV collagen lattice built upon the noncovalently associated laminin network.
- Within different tissues and during development, expression of unique members or isoforms of the collagen IV and laminin families imparts diversity to tissue-specific basement membranes and the many structures and functions that it supports.
- Basement membranes define epithelial cell polarity and support cellular differentiation. They are also filters, cellular anchors, and substrates for newly migrated epidermal cells after injury, and they help re-form neuromuscular junctions after nerve damage. Basement membranes determine cell shape, contribute to developmental morphogenesis, and provide a repository for growth factors and chemotactic peptides.

Provisional Matrix

Provisional matrix is the temporary extracellular milieu of soluble plasma- and tissue-derived components that accumulate at sites of injury. *Plasma-derived provisional matrix*

proteins include *fibrinogen, fibronectin, thrombospondin (TS), and vitronectin.* Other components, such as hyaluronan, tenascin, and fibronectin are made locally. These molecules associate with fibrin clots and platelets, and with pre-existing stromal matrix to limit blood/fluid loss. Provisional matrix is a loosely woven substrate that supports migration of leukocytes, endothelial cells, and fibroblasts to the wound site. The platelet thrombus also contains growth factors, most prominently PDGF. Fibrin clots form, the provisional matrix is internally stabilized, and it binds to adjacent stromal matrix by transglutaminase (factor XIII)-generated cross-links. In addition, factor XIII stabilizes the fibrin clot. Tissue transglutaminases 1 and 2 promote wound remodeling and skin regeneration.

Stromal (Interstitial Connective Tissue) Matrix

Connective tissue, also called **stroma** or **interstitium,** forms a mechanical continuum between tissue elements such as epithelia, nerves, and blood vessels, and confers resistance to compression or tension. Stroma is also important for cell migration and as a medium for storage and exchange of bioactive proteins.

Connective tissue comprises ECM and resident cells which synthesize matrix. These are mainly mesenchymal cells: fibroblasts, myofibroblasts, adipocytes, chondrocytes, osteocytes, and vascular endothelial cells. Bone marrow-derived cells (e.g., mast cells, macrophages, transient leukocytes, and mesenchymal progenitor cells) are also present.

Stroma mostly contains fibers from multiple members of the large family of collagen molecules (Table 3-2). Type I collagen is the major constituent of bone, skin, tendons, ligaments, and other structures requiring high tensile strength. Type III collagen promotes finer, more extensible fibrils, is also found in skin, and is prominent in blood vessel walls. Type II collagen predominates in cartilage. Elastic fibers, which impart elasticity to skin, large blood vessels, and lungs, are composite structures made of elastin and microfibrillar scaffolding proteins such as fibrillin and fibulin. The so-called **ground substance,** which fills much of the stroma that is not occupied by fibrous proteins, contains glycosaminoglycans (GAGs), proteoglycans, matricellular proteins, and fibronectin. These are important in many biologic functions of connective tissue and support and modulate cell attachment, migration, and differentiation.

Collagens

Collagen is the most abundant protein in the animal kingdom; it is essential for the structural integrity of tissues and organs. If its synthesis is reduced, delayed, or abnormal, wounds fail to heal, as in scurvy or nonhealing wounds. Excess collagen deposition leads to **fibrosis.** Abnormal fibrosis leads to hypertrophic scars, connective tissue diseases such as scleroderma and keloids. Scarring can compromise some tissue functions in many organs, such as the kidney, lung, heart, and liver.

Collagens are the major constituents of connective tissue in all organs: most notably cornea, arteries, dermis, cartilage, tendons, ligaments, and bone. There are at least 28 genetically distinct types of collagen molecules (designated I to XXVIII). Each is formed by three type-specific α-chains that make homo- or hetero-trimeric helices. Some collagen types have multiple α-chains and therefore different isoforms. Other proteins, not classified as collagens, also contain rigid

TABLE 3-1

BASEMENT MEMBRANE CONSTITUENTS AND ORGANIZATION

Basement Membrane Components	Chains	Molecular Structure	Molecular Associations	Basement Membrane Aggregate Form
Perlecan (heparan sulfate proteoglycan)	1 protein core 3 heparan sulfate GAG chains	GAG chains	Laminin, collagen IV, fibronectin, growth factors (VEGF, FGF), chemokines	
Laminin	16 isoforms Heterotrimers with α-, β-, γ-chains 5 α-chains, 3 β-chains, 3 γ-chains		Integrin, dystroglycan, and other receptors on a variety of cells (epithelium, endothelium, muscle, Schwann cells, adipocytes) Forms self-associated noncovalent network that organizes basement membranes Laminin, nidogen/entactin, perlecan, agrin, fibulin	
Nidogen/entactin	2-member family monomeric		Collagen IV, laminin, perlecan, fibulin Stabilizes basement membrane through association of laminin and collagen IV networks	
Collagen IV	≥3-member family Heterotrimers Chains selected from 2 or 3 of 6 unique α-chains	3 single chains form α-helical tail of collagenous regions and association of the 3 globular regions	Integrin receptors on many cells Forms covalent self-associated network Collagen IV, perlecan nidogen/entactin, SPARC	

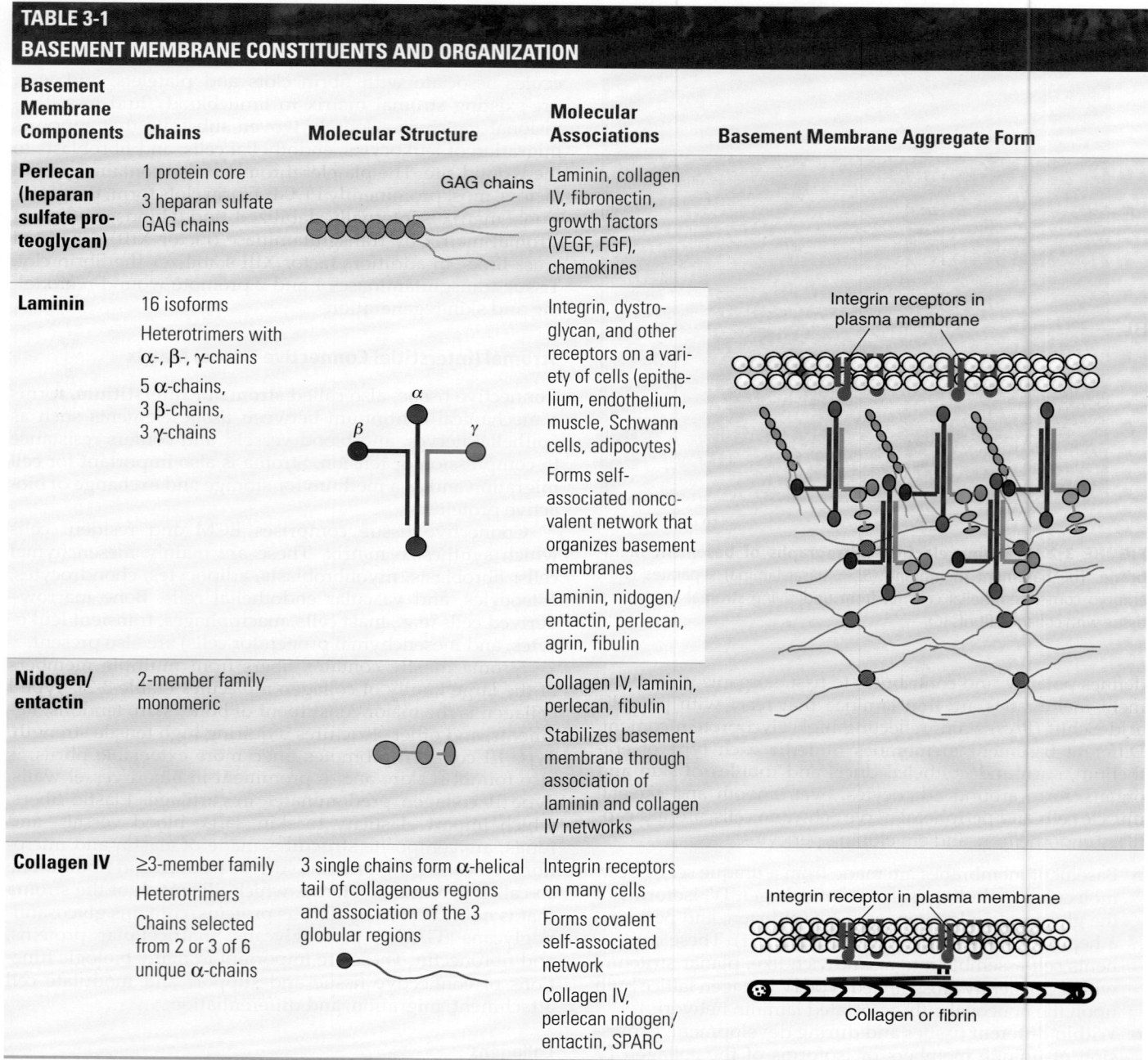

FGF = fibroblast growth factor; GAG = glycosaminoglycan; SPARC = secreted protein acidic and rich in cysteine; VEGF = vascular endothelial growth factor.

triple-helical domains of varying length and continuity. All collagen α-chains have at least one domain with a repeating α-helical sequence, usually Gly-X-Y, in which every third amino acid is glycine and X and Y are often proline or its posttranslational derivative, hydroxyproline. Formation and stability of the triple-helical structure requires this canonical collagen sequence, with its glycine repeat. It also requires ascorbate-dependent formation of hydroxyproline. Residues of lysine, hydroxylysine, and histidine are distributed along the triple-helical molecule to enable the formation of tissue-specific, intra- and intermolecular, covalent cross-links in fibrillar collagens. The continuous, uninterrupted,

cross-linked triple-helical α-chains are the main structure of stiff, fibrillar collagens. Nonfibrillar collagens contain interrupted, flexible, noncollagenous domains which may even make up the major portion of the protein. Collagen family members have important structural functions, but they also affect cell differentiation, growth, migration, and matrix morphogenesis through interaction with integrin and discoidin domain transmembrane receptors, while defining the mechanical environment.

Collagen synthesis exemplifies complex posttranslational protein modifications that yield highly insoluble molecular assemblies. Soluble procollagen molecules are formed by

TABLE 3-2
COLLAGEN MOLECULAR COMPOSITION AND STRUCTURE

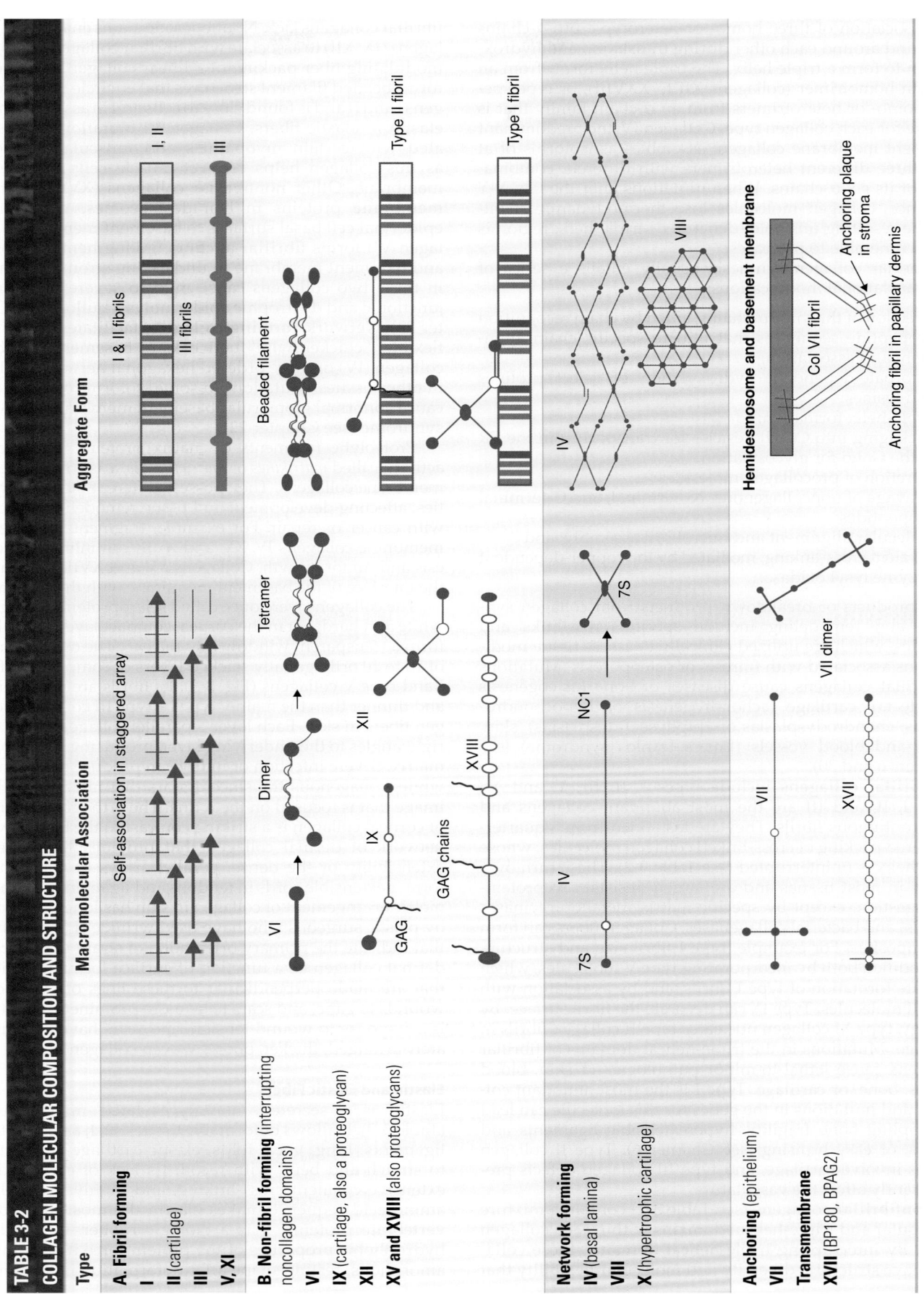

Type	Macromolecular Association	Aggregate Form

A. Fibril forming
I
II (cartilage)
III
V, XI

Self-association in staggered array

I & II fibrils — I, II
III fibrils — III

B. Non-fibril forming (interrupting noncollagen domains)
VI
IX (cartilage, also a proteoglycan)
XII
XV and XVIII (also proteoglycans)

Dimer → Tetramer — Beaded filament
VI
IX — GAG
XII
XVIII — GAG chains

Type II fibril
Type I fibril

Network forming
IV (basal lamina)
VIII
X (hypertrophic cartilage)

7S — IV — NC1
7S

IV
VIII

Anchoring (epithelium)
VII

VII — VII dimer

Hemidesmosome and basement membrane

Col VII fibril
Anchoring plaque in stroma
Anchoring fibril in papillary dermis

Transmembrane
XVII (BP180, BPAG2)

XVII

self-association of three homo- or heterotypic pro-α-chains that wind around each other during translation and hydroxylation to form a triple helix. The triple helix forms from an α-chain homotrimer (collagens XII to XXVIII), or type-specific homo- or heterotrimers from an α-chain family that is unique for each collagen type. Collagen IV, the predominant basement membrane collagen, assembles as isoforms of at least three different heterotrimers with different combinations of its six α-chains. When mutations alter the Gly-X-Y sequence, collagen molecules lose thermodynamic stability. The resulting unstable (denatured) triple-helix region is more vulnerable to proteases.

Fibrillar collagen synthesis usually entails a series of posttranslational modifications:

1. selection of the three α-chains, aided by chain recognition propeptide sequences that initiate specific chain alignment and association;
2. ascorbate-dependent hydroxylation of select prolines and lysines;
3. triple-helix formation;
4. packaging into COPII vesicles for transport from the ER to the Golgi for glycosylation;
5. secretion of procollagen molecules;
6. cleavage of noncollagenous, N- terminal, and C-terminal propeptides;
7. molecular alignment and microfibril assembly; and
8. covalent cross-linking, mediated by the copper-dependent enzyme lysyl oxidase.

Byproducts or breakdown products from collagen synthesis and remodeling include specific cross-links and peptides, which are utilized clinically to assess tissue modifications associated with fibrosis or osteoporosis. Mutations of fibrillar collagens cause diseases of bone (osteogenesis imperfecta), cartilage (achondrogenesis or hypochondrogenesis, chondrodysplasias or epiphyseal dysplasias), skin, joints, and blood vessels (Ehlers–Danlos syndrome) (see Chapters 6 and 30).

Fibrillar collagens include types I, II, III, V, and XI. Types I, II, and III are the most abundant collagens and form continuous fibrils. They are fashioned from a quarter-staggered packing of cross-linked collagen molecules, whose triple helix is uninterrupted (see Table 3-2). These turn over slowly in most tissues and are largely resistant to proteinase digestion, except by specific matrix metalloproteinases (MMPs) and bacterial collagenases. Collagen fibers can form as composites. For example, type I fibril size and structure are modified both by incorporating type V molecules, which nucleate formation of type I fibrils, and by association with type III molecules. Type IX can decorate the fibril surface. By analogy, type XI collagen nucleates type II collagen fibrils in cartilage. Mutations in the triple-helical domains of fibrillar collagens cause lethal-to-minor pathologies in skin, blood vessels, bone, or cartilage. Type I is the most abundant collagen, and mutations in the genes for this molecule can lead to crippling bone fragility, hyperextensible ligaments and dermis, or easy bruising (see Chapter 6). Type II collagen defects involve cartilage, and type III collagen defects predominantly affect the vasculature.

Nonfibrillar collagens (see Table 3-2) contain a mixture of globular and triple-helical domains within each collagen chain. By interrupting triple-helical domains, these collagens have structural diversity and molecular flexibility that fibrillar collagens lack. Nonhelical domains enable small collagens (IX, XII) to associate with fibrillar collagen fibers, thus modulating fiber packing of a linear collagen. Collagen VI forms beaded filament structures that encircle fibrillar collagens I and II and is found close to cells and in association with elastin in elastic fibers. Collagen VI mutations are associated with certain myopathies and muscular dystrophy, as this collagen helps connect muscle cells to basement membrane. Other nonfibrillar collagens (XVII) are **transmembrane** proteins in hemidesmosomes, which attach epidermal cell basal surfaces to basement membranes. Collagen VII forms **fibrillar anchors** linking hemidesmosome and basement membrane to underlying stroma. Mutations in these two collagens cause mild to severe blistering in junctional and dystrophic epidermolysis bullosa (see Chapter 28). **Network-forming collagens** facilitate formation of flexible, "chicken-wire" networks of basement membrane collagen (IV) or more ordered hexagonal networks (VIII, X) in other tissues. Mutations in some isoforms of collagen IV cause abnormal glomerular basement membranes in Alport syndrome (see Chapter 22).

Proteolytic fragments of matrix proteins with biologic activity, called *matrikines* or *matricryptins*, arise from basement membrane collagens. They possess different biologic properties, affecting development and tissue remodeling associated with cancer or repair. For example, fragments of basement membrane collagens IV, XV, and XVIII can inhibit angiogenesis and tumor growth. Collagens XV and XVIII are found at the interface of the basement membrane with the stroma.

The collagens were once called scleroproteins, being both white and hard; yet in the cornea, compact layers of collagen form a transparent window into the eye. The cornea consists of 10 to 20 orthogonally stacked layers of composites of type I and type V collagens (Fig. 3-3). Its fibrils are very uniform and thinner than the mainly type I + type III composite collagen fibers in skin. Each layer's parallel collagen fibers are at right angles to the underlying layer, producing a transparent matrix. Severe infection or injury can produce disorganized, white, collagenous translucent scars that interfere with the image that is focused on the retina. The orthogonal structure of corneal collagen is a striking contrast to the basket-weave network of dermal collagen that provides limited tissue extensibility or the dense, parallel arrays of collagen that form inextensible cords in tendons and ligaments. The asymmetric arrangement of collagen in skin has long been known by plastic surgeons who have used wrinkle (Langer's) lines that indicate the primary orientation of strain in underlying dermal collagen as a function of surface location. Incisions that are made perpendicular to these lines of strain cause wounds to gape, and scars to be more prominent. Scar tissue is a response to wound tension, and scars have inappropriately arranged, thicker, poorly woven collagen fibers.

Elastin and Elastic Fibers

Elastin is a secreted, non-glycosylated matrix protein (Table 3-3). It allows deformable tissues such as skin, uterus, ligaments, lung, vocal folds, elastic cartilage, and arteries to stretch and bend with recoil. Its lack of carbohydrate, extensive covalent cross-linking, and highly hydrophobic amino acid sequence makes elastin the most insoluble of vertebrate proteins. It is a biologic rubber, in which the hydrophobic properties of the protein force it back into its amorphous, resting shape after deformation in an aqueous

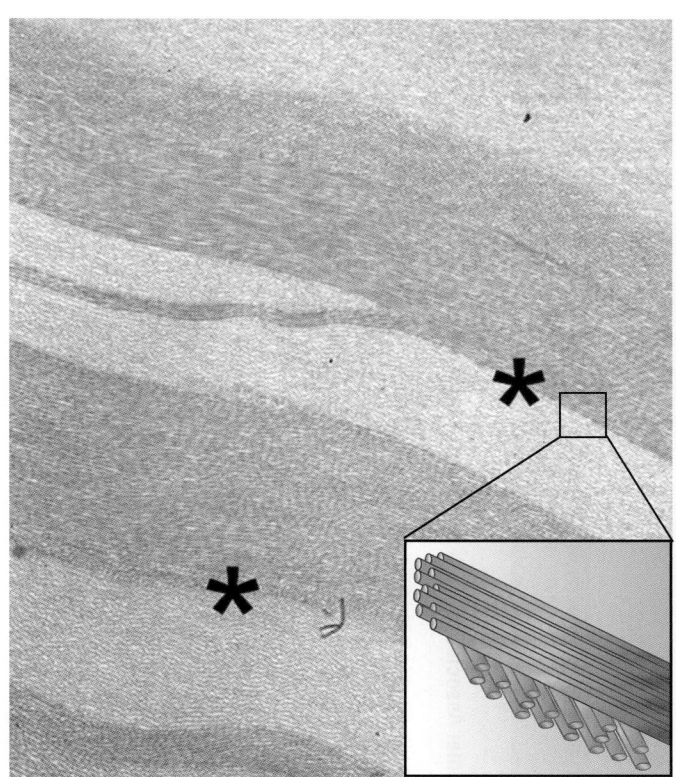

FIGURE 3-3. Human cornea, near center. Collagen fibers are highly organized in the cornea. Multiple plywood-like arrays of collagen fibers are of similar width and layers with distinct orientation are sharply demarcated between asterisks (*). This precise, unique matrix organization, layers of highly ordered collagen bundles at oblique, nearly perpendicular angles, is critical to the transparency and refractive index of the cornea.

environment. The elastic fiber is crucial for several vital tissues to function. This extremely durable protein is largely deposited during development and not efficiently replaced during repair of tissues such as skin and lung. Emphysema is characterized by loss of lung recoil due to degradation and dysfunctional replacement of alveolar elastin. The absence, impaired assembly or slow accumulation of functional elastin after damage to skin or lung is compensated, in part, by the fact that elastic fibers are extremely resistant to proteolysis and turn over slowly. Still, functional elastic fibers degenerate over time, particularly in skin, which leads to dermal atrophy, wrinkling, and loss of dermal suppleness. Excess sun exposure increases abnormal *elastotic* material that, together with age-related collagen loss, accumulates in the dermis, causing skin to become thick and coarse, furrowed with wrinkles.

Elastin turns over very little. Its durability reflects its (1) hydrophobicity, (2) extensive covalent cross-linking (mediated by lysyl oxidase, the same enzyme that cross-links collagen), and (3) resistance to most proteolytic enzymes, except elastases. Elastin formed during repair may not be appropriately arranged, a feature that is crucial to pulmonary and arterial physiology. In contrast to loss of functional elastic fibers in injured skin and lung, in hypertension, arterial wall smooth muscle cells rapidly form new concentric elastic lamellae. Furthermore, inelastic veins that are transplanted in coronary artery bypass surgery undergo *arterialization* and rapidly generate new elastic lamellae. Thus, elastin synthetic capabilities of vascular smooth muscle differ greatly from those of dermal or lung fibroblasts.

Elastic fibers form when their secreted, soluble elastin precursor (tropoelastin) condenses onto a complex of several microfibrillar glycoproteins after secretion. The best characterized microfibrillar protein is **fibrillin** (see Table 3-3). In Marfan syndrome, mutated, abnormal fibrillin binds poorly, with reduced biomechanical TGFβ activation. This pleomorphic syndrome may entail dissecting aortic aneurysms, scoliosis, and disproportionately long limbs (see Chapter 6). Mutations in another microfibrillar protein, **fibulin,** can cause a generalized elastin defect, cutis laxa.

Matrix Glycoproteins

Matrix glycoproteins, or matricellular proteins, contribute essential biologic functions to basement membrane and connective tissue stroma. These are generally large (150,000 to 1,000,000 kDa), multimeric, multidomain macromolecules with long arms that bind other matrix molecules and support or modulate cell attachment. Matrix glycoproteins help to (1) organize tissue topography, (2) support cell migration, (3) orient cells, and (4) induce cell behavior. The principal matrix glycoprotein of basement membrane is **laminin,** and that of stromal connective tissue is **fibronectin.**

LAMININS: The laminins are a versatile family of basement membrane glycoproteins whose cross-like structure is formed by products of three related gene subfamilies to form α, β, and γ heterotrimers (see Table 3-1). There are 18 known laminin isoforms, which assemble intracellularly from varying combinations of the five α-, three β-, and three γ-chains. Once secreted, some laminin trimers are further processed by proteinases. Laminin molecules self-polymerize into sheets that initiate basement membrane formation by associating with type IV collagen sheets and other basement membrane molecules. Expression of laminin isoforms in specific tissues contributes to the heterogeneity of tissue morphology and

TABLE 3-3
NONCOLLAGENOUS MATRIX CONSTITUENTS OF STROMA

Stromal Connective Tissue Components	Chains	Molecular Structure	Molecular Associations	Tissue Structures
Fibronectin	Dimeric protein. Chains chosen from ~20 splice variants of 1 gene	(fibrin, collagen, heparin cells, heparin, fibrin, RGD, N, C)	Integrin receptors of many cells (RGD-binding site). Plasma fibronectin is soluble. Cellular fibronectin can self-associate into fibrils at cell surface and also binds collagen, heparin, decorin, fibrin, certain bacteria (opsonin), LTBPs	Cell cytoplasm; Integrin receptor in plasma membrane; Collagen or fibrin
Elastin	Monomer with several splice variants, 1 gene	Elastin cross-links to form fiber	Self-association to form cross-linked amorphous fibers. Formed on scaffold of microfibrillar polymers	Elastin fiber with microfibril polymers
Fibrillins	Large glycoproteins—most common microfibrils needed for elastin fiber assembly		Forms beaded polymer. Other microfibrillar proteins: LTBPs, fibulins, emilins, MAGP 1 and 2, lysyl oxidase	
Versican (hyaluronan-binding proteoglycans)	Family of 4 related genes. Aggrecan found in cartilage. Protein core decorated with 10–30 chondroitin sulfate and dermatan sulfate GAG chains	CS	Proteoglycans linked to hyaluronan via link protein to form very large composite structure	Hyaluronan
Decorin (small leucine-rich proteoglycans)	1 protein core, 1 gene. 1 chondroitin sulfate or dermatan sulfate GAG chain. Biglycan and fibromodulin structurally related, genetically distinct		Collagens I and II, fibronectin, TGFβ, thrombospondin	Collagen I or II

GAG = glycosaminoglycan; LTBPs = latent transforming growth factor-β–binding proteins; MAGP = microfibril-associated growth protein; RGD = Arg-Gly-Asp; TGFβ = transforming growth factor-β.

functions, in part by supporting cell attachment via binding to membrane sulfated glycolipids and transmembrane receptors. These cell attachments concentrate laminin and construct the framework on which other basement membrane molecules accumulate. Laminin binds both heparan sulfate proteoglycans (see below) in basement membranes and heparan sulfate side chains on transmembrane syndecans. Cells bind to laminin via several integrins, as well as muscle dystroglycan and Lutheran blood grouping receptors, which may be involved in red cell release from bone marrow during hematopoiesis. Muscle cell dystroglycan receptor complexes bind basement membrane laminin, and mutations in either the receptor or laminin cause different forms of muscular dystrophy (see Chapter 31). Appropriate proteolytic processing of the epidermal laminin isoform is critical for normal epidermal function and wound reepithelialization. Epidermal integrity is stabilized at the basal surface by hemidesmosomes, which arise when basement membrane laminin binds epithelial integrin (integrin $\alpha_6\beta_4$), and involve transmembrane collagen XVII and subepithelial collagen VII. The latter is the *anchoring fibril* that connects the epidermal cell and basement membrane to dermal connective tissue. Mutations in epidermal laminin, the appropriate integrin, collagen VII or XVII (see above), yield different forms of a potentially fatal skin blistering disease, **epidermolysis bullosa** (see Chapter 28).

FIBRONECTINS: Fibronectins are versatile, adhesive glycoproteins that are widely distributed in stromal connective tissue and deposited in wound provisional matrix (see Table 3-3). Fibronectin chains form a V-shaped homo- or heterodimer linked at the C terminus by two disulfide bonds. Specific fibronectin domains bind bacteria, collagen, heparin, fibrin, fibrinogen, and the cell matrix receptor integrin. Indeed, the integrin receptor family has been partly defined by studies showing its specific binding to fibronectin. The multifunctional dimer links matrix molecules to one another or to cells. Blood clots (thrombi) support cell migration due to their high concentration of plasma-derived fibronectin that connects fibrin strands. This complex is further stabilized by cross-linking with factor XIII (transglutaminase) to other provisional and dermal matrix components.

There are two forms of fibronectin, encoded by one gene but synthesized by different cells: an insoluble, tissue-derived form; and a soluble, hepatocyte-derived, plasma form. Alternative splicing may generate up to 24 variant fibronectins. Thrombus-bound fibronectin supports platelet adhesion. It also promotes keratinocyte attachment and migration during reepithelialization by interacting with collagen and augmenting binding to collagen fibers. Fibronectin synthesized by mesenchymal cells, like fibroblasts, is assembled into insoluble fibrils with the aid of integrins and collagen fibrils. Polymerized cellular fibronectin is found in granulation tissue and loose connective tissue. Blood coagulation and reepithelialization of skin wounds are unaffected by deletion of plasma fibronectin, suggesting that cellular fibronectin and other factors can compensate for its absence.

Glycosaminoglycans

GAGs (historically called mucopolysaccharides) are long, linear polymers of specific repeating disaccharides, each with a uronic acid. GAG chains are distinguished by the disaccharide subunits in the polymer. The chains are negatively charged, because of carboxylate groups and, excepting hyaluronan, by modification with N- or O-linked sulfate groups. Epimerization and diversity in modifications (e.g., acetylation and sulfation) allow GAGs to be exceptionally diverse and functionally specific. When sulfated GAG chains are O-linked to serines of protein cores, to form **proteoglycans** (see below).

GAGs are degraded by lysosomes, and deficiencies in lysosomal hydrolases cause GAGs to accumulate intracellularly. Consequent *mucopolysaccharidoses* (see Chapter 6) are diverse storage disorders of connective tissue that impact many different tissues and significantly decrease life expectancy.

Hyaluronan

Hyaluronan (**hyaluronic acid**, HA) is the only GAG that does not covalently bind a protein. HA is a linear polymer of 2,000 to 25,000 disaccharides of glucosamine and glucuronic acid. Its negative charge makes hyaluronan very hydrophilic. Hyaluronan can associate with protein cores of proteoglycans that contain hyaluronan-binding regions and with hyaluronan-binding proteins at the cell surface. Certain proteoglycans associate noncovalently along the hyaluronan backbone via a link protein to form large, space-filling, hydrophilic hyaluronan/proteoglycan composites. The proteoglycans **aggrecan** and **versican** (see Table 3-3) are found in cartilage and stromal tissues, respectively. The viscosity of free hyaluronan in solution imparts resilience and lubrication to joints and connective tissue, and their accumulation around cells as part of the glycocalyx facilitates cell migration through the ECM.

Hyaluronan is highly prevalent in less-dense stromas of embryonic and fetal development, and it is added early to provisional matrix. The negatively charged carboxylate backbone of hyaluronan binds large amounts of water, creating a viscous gel that increases matrix turgor and facilitates cell migration. As a biomaterial, hyaluronan can be chemically modified to act as a temporary dermal filler, joint lubricant, or replacement for vitreous humor. Unlike other secreted macromolecules, hyaluronan synthesis occurs at the cell surface. Cells also express several types of hyaluronan receptors. Pericellular hyaluronan increases during dynamic tissue remodeling associated with inflammation, wound repair, morphogenesis, and cancer. For wound healing to resolve, inflammatory monocytes with hyaluronan-binding CD44 receptors remove pericellular and excess interstitial hyaluronan, together with hyaluronidases. Reduced hyaluronidase activity in fetal wounds may reduce inflammation and favor less scar formation.

Proteoglycans

Proteoglycans are a diverse family of proteins with varying numbers, types, and sizes of attached GAG chains linked by O-glycosidic bonds to serines or threonines in a core protein. They have higher carbohydrate content than matrix glycoproteins and, though not branched, show substantial diversity via carbohydrate modifications, such as sulfation, unique linkages, and varying sequences. Common GAGs include chondroitin sulfate, keratan sulfate, and heparan sulfate, which may each be present in a single proteoglycan at differing frequencies. Individual proteoglycans whose names are designated by the core protein can differ widely in number and choice of GAG chains, as well as tissue distribution.

Proteoglycans participate in matrix organization, structural integrity, and cell attachment. Though their protein core often has biologic activity, the properties of several proteoglycans are largely mediated by the GAG chains. The strongly charged heparan sulfate GAG chains of basement membrane (perlecan, collagen XVIII) and cell receptor proteoglycans (syndecan, glypican) modulate availability and actions of heparin-binding growth factors, such as **vascular endothelial growth factor (VEGF)**, **fibroblast growth factor (FGF)**, and **heparin-binding epidermal growth factor (HB-EGF)**. PDGF also binds these highly charged molecules weakly. A group of small proteoglycans, which share a core protein domain of leucine-rich repeats, regulates TGFβ activity and fibril formation in collagens I and II (see Table 3-3). Sequestered growth factors are released when heparanase and other hydrolases degrade proteoglycans. Tissue expression of ECM proteins and proteoglycans is shown in Table 3-4.

TABLE 3-4
TISSUE EXPRESSION OF EXTRACELLULAR MATRIX MOLECULES

Tissue or Body Fluid	Primary Mesodermal Cell	Prominent Collagen Types	Noncollagenous Matrix Proteins	Glycosaminoglycans Proteoglycans (PGs)
Plasma			Fibronectin, fibrinogen, vitronectin	Hyaluronan
Dermis **Reticular/papillary** **Epidermal junction**	Fibroblast	I, III, V, VI, XII, XXIV, XXIX, VII, XVII (BP180), anchoring fibrils, hemidesmosome	Fibronectin, elastin, fibrillin	Hyaluronan, decorin, biglycan, versican
Muscle	Muscle cell	I, III, V, VI, VIII, XII, XV, XXII	Fibronectin, elastin, fibrillin	Aggrecan, biglycan, decorin, fibromodulin
Peri-, epimysium **Aortic media/adventitia**	Fibroblast			
Tendon	Fibroblast	I, III, V, VI, XII, XXII	Fibronectin, tenascin (myotendon junction), elastin, fibrillin	Decorin, biglycan, fibromodulin, lumican, versican
Ligament	Fibroblast	I, III, V, VI	Fibronectin, elastin, fibrillin	Decorin, biglycan, versican
Cornea	Fibroblast	I, II, III, V, VI, XII, XXIV		Lumican, keratocan, mimecan, biglycan, decorin
Cartilage	Chondrocyte hypertrophic cartilage	II, IX, VI, VIII, X, XI, XXVII	Anchorin CII, fibronectin, tenascin	Hyaluronan, aggrecan, biglycan, decorin, fibromodulin, lumican, perlecan (minor)
Bone	Osteocyte	I, V, XXIV, XIII	Osteocalcin, osteopontin, bone sialoprotein, SPARC (osteonectin)	Decorin, fibromodulin, biglycan
Nervous system: **CNS, PNS (including Schwann cell basement membrane)**	Neurons, neurologic cells	I–IX; XI–XIX; XXI–XXIII; XXV, XXVII, XXVIII, XXIX	Laminins, nidogen/entactin, tenascin, thrombospondin	Chondroitin sulfate containing proteoglycans, heparan sulfate containing proteoglycans (agrin, perlecan)
Basement membrane zones	Epithelial (most organs, e.g., kidney), endothelial (capillaries), adipocytes, Schwann cell, muscle cells (endomysium), pericytes, neuromuscular junction	IV, XV, XVIII	Laminins, nidogen/entactin	Heparan sulfate proteoglycans, perlecan Collagen XVIII (vascular), agrin (neuromuscular junctions)

CNS = central nervous system; PNS = peripheral nervous system; SPARC = secreted protein acidic and rich in cysteine.

Remodeling Is the Long-Lasting Phase of Repair

As repair proceeds, inflammatory infiltrates wane, and capillary formation crescendos, then declines. During normal remodeling, fibroblasts rapidly increase and then drop as equilibrium between collagen deposition and degradation is restored. MMPs are the main remodeling enzymes, while neutrophil-derived **cathepsins** and **serine proteases** are also present at the early phase of wound debridement or in cases of persistent infection. Unlike the broader diffusion of inflammatory cell proteinases, the activities of MMP, and a family of metalloendopeptidases that traverse cell membranes, **ADAM (a disintegrin and metalloprotease)** are highly localized to allow precise remodeling. MMPs belong to a superfamily of proteinases with zinc at the catalytic site (metzincins). These include other subfamilies containing ADAM and ADAM with **thrombospondin motifs** (**ADAMTS**; see Chapter 26). Members of the metzincin superfamily are key regulators in tissue during times of change such as development or remodeling. The activity of these proteases is regulated, in part, by a family of secreted molecules: **tissue inhibitors of metalloproteinases (TIMPs)**.

MMPs are a large family of 23 proteinases with overlapping specificities. They enable cells to migrate through stroma by degrading matrix proteins, and so are central to wound healing (see Table 3-3) and other processes, like tumor invasiveness, that require cell motility through ECM. They participate in cell–cell communication and activation or inactivation of bioactive molecules (e.g., immune system components, matrix fragments, growth factors) and influence cell growth and apoptosis. MMPs are synthesized as inactive proenzymes (zymogens). Many secreted MMPs require extracellular activation by previously activated MMPs, such as MMP-3, MMP-14 or serine proteinases. The six membrane-anchored MMPs are activated while anchored at the cell surface. They are attached via a small cytoplasmic tail or, for two of them, via a glycosylphosphatidylinositol (GPI) anchor. Secreted MMPs are named sequentially (e.g., MMP-1, MMP-2); membrane-type MMPs are MT1-, 2-, etc., MMPs (e.g., MT1-MMP). Cell surface activities of MT1- and MT2-MMPs are important for cell migration and invasion. MMPs were originally named by their substrates (e.g., collagenase, stromelysin, gelatinase). However, MMPs cleave diverse extracellular substrates, many of which are degraded by multiple MMPs. As with integrins, such redundancy emphasizes these molecules' in regulation by activating, deactivating, and shedding of substrates. *The list of molecules needed for wound healing is indistinguishable from the list of MMP substrates* and include:

- Clotting factors
- ECM proteins
- Latent growth factors and growth factor–binding proteins
- Receptors for matrix molecules and cell–cell adhesion molecules
- Immune system components
- Other MMPs, other proteinases, and proteinase inhibitors
- Chemotactic molecules

Most MMPs are tightly regulated at the transcriptional level, except for MMP-2 (gelatinase A), which is often constitutively expressed and activated at the cell surface by complexing with MT1-MMP (MMP-14). MMP transcription is regulated by:

1. integrin signaling;
2. cytokine and growth factor signaling;
3. binding to certain matrix proteins; or
4. tensional force on the cell surface or the adjacent ECM.

Several MMP activities support remodeling and resolution phases of wound healing. MT1-MMP and MT2-MMP may aid cell migration and invasion together with integrins, or activate TGFβ. MMP-1 associates with $\alpha_2\beta_1$ integrin, facilitating dermal keratinocyte migration on collagen during reepithelialization of open wounds. Integrins bind the cell to the collagen substrate, and MMP-1 cleaves collagen to enable cell release and migration. Membrane-associated proteoglycans (**syndecans**, CD44) also bind and regulate MMP bioavailability and activity. In addition to affecting cell–cell adhesion and release, MMPs activate or inactivate bioactive matrix molecules, such as growth factors, chemokines, growth factor–binding proteins, angiogenic/antiangiogenic factors, and bioactive, cryptic fragments of collagens and proteoglycans (**matrikines**).

Secreted MMPs act largely near cell surfaces, with localization and precision determined by local activation, limited diffusion/sequestration, substrate specificity, and a barrier of MMP inhibitors. These secreted proteins include the family of TIMPs and the generic, plasma-derived proteinase inhibitor, α_2-macroglobulin. At the cell surface, ADAMs act surgically to shed ectodomains of growth factors, chemokines, and receptors on cell or neighboring cell surfaces. The ADAMTS family members are released and activated by cleavage of the TS domain, cleaving substrates like aggrecan, a large proteoglycan of cartilage, and von Willebrand factor.

Cytokines and Matrix Stimulate Cell Proliferation

Within hours to days after injury, there is a dramatic, transient increase in cellularity that replaces lost tissue. Cell proliferation and migration initiate and promote formation of granulation tissue, a specialized, highly vascularized tissue that forms transiently during repair (see below). Cells comprising granulation tissue derive from ephemeral cell populations, including circulating leukocytes, and by infiltration of adjacent, resident capillary endothelial and mesenchymal cells (fibroblasts, myofibroblasts, pericytes, and smooth muscle cells). Local and marrow-derived progenitor cells, which share some properties of leukocytes, can also populate wounds, potentially differentiating into (transient) endothelial and fibroblast populations. Terminally differentiated cells (e.g., cardiac myocytes, neurons) do not, for the most part, contribute to early repair or regeneration (see below).

Growth factors and small chemotactic peptides (chemokines) that are released by local and circulating cells provide soluble autocrine and paracrine signals for cell proliferation, differentiation, and migration. Signals from soluble factors in association with ECM also work collectively to influence cell behavior.

Cell activities in healing wounds—proliferation, migration, and altered gene expression—are largely initiated by three receptor systems that share integrated signaling pathways:

- **Protein tyrosine kinase receptors** for peptide growth factors
- **G-protein–coupled receptors** for chemokines and other factors
- **Integrin receptors** for ECM

These receptors act in concert to direct cell behavior. These distinct receptor families are influenced by the mechanical environment, primarily via integrin-mediated binding to

ECM. These receptors may bind different types of ligands, but they signal through cascading and intersecting intracellular pathways. These routes amplify the messages, often activating similar processes that affect cytoskeletal organization and gene expression. Even different processes, such as proliferation, differentiation, and migration, may share signals, for example, those that initiate cytoskeletal changes. Intracellular signaling to regulate cell growth, survival, and proliferation is complex beyond the scope of the current discussion. What is important is to understand that integrated signals from all these systems govern tissue responses.

REPAIR

Wound Healing Follows a Defined Sequence

The predominant mode of adult repair results in scar formation. Since wounds in the skin and extremities are easily accessible, their healing has been studied extensively. Healing within hollow viscera and body cavities, though less accessible for study, generally parallels the repair sequence in skin (Figs. 3-4 and 3-5).

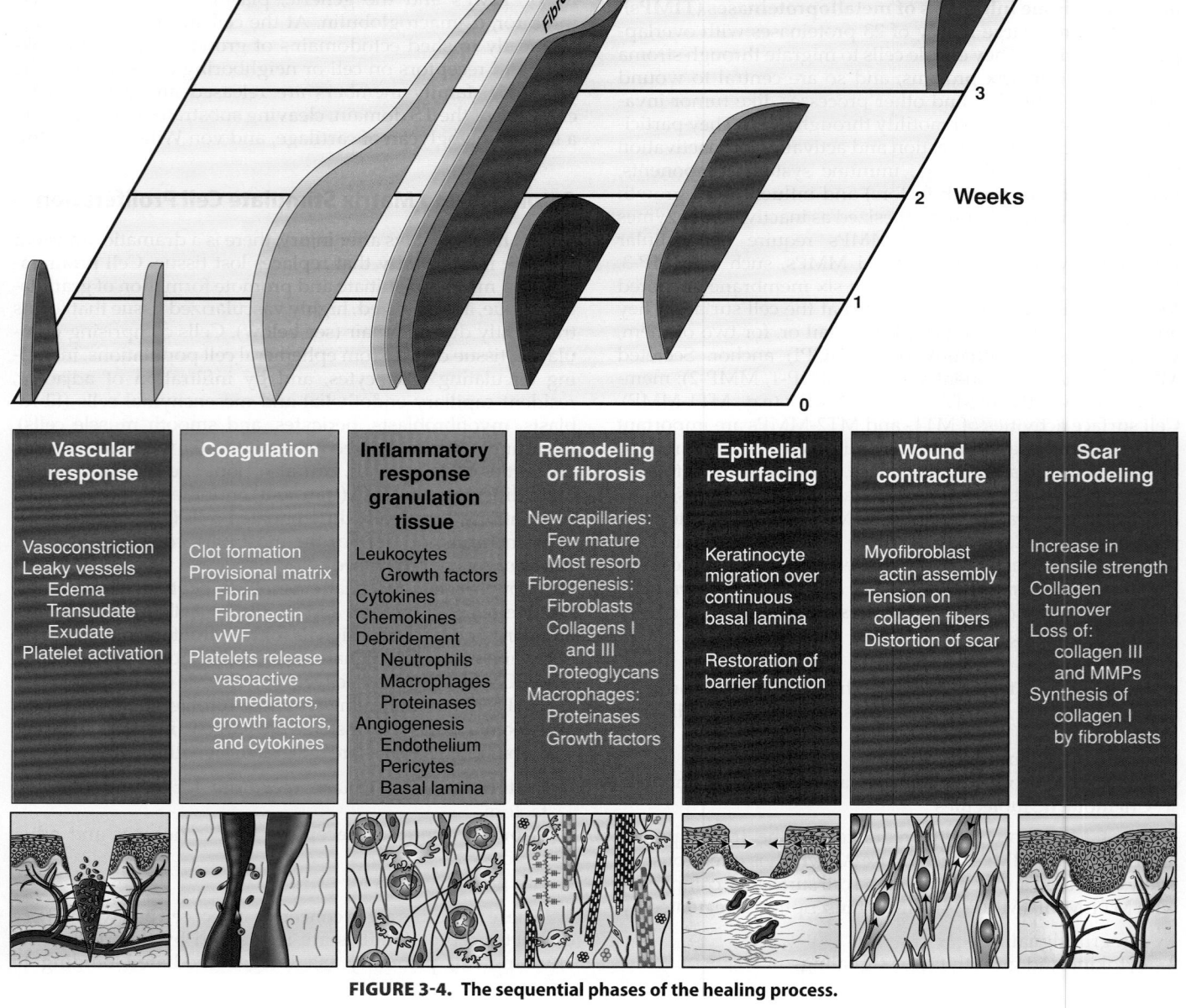

FIGURE 3-4. The sequential phases of the healing process.

Vascular response	Coagulation	Inflammatory response granulation tissue	Remodeling or fibrosis	Epithelial resurfacing	Wound contracture	Scar remodeling

Vasoconstriction
Leaky vessels
  Edema
  Transudate
  Exudate
Platelet activation
	Clot formation
	Provisional matrix
	  Fibrin
	  Fibronectin
	  vWF
	Platelets release
	  vasoactive
	  mediators,
	  growth factors,
	  and cytokines
		Leukocytes
		  Growth factors
		Cytokines
		Chemokines
		Debridement
		  Neutrophils
		  Macrophages
		  Proteinases
		Angiogenesis
		  Endothelium
		  Pericytes
		  Basal lamina
			New capillaries:
			  Few mature
			  Most resorb
			Fibrogenesis:
			  Fibroblasts
			  Collagens I
			    and III
			  Proteoglycans
			Macrophages:
			  Proteinases
			  Growth factors
				Keratinocyte
				migration over
				continuous
				basal lamina
				
				Restoration of
				barrier function
					Myofibroblast
					actin assembly
					Tension on
					collagen fibers
					Distortion of scar
						Increase in
						  tensile strength
						Collagen
						  turnover
						Loss of:
						  collagen III
						  and MMPs
						Synthesis of
						  collagen I
						  by fibroblasts

2–4 days

Thrombus

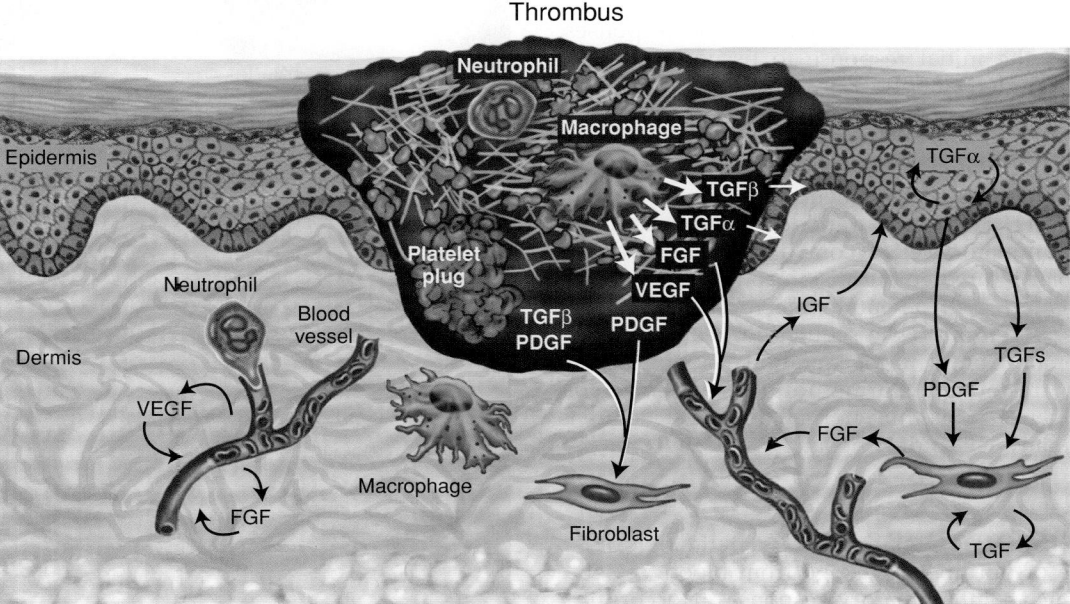

4–8 days

Thrombus

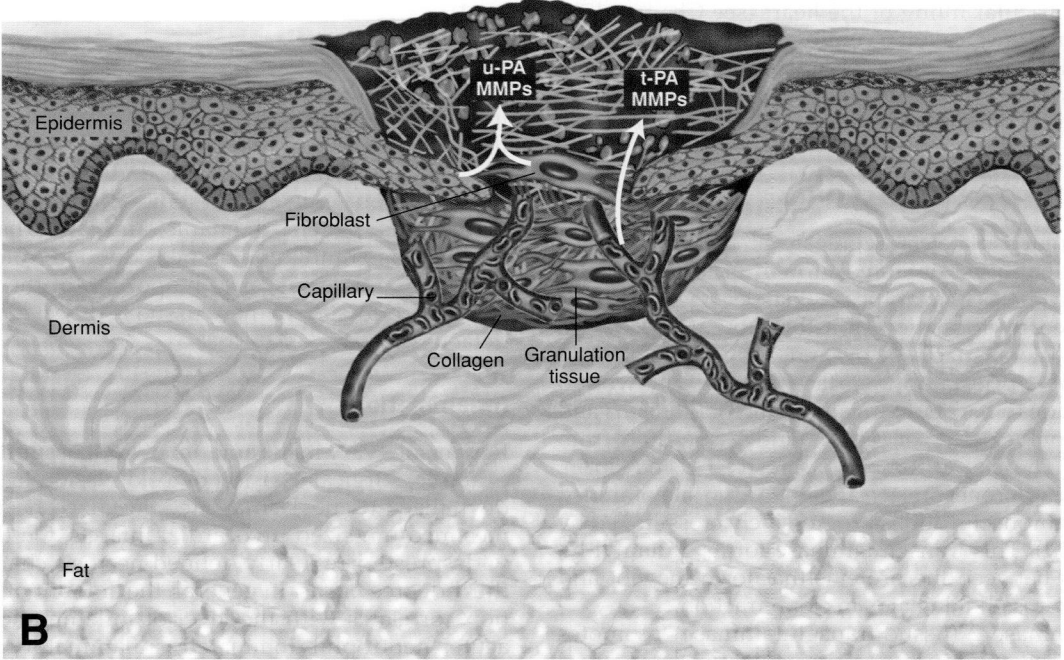

FIGURE 3-5. Cutaneous wound healing. A. 2–4 days. Growth factors controlling migration of cells are illustrated. Extensive redundancy is present, and no single growth factor is rate limiting. Most factors have multiple effects, as listed in Table 3-6. Growth factor signals first arise from degranulating platelets, but activated macrophages, resident tissue cells, injured epidermis, and the matrix itself release a complex interplay of interacting signals. **B. 4–8 days.** Capillary blood vessels invade and proliferate within the provisional matrix, and the epidermal keratinocytes advance along the granulation tissue below the thrombus. The upper, acellular portion of the wound site will become an eschar or scab. Fibroblasts deposit a collagen-rich matrix. *FGF* = fibroblast growth factor; *IGF* = insulin-like growth factor; *MMPs* = matrix metalloproteinases; *PDGF* = platelet-derived growth factor; *TGF* = transforming growth factor; *t-PA* = tissue plasminogen activator; *u-PA* = urokinase-type plasminogen activator; *VEGF* = vascular endothelial growth factor.

Outcomes of Injury Include Repair With Restoration or Regeneration

Repair and restoration follow inflammatory responses. Inflammation is the initial response to tissue injury (see Chapter 2). To understand how inflammation influences repair, it is useful to review the various possible outcomes of acute inflammation.

Transient acute inflammation may resolve completely: locally injured parenchymal elements regenerate without significant scarring. Thus, after a moderate sunburn, occasional acute inflammatory cells accompany transient vasodilation under solar-injured epidermis. In contrast, *progressive* acute inflammation, with eventual macrophage-predominant infiltrates, is central to the sequence of collagen elaboration and repair. Complete regeneration—as opposed to the more usual restoration during adult repair—may follow injury to liver or bone: thus, normal hepatic structure is replaced after many self-limited hepatic insults.

PATHOLOGY: Organization is a pathologic outcome of fibrinogen leakage from blood vessels during an inflammatory response. It occurs in serous cavities, like the peritoneum: when fibrin strands are not degraded, they form a provisional matrix. The provisional matrix becomes fibrous (granulation) tissue after connective tissue cells, inflammatory cells, and capillaries invade. In pericarditis, fibroblasts invade the provisional fibrin matrix and secrete and organize a collagenous ECM among fibrin strands, thus binding visceral and parietal pericardium together (Fig. 3-6). This constricts ventricular filling of the heart (see Chapter 17) and may require surgical intervention. In the peritoneum, fibrin strands may become organized as **adhesions** (threads of collagen) after intra-abdominal surgery, can trap loops of bowel, and cause intestinal obstruction.

Thrombosis

Shortly after injury, platelets aggregate at the wound site, releasing an initial burst of stored growth factors and cytokines, initiating the healing process. Platelet aggregation is quickly followed by formation of a thrombus (clot), which provides a provisional matrix below and, above, a visible **scab** or **eschar** when it dries atop a surface wound. The wound thrombus provides a barrier to invading microorganisms and is essential to prevent loss of plasma and tissue fluid from injury vessels. The clot/thrombus is mostly plasma fibrin, but is also rich in fibronectin (see above). At the site of injury, fibrin binds to fibronectin and is progressively cross-linked by factor XIII (FXIII). This transglutaminase forms glutamyl-lysine cross-links between the proteins that form the clot and ECM proteins. Cross-linking aids in clot retraction.

Transglutaminase 2 (tissue transglutaminase) promotes cell adhesion, cell migration, and organization of wound ECM by (1) interlinking matrix proteins such as fibrinogen, fibronectin, collagen, and vitronectin; (2) providing local tensile strength; and (3) maintaining closure as the new matrix evolves. Balanced production of this provisional matrix is critical to proper repair. Excess transglutaminase may cause undue scarring, while deficiencies of the FXIII lead to poor wound healing and bleeding. Over time, the

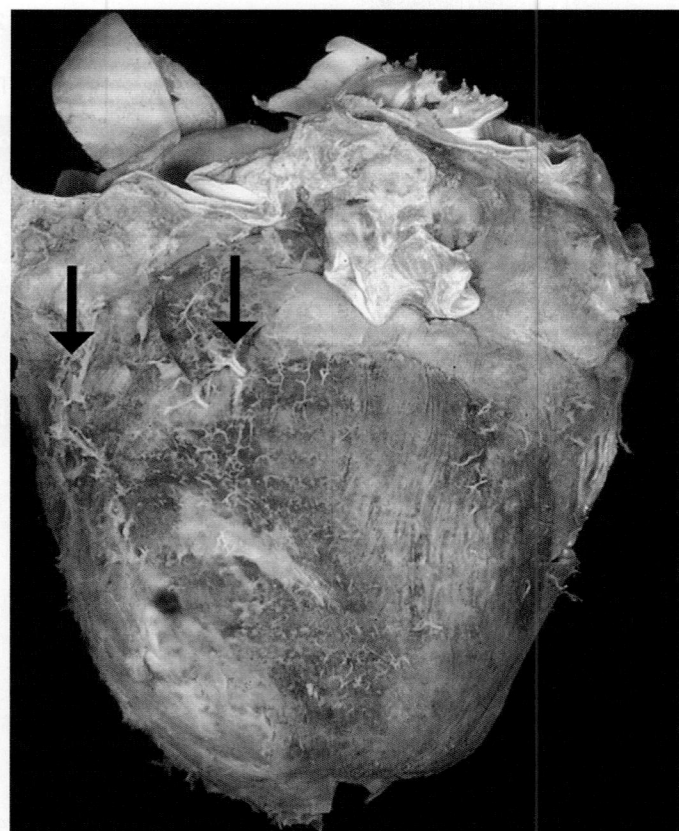

FIGURE 3-6. Organized strands of collagen in constrictive pericarditis (*arrows*). Excess collagen distorts the biomechanical properties of the heart.

internal (non-desiccated) part of the provisional matrix is transformed into granulation tissue by invasion of mononuclear cells, connective tissue, and vascular cells, while the outer portion (eschar) is a temporary repository for spent neutrophils, platelet remnants, and killed bacteria. During healing, the granulation tissue is divided from the eschar by migrating epidermis, and the portion of the thrombus that is not repopulated by new tissue is digested. The scab then detaches.

Inflammation

Repair sites vary in the amount of local tissue destruction. For example, surgical excision of a skin lesion leaves little or no devitalized tissue. Demarcated, localized necrosis accompanies medium-sized myocardial infarcts. On the other hand, widespread, irregularly defined necrosis characterizes large third-degree burns. In general, the amount of tissue destruction correlates with the level of inflammation. Initially, an acute, neutrophil-dominated, inflammatory response predominates. Neutrophils flood the wound as long as necrotic material or bacterial infection persists. These elements must be removed for repair to progress. Before granulation tissue appears, exudative, spent neutrophils may form pus or become trapped in the eschar. Fibronectin, **matricryptins**, chemokines, activated complement, and cell debris are early chemotactic elements for macrophages and fibroblasts (Figs. 3-5 and 3-7).

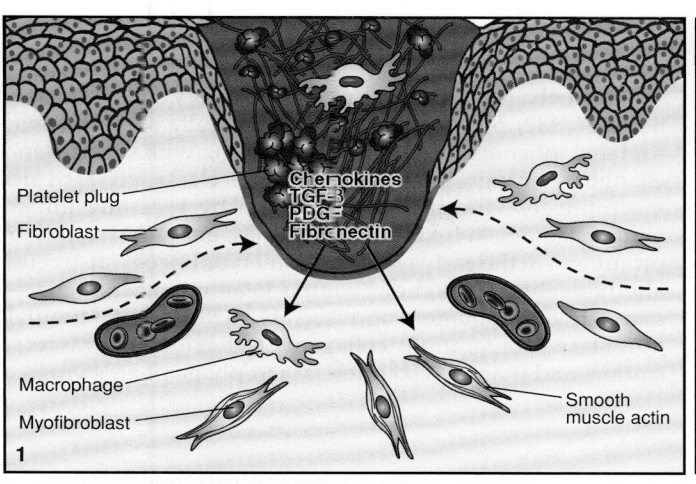

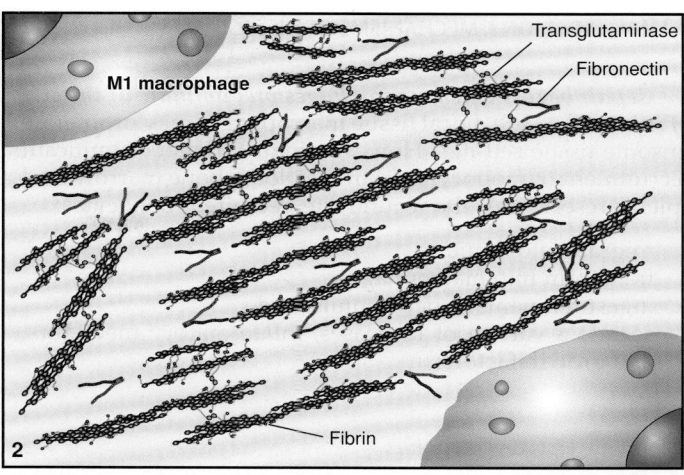

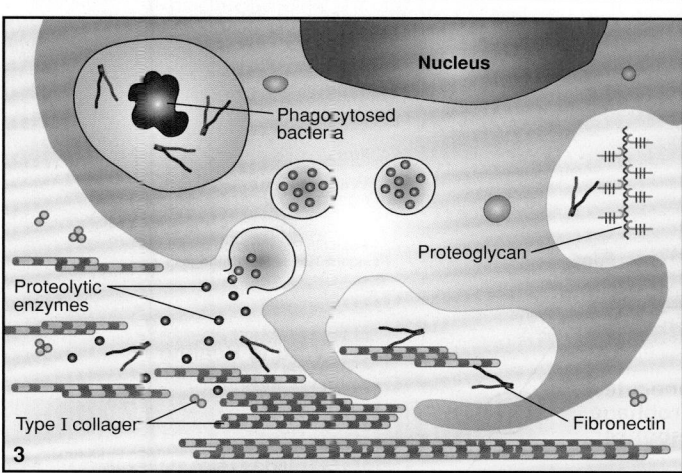

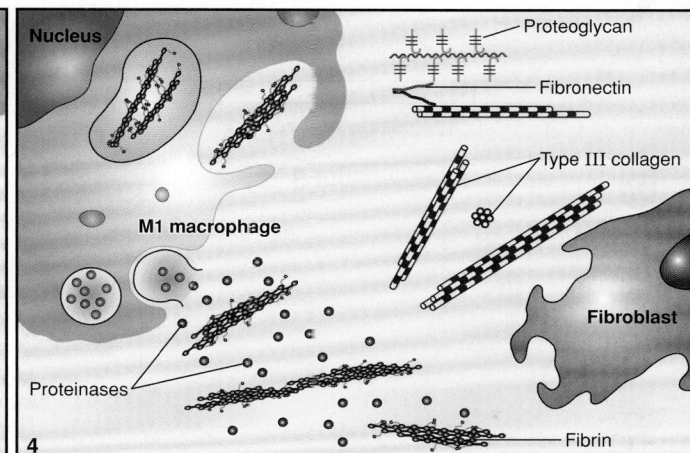

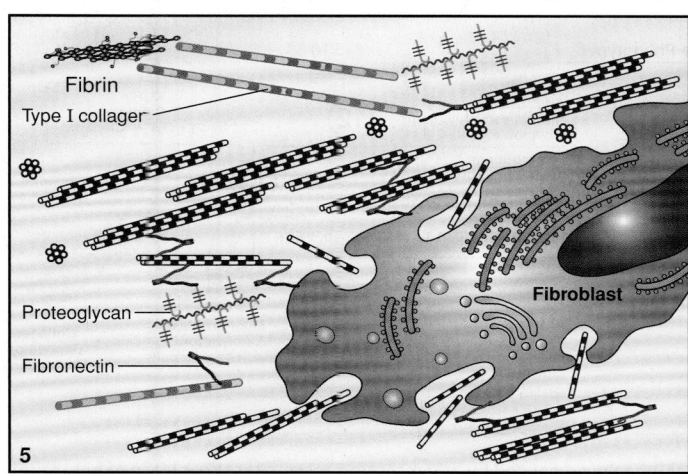

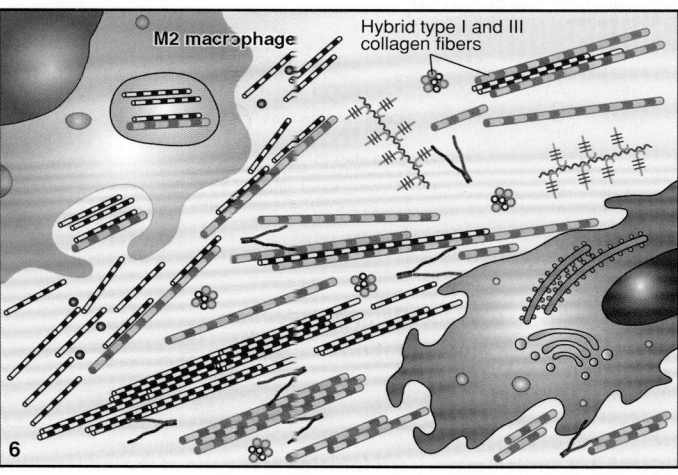

FIGURE 3-7. **Summary of the healing process. 1. Inflammatory cell migration.** A low-power view of the wound site depicts the mobilization of macrophages, fibroblasts, and smooth muscle actin–containing myofibroblasts as they migrate to the wound from the surrounding tissue into the provisional matrix. Fibronectin, growth factors, chemokines, cell debris, and bacterial products are chemoattractants for a variety of cells that are recruited to the wound site (2–4 days). The initial phase of the repair reaction typically begins with hemorrhage into the tissues. **2.** A **fibrin clot** forms from plasma and platelets, and it fills the gap created by the wound. Fibronectin from the extravasated plasma binds fibrin, collagen, and other extracellular matrix components within fibrin strands that are cross-linked by the action of transglutaminase (factor XIII). This cross-linking provides a provisional mechanical stabilization of the wound (0–4 hours) and a substrate for integrin-dependent cell migration. Neutrophils rapidly infiltrate in the presence of chemotactic signals from bacteria or damaged tissue. **3. Macrophages** recruited to the wound area further process cell remnants and damaged extracellular matrix. The binding of fibronectin to cell membranes, collagens, proteoglycans, DNA, and bacteria (opsonization) facilitates phagocytosis by these macrophages and contributes to the removal of debris (1–3 days). **4.** During the intermediate phase of the repair reaction, recruited **fibroblasts** deposit a new extracellular matrix at the wound site that is initially enriched in type III collagen and hence finer collagen fibers. Concurrently, the fibrin clot is cleared by a combination of extracellular proteolysis and phagocytosis (2–4 days). **5.** Together with fibrin removal by macrophages, there is continued fibroblast production of a **temporary matrix** including proteoglycans, glycoproteins such as polymerized cellular fibronectin and fibers enriched in type III collagen (2–5 days). Integrin receptors aid in the assembly of fibronectin complexes, and both integrins and fibronectin help assemble collagen fibrils. **6. Final phase of the repair reaction.** Fibroblasts progressively convert to production of thicker, stiffer collagen fibers that are enriched in type I collagen and the temporary, thinner collagen III–enriched fibers are turned over, leading to the stronger definitive matrix (5 days to weeks). Many other matrix molecules are involved in the assembly of the collagen network.

Repair begins when macrophages predominate at the site of injury (Fig. 3-8). Local tissue macrophages may proliferate in some tissue settings. However, injury triggers significant recruitment of monocytes from the blood, bone marrow, and splenic reserves. At the wound site, recruited monocytes:

1. migrate into tissue;
2. transform into macrophages;
3. ingest remnants of neutrophils; and
4. secrete a variety of proteases, inflammatory mediators, and growth factors.

Macrophages can assume proinflammatory (M1) or "wound healing" (M2) phenotypes, though, practically speaking, macrophage phenotypes are a continuum, with the balance changing through the process. M1—or classically activated macrophages—increase inflammation by secreting inflammatory factors, cytokines, chemokines, and MMPs, and are prominent in the early wound. M2 macrophages—also called alternatively activated or "wound healing" macrophages—dampen inflammation and secrete factors that stimulate fibroblast proliferation, collagen production, neovascularization, and wound resolution. Macrophage phagocytosis of

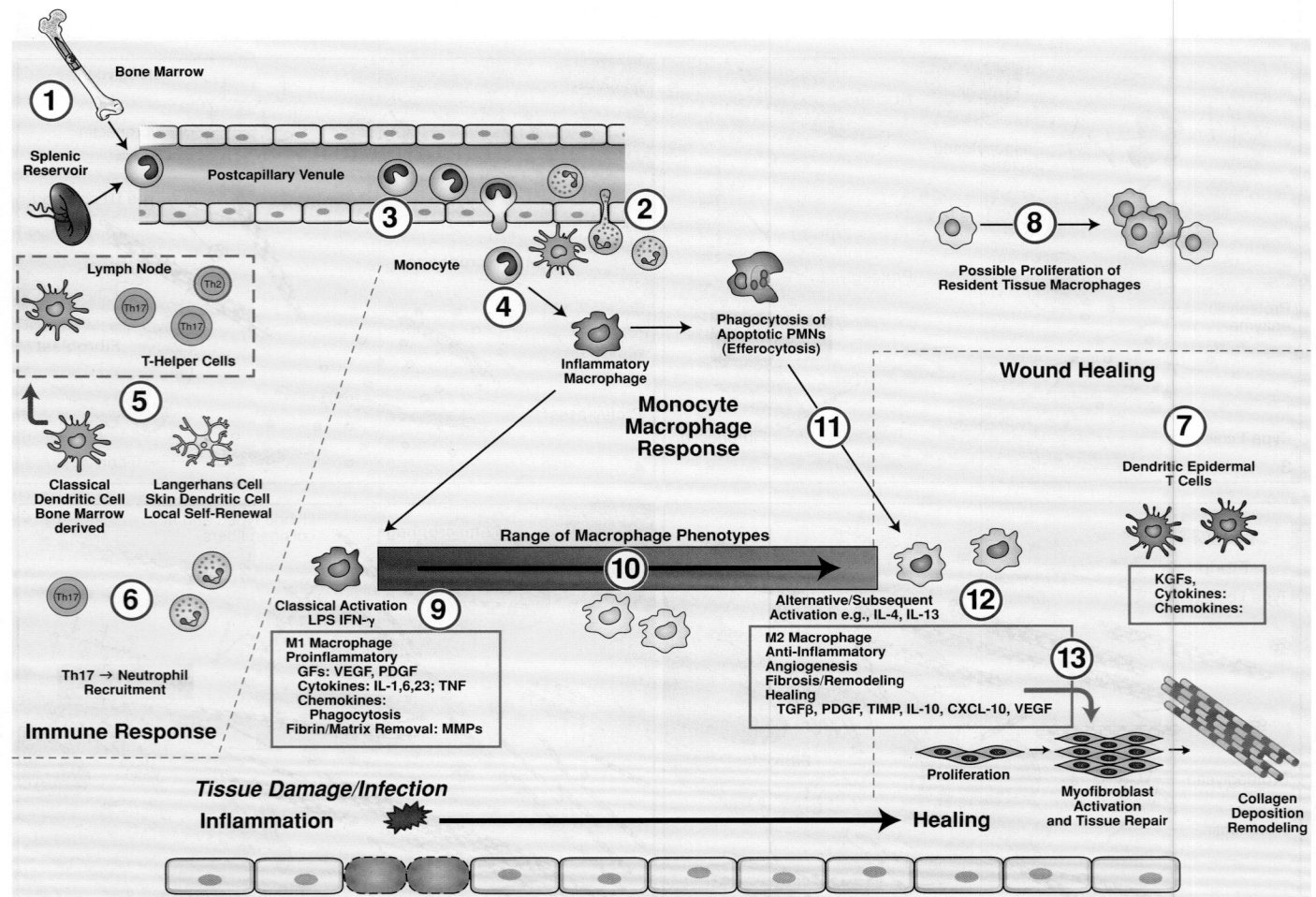

FIGURE 3-8. Inflammatory cell function at the site of the wound. Chemokine release, caused by inflammation, stimulates the release of neutrophils and monocytes from bone marrow (1). Monocytes may also be recruited from a reservoir in the subcapsular red pulp of the spleen (1). Neutrophils, normally absent in tissue, quickly enter sites of injury in response to local chemoattractant gradients (2). Monocytes and dendritic cells (DCs) have separate and shared paths of differentiation and often have shared markers but different functions; plasticity is a feature of both cell types. Classic dendritic cells populate tissue from bone marrow. A resident population, called Langerhans cells, which resemble resident tissue macrophages and arise prenatally from a macrophage population are also present in skin. Monocytes entering tissue (3) initially develop the phenotype of an inflammatory/M1 macrophage (4). Dendritic cells phagocytose antigen and migrate (5) to a local lymph node to engage the lymphocytes, stimulating an adaptive immune response. During the early response, Th17 cells secrete interleukin-17, attracting more neutrophils (6). Dendritic epidermal T cells respond to signals from injured keratinocytes, producing growth factors to support tissue repair (7). Resident tissue macrophages have been shown to proliferate in some tissues (8); however, the bulk of macrophages arise from monocytes that migrate from the circulation into the site of injury (3). Recruited macrophages are M1 macrophages, activated by interferon and infectious particles. They are proinflammatory and secrete cytokines, growth factors, chemokines, and matrix metalloproteinases (9) to attract more inflammatory cells and stimulate breakdown and removal of infectious agents and debris. Over time, the macrophages at the wound site become a mixture of transitional (10) phenotypes. As macrophages phagocytose apoptotic neutrophils (11) and the cytokine environment transitions, the anti-inflammatory M2 macrophage (12) begins to predominate. Under this influence, angiogenesis and fibrogenesis prevail as the restorative process initiates. Fibroblasts accumulate, and under the influence of macrophage-derived transforming growth factor-β (TGFβ), a portion of these cells transform into myofibroblasts, leading to increased collagen and matrix synthesis, mechanical tension, and contraction of the wound (13).

apoptotic neutrophils induces macrophage transition from M1 to M2 phenotype, thus switching from inflammatory to reparative activity in the wound bed.

DCs, which may derive from monocytes, play several roles in wound healing. To suppress infection, DCs take up antigens and migrate to lymph nodes where they activate adaptive immunity. They can also modulate immune responses in wounds by producing pro- and anti-inflammatory mediators, and so may influence the M1/M2 ratio. As well, DCs can secrete molecules that promote repair, such as TGFβ.

DETCs respond to signals from injured epithelial cells and secrete factors that stimulate repair. These factors include keratinocyte growth factors (KGF-1, KGF-2), cytokines, and chemokines. DETCs play an important role in skin repair, and impaired healing with advancing age may reflect altered DETC function.

Granulation Tissue

Granulation tissue is a transient, specialized tissue that replaces the provisional matrix. Like a placenta, it is only present where and when needed (Fig. 3-9). Microscopically, granulation tissue is formed by fibroblasts, leukocytes, and new capillaries invading the provisional matrix.

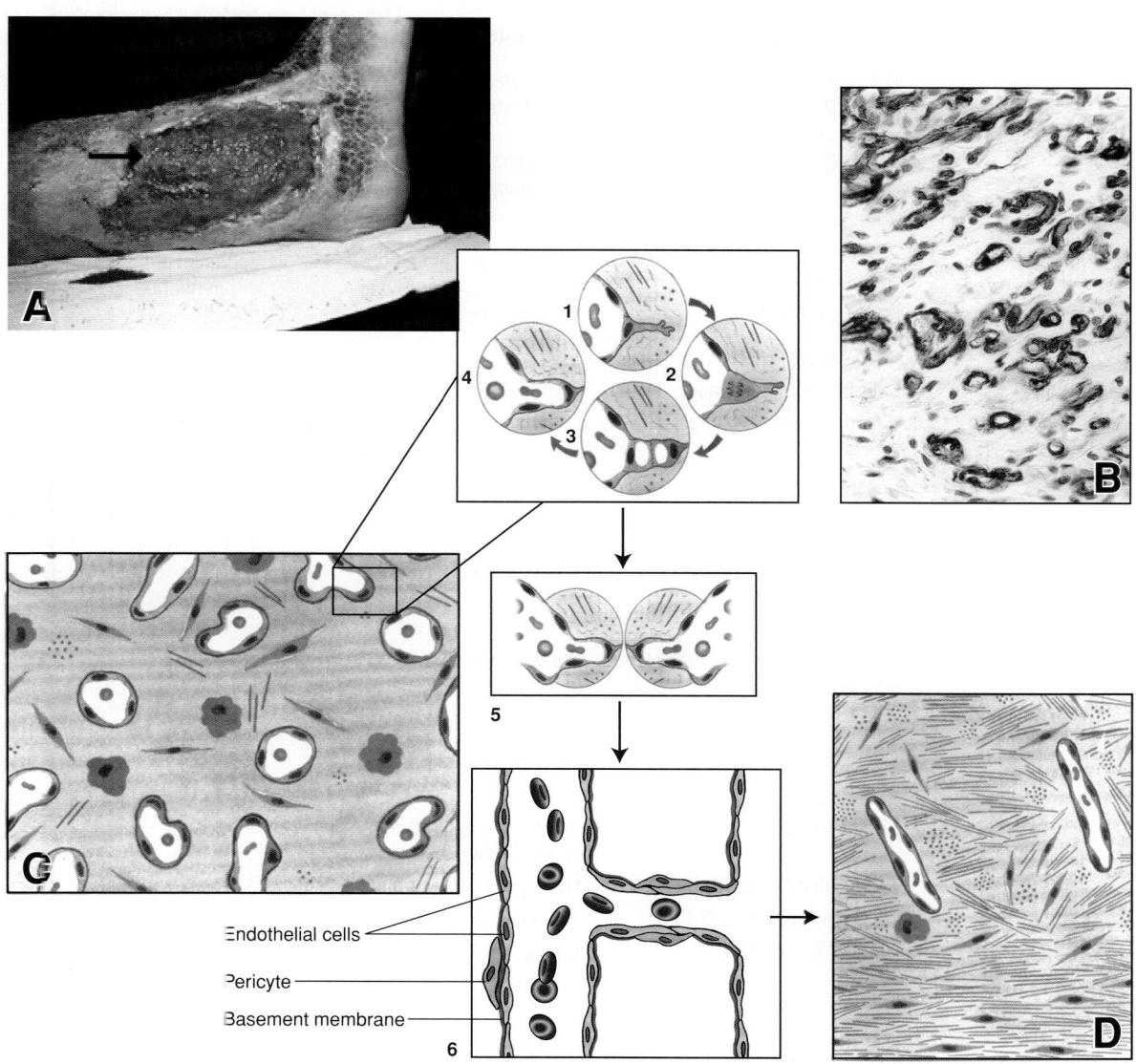

Endothelial cells
Pericyte
Basement membrane

FIGURE 3-9. Granulation tissue. A. A venous stasis leg ulcer illustrates the cobbled appearance of exposed granulation tissue. **B.** A photomicrograph of granulation tissue shows thin-walled capillary sprouts immunostained to highlight the basement membrane collagens. The infiltrating capillaries penetrate a loose connective tissue matrix containing mesenchymal cells and occasional inflammatory cells. **C.** Granulation tissue has two major components: stromal cells and proliferating capillaries. Initially, capillary sprouts of granulation tissue are a key feature, growing in a loose matrix in the presence of fibroblasts, myofibroblasts, and macrophages. The macrophages are derived from monocyte migration to the wound site. The fibroblasts derive from adjacent connective tissue or possibly from circulating fibrocytes and mesenchymal stem cells; myofibroblasts derive from fibroblasts, fibrocytes, or pericytes; and the capillaries arise primarily from adjacent vessels by division of the lining endothelial cells (steps 1–6), in a process termed ***angiogenesis.*** Endothelial cells put out cell extensions, called ***pseudopodia,*** that grow toward the wound site. Cytoplasmic flow enlarges the pseudopodia, and eventually the cells divide. Vacuoles formed in the daughter cells eventually fuse to create a new lumen. The entire process continues until the sprout encounters another capillary sprout, with which it will connect. At its peak, granulation tissue is the most richly vascularized tissue in the body. **D.** Once repair has been achieved, most of the newly formed capillaries undergo apoptosis, leaving a pale, avascular scar rich in collagen.

TABLE 3-5
EXTRACELLULAR SIGNALS IN WOUND REPAIR

Phase	Factor(s)	Source	Effects
Coagulation	XIIIa	Plasma	Cross-linking of fibrin thrombus
	TGFα, TGFβ, PDGF, ECGF, FGF	Platelets	Chemoattraction and activation of subsequent cells
Inflammation	TGFβ, chemokines	Neutrophil, M1 macrophages, endothelial cells	Attract monocytes and fibroblasts; differentiate fibroblasts and stem cells
	TNFα, IL-1, IL-6, CXCL12, CX3CL1, PDGF		
Granulation tissue formation	FGF-2, TGFβ, HGF	Keratinocytes, monocytes then fibroblasts	Various factors are bound to proteoglycan matrix
Angiogenesis	VEGFs, FGFs, HGF, angioprotein-1/2, PDGF, PEDF, Sprouty2	Monocytes, macrophages, fibroblasts, endothelial cells	Development of blood vessels Pericyte growth
Contraction	TGFβ$_1$, β$_2$	Macrophages, fibroblasts, keratinocytes	Myofibroblasts differentiate, bind to each other and to collagen and contract
Reepithelialization	KGF-1/2 (FGF-7/10), HGF, EGF, HB-EGF, TGFα, activin, TGFβ$_3$, CXCL10, CXCL11	Macrophages, platelets, fibroblasts, keratinocytes, endothelial cells	Epithelial proliferation, migration, and differentiation
Maturation, fibroplasia, arrest of proliferation	TGFβ$_1$, PDGF, CTGF, IL-27, IL-4, CX3CL1, thrombospondin	M2 macrophages, fibroblasts, keratinocytes	Accumulation of extracellular matrix, fibrosis, tensile strength
	Heparan sulfate proteoglycan (HSPG)	Endothelium	HSPG: capture of TGFβ, VEGF, and basic FGF in basement membrane
	Decorin proteoglycan	Secretory fibroblasts	Decorin: capture of TGFβ, stabilization of collagen structure, downregulation of migration, proliferation
	Interferon, CXCL10, CXCL11	Plasma monocytes	Suppresses proliferation of fibroblasts and endothelial cells and accumulation of collagen
	Increased local oxygen, decreased mechanotransduction	Repair process	Suppression of release of cytokines
Resolution and remodeling	PDGF-FGF, TGFβ, interleukins	Platelets, fibroblasts, keratinocytes, macrophages	Regulation of MMPs and TIMPs Remodeling by restructuring of ECM (e.g., collagen III replaced by collagen I)
	MMPs, t-PAs, u-PAs	Sprouted capillaries, epithelial cells, fibroblasts	
	Tissue inhibitors of MMPs	Local, not further defined	Balance the effects of MMPs in the evolving repair site
	Signals for arrest: CXCL11 or IP-9, CXCL10 or IP-10	Basal keratinocytes	Reduce cellularity CXCR3 signals
		Neovascular endothelium	Reduced migration and proliferation of fibroblasts, endothelial cells, increased migration of keratinocytes

CTGF = connective tissue growth factor; CXCL10 and 11 = CXC-type chemokine ligand 10 and 11; ECGF = endothelial cell growth factor; ECM = extracellular matrix; EGF = epidermal growth factor; FGF = fibroblast growth factor; HB-EGF = heparin-binding EGF; HGF = hepatocyte growth factor; IL = interleukin; IP = interferon-γ–inducible protein; KGF = keratinocyte growth factor (FGF-7); MMPs = matrix metalloproteinases; PDGF = platelet-derived growth factor; TGF = transforming growth factor; TIMP = tissue inhibitor of metalloproteinase; TNF = tumor necrosis factor; t-PA = tissue plasminogen activator; u-PA = urokinase-type plasminogen activator; VEGF = vascular endothelial growth factor.

Development of ECM follows, and the initially leaky, single cell–lined capillaries mature as pericytes surround and stabilize them.

Recruitment of monocytes to the site of injury by chemokines and fragments of damaged matrix is key to this process. As activated macrophages progressively shift from a proinflammatory M1 phenotype to a more reparative M2 phenotype(s), they release growth factors and cytokines (Table 3-5, and see below) that promote angiogenesis, activate fibroblasts to form new stroma, and support degradation and removal of the provisional matrix.

Granulation tissue is rich with capillaries and fluid, leading to an abundant supply of immunoglobulins, antibacterial peptides **(defensins),** and growth factors. It is highly resistant to bacterial infection, allowing surgeons to create anastomoses at such nonsterile sites as the colon, where one-third of fecal contents are bacteria.

Fibroblast Proliferation and Matrix Accumulation

Fibroblasts are key early responders to injury. These collagen-secreting cells (Fig. 3-10) are activated by cytokines, particularly EGF, PDGF, FGF, TGFβ, and the biomechanical environment. Fibroblasts participate in inflammatory, proliferative, and remodeling phases of wound repair. They can further differentiate to contractile myofibroblasts (Fig. 3-11), which are characterized by abundant stress fibers containing α-smooth muscle actin and high levels of fibrillar collagen expression. Resident fibroblasts at the wound site proliferate, but the bone marrow can also contribute cells that assume a fibroblast phenotype. Such cells include mesenchymal stem cells (MSCs) and fibrocytes; the latter has been suggested as a contributor to fibrosis and scar formation. Marrow-derived fibroblast-like cells are recruited to wounds, but do not appear to become a permanent part of the connective tissue.

Early granulation tissue matrix, which is largely derived from fibroblasts, contains high concentrations of hyaluronan, proteoglycans, glycoproteins, and fine fibers of type III collagen (see Figs. 3-4 and 3-5). Fibroblasts in the wound change from oval to bipolar as they begin to produce collagen (see Figs. 3-7 and 3-10) and other matrix proteins, like fibronectin, and develop contractile properties. Diverse, successive lineages of fibroblasts are activated during repair and resolution. Initial secretion of type III collagen is rapidly overwhelmed by type I collagen, which promotes the assembly of larger-diameter fibrils to provide greater tensile strength. Eventually, the matrix resumes its original composition of predominantly type I collagen and 15% to 20% type III collagen. The rate of matrix accumulation peaks at 5 to 7 days, depending on the tissue. This process is strongly influenced by production of TGFβ, which increases synthesis of collagen, fibronectin, TIMPs, and other matrix proteins, while decreasing MMP transcription and matrix degradation. Extracellular cross-linking of newly synthesized collagen progressively increases wound strength, which improves over weeks to months as the wound matures.

Growth Factors in Wounds

Interactions among growth factors, other cytokines, and MMPs are illustrated in Tables 3-6 and 3-7. Each signal has a predominant function in repair, but many pathways are redundant. Specificity derives from (1) selective expression from members of large families (e.g., FGF, TGFβ), (2) temporal expression of different tyrosine kinase receptors and isotypes in unrelated cell populations, (3) variation in response pathways or intensity by distinct receptors, and (4) latency or activation of growth factors (see Table 3-5). Tables 3-6 and 3-7 show how growth factors control specific events in repair.

Several growth factor ligands are presented to their (tyrosine kinase) receptors by local release from ECM components, notably heparan sulfate proteoglycan and matricellular and microfibrillar proteins. Equally important in growth factor

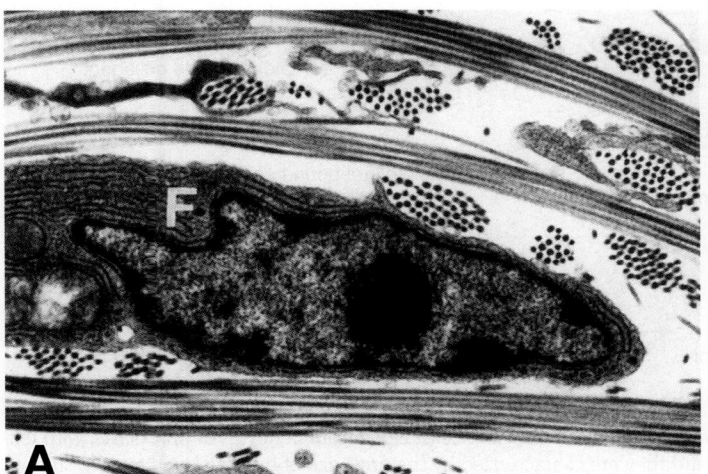
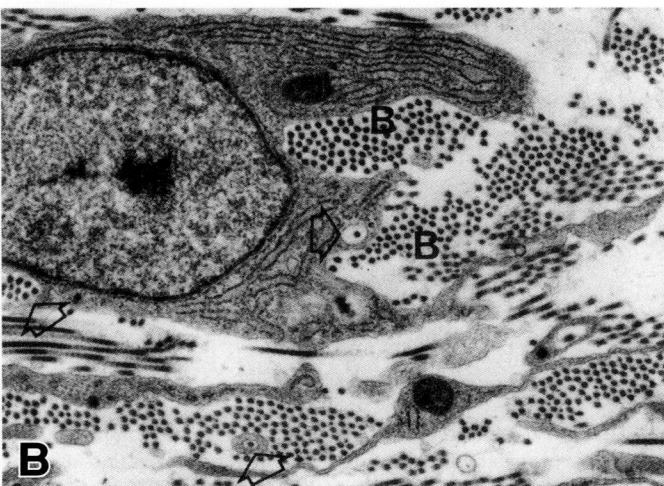

FIGURE 3-10. Fibroblasts and collagen fibers. A. Chick embryo fibroblast (*F*) lying between collagen fibers. The collagen fibers are seen as crosswise strands traversing the field and along the long axis, at a right angle, as *dots*. **B.** A chick embryo dermal fibroblast with abundant endoplasmic reticulum consistent with secretory activity and cell surface–associated collagen fibril bundles (*B*); some bundles are enveloped by fibroblast membrane and cytoplasm, indicating that collagen fibers can be assembled and extruded from long cellular processes (fibropositors; *arrows*). The fibrils are visualized in cross-section as *dots*.

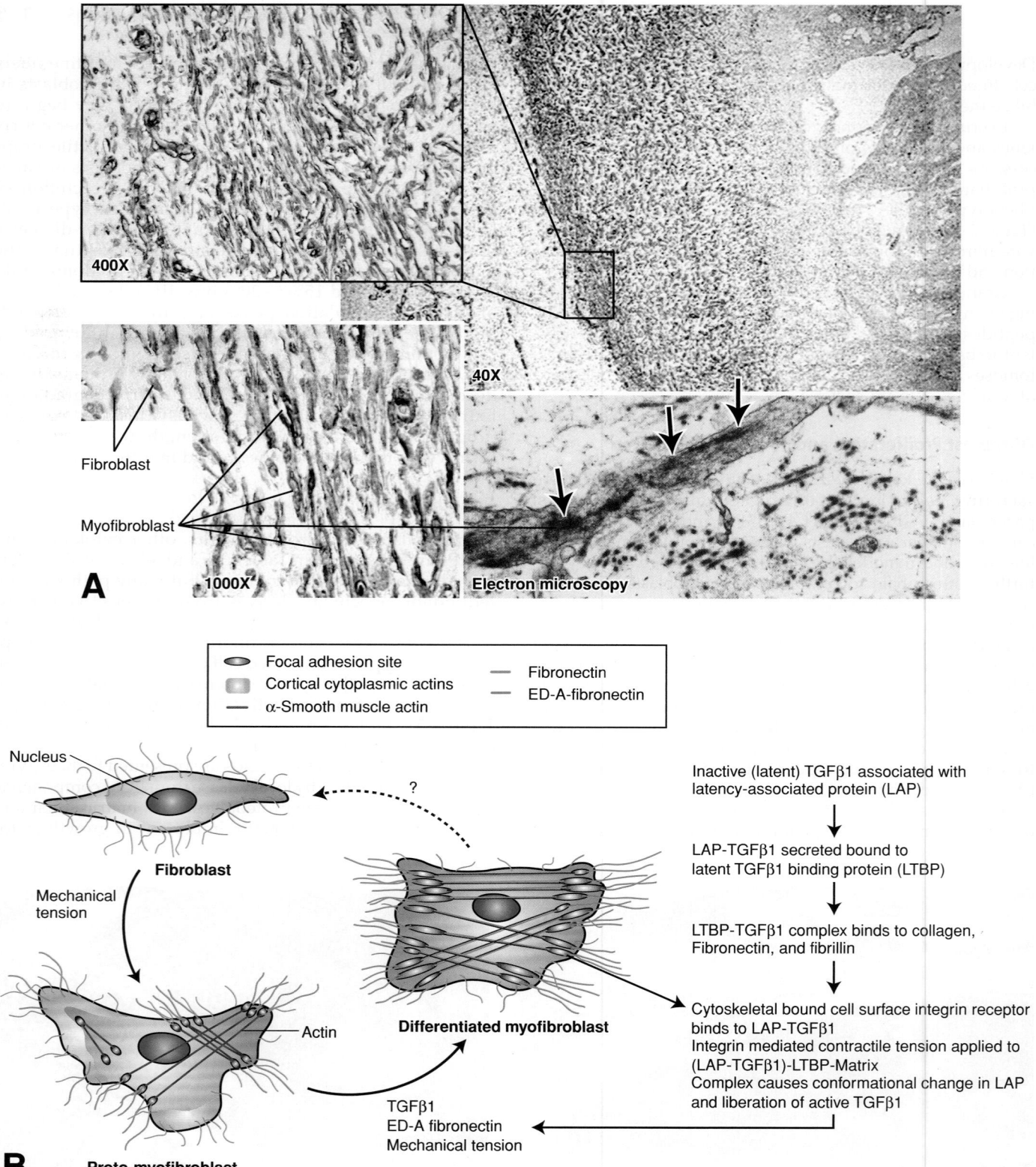

FIGURE 3-11. Myofibroblasts. Myofibroblasts have an important role in the repair reaction. These cells derive from pericytes or fibroblasts, with features intermediate between those of smooth muscle cells and fibroblasts, and they are characterized by the presence of discrete bundles of α-smooth muscle actin in the cytoplasm (*arrows*). Their clustered integrin receptors adhere tightly to and aid in formation of insoluble fibrils of cellular fibronectin, which align the cytoskeleton and bind collagen fibers, generating contractile forces important in wound contraction. **A. Myofibroblasts stained with anti–smooth muscle actin** can be viewed by light microscope at different magnifications. A band of cells (nuclei stain blue, α-smooth muscle actin stains brown) are stained in the papillary dermis of an ulcerated skin wound. Pericytes that surround capillaries also contain α-smooth muscle actin. α-Smooth muscle actin is seen in dense bundles by electron microscopy (*arrows*). **B. Development of myofibroblasts** from fibroblast and a model involving increased matrix production and matrix stiffness, leading to increased cytoskeletal contractility that activates matrix-bound latent transforming growth factor-β (TGF-β), hence creating a positive feedback system that magnifies matrix deposition and contractility. It is thought that this loop is normally interrupted by the phenomenon of tensional homeostasis, a biochemical set point.

TABLE 3-6

GROWTH FACTORS CONTROL VARIOUS STAGES IN REPAIR

Attraction of Monocytes/ Macrophages	PDGFs, FGFs, TGFβ, MCP-1 (CCL2)
Attraction of fibroblasts	PDGFs, FGFs, TGFβ, CTGF, EGFs, SDF-1
Proliferation of fibroblasts	PDGFs, FGFs, EGFs, IGF, CTGF
Angiogenesis	VEGFs, FGFs, HGF
Collagen synthesis	TGFβ, PDGFs, IGF, CTGF
Collagen secretion	PDGFs, FGFs, CTGF
Epithelial migration and proliferation	KGF, TGFα, HGF, IGF of epithelium– epidermis
Resolution of repair	IP-9 (CXCL11), IP-10 (CXCL10), PEDF, Sprouty2

CCL2 = C-type chemokine ligand 2; CTGF = connective tissue growth factor; CXCL10 and 11 = CXC-type chemokine ligand 10 and 11; EGF = epidermal growth factor; FGF = fibroblast growth factor; HGF = hepatocyte growth factor; IGF = insulin-like growth factor; IP-9/10 = interferon-γ–inducible protein 9/10; KGF = keratinocyte growth factor; MCP-1 = macrophage chemotactic protein-1; PDGF = platelet-derived growth factor; PEDF = pigment epithelium–derived factor; SDF-1 = stromal cell–derived factor-1; TGF = transforming growth factor; VEGF = vascular endothelial growth factor.

TABLE 3-7

GROWTH FACTORS, ENZYMES, AND OTHER FACTORS REGULATE PROGRESSION OF REPAIR AND FIBROSIS

Secretion of Collagenase	PDGF, EGF, IL-1, TNF, Proteases
Movement of surface and stromal cells	t-PA (tissue plasminogen activator) u-PA (urokinase-type plasminogen activator) Elastase MMPs (matrix metalloproteinases) MMP-1 (collagenase 1) MMP-2 (gelatinase A) MMP-3 (stromelysin 1) MMP-8 (collagenase 2) MMP-9 (gelatinase B) MMP-13 (collagenase 3) MT1-MMP (MMP-14; membrane bound) MMP-19
Maturation or stabilization of blood vessels	Angiopoietins (Ang1, Ang2); PDGF; HIF-1, PEDF, Sprouty2
Inhibition of collagenase production	TGFβ
Increase of TIMP production	
Reduction in collagen production and turnover	Reduction in mechanotransduction feedback and release/activation of latent TGFβ
Collagen cross-linking and maturation	Lysyl oxidase, integrin receptors, fibronectin polymers, small proteoglycans

EGF = epidermal growth factor; HIF-1 = hypoxia-inducible factor-1; IL = interleukin; PDGF = platelet-derived growth factor; PEDF = pigment epithelium–derived factor; TGF = transforming growth factor; TIMP = tissue inhibitor of metalloproteinases; TNF = tumor necrosis factor.

signaling are cell surface proteoglycans, which weakly tether the signal molecule and integrins that place receptor binding into a biochemical context by linking the ECM with the cell interior. The signals generated by these interactions are confined, persistent, and concentrated.

Growth factors expressed or mobilized early in wound responses (VEGF, FGF, PDGF, EGF, keratinocyte growth factor [KGF, FGF-7], and others) support migration, recruitment, and proliferation of cells involved in fibroplasia, reepithelialization, and angiogenesis. Growth factors that peak later (TGFβ, insulin-like growth factor 1 [IGF 1]) sustain the maturation phase, growth, and remodeling of granulation tissue. Tissue restoration is driven by complex, interactive signaling networks, which, in cooperation with matrix, support self-renewal, maintenance, and differentiation of progenitor cells.

Experimentally, wound outcomes can be improved by adding various growth factors exogenously. However, translating these observations to clinical application has been only marginally successful. Applying a single growth factor topically in a bolus does not consistently improve healing in problematic wounds, compared to more conventional chronic wound management. Limited success results, in part, from the lack of responsiveness of the target tissue and wound diagnosis. Progress in cell culture, matrix, and growth factor biology has sped the engineering of cultured skin substitutes that express or can be genetically engineered to express many growth factors, which—in combination—can improve clinical outcomes in chronic wounds. Cellular therapy, that is, adding activated cells to a wound, also shows clinical promise.

Angiogenesis

Growth of Capillaries

At its peak, granulation tissue has more capillaries per unit volume than any other tissue. Restoring the capillary bed is essential for delivery of oxygen and nutrients. New capillaries form by angiogenesis (i.e., sprouting of endothelial cells from pre-existing capillary venules; see Chapter 5) (see Fig. 3-9) and create the granular appearance for which the tissue is named. Less often, new blood vessels form de novo from angioblasts (endothelial progenitor cells [EPCs]). The latter process, known as **vasculogenesis** (see Chapter 5), mainly occurs during ontogeny.

Angiogenesis in wound repair is tightly regulated. It is activated by local release of cytokines and growth factors, and loss or disruption of basement membranes around endothelium and pericytes. The latter phenomenon occurs at sites where endothelial cells migrate into the provisional matrix. This passage is an invasive process that requires cooperation of plasminogen activators, matrix MMPs, and integrin receptors. Proliferation and assembly of endothelial cells support growth of new capillaries (see Fig. 3-9). Recruited mononuclear, bone marrow–derived EPCs may also support growing vessels.

Soluble ligands direct cell migration into a wound site. Cells follow the concentration gradients of cytokine signals (by **chemotaxis**). They respond to inherent signals from matrix substrates (by **haptotaxis**), and adhesive and mechanical signals from matrix (**durotaxis** or **mechanotaxis**). Once capillary endothelial cells are immobilized, cell–cell contacts form and an organized basement membrane develops around the nascent capillary. At first, the capillary bed formed within the healing wound is significantly more dense than in normal tissue. Many provisional capillaries are tortuous and malformed, leaky and poorly perfused. Their leakiness leads to edema. As the wound resolves, an interplay between endothelial cells and pericytes occurs. Endothelial association with pericytes and signals from angiopoietin 1, TGFβ, and PDGF help to establish mature, nonleaky capillaries. Those capillaries which do not mature fully are removed by apoptosis. Regression and pruning of capillary beds is mediated by specific anti-angiogenic mediators, including PEDF and Sprouty2, which are produced in the late proliferative phase of healing.

While many proangiogenic mediators are produced in wounds, it is mainly VEGF that stimulates wound angiogenesis. VEGF production is triggered by hypoxia, via the transcription factor, hypoxia-inducible factor-1α (HIF-1α; see Chapter 5). Activated macrophages and endothelial cells produce VEGF, and wound epidermal cells release it in response to KGF (FGF-7) secreted by dermal cells. Because the chief target of VEGF is endothelial cells, this molecule is critical for embryonic vascular development and angiogenesis, endothelial survival, differentiation, and migration. Splice variants of VEGF concentrate along soluble and matrix-bound gradients to ensure appropriate vessel branching.

In addition to active growth factor production in wounds, the ECM produces growth factors to support angiogenesis. Growth factor binding to heparan sulfate, containing GAG chains on proteoglycans of basement membrane, and to syndecan receptors is crucial to angiogenesis. Association with heparan sulfate chains affects the availability and action of growth factors and vessel pattern formation by (1) creating a storage reservoir of VEGF and basic FGF within capillary basement membranes and (2) using cell surface proteoglycan receptors to regulate VEGF and FGF receptor congregation, signal delivery, and intensity.

Beyond growth factor receptors, surface integrin receptors are important components of angiogenic responses. These receptors sense changes in ECM and react by modulating cellular responses to growth factors. Quiescent endothelial cells that are exposed to growth factors, or that lose an organized basement membrane, express new integrins that modulate their migration on provisional matrix proteins. Capillary sprouting relies principally on β_1-type integrins. Survival and spatial organization of the capillary network are regulated by other integrins, such as $\alpha_v\beta_3$, which respond to the composition and structure of their ECM ligands. Without appropriate matrix or sufficient growth factor signaling, endothelial cells are vulnerable to apoptosis.

Reepithelialization

Epidermal integrity protects against infection and fluid loss. The epidermis constantly renews itself by mitosis of stem cells that reside in the basal layer. Squamous cells then cornify or keratinize as they mature, moving outward, toward the surface, from where they are eventually shed.

Maturation requires an intact layer of basal cells, in direct contact with each other and with the basement membrane (Fig. 3-1.5). As it becomes reestablished, the epidermal barrier separates the scab from the newly formed granulation tissue. Afterward, the epidermis resumes its normal cycle of vertical maturation and shedding.

Epithelial cells in the skin and many hollow organs cover or close wounds in two ways:

1. migrating to cover damaged surfaces or
2. less often, in minor abrasions, by **purse-string closure**, a cinching process that augments fibroblast/myofibroblast-mediated wound contraction.

Skin provides an intensively studied example of epithelial repair, since there are complex differentiation patterns in the epidermal surface itself, the hair follicle, and the sweat glands. These cells normally bind basement membrane laminin by hemidesmosome protein complexes containing $\alpha_6\beta_4$ integrin. Several collagens, namely, types XVII (BP180) and VII, the latter also called **anchoring fibril** (see Table 3-2), are associated with the hemidesmosome complex. The anchoring fibril connects the hemidesmosome–basement membrane complex to the dermal connective tissue collagen fibers. Mutations in these components, or autoantibodies against one of them, may cause blistering diseases (see Chapter 28).

Epithelial cells are connected at their lateral edges by **tight junctions** and **adherens junctions** made of cadherins: calcium-dependent, integral membrane proteins that form extracellular cell–cell connections and anchor intracellular cytoskeletal connections. In adherens junctions, they bind stable actin bundles to a cytoplasmic complex of α-, β-, and γ-catenins. A girdle of actin encircles epithelial cytoplasm, creating lateral tension and strength, called the **adhesion belt**. *The shape and strength of epithelial sheets result from the strength of cytoskeletal association with basement membrane and intercellular connections.*

If cell–cell contact is disrupted, basal **epidermal keratinocytes** must reestablish contact with other basal cells, which they do mainly by cellular migration along the provisional matrix. They do this by transiently assuming a migratory phenotype (**EMT**; see Chapter 5), dividing and contributing important cytokines (interleukin-1 [IL-1], VEGF, TGFα, PDGF, TGFβ) that initiate healing and local innate immune responses. At the same time, adjacent progenitor cells in the basal layer, hair follicles, or sweat glands undergo mitosis, resulting in a thickened (hypertrophic) and less differentiated epidermis. If the basement membrane is lost, cells come in contact with unfamiliar stromal or provisional matrix components, which stimulates cell locomotion and proteinase expression. As a result, β_1 integrins that recognize stromal collagens shift from the lateral to the basal epithelial surface. Keratinocytes at the leading edge of the wound margin become migratory and secrete MMPs. These enzymes facilitate their detachment from the basement membrane and remodeling of the granulation tissue surface. Cells migrate along soluble chemical gradients (**chemotaxis**), due to matrix concentrations or adhesion (**haptotaxis**) and matrix pliability or stiffness (**durotaxis**).

Epithelial motility is activated by assembly of actin fibers at focal adhesions organized by integrin receptors. Distinct sets of integrins bind components of the wound—stromal or basement membrane matrices—and direct the migrating cells along the margin of viable dermis. Movement through cross-linked fibrin within the granulation tissue also requires activation of plasmin from plasminogen to degrade fibrin. In addition to degrading fibrinogen and fibrin, plasmin activates specific MMPs. Proteolytic cleavage of stromal collagens I and III and laminin at focal adhesion contacts can release cell adhesion or enable keratinocyte migration. Migrating keratinocytes later resume their normal phenotype. They become less hypertrophic after re-forming a confluent layer and attaching to their newly formed basement membrane.

Wound Contraction

Open wounds contract and deform as they heal, depending on the degree of attachment to, and compliance of, underlying connective tissue structures. A central role in wound contraction and fibrosis is played by the **myofibroblast** (Fig. 3-11). Compared to collagen-secreting fibroblasts, myofibroblasts contain abundant actin stress fibers (particularly α-smooth muscle actin), desmin, vimentin, and a particular fibronectin splice variant (ED-A) that forms polymerized cellular fibronectin. Myofibroblasts respond to mechanical forces and agents that cause smooth muscle cells to contract or relax. In short, they look like fibroblasts but act like smooth muscle cells. In addition to differentiating from fibroblasts, wound myofibroblasts may come from circulating, marrow-derived fibrocytes and from EMT in the lung and kidney. They may also arise from closely related cells in the wound environment, for example, perivascular- or perisinusoidal-like pericytes, mesangial cells in the glomerulus, and stellate cells in the liver. *Together with fibroblasts, myofibroblasts contribute to normal wound contraction and become more prevalent in deforming, pathologic wound contracture.*

Myofibroblasts usually appear about the third day of wound healing, in parallel with the sudden appearance of contractile forces, which then gradually diminish over the next several weeks. These cells are associated with increased type I collagen and are prevalent in fibrosis and hypertrophic scars, particularly burn scars. Myofibroblasts and fibroblasts (and other mesenchymal cells) sense the stress on integrin receptors exerted by ECM stiffness. The underlying, intracellular focal adhesion complexes ultimately activate Rho kinase, triggering myofibroblast contraction via intracellular actin stress fibers. Cell contraction impacts the ECM via integrins, facilitating biomechanical TGFβ activation by dissociating it from latent TGFβ-binding proteins or fibrillin. This then reinforces the fibrotic response. Myofibroblasts extend their contractile effects through specific cell–cell interconnections.

Resolution of Repair and Wound Strength

The signals that dictate inflammatory and proliferative phases of healing are reasonably well understood, but how wound repair winds down is not well defined. Improving oxygenation as repair progresses and reduced matrix turnover may trigger the end of the proliferative process. Recent evidence suggests that cytokines that bind to CXCR3 receptor may be important for regression of granulation tissue and limiting scarring. Specific wound termination signals, including anti-angiogenic proteins and ECRG4 tumor suppressor, may also participate in resolving healing. Finally,

increased storage and decreased release of growth factors may stabilize the matrix, which may then transmit mechanical signals that reduce the effects of growth factors, leading to tensional homeostasis. Granulation tissue eventually becomes scar tissue, as the equilibrium between collagen synthesis and breakdown comes into balance within weeks of injury. Fibroblasts continue to alter scar appearance for several years.

ECM remodeling in the wound bed may continue for a year or more. Despite this, skin incisions and surgical anastomoses in hollow viscera ultimately only reach 75% to 90% of the strength of the unwounded site. Tensile strength increases rapidly by 7 to 14 days, yet by the end of 2 weeks the wound still has a high proportion of type III collagen and only about 20% of its ultimate strength. Most of the strength of the healed wound results from synthesis and intermolecular cross-linking of type I collagen during remodeling. A 2-month-old incision, although healed, is still obvious. Incision lines and suture marks are distinct, vascular, and red. By 1 year, the incision is white and avascular, but usually still identifiable. As the scar fades further, it is often slowly deformed into an irregular line by stresses in the skin.

REGENERATION

Regeneration returns injured tissues or lost appendages to their original states. Tissue homeostasis, repair, and regeneration require populations of stem or progenitor cells that can replicate and differentiate.

The adult human body contains hundreds of types of well-differentiated cells, yet it maintains the remarkable potential, in the healthy state, to sustain its form and function by replenishing dying cells. It also heals itself by recruiting or activating cells that repair or regenerate injured tissue. The bone marrow continuously produces a wide variety of blood cells from resident stem cells. Epithelial cells in the skin and digestive tract turn over rapidly. However, tissue remodeling is much slower in most other adult tissues. Some forms of regeneration may partially recapitulate embryonic morphogenesis from pluripotent stem cells. In general, regeneration in adults after injury is overwhelmed by inflammation; so fibrosis restores tissue integrity at the expense of tissue organization. The potential to replenish or regenerate tissues depends upon small numbers of long-lived, less differentiated **stem cells** that replicate slowly, self-renew, and produce clonal progeny that rapidly divide and differentiate into more specialized derivatives. Stem cells in most tissues, including bone marrow, epidermis, intestine, and liver, maintain sufficient developmental plasticity to orchestrate tissue-specific regeneration.

Embryonic and Adult Stem Cells Are Key to Regeneration

Embryonic stem (ES) cells, up to the stage of preimplantation blastocyst, can differentiate into all the cells of adult organisms *and* maintain small populations of partially differentiated stem cells. Hence, ES cells are pluripotent. The concept of **stemness** has been revolutionized by the discovery that three to four regulators of transcription patterns active in ES cells are enough to restore pluripotency in differentiated cells from adult tissues: induced pluripotential stem

[iPS] cells that can then be conducted down a wide variety of developmental pathways. Postnatal progenitor/stem cells, which are able to divide indefinitely without terminally differentiating, inhabit many adult tissues, and including tissues that do not normally regenerate. These **adult stem cells** may inhabit a specific tissue or be recruited to sites of injury from circulating cells of bone marrow origin. Nonetheless, the presence of stem cells in most tissues underscores the importance of a permissive and supportive environment

for stem cell–driven replacement or regeneration (Table 3-8). Multipotential stem cells of adult tissues have more restricted ranges of differentiation than do ES cells, but they have potential clinical utility, since they can be isolated from autologous tissue (e.g., adipose, skeletal muscle, or bone marrow), reducing concerns of immunologic rejection after implantation.

Adult stems cells have been challenging to identify and categorize because similar stem cells may be present

TABLE 3-8
ADULT STEM CELLS DESCRIBED IN MAMMALS

Cell Type	Cell Source and Stability	Tissue Stem Cell and Role
Bone marrow–derived stem cells	Hematopoietic stem cells (HSCs)	HSCs—hematopoiesis, formation of all blood system cells
	Mesenchymal stem cells (MSCs)[a]	MSCs—replenish non-blood cells of bone and bone marrow, provide HSC niche and potential source of progenitor cells for certain other tissues
Adult tissue stem cells except connective tissue (some may be bone marrow derived)	*Constantly renewing (labile) cells*	Epidermis: unipotent basal keratinocyte basal stem cell and multipotent stem cells of hair follicle bulge and sebaceous gland
	—Epithelial and epithelial-like cells of epidermis and gut (ectoderm or endoderm derived)	Gut: multipotent columnar cells of small and large intestine crypt base
		Cornea: corneal epithelial stem cells are located in the basal layer of the limbus between the cornea and the conjunctiva (corneal stromal stem cells are similarly located but beneath the epithelial basement membrane)
	Persistent (stable) cells in tissues with less turnover	Liver: compensatory hepatocyte hyperplasia for maintenance, for regeneration, and in response to surgical resection (other liver cells also divide); hepatic stem cells, DNA markers in label retention studies are seen in cells in the canals of Hering, intralobular bile duct cells, peribiliary null cells, and peribiliary hepatocytes
	—Epithelial, parenchyma, neural (endoderm or ectoderm derived)	Lung: putative lung bronchioalveolar progenitor or stem cells that form bronchiolar Clara cells and possibly alveolar cells. Some evidence for alveolar epithelial type II progenitor cells
		Ear: mammalian cochlea are not known to regenerate sensory hair cells, though some nonmammalian vertebrates do. Human mesenchymal stem cells have been differentiated to hair cells and auditory neurons in vitro
		Neural stem cells: multipotent, thought to be ependymal cells or astrocytes; subventricular zone of the lateral ventricle (possibly inactive in adult humans); subgranular zone of dentate gyrus of the hippocampus. Other potential sites are the olfactory bulb and subcallosal zone under the corpus callosum.
Connective tissue or mesenchymal stem cells outside bone marrow	*Mesoderm derived*	Skeletal: satellite cells—between sarcolemma and overlying basement membrane of myofiber—also derived from pericytes or bone marrow mesenchymal stem cells
	Progenitors of connective tissue cells; isolated from several tissues, although bone marrow origin cannot be excluded	Adipose: fat is a rich source of multipotential mesenchymal cells
		Kidney: there are findings supportive of kidney renal tubular and parietal epithelial podocyte (Bowman capsule) stem/progenitor cells. Cells of the kidney are of mesodermal origin, with the possible exception of the endothelial cell
	Muscle cells	Cardiac: cardiac progenitor or stem cells—multipotent cardiomyocytes capable of maintaining homeostasis, limited differentiation and proliferation after ischemic injury; bone marrow mesenchymal stem cells

[a]These may be the same as multipotent adult progenitor cells (MAPCs), which represent bone marrow stromal cells whose differentiation is influenced by in vitro growth conditions. These cells are capable of seeding tissues outside the bone marrow by one or more several possible processes: (a) specific progenitors or multipotent progenitors, (b) transdifferentiation, (c) cell fusion, and (d) dedifferentiation.

in diverse tissues, which themselves may contain more than one type of stem cell. Also, many derive from the bone marrow, and so are dispersed. More recently, new, lineage-specific protein markers help to define stem cells by common properties that reflect their exquisite regulation, including:

- Replicative immortality, avoiding senescence, maintaining genomic integrity
- Capacity to intermittently undergo division or to remain quiescent
- Ability to propagate by self-renewal and differentiation of daughter cells
- Absence of lineage markers
- Sometimes, specific anatomic localization
- Growth and transcription markers common to uncommitted cells

Self-Renewal

Self-renewal is the defining property of adult stem cells and of early ES cells in vivo. The definition of a stem cell depends on its ability to differentiate into multiple cell types. Stem cells self-renew by asymmetric cell division, which produces a new stem cell and a daughter **progenitor cell** that can proliferate transiently and differentiate. Unlike stem cells, progenitor cells (transit amplifying cells) have little or no capability for self-renewal.

Stem Cell Differentiation Potential

The ability of ES cells to differentiate into all lineages diminishes as embryos develop. Cells from the zygote and the first few divisions of the fertilized egg are **totipotent;** each can form any of about 200 different cell types in the adult body and the cells of the placenta. Nuclei of adult somatic cells can be totipotent, as dramatically proven by nuclear transplantation cloning experiments in amphibians and now several species of domesticated mammals. However, this should not be confused with stem cell potency.

ES cells derived from the inner cell mass of blastocysts are **pluripotent**—that is, they may differentiate into nearly all cell lineages among the three germ layers. Pluripotent stem cells of postfertilization zygotes, such as neural crest cells, may differentiate into many cell types, but are lineage restricted. Somatic cells can now be converted into totipotent iPS cells, which may potentially generate new tissues from the same individual. Postembryonically, implanted ES cells can also form teratomas due to unregulated differentiation. Adult cells that self-renew throughout the individual's lifetime are **multipotent,** that is, able to differentiate into several cell types within one lineage or one germ layer. **Hematopoietic stem cells (HSCs)**, for example, are lineage restricted; they can form all the cells found in blood (Table 3-8). Marrow stromal cells (also called **mesenchymal stem cells [MSCs]**) are multipotent stem cells in bone marrow that can mobilize into the bloodstream and travel to injured organs. MSCs can be coaxed to differentiate into multiple mesoderm-derived cell types in vitro (adipocytes, chondrocytes, osteoblasts, myoblasts, fibroblasts). MSCs from cord blood and connective tissues, particularly adipose tissue, may act as progenitors for tissue repair.

Tissue-specific cells support renewal as multipotent stem cells or as progenitor cells. Progenitor cells are **stable cells** that differ from stem cells in lacking self-renewal; however, they can differentiate and proliferate rapidly. They are sometimes called **unipotent** stem cells, as exemplified by interfollicular basal skin keratinocytes, although other skin cells may be multipotent or oligopotent. An example is the more versatile bulge stem cells of the hair follicle, which are able to reconstitute hair follicles and sebaceous glands, and contribute to repair of epidermis. Intestinal epithelium turns over rapidly and is replenished by intestinal stem cells that reside in the crypts of Lieberkühn. Mature differentiated hepatocytes regenerate liver after partial hepatectomy. However, stem, or progenitor, cells may drive liver regeneration after damage by viral hepatitis or toxins. "Oval cells," in terminal ductal cells in the canal of Hering are probably responsible: they have characteristics of both hepatocytes (α-fetoprotein, albumin) and bile duct cells (γ-glutamyl transferase, duct cytokeratins).

In addition to normal differentiation pathways within a single tissue, cells of one tissue may **transdifferentiate** into cells of another tissue. In adults, injured epithelium (renal tubules, pulmonary) may transform into fibroblasts under the influence of cytokines such as TGFβ, adding to scarring and fibrosis; cardiac endothelial cells may do the same. This phenomenon, EMT (see above) is also important in tumor invasion.

Bone marrow contains hematopoietic, mesenchymal, and endothelial stem cells, providing a multifaceted regenerative capacity. Bone marrow stem cells, which are created during embryonic development, replenish the bone marrow mesenchyme and the hematopoietic population. Circulating EPCs from bone marrow facilitate angiogenesis. Likewise, bone marrow–derived MSCs can populate repairing tissues in many distant sites (see Table 3-8).

Influence of Environment on Stem Cells

Stem cells exist in **microenvironments** or **niches** that provide sustaining signals from ECM and neighboring cells that limit their differentiation and ensure that they perpetuate themselves while controlling cell number, fate, and motility. These niches rely on basement membrane matrix molecules, plus proximity to mesenchymal cells, chemokines, growth factors, and differentiation mediators. The mere presence of adult stem cells or progenitor cells is not sufficient for tissue regeneration after injury. Many tissues contain resident progenitor cells yet do not heal by regeneration. The method of repair is also influenced by growth factors, cytokines, proteinases, and the composition of the ECM.

Whether a wound is repaired by regeneration—or scarring and fibrosis—is at least in part determined by the concentration, duration, and composition of environmental signals present during inflammation. The process is strongly influenced by many types of leukocytes, including macrophages, mast cells, and T lymphocytes. The continuous regeneration of adult epidermis or intestinal epithelium generally occurs without inflammation and within an innate ECM. In such instances, normal structures and architecture are assembled without fibrosis or scarring. Wounds rapidly shift to an inflammatory response and a matrix expression profile that emphasizes protection (scarring) rather than perfection (regeneration). Spinal cord injury, for example, provides a particularly difficult challenge. Injury-induced cellular reactions cause neurons, glial cells, and oligodendrocytes to die. Further inflammatory damage results in glial scar development by astrocytes, which release chondroitin sulfate proteoglycans and proteins that block axonal growth. Current strategies for regeneration rest upon the possibility that transplantation or stimulation of an appropriate stem cell population might reestablish normal tissue function and prevent scarring. Fibrosis, an urgent response that preserves mechanical integrity after tissue damage, is a key impediment to regeneration.

Differentiated Cells Can Revert to Pluripotency

Cell differentiation involves controlled regulation of gene expression. This occurs via **epigenetic modulation** of gene expression (see Chapter 5) that reduces expression of pluripotency-related genes, and increases expression of lineage development genes.

Epigenetic modifiers stabilize and restrict transcriptional states as necessary for cell differentiation. Interplay between epigenetic modifiers and lineage-determining transcription factors is necessary for progressive differentiation states in a cell lineage. Differentiation is controlled at many levels, and may involve cell–cell contact and extracellular signals, but coactivation and coregulation of transcription factors associated with potency or lineage and epigenetic modifications are also key to the final state of a cell.

Cells Can Be Classified by Their Proliferative Potential

Cell populations divide at different rates. Some mature cells never divide, while others cycle repeatedly.

LABILE CELLS: Labile cells occur in tissues that are in a constant state of renewal. Tissues in which over 1.5% of cells are in mitosis at any one time are composed of labile cells. However, stable cells are also constituents of labile tissues with high rates of cell turnover. Labile epithelial tissues that typically form physical barriers between the body and the external environment self-renew constantly—for example, epidermis, cornea, and epithelia of the GI, respiratory, reproductive, and urinary tracts. Hematopoietic cells of the bone marrow and lymphoid organs involved in immune defense are also labile. *If stem cells survive, tissues composed of labile cells often can regenerate after injury.*

STABLE CELLS: Stable cells populate tissues that normally renew very slowly, but contain progenitor cells that can respond rapidly after tissue loss. Liver, bone, and proximal renal tubules contain stable cell populations in which <1.5% of cells are in mitosis. Stable tissues (e.g., endocrine glands, endothelium, and liver) do not have conspicuous stem cells. These cells require an appropriate stimulus, such as stress or injury, to divide. *The potential to replicate, not the number of steady-state mitoses, determines an organ's regenerative capacity.* For example, the liver is a stable tissue with very infrequent mitosis, but it rapidly recovers by hepatocyte hyperplasia after losing up to 75% of its mass.

PERMANENT CELLS: Permanent cells are terminally differentiated. They have no capacity to regenerate, and do not enter the cell cycle. Traditionally, neurons, chondrocytes, cardiac myocytes, and cells of the lens have been considered permanent cells. Cardiac myocytes and neurons may be replaced from progenitors, but not from division of pre-existing cardiac myocytes or mature neurons. Permanent cells do not divide, but they do renew their organelles. The extreme example of permanent cells is the lens of the eye. Every lens cell generated during embryonic development and postnatal life is preserved in the adult without turnover of its constituents.

CONDITIONS THAT MODIFY REPAIR

Local Factors May Influence Healing

Location of the Wound

In addition to its size and shape, a wound's location also affects healing. If scant tissue separates skin and bone (e.g., over the anterior tibia or the cranium), a wound in the skin cannot contract. Skin lesions in such areas, as well as extensive burns, often require skin grafts because their edges cannot be apposed. Complications such as infection, obesity, diabetes, chemotherapy, glucocorticoids, or ionizing radiation, also slow repair processes.

Blood Supply

Compromised circulation is a common cause of chronic wounds. Leg wounds often heal poorly, or may even require amputation, because advanced peripheral vascular atherosclerosis (see Chapter 16) and defective angiogenesis compromise local blood supply and impede repair. Similarly, poor venous return may both cause skin to break down and hinder reepithelialization. Bed/pressure sores (decubitus ulcers) result from prolonged, localized, dependent pressure that diminishes both arterial and venous blood flow and causes intermittent ischemia. Limited diffusion capacity, as in joint (articular) cartilage, prevents vigorous inflammatory responses, so that articular cartilage repairs poorly after progressive, age-related wear and tear. Coagulation defects, thrombocytopenia, and anemia impede repair. Local thrombosis decreases platelet activation, reducing the supply of growth factors and limiting the healing cascade. Decreased tissue oxygen in severe anemia also interferes with repair.

Aging and Systemic Factors

Stem cell reserves—and, not coincidentally, healing capacity—decline with age, and aged cells show senescence-associated secretory phenotype, with altered cytokine profiles (see Chapter 10). This varies with tissues: a 90-year-old's skin has reduced collagen and elastin, and so heals slowly, but their colon resection or cataract extraction will heal normally because the bowel and eye are practically unaffected by age.

Exogenous corticosteroids retard wound repair by inhibiting collagen and protein synthesis, and also suppress both destructive and constructive aspects of inflammation. Chemotherapeutic agents can impair healing by limiting inflammatory responses.

Fibrosis and Scarring Contrasted

Successful wound repair with localized, transient scarring promotes rapid resolution of local injury while restoring mechanical integrity. Scars reflect altered organization of matrix (i.e., collagen fibers) compared to normal, surrounding tissue. They vary in size, and may be larger than the wound site, depending on the nature of the wound and its treatment. Scarring occurs particularly where there is greater mechanical movement and tension, such as over limb joints. It is triggered by traumatic injury, and restores lost tissue integrity.

Some chronic diseases, including many autoimmune diseases (e.g., scleroderma, rheumatoid arthritis; see Chapter 11), can arise from inappropriate and persistent inflammation, which progresses to diffuse and progressive fibrosis, or continued and excessive deposition of matrix proteins, especially collagen. Repeated exposure to irritants (e.g., inhaled smoke or silica particles) may cause pulmonary fibrosis. Whatever its origin, inflammatory and noninflammatory processes may cause fibrosis in many organs and tissues, including the heart, lungs, kidneys, joints, and soft tissues.

Ongoing insult or inflammation, mediated via the interplay of M1 macrophages and T-helper (Th2, Th17) lymphocytes, results in persistently high levels of cytokines (IL-1β, IL-6, TNFα), fibrogenic growth factors (TGFβ), and locally destructive enzymes, such as MMPs. Resolution of a fibrogenic response is associated with M2 macrophages and, in some studies, Th1 and T_{reg} cells. Fibrotic reaction, once initiated, may resolve if the initiating triggers are removed. However, fibrosis further alters matrix composition, stiffness, and mechanical stress, propagating fibroblast conversion to myofibroblasts and further matrix production. Matrix composition changes from provisional matrix during fibrogenesis and remodeling in response to mechanical stress, providing opportunities for a matrix that supports continued fibrosis.

Uncontrolled fibrosis self-perpetuates, even without continued inflammation: Myofibroblasts produce ECM and activate latent TGFβ that is stored in the matrix. The nonstructural ECM protein, osteonectin/BM-40/SPARC (secreted protein acidic and rich in cysteine), is secreted into the extracellular space (matricellular protein) during development and fibrosis. **SPARC** dissociates collagen from the cell surface by competing with binding of fibrillar collagens to the cellular DDR. It may encourage further collagen secretion and deposition. Similarly, osteopontin is associated with persistent fibrosis in several organs. Regardless of the underlying mechanism, fibrosis in parenchymal organs such as the heart, lungs, kidney, or liver disrupts normal architecture and impedes function. Disordered collagen replaces functional units (contractile muscle, alveoli, hepatic lobules, or renal glomeruli). Such fibrosis and resulting dysfunction are largely irreversible. Correction requires removing the inciting stimulus by treatment, for example, to suppress rheumatoid joint inflammation, and so minimize tissue damage. Otherwise, tissue architecture and mechanics are so impaired that regenerative processes cannot reverse the injury.

Fibrosis is the pathologic consequence of persistent injury and causes loss of function. It is an abnormal process that develops from persistent or impaired normal processes. Often it is the final common result of diverse diseases or injuries, the causes of which cannot be ascertained from the end result.

Prevention of fibrosis requires either blocking the stimulus of matrix production or increasing the level of matrix degradation. TGFβ and connective tissue growth factor (CTGF, CCN-2) regulate matrix production and have been associated

with fibrotic connective tissue diseases. TGFβ has many activities besides activation of matrix synthesis, and therapeutic blockade has thus far been unsuccessful. Fibrosis is also regulated by cytokines, growth factors, Wnt/β-catenin signaling, and microRNAs. Approaches to controlling fibrotic progression to end-stage kidney disease have targeted profibrotic factors such as TGFβ and plasminogen activator inhibitor-1 (PAI-1). Inhibiting PAI-1 activates plasminogen. As a result, plasmin degradation of ECM increases, directly or by activating MMPs. Interestingly, inhibition of PAI could also reduce **intra-abdominal adhesions,** which are a persistent problem of abdominal surgery and an important cause of intestinal obstruction. These adhesions are initiated by fibrin deposition when mesothelial lining is disrupted or heals ineffectively. If plasmin does not dissolve the fibrin matrix within a few days, the provisional matrix is invaded by fibroblasts and eventually transformed into a permanent fibrotic adhesion, with collagen, capillaries, and nerves.

The fibrotic process may not resolve merely from reducing activating signals or developing appropriate levels of tensile strength and elasticity. Members of the CXCL3 family of cytokines—like interferon-γ–inducible protein 9 (IP-9 or CXCL11) and IP-10 (or CXCL10)—are produced by fibroblasts, and epithelial and other cells. Increases in these proteins are associated with reduced fibrosis, while their absence can lead to exaggerated scarring.

Specific Sites Show Different Repair Patterns

Skin

Successful healing in the skin involves repair, primarily dermal scarring and regeneration, mainly of the epidermis, innervation, and vasculature. The salient features of primary and secondary healing are shown in Figure 3-12.

Primary healing occurs when the surgeon closely approximates the edges of a wound. The actions of myofibroblasts are minimized owing to the lack of mechanical strain, and regeneration of the epidermis is optimal, since epidermal cells need to migrate only a minimal distance. Nevertheless, some scarring often occurs.

Secondary healing proceeds when a large area of hemorrhage and necrosis cannot be totally corrected surgically. Granulation tissue formation is extensive. Myofibroblasts contract the wound and restore mechanical integrity by depositing extensive ECM.

The method and success of healing after a burn wound depend on the depth of the injury. If it does not extend lower than the upper dermis, stem cells from sweat glands and hair follicles regenerate the epidermis. If deep dermis is affected, its regenerative elements are destroyed and surgery with epidermal or keratinocyte grafts is necessary to cover or heal the wound site and reduce scarring and severe contractures. In this case, epidermal appendages (follicles, sweat glands) are not regenerated, although cytokines produced by the grafted epidermis may contribute to the improved outcome.

Oral Mucosa

Oral mucosa consists of nonkeratinizing stratified epithelium overlying a connective tissue base, the lamina propria. It resembles skin, albeit without skin appendages like hair follicles and sweat glands. However, oral mucosa heals

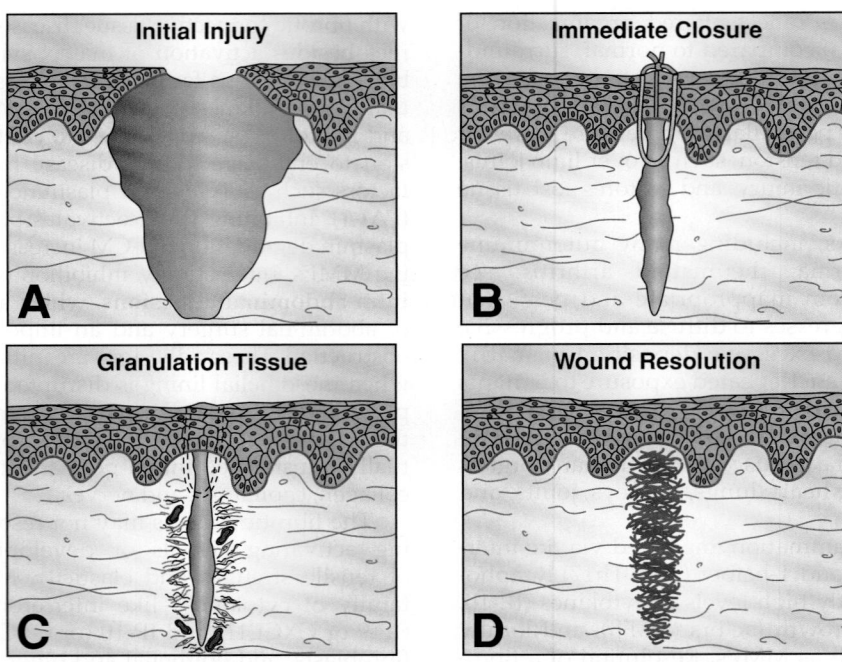

HEALING BY PRIMARY INTENTION (WOUNDS WITH APPOSED EDGES)

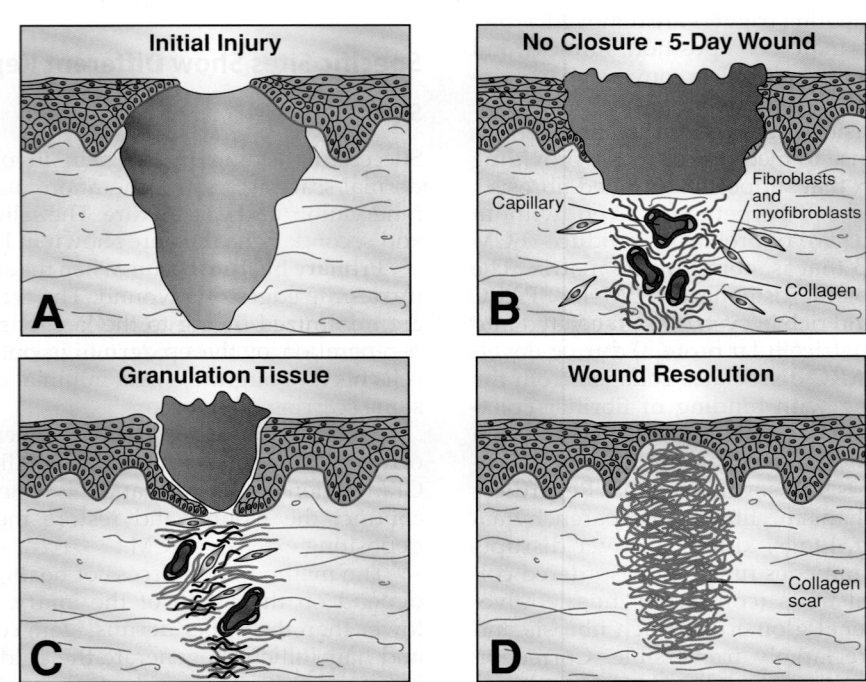

HEALING BY SECONDARY INTENTION (WOUNDS WITH SEPARATED EDGES)

FIGURE 3-12. Top. Healing by primary intention. A. An initial open, incised wound **(B)** with closely apposed wound edges is held together with a suture, leading to minimal tissue gaping or loss. **C.** There is decreased granulation tissue. Such a wound requires only minimal cell proliferation and neovascularization to heal. **D.** The result is a narrow, linear scar. **Bottom. Healing by secondary intention. A.** A gouged wound that remains or is left to remain open. The edges remain far apart and there is substantial tissue loss. **B.** The healing process requires wound contraction (mechanical strain), extensive cell proliferation, matrix accumulation, and neovascularization (granulation tissue) to heal. **C.** The wound is reepithelialized from the margins, and collagen fibers are deposited throughout the granulation tissue. **D.** Granulation tissue is eventually resorbed, leaving a large collagenous scar that is functionally and esthetically imperfect.

extremely rapidly with minimal scarring. Hypertrophic scars and keloids are quite rare in the oral cavity. Healing in the oral mucosa includes reduced inflammation, decreased—but more functional—angiogenesis, and a more limited genomic response than skin. The difference between skin and oral mucosa injury responses reflects intrinsically different behaviors of their epithelial cells and fibroblasts. For example, compared to skin epithelium, oral epithelial cells exposed to hypoxia produce significantly less inflammatory mediators, and thus are more programmed for rapid healing response with better tissue fidelity than skin. In addition, the moist environment of the mouth, growth factor–rich saliva, and abundant local epithelial stem cells contribute to the enhanced healing capacity of oral mucosa.

Cornea

Corneal stratified squamous epithelium differs from skin in its stromal organization, vascularity, and cellularity. Like skin, cornea is continually renewed by a stem cell population, at the periphery of the corneal limbus (margin). Superficial epithelial damage that does not involve stroma heals by keratinocyte migration and replication without scarring. Stem cells from the limbus can be expanded in vitro and transplanted to eyes injured by surface chemical or thermal burns. Chemical, infectious, surgical, or traumatic injury to the corneal stroma results in scarring due to distortion of the precisely arranged collagen fibers, effectively blinding the eye. Parenthetically, the cornea, because of its relative avascularity, was the first organ or anatomic structure to be successfully transplanted. Trachoma, an inflammatory response to infection with *Chlamydia trachomatis,* causes corneal scarring and opacity, and is the world's most common cause of blindness (see Chapter 33).

Liver

Adult livers have remarkable regenerative capacity, even though virtually all hepatocytes are in G_0. After resection, they enter the cell cycle and the liver regenerates by compensatory hyperplasia. The conditions necessary for hepatic regeneration are complex (see Chapter 20). Suffice it here to say that regeneration ceases when the normal ratio of liver to total body weight is reestablished; the molecular switch that regulates this ratio is unknown but may involve a kinase cascade, the *Hippo* pathway, that controls organ size.

Unlike acute liver injury (see above), in which cells resident in bile ducts may regenerate parenchyma, in chronic liver injury—as in chronic viral hepatitis or alcoholism—broad collagenous scars develop in the hepatic parenchyma. This is **cirrhosis** of the liver (Fig. 3-13). Hepatocytes form regenerative nodules that lack central veins and expand to obstruct blood vessels and bile flow. Architectural disarray impairs liver function, even if hepatocyte numbers are adequate, and hepatic insufficiency develops that can only be rectified by liver transplantation.

Kidney

Removal of one kidney (nephrectomy) leads to compensatory hypertrophy of the remaining kidney. If renal injury, such as acute kidney injury due to nephrotoxins or ischemia, is not extensive and the ECM framework, especially the basement membrane, is intact, tubular epithelium regenerates. In most renal diseases, however, the matrix is disrupted, so regeneration is incomplete and scars form. The regenerative capacity of renal tissue is maximal in cortical tubules and less in medullary tubules. Podocyte hypertrophy or regeneration is possible in some diseases like diabetes or chronic nephropathy, if scarring and disease are reversed with pancreatic transplants or inhibition of angiotensin-converting enzyme. Recent data suggest that tubule repair occurs from proliferation of endogenous, multipotent tubular stem cells.

Cortical Renal Tubules
Tubular epithelium normally turns over and cells are shed into the urine. No reserve cell has been identified, and replacement involves simple division. The outcome of injury

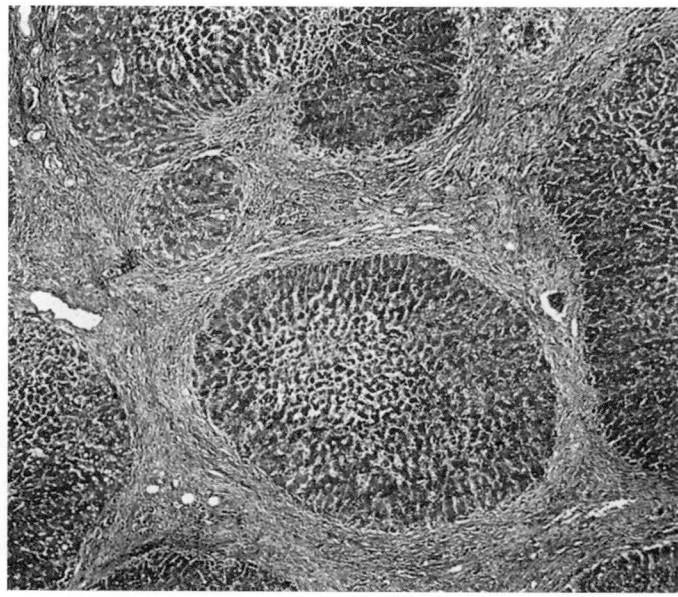

FIGURE 3-13. Cirrhosis of the liver. The consequence of chronic hepatic injury is the formation of regenerating nodules separated by fibrous bands. A microscopic section shows regenerating nodules (*red*) surrounded by bands of connective tissue (*blue*).

hinges on the integrity of the tubular basement membrane. As long as it remains continuous, surviving tubular cells near a wound flatten, acquire a squamous-like appearance, and migrate into the injured area along the basement membrane. Mitoses are frequent, and occasional epithelial clusters project into the lumen. The flattened cells soon become more cuboidal, and differentiated cytoplasmic elements appear. Tubular morphology and function return to normal in 3 to 4 weeks.

Tubulorrhexis

If tubulorrhexis—tubular basement membrane rupture—occurs, the response resembles that described above (with intact membrane), save that interstitial changes are more prominent. Fibroblasts proliferate and deposit more ECM, and tubular lumina collapse. Some tubules will regenerate; others will become fibrotic, with consequent focal losses of functional nephrons.

Medullary Renal Tubules

Medullary diseases of the kidney are often associated with extensive necrosis, which involves tubules, interstitium, and blood vessels. Necrotic tissues slough into the urine. Healing by fibrosis causes urinary obstruction within the kidney. Although there is some epithelial proliferation, there is no significant regeneration.

Glomeruli

Glomeruli do not regenerate. Necrosis of glomerular endothelial or epithelial cells, whether focal, segmental, or diffuse, heals by scarring (Fig. 3-14). Mesangial cells are related to smooth muscle cells and have some capacity for regeneration. After unilateral nephrectomy, glomeruli in the remaining kidney enlarge by both hypertrophy and hyperplasia. Podocyte progenitor cells in Bowman capsule may replace lost podocytes.

Lung

Respiratory tract lining epithelium can regenerate to some degree if underlying matrix is intact. Superficial injuries to tracheal and bronchial epithelia heal by regeneration from adjacent epithelium. The progenitor cells have not been clearly identified, but bronchoalveolar stem cells or alveolar epithelial type II progenitors are candidates. Bone marrow–derived stem cells may also take residence in the lung. The outcome of alveolar injury ranges from complete recovery of structure and function to incapacitating fibrosis. As with the liver, the degree of cell necrosis and extent of damage to the ECM determine the outcome (Fig. 3-15).

Alveolar Injury With Intact Basement Membranes

Alveolar injury due to infections, shock, oxygen toxicity, etc. causes variable alveolar cell death. Alveoli are flooded with an inflammatory exudate rich in plasma proteins. As long as the alveolar basement membrane is intact, healing occurs by regeneration. Neutrophils and macrophages clear the alveolar exudate, but if they fail to do so, it is organized by granulation tissue, and intra-alveolar fibrosis results. Alveolar type II epithelial cells or pneumocytes (the alveolar reserve cells) migrate to denuded areas and divide to form cells with features intermediate between type I and type II pneumocytes. These cells cover the alveolar surface and establish contact with other epithelial cells. When mitosis stops, the cells differentiate into type I pneumocytes. Bone marrow–derived cells or putative lung bronchoalveolar progenitor or stem cells may participate by differentiating into bronchiolar Clara cells and alveolar cells (see Table 3-8).

Alveolar Injury With Disrupted Basement Membranes

Extensive alveolar basement membrane damage evokes scarring and fibrosis. Mesenchymal cells from alveolar septa proliferate and differentiate into fibroblasts and myofibroblasts. Macrophage products induce fibroblast proliferation. The myofibroblasts and fibroblasts migrate into alveolar spaces. There they secrete ECM components, mainly type I collagen and proteoglycans, to produce pulmonary fibrosis. In emphysema (see Chapter 18), airspaces enlarge and alveolar walls are destroyed. Ineffective replacement of elastin leads to irreversible loss of tissue resiliency and function.

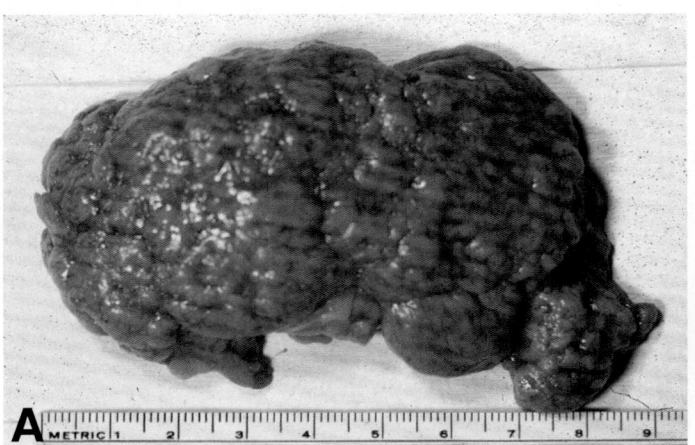
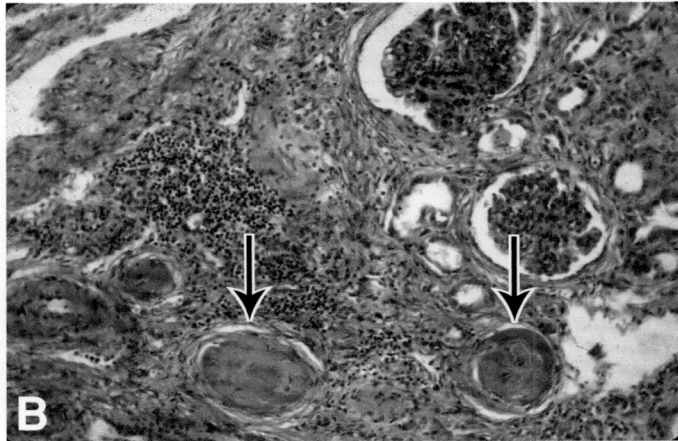

FIGURE 3-14. Scarred kidney. A. Repeated bacterial urinary tract infections have scarred the kidney. **B.** Many glomeruli have been destroyed and appear as circular scars (*arrows*).

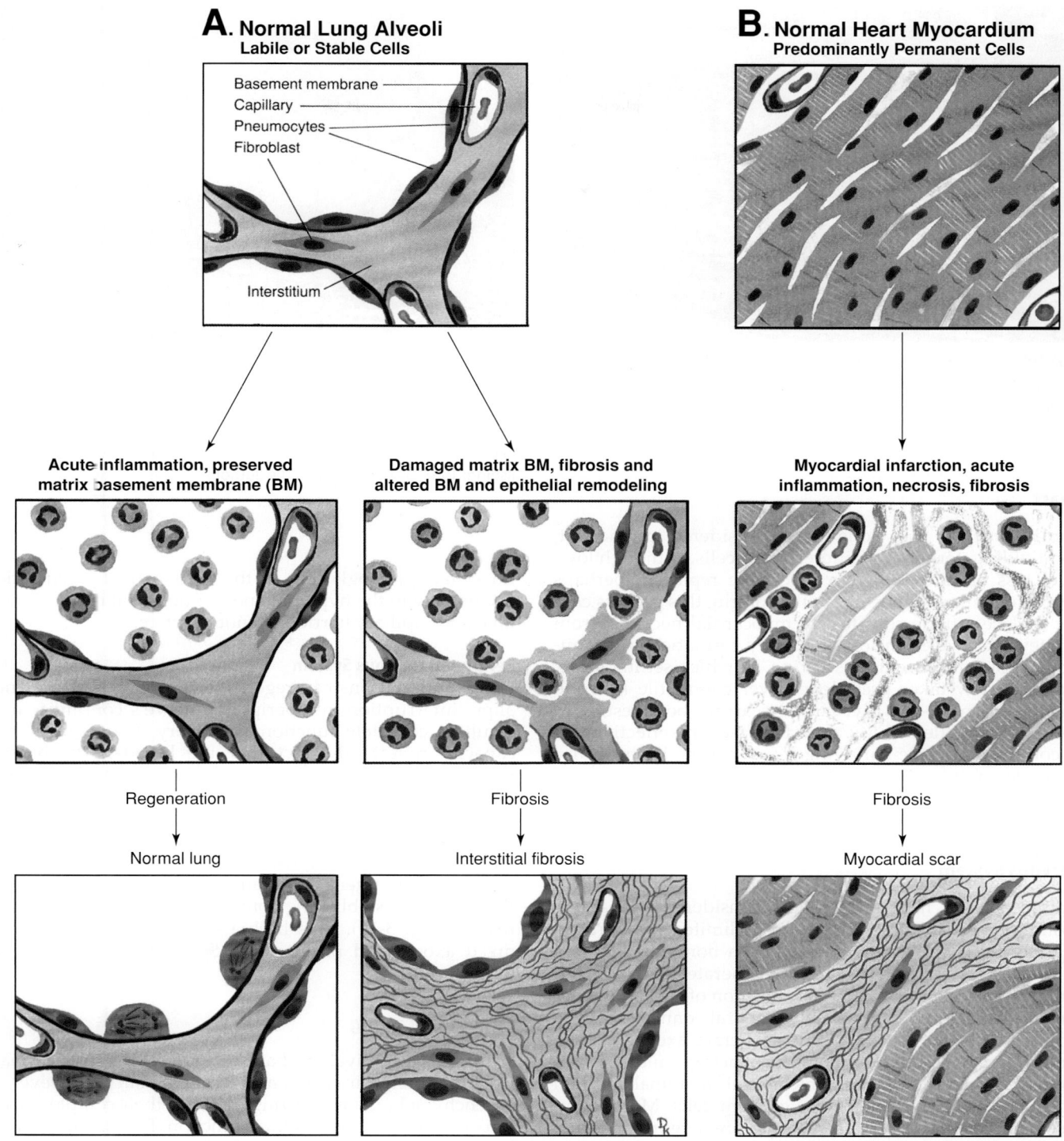

FIGURE 3-15. Examples of fibrotic and regenerative repair. A. The lung alveoli are lined with type I and type II epithelial cells (pneumocytes) that lie on a basement membrane. If the basement membrane remains intact following lung damage, there is rapid reepithelialization and return to normal lung architecture. If the basement membrane is damaged, type II epithelial cells proliferate on the underlying extracellular matrix, and fibroblasts and myofibroblasts are recruited to deposit a collagen-rich matrix, leading to fibrosis. **B.** Though small numbers of cardiac stem cells have been described, regeneration of myocardium is rarely observed. By and large cardiomyocytes are terminally differentiated and not capable of renewal. Myocardial damage due to infarction and acute inflammation is repaired by fibrosis and scar formation, increasing chances of arrhythmia or heart failure.

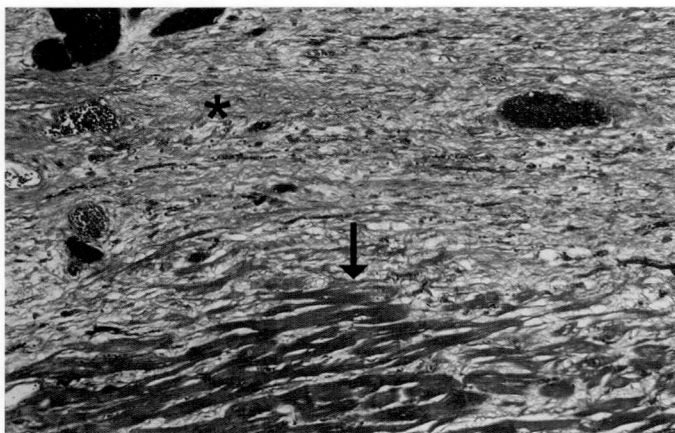

FIGURE 3-16. Myocardial infarction. A section through a healed myocardial infarct shows mature fibrosis (*) and disrupted myocardial fibers (*arrow*).

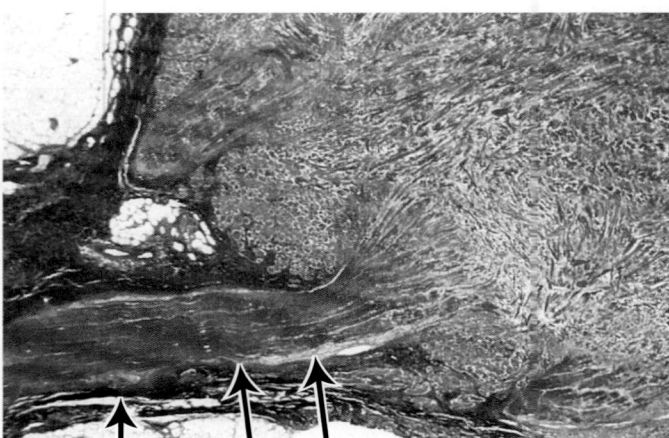

FIGURE 3-17. Traumatic neuroma. In this photomicrograph, the original nerve (*arrows*) enters the neuroma. The nerve is surrounded by dense collagenous tissue, which appears *dark blue* with this trichrome stain. Excessive repair obstructs axonal reconnection. (From Okazaki H, Scheithauer BW. *Atlas of Neuropathology.* New York: Gower Medical Publishing; 1988. By permission of the author.)

Heart

Cardiomyocytes had long been considered permanent, nondividing, terminally differentiated cells. Although low-level loss of cardiac myocytes can be replaced, perhaps from progenitors of one or another origin, this process cannot replace muscle cells lost to myocardial necrosis, from whatever cause. Such losses heal by formation of granulation tissue and eventual scarring, in which setting structural integrity takes precedence over contractile function (Figs. 3-15 and 3-16). Myocardial scarring both results in loss of contractile activity, and decreases the effectiveness of contraction in the surviving myocardium. With cardiac ischemia or infarction, and often in other organs, healing results in scarring despite the presence of cells with a regenerative capacity.

Nervous System

Mature neurons have always been considered permanent, postmitotic cells. While the brain has limited regenerative capacity from stem cells, derived from bone marrow and perhaps other sources, the CNS regenerates poorly. After trauma, only regrowth and reorganization of surviving neuronal cell processes can reestablish neural connections. The peripheral nervous system can regenerate axons, but the central nervous system cannot. The olfactory bulb and hippocampal dentate gyrus regions of adult mammalian brain regenerate via neural precursor or stem cells. Multipotent precursor cells have also been seen elsewhere in the brain, raising hope that repair of neural circuitry may eventually be possible (see Table 3-8).

Central Nervous System

Damage to the brain or spinal cord is followed by growth of capillaries and gliosis (i.e., inflammatory immune cell response, astrocytic and microglial proliferation). Gliosis in the CNS is the equivalent of scar formation elsewhere; once established, it is permanent. In spinal cord injuries, axonal outgrowth can occur up to 2 weeks after injury. After that, gliosis has taken place and axonal regeneration is prevented by release of myelin-associated glycoprotein and chondroi-

tin sulfate proteoglycans. In the CNS, axonal regeneration occurs only in the hypothalamo-hypophyseal region, where glial and capillary barriers do not interfere.

Peripheral Nervous System

Peripheral neurons can regenerate axons, and if the ends align, interruption in a peripheral nerve's continuity may result in complete functional recovery. This regenerative capacity reflects the fact that the blood–nerve barrier, which would insulate peripheral axons from extracellular fluids, is not restored for 2 to 3 months. As well, Schwann cell basement membranes guide regeneration, as basement membrane laminin and nerve growth factor (NGF) guide and stimulate neurite growth. If, however, cut ends are not in perfect alignment or inflammation or scarring prevents them from reestablishing continuity, a traumatic neuroma results (Fig. 3-17). This bulbous lesion contains disorganized axons, and proliferating Schwann cells and fibroblasts.

Effects of Scarring

Scarring is a survival mechanism, with roles in tissue repair, isolating foreign invaders and limiting injury. However, in parenchymal organs, scarring modifies their complex structure and never improves their function. For example, in the heart, the scar of a myocardial infarction prevents cardiac rupture, but reduces total contractile tissue and interferes with the contraction efficiency of remaining cardiac myocytes. Extensive postinfarction scarring may itself cause congestive heart failure (see Chapter 17). Similarly, an aorta that is weakened and scarred by atherosclerosis is prone to dilate as an aneurysm (see Chapter 16). Scarred mitral and aortic valves injured by rheumatic fever are often stenotic, regurgitant, or both, leading to congestive heart failure. Persistent inflammation within the pericardium produces fibrous adhesions, which result in constrictive pericarditis and heart failure.

Pulmonary alveolar fibrosis causes respiratory failure. Peritoneal infection, or even surgery, may create adhesions that obstruct the intestines. After immunologic injury, collagenous scars replace glomeruli and, if extensive, lead to kidney failure. Cutaneous scarring after burns or surgery may severely limit mobility and produce unsatisfactory cosmetic results. Therapeutic intervention seeks both to create optimum conditions for constructive scarring and to prevent pathologic overshoot of this process.

Wound Repair Is Often Suboptimal

Abnormalities in any of the three healing processes—repair, contraction, and regeneration—yield unsuccessful or prolonged wound healing. The surgeon's skill is often of critical importance.

Deficient Scar Formation

Inadequate formation of granulation tissue or an inability to form a suitable ECM leads to deficient scar formation and its complications.

Wound Dehiscence and Incisional Hernias
Dehiscence (a wound-splitting open) occurs most often after abdominal surgery, and can be life threatening. Increased mechanical stress on an abdominal wound from vomiting, coughing, pathologic obesity or bowel obstruction may cause that wound to dehisce. Metabolic deficiency, hypoproteinemia, and general inanition such as often accompanies metastatic cancer and other terminal conditions, may predispose to dehiscence. **Incisional hernias** of the abdominal wall are defects caused by weak surgical scars because of insufficient ECM deposition or inadequate collagen matrix cross-linking. Loops of intestine may become trapped within incisional hernias.

Ulceration
Wounds can ulcerate if intrinsic blood supply is poor or vascularization during healing is insufficient. Backpressure from incompetent venous valves can cause stasis ulcers, which are common and often occur on the lower leg (see Chapter 16). Arterial insufficiency, due to severe atherosclerosis can cause ulcers, frequently on the lower leg or the foot. In diabetes, cutaneous ulcers develop for several reasons: diabetes limits poor arterial and capillary blood supply, at the same time it reduces expression of, and cellular responsiveness to, growth factors. Trauma, pressure, or diabetic neuropathy may blunt pain sensation and lead to nonhealing wounds. **Decubitus ulcers** are commonly seen in patients immobilized in beds or wheelchairs. Constant pressure on skin over a bony prominence can cause local infarction within 2 to 3 hours. Age-related thinning of the skin and subcutaneous fat can exacerbate this response. These ulcers can be both broad and deep, with infection penetrating deep into the connective tissue.

Excessive Scar Formation in the Skin

Excessive ECM deposition—largely excessive collagen—at a wound site may cause hypertrophic scars or keloids. **Keloids** are exuberant scars that tend to progress beyond the site of initial injury and recur after excision (Fig. 3-18), resembling benign tumors. They are unsightly. Attempts at surgical repair are always problematic, often generating a still larger keloid. Keloids occur mainly during adolescence and early adulthood, and mainly on the upper trunk, neck, and head, but not the scalp. This distribution reflects the (epigenetic) heterogeneity of fibroblast populations in different locations. Dark-skinned individuals are more often affected, suggesting a genetic predisposition. Unlike normal scars, keloids are less responsive to glucocorticoids; local administration of 5-fluorouracil has been effective.

Hypertrophic scars, on the other hand, are not associated with race or heredity, and their severity can decline with age. These scars are confined to wound margins, and often develop in association with unrelieved mechanical stress. Hypertrophic scars are reddish, indicating hypervascularity. They are pruritic, which suggests that local mast cells are releasing excessive histamine.

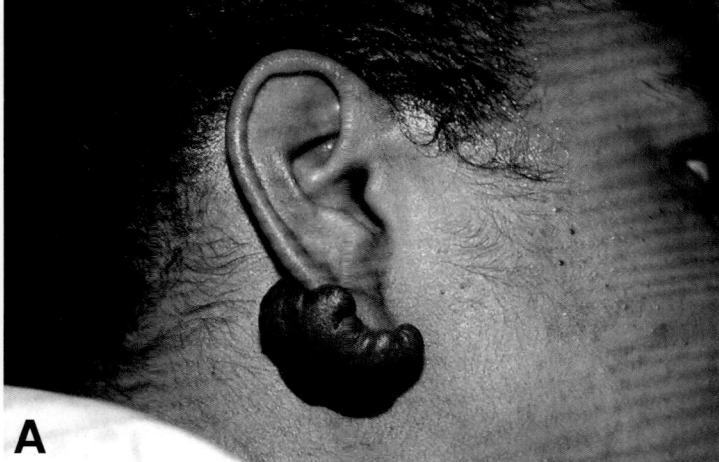 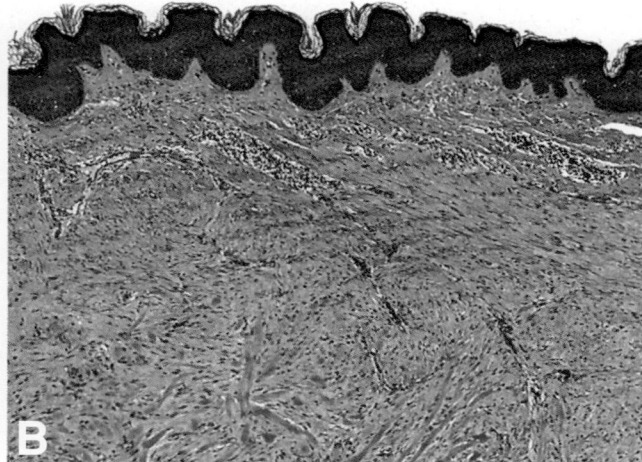

FIGURE 3-18. Keloid. A. A light-skinned black woman developed a keloid as a reaction to having her earlobe pierced. **B.** Microscopically, the dermis is markedly thickened by the presence of collagen.

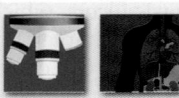 **PATHOLOGY; PATHOPHYSIOLOGY:** Histologically, hypertrophic scars and keloids both have broad and irregular collagen bundles, with more capillaries and fibroblasts than a normal scar of the same age. Collagen synthesis and numbers of reducible cross-links remain excessively high, suggesting "maturation arrest," or block, in healing. Observed overexpression of fibronectin supports this hypothesis. Mechanisms that can contribute include stress-related activation of matrix-bound, latent TGFβ and activation of fibrogenic signaling from macrophages.

Excessive Contraction

A decrease in a wound/scar's size requires fibroblasts, myo-fibroblasts, cell–cell contacts, and sustained cell contraction. Exaggeration of these is **contracture**, and causes severe deformity of the wound and surrounding tissues. Interestingly, regions that normally show minimal wound contraction (e.g., palms, soles) are prone to develop contractures. Contractures are particularly conspicuous when serious burns heal, and can be severe enough to compromise joint movements. In the gut, contractures (strictures) can obstruct passage through the esophagus or intestines.

Several diseases entail contractures and irreversible fibrosis of the superficial fascia, including Dupuytren contracture (palmar contracture), Lederhosen disease (plantar contracture), and Peyronie disease (contracture of the cavernous tissues of the penis). These often occur without known precipitating injury, even though the basic process is similar to contracture in wound healing.

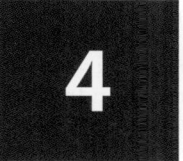

4 Immunopathology

Jeffrey S. Warren, David S. Strayer

Biology of the Immune System

Higher vertebrate immune systems have evolved to protect hosts (and species) from microbial invasion; they are multifaceted and highly regulated, with many cross-system interactions. Beyond microorganisms, other agents including toxins, chemicals, drugs, multicellular parasites and transplanted foreign tissues can elicit responses. The immune system has two arms: innate immunity, which is a ready-made, rapid-response initial line of defense; and adaptive immunity, which is both powerful and specific, which can ramp up dramatically, and generate memory and heightened intensity upon reexposure to a particular agent. Familiar examples of adaptive immunity include responses to infections and vaccinations. It is important to consider innate and adaptive immunity in the context of inflammation, cell injury, and cell death. Inflammation is a largely stereotyped response to insult: whether microbial infection, physical trauma, ischemia–reperfusion, or others (see Chapter 2). Immune responses can lead to tissue- and organ-specific pathology sequelae to infections, hypersensitivity reactions, autoimmune diseases, and transplantation. Defects in either the innate or adaptive systems can lead to increased susceptibility to infections. Understanding of both acquired and genetic–molecular defects has provided great insight into the pathophysiology of autoimmune and immunodeficiency diseases.

INNATE AND ADAPTIVE IMMUNITY

Innate immunity is a first-line defense system. It encompasses barriers such as regionally adapted epithelia (e.g., thick keratinized skin, ciliated respiratory epithelium), chemical–mechanical surface coatings (e.g., antibacterial peptides, mucus) and indigenous microbial flora (microbiome) that compete with potential pathogens and shape host immune responses. Cell surface, endosomal, cytosolic, and soluble extracellular mediator molecules bind targets through mechanisms independent of specific B- and T-lymphocyte–mediated antigen recognition. This distribution of defense molecules forms a monitoring system that defends against extracellular, intraendosomal, and cytosolic pathogens.

The innate system includes hundreds of germline-encoded **pattern recognition receptors (PRRs)** and antimicrobial peptides (AMPs). PRRs are widely distributed among various types of cells. Because of their distribution throughout many tissues (and subcellular compartments), they help protect essentially every route of entry against a vast array of microorganisms. The innate system also includes many specialized host defense cell types (e.g., neutrophils, **innate lymphoid cells [ILCs]**, lymphoid cells without the highly variable antigen-binding structures found on "standard" B and T lymphocytes).

Adaptive immunity encompasses specialized **antigen-presenting cells (APCs)** and **clonal lymphocytes** (B and T cells) that bear, and/or secrete, molecules (**T-cell receptors [TCR]**, **antibodies**) which specifically bind discrete foreign structures (antigens/epitopes). Unlike the innate system, an individual's B- and T-lymphocyte armamentaria can recognize and distinguish many millions of different antigens/epitopes. The vast diversity of adaptive system receptors largely results from recombination of multiple discrete blocks of DNA. Adaptive immunity encompasses generative lymphoid organs (bone marrow, thymus) that produce mature but naive immune cells, secondary lymphoid structures (lymph nodes, spleen, regionally adapted lymphoid tissues) that facilitate the colocalization and concentrated exposure of foreign antigens to immune cells and tertiary lymphoid tissues (see below).

The efficiency of adaptive immunity is dramatically enhanced by long-lived memory lymphocytes and cell trafficking and recirculation (via lymphatics and blood vessels) orchestrated by soluble chemotactic factors and location-specific intercellular adhesion molecules. This systemically integrated system enables the relatively few lymphocytes that express a particular antigen receptor to interact efficiently with individual target molecules among the vast variety of incoming antigens. The abilities of APCs to interact with T cells to initiate immune responses and of antigen-specific cytotoxic T-effector cells to kill (e.g., virus-infected) host cells each require compatible cell-to-cell surface molecules (histocompatibility molecules; human leukocyte antigens) encoded by genes of the **major histocompatibility complex (MHC)**.

Innate Immunity Entails Barriers, Pattern Recognition Responses, and Specialized Cells

The innate immune system appeared in evolution 200 to 300 million years before adaptive immunity, and evolved in concert with microorganisms as the latter developed ways to circumvent host defenses. Innate system defenses are mediated by inflammation (see Chapter 2) and/or antiviral

effector mechanisms. Resident and recruited phagocytes and redundant sets of soluble mediators respond quickly to agents that penetrate outer defenses. The innate system distinguishes self from nonself far less precisely than does adaptive immunity. *Germline-encoded receptors recognize and bind categories of structures* (**pathogen-associated molecular patterns [PAMPs]**) *present on the surfaces of microbes—but not on healthy host cells.* PRRs are far less diverse (hundreds of patterns) than are antibodies and TCRs (millions of specificities) and are not clonal (i.e., each is identical on all cell types). PRRs of the innate system are diverse, redundant, and counter both extracellular and intracellular invaders. Through recognition of **damage-associated molecular patterns (DAMPs)**, the innate system also eliminates damaged host cells and triggers tissue repair (see Chapters 2 and 3). Finally, the innate system connects functionally with many levels of the adaptive system.

Whether cutaneous, respiratory, gastrointestinal or urothelial, barrier epithelial cells are held together by tight junctions and have region-specific adaptations (e.g., keratin layers, cilia, mucus production) that enhance their defensive functions. Chemical defenses include low pH (e.g., skin, gastric juice) and secreted **AMPs** and lytic enzymes (e.g., **lysozyme**). Across the animal kingdom, there are more than 1,000 different AMPs. Human AMPs include **defensins**, **cathelicidins**, **bacterial permeability-increasing proteins**, some **chemokines**, and C-terminal keratin fragments. Human defensins are 18- to 45-amino acid cationic peptides, made by diverse leukocytes and epithelial cells (skin, respiratory, gastrointestinal), and classified into α and β families based on the locations of conserved cysteine residues. They bind microbes in which they form pore-like cell membrane defects. More structurally diverse, cathelicidins are 12- to 80-amino acid peptides made by neutrophils, activated macrophages, and barrier cells. The physical and biochemical barriers of innate immunity are backed by phagocytes as well as nonphagocytic ILCs (including **natural killer [NK] cells**), mast cells, and other specialized lymphocytes with limited antigen receptor diversity.

PRRs recognize PAMPs and DAMPs—but not healthy mammalian cells—and thus "see" such patterns as nonself (Table 4-1). DAMPs, also called **alarmins** or danger signals, are revealed by injured or dying cells and, on occasion, by activated immune cells, whether the result of infection, trauma, or other injury. The multicompartment anatomic distribution of PRRs reflects their varied roles in innate host defense. Beyond the scope of this chapter, there have been great advances in understanding signal-transduction pathways and downstream mediator cross talk.

Cell Surface and Endosomal PRRs

Toll-like receptors (TLRs) are leucine-rich transmembrane proteins that occur throughout the animal kingdom (Fig. 4-1). TLRs form homodimers (and sometimes heterodimers) when they bind PAMPs and DAMPs and in many cell types are expressed selectively on either plasma or endosomal membranes (Table 4-2). Plasma membrane TLRs (TLR1, -2, -4, -5, -6) recognize surface moieties of extracellular microbes (e.g., bacterial **lipopolysaccharides [LPSs]**, lipopeptides, flagellin, bacterial peptidoglycan), while endosomal TLRs (TLR3, -7, -8, -9) recognize microbial nucleic acid (e.g., double-stranded RNA [dsRNA], single-stranded RNA [ssRNA], cytidine-guanidine dinucleotide [CpG] DNA). Defects in

TABLE 4-1
PATHOGEN-ASSOCIATED (PAMPs) AND DAMAGE-ASSOCIATED MOLECULAR PATTERNS (DAMPs)

	Molecular Moiety (Examples)	Microbe Type
PAMPs		
Cell wall lipids	Lipopolysaccharide (LPS)	Gram-negative bacteria
	Teichoic acid	Gram-positive bacteria
Cell wall carbohydrates	Mannans	Fungi
	Glucans	
Cell surface proteins	Flagellin	Bacteria
	Pilin	
Microbial nucleic acids	ssRNA	Viruses
	dsRNA	Microorganisms
	CpG sequences	
DAMPs		
Stress-induced proteins	Heat-shock proteins (HSPs)	N/A
Nuclear proteins	High-mobility group box 1	N/A
Crystals	Monosodium urate	N/A

CpG = cytidine-guanidine dinucleotide; dsRNA = double-stranded RNA; N/A = not applicable; ssRNA = single-stranded RNA.

endosomal TLR localization and function have been identified as a cause of immunodeficiency. Once foreign invaders, whether extra- or intracellular, activate them, transduced signals drive expression of proinflammatory genes (e.g., cytokines, chemokines, endothelial adhesion molecules,

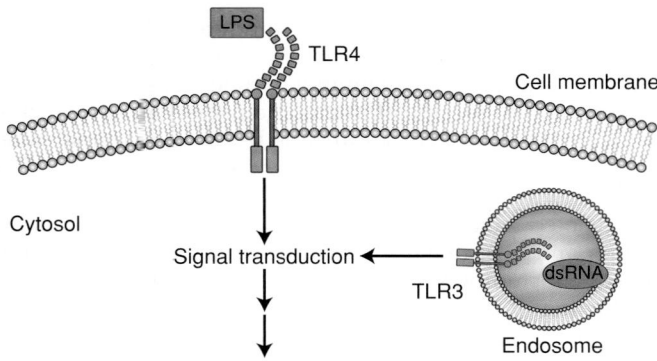

FIGURE 4-1. Toll-like receptors (TLRs) form transmembrane dimers that bind pathogen-associated molecular patterns (PAMPs) on the outer surfaces of cells and on the inner surfaces of phagocyte endosomes. Plasma membrane TLRs (e.g., TLR4) mediate defense against extracellular pathogens (e.g., pyogenic bacteria) and endosomal TLRs (e.g., TLR3) mediate defense against intracellular pathogens (e.g., viruses). In both cases, signal transduction leads to a variety of proinflammatory and/or antiviral cellular responses. Extracellular and intraendosomal PAMP recognition domains contain leucine-rich repeat sequences. *LPS* = lipopolysaccharide.

TABLE 4-2
PATTERN RECOGNITION MOLECULES

	Cellular/Anatomic Location	Examples
Membrane Associated		
Toll-like receptors (TLRs)	Plasma membranes	TLR1, -2, -4, -5, -6
	Endosomal membranes	TLR3, -7, -8, -9, -10[a]
C-type lectin-like receptors	Plasma membrane	Mannose receptor
Scavenger receptors	Plasma membrane	CD36 (Platelet gpIIIb)
N-formyl peptide receptors	Plasma membrane	N-formyl peptide receptor
Cytosolic		
NOD-like receptors (NLRs)	Cytosol	NOD1/2
RIG-like receptors (RLRs)	Cytosol	RIG-1
Soluble		
Natural antibodies (IgM)	Plasma	IgM antiphosphorylcholine
Complement	Plasma	C3, C1qrs[b]
Pentraxins	Plasma	C-reactive protein, Amyloid P, Pentraxin 3
Collectins	Plasma/alveoli	Mannose-binding lectin, Surfactant protein, SP-A
Lectins	Plasma	Ficolin -1, -2, -3, Galectins

[a]The function of TLR10 is unknown.
[b]C1qrs spans Fc domains of fixed immunoglobulin molecules and binds directly to some pattern-associated molecular patterns.
IgM = immunoglobulin M; NOD = nucleotide oligomerization domain–containing protein; RIG = retinoic acid–inducible gene.

costimulatory molecules) and/or antiviral genes (e.g., type I interferons [IFNs]). Accessory molecules (e.g., LPS-binding protein, CD14, MD2) may enhance TLR-mediated cell activation by a PAMP.

Additional types of cell surface PRRs also participate in innate host defense (Table 4-2). C-type (calcium-dependent) **lectin receptors** bind carbohydrate moieties (e.g., β-glucans, mannose) characteristic of microorganisms but not mammals, thus conferring distinction of nonself from self. The best-studied C-type lectin receptors are **dectin**-1, dectin-2, and the **mannose receptor (CD206)**. Dectin-1 and dectin-2 bind β-glucan and mannose-rich oligosaccharides expressed by the yeast and hyphal forms, respectively, of *Candida albicans*. Scavenger receptors bind many cell surface moieties, mediate uptake of oxidized lipoproteins, and facilitate microbe phagocytosis. Finally, ***N*-formyl peptide receptors** are 7-span transmembrane GTP-binding proteins expressed by phagocytes. *N*-formyl peptides are only made by bacteria (and within mitochondria); engagement activates cells and chemotaxis.

Cytosolic PRRs

NOD-like (<u>n</u>ucleotide <u>o</u>ligomerization <u>d</u>omain–containing protein) receptors, **RIG-like** (<u>r</u>etinoic acid–<u>i</u>nducible <u>g</u>ene I) receptors, and cytosolic DNA sensors, all distinct from cell surface and endosomal receptors, monitor the cytosolic compartment (Table 4-2) and connect to activation pathways for inflammation and/or **type I IFN** generation. Nearly two dozen NOD-like receptors (NLRs) have been identified. Like TLRs, NLR proteins possess a leucine-rich microbial recognition domain. Other functional domains allow formation of oligomeric multiunit signaling complexes. NOD1 and NOD2 (expressed in gut epithelial cells and phagocytes) are important in innate responses to GI pathogens like *Helicobacter* and *Listeria*. Mutations that affect the NOD-like receptor P3 (NLRP3) pyrin effector domain are associated with hereditary periodic fever syndromes. Finally, some crystalline substances like monosodium urate also act via NLRs to trigger an inflammatory response with assembly and activation of the "**inflammasome**" (see Chapter 1).

RIG-like receptors (RLRs) sense cytosolic viral RNA and elicit antiviral type I IFNs. Cytosolic DNA sensors encompass a heterogeneous group of proteins that recognize DNA and trigger inflammasome assembly, type I IFN production and/or autophagy (see Chapter 2).

Table 4-2 also lists soluble high–molecular-weight pattern recognition molecules. Members of each group are active in plasma and extracellular tissue fluid and contain several extended PAMP ligand-binding domains. Natural immunoglobulin M (IgM) antibodies and the complement protein complex C1qrs are most familiar. Pentameric IgM can span adjacent antigen epitopes and fix complement. C1qrs spans adjacent Fc domains of surface-bound immunoglobulin (Ig) molecules, thus initiating the classical complement pathway and functionally linking the adaptive immune system (antibodies) to the complement system. C1qrs and C3-derived moieties also directly bind microbial structures and thus are components of innate immunity. **Pentraxins**, including C-reactive protein, contain five extended binding domains. **Collectins** include **mannose-binding lectin**, a key mediator of the most recently discovered third (nonclassical, nonalternative) complement pathway and the pulmonary alveolar surfactant proteins, SP-A and SP-D. **Ficolins** possess structural homology to C1qrs and collectins, and bind PAMPs on Gram-positive bacteria surfaces. Over a dozen **galectins** (which bind β-galactoside sugars) have been described.

Cells of the Innate Immune System

With few exceptions, ILCs resemble resting B and T lymphocytes morphologically. (NK cells contain cytoplasmic granules and so are called "**large granular lymphocytes**.") Bone marrow-derived, ILCs arise from a common precursor that expresses the transcription factor, Id2. In turn, Id2$^+$ precursor cells can differentiate into ILC1, ILC2, or ILC3 subsets which differ in their transcription factors, required growth factors, elaborated cytokines and their roles in host defense (Table 4-3).

TABLE 4-3
INNATE LYMPHOID CELLS (ILCs)

Subset	Transcription Factors	Cytokines Produced	Function
ILC1	T-bet	Interferon-γ	Antiviral defense
ILC2	GATA-3	IL-5 IL-3	Allergic response
ILC3	RORγT	IL-17 IL-22	Intestinal barrier function

IL = interleukin.

ILCs do not express Igs or TCRs and each subset contains subtypes, the best understood of which are NK cells—a type of ILC1 that defend against intracellular viruses and bacteria and participate in antitumor surveillance. All NK cells express CD56; most express CD16; none express T-lymphocyte–restricted CD3. NK cells constitute about 10% of peripheral blood lymphocytes and kill target cells via the same cytotoxic mechanisms as CD8$^+$ T cells, via antibody-dependent cellular cytotoxicity (ADCC) and indirectly via production of IFN-γ which in turn activates macrophages (see below).

A complex set of counterbalancing host target cell activating and inhibitory receptors regulate NK cells. The most numerous NK cell inhibitory receptors are <u>k</u>iller cell <u>im</u>munoglobulin-like <u>r</u>eceptors (KIRs). KIRs bind several different MHC class I molecules. Other NK cell-inhibitory receptor classes include leukocyte Ig-like receptors (LIRs) and lectins such as CD94/NKG2A. These inhibitory receptor types also engage MHC class I molecules. Downregulating host cell MHC class I molecules tips the balance toward NK cell-mediated lysis. Activating NK cell receptors are also diverse; they recognize many ligands, some expressed on normal cells and others on stressed, injured, infected, or transformed host cells. Major NK cell-activating receptors include KIRs, lectins, and CD16 which binds IgG antibody via its Fc domain and initiate ADCC.

Finally, there are some less well understood B and T lymphocytes which express antigen receptors (like "standard" B and T cells) but recognize limited numbers of structures that are common to groups of microorganisms. These members of the innate host defenses include B-1 cells, marginal-zone B cells, γδ T lymphocytes, intraepithelial T cells with αβ TCRs, and the so-called invariant NKT cells.

As noted, innate system pathways facilitate acute inflammation and host defense via antiviral responses. A variety of PRRs, including several TLRs, NLRs, and RLRs, mediate production of type I IFNs (IFN-α and IFN-β). Type I IFNs upregulate class I MHC molecules on potential target cells for cytotoxic T lymphocytes, increase cytotoxic activities of NK cells and cytotoxic T lymphocytes, facilitate conversion of naive T cells to Th1-helper cells, increase intranodal lymphocyte sequestration and, via type I IFN receptor, induce host cell resistance to viruses. Finally, the activated innate immune system also facilitates adaptive immune responses by inducing the "second signal" (e.g., CD80 [B7-1], CD86 [B7-2]) needed in antigen-induced responses, via conversion of naive T-helper cells into Th1 and Th17 effector cells and by stimulating lymphocyte proliferation and differentiation by upregulating key cytokines.

CELLS AND TISSUES OF THE IMMUNE SYSTEM

Cells of the immune and hematopoietic systems are derived from **multipotent hematopoietic stem cells (HSCs)**. Near the end of the first month of embryogenesis, HSCs first appear in the extraembryonic erythropoietic islands adjacent to the yolk sac. At 6 weeks, hematopoiesis shifts largely to fetal liver and then bone marrow. The latter begins at 2 months and by 6 months has completely shifted to bone marrow. By 8 weeks' gestation, lymphoid progenitors derived from HSCs circulate to the thymus where they differentiate into mature but naive T lymphocytes. ("Naive" indicates that the lymphocytes have not yet been exposed to foreign antigens.) Lymphoid progenitors destined to become B cells differentiate first within fetal liver (8 weeks) and later within bone marrow (12 weeks).

A structurally ordered microenvironment (e.g., thymic epithelium, bone marrow stromal cells, growth factors) is critical to thymus-derived T-lymphocyte and marrow-derived B-lymphocyte development. Thymus and bone marrow are "generative" lymphoid organs. Mature lymphocytes exit the thymus and bone marrow and "home" to peripheral lymphoid tissues (e.g., lymph nodes, spleen, skin, submucosa). Colonization of peripheral lymphoid tissues by mature B and T lymphocytes and the rapid deployment and recirculation of mature lymphocytes to different, often remote, parts of the immune system are both anatomically specific. Lymphocyte homing and recirculation are orchestrated by a series of complementary leukocyte and endothelial surface molecules that include site-specific **selectins** and **addressins** (see below). Lymphocyte development and homing/recirculation are fundamental to understanding immune responses, immunodeficiency states, regional host defense and the underpinnings of modern therapeutics (e.g., HSC transplantation and therapeutic antibodies that block lymphocyte–endothelial adhesion or lymphocyte egress from lymphoid organs).

Immune system cells express many surface molecules important in differentiation and cell-to-cell communication. These surface molecules are also markers of cell identity (e.g., CD4+ lymphocytes in AIDS monitoring). Currently, 300 different molecules have been assigned cluster of differentiation or cluster designation (CD) numbers by the International Workshop on Human Leukocyte Differentiation Antigens.

HSCs Are the Progenitors to Cells of the Immune System

Multipotent HSCs account for 0.01% to 0.1% of nucleated bone marrow cells, show characteristic flow cytometric light-scattering properties, can self-renew, usually express CD34 and c-KIT (CD117) cell surface proteins, and lack cell surface markers characteristic of more mature cells (a condition called "LIN–"). Developing HSCs differentially express more than 2,000 genes. Stem cells cycle, replicate, and give rise to lineage-committed progenitor cells. As progenitor cells differentiate into lymphocytes, erythrocytes, neutrophils, etc., they lose proliferative capacity (Fig. 4-2). Prevailing models of hematopoiesis/lymphopoiesis suggest that primitive stem cells give rise to committed progenitors (the hierarchical model) or can develop either into progenitor cells and back into stem cells (the cell cycle or continuum model).

CD34+ HSCs account for 0.01% to 0.1% of peripheral blood mononuclear cells. Bone marrow and blood HSCs are heterogeneous in terms of expressing lymphocyte or myeloid markers, activation antigens, and capacity to engraft bone marrow. Peripheral blood HSC infusion into transplant recipients reconstitutes marrow faster than do marrow-derived HSCs. In clinical HSC transplantation, donors receive recombinant growth factors before HSC harvest, a practice that increases harvested HSCs, decreases time to engraftment, and improves engraftment rates. The differential efficacy of peripheral blood versus marrow HSCs in leukemia patients is not decided, and *ex vivo* HSC manipulations to improve engraftment are an active area of research.

The primary branch point in differentiation is between lymphoid and myeloid progenitors (Fig. 4-2). The former ultimately give rise to T lymphocytes, B lymphocytes, and ILCs, while the latter become granulocytic, erythroid, monocytic-dendritic, and megakaryocytic colony-forming units (GEMM-CFUs). **Colony-forming units (CFUs)** are cells that give rise to specified populations of derivative cells, like granulocytes, monocytes, etc. Downstream CFUs become increasingly lineage specific, for example, CFU-GM (granulocyte-monocyte), CFU-Eo (eosinophil), and CFU-E (erythrocyte).

Lymphocytes

Committed lymphoid progenitor (CLP) cells give rise to **B lymphocytes**, **T lymphocytes**, and ILCs (Fig. 4-3). Lymphocytes constitute 25% to 30% of blood leukocytes; about 80% T cells, 10% B cells, and 10% ILCs (mostly NK cells). Comparing blood and lymphoid tissues, the relative proportions of lymphocyte types vary: unlike the blood, only 30% to 40% of splenic and bone marrow lymphocytes are T cells.

T Lymphocytes

T cells are categorized into subpopulations, based on their specialized functions, surface CD molecules and, in some cases, subtle morphologic features. Lymphoid progenitor cells destined to become T cells exit the marrow and migrate to the thymus where both α/β and γ/δ T lymphocytes are formed (Fig. 4-4). Thymic epithelium and stroma determine the microenvironment. The developing thymus is colonized by progenitors that give rise to T cells, macrophages, and **dendritic cells (DCs)**. The cortex contains a meshwork of epithelial cell processes that surround groups of immature thymocytes bearing both CD4+ and CD8+ surface molecules. As T lymphocytes mature, they percolate into the thymic medulla where, in close proximity to nested groups of epithelial cells, they form more mature cells that are either CD4+ or CD8+ (Fig. 4-4).

The thymic corticomedullary junction contains marrow HSC-derived macrophages and DCs. Much of the positive selection of thymocytes occurs in the cortex; negative selection tends to occur through exposure of developing (immature) thymocytes to corticomedullary DCs. *In positive selection, transient, low-affinity binding of cell surface TCRs to a person's own MHC class I or II molecules prevents cell death. Negative selection is the converse process; high-affinity TCR-mediated antigen binding in the context of one's own MHC class I or II molecules results in cell death by apoptosis. Self-antigens are presented by thymic medullary epithelial cells (TMECs). These two processes are pivotal to T-cell development, ensuring*

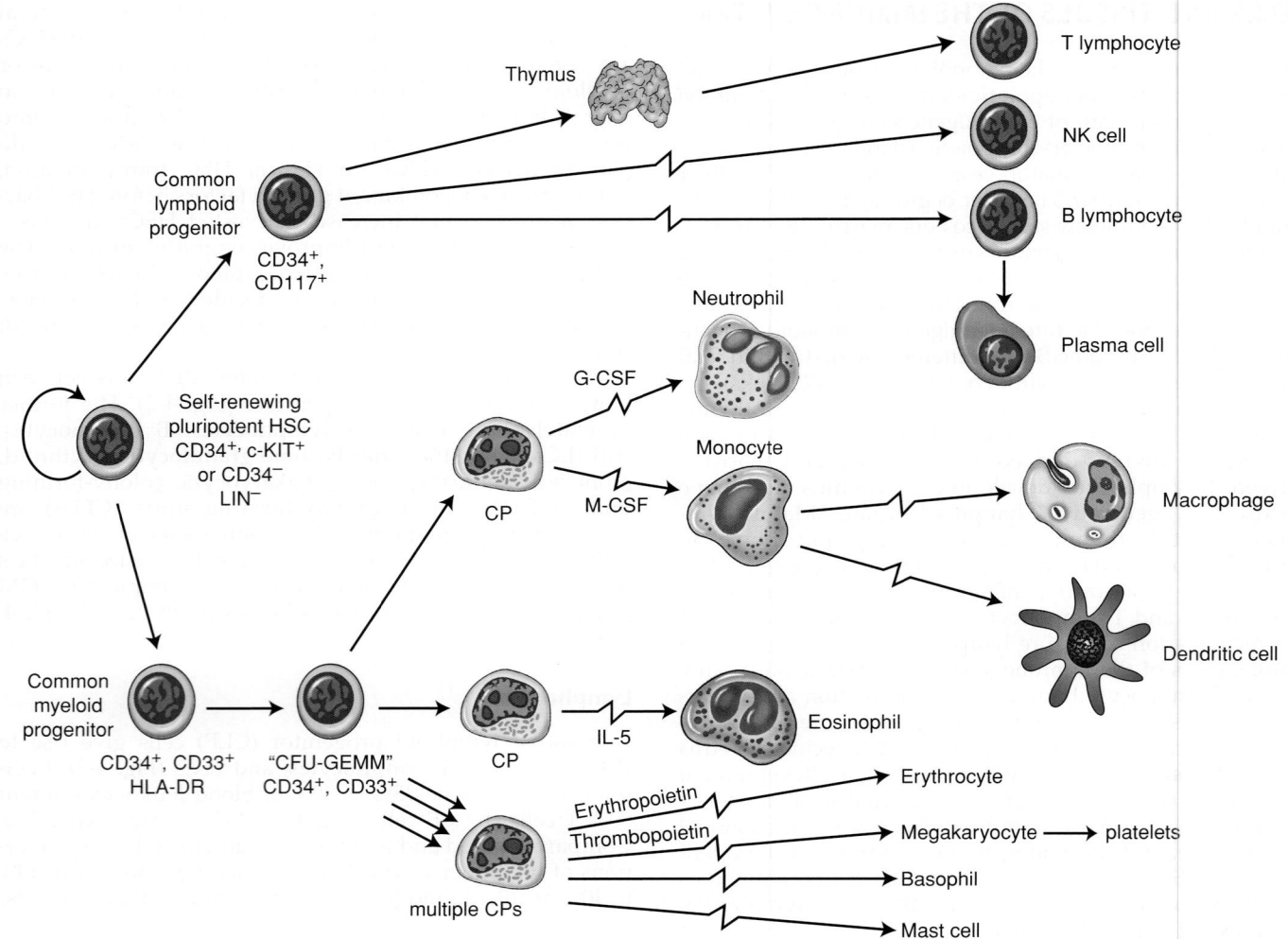

FIGURE 4-2. Pluripotent hematopoietic stem cells (HSCs) differentiate into either common lymphoid or myeloid progenitors and, in the case of myeloid cells, into lineage-specific colony-forming units (CFUs). Under the influence of an appropriate microenvironment and growth factors (e.g., erythropoietin, thrombopoietin), committed precursors (CPs) give rise to definitive cell types. Lymphoid progenitors are precursors of innate lymphoid cells (ILCs), T lymphocytes, and B lymphocytes. B lymphocytes give rise to plasma cells. *CD* = cluster designation; *GEMM-CFUs* = g̲ranulocytic, e̲rythroid, m̲onocytic-dendritic, and m̲egakaryocytic colony-forming units; *HLA* = human leukocyte antigen; *LIN–* = lineage-negative. "Colony-forming unit" refers to an in vitro bioassay.

that mature T cells can interact with the host cells but not so as to generate excessive self-reactivity (see Autoimmunity below, Chapter 11).

Lineage-specific differentiation and thymic selection of T cells are key to understanding immune responses and autoimmunity, respectively. Thymic T-lymphocyte maturation includes a series of linked processes. Developing T cells recombine dispersed gene segments that encode heterodimeric α/β or γ/δ TCRs. α/β cells serially progress through developmental stages: first CD4⁻/CD8⁻, then CD4⁺/CD8⁺, and then either CD4⁺/CD8⁻ or CD4⁻/CD8⁺ (Fig. 4-4). Most CD4⁺/CD8⁻ T cells function as helper cells, while most CD4⁻/CD8⁺ T cells are cytotoxic. Genetic defects in various developmental steps lead to immunodeficiency disorders and monogenic autoimmune disorders.

Naive T lymphocytes exit the thymus and populate secondary lymphoid tissues. In the thymus, antigen-specific TCRs are formed and expressed in conjunction with **CD3**, an essential accessory molecule (see below). Nearly 95% of circulating T lymphocytes express α/β TCRs and either CD4

or CD8. About 5% of T cells express γ/δ TCRs plus CD3, but lack both CD4 and CD8.

B Lymphocytes

B cells mature from CLP cells in bone marrow via several stages: pro-B lymphocytes, with unrecombined (germline) DNA and no-surface Ig; pre-B lymphocytes, which express an "early" antigen receptor (μ heavy chain plus an invariant surrogate light chain); immature B cells, which express a recombined H chain gene plus κ or λ messenger RNA (mRNA) and membrane IgM κ or λ; and finally, mature but naive B lymphocytes, which coexpress surface IgM and IgD. CD5⁺ B-1 and marginal zone CD5⁻ B cells develop from immature B lymphocytes via a different program from IgM/IgD B cells. B cells differentiate in the marrow into mature B cells and sometimes further into antibody-secreting plasma cells. The microenvironments of fetal liver and bone marrow are critical to B-cell development. In both sites, only B lymphocytes that survive pass through the multiple steps necessary to produce surface Ig. Conversely, if a surface Ig binds too avidly

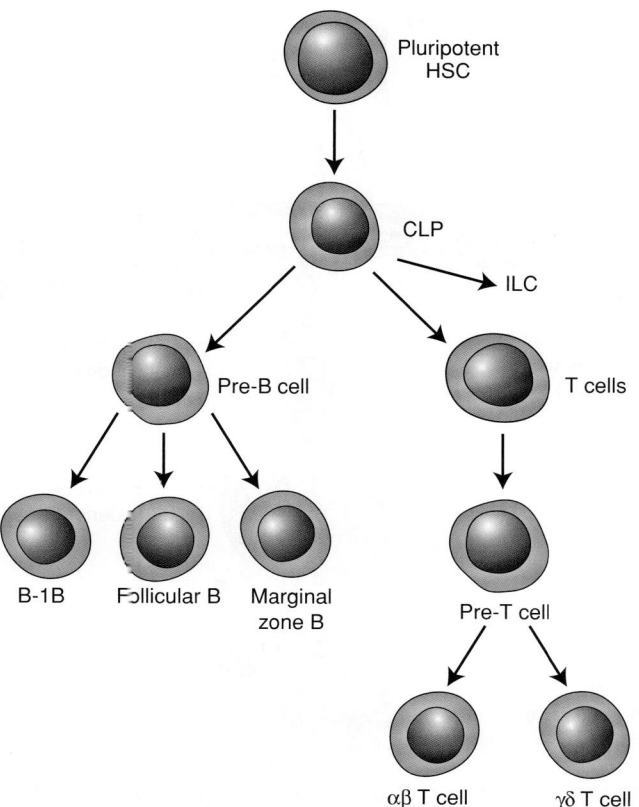

FIGURE 4-3. Pluripotent hematopoietic stem cells (HSCs) give rise to B and T lymphocytes—including their subsets. The common lymphoid progenitor (CLP) gives rise to B lymphocytes, T lymphocytes, and ILCs. (Fig. 4-2 depicts how HSCs and CLPs fit into the larger hematopoietic and lymphopoietic development schemes.) Commitment of CLPs to the B-lymphocyte lineage is triggered by E2A and EBF transcription factors followed by Pax5. In turn, commitment of CLPs to T lymphocytes is triggered by Notch 1, GATA3, and other (not shown) transcription factors. (ILC development is described in the text.)

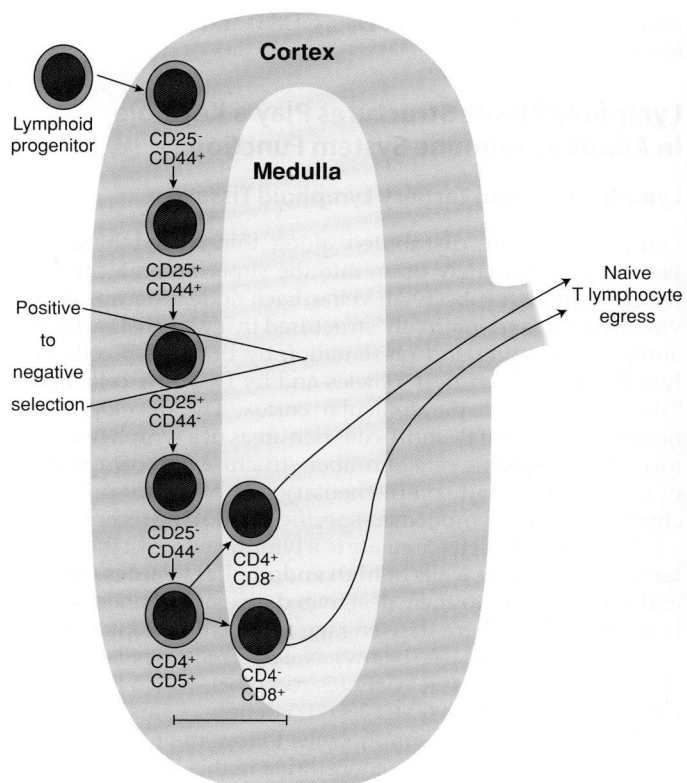

FIGURE 4-4. Lymphoid progenitors give rise to mature but naive T lymphocytes. Lymphocytes destined to become T lymphocytes migrate to the thymus where they express either α/β or γ/δ TCRs. As thymocytes percolate through the cortex and then medulla, they are positively and negatively selected. Most α/β T lymphocytes emerge as either CD4$^+$/CD8$^-$ helper cells or CD4$^-$/CD8$^+$ cytotoxic cells.

to self-antigens, developing B cells are eliminated. Analogous to T cells, B lymphocytes express a surface antigen-binding receptor: cell membrane immunoglobulin (mIg) with the same antigen-binding specificity as the soluble antibody that corresponding terminally differentiated plasma cells (see below) will ultimately secrete.

Mononuclear Phagocytes, Antigen-Presenting Cells, and Dendritic Cells

Mononuclear phagocytes, chiefly monocytes, comprise 5% to 10% of white blood cells. Circulating monocytes give rise to resident tissue macrophages including, among others, Kupffer cells (liver), alveolar macrophages (lung), and microglial cells (brain). Monocytes and macrophages express specific cell surface host defense molecules. These include MHC class II molecules, CD14 (which binds bacterial LPS and can trigger cell activation), several types of Fc Ig receptors, TLRs and other PRRs, adhesion molecules, and diverse cytokine receptors that help to regulate monocyte/macrophage function. Activated macrophages produce cytokines and soluble mediators of host defense (e.g., **IFN-γ**, interleukin-1β [IL-1β], tumor necrosis factor [TNF], complement proteins).

APCs, defined by their function and derived from HSCs, acquire the capacity to present processed antigen to T

lymphocytes in the context of cell-to-cell histocompatibility. Monocytes, macrophages, DCs and, under some conditions, B lymphocytes, endothelial cells, and epithelial cells can be APCs. Several cytokines can upregulate MHC class II molecules on APCs, a process that increases the efficiency of antigen presentation. In some locations, APCs are highly specialized for this function, for example, specialized APCs (**follicular dendritic cells [FDCs]**) in B-cell–rich follicles of lymph nodes and spleen. In these sites, APCs trap antigen–antibody complexes by engaging antibody and complement via Fc and C3b receptors. In lymph nodes, immune complexes arrive via afferent lymphatics, and in spleen, via blood (see below). FDC antigen presentation leads to generation of memory B cells.

DCs are specialized APCs whose name, "dendritic," reflects their spider-like appearance. They are present in B lymphocyte–rich lymphoid follicles, thymic medulla, and many peripheral sites, including intestinal lamina propria, lung, genitourinary tract, and skin. Peripherally located DCs are less mature than APCs found in lymphoid follicles and express lower densities of accessory cell activation molecules (CD80 [B7-1], CD86 [B7-2]) than do mature DCs. Epidermal Langerhans cells, for example, are peripheral APCs. Upon exposure, Langerhans cells engulf antigen, migrate to regional lymph nodes via afferent lymphatics, and differentiate into more mature DCs. Langerhans cell–derived DCs express high densities of MHC class I and II molecules and costimulatory molecules (CD80, CD86) and present antigens efficiently to T cells.

Lymphoid Tissue Structures Play a Key Role in Adaptive Immune System Function

Lymph Nodes and Tertiary Lymphoid Tissues

Lymph nodes are distributed along thin-walled lymphatic vessels that ultimately drain into the superior vena cava, via the right and left subclavian veins. Each node is encapsulated, vascularized, and internally structured in a way that facilitates antigen processing and presentation by FDCs to B cells in B lymphocyte-rich cortical follicles and by DCs to T cells in the T-lymphocyte–rich parafollicular cortex. The developmental organization of the B- and T-cell–rich areas of a lymph node follows region-specific reticulin fiber structure, the composition of stromal cells, and complementary sets of locally produced chemokines and lymphocyte-specific chemokine receptors.

Naive B and T cells circulate to a lymph node, exit the vascular space across the walls of **high endothelial venules (HEVs)**, and then migrate to their designated areas. Lymphocytes are home to HEVs where they engage in specific receptor-ligand binding interactions (see below). Naive B cells express CXCR5 chemokine receptor ("R" denotes receptor), which binds specifically to chemokine CXCL13 ("L" denotes ligand) which is produced by FDCs. B lymphocytes follow the follicle-centric CXCL13 gradient and thus concentrate in this region. In parallel, naive T cells express CCR7, which binds CCL19 and CCL21 produced by stromal and DCs in the paracortical T region.

Lymph node antigen processing starts with size-dependent sorting that relies on microanatomic features depicted in Figure 4-5. DCs that have phagocytized proteins, microbes, and particulates elsewhere (e.g., skin) migrate via afferent lymphatics into regional lymph nodes and then to the node's T-cell zone, where antigens are processed and presented. Soluble lymph-borne substances such as intact viruses or high–molecular-weight particles/molecules also enter lymph nodes via afferent lymphatics. Within the subcapsular sinus, viruses, particles and high–molecular-weight molecules are engulfed by macrophages/DCs that process and present antigen to cortical B cells which make antibody. Lower–molecular-weight molecules (which cannot penetrate the impermeable lymph node sinus floor) flow down tubular structures—fibroblastic reticular cell (FRC) conduits—where they encounter DC processes intercalated between FRC cells along the conduits. Here, molecules are taken up, processed by the DCs, and presented to T lymphocytes (Fig. 4-5). Nodal structure and function thus sorts incoming agents/molecules, optimizing antigen presentation to either B or T cells, which, in turn, constitute key pivot points in initiating adaptive immune responses.

Tertiary lymphoid tissues (organs), also called ectopic lymphoid tissues, are organized collections of lymphocytes, DCs, HEVs, and fibroblastic reticular conduits that resemble lymph nodes but are outside of encapsulated nodes. Formation is directed by the same mediators involved in lymph node development. Tertiary lymphoid tissues are formed in autoimmune conditions, chronic infections, some cancers, and graft rejection. Their functions are not understood.

Spleen

The spleen initiates adaptive immune responses to blood-borne antigens and removes aged and damaged red blood

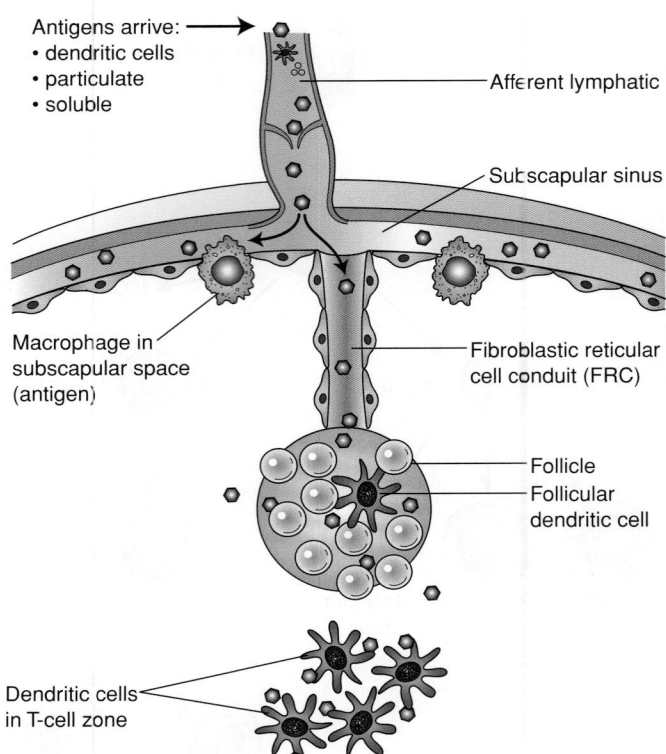

FIGURE 4-5. Potential antigens enter lymph nodes via afferent lymphatic vessels; carried in migratory DCs or as free soluble (large or small) particles or molecules. Within the subcapsular sinus, higher–molecular-weight particles/molecules are engulfed by subcapsular macrophage/DCs, while lower–molecular-weight molecules flow down fibroblastic reticular cell (FRC) conduits where they are pinocytosed via DC processes.

cells, circulating immune complexes and opsonized microbes. As asplenic patients are highly susceptible to infection by encapsulated bacteria, the spleen is particularly important for development of antibody-mediated immunity. Induction of adaptive immunity in the spleen occurs in the lymphocyte-rich white pulp, while particle clearance occurs in the red pulp (Fig. 4-6). White pulp lymphocyte aggregates are organized

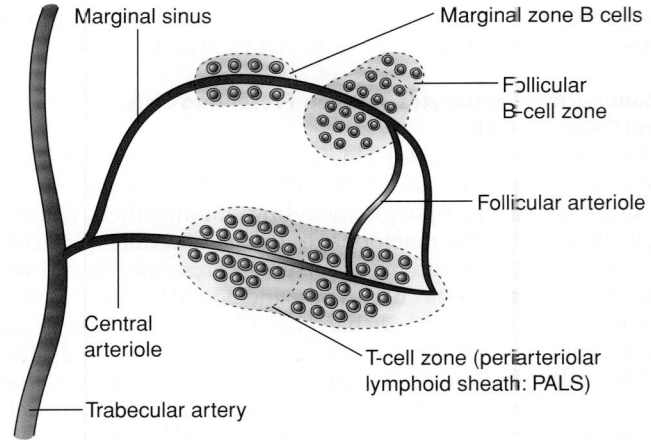

FIGURE 4-6. Splenic white pulp includes a sheath of T lymphocytes wrapped around and along central arterioles, collections of B lymphocytes around and along the marginal sinuses (marginal zone B cells), and follicular B-cell aggregates.

into T- and B-cell–rich zones, where local stromal cells and APCs elaborate the same chemokines (CXCL13 for B cells, CCL19 and CCL21 for T cells) that direct analogous lymph node structure. Periarteriolar T-cell zones of the splenic white pulp contain filtration conduits lined by FRC-like cells. Marginal zone B cells have a limited antigen receptor repertoire, while follicular B cells exhibit the whole range of antibody receptor diversity. Blood-borne particles (including microbes) may be delivered to marginal zone B cells via circulating **plasmacytoid DCs**, and soluble antigens (particularly polysaccharides) may bind marginal zone macrophages directly and then are engaged by nearby B cells.

Thymus

The bilobed thymus, in the anterior mediastinum before it undergoes involution, is the site of T-lymphocyte maturation. Individual thymic lobules are organized into highly cellular cortex and less cellular medulla. Thymic lymphocytes (thymocytes) originate in the bone marrow as progenitors committed to T-cell development. Maturation occurs as the cells percolate first through the cortex and then the medulla, before exiting.

Antibodies and T-Cell Receptors Mediate Adaptive Immunity

Antibodies

Antibody function was recognized more than a century ago when serum from animals previously exposed to attenuated diphtheria toxin specifically protected naive animals from live diphtheroid bacteria. Secreted by plasma cells and B lymphocytes, soluble Ig molecules bind many complementary antigens with high affinity and specificity. They recognize diverse biologic (and nonbiologic) molecules including proteins, carbohydrates, lipids, nucleic acids, and others. The specific part of an antigen to which an Ig molecule binds is an "**epitope**." Antibody–antigen interactions differ from TCR–antigen interactions in that the latter, with few exceptions, involve only processed peptide antigens and occur in the context of MHC molecule compatibility. The various Ig isotypes have different effector functions. Membrane-bound Igs are receptors that mediate B-lymphocyte activation when they bind antigen. Secreted and membrane Igs consist of paired light (L) chains and heavy (H) chains that together form antigen-binding sites (Fig. 4-7). An individual's repertoire of Ig molecules covers a huge range of antigen-binding specificities (10^7 to 10^9), and binding affinities ($K_d = 10^7$ to 10^{11} M). The broad range of specificities is determined by hypervariability of amino acid sequence within the so-called complementarity-determining regions (CDRs) of the antigen-binding V_L and V_H domains (Fig. 4-7). The high degree of variability is generated via highly regulated and stereotyped somatic recombination of physically separated germline segments of DNA that encode different portions of the variable domains. Additional variability is generated by high rates of point mutation and by addition and/or deletion of nucleotides at sites where the above-mentioned gene segments are joined together.

Ig isotypes include IgG, IgA, IgM, IgE, and IgD, each defined by its H-chain gene segments. Antibodies also include light chains, either κ or λ, determined by L-chain gene segments (Table 4-4). Heavy chains guide function

TABLE 4-4

IMMUNOGLOBULIN ISOTYPES AND FUNCTIONS

Isotype	Subtypes	Secreted Form	Functions
IgG	IgG 1, 2, 3, 4	Monomer	Complement fixation Opsonization ADCC Neutralization
IgA	IgA 1, 2	Dimer, monomer	Mucosal immunity
IgM	None	Pentamer	Naive B cell Complement fixation
IgE	None	Monomer	Immediate hypersensitivity
IgD	None	Not secreted	Naive BCR

ADCC = antibody-dependent cellular cytotoxicity; BCR = B-cell receptor; Ig = immunoglobulin.

(Table 4-4). The role of secreted antibodies (e.g., complement fixation, Fc receptor binding, etc.) is determined by Fc region interactions (Fig. 4-7).

Ig molecules are expressed clonally: a given B cell or plasma cell produces many millions of identical intact Ig molecules. During T-cell–dependent humoral immune responses to protein antigens, high-affinity Igs can be generated through somatic mutation of V-region genes in antigen-stimulated B cells. As a humoral immune response evolves, subsets of B lymphocytes that bind a particular antigen with the greatest affinity proliferate and differentiate into plasma cells. Thus, subsequent selections of B cells (via antigen binding) produce increasingly high-affinity antibodies. This

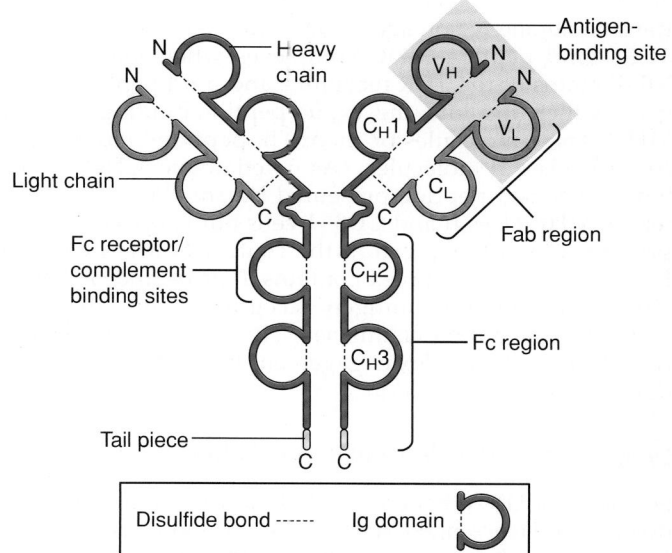

FIGURE 4-7. Schematic structure of immunoglobulin molecule (IgG). Immunoglobulin molecules consist of disulfide-linked pairs of heavy chains and light chains. Antigen-binding sites (2 for IgG) are determined by the highly variable VH and VL Ig domains located at the N-terminal portions of the structure. "Fab" refers to <u>a</u>ntigen-<u>b</u>inding fragment and "Fc" refers to <u>c</u>rystallizable <u>f</u>ragment.

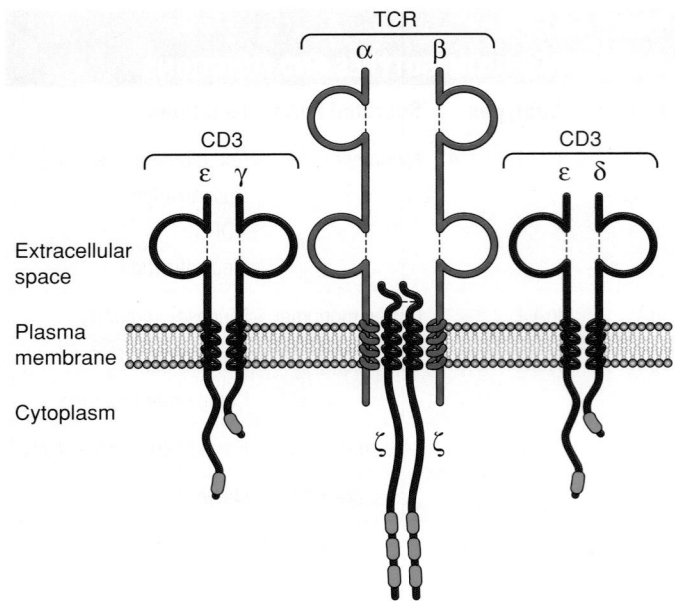

FIGURE 4-8. The T-cell receptor (TCR) consists of noncovalently linked α- and β-chains that each contain a transmembrane domain. The TCR complex includes two ζ-chains and two CD3 subunits ε/γ and ε/δ. TCRs recognize antigen presented in the context of class I human leukocyte antigen (HLA) or class II HLA.

process generates a population of antibody molecules that over time show progressively higher average affinities. Such "**affinity maturation**" is important for an effective humoral immune response.

T-Cell Receptors

Most TCRs consist of paired α- and β-chains that each have an *N*-terminal variable (V) domain, a constant (C) region, a transmembrane region and a cytosolic C-terminus (Fig. 4-8). TCRs bind peptide–MHC complexes where the Vα and Vβ domains of the TCR recognize and bind peptide (antigen), which fits into the α_1/α_2 peptide-binding cleft of MHC class I molecules or the α_1/β_1 peptide-binding cleft of MHC class II molecules. (As noted above, CD4+ T cells bind processed peptide presented by an APC in the context of MHC class II and CD8+ T cells bind surface peptide presented by a target cell in the context of MHC class I.) In turn, the TCR complex contains TCR α- and β-chains, which contribute to antigen recognition and the CD3 γ, δ, and ε signaling chains as well as the ζ–homodimer (Fig. 4-8). TCR complex engagement leads to signal transduction and cell activation.

Lymphocyte Trafficking and Recirculation

Segments of DNA that encode TCR and Ig antigen-binding domains are rearranged in developing T and B cells, respectively, to form "new" genes. This combinatorial process and the other previously mentioned diversity-generating mechanisms, generate vast numbers of different antigen receptors. Adults possess about 10^{12} lymphocytes, only 10% of which circulate at a given time. Despite the large number of lymphocytes, the subset with any specific antigen receptor is relatively small. Body surfaces that serve as portals of entry for foreign invaders are very large (e.g., skin, 2 m²; respiratory tract, 100 m²; GI tract, 400 m²). Lymphocyte trafficking is fundamental to host defenses, because it allows relatively small numbers of any subset of antigen-specific lymphocytes to move to sites of "need." Lymphocyte trafficking is a high-flux process by which individual lymphocytes pass through a given lymph node, on average, once daily. It entails homing and recirculation, enables rapid, flexible and widespread distribution of lymphocytes, and a means of focusing specific immunologic processes at anatomically discrete sites (e.g., lymph node cortex).

After completing early development, naive B and T cells circulate via the vascular system to secondary lymphoid tissues (e.g., spleen, lymph nodes, mucosa-associated lymphoid tissues [MALT] [e.g., Peyer patches]). As noted, lymphocyte trafficking through lymph nodes occurs through HEVs which express adhesion molecules that mediate lymphocyte binding. The cuboidal shape of HEV cells reduces flow-mediated shear forces and specialized intercellular connections facilitate egress of lymphocytes from the vascular space. Lymphocytes that do not find a cognate antigen as they percolate through secondary lymphoid tissues reenter the circulation through efferent lymphatics. Naive lymphocytes have a finite life span maintained by receptor-mediated signals. For example, B cells are engaged via B-cell receptors (surface Ig) and B-cell activity factor (BAFF) receptors.

In contrast, lymphocytes that meet an antigen leave the secondary lymphoid tissue, enter the circulation via lymphatics, then preferentially bind and migrate into peripheral tissues (e.g., lymph nodes or MALT) from which the activating antigen was introduced. Hence, there are at least two major circuits, namely, lymph node and mucosa-associated. Within the mucosa-associated system, nonnaive lymphocytes can distinguish among the gut, respiratory, and genitourinary tracts. Lymphocyte (and neutrophil) homing to sites of inflammation is mediated by different sets of leukocyte and endothelial cell adhesion molecules (see Chapter 2). The best-understood adhesion molecules involved in lymphocyte-lymphoid tissue trafficking include **L-selectins** (on lymphocytes) and **peripheral lymph node addressins (PNAds)** that act as attachment sites for lymphocytes. Among others, the addressins include mucosal addressin cell adhesion molecule-1 (MadCAM-1), glycosylation-dependent cell adhesion molecule-1 (GlyCAM-1), and CD34.

MAJOR HISTOCOMPATIBILITY COMPLEX

The discovery that sera of multiparous women and multiply transfused patients contain antibodies against foreign blood leukocytes led to identification of a system of cell surface proteins—**human leukocyte antigens (HLAs)**—which were first identified on leukocytes and are expressed in high concentrations on lymphocytes, but are present on all nucleated cells.

HLAs (or, **histocompatibility antigens**) orchestrate cell–cell interactions fundamental to adaptive immune responses. They are also major immunogens and thus targets in transplant rejection. The MHC encodes these cell surface proteins, which include class I, II, and III antigens. (Class III includes certain complement components and cytokines that are not HLAs per se.)

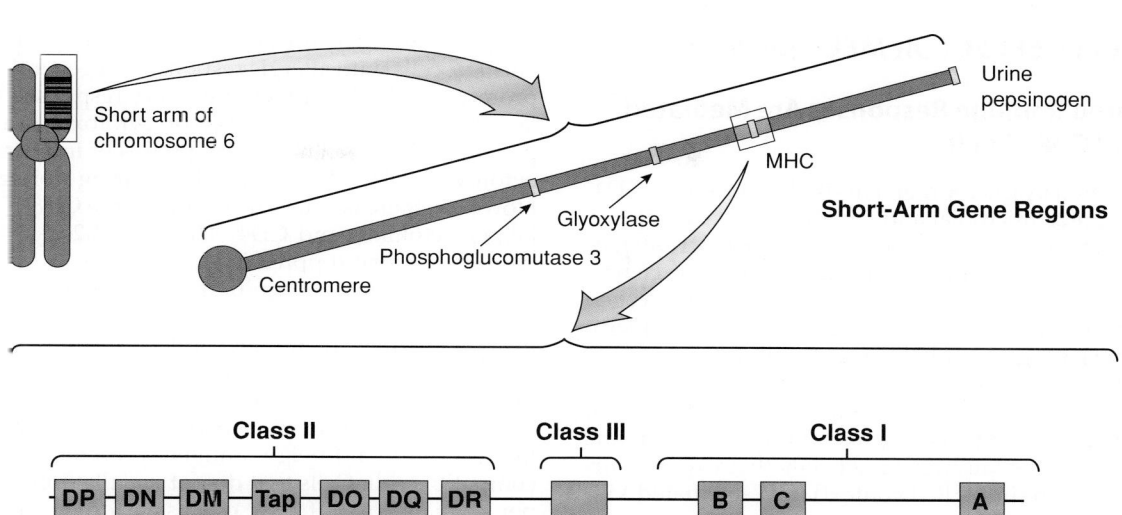

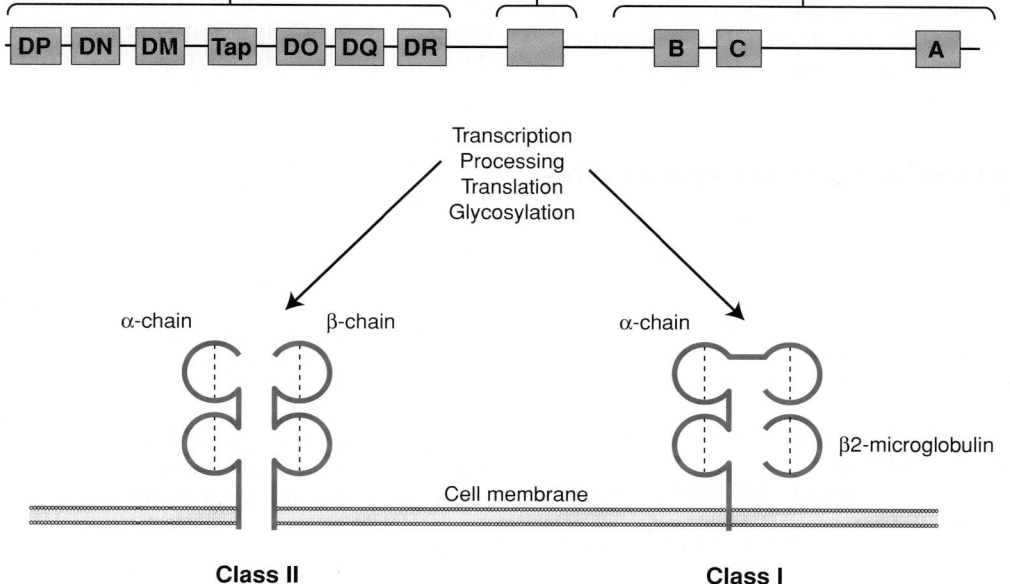

FIGURE 4-9. The highly polymorphic loci that encode major histocompatibility antigens are located on the short arm of chromosome 6. Class I and class II molecules exhibit different structures, but each participates in fundamentally important cell–cell interactions. Class III genes encode some complement components that are not strictly histocompatibility antigens.

Molecules structurally resembling "traditional" MHC class I and II molecules are encoded beyond the specific MHC region on the short arm of chromosome 6 (Fig. 4-9). Among these, MHC-1b and CD1d can activate the so-called NK T cells. The latter resemble both NK cells and T lymphocytes. Other nontraditional MHC class I molecules (e.g., HLA-E, -F, and -G) are less well understood. Some may regulate NK cell activity.

Class I MHC Molecules Are Encoded by A, B, and C MHC Regions

Class I MHC genes (Fig. 4-9) encode molecules expressed in virtually all tissues; heterodimers consisting of a 44-kDa polymorphic transmembrane glycoprotein and a 12-kDa nonpolymorphic molecule, β_2-microglobulin. The latter has no membrane component, and is noncovalently associated with the larger heavy chain. Structural polymorphism occurs primarily in the extracellular domains of the α-chain. MHC class I alleles are expressed codominantly, so tissues have class I molecules inherited from each parent. These antigens are recognized by **cytotoxic T cells (CTLs)** during graft rejection and T-lymphocyte–mediated killing of virus-infected host cells.

Class II MHC Molecules Are Encoded in MHC D

Multiple D region loci encode class II MHC: DP, DN, DM, DO, DQ, and DR (Fig. 4-9). These structurally similar molecules are expressed mainly on antigen-presenting cells. Class II molecules, also called "Ia" (immunity-associated) antigens, are heterodimers of two noncovalently linked transmembrane glycoproteins: a 29-kDa α-chain with two disulfide bonds and a 34-kDa β-chain with one disulfide bond. The extracellular domain is the major site of class II variability. Like class I, D alleles are codominantly expressed.

Recently, the WHO revised nomenclature to accommodate high-resolution DNA sequencing, rather than the older serologically defined designations. For example, the former HLA-B27 became B*2701-2725, with B*2701, B*2702, B*2703, etc., encompassing 25 different B27 molecules (each defined by DNA sequence).

IMMUNE CELL EFFECTOR MECHANISMS

Cell-Mediated Immune Responses Are Mediated by CD4+ and CD8+ T Cells

They are triggered by microorganisms within host cells. CD4+ Th1 cells recognize microbial antigens and secrete cytokines (IFN-γ) that activate macrophages. Activated macrophages ingest microorganisms and kill through a series of chemical reactions that involve enzymes and both reactive oxygen and nitrogen intermediates. CD4+ Th2 cells recognize microbial (and other) antigens and promote B-cell differentiation, antibody production, Ig isotype switching, and IgE production. Finally, CD4+ Th17 cells induce neutrophils to kill microorganisms by phagocytosis, oxidation, and enzymatic digestion. CD8+ CTLs kill host target cells that express surface foreign antigen (in MHC I context). CTL-mediated killing occurs via the perforin/granzyme pathway and/or by producing IFN-γ and subsequently activating macrophages.

Immunoglobulins Are Produced by B Lymphocytes and Plasma Cells

Antibodies define humoral immunity (Table 4-4). Effector functions include:

- steric blockade (e.g., antibody to HIV type 1 prevents its binding to T-cell CD4 molecules)
- binding and Fc-mediated clearance by mononuclear phagocytes
- binding and Fc-mediated **antibody-dependent cell-mediated cytotoxicity (ADCC)**
- Fc binding and cell activation (e.g., IgE tightly bound to mast cells via Fcε receptor)
- mast cell activation triggered by allergen binding to cytophilic IgE
- Ig-mediated complement fixation

Pentavalent IgM and properly spaced IgG molecules (IgG subclasses 1, 2, and 3) effectively bind (fix) C1qrs, activating the classical complement cascade and generating its attendant proinflammatory mediators (e.g., C3a, C3b, C5a, membrane attack complex [MAC]) (see Chapter 2).

INTEGRATED IMMUNE RESPONSES

T-Lymphocyte Interactions

T lymphocytes recognize specific antigens, usually proteins or haptens bound to proteins. T cells undergo activation when engaged via their TCR in the context of processed antigen presented by an MHC-identical (histocompatible) APC. Exogenous signals are delivered by cytokines. CD4+ and CD8+ T-cell subsets have multiple regulatory and effector functions. Regulatory functions include augmentation or suppression of immune responses, usually via secretion of specific helper or suppressor cytokines. Effector functions include secretion of proinflammatory cytokines and killing cells that express foreign or altered membrane antigens.

CD4+ T cells, and possibly CD8+ T cells, can be further distinguished by the types of cytokines they produce. Helper type 1, or "Th1," cells produce IFN-γ and IL-2, while helper type 2, or "Th2," cells secrete IL-4, IL-5, and IL-10. Th1 lymphocytes are associated with cell-mediated phenomena and Th2 cells with allergic responses. In general, CD4+ T cells promote antibody and inflammatory responses. CD8+ T cells largely exert suppressor and/or cytotoxic functions. Suppressor cells inhibit activation phases of immune responses; cytotoxic cells kill target cells bearing foreign antigens. However, there is some overlap, as some CD8+ T cells secrete helper cytokines and CD4+ Th1 and Th2 cells can mediate cross-regulatory suppression.

T-cell antigen recognition requires antigen to be presented at the surfaces of other cells in association with a histocompatible membrane protein (Figs. 4-8 and 4-9). As noted, T cells bear membrane receptor complexes (α/β TCRs plus CD3 accessory molecules) on their surfaces (Figs. 4-8 and 4-9). For maximal response, TCR-CD3 complex must interact with a foreign antigen presented by an MHC-compatible cell. Cells that do not usually "present" antigens per se may do so if they express a foreign or altered self-protein in association with an appropriate MHC molecule on their surface.

CD8+ cells (CTLs) recognize antigens in conjunction with HLA class I molecules; CD4+ cells (T-helper cells) recognize antigens together with class II molecules. Cell membrane CD4 and CD8 molecules of α/β T cells help stabilize binding interactions. γ/δ T cells may also acquire CD8 outside the thymus, then use class I antigens for binding target cells. Foreign class I and class II molecules, which are histoincompatible with the host (e.g., foreign MHC on transplanted tissues), are themselves potent immunogens and can be recognized by host T cells. This is why optimal tissue transplantation requires that donor and recipient be HLA matched. In addition to binding foreign peptides presented by MHC molecules to the TCR complex, other receptor–ligand interactions must occur for maximal lymphocyte activation. A CD4+ T cell becomes a fully activated effector cell when stimulated via the TCR complex and "accessory" receptors (CD28 and cytotoxic lymphoid line [CTLL]-4), which engage costimulatory molecules (e.g., CD80 [B7-1, CD86 [B7-2]). In turn, an activated T-helper cell recognizes an antigen-specific B cell via its receptor. T-helper cells then provide costimulatory and regulatory signals, such as CD40 ligand and "helper" cytokines (e.g., IL-4, IL-5).

Mature B Cells Are Mainly Resting, Awaiting Activation by Foreign Antigens

B-cell activation requires cross-linking of mIg receptors via antigens presented by accessory cells and/or interactions with membrane molecules of helper T cells via a mechanism called cognate T cell–B cell help. This stimulus triggers B-cell proliferation and clonal expansion, amplified by cytokines from accessory cells and T cells. If there is insufficient additional signal, proliferating B cells return to a resting state and enter the memory cell pool. These events occur largely in lymphoid tissues. B cells proliferate in germinal centers, where they undergo further somatic gene rearrangements to generate cells that produce the various Ig isotypes and subclasses (Table 4-4).

T cells also influence B-cell differentiation. In the presence of antigen, T cells produce cytokines that stimulate isotype switching or induce proliferation of previously isotype-committed populations. For example, IL-4 induces switching to IgE isotype.

The ultimate stage of B-cell differentiation into antibody-synthesizing plasma cells requires exposure to additional T-lymphocyte products (e.g., IL-5, IL-6), especially for protein antigens. However, some polyvalent agents (called polyclonal B-cell activators) may induce B-cell proliferation and differentiation into plasma cells directly, bypassing B-cell growth and differentiation factors. These activators, which include various viral and bacterial products, do not interact with antigen-binding sites: they are not specific antigens.

The predominant Ig isotype produced during an immune response changes with age. Newborns mainly produce IgM. Older children and adults initially produce IgM following antigenic challenge but rapidly shift toward IgG synthesis.

IMMUNOLOGICALLY MEDIATED TISSUE INJURY

While a variety of foreign substances (e.g., viruses, bacteria) provoke protective responses, those immune responses can lead to harmful consequences, if immunologically triggered inflammation attacks the body's own tissues. For example, while ingesting and destroying bacteria, phagocytic cells (neutrophils and macrophages) often cause injury to surrounding tissue (see Chapter 2). An immune response that leads to tissue injury is broadly called a hypersensitivity reaction. Many diseases are categorized as immune disorders or immunologically mediated conditions, in which an immune response to a foreign or self-antigen causes injury. Immune- or hypersensitivity-mediated diseases are common and include hives (urticaria), asthma, hay fever, hepatitis, glomerulonephritis, and arthritis.

Hypersensitivity reactions are classified according to immune mechanism (Table 4-5). Type I, II, and III hypersensitivity reactions all involve antibodies specific for exogenous (foreign) or endogenous (self) antigens. (An exception includes a subset of type I reactions.) Antibody isotype influences the mechanism of tissue injury.

- Type I, or immediate-type hypersensitivity, reactions: The Fc domain of IgE binds high-affinity receptors on mast cells and/or basophils. Subsequent antigen binding and cross-linking of IgE trigger rapid (immediate) release of products from these cells, leading to the characteristic manifestations of urticaria, asthma, and anaphylaxis.
- Type II hypersensitivity reactions: IgM or IgG antibody is formed against an antigen, usually a cell surface protein. Less commonly, the antigen is an intrinsic structural component of the extracellular matrix (e.g., basement membrane). Such antigen–antibody coupling fixes complement, which attracts neutrophils that lyse the cell (cytotoxicity) or damages the extracellular matrix. In some type II reactions, other antibody-mediated effects are operative.
- Type III hypersensitivity reactions: The antibody responsible for tissue injury is also usually IgM or IgG, but the mechanism of tissue injury differs. Antigen circulates in the vascular compartment until it is bound by antibody. Resulting immune complexes deposit in tissue where complement activation recruits leukocytes, which mediate tissue injury. In some type III reactions, antibody binds previously deposited antigen (called "planted" antigen) in situ.
- Type IV, cell-mediated or delayed-type, hypersensitivity reactions: Antigen activates T lymphocytes, usually with the help of macrophages, causing release of products by these cells, leading to tissue injury.

Many immunologic diseases are mediated by more than one type of these reactions. For example, in hypersensitivity pneumonitis, lung injury from inhaled fungal antigens involves types I, III, and IV reactions.

IgE-Mediated Hypersensitivity Reactions (Type I)

Immediate-type hypersensitivity entails localized or generalized reactions that occur within minutes of exposure to an antigen or "allergen" to which the person has been previously sensitized. Clinical manifestations depend on the site of antigen exposure and extent of sensitization. For example, a reaction involving the skin appears as a characteristic local "wheal and flare," or urticaria. When the conjunctiva and upper respiratory tract are involved, sneezing

TABLE 4-5		
MODIFIED CELL AND COOMBS CLASSIFICATION OF HYPERSENSITIVITY REACTIONS		
Type	**Mechanism**	**Examples**
Type I (anaphylactic type): immediate hypersensitivity	IgE antibody–mediated mast cell activation and degranulation Non-Ig mediated	Hay fever, asthma, hives, anaphylaxis Physical urticarias
Type II (cytotoxic type): cytotoxic antibodies	Cytotoxic (IgG, IgM) antibodies formed against cell surface antigens; complement usually involved Noncytotoxic antibodies against cell surface receptors	Autoimmune hemolytic anemias, Goodpasture disease Graves disease
Type III (immune complex type): immune complex disease	Antibodies (IgG, IgM, IgA) formed against exogenous or endogenous antigens; complement and leukocytes (neutrophils, macrophages) often involved	Autoimmune diseases (SLE, rheumatoid arthritis), many types of glomerulonephritis
Type IV (cell-mediated type): delayed-type hypersensitivity	Mononuclear cells (T lymphocytes, macrophages) with interleukin and lymphokine production	Granulomatous disease (tuberculosis), delayed skin reactions (poison ivy)

Ig = immunoglobulin; SLE = systemic lupus erythematosus.

IMMUNOPATHOLOGY

and conjunctivitis result (hay fever or allergic rhinitis). In their generalized and most severe form, immediate hypersensitivity reactions cause bronchoconstriction, airway obstruction, systemic vasodilation and circulatory collapse, as seen in anaphylactic shock. There is a high degree of genetically determined variability in susceptibility to type I hypersensitivity reactions; susceptible individuals are termed "atopic."

In type I reactions IgE antibodies (formed by a CD4+, Th2 T-cell–dependent mechanism) bind avidly to mast cell and basophil Fcε receptors. High avidity ($K_d = 10^{-15}$ M) of IgE binding accounts for the term "cytophilic" antibody. Once a specific allergen elicits IgE, a person is sensitized; subsequent exposures to that allergen or a cross-reacting epitope induce immediate hypersensitivity reactions. Subsequent exposure to that antigen typically induces more IgE, rather than antibodies of other classes.

IgE can persist for years bound to Fcε receptors on long-lived mast cells and basophils. When the antigen (allergen) binds the Fab region of the IgE and cross-links at least two adjacent IgE antibody molecules, it activates the mast cell or basophil (Fig. 4-10). Released inflammatory mediators cause type I hypersensitivity reactions.

Other agents besides antibodies may activate mast cells and basophils. Some people develop urticaria after exposure to an ice cube (physical urticaria) or pressure (dermographism). The complement-derived anaphylatoxic peptides, C3a and C5a, can directly stimulate mast cells by a different receptor-mediated process (Fig. 4-10). These cell-activating events trigger release of stored granule constituents and rapid synthesis and release of other mediators. Some compounds, such as melittin (from bee venom), and some drugs (e.g., morphine) activate mast cells directly.

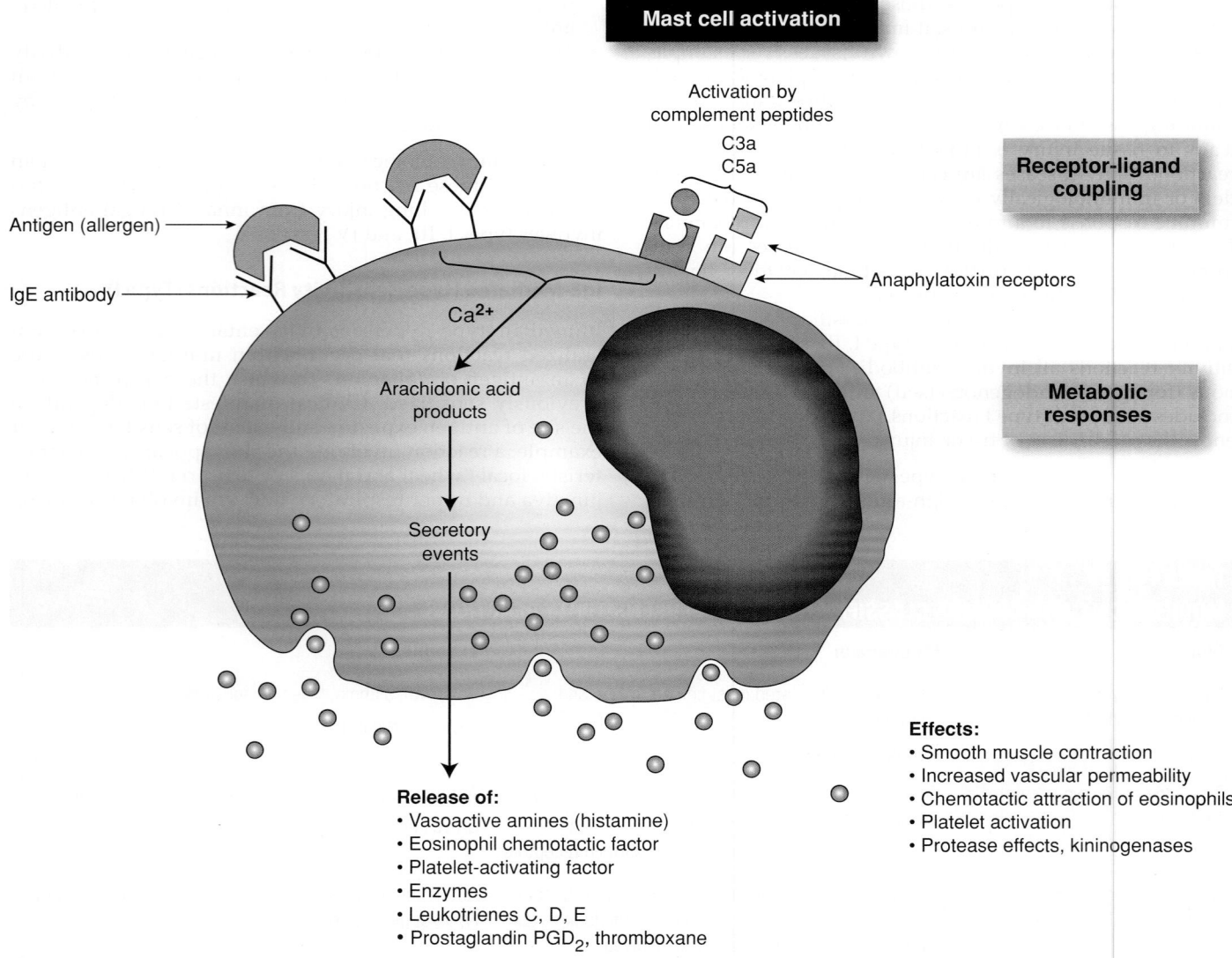

FIGURE 4-10. **In a type I hypersensitivity reaction, antigen (allergen) binds to cytophilic surface IgE displayed on a mast cell or basophil and triggers cell activation and release of a cascade of proinflammatory mediators.** Mast cells and basophils can also be activated by anaphylatoxins like C3a and C5a, as well as some physical stimuli (e.g., cold). These mediators are responsible for smooth muscle contraction, edema formation, and the recruitment of eosinophils. Ca^{2+} = calcium ion; Ig = immunoglobulin; PGD_2 = prostaglandin D_2.

Regardless of how mast cell activation is initiated, a rise in cytosolic free calcium triggers generation of cAMP, activation of several metabolic pathways within the mast cell and secretion of preformed and newly synthesized mediators. Mediators stored in granules are released within minutes and act rapidly.

Histamine, one of those granule constituents, induces constriction of vascular and nonvascular smooth muscle, causes microvascular dilation, and increases venule permeability. These effects are largely mediated through H_1 histamine receptors. It also increases gastric acid secretion through H_2 histamine receptors and provokes the cutaneous wheal-and-flare reaction. In the lungs, histamine causes bronchospasm, vascular congestion, and edema. Other preformed products released from mast cell granules include heparin, a series of neutral proteases (PRs) (trypsin, chymotrypsin carboxypeptidase, and acid hydrolases) and factors chemotactic for neutrophils and eosinophils. Eosinophil accumulation is characteristic of immediate hypersensitivity.

Cytokines from mast cells, other recruited inflammatory cells, and even indigenous cells (e.g., epithelium) mediate the "late phase" of immediate hypersensitivity. Late-phase responses typically last 2 to 24 hours, and are marked by a mixed inflammatory infiltrate. Many cytokines—including IL-1, IL-3, IL-4, IL-5, IL-6, TNFα, granulocyte-macrophage colony-stimulating factor (GM-CSF) and macrophage inflammatory protein (MIP)-1α and MIP-1β—mediate these responses.

Mast cell activation also increases synthesis of arachidonic acid pathway products formed after activation of phospholipase A_2. Products of **cyclooxygenase** (prostaglandins D_2, E_2, and F_2 and thromboxane) and **lipoxygenase** (leukotrienes B_4, C_4, D_4, E_4) are also produced. Arachidonic acid derivatives, generated by a variety of cell types, induce smooth muscle contraction, vasodilation, and edema. Leukotrienes C_4, D_4, and E_4, previously known as "slow-reacting substances of anaphylaxis" (SRS-As), are important in the delayed bronchoconstriction phase of anaphylaxis. Leukotriene B_4 is a potent chemotactic factor for neutrophils, macrophages, and eosinophils.

Another inflammatory mediator synthesized by mast cells is **platelet-activating factor (PAF)**, a lipid derived from membrane phospholipids. PAF is a neutrophil chemotaxin, and strongly triggers platelet aggregation and release of vasoactive amines. It also can activate all types of phagocytic cells.

Activated Th2 T cells produce cytokines that have important roles in allergic responses. This subset releases IL-4, IL-5, and IL-13, stimulating IgE production and increasing numbers of mast cells and eosinophils. In allergy-prone people, a similar response occurs via T cells that produce IL-4, IL-6, and IL-2 concentrations of which are also increased in allergic individuals. These people produce reduced levels of IFNγ, which normally suppresses development of Th2 cells and subsequent production of IgE.

In summary, in type I (immediate) hypersensitivity reactions, specific cytophilic IgE antibody binds via its Fc domain to high-affinity Fcε receptors on basophils and mast cells, and reacts with a specific antigen (allergen). Activated mast cells and basophils release preformed (granule) products and synthesize mediators that cause the classic manifestations of immediate hypersensitivity and the late-phase reaction.

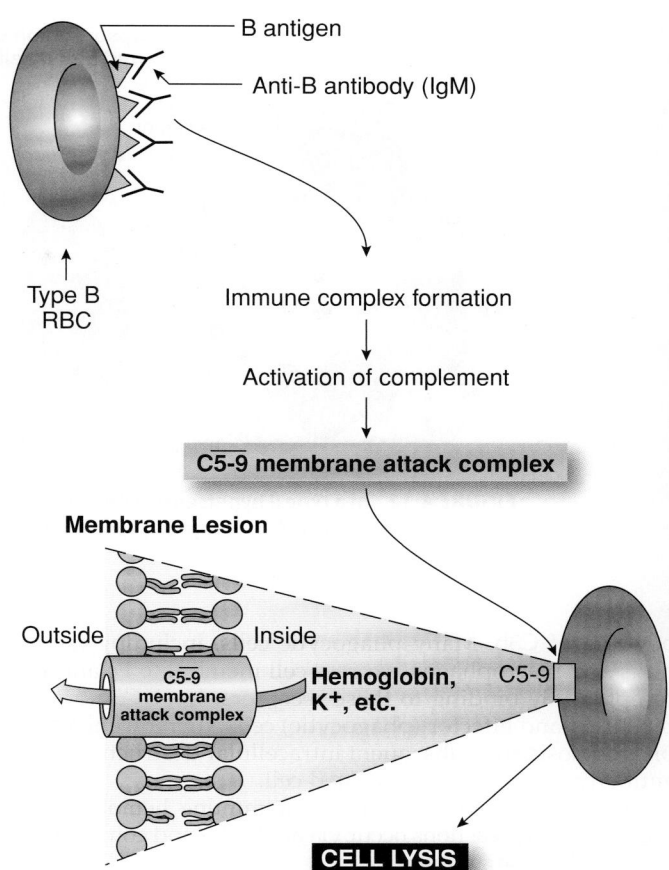

FIGURE 4-11. In a type II hypersensitivity reaction, binding of IgG or IgM antibody to an immobilized antigen promotes complement fixation. Activation of complement leads to amplification of the inflammatory response and membrane attack complex (MAC)-mediated cell lysis. *Ig* = immunoglobulin, K^+ = potassium ion; *RBC* = red blood cell.

IgM- and IgG-Mediated Hypersensitivity Reactions (Type II)

IgM and IgG mediate most type II reactions. These Ig isotypes fix complement via their Fc domains. There are several antibody-dependent mechanisms of tissue injury. Prototypic antibody-mediated erythrocyte cytotoxicity is illustrated in Figure 4-11. IgM or IgG binds an antigen on the erythrocyte membrane. At sufficient density, bound Ig fixes complement via C1q and triggers the classical pathway (see Chapter 2). Activated complement can destroy target cells directly, via C5b-9 complexes (Fig. 4-11). The C5b-9 **MAC** inserts like the staves of a barrel into the plasma membrane, forming holes (ion channels) and lysing cells. This mechanism is active in certain autoimmune hemolytic anemias due to antibodies against red blood cell group antigens. In some transfusion reactions that result from major blood group incompatibilities, intravascular hemolysis occurs through activation of complement.

Complement and antibody molecules can also destroy target cells by opsonization. Phagocytes that express Fc or C3b receptors bind target cells coated (opsonized) with Ig and/or C3b molecules (Fig. 4-12). Complement activation near a target cell surface leads to formation and covalent

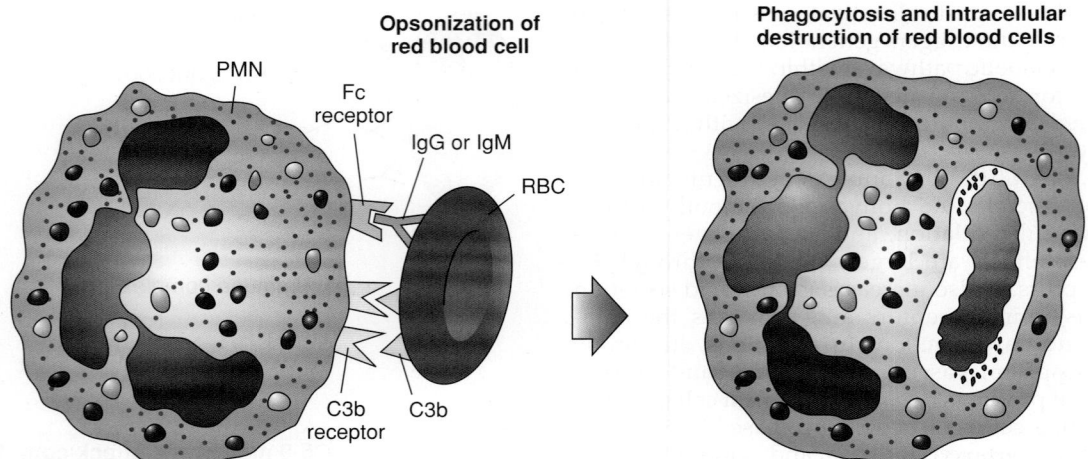

FIGURE 4-12. In a type II hypersensitivity reaction, opsonization by antibody or complement leads to phagocytosis via either Fc or C3b receptors, respectively. *Ig* = immunoglobulin; *PMN* = polymorphonuclear leukocyte; *RBC* = red blood cell.

bonding of C3b. Many phagocytic cells, including neutrophils and macrophages, express cell membrane Fc and C3b receptors. By binding to these receptors, Ig or C3b bridges the target and effector (phagocytic) cells, thereby enhancing phagocytosis and subsequent intracellular destruction of the antibody- or complement-coated cell.

Some transfusion reactions, autoimmune hemolytic anemias, and drug reactions occur via antibody- and complement-mediated opsonization.

ADCC does not require complement, but rather involves cytolytic leukocytes that attack antibody-coated target cells after binding via Fc receptors. ADCC effectors, phagocytes, and NK cells, synthesize homologs of terminal complement proteins (e.g., perforins), which participate in cytotoxic events (see above) as effector cells in ADCC. Antibody alone is only rarely directly cytotoxic. In cases involving primarily lymphoid cells, apoptosis is activated. ADCC is implicated in the pathogenesis of some autoimmune diseases (e.g., autoimmune thyroiditis).

In some type II reactions, antibody binding to a specific target cell receptor does not lead to cell death but rather to a functional change. For example, autoantibodies against cell surface receptors (Fig. 4-13) may stimulate or inhibit cell activation. In Graves disease, autoantibody against thyroid-stimulating hormone (TSH) receptors on thyroid cells elicits thyroxine production and causes thyrotoxicosis. In myasthenia gravis, antibodies to acetylcholine receptors on postsynaptic membranes inhibit effective synaptic transmission and cause patients to suffer from muscle fatigue.

In some type II-mediated diseases, antibodies against structural connective tissue components evoke destructive local inflammation. In Goodpasture syndrome, for example,

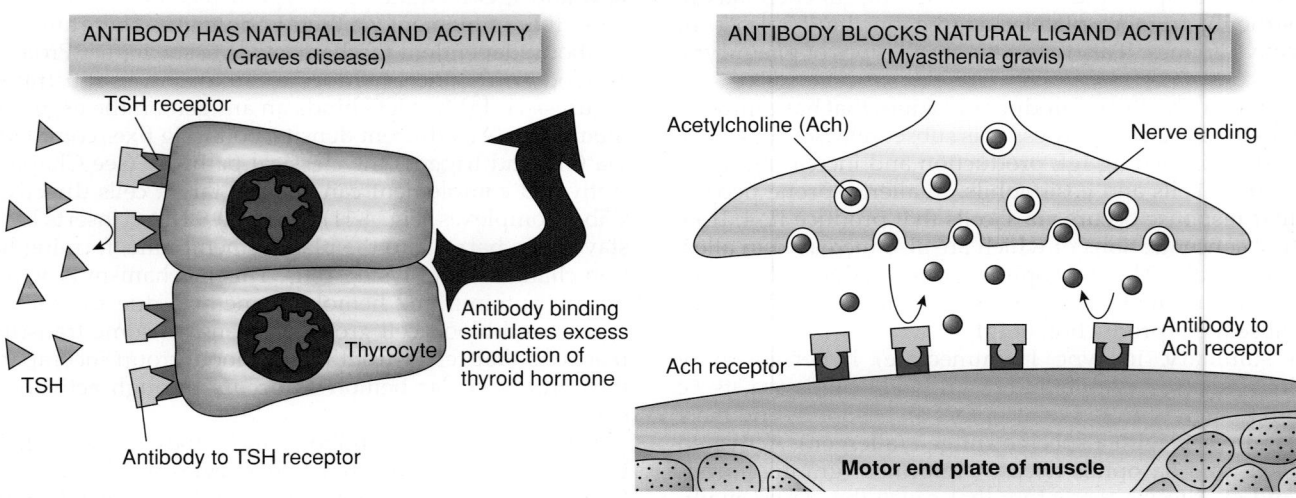

FIGURE 4-13. In a type II hypersensitivity reaction, antibodies bind to a cell surface receptor and induce activation (e.g., thyroid-stimulating hormone [TSH] receptors in Graves disease) or inhibition/destruction (e.g., acetylcholine receptors in myasthenia gravis).

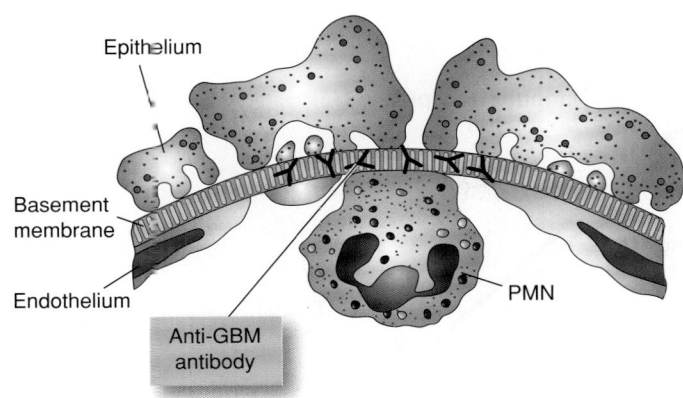

Epithelium

Basement
membrane

Endothelium

Anti-GBM
antibody

PMN

FIGURE 4-14. Goodpasture syndrome involves a type II hypersensitivity reaction in which antibody binds to a structural antigen, activates the complement system, and leads to the recruitment of tissue-damaging inflammatory cells. Several complement-derived peptides (e.g., C5a) are potent chemotactic factors. *GBM* = glomerular basement membrane; *PMN* = polymorphonuclear leukocyte.

antibody binds a noncollagenous domain of type IV collagen, which is a major component of pulmonary and glomerular basement membranes (Fig. 4-14). Local complement activation results in neutrophil chemotaxis and activation, tissue injury and pulmonary hemorrhage, and glomerulonephritis. Direct complement-mediated damage to glomerular and alveolar basement membranes via MAC may also occur.

In summary, type II hypersensitivity reactions are directly or indirectly cytotoxic via actions of antibodies against antigens on cell surfaces or in connective tissues. Complement participates in many of these events. It may mediate lysis directly, or indirectly by opsonization and phagocytosis, or by chemotaxis of phagocytes, which produce a variety of tissue-damaging products. Complement-independent reactions, such as ADCC, also play a role in type II hypersensitivity.

Immune Complex Reactions (Type III)

In the presence of circulating antigen, specific IgM, IgG, or occasionally IgA deposits in a tissue can cause type III responses. Physicochemical characteristics of the immune complexes, such as size, charge and solubility, in addition to Ig isotype, determine if and where an immune complex deposits in tissue and fixes complement. Circulating immune complexes do not necessarily cause tissue injury: their physicochemical properties often differ from complexes that deposit in tissues.

Immune complexes cause many human diseases. Examples include cryoglobulinemic vasculitis associated with hepatitis C infection, Henoch–Schönlein purpura with IgA deposits at sites of vasculitis, and systemic lupus erythematosus (SLE) (anti–double-stranded DNA in vasculitic lesions). Immune complexes elicit inflammatory responses by activating complement and recruiting neutrophils and monocytes. These activated phagocytes release tissue-damaging PRs and ROS (see Chapter 2).

Sometimes, vascular permeability determines where circulating immune complexes localize. Diseases associated with immune complex deposition are inflammatory diseases of connective tissue, such as SLE and rheumatoid arthritis,

some types of vasculitis, and many varieties of glomerulonephritis (see Chapters 11, 16, and 22).

Serum sickness is an acute, usually self-limited disease that typically occurs 6 to 8 days after administration of a foreign protein or a compound that binds to and thus modifies a native protein. Human serum sickness is uncommon but can occur in patients given foreign proteins as therapies (e.g., equine antilymphocyte globulin). It is characterized by fever, arthralgias, vasculitis, and acute glomerulonephritis. In experimental acute serum sickness, serum levels of exogenously injected antigen remain constant until about day 6, after which they fall rapidly (Fig. 4-15). At the same time, immune complexes (with IgM or IgG bound to antigen) appear in the circulation. Some circulating complexes, rendered more soluble by interacting with complement which increases tissue deposition, deposit in tissues such as renal glomeruli and blood vessel walls. Immune complexes fix complement, leading to generation of C3a and C5a, which increase vascular permeability.

Immune complexes deposited in tissue may trigger inflammatory responses. They activate complement, forming C5a, which is a potent neutrophil chemoattractant. Other neutrophil chemotaxins include leukotriene B_4 and IL-8. Neutrophil adherence and migration into sites of immune complex deposition involve a series of cytokine-mediated adhesive interactions (see Chapter 2). Several cytokines are implicated in this response. Early production of IL-1 and TNFα upregulates endothelial cell adhesion molecules and production of other proinflammatory cytokines, including **platelet-derived growth factor (PDGF)**; transforming growth factor-β (TGFβ); and IL-4, IL-6, and IL-10, which modulate activation of leukocytes and fibroblasts. Not all cytokines are proinflammatory; IL-10, in particular, downregulates inflammatory responses.

Contact with, and ingestion of, immune complexes activate recruited neutrophils. Activated cells release inflammatory mediators, including PRs, ROS, and arachidonic acid products, which collectively produce tissue injury.

In the **Arthus reaction**, an experimental model of vasculitis, immune complexes evoke localized injury (Fig. 4-16). In an individual previously immunized against an antigen, local injection of that antigen into the skin evokes this reaction in dermal blood vessels. Circulating antibody and locally injected antigen diffuse down concentration gradients toward each other to form complex deposits in walls of small blood vessels. Resulting vascular injury is caused by activated complement and recruited neutrophils with their proinflammatory mediators. These lesions develop over 2 to 10 hours. Affected vessel walls have many neutrophils and are damaged, with edema and hemorrhage into surrounding tissue. The presence of fibrin creates the classic appearance of immune complex–induced vasculitis, namely, fibrinoid necrosis. Although it is an experimental model, it recapitulates many human vasculitides (e.g., certain drug reactions).

Type III hypersensitivity reactions are immune complex–mediated injuries. Antigen–antibody complexes may either form in situ, or in the circulation and then deposit in the tissues. Immune complexes fix complement, which leads to recruitment of neutrophils and monocytes. These activated inflammatory cells release potent inflammatory mediators, and are directly responsible for injury (Fig. 4-16). Autoimmune diseases such as SLE and many types of glomerulonephritis, are mediated by this mechanism.

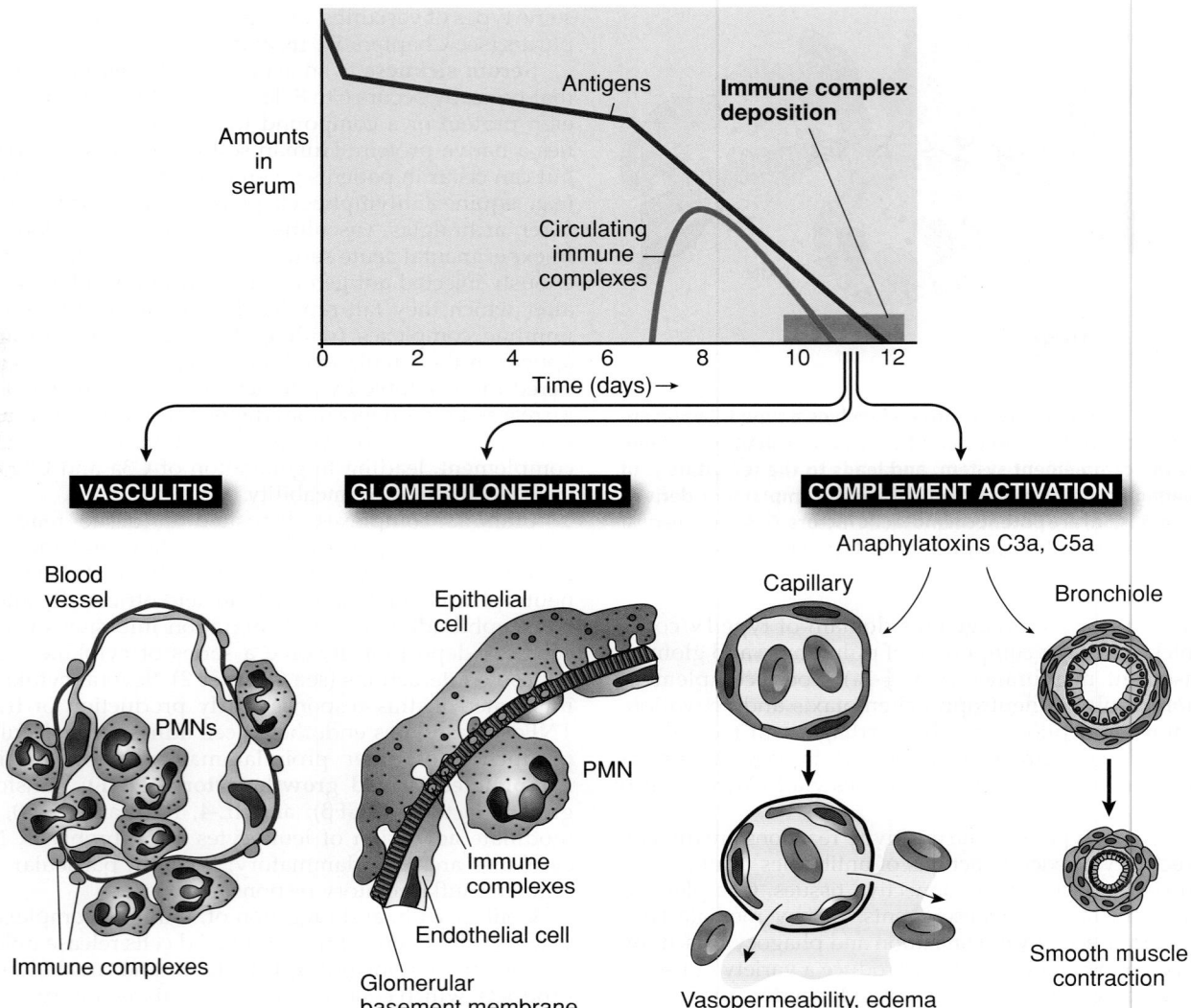

FIGURE 4-15. In type III hypersensitivity, immune complexes are deposited and can lead to complement activation and the recruitment of tissue-damaging inflammatory cells. This schematic illustrates the series of events that occur in acute serum sickness. The ability of immune complexes to mediate tissue injury depends on size, solubility, net charge, and ability to fix complement. *PMN* = polymorphonuclear leukocyte.

Cell-Mediated (Delayed-Type) Hypersensitivity Reactions (Type IV, DTH)

Type IV reactions often occur together with antibody reactions, which can make them difficult to distinguish. The type of tissue response is largely determined by the nature of the inciting agent. DTH is usually a tissue reaction, mainly involving lymphocytes and mononuclear phagocytes, occurring in response to soluble protein antigen and reaching peak intensity after 24 to 48 hours. A common example is the contact response to poison ivy. Although the chemical ligands in poison ivy (e.g., urushiol) are not proteins, they bind covalently to cell proteins and generate products that are recognized by antigen-specific lymphocytes.

In delayed-type hypersensitivity reactions (Fig. 4-17), foreign protein antigens or chemical ligands first *interact with accessory cells that express class II HLA molecules* (Fig. 4-17A). Accessory cells (macrophages, DCs) secrete IL-12, which,

along with processed and presented antigen, activate $CD4^+$ T cells (Fig. 4-17B). Activated $CD4^+$ T cells secrete IFNγ and IL-2, which respectively activate more macrophages and elicit T-lymphocyte proliferation (Fig. 4-17C). Protein antigens are actively processed into short peptides within macrophages' phagolysosomes and presented on the cell surface with class II HLA molecules. Processed and presented antigens recognized by MHC-restricted, antigen-specific $CD4^+$ T cells become activated and, as Th1 cells, synthesize various cytokines. These cytokines then recruit and activate lymphocytes, monocytes, fibroblasts, and other inflammatory cells. If the antigenic stimulus is eliminated, the reaction spontaneously resolves after about 48 hours. If the stimulus persists (e.g., poorly biodegradable mycobacterial cell wall components), an attempt to sequester the inciting agent may result in a granulomatous reaction (see Chapter 2).

Another mechanism by which T cells (especially $CD8^+$) mediate tissue damage is direct lysis of target cells (Fig. 4-18).

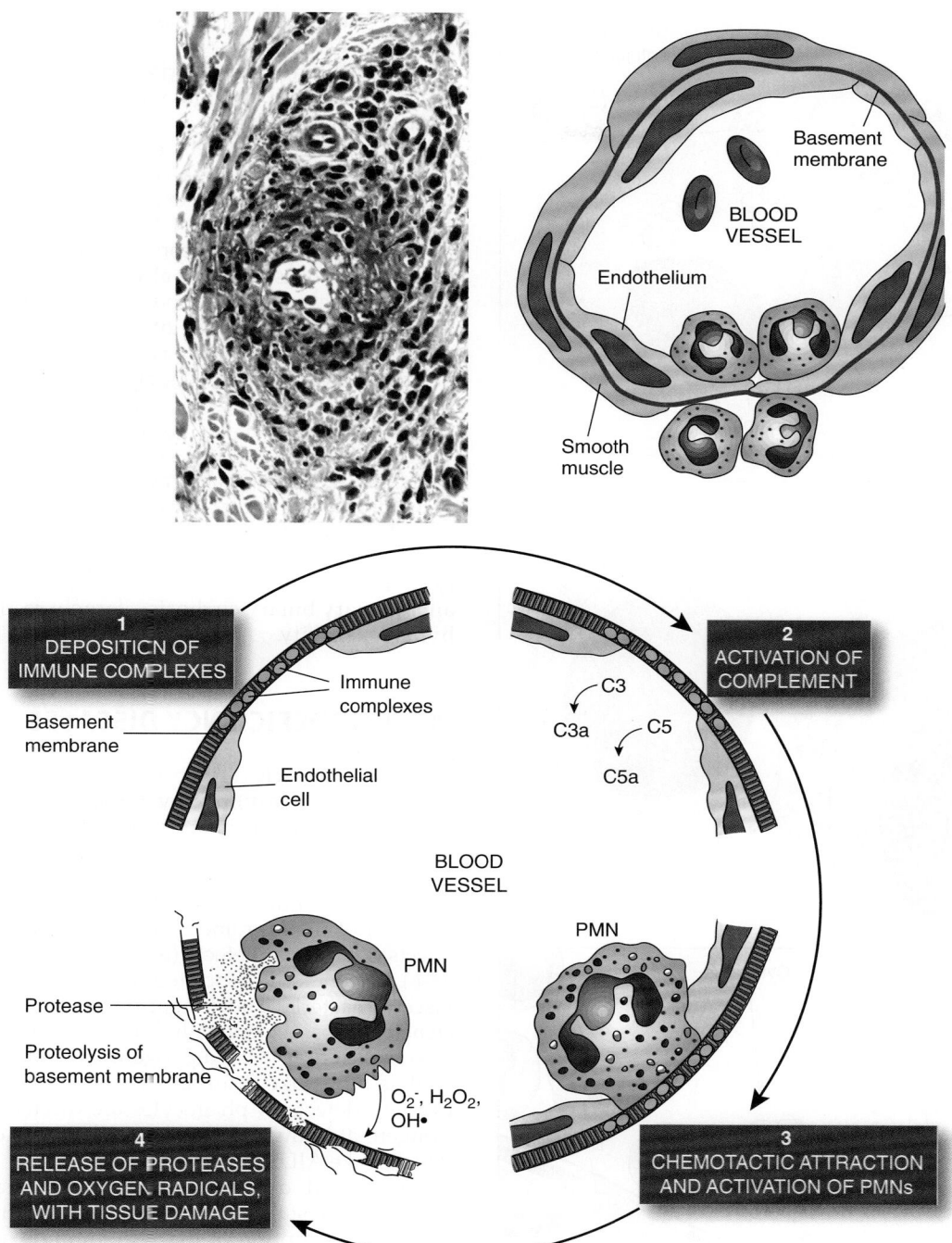

FIGURE 4-16. The Arthus reaction is a type III hypersensitivity reaction characterized by the deposition of immune complexes and the induction of an acute inflammatory response within blood vessel walls. Some vasculitic lesions exhibit fibrinoid necrosis. H_2O_2 = hydrogen peroxide; O_2^- = superoxide anion; $OH\bullet$ = hydroxyl radical; *PMN* = polymorphonuclear leukocyte.

This mechanism is important in destroying and eliminating cells infected by viruses, transplanted tissues, and possibly, tumor cells.

Unlike DTH, cytotoxic CD8+ T cells (CTLs) specifically recognize target antigens *in the context of class I MHC*. Foreign antigens are actively presented together with self-MHC. In graft rejection, foreign MHC antigens are themselves potent activators of CD8+ T cells. Once activated by antigen, CTL proliferation is abetted by helper cells and mediated by soluble growth factors such as IL-2 (Fig. 4-18C). The population of antigen-specific cytotoxic cells thus expands. Cell killing occurs via several mechanisms (Fig. 4-18D; see Chapter 1). CTLs secrete perforins that form channels in target cell membranes and introduce granzymes that activate intracellular caspases, leading to apoptosis. CTLs can also kill targets by engaging Fas ligand (FasL, on the CTL) and

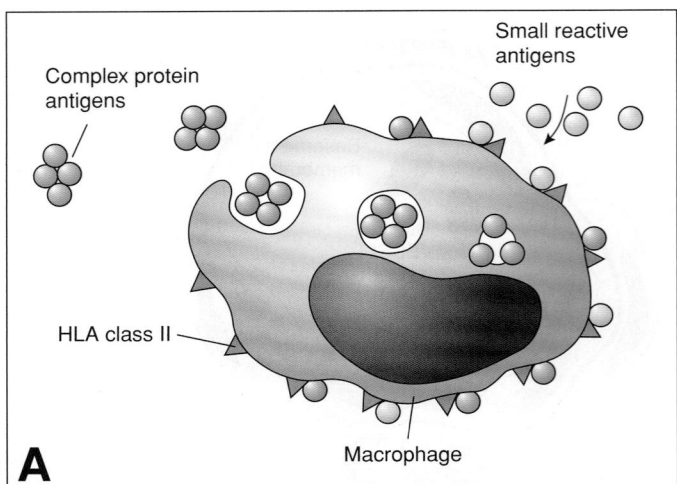

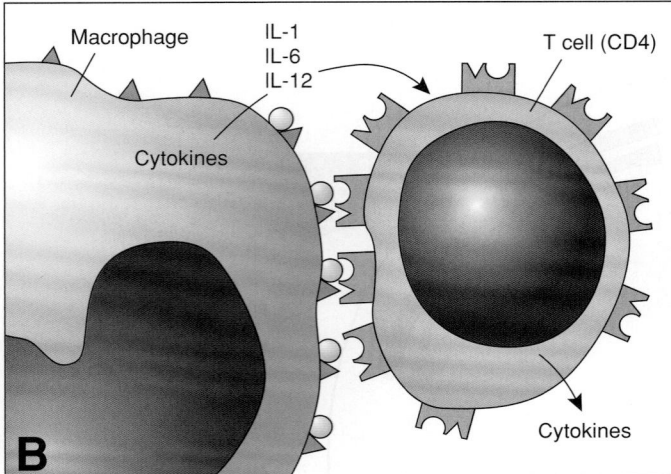

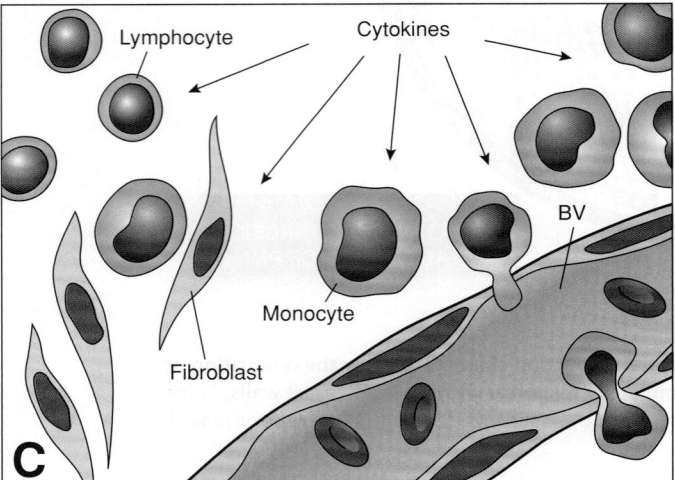

FIGURE 4-17. In a type IV (delayed-type) hypersensitivity reaction, complex antigens are phagocytized, processed, and presented on macrophage cell membranes in conjunction with class II MHC antigens. Antigens are in turn recognized via T-cell receptors (TCRs) expressed on histocompatible T lymphocytes. **A.** Antigen-specific, histocompatible, cytotoxic T lymphocytes bind presented antigens and are activated. **B, C.** Activated cytotoxic T cells secrete cytokines that amplify the response. *BV* = blood vessel.

Fas (on the target). FasL-Fas interaction triggers apoptosis of the Fas-bearing cell.

The defining characteristics of NK cells have been described, but the extent to which they participate in tissue-damaging reactions is unclear. Some evidence indicates that NK cells exert both effector and immunoregulatory functions. NK cells can recognize a variety of targets including membrane glycoproteins expressed by some virus-infected cells and tumor cells (Fig. 4-19). NK cells bind to target cells through membrane receptors and deliver molecular signals that result in lysis. NK cells also express membrane Fc receptors, which can bind antibodies and mediate cell killing by ADCC. NK cell activity is influenced by a variety of mediators. For example, it is increased by IL-2, IL-12, and IFNγ and decreased by several prostaglandins.

In type IV hypersensitivity reactions, antigens processed by macrophages are presented to antigen-specific T lymphocytes. These become activated and release mediators that recruit and activate lymphocytes, macrophages, and fibroblasts. Injury is caused by T cells, macrophages, or both. No antibodies are involved. Chronic inflammation associated with autoimmune diseases—including type 1 diabetes, chronic thyroiditis, Sjögren syndrome, and primary biliary cirrhosis—largely results from type IV hypersensitivity.

IMMUNODEFICIENCY DISEASES

Immunodeficiencies are classified as congenital (primary) or acquired (secondary), and by the host defense defect. The former are inherited. Primary immunodeficiencies are broadly classified as B-cell or humoral, T-cell or cellular defects of phagocytes or of the complement system. This scheme is useful, but it should be recognized that a primary defect in one part of the immune system may have farther-reaching effects. Phagocyte defects (e.g., chronic granulomatous disease) are generally associated with cutaneous, soft tissue and visceral bacterial and fungal infections. Complement deficiencies are associated with recurrent and/or severe bacterial infections (encapsulated pyogenic bacteria and Neisseria) as well as lupus-like disorders. Disorders of complement and primary defects of phagocytes are discussed in Chapter 2. Congenital immunodeficiencies are rare. Acquired immune deficits, like AIDS, however are not.

Functional defects in lymphocytes can be localized to particular stages in the ontogeny of the immune system, or interruption of discrete immune activation events (Fig. 4-20). Detailed classifications primary immunodeficiency disorders are available elsewhere. This section aims to introduce examples of prototypic primary immunodeficiency diseases.

Primary Antibody Deficiencies Predispose to Recurrent Bacterial Infections

Humoral (antibody) deficiencies are marked by subnormal serum concentrations of either all or specific isotypes of Igs. There are several isotype and subclass deficiencies including selective deletions of Ig H chains and selective loss of L-chain expression (Table 4-6). Some patients have normal antibody levels but cannot make antibodies against specific antigens, usually polysaccharides. Clinical manifestations are highly

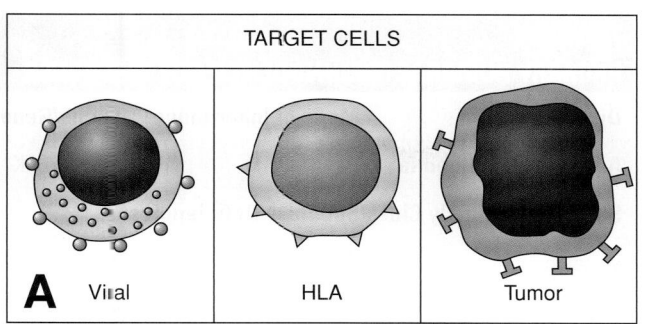

TARGET CELLS

A Viral | HLA | Tumor

TARGET ANTIGENS
• Virally coded membrane antigen
• Foreign or modified histocompatibility antigen
• Tumor-specific membrane antigens

B T-helper (CD4) | T-Cytotoxic (CD8)

RECOGNITION OF ANTIGEN BY T CELLS
• T-helper cells recognize antigen plus class II molecules
• T-cytotoxic/killer cells recognize antigen plus class I molecules

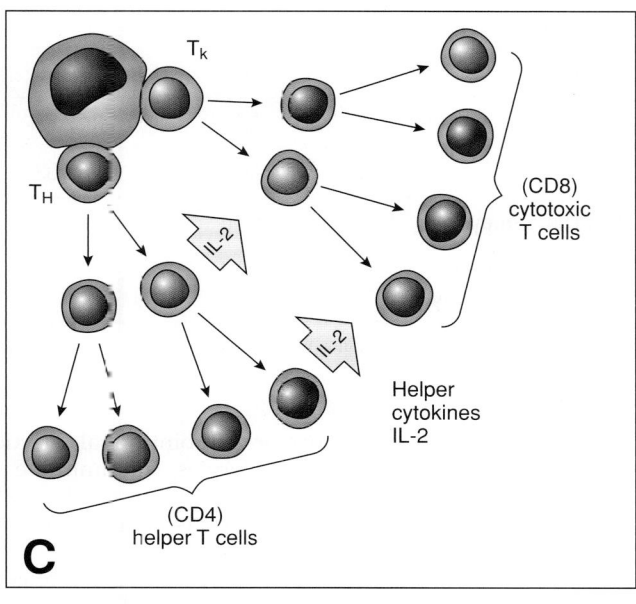

T_k

T_H

IL-2

IL-2

(CD8) cytotoxic T cells

Helper cytokines IL-2

C (CD4) helper T cells

ACTIVATION AND AMPLIFICATION
• T-helper cells activate and proliferate, releasing helper molecules (e.g., IL-2)
• T-cytotoxic/killer cells proliferate in response to helper molecules

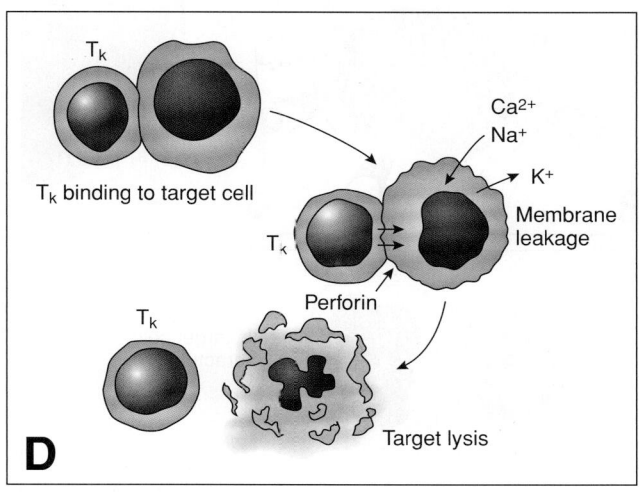

T_k

T_k binding to target cell

T_k

T_k

Ca^{2+}
Na^+

K^+

Membrane leakage

Perforin

Target lysis

D

TARGET CELL KILLING
• T-cytotoxic/killer cells bind to target cell
• Killing signals perforin release and target cell loses membrane integrity
• Target cell undergoes lysis

FIGURE 4-18. In T-cell–mediated cytotoxicity, potential target cells include (A) virus-infected host cells, malignant host cells, and foreign (histoincompatible transplanted) cells. B. Cytotoxic T lymphocytes recognize foreign antigens in the context of human leukocyte antigen (HLA) class I molecules. **C.** Activated T cells secrete lytic compounds (e.g., perforin and other mediators) and cytokines that amplify the response. **D.** Apoptosis (target cell killing) is mediated by perforin and involves influx of Ca^{2+} (calcium ion) and Na^+ (sodium ion) and efflux of K^+ (potassium ion). *IL* = interleukin.

variable: some patients suffer from life-threatening bacterial infections, varying from meningitis to mucosal infections, while others are asymptomatic. Several types of viral infections may also occur (e.g., CNS echovirus infections).

Bruton X-Linked Agammaglobulinemia

First described in 1952, Bruton X-linked agammaglobulinemia (XLA) often presents in boys younger than 1 year, when protective maternal antibody levels have declined. Up to 10% of XLA patients do not present until they are teenagers. Studies suggest that up to 10% of adults diagnosed with "common variable immunodeficiency (CVID)" (see below) actually have XLA. Patients develop recurrent mucosal

infections (e.g., sinusitis, bronchitis), pyoderma, meningitis, and septicemia. Severe hypogammaglobulinemia involves all Ig isotypes. Some patients develop viral hepatitis or chronic enterovirus infections of the CNS or large joints. Immunization with live attenuated poliovirus can lead to paralytic poliomyelitis. About 1/3 of XLA patients develop a poorly understood form of arthritis, possibly due to enteroviruses or *Ureaplasma*.

There are no mature B cells in peripheral blood or plasma cells in lymphoid tissues. Pre-B cells, however, can be detected. The genetic defect, on the long arm of the X chromosomes (Xq21.22), inactivates the gene for B-cell tyrosine kinase (**Bruton tyrosine kinase**), an enzyme critical to B-lymphocyte maturation (Table 4-6).

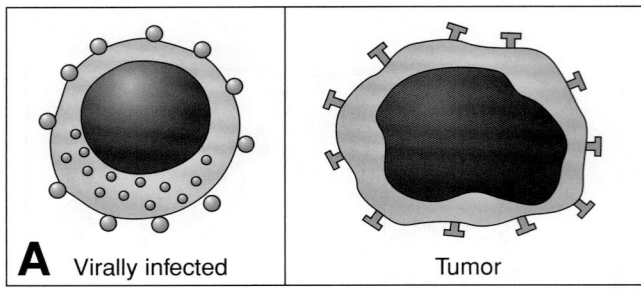

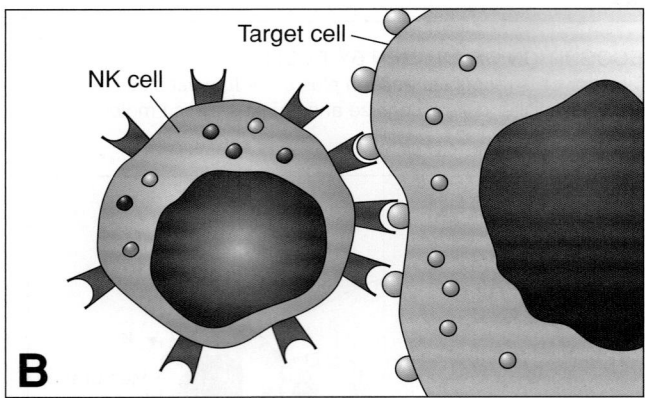

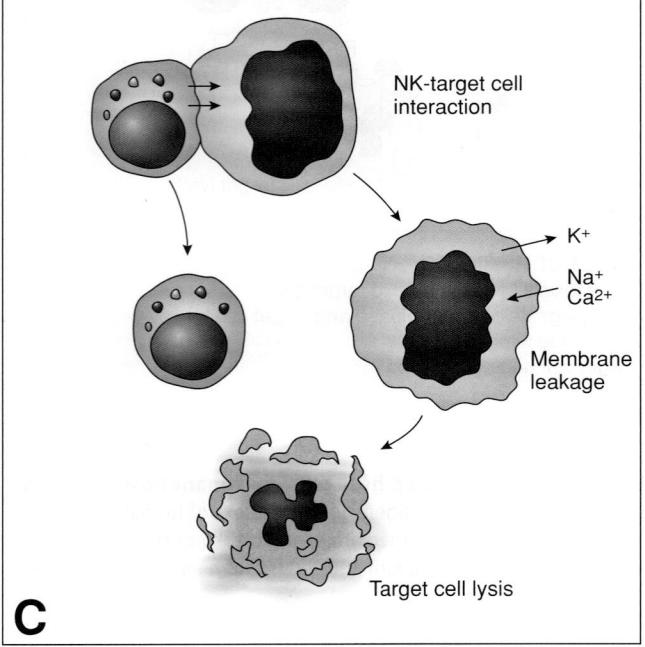

FIGURE 4-19. In NK-cell–mediated cytotoxicity, potential target cells include virus-infected and neoplastic cells. NK cells bind target cells (A), are activated (B), and secrete lytic compounds (C). NK cells bind to target cells that express decreased numbers of surface human leukocyte antigen (HLA) class I molecules. Ca^{2+} = calcium ion; K^+ = potassium ion; Na^+ = sodium ion.

Selective IgA Deficiency

In this common primary immunodeficiency syndrome, serum levels of IgM and IgG are normal, while serum and secretory concentrations of IgA are very low or undetectable. Incidence ranges from 1:18,000 in Japan to 1:400 among northern Europeans. Patients are often asymptomatic but may present with

TABLE 4-6
PRIMARY HUMORAL IMMUNODEFICIENCY DISORDERS

Disease	Mode of Inheritance	Locus/Gene
Agammaglobulinemia	XL	Xq21.3/BTK
Selective Antibody Class/Subclass Deficiencies		
γ_1 isotype	AR	14q32.33
γ_2 isotype	AR	14q32.33
Partial γ_3 isotype	AR	14q32.33
γ_4 isotype	AR	14q32.33
IgG subclass ± IgA deficiency	?	
α_1 isotype	AR	14q32.33
α_2 isotype	AR	14q32.33
ε isotype	AR	14q32.33
IgA Deficiency	Varied	—
Common Variable Immunodeficiency	Varied	—

AR = autosomal recessive; BTK = Bruton tyrosine kinase; Ig = immunoglobulin; XL = X-linked.

chronic or recurrent respiratory or gastrointestinal infections. Symptomatic patients develop allergies, autoimmune diseases, and collagen vascular disorders and are at risk for allergic, occasionally anaphylactic, reactions to IgA-containing transfused blood products.

Patients with IgA deficiency have circulating B cells that coexpress IgA, IgM, and IgD; their varied and poorly understood defects prevent IgA synthesis and secretion (Table 4-6). There may be a common origin with CVID (see below). Some cases have been linked to drug exposures (e.g., phenytoin, D-penicillamine) and some to deletions or defects in chromosome 18. Patients with concomitant IgG subclass deficiencies are more likely to be clinically affected.

Common Variable Immunodeficiency

CVID is a heterogenous group of disorders with severe hypogammaglobulinemia and attendant infections (Table 4-6), apparently due to a variety of defects in B-lymphocyte maturation or in T cells that regulate B-lymphocyte maturation. Some relatives of patients with CVID have selective IgA deficiency. Affected patients present with recurrent severe pyogenic infections, especially pneumonia and diarrhea, the latter often due to infection with *Giardia lamblia*. Recurrent Herpes simplex virus attacks are common; Herpes zoster develops in 1/5 of patients.

CVID appears years to decades after birth, with a mean age at onset of 25 years. It affects between 1:50,000 and 1:200,000 people. Inheritance patterns vary. There are several maturational and regulatory defects of the immune system. Cancers are increased in CVID, including a 50-fold greater incidence of gastric cancer. Interestingly, lymphoma

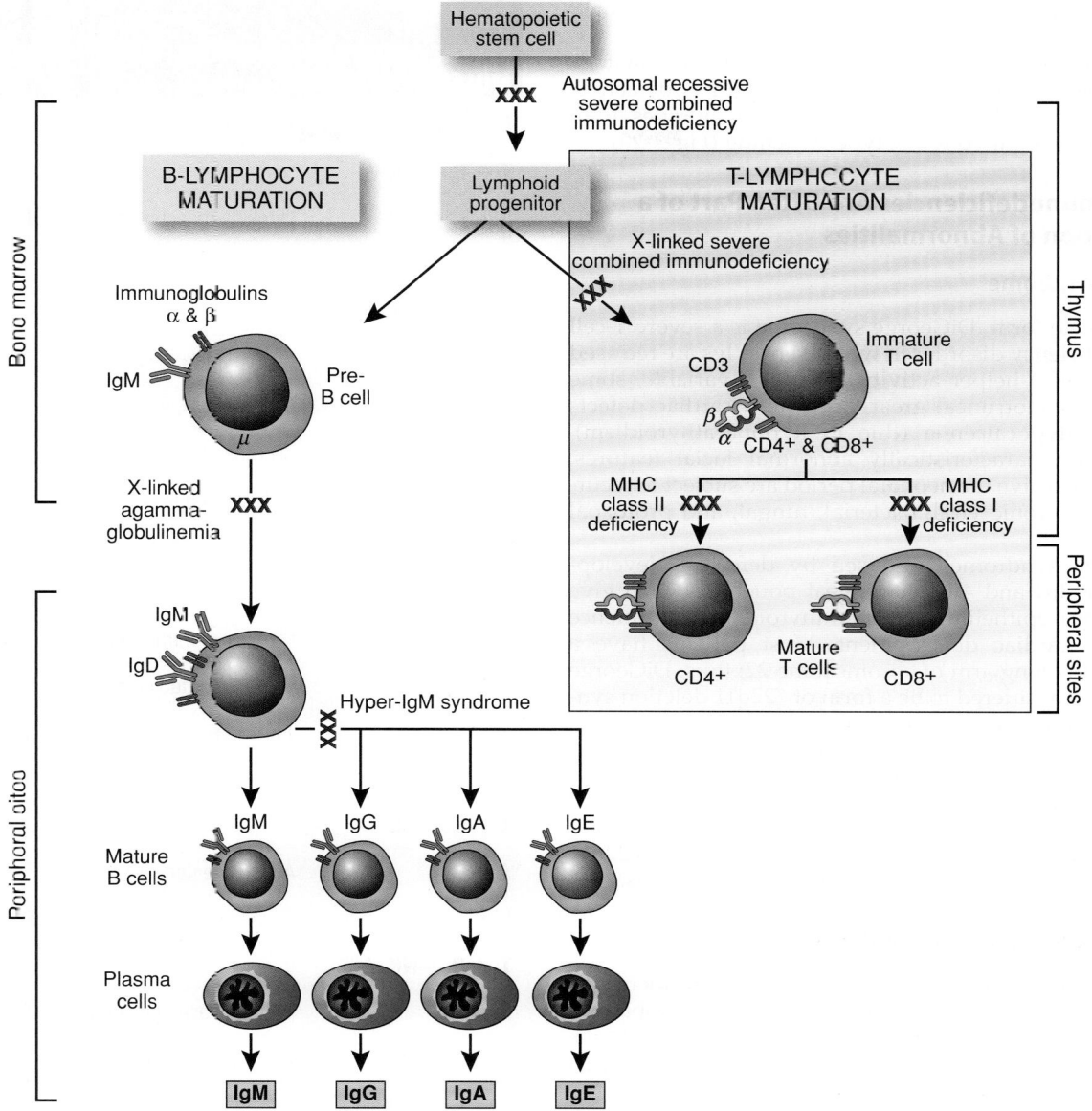

FIGURE 4-20. Hematopoietic stem cells give rise to lymphoid progenitor cells that, in a predetermined manner, populate either the bone marrow or thymus. More than 200 primary immunodeficiency disorders have been characterized at the genetic and/or molecular levels. In a number of immunodeficiency disorders, a discrete molecular defect results in a form of "maturational arrest" in the development of fully differentiated and functional lymphocytes. The identification of specific molecular lesions has hastened diagnostic evaluation and mechanistic understanding.

is 300 times more common in women with this disease than in affected men. Malabsorption due to lymphoid hyperplasia and inflammatory bowel diseases is more common than in the general population. Patients are also more susceptible to other autoimmune disorders, including hemolytic anemia, neutropenia, thrombocytopenia, and pernicious anemia.

Transient Hypogammaglobulinemia of Infancy

In some infants, prolonged hypogammaglobulinemia occurs once maternal antibodies reach their nadir. Some affected children develop recurrent infections and require therapy, but all eventually produce antibodies. Affected infants have mature

B cells that are temporarily unable to produce antibodies. The defect is not well understood but may represent delayed helper T-cell signal-generating capacity.

Hyper-IgM Syndrome

Hyper-IgM (HIM) syndrome is often classified as a humoral immunodeficiency because Ig production is disordered. Blood IgG, IgA, and IgE are subnormal, but IgM is elevated. There is an X-linked form that results from defects in CD40 ligand type 1 (HIM) and an autosomal recessive form due to defects in CD40 (type 3 HIM). Infants with X-linked disease suffer pyogenic and opportunistic infections, especially with *Pneumocystis jiroveci* (formerly *Pneumocystis carinii*), and also tend to develop autoimmune diseases involving the formed elements of blood.

Circulating B cells bear only IgM and IgD. The "switch" to other heavy-chain isotypes from IgD/IgM is defective. Interaction of CD40 receptor on B-cell membranes with CD40 ligand is required for isotype switching (Fig. 4-20).

T-Cell Immunodeficiencies Are Often Part of a Constellation of Abnormalities

DiGeorge Syndrome

In its complete form, DiGeorge syndrome is a severe T-cell immunodeficiency disorder in which serum Igs are reduced due to lack of T-helper activity. Although variable, some infants have conotruncal great vessel and cardiac defects and severe hypocalcemia (due to hypoparathyroidism). Others show characteristically abnormal facial features. Infants who survive the neonatal period are subject to recurrent and/or chronic viral, bacterial, fungal, and protozoal infections.

DiGeorge syndrome is caused by defective development of the 3rd and 4th pharyngeal pouches, which give rise to thymic epithelium and parathyroids, and influence conotruncal cardiac development. Most patients have a deletion in the long arm of chromosome 22; thus, DiGeorge syndrome is considered to be a form of "22q11 deletion syndrome." Without a functional thymus, T-cell maturation stops at the pre–T-cell stage. The immune defect has been corrected by transplanting thymic tissue.

Most patients have "partial" DiGeorge syndrome, and have a small remnant of thymus. With time, many recover T-cell function without treatment. Some patients with 22q11 mutations suffer only from conotruncal cardiac defects.

Chronic Mucocutaneous Candidiasis

CMC results from impaired T-cell function, with increased susceptibility to *Candida* infections and endocrinopathies (hypoparathyroidism, Addison disease, diabetes mellitus). Most T-cell functions are intact, but responses to *Candida* antigens are impaired.

A series of defects in T-cell development are involved. Patients react to *Candida* antigens differently from normal individuals. Unlike normal responses in which Th1 (IL-2/IFNγ) cells predominate and effectively control candidal infections, affected patients mount a less effective Th2 (IL-4/IL-6)-helper cell response.

Combined Immunodeficiency Diseases Vary in Severity

Severe combined immunodeficiencies are conspicuously heterogenous and are often life threatening (Table 4-7).

Severe Combined Immunodeficiency

Severe combined immunodeficiency (SCID) diseases include several disorders of development and function. Affected patients present in the first few months of life with recurrent, often severe infections, diarrhea, and failure to thrive. Some forms of SCID have nonimmunologic developmental defects. SCID is usually fatal within the first year of life without HSC transplantation to provide an immune system.

TABLE 4-7

SEVERE COMBINED IMMUNODEFICIENCY (SCID): MOLECULAR LESIONS[a]

Disease	Locus/Gene
T–/–B+/–NK–/–	
IL2RG	Cytokine receptor common γ-chain
JAK3	Tyrosine kinase JAK3
T–/–B+/–NK+/–	
CD3D	CD3 complex, δ subunit
CD3E	CD3 complex, e subunit
CD3G	CD3 complex, γ subunit
CIITA	MHC class II transactivator
RFXANK	MHC class II transactivator
FRX5	MHC class II transactivator
RXAP	MHC class II transactivator
ZAP70	TCR-associated protein of 70 kDa
TAP1	Transporter-associated antigen processing 1
TAP2	Transporter-associated antigen processing 2
T–/–B–/–NK–/–	
ADA	Adenosine deaminase
PNP	Purine nucleoside phosphoacylase
T–/–B–/–NK+/–	
RAG1	Recombinase-activating gene 1
RAG2	Recombinase-activating gene 2

[a]This is a partial list of SCID disorders.
MHC = major histocompatibility complex; TCR = T-cell receptor.

T-cell development and/or function are defective. In some types, B-cell development is also affected. Since B cells need T-cell–derived signals for optimal antibody production, most patients have defective cellular and humoral immunity. NK cell development and function are variably affected. There are several categories of SCID (Table 4-7).

The most common form of SCID in the United States (50% of cases) is due to mutations in IL2RG. This gene encodes the cytokine receptor common γ-chain, which is shared by receptors for IL-2, IL-4, IL-7, IL-9, IL-15, and IL-21. Defects result in complete absence of T cells and NK cells (90% of cases) but normal numbers of B cells. Ig production is severely impaired because of the T-cell defect. Signaling downstream of the common γ-chain IL receptors requires activation of JAK3 tyrosine kinase (Janus kinase 3). Not surprisingly, T–/–B+/–NK– SCID patients with mutations in JAK3 have been identified.

MOLECULAR PATHOGENESIS: More than a dozen molecular lesions have been described in T–/–B+/–NK+ SCID patients. For instance, mutations in genes (CD3D, CD3E, CD3G) that encode each subunit (δ, ε, γ) of the TCR-associated CD3 complex are known. These patients all show defects in T-lymphocyte function, but clinical features vary. Another group of T–/–B+/–NK+ SCID patients lack CD4+ T cells in association with various defects in expression of MHC class II molecules. Yet another group of T–/–B+/–NK+ SCID patients are deficient in CD8+ T cells. Among this group of patients, mutations in ZAP70, TAP1 and TAP2 have been described. ZAP70 (TCR-associated protein of 70 kDa) is a tyrosine kinase involved in TCR signaling; TAP1 and TAP2 are required for shuttling of cytosolic peptide onto naive HLA class I molecules for subsequent presentation to TCRs.

Mutations in the genes for enzymes in the purine nucleotide salvage pathway, adenosine deaminase (ADA) and purine nucleoside phosphorylase (PNP), result in T–/–B–/–NK– SCID. Accumulation of toxic purine metabolites leads to death of immature, proliferating lymphocytes (and other cell types). ADA deficiency accounts for 15% of all SCID patients in the United States. PNP deficiency is very rare.

Rare patients with T–/–B–/–NK+ SCID possess mutations within genes for DNA-binding proteins involved in Ig and TCR gene rearrangement. Some patients suffer from radiation sensitivity in addition to immunodeficiency.

Molecular lesions are known in approximately 95% of patients with SCID. Additional molecular lesions may account for the remaining 5%.

AUTOIMMUNITY

Autoimmunity is fundamentally a physiologic process that helps regulate immune system function. Disrupted "normal" regulatory mechanisms can lead to uncontrolled autoantibody production and/or abnormal cell–cell recognition, which cause tissue injury and autoimmune diseases. Specific autoantibodies, if present and integral to disease development, are useful in diagnosing autoimmune diseases. Prototypic examples of causal linkage between immune response and disease include myasthenia gravis (see above: antibodies disrupt postsynaptic acetylcholine receptors) and type 1 diabetes (CTLs kill pancreatic β-cells). Autoimmune diseases may be organ specific or generalized. There are several very rare monogenic autoimmune diseases that have provided insight into both autoimmunity and immune system regulation.

In Autoimmune Diseases, the Immune System Fails to Discriminate Between Self and Nonself Adequately

Immune tolerance occurs when there is no measurable (or clinically harmful) immune response to a specific previously presented antigen. Normally, people are tolerant to self-antigens. An abnormal or injurious autoimmune response to self-antigens implies loss of immune tolerance. Tolerance to self-antigens is an active process and requires contact between self-antigens and immune cells. During fetal development, tolerance is readily established to antigens that otherwise trigger vigorous immune responses in adults. Several mechanisms induce and maintain tolerance, actively and continuously, blocking and aborting potentially harmful immune responses constantly. Tolerance to an antigen is partly related to the dose of antigen administered.

During immune development, both central and peripheral mechanisms cause tolerance. In **central tolerance**, self-reactive immature T and B cells are "deleted" or changed during their maturation in the "central" thymus and bone marrow, respectively.

Developing T cells that recognize self-peptides presented by TMECs (in the context of compatible MHC) with high binding affinity undergo negative selection and die by apoptosis. The autoimmune regulator (**AIRE**) **protein** is involved in expression of peripheral tissue-restricted self-antigens within the thymus, and so is important in central expression of peripheral self-antigens to which the individual becomes tolerant. Mutations in AIRE cause autoimmune polyendocrinopathy.

In the bone marrow, similar negative selection occurs in B cells. As well, engagement of self-antigens by developing marrow B cells can reset antigen receptor gene rearrangement through a process called "receptor editing." These reprogrammed B cells thus do not recognize self. CD4+ regulatory T cells (T_{reg}) also develop.

Peripheral tolerance regulates T cells that escape intrathymic negative selection. Mature T lymphocytes are held in check in the periphery via anergy, suppression and/or activation-induced cell death. Anergy occurs when T lymphocytes bind antigen presented by APCs without the second signal, normally provided by CD80/B7-1 and CD86/B7-2 (see above) on the APC via CD28 on the T cell. Thus, the milieu in which antigens are presented to T cells helps determine immunity or tolerance.

Downstream T-cell inactivation/unresponsiveness (anergy) entails at least two mechanisms. Immune responses are suppressed by a population of regulatory T cells generated in response to exposure to self-antigens. These CD4+ T_{reg}s constitutively express CD25 (β-chain of high-affinity IL-2 receptor) and express FOXp3 transcription factor. Mutations and polymorphisms affecting CD25, IL-2R, or FOXp3 result in autoimmune disorders. Finally, CD4+ T cells and self-reactive B cells can be deleted by several activation-initiated mechanisms. In some situations, antigens are ignored; the mechanism(s) for this process are poorly understood.

Theories of Autoimmunity

There are several, not mutually exclusive, explanations for autoimmune diseases.

Inaccessible Self-Antigens
An immune reaction may develop against self-antigens not normally "accessible" to the immune system. Intracellular antigens are generally not exposed or released until infection and/or tissue injury "releases" or "exposes" them. At that time, an immune response develops (e.g., antibodies against spermatozoa, lens tissue, and myelin). Whether such autoantibodies directly induce injury is another matter. For example, there is no evidence that antisperm antibodies induce generalized injury, aside from a localized orchitis.

Thus, autoantibodies may form against normally "sequestered" antigens but are infrequently pathogenic.

Abnormal T-Cell Function

Autoimmune reactions may develop due to T-cell abnormalities. As noted, several mutations and/or polymorphisms are linked to autoimmune disease. Altered numbers or functional activities of helper or suppressor T cells could thus influence one's ability to mount an immune response. Defective or abnormal suppressor function, particularly in T cells, occurs in many autoimmune diseases, including primary biliary cirrhosis, thyroiditis, multiple sclerosis, myasthenia gravis, rheumatoid arthritis and scleroderma (see Chapter 12). Defective suppressor T-cell activity also occurs in people who have no evidence of autoimmune disease. Thus, the key question is how—or if—observed altered suppressor T-cell functions cause these diseases or are epiphenomena.

Helper T cells are defined by their role in antigen-specific B-cell activation; but their function may also be abnormal and autoreactive in autoimmune disease.

Tolerance may be abrogated by environmental influences, sometimes in antigen nonspecific ways. Drugs and other agents may trigger epigenetic changes, for example, DNA hypomethylation. This may upregulate leukocyte function antigen-1 (LFA-1) and cause B-cell activation independently of antigen. Drug-induced lupus exemplifies T-cell autoreactivity without antigen specificity. Exposure to modified antigens may also break tolerance, so that helper cells are activated and trigger B cells. This occurs when an antigen is partially degraded or complexed with a carrier protein. Thus, antibodies recognize partially degraded connective tissue proteins such as collagen or elastin in some rheumatologic diseases. In some drug-induced hemolytic anemias, antibody against a drug causes hemolysis when the drug binds to erythrocyte membranes.

Molecular Mimicry

Some foreign antigens elicit antibodies that cross-react with self-antigens. Helper T cells acting "correctly," do not induce autoantibodies. However, the efferent limb of the immune response, whose reactivity is against the foreign antigen, turns around and attacks the similarly structured self-antigen. Thus, in rheumatic fever, antibodies versus streptococcal antigens cross-react with molecules in the heart—molecular mimicry.

Polyclonal B-Cell Activation

In polyclonal B-cell activation, B lymphocytes are directly activated by complex substances that contain many antigenic sites (e.g., bacterial cell walls and viruses). Bacterial, viral, and parasitic infections may thus elicit rheumatoid factor in rheumatoid arthritis, anti-DNA antibodies in SLE and other autoantibodies. Such scattergun stimulation of antibody responses may also lead to autoantibodies.

Insights From Immune-Related Adverse Events Associated With Immune Checkpoint Blockade and Monogenic Autoimmune Diseases

In recent years, survival of patients with several solid organ cancers has improved through **immune checkpoint blockade (ICB)**, a therapy that increases antitumor immunity by inhibiting intrinsic downregulation of immunity. Monoclonal antibodies that block **cytotoxic T-lymphocyte antigen 4 (CTLA-4)**, **programmed death 1 (PD-1)** and **PD-1 ligand (PD-L1)** have all been effective. Immune-related adverse events associated with ICB resemble those of idiopathic autoimmune diseases, with many organ systems involved: the most common being endocrine tissue, liver, skin, and the GI tract. While individuals' manifestations may vary, these observations have provided new insights into pathophysiology of autoimmune disease.

Very rare monogenic autoimmune syndromes are clinically important per se, but they have also provided valuable insight into autoimmunity and immune system regulation. In each example, there are functional linkages between a discrete monogenic lesion and downstream autoimmunity. Pathophysiologic mechanisms that lead to disease are multifaceted. Discrete defects in innate immunity appear more likely to result in systematic manifestations while defects in adaptive immunity are more likely to result in organ system–specific disease. Examples include C1q deficiency, Aicardi–Goutieres syndrome, autoimmune lymphoproliferative syndrome (ALPS), ALPS-related disorders, immune dysregulation–polyendocrinopathy, and X-linked (IPEX) and autoimmune polyglandular syndrome type 1 (APS1, previously APECED).

Tissue Injury in Autoimmune Diseases

Autoimmune diseases have traditionally been considered to be prototypical immune complex diseases, with immune complexes forming in the circulation or in tissues. Thus, type II (cytotoxic) and type III (immune complex) hypersensitivity reactions explain most autoimmune tissue injury. But of course the story is more complicated. In some autoimmune diseases, for example, T cells sensitized to self-antigens (such as thyroglobulin) cause tissue injury directly (type IV reaction).

In ADCC, antibodies against cell membrane antigens can destroy such antigen-bearing cells. Thus, antibodies to parietal cell H^+/K^+-ATPase contribute to development of atrophic gastritis—but not in all patients, as many people have antiparietal cell antibodies but do not develop gastritis.

Not all autoantibodies cause disease via cytotoxicity. In antireceptor antibody diseases, like Graves disease and myasthenia gravis (see above), antibody-bound cells are not killed (however, anti-acetylcholine antibodies may lead to postsynaptic cell membrane damage). Antibodies against insulin receptors in acanthosis nigricans and ataxia telangiectasia cause some patients to develop extremely insulin-resistant diabetes.

Type III hypersensitivity reactions (immune complex disease) explain tissue injury in some autoimmune diseases (e.g., SLE). DNA–anti-DNA complexes formed in the circulation (or at local sites) deposit in tissues, induce inflammation, and injure tissues (e.g., vasculitis, glomerulonephritis) (see Chapter 11). For many autoimmune diseases, clinical manifestations are systemic, with many organs and tissues affected. However, cytotoxic (type II–mediated) autoimmune antibody reactions are mostly organ specific.

TRANSPLANTATION IMMUNOLOGY

Donor MHC-encoded antigens are immunogenic molecules that can stimulate rejection of transplanted tissues. Optimal graft survival occurs when recipient and donor are closely matched for major HLAs. In practice, an exact HLA match is uncommon, except between monozygotic twins. Thus, organ transplantation necessitates subsequent immunosuppressive therapy and vigilant monitoring of graft function. Therapeutic advances have greatly improved transplant success rates, even when there is some histoincompatibility. When host-versus-graft immune reactions (rejection) occur, a combination of immune mechanisms may injure the graft.

Both T-cell–mediated and antibody-mediated reactions may contribute to transplant rejection. Within the graft, APCs, specifically those bearing foreign MHC molecules, are recognized by host CD8$^+$ CTLs, which mediate tissue injury, and host CD4$^+$ T-helper cells, which augment antibody production, induce IFNγ production, and activate macrophages. In turn, IFNγ enhances MHC expression, amplifying the immune response and resulting tissue injury. Host APCs also process foreign donor antigens, leading to CD4$^+$-mediated DTH and CD4$^+$-mediated antibody production.

Solid organ transplant rejection reactions are usually categorized as "hyperacute," "acute," and "chronic" based on the clinical tempo of the response and pathophysiologic mechanism involved. However, in practice, features often overlap, creating diagnostic ambiguity. Assessment of transplant rejection is further complicated by the toxicity of immunosuppressive drugs,

potential mechanical problems (e.g., vascular thrombosis), and recurrence of original disease (e.g., some types of glomerulonephritis). The next sections illustrate rejection in the context of renal transplantation. Similar responses occur in other transplanted tissues, although rejection as applied to each tissue type has its own unique features.

Hyperacute Rejection Occurs Within Minutes of Transplantation

Hyperacute kidney rejection may be so fast that it occurs intraoperatively and manifests as a sudden cessation of urine output, darkening of the graft, and rapid development of fever and pain at the graft site. This form of rejection is triggered by preformed anti-HLA antibodies and generation of complement activation products, including chemotactic and other inflammatory mediators. Hyperacute rejection is catastrophic, necessitating prompt surgical removal of the grafted kidney. Histologic features include vascular congestion, fibrin–platelet thrombi within capillaries, neutrophilic vasculitis with fibrinoid necrosis, prominent interstitial edema, and neutrophil infiltrates (Fig. 4-21A). It is fortunately distinctly uncommon with adequate pretransplantation antibody screening.

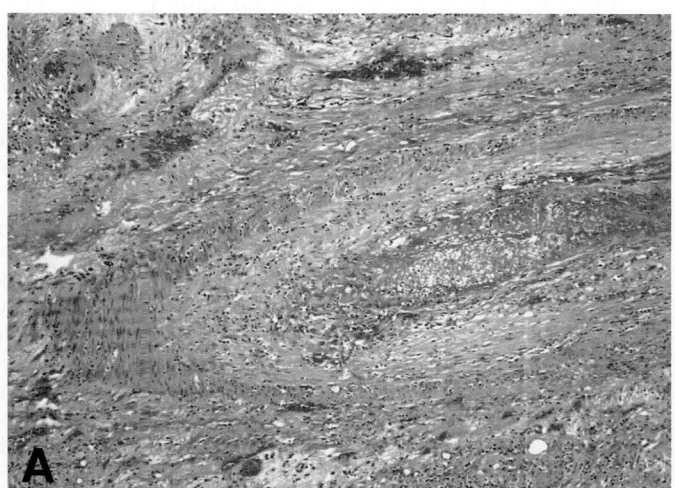

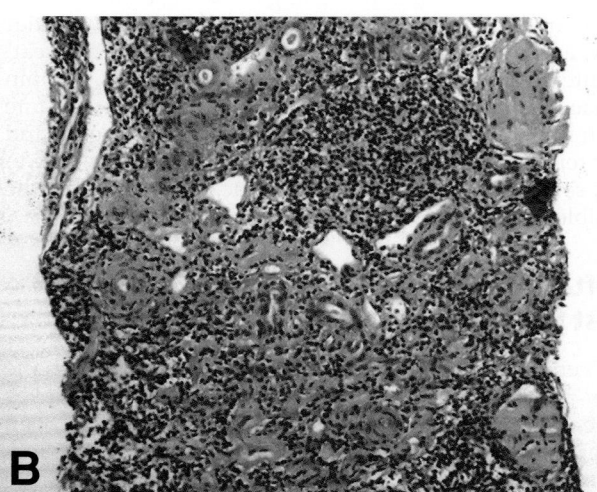

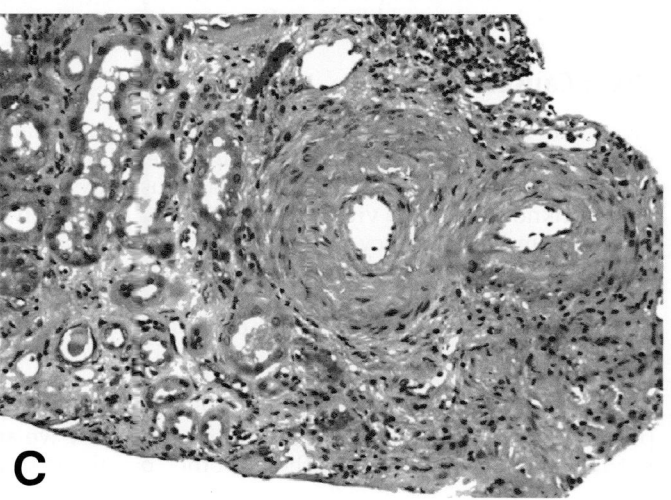

FIGURE 4-21. There are three major forms of renal transplant rejection. A. Hyperacute rejection occurs within minutes to hours after transplantation and is characterized, in part, by neutrophilic vasculitis, intravascular fibrin thrombi, and neutrophilic infiltrates. **B.** Acute cellular rejection occurs within weeks to months after transplantation and is characterized by tubular damage and mononuclear leukocyte infiltration. **C.** Chronic rejection is observed months to years after transplantation and is characterized by tubular atrophy, patchy interstitial mononuclear cell infiltrates, and fibrosis. In this example, arteries show fibrointimal thickening.

Acute Rejection Usually Occurs Weeks to Months After Transplantation

In acute renal graft rejection, azotemia and oliguria begin abruptly, sometimes with fever and graft tenderness. Acute rejection usually involves cell-mediated *and* humoral tissue damage. If detected early, it can be reversed with immunosuppressive therapy. Needle biopsy is often needed to differentiate acute rejection from acute kidney injury or toxicity from immunosuppressive drugs. Findings vary depending on whether the process is mainly cellular or humoral. In acute cellular rejection, interstitial lymphocyte and macrophage infiltration, edema, lymphocytic tubulitis, and tubular necrosis occur (Fig. 4-21B). In the acute humoral form, sometimes called rejection vasculitis, vascular damage predominates, with arteritis, fibrinoid necrosis, and thrombosis. Blood vessel involvement is an ominous sign that usually portends resistance to therapy.

Chronic Rejection Follows Transplantation by Months to Years

Such patients typically develop progressive azotemia, oliguria, hypertension, and weight gain over a period of months. Chronic rejection may be due to repeated episodes of cellular rejection, either asymptomatic or clinically apparent. Arterial and arteriolar intimal thickening cause vascular stenosis or obstruction, thickened glomerular capillary walls, tubular atrophy, and interstitial fibrosis (Fig. 4-21C). There are scattered interstitial mononuclear infiltrates. Tubules contain proteinaceous casts. Chronic rejection is an advanced state of organ injury and does not respond to therapy. Acute and chronic rejection may overlap histologically and may vary in degree, so that unambiguous pathologic distinction may be impossible.

In Graft-Versus-Host Disease, Donor Cells React Against the Recipient

The advent of transplantation of allogeneic (donor) bone marrow or HSCs harvested from peripheral blood makes possible treatment of diseases that had previously been considered terminal or untreatable. In order for transplanted marrow/HSCs to engraft in the new host, the recipient's bone marrow and immune system must be conditioned (usually ablated) by cytotoxic drugs, sometimes plus radiation.

Graft-versus-host disease (GVHD) may be acute or chronic. If there are immunocompetent lymphocytes in the HSC preparation, these donor cells may react against—reject—the recipient and, acute GVHD results. If, instead, the transplant contains donor lymphoid progenitors, these may differentiate after transplantation and elicit a more chronic form of GVHD. Passenger lymphocytes may also mediate GVHD if a severely immunodeficient patient receives a solid organ containing many "passenger" lymphocytes, or is transfused with blood products containing viable HLA-incompatible lymphocytes.

The major organs affected in GVHD are skin, GI tract, and liver. The skin and intestines show mononuclear cell infiltrates and epithelial cell necrosis. In the liver, GVHD entails peri-portal inflammation, damaged bile ducts and hepatocyt

injury. Clinically, acute GVHD presents with rash, diarrhea, abdominal cramps, anemia, and liver dysfunction. In chronic GVHD, there are dermal sclerosis, sicca syndrome (dry eyes and mouth due to chronic inflammation of lacrimal and salivary glands), and immunodeficiency. Treatment of GVHD requires immunosuppression. Patients, especially those with chronic GVHD, may be at a higher risk for potentially life-threatening opportunistic infections (e.g., invasive aspergillosis).

HIV/AIDS

ACQUIRED IMMUNODEFICIENCY SYNDROME

On June 5, 1981, an article appeared in *Morbidity and Mortality Weekly Report*, or *MMWR*, entitled, "Pneumocystis pneumonia—Los Angeles." Soon thereafter, on July 3, another article in *MMWR*, followed, "Kaposi's sarcoma and Pneumocystis pneumonia among homosexual men—New York City and California," then, again, on August 28, in *MMWR*, "Follow-up on Kaposi's sarcoma and Pneumocystis pneumonia." There followed, on December 10, an article by Gottlieb et al., in *The New England Journal of Medicine*, entitled, "*Pneumocystis carinii* pneumonia and mucosal candidiasis in previously healthy homosexual men: Evidence of a new acquired cellular immunodeficiency" (305(24):1425–1431;1981).

These communications described a small number of cases of a previously unknown syndrome. They heralded something unthinkable: a brand new terrifying and mysterious epidemic, caused by an unrecognized agent, capable of killing young people who should, by all criteria known at the time, be robust and resilient.

As investigators sought an explanation, contemporary medical practitioners began seeing strange constellations of infections that we had not seen before in seemingly healthy, young adults: *P. carinii* (now, *P. jiroveci*) pneumonia, disseminated *Mycobacterium avium-intracellulare (MAI)*, systemic cytomegalovirus (CMV), other opportunistic agents (Cryptococcus, Toxoplasma, Cryptosporidia, and others) which we had mostly seen in neonates, patients severely immunocompromised by treatment for malignancies or those with an inherited immune deficiency. And, there was the puzzling seeming epidemic of Kaposi sarcoma (KS) in young men—a tumor mostly seen in old Eastern European men.

HIV-1 Causes AIDS

Two years later, in back-to-back articles in *Science*, the laboratories of Robert Gallo and Luc Montagnier established that this mysterious and horrible disease was caused by a previously unknown human virus, which came to be known as human immunodeficiency virus type I (HIV-1). The disease it caused became acquired immunodeficiency syndrome (AIDS). It turns out that HIV-1, and its effects on the immune system, explained the constellations of clinical presentations and cataclysmic clinical evolution with which we became all too familiar in the years that followed.

The biology of HIV-1 and evolution of AIDS (see below) provide lessons in the dangers of smugness, in how we are not insulated from diseases afflicting other people or from zoonotic diseases, in how much we can know about an etiologic agent, how much we can study it in people and animal models, and yet how much we can fail to understand or anticipate.

Early Human HIV Infections Were Unreported

It turns out, of course, that there were harbingers of this disease. They just went unnoticed. The exact beginning of this human epidemic is uncertain, but unreported human HIV infections almost certainly occurred at least as early as 1902. The North American epidemic probably began in Haiti in 1966 and a single transmission event led to its spread to the United States about 5 years later.

The explosion that followed was just brewing at the time of the *MMWR* reports. About 2 years after the virus was first described in 1983, a blood test for it became available. In the interim, HIV-1–positive blood and blood products were in mainstream supplies. As a result, not only were men who had sex with men (MSM) at risk to contract the disease, so also did other people, including IV drug abusers, women who had sex with carriers, and people who received blood transfusions or products.

 EPIDEMIOLOGY: HIV began as a variant of a simian lentivirus that infected monkeys and apes. Initial human infections probably reflected several different transmission events, and occurred among Africans who ate meat from those animals. Human HIV-1 infections reflect 4 separate transmissions: 3 in which chimpanzees were the source of the virus, with gorilla(s) being the source in the fourth. The source of HIV-2 was a sooty mangabey.

These different origins resulted in different viral groups. One chimpanzee-derived strain (called Group M) appears to have caused the worldwide human epidemic, starting a century ago. Other groups of HIV-1 and HIV-2 tend to predominate in specific parts of the world.

WHO estimates that 36.7 million people were living with HIV/AIDS by late 2016, up from 31 million in 2002. Most (25.6 million) live in sub-Saharan Africa, and most of those are women. Only about 60% of those infected with HIV are aware of their condition. In 2016, 1.8 million people acquired new HIV infection, compared to 3.3 million in 2002. Further, as of July 2017, 20.9 million people were receiving antiretroviral therapy (ART, see below), compared to 15.8 million in June 2015, 7.5 million in 2010, and under 1 million in 2000. Mortality from HIV/AIDS is declining: the disease killed about 1 million people in 2016, a 48% decrease from 1.9 million deaths 11 years previously. *These statistical trends document that people infected with HIV are living longer: the advent of ART has transformed HIV infection from an inexorably fatal illness to chronic condition that may allow a semblance of a normal life expectancy.*

HIV-1 Is Transmitted by Sexual Activity and Bodily Fluids

HIV-1 is present in blood, semen, vaginal and endocervical secretions, breast milk, and cerebrospinal fluid of infected patients, both within lymphocytes and as free virus. Blood virus concentration is a factor in the likelihood of transmission, as are (separately) seminal and endocervical viral loads. Thus, an infected person can spread HIV-1 to sexual partners, drug users who share needles, recipients of blood products, and via breast milk to nursing infants.

Free virus or virus-infected cells may transmit infection. Virus and virus-bearing lymphocytes in semen may enter through tears in the rectal mucosa, particularly in anal-receptive MSM partners. HIV-1 can also infect intestinal and oral epithelial cells directly, and can pass, via **transcytosis**, that is, passing through these epithelial cells to underlying lymphoid tissues.

In heterosexual contact, male-to-female transmission is more likely than the reverse, perhaps because there is more HIV in semen than in vaginal fluid. Coexisting genital lesions facilitate virus entry. HIV infections are less common in circumcised men, possibly since the foreskin is less well keratinized than other parts of the penis and has a higher concentration of cutaneous DCs (Langerhans cells, see below).

Nonsexual, casual exposure to infected people does not transmit the virus. In fact, <1% of health care workers who sustained "needlesticks" or other accidental exposures to blood from HIV-positive patients became infected with HIV-1. Immediate postexposure antiretroviral prophylaxis is available (see http://www.cdc.gov/hiv/resources/guidelines for details).

Decreases in documented new infections (see above) generally represent lower rates of heterosexual transmission. Incidence of new infections among MSM has been stable.

HIV-1 BIOLOGY AND HOW IT CAUSES DISEASE

HIV-1 is an extraordinarily successful human pathogen. Several important factors contribute to the pathogenesis and consequences of HIV-related disease and our efforts to control it:

- the virus' resilience, which reflects its peculiar biology
- the cell populations it targets
- immune stimulation, then exhaustion, and long-term inability of immune responses to clear the infection
- consequences of therapy, including drug toxicities and virus latency and reservoirs
- diseases that occur because of HIV-1 infection but are not directly due to the virus itself

The Biology of HIV-1 Has Driven Its Success as a Pathogen

 MOLECULAR PATHOGENESIS: HIV-1 belongs to the lentivirus group of retroviruses. Although animal lentiviruses had been recognized for a century, medicine had had little awareness of, or contact with, human lentiviruses.

HIV-1 virions carry the virus' RNA genome, plus important proteins, in a virus-encoded capsid. Key virus proteins inside virions are reverse transcriptase (RT), which makes a DNA copy (cDNA, provirus), of the virus' RNA genome, integrase (IN), which integrates that copy into host DNA, and PR, which mediates virion maturation. An envelope grudgingly provided by the productively infected host cell surrounds this parcel, with two additions: viral envelope (Env) glycoproteins, gp120 and gp41. Molecular events in the virus' replicative cycle are illustrated in Figure 4-22:

1. **Binding:** Either free HIV-1 or an infected cell may introduce HIV-1 RNA into naive targets. Envelope gp120 on either binds CD4, plus a specific β-chemokine receptor, which initially is CCR5. (Later generations of virus may use CXCR4 or other related receptors instead.) C-type lectin receptors, for example, **DC-SIGN** (largely on DCs) may mediate virus entry.
2. **Internalization:** After HIV-1 binds a hapless target cell's plasma membrane, its Env glycoproteins change conformation. The virion genome, plus IN and RT, enters.
3. **DNA synthesis:** RT catalyzes reverse transcription, making HIV's single-stranded RNA genome into double-stranded DNA, or provirus. *This step is critical. HIV-1's RT lacks an editing function, so reverse transcription creates a huge number of mutations.* A high percentage of viral progeny are therefore defective (i.e., noninfectious). This error-prone viral genome replication also provides HIV-1 with enormous evolutionary adaptability: Since it generates so many mutant viral genomes constantly, the virus evolves continually and can adapt to almost any selective stress or pressure. Coreceptor usage, antigenicity, tropisms, antiviral drug resistance, and other traits are always changing.
4. **Integration:** HIV-1 provirus DNA can enter nuclei of resting cells, which is very uncommon among retroviruses. How this occurs is not well understood, but a combination of IN plus provirus plus other virus components probably mediates proviral transit through nuclear membranes, whereupon IN catalyzes proviral integration into cellular DNA.
5. **Replication and spread:** Host transcription factors (especially NF-κB, see Chapter 5), in conjunction with HIV-1 Tat and Rev proteins, mediate transcription of integrated proviral DNA. Several transcripts result: an unspliced whole-genome transcript and multiple different spliced transcripts. The latter encode specific viral proteins. The resulting capsid-enclosed virion assembles and buds from the cell membrane, a part of which becomes the virus' envelope. Viral budding is not the end of the process, however, as some HIV-1 proteins, particularly gp160 envelope, must be processed by HIV-1 PR, for resulting particles to be infectious. The infected cell, or free virus, binds another cell and the cycle repeats.

About 1% of Caucasians are homozygous for asymptomatic deletions in the CCR5 gene (the major mutation being a 32-base-pair deletion, causing a frameshift leading to a premature stop codon and a truncated, inactive protein product). These people may remain uninfected despite extensive exposure. Heterozygosity for mutant CCR5 alleles (≈20% of whites) affords partial protection; if infections occur, they tend to be milder. The mutant allele is largely absent in other races.

A basic understanding of the HIV-1 constituents and their roles in the infectious cycle helps to appreciate current approaches to ART. Most first ART regimens target two key viral proteins: RT (with multiple inhibitors) plus either PR or IN (see below).

PATHOPHYSIOLOGY: Initial infection: portal of entry. HIV may enter the body through several portals, the most efficient (except for direct inoculation of blood products) being the GI tract. Infants acquire HIV infection from their mothers by ingesting blood and cervical mucus during birth, or breast milk during feeding. During anal-receptive homosexual and heterosexual intercourse, infection starts with the colonic mucosa.

In orally acquired infection (e.g., via breastfeeding), virions traverse oropharyngeal mucosal cells by **transcytosis**. This is more effective in neonates than in adults, probably because endogenous defense molecules, like defensins, protect adult oral mucosa. Colonic mucosa is a key entry point in adults, especially for cell-associated virus. HIV-infected lymphocytes traverse colorectal mucosal cells by transcytosis, which delivers them to underlying lymphoid tissues. These epithelial cells do not have surface CD4, but HIV binds to them via galactosylceramide and chemokine receptors for transcytosis.

(Cervical and endocervical cells also allow transcytosis, but mucus substantially limits their accessibility to HIV.)

Initial infection: target cells. HIV's principal cellular targets at sites of entry are dendritic cells (DCs), which it reaches after traversing whatever epithelial surface interfaces with the source of virus. DCs express HIV receptors CD4, CCR5, and CXCR4 plus two additional cell surface proteins, CD209 (**DC-SIGN**) and **Siglec-1**, which boost HIV-1 entry. The virus may also infect some non-CD4$^+$ cells, such as astrocytes and renal epithelium, but such infections occur secondarily, after virus dissemination.

HIV-1's preferred target cells are activated CD4$^+$ T lymphocytes. Therefore, viral transit through mucosal surfaces and entry into DCs have several consequences, all of which serve this purpose:

- the virus need not replicate in DCs, but infectious virions persist stably in them for months
- DCs process virus antigens and present them to T cells, activating the lymphocytes and triggering an immune response
- DCs may transfer virions to CD4$^+$ T lymphocytes
- A subset of DCs (plasmacytoid DCs, or pDCs) produce type I interferon

Each of these characteristics of HIV-1–DC interaction helps promote HIV-1 infection. To succeed in its infectious quest, HIV must achieve several important goals. It must:

1. infect, replicate in, and disseminate from its favored cells (activated CD4$^+$ T cells)
2. generate an ever-enlarging pool of such cells, to have more infectious targets
3. evade immune defenses
4. establish reservoirs, to facilitate reactivation, should that be necessary
5. generate sufficient heterogeneity to facilitate (assure) survival in a hostile environment

HIV achieves these goals by establishing a state of perpetual immune system stimulation (Fig. 4-23). **The diverse arms of innate and adaptive immune systems are in a perpetual state of activation, which eventually leads to exhaustion.** *Paradoxically, despite their high level of activity, their ability to respond to specific stimuli is crippled.*

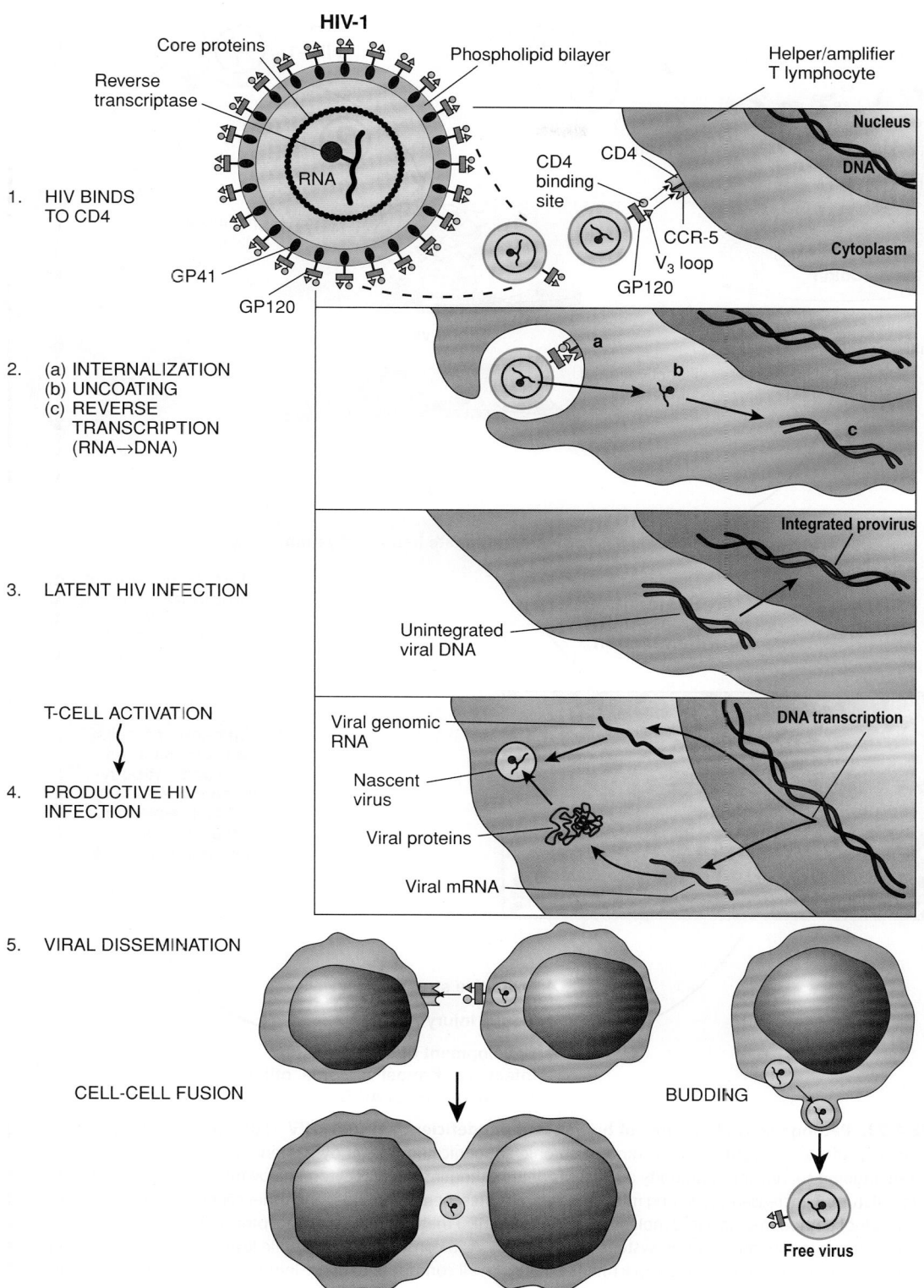

HIV-1

Core proteins
Reverse transcriptase
Phospholipid bilayer
Helper/amplifier T lymphocyte

RNA

1. HIV BINDS TO CD4

Nucleus
DNA
CD4 binding site
CD4
CCR-5
Cytoplasm
V_3 loop
GP120

GP41
GP120

2. (a) INTERNALIZATION
   (b) UNCOATING
   (c) REVERSE TRANSCRIPTION (RNA→DNA)

a
b
c

3. LATENT HIV INFECTION

Integrated provirus
Unintegrated viral DNA

T-CELL ACTIVATION

4. PRODUCTIVE HIV INFECTION

Viral genomic RNA
Nascent virus
Viral proteins
Viral mRNA

DNA transcription

5. VIRAL DISSEMINATION

CELL-CELL FUSION

BUDDING

Free virus

FIGURE 4-22. The life cycle of human immunodeficiency virus-1 (HIV-1) is a multistep process that includes (1) binding CD4 receptor in conjunction with chemokine receptor (e.g., CCR5); (2) internalization, uncoating and reverse transcription; (3) integration into host DNA as a provirus where it persists in a state of latency; (4) replication in concert with host T-cell activation; and (5) dissemination.

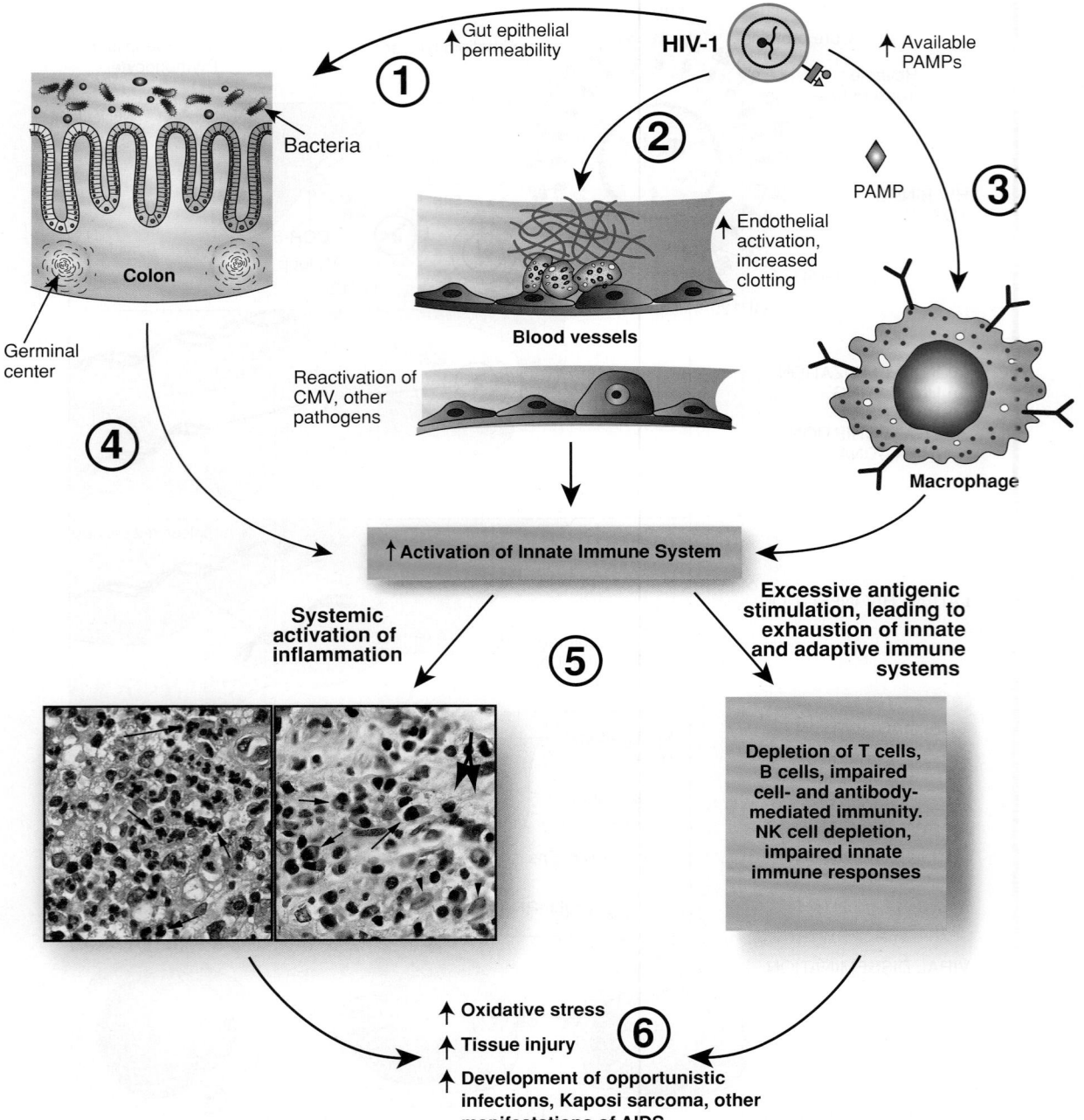

FIGURE 4-23. Pathogenesis of features of human immunodeficiency virus-1 (HIV-1) infection. 1. HIV-1 infection impairs the barrier function of the gut epithelium, leading to chronic antigenic stimulation by bacteria and other microbes in the gut lumen. **2.** Impaired ongoing surveillance immunity against resident pathogens, such as cytomegalovirus (CMV), leads to reactivation, shown here in vasculature. **3.** Increased circulating microbial antigens present macrophages and other cells of the innate immune system with excessive levels of pathogen-associated molecular patterns (PAMPs) that stimulate their receptors (PRRs) on these cells. **4.** These factors combine to activate the innate immune system excessively. **5.** As a consequence, systemic levels of inflammatory responses, tissue factor triggering of clotting, and T-cell compartment exhaustion all contribute to tissue injury. **6.** Continuing production of HIV-1 antigens and virus particles leads to increased oxidative stress, depleting antioxidant reserves and accelerating many types of tissue injury.

Gut-associated lymphoid tissue (GALT) is a huge pool of lymphocytes and DCs, and a key target and reservoir for HIV-1. Virus replication in GALT triggers massive outpouring of inflammatory mediators, leading to local inflammation. In parallel, HIV directly destroys GALT's protective effectiveness. Enterocyte apoptosis increases. These forces collectively weaken the mucosal shield that keeps bacteria and their products (like LPS) away from circulation. Bacterial products flood the circulation, further stimulating an already overcommitted immune system.

Inflammatory responses (Figs. 4-23 and 4-24) to HIV and LPS stimulate regulatory T cells to make TGFβ, which activates resident fibroblasts in lymph nodes and

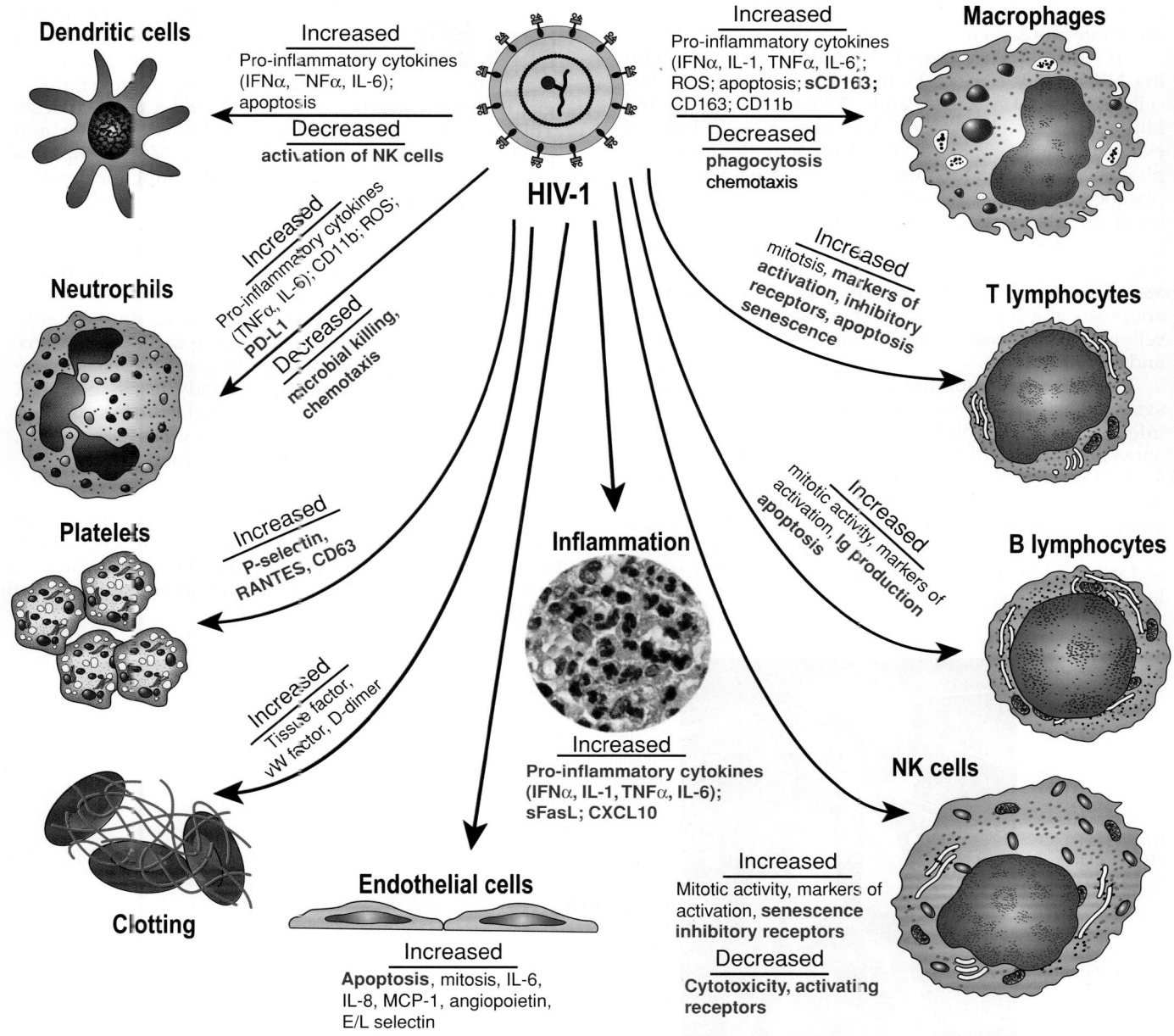

FIGURE 4-24. Cells involved in immune and inflammatory responses, as well as clotting, that are activated and affected during HIV-1 infection. Dysfunctions that often persist in the face of ART are highlighted.

other lymphoid tissues (e.g., GALT) to deposit collagen. This scarring distorts lymphoid tissue architecture, misdirecting circulating T-cell traffic: impairing homing to paracortical zones, disrupting contact with APCs, and limiting access to survival-promoting cytokines (like IL-7). Fibrosis also impairs B-cell function, preventing interaction with APCs and interfering with germinal center formation.

HIV-stimulated immune responses, humoral and cytotoxic, may transiently decrease viral load but actually perpetuate infection. In addition to causing immune exhaustion, they complement the virus' high mutation rate, and so select continuously for antibody- and CTL-resistant variants. The immune system is further handicapped in playing catch-up ball with an ever-changing set of viral antigens because HIV stimulates PD-1 (programmed cell death, see above) expression on virus-specific lymphocytes.

HIV infection greatly depletes and destroys CD4$^+$ T cells and limits their generation. Much of this occurs in the GALT early in infection. T_H17 cells and mucosal T cells, particularly, are lost. Altered GALT structure impairs the ability of T-cell survival factor, IL-7, to reach T cells, diminishing both CD4$^+$ and CD8$^+$ T-lymphocyte numbers. Reduced IL-2 production limits CTL-mediated killing. Thus, patients with AIDS cannot generate antigen-specific cytotoxic T cells to clear other infectious agents.

HIV also weakens innate immunity, greatly impairing NK activity (Figs. 4-23 and 4-24). About half of NK cells express CD4, CCR5, and CXCR4. HIV infects and kills these cells. Remaining NK cells show features of exhaustion and impaired killing capacity. Mononuclear phagocyte (monocytes, macrophages) chemotactic and phagocytic activities is feeble, but they elaborate high levels of proinflammatory cytokines (e.g., TNFα, IL-1, IL-6) and chemokines. Neutrophils, similarly, appear to be activated, and make some of the same inflammatory mediators. They produce **PD-1 ligand (PD-L1)**, and undergo apoptosis at a high rate. Diverse innate immune system cells express increased PD-L1, which magnifies lymphoid and other cell loss.

HIV activates endothelial cells and the coagulation system. Drivers of endothelial cell activation in HIV infection include proinflammatory cytokines mentioned above, and several HIV-1 gene products (Figs. 4-23 and 4-24). Proinflammatory conditions activate endothelial cells, which boost inflammation, in a vicious circle. In tandem, HIV fosters a procoagulant milieu, with increased levels of platelets and coagulation activators (e.g., tissue factor) and lower levels of thrombolytic and anticoagulant molecules.

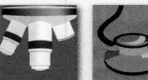

PATHOLOGY; CLINICAL FEATURES: Within 2 to 3 weeks of exposure, an acute, usually self-limited flu-like illness develops—acute retroviral syndrome—with fever, myalgia, lymphadenopathy, sore throat, and a macular rash. This resembles infectious mononucleosis clinically, and predates the appearance of antibodies. Most symptoms resolve within 2 to 3 weeks, although lymphadenopathy, fever, and myalgia may persist for a few months. Less often, patients develop neurologic symptoms suggesting encephalitis, aseptic meningitis, or a neuropathy. Seroconversion occurs 1 to 10 weeks after this acute illness starts. There are several laboratory tests to detect HIV-1 infection. CDC recommends a combined antigen/antibody test, which can detect all but the earliest infections. A test for HIV-1 nucleic acid may be used, if clinical suspicion is high and the antigen/antibody test is negative. Most patients recover from this initial illness as their immune system counterattacks with CTLs (see above), though a few may progress rapidly to frank AIDS.

A period of latency follows, while immune function wanes for about 10 years before impairment becomes life threatening. If symptoms go unrecognized or untreated, the outcome will eventually be extreme immunodeficiency, with fatal complications (Fig. 4-25).

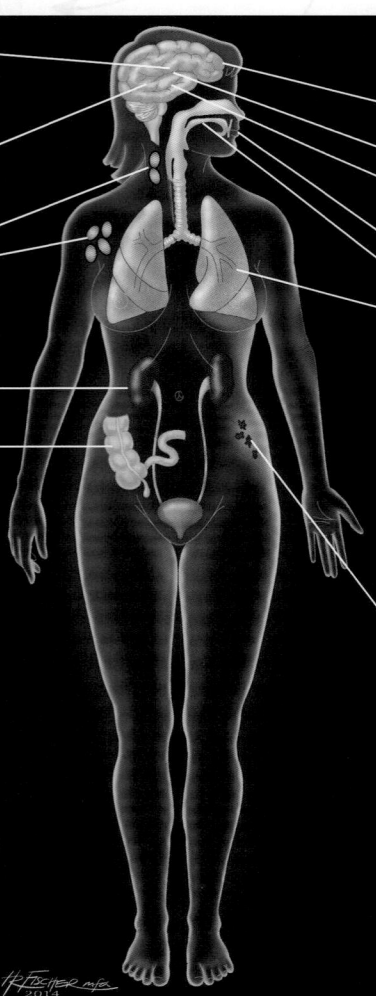

AIDS dementia (HAND)

LYMPHOID DISEASE
CNS lymphoma
Persistent generalized lymphadenopathy
B-cell lymphoma

AIDS nephropathy

DIARRHEA
Protozoa:
Cryptosporidium
Isospora belli
Giardia lamblia
Bacteria:
M. avium-intracellulare
Viruses:
CMV

OPPORTUNISTIC INFECTIONS
CNS
Cryptococcal meningitis
Toxoplasmosis
Papovavirus (PML)

MUCOCUTANEOUS
Herpes simplex
Candidiasis

PNEUMONIA
Pneumocystis
Mycobacterium avium intracellulare
CMV
COPD

SKIN
Staphylococcus
Scabies
HPV
Molluscum contagiosum
Kaposi sarcoma

FIGURE 4-25. Human immunodeficiency virus-1 (HIV-1)–mediated destruction of the cellular immune system results in AIDS. The infectious and neoplastic complications of AIDS can affect practically every organ system. *CNS* = central nervous system; *HPV* = human papillomavirus.

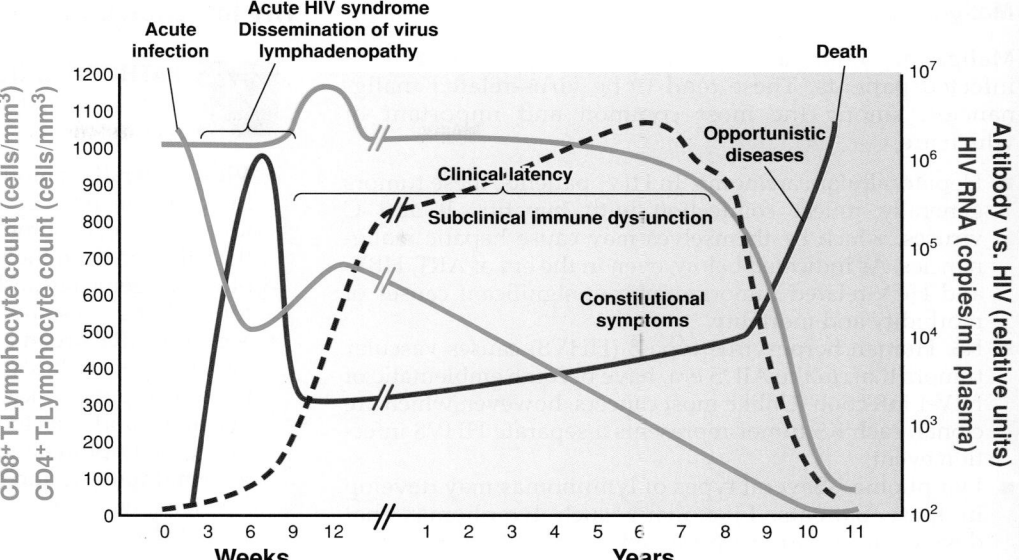

FIGURE 4-26. Generalized time course of human immunodeficiency virus-1 (HIV-1) infection. Infection occurs at the time indicated. The eclipse period, between the acute exposure and the beginning of symptoms and detectability, depends on the route of exposure. Important events in the development of HIV-1 infection are shown, including the clinical syndrome, virus loads, and CD4+ and CD8+ lymphocyte population dynamics over time.

Persistent generalized lymphadenopathy persists for months, mostly affects axillary, inguinal, and posterior cervical nodes. Biopsy shows reactive, nondiagnostic, follicular hyperplasia. Ongoing lymphoproliferative responses cause many of the long-term effects of HIV, even in patients treated with ART (see below).

Most patients infected with HIV express detectable viral RNA, antigens, and antibodies within months, the lag time varying with route of exposure. After an initial period of intense viremia with very high blood viral loads, and a corresponding sharp drop in absolute CD4+ T-cell counts (Fig. 4-26), immune recognition begins, with vigorous CTL responses. Viral loads drop. CD4+ T-cell counts begin to climb.

Virus continues to replicate, but is constrained by the immune response. The immune system and HIV eventually enter into a sort of uneasy equilibrium, playing a cat-and-mouse game, with new antigenic viral variants emerging, then eliciting immune responses, which select for other substrains. During this period, circulating HIV-1 viral loads stay fairly constant at the "viral set point," and patients are generally asymptomatic. However, HIV-1 evolves rapidly within each host, and represents a continually moving antigenic target for the immune system.

Eventually CD4+ T-cell counts decline. Patients generally become symptomatic with nonspecific constitutional symptoms and opportunistic infections when CD4+ counts fall below 500/μL. Once CD4+ levels reach 150/μL, with CD4:CD8 ratios l<0.8, the disease progresses rapidly, with opportunistic infections, KS, and virus-related lymphoproliferative disorders (see Chapter 26).

Neurologic disease is common. HIV enters the brain very shortly after initial infection, and resides there in several cell populations, including macrophages, microglia, and astrocytes. Although HIV does not infect neurons, its gene products diffuse from infected cells and are highly toxic to neurons. Untreated and treated HIV infections are associated with neurologic syndromes (**HIV-associated neurologic disease, or HAND,** see Chapter 32).

Diverse Secondary Diseases May Complicate HIV Infection

Infectious Agents

Many other infections cause disease in HIV-1–infected patients, for example, hepatitis viruses. They also include opportunistic diseases that complicate immune or other compromise as HIV-1 infection progresses. These are many, and cannot all be described here, but several deserve specific mention:

- *Pneumocystis.* Now called *P. jiroveci,* but originally *P. carinii,* this agent causes a particular type of pneumonia in people with compromised defense systems (see Chapter 9).
- *Mycobacterium tuberculosis* and *MAI.* These exist mainly within phagocytic cells. Effective cell-mediated immune responses, such as are severely impaired by HIV-1 infection, are needed to control them. They may cause pneumonia or systemic infection. The AIDS epidemic has accelerated emergence and spread of multidrug-resistant strains of *M. tuberculosis,* even among immunocompetent hosts.
- Central nervous system (CNS) infections. Important CNS infectious agents in HIV/AIDS patients include Cryptococcus and Toxoplasma, as well as such viral diseases as progressive multifocal leukoencephalopathy (see Chapter 32).
- Digestive tract infections. Many agents, including protozoa (e.g., Cryptosporidium), diverse gut-tropic bacteria (e.g., Salmonella), cause gastrointestinal complications. In addition, hepatotropic viruses, such as HBV and HCV, commonly complicate HIV-1 infection.
- CMV. Infections with CMV, in the GI tract or elsewhere, commonly complicate AIDS, especially when CD4+ T-cell counts are very low.
- Fungal infections. Both surface and deep infections with diverse fungi, particularly Candida and Aspergillus, commonly complicate HIV/AIDS.

Malignancies

Malignant tumors are common complications in HIV-1–infected patients. These tend to be virus-related malignancies, among the most common and important of which are:

- Hepatocellular carcinoma. In HIV⁺ patients, these tumors generally reflect coinfection with hepatitis B and C viruses, which by themselves may cause hepatic malignancies. As indicated below, even in the era of ART, HBV- and HCV-related tumors represent significant causes of morbidity and mortality.
- KS. Human herpesvirus type 8 (HHV8) causes vascular tumors that, in the AIDS era, have become emblematic of HIV-1 infection. Unlike most cancers, however, which are clonal, each KS tumor represents a separate HHV8 infection event.
- Lymphomas. Several types of lymphomas may develop in these patients. Like many such lymphomas that develop in immunosuppressed people, these are often virus-induced. HHV8 is associated with **Castleman disease** and an otherwise rare tumor, called **primary effusion lymphoma**. Epstein–Barr virus (EBV)–related B-lymphoproliferative diseases, such as also develop in immunosuppressed transplant recipients, may also occur.

ANTIRETROVIRAL THERAPY AND HIV-RELATED DISEASE IN THE ART ERA

Current ART regimens generally include variable combinations of (usually two) nucleoside RT inhibitors (NRTIs), plus a nonnucleoside RT inhibitor (NNRTI), plus either PR or IN inhibitors.

What Has ART Done?

Sometimes called **highly active antiretroviral therapy (HAART)**, ART has been broadly effective, and has improved HIV⁺ patients' lives, immune function, and health immeasurably. ART effectiveness rests on the premise (not unlike cancer chemotherapy) that a rapidly evolving infectious agent may best be treated by simultaneously attacking several points of its replicative cycle at by targeting HIV-1–encoded proteins.

Immune System Status and Circulating Viral Load

As treatment regimens have become less toxic, more widely available and easier to manage, HIV-1 infection has become a different disease. Generally, plasma viral loads decline to undetectable levels in a few months. Blood CD4⁺ T cells mostly—but variably, and more slowly—return to, or approach, normal numbers.

Opportunistic infections and many other manifestations of AIDS are much less common in people who comply with their prescribed therapy. What used to be an almost inexorably fatal, terrifying disease became a chronic condition that required attention (like, e.g., hypertension or diabetes) but did not portend inevitable doom. (However, see Immune Reconstitution Syndrome, below.)

HIV Infection Continues Despite ART

 PATHOPHYSIOLOGY: The reality of HIV infection in the ART era reflects several important factors:

- **Viral diversity among anatomic sites:** When HIV-1 infects someone, it spreads widely (see above). Its rapidly mutating genome generates many genetic variants that diverge from the original inoculum and from each other antigenically and biologically. These may provide for evolving resistance—often partial—to ART agents.
- **Variable ART organ and cell penetration:** ART drugs' variable penetrability in some surprising sites facilitates virus persistence, including persistent replication. Locations and infected cell types in which drug levels may be suboptimal include:
  - **hematopoietic and lymphoid organs** (bone marrow, spleen, lymph nodes) where concentrations of some ART drugs may not be optimally effective
  - **CNS** (macrophages, astrocytes, microglia, T cells), where the blood–brain barrier and P-glycoprotein drug efflux pumps limit organ and cellular drug concentrations
  - **GI tract** (epithelia, DCs, T cells, macrophages), with poor drug penetration, particularly in distal small and large intestines
  - **liver** (DCs, Kupffer cells, sinusoidal lining and stellate cells, hepatocytes) where fibrosis may alter drug clearance and accessibility to infected cells
  - **genital tract** (DCs, mucosal cells, germ cells, T cells) where some drug concentrations are suboptimal. Testes may not allow adequate access to some drugs
  - **respiratory tract** (DCs, epithelial cells, alveolar and other macrophages) shows low drug concentrations in alveolar fluids
  - **kidneys** (tubular epithelium): Epithelial cells affected early after infection may harbor virus and shed it into the urine for years
- **Reservoirs of HIV infection and HIV-1 persistence:** Blood CD4⁺ T-cell counts and plasma virus loads do not tell the whole story: ART does not eliminate the virus. HIV-1 genomes endure. They integrate into cellular DNA of many long-lived cells, particularly memory T cells, astrocytes, hematopoietic precursor cells and macrophages, where they may continue low level replication or become latent and await reactivation. Infected cells survive in diverse anatomic sites for the individual's lifetime, at least with currently available approaches (Fig. 4-27). From these sites and cells, the virus may reseed the periphery if resistant strains emerge or if patient compliance with treatment falters. Viral genome diversity among the different sites contributes to this threat. It also contributes to ongoing disease (see below).

In this context, it should be noted that some patients on ART, with undetectable virus and normal CD4⁺ T-cell counts in their blood, may still shed virus. Detectable virus may be present in their cervical fluid, semen, and CSF.

- **Smoldering vestiges of the same processes that drive progression to AIDS:** It must be emphasized that the same processes that contribute to progression of HIV-1 infection to AIDS are still active—albeit usually

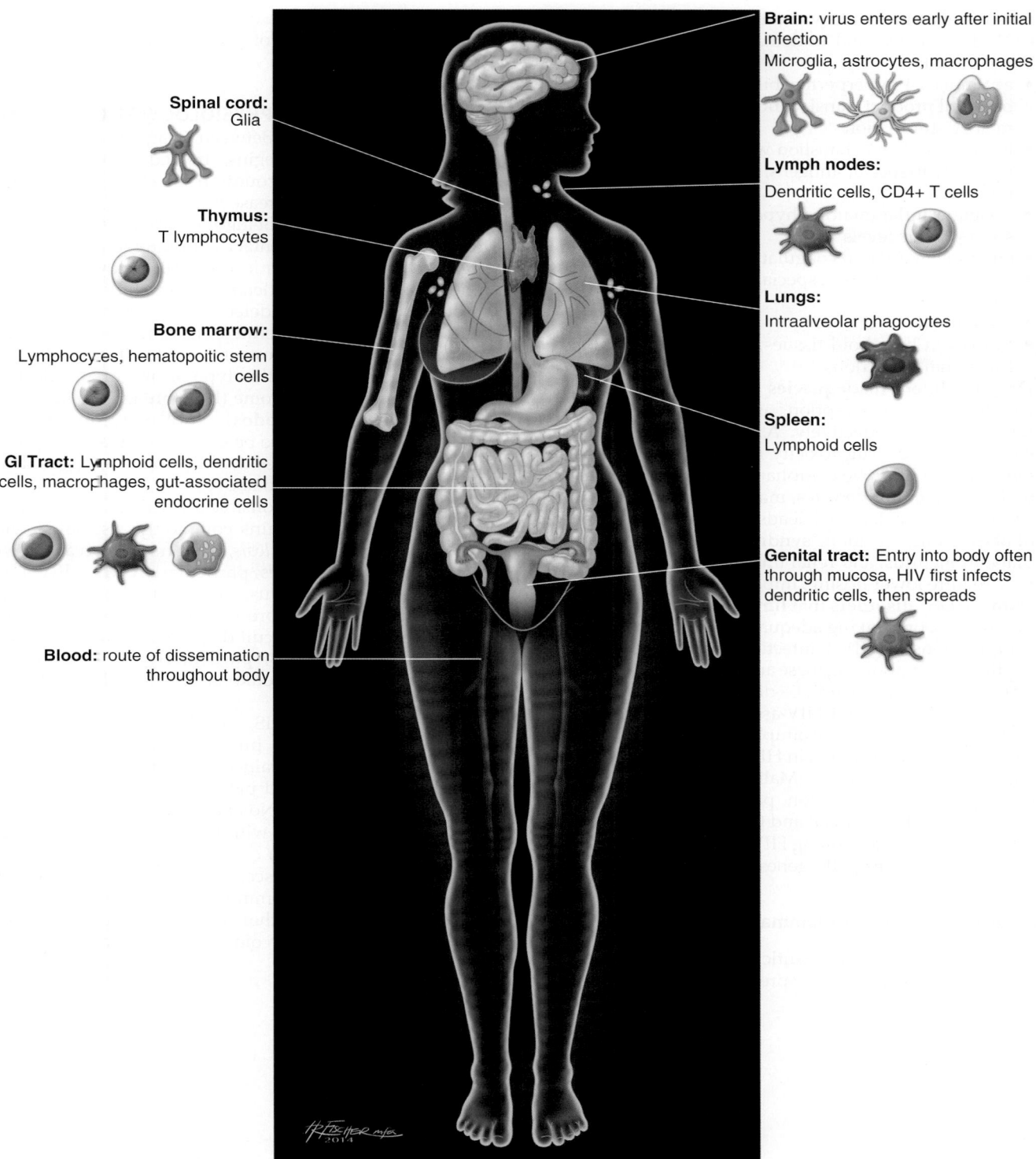

Brain: virus enters early after initial infection
Microglia, astrocytes, macrophages

Lymph nodes:
Dendritic cells, CD4+ T cells

Lungs:
Intraalveolar phagocytes

Spleen:
Lymphoid cells

Genital tract: Entry into body often through mucosa, HIV first infects dendritic cells, then spreads

Spinal cord:
Glia

Thymus:
T lymphocytes

Bone marrow:
Lymphocytes, hematopoitic stem cells

GI Tract: Lymphoid cells, dendritic cells, macrophages, gut-associated endocrine cells

Blood: route of dissemination throughout body

FIGURE 4-27. Where HIV-1 hides, both during acute infection and in the context of ART. The organ locations and cell types which harbor HIV-1 early in the course of infection, and in which HIV-1 may persist despite ART that is effective in controlling peripheral blood viral load and restoring CD4⁻ T-cell numbers.

muted—even in people with adequate peripheral blood $CD4^+$ T-cell levels and undetectable blood virus load. These include:

- gut mucosal hyperpermeability and consequent gut bacterial product translocation and excessive inflammatory stimulation
- immune system exhaustion with inadequate immune responses to specific antigens, impaired innate immune function
- systemic inflammatory hyperactivation and excessive cytokine levels
- endothelial cell and coagulation abnormalities
- comorbid infections, especially with HBV and HCV (see below)
- impaired liver function
- fibrosis in lymphoid tissues, with architectural and functional distortions

- **Drug treatment inadequacies and toxicities:** ART has evolved since its inception, and targets more HIV-1 functions more effectively. A key improvement has been decreased drug toxicity and easier dosing regimens, which improve compliance. However, any drug regimen, taken for decades, may carry cumulative toxicities. In particular, ART leads to increased incidence of obesity and metabolic syndrome, insulin resistance, diabetes mellitus, and renal impairment. Liver toxicity may require lower dosing, impairing antiviral efficacy.

- **"Non-AIDS" disorders that limit longevity and impair health:** In people taking adequate ART, other non-AIDS complications of HIV-1 infection cause about half of deaths. Principal among these are cardiovascular—especially ischemic myocardial—disease, renal, neoplastic and liver diseases, and HIV-associated neurocognitive disorders (HAND). For example, ischemic cardiac disease is 50% more common in HIV^+ patients than in comparable uninfected people. Malignancies, especially, are disproportionately common, particularly those due to EBV, HPV, and hepatitis B and C viruses. Some of these reflect comorbidities among HIV^+ patients, while others have more complex pathogenesis.

Immune Reconstitution Inflammatory Syndrome

ART has engendered an unanticipated consequence: the complications of sudden widespread suppression of HIV-1 replication, reconstitution of immune function. This syndrome affects about 1/6 of patients, usually shortly after ART begins.

PATHOPHYSIOLOGY; ETIOLOGIC FACTORS: Between 3 and 6 months after ART begins, treated patients recover peripheral lymphocyte counts from HIV-1–caused suppression, the sudden increase in $CD4^+$ and $CD8^+$ memory cells can be dangerous. Being memory cells, their repertoire reflects previous contact with foreign antigens. The presence of unresolved infections (see below) then magnifies these populations, leading to exaggerated immune responses. A postulated defect in immunoregulatory T_{reg} cells may lead to exaggerated activation of pre-existing memory cells and their conversion into effector cells.

Lurking triggers for this type of immune reconstitution inflammatory syndrome (IRIS) are largely infectious agents. The so-called paradoxical IRIS occurs in the face of what had been thought to be effectively treated opportunistic infections, when residual microbial antigens drive the T-cell responses noted above.

Pathogens often responsible for IRIS include many of the usual suspects: villains commonly associated with AIDS, such as *M. tuberculosis*, *MAI*; fungi such as *Cryptococcus neoformans*; viruses, particularly CMV, HBV, HSV and Varicella-zoster virus; and *P. jiroveci*. These may present atypically and present vexing problems in differential diagnosis. Difficult diagnostic problems in IRIS involve CNS infections, particularly JC virus-related progressive multifocal leukoencephalopathy (PML, see Chapter 32).

A second type of IRIS, called the unmasking form, reflects the ability of a previously unsuspected infection to stimulate unrestrained inflammation. In general, IRIS due to undiagnosed pathogens occurs sooner than the paradoxical form. (Notably, IRIS may also complicate recovery of patients with hematologic malignancies, without HIV-1 infection.)

Additionally, recrudescent autoimmune diseases may trigger IRIS. The most common of these is Graves disease (see Chapter 27), but other autoimmune diseases have also been implicated. Sarcoidosis may also act as an initiator for this syndrome.

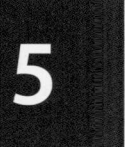

5 Neoplasia

David S. Strayer

The Pathology of Neoplasia

A neoplasm (Greek, *neo,* "new," plus *plasma,* "thing formed") is an autonomous growth that has escaped normal restraints on cell proliferation and accumulation. It may show variable resemblance to its tissue of origin, which usually allows conclusions about tumors' sources and potential behavior. As most neoplasms occupy space, they are often called **tumors** (Gr., *swelling*). Tumors that remain localized are considered **benign,** while those that spread to distant sites are called **malignant,** or **cancer.** The neoplastic process entails both cell proliferation and variably modified phenotypic differentiation by involved cell types. In this sense, cancers may be viewed as a burlesque of normal development.

Cancer is an ancient disease. Prehistoric evidence of bone tumors, and early writings from India, Egypt, Babylonia, and Greece mention the disease. Hippocrates reportedly distinguished benign from malignant growths, and coined the term *karkinos,* from which our term **carcinoma** derives. He described breast cancer, and in the 2nd century AD, Paul of Aegina commented on its frequency.

Incidence of neoplastic disease increases with age, and longer life spans in modern times enlarge the population at risk. In previous centuries, humans did not live long enough to develop many cancers that are particularly common in middle and old age, such as those of the prostate, colon, pancreas, and kidney.

If we remove tobacco-related cancer deaths from the statistics, overall age-adjusted cancer death rates have been decreasing. In part, this reflects improved early detection techniques (e.g., Pap smears, colonoscopy).

Neoplasms are derived from cells that normally can multiply. Thus, mature neurons and cardiac myocytes do not give rise to tumors. A tumor may mimic its tissue of origin to a variable degree. Some closely resemble their parent structures (e.g., hepatic adenomas) while others appear so primitive that the tumor's origin is uncertain.

BENIGN VERSUS MALIGNANT TUMORS

Although there are exceptions, benign tumors basically neither penetrate (invade) adjacent tissue borders, nor spread (metastasize) to distant sites. They remain as localized overgrowths where they arise. Benign tumors tend to be better differentiated than malignant ones—that is, they more closely resemble their tissue of origin. *By contrast, malignant tumors invade contiguous tissues and metastasize to distant sites, where subpopulations of malignant cells take up residence, multiply, and again invade surrounding areas.*

That said, **the terms benign and malignant reflect a tumor's biologic behavior rather than its morphologic characteristics.** Generally, benign tumors spare the patient, while malignant ones can kill. However, biologically benign tumors in critical locations can be deadly. A benign intracranial meningeal tumor (meningioma) may be fatal if it exerts pressure on an important brain structure. A tiny benign ependymal cell tumor (ependymoma) in the third ventricle can block cerebrospinal fluid circulation and so cause lethal hydrocephalus. A benign left atrial myxoma may precipitate sudden death by blocking the mitral valve orifice. Rarely, a hormonally active, biologically benign pancreatic insulinoma can be life threatening if it causes sudden hypoglycemia, or a pheochromocytoma

in the adrenal medulla may trigger a hypertensive crisis. Conversely, some malignant tumors (e.g., of the thyroid or prostate) grow so slowly that they never pose a threat to life.

Tumor histology usually allows categorization as benign or malignant. However, biologic behavior does not necessarily correlate with pathologic appearance. Some tumors that look histologically malignant may not metastasize or be able to kill a patient: basal cell carcinomas of the skin may invade subjacent structures locally but rarely metastasize and are not life threatening. On the other hand, some histologically benign tumors may be lethal. Aggressive meningiomas do not metastasize but may be locally invasive and cause death by compromising vital structures. It is important to note that for many endocrine tumors, for example, pancreatic islet cell tumors, histologic appearance does not predict metastatic potential, and a tumor's biologic benignity or malignancy is only clear if it does or does not metastasize.

TUMOR CLASSIFICATION

Classification paradigms are only useful to the extent that they are predictive. Tumor nosology combines many factors that impact on this point: historical concepts, technical jargon, location, origin, descriptive modifiers, and predictors of biologic behavior. Although the language of tumor classification is neither rigidly logical nor consistent, it still serves as a reasonable mode of communication.

HISTOLOGIC DIAGNOSIS OF MALIGNANCY

Essentially, labeling a tumor as benign or malignant constitutes a prediction of its eventual biologic behavior and possible clinical outcome. The criteria used to predict a tumor's biologic nature are not based on scientific principles but rather on accumulated experience and historical correlations between histologic and cytologic patterns and clinical courses. The differentiation between benign and malignant tumors generally poses few problems; some cases require additional study before an accurate diagnosis is secure. However, there will always be tumors that defy the diagnostic skills and experience of any pathologist; in these cases, the correct diagnosis must await the clinical outcome. *Remember that the definition of a benign tumor resides above all in its inability to invade adjacent tissue and to metastasize.*

The Primary Descriptors of All Tumors Are Their Cells of Origin

Although historically the suffix "oma" applied to benign tumors, current terminology is so varied that tumor names do not specify biologic behavior with any precision. Melanomas, mesotheliomas, and seminomas are all highly malignant even though they carry the suffix "oma." Hamartomas are not even true neoplasms but disorganized developmental medleys of multiple structures.

This lax use of the word "oma" notwithstanding, with regard to cancers a bit more stringency applies. "Carcinoma" designates a malignant proliferation of epithelial cells and "sarcoma" refers to malignancies of mesenchymal origin. These terms are not necessarily all-inclusive, since most malignant proliferations of blood-forming organs are leukemias and lymphoid malignancies are lymphomas. Finally, eponyms

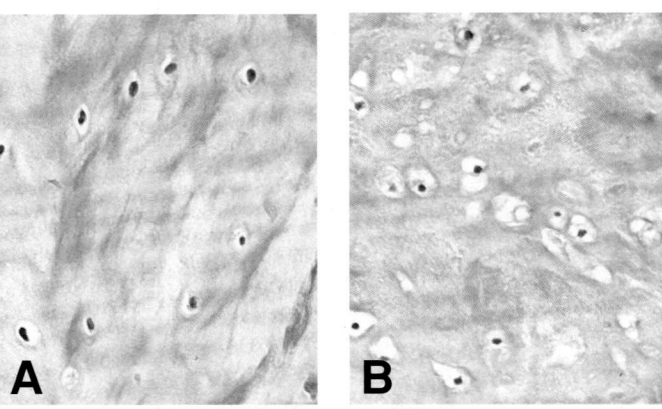

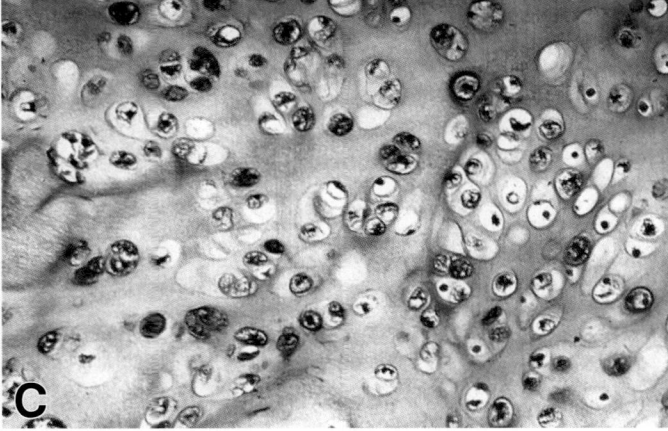

FIGURE 5-1. Cartilaginous lesions. A. Normal cartilage. **B.** A benign chondroma closely resembles normal cartilage. **C.** Chondrosarcoma of bone. The tumor is composed of malignant chondrocytes, which have bizarre shapes and irregular hyperchromatic nuclei, embedded in a cartilaginous matrix. Compare with **A** and **B**. (Reprinted from Bullough PG, Vigorita VJ. *Atlas of Orthopaedic Pathology.* New York: Gower Medical Publishing; 1984. Copyright © 1984 Elsevier. With permission.)

often refer to tumors of historically dubious histogenesis, such as Hodgkin disease, Ewing sarcoma.

Some histologic features that are useful in distinguishing benign from malignant tumors include:

- **Cellular atypia,** that is, the extent to which a tumor's appearance departs from that of its normal tissue or cellular counterparts. An example is the comparison between normal cartilage, a chondroma (benign) and a chondrosarcoma (malignant) (Fig. 5-1). The magnitude of cellular atypia (or, anaplasia) generally correlates with a tumor's aggressiveness. Cytologic evidence of anaplasia includes (1) variation in the size and shape of cells and nuclei **(pleomorphism)**; (2) enlarged and hyperchromatic nuclei with coarsely clumped chromatin and prominent nucleoli; (3) atypical mitotic figures (i.e., more complex than bipolar figures); and (4) bizarre cells, including tumor giant cells (Fig. 5-2).
- **Mitotic activity:** Many malignant tumors show high mitotic rates, identifiable as abnormally high numbers of mitotic figures. For of some tumors (e.g., leiomyosarcomas), finding even a few mitoses is sufficient to diagnose malignancy. Nonetheless, not all situations require such obvious proliferative activity to call a tumor malignant.
- **Growth pattern:** This is a variably useful determinant of malignancy. Malignant neoplasms often show disorganized growth: as sheets of cells, whorls, papillary structures, rosettes, often arrayed around blood vessels, etc. Compromised blood supply to some malignant tumors may cause ischemic necrosis.
- **Invasiveness,** particularly into blood vessels and lymphatics, helps identify malignancies. In some circumstances (e.g., follicular thyroid cancer), local invasion is important to make a diagnosis of malignancy.
- **Metastases** identify a tumor as malignant. If a diagnosed primary cancer did not precede a metastatic lesion, the tumor's origin may not be readily apparent from histologic characteristics alone. In such cases, tissue-related tumor markers may establish the correct origin.

Generalizations are just that: they are usually applicable, but at times must be used cautiously. Thus, **nodular fasciitis** is a reactive proliferation of connective tissue cells (Fig. 5-3) that may appear more alarming histologically than many fibrosarcomas, and misdiagnosis can lead to unnecessary surgery. Conversely, well-differentiated endocrine adenocarcinomas may be pathologically identical to benign adenomas.

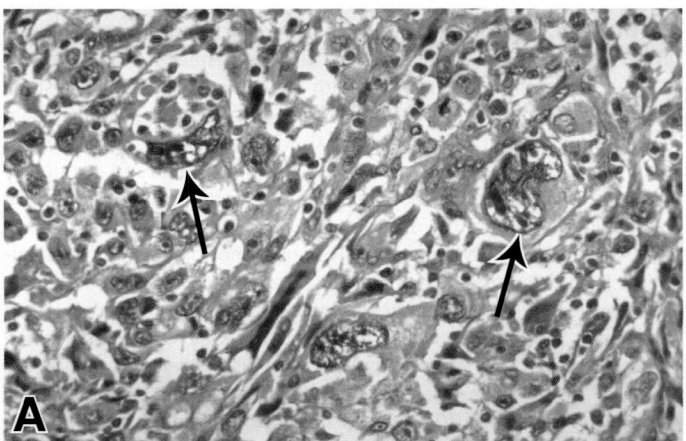

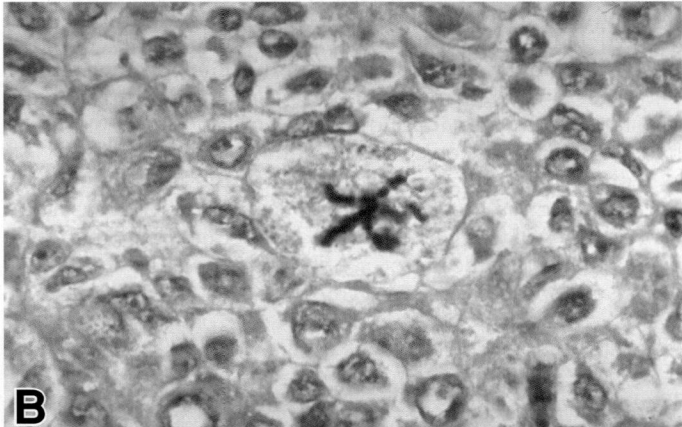

FIGURE 5-2. Anaplastic features of malignant tumors. A. The cells of this anaplastic carcinoma are highly pleomorphic (i.e., they vary in size and shape). The nuclei are hyperchromatic and are large relative to the cytoplasm. Multinucleated tumor giant cells are present (*arrows*). **B.** A malignant cell in metaphase exhibits an abnormal mitotic figure.

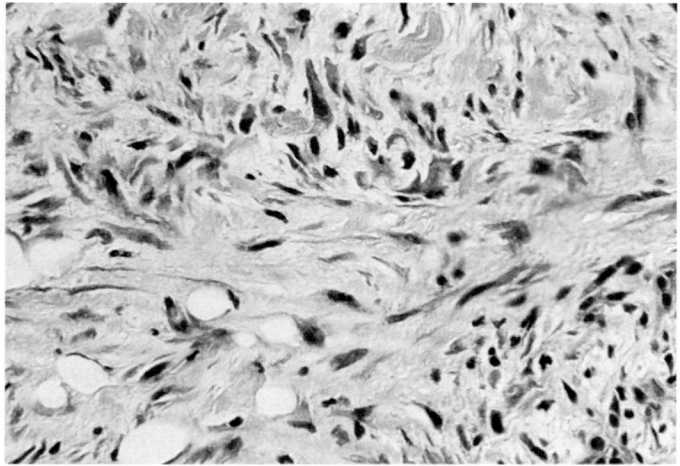

FIGURE 5-3. Nodular fasciitis. This cellular reactive lesion contains atypical and bizarre fibroblasts, which may be mistaken for a fibrosarcoma.

Marker Studies Help to Identify Tumor Origin

Tumor Markers

Tumor markers are gene products of neoplasms that are detected in or on tumor cells themselves, or in body fluids. Their utility requires that tumor cells retain gene expression patterns characteristic of their organ or cell of origin, or that they synthesize specialized substances associated with tumors of a particular origin. Determining cell lineage is more than an academic exercise: therapies are often based on identification.

Immunologic (immunohistochemistry, flow cytometry) techniques (Fig. 5-4) and molecular studies (in situ hybridization, gene expression profiling, and sequencing) help make these determinations. Diagnostically useful markers include immunoglobulins, fetal proteins, enzymes, hormones, and cytoskeletal and junctional proteins. Identified markers that are useful for tissue and tumor profiling are increasing rapidly.

Tumor-associated antigens are also used in other ways. Blood levels of tumor antigens, as assayed by immunologic and other techniques, help clinicians to follow tumor progression and development of metastases after a primary neoplasm has been treated. Examples include carcinoembryonic antigen (CEA) for gastrointestinal tumors, cancer antigen (CA) 125 for ovarian carcinoma, and prostate-specific antigen (PSA) for prostate cancer. Blood levels for tumor-produced substances may help in following a tumor's course, but have had less success as tools for population screening.

Some tumor antigens help to guide important therapeutic decisions (e.g., estrogen/progesterone receptors in breast cancer and Bcr-Abl for chronic myeloid leukemia). They may also be useful therapeutic targets: antibodies target HER2/neu for breast and other cancers, and CD20 for B-cell lymphomas.

Electron Microscopy

Tumor marker studies have almost entirely replaced electron microscopy (EM) in tumor analysis. Still, EM may detect specialized structures that characterize tumors derived from certain organs and cell types and differentiate them from others with which they may be confused—carcinomas often

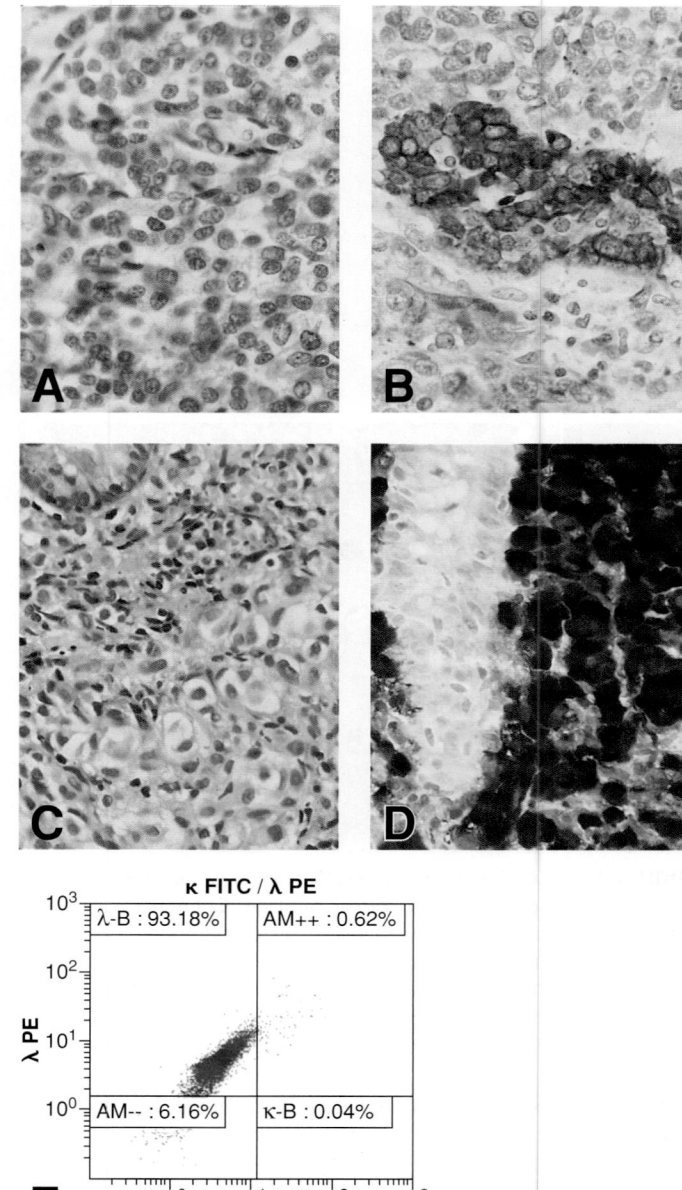

FIGURE 5-4. Tumor markers in the identification of undifferentiated neoplasms. A. A poorly differentiated metastatic bladder cancer is difficult to identify as a carcinoma with the hematoxylin and eosin stain. **B.** Positive immunostaining for cytokeratin of the tumor depicted in **A**, which identifies it as a carcinoma. **C.** A metastasis to the colon of an undifferentiated malignant melanoma is not pigmented, and its origin is unclear. **D.** Immunoperoxidase stain of the tumor in **C** showing that the cells express S-100 protein, a commonly used marker for cells of melanocytic origin. **E.** Flow cytometric analysis of monoclonal lymphoid population. Each **dot** represents an individual cell, 10,000 cells counted in all. Cells are treated simultaneously with two different antibodies conjugated to different fluorophores (here, FITC-labeled anti-κ L chain and PE-labeled anti-λ L chain). x-axis shows population of cells bearing cell surface κ L chains; y-axis shows cells bearing λ L chain. This monoclonal population is κ-negative, λ-positive. FITC = fluorescein isothiocyanate; PE = phycoerythrin.

have desmosomes and specialized junctional complexes that are not typical of sarcomas or lymphomas; melanomas have melanosomes or premelanosomes.

INVASION AND METASTASIS

Almost all malignant tumors can invade locally and metastasize to distant sites. These features cause the vast majority of cancer-related deaths; the primary tumor itself (e.g., breast or colon cancer) is generally not itself fatal, and is usually amenable to surgical resection.

Direct Extension Damages Involved Organs and Adjacent Tissues

Most carcinomas begin as localized growths that are confined to the epithelium where they arise. As long as these early cancers do not penetrate the underlying epithelial basement membrane, they are **carcinomas in situ** (Fig. 5-5). Because they have not invaded, these tumors are invariably curable. When in situ tumors extend through the underlying basement membrane, they can invade neighboring tissues and involve blood and lymphatic vessels to metastasize. When cancers arise from cells that are not bound by a basement membrane—such as connective tissue cells, lymphoid elements, and hepatocytes—no in situ stage is defined.

Malignant tumors that grow within a tissue of origin may also spread beyond the borders of that organ, and involve adjacent tissues. A tumor's growth may be so extensive that it causes a functional deficit of the organ. Ocular tumors may impair vision. Or, they may be life threatening by spreading to vital parts of an organ, as with astrocytomas that infiltrate

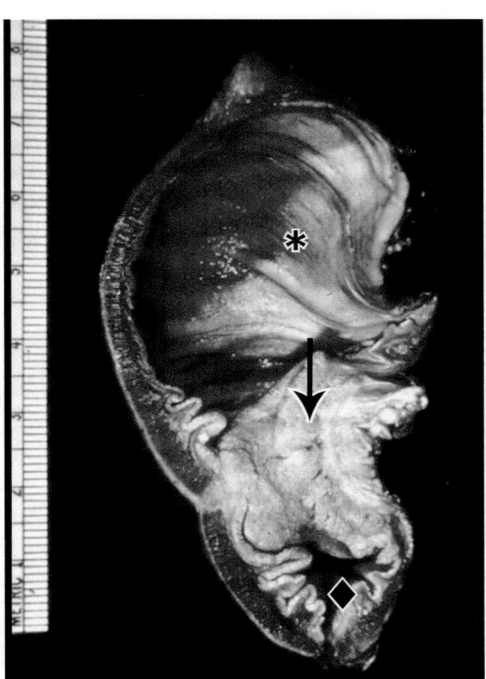

FIGURE 5-6. Adenocarcinoma of the colon with intestinal obstruction. The lumen of the colon at the site of the cancer is narrow (*arrow*). The colon above the obstruction is dilated (*). The colon distal to the stricture is normal caliber (♦).

the brain and they compromise vital regions, or a colon cancer that obstructs the large intestine (Fig. 5-6).

Tumors' invasive growth pattern may secondarily impair an adjacent organ. Cervical carcinoma may grow to obstruct ureters. When tumors invade vital structures, they can cause fistulas and hemorrhage: lung cancers may cause bronchopleural fistulas if they penetrate a bronchus or exsanguinating hemorrhage if they erode a blood vessel. The agonizing pain of pancreatic carcinomas results from direct tumor extension into the celiac nerve plexus. Tumor cells that reach serous cavities (e.g., the peritoneum or pleura) spread easily by direct extension, as when an ovarian cancer seeds the peritoneal cavity (Fig. 5-7).

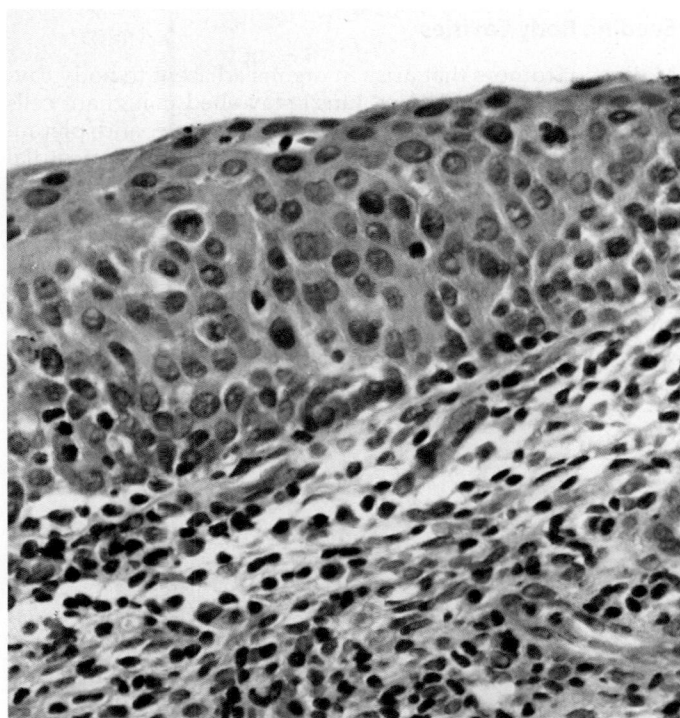

FIGURE 5-5. Carcinoma in situ. A section of the uterine cervix shows neoplastic squamous cells occupying the full thickness of the epithelium, yet confined to the mucosa by the underlying basement membrane.

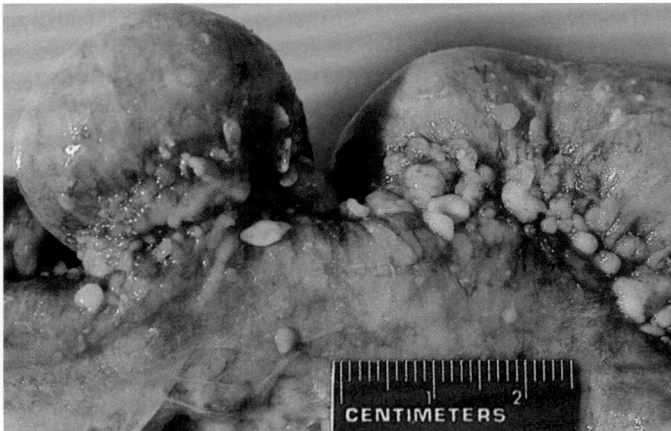

FIGURE 5-7. Peritoneal carcinomatosis. The mesentery attached to a loop of small bowel is studded with small nodules of metastatic ovarian carcinoma.

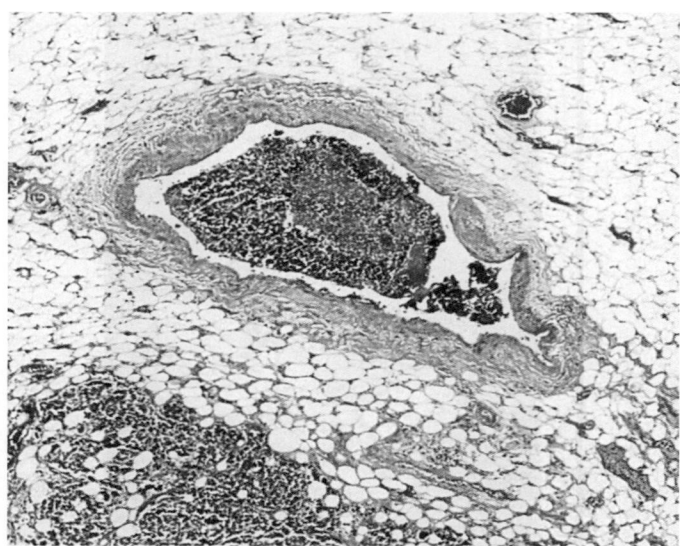

FIGURE 5-8. Hematogenous spread of cancer. A malignant tumor **(bottom)** has invaded adipose tissue and penetrated into a small vein.

Metastatic Spread Is the Most Common Cause of Cancer Deaths

Migration of malignant cells from one site to another—noncontiguous—site is metastasis (Greek, "displacement"). Invading malignant tumors come into contact with blood and lymphatic vessels, which they can also penetrate, and through which they spread to distant sites. They may also reach body cavities (e.g., pleural space), and so spread via those routes as well.

Hematogenous Metastases

Cancer cells often invade capillaries and venules, but not thicker-walled arterioles, arteries, or venules. Before they can form viable metastases, circulating tumor cells (CTCs) must lodge in the vascular bed at the target site (Fig. 5-8). There, they attach to, and then traverse, blood vessel and lymphatic walls. Often, patterns of blood or lymph flow at the primary tumor's origin determine the distribution of initial metastases. Thus, abdominal tumors from organs whose venous drainage is into the hepatic portal system tend to cause liver metastases; other tumors whose organs drain into systemic veins, and through the vena cava to the lungs will metastasize to the lungs. Breast cancers first spread to regional lymph nodes, which is the path of lymphatic flow. Extensive early tumor cell dissemination, or secondary spread from early metastatic foci, may cause more widespread disease (Fig. 5-9).

Lymphatic Metastases

Only large lymphatic channels have basement membranes; lymphatic capillaries lack them, which makes it easier for tumor cells to penetrate those smaller lymphatics. Once the cells are inside these vessels, they go with the flow: to regional draining lymph nodes. There, they lodge first in marginal (subcapsular) sinuses, and then extend throughout the node. Lymph nodes with metastatic deposits may expand to many times their normal size, even exceeding the diameter of the primary lesion (Fig. 5-10).

Breast cancers exemplify this type of spread. Initial metastases are almost always lymphatic. Patients' prognoses and

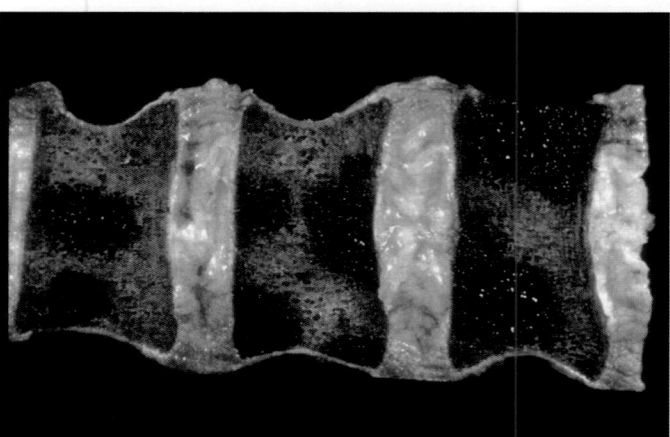

FIGURE 5-9. Multiple pigmented metastases in the vertebral bodies in a patient who died of malignant melanoma. (From Bullough PG, Boachie-Adjei O. *Atlas of Spinal Diseases*. New York: Gower Medical Publishing; 1988. Copyright Lippincott Williams & Wilkins.)

treatments depend heavily on the extent of these regional lymphatic metastases. Cancers arising laterally in the breast generally spread to axillary lymph nodes; those arising in the medial portion drain to internal mammary nodes, within the thorax.

The first sign of a tumor may be lymphatic metastases far from the primary tumor. For example, some abdominal cancers may first present as an enlarged supraclavicular node.

Lymphatic drainage tends to reflect embryologic origin. Testes develop in the abdominal cavity and migrate to the scrotum during fetal development. As a result, testicular cancers typically spread to abdominal periaortic nodes, and not inguinal nodes, which drain the scrotum.

Seeding Body Cavities

Malignant tumors that arise in organs adjacent to body cavities (e.g., ovaries, GI tract, lung) may shed malignant cells into these spaces, particularly the peritoneal and pleural cavities. Occasionally, tumors may also seed the pericardial

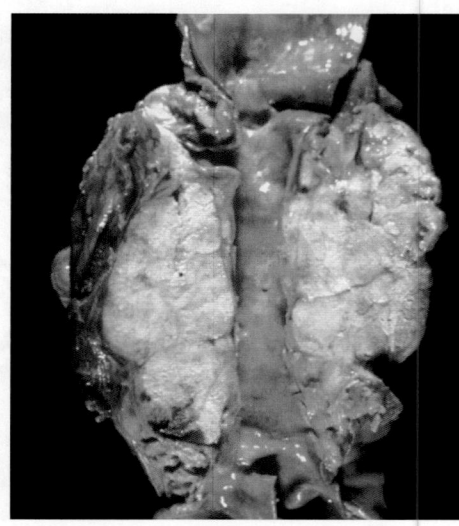

FIGURE 5-10. Metastatic carcinoma in periaortic lymph nodes. The aorta has been opened and the nodes bisected, showing large masses of metastatic prostatic carcinoma.

cavity, joint spaces, and the subarachnoid space. Once in those spaces, tumors grow in masses and may cause fluid accumulation (e.g., malignant ascites), sometimes in very large quantities. Some mucinous adenocarcinomas may also secrete mucin into these locations.

Organ Tropisms of Metastases

For over a century, doctors understood that metastatic patterns were not random. In 1889, Paget proposed that tumor cell spread to specific secondary sites depends on compatibility between the tumor cells (the seed) and favorable microenvironmental factors in the secondary site (the soil). Breast, prostate, and thyroid cancers spreading to bone, suggests an organ tropism—a favored "soil." Conversely, despite their size and abundant blood flow, neither the spleen nor skeletal muscle is a common site for metastases. Tumor-associated stromal cells may, in fact, "plow the road" for tumor cells to lodge in particular sites (see below).

STAGING AND GRADING OF CANCERS

Cancer Staging Describes How Far a Tumor Has Spread

In order to predict how a malignant tumor is likely to behave, and to establish criteria for therapy, many cancers are staged. Specific assessment protocols help identify where tumor has spread detectably. Choice of surgical approach and additional treatment modalities, often reflects a cancer's stage. Moreover, our understanding of cancer survival is also based on tumor stage at the time of diagnosis. Staging criteria vary greatly, depending on tumor type and organ of origin. Common criteria include:

- Tumor size
- Extent of local growth, whether it remains within or has spread out of the organ
- Presence and number of lymph node involvement
- Presence and locations of distant spread

In the international **TNM cancer staging** systems, in which "T" denotes the size and local extent of the primary tumor, "N" reflects the extent of regional node metastases and "M," the presence of distant metastases. A breast cancer that is T3N2M0 is a large primary tumor (T3) that involves axillary lymph nodes moderately (N2), but has not detectably spread to distant sites (M0). Specific definitions of each category vary from tumor type to tumor type, and may be quite complex. Some tumors, like hematologic malignancies, are staged according to different systems. Tumor spread is often designated more compactly as stage I, II, III, or IV, often with substages.

Cancer Grading Reflects Tumor Architecture and Cytology

It is axiomatic, if not necessarily universal, that tumors that recapitulate cytologic and histologic features of their origins tend to be less aggressive, while those that represent their roots less well are more malignant. Well-differentiated tumors are thus "low grade" and poorly differentiated neoplasms are "high grade." Cytologic and histologic grading, which are necessarily subjective and at best semiquantitative, are based on the degree of anaplasia and on the number of proliferating cells. Degrees of anaplasia reflect tumor cell size, shape and uniformity, as well as and the extent of organ-like features, such as gland-like structures in adenocarcinomas. Well-differentiated tumors have a lot of such structures. Poorly differentiated tumors do not, and show little resemblance to their normal counterparts.

Evidence of rapid growth includes (1) large numbers of mitoses, (2) atypical (i.e., not bipolar, see above) mitoses, (3) nuclear pleomorphism, and (4) tumor giant cells. Most grading schemes classify tumors into three or four grades of increasing malignancy (Fig. 5-11). Cytologic grade and biologic behavior do not invariably correlate: tumors of low cytologic grade may be very aggressive. In this sense, staging—which reflects a tumor's actual behavior in that patient—is more important and helpful than grading in predicting a tumor's course and influencing therapeutic decisions.

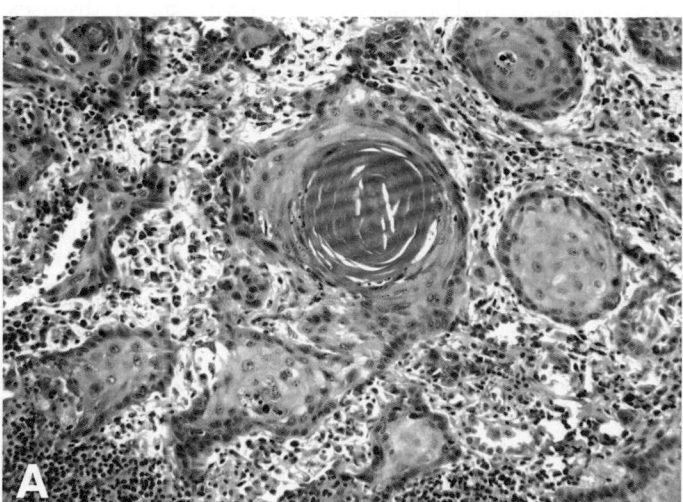
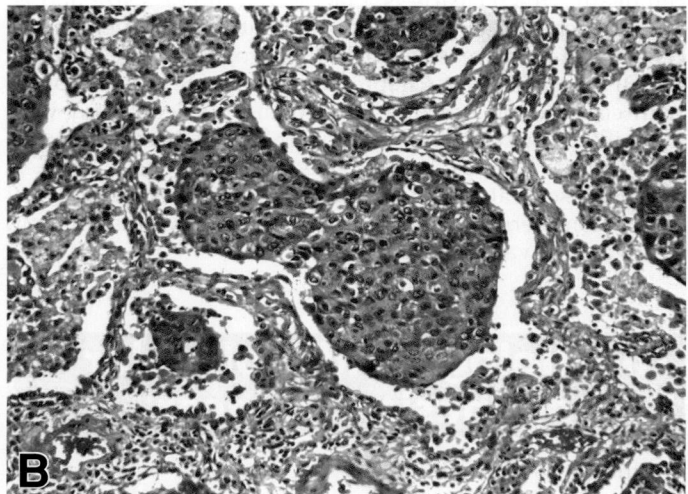

FIGURE 5-11. Cytologic grading of squamous cell carcinoma (SCC) of the lung. A. Well-differentiated (grade 1) SCC. Tumor cells closely resemble normal squamous cells and make keratin, as evidenced by epithelial pearls. **B.** Poorly differentiated (grade 3) SCC. The malignant cells are difficult to identify as being of squamous origin.

Tumor Doubling Time Reflects How Fast Tumors Grow and Influences Prognosis

Tumors enlarge over time. The interval needed for a tumor to double in volume is *tumor doubling time (DT)*, which usually reflects serial radiographic studies or, in some cases, blood levels of tumor markers, over time. Internal cancers are usually first detected clinically when they are about 1 cm^3 ($\approx$1 g). This corresponds to 10^8 to 10^9 cells. As most cancers start from a single cell, cell numbers have doubled at least 30 times to reach this size. Thus, *cancers are already far advanced when they are initially detected clinically*. Because tumor cell death rate and cell cycle kinetics vary between different tumor types, among tumors of the same type from person to person and among different metastases in the same patient, actual DTs generally fall within certain ranges that reflect these factors for any particular patient's cancer. If, for example, blood markers (e.g., circulating tumor antigens) or tumor sizes (e.g., pulmonary metastases on chest radiographs) have been followed over time, these may provide the clearest insight into a tumor's growth rate in any given person.

Different individual tumors, and different tumor types, vary greatly in their growth rates. As a rule, solid epithelial tumors grow less rapidly than do hematologic and mesenchymal malignancies. Many studies over the last 25 years, often focusing on either primary or metastatic tumors in the liver or lung, have reported highly variable results. In general, mean DTs for most solid epithelial tumors studied varies from 2 months to 4 months, with very wide ranges, sometimes exceeding 1 year. Some reported evidence suggests that smaller tumors may double slightly more quickly, on the average, than do larger tumors. Although many situations do not lend themselves to following primary or metastatic tumors for months radiographically or serologically without therapeutic intervention, such studies are the most effective way to assess how fast an individual tumor is doubling.

DT does not necessarily correlate with histologic evaluation of tumor cell growth fraction (i.e., the proportion of cells that are actively cycling), for several reasons. The duration of mitosis in cancer cells may be prolonged, so that numbers of mitotic figures in a tissue section may not correlate with overall growth. Also, mitotic activity does not account for tumor cell death, which clearly is a factor in a tumor's size and is better reflected by the parameters mentioned above. Tumor cells die for many reasons, including programmed cell death (PCD) (apoptosis, **see Chapter 1**); inadequate blood supply, with consequent ischemia; inadequate nutrients; and vulnerability to specific and nonspecific host defenses.

Tumor DT tends to correlate with prognosis. Studies involving several different tumor types, and reporting with careful long-term follow-up, have often shown that patient survival may vary according to DT.

The Biology and Molecular Pathogenesis of Cancer

Normal cells do not multiply, accumulate, or spread of their own accord. Even those that divide the most rapidly (e.g., myelocytes, intestinal mucosal cells) do so under tight control. Cancers arise from accumulated genomic and gene expression changes that begin with a single cell. With repeated cell division, mutations accrue. Eventually, the cell's progeny escape growth control, continue to acquire more mutations, invade locally, and spread through vascular and lymphatic channels.

NORMAL PROCESSES THAT REGULATE CELLS AND INHIBIT ONCOGENESIS

Cancer develops because of changes in cellular genes and gene expression. These changes cause tumors to develop and, often, spread. Critical cellular processes, which are closely related and often intertwined, protect from these developments: including antioxidants, cell cycle regulation, DNA repair, apoptosis, telomerase. The next sections describe how these defenses operate, how they can be—and are—subverted during oncogenesis, and what clues they may offer for treating patients with cancer.

What is a gene? A century before the discovery of the structure of DNA, Gregor Mendel described discrete units of heredity that were later called genes. As the genetic code became clearer, the term "gene" came to signify a DNA string that encoded a protein's amino acid sequence. Nothing is that simple. Our understanding of what constitutes a gene is now being rethought, because parts of the genome once thought to be "noncoding" are now known to produce new classes of RNAs that influence gene expression. Moreover, we are deciphering complex regulatory DNA sequences, which may be adjacent to, far from, and even within protein-coding sequences. Current ideas of what constitutes a gene entail interdependent structures and layers and webs of control that incorporate DNA sequences, diverse RNAs, regulatory proteins, and complex signaling apparati. Thus, the precise definition of a gene remains unsettled.

Mutations and polymorphism: The vast majority (99.6%) of DNA base pairs in somatic cells are identical throughout the human race; two people differ on the average by about 2.4×10^7 base pairs out of $\approx 3 \times 10^9$ base pairs. Variations in DNA sequences may be caused by changes in germline DNA or somatic mutations, such as single nucleotide substitutions, translocations or insertions, or deletions of one or more nucleotides. **Polymorphisms** are variations in DNA sequence that are not associated with known diseases. **Mutations** are comparable genetic changes that contribute to disease. (Mechanisms and types of DNA sequence variations are described in **Chapter 6**.)

The Normal Cell Cycle Drives Cellular Proliferation

In most malignancies, cells proliferate differently from normal cells: forces that drive and restrain normal cell division no longer drive, or regulate, proliferation. Thus, to understand cancer growth, one must understand how normal cells cycle. We focus here on those aspects of the cell cycle that commonly go awry in tumor development.

Phases of the Cell Cycle

Cells may be cycling or quiescent. Cells that replicate continuously (e.g., intestinal mucosa, hematopoietic progenitor cells) always transition from mitosis (M phase) to G_1, the latter leading to further cell division. Cells that divide infrequently (e.g., liver cells) are mostly quiescent, in G_0 phase. They replicate their DNA in S phase, where DNA replicates.

G₂ follows S. Ultimately, cells undergo mitosis (M phase). After mitosis, they again enter G₁ if they are in an actively cycling mode (Fig. 5-12A).

Cyclins and Cyclin-Dependent Kinases Driving Cell Cycle

A cell's progress through the proliferative cycle requires two classes of regulatory molecules, **cyclins** and **cyclin-dependent kinases (CDKs)** (Fig. 5-12A). These form a series of dimeric complexes that drive cell proliferation. Once a cell is stimulated to divide (e.g., by growth factors, see below), D-type cyclins are activated first. They complex with two CDKs (4, 6). Then, cyclin E-CDK2 complexes form. Together with the cyclin D-CDK4/6 complexes, they drive the cell into S phase. Other cyclins, A and then B, bind CDKs (1, 2) and push the cycle to completion. CDK complexes with cyclins D and E help to inactivate the retinoblastoma protein (pRb, see below).

Regulation of Cyclins and CDKs Provides Critical Protection Against Tumor Development

Considering their role in driving cell proliferation, it is not surprising that cells regulate cyclin and CDK activities carefully. This occurs in several ways (Fig. 5-12B).

Limiting Cyclin Availability

CDKs require activation by cyclins. Thus, cyclin availability limits CDK activity. Levels of most cyclins fluctuate with the cell cycle: most are synthesized only when needed, and then, when the cell has passed that part of its cycle, the cyclin is ubiquitinated and degraded by proteasomes (**see Chapter 1**).

CDK Inhibitors

Several families of CDK inhibitors (CKIs) strongly inhibit cell proliferation and so collectively represent important protection against oncogenesis. Not surprisingly, then, genes for CKIs are commonly mutated in human cancers. CKIs mostly act by binding binary cyclin–CDK complexes, or themselves binding CDKs and preventing their activation by cyclins. The three major families of CKIs are:

- INK4 proteins bind and inhibit CDKs 4 and 6, and prevent them from complexing cyclin D. INK4 CKIs thus block cell cycle progression in G1. There are several INK4 proteins: p15, p16, p18, and p19. The same gene that encodes p16^NK4a also encodes p14^ARF, but as an alternate reading frame (i.e., ARF). These proteins play important roles in regulating both CDKs and MDM2 (**see Chapter 1** and below).
- Cip/Kip proteins bind and strongly block CDK2 and, to a lesser extent, CDK1. Thus, they take up where the INK4 family leaves off, and inhibit the rest of the cell cycle. The best understood of the Cip/Kip proteins is p21^CIP (also called p21^WAF1).
- Rb family members (see below) also inhibit CDK2.

CKI expression can be triggered by senescence, contact inhibition, extracellular antimitogenic factors (e.g., transforming growth factor-β [TGFβ]) and the tumor suppressor protein p53 (see below).

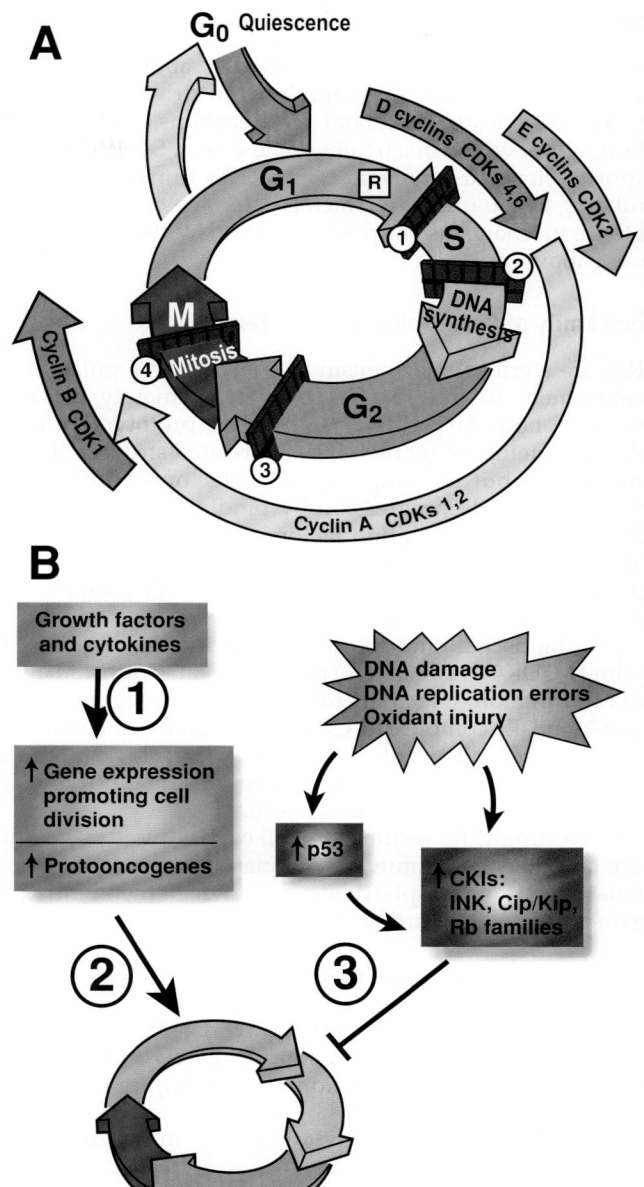

FIGURE 5-12. A. Normal cell cycle and the cyclins and CDKs that drive it. The phases of the cell cycle, with key check points (1–4) indicated. R is the restriction point (see text). D cyclins, complexed with CDKs 4 and 6, drive passage through G₁ and into early S phase. E cyclins, together with CDK2, overlap D cyclins at early in S phase. Cyclin A, bound to CDKs 1 and 2, drives the cell through S and G₂ phases, into M phase. Finally, cyclin B, together with CKD1, overlaps cyclin A in late G₂, and directs the cell through mitosis (M phase). The cell may exit active cycling from G₁ and enter G₀. **B. Activation and inhibition of the cyclins. 1. Activation.** Cells receive signals via growth factors, cytokines, etc. **2.** These trigger cell proliferation by increasing expression of genes that promote cell cycle progression, including a number of proto-oncogenes. **3. Inhibition.** Many stimuli, including errors in DNA replication, DNA damage, internal and external inhibitory signals of many kinds, may counteract the activating signals in **1**. These may do so by activating p53. Whether via p53 or otherwise, these inhibitors increase production and activity of cyclin kinase inhibitors (CKIs) and other inhibitors, for example, the INK family of proteins, CIP and KIP, and Rb. These families of CKIs block all the steps listed in **A**.

Other Forms of Inhibition of Cyclin–CDK Activities

In addition to mechanisms mentioned above, cells limit the ability of cyclin–CDK complexes to drive proliferation by selective posttranslational modifications, largely phosphorylation, which inactivates some CDKs. Specific nuclear export systems also prevent cyclin–CDK dimers from accumulating in the nucleus, which is their site of activity. Both of these mechanisms support regulation by the other means noted above.

The Family of Retinoblastoma Proteins

pRbs are a critical mechanism by which cells regulate their commitment to mitosis. These proteins mainly act near the $G_1 \rightarrow S$ boundary. P105^{Rb} (pRb) is the prototype of these related proteins. Other members are related structurally and functionally, but for simplicity, we refer only to pRb. pRb inhibits cell cycle progression by binding members of the E2F family of transcription factors. These factors drive cell entry into, and transit through, S phase by triggering transcription of cyclins A and E, as well as other proteins that promote DNA replication.

pRb binds E2F and blocks its activity. The complex of cyclin D-CDK4/6 (see above) phosphorylates pRb and alters its conformation, which liberates E2F. E2F-upregulated cyclins (A and E) complex to CDK2 and again phosphorylate pRb. This second event allows the cell cycle to progress (Fig. 5-13). The Rb system thus integrates many of the signals that control cell cycle progression.

Interestingly, Rb resumes its cell cycle inhibitory activity once cell division culminates: in anaphase, a protein phosphatase (PP1) dephosphorylates pRb, which then binds E2F again and prevents further division.

Landmark Transitions in the Cell Cycle

The major cell cycle transitions are $G_1 \rightarrow S$ and $G_2 \rightarrow M$. Cells pass from $G_1 \rightarrow S$ when complexes involving cyclins A and E overwhelm inhibition by Cip/Kip family members. Cells progress from $G_2 \rightarrow M$ when cyclin B-CDK1 complexes are activated by removing inhibitory phosphorylation of CDK1.

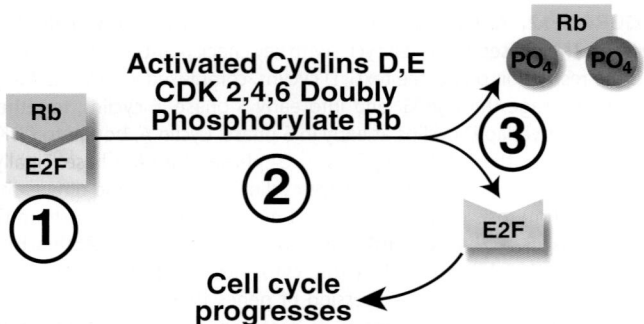

FIGURE 5-13. Role of cyclins and CDKs in removing pRb-mediated blockade of cell cycle progression. 1. Normally, Rb protein (pRb) binds E2F transcription factor and keeps E2F inactive. E2F must be freed for cell division to proceed. **2.** Activated cyclins D and E, plus CDKs 2, 4, and 6, phosphorylate then hyperphosphorylate pRb. **3.** This induces a conformational change so that pRb releases E2F, which is now free to direct transcription of proteins that help cell division to proceed.

Cell Cycle Checkpoints

Several **checkpoints** regulate cell cycle transit from one phase to another. These are points when cell cycle progression can be arrested, should the need arise (Fig. 5-12A). There are checkpoints in G_1, before entry into S, during S, and in G_2 before entry into M. These are activated by DNA damage. Others, during S phase and during M phase, are activated differently (see below).

Checkpoints Activated by DNA Damage

Safeguarding the integrity of the cell's DNA requires ceaseless vigilance (see below for details). However, once DNA damage is sensed (by ataxia-telangiectasia mutated [**ATM**] and ATM and Rad3-related [**ATR**] proteins, see below), p53 is activated (Fig. 5-14). If the cell is in G_1, p53 directs increased Cip/Kip CKI production, blocking further progress in cell division. If the cell is in G_2, there are two means by which cycling is arrested. First, two related checkpoint kinases (**Chk1**, **Chk2**, see below) block cell cycle progression immediately. These kinases are also responsible for blocking the cycle at the S-phase DNA damage checkpoint as well. In addition, p53 downregulates cyclin B and cdk1.

Restriction Point

During G_1, the cell commits itself to enter S phase at the **restriction point (R,** see Fig. 5-12A): the cell decides whether to proceed with mitosis and crosses the Rubicon— or not. Beyond the R point, external forces no longer drive or inhibit mitosis, that is, cell proliferation is only driven or stopped by intracellular mechanisms. Cyclin D-CDK4/6 phosphorylation of pRb, with consequent release of E2F (see above) activate the R point, to facilitate mitosis. *Loss of R-point control occurs in many cancers and deregulates progression through the cell cycle.*

Other Checkpoints

The duration of the proliferative cycle is finite. On occasion, the cell dawdles (usually because of exposure to a toxic agent) in S phase. Should that happen, nature loses its patience and activates **Chk1** to block mitotic separation of incompletely duplicated chromosomes. This is called the **replication checkpoint**.

During M phase, there are elaborate controls to ensure that daughter cells each receive the correct complement of chromosomes. Thus, sensors at the points (kinetochores) where chromosomes attach to the mitotic spindle may activate a **spindle integrity checkpoint** if they sense that segregation is unbalanced or inaccurate. An additional mechanism involves an important enzyme, **Aurora B kinase**, which assures that the kinetochore binds the mitotic spindle effectively, and so prevents improper segregation of chromosomes.

p53 Is a Key Cell Cycle Regulator

As mentioned in **Chapter 1**, p53 has been called "the guardian of the genome." It coordinates cellular responses to DNA damage, activates G_1/S and G_2/M checkpoints, and initiates apoptosis. Mechanisms underlying these p53 activities include:

1. Normally, p53 is kept at low levels by MDM2, an E3 ubiquitin (Ub) ligase that polyubiquitinates p53, causing its proteasomal degradation (Fig. 5-14A, **see Chapter 1**).

A

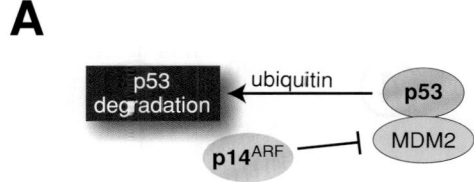

B

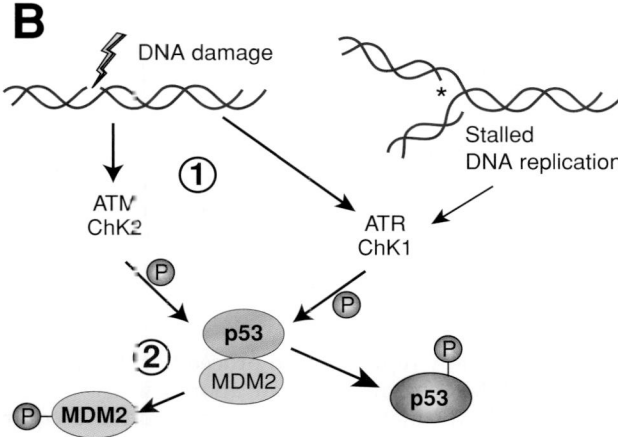

C

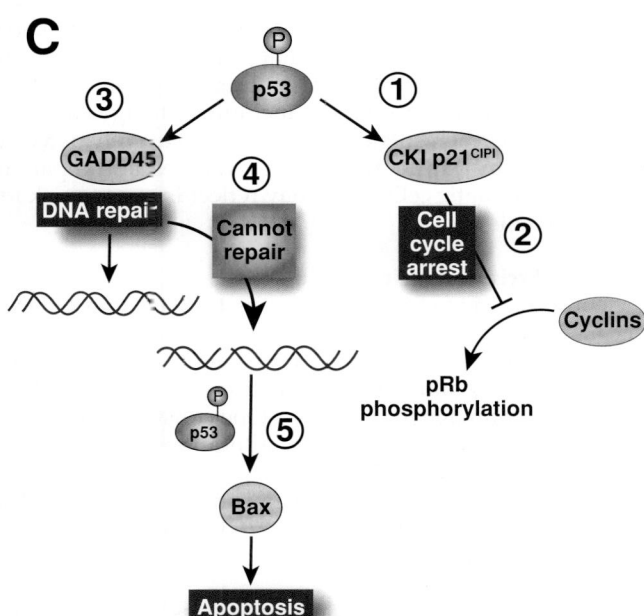

2. DNA damage or stalled DNA replication are recognized by the protein kinases **ATM** and **ATR**. In combination with **Chk2** and **Chk1**, respectively, they phosphorylate p53.
3. Phosphorylated p53 dissociates from MDM2 (Fig. 5-14B) and translocates to the nucleus, where it further promotes cell cycle arrest by increasing production of p21^{Cip1}, a member of the Cip/Kip family of CKIs (Fig. 5-14C).
4. P21 blocks cell cycle progression by preventing pRb phosphorylation. When a cell cycle checkpoint is activated, the cell cycle pauses to permit DNA repair.
5. If DNA is repaired, the block is removed and the cell cycle proceeds (Fig. 5-14C).
6. If DNA cannot be repaired, p53 triggers apoptosis (Fig. 5-14C).

Many tumor cells have mutations in genes that control cell cycle transit. Further, whether or not these genes are mutated, many antineoplastic agents target cell cycle–related genes to try to limit the ability of cancer cells to divide. Mutations in cyclins or CDKs, for example, may render cancer cells impervious to regulatory activities described above. Other alterations, in regulatory proteins like Cip/Kip CKIs or pRb, may impair one or another aspect of their ability to limit cell cycle progression.

DNA Repair Protects Cellular Genomes From Genotoxic Stresses

There are one hundred trillion (10^{14}) cells in the human body. Their DNA is under relentless assault by internal and exogenous stresses, including environmental chemicals, ultraviolet and ionizing radiation, free radicals, and an intracellular milieu that may breakdown the chemical bonds that hold DNA together. Cellular DNA is further at risk from the infidelity of DNA polymerases. Cells maintain genomic stability via diverse mechanisms that vigilantly detect and repair such damage. In addition, these systems also communicate with cell cycle checkpoint regulators (see above) and apoptosis triggers, all in an effort to prevent mutations from being transmitted to daughter cells. Collaborations among diverse proteins restore genomic integrity after such DNA modifications as single- and double-strand breaks (DSBs), single nucleotide substitutions, base insertions and deletions of variable lengths, and other perturbations of orderly and correct double-stranded DNA structure.

The importance of understanding these mechanisms extends beyond their roles in homeostasis and, if impaired, tumorigenesis. DNA repair systems may also protect tumors from genotoxic therapies. In this sense, they represent a key facet of tumor resistance to treatment and, therefore, important targets for current drug development.

DNA Repair Pathways

DNA damage may occur any time in the cell cycle, be caused by diverse insults, and reflect many types of alterations in DNA structure. Maintaining cell's genomic integrity thus requires a plethora of DNA repair mechanisms (Fig. 5-15).

Mismatch Repair

Mismatch repair (MMR) mainly repairs errors in DNA replication. Estimates of base mismatches per mitosis vary, and are different in somatic cells, compared to germline cells.

FIGURE 5-14. Connections between DNA damage and replication stress to cell cycle arrest, via p53. A. MDM2 is an E3 ubiquitin ligase that, under normal circumstances, binds p53 and directs its inactivation. P14^{ARF} inhibits this interaction. **B. 1.** DNA damage and other interference with DNA replication activate ATM (ataxia-telangiectasia mutated) and ATR (ATM and Rad3-related) kinases. ATM activates Chk2; ATR activates Chk1. **2.** Both phosphorylate p53, releasing it from bondage to MDM2. **C.** Activated p53 does two things. **1.** It binds to DNA and upregulates transcription of several genes, including cyclin-dependent kinase inhibitor (CKI) p21$^{CIP1/WAF1}$, (**2**) which, in turn, induces cell cycle arrest by preventing release of E2F from pRB. **3.** P53 also activates GADD45, which promotes DNA repair. **4.** Should DNA repair not be possible, p53 directs increased transcription of the proapoptotic protein Bax. **5.** Increased Bax triggers apoptosis.

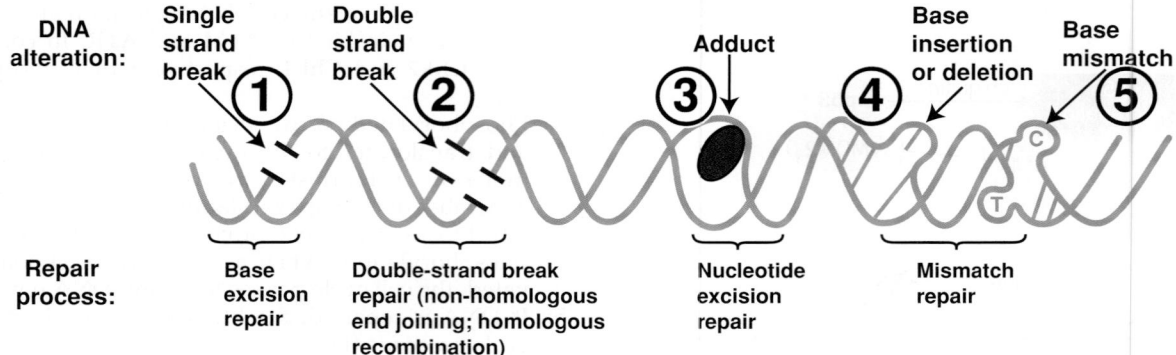

FIGURE 5-15. DNA damage and the mechanisms that repair DNA damage. Most forms of localized DNA damage are either (1) single-strand breaks; (2) double-strand breaks; (3) DNA adducts; (4) base insertions or deletions; or (5) base mismatches. The mechanisms that repair these insults are respectively (1) base excision repair; (2) double-strand break repair; (3) nucleotide excision repair; and (4) and (5) mismatch repair. Some tumor types that arise from dysfunctional DNA repair mechanisms are indicated in conjunction with the mechanisms that tend to malfunction in those tumors.

The human genome is about 3×10^9 DNA base pairs. For one somatic cell division, the DNA duplication error rate is 1 miscopied base per 10^9 bases. In germ cells, it is even lower, about 1 miscopied base in 10^{11}. The polymerases that replicate human DNA (Pol δ and ε) edit as they go, but still make 1 base mistake/10^{4-5}. The difference between polymerase editing errors and the final product, 4 to 5 orders of magnitude, reflects the effectiveness of MMR (Fig. 5-16).

MMR includes two overlapping systems, one of which mainly corrects single-base mismatches, and another that fixes insertions and deletions due to polymerase slippage during DNA replication. Errors are recognized and repaired by a family of enzymes (e.g., MSH6, MSH2) (Fig. 5-16) that stop DNA replication at the G_2/M checkpoint, correct the

mistake, then allow replication to proceed. If the damage is irreparable, MMR enzymes activate apoptosis.

Defective MMR may be inherited or acquired. Acquired defects in MMR may reflect mutations that develop in somatic cells over time, or epigenetic silencing (see below) of part of the MMR system. An important indicator of defective MMR is **microsatellite instability**. Microsatellites are short (up to 6 base pairs) sequences that may be repeated up to 100 times. They are common in the human genome and are inordinately prone to mutation, including changes in numbers of repeats. Microsatellite mutations are usually detected and repaired by MMR. If, however, they escape repair in germline or somatic cells, they may reflect increased risk for cancer (see below).

Nucleotide Excision Repair

Nucleotide excision repair (NER) corrects distortions of DNA helical structure, such as are caused by bulky DNA adducts, base oxidation by ROS derived from mitochondria or other sources, or by UV and ionizing radiation (see Table 5-1). NER detects DNA damage in two ways. One constantly scans the genome and the other identifies alterations that interfere with RNA transcription. Inherited defects in NER detection systems are associated with human cancer syndromes. The scanning pathway is deficient in xeroderma pigmentosum, and the transcription-coupled mechanism is impaired in Cockayne syndrome.

Once either NER pathway recognizes a defect, both repair it similarly, using an enzyme called ERCC1, which is of considerable practical importance. If tumor cells can repair DNA effectively, they are more resistant to chemotherapies that target DNA. For some tumors, ERCC1 activity (or lack thereof) helps predict cancer cells sensitivity to chemotherapy with such DNA-damaging agents as *cis*-platinum.

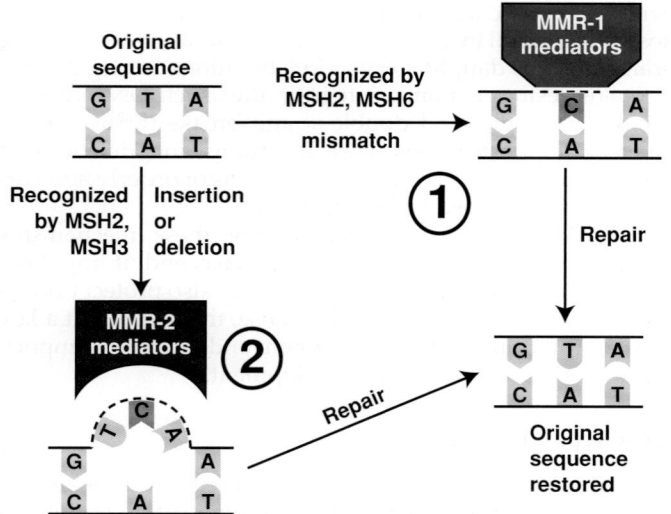

FIGURE 5-16. Mediators of mismatch repair (MMR). 1. A DNA single-base mismatch (here, a *C* is present where a *T* should be) is recognized by two proteins, MSH2 and MSH6. These recruit a group of MMR repair enzymes which correct the defect. **2.** If the mispairing is due to a small insertion or deletion, a second group of MMR enzymes, MSH2 and MSH3, recognize the mistake and recruit another group of MMR mediators to correct the defect and restore the correct sequence.

Base Excision Repair

Base excision repair (BER) is related to NER, and the two overlap somewhat in the types of DNA damage for which they are responsible (see Table 5-1). BER mostly repairs chemical injury to DNA bases, such as hydrolysis of base-sugar bonds, single-strand breaks, and small chemical changes in base structure. These alterations occur

TABLE 5-1		
TYPES OF DNA DAMAGE, THEIR COMMON CAUSES, AND THE RESPECTIVE REPAIR PATHWAYS		
Type of Damage	**Causes**	**Repair Pathway**
Base oxidation	Mitochondrial ROS	NER, BER
	Phagocyte-generated oxidants	
	UV and ionizing radiation	
	Smoking	
Other base modifications	Chemotherapeutic drugs	BER
	Neutrophil bactericidal enzymes	
	Cigarette smoke	
	Other environmental chemicals	
Alterations Perturbing DNA Architecture		
Additions	Errors in transcription	NER
	ROS	
	UV light	
Interstrand DNA cross-links	Ionizing radiation	Other[a]
	Arrested DNA replication	
	Environmental chemicals	
Single-strand nicks	ROS	BER, NER
	Ionizing radiation	
	Spontaneous loss of sugar–phosphate bonding	
Double-strand breaks	Arrested DNA replication	HR, NHEJ
	Ionizing radiation	
	Chemical damage	

[a]Other mechanisms include Fanconi-related repair pathways.

BER = base excision repair; HR = homologous recombination; NER = nucleotide excision repair; NHEJ = nonhomologous end joining.

frequently: 10^4 times/cell/day, and mostly reflect changes due to environmental and other chemicals, ROS, and UV and ionizing radiation. Inherited defects in BER have not been described.

Double-Strand Break Repair

DSBs may be caused by ROS or ionizing radiation, or during DNA replication if replication stalls at a single-strand break (see Table 5-1). Such lesions often cause chromosome rearrangements, especially when they occur, as they often do, in clusters.

Two related enzymes, ATM and ATR (see above, Fig. 5-14), are the sensors for DSBs. Each recognizes different types of DSBs. ATM identifies those caused by DNA damage (e.g., ionizing radiation). Once activated, ATM recruits **Chk2**. ATR detects single-stranded DNA at stalled replication forks, whereupon it activates **Chk1** (see above). Both resulting complexes, ATM/**Chk2** and ATR/**Chk1**, phosphorylate p53 and so activate cell cycle checkpoints, halting cell division until the break is fixed. DSBs are repaired either by **nonhomologous end joining (NHEJ)** or by **homologous recombination (HR)**.

In HR, which is mostly active in S and G_2 phases, the sister chromatid or homologous chromosome serves as a template to reproduce the original sequence. This can cause two major types of genome alterations. First, if the homologous chromosome serves as a template, allelic differences between the two chromosomes may be lost (loss of heterozygosity, LOH, see below). Second, since repetitive sequences are abundant in the human genome, repair of a break that occurs among repetitive sequences of one chromosome may lead HR to use an identical repetitive sequence, but which is on a nonhomologous chromosome, as a template for recombination. This generates a translocation. Several genes (e.g., BRCA1, BRCA2, PALB2) whose protein products participate in HR may be mutated or inactivated (see below) in inherited cancer susceptibility syndromes, via somatic mutation or because of epigenetic changes.

NHEJ repairs DSBs by rejoining the broken ends. NHEJ thus restores DNA integrity but may not regenerate the original sequence (depending on the nature of the break). Furthermore, there is no guarantee that the ends that are so joined are in fact broken ends of the same chromatid, in which case, translocations may result.

Unlike HR, NHEJ operates throughout the cell cycle. It is more efficient than HR, and uses the Ku proteins (Ku70, Ku80), which are among the most abundant protein species within cells. NHEJ is the mechanism that mediates V(D)J recombination to generate antibody diversity in B lymphocytes (**see Chapter 4**).

NHEJ generally works well, and with few errors. However, it does not easily account for the original base order of the DNA sequences it joins. If there are multiple, clustered DSBs, NHEJ may link noncontiguous DNAs. NHEJ is not affected in any known inherited predispositions to developing cancer, nor is it commonly associated with oncogenesis.

HALLMARKS OF CANCER

Most tumors begin as a single cell, which acquires malignant characteristics. In the process, that cell's behaviors change, mostly—but not totally—reflecting accumulated mutations. Genomic analyses show that human tumors carry a great many mutations, some of which are critical for tumor development, some of which are not. Still, these genetic changes, as important as they are, tell only part of a story that has become much more complex than was originally imagined.

"Driver" Mutations Propel Tumor Development

There are relatively few such drivers. Some affect genes that encode proteins; others alter so-called noncoding sequences, which include regulatory regions and areas encoding a wide variety of untranslated RNAs (see below). Thus, our idea of driver mutations should be broad and inclusive, and accommodate the complexities of regulation of gene expression and action.

Other mutations—"passengers" or "hitchhikers"—seem to be along for the ride. Their role(s) in tumor development and progression, if any, is mostly unknown.

Malignant Cells Differ in Several Ways From Their Normal Cousins

There are currently eight **hallmark** activities by which cells of solid cancers differ from their normal counterparts. (Hematologic cancers develop and spread differently, and so share some, but not all, of these characteristics.) To understand oncogenesis and how cancer-related processes are being targeted therapeutically, the following hallmarks, or attributes, of malignant tumors should be appreciated:

- **Signaling that sustains cell proliferation.** When normal cells enter and progress through the cell cycle (see above), highly regulated signals guide and check all of their activities. Cancer cells, however, march to their own drummers and determine their own destinies. Their mitotic activities proceed independently of normal restraints.
- **Avoiding normal growth regulators.** Normal cells and tissues cannot grow indefinitely: many forces—from intracellular viability and mitosis regulators, to cell–cell contacts, to inhibitory cytokines—restrain any tendencies toward proliferative exuberance. Cancer cells are generally insensitive to those restraints.
- **Evasion of PCD.** In normal cells, such factors as genomic instability, poor anchorage, and inhospitable cellular microenvironments may trigger PCD (**see Chapter 1**). Cancer cells often develop strategies to circumvent suicide programs.
- **Cellular immortalization.** While normal cells have limited replicative potential before they stop dividing (senescence) or die, cancer cells can multiply indefinitely. They evade senescence and keep their youthful biosynthetic and reproductive vigor.
- **Stimulating blood vessel growth.** Solid tumors require huge supplies of nutrients and oxygen in order to grow. Blood vessels deliver. Tumor cells and their neighbors secrete molecules that stimulate angiogenesis, that is, new blood vessel formation.
- **Invasion and metastasis.** Solid tumor masses do not usually kill by growing large. They kill by metastasizing widely. Tumor cells thus must escape the shackles of their anchorage to adjacent cells and to basement membrane, traverse intervening connective tissue, enter blood and lymphatic vessels, identify distant homesteads for implantation, exit the vasculature, then establish colonies far from their origin.
- **Altered bioenergetics.** Cancer cells generally favor glycolysis over oxidative phosphorylation for ATP generation. This change requires that they import and use more glucose, which in turn affects their metabolism and that of neighboring cells.
- **Immune avoidance.** Accumulated data show that the immune system may protect from tumor development and progression. However, cells of at least some tumors protect themselves by actively suppressing host immune defenses.

Processes That Facilitate Tumor Growth and Spread

Several oncogenic mechanisms play supporting roles in developing and maintaining many cancers. To a variable extent, these are active in almost all tumors.

- **Genomic instability.** Most human cancer cells generate random mutations far faster than do their normal counterparts. This allows tumor cells to evolve quickly, to adapt to changing environments, and to optimize their own maintenance and progression.
- **Inactivation of tumor suppressors.** Normally, strong regulators limit cell cycle transit, maintain genomic stability, and control other key functions. These restraints affect most of the attributes mentioned above, as well as associated facilitating processes described below. For a tumor to succeed, it must evade or inactivate these suppressors.
- **Inflammation.** Inflammatory cells infiltrate most developing solid tumors and secrete factors that facilitate tumor development and progression. Nontransformed cells near cancers thus provide a microenvironment that accommodates tumor growth.

In considering how cells become malignant, and how the tumors that they engender grow and spread, it is not enough to limit one's scope to genomic alterations in tumor cells. The situation is far more complex—and therefore daunting—than that. In addition to generating and accumulating multiple mutations, tumor cells show **altered epigenetic regulation** (see below), in which changes arise that are independent of the DNA sequences whose activities and products are being controlled. In addition, tumor cells reprogram the activities of their neighboring nontumor cells. The complexity of these nefarious interactions is also important in facilitating and maintaining tumor growth, development, spread, and protection.

Interrelated though they are, cancer hallmarks are conceptually distinct. Further, every tumor evolves differently, so that certain attributes and genes may characterize one tumor differently from others, or may suppress oncogenesis in one context but encourage it in another.

Tumor Cells Evade Cell Cycle Control

Tumor cell mutations that activate and inactivate certain genes allow cancer cells to escape from regulated cycling. Generally, activating mutations that stimulate passage through the cell cycle occur in genes affected called oncogenes (actually, proto-oncogenes, see below). Inactivating mutations usually prevent inhibitory influences that we call tumor suppressors (see below).

Oncogenes

Early research on tumor-causing retroviruses showed that transferring particular viral genes made normal cells behave like cancer cells. These viral genes were designated oncogenes. Later studies used similar genes from human cancer cells to impart a transformed phenotype to normal recipient cells. Some of these transforming human tumor genes that stimulated cellular proliferation turned out to be mutant versions of normal human genes (**proto-oncogenes**). To minimize confusion, transforming viral genes begin with v- (e.g., v-*myb*), and their cellular cousins with a c- (e.g., c-*myb*).

Mechanisms That Drive Cell Proliferation

One or more genes that stimulate cell multiplication are often dysregulated or mutated during oncogenesis. They act in biochemical pathways that guide entry into and through the cell cycle. These include (see Fig. 5-17):

- Growth factors
- Cell membrane receptors

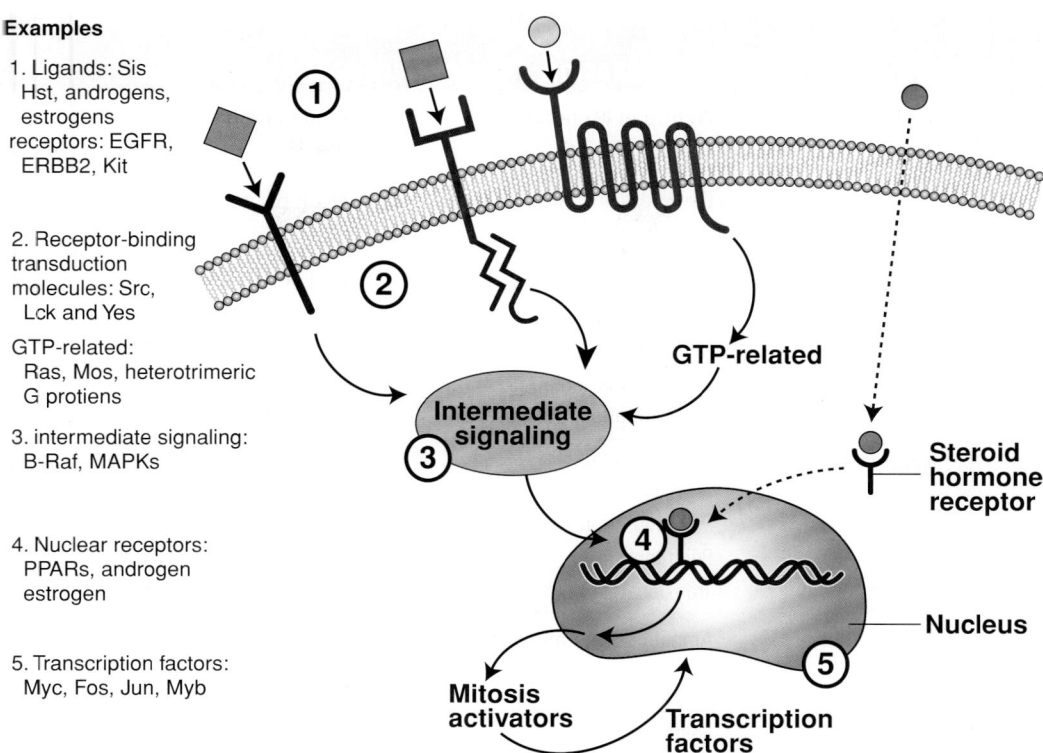

Examples

1. Ligands: Sis
   Hst, androgens,
   estrogens
   receptors: EGFR,
   ERBB2, Kit

2. Receptor-binding
   transduction
   molecules: Src,
   Lck and Yes

   GTP-related:
   Ras, Mos, heterotrimeric
   G protiens

3. intermediate signaling:
   B-Raf, MAPKs

4. Nuclear receptors:
   PPARs, androgen
   estrogen

5. Transcription factors:
   Myc, Fos, Jun, Myb

FIGURE 5-17. Signaling paradigms in cellular transformation. 1. Extracellular ligands bind to cell membrane receptors. **2.** One of several pathways of signaling is then activated. The receptor itself can activate intracellular signaling (**left**). A protein that binds to the activated receptor may trigger intracellular signaling (**center**). The receptor may be a G-protein–coupled receptor, which stimulates guanine nucleotide–related signaling. Or, the ligand may traverse the cell membrane to activate receptors within the cytosol directly, without a cell membrane intermediate (**far right**). **3.** In the first three cases, cellular intermediates of many types are activated. **4.** These intermediates enter the nucleus and recognize DNA sequences, usually in promoter regions of relevant genes. **5.** The result for all pathways is activation of transcription, particularly of proteins that help take the cell through the cell cycle. Shown at the left are examples of proto-oncogenes and other cellular products that act in each capacity.

- Intracellular signal transduction intermediates
- Nuclear receptors
- Transcription factors

Growth Factor–Related Signaling and Oncogenesis

Normal cells proliferate when demand for more cells stimulates factors that drive mitosis and that overcome cell cycle regulators (see above). For cancer cells to multiply without restraint, they must divide independently of outside stimulatory influences. They achieve this by mimicking those influences. To understand how this occurs, one must first review how receptor-ligand interactions drive mitosis, as illustrated in the general schematic in Figure 5-17.

Tumor-driving mutations may occur at any step of this process. Those mutations drive cellular proliferation without the normal restraints that match cell numbers to the body's needs.

Ligands, Their Receptors, and Cell Proliferation

Ligands. In general, the role of external ligands reflects an ongoing need of normal cells and, often, developing tumor cells, for exogenous stimulation to activate and maintain proliferation. Some ligands may drive cell multiplication early in oncogenesis, with tumor cells eventually becoming independent of those ligands, due to changes in, for example,

receptors or other molecules. Sometimes, developing (or developed) tumor cells themselves produce these ligands, as an autocrine trigger to proliferation. Some such stimulatory molecules are overexpressed as oncoproteins, mostly because of gene amplification (see Table 5-2).

Receptors. Several main classes of receptors stimulate or inhibit cell proliferation (see Table 5-3). Except for steroid hormone receptors, these are cell membrane molecules that respond to external ligands. Receptor-ligand interactions trigger changes in the receptors, which become docking sites for one or more intracellular signaling networks.

The changes that ligands elicit in receptors reflect the specifics of the receptor:

- **Receptor tyrosine kinases (RTKs)** possess intrinsic tyrosine kinase activity that causes the receptor to phosphorylate itself, a nearby duplicate RTK and, perhaps, other molecules as well, after it binds its ligand.
- **Nonkinase receptors** may undergo structural rearrangements upon ligand binding. This makes them receptive to initiating downstream signaling (see below). These types of receptors often associate with nonreceptor tyrosine kinases (**NRTKs**, see below), which mediate further signaling.
- **G-protein–coupled receptors (GPCRs)** are common signaling activators. After binding their ligands—which

TABLE 5-2

COMMON ONCOPROTEINS THAT DRIVE CELL PROLIFERATION, THEIR ACTIVITIES AND ACTIVATION

Activity	Name of Protein	Nature of Mutation	Explanation
Ligand	Hst	Amplification	Growth factor in FGF family
	Sis	Derepression (autocrine stimulation)	PDGF, β subunit
	FGF3	Amplification	
RTK	Kit	Activating point mutation	Receptor for stem cell factor
	Her2/neu (ErbB2)	Amplification	Constitutively activated
	EGFR	Mutations, amplification	Constitutively activated
	Met	Translocation	HGF receptor
	Ret	Point mutation, translocation	Constitutively activated
Intracellular signaling intermediate	Ras (K-Ras, N-Ras, H-Ras)	Point mutation	GTP-binding protein, three different *RAS* genes, activated in different settings
	B-Raf	Point mutation	Tyrosine kinase
	Src	Point mutation	Tyrosine kinase
	Abl	Translocation	Mutant protein, Bcr-Abl
Transcription factor	Myc (c-Myc, N-Myc, L-Myc)	Amplification, translocation	Directs transcription of up to 15% of human genes
	Fos	Amplification	Part of AP-1, with Jun
	Myb	Point mutations	Promotes hematopoietic stem cell proliferation
	Rel	Amplification, point mutations	Member of NF-kB family, expressed mainly in lymphocytes
	Ets	Translocation	Large family; fusion products may drive tumorigenesis

FGF = fibroblast growth factor; PDGF = platelet-derived growth factor; RTK = receptor tyrosine kinase.

may be diverse types of molecules—GPCRs change conformation. In so doing, they activate GTP-related nucleotide exchange factors (GEFs, see below). Some GPCRs transduce mitogenic signals triggered by ligands like prostaglandins, endothelin, and thrombin. GPCRs may be amplified in cancers or they may mediate stimulatory autocrine or paracrine signals.

TABLE 5-3

TYPES OF SIGNAL-TRANSDUCING RECEPTORS IMPORTANT IN TUMORIGENESIS

Receptor Category	Prototypical Ligands
Tyrosine kinase (RTK)	EGF, IGF-1, Insulin
G-protein–coupled receptor (GPCR)	Prostaglandins, RANTES, SDF-1
Nuclear receptors	Androgens, estrogens, other steroid hormones
Serine/threonine kinases	TGFβ
Kinase-associated receptors	GH, TcR, IL-2
Extracellular matrix receptors	Fibronectin, collagen, laminin

EGF = epidermal growth factor; GH = growth hormone; IGF-1 = insulin-like growth factor-1; IL-2 = interleukin-2; RANTES = CCL5, a ligand for CCR5; SDF-1 = CXCL12, stromal-derived factor-1 (CXCR4 ligand); TcR = T-cell receptor; TGFβ = transforming growth factor-β.

Signaling activated by receptor-ligand interactions varies. Many activated receptors are platforms for other proteins, like NRTKs, which often phosphorylate themselves and nonkinase receptors. The cell membrane complex thus formed recruits signaling intermediates and activates diverse downstream signaling pathways.

Receptor proteins are among the most important transforming proteins. They are widely implicated in oncogenesis (Table 5-3), *and often drive oncogenesis via mutations that activate them constitutively, so they no longer need their ligands to drive proliferation.*

Signaling After Receptor Activation

Receptor-ligand binding stimulates downstream signaling pathways. If an RTK or NRTK is involved, the subsequent set of signaling intermediates use **SH2 domains** (for Src-homology-2) to recognize phosphorylated tyrosine(s). SH2 domains bind specific phosphotyrosines on the specific RTK or NRTK.

What follows depends on many factors, including the type of receptor activated, if its activation entails tyrosine kinase activity, and the molecular species that immediately follow. Pathways that may be set in motion include:

- **Ras.** The three members of the Ras family (K-Ras, N-Ras, H-Ras) are small guanine nucleotide–binding proteins that may be activated by tyrosine kinases via a linker protein, usually **Grb2**. To understand activated Ras and Ras-related oncogenesis, the Ras cycle should be appreciated (Fig. 5-18). Ras binds GDP and GTP. Ras is active when it binds GTP. GTP binding is catalyzed by a **guanine**

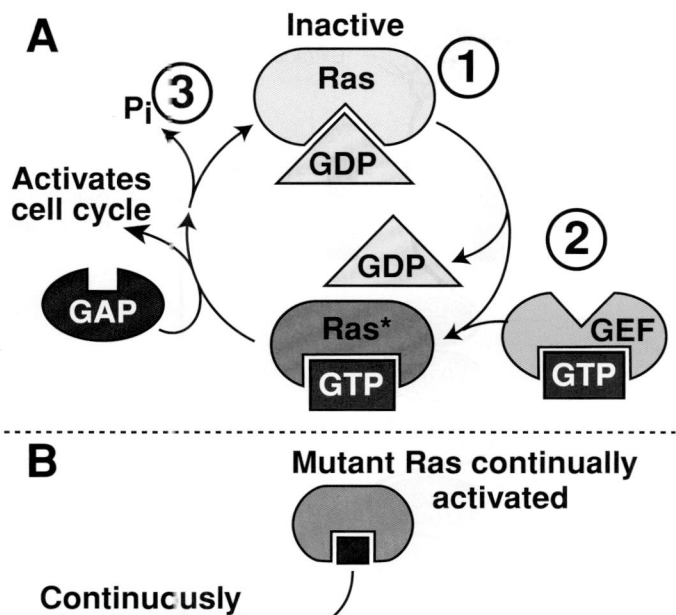

FIGURE 5-18. Mechanism of action of Ras. A (upper). Normal. The Ras protein, p21^{Ra}, exists in two conformational states, determined by the binding of either guanosine diphosphate (GDP) or guanosine triphosphate (GTP). **1.** Normally, most of the p21^{Ras} is in the inactive GDP-bound state. **2.** An external stimulus, or signal, triggers the exchange of GTP for GDP, an event that converts Ras to the active state. **3.** Activated p21^{Ras}, which is associated with the plasma membrane, binds GTPase-activating protein (GAP) from the cytosol. The binding of GAP has two consequences. In association with other plasma membrane constituents, it initiates the effector response. At the same time, the binding of GAP to Ras GTP stimulates by about 100-fold the intrinsic GTPase activity of Ras, promoting hydrolysis of GTP to GDP and the return of Ras to its inactive state. **B (lower).** Mutated Ras protein is locked into the active GTP-bound state because of an insensitivity of its intrinsic GTPase to GAP or because of a lack of the GTPase activity itself. As a result, the effector response is exaggerated, and the cell is transformed.

nucleotide exchange factor (**GEF**, also see above), which is in turn activated when Grb2 recognizes phosphorylated tyrosines (see above). A **GTPase-activating protein** (**GAP**) directs Ras GTPase activity. This activates downstream signaling and converts Ras GTP to Ras GDP, its quiescent state. Many malignant tumors carry a mutated form of Ras, which does not undergo deactivation and is constitutively turned on.

Many GPCRs stimulate a similar type of response, but via a different group of intermediates, called **heterotrimeric G proteins**. Unlike Ras, these G proteins tend not to be mutated in cancers. Rather, they may be overexpressed, achieving a comparable effect, that is, constitutive triggering downstream signaling.

- **PI3 kinase.** This family of enzymes (**see Chapter 1**) is generally activated by RTKs and GPCRs. Family members add a phosphate group to the lipid, **phosphatidylinositol**, to create phosphatidylinositol-3-phosphate (PI(3)P), and more heavily phosphorylated derivatives such as PI(3,4,5)P$_3$. These mediate many proliferation-related (see below) and cell survival reactions.

- **Phospholipase C.** This family of enzymes is commonly activated by diverse types of receptors, especially GPCRs, but also others. They cleave certain phospholipids and help generate inositol phosphate signaling intermediates and diacylglycerol. These both may drive cellular multiplication via, respectively, calcium-signaling pathways and **protein kinase C (PKC)**.

- **Mitogen-activated protein kinases (MAPKs).** These enzymes trigger cell proliferation via many different types of signaling reactions. MAPKs may be activated variously by upstream proteins like Ras, by GPCRs, or by other mechanisms. Some very important driver mutations for malignancy (e.g., b-Raf) occur among these proteins, frequently leading to constitutive activation. Typically, MAPK cascades involve three sequential species, one activating the next. Consequences of MAPK stimulation are diverse, and there is extensive cross talk between these and other signaling intermediates.

Transforming Growth Factor-β and Other Cytokines

TGFβ, an extracellular cytokine in the microenvironment of cancer cells that triggers important regulatory pathways, is an example of cell communication mediators that strongly influence the pathogenesis of tumors. It is important in oncogenesis, although cell and tissue responses to it depend on context (Table 5-4). Normally, TGFβ tends to suppress tumor development by modulating cell proliferation, survival, adhesion, and differentiation. It also inhibits mitogenesis induced by constituents of the extracellular matrix (ECM) (see above).

TABLE 5-4	
TRANSFORMING GROWTH FACTOR-β (TGFβ) AND CANCER	
Promotes	**Inhibits**
Normal Tumor–Suppressive Effects	
Apoptosis	Inflammation
Differentiation	Mitogenesis induced by extracellular matrix
Maintenance of cell number	
Failure of Tumor Suppression	
Autocrine mitogens	Immune surveillance
Motility	
Invasion and Metastasis	
Recruitment of myofibroblasts	
Malignant cell extravasation	
Modification of microenvironment	
Mobilization of osteoclasts	

Normally, TGFβ compels homeostasis and exerts tumor-suppressive activity through effects on the target cells themselves or the extracellular matrix.

Failure of this activity by TGFβ permits production of growth factors, evasion of immune surveillance, and establishment of factors that facilitate tumor cell invasion and metastasis.

However, frankly malignant cells often acquire the capacity to evade or even to manipulate TGFβ pathways for their own wicked ends. Consequent abnormal TGFβ pathway signaling may actually stimulate tumor cell proliferation, facilitate their evasion of host defense mechanisms (see below), and promote invasion and metastasis.

Cancer cells may develop the ability to circumvent TGFβ–related suppressive activity via mutations in genes for TGFβ receptors, or by interfering with downstream signaling by mutation or by promoter methylation of key proteins. In such settings, cancer cells can hijack TGFβ regulatory activities to advance their needs, such as tumor growth, invasion, and metastasis. Loss of TGFβ suppressor function via inactivating mutations of genes in its core pathway occurs in many cancers.

Overexpression of other cytokines (e.g., **granulocyte/monocyte colony-stimulating factor [GM-CSF]** and **interleukin-3 [IL-3]**) may contribute to tumor development, especially for hematopoietic malignancies.

Steroid Hormones

Some three centuries ago, the Italian physician Ramazzini observed that nuns had a particularly high incidence of breast cancer. This phenomenon is now known to reflect unopposed estrogen stimulation of breast epithelium, uninterrupted by pregnancy and lactation. Both estrogens and progesterone bind to specific cytoplasmic receptors. Resulting hormone–receptor complexes are then translocated to the nucleus, where they act as transcription factors that foster proliferation of responsive cells. Antiestrogen therapy for hormone receptor–positive tumors reduces risk of recurrence after surgery. Other nuclear receptors identified in breast cancer bind androgens, corticosteroids, vitamins A and D, fatty acids, and some dietary lipids. Interactions of these signaling pathways with each other and with other signaling pathways are very complex, and not well understood.

Androgen influence is most conspicuous in prostate cancer, in which they stimulate growth by binding to the androgen receptor. This receptor pathway engages in cross talk with other important pathways that affect the cell cycle, apoptosis, and differentiation. Such interactions involve EGF, IGF-1, FGF, VEGF, TGFβ, and other important signaling species. Removing androgen stimulation, whether by surgical or pharmacologic means, inhibits prostate cancer growth, although most tumors eventually become androgen insensitive.

Membrane-Bound Mucins

Far from being simply extracellular molecules that establish an interface between epithelial surfaces and the exterior, membrane-bound mucins (MUCs) comprise a large family of glycoproteins that are overproduced in a variety of cancers. Extracellular domains of these MUCs lubricate and protect the cell surface. The cytoplasmic domains of these transmembrane glycoproteins act as scaffolds for interaction with signaling molecules that influence cell proliferation and survival (Fig. 5-19). In this sense, the large majority of breast cancers overexpress MUC1, as do many malignancies of the colon, ovary, pancreas, and lungs.

Interaction Among Intermediate Signaling Pathways

Whether elicited by receptor-ligand interactions or by a constitutively activating driver mutation, signaling avenues

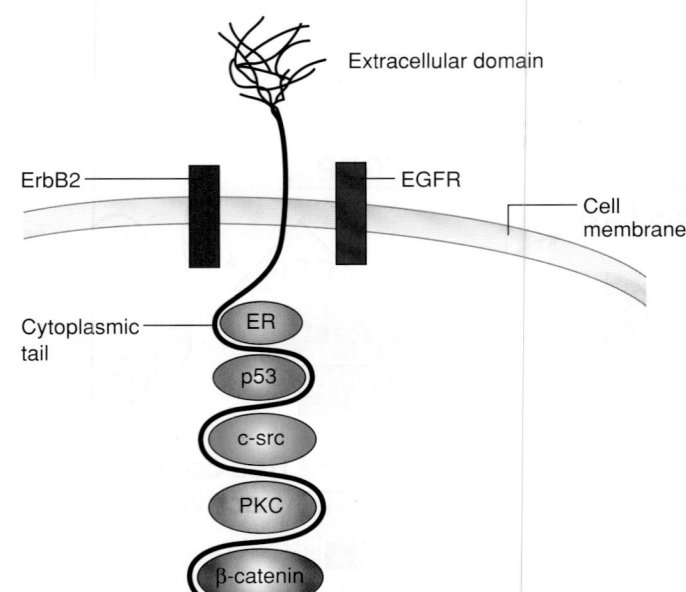

FIGURE 5-19. Membrane-bound mucins with important signaling molecules. *EGFR* = epidermal growth factor receptor; *ER* = estrogen receptor; *PKC* = protein kinase C.

discussed above, and many others, interconnect extensively. This fact endows them with baffling complexity, challenging those trying to understand how cells sustain proliferation and those seeking specific targets for therapy. *Because of these complexities, the consequences of unrestrained activation of a given gene are not always predictable.* A mutant protein may drive proliferation in one cell type, apoptosis in another, and differentiation in a third.

Transcriptional Activation

In the end, a key element of cancer cells' unrestrained proliferation is the array of genes whose transcription is activated or repressed. Whatever the upstream driver mutations are, transcription factors sit at the end of the *afferent* limb of processes that drive uncontrolled mitosis, and these factors generally increase production of wild-type proteins. Driver mutations involving transcription factors typically increase their activity by placing them—for example, via translocation—under the control of more vigorous or more active promoters. Among the best known, and most commonly inculpated, of the many transcription factors implicated in oncogenesis are:

- **Myc.** A ubiquitous transcription factor which may control transcription of as many as 10% to 15% of human genes, c-Myc and its cousins, N-Myc and L-Myc, are key to development of many tumors. Among its functions, Myc pushes cellular proliferation, favors stemness (see cancer stem cells [CSCs], below), increases energy production, and facilitates tumor cell invasiveness. If p53 and other cell death effectors are intact, Myc may also activate cell death programs.
- **Fos and Jun.** Together, these proteins form activation protein-1 (**AP-1**) transcription factor. Increased AP-1 activity generally results from increased signaling via several pathways, including MAPK and the PKC family (PKC, see above), and promotes cellular proliferation and

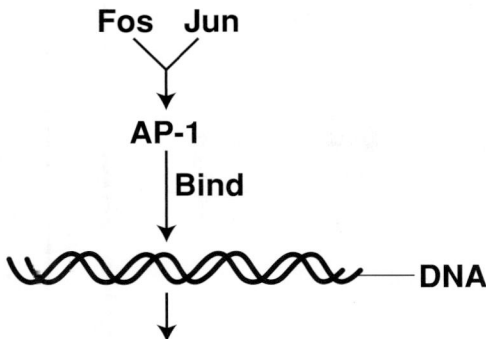

FIGURE 5-20. AP-1 complex. The AP-1 transcription factor complex is formed by the protein products of two proto-oncogenes, Fos and Jun. When these factors form a heterodimer, they bind DNA and direct transcription of genes whose products are involved in cell proliferation, tumor cell invasion and metastasis, angiogenesis, and inhibiting apoptosis.

survival (Fig. 5-20). AP-1 also represses expression of tumor suppressors like p53 (see below).

- **Androgen and estrogen receptors.** These cytoplasmic receptor proteins are both receptors and transcription factors. They bind their cognate ligands in the cytosol, whereupon they translocate to the nucleus, and act as transcription factors. Depending on the cell type, steroid sex hormone receptors may elicit cell proliferation. Thus, estrogen receptors stimulate ductal epithelial proliferation, which is often important in breast tumorigenesis. Similarly, androgens stimulate prostate tumor cells to proliferate.

As noted above, tumor cells may stimulate their own proliferation via autocrine mechanisms. They may themselves produce the requisite androgens or estrogens that drive proliferation mediated by these and similar receptors. Cancer progression may thus be independent of exogenous sources of stimulatory hormones, allowing tumors to resist hormone antagonist therapies.

Thus, whether by gene amplification, point mutation, translocation, or other mechanisms (see genomic instability, below), tumor cells proliferate heedless of the regulatory chains that limit normal cells. Other restraints, however, still face them.

Senescent Cells Are Viable but Can No Longer Divide

Such cells are metabolically active but do not proliferate. Cellular senescence occurs when cells exhaust their ability to proliferate. As such, it is a major defense against tumor development, to which many key mechanisms contribute.

Mediators of Cellular Senescence

Clearly, for malignant cells to indulge in endless proliferation, they must neutralize a mechanism that limits the number of mitoses they may undergo. The senescent phenotype entails increased formation of heterochromatin (**senescence-associated heterochromatin formation, SAHF**), in which certain proteins are modified, leading them to bind chromosomal DNA and impede transcription of E2F-activated genes that mediate cell multiplication (see above). Effectors of senescence include:

- **Telomere depletion.** Telomeres are tandem repeats of TTAGGG sequences at the 3′ end of chromosomal DNA strands, followed by an unpaired single DNA strand. With each cell division, telomere length decreases, triggering a series of processes (see below) that abrogate proliferation.
- **Shelterin.** This heteromeric protein has multiple functions, among which are regulating telomerase (see below), capping and protecting chromosome ends, and assuring that telomere depletion leads to senescence.
- **DNA damage response (DDR).** Exposed chromosomal ends can activate DNA damage–sensing proteins ATR and ATM (see above). These activate p53, pRb, and cdc25. The cell stops dividing until DNA damage is fixed or the cell enters senescence or apoptosis pathways. This mechanism is critical to oncogene-induced senescence (OIS, see below).
- **Tumor suppressors.** The intimacy between several critical proteins and cell cycle blockage is important in forcing cells into a senescent phenotype. Key among these proteins are p16^{INK4a} and pRb, which induce certain proteins to associate with the cell's DNA. This results in SAHF and gene silencing.
- **Oxidative stress.** Senescence can be delayed in cultured cells by decreasing ambient oxygen. Conversely, it can be hastened by adding oxidants like H_2O_2 to the culture. Activation of some oncoproteins, like RAS, increases oxidative stress. Resulting increases in ROS may trigger p38 MAPK signaling and activate ATM.
- **Cytokines.** Cells secrete factors, including IL-6 and IL-8, that help trigger the senescent phenotype. Together with their receptors, they help to establish and maintain senescence. Their participation led to the descriptive designation, secretion-associated senescent phenotype (SASP). Transcriptional regulation that these cytokines elicit inhibits cellular proliferation and promotes senescence.

Telomeres and Telomerase

Telomeres function as powerful tumor suppressors. These complex structures, which include shelterin protein caps that bind the ends of DNA sequences, regulate the number of mitoses cells may undergo. With each mitosis, telomeres shorten by 50 to 100 bp. Shelterin then regenerates the 3′ unpaired overhang. In normal cells, where p53 and pRb pathways are intact, shortened telomeres activate cell cycle checkpoints and cell division ceases. This is called replicative senescence (Fig. 5-21). The cell remains in G_0 (senescence) or dies. Telomere length limits the number of mitoses, and so the number of potentially error-prone cycles of DNA replication. It thus represents a key tumor suppressor mechanism.

There are, however, some cell types which engage in repeated mitosis, and for which telomere-activated senescence or apoptosis is not an attractive fate. For these cells (e.g., colon crypt epithelium), as for some cells during embryogenesis, **telomerase** preserves telomere length and

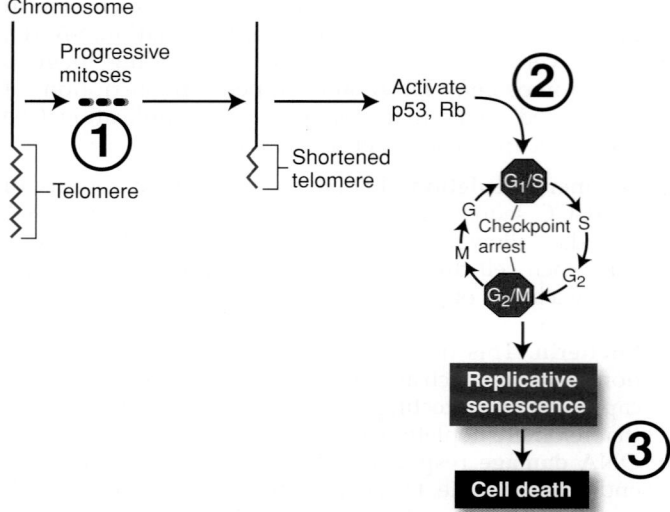

FIGURE 5-21. **The sequence of events resulting from DNA instability as a result of telomere shortening and leading to cell death.** This sequence occurs when the tumor suppressors p53 and Rb are intact. **1.** Progressive telomere shortening activates p53 and Rb. **2.** This leads to cell cycle arrest at the G1/S and G2/M checkpoints. **3.** Consequent replicative senescence triggers cell death programs.

so allows continuous replenishment of derivative cell populations. This enzyme is a complex ribonucleoprotein reverse transcriptase, which replenishes telomeres in cells that must undergo many cycles of mitosis.

Telomerase is inactive in all but a few adult cell types. Thus, if cell cycle checkpoints are impaired or inactive in a dividing cell, when telomeres reach a critical size, they become uncapped and may be subject to DNA "repair" by nonhomologous end joining (NHEJ). Resulting NHEJ may fuse the exposed ends of sister chromatids or nonhomologous chromosomes. As the cell cycle progresses, this fusion generates a chromosome "bridge," as fused DNA strands are pulled apart during anaphase. As daughter cells separate, complex mechanisms may cause resulting heterocentric chromosomes to break, leading to further recombination (Fig. 5-22).

Aneuploidy, gene and chromosome segment duplications and translocations and other genomic aberrations result. This is **telomere crisis**. While these changes may help incipient tumors to develop and generate mutations that allow them to become even more malignant, they also lead to high levels of chromosomal instability (CI) and so impair the viability of daughter cells. As a result, tumors tend to reactivate telomerase. That is, tumor cells improve DNA replicative efficiency if they protect telomeres. A high level of this activity protects the cancer cell by suppressing the development of further, potentially lethal, CI. *Thus, telomerase activation permits—but does not directly cause—the emergence of cancer* (Fig. 5-23).

Of the several components of telomerase, the limiting factor is production of the protein part of the enzyme, TERT. The *TERT* gene is therefore expressed in >90% of human tumors, which makes it the single most common gene expression abnormality in human cancer. *TERT* reactivation may entail diverse mechanisms. Among the best understood are mutations in the gene's promoter, which allow binding and activation by a ubiquitous family of transcription factors.

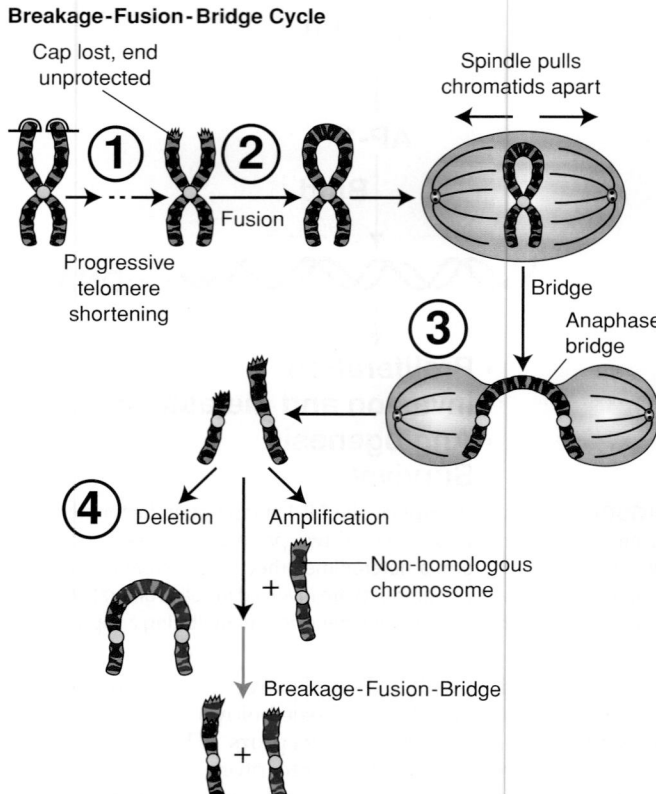

FIGURE 5-22. **The genesis of telomere-related chromosome breakage. 1.** In the absence of telomerase, extensive cell proliferation leads to unprotected telomere ends. **2.** These are "repaired" by fusion of telomeres between sister chromatids, creating a bridged structure like a tongs. **3.** During anaphase, the spindles attached to the two centromeres pull the now-attached chromatids apart, resulting in abnormal chromosomes. **4.** Further production of chromosome ends without telomeres may cause the cycle to repeat itself.

Some aspects of telomerase production may involve mTOR activation (**see Chapter 1**). In particular, data suggest that mTOR facilitates translation of TERT mRNA, and that mTOR inhibitors may decrease TERT protein—but not mRNA—levels.

Oncogene-Induced Cellular Senescence

The vast majority of cells that develop oncogenic mutations never become cancers. Such mutations occur several times per minute in people, which contrasts with the relative infrequency of cancer in a human life span. OIS is a major barrier tumorigenesis (Fig. 5-24). OIS constrains tumor development for many types of cancer. Consistent with this role for OIS, oncogene activation stimulates tumor suppressors such as p53 and Rb.

If an oncogene mutation (e.g., activated Ras) triggers cell proliferation in cells with intact p53 and pRb, irreversible growth arrest (i.e., senescence) follows. This fate could be avoided by crippling p53 and pRb pathways. Thus, OIS is a potent tumor inhibitor (Fig. 5-24). Activating alterations in other oncogenes also induce OIS in vivo. Active OIS mechanisms distinguish between many benign and malignant tumors, as well as between "premalignant" cell proliferations and frankly malignant ones. That is, benign tumor cells

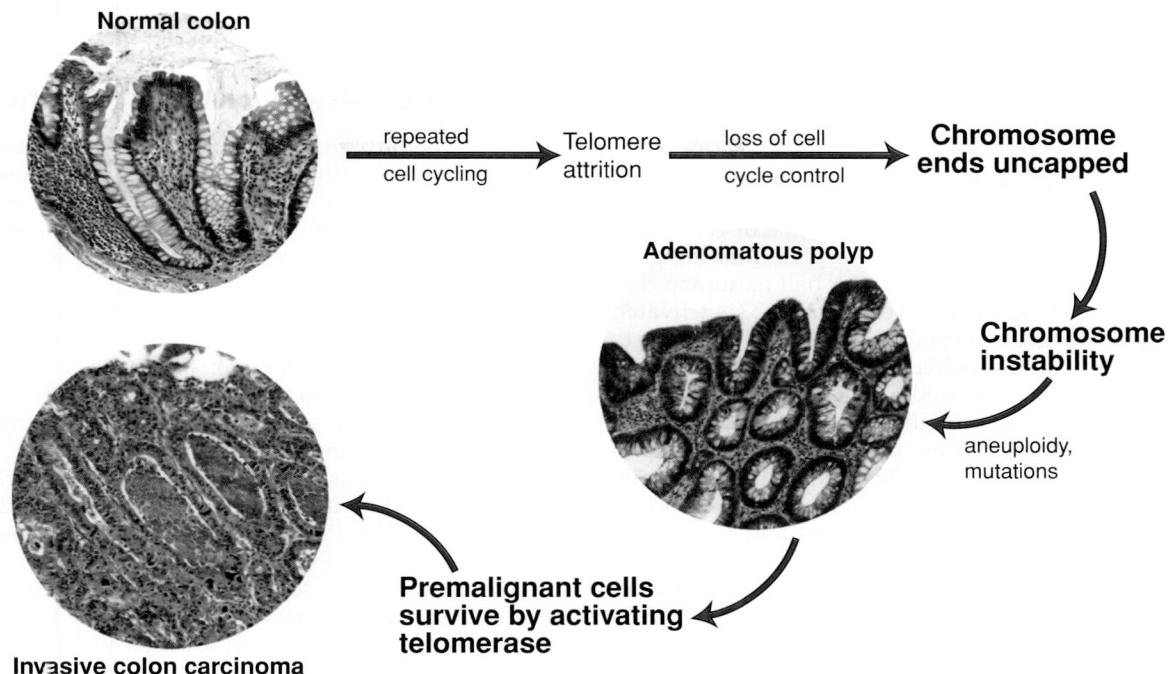

FIGURE 5-23. Role of telomere attrition and subsequent telomere activation in carcinogenesis. Normal colonic mucosa features continuous epithelial renewal, with resulting shortening of telomeres, which leads to uncapping of chromosomal ends. Accumulated DNA damage may impair cell cycle control, allowing development of a variety of mutations. At first, a benign accumulation of colonic epithelial cells (i.e., a colonic adenomatous polyp [or tubular adenoma; see Chapter 19]) grows. The preservation of abnormal cells by telomerase activation allows further mutation to occur and eventuates in malignant transformation.

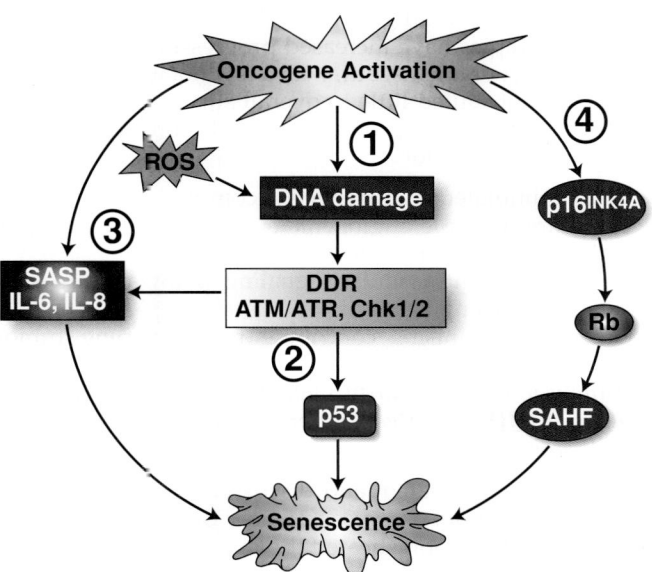

FIGURE 5-24. Oncogene-induced senescence (OIS). Oncogenic stress can elicit cellular responses that eventuate in cellular senescence. **1.** Excessive cell division a result, for example, of oncogene activation, causes oxidative stress and DNA damage to accumulate. **2.** As a consequence, the DNA damage response (DDR) is activated, with p53 expression blocking cell cycle progression. **3.** The same DDR may also activate the senescence-associated secretory phenotype (SASP), which leads affected cells to secrete cytokines that maintain the senescent state (IL-6, IL-8). SASP can also be activated directly by the excessive oncogene activity. **4.** Oncogene activation may directly activate the tumor suppressor p16^{INK4A}, which in turn activates Rb. This leads to the formation of senescence-associated heterochromatin (SAHF), which restricts expression of cell cycle drivers.

can senesce, but advanced malignant tumor cells do not, as exemplified by the fact that benign tumors may respond to IL-8–induced senescence (see above), while their malignant counterparts do not. OIS thus helps prevent benign proliferations from becoming cancers.

In addition to telomerase activation, there are alternative mechanisms of telomere maintenance which may be activated in tumor cells. Once a cell manages to avoid senescence after oncogene activation, however it may do that, it is considered immortal, and may proliferate indefinitely. Thus, loss of those tumor suppressor activities that contribute to cellular senescence is important for emerging cancer cells to become full-fledged tumors.

Programmed Cell Death Prevents Oncogenesis

The total number of cells in any organ reflects a balance between cell division and cell death. Interference with this intricate equilibrium can lead to tumor development. Cell death programs encompass several different pathways (**see Chapter 1**), dysfunction of which is often a fundamental requirement for tumor development. The best understood of these is apoptosis, and its cousin, anoikis.

Apoptosis as an Inhibitor of Cancer

As mentioned above and in **Chapter 1**, apoptosis eliminates damaged or abnormal cells. Apoptotic pathways are activated by errors in DNA replication or repair, detected genetic or metabolic instability, loss of anchoring connections to ECM (**anoikis**) and other stimuli. Since many tumor cell attributes can trigger PCD, tumorigenesis requires that those cells evolve mechanisms to disable apoptosis. There are many known pro- and antiapoptotic proteins that interact in a head-spinning number of ways. To make this topic understandable, we use illustrative examples. Cancers may avoid PCD by impairing proapoptotic activities and/or by augmenting prosurvival functions.

Fighting the Forces of Death

There are many participants in the programs of cell death. The best known is p53, and it is no surprise that the gene for this protein, *TP53*, is mutated in over half of human cancers (see below). As the key angel of cell death, p53 is activated when oncogenic danger is sensed, for example, if damage to cellular DNA cannot be repaired (**see Chapter 1**). Wearing several of its many hats, activated p53 increases transcription of proapoptotic Bcl-2–like proteins and downregulates their prosurvival cousins. In addition, p53 is a BH3-only protein (**see Chapter 1**) and so may meddle directly in Bcl-2 family affairs by binding, for example, prosurvival Bcl-2 or Bcl-xL to force them to release proapoptotic Bad and Bax. These later activate effector caspases and cause the cell to die. It is worth recalling that apoptosis does not elicit florid, cytokine-rich inflammatory responses. Rather, apoptotic cells pass from the world not with a bang but with a whimper—they are quietly removed by macrophages.

Along similar lines, anoikis is a form of apoptosis that is activated when epithelial cell membrane integrins no longer bind their appropriate ECM partners (**see Chapter 1**). Integrins mediate prosurvival signals. When they detach from their extracellular ligands, cells are excessively susceptible to all manners of proapoptotic stimuli. Also, unligated integrins may activate caspase 8 directly. However, in some cancer cells, unbound integrins can maintain survival signaling and so protect from PCD.

The prototypical example of tumor effectiveness of inhibiting apoptosis is follicular lymphoma (**see Chapter 26**). There, the prosurvival protein, Bcl-2, is constitutively activated by a translocation t(8;14) that places its expression under the control of the immunoglobulin heavy-chain promoter. As a result, the normal equilibrium between B-lymphocyte life and death is altered in favor of the former, thus allowing accumulation—or, perhaps, more to the point, insufficient elimination—of excess neoplastic B cells.

Some other tumor types, including lung cancer and non-Hodgkin lymphoma, also express excess Bcl-2. Chromosomal translocation is not the only mechanism by which tumor cells increase Bcl-2 expression. They may suppress production of microRNAs (miRNAs) that repress Bcl-2 expression. Similarly, any impairment of p53 function can increase Bcl-2 production and decrease expression of proapoptotic Bcl-2 binding partners (**see Chapter 1**) and so promote tumor formation.

The issue of PCD and cancer is further complicated by **oncogene-mediated apoptosis**. For example, although Myc transcription factor is generally considered to be oncogenic, if PCD pathways are intact, Myc overproduction induces a default apoptosis pathway. Thus, promotion of cell proliferation by deregulated Myc expression is usually balanced by increased apoptosis. Induction of apoptosis by Myc acts as a molecular safety valve to block cancer development. If Myc-stimulated tumors are to develop, some cells overproducing Myc must also inactivate PCD, whether by overexpressing antiapoptotic proteins or by inactivating apoptosis mediators like p53.

This example illustrates the complexity inherent in the control of apoptosis in cancer development.

Tumors Induce New Blood Vessel Formation

Tumors generally grow faster than do normal tissues, and so consume more nutrients and oxygen. As new growths (neoplasms), tumors' vascular supply is not established, but must be coaxed into existence from pre-existing vessels. From these simple observations, the idea of a drama, called **tumor angiogenesis**, grew. A cytokine, dubbed, "tumor angiogenesis factor," was postulated as the villain.

The evil angiogenic factor was renamed: **vascular endothelial growth factor (VEGF)**. Produced and secreted by tumor cells, it bound to receptors on endothelial cells (ECs), stimulated capillary sprouting from pre-existing vasculature, and elicited new vessels to feed the tumor. The stage was set. A plot was to unfold: the tumor's wicked plans would be foiled by inhibiting VEGF and so blocking tumor angiogenesis. The inescapable denouement was decided: tumors would halt in their tracks.

According to this script, suppressing VEGF-stimulated angiogenesis would starve and suffocate tumors. Many pharmaceuticals were devised to target VEGF-driven angiogenesis, with great optimism. Antibodies to VEGF could prevent the cytokine from reaching its receptor; inhibiting VEGF receptor could block VEGF-triggered signaling; targeting downstream intermediates could stop EC activation. Best yet, since these therapies aimed at nonneoplastic ECs, the genetic plasticity of cancer cells could not rescue their servile vasculature from inhibition. What could go wrong?

Actually, a lot could go wrong. And did. To date, antiangiogenic therapies have increased progression-free survival for many cancer patients, but, with a few notable exceptions, they have contributed little to overall survival and perhaps even helped tumors to grow and spread more aggressively. Reasons for this include:

- VEGF-stimulated angiogenesis is complex and imperfect
- There are multiple angiogenic cytokines, with multiple, and promiscuous, receptors
- Networks of intracellular signaling pathways are activated during angiogenesis
- Diverse mechanisms contribute to developing tumor blood supply
- *Perhaps most importantly, hypoxia and <u>hypoxia-inducible factor-1 (HIF-1)</u> protect tumor viability and enhance its malignancy*

These are interrelated, and discussed below. They shed light on how tumors progress and how they can stubbornly resist increasingly sophisticated therapies.

VEGF-Stimulated Tumor Angiogenesis

Normal capillary ECs contact each other via tight junctions and rest on continuous basement membranes. Such vessels tend to follow fairly direct courses through tissue, to become venules. They are made, whether during embryogenesis or following injury, by balanced combinations and sequences of soluble factors that allow vessels to form and then mature. As a result, blood delivery is orderly and fluid leakage is minimal.

VEGF-stimulated capillary formation occurs by sprouting angiogenesis (see below). Physiologically, this is followed by a maturational sequence whereby the various components mentioned above are produced or recruited. This is not what happens when tumor-produced VEGF stimulates blood vessel formation. Tumor-induced sprouting angiogenesis produces imperfect, leaky, poorly formed capillaries.

Briefly, the following steps occur during this process:

1. ECs, stimulated by VEGF, dissolve intercellular connections and basement membrane.
2. Migrating "tip cells" make filopodia, and produce **matrix metalloproteinases (MMPs)** to help them migrate through the **ECM**, up the gradient toward the source of VEGF. This endothelial–mesenchymal transition resembles the epithelial–mesenchymal transition (EMT) which is part of tumor metastasis (see below).
3. These cells are followed by "stalk cells," which support and sustain tip cell migration.
4. Continued VEGF production impedes maturation, counteracts other maturation-related cytokines, limits basement membrane investiture and adequate recruitment of pericytes to stabilize the blood vessel.
5. Consequently, the tumor vessel is leaky and tortuous, and provides oxygen and nutrients less effectively than do capillaries in normal tissues. That is, the hypoxic condition that stimulates VEGF production to begin with (see below) continues. This leakiness elevates extracellular fluid pressure, impeding diffusion of chemotherapeutic drugs into the tumor. It also facilitates tumor cell invasion and metastasis.

The VEGF Family of Cytokines

VEGF is not one cytokine, but a family of related proteins, some of which have multiple forms. VEGF-A is the best understood. In the context of hypoxia, cells (including tumor cells) express **hypoxia-inducible factors** (HIFs, see below), particularly **HIF-1**. HIF-1 is a transcription factor that stimulates many genes, including VEGFs. VEGF-A binds multiple receptors, such as VEGFR2, and activates multiple cascades of downstream signaling (Fig. 5-25). As shown, the consequences are diverse and contribute to subverting otherwise physiologic EC processes to serve the tumor's purposes.

Multiple Cytokine Mediators of Tumor Angiogenesis

In addition to the VEGF family of factors, an array of other cytokines stimulate and facilitate tumor vascularization. These include VEGF-like proteins, angiopoietins, growth factors, and enzymes (Table 5-5). Not all derive from tumor cells themselves, but may be made by other tumor-associated cell populations (Fig. 5-26).

Blood Supply to Tumors Beyond Sprouting Angiogenesis

Tumors secure vascular access by multiple means, independently of sprouting angiogenesis. Other mechanisms include:

1. Intussusceptive microvascular growth (IMG)
2. Vascular co-option
3. Stimulating endothelial progenitor cells (EPCs) to produce new vessels
4. Vasculogenic mimicry (VM)
5. The role of **CSCs** in tumor blood vessel formation

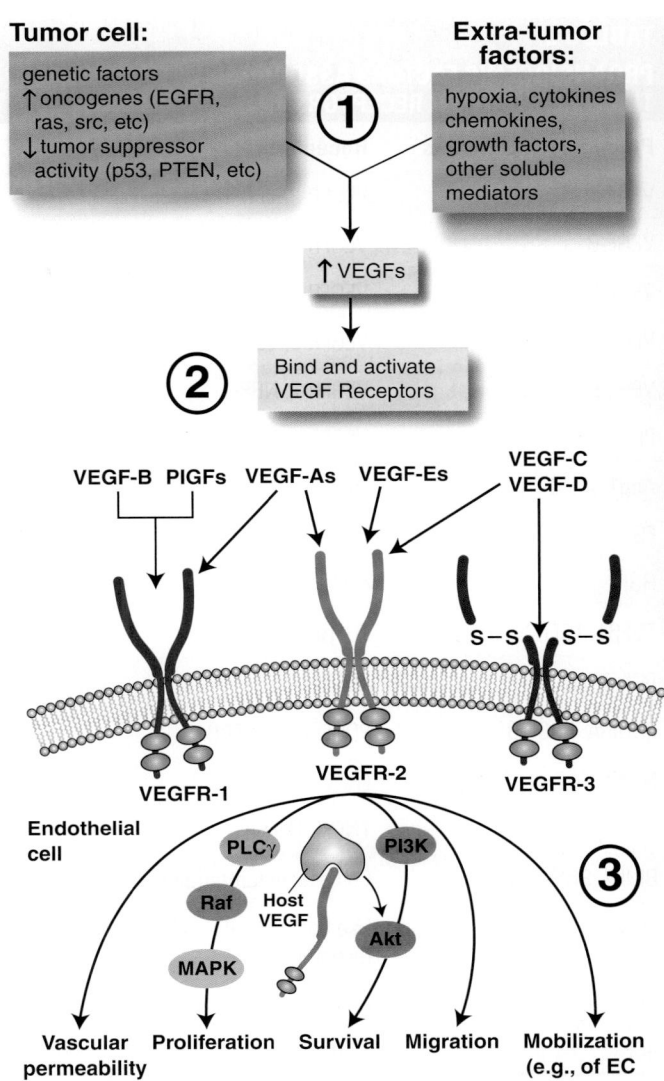

FIGURE 5-25. The VEGF system and its effects. 1. Under the influence of factors generated by tumor cells (left; increased expression of certain oncogenes or decreased activity or tumor suppressors) or coming from other sources (tumor-related stroma, external environment, etc.), several vascular endothelial growth factors (VEGFs) are produced. **2.** These bind the several VEGF receptors, the principal of which is VEGFR-2. **3.** Downstream signaling from these receptors has diverse effects on vascular endothelium, including increasing vascular permeability, activating cell proliferation and survival mechanisms, inducing inmigration of endothelial cells, and mobilizing progenitor cells to the area, to help form new blood vessels.

These different mechanisms are illustrated in Figure 5-27, and described briefly below.

Intussusceptive Microvascular Growth

In IMG, a capillary wall lining grows into the blood vessel's lumen and divides the vessel into two. This entails basement membrane degradation, which is followed by formation of a new basement membrane from ECM materials brought into the evolving bifurcation. The new structure then recruits an investiture of pericytes and myofibroblasts. Like sprouting angiogenesis, IMG may occur under physiologic circumstances (Fig. 5-27, left frame).

TABLE 5-5
PROANGIOGENIC FACTORS ASSOCIATED WITH TUMORS AND THEIR RECEPTORS

Proangiogenic Factors	Receptors
VEGF-A	VEGFR-2, VEGFR-1, NRP-1, NRP-2
VEGF-B	VEGFR-1, NRP-1
VEGF-C	VEGFR-3, VEGFR-2, NRP-2
VEGF-D	VEGFR-3, VEGFR-2, NRP-2
VEGF-Es	VEGFR-2, NRP-1
PlGF	VEGFR-1, NRP-1, NRP-2
Ang1, Ang4	Tie2
FGF2	FGFR2, FGFR3
HGF	c-Met
TGFβ1, TGFβ2, TGFβ3	TGFβR2
EGF, TGFα	EGFR
PDGF-A, PDGF-B	PDGFRα, PDGFRβ
MMP	LRP
TNFα	TNFRI, TNFRII
BMP2, BMP4, BMP6	Complex heterotetrameric receptors
Ephrins	Use both cognate and other EGFR-like receptors
SDF-1 (CXCL12)	CXCR4
SCF	c-Kit

Ang = angiopoietin; BMP = bone morphogenic protein; EGF = epidermal growth factor; FGF = fibroblast growth factor; HGF = hepatocyte growth factor; MMP = matrix metalloproteinases; NRP = neuropilin; PDGF = platelet-derived growth factor; PlGF = placental growth factor; SCF = stem cell factor; SDF-1 = stromal-derived factor-1; TGF = transforming growth factor; TNF = tumor necrosis factor; VEGF = vascular endothelial growth factor.

This mechanism entails very little EC proliferation, and occurs rapidly. Tumors that have received radiation or antiangiogenic therapy have been shown to switch from sprouting angiogenesis to IMG in vivo. Further, because IMG-formed vessels include fully formed basement membranes and adventitial cells, they are better formed and structurally more sound. Multiple cytokines, including VEGFs, PDGF, FGF2, Ang-1, and erythropoietin facilitate this type of vessel growth.

Vascular Co-Option

In this scenario, tumor cells essentially take over normal blood vessels serving the tissue in which the tumor is growing and subvert that vessel to supply the tumor. This does not entail new vessel formation, but simply diverting an existing vessel to the cancer's needs. Primary or metastatic tumors involving highly vascular organs—such as the liver, lungs, and brain—are most likely to use this mechanism. For co-option to work well, the tumor must mimic the architecture of the host tissue. Thus, a colon carcinoma metastatic to

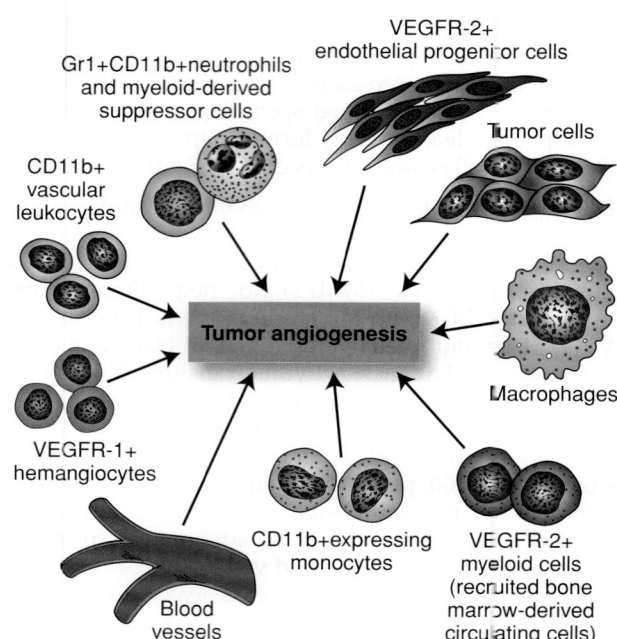

FIGURE 5-26. Diverse populations of bone marrow–derived cells that participate in angiogenesis. Circulating cells derived from bone marrow progenitors contribute to the development of tumor-related blood vessels. These include macrophages, early cells in the myeloid (neutrophil) series as well as neutrophils and myeloid-derived suppressor cells, endothelial progenitor cells, and tumor cells themselves.

the liver would grow along hepatic sinusoids and replace hepatocytes that had previously been there.

Recruitment of EPCs

In postembryonic life, bone marrow–derived EPCs persist in the marrow. These CXCR4-bearing cells inhabit that SDF-1 (CXCL12)–rich environment. Influenced by VEGF-stimulated MMP9, EPCs leave the bone marrow. As indicated above, tumors produce SDF-1, which stimulates these errant EPCs to migrate toward the tumor and contribute to ongoing tumor blood vessel formation.

Vasculogenic Mimicry

Tumor cells possess great plasticity in expressing their neoplastic phenotype and may themselves line vascular spaces. This mechanism of tumor vascularization requires extensive remodeling of connective tissue by the tumor, which occurs under the influence of MMPs 2 and 4. These cleave an ECM component (lamin-5γ2), to produce fragments that stimulate tumor cell migration and invasion.

The tumor cells then mimic vascular endothelium. In lining such blood vessels, tumor cells are in direct contact with circulating blood, which facilitates tumor metastasis. Because of the phenotypic plasticity involved, it should come as no surprise that CSCs may participate in VM.

This happens not infrequently in malignant melanomas and glioblastomas, but occurs with many other types of malignancies as well. The presence of VM indicates a poor prognosis.

Role of CSCs in Tumor Blood Vessel Formation

CSCs are the cells that remake a tumor after treatment with radiation or chemotherapy (see below). They carry cell

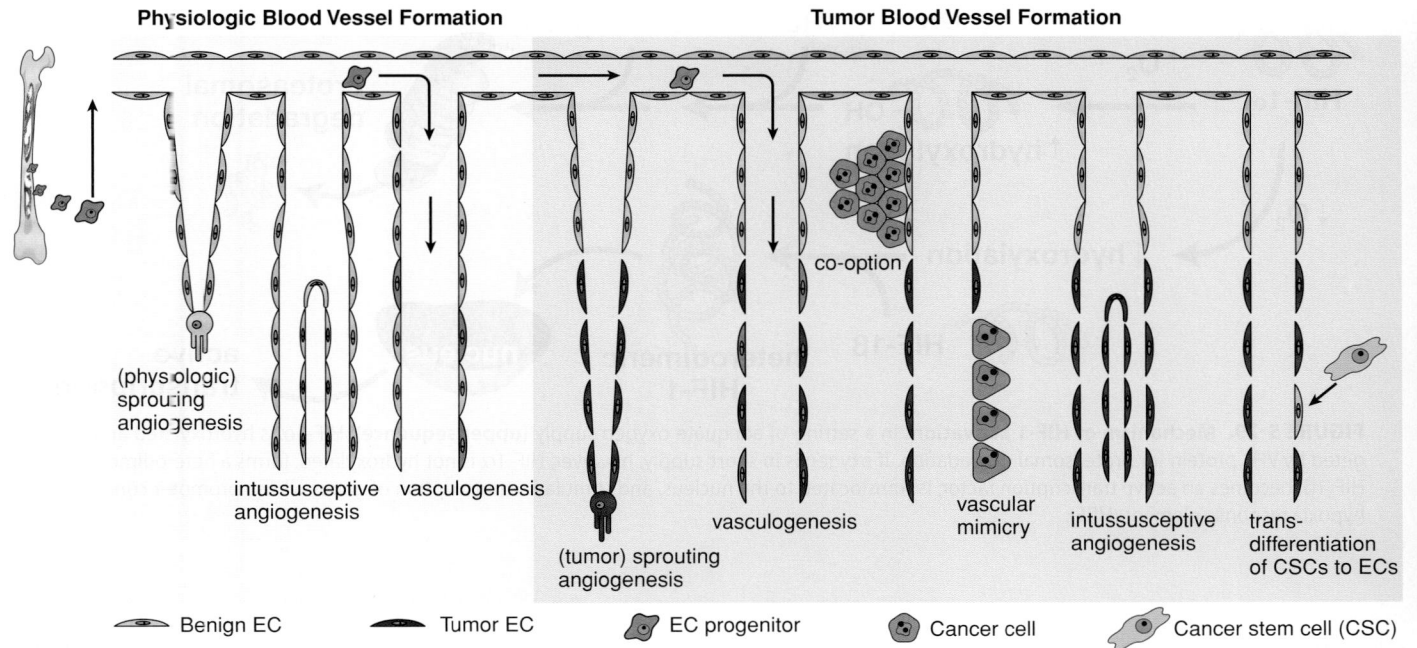

FIGURE 5-27. Mechanisms of Physiologic and Tumor Vascularization. Physiologic (left). In normal settings, increased vascularity generally occurs by three basic mechanisms, which are sprouting angiogenesis, intussusceptive angiogenesis, and vasculogenesis, as described in the text. **Tumors (right).** Tumors may exploit these three mechanisms, but may also utilize other approaches to ensuring adequate nutrient and oxygen supply, including co-option of vascular structures previously committed to normal structures and differentiation of CSCs into endothelial cells (see text).

membrane markers CD133 and CD44 (VE-cadherin). CSCs may differentiate directly into blood vessel cells, including ECs and pericytes, as an additional mechanism of VM. This occurs in a variety of tumors. For some tumors, most pericytes may come from CSCs. CSCs are associated with high levels of VEGF and SDF-1, which (see above) stimulate EPCs to migrate to the tumor to make new vessels.

Hypoxic Environments Sustain Tumor Survival and Spread

When oxygen supplies are compromised, cells respond by producing **HIF-1**. The consequences of this simple survival mechanism for normal tissues include improved vascularization (e.g., of an ischemic myocardium). In the case

of tumor cells exposed to hypoxia, HIF-1 does much more than to stimulate increased blood supply. It has far-reaching impact on many aspects of the tumor–patient relationship, including stimulating tumor growth, spread, aggressiveness, and resistance to therapies (Fig. 5-28). Mechanisms underlying these phenomena are described below.

HIF-1

HIF-1 is a heterodimer of two subunits: HIF-1β, which is expressed constitutively, and HIF-1β, which responds to O_2 concentration. Both are cytoplasmic proteins. In situations of high (physiologic) oxygen tension, HIF-1β is modified by hydroxylation of specific proline and asparagine residues. This modification recruits VHL tumor suppressor protein,

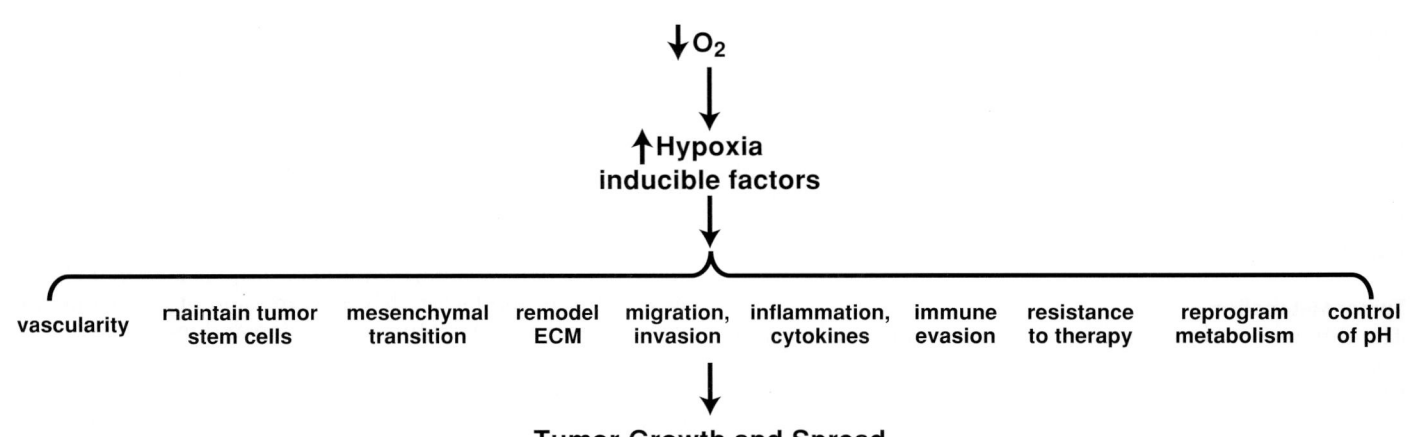

FIGURE 5-28. Hypoxia and its effects on tumor behavior.

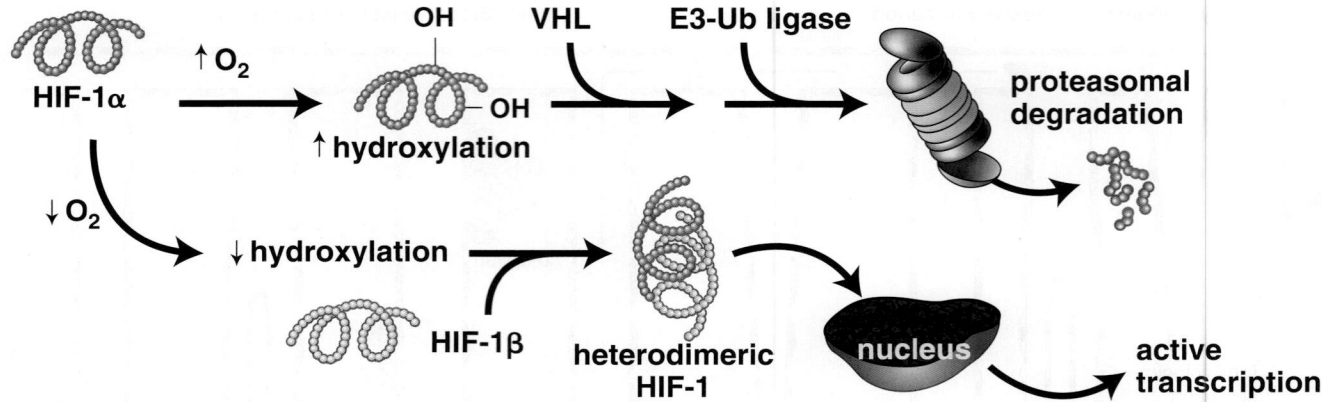

FIGURE 5-29. Mechanism of HIF-1 activation. In a setting of adequate oxygen supply (**upper sequence**), HIF-1α is hydroxylated and targeted by VHL protein for proteasomal degradation. If oxygen is in short supply, however, HIF-1α is not hydroxylated, forms a heterodimer with HIF-1β, becomes an active transcription factor, is translocated to the nucleus, and stimulates transcription of genes whose promoter contains a hypoxia response element (HRE).

which then recruits an E3 Ub ligase (**see Chapter 1**), leading to HIF-1β proteolytic degradation (Fig. 5-29).

If, on the other hand, oxygen tension is low, HIF-1α is not hydroxylated and degraded, but binds to HIF-1β. Resulting active, heterodimeric HIF-1 translocates to the nucleus, where it binds gene promoters containing hypoxia-responsive elements and activates transcription of responsive genes, which include those mediating:

- angiogenesis
- metabolic reprogramming
- facilitating tumor spread by effects on ECM, EMT, cell motility, invasion, metastasis
- CSC survival and numbers
- immune evasion
- resistance to therapeutic interventions

Each will be addressed in turn. In considering (see below) how HIF-1 affects tumor survival, growth, and resilience, it is worth bearing in mind that use of antiangiogenic therapies may elicit or magnify tumor hypoxic responses, and so may follow the law of unintended consequences.

Angiogenesis

As indicated above, tumor hypoxia triggers transcriptional activation mediated by HIF-1. Among the genes whose expression increases in this way are VEGFs, angiopoietins, SCF, PDGFs, PlGF, and SDF-1 (CXCL12). It bears emphasis, in this vein, that sprouting angiogenesis elicited in this fashion is less efficient than physiologic angiogenesis, and yields immature and abnormal blood vessels that only marginally supply tumors' needs. The result of this is continued tumor hypoxia, with all the consequences listed.

Tumor Metabolism

The differences between metabolic patterns in tumors and normal tissues are addressed later. This discussion focuses how HIF-1 reprograms tumor cell metabolism, and how that reprogramming affects tumor resilience and survival. *These effects decrease tumor cell dependence on oxygen and protect them from the effects of this metabolic change:*

1. decreasing mitochondrial electron transport chain (ETC) activity: HIF-1 upregulates genes (e.g., for miR-210) that inhibit oxidative phosphorylation by directly interfering with the process and by impeding production of ETC components. Simultaneously, there is evidence that HIF-1 improves ETC efficiency.
2. increased mitophagy and decreased mitochondrial biogenesis: HIF-1 accelerates removal of damaged mitochondria and impedes generation of new mitochondria. This lowers both cellular respiration and ETC generation of ROS.
3. increased reliance on glucose and glycolysis for energy generation: Glycolysis becomes the main source of energy, as well as of building blocks for new cells. HIF-1 increases production of GLUT1 glucose transporter and glycolytic enzymes, and facilitates glycogen production from glucose not immediately needed.
4. decreased fatty acid oxidation: Fatty acid uptake increases and fatty acids are redirected to serve as building blocks for cellular proliferative activity.
5. pH and redox balance: Glycolysis produces pyruvate, and HIF-1 upregulates expression of lactate dehydrogenase (LDH) isomers, which converts pyruvate to lactate. HIF-1 also increases transporters to export lactate, ion exchangers to export H and carbonic anhydrase, to protect from pH and redox imbalances.

Decreased reliance on oxygen has a further effect of limiting the effectiveness of radiation therapy, which relies in part on ROS to kill tumor cells.

Tumor Spread

HIF-1 helps orchestrate all steps of the process of tumor invasion and dissemination. These steps are discussed in more detail below. Here, it should be emphasized that HIF-1, as a transcription factor, drives expression of genes that are central to all aspects of tumor invasion and metastasis.

Hypoxia and Cancer Stem Cells

Cancer stem cells (CSCs, see below) mediate cancer resilience and survival; HIF-1 helps mediate CSC resilience and survival. CSCs are pluripotent and dedifferentiated.

HIF-1–activated genes OCTA, NANOG, and others, mediate this phenotype. Simultaneously, HIF-1–upregulated expression of IL-6 and IL-8 helps to enrich tumors in CSCs in the face of cytotoxic chemotherapy, just as HIF-1 upregulation of drug-exporting functions (multidrug resistance genes, or MDR) facilitates CSC survival during therapy (see below). Another hypoxia-responsive gene, CD47, helps perpetuate stemness and protect CSCs from innate host antitumor responses. Some of these effects are indirect, in settings in which HIF-1 activates transcription of secondary (and tertiary) transcription factors that in turn increase expression of genes that sustain CSCs.

Immune Evasion

Tumors thrive in part because they can avoid destruction by cells of innate and adaptive immune systems (**see below and Chapter 4**). HIF-1 plays an important role in both. It upregulates tumor cell expression of CD47, which blocks macrophage-mediated tumor cell phagocytosis. HIF-1 promotes cancer cell expression of PD-L1, which protects them from T-cell–mediated cytolysis. It also stimulates migration of myeloid-derived suppressor cells (MDSCs) and regulatory T cells (Treg), which inhibit cytotoxic T-cell activity. Interestingly, HIF-1 expression in macrophages is important in driving their T-cell suppression.

This story of tumor angiogenesis illustrates the complexity of tumor survival mechanisms. Tumors clearly have at their disposal diverse, redundant, and alternative ways of sustaining their activities. Many of the mechanisms discussed in this one section represent multiple, quite different, pathways to a goal (e.g., oxygen supply). Further, many are triggered by changes in tumor environment (e.g., hypoxia) or epigenetics. As such, tumors can access them quickly, without the time-consuming need to have generated subclones carrying specific mutations and then for a selective pressure to allow those cells in subclones to outcompete cells lacking those mutations.

This story also illustrates potential unforeseen consequences that may await when we believe we understand a phenomenon, treat patients based on that assumption, and then discover otherwise. Antiangiogenic therapies, applied with the intention of using induced hypoxia to kill tumors, may do the unanticipated—they may stimulate tumor growth, spread, virulence and resistance to therapy.

Most Tumor Lethality Reflects Invasion and Metastasis

Over 90% of cancer deaths occur because tumors invade and metastasize. While we know a lot about tumorigenesis, metastasis remains poorly understood. What is clear is that invasion and dissemination are multistep processes, involving major phenotypic and behavioral changes in tumor cells and tumor-associated cells. Many of these changes are epigenetic (see below) and so are highly plastic and rapidly changeable.

Among the steps in tumor invasion and metastasis are (Fig. 5-30):

1. Traversing the basement membrane underlying the in situ tumor
2. Moving through subjacent connective tissue
3. Surviving in the circulation

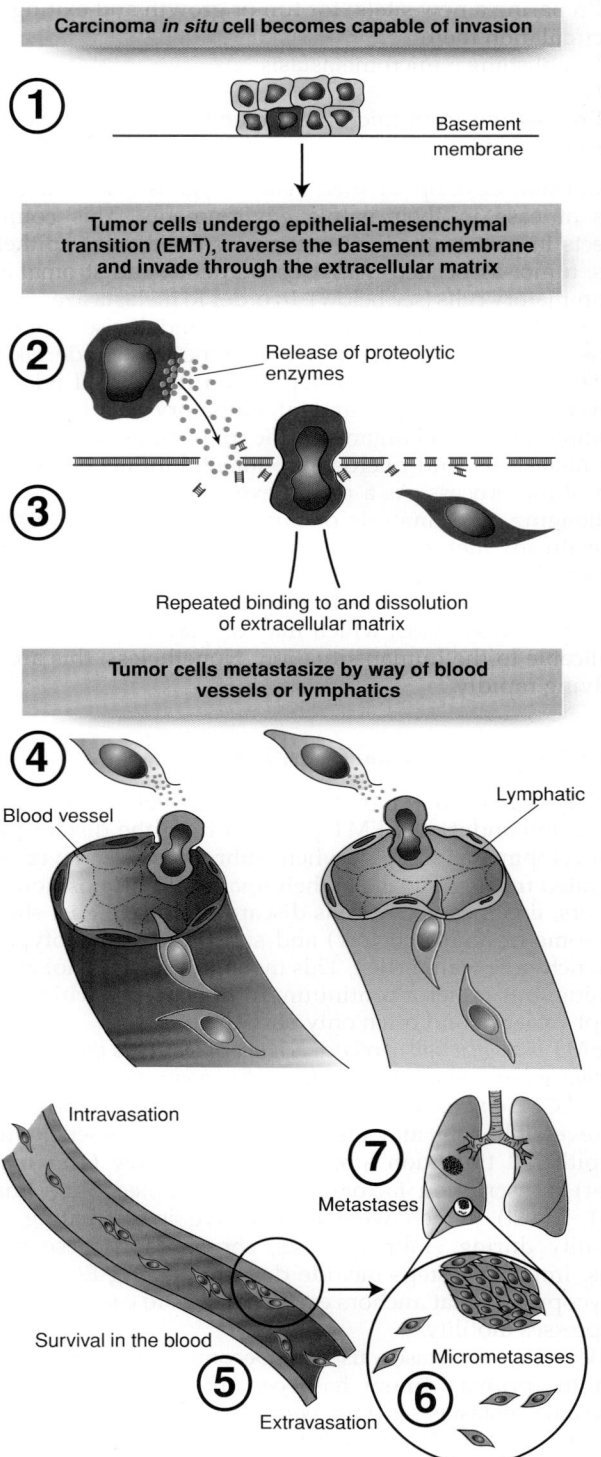

FIGURE 5-30. Mechanisms of tumor invasion and metastasis. 1. Tumor cells first acquires the ability to bind ECM components, by expressing several adhesion molecules. **2.** The tumor undergoes epithelial-mesenchymal transition (EMT) and traverses the basement membrane. **3.** Proteolytic enzymes released from the tumor cells, degrade the ECM. **4.** After moving through the extracellular environment, the invading cells penetrate blood vessels and lymphatics similarly. **5.** After surviving in the circulation, tumor cells exit the vascular system. **6.** They establish micrometastases at that site. **7.** These micrometastases grow into gross masses of metastatic tumor.

4. Preparing a new site(s) for tumor growth and exiting the circulation there
5. Establishing a micrometastasis
6. Dormancy
7. Progressing from micrometastatic foci into macroscopic tumor masses

Cancers develop in their native organs, the malignant cells at ease in their native environments. This comfort reflects in part to their interactions with adjacent epithelial cells, tumor-associated matrix constituents, and stromal and inflammatory cells (see below). In order to metastasize, cancer cells must dissolve many of those bonds and devise a commodious ecosystem at a distant site. This is no small undertaking.

The processes involved depend on tumor–cell relationships with nearby stroma and inflammatory cells, circulation dynamics, ECM and organ-specific contributions to invasion and metastasis, and microenvironmental influences at each step of the process. As a result, experimental study is very challenging, and analysis of human samples after tumors have already metastasized often does not shed light on how metastasis has come to pass. Some of our understanding reflects inferences drawn from specific in vitro and animal experimental systems, which may or may not be generally applicable to the human situation. Nonetheless, this area is evolving rapidly.

Epithelial–Mesenchymal Transition

EMT is central to tumor invasion and metastasis. Tumor cells commandeer the EMT program from the distant past, in developmental biology, when embryonic germ layer cells migrated from primordia to their final anatomic positions. In cancers, this means that cells discard their epithelial shackles (some or all, see below) and substitute a phenotype of mesenchymal wanderlust. This metamorphosis is not all-or-nothing, but rather a continuum of phenotypes which cells adopt variably, and often only partially.

EMT is a collection of related behavioral patterns that lead cells to remove intercellular bonds, digest basement membranes, rearrange ECM, and navigate through that matrix. EMT programs are reversible: cells may undergo the reverse, mesenchymal-to-epithelial transition afterward. Several key (and many other) transcription factors (colorfully named Slug, Snail, Zeb1, Twist), which were once active in mediating cell mobility during embryogenesis, choreograph these functions. Important steps include downregulating E-cadherin, a glycoprotein that anchors epithelial cells to each other and suppresses motility.

Because metastases usually become clinically evident after the primary tumor has been discovered (and, often, removed), metastasis is often perceived as a late occurrence—spread from an already substantial primary tumor. However, this appears not to be the case, at least for many tumors. Instead, EMT is often activated early during tumor development. Cells may even show EMT features while still preneoplastic. Thus, metastases too small to be apparent are frequently in place even before the primary tumor comes to clinical attention.

What Elicits EMT?

Tumor cells express EMT programs under the influence of factors derived both from tumor cells and from tumor-associated cells—adjacent inflammatory, connective tissue, vascular, and similar cells. Some are conveyed as soluble mediators, or as membrane-bound vesicles—exosomes (see below)—from tumor or associated cells. Cellular phenotypes and many soluble mediators that activate EMT in developing tumors resemble those in healing wounds (see **Chapter 3**), in which tumor-associated nonneoplastic cell types participate. EMT-stimulating substances, delivered as soluble cytokines or by exosomes include cell membrane molecules, like **Notch-1** and **Wnt family** proteins, signaling molecules such as β-catenin and AKT, cytokines like IL-6, TGFβ, TNFα, and others. These reversibly reactivate EMT programs that had been quiescent in cancer cells since embryogenesis.

Tumor Cell Migration in Clusters

Cancer cells may invade individually, but often do so as heterogeneous nests of variably cohesive cells. Central cells in these packs continue to express epithelial E-cadherin which helps them to remain bound to each other. The lead cells of these groups may be either tumor cells or tumor-associated stromal cells, which secrete enzymes that help clear a path through the connective tissue to help the squad of invading tumor cells migrate.

Among these intrusive clusters are cells with a **CSC** phenotype (see below), which are therapy-resistant and which are key to effective metastasis. Phenotypic diversity among collectives of invading cells allows a division of labor that appears to be critical for the ability to establishing metastatic foci, for which purpose the ability to retain and resume epithelial phenotype appears to be obligatory.

Tumor-Associated Cells

Nonneoplastic cells associated with tumors constitute about half of all cells within tumor masses. They include macrophages, leukocytes, fibroblasts, vascular ECs, neuronal cells, and fat cells (Fig. 5-31). Many of these resided originally

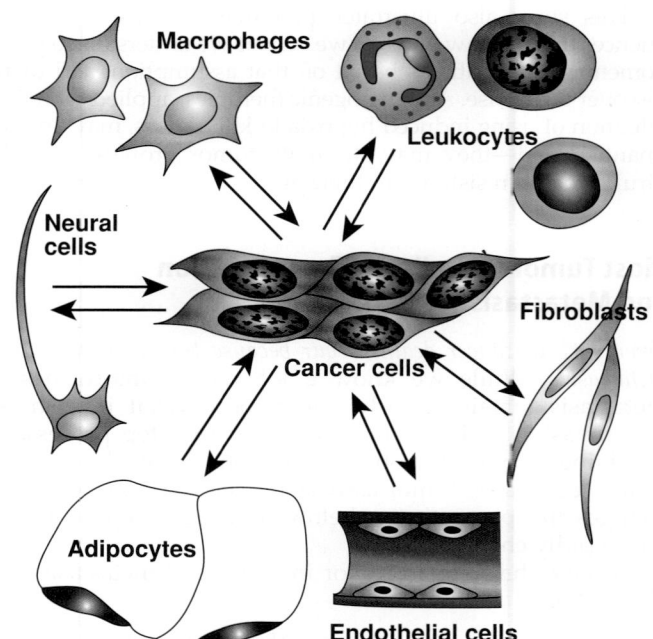

FIGURE 5-31. The cancer cell ecosystem. The developing tumor cells interact with the nonmalignant cells in their environment via production of soluble and other mediators.

in the ECM, but others are of bone marrow origin and are recruited to the site of the expanding tumor. All of these non-tumor cells can influence the behavior of the cancer, both at its site of origin and at locations of metastases.

The Contributions of Tumor Stroma

Stimulation of tumor cell invasiveness by nearby stromal elements plays an important role in the ability of cancer cells to breach the basement membrane and traverse underlying connective tissues. Tumors co-opt normal stromal cell functions, trigger inflammatory reactions, and recruit additional cells to the area of the developing malignancy to further subvert anatomic and other barriers to invasion. Perversely, components of inflammatory and wound repair processes **(see Chapters 2, 3, and 4)** that protect against, for example, pathogens are then brought to bear to render the individual susceptible to cancer cell invasiveness. *The players in inflammatory and wound healing that are observed nearby tumors are orchestrated by the developing cancers themselves* (Fig. 5-32) *and should not be misconstrued as protecting the host.*

- *MMPs.* These are a family of endopeptidases that are normally regulated by tissue inhibitors of MMPs (TIMPs). MMPs are synthesized and secreted by normal cells during physiologic tissue remodeling, at which times the balance between MMPs and TIMPs is strictly regulated. By contrast, invasive and metastatic phenotypes of cancer cells are characterized by dysregulation of the MMP-TIMP balance.

- *Lysyl oxidase (LOX).* This secreted enzyme helps establish cross-links among collagens and elastins. LOX increases ECM rigidity, and facilitates tumor cell migration. It also helps retain bone marrow–derived tumor-associated cells to areas of tumor establishment and growth.

In many tumors, invasiveness correlates directly with increased MMP expression. In many of these same tumors, TIMPs are decreased. MMPs in invading cancers may be produced by the tumor cells themselves, by surrounding stromal cells or both, depending on the particular neoplasm. MMPs secreted by stromal cells may be bound to integrins on the surface of the tumor cells, thus providing particularly high local concentrations of protease activity precisely where the tumor needs it in order to invade. Deregulated MMP activity permits cancer cells to enter and traverse the ECM.

Tumor cell motility is enhanced by upregulation of CXCR4 chemokine receptor in cancer cells at the invasion front. Interestingly, the invading cells induce nearby stromal cells to secrete SDF-1 (also called CXCL12), the ligand for this receptor.

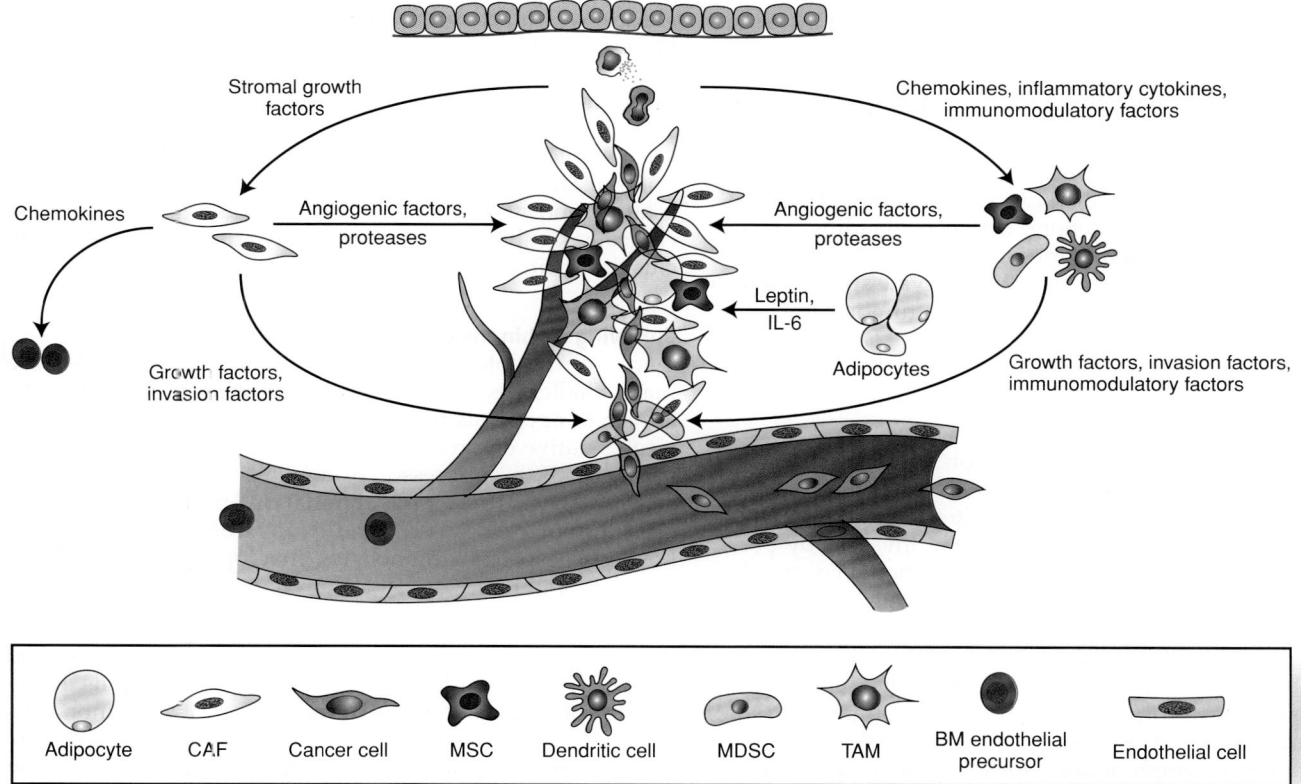

FIGURE 5-32. Tumor cell–stromal interactions involved in invasion and metastasis. Stroma adjacent to tumor is critical to the survival of tumor cells in place and to their dissemination. Such "cancerized stroma" contains bone marrow–derived elements (see Fig. 5-26), including myeloid-derived suppressor cells (MDSCs), dendritic cells, tumor-associated macrophages (TAMs), fibroblasts, adipocytes, and endothelial cells. Cytokines, chemokines, and other mediators produced by tumor cells, as well as influences of tissue destruction and hypoxia, recruit TAMs, MDSCs, cancer-associated fibroblasts (CAFs), and mesenchymal stem cells (MSCs). MDSCs and TAMs are present at the invading tumor front—points where the basement membrane is being broken down and the tumor cells are infiltrating the stroma. These cells produce angiogenic factors, proteases, and other factors that promote tumor invasion. CAFs produce similar facilitators, and bring marrow-derived blood vessel precursor cells to generate new blood vessels.

- **Marrow-derived suppressor cells (MDSC).** Tumors recruit these cells from the blood and bone marrow. They are at the edges of developing tumors and affect host responses to tumors (see below). MDSCs also secrete MMPs, which help to degrade basement membrane and ECM. They stimulate angiogenesis by secreting VEGF and PDGF.
- **Tumor-associated macrophages (TAMs).** These cells congregate at areas in which the basement membrane is breaking down. Like MDSCs, they secrete proteases, particularly urokinase plasminogen activator (uPA), which converts plasminogen to plasmin. The latter, in turn, helps digest type IV collagen in basement membranes. TAMs also produce cathepsin proteases in response to IL-4 made by tumor cells, further augmenting tumor invasiveness.
- **Carcinoma-associated fibroblasts (CAFs).** Like TAMs, CAFs produce proteases that facilitate tumor cell invasion. They also synthesize growth factors and angiogenic factors, and recruit precursor cell from the marrow, to become vascular endothelium.
- **Adipocytes.** The stroma in which many tumors arise contains adipocytes. Cross talk between these cells and tumor cells facilitates early stromal invasion by the malignant cells. Fat cells near tumors often express a particular MMP that assists cancer cell in traversing surrounding connective tissues. Adipocyte-derived IL-6 stimulates tumor cell invasiveness. Leptin produced by adipocytes (**see Chapter 13**) induces macrophages to secrete proinflammatory cytokines, which, in turn, promote invasion and metastasis.
- **Lymphocytes.** T cells may facilitate tumor invasiveness via TAMs. CD4+ lymphocyte-activated TAMs can elicit EGFR-related activation in some types of cancers.

The combination of these and other elements by developing tumors is sometimes called cancerized stroma. It should be noted that many interactions between invading cancer cells and their stromal accessories in crime constitute a positive feedback loop: tumors recruit and activate stromal cells, which repay the favor by magnifying the tumor's invasive tendencies.

Invading the Circulation

Invading cells penetrate lymphatic or vascular channels. **Intravasation** (penetration into blood vessels) provides a route for migration to faraway body sites. Tumor-associated capillaries (see above) are not completely invested by pericytes, show increased permeability, and remodel constantly. In addition, TAMs produce EGF and tumor cells secrete CSF-1, both of which enhance intravasation. MMPs 1 and 2, as well as other tumor and stromal cell products, increase tumor-induced blood vessel leakiness and facilitate their invasion.

Lymphatic invasion conducts tumor cells' transfer to the lymph nodes, where they generally remain in place. Collective cell migration to lymph nodes appears to be independent of spread through blood vessels, and each may be the preferred mode of dissemination for specific tumors. In lymph nodes, communications between lymphatics and venous tributaries may allow the cells access to the systemic blood circulation.

Circulating Tumor Cells

CTCs are tumor cells that are in the bloodstream. While their role in metastasis is debatable, they are useful in assessing

tumor burden and, perhaps more importantly, tumor persistence after therapy, as well as response to treatment. They are among three tumor products that are assayed in the blood, the others (**see Chapter 35**) being **cell-free DNA (cfDNA)** and **exosomes**, which are vesicles derived from tumor cells and contain tumor DNA, RNA, and/or protein.

CTCs are harvested from blood, or sometimes, from the bone marrow, and identified by their cell membrane epithelial markers, usually epithelial cell adhesion molecule (EpCAM) or epithelial cytokeratins (CKs). They are commonly used to assess prognosis and follow tumors during therapy. Other means of identification, whether by protein or RNA analysis, have been used, and specific modifications of this approach have been used to quantify CSCs (see below) and cancer cells that express mesenchymal markers in the blood.

CTCs have broad biologic significance. They offer fertile material for studying cancer progression. Also, specific circulating cell populations may be helpful in assessing risk for metastatic disease, or development of metastatic recurrences: in particular, circulating host cell types that help form premetastatic niches (see below) or CSCs, which are felt to be the cells that initiate tumor metastases.

As indicated, CTCs include individual cells and cell clusters. Since they are assayed in peripheral blood and bone marrow, they must be able to pass through pulmonary capillaries, which act as a filtration system. Although lung capillaries may be as small as 8 μm in caliber, which is smaller than both single tumor cells and cell clusters, both may pass through even these small vessels. Cell clusters can do so by stringing themselves out, single file.

The role of individual CTCs in generating metastases is unclear. The efficiency with which single CTCs become metastatic deposits is very low. Most opinion now holds that clinically significant metastases derive from CSC-containing clusters of circulating cells.

Surviving Within the Circulation

Once in the bloodstream, circulating cancer cells face many challenges. They must avoid anoikis (**see Chapter 1**), a form of apoptosis triggered by loss of ECM anchors from a cell's native environment. Some cells achieve this by activating TrkB, a suppressor of anoikis. They must, as well, survive shear stress and elimination, particularly by NK cells. Tumor cells survive and extravasate with the help of host cells, especially monocytes/macrophages, neutrophils, platelets, and ECs.

- **Platelets.** Tissue factor on CTC membranes facilitates platelet binding. This can trigger localized or widespread coagulation, in addition to coating the tumor cells. Platelets themselves can surround and protect tumor cells from recognition and elimination by NK cells, in part by secreting TGFβ and PDGF, which impair NK function (Fig. 5-33). Platelet-derived TGFβ can also activate tumor cell NF-κB signaling, which reinforces EMT. ATP from platelet granules also increases vascular permeability and CTC adherence to vascular endothelium.
- **Neutrophils.** Polymorphonuclear granulocytes may both kill CTCs and facilitate their survival in, and exit from, the circulation. They are attracted, at least in part, to CTCs by soluble mediators elaborated by platelets.

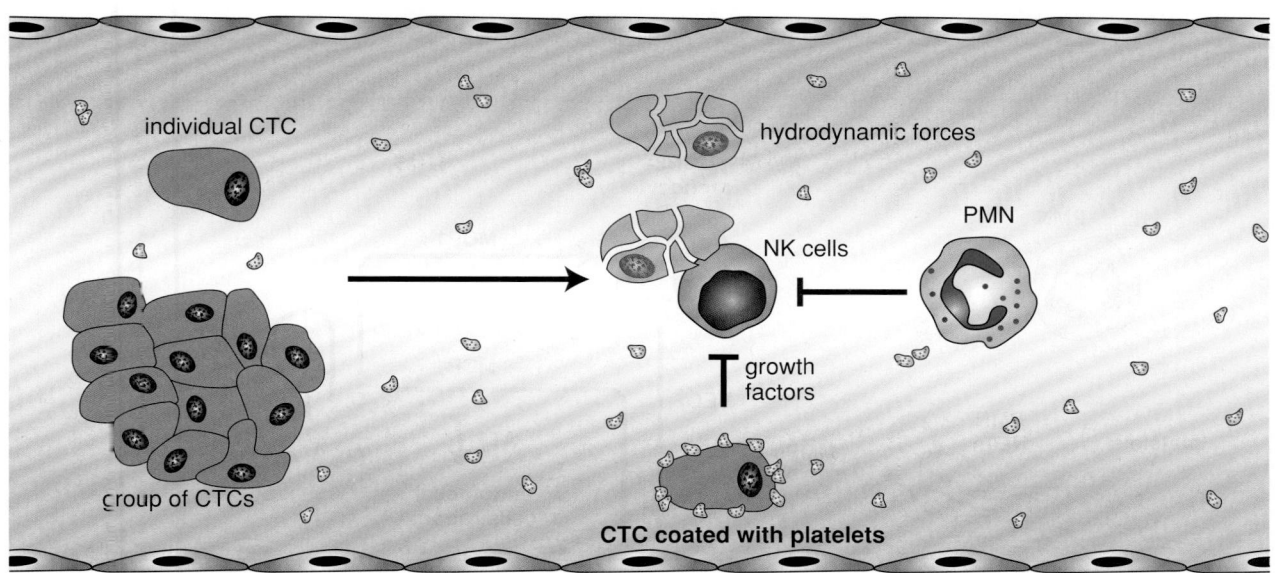

FIGURE 5-33. Circulating tumor cells. Individual CTCs and clusters circulate, and encounter both cells that can destroy them and cells, especially platelets and neutrophils, that protect them.

Neutrophil extracellular traps (NETs, **see Chapter 1**) trap tumor cells and help them survive in close proximity to endothelium and hepatic sinusoid lining cells (see below). They also protect CTCs from lysis by NK cells and CD8+ T cells.

Extravasation (Trans-Endothelial Migration)

When tumor cells leave the bloodstream, whether they are traveling singly or as clusters, they must adhere to and traverse vascular endothelium, into surrounding tissues. Neutrophils and platelets, again, as well as monocytes, abet this process.

■ Factors that promote *trans*-endothelial migration (TEM). For CTCs, invested or not with platelets, fibrin, etc., to leave the circulation, several factors must participate: adhesion to vascular endothelium, increased endothelial permeability, and migration into perivascular tissue. An additional factor, the premetastatic niche to which tumor cells home, is discussed below.
■ Adherence to the endothelium. NETs, DNA released from neutrophils adherent to vascular lining, trap tumor cells and help tether them to the vessel wall. Neutrophil-derived MMPs also help tumor cells traverse basement membranes. Platelets adherent to CTCs release ATP, which increases vascular permeability, and other cytokines (TGFβ, PDGF), which stimulate tumor cells to make other cytokines that enhance vessel leakiness (Fig. 5-34).
■ Monocytes. Tumor and other host cells also release monocyte chemotactic protein-1 (MCP-1, also called CCL2). This binds CCR2 at the surface of a subclass of monocytes (inflammatory monocytes), stimulating them to release VEGF. Both VEGF and CCL2 cause ECs to retract, creating channels through which tumor cells can pass. These monocytes mature into macrophages, which can facilitate establishment and growth of metastatic deposits.

■ Necroptosis. TGFβ from platelets stimulates this cell death program (**see Chapter 1**), which causes EC death, further facilitating TEM.

Metastatic colonization obviously differs from organ to organ, depending on the tightness of endothelial–endothelial cell junctions. Sinusoidal organs like the liver or bone marrow pose less formidable barriers than does the brain, for example.

Premetastatic Niches

CTCs do not exit the bloodstream randomly, but rather home to areas of the body that are commodious to their survival. These areas—premetastatic niches—are nests constructed under the direction of tumor-derived mediators, for CTCs to use to make metastases. There are two kinds of premetastatic niches: (1) pre-existing and (2) induced.

Pre-Existing Premetastatic Niches

There are pre-existing sites in which metastatic tumor cells establish themselves comfortably. The paradigm of such a site is the endosteal osteoblastic niche in the bone marrow. Normally, osteoblasts and hematopoietic stem cells (HSCs) inhabit this nook. Metastatic tumor, either single disseminated cancer cells (DTCs) or as small micrometastatic clusters, can displace HSCs from this cubbyhole and may persist there indefinitely, quietly (see Tumor Dormancy, below), under the influence of antiproliferative signals. In at least some cases, tumor cell expression of E-cadherin interacts with osteoblast N-cadherin to help establish the metastatic focus. Other such pre-existing niches probably exist elsewhere.

Induced Premetastatic Niches

Specifics of site preparation vary from organ to organ and tumor to tumor. However, certain generalizations apply. Tumors induce premetastatic niches by stimulating ECM remodeling, angiogenesis, proliferation, and recruitment

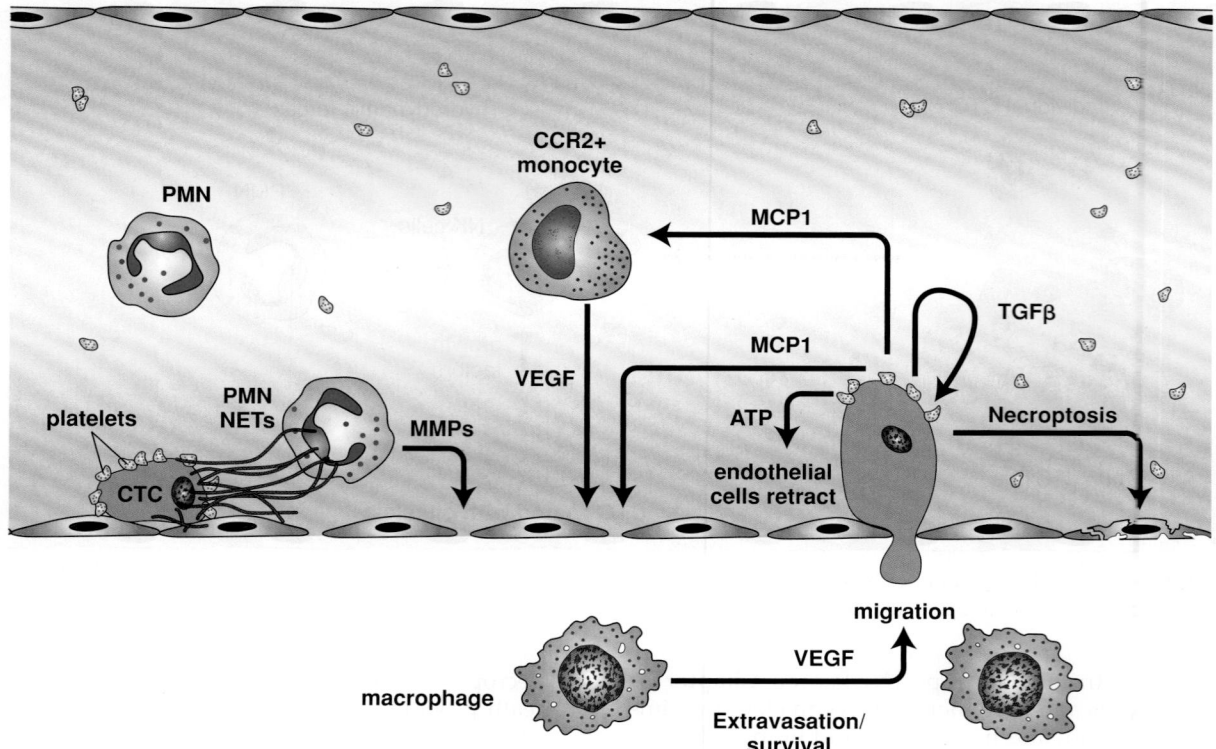

FIGURE 5-34. Mechanisms of CTC arrest in, and exit from, the circulation. CTCs may become entwined in neutrophil NETs, which facilitates their lodgment in the circulation. They may also reach vessels too narrow to traverse. The CTCs and their companion cells (platelets, neutrophils) then secrete cytokines that are recognized by endothelial cells, monocytes, extravascular macrophages, and the CTCs themselves to increase vascular permeability and facilitate cell migration through vessel walls into the surrounding tissue.

of key stromal cells (Fig. 5-35). Recruiting EPCs (see above) promotes angiogenesis, and bringing marrow-derived cells to the premetastatic niche serves diverse functions, including protecting tumor cells from elimination by innate and adaptive immune mechanisms. Revamping the ECM entails activating and generating myofibroblasts, to reconnect existing ECM constituents and stimulate production of others, depending on the tumor type and organ location.

These activities are orchestrated by tumor cells and their attendant stroma via soluble mediators secreted by tumors themselves, particularly TGFβ, and by **tumor-derived exosomes (TDEs)**. By virtue of their membrane constituents, especially specific integrins, exosomes released by tumor cells help direct these functions in sites of future metastatic colonization. Interestingly, exosomes released by stromal cells may also facilitate tumor cell adaptation to their new home.

Inefficiency of Metastasis

Although estimates vary greatly, patients' tumors release CTCs at rates approximating 1,000/g tumor/hr. From all these cells, very few clinically significant metastases emerge. That is, metastasis is an extraordinarily inefficient process. Just how inefficient it is, is unclear. Published estimates in animal models are on the order of 1 per 100,000,000 CTCs. Given the general resilience of tumors in the face of massive pharmacotherapy, this may be surprising, but the ability to

form viable metastases is generally thought to reside solely in CSCs. These cells (see below), are a tiny proportion within primary tumors and among CTCs.

Micrometastases and Tumor Dormancy

The traits that tumor cells need to metastasize are generally distinct from those needed to establish unrestrained clonal proliferation. Extensive analyses of primary tumors and metastases derived from them, even years later, have not identified distinguishing genetic alterations. As indicated above, for many tumors, metastasis appears to be an early event. EMT is followed by the reverse process (mesenchymal–epithelial transition) once metastatic foci form. These observations suggest that many of the behavioral changes needed for metastasis are epigenetic (see below), not genetic. The fact that chromatin structure in metastases tends to differ from that in their original primary tumors supports this possibility.

Once the planets align for a CSC(s) to establish itself and its cellular progeny at a distant site, a micrometastasis is in place. What happens next? Cells in the focus may follow one of several fates (Fig. 5-36):

1. They may die, whether by apoptosis, anoikis, immune elimination, or some other mechanism.
2. They may become dormant and remain so.
3. They may become dormant and eventually reactivate.
4. They may continue to proliferate.

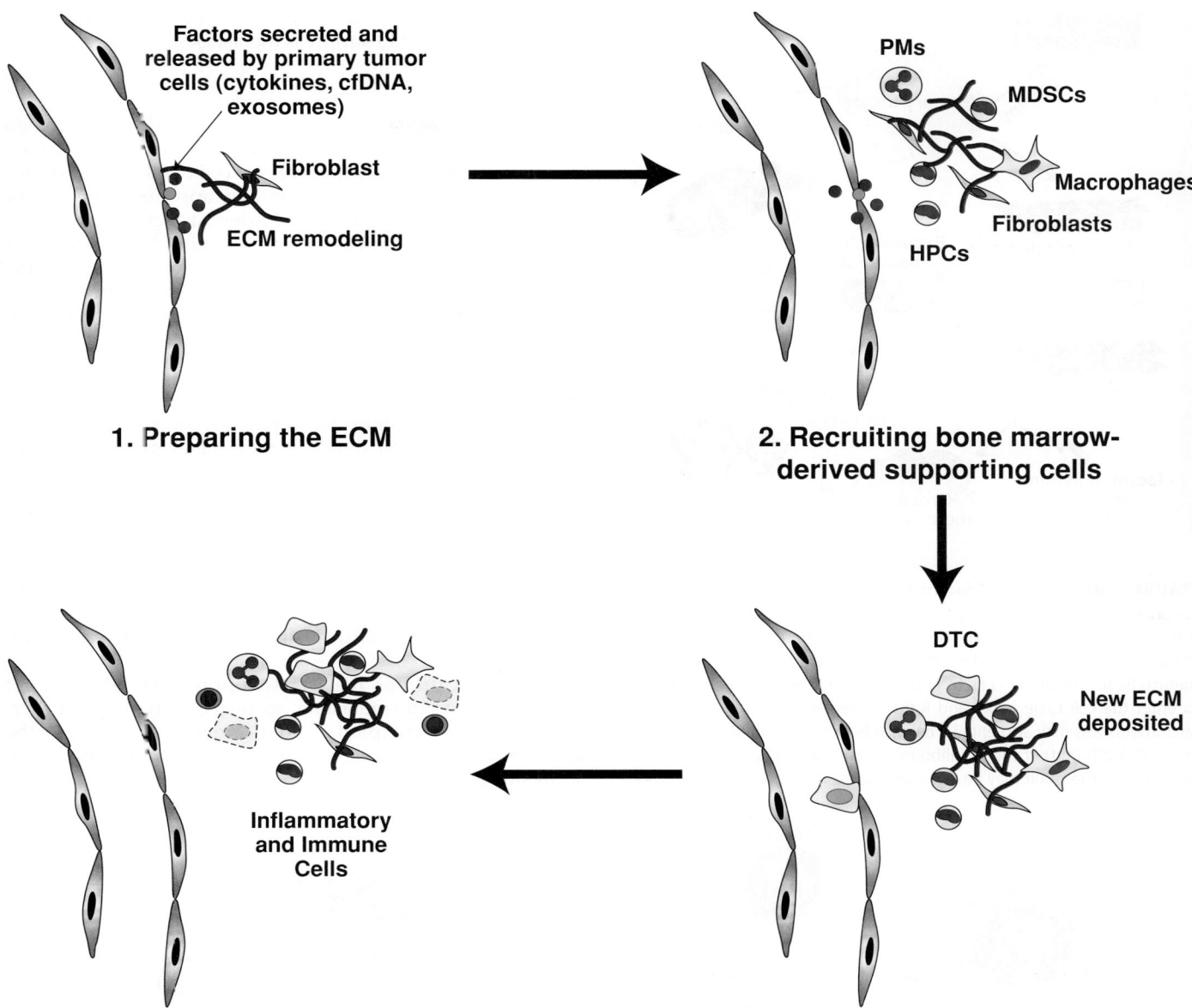

1. Preparing the ECM

2. Recruiting bone marrow-derived supporting cells

3. CTCs become DTCs

4. Micrometastasis becomes established

FIGURE 5-35. Formation and development of premetastatic niches. 1. Factors produced by tumor cells, whether packaged in microvesicles or soluble, cause alterations in ECM in areas that will become foci of metastatic disease. **2.** Various cells originating in the bone marrow migrate to the site. **3.** CTCs arrive at the location (and are then called DTCs, or disseminated tumor cells). They trigger additional ECM modifications. **4.** Developing micrometastases manipulate the immune system to support and sustain tumor growth, and a macrometastasis forms. (An alternative fate is that the micrometastasis becomes dormant, which is not shown here.)

Dormancy

For micrometastases, dormancy is not suspended animation, but rather an equilibrium between a low level of cell proliferation and a low level of cell death (Fig. 5-37). Tumor cells must survive. Proliferation may be put aside for later (or, often, never). Diverse survival paradigms are known, often specific for the organ location and tumor type.

Factors favoring dormancy include ECM–tumor cell interactions that only signal proliferation weakly. For example, low levels of integrin β_1 binding to ECM may generate attenuated signaling via focal adhesion kinase

(FAK) into the cell's ERK pathway. At the same time, dormancy signals of many kinds may preferentially stimulate p38 MAPK, arresting the cell in G_0/G_1 of the cell cycle. In some settings, niche-specific signals (e.g., thrombospondin-1 [TSP-1] in perivascular niches) may sustain dormancy. Survival may be protected by other signaling mechanisms, again depending on the location of the micrometastasis.

Simultaneously, tumor cells in micrometastatic deposits may sustain an equilibrium with host recognition systems. They may downregulate cell membrane molecules that

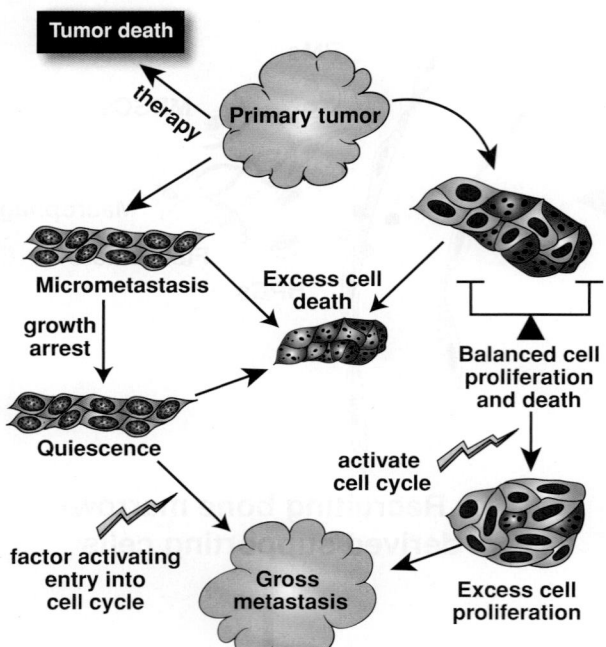

FIGURE 5-36. The fate of foci of cancer micrometastases. A primary cancer may be killed by therapies, such as radiation or chemotherapy, or it may be surgically removed. The tumor may produce a grossly evident metastasis. A number of factors may cause minute, clinically inapparent, metastatic foci of tumor cells to enter G_0 (*green*), but may be reactivated to enter the cell cycle (*blue*) and form a clinically detectable metastasis. Micrometastasis may also entail a balance between cell proliferation (*blue*) and cell death (*red*). If this equilibrium is disturbed in favor of tumor cell proliferation, the result may be a grossly evident mass of metastatic tumor.

activate NK cells. At the same time, they must evade CD8+ T cells, which tend to suppress metastases.

Exiting Dormancy

Micrometastatic colonies may awaken from dormancy when they have adapted to their new environment so that they can sustain proliferation in excess of cell death. This requires a low level of cell proliferation and appears to be a very inefficient process. Sometimes, external factors may drive activation. Thus, neovascularization-stimulated sprouting vascular tips (see above) secrete cytokines that overcome TSP-1–induced dormancy in micrometastases in perivascular niches. Inflammation may also trigger escape from micrometastatic dormancy.

Implications of Dormancy

The dynamics of tumor dormancy are complex. Cells from micrometastases and dormant metastases may themselves metastasize or even reseed original tumor sites, as illustrated in Figure 5-38.

In patients without clinical evidence of metastatic disease, adjuvant therapies often follow tumor resection. Such treatments seek to eliminate undetected micrometastases, but are often of short duration and tend to work best against rapidly proliferating cells. Dormant micrometastases and CSCs are relatively impervious to such adjuvant approaches.

There are, further, metastasis suppressors, which target various steps in the metastatic sequence. Future cancer therapies may need to exploit tumor dormancy and enhance the forces that naturally keep tumors in check, to improve long-term survival.

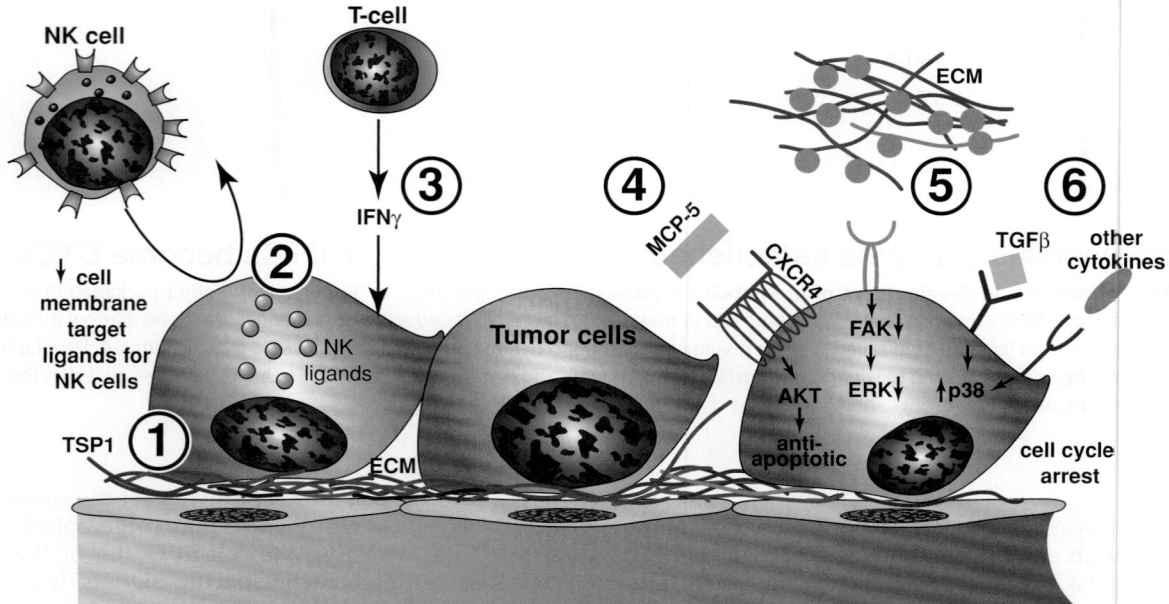

FIGURE 5-37. Factors facilitating and sustaining DTC dormancy. 1. DTCs can occupy perivascular (or bone marrow, not shown) sites that facilitate their persistence in a dormant state. Thrombospondin-1 (TSP1) in perivascular connective tissue of mature blood vessels facilitates dormancy. **2.** Tumor cells circumvent NK-mediated destruction by downregulating NK cell ligands. **3.** T-cell–derived IFNγ also promotes DTC quiescence. **4.** Dormancy signaling entails both survival and quiescence signaling. Thus, MCP-5 (also called CXCL12) from the microenvironment signals through Src and AKT to promote survival. **5.** Disturbed ECM alters integrin-related signaling and lowers focal adhesion kinase (FAK) and ERK activation, which, **(6)** when combined with signals from TGFβ and other dormancy-promoting cytokines, prevents entry into the cell cycle.

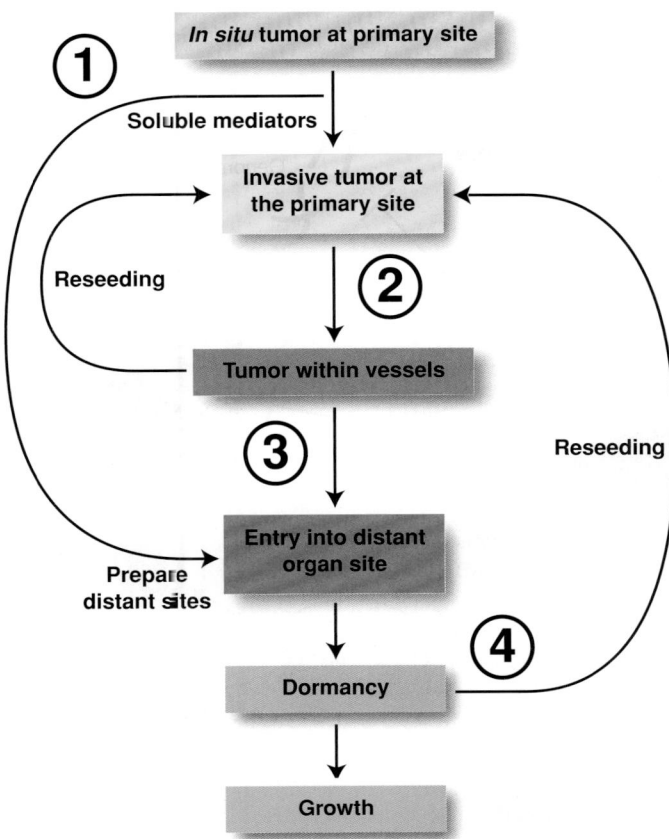

FIGURE 5-38. The sequence of events in tumor invasion and metastasis. **1.** An *in situ* tumor develops at the primary site. The tumor and its subjacent stromal cells secrete soluble mediators that prepare a distant site for eventual colonization by metastatic tumor. **2.** The local tumor becomes invasive, and traverses the intervening tissue to invade blood vessels. **3.** Once within blood vessels, tumor cells may home back to their original site of origin (reseeding) or establish themselves at a distant site, the suitability of which has been facilitated by preparative activity (**1**). **4.** Once in a distant site, the tumor may either reseed its site of origin, it may become dormant or it may grow.

TUMOR SUPPRESSORS

Tumor suppressors are a very large and diverse group of cellular functions, carried out via many different pathways and mediators. Suppressors exist for all the cancer attributes mentioned above (immortalization, evading PCD, etc.) and those companion tumor characteristics (genomic instability, altered metabolism, etc.) described below. This section is organized according to the tumor attributes listed above, and highlights how tumor suppression works and the nature of many different molecules, and the diverse types of molecules, that carry the burden of these functions.

Tumor suppression is an amalgam of processes. Some of these processes are inherent in particular molecules, for example, cell cycle regulation and Rb, or the intrinsic pathway of apoptosis and Bax. It is tempting to confuse functions with the mediators of those functions, a logical jump that is made all the time. But, like that extra scoop of ice cream, this temptation should be resisted, and to remember that tumor suppression is defined by function, not by structure. One tumor suppressor function may be executed by several

different molecules, and one molecule may have multiple functions.

There are almost infinite variations on the themes of tumor suppression. Many tumor suppressors only inhibit development and spread of some types of tumors. Still others—for example, WT1—act as tumor suppressors in some circumstances but as oncogenes in others. Some molecules may execute their duties in some settings, but not always. Further, some tumor suppressors (like p53), if mutated, not only fail to inhibit tumor development, but may actively facilitate it and inactivate other tumor suppressors. This fluidity should be kept in mind, even as tumor suppressors are presented as static structures, for example, PTEN, VHL. This may facilitate understanding how they work, the processes they antagonize, and what goes awry when they are mutated or inactivated, but is only part of the picture.

The student should be mindful of this complexity, as it may come in handy when dealing with one of Nature's most vexing principles, the law of unintended consequences. That is, it may help in appreciating that, for example, therapeutic manipulations conceived with seemingly ironclad theoretical logic so as to produce a particular result may yield consequences quite different from expectations (see above).

Tumor Suppressor Mechanisms Protect From Oncogenesis by Inhibiting Every Tumor Attribute

Cells possess complex mechanisms that guard against tumor development. The molecular guardians responsible for this protection are tumor suppressors and the genes that encode them, tumor suppressor genes (TSGs). Major activities of tumor suppressors are illustrated in Figure 5-39. If an incipient tumor is to develop successfully, it must generally inactivate or circumvent multiple TSGs or their products.

There are many TSGs, with many functions and mechanisms of action. Some tumor suppressors have multiple activities and targets. Some are not proteins, but may be untranslated RNAs (see below). And some are part-time tumor suppressors and part-time oncogenes. In light of this considerable complexity, we focus here on key concepts in understanding how important aspects of tumor suppression work, the ways in which tumor suppressors are circumvented, and how tumors arise once suppressor activities go awry. The protective activities of tumor suppressors are illustrated below for each of the major cancer attributes (see above).

Tumor Suppressors Regulate Cellular Proliferation

There are several important mechanisms that limit cell division. As noted above, extracellular molecules and their cell membrane receptors interact to trigger intracellular signaling via multiple pathways (Fig. 5-40). These include activation of PI-3 kinase (PI3K, see above), which phosphorylates phosphatidylinositol-4,5-bisphosphate (PIP2) to phosphatidylinositol-3,4,5-trisphosphate (PIP3). PIP3 activates downstream signaling via Akt and mTOR, to drive cell division. A key tumor suppressor protein, PTEN, dephosphorylates PIP3, and so undoes activation initiated by extracellular mitogenic signaling (Fig. 5-41). PTEN is a major tumor suppressor, second only to p53 in the frequency with which loss of its function occurs in human cancers.

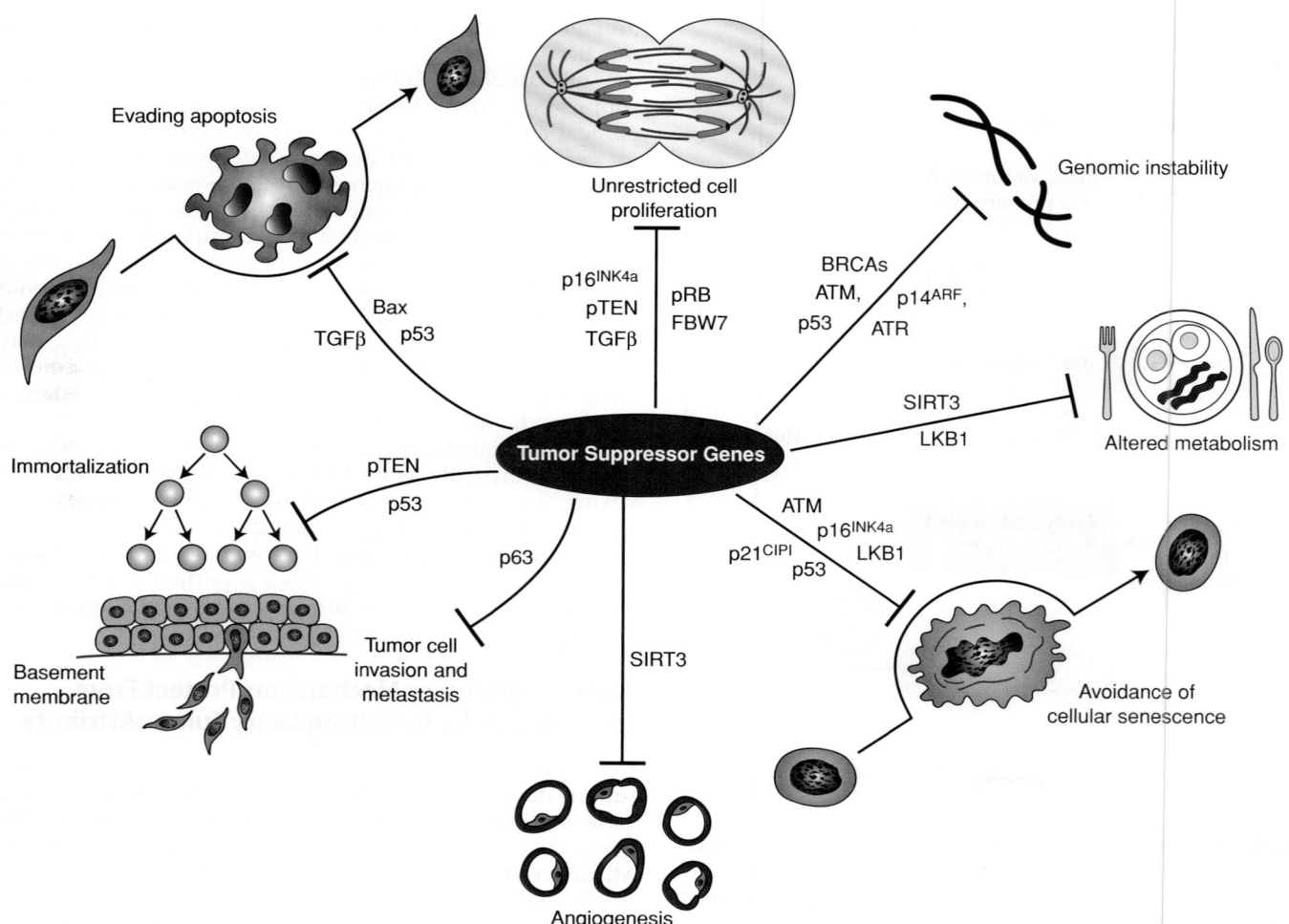

FIGURE 5-39. Tumor-related activities that are targeted by important tumor suppressor genes and representative tumor suppressors involved. The major hallmarks of malignant tumors each is antagonized by multiple tumor suppressor gene products. Those hallmarks, and the tumor suppressor activities that work against them, are illustrated here.

Many tumor suppressors act downstream from receptor-ligand interactions. Key tumor suppressor targets include the various transitions in the cell cycle (see above) and activation/inactivation of gene transcription. Thus, pRb blocks cell cycle transit unless it is hyperphosphorylated to release E2F transcription factor that drives cell division. The enzymes that phosphorylate pRb (CDKs 2, 4, 6, complexed with various cyclins, see above) are inhibited by p16^{INK4a} and p21^{WAF1} tumor suppressors. Phosphorylated pRb, however, may be dephosphorylated, restoring its ability to block E2F.

E2F-mediated transcription of many genes that drive cell division (e.g., c-*myc*) is powerfully inhibited by TGFβ. TGFβ binds its receptor to activate intermediary signaling molecules called Smads (Fig. 5-42A). Smad4 is a key effector of TGFβ-induced transcriptional activity. It first blocks transcription of c-*myc* proto-oncogene, thus inhibiting cell cycle transit and allowing Smad4 to upregulate expression of genes that block cell division, p16^{INK4a} and p21^{WAF1} (Fig. 5-42B). TGFβ signaling is among the most potent endogenous mechanisms that inhibit cell division and is commonly mutated in human cancers. (Note, however, its role in facilitating metastasis, see above.)

Tumor suppressors also inhibit cell division at stages after transcriptional activation or repression. Thus, TGFβ signaling activates molecules that impede translation of mRNAs for proteins that drive cell cycle progression. Another tumor suppressor, FBW7, is part of a ubiquitin ligase complex that eliminates many proteins that drive cell division, such as Myc, Cyclin E, and Jun.

Many other tumor suppressors, far too numerous to mention, also regulate cell division. The above descriptions illustrate the diversity of mechanisms that protect the organism from runaway cell proliferation.

Programmed Cell Death Destroys Cells at the Cusp of Becoming Dangerous

Several signaling networks that culminate in cell death were described in **Chapter 1**. They all protect from tumor development, but the most critical of these is the PCD pathway that is activated by altered DNA structure. This pathway contains several key participants—including ATM and ATR (see above), and most critically, p53.

The p53 tumor suppressor is a principal mediator of growth arrest, senescence, and apoptosis (Fig. 5-14). In response to

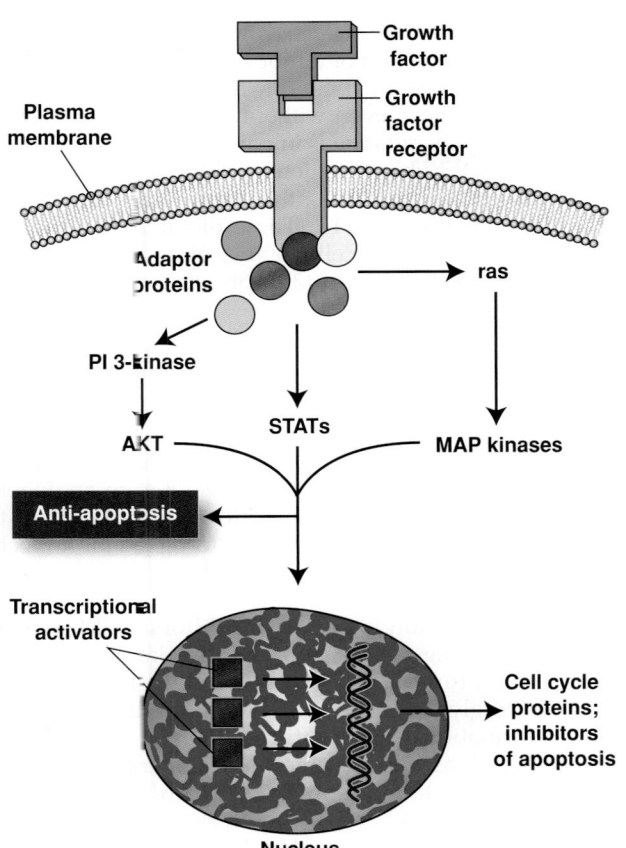

FIGURE 5-40. Signaling pathways controlling proliferation and apoptosis. When their ligands activate growth factor receptors, they recruit adaptor proteins and activate a series of intracellular signaling molecules, leading to transcriptional activation of proteins that promote cell cycle progression and inhibit apoptosis.

DNA damage, oncogenic activation of other proteins and other stresses (e.g., hypoxia), p53 levels rise and prevent cells from entering the S phase of the cell cycle, thus allowing time for DNA repair to take place. P53 thus acts as a "guardian of

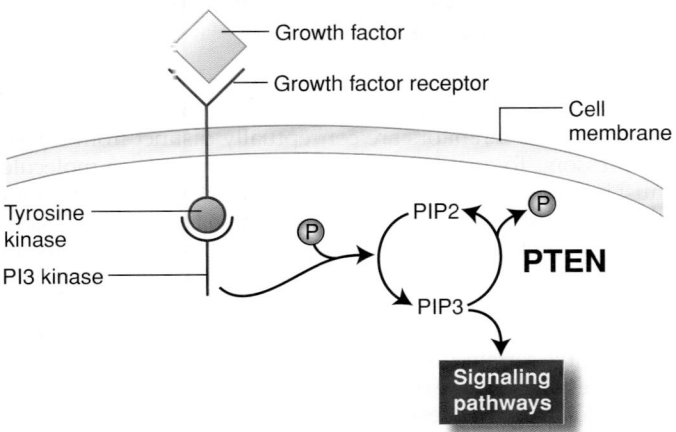

FIGURE 5-41. Signaling function of PTEN. Normal binding of a growth factor to its receptor leads to phosphorylation of phosphatidylinositol-bisphosphate (PIP2) to produce the important signaling molecule phosphatidylinositol-trisphosphate (PIP3). The level of PIP3 is regulated by its dephosphorylation by PTEN.

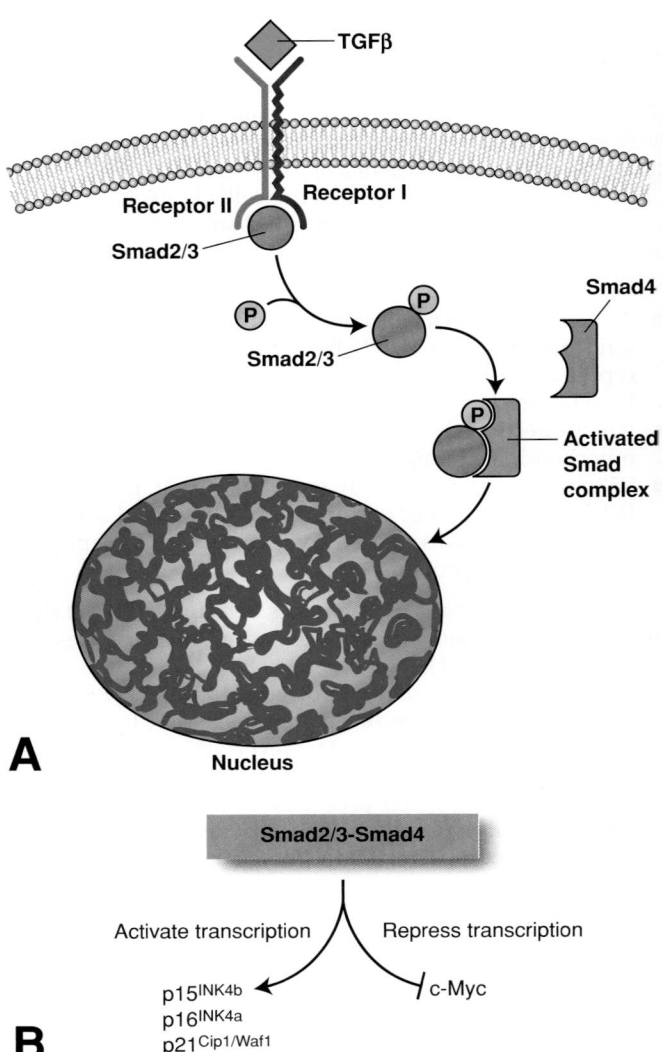

FIGURE 5-42. TGFβ as a tumor suppressor. A. Signaling. Transforming growth factor-β binds its heteromeric receptor to phosphorylate and so activates SMADs 2 and 3. These bind SMAD4, to form an activated SMAD complex that translocates to the nucleus to mediate transcriptional activation and repression. **B. Consequences.** SMAD2/3–SMAD4 complex activates transcription of cell cycle suppressors, as shown, and represses transcription of the proliferation activator c-*Myc*.

the genome" by restricting uncontrolled cellular proliferation when cells with abnormal DNA might propagate.

Acquired mismatches in DNA bases are detected by ATM if they occur in resting cells damaged by, for example, radiation or oxidative damage, or by ATR if they occur during DNA replication (see above). These proteins then activate one of two kinases, Chk2 or Chk1, respectively. The latter phosphorylates p53 (above and Fig. 5-14), causing it to dissociate from its inhibitor, MDM2, and activating the p53 damage response.

In addition, p53 is a transcription factor that promotes expression of other genes involved in controlling cell cycle progression and apoptosis. DNA damage and other stresses (e.g., hypoxia) upregulate the expression of p53, which in turn enhances the synthesis of CKIs. The latter inactivates cyclin/CDK complexes, thus leading to cell arrest at the G_1/S checkpoint. Cells arrested at this checkpoint may either: (a) repair the DNA damage and then reenter the cycle, or (b) undergo apoptosis. P53-stimulated gene transcription results in the synthesis of proteins (CIP1, GADD45) (Fig. 5-14) that enhance DNA repair by binding proliferating cell nuclear antigen (PCNA, see above). Thus, *upregulation of p53 as a tumor suppressor has two important and related consequences: arrest of cell cycle progression and promotion of DNA repair.*

If it is not possible to return the cell's DNA to its correct sequence, p53 may then trigger cell death, which it may do in several ways (**see Chapter 1**). Largely, p53 activates the intrinsic apoptosis pathway by:

- As a transcription factor, it increases production of proapoptotic proteins (e.g., Bad, Bax, PUMA, and others) and represses transcription of prosurvival proteins (e.g., Bcl-2, Bcl-xL, Mcl-1).
- It may directly activate cytosolic Bax, which in turn moves into mitochondria and triggers release of cytochrome C (CytC).
- P53 may act as a BH3-only (**see Chapter 1**), proapoptotic Bcl-2 family member by directly binding to Mcl-1, therefore freeing Bak to release CytC and other proapoptotic mitochondrial proteins.

By whatever means p53 activates apoptosis, the cell death program is executed by caspases, especially caspases 3, 6, and 7 (**see Chapter 1**).

The issue of apoptosis and protection from cancer is further complicated **oncogene-induced apoptosis**. Myc transcription factor drives cell proliferation. However, activated Myc can be a blessing in disguise. It also induces a default apoptosis pathway. That is, deregulated production of Myc promotes cell proliferation but is usually balanced by increased apoptosis. Myc-induced apoptosis acts as a "molecular safety valve" that blocks cancer development. If Myc-stimulated tumor development is to occur, cells producing Myc at high levels must also overcome PCD-inducing mechanisms by overexpressing Bcl-2 or other antiapoptotic proteins.

Tumor Suppressors and Senescence

No single paradigm explains all of OIS. The centrality of DDR via Rb and p53 is generally accepted, but senescence entails complex signaling (Fig. 5-24), perturbation of any member of which could facilitate development of malignancy.

As described above, ongoing telomere shortening in normal cells eventually leads to senescence. Tumor suppressor activities that elicit senescence are critical defenses against oncogenesis. They include components of the DDR system, such as ATM, ATR, Chk 1 and 2, the cell cycle regulators, p53 and Rb, and many others.

Inhibitors of Tumor Angiogenesis Limit Tumor Growth

There are many potent endogenous suppressors of tumor-related blood vessel growth:

- **VHL.** This protein is part of a ubiquitin ligase that targets HIFs (see above and **Chapter 1**) for degradation. Inactivation of VHL impairs Ub conjugation of HIF-1α, in turn increasing HIF-1α concentration (see above). This angiogenic transcription factor facilitates cell adaptation to low oxygen environments. Such adaptations include (1) increasing glucose intake for anaerobic glycolysis, (2) stimulating angiogenesis (VEGF; see above), and (3) activating several critical growth factors.

The tumorigenicity associated with VHL inactivation largely reflects HIF-1α promotion of tumor growth. Interestingly, similar activation of HIF-1α occurs in the often oxygen-starved cores of many tumors, even without VHL mutation. In those settings, HIF-1α degradation is impaired by decreased activity of a cofactor for the ubiquitination reaction.

Normal VHL protein has other tumor suppressor activities, independent of HIF-1α. These include (1) promoting apoptosis, (2) increasing cellular immobilization by adherence to matrix proteins, and (3) repressing certain cell activation responses.

- **NOTCH.** Although important stimulators of embryonic blood vessel development, the NOTCH family of EC receptors, together with their cognate cell surface-bound ligands (especially DLL4) inhibits tumor angiogenesis. In fact, VEGF stimulation elicits DLL4 production as a negative feedback mechanism. Its conversion to angiogenesis inhibitor in postembryonic life notwithstanding, the NOTCH/DLL4 system is thought to represent a mechanism by which tumors outwit VEGF-targeted antiangiogenic therapies (see above).
- **ECM and other angiogenesis inhibitors.** ECM constituents and clotting factors, and their breakdown products, all suppress tumor angiogenesis. **TSP-1**, derived from a large ECM glycoprotein, is a powerful inhibitor of blood vessel formation. **Angiostatin**, a breakdown product of plasminogen, as well as numerous fragments of ECM constituents (endostatin, inhibin, and many others) restrain tumor-related blood vessel growth as well.
- **P53.** While p53 is not known to interfere with tumor angiogenesis itself, it upregulates TSP-1 expression and so has a strong antitumor angiogenic function. TSP-1 inhibition of tumor angiogenesis is a casualty of loss of p53.
- **SIRT.** Sirtuin deacetylases are important in stress responses and longevity. One of the sirtuins, SIRT3, increases the mitochondrial antioxidant, MnSOD (**see Chapter 1**). As a result, mitochondria produce less reactive oxygen (ROS), causing decreased HIF-1α activity and thus decreased angiogenesis.

For Each Step in Invasion and Metastasis, There Are Antagonists That Hinder the Ability of Tumors to Spread

Just as the body arrays its defenses to prevent cancers from arising, it has mechanisms to impede invasion and metastasis. Metastasis inhibitors are conceptually distinct from tumor suppressors. To qualify as a metastasis suppressor, a molecule must impede invasion- or metastasis-related behaviors without necessarily affecting growth and survival of the primary lesion. About 30 metastasis suppressor proteins are known, plus an increasing number of miRNAs (see below) that show metastasis suppressor activity. Some suppressors act at multiple steps, while others are known to act at only one. Also, some molecules may inhibit certain processes in some tumors or tumor types but have the opposite effects in others. Finally, there are some molecules that suppress metastasis *and* separately inhibit the primary tumor (e.g., proapoptotic, antiproliferative).

Impairing EMT

Cadherins are a family of cell–cell adhesion molecules, the best-characterized of which is E-cadherin. It is expressed on the surface of all epithelia and mediates cell–cell adhesion by mutual **zipper** interactions. **Catenins** (α, β, γ) are proteins that interact with the intracellular domain of E-cadherin and link it mechanically to the cytoskeleton, which is essential for effective epithelial cell interactions. Overall, cadherins and catenins are critical in suppressing invasion and metastasis. Most carcinomas show reduced expression of both E-cadherin and catenins, due largely to downregulation by the transcription factors mentioned above, Snail, ZEB1, etc. The miRNAs, miR-101 and the miR-200 family, help maintain epithelial phenotype. The latter does so by repressing ZEB1 and ZEB2 levels, thus relieving their repression of E-cadherin levels (see above). (Nothing, of course, is so simple: the ZEBs also downregulate miR-200.)

Not to be outdone, TGFβ, which is an inhibitor of tumorigenesis, is also a promoter of metastasis. It acts in part by downregulating miR-200s. As a result, in most carcinomas, loss of E-cadherin is associated with development of an invasive and aggressive phenotype. Clinically, there is an inverse correlation of levels of E-cadherin with tumor grade and patient mortality. Interestingly, β-catenin also binds to the APC gene product, independently of its interaction with E-cadherin and α–catenin. Mutations in either the APC or β-catenin gene are implicated in the development of colon cancer (see later and **Chapter 19**).

Inhibitors of Tumor Cell Invasiveness

- **Nm23-H1.** This was the first metastasis suppressor discovered. Its mechanism(s) of action is still not fully understood, but it inhibits tumor cell motility. Nm23-H1 achieves this by blocking cellular mobility signaled by Ras-related cell activation pathways.
- **P63.** This member of the p53 family of tumor suppressors (see below) helps to restrain cellular invasiveness. P63 is often expressed in some in situ carcinomas, for example, in prostate and breast. It is often repressed or lost in aggressive, metastatic carcinomas. Furthermore, mutants of p53 (see below) may bind and inactivate p63 by forming heterotetramer aggregates. Acting as a transcriptional regulator, p63 also upregulates expression of certain genes that inhibit metastasis (e.g., miR-130B).
- **miR-31.** Movement through connective tissue is a key function of tumor cells after EMT. This passage depends on the ability of cells to wiggle through the ECM, which in turn depends on integrin-α5 to mediate EMT and RhoA, to help direct ameboid movement. These invasive characteristics are inhibited by miR-31 (see below).

Suppressors of Intravasation

Notch inhibits tumor angiogenesis (see above). Mechanisms that impede intravasation also involve Notch. Thus, a protein called Aes (for amino-terminal enhancer of split) helps to inhibit migration of tumor cells through vascular walls, via signaling networks that include Notch activation.

Limiting Tumor Cell Survival in the Circulation

Life for a tumor cell as a vagabond is no simple matter. Anoikis (**see Chapter 1**) is a form of apoptotic cell death triggered by loss of cells' usual liaisons with familiar ECM constituents.

To add to the dangers of a cell's metastatic pilgrimage, many ECs express a Duffy blood group glycoprotein, DARC. Upon recognizing KAI1 on tumor cell membranes, DARC triggers senescence programs, thus condemning the wandering tumor cell to a short, sterile existence. In addition, cells of the innate immune system can trigger cell death programs via TRAIL and CD95 (**see Chapter 1**).

As mentioned above, tumor cells tend to be significantly larger than the caliber of many vascular spaces they encounter. This disparity can stimulate cells lining liver sinusoids to secrete nitric oxide (NO). NO triggers apoptosis in the overly large tumor cells trying to slog their way through channels that are too small for them.

Impeding Extravasation

The versatile miR-31 (see above), which inhibits tumor cell invasiveness, also blocks extravasation. This miRNA targets both integrin-5α and RhoA in the process.

Metastatic Colonization

Colonization and subsequent growth are the major rate-limiting processes in metastasis (see above). Several documented and likely suppressors act at this point, including **KISS1** and its receptor, **KISS1R**. This pair derives their names from their discovery in Hershey, PA, home of chocolate kisses. KISS1, made by tumor cells, binds its cell membrane receptor, KISS1R, triggering tumor cell apoptosis (a kiss of death).

Other suppressors of metastatic colonization include GATA3 in breast cancers, which promotes cellular differentiation and impedes multiplication, and Psap in prostate cancers, which induces stromal cell production of the antiangiogenic substance TSP-1 (see above). MiR-31 also inhibits the ability of cancer cells to colonize distant sites effectively.

Many metastasis suppressors have documented antimetastatic function but the mechanism(s) by which these properties are exerted are uncertain. Once a primary tumor is removed, almost all therapy is aimed at suppressing metastases. Thus, it is not surprising that activating endogenous metastasis–suppressive functions and trying to mimic them pharmacologically represent key targets of pharmaceutical investigation.

Diverse Mechanisms Compromise the Effectiveness of Tumor Suppressors

Of course, despite the body's best efforts, tumors still develop. In order to do so, they must inactivate or circumvent the formidable defenses described above. There are several mechanisms by which this treachery occurs:

- LOH
- Spontaneous mutation
- Dominant negative mutations
- Fragile site translocations
- Altered levels or activities of tumor suppressor proteins
- Functional blockade by other related proteins
- Epigenetic changes that alter tumor suppressor expression or function

These mechanisms are described and illustrated below. Epigenetic changes in cancer are discussed later.

Retinoblastoma Gene and Loss of Heterozygosity

Retinoblastoma is a rare childhood cancer, about 40% of which cases reflect a germline mutation; the remainder are sporadic. In patients with the hereditary form, all somatic cells carry a single missing or mutated allele of the *Rb* gene on the long arm of chromosome 13. The retinoblastoma tumors they develop, however, lack both *Rb* gene alleles. The protein product of this Rb gene, p105^{Rb}, *is a critical checkpoint in the cell cycle, and inactive* Rb *proteins permit unregulated cell proliferation.*

Loss of Heterozygosity

A child with hereditary retinoblastoma is *heterozygous* at the *Rb* locus. He inherits one defective *Rb* allele, plus one wild-type allele (Fig. 5-43). This heterozygous state is not associated with any observable changes in the retina, because 50% of the *Rb* gene product in the heterozygous child is sufficient to prevent a retinoblastoma. *However, heterozygosity in some TSGs is unstable, because a subsequent, randomly acquired, deletion or mutation may inactivate the remaining normal Rb allele.* If that occurs, no Rb tumor suppressor function remains to protect from unregulated cell proliferation. The child then develops a retinoblastoma. Thus, *even though the child inherits a heterozygous Rb genotype, susceptibility to retinoblastoma is inherited in a dominant fashion: it is the heterozygote who develops the tumor.*

Precisely, the same susceptibility to LOH occurs if there is an acquired *Rb* mutation: cells carrying the newly acquired mutation become similarly susceptible to inactivation of the remaining *Rb* allele.

The principle, then, is that the presence of one mutant *Rb* TSG predisposes to eventual LOH and consequent development of malignancy. A mutation in one allele (whether inherited or acquired) facilitates clonal expansion of cells

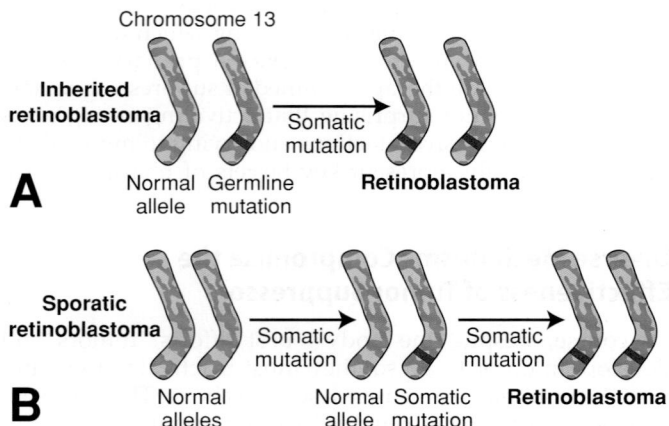

FIGURE 5-43. The "two-hit" origin of retinoblastoma. A. A child with the inherited form of retinoblastoma is born with a germline mutation in one allele of the *RB* gene, at the long arm of chromosome 13. One mutation is not sufficient for tumorigenesis, but the absence of 2 wild-type alleles weakens protection from tumor development if the remaining allele becomes altered. A second somatic *RB* gene mutation in the retina leads to inactivation of the remaining functioning *RB* allele and subsequent development of a retinoblastoma. **B.** In sporadic cases of retinoblastoma, a child is born with two normal *RB* alleles. Tumor development requires two independent somatic mutations to inactivate all *RB* gene function and allow a neoplastic clone.

bearing a mutation in the other allele. This fact underscores an essential paradox of TSGs: even if a wild-type phenotype is dominant, heterozygous cells are at high risk for LOH and become homozygous mutant cells, with tumor development likely to ensue.

While Rb is named for its signature tumor, an inherited *Rb* mutation affects every cell in the body and confers a more general increase in malignancies. Such patients have a 200-fold increased risk of developing mesenchymal tumors in early adult life. As well, *Rb* is not infrequently mutated in sporadic tumors, including 70% of cases of osteosarcoma and in many instances of small-cell lung cancer; carcinomas of the breast, bladder, pancreas, and other organs.

There are many types of *Rb* mutations, including point mutations, insertions, deletions, and translocations. Epigenetic events, such as promoter hypermethylation (see below), may also reduce *Rb* expression and contribute to a tumorigenic phenotype.

p53, Acquired Point Mutations, and Dominant Negative Mutants

The *TP53* gene is on the short arm of chromosome 17, and its protein product, p53, is present in virtually all normal tissues. *TP53* is deleted or mutated in 75% of human colorectal cancers and frequently in carcinomas of the breast, lung (small cell), liver, brain (astrocytomas), and many others. *In fact, mutations of* TP53 *are the most common genetic change in human cancer.* Inactivating mutations in human cancers are largely missense mutations that impair the ability of p53 to bind to DNA (Fig. 5-44A). Affected cells may then progress through the cell cycle despite having damaged DNA. While in some cancers both *TP53* alleles are inactivated by the mechanism described above, this is not always the case. Often, one mutant *TP53* gene is sufficient.

Active p53 protein is a homotetramer: a composite of four individual p53 proteins (Fig. 5-44B). Each allele of *TP53* contributes a homodimer of p53 proteins. These homodimers assort randomly to form homotetramers. *For the complex to be active, all p53 subunits must be functional* (Fig. 5-44C). One mutant p53 subunit (which, actually, would be one mutant pair, as each dimer is from one allele) therefore can inactivate the whole tetramer (Fig. 5-44C). This situation—when a protein product of a mutant allele inactivates that of the wild-type allele—the mutant is **dominant negative**. A cell with a mutant *TP53* allele (i.e., a heterozygote) would have a growth advantage over normal cells, and so predominate in vivo with a high risk of then becoming cancerous.

Additional Mechanisms of Inactivating p53

As p53 is so intensively studied, much of the diversity of mechanisms by which tumor suppression can be inactivated has been uncovered for this protein. Normally, the E3 ubiquitin ligase, MDM2, binds to and regulates p53 activity. The MDM2–p53 complex blocks p53 function and targets it for degradation via the ubiquitin-proteasome pathway (UPS, **see Chapter 1**). In turn, p14^{ARF} inhibits MDM2 (see above).

Some cancers in which both *p53* alleles are structurally normal may overexpress MDM2, consequently increasing p53 degradation. Other tumors in which p53 is intact do not express functional p14^{ARF}, and so allow unopposed

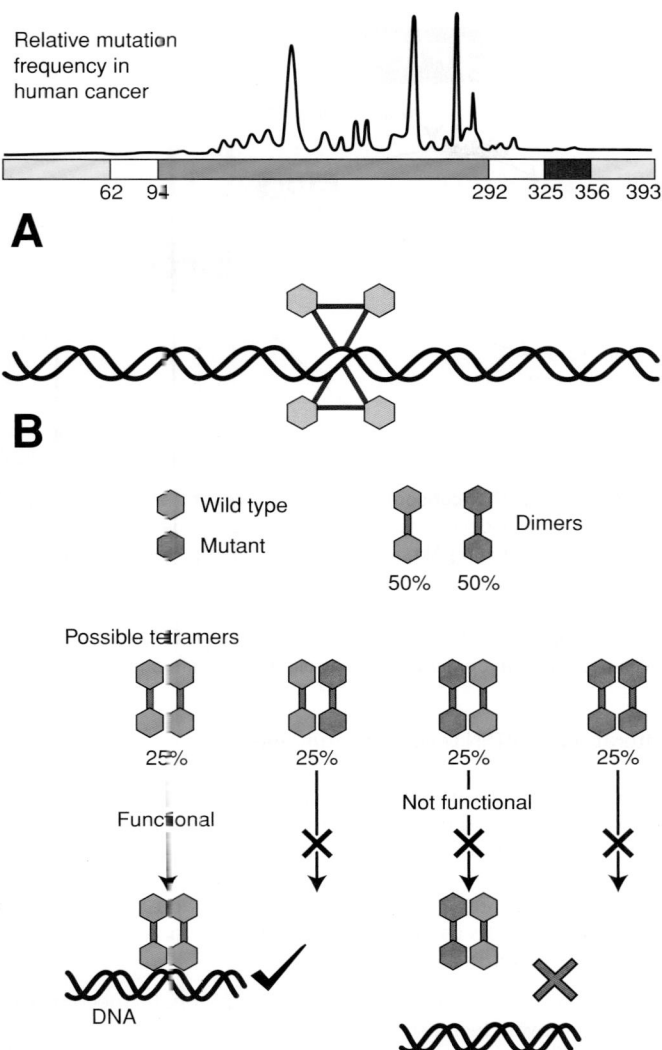

Relative mutation frequency in human cancer

62 94   292 325 356 393

A

B

Wild type
Mutant

Dimers

50%   50%

Possible tetramers

25%   25%   25%   25%

Functional   Not functional

DNA   DNA

C

FIGURE 5-44. Mutations in *TP53*, stoichiometry of impaired function of p53 tumor suppressor. A. Locations and frequency of mutations in different p53 protein regions. P53 protein has multiple domains, the largest of which is the DNA-binding domain. That is where the vast majority of known mutations in p53 are located. **B. p53 binding to DNA.** To regulate transcription, p53 binds DNA as a tetramer, composed of two dimers. Each dimer is the product of one of the two alleles of the *TP53* gene. **C. Consequences of heterozygous mutation in *TP53* gene.** If one of the two alleles of the *TP53* is mutant, the p53 protein dimer derived from that mutant gene is completely mutant (and hence inactive). The other is wild type (and hence active). However, as p53 transcriptional activity requires a fully functional tetramer, and as the sorting of the dimers into a tetramer is random, 3/4 of resulting tetramers will be inactive, as shown. Thus, one mutant allele of p53 inactivates 3/4 of p53 activity.

MDM2-mediated proteolysis of p53. As in the case of *Rb*, certain DNA viral products in tumors (e.g., HPV E6, see below) bind p53 and promote its degradation. In addition to many feedback loops there are posttranslational modifications (phosphorylation, acetylation, etc.), natural antisense transcripts, binding proteins, and small regulatory RNAs. It is no

surprise, then, that *most human cancers either have inactivating mutations of* TP53 *or abnormalities in the proteins that regulate p53 activity.*

P53 directs cell cycle arrest, apoptosis, and cellular senescence, but these activities are only a part of a more complex tapestry of p53 functions. It also oversees responses to metabolic stress; regulates autophagy, redox state, ROS production; and promotion and limitation of longevity.

The p53 Family

Like a gathering of relations among whom one is the most boisterous, the family of p53-like proteins has largely been dominated by its most conspicuous member—that is, p53. However, there are several important cousins, p63 and p73, and some derivative proteins that deserve mention. Just as the region on chromosome 17 that encodes p53 is often mutated or deleted in human cancers, so are the regions on chromosomes 1 and 3 where p73 and p63 reside, respectively. If p63 and p73 are intact, they may partly compensate for loss of p53. Both are tumor suppressors in their own rights, with functions that partly overlap, and that are partly distinct from, those of p53. P63 is a transcriptional regulator, directly increasing levels of the proapoptotic proteins, CD95 (FasR, **see Chapter 1**) and Bax. It is also important for effective chemotherapy using agents like *cis*-platinum.

There are many variants of each of these proteins. These may affect the protection afforded by these three proteins in diverse ways (see below).

Treacherous Mutant p53

Interestingly, the mischief of mutant p53 molecules extends far beyond simple inactivation of tumor suppressor function. *The aberrant protein also functions as an oncogene, modulating gene transcription.* It also protects cells from apoptosis. Mutant p53 may activate proinflammatory cytokines and ECM modulators. It blocks ATM-mediated (see above) protection against double-stranded DNA breaks. A common denominator underlying the effects of mutant p53 is its widespread stimulation of genes involved with cell proliferation. Moreover, mutant p53 activates cellular mechanisms that mediate resistance to chemotherapeutic drugs. In many cases, including tumors of the hematopoietic system, breast, urinary bladder, and head and neck, mutant p53 is associated with a poorer prognosis. Along these lines, some splice variants of p53 and p73, particularly those lacking *N*-terminal domains, appear to inhibit aspects of their tumor suppressor activities and to act in part as oncogenes.

Fragile Site Translocations

The human genome contains a number of more or less universally shared **fragile sites** (CFS) that are inordinately structurally unstable. (Small percentages of people, 5% or less, also have rare fragile sites susceptible to the same fragility.) Gene amplification, chromosomal translocations, sister chromatid exchanges, deletions, and other kinds of chromosomal malfunctions occur inordinately often at these sites. This instability may be implicated in tumor development, via resultant loss of TSG integrity.

The most active CFS is called FRA3B, and deletions or translocations there are associated with many human malignancies, including solid tumors and leukemias. A gene that is often inactivated or deleted in that setting is the **fragile histidine triad (FHIT)** tumor suppressor. It encodes a protein that cleaves certain nucleotides into adenosine monophosphate (AMP) and adenosine diphosphate (ADP), but it is not clear how much its tumor suppressor activity relates to this enzymatic function. Unlike most tumor suppressors except for APC, FHIT protein does not bind DNA. Rather, it (like APC) enhances microtubule assembly. It is also felt to promote apoptosis via caspase-8 activation (**see Chapter 1**). Lack of *FHIT* expression is associated with enhanced resistance to apoptosis. FRA3B alterations are particularly common in human cancers associated with environmental carcinogens.

Other important tumor suppressors that are commonly inactivated during genomic alterations involving CFSs include Wwox, Parkin, and caveolin-1. The gene encoding Wwox spans FRA16D common fragile site. Wwox is important in growth regulation and some forms of apoptosis. Levels of this protein are decreased in most human malignancies. Parkin, an E3 ubiquitin ligase is important in autophagy (see later and **Chapter 1**), and is often lost in certain solid tumors. **Caveolin-1** is one of two tumor suppressors (the other being testin) at FRA7G. Caveolins regulate several cellular functions, including signal transduction. This site is often lost in many solid and hematopoietic tumors.

Altered Levels of Tumor Suppressor Proteins and/or Activity

It would be tempting to understand loss of effective tumor suppression as basically a matter of altered TSG structure, or LOH. It would also be wrong. For some important tumor suppressors, the critical parameter is the level of tumor suppressor activity, the presence or absence of mutations being important mainly in determining protein level. Such a tumor suppressor is **phosphatase and tensin homolog (PTEN) detected on chromosome 10**.

PTEN Function

PTEN is a phosphatase that dephosphorylates proteins and lipids. It regulates many pathways that connect growth factor–triggered signals from cell surface receptors to nuclear transcription factors that mediate many cellular functions. PTEN dephosphorylates the highly active signaling intermediate, PIP3, to its inactive 3,4-bisphosphate (PIP2) form. In so doing, PTEN inhibits the AKT-mTOR pathway (Figs. 5-41 and 5-45). As well, PTEN and p53 physically interact and regulate each other. PTEN may be necessary for p53 to be functional, and protects p53 from Mdm2-mediated degradation. Overall, both by virtue of its lipid phosphatase and other activities, *PTEN protein is critical for DNA damage repair, apoptosis, regulating cell cycle progression, maintaining epithelial polarity, and inhibiting EMT. It also regulates cell metabolism to limit glycolysis, as opposed to oxidative phosphorylation* (see later).

PTEN protein is normally maintained at a steady, high concentration. Thus, anything that changes PTEN protein levels even slightly, whether inactivation of one or both alleles, altered promoter activity or other epigenetic or post-translational change, may lower PTEN protein concentration to a point where it is unable to regulate PIP3 effectively. Decreased PTEN activity permits PIP3 to accumulate and constitutively activate diverse signaling pathways involved in cell proliferation and survival, which are key in cancer development.

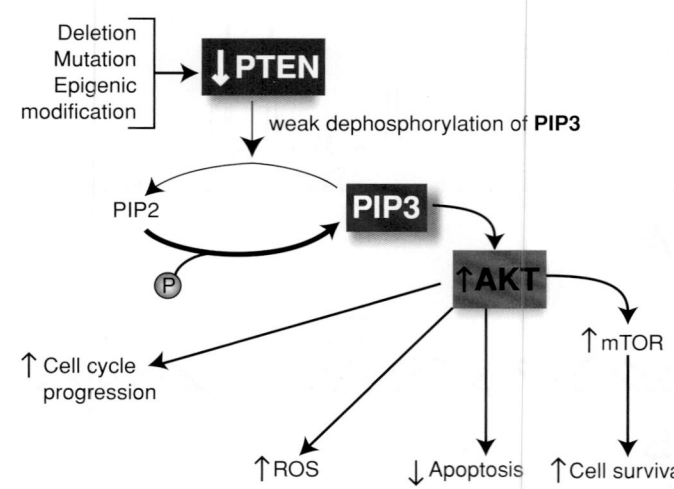

FIGURE 5-45. The consequences of decreased PTEN activity. If activity of PTEN is decreased by mutation or by epigenetic means, PIP3 accumulates, activating Akt, a central signaling intermediate. As a result, certain regulators—p27, Bad, and FOXO—are not activated, thus promoting cell cycle progression and decreasing apoptosis. At the same time, activation of mTOR stimulates cell survival. Loss of PTEN activity therefore facilitates the development of uncontrolled cell proliferation and cancer.

Alterations in PTEN Levels and Function

PTEN is the second most frequently mutated gene in human cancers, after p53. However, the key to its tumor suppressor activity is the level of PTEN activity: even small decreases in PTEN activity may allow some tumors to develop.

There are many mechanisms, and many points in the pathway from gene to functional PTEN activity, at which levels of that activity are subject to up-, or mostly, downregulation (Fig. 5-46):

- **Regulation of transcription.** Several epigenetic mechanisms (see below) decrease levels of transcription of the *PTEN* gene. These include altered histone structure and promoter DNA methylation. Concentrations of proteins that increase or decrease promoter activity are also important.
- **miRNAs** (see below) bind mainly the 3′ untranslated region (UTR) of PTEN mRNA and may cause that transcript to be degraded, or prevent its translation.
- **Pseudogene transcripts as decoys.** A gene, called *PTENP1*, which does not code for a protein, produces an untranslated RNA that closely resembles PTEN mRNA. This transcript is representative of a class of transcripts called **competing endogenous RNAs (ceRNAs)**. Sequence homology between the PTENP1 ceRNA and the PTEN mRNA allows the former to bind to miRNAs that would otherwise target and inhibit PTEN transcripts. The likely significance of this decoy to tumor suppression is illustrated by the fact that *PTENP1* gene is commonly lost in some human cancers, leading to lower PTEN protein levels in such tumors.
- **Protein modifications.** Known posttranslational modifications of PTEN protein can inactivate it (acetylation, oxidation), target it for degradation (polyubiquitination), direct it to subcellular sites where its activity is particularly needed (monoubiquitination) or reverse inactivating modifications (e.g., SIRT1 deacetylates PTEN).

This intricacy and diversity of systems that control levels of active PTEN protein keep its functionality in normal

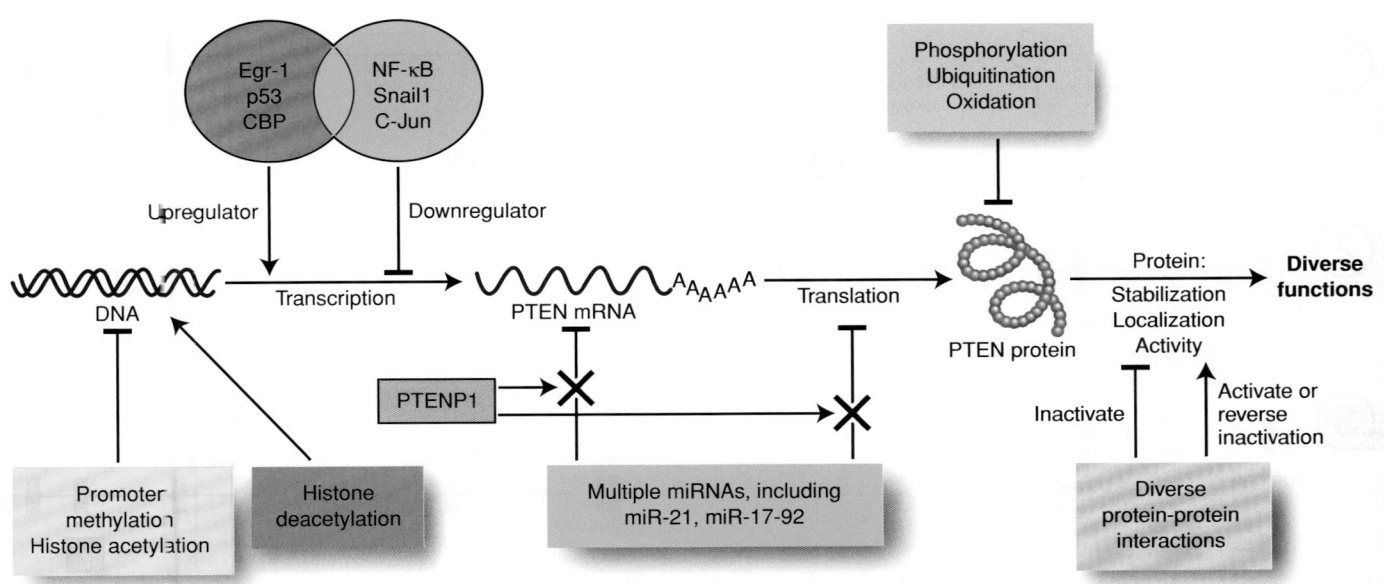

FIGURE 5-46. Regulation of levels of PTEN expression and activity. PTEN is a fundamental regulator of many cellular activities involved in oncogenesis (see Fig. 5-45). Levels of PTEN expression and activity are crucial to cellular homeostasis. PTEN can be regulated by multiple mechanisms, as illustrated here, from altered transcription to mRNA stability to protein modifications.

tissues within very narrow tolerances. Data suggest that a decrease of only 20% in PTEN levels contributes to oncogenesis. In this context, some tissues (e.g., endometrium, hematopoietic) are more susceptible than others (e.g., prostate) to tumorigenesis when PTEN activity is slightly reduced. These observations underscore two important facts: (1) small changes in levels of a tumor suppressor protein may significantly impair its protective tumor suppressor function, in the absence of an inactivating mutation in the TSG itself; and (2) different tissues vary greatly in their susceptibility (see below) to oncogenic stimuli—be they decreased tumor suppression or increased tumor promotion.

PTEN is not the only such protein to which these conclusions apply. Protection afforded by several tumor suppressors, like the breast cancer susceptibility proteins BRCA1 and BRCA2, is observed when one allele is mutant while the other is still active, and so does not necessarily require LOH.

Alternate or Aberrant Forms of Tumor Suppressors

Mechanisms

A single gene may encode multiple proteins, independent of alterations in DNA structure. Among the most important mechanisms for this are alternate splicing and multiple promoters (Fig. 5-47). About 95% of human genes with multiple exons are known to be spliced in multiple ways, generating proteins of different sizes, often with different amino acid sequences and different functions.

Two characteristically important aspects of alternative splicing are shown in Figure 5-47. What is important is that the same genomic DNA sequence encodes multiple individual proteins. Alternative splice donor and acceptor sites may cause an entirely, or partially, different protein to be produced, depending on whether resulting mRNAs are in frame or not, compared to the original, "classical," transcript and its derivative protein.

Alternatively, transcription may be initiated from a second promoter (often designated P2). This may yield a

protein homologous to the "classical protein," yet truncated at its amino terminus. Such amino-terminal variants are often designated, ΔN. Of course, these two mechanisms may operate in tandem to produce a plethora of proteins of different sizes, compositions, and degrees of homology.

Factors that determine how splicing occurs, what sites are suitable donors and acceptors, etc., are quite complex. They involve many participant molecules. Some of these are tissue specific, so that different mRNA alternatives and resulting variant proteins may be dissimilar in different cell or tissue types.

Alternative Splicing, Tumor Suppression, and Interference With Tumor Suppression

Alternative splicing, etc., is important in generating specific tumor suppressor proteins, in determining their ability to protect from cancer and the spread of cancer, regulating tumor suppression, and escape from tumor suppression.

The ARF-INK4 Locus. One of nature's more impressive mistakes was to have concentrated three major (and several minor) tumor suppressors at the same locus (Fig. 5-48A). This renders them all simultaneously susceptible to elimination with a single deletion event. Even worse, these tumor suppressors can all be turned off by a single interaction between a repressor protein and one specific area in the gene complex. Thus, p14^{ARF}, p15^{INK4b}, and p16^{INK4a} (see above) are all encoded at chromosome 9p21. Loss of this locus is very common in human cancers, and leads to deregulation of Rb-related cell cycle control and excessive inhibition of p53 (Fig. 5-48A).

The three tumor suppressor transcripts are all driven by different promoters, p15^{INK4b} being upstream of the others. P14^{ARF} (ARF = alternate reading frame) and p16^{INK4a} share some exons (see Fig. 5-48A), but shared coding sequences are in different reading frames. Thus, these protein products of the same gene have no sequence homology.

Despite having different promoters, all three open reading frames share a common repressor site (Fig. 5-48B). The

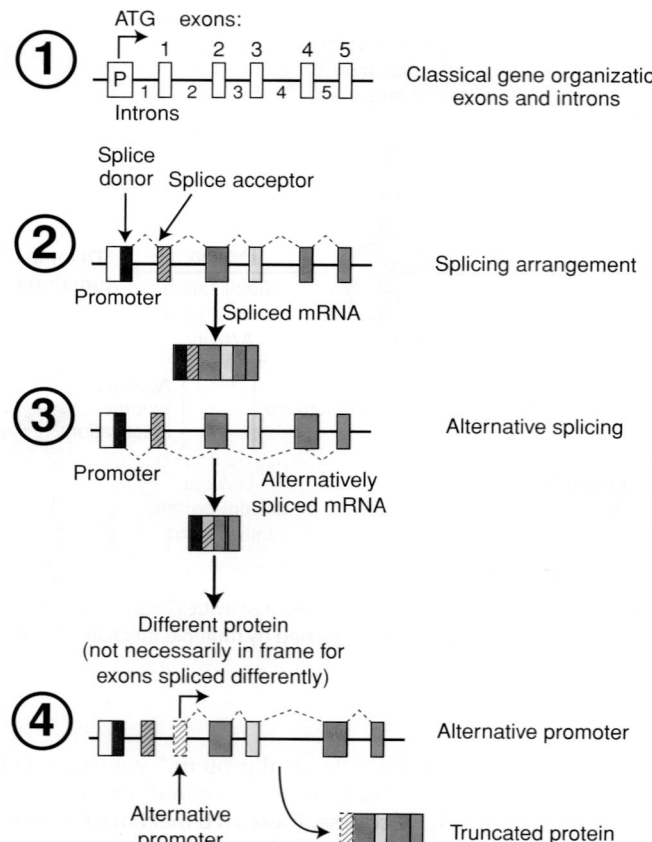

FIGURE 5-47. How alternate splicing affects a gene's products and their activities. RNA splicing is an important mechanism by which gene activity is controlled. It is illustrated here. **1.** The organization of exons and introns in a hypothetical gene is shown. **2.** Transcribed RNAs are spliced: a splice "donor" site at the 3′ end of one exon is linked to a splice "acceptor" site at the 5′ end of the following exon, with the RNA corresponding to the intervening intron removed. The result is an mRNA that is exported from the nucleus for translation by ribosomes. **3.** However, there may be alternative splice donor and acceptor sites at different points within the several exons, so that an entirely different mRNA may be generated. The resulting protein may have variable sequence homology to the protein produced in **2**, depending on whether the alternate splice sites result in an mRNA that is in frame with the original or not. **4.** Another strategy for generating a different protein from the same gene is alternate promoters. In this situation, a promoter different from the promoter in **2** mediates transcriptional activation, and transcription begins from a completely different site in the DNA sequence. The result may be a partial protein, a protein that is spliced differently from the original (in **2**) and thus potentially completely different, or some variation thereof.

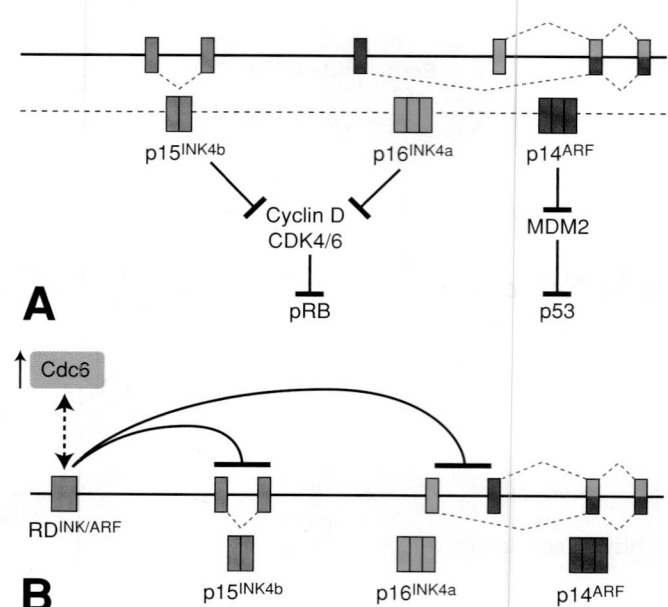

FIGURE 5-48. Multiple tumor suppressors from one locus. A. The organization of the INK/ARF locus. This gene encodes three major and different tumor suppressors, as shown. p15^INK4b and p16^INK4a are both critical regulators of cyclin D and CDKs 4 and 6. p15 is transcribed separately from p16. However, p16 and p14^ARF (ARF stands for alternate reading frame) coding sequences overlap. Due to alternate splicing (see Fig. 5-44), their coding sequences are totally different. The functions of p16 and p14 are also distinct, as shown. **B.** The area RD^INK/ARF represents a region 5′ to the transcriptional start sites that is the target for Cdc6-mediated transcriptional silencing of all of these proteins. All three tumor suppressors are silenced by Cdc6, however, as Cdc6 binds the promoter for p15 and recruits histone deacetylases to the entire gene complex, inhibiting transcription of all three tumor suppressors.

repressor protein, Cdc6, binds a common site and simultaneously extinguishes expression of all three critical tumor suppressors.

An additional mechanism of tumor suppression is exemplified at this locus, that is, **long, noncoding RNAs (lncRNA,** see below). An important lncRNA, called ANRIL, suppresses expression of p15^INK4b, and is particularly important in some leukemias and prostate cancers.

p53 and Its Cousins. As mentioned above, p53 is the most prominent member of a family of tumor suppressors with diverse functions. All of them are transcriptional activators

and repressors, and all inhibit one or more cancer attributes (see above). Like p53, p63 and p73 are active in this mode as homotetramers. The p53/p63/p73 story is more complex than that, however. Each of these genes encodes multiple transcripts, for which diverse, sometimes antagonistic, functions have been identified.

The best understood of these variants are shortened transcripts, generated by alternative splicing and/or different internal promoters. These variant mRNAs encode proteins lacking variable amounts of the full-length proteins. Transcriptionally deficient forms of each family are known: ΔNp53, ΔNp63, ΔNp73. Many splice variants, designated with α, β, etc., are also known. These ΔNs and splice variants may oligomerize with the full-length proteins, to form transcriptionally inactive tetramers. Furthermore, these variants, especially the ΔN variants, can bind to promoters normally activated by the full-length proteins (e.g., proapoptotic proteins such as Bax, Puma) and block access to these promoters by wild-type proteins (Fig. 5-49). The existence of multiple additional promoters and many splice variants for each protein further complicates matters.

Nonetheless, ratios of full length: ΔN variants are tightly regulated in normal tissues. Although p63 and p73 genes are not often mutated in cancers, the ΔN forms of p53 family member proteins are upregulated—or ΔN:full-length ratios altered—in many tumors. For example, ΔNp63 predominance

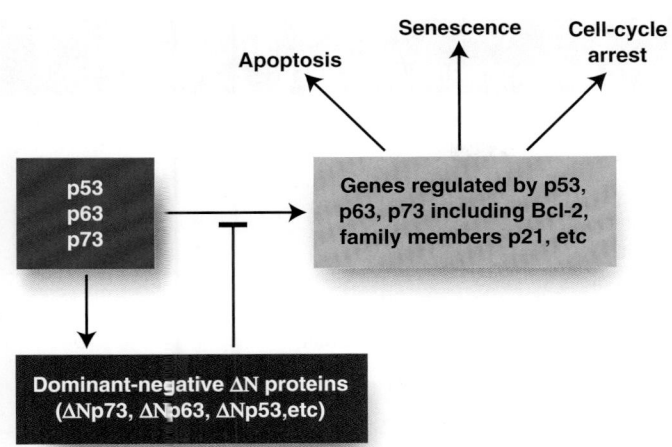

FIGURE 5-49. The isoforms of the members of the p53 family and their interactions. All members of the p53 tumor suppressor protein family have alternate isoforms deleted at their amino termini (ΔN), which act as dominant negative proteins, and impede the transcriptional and other activities of the full-length p53, p63, and p73.

is associated with poor response to certain chemotherapies that target DNA and may portend poor prognosis.

Thus, complex as it is, the availability of alternate transcripts, and resulting variants or different proteins, encoded by the same locus represents an important means by which cancers can evade tumor suppression mechanisms.

INHERITED CANCER SYNDROMES

Cancer syndromes attributed to inherited mutations make up only 1% of human cancers. These mutations mainly involve tumor suppressor and DNA repair genes. As discussed above for *Rb*, inheritance of a single mutated allele of a TSG results in a heterozygous state, and high risk for LOH (i.e., inactivation of the normal allele). What is inherited in this setting is a high degree of susceptibility to developing cancer. The germline genotype of such people is heterozygous, but both tumor suppressor alleles are inactivated in the tumors that develop.

Hereditary tumor syndromes can be arbitrarily divided into three categories:

1. Inherited malignant tumors (e.g., Rb, WT, many endocrine tumors)
2. Inherited tumors that remain benign or have a malignant potential (e.g., APC)
3. Inherited syndromes associated with a high risk of malignant tumors (e.g., Bloom syndrome, ataxia-telangiectasia)

These syndromes highlight tumor suppressor activities and the genes that cause them. However, many inherited syndromes entail a spectrum of tumors different from what the significance of the mutated gene(s) would suggest. For example, decreased PTEN is very common in many malignancies (see above) but germline loss of PTEN (Cowden syndrome) is mainly associated with benign hamartomas.

Bear in mind that inherited defects in tumor suppression are fortunately rare. However, they help to identify tumor suppressors, delineate how the affected TSG products act, and identify mechanisms of tumor suppressor inactivation. Acquired impairments in tumor suppression are common.

Many more TSGs are known than can be described here, and their numbers are increasing. In addition, inherited mutations in TSGs are responsible for many named tumor susceptibility syndromes, some representative examples of which are listed in Table 5-6. Most of these are discussed in chapters dealing with specific organs.

Some disorders, called **phakomatoses** (e.g., tuberous sclerosis, neurofibromatosis), are difficult to classify. These have both developmental and neoplastic features. Tumors associated with these syndromes mostly involve the nervous system.

Only a small proportion of cancers show mendelian inheritance, but certain malignancies undeniably tend to run in families. For many tumors, other family members of an affected person have two- to threefold increased risk of developing that type of cancer. This predisposition is particularly marked for cancers of the breast and colon, but is also exemplified in the interplay of heredity and environment. Thus, smokers who are closely related to someone with lung cancer have a higher risk of developing lung cancer than do smokers without this familial background.

Organ Specificity in Inherited Cancer Syndromes

Many of the inherited germline mutations cited above (e.g., *BRCA1* or *VHL* genes) lead to specific tumor syndromes. However, it remains unclear why alterations in certain genes tend to affect some organs but not others. Thus, the importance of BRCA1 in repair of DNA DSBs is well established, but it is unknown why germline *BRCA1* mutations lead mainly to breast and ovarian cancers and not others, and why women are more profoundly affected than men.

GENETIC INSTABILITY IN CANCER

Oncogenesis involves extensive genetic changes, among which genomic instability is central. Although not universal in tumors, CI entails translocations, additions or deletions of entire chromosomes, or portions thereof, and yields variable cellular karyotypes. CI may result in **aneuploidy** (abnormal chromosome number), **gene amplification** (increased copy number of a gene), and LOH (loss of one allele of a pair).

LOH may follow loss of a whole chromosome, deletion of a bit of DNA bearing the gene in question, or inactivation of that gene. As a result, the remaining allele is the only one for that locus and controls the phenotype. If that remaining allele is rendered abnormal, the lack of a second allele to compensate means that its abnormal phenotype is unopposed. Moreover, the phenotype of the remaining allele may facilitate tumorigenesis. Typically, about one-fourth of alleles are lost in malignancies.

Three Main Mechanisms Alter Activation of Cellular Genes

There are three general mechanisms by which proto-oncogenes become activated:

- A mutation in a proto-oncogene leads to **production of an abnormal protein**.
- Increased expression of a proto-oncogene causes **overproduction of a normal gene product**.
- Activation or expression of proto-oncogenes is regulated by numerous autoinhibitory mechanisms that

TABLE 5-6

SELECTED EXAMPLES OF HEREDITARY CONDITIONS PREDISPOSING TO INCREASED RISK OF CANCER

Syndrome	Gene	Predominant Malignancies	Gene Function	Inheritance[a]
Chromosomal Instability Syndromes				
Bloom syndrome	BLM	Many sites	DNA repair	R
Fanconi anemia	?	Acute myelogenous leukemia	DNA repair	R
Hereditary Skin Cancer				
Familial melanoma	CDKN2 (p16)	Malignant melanoma	Cell cycle regulation	D
Xeroderma pigmentosum	XP group	Squamous cell carcinoma of skin; malignant melanoma	DNA repair	R
Endocrine System				
Multiple endocrine neoplasia (MEN) type 1	MEN1	Pancreatic islet cell tumors	Transcriptional regulation	D
MEN type 2	RET	Thyroid medullary carcinoma; pheochromocytoma (MEN type 2A)	Receptor tyrosine kinase; cell cycle regulation	D
Breast Cancer				
Breast/ovary cancer syndrome	BRCA1	Carcinomas of ovary, breast, fallopian tube and prostate	DNA repair	D
Site-specific breast cancer	BRCA2	Female and male breast carcinoma; carcinomas of prostate, pancreas, and ovary	DNA repair (Fanconi pathway)	D/R
Breast cancer	PALB2	Breast, pancreas	DNA repair (Fanconi pathway)	D/R
Nervous System				
Retinoblastoma	RB	Retinoblastoma	Cell cycle regulation	D
Phakomatoses				
Neurofibromatosis type 1	NF1	Neurofibrosarcomas; astrocytomas; malignant melanomas	Regulator of Ras-mediated signaling	D
Neurofibromatosis type 2	NF2	Meningiomas; schwannomas	Regulator of cytoskeleton	D
Gastrointestinal System				
Familial adenomatous polyposis	APC	Colorectal carcinoma	Cell cycle regulation; migration and adhesion	D
Hereditary nonpolyposis colorectal carcinoma (HNPCC; Lynch syndrome)	hMSH2, hMSH6, MLH1, hPMS1, hPMS2	Carcinomas of colon, endometrium, ovary, and bladder; malignant melanoma	DNA repair	D
Peutz–Jeghers syndrome	LKB1/STK11	Stomach, small bowel, and colon carcinomas	Serine threonine kinase	D
Kidney				
Wilms tumor	WT	Wilms tumor	Transcriptional regulation	D
von Hippel–Lindau	VHL	Renal cell carcinoma	Regulator of adhesion	D
Multiple Sites				
Li–Fraumeni syndrome	TP53	Breast carcinoma; soft tissue sarcomas; brain tumors; leukemia	Transcriptional regulation	D
Ataxia-telangiectasia	ATM	Lymphoma; leukemia	Cell signaling and DNA repair	R

[a]D, autosomal dominant; R, autosomal recessive.

ATM = ataxia-telangiectasia mutated (gene); cAMP = cyclic adenosine 3′,5′-monophosphate; PTEN = phosphatase and tensin homolog; TGFβ = transforming growth factor-β.

safeguard against inappropriate activity. Many mutations in proto-oncogenes render them **insensitive to normal autoinhibitory and regulatory constraints** and lead to constitutive activation.

The converse processes apply to inactivation of tumor suppressors (see above). That is: (1) mutations may produce an abnormal protein that lacks or interferes with tumor suppression; (2) they become ineffective if a regulatory target is overexpressed, overwhelming a normally expressed suppressor; or (3) their expression is impaired, whether by regulatory mutation or epigenetic inactivation.

Multiple Mechanisms Generate Genetic Instability

Several mechanisms of genetic instability contribute to tumorigenesis. These include: (1) point mutations; (2) translocations; (3) amplifications and deletions; and (4) loss or gain of whole chromosomes. These types of instability occur in many ways. Among the most important is the loss—whether by inheritance, mutation, or epigenetic inactivation—of proteins that protect cells from mutations. These include cell cycle regulatory proteins (checkpoints, proofreaders, mitosis-related chromosomal sorting proteins, etc.) and proteins that mediate DNA repair functions.

Role of Defects in DNA Repair Systems

Part of our understanding of how defects in DNA repair contribute to oncogenesis comes from observations made in familial cancer syndromes. For example, a type of colon cancer syndrome, hereditary nonpolyposis colon cancer (HNPCC, Lynch syndrome), entails a 75% lifetime risk for colon cancer. The large majority of HNPCC patients have mutations in *MLH1* or *MSH2* DNA MMR enzymes (see above).

Xeroderma pigmentosum (XP), a hereditary syndrome in which enhanced sensitivity to UV light predisposes to skin cancer, reflects defects in NER enzymes. Most cases of some common forms of spontaneous lung cancer, entail acquired mutations in proteins that mediate NER.

Double-Strand Break Repair and Cancer

As mentioned above, detection of DSBs and initiation of repair processes involves the ATM protein. Mutations in ATM and other enzymes involved in DSB repair are associated with a high frequency of malignant tumors.

Point Mutations

Although humans have evolved highly efficient mechanisms to recognize and repair point mutations, single-base changes do occur normally, at rates of 10^{-9}/base/cell division in somatic cells and 10^{-11} in germ cells. Advanced DNA sequencing techniques detect many of these single-base changes—called **single nucleotide polymorphisms**, or **SNPs**—in tumors.

Activation by Point Mutation

Conversion of proto-oncogenes into oncogenes may involve (1) point mutations, (2) deletions, or (3) chromosomal translocations. The first oncogene identified in a human tumor was activated *HRAS* in a bladder cancer. This gene had a remarkably subtle alteration—a point mutation in codon 12, which

changed a glycine to a valine in H-ras protein. Subsequent studies of other cancers revealed point mutations involving other *HRAS* codons, suggesting that these positions are critical for the normal function of the Ras protein. Many alterations in other growth-regulatory genes have since been described.

Activating, or gain-of-function, mutations in proto-oncogenes are usually somatic rather than germline alterations. Germline mutations in proto-oncogenes, which are known to be important regulators of growth during development, are ordinarily lethal in utero. There are exceptions to this rule. For example, mutant c-*ret* causes certain heritable endocrine cancers, and c-*met*, which encodes hepatocyte growth factor receptor, is associated with a hereditary form of renal cancer.

Chromosomal Translocation

In chromosomal translocations, a piece of one chromosome joins with a part of another. These rearrangements contribute to tumorigenesis in one of two main ways. Sometimes they place a normal gene, like a proto-oncogene, under the control of a promoter that is regulated less effectively than the native proto-oncogene promoter.

Activation by Chromosomal Translocation

In 75% of patients with Burkitt lymphoma (see below and **Chapter 26**), c-*myc*, which drives cell cycle progression, is translocated from its regulated site on chromosome 8 to a position on chromosome 14 (Fig. 5-50). This change changes control of c-*myc* expression to a promoter for immunoglobulin heavy chains (IgH). As a result, c-*myc* is driven by immunoglobulin promoter/enhancer sequences and consequently is expressed constitutively in B lymphocytes, rather than in a regulated manner. In 25% of patients with Burkitt lymphoma, the c-*myc* proto-oncogene remains on chromosome 8 but is activated by translocation of immunoglobulin light-chain genes (IgL) from chromosome 2 or 22 to the 3' end of the c-*myc* gene. In either case, these chromosomal translocations do not create a novel protein but stimulate

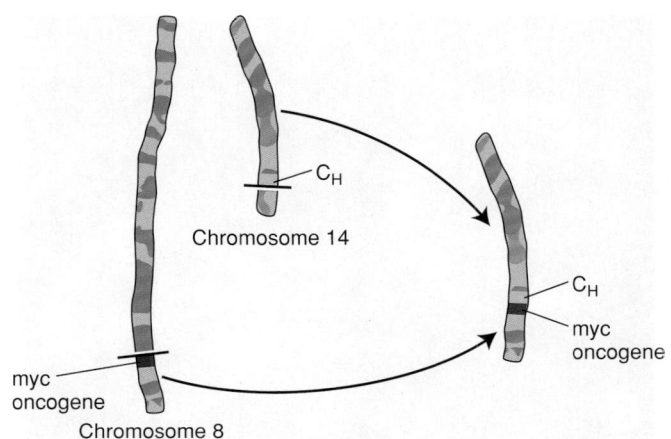

FIGURE 5-50. Schematic representation of the t(8;14) translocation in Burkitt lymphoma (BL). In BL, chromosomal breaks involve the long arms of chromosomes 8 and 14. The c-*myc* gene on chromosome 8 is translocated to a region on chromosome 14 adjacent to the gene coding for the constant region of an immunoglobulin heavy chain (C_H). Expression of c-*myc* is enhanced by its association with promoter/enhancer regions of the actively transcribed immunoglobulin genes.

overproduction of a normal gene product. In Burkitt lymphoma, excessive expression normal c-*myc*, probably in association with other genetic alterations, leads to the emergence of a dominant B-cell clone, driven relentlessly to proliferate as a monoclonal neoplasm. Many other hematopoietic malignancies, lymphomas, and solid tumors reflect activation of oncogenes by chromosomal translocation. Although some malignancies are **initiated** by chromosomal translocations, myriad chromosomal abnormalities take place (translocations, breaks, aneuploidy, etc.) during **progression** of many cancers.

Translocation Generating a New Protein

Chromosomal translocation may cause a new, abnormal protein to be produced. Part of one chromosome, including part or all of the coding region from a protein, moves to another chromosome, into the coding region of another gene. The result is a new protein, sharing sequence homology with both original ones, but active in driving oncogenesis in a way that the originals are not.

The first—and still best-known—example of a hybrid protein resulting from chromosomal translocation in a human cancer is the **Philadelphia chromosome** in 95% of patients with chronic myelogenous leukemia (CML, Fig. 5-51). In this situation, c-*abl* proto-oncogene on chromosome 9 is translocated to chromosome 22, into the breakpoint cluster region (BCR). There, c-*abl* coding sequences unite with BCR to produce a hybrid oncogene that encodes an aberrant protein

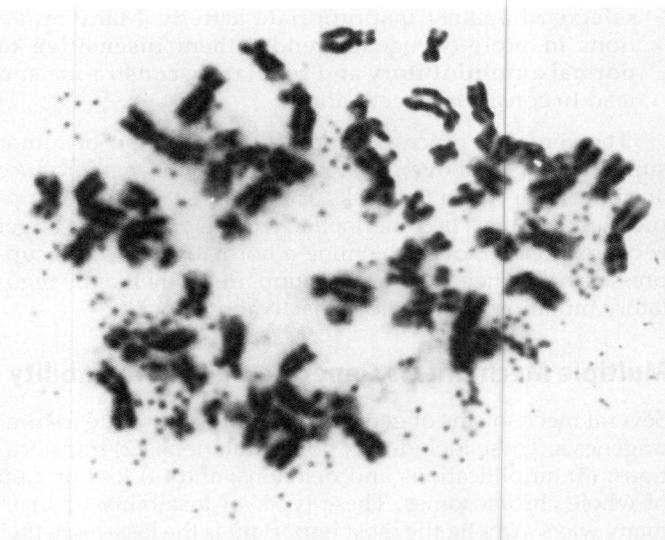

FIGURE 5-52. Double minutes in human cancers. Double minutes in a karyotype of a soft tissue sarcoma appear as multiple small bodies.

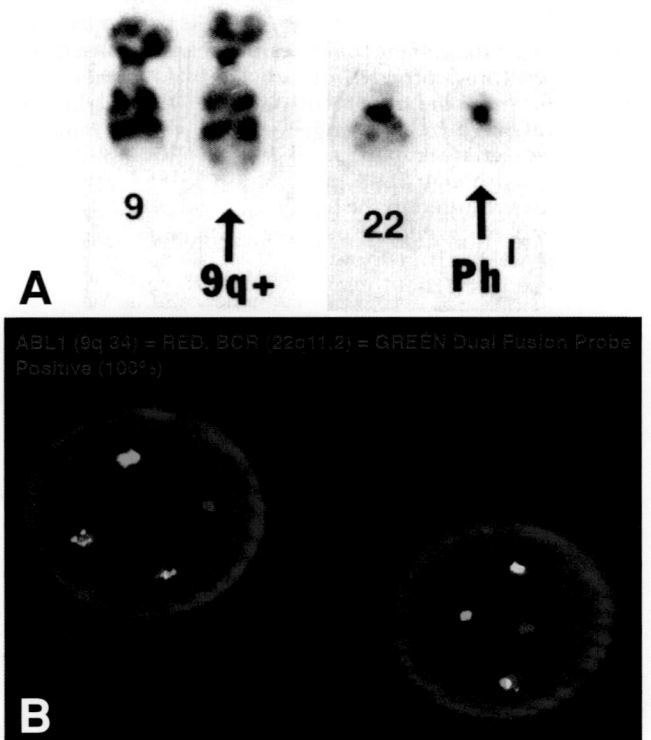

FIGURE 5-51. The t(9;22) translocation in chronic myelogenous leukemia. A. The shortened chromosome 22 and the longer chromosome 9 shown on the translocated chromosomes. B. Fluorescence in situ hybridization (FISH). This assay shows the fusion chromosome using a *red* ABL chromosome 9 probe and a *green* BCR chromosome 22 probe, which join to make a *yellow* signal. Two tumor cells are shown. Each has one normal chromosome 9 and one normal chromosome 22.

with very high tyrosine kinase activity and provides potent mitogenic and antiapoptotic signals. Bcr-Abl protein, from the Philadelphia chromosome translocation, exemplifies how chromosomal rearrangements may generate a novel chimeric (fusion) protein. This novel protein provides a target for highly effective pharmacotherapy for CML.

Amplifications and Deletions

Genetic amplifications are duplications of variable-sized regions of chromosomes. Cytogenetically, such modifications appear as small DNA fragments that are not part of any chromosome, called "double minutes" (Fig. 5-52), or as increased signal intensity when fluorescent probes for specific regions hybridize with chromosomes. In tumors, such changes may provide survival advantages if they affect oncogenes, drug resistance genes, or related nefarious characters within the genomic fragments.

Activation by Gene Amplification

The *ERBB2* proto-oncogene is amplified in up to a third of breast and ovarian cancers. The *ERBB2* gene (also called *HER2/neu*) encodes a receptor-type tyrosine kinase that structurally resembles EGF receptor. *ERBB2* amplification in those cancers (Fig. 5-53) correlates with poorer overall survival and decreased time to relapse. In this context, an antibody targeted against HER2/neu (trastuzumab) is used as adjunctive therapy for breast cancers that overexpress this protein.

Inactivation by Deletion

Deletions, naturally, are lost chromatin—from tiny pieces to whole arms of chromosomes. Just as amplifications come to attention when they occur at sites of oncogenes, so do deletions that affect TSGs.

Alterations in Chromosome Number

Addition or loss of whole chromosomes generally occurs during mitosis and probably reflects defective mitotic

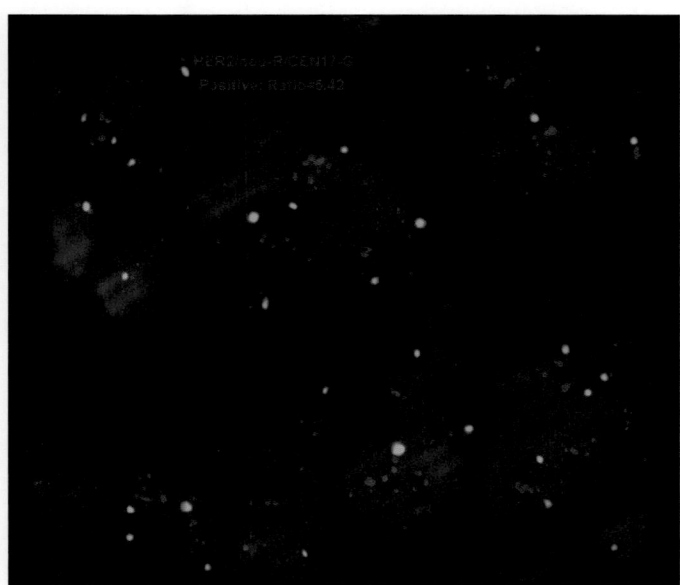

FIGURE 5-53. *ER3B2* **amplification in human cancers.** ERBB2 amplification in a human breast cancer (FISH), showing the multiple copies (*red fluorescence*) as minute bodies. As a chromosome control, a green probe for chromosome 17 is shown.

spindle binding to chromosomal kinetochores (see above), possibly when the Aurora B kinase apparatus malfunctions (see above). Chromosomes then attach too avidly to mitotic spindles and fail to separate and segregate normally.

Almost all solid tumors have abnormal karyotypes. Tumors often lose one copy of chromosome 10, where the gene for PTEN (see above) resides, or possess extra copies of chromosomes that carry particular oncogenes.

Chromosomal loss may also occur with diploid karyotypes. One copy of each chromosome derives from each parent. If, for any particular chromosome pair, one parent's chromosome is lost, the other parent's copy of that chromosome may be duplicated and replace the one that was lost. That is, the cell has two copies of one parent's chromosome instead of one copy from each parent. The resulting copy-neutral loss of heterozygosity (CN-LOH) is called **uniparental disomy (see Chapter 6)**, and is common in many malignancies. CN-LOH has prognostic significance in several cancer types, such as acute myeloid leukemias.

EPIGENETIC MECHANISMS IN CANCER

Most of our appreciation of carcinogenesis comes from studying changes in the DNA sequences that encode proteins—whether oncogenes, tumor suppressors, or others. These are easily studied experimentally, and readily understandable. However, as noted above, mutations that yield mutant or dysfunctional proteins, or abolish some proteins altogether do not adequately explain tumorigenesis. Other forces are at work, which influence cell behavior at least as profoundly as do DNA codons themselves.

Epigenetics, then, encompasses diverse mechanisms that control gene expression, independently of the DNA sequences encoding the protein(s) in question. These physiologic processes are integral to normal cell equilibrium. *No individual modality necessarily promotes or suppresses cancer, but*

all may act both to inhibit tumor development and to promote it. The net result depends on the specific gene(s) involved and how they are affected. Epigenetic mechanisms interact with each other. They are complex, interwoven, and layered, so that effects of one may require others to participate.

Multiple Epigenetic Mediators Influence Tumorigenesis

> "… there is nothing either good or bad, but thinking makes it so." —Hamlet II:2

Epigenetics mostly determines whether—and how much—protein is produced, and, to a lesser extent, that protein's structure. It is the direct action of the epigenetic change and the function of the protein that determine the consequences. The biologic results of altered epigenetics depend on whether the alteration up- or downregulates the target gene, and function of that gene. A base change in a gene's promoter may impair transcription factor binding and so decrease expression. Or, it may add a new transcription factor–binding site and so increase expression. The nature of the gene's product then determines whether the effect is pro- or antitumorigenic.

To understand how epigenetic influences contribute to tumor development, one should appreciate the diversity of these influences. These are summarized in Table 5-7. These influences may overlap, so that, for example, methylation of the promoter (see below) of a gene that encodes an miRNA may decrease the amount of that miRNA. If that miRNA in turn decreases translation of a gene encoding (again, for example) an oncogene, then levels of that oncogene protein would increase.

Rather than try to understand each of these different mechanisms, it is more important to appreciate their diversity and complexity, and the plasticity of regulatory mechanisms that may be activated during oncogenesis. *Epigenetic mechanisms orchestrate many physiologic processes, like embryogenesis, and normally function to prevent tumors. In those settings, they stimulate scant investigative or clinical attention. However, when they are dysfunctional or run amok, they may, among other things, drive or facilitate tumor development. Then, they stimulate interest.* Multiple influences (see below) may trigger their contribution to tumorigenesis, but collectively epigenetics are key determinants of tumor development and evolving targets for therapeutic intervention.

DNA and Histone Modifications Regulate Promoter Activity

How much of a specific protein a cell possesses or makes can be at least as important as that protein's structure in determining how well it, for example, repairs DNA or drives mitosis. Transcriptional activity is among the most basic determinants of how much protein is made. Transcription in turn depends on multiple factors, including promoter activity. Common histone and DNA modifications which affect transcriptional activity are illustrated in Figure 5-54.

Methylating and Demethylating Enzymes

DNA and histone methylation are mediated by DNA methyltransferases (DNMTs) and histone methyltransferases

TABLE 5-7
BASIC EPIGENETIC MECHANISMS

A. Involving the Gene to Be Expressed

Processes/Structures Involved	Effect
DNA methylation and demethylation Histone methylation and demethylation Histone acetylation and deacetylation Nucleosome positioning	Levels of transcription

Noncoding sequences in the expressed gene

Promoter	Levels of transcription
Enhancer	Levels of transcription
Splice sites (donor/acceptor)	Multiple effects, including protein structure
Introns	Multiple effects
Synonymous mutations	Multiple effects, including altered translation, RNA stability, splicing
5′ UTR 3′ UTR	mRNA stability, processing, translation

B. Reflecting Changes in Other Genes

Processes/Structures Involved	Effect
Genes for noncoding RNAs	
MicroRNAs Long noncoding RNAs Protein-interacting RNAs	Many processes, including transcript stability, translation, protein structure
Genes encoding proteins regulating RNA	
Splicing enzymes IRES and upstream orfs RNA-binding proteins	RNA sequence, protein structure, translation, RNA stability
Genes encoding proteins regulating transcription	
Transcription factors Repressors	Level of transcription
Proteins regulating DNA structure	
Insulators	Independence of gene expression from factors influencing neighboring genes

(HMTs), respectively. Both sets of enzymes use S-adenosyl methionine (SAM) as a methyl donor. As illustrated in Figure 5-54, SAM for all these reactions is generated from extracellular supplies of folate and methionine.

DNA and histone demethylation, similarly, follow parallel paths. **Jumonji-C domain–containing histone demethylases (JHDMs)** catalyze most histone demethylation. A group of enzymes called **ten–eleven transloca-tion enzymes (TETs)** catalyze DNA demethylation. Both

sets of enzymes depend on ascorbate and **α-ketoglutarate (αKG)**.

Promoter Methylation and Demethylation

Because molecular techniques to study DNA methylation were available long ago, our understanding of promoter methylation is deeper than that of many other epigenetic influences. **CpG** dinucleotides—CpG islands ("p" denoting

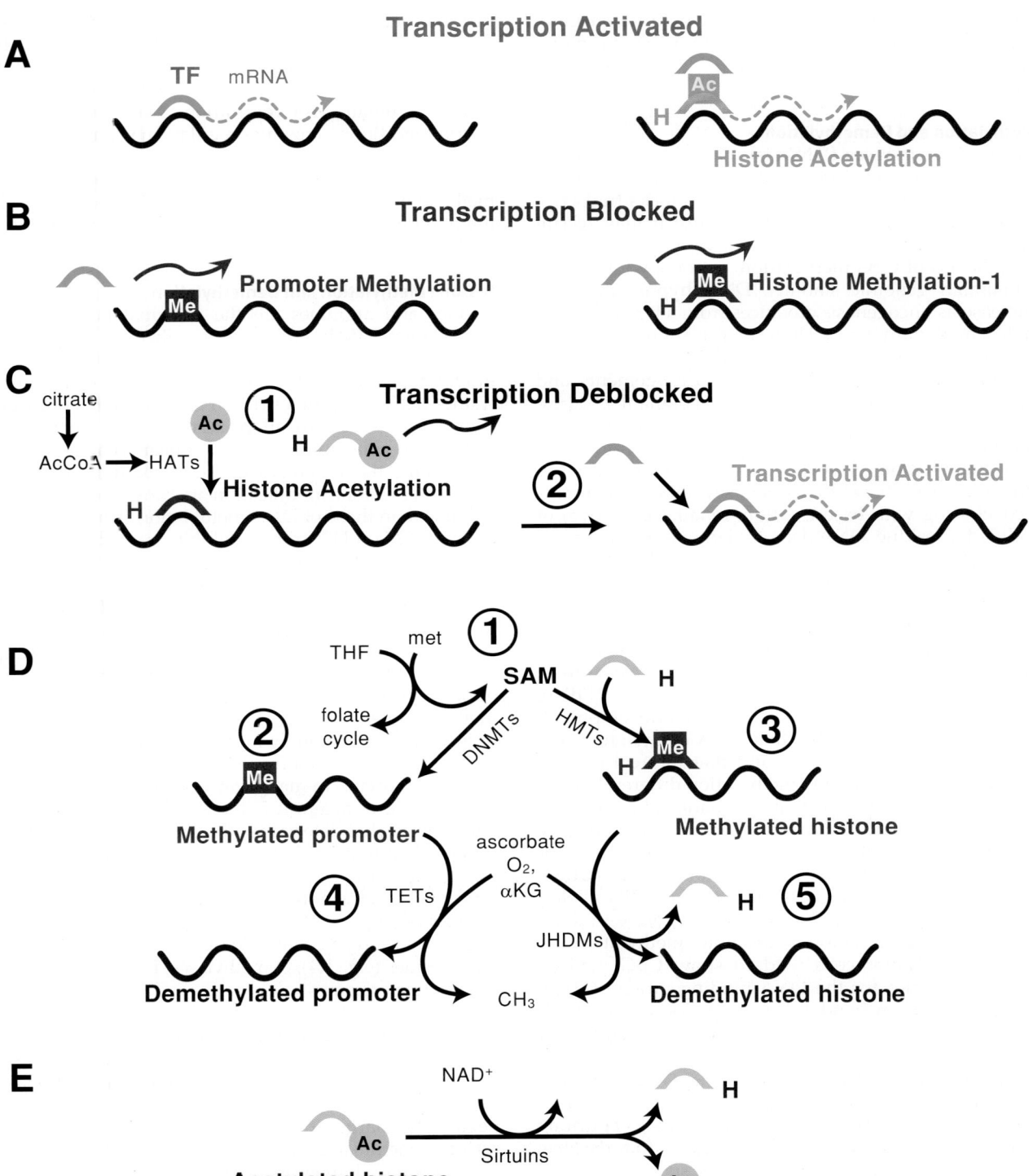

FIGURE 5-54. Transcriptional regulation. A. Normally, a transcription factor (TF) binds a promoter, and initiates transcription (**left**). Acetylation of a histone tends to facilitate transcription (**right**). **B.** Transcription is generally impeded by methylation of a promoter or a promoter-binding histone. **C.** If an obstructing histone is acetylated, as indicated, transcription is deblocked. **D.** The mechanics of promoter and histone methylation and demethylation are shown. S-adenosyl methionine is central to both promoter and histone methylation, as shown, by providing the methyl group to be transferred to DNA by DNA methyltransferases (DNMTs, left upper), with folate as a participant, or to histones by histone methyltransferases (HMTs, right upper). Demethylation reactions (lower frames) are catalyzed by enzymes that require ascorbate, α-ketoglutarate (αKG), and oxygen. Ten–eleven translocation enzymes (TETs) demethylate promoters; Jumonji-C domain–containing histone demethylases (JHDMs) demethylate histones. **E.** Acetylated histones (which, unlike methylated histones, increase transcription of the gene(s) in question) may be deacetylated (thereby silencing the gene) in an NAD⁺-dependent reaction by sirtuins (**see** Chapter 1).

the interbase phosphodiester bond)—are distributed inhomogeneously in the genome. They predominate in promoter regions of many genes and in repetitive DNA sequences, like **transposable elements** (see below).

DNA Methylation and Demethylation

DNA methyltransferases (DNMTs) may transfer a methyl group to CpG cytosines. CpG promoter methylation generally decreases gene expression, because it blocks transcription factor–binding promoters and because it may recruit transcriptional suppressors to the site. Normal cells tend to have high levels of CpG methylation, genome-wide, which helps maintain genomic stability. DNA hypomethylation may increase as oncogenesis advances from a benign proliferation to a malignant tumor. Undermethylation destabilizes DNA structure, favors genomic instability, and facilitates chromosomal deletions, translocations, rearrangements, and aneuploidy, all of which contribute to malignant progression. Transposable DNA sequences are particularly prone to translocation when hypomethylated.

DNA methylation is reversible. TET-catalyzed DNA demethylation (see above) may entail several cycles of reactions, concluding with base excision/repair (see above) of the modified C residue. DNA demethylation is important for maintaining DNA structure and regulating transcription.

Hypomethylation is particularly prominent in repetitive DNA sequences, exons, and introns of protein-encoding genes. Decreased methylation of genes associated with cell proliferation may increase transcription of such genes. The same principle applies to latent human tumor viruses (e.g., human papillomavirus [HPV], Epstein–Barr virus [EBV]), hypomethylation of which may lead to tumor development.

It is important to remember that DNA methylation patterns in tumors show specificity, and that the real issue is that tumor cells distribute CpG methylation differently from normal cells. Tumors often use this mechanism to inactivate **TSG** transcription, and methylation of TSGs is generally more common than mutations as a way tumors evade suppression. CpG methylation may also complement mutation, to complete inactivation of both of a pair of TSG alleles. FHIT, p15^{INK4b}, and BRCA1 TSGs (see above) are especially susceptible to downregulation by promoter methylation.

Furthermore, tumor cells tend to show CpG methylation at binding sites for the DNA-binding protein **CTCF**. This protein acts as an **insulator**. It forms loops—of which there are thousands—in genomic DNA to protect genes from enhancer-mediated transcriptional orchestration directed at other nearby genes. Methylation blocks CTCF binding, removing the protection provided by CTCF's insulator function and subjecting normally insulated genes to spurious regulation. Thus, the fundamental principle is that *the basic alteration is **aberrant methylation**, and is site-specific. CpG methylation patterns in every tumor and every gene are different.*

Histone Modifications

Chromatin is a complex of DNA and proteins that promotes DNA stability and allows it to fit in a small space (the nucleus). It contains repeating units, **nucleosomes** (see below), periodically spaced structures with a combination of four histone proteins (H2A, H2B, H3, H4), wrapped in DNA. Covalent alterations to histones include methylation, acetylation, ubiquitination, phosphorylation, and others. These require specific histone-modifying enzymes, and are reversible. What histone methylases (HMTs) do can be undone by histone demethylases (JHDMs). Histone acetylation (by HATs) can be reversed by histone deacetylases (Sirtuins, HDACs). Covalent changes to histone structure control DNA transcription, repair, and replication. Not surprisingly, then, histone-modifying enzymes regulate many activities, including oncogenesis.

Histone modifications are more complex than CpG methylation-related changes in DNA. There are basically two main types: methylation/demethylation and acetylation/deacetylation.

Histone Methylation and Demethylation

Lysines and arginines are the principal targets of histone methylation. HMTs and JHDMs utilize the same metabolic substrates (SAM; ascorbate/αKG, respectively) as their DNA-modifying cousins (Fig. 5-54). However, there are many lysines (K) and arginines (R) on the several histones, and the consequences of methylation, etc. depend on where (on which histone, on what amino acids, and near what gene) and how many times the amino acid(s) is(are) methylated. The consequences of histone modification are consequently much more variable than those of DNA methylation. Thus, triple methylation of K27 on H3 strongly inhibits transcription. But triple methylation of K4 on H3 stimulates transcription.

In some cases, a specific transcriptional repressor complex, the **polycomb repressor complex-2** (PRC2), is recruited to promoters to be inactivated. This complex triply methylates a specific residue (K27) on H3 and silences transcription. If a different H3 lysine is methylated by different means, the opposite (transcriptional activation) may occur. The histone methylating enzyme, **EZH2**, is part of PRC2. Cells may gain or lose EZH2 function by mutation or by altered levels of an miRNA that inhibits it (miR-101). Altered EZH2 function or expression occurs in many cancers and correlates with poor prognosis. But, again, it is the context in which such alterations occur that determines the consequences: gain of function EZH2 mutations help drive B-lymphoma development, by blocking transcription of differentiation-related genes; but EZH2 inactivation contributes to other malignancies.

Everything that PRC2 can do, other enzymes can undo. These other enzymes include histone methylases that target other lysines (e.g., K4), demethylases, HATs and nucleosome-remodeling enzymes.

Histone Acetylation and Deacetylation

Histone acetylation tends to open chromatin (see below) and is generally associated with increased transcriptional activity. Positively charged histone K moieties, associate with negatively charged nucleic acids to impede access of transcription factors to underlying DNA. Acetylation neutralizes those positive charges and causes the histone–DNA relationship to dissociate.

Histone deacetylation causes chromatin condensation, making it inaccessible for transcription, and so is associated with transcriptional silencing. Histone deacetylating enzymes (Sirtuins, HDACs) are often dysregulated (up or down) in cancers, causing TSG silencing and derepression of oncogenes.

The combination of histone modifications and DNA methylation is an intricate regulatory web. This network functions physiologically in regulating many biologic and even behavioral functions. Its disruption plays an important role in oncogenesis.

Connections Among Histone and DNA Modifications

Histone methylases may recruit DNA methylases (DNMTs) to a gene to be silenced. DNMTs, in turn, can bring HDACs to these sites to deacetylate histones and silence expression. These relationships are complex, however. In some cases, DNA methylation appears to precede histone methylation and deacetylation, and vice versa. Thus, the three processes are linked, but the sequence of events and the final status of the DNA and histones at a site are probably all specific for individual genes.

Nucleosome Positioning, Histone Composition, and Gene Activity

Chromatin structure is dynamic, and fluctuates as cells' needs vary. Nucleosomes tend to leave open those parts of genes where transcriptional machinery drives gene expression, and again where that apparatus releases the DNA at the end of transcription. Remodeling complexes busily modify nucleosome position and composition, causing nucleosomes to slide or be removed, as needed to tailor gene expression to changing cellular circumstances.

Synchronizing nucleosome positioning entails incorporating modified or variant histones into chromatin. These also substitute for their more conventional cousins on an ongoing basis, and strongly influence the susceptibility or resistance of associated DNA to silencing by CpG methylation. Such histones help to determine nucleosome positioning itself. Continuing modification of histone proteins, as well, is part of the dynamic of chromatin remodeling.

Nucleosome remodeling enzymes, such as those of the SW1/SNF complex, are very commonly mutated in human malignancies. When they are inactivated or repressed by EZH2, failure to position nucleosomes correctly downregulates genes driving differentiation. Clinical trials of genes EZH2 inhibitors, with the goal of upregulating SW1/SNF genes and driving differentiation, are in progress.

Epigenetic Influences on Oncogenesis Entail Altered Noncoding DNA Structure and Nonstructural Modifications of Gene Expression

About 2% of the human genome codes for proteins. The remainder includes regulatory sequences of many types and genes that encode untranslated RNA species. Changes in both the structures and activities of these DNA sequences that do not encode proteins are key drivers and important contributors to tumor development. The diverse effects of such changes are summarized in Table 5-7. As noted above, the complexity of these, the complexity of their connections with each other, and the importance of the context in which the settings occur all make generalization impossible. Therefore, this section describes briefly the main epigenetic factors that contribute to tumor development and how they do so.

MicroRNAs Are Long, Noncoding Regulatory RNAs

Not too long ago, researchers noticed that a specific area in a B-lymphocytic leukemia (**see Chapter 26**) tended to be disrupted, but the affected region did not code for any known protein. On further analysis, they found that the disrupted gene encoded—not a protein, but—a tiny RNA species that acted as a tumor suppressor. Loss of that **miRNA** tumor suppressor was linked to development of that type of leukemia. Since then, over 1,000 miRNAs have been discovered. They are tumor suppressors, oncogenes, regulators having nothing to do with oncogenesis, etc.

Generation and Actions of miRNAs

miRNAs may be encoded anywhere in the genome: intergenic DNA, introns, exons, 3′ UTRs, etc. They are usually transcribed by RNA polymerase II (pol II), the same enzyme that transcribes protein-encoding genes. Initial transcripts that will eventually become miRNAs are processed to precursor miRNAs about 70 bases long. These are exported (Fig. 5-55) to the cytosol, where they are processed further to become single strands about 22 bases long and are incorporated into an **RNA-induced silencing complex (RISC)**. RISC includes an enzyme (**Argonaute**, or **Ago**) that can cleave target mRNAs.

If an miRNA's recognition sequence (bases no. 2–8) matches an mRNA—usually the 3′ UTR—perfectly or nearly perfectly, Ago may degrade the targeted transcript. If miRNA complementarity for an mRNA is imperfect, translation of the latter is blocked without degrading the target mRNA. miRNAs are thus promiscuous: any individual miRNA may regulate many different transcripts.

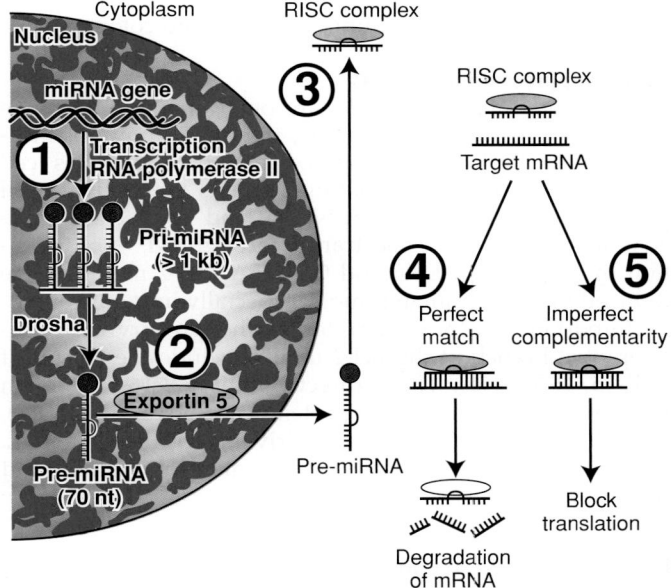

FIGURE 5-55. Production, modification, and activities of micro-RNAs. 1. Most miRNAs are transcribed by RNA polymerase II, the same enzyme that transcribes mRNAs for protein production. **2.** However, the original transcript, which is often >1 kb in length (pri-miRNA) is processed by an enzyme, Drosha, to a shorter form, which is called a pre-miRNA. **3.** This form is exported from the nucleus. In the cytosol, it joins an RNA-induced silencing complex (RISC), where the pre-miRNA is tailored further to the final miRNA by an enzyme called Dicer. A member of this complex, a protein called Argonaute, or Ago, can cleave targeted mRNAs. The nature of the effect of miRNAs depends on the extent of complementarity with a particular mRNA. **4.** If the nucleotides no. 2–8 of the miRNA align with the 3′ untranslated region of a target perfectly, the target is digested and degraded. **5.** If, on the other hand, the complementarity is imperfect, the miRNA inhibits translation of the target mRNA.

miRNAs and Cancer

MiRNAs orchestrate many activities, for example, embryogenesis, development, cell cycling, differentiation, apoptosis, and maintaining stem cell pluripotency ("stemness"). They also regulate many steps in oncogenesis—inhibiting tumor suppressor proteins or as tumor suppressors themselves. In the latter mode, they may target and block oncogene transcripts directly, for example. They may also act as oncogenes. Their activities may depend on the setting: an miRNA species, or clusters of related species, may promote tumor development in some tissues but suppress it in others. This context-dependence recalls the ambidexterity of some proteins that may be tumor suppressors sometimes and tumor activators at other times (see above).

miRNAs That Promote Oncogenesis

Because pro-oncogenic miRNAs are as diverse as proto-oncogene–encoded proteins, they are illustrated, rather than enumerated, here. A cluster of homologous miRNAs, miR-17-92, is commonly increased in certain hematologic cancers. They protect cells from oncogene-induced apoptosis (see above) by tightly regulating Myc-induced proliferation. They also block the proapoptotic protein Bim (**see Chapter 1**), PTEN tumor suppressor, and $p21^{WAF1/CIF1}$ cell cycle regulator (see above). Other miRNAs suppress other diverse TSGs, including miR-21, which targets p53, TGFβ signaling, and PTEN pathways and—depending on the cell type—other antioncogenic pathways. miR-21 is overexpressed in many human tumors, including lung, pancreas, and colon cancers.

Tumor Suppression by miRNAs

Just as many, many miRNAs are oncogenic, so many are tumor suppressors. For example, the Let-7 family of miRNAs, with 12 highly conserved members impedes cell proliferation by downregulating proteins that activate cell proliferation, such as KRAS, NRAS, and Myc. These miRNAs also block cell cycle transit through G1 → S transition by inhibiting CDK6 and CDC25A. Let-7 members are reduced in many human tumors, especially lung cancers.

Important miRNAs that target the prosurvival (antiapoptotic) branch of the Bcl-2 family include the cluster of miR-15/16 species. These directly inhibit Bcl-2, the main mitochondrial antiapoptotic protein (see above, **Chapter 1**), as well as important cell cycle drivers—cyclins D and E. miR-15/16 are often decreased or absent in solid tumors and certain lymphomas.

Regulatory Roles of Long, Noncoding RNAs

Many DNA sequence changes associated with cancer and other diseases occur within the regions that encode long, untranslated RNAs. *These **long noncoding RNAs (lncRNAs)** are defined as RNAs, either primary or spliced transcripts, that do not fit into recognized classes such as structural, protein-coding or small RNAs.* LncRNAs may be quite large, often 1,000s or 10,000s of bases. As with miRNAs, DNA sequences almost anywhere can encode lncRNAs, including intergenic regions, introns, exons, even antisense to coding regions. A recent compendium lists over 48,000 lncRNAs, and others probably remain undiscovered. However many there are, they are very low in abundance, poorly understood, and poorly characterized. They do, though, play many important regulatory epigenetic roles, including processing of small RNAs,

controlling transcription, acting as organizers, decoys, signal transducers and scaffolds that bind to proteins, DNA, or other RNAs. For example, inactivation of one of the pair of X chromosomes in females is the work of an lncRNA called Xist. LncRNAs also help direct chromatin remodeling and DNA methylation, and determine the stability and fate of protein-coding RNAs.

The PTENP1 lncRNA (see above) acts as decoys for regulatory miRNAs, that is, as alternative targets for degradative miRNAs, allowing their protein-coding tumor suppressor cousin (here, PTEN mRNA) to survive unmolested. Given the range of their functions, it is not surprising that, like miRNAs, many lncRNAs are known to be up- and downregulated in human malignancies.

Other Epigenetic Regulators That Are Distorted in Cancers

The discussion above touches on some well-understood epigenetic regulators. Additional important, but less well understood, epigenetic contributors to tumor behavior are addressed below and illustrated in Figure 5-56.

Regulatory Regions

Regulatory regions of genes are generally noncoding DNA sequences that control levels of gene transcription.

- **Promoters.** Mutations in promoter regions directly affect transcriptional efficiency by affecting transcription factor (TF) binding. These may include mutations that reduce TF binding, and so decrease transcription. Altered promoter region sequences may generate a new TF binding site, and so increase transcription.

Genomic rearrangements may place the coding sequence of a gene under the control of a promoter not normally its own. Thus, c-*myc* translocations in Burkitt lymphoma place that mitotic activator under the control of immunoglobulin gene promoters.

- **Enhancers.** As with promoters, altered enhancer element sequences may increase or decrease transcriptional activity.
- **Insulators.** Protein insulators were mentioned above. Insulator DNA sequences function to isolate genes from the influences of regulatory elements that affect other genes. Thus, mutations in insulators may cause a gene to be upregulated under the control of an enhancer for a nearby, but unrelated, gene.
- **5′ UTR.** The structure of mRNA 5′ UTRs affects translation by the structure of its 5′ cap, and impacts mRNA stability in several ways. Increased mRNA stability, for example, may impede access to the mRNA by ribosomal recognition structures, and so decrease translation.
- **IRES structure.** Internal ribosomal entry signals (IRES) allow for translation of mRNAs independently of 5′ caps, particularly in stressed cells. These may generate polycistronic transcripts—mRNAs that encode more than one protein. In this setting, a mutation that generates an IRES, that generates a new upstream orf or that affects the upstream orf sequence may increase or decrease the efficiency of translation for the downstream orf. mRNA degradation may be accelerated.

Coding Sequences and Introns
- **Synonymous mutations.** These are mutations that change a coding DNA sequence, but do not change the amino acid encoded. Such mutations reflect the degeneracy of

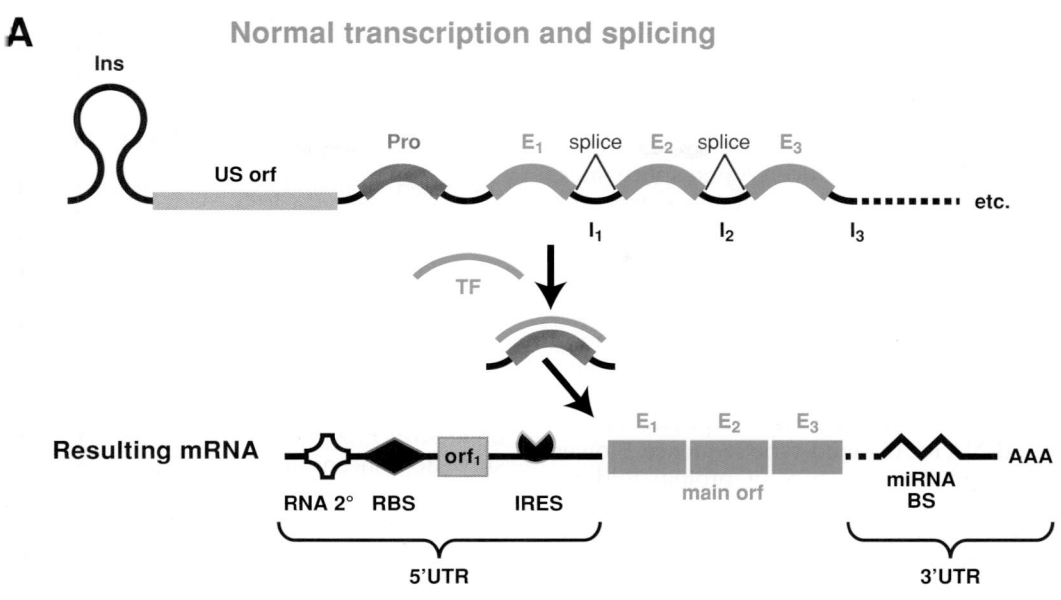

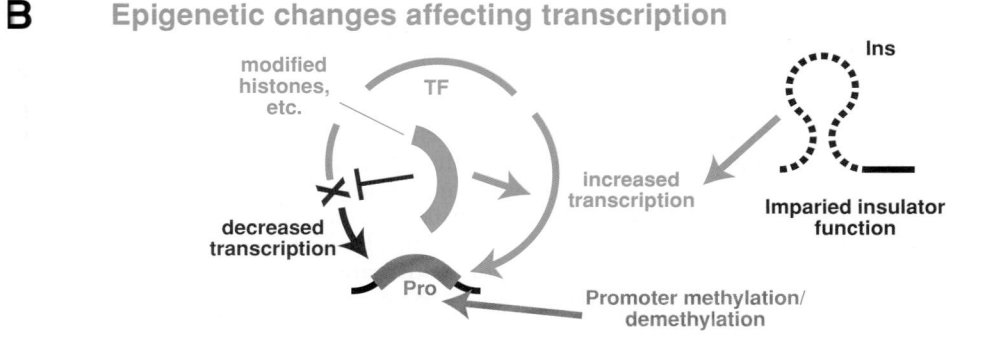

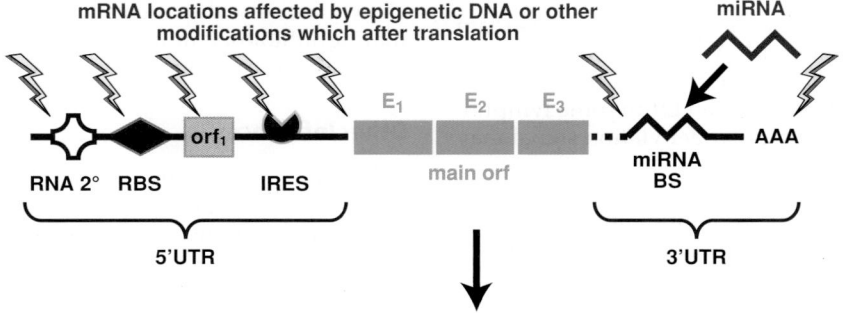

increased or decreased translation
altered speed of translation
altered transcript stability
altered orf structure due to aberrant splicing
altered protein structure

FIGURE 5-56. Transcription, splicing, and translation, and how epigenetic influences affect them. A. Normal transcription of a gene reflects multiple influences that do not affect the amino acid sequence of the main protein product: insulators (Ins), upstream open reading frames (US orfs), promoters (Pro), splice sites, and downstream sequences. When a transcription factor (TF) binds a promoter, transcription is triggered. Introns (I) are excised from the resulting mRNA, which will still include secondary structure, a ribosomal-binding site, internal ribosomal entry site (IRES, if a polycistronic transcript), and other sequences in the 3′ untranslated region (UTR), including possible sites for miRNA binding and a poly-A tail. **B.** Epigenetic changes that may influence transcription include altered DNA-binding proteins (e.g., histones), DNA methylation and demethylation, which (depending on the nature of the alteration) may up- or downregulate transcription, and alter TF binding, altered insulator function. **C.** Epigenetic changes that affect mRNA structure (without altering main orf amino acid sequence) are illustrated here, and include changes in mRNA structure in the 5′ and 3′ UTRs.

the genetic code, in which more than one trinucleotide sequence may encode a particular amino acid. Synonymous DNA sequence changes may have major impact on gene products in several ways.

They may alter mRNA splicing in any of several ways. Synonymous mutations may introduce cryptic splice sites, changing mRNA—and thus product protein—structure. Some exons may be deleted from the mRNA and others may have a different sequence. An altered splice donor or acceptor site may cause exons to be skipped.

Even without splicing anomalies, synonymous base changes may affect message stability. miRNA binding may be increased or decreased, affecting both translation and mRNA stability. Or, translation may be slowed, if the tRNA corresponding to the new trinucleotide sequence is less abundant than the tRNA for the wild-type sequence. Slower translation may change the dynamics of protein folding, leading to conformational changes in protein structure.

Finally, if the gene encodes overlapping orfs, a mutation that is synonymous in one orf may cause an amino acid change in another.

- **Intron sequences.** Like synonymous base changes, altered intron sequences may create or destroy splice sites. In addition, introns contain elements that specify splicing. Mutations in these splicing regulatory elements and "branch points" (which interact with 5′ ends of downstream exons) may alter splice sites so as to include part of an intron as an exon, or to exclude part of an exon (Fig. 5-56).
- **3′ UTR.** Like the 5′ UTR, this region also affects transcript stability and translational efficiency. Altered 3′ UTR sequences may have other consequences, though. Since miRNAs mostly target 3′ UTRs, a base change could increase or decrease inhibitory miRNA binding. (Thus, a mutation in the KRAS 3′ UTR decreases binding by Let-7 miRNA, increasing KRAS mRNA longevity and protein levels.)

Changes in 3′ UTR sequence may insert an upstream polyadenylation site to the mRNA, which may increase message stability (e.g., by decreasing miRNA binding) and protein levels. This happens with cyclin D1 in some lymphomas. Alternatively, a premature polyadenylation signal may truncate the protein.

The intricacy of epigenetic control over normal cellular processes should, by this point, be abundantly evident, as should the limitations of our understanding of it. *It cannot be emphasized too strongly that the devil is always in the details, and that overarching generalizations about how tumors develop may be conceptually useful but often break down when applied to specific situations. Tumor development, progression, and dissemination all entail extensive disequilibrium at every level of epigenetic activity.* Always, one should remember that each gene is affected differently and the results of such alterations always depend on the specific genes, and how they are affected.

Environmental Stimuli Shape Epigenetic Regulators

The epigenome is highly dynamic, and responds to modulation by influences in the cell's milieu. How these factors influence epigenetics is largely obscure. But what is known suggests that this impact may be fundamental to how tumors arise and spread. Known environmental influences on epigenetics include inflammation, nutrition and metabolism, physical and other stresses, hypoxia and aging (Fig. 5-57).

Metabolic Influences on Epigenetic Remodeling

As noted above, DNA and histone-modifying reactions require that certain cofactors and reaction participants be present. Although mutations in, for example, regulatory elements of the genes encoding transcription factors and methylating enzymes may alter these enzymes' activities, they represent only a small minority of tumor-related methylation, acetylation, etc., aberrations. The majority reflect dietary and other metabolic influences. Folate, αKG, ascorbate (vitamin C), acetyl CoA, and other contributors are obligatory. Enzymes mediating these reactions are very sensitive to concentrations of these substances. For example, butyrate generated by colonic bacteria may inhibit histone deacetylases. In some cases, carbon donors and other participants (e.g., citrate, Ac-CoA, αKG) are constituents of the Krebs cycle and need to be replenished after use in epigenetic reactions.

Inflammation and Epigenetics

It has long been known that chronic inflammatory conditions are associated with tumor development, whether in the stomach (*Helicobacter pylori*), the colon (ulcerative colitis), the esophagus (Barrett esophagus), or elsewhere. These inflammatory conditions are often associated with epigenetic alterations which can be mitigated with anti-inflammatory treatments. How an inflammatory milieu stimulates epigenetic modifications is not well understood. In part, it reflects the oxidant-rich environment created by inflammatory cells, with increased production of ROS/RNS (**see Chapter 1**) and proinflammatory cytokines and other mediators that affect at least some relevant enzymes. Thus, reactive radicals, proinflammatory prostaglandins, and IL-1β stimulate DNMT activity. IL-6 increases DNMT activity by downregulating inhibitory miRNAs. Nitric oxide activates HDACs. Free radical scavengers prevent some of these effects.

Other Influences

The mechanisms behind some other environmental factors that modify epigenetic regulators are very poorly understood. Hypoxia, for example, suppresses DNA methylation. Aging, similarly, leads to progressive genome-wide DNA demethylation, with increased methylation of DNA in CpG islands, very much as is seen in tumors. This pattern correlates so well with chronologic age that DNA methylation patterns in 353 CpGs have been called an "epigenetic clock." Senescence is also associated with altered chromatin organization and histone modifications. Some syndromes that cause premature aging may produce the same types of changes.

Stress and Epigenetic Modifications

Nutritional, emotional, and other stresses may also correlate with DNA methylation patterns. Severe trauma (e.g., maternal depression) and other stressors that occur early in life may cause durable gene-selective changes in DNA methylation in children. These patterns of DNA methylation parallel senescence-related patterns.

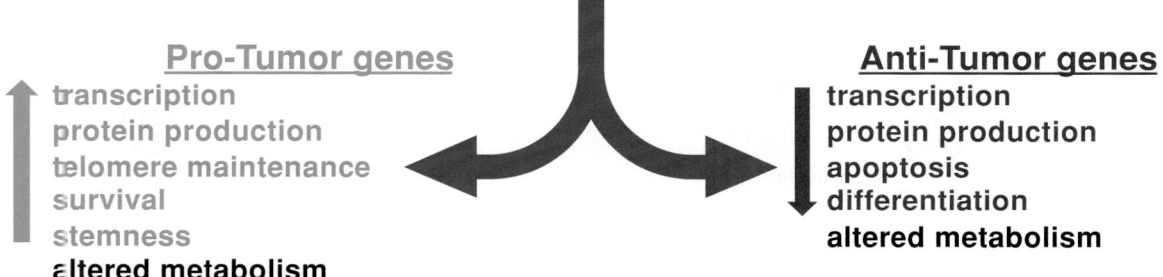

Triggers for Epigenetic Alterations

DNA sequence intact
Stresses (physical, emotional)
Inflammation
Nutrition and metabolism
Hypoxia
Aging

DNA sequence altered
introns
intergenic DNA
promoter
enhancer
insulator
5' UTR
3' UTR
noncoding RNAs
regulatory genes
splice sites

Direct Consequences
decreased/increased gene transcription
decreased/increased mRNA stability
decreased/increased protein production
decreased/increased binding of untranslated RNAs
aberrant open reading frames

Pro-Tumor genes
transcription
protein production
telomere maintenance
survival
stemness
altered metabolism

Anti-Tumor genes
transcription
protein production
apoptosis
differentiation
altered metabolism

FIGURE 5-57. Triggers for epigenetic alterations. These may entail environmental and other effects that do not alter DNA sequences, or they may entail altered noncoding DNA sequences of the gene(s) in question. Direct consequences of these changes may, depending on the specific changes, positively or negatively impact multiple processes relating to mRNA production, structure, and stability. Generally, oncogenic epigenetic alterations tend to upregulate gene activities that contribute to tumorigenesis and downregulate tumor suppressor activities.

Some of these alterations may reflect the activity of glucocorticoids. These stress-induced hormones have been shown to affect DNA methylation in two mutually reinforcing ways: (1) they interfere with cellular mechanisms that maintain and perpetuate DNA methylation; (2) they upregulate enzymes that catalyze DNA demethylation (e.g., TET transcriptional activators, see above).

Epigenetic regulators are central to normal cellular equilibrium. They become unbalanced during carcinogenesis, but unevenly so: generally, opposite changes in these regulators affect tumor suppressors, as compared to tumor-promoting genes. Because epigenetic effects often reflect the influence of the cellular milieu, they can change readily and be up- or downregulated to reflect fluctuations in the environment in which tumors develop and spread. This plasticity endows tumor cells with a nongenetic adaptive mechanism that gives such cells selective advantages without requiring permanent genomic changes. Thus, epigenetic modifiers are both important

and complex: as central as they are to tumor development and spread, there is as yet no single general principle that applies to all aspects of epigenetic regulation.

CANCER CELL METABOLISM

A cell's metabolic activities support that cell's functions. All cells generate energy, in the form of ATP, from carbon-containing substrates. They also produce the materials they need to repair damage, to support their operations, and (in some cases) produce daughter cells. The proportions of cells' metabolic pathways devoted to these different pursuits depend on what the cell does. Since cancer cells generally differ greatly from their normal cousins in their reconstructive, proliferative, and other activities, their metabolism reflects these differences. The divergent metabolic paths between normal and malignant cells are currently being studied as potential therapeutic levers to treat tumors.

To understand current perspectives on cancer cell metabolism and the possible therapeutic tools it may offer, we should review briefly normal cell metabolism, focusing on key areas in which normal and malignant cells are known to differ. Most of these metabolic functions begin with carbon sources, that are used to generate energy and build cellular constituents.

Normal Cell Metabolism Favors ATP Generation

Normal cells utilize glucose as their main (but not only, see below) carbon source, both to produce ATP and to synthesize macromolecules. Cells derive ATP and biosynthetic building blocks from glucose (Fig. 5-58) via cytosolic and mitochondrial reactions including:

- **Glucose entry.** Glucose enters cells via transporters, the best understood being GLUT1 (Fig. 5-58A), although GLUT2, GLUT3, and GLUT4 may also participate.
- **Aerobic glycolysis.** These enzymatic reactions transform glucose, via glucose-6-phosphate to pyruvate and generate two net ATPs.
- **Pyruvate.** This product of aerobic glycolysis is the lynchpin of metabolism in normal and malignant cells. Pyruvate may be converted to lactate, via lactic dehydrogenase-A (LDH-A). Or, it may enter mitochondria, where pyruvate dehydrogenase (PDH) may convert it to acetyl-coenzyme A (Ac-CoA, see below). Pyruvate may enter the tricarboxylic acid (TCA) cycle after conversion to oxaloacetate or after conversion to Ac-CoA (Fig. 5-58B).

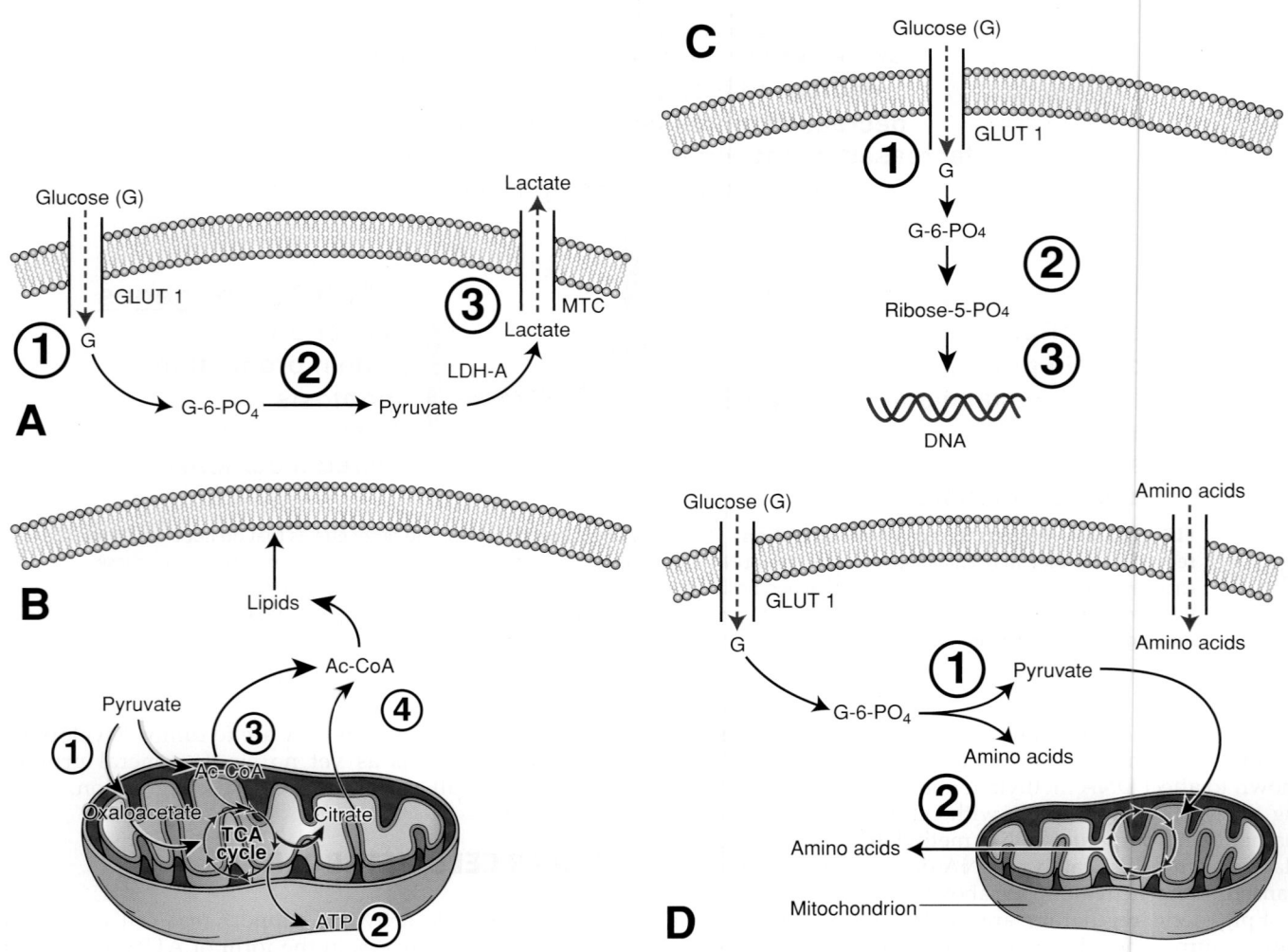

FIGURE 5-58. Cell metabolism. A. Glucose entry. 1. Entry of glucose (G) into the cell is mediated by the glucose transporter, GLUT1. Upon entry, it is converted to glucose-6-phosphate. **2.** Most of the latter is metabolized by glycolysis, which leads to production of pyruvate. Pyruvate, in turn is converted by lactic dehydrogenase-A (LDH-A) to lactate. **3.** Lactate is exported from the cell by a transporter called MTC. **B. Pyruvate utilization in mitochondria. 1.** Some of the pyruvate generated from glucose metabolism enters mitochondria, to become oxaloacetate and to join of the tricarboxylic acid (TCA) cycle. **2.** This drives oxidative phosphorylation to produce adenosine triphosphate (ATP). **3.** Pyruvate may be converted as well to acetyl coenzyme A (acetyl-CoA). **4.** Either this Acetyl-CoA, or citrate from the TCA cycle, is exported to the cytosol, where it is incorporated into lipids. **C. Incorporation into DNA. 1.** Glucose-6-phosphate undergoes a number of enzymatic alterations. **2.** It is a precursor for ribose-5-phosphate (Ribose-5-PO4). **3.** This later enters the nucleus and is an important building block in nucleic acid synthesis. **D. Incorporation into amino acids. 1.** G-6-phosphate metabolism products may be directly converted into certain amino acids. **2.** Alternatively, after pyruvate enters mitochondria, products of the TCA cycle may be converted into amino acids.

- **Ribose-5-phosphate.** This sugar is derived from glucose-6-phosphate, and is then incorporated into nucleic acids (Fig. 5-58C).
- **Ac-CoA.** PDH converts mitochondrial pyruvate to Ac-CoA, which may enter the TCA cycle, where oxidative phosphorylation eventually produces 36 ATPs (Fig. 5-58D) Ac-CoA may also exit mitochondria to participate in lipid biosynthesis.
- **Amino acid synthesis.** Many amino acids enter the cell via cell membrane transporters. Essential amino acids, which humans cannot synthesize, must derive from foodstuffs. Other amino acids, however, can be synthesized by cells from pyruvate or its metabolites that are part of, for example, the TCA cycle.

Glucose metabolism therefore provides cells with much more than just energy. It furnishes key building blocks for virtually all types of cellular structural and functional constituents.

Signals Involved in Glucose Uptake and Utilization

Cells import glucose (and other carbon sources, see below) in response to both intracellular and extracellular signals. Many of these signals are significantly altered in cancers, contributing to tumor cells' deviant metabolism.

Exogenous signals. The key outside regulators of cellular metabolism are insulin and insulin-like growth factor-1 (IGF-1). Upon binding their receptors, these hormones activate intracellular signals that drive many of the processes and mediators involved in oncogenesis. This may, in part, explain the fact that people with type II diabetes, who have high circulating insulin levels, tend to develop cancer more than other people.

Endogenous mediators. At the center of the intracellular response is Akt (Fig. 5-59A). By virtue of the many pathways downstream from Akt (see above and **Chapter 1**), the cell is protected from apoptosis, stimulated to proliferate, etc. Akt function is antagonized by PTEN tumor suppressor. Regarding metabolism, mTOR is the key downstream effector of Akt. This protein stimulates production of amino acid transporters and important of amino acids (Fig. 5-59B). It also stimulates lipid and protein synthesis. C-*myc*, also upregulated by IGF-1, increases production of GLUT1 and importation of glucose, as well as glutamine (Gln) transport and LDH production (see below).

Tumor Metabolism Is Heterogeneous and Relies Heavily on Glucose for Biosynthesis as Well as for Energy

Cancer cells have different needs from normal cells. As they usually proliferate much faster than their normal cousins, they must synthesize structural components for soon-to-be daughter cells at rates that sustain their mitotic activity. Thus, protein, lipid, etc., synthesis must march to a much faster drummer than normal.

More so than normal cells, tumor cells tend to generate energy by cytosolic aerobic glycolysis in the cytosol, yielding pyruvate plus 2 ATPs, instead of mitochondrial oxidative phosphorylation, which generates 36 ATPs, CO_2, and H_2O. This effect, which is named after Otto Warburg, who first described it, presents a seeming paradox between tumor cells' greater metabolic needs and their preference for

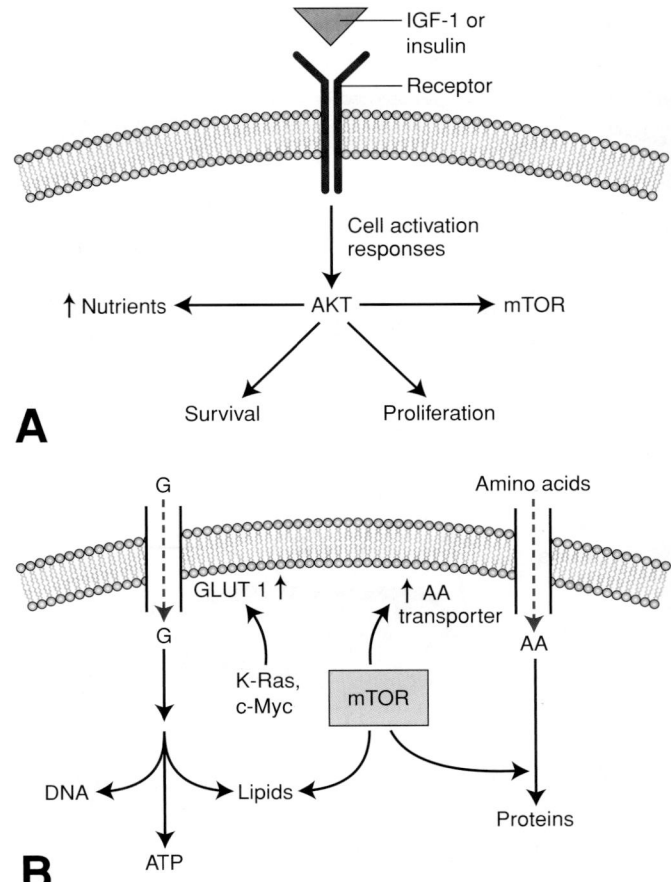

FIGURE 5-59. Effects of metabolic activation on cancer cell metabolism. A. IGF-1 activation. When IGF-1 or insulin binds its receptor, it activates Akt, which in turn elicits many downstream responses. Among the key mediators of Akt effects on cancer cell metabolism is mTOR. **B. Consequences of mTOR activation for cancer cell metabolism.** Operating in tandem with K-Ras- and c-Myc-activated increases in GLUT1 glucose transporter, mTOR increases synthesis of lipids. It also increases the activity of cell membrane transporters so that increased amino acids are available to support the increased proteosynthetic needs of cancer cells.

a pathway that yields much less energy. However, pyruvate contributes to protein, lipid, and other macromolecular synthesis. Furthermore, lactate generated by LDH from pyruvate (Fig. 5-58) may be exported (or imported, see below) via cell membrane **monocarboxylate transporters (MCTs)**.

Like an athlete who uses an array of different power bars, tumor cells can also generate energy from multiple carbon sources (Fig. 5-60). Lactate, excreted by some tumor and other cells via MCT4, may be imported via related MCT channels. LDHA converts this lactate back into pyruvate, for use in the several ways described above. Acetate may also be taken up by tumor cells, and made into Ac-CoA, to be used mostly for lipid synthesis. Fatty acids, taken up by tumor cells, may undergo β-oxidation to generate mitochondrial Ac-CoA. Another important energy source for cancer cells is Gln, which is converted to αKG, a TCA intermediate. Although normal cells, depending on their functions, may also exploit these other molecules similarly, cancer cells have turned this multiplicity of carbon sources into an art form.

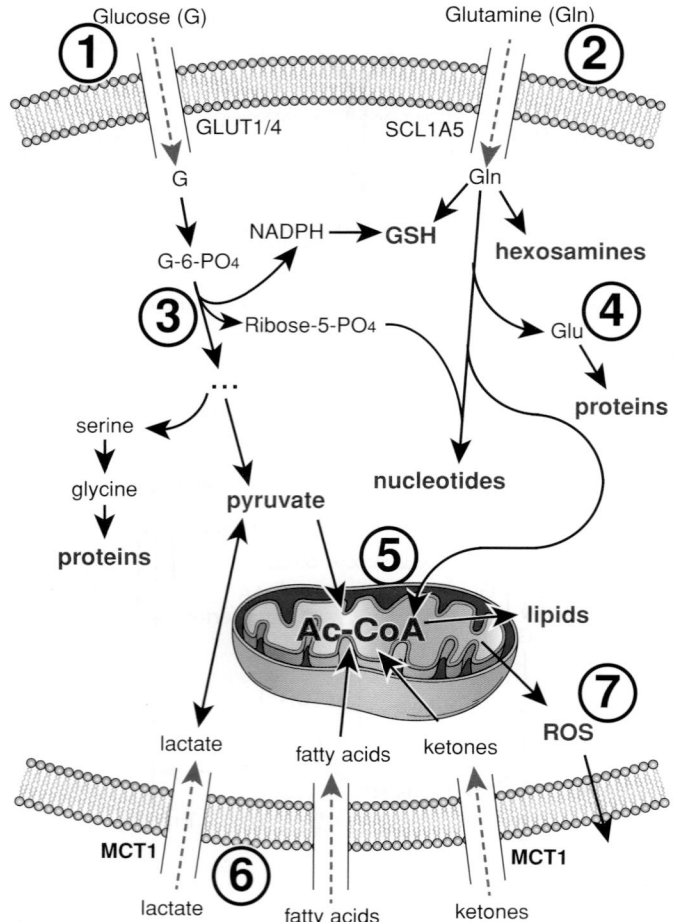

FIGURE 5-60. Metabolic alterations in cancer cells and their contribution to oncogenesis. 1. Tumor cells upregulate glucose importation by increasing levels of glucose transporters, especially GLUT1 and GLUT4. **2.** They also import more glutamine by upregulating glutamine transporters (SCL1A5). **3.** Glucose is phosphorylated, to provide progenitors for nucleotide and protein synthesis, as well as pyruvate, which can be utilized by mitochondria for multiple purposes. It is also used to generate NADPH. **4.** Glutamine can be converted to glutathione (GSH), as can the NADPH from **3**, to detoxify free radicals generated by tumor cells' increased metabolism. It can also be used to generate nucleotides, proteins, and hexosamines for glycosylating macromolecules. **5.** In mitochondria, these precursors may be used to produce acetyl coenzyme A (Ac-CoA), which may be converted into lipids. **6.** Monocarboxylate transporters (MCT1) import lactate and ketones from supporting tumor-associated cells. These may be used in mitochondria, along with additionally imported fatty acids, to generate more Ac-CoA. **7.** Enhanced mitochondrial activity in tumor cells generates ROS, which are exported.

Multiple Sources of Materials for Biosynthesis

These alternative sources of energy also play key roles in tumor cell biosynthetic activities that create new cells (Fig. 5-60). Thus, just as glucose metabolism generates building blocks of proteins, lipids, and nucleotides, other substances imported by tumor cells do so as well. Gln, in addition to supporting ATP generation, helps to generate antioxidants (GSH) and hexosamines to glycosylate proteins. Converted to glutamate (Glu), it helps build proteins. Enzymatic conversion to citrate and pyruvate both sustain ATP generation and provide biosynthetic precursors for lipid

biosynthesis. Particularly in settings of low oxygen tension, Gln is a major source of cellular ATP. Patients with advanced cancers, not coincidentally, tend to have elevated blood Glu.

Ketone bodies, especially acetoacetate, short-chain fatty acid acetates, and β-hydroxybutyrate, are important products of catabolism that are produced, and imported by tumor and adjacent cells in nutrient- and oxygen-poor environments. These secreted ketones may help protect tumors from host responses. They also are sources of NADP and NADPH for ATP generation, pathways that are controlled by AMPK (**see Chapter 1**), and are involved in tumor cell motility and metastasis.

Tumor Metabolism Reflects Cell–Cell Collaboration in the Cancer Ecosystem

Pathologists have observed for many years that mononuclear inflammatory cells often accompany cancers (Fig. 5-61). Once an understanding of the role of lymphocytes in immune function had developed, it was a short step to conclude that these lymphocytes (and other cells) were part of a host response to the presence of tumor. The conclusion that tumors produced antigens that elicited such a response was seemingly inescapable. However, the roles of these infiltrating lymphocytes are, in fact, generally much different from what had been imagined: in many respects, they help support and sustain the tumor's metabolic activities.

The metabolic environment in which tumors grow and spread is not homogeneous, either in terms of the tumor cells themselves or in terms of nontumor stromal cells. These elements combine to produce a setting, seemingly orchestrated by tumor cells, in which metabolic products of both slowly growing tumor cells and tumor-related stromal cells contribute to the ability of rapidly growing tumor cells to thrive. These relationships are illustrated in Figure 5-62.

Metabolic Gradients and Heterogeneity in Tumors

There is a gradient of cancer cell metabolism: tumor cells near blood vessels feast on a diet high in nutrients and oxygen.

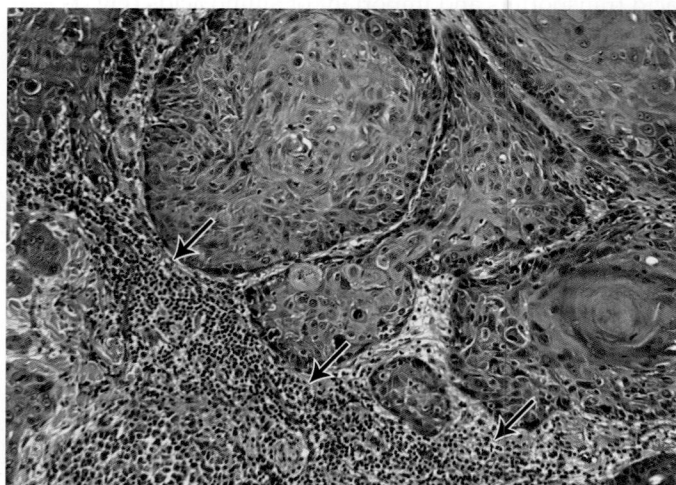

FIGURE 5-61. Mononuclear infiltrate adjacent to a squamous cell carcinoma. Extensive mononuclear cell (*arrows*) composed mostly of lymphocytes infiltrates a primary squamous cancer (**above**) in the skin. The mononuclear infiltrate may serve to nourish and support tumor growth.

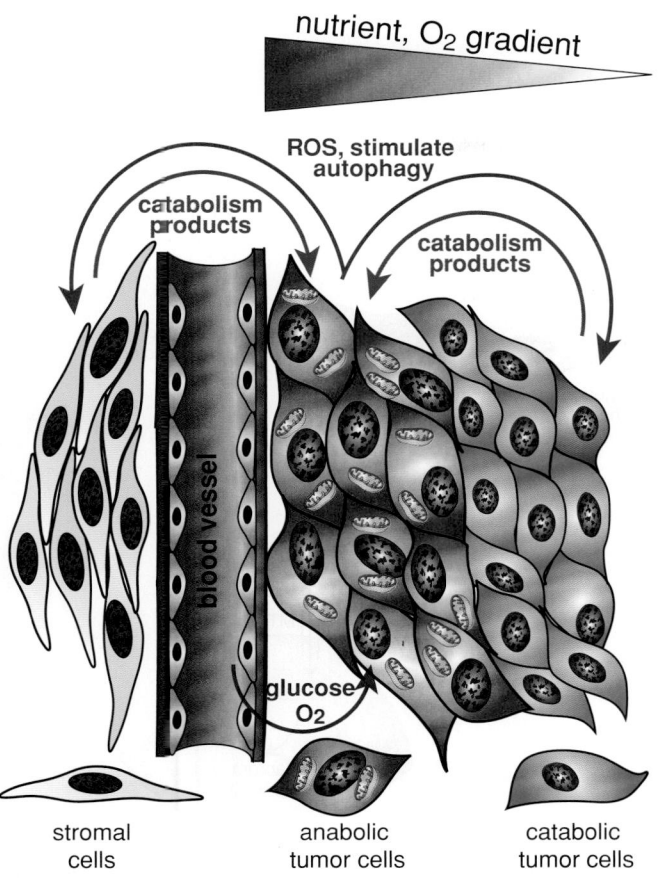

nutrient, O₂ gradient

ROS, stimulate autophagy

catabolism products

catabolism products

blood vessel

glucose O₂

stromal cells

anabolic tumor cells

catabolic tumor cells

FIGURE 5-62. How tumor cells exploit metabolism of each other and tumor-associated cells to enhance their growth. Not all tumor cells metabolize the same way. Tumor cells nearest blood vessels behave most like normal cells metabolically: they generate ATP most by oxidative phosphorylation and show generally anabolic metabolic activity, to generate more progeny. They cannibalize catabolic products from tumor cells that are farther from oxygen and nutrients, in which they also stimulate autophagy, so as to provide themselves with more nutrients. They also orchestrate net catabolic metabolism in tumor-associated stromal cells for the same purpose.

These cells can generate ATP by oxidative phosphorylation, are robust, and aggressive. In this process, they generate considerable ROS. This high level of oxidative stress stimulates two important processes in neighboring tumor cells, which are farther from blood vessels and cannot sustain mitochondrial metabolism, and also in tumor-associated stromal cells: autophagy and glycolytic metabolism. Both autophagy and glycolysis generate catabolic substrates that those cells export and well-oxygenated, well-fed cancer cells import (see Fig. 5-60).

As a result, rapidly metabolizing tumor cells manipulate surrounding cell populations to feed their proliferative ambitions.

Stromal Cell Responses to Tumor Cell–Derived Triggers

Neighboring cells participate in the process as well. Oxidative stress created by rapidly metabolizing tumor cells, leads stromal cells and oxygen-starved tumor cells to respond via a sequence of events that further impairs mitochondrial function. This then increases their ROS levels. Increased ROS

damages these cells' mitochondria, magnifying ROS production, and impairing mitochondrial function even more, in a vicious cycle (Fig. 5-63A). Resulting ROS generated by these cells enhance genomic destabilization in nearby tumor cells.

Mitochondrial injury that stromal cells sustain in this process eventually leads to autophagic destruction of the damaged organelles (mitophagy, **see Chapter 1**). Deprived of much of the machinery of oxidative phosphorylation, stromal cells engage in more aerobic glycolysis. They therefore produce and export more lactate (see above), which is used as a source of energy and a biosynthetic substrate by nearby cancer cells, as detailed above (Figs. 5-62 and 5-63B). Therefore, tumor cells induce metabolic alterations in their malignant and nonmalignant neighbors that cause oxidant injury and autophagy, and supply tumor cells with abundant lactate and ketone bodies for use in sustaining multiple nefarious cancer cell activities.

Tumor Suppressors Regulate Metabolism

The ability of oncoproteins to accelerate anabolism is normally balanced by the effectiveness of tumor suppressors in preventing runaway metabolism:

- **VHL.** This E3 ubiquitin ligase component directs polyubiquitination—and thence degradation—of HIF-1α. VHL thus prevents HIF-1α from redirecting cell energy production toward glycolysis.
- **PTEN.** Activation of mTOR leads to enhanced glycolysis, among other things, as a direct consequence of increased Akt triggering of PI3K (see above). PTEN strongly inhibits PI3K. It thus decreases mTOR activity, reduces HIF-1α, and limits GLUT1 production (Fig. 5-64). Because it inhibits HIF-1α, PTEN also prevents HIF-1α–induced blockage of mitochondrial use of pyruvate to drive the TCA cycle forward.
- **p53.** In addition to its many other regulatory functions, p53 controls and directs cellular metabolism (Fig. 5-65). It has been suggested, in fact, that the main reason for the Warburg phenomenon is that many tumors inactivate p53. *It is instructive both to view p53 activities as directing certain energy-producing functions, and to appreciate how loss of p53 activity (e.g., by mutation) affects all of these activities.* When p53 is activated by AMPK in response to metabolic stress, it:
  - upregulates a glycolysis regulator, TP53-induced glycolysis regulator (**TIGAR**) that blocks aerobic glycolysis and shunts its intermediates to other pathways
  - decreases glucose transporter (mainly GLUT1) synthesis, decreasing glucose entry into cells
  - blocks NF-κB, thus hindering its direct and indirect activation of glycolysis (NF-κB upregulates HIF-1α)
  - increases synthesis of a stimulator of cytochrome oxidase, **SCO₂**, which then increases mitochondrial electron transport and thus
  - increases pyruvate and Gln importation into mitochondria and incorporation into the TCA cycle by upregulating PDH
  - lowers c-Myc levels by activating miR-145, a direct inhibitor of c-Myc; this, in turn, decreases c-Myc–stimulated HIF-1α production and increases oxidative phosphorylation
  - indirectly impedes fatty acid biosynthesis
  - upregulates molecules that can trigger autophagy (see below)

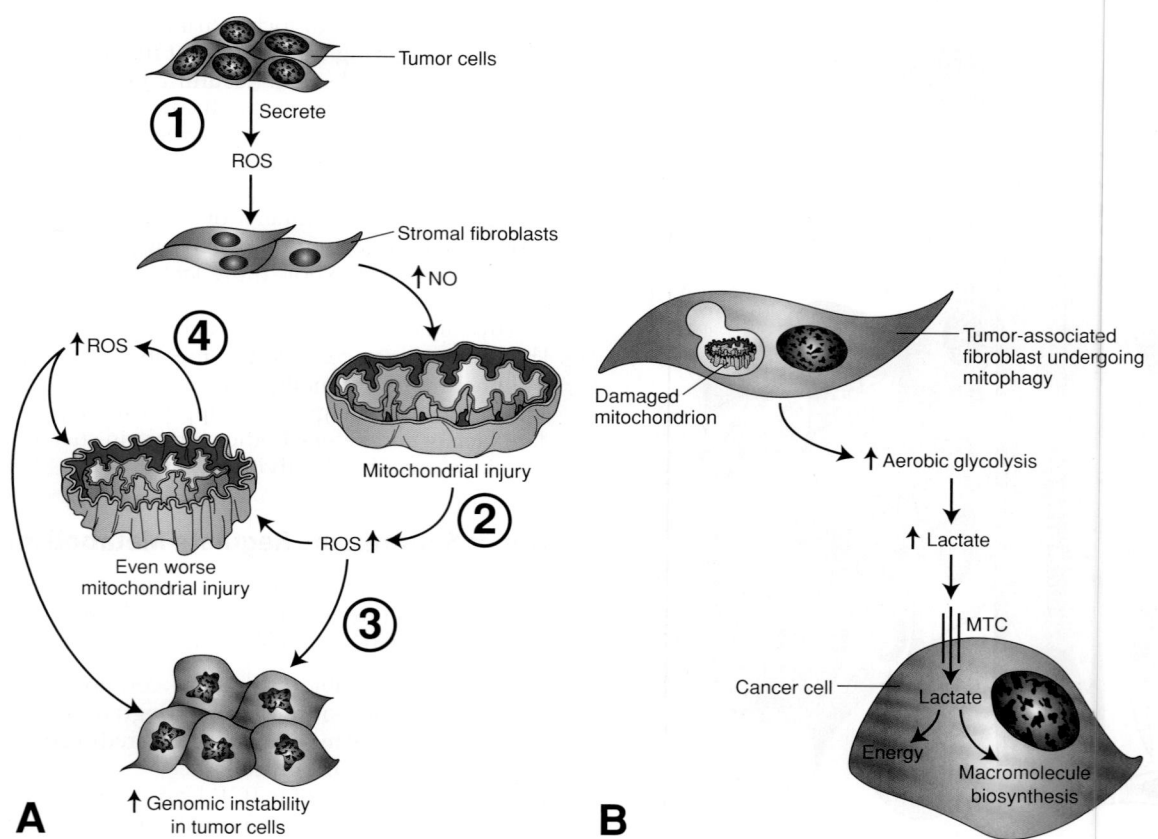

FIGURE 5-63. Stromal cell responses to tumor cell–derived signals. A. Role of ROS. Tumor cells manipulate stromal cells so as to augment tumor cell metabolic activity. **1.** Reactive oxygen species (ROS) elaborated by tumor cells stimulate stromal cells to increase their production of nitric oxide (NO). This NO causes mitochondrial injury in the stromal cells. **2.** As a result, stromal cells generate excessive ROS. **3.** Increased stromal cell ROS generates more oxidative injury in neighboring cancer cells, leading to increased genomic instability in the tumor. **4.** Increased stromal cell ROS also increases stromal cell mitochondrial injury, creating a vicious circle and magnifying tumor cell genomic instability. **B. Altered metabolism in tumor-associated fibroblasts.** Mitochondrial damage in tumor-associated fibroblasts leads to autophagy of damaged mitochondria (mitophagy). Resulting loss of mitochondria directs more fibroblast metabolism toward glycolysis, producing lactate, which is secreted by the stromal cells. Lactate is taken up by tumor cells, via MTC and used for macromolecule biosynthesis and other tumor cell metabolic activities.

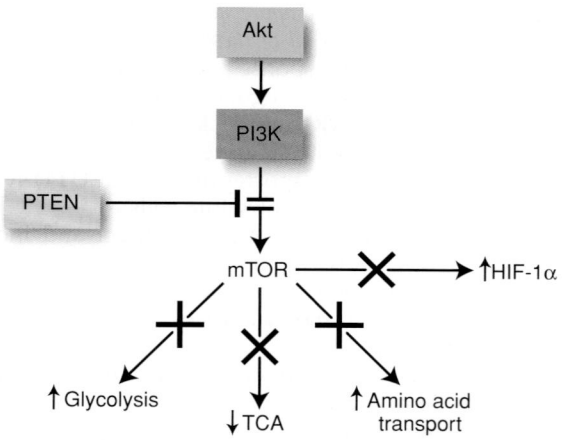

FIGURE 5-64. PTEN controls cellular metabolism and is a suppressor of the metabolic changes that power cancer cell activity. PTEN downregulates mTOR by dephosphorylating PIP3 (see Fig. 5-41). All downstream effects of mTOR are thus restricted: upregulation of HIF-1α, increased glycolysis, increased amino acid transport, and decreased TCA activity. Thus, PTEN's regulation of mTOR makes it impossible for cancer cells to generate the biosynthetic building blocks they need to sustain proliferation.

The net metabolic effect of p53, acting in all of these ways, is to shunt energy production away from glycolysis and toward oxidative phosphorylation. Thus, loss of p53 facilitates tumor cell metabolism.

P53-related metabolic protection is triggered by a sequence of events in which AMPK is activated. AMPK directly inhibits mTOR (see above). This may be a mechanism by which metformin, which stimulates AMPK, inhibits tumors.

■ **Isocitrate dehydrogenase (IDH).** This TCA enzyme has turned out to be a potent tumor suppressor. One allele of IDH is mutated in a high percentage of malignant gliomas (**see Chapter 32**), and in myelodysplastic syndromes (MDS, **see Chapter 26**). The oncogenic mutation results in a gain of function alteration which generates large amounts of a new product (R-2-hydroxyglutarate, or R2HG). R2HG directly inhibits the TET family of DNA hydroxylases and also a family of histone demethylases (see above). The result is that TET2-related histone demethylation and 5-methylcytosine hydroxylation (see above) are not available to protect from downregulation of TSG promoters by CpG and histone methylation, such as occurs during oncogenesis. This inactivation of TET tumor suppressors facilitates tumor development.

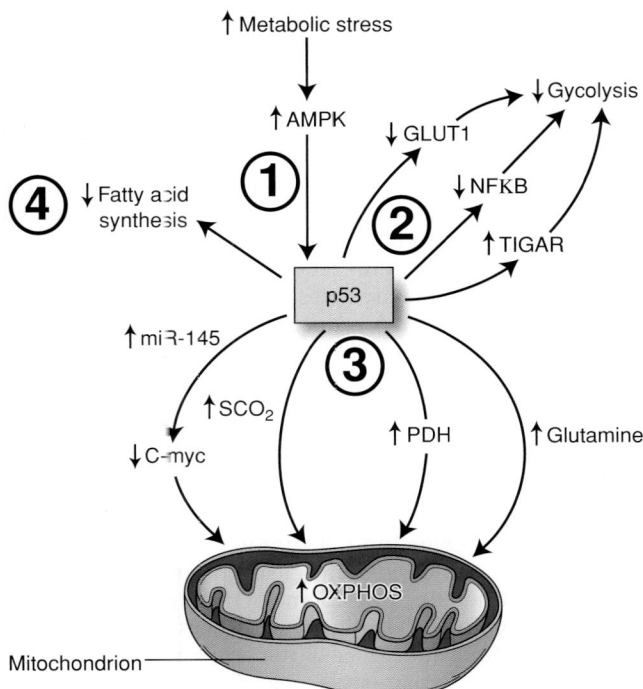

FIGURE 5-65. P53 regulation of cellular metabolism. In addition to its other functions, P53 is a critical metabolic regulator. It prevents cancer cells from achieving their malignant potential by multiple pathways. **1.** P53 is activated by the increased metabolic stress attendant to increased cellular proliferation. This activates AMP-protein kinase (AMPK), which in turn activates p53. **2.** P53 directly downregulates transcription of GLUT1 and NF-κB. It also upregulates TP53-induced glycolysis regulator (TIGAR), which impedes glycolysis and directs glycolytic intermediates into other pathways. **3.** It increases TCA cycle activity in several ways. P53 upregulates SCO$_2$, a stimulator of cytochrome oxidase that directly increases mitochondrial electron transport. It also increases pyruvate and glutamine incorporation into the TCA by upregulating pyruvate dehydrogenase (PDH). As well, it upregulates miR-145 which directly downregulates c-Myc and so prevents Myc-mediated metabolic effects (see Fig. 5-49). **4.** As well, p53 downregulates a key enzyme that mediates fatty acid synthesis.

CANCER STEM CELLS AND TUMOR HETEROGENEITY

Most Cancers Derive From a Single Cell

This conclusion is best established for proliferative disorders of the lymphoid system, in which clonality is easiest to assess. Neoplastic plasma cells in multiple myeloma produce a single immunoglobulin species, unique to each patient and consistent in that patient over time. Monoclonal T-cell receptor (TCR) and Ig gene rearrangements, as well as monoclonal cell surface markers, establish monoclonal origin for many lymphoid malignancies. Cells of B-cell lymphomas exclusively carry either κ or λ light chains on their surfaces, while polyclonal lymphoid proliferations—which are almost always benign—contain a mixture of cells, some with κ, and some λ, light chains.

Monoclonality has also been demonstrated for many solid tumors. One of the best examples of this principle utilized glucose-6-phosphate dehydrogenase (G6PD) in women who were heterozygous for its two isozymes, A and B (Fig. 5-66). These isozymes are encoded by genes on

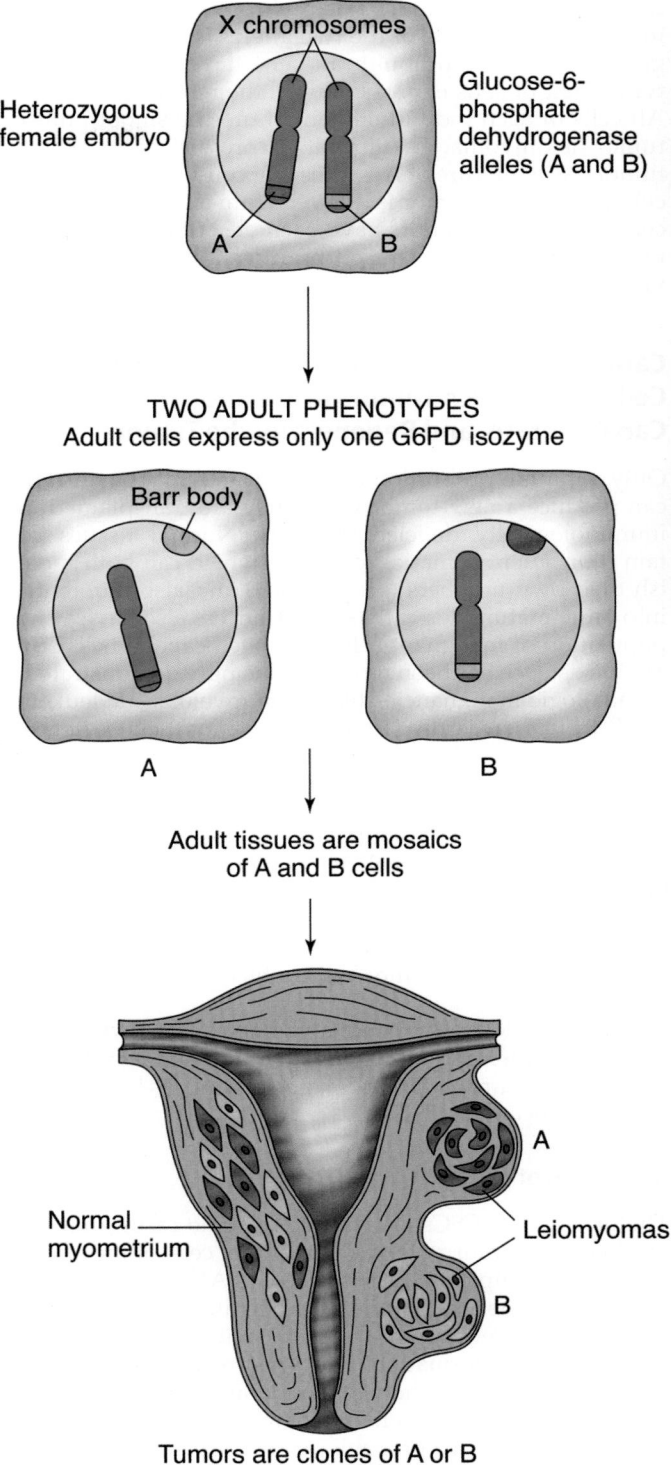

FIGURE 5-66. Monoclonal origin of human tumors. Some females are heterozygous for the two alleles of glucose-6-phosphate dehydrogenase (G6PD) on the long arm of the X chromosome. Early in embryogenesis, one of the X chromosomes is randomly inactivated in every somatic cell and appears cytologically as a Barr body attached to the nuclear membrane. As a result, the tissues are a mosaic of cells that express either the A or the B isozyme of G6PD. Leiomyomas of the uterus have been shown to contain one or the other isozyme (A or B) but not both, a finding that demonstrates the monoclonal origin of the tumors.

the X chromosome. Since one X chromosome is randomly inactivated, only one of the two alleles is expressed in any given cell. Thus, although all cells have the same genotypes, half of cells express only A; the rest express only B. All cells of each individual benign uterine smooth muscle tumor (leiomyoma, or "fibroid") express either A or B. No tumor has a mixture of A-expressing cells and B-expressing cells. Thus, each tumor is derived from a single progenitor cell. Oligoclonal tumors have been described, but they are rare and are usually caused by infection with oncogenic viruses (see below).

Cancer Stem Cells Are Primordial Malignant Cells From Which Tumors Arose and Which Can Generate, and Regenerate, the Tumors

Only a minute proportion of the cells in a malignant tumor can produce a new tumor when they are transplanted into immunologically deficient animals. Normal tissues contain pluripotent somatic stem cells, which can both replenish their own numbers (self-renewal) and also differentiate into more mature derivative cells. Cancers also have a small population of malignant cells with such capabilities: **CSCs**. Their existence has been most convincingly demonstrated in hematologic malignancies like acute myeloblastic leukemia (AML), but there is also strong evidence for their existence in an increasing number of solid tumors.

In AML, far less than 1% of leukemic cells express HSC membrane markers (CD34$^+$, CD38$^-$). Only these cells among the entire leukemic population can reestablish leukemia in an appropriate transplant recipient host. Comparable, but not identical, data have been obtained from studies of cancers of the breast, colon, and brain, in which different markers identify CSC-rich cell populations and exclude the vast majority of tumor cells, which cannot recapitulate tumorigenesis.

CSCs are defined functionally. Their respective markers allow us to identify populations that are enriched for stem cells, but not pure CSCs. Only some of the cells in those populations function as CSCs.

Derivation of CSCs

The origin(s) of CSCs are murky. In some cases, they may originate from pluripotent somatic stem cells of the affected organ, for example, HSCs in the case of AML (Fig. 5-67A). In other cases, lineage-committed progenitor cells may be the culprits. Such cells are multipotent, but not pluripotent, at the time of transformation. They may reacquire a degree of "stemness," allowing them to repopulate their own numbers and to differentiate into more committed cells (Fig. 5-67B). Therefore, CSCs can probably arise both from tissue stem cells and from their slightly differentiated immediate progeny. Lurking within the tumor, they function as a reservoir of cells that continue to provide more differentiated tumor cells and that can regenerate the entire tumor, should that become necessary.

Tumor Cells Derived From CSCs

Although almost all tumors begin as a clone of neoplastic cells, their cells vary considerably in appearance (Fig. 5-68) and behavior as they grow. This diversity among tumor cells

has broad implications for tumor progression and dissemination, as well as for response—and resistance—to chemotherapy. Several theories, which are not necessarily mutually exclusive, and which all may apply to some cases, have been proposed to account for the development of phenotypic diversity of cells in tumors.

It is critical to understand that these derivative cells comprise the overwhelming majority of tumor bulk. Treatments that reduce tumor volume mostly target these cells, and consequent reduced tumor volume reflects the susceptibility of these cells—not CSCs—to the therapies employed. However, as will become clear (see below) reduced tumor volume does not equate with elimination of CSCs, nor does it necessarily impair the ability of CSCs to regenerate the tumor after treatment.

Clonal Evolution

The original explanation of tumor heterogeneity holds that tumor cells progressively accumulate new mutations as they proliferate. Over time, a tumor in which many cells are dividing can thus generate a potpourri of genetically related—but different—cells. Some of these cells may be destined for ignominious death, while others may flourish as genetically distinct subclones of the original malignant cells (Fig. 5-67A). Darwinian-style selection—whether due to localized hypoxia, differences in proliferation rates, potential for invasion and metastasis, therapy, etc.—determines which subclones will succeed and which will perish, which will metastasize and which will remain localized, which will be mitotically active and which will be quiescent.

Epigenetic Cancer Cell Plasticity

Cancer's evil machinations have led to even more devious ways for tumors to maintain themselves and to grow and spread. Thus, some tumors (e.g., malignant melanomas) adapt to the progressive challenges to survival and dissemination via epigenetic changes (e.g., by upregulating noncoding RNAs, or expressing proteins that modify histones) (Fig. 5-69). A mass of slowly proliferating tumor cells may alternate rapidly among different epigenetic states, and so fluctuate between the ability to reconstitute a tumor (stem cell-like) and the lack of such ability. Such deviousness allows diverse populations of tumor cells to alternate from stemness—slowly dividing, tumor-reconstituting cells—to rapidly dividing, nonreconstituting cells. *Such metamorphoses require no further mutations.*

The implications of epigenetic plasticity are substantial. Tumors may represent constantly shifting therapeutic targets, with incredible plasticity in adapting to a changing chemotherapeutic milieu because they can shift phenotypes rapidly to evade antineoplastic drugs, and then to shift back to reemerge from a defensive posture and reassert an aggressive nature—all without changing genotype.

The Significance of CSCs

CSCs are not merely an experimental curiosity. They are the cells from which many human tumors arise. They divide infrequently, which allows them to evade destruction by cytotoxic chemotherapeutic agents that preferentially target rapidly dividing cells. Thus, chemotherapy or radiotherapy may destroy the vast bulk of rapidly dividing cells in a malignant tumor mass, but residual CSCs may survive to regenerate the cancer.

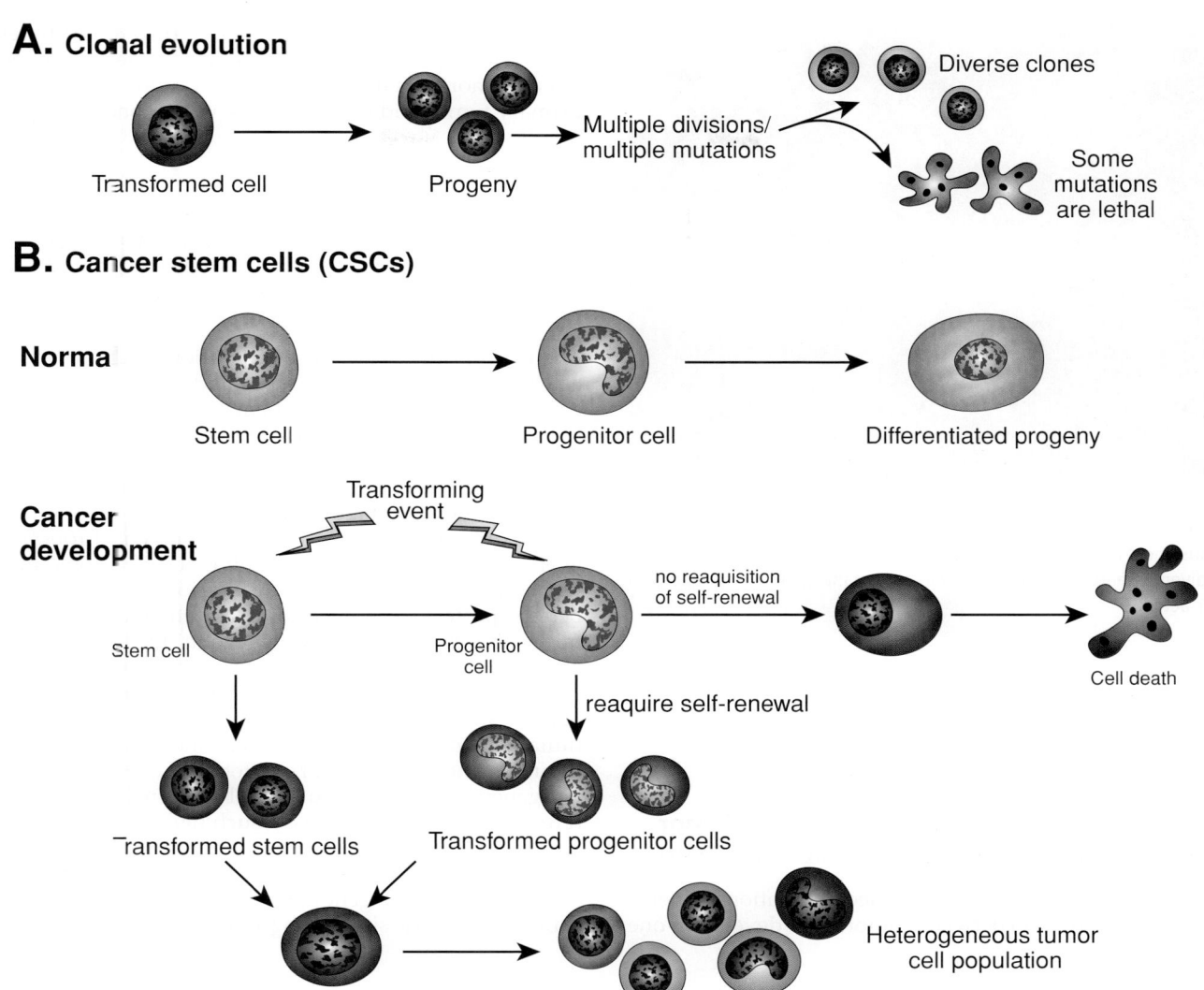

A. Clonal evolution

Transformed cell → Progeny → Multiple divisions/ multiple mutations → Diverse clones / Some mutations are lethal

B. Cancer stem cells (CSCs)

Normal

Stem cell → Progenitor cell → Differentiated progeny

Cancer development

Transforming event

Stem cell → Progenitor cell → no reaquisition of self-renewal → → Cell death

reaquire self-renewal

Transformed stem cells

Transformed progenitor cells

CSCs → Heterogeneous tumor cell population

FIGURE 5-67. Tumor stem cells and tumor heterogeneity. A. Linear progression of tumor clonal evolution. Proliferating cancer progenitor cells eventually develop a variety of mutations, with different individual cells acquiring different mutations, leading to heterogeneity in the tumor cell population. Some such mutations are inconsistent with cell survival, while others facilitate cancer progression. This model is most consistent with critical enabling primordial mutations in a stem cell that must be retained throughout subsequent tumor evolution. **B. Cancer stem cells and progenitor cells.** Normally (*above*), stem cells give rise to committed progenitor cells. These then produce terminally differentiated cells. An oncogenic stimulus (*below*) to a stem cell may lead to an expanded pool of transformed stem cells. These become cancer stem cells (CSCs). Alternatively, the oncogenic stimulus may affect a committed progenitor cell. If the latter recapitulates a program of self-renewal, the resulting transformed progenitor may become a CSC. If it does not activate the self-renewal program, resulting differentiated progeny will be produced and eventually die. CSCs generated either via transformation of stem cells or transformation of committed progenitors may then be the antecedents of a heterogeneous malignant cell population.

Even more significantly, CSCs in many ways are closer to their normal tissue counterparts than to the cells that comprise the bulk of the tumor. They may be far more capable of, for example, repairing DNA damage than their more aggressive derivative cells. Also, because they proliferate less, they rely less on mutant cell activation signaling pathways and resemble normal cells more than do their highly mitotically active progeny. The main determinants of their survival allow them to persevere better through treatments—even kinase inhibitors—that kill the rapidly dividing cells that comprise the vast majority of the tumor. Radiating a glioblastoma may destroy the vast majority of tumor cells, but CSCs are radioresistant. Their numbers, as a percentage of

remaining viable tumor cells, increase after radiation. They survive and repopulate the tumor. In this sense, therapy may destroy 99.9%, or 99.99% of a tumor, shrink its mass correspondingly, provide several more months of life, but not change the outcome.

CSCs have evolved to repair DNA damage and mutations, preserve telomeres, and evade apoptosis and senescence. Tumor stem cells are thus better suited to survive cytotoxic therapy that is likely to kill the normal tissue stem cells from which the CSCs probably derive.

It is therefore critical to bear in mind that the goal of tumor therapy is not to eliminate the bulk of the tumor, but to save the patient's life. The latter requires approaches that are effective

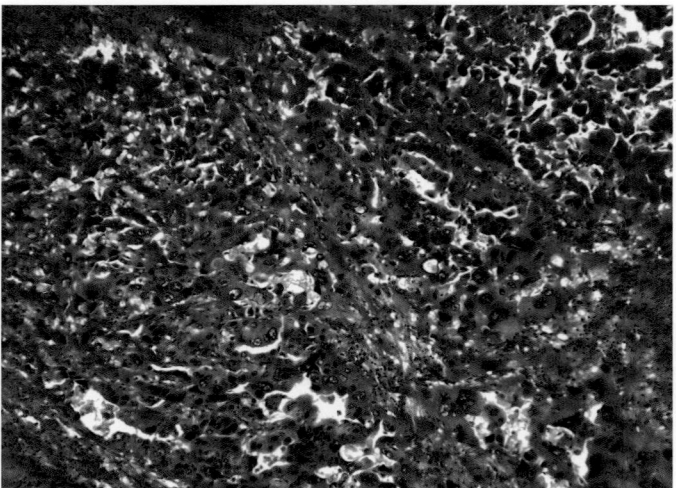

FIGURE 5-68. Phenotypic diversity in human tumors. Human tumor cells show great heterogeneity in their appearance, proliferative activity, etc. Thus, most human tumors are mixtures of small and large cells, often with diverse shapes, varying nuclear appearances, and differences in mitotic activity.

against CSCs because it is these cells, and not the aggregate of their highly proliferating progeny, that will regenerate the tumor after cytoreductive or other therapy. The CSCs, then, are the true enemies; it is they that will kill the patient.

Tumors Are Both Heterogeneous Within a Tumor and Between Different Tumors of the Same Type

Thus, **intertumor heterogeneity** reflects variation (genetic, epigenetic, phenotypic) between tumors that develop in one

patient and those that arise in others. **Intratumor heterogeneity** refers to variation in the same parameters among different tumor cells and areas at one location, and between a primary tumor and its metastases, within one patient.

Intertumor Heterogeneity

Walter Donovan: "… we're on the verge of completing a quest that began [many] years ago. We're just one step away."
Indiana Jones: "That's usually when the ground falls out from underneath your feet."
—Indiana Jones and the Last Crusade

There are distinct patterns of alterations that are both characteristic of certain tumor types and that offer useful therapeutic targets, at least for hematologic malignancies. For example, almost every case of Burkitt lymphoma has chromosome rearrangements involving the MYC gene on chromosome 8. These tumors seem to follow the paradigmatic sequence shown in Figure 5-67A: one initial set of mutations triggers the tumor and is needed to carry it through whatever follows. Similarly, almost all cases of chronic myeloid leukemia show the t(9;22) translocation to generate mutant bcr-abl protein. The successful targeting of bcr-abl epitomizes the goal of developing agents that are specific for mutations which are necessary for tumor survival.

As comforting as this paradigm is for hematologic malignancies (at least selected ones), the situation for characteristic mutations in solid tumors has been more problematic. Even though some studies that have focused on selected individual genes have found mutational patterns, these studies in retrospect may have exercised such high levels of selectivity that many other, perhaps more important, mutations were not detected. More extensive genetic analysis of the protein coding parts of the genome (whole-exome sequencing) has shown wide diversity among individual solid tumors. One

Epigenetic cancer cell plasticity

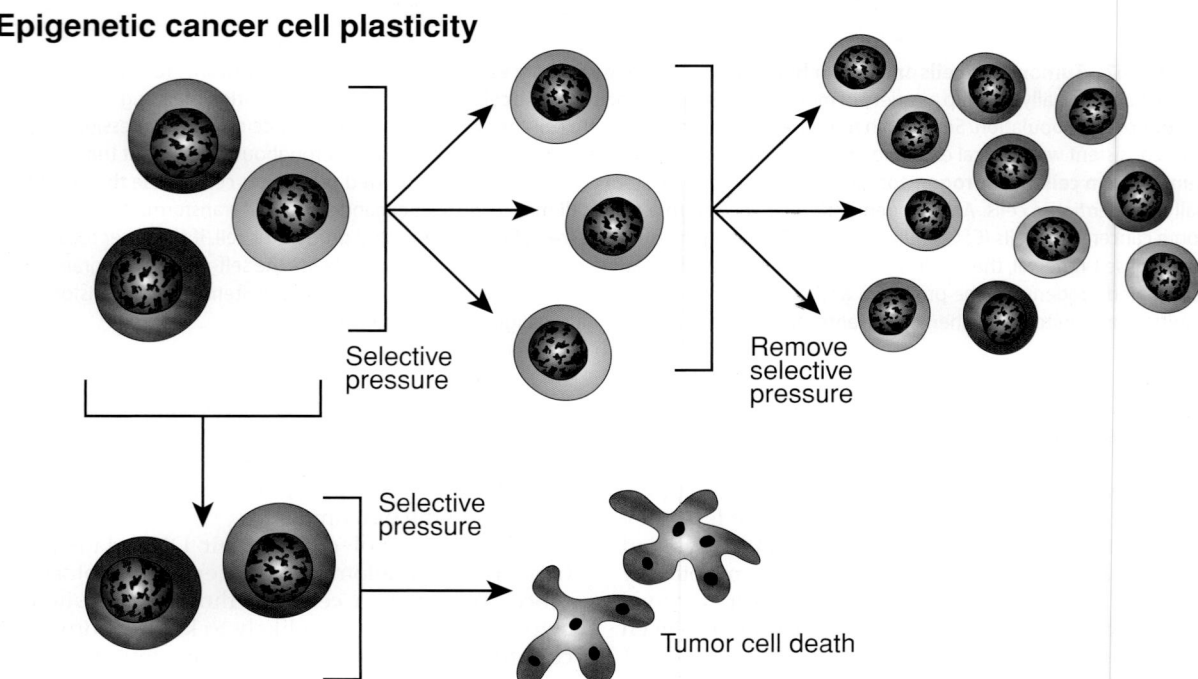

FIGURE 5-69. Nonheritable epigenetic modification. Epigenetic changes in cell populations may lead to tumor progression or cell death. These changes may be retained, or readily discarded, as selective pressures dictate.

study of almost 200 lung cancers showed that only 4 genes were mutated (all SNPs, or point mutations) in >10% of tumors, and 15% of tumors showed no structural changes in proteins at all.

Our increasing awareness of the roles of untranslated RNAs in human cancer (see above) underscores this problem. The wider a net we cast, the more we find and the more restricted the applicability of the simple stepwise model shown in Figure 5-67A appears to be. The extensive intratumor and tumor-to-tumor diversity (e.g., Fig. 5-69) in patterns of genetic changes in solid tumors underscores the potential complexity of developing effective targeted therapies.

Intratumor Heterogeneity

In addition to variability of one tumor type from one person's tumor to someone else's tumor, all models predict that there will be variability within the tumor of a single individual. If a stochastic (i.e., random) mutation model (e.g., Fig. 5-69) applies to solid tumor evolution, rather than a linear stepwise model in which all cells progressively evolve from identically altered progenitors (as in Fig. 5-67A), one would expect cells of any individual tumor to be highly heterogeneous, one to the other.

Although only a few such studies have been reported, they generally confirm our worst fears along these lines. It is clear that, at least for some solid tumors, variability is enormous. In one study of renal cell carcinomas, multiple biopsies of a single tumor mass showed that only 34% of protein-coding genetic alterations were concordant *between different pieces of that one tumor mass*. When analyses also included metastases, or comparison of pre- and posttreatment tumor samples, concordance was even lower.

Therefore, sophisticated tools to analyze tumors have not exactly allowed us to impose a man-made paradigm—either analytical or therapeutic—on the field of cancer biology. Rather, these technologies have illuminated the fact that cancers, especially solid ones, are highly diverse genetically and that each patient's individual tumor presents a vast, nonuniform array of mutations. When patient-to-patient variations in tumor genotypes are considered, it is clear that tumors are incredibly more complicated than we had imagined. We are only beginning to lift the veil on that heterogeneity.

THE IMMUNE SYSTEM AND CANCER

The immune system distinguishes self from nonself molecules, and is generally very effective in avoiding autoimmunity and in combating infectious agents (**see Chapters 4 and 11**). As noted above, oncogenesis usually entails extensive alteration of cellular DNA, generating proteins whose structures the body had not previously encountered. These tumor-related antigens should be expected to trigger effective adaptive immune responses, leading to generation of cytotoxic T lymphocytes (CTLs) and other killer cells. And tumors should be destroyed in their infancy.

Undoubtedly, many are. However, the success of cancers in growing and spreading testifies to their dexterity in avoiding such elimination and ability to thrive in an environment that would seem to have been designed to prevent just such an event. The discussion below highlights current thinking on how tumors manipulate normal immune regulatory mechanisms.

Tumors recruit suppressor cells, both of lymphocytic (e.g., Tregs) and other MDSCs, macrophages, and others. They also secrete cytokines and other substances that impair immune elimination of tumors. These include TGFβ, IL-10, ROS, and NO.

T-Cell Responses Both Activate and Inhibit Cytotoxic Activities

To understand how tumor cells manage to thrive in an environment that should be hostile, one must first understand certain aspects of how **CTLs (see Chapter 4)** are normally activated and inhibited.

CTL Generation

To generate CTL responses, several signals are necessary. First, an antigen-presenting cell (APC) must present an antigen associated with major histocompatibility complex (MHC), for recognition by the TCR. A second, costimulatory signal is also required, and is usually supplied when T-cell membrane CD28 binds an APC membrane molecule, either **CD80** or **CD86** (also called **B7-1** and **B7-2**). This combination activates the T cell, which will then produce IL-2 (**see Chapter 4**) and begin to proliferate (Fig. 5-70A).

Resting APCs do not express the B7 molecules, but are stimulated to do so when activated. If a TCR sees an antigen but not the costimulatory signal, it becomes unresponsive (anergic) to that antigen. Anergy may also result in other situations.

CTLA-4

As often happens, when CTLs are activated, modulatory or inhibitory activities are also activated. In resting T cells, cytotoxic T-lymphocyte antigen-4 (CTLA-4, or CD152) resides in a cytoplasmic vesicle. When the cell is activated by antigen plus costimulator, CTLA-4 translocates to the cell membrane. Like CD28, CTLA-4 binds B7s on APCs, only with far higher avidity. It then outcompetes CD28 for B7 molecules on APC membranes and downregulates CTL activation (Fig. 5-70B). IL-2 production and T-cell proliferation and survival decrease. The extent of CTLA-4 translocation to the T-cell membrane is proportional to the activating signal, so strong T-cell activation leads to high CTLA-4 cell membrane concentrations. CTLA-4 inhibition of CTL activation occurs mainly in secondary lymphoid organs (e.g., lymph nodes), and largely suppresses the activation phase of cytotoxic responses.

CTLA-4 does this in several ways (Fig. 5-71). It:

- binds B7s more avidly than CD28, and so outcompetes the latter for B7 binding
- generates inhibitory signals of several kinds. When it binds B7, CTLA-4 activates tyrosine phosphatases, which dephosphorylate antigen-bound TCR, blocking downstream signaling via several pathways, including Ras and tyrosine kinases
- inhibits transcription of IL-2
- induces APCs to internalize B7s (*trans*-endocytosis), further impeding T-cell activation
- decreases AKT activation (**see Chapter 1**), without directly affecting PI3K
- stimulates APCs to secrete indoleamine 2,3-dioxygenase (IDO), which depletes T-cell tryptophan and severely limits T-cell proliferative ability

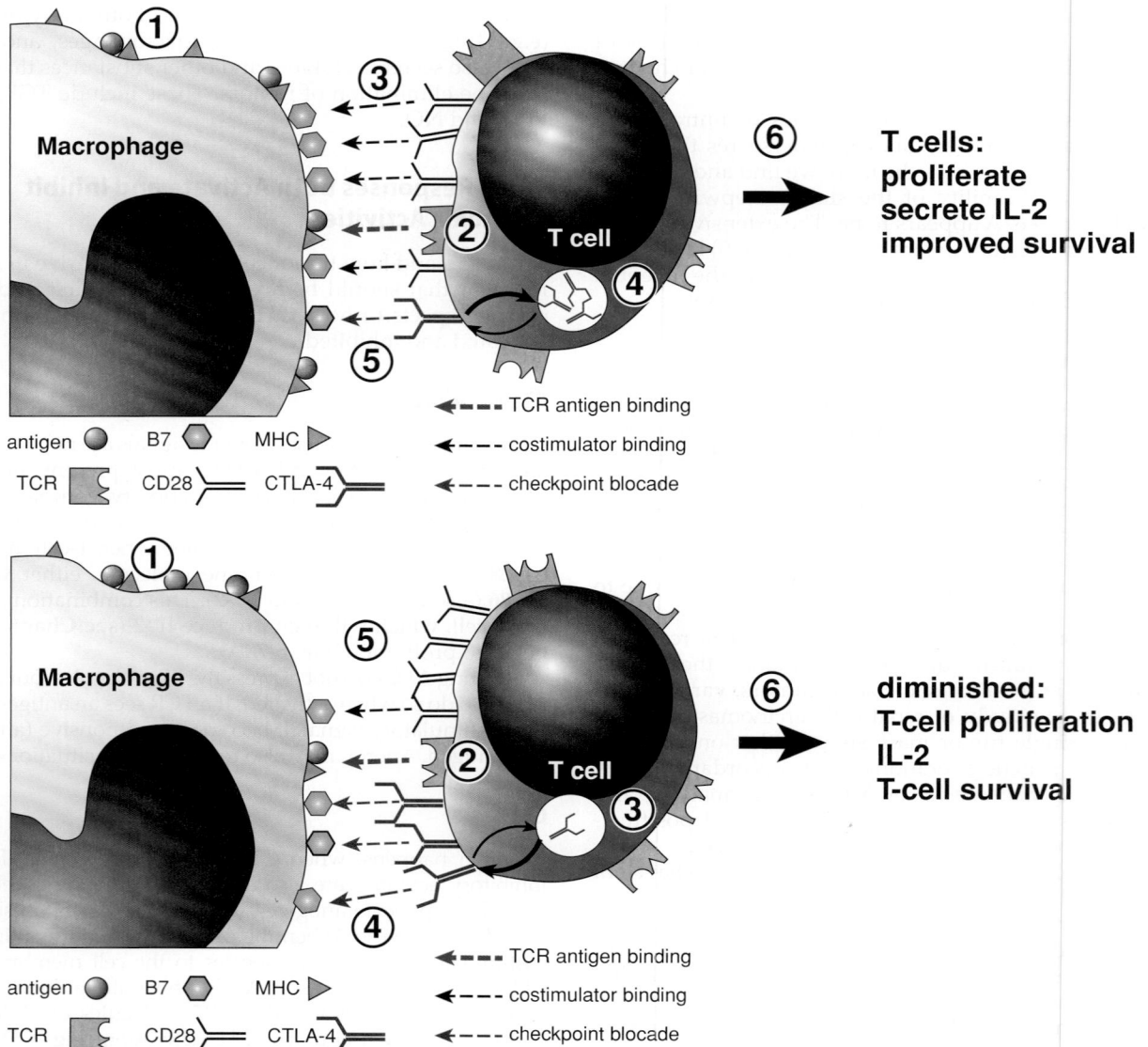

FIGURE 5-70. Generation of effector T cells and their inhibition by CTLA-4. A. Producing CTLs. 1. Antigen-presenting cells (APCs, here, macrophages) present antigen to a T cell in the context of self-MHC. **2.** T-cell receptors recognize this presentation. **3.** T-cell stimulation requires that T-cell CD28 bind a costimulatory molecule, either B7-1 or B7-2, on the APC surface. **4.** Part of the T-cell response is to recruit CTLA-4 from cytoplasmic vesicles to the cell membrane. **5.** If the immune response is to be fruitful, a small amount of CTLA-4 is brought to the cell membrane, and does not prevent T-cell activation. **6.** T cells so activated proliferate, produce IL-2, and generate prosurvival signals. **B. Inhibiting CTL activation. 1.** However, the same process can lead to anergy, in which case antigen is presented in the context of MHC. **2.** TCR recognizes this combination. **3.** However, CTLA-4 trafficking from the cytoplasmic vesicle is greater than in **A**, and a large amount of CTLA-4 reaches the cell membrane. **4.** There, it recognizes B7 molecules at higher affinity than does CD28, **5.** preventing adequate interaction between B7 and CD28 to activate the T cell. **6.** This leads to impaired T-cell survival and proliferation.

Regulatory T lymphocytes (Tregs) also express CTLA-4 constitutively. Treg CTLA-4, possibly because it sequesters B7s and/or because it promotes B7 internalization, is considered to be important to their immunomodulatory function.

CTLA-4, like PD-1 (see below), is important in normal immune physiology. Naturally occurring polymorphisms in CTLA-4 are associated with various autoimmune diseases, including systemic lupus, rheumatoid arthritis, and others (**see Chapter 11**). It may also help mediate allograft acceptance.

PD-1, PD-L1, and PD-L2

Programmed cell death-1 (PD-1, or CD279) is a T-cell membrane receptor that helps induce anergy and also inhibits effector functions of activated CTLs. In the former case, T cells that do not receive full activation signals (see above) upregulate PD-1 and become anergic. In the latter case, PD-1 acts at the site of CTL target cell killing. Once PD-1 is activated by either of its two ligands (PD-L1, PD-L2), it blocks CTL effector functions. T cells proliferate and survive less. Further, they produce less IFNγ, TNFα, IL-2, IL-4, and IL-10.

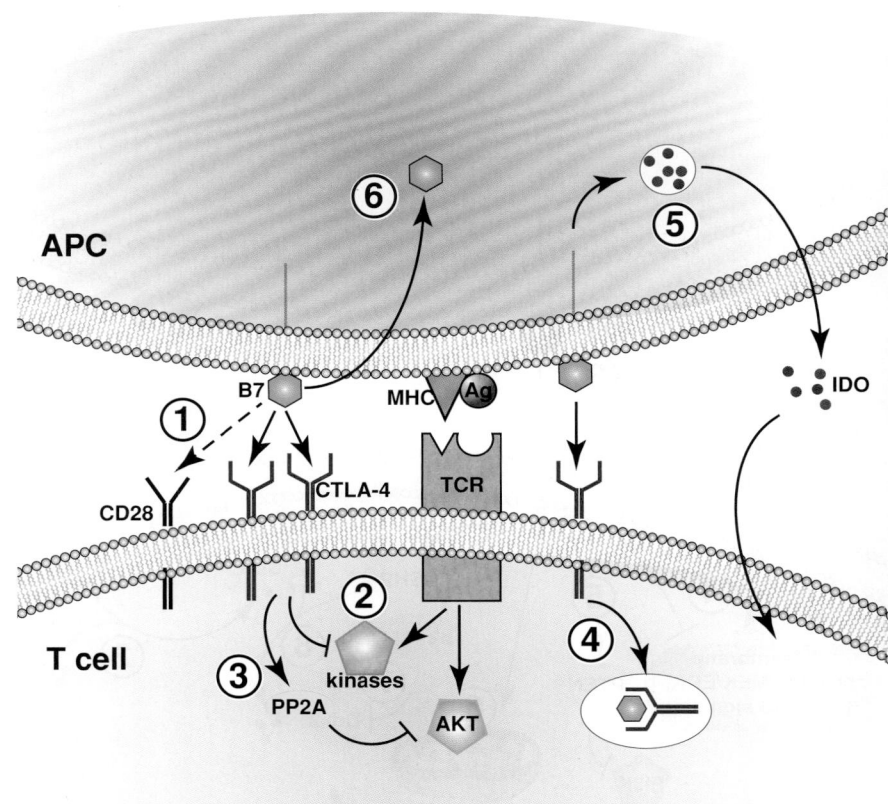

FIGURE 5-71. Mechanisms of CTLA-4 inhibition of immune effector responses. CTLA-4 inhibits effector T-cell responses in several ways. **1.** Its higher affinity for B7 ligands on APC membranes allows it to outcompete CD28 for binding to this costimulatory molecule. **2.** On binding B7s, it activates protein phosphatases, for example, SHP-2, which dephosphorylate kinases (e.g., LCK) and Ras-related signaling, which are activated by TCR. **3.** It activates protein phosphatase PP2A, which dephosphorylates AKT and thus blocks T-cell proliferation. **4.** It internalizes bound B7s, making them unavailable to bind CD28. **5.** It induces APCs to secrete indoleamine 2,3-dioxygenase (IDO), which depletes T-cell tryptophan and blocks T-cell proliferation. **6.** CTLA-4 also stimulates APC cells to endocytose B7 (*trans*-endocytosis), thus decreasing total available B7 at APC cell membranes.

PD-1 are low or nonactivated T cells, but increase when antigen binds the TCR, and so characterizes activated T cells. It is also present at the cell membranes of B cells, myeloid and NK cells, and γδT cells.

Like CTLA-4, PD-1 is important in limiting the severity of cytotoxic immune responses. Animals lacking PD-1 have exaggerated tissue destruction during viral infections, and are susceptible to developing autoimmune diseases.

PD-L1 and PD-L2

PD-L1, which is the most commonly studied ligand for PD-1, is expressed on both hematopoietic and nonhematopoietic cells. Among the latter, many epithelial cells express PD-L1, particularly after stimulation with IFNγ. Tumorigenic signaling (see below) also upregulates PD-L1. PD-L2 is less ubiquitous and occurs mainly on dendritic cells and monocytes, but can be induced on other cell types.

Mechanism of PD-1 Action

When TCR binds antigen, it activates tyrosine kinases (e.g., LCK). These phosphorylate the cytoplasmic tail of CD3. Once either of its two known ligands binds and activates PD-1, it acts via its immunoreceptor tyrosine-based inhibitory motif (ITIM). ITIM activates tyrosine phosphatases, particularly SHP-2, which dephosphorylate CD3, and block downstream CTL activation signaling (Fig. 5-72).

Activated PD-1 decreases T-cell responses in many ways, and additional study will undoubtedly uncover many more. It:

- increases PTEN protein levels and inhibits PI3K, which is important in stimulating cell proliferation and transcription
- blocks cell cycle progression, as well, by decreasing ubiquitination (and so, degradation) of the tumor suppressor protein, p27^{Kip1}. In so doing, it inhibits Cdk2 activity and blocks cell cycle progression
- further impedes T-cell proliferation by blocking signaling through MEK/Erk and PLCγ/Ras pathways
- facilitates development of anergy when T cells are presented with antigen in the absence of facilitating signals from an inflammatory environment

Interestingly, PD-1 reprograms cellular metabolism. Activated T cells tend to utilize glycolysis to generate energy. Quiescent T lymphocytes, on the other hand, prefer oxidative phosphorylation. PD-1 upregulates fatty acid β-oxidation (FAO), which favors oxidative phosphorylation and inhibits glycolysis. FAO also characterizes Tregs and memory—as opposed to active—T cells. In this regard, TGFβ stimulates Treg generation, and PD-1 lowers the threshold for cell responses to TGFβ, thus favoring naive T-cell differentiation into Tregs.

Tumor Cells Generate High Levels of PD-1 Ligands

With this background, we return to tumors. Many tumors generate high levels of PD-1 ligands. Levels of PD-L1 in human tumors are associated with poor prognosis, more extensive metastases, and resistance to therapies. Many

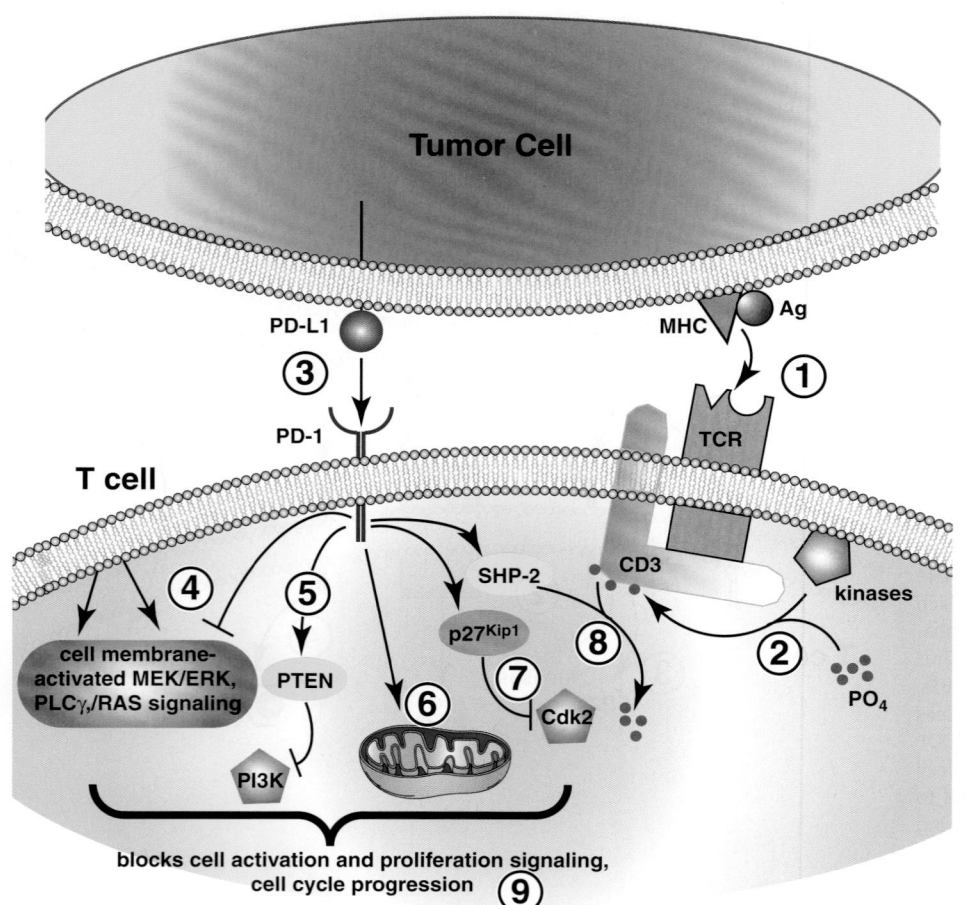

FIGURE 5-72. Immune checkpoint inhibition by PD-1/PD-L1. 1. T lymphocytes recognize tumor-related antigens on the cell membranes of cancer cells. **2.** This leads to a series of cell activation reactions, including phosphorylation of the cytoplasmic portion of TCR-bound CD3. **3.** Tumor cells produce ligands for T-cell membrane receptor, PD-1 (see Fig. 5-73), mostly PD-L1. **4.** This interaction inhibits diverse pathways of T-cell activation, including Ras and other cell membrane-activated cascades. **5.** Activated PD-1 increases PTEN, which inhibits PI3K. **6.** It also alters cellular metabolism to favor oxidative phosphorylation, rather than glycolysis. **7.** Degradation of p27^{Kip1} is blocked, which increases p27^{Kip1} in the cytosol, blocking Cdk2 and preventing cell cycle progression. **8.** PD-1–activated SHP-2 phosphatase dephosphorylates—and so inactivates—phosphorylated CD3. **9.** All these activities have the collective effect of blocking effector T-cell activation and proliferation.

different triggers and pathways stimulate tumor production of PD-L1 (Fig. 5-73). In many cases, oncogenic mutations that are integral to tumor generation upregulate PD-L1 production. The MAPK signaling pathway, mutation-generated activation of which is integral to development of many tumors, stimulates PD-L1 production. Thus, activating mutations of *BRAF* and EGFR stimulate MAPK, which increase PD-L1 transcription. Some chemotherapeutic drugs may do the same, for example, cisplatin.

PTEN tumor suppressor is frequently impaired or mutated in tumorigenesis, causing overactivity of PI3K/AKT pathways, which also increase PD-L1 expression. Interestingly, this may occur both at transcriptional and translational levels.

Other factors, reflecting environmental, genetic and epigenetic stimuli, also contribute to increasing PD-L1 production on tumor cells. Hypoxia, which induces HIF-1α (see above), stimulates transcriptional activity at the PD-L1 promoter. Other transcription factors that act similarly include STAT3 and NF-κB, both of which are commonly part of the increased cellular proliferative machinery in tumor development.

Finally, epigenetic factors contribute to upregulation as well. Thus, a plethora of miRNAs normally prevent translation of the PD-L1 transcript. Many of these, including miR-513, miR-570, miR-34a, and miR-200, are mutated in diverse tumors and contribute to overexpression of PD-L1.

Coinhibitory Pathways as Therapeutic Targets

Needless to say, the centrality of immune suppressor mechanisms—particularly those that impede CTL generation and activity—to tumor survival makes them important targets for therapeutic manipulation. This is a rapidly evolving field, with new and ingenious approaches to enhancing antitumor immunity being introduced all the time. To date, considerable progress has been shown in improving therapeutic outcomes in melanomas and other tumors. One looks

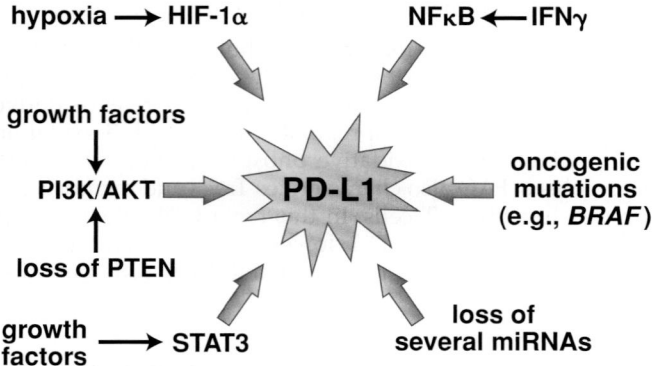

FIGURE 5-73. Pathways causing tumor cells to increase cell membrane PD-L1. Multiple intrinsic factors that are associated with tumorigenesis and extrinsic factors that reflect changing facets of tumor cells' microenvironments upregulate PD-L1 production and protect tumor cells from immune elimination.

forward to continued improvement in this area. At the same time, because such moieties as CTLA-4 and PD-1 are important regulators of cell-mediated immunity, their inhibition sometimes entails problematic toxicities.

Agents Implicated in Causing Cancer

The general mechanisms underlying the development of neoplasia caused by infectious or environmental agents are summarized in Figure 5-74.

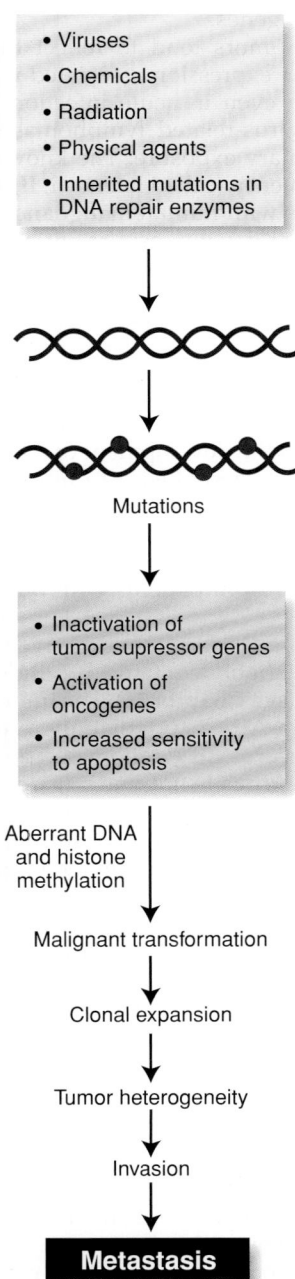

- Viruses
- Chemicals
- Radiation
- Physical agents
- Inherited mutations in DNA repair enzymes

Mutations

- Inactivation of tumor supressor genes
- Activation of oncogenes
- Increased sensitivity to apoptosis

Aberrant DNA and histone methylation

Malignant transformation

Clonal expansion

Tumor heterogeneity

Invasion

Metastasis

FIGURE 5-74. Summary of the general mechanisms of cancer.

INFECTIOUS AGENTS AND HUMAN CANCER

Most focus on infections and human cancer reflects the important role of viruses in oncogenesis, and the identifiable contributions of specific viral genes to tumor development. However, in recent years, mechanisms of nonviral infectious carcinogenesis have been elucidated, thus shedding light on other agents as well.

Only a Few Viruses Are Known to Cause Human Cancer

Viruses are responsible for about 15% of cancers. The strongest associations involve:

- Human T-cell leukemia virus type I (HTLV-I) **(RNA retrovirus)** and T-cell leukemia/lymphoma
- Hepatitis B virus (HBV, **DNA**) and hepatitis C virus (HCV, **RNA**) and primary hepatocellular carcinoma (HCC)
- HPV **(DNA)** and carcinomas of the cervix, anus, and vulva, and some oropharyngeal cancers
- EBV (DNA) and certain forms of lymphoma and nasopharyngeal carcinoma
- Human herpesvirus 8 (HHV 8, **DNA**) and Kaposi sarcoma (KS)

Globally, HBV, HCV, and HPV account for 80% of virus-related human cancers.

HTLV-1, the Only Retrovirus Known to Cause a Human Cancer

The rare adult T-cell leukemia is endemic in southern Japan and the Caribbean basin, and occurs sporadically elsewhere. The etiologic agent, HTLV-I, is tropic for $CD4^+$ T lymphocytes and has also been incriminated in several neurologic disorders. It is estimated that leukemia develops in 3% to 5% of HTLV-I–infected people and then only after a latent period of 30 to 50 years. A closely related virus, HTLV-II, has been associated with only a few cases of lymphoproliferative disorders.

The HTLV-I genome contains no known oncogene and does not integrate at specific sites in the host DNA. The viral transcriptional activator, Tax, appears to mediate HTLV-I oncogenicity. Tax both drives transcription of viral genes and promotes the activity of other genes involved in cell proliferation, such as NF-κB and IL-2 receptor. It also downregulates p53 and the cell cycle control protein, $p16^{INK4a}$. Since HTLV-I–induced lymphocyte proliferation in vitro is initially polyclonal and only later monoclonal, Tax probably begins a process that requires additional genetic events for a complete malignant phenotype to develop.

HBV, HCV, and Hepatocellular Carcinomas

Epidemiologic studies have established a strong link between primary HCC and chronic infection with HBV, a DNA virus, and HCV, an RNA virus (**see Chapter 20**). Two mechanisms have been invoked to explain virus-related hepatocarcinogenesis. One theory holds that the inability of some people to clear these infections leads to continued hepatocyte proliferation due to ongoing liver injury, and eventually causes malignant transformation. However, a small subset of patients with HBV infection develop HCCs in noncirrhotic livers. A second theory implicates a virally encoded protein in the pathogenesis of HBV-induced liver cancer. Transgenic mice expressing HBx, a small viral regulatory protein, develop liver cancer, but without evident pre-existing liver cell injury and inflammation. The *HBx* gene product upregulates several cellular genes. It also binds and inactivates p53. The underlying mechanisms in HBV-induced carcinogenesis remain unsettled.

It has not been shown that HCV is directly oncogenic. HCCs, when they develop in HCV-infected patients, tend to do so 20 or more years after primary infection, and then usually in the context of cirrhosis and chronic liver injury. However, some data suggest that HCV core protein may contribute to the development of HCC, and one of the HCV nonstructural proteins activates NF-κB.

DNA Viruses in Human Tumors

Several DNA viruses (mainly HPV, EBV, HBV, HHV8) are incriminated in human cancers. Unlike animal retroviruses which carry oncogenes that are homologous to human genes (proto-oncogenes), transforming genes of oncogenic DNA viruses show virtually no homology to cellular genes. Rather, the paradigm of oncogenicity among human oncogenic DNA viruses is genes that encode protein products that bind to, and inactivate, products of TSGs (e.g., Rb, p53).

Human Papillomavirus

HPVs induce lesions in humans that progress to squamous cell carcinoma (**see Chapters 23 and 24**). The full HPV productive cycle occurs only in squamous cells. Over 170 distinct HPV serotypes are known, most being associated with benign squamous epithelial lesions, including warts, laryngeal papillomas, and condylomata acuminata (genital warts) of the vulva, penis, and perianal region. Cutaneous warts invariably remain benign, but genital warts may rarely show malignant change. HPV, especially HPV 16, has been identified in many head and neck squamous cell carcinomas, especially those of the tonsils and oropharynx (**see Chapter 29**), and laryngeal papillomatosis in young children is associated with maternal infection with genital wart–causing HPV serotypes. In a rare hereditary disease called **epidermodysplasia verruciformis**, HPV-related warts may progress to squamous carcinoma. At least 20 HPV types are associated with cervical cancer, 70% of which are caused by serotypes 16 and 18 (**see Chapter 24**). Multivalent HPV vaccines protect from some wart–causing and most cancer-related HPV types.

The major oncoproteins encoded by HPV are E6, E7, and E5. E6 binds to p53 and targets it for degradation. It also activates telomerase expression and promotes tumor development via other mechanisms, independent of p53. E7 binds to pRb and releases its inhibitory effect on E2F transcriptional activity, allowing cell cycle progression. E6 and E7 of non–cancer-causing strains of HPV do not have these activities. E5 can activate the epidermal growth factor receptor. During the last half century, a cell line derived from cervical cancer, *HeLa cells*, has maintained worldwide popularity in the study of cancer. HeLa cells express HPV-18 E6 and E7, and, even after many years of in vitro passaging, inactivation of these oncoproteins results in growth arrest.

Epstein–Barr Virus

EBV is a HHV that is so widely disseminated that 95% of adults in the world have antibodies to it. It infects B lymphocytes and transforms them into lymphoblasts. In a small proportion of primary EBV infections, this lymphoblastoid transformation manifests clinically as infectious mononucleosis (**see Chapter 9**), a short-lived benign lymphoproliferative disease.

EBV is also intimately associated with certain human cancers. A number of EBV genes are implicated in lymphocyte immortalization, including Epstein–Barr nuclear antigens (EBNAs), certain untranslated nuclear EBV RNAs, called EBER1 and EBER2, and latency-associated membrane proteins (LMPs). EBV also encodes about 40 miRNAs, some of which activate or repress specific cellular genes. LMP1 interacts with cellular proteins that normally transduce signals from the TNF receptor, but it does not trigger apoptosis. Rather, it activates NF-κB and other cell division–associated signaling molecules. Generally, EBV-related tumors are ascribed to the activities of the virus' latency-associated genes.

EBV-induced tumors tend to reflect the establishment of patterns of gene expression associated with viral latency. This may happen even in acute infection. EBV, in fact, is unusual in that virus-related lymphomas (see below) can occur during primary exposure. The known three different patterns of EBV latency (called latency I, II, and III) have different associations with human malignancies. However, the human tumors that develop as a result all appear to entail viral orchestration of the same types of cancer hallmark traits (see above) that characterize sporadic cancers that occur independently of such infections.

PATHOPHYSIOLOGY: *BURKITT LYMPHOMA:* EBV was the first virus to be unequivocally linked to the development of a human tumor. In 1958, Denis Burkitt described a form of childhood lymphoma in a geographical belt across equatorial Africa, which he suggested might have a viral etiology. A few years later, Epstein and Barr discovered viral particles in cell lines cultured from patients with Burkitt lymphoma (BL).

African BL is a B-cell tumor, in which the neoplastic lymphocytes invariably contain EBV and manifest EBV-related antigens (**see Chapter 26**). The tumor has also been recognized in non-African populations, but in those cases only about 20% carry EBV genomes. The localization of BL to equatorial Africa is not understood, but prolonged stimulation of the immune system by endemic malaria may be important. Normally, EBV-stimulated B-cell proliferation is controlled by suppressor T cells. Inadequate T-cell responses are often reported in chronic malarial infections. These might allow unrestrained B-cell proliferation and so facilitate further genetic changes that may eventuate in lymphoma. One such change is translocation in which c-*myc* expression is driven by an immunoglobulin promoter. In addition, EBV proteins inhibit apoptosis and activate signaling pathways involved in cell proliferation. Therefore, the multistep pathogenesis of African BL may be viewed as follows:

1. Infection and polyclonal lymphoblastoid transformation of B cells by EBV
2. Proliferation of B cells and inhibition of suppressor T cells induced by malaria
3. C-*myc* by translocation in a single B cell, with effects on other signaling pathways

4. Uncontrolled proliferation of a resulting clone of malignant B lymphocytes

NASOPHARYNGEAL CARCINOMA: Nasopharyngeal carcinoma is a variant of squamous carcinoma that is particularly common in certain parts of Asia. EBV DNA and EBNA are present in virtually all of these cancers. Epithelial cells may be exposed to EBV via infected lymphocytes traveling through lymphoid-rich epithelium. One of the EEV proteins in this tumor has been shown to activate the EGF receptor signaling. Fortunately, 70% of patients with this disease are cured by radiation therapy alone.

OTHER EBV–ASSOCIATED TUMORS: EBV markers have been identified in about half of cases of classical Hodgkin lymphoma, in which the virus infects Reed–Sternberg cells. A number of T-cell and NK lymphomas have also been found to harbor EBV, as well as 5% of gastric carcinomas.

POLYCLONAL LYMPHOPROLIFERATION IN IMMUNODEFICIENT STATES: EBV-induced B-cell proliferative disorders may complicate congenital or acquired immunodeficiencies. These diseases are clinically and pathologically indistinguishable from other malignant lymphomas, but are mostly polyclonal. Lymphoid neoplasia occurs in immunosuppressed renal transplant recipients 30 to 50 times more often than in the general population. Almost all lymphoproliferative diseases associated with organ transplantation, and congenital or acquired immunodeficiencies (especially AIDS) involve EBV. Monoclonal lymphomas may occasionally develop in a patient with an EBV-induced lymphoproliferative disorder.

Human Herpesvirus 8

KS is a vascular tumor that was originally described in elderly eastern European men and later observed in sub-Saharan Africa (**see Chapter 16**). It is now the most common neoplasm associated with AIDS. HHV8, also known as KS-associated herpesvirus (KSHV), is present in virtually all KS lesions, whether from HIV-positive or HIV-negative patients, and appears to be necessary—but not sufficient—for development of KS.

Other, unidentified, factors contribute. Many more people who are HHV8-positive than ever develop KS. In the United States, about 6% of the population carries HHV8, and 60% to 80% of the black population in sub-Saharan Africa is seropositive for HHV 8, but the risk of developing KS is miniscule compared to these percentages. Furthermore, among HIV-1–positive people, the risk of KS is greatest when HIV-1 infection was acquired via sexual transmission, rather than by transfusion or by a baby from an infected mother.

In addition to infecting the spindle cells of KS, HHV8 is lymphotropic and has been implicated in two uncommon B-cell lymphoid malignancies, namely, **primary effusion lymphoma** and **multicentric Castleman disease** (**see Chapter 26**).

Like other DNA viruses, the HHV8 viral genome encodes proteins that interfere with the p53 and Rb tumor suppressor pathways. Some viral proteins also inhibit apoptosis, and act in multiple ways to accelerate cell cycle transit. HHV8 encodes an inhibitor of IκB, the normal regulator of NF-κB. As a result, HHV8 infection is associated with unrestrained activation of NF-κB. Development and progression of KS seems to entail interdependence between lytic HHV8 infection and latently infected cells. Thus, antiviral drugs that inhibit HHV8 lytic infection provide strong protection from the development of KS.

Other DNA Viruses

A very uncommon skin tumor, Merkel cell carcinoma, is associated with **Merkel cell polyomavirus (MCPyV)**. MCPyV genomes integrated into cellular DNA have been identified in most of these tumors. However, as with some other viruses, the percentage of the population showing serologic evidence of infection is far greater than the frequency of Merkel cell carcinoma.

Other viruses have been suggested to be associated with human cancers over the years, but with little or no verifiable data to substantiate those assertions. SV40, which causes tumors in some rodents, is a case in point: after extensive study, there are no reproducible experimental or epidemiologic data to support the contention that SV40 is oncogenic for humans.

Enormous interspecies differences in susceptibility to virus infection and oncogenicity, and past experience, underscore the dangers of excessive gullibility and accepting seemingly reasonable associations as a substitute for hard data. Careful studies and independent verification are obligatory before inculpating any agent as a cause of human cancer.

Helicobacter pylori Is a Bacterial Gastric Carcinogen

H. pylori was discovered in 1984, and linked to upper GI ulcerative disease (**see Chapter 19**). It is now known to cause at least 3/4 of the world's 723,000 yearly gastric cancer deaths. **CagA** bacterial protein is the principal malefactor. A complex bacterial structure, T4SS, delivers CagA and other bacterial products into gastric epithelial cells. CagA then acts via multiple pathways to stimulate oncogenesis and inflammation. It activates Shp-2 phosphatase (see above), which weakens intercellular adhesion by dephosphorylating FAK. This alters cell polarity and increases mobility. CagA also turns on **PKCδ**. This stimulates Ras-mediated signaling through the B-Raf/Erk pathway, to increase NF-κB. Multiple other CagA-activated pathways also converge on NF-κB, which orchestrates *H. pylori*-stimulated cell proliferation, inflammation (by activating IL-8 promoter) and cell motility and invasiveness.

Aflatoxin Is a Fungal Protein That Is a Potent Hepatocarcinogen

Aflatoxin B_1 is a natural product of the fungus *Aspergillus flavus*. Aflatoxin B_1 is metabolized (see below) to an epoxide, which binds DNA covalently. Aflatoxin B_1 is among the most potent liver carcinogens known. Since *Aspergillus* spp. are ubiquitous, *A. flavus* contamination of foods, particularly peanuts and grains, may generate significant amounts of aflatoxin B_1. It has been suggested that aflatoxin-rich foods may contribute to the high incidence of liver cancer in parts of Africa and Asia. Interestingly, both experimental aflatoxin-induced tumors in rodents and exposed to aflatoxin B_1 and human liver cancers in areas of high dietary concentrations of aflatoxin carry the same p53 mutation.

CHEMICAL CARCINOGENESIS

The field of chemical carcinogenesis originated some two centuries ago in descriptions of an occupational disease (this was not the first recognition of occupation-related cancer, since a specific predisposition of nuns to breast cancer was appreciated even earlier). Sir Percival Pott gets credit for relating cancer of the scrotum in chimney sweeps to a specific chemical exposure: soot. Today we realize that other products of the combustion of organic materials are responsible for a man-made epidemic of cancer, especially, lung cancer in those exposed to cigarette smoke (**see Chapter 8**).

The first experimental chemical carcinogenesis was reported in 1915, with skin cancers in rabbits painted with coal tar. Since then, the list of organic and inorganic carcinogens has grown exponentially. Yet, curiously, many compounds known to be potent carcinogens are relatively chemically inert. *The solution to this riddle became apparent in the early 1960s, when it was shown that many chemical carcinogens require metabolic activation before they can react with cell constituents.* These data, since extended extensively to many compounds, highlight the complexity of chemical carcinogenesis.

Chemical Carcinogens Are Mostly Mutagens

Causal links between chemical exposures and human cancers are difficult to establish convincingly. Epidemiologic studies, which are commonly cited, have many inherent drawbacks, including uncertainties in estimated doses, population variability, long and variable latency, and reliance on clinical and public health records of questionable accuracy. Consequently, studies involving animals are legally required before a new drug is introduced. Yet, the huge increase in the numbers of chemicals synthesized every year makes even this method cumbersome and expensive. Reproducible and reliable screening assays for potential carcinogenic activity have therefore centered on relationships between carcinogenicity and mutagenicity.

A **mutagen** *is an agent that can permanently alter a cell's genome.* One test (Ames) uses frameshift mutations and base-pair substitutions in bacterial cultures. Others look for mutations, unscheduled DNA synthesis, and DNA strand breaks in cultured rodent or human cells. About 90% of known carcinogens are mutagenic in these systems. Moreover, most, but not all, mutagens are carcinogenic. This correlation between carcinogenicity and mutagenicity presumably occurs because both reflect DNA damage. Although not infallible, in vitro mutagenicity assays are valuable tools in screening chemicals for carcinogenic potential.

Chemical Carcinogenesis Is a Multistep Process

Studies of chemical carcinogenesis in experimental animals have shed light on the distinct stages in the progression of normal cells to cancer. Long before the genetic basis of cancer was appreciated, studies found that a single application of a carcinogen to a mouse's skin did not, by itself, produce cancer. However, adding a local proliferative stimulus (a noncarcinogenic irritating chemical) allowed tumors to appear. The first effect was called **initiation**. The action of the second, noncarcinogenic chemical was **promotion**. *Chemical carcinogenesis is a multistep process that involves numerous mutations:*

1. **Initiation** likely represents a mutation in a single cell.
2. **Promotion** reflects an initiated cell's clonal expansion, in which the mutation has conferred a growth advantage, but altered cells still require the continued presence of the promoting stimulus. This stimulus may be a chemical or physical agent, or endogenous stimulation (e.g., hormonal [breast, prostate]).
3. **Progression** is the stage in which growth becomes autonomous (i.e., independent of both added carcinogen and promoter). By this point, enough cellular changes have accrued to immortalize cells.
4. **Cancer** is the consequence of this sequence, and develops when the cells acquire the capacity to invade and metastasize.

The morphologic changes that reflect this progression in humans are best seen in accessible epithelia, such as those of the skin, cervix, and colon, which can be sampled repeatedly. Initiation has no morphologic counterpart, but *promotion and progression are represented by the sequence of hyperplasia, dysplasia, and carcinoma in situ.*

Chemical Carcinogens Usually Undergo Metabolic Activation

The International Agency for Research in Cancer (IARC) lists 109 chemicals as human carcinogens, 82 as probable, and 302 as possible human carcinogens. Chemicals cause cancer either directly or, more often, after metabolic activation. Direct-acting carcinogens are inherently reactive enough to bind covalently to cellular macromolecules. A number of highly reactive compounds, such as nitrogen mustard, and certain metals are in this category. Most organic carcinogens, however, require enzymatic conversion to an ultimate, more reactive compound, usually by cellular drug metabolism and detoxification systems. Many cells, but particularly liver cells, have enzyme systems that can convert procarcinogens to their active forms. Yet, each carcinogen has its own spectrum of target tissues, often limited to a single organ. The basis for organ specificity in chemical carcinogenesis is not well understood.

 PATHOPHYSIOLOGY: *POLYCYCLIC AROMATIC HYDROCARBONS:* These are originally derived from coal tar, and are among the most extensively studied carcinogens. This class includes compounds as benzo(a)pyrene, 3-methylcholanthrene, and dibenzanthracene. These have a broad range of targets and generally produce cancers at the site of application. The specific type of cancer produced varies with the route of administration.

Polycyclic hydrocarbons, many of which are present in cigarette smoke, are metabolized by cytochrome P450-dependent mixed function oxidases to electrophilic epoxides, which then react with proteins and nucleic acids. Epoxide formation depends on the presence of an unsaturated carbon–carbon bond. For example, vinyl chloride, the simple two-carbon molecule from which the widely used plastic polyvinyl chloride is synthesized, is metabolized to an epoxide which mediates its carcinogenic properties. Workers exposed to vinyl chloride monomer later develop hepatic angiosarcomas.

ALKYLATING AGENTS: Many chemotherapeutic drugs (e.g., busulfan cyclophosphamide, cisplatin) are alkylating agents that transfer alkyl groups (methyl, ethyl, etc.) to macromolecules, including guanines within DNA. They destroy cancer cells by damaging DNA, but also injure normal cells. Thus, alkylating chemotherapy carries a significant risk of solid and hematologic malignancies at a later time.

AROMATIC AMINES AND AZO DYES: Aromatic amines and azo dyes, unlike polycyclic aromatic hydrocarbons, are not ordinarily carcinogenic at the point of application. However, they commonly produce bladder and liver tumors, respectively, when fed to experimental animals. Both aromatic amines and azo dyes are primarily metabolized in the liver. The liver metabolizes aromatic amines to hydroxylamino derivatives, and conjugates these to glucuronic acid. Unfortunately, the glucuronides are hydrolyzed in the bladder, releasing those hydroxylamines. Occupational exposure to aromatic amines in the form of aniline dyes has resulted in bladder cancer.

NITROSAMINES: Nitrosamines are potent carcinogens in primates, but their role in human cancer is unclear. Geographic and epidemiologic overlap between nitrosamine and nitrite consumption suggests possible roles in esophageal and other GI cancers. Nitrosamines are activated by hydroxylation, followed by formation of a reactive alkyl carbonium ion.

METALS: Several metals or metal compounds can induce cancer. Divalent metal cations, such as nickel (Ni^{2+}), lead (Pb^{2+}), cadmium (Cd^{2+}), cobalt (Co^{2+}), and beryllium (Be^{2+}), are electrophilic and can react with macromolecules. In addition, metal ions react with guanine and phosphate groups of DNA. Metal ions such as Ni^{2+} can depolymerize polynucleotides. Some metals can bind purine and pyrimidine bases. Most metal-induced cancers occur in an occupational setting (**see Chapter 8**).

Endogenous and Environmental Factors Influence Chemical Carcinogenesis

Many factors affect the outcome of chemical exposures in experimental animals—species and strain, age and sex, hormonal status, diet, and the presence or absence of inducers of drug-metabolizing systems and tumor promoters. Such factors may also play a role in individual variability in human epidemiologic studies.

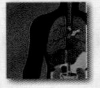 **PATHOPHYSIOLOGY:** *CARCINOGEN METABOLISM:* **Mixed-function oxidases** are a family of enzymes that oxidize two different substrates at once. In mice, the levels of these enzymes correlate with sensitivity to chemical carcinogens, theoretically reflecting enzymatic activation of procarcinogens to carcinogens. These correlations have yet to prove informative in human studies, however.

SEX AND HORMONAL STATUS: These factors affect susceptibility to chemical carcinogens but are highly variable and not readily predictable. Experimental animals often show sex-linked susceptibility to carcinogenic effects of certain chemicals. However, how and whether gender and hormones affect chemical carcinogenesis in humans is not clear.

DIET: Diet can affect levels of drug-metabolizing enzymes. Experimentally, low-protein diets reduce the hepatic mixed-function oxidase activity, and so decrease sensitivity to hepatocarcinogens. This is a double-edged sword, however: increased renal tumors in mice accompany diet-related decreased incidence of dimethylnitrosamine-related liver tumors.

PHYSICAL CARCINOGENESIS

The physical agents of carcinogenesis discussed here are UV light, asbestos, and foreign bodies. Radiation carcinogenesis is discussed in Chapter 8.

Ultraviolet Radiation Causes Skin Cancers

Among fair-skinned people, a glowing tan is commonly considered a healthy sign of a successful holiday. However, solar radiation causes considerable underlying tissue damage. Its harmful effects were recognized long ago, when ladies shielded themselves from the sun with parasols to maintain a "roses-and-milk" complexion and prevent wrinkles. Tanned complexions have been accompanied by cosmetic deterioration of facial skin and by an increased incidence of the major skin cancers.

Cancers attributed to sun exposure, namely, basal cell carcinoma, squamous carcinoma, and melanoma, occur mainly in paler people. Melanin pigment absorbs UV radiation, and so protects the skin of darker people. In fair-skinned people, the areas exposed to the sun are most prone to develop skin cancers, and there is a direct correlation between total exposure to sunlight and the incidence of skin cancer.

UV is short-wavelength electromagnetic radiation just beyond visible violet in the spectrum. Only certain parts of the UV spectrum are associated with tissue damage. *At wavelengths between 290 and 320 nm, UV radiation inactivates enzymes, inhibits cell division, and induces mutations, cell death, and cancer.*

Pyrimidine Dimers

Most importantly, UV radiation promotes DNA **pyrimidine dimer** formation. This type of DNA damage is not seen with any other carcinogen. Such dimers may form between thymine and thymine, between thymine and cytosine, or between cytosine pairs alone. Dimer formation leads to a cyclobutane ring, which distorts the phosphodiester backbone of the double helix in the region of each dimer. Unless efficiently eliminated by the nucleotide excision repair pathway, genomic injury produced by UV radiation is mutagenic and carcinogenic.

Xeroderma Pigmentosum

XP is an autosomal recessive disease that exemplifies the centrality of DNA repair in protecting against the harmful effects of UV radiation. In XP, sensitivity to sunlight is accompanied by a high incidence of skin cancers, including basal cell carcinoma, squamous cell carcinoma, and melanoma. Both neoplastic and nonneoplastic disorders of the skin in XP reflect impaired excision of UV-damaged DNA.

Asbestos Causes Mesothelioma and Lung Cancer

Asbestos, a material widely used in construction, insulation, and manufacturing, is a family of related fibrous silicates, which are classed as "serpentines" or "amphiboles." Serpentines, of which chrysotile is the only example of commercial importance, occur as flexible fibers; the amphiboles, represented principally by crocidolite and amosite, are firm narrow rods.

The characteristic tumor associated with asbestos exposure is malignant mesothelioma of the pleural and peritoneal cavities. This cancer, which is exceedingly rare in the general population, occurs in 2% to 3% (in some studies even more) of heavily exposed workers. The latent period—the interval between exposure and the appearance of a tumor—is usually about 20 years but may be twice that figure. Mesotheliomas of both pleura and peritoneum reflect the close contact of these membranes with asbestos fibers transported to them by lymphatic channels.

The pathogenesis of asbestos-associated mesotheliomas is unclear. It is not totally certain whether cancers related to asbestos exposure (**see Chapters 8 and 18**) are examples of chemical carcinogenesis, of physically induced tumors, or both. Thin crocidolite fibers are associated with much greater risk of mesothelioma than are shorter and thicker chrysotile fibers. There is increasing evidence that the surface properties of asbestos fibers are important in their carcinogenic properties.

Asbestos exposure also increases the risk of lung cancer, independent of cigarette smoking. Together, cigarette plus asbestos exposures synergize to greatly magnify lung cancer incidence. Both experimental and anecdotal epidemiologic studies suggest that asbestos in drinking water may increase incidence of digestive system cancers.

SYSTEMIC EFFECTS OF CANCER ON THE HOST

The symptoms of cancer usually reflect local effects of the primary tumor mass or its metastases. However, in some patients, cancers produce remote effects not attributable to tumor invasion or to metastasis. Collectively, these are **paraneoplastic syndromes**. Such effects are rarely lethal, but they may dominate the clinical course. It is important to recognize these syndromes for several reasons. First, a paraneoplastic syndrome may be the first clinical manifestation of a malignant tumor. Second, they may be mistaken as indicating advanced metastatic disease, and so lead to inappropriate therapy. Third, paraneoplastic symptomatology itself may be disabling, and treating those symptoms may provide important palliation to suffering patients. Finally, levels and effects of tumor products that cause paraneoplastic syndromes may provide a way to monitor the tumor's course and the effectiveness of therapies.

Most paraneoplastic manifestations manifest as involvement of one or another organ system, and are discussed in the chapters specific for individual organs. But there are also important systemic effects.

Fever

It is not uncommon for cancer patients to present initially with fever that cannot be explained by an active infection. Cancer-related fever correlates with tumor growth, disappears after treatment, and reappears on recurrence. Any tumor may cause fever, although febrile presentations are particularly common with Hodgkin and other lymphomas. Tumor cells may themselves release pyrogens or inflammatory cells in the tumor stroma can produce IL-1.

Anorexia and Weight Loss

Anorexia (weight loss) and cachexia are very common in patients with cancer, often appearing before a malignancy becomes apparent. For example, a small asymptomatic pancreatic cancer may be suspected only on the basis of progressive and unexplained weight loss. Although cancer patients often eat less because of anorexia and abnormalities of taste, decreased dietary intake does not explain the profound wasting so common among these people. The mechanisms responsible for this phenomenon are poorly understood. It is known, however, that unlike starvation, which is associated with a lowered metabolic rate, cancer is often accompanied by an elevated metabolic rate. TNFα and other cytokines (IFNs, IL-6) can produce a wasting syndrome in experimental animals.

EPIDEMIOLOGY OF CANCER

Cancer accounts for one-fifth of the total mortality in the United States and is the second leading cause of death after ischemic cardiovascular diseases. For most cancers, death rates in the United States have largely remained flat for more than half a century, with some notable exceptions (Fig. 5-75). The death rate from cancer of the lung among men rose dramatically from 1930, when it was an uncommon tumor, to the present, when it is by far the most common cause of death from cancer. As discussed in Chapter 8, the entire epidemic of lung cancer deaths is attributable to smoking. Among women, smoking did not become fashionable until World War II. Considering the time lag between starting smoking and development of lung cancer, it is not surprising that the increased death rate from lung cancer in women did not become significant until after 1965. Lung cancer is now by far the most common cause of cancer deaths among women. For unknown reasons, cancer of the stomach, which in 1930 was by far the most common cancer killer in men, and the second most common cause of cancer deaths in women, has shown a remarkable and sustained decline in frequency. The conspicuous decline in the death rate from cancer of the uterus (corpus plus cervix), probably reflects better screening, diagnostic techniques, and therapies. Overall, after decades of steady increases, age-adjusted mortality from all cancers has been fairly flat.

Individual cancers have their own age-related profiles, but for most, increased age is associated with an increased incidence. The most striking example of the dependency on age is carcinoma of the prostate, the incidence of which increases 30-fold from age 50 to 85. Certain neoplastic diseases, such as acute lymphoblastic leukemia in children and testicular cancer in young adults, show different age-related peaks of incidence (Fig. 5-76).

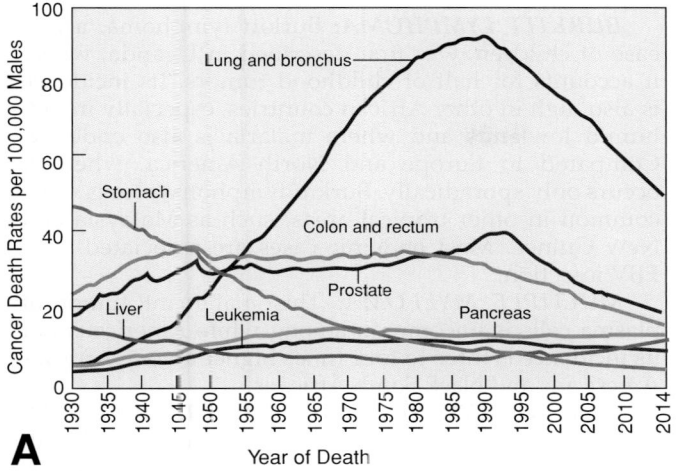

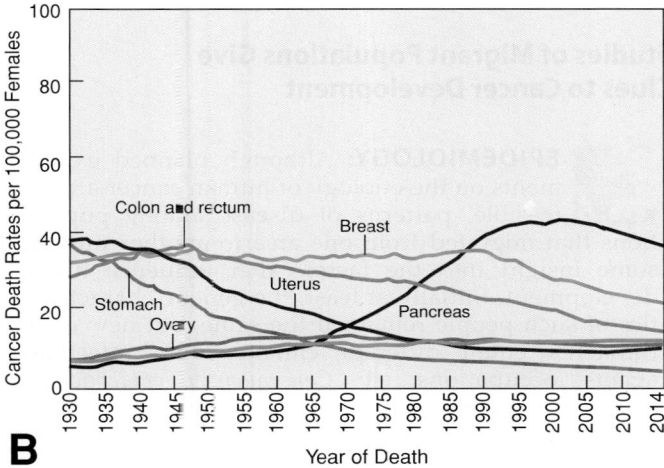

FIGURE 5-75. Cancer death rates in the United States, 1930 to 2002, among men (A) and women (B). (From US Mortality Data, 1960 to 2005, US Mortality Volumes, 1930 to 1959. National Center for Health Statistics, Centers for Disease Control and Prevention, 2008.)

Geographic and Ethnic Differences Influence Cancer Incidence

EPIDEMIOLOGY: Some cancers show striking differences between different populations and locations. Sometimes, these associations shed light on the etiologies of these tumors. Sometimes, they reflect definable environmental or genetic differences among people. Sometimes, though, these differences add to the mystery of what causes cancers:

NASOPHARYNGEAL CANCER: Nasopharyngeal cancer is rare in most of the world except for certain regions of China, Hong Kong, and Singapore.

ESOPHAGEAL CARCINOMA: Esophageal carcinoma is extremely rare among Mormon women in Utah but is ≈300 times more common among women in northern Iran. People in the so-called Asian esophageal cancer belt, which stretches from Turkey to eastern China, have very high rates of esophageal cancer. Interestingly, in this region, as the incidence rises, the proportional excess in males decreases; in some parts of this high-incidence area, there is a female excess. The disease is also more common in certain regions of sub-Saharan Africa and among African-Americans. Esophageal cancer disproportionately affects poor people in many areas of the world, and the combination of alcohol abuse and smoking is associated with a particularly high risk.

STOMACH CANCER: The highest incidence of stomach cancer is in Japan, where it is almost 10 times more common than among white Americans. It also occurs more frequently in Latin American countries, particularly Chile. Stomach cancer is also common in Iceland and eastern Europe.

COLORECTAL CANCER: The incidence of colorectal cancer is highest in the United States, where it is 3 to 4 times more common than in Japan, India, Africa, and Latin America. The basis for this difference, about which much has been speculated, remains unclear.

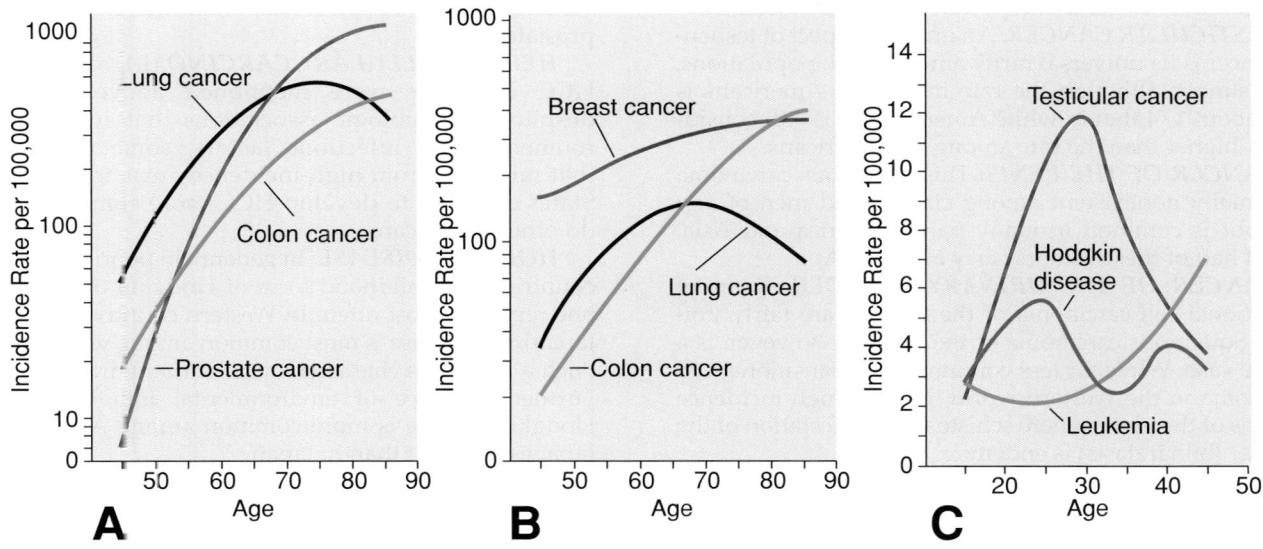

FIGURE 5-76. Incidence of specific cancers as a function of age. A. Men. **B.** Women. **C.** Testicular cancer in men and Hodgkin disease and leukemia in both sexes. The incidence of these cancers in **C** peaks at younger ages than do those in **A** and **B**.

LIVER CANCER: There is a strong correlation between the incidence of primary HCC and the prevalence of HBV and HCV (see above). Regions endemic for both diseases include large parts of sub-Saharan Africa and most of Asia, Indonesia, and the Philippines. Hepatitis viruses may not be the only culprits in these regions: levels of aflatoxin B_1 are high in the staple diets of many of the high-risk areas.

SKIN CANCER: As noted above, the rates for skin cancers vary with skin color and sun exposure. Thus, rates are particularly high in northern Australia, where the population is principally of English origin and sun exposure is intense. Skin cancer is also more common among the white population of the American Southwest. The lowest rates are found among people with darker skin (e.g., Japanese, Chinese, and Indians). Rates among black Africans may exceed those for Asians, despite their heavily pigmented skin, because they develop more melanomas of the soles and palms.

BREAST CANCER: Adenocarcinoma of the breast, the most common female cancer in many parts of Europe and North America, shows wide geographic variation. Among African and Asian populations, breast cancer is 1/5 to 1/6 as common as in Europe and the United States.

CERVICAL CARCINOMA: There are striking differences in the incidence of squamous carcinoma of the cervix between ethnic and different socioeconomic groups. In general, cervical cancer occurs more frequently in women who are more sexually active, reflecting the fact that this tumor is almost always associated with HPV infection (**see Chapter 24**).

CHORIOCARCINOMA: Choriocarcinoma is an uncommon cancer of trophoblastic differentiation. It occurs mainly in women, after a pregnancy, but can also occur as a testicular tumor in men. It is particularly common in the Pacific rim of Asia (Singapore, Hong Kong, Japan, and the Philippines).

PROSTATIC CANCER: Prostatic cancer is quite uncommon among Asian men, particularly Japanese, while the highest rates described are in African-Americans, in whom the disease occurs about 25 times more frequently. The incidence in American and European whites is intermediate.

TESTICULAR CANCER: An unusual aspect of testicular cancer is its universal rarity among black populations. Interestingly, although the rate in African-Americans is only about 1/4 that in white Americans, it is still considerably higher than the rate among black Africans.

CANCER OF THE PENIS: This squamous carcinoma is virtually nonexistent among circumcised men of any race but is common in many parts of Africa and Asia. About half of these tumors carry HPV DNA.

CANCER OF THE URINARY BLADDER: Rates of transitional cell carcinoma of the bladder are fairly uniform. Squamous carcinoma of the bladder, however, is a special case. While far less common than transitional cell carcinoma in the Western world, it has a high incidence in areas of the globe where schistosomal infestation of the bladder (bilharziasis) is endemic.

BURKITT LYMPHOMA: Burkitt lymphoma, a disease of children, was first described in Uganda, where it accounts for half of childhood tumors. Its incidence is also high in other African countries, especially in hot, humid lowlands and where malaria is also endemic. Compared to Europe and North America, where it occurs only sporadically, Burkitt lymphoma also is more common in other tropical areas, such as Malaysia and New Guinea. Most endemic cases are associated with EBV infection.

MULTIPLE MYELOMA: This malignant tumor of plasma cells is uncommon among white Americans but its incidence is three to four times higher among African-Americans and black South Africans.

CHRONIC LYMPHOCYTIC LEUKEMIA (CLL): CLL is common among elderly people in Europe and North America but is considerably less common in Japan.

Studies of Migrant Populations Give Clues to Cancer Development

EPIDEMIOLOGY: Although planned experiments on the etiology of human cancer are not feasible, patterns of disease among populations that migrated from one area to another provide some insight into the factors that influence tumor development. Initially at least, the genetic characteristics of such people remained the same, but new environments entail different climate, diet, infectious agents, occupations, etc. *Consequently, epidemiologic studies of migrant populations have provided many intriguing clues to the factors that may influence the pathogenesis of cancer.*

COLORECTAL, BREAST, ENDOMETRIAL, OVARIAN, AND PROSTATIC CANCERS: Emigrants from low-risk areas in Europe and Japan to the United States increase their risk of colorectal cancer. Moreover, their offspring often approach the incidence levels of the general American population. This rule for colorectal cancer also prevails for cancers of the breast, endometrium, ovary, and prostate.

HEPATOCELLULAR CARCINOMA: Patterns of HCC incidence were mentioned above. However, despite epidemiologic associations that suggest environmental and infectious factors, some populations that migrated from high-incidence areas to the United States continue to develop HCC more commonly than do other Americans.

HODGKIN DISEASE: In general, in poorly developed countries, the childhood form of Hodgkin disease is the one reported most often. In Western countries (except in Japan), the disease is most common among young adults. Such a pattern is characteristic of certain viral infections. Further evidence of environmental influence is that Hodgkin disease is more common among Americans of Japanese descent than in Japan.

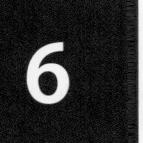

6

Genetic and Developmental Disorders

Christine R. Bryke, Gordana Raca

INTRODUCTION

Diseases with a genetic basis account for a sizable proportion of human suffering and death. Although individual genetic diseases are mostly rare, combined they affect millions of people worldwide. Three to 5% of infants are born with a birth defect or other genetic problem. However, by 1 year of age 6% to 7% genetic or developmental problems—reaching 12% to 14% by school age. Recent advances in molecular and cytogenetic technologies have facilitated clinical characterization of diseases of the roughly 3 billion nucleotides in the human genome.

Humans have about 20,000 protein-coding genes, occupying <2% of the genome. Most of these genes are also present in other organisms, from yeast to lower mammals. The remaining vast majority of human genome DNA, then, adds the remarkable complexity that ultimately determines the human species, and includes many genes that are transcribed into RNA molecules, like microRNAs and long noncoding RNAs. These are important in regulating gene function, organizing chromosome architecture and controlling epigenetic inheritance.

It has been estimated that the genomes of all *healthy* individuals are heterozygous for several recessive mutations which, if they were homozygous, would cause severe genetic disease. In addition, we all have at least a few hundred protein-altering gene sequence variants, but simply having a potential disease-causing mutation does not inevitably produce disease. As we will see in this chapter, disease expression ultimately depends upon the type of protein encoded by a mutated gene, the type of mutation, mutated gene dosage, and complex interactions among genetic, epigenetic and environmental factors.

This chapter begins with cytogenetics: the analysis of chromosome structure and function, and chromosomal disorders. Single gene disorders follow, and then sections on congenital anomalies and developmental diseases of infancy and childhood. Many disorders in the latter two sections have chromosomal, copy number variant, single gene and/or environmental etiologies. Premature birth also causes significant diseases in infancy and childhood.

CYTOGENETICS

Cytogenetics is the study of chromosomes and their abnormalities. Cytogenetic analysis was among the earliest approaches to analyzing genetic material. It helped elucidate the genetic basis of constitutional diseases and cancer. Newer methods tie cytogenetics to molecular genetics—**Fluorescence In Situ Hybridization (FISH)** and array-based **Comparative Genomic Hybridization (aCGH)**—and have increased the scope and power of chromosome analysis.

Chromosomal abnormalities are relatively common, and contribute significantly to morbidity and mortality among children. Gross chromosome aberrations occur in 1 per 200 newborns, but are far more frequent in fetuses that do not survive to term. At least half of first trimester spontaneous abortions contain an abnormal chromosomal complement.

Human DNA Contains 2.9 Billion Base Pairs in 46 Chromosomes

Human chromosomes bind to histone and non-histone proteins. As **diploid organisms**, people inherit **haploid** sets of genes (organized into 23 chromosomes) from each parent, and thus, have 2 copies of every gene in the genome (except genes on the X and Y chromosomes in males). When uncoiled the total length of human DNA molecules reaches 4 cm, meaning that DNA has to be tightly wound to fit in the nucleus. An extended DNA double helix undergoes an 8,000-fold compaction to make a metaphase chromosome (Fig. 6-1). Condensation of DNA chromatin fibers that exist during interphase into metaphase chromosomes allows correct segregation and recombination of genetic material during cell division.

Chromosomes Segregate During Cell Division

Clinically important numerical chromosome abnormalities typically arise through segregation errors. To understand these diseases, one must understand how chromosomes segregate. There are important differences in chromosome segregation into daughter cells in somatic cell division, **mitosis**, compared to germ cell division during gametogenesis, **meiosis**.

Mitosis

Mitosis normally produces two daughter cells identical to the original parent cell in chromosome number and genetic content. Mitosis maintains a diploid (2n) number of chromosomes in daughter cells. Nuclear DNA replicates during the S (synthesis) phase of the cell cycle, which always precedes mitosis (see Chapter 5). At the start of mitosis, each chromosome has two identical DNA molecules organized into symmetrical chromatids. During mitosis, chromosomes first condense, then thicken (prophase) and then align to the metaphase plate by attaching their centromeres to **mitotic spindle** fibers (**metaphase**). The two chromatids of each chromosome separate (**anaphase**) as the mitotic spindle pulls them toward opposite poles of the dividing cell and congregate at opposite ends (**telophase**). The result is two daughter cells, each with the same chromosome number and DNA content as the parent cell (Fig. 6-2).

Meiosis

Meiosis, or cell division among male and female germline cells, results in gametes with half the diploid (haploid) chromosome content (23 chromosomes including either an X or a Y sex chromosome). Meiosis consists of two consecutive divisions (meiosis I and II), but DNA replication only occurs before meiosis I. No S-phase intervenes between meiosis I and meiosis II. At the outset of meiosis I, each chromosome consists of two chromatids, and **homologous chromosomes** (i.e., the copies of each chromosome inherited from both parents) align into pairs, called **bivalents**. At this time sister chromatids engage in crossing over that results in recombination (exchange) of genetic material. Individual chromosomes from each bivalent randomly then segregate into daughter

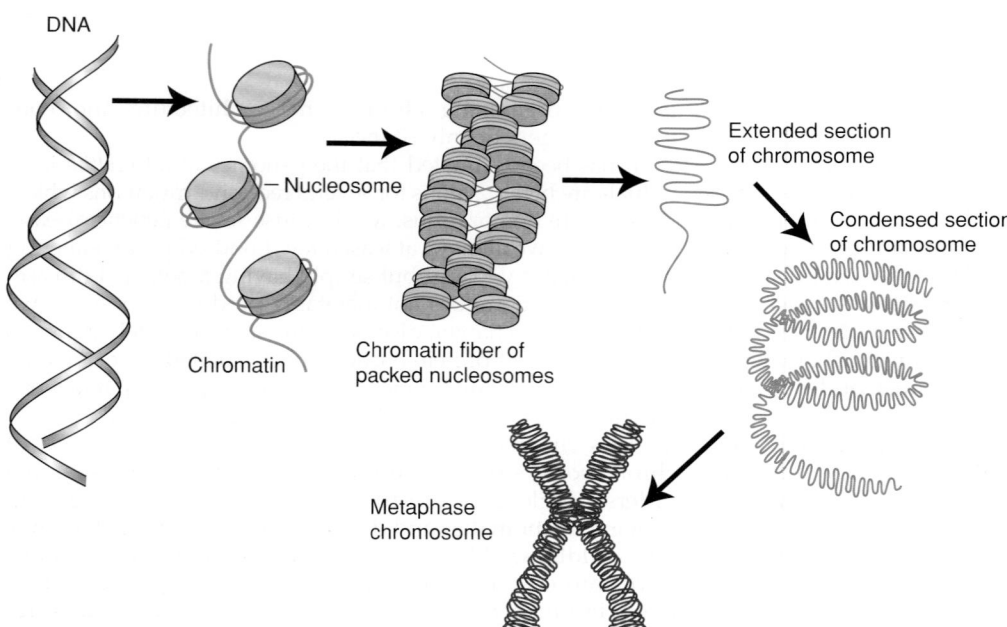

DNA

Nucleosome

Chromatin

Chromatin fiber of packed nucleosomes

Metaphase chromosome

Extended section of chromosome

Condensed section of chromosome

FIGURE 6-1. Levels of organization of chromatin. Naked DNA molecules are wrapped around histones to form nucleosomes, which represent the lowest level of chromatin organization. Nucleosomes are organized into 30-nm fibers, which in turn are organized into looped domains. When cells prepare for mitosis, the loops become further compacted into mitotic chromosomes. (Adapted with permission from Widnell CC, Pfenninger KH. *Essential Cell Biology*. Baltimore, MD: Williams & Wilkins; 1990:47.)

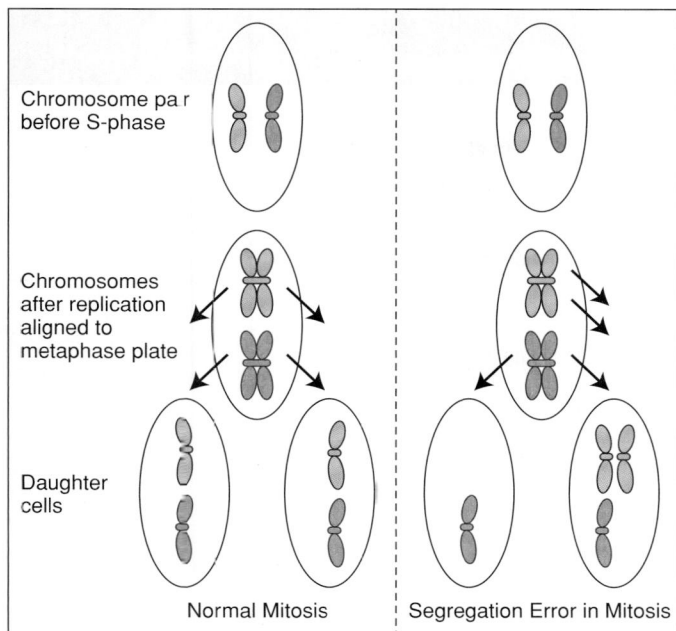

FIGURE 6-2. Normal and aberrant chromosome segregation in mitosis. Only one chromosome pair is represented. After DNA replication each chromosome consists of two chromatids which segregate into daughter cells. Normal segregation is shown on the left. The chromosome number is identical between the parent cell and daughter cells. A segregation error is depicted on the right. Both chromatids of one of the chromosomes move to the same daughter cell. This results in a cell with trisomy for that particular chromosome and a cell with monosomy for the same chromosome.

cells, thus halving of the chromosome number from diploid (2n) to haploid (n). In meiosis II, the chromatids separate into daughter cells and preserve the same (haploid) chromosome number (Fig. 6-3). The **recombination** of genetic material and **random segregation of homologous chromosomes** that occur during meiosis I contribute to a vast potential for genetic variability between resulting gametes, and thus in the progeny.

There are important differences in meiosis between males and females. Male meiosis is a continuous process starting at puberty in seminiferous tubules of the testes, and continuing throughout life. It produces millions of spermatozoa daily. In females, the process begins around the 12th week of fetal life: germ cells enter meiosis but stop early in meiosis I. They only resume the process many years later. Each month after the female reaches puberty, several germ cells are stimulated to proceed with meiosis, but typically only one completes the process to become a mature ovum. Some female germ cells may take over 40 years to complete meiosis. This extended progression of female meiosis may explain why errors in chromosome segregation and resulting numerical chromosome abnormalities occur more frequently in female, rather than male, gametogenesis, and why their incidence increases with advanced maternal age (see Numerical Chromosome Abnormalities below).

Chromosome Studies Using Conventional Cytogenetic Methods Require Dividing Cells

Cell Culture, Chromosome Spread Preparation

To identify chromosome numbers and structures, cells (typically, blood T lymphocytes) are stimulated to divide, arrested in metaphase, then stained with Giemsa (G-banding). This technique produces chromosome-specific patterns. Lightly stained chromosome regions (light bands) correspond to gene rich "active" chromatin (euchromatin). Darkly stained regions (dark bands), inactive chromatin (heterochromatin), are gene poor. Microscopic examination identifies numerical and structural abnormalities.

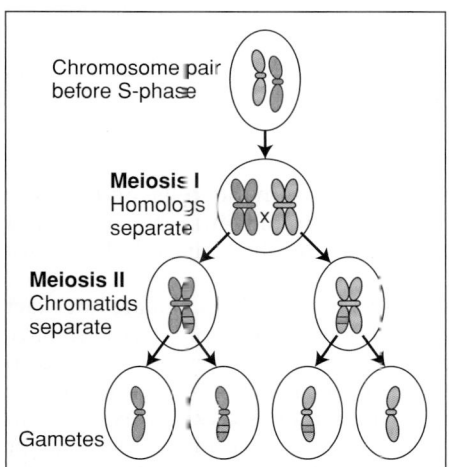
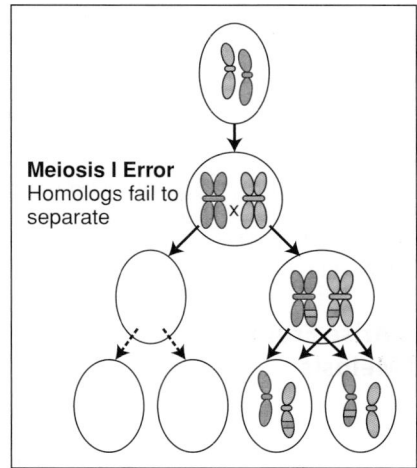
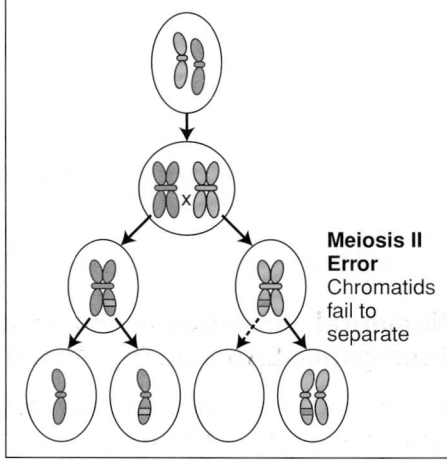

FIGURE 6-3. Normal and aberrant chromosome segregation in meiosis. Only one chromosome pair is represented. Simplified scheme of normal chromosome segregation in meiosis is depicted on the left. DNA replication occurs before meiosis I and each chromosome then consists of two chromatids. In meiosis I, homologous chromosomes from each pair separate into daughter cells, thus reducing the chromosome number from 46 to 23. During meiosis I pairing (synapsis) and recombination (crossing-over) occur between chromatids of homologous chromosomes. In meiosis II, chromatids from each chromosome separate into individual gametes, maintaining the number of chromosomes at 23 (haploid). **Segregation error in meiosis I** is depicted in the middle. Two homologous chromosomes migrate to the same daughter cells. After segregation of chromatids in meiosis II this results in gametes with two different copies of a specific chromosome. **Segregation error in meiosis II** is depicted on the right. Homologs segregate normally in meiosis I, but chromatids of one chromosome fail to segregate in meiosis II. This results in gametes with two copies of the same chromosome.

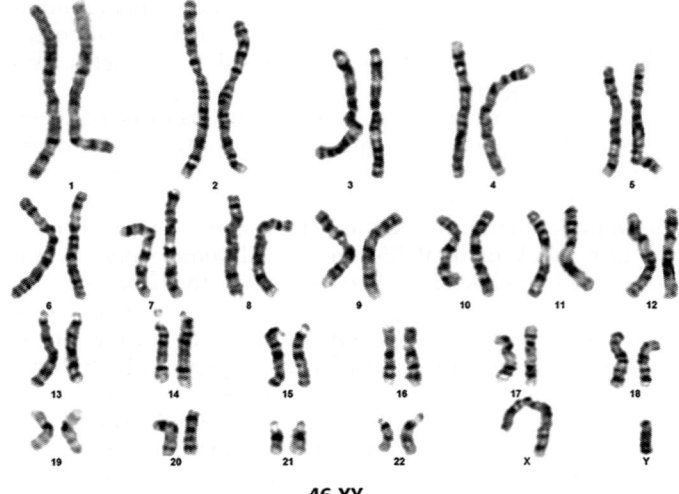

46,XY

FIGURE 6-4. G-banded karyogram of a normal male karyotype.

Chromosomes Are Classified by Centromere Length and Position

Centromeres are constrictions where the mitotic spindle attaches during mitosis. Their location divides a chromosome into arms. The chromosome's short arm is designated **p** (from French, *petite*), and the long arm is **q**. Chromosomes 13, 14, 15, 21, and 22 are **acrocentric**, with very short p arms consisting of stalks and satellites with noncoding repetitive sequences. In a **karyogram**, homologous chromosome pairs are lined up according to their size and centromere position from largest to smallest) (Fig. 6-4).

According to International System for Human Cytogenetic Nomenclature (ISCN) (Table 6-1) convention, karyotypes are described by sequentially listing:

Total number of chromosomes
Sex chromosome complement
Detected abnormalities in the ascending chromosome order

A plus sign (+) before the number of the affected chromosome designates gain of an entire chromosome. A minus sign (–) denotes a loss of a chromosome. Deletion of a part of a chromosome is designated by del, and duplication by dup, followed by the band location of the deleted or duplicated material on the affected chromosome arm: every light and dark G-band has a unique number assigned by the ISCN (Fig. 6-5).

Numerical Chromosome Abnormalities Arise From Segregation Errors During Mitosis and Meiosis

Genesis and Classification of Numerical Chromosome Abnormalities

Most abnormalities in chromosome number arise from nondisjunction, in paired chromosomes (bivalents) or chromatids fail to separate and move to opposite poles of a dividing cell (see Figs. 6-2 and 6-3). Such errors may involve individual chromosomes or the entire chromosome set. Any multiple of the haploid number of chromosomes (n) is referred to as euploid (2n is diploid, 3n is triploid, 4n is tetraploid etc.). For example, many normal liver cells have two times the diploid

TABLE 6-1 CYTOGENETIC NOMENCLATURE	
Numerical designation of autosomes	1–22
Sex chromosomes	X, Y
Whole chromosome gain	+
Loss of a chromosome	–
Short chromosome arm	p
Long chromosome arm	q
Separates different clones	/
Translocation	t
Deletion	del
Duplication	dup
Inversion	inv
Derivative chromosome (from a rearrangement)	der
Isochromosome	i
Ring chromosome	r
Representative Karyotypes	
Male with trisomy 21 (Down syndrome)	47,XY,+21
Female with robertsonian translocation between chromosomes 14 and 21	45,XX,der(14;21) (q10;q10)
Cri du chat syndrome (male) with a deletion of the short arm of chromosome 5 starting at band p14	46,XY,del(5)(p14)
Male with ring chromosome 19	46,XY,r(19) (p13.3q13.3)
Monosomy X (Turner syndrome)	45,X
Mosaic Klinefelter syndrome	47,XXY/46,XY

chromosome number of other somatic cells and so are euploid or, more specifically, tetraploid (4n). If the number of full sets of chromosomes is greater than diploid, the karyotype is polyploid.

Karyotypes with chromosome numbers that are not exact multiples of the haploid number are aneuploid. Aneuploidy is common in samples from early pregnancy loss, and is also frequently observed in cancer cells. Lack of one chromosome of a homologous pair is called monosomy. For example, in Turner syndrome there is a single X chromosome (45,X or monosomy X). In contrast, the presence of an extra copy of a chromosome is called trisomy; in Down syndrome, there are three chromosomes 21 (47,XX,+21 or trisomy 21).

Nondisjunction can occur between sister chromatids during mitosis. In meiosis it can affect bivalents (homologous chromosomes) in meiosis I or sister chromatids in meiosis II. Nondisjunction in somatic cells leads to one daughter cell with trisomy (2n + 1) and the other with monosomy (2n – 1) for the affected chromosome pair, but cells with monosomy

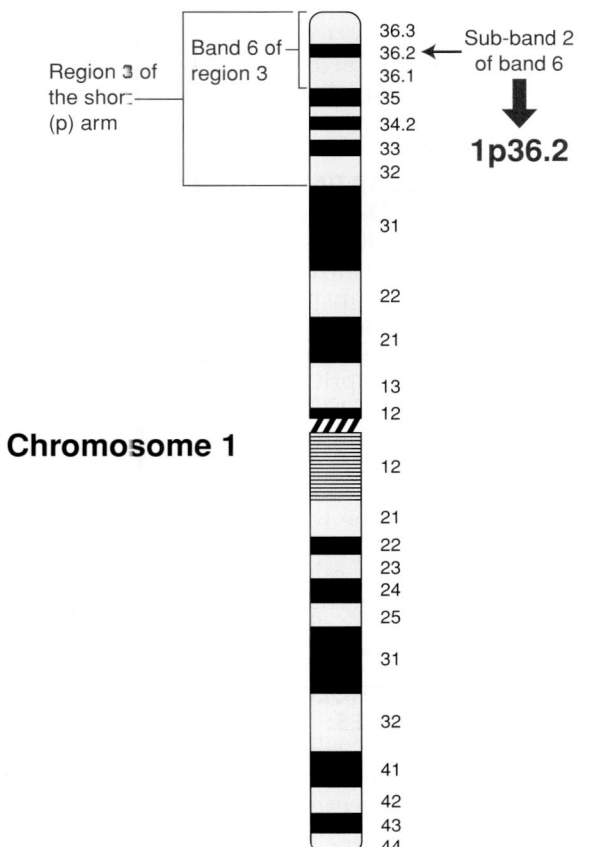

Region 3 of the short (p) arm

Band 6 of region 3

36.3
36.2 ← Sub-band 2 of band 6
36.1
35
34.2
33
32

1p36.2

31

22

21

13

12

Chromosome 1

12

21
22
23
24
25

31

32

41
42
43
44

FIGURE 6-5. Numbering of regions, bands and sub-bands on chromosomes allows precise designation of breakpoint locations of structural abnormalities.

are often less viable and may be out-competed by normal and trisomic cells. If somatic (mitotic) nondisjunction occurs early in embryogenesis, affected people may have two or more karyotypically different cell lines; this is called mosaicism (see below), and may involve autosomes or sex chromosomes. The patient's resulting appearance (phenotype) depends on the specific chromosome involved and the extent of mosaicism (the ratio of abnormal to normal cells in different tissues). Nondisjunction during gametogenesis produces aneuploidy in germ cells (gametes). Fertilization of a gamete which has two copies of the same chromosome (n + 1) will yield an embryo with trisomy for that chromosome. Fertilization of a gamete that lacks a chromosome entirely (n − 1) results in an embryo with monosomy, which will likely be nonviable unless the monosomy involves the X chromosome.

Numerical Chromosome Aberrations in Prenatal Samples

Most numerical chromosomal abnormalities are incompatible with life. Aneuploidy and polyploidy are common in early embryos and are usually lethal, resulting in spontaneous abortion (SAB). About half of SABs have a chromosomal abnormality. Chromosomal abnormalities identified in newborns typically have less genetic imbalance than those in early SABs, allowing survival in utero. The most common chromosomal abnormalities in SABs are, in descending order of frequency monosomy X, triploidy (Fig. 6-7) and trisomies 16 and 22. SABs tend to occur earlier if larger chromosomes

are trisomic, or if there is significant loss of genetic material (e.g., autosomal monosomies).

Monosomy X (45,X) may be compatible with life and is even associated with a relatively mild abnormal postnatal phenotype (see Turner syndrome below), but over 95% of 45,X embryos are lost during pregnancy. Absence of an X chromosome in males (45,Y) invariably leads to early abortion. At birth, the other common numerical chromosomal abnormalities are trisomy 21 (most frequent), 18, 13, and X or Y (47,XXX; 47,XXY; and 47,XYY).

Autosomal trisomies lead to severe developmental abnormalities and affected fetuses usually die during pregnancy or shortly after birth. Trisomy 16, for example, is common in early embryos but hardly ever detected in newborns, as it is nearly always lethal in utero. Trisomy 21, and to a lesser extent trisomies 13 and 18 are the only human autosomal trisomies which, in nonmosaic form, allow longer survival. Gain of additional copies of sex chromosomes (X and Y) may result in nonlethal abnormal development.

Numerical Aberrations of Autosomes

Trisomy 21: Down Syndrome

EPIDEMIOLOGY AND ETIOLOGIC FACTORS: Trisomy 21 is the most common chromosome abnormality among live born infants and the most frequent genetic cause of intellectual disability. It occurs in about 1 in 800 newborns, meaning that approximately 5,300 children with Down syndrome are born in the United States yearly and that 200,000 people in the country have this disorder.

Nondisjunction, typically in meiosis I of maternal gametogenesis in a woman of normal karyotype, accounts for the majority (≈95%) of people with trisomy 21. **Incidence of trisomy 21 rises dramatically with increasing maternal age.** In her early 20s a woman's risk of having a Down syndrome infant is ≈1/1,000, rising to 1/500 in her early 30s it is approximately 1/500, and 1/20 by age 45 (Fig. 6-6). Still, 80% of children with Down syndrome are born to mothers under 35, because the most pregnancies occur in among these younger women.

About 4% of Down syndrome patients have additional chromosome 21 material as an unbalanced robertsonian translocation involving a third chromosome 21 and another acrocentric chromosome, commonly chromosome 14 (see Fig. 6-12B), not as a separate extra chromosome. This mechanism for Down syndrome is not related to maternal age, but is usually inherited from one parent, who is a balanced translocation carrier (see Structural Chromosome Abnormalities below). This distinction is important for recurrence risk assessment. In nontranslocation cases of trisomy 21, the risk for having another child with trisomy is slightly, but not significantly higher than the general population risk. However, there is a one in three chance of Down syndrome among offspring of a carrier of such a balanced robertsonian translocation. In practice, the actual incidence is 10% to 15% with a maternal translocation and under 5% if the father is the carrier, the difference reflecting selection against unbalanced gametes and early loss of most embryos with trisomy 21.

About 1% of patients with trisomy 21 have mosaicism, from mitotic nondisjunction of chromosome 21 early

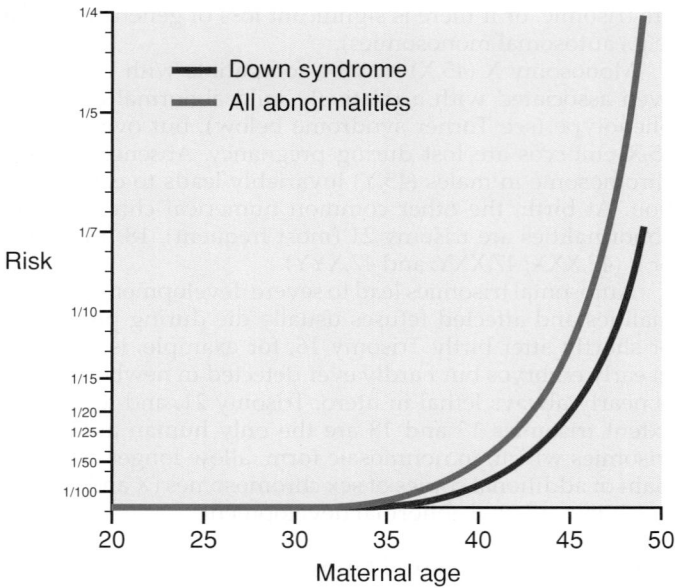

Risk

- Down syndrome
- All abnormalities

Maternal age

FIGURE 6-6. The risk of a woman to carry a fetus with a chromosome abnormality increases with maternal age. This risk dramatically increases after age 35. The *red line* indicates the Down syndrome risk and the *blue line* indicates the risk for all fetal chromosome abnormalities combined. (Data from Hook EB, Cross PK, Schreinemachers DM. Chromosomal Abnormality Rates at Amniocentesis and in Live-Born Infants. *JAMA*. 1983;249(15):2034–2038.)

during embryogenesis. Clinical manifestations in such cases vary, depending on the proportion of abnormal cells, but are typically milder than with nonmosaic trisomy.

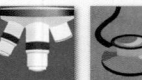 **MOLECULAR PATHOGENESIS:** The pathogenesis of the Down syndrome manifestations presumably relates to increased dosage of genes on chromosome 21, but which genes are responsible is unknown. Studies of rare patients who have duplications of only part of chromosome 21 rather than an extra copy of the entire chromosome suggest that a 4 Mb region in band 21q22.2 may be the culprit. It is known as the **Down syndrome critical region** (DSCR). A strong candidate gene for Down syndrome cognitive deficits is *DYRK1A*, which encodes a dual-specificity tyrosine phosphorylation-regulated kinase (DYRK). *RCAN1* (regulator of calcineurin 1), another gene within DSCR encodes a protein that is overexpressed in the brain of Down syndrome fetuses and inhibits calcineurin-dependent signaling pathways, possibly affecting CNS development.

PATHOLOGY AND CLINICAL FEATURES: The Down syndrome phenotype includes dysmorphic features, congenital malformations and other health problems, but not all of these occur in each affected individual (Fig. 6-7).

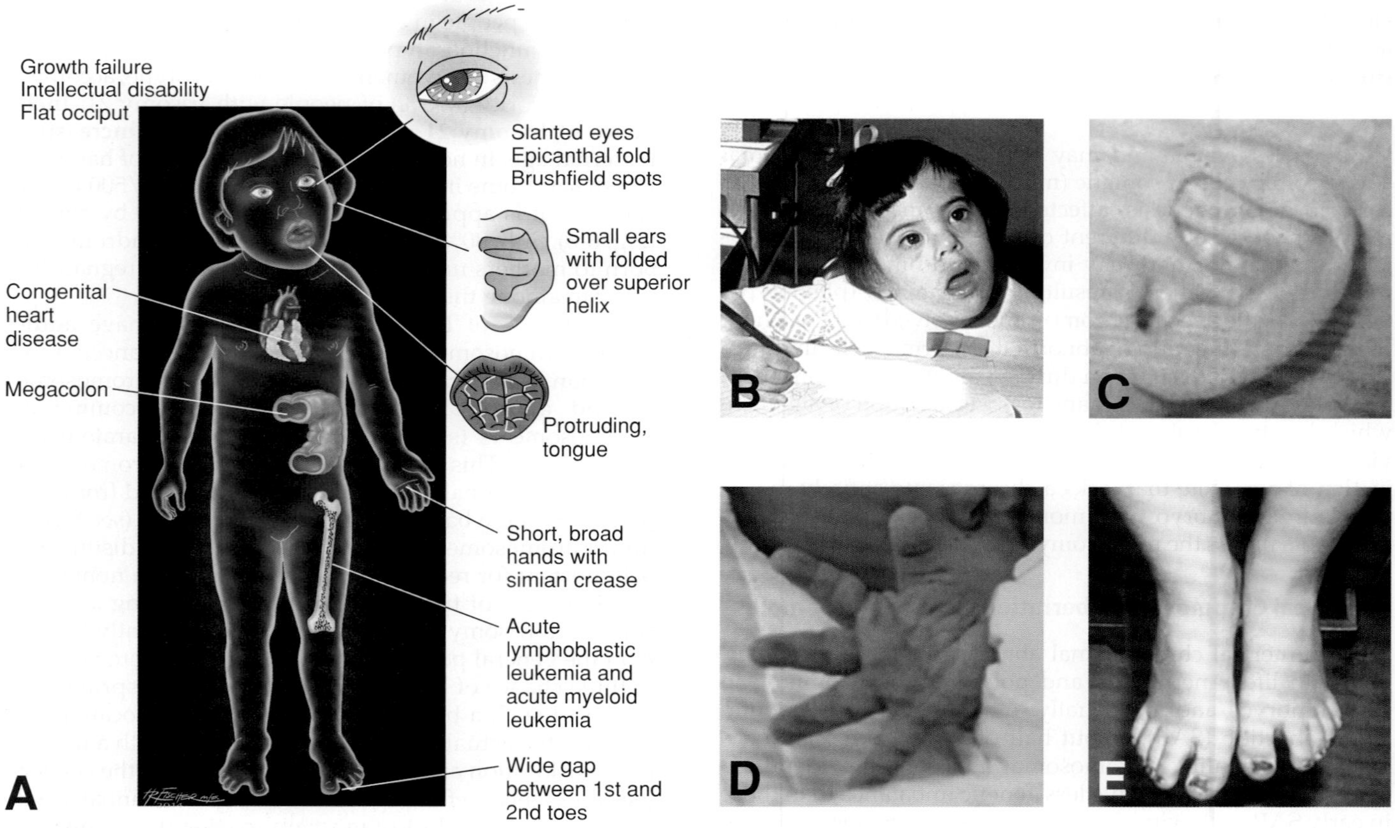

Growth failure
Intellectual disability
Flat occiput

Slanted eyes
Epicanthal fold
Brushfield spots

Small ears with folded over superior helix

Congenital heart disease

Megacolon

Protruding, tongue

Short, broad hands with simian crease

Acute lymphoblastic leukemia and acute myeloid leukemia

Wide gap between 1st and 2nd toes

FIGURE 6-7. A. Typical Down syndrome features. B. Young girl with upslanting palpebral fissures, epicanthal folds and open mouth with protruding tongue. **C.** Infant with small ear with folded superior helix. **D.** Newborn with small hand with single transverse palmar crease. **E.** Adolescent girl with wide space between 1st and 2nd toes.

Infants with trisomy 21 are usually recognized at birth by their hypotonia (low muscle tone) and characteristic **craniofacial features,** including brachycephaly (rounder cranial contour than usual), upslanting palpebral fissures, epicanthal folds (small pleats of skin at the inner canthi), small ears with folded over superior helices, Brushfield spots (white speckles on the irides), open mouth with protruding tongue, and redundant skin at the nape of the neck. Characteristic **skeletal changes** include short stature, shortened long bones of the chest and extremities. Their hands are broad and short with a single transverse palmar crease and the fifth finger often curves inward due to hypoplasia of the middle phalanx.

Congenital anomalies: Half of newborns with Down syndrome have **cardiac malformations,** with even higher incidence in aborted fetuses: atrioventricular canal, ventricular and atrial septal defects, tetralogy of Fallot, and patent ductus arteriosus. **GI tract** anomalies include duodenal atresia, Hirschsprung disease (megacolon), and imperforate anus.

Cognitive impairment: Cognitive impairment is universal, but is variably severe. Most are mildly to moderately intellectually disabled, with IQs between 50 and 70, or 35 to 50, respectively. Adults often show further cognitive decline, beyond their congenital intellectual disability. By age 40, most develop neuropathologic and functional changes typical of Alzheimer disease (see Chapter 32).

Hematologic abnormalities: *The risk of leukemia (lymphoid and myeloid) in Down syndrome children under 15 years is 10- to 20-fold higher than in normal children.* Under age 4, acute myeloic leukemia predominates, although acute lymphoblastic leukemia is more common in non–Down syndrome children of this age. Transient abnormal myelopoiesis (TAM), characterized by leukocytosis with blasts and other immature myeloid cells in the blood, occurs in 10% to 20%. This condition usually resolves spontaneously. However, up to 25% of infants with TAM later develop acute megakaryoblastic leukemia (AMKL). AMKL may also occur in young children with trisomy 21 without prior history of TAM.

Immunologic impairments may result in increased susceptibility to infection, autoimmune disorder, and malignancies.

Most females with Down syndrome are fertile, but 40% of their progeny had trisomy 21. Down syndrome men are invariably sterile, owing to arrested spermatogenesis.

Life expectancy: Survival in the first decade of life largely reflects the presence (15% mortality) or absence (5%) of congenital heart disease. Life expectancy in patients who reach age 10 is about 55 years, which is at least 20 years less than the general population. Only 10% of trisomy 21 patients reach age 70.

Other Autosomal Trisomies

Trisomy 18 (Edwards syndrome) is the second most common autosomal trisomy in live births, occurring in 1 of 5,000 newborns. Like trisomy 21, incidence increases with advancing maternal age, because meiotic nondisjunction is more common in older women. Most affected infants are female (3:1). Newborns have severe **intrauterine growth restriction (IUGR),** hypertonia (increased muscle tone), abnormal skull and limb structure and severe neurologic impairment often with apnea and bradycardia. Congenital anomalies may involve any organ system, and cardiac defects occur in most cases. Anomalies of the brain, GI tract, and kidneys are common. Given how severe these anomalies are, 95% of fetuses with trisomy 18 abort spontaneously. About half of trisomy 18 newborns die within 1 week, and 90% die within a year. Trisomy 18 may occur as a mosaic with more moderate phenotypes and longer viability.

Trisomy 13 occurs in 1 per 16,000 births. Sporadic trisomy 13, like other autosomal trisomies correlates with increased maternal age. However, like trisomy 21, a third copy of chromosome 13 can be present because of an inherited unbalanced **robertsonian translocation** (see below), unrelated to maternal age and with important implications for recurrence risk. Multiple congenital anomalies and severe neurologic impairment are characteristic. Affected infants often have a narrow sloping forehead, anomalous ears and a classic triad of cleft lip and/or palate, microphthalmia, and postaxial polydactyly. Over 50% of these newborns have holoprosencephaly, scalp defects, cardiac malformations, omphalocele, cystic kidneys, abnormal genitalia, and club feet. Most trisomy 13 fetuses die in utero, and >90% who are born alive will die within the first year.

Function and Numerical Aberrations of Sex Chromosomes

Role of X and Y in Sex Determination

Human X and the Y chromosome differ substantially. The X chromosome contains about 2,000 genes and is intermediate in size, while the Y chromosome is much smaller and only has ~80 genes mostly related to sex determination and spermatogenesis.

This difference between these chromosomes is the basis of sex (gender) determination: males have one of each, while females have two X's. Sex phenotype always reflects the presence or absence of a Y chromosome. For example, sex-chromosome aneuploidies, people with 47,XXY and 47,XYY karyotypes are males, while those who are 45,X and 47,XXX are females.

One gene on the Y chromosome, SRY, the sex-determining region of the Y, is the master regulator of sex determination. Just this locus is sufficient to cause male development. The intron-less *SRY* gene encodes a transcription factor of the *SOX* (SRY-like box) family of DNA-binding proteins. *SRY* expression activates a testis-forming pathway at about 7 weeks of development of male embryos. Before this point, the embryonic gonad is "indifferent," that is, it can develop into either a testis or an ovary. Without *SRY,* a different set of proteins activates the ovary-forming pathway. Mutations that disrupt *SRY* lead to XY females, while translocations that move *SRY* to an X chromosome produce XX males. In addition to sex determination, the Y chromosome regulates spermatogenesis. A small proportion of infertile men with azoospermia or severe oligospermia have small deletions in key spermatogenesis loci of the Y chromosome.

X Inactivation in Females

With the X chromosome being much larger and containing more genes than the Y, females have two copies of hundreds of genes that of which males have only one. In mammalian females, X-chromosome inactivation (XCI) redresses this imbalance: females transcriptionally silence one of their two X's in each cell. The inactivated X chromosome condenses into a compact structure called a **Barr body,** and rests stably silent, with its gene control regions extensively methylated.

MOLECULAR PATHOGENESIS: A non–protein-coding RNA gene, *XIST*, which maps in the Xq13.2 region, is expressed only by the inactive X-chromosome and mediates its repression. On the active X, another non–protein-coding RNA—*TSIX* ("*XIST*" backward)—is transcribed in the opposite (antisense) direction relative to *XIST*. This *XIST* antisense partner prevents *XIST* transcription, preventing X-inactivation in *cis* (on that same X).

X inactivation occurs randomly in the early female embryo; either the maternal or the paternal X chromosome have an equal chance of becoming inactivated. Once established, X chromosome inactivation is permanent and transmitted to progeny cells, so paternally or maternally derived inactivated X chromosomes are propagated clonally. All females are thus mosaic, expressing paternal X chromosome genes in some cells and maternal X chromosome genes in other cells (Fig. 6-8). Such mosaicism for X-linked glucose-6-phosphate dehydrogenase (G6PD) was key in demonstrating the monoclonal origin of neoplasms (see Chapter 5).

A small set of X-linked genes escape inactivation and continue to be expressed by both X chromosomes. In addition, X and Y chromosomes both carry two small regions of homology known as **pseudoautosomal regions**, and all pseudoautosomal genes escape X-inactivation. Pseudoautosomal region 1 (PAR1) is ~2 Mb in size and maps to the ends of X and Y short arms. Pseudoautosomal region 2 (PAR2) is ~320 kb, and maps to the ends of the long arms of the sex chromosomes (Fig. 6-9). In male meiosis, pairing and recombination between the sex chromosomes can only occur within pseudoautosomal regions, and typically happens within PAR1. Only 95% of the human Y chromosome is unable to recombine and is passed on to the next generation relatively intact. For this reason, the Y chromosome can be used for investigating male human evolution.

Both males and females have two functional copies of genes in pseudoautosomal regions, and so may show gene dosage effects in sex chromosome aneuploidies. Patients with Turner syndrome (45,X) are haploinsufficient for these genes; those with more than two X chromosomes (e.g., Klinefelter syndrome (47,XXY) and triple X syndrome (47,XXX) have more than two functional copies. A gene in this region, *SHOX*, is associated with height, and its haploinsufficiency in Turner syndrome may explain the short stature characteristic of the syndrome. Extra copies of *SHOX* may explain the increased stature in 47,XXY, 47,XXX, and other sex chromosome aneuploidy conditions.

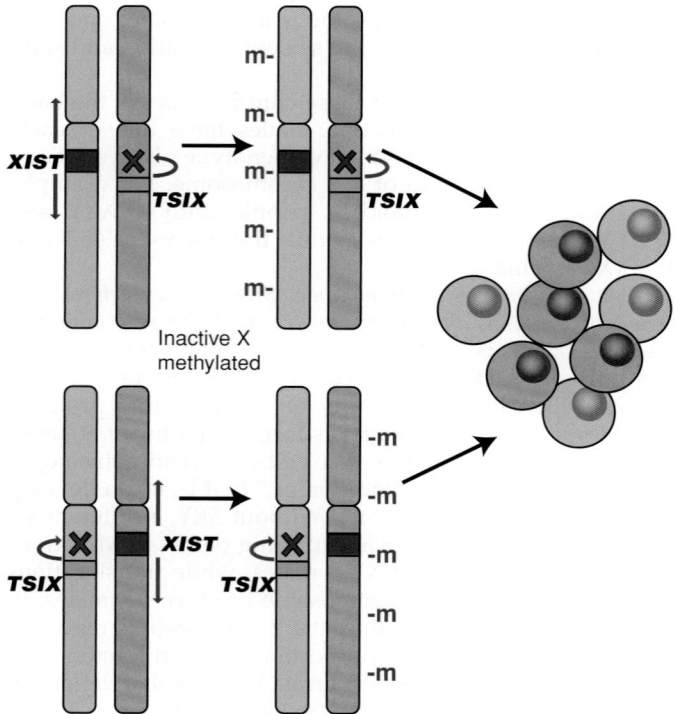

FIGURE 6-8. Mechanism of random X-inactivation. Maternally derived (*blue*) X chromosomes or paternally derived (*purple*) X chromosomes are inactivated at random independently in each cell early in embryogenesis. Inactivation is established by expression of the *XIST* gene and coating of the inactive X by *XIST* RNA. On the active X, activation of *TSIX* prevents *XIST* expression. Once established, X inactivation is maintained by methylation (m) of DNA cytosine residues. In mature tissue the resulting mosaicism reflects roughly equal proportions of maternally derived and paternally derived active X chromosomes, but in some cases the distributions can be skewed.

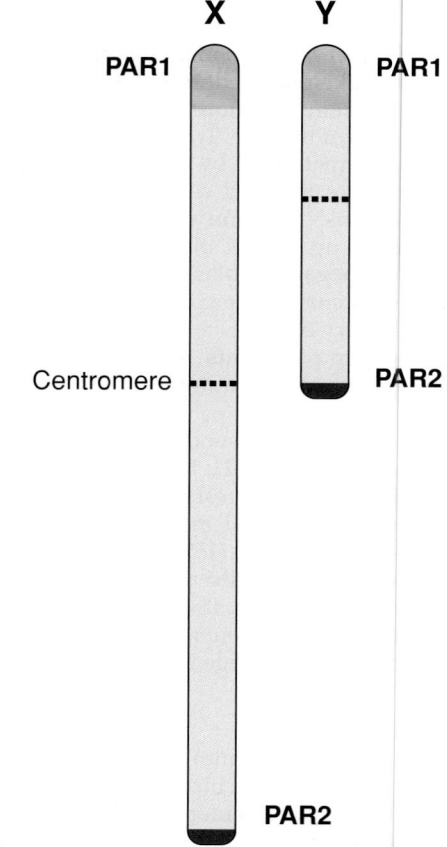

FIGURE 6-9. Pseudoautosomal regions are the regions of homology between the X and the Y chromosomes. The pseudoautosomal region 1 (PAR1) is ~2 Mb in size and maps to the ends of the X and Y short arms. The pseudoautosomal region 2 (PAR2) spans only ~320 kb and maps to the ends of the long arms of the X and the Y.

Klinefelter Syndrome (47,XXY)

  ETIOLOGY FACTORS AND EPIDEMIOLOGY: Males with Klinefelter syndrome have one Y chromosome and two or more X chromosomes. They are infertile due to hypogonadism. Klinefelter syndrome occurs in 1 per 500 to 1,000 male newborns and so is an important cause of male infertility. The additional X chromosome(s) results from meiotic nondisjunction during maternal or paternal gametogenesis. In half of cases, nondisjunction in paternal meiosis I leads to sperm with both X and Y chromosomes. Fertilization of a normal egg by such a sperm yields a 47,XXY karyotype.

MOLECULAR PATHOGENESIS: Most men with Klinefelter syndrome (80%) have one extra X chromosome (47,XXY). A minority are mosaics (46,XY/47,XXY) or have more than two X chromosomes (48,XXXY). *Regardless of how many supernumerary X chromosomes (even up to four), the Y chromosome ensures male phenotype.* Mosaics may be more mildly affected. Additional X chromosomes correlate with a more abnormal phenotype and intellectual disability despite inactivation of the extra X chromosomes, presumably due to the genes that escape inactivation.

CLINICAL FEATURES: Male newborns with a 47,XXY karyotype are phenotypically normal, with normal male external genitalia and no dysmorphic features. Children with Klinefelter syndrome tend to be tall and thin, with narrow shoulders and chest and relatively long legs (eunuchoid body habitus) (Fig. 6-10). Normal testicular growth and masculinization do not occur at puberty, and testes remain small. The penis is often normal in size. Gynecomastia and a female pattern of pubic hair are also observed. Azoospermia results in infertility. These changes reflect hypogonadism and a resulting lack of androgens. Serum testosterone is low to normal, but LH and FSH are quite high, indicating normal pituitary function. High circulating estradiol levels increase the estradiol-to-testosterone ratio, which determines the degree of feminization. Treatment with testosterone results in virilization, but does not restore fertility. Klinefelter syndrome individuals are at increased risk for learning disabilities, autism, psychiatric disorders, and social problems. Klinefelter syndrome is often diagnosed after puberty, during evaluation for gynecomastia or infertility, or in childhood due to learning and/or behavioral problems.

PATHOLOGY: After puberty, the intrinsically abnormal testes do not respond to gonadotropin stimulation and later show regressive changes. Seminiferous tubules show atrophy, hyalinization, and peritubular fibrosis. Germ cells and Sertoli cells are usually absent and the tubules become dense cords of collagen. Leydig cells are usually increased in number and are functionally impaired.

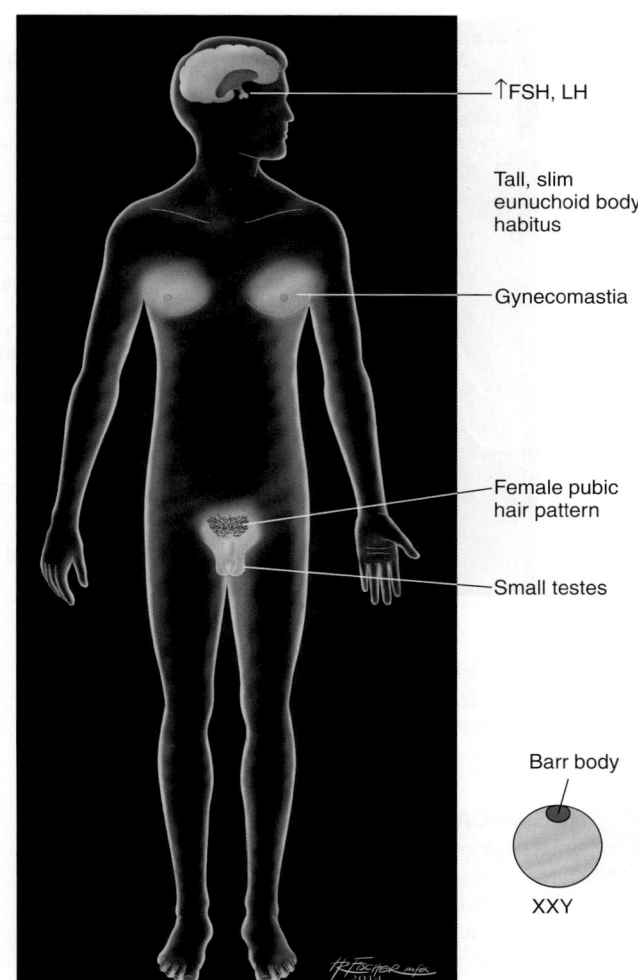

FIGURE 6-10. Clinical features of Klinefelter syndrome.

The XYY Male

A 47,XYY karyotype occurs once in roughly 1,000 male newborns, and results from paternal meiotic nondisjunction. These males are tall, and may have learning and behavioral problems. Many have large teeth and nodulocystic acne. They have normal pubertal development and most are fertile. Many 47,XYY males remain undiagnosed due to the mild phenotype. Despite initial reports propensity, these people are not prone to more aggressive or criminal behavior, although they may show more antisocial behavior, poorer academic performance, and lower socioeconomic status.

Turner Syndrome

  ETIOLOGIC FACTORS AND EPIDEMIOLOGY: Turner syndrome is a spectrum of abnormalities derived from **complete or partial X chromosome monosomy in a phenotypic female**. It occurs in 1 in 2,500 newborn females, and does not correlate with maternal age. In 3/4 of cases, the single X chromosome is of maternal origin, so the meiotic error is usually paternal. The 45,X karyotype is one of the most common aneuploids in human conceptuses, but 95% abort spontaneously. It is unclear why monosomy X is lethal

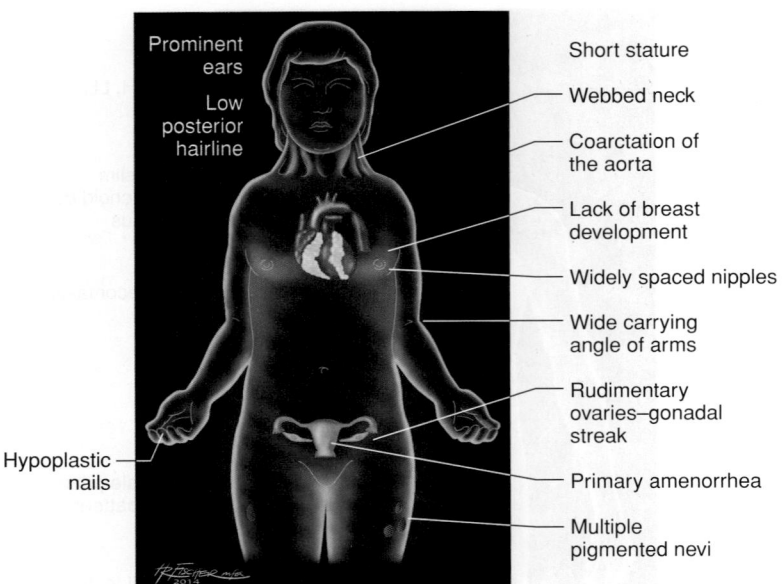

FIGURE 6-11. Clinical features of Turner syndrome.

during fetal development, but it is possible that a normal dosage of pseudoautosomal genes may be important for survival of embryos.

CLINICAL FEATURES: Short stature and primary hypogonadism (gonadal dysgenesis) are the main features of Turner syndrome (Fig. 6-11). Most affected women are less than 5 ft (152 cm) tall and have no breast development and primary amenorrhea. About 15% to 30% either have initial breast development followed by pubertal arrest, or complete puberty followed by secondary amenorrhea. These females often have mosaic karyotypes. **Dysmorphic features** include a short, webbed neck (pterygium coli); low posterior hairline; wide carrying angle of the arms (cubitus valgus); broad shield-like chest with widely spaced nipples; hypoplastic hyperconvex fingernails; facial abnormalities, including a small mandible, prominent ears and epicanthal folds. Pigmented nevi may become numerous and prominent with age. **Cardiovascular anomalies** are common, 15% have aortic coarctation; bicuspid aortic valve occurs in up to 30%. Some patients have essential hypertension, and dissecting aortic aneurysm is an uncommon, but serious complication. **Renal anomalies** include horseshoe kidney and malrotation. Women with Turner syndrome have an increased risk for chronic autoimmune thyroiditis and goiter. Intelligence is usually within the normal range, but some may have specific neurocognitive deficits, such as problems with visuospatial organization or nonverbal learning disability.

MOLECULAR PATHOGENESIS: About half of Turner individuals lack an entire X chromosome (monosomy X). The others either are mosaic for cells with monosomy (45,X) and normal (46,XX) cells, or have structural aberrations causing partial X chromosome loss, such as isochromosome of the long arm, translocations and deletions. Patients with a mosaic karyotype

(45,X/46,XX) tend to have a milder phenotype and may be fertile. About 5% of patients have 45,X/46,XY mosaic karyotype, which arises by mitotic nondisjunction in a male zygote. Such individuals have a 20% risk of developing a germ cell cancer and should have prophylactic removal of their abnormal gonads.

PATHOLOGY: Ovaries in Turner syndrome patients usually contain small amounts of connective tissue with no or only a few atretic follicles (streak ovaries). Such gonadal dysgenesis may reflect accelerated apoptosis, rather than abnormal germ cell formation. Normal fetal ovaries each contain 7 million oocytes, less than half of which survive until birth. Loss of oocytes continues, so that by menarche normal females have only about 5% (400,000). Ovaries of fetuses with Turner syndrome contain oocytes at first but lose them rapidly such that none remain by 2 years of age. The ovaries become fibrous streaks, but the uterus, fallopian tubes, and vagina develop normally. Interestingly, some women who enter menopause prematurely show deletions of part of the long arm of one of their X chromosomes.

Females With Multiple X Chromosomes

A triple X karyotype (47,XXX) occurs about 1 in 1,000 newborn girls. 47,XXX women are usually physically normal and fertile and most have normal intelligence. Some may have learning and/or psychological problems. It is estimated that most such people are never diagnosed. Females with 4 and 5 X chromosomes are rare; virtually all are cognitively impaired.

Breakage and Incorrect Rejoining Alter Chromosome Structure

Chromosome breaks can occur spontaneously, or after exposure to clastogenic agents, such as viruses, radiation or various chemicals.

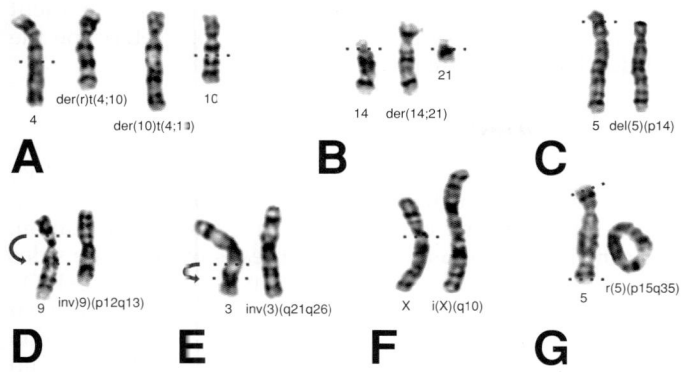

FIGURE 6-12. Examples of structural chromosome abnormalities.
A. A **reciprocal translocation** involves breaks on two chromosomes, with exchange of the acentric segments to form two derivative chromosomes.
B. A **robertsonian translocation** occurs when two acrocentric chromosomes (13–15, 21, and 22) break near their centromeres, after which the long arms fuse to form one large derivative chromosome. **C. Deletion** of a portion of a chromosome leads to loss of genetic material and a shortened chromosome. An **inversion** requires two breaks in a single chromosome. With flipping and rejoining of the intervening segment. **D.** If the breaks are on opposite sides of the centromere, the inversion is **pericentric. E.** It is **paracentric** if the breaks are on the same arm. **F.** An **isochromosome** arises from faulty centromere division, which leads to two copies of the long arm joined at the centromere and deletion of the short arm, or the reverse with two copies of the short arm joined at the centromere and deletion of the long arm (not depicted). **G.** A **ring chromosome** involve breaks of both telomeric portions of a chromosome, deletion of the acentric fragments and fusion of the remaining short and long arms.

Chromosome Translocations

There are two major types of chromosomal translocations, reciprocal and robertsonian. In **reciprocal translocations** two chromosomes exchange genetic material (Fig. 6-12A). Translocations are denoted with "t," with the involved chromosomes listed in ascending order. For example, a translocation between chromosomes 4 and 10 is written as t(4;10). Sites of translocation breakpoints follow in a second set of parentheses with the breakpoint of the lower number chromosome first. Thus, t(4;10)(q23;q22) means that breaks occurred in band q23 on chromosome 4 and band q22 on chromosome 10, and the chromosomal regions distal from the breakpoint sites were swapped between the two chromosomes. The abnormal chromosomes that result from a translocation are referred to as **derivative** chromosomes. In the present example the derivative chromosomes are der(4)t(4;10)(q23;q22) and der(4)t(4;10)(q23;q22), shortened as der(10)t(4;10) and der(10)t(4;10) in Figure 6-12A.

Reciprocal translocations are **balanced** if there is no net loss or gain of genetic material. Balanced translocations rarely disrupt vital genes; carriers of balanced translocations are usually phenotypically normal. One in 500 people has a balanced reciprocal translocation. Reciprocal translocations can be inherited in a balanced form, but can also lead to unbalanced karyotypes in the offspring who as the result may show severe phenotypic abnormalities. Complete pairing of translocated segments during meiosis in a carrier parent requires formation of a cross-like structure (quadriradial) between the two translocated chromosomes and their two normal homologs (Fig. 6-13A). Unlike a normal bivalent, which typically resolves by chromosomes migrating to

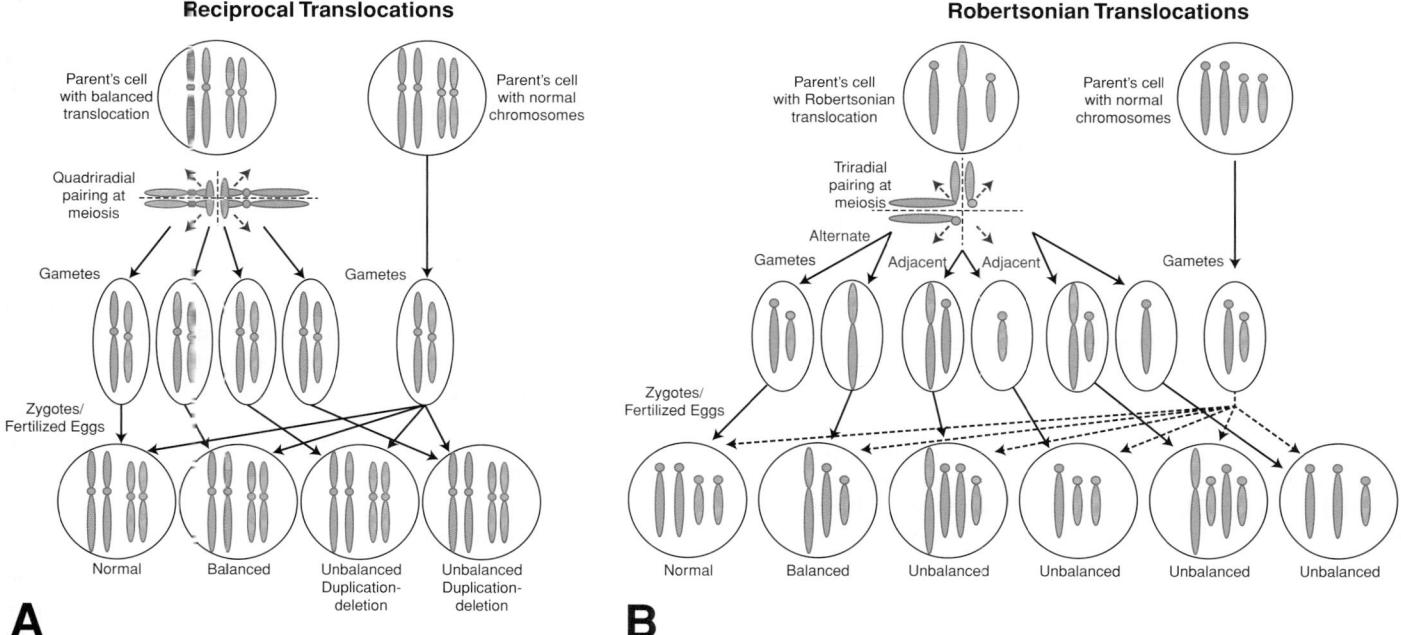

FIGURE 6-13. Meiotic Segregation of Translocations. A. Reciprocal translocation with gametes with four segregation combinations (normal, balanced, and two unbalanced). In a translocation carrier, cells contain pairs of homologous chromosomes each of which consists of one normal chromosome and one that carries a translocation. During meiosis, instead of the normal pairing into two bivalents, a quadriradial structure, containing all four chromosomes, is formed. In this circumstance, the chromosomes can segregate along different planes of cleavage (*dotted lines*). In addition, the chromosomes can segregate diagonally (*arrows*). Different gametes can be produced as a result, some of which are unbalanced and can result in affected progeny. **B. Robertsonian translocation** with triradial pairing produces gametes with six segregation combinations (normal, balanced, two trisomic and two monosomic).

opposite poles of the cell, chromosomes in a quadriradial may segregate along several different planes, potentially yielding gametes with unbalanced chromosome complements. Upon fertilization, resulting zygotes may exhibit partial trisomy and monosomy for segments of the translocated chromosomes (Fig. 6-13A). Reciprocal translocations can also be acquired and result in cancer-producing gene fusions (see FISH below).

In **robertsonian translocations** (centric fusions) the long arms of two acrocentric chromosomes fuse at their centromeres (Fig. 6-12B), to form one large chromosome. The short arms are lost, but since they are composed of highly redundant genes for ribosomal RNA their loss does not result in an abnormal phenotype. Carriers have 45 chromosomes and are usually phenotypically normal. However, they have an increased risk for pregnancies with a trisomic fetus and/or recurrent miscarriages due to unbalanced chromosome complements (Fig. 6-13B). Robertsonian translocations occur in about 1 per 1,000 people, and most often involve chromosomes 13 + 14, and 14 + 21. Maternal transmission is more common since male carriers are often less fertile.

Chromosomal Deletions and Duplications

A deletion is a loss, while a duplication is a gain of part of a chromosome (Fig. 6-12C). By definition, such chromosome alterations are unbalanced, with a loss or gain of genes localized within affected chromosome segments. Clinical phenotypes caused by deletions or duplications of specific chromosomal regions are sometimes called **"contiguous gene syndromes"** to denote that the multiple clinical features of a particular chromosomal syndrome are caused by abnormal dosage of genes lying on a chromosome in proximity to one another. However, many genes can tolerate changes in expression levels, and one copy of a gene provides normal function. There is only a subset of genes whose expression level is tightly regulated, with increased or decreased dosage causing abnormal development. Therefore, even if a deletion or duplication affects dozens of genes, clinical phenotypes may reflect altered expression of only a few dosage-sensitive genes.

Only deletions and duplications ≥5 Mb are easily detected by visualizing metaphase chromosomes. However, many disease causing deletions and duplications, at <5 Mb (microdeletions and microduplications) are too small to be detected this way. These are diagnosed with higher-resolution methods, including FISH and chromosomal microarray analysis (CMA) (see below).

Deletions and duplications often originate by breaks occurring at random locations on chromosomes, so that the exact size of a deleted or duplicated region differs in individual patients. However, such patients will share clinical features of a particular **"contiguous gene syndrome"** if their deletions (duplications) involve the same or overlapping sets of dosage sensitive genes. One of the best-known examples is **Cri-du-chat syndrome or 5p- syndrome** due to deletion of a terminal portion of the short arm of chromosome 5 (Fig. 6-12C). The condition is recognized by the distinctive high-pitched cry of the affected newborn (often described as resembling the cry of a kitten). Clinical features include microcephaly, low birth weight, hypotonia, delayed development, and intellectual disability. 5p- patients have a dysmorphic round face with widely set eyes (hypertelorism), low-set ears and a small jaw. Some have heart defects.

The size of the deleted 5p- segment differs from patient to patient, deleted bands 5p15.2 and 5p15.3 determine the **Cri-du-chat syndrome** phenotype.

Chromosomal Inversions

In chromosomal inversions, a chromosome breaks at two points, the segment between the breakpoints inverts and reintegrates into the chromosome in inverted orientation. **Pericentric inversions** result from breaks on opposite sides of the centromere and include the centromere (Fig. 6-12D). **Paracentric inversions** involve breaks on the same arm of the chromosome and do not involve the centromere region (Fig. 6-12E). Inversions are usually not associated with gain or loss of chromosomal material and inversion carriers are usually phenotypically normal. However, some inversions impair infertility, cause pregnancy loss, and increase risk of children with unbalanced karyotypes. This is explained by an unusual loop mechanism through which pairing and recombination occur between the inverted chromosome and its normal homolog during meiosis, which can result in unequal crossing over. Small pericentric inversions are often inherited without phenotypic consequences. Up to 1% of the population has inv(9)(p12q13), a small pericentric inversion of chromosome 9, which is considered a normal polymorphism (benign normal variant) in the population (Fig. 6-12D).

Isochromosomes

Isochromosomes are abnormal chromosomes with two identical arms, and are formed by faulty centromere division, where the replicating chromosomes split by transverse rather than the normal longitudinal axis (Fig. 6-12F). The most common clinical condition involving an isochromosome is **Turner syndrome**, where 15% of affected females have an isochromosome composed of either short or long arms of the X chromosome i(X)(q10), isochromosome of the long arm is most common. Isochromosomes are also frequently observed in hematologic malignancies.

Ring Chromosomes

Ring chromosomes form by breaks involving both telomeric ends of a chromosome, deletion of the acentric (without a centromere) fragments and end-to-end fusion of the remaining centric portion of the chromosome (Fig. 6-12G). The abnormal phenotype of a patient carrying a ring chromosome is due to loss of genes in the deleted telomeric regions of that chromosome, rather than to the formation of a ring structure itself.

Marker Chromosomes

Marker chromosomes are composed of chromosome material of unknown origin as a result of unbalanced chromosome rearrangements. Their identity can often be determined with molecular cytogenetic techniques (see below).

Microdeletions and Microduplications Occur in Repeat Regions Flanking Unique Sequences

They involve the same or very similar chromosomal regions in many unrelated patients, and arise through a molecular

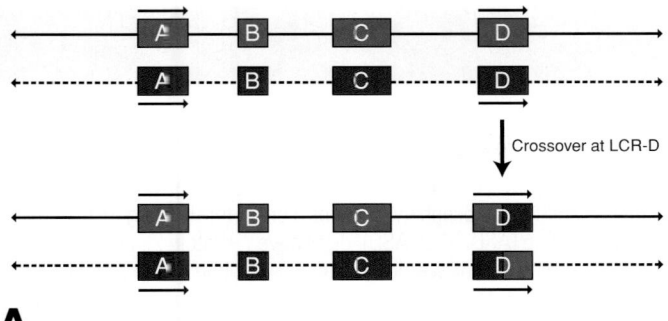

A. Normal recombination event

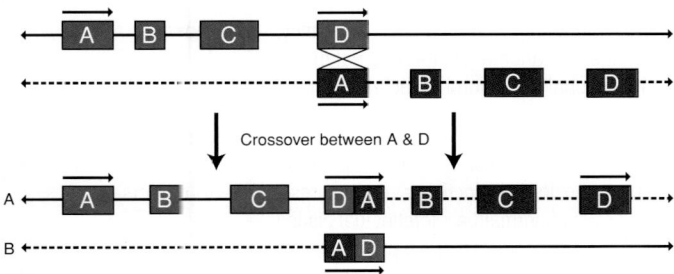

B. Misalignment followed by recombination

FIGURE 6-14. Non-allelic homologous recombination. Recurrent microdeletions and microduplications arise through the mechanism of non-allelic homologous recombination (NAHR). Due to their high homology, low copy repeats (LCRs), A-D, can misalign during pairing of homologous chromosomes in meiosis. If crossover occurs between misaligned LCRs, the sequences between hose LCRs will be duplicated on one, and deleted on the other, recombinant chromosome (panel B at the bottom). (From Emanuel BS, Saitta SC. *Nat. Rev. Genet.* 2007;8:869–883.)

mechanism that does not involve random chromosome breaks. Flanking repeat blocks vary from several hundred kb to several Mb. They are highly homologous, which makes them prone to misalign during homologous chromosome pairing in meiosis. If crossing over occurs within misaligned low copy repeats (unequal crossing over), the two non-sister chromatids will recombine at an incorrect location and one of the chromatids will acquire a duplication of the intervening sequence, while the corresponding segment will be deleted on the other chromatid (Fig. 6-14). This is called **non-allelic homologous recombination (NAHR)**, and causes many recurrent microdeletion and microduplication syndromes (Table 6-2). Some of the most common and best characterized microdeletion syndromes that originate through NAHR are DiGeorge/velocardiofacial syndrome, caused by a deletion in chromosome 22 (q11.21), and Williams syndrome, due to a deletion in chromosome 7 (q11.23).

DiGeorge/velocardiofacial syndrome/22q11.21 deletion syndrome, at 1 in 4,000 live births, is the commonest microdeletion syndrome. It features diverse cardiovascular anomalies, hypoplastic thymus resulting in T-cell deficit and immunodeficiency, and hypocalcemia from parathyroid hypoplasia. Facial dysmorphology and intellectual disability are also common. However, clinical features are variable and may be so mild that some adult patients are ascertained only after a more severely affected child is born. Individuals with velocardiofacial syndrome often have cleft hard or soft

palate with velopharyngeal incompetence and other facial abnormalities, cardiac defects, and psychiatric and intellectual problems. Since DiGeorge syndrome and velocardiofacial syndrome reflect the same microdeletion of chromosome 22 they are now combined into a single diagnostic entity.

 MOLECULAR PATHOGENESIS: DiGeorge/velocardiofacial syndrome reflects a 3-Mb deletion in chromosome region 22q11.21, arising through NAHR. Many of the abnormalities associated with the syndrome result from an abnormal developmental sequence in the embryonic pharyngeal arches and pouches which contribute to the morphogenesis of the thymus, thyroid, parathyroids, maxilla, mandible, aortic arch, cardiac outflow tract, and external/middle ear. Candidate genes responsible for this syndrome include *TBX1* (T-box transcription factor) and *CRKL* (V-CRK avian sarcoma virus CT10 oncogene homolog-like). Since the causative deletions are below the resolution of conventional cytogenetic analysis, the diagnosis of the 22q11.21 deletion syndrome is typically made by molecular cytogenetic methods, either FISH or CMA (see below). More than 90% of the probands have a de novo deletion of 22q11.21, but in 10% of the cases the deletion is inherited from a parent. Parental testing is thus indicated for recurrence risk assessment.

Fluorescence In Situ Hybridization (FISH) Uses DNA Probes to Visualize Specific DNA Regions

FISH can visualize specific chromosomal regions and enumerate multiple such regions simultaneously, by an array of fluorophores with different fluorescence characteristics, each attached to a different DNA probe. A FISH signal highlights the targeted region in a patient's cells. For example, in a normal individual hybridization with a probe for the DiGeorge/velocardiofacial syndrome critical region in 22q11.21 should show two signals per nucleus. A single probe signal would confirm that a patient has DiGeorge/velocardiofacial syndrome due to deletion of the critical region for the syndrome on one of his or her chromosomes 22. FISH probes are available to detect many of the microdeletion and microduplication syndromes (Table 6-2) in a similar fashion.

FISH is a common tool in prenatal diagnosis, as well as in other settings (see below and Chapter 5). A panel of probes for chromosomes 13, 18, 21, X and Y, applied to amniotic fluid or chorionic villi rapidly tests fetal cells for autosomal trisomies and numerical sex chromosome abnormalities (Fig. 6-15).

FISH routinely assists genomic analysis of some human malignancies (see Chapter 5). For example, in chronic myelogenous leukemia a translocation between chromosomes 9 and 22: t(9;22)(q34;q11.2) joins two genes, *ABL1* on chromosome 9, with *BCR* on chromosome 22, generating an abnormal protein kinase (see Chapters 5 and 26).

FISH allows hundreds of cells to be analyzed rapidly, and so it can detect abnormalities in low percentages of cells (low level mosaicism). Thus, FISH is commonly used to detect possible minimal residual disease post-chemotherapy for leukemia and lymphoma, when infrequent cytogenetically abnormal malignant cells may intermingle with many normal cells. It also can be used to detect gene amplification, for example, certain cancers have multiple copies of *ERBB2* gene (see Chapters 5 and 25).

TABLE 6-2
MICRODELETION SYNDROMES

Syndrome	Cytogenetic Location	Mechanism	Size	Main Clinical Features	Important Genes
Wolf-Hirschhorn	4p16.3	Nonrecurrent breakpoint	Variable	Pre- and postnatal growth restriction, significant intellectual disability, microcephaly, seizures, congenital heart disease (ASD, VSD, ASD), distinctive facial features with a "Greek warrior helmet" appearance due to high forehead, prominence of the glabella, hypertelorism, high and arched eyebrows, epicanthal folds, and downturned corners of the mouth	NSD2 (Nuclear Receptor–Binding SET Domain Protein 2), LETM1 (Leucine Zipper And EF-Hand Containing Transmembrane Protein 1)
Cri-du-chat	5p15.3	Nonrecurrent breakpoint	Variable	Characteristic mewing cry (cri du chat) in infancy, multiple congenital anomalies, intellectual disability, microcephaly, dysmorphic facial features	Unknown
Williams	7q11.23	NAHR	1.5 Mb	Cardiovascular disease (elastin arteriopathy, peripheral pulmonary stenosis, supravalvular aortic stenosis, hypertension), distinctive facial features connective tissue abnormalities, intellectual disability (usually mild), a specific cognitive profile, unique personality characteristics, growth abnormalities and endocrine abnormalities (hypercalcemia, hypercalciuria, hypothyroidism, and early puberty)	ELN (Elastin) responsible for elastic tissue defects, heart defects
Wilms tumor-aniridia (WAGR)	11p13	Nonrecurrent breakpoint	Variable	WAGR is an acronym for a group of abnormalities that include Wilms tumor, Aniridia, Genitourinary anomalies, and mental Retardation. Wilms tumor in ~50% of patients, intellectual disability ranging from severe to mild, eye anomalies (aniridia, cataracts, glaucoma, and nystagmus), genitourinary abnormalities (cryptorchidism in males, streak ovaries and bicornuate uterus in females, ambiguous genitalia in males and females).	WT1 (Wilms Tumor 1) responsible for Wilms tumor; PAX6 (Paired Box 6) responsible for aniridia.
Prader–Willi	15q11.2-q13.1	NAHR-paternal deletion	4 Mb	Severe hypotonia and feeding difficulties in early infancy, excessive eating in later infancy and gradual development of morbid obesity (unless eating is externally controlled), developmental delay/cognitive impairment, distinctive behavioral phenotype (temper tantrums, stubbornness, manipulative behavior, and obsessive-compulsive characteristics), hypogonadism, short stature is common (if not treated with growth hormone), characteristic facial features	Unknown; likely combined effects of multiple gene
Angelman	15q11.2-q13.1	NAHR-maternal deletion	4 Mb	Severe developmental delay/intellectual disability, severe speech impairment, ataxia, seizures, behavioral changes (inappropriate happy demeanor, frequent laughing and smiling, excitability)	UBE3A (Ubiquitin Protein Ligase E3A)
Smith–Magenis	17p11.2	NAHR	3.7 Mb	Distinctive facial features, developmental delay/cognitive impairment (mild to moderate), behavioral abnormalities (significant sleep disturbance, stereotypies (self-hugging), and maladaptive and self-injurious behaviors including self-hitting, self-biting, and/or skin picking, inserting foreign objects into body orifices and yanking fingernails and/or toenails)	RAI1(Retinoic Acid Induced 1)

GENETIC AND DEVELOPMENTAL DISORDERS

TABLE 6-2

MICRODELETION SYNDROMES (*CONTINUED*)

Syndrome	Cytogenetic Location	Mechanism	Size	Main Clinical Features	Important Genes
Miller–Dieker	17p13.3	Nonrecurrent breakpoint	Variable	Lissencephaly (agyria or pachygyria) by brain MRI, profound intellectual disability, seizures, distinctive facial features, feeding difficulties, growth retardation, impaired motor abilities	PAFAH1B1 (Platelet Activating Factor Acetylhydrolase 1b Regulatory Subunit 1) responsible for neuronal migration defect
DiGeorge/VCFS	22q11.21	NAHR	3 Mb	Congenital heart disease (conotruncal malformations including tetralogy of Fallot, interrupted aortic arch, VSD, and truncus arteriosus), palatal abnormalities (velopharyngeal incompetence, submucosal cleft palate, bifid uvula, cleft palate), characteristic facial features, learning difficulties, immune deficiency, hypocalcemia	TBX1 (T-Box 1) implicated in cardiac anomalies; CRKL (CRK Like Proto-Oncogene, Adaptor Protein)

Microarrays Allow Testing for Large Numbers of Copy Number Abnormalities

Chromosomal microarrays (CMAs) allow genome-wide detection of copy number abnormalities (deletions and duplications) with very high resolution (down to 50 kb) using hundreds of thousands to millions of fluorescent DNA probes. CMA panels typically provide genome-wide backbone coverage, plus high-density coverage for clinically relevant haploinsufficient genes and microdeletion/microduplication syndrome regions. CMAs detect disease-causing deletions and duplications using **comparative genomic hybridization (CGH)**. Fluorescence scanning measures signal intensities from each probe-patient DNA complex, which data are then compared with a normal sample to detect abnormalities (increases or decreases) in the intensity of the patient's signal.

CMA has dramatically increased the diagnostic yield for chromosomal copy number abnormalities over routine metaphase chromosome analysis, and is now a first-tier clinical diagnostic test to evaluate individuals with: (1) apparently nonsyndromic developmental delay and/or intellectual disability; (2) autism spectrum disorders; and (3) multiple congenital anomalies not specific to a well-delineated chromosomal or single gene syndrome.

Copy Number Variants (CNVs)

A CNV is a stretch of genomic DNA (from kilobases [kb] to megabases [Mb]) present in more than or less than two copies. As analytical techniques become increasingly sophisticated and sensitive, they have detected copy number changes of unknown clinical significance. Thus, CMA determined that human CNVs are much more common than

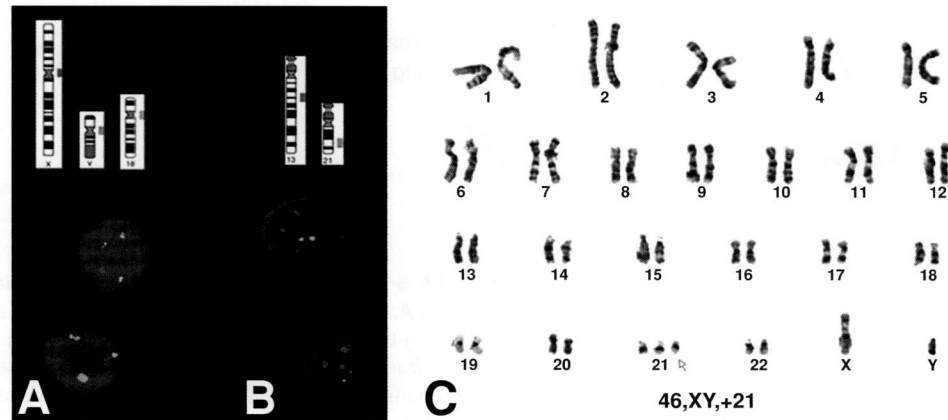

FIGURE 6-15. Prenatal FISH analysis performed on interphase amniocytes is positive for a male fetus with trisomy 21 and a clinical diagnosis of Down syndrome. A. Hybridization with centromere probes for chromosomes X and Y and 18 in green, red, and aqua, respectively, shows a probe signal pattern consistent with an XY sex chromosome complement and two chromosomes 18. **B.** Hybridization with probes for loci on chromosome 13 in green and chromosome 21 in red. The probe signal pattern is consistent with two copies of chromosome 13 and three copies of chromosome 21. **C.** The 47,XY,+21 karyotype of a metaphase cell from the same amniotic fluid sample confirms the FISH diagnosis.

previously appreciated. They are widespread in the human genome and are a significant source of human genetic variation accounting for population diversity and human disease. A recent estimate of the proportion of the human genome that is structurally variable (i.e., benign CNVs) is in the order of ~5% to 10%. The majority (>95%) of benign CNVs in humans are <100 kb in size and are typically inherited from a phenotypically normal parent. Databases that catalog common benign CNVs are an important resource for interpreting the clinical significance of CNVs detected by CMA testing. If a CNV does not involve a region known to be associated with a cytogenetic syndrome and does not correspond to one of the benign variants in population databases, its clinical significance can be unclear, and depends on whether it spans known dosage-sensitive genes or regulatory sequences. Large and de novo CNVs are more likely to cause disease. Parental testing may facilitate interpretation.

SINGLE GENE DISORDERS

Thousands of **single gene**, or **Mendelian**, **disorders** have been identified. Although individually rare, collectively, they contribute significantly to morbidity and mortality, especially among children.

DNA Sequence Variants May Involve Single Nucleotides or Whole Chromosomes

Terminology of Sequence Alterations

Changes that affect germ cells are transmitted to the individual's offspring, and may give rise to inherited diseases. DNA alterations that arise in somatic cells are not heritable, but can be associated with diseases nonetheless. The term, **mutation,** was applied to a disease-causing change, while **polymorphism** was indicated a non–disease-causing change, or a change found in 1% or more people in the population. Current guidelines recommend using terms like **sequence variant** or **sequence alteration**, plus attributes like benign or pathogenic to indicate predicted functional consequences of observed sequence changes. Both in research and in clinical testing, sequence variants are determined relative to accepted human genome references from the National Center for Biotechnology Information (NCBI) and the European Bioinformatics Institute.

Common types of DNA variants (Fig. 6-16) include:

- **Single nucleotide variants (SNVs) or point mutations** occur when one genomic DNA base replaces another. If this happens within the coding region (the part of the gene that is translated into a protein), there are three possible consequences:

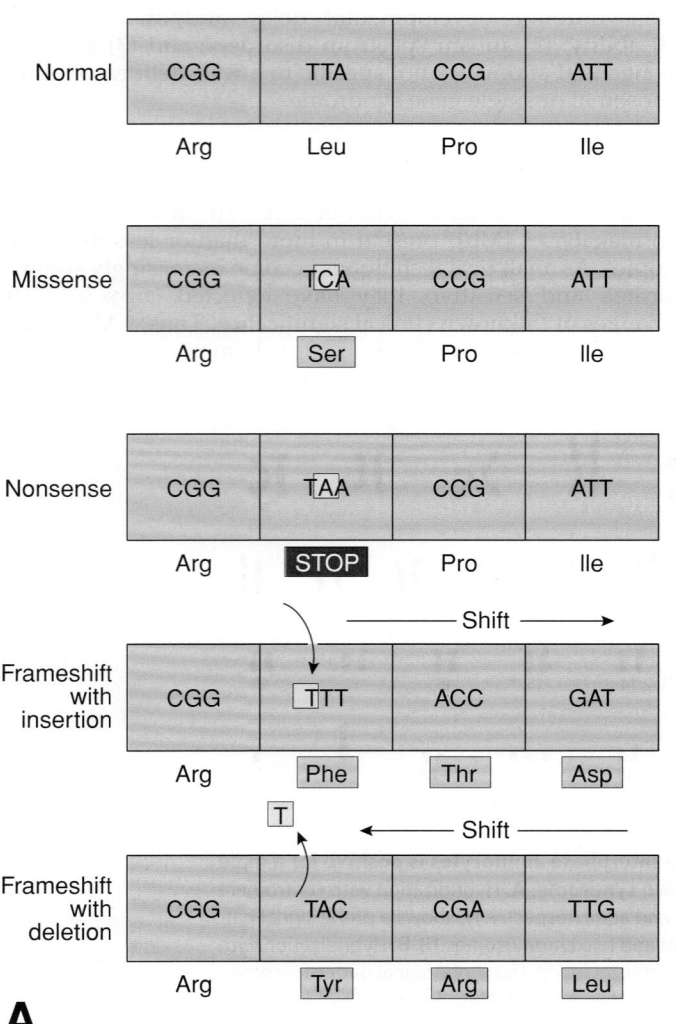

A

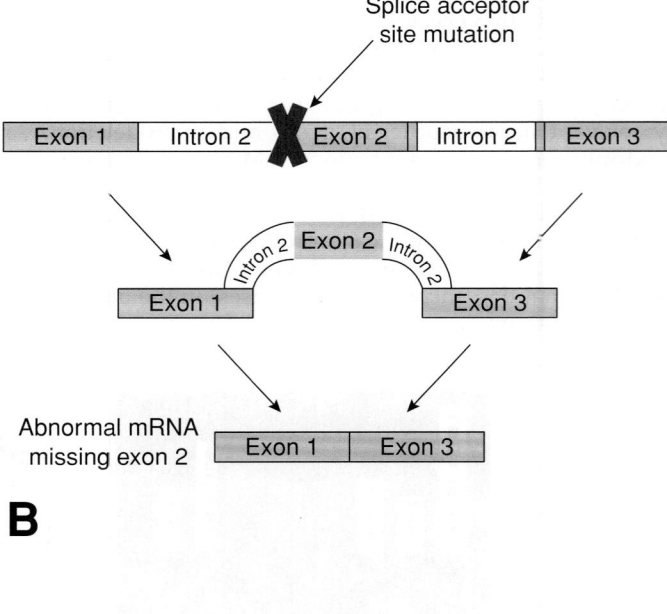

B

FIGURE 6-16. Possible effects of sequence variants on an encoded protein. A. A normal (wild type) sequence encoding a stretch of four amino acids (Arg-Leu-Pro-Ile) is depicted on the top. With a missense variant, a change from T to C transforms the codon for leucine (Leu) to serine (Ser). With a nonsense variant, a change from T to A converts the leucine codon to a stop codon. With a frameshift variant, insertion of a T results in a shift in the reading frame to the right, thus changing the sequence of all subsequent amino acids. Conversely, deletion of a T shifts the reading frame one base to the left and also changes the sequence of subsequent amino acids. Arg = arginine; Asp = aspartate; Ile = isoleucine; Phe = phenylalanine; Pro = proline; Thr = threonine; Tyr = tyrosine. **B.** Effects of a pathogenic splicing variant: a sequence change disrupts the canonical splice acceptor site before exon 2. This results in skipping of the exon and an abnormal mRNA product.

- A **synonymous variant (mutation)** changes the **codon** (the trinucleotide encodes a specific amino acid during protein synthesis), but the resulting sequence still encodes the same amino acid. This reflects the degeneracy of the genetic code. For example, CGA and CGC both code for arginine. Synonymous variants may not change amino acid code, but they still may have functional implications by affecting mRNA splicing or altering gene expression.
- A **missense variant (mutation)** alters the codon, to specify a different amino acid, thereby changing the protein sequence. In sickle cell anemia, an adenine-to-thymine base change in the β-globin gene replaces a codon for glutamic acid (GAG) with a codon for valine (GTG). Missense variants account for about 75% of base changes in coding regions. Their functional consequences vary. Some are completely benign, but others may impede or destroy protein function, or alter its folding, trafficking, and stability.
- A **nonsense variant (mutation)** (4% of SNVs in coding regions) changes a codon for an amino acid to one of the three termination codons (TAG, TAA, or TGA), stopping translation and so yielding a truncated protein. For example, TAT codes for tyrosine, but TAA is a stop codon.
- **Frameshift variants (mutations).** Amino acids are encoded by trinucleotide sequences. If the number of bases in a gene is changed by insertion or deletion, and if the number of bases added or lost is not a multiple of 3, the reading frame of the message is changed. Thus, although the sequence downstream of the insertion or deletion site is unchanged, it will encode a different amino acid sequence. A change in a protein reading frame often leads to an unscheduled termination signal, and produces an altered and truncated protein.
- **Splicing variants (mutations)** are changes (substitutions, deletions, or insertions) of nucleotides at the specific boundaries of exons and introns (splice sites) where **splicing** occurs as precursor messenger RNAs are processed into mature mRNAs. Splice site changes can disturb RNA splicing, and cause loss of exons or inclusion of introns and an altered protein-coding sequence.
- **Large deletions.** Deletions that remove a portion or an entire coding region of a dosage-sensitive gene are relatively common causes of single gene disorders. Deletions of larger regions (hundreds and thousands of kilobases) and include multiple genes result in **contiguous gene deletion syndromes** (see above).
- **Expansions of unstable trinucleotide repeat sequences.** Trinucleotide repeats are 3-bp repetitive sequences in the human genome. They occur at many places in the genome. Some within coding or regulatory gene regions are responsible for a specific class of genetic disorders known as triplet-repeat diseases. The number of repeat copies at many such loci varies among individuals, reflecting allelic polymorphism of the genes in which these repeats are found. Typically, the number of repeats below a particular threshold does not change during mitosis or meiosis; however, above this threshold, repeats become unstable and can contract or, much more commonly, expand in meiosis. People carrying an "unstable" allele of a trinucleotide repeat in a particular gene are at risk of having children affected by the corresponding trinucleotide repeat disorder, as unstable repeats can undergo

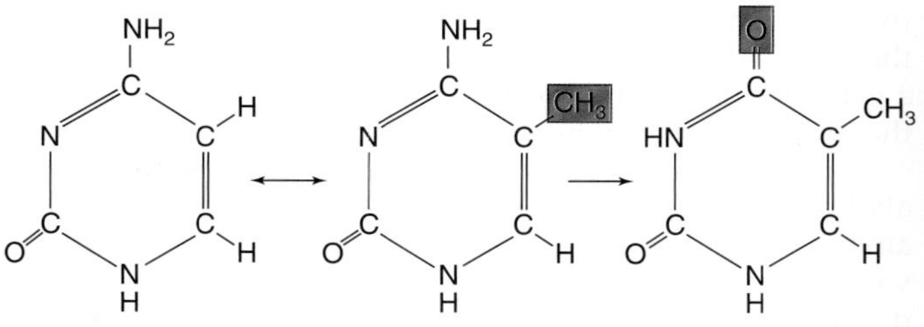

FIGURE 6-17. Generation of C to T substitutions in genomic DNA through spontaneous deamination of 5-methylcytosine. Cytosine residues in genomic DNA are often methylated as a mechanism to regulate (inhibit) gene expression. However, 5-methylcytosine residues can undergo spontaneous deamination which converts them into thymine.

large expansions in meiosis. They may reach a point at which they disrupt the function of the gene where they reside. Several trinucleotide expansion disorders are known (see below).

Mutation Hotspots

Certain regions of the genome mutate at more than others. These hotspot DNA sequences are usually inherently instable. In addition to trinucleotide repeats which tend to change in length, *hypermutable sites* may engage in unequal crossing over, or be predisposed to single nucleotide substitutions. The best-characterized hotspots for single nucleotide substitutions are dinucleotides, where a cytosine (C) occurs next to a guanine (G) in the linear base sequence, with an intervening phosphate, designated CG (or CpG, meaning C-PO$_4$-G).

The Cs in CpG dinucleotides can be methylated to 5-methylcytosine. CpG methylation typically represses gene expression. Regions of the genome with higher concentrations of CpGs are called CpG islands, and are found in many promoter regions, where their methylation can serve as a signal to shut down that particular gene's expression. However, methylated cytosines can undergo spontaneous deamination to thymine (Fig. 6-17). If that occurs in germ cells, it can become a fixed, heritable sequence change.

Single Gene Disorders May Be Dominant or Recessive, Autosomal or X-Linked

A segment of DNA at a particular location on a chromosome is a **locus**, or, if it contains a gene, a **gene locus**. Alternative variants of a gene are **alleles**. Most genes have a single prevailing allele in most individuals: a **common** or **wild-type** allele. **Variant** or **mutant** alleles differ from wild-type alleles by having a permanent change in DNA sequence or arrangement. If there are at least two relatively common alleles at a locus in the population, the locus **polymorphic**.

Each person normally has a pair of homologous chromosomes (see above). If someone has identical alleles at a particular locus on both chromosomes in a homologous pair, he or she is **homozygous** (or a **homozygote**). If that locus on someone's two homologous chromosomes have different alleles, *and* if one is a common (wild-type) allele and one a variant (mutant) allele, that person is **heterozygous** (or **heterozygote**). A **compound heterozygote** is somebody with two different variant (mutant) alleles at a particular locus. In the special case when a male has a variant (mutant) allele for a gene on the X chromosome, and there is no other copy of that gene in the genome, he is **hemizygous**.

Single genes disorders are determined by pathogenic alleles (variants) of a gene at a single locus. Clinical features among individuals affected with single gene disorders can vary, even within the same family, especially with autosomal dominant disorders. Some individuals inherit the mutant gene but are phenotypically normal or near normal. This phenomenon is called reduced **penetrance**. In contrast, if a mutant allele shows a broad range of clinical manifestations, from mild to very severe, the situation is called variable **expressivity**. The molecular bases for reduced penetrance and variable expressivity are poorly understood; both are probably influenced by an individual's overall genetic background and environmental factors.

Autosomal Dominant Disorders

If only one mutated allele is sufficient to cause disease when its paired allele on the homologous autosome is normal, the trait or the disorder is considered to be dominant. In autosomal dominant conditions (Fig. 6-18):

- Males and females are equally affected, as the responsible genes are on autosomes. Father-to-son transmission (which is absent in X-linked disorders) may occur.
- Proportions of normal and diseased offspring of individuals with the disorder are about equal, since an affected parent has a 50% chance to transmit the abnormal allele with each pregnancy.
- Assuming complete penetrance (i.e., all individuals who carry a pathogenic variant have disease, see above),

unaffected members of a family do not transmit the trait to their offspring.
- Unless the disease is the result of a new mutation in an affected individual, everyone in a family with the disease has an affected parent.

New Mutations Versus Inherited Mutations

As noted above, autosomal dominant diseases may result from a new mutation in an individual rather than from a mutation inherited from an affected parent. However, future generations of offspring of someone with a *new* dominant mutation have a 50% risk for the disease. *If a disease impairs fertility, it becomes more likely that affected people will represent new mutations.* A person with a dominant mutation that causes 100% infertility would have to have a new mutation. If reproductive capacity is only partly impaired, the proportion of new mutations would be correspondingly lower. For example, **tuberous sclerosis** is an autosomal dominant condition in which cognitive impairment severely limits reproductive potential; new mutations account for 80% of cases. If a dominant disease has little effect on fertility (e.g., familial hypercholesterolemia), virtually all affected individuals will have pedigrees showing classic autosomal dominant transmission.

 MOLECULAR PATHOGENESIS: There are several major mechanisms by which a single mutant allele may cause disease even when the other allele is normal.

- **Haploinsufficiency.** If the gene product is rate limiting in a complex metabolic network (e.g., a receptor, regulatory factor or an enzyme), having half of the normal amount of gene product may be insufficient for a normal

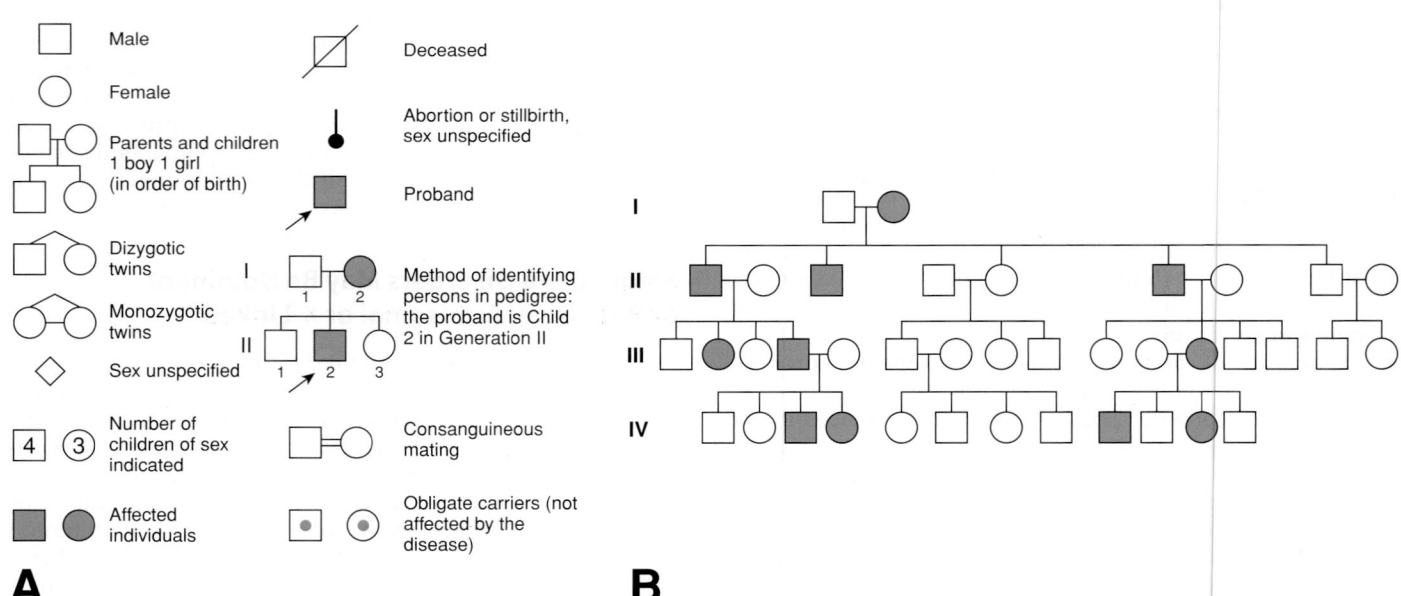

A   **B**

FIGURE 6-18. **A. Definition of pedigree symbols.** Males = squares; females = circles. A line drawn between a square and a circle represents a mating of that male and female. Two lines drawn between a square and a circle indicate a consanguineous mating in which the two individuals are related. Children from the same parents are connected to a horizontal line (sibship line) by short vertical lines. The children of a sibship are always listed in order of birth with the oldest on the left. Other conventions concerning twins, identification of probands and deceased individuals, affected individuals, and nonaffected obligate carriers are shown in the figure. **B. Autosomal dominant inheritance.** Heterozygotes are symptomatic and can transmit the trait to the next generation. Both males and females are affected.

phenotype. Thus, familial hypercholesterolemia is caused by inadequate low-density lipoprotein (LDL) uptake receptors on hepatocytes.

- **Gain of function mutations.** A mutation may change the gene product so that its original functionality is increased (enhanced activation) or replaced by a different and abnormal function. Mutations in *RET* proto-oncogene in families with **multiple endocrine neoplasia type 2** increase the tyrosine kinase activity of the RET protein, thus stimulating cell proliferation and increasing probability of malignant transformation of endocrine cells. In achondroplasia, mutations in *FGFR3*, the fibroblast growth factor (FGF) receptor 3 gene increase receptor activity; since this receptor downregulates bone growth, its increased activity leads to severely shortened bones and dwarfism.
- **Dominant negatives.** Mutations in genes for structural proteins (e.g., collagens, cytoskeletal constituents) often result in abnormal proteins that are not only nonfunctional themselves, but also antagonize the products of the wild-type alleles. For example, a product of the mutant allele may disrupt molecular interactions between subunits of a protein polymer, and compromise its stability and function. This mechanism of action is exemplified by osteogenesis imperfecta (see below) and hereditary spherocytosis (see Chapter 26).

Autosomal Recessive Disorders

Most genetic metabolic diseases show autosomal recessive inheritance: clinical manifestations only occur if both alleles of the causative gene carry a pathogenic variant. Features of these disorders (Fig. 6-19) include:

- Both parents of an affected person are usually heterozygous for the trait and are clinically normal.
- Autosomal recessive traits are transmitted equally to males and females.
- An unaffected heterozygous parent has a 50% chance of passing on the mutant allele with each pregnancy, while a homozygous affected individual will always pass on a mutant allele with each pregnancy.
- **Most mutant genes responsible for autosomal recessive disorders are rare in the general population, since affected individuals often fail to reproduce and transmit abnormal alleles.** However, a few autosomal recessive diseases, for example, sickle cell anemia, cystic fibrosis (CF), and spinal muscular atrophy are relatively common.
- The more infrequent the mutant gene is in the general population, the lower the chance that unrelated parents carry the trait. Consequently, **many rare autosomal recessive disorders are concentrated in offspring of consanguineous parents** who are more likely than unrelated individuals to carry the same mutant gene.
- With each pregnancy, carrier parents have a 25% risk for a child to be homozygous for the mutant gene and affected, a 50% chance for an unaffected heterozygous child, and a 25% chance that the child will be unaffected and not carry the mutant gene. Thus, 2/3 of unaffected offspring are heterozygous carriers.
- Symptoms of autosomal recessive disorders tend to be more consistent within families than in autosomal dominant diseases. Recessive traits typically present in

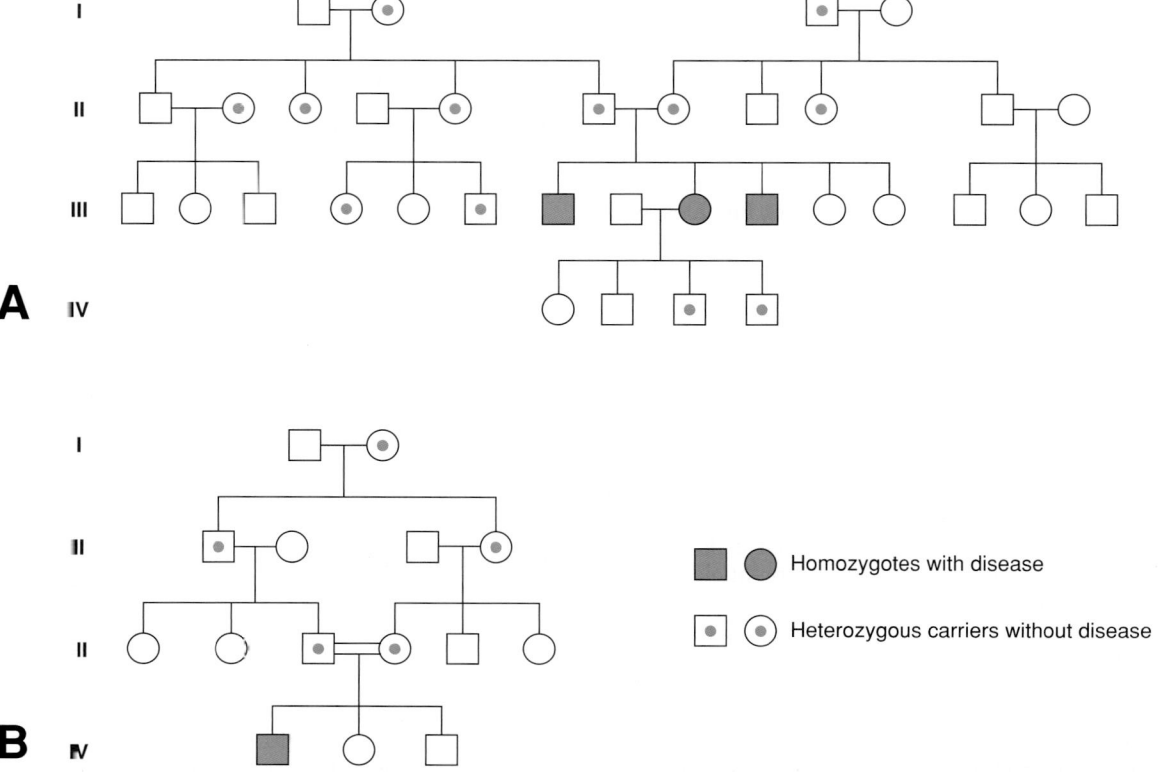

FIGURE 6-19. Typical pedigrees showing autosomal recessive inheritance. Symptoms of the disease appear only in homozygotes, both male and female, who result from the mating of asymptomatic heterozygotes. In family A the asymptomatic heterozygous parents are unrelated and in family B they are consanguineous.

childhood with similar severity among affected siblings, while dominant disorders show more variable age of onset and severity of symptoms.

- Variability in clinical expression between families with some autosomal recessive diseases may reflect residual functionality of the affected protein. This is in part because the specific mutation in one family may differ from the mutation in that gene in another family. Thus, there may be: (1) differences in disease severity, (2) age at onset, or (3) possibly acute and chronic forms of the disease.

MOLECULAR PATHOGENESIS: Most known recessive disorders reflect mutations that reduce or eliminate the function of the gene product: **loss-of-function** mutations. For example, many recessive diseases are caused by mutations that impair or eliminate the function of an enzyme. Enzyme deficiencies are typically inherited as recessive diseases because most enzymes have functional stoichiometric advantages: they operate within cells at substrate concentrations well below saturation. Even if one allele is inactivated by mutation, enough protein is produced by the remaining functional allele for normal physiologic function, so heterozygous people are phenotypically normal. Loss of both alleles, however, in a homozygous individual causes complete loss of enzyme activity and results in disease.

X-Linked Disorders

X-linked traits are determined by genes on the X chromosome, and their expression is different in males and females. Males, having one X chromosome, are hemizygous for such traits, and typically express them regardless of whether the trait is dominant or recessive. X-linked traits are only transmitted from mother to son. Even a symptomatic father transmits only a Y chromosome to his male offspring, but he always transmits his abnormal X chromosome to his daughters, who are therefore obligate carriers. Females, with two X chromosomes, may be homozygous or heterozygous at the DNA level for a variant determining a given trait, but functionally express only one of the alleles in individual cells due to X-inactivation (lyonization, see above). X-linked disorders thus do not perfectly follow either dominant or recessive inheritance patterns. Their expression can be highly variable in females, dependent on X-inactivation patterns. While X-inactivation is normally random, in some X-linked disorders affected females have skewed patterns of X chromosome inactivation that favor the X chromosome with the wild-type allele, possibly because the mutant gene on an active X chromosome may be lethal, so that cells with an active X chromosome carrying the wild-type allele survive better. For many disorders caused by mutations in X-linked genes that are subject to X-inactivation, females have been described that show unusually severe or mild phenotypes because of extreme non-random patterns of X-inactivation that occurred for a variety of reasons. Despite the ambiguities and complexities due to hemizygosity in males and skewed X-inactivation in females, the terms, **X-linked recessive** (if carrier females are typically healthy) and **X-linked dominant** (if females with one mutant allele tend to be affected) persist (Fig. 6-20).

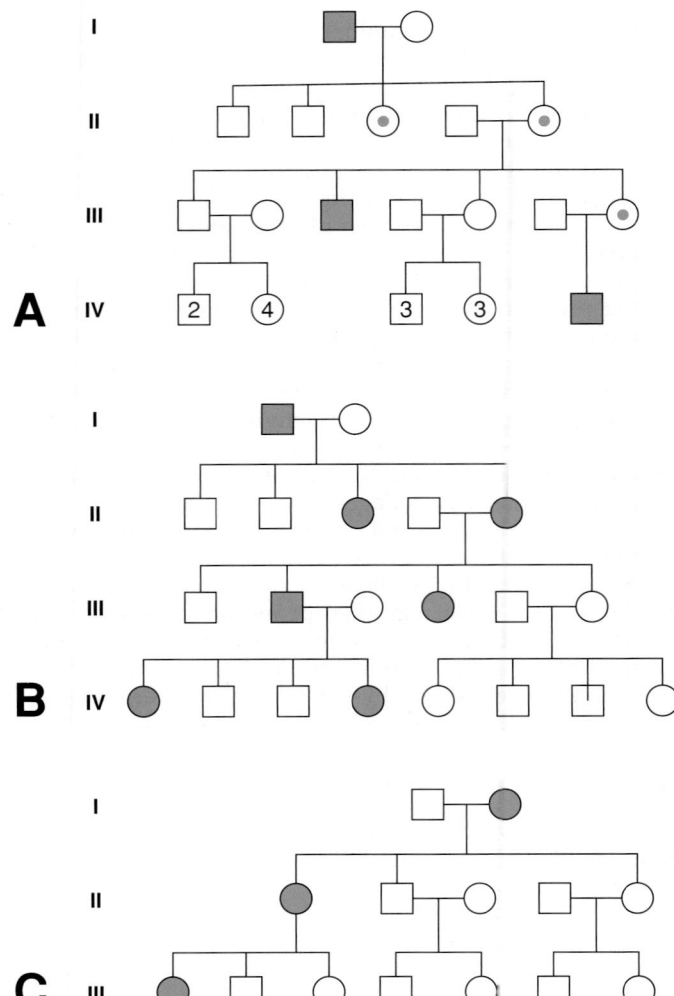

FIGURE 6-20. X-linked inheritance. For X-linked disorders, a woman can transmit the trait equally to sons and daughters; men transmit the trait only to their daughters. **A.** Pedigree demonstrating inheritance of an X-linked recessive disorder. Only males are affected; all daughters of affected men are asymptomatic carriers. Asymptomatic men do not transmit the trait. A disorder is transmitted from an affected male through female carriers to an affected grandson and great-grandson. Clinical expression of the disease skips a generation. **B.** Transmission of an X-linked dominant disorder. A heterozygous woman transmits the trait equally to males and females; men transmit the trait only to their daughters. Asymptomatic males and females do not carry the trait. **C.** Transmission of an X-linked dominant disorder that is lethal in males during the prenatal period. The pedigree only shows affected females, and they will usually have more female than male children.

X-Linked Recessive Traits

Well-known X-linked recessive disorders include Duchenne–Becker muscular dystrophy, Fragile X syndrome, hemophilia, and other diseases (see Table 6-3). The characteristics of this mode of inheritance are:

- Sons of women who are asymptomatic carriers have a 50% chance of inheriting the disease. Daughters are not symptomatic, but 50% of daughters will be carriers.
- All daughters of affected men are asymptomatic carriers, but sons of these men do not have the trait and cannot transmit it to their children.

TABLE 6-3
REPRESENTATIVE X-LINKED RECESSIVE DISORDERS

Disorder	Frequency	Inheritance	Gene	Chromosomal Location
Duchenne and Becker muscular dystrophy	1/3,500–5,000 newborn male	XLR	*DMD*	Xp21.1-p21.2
Fragile X syndrome	1/4,000 males 1/8,000 females	XLR	*FMR1*	Xq27.3
Hemophilia A (Factor VIII Deficiency)	1/4,000–5,000 males	XLR	*F8*	Xq28
Hemophilia B (Factor IX Deficiency)	1/20,000 males	XLR	*F9*	Xq27.1
Glucose-6-phosphate dehydrogenase deficiency	400 million people worldwide; more common in certain parts of Africa, Asia, the Mediterranean, and the Middle East	XLR	*G6PD*	Xq28
Lesch–Nyhan syndrome	1/380,000 newborns	XLR	*HPRT1*	Xq26.2-q26.3
X-linked agammaglobulinemia	1/200,000 newborns	XLR	*BTK*	Xq22.1
X-linked severe combined immuno-deficiency	1/50,000–100,000 newborns	XLR	*IL2RG*	Xq13.1
Fabry disease	1/40,000–60,000 males	XLR	*GLA*	Xq22.1
Adrenoleukodystrophy	1/20,000–50,000 individuals	XLR	*ABCD1*	Xq28
Menkes syndrome	1/100,000 newborns	XLR	*ATP7A*	Xq21.1

XLR = X-linked recessive.

- An X-linked recessive disease diagnosed in a male thus skips the next generation, but can be transmitted to his grandsons through his carrier daughters.
- Symptomatic females can result from (1) a mutant allele on the single X chromosome in a female with Turner syndrome, (2) a rare mating of an affected man with an asymptomatic heterozygous woman, or (3) extremely skewed lyonization with inactivation of the normal X chromosome.
- A significant proportion of isolated cases are due to a new mutation in the affected male (Fig. 6-20A).

X-Linked Dominant Traits

X-linked dominance refers to expression of a trait both in heterozygous females and hemizygous males. X-linked dominant disorders are rare; examples include familial hypophosphatemic rickets, Rett syndrome, and incontinentia pigmenti. Clinical disease tends to be less severe and more variable in heterozygous females than in hemizygous males because heterozygous females may have skewed patterns of X chromosome inactivation (see above), that favor an active X chromosome carrying the wild-type allele. Males with many of these disorders do not survive or survive poorly, with very severe disease. The genes causing such conditions may be so critical to development that their mutations do not allow hemizygous males who have only one X chromosomes to survive. Embryonic lethality in males, may lead to increased rates of pregnancy loss in women carrying X-linked dominant mutations.

The distinctive features of X-linked dominant disorders are:

- Females are affected twice as often as males.

- Heterozygous women have a 50% chance with each pregnancy to transmit disease to their children, both male and female.
- A man with a dominant X-linked disorder transmits it to all of his daughters and none of his sons (Fig. 6-20B,C).

Inborn Errors of Metabolism Are Often Monogenic Mutations Affecting Enzymes in Key Biochemical Pathways

A biochemical pathway is a series of enzymatic reactions, mediated by different enzymes, each encoded by a specific gene. A typical pathway (below) can be depicted as enzymatic conversion of substrate (A) via intermediate metabolites (B and C) to a final product (D).

Enzymes: 1 → 2 → 3
A → B → C → D
initial substrate / intermediary metabolites / end-product(s)

A single gene defect that diminishes activity of one enzyme in the series can lead to:

- **Failure to complete a pathway, and deficiency of the final product:** The end-product (D) is not formed since an enzyme needed to complete a metabolic sequence is missing

$$A \to B \to C - // \to (D) (\downarrow)$$

An example of failure to complete a metabolic pathway is albinism, a pigment disorder due to a deficiency of tyrosinase, which converts tyrosine to melanin (via an intermediate, dihydroxyphenylalanine [DOPA]). Without tyrosinase, the melanin end-product is not formed, and the affected person completely lacks the pigment, which primarily manifests in the eyes, skin, and hair.

- **A toxic unmetabolized substrate accumulates:** If the enzyme (i.e., #1) that converts the initial substrate to the first intermediary metabolite is missing, substrate A accumulates in excess, causing toxicity.

$$A (\uparrow) \, // \rightarrow B (\downarrow) \, C (\downarrow) \, D (\downarrow)$$

In phenylketonuria, phenylalanine hydroxylase deficiency allows dietary phenylalanine to accumulate and reach toxic levels that interfere with postnatal brain development and cause severe cognitive impairment.

- **An intermediary metabolite accumulates:** Normally, an intermediary metabolite is processed quickly into the final product, and so is usually present only in tiny amounts, accumulates in large quantities if the enzyme (here #2) for its metabolism is lacking.

$$A \rightarrow B (\uparrow) \, // \rightarrow C (\downarrow) \, D (\downarrow)$$

In **alkaptonuria,** a defect in homogentisate 1,2-dioxygenase (HGD), allows homogentisic acid, an intermediate product in the tyrosine degradation pathway, to accumulate. This acid and its oxidative products accumulate in blood and connective tissues, causing ochronosis (bluish-black pigmentation in connective tissue) and arthritis of the spine and larger joints.

- **An alternative pathway dominates:** Often, intermediate metabolites from many metabolic pathways may also be substrates for other pathways, leading to other final products. If an enzyme defect causes an intermediate metabolite to build up abnormally, the excess may be shunted into an alternative pathway allowing a different end-product to accumulate abnormally.

$$A \rightarrow B (\uparrow) \, // \rightarrow C (\downarrow) \, D (\downarrow)$$
$$\downarrow$$
$$E (\uparrow)$$

In congenital adrenal hyperplasia, 21-hydroxylase deficiency prevents normal glucocorticoid and mineralocorticoid biosynthesis. Overproduced precursors are then shunted into the pathway of androgen biosynthesis, generating abnormally high androgen levels and in utero virilization of affected female fetuses.

Inherited Defects in Synthesis and Degradation May Affect Many Amino Acids

This is a large group of diseases that vary in severity from lethal in early childhood to clinically insignificant (Table 6-4). Examples below focus on defects in phenylalanine and tyrosine metabolism.

Phenylalanine Hydroxylase Deficiency (Phenylketonuria, PKU)

In PKU high circulating levels of phenylalanine cause profound, irreversible intellectual disability if untreated. The incidence is 1 per 5,000 to 10,000 among white and Asian populations, but varies widely in different geographic areas.

Phenylalanine is an essential amino acid, derived exclusively from the diet. It is oxidized to tyrosine in the liver by phenylalanine hydroxylase (PAH) (Fig. 6-21). PAH deficiency leads to hyperphenylalaninemia. Phenylalanine causes the neurologic damage central to this disease. The exact mechanism of neurotoxicity in PKU is uncertain. The risk of adverse outcome depends on the degree of PAH deficiency.

TABLE 6-4

REPRESENTATIVE INBORN ERRORS OF AMINO ACID METABOLISM

Amino Acid Metabolism Disorder	Enzyme	Frequency	Inheritance	Gene	Chromosome Location
Phenylketonuria (hyperphenylalaninemia)	Phenylalanine hydroxylase	1/5,000–10,000	AR	PAH	12q23.2
Tetrahydrobiopterin (BH$_4$) deficiency	Dihydropteridine reductase	1/500,000–1,000,000	AR	QDPR	4p15.32
Tyrosinemia, type 1	Fumarylacetoacetate hydrolase	1/100,000 1 in 1,846 in the Saguenay–Lac St. Jean region of Quebec	AR	FAH	15q25.1
Alkaptonuria	Homogentisate 1,2-dioxygenase	1/250,000	AR	HGD	3q13.33
Maple syrup urine disease (branched chain ketoacidemia)	Branched-chain alpha-keto-acid dehydrogenase complex (BCKD) α-chain, BCKD β-chain, BCKD E2 component, dihydrolipoamide dehydrogenase, BCDK kinase	1/185,000 1/380 in Old Order Mennonites	AR	BCKDHA BCKDHB DBT DLD BCKDK	19q13.2 6q14.1 1p21.2 7q31.1 16p11.2
Histidinemia	Histidase	1/8,600–90,000	AR	HAL	12q23.1

AR = autosomal recessive.

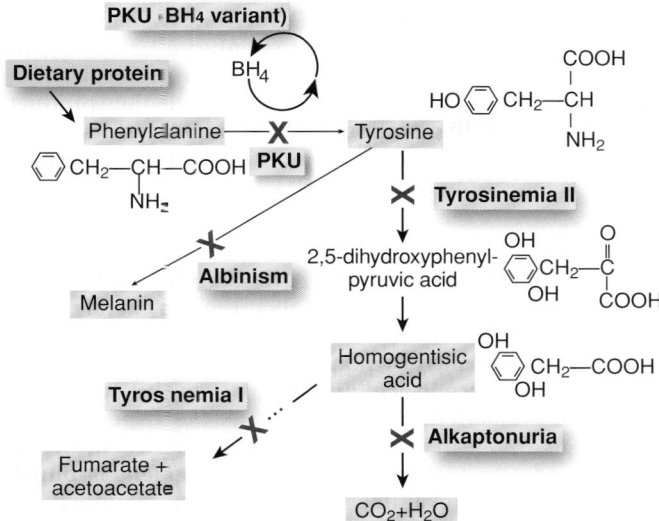

FIGURE 6-21. Diseases caused by disturbances of phenylalanine and tyrosine metabolism. 1. Classic phenylketonuria is caused by deficiency in phenylalanine hydroxylase (PAH) which oxidizes phenylalanine to tyrosine in the liver. 2. Hyperphenylalaninemia related to BH$_4$ deficiency is caused by impaired synthesis or recycling of tetrahydrobiopterin (BH$_4$), which is a necessary cofactor for PAH. 3. Tyrosinemia type I is caused by deficiency of fumarylacetoacetate hydrolase, which is the last enzyme in the catabolic pathway that converts tyrosine to fumarate and acetoacetate. 4. Tyrosinemia type II results from deficiency of tyrosine transaminase which converts tyrosine to p-hydroxyphenylpyruvate. 5. Alkaptonuria is caused by a defect in the enzyme homogentisate 1,2-dioxygenase (HGD), which catalyzes another step in tyrosine degradation.

 MOLECULAR PATHOGENESIS: Classic PKU is an autosomal recessive disorder caused by mutations in the *PAH* gene at 12q23.2. There are many different disease-causing missense, nonsense, frameshift, and splice variants in *PAH*. Variants that confer the most severe phenotypes appear to abolish PAH activity completely. Missense pathogenic variants usually allow some residual enzyme activity, and so lead to milder disease than in classic PKU. People with under 1% of normal PAH activity generally have a PKU phenotype. Those with over 5% have mutations that only partly abolish the enzyme activity. They have non-PKU hyperphenylalaninemia, do not suffer neurologic damage and develop normally.

Tetrahydrobiopterin (BH$_4$) Deficiency

Hyperphenylalaninemia may also result from impaired synthesis or recycling of tetrahydrobiopterin (BH4), the cofactor required for phenylalanine hydroxylation by PAH (Fig. 6-21). BH4 deficiency can reflect impaired synthesis, or insufficient dihydropteridine reductase (DHPR), the enzyme that reduces dihydrobiopterin (BH2) to the active tetrahydro form (BH4). Infants with BH4 deficiency are phenotypically identical to those with classic PKU at first, but later develop additional symptoms likely due to abnormal synthesis of other products that require BH4, including the neurotransmitters dopamine (tyrosine hydroxylase dependent) and serotonin (tryptophan hydroxylase dependent). Thus, brain damage in BH4 deficiency most likely involves more than a simple elevation in phenylalanine levels.

 CLINICAL FEATURES: PKU illustrates how genetics and environment interact to cause disease: a genetic defect only causes disease with dietary exposure to phenylalanine. Affected infants appear normal at birth, but developmental delay is evident within months. Infants with PKU tend to have fair skin, blond hair, and blue eyes, because they cannot convert phenylalanine to tyrosine, and so have reduced melanin synthesis. They exude a "mousy" or "musty" odor, owing to excretion of phenylacetic acid in the urine.

The main treatment for classic PKU patients is a strict phenylalanine-restricted diet supplemented by a medical formula containing amino acids and other nutrients. In the United States, the current recommendation is that the PKU diet be maintained for life. Patients who are diagnosed early and maintain a strict diet can have a normal life span with normal mental development. However, normal neurocognitive and psychosocial development and growth require that the diet be supplemented with amino acids.

In developed countries, broad implementation of newborn screening had made classical PKU more of historical interest than a significant concern. Expectant mothers who are homozygous for PKU (maternal PKU) must restrict phenylalanine intake while pregnant for the fetus to avoid complications of maternal hyperphenylalaninemia. Infants exposed to high levels of phenylalanine in utero show microcephaly, mental and growth retardation and cardiac anomalies due to teratogenic effects of high phenylalanine levels.

Tyrosinemia

Tyrosinemia is a collective name for autosomal recessive disorders involving tyrosine metabolism. These are characterized by abnormally high levels of tyrosine in blood and urine. There are three main types, each caused by mutations in different genes. Type I is the most severe form. It occurs in 1 per 100,000 people, but is more common in Norway and Quebec's Saguenay–Lac St. Jean region. Type I tyrosinemia is caused by deficiency of fumarylacetoacetate hydrolase (FAH). It manifests as acute liver disease in early infancy, or as a more chronic liver, kidneys and brain disease in children.

 MOLECULAR PATHOGENESIS: The FAH gene (*FAH*) located in 15q25.1 is the final enzyme in the catabolic pathway that converts tyrosine to fumarate and acetoacetate (Fig. 6-21). The enzyme is deficient in both acute and chronic forms of type I tyrosinemia, but in the former, it is completely inactive, while patients with the chronic disease have variable levels of residual enzyme activity. Due to the block in the final stage of its catabolism, tyrosine and its degradation products are elevated in blood and tissues, and shunted into production of abnormal metabolites. Cell injury in hereditary tyrosinemia is attributed to abnormal toxic metabolites, succinylacetone and succinyl acetoacetate.

 CLINICAL FEATURES: Analysis of amniotic fluid for succinylacetone or fetal cells for mutations in *FAH* (if both pathogenic variants in a family are known) establishes the diagnosis prenatally. Severe type I tyrosinemia manifests in the first few months of life as hepatomegaly, edema, failure to thrive and a cabbage-like odor. If untreated, infants die within a few months, typically of hepatic failure. The less severe form presents later in the first year with liver dysfunction and renal tubular dysfunction (Fanconi syndrome), with growth failure, rickets and neurologic abnormalities. Hepatocellular carcinoma occurs in more than a third of patients. Untreated children usually die before 10 years of age, from liver failure, neurologic crisis, or hepatocellular carcinoma.

At present, the diagnosis is typically suspected based on the results of newborn screening, and confirmed by biochemical and molecular testing. Treatment with nitisinone (Orfadin®), which blocks enzymes in the tyrosine degradation pathway, prevents toxic metabolites from accumulating. Because nitisinone increases blood tyrosine, dietary management with controlled intake of phenylalanine and tyrosine should begin immediately after diagnosis. This regimen allows >90% survival, normal growth, improved liver function, prevents cirrhosis, corrects renal tubular acidosis, and improves secondary rickets. Liver transplantation, once the only definitive treatment, is now reserved for children with severe liver failure at presentation who do not respond to nitisinone therapy or have hepatic malignancy. Liver transplantation corrects hepatic metabolic abnormalities and prevents the neurologic crises.

Alkaptonuria (Ochronosis)

This rare autosomal recessive disease affects 1 in 250,000 to 1,000,000 people worldwide, but is more common in Slovakia and the Dominican Republic. It has greater historical than clinical significance: reports of Garrod and others 100 years ago of the inheritance of alkaptonuria helped establish the idea of hereditary inborn errors of metabolism.

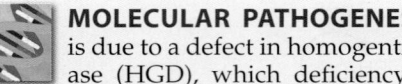 **MOLECULAR PATHOGENESIS:** Alkaptonuria is due to a defect in homogentisate 1,2-dioxygenase (HGD), which deficiency prevents catabolism of homogentisic acid (HGA), an intermediate product in the tyrosine degradation pathway. HGA and its oxide, alkapton, accumulate in the blood and are excreted in urine in large amounts (Fig. 6-21).

 PATHOLOGY AND CLINICAL FEATURES: Patients with alkaptonuria excrete urine that darkens rapidly on standing, because of a pigment formed by nonenzymatic HGA oxidation to benzoquinone acetic acid. In long-standing alkaptonuria, a similar pigment deposits in many tissues, especially the sclerae, cartilage in many areas (ribs, larynx, trachea), tendons, and synovial membranes. The pigment is bluish black on visual examination, but is brown under the microscope (hence the term **ochronosis** [color of ocher] coined by Virchow). A degenerative and frequently disabling **arthropathy** ("ochronotic arthritis"). affecting particularly the spine and larger joints, may develop after years of alkaptonuria. Despite affecting many organs, alkaptonuria does not reduce longevity. The diagnosis is based on the detection of a significant amount of HGA in the urine. In addition to management of symptoms and dietary restriction of phenylalanine and tyrosine, pharmacologic treatment with nitisinone, which is approved for tyrosinemia type I (see above) and blocks enzymes in the tyrosine degradation pathway, has shown promising results in clinical trials.

Urea Cycle Disorders (UCD)

The urea cycle provides clearance of waste nitrogen from protein turnover (Fig. 6-22). The urea cycle removes nitrogen from the blood and converts it to a soluble nontoxic

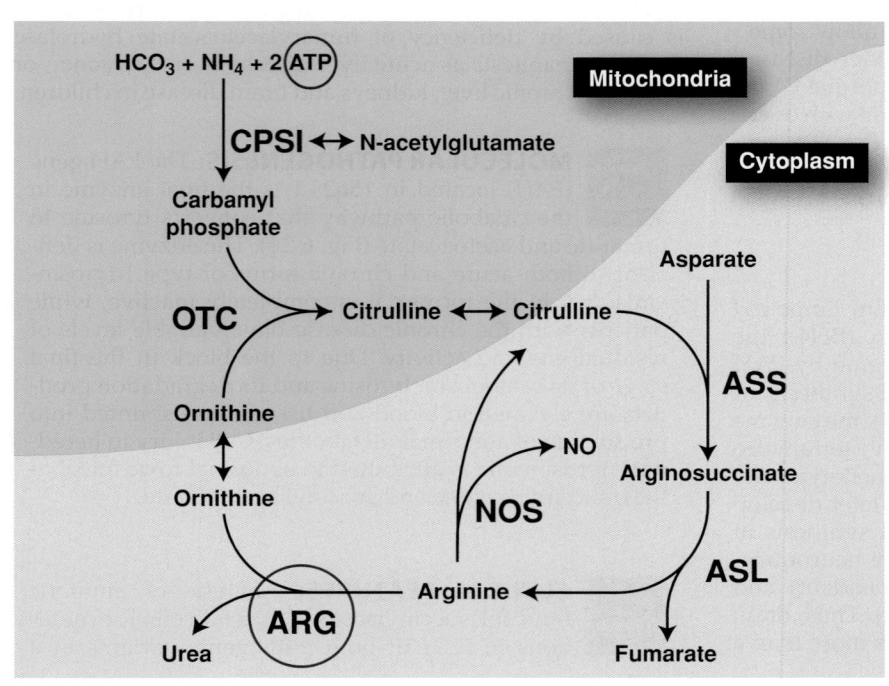

FIGURE 6-22. Schematic representation of the urea cycle. A series of biochemical steps removes waste nitrogen resulting from protein turnover by converting it into urea, a soluble nontoxic compound that is excreted in the urine. Deficiency of any of the urea cycle enzymes results in accumulation of nitrogen in the form of ammonia, which is a highly toxic substance. In addition to its role in ammonia removal, the urea cycle serves as the sole source of endogenous production of the amino acids arginine, ornithine, and citrulline.

TABLE 6-5
UREA CYCLE DEFECTS

Disorder	Incidence	Inheritance	Gene	Chromosomal Location
Carbamoyl phosphate synthetase I deficiency	1/150,000–200,000; 1/800,000 in Japan	AR	CPS1	2q34
Ornithine transcarbamylase deficiency	1/14,000–77,000	XL	OTC	Xp11.4
Argininosuccinate synthase 1 deficiency (Citrullinemia)	1/57,000	AR	ASS1	9q34.11
Argininosuccinate lyase deficiency	1/70,000	AR	ASL	7q11.21
Arginase deficiency	1/300,000–1,000,000	AR	ARG1	6q23.2
N-acetylglutamate synthase deficiency	<1/2,000,000	AR	NAGS	17q21.31

AR = autosomal recessive; XLR = X-linked recessive.

Complete deficiency of any of the urea cycle enzymes results in hyperammonemia, irreversible brain damage, coma and/or death.

Estimated incidence of urea cycle disorders collectively is 1/30,000.

compound urea, which is then excreted in the urine. In urea cycle disorders, nitrogen accumulates as ammonia, which is highly toxic. Hyperammonemia (elevated blood ammonia) can cause irreversible brain damage, coma, and death.

In addition to its role in ammonia removal, the urea cycle is the sole endogenous source producing the amino acids arginine, ornithine, and citrulline. It occurs in the liver and requires participation of multiple catalytic enzymes, cofactors, and amino acid transporters; a defect in any of these important components of the cycle may cause a UCD (Table 6-5). The incidence of UCDs is estimated to be at least 1/30,000 births; partial defects may make the number much higher. The severity of a urea cycle defect reflects the position of the defective protein in the pathway and the amount of its functional enzymatic activity.

 PATHOPHYSIOLOGY: Severe deficiency or total absence of activity of any of the first four enzymes in the pathway or production of the cofactor N-acetylglutamate causes ammonia and other precursor metabolites to accumulate during the first days of life. Because there are no alternative systems for ammonia clearance, complete disruption of the urea pathway results in the rapid accumulation of ammonia and development of related symptoms. Complete deficiencies in urea cycle enzymes thus present in the newborn period, accentuated by the immaturity of the neonatal liver. Affected infants appear normal at birth but rapidly develop cerebral edema and related signs of lethargy, anorexia, hyper- or hypoventilation, hypothermia, seizures, neurologic posturing, and coma. Ammonia can cause brain damage via several mechanisms, a major component being cerebral edema due to rapid accumulation of ammonia and other precursor metabolites. In milder (or partial) urea cycle enzyme deficiencies, ammonia accumulation may be triggered at almost any time of life by illness or stress (e.g., surgery, prolonged fasting, the peripartum period), resulting in multiple mild elevations of plasma ammonia concentration.

 CLINICAL FEATURES: Although clinical manifestations among specific UCDs vary, hyperammonemic episodes are commonly marked by loss of appetite, vomiting, lethargy, and behavioral abnormalities. Sleep disorders, delusions, hallucinations, and psychosis may occur. The diagnosis is established through biochemical evaluation for elevated plasma ammonia concentration.

Treatment of acute manifestations aims to normalization of plasma ammonia levels rapidly, replace deficient urea cycle intermediates, treat the catabolic state with calories from glucose, fats and essential amino acids and use intravenous fluids to reduce risk for neurologic damage. Subsequent treatment is tailored to the specific urea cycle disorder. Although delayed treatment is dangerous, rapid identification and current treatment strategies have improved survival dramatically.

Ornithine Transcarbamylase (OTC) Deficiency

Ornithine transcarbamylase deficiency is the most common UCD. OTC converts carbamoyl phosphate and ornithine into citrulline, and is the final enzyme in the proximal portion of the urea cycle. OTC deficiency is an X-linked recessive defect, unlike other UCDs which are autosomal recessive. OTC thus occurs as a severe neonatal-onset disease in males; females may remain unaffected, although about 15% of carrier females develop hyperammonemia during their lifetime and many require chronic medical management for hyperammonemia. However, carrier females who lacked symptoms of overt hyperammonemia have deficiencies in executive function.

CLINICAL FEATURES: Males with severe neonatal-onset OTC deficiency are typically normal at birth but become symptomatic from hyperammonemia on day 2 to 3 of life. In severely affected individuals, ammonia concentrations increase rapidly, causing ataxia, lethargy, and death without rapid intervention. After successful treatment of neonatal hyperammonemic coma, infants can easily become hyperammonemic again despite appropriate treatment; they typically require liver transplant by age 6 months. Males and heterozygous females with post–neonatal-onset (partial) OTC deficiency can present from infancy to late childhood, adolescence, or adulthood. No matter how mild the disease, a hyperammonemic crisis can be precipitated by stressors and become a life-threatening event at any age and in any situation. Typical neuropsychological complications include developmental delay, learning disabilities, intellectual disability, attention-deficit hyperactivity disorder (ADHD), and executive function deficits.

Inborn Errors of Carbohydrate Metabolism Reflect Failure to Degrade or Synthesize Carbohydrates

Carbohydrates are divided into monosaccharides (glucose, galactose, and fructose), disaccharides (lactose and saccharose), oligosaccharides, and polysaccharides (glycogen and amylase/starch). Defective carbohydrate metabolism includes disorders of monosaccharide transport and anabolism, impaired digestion of dietary disaccharides, glycogen metabolism disorders, and disorders of gluconeogenesis. Of these, galactosemia and hereditary fructose intolerance are the most common (Table 6-6). Abnormalities of glycogen synthesis and degradation are described with lysosomal storage diseases (see below).

Galactosemia (Galactose-1-Phosphate Uridylyltransferase Deficiency)

EPIDEMIOLOGY: The frequency of **classic galactosemia** in the United States is roughly 1/30,000–60,000. It is an autosomal recessive

trait, and occurs in all races and ethnic groups, but is more common among Caucasians, and less among Asians.

MOLECULAR PATHOGENESIS: As a component of the milk sugar lactose, galactose is an important nutrient for newborn infants and young children. In human breast milk, the lactose content is about 7g/dL, and lactose may provide as much as 40% of a newborn's caloric intake. Galactose is also a constituent of many glycoproteins, glycolipids, and mucopolysaccharides.

The principal pathway for galactose metabolism has three steps: (1) galactose is phosphorylated to galactose-1-phosphate (Gal-1-P) by galactokinase, (2) Gal-1-P is exchanged by a transferase for the glucose-1-phosphate moiety of uridine diphosphate glucose (UDP-Glu) to form UDP-galactose (UDP-Gal), and (3) UDP-Gal is converted by an epimerase to UDP-Glu. A deficiency of involved enzymes causes, respectively, galactokinase deficiency (galactosemia II), galactose-1-phosphate uridylyltransferase (GALT) deficiency (galactosemia I) and UDP galactose-4-epimerase deficiency (galactosemia III) (Fig. 6-23). GALT deficiency (G/G, galactosemia I or classic galactosemia, defined as GALT activity below 5% and Gal-1-P buildup greater than 20 mg/dL), is the most prevalent.

Molecular testing can differentiate severe, loss-of-function mutations (G alleles) from decreased-function (hypomorphic) alleles. The most frequent of the latter are Duarte alleles, which have two forms: Duarte-1 (higher activity) and Duarte-2. Because Duarte variants are relatively common, compound heterozygotes with one

TABLE 6-6
DISORDERS OF CARBOHYDRATE METABOLISM

Disorder	Deficient Enzyme	Clinical Features	Frequency	Inheritance	Gene	Chromosomal Location
Galactosemia Type I classic galactosemia (severe)	Galactose 1-phosphate uridylyltransferase	Feeding difficulty, lethargy, failure to thrive, sepsis, liver disease, jaundice, cataracts	1/30,000–60,000 newborns	AR	*GALT*	9p13.3
Galactosemia Type II (mild)	Galactokinase 1	Cataracts in infancy	1/100,000 newborns	AR	*GALK1*	17q25.1
Galactosemia Type III (mild to severe)	Uridine diphosphate galactose-4-epimerase	Cataracts, delayed growth and development, intellectual disability, liver disease, and kidney problems	Rare	AR	*GALE*	1p36.11
Hereditary fructose intolerance	Aldolase B	Nausea, bloating, abdominal pain, diarrhea, vomiting, and hypoglycemia after ingesting fructose; failure to thrive, liver and kidney damage with chronic fructose exposure	1/20,000–30,000 worldwide	AR	*ALDOB*	9q31.1
Glycogen storage diseases (see Table 6-8)						

AR = autosomal recessive.

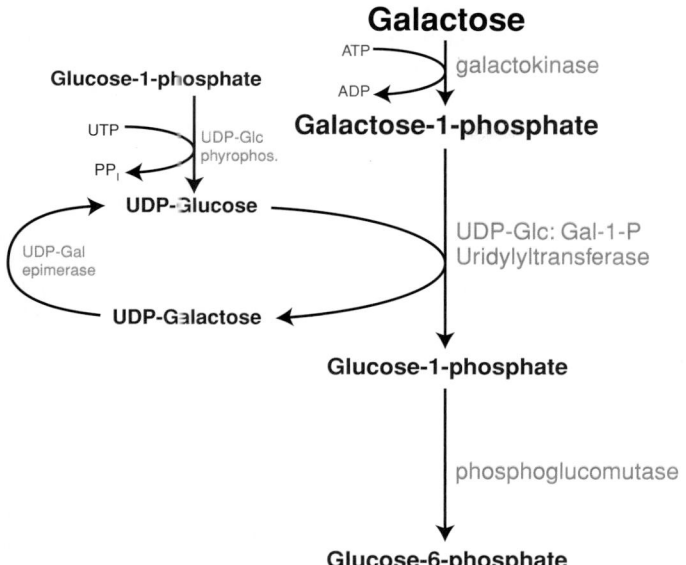

FIGURE 6-23. Galactose metabolism. There are three main steps in the metabolism of galactose: (1) galactose is phosphorylated to galactose-1-phosphate by galactokinase, (2) galactose-1-phosphate is exchanged for the glucose-1-phosphate moiety of uridine diphosphate glucose (UDP-glucose) to form uridine diphosphate galactose (UDP-galactose); the released glucose-1-phosphate feeds into the glucose pathway, and (3) the formed UDP-galactose is converted to UDP-glucose by UDP-galactose-4-epimerase.

Duarte allele and one loss-of-function allele are common, and have about 25% of normal enzyme activity.

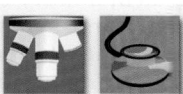 **PATHOLOGY AND CLINICAL FEATURES:** In the classic form, affected infants appear normal at birth, but experience a rapid and devastating decline after drinking breast milk or milk formula, which are high in galactose. Acute symptoms can progress within days from jaundice, vomiting, and diarrhea to failure to thrive, hepatomegaly, and *E. coli* sepsis. Untreated, affected infants often die in the neonatal period. Some patients, have much milder disease and may even escape early detection. Late clinical manifestations in both untreated and treated patients include hypergonadotropic hypogonadism in about 80% of affected women, speech defects in about half and, less often neurologic sequelae. Heterozygotes (carriers), and Duarte variant (D/G) who typically have 25% of normal GALT enzyme activity, show little to no symptoms, slightly elevated metabolites and do not need intervention.

Population newborn screening for galactosemia allows identification of affected newborns before they became critically ill. Treatment aims to minimize accumulation of galactose and its metabolites by replacing milk and milk-containing products with milk substitutes (casein hydrolysates, soy formulas). A galactose-free diet is the basis of treatment, but supplementary measures are often required in neonates to correct secondary manifestations, like hyperbilirubinemia, hypoprothrombinemia, sepsis

with gram-negative organisms and anemia. Patients treated in early infancy can achieve low to normal intelligence scores, but despite dietary lactose restriction, many patients still have learning and/or behavioral problems later in life. Children with Duarte variants do not need a restrictive diet; although they present with elevated levels of galactose metabolites, they have normal levels of erythrocyte Gal-1-P.

Hereditary Fructose Intolerance (HFI)

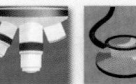 **EPIDEMIOLOGY:** The frequency of HFI in the general population is uncertain because many patients remain unrecognized. In some European countries (Switzerland), incidence may reach 1 in 20,000.

MOLECULAR PATHOGENESIS: Fructose is a monosaccharide found in honey, fruits, vegetables, and plants. It combines with glucose to form sucrose. Ingested sucrose is hydrolyzed by intestinal sucrase to glucose and fructose. The liver plays a dominant role in fructose metabolism by converting it into glycolytic intermediates: **fructokinase**-catalyzed phosphorylation to fructose-1-phosphate (F-1-P), which is further metabolized to glycolytic intermediates D-glyceraldehyde and dihydroxyacetone phosphate by F-1-P aldolase or aldolase B. *The biochemical defect in HFI is a deficiency of liver F-1-P aldolase (aldolase B).* Lacking aldolase B activity causes F-1-P to accumulate. In addition to its immediate toxicity, F-1-P excess inhibits gluconeogenesis and causing hypoglycemia, and interferes with ATP regeneration.

PATHOLOGY AND CLINICAL FEATURES: Affected individuals are asymptomatic and healthy, if they do not ingest foods containing fructose or any of its common precursors, sucrose and sorbitol. Symptoms appear when the person ingests these substances. In the past, infants often became symptomatic when they were fed formulas sweetened with fructose or sucrose (which are not common in formulas today). Symptoms such as vomiting, nausea, restlessness, pallor, sweating, trembling, and lethargy can also first present when infants are introduced to fruits and vegetables. The symptoms can progress to apathy, coma, and convulsions if the source is not recognized early. A dietary history will often reveal an aversion to fruit and other foods high in fructose. Interestingly, most adult patients do not have any dental caries, probably because they avoid eating sucrose and fructose. HFI is not clinically devastating, but deaths are reported in infants and children as a result of the metabolic consequences of HFI.

HFI may be suspected on clinical grounds, but laboratory confirmation is necessary. Treatment entails dietary exclusion of foods containing fructose and its precursors sucrose or sorbitol. Prognosis for treated patients is good. Liver and kidney damage is reversed, and neurologic deficits are uncommon.

Lysosomal Storage Diseases Reflect Mutations Impairing Lysosomal Function

Lysosomes (see Chapter 1) serve to degrade material taken up from outside the cell, to remove intracellular aggregates and to digest obsolete organelles. Lysosomal digestive enzymes, **acid hydrolases** operate optimally at low pH (pH 3.5 to 5.5), which is maintained by an ATP-dependent proton pump in the lysosomal membrane. Lysosomal enzymes degrade virtually all types of organic macromolecules including lipids, glycoproteins, and mucopolysaccharides. Extracellular macromolecules that are internalized by endocytosis or phagocytosis and intracellular constituents that are subjected to autophagy are digested in lysosomes to their basic components. End-products are recycled for biosynthetic and other purposes.

Lysosomal degradative enzymes include nucleases, proteases, glycosidases, lipases, phosphatases, sulfatases, and phospholipases. Deficiency in any of these acid hydrolases can prevent catabolism of the normal macromolecular substrate of that enzyme. As a result, undigested substrates accumulate in, and engorge lysosomes, expanding the lysosomal compartment of the cell. Resulting lysosomal distention impairs other critical cellular activities, particularly in the brain and heart, and can lead to poor cellular function or cell death.

Lysosomal storage diseases are classified by the material retained in the lysosomes (Table 6-7): accumulated sphingolipids cause **sphingolipidoses**; mucopolysaccharides (glycosaminoglycans) lead to **mucopolysaccharidoses**, etc. Over 50 lysosomal storage diseases are known, but only the most important examples are discussed here.

Glycogen Storage Diseases (Glycogenoses)

At least 14 inherited disorders are characterized by glycogen accumulation, mainly in liver, skeletal muscle, and heart (Table 6-8). Each disease reflects a deficiency of one of the enzymes involved in glycogen metabolism (Fig. 6-24). Except for the X-linked phosphorylase kinase deficiency, all are autosomal recessive traits, with a collective incidence of 1 in 20,000 to 25,000 births.

Glycogen is a large branched glucose polymer (20,000 to 30,000 glucose moieties per molecule) that is stored in most

TABLE 6-7
LYSOSOMAL STORAGE DISEASE GROUPS

Disease Groups[a]	Accumulated Substrate
Mucopolysaccharidoses	Mucopolysaccharides (glycosaminoglycans)
Mucolipidoses	Complex carbohydrates and lipids
Sphingolipidoses	Sphingolipids
Gangliosidoses	Gangliosides
Neuronal ceroid lipofuscinoses	Lipopigment (lipofuscin)
Glycogen storage diseases	Glycogen

[a]Lysosomal storage diseases are grouped by the class of undigested intermediate substrate that accumulates in lysosomes.

cells as a ready source of energy during fasting. Liver and muscle are particularly rich in glycogen, these two organs use it differently. The liver stores glycogen, not for its own use, but rather to supply glucose quickly to the blood for use in other organs, particularly the brain. Skeletal muscle uses glycogen as a local energy source when oxygen or glucose supplies drop.

Glycogen is degraded by several enzymes, deficiency of any of which leads to its accumulation. Regulation of hepatic glycogen degradation (glycogenolysis) is complex. The best understood mechanism involves activation of adenylate cyclase by glucagon and epinephrine. This increases cAMP levels in the cytosol, leading to activation of phosphorylase kinase (PK), which in rapid sequence phosphorylates and activates phosphorylase. Phosphorylase acts upon the termini of glycogen chains, liberating glucose-1-phosphate. Debrancher enzyme removes branch points and liberates free glucose (Fig. 6-24).

Organ involvement in glycogen storage disorders depends upon the specific enzyme defect. Some glycogen storage diseases mainly affect the liver; others principally cause cardiac or skeletal muscle dysfunction. Symptoms of these diseases may reflect accumulation of glycogen itself (Pompe disease, Andersen disease) or lack of the glucose normally derived from glycogen degradation (von Gierke disease, McArdle disease). Representative glycogen storage diseases are described below.

Von Gierke Disease (Type IA Glycogenosis)
Von Gierke disease is caused by deficiency of glucose-6-phosphatase, which converts glucose-6-phosphate to glucose and is important in glycogenolysis and gluconeogenesis. In affected individuals, glycogen accumulates in the liver, and symptoms reflect the inability of the liver to convert glycogen to glucose, leading to hepatomegaly and hypoglycemia. The disorder usually presents in infancy or early childhood, with marked hepatomegaly and symptoms of hypoglycemia. More severely affected infants and children are prone to severe lactic acidosis during minor infections. Untreated children have significant growth retardation. Treatment aims to maintain euglycemia by frequent feedings of carbohydrate, and dietary supplementation with uncooked cornstarch. Although mortality during childhood was once high, the prognosis now is generally good for normal mental development and longevity.

Pompe Disease (Type IIA Glycogenosis)
Pompe disease is a lysosomal storage disease that involves virtually all organs. Its most severe infantile form is characterized by muscle weakness, with death from heart failure in the first year of life. Juvenile and adult variants are less common and have better prognoses. Incidence is 1 in 40,000 for infantile GSD II, and 1 in 60,000 for adult GSD II. Normally, a small proportion of cytoplasmic glycogen is degraded within lysosomes after an autophagic sequence. Type II glycogenosis is caused by defects in this process of lysosomal glycogen degradation, due to mutations in the *GAA* gene which encodes lysosomal acid α-glucosidase (also called acid maltase). Enzyme deficiency causes undegraded glycogen to accumulate in lysosomes of diverse cell types. Patients do not develop hypoglycemia, because the main metabolic pathways of glycogen synthesis and degradation are intact.

TABLE 6-8
GLYCOGEN STORAGE DISEASES (GLYCOGENOSES)

Disorder	Disease	Deficient Enzyme	Clinical Features	Frequency	Inheritance	Gene	Chromosomal Location
GSD 0		Muscle glycogen synthase	Hypoglycemia, muscle pain and weakness or episodes of fainting (syncope) following moderate physical activity, long QT syndrome	Unknown	AR	GYS1	19q13.33
		Liver glycogen synthase				GYS2	12p12.1
GSD I	von Gierke disease	Glucose 6-phosphatase (GSD Ia)	Hypoglycemia, lactic acidosis, hyperuricemia, hyperlipidemia, hepatomegaly, short stature, thin extremities, (type Ib—neutropenia, inflammatory bowel disease, oral problems)	1/100,000 (both types combined)	AR	G6PC	17q21.31
		Glucose 6-phosphate translocase (GSD Ib)				SLC37A4	11q23.3
GSD II	Pompe disease	Acid α-glucosidase (acid maltase)	Myopathy, hypotonia, hepatomegaly, cardiac failure	1/40,000 (infantile-onset) 1/60,000 (late-onset)	AR	GAA	17q25.3
GSD III (types IIIa-d)	Cori disease	Glycogen debranching enzyme	Mainly affects liver and muscle (skeletal and cardiac), hypoglycemia, hyperlipidemia, elevated liver enzymes, hepatomegaly	1/100,000 in US 1/5,400 in North African Jewish	AR	AGL	1p21.2
GSD IV	Andersen disease	Glycogen branching enzyme	Mainly affects liver and muscle (skeletal and cardiac), severity ranges from the fatal perinatal neuromuscular type to the childhood neuromuscular type	1/600,00–800,000 worldwide	AR	GBE1	3p12.2
GSD V	McArdle disease	Myophosphorylase	Fatigue, muscle pain, cramps within first few minutes of exercise (exercise intolerance), rhabdomyolysis	1/100,000	AR	PYGM	11q13.1
GSD VI	Hers disease	Liver glycogen phosphorylase	Hepatomegaly, hypoglycemia, lactic acidosis, symptoms vary and improve with age	Rare; 1/1,000 in Old Order Mennonites	AR	PYGL	14q22.1
GSD VII	Tarui disease	Phosphofructo-kinase	Results in muscle breakdown with exercise, myoglobinuria, hyperuricemia, jaundice, cardiomyopathy	Rare	AR	PFKM	12q13.11
GSD IX		Phosphorylase b kinase (α1-subunit)	Hepatomegaly, slow growth, hypoglycemia and ketosis with fasting, delayed motor development, delayed puberty, exercise intolerance in some	1/100,000	XLR	PHKA1	Xq13.1
		Phosphorylase b kinase (α2-subunit)			XLR	PHKA2	Xp22.13
		Phosphorylase b kinase (β-subunit)			AR	PHKB	16q12.1
		Phosphorylase b kinase (γ2-subunit)			AR	PHKG2	16p11.2

AR = autosomal recessive; XLR = X-linked recessive.

Without enzyme replacement therapy, patients with infantile-onset Pompe disease die from cardiorespiratory failure or respiratory infection. For people with late-onset Pompe disease, prognosis depends on age of onset: later onset generally means slower disease progression. Ultimately, prognosis depends on the extent of respiratory muscle involvement. Enzyme replacement therapy via infusion of recombinant acid α-glucosidase is current definitive treatment for Pompe disease.

McArdle Disease (Type V Glycogenosis)
In **McArdle disease**, glycogen accumulates in skeletal muscles, due to a lack of muscle phosphorylase, the enzyme that releases glucose-1-phosphate from glycogen. The disorder

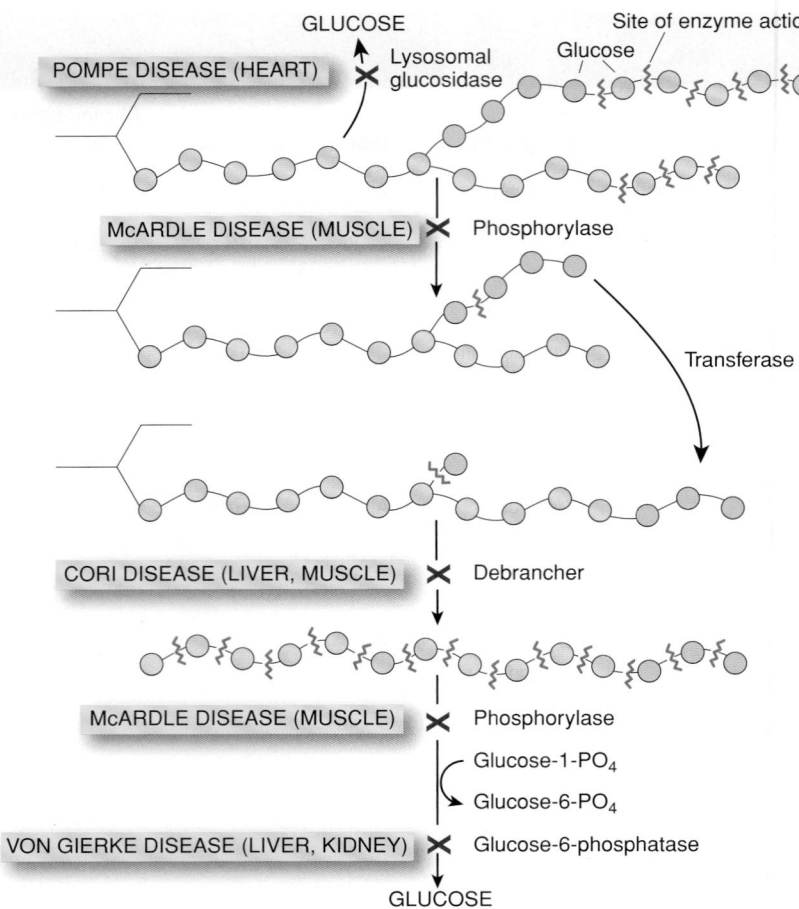

FIGURE 6-24. Sequential catabolism of glycogen and enzymes that are deficient in various glycogenoses. Glycogen is a long-chain branched polymer of glucose residues connected by α-1,4 linkages, except at branch points, where an α-1,6 linkage is present. Phosphorylase hydrolyzes α-1,4 linkages to a point three glucose residues distal to an α-1,6–linked sugar. These three glucose residues are transferred to the chain linked by α-1,4 bonds, by the bifunctional debrancher enzyme amylo-1,6-glucosidase. Subsequently, the same enzyme removes the α-1,6–linked sugar at the original branch point. This creates a linear α-1,4 chain, which is degraded by phosphorylase to glucose-1-phosphate. Following the conversion to glucose-6-phosphate, glucose is released by the action of glucose-6-phosphatase. A small proportion of glycogen is totally degraded within lysosomes by acid α-glucosidase. Red x's indicate a metabolic block and its associated glycogen storage disease.

is caused by mutations in the gene for myophosphorylase, *PYGM*. A large number of different mutations, which vary among ethnic groups, are implicated. Symptoms usually appear in adolescence or early adulthood. Patients have muscle cramps and spasms during exercise, which may lead to myocytolysis and myoglobinuria, as a result of deficient energy production in muscle. Aerobic exercise and high-protein diets have been effective treatment for some patients.

Sphingolipidoses

Sphingolipidoses are lysosomal storage diseases in which lipids derived from turnover of obsolete cell membranes accumulate (Table 6-9). The primary component of sphingolipids is sphingosine, an 18-carbon amino alcohol with an unsaturated hydrocarbon chain. Sphingolipids are classified by the nature of the side residues attached to sphingosine, including cerebrosides, sphingomyelin, and gangliosides (Fig. 6-25). These are degraded within lysosomes by complex pathways, producing sphingosine and fatty acids (Fig. 6-26). Deficiencies of acid hydrolases that mediate specific steps in these pathways lead to accumulation of undigested intermediate substrates in lysosomes.

Tay–Sachs Disease (TSD)

TSD, or hexosaminidase A deficiency, is a severe infantile form of a class of lysosomal storage diseases called GM2-gangliosidoses. Named for Warren Tay, a British ophthalmologist, and Bernard Sachs, an American neurologist, it

is the most common of GM2-gangliosidoses. Other GM2-gangliosidoses (**Sandhoff disease** and **GM2-gangliosidosis, AB variant**) are very rare, but resemble TSD clinically. In these diseases a glycosphingolipid abundant in cell membranes (a ganglioside called GM2) deposits in CNS neurons, because of faulty lysosomal degradation.

EPIDEMIOLOGY: Tay–Sachs disease is an autosomal recessive trait, mainly occurring in Ashkenazi Jews and French Canadians, among whom the carrier rate is about 1 in 30. One if 4,000 live newborns is an affected homozygote. The incidence in non–Jewish Americans is <1 in 100,000. Although carrier frequency in Ashkenazi Jews is similar to that in French Canadians, the two groups harbor different mutations. Interestingly, Cajuns of southern Louisiana carry the mutation seen mostly in Ashkenazi Jews, which has been traced back to a founder couple in 18th-century France. Screening programs for heterozygous Ashkenazi Jews have reduced incidence of TSD by 90%.

MOLECULAR PATHOGENESIS: Gangliosides are glycosphingolipids with a ceramide (sphingosine + fatty acid) and an oligosaccharide chain that contains *N*-acetylneuraminic (sialic) acid (Fig. 6-25). They occur in the outer leaflet of animal cell membranes,

TABLE 6-9
SPHINGOLIPIDOSES

Disorder	Clinical Features	Deficient Enzyme	Frequency	Inheritance	Gene	Chromosomal Location
Tay–Sachs disease (GM2-gangliosidosis)	Loss of developmental skills starting at 3–6 months, hypotonia, seizures, retinal cherry red spot, death in early childhood	Hexosaminidase A	1/4,000 in Ashkenazi Jews, French Canadians, Old Amish and Louisiana Cajun <1/100,000 in others	AR	*HEXA*	15q23
Gaucher disease type 1	Nonneuropathic, hepatosplenomegaly, anemia, thrombocytopenia, bone problems	β-glucocerebrosidase	Type 1 1/500–1,000 in Ashkenazi Jews Other types 150,000–100,000	AR	*GBA*	1q2
Gaucher disease type 2	Similar to type 1 and CNS abnormalities (abnormal eye movements, seizures, brain damage)					
Gaucher disease type 3	Similar to type 2 but with later onset and slower progression					
Gaucher disease Perinatal lethal	Hydrops, ichthyosis, hepatosplenomegaly, distinctive facial features, severe neurologic problems					
Niemann–Pick disease type A	Infantile form, hepatosplenomegaly, failure to thrive, developmental regression, interstitial lung disease, retinal cherry red spot, death in early childhood	Acid sphingomyelinase	Type A 1/40,000 Ashkenazi Jews Types A and B 1/250,000 in other population	AR	*SMPD1*	11p15.4
Niemann–Pick disease type B	Similar to type A but with later onset and slower progression, survival into adulthood					
Niemann–Pick disease types C1 and C2	Childhood onset, ataxia, vertical supranuclear gaze palsy, dystonia, severe liver and interstitial lung disease, difficulty with speech and swallowing, intellectual decline, seizures, survival into adulthood	NPC intracellular cholesterol transporters 1 (type C1) and 2 (type C2)	Types C1 and C2 1/150,000 most common in French Acadians in Nova Scotia	AR	*NPC1* *NPC2*	18q11.2 14q24.3

AR = autosomal recessive.

particularly in brain neurons. Lysosomal catabolism of ganglioside GM2, 1 of 12 known gangliosides in the brain, requires β-hexosaminidases (A and B). β-hexosaminidase A has one α-subunit, encoded by the *HEXA* gene in 15q23-24 plus one β-subunit, encoded by the *HEXB* gene in 5q13.3. β-hexosaminidase B has two β-subunits. Mutations in the *HEXB* gene thus cause deficiency of both β-hexosaminidase A and B. In addition, both β-hexosaminidases need GM2 ganglioside activator protein for their function, and deficiency of that activator can also cause clinical disease.

TSD is due to mutations in *HEXA*. Many *HEXA* mutations occur at significant frequencies in specific populations. TSD in Ashkenazi Jews usually results from a 4-nucleotide insertion in exon 11 of *HEXA*. Over 2/3 of Ashkenazi Jewish carriers of TSD (about 2% of that population) have this mutation. β-subunits are synthesized normally and associate to form hexosaminidase B dimers, levels of which are normal or increased in TSD.

Sandhoff disease is caused by mutations in *HEXB*. **GM2-gangliosidosis, AB variant** results from defective synthesis of GM2 ganglioside activator protein, despite

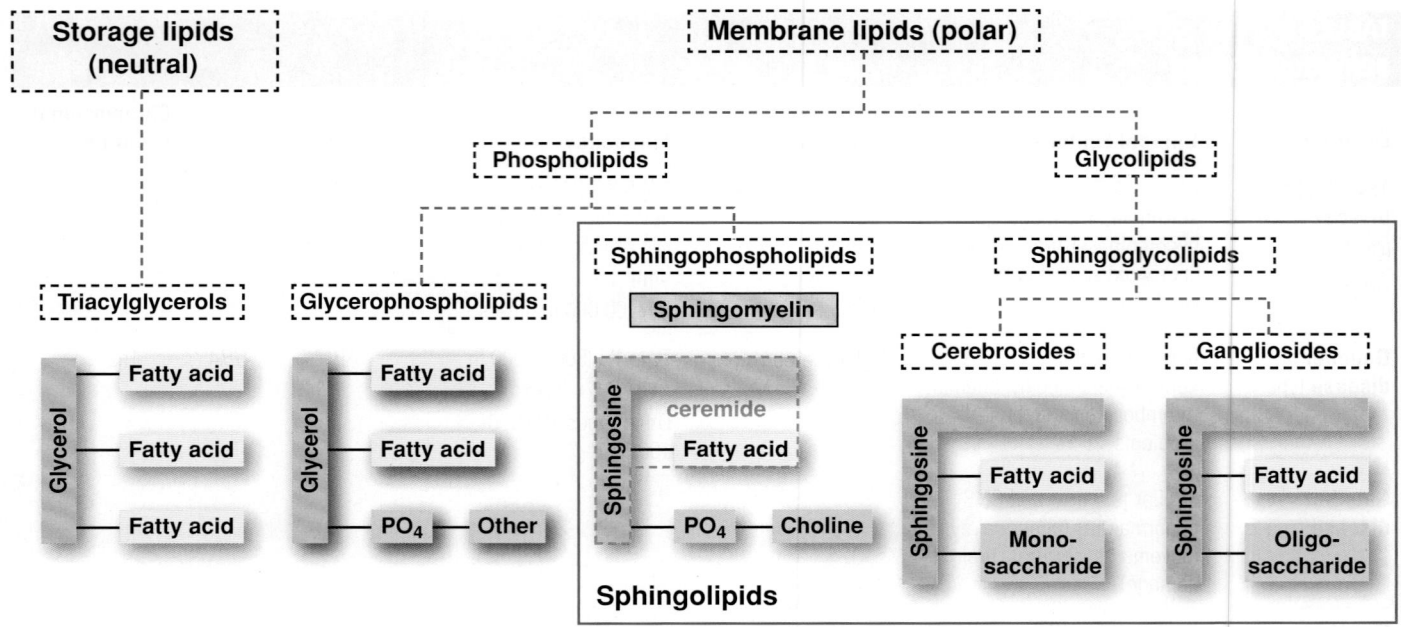

FIGURE 6-25. Different types of lipids based on composition and function. Nonpolar nonsoluble lipids (triacylglycerols) mostly provide energy reserves, while different types of polar lipids mainly serve as structural components of biologic membranes. One class of lipids abundant in biologic membranes are glycerophospholipids, which have fatty acids linked to carbons 1 and 2 of the glycerol backbone. Phosphate is linked to carbon 3, while one of several possible substituents is linked to the phosphate moiety. Sphingolipids are another large class of polar lipids that rather than glycerol have an 18-carbon amino-alcohol sphingosine as the backbone. The simplest sphingolipids are the ceramides, which contain a sphingosine plus a fatty acid. The other sphingolipids are derivatives of ceramides. Sphingomyelins are the only phosphorus-containing sphingolipids, and have a phosphate and choline or phosphate and ethanolamine attached to ceramide. Glycosphingolipids are a large group of sphingolipids in which a simple or more complex sugar molecules are attached to ceramides.

normal activities of both hexosaminidases. This activator is encoded by *GM2A* at 5q33.1.

PATHOLOGY: GM2-ganglioside accumulates in lysosomes of all organs in TSD disease, but it is most prominent in brain neurons and retinal cells. The size of the brain varies with the length of survival of affected infants. Early lethal cases are marked by brain atrophy, but the organ weight may be as much as doubled in those who survive beyond a year. Neurons are markedly distended with stored undegraded gangliosides, membranous cytoplasmic bodies of concentric

whorls of lamellar structures (Fig. 6-27). As the disease progresses, neurons are lost and lipid-laden macrophages accumulate in cortical gray matter. Eventually, gliosis becomes prominent and myelin and axons in the white matter die. Pathologies of the other GM2-gangliosidoses are similar, but usually less severe.

CLINICAL FEATURES: The phenotypes of hexosaminidase A deficiency include the (1) acute infantile form (TSD) with rapid progression and early death, (2) juvenile (subacute) form with later onset and survival into late childhood or adolescence, and

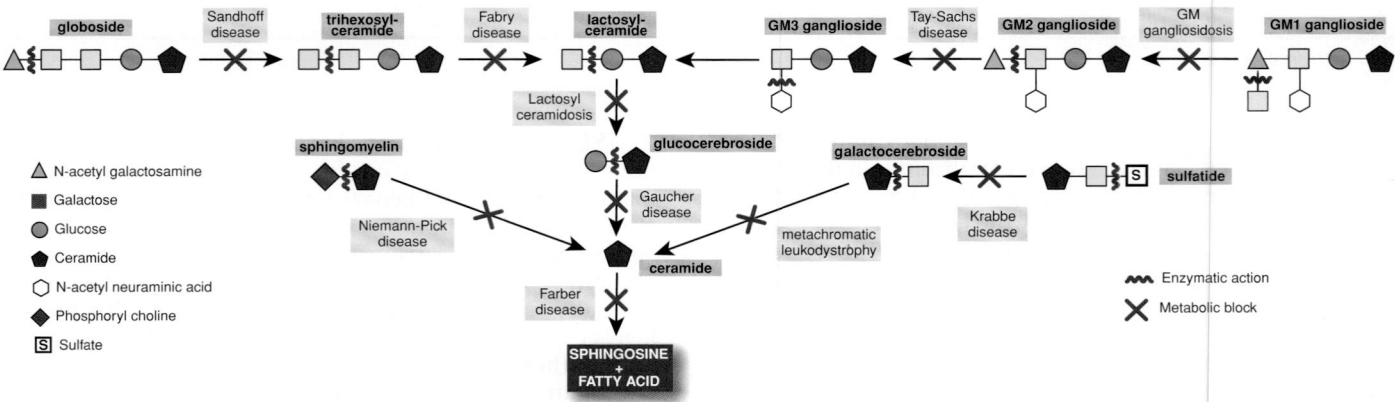

FIGURE 6-26. Disturbances of sphingolipid degradation in various sphingolipidoses.

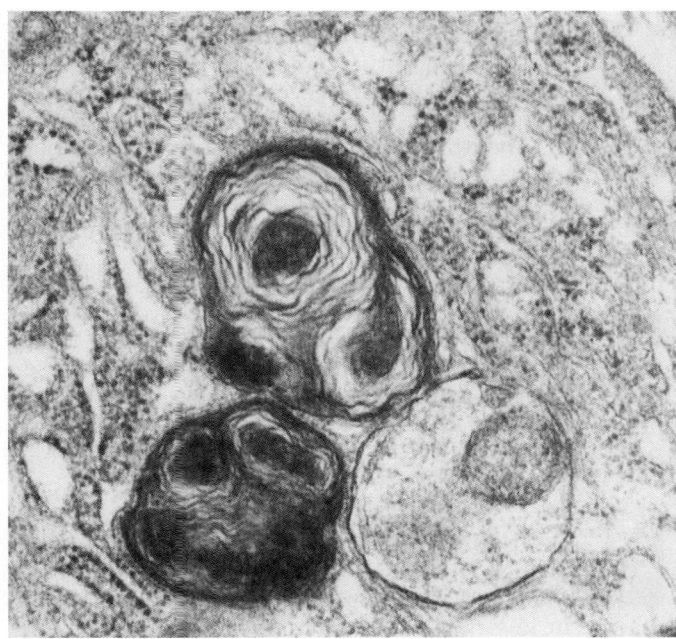

FIGURE 6-27. Tay–Sachs disease. An electron micrograph of a neuron showing lysosomes filled with whorled undegraded membranes.

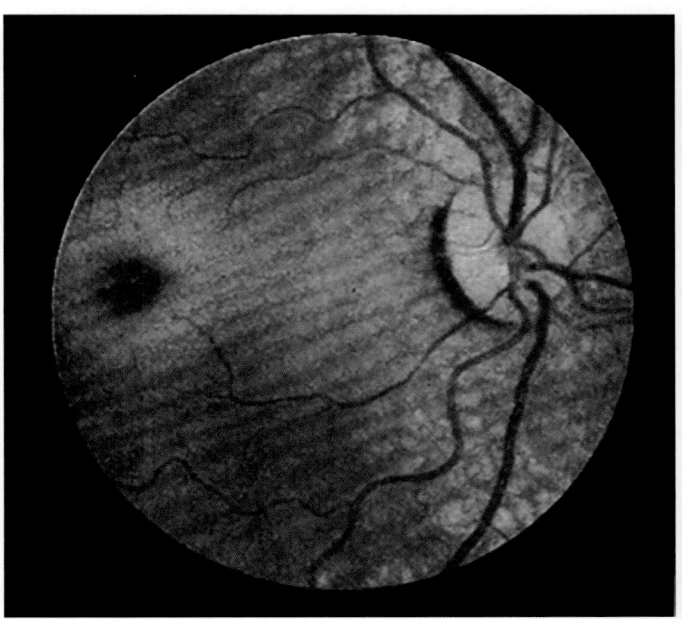

FIGURE 6-28. Macular cherry-red spot of Tay–Sachs disease and other sphingolipidoses. Sphingolipids accumulate in the retinal ganglion cells in the perifoveal area of patients with sphingolipidoses causing the perifoveal area to appear pale. The fovea, which has no ganglion cells, retains its "cherry red" color.

(3) chronic, adult-onset form with long-term survival. Levels of residual HEXA activity vary inversely with the severity of the disease: the lower the HEXA activity level, the more severe the phenotype. TSD presents between 6 and 10 months of age with progressive weakness, hypotonia, and decreased attentiveness. Motor and mental deterioration, often with generalized seizures, follow rapidly. Vision is seriously impaired. Retinal ganglion cell involvement is detected by ophthalmoscopy as a **cherry-red spot** in the macula (Fig. 6-28). This feature reflects the pallor of the affected cells, which enhances the prominence of blood vessels underlying the central fovea. Most children with TSD die before 4 years of age. There is currently no effective treatment for TDS or the other GM2-gangliosidoses.

Niemann–Pick Disease (NPD)

NPD is a form of sphingolipidosis in which catabolism of a cell membrane sphingolipid, **sphingomyelin** is dysfunctional. In these patients, excess sphingomyelin accumulates in macrophage lysosomes in many cells, especially in the liver and brain.

There are several NPD variants. Type A appears in infancy, with hepatosplenomegaly and progressive neurodegeneration. Patients die by 3 years of age. Type B is more variable, with hepatosplenomegaly, minimal neurologic symptomatology, and survival to adulthood. NPD type C is biochemically and genetically distinct from NPD types A and B, and is clinically characterized by variable severity and age of onset.

EPIDEMIOLOGY: The incidence of NPD type A is 1 in 40,000 among Ashkenazi Jews. In all other populations, both types A and B NPD occur in 1 in 250,000. For type C, incidence is 1 in 150,000.

MOLECULAR PATHOGENESIS: Sphingomyelin is a membrane phospholipid made of sphingosine (a long-chain amino alcohol), phosphorylcholine, and a fatty acid (Fig. 6-25). It is especially abundant in the myelin sheaths of nerve axons, and represents up to 14% of phospholipids of the liver, spleen, and brain. The metabolic defects in NPD type A and B reflect different mutations in the *SMPD1* gene at 11p15.4, which encodes acid sphingomyelinase, the lysosomal enzyme that hydrolyzes sphingomyelin to ceramide and phosphorylcholine. In NPD type A enzyme activity is completely absent and in type B it is partially lacking. In type C, most affected individuals carry pathogenic variants in the *NPC1* gene and rare patients have mutations in the *NPC2* gene. NPC1 is not an enzyme but appears to function as a transporter in the endosomal-lysosomal system, which moves large water-insoluble molecules through the cell. The protein encoded by the *NPC2* gene seems to cooperate with NPC1 protein in molecular transport. Disruption of this transport system in patients with NPD type C causes abnormal accumulation of lipid molecules in lysosomes. *NPC1* and *NPC2* gene products mainly help transport cholesterol and glycolipids rather than sphingomyelin.

PATHOLOGY: The characteristic storage cell in NPD is a foam cell— an enlarged (20 to 90 μm) macrophage whose cytoplasm is distended by uniform vacuoles containing sphingomyelin and cholesterol (Fig. 6-29). Foam cells are particularly abundant in the spleen, lymph nodes, and bone marrow but also occur

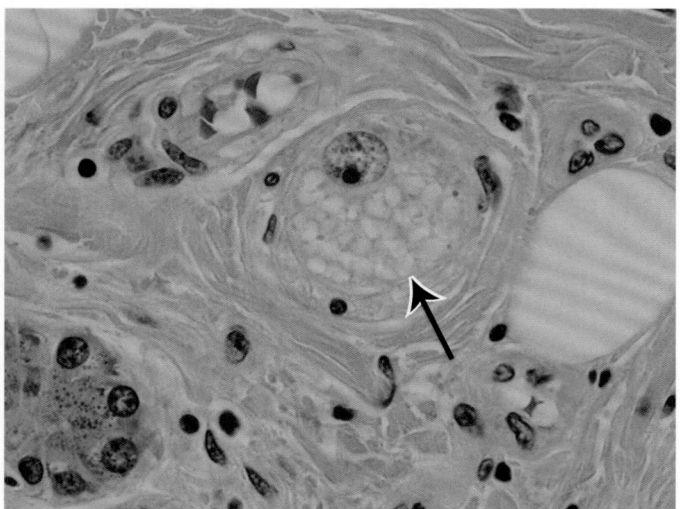

FIGURE 6-29. Niemann–Pick disease foam cell in pancreas, an enlarged (20 to 90 μm) macrophage whose cytoplasm is distended by uniform vacuoles containing sphingomyelin and cholesterol. (Photomicrograph courtesy of David Suster, MD.)

in the liver, lungs, and GI tract. These cells diffusely infiltrate lymphoid organs, often causing massive splenic enlargement by expanding the red pulp expansion, enlarging lymph nodes and displacing hematopoietic elements from the bone marrow. The liver is enlarged by stored sphingomyelin and cholesterol in lysosomes of Kupffer cells and hepatocytes.

The brain is atrophied and in severe cases may be half of normal weight. Neurons are distended by vacuoles containing the same stored lipids found elsewhere in the body. In advanced cases, neuron loss is severe and may be accompanied by demyelination. All children with NPD type A have cherry-red retinal spots, as in TSD.

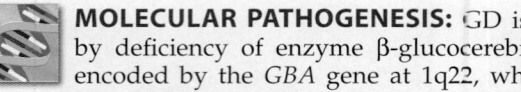

CLINICAL FEATURES: NPD type A manifests in early infancy, with progressive hepatosplenomegaly, interstitial lung disease, and psychomotor retardation. Death before 3 years of age is usually due to neurologic damage. Patients with NPD type B present in childhood and have marked hepatosplenomegaly and pulmonary infiltration with sphingomyelin-laden macrophages that eventually impairs respiratory function. However, these patients have few neurologic symptoms and may survive into adulthood. Symptoms of NPD type C can appear at any time, patients typically present in mid-to-late childhood with the insidious onset of ataxia, vertical supranuclear gaze palsy, and loss of cognitive function. Adults are more likely to present with dementia or psychiatric symptoms.

Gaucher Disease (GD)

GD encompasses varies a disease that is lethal in the perinatal period to asymptomatic. It is characterized by accumulation of glucosylceramide (with glucose as the monosaccharide attached to ceramide), mainly in macrophage lysosomes (Fig. 6-25).

MOLECULAR PATHOGENESIS: GD is caused by deficiency of enzyme β-glucocerebrosidase, encoded by the *GBA* gene at 1q22, which converts glucocerebroside into glucose and ceramide (Fig. 6-26). Abnormal alleles include missense and nonsense variants, splice junction variants, deletions and insertions of one or more nucleotides and complex alleles resulting from gene conversion or recombination with the downstream pseudogene. Diverse mutations may cause each of the clinical types of the disease (see below), although the molecular basis for the phenotypic differences remains unclear. Diagnosis, regardless of type, requires demonstration of deficient β-glucocerebrosidase enzyme activity in nucleated cells (usually blood leukocytes). Molecular testing provides additional confirmation by identifying two disease-causing alleles in *GBA*.

PATHOLOGY: The hallmark of Gaucher disease is the presence of **Gaucher cells.** These lipid-laden cells come from resident macrophages, may occur in virtually any organ but are most abundant in the red pulp of the spleen, liver sinusoids, lymph nodes, lungs, and bone marrow. In variants of Gaucher disease with CNS involvement, Gaucher cells originate from periadventitial cells in Virchow–Robin spaces. The incompletely metabolized glucosylceramide that accumulates in Gaucher cells derives principally from catabolism of membranes of senescent leukocytes, which are rich in cerebrosides. In the CNS, accumulated glucosylceramide is believed to originate from the turnover of membrane gangliosides, and neuronal cell death may be the basis of neurologic involvement.

Gaucher cells are large (20 to 100 μm), with eccentric nuclei. Their clear cytoplasm (Fig. 6-30) has a characteristic fibrillar appearance, resembling wrinkled tissue paper and staining intensely positively with periodic acid–Schiff (PAS) stain. The material is stored in enlarged lysosomes and appears as parallel layers of tubular structures.

Splenomegaly is virtually universal in Gaucher disease. In adult forms of the disease, spleens may weigh up to 10 kg. The cut surface of the enlarged spleen is firm

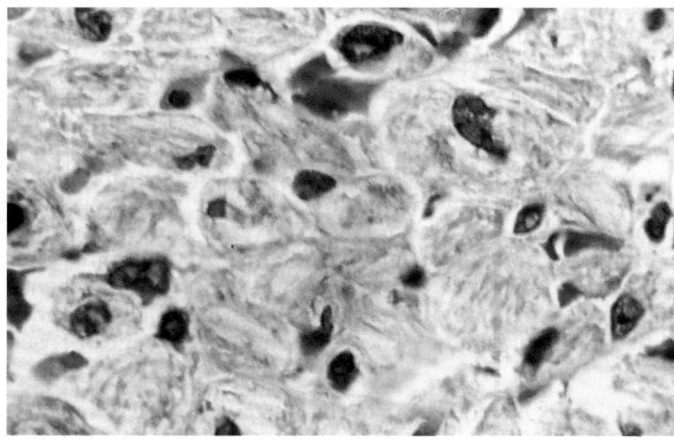

FIGURE 6-30. The spleen in Gaucher disease. Typical Gaucher cells have eccentrically located nuclei and abundant cytoplasm that resembles wrinkled tissue paper.

and pale, often with sharply demarcated infarcts. The red pulp shows nodular and diffuse infiltrates of Gaucher cells and moderate fibrosis.

The liver is usually enlarged by Gaucher cells within sinusoids, but hepatocytes are not affected. In severe cases, hepatic fibrosis and even cirrhosis may ensue. Bone marrow involvement varies but leads to radiologic abnormalities in 50% to 75% of cases. Gaucher cells may also be found in many other organs, including lymph nodes, lungs, endocrine glands, skin, GI tract and kidneys, but symptoms reflecting involvement of these organs are uncommon.

In infantile (neuronopathic) forms of the disease, Gaucher cells are also seen in the brain parenchyma, where they may stimulate gliosis and microglial nodules.

 CLINICAL FEATURES: GD is classified into three forms, based on the age at onset and degree of neurologic involvement:

- **Type 1 (non-neuronopathic Gaucher disease):** This variant is the most common lysosomal storage disease. It occurs in 1 per 40,000 to 60,000 in the general population. But, among Ashkenazi Jews the carrier rate is 1 in 12 and disease prevalence is 1 in 500 to 1,000. Age at onset varies from infancy to old age. The severity of clinical manifestations also varies widely. Most patients are diagnosed in adulthood, and present with painless splenomegaly and complications of hypersplenism including anemia, leukopenia, and thrombocytopenia. Hepatomegaly is common, but clinical liver disease is infrequent. Skeletal involvement, manifesting as bone pain, pathologic fractures and arthritis can cause disability severe enough to confine a patient to a wheelchair.
- **Type 2 and Type 3 (neuronopathic Gaucher disease):** Individuals affected with GD who have CNS involvement in addition to the problems described above are classified as type 2 or type 3 GD based on the age of onset of neurologic signs and symptoms and the rate of disease progression. Type 2 GD is more severe, with disease manifesting in infants, who show a classic triad of trismus (spasm of the jaw muscles causing the mouth to remain tightly closed), strabismus (eyes appear to be looking in different directions) and backward flexion of the neck. Seizures also occur. Further neurologic deterioration rapidly ensues and most patients die by age 3 years. Individuals with type 3 GD may present before age 2 years, but often have a more slowly progressive course, with life span extending into the third or fourth decade in some cases. The distinction between types 2 and 3 GD is not absolute and neuronopathic GD represents a phenotypic continuum.
- Additional types of GD include a perinatal lethal form with hydrops fetalis, hepatosplenomegaly, skin and neurologic abnormalities, and a cardiovascular type that primarily affects the heart, causing valvular calcification.

Enzyme replacement therapy (ERT) is available for GD, and provides sufficient exogenous enzyme to overcome the catabolic block, clear stored substrate, and reverse hematologic and liver/spleen involvement. Bone marrow transplantation (BMT), once used for individuals with severe chronic neurologic involvement (GD type 3), has largely been superseded by ERT. Prenatal diagnosis, whether by measuring β-glucosidase activity, or prenatal DNA testing are **routinely available**.

Mucopolysaccharidoses (MPSs)

MPSs are lysosomal diseases in which **glycosaminoglycans (mucopolysaccharides)** accumulate in many organs. All are inherited as autosomal recessive traits, except for Hunter syndrome, which is X-linked recessive. These rare diseases are caused by deficiencies in lysosomal enzymes that catabolize glycosaminoglycans (Fig. 6-31). The six abnormal MPS phenotypes vary with the specific enzyme deficiency (Table 6-10).

 MOLECULAR PATHOGENESIS: Glycosaminoglycans (GAGs) are large polymers of repeating **disaccharide** units containing N-acetylhexosamine plus a hexose or hexuronic acid. Either disaccharide may be sulfated. The accumulated GAGs (**dermatan sulfate, heparan sulfate, keratan sulfate,** and **chondroitin sulfate**) in MPSs all derive from cleavage of proteoglycans, which are important extracellular matrix constituents. GAGs are degraded stepwise by removing sulfates or sugar residues. Thus, a deficiency in any one of the glycosidases or sulfatases causes undegraded GAGs to accumulate and causes an MPS. An exception is Sanfilippo C disease, in which an N-acetyltransferase is lacking, leading to heparan sulfate deposition.

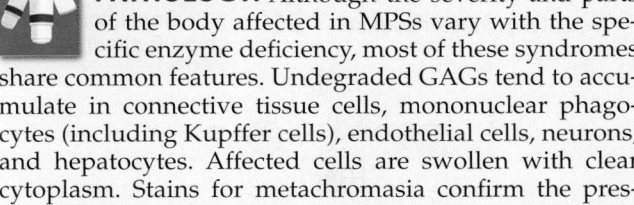 **PATHOLOGY:** Although the severity and parts of the body affected in MPSs vary with the specific enzyme deficiency, most of these syndromes share common features. Undegraded GAGs tend to accumulate in connective tissue cells, mononuclear phagocytes (including Kupffer cells), endothelial cells, neurons, and hepatocytes. Affected cells are swollen with clear cytoplasm. Stains for metachromasia confirm the presence of GAGs. Enlarged lysosomes contain granular or striped material. The most critically involved sites include the CNS, skeleton and heart, but hepatosplenomegaly and corneal clouding are common.

- Initially, the **CNS** only accumulates GAGs, but as disease advances, there is extensive neuronal death and gliosis, leading to cortical atrophy. Communicating hydrocephalus, due to meningeal involvement, is common.
- **Skeletal deformities** reflect GAG accumulation in chondrocytes, which eventually interferes with normal endochondral ossification. Abnormal foci of osteoid and woven bone are common in the deformed skeleton.
- **Cardiac** involvement is often severe, with thickened, distorted valve leaflets, chordae tendineae, and endocardium. Coronary arteries are often narrowed due to proliferation of intimal smooth muscle cells containing GAG deposits.
- **Hepatosplenomegaly** is secondary to distention of Kupffer cells and hepatocytes, and accumulation of GAG-filled macrophages in the spleen.

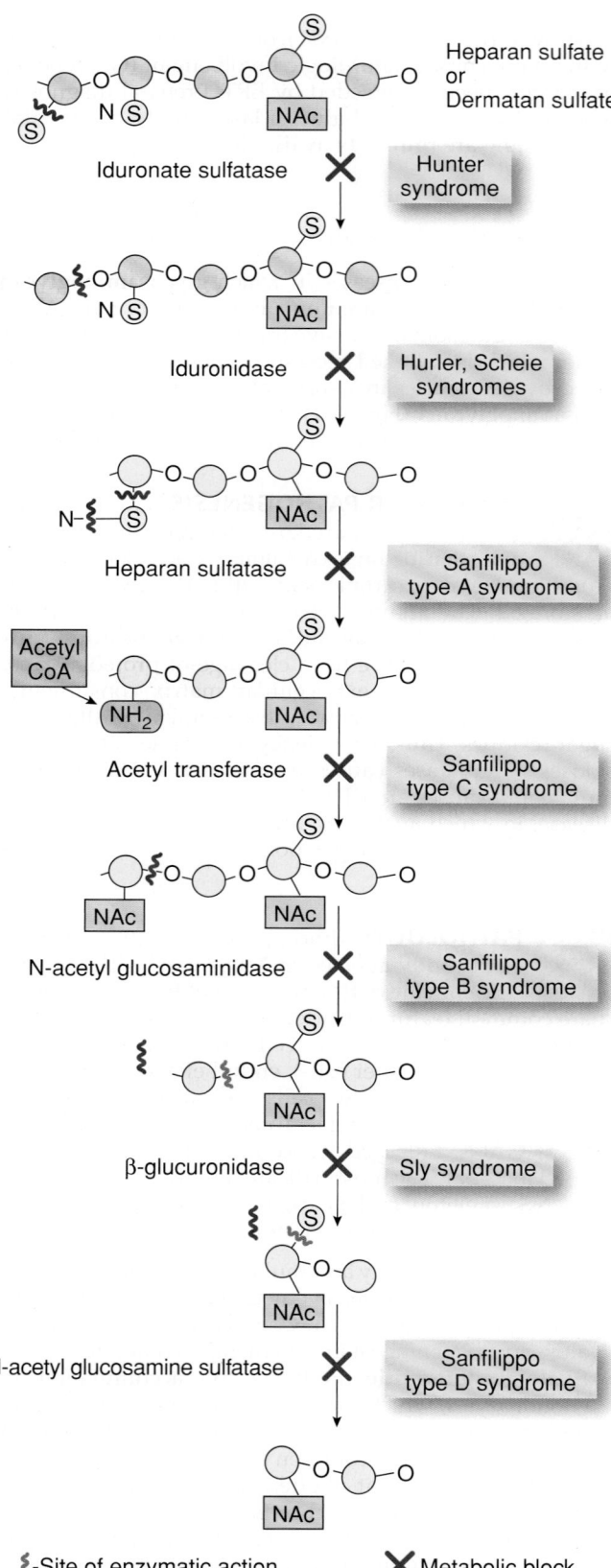

§ -Site of enzymatic action ✗ Metabolic block

FIGURE 6-31. Metabolic blocks in mucopolysaccharidoses. Deficiency in the enzymes involved in the degradation of glycosaminoglycans results in the various mucopolysaccharidoses. Acetyl CoA = acetyl coenzyme A; NAc = *N*-acetyl moiety.

MPS I exemplifies the MPSs. Once separated into three syndromes based on severity of symptoms, it is now considered either severe (originally called **Hurler syndrome**) or attenuated. MPS I is caused by α-L iduronidase (IDUA) deficiency. Heparan sulfate and dermatan sulfate accumulate in various tissues. The enzyme defect is caused by homozygous or compound heterozygous mutations in the *IDUA* gene located in 4p16.3.

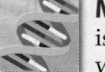 **CLINICAL FEATURES:** In severe MPS I, an umbilical hernia may be present at birth and symptoms appear at 6 months to 2 years. Children typically show macrocephaly (large head) skeletal deformities, hepatosplenomegaly, coarse facies, macroglossia (enlarged tongue), and joint stiffness. Multiple skeletal abnormalities, called *Dysostosis multiplex* in aggregate, can be seen on radiographs. Affected children have deeply hoarse voices, due to accumulated GAGs in their vocal cords. They also suffer developmental delay, hearing loss, corneal clouding, and progressive cognitive deterioration, as well as increased intracranial pressure, due to communicating hydrocephalus. Most patients with severe MPS I die from recurrent pulmonary infections and cardiac complications before 10 years of age. People with the attenuated form of MPS I often live into adulthood and may not have a shortened lifespan. Some, but not all, have intellectual deficits. With both types of MPS I, airway obstruction and heart disease are the major causes of mortality.

The diagnosis is established in a proband with suggestive clinical and laboratory findings by detecting deficient lysosomal α-L-iduronidase activity or identifying biallelic pathogenic *IDUA* gene variants by molecular genetic testing.

Hematopoietic stem cell transplantation (HSCT) is standard of care for children with severe MPS I. Outcomes depend on the patient's age and disease burden at the time of diagnosis. HSCT can increase survival, improve growth, reduce facial coarseness and hepatosplenomegaly, improve hearing and alter the course of cardiac and respiratory manifestations. HSCT has less beneficial effects on skeletal and joint problems, or corneal clouding. Enzyme replacement therapy (ERT) is used for non-CNS aspects of MPS I and improves liver size, linear growth, joint mobility, breathing, and sleep apnea in patients with milder disease.

Mendelian Diseases That Affect Cell Membrane Proteins May Affect Receptors and Transport Proteins

Achondroplasia

Achondroplasia, which occurs in 1 in 15,000 to 40,000 newborns, is an autosomal dominant disorder characterized by disproportionate small stature. All cases reflect activating, gain of function mutations in the fibroblast growth factor receptor 3 (*FGFR3*) gene at 4p16.3.

MOLECULAR PATHOGENESIS: FGFR3 protein is a membrane-spanning tyrosine kinase receptor with an extracellular ligand-binding domain, a transmembrane domain and an intracellular catalytic

TABLE 6-10
MUCOPOLYSACCHARIDOSES

Type	Disease	Deficient Enzyme	Clinical Features	Frequency	Inheritance	Gene	Chromosomal Location
MPS I	Hurler syndrome (severe and attenuated forms)	α-L-iduronidase	Organomegaly, macrocephaly, coarse facial features, corneal clouding, cardiac valve thickening, dysostosis multiplex, spinal stenosis, decline in intellectual function, death in childhood (severe form), normal intelligence and longevity (attenuated form)	1/100,000 (severe form) and 1:500,000 (attenuated form)	AR	*IDUA*	4p16.3
MPS II	Hunter syndrome (severe and mild forms)	Iduronate-2-sulfatase	Similar to MPS 1	1/100,000–170,000 males	XLR	*IDS*	Xq28
MPS III	Sanfilippo syndrome (types IIIA-D)	N-acetylglucosamine-6-sulfatase	Similar, but less pronounced than MPS I and II, primarily affects brain and spinal cord, progressive intellectual disability, early death	1/70,000 (all types combined)	AR	*GNS*	12q14.3
		N-acetyltransferase α-N-acetylglucosaminidase sulfamidase				*HGSNAT* *NAGLU* *SGSH*	8p11.21-p11.1 17q21.2 17q25.3
MPS IV	Morquio	N-acetylgalactosamine 6-sulfatase β-galactosidase	Skeletal deformities, odontoid process hypoplasia, corneal clouding, mildly coarse facial features, reduced life expectancy	1/200,000–300,000	AR	*GALNS* *GLB1*	16q24.3 3p22.3
MPS VI	Maroteaux-Lamy	Arylsulfatase B	Similar to MPS I	1/250,000–600,000	AR	*ARSB*	5q14.1
MPS VII	Sly	β-glucuronidase	Hydrops fetalis (most severe form), similar to MPS I	1/250,000	AR	*GUSB*	7q11.21

AR = autosomal recessive, XLR = X-linked recessive.

domain. Upon binding various FGFs, the receptor dimerizes, transactivating tyrosine kinase function and transphosphorylating tyrosine residues. These modifications trigger several downstream signaling pathways which ultimately slow chondrocyte proliferation and differentiation. Almost all people with achondroplasia have one of two pathogenic *FGFR3* variants, both of which lead to the same amino acid change (p.Gly380Arg). This change constitutively activates FGFR3, slowing chondrocyte proliferation and differentiation, and stifling bone growth.

 CLINICAL FEATURES: Patients with achondroplasia have short stature with short arms and legs, macrocephaly, characteristic facial features

with frontal bossing and midface retrusion, exaggerated lumbar lordosis, limitation of elbow extension and rotation, bow legs, brachydactyly (short fingers), and trident appearance of the hands. Average adult height for men is 131 ± 5.6 cm (4′4″), and for women, 124 ± 5.9 cm (4′). Intelligence is normal unless hydrocephalus or other CNS complications occur. Common complications include compression of the craniocervical junction, obstructive sleep apnea, and middle ear dysfunction. Achondroplasia is diagnosed by characteristic clinical and radiographic findings, with molecular genetic confirmation. Most (≈80%) parents of affected individuals have average stature, so that disease usually reflects a de novo pathogenic variant. Advanced paternal age appears to increase risk of such mutations.

Familial Hypercholesterolemia

Familial hypercholesterolemia is an autosomal dominant disorder characterized by increased blood LDLs and cholesterol deposition in arteries, tendons, and skin. It is one of the most common autosomal dominant disorders: in its heterozygous form, it affects 1 in 500 adults in the United States, causing striking acceleration of atherosclerosis and its complications.

 MOLECULAR PATHOGENESIS: Familial hypercholesterolemia results from pathogenic variants in the LDL receptor *LDLR* gene in 19p13.2. The gene encodes a receptor that removes cholesterol-rich LDL particles from the blood.

Endogenous cholesterol synthesized in hepatocytes is initially released into the blood in the form of triglyceride-rich very low-density lipoprotein (VLDL). Within adipose tissue and muscle capillaries, VLDL particles undergo lipolysis; their triglyceride content is reduced and cholesteryl esters increase, transforming them at first into intermediate-density lipoprotein (IDL), then ultimately into LDL particles. Most of the IDL and 2/3 of resultant LDL particles are metabolized via the LDL receptor pathway. The LDL receptor (LDLR) binds apolipoproteins B-100 and E found in both LDLs and IDLs. Upon receptor binding, IDL and LDL particles are endocytosed in clathrin-coated pits. Once inside the cell, these endocytic vesicles fuse with lysosomes. LDL molecules are then enzymatically degraded, ultimately releasing free cholesterol into the cytosol. In addition to being used for membrane synthesis, this internalized cholesterol suppresses endogenous cholesterol synthesis by inhibiting the enzyme 3-hydroxy-3-methylglutaryl–coenzyme A reductase (HMG-CoA reductase), which is encoded by *HMGCR* in 15q13.3, and is the rate-limiting enzyme in cholesterol biosynthesis. LDL particles that are not removed from the blood via the LDLR pathway are bound by scavenger receptors in cells of the mononuclear–phagocyte system.

The LDLR is normally made in the endoplasmic reticulum (ER), transferred to the Golgi and transported to the cell surface, where it resides in clathrin-coated pits. Once it binds LDL, the receptor and its ligand are internalized by receptor-mediated endocytosis and processed in lysosomes. *LDLR* mutations may interfere with different steps of this process:

- **Class 1 variants** have large deletions in the gene, so the ER fails to synthesize nascent LDLR protein (null alleles).
- **Class 2 variants** fail to transfer LDLR from the ER to the Golgi (transport-defective alleles), preventing receptor molecules from reaching the cell surface.
- **Class 3 variant** LDLR have defective ligand-binding domain (binding-defective alleles).
- **Class 4 variant** receptors bind LDL particles normally, but cannot cluster in coated pits, and so show impaired LDLR endocytosis (internalization-defective alleles).
- **Class 5 variants** cause LDL–LDLR complexes to remain in endosomes, so receptors are unable to recycle to the plasma membrane (recycling-defective alleles).

Hepatocytes are the main cells expressing LDLR: the liver removes roughly 70% of LDL from the blood.

After LDLs bind to LDLR, they are internalized and processed in lysosomes, freeing cholesterol for further metabolism. If LDL receptor function is impaired, high levels of LDLs continue to circulate. They are taken up by scavenging tissue macrophages, which accumulate to form atheromas—occlusive arterial plaques—and xanthomas—papules or nodules of lipid-laden macrophages (see Chapter 16).

 CLINICAL FEATURES: Heterozygous and homozygous familial hypercholesterolemia are distinct clinical syndromes, showing a clear gene-dosage effect. In heterozygotes, total blood cholesterol is elevated at birth (mean, 350 mg/dL; normal, <200 mg/dL in adults). Tendon xanthomas develop in half of patients before age 30, and symptoms of coronary heart disease often occur before age 40. In homozygotes, blood cholesterol content is extremely high (600 to 1,200 mg/dL). Virtually all patients have tendon xanthomas and generalized atherosclerosis in childhood. Untreated homozygotes typically die of myocardial infarction before age 30. Treatment of heterozygotes with statins has significantly reduced coronary heart disease morbidity and mortality to levels like those in the general population.

Cystic Fibrosis

Cystic fibrosis (CF) exemplifies dysfunction of a cell membrane transport protein. It is an autosomal recessive multisystem disease affecting epithelia of the respiratory tract, exocrine pancreas, intestine, hepatobiliary system, and exocrine sweat glands. Thick, sticky mucus builds up and slowly damages these organs. The defect is in the chloride channel, the CF transmembrane conductance regulator (CFTR).

 EPIDEMIOLOGY: CF is the most common life-limiting autosomal recessive disorder in people of northern European background, in whom disease incidence is 1 in 2,500 to 3,500 live births, and carrier frequency is 1 in 28. It is much less common in other populations (1 in 15,000 African Americans; 1 in 31,000 Asian Americans).

 MOLECULAR PATHOGENESIS: The *CFTR* gene, at 7q31.2, encodes a 1,480 amino acid chloride ion transporter in most epithelial cells. Two ATP-hydrolyzing domains power CFTR transporter function, two domains anchor it as a transmembrane protein and it has two R-domains with phosphorylation sites for cAMP-dependent protein kinase A (PKA) regulate chloride channel activity. Its level of activity depends on the balance between kinase (phosphorylation) and phosphatase (dephosphorylation) activities.

The most common *CFTR* mutation among Caucasians is loss of three base pairs, which deletes a phenylalanine (F) residue at position 508 (ΔF_{508}), generating an abnormally folded protein that cannot be transported to the cell membrane, and so is degraded. ΔF_{508} accounts for 70% of

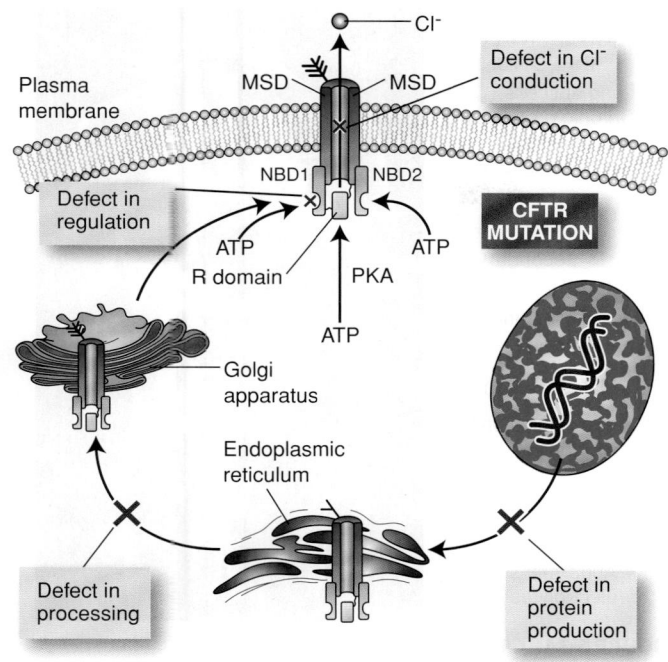

FIGURE 6-32. Cellular sites of disruption in the synthesis and function of the cystic fibrosis transmembrane conductance regulator (CFTR) in cystic fibrosis. ATP = adenosine triphosphate; Cl⁻ = chloride ion; MSD = membrane-spanning domain; NBD = nucleotide-binding domain; PKA = protein kinase A.

CFTR mutations in Caucasians. Mutations in *CFTR* that disturb chloride channel function fall into several functional groupings (Fig. 6-32):

I. **Failure of CFTR synthesis:** Mutations that lead to premature termination signals interfere with synthesis of full-length CFTR protein. As a result, no CFTR-mediated chloride secretion occurs in involved epithelia.

II. **Failure of CFTR transport to the plasma membrane:** Some mutations (including ΔF_{508}) prevent proper folding of the mutant protein, which is then targeted for proteasomal degradation (see Chapter 1).

III. **Defective ATP binding to CFTR:** Certain mutations that affect ATP-binding domains allow CFTR proteins to reach the plasma membrane, but interfere with channel regulation; these limit, but do not abolishing, chloride secretion.

IV. **Defective chloride secretion by mutant CFTR:** Mutations in the channel pore inhibit chloride secretion.

The relationship between these genotypes (>1,500 known mutations) and CF clinical severity is complex, and not always consistent. The best correlation relates to pancreatic insufficiency. Severe forms of the disease typically include pancreatic insufficiency (85% of cases), while pancreatic function is preserved in milder cases. Severely affected patients generally have class I (lack of CFTR synthesis) or class II (defective protein processing) mutations. Milder forms of CF have class III (defective channel regulation) and class IV (defective chloride conductance) mutations.

PATHOPHYSIOLOGY: Mutations in *CFTR* render affected epithelial membranes relatively impermeable to chloride ions, but the impact of this defect is tissue-specific. The major function of CFTR protein in sweat gland ducts is to reabsorb luminal chloride ions and augment sodium reabsorption through a separate epithelial sodium channel. Therefore, loss of CFTR function in the sweat ducts leads to decreased reabsorption of sodium chloride and production of hypertonic ("salty") sweat.

CFTR functions differently in respiratory and intestinal epithelia. It supports active secretion of chloride ions. At these sites, CFTR mutations reduce chloride secretion into the lumen. This is accompanied by increased active luminal sodium absorption, and both of these ion changes increase passive water reabsorption from the lumen, lowering the water content of the surface fluid layer-coating mucosal cells. This dehydration increases fluid viscosity, hindering mucociliary action, causing concentrated, thick secretions to obstruct air passages and predispose to recurrent pulmonary infections.

PATHOLOGY: Pathologic consequences of CF reflect abnormally thick mucus, which obstructs airway lumina, pancreatic and biliary ducts and fetal intestine. CF affects multiple organs that produce exocrine secretions.

Respiratory tract: Lung disease causes most morbidity and mortality in CF. It begins as obstruction of bronchioles by mucus, with secondary bronchiolar infection and inflammation. Recurrent cycles of obstruction and infection lead to chronic bronchiolitis and bronchitis, which increase in severity as disease progresses, and may lead to secondary pulmonary hypertension. Bronchial mucous glands undergo hypertrophy and hyperplasia, and airways are distended by thick, tenacious secretions. Widespread bronchiectasis is apparent by age 10 and often earlier. Late in the disease, large bronchiectatic cysts and lung abscesses are common.

Pancreas: Most patients (85%) with CF have a form of chronic pancreatitis, and in long-standing cases, little or no functional exocrine pancreas remains. Inspissated secretions in central pancreatic ducts produce secondary dilation and cystic change of distal ducts. Recurrent pancreatitis causes loss of acinar cells and extensive fibrosis so that the gland may become simply cystic fibroadipose tissue containing islets of Langerhans. The finding of pancreatic cysts and fibrosis led to the disease name of CF (Fig. 6-33). Pancreatic islets may be damaged if CF is long-standing.

Liver: Thickened mucous secretions in the intrahepatic biliary system obstruct bile flow and lead to focal secondary biliary cirrhosis. This occurs in 1/4 of patients at autopsy. Concentrated secretions clog bile ducts and ductules. Hepatic lesions, which include chronic portal inflammation and septal fibrosis, are in some cases (<5%) sufficiently widespread to lead to clinical manifestations of biliary cirrhosis.

GI tract: Shortly after birth, a normal neonate passes the intestinal contents that have accumulated in utero (meconium). The most important gut lesion in CF is **meconium ileus**, small bowel obstruction in newborns due

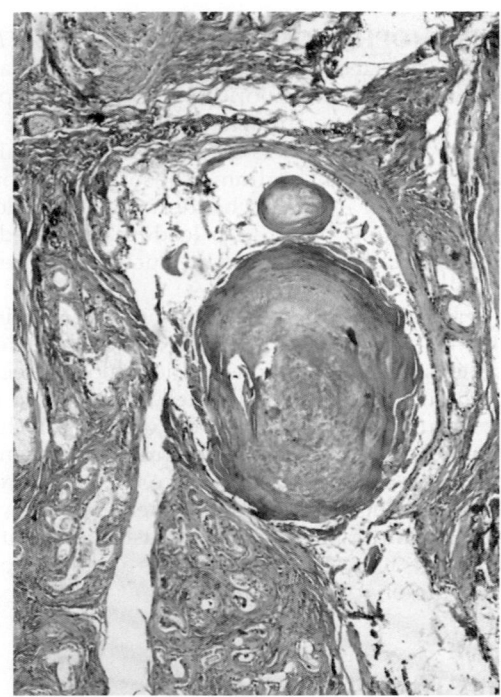

FIGURE 6-33. Intraductal concretion and acinar atrophy in the pancreas of a patient with cystic fibrosis.

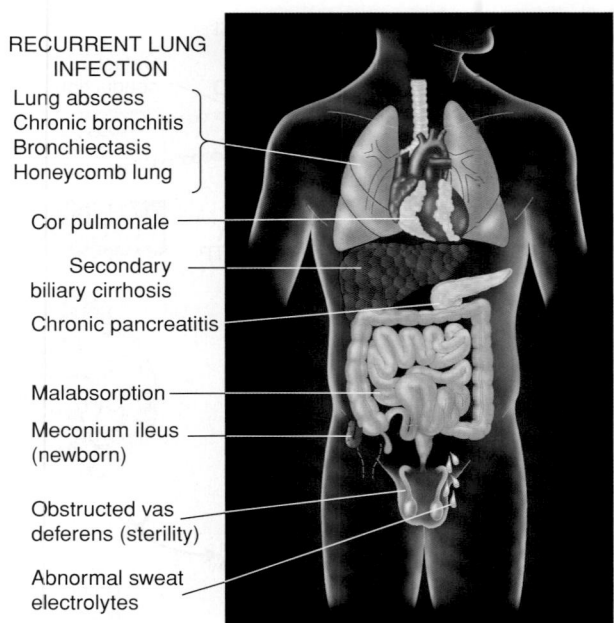

FIGURE 6-34. Clinical features of cystic fibrosis.

to failure to pass meconium in the first few days of life. This occurs in ≈10% of newborns with CF, due to failure of pancreatic secretions to digest meconium, possibly augmented by the greater viscosity of small bowel secretions.

Reproductive tract: The large majority of men with CF are infertile as a result of congenital bilateral absence of the vas deferens due to luminal obstruction by inspissated secretions early in life, even in utero.

 CLINICAL FEATURES: Clinical manifestations of CF are many and variable, range from mild to severe and vary from being present at birth to beginning later in life (Fig. 6-34).

Respiratory symptoms begin with cough, which becomes productive of large amounts of tenacious and purulent sputum. Repeated infectious bronchitis and bronchopneumonia become progressively more frequent, leading to chronic dyspnea. Respiratory failure and cardiac complications of pulmonary hypertension (cor pulmonale) develop with time.

The most common respiratory tract pathogens in CF are *Staphylococcus* and *Pseudomonas* spp. As the disease advances, *Pseudomonas* may be the only organism cultured from the lung. Recovery, particularly of mucoid *Pseudomonas* sp. from the lungs of a child with chronic pulmonary disease is virtually diagnostic of CF. Infection with *Burkholderia* (formerly *Pseudomonas*) cepacia is associated with **cepacia syndrome,** a commonly fatal pulmonary infection that causes necrotizing pneumonia, worsening respiratory failure, and bacteremia that is highly resistant to antibiotics.

Failure of pancreatic exocrine secretion leads to fat and protein malabsorption, causing bulky, foul-smelling

stools (**steatorrhea**), nutritional deficiencies, and growth retardation. CF-related diabetes mellitus may develop.

Gastrointestinal. Affected newborns may have distended abdomens and bowel obstruction due to meconium ileus, which may be suspected before birth if fetal echogenic (brighter than usual) bowel is seen on second trimester ultrasound.

Liver disease usually presents by age 10 years, with hepatomegaly, elevated serum hepatic enzyme levels, and/or liver ultrasound abnormalities other than hepatomegaly. Liver disease is reported in ≈10% of CF patients.

Fertility. Almost all males with CF are infertile because congenital absence of the vas deferens causes azoospermia. Women with CF are fertile, but a few have abnormal cervical mucus that may contribute to infertility. Others with severe illness and reduced body mass index may be anovulatory.

Diagnosis and treatment. Sweat chloride tests showing increased electrolytes in sweat, supported by genetic studies that show disease-causing mutations (typically by whole gene sequencing), establish the diagnosis. Many states screen newborns for CF, using elevated pancreatic trypsinogen as the initial screen, followed by molecular testing for common *CFTR* mutations.

Treatment for CF focuses on **postural drainage** of airways, antibiotics, and pancreatic enzyme supplementation. Some patients undergo lung transplantation. Although CF patients once rarely survived beyond adolescence, with current treatments, their life expectancy is nearing 40 years.

Some Mendelian Diseases Affect Intracellular Structural Proteins or Key Extracellular Matrix Components

Common disorders belonging to this group are listed in Table 6-11. Representative diseases in this group of disease are described below.

TABLE 6-11
DISORDERS INVOLVING DEFECTS IN STRUCTURAL PROTEINS

Disorder	Clinical Features	Frequency	Inheritance	Gene	Chromosomal Location
Marfan syndrome	Tall stature, arachnodactyly, ectopia lentis, aortic rupture	1/5,000	AD	FBN1	15q21.1
Ehlers–Danlos syndrome[a,c] Classical type (I and II)[b]	Soft velvety hyperelastic skin with abnormal scarring, easy bruising	1/20,000–40,000	AD	COL5A1 COL5A2	9q34.3 2q32.2
Ehlers–Danlos syndrome Hypermobility type (III)	Unusually large range of joint motion, unstable joints prone to dislocation and pain, easy bruising	1/5,000–20,000	AD	unknown	unknown
Ehlers–Danlos syndrome Vascular type (IV)	Life-threatening rupture of blood vessels, intestine or gravid uterus	1/250,000	AD	COL3A1	2q32.2
Ehlers–Danlos syndrome Kyphoscoliotic type (VIA)	Severe, progressive curvature of the spine	Rare	AD	PLOD1 FKBP14	1p36.22 7p14.3
Ehlers–Danlos syndrome Arthrochalasia type (VIIA, VIIB)	Severe joint hypermobility, congenital hip dislocation, fragile hyperextensible skin, hypotonia, and kyphoscoliosis	Rare	AD	COL1A2 COL1A1	7q21.3 17q21.33
Ehlers–Danlos syndrome Dermatosparaxis type (VIIC)	Soft, fragile skin that sags and wrinkles; easy bruising; and distinctive facial features	Rare	AD	ADAMTS2	5q35.3
Osteogenesis imperfecta Type I (mild)	Mild bone fragility with several fractures of long bones with minimal trauma, rate of fractures decreases after puberty, minimal deformity, normal stature. blue sclera, hearing loss in adulthood	1/10,000–20,000 live births (combined incidence of all types) types I and IV are the most common	AD	COL1A1 COL1A2 These account for 90% of all cases of OI of all types	7q21.3 17q21.33
Osteogenesis imperfecta Type II (perinatal lethal)	Severe with multiple fractures with deformity at birth, neonatal death due to small chest and respiratory insufficiency		AD (new mutation)		
Osteogenesis imperfecta Types III–IV (moderate–severe)	Moderate to severe bone fragility with multiple fractures, some at birth, progressive limb and spine deformity, variable short stature, some wheelchair bound, blue sclera, dentinogenesis imperfecta, hearing loss in adulthood		AD, AR (some cases)		

AD = autosomal dominant; AR = autosomal recessive.
[a]Although all types of Ehlers–Danlos syndrome affect the joints and skin, additional features vary by type. 6 of the 19 types in the 2017 EDS classification are listed here.
[b]Former classification types.
[c]Combined prevalence of all types of Ehler–Danlos syndrome 1/5,000 worldwide.

Marfan Syndrome

Marfan syndrome is an autosomal dominant disorder of connective tissue that primarily involves the skeletal, ocular, and cardiovascular systems. Affected people may experience sudden death from aortic aneurysm and dissection (see Chapter 16). The disease is highly variable clinically, ranging from isolated features affecting one or a few systems, to severe and rapidly progressive multiorgan disease. About 75% of patients with Marfan syndrome have an affected parent, while the others 25% have a de novo pathogenic variant. The worldwide prevalence of Marfan syndrome is about 1 in 5,000, and with no apparent ethnic, racial group or gender preference.

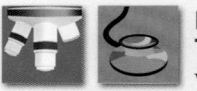

MOLECULAR PATHOGENESIS: Marfan syndrome is caused by pathogenic variants in *FBN1*. This gene at 15q21.1, encodes **fibrillin-1**, an extracellular matrix glycoprotein which is the key component of **microfibrils**. Microfibrils are large thread-like structures that serve as scaffolds for elastin deposition during embryonic development. Thereafter, they remain as a component of elastic tissues. Although microfibrils are widely distributed in the body, they are particularly abundant in the aorta, ligaments, and ciliary zonules that support the ocular lens, which are all prominently affected in Marfan syndrome. Microfibrils participate in elastic matrix formation and homeostasis, and in matrix-cell attachments in regulating some growth factors.

PATHOPHYSIOLOGY: The pathogenesis of Marfan syndrome is complex. *FBN1* mutations of several types—nonsense, frameshift, splice site, missense—are known. Loss-of-function alleles may lead to haploinsufficiency. In some cases, disease related to missense mutations may reflect dominant negative effects. Regardless of mutation type, residual fibrillin-1 protein levels in affected tissues were found to be much less than the 50% that would be consistent with a haploinsufficiency model.

Although some features of Marfan syndrome may reflect structural failure of connective tissues due to inadequate or insufficient microfibrils, other factors appear to contribute. Thus, microfibril loss due to *FBN1* mutations causes abnormal and excessive activation of transforming growth factor-β (TGFβ). Fibrillin binds and sequesters TGFβ (see Chapters 2, 3, and 5), and so controls its bioavailability. TGFβ signaling regulates extracellular matrix formation during tissue repair or remodeling: higher levels of TGFβ ligand caused by loss of microfibrils in Marfan syndrome thus should cause a failure of connective tissue repair/remodeling processes. For example, TGFβ upregulates expression of elastase and many matrix-metalloproteases (MMPs), leading to enhanced elastin degradation and disintegration of elastic fibers. MMP overproduction reduces connective tissue elasticity and weakens the aortic wall. In early clinical studies, TGFβ antagonists, for example, angiotensin II receptor blockers, have shown efficacy in preventing cardiovascular complications.

PATHOLOGY AND CLINICAL FEATURES: Skeletal system: Individuals with Marfan syndrome are typically tall and thin, with greater lower body segment length (measured from pubic bone to floor) than upper body segment length (measured from pubic bone to top of head) due to abnormally long limbs. Their arm span is almost always greater than their height. In addition to long thin extremities and **arachnodactyly** (spider-like fingers and toes), they usually have a long narrow face, a high arched palate and crowded teeth (Fig. 6-35). Disorders of the ribs causing **pectus excavatum** (concave sternum) or **pectus carinatum** (pigeon breast) are frequent.

Spontaneous pneumothorax is not uncommon. Tendons, ligaments, and joint capsules are weak, leading to hyperextensibility of the joints (double-jointedness), dislocations, hernias, and often scoliosis or kyphosis. Dural ectasia, an outpouching of the dura around the spinal cord and brain, can result in pain in the back, abdomen, legs, or head.

Cardiovascular system: The aortic tunica media is weak, leading to variable dilation of the ascending aorta and a high incidence of **dissecting aneurysms**, usually of the ascending aorta. These may rupture into the pericardial cavity or extend down the aorta and rupture into the retroperitoneal space. Dilation of the aortic annulus results in aortic regurgitation, which may be severe enough to produce angina pectoris and congestive heart failure. The mitral valve typically has redundant leaflets and chordae tendineae—leading to mitral valve prolapse syndrome. Histologically, the aorta shows marked fragmentation and loss of elastic fibers (see Chapter 7), with increased metachromatic mucopolysaccharide, which may accumulate in discrete pools. These features are sometimes called *cystic medial necrosis* of the aorta. Cardiovascular complications are the most common cause of death in affected individuals.

Eyes: Ocular changes are common. These include upward dislocation of the lens (ectopia lentis) and myopia due to elongation of the eye.

Untreated men with Marfan syndrome usually die in their 30s of aortic aneurysm rupture, and untreated women often die in their 40s. There is no cure, but life expectancy has increased significantly in recent decades. Antihypertensive therapy and surgical replacement of the ascending aorta and aortic valve with prosthetic grafts have significantly improved longevity. With proper management of cardiovascular disease, the life expectancy with Marfan syndrome approaches that of the general population.

Ehlers–Danlos Syndrome (EDS)

EDS is a collective term for a group of clinically and genetically heterogeneous inherited disorders of connective tissue characterized by remarkable cutaneous hyperelasticity and fragility, joint hypermobility, and often a bleeding diathesis. Different forms are inherited as autosomal dominant, autosomal recessive or X-linked traits, depending on the specific gene and mutation involved. Worldwide prevalence of all types of EDS is approximately 1 in 5,000.

MOLECULAR PATHOGENESIS: Collagen is the main extracellular structural protein in connective tissues. Most EDS types entail inherited alterations in genes affecting the structure, synthesis, and processing of different forms of collagen. As the main connective tissue constituent, collagen is the body's most abundant single protein, comprising 25% to 35% of the whole-body protein content. At least 16 different types of collagen are known, the most common being types I, II, and III. Collagen proteins are triple helices, generally with two identical chains (α1) plus another chain with slightly different composition (α2). Normal formation of collagen triple helices requires modifying the collagen chains by

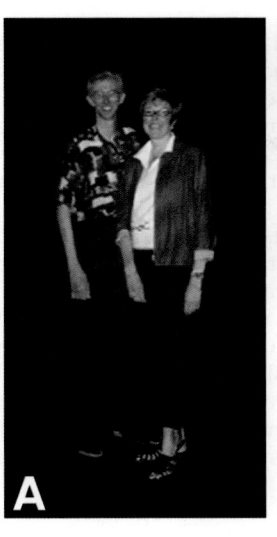
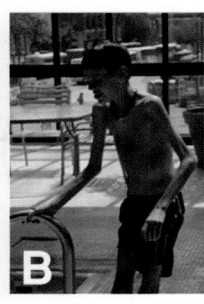
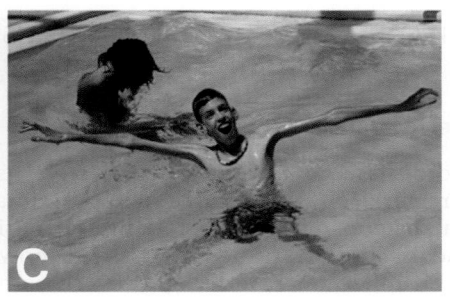

FIGURE 6-35. Features of Marfan syndrome. A. Very tall man and woman with long thin extremities as a result of Marfan syndrome. **B,C.** Tall thin boy with Marfan syndrome. His sternum dips inward slightly (mild pectus excavatum) and he has a very wide arm span and long slender fingers (arachnodactyly). (Courtesy of The Marfan Foundation www.marfan.org.)

adding hydroxyl groups to prolines and lysines, followed by glycosylation. Thus, in addition to abnormalities in collagen genes themselves, some forms of EDS are caused by defects in enzymes involved in modification and assembly of collagen fibers. Deficient or defective collagen weakens supporting structures in the skin, joints, arteries, and internal organs in EDS patients.

The 2017 classification of EDS defines 13 types, based upon clinical features, mode of inheritance, and biochemical and genetic findings. Pathogenic variants in 19 genes are involved.

The best recognized types of EDS are:

- Classical (previously, EDS types I and II)
- Hypermobile (previously, EDS type III)
- Vascular (previously EDS, type IV)

Some other less common, but well characterized, types include kyphoscoliotic (EDS type VI), arthrochalasia (EDS type VIIA and B), and dermatosparaxis (EDS type VIIC).

Classical EDS forms a continuum of clinical findings. It is inherited in autosomal dominant fashion and is caused by pathogenic variants in *COL5A1* gene in 9q34.3 or, less frequently, *COL5A2* gene in 2q32.2, encoding type V collagen. Pathogenic *COL5A1* and *COL5A2* variants, identified by molecular testing in more than 50% of patients with classic EDS, include loss-of-function mutations resulting in haploinsufficiency, as well as missense dominant-negative mutations. Type V collagen is a quantitatively minor fibrillar collagen that is widely distributed in skin, bone, tendon, and elsewhere. Patients typically have skin hyperextensibility, abnormal wound healing with atrophic scars and generalized joint hypermobility. Their skin, which is often fragile, can be stretched several centimeters. Joint hypermobility allows unusual extension and flexion which may lead to subluxation or dislocation of joints.

Hypermobile EDS is inherited as an autosomal dominant. Its molecular basis remains unknown. Patients often have soft velvety skin, increased range of joint motion, unstable joints prone to dislocation, chronic musculoskeletal pain, and easy bruising.

Vascular EDS is inherited in autosomal dominant fashion and is the most serious EDS subtype. It is caused by mutations in the *COL3A1* gene in 2q32.2, which codes for type III collagen α-chain. The type III procollagen molecule is a homotrimer, and is a major structural component of skin, blood vessels, and hollow organs. The presenting signs in most affected young adults include arterial rupture or dissection, sigmoid colon perforation, or third trimester uterine rupture (without a previous cesarean delivery). Patients may also have thin, translucent skin, easy bruising, characteristic facial features (small chin, thin nose and lips, sunken cheeks). About 25% of patients with vascular EDS experience significant complications by age 20, and over 75% develop life-threatening problems or die before age 40.

Kyphoscoliotic EDS is a recessive disorder caused by mutations in *PLOD1* gene in 1p36.22, and resulting in lysyl hydroxylase deficiency. Lysyl hydroxylase is a collagen-modifying enzyme that cross-links collagen trimers, and so increases collagen strength. Patients have hypotonia, congenital or early-onset kyphoscoliosis, and generalized joint hypermobility. Hyperextensible skin, easy bruising, rupture of medium size arteries, and several other medical problems may occur.

Arthrochalasia EDS is caused by mutations in *COL1A1* in 17q21.33 or *COL1A2* in 7q21.3 causing type I collagen structural defects. It often presents with congenital bilateral hip dislocation. Generalized joint hypermobility and hyperextensible skin are common. Muscle hypotonia and kyphoscoliosis may be seen.

Dermatosparaxis EDS is inherited in an autosomal recessive fashion and is due to mutations in the *ADAMTS2* gene in 5q35.3, resulting in deficiency of a peptidase involved in processing pro-collagen fibers. Patients show extreme skin fragility with congenital or postnatal skin tears, characteristic facies, poor growth, sagging skin with excessive folds at wrists and ankles, severe bruisability with risk for subcutaneous hematomas and large hernias.

Many people with clinical abnormalities suggesting EDS have a constellation of findings that do not exactly fit any recognized EDS type. Clinical and molecular study of such cases is likely to expand the classification of EDS even further.

Osteogenesis Imperfecta (OI)

OI, or brittle bone disease, is a group of connective tissue diseases characterized by fractures with minimal or absent trauma, osteopenia, variable dentinogenesis imperfecta (DI) and, in adult years, hearing loss. OI shows autosomal dominant inheritance, although rare cases be autosomal recessive. Currently at least eight types of OI are described, based on clinical features and molecular findings.

MOLECULAR PATHOGENESIS: OI is caused by pathogenic variants in *COL1A1* or *COL1A2* genes, which encode α1 and α2 chains of collagen type I. Milder forms of OI result from variants that encode premature termination codons, express less mRNA or produce less collagen I protein. More severe forms of the disease are caused by point mutations that disrupt type I collagen α-helices by converting glycines that occupy every third amino acid position into bulkier amino acids. Mutations associated with the most severe forms of the disease are typically de novo, while less severe mutations are often inherited from nonsymptomatic or mildly affected parents. For example, about 60% of classic nondeforming OI cases are de novo, while virtually all perinatally lethal OI are de novo. However, gonadal mosaicism is frequent, and may be present in 3% to 5% of cases.

PATHOPHYSIOLOGY: Type I collagen is a heterotrimer, with two α1 chains and one α2 chain. Collagen I chains have a repetitive amino acid composition in which glycine, the smallest amino acid, occupies every third position. Glycine positioning in type I collagen assures proper chain folding. If a different amino acid is substituted, triple helix propagation is delayed, additional post-translational modifications occur and some assembled trimers are never secreted. In addition to glycine substitutions, alterations in the C-terminus and certain deletions can disrupt formation of mature type I collagen fibrils.

PATHOLOGY AND CLINICAL FEATURES: The four traditional types of *COL1A1/2*-related OI based on clinical presentation and radiographic findings are: type I-classic nondeforming OI with blue sclerae, type II-perinatally lethal OI, type III-progressively deforming OI, and type IV-common variable OI with normal sclerae (see Chapter 30).

Type I OI is characterized by a normal appearance at birth, but fractures of many bones occur during infancy and when the child learns to walk. Such patients have been described as being "fragile as a china doll." Bowing of the femur and tibia and kyphoscoliosis are common. Deficiency in collagen makes sclerae translucent, allowing partial visualization of the choroid. These children also have translucent teeth with an opalescent appearance (dentinogenesis imperfecta) due to hypoplasia of dentin and pulp. Hearing loss due to otosclerosis first appears in the third decade. Type I collagen is normally formed, but is reduced in amount by null mutations.

Type II OI with innumerable fractures, is usually fatal in utero or shortly after birth. Affected infants have a poorly mineralized calvarium, large fontanels, shallow orbits, a small nose, and deep blue sclera. Brain development is abnormal. Chest circumference is small and the limbs are short and bent. Those who are born alive usually die of respiratory failure within their first month. Abnormal forms of collagen resulting from glycine substitution are responsible. Most are due to severe de novo mutations.

Type III OI causes progressive deformities. It is ordinarily detected at birth by the baby's short stature and misshapenness due to fractures in utero. Dentinogenesis imperfecta and hearing loss are common. Severe kyphoscoliosis can sometimes lead to early death from respiratory compromise. Most cases are due to autosomal dominant de novo mutations in *COL1A1* and *COL1A2*, but occasional cases are inherited as autosomal recessives, due to mutations in other genes associated with OI.

Type IV OI is characterized by normal to moderate short stature with significant bone deformity, dentinogenesis imperfecta, and normal sclerae. Most of these cases are due to autosomal dominant mutations in *COL1A1* and *COL1A2*, although some have autosomal recessive inheritance due to mutations in other genes associated with OI.

Duchenne/Becker Muscular Dystrophy

Duchenne/Becker muscular dystrophy (see Chapter 31) is a muscle disease caused by pathogenic variants in the *DMD* gene in Xp21.2-p21.1 which encodes the protein dystrophin. It is inherited as an X-linked recessive disorder, so most patients are male. Females are rarely affected except in cases of Turner syndrome or as a consequence of extremely skewed X-inactivation or structural abnormalities of the X chromosome.

MOLECULAR PATHOGENESIS: Dystrophin is a membrane-associated protein present in muscle cells and some neurons. The *DMD* gene is one of the largest genes in the genome; spanning 2.2Mb of DNA and comprising 79 exons. Pathogenic *DMD* alleles are highly variable, and include deletions of the entire gene, deletions or duplications of one or more exons, small deletions and insertions of bases resulting in frameshifts and premature termination or single-base changes. Pathogenic *DMD* variants that lead to lack of dystrophin expression tend to cause Duchenne muscular dystrophy, which is a more severe form of the disease. Variants that lead to abnormal quality or quantity of dystrophin cause a milder form of the disease, Becker muscular dystrophy. These are discussed in detail in Chapter 31.

Inherited Defects in Tumor Suppressor Genes Predispose to Tumor Development

Inherited mutations that alter tumor suppressor gene functions underlie disorders in which tumors feature prominently. Resulting tumor syndromes are many, and are diverse. Basic mechanisms leading to tumorigenesis in these settings are discussed in detail in Chapter 5, and are not recapitulated here. Many of these inherited tumor predisposition syndromes affect mainly specific organ systems (e.g., Familial Polyposis Coli, Fanconi Anemias, BRCA syndromes, Hereditary Retinoblastoma, and many others). These are addressed in Chapter 5 and in chapters covering the most affected organ systems (e.g., the GI tract in Chapter 19, the eye in Chapter 33, and the breast in Chapter 25). The neurofibromatoses are presented here as an example.

The neurofibromatoses include two distinct autosomal dominant disorders, NF1 and NF2. In these, multiple neurofibromas, benign Schwann cell tumors of peripheral nerves (see Chapter 31), develop. Other cells of neural crest origin affected in these disorders include melanocytes and endoneurial fibroblasts, and both diseases, but especially NF1, involve abnormal pigmentation. Despite superficial similarities, NF1 and NF2 have separate genetic origins (see below).

Neurofibromatosis Type I (von Recklinghausen Disease)

Neurofibromatosis type I (NF1) occurs 1 in 4,000 people of all races, and so is one of the more common autosomal dominant disorders. It was first described in 1882 by von Recklinghausen, but references to it can be found as early as the 13th century. It is characterized by neurofibromas, **café au lait spots**, **Lisch nodules**, axillary and inguinal freckling, optic nerve gliomas and skeletal abnormalities (Fig. 6-36). Half of the cases are sporadic rather than inherited.

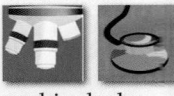 **MOLECULAR PATHOGENESIS:** NF1 is caused by germline loss of function mutations in the 374Kb *NF1* gene in 17q11.2. It encodes the protein neurofibromin, a member of a family of guanosine triphosphatase (GTPase)-activating proteins (GAPs), which inactivate N-Ras (see Chapter 5). *NF1* is a classic tumor suppressor gene. Loss of its function results in loss of GAP activity and uncontrolled N-Ras activation, which greatly increases risk of developing neurofibromas and other benign and malignant tumors. The fact that half of NF1 cases occur de novo probably reflects the high spontaneous mutation rate of *NF1* (100× the rate for many other genes). There are over 1,000 known mutations in *NF1*. A more severe phenotype occurs in patients with complete deletion of *NF1* and sometimes adjacent genes as well.

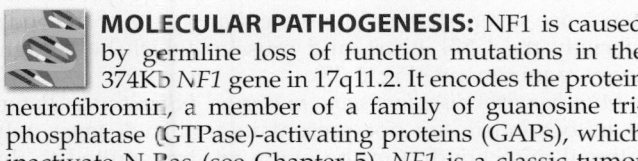 **PATHOLOGY AND CLINICAL FEATURES:** Clinical manifestations of NF1 vary widely among affected individuals and include:

Café au lait spots: These are usually the first manifestation of NF1 and begin to appear in early childhood. Normal people may have occasional light brown skin patches, but ≥95% of people with NF1 have six or more

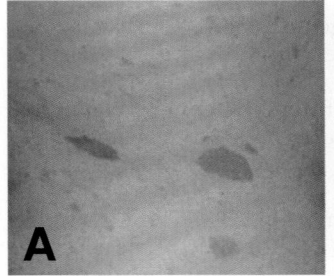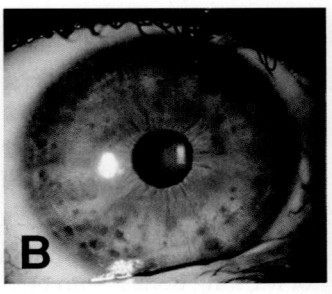
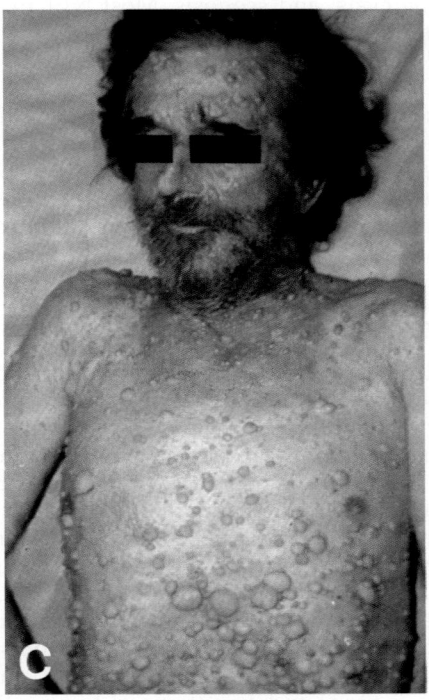

FIGURE 6-36. Features of neurofibromatosis type 1. A. Café au lait spots. **B.** Lisch nodules. **C.** Multiple cutaneous neurofibromas on the face and trunk.

such lesions. Café au lait spots are flat ≥5 mm nonraised areas of light hyperpigmentation that increase in number and size with age (Fig. 6-36A). They tend to be ovoid, with the longer axis parallel to a cutaneous nerve. Freckles in the axilla and groin appear in late childhood.

Neurofibromas: Over 90% of patients with NF1 have cutaneous and subcutaneous neurofibromas by late childhood or adolescence. They are soft, pedunculated masses, usually ≥1 cm in diameter (Fig. 6-36C). They may become quite large (up to 25 cm). These benign tumors increase in number with age and may exceed 500. Subcutaneous neurofibromas are soft nodules along the course of peripheral nerves.

Plexiform neurofibromas only occur in the context of NF1. They are benign tumors that usually arise from multiple large peripheral nerves as bulging and deforming masses. Occasionally they involve cranial or intraspinal nerves (see Chapter 31). In 3% to 5% of NF1 patients, a malignant peripheral nerve sheath tumor—also called malignant schwannoma or neurofibrosarcoma—will develop in a plexiform neurofibroma. NF1 patients have increased risk for other neurogenic tumors, such as meningiomas, optic gliomas, and pheochromocytomas.

Lisch nodules: Over 90% of patients with NF1 have small pigmented nodules of the iris which begin to appear in childhood. These are masses of melanocytes (Fig. 6-36B) that are believed to be hamartomas and do not affect vision.

Skeletal lesions are common in NF1. These include sphenoid bone malformations and thinning of the cortices of the long bones, with bowing and pseudarthrosis of the tibia, bone cysts, and scoliosis. Most NF1 patients have short stature and macrocephaly.

Mild intellectual impairment is common in NF1, as is ADHD.

Leukemia: Risk of myeloid leukemias in children with NF1 is a few hundred times the normal population risk. They are specifically at risk of juvenile myelomonocytic leukemia, which is very rare in non-NF1 individuals. In some patients, both alleles of *NF1* are mutated in leukemic cells.

Neurofibromatosis Type II (Central Neurofibromatosis)

NF2 syndrome is defined by bilateral acoustic neuromas, also known as vestibular schwannomas, which are benign tumors of the eighth cranial nerve. Meningiomas and gliomas are also commonly present. NF2 is much rarer than NF1, occurring in 1 in 33,000 people. Most patients have bilateral acoustic neuromas, but a unilateral VIII nerve tumor may occur with two or more of: neurofibroma, meningioma, glioma, schwannoma, or juvenile posterior lenticular opacity. Although they can become evident at any age, signs and symptoms of NF2 usually appear in adolescence or young adulthood. The most frequent early symptoms of vestibular schwannomas are hearing loss, tinnitus, and problems with balance. Signs and symptoms of tumors that develop elsewhere in the nervous system, vary according to their location.

MOLECULAR PATHOGENESIS: NF2 is caused by mutations in *NF2* tumor suppressor gene in 22q12.2, encoding the merlin protein, also known as schwannomin. Merlin, which is produced in the nervous system, particularly in Schwann cells, is a member of a superfamily of proteins that link the cytoskeleton to the cell membrane. In addition to a germline *NF2* mutation, tumors in NF2 also commonly show monosomy 22, deletion of 22q12.2 or copy number neutral loss of heterozygosity of chromosome 22.

Many Diseases Are Inherited via Non-Mendelian Mechanisms

Gonadal Mosaicism

If phenotypically, genetically normal parents bear a child with an autosomal dominant disorder the child's disease is considered to have arisen via spontaneous de novo mutation. In this situation the risk that subsequent children of these parents will be affected by that mutation is low, but it is not zero. The small residual risk is due to the possibility of **gonadal (germline) mosaicism**. As mentioned above,

mosaicism is the presence in an individual of at least two genetically different cell lines that are derived from the same zygote. Occasionally, an unaffected parent is mosaic for the mutation responsible for his or her child's genetic disorder. If the cells with the mutation are largely confined to the gonads, the parent will not show signs of the disorder, but may pass the mutant gene on to additional children. Gonadal mosaicism can also be seen with X-linked disorders such as Duchenne muscular dystrophy (see Chapter 31). The causative gene mutation found in a son may not be present in the mother's blood, but might exist in some of her egg cells, putting her at risk to have another affected son.

Mitochondrial Disorders

As discussed above, the vast majority of genes in cells reside on nuclear chromosomes, and are inherited in a Mendelian fashion. A few genes are located on mitochondrial DNA (mtDNA). Proteins found in mitochondria may be encoded by nuclear or mitochondrial genes. Although most mitochondrial respiratory chain proteins are encoded by nuclear genes, a small but important fraction is encoded by mtDNA. Mitochondrial disorders result from mutations in the mitochondrial genome, and do not follow Mendelian inheritance. All of these disorders are rare (see Table 6-12 for representative examples).

The mitochondrial genome is a circular DNA molecule with 37 genes that encode 13 subunits of enzymes involved in oxidative phosphorylation, 2 ribosomal RNAs and 22 transfer RNAs required to translate transcripts of polypeptides encoded by mtDNA. Each mitochondrion has 2 to 10 mtDNA molecules, and cells have 100 to 10,000 mitochondria. Different tissues need different amounts of ATP, which correlate with the number of mitochondria and mtDNA molecules per cell. Because mitochondria in all cells produce ATP, mtDNA mutations that disrupt energy production often cause severe disease involving many parts of the body, especially the CNS, heart, and muscles which have high-energy requirements (Fig. 6-37).

Mitochondrial disorders show **maternal inheritance**. Paternal mitochondria are not present in fertilized eggs: only maternal mitochondria in the ovum are transmitted to the next generation. All children, both male and female, of a woman who has an mtDNA mutation will likely inherit the mutation. A man with an mtDNA mutation will not transmit that mutation to his offspring. Figure 6-38 shows a typical pedigree of a family with several members affected with Leber hereditary optic neuropathy (see below). Inheritance of the disorder is only through females and no affected male transmits it. Affected individuals may exhibit various degrees of severity of the disorder depending upon the proportion of mitochondria that carry the mutant mtDNA they inherit.

MOLECULAR PATHOGENESIS: Before cell division, each of the many copies of mtDNA in all mitochondria in a cell replicate themselves. These mtDNA molecules randomly segregate into the newly synthesized mitochondria, which in turn randomly segregate into the daughter cells, in a process called **replicative segregation**. When a mutation in the mitochondrial genome first occurs it is in a single mtDNA molecule in one mitochondrion. When that cell divides, all mtDNA molecules replicate and the mitochondrion undergoes fission, wild-type and mutant mtDNA molecules are randomly distributed among daughter mitochondria, which by chance contain different proportions of wild-type and mutant mtDNA molecules, which is called **heteroplasmy**. The cell, which now contains mitochondria with various proportions of wild-type and mutant mtDNA, in turn randomly distributes those mitochondria to its daughter cells. Occasionally, by chance, all mitochondria in a daughter cell have only normal mtDNA molecules or only mutant mtDNA molecules, which is called **homoplasmy**. As not all mitochondria in the original ovum will carry mutant mtDNA, mitochondrial diseases vary among tissues and individuals,

since phenotypic expression of an mtDNA mutation depends upon the relative proportions of normal and mutant mtDNA in an individual's cells of different tissues in the body (Fig. 6-39).

Leber hereditary optic neuropathy (LHON) was the first mitochondrial disorder described. It is characterized by rapid painless bilateral loss of central vision in young people due to optic atrophy. Symptoms usually have onset between 15 and 35 years of age. Mitochondria of affected individuals are largely homoplasmic for mutated mtDNA. Three mutations, the most common of which is substitution m.11778A>G in the *ND4* subunit of electron transport chain complex I, account for >90% of cases of LHON.

Myoclonic epilepsy with ragged red muscle fibers (MERRF) exemplifies a heteroplasmic mitochondrial

TABLE 6-12
REPRESENTATIVE MITOCHONDRIAL DISORDERS

Disorder	Clinical Features	Frequency[a]	Inheritance	Gene(s)	Mitochondrial Chromosomal Location
Leber hereditary optic neuropathy (LHON)	Progressive blurring and clouding of central vision due to optic nerve death with usual onset in late teens and 20s	Unknown in most populations. 1/30,000–50,000 in northeast England and Finland	Maternal Largely homoplasmic	*MT-ND1* *MT-ND4* *MT-ND4L* *MT-ND6* (70% of cases)	3,307–4,262 10,760–12,137 10,470–10,766 14,149–14,673
Myoclonic epilepsy with ragged-red fibers (MERRF)	Onset in childhood or adolescence of myoclonus, myopathy, spasticity, seizures, ataxia, peripheral neuropathy, intellectual deterioration, hearing loss, optic atrophy, cardiomyopathy (in some patients)	Rare	Maternal Heteroplasmic	*MT-TK* (80% of cases) *MT-TL1* *MT-TH* *MT-TS1*	8,295–8,364 3,230–3,304 12,138–12,206 7,446–7,514
Mitochondrial encephalomyopathy, lactic acidosis, and stroke-like episodes (MELAS)	Onset most often in childhood, muscle weakness and pain, headaches, anorexia, vomiting, seizures, stroke-like episodes, lactic acidosis	Rare, but most common of the mitochondrial disorders	Maternal Heteroplasmic	*MT-TL1* *MT-ND1* *MT-ND5* *MT-TH* *MT-TV*	3,230–3,304 3,307–4,262 12,337–14,148 12,138–12,206 1,602–1,670
Kearns–Sayre syndrome	Onset before age 20 of external ophthalmoplegia, ptosis, pigmentary retinopathy, loss of vision, cardiac conduction disturbance, ataxia, elevated CSF protein, muscle weakness, renal disease, hearing loss, dementia	1–3/100,000	Generally sporadic, likely due to maternal gonadal mosaicism Heteroplasmic	Single large deletions (1,000–10,000 bp), most common is 4,997 bp deletion that includes 12 mitochondrial genes	
Leigh syndrome (~20% is due to mitochondrial gene mutation, ~80% due to mutant nuclear genes with Mendelian inheritance)	Progressive psychomotor regression with onset in infancy or early childhood, lactic acidosis and high lactate level in CSF, characteristic lesion on MRI in basal ganglia, cerebellum and brainstem, hypertrophic cardiomyopathy, respiratory failure, death in 2–3 years	1/40,000 newborns, more common in Saguenay Lac–Saint–Jean region of Quebec and Faroe Islands	Maternal Heteroplasmic	*MT-ATP6*	8,527–9,207

[a]As a disease group mitochondrial disorders affect 1/4,000–5,000 worldwide.

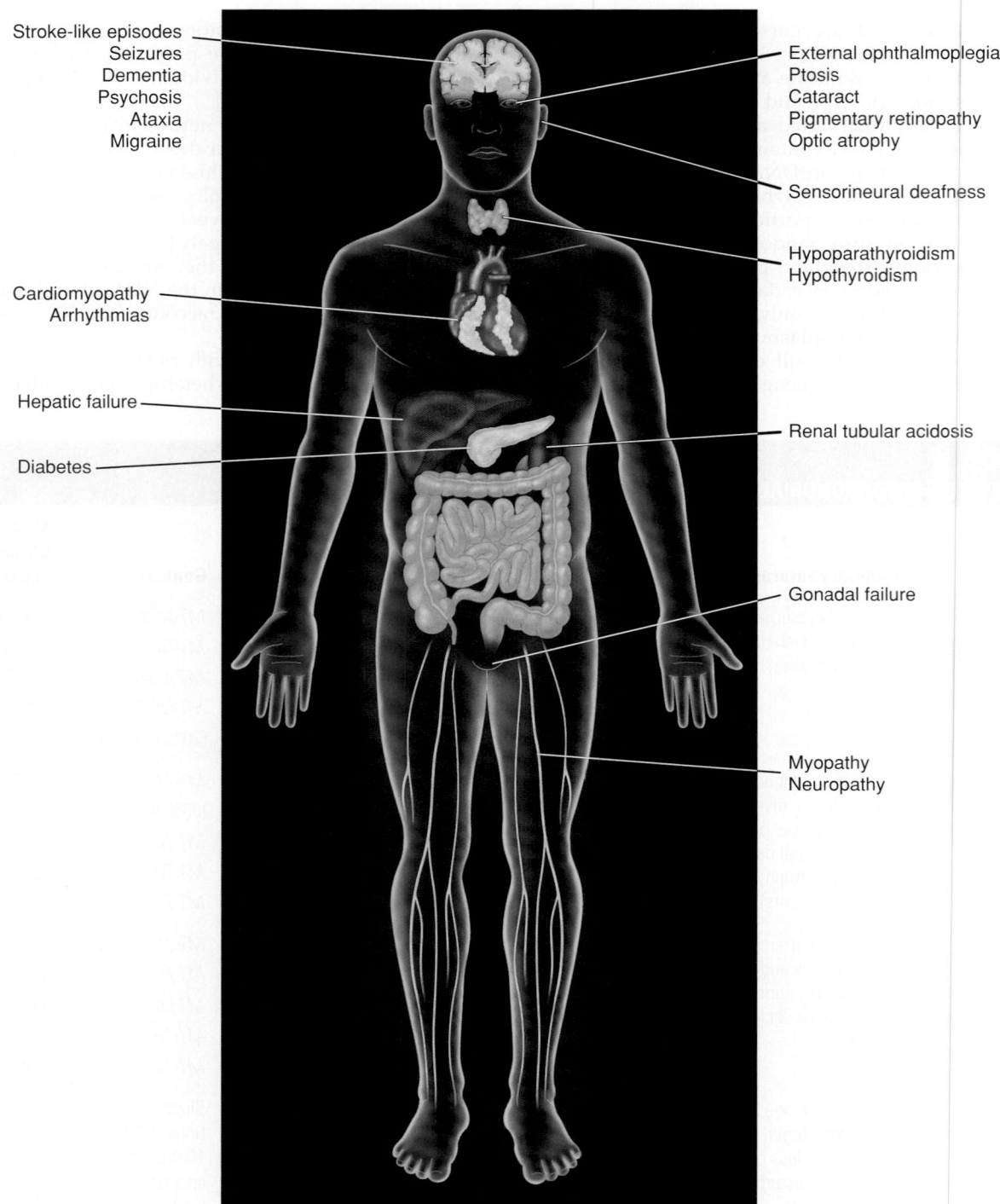

FIGURE 6-37. Mutations in mitochondrial DNA may affect a range of tissues and produce a range of clinical phenotypes.

disorder. It is due to point mutations, most commonly m.8344A>G, in the gene *MT-TK*, a mitochondrial tRNA for lysine, mt-tRNA$^{(Lys)}$. In addition to epilepsy and abnormal muscle fibers, patients with MERRF usually have myopathy, ataxia, sensorineural deafness, and dementia.

The rate of mtDNA mutation is much higher than that of nuclear DNA, due (at least in part) to less efficient mtDNA repair. As mutations in both nuclear and mitochondrial DNA accumulate with age, many diseases of aging are caused in part by defects in mitochondrial function. Since mitochondria process oxygen and produce

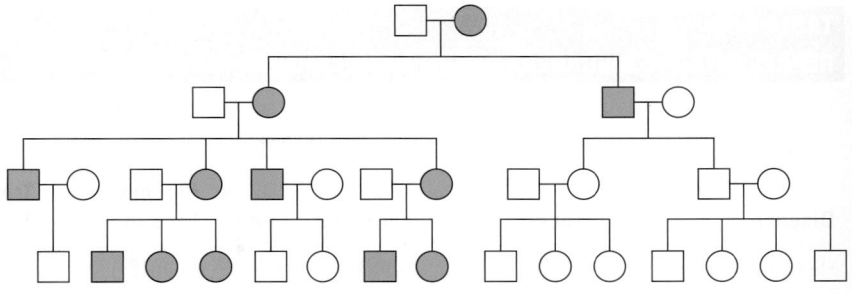

FIGURE 6-38. Four generation pedigree of a family with Leber hereditary optic neuropathy, a form of blindness with onset in young adults. Affected individuals have a His340Arg mutation in the *ND4* mitochondrial gene. Inheritance is only maternal. All the progeny of an affected female inherit the disorder and are affected to various degrees of severity, while none of the progeny of an affected male inherit the disorder.

ATP, mitochondrial dysfunction can contribute to complex diseases in older adults including type 2 diabetes, Parkinson disease, atherosclerotic heart disease, stroke, Alzheimer disease, and cancer.

Disorders due to Trinucleotide Repeat Expansion

In Mendelian inheritance, once mutation that causes a disorder occurs, it is stably transmitted from one generation to the next. In contrast, a group of genetic disorders are due to **dynamic mutations**, which change as they are passed on. The genes for these disorders have segments of DNA with tandem repeating units of three or more nucleotides (usually three) such as CAG or CCG. Wild-type alleles of these genes are **polymorphic**, that is, the number of trinucleotide repeats varies among normal people. The number of sequential repeats may increase gradually as they are passed from generation to generation, eventually reaching a size range where they are unstable and may undergo a marked disease-producing expansion. Huntington disease, fragile X syndrome, myotonic dystrophy, and Friedreich

ataxia are examples of trinucleotide repeat expansion disorders (Table 6-13).

Huntington Disease (HD)

HD is a well-known autosomal dominant disorder in which there is degeneration of the striatum and the cortex of the brain. Symptoms of chorea, dystonia, change in personality, and gradual loss in cognition, typically first appear in midlife and eventually cause death.

MOLECULAR PATHOGENESIS: Normally, there are 26 or fewer CAG repeats in the *HTT* gene which encodes the protein **huntingtin**. Individuals with Huntington disease usually have 40 or more repeats, averaging 46 repeats. People with 36 to 39 repeats may develop symptoms late in life, or not at all. The age of symptom onset depends on how many CAG repeats someone carries. In general, the more repeats, the earlier in life symptoms begin, a phenomenon known as **anticipation**. Children may inherit a CAG repeat number that is within the affected range from a young parent

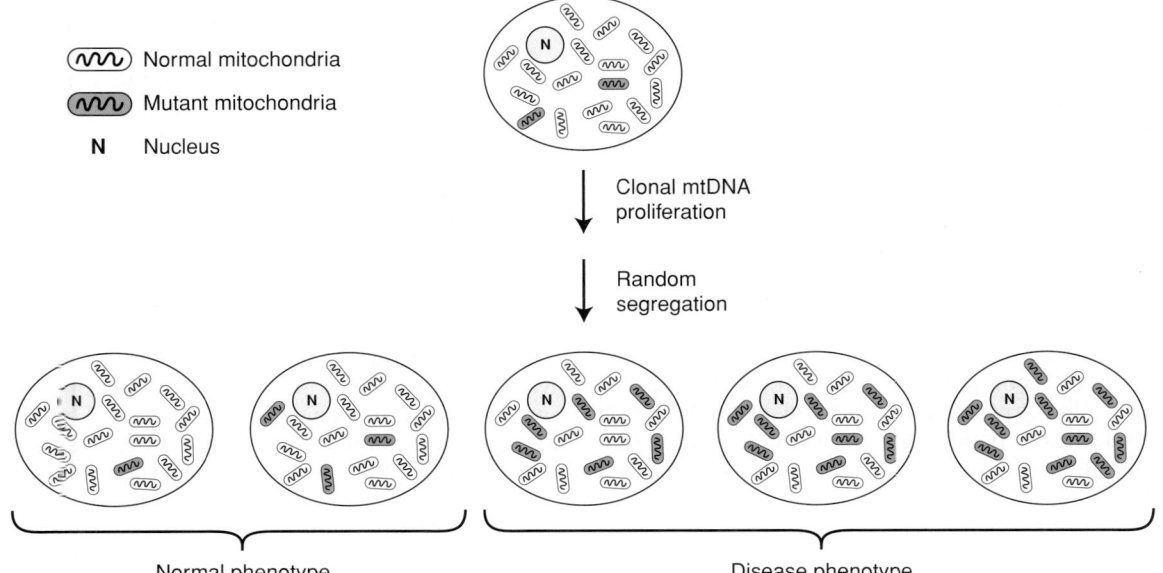

FIGURE 6-39. Replicative segregation of a heteroplasmic mitochondrial mutation. Daughter cells with wide variation in the proportion of normal and mutant mitochondria are produced by multiple rounds of mitosis with random segregation of mutant and normal mitochondria. When the proportion of mutant mitochondria exceeds a certain threshold, cell and tissue dysfunction results.

TABLE 6-13

REPRESENTATIVE DISORDERS DUE TO TRINUCLEOTIDE REPEAT EXPANSION

Disease	Frequency	Inheritance	Gene	Chromosome Location	Trinucleotide Sequence	Normal Number of Repeats	Premutation Number of Repeats (Mutable Normal)	Full Mutation Number of Repeats
Huntington disease	3–7/100,000 European descent	AD	HTT	4p16.3	CAG	≤26	27–35	≥36 36–39 reduced penetrance
Fragile X syndrome	1/4,000 males 1/8,000 females	XL	FMR1	Xq27.3	CGG	5–44 (45–54 gray zone)	55–200	≥200
Myotonic dystrophy I	1/8,000	AD	DMPK	19q13.32	CTG	5–34	35–49	50–2,000
Friedreich ataxia	1/40,000 in the US	AR	FXN	9q21.11	GAA	6–33	34–65	66–1,300
Spinocerebellar ataxia, type 3 (most common type of SCA among numerous types)	All SCAs are rare.	AD	ATXN3	14q32.12	CAG	12–43	44–52	52–87
Kennedy disease (spinal bulbar muscular atrophy)	1/150,000 males	XL	AR	Xq12	CAG	≤34	35–37	≥38

AD = autosomal dominant; AR = autosomal recessive; XLR = X-linked recessive.

who is not yet showing signs of the disorder. Alternatively, a parent with 35 to 40 CAG repeats, which may or may not result in HD in his or her lifetime, may pass on a CAG repeat string that has expanded during gametogenesis into the affected range. In addition, CAG repeats at the upper limit of normal in the premutation range (29 to 35) may increase during meiosis to 40 or more. Expansion of the gene for HD occurs mostly during male gametogenesis. A juvenile severe early-onset form of HD with a very high number of CAG repeats is always paternally inherited.

Fragile X Syndrome (FXS)

FXS, one of the many autism spectrum disorders, is the most common heritable type of moderate intellectual disability. It entails a fragile site in the distal long arm of the X chromosome, in which chromatin does not condense properly during mitosis. The syndrome is inherited in an X-linked fashion with reduced penetrance in females (Fig. 6-40). Affected individuals often have a long narrow face, prominent jaw, large ears, and flexible fingers. Affected males have large testes (macroorchidism).

MOLECULAR PATHOGENESIS: FXS is caused by massive unstable expansion of the CGG trinucleotide repeat in the 5′ untranslated region of the *FMR1* gene on Xq27.3. This leads to excessive cytosine

methylation in the *FMR1* promoter, in turn inhibiting gene expression. Too little of the encoded protein, FMRP, is produced. The normal number of CGG repeats is ≤55. FXS patients with a "full" mutation have >200 repeats, and may have thousands of repeats. From 56 to 200 CGG repeats represents the premutation stage. Expansions in this range are unstable and tend to undergo further expansion into the "full" mutation range during maternal gametogenesis. Expansion risk increases dramatically with increasing premutation repeat number. Although premutation carriers are cognitively normal, males are at risk for adult-onset ataxia and females for premature ovarian failure.

Myotonic Dystrophy

Myotonic dystrophy is a relatively common form of autosomal dominant muscular dystrophy (see Chapter 31). There are two very similar types. Myotonic dystrophy 1 (DM1; also called Steinert disease), is characterized by progressive myotonia (prolonged muscle contractions), muscle weakness and wasting, cardiac conduction defects, cataracts, testicular atrophy, and insulin resistance. The severe congenital form of DM1 also includes intellectual disability and contractures of the extremities. Affected newborns often have marked hypotonia that may cause life-threatening respiratory and feeding difficulties. DM1 occurs in approximately 1 in 8,000 people worldwide.

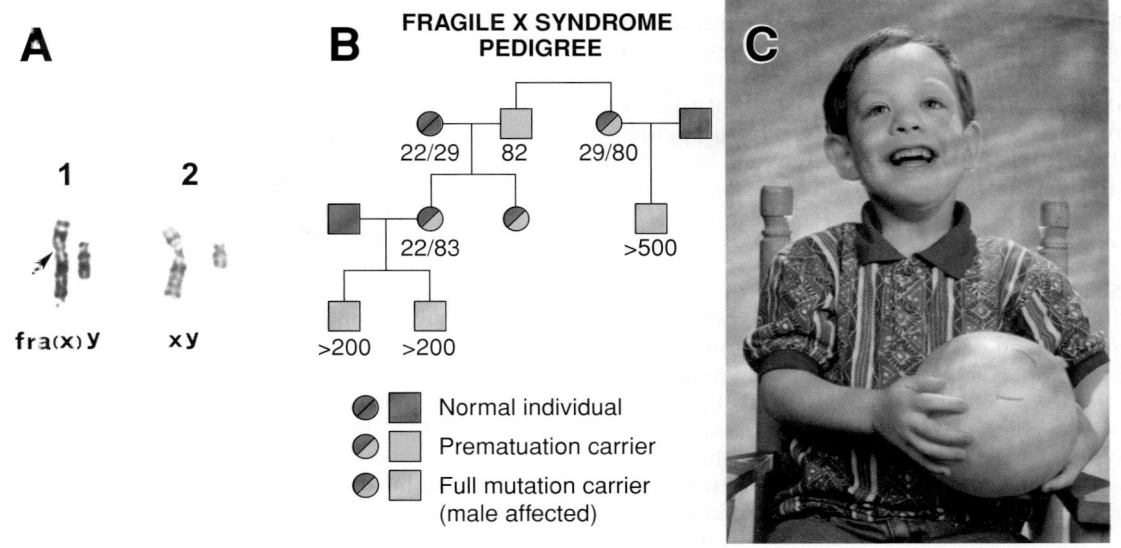

FIGURE 6-40. Fragile X syndrome. A. Fragile X chromosome (1), compared to normal (2). Note the *arrow* demonstrates the nonstaining gap at Xq23.1. **B.** Pedigree showing the inheritance pattern of fragile X syndrome. The number of copies of the CGG trinucleotide repeat on each X chromosome is below selected each family members. CGG repeat expansion occurs primarily during female meiosis. When the number of repeats exceeds ~200, the clinical syndrome is manifested. Individuals shaded blue carry a premutation and are asymptomatic, as are normal individuals who are shaded in orange. **C.** Boy with fragile X syndrome who has the characteristic macrocephaly, prominent forehead, elongated face, large ears, and prominent chin. He also has macroorchidism, intellectual disability and autistic behavior.

MOLECULAR PATHOGENESIS: DM1 is caused by abnormal expansion of the CTG trinucleotide repeat in the 3′ noncoding region of the *DMPK* gene on chromosome 19q13.32. People with 5 to 35 CTG repeats are normal; those with 50 to 2,000 repeats are affected. Premutation carriers with 36 to 49 repeats are usually asymptomatic, but are at risk to pass on expanded repeats that are in the affected range to their offspring. Myotonic dystrophy 2, caused by a CCTG tetranucleotide repeat expansion in the *CNBP* gene on 3q21.3, resembles DM1 clinically, but lacks the severe congenital presentation.

Friedreich Ataxia

Friedreich ataxia **(FA)** is an autosomal recessive neurodegenerative disorder characterized by ataxia, muscle weakness, impaired vision, hearing loss, slurred speech, cardiomyopathy, scoliosis, and diabetes mellitus.

MOLECULAR PATHOGENESIS: The *FXN* gene on chromosome 9q21.11 encodes **frataxin**, which binds iron and is required to synthesize the iron–sulfur clusters needed for mitochondrial function in nerve and muscle cells. Abnormally long GAA trinucleotide repeats in intron 1 of *FXN* causes impaired transcriptional elongation and thus loss of frataxin function. The normal number of GAA repeats in FXN is 6 to 33, but people with FA have 66 to 1,300. Those with 34 to 65 are premutation carriers, and can pass on an expanded GAA repeat in the affected range to their children. Because FA is an autosomal recessive disorder, affected individuals must have GAA repeat expansions in both *FXN* genes. The length of the GAA trinucleotide repeat is related to the age of onset of FA symptoms, the severity of symptoms, and the rate of progression. Patients with <300 GAA repeats tend to show symptoms after age 25. Those with larger GAA expansions are affected earlier and generally have more severe disease.

Genomic Imprinting Disorders

MOLECULAR PATHOGENESIS: Genomic imprinting is a normal epigenetic process that involves selective inactivation of certain genes via CpG methylation (see above) in a manner that depends on a parent of origin. Not all of the genes on autosomal chromosomes are transcribed from both alleles. Genes expressed only on one of the parental chromosomes (paternal or maternal) are said to be "imprinted." The exact number of imprinted genes is unknown, but several hundred autosomal genes are felt to be normally transcribed only from the maternally inherited allele, while a few hundred other genes are transcribed only from the paternally inherited allele. The other allele is silenced via methylation and other epigenetic mechanisms. Epigenetic modifications are erased in gonadal cells, and sperm or ovum-specific epigenetic marks are then re-established before fertilization. Different epigenetic modifications on the paternal and maternal chromosomes are then transmitted through mitosis to all somatic cells. Some chromosomal regions may contain only one imprinted gene, while others may have a cluster of multiple imprinted genes. If a normal allele is inactivated and a lack of function allele is imprinted, a disease phenotype may arise. Prader–Willi syndrome (PWS) and Angelman syndrome illustrate how genomic imprinting causes human disease.

Prader–Willi Syndrome

PWS occurs in approximately 1 in 10,000 to 30,000 newborns. It presents in the neonatal period with hypotonia, feeding difficulty and hypoplastic genitalia in males. Paradoxically, in early childhood the feeding problems transition to difficult to control hyperphagia with indiscriminate eating habits that lead to obesity. Affected individuals have short stature, small hands and feet, mild to moderate intellectual disability, behavioral problems, and fair hair and skin coloring (Fig. 6-41A).

MOLECULAR PATHOGENESIS: PWS is due to lack of expression of a region of genes on the proximal long arm of the paternal chromosome 15, including the snoRNA (small nucleolar RNA) gene cluster that is involved in modifications of ribosomal RNAs. Approximately 70% of cases are due to deletion of 15q11.2-q13 from the paternally inherited chromosome 15. The maternal genes in this region are normally inactive and, despite deletion of the active paternal allele, remain silenced. Maternal uniparental disomy (to be discussed below) can also result in nonexpression of the snoRNA gene cluster and cause PWS.

Angelman Syndrome

Angelman syndrome (AS), once called happy puppet syndrome, is less common than PWS. It is mainly a neurologic

disorder, with an apparent happy demeanor, ataxia and jerking arm movements, microcephaly, a large mouth, widely spaced teeth, prominent jaw, little or no speech, severe intellectual disability, and seizures (Fig. 6-41B).

MOLECULAR PATHOGENESIS: AS is due to lack of expression of the *UBE3A* (ubiquitin-protein ligase E3A) gene on the proximal long arm of chromosome 15. In specific parts of the brain, the paternal gene is inactive, and expression is from the maternal chromosome 15. Elsewhere in the body, both parental genes are expressed. Approximately 70% of cases of AS are due to deletion of 15q11.2-q13 from the maternal chromosome 15. The paternal *UBE3A* gene in this part of the brain is normally inactive and remains silenced despite deletion of the maternal copy. Paternal **uniparental disomy** (see below) can also result in nonexpression of *UBE3A*.

Mutations in the imprinting center in the 15q11.2-q13 region may also result in both PWS and AS, and account for 2% to 3% of both disorders.

A normal individual inherits one chromosome of each homologous pair from each parent. Occasionally, both chromosomes of a homologous pair are from one parent, with no contribution from the other parent. This situation is known as **uniparental disomy** and can result in an abnormal phenotype if imprinted genes are present on the uniparental disomic chromosomes. For example, an infant who has inherited both chromosomes 15 from its mother will have PWS. This is because no paternal allele with an active PWS gene region is present and both maternally inherited chromosomes 15 have inactive PWS gene region. AS, on the other hand, will occur in people who inherit both chromosomes 15 from their fathers. No maternal allele with an active *UBE3A* gene is present and both paternally inherited chromosomes 15 have an inactive *UBE3A* gene. Figure 6-42 depicts imprinting mechanisms that can produce PSW and AS.

PWS is more common than AS because of **zygote rescue**. A zygote may have three copies of a chromosome due to maternal nondisjunction, which, as mentioned earlier in the chapter, occurs more frequently with advanced maternal age. Usually a trisomic pregnancy will spontaneously abort early in the first trimester. However, occasionally one of the trisomic chromosomes will be lost in an early cell division of the embryo, allowing the pregnancy to continue. If the trisomic chromosome lost was paternally inherited, the embryo will now have two homologous maternal chromosomes. If zygote rescue occurs with loss of a paternal chromosome 15 in a pregnancy that started with trisomy 15, the product of the pregnancy will be an infant with PWS. Duplication of a chromosome in a zygote with a monosomic chromosome can also lead to uniparental disomy. Up to 1% of viable pregnancies carry uniparental disomy for at least one chromosome.

Paternal uniparental disomy for chromosome 11 is a mechanism that can cause **Beckwith–Wiedemann syndrome (BWS)**. Another cause is duplication of 11p15 which contains an imprinted region on the short arm of chromosome 11. BWS is characterized by overgrowth, organomegaly,

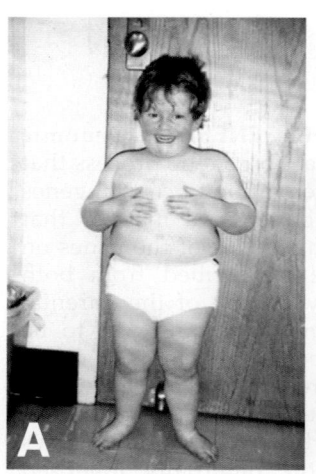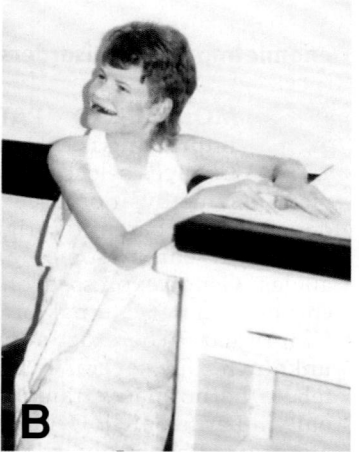

FIGURE 6-41. A. Young boy with **Prader–Willi syndrome**. Note the obesity and small hands and feet. He also had hypoplastic genitalia, a voracious appetite and moderate intellectual disability. **B.** Girl with **Angelman syndrome**. Note the happy demeanor and large mouth with widely spaced teeth. She had no speech, an unsteady gait and severe intellectual disability. Both syndromes are due imprinting abnormalities of the proximal 15q.

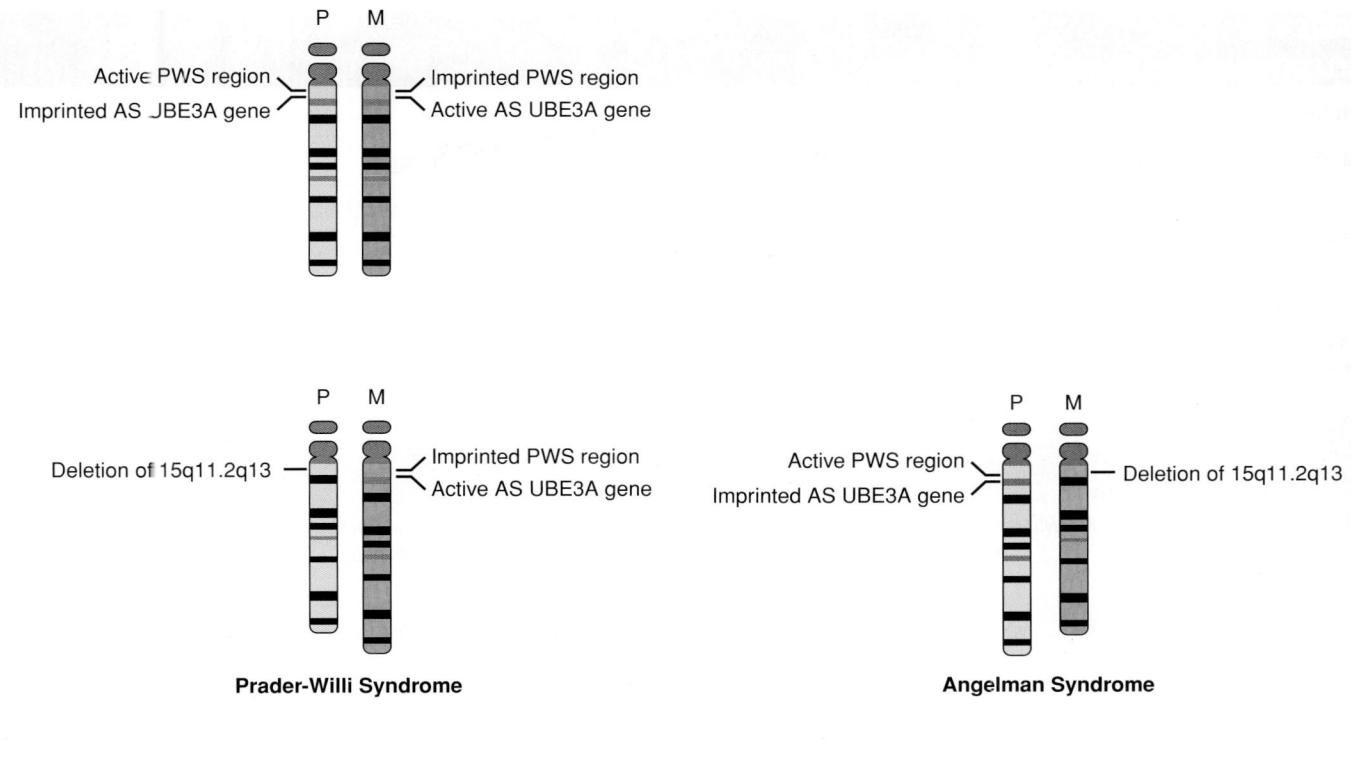

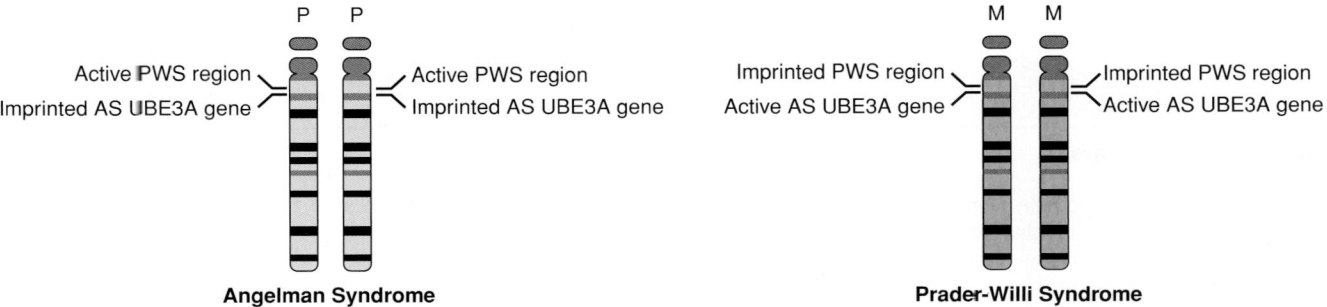

FIGURE 6-42. Imprinting mechanisms that result in Prader–Willi syndrome (PWS) and Angelman syndrome (AS). Upper. Chromosomes 15 of normal individuals. On the paternally inherited (P) chromosome 15 the PWS region is active and the UBE3A gene of AS is imprinted (inactive). On the maternally inherited (M) chromosome 15 the PWS region is imprinted and the UBE3A gene is active. **Middle.** PWS results when the paternally inherited chromosome 15 has a deletion of 15q11.2-q13 and AS results when the maternally inherited chromosome 15 has the same deletion. **Below.** PWS can also result if both chromosomes 15 have been inherited from the mother. AS can also result if both chromosomes 15 have been inherited from the father.

asymmetry, coarse facies, neonatal hypoglycemia and increased risk for Wilms tumor, hepatoblastoma, and adrenal cortical carcinoma.

Molecular Diagnostic Methods Help Establish Genetic Correlates of Disease

Recent years have witnessed a tremendous increase in the power and applicability, and in clinical use, of molecular diagnostic technologies. Some of these, like FISH, are mentioned above; while others are described below (see Tables 6-14, 6-15) and in other chapters.

CONGENITAL ANOMALIES

Congenital anomalies, or birth defects, are alterations in the form or size of one or more parts of the body. They result from disturbed morphogenesis, and cause significant morbidity and mortality in infancy and early childhood. Worldwide, at least 1 in 50 newborns has a major congenital anomaly. Anomalies may have an intrinsic (genetic) or extrinsic (environmental) etiology, or both. Often, the cause of an anomaly is not known, and by default is considered to be multifactorial until a definitive genetic or environmental cause is found.

Many birth defects reflect genetic changes discussed above, including chromosome abnormalities (≈25%), copy

TABLE 6-14

SELECTED MOLECULAR DIAGNOSIS METHODS

Methods for Targeted Mutation Testing

Method	Application	Principle	Advantages	Disadvantages
Restriction Fragment Length Analysis of PCR fragments	Selected known variants	Sequence variants change a restriction enzyme recognition site and length of restriction fragments	Fast and affordable	Depends on a change in a recognition site; concern for errors due to restriction enzyme failure
Allele-specific PCR amplification	Known variants	Specific primers are designed for the mutant and wild-type alleles	Fast and affordable	Specific primers can be difficult to design
Single-base extension (SBE)	Known variants	Primer extension for one position using labeled nucleotide terminators	Limited multiplexing possible	Requires high-resolution electrophoresis equipment
Oligonucleotide Ligation Assay (OLA)	Known variants	Differential ligation of the probes that is perfectly complementary to the target DNA	Allows multiplexing, relatively cheap	Concern for errors due to ligation failure
Allele-specific oligonucleotide (ASO) assay-dot blot	Known variants	Utilizes hybridization of labeled allele-specific probes to target region amplified in patients' samples and applied to duplicate support membranes as Dot blots	Allows multiplexing, relatively cheap	Laborious and cannot differentiate between correct hybridization and cross hybridization.
Allele-specific oligonucleotide (ASO) assay-reverse dot blot	Known variants	Reverse approach relative to the "dot-blot" based on immobilizing allele-specific oligonucleotide probes on a nylon membrane rather than the individual DNA samples	Allows multiplexing, relatively cheap	Laborious and cannot differentiate between correct hybridization and cross hybridization

Sequencing-Based Assays

Sanger sequencing	Single-gene sequencing for Mendelian disorders caused by one specific gene	Primer extension with incorporation of fluorescently labeled nucleotide terminators and fragment separation	Well established, high accuracy	Low throughput and labor intensive
Next generation sequencing (NGS) gene panels	Genetic disorders that can be caused by multiple genes	Simultaneous sequencing by NGS of all known genes implicated in a particular disorder	More efficient and cheaper than sequential Sanger sequencing	Separate analysis has to be conducted for exon-level deletions and duplications
Clinical exome sequencing	Patients with nonspecific or complex phenotype which do not fit an identifiable diagnosis	Simultaneous sequencing of all protein coding genes (exome) by NGS	More effective than sequential testing for patients with complex phenotypes	Some genes and regions not fully covered; some frameshift variants hard to detect; does not test for gene deletions and duplications; complex analysis and interpretation
Whole genome sequencing	Patients with nonspecific or complex phenotype which do not fit an identifiable diagnosis	Sequencing of the entire genome	Has capacity to reveal noncoding (regulatory variants and structural genomic aberrations	Complex analysis, relatively expensive and not widely available, limited ability to interpret regulatory variants

TABLE 6-14

SELECTED MOLECULAR DIAGNOSIS METHODS (*CONTINUED*)

Method	Application	Principle	Advantages	Disadvantages
Gene Deletions and Partial Gene Deletion Testing				
Real-time quantitative PCR	Partial (exon level) deletions and duplications	Quantitative PCR measures the amount of target sequence and compares to a housekeeping gene	Widely available, custom assays for any gene of interest easy to design	Not robust, can be affected by DNA quality
Multiplex Ligation-dependent Probe Amplification (MLPA)	Partial (exon level) deletions and duplications	Involves annealing of two adjacent oligonucleotides to a segment of genomic DNA followed by ligation with product amount corresponding to the amount of the target, PCR amplification and size separation to characterize copy number	Predesigned kits for genes of interest; relatively inexpensive	Not robust, can be affected by DNA quality
Custom copy number (DNA) arrays	Partial (exon level) deletions and duplications	Hybridization signal from patient sample to the probes on the array compared to reference samples	Custom arrays can be designed to test for many genes of interest simultaneously	Both arrays and hybridization equipment are expensive

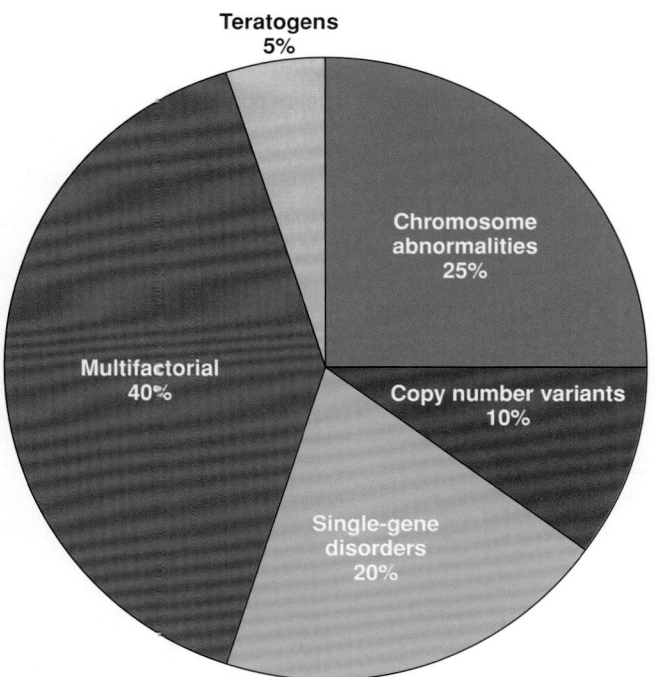

FIGURE 6-43. Relative contribution of the causes of congenital anomalies.

Teratogens 5%

Chromosome abnormalities 25%

Multifactorial 40%

Copy number variants 10%

Single-gene disorders 20%

category are injurious levels of metabolites present due to poorly controlled maternal metabolic disorders and infections. The relative distribution of the causes of congenital anomalies is shown in Figure 6-43.

Congenital Anomalies May Result From Errors of Morphogenesis

During embryonic development cells (1) divide and proliferate, (2) differentiate and acquire novel functions or structures, (3) migrate within the embryo, and (4) undergo programmed cell death (apoptosis). Various combinations of these four basic cellular processes at different times bring about growth and morphogenesis. The creation of a normal size human embryo with all its organs normally formed and positioned is tightly controlled by orderly regulation of developmental genes, each activated or silenced at the appropriate times. During the first 2 weeks of development post conception the fertilized egg is cleaved to become a collection of **blastomeres**, then a **morula**, followed by a **blastocyst**. Approximately 5 to 6 days after fertilization, the blastocyst hatches out of its **zona pellucida** and begins implanting into the endometrium. This is followed by **gastrulation** with formation of endoderm, ectoderm, and mesoderm. The major axes of the embryo result from complicated movements of these germ layers. Establishment of the basic body plan and initiation of the nervous system ensue, followed by organogenesis during weeks 4 to 8 (Fig. 6-44). The influences mentioned above may upset this intricate sequence of events to result in congenital anomalies.

Blastomeres are equipotent and interchangeable; loss of a single blastomere at this stage does not have adverse consequences. In fact, during preimplantation genetic diagnosis to determine whether an embryo is suitable for implantation after in vitro fertilization, a blastomere is removed from an eight-cell blastocyst for cytogenetic or molecular analysis.

number variants (up to 10%) and single gene mutations (20%). Some may either be inherited or result from a de novo mutation in an autosomal dominant gene. Approximately 40% of congenital anomalies have no identifiable cause, but recur in families of affected children with a higher frequency than in the general population—these are considered multifactorial. The remaining 5% probably result from exposure to teratogens, including drugs, alcohol, chemicals, and radiation. Also included in this

TABLE 6-15

SYMBOLS AND EXAMPLES ILLUSTRATING INTERNATIONALLY ACCEPTED HUMAN GENOME VARIATION SOCIETY (HGVS) NOMENCLATURE FOR MOLECULAR VARIANTS (2016 UPDATE)

Reference Sequences

c.	coding DNA reference sequence
g.	genomic reference sequence
m.	mitochondrial reference sequence
n.	noncoding RNA reference sequence (gene producing an RNA transcript but not a protein)
r.	RNA reference sequence
p.	protein reference sequence

Nomenclature Abbreviations and Symbols

"del" deletion	"inv" inversion	"t" translocation	">" "changes to" (substitution)
"dup" duplication	">" substitution	"*" translation termination (stop) codon	":" separates the description of a reference sequence and the actual description of a variant
"ins" insertion	"con" conversion	"_" nucleotide numbering, used to indicate a range	" = " indicates identity to reference sequence

Examples of Nomenclature on cDNA and Protein Level

cDNA change	Interpretation	Protein change	Interpretation
c.262A>G	adenine at the cDNA position 262 is replaced by guanine	p.Asn88Asp	asparagine at the protein position 88 is replaced by aspartic acid
c.1534G>T	guanine at the cDNA position 1534 is replaced by thymine	p.Glu512*	glutamic acid at the protein position 512 is replaced by a stop codon
c.142_143delAT	deletion of nucleotides A and T at cDNA positions 142 and 143	p.Ile48Lysfs*2	Frameshift that results in substitution of isoleucine at the protein position 48 with lysine and a stop codon 3 positions downstream of the deletion site
c.363+1G>A	guanine in the intron immediately after the cDNA position 363 replaced by adenine (changes the canonical splice site)	p.?	Protein effects unknown (variant is predicted to affect splicing but that has to be tested by functional studies)

Examples of Complete Nomenclature for Different Variant Types in the CFTR Gene

Missense variant: NM_000492.3 (*CFTR*):c.224G>A (p.Arg75Gln)
Truncating variant (stop codon): NM_000492.3 (*CFTR*):c.115C>T (p.Gln39*)
Truncating variant (frameshift): NM_000492.3 (*CFTR*):c.174_177del (p.Asp58Glufs*32)
Splicing variant: NM_000492.3 (*CFTR*):c.164+1G>A (p.?)

Genetically normal embryos consisting of the remaining seven blastomeres are then selected for implantation in the mother (Fig. 6-45).

Separation of blastomeres in the first 3 days after conception, or of the inner cell mass of a blastocyst at 4 to 7 days, can result in identical twins. An insult causing separation after 7 days can result in conjoined twins. Conjoined twins may be asymmetric with one well developed and the other rudimentary or hypoplastic. The latter is always abnormal, and sometimes resides within the body of the better-developed twin (*fetus in fetu*). Some congenital teratomas, especially in the sacrococcygeal area, are actually an asymmetric conjoined twin.

Congenital Anomalies Fall Into Three Major Groups

Malformations are congenital anomalies that are due to an *intrinsic developmental disturbance*, a primary error of morphogenesis of an organ or tissue. They may occur as an

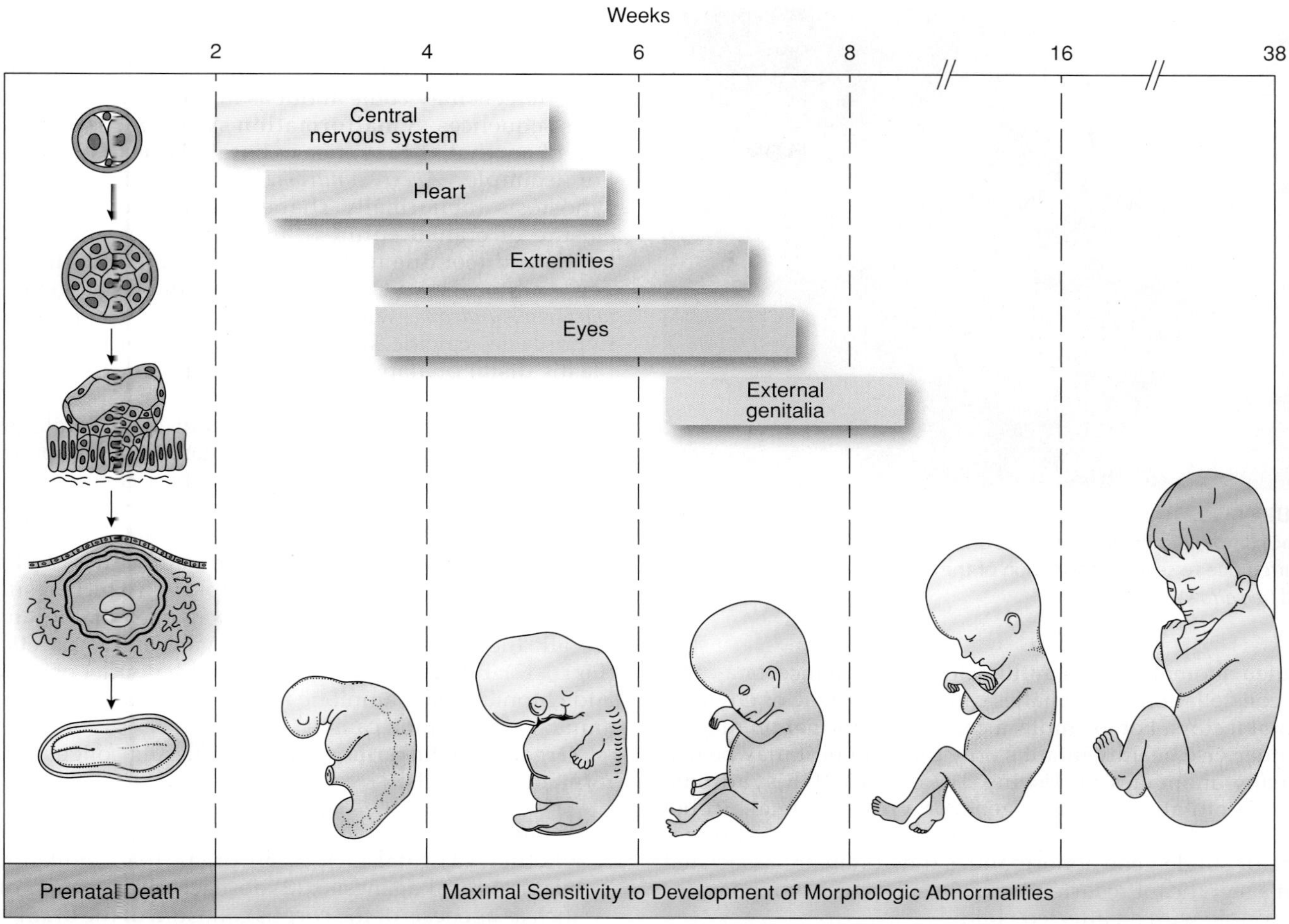

FIGURE 6-44. Sensitivity of specific organs to teratogenic agents at critical stages of embryogenesis. Exposure to adverse influences in the preimplantation and early post implantation stages of development during the first 2 weeks post conception (far left) either leads to early prenatal death or does not harm the embryo. Later, periods of maximal sensitivity to teratogens (horizontal bars) vary for different organ systems, but overall are limited to the first 8 weeks of pregnancy.

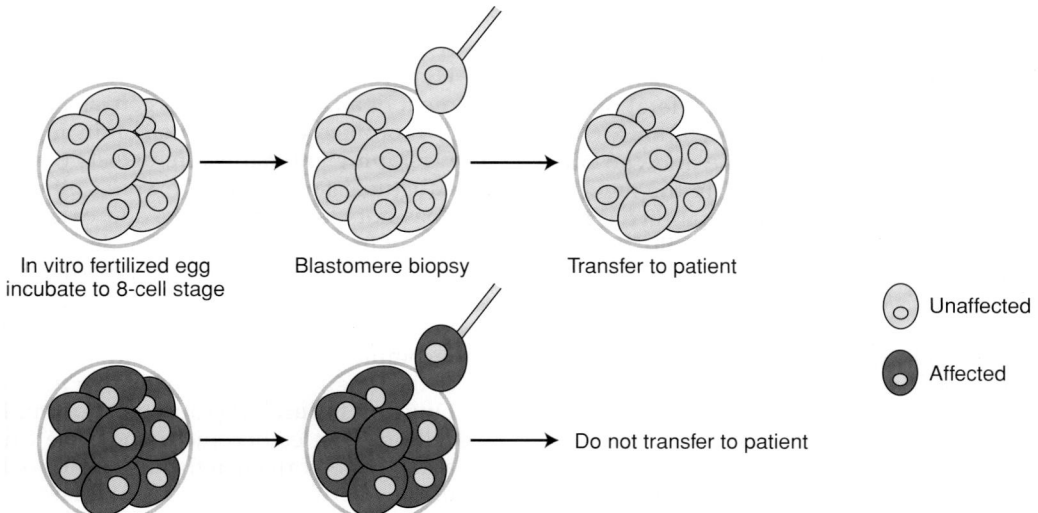

FIGURE 6-45. Preimplantation genetic diagnosis via blastomere biopsy. After in vitro fertilization the fertilized egg is incubated for 3 days until the 8- to 16-cell stage of development. A single blastomere is removed and undergoes genetic testing for a chromosomal abnormality or a single-gene disorder. Only those early embryos that are found to be unaffected will be transferred to the patient. The blastomeres are still pluripotent at this stage and the loss of a blastomere will not adversely affect the development of the embryo.

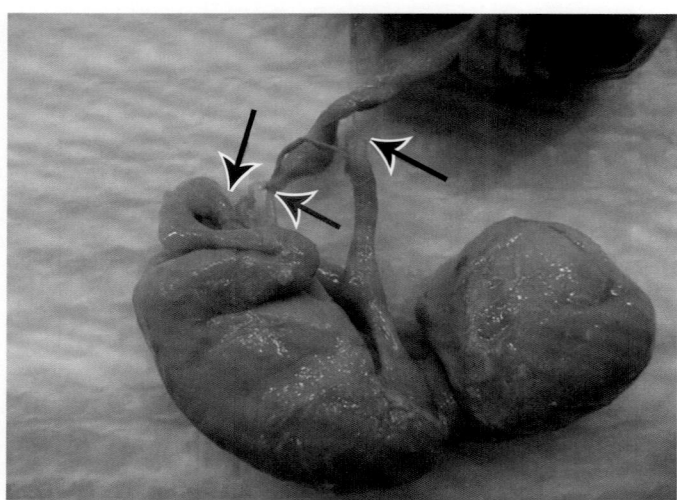

FIGURE 6-46. Twelve weeks gestation fetus with distal limb defects due to encircling and constricting strands of amnion (*black arrows*). Fetal death occurred due to severe constriction of the umbilical cord by an amniotic band (*red arrow*).

isolated anomaly due to multifactorial inheritance, or as part of a constellation of anomalies caused by genetic or environmental factors. For example, a cardiac malformation may be an otherwise healthy infant's only problem or it may be one of many anomalies in trisomy 21, or **CHARGE syndrome** due to a mutation in *CHD7* gene, or a result of fetal alcohol syndrome. Because many malformations are due to chromosome or single gene abnormalities they often are associated with a significant recurrence risk in subsequent pregnancies of a couple with an affected child.

Deformation is an *extrinsic disturbance* in morphogenesis that involves localized or generalized compression of the fetus usually due to uterine constraint late in pregnancy. In the third trimester all fetuses experience some compression as rapid fetal growth outpaces uterine enlargement and the volume of amniotic fluid that cushions the fetus decreases. Risk factors for excessive compression and deformation include leiomyomas, bicornuate uterus, first pregnancy, oligohydramnios (severely reduced amount of amniotic fluid), abnormal fetal presentation, twin and higher-order multiple gestations. Clubfoot due to deformation is usually flexible and can often be successfully corrected by serial casting in the newborn period. In contrast, clubfoot due to malformation has been present throughout gestation, is usually not flexible and requires surgical correction.

Disruption is an *extrinsic disturbance* in morphogenesis in which a previously normally formed organ or anatomic region is damaged by an intrauterine factor. Amniotic band syndrome is a common example of congenital anomalies caused by disruption. The amniotic sac may rupture producing bands of amnion that can encircle parts of the fetus, often the extremities. With fetal movement the bands may constrict a fetal part tightly and disrupt or amputate the limb distal to the constriction (Fig. 6-46).

Congenital Anomaly Terminology

In **pleiotropy**, a single underlying etiology (see above) causes anomalies of more than one organ system in different parts of the embryo or in multiple structures that arise at different times during intrauterine development. Depending on how the agent produces its damaging effect, pleiotropic birth defects may come about as malformation syndromes or as sequences. A **malformation syndrome** is a constellation of anomalies that arise in parallel due to one etiology. For example, *Apert syndrome*, characterized by craniosynostosis (abnormally shaped skull due to premature closure of cranial sutures), unusual facies and hoof-like hands and feet due to syndactyly (fusion of digits) of fingers and toes, result from mutations in *FGFR2* gene. *Fetal warfarin syndrome* with low birth weight, marked nasal hypoplasia, calcific stippling of the skeleton, and hypoplastic distal phalanges is due to prenatal exposure to the anticoagulant warfarin (Coumadin).

A **sequence** occurs when a mutant gene, teratogen, or other trigger only affects a single organ system at one point in time, and that perturbation triggers a cascade of additional anomalies elsewhere in the fetus. In the *Potter sequence* (Fig. 6-47), external signs of excessive fetal compression (flat face, large ears, clubfeet, finger contractures, and loose redundant skin), pulmonary hypoplasia (which results in neonatal death) and morphologic changes of the amnion are all due to oligohydramnios, regardless of its etiology (Fig. 6-47). Bilateral renal aplasia, bladder outlet obstruction and chronic leak of amniotic fluid due to a disruption of the amnion are common causes.

Organ-specific terms used in discussing congenital malformations include:

- **Agenesis** is complete absence of an organ primordium, whether: (1) total lack of an organ (e.g., unilateral or bilateral renal agenesis); (2) absence of part of an organ, such as agenesis of the corpus callosum of the brain; or (3) lack of a specific cell type(s) in an organ, such as absence of testicular germ cells in congenital Sertoli cell–only syndrome.
- **Aplasia** is persistence of an organ rudiment, or anlage, without the mature organ. In pulmonary aplasia, for example, the main bronchus ends blindly in a nondescript mass of rudimentary ducts and connective tissue.
- **Hypoplasia** is reduced size due to incomplete development of all or part of an organ, as in micrognathia (small jaw) or microcephaly (small brain and head).
- **Dysraphic anomalies** are defects caused when apposed structures fail to fuse. In spina bifida, the spinal canal does not close completely, and overlying bone and skin do not fuse, leaving a midline defect.
- **Involution failures** denote persistence of embryonic or fetal structures that normally involute during development. Thus, a persistent thyroglossal duct results from incomplete involution of the tract that connects the base of the tongue with the developing thyroid.
- **Division failures** are caused by incomplete programmed cell death in embryonic tissues (see Chapter 1). Fingers and toes are formed at the distal ends of limb buds by loss of cells between cartilage-containing primordia. If these cells do not undergo apoptosis, digits are conjoined or incompletely separated (syndactyly).
- **Atresia** describes incomplete formation of a normal body orifice or tubular passage. Many hollow organs begin as cell strands and cords whose centers undergo apoptosis to form a central cavity or lumen. Esophageal atresia

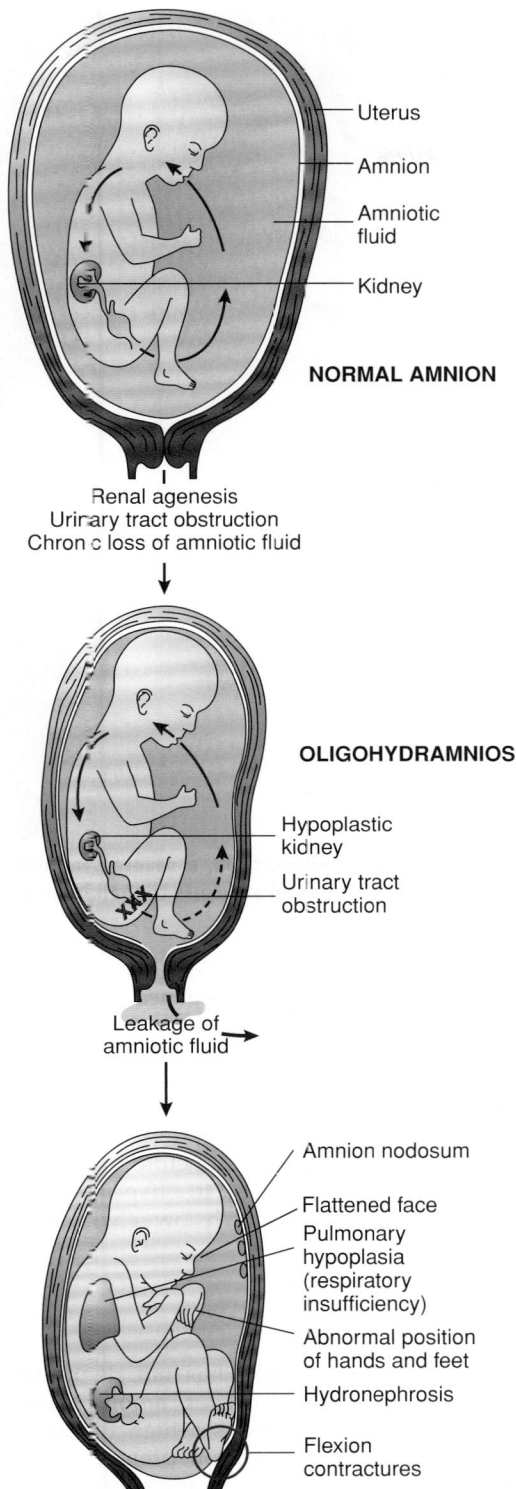

is characterized by localized absence of the lumen, which was not fully established in embryogenesis.

■ **Dysplasia** is caused by abnormal histogenesis. (This context is different from "dysplasia" in precancerous epithelial lesions [see Chapters 1, 5].) In tuberous sclerosis abnormal aggregates of normally developed brain cells are arranged into grossly visible "tubers."

■ **Ectopia, or heterotopia,** is a normally formed organ not in its normal anatomic location. Thus, heterotopic parathyroid glands may be within the thymus in the anterior mediastinum or a normally formed kidney may be one in the pelvis.

Teratogens Are Agents That Can Cause Developmental Anomalies

Teratogens may be drugs, chemicals, radiation, metabolites due to maternal metabolic disorders and infections (Table 6-16). In general, insults due to teratogen exposure in the first 2 weeks post-conception either result in death of the conceptus, especially those that occur before implantation, or do not harm the pregnancy (Fig. 6-44). Such early pregnancy loss often goes unnoticed or is misconstrued as heavy delayed menstrual bleeding.

Complex developmental abnormalities affecting multiple organ systems are usually due to insults during early

FIGURE 6-47. Potter sequence. The fetus normally swallows and, in turn, excretes urine, thus maintaining a normal volume of amniotic fluid. In the face of a urinary tract anomaly (e.g., renal agenesis or urinary tract obstruction) or amniotic fluid leak, the volume of amniotic fluid becomes greatly reduced, a situation called **oligohydramnios**. Oligohydramnios results in a spectrum of congenital anomalies known as **Potter sequence**, which includes pulmonary hypoplasia, limb contractures, and flattened face and ears. The amnion has a nodular appearance known as amnion nodosum.

TABLE 6-16
REPRESENTATIVE TERATOGENS

Teratogens

Drugs and chemicals
- Alcohol
- Thalidomide
- Phenytoin
- Isotretinoin
- Warfarin
- Androgens
- Folic acid antagonists
- Others

Radiation

Maternal diseases
- Diabetes
- Other endocrinopathies
- Phenylketonuria

Uterine/placental infection
- Toxoplasmosis
- Rubella
- Cytomegalovirus
- Herpes simplex virus
- Varicella-zoster virus
- Treponema pallidum (syphilis)
- Parvovirus B19 (fifth disease, slap cheek disease)
- Human immunodeficiency virus
- Enteroviruses
- Zika virus

organogenesis—through the end of the eighth week of pregnancy. This developmental stage of primordial organ system formation is susceptible to malformation due to the influence of a chromosome imbalance, a mutant gene, or a teratogen (Fig. 6-44).

Risk of teratogenesis also depends on dose. Teratogenic drugs may inhibit crucial enzymes or receptors, interfere with formation of mitotic spindles or impair energy production, thus inhibiting metabolic steps critical for normal morphogenesis. Mechanisms of teratogenesis are specific for each agent and may depend upon the genotypes (e.g., drug metabolizing abilities) of both the fetus and the mother. Teratogenic agents often cause specific patterns of congenital anomalies (see below), and rarely cause major errors of morphogenesis after the third month of pregnancy. However, functional and, to a lesser degree, structural abnormalities may occur in children exposed to exogenous teratogens during later trimesters. Although organs are formed by the end of the first trimester, most restructure and mature at prescribed rates. For example, the CNS attains functional maturity several years after birth and remains susceptible to adverse exogenous influences for this interval.

Drugs

Thalidomide is the classic example of a teratogenic drug. It was widely used in Europe in the 1950s to treat morning sickness in pregnancy. It was eventually found to be the cause of severe bilateral limb reduction defects seen in a large number of infants in Europe (Fig. 6-48). Typically, limbs were short and malformed, resembling a seal's flippers (phocomelia), or sometimes completely missing (amelia). Thalidomide, a derivative of glutamic acid, is teratogenic between days 28 and 50 of gestation. It impairs limb growth by blocking angiogenesis. (These same properties make it useful for treating certain malignancies.) The tissue-specific teratogenic effect of thalidomide (and its anti-neoplastic activity) may reflect the fact that there are multiple angiogenic pathways (see Chapter 5), only some of which are thalidomide-sensitive. Thalidomide is not teratogenic in rodents; *thus, just because a drug is not teratogenic in laboratory animals does not necessarily establish that it is innocuous for humans.* Without adequate, well-controlled human studies on a particular agent, a prescribing physician contemplating treating a pregnant woman should consider potential risks to the developing fetus.

About 10T of children born to mothers taking the antiepileptic drug, **hydantoin** (Dilantin), during pregnancy may show **fetal hydantoin syndrome**, with characteristic facial features with wide-set eyes, a broad depressed nasal bridge and occasionally cleft lip and palate. They also may have hypoplastic nails and digits, congenital heart defects, and neurodevelopmental problems. The spectrum of syndromes associated with prenatal exposure to such antiepileptics is broad. The mechanism by which hydantoin and other antiepileptic drugs cause malformations is thought to involve their metabolism by epoxide hydrolase. Genetic variability among maternal and fetal genes encoding the enzyme may increase susceptibility.

Isotretinoin (13-cis-retinoic acid), an oral medication used to treat treatment acne, was recognized as a human teratogen. Several exposed infants had craniofacial, cardiac, CNS, and thymic anomalies. Some were stillborn and those

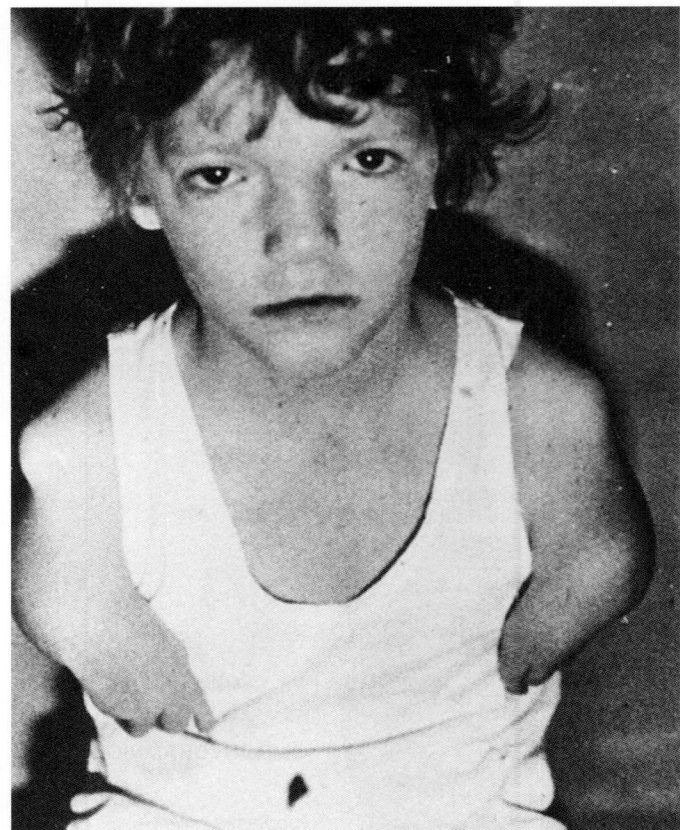

FIGURE 6-48. Child with phocomelia, a severe symmetrical limb reduction defect, due to prenatal exposure to thalidomide.

that survived had subnormal intelligence. This constellation of birth defects is now known as *retinoic acid embryopathy.* Isotretinoin is a retinoid that closely resembles retinoic acid, a natural vitamin A derivative that plays an important role in embryonic development. Offspring of women who take isotretinoin after day 15 post fertilization have a 35% risk for malformations. Stopping the drug before the third week of pregnancy carries no known risk to offspring. The risk for congenital malformations is much lower with topical retinoids such as tretinoin.

Chemicals

Nicotine from cigarette smoke has not definitively been shown to be teratogenic. However, among women who smoke during pregnancy there is a high rate of placental abnormalities, spontaneous abortion, premature labor, low–birth-weight infants (see Chapter 8) and sudden infant death syndrome (SIDS, see below).

Prenatal exposure to **alcohol** is a leading preventable cause of birth defects and developmental disabilities. Harm caused by intrauterine exposure to alcohol was noted in biblical times and was reported during the historic London gin epidemic (1720–1750). However, a specific syndrome was not defined until 1968. The incidence of *fetal alcohol syndrome* (FAS) ranges from 0.2 to 2.0 cases per 1,000 live births in the United States, but may be as high as 20 to 150 cases per 1,000 in populations with high rates of alcoholism. FAS is the extreme end of *fetal alcohol spectrum disorder*, which includes pre- and postnatal growth retardation, microcephaly, CNS abnormalities, cardiac septal defects, minor joint contractures, small distal phalanges, and psychomotor disturbances. Characteristic facial dysmorphology includes short palpebral fissures, maxillary hypoplasia, a smooth philtrum (slightly folded area between base of nose and upper lip), and thin lips. A minority of children affected by maternal alcohol abuse show the full FAS spectrum. Mild mental deficiency and emotional disorders related to fetal alcohol effect are far more common than full-blown FAS. One-fifth of children with FAS have intelligence quotients below 70, and 40% are between 70 and 85. Even those with normal intelligence, tend to show short memory spans, impulsive behavior, and emotional instability (see Chapter 8). Those with full FAS are often born to frankly alcoholic mothers who drank 8 to 10 alcoholic beverages per day of gestation, while those with mild findings were often exposed to 2 drinks per day. Heavy alcohol consumption during the first trimester of pregnancy is particularly dangerous. The mechanism by which alcohol damages the developing fetus is poorly understood.

Radiation

Birth defects, especially those involving the CNS, can result if a fetus receives a large **radiation** dose (exceeding the exposure from 500 chest x-rays) between 2 and 18 weeks of gestation. The fetus will also have an increased risk for cancer later in life. Fetuses in the 8- to 18-week stage of pregnancy exposed to the atomic bombs dropped on Hiroshima and Nagasaki were found to have a high rate of brain damage that resulted in lower IQs and even severe mental retardation. They also suffered stunted growth and an increased rate of other birth defects. As a group they were 4% shorter than the general population.

Maternal Metabolic Disease

High serum levels of glucose are teratogenic. Infants of mothers with **diabetes mellitus** have a significantly increased risk for congenital malformations, the risk correlating strongly with the degree of hyperglycemia in the periconceptional period. Overall risk for a major malformation is about 5% and is approximately 10% if a pregnant woman requires insulin therapy. The types of major congenital anomalies induced by *diabetic embryopathy* include orofacial clefts and heart, neural tube, and limb defects. Sacral agenesis/caudal dysplasia (lack of fetal development of the caudal spine and corresponding segments of the spinal cord) is rare in the general population but highly associated with maternal diabetes, which accounts for 15% to 25% of cases.

All children of women with **phenylketonuria** (PKU) are obligate heterozygotes and as carriers would be expected to be unaffected with the disorder. However, those born to mothers not receiving dietary treatment are severely intellectually impaired. Many have microcephaly, poor growth, and cardiac malformations. This is due to the highly teratogenic effect of elevated phenylalanine in the maternal circulation. Therefore, it is very important that a PKU woman who is considering pregnancy be on a low-phenylalanine diet before conceiving, and throughout pregnancy.

Intrauterine or Peripartum Infections Are Important Causes of Fetal and Neonatal Complications

A prenatally infected neonate may have congenital anomalies, poor growth, and abnormal clinical and laboratory findings.

TORCH Complex

TORCH complex is an acronym for congenital infections that were grouped together because they have similar neonatal signs and symptoms, most commonly rash and ocular abnormalities (Fig. 6-49). The TORCH infections: Toxoplasmosis, Other (syphilis), Rubella, Cytomegalovirus, and Herpes simplex virus affect 1% to 5% of all liveborn infants in the United States. The TORCH complex concept was originally put forth to remind obstetricians and pediatricians that these fetal and newborn infections may be indistinguishable from one another and that "TORCH titers" (antibody testing for all TORCH infectious agents) should be performed in suspected cases because prompt diagnosis is crucial to initiating therapy and optimal outcome.

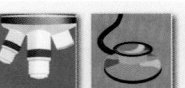 **PATHOLOGY AND CLINICAL FEATURES:** Clinical and pathologic findings in symptomatic newborns with TORCH infections vary. Only a minority show the entire

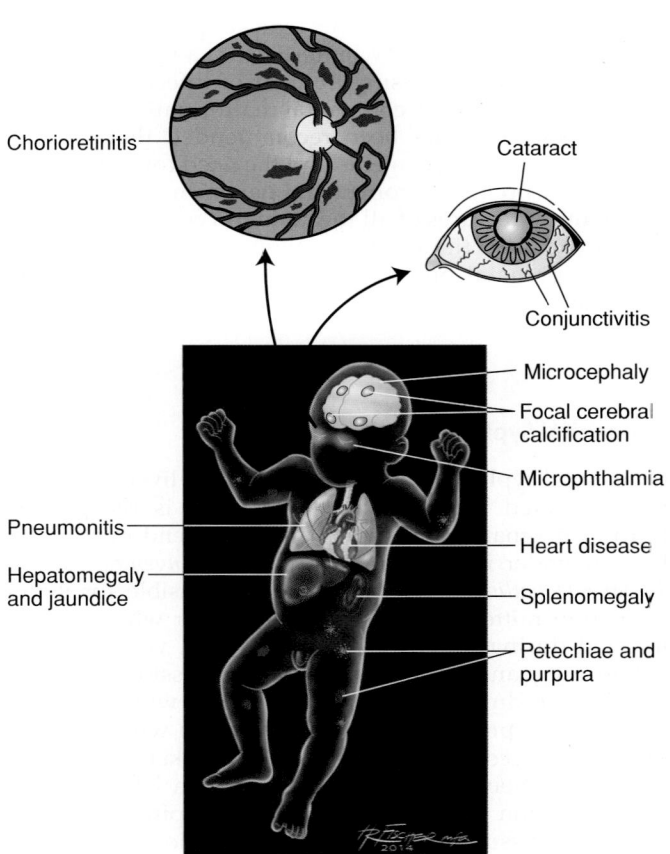

FIGURE 6-49. TORCH complex. Children infected in utero with toxoplasma, rubella virus, cytomegalovirus, or herpes simplex virus show similar effects.

spectrum of abnormalities (Fig. 6-49). Growth retardation and abnormalities of the brain, eyes, liver, hematopoietic system, heart, and skin are common.

CNS lesions are the most serious changes in TORCH-infected children. In acute encephalitis, foci of necrosis are initially surrounded by inflammatory cells. Later these lesions calcify, most prominently in congenital toxoplasmosis. Microcephaly, hydrocephalus, and small abnormally shaped gyri and sulci (microgyria) are common. Radiologically, abnormal cerebral cavities (porencephaly), missing olfactory bulbs and other major brain defects may occur. Severe CNS injury may entail psychomotor retardation, neurologic defects, and seizures.

Ocular defects may also be prominent, particularly with rubella infection, in which over 2/3 of patients have cataracts and microphthalmia. Glaucoma and retinal malformations (coloboma) may occur. Choroidoretinitis, usually bilateral, is common with rubella, Toxoplasma, and CMV. Keratoconjunctivitis is the most common eye lesion in neonatal herpes infection.

Cutaneous findings that may be present include petechiae and purpura.

Cardiac anomalies occur in children with the TORCH complex, most often with congenital rubella infection, and include patent ductus arteriosus and septal defects. Pulmonary artery stenosis and complex cardiac anomalies are occasionally seen.

The "O" in TORCH has now been broadened to include varicella-zoster virus (chickenpox), parvovirus B19 (fifth disease), HIV, enterovirus, and Zika virus. Because of the increasing number of infectious agents now known to cause congenital malformations, a diagnostic approach has been recommended that reflects the diversity of such agents and the need for physicians caring for pregnant women and newborns to recognize the clinical features of all the common congenital infections. Because the damage involved is largely irreparable, prenatal prevention is the best approach. The specific agents of the TORCH complex are discussed in detail in Chapter 9.

Congenital Syphilis

Congenital syphilis affects about 1 in 2,000 liveborn infants in the United States, and the incidence is rising. One-third of pregnancies in syphilitic women end in stillbirth, the remainder in liveborn infants with *congenital syphilis*. *Treponema pallidum*, the bacterium responsible for syphilis, is transmitted to the fetus by a mother who had been infected during pregnancy or, potentially, within 4 years before pregnancy. Transplacental transmission can occur at any time during gestation, but occurs with increasing frequency as pregnancy advances. Women with untreated primary or secondary syphilis are more likely to transmit syphilis to their fetuses than women with latent disease. Early infection usually causes abortion. Spirochetes grow in all fetal tissues and clinical manifestations result from the inflammatory response. The severity of the manifestations is variable and depends upon the timing of intrauterine infection.

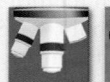 **PATHOLOGY AND CLINICAL FEATURES:** Children with congenital syphilis may appear normal at birth or show signs and symptoms of the TORCH complex. The lesions in symptomatic infants, including granulomas called **gummas**, teem with spirochetes and show perivascular infiltrates of lymphocytes and plasma cells. Many infants are asymptomatic and only develop stigmata of congenital syphilis in the first few months or years of life. Late symptoms of congenital syphilis appear after many years and reflect slowly evolving tissue destruction and repair.

Signs and symptoms of congenital syphilis include:

- **Rhinitis:** A conspicuous mucopurulent nasal discharge, "snuffles," is almost always present as an early sign of congenital syphilis. Nasal mucosa is edematous and tends to ulcerate, leading to nosebleeds. Destruction of the nasal bridge eventually results in flattening of the nose, the so-called **saddle nose**.
- **Skin:** A maculopapular rash is common early in congenital syphilis. It usually affects palms and soles (as in secondary syphilis of adults), although it may cover the entire body or any part of it. Cracks and fissures **(rhagades)** occur around the mouth, anus, and vulva. Flat raised plaques **(condylomata lata)** around the anus and female genitalia may develop early or after a few years.
- **Visceral organs:** A distinctive pneumonitis, with pale hypocrepitant lungs **(pneumonia alba),** may develop in the neonatal period. Hepatosplenomegaly, anemia, and lymphadenopathy may also occur in early congenital syphilis.
- **Teeth:** Buds of incisors and sixth-year molars develop early in postnatal life, at a time when congenital syphilis is particularly aggressive. Thus, permanent incisors may be notched **(Hutchinson teeth)** and molars malformed **(mulberry molars)**.
- **Bones:** Periosteal inflammation with new bone formation **(periostitis)** is common, especially in the anterior tibia, which may bow outward **(saber shins)**.
- **Eye:** Progressive corneal vascularization **(interstitial keratitis)** may occur as early as 4, and as late as 20, years of age. The cornea eventually scars and becomes opaque.
- **Nervous system:** The nervous system is commonly involved. Symptoms start in infancy or after the first year. **Meningitis** predominates in early congenital syphilis, causing convulsions, mild hydrocephalus, and intellectual disability. **Meningovascular syphilis** is common later and may lead to deafness, intellectual disability, paresis, and other complications.
- **Hutchinson triad** is a combination of deafness, interstitial keratitis, and notched incisor teeth.

Clinical findings and a history of maternal syphilis, suggest the diagnosis, but serologic testing to confirm active infection may not be definitive since newborns, in addition to receiving the treponemes, have also received maternal antibody transplacentally. Penicillin is the drug of choice for intrauterine and postnatal syphilis. If given prenatally, or in the first 2 years of postnatal life, most symptoms of congenital syphilis will be prevented.

MULTIFACTORIAL INHERITANCE

Some congenital anomalies such as congenital heart disease (the most common structural birth defect, see Chapter 17), cleft lip and palate, pyloric stenosis, hypospadias, neural tube defects, congenital dislocated hip, and aganglionic megacolon (Hirschsprung disease) may occur alone or as one of multiple anomalies in a chromosomal, copy number variant, single gene or teratogen malformation syndrome. When any of these is an isolated anomaly, it has **multifactorial inheritance**. Like most normal human traits, such as height, hair color and body habitus, isolated congenital anomalies are not simple dominant or recessive Mendelian attributes. Many result from interplay between multiple genes and environmental, epigenetic and other factors. Similarly, many chronic disorders that occur later in life—diabetes, atherosclerosis, hypertension, arthritis, many forms of cancer—"run in families," and have multifactorial inheritance (Table 6-17). The number of involved genes for any particular defect is not known. However, cleft lip with or without cleft palate is thought to be due to two to eight genes acting in a multiplicative fashion in concert with environmental factors. The situation for other congenital malformations with multifactorial inheritance is likely similar.

The risk of any multifactorial anomaly is estimated from the number of relatives affected, the severity of their disease and statistical projections based on population analyses. The probability of a multifactorial disorder in first-degree relatives of someone with the disorder is usually only about 5% to 10%, and is much lower in second-degree relatives. Risk increases with the number of affected family members and disease severity. If there is an altered sex ratio in the incidence of a multifactorial anomaly, as a rule, the recurrence risk is higher in families where the affected member is of the less commonly affected sex.

Isolated **cleft lip and cleft palate** exemplify multifactorial inheritance. At the 35th day of gestation, the embryonic frontal prominence fuses with the maxillary process to form the upper lip. Many genes control this process, and disturbances

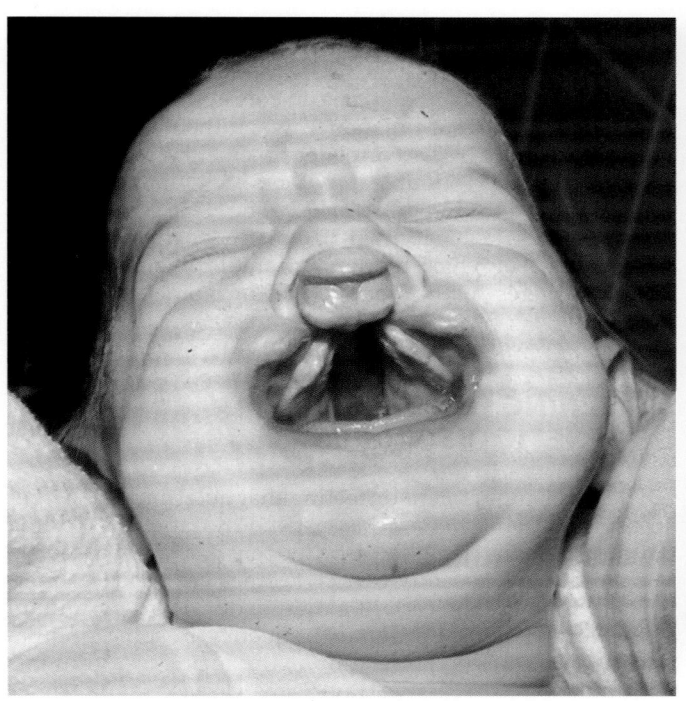

FIGURE 6-50. Infant with bilateral cleft lip and palate.

in gene expression (hereditary and environmental) may interfere with proper fusion, causing cleft lip with or without cleft palate (Fig. 6-50). The incidence of cleft lip with or without cleft palate, is about 1 per 1,000 live births. If one child is born with a cleft lip, the chances are 4% that a second child in the same family will have the same defect. If two children are affected, the risk of cleft lip in subsequent children of the family becomes 9%. The more severe the defect, the greater the probability of transmitting cleft lip. Furthermore, since 75% of cases of cleft lip occur in boys, the sons of women with cleft lip have a 4-fold higher risk for the defect than do sons of affected fathers.

CNS malformations are discussed in detail in Chapter 32. **Neural tube defects** (NTDs), anencephaly and spina bifida, are devastating congenital anomalies to which two factors contribute: one major environmental factor (lack of dietary folate) and one major genetic factor (a homozygous missense variant in the *MTHFR* gene). **Anencephaly**, congenital absence of the cranial vault, is a **dysraphic defect** of neural tube closure, in which cerebral hemispheres are completely missing or reduced to small disorganized tissue masses. Affected infants are stillborn or die shortly after birth; approximately 2/3 are female. **Spina bifida** is due to failure of fusion of the vertebral arches resulting in exposure of part of the spinal cord and meninges, typically in the lumbar region. Other related defects include **meningocele** and **myelomeningocele**, in which part of the meninges or meninges plus spinal cord, respectively, protrude through the open spine.

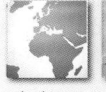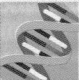 **EPIDEMIOLOGY AND MOLECULAR PATHOGENESIS:** Risk of NTDs varies with country, ethnicity, socioeconomic status, and time of year. It is roughly 10 in 10,000 births in

TABLE 6-17

REPRESENTATIVE DISORDERS WITH MULTIFACTORIAL INHERITANCE

Adults	Children[a]
Hypertension	Pyloric stenosis
Atherosclerosis	Isolated cleft lip and/or palate
Diabetes, type 2	Isolated congenital heart disease
Allergic diathesis	Neural tube defects
Psoriasis	Hypospadias
Schizophrenia	Congenital hip dislocation
Ankylosing spondylitis	Hirschsprung disease
Gout	

[a]Refers to congenital anomalies that are not a component of a chromosomal, copy number variant, single-gene or teratogen malformation syndrome.

Europe and 5 in 10,000 births in the United States. These rates are much lower since the 1980s, when women began taking folate supplements before conception and during the first 2 months of pregnancy, when the neural tube is forming. Risk of NTDs correlates inversely with maternal folate levels and is double if mothers are homozygous for a missense variant in the *MTHFR* gene. This gene variant encodes a less stable form of 5,10-methylenetetrahydrofolate reductase, which hinders tetrahydrofolate recycling and interferes with methylation of homocysteine to methionine.

SCREENING FOR CARRIERS OF GENETIC DISORDERS

Carrier screening is genetic testing that determines whether an asymptomatic person has a gene mutation associated with a particular genetic disorder that may be passed on to a child. Until recently carrier testing was based primarily on ethnicity. For certain single gene disorders mutant alleles are present at a higher frequency in some populations than in others. For example, the incidence of infants with autosomal recessive Tay–Sachs disease is 100 times higher among Ashkenazi Jews than in most other populations. In the 1970s, heterozygote screening by measuring hexosaminidase A activity in Ashkenazi Jews was the first population-based carrier screening. Molecular analysis eventually replaced enzyme activity-based testing, and now includes panel of molecular tests for several relatively rare genetic disorders that are more common in the Ashkenazi Jewish population.

Carrier screening has expanded greatly. There are now gene sequencing panels that test up to several hundred genetic conditions simultaneously. It is recommended that the disorders included in these extensive panels have a carrier frequency of 1 in 100 or greater, a significant detrimental effect on the quality of life, and onset early in life. These panels are now offered to all pregnant patients because many genetic conditions are not limited to a single ethnic group, a growing number of Americans are of mixed race or uncertain ethnic background and cost is relatively low due to advances in molecular diagnostic technologies.

PRENATAL DIAGNOSIS FOR GENETIC DISORDERS

Prenatal diagnosis includes *screening* as well as *diagnostic testing*. High-resolution real-time **ultrasonography** (US) is routinely used to assess fetal age, multiple gestations and fetal viability, and to screen for possible congenital malformations. If a malformation is detected or suspected on a routine US study, a detailed fetal US is done to look for possible additional fetal anomalies that may indicate a syndrome causing multiple malformations (see above). Diagnostic testing is then often performed. In addition to abnormal ultrasound findings, indications for diagnostic prenatal genetic testing include:

- Advanced maternal age
- Abnormal maternal serum screen results

- Parents have positive carrier screening results
- Parent is a balanced translocation carrier
- Family history of previous child with a genetic disorder

Chorionic villus sampling (CVS) and **amniocentesis** are procedures to obtain cells of fetal origin for genetic testing. CVS involves transcervically or transabdominally removing a small amount of chorionic villi from the placenta with ultrasound guidance, generally at 10 to 13 weeks of gestation. Amniocentesis involves transabdominally inserting a needle into the amniotic sac to remove a sample of amniotic fluid, usually at 16 or more weeks of gestation. Chorionic villus cells and amniotic fluid cells can be examined with one or more methodologies (see above). There are now over 2,000 single gene disorders for which prenatal genetic testing is available.

Other noninvasive prenatal screening tests include measuring various pregnancy-derived proteins and hormones (*analytes*) whose levels are altered in maternal serum when a fetus has an autosomal trisomy or an open neural tube defect (NTD). Elevated maternal serum α-fetoprotein (MSAFP) measured at 16 to 20 weeks of gestation indicates that a fetal open NTD may be present and that detailed US examination to investigate the possibility is warranted. Several other noninvasive tests and screening panels on maternal blood are available for first and second trimester assessments.

The discovery that maternal blood contains circulating cell-free fetal DNA allows *noninvasive prenatal screening* (NIPS), which is highly sensitive for detecting fetal chromosome abnormalities (e.g., sensitivity of >99% and a <1% false-positive rate specificity) for detecting fetal trisomy 21. Other autosomal trisomies and sex chromosome aneuploidies can also be assessed by this method. NIPS is expected to replace prenatal screening based on analyte measurement in maternal serum.

DISEASES OF INFANCY AND CHILDHOOD

Infants and children may be affected by diseases that are unique to their particular age group and are not seen in adults. The period from birth to puberty has traditionally been subdivided into several different stages.

- Newborn—birth to 1 month
- Infant—the first year
- Early childhood—1 to 4 years
- Late childhood—5 to 14 years

Each of these periods has its own anatomic, physiologic, and immunologic characteristics that determine which diseases occur and how they manifest. Table 6-18 shows that the major causes of death in the neonatal period and infancy differ greatly from those in the other pediatric age groups. Congenital anomalies and chromosome abnormalities are the leading cause of mortality in the first year of life. Disorders related to short gestation and low birth weight are also important causes of mortality early in life. In older children, there are other, more common, causes of death.

Prematurity and Intrauterine Growth Restriction Contribute to Low Birth Weight

Infants who are born earliest and are smallest have the greatest risk for mortality. Those who survive have a significant

TABLE 6-18
CAUSES OF DEATH IN CHILDREN

Causes of Death	Rate per 100,000 Population
Neonates and Infants (0–12 months)	
Congenital malformations, deformations, and chromosomal abnormalities	119.0
Disorders related to prematurity and low birth weight, not elsewhere classified	104.6
Newborn affected by maternal complications of pregnancy	39.5
Sudden infant death syndrome	38.6
Accidents (unintentional injuries)	29.1
Newborns affected by complications of placenta, cord and membranes	24.2
Bacterial sepsis of newborn	13.6
Respiratory distress of newborn	11.5
Disease of the circulatory system	11.1
Neonatal hemorrhage	11.1
Necrotizing enterocolitis of newborn	9.5
1–4 years	
Accidents (unintentional injuries)	7.6
Congenital malformations, deformations, and chromosomal abnormalities	2.5
Assault (homicide)	2.3
Malignant neoplasms	2.0
Diseases of the heart	0.9
5–9 years	
Accidents (unintentional injuries)	3.6
Malignant neoplasms	2.1
Congenital malformations, deformations, and chromosomal abnormalities	0.9
Assault (homicide)	0.6
Diseases of the heart	0.3
10–14 years	
Accidents (unintentional injuries)	3.6
Intentional self-harm (suicide)	2.1
Malignant neoplasms	2.0
Congenital malformations, deformations, and chromosomal abnormalities	0.8
Assault (homicide)	0.8

Causes are listed in decreasing order of frequency. Rates are per 100,000 population in the specified demographic. Based on data of the Centers for Disease Control, National Center for Health Statistics, National Vital Statistics System, Mortality 2014. Data collected for 2014 and released 2017. www.cdc.gov/nchs/nvss/mortality_tables.htm

chance for chronic medical problems and poor neurodevelopmental outcome with cognitive abnormalities and motor deficits. This risk is inversely related to gestational age and birth weight. Babies born very preterm (<32 weeks) or at a very low birth weight (<1,500 g) have about 100 times greater risk of dying in the first year of life, compared to full-term and non–low birth weight infants. Most infant deaths occur among the <2% of infants born very prematurely or at very low birth weight. Even late preterm or moderately low–birth-weight babies have higher morbidity and mortality than do full-term and normal birth weight babies.

A Premature Baby Is one Born Before the 37th Week of Gestation

Human pregnancy normally lasts 40 ± 2 weeks (from the first day of the last menstrual period). An infant is considered full-term if delivered at the completion of the 37th week or later. Every year worldwide 15 million babies are born prematurely. In 2016, the preterm birth rate in the United States was 10%. Among non-Hispanic black women this rate was 14%, that is, about 50% higher among non-Hispanic white women (9%).

Risk factors for preterm delivery include: preterm premature rupture of placental membranes, intrauterine infection, uterine structural abnormalities, cervical incompetence, and placental abnormalities (see Chapter 14). Twins and higher-order multiple gestations also entail increased risk of prematurity. Often no cause for early delivery is identified.

The medical problems of premature infants frequently result from organ immaturity. Immaturity of the lungs often results in **neonatal respiratory distress syndrome** (**NRDS**, see below). Premature livers are deficient in **glucuronyl transferase**, resulting in reduced ability to conjugate bilirubin which often leads to **neonatal jaundice**. This enzyme deficiency is aggravated by the rapid destruction of fetal erythrocytes that normally occurs in the neonatal period and increases the supply of bilirubin. Incomplete brain development in premature infants often contributes to feeding difficulties and recurrent apnea and bradycardia.

The Apgar Score

The Apgar score reflects a newborn's clinical appearance soon after birth (Table 6-19). At 1 and 5 minutes after birth, a newborn's color, heart rate, respiration, muscle tone, and reflex irritability are assessed and assigned a score of 0, 1, or 2 for each parameter. About 90% of newborns have Apgar scores of 7 to 9, are spontaneously breathing have good muscle tone and pink color and usually do not require medical intervention. Neonates with lower scores often require further evaluation and intervention. They may be premature or growth restricted, and may have or will develop one of the medical problems mentioned below. Ten percent of all neonates require some type of resuscitative measures after birth.

Intrauterine Growth Restriction May Affect Infants Born at any Gestational Age

Most term newborns weigh 3,300 ± 600 g (7+ lb, with a normal range of approximately 5½ to 10 lb). At any point in

TABLE 6-19
APGAR SCORE

Sign	0	1	2
Color	Blue or pale	Acrocyanotic (blue hands and feet)	Completely pink
Heart Rate	Absent	<100 per minute	>100 per minute
Respiration	Absent	Weak cry Hypoventilation	Good, crying
Muscle Tone	Limp	Some Flexion	Active motion
Reflex Irritability	No response	Grimace	Cry or active withdrawal

An infant's color, heart rate, reflex irritability, muscle tone, and respiration are assessed at 1 and 5 minutes after birth.

gestation, an infant's birth weight may be appropriate for gestational age (AGA), small for gestational age (SGA, <10th percentile), or large for gestational age (LGA, >90th percentile). Maternal gestational diabetes is a common cause of an LGA infant. Rare causes of LGA include syndromes such as BWS (see below).

IUGR occurs when fetal growth is decreased and does not meet the appropriate intrauterine growth potential. Obstetricians use the term when fetal growth decreases to less than 10% of the expected fetal weight based on gestational age due to the fetal environment. Depending upon the cause and severity, infants may be at increased risk for neurologic dysfunction, intellectual impairment, and other problems. In addition, IUGR infants often suffer perinatal depression and meconium aspiration due to an intolerance of labor.

 ETIOLOGIC FACTORS: IUGR may be due to maternal, placental, or fetal abnormalities. Long-standing maternal insulin-dependent diabetes, chronic hypertension, and preeclampsia (see Chapter 14) are common causes of decreased placental blood flow which leads to IUGR. Placental abnormalities that may lead to IUGR include small placental size and vascular anomalies such as single umbilical artery, abnormal umbilical cord insertion, and placental hemangioma (see Chapter 14). Placental thrombosis and infarction as well as placenta previa and placental abruption may also lead to a poorly grown fetus. Placental causes of IUGR often result in disproportionate (asymmetric) growth restriction with relative sparing of fetal brain growth. If the fetus develops an infection (i.e., TORCH infection) or is exposed to a teratogen, intrauterine growth can be inhibited.

Fetal growth failure due to intrinsic fetal etiologies (see above) is usually evident early in the pregnancy. Affected infants will often be born small but proportionate.

Neonatal Respiratory Distress Syndrome Is due to Surfactant Deficiency

Neonatal RDS is the most common cause of respiratory distress in preterm newborns. Its incidence varies inversely with gestational age and birth weight. Between 2003 and 2007, 93% of preterm infants born <28 weeks of gestation had RDS. In contrast, the incidence of RDS was 10.5% in infants born at 34 weeks of gestation. Improvements in management of this disorder have dramatically decreased the death rate due to respiratory insufficiency.

 ETIOLOGIC FACTORS: The cause of neonatal RDS is surfactant deficiency. Pulmonary surfactant is a soap-like substance that reduces intraalveolar surface tension and allows alveoli to remain expanded during expiration. Surfactant is produced by type II pneumocytes and is approximately 90% phospholipids and 10% proteins. The main phospholipid is dipalmitoyl phosphatidylcholine (DPPC, lecithin). Sphingomyelin and phosphatidylglycerol are also present. Two groups of proteins associate with these lipids in surfactant. One group includes hydrophilic glycoproteins SP-A and SP-D, which are involved in pulmonary innate immunity. The other group includes hydrophobic surfactant proteins SP-B and SP-C, which act with surfactant phospholipids to reduce surface tension at the alveolar lining. Alveoli with reduced surface tension require less effort to remain open and aerated. After the 35th week of pregnancy the production of surfactant by type II fetal pneumocytes accelerates (Fig. 6-51). Surfactant is released into the amniotic fluid, which can be sampled by amniocentesis to assess fetal lung maturity. A lecithin/sphingomyelin ratio over 2:1 predicts extra-uterine survival without RDS.

 PATHOPHYSIOLOGY: A high inspiratory pressure during the first breath after birth is required to expand the lungs. If a normal amount of surfactant is present, a newborn's lungs retain about 40% of their residual air volume with the initial breath. If there is insufficient surfactant, each successive breath, causes the lungs to collapse, so the infant has to exert as much energy with each successive breath to keep alveoli open as with the first breath.

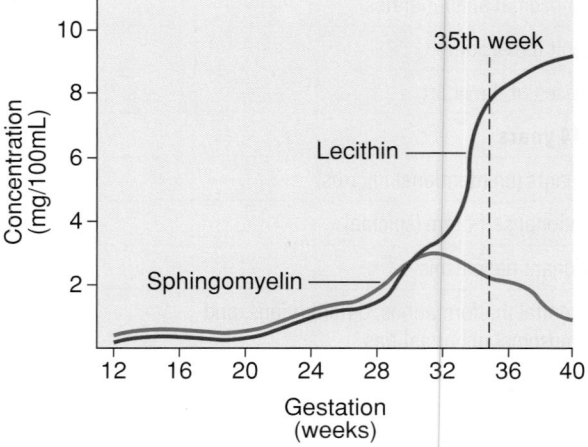

FIGURE 6-51. Changes in amniotic fluid composition during pregnancy. Lecithin is the predominant phospholipid in amniotic fluid.

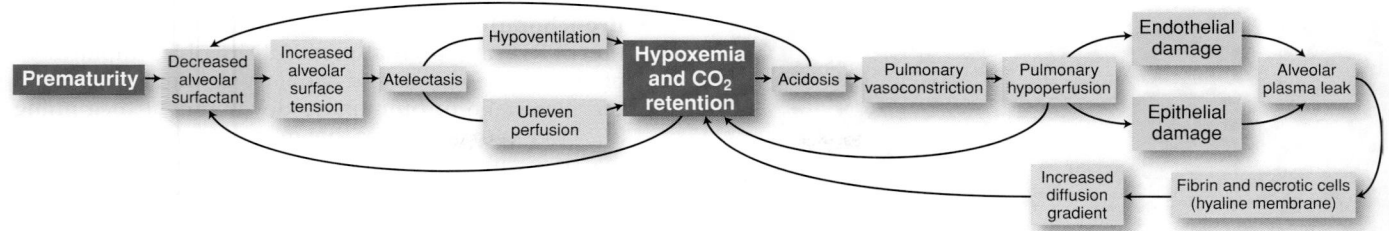

FIGURE 6-52. Pathophysiology of neonatal respiratory distress syndrome. Alveolar cells of premature infants do not produce a sufficient amount of surfactant to prevent atelectasis which leads to hypoventilation and uneven perfusion. The hypoxia and CO_2 retention that result lead to acidosis which leads to pulmonary vasoconstriction and pulmonary hypoperfusion which cause endothelial and epithelial cell damage. Plasma then leaks into the alveoli and coagulates as fibrin which, with necrotic cells, forms a hyaline membrane which increases the diffusion gradient of O_2 and CO_2 and worsens the hypoxemia and hypercarbia. A vicious cycle is created unless therapeutic intervention with mechanical ventilation, supplemental O_2, and exogenous surfactant is instituted.

Adding to this problem is the fact that the newborn chest wall is quite pliable and sucks in with the downward movement of the diaphragm with each breath. The result is stiff, atelectatic lungs that have uneven perfusion and hypoventilation which causes hypoxia and carbon dioxide retention. The ensuing acidosis can impair surfactant synthesis and release, and cause pulmonary vasoconstriction, exacerbating pulmonary hypoperfusion. Insufficient blood flow leads to alveolar endothelial and epithelial cell damage, causing plasma to leak into alveoli. Deposits of fibrin and necrotic cells in the alveolar spaces form a hyaline membrane. This hyaline membrane increases the diffusion gradient, causing and further hypoxemia and CO_2 retention and creating a vicious cycle (Fig. 6-52). Without intervention the infant will die.

CLINICAL FEATURES: Typically, premature infants with RDS develop respiratory distress soon after birth, with chest retractions, tachypnea, and cyanosis. Breath sounds are decreased and may be coarse. Chest radiographs show characteristic "ground-glass" appearance with uniform minute reticulogranular densities and air bronchograms (Fig. 6-53). As infants are hypoxic, they are given high concentrations of inspired oxygen and mechanical ventilation to maintain adequate oxygenation. This makes the ongoing lung injury worse and also puts the retina at risk for damage (see below).

Hormones, growth factors and gene mutations affect surfactant production. Thus, glucocorticoids increase surfactant synthesis and release. In utero stress increases cortisol release and explains why the risk of RDS is lower in infants with IUGR: many of these are under chronic stress during gestation. The stress of labor also increases surfactant production, so cesarean sectioning before the onset of labor, increases risk for RDS. Insulin counteracts the effects of corticosteroids, explaining in part why infants of diabetic mothers are at increased risk for RDS. These infants produce more insulin, to compensate for the higher glucose content of maternal blood from which they are nourished.

Lack of surfactant may rarely be due to mutations in the *SFTPB* and *SFTBC* genes which encode the hydrophobic surfactant proteins, SP-B and SP-C, or in the *ABCA3* gene which codes the ATP-binding cassette transporter responsible for transporting surfactant phospholipids and proteins to the alveolar space. Full-term infants with two mutant alleles in any of these genes will develop severe respiratory failure and die, unless lung transplantation is performed.

PATHOLOGY: Grossly, the lungs in neonatal RDS are dark red-purple and airless. Microscopically, many alveoli are collapsed and have thick walls. Capillaries are congested and lymphatics are filled with proteinaceous material. Alveolar ducts and terminal bronchioles are dilated and lined with conspicuous hyaline membranes: eosinophilic, fibrin-rich, amorphous structures with cellular debris from necrotic type II pneumocytes and proteinaceous edema fluid (Fig. 6-54). Hence, the original term **hyaline membrane disease** for RDS.

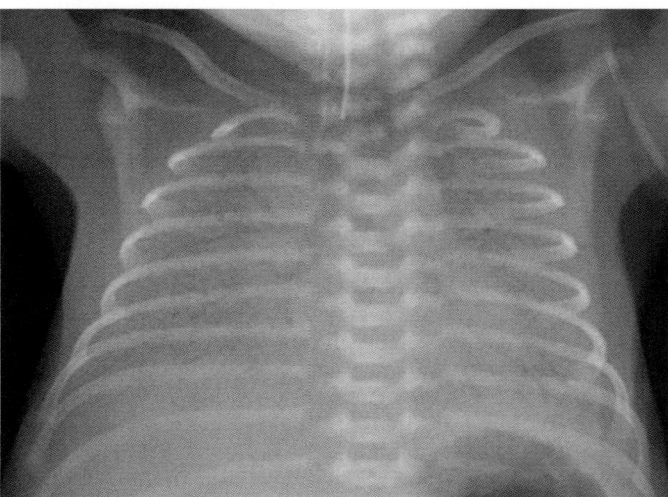

FIGURE 6-53. Chest x-ray of a premature infant with respiratory distress syndrome showing lung fields with uniform minute reticulogranular densities (ground-glass appearance) and air bronchograms. (Image courtesy of neonatologist Dara Brodsky, MD.)

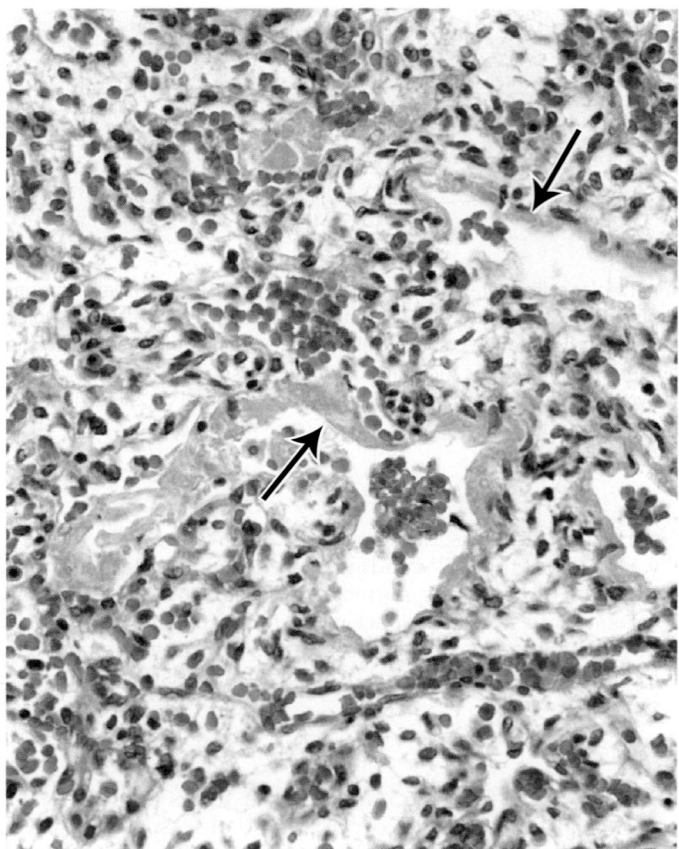

FIGURE 6-54. **The lung in respiratory distress syndrome of the neonate.** Alveoli are atelectatic, and dilated alveolar ducts are lined by fibrin rich hyaline membranes (*arrows*).

Therapeutic advances in recent decades have dramatically improved survival of infants with RDS. If labor threatens a preterm pregnancy, corticosteroids given to the mother hasten fetal lung maturation and surfactant production. Animal-derived surfactants (porcine or bovine) administered to the premature infant, plus improved ventilatory therapy, minimize barotrauma and supplemental oxygen concentration. The morbidity associated with RDS has decreased with modern therapy. Retinopathy of prematurity, bronchopulmonary dysplasia, and patent ductus arteriosus, which result from treatment of RDS have fortunately become less common and often less severe than before.

- **Retinopathy of prematurity (ROP),** or retrolental fibroplasia, was once the leading cause of infant blindness in the United States and other developed countries. The high inspired oxygen levels used to treat RDS markedly decreased the proangiogenic cytokine, VEGF (see Chapter 5). When a baby recovering from RDS is weaned to room air which has only 21% oxygen, VEGF levels rebound, inducing retinal blood vessels to proliferate (neovascularization), the hallmark lesion of ROP. Retinal scarring and detachment and a fibrovascular mass behind the lens may ensue causing blindness (see Chapter 33). Use of surfactant, which has allowed reduced supplemental oxygen therapy, and decreased the incidence of ROP.

- **Bronchopulmonary dysplasia (BPD)** is a late complication of RDS and prematurity. BPD involves impairment of alveolar septation and capillary configuration at the saccular stage of pulmonary development (beginning at 24 weeks of gestation) that may potentially be reversible. It is caused by chronic mechanical ventilation and the high percentage of supplemental oxygen required in premature infants with RDS. The longer the exposure to these interventions and the younger the infant's birth gestational age, the higher the risk of BPD. Positive pressure ventilation may overstretch delicate developing alveoli and high levels of inspired oxygen are toxic to alveoli. The less developed the lungs are, the more likely they are to be damaged. Thus, BPD is common in very premature infants and unusual in infants born after 32 weeks of gestation. Proinflammatory cytokines such as interleukins IL-1β, IL-6, and IL-8 and TNFα also play a role in the development of BPD. Radiographs of the lungs show a sponge-like appearance, with small lucent areas of enlarged terminal airspaces alternating with denser pulmonary tissue (Fig. 6-55). The bronchiolar epithelium is hyperplastic, with bronchial and bronchiolar squamous metaplasia. Atelectasis, interstitial edema and thickening of alveolar basement membranes are also seen. BPD is a chronic disease; affected infants may continue to require oxygen supplementation into their second or third years of life, and some degree of respiratory impairment may persist, even into adolescence and beyond.

- **Patent ductus arteriosus (PDA):** During fetal life the ductus arteriosus, which connects the pulmonary artery to the aorta, diverts oxygenated blood from the lungs to the general circulation. It closes shortly after birth in healthy full-term infants in response to decreased pulmonary vascular resistance, increased arterial oxygenation

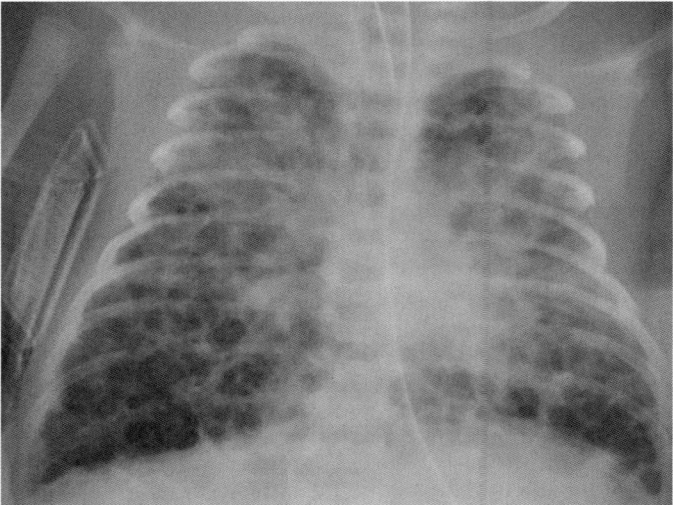

FIGURE 6-55. Chest x-ray of a premature infant with bronchopulmonary dysplasia (BPD) showing lung fields which show a sponge-like appearance, with small lucent areas of enlarged terminal airspaces alternating with denser pulmonary tissue. (Image courtesy of neonatologist Dara Brodsky, MD.)

and a decreased local level of prostaglandin E2. Closure is delayed in infants with hypoxia due to RDS or congenital heart disease (see Chapter 17). If PDA persists, the recovery from the pulmonary disease reduces pulmonary arterial pressure, so the higher pressure in the aorta reverses the direction of blood flow in the ductus, and creates a persistent left-to-right shunt. Congestive heart failure follows, and medical or, in severe cases, surgical treatment of the patent ductus may be needed.

Other Disorders Associated With Prematurity

Intraventricular hemorrhage (IVH) is an important cause of brain injury in premature infants, especially in neonates <32 weeks of gestation or under 1,500 g birth weight. The periventricular germinal matrix in the preterm neonatal brain is particularly vulnerable to hemorrhage because dilated, thin-walled veins in this area are more permeable in settings of hypoxia and/or increased venous pressure. Bleeding may extend into the lateral ventricle by disrupting the ependymal lining (Fig. 6-56). IVH severity depends on whether bleeding is confined to the germinal matrix region or extends into adjacent ventricles or white matter. The incidence of IVH has declined over the past few decades, with improved treatment of RDS. This is partly due to maternal antepartum steroid administration and postnatal neonatal management that avoids high swings in blood pressures.

Necrotizing enterocolitis (NEC): NEC is the most common gastrointestinal emergency in newborns. In the United States, the incidence is 1 to 3 per 1,000 live births. It is most common among premature infants, its incidence being inversely proportional to gestational age. About 6% to 7% of neonates weighing under 1,500 g develop NEC.

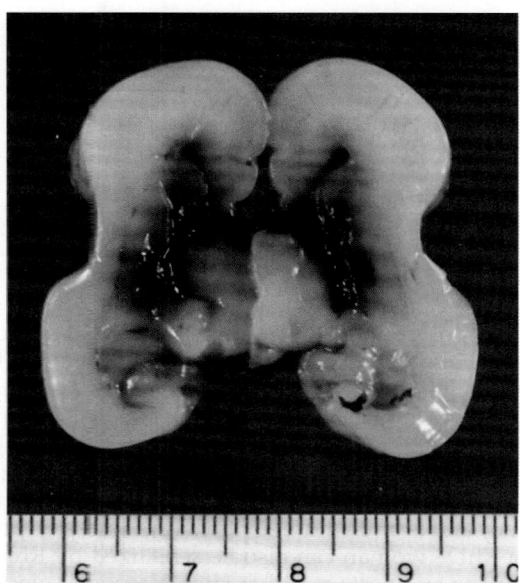

FIGURE 6-56. I ntraventricular hemorrhage with extension into the brain parenchyma in a premature neonate with respiratory distress syndrome.

 PATHOPHYSIOLOGY: NEC involves ischemic necrosis of the intestinal mucosa, with inflammation, invasion of enteric gas-forming bacteria and dissection of gas into the muscularis and portal venous system. Immaturity of the GI tract, with impaired mucosal defenses, intestinal motility, and function may predispose preterm infants to NEC. The pathogenesis of NEC remains uncertain, but is likely to be multifactorial in a susceptible host. Prematurity, infectious agents often introduced by enteral feeding, severe anemia and inflammatory mediators such as tumor necrosis factor (TNF), platelet-activating factor (PAF), and several interleukins are likely etiologic factors. Hypoxia may weaken the immature neonatal intestinal mucosa and allow bacteria invasion, which along with PAF and other inflammatory mediators, may result in increased mucosal permeability by weakening intercellular tight junctions and promoting apoptosis of enterocytes. Transluminal migration of gut bacteria then sets up a vicious cycle of inflammation, mucosal necrosis and entry of additional bacteria leading eventually to sepsis and shock.

 PATHOLOGY: Any section of the bowel may be involved, but the terminal ileum, cecum, and right colon are most affected. The distended bowel segment is congested and friable and may be gangrenous and perforated. Mucosal or transmural coagulative necrosis, ulceration, bacterial colonization, and bubbles of gas in the submucosa are characteristic. Shortly after an acute episode reparative changes like granulation tissue and fibrosis may be observed. NEC can be successfully managed conservatively when it is not severe. However, in severe cases, necrotic sections of bowel require surgical resection. The perinatal mortality associated with NEC is high. Infants who survive may have digestive problems from a short gut or intestinal strictures from fibrosis due to healing.

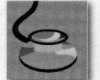 **CLINICAL FEATURES:** NEC starts with bloody stools and abdominal distention, followed by hypotension and impending circulatory collapse and death. Abdominal x-rays show loops of distended bowel with **pneumatosis intestinalis**, which is gas within the intestinal wall. Full blown cases with bowel perforation and peritonitis also show **pneumoperitoneum**, or free air in the abdomen.

Newborns, Especially Premature Newborns, Are at High Risk for Severe Infection

Premature infants have very immature immune systems, and lack maternal antibodies that would have been passively acquired late in the third trimester. Perinatal infections acquired transcervically are called *ascending infections*, and those acquired transplacentally are *hematologic infections*.

 ETIOLOGIC FACTORS: Most bacterial and a few viral infections such as herpes simplex type II reach the fetus or neonate transcervically.

Preterm or term prolonged rupture of membranes allows—or is caused by—ascending infection by bacteria that are normally present in the maternal cervicovaginal canal. Microorganisms can then reach the fetus in utero by inhalation of infected amniotic fluid or by delivery through an infected birth canal. Infected neonates may then develop pneumonia, sepsis and/or meningitis within a few days after birth. The most common cause of these serious infections in the early newborn period is Group B *Streptococcus*. Later-onset sepsis presents with signs of infection one to several weeks after delivery. It is often due to microorganisms, such as *Listeria* and *Candida*, with longer latency between the time of fetal or newborn exposure and appearance of symptoms.

Most viral and parasitic infections and a few bacterial infections such as *Treponema*, are acquired transplacentally through hematologic spread via chorionic villi at any time during gestation. TORCH infections are acquired in this manner. HIV and hepatitis B infection can be passed on to the neonate at the time of delivery.

In Fetal Hydrops, Fluid Accumulates in Soft Tissues and Body Cavities

Some affected infants have mild generalized edema or localized fluid collections, such as ascites, pleural effusion, or cystic hygroma (cervical lymphangioma). *Hydrops fetalis* describes the most severe and generalized form of the condition. Affected infants may be stillborn, or die shortly after birth. Those with milder disease may survive with unfortunate sequela or experience complete recovery. Fetal hydrops has immune and nonimmune etiologies and can vary from mild generalized edema to anasarca. **Immune hydrops** is caused by fetal hemolytic anemia due to blood group, usually Rh, incompatibility between a fetus and the mother. **Nonimmune hydrops** has many etiologies (Table 6-20). With the advent of effective prophylactic therapy for maternal–fetal Rh incompatibility, nonimmune hydrops has become much more common and is often a diagnostic challenge due to the myriad of possible etiologies.

Immune Hydrops

Blood group antigen incompatibility between a pregnant woman and the fetus can cause hemolysis in the fetus, resulting in immune hydrops in severe cases. Such an immune response may occur when a fetus inherits paternal red blood cell antigens to which the pregnant woman has antibodies that cross the placenta. Only antibodies to RhD and ABO antigens cause significant hemolysis and approximately 90% of immune hydrops is due to RhD incompatibility.

RhD Incompatibility

The disorder was first recognized by Hippocrates but was not explained until 1940, when Rh (Rhesus) antigen on erythrocytes was identified (Fig. 6-57). Fetal red blood cells enter the maternal circulation at delivery and late in the third trimester when the cytotrophoblast barrier wanes. RhD+ fetal RBCs induce an RhD– mother to produce anti-RhD+ antibodies. These pass through the placenta into the fetus. The initial response in a first pregnancy is maternal anti-RhD+ IgM antibodies that cannot cross the placenta to the fetus.

TABLE 6-20
SELECTED ETIOLOGIES OF NONIMMUNE FETAL HYDROPS
Cardiovascular
Malformations
Tachyarrhythmias
High output failure due to fetal or placental vascular tumors
Chromosomal
45,X Turner syndrome
Trisomy 21, Down syndrome
Hematologic (Anemia)
Homozygous α-thalassemia
Parvovirus B19 infection
Twin Gestation
Twin to twin transfusion
Acardiac twin
Infections
Cytomegalovirus
Toxoplasmosis
Syphilis
Mendelian Syndromes
Noonan syndrome
Osteogenesis imperfecta
Multiple pterygium syndrome
Malformations
Diaphragmatic hernia
Congenital cystic adenomatoid malformation of lung
Gastrointestinal and Genitourinary Tract Malformations
Metabolic Disorders

However, the IgG anti-RhD+ that is eventually produced can pass through the placenta to subsequent fetuses. In later pregnancies with an RhD+ fetus there is a brisk maternal anti-RhD+ IgG antibody response that can cause significant fetal RBC hemolysis and risk for hydrops due to congestive heart failure as a consequence of severe anemia (Fig. 6-57). This explains why immune hydrops is uncommon in a first pregnancy and is often more severe with successive pregnancies. An RhD– woman can also be sensitized by RhD+ fetal RBCs during an abortion, either spontaneous or elective, or, for example, inadvertent transfusion with RhD+ blood.

The maternal antibody response depends on how much RhD antigen is presented to the RhD– mother. Usually

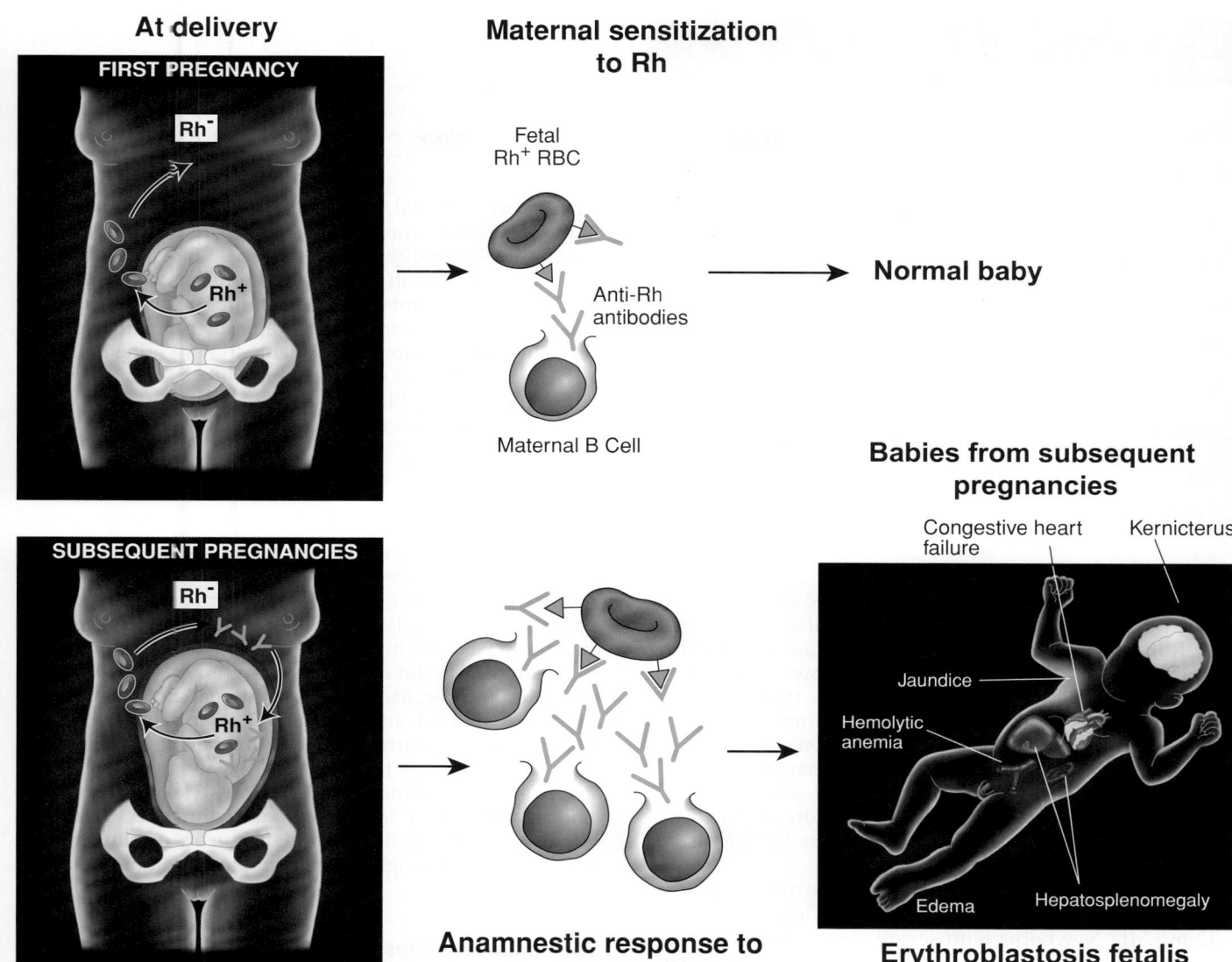

FIGURE 6-57. Pathogenesis of erythroblastosis fetalis due to maternal–fetal Rh incompatibility. Immunization of an Rh-negative mother with Rh-positive fetal erythrocytes in the first pregnancy leads to formation of IgG anti-Rh antibodies. In subsequent pregnancies these antibodies cross the placenta and damage the Rh-positive fetus by destroying fetal erythrocytes.

an initial fetomaternal bleed of >1 mL of RhD+ fetal RBCs is required. A much smaller subsequent exposure to fetal RhD antigen will boost maternal antibody titer. Maternal immunocompetency is also a factor. Women with AIDS may not make antibodies to RhD. In addition, simultaneous ABO incompatibility protects against RhD immunization, because fetal RBCs are quickly coated with antibody and removed from the mother's circulation by pre-existing anti-A or anti-B IgM antibodies that cannot cross the placenta.

The distribution of Rh antigens varies among ethnic groups. Of Caucasians 15% are RhD–, but only 8% of African Americans. The vast majority of Asians and Native Americans are RhD+. By contrast, 35% of Basque people, among whom the RhD– phenotype may have arisen, are RhD– (Table 6-21).

However, many Rh-negative women who are exposed to significant amounts of fetal RhD+ blood do not mount a substantial immune response. Even after multiple pregnancies, only 5% of RhD-negative women deliver infants with immune hydrops.

PATHOPHYSIOLOGY: Anemia and jaundice are the major consequences of excessive destruction of RBCs in the newborn, the severity of each depending upon the extent of hemolysis and the gestational age of the neonate. Increased RBC production may be adequate to maintain near-normal numbers of RBCs if hemolysis is mild. However, severe hemolysis can result in significant anemia which may cause hypoxic heart and liver injury, leading to cardiac failure and decreased plasma protein synthesis, respectively. Increased circulatory hydrostatic pressure due to heart failure, combined with decreased plasma oncotic pressure because of low

TABLE 6-21

DISTRIBUTION OF Rh ANTIGENS AMONG ETHNIC GROUPS

Ethnic Group	Percent of Population Rh D (%)
Basque	30–35
Caucasian (N. American and European)	15
African American	8
African	4–6
Indian	5
Native American and Inuit Eskimo	1–2
Japanese	0.5
Thai	0.3
Chinese	0.3

plasma protein levels leads to generalized edema, which may progress to anasarca and *hydrops fetalis*.

RBC destruction causes unconjugated hyperbilirubinemia which is exacerbated by the low level of bilirubin uridine diphosphate glucuronyl transferase in the immature fetal/neonatal liver. The immature fetal/neonatal blood–brain barrier also allows passage of unconjugated bilirubin into the brain, where it binds lipids in the basal ganglia, pontine nuclei, and cerebellar nuclei and gives these structures a yellowish hue. The ensuing neurologic damage is known as *kernicterus* or bilirubin encephalopathy.

Premature infants are more vulnerable to hyperbilirubinemia and may develop kernicterus at levels as low as 12 mg/dL. Newborns with severe kernicterus have loss of the normal startle reflex and exhibit athetoid movements, which progress to lethargy and death in 75% of cases. Most surviving infants have severe **choreoathetosis** and intellectual impairment; a minority are less severely affected and show some motor and intellectual deficits.

CLINICAL FEATURES: Exchange transfusions may keep serum bilirubin at a nondamage producing level. The need for exchange transfusion has been greatly reduced by phototherapy, which converts toxic unconjugated bilirubin into nontoxic water-soluble pyrroles that are readily excreted in the urine. Administration of intravenous Ig may also slow progression of indirect hyperbilirubinemia, but infants are still at risk of anemia for the next few weeks.

The incidence of erythroblastosis fetalis due to Rh incompatibility has markedly declined (<1% of women at risk) since the use of anti-D immune globulin, starting about 50 years ago. In every pregnancy of RhD– pregnant women, it is administered at 28 weeks of gestation and within 72 hours after delivery to reduce risk of hemolytic disease in Rh+ newborns and in subsequent pregnancies.

It is also given after spontaneous and elective abortions, amniocentesis, and chorionic villus sampling.

Anti-D immune globulin binds to and neutralizes antigenicity of fetal cells that may have entered maternal circulation, and prevents development of maternal anti-RhD antibodies. Once alloimmunization has occurred, anti-RhD immune globulin cannot prevent or reduce the severity of fetal/neonatal hemolytic disease. Anti-D immune globulin prophylaxis has made erythroblastosis fetalis a rare condition. RhD+ fetuses with severe hemolytic disease due to maternal alloimmunization can be treated with intrauterine Rh– red blood cell transfusion via the umbilical cord and therapeutic premature delivery. Prenatal diagnosis is available to determine the fetal *RHD* genotype and ultrasound monitoring of fetal middle cerebral artery blood flow velocity as an indirect measure of fetal anemia to determine when interventions are necessary.

ABO Incompatibility

ABO incompatibility is present in 20% to 25% of gestations, but clinically significant hemolytic disease of the newborn is uncommon. About 10% of such infants show laboratory evidence of hemolysis, which is severe enough to necessitate therapy in 0.5%. In most infants with ABO incompatibility, mild jaundice is the only clinical sign. Fetal RBC destruction is limited because: (1) most maternal anti-A and anti-B antibodies are IgM, and do not cross the placenta, (2) A and B antigens are poorly expressed on newborn RBCs, and (3) many other cell types express A and B antigens and absorb some of the maternal antibody, so less is available to bind to and destroy fetal/neonatal erythrocytes. Firstborns can be affected and there is no effective protection against the potential, although usually minimal, hemolysis due to ABO incompatibility.

Nonimmune Hydrops

The major causes of nonimmune hydrops include fetal heart abnormalities, chromosome aberrations, and fetal anemia. Cardiac malformations and arrhythmias can cause intrauterine heart failure and hydrops. Turner syndrome due to a 45,X karyotype and trisomies 21 and 18 are the most common chromosomal causes of nonimmune hydrops, often with an accompanying heart defect or large lymphatic tumors, called **cystic hygromas**. Fetal anemia not caused by Rh or ABO antibodies can result in hydrops. In Southeast Asia the most common cause of nonimmune hydrops is severe fetal anemia due to homozygous α-thalassemia, which results when all four α-globin genes are deleted (Fig. 6-58 and Chapter 26).

Another important cause of significant fetal anemia is transplacental infection by parvovirus B19. The virus replicates after entering fetal erythroid precursors (normoblasts), leading to apoptosis of red cell progenitors and red cell aplasia. In hydropic stillborns with parvovirus infection intranuclear inclusions can be seen in bone marrow and circulating erythroid precursors. Monozygous twin pregnancies with twin-to-twin transfusion that takes place through placental vascular anastomoses between the two circulations accounts for about 10% of nonimmune hydrops. Certain single gene malformation syndromes, isolated malformations, and metabolic disorders may also cause hydrops.

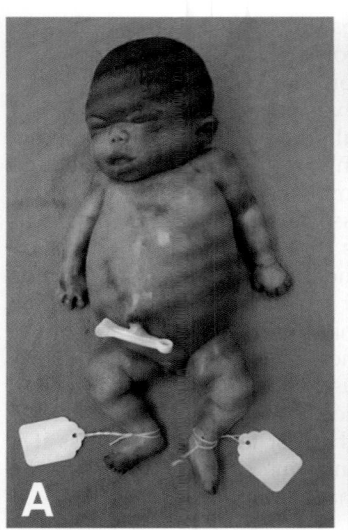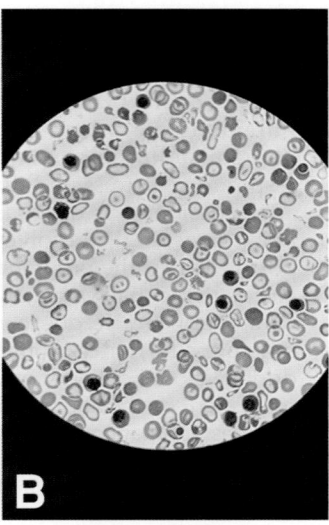

FIGURE 6-58. A. Deceased hydropic premature Asian infant with homozygous α-thalassemia. **B.** Umbilical cord blood smear showing marked hypochromia and anisopoikilocytosis due to deletion of all four α-globin genes.

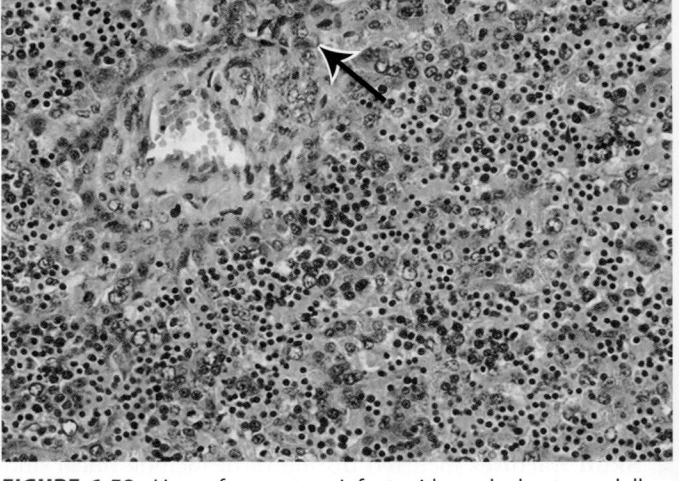

FIGURE 6-59. Liver of premature infant with marked extramedullary erythroid hematopoiesis due to fetal anemia. Increased hemosiderin pigment (*arrow*) reflects high red cell turnover.

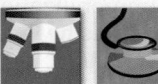 **PATHOLOGY AND CLINICAL FEATURES:** The underlying etiology and severity of the disease determine the clinical pathologic features in a fetus or neonate with hydrops. A chromosome abnormality may be the etiology if dysmorphic features are present. Autopsy may show that a heart defect is the cause of the hydrops. If the abnormal fluid accumulation is due to fetal anemia, both the hydropic fetus and the enlarged edematous placenta will exhibit characteristic pallor and there is hepatosplenomegaly secondary to cardiac failure. In immune hydrops due to Rh incompatibility and in nonimmune hydrops due to homozygous α-thalassemia there is compensatory erythroid hyperplasia in the bone marrow and extramedullary hematopoiesis in liver, spleen, lymph nodes, and sometimes other tissues (Fig. 6-59). These infants have large numbers of erythroblasts and other erythroid precursors in their blood, due to markedly increased hematopoiesis. This state is *erythroblastosis fetalis*. In severe immune hydrops with hemolysis deceased neonates may be icteric and their brains edematous and bright yellow upon sectioning, particularly basal ganglia, thalamus, cerebral gray matter, and cerebellum.

Inborn Errors of Metabolism Often Present in the Newborn Period

They should always be considered when a neonate has feeding difficulty and lethargy. Laboratory findings reflect the specific metabolic block and may include acidosis, hypoglycemia, and hyperammonemia. Prompt diagnosis and treatment can be lifesaving and prevent neurologic damage caused by accumulation of toxic metabolites.

Birth Injuries Impair a Newborn's Functional or Structural Integrity

Such injuries are defined as being due to an adverse event that occurred around the time of birth. Injury may occur during labor, delivery or after delivery in newborns who require resuscitation. They range from minor self-limited problems to severe injuries that may lead to significant morbidity or mortality. Some birth injuries are the result of obstetric manipulation, but many are due to unavoidable events in routine deliveries. The incidence of birth injuries—about 2% in singleton, vaginal, head-first deliveries and 1% in cesarean sections—has declined with improvements in prenatal diagnosis and obstetrical and neonatal care. Cephalopelvic disproportion, which can lead to dystocia (difficult labor), plays a role in many birth injuries.

Risk factors involving the fetus include fetal macrosomia, prematurity, and presentation other than vertex for vaginal delivery. Larger infants experience more birth injuries. Maternal risk factors include size of the mother and the presence of pelvic anomalies. Maternal obesity increases the risk of birth injuries, possibly because of greater use of instrumentation during deliveries and a tendency toward LGA infants. Small maternal stature is also a risk factor, as is delivery of primigravidas. Birth trauma is less frequent with cesarean deliveries, although the most common injury with this mode of delivery is fetal laceration.

Soft Tissue Injury

The most common birth injuries are soft tissue injuries, including bruising, petechiae, subcutaneous fat necrosis, and lacerations. Most of these are self-limiting. Bruising and petechiae are usually on the presenting part of the neonate's body, the head and face for vertex deliveries and the genitalia for breech deliveries. Subcutaneous fat necrosis, which presents as firm erythematous, flesh colored or blue nodules or plaques that appear a week or 2 after delivery, is uncommon and is due to ischemic necrosis from sustained pressure on subcutaneous adipose tissue during labor and delivery. Fetal laceration is the most common birth injury after cesarean delivery, and readily heals with application of sterile strips.

Cranial Injury

Cranial injuries at birth include:

- **Caput succedaneum** is scalp edema and occasionally bleeding above the periosteum caused by prolonged engagement of the fetal head in the birth canal or after vacuum extraction. Unlike cephalohematoma, it extends across the suture lines. Swelling disappears rapidly without treatment and is of little clinical concern.
- **Cephalohematoma** is subperiosteal hemorrhage caused by rupture of vessels beneath the periosteum of a single cranial bone, usually the parietal or occipital bone. It presents as swelling that does not cross suture lines. It is estimated to occur in 1% to 2% of deliveries, and is much more common with the use of forceps or vacuum extraction. Most cephalohematomas resolve without complication and require no treatment.
- **Skull fractures** incurred during birth include linear and depressed fractures. Linear fractures are often asymptomatic, heal without intervention and are not associated with neurologic sequela. Depressed fractures with inward buckling of a skull bone are frequently associated with forceps-assisted delivery or impact of the fetal head on the maternal pelvic bones during unassisted vaginal delivery. Depressed fractures have an increased risk of intracranial bleeding and may require neurosurgical repair if they are depressed more than 1 cm. Unlike most cranial fractures, those of the occipital bone often extend through the underlying venous sinuses and may produce fatal hemorrhage.
- **Intracranial hemorrhage** is one of the most dangerous birth injuries and may be traumatic, secondary to asphyxia or a result of an underlying bleeding diathesis. Intracranial hemorrhages, in decreasing order of frequency, include subdural, subarachnoid, epidural, intraventricular, intracerebral, and intracerebellar hemorrhages. Affected neonates often present with apnea, respiratory depression and seizures 24 to 48 hours after delivery. Prognosis depends on the extent of bleeding. Traumatic intracranial hemorrhage may occur in the setting of significant cephalopelvic disproportion, precipitous delivery, breech presentation, prolonged labor, or forceps-assisted delivery. These traumas can result in laceration of the falx cerebri or tentorium cerebelli that involve the vein of Galen or the venous sinuses. Anoxic injury from asphyxia, particularly in premature infants, is often associated with intraventricular hemorrhage. Massive hemorrhage is often rapidly fatal. Surviving infants may recover completely or have long-term neurologic impairment.

Peripheral Nerve Injury

Nerve injuries that can be seen at birth include:

- **Brachial palsy** presents with varying degrees of paralysis of a newborn's arm. It can be caused by extreme lateral traction on the neonatal shoulder, during delivery of the shoulder in vertex presentations and the head in breech presentations. This can injure or transect the brachial plexus by stretching its cervical nerve roots. If the nerves are severed, impairment may be permanent. Function may return within a few months if the palsy results from edema and hemorrhage. Many cases of brachial palsy occur without shoulder dystocia. Possible risk factors include those that lead to cephalopelvic disproportion, for example, maternal diabetes and fetal macrosomia, fetal malposition, abnormal labor, operative vaginal delivery, and previous pregnancy complicated by shoulder dystocia or neonatal brachial plexus palsy.
- **Phrenic nerve injury** results in paralysis of a hemidiaphragm and usually presents on the first day of life with respiratory distress and diminished breath sounds on the affected side. It is often associated with brachial plexus palsy. It generally resolves in 6 to 12 months with supportive care if the phrenic nerve has not been transected.
- **Facial nerve palsy** usually presents as unilateral flaccid paralysis of the face, due to injury to the seventh cranial nerve from pressure from a prominent maternal sacral promontory during labor or delivery, or use of forceps. There is decreased movement on the affected side of the infant's face. It usually resolves spontaneously in the first few weeks, unless it is due to a developmental syndrome such as facio-auriculo-vertebral dysplasia (Goldenhar syndrome).

Fractures

The *clavicle* is most vulnerable to fracture during delivery, followed the *humerus*. Clavicular fractures usually follow difficult vaginal delivery, but can be seen in infants born by nontraumatic vaginal or cesarean deliveries. Immobilization of the arm and shoulder usually allows for complete healing. Fractures of other long bones are rare, but heal well.

Sudden Infant Death Syndrome (SIDS) Is Sudden, Unexplained Death in the First Year of Life

As defined by the National Institute of Child Health and Human Development, SIDS deaths should be unexplained after a thorough case investigation, including a complete autopsy, examination of the death scene and review of the clinical history. A diagnosis of SIDS is made only after excluding other specific causes of sudden death (Table 6-22). *Sudden unexpected infant death* (SUID) is often used to describe all unexpected infant deaths, including those that have an explanation and those that do not. Unexplained SUID includes cases considered SIDS by the medical examiner, as well as some cases that are not considered SIDS but lack a definitive explanation due to uncertain circumstances. As predisposing factors and environmental, biochemical, structural and genetic etiologies have been identified, the number of infant deaths that truly have no identifiable pathogenesis has diminished.

EPIDEMIOLOGY: After the neonatal period, SIDS is the leading cause of death in the first year of life. In this age bracket, 1/3 of deaths are due to SIDS, of which 90% happen before 6 months of age (peak incidence, 2 to 4 months). The male:female ratio is approximately 1.5. Most SIDS deaths occur during periods associated with sleep. Typically, SIDS infants were apparently healthy babies who went to sleep without any hint of the impending calamity and did not wake up.

Infants who slept prone or on their sides were found to have a much higher incidence of SIDS than those who slept supine. A worldwide "Back to Sleep" campaign beginning in 1992, encouraged parents to place infants on their backs for sleep, and rapidly lowered the rate of SIDS by more than half. Other improvements in prenatal and neonatal care were also instituted around that time.

TABLE 6-22
DISORDERS FOUND IN INFANTS WITH SUID THAT CAN MIMIC SIDS

General

Sepsis (including meningococcemia)

Asphyxiation (accidental or deliberate)

Anaphylaxis

Metabolic decompensation

Hyperthermia

Poisoning

Inborn errors of metabolism (including fatty acid oxidation disorders) (MCAD, LCHAD, SCHAD mutations)

Abnormal inflammatory responsiveness (partial deletions in C4a and C4b)

Blood

Sickle cell disease in crisis

Heart

Subendocardial fibroelastosis

Congenital heart defects (especially aortic stenosis)

Viral myocarditis

Long QT syndrome (SCN5A and KCNQ1 mutations)

Histiocytoid cardiomyopathy (MTCYB mutations)

Lungs

Pneumonia

Bronchiolitis

Tracheal Bronchiolitis, severe

Aspiration or airway obstruction

Idiopathic pulmonary hypertension

Kidney

Pyelonephritis

Gastrointestinal Tract

Enterocolitis with Salmonella, Shigella, or pathogenic E. coli

Liver

Hepatitis

Pancreas

Pancreatitis

Boric acid poisoning

Cystic fibrosis

Adrenal

Congenital adrenal hyperplasia

Brain

Encephalitis

Trauma (skull fracture, cerebral edema, subdural hematoma)

Arteriovenous malformation with bleeding

Modified from Disorders That Can Mimic SIDS, UpToDate, 20 January, 2018.

Incidence of SIDS in the United States was 12 in 10,000 live births in 1992 when the American Academy of Pediatrics first endorsed the supine sleeping position. By 2006, the rate was 5.6 in 10,000 live births, and in 2013 it was 4.0 per 10,000 live births. SIDS still causes 1,560 infant deaths annually in the United States, of which 15% to 20% occur in child care settings. The rate of SIDS in black and American Indian/Alaskan Native children is two to three times the national average. Reducing the risk of SIDS remains an important public health priority.

Risk factors: A number of retrospective studies have identified maternal, infant, and sleeping environment risk factors for SIDS. One or more risk factors are present in 95% of SIDS cases.

Maternal risk factors:

- Age younger than 20 years
- Maternal cigarette smoking
- Late or no prenatal care
- Maternal alcohol consumption
- Maternal use of illicit drugs

The two most significant maternal risk factors for SIDS are teenage motherhood and maternal cigarette smoking. Risk of SIDS increases with the amount smoked. Prenatal exposure to smoking poses the highest risk. In addition, babies exposed to secondhand smoke have a higher risk for SIDS than do those not exposed to it. Infants of mothers who smoked during gestation show abnormal cardiovascular responses to stimuli such as hypoxia and hypercarbia. Maternal drug and alcohol abuse during and after pregnancy and all of the adverse phenomena associated with substance abuse also increase risk for SIDS. Pregnancy complications such as elevated maternal α-fetoprotein, premature rupture of membranes, placenta previa, and abruptio placenta are also risk factors for SIDS independent of their association with preterm delivery.

Infant risk factors:

- Prematurity
- Low birth weight
- Male sex
- Previous siblings were SIDS victims
- Twins
- Recent respiratory infection

Preterm infants and SGA infants have higher risk for SIDS than do term or AGA infants. Siblings of SIDS victims have a small increased risk for SIDS over the general infant population. This is likely due to a combination of epidemiologic and biologic factors that are difficult to sort out. In some sibling SIDS cases child abuse or an undiagnosed inborn error of metabolism may have been responsible for the deaths. Twins have a higher risk for SIDS than singletons, even factoring in the fact that twins have higher rates of prematurity and low birth weight. SIDS occurs more in male than female babies. Many SIDS victims have had a respiratory infection a few weeks before their death, but the rate of respiratory infections in control infants is similar and no single causative microorganism has been identified.

Sleeping environment risk factors:

- Prone or side sleeping
- Soft sleeping surface
- Bed-sharing
- Overheating

In addition to the prone sleeping position discussed above, environmental factors can increase an infant's risk for SIDS. These include a soft sleeping surface and bedding items such as blankets, pillows, stuffed toys, and crib bumper pads that can inadvertently lead to suffocation. Bed sharing with parents increases the risk for SIDS, as does overheating due to a high room temperature or excessive clothing and blankets, and swaddling.

Factors that are not associated with SIDS include a history of apnea, breathing pattern abnormalities, or other apparent life-threatening events, like choking or turning blue. Standard cardiorespiratory monitors do not reduce risk of SIDS risk.

PATHOLOGY: There are some morphologic findings in babies who have died of SIDS. They are often of unknown significance, subtle and not present in every case. The lungs are often grossly congested, showing vascular engorgement with or without pulmonary edema. The most common finding is petechiae on the thymus, epicardium, and parietal and visceral pleura. Because these findings are also seen in babies with explained SUID they probably are agonal events. Microscopic signs of recent infections in the larynx and trachea are common, but are not severe enough to cause death and, as noted above, no common causative microorganism(s) has been identified.

Periadrenal brown fat and persistent hepatic extramedullary hematopoiesis may be present, possibly reflecting delayed development, chronic intermittent hypoxia, or long-standing stress. Brainstem and cerebellar astrogliosis can be seen, and some SIDS infants have shown hypoplasia of the arcuate nucleus and other areas of the brainstem that regulate ventilatory and blood pressure responses to hypoxia and hypercarbia. In true SIDS cases, postmortem examination does not reveal a clear cause of death. A thorough autopsy done to exclude other possible etiologies of SUID, such as unsuspected infection, congenital anomaly, genetic disorder or child abuse, reveals an unexpected cause of death in ~20% of SUID babies. Several rare genetic conditions such as fatty acid oxidation defects and cardiac channelopathies (see Chapters 1 and 17) that may cause arrhythmias have been discovered as causes of SUID (see Table 6-22).

PATHOPHYSIOLOGY: The evolution of SIDS is unknown, probably different from one patient to the next and probably entails a confluence of events. It is most likely a multifactorial disorder, with different types of contributing factors that vary from case to case. In this scenario, a combination of simultaneous chance events causes an infant's death, where any individual factor would not have been lethal. Extrinsic stressors or triggering events would include obstruction of airflow, a respiratory infection or overheating. The impact of these influences would dovetail with an infant's intrinsic underlying vulnerabilities, such as developmentally abnormal brainstem neurotransmitter networks that regulate arousal and autonomic control of cardiorespiratory function. This brainstem circuitry develops rapidly in the first months of life. Some experimental data point to the laryngeal chemoreflex which causes apnea, bradycardia and cardiovascular collapse in young, maturing mammals upon exposure of the laryngeal mucosa to acidic and/or organic stimuli.

SIDS infants may have abnormal neurotransmitter activity. Prenatal nicotine exposure via maternal cigarette smoking can cause hypoxic fetal brain injury from reduced uteroplacental blood flow. It is also associated with abnormal nicotinic receptor binding in some SIDS victims. Brainstem neurotransmission may be dysfunctional, for example, medullary serotoninergic transmission and GABA (γ-aminobutyric acid) receptors. Very recently, a significant developmental abnormality of the SP/NK1R (neuropeptide substance P and its tachykinin/neurokinin-1-receptor) system has also been identified. Mutations and/or polymorphisms in genes for these and other neurotransmitters, receptors and related proteins and enzymes involved in medullary homeostatic control may lead to suboptimal, perhaps lethal, responses to external stressors. Such genetic variants could explain how siblings of SIDS victims have increased risk for SIDS.

NEOPLASMS OF INFANCY AND CHILDHOOD

Tumor-Like Conditions Include Displaced Tissues and Cells

Hamartomas are focal, benign overgrowths of one or more mature cellular elements of a normal tissue, often arranged irregularly. They are characteristic in some inherited syndromes, like tuberous sclerosis complex. Some hamartomas have a clonal chromosome abnormality, and so may be classified as true neoplasms.

Choristoma, also called **heterotopia,** is a small aggregate of well-developed, normally organized tissue in an aberrant location. Pancreatic rests in the walls of the GI tract and adrenal tissue in the renal cortex are examples. These are not true tumors.

Vascular Proliferations Are the Most Common Benign Pediatric Tumors

Hemangiomas are benign tumors of blood vessels, usually capillaries. They vary in size and location, and are the most common tumor in childhood. Whether they are true neoplasms is unclear, but many appear shortly after birth and regress by age 10 years. Large, rapidly growing hemangiomas, especially on the head or neck, may occasionally cause serious problems by compressing airways, eyes, or other important structures.

Port wine stains are large flat congenital capillary hemangiomas of the skin of the face and scalp. They are a defining feature of **Sturge–Weber syndrome** and are often disfiguring, giving the affected area a dark crimson color. Unlike many small hemangiomas, they persist for life.

Lymphangiomas are poorly circumscribed collections of dilated lymphatic channels, separated by fibrous septa. They are usually present at birth and enlarge rapidly thereafter. Most occur on the head and neck, but the floor of the mouth, mediastinum, and buttocks are not uncommon sites. They may be unilocular or multilocular, and have thin, transparent walls and contain straw-colored fluid. Whether lymphangiomas are developmental malformations or neoplasms is unclear. Lymphangiomas do not regress spontaneously, and are generally resected.

Sacrococcygeal teratoma, a rare germ cell tumor that occurs in 1 in 40,000 live births, is the most common solid neoplasm in the newborn. Over 75% occur in girls, particularly in twins. They usually present at birth as masses near the sacrum and buttocks. They may be large, lobulated tumors, sometimes as large as the infant's head. Half grow externally and may be connected to the body by a stalk. Some have both external and intrapelvic components, and a few are entirely in the pelvis. Sacrococcygeal teratomas contain multiple tissues, particularly of neural origin. Most (90%) that are detected before 2 months of age are benign, but up to half of those found later in life are malignant. Associated congenital anomalies of vertebrae, the genitourinary system, and the anorectum are common. These lesions should be resected promptly.

Pediatric Malignancies Mostly Derive From Embryonic Mesoderm

Malignancies in children 1 to 15 years old occur in 1.3 per 10,000 children per year. However, cancer is a leading cause of death from disease in this age group, accounting for 10% of deaths in children, and exceeded only by accidental trauma (and suicide in adolescents). Unlike adults, in whom most cancers are of epithelial origin (e.g., lung, colon, and breast carcinomas), most childhood malignancies arise from hematopoietic, nervous, and soft tissues (Fig. 6-60). Almost half are lymphomas and acute leukemias. The latter, particularly acute lymphoblastic leukemia, comprise 1/3 of childhood cancers. Most of the rest are neuroblastoma, brain tumors, Wilms tumor, retinoblastoma, bone cancers, and soft tissue sarcomas.

Mortality is determined by the intrinsic behavior of a tumor and its response to therapy, but overall, the death rate for childhood cancers is 1/3 of the incidence. Occasionally tumors are evident at birth, and so obviously developed in utero. In addition, abnormally developed organs, persistent organ primordia and displaced organ rests may undergo neoplastic transformation. Many childhood cancers are part of genetic disorders, for example, defects in DNA repair pathways or mutations in tumor suppressor genes (see Chapter 5). Table 6-23 lists examples of chromosome abnormalities and single gene syndromes that have a strong disposition for pediatric cancers.

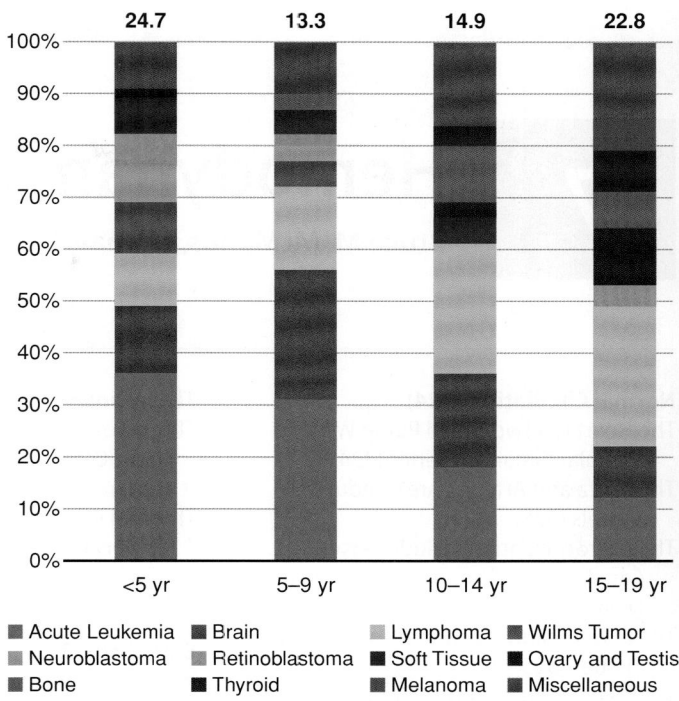

FIGURE 6-60. Distribution of childhood malignant tumors according to age and primary site. At the top of each age bracket column is the combined rate of all pediatric cancers per 100,000 children.

Genetic influences in the development of childhood tumors are well studied for some of these tumors, like retinoblastoma and Wilms tumor. Interactions of heritable and environmental factors in the pathogenesis of malignancies are discussed in Chapter 5, and individual cancers of childhood are discussed in detail in chapters on their respective organs.

ACKNOWLEDGMENTS

The authors of Chapter 6 would like to thank Anthony Garber, PhD for editorial assistance and Nancy Hsu, MS and Andrew Powell, MA, CPA for their help with figure creation. They also wish to thank Dara Brodsky, MD for review of the Diseases of Infancy and Childhood section and Hannah Kinney, MD for review of the section on Sudden Infant Death Syndrome.

TABLE 6-23			
REPRESENTATIVE SYNDROMES WITH PREDISPOSITION FOR PEDIATRIC TUMORS			
Disorder	**Main Clinical Features**	**Malignancy**	**Altered Gene(s)**
11p- syndrome (WAGR syndrome)	Aniridia, genitourinary malformations and mental retardation	Wilms tumor	Deletion of *WT1*
13q- syndrome	IUGR, microphthalmia, hypertelorism, cardiac and brain malformations, absent thumbs	Retinoblastoma, osteosarcoma	Deletion of *RB1*
Gorlin syndrome (Basal cell nevus syndrome)	Broad facies, jaw cysts, basal cell nevi, rib anomalies, calcified falx cerebri	Basal cell carcinomas, medulloblastoma	*PTCH1* mutations
Beckwith–Wiedemann syndrome	Overgrowth, hemihypertrophy, organomegaly, coarse facies with macroglossia	Wilms tumor, hepatoblastoma, adrenal carcinoma	*CDKN1C, H19, IGF2, KCNQ10T1* methylation abnormalities

7 Hemodynamic Disorders

Bruce M. McManus, Michael F. Allard, Bobby Yanagawa

NORMAL CIRCULATION

Normal function and metabolism of organs and cells depend on an intact circulatory system for continuous delivery of oxygen, nutrients, hormones, electrolytes and water, as well as for removal of metabolic waste and carbon dioxide. The circulatory system is a vascular conduit with a muscular pump that drives blood to organs and tissues which returns to the heart to complete the circuit. Delivery and elimination at the cellular level are controlled by exchanges between the intravascular space, interstitial space, cellular space, and lymphatic space, which occur via the smallest-diameter blood vessels in the body (the microcirculation).

The Heart Is a Two-Sided Pump With Vascular Circuits in Series

In this series circuit, the amount of blood handled by the right ventricle, which pumps blood to the lungs (pulmonary circulation), must, over time, exactly equal the amount of blood going through the left ventricle, which distributes blood to the body (systemic circulation). The hemodynamically important parameters are cardiac output, perfusion pressure, and peripheral vascular resistance.

- **Cardiac output** is the volume of blood pumped by each ventricle per minute and represents the total blood flow in pulmonary and systemic circuits. Cardiac output is the product of heart rate and stroke volume and, together with **cardiac index**, adjusted for body surface area (in square meters), are indicators of ventricular function.
- **Perfusion pressure** (also called **driving pressure**) is the difference in dynamic pressure between two points along a blood vessel. Blood flow to any segment of the circulation ultimately depends on arterial driving pressure. However, each organ can autoregulate flow based on hormonal, neural, metabolic, and hemodynamic factors.

- **Peripheral vascular resistance** is the sum of the factors that determine regional blood flow in each organ. Arterioles determine 2/3 of the resistance in the systemic vasculature.

The sum of all regional flows equals the **venous return**, which in turn determines the cardiac output. Assessing the heart's response to inflow (preload) and outflow (afterload) relies on cardiac reflexes, cardiac muscle integrity, and neurohormonal regulation.

The Aorta and Arteries Are Conducting Vessels

The aorta and arteries transport blood to the organs, and convert pulsatile flow into sustained regular flow. The latter function derives from the elastic properties of the aorta and the resistance of arteriolar sphincters.

The Microcirculation Includes Arterioles, Capillaries, and Venules <100 µm in Diameter

Arteriolar blood enters capillaries, which freely anastomose with each other (Fig. 7-1), either directly or through metarterioles. Capillary length, measured from terminal arteriole to collecting venule, ranges from 0.1 to 3 mm, averaging 1 mm. However, because of capillaries' extensive anastomotic network, the path length blood cells travel through capillaries may be longer, allowing for microvascular exchange of substances. The large aggregate surface area of capillaries determines that velocity is low, which further enhances microvascular exchange (Fig. 7-2). Capillary density also influences microvascular exchange by affecting the diffusion distance. For example, in tissues with high oxygen demands, like the heart, capillary density is very high. Entry into the capillary system is guarded by precapillary sphincters, except for thoroughfare channels, which bypass capillaries and are always open. Not all capillaries are open simultaneously, so blood flow can be increased by recruiting additional capillaries. The sum of blood flow through a capillary bed, the thoroughfare channels, and the arteriovenous anastomoses determines regional blood flow.

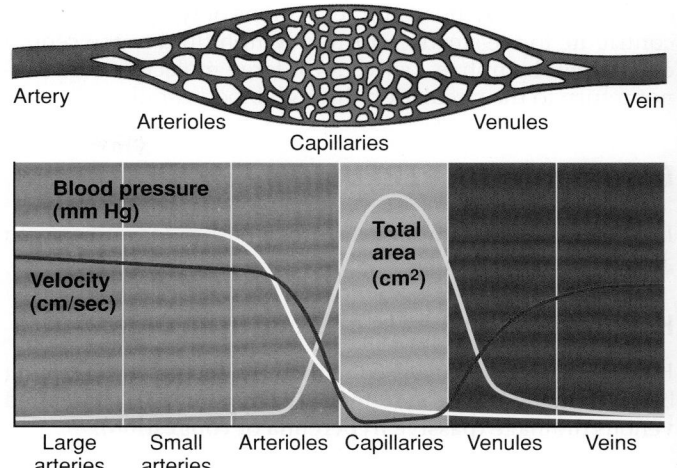

FIGURE 7-2. Blood pressure, velocity, and total area within the circulatory system. Note that the higher resistance due to diameter reduction in the arterioles results in a drop in perfusion pressure; the capillary network constitutes the vast majority of vascular surface area and the venous system is a low-pressure, high-capacitance structure with a series of valves to prevent retrograde flow.

Exactly how an organ regulates blood flow according to its metabolic needs is unclear, but oxygen demand and blood flow are linked. In the heart, blood flow is adjusted on a second-to-second basis. Factors that mediate and link metabolic vasodilation to cellular metabolism include adenosine, other nucleotides, nitric oxide, certain prostaglandins, carbon dioxide, and pH. The microcirculation is an important contributor to all forms of hyperemia and edema, and is a target in septic shock (see below). Vasoregulation in conducting arteries, resistance arteries, and veins relies on delicate interactions between blood, endothelium, smooth muscle cells, and surrounding stroma.

The Endothelium Separates the Blood and Tissues

Endothelial cells are important for anticoagulation, transfer of substances from blood to tissue and back, regulating vessel tone (particularly for resistance arteries), and controlling vascular permeability (**see Chapters 2 and 16**).

Veins and Venules Return Blood to the Heart

Blood from the capillaries enters venules and, eventually, veins on its route back to the heart. Veins are also a blood reservoir; veins contain 64% of total blood volume.

The Interstitium Is 15% of Total Body Volume

The interstitial fluid between cells facilitates nutrient delivery and waste removal. Most interstitial water is bound to a dense network of glycosaminoglycans.

Lymphatics Reabsorb Interstitial Fluid

Interstitial fluid reenters the circulation at the venous end of capillaries; a small portion is drained through lymphatics. Lymphatic capillaries conduct lymph from the periphery to the central venous system via the thoracic duct. Normal

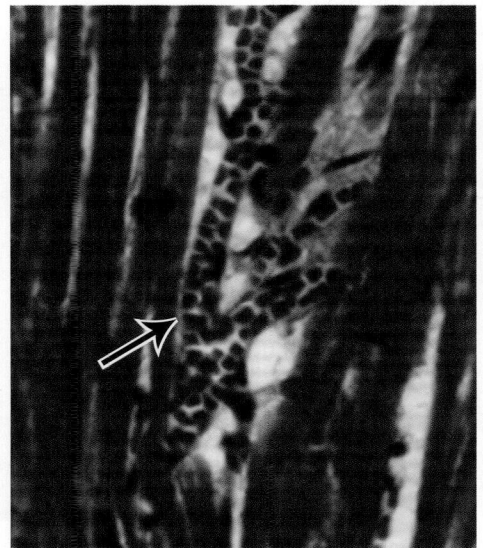

FIGURE 7-1. Microcirculation. Photomicrograph of myocardium showing capillaries and venules (*arrow*).

oscillatory constrictions and relaxations of lymphatic vessels contribute to the steady return of lymph fluid to the central circulation. Lymph is a solvent for large molecules that cannot return to the circulation through blood capillaries.

DISORDERS OF PERFUSION

In hemodynamic disorders, disturbed perfusion causes organ and cellular injury.

Hyperemia Is an Excess of Blood in an Organ

Hyperemia may be caused either by increased incoming blood from the arterial system (**active hyperemia**) or impaired venous drainage (**passive hyperemia** or **congestion**).

Active Hyperemia

Active hyperemia is augmented supply of blood to an organ. It is usually a physiologic response to increased functional demand, as in the heart and skeletal muscle during exercise. Skeletal muscle may increase its blood flow (and thus oxygen delivery) 20-fold during exercise. The increased blood supply occurs by arteriolar dilation and recruitment of unperfused capillaries. Neurogenic and hormonal influences play a role in active hyperemia (e.g., the menopausal flush). Although the utility of vasodilation in these examples is not clear, skin hyperemia during fever serves to dissipate heat.

The most striking active hyperemia occurs in association with inflammation. Vasoactive substances released by inflammatory cells (**see Chapter 2**) cause blood vessels to dilate; in the skin, this contributes to classic "tumor, rubor, and calor" (swelling, redness, heat) of inflammation. In pneumonia, for example, alveolar capillaries become engorged with erythrocytes as a hyperemic response to inflammation. Because inflammation can also increase capillary permeability and even damage endothelial cells, inflammatory hyperemia is often accompanied by edema and local extravasation of erythrocytes.

Reactive hyperemia occurs after temporary interruption of blood supply (ischemia). Active hyperemia follows when the obstruction eases, probably because ischemic tissue injury causes release of inflammatory agents like adenosine. The magnitude and duration of hyperemia are proportional to the period of occlusion until a plateau of hyperemic response is reached.

Passive Hyperemia (Congestion)

Congestion occurs when an organ is engorged with venous blood. Acute passive congestion is clinically a consequence of acute left or right ventricular failure. In left ventricular failure, blood backs up into the lungs, causing a transudate to accumulate in alveoli—**pulmonary edema**. Acute right ventricular failure causes the liver to become severely congested.

Generalized increases in venous pressure, typically from chronic heart failure, lead to slower blood flow and consequently increased blood volume in many organs, including liver, spleen, and kidneys. Heart failure from rheumatic mitral stenosis was once a common cause of generalized venous congestion, but such cases are now unusual. Congestive heart failure due to coronary artery disease and

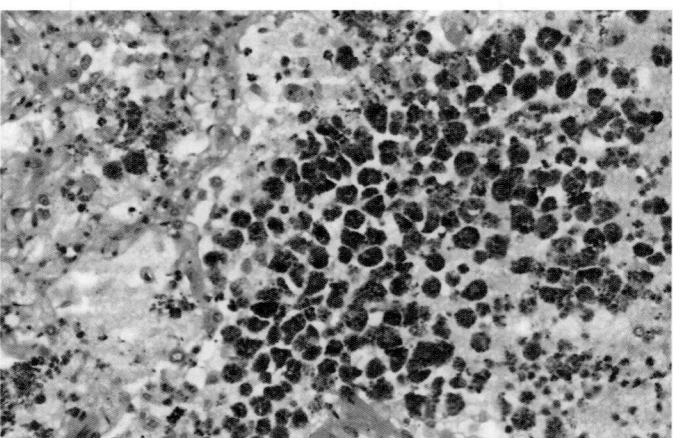

FIGURE 7-3. Passive congestion of lung. Hemosiderin-laden macrophages in the lung of a patient with congestive heart failure.

hypertension, and right-sided failure due to pulmonary disease, are now more common.

Passive congestion may also be confined to a limb or an organ because of more localized obstruction to venous drainage. Thus, deep venous thrombosis (DVT) of the leg veins causes lower extremity edema, and thrombosis of hepatic veins (Budd–Chiari syndrome) leads to secondary chronic passive hepatic congestion.

LUNGS: In chronic left ventricular failure, the left heart cannot pump out the blood flowing in from the lungs, creating back pressure and chronic passive pulmonary congestion. As a result, alveolar capillaries experience increased pressure and become engorged with blood. This increased pressure has four major consequences:

- Microhemorrhages cause bleeding into alveolar spaces, where erythrocytes are phagocytosed and degraded by alveolar macrophages. Released iron, in the form of hemosiderin, remains in these macrophages, consequently called "heart failure cells" (Fig. 7-3).
- Fluid is forced from the capillaries into alveolar airspaces, resulting in pulmonary edema (Fig. 7-4), which impedes gas exchange in the lung.

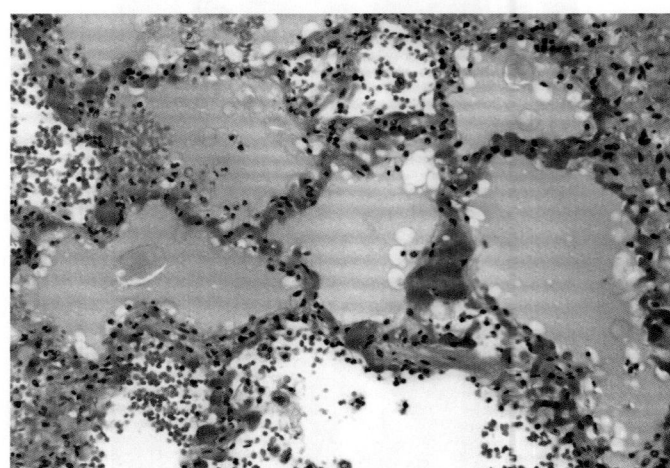

FIGURE 7-4. Pulmonary edema. A patient with congestive heart failure shows pink-staining fluid in the alveoli. (Courtesy of UBC Pulmonary Registry, St. Paul's Hospital.)

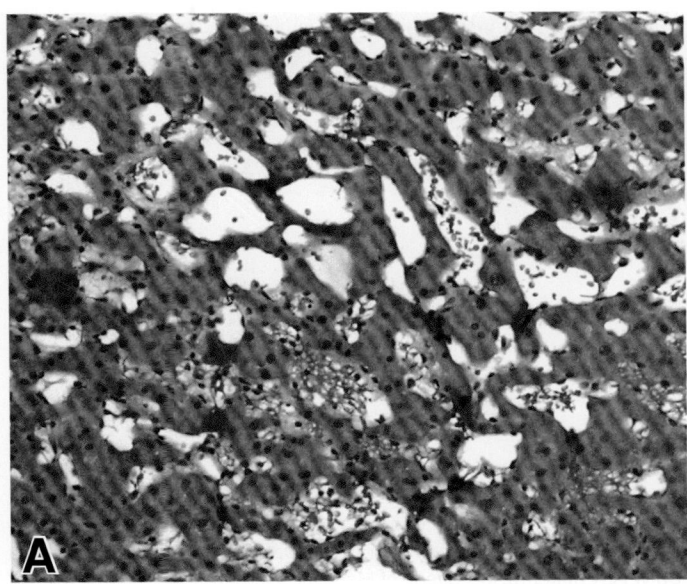

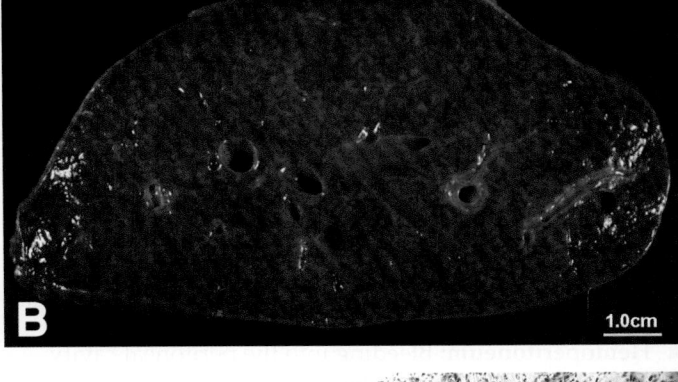

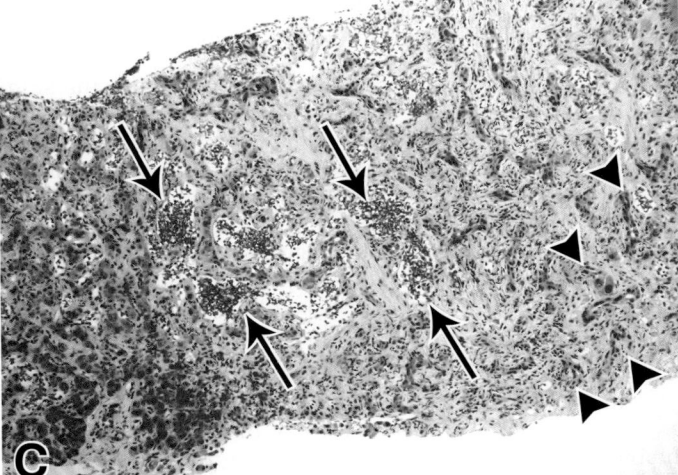

FIGURE 7-5. Passive congestion of liver. A. A photomicrograph of liver shows dilated centrilobular sinusoids. The intervening plates of hepatocytes exhibit pressure atrophy. **B.** A gross photograph of liver shows nutmeg appearance, reflecting congestive failure of the right ventricle. **C.** Late changes in chronic passive congestion characterized by dilated sinusoids (*arrows*) and fibrosis (note the blue staining of collagen in this trichrome stain). Proliferated bile ducts are on the **right** (*arrowheads*).

- The pulmonary interstitium becomes fibrotic. The combination of fibrosis and iron makes the lungs firm and brown (**brown induration**).
- **Pulmonary hypertension** occurs when the back pressure is transmitted to the pulmonary arterial system. This may lead to right-sided heart failure, and then generalized systemic venous congestion.

LIVER: The hepatic veins empty into the vena cava just inferior to the heart, so the liver is particularly vulnerable to acute or chronic passive congestion (**see Chapter 20**). In hepatic lobules, central veins become dilated, the increased pressure is transmitted to the sinusoids, which also dilate. Centrilobular hepatocytes undergo pressure atrophy (Fig. 7-5). The cut surface of a chronically congested liver has dark foci of centrilobular congestion, surrounded by paler unaffected peripheral portions of the lobules. The resulting reticulated appearance resembles a cross section of a nutmeg ("nutmeg liver") (Fig. 7-5). In extreme cases, with acute right ventricular failure, frank hemorrhagic necrosis of hepatocytes in centrilobular zones is conspicuous. Prolonged hepatic venous congestion eventually leads to thickening of central veins and centrilobular fibrosis. Only in the most extreme cases of venous congestion (e.g., constrictive pericarditis or tricuspid stenosis) is the fibrosis sufficiently generalized and severe to justify the label **cardiac cirrhosis**.

SPLEEN: Increased intravascular pressure in the liver, from cardiac failure or intrahepatic obstruction to blood flow (e.g., cirrhosis), generates higher back pressure in the hepatic portal vein (formed from the superior mesenteric and splenic veins) and causes splenic congestion. The organ becomes enlarged (250 to 750 g; normal, 150 g) and tense; the cut section oozes dark blood. Such an enlarged spleen may be overactive—**hypersplenism**—sequestering blood elements excessively (e.g., thrombocytopenia). Long-standing congestion may cause diffuse splenic fibrosis, with iron-containing, fibrotic, and calcified foci of old hemorrhage (Gamna–Gandy bodies).

EDEMA AND ASCITES: Venous congestion impedes blood flow through the capillaries, increasing hydrostatic pressure and promoting edema formation. Pulmonary edema primarily accumulates in left heart failure, and peripheral edema in dependent areas—legs and feet in ambulatory patients and the back in bedridden patients—mostly accumulates in right heart failure. **Ascites** is fluid accumulation in the peritoneal space. It reflects (among other factors) lack of tissue rigor, that is, insufficient countervailing external pressure to oppose hydrostatic pressure within the blood vessels.

Hemorrhage Is Blood Exiting the Vascular Compartment

Bleeding may be internal (within the body) or external. The most common and obvious cause of hemorrhage is trauma.

Yet other dramatic causes include rupture of aortic aneurysm and rupture of cerebral aneurysm (berry aneurysm) causing subarachnoid hemorrhage (**see Chapter 32**). Infections (e.g., pulmonary tuberculosis) and invasive tumors may erode blood vessels and cause hemorrhage.

Hemorrhage is described by its clinical presentation, location, and appearance:

- **Hematoma:** Hemorrhage into soft tissue. Such collections of blood can be merely painful, as in a muscle bruise, or fatal, if located in the brain.
- **Hemothorax:** Hemorrhage into the pleural cavity.
- **Hemopericardium:** Hemorrhage into the pericardial space.
- **Hemoperitoneum:** Bleeding into the peritoneal cavity.
- **Hemarthrosis:** Bleeding into a joint space.
- **Purpura:** Diffuse superficial hemorrhages in the skin, up to 1 cm in diameter.
- **Ecchymosis:** A large superficial hemorrhage in the skin (Fig. 7-6). It is purple at first, then turns green, then yellow before resolving. This sequence reflects progressive oxidation of bilirubin released from the hemoglobin of degraded erythrocytes. A good example of an ecchymosis is a "black eye."
- **Petechiae:** Pinpoint hemorrhages, usually in the skin or conjunctiva (Fig. 7-7). These represent capillary or arteriole rupture, and occur in coagulopathies or vasculitis. Petechiae may also be produced by microemboli from infected heart valves (bacterial endocarditis).

Damage to capillaries can also cause hemorrhage, as when blunt trauma creates a bruise (**ecchymosis**). Increased pulmonary venous pressure may cause blood extravasation from pulmonary capillaries. In scurvy (**see Chapter 8**), defective supporting connective tissue structures cause increased capillary fragility and predispose to bleeding. Capillaries are fragile. An intact clotting system is necessary to contain blood within the intravascular space, otherwise the minor trauma of normal movement would cause extensive bruising. This is illustrated in people with severely decreased circulating platelets

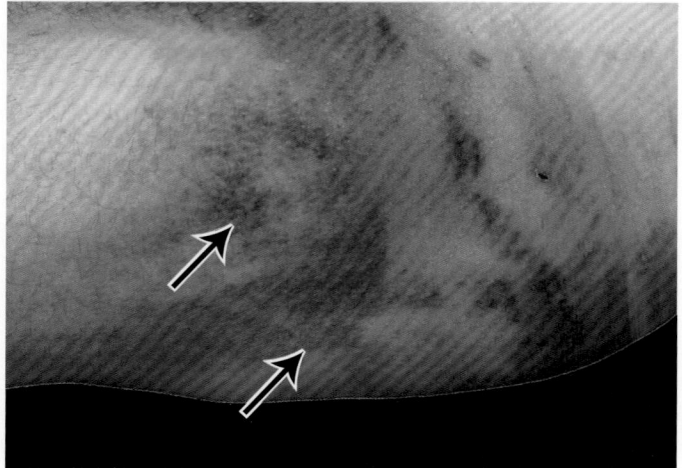

FIGURE 7-6. Ecchymosis. Superficial diffuse hemorrhage (*arrows*) on the thigh caused by blunt force trauma. (Courtesy of Dr. Charles Lee, University of British Columbia, Department of Pathology and Laboratory Medicine.)

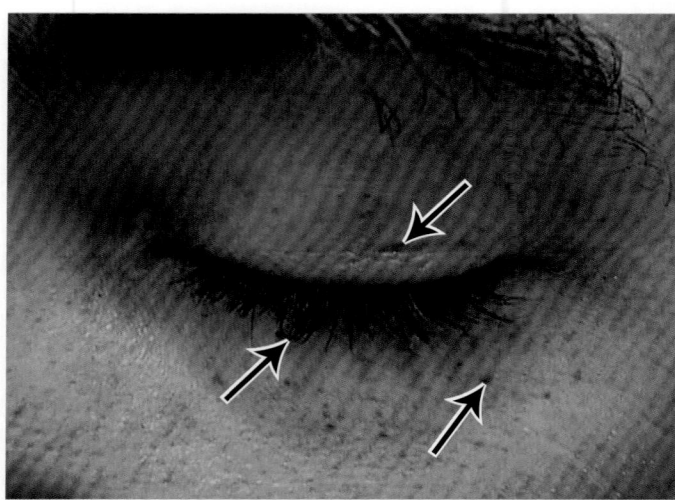

FIGURE 7-7. Petechiae. Periorbital microhemorrhages (*arrows*) appear as punctate red foci. (Courtesy of Dr. Greg J. Davis, Department of Pathology, University of Kentucky College of Medicine.)

(**thrombocytopenia**) or a coagulation factor deficiency (e.g., factor VIII in hemophilia A or von Willebrand factor in von Willebrand disease, **see Chapter 26**), who hemorrhage without apparent trauma.

Gastrointestinal hemorrhage from a peptic ulcer (arterial hemorrhage) or esophageal varices (venous hemorrhage) may result in large amounts of fresh blood filling the GI tract.

Genetic Polymorphisms Affect Coagulation and Responsiveness to Anticlotting Drugs

 MOLECULAR PATHOGENESIS: Rare, well-characterized, highly penetrant, monogenic causes of coagulopathies include von Willebrand disease and hemophilias. Hereditary factors control circulating levels of several coagulation cascade proteins, including plasminogen activator inhibitor-1, factor XIII, factor VII, fibrinogen, and tissue plasminogen activator.

Similarly, there are significant individual genetic variations on the action of drugs that inhibit thrombus formation. **Warfarin** is an anticoagulant with a narrow therapeutic index and greater than 10-fold variability in dose requirements. Clinically, this necessitates regular measurements of the **international normalized ratio (INR)**. *This depends on genetic variants of the metabolic enzyme cytochrome P450 2C9 (CYP2C9) and vitamin K epoxide reductase complex 1 (VKORC1). Variants CYP2C9*2 or CYP2C9*3 increase metabolic clearance of warfarin. Among VKORC1 mutations, −1639G>A is the strongest predictor of warfarin dose requirements. A thienopyridine antiplatelet agent, clopidogrel, is a prodrug that requires hepatic activation by cytochrome P450 (CYP) enzymes. Genetic polymorphisms in CYP2C19 can cause clopidogrel resistance. Newer thienopyridines, such as ticagrelor and prasugrel, are not CYP dependent and so act more rapidly and consistently.*

THROMBOSIS

Thrombosis is formation of an aggregate of coagulated blood containing platelets, fibrin, and entrapped cellular elements within a vascular lumen. A **thrombus** adheres to vascular endothelium and should be distinguished from a simple blood clot, which reflects only activation of coagulation and can form in vitro or postmortem. A thrombus also differs from a hematoma, which results from hemorrhage and then clotting outside the vascular system. Venous and arterial thromboses tend to be triggered differently, but they share commonalities in risk factors, suggesting some mechanistic overlap. Here we present the causes and consequences of thrombosis in these different vascular sites.

Thrombosis in the Arterial System Is Most Often Associated With Atherosclerosis

 ETIOLOGIC FACTORS: The vessels most commonly involved in arterial thrombosis are those most often affected by atherosclerosis: the coronary, cerebral, mesenteric and renal arteries, and arteries of the legs. Less commonly, arterial thrombosis occurs in other settings, including inflammation of arteries (arteritis), trauma, and blood disorders. Thrombi are common in aortic aneurysms (Fig. 7-8), in which the distortion of blood flow, combined with intrinsic vascular disease, promotes thrombosis. Risk factors for thrombosis include metabolic syndrome, which typically includes obesity, hyperglycemia, insulin resistance, dyslipidemia and hypertension; advanced age; tobacco use; previous thrombosis; cancer; and immobilization after surgery or leg casting.

 PATHOPHYSIOLOGY: Arterial thrombi mainly develop in three settings:

- **Endothelial damage,** usually by atherosclerosis, disturbs the anticoagulant properties of the vessel wall and serves as a nidus for platelet aggregation and fibrin formation.
- **Alterations in blood flow,** whether from turbulence in an aneurysm or at sites of arterial bifurcation, favors thrombosis, as does slowing of blood flow in narrowed arteries.
- **Increased coagulability** occurs in certain hematologic diseases, like promyelocytic leukemia or polycythemia vera, or in association with some cancers.

MOLECULAR PATHOGENESIS: Genetic studies of arterial thrombosis have not identified specific genetic factors with a large population-attributable risk, probably because atherosclerosis and atherosclerotic plaque rupture or erosion are complex, multifactorial processes. The most consistent genetic associations with arterial thrombosis are with factor VII and fibrinogen. Hyperhomocysteinemia is also associated with coronary artery disease and cardiac ischemic events.

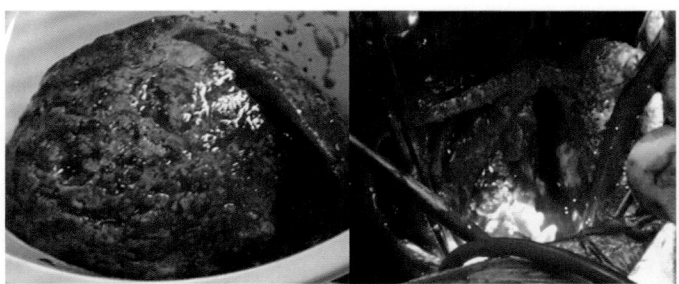

FIGURE 7-8. A large, white, platelet-rich arterial thrombus (left panel) from a fusiform thoracoabdominal aortic aneurysm (right panel) and the remaining aneurysmal and thickened, fibrotic adventitia. (Courtesy of Dr. Paul Haser, University Hospital Centre in Moncton, Department of Surgery.)

PATHOLOGY: Arterial thrombi attached to vessel walls are soft, friable, and dark red at first, with fine alternating bands of yellowish platelets and fibrin, the lines of Zahn (Fig. 7-9). They then have several possible fates.

- **Lysis,** owing to the potent thrombolytic activity of the blood.
- **Propagation** (i.e., increase in size), as the thrombus acts as a focus for further thrombosis.
- **Organization,** the eventual invasion of connective tissue elements, which causes a thrombus to become firm and grayish white (Fig. 7-9).
- **Canalization,** by which new lumina lined by endothelial cells form in an organized thrombus (Fig. 7-10). Its functional significance is often unclear.
- **Embolization,** when part or all of the thrombus becomes dislodged, travels through the circulation, and lodges in a blood vessel some distance from the site of thrombus formation (see below for further discussion).

The organized structure of a thrombus reflects a tight interaction between platelets and fibrin and differs in appearance from a postmortem clot or one formed in a test tube. The question of whether a clot is formed during life

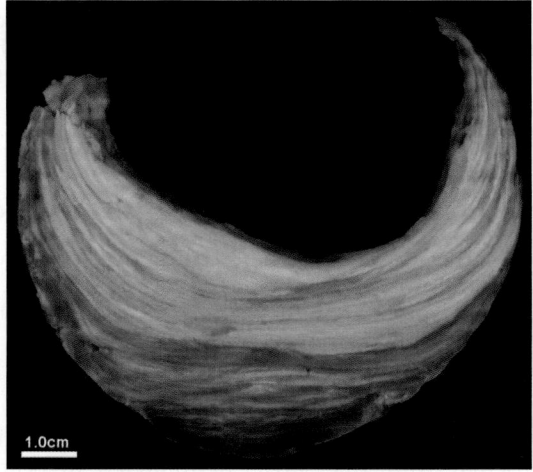

FIGURE 7-9. Arterial thrombus. Gross photograph of a thrombus from an aortic aneurysm shows the laminations of fibrin and platelets known as the lines of Zahn.

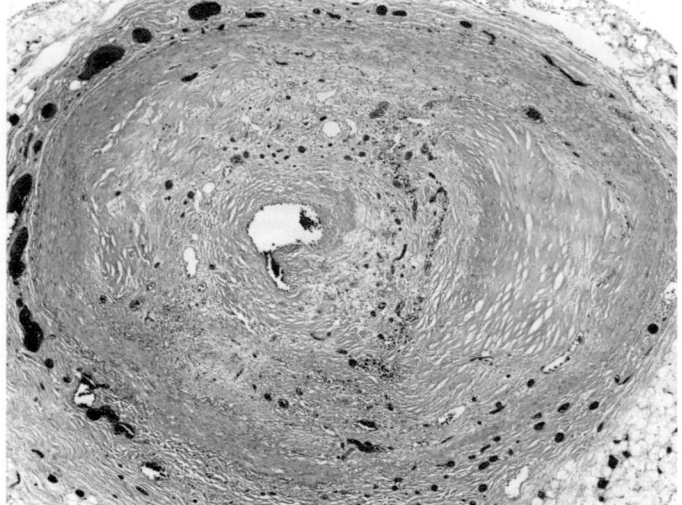

FIGURE 7-10. Canalization of thrombus. Photomicrograph of the left anterior descending coronary artery shows severe atherosclerosis and canalization.

(antemortem clot) or after death (postmortem clot) is often important in a medical autopsy and in forensic pathology. Lines of Zahn stabilize a thrombus formed during life.

In contrast, postmortem clots are more gelatinous. They develop in stagnant blood, where gravity fractionates the blood. The part of the clot containing many red blood cells has a reddish, gelatinous—often called "currant jelly"—appearance. The overlying clot is firmer and yellow-white, representing coagulated plasma without red blood cells. It is called "chicken fat" because of its color and consistency.

CLINICAL FEATURES: *Arterial thrombosis due to atherosclerosis is the most common cause of death in industrialized countries.* Since most arterial thrombi occlude vessels, they often cause ischemic necrosis, or **infarction,** of tissue supplied by that artery. Thus, thrombosis at a coronary or cerebral arterial plaque (Fig. 7-11) results in **myocardial infarction** (heart attack) or **cerebral infarction** (stroke), respectively. Other end arteries often affected by atherosclerosis and thus susceptible to atherosclerosis-triggered thrombosis include mesenteric (intestinal infarction) and renal arteries (kidney infarcts), and arteries of the leg (ischemic leg and gangrene).

Thrombi in the Heart Develop on the Endocardium

As in the arterial system, where endothelial damage may lead to thrombosis, in the heart, endocardial injury, especially when combined with changes in blood flow, may cause mural thrombosis (i.e., a thrombus adhering to the underlying cardiac wall). Disorders in which mural thrombosis occurs include:

- **Myocardial infarction:** Mural thrombi adhere to the left ventricular wall, over areas of infarcted myocardium, because injured endocardium and the altered blood flow associated with an akinetic or dyskinetic segment of the myocardium predispose to thrombus formation.

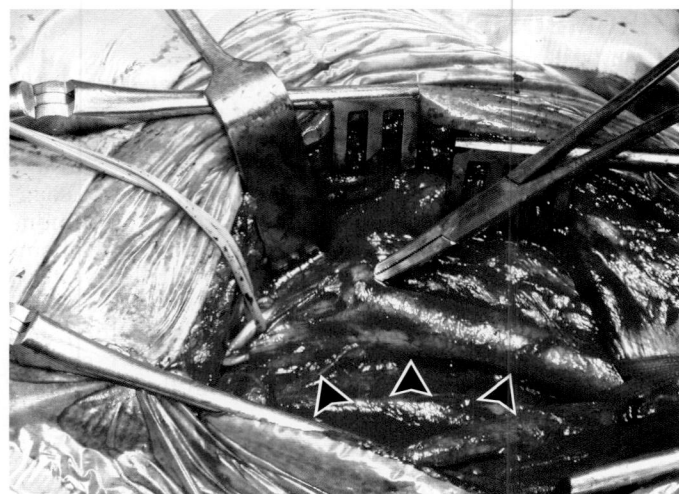

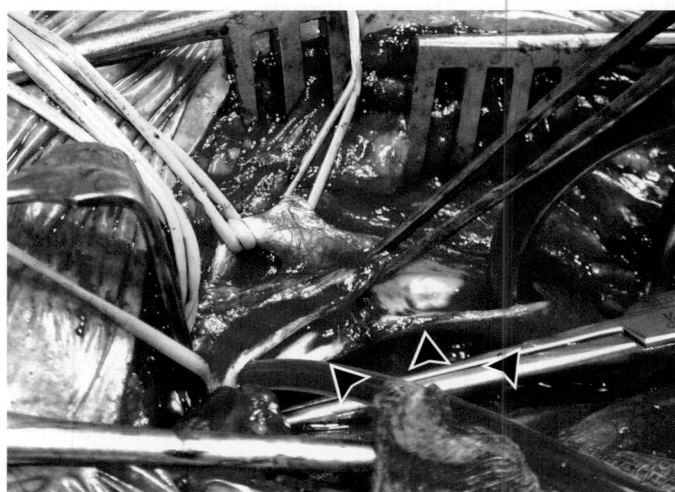

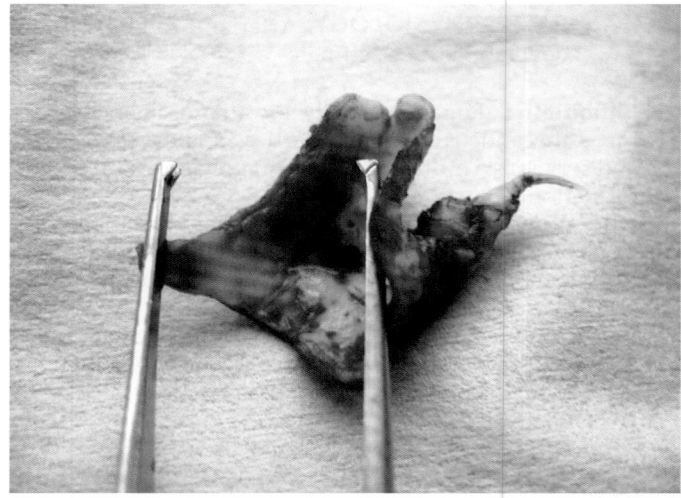

FIGURE 7-11. Endarterectomy. Intraoperative image of a carotid artery (**above**, *arrowheads*) postarteriotomy displaying a near-occlusive atherosclerotic plaque in situ (**middle**, *arrowheads*) and the atherosclerotic plaque itself after carotid endarterectomy (**below**).

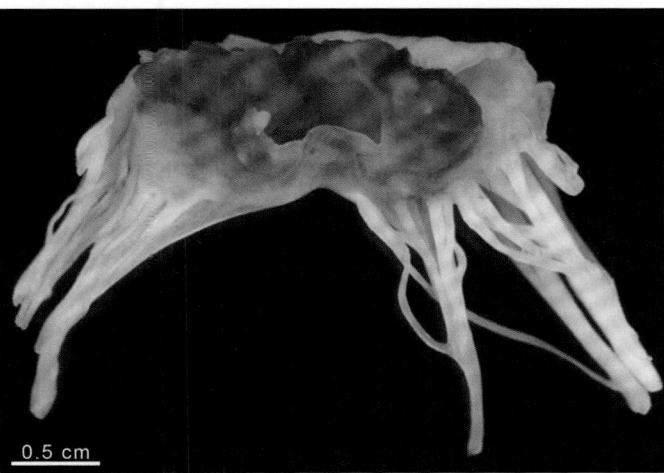

FIGURE 7-12. Endocarditis. The anterior leaflet of the mitral valve is damaged by a friable bacterial vegetation.

- **Atrial fibrillation:** Irregularly irregular atrial activity (atrial fibrillation, **see Chapter 17**) stalls atrial blood flow, which facilitates mural thrombus formation, most often in the left atrial appendage.
- **Cardiomyopathy:** Primary myocardial diseases are associated with mural thrombi in the left ventricle, presumably because of endocardial injury and altered hemodynamics associated with poor myocardial contractility.
- **Endocarditis:** Small thrombi, **vegetations,** may develop on cardiac valves, usually mitral or aortic, that are damaged by inflammation (e.g., in lupus erythematosus) or bacterial infection (bacterial endocarditis, **see Chapter 17**) (Fig. 7-12). In chronic wasting states, as advanced cancer, large, friable vegetations may form on cardiac valves (marantic endocarditis), possibly reflecting a hypercoagulable state.

The major complication of thrombi anywhere in the heart is detachment of fragments and their lodging in blood vessels at distant sites **(embolization)**.

Thrombosis in the Venous System Is Multifactorial

Thrombi occurring in veins (once called thrombophlebitis or phlebothrombosis), is now called **DVT**, reflecting the most common manifestation of the disorder: thrombosis of the deep veins of the legs.

 ETIOLOGIC FACTORS: DVT is caused by the same factors that favor arterial and cardiac thrombosis—endothelial injury, stasis, and a hypercoagulable state. Conditions favoring DVT development include:

- **Vascular stasis** (heart failure, chronic venous insufficiency, postoperative immobilization, prolonged bed rest, hospitalization, and travel)
- **Injury and inflammation** (trauma, surgery, childbirth, infection)
- **Hypercoagulability** (hyperestrogenemia due to exogenous hormones, late pregnancy [etc.], cancer, inherited thrombophilic disorders [**see Chapter 26**])
- **Advanced age** (venous varicosities, phlebosclerosis)
- **Sickle cell disease (see Chapter 26)**

 MOLECULAR PATHOGENESIS: Genetic factors account for 60% of the risk for DVT. Epidemiologic data from the United States demonstrated that African-Americans are more susceptible to development of DVT than are whites, who in turn are more susceptible than Asian and Hispanic Americans. The most common gene variant associated with venous thrombosis is factor V Leiden, which causes poor inactivation and anticoagulant responses to activated protein C. Another common but mild risk factor is the prothrombin G20210A mutation. Deficiencies in proteins C and S and antithrombin are rare but strong risk factors for DVT. Any single SNP or combination of such SNPs can carry an increased risk of venous thromboembolic episodes in childhood and adolescence.

 PATHOLOGY: Most (>90%) venous thrombosis occurs in deep veins of the legs; and most of the rest usually involve pelvic veins. Generally, DVTs begin in calf veins, often in sinuses above venous valves. After that, venous thrombi may:

- **Lyse:** They may stay small, eventually be lysed, and pose no further danger.
- **Organize:** Many undergo organization, like those of arterial origin. Small, organized venous thrombi may be incorporated into the vessel wall; larger ones may undergo canalization, with partial restoration of venous drainage.
- **Propagate:** Venous thrombi often elicit further thrombosis and so enlarge proximally to involve the larger iliofemoral veins (Fig. 7-13).
- **Embolize:** Large venous thrombi or those that have propagated proximally are a significant hazard to life: they, or fragments of them, may dislodge and be carried to the lungs as pulmonary emboli.
- **Limit blood flow:** In severe cases, complete or near-complete venous obstruction in a limb may result in

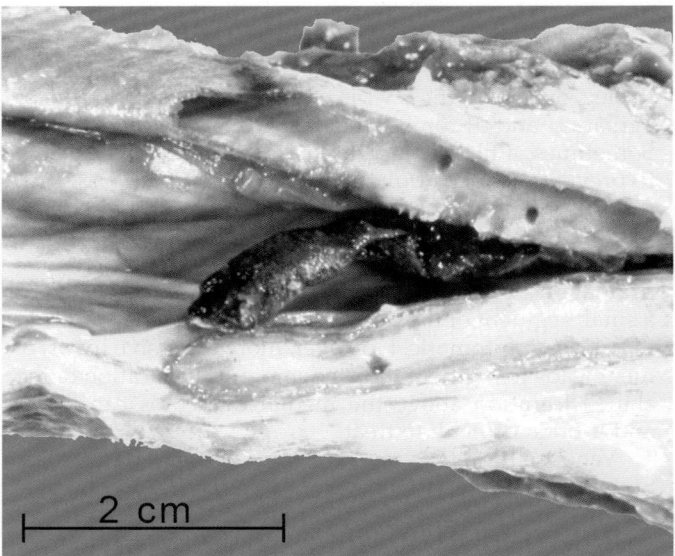

FIGURE 7-13. Venous thrombus. The femoral vein has been opened to reveal a large thrombus within the lumen.

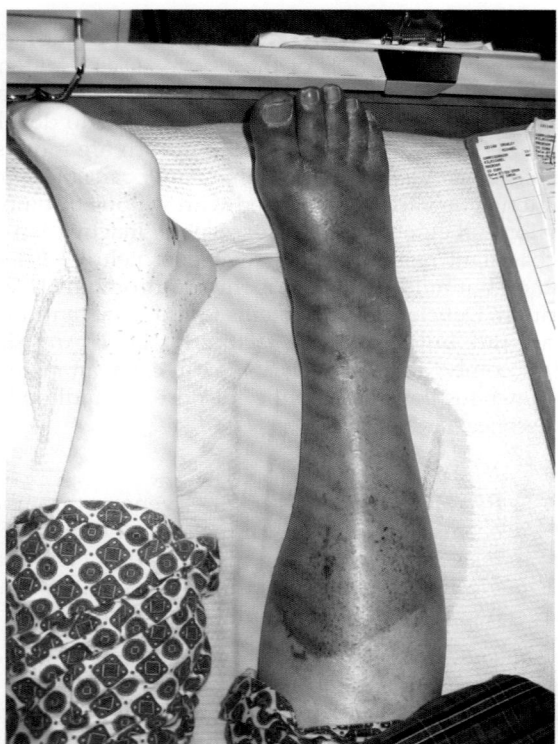

FIGURE 7-14. Phlegmasia cerulea dolens in the right foot. The cause is venous obstruction due to deep vein thrombosis and is associated with cyanosis, edema, swelling, and pain.

phlegmasia cerulea dolens, characterized by pain, swelling, edema, and cyanosis (Fig. 7-14).

CLINICAL FEATURES: Small thrombi in calf veins are ordinarily asymptomatic, and even larger thrombi in the iliofemoral system may cause no symptoms. Some patients have calf tenderness, often associated with forced dorsiflexion of the foot **(Homan sign)**. Occlusive thrombosis of femoral or iliac veins leads to severe congestion, edema, and cyanosis of the leg. Symptomatic DVT is treated with systemic anticoagulants, and thrombolytic therapy in selected cases. Sometimes, a filter is inserted into the inferior vena cava to prevent recurrent pulmonary embolization (PE).

The function of venous valves is always impaired in a vein subjected to thrombosis and organization. As a result, chronic deep venous insufficiency (i.e., impaired venous drainage) is virtually inevitable. If a lesion is restricted to a small segment of the deep venous system, the condition may be asymptomatic. However, more extensive involvement leads to pigmentation, edema, and induration of leg skin. Ulceration above the medial malleolus can occur and is often difficult to treat.

Venous thrombi elsewhere may be very dangerous. Superior mesenteric vein thrombosis can cause hemorrhagic small-bowel infarction; thrombosis of cerebral veins can limit cerebral blood flow; hepatic vein thrombosis (Budd–Chiari syndrome, **see Chapter 20**) can destroy the liver. All of these may be fatal.

EMBOLISM

Embolism is passage of any material that can lodge in a blood vessel and obstruct its lumen through venous or arterial circulation. The most common embolus is a thromboembolus— a clot, or part of a clot, that is formed at one location and then travels to a distant site.

Pulmonary Arterial Embolism Is Potentially Fatal

Pulmonary thromboemboli are seen in over half of autopsies, and occur in 1% to 2% of postoperative patients over 40. Risk of postsurgical PE increases with advancing age, obesity, length and type of operative procedure, postoperative infection, cancer, and pre-existing venous disease.

Most PEs (90%) arise from deep veins of the legs; most fatal ones form in iliofemoral veins (Fig. 7-15). Only half of patients with such emboli have signs of DVT. Some thromboemboli arise from the pelvic venous plexus, and others from the right side of the heart or around indwelling lines in systemic veins or pulmonary artery. The upper extremities are rarely sources of thromboemboli.

CLINICAL FEATURES: The clinical features of pulmonary embolism reflect the size of the embolus, the patient's health, and whether embolization occurs acutely or chronically. Acute pulmonary embolism may:

- Be **asymptomatic** and small
- Cause **transient dyspnea and tachypnea** without other symptoms
- Lead to **pulmonary infarction**, with pleuritic chest pain, hemoptysis, and PE
- Trigger **cardiovascular collapse** with **sudden death**

Chronic PE, with multiple (usually asymptomatic) emboli lodging in small arteries of the lung, can lead to pulmonary hypertension and right-sided heart failure, a syndrome known as chronic thromboembolic pulmonary hypertension (Figs. 7-16 and 7-17; see below).

Massive Pulmonary Embolism

One of the most dramatic calamities complicating hospitalization is the sudden collapse and death of a patient who had appeared to be well on the way to an uneventful recovery. The cause of this catastrophe is often massive PE from a large DVT from a lower extremity. Classically, when a postoperative patient gets out of bed for the first time, the muscular activity dislodges part of a thrombus that had formed because of venous stasis during prolonged bed rest. Excluding deaths related to surgery itself, PE is the most common cause of death after major orthopedic surgery and is the most frequent nonobstetric cause of postpartum death. It also is a common cause of death in patients with chronic heart and lung diseases or subjected to prolonged immobilization for any reason. Inactivity associated with air travel can also lead to venous thrombosis and, occasionally, sudden death from a PE.

A large PE may lodge at the bifurcation of the main pulmonary artery **(saddle embolus)** and obstruct blood flow to both lungs (Fig. 7-18). Large lethal emboli may also block right or left main pulmonary arteries or their first branches.

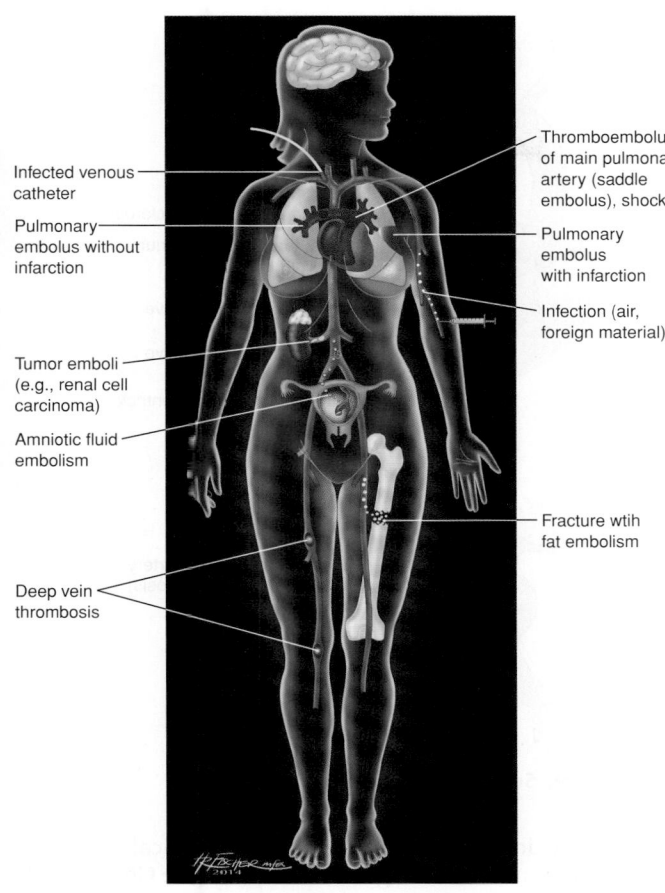

FIGURE 7-15. Sources and effects of venous emboli.

Labels on figure:

Infected venous catheter

Pulmonary embolus without infarction

Tumor emboli (e.g., renal cell carcinoma)

Amniotic fluid embolism

Deep vein thrombosis

Thromboembolus of main pulmonary artery (saddle embolus), shock

Pulmonary embolus with infarction

Infection (air, foreign material)

Fracture wtih fat embolism

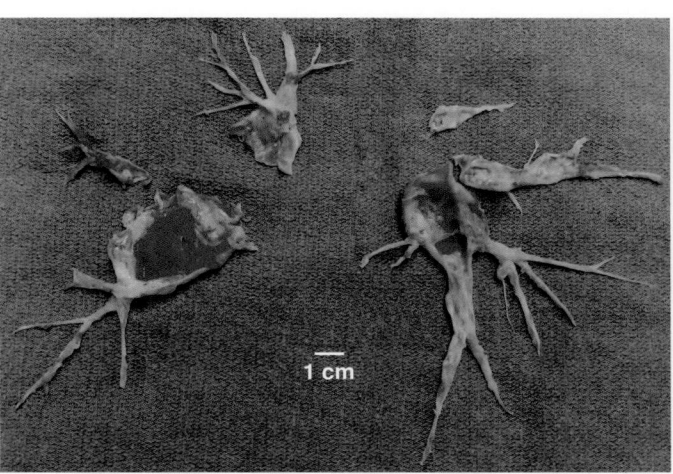

FIGURE 7-17. **Intraoperative image of surgically resected, platelet-rich, white neointimal plaque from bilateral pulmonary arteries in a patient with chronic thromboembolic pulmonary hypertension.** The plaque is removed intact from the lobular, interlobular, segmental, and subsegmental pulmonary arteries. (The intact courtesy of Dr. Marc De Perrot and Dr. Laura Donahoe, Toronto General Hospital, Division of Thoracic Surgery.)

Multiple smaller emboli that lodge in secondary branches may also be fatal. With acute obstruction of more than half of the pulmonary arterial tree, the patient often experiences immediate severe hypotension (or shock) and death.

The hemodynamic consequences of massive PE are acute right ventricular failure from sudden obstruction of outflow

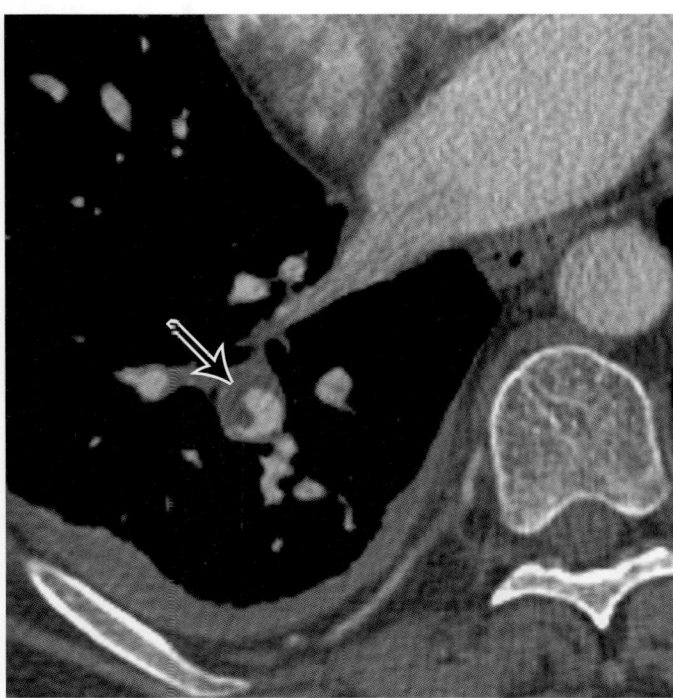

FIGURE 7-16. **Contrast-enhanced computed tomographic image of chronic pulmonary embolism.** A low-attenuation (*dark*) nonocclusive thrombus is seen ⁿ a right segmental pulmonary artery (*arrow*).

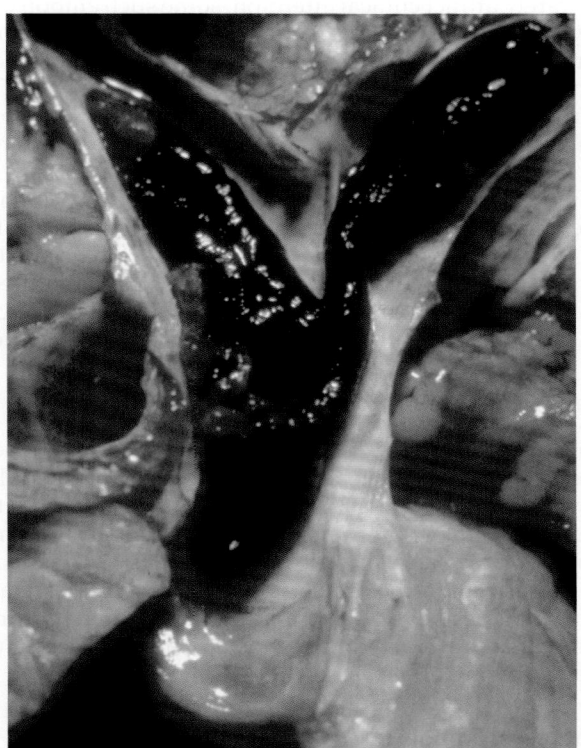

FIGURE 7-18. **Pulmonary embolism.** The main pulmonary artery and its bifurcation have been opened to reveal a large saddle embolus. (Courtesy of Dr. Greg J. Davis, Department of Pathology, University of Kentucky College of Medicine.)

and pronounced reduction in left ventricular cardiac output, due to loss of right ventricular function. Consequent low cardiac output leads to sudden hypotension.

Pulmonary Infarction

Small pulmonary emboli are not ordinarily lethal. They tend to lodge in peripheral pulmonary arteries and sometimes (15% to 20% of PEs) cause lung infarcts.

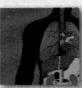 **PATHOPHYSIOLOGY:** Normally, the lung's dual blood supply—from the pulmonary and bronchial systems—protects it from ischemia. Pulmonary infarction usually occurs in the setting of congestive heart failure or chronic lung disease, because one or the other branch of that dual circulation is compromised. Since the bronchial artery supplies blood to necrotic areas, pulmonary infarcts are typically hemorrhagic. They tend to be pyramidal, with the base of the pyramid at the pleural surface. Patients develop cough, stabbing pleuritic pain, shortness of breath, and occasional hemoptysis. Pleural effusion, often bloody, is common. With time, the blood in the infarct is resorbed, and the center of the infarct becomes pale. Granulation tissue forms on the edge of the infarct, after which it is organized to form a fibrous scar.

Pulmonary Embolism Without Infarction

Most (75%) small pulmonary emboli do not produce infarcts, because of the lung's dual blood supply. Although they rarely attract clinical attention, some such emboli cause a syndrome of dyspnea, cough, chest pain, and hypotension. Rarely (3%), recurrent small pulmonary emboli cause pulmonary hypertension by mechanical blocking of the arterial bed. This causes reflex vasoconstriction and bronchial constriction due to release of vasoactive substances, and may limit the functional pulmonary vascular bed.

In the clinical syndrome of "**partial infarction**," patients have clinical and radiologic findings of pulmonary infarction from thromboembolism, but the lesion resolves without leaving a scar. Hemorrhage and necrosis occur in the affected area, but the tissue framework remains. Collateral circulation maintains tissue viability and allows it to regenerate.

Fate of Pulmonary Thromboemboli

Small pulmonary emboli may completely resolve, depending on (1) the embolic load, (2) the adequacy of the pulmonary vascular reserve, (3) the state of the bronchial collateral circulation, and (4) thrombolysis. Alternatively, thromboemboli organize and leave strings of fibrous tissue attached to a vessel wall in the lumen of pulmonary arteries. Radiographic studies have shown that half of pulmonary thromboemboli are resorbed and organized within 8 weeks, with little narrowing of the vessels.

Paradoxical Embolism

If emboli that arise in the systemic venous circulation bypass the lungs by traveling through an incompletely closed foramen ovale, they may enter the left-sided circulation and block flow through systemic arteries. Since left atrial pressure usually

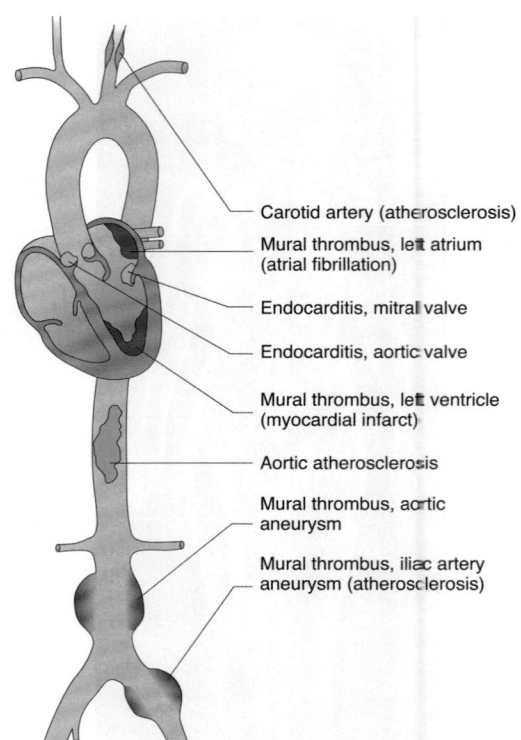

FIGURE 7-19. Sources of arterial emboli.

- Carotid artery (atherosclerosis)
- Mural thrombus, left atrium (atrial fibrillation)
- Endocarditis, mitral valve
- Endocarditis, aortic valve
- Mural thrombus, left ventricle (myocardial infarct)
- Aortic atherosclerosis
- Mural thrombus, aortic aneurysm
- Mural thrombus, iliac artery aneurysm (atherosclerosis)

exceeds that in the right, most such paradoxical embolism occurs in the context of a right-to-left shunt (see **Chapter 17**).

Systemic Arterial Embolism Often Causes Infarcts

Thromboembolism

The heart is the most common source of arterial thromboemboli (Fig. 7-19), which usually arise from mural thrombi (Fig. 7-20) or diseased valves. These emboli tend to lodge at points where vessel lumens narrow abruptly (e.g., at bifurcations or near atherosclerotic plaques). The viability of tissue

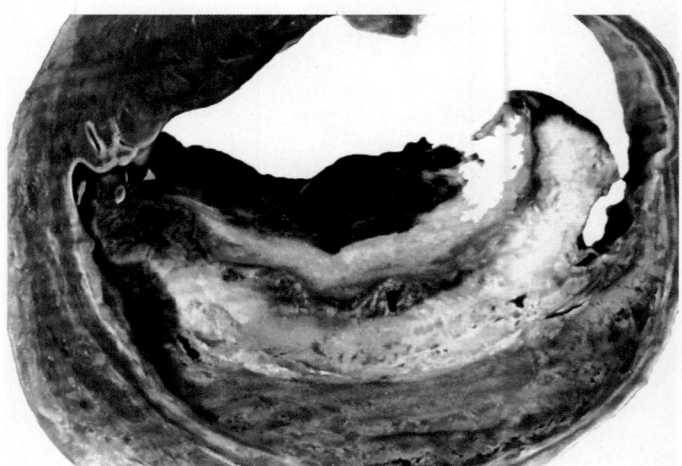

FIGURE 7-20. Mural thrombus of the left ventricle. A laminated thrombus adheres to the endocardium overlying a healed aneurysmal myocardial infarct.

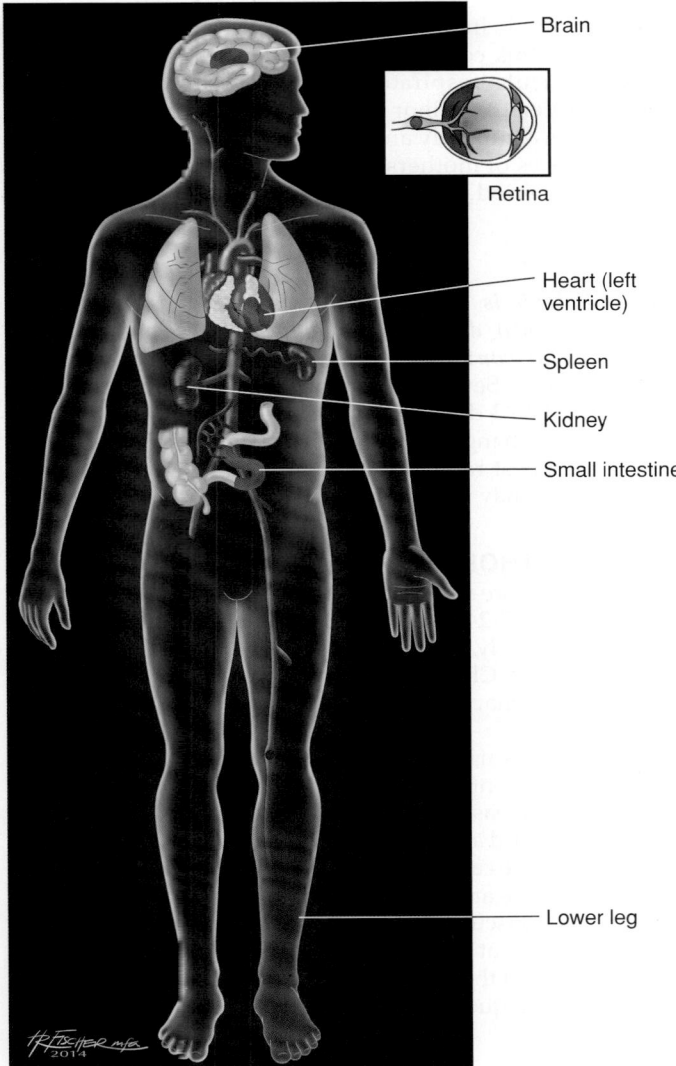

FIGURE 7-21. Common sites of infarction from arterial emboli.

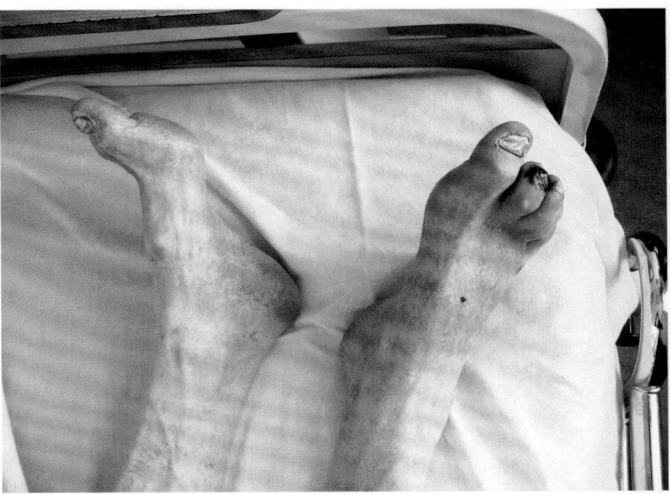

FIGURE 7-22. Acute ischemic right foot. A condition of sudden poor arterial perfusion, usually the consequence of acute thrombosis of an atherosclerotic plaque or embolism. This foot has a red dusky hue with second-toe necrosis. Symptoms may include pain, paresthesia, and paralysis.

supplied by the vessel depends on the available collateral circulation and the fate of the embolus itself. Thromboemboli may propagate locally and cause more severe obstruction, become absorbed into the vessel wall, fragment or lyse. Organs that suffer most from arterial thromboembolism (Fig. 7-21) include:

- **Brain:** Arterial emboli to the brain cause ischemic necrosis (strokes).
- **Intestine:** In the mesenteric circulation, emboli cause bowel infarction, which manifests as an acute abdomen and requires immediate surgery.
- **Legs:** Embolism to an artery of the leg leads to sudden pain, absence of pulses, and a cold limb (Fig. 7-22). In some cases, the limb may require amputation.
- **Kidney:** Renal artery embolism may infarct an entire kidney but more commonly causes small peripheral infarcts.
- **Heart:** Coronary artery embolism causing myocardial infarction is rare.

Air Embolism

Air may enter the venous circulation through neck wounds, thoracentesis or punctures in great veins during invasive procedures or intraoperatively during cardiac surgery. Small amounts of circulating air as bubbles are of little consequence, but quantities of 100 mL or more can result in sudden death. Air bubbles tend to coalesce and physically obstruct blood flow in the right side of the heart, pulmonary circulation, and brain. Histologically, air bubbles appear as empty spaces in capillaries and small pulmonary vessels.

People exposed to increased atmospheric pressure, such as scuba divers and workers in underwater occupations (e.g., tunnels, drilling platform construction), may develop **decompression sickness**, a unique form of gas embolism. After descent, large amounts of inert gas (nitrogen or helium) dissolve in body fluids. When the diver ascends, this gas is released from solution and exhaled. However, if ascent is too rapid, gas bubbles form in the circulation and within tissues, obstructing blood flow and directly injuring cells. Air embolism is the second most common cause of death in sport diving (drowning is the first).

CLINICAL FEATURES: Acute decompression sickness, "the bends," is characterized by temporary muscular and joint pain, due to small-vessel obstruction in these tissues. However, severe involvement of cerebral blood vessels may cause coma or even death.

Caisson disease is decompression sickness in which vascular obstruction causes multiple areas of ischemic (avascular) necrosis of bone, particularly in the femoral head, tibia, and humerus. This complication was originally described in construction workers in diving bells (caissons).

Amniotic Fluid Embolism

Amniotic fluid containing fetal cells and debris may enter the maternal circulation through open uterine and cervical veins. This rare, but potentially catastrophic, maternal complication of childbirth usually occurs at the end of labor. Amniotic fluid emboli are composed of the solid epithelial constituents

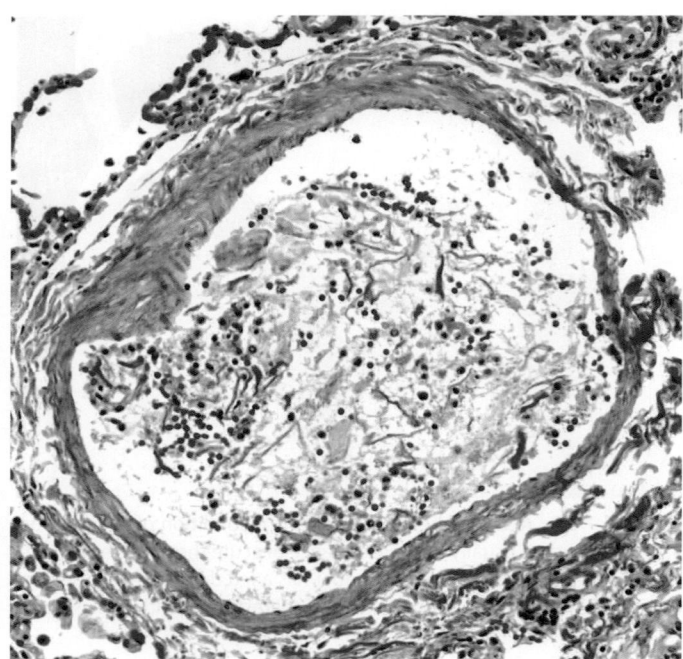

FIGURE 7-23. Amniotic fluid embolism. A section of lung shows a pulmonary artery filled with epithelial squames. (Courtesy of Dr. Sean Kelly, Office of Chief Medical Examiner of the City of New York.)

(squames) contained in the amniotic fluid (Fig. 7-23). Such emboli may also initiate potentially fatal consumptive coagulopathy (**see Chapter 26**) as amniotic fluid contains high thromboplastin activity.

CLINICAL FEATURES: Amniotic fluid embolism can be dramatic, with sudden onset of cyanosis and shock, followed by coma and death. If the mother survives this acute episode, she may die of

disseminated intravascular coagulation. Should she overcome this complication, she is still at high risk to develop **acute respiratory distress syndrome** (ARDS, **see Chapter 18**). Minor amniotic fluid embolism probably occurs commonly and is asymptomatic, as suggested by autopsies of mothers who died of other causes in the perinatal period.

Fat Embolism

Fat embolism is the release of emboli of fatty marrow (Fig. 7-24) into damaged blood vessels following severe trauma to fat-containing tissue, particularly accompanying bone fractures. Severe fat embolism induces **fat embolism syndrome** 1 to 3 days after the injury, with respiratory failure, mental changes, thrombocytopenia, and widespread petechiae. Chest radiography reveals diffuse opacity of the lungs, which may progress to a "whiteout" typical of ARDS.

PATHOLOGY: At autopsy, innumerable fat globules are seen in the microvasculature of the lungs (Fig. 7-24) and brain and sometimes other organs. Morphologically, the lungs typically exhibit the changes of ARDS (**see Chapter 18**). Lesions in the brain include cerebral edema, small hemorrhages, and occasionally microinfarcts.

Fat embolism is usually considered a direct consequence of trauma: fat enters ruptured capillaries at a fracture site. However, increased tissue pressure from hemorrhage into the marrow and also subcutaneous fat may raise interstitial pressure above capillary pressure, and force fat into the circulation. There are other uncertainties. There is more fat in pulmonary vasculature than can be accounted for by simple transfer of fat from peripheral depots, and the chemical composition of the fat in the lung differs from that in tissue. Finally, the frequencies of fat and bone marrow embolism differ.

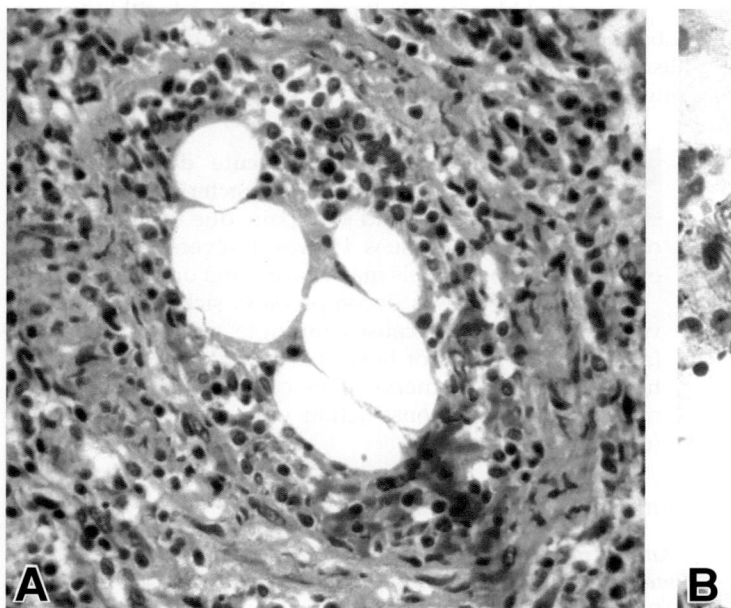
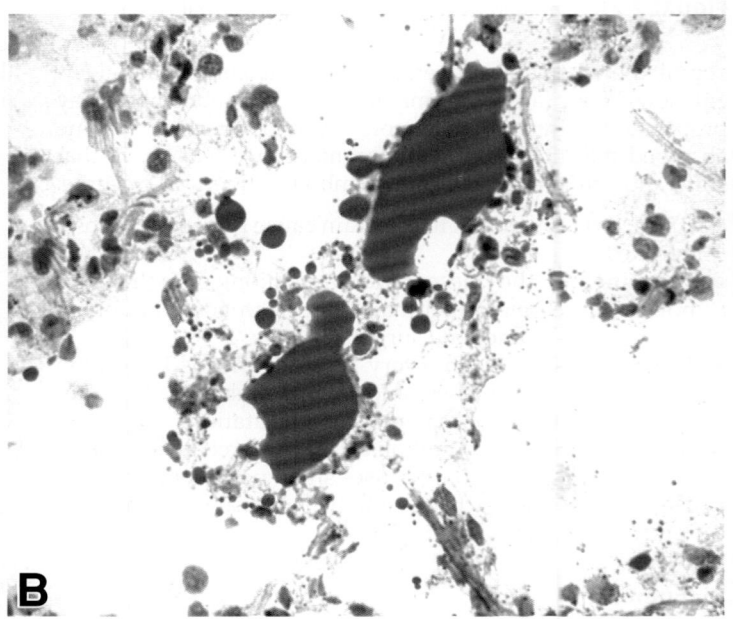

FIGURE 7-24. Fat embolism. A. The lumen of a small pulmonary artery is occluded by a fragment of bone marrow consisting of fat cells and hematopoietic elements. **B.** A frozen section of lung stained with Sudan red shows capillaries occluded by red-staining fat emboli.

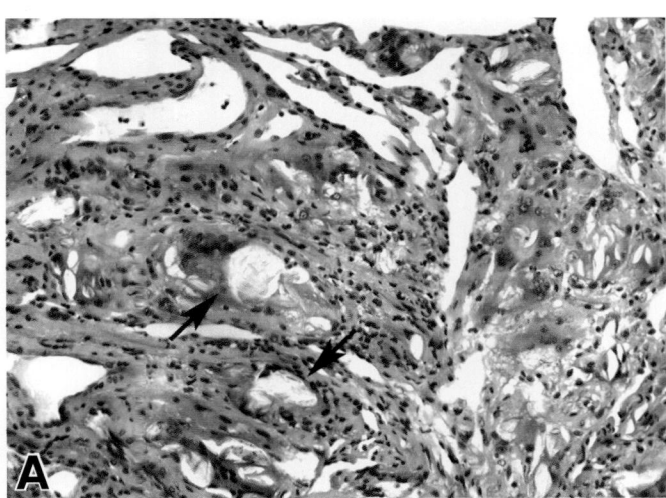
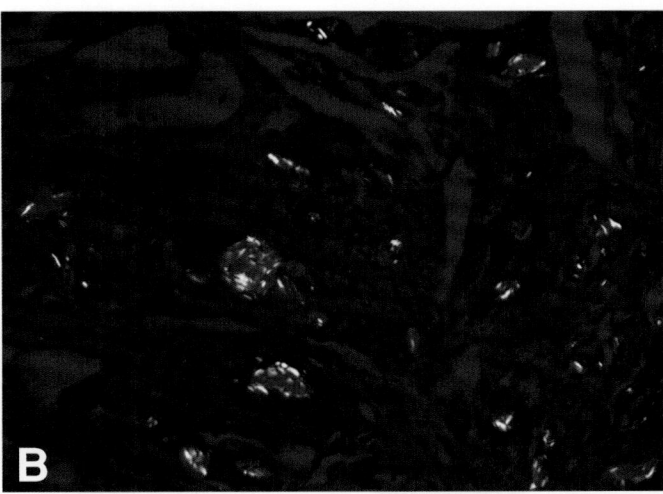

FIGURE 7-25. **Talc emboli.** A section of lung from an intravenous drug abuser shows talc particles (*arrows*) before (**A**) and after (**B**) polarization of light.

Bone Marrow Embolism

Bone marrow emboli to the lungs, complete with hematopoietic cells and fat, are often found at autopsy when cardiac resuscitation fractures the sternum and ribs. They also occasionally occur after fractures of long bones. In most cases, no symptoms are attributed to such bone marrow embolism.

Miscellaneous Pulmonary Emboli

Intravenous drug abusers who use talc as a carrier for illicit drugs may introduce it into the lung via the bloodstream. **Talc emboli** produce granulomatous responses in the lungs (Fig. 7-25). **Cotton emboli** are surprisingly common and are due to cleansing of the skin prior to venipuncture. In **schistosomiasis,** parasite ova may embolize from bladder or gut to the lungs, where they incite a foreign body granulomatous reaction. **Tumor emboli** are occasionally seen in the lung during hematogenous dissemination of cancer.

INFARCTION

Infarction is the process during which coagulative necrosis develops distal to occlusion of an end artery. The necrotic zone is an **infarct**. Infarcts of vital organs such as heart, brain, and intestine are serious medical conditions and are major causes of morbidity and mortality. If the victim survives, the infarct heals with a scar. Partial arterial occlusion (i.e., stenosis) occasionally causes necrosis, but it more commonly leads to atrophic changes associated with chronic ischemia. For example, in the heart, these changes include vacuolization of cardiac myocytes, atrophy, loss of muscle cell myofibrils, and interstitial fibrosis.

PATHOLOGY: The appearance of an infarct depends on its location and age. After arterial occlusion, the area supplied by the vessel rapidly becomes swollen and deep red. Vascular dilation and congestion, and occasionally interstitial hemorrhage, are present. Subsequently, several types of infarcts are distinguishable by gross examination.

Pale infarcts are typical in the heart, kidneys, and spleen (Fig. 7-26), although certain renal infarcts may be cystic. **Dry gangrene** of the foot or leg due to arterial occlusion (often noted in diabetes) is actually a large pale infarct (Fig. 7-27). Within 1 to 2 days after the initial hyperemia, an infarct becomes soft, sharply delineated, and light yellow (Fig. 7-28). Its border tends to be dark red, reflecting hemorrhage into surrounding viable tissue. Such pale infarcts show uniform coagulative necrosis.

Red infarcts may result from either arterial or venous occlusion and also contain coagulative necrosis. However, they also show bleeding into the affected area from adjacent vessels. *Red infarcts occur mainly in organs with dual blood supplies,* such as the lung, or those with extensive collateral circulation (e.g., small intestine, brain). In the heart, a red infarct occurs after an infarcted area is reperfused, which may occur after spontaneous or with therapeutically induced lysis of an occluding thrombus. Red infarcts are sharply circumscribed, firm, and dark red to purple (Fig. 7-29). For several days, acute inflammatory cells infiltrate the necrotic area from the viable border. Cellular debris is phagocytosed and digested by neutrophils, and later by macrophages. Granulation

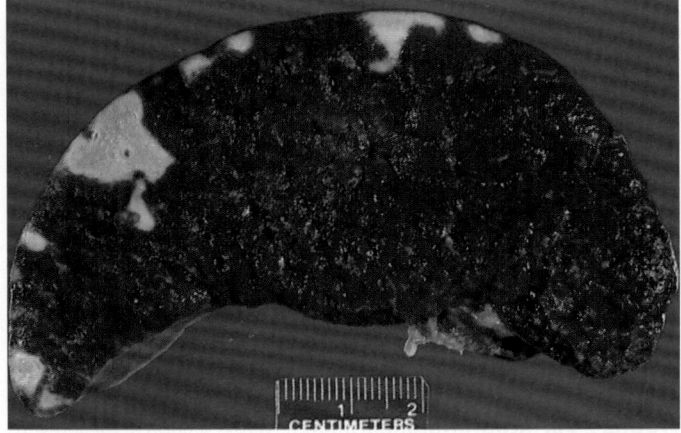

FIGURE 7-26. **Spleen infarcts.** A cut section of spleen displays multiple pale, wedge-shaped infarcts beneath the capsule.

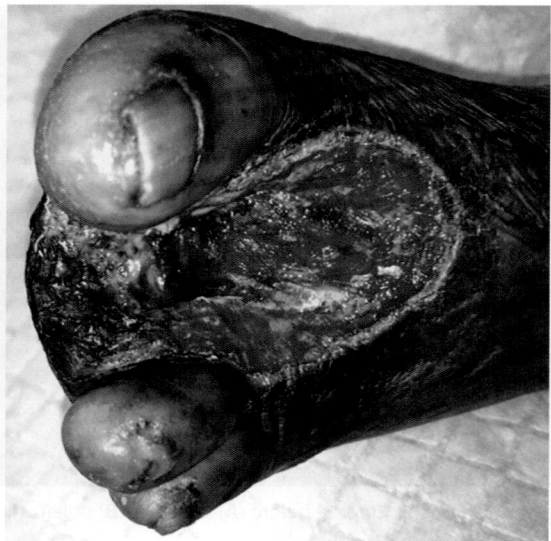

FIGURE 7-27. Dry gangrenous foot in a patient with end-stage diabetic foot ulcer with amputation of second and third toes with debridement of devitalized tissues. The remainder of the foot has severe ischemic skin changes but the soft tissues are well-perfused as evidenced by the pink color. (Courtesy of Dr. Paul Haser, University Hospital Centre in Moncton, Department of Surgery.)

tissue eventually forms, to be replaced ultimately by a scar. In a large infarct of an organ such as the heart or kidney, the necrotic center may remain inaccessible to inflammatory infiltration, and may persist for months. In the brain, an infarct typically undergoes liquefactive necrosis and may become a fluid-filled cyst, which is referred to as a **cystic infarct** (Fig. 7-30).

Septic infarction results when the necrotic tissue of an infarct contains pyogenic bacteria and is, or becomes, infected. Pulmonary infarcts are not uncommonly infected, presumably because necrotic tissue offers little resistance to inhaled bacteria. Emboli arising from bacterial endocarditis are themselves infected, and resulting infarcts are often septic. A septic infarct may become a frank abscess (Fig. 7-31).

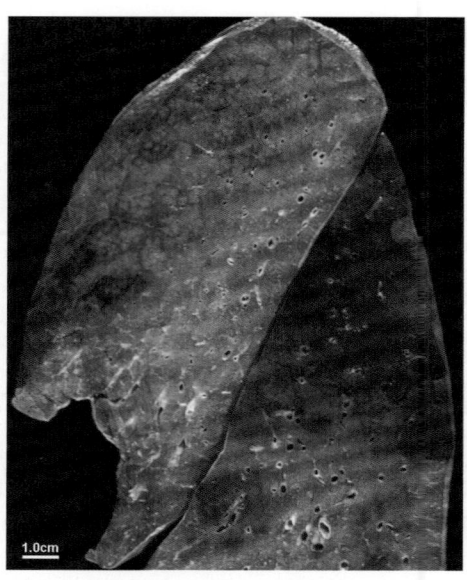

FIGURE 7-29. Red infarct. A sagittal slice of lung shows a hemorrhagic infarct in upper segments of the lower lobe.

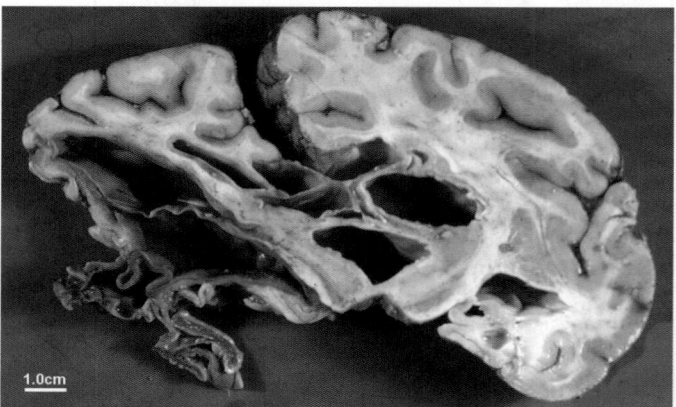

FIGURE 7-30. Cystic infarct. A cross section of brain in the frontal plane shows a healed cystic infarct. (Courtesy of Dr. Ken Berry, Department of Pathology, St. Paul's Hospital.)

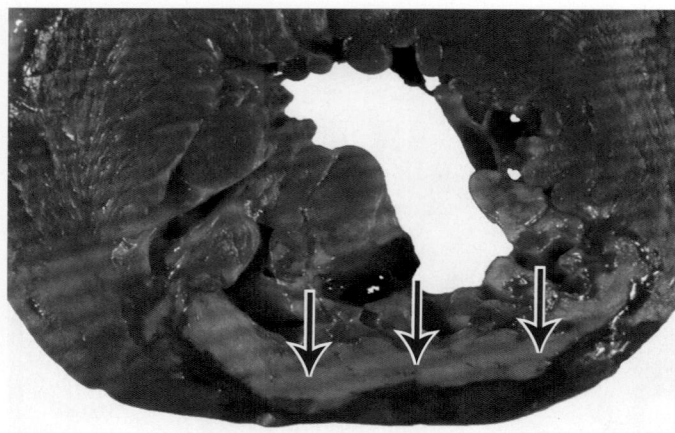

FIGURE 7-28. Acute myocardial infarct. A cross section of the left ventricle reveals a sharply circumscribed, soft, yellow area of necrosis in the posterior free wall (*arrows*).

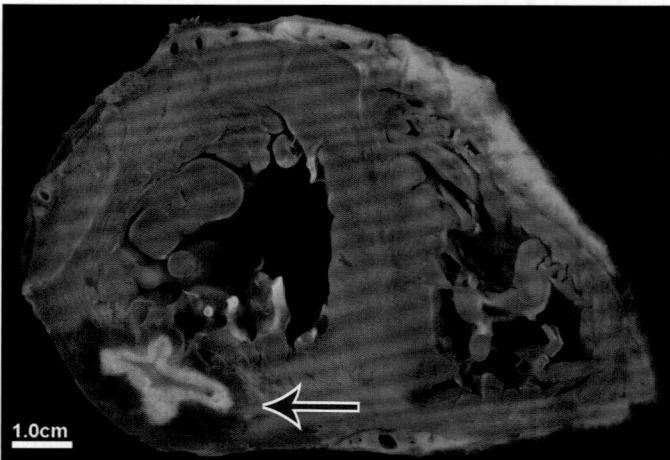

FIGURE 7-31. Septic infarct. A myocardial abscess (*arrow*) within the left ventricular free wall was due to infection with *Staphylococcus aureus*.

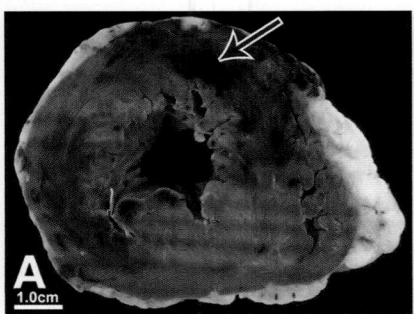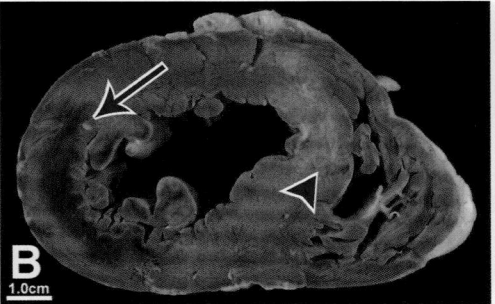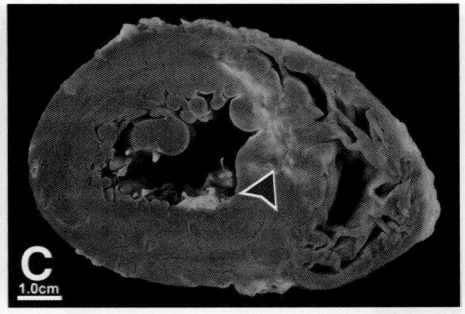

FIGURE 7-32. Myocardial infarct. Transverse sections of ventricular myocardium show (**A**) reperfused, (**B**) acute (*arrow*) and healed (*arrowhead*) together, and (**C**) a healed infarct white scar (*arrowhead*) in the anterior ventricular septum. Reperfusion is typically associated with hemorrhage as in **A** (*arrow*) and **B** (*arrow*).

Infarction in Certain Organs Is Often Fatal

Myocardial Infarcts

Myocardial infarcts can be transmural or subendocardial. A transmural infarct results from complete occlusion of a major extramural coronary artery. Subendocardial infarction reflects prolonged ischemia caused by partially occluding, atherosclerotic, stenotic coronary artery lesions when tissue oxygen requirement exceeds supply. This happens in, for example, shock, hypoxia, or severe tachycardia (rapid pulse). A myocardial infarct may be pale or red, depending on the extent of reflow of blood into the infarcted area (Fig. 7-32).

Pulmonary Infarcts

About 10% of pulmonary emboli cause clinical symptoms of lung infarction, usually after occlusion of a middle-sized pulmonary artery. Infarction occurs only if circulation from bronchial arteries is inadequate to compensate for supply lost from the pulmonary arteries. This occurs often in congestive heart failure, although stasis in the pulmonary circulation may contribute. Hemorrhage into the alveolar spaces of the necrotic lining tissue occurs within 48 hours.

Cerebral Infarcts

Infarction of the brain may follow local ischemia or a generalized reduction in blood flow. The latter often results from systemic hypotension, as in shock, and produces **watershed infarcts**, at the border zones between the distributions of the major cerebral arteries. If prolonged, severe hypotension can cause widespread brain necrosis. Occlusion of a single vessel in the brain (e.g., after an embolus has lodged) causes a well-defined area of ischemia and necrosis. This type of cerebral infarct may be pale or red, the latter being common with embolic occlusions. Occlusion of a large artery causes a wide area of necrosis, which may ultimately resolve as a large fluid–filled cavity in the brain (cystic infarct).

Intestinal Infarcts

The earliest tissue changes in intestinal ischemia are necrosis at the tips of the villi in the small intestine and necrosis of the superficial mucosa in the large intestine. In either case, more severe ischemia causes hemorrhagic necrosis of the submucosa and muscularis but not the serosa. Small mucosal infarcts heal within a few days, but more severe injury leads to ulceration. These ulcers can eventually reepithelialize. However, large ulcers are repaired by scarring, which may cause strictures. Severe transmural necrosis leads to massive bleeding or bowel perforation, complications that often result in irreversible shock, sepsis, and death.

EDEMA

Edema is excess fluid in interstitial tissue spaces, which may be local or generalized. **Local edema** in most instances occurs with inflammation, the "tumor" of "tumor, rubor, and calor." Local edema of a limb, usually the leg, results from venous or lymphatic obstruction. Burns cause prominent local edema by altering local vascular permeability. Local edema may be a prominent component of an immune reaction, for example, urticaria (hives) or edema of the epiglottis or larynx (angioneurotic edema).

Generalized edema, affecting visceral organs and the skin of the trunk and lower extremities (Fig. 7-33), reflects a global disorder of fluid and electrolyte metabolism, most often due to heart failure. Generalized edema also occurs in nephrotic syndrome, when serum protein is lost into the urine (**see Chapter 22**), and when albumin production is low (e.g., cirrhosis). **Anasarca** is extreme generalized edema, with conspicuous fluid accumulation in subcutaneous tissues, visceral organs, and body cavities. Edema may accumulate in body spaces, such as the pleural cavity (**hydrothorax**), peritoneal cavity (**ascites**), or pericardial space (**hydropericardium**).

Interstitial Fluid Dynamics Depend on Starling Forces

Formation and retention of interstitial fluid reflects capillary filtration and reabsorption (Starling forces). The internal, or hydrostatic, pressure in arteriolar segments of capillaries is 32 mm Hg. In the middle of the capillary, it is 20 mm Hg. Since interstitial hydrostatic pressure is only 3 mm Hg, there is an outward fluid filtration of 14 mL/min. Hydrostatic pressure is opposed by plasma oncotic pressure (26 mm Hg), causing osmotic reabsorption at 12 mL/min at the venous end of the capillary. Thus, interstitial fluid is formed at the rate of 2 mL/min, and then is reabsorbed by the lymphatics. In equilibrium, there is thus no net fluid gain or loss in the interstitium.

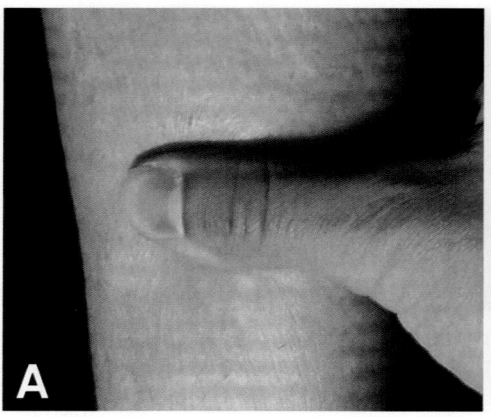
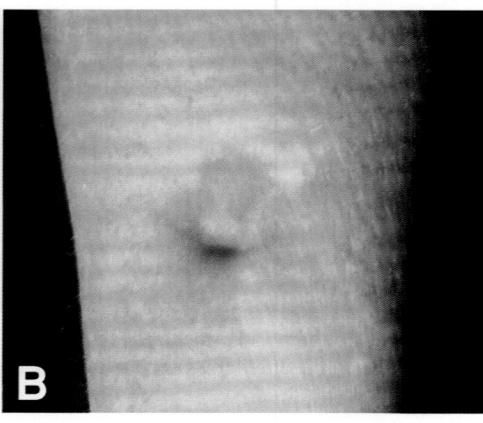

FIGURE 7-33. Pitting edema of the leg. A. In a patient with congestive heart failure, severe edema of the leg is demonstrated by applying pressure with a finger. **B.** The resulting "pitting" reflects the inelasticity of the fluid-filled tissue.

Sodium and Water Metabolism

Water represents 50% to 70% of body weight and is divided between intracellular and extracellular fluid (ECF) spaces, the latter being further divided into interstitial and vascular compartments. The interstitium contains about 75% of **ECF**.

The Role of Sodium Retention in Edema

Total body sodium is the principal determinant of ECF volume because it is the major cation in the ECF. In other words, increased total body sodium must be balanced by more extracellular water to maintain constant osmolality. Control of ECF volume depends largely on regulation of renal sodium excretion, which is influenced by (1) **atrial natriuretic factor (ANF)**, (2) the **renin–angiotensin system** of the **juxtaglomerular apparatus**, and (3) sympathetic nervous system activity (**see Chapter 22**).

When peripheral edema first appears clinically, ECF volume has already expanded by at least 5 L. Mechanisms of edema formation and representative disorders associated with them are summarized in Figure 7-34 and Table 7-1.

Edema Caused by Increased Hydrostatic Pressure

Unopposed increases in hydrostatic pressure increase fluid extrusion into the interstitial space, leading to its retention as edema. This is prominent in heart failure, when back pressure in the lungs due to left ventricular failure causes acute pulmonary edema and secondary right-sided heart failure, and contributes to systemic edema. Similarly, back pressure caused by venous obstruction in the lower extremity causes edema of the leg. Obstruction to portal blood flow in cirrhosis of the liver contributes to formation of abdominal fluid (ascites).

Edema Caused by Decreased Oncotic Pressure

The concentration of plasma proteins, especially albumin, largely determines the difference in pressure between intravascular and interstitial compartments. Any condition that lowers plasma albumin levels, whether it is loss through the kidneys in nephrotic syndrome, reduced synthesis in chronic liver disease or severe malnutrition, tends to promote generalized edema.

Edema Caused by Lymphatic Obstruction

Normally, more fluid is filtered into the interstitial spaces than is reabsorbed into the vascular bed. The excess interstitial fluid is removed by lymphatics. Thus, obstruction to lymphatic flow leads to localized edema. Lymphatic channels can be obstructed by: (1) malignant neoplasms, (2) scarring following inflammation or irradiation, and (3) surgical disruption. For instance, inflammatory responses to filarial worms (bancroftian and malayan filariasis; **see**

TABLE 7-1	
DISORDERS ASSOCIATED WITH EDEMA	
Increased Hydrostatic Pressure	
Arteriolar dilation	Inflammation
	Heat
Increased venous pressure	Venous thrombosis
	Congestive heart failure
	Cirrhosis (ascites)
	Postural inactivity (e.g., prolonged standing)
Hypervolemia	Sodium retention (e.g., decreased renal function)
Decreased Oncotic Pressure	
Hypoproteinemia	Nephrotic syndrome
	Cirrhosis
	Protein-losing gastroenteropathy
	Malnutrition
Increased Capillary Permeability	Inflammation
	Burns
	Adult respiratory distress syndrome
Lymphatic Obstruction	Cancer
	Postsurgical lymphedema
	Inflammation

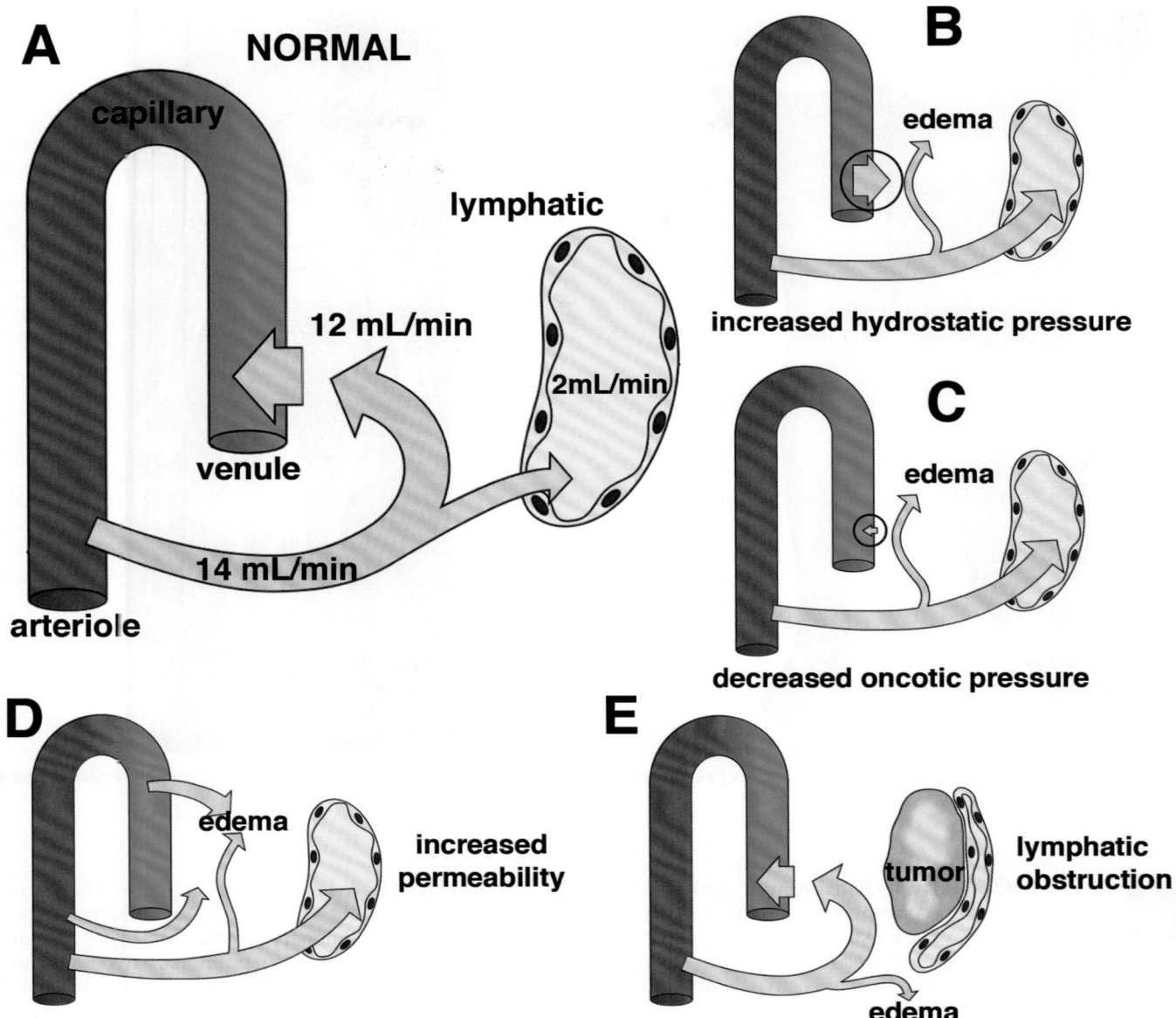

FIGURE 7-34. The capillary system and mechanisms of edema formation. A. Normal. The differential between the hydrostatic and oncotic pressures at the arterial end of the capillary system is responsible for the filtration into the interstitial space of approximately 14 mL of fluid per minute. This fluid is reabsorbed at the venous end at the rate of 12 mL/min. It is also drained through the lymphatic capillaries at a rate of 2 mL/min. Proteins are removed by the lymphatics from the interstitial space. **B. Hydrostatic edema.** If the hydrostatic pressure at the venous end of the capillary system is elevated, reabsorption decreases. As long as the lymphatics can drain the surplus fluid, no edema results. If their capacity is exceeded, however, edema fluid accumulates. **C. Oncotic edema.** Edema fluid also accumulates if reabsorption is diminished by decreased oncotic pressure of the vascular bed, owing to a loss of albumin. **D. Inflammatory and traumatic edema.** Edema, either local or systemic, results if the vascular bed becomes leaky following injury to the endothelium. **E. Lymphedema.** Lymphatic obstruction causes the accumulation of interstitial fluid because of insufficient reabsorption and deficient removal of proteins, the latter increasing the oncotic pressure of the fluid in the interstitial space.

Chapter 9) can obstruct lymphatics, and produce massive lymphedema upstream of the obstruction **(elephantiasis)** (Fig. 7-35). Radical mastectomies remove axillary lymph nodes and may obstruct lymphatic flow, to cause lymphedema of the arm.

Lymphatic edema fluid, unlike other forms of edema, has high protein content, since lymph is the vehicle by which proteins and interstitial cells are returned to the circulation. Such increased protein concentration may stimulate dermal fibrosis in people with chronic edema (indurated edema).

Congestive Heart Failure Results From Inadequate Cardiac Output

About 5 to 6 million people in the United States suffer from congestive heart failure, of whom 15% die annually. Half of patients with congestive heart failure who require hospital admission will die within 1 year. In the United States, this disorder is most commonly associated with ischemic heart disease, although virtually any chronic cardiac disorder may lead to congestive heart failure (**see Chapter 17**).

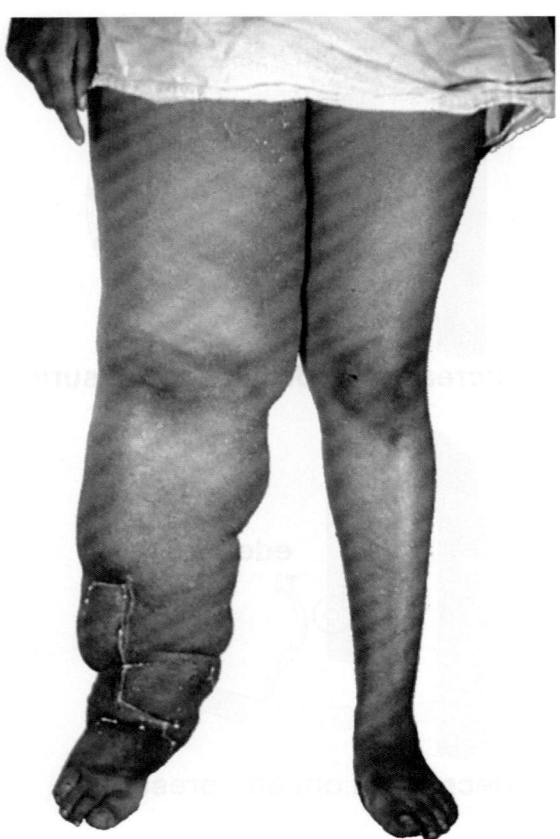

FIGURE 7-35. Edema secondary to lymphatic obstruction. Massive edema of the right lower extremity (elephantiasis) in a patient with obstruction of lymphatic drainage.

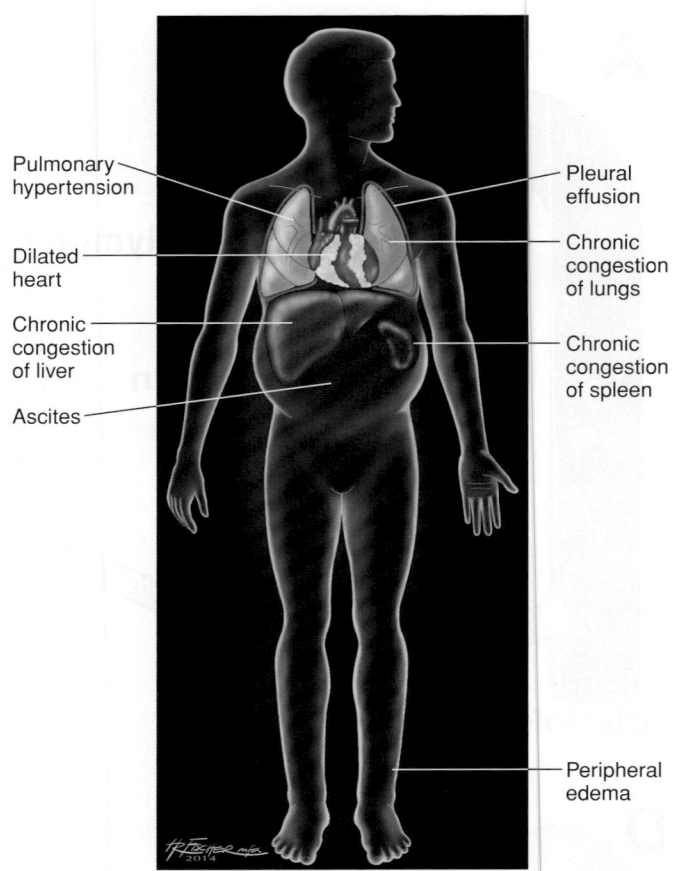

FIGURE 7-36. Pathologic consequences of chronic congestive heart failure.

 PATHOPHYSIOLOGY: Both systolic and diastolic dysfunction contribute to the low cardiac output and high ventricular filling pressure characteristic of congestive heart failure.

Inadequate cardiac output in congestive heart failure decreases glomerular filtration, leading to increased renin secretion. The latter activates angiotensin, inducing aldosterone release, subsequent sodium reabsorption, and fluid retention. Furthermore, reduced hepatic blood flow impairs aldosterone catabolism, further raising its concentration in the blood. As a compensatory mechanism, increased fluid volume preserves an adequate intracardiac pressure. In addition, increased sympathetic discharge leads to augmented levels of catecholamines, which stimulate cardiac contractility and further counteract the impairment in cardiac performance. At the same time, atrial distention because of the increased blood volume promotes release of atrial natriuretic peptide, which stimulates renal sodium excretion.

Over time, these compensatory mechanisms fail, in which case renal sodium retention again becomes important. Further expansion of plasma volume increases pulmonary and systemic venous pressure, thus increasing hydrostatic pressure in the respective capillary beds. The increased capillary pressure, together with decreased plasma oncotic pressure, results in the edema of congestive heart failure.

 PATHOLOGY: Left ventricular failure is associated principally with passive congestion of the lungs and pulmonary edema (Fig. 7-36). When chronic, these conditions result in pulmonary hypertension and eventual failure of the right ventricle. Right ventricular failure is characterized by generalized subcutaneous edema (most prominent in dependent parts of the body) and ascites. The liver, spleen, and other splanchnic organs are typically congested. At autopsy, the heart is enlarged and its chambers dilated.

 CLINICAL FEATURES: The effects of heart failure depend on which ventricle is failing, recognizing that both may be failing simultaneously. Patients in left-sided heart failure complain of shortness of breath **(dyspnea)** on exertion and when recumbent **(orthopnea)**. They may be awakened from sleep by sudden episodes of shortness of breath **(paroxysmal nocturnal dyspnea)**. Physical examination usually reveals distended jugular veins. Those with right-sided failure have pitting edema of the legs and an enlarged and tender liver. When ascites is present, the abdomen is distended. Patients in congestive heart failure with pulmonary edema have crackling breath sounds **(rales)** caused by expansion of fluid-filled alveoli.

In Pulmonary Edema, Fluid Fills the Airspaces and Interstitium of the Lung

Pulmonary edema leads to decreased gas exchange in the lung, causing hypoxia and carbon dioxide retention (**hypercapnia**).

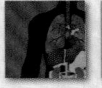 **PATHOPHYSIOLOGY AND CLINICAL FEATURES:** The lung is a loose tissue with little connective tissue support. Normal lungs do not develop edema because of:

- Low perfusion pressure in lung capillaries, due to low right ventricular pressure
- Effective drainage of the pulmonary interstitial space by lymphatics, which are under a slightly negative pressure and can accommodate up to 10 times the regular lymph flow
- Tight cell–cell junctions between endothelial cells, which limit capillary permeability

Pulmonary edema results when these protective mechanisms are disturbed. The most common causes of pulmonary edema entail hemodynamic alterations in the heart that increase pulmonary capillary perfusion pressure and block effective lymphatic drainage. In acute lung injury associated with adult respiratory distress syndrome, inhalation of toxic gases, aspiration of gastric contents, viral infections and uremia, destruction of endothelial cells or disruption of their tight junctions increases pulmonary capillary permeability (**see Chapter 18**).

Pulmonary edema may be interstitial or alveolar. Interstitial edema is the earliest phase and is an exaggeration of normal fluid filtration. Lymphatics become distended and fluid accumulates in the interstitium of lobular septa and around veins and bronchovascular bundles. Radiologically, there is a reticulonodular pattern, more marked at lung bases. Lobular septa become edematous and produce linear shadows ("**Kerley B lines**") on chest radiographs. Edema results in shunting of blood flow from the lung bases to the upper lobes. Airflow resistance increases because of edema in the bronchovascular tree. Patients are often asymptomatic in this early stage.

When the fluid exceeds the capacity of the interstitial space, it accumulates within alveoli as **alveolar edema**. At this stage, a radiologic alveolar pattern is seen, usually worse in central portions of the lung and in lower zones. Dyspnea and coughing become prominent. If edema is severe, the patient expectorates large amounts of frothy pink sputum. Hypoxemia manifests as cyanosis. Bubbly rales are heard. In extreme cases, frothy fluid is coughed up or wells up out of the trachea.

Pulmonary function is restricted in severe congestion and interstitial pulmonary edema because fluid accumulation in interstitial space reduces pulmonary compliance, stiffening the lung. Thus, increased effort is required to maintain ventilation. Thickened alveolar walls impair oxygen and CO_2 exchange, especially decreasing oxygen, particularly the former, resulting in hypoxia with near-normal carbon dioxide levels. Mismatch between ventilation (which is reduced) and perfusion (which persists) causes hypoxemia in patients with pulmonary edema.

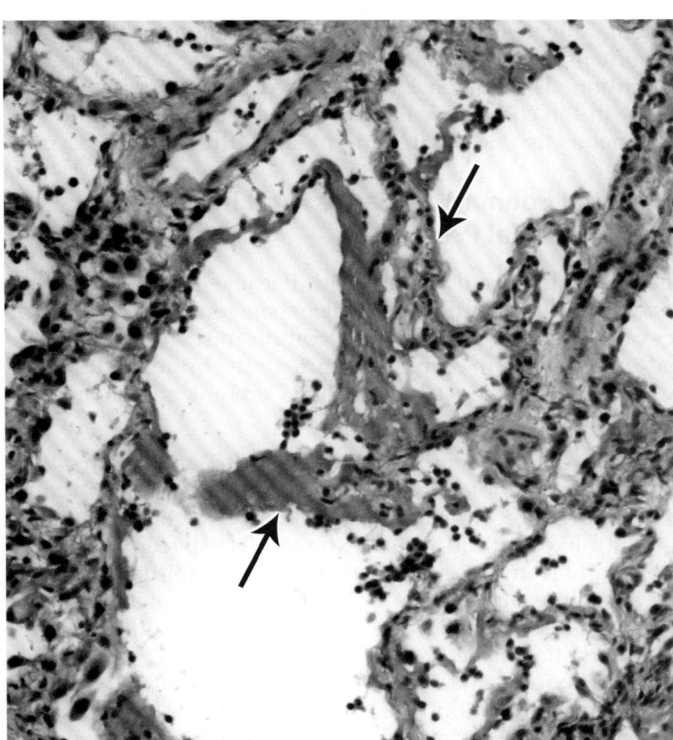

FIGURE 7-37. Pulmonary edema due to diffuse alveolar damage. A section of lung shows hyaline membranes (*arrows*) in alveoli. (Courtesy of UBC Pulmonary Registry, St. Paul's Hospital.)

PATHOLOGY: Edematous lungs are severely congested: their alveolar capillaries and alveoli are filled with a homogeneous, pink-staining fluid permeated by air bubbles (Fig. 7-4). If pulmonary edema is caused by alveolar damage, cell debris, fibrin, and proteins form films of proteinaceous material in the **alveolar—hyaline membranes** (Fig. 7-37).

Edema in Cirrhosis of the Liver Is Commonly an End-Stage Condition

Cirrhosis of the liver is often accompanied by ascites and peripheral edema (**see Chapter 20**). Liver scarring obstructs portal blood flow into the liver, causing portal hypertension and increasing splanchnic circulation hydrostatic pressure. Decreased hepatic synthesis of albumin due to parenchymal injury compounds the problem. Resulting accumulation of peritoneal fluid decreases effective blood volume and leads to renal sodium retention, as in congestive heart failure. Chronic liver disease itself may also cause renal sodium retention. Subsequent expansion of ECF volume accentuates ascites and edema, thus establishing a vicious circle. Increased transudation of lymph from the liver capsule augments abdominal fluid accumulation.

The Nephrotic Syndrome Reflects Massive Proteinuria

In nephrotic syndrome, the magnitude of protein loss in the urine exceeds the rate at which it can be replaced by the liver (**see Chapter 22**). Plasma proteins—especially albumin—decrease, reducing plasma oncotic pressure. This promotes edema, decreases blood volume, stimulates the renin–angiotensin–aldosterone mechanism, and causes sodium retention. The edema is generalized but appears preferentially in soft connective tissues, the eyes, the eyelids, and subcutaneous tissues. Ascites and pleural effusions also occur.

Cerebral Edema May Cause Fatal Increases in Intracranial Pressure

Edema of the brain is dangerous because the rigidity of the cranium allows little room for expansion. Increased intracranial pressure from edema compromises cerebral blood supply, distorts the gross structure of the brain, and impairs CNS function (**see Chapter 32**). Cerebral edema may be vasogenic, cytotoxic, or interstitial.

- **Vasogenic edema** is most common, and occurs with trauma, neoplasms, encephalitis, abscesses, infarcts, hemorrhage, and toxic brain injury (e.g., lead poisoning). Excess fluid in the extracellular space of the brain results from increased vascular permeability, mainly in the white matter. The tight endothelial junctions of the blood–brain barrier are disrupted and fluid enters the interstitial space.
- **Cytotoxic edema** is equivalent to hydropic cell swelling (i.e., accumulation of intracellular water). It is usually a response to cell injury, for example, following ischemia. Cytotoxic cerebral edema preferentially affects the gray matter.
- **Interstitial edema** is a consequence of hydrocephalus, in which fluid accumulates in the cerebral ventricles and periventricular white matter.

Edematous brains are soft and heavy, with flattened gyri and narrowed sulci. Because of altered brain function, patients with cerebral edema suffer vomiting, disorientation, and convulsions. Severe cerebral edema may lead to fatal herniation of the cerebellar tonsils.

Fluid Accumulates in Body Cavities as Extensions of the Interstitial Space

The Pleural Space

Pleural effusion (fluid in the pleural space) is a straw-colored transudate of low specific gravity that contains few cells (mainly exfoliated mesothelial cells). It usually reflects a generalized tendency to form edema, for example, in diseases like nephrotic syndrome, hepatic cirrhosis, and congestive heart failure. Pleural effusion is also a frequent response to an inflammatory process or tumor in the lung or on the pleural surface.

The Pericardium

Fluid may accumulate in the pericardial sac from either hemorrhage (**hemopericardium**) or pericardial injury (**pericardial effusion**). Pericardial effusions occur with infections, metastasis, uremia, and systemic lupus erythematosus. They also occasionally occur after cardiac operations (**postpericardiotomy syndrome**) or radiation therapy.

Pericardial fluid may accumulate rapidly (e.g., with hemorrhage from a ruptured myocardial infarct, dissecting aortic aneurysm, or trauma). In such cases, pericardial cavity pressure rises quickly to exceed the filling pressure of the heart, which is called **tamponade** (Fig. 7-38). The resulting

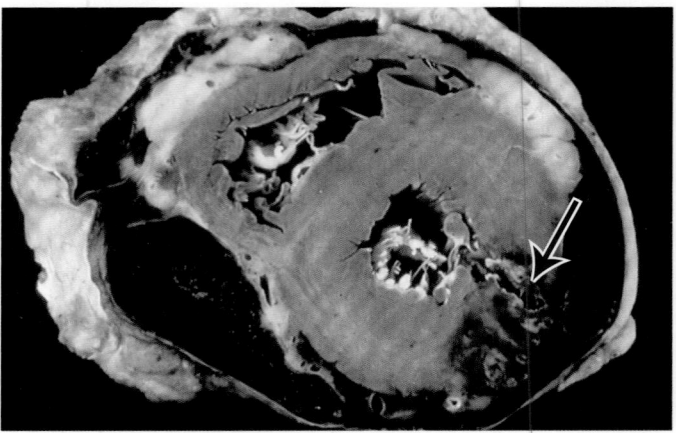

FIGURE 7-38. Cardiac tamponade. A cross section of the heart shows rupture of a myocardial infarct (*arrow*) with the accumulation of a large quantity of blood in the pericardial cavity.

precipitous decline in cardiac output is often fatal. The pericardial sac is fibrous and fairly rigid, but it can adjust if fluid accumulates slowly. Thus, the pericardium can accommodate only 90 to 120 mL if it accumulates rapidly, but a liter or more of fluid if the process is gradual.

Peritoneum

Peritoneal effusion, or **ascites**, is mainly caused by cirrhosis (see above), abdominal tumors, pancreatitis, cardiac failure, nephrotic syndrome, and hepatic vein obstruction (Budd–Chiari syndrome). Obstruction of the thoracic duct by cancer may cause **chylous ascites**, a milky effusion with a high fat content.

Patients with severe ascites may accumulate many liters of fluid and have hugely distended abdomens. Complications of ascites reflect increased abdominal pressure and include anorexia and vomiting, reflux esophagitis, dyspnea, ventral hernia, and leakage of fluid into the pleural space.

FLUID LOSS AND OVERLOAD

Excessive fluid loss (dehydration) and fluid overload are clinical situations that cause hemodynamic disorders; alterations in osmolality and the quantity of fluid in intravascular, interstitial, and cellular spaces may affect perfusion or delivery of substrates, electrolytes, or fluids.

In Dehydration, Available Fluid Is Not Available to Fill the Body's Fluid Compartments

Dehydration results from insufficient fluid intake, excessive fluid loss, or both. Water loss may exceed intake in cases of vomiting, diarrhea, burns, excessive sweating, and diabetes insipidus. When excessive fluid loss occurs, fluid recruited from the interstitial space enters the plasma. Fluids in the cells and within the interstitial and vascular compartments become more concentrated, particularly if there is a preferential loss of water, for example, with inappropriate secretion of antidiuretic hormone in diabetes insipidus. Patients with burns, vomiting, excessive sweating, or diarrhea lose both fluid and electrolytes.

Clinically, only dryness of the skin and mucous membranes is noted initially, but as dehydration progresses, skin turgor is lost. If dehydration persists, **oliguria** (reduced urine output) occurs to compensate for fluid loss. With more severe fluid loss, water shifts from the intracellular space to the extracellular space, leading to severe cell dysfunction, particularly in the brain. Shrinkage of brain tissue may rupture small vessels and cause bleeding. Systemic blood pressure (BP) falls with continuous dehydration, and declining perfusion eventually leads to death.

In Overhydration, Fluid Intake Exceeds Renal Excretory Capacity

If renal function is adequate, overhydration is rare. Fluid overload today occurs mostly with excess iatrogenic intravenous fluid administration. The most serious effect of such fluid overload is induction of cerebral edema or congestive heart failure in patients with cardiac dysfunction.

BLOOD PRESSURE CONTROL

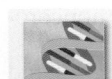 **MOLECULAR PATHOGENESIS:** Data from twin and family studies indicate that genetics accounts for some 30% of blood pressure (BP) regulation. This finding may also account for the huge variation in patients' responses to BP-lowering medication. Human genetic linkage and whole genome association studies have identified diverse mutations in key BP regulators. Prominent are genes of the renin–angiotensin system, which regulates vasoconstriction and sodium and water balance. SNPs in genes encoding angiotensin, angiotensin-converting enzyme (ACE), angiotensin II receptor, renin and renin-binding protein are associated with altered BP control. Hypertension has been associated with SNPs in the vasoconstrictor endothelin and its receptor, the vasodilator nitric oxide synthase, and endothelial sodium channel subunits. Polymorphisms of β-adrenergic receptors 1 and 2 have been associated with hypertension and altered response to β-agonists.

Shock

Shock is a profound hemodynamic and metabolic disturbance in which the circulatory system fails to supply the microcirculation adequately, with consequent inadequate perfusion of vital organs. In this often catastrophic circumstance, tissue perfusion, oxygen delivery, and metabolic waste removal do not meet tissue demands. **Shock** encompasses all the reactions that occur in response to such disturbances. In uncompensated shock, rapid circulatory collapse leads to impaired cellular metabolism and death. However, in many cases, compensatory mechanisms sustain the patient, at least for a while. When these adaptations fail, shock becomes irreversible. Shock is a major cause of morbidity and mortality in intensive care units, and despite endeavors to suppress portions of the immune response, the outcome of shock has been unchanged in the past 50 years.

Shock is not synonymous with low BP, although hypotension is often part of shock syndrome. *Hypotension is actually a late sign in shock and indicates failure of compensation.* At

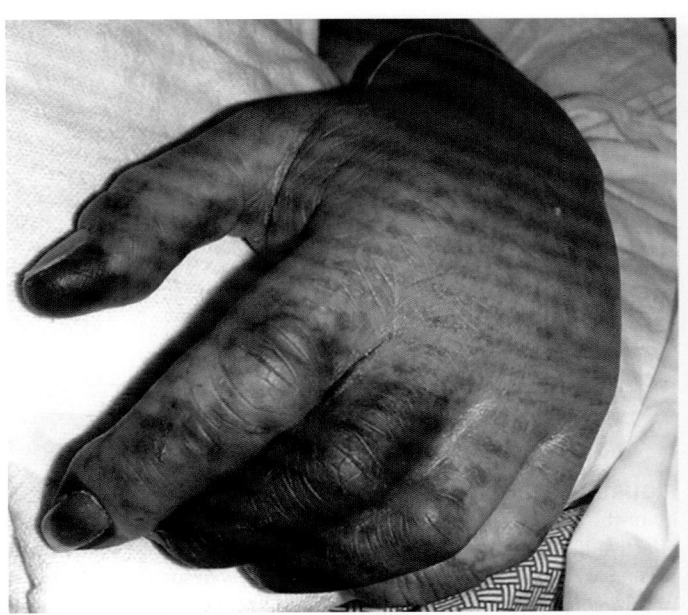

FIGURE 7-39. Ischemic and necrotic hand in a critically ill patient with shock and high-dose vasopressor use. Ischemic limb necrosis is symmetric with involvement of all fingers bilaterally. (Courtesy of Dr. Paul Haser, University Hospital Centre in Moncton, Department of Surgery.)

the same time that peripheral blood flow falls below critical levels, extreme vasoconstriction can maintain arterial BP. The distinction between shock and hypotension is important clinically because rapid restoration of systemic blood flow is the primary goal in treating shock. When BP alone is raised with vasopressive drugs, systemic blood flow may actually be dramatically diminished, particularly to the peripheries (Fig. 7-39).

 PATHOPHYSIOLOGY: Decreased perfusion in shock most often results from decreased cardiac output, reflecting: (1) either the heart's inability to pump normal venous return (**cardiogenic shock**) or (2) decreased venous return due to decreased effective blood volume (**hypovolemic shock**). Systemic vasodilation, with or without increased vascular permeability, causes the other broad category of shock: **distributive shock**, which has several key subcategories: **septic shock, anaphylactic shock,** and **neurogenic shock** (Fig. 7-40).

- **Cardiogenic shock** is caused by myocardial pump failure, most often after massive myocardial infarction. Disorders that prevent left or right heart filling reduce cardiac output, resulting in "obstructive" shock. Such conditions include PE and cardiac tamponade (Fig. 7-38).
- **Hypovolemic shock** occurs when loss of fluid causes pronounced decreases in blood or plasma volume. Hemorrhage, fluid loss from severe burns, diarrhea, excessive diuresis, perspiration, and trauma all lose fluid, and can trigger hypovolemic shock. Burns or trauma directly damage the microcirculation, increasing vascular permeability.
- **Septic shock** is caused by severe systemic microbial infections. The pathogenesis of septic shock is complex (**see Chapter 12** and below).

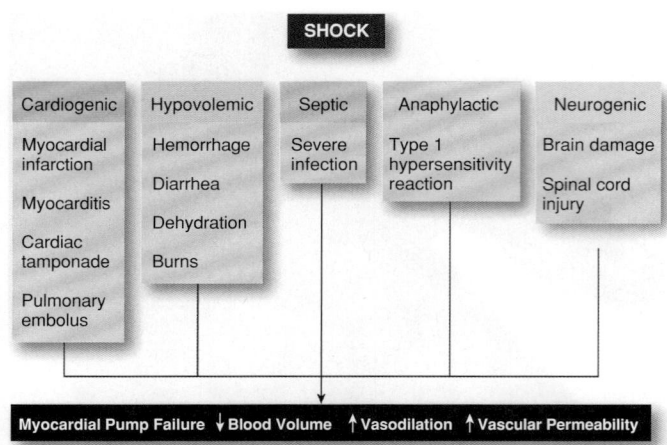

FIGURE 7-40. Classification of shock. Shock results from (1) an inability of the heart to pump adequately (cardiogenic shock), (2) decreased effective blood volume as a consequence of severely reduced blood or plasma volume (hypovolemic shock), or (3) widespread vasodilation (septic, anaphylactic, or neurogenic shock). Increased vascular permeability may complicate vasodilation by contributing to reduced effective blood volume.

■ **Anaphylactic shock** may follow systemic type I hypersensitivity reactions, with widespread vasodilation and increased vascular permeability.

■ **Neurogenic shock** can follow acute brain or spinal cord injury, which impairs neural control of vasomotor tone and causes generalized vasodilation.

In both anaphylactic and neurogenic shock, redistribution of blood to the periphery, with or without increased vascular permeability, reduces the effective circulating blood and plasma volume. This ultimately leads to the same consequences as in hypovolemic shock.

In hypovolemic and cardiogenic shock, lower cardiac output and resultant decreased tissue perfusion are key steps in the progression from reversible to irreversible shock. Cellular hypoxia often follows initial decreases in tissue perfusion. Such changes do not cause irreversible injury at first, but they trigger a vicious circle of decreased tissue perfusion and more cell injury via:

■ Endothelial injury: hypoxia from poorer tissue perfusion and increased vascular permeability allow fluid to exit the vascular compartment.

■ Increased exudation of fluid from the circulation reduces (a) blood volume, (b) venous return, and (c) cardiac output, thus aggravating hypoxic cell injury.

■ Decreased renal and skeletal muscle perfusion causes metabolic acidosis, which in turn further decreases cardiac output and tissue perfusion.

■ Diminished perfusion of the heart injures myocardial cells and impairs their ability to pump blood, further reducing cardiac output and tissue perfusion.

Septic Shock Is a Severe, Dysregulated Response to Infection

It is an endpoint of a spectrum that includes *systemic inflammatory response syndrome (SIRS)*, circulatory collapse, and functional impairment of multiple organ systems (see below). SIRS is a hypermetabolic state defined by two or more signs of systemic inflammation: fever, tachycardia, tachypnea, leukocytosis or leukopenia, in the setting of a known cause of inflammation. **Septic shock** is defined as clinical SIRS so severe that it causes organ dysfunction and hypotension. The pathophysiology of septic shock is addressed in Chapter 12.

Septicemia with gram-negative organisms is the most common cause of septic shock, followed by gram-positive and fungal infections. The most common primary sources of infection are pulmonary, abdominal, and urinary.

Multiple Organ Dysfunction May Be an End Result of Shock

Improved early treatment of shock and sepsis has allowed patients to survive long enough to manifest a new problem, progressive deterioration of organ function. Almost all septic shock patients suffer from dysfunction of at least one organ. However, multiple organ dysfunction occurs in one-third of patients with septic shock, trauma or burns, and a quarter of those with acute pancreatitis. Whatever the trigger, the mortality of multiple organ dysfunction in the context of shock exceeds 50%; it is responsible for most deaths in noncoronary intensive care units in the United States.

The acute response to sepsis entails poorly regulated inflammatory and immune mechanisms which differ greatly from individual to individual. The net result is shutdown of noncritical systems and an overall catabolic state. Proinflammatory mediators may predominate in SIRS, but counterinflammatory factors are important in some patients. It is now thought that following bacterial infection, the initial inflammation and septic shock characteristic of SIRS may follow a stage of anergy and immune repression.

Vascular Compensatory Mechanisms

Changes in the macrovascular and microvascular circulation are at least partly responsible for variable organ injury in SIRS. Compensatory mechanisms in shock shift blood flow away from the periphery, so as to maintain flow to the heart and the brain. These responses involve sympathetic nervous release of endogenous vasoconstrictors and hormones, and local vasoregulation. These lead to increased cardiac output by increasing heart rate and myocardial contractility while constricting arteries and arterioles.

■ **Increased sympathetic discharge** augments catecholamine release by the adrenal medulla. Skeletal muscle, splanchnic bed and skin arterioles respond to increased sympathetic discharge; cardiac and cerebral arterioles are less reactive. Thus, increased sympathetic tone redirects blood flow from the periphery to the heart and brain. The marked arteriolar vasoconstriction reduces capillary hydrostatic pressure and decreases interstitial fluid. This facilitates an osmotic fluid shift from the interstitium into the vascular system. This sympathetic–adrenal response can completely compensate for blood loss of 10% of intravascular volume. With a greater volume deficit, cardiac output and BP are affected and blood flow to tissues is reduced.

■ **The renin–angiotensin–aldosterone system** stimulates sodium and water reabsorption, thus helping to maintain intravascular volume. Pituitary antidiuretic hormone secretion similarly increases renal water retention.

- **Vascular autoregulation** responds to hypoxia and acidosis by preserving regional blood flow to vital organs, particularly the heart and brain, by vasodilation in coronary and cerebral circulations. Vasoconstriction mediated largely by α-adrenergic receptors in mesenteric venules and veins helps maintain cardiac filling and arterial pressure. Circulation to organs such as skin and skeletal muscle, which are less sensitive to hypoxia, is not so tightly autoregulated.

Genetic Polymorphisms in Toll-Like Receptors and Tumor Necrosis Factor Participate in the Pathogenesis of Septic Shock

MOLECULAR PATHOGENESIS: Epidemiologic studies have shown that death from infection correlates more strongly with genetic background than do cardiovascular disease or cancer. Gene mutations in several cytokines, cell surface receptors, and other circulating markers have been associated with susceptibility to sepsis. Toll-like receptor (TLR) pattern recognition receptors (PRRs) recognize pathogen-associated microbial patterns (PAMPs, **see Chapters 2 and 12**) and so are critical in triggering innate immune responses. TLR4 is critical for recognizing gram-negative bacterial lipopolysaccharides. A mutation of TLR4 (aspartic acid to glycine at amino acid 299) has been linked to development of septic shock in a number of studies. TLR4 also participates in exacerbating endotoxin responses, and in sepsis, polymorphisms in TLRs and other PRRs may help explain why patients respond so differently to a given infective agent.

PATHOLOGY: Shock is associated with specific changes in a number of organs (Fig. 7-41), including acute renal tubular necrosis, ARDS, liver failure, depression of host defense mechanisms, and heart failure. Interestingly, paracrine cross talk from molecules in one injured organ, such as proinflammatory mediators from the lung, can affect distant organ injury.

Heart

Cardiac systolic and diastolic dysfunction occurs during septic shock, probably secondary to paracrine injury and possibly hypoperfusion. The heart shows petechial hemorrhages of the epicardium and endocardium. Necrotic foci in the myocardium vary from loss of single fibers to large areas of necrosis. Prominent contraction bands are visible by light or electron microscopy. Flattened areas of the intercalated disk indicate cell swelling, and invagination of adjacent cells is thought to be a catecholamine-induced lesion.

Kidney

Acute tubular necrosis (ATN, acute renal failure), a major complication of shock, has three phases: (1) **initiation**, from the onset of injury to the beginning of renal failure; (2) **maintenance**, from the start of renal failure to a stable, reduced renal function; and (3) **recovery**. In those who survive an episode of shock, recovery phase begins about 10 days after its onset and may last up to 8 weeks.

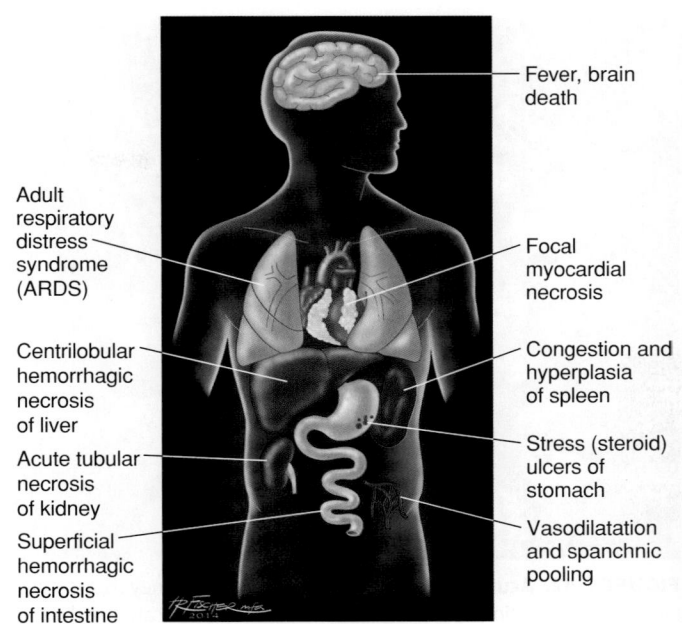

FIGURE 7-41. Complications of shock.

Renal blood flow is limited to 1/3 of normal after the acute ischemic phase, and is even more restricted in the outer cortex. Arteriolar constriction reduces filtration pressure, thus lowering the amount of filtrate and contributing to oliguria. Interstitial edema occurs, possibly through a process called **backflow**. Excessive vasoconstriction is also related to stimulation of the renin–angiotensin system.

PATHOLOGY: In acute renal failure, the kidney is large, swollen, and congested, although the cortex may be pale. A cross section reveals blood pooling in the outer stripe of the medulla. Microscopically, fully developed acute tubular necrosis is evidenced by dilation of the proximal tubules and focal necrosis of cells (Fig. 7-42). Often, pigmented casts in tubular lumina indicate leakage of hemoglobin or myoglobin. Coarse "ropy" casts are seen in the distal nephron and distal convoluted tubules. Interstitial edema is prominent in the cortex, and mononuclear cells accumulate within tubules and surrounding interstitium (**see Chapter 22**).

Lung

Once severe (prolonged shock takes hold), injury to alveolar walls can lead to **shock lung**, which is a cause of ARDS (**see Chapter 18**). The sequence of changes is mediated by neutrophils, and includes interstitial edema, necrosis of endothelial and alveolar epithelial cells, and formation of intravascular microthrombi and hyaline membranes lining the alveolar surface.

PATHOLOGY: In ARDS, the lungs are firm and congested, and a frothy fluid often exudes from the cut surface. Interstitial edema starts around peribronchial connective tissue and lymphatics, then fills the interstitial connective tissue. At first, a large fluid volume drains into pulmonary lymphatics. If removal of this

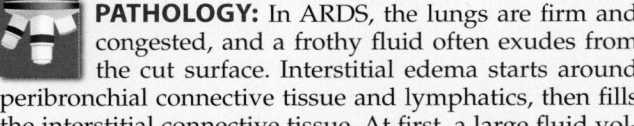

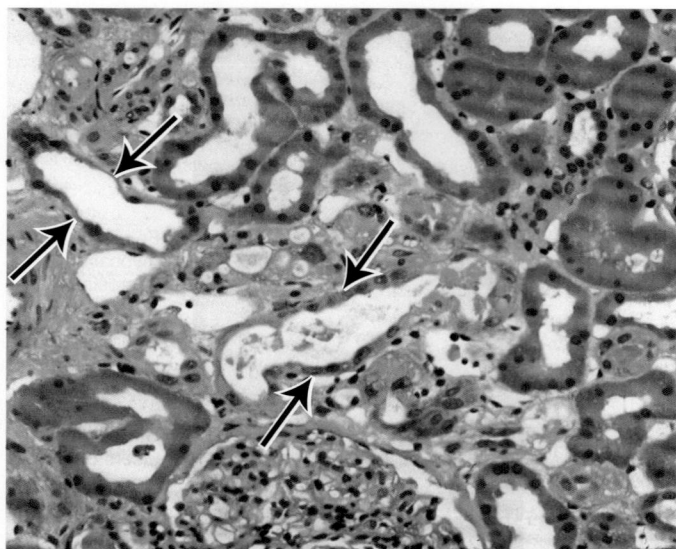

FIGURE 7-42. Acute tubular necrosis. A section of kidney shows swelling and degeneration of tubular epithelium. *Arrows* indicate the thinned and damaged epithelium. (Courtesy of Dr. Alex Magil, Department of Pathology, St. Paul's Hospital.)

fluid becomes inadequate, or if the balance of forces that keep the fluid in the interstitial space is disturbed, alveolar edema develops.

Shock-induced lung injury leads to alveolar hyaline membranes (Fig. 7-37), which also frequently line alveolar ducts and terminal bronchioles. These changes may heal entirely, but in half of patients, repair causes alveolar wall thickening. Type II pneumocytes proliferate and line alveoli, replacing damaged type I pneumocytes. Fibrous tissue proliferates as the alveolar exudate organizes. These chronic changes may result in persistent respiratory distress and even death. Shock lung and ARDS are more fully discussed in Chapter 18.

Gastrointestinal Tract

Shock often results in diffuse gastrointestinal hemorrhage. Gastric mucosal erosions and superficial ischemic necrosis in the intestines are the usual sources of this bleeding. Interruption of the barrier function of the intestine may result in septicemia. More severe necrotizing lesions contribute to deterioration in the final phase of shock.

Liver

In patients who die in shock, the liver is enlarged and has a mottled cut surface that reflects marked centrilobular pooling of blood. The most prominent histologic lesion is centrilobular congestion and necrosis. The reason centrilobular hepatocytes show increased sensitivity to shock is not completely clear, and may not simply be

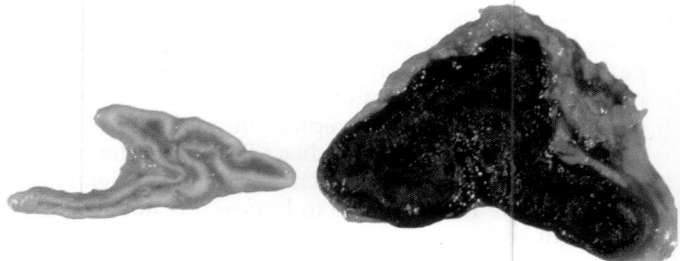

FIGURE 7-43. Waterhouse–Friderichsen syndrome. A normal adrenal gland (*left*) in contrast to an adrenal gland enlarged by extensive hemorrhage (*right*), obtained from a patient who died of meningococcemic shock.

their greater distance from the portal tract blood supply (**see Chapter 20**).

Pancreas

The splanchnic vascular bed, which supplies the pancreas, is particularly affected by impaired circulation during shock. Resulting ischemic damage to the exocrine pancreas unleashes activated catalytic enzymes and causes acute pancreatitis, a complication that further promotes shock.

Brain

Although septic patients often develop clinical encephalopathy, brain lesions are rare in SIRS and shock. There may be microscopic hemorrhages, but patients who recover do not ordinarily have neurologic deficits. In severe cases, particularly in people with cerebral atherosclerosis, hemorrhage and necrosis may appear in the region between the terminal distributions of major arteries, the so-called **watershed infarcts** (**see Chapter 32**).

Adrenals

In severe shock, adrenal glands exhibit conspicuous hemorrhage in the inner cortex. Although the hemorrhage is often focal, it can be massive and may be accompanied by hemorrhagic necrosis of the entire gland, as seen in the **Waterhouse–Friderichsen syndrome** (Fig. 7-43), typically associated with overwhelming meningococcal septicemia (**see Chapter 27**).

Host Defenses

Changes in immune function and host defenses in shock are not well understood, but patients who survive the acute phase of shock don't infrequently succumb to subsequent overwhelming infection. Several factors may well interact, namely, ischemic colitis, tissue trauma, and immune and metabolic suppression of host defenses. Humoral immunity and phagocytic activity by leukocytes and macrophages are both depressed, but the mechanisms underlying these effects are not clear.

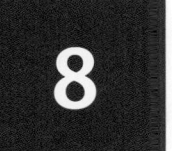

8 Environmental and Nutritional Pathology

David S. Strayer, Emanuel Rubin

Environmental pathology is the study of human diseases caused by harmful environmental exposures, impairing human physiology and causing deficiencies of vital substances. Such exposures may reflect constituents of the external environment (e.g., air pollution, ultraviolet [UV] irradiation), foreign materials an individual consumes—by ingestion, smoking, or other routes—or occupational hazards. Heightened awareness of the impact of accelerating climate change, pollution, and iatrogenic and other medications on human health and safety makes this topic particularly pressing.

Environmental and Occupational Exposures

POLLUTION

Awareness of potential hazards posed by harmful chemicals in the environment is not new. In the 12th century, Maimonides wrote:

Comparing the air of cities to the air of deserts is like comparing waters that are befouled and turbid to waters that are fine and pure. In the city, because of the height of its buildings, the narrowness of its streets and all that pours forth from its inhabitants, the air becomes stagnant, turbid, thick, misty and foggy.... Wherever the air is altered...men develop dullness of understanding, failure of intelligence and defects of memory.

Worldwide, 8.5 to 9 million premature deaths—about one-sixth of all deaths—result from pollution. This total far exceeds that attributable to the second most important risk factor, which is tobacco smoking (see below). Air, water, soil, occupational, and heavy metal pollution sources all contribute. Air pollution is inextricably intertwined with climate change. Thus, the combination of biomass burning and fossil fuel combustion generates about 85% of airborne particulates and contributes substantially to climate change–related gases. Climate change (see below) also magnifies the harmful impact of air pollution.

TABLE 8-1

INCREASED MORBIDITY AND MORTALITY AS A FUNCTION OF PARTICULATE AIR POLLUTION (RESULTS OF REPRESENTATIVE STUDIES)

Type of Exposure	Health Consequence	Relative Increase in Incidence of Death and Disease (%)
Acute	Cardiovascular death	0.68[a]
	Ischemic cardiac disease	0.7[a]
	Heart failure	0.8[a]
	Acute attacks of asthma (children)	1.2[a]
	Acute attacks of asthma (adults)	1.1[a]
	Total lung (including asthma and COPD)	0.9[a]
	Acute myocardial infarction	4.5[b]
	Acute myocardial infarction	48[c]
Chronic	Cardiovascular death	12–76[d]
	Atherosclerosis	4[d]
	Venous thromboembolism	70[e]

COPD = chronic obstructive pulmonary disease.
[a]Per every 10 μg/m³ increase in PM_{10}, 1 day before the event.
[b]Per every 10 μg/m³ increase in $PM_{2.5}$ acutely.
[c]Per every 25 μg/m³ increase in $PM_{2.5}$ acutely.
[d]Per every 10 μg/m³ increase in $PM_{2.5}$.
[e]Per every 10 μg/m³ increase in PM_{10}.

No country, age group, or geographic region is immune to pollution-related mortality, but poorer countries, the elderly, and infants bear the greatest burden.

Air Pollution Is the Major Cause of Pollution-Related Deaths

Harmful chemicals are ubiquitous in the air and have considerable potential for causing disease, depending on the agent in question and type and chronicity of exposure. Table 8-1 lists examples of the health consequences of airborne pollutants.

The World Health Organization (WHO) finds that air pollution is responsible for 6.5 million lives lost worldwide annually.[1] The most important air pollutants are those that are generated by combustion of fossil fuels, industrial and agricultural processes, and so forth. The principal contributors to human disease among these are particulates, especially carbon particles. In addition, noxious and irritant gases **sulfur dioxide** (SO_2), **oxides of nitrogen**, carbon monoxide (CO), and **ozone** are important constituents of polluted air.

[1]Estimated 4.3 million deaths from household air pollution and 3.7 million deaths from ambient air pollution for 2012. These deaths include acute lower respiratory disease, chronic obstructive lung disease, ischemic heart disease, stroke, and lung cancer, according to the WHO, March 24, 2014.

Carbon Particulates

Carbon **particulates** in urban air and certain industrial settings are responsible for considerable human morbidity and mortality. Although the composition and sources of particulate matter vary widely, exhaust from diesel fuel combustion is the single largest source of carbon particles in urban air.

Particulates vary in size, composition, and origin. They fall into three categories, according to their aerodynamic diameter (AD): those between 2.5 and 10 μm (PM_{10}) are coarse particulates; those under 2.5 μm in AD are fine, designated $PM_{2.5}$; and the smallest, ultrafine particles ($PM_{0.1}$) are under 0.1 μm (or 100 nm).

The ability of PM to cause disease (see below) is a function of the toxic and carcinogenic combustion products they carry. Although polycyclic aromatics (PAHs) were once thought to be the most potent of these, it is now clear that nitrated compounds (nitroarenes) are even more dangerous. When these chemicals, bound to carbon particles, are breathed in, their disposition is a function of where the particles localize. Carbon particles have different abilities to deliver these toxic chemicals and have different pathogenetic properties based on their size (Fig. 8-1). PM_{10} particles mostly settle in the conducting airways of the tracheobronchial tree. Fine particles ($PM_{2.5}$) penetrate more deeply into the lungs because of their smaller size. These find their way to small terminal airways and alveoli. Ultrafine particles ($PM_{0.1}$, <100 nm) penetrate

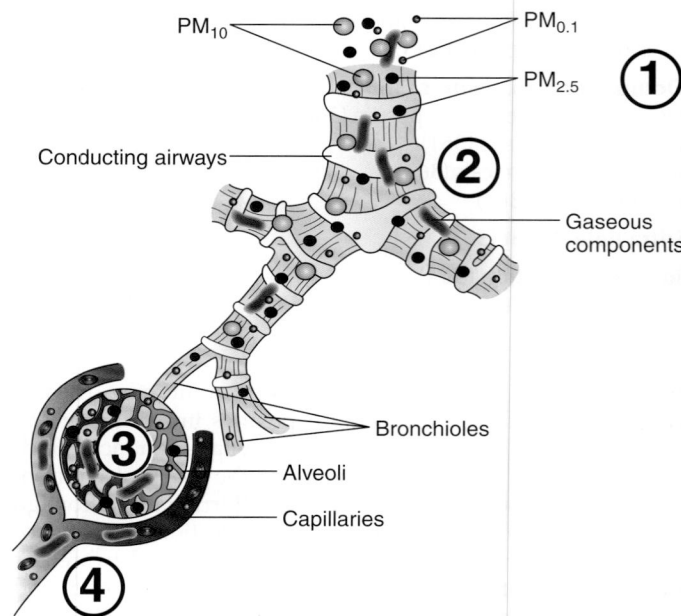

FIGURE 8-1. Fate of inspired pollutant particles. 1. Urban and industrial atmospheric pollution includes gases and particulate carbon (PM) of various sizes. PM_{10} species (coarse particles) have aerodynamic diameter (AD) between 2.5 and 10 μm. $PM_{2.5}$ (fine particles) have AD less than 2.5 μm, and ultrafine particles ($PM_{0.1}$) have AD less than 0.1 μm. **2.** PM_{10} particles are largely trapped by mucus and cilia in conducting airways. Smaller particles and gases pass through these airways. **3.** $PM_{2.5}$ particles deposit in terminal conducting airways and alveoli, where they are commonly engulfed by macrophages and elicit inflammatory responses. **4.** Ultrafine particles ($PM_{0.1}$) and gases may pass through alveolar walls to enter the capillary circulation and then disseminate throughout the body. $PM_{0.1}$ particles may also deposit in alveolar walls.

very deeply. They have a high surface area to mass ratio (which allows for greater potential delivery of noxious components). These can traverse alveolar walls, pass through alveolar capillaries, enter the bloodstream, and disseminate throughout the body (Fig. 8-1).

Fine Particulates

Among these, the consequences of exposure to fine particulates (PM$_{2.5}$) are best documented. They are strongly linked to pulmonary and cardiac diseases, as well as such systemic cardiovascular conditions as stroke. The former include obstructive lung diseases and lung cancer. Among the latter are overall cardiac mortality as well as ischemic cardiac diseases, hypertension, heart failure, and disturbances of rhythm. Mechanisms related to PM$_{2.5}$ and other particles are discussed below. Other, less well-established, associations have also been identified in some studies, relating to diabetes, neurologic and neurodegenerative diseases, poorer outcomes of pregnancy, and others.

Duration of Exposure

Many epidemiologic studies establish that both short-term and extended exposures to particulate air pollutants are associated with morbidity and increased mortality. The latter is evident as both increased overall death rates and more deaths from cardiovascular diseases and cancer. Short- and long-term studies document excess mortality and dose–response relationships between particulate concentrations and sizes on the one hand and both disease and death from cerebrovascular, peripheral vascular, cardiopulmonary, and neoplastic causes on the other.

Short-term exposure to particulates. Studies of short-term human exposure examine transient spikes in ambient air pollution occur and, together with particle sizes, are correlated with morbidities and mortality. In such analyses, particulate concentrations correlate with disease and death that involve cardiac, vascular, thrombotic, and short-term autonomic nervous system abnormalities (Fig. 8-2). Daily death rates increase between 0.2% and 0.6% per 10-μg/m^3 elevation in PM$_{10}$. Outcomes include acute myocardial

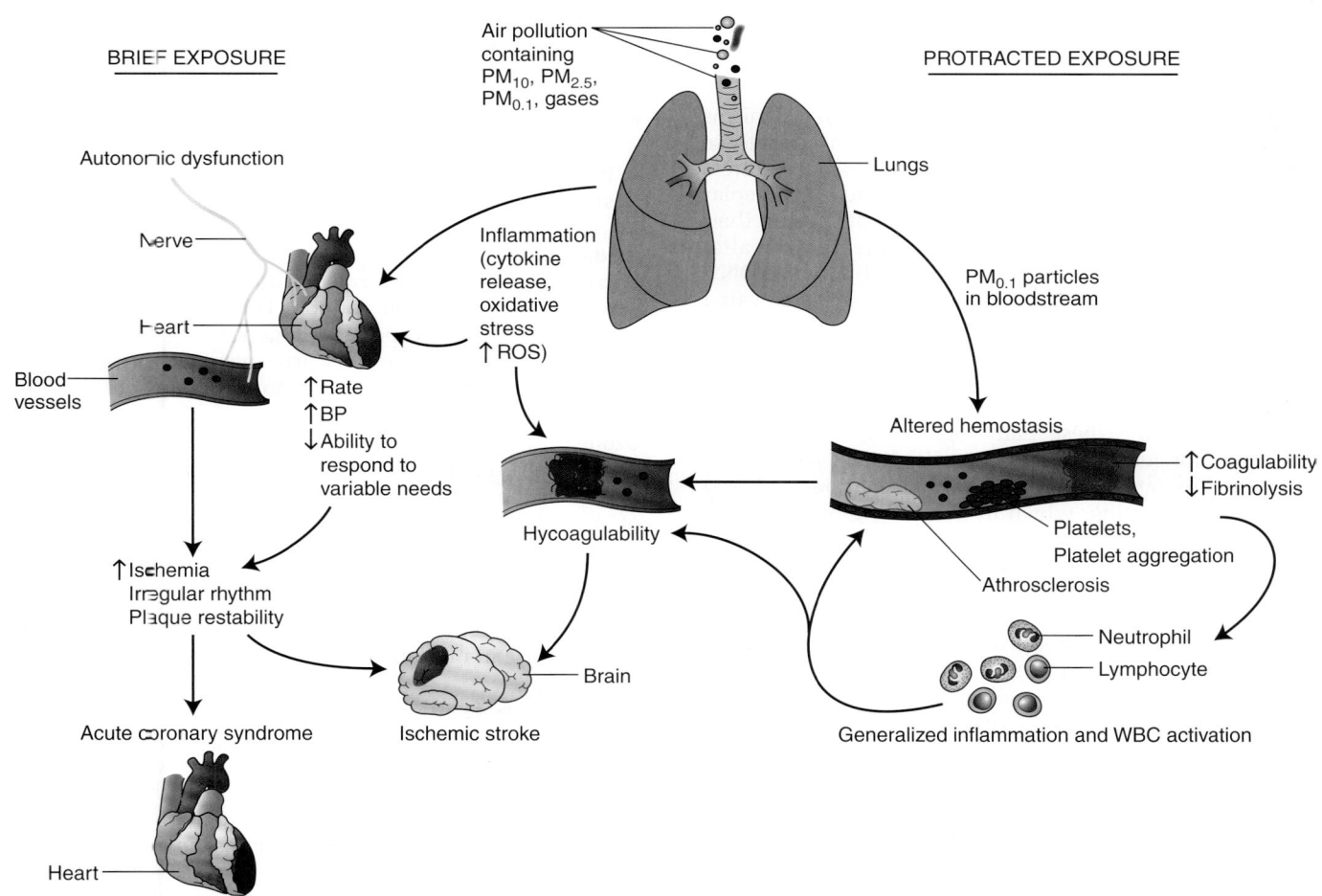

FIGURE 8-2. Pathophysiology relating to cardiovascular and thrombotic consequences of particulate air pollution. These are divided into the consequences of short-term exposure and more extended exposure to particulate air pollution. Carbon particles, especially fine and ultrafine particles, carry toxic and oxidant chemical products of combustion to the distal lungs and the circulation (hence to blood vessels and the entire body). These affect autonomic responses, elicit inflammation, and alter the balance of thrombotic and thrombolytic activities and thus impair hemostasis. The likely pathophysiologic mechanisms mediating the consequences of these derangements after both immediate exposure and protracted exposure are indicated. BP = blood pressure; ROS = reactive oxygen species.

infarction, thromboembolism, ischemic stroke, arrhythmias, and other related cardiac and vascular diseases.

In addition, short-term exposure to particulates has a strong impact on respiratory illnesses. Documented associations include acute exacerbations of preexisting asthma in children and adults, as well as increased hospital admissions for people who have chronic obstructive pulmonary disease (COPD; **see Chapter 18**). Particulates measured in these studies were principally PM_{10} and $PM_{2.5}$.

Extended exposure to particulates. Longer-term studies document associations between PM_{10} and $PM_{2.5}$ levels and lung cancer and more protracted indices of cardiovascular disease. For example, a large study conducted under the auspices of the American Cancer Society showed an average 13% increased risk of lung cancer for each $10\text{-}\mu g/m^3$ increase in $PM_{2.5}$. Increased levels of larger particulates also correlated with higher rates of lung cancer. Other cancers, including bladder tumors and lymphomas, have been linked as well to occupational exposure to diesel fumes.

In addition to neoplastic diseases, long-term studies of the toxicity of particulate pollution have shown accelerated atherogenesis (see above). These nonrespiratory consequences of particulates are documented for $PM_{2.5}$ and also reflect the ability of ultrafine particles to enter the systemic blood circulation (see below).

PATHOPHYSIOLOGY: The principal mechanisms by which carbon particulate pollution exerts these effects relate to inflammation and oxidative stress (Fig. 8-2). Carbon particles are phagocytosed by alveolar macrophages and endothelial cells, thus delivering their toxic and irritating cargoes into cells where they can alter intracellular oxidant concentrations and modify DNA structure. Generalized inflammatory activity is elevated because of delivery of oxidant chemicals, particularly by $PM_{0.1}$ particles.

Lung-related oxidant stress is a product of chemicals bound to larger particles ($PM_{2.5}$, PM_{10}). Postulated mechanisms mediating these pathologies triggered by both short- and longer-term exposures to high levels of particulates are illustrated in Figure 8-2. Inflammation-mediated activation of clotting, which in this setting often accompanies inhibition of fibrinolysis, plays a large role in these phenomena. For example, reactive oxygen species (ROS) facilitate platelet aggregation and fibrin formation at nearby atherosclerotic plaques. Resultant inflammatory cell infiltration can destabilize such plaques and lead to acute cardiac events (ACEs).

In utero exposure affects developing infants. Intrauterine growth retardation (IUGR) is more common if mothers are exposed to high levels of particulates (PM_{10}, $PM_{2.5}$). Also, PAH–DNA adducts are increased in babies born after such exposures, more in newborns who were exposed in utero than in their mothers. Gestating human embryos thus may be more susceptible to chemical DNA alterations than are adults.

MOLECULAR PATHOGENESIS: Genetic polymorphisms—particularly for genes encoding antioxidant enzymes—probably affect susceptibility to, and development of, diseases related to air pollution. A cohort of asthmatic children in Mexico City, whose disease exacerbations correlated with levels of fine particulates, was found to have mutations in glutathione *S*-transferase (GST), an enzyme that metabolizes a variety of toxins and that can detoxify ROS. Treating these children with antioxidant vitamins C and E led to clinical improvement. Patients with mutations in *GSTP1* and *GSTM1* genes have much higher levels of IgE, and they release more histamine in response to allergen challenge during exposure to diesel exhaust.

Mutant forms of other antioxidant enzymes render people increasingly susceptible to airway disease caused by airborne particulates. Among these enzymes is heme oxygenase-1 (*HMOX1*) and NAD(P)H:quinone oxidoreductase (*NQO1*). Polymorphisms in inflammation-related genes *TLR2* and *TLR4*, encoding toll-like receptors (**see Chapters 2** and **4**), may also affect the pathogenicity of carbon particulates.

Gases Associated With Air Pollution

Sulfur Dioxide

Sulfur dioxide **(SO_2)** is highly irritative and may be oxidized to sulfuric acid. SO_2 is mainly derived from burning fossil fuels. Acute exposure causes bronchoconstriction and respiratory tract inflammation. Chronic experimental exposure to high SO_2 levels may cause a chronic bronchitis–like syndrome, but it is not clear that there are significant sequelae of human exposure to concentrations of SO_2 normally found in smog.

Oxides of Nitrogen

Nitrogen oxides are generally written NO_x because they are mixtures of several compounds. They, as well, come from burning fossil fuels, especially in generating electricity. NO_x are oxidants and respiratory irritants that induce airway hyperreactivity upon acute exposure.

Ozone

Tropospheric **ozone** (i.e., ozone near the ground as opposed to that in the upper atmosphere) largely reflects the action of sunlight on NO_2, especially on warm, sunny days. It is a strong oxidant that causes respiratory (cough, dyspnea) and nonrespiratory (nausea, headache) symptoms on acute exposure. Chronic exposure to ozone in smog may lead to deterioration in pulmonary function and a slight but significant increase in mortality.

Carbon Monoxide

CO is an odorless and nonirritating gas that results from incomplete combustion of organic substances. Its affinity for hemoglobin is 240 times greater than that of oxygen. CO thus binds preferentially to hemoglobin to form carboxyhemoglobin. It also increases the affinity of remaining heme moieties for oxygen so that oxygen does not dissociate from such hemoglobin in the tissues as readily as it should. This further impairs oxygen delivery to tissues. As a result, hypoxia in CO poisoning exceeds what can be attributed to loss of oxygen-carrying capacity alone.

Atmospheric CO mainly comes from automobile exhaust and does not pose a health problem. Carboxyhemoglobin concentrations under 10% are common in smokers and ordinarily do not produce symptoms. Indoor combustion, however, especially from space heaters, can generate much higher CO concentrations, which can be hazardous. Concentrations up to 30% cause headache and mild exertional dyspnea. Higher levels of carboxyhemoglobin lead to confusion and lethargy. Above 50%, coma and convulsions ensue. Levels greater than 60% are usually lethal. In fatal CO poisoning, carboxyhemoglobin in superficial capillaries gives the skin a characteristic cherry-red color. People who survive severe CO poisoning may have residual brain damage, including subtle intellectual deficits, memory loss, or extrapyramidal symptoms (e.g., parkinsonism). Treatment of acute CO poisoning, as in people who attempt suicide or are trapped in fires, is inhaling 100% oxygen.

Harmful effects of long-term exposure to low levels of CO have been difficult to substantiate. However, in patients with ischemic heart disease, concentrations of carboxyhemoglobin below 5% to 8% (often seen in smokers) may predispose to exertional angina and cause changes in electrocardiograms.

Environmental Tobacco Smoke Is Harmful to Nonsmokers

Involuntary exposure to tobacco smoke in the environment—which is variably called secondhand or sidestream smoke, passive smoking, or environmental tobacco smoke (ETS)—is a risk factor for some diseases in nonsmokers (Table 8-2). *Nonsmoking spouses of smokers have approximately a 20% to 30% increased risk of lung cancer.* The WHO and the U.S. Environmental Protection Agency (EPA) classify ETS as a carcinogen and recognize that it is responsible for some lung cancers occurring in nonsmokers. Data also suggest that ETS is associated with an increased risk of breast cancer in premenopausal women who do not smoke. There are other associations between ETS and human tumors—of the upper respiratory tract and elsewhere—but these connections are more tentative.

Cardiovascular and metabolic consequences of ETS exposure are legion. Healthy nonsmoking adults exposed to ETS develop abnormalities in low-density lipoprotein cholesterol (LDL-C) and lipid peroxidation and their macrophages accumulate excess LDL-C. There are also reports linking ETS and elevated blood pressure.

The range of diseases significantly associated with ETS has been studied in many prospective and retrospective reports, and underlying pathophysiology has been investigated and continues to be examined. These are illustrated in Figure 8-3.

Effects of ETS on Children

Four of 10 American children of school age (about 24 million children), and one-third of adolescents, are subject to ETS, in large part because their parents smoke. The consequences of this exposure are considerable and include accelerated development of atherosclerosis, as well as its circulatory consequences. Children subject to ETS also tend to develop other cardiovascular risk factors, which include insulin resistance, abnormal autonomic cardiovascular function, obesity, and dyslipidemias more often than nonexposed children.

Children born of cigarette-smoking mothers have been reported to be more susceptible to several respiratory diseases, including respiratory infections and otitis media. Infants whose parents smoke develop respiratory illnesses more often than other children and are hospitalized more often. Several studies have reported reduced indices of pulmonary function among children of smokers and exacerbation of preexisting asthma. ETS is associated with an increased risk for sudden infant death syndrome (SIDS) as well (see below).

Cardiovascular Effects of ETS on Children

The impact of childhood ETS on the vascular system varies with the child's age and the dose and duration exposure. Children experience disordered circulation. Flow-mediated changes in vascular tone are impaired, reflecting altered endothelial cell release of vasodilatory nitric oxide. This dysfunction persists for years beyond the time of exposure.

Furthermore, childhood and in utero ETS affects children's heart rates and is associated with tachycardia and impaired responsiveness to stimuli that can increase or decrease pulse rates. For reasons that are unclear, males are more susceptible to this problem than are females.

In Utero Exposure to Tobacco Smoke Causes Lasting Harm

Maternal cigarette smoking impairs the development of the fetus. Infants born to women who smoke during pregnancy are, on average, 200 g lighter than infants born to comparable women who do not smoke. *These infants are not born preterm but rather are small for gestational age at every stage of pregnancy.* In fact, 20% to 40% of the incidence of low birth weight can be attributed to maternal cigarette smoking (Fig. 8-4), reflecting direct retardation of fetal growth.

TABLE 8-2
HEALTH CONSEQUENCES OF ENVIRONMENTAL TOBACCO SMOKE

Cancer	During Childhood	Cardiac and Vascular	Respiratory and Other	During Pregnancy
Lung	New cases of asthma	Acute myocardial infarction	New cases of asthma	Stillbirth
Breast	Acute otitis media	Ischemic stroke	Pulmonary infections	IUGR
	Pulmonary infections	Sudden cardiac death	COPD	SIDS
		Angina	Stroke	Neurologic and behavioral disorders
				Preterm delivery

COPD = chronic obstructive pulmonary disease; IUGR = intrauterine growth retardation; SIDS = sudden infant death syndrome.

Children   **Adults**

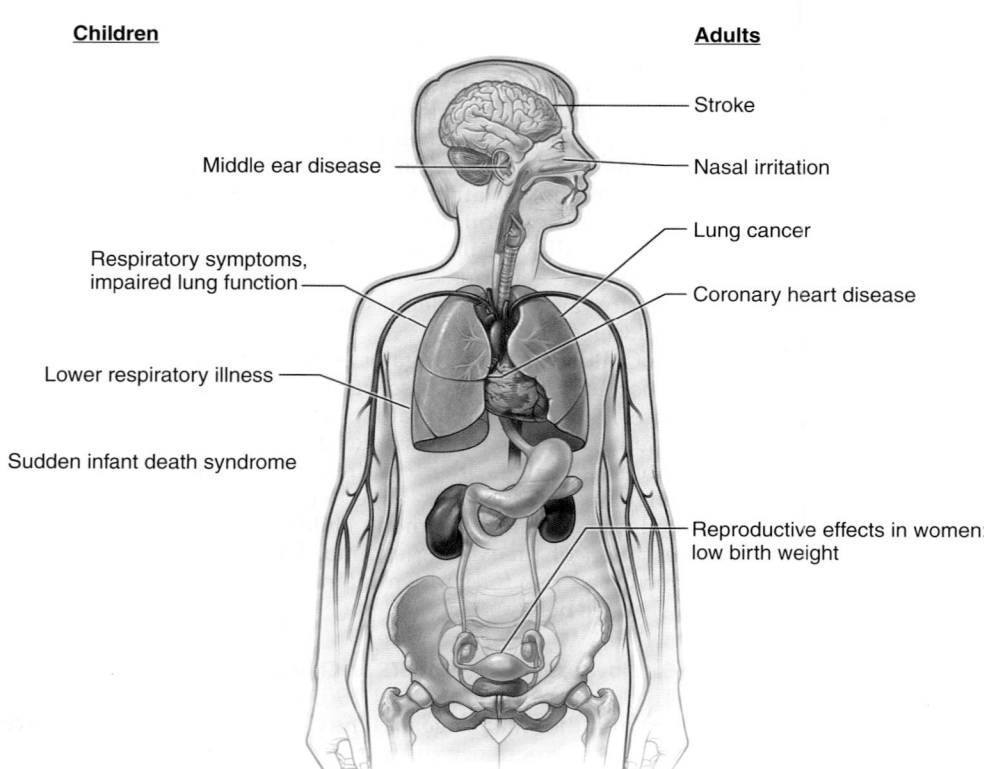

FIGURE 8-3. Complications of environmental tobacco smoke. (From U.S. Department of Health and Human Services. *The Health Consequences of Smoking: 50 Years of Progress. A Report of the Surgeon General.* Atlanta, GA: U.S. Department of Health and Human Services, Centers for Disease Control and Prevention, National Center for Chronic Disease Prevention and Health Promotion, Office on Smoking and Health; 2014.)

This decrease in birth weight does not translate into thinness later in life. Quite the contrary, in utero smoke exposure increases the frequency of overweight children by 60% at 4 years of age and increases the likelihood of obesity in adolescents. Such exposure also decreases high-density lipoprotein levels in children and has been linked to increased lipid peroxidation and metabolic syndrome later in life.

The harmful consequences of maternal cigarette smoking on the fetus are illustrated by its effect on the uteroplacental unit. Perinatal mortality is higher among offspring of smokers; the increases ranging from 20% among progeny of women who smoke less than a pack per day to almost 40% among offspring of those who smoke more than 1 pack per day, with the excess mortality reflecting problems related to the uteroplacental system. Incidences of abruptio placentae, placenta previa, uterine bleeding, and premature rupture of membranes are all increased (Fig. 8-5; **see Chapter 12**). These complications of smoking tend to occur at times when the fetus is not viable or is at great risk (i.e., 20–32 weeks of gestation).

Substantial evidence indicates that maternal cigarette smoking inflicts lasting harm on children and impairs physical, cognitive, and emotional development. Thus, these children showed measurable deficits in physical growth, intellectual maturation, and emotional development. In utero exposure to maternal cigarette smoking has been shown to increase several-fold the risk of certain types of attention-deficit/hyperactivity disorder (ADHD) in children. Deficits in cognitive and auditory functions related to smoking during pregnancy may persist for years and are detectable well into adolescence. Boys appear to be generally more vulnerable than girls to many of the psychosocial problems resulting from perinatal exposure to maternal cigarette smoking.

Furthermore, maternal smoking during pregnancy greatly increases (approximately fourfold in a recent study) the risk of SIDS (**see Chapter 6**). This is thought to represent mainly the consequences of prenatal exposure to maternal smoking since the increase in risk for SIDS if the father smokes, but not the mother, is much less (about 1.5-fold).

In the most comprehensive study to date, 17,000 children born during 1 week in Great Britain were studied at the ages of 7 and 11 years. Children of mothers who smoked 10 or more cigarettes a day during pregnancy were, on average,

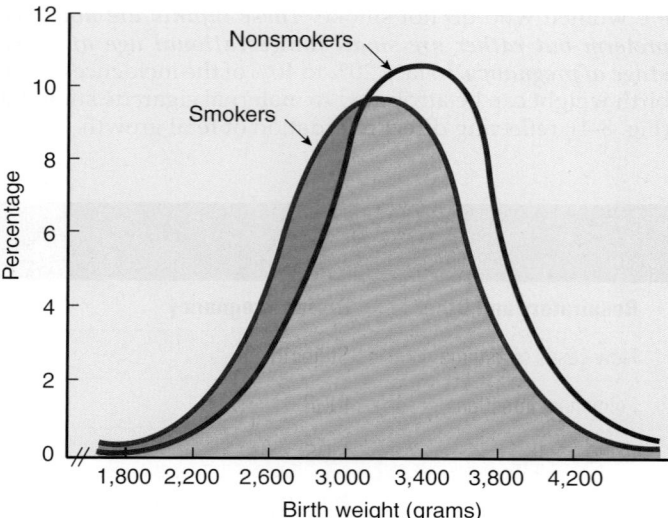

FIGURE 8-4. **Effect of smoking on birth weight.** Mothers who smoke give birth to smaller infants. In particular, the incidence of babies weighing less than 3,000 g is increased significantly by smoking.

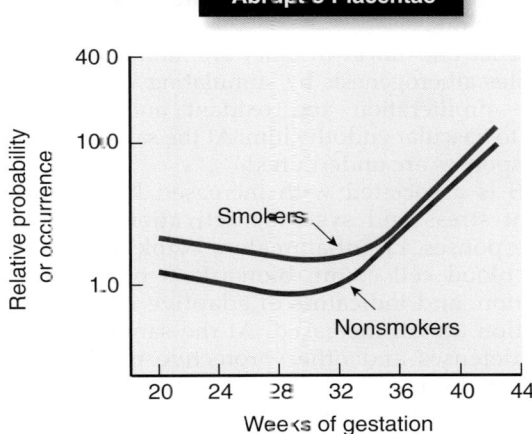

Abruptio Placentae

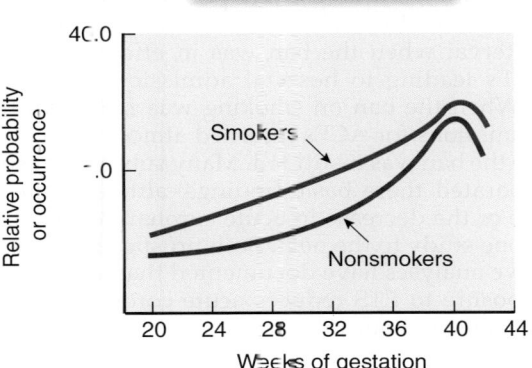

Placenta Previa

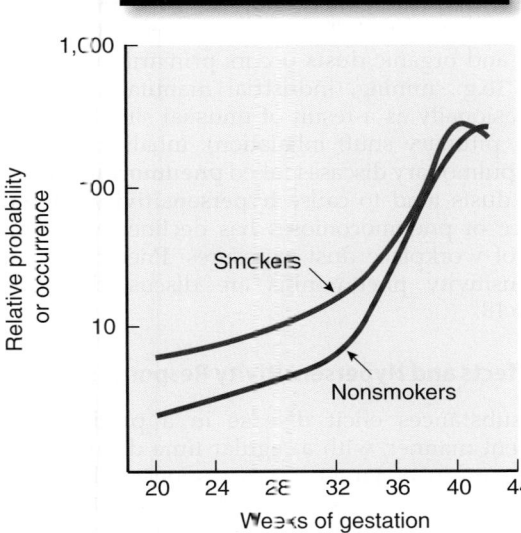

Premature rupture of membranes

FIGURE 8-5. Effect of smoking on the incidence of abruptio placentae (top), placenta previa (middle), and the premature rupture of amniotic membranes (bottom). In each, the ordinate shows the probability of one of three complications of the third trimester of pregnancy. Note that it is a logarithmic scale. Smoking increases the probability of abruptio placentae and premature rupture of the amniotic membranes prior to 34 weeks of gestation, at which time the fetus is still premature. Smoking increases the risk of placenta previa up to 40 weeks of gestation.

1.0 cm shorter than children of nonsmoking mothers and 3 to 5 months behind in reading, mathematics, and general intellectual ability. Moreover, the extent of the deficits was proportional to the number of cigarettes smoked during pregnancy.

ETS Correlates With Cardiovascular and Cerebrovascular Diseases

There is a very strong connection between ETS and an increased risk of coronary artery disease, acute coronary events, and sudden death. Many reports substantiate this association, in addition to a considerable number of controlled physiologic studies that address mechanisms involved (see below). The magnitude of increased risk is in the range of 25% to 30%, is dose dependent, and is disproportionate to the level of smoke exposure if compared to smokers.

A similar correlation exists between ETS and stroke. Many epidemiologic studies have documented that cerebrovascular accidents occur significantly more often in the context of ETS exposure.

 ETIOLOGIC FACTORS: ETS differs from mainstream smoke and represents about three-fourths of the smoke generated by cigarettes. Chemicals contained in ETS may differ both in amount and in potential toxicity from mainstream smoke. Some important chemicals present in ETS in far higher levels than in mainstream smoke are listed in Table 8-3. Some ETS constituents may dissipate rapidly, whereas others may contaminate surfaces and lead to continued exposure.

TABLE 8-3

EXAMPLES OF TOXIC CHEMICALS THAT ARE MORE ABUNDANT IN ETS THAN IN MAINSTREAM SMOKE

Chemical	Approximate Ratio in ETS vs. Mainstream Smoke
Benzene	5 to 10
Oxides of nitrogen	4 to 10
Formaldehyde	0.1 to 50
Acrolein	8 to 15
Nicotine	2.6 to 3.3
Ammonia	40 to 170
Nitrosamines	0.6 to 100
Cadmium	7.2
Polyaromatic hydrocarbons	1.3 to 1.9
Nickel	13 to 30
Nicotine	2.6 to 3.3
Pyridine	6.5 to 20
Polonium	1 to 4

ETS = environmental tobacco smoke.

PATHOPHYSIOLOGY: The products of cigarette combustion that passive smokers are exposed to are not the same as those that active smokers breathe in. Some of the toxins and carcinogens in mainstream smoke are the same as in ETS. However, unlike mainstream smoke, environmental smoke also includes products of combustion at the ends of lit cigarettes, where hotter temperatures generate higher levels of toxic and carcinogenic combustion products. These include nitrosated and nitrated hydrocarbons and aromatic and polycyclic compounds that do not characterize mainstream smoke. There is a documented exposure–risk relationship in ETS-related disease, the magnitude of which differs between men and women. In some studies, women exposed to secondhand smoke for extended periods (e.g., at home) suffer more from ACEs due to ETS. Furthermore, ETS-related ACEs are significantly more likely to predispose to subsequent coronary events; again, the probabilities reflect levels of exposure to ETS.

Although some observers have persisted in arguing otherwise, *there is overwhelming pathophysiologic mechanistic substantiation that ETS poses considerable danger to the heart and circulation* (Table 8-4). The ability of the heart rate to adjust to changes in demand is compromised by short-term (5–60 minutes) exposure to ETS, as is the functionality of the microvasculature and the left ventricle. As a result, exercise tolerance is greatly diminished. Short exposures to sidestream smoke substantially impair antioxidant defenses and similarly hinder parasympathetic adaptive responses to fluctuating demand for cardiac output. Many of these observations have been made in healthy young adults and highlight that ETS is pathogenic even in the absence of predisposing conditions.

Platelet and fibrin thrombi are stimulated. ETS also promotes atherogenesis by stimulating vascular smooth muscle proliferation and oxidant and inflammatory injury to vascular endothelium. At the same time, reparative responses are undermined.

ETS is associated with increased body burden of oxidant stress and systemic activation of inflammatory responses. Proinflammatory cytokines, circulating white blood cell count, biomarkers of inflammatory activation, and indicators of adaptive immune system activation are all increased. At the same time, antioxidant defenses and other protective mechanisms are often impaired.

Studies of the consequences of outlawing smoking in public places illustrate the strongest links between ETS and acute coronary morbidity and mortality. In one report, the city of Helena, Montana, banned cigarette smoking in workplaces and public places. This ban was overturned by court order 6 months later. During the interval when the ban was in effect, the number of ACEs leading to hospital admission decreased by 40%. When the ban on smoking was removed, hospital admissions for ACEs returned almost to levels seen before the ban was instituted. Many subsequent studies corroborated these basic findings, although the magnitude of the decrease in acute coronary events differs from one study to the next. Both prospective and retrospective analyses have documented that lowering public exposure to ETS reduces acute coronary events by an average of about 15%.

TABLE 8-4

EFFECTS OF ENVIRONMENTAL TOBACCO SMOKE ON THE HEART AND BLOOD

Magnification of atherogenesis

Higher levels of oxidant stress

Enhanced proliferation of arterial smooth muscle

Amplification of oxidation of LDL

Increased WBC adhesion to blood vessel walls

Higher levels of platelet aggregation

Impaired ability to adapt heart rate to fluctuations in demand

Depressed left ventricle function

Heightened inflammatory responses

Intensified platelet activation

Increased thrombogenesis

Poorer exercise tolerance

Reduced ability of arteries to dilate

LDL = low-density lipoprotein; WBC = white blood cell.

Toxic Substances Enter the Body via Many Routes

Environmental dusts are among the most important chemical hazards to which humans are exposed. Inhalation of mineral and organic dusts occurs primarily in occupational settings (e.g., mining, industrial manufacturing, farming) and occasionally as a result of unusual situations (e.g., bird fanciers, pituitary snuff inhalation). Inhaling mineral dusts leads to pulmonary diseases called **pneumoconioses**, whereas organic dusts tend to cause **hypersensitivity pneumonitis**. Incidence of pneumoconioses has declined with improved control of workplace dust exposures. Pneumoconioses and hypersensitivity pneumonitis are discussed in detail in Chapter 18.

Toxic Effects and Hypersensitivity Responses

Many substances elicit disease in a predictable, dose-dependent manner, with a regular time delay and a reproducible pattern of target organ responses. In these cases, pathologies of injured tissues are predictable. Disease caused by some other agents is unpredictable, showing (1) great variability in their ability to produce disease, (2) irregular lag times before injury is apparent, (3) no dose dependency, and (4) lack of reproducibility. In general, **predictable dose–response reactions** reflect direct actions of a compound or its metabolite on a tissue—a "toxic" effect. The second, **unpredictable type of reaction** often reflects "hypersensitivity," whether it involves an immunologic response or other type of idiosyncratic side effect.

Toxic Metal Exposures May Be Environmental

Lead Toxicity

EPIDEMIOLOGY: Lead is a ubiquitous heavy metal that is common in the environment of industrialized countries. It was used extensively in paints, plumbing, solder, and gasoline. Lead-based paints and leaded gasoline delivered large amounts of lead to the environment for much of the 20th century. Most dwellings built before 1940 had lead-containing paint on the interior and exterior walls, putting children at significant risk for chronic lead poisoning. Atmospheric lead in the form of dust derived from the combustion of lead-containing gasoline. Most countries have banned lead-containing gasoline. Still, lead leaching from old water pipes has led to crises of unsafe drinking water in several American cities, most vividly publicized in Flint, Michigan, putting large populations at risk for overexposure.

In the last 40 to 50 years, lead production has increased more than twofold, largely for battery manufacture and recycling. Children and adults living near point sources of environmental lead contamination, such as smelters, are exposed to even higher levels of lead.

PATHOPHYSIOLOGY: Lead is absorbed through the lungs or, less often, the gastrointestinal (GI) tract and skin. Once in the blood, it rapidly equilibrates with the plasma and erythrocytes and is excreted by the kidneys. A portion of blood lead remains freely diffusible. It readily crosses the blood–brain barrier, and concentrations in the brain, liver, kidneys, and bone marrow are directly related to its toxic effects. It binds sulfhydryl groups and interferes with the activities of zinc (Zn)-dependent enzymes. As well, it interferes with enzymes involved in the synthesis of steroids and cell membranes.

Bones, teeth, nails, and hair represent a tightly bound pool of lead that is not generally regarded as harmful. With chronic exposure, 90% of the total body lead burden is in the bones. During metaphyseal bone formation in children, lead and calcium are deposited to produce the increased bone densities ("lead lines") seen radiographically at the metaphysis, thus providing a simple method of detecting increased body stores of lead in children.

Lead toxicity affects both children and adults. Lead may pass through the placenta and be present in breast milk. The effects of childhood lead exposure are currently mostly neurodevelopmental. Such toxicities occur even at the lowest lead concentrations, causing psychosocial and behavioral problems, cognitive impairment, attention-deficit disorders, and other behavioral pathologies.

Anemia is a cardinal sign of lead intoxication. Lead disrupts heme synthesis in bone marrow erythroblasts by inhibiting δ-aminolevulinic acid dehydratase, the second enzyme in de novo heme synthesis. It also inhibits ferrochelatase, which incorporates ferrous iron into the porphyrin ring. Resulting impaired heme synthesis causes a microcytic and hypochromic anemia such as that seen in iron deficiency (**see Chapter 26**), in which heme synthesis is also impaired. Erythrocytes in lead

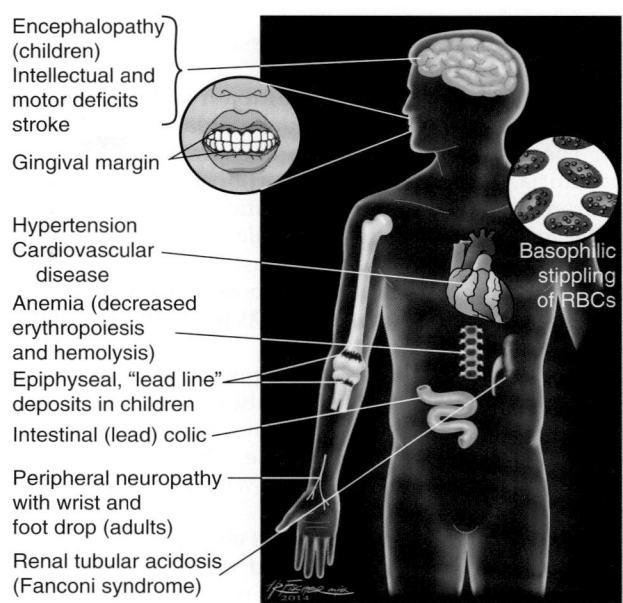

Encephalopathy (children)
Intellectual and motor deficits stroke
Gingival margin

Hypertension
Cardiovascular disease
Anemia (decreased erythropoiesis and hemolysis)
Epiphyseal, "lead line" deposits in children
Intestinal (lead) colic

Peripheral neuropathy with wrist and foot drop (adults)
Renal tubular acidosis (Fanconi syndrome)

Basophilic stippling of RBCs

FIGURE 8-6. Complications of lead intoxication. RBC = red blood cell.

intoxication also show prominent basophilic stippling, reflecting clustering of ribosomes. Red blood cell life span is decreased; thus, lead intoxication leads to anemia due to ineffective hematopoiesis and accelerated erythrocyte turnover.

PATHOLOGY: Classic lead overexposure is rarely seen in the United States nowadays. It affects many organs, but its major toxicities affect (1) the nervous system, (2) kidneys, (3) cardiovascular system, and (4) hematopoiesis (Fig. 8-6).

CLINICAL FEATURES: *NEUROTOXICITY. In children, lead toxicity mainly manifests as brain-related dysfunction. Adult lead neurotoxicity tends more to be present as peripheral neuropathy.* Children with lead encephalopathy are typically irritable and ataxic. They may convulse or display altered states of consciousness, from drowsiness to frank coma. Children with blood lead levels above 80 µg/dL, but with concentrations lower than those in children with frank encephalopathy (120 µg/dL), show milder central nervous system (CNS) symptoms such as clumsiness, irritability, and hyperactivity.

In **lead encephalopathy**, the brain is edematous, with flattened gyri and compressed ventricles. There may be herniation of the uncus and cerebellar tonsils. Microscopically, congestion, petechial hemorrhages, and foci of neuronal necrosis are seen. Diffuse astrocytic proliferation in both the gray and white matters may accompany these changes. Vascular lesions in the brain are particularly prominent, with capillary dilation and proliferation.

Peripheral motor neuropathy is the most common manifestation of lead neurotoxicity in the adult, typically affecting the radial and peroneal nerves and resulting in **wrist drop** and **foot drop**, respectively. Lead-induced neuropathy is probably also the basis of paroxysms of GI pain known as **lead colic**.

NEPHROPATHY. **Lead nephropathy** reflects the toxic effect of the metal on the proximal tubular cells of the kidney. The resulting dysfunction is characterized by aminoaciduria, glycosuria, and hyperphosphaturia (Fanconi syndrome). Such functional alterations are accompanied by the formation of inclusion bodies in the nuclei of the proximal tubular cells. These inclusions are characteristic of lead nephropathy and are composed of a lead–protein complex containing more than 100 times the concentration of lead in the whole kidney.

CARDIOVASCULAR. Lead exposure in adults causes diverse cardiovascular complications, including high blood pressure, peripheral vascular disease, arrhythmias, stroke, and ischemic heart disease. These consequences have been documented in adults with blood lead levels of 5 μg/dL.

Lead poisoning is treated with chelating agents such as ethylenediaminetetraacetic acid (EDTA), either alone or in combination with dimercaprol (BAL). Both the hematologic and renal manifestations of lead intoxication are usually reversible; alterations in the CNS are generally irreversible.

Laboratory diagnosis is made by demonstrating high blood levels of lead and increased free erythrocyte protoporphyrin. Elevated urinary excretion of δ-aminolevulinic acid and decreased levels of aminolevulinic acid dehydratase in erythrocytes are confirmatory.

EFFECTS OF CHRONIC EXPOSURE TO LOW LEAD LEVELS: Because of effective environmental legislation in the United States, ambient levels of lead have fallen significantly: Blood levels in the general population of the United States decreased from an average of 16 μg/dL in 1976 to 1.0 μg/dL in 2000. It has been established that cumulative exposure to lead is best measured in bone, rather than in blood. The latter lead levels reflect more ongoing exposure. Thus, elevated bone levels of lead have been correlated with adult hypertension, whereas no relationship has been established with blood levels. This decline in mean blood lead levels led to the near elimination of lead-related childhood fatalities and encephalopathy. Nonetheless, low-level lead exposure in children may still permanently impair cognitive performance. The WHO has indicated that "there is no known level of lead exposure that is considered safe." Efforts to reduce environmental lead decreased the percentage of children in the United States with blood levels of 10 μg/dL or more from 88% in the 1970s to 4.4% in the 1990s. However, high blood lead concentrations remain a problem among poor, mainly urban, children.

Mercury

Inorganic mercury has been used since prehistoric times and has been known to be an occupation-related hazard, at least since the Middle Ages, and continues to represent a hazard, especially to people engaged in mining gold. In recent years, it has become clear that organic mercury also represents a great risk to human health. Occupational mercury poisoning still occurs, but there has been increasing concern over the potential health hazards of mercury contaminating ecosystems, especially after several outbreaks of methylmercury poisoning. Local inhabitants in Minamata Bay, Japan, in the 1950s and then in Niigata developed severe, chronic organic mercury intoxication. This poisoning was traced to the consumption of fish contaminated with mercury that had been discharged into the environment as the effluents from a fertilizer factory and a plastic factory. Children exposed in utero showed delayed developmental milestones and abnormal reflexes despite the fact that fetal exposure was estimated to be one-fifth to one-tenth that in adults.

Mercury released into the environment may be bioconcentrated and enter the food chain. Bacteria in bays and oceans convert inorganic mercury compounds from industrial wastes into highly neurotoxic organomercurials. These compounds are then transferred up the food chain and are eventually concentrated in the large predatory fish (e.g., tuna, pike) that make up a substantial part of the diet in many countries.

Unlike inorganic mercury, which is not efficiently absorbed by the gut, organic mercurial compounds are readily taken up because they are lipid soluble. Inorganic and organic mercury is preferentially concentrated in the kidney, and methylmercury also distributes to the brain. *The kidney is the principal target of the toxicity of inorganic mercury, but the brain is damaged by organic mercurials.*

Claims that mercuric preservatives in vaccines cause autism or other neurologic complications have been proven false.

NEPHROTOXICITY: At one time, mercuric chloride was widely used as an antiseptic and acute mercuric chloride poisoning was much more common; the compound was ingested by accident or to commit suicide. Resulting **proximal tubular necrosis** led to oliguric renal failure. Mercurial diuretics were also widely prescribed in the past, and chronic mercury nephrotoxicity was a not uncommon complication of their long-term use. Nowadays, chronic mercurial nephrotoxicity is almost always a consequence of long-term industrial exposure. Proteinuria is common in chronic mercurial nephrotoxicity, and there may be a nephrotic syndrome with more severe intoxication. Pathologically, there is a membranous glomerulonephritis with subepithelial electron-dense deposits, suggesting immune complex deposition.

NEUROTOXICITY: The neurologic effects of mercury are manifested as a constriction of visual fields, paresthesias, ataxia, dysarthria, and hearing loss. Pathologically, there is cerebral and cerebellar atrophy. Microscopically, the cerebellum shows atrophy of the granular layer, without loss of Purkinje cells and spongy softening in the visual cortex and other cortical regions.

Iron

Iron-deficiency anemia is a common disease, particularly in premenopausal women. Oral iron preparations mostly contain ferrous sulfate, which is absorbed by the gut mucosa and then converted to the trivalent iron. Acute ferrous sulfate poisoning from accidental ingestion occurs mainly in little children. As little as 1 to 2 g of ferrous sulfate may be lethal, but most fatal cases follow ingestion of 3 to 10 g. Hemorrhagic gastritis and acute liver necrosis have been most prominent at autopsy.

Long-term, excessive dietary iron intake does not ordinarily lead to abnormal iron accumulation. South African Bantus have a significant incidence of iron overload, which has been attributed to a diet very high in iron, largely derived from iron drums used to prepare homemade beer. The acidic pH of these brews readily solubilizes the iron, and their low alcohol content allows large volumes to be consumed. A large proportion of the excess iron accumulates in the liver, and the degree of siderosis correlates with the presence of cirrhosis. There is also a high incidence of diabetes and heart disease in this "Bantu siderosis."

A similar syndrome has been noted in some African Americans and is attributed to a mutation in the gene for ferroportin (*SLC4A1*). This genetic abnormality may predispose affected people to iron overload (**see Chapter 20**).

CLIMATE CHANGE

Temperatures in the Earth's lower atmosphere have increased about 1°C worldwide since the late 19th century. Parallel changes in upper ocean temperatures have also occurred.

Climate Change Mostly Reflects the Consequences of Fossil Fuel Combustion

Accumulation of greenhouse gases in the atmosphere, especially CO_2, methane, and nitrous oxide, is responsible. *These gases derive mostly from fossil fuel combustion, with additional contributions from agricultural activities. Thus, climate change is anthropogenic, that is, human activity is the principal cause.*

Currently documented effects of climate change are profound, and temperatures are expected (by the WHO) to continue to rise an additional 1.4° to 5.8°C by year 2100. The US government, in the Fourth National Climate Assessment (2018), projects a total increase in global air temperatures of 5°C by 2100 compared to preindustrial temperatures.

The Potential Risk of Climate Change

To understand the magnitude of the potential effects of climate change, it is worth considering that a 4° to 7°C total increase in global temperatures triggered—it is felt—by volcanic release of massive amounts of greenhouse gases (particularly CO_2) led to cataclysmic global climatic changes, including 2 million years of torrential rains, causing worldwide extinction of vast numbers of species during the Carnian Pluvial Episode (or Event, CPE), about 234 million years ago. (Parenthetically, this episode paved the way to the rise of dinosaurs.)

We are, fortunately, not at this point yet. But the impact of this unfolding, largely man-made environmental situation on human health and disease is already noticeable and is only likely to become much more so as climate change continues.

Climate Change Impacts Human Health Directly and Indirectly

Climate change, it should be noted, entails not only warmer global temperatures but also more severe weather—warm and cold; wet and dry—across the globe. Direct effects of climate change include the consequences of severe weather (storms, drought, floods, and extreme temperatures). Indirect effects include the effects of these factors on the environment, their ramifications for human societies, and

consequent changes in disease patterns. As such, they are more subtle but no less consequential: adulteration of water quality, effects on air pollution, agriculture and land use, and changes in plant, insect, and animal life that reflect adaptation to warmer temperatures.

Not all human populations are affected equally, though all are affected. People living in less developed countries, with less stringent sanitation and more marginal food supply, are at greater risk. The elderly and the very young, wherever they are, are also more vulnerable.

Direct Effects of Climate Change on Human Health

Hot days in summer have increased. Briefly, from 1970 to 2017, in the 50 largest US cities, the number of days in which summer temperatures exceeded the 30-year average for each individual city increased from 37.5 ± 1.2 to 55.2 ± 0.9 ($P \ll .0001$) (Fig. 8-7). Increased temperatures correlate with increased hospital visits and admissions for respiratory ailments, as well as frequency of myocardial infarction and congestive cardiac failure.

Other direct effects of climate change on human health include exacerbation of air pollution. Higher temperatures increase airborne particulates of all sizes and ozone. Short-term spikes in mortality, mainly from cardiovascular and respiratory diseases, correlate with increases in ozone concentrations. Particulate pollution, particularly $PM_{2.5}$ and $PM_{0.1}$, is dangerous in itself—accelerating atherosclerosis and increasing vascular inflammation and myocardial infarction (see above)—but high temperatures exacerbate particulate lethality.

Infectious Diseases and Climate Change

Increased temperature and fluctuations in rainfall alter the range of insect vectors that carry human diseases. Such associations have been reported for malaria and dengue fever. Changing patterns of migration of animal reservoirs for vector-spread diseases are also changing the incidence and enlarging geographic areas affected by such

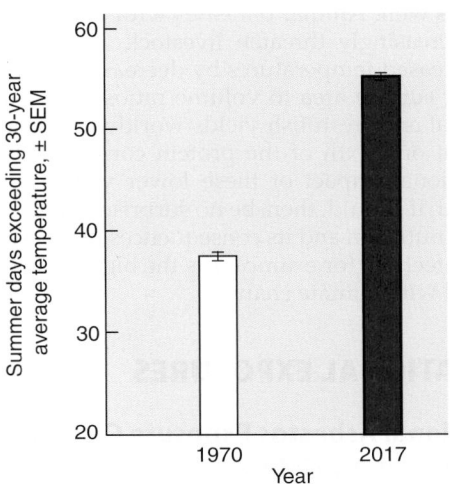

FIGURE 8-7. Summer temperatures in US cities. Number of summer (June 1–August 31) days exceeding the 30-year (1980–2010) average temperature for each city, for the 50 largest cities in the United States, comparing 1970 and 2017. Data shown are $\pm$ SEM. The difference between 1970 and 2017 is statistically significant (Student 2-tailed *t* test), $P < 10^{-12}$.

zoonotic infections as West Nile virus and Lyme disease (**see Chapter 9**).

Some bacteria multiply more rapidly in warmer settings. This is particularly true of *Salmonella* and *Vibrio*. Cholera outbreaks have occurred recently farther north than the disease had previously been recorded.

Indirect Effects of Climate Change on Human Health

Increased temperatures lead to changes in the environment that have had, and undoubtedly will have even more, substantial effects on people's health. Thus, heat waves leave forestlands parched and susceptible to fire. In one such situation, near Moscow in 2010, huge forest fires caused increased wind-spread particulate pollution that led to an estimated 11,000 additional deaths.

Increased incidence of severe storms and rising sea levels has impacted food and water supplies in many ways. Spillage of seawater into aqueducts has contaminated fresh water supplies, contributed to people using less safe sources of drinking water, and led to an increased incidence of diarrheal diseases. This problem is further exacerbated by the increasing range of certain tree-destroying insects (shifting northward about 2–3.5 km/yr since the 1960s), which have wreaked havoc on trees. Millions of acres of forests have been destroyed in the last 25 years for this reason. Loss of these trees' watershed and soil control functions impairs food growth because of soil erosion and further damages the quality of the water supply.

Yields of many crops have declined not only because of inconsistent cycles of rain and drought but also because of warmer temperatures that alter plants' fertility cycles. Thus, adaptive changes in the geographic ranges of pollinating insects have led to poorer plant pollination. Shorter cold spells in the winter have caused male and female flowers to develop asynchronously, also decreasing pollination. Correspondingly, fruit yields have decreased worldwide. In parallel, global wheat and other grain production has declined considerably in the past 35 years.

Finally, animals, particularly those used for food, are affected as well. Animal parasites with broader geographic ranges increasingly threaten livestock. Animals are adapting to increased temperatures by decreasing body mass (i.e., increasing surface area to volume ratios). This has reduced commercial and fresh fish yields worldwide. Since fish provide about one-sixth of the protein consumed by humans, the nutritional impact of these lower yields is potentially substantial. It should, then, be no surprise that the WHO considers malnutrition and its consequences (increased susceptibility to infection, for example) as the biggest health concern associated with climate change.

OCCUPATIONAL EXPOSURES

Occupational Asbestos Exposure Causes Lung and Other Cancers and Fibrotic Lung Disease

Asbestos, in many ways, is a prototypical occupational disease-causing agent. Most exposure and disease derive from the workplace—in asbestos workers and their families. Its relationship with at least some human diseases is well established, and it is likely to be causally linked to others as additional studies become available. Like many other environmental agents, its mechanisms of action (see below) are both unique to the substance and in need of further elucidation.

Types of Asbestos

Asbestos is a family of naturally occurring minerals that share diverse fibrous silicate structures. There are two major types of asbestos fibers: amphibole and serpentine. The former, which comprises crocidolite, amosite, tremolite, and others, is more harmful to human health than the latter, which contains only chrysotile. But both types of fibers cause disease and should be considered both fibrogenic and carcinogenic.

Sources of Asbestos Exposure

Asbestos fibers' relative stability, resistance to heat and fire, and malleability led to extensive industrial uses, particularly for construction, insulation, and surfacing. In the United States, they were exploited extensively for these and other uses. Beginning in the 1970s, asbestos was removed from some consumer products, and in 1989, the U.S. EPA prohibited new uses of asbestos. Previously established uses, however, continue.

Most contact with asbestos occurs among people with occupational exposure. In that context, it is generally inhaled, with the respiratory tract consequently being the main organ system affected. Family members of people with occupational exposures are also susceptible to asbestos-related diseases, particularly mesothelioma (**see below and Chapter 18**), most likely because of asbestos fibers carried in workers' clothes and on their bodies.

Pathogenetically significant asbestos exposures may potentially occur in nonoccupational settings. Since asbestos is a natural mineral, it may appear in drinking water, and some studies' data suggest that ingesting asbestos in drinking water may be associated with digestive tract cancers (see below). Other exposures, such as nonoccupational airborne exposures in the vicinity of asbestos mines or in heavy traffic (due to asbestos aerosolized from brake linings), have also been documented.

Asbestos Exposure and Diseases Caused by Asbestos

Several different diseases, and types of diseases, have been linked with asbestos exposure (Table 8-5). Occupational exposure to all types of asbestos is causally associated with both malignant and nonmalignant diseases. Disease development is dose dependent: Duration and intensity of asbestos exposure correlate with the incidence of these diseases, independently of other risk factors (e.g., smoking) or identifiable confounding influences. In most cases, there is a lag time of 10 to 40 years between exposure and clinically evident disease.

The best and most abundant data, because of the route of greatest exposure and the focus of research, relate to lung and pleural diseases: asbestosis, lung cancer, pleural caps and effusions, and mesothelioma. Other data are becoming increasingly available with time. The U.S. National Cancer Institute recognizes that laryngeal and ovarian cancers are related to asbestos exposure. Good studies support the likelihood that cancers of the esophagus and the colon and

TABLE 8-5
DISEASES LINKED TO ASBESTOS EXPOSURE

Disease	Organ and Site Affected
Asbestosis	Lung parenchyma
Inflammation	Pleural effusion
Pleural caps	Pleural surface of lung
Mesothelioma	All mesothelial surfaces, particularly pleural, but also peritoneal and pericardial
Epithelial cancers	Lung[a] Larynx[a] Ovary[a] Esophagus[b] Colon and rectum[b]

[a]Listed by federal and international agencies; generally accepted.

[b]Controversial, IOM study of 2006 (Committee on Asbestos, Institute of Medicine of the National Academies. *Asbestos: Selected Cancers*. Washington, DC: The National Academies Press; 2006) did not reach conclusion for lower exposures but indicated correlations for higher levels of exposure; subsequent studies suggest a relationship between these tumors and asbestos exposure.

rectum are also increased in people with occupational exposure to asbestos. Associations between asbestos and several other malignancies have been suggested (pancreas, pharynx, kidney) by some studies, but those links—if they exist—remain to be clarified.

PATHOPHYSIOLOGY: The mechanism(s) by which asbestos causes tissue injury and tumors are only partly understood. Most studies relate to the effects of asbestos on the lung and the mesothelium. The extent to which results of these studies can be generalized to other tissues is unclear. Nonetheless, several key considerations connect patterns of asbestos-induced tissue injury and disease.

Physical parameters. Asbestos particles are fibers, mostly shaped like splinters. Tissue injury is a direct function of tissue burden of fibers, which, in turn, is a function of fiber diameter and length. These parameters determine how deeply fibers penetrate the lungs, and beyond, as well as their disposition once there. Only fibers <10 μm long and <0.4 μm thick reach alveoli. Longer fibers tend to deposit in airways and, because they may be variably phagocytosed by macrophages (≈15–20 μm in size), may persist where they land. These are most carcinogenic and, if they exceed 20 μm, may cause asbestosis. Fibers <6 μm long may penetrate lung structures and reach lymph nodes and distal organs.

Inflammation and ROS. Once they settle in the lung, fibers incite inflammatory responses, with macrophages or neutrophils predominating, depending on particle dose and size. These cells ingest the long, thin fibers with difficulty. Respiratory bursts, which generate damaging free radicals (mostly ROS, **see Chapters 1 and 2**), are part of these cells' responses to foreign materials. All asbestos particles contain iron, and iron-catalyzed ROS (see Fenton,

Haber-Weiss reactions, Chapter 1) magnify the tissue damage caused by the inflammatory cells themselves.

Fibrogenesis. The inflammatory response to asbestos, magnified by the mechanisms mentioned above, leads to release of cytokines, especially TGFβ, TNFα, and IL-1β, which stimulate fibroblast to produce collagen. Because of the size of many fibers, they persist where they are deposited, and continue to stimulate both fibrosis and inflammation, with ROS. These reactive species (plus reactive nitrogen and alkoxyl radicals) are thought to mediate much of asbestos-related damage.

Apoptosis. Increased free radicals stimulate the intrinsic pathways of apoptosis (**see Chapter 1**). The link between these two is complex, involving several intertwined pathways, but they lead to endoplasmic reticulum calcium release, mitochondrial cytochrome C release, and activation of caspases 3 and 9. Countervailing forces are also activated: Mitochondria respond to these stimuli by producing aconitase and oxoguanine glycosylase-1, which prevent apoptosis.

DNA damage. ROS damage DNA, particularly by oxidizing guanine to 8-hydroxyguanine. This triggers the DNA damage response, including activated p53, further contributing to apoptosis.

Oxidant injury and oncogenesis. Interestingly, these forces also activate cellular signaling mechanisms such as those that are often implicated in oncogenesis (**see Chapter 5**). Oxidant stress may trigger MAPK pathways to stimulate NF-κB and AP-1 transcriptional activators and cell proliferation. In addition, asbestos fibers may directly activate cell membrane receptors, such as EGFR. Continued exposure, inflammation, and epithelial and mesothelial cell proliferation contribute to tumor development.

Industrial Exposures May Involve Heavy Metals and Organic and Other Toxins

Cyanide

Prussic acid (HCN) is the classic murderer's tool in detective fiction, where the smell of bitter almonds (*Prunus amygdalus*) betrays the crime. Cyanide blocks cell respiration by reversibly binding to mitochondrial cytochrome oxidase, the terminal acceptor in the electron transport chain, which is responsible for reducing molecular oxygen to water. The pathologic consequences are similar to those produced by any acute global anoxia.

Arsenic

The toxic properties of arsenic have been known for centuries. Arsenic-containing compounds have been widely used as insecticides, weed killers, and wood preservatives. Arsenicals may also contaminate soil and leach into ground water as a result of naturally occurring arsenic-rich rock formations, from coal burning, or from the use of arsenical pesticides. As with mercury, there is evidence for its bioaccumulation along the food chain.

Acute arsenic poisoning is almost always the result of accidental or homicidal ingestion. Death is due to **CNS toxicity**. Chronic arsenic intoxication affects many organ systems. It is characterized initially by such nonspecific symptoms as malaise and fatigue. Eventually,

GI, cardiovascular, and hematologic dysfunctions become evident. Both encephalopathy and peripheral neuropathy develop. The latter is characterized by paresthesias, motor palsies, and painful neuritis. **Cancers of the skin, respiratory tract,** and **GI tract** have been attributed to industrial and agricultural exposures to arsenic. In some parts of the world, exposure of workers in rice paddies to arsenic in the ground water has been associated with skin cancers. Rare cases of hepatic angiosarcomas have been related to chronic arsenic exposure.

Cadmium

Cadmium is often inhaled as part of mainstream cigarette smoke. It is also used in ever-increasing quantities in manufacturing alloys, producing rechargeable batteries, and electroplating other metals (e.g., automobile parts and musical instruments). It is a plasticizer and a pigment. Cadmium oxide fumes are released in the course of welding steel parts previously plated with a cadmium anticorrosive. It accumulates in the human body, with a half-life of over 20 years, and since it is rarely recycled, its increased industrial use is of concern. The main routes of exposure for the general population are ingestion and inhalation. Both plant- and animal-derived foodstuffs may contain substantial levels of cadmium.

Short-term cadmium inhalation irritates the respiratory tract, with pulmonary edema the most dangerous result. Chronic cadmium intoxication mainly affects the lungs and the kidneys and, to a lesser extent, the skeletal and vascular systems. Although the confounding effects of smoking complicate interpretation of some of these studies, chronic obstructive lung disease, cardiovascular disease, and cancers of the lungs, cervix, pancreas, and prostate are significantly associated with chronic cadmium exposure. Proteinuria, which reflects tubular rather than glomerular damage, has been the most consistent finding in cadmium workers with renal damage.

Chromium

Chromium (Cr) is used extensively in several industries, including metal plating and some types of manufacturing. Although it occurs in any number of oxidation states, only Cr(III) and Cr(VI) are commonly used industrially. Toxicity is usually a result of Cr(VI) inhalation, and the consequences of exposure depend on the solubility of the specific salt. Although acute intoxication is known, it is chronic exposure that is most problematic.

Cr(VI) is causes free radical–related damage and is highly genotoxic. People who chronically inhale salts of hexavalent chromium have an increased risk of lung, sinus, and nasal malignancies. The less-soluble chromate salts are generally more potent pulmonary carcinogens, particularly zinc chromate.

Nickel

Nickel is a widely used metal in electronics, coins, steel alloys, batteries, and food processing. Dermatitis ("nickel itch"), the most frequent effect of exposure to nickel, may occur from direct contact with metals containing nickel, such as coins and costume jewelry. The dermatitis is a sensitization reaction; the body reacts to nickel-conjugated proteins formed following the penetration of the epidermis by nickel ions. Exposure to nickel, as to arsenic, increases the risk of development of specific types of cancer. Epidemiologic studies have demonstrated that workers who were occupationally exposed to nickel compounds, especially $NiCl_2$, have an increased incidence of lung cancer and cancer of the nasal cavities.

Cobalt

Acute occupational inhalation of cobalt leads to acute respiratory distress syndrome (ARDS, **see Chapter 18**). Cobalt was once added to beer to enhance foaming qualities, but excessive imbibing of cobalt-containing beers caused a degenerative disease of heart muscle (cardiomyopathy; **see Chapter 17**). When cobalt was removed from the beer, the cardiomyopathy disappeared, leaving only toxicities due to alcohol itself (see below). Metal-on-metal joint replacements may rarely be associated with cobalt toxicity (prosthetic hip-associated cobalt toxicity, or PHACT), with diverse manifestations including neuropathies and endocrinopathies. Inhaled cobalt salts (especially $CoSO_4$) can trigger oxidative stress and so are considered genotoxic at high concentrations, but there are no known links to human cancers.

Radioactive Elements

Elements whose radioactive isotopes are potentially hazardous include radium, strontium, uranium, plutonium, thorium, and iodine. Chronic toxicities relate principally to radiation-induced carcinogenesis. The individual tumors reflect the organ localization of the elements and are discussed in the chapters that address specific organ pathology.

Volatile Organic Solvents and Vapors

These are widely used in industry. With few exceptions, exposures to these compounds are by inhalation and reflect to be industrial or accidental and represent short-term dangers rather than long-term toxicities.

- **Chloroform ($CHCl_3$) and carbon tetrachloride (CCl_4):** These solvents are CNS depressants (anesthetics) and impair the heart and blood vessels but are better known as hepatotoxins. Both, but classically CCl_4, cause acute hepatic necrosis, fatty liver, and liver failure in large doses.
- **Trichloroethylene (C_2HCl_3):** A ubiquitous industrial solvent, trichloroethylene in high concentrations depresses the CNS but hepatotoxicity is minimal. There is no evidence of diseases in humans even after ordinary long-term industrial exposure.
- **Methanol (CH_3OH):** Because methanol, unlike ethanol, is not taxed, it has been used as a substitute for ethanol or as an adulterant of alcoholic beverages. Methanol inebriation resembles that produced by ethanol but is followed by GI symptoms, visual dysfunction, seizures, coma, and death. The major toxicity of methanol is believed to arise from its metabolism, first to formaldehyde and then to formic acid. Metabolic acidosis is common after methanol ingestion. The most characteristic lesion of methanol toxicity is necrosis of retinal ganglion cells and subsequent degeneration of the optic nerve, leading to blindness.

Severe poisoning may lead to lesions in the putamen and globus pallidus.

- **Ethylene glycol (HOCH$_2$CH$_2$OH):** Ethylene glycol exposure is usually due to ingestion. It is commonly used in antifreeze and has been consumed by chronic alcoholics as a substitute for ethanol for many years. It has been used to adulterate wines because of its sweet taste and solubility. Its toxicity largely reflects its metabolites, particularly oxalic acid, and occurs within minutes of ingestion. Metabolic acidosis, CNS depression, nausea and vomiting, and hypocalcemia-related cardiotoxicity occur. Oxalate crystals in renal tubules and oxaluria are often noted and may cause renal failure.

- **Gasoline and kerosene:** These fuels are mixtures of aliphatic hydrocarbons and branched, unsaturated, and aromatic hydrocarbons. Chronic exposure is by inhalation. Despite prolonged exposure to gasoline by gas station attendants, auto mechanics, and so forth, there is no evidence that inhalation of gasoline over the long term is particularly injurious. Acutely, gasoline is an irritant but inhalation really causes only systemic problems in very high concentrations. Increased use of kerosene for home heating leads to accidental poisoning of children.

- **Benzene (C$_6$H$_6$):** Benzene is the prototypic aromatic hydrocarbon. It is one of the most widely used chemicals in industrial processes, being a solvent and a starting point for innumerable syntheses. It is also a constituent of fuels, accounting for as much as 3% of gasoline. Virtually all cases of acute and chronic benzene toxicity have occurred as industrial exposures (e.g., in shoemakers and workers in shoe manufacturing, which once entailed heavy exposure to benzene-based glues).

- Acute benzene poisoning primarily affects the CNS, and death results from respiratory failure. However, the long-term effects of benzene exposure, in which the bone marrow is the principal target, have attracted the most attention. Marrow **hypoplasia** or **aplasia**, with **pancytopenia**, may develop. **Aplastic anemia** usually occurs while workers are still exposed to high concentrations of benzene. Many people with benzene-induced anemias develop **myelodysplastic syndromes, acute myeloblastic leukemia, erythroleukemia,** or **multiple myeloma,** either during ongoing exposure to benzene or after a variable latent period after the worker leaves the hazardous environment. Some cases of acute leukemia have occurred without a prior history of aplastic anemia. Occasionally, chronic myeloid and chronic lymphocytic leukemias are reported but their causal link to benzene exposure is weaker than that with acute leukemias. Overall, workers exposed to the highest atmospheric concentrations of benzene have a 60-fold increased risk of leukemia.

- Both gasoline and tobacco smoke contain benzene, and both contribute to increased benzene levels in urban air. The consequent contribution of such benzene concentrations to hematologic diseases is speculative.

- The toxic effects of benzene are related to its metabolites, which derive from cytochrome P450 degradation of the parent compound. Although chemically closely related and also widely used as solvents, toluene and xylenes have not been incriminated as causing hematologic abnormalities, possibly because they are metabolized via different pathways.

Agricultural Chemicals May Be Toxic During Acute Exposure or by Cumulative Effects

Pesticides, fungicides, herbicides, fumigants, and organic fertilizers are crucial to the productivity of modern agriculture. However, many of these chemicals persist in soil and water and may pose a potential long-term hazard. Exposure to industrial concentrations or inadvertently contaminated food can cause severe acute illness. Children are particularly susceptible and may ingest home gardening preparations.

Pesticides

Organochlorine pesticides, such as DDT (dichlorodiphenyltrichloroethane), chlordane, and others, have caused concern because they accumulate in soils and in human tissues and break down very slowly. High levels of any such pesticide can be harmful to humans in acute exposures, but the side effects of chronic contact with the materials and their buildup are of greatest interest. Many of these compounds act as weak estrogens, the consequences of which are as yet unclear. Some of these compounds, such as aldrin and dieldrin, have been associated with tumor development, but the acute toxicity of most organochlorine insecticides relates to inhibition of CNS γ-aminobutyric acid (GABA) responses.

Symptoms of acute toxicity often reflect the toxin's mode of action. For example, organophosphate insecticides, which have largely replaced organochlorine compounds, are acetylcholinesterase inhibitors that are readily absorbed through the skin. Thus, acute toxicity in humans mainly involves neuromuscular disorders such as visual disturbances, dyspnea, mucous hypersecretion, and bronchoconstriction. Death may result from respiratory failure. In the United States, 30 to 40 people die annually of acute pesticide poisoning. Long-term exposure to substantial concentrations produces symptoms such as those of acute exposure.

Human exposure to herbicides is not infrequent. Among the best known of these is paraquat. Occupational exposure to paraquat is usually via the skin, although toxicity from ingestion and inhalation has been documented. The compound is very corrosive and causes burns or ulcers wherever it comes in contact. It is transported actively to the lung, where it can damage pulmonary epithelium, causing edema and even respiratory failure. High-level exposures may lead to death from cardiovascular collapse; lower doses may cause pulmonary fibrosis and, ultimately, death.

Aromatic Halogenated Hydrocarbons

The halogenated aromatic hydrocarbons that have received considerable attention include (1) the polychlorinated biphenyls (PCBs); (2) chlorophenols (pentachlorophenol, used as a wood preservative); (3) hexachlorophene, previously used as an antibacterial agent in soaps; and (4) the dioxin TCDD (2,3,7,8-tetrachlorodibenzo-p-dioxin), a by-product of the synthesis of herbicides and hexachlorophene and therefore a contaminant of these preparations that has not been produced intentionally.

In 1976, an industrial accident in Seveso, Italy, exposed many people to 6 metric tons of gaseous cloud containing about 1 kg of TCDD. Acute effects included peripheral neuropathy, evidence of liver damage, and chloracne. Exposed population showed excess mortality from diabetes and respiratory and cardiovascular diseases, as well as an increased risk of lymphomas, hematologic malignancies, and breast cancer, with a significantly higher frequency of all cancers combined. Chronic PCB exposure entails an increased likelihood of obesity, hypertension, diabetes, and other endocrine dysfunction, perhaps related to higher levels of oxidative stress and inflammation.

Biologic Toxins Are Organisms and Their Nonviable Components

These toxins are mostly of microbial, algal, plant, protozoan, arthropod, or mammalian origin. They include whole organisms, intact particulate, or soluble products of those organisms (e.g., exotoxins), released aerosols and gases, and fragments of organisms. Unlike hypersensitivity (Chapter 4) and infectious (Chapter 9) reactions, toxic reactions tend to be dose dependent and generally entail substantially higher levels of exposure (about 10-fold) than hypersensitivity or infections.

Organic Dust Toxic Syndrome

Organic dust toxic syndrome (**ODTS**) is a systemic reaction to the direct toxicities of many substances. These are often of fungal or bacterial origin. Flu-like symptoms begin about 4 to 8 hours after exposure: dyspnea, chest tightness, fever, myalgias, dry cough, fatigue, and leukocytosis. Generally, chest radiographs, blood gases, and pulmonary function are normal. Symptoms resolve in a few days.

Dust particles responsible for these symptoms are generally between 2 and 4 μm in diameter and deposit in terminal airways and alveoli. These elicit the greatest levels of macrophage-derived inflammatory cytokines. Exposures relate particularly to swine handling.

Other Toxic Biologic Products

Bacterial endotoxins, which are lipopolysaccharide constituents of gram-negative cell walls that are often complexed with proteins and phospholipids, may cause considerable inflammation. *Enterobacter, Pasteurella, Bacillus, Vibrio, Corynebacterium,* and *Pseudomonas* species are commonly responsible. On inhalation, these compounds elicit profuse pulmonary inflammation, involving release of inflammatory mediators (TNFα, IL-1, etc.), causing fever, pneumonitis, and pulmonary edema. Unlike other organic dusts, flu-like syndromes associated with endotoxin-containing dusts usually are associated with altered pulmonary function tests.

In addition, gram-positive bacterial products, in the form of muramic acid–containing **peptidoglycans**, comprise a high percentage of biologic materials in some pathogenic organic dusts. Other agents that elicit ODTS include *Actinomycetes, Aspergillus, Stachybotrys, Penicillium,* and *Fusarium* species. The latter agents are fungi, which are particularly abundant in water-damaged buildings and moist warm environments. Their mycotoxins include trichothecenes and β-1,3-glucans, which may elicit disease by ingestion and inhalational routes.

Gaseous products of plants and animals in confinement may also be toxic, including oxides of nitrogen (NO_x), H_2S, and ammonia. These are common products of decomposition of manure and the action of moisture and microorganisms on grains.

One particular toxin produced by *Aspergillus flavus* and *Aspergillus parasiticus,* called **aflatoxin**, is highly hepatotoxic and is recognized as a potent hepatocarcinogen. There are several known varieties of aflatoxin.

Biologic toxins are of considerable concern because of possible weaponization for use in biologic warfare (**see Chapter 9**).

ULTRAVIOLET LIGHT

UV light is beyond the visible range of solar electromagnetic emissions and is subdivided into UV-A, UV-B, and UV-C (320–400, 280–320, 200–280 nm, respectively). UV-C radiation is ionizing: It can act as a mutagen and is a leading cause of skin cancer (**see Chapters 5 and 28**). UV-B radiation stimulates endogenous production of previtamin D3, a precursor for vitamin D, from a cholesterol derivative.

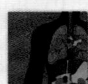 **PATHOPHYSIOLOGY:** UV-B radiation promotes keratinocyte injury via several mechanisms. It causes DNA adducts that are removed by nucleotide excision-repair (NER) mechanisms (**see Chapter 1**). This activates cell-cycle checkpoints and DNA repair. NER works via single-stranded DNA intermediates, which are inherently more fragile than double-stranded DNA, and so susceptible to recombination. This is particularly problematic if NER mechanisms are impaired because in that case DNA repair then generates larger single-stranded intermediates to be repaired by other mechanisms.

UV radiation, particularly UV-B, causes inflammatory reactions, as part of which the proinflammatory cytokine, TNFα, is produced. There is evidence suggesting that TNFα inhibits the G2/M cell-cycle checkpoint (by a mechanism involving Akt and mTOR) and so prevents DNA repair. Thus, the combination of UV-related DNA injury, inflammation, and DNA repair mechanisms gone awry may help explain the carcinogenic effects of UV radiation.

IONIZING RADIATION

Ionizing radiation is electromagnetic, and particle emissions can ionize—that is, remove electrons from atoms and molecules. This includes UV-C, x-rays, and gamma radiation, as well as alpha and beta particles. It does not include lower-energy UV irradiation, visible light, infrared radiation, or microwave radiation.
Radiation is quantitated in several ways:

- **A roentgen** is a measure of radiant energy emission and reflects the amount of ionization produced in air.
- **A rad** measures energy absorption, which is the biologically more important parameter. It is energy, expressed as ergs, absorbed by a tissue, and 1 rad is defined as 100 ergs absorbed per gram of tissue.
- **A gray** (Gy) corresponds to 100 rads (1 joule/kg of tissue). A centigray (cGy) is equivalent to 1 rad.
- **The rem** was introduced to describe the biologic effect caused by a rad of high-energy radiation since low-energy particles produce more biologic damage than gamma or x-rays.
- **A sievert** (Sv) is a unit for measuring health effects, particularly for small amounts of ionizing radiation. 1 Sv = 1 joule/kg tissue. It is derived from the dose in Gy,

multiplied by a quality factor Q. Thus, 1 Sv is the equivalent in biologic effectiveness to 1 Gy of gamma rays.

For the purposes of this discussion of radiation-related pathology, rad, Gy, rem, and sievert are considered comparable.

PATHOPHYSIOLOGY: At the cellular level, radiation essentially has two effects: (1) acute cell killing; and (2) genetic damage. Radiation-induced cell death is considered to be caused by the acute effects of radiolysis of water (**see Chapter 1**). Consequent production of ROS may lead to lipid peroxidation, membrane injury, and possibly interaction with macromolecules of the cell. Genetic damage to the cell caused indirectly by a reaction of DNA with oxygen radicals is expressed either as mutation or as reproductive failure. Both mutation and reproductive failure may lead to delayed cell death, and mutation is involved in radiation-induced neoplasia.

Different tissues are differently sensitive to radiation. A tissue's vulnerability to radiation-induced damage depends on its proliferative rate, which, in turn, correlates with the natural life span of the constituent cells. Thus, the intestine and hematopoietic bone marrow are far more vulnerable than are less mitotically active tissues such as bone and brain. DNA damage in long-lived, nonproliferating cells does not necessarily impair their function or viability because reproductive and metabolic properties are separate. On the other hand, short-lived, actively proliferating cells, such as intestinal crypt cells or hematopoietic precursors, must be rapidly replaced by progeny of dividing precursor cells. If radiation-induced DNA damage prevents these cells from undergoing mitosis, mature cells are not replaced and the tissue loses function.

It is important to distinguish between whole-body irradiation and localized irradiation. Except for unusual circumstances, as in the high-dose irradiation that precedes bone marrow transplantation, significant levels of whole-body irradiation result only from industrial accidents or from nuclear weapons explosions. Localized irradiation is an inevitable by-product of any diagnostic radiologic procedure, and it is the intended result of radiation therapy. Rapid somatic cell death occurs only with extremely high radiation doses, well in excess of 10 Gy. It is morphologically indistinguishable from coagulative necrosis from other causes (**see Chapter 1**). Irreversible damage to the replicative capacity of cells involves far lower doses, possibly only 50 cGy.

High-Dose, Whole-Body Irradiation Injures Many Organs

Fortunately, human exposure to high doses of whole-body irradiation is very rare and most of our information has been derived from studies of Japanese atom bomb survivors. Additional information comes from the studies of people exposed in the accident at the Chernobyl nuclear power plant in Ukraine in 1986.

Since comparable doses of radiant energy are transmitted to all organs in whole-body irradiation, development of the different acute radiation syndromes reflects the dissimilarities in vulnerability of the target tissues (Fig. 8-8).

- **300 cGy:** At this dose of whole-body radiation, a syndrome characterized by **hematopoietic failure** develops within 2 weeks. After initial depletion of circulating lymphocytes, a progressive decrease in formed elements of the blood eventually leads to bleeding, anemia, and infection. The last is often the cause of death.

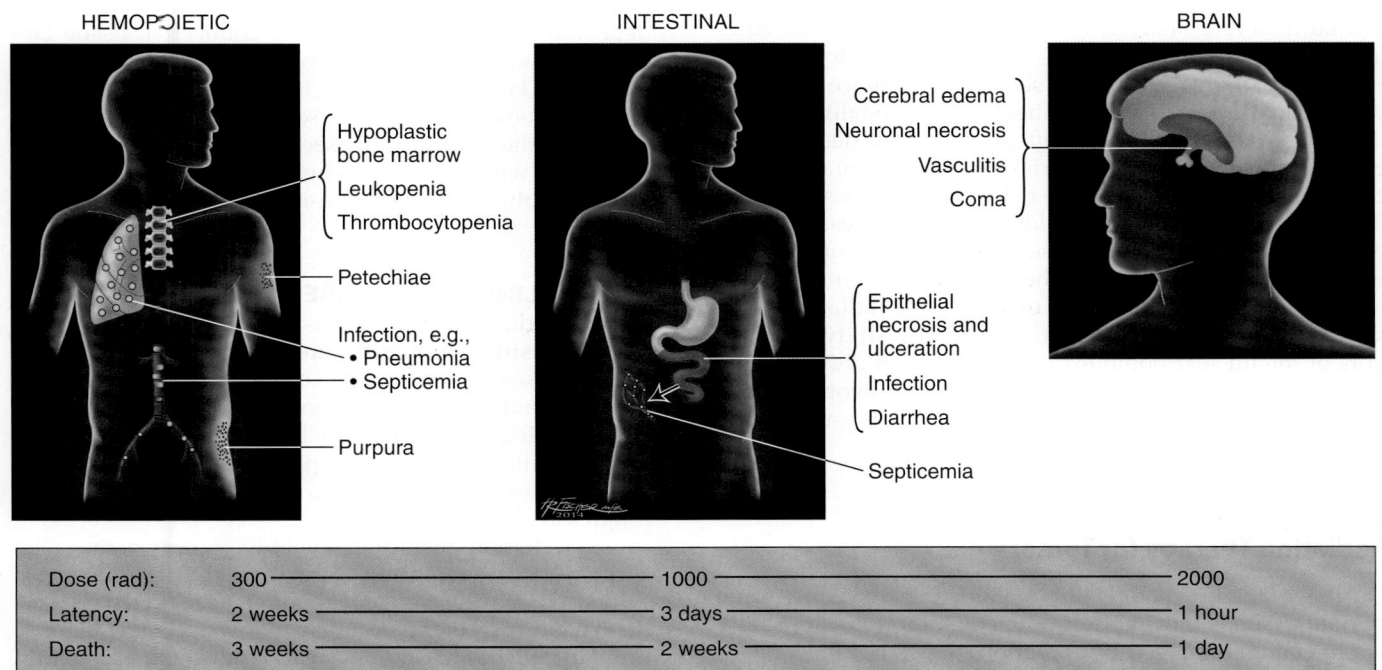

Dose (rad):	300	1000	2000
Latency:	2 weeks	3 days	1 hour
Death:	3 weeks	2 weeks	1 day

FIGURE 8-8. Acute radiation syndromes. At a dose of approximately 300 rads of whole-body radiation, a syndrome characterized by hematopoietic failure develops within 2 weeks. In the vicinity of 1,000 rads, a gastrointestinal syndrome with a latency of only 3 days is seen. With doses of 2,000 rads or more, disease of the central nervous system appears within 1 hour and death ensues rapidly.

- **10 Gy:** At these levels, the main cause of death is related to the **digestive tract**. GI symptoms occur through the entire dose range of whole-body exposures. At higher levels, the entire GI epithelium is destroyed within 3 days (i.e., the normal life span of villous and crypt cells). As a result, fluid homeostasis of the bowel is disrupted and severe diarrhea and dehydration ensue. Moreover, the epithelial barrier to intestinal bacteria is breached; gut organisms invade and disseminate throughout the body. Septicemia and shock kill the victim.

- **20 Gy:** With whole-body doses of 20 Gy and above, CNS damage causes death within hours. In most cases, endothelial injury leads to loss of the integrity of the blood–brain barrier, causing cerebral edema. At extreme doses, radiation necrosis of neurons occurs, followed by convulsions, coma, and death.

FETAL EFFECTS: The effects of whole-body irradiation on the human fetus have been documented in studies of Hiroshima nuclear bomb survivors. Pregnant women exposed to 25 cGy or more gave birth to infants with reduced head size, diminished overall growth, and mental retardation.

Children exposed to therapeutic doses of radiation between the 3rd and 20th weeks of gestation showed growth retardation and microcephaly. Other effects of irradiation in utero include hydrocephaly, microphthalmia, chorioretinitis, blindness, spina bifida, cleft palate, clubfeet, and genital abnormalities. Experimental and human studies suggest that major congenital malformations are very unlikely at doses below 20 cGy after day 14 of pregnancy. However, lower doses may produce more subtle effects, such as decreased mental capacity. *To protect against such a possibility, the established maximum permissible dose of radiation to the fetus from exposure of the expectant mother is far below the known teratogenic dose.*

GENETIC EFFECTS: Most data on which predictions of human genetic effects are based are derived from experimental data and analysis of nuclear bomb survivors. After long-term follow-up, survivors of the nuclear detonations at Hiroshima and Nagasaki have shown no evidence of genetic damage in the form of either congenital abnormalities or heritable diseases in subsequent offspring or their descendants. In experimental animals, the risk of induced mutation per cGy is at most 0.5% to 5% of the risk of spontaneous mutation (the spontaneous risk of mutation in humans is estimated to be 10% of live births). By extension, 20 to 200 cGy of radiation would approximately double the spontaneous mutation rate.

AGING: There is to date no evidence that radiation exposure leads to premature aging. A mortality study of survivors of the nuclear bomb explosions in Japan did not show excess mortality beyond that attributable to neoplasia, nor is there any evidence of acceleration in disease among the survivors in any part of the age range.

Localized Radiation Injury May Follow Radiation Therapy for Tumors

During radiation therapy for malignant neoplasms, some normal tissue is inevitably irradiated. Although almost any organ can be damaged by radiation, the skin, lungs, heart, kidney, bladder, and intestine are susceptible and difficult to shield (Fig. 8-9). The immense reserve capacity of the hematopoietic system limits functional damage due to localized irradiation of the bone marrow.

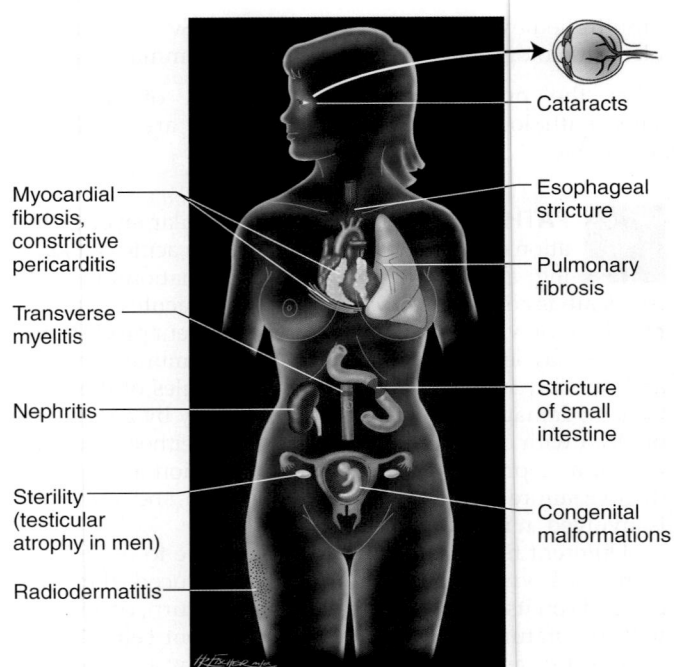

FIGURE 8-9. The nonneoplastic complications of radiation.

PATHOLOGY: Persistent damage to radiation-exposed tissue reflects (1) compromise of the vascular supply and (2) fibrotic repair reaction to acute necrosis and chronic ischemia. Radiation-induced tissue injury predominantly affects small arteries and arterioles. Endothelial cells are the most sensitive elements in blood vessels and show swelling and necrosis in the short term. With time, vascular walls become thickened by endothelial cell proliferation and subintimal deposition of collagen and other connective tissue elements. Striking vacuolization of intimal cells (foam cells) is typical. Fragmentation of the internal elastic lamina, loss of smooth muscle cells, scarring in the media, and fibrosis of the adventitia are seen in small arteries. Bizarre fibroblasts with large hyperchromatic nuclei are common and probably reflect radiation-induced DNA damage.

CLINICAL FEATURES: Acute necrosis from radiation presents as **radiation pneumonitis, cystitis, dermatitis**, and **diarrhea from enteritis**. Chronic disease is characterized by **interstitial fibrosis** in the heart and lungs, esophageal and intestinal **strictures**, and **constrictive pericarditis**. Chronic **radiation nephritis**, which simulates malignant nephrosclerosis, is primarily a vascular disease that leads to severe hypertension and progressive renal insufficiency.

As radiation therapy inevitably traverses the skin, it often causes **radiation dermatitis**. Initial damage is evidenced by blood vessel dilation, recognized as **erythema**. Necrosis of the skin may follow and may linger as **indolent ulcers** that do not heal because the epithelium cannot regenerate. Impaired wound repair in irradiated tissues may pose serious problems for surgeons operating in those areas. **Poorly healed** or **dehisced wounds** or

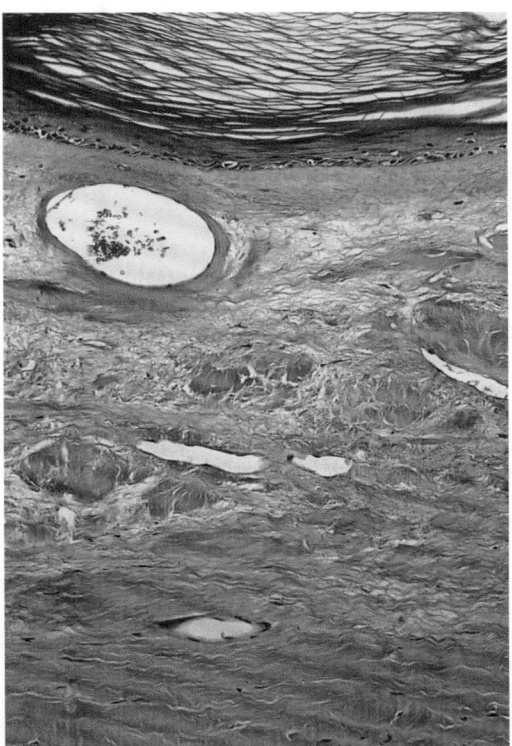

FIGURE 8-10. Chronic radiation dermatitis. The epidermis is atrophic. The dermis is densely fibrotic and contains dilated superficial blood vessels.

persistent ulcers often require full-thickness skin grafts. **Chronic radiation dermatitis** results from repair and revascularization of the skin and is characterized by atrophy, hyperkeratosis, telangiectasia, and hyperpigmentation (Fig. 8-10).

The **gonads,** both testes and ovaries, are similar to other tissues in their dependence on continuous cell cycling and are exquisitely radiosensitive. Acute inhibition of mitosis in the testis causes loss of spermatogonia, the germinal stem cells. The combination of radiation-induced vascular injury and direct damage to the germ cells leads to progressive atrophy of seminiferous tubules, peritubular fibrosis, and loss of reproductive function. Interstitial and Sertoli cells do not cycle rapidly and so persist, thus preserving normal hormonal status. Comparable injury occurs in irradiated ovaries: Follicles become atretic, and the organ eventually becomes fibrous and atrophic.

Cataracts (lenticular opacities) may be produced if the eye lies in the path of the radiation beam. **Transverse myelitis** and paraplegia occur when the spinal cord is unavoidably irradiated during treatment of certain thoracic or abdominal tumors. **Vascular damage in the cord** may bring about localized ischemia.

High Doses of Radiation Cause Cancer

The evidence that radiation can lead to cancer is incontrovertible and comes from many sources (Fig. 8-11). In the early part of the 20th century, scientists and radiologists tested their x-ray equipment by placing their hands in the path of the beam. As a result, they developed basal and squamous cell carcinomas of the exposed skin. In addition, early instruments were not well shielded and the hazards associated with fluoroscopy were not appreciated. Radiologists of that era suffered an unusually high incidence of leukemia. This situation has been rectified with the use of modern shielding and protective equipment.

An unusual occupational exposure to radiation occurred among workers who painted radium onto watches to create luminous dials. These workers often licked their paint brushes to produce a point and so ingested the radium. Since the body handles radium as it does in the case of calcium, it subsequently localized in their bones, exposing them to a long-lived isotope that persisted in their bones indefinitely. These people experienced a high incidence of cancer of the bone and of the paranasal sinuses. Another example of occupational exposure to a radioactive element is the high rate of lung cancer in uranium miners who inhaled radioactive dust and radon gas. Chronic exposure to radon caused lung cancer with substantially increased frequency in these miners, whether they smoked or not.

Iodine is concentrated by the thyroid. Inhaled or ingested radioactive iodine isotopes expose the thyroid to highly concentrated radioactivity. An explosive increase in the incidence of thyroid cancer among children in geographical areas contaminated by the nuclear catastrophe at Chernobyl in Ukraine in 1986 has been linked to release of radioactive iodine isotopes in that incident.

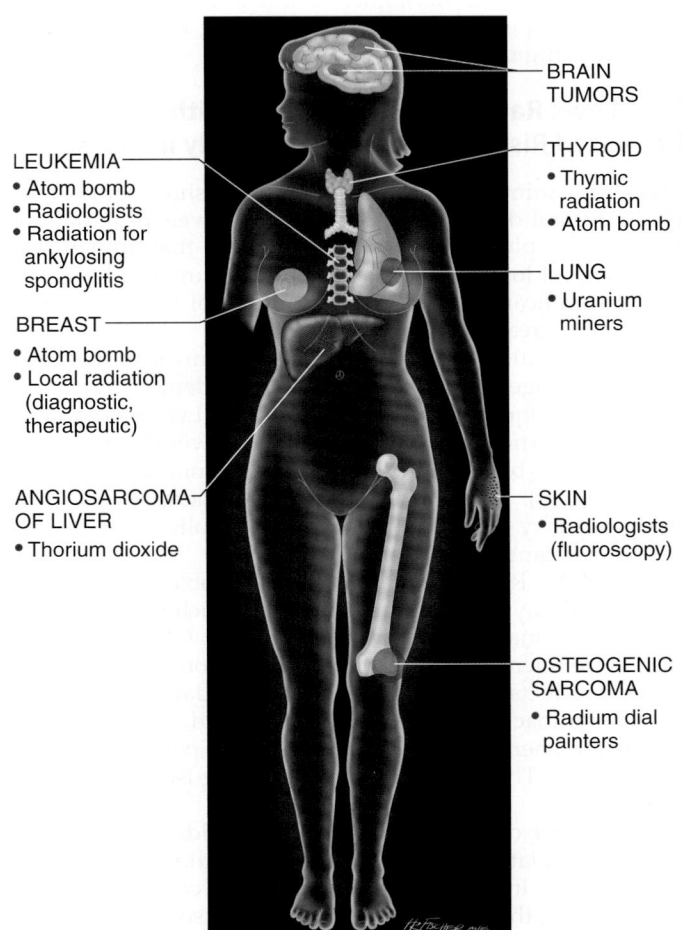

FIGURE 8-11. Radiation-induced cancers.

The survivors of the nuclear bomb explosions in Japan had a more than 10-fold increase in the incidence of leukemia, which peaked 5 to 10 years after exposure and then declined to background rates. Two-thirds were cases of acute leukemia; the remainder were of chronic myeloid leukemias. Chronic lymphocytic leukemia, which is uncommon in Japan, did not increase. The risk of multiple myeloma increased fivefold, and the incidence of lymphoma increased slightly. The frequency of solid tumors was clearly increased for the breast, lung, thyroid, GI tract, and urinary tract, although not as much as for leukemia. The development of radiation-related malignant tumors, including leukemia, showed a dose–response relationship.

Iatrogenic Radiation Exposure and Cancers

The risk of **solid tumors**, especially breast cancer, is particularly high among adult women who were treated during childhood with thoracic radiation for Hodgkin disease. They have almost a 20-fold increased risk of developing a second neoplasm due to the radiation. In Great Britain, patients with ankylosing spondylitis were once treated with low-dose spinal irradiation. They later developed aplastic anemia, acute myelogenous leukemia (AML), and other tumors with a high frequency. An increase in brain tumors occurred in people who had received cranial irradiation for tinea capitis infection of the scalp in childhood. Thorium dioxide (Thorotrast), which is avidly ingested by phagocytic cells, was once used for radionuclide imaging. This long-lived radioisotope persisted in the liver, leading to development of hepatic angiosarcomas.

Low-Level Radiation Is Associated With an Increased Risk of Cancers, Particularly in Children

Data from animal studies and cell culture show some DNA chromosomal damage even at very low levels of radiation. Large-scale epidemiologic studies indicate that human risk in settings of low levels of radiation exposure may be statistically significant even as the magnitude of that risk is not necessarily great.

Thus, a study of almost 120,000 US nuclear workers, whose average exposure was 20 mSv, demonstrated an increased frequency of many cancers. Lymphoma and myeloma, particularly, were increased, as were tumors considered not to be related to smoking (e.g., bone, breast, CNS, thyroid, skin). The magnitude of those increases was not large, but they were dose related, and results were statistically significant.

RADON: Radon is a radioactive noble gas formed from the decay of uranium 238 (^{238}U), which occurs in soil and rock formations. Radon itself is inert. Concerns about the environmental hazards of radon focus on its radioactive decay products, which are called radon daughters. These include radioactive isotopes of bismuth, lead, and polonium, which are chemically active and bind to particulates and lung tissues. The half-life of the α-emitting isotope, ^{218}Po, is 103 years.

A number of very large studies of children exposed to low-level radiation have been reported. Although they vary, as expected, in specifics and in overall conclusions, the trend among those studies supports the association of low-level childhood exposure to radiation with development of childhood leukemias and CNS malignancies. For example,

a study of over 2,000,000 Swiss children demonstrated a significantly increased incidence of leukemia and CNS tumors, in a dose-related fashion, due to exposure to radiation from natural sources (radon, terrestrial gamma irradiation, etc.).

Microwave Radiation, Electromagnetic Fields, and Ultrasound Are Not Ionizing

Microwaves, produced by ovens, radar, and diathermy, are electromagnetic waves that penetrate tissue but do not produce ionization. Unlike x-rays and gamma radiation, absorption of microwave energy produces only heat and not light. The activation energy of radiofrequency and microwave radiation is too low to modify chemical bonds or alter DNA. Thus, exposure to microwave radiation under ordinary circumstances is highly unlikely to produce any injury. A study of 20,000 radar technicians in the Navy who were chronically exposed to high levels of microwave radiation failed to detect any increased incidence of cancer. Similarly, nonionizing electromagnetic fields, as occur nearby high-voltage electric lines, have not been found to increase the incidence of leukemia or other cancers.

Ultrasound, air vibrations above the audible range, produces mechanical compression but no ionization. Highly focused and energetic ultrasound devices can disrupt tissues in vitro during chemical analysis and while cleaning various surfaces, including teeth. However, there is no reason to believe that diagnostic ultrasound or accidental exposure to any industrial ultrasound device results in any measurable harm.

Diseases due to Agents Consumed

SMOKING

Tobacco smoking is the single largest preventable cause of death in the United States. *About 480,000 premature deaths per year—about one-fifth of the total—occur because of smoking.* The Surgeon General in 2014[2] incriminated tobacco in 48% of cancer deaths, 19% of deaths from cardiovascular and metabolic diseases, 61% of deaths from nonmalignant lung diseases, and 8% of perinatal deaths (see above regarding ETS). Smoking shortens life expectancy, and overall mortality is proportional to the amount and duration of cigarette smoking, commonly quantitated as "pack-years" (Fig. 8-12). Thus, someone who smokes two packs of cigarettes a day at the age of 30 years will live an average of 8 years less than a nonsmoker.

Smoking-related illness affects men and women about equally. Thus, smoking-related illnesses reflect the amount smoked, not the gender of the smoker. Mortality from lung cancer, almost all of which is related to cigarette smoking, exceeds that from cancers of the breast and prostate, which are the most common cancers of women and men, respectively, in the United States. The excess mortality

---

[2]*The Health Consequences of Smoking—50 Years of Progress: A Report of the Surgeon General.* Rockville, MD: U.S. Department of Health and Human Services; 2014.

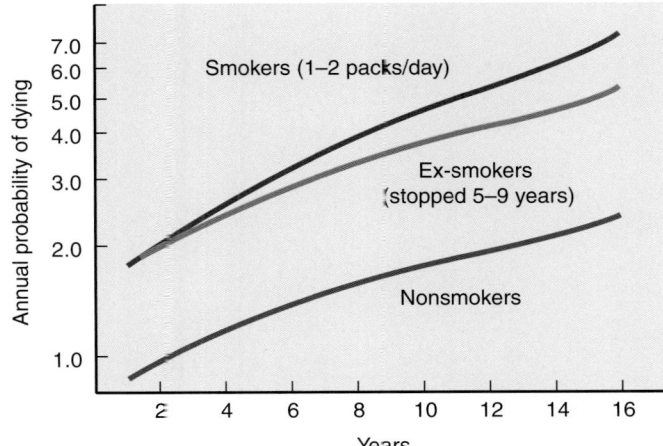

FIGURE 8-12. The risk of dying in smokers and nonsmokers. Note that the annual probability of an individual dying, indicated on the ordinate, is a logarithmic scale. Individuals who have smoked for 1 year have a twofold greater probability of dying than a nonsmoker, whereas those who have smoked for more than 15 years have more than a threefold greater probability of dying.

associated with cigarette smoking declines after one quits smoking: By 15 years of abstinence from cigarettes, mortality in ex-smokers from all causes approaches that of people who have never smoked. Cancer mortality among those who smoke only cigars or pipes is somewhat greater than that of the nonsmoking population. Smokeless tobacco (snuff, chewing tobacco) entails little, if any, increased risk of malignancy. However, the health risks associated with smoking electronic cigarettes ("vaping"), particularly among adolescents, have recently come to the fore. The US Surgeon General declared (September 2018) that nicotine in those e-cigarettes has harmful effects on brain function and development.

The major diseases responsible for excess mortality reported in cigarette smokers are, in order of frequency, many types of cancers, cardiovascular and metabolic diseases, and chronic pulmonary diseases. Cancers of the oral cavity, larynx, esophagus, pancreas, bladder, kidney, colon, liver, and cervix are all more common in smokers than in nonsmokers. Also, smokers show excess mortality from tuberculosis, atherosclerotic aortic aneurysms, and peptic ulcers. The effects of cigarette smoking on the organs of smokers are illustrated in Figure 8-13.

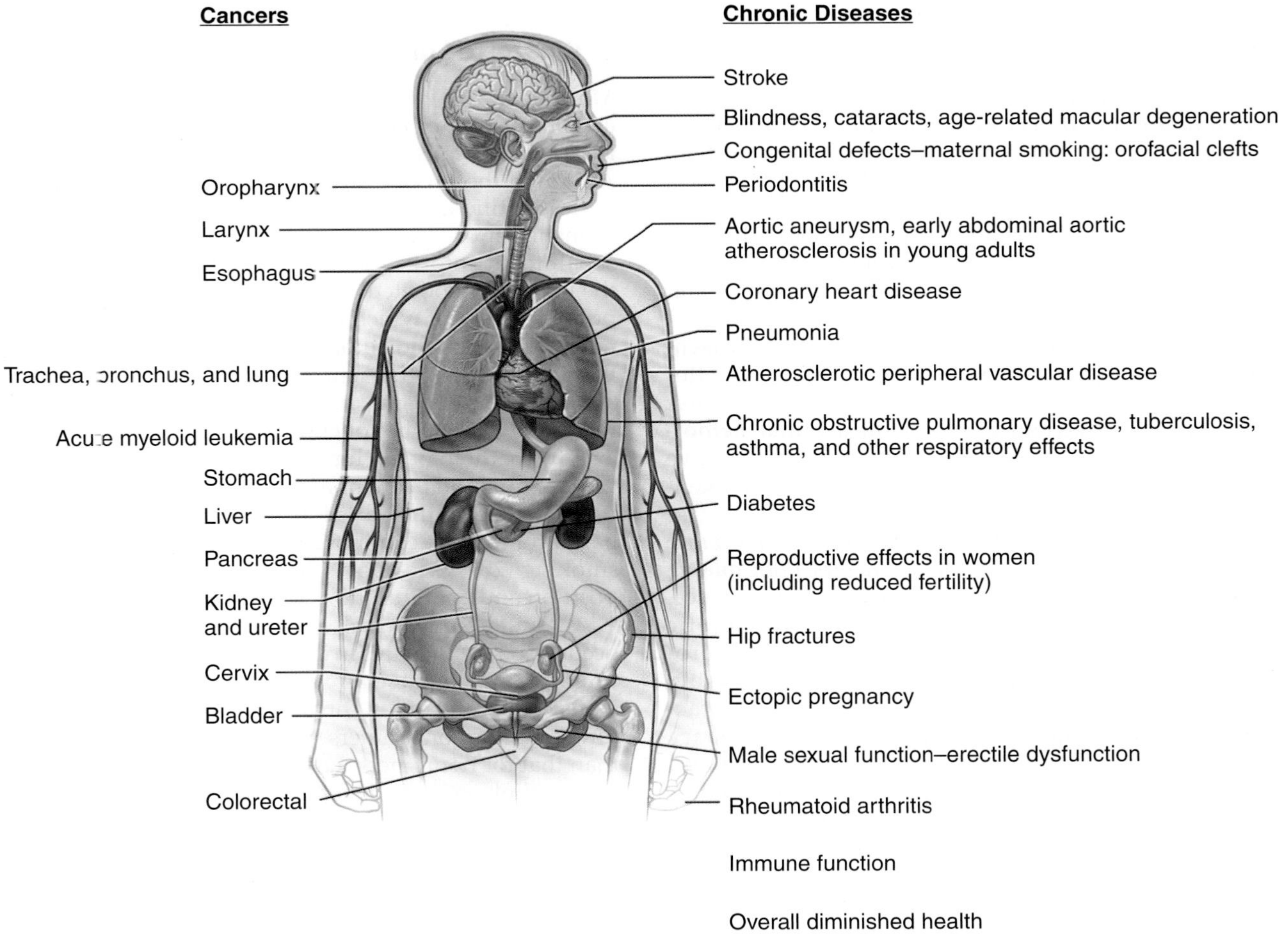

Cancers

Oropharynx
Larynx
Esophagus
Trachea, bronchus, and lung
Acute myeloid leukemia
Stomach
Liver
Pancreas
Kidney and ureter
Cervix
Bladder
Colorectal

Chronic Diseases

Stroke
Blindness, cataracts, age-related macular degeneration
Congenital defects–maternal smoking: orofacial clefts
Periodontitis
Aortic aneurysm, early abdominal aortic atherosclerosis in young adults
Coronary heart disease
Pneumonia
Atherosclerotic peripheral vascular disease
Chronic obstructive pulmonary disease, tuberculosis, asthma, and other respiratory effects
Diabetes
Reproductive effects in women (including reduced fertility)
Hip fractures
Ectopic pregnancy
Male sexual function–erectile dysfunction
Rheumatoid arthritis
Immune function
Overall diminished health

FIGURE 8-13. Organs affected by active cigarette smoking. (From U.S. Department of Health and Human Services. *The Health Consequences of Smoking: 50 Years of Progress. A Report of the Surgeon General.* Atlanta, GA: U.S. Department of Health and Human Services, Centers for Disease Control and Prevention, National Center for Chronic Disease Prevention and Health Promotion, Office on Smoking and Health; 2014.)

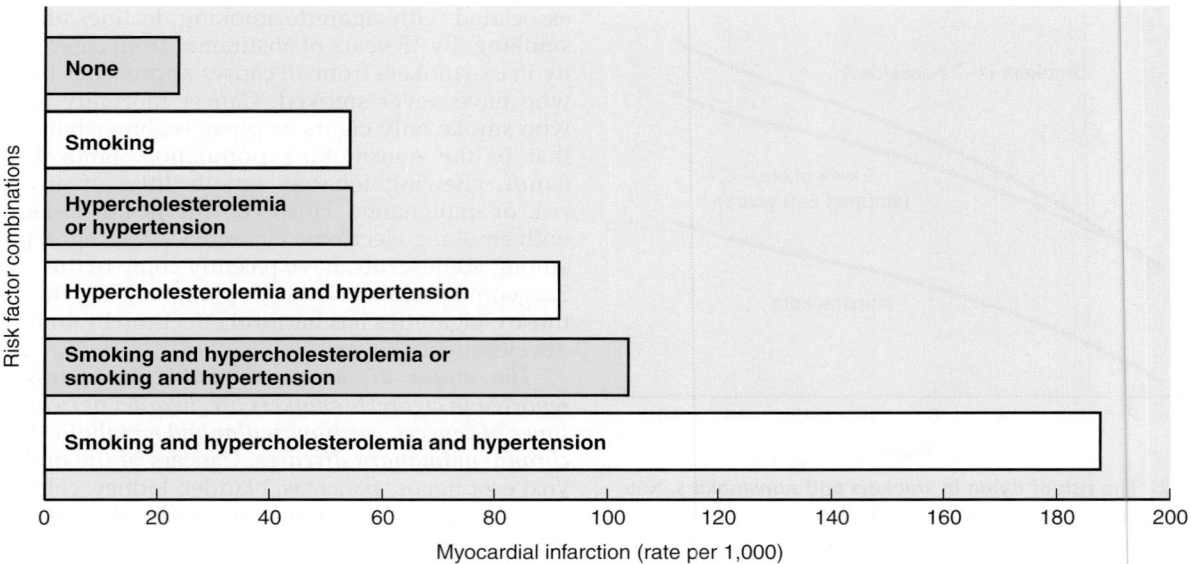

FIGURE 8-14. The risk of myocardial infarction in cigarette smokers. Smoking is an independent risk factor and increases the risk of a myocardial infarction to about the same extent as does hypertension or hypercholesterolemia alone. The effects of smoking are additive to those of these other two risk factors.

Cardiovascular Disease Is a Major Complication of Smoking

Cigarette smoking is a major independent risk factor for myocardial infarction. It acts synergistically with other risk factors such as elevated blood pressure and blood cholesterol levels (Fig. 8-14). Smoking precipitates initial myocardial infarction, increases the risk for second heart attacks, and impairs survival after a heart attack among those who continue to smoke. It also contributes to development of atherosclerotic plaques leading to ischemia and arrhythmias and increasing the incidence of sudden cardiac death.

Cigarette smoking is an independent risk factor for **ischemic stroke**. The risk correlates with the number of cigarettes smoked and declines when one stops smoking. Tobacco use also increases risk of certain forms of **intracranial hemorrhage**. The combination of smoking and oral contraceptive (OC) use in women older than 35 years increases the likelihood of **myocardial infarction** and stroke.

Atherosclerosis of the coronary arteries and aorta is more severe and extensive among cigarette smokers than among nonsmokers, and the effect is dose related. As a consequence, cigarette smoking is a strong risk factor for **atherosclerotic aortic aneurysms**. The incidence and severity of **atherosclerotic peripheral vascular disease** are also remarkably increased by smoking. Smoking is also a major risk factor for **coronary vasospasm**. It disturbs regional coronary blood flow in patients with coronary artery disease and lowers the threshold for ventricular fibrillation and cardiac arrest in patients with established ischemic heart disease. Smoking-related pharmacologic actions of nicotine itself, carbon monoxide, reduced plasma high-density lipoprotein levels, increased plasma fibrinogen levels, and higher leukocyte counts may predispose to myocardial infarction.

Buerger disease, a peculiar inflammatory and occlusive disease of the lower leg vasculature, occurs almost only in heavy smokers (**see Chapter 16**).

Lung Cancer Is Largely a Disease of Cigarette Smokers

More than 85% of deaths from lung cancer, the single most common cause of cancer death in both men and women in the United States, are due to cigarette smoking (Fig. 8-15). Although the precise offenders in cigarette smoke have not been identified, cigarette smoke is toxic and carcinogenic to bronchial mucosa. Passing cigarette smoke through a filter separates it into gas and particulate phases. Cigarette tar, the material deposited on the filter, contains over 3,000 compounds, many of which have been identified as carcinogens, mucosal toxins, and ciliotoxic agents. Compounds with similar harmful properties are found in the gas phase, but they are fewer. Among smokers, the risk of lung cancer is directly related to the number of cigarettes smoked.

The pathology of lung cancers has changed over the years. Squamous carcinoma was once predominant, but it has declined with reduction in smoking. Adenocarcinoma has become more common. The Surgeon General's report on smoking (2014, see above) links this to changes in the composition and configuration of cigarettes.

Cigarette smoking also acts synergistically with certain occupational exposures in inducing **lung cancer**. For instance, uranium miners have an increased rate of lung cancer, presumably because they inhale radon daughters. The rate of lung cancer among miners who smoke is considerably higher than that for nonminers who smoke similarly. Also, although heavy smokers in the general population have 20-fold greater risk of lung cancer than nonsmokers, asbestos workers with interstitial pulmonary fibrosis (see above) who smoke heavily have a risk over 60 times that of nonsmokers.

■ **Cancers of the lip, tongue, and buccal mucosa** occur mainly (>90%) in tobacco users. All tobacco use—cigarette, cigar, and pipe smoking, as well as tobacco chewing—expose the oral cavity to the compounds found in raw tobacco or tobacco smoke.

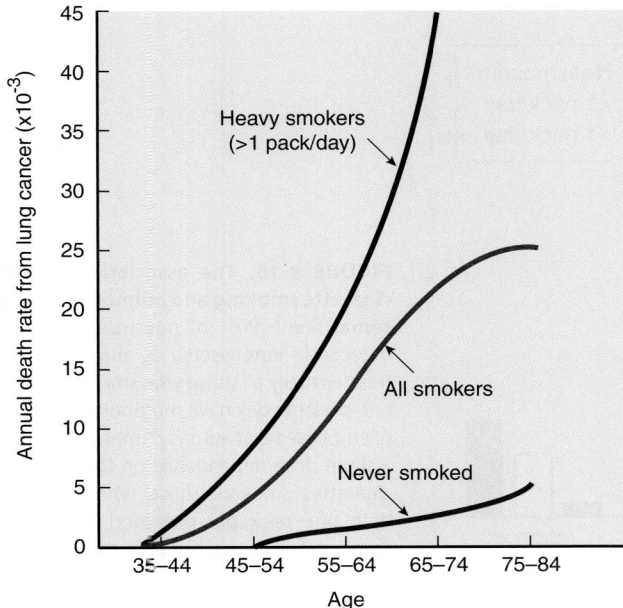

FIGURE 8-15. Death rate from lung cancer among smokers and nonsmokers. Nonsmokers exhibit a small, linear rise in the death rate from lung cancer from the age of 50 years onward. In contrast, those who smoke more than one pack per day show an exponential rise in the annual death rate from lung cancer starting at about the age of 35 years. By the age of 70 years, heavy smokers have about a 20-fold greater death rate from lung cancer than nonsmokers.

- **Laryngeal cancer** is similarly related to cigarette smoking. White male smokers have a 6 to 13 times greater death rate from laryngeal cancer than nonsmokers.
- **Cancer of the esophagus** in the United States and Great Britain is estimated to result from smoking in 80% of cases.
- **Bladder cancer** causes death in cigarette smokers twice as much as in nonsmokers. In fact, 30% to 40% of bladder cancers are attributable to smoking. As with most tobacco-related disorders, there is a clear dose–response relationship between incidence of bladder cancer and pack-years of cigarette smoking.
- **Carcinoma of the kidney** is increased 50% to 100% among smokers. A modest increase in cancer of the renal pelvis has also been documented.
- **Pancreatic cancer** has increased steadily in incidence, due, at least in part, to cigarette smoking. The risk ratio in male smokers for adenocarcinoma of the pancreas is two- to threefold, and a dose–response relationship exists. Men who smoke over 2 packs a day have a fivefold greater risk of pancreatic cancer than nonsmokers.
- **Cancer of the uterine cervix** is significantly more common in smokers. It has been estimated that about 30% of cervical cancer mortality is associated with smoking.
- **AML** in men occurs about twice as frequently as in male nonsmokers.
- **Colon and rectum cancers** are more common in active smokers, particularly heavy smokers, than in nonsmokers. The relative risk (RR, the ratio of risk for smokers compared to nonsmokers) is about 1.25. Smokers also have an increased risk for colonic adenomatous polyps,

which are premalignant precursors of adenocarcinomas (RR ≈ 1.5).
- **Liver cancers** may be caused by many environmental influences, such as hepatitis viruses and aflatoxin (**see above and Chapters 9 and 20**). However, cigarette smoking increases the risk of developing hepatic malignancies (RR ≈ 1.6) independently of other known risk factors.
- **Breast cancer** has been linked to cigarette smoking in active smokers and people exposed to ETS (see above). This association is best documented for premenopausal women. There is a relationship between risk for tobacco-related breast cancer and rapid acetylator phenotypes for the enzyme N-acetyltransferase-2.
- **Ovarian tumors** are more tenuously linked to tobacco smoking. A slightly increased incidence of borderline mucinous tumors of the ovary with cigarette smoking is reported. No such relationship is reported for other types of ovarian tumors.

Smokers Are at Higher Risk for Certain Nonneoplastic Diseases

- **Chronic bronchitis and emphysema** occur mostly in cigarette smokers. Incidence of these diseases is a function of the number of cigarettes smoked (Fig. 8-16; **see Chapter 18**).
- **Peptic ulcers** are 70% more common in male cigarette smokers than in nonsmokers.
- **Diabetes mellitus** type II occurs 30% to 40% more often in smokers. Several different mechanisms may contribute to this effect, including nicotine-related insulin resistance and β-cell apoptosis, increased central adiposity, and altered metabolism of estrogens and androgens in smokers.
- **Tuberculosis** is more severe in smokers, who are at an increased risk for its recrudescence and for tuberculosis-related death.
- **Asthma** incidence and exacerbations are increased in smokers compared to nonsmokers.
- **Impaired immune function,** affecting both innate and adaptive arms of the immune system, affects smokers. These effects are complex and difficult to summarize briefly but reflect cigarette smoke's pro-oxidant effects and specific responses induced by individual smoke components. However, although smoke acts as an irritant, it also impairs innate immune system recognition and other responses to pathogens, so smokers have an increased risk of respiratory infections. Cigarette smoke also alters T- and B-cell–mediated immune functions.
- **Seropositive rheumatoid arthritis** occurs more often among cigarette smokers.
- **Osteoporosis** in women is exacerbated by tobacco use. Women who smoke a pack of cigarettes daily during their reproductive period have a 5% to 10% deficit in bone density at menopause. This deficit is enough to increase the risk of bone fractures.
- **Thyroid diseases** are linked to cigarette smoking, especially Graves disease, and particularly when hyperthyroidism is complicated by exophthalmos.
- **Ocular diseases,** particularly macular degeneration and cataracts, are reported more frequently in smokers.
- **Brain development** may be impaired by nicotine in adolescent smokers.

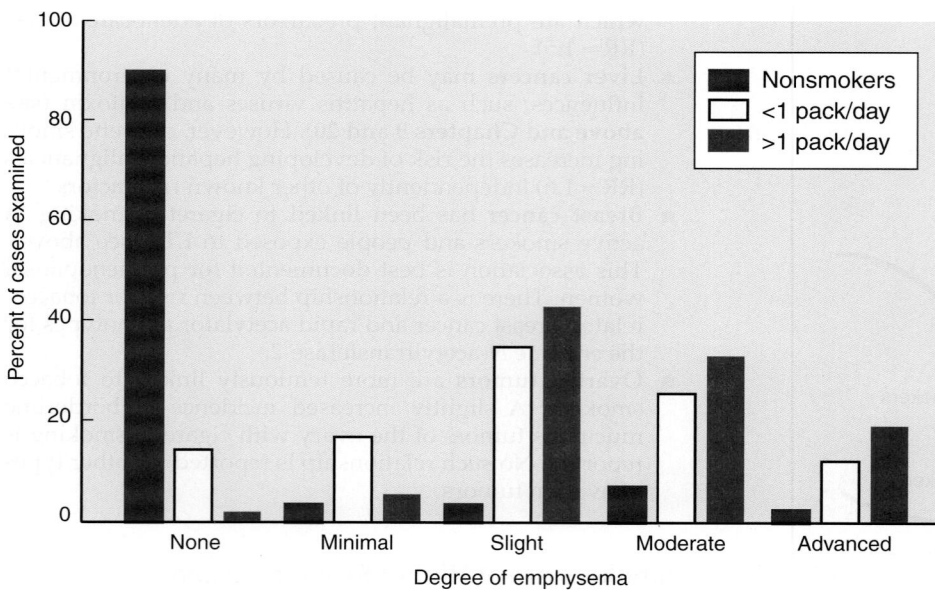

FIGURE 8-16. The association between cigarette smoking and pulmonary emphysema. Some 90% of nonsmokers have no detectable emphysema at autopsy. In contrast, virtually all those who smoke more than one pack per day have morphologic evidence of emphysema at autopsy. Emphysema shows a slight dose dependence on the number of cigarettes smoked. Those who smoke less than one pack per day tend to have less severe emphysema, but 85% to 90% of such smokers have some emphysema at autopsy.

Smoking Impairs Reproductive Function

Men who smoke are more susceptible to erectile dysfunction. Smoking women undergo **menopause earlier** than do nonsmokers, possibly because of the effects of tobacco on estrogen metabolism.

PATHOPHYSIOLOGY: In the liver, estradiol is hydroxylated to estrone, which then enters one of two irreversible metabolic pathways. In one, 16-hydroxylation leads to production of estriol, a potent estrogen. In the other, 2-hydroxylation yields methoxyestrone, which lacks estrogenic activity. In female smokers, the latter pathway (which leads to the inactive metabolite) is stimulated. Consequently, circulating levels of estriol, the active estrogen, are reduced. The increased incidence of postmenopausal osteoporosis in smokers has been attributed to decreased estriol levels. (Smoking stimulates same type of estrogen metabolism in men.)

ALCOHOLISM

Chronic alcoholism has been defined as regular intake of sufficient alcohol to injure a person socially, psychologically, or physically. Ethanol addiction entails dependence and withdrawal symptoms and leads to both acute and chronic toxic effects of alcohol on the body.

EPIDEMIOLOGY: There are about 15 to 18 million alcoholics in the United States, about one-tenth of the population at risk. The proportion is even higher in some other countries. Certain ethnic groups, such as Native Americans and Eskimos, have high rates of alcoholism, whereas others, such as Chinese and Jews, are less afflicted. Alcoholism is more common in men, but the number of female alcoholics has been increasing.

CLINICAL FEATURES: There are no firm rules, but for most people, daily consumption of more than 45 g of alcohol should probably be discouraged and 100 g or more a day may be dangerous (10 g alcohol = 1 oz, or 30 mL, of 86 proof [43%] spirits).

The short-term effects of alcohol on the brain are familiar to most people, but the mechanism of inebriation is not understood. Like other anesthetic agents, alcohol is a CNS depressant. However, it is such a weak anesthetic that it must be drunk by the glassful to exert any significant effect. In a normal person, characteristic behavioral changes can be detected at low alcohol concentrations (below 50 mg/dL). Levels above 80 mg/dL are usually associated with slower reaction times and gross incoordination and in American jurisdictions are considered legal evidence of intoxication while driving a motor vehicle. At levels above 300 mg/dL, most people become comatose, and at concentrations above 400 mg/dL, death from respiratory failure is common. In humans, the LD_{50} (median lethal dose) is about 5 g of alcohol per kilogram of body weight.

The situation is somewhat different in chronic alcoholics, who develop CNS tolerance to alcohol. Such individuals may easily tolerate blood alcohol levels of 100 to 200 mg/dL; in fatal automobile accidents, blood levels of 500 to 600 mg/dL or more have been found by medical examiners. The mechanism underlying tolerance has not been established.

Acute alcohol intoxication is dangerous. Some 28% of fatalities from motor vehicle accidents involve alcohol—currently, about 10,500 deaths annually in the United States. Alcoholism is also a major contributor to fatal home accidents, death in fires, and suicide.

Many chronic diseases associated with alcoholism were once attributed to malnutrition. Some alcoholics do suffer from nutritional deficiencies, such as thiamine deficiency (Wernicke encephalopathy) or folic acid deficiency (megaloblastic anemia), but *most alcoholics have adequate diets and most alcohol-related disorders reflect*

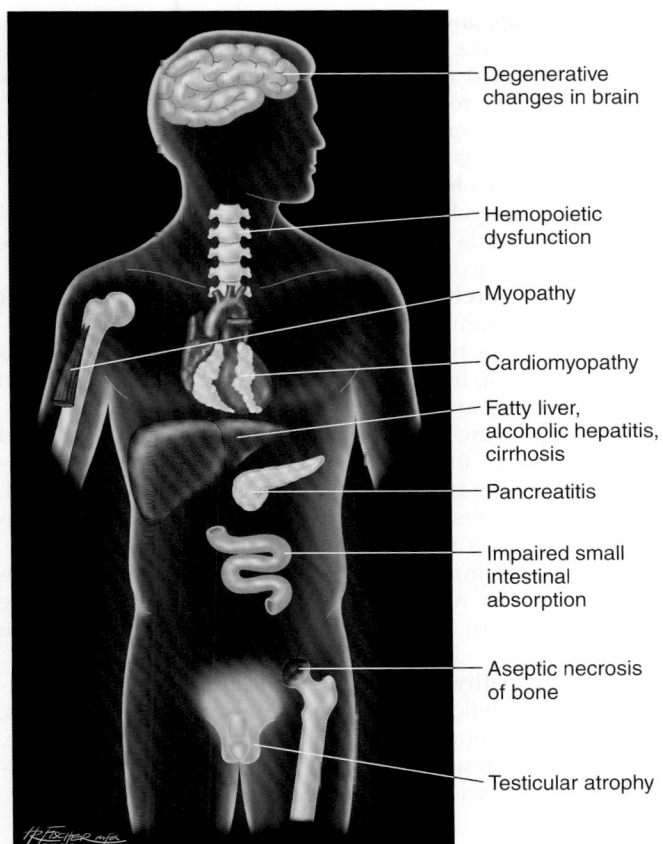

- Degenerative changes in brain
- Hemopoietic dysfunction
- Myopathy
- Cardiomyopathy
- Fatty liver, alcoholic hepatitis, cirrhosis
- Pancreatitis
- Impaired small intestinal absorption
- Aseptic necrosis of bone
- Testicular atrophy

FIGURE 8-17 Complications of chronic alcohol abuse.

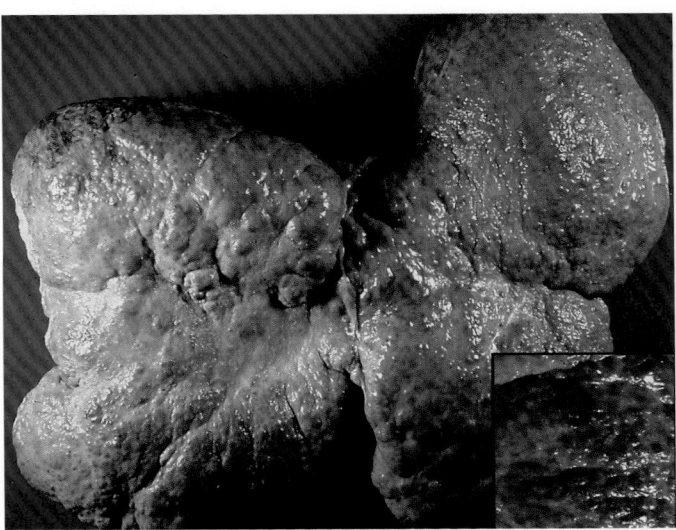

FIGURE 8-18. Cirrhosis of the liver in a chronic alcoholic. The surface displays innumerable small nodules of hepatocytes separated by interconnecting bands of fibrous tissue. These are highlighted in the higher magnification in the inset (lower right).

the toxic effects of alcohol alone. Diseases associated with alcoholism are discussed in detail in chapters dealing with individual organs; this discussion focuses on the spectrum of alcohol-related disease (Fig. 8-17).

Alcohol Impairs Functionality of Many Organs

Liver

Alcoholic liver disease, the most common medical complication of alcoholism, has been known for thousands of years and accounts for a large proportion of cases of cirrhosis of the liver (Fig. 8-18) in industrialized countries. The nature of the alcoholic beverage is largely irrelevant; consumed in excess, beer, wine, whiskey, hard cider, etc., all produce cirrhosis. Only the total dose of alcohol itself is relevant.

Pancreas

Both acute and chronic pancreatitides are complications of alcoholism, but they may be consequences of other disease processes as well (**see Chapter 23**). **Chronic calcifying pancreatitis**, on the other hand, is an unquestioned result of alcoholism and an important cause of incapacitating pain, pancreatic insufficiency, and pancreatic stones.

Heart

Alcohol-related heart disease was recognized over a century ago in Germany as "beer drinker's heart." This myocardial

degeneration, called **alcoholic cardiomyopathy**, is a form of dilated cardiomyopathy and leads to low-output congestive heart failure (**see Chapter 17**). Alcoholics' hearts also seem to be more susceptible to arrhythmias. Many cases of sudden death in alcoholics are probably caused by sudden, fatal arrhythmias.

In this context, moderate alcohol consumption, or "social drinking" (one to two drinks a day), provides significant protection against coronary artery disease (atherosclerosis) and its consequence, myocardial infarction. Similarly, compared with abstainers, social drinkers have a lower incidence of ischemic stroke.

Skeletal Muscle

Muscle weakness, particularly of proximal muscles, is common in alcoholics (**see Chapter 31**). Chronic alcoholics have many changes in skeletal muscles, from mild changes in muscle fibers detectable only by electron microscopy to severe, debilitating chronic myopathy, with degeneration of muscle fibers and diffuse fibrosis. Rarely, **acute alcoholic rhabdomyolysis**—necrosis of muscle fibers and release of myoglobin into the circulation—occurs. This sudden event can be fatal because of renal failure secondary to myoglobinuria.

Endocrine System

In male alcoholics, feminization and loss of libido and potency are common. Breasts may become enlarged (gynecomastia), body hair is lost, and a female distribution of pubic hair (female escutcheon) develops. Some of these changes reflect impaired hepatic estrogen metabolism due to chronic liver disease, but many of the changes—particularly testicular atrophy—occur even without liver disease. Chronic alcoholism leads to lower circulating testosterone levels because of a complex interference with the pituitary–gonadal axis, possibly complicated by accelerated hepatic metabolism of testosterone. Alcohol has a direct toxic effect on the testes;

thus, male sexual impairment is one of the prices exacted by alcoholism.

Gastrointestinal Tract

Since esophageal and gastric mucosae may be exposed to 10 M ethanol, it is not surprising that these organs suffer alcohol's direct toxic effects. Such mucosal injury is potentiated by hypersecretion of gastric hydrochloric acid stimulated by ethanol. **Reflux esophagitis** may be particularly painful, and peptic ulcers are also more common in alcoholics. Violent retching may lead to tears at the gastroesophageal junction **(Mallory–Weiss syndrome)**, sometimes severe enough to cause exsanguinating hemorrhage **(see Chapter 19)**. Small intestine mucosal cells are also exposed to circulating alcohol and develop diverse absorptive abnormalities. Alcohol inhibits active transport of amino acids, thiamine, and vitamin B_{12}.

Blood

Megaloblastic anemia is not uncommon among alcoholics. It reflects the facts that alcoholics often have dietary folate deficiency, plus the facts that alcohol both impairs folic acid absorption in the small intestine and is a weak folic acid antagonist. In addition, chronic ethanol intoxication leads directly to **increased erythrocyte mean corpuscular volume**. In alcoholic cirrhosis, the spleen is often enlarged because of portal hypertension, in which case, **hypersplenism** may cause **hemolytic anemia**. Transient **thrombocytopenia** is common after acute alcohol intoxication and may cause bleeding. Ethanol impairs platelet aggregation, further contributing to bleeding.

Bone

Chronic alcoholics, particularly postmenopausal women, are at an increased risk for **osteoporosis**. Alcohol inhibits osteoblast function, but the precise mechanism of alcohol-induced accelerated bone loss is not understood. Interestingly, moderate alcohol intake seems to protect from osteoporosis. Male alcoholics have an unusually high incidence of **aseptic necrosis of the head of the femur**, the mechanism for which is also obscure.

Immune System

Alcoholics are prone to many infections (particularly pneumonias) with organisms that are unusual in the general population, such as *Haemophilus influenzae*. They have an increased incidence of sepsis and ARDS. Alcohol hinders the body's physical barrier functions, including gut mucosa and respiratory ciliary clearance, impairs innate and adaptive immunity and other defenses, and interferes with tissue recovery from injury.

Nervous System

Cerebral cortical atrophy is common in alcoholics and may reflect direct alcohol toxicity **(see Chapter 32)**. Alcohol-related brain diseases often reflect nutritional deficiencies that are common in alcoholics.

- **Alcohol-related dementia (ARD)** entails progressive loss of cognitive and intellectual functions, not generally affecting memory. Decreases in the prefrontal, corpus callosum, and cerebellar white matter are characteristic.

These losses, and clinical signs, may be partly reversible with abstinence. Alcohol-induced inhibition of *N*-methyl-D-aspartic acid (NMDA) receptors, leading to oxidative stress, may be responsible.

- **Wernicke encephalopathy**, with confusion, ataxia, and neuropathies, is due to thiamine deficiency (see below) and affects alcoholics (and others) with poor diet.
- **Korsakoff psychosis** entails amnesias, apathy, and confabulation. It is poorly understood and may reflect the interplay of alcoholism and thiamine deficiency.
- **Alcoholic cerebellar degeneration** differs from other acquired or familial cerebellar degeneration by the uniformity of its manifestations. Progressive unsteadiness of gait, ataxia, incoordination, and reduced deep tendon reflex activity are present.
- **Central pontine myelinolysis (CPM)** is apparently caused by electrolyte imbalance—usually after electrolyte therapy following an alcoholic binge or during withdrawal. In CPM, progressive weakness of bulbar muscles eventuates in respiratory paralysis.
- **Amblyopia** (impaired vision) occurs occasionally in alcoholics. It may reflect alcohol-related decreases in tissue vitamin A, but other vitamin deficiencies may also be involved.
- **Polyneuropathy** is common in chronic alcoholics. It usually reflects deficiencies of thiamine and other B vitamins, but a direct neurotoxic effect of ethanol may play a role. The most common complaints include numbness, paresthesias, pain, weakness, and ataxia.

Fetal Alcohol Syndrome Results From Alcohol Abuse in Pregnancy

Infants born to mothers who consume excess alcohol during pregnancy may show a cluster of abnormalities that together constitute the fetal alcohol syndrome. These include growth retardation, microcephaly, facial dysmorphology, neurologic dysfunction, and other congenital anomalies. About 6% of the offspring of alcoholic mothers manifest the full syndrome. More often, fetal exposure to high concentrations of ethanol leads to less severe abnormalities, prominent among which are mental retardation, IUGR, and minor dysmorphic features **(see Chapter 6)**. Alcohol is an antagonist of NMDA and GABA-mimetic neurotransmitters and can trigger neuron apoptosis.

Alcohol Increases the Risk of Some Cancers

Cancers of the oral cavity, larynx, and esophagus occur more often in alcoholics than in the general population. As most alcoholics are also smokers, the differential contributions of ethanol and cigarette smoke to these observed increases are not well defined. The risk of hepatocellular carcinoma is increased in patients with alcoholic cirrhosis. Although the issue remains contentious, alcohol consumption is associated with an increased risk of breast cancer in a dose-dependent fashion.

The Mechanisms by Which Alcohol Injures Tissues Are Not Understood

The pathogenesis of ethanol-induced organ damage remains obscure. In a number of experimental settings, ethanol and its metabolites have been shown to have harmful effects on cells.

Among these are changes in redox potential (NAD/NADH ratio). In addition, ethanol may lead to formation of unusual compounds such as the first metabolite of ethanol oxidation, acetaldehyde, protein adducts, fatty acid ethyl esters, and phosphatidyl ethanol. It also increases production of ROS (see Chapter 1) and tends to intercalate between phospholipids within biologic membranes and so it disturbs them. Moreover, ethanol has pleiotropic effects on cellular signaling and may promote apoptosis under some circumstances. The relationship of this effect to cell injury requires further study.

DRUG ABUSE

Drug abuse is a compulsive behavior in which an individual persists in repeatedly taking a substance regardless of possible harm. For the most part, this involves agents that alter mood and perception, for example, (1) opiates (heroin, morphine); (2) depressants (barbiturates, tranquilizers, alcohol); (3) stimulants (cocaine, amphetamines) and psychedelic drugs (phencyclidine [PCP], lysergic acid diethylamide [LSD]); and (4) inhalants (amyl nitrite, organic solvents such as those in glue). It also includes habituation to, and excessive use of, prescription drugs. The Centers for Disease Control and Prevention (CDC) estimates that drug overdoses caused over 63,000 deaths in 2016 in the United States.

Illicit Drugs Are Responsible for Many Pathologic Syndromes

Medicinal Opioids and Heroin

Consumption of prescription opioids and heroin, orally and intravenously, is a severe problem in the United States. The CDC estimates that over 42,000 deaths in 2016 in the United States resulted from prescription and illegal opioids. The ready availability of potent prescription opioids such as oxycodone, fentanyl, hydromorphone, and others fueled this epidemic.

 MOLECULAR PATHOGENESIS: Opioids act by stimulating endogenous G protein–coupled opiate receptors, the most important of which is the μ receptor. This activates a signaling pathway leading to dopamine release in the nucleus accumbens, which is felt to mediate the drug-induced euphoria. Different opioids differ in lipid solubility and affinity for the μ receptor.

In addition to the "high," some opioids—for example, heroin—cause a negative feeling. It is reported that some prescription opioids (e.g., oxycodone) do not do this, which may account, in part, for their popularity. Oxycodone, usually combined with acetaminophen, is an opiate alkaloid with both stimulant and analgesic properties. The strongest effect is achieved by intravenous administration. Fentanyl is an opiate similar to morphine but is up to 100 times more potent. Its illicit use involves injection or oral intake, and it is associated with a high risk of addiction.

As prescription sources of these opioids become more carefully regulated, habituated people have turned to illicit sources and to heroin. Therefore, although the number of people reporting taking prescription opioids for nonmedical purposes has leveled off recently, heroin use has increased greatly. Overdoses are characterized by hypothermia, bradycardia, and respiratory depression.

Stimulants

Cocaine

Cocaine is an alkaloid derived from coca leaves. The freebase form of cocaine is hard and is far more potent than coca leaves. It may be taken by sniffing, by smoking, as intravenous injection, or orally. An even more potent form of cocaine ("crack") is generally smoked. The half-life of cocaine in the blood is about 1 hour.

Cocaine acts by interfering with dopamine reuptake. Cocaine users report extreme euphoria and heightened sensitivity to a variety of stimuli. However, with addiction, paranoid states and conspicuous emotional lability occur. Overdose leads to anxiety and delirium and occasionally to seizures. Cardiac arrhythmias and other effects on the heart may cause sudden death in otherwise apparently healthy people. Chronic cocaine users may develop a potentially fatal dilated cardiomyopathy.

Amphetamines

Amphetamines, mainly methamphetamine, are sympathomimetic and resemble cocaine in their effects, although they have a longer duration of action. Methamphetamines are most commonly used as "crystal meth," which is easily produced in home laboratories by hydrogenation of ephedrine or pseudoephedrine and is a major public health problem in the United States. It is inhaled (snorted) or smoked. The most serious complications of amphetamines include severe psychiatric instability, seizures, tachycardia and arrhythmias, and hyperthermia. Amphetamine use has been reported to lead to CNS vasculitis, and both subarachnoid and intracerebral hemorrhages have been described.

Hallucinogens

Hallucinogens are a group of chemically unrelated drugs that alter perception and sensory experience.

PCP is an anesthetic agent that has psychedelic or hallucinogenic effects. As a recreational drug, it is known as "angel dust" and is taken orally, intranasally, or by smoking. Its anesthetic properties diminish capacity to perceive pain and therefore may lead to self-injury and trauma. Other than its behavioral effects, PCP produces tachycardia and hypertension. High doses result in deep coma, seizures, and even decerebrate posturing.

LSD is a hallucinogenic drug whose popularity peaked in the late 1960s and is little used nowadays. It causes perceptual distortion, interferes with logical thought, alters time perception, and induces a sense of depersonalization. "Bad trips" are characterized by anxiety and panic and objectively by sympathomimetic effects that include tachycardia, hypertension, and hyperthermia. Large overdoses cause coma, convulsions, and respiratory arrest.

Organic Solvents

Recreational inhalation of organic solvents (fingernail polish, glues, plastic cements, and lighter fluid) is not uncommon, particularly among adolescents. Among the active ingredients are benzene, carbon tetrachloride, acetone, xylene, and toluene. Many of these compounds are also industrial solvents and reagents and so chronic low-level occupational exposure occurs. All are CNS depressants, although early effects (e.g., with xylene) may be excitatory. Acute intoxication

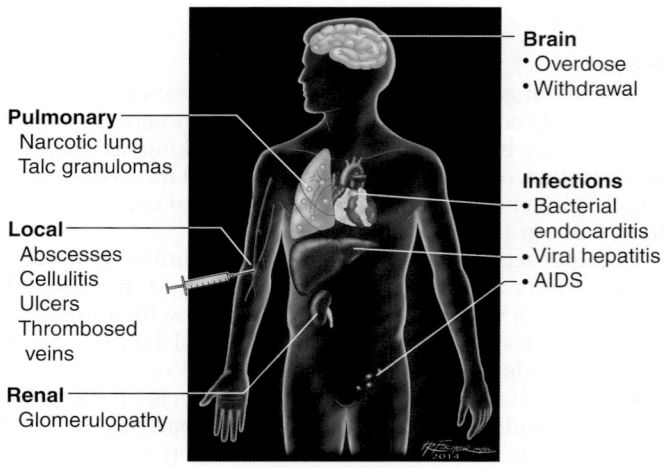

FIGURE 8-19. Complications of intravenous drug abuse.

with organic solvents resembles inebriation with alcohol. Large doses produce nausea and vomiting, hallucinations, and eventually coma. Respiratory depression and death may follow. Chronic exposure to, or abuse of, organic solvents may result in damage to the brain, kidneys, liver, lungs, and hematopoietic system. Benzene, for example, is a bone marrow toxin and has been associated with the development of AML.

Intravenous Drug Abuse Has Many Medical Complications

Apart from pharmacologic or physiologic effects of substance abuse, the most common complications are caused by introducing infectious organisms by a parenteral route. Most occur at the site of injection: cutaneous abscesses, cellulitis, and ulcers (Fig. 8-19). When these heal, "track marks" persist and these areas may be hypopigmented or hyperpigmented. Thrombophlebitis of veins draining sites of injection is common. Intravenous introduction of contaminating bacteria may lead to septic complications in internal organs. Bacterial endocarditis, often involving *Staphylococcus aureus*, occurs on both sides of the heart (Fig. 8-20) and may cause pulmonary,

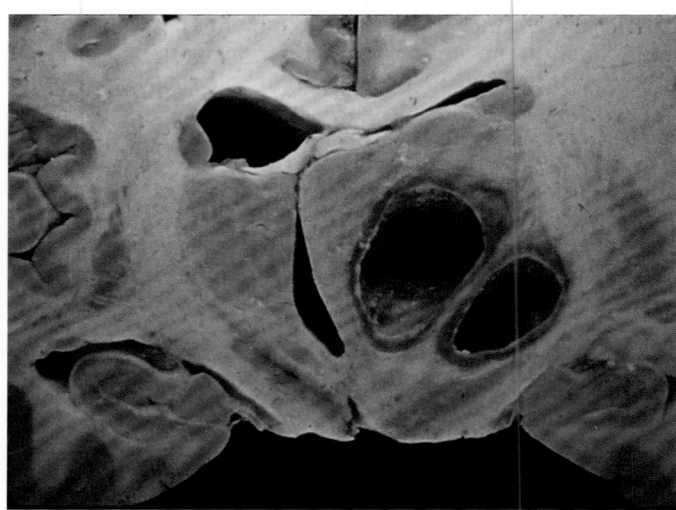

FIGURE 8-21. Brain abscess. Cross section of the brain of an intravenous drug abuser showing two encapsulated cavities. (From Okazaki H, Scheithauer BW. *Atlas of Neuropathology*. New York: Gower Medical Publishing; 1988. By permission of the author.)

renal, and intracranial abscesses, meningitis, osteomyelitis, and mycotic aneurysms (Fig. 8-21).

Intravenous drug abusers are at very high risk for viral diseases and their complications, such as AIDS and hepatitis B and C. A focal glomerulosclerosis ("heroin nephropathy") is characterized by immune complexes and has been ascribed to an immune reaction to impurities that contaminate illicit drugs.

Intravenous injection of talc, which is used to dilute pure drug, is associated with the appearance of foreign body granulomas in the lung (Fig. 8-22). These may be severe enough to lead to interstitial pulmonary fibrosis.

Drug Addiction in Pregnant Women Poses Risks for the Fetus

Maternal drug use may cause addiction in their newborns, who often develop full-blown withdrawal. Moreover, drug

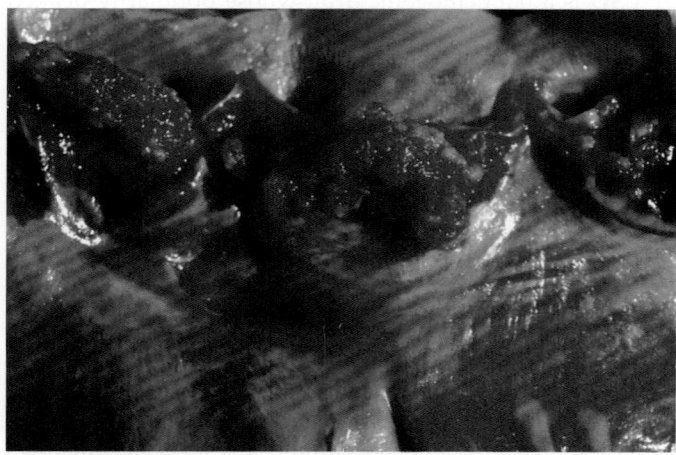

FIGURE 8-20. Bacterial endocarditis. The aortic valve of an intravenous drug abuser displays adherent vegetations.

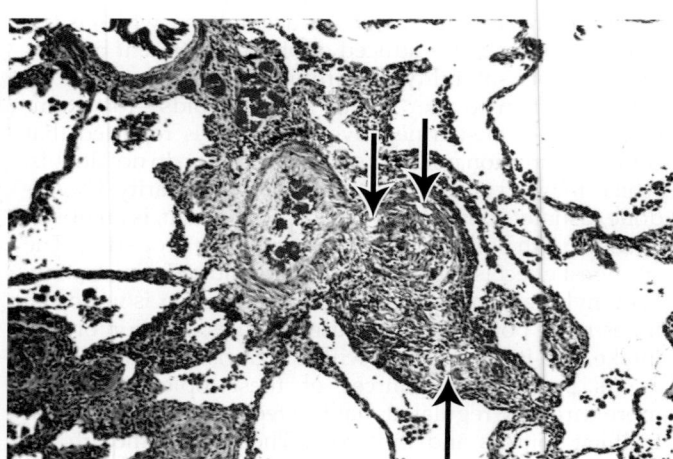

FIGURE 8-22. Talc granulomas in the lung. A section of lung of an intravenous drug abuser viewed under polarized light reveals a granuloma adjacent to a pulmonary artery. The refractile material (*arrows*) is talc that was used to dilute the drug prior to its intravenous injection.

withdrawal developing in the fetus during labor may cause excessive fetal movements and increased oxygen demand, which predisposes to intrapartum hypoxia and meconium aspiration. If labor occurs when maternal drug levels are high, the infant is often born with respiratory depression. Mothers who are addicted to drugs have higher rates of toxemia of pregnancy and premature labor.

Developing fetuses are at risk in other ways. Thus, pregnant women who use cocaine more commonly experience placental abruption and premature labor. Infants born to such mothers are prone to be low birth weight, to have one of an array of CNS and other anomalies, and to show impaired brain function after birth. Maternal heroin addiction increases risks of abnormalities of pregnancy and premature birth. It is also associated with a large number of postnatal problems (in addition to heroin withdrawal), including SIDS, neonatal respiratory distress syndrome, and developmental retardation. Maternal abuse of other substances (e.g., amphetamines and hallucinogens) also leads to variably severe fetal and postnatal disorders.

IATROGENIC INJURIES

Medical errors are defined by Makary and Daniel (*BMJ* 2016;353:i1239) as including:

- Unintended deed, whether of commission or omission
- A course of action that does not attain its intended result
- Incomplete or inadequate performance of a course of action
- Improper choice of a strategy to reach a particular goal
- Variance from correct course of care

The magnitude of the problem so defined is difficult to know with any accuracy, but a conservative estimate by the same authors is that medical errors cause over 250,000 deaths in the United States annually, constituting the third most common cause of death.

Iatrogenic Drug Injuries Are Unintended Consequences of Prescribed Drugs

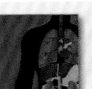 **EPIDEMIOLOGY:** Adverse drug reactions, or events (ADEs), are surprisingly common and are increasing. They are present at the time of admission to hospitals in about 5% of cases and develop subsequently in about 2% of hospitalized patients. Not surprisingly, patients older than 65 years, who take more medications and do so more often, are most affected. Children are least affected. Beyond that, the incidence of ADEs is relatively uniform across income levels, both for those occurring during the hospital stay and for those present at the time of admission. Of the former, the mortality rate is 3.9%, whereas of the latter, it is 3.2%.

The risk of an adverse reaction increases proportionately with the number of different drugs. Because they are so ubiquitously prescribed, drugs represent a significant environmental hazard. Untoward effects of drugs result from (1) overdose, (2) exaggerated physiologic responses, (3) a genetic predisposition, (4) hypersensitivity, (5) interactions with other drugs, and (6) other unknown factors. The characteristic pathologic changes associated with

drug reactions are treated in chapters dealing with specific organs.

The drugs most often associated with such adverse events include antibiotics, antineoplastic and antiallergy agents, hormones (including insulin), and analgesics, but drugs in any therapeutic category may be involved. Symptoms may vary from mild rashes to severe, fatal organ failures.

Stevens–Johnson Syndrome and Related Reactions

Because of the diversity of agents, presentations, and consequences, it is impossible to generalize as to how ADEs present or the mechanisms by which they occur. One important and relatively common adverse reaction is **Stevens–Johnson Syndrome (SJS)**, which is part of a spectrum of erythema multiforme–like reactions (**see Chapter 28**).

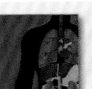 **PATHOPHYSIOLOGY:** SJS may occur following many drug exposures, including anticonvulsants, antibiotics, analgesics, and many others. It may also follow certain infections. SJS is generally considered to represent an aberrant cytotoxic T-lymphocyte (CTL)– and NK-mediated reaction. The inciting agent (e.g., drug) associates, often apparently noncovalently, with a T-cell receptor or HLA molecule, triggering CTL and NK responses that target keratinocytes. A genetic predisposition has been documented for certain HLA haplotypes. Proinflammatory cytokines, such as TNFα, IFNγ, and others, cause keratinocyte apoptosis and blistering reactions (Fig. 8-23).

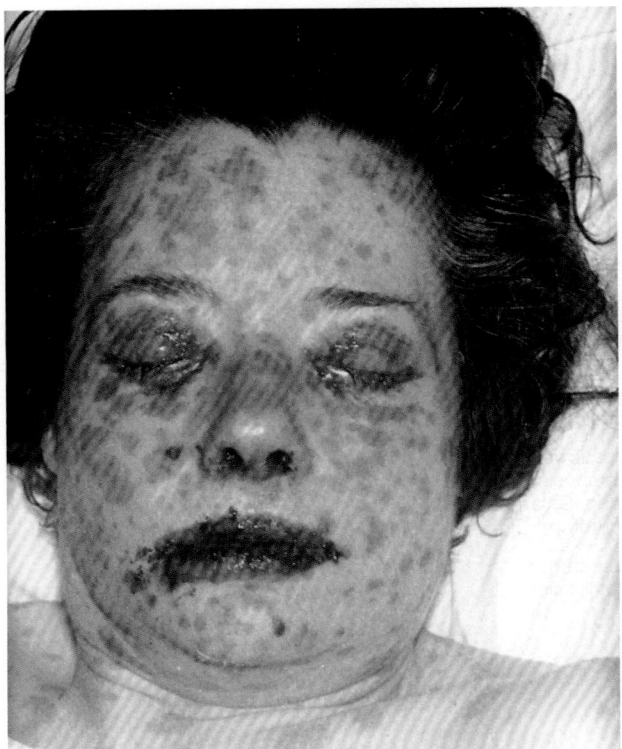

FIGURE 8-23. Erythema multiforme secondary to sulfonamide therapy. (From McKee PH. *Pathology of the Skin.* New York: Gower Medical Publishing; 1989. Copyright Lippincott Williams & Wilkins.)

CLINICAL FEATURES: Because these are mostly CTL-mediated reactions, their clinical onset may be quite delayed (sometimes a month or more) compared to the triggering exposure. Thus, it may be very difficult to establish a link between the stimulus and the presentation. Clinical presentations and courses are highly variable (**see Chapter 28**), but SJS usually starts with flu-like symptoms, with the characteristic cutaneous and mucosal eruptions thereafter. Beyond discontinuing exposure (if ongoing) to the inciting drug, there is little consensus as to optimal therapy. Severe cases of SJS may evolve into multiorgan failure, which carries a high fatality rate.

PHARMACOLOGIC HORMONES

Oral Contraceptives Carry a Small Risk of Complications

Orally administered hormonal contraceptives (OCs) are now the most commonly used method of birth control in industrialized countries. Current formulations vary but mostly are combinations of synthetic estrogens and steroids with progesterone-like activity. They act either by inhibiting the gonadotropin surge at midcycle, thus preventing ovulation, or by preventing implantation by altering the phase of the endometrium. Most complications of OCs involve either the vasculature or reproductive organs (Fig. 8-24).

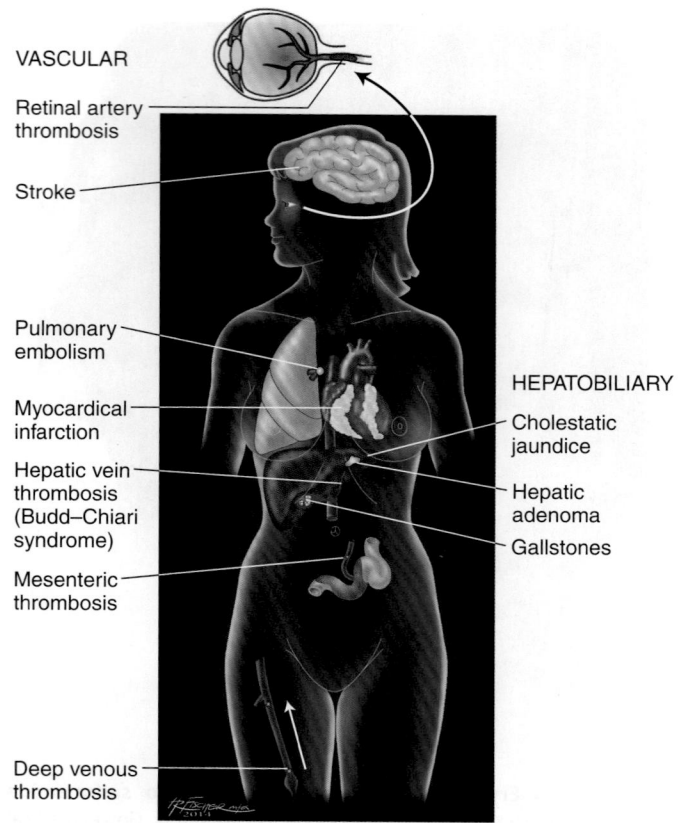

FIGURE 8-24. Complications of oral contraceptives.

Vascular Complications

Venous thromboembolism (VTE) is a recognized complication of OC use, the risk being about four times that in nonusers. This risk, about seven incidents per 10,000 woman-years, is substantially lower than the risk of VTE in pregnancy. As a consequence, the risk of thromboembolism is correspondingly increased. Obesity, a family history of venous thrombosis, and smoking magnify the risk of VTE with OCs, as do coexisting disorders that increase clotting (thrombophilia).

The risk of arterial thrombotic events in women taking OCs is also increased. Thus, both myocardial infarction and thrombotic stroke are reported to be increased in some studies.

Neoplastic Complications and Benefits

Tumors of several of the female reproductive organs, especially ovary, endometrium, and breast, are strongly influenced by female hormones. Repeated epidemiologic studies indicate that OC use decreases risk of ovarian and endometrial cancers substantially, presumably because of suppression of the production of pituitary gonadotropins. Decreased risk of colorectal and hematopoietic tumors has also been reported among women taking OCs.

Breast Cancer and OCs

There is a very large, mostly observational, literature relating to the question of whether women taking OCs are at greater risk for developing breast cancer. Most—but not all—current literature does not support the conclusion that using modern formulations of OCs increases risk of breast cancer.

Squamous carcinoma of the cervix may be somewhat increased in association with long-term (>5 years) OC use.

Lung cancer risk among women who smoke when beginning OC use has been reported to be higher than that among nonsmoking OC users and non-OC users.

Liver lesions noted in some older studies, including hepatic adenomas and hepatocellular carcinomas, have not been reported with more recent OC preparations.

Other Complications

Use of OCs has been associated with an increased incidence of Crohn disease and ulcerative colitis. The mechanism of this connection is not clear.

Reported Risks of Postmenopausal Hormone Replacement Therapy Vary With the Formulation, Age When Treatment Begins, and Duration of Treatment

As complex as the aforementioned analysis of the risks of OC use is, that for hormone replacement therapy (HRT) is far more so. As with OCs, results of different studies vary with all the variables indicated and are not at all consistent from one to the next. A clear consensus seems not to exist. Data from the Women's Health Initiative (WHI), which were interpreted as showing increased risk, particularly of breast cancer, from HRT, had a huge impact. Reinterpretation of these data has mitigated those conclusions considerably, but, as stated, there seems to be no clear conclusion.

Rather than rehash the controversy, the following conclusions are supported by most recent studies:

- Postmenopausal HRT containing estrogens only (of varying formulations) appears not to be associated with an increased risk of breast cancer. Combined estrogen–progestogen formulations are more controversial and may entail increased risk.
- There is little unequivocal evidence that HRT has any negative effect on death from all causes, including all cancers, coronary heart disease, and stroke.
- HRT begun around the time of menopause, with estrogen-only formulations, and continued for relatively short duration provides relief from symptoms and some consequences (e.g., hip fractures) of menopause.
- There is an increased risk of VTE with HRT but not necessarily with all preparations, routes of administration, or age groups.

Other Forms of Hormone Replacement

There are scant data regarding the risks of other forms of HRT. Androgen production in men declines with age, resulting in loss of muscle mass, increased adiposity, and other problems. However, testosterone replacement therapy for age-related decline in muscular strength, sexual performance, and other parameters remains controversial. Although prostate cancer in men is often hormonally sensitive, there are few studies reporting the incidence of prostate or other cancers in men receiving androgen replacement treatments.

Growth hormone (GH) replacement is used in people who lack adequate GH. Although many tumors require GH for their growth, there is no evidence that people given GH replacement are more susceptible to developing tumors than other people of their age. GH is being suggested as providing a possible benefit in older people with age-related decreases in skeletal muscle mass. To date, there is little evidence of adverse consequences, although the question of GH-induced insulin resistance remains.

Temperature, Altitude, and Related Injuries

THERMAL REGULATORY DYSFUNCTION

Hypothermia Is Body Temperature Below 35°C

Hypothermia can result in systemic or focal injury, the latter exemplified by **trench foot** or **immersion foot.** In localized hypothermia of these types, actual tissue freezing does not occur. **Frostbite,** in contrast, involves the crystallization of tissue water.

Generalized Hypothermia

Hypothermia may occur in a number of settings, including immersion in cold water or exposure to extremely cold air temperatures, especially after taking agents that impair thermoregulation, such as alcohol and some drugs. Perhaps, the best studied cause of hypothermia is cold water immersion.

 PATHOPHYSIOLOGY: Acute immersion in water at 4° to 10°C reduces central blood flow. Coupled with decreased core body temperature and cooling of the blood perfusing the brain, this results in mental confusion. Tetany makes swimming impossible. Furthermore, increased vagal discharge leads to premature ventricular contractions, ventricular arrhythmias, and even fibrillation.

Attempting to increase heat production, the immersed body immediately responds by increasing muscle activity and oxygen consumption. However, energy available for sustained warming is limited. Within 30 minutes, fatigue and heat loss from direct conduction via the whole skin surface cause core temperature to fall. Peripheral vasoconstriction to conserve heat increases sympathetic neural discharge, resulting in increased heart and basal metabolic rates and shivering. When core temperature reaches under 35°C, respiratory rate, heart rate, and blood pressure decline because of reduced functional reserve.

With prolonged cooling, "cold-induced" diuresis increases blood viscosity, decreasing oxygen–hemoglobin association and cardiac stroke volume. Death ensues from cardiac arrhythmia or sudden cardiac arrest.

Hypothermia is used safely for some patients undergoing open-heart surgery. With careful pharmacologic control, prolonged periods of lower body temperature can be achieved with no residual harm.

Although there are no specific morphologic changes in those who die from hypothermia, the skin shows red and purple discolorations, ears and hands swell, and there are irregular vasoconstriction and vasodilation. Areas of cardiac myocytolysis are seen. Lungs may show pulmonary edema and intra-alveolar, intrabronchial, and interstitial hemorrhages.

Focal Thermal Alterations

Local reduction in tissue temperature, particularly in the skin, causes vasoconstriction. Tissue water crystallizes if circulation cannot counter persistent thermal loss. When freezing occurs slowly, ice crystals form within tissue cells and in the interstitial space. Macromolecules denature, and ice disrupts cellular membranes. If freezing is rapid, a gel-like structure forms within the cell without water crystals. This gel reduces mechanical and chemical injuries. However, severe injury occurs on thawing: The gel transforms into a crystal, causing mechanical disruption of membrane structures.

Injury to the endothelial lining of capillaries and venules alters small vessel permeability, leading to plasma extravasation, localized edema and blisters, and inflammation. Endothelial damage leads to local thrombosis, and changes caused by altered permeability are prominent. Vascular occlusion often leads to gangrene.

Hyperthermia Means an Increase in Body Temperature

Hyperthermia also injures the vascular endothelium, increasing vascular permeability and causing edema and blisters. The degree of injury depends on the extent of temperature elevation and how quickly it is reached. Small increases in body temperature increase the metabolic rate. However, above a certain limit, enzymes denature and other proteins precipitate and "melting" of lipid bilayers of cell membranes takes place.

Systemic Hyperthermia

Increased body core temperature, or **fever**, occurs because of (1) increased heat production, (2) decreased elimination of heat from the body (reflecting an aberrant response of the thermal regulatory center), or (3) damage to the thermal regulatory center itself. Hyperthermia can also occur because heat is conducted into the body faster than the system can clear it.

A body temperature above 42.5°C leads to general vasodilation, inefficient cardiac function, and altered respiration. Isolated heart–lung preparations fail at about that temperature, suggesting an inherent limitation in the cardiovascular system and perhaps in the myocardial cells themselves. *In general, systemic temperature elevations above 42°C (107.6°F) are not compatible with life.*

During infectious and inflammatory responses, several cytokines, including IL-1, IL-6, and TNFα, interact with parts of the hypothalamus at the roof of the third ventricle and apparently reset the body's "thermostat" to permit a higher body core temperature. For mild pyrogens, parasympathetic activation may be involved. Few, if any, defined pathologic changes are associated with fever alone.

CLINICAL FEATURES: Physical findings include increased heart and respiratory rates, peripheral vasodilation, and diaphoresis, all recognized mechanisms for thermal regulation. The CNS may respond with irritability, restlessness, and (particularly in children) convulsions. Nocturnal temperature elevations with "night sweats" are a feature of pulmonary granulomatous infection (especially tuberculosis) and are also observed in lymphoproliferative diseases. Prolonged temperature elevation can produce wasting, principally because of an increased metabolic rate.

Malignant hyperthermia is a thermal alteration, accompanied by a hypermetabolic state and often by rhabdomyolysis (muscle necrosis), which occurs after anesthesia in susceptible people. This autosomal dominant disorder is associated with at least 70 different mutations in the gene for the sarcoplasmic reticulum ryanodine receptor (*RYR1*). A less common mutation causing malignant hyperthermia occurs in the gene for the α-subunit of the L-type voltage-gated calcium channel (*CACNA1S*). Muscle damage is caused by an abnormally high calcium concentration produced by accelerated release of Ca^{2+} through the mutant calcium release channel. Treatment with dantrolene, which binds the ryanodine receptor, reduces mortality from malignant hyperthermia to less than 10%.

Heat stroke is a form of hyperthermia that occurs at very high ambient temperatures and is not mediated by endogenous pyrogens. It reflects impaired thermal regulatory cooling responses and characteristically occurs in infants, young children, and the elderly. Often it is associated with an underlying chronic illness and use of diuretics, tranquilizers that may affect the hypothalamic thermal regulatory center, or drugs that inhibit perspiration. Another form of heat stroke is seen in healthy men during unusually vigorous exercise due, in part, to lactic acidosis, hypocalcemia, and rhabdomyolysis. Almost one-third of patients with exertional heat stroke develop myoglobinuric acute renal failure. Heat stroke is not amenable to treatment with standard antipyretics but requires external cooling and fluid and electrolyte replacement.

ALTITUDE-RELATED ILLNESSES

High-altitude illness is rare, largely because mountain climbers tend to acclimatize before they reach extreme altitudes. Andean communities at 400 to 4,300 m survive because their inhabitants develop increased hematocrits to improve oxygen delivery. However, prolonged stays at 5,500 to 6,000 m causes weight loss, difficulty sleeping, and lethargy, perhaps because 75% to 90% of available oxygen is needed simply for the effort of inspiration. Physical activity at these elevations leads to decreased partial pressure of arterial oxygen.

Acclimation to high altitudes includes more (1) capillaries per unit volume of brain, muscle, and myocardium; (2) myoglobin within tissues; (3) mitochondria per cell; and (4) hematocrit. Erythrocyte 2′,3′-diphosphoglycerate increases, which enhances oxygen delivery to tissues. Minor effects of high altitude include systemic edema, retinal hemorrhages, and flatulence. The more serious nonfatal diseases are acute and chronic mountain sickness and high-altitude deterioration. Fatal **high-altitude pulmonary edema** and **high-altitude encephalopathy** may ensue.

- **High-altitude systemic edema** results from asymptomatic increases in vascular permeability, particularly in hands, face, and feet. It may, in part, reflect endothelial cell responses to hypoxia and is more common among women. On return to lower altitude, diuresis causes the edema to disappear.
- **High-altitude retinal hemorrhage** occurs in 30% to 60% of people sleeping above 5,000 m. At first, retinal vessels engorge and become tortuous. Optic disc hyperemia and multiple flame-shaped hemorrhages subsequently occur. These changes are reversible.
- **High-altitude flatus:** Changes in external pressure and production of intestinal gas cause intestinal luminal contents to expand, leading to increased flatus at altitudes above 3,500 m. No medical disease attends these changes.
- **Acute mountain sickness** is rare below 2,500 m but occurs to some degree in nearly everyone at 3,000 to 3,600 m. Headache, lassitude, anorexia, weakness, and difficulty sleeping are symptoms, which are caused by hypoxia-induced shifts in plasma fluid to the interstitial space. Increasing respiratory rate allows some improvement, and descent to lower altitudes is indicated. Exacerbations may occur, frequently at lower altitudes, with severe symptoms. Acetazolamide (a carbonic anhydrase inhibitor) and dexamethasone are useful for preventing acute mountain sickness.
- **High-altitude deterioration:** Generally occurring at very high elevations (≥5,500 m), high-altitude deterioration presents as decreased physical and mental performance. Chronic hypoxia, inadequate fluid intake, inadequate nutrition, decreased plasma volume, and hemoconcentration are aggravating factors.

- **High-altitude pulmonary edema and cerebral edema:** Serious high-altitude problems, including pulmonary edema and cerebral edema, can occur with a rapid ascent to heights over 2,500 m, particularly in susceptible people who have difficulty sleeping at higher altitudes. Tachycardia, right ventricular overload, and marked reduction in arterial oxygen pressure occur, without changes in pH or carbon dioxide retention. Radiography reveals a characteristic patchy pulmonary infiltrate. Pulmonary hypertension is common in such patients, possibly due to hypoxic vasoconstriction and intravascular thrombosis. Eventually, cardiac output and systemic blood pressure fall. The precapillary arterioles dilate, increasing capillary bed pressure and inducing interstitial and alveolar edema. Autopsy findings include severe confluent pulmonary edema and proteinaceous alveolar exudates and hyaline membranes. Capillary obstruction by thrombi, cardiac dilatation, and enlarged pulmonary arteries are common.
- **High-altitude encephalopathy** is characterized by confusion, stupor, and coma. Autopsies reveal cerebral edema and vascular congestion. A proposed mechanism is severe cerebral hypoxia, with inhibition of the sodium pump and resultant intracellular edema.

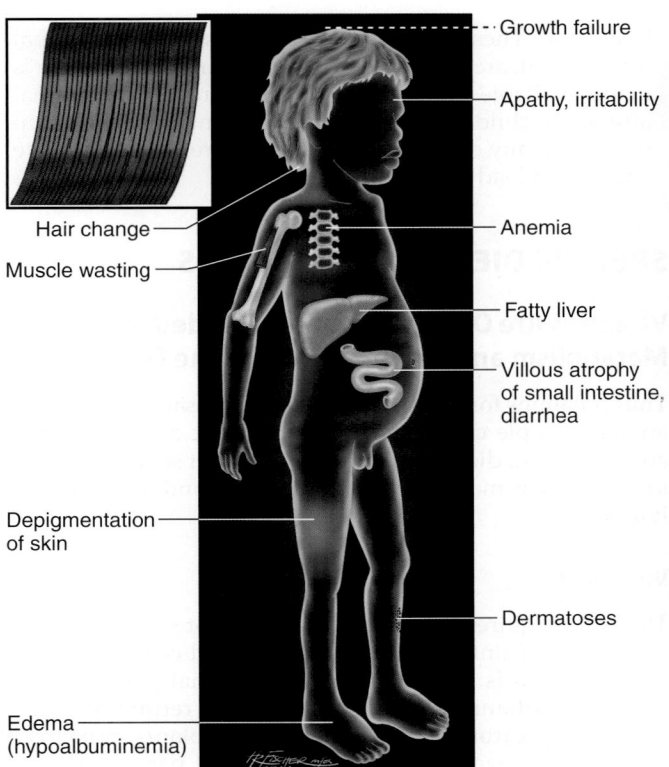

FIGURE 8-25. Complications of kwashiorkor.

Nutritional Disorders

MALNUTRITION

Starvation or Specific Deficiencies May Cause Protein–Calorie Malnutrition

Definitions

Marasmus is a deficiency of calories from all sources. **Kwashiorkor** is a form of malnutrition in children caused by a diet deficient in protein alone.

Marasmus

Global starvation—that is, a deficiency of all elements of the diet—leads to marasmus. The condition occurs throughout the nonindustrialized world, particularly when breastfeeding stops, and a child must subsist on a calorically inadequate diet. Consequences include decreased body weight and subcutaneous fat, a protuberant abdomen, muscle wasting, and a wrinkled face. In general, the child resembles a "shrunken old person." Visceral organs, especially the heart and liver, show wasting and increased lipofuscin pigment. Edema is absent. Pulse, blood pressure, and body temperature are low; diarrhea is common. Since immune responses are impaired, the child suffers from frequent infections. An important consequence of marasmus is **growth failure**. If these children do not receive adequate food in childhood, they will not reach their full potential stature as adults. Severe marasmus, if accompanied by iron-deficiency anemia in early childhood when the brain is developing, may lead to permanent intellectual deficit.

Kwashiorkor

Kwashiorkor (Fig. 8-25) results from a **deficiency of protein** in diets relatively high in carbohydrates. It is among the most common diseases of infancy and childhood in the non-industrialized world. Like marasmus, it usually occurs after an infant is weaned when a protein-poor diet, consisting principally of staple carbohydrates, replaces mother's milk. There is generalized growth failure and muscle wasting, as in marasmus, but subcutaneous fat is normal since caloric intake is adequate.

Unlike children with marasmus, who are usually alert and lack edema or organomegaly, those with kwashiorkor are usually very apathetic, are severely edematous, and show hepatomegaly. Skin depigmentation and "flaky paint" lesions appear, and the face, extremities, and perineum are dry and hyperkeratotic. Hair becomes sandy or reddish color; a characteristic linear depigmentation of the hair ("flag sign") characterizes particularly severe periods of protein deficiency.

The abdomen is distended because of flaccid abdominal muscles, hepatomegaly, and ascites due to hypoalbuminemia. Viscera are generally atrophic, and intestinal villous atrophy may impair nutrient absorption. Diarrhea is common. Anemia is the rule, but it is not generally life-threatening. The nonspecific effects on growth, pulse, temperature, and the immune system are like those in marasmus. Some studies suggest that kwashiorkor impairs both physical and intellectual development.

PATHOLOGY: The liver in kwashiorkor is conspicuously fatty, and lipid accumulation may displace hepatocyte nuclei to the periphery. Adequate dietary carbohydrate provides lipid for the hepatocyte, but inadequate dietary protein limits synthesis of enough apoprotein carrier to transport lipid from the liver cell. These changes, except possibly intellectual impairment, are fully reversible when sufficient protein is made available. In fact, the fatty liver reverts to normal after early childhood even if the diet remains deficient in protein. In any event, hepatic changes are not progressive and do not lead to chronic liver disease.

SPECIFIC DIETARY DEFICIENCIES

Vitamins Are Organic Catalysts Needed for Normal Metabolism and Available Only in the Diet

Thus, vitamins for one species are not necessarily vitamins for another. People cannot synthesize ascorbic acid (vitamin C) and so require dietary ascorbate to prevent scurvy, but most lower animals make their own vitamin C and do not require it in food.

Vitamin A

The body requires fat-soluble vitamin A for skeletal maturation and to maintain epithelial linings and cell membranes. In addition, it is a key constituent of retinal photosensitive pigments. Vitamin A occurs naturally as **retinoids** or as a precursor, **β-carotene**, which is found in plants, principally leafy, green vegetables. Fish livers are a particularly rich source of vitamin A (retinoids).

Vitamin A is also important for immune and nonimmune defenses, and its deficiency is associated with poor resistance to infection. Administration of vitamin A to deficient people reduces overall mortality. In underdeveloped countries, vitamin A supplementation in pregnant women and their children has reduced infant mortality.

Metabolism

The intestinal mucosa converts dietary β-carotene to retinoids, which are absorbed with chylomicrons. The liver stores 90% of the body's vitamin A. If diarrhea or insufficient dietary limits fat absorption (e.g., diarrhea, anorexia), vitamin A absorption decreases.

Vitamin A Deficiency

Vitamin A deficiency is uncommon in developed countries but is a significant health problem in poorer areas, including much of Africa, China, and Southeast Asia.

PATHOLOGY: *Deficiency of vitamin A causes squamous metaplasia, especially in glandular epithelium* (Fig. 8-26). Consequently, keratin debris blocks sweat and tear ducts. Squamous metaplasia is common in the trachea and bronchi, impairing their clearance function and predisposing to bronchopneumonia, which may be fatal. Other columnar epithelia may be similarly affected, so limited clearance functions of the renal pelvis, pancreatic ducts, uterus, and salivary glands may lead to stasis and infection. In the renal pelvis, for example, kidney stones may develop. Occluded sebaceous ducts may lead to **follicular hyperkeratosis**. As deficiency worsens, there is squamous metaplasia of conjunctival and tear duct epithelia, leading to **xerophthalmia**, dryness of the cornea, and conjunctiva. The cornea becomes softened

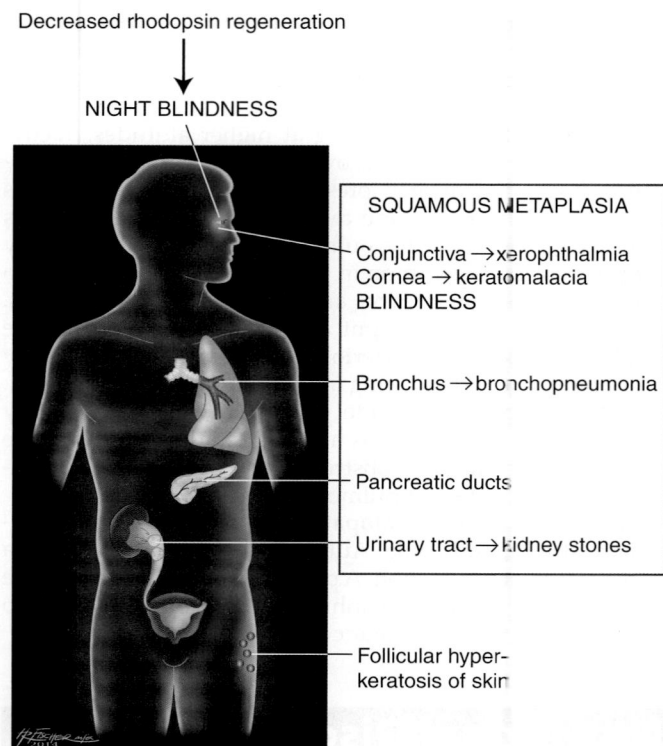

FIGURE 8-26. Complications of vitamin A deficiency.

(**keratomalacia,** Fig. 8-27) and susceptible to ulceration and bacterial infection, which may lead to blindness.

CLINICAL FEATURES: The earliest sign of vitamin A deficiency often is poor vision in dim light. Vitamin A is a necessary component in retinal rod pigment and is active in light transduction. Its aldehyde, retinal, degrades when it generates light signals, so a continuous supply of vitamin A is required for night vision.

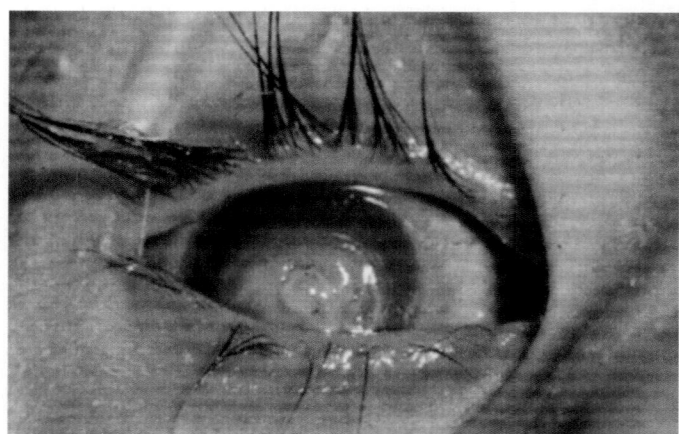

FIGURE 8-27. Keratomalacia in vitamin A deficiency. (From Shils ME, Shike M, Ross AC, et al., eds. *Modern Nutrition in Health and Disease.* 10th ed. Philadelphia, PA: Lippincott Williams & Wilkins; 2006:38 1C.)

TABLE 8-6 B VITAMINS	
Vitamin	Biochemical Name
B$_1$	Thiamine
B$_2$	Riboflavin
B$_3$	Niacin
B$_5$	Pantothenic acid
B$_6$	Pyridoxine
B$_7$	Biotin
B$_9$	Folic acid
B$_{12}$	Cyanocobalamin

Vitamin A Toxicity

Vitamin A poisoning usually reflects overenthusiastic administration of vitamin supplements. Early Arctic explorers were said to have experienced vitamin A toxicity because they ate polar bear liver, which is particularly rich in vitamin A. Hepatosplenomegaly are common, and these organs show lipid-laden macrophages. In the liver, vitamin A is also present in hepatocytes and prolonged hypervitaminosis A may rarely cause cirrhosis. Bone pain and neurologic symptoms, such as hyperexcitability and headache, may be presenting symptoms. Symptoms disappear when vitamin A consumption returns to normal. Excessive carotene intake is benign and simply stains the skin yellow, which may be mistaken for jaundice.

Synthetic retinoic acid derivatives are now used pharmacologically for several purposes. Retinoic acid and a high dietary intake of vitamin A are especially dangerous in pregnancy, because they are potent teratogens. Excess vitamin A intake leads to reduced bone mineral density and an increased incidence of bone fractures.

Vitamin B Complex

Vitamins in the B group of water-soluble vitamins are numbered 1 through 12, but only eight are distinct vitamins (Table 8-6).

Thiamine (B$_1$)

When originally discovered, vitamin B was defined as a water-soluble extract in rice polishings that cured beriberi. Thiamine was that factor. It is an essential cofactor in the activity of several enzymes crucial to energy metabolism, mainly in the tricarboxylic acid (Krebs) cycle. Beriberi was classically seen in the Orient, where the staple food was polished rice shorn of thiamine during processing. With increased awareness and improved nutrition, it is less common now. In Western countries, beriberi occurs in alcoholics and in wasting diseases (see below).

 CLINICAL FEATURES: *The cardinal symptoms of thiamine deficiency are polyneuropathy, edema, and cardiac failure* (Fig. 8-28). The syndrome is classically divided into **dry beriberi**—with mainly neuromuscular symptoms paresthesias, depressed

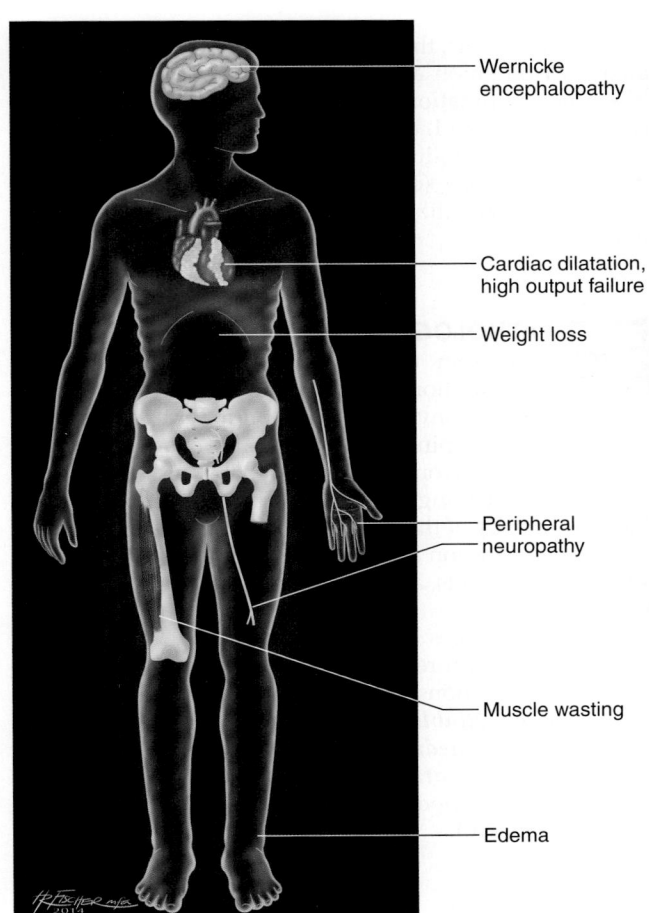

FIGURE 8-28. Complications of thiamine deficiency (beriberi).

reflexes, and weakness and muscle atrophy in the extremities—and **wet beriberi**, with generalized edema, a reflection of severe congestive failure.

In chronic alcoholics, CNS involvement causes Wernicke encephalopathy, with progressive **dementia, ataxia, and ophthalmoplegia** (paralysis of extraocular muscles). Korsakoff psychosis, a thought disorder caused by inadequate thiamine, often accompanies Wernicke syndrome (as Wernicke–Korsakoff syndrome), with confusion, memory impairment, and the neurologic signs listed above.

PATHOPHYSIOLOGY: Wernicke–Korsakoff syndrome may occur in simple dietary deficiency of thiamine. However, it also occurs in alcoholics and patients with wasting diseases, whether or not dietary thiamine intake is adequate. Alcohol decreases intestinal thiamine absorption by decreasing expression of thiamine transporters and increases its renal excretion. It also reduces hepatic thiamine storage and directly interferes with thiamine-dependent enzymes.

Similarly in many chronic diseases, such as advanced cancer, vomiting and malabsorption limit effective intake, whereas its overuse by certain aggressive cancers may limit supplies for normal tissues. Electrolyte abnormalities, for example, hypomagnesemia, may limit its biochemical effectiveness.

In wet beriberi, the basic lesion is uncontrolled, generalized vasodilation and peripheral arteriovenous shunting. This combination causes a compensatory increase in cardiac output and, eventually, a large dilated heart and congestive heart failure. In a patient without documented metabolic disease (e.g., hyperthyroidism), high-output failure and generalized edema strongly suggest thiamine deficiency.

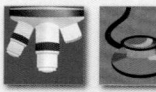 **PATHOLOGY:** There is no pathognomonic change in the peripheral nerves, but myelin degeneration—which often begins in the sciatic nerve and then involves other peripheral nerves and sometimes the spinal cord itself—is characteristic. In advanced cases, axon fragmentation may be seen.

The most striking lesions in Wernicke encephalopathy include atrophy of the mamillary bodies and surrounding areas. Degeneration and loss of ganglion cells, rupture of small blood vessels, and ring hemorrhages are seen in the brain.

Cardiac changes, which include flabby myocardium, edema, and a mixture of myofiber hypertrophy and degeneration, are also nonspecific.

The most reliable diagnostic test for thiamine deficiency is an immediate and dramatic response to parenteral administration of thiamine. Measurements of thiamine in the blood and erythrocyte transketolase activity are also useful.

Riboflavin (B₂)

Riboflavin is found in many plant and animal sources. It is important for synthesis of flavin nucleotides, which act in electron transport and other energy transfer reactions. Symptomatic riboflavin deficiency is uncommon and usually occurs in debilitated patients and poorly nourished alcoholics. Deficiencies of thiamine, riboflavin, and niacin are unusual in industrialized countries because bread and cereals are fortified with these vitamins. Occasionally, mild riboflavin deficiency develops during pregnancy and lactation or during rapid growth in childhood and adolescence, when increased demands may be combined with moderate nutritional deprivation.

PATHOLOGY AND CLINICAL FEATURES: Riboflavin deficiency, when occurs, is almost always seen in conjunction with deficiencies of other water-soluble vitamins. It manifests mainly as lesions of facial skin and corneal epithelium. **Cheilosis**—fissures in the skin at the angles of the mouth—is characteristic (Fig. 8-29). These cracks in the skin may be painful and often become infected.

Hyperkeratosis and a mild chronic dermatitis may accompany **seborrheic dermatitis**, the latter giving the skin on the cheeks and behind the ears a greasy, scaling appearance. Mucosal atrophy leaves the tongue smooth and magenta. **Corneal interstitial keratitis** may lead to corneal opacification and ulceration. The pathogenesis of these lesions is not understood. There is no known toxicity from ingesting large amounts of riboflavin.

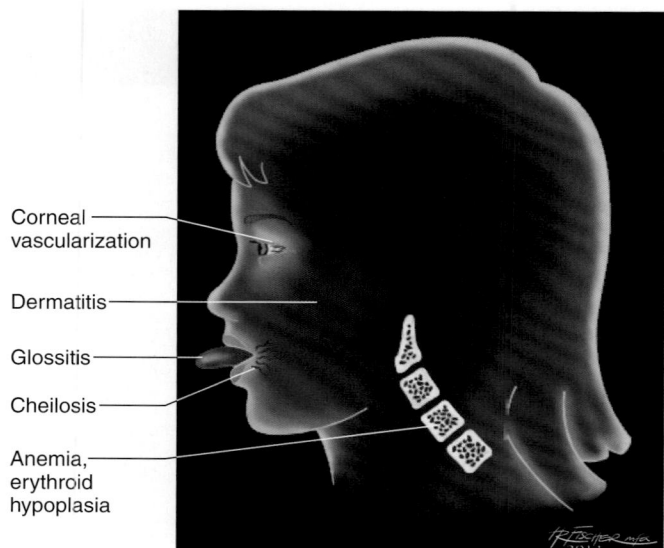

Corneal vascularization
Dermatitis
Glossitis
Cheilosis
Anemia, erythroid hypoplasia

FIGURE 8-29. Complications of riboflavin deficiency.

Niacin (Nicotinic Acid, B₃)

Niacin is consumed from dietary sources or produced from tryptophan. It is converted to nicotinamide, which helps form NAD. NAD and its phosphorylated derivative, NADP, are important in intermediary metabolism and many redox reactions. Animal protein, as in meat, eggs, and milk, is high in tryptophan and so is a good source of endogenously synthesized niacin. Niacin is also available in many grains.

 PATHOPHYSIOLOGY: Pellagra (Ital., "rough skin") is clinical niacin deficiency. Nowadays, it occurs mainly in people with chronic wasting diseases and poorly nourished alcoholics. People who do not eat enough protein may be deficient in tryptophan. In combination with inadequate exogenous niacin, they may develop mild pellagra. Malabsorption of tryptophan, as in **Hartnup disease**, or excessive diversion of tryptophan for serotonin synthesis in the carcinoid syndrome may also cause mild symptoms of pellagra. Inadequate pyridoxine and riboflavin intake increases dietary niacin requirements because these cofactors are required for niacin biosynthesis from tryptophan. Pellagra may occur where corn (maize) is the staple food, because niacin in corn is poorly chemically available. Native Americans, who soaked corn in alkali, which broke down cell walls, did not develop pellagra, but Europeans, who imported corn and did not pretreat it, did. (Corn is also a poor source of tryptophan.)

  PATHOLOGY AND CLINICAL FEATURES: Hyperkeratosis, vascularization, and chronic inflammation occur in affected skin and mucous membranes of the mouth and vagina, with subcutaneous fibrosis and scarring in late stages. In the mouth, inflammation and edema create a large, red tongue, resembling raw meat. Pellagra is characterized by the three "Ds" of niacin deficiency: **dermatitis, diarrhea,** and **dementia** (Fig. 8-30).

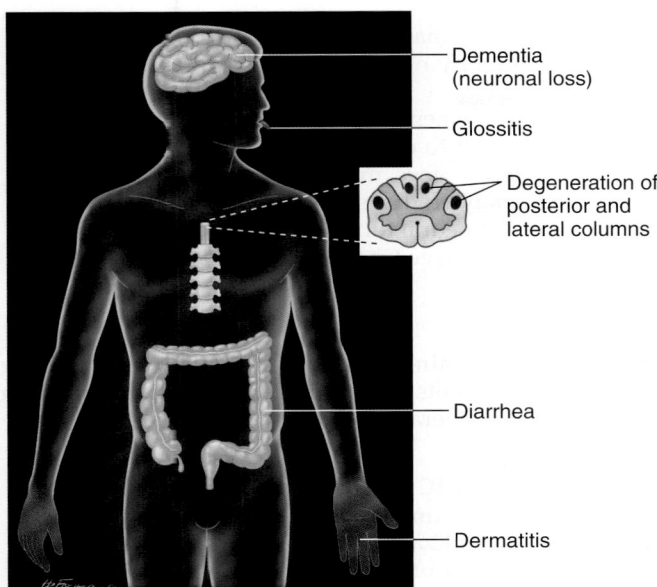

FIGURE 8-30. Complications of niacin deficiency (pellagra).

Light-exposed skin, for example, the face and the hands (glove dermatitis), or areas subject to pressure, such as knees and the elbows, have a rough, scaly dermatitis (Fig. 8-31). Lesions are discrete, with areas of pigmentation and depigmentation.

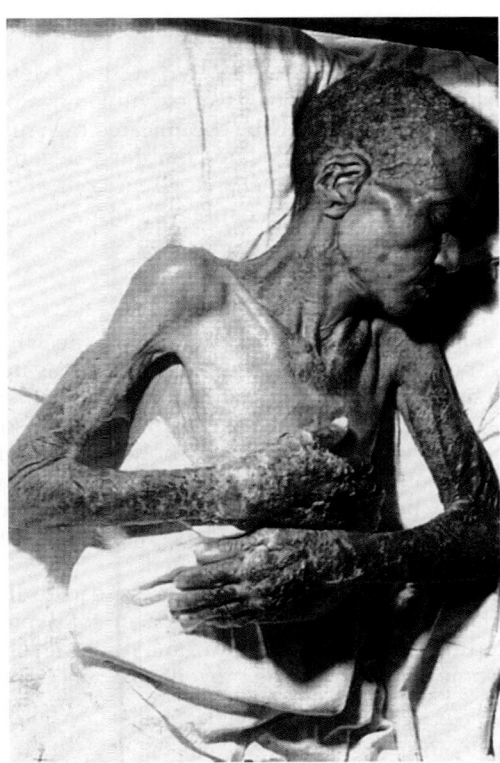

FIGURE 8-31. Pellagra. Dermatitis in sun-exposed areas of the arms and around the neck in an elderly woman. (From Shils ME, Shike M, Ross AC, et al., eds. *Modern Nutrition in Health and Disease*. 10th ed. Philadelphia, PA: Lippincott Williams & Wilkins; 2006:Fig. 38.2C.)

Mucosal atrophy and ulceration throughout the GI tract cause chronic, watery diarrhea. Dementia, characterized by aberrant ideation bordering on psychosis, reflects degeneration of cortical ganglion cells. Myelin degeneration of tracts in the spinal cord resembles the subacute combined degeneration of vitamin B_{12} deficiency. In severe, long-standing pellagra, the fourth **"D"** is death.

In pharmacologic doses, niacin supplements decrease blood LDL-C and increase high-density lipoprotein cholesterol (HDL-C) and so may be useful in preventing atherosclerosis.

Pantothenic Acid (B₅)

Pantothenic acid is a component of coenzyme A (CoA) and is essential for biosynthesis of fatty acids and certain peptides. Major sources of pantothenic acid include beef, chicken, liver, eggs, grains, and a number of vegetables.

Pantothenic acid deficiency is very uncommon, except in severe malnutrition. The syndrome features behavioral, neurologic, and GI disturbances.

There are no known adverse effects of overconsumption of pantothenic acid.

Pyridoxine (B₆)

Vitamin B_6 occurs naturally in three forms: pyridoxine, pyridoxal, and pyridoxamine, grouped for convenience as pyridoxine. They occur widely in vegetable and animal foods. Vitamin B_6 is a coenzyme in many metabolic pathways, including those related to amino acids, lipids, methylation and decarboxylation, gluconeogenesis, heme, and neurotransmitters.

EPIDEMIOLOGY: Inadequate dietary intake of vitamin B_6, as measured by blood levels, is not uncommon among older people and especially those with chronic addictions, such as alcoholism. Infants fed poorly prepared powdered formula in which pyridoxine was destroyed during preparation suffer from convulsions.

Pyridoxine functions as an antioxidant and thus an anti-inflammatory agent. Perhaps, as a result, epidemiologic studies suggest that higher vitamin B_6 levels may help protect from several malignancies, particularly cancers of the colon and rectum, pancreas, and lung. Among these, the inverse relationship between vitamin B_6 levels and colorectal cancer is the best documented.

MOLECULAR PATHOGENESIS: Pyridoxal 5'-phosphate (PLP) is a cofactor for many enzymes. A higher demand for the vitamin, as may occur in pregnancy, may lead to a secondary deficiency state. Of particular concern is the deficiency of pyridoxine that follows prolonged medication with a number of drugs, particularly isoniazid, levodopa, and penicillamine. Isoniazid, for example, inhibits the enzyme pyridoxal phosphokinase, lowering PLP levels. It also increases renal PLP excretion.

CLINICAL FEATURES: *The main symptoms of vitamin B6 deficiency are neurologic, consistent with its role in the formation of the neurotransmitter GABA.* A seizure disorder, particularly in infants and children, accompanied by diarrhea or anemia, may suggest such a condition. Pyridoxine deficiency may present as microcytic, hypochromic anemia, which can be confused with iron deficiency, save that iron stores are adequate. Severe vitamin B6 deficiency may present as a peripheral neuropathy.

Excessive vitamin B6 consumption has been linked to development of peripheral neuropathy.

Biotin (B7)

Biotin is mostly found in meats and cereals, where it is largely bound to protein. It is an obligatory cofactor for five carboxylases that participate in intermediary metabolism, including the Krebs cycle.

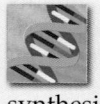 **EPIDEMIOLOGY: Biotin deficiency** may occur in people who consume large amounts of raw eggs, in those with prolonged malabsorption, and in children with severe protein–calorie malnutrition. Chronic administration of anticonvulsant drugs can also deplete biotin.

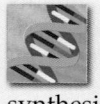 **CLINICAL FEATURES:** Symptoms of biotin deficiency include seborrheic and eczematous rashes. Adults may show lethargy, hallucinations, and paresthesias. In infants, hypotonia and developmental delay have been reported.

There are no known adverse consequences of high-dose biotin administration.

Folic Acid (B9)

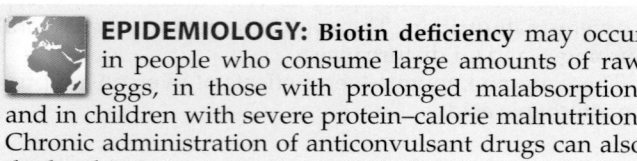 **MOLECULAR PATHOGENESIS:** Folic acid is a heterocyclic derivative of glutamic acid and is a methyl group donor, especially in nucleotide synthesis. Together with vitamin B12 (see below), it is a key cofactor in methylation reactions. Particularly, folate-dependent conversion of homocysteine to methionine is needed to generate *S*-adenosylmethionine (SAM, **see Chapter 5**). SAM is a key methyl donor in the synthesis of neurotransmitters (norepinephrine to epinephrine), phospholipids (phosphatidylethanolamine to phosphatidylcholine), methylated nucleotides, and histones. Folate is reduced by **dihydrofolate reductase (DHFR)** to **tetrahydrofolate (THF)**. THF participates in purine and pyrimidine metabolism.

FOLATE DEFICIENCY: Both folic acid and vitamin B12 (see below) participate in the pathway to produce methionine (see above), and the importance of SAM in many biochemical reactions explains the overlap in manifestations of folate and B12 deficiencies (e.g., megaloblastic anemia; **see Chapter 26**).

Folate is present in almost all foods, including meat, dairy products, seafood, cereals, and vegetables. Deficiency is thus usually a consequence of a generally poor diet or as in malabsorption syndromes. Because it occurs in so many nutrients, isolated folate deficiency is rare.

Folate supplements given during early pregnancy have been shown to decrease the incidence of fetal neural tube defects. Since mandated folate fortification of cereal and grain products in the United States in 1998, the incidence of neural tube defects among newborns has decreased greatly (**see Chapter 6**).

Cyanocobalamin (B12)

Deficiency of vitamin B12 is almost always seen in pernicious anemia. It results from impaired absorption of vitamin B12 due to one of several etiologies.

 ETIOLOGIC FACTORS: Since vitamin B12 is found in almost all animal protein, including meat, milk, and eggs, dietary deficiency is seen only in rare cases of extreme vegetarianism and then only after many years of a restricted diet. Parasitization of the small intestine by the fish tapeworm *Diphyllobothrium latum* (from undercooked fish) may lead to vitamin B12 deficiency because the parasite absorbs the vitamin in the gut lumen. Absorption of vitamin B12 occurs in the terminal ileum and requires the action of intrinsic factor, which is produced by gastric parietal cells. Thus, atrophic gastritis, which destroys parietal cells, or diseases of the terminal ileum (e.g., Crohn disease) impair cyanocobalamin absorption and may cause pernicious anemia.

 CLINICAL FEATURES: Vitamin B12 deficiency may cause pernicious anemia, a megaloblastic condition that may be complicated by neurologic manifestations, called subacute combined degeneration of the spinal cord. Comprehensive discussions of vitamin B12 deficiency are found in Chapters 26 and 32.

Choline

Choline is an amine found in many foods, especially wheat products, peanuts, soybeans, fish, and meat. It is necessary for lipid signaling, transport, and metabolism, membrane synthesis, and cholinergic neurotransmission. It also participates in methyl group transfer reactions. Since there is an endogenous pathway for choline biosynthesis, it was not considered to be an essential human nutrient. However, choline deficiency syndromes have been identified and adequate dietary levels are now established.

Experimentally, choline-deficient diets lead to liver and muscle damage. Patients maintained on total parenteral nutrition due to short bowel syndrome often develop liver disease, some of which can be prevented by choline supplementation.

Vitamin C (Ascorbic Acid)

The effects of vitamin C deficiency—**scurvy**—were described 5,000 years ago in Egyptian hieroglyphs and were mentioned by Hippocrates in 500 BC.

PATHOPHYSIOLOGY: Ascorbic acid is a water-soluble vitamin that is a powerful biologic reducing agent involved in many oxidation/reduction reactions and in proton transfer. It is important for chondroitin sulfate synthesis and for proline hydroxylation to form the hydroxyproline of collagen. It serves many other functions: It prevents oxidation of THF and increases iron absorption from the gut. Without vitamin C, biosynthesis of certain neurotransmitters is impaired, reducing dopamine β-hydroxylase activity. Wound healing and immune functions also require ascorbic acid. The best dietary sources of vitamin C are citrus fruits, green vegetables, and tomatoes.

Scurvy is clinical vitamin C deficiency. This was first shown when the British navy distributed limes to its sailors and, in so doing, prevented scurvy (hence the name "limey" for British seamen). In industrialized countries, scurvy is now a disease of people afflicted with chronic diseases who do not eat well, the neglected aged, and malnourished alcoholics but is not uncommon in poorer countries, where it may coexist with other forms of malnutrition. The stresses of cold, heat, fever, or trauma (accidental or surgical) increase the need for vitamin C. Mild depression of ascorbic acid levels also occurs in cigarette smoking, tuberculosis, rheumatic fever, and other debilitating disorders. About 3% of the body's ascorbic acid is catabolized per day.

PATHOLOGY: *Vitamin C deficiency impairs collagen synthesis so that collagen that is produced lacks tensile strength* (Fig. 8-32). Within 1 to 3 months, subperiosteal hemorrhages cause bone and joint pain, as well as petechial hemorrhages, ecchymoses, and purpura, particularly after mild trauma or at pressure points. Perifollicular hemorrhages in the skin are particularly typical of scurvy. In advanced cases, swollen, bleeding gums are characteristic. Alveolar bone resorption results in loss of teeth. Wound healing is poor, and previously healed wounds undergo dehiscence. Anemia may ensue from prolonged bleeding, impaired iron absorption, or associated folate deficiency.

Scurvy in children leads to growth failure, and collagen-rich structures such as teeth, bones, and blood vessels develop abnormally. Effects on developing bone are conspicuous and relate principally to impaired function of osteoblasts (**see Chapter 30**). In addition, **scorbutic patients** have difficulty walling-off infections to form abscesses; as a result, infections spread more easily. The diagnosis is confirmed by finding low serum levels of ascorbic acid.

Ingesting large amounts of vitamin C is not known to be harmful even as it may not help prevent upper respiratory infections.

Vitamin D

Vitamin D first appeared on the Earth 500,000,000 years ago, in ocean-dwelling phytoplankton, in which it may have functioned to absorb UV irradiation or act as a photochemical signal. During evolution, terrestrial vertebrates became dependent on it to sustain their bony skeletons.

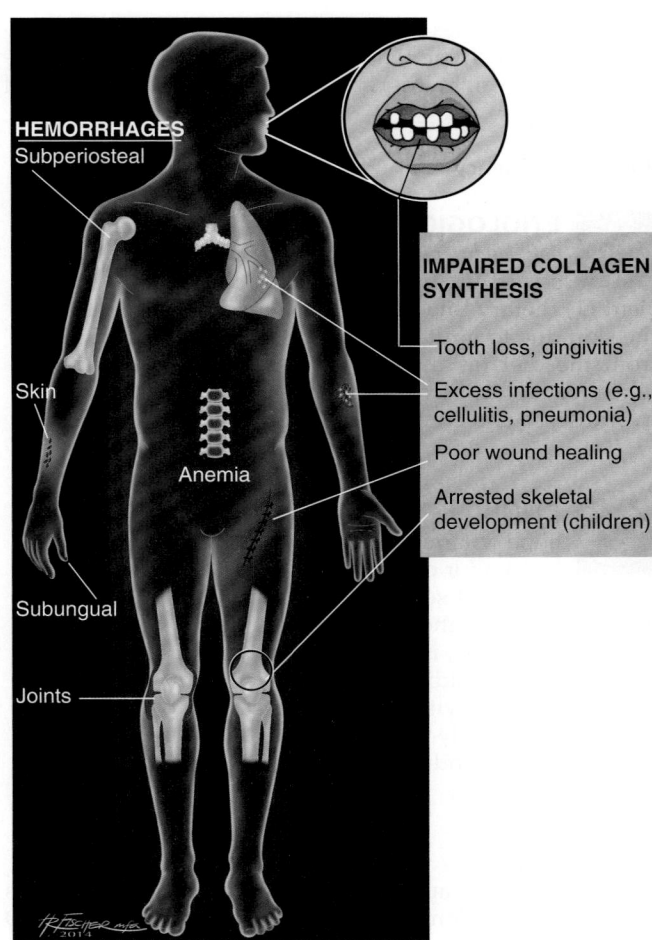

FIGURE 8-32. Complications of vitamin C deficiency (scurvy).

Vitamin D is a fat-soluble steroid with two forms: vitamin D_3 (cholecalciferol) and vitamin D_2 (ergocalciferol), both of which are equally potent in humans. Vitamin D_3 is made in the skin. Vitamin D_2 is derived from plant ergosterol and absorbed in the jejunum along with fats. In the blood, it binds an α-globulin (vitamin D–binding protein). *For biologic potency, vitamin D must be hydroxylated to active metabolites in the liver and kidneys. Its active form promotes small intestinal calcium and phosphate absorption and may directly influence mineralization of bone.*

Tissues not related to calcium metabolism have nuclear receptors for $1,25(OH)_2$-vitamin D. Accordingly, there are many studies purporting to examine the relationship between (a) vitamin D deficiency and many diseases; and (b) protective effects (if any) of vitamin D supplementation for those diseases. Parsing fact from hype in this context is very challenging. Correlations undoubtedly exist between low vitamin D levels and increased occurrence of many diseases, including cardiovascular, neoplastic, psychiatric, and inflammatory diseases. Randomized controlled studies of people who are not per se vitamin D–deficient tell somewhat different stories. With considerable variation among studies, vitamin D supplementation in people who are not deficient to begin with may well have significantly reduced respiratory infections, depression, and all-cause mortality. Other positive outcomes that have been suggested by observational studies (reduced incidence of cancer, cardiovascular disease, hypertension, low birth weight and diabetes, improved weight loss) are not supported by randomized clinical trials.

Vitamin D Deficiency

 ETIOLOGIC FACTORS: *In children, vitamin D deficiency causes* **rickets**; *in adults,* **osteomalacia** *occurs.* Vitamin D deficiency results from insufficient (1) dietary vitamin D, (2) vitamin D production in the skin due to limited sunlight exposure, (3) absorption from the diet (as in fat malabsorption syndromes), or (4) conversion to bioactive metabolites. The last occurs in liver disease and chronic renal failure.

 CLINICAL FEATURES: Bone lesions in childhood vitamin D deficiency (rickets) have been known for centuries and were common in Western industrialized societies until recently. It was a problem that affected the urban poor much more than their rural counterparts, in part because of differences in sunlight exposure. Addition of vitamin D to milk and many processed foods, vitamin administration to young children, and generally improved nutrition have made rickets a curiosity in industrialized countries. **See Chapter 26** for more details.

Hypervitaminosis D

The most common cause of hypervitaminosis D is the excess vitamin consumption. Abnormal conversion of vitamin D to biologically active metabolites happens occasionally in granulomatous diseases such as sarcoidosis. In cases when calcium malabsorption is corrected, target tissue sensitivity to vitamin D may be increased.

PATHOLOGY: The initial response to excess vitamin D is **hypercalcemia**, which leads to nonspecific symptoms—weakness and headaches. Increased renal calcium excretion results in **nephrolithiasis** or **nephrocalcinosis. Ectopic calcification** in other organs, such as blood vessels, heart, and lungs, may occur. Infants are particularly susceptible to excess vitamin D, and if the condition is not corrected, they may develop premature arteriosclerosis, supravalvular aortic stenosis, and renal acidosis.

Vitamin E

Vitamin E is an antioxidant that (experimentally at least) protects membrane phospholipids from free radical–related lipid peroxidation. This fat-soluble vitamin occurs, principally as α-tocopherol, in many dietary constituents, especially corn and soybeans.

Dietary vitamin E deficiency can occur in children because of mutations in the α-tocopherol transfer protein. In adults, various malabsorption syndromes may be responsible. Vitamin E deficiency may present clinically as spinocerebellar ataxia, skeletal myopathy, and pigmented retinopathy.

In premature infants, hemolytic anemia, thrombocytosis, and edema have been associated with vitamin E deficiency. Vitamin E therapy may improve hemolytic anemia in premature newborns and reduce the severity—but not the incidence—of retrolental fibroplasia. It is reported to retard development of cirrhosis in infants with congenital biliary atresia. Experimentally, it also inhibits (1) platelet aggregation, (2) conversion of dietary nitrites to carcinogenic nitrosamines, (3) prostaglandin synthesis, and (4) toxins that act by generating ROS. Applicability to human disease is unclear, as attempts to use vitamin E pharmacologically to prevent cancer and coronary artery disease have been unsuccessful.

Vitamin K

Vitamin K is a fat-soluble material that occurs in two forms: vitamin K_1, from plants, and vitamin K_2, which is mostly made by normal intestinal bacteria. It is abundant in green leafy vegetables; liver and dairy products contain smaller amounts.

TABLE 8-7 AMINO ACIDS	
Amino Acid	**Nature of Requirement**
Alanine (A)	Nonessential
Arginine (R)	Nonessential
Asparagine (N)	Nonessential
Aspartic acid (D)	Nonessential
Cysteine (C)	Conditionally essential
Glutamic acid (E)	Nonessential
Glutamine (Q)	Nonessential
Glycine (G)	Nonessential
Histidine (H)	Conditionally essential
Isoleucine (I)	Essential
Leucine (L)	Essential
Lysine (K)	Essential
Methionine (M)	Essential
Phenylalanine (F)	Essential
Proline (P)	Nonessential
Serine (S)	Nonessential
Threonine (T)	Essential
Tryptophan (W)	Essential
Tyrosine (Y)	Conditionally essential
Valine (V)	Essential

PATHOPHYSIOLOGY: Dietary vitamin K deficiency is very uncommon in the United States but may occur in anorexic patients who consume little or no fat. Vitamin K deficiency occurs in severe fat malabsorption, as in sprue and biliary tract obstruction. Destruction of intestinal flora by antibiotics may also result in vitamin K deficiency. Newborn infants are frequently vitamin K–deficient because the vitamin is not transported well across the placenta and the newborn's sterile gut does not have bacteria to produce it. *Vitamin K confers calcium-binding properties to certain proteins and is important for activities of four clotting factors: prothrombin, factor VII, factor IX, and factor X. Deficiency, then, can be serious since it can lead to, or potentiate, severe bleeding. Parenteral vitamin K therapy is rapidly effective.*

Amino Acids

Of the 20 amino acids in human proteins, no pathways exist for the synthesis of 8, or possibly 9, amino acids (the additional amino acid being histidine). Amino acids that must come from the diet are **essential amino acids**. Humans can synthesize nine **nonessential amino acids** from simple precursors. Finally, synthesis of two amino acids (cysteine and tyrosine) is limited under certain conditions or when adequate quantities of precursors are limited (Table 8-7).

Deficiency of essential amino acids manifests as protein deficiency (kwashiorkor; see above).

Essential Trace Minerals Are Mostly Components of Enzymes and Cofactors

Essential trace minerals include iron, copper, iodine, zinc, cobalt, selenium, manganese, nickel, chromium, tin, molybdenum, vanadium, silicon, and fluorine. Dietary deficiencies of these minerals are clinically important in the case of iron and iodine (**see Chapters 26 and 27**).

Chronic zinc deficiency has been reported in Iran and Egypt to result in hypogonadal dwarfism in boys. Affected children usually consume clay, which may bind zinc, but they also may have protein deficiency. An inherited disorder of zinc metabolism, **acrodermatitis enteropathica**, which is a chronic form of zinc deficiency, is characterized by diarrhea, rash, hair loss, muscle wasting, and mental irritability. Similar symptoms are seen in acute zinc deficiency associated with total parenteral nutrition. Zinc deficiency also occurs in diseases that cause malabsorption, such as Crohn disease, celiac disease, cirrhosis, and alcoholism.

Dietary copper deficiency is rare but may occur in certain inherited disorders, in malabsorption syndromes, and during total parenteral nutrition. It causes microcytic anemia, but megaloblastic changes are also described.

Manganese deficiency causes poor growth, skeletal abnormalities, reproductive impairment, ataxia, and convulsions. Industrial exposure to excess manganese causes symptoms closely related to those of parkinsonism.

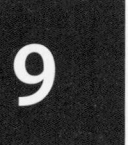

9 Infectious and Parasitic Diseases

David A. Schwartz

THE TOLL OF INFECTIOUS DISEASES

Perhaps the greatest scourge to humankind, the diverse group of disorders collectively known as the infectious diseases have caused more pain, suffering, disability, and premature death than any other group of diseases in history and continue to be significant causes of morbidity and mortality worldwide. The impact of infectious diseases is greatest in low- and middle-income countries, where millions of people, mostly children under 5 years, die of treatable or preventable infections. Even in developed countries of Europe and North America, mortality, morbidity, and loss of economic productivity from infectious diseases are enormous. In the United States, infectious diseases annually cause over 200,000 deaths, more than 50 million days of hospitalization, and almost 2 billion days lost from work or school. It is estimated that smallpox claimed between 300 and 500 million human lives during the 20th century alone. Although smallpox has been eradicated from the natural environment, many other infectious agents continue to claim millions of lives each year. Tuberculosis, malaria, childhood diarrhea, and human immunodeficiency virus (HIV)/acquired immunodeficiency disease (AIDS) continue to ravage the developing world, taking millions of lives each year. Infectious diseases are an important cause of global maternal, infant and child morbidity and mortality, including in those high-income countries where there is an increasing trend towards non-vaccination. Even in industrialized nations, the morbidity and mortality from infectious disease is still substantial. In the United States, sepsis alone causes an estimated 200,000 deaths per year.

Despite the untold past and present (and, undoubtedly, future) misery for which these diseases are responsible, past accomplishments of individuals great and small illustrate how contributions can be made in this area to alleviate human suffering: Edward Jenner's use of cowpox (vaccinia) virus in 1798 to immunize against smallpox; John Snow's removal of the Broad Street pump handle which ended the 1854 London cholera outbreak; the discovery in 1843 by Oliver Wendell Holmes, Sr., that simply washing hands between patients could dramatically reduce the incidence of puerperal fever. All these discoveries were made before an understanding of causation of these illnesses existed. That knowledge came with the work of Koch, Pasteur, Lister, and Ehrlich, who established the field of microbiology which led directly to identification of agents responsible for many infectious diseases, establishment of effective standards of antisepsis and, eventually, the discovery and development of antibiotics to treat common bacterial, fungal, helminthic, and protozoal diseases.

By the 1970s it almost seemed that advanced antibiotics, improved sanitation and vaccination might finally conquer infectious diseases. Unfortunately, that was not to be, as tremendous problems were lurking: Legionnaires disease was discovered in 1976, followed, in 1981, by the first reports of HIV-1/AIDS. Many other infections have emerged (see below) since then, for which we currently have little treatment and no cures: Ebola virus, severe acute respiratory syndrome (SARS), drug-resistant tuberculosis, pandemic strains of influenza virus, carbapenem-resistant enterobacteriaceae (CRE), and others. Three diseases resulting from infectious agents are ranked in the top 10 causes of death worldwide—lower respiratory infections, diarrheal diseases, and tuberculosis. In lower income countries, malaria and AIDS still remain among the top causes of deaths. The emergence of the Ebola virus epidemic in West Africa and later in Democratic Republic of the Congo, and the global Zika virus pandemic, remind us that emerging infections remain an unsolved global public health priority. The recent concern over these and other infectious diseases underscores the facts that the potential for future infectious threats to human existence is real, animal reservoirs of microbes that can be transmitted to humans are bottomless and vigilance can never be relaxed. Finally, the possibility that people may seek to use infectious agents as weapons of warfare should dispel any complacency we have developed that we are safe from these pathogens.

Infectious Diseases Are Disorders in Which Tissue Damage or Dysfunction Results From an Invading Transmissible Agent

These diseases represent many of the familiar taxa: bacteria, fungi, protozoa, and various parasitic worms. Yet some infectious agents do not qualify as completely independent organisms. Viruses cannot replicate by themselves and are obligate intracellular parasites that hijack the replicative machinery of susceptible cells. Likewise, prions, the class of proteinaceous infectious agents, lack nucleic acids and clearly represent a different infectious disease paradigm.

There is great diversity in how various infectious diseases are acquired. Many of these diseases, such as influenza, syphilis and tuberculosis, are contagious, that is, transmissible from person to person. Many infectious diseases, like legionellosis, histoplasmosis, and toxoplasmosis, are not contagious but are rather acquired from the environment. *Legionella* species bacteria normally replicate in aquatic amebas but can infect humans via aerosolized water or through microaspiration of contaminated water. Other infectious agents come from diverse sources, including animals, insects, soil, air, inanimate objects, and the endogenous microbial flora of the human body.

Certain retroviruses have actually been incorporated into the human genome and pass from generation to generation. Their function is unclear but they may activate during placentation, suggesting that they may have facilitated evolution of placentation.

BASIC CONCEPTS

Virulence Is a Characteristic That Allows an Organism to Cause Disease

To do this, an organism must (1) gain access to the body, (2) avoid multiple host defenses, (3) adapt to growth in a human, and (4) exploit human resources. Virulence reflects both the structures inherent to the offending microbe and the interplay of those factors with host defense mechanisms.

Diverse Host Defenses Protect the Body From Infections

For an infectious agent to succeed, it must overcome diverse hurdles, including anatomic barriers (skin), filtration and flushing systems (tears, nasopharyngeal filters), clearance mechanisms (secretions of many organ systems), hostile chemical environments (lysozyme, gastric acid, bile), established competition (commensal gut flora) and, once all these have been overcome, the cellular and soluble components of the innate and adaptive immune systems.

Age Is an Important Determinant of Susceptibility to, and Outcome of, Many Infections

Infections that affect developing fetuses *in utero* illustrate how age affects the outcomes of infectious exposures. Some organisms produce more severe disease *in utero* than in children or adults. Infections of the fetus with cytomegalovirus (CMV), rubella virus, parvovirus B19, and *Toxoplasma gondii* interfere with fetal development. Primary Zika virus infection of adults is asymptomatic in 80% of cases and mildly symptomatic in 20%, but it can cause perinatal death, microcephaly and a congenital fetal malformation syndrome in infected fetuses. Normally, maternal IgG generated by a specific previous infection crosses the placenta and protects the fetus. However, during primary infection in a pregnant woman who lacks neutralizing antibody, certain pathogens may cross the placenta. Although such infections are usually subclinical or mild in the mother, fetal infection can produce minimal damage, major congenital abnormalities or death, depending on the organism and timing of exposure.

Age also affects the courses of common illnesses, like viral and bacterial diarrheas. In older children and adults, these infections cause discomfort and inconvenience, but are rarely severe. Outcomes can be different in children under 3 years, who cannot compensate for rapid volume loss resulting from profuse diarrhea. The United Nations Children's Fund (UNICEF) estimates that diarrheal diseases account for 8% of deaths of children under 5 years globally—over 1,300 daily, and about 480,000 annually.

Mycobacterium tuberculosis, which produces severe, disseminated tuberculosis in children under 3 years, probably because their cell-mediated immune systems are not mature. Older people fare much better.

Maturity, however, is not always an advantage in infections. Epstein–Barr virus (EBV) infections are more likely to be symptomatic in adolescents and adults than in younger children. Varicella-zoster virus, which causes chickenpox, produces more severe disease in adults, who are more likely to develop viral pneumonia.

Elderly patients tend to fare worse with almost all infections than younger ones. Common respiratory illnesses such as influenza and pneumococcal pneumonia are more often fatal in those older than 65 years of age. An example of the susceptibility of the aged to infectious disease occurred during the 2002–2003 outbreak of the newly emergent SARS coronavirus—the case fatality rate was less than 1% for people under 24 years, but was over 50% for those 65 and older.

Human Behaviors Often Determine Exposure to Infectious Agents

Occupational and environmental exposures among farmers, herders, and meat processors to pathogens lead humans to contract brucellosis and Q fever, which are primarily bacterial diseases of domesticated farm animals. Parasites that enter the skin do so when people swim or stand in infested waters (schistosomiasis) or walk barefoot in humid soil (hookworm, *Strongyloides stercoralis*). Some such diseases result from eating undercooked fish (anisakiasis and diphyllobothriasis), meat (toxoplasmosis), or improperly canned food (botulism).

Sexually transmitted diseases—syphilis, gonorrhea, HPV, urogenital chlamydial infections, AIDS, and others—are transmitted mainly by sexual contact. The risk of acquiring sexually transmitted diseases increases with the type and number of sexual encounters.

As human behaviors change, there are new possibilities for infectious diseases. The agent of Legionnaires disease is common in the environment, but causes human infections through aerosols generated by cooling plants, faucets, and humidifiers. Some ritual or traditional behaviors may also promote disease, including coating umbilical cord stumps with dirt (which may contain *Clostridium tetani* spores), or exposure to fecal material which may contain *Taenia solium*, causing cysticercosis). Funerary practices in West Africa exacerbated the spread of Ebola virus to people residing in rural areas and, for the first time, into cities.

People With Compromised Defenses Tend to Contract More, and More Severe, Infections

Impaired host defenses (see above) increase the numbers and severity of infections. Trauma or burns can disrupt epithelial surfaces, allowing access to invasive bacteria or fungi. Injury to mucociliary airway clearance, as in smoking or influenza, impedes elimination of inhaled organisms and predisposes to bacterial pneumonia. Congenital absence of certain complement components (C5–C8) prevents formation of fully functional membrane attack complexes and permits disseminated, and often recurrent, *Neisseria* infections (see Chapter 2). Some diseases (e.g., diabetes mellitus), or medications (chemotherapeutic drugs, steroids) may interfere with neutrophil production or function and increase the likelihood and severity of bacterial infection or invasive fungal infections.

Impaired inflammation or immune function, whether due to cytotoxic and immunosuppressive therapies, debilitation or AIDS, leaves people unable to protect themselves from infections. Compromised hosts become infected more easily, often with organisms that are innocuous to normal people. For example, chemotherapy patients deficient in neutrophils may develop life-threatening bloodstream infections with commensal microorganisms that normally populate the skin and GI tract.

Organisms that mainly cause disease in hosts with impaired defenses are **opportunistic pathogens**. Many are part of normal endogenous human or environmental microbial flora, and take advantage of inadequate defenses to attack more violently and concertedly.

Viral Infections

Viruses range from 20 to 300 nm, with RNA or DNA inside a protein shell. Some also have lipid membrane envelopes. *Viruses do not engage in metabolism or reproduction independently, and thus are obligate intracellular parasites: they require living cells in order to replicate.* After invading cells, viruses commandeer the cells' biosynthetic and metabolic systems in order to produce virus-encoded nucleic acids and proteins.

Viruses often cause disease by killing infected cells, but many do not. For example, rotavirus, a common cause of diarrhea, interferes with the function of infected enterocytes without immediately killing them. It prevents enterocytes from making proteins that transport molecules from the intestinal lumen and so causes diarrhea.

Viruses may also promote release of chemical mediators that elicit inflammatory or immune responses. The symptoms of the common cold are due to release of bradykinin from infected cells. Other viruses cause cells to proliferate and form tumors. Human papillomaviruses (HPVs), for instance, cause squamous cell proliferative lesions, which include common warts and certain cancers.

Some viruses infect and persist in cells without interfering with cellular functions, a process known as **latency**. Latent viruses can emerge to produce disease years after the primary infection. Opportunistic infections are frequently caused by viruses that have established latent infections. CMV and herpes simplex viruses (HSVs) are frequent opportunistic pathogens that are commonly present latently, then emerge in people with impaired cell-mediated immunity.

Finally, some viruses integrate into their genomes or remain as episomes, and cause affected cells to generate tumors. Thus, EBV causes endemic Burkitt lymphoma in Africa, and other tumors in different settings, and human T-cell leukemia virus 1 (HTLV-1, see Chapter 5) causes a form of T-cell lymphoma.

This section is divided into diseases caused by RNA viruses and those caused by DNA viruses. This division reflects fundamental differences in the biology of these agents. Some viruses with highly organ-specific tropisms are not described here in detail, but are addressed in chapters that deal with the main target organs: thus, HIV (see Chapter 4), hepatitis B and C (see Chapter 20), etc.

RNA VIRAL INFECTIONS

A key difference between some RNA viruses and many DNA viruses is that viral polymerases (e.g., HIV-1, hepatitis C virus [HCV]) do not proofread the strand being synthesized. This has two important consequences. First, the mutation rate—and thus the plasticity of these viruses in circumventing

therapies—is very high. Second, a greater percentage of daughter virions are inactive.

The Common Cold Is the Most Common Viral Disease

The common cold (coryza) is an acute, self-limited upper respiratory infection caused by various RNA viruses, including over 110 distinct rhinoviruses and several coronaviruses. Colds are frequent and worldwide in distribution. They spread from person to person via infected secretions. Infection is more likely during winter months in temperate areas, and during rainy seasons in the tropics, when spread is facilitated by indoor crowding. In the United States, children usually suffer six to eight colds per year and adults two to three. Overall, rhinoviruses cause from 10% to 40% of colds, coronaviruses 20%, and respiratory syncytial virus (RSV) 10%.

The viruses infect nasal respiratory epithelial cells, causing increased mucus production and edema. Rhinoviruses and coronaviruses have a tropism for respiratory epithelium and reproduce optimally at temperatures well below 37°C (98.6°F). Thus, infection remains confined to the cooler passages of the upper airway. Infected cells release chemical mediators, such as bradykinin, which produce most of the symptoms associated with colds: increased mucus production, nasal congestion, and eustachian tube obstruction. Resulting stasis may predispose to secondary bacterial infection and lead to bacterial sinusitis and otitis media. Rhinoviruses and coronaviruses do not destroy respiratory epithelium and produce no visible alterations. Clinically, the common cold is characterized by rhinorrhea, pharyngitis, cough, and low-grade fever. Symptoms last about a week.

Influenza May Predispose to Bacterial Pneumonia

Influenza is an acute, usually self-limited, infection of upper and lower airways, caused by influenza virus. These are enveloped, single-stranded RNA viruses.

 EPIDEMIOLOGY: There are three distinct types of influenza virus—types A, B, and C—that cause human disease, but influenza A is by far the most common and causes the most severe disease. Ten to 40 million cases of influenza occur annually in the United States, causing over 40,000 deaths. Influenza is highly contagious, and epidemics often spread around the world. New strains emerge regularly, often from animal hosts, infect humans in parts of the world where humans and animals live in close contact and then disseminate rapidly. Influenza strains are identified by their type (A, B, C) serotype of their hemagglutinin (H) and neuraminidase (virus subtype), their geographic site of origin, strain number, and year of isolation (Fig. 9-1). Thus, the avian influenza virus ("bird flu") strain that emerged in 2003 and spread around the globe up to 2016–2017 is designated A(H5N1). In 2009, a novel influenza A virus, designated H1N1 ("swine flu"), emerged in Veracruz, Mexico, and swiftly spread globally as a pandemic infection. H1N1 was very serious: It caused approximately 10,000 deaths in the United States alone within 7 months of first being identified and over 284,000 deaths worldwide by the end of the pandemic in 2009. It produced significant mortality in infected children

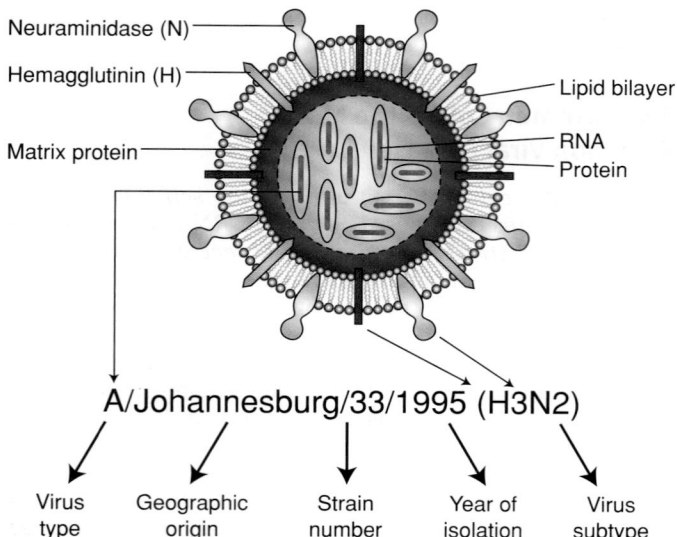

A/Johannesburg/33/1995 (H3N2)

Virus type — Geographic origin — Strain number — Year of isolation — Virus subtype

FIGURE 9-1. Nomenclature of influenza virus strains. The virus type (A, B, or C) is based on nucleoprotein characteristics encoded by the NP gene of the virus. The H classification is based on the hemagglutinin (most commonly H1, H2, or H3, also H5) encoded by the HA gene. The N classification is based on the type of neuraminidase (N1 or N2) encoded by the NA gene.

and pregnant women. Beginning in 2013, a newly strain of avian flu virus, H7N9, was identified in China and was responsible for human deaths. In 2019, a severe strain of flu A virus, H3N2, accounted for almost 50% of cases of influenza in the United states.

Because epidemic influenza virus antigens change so often, host immunity that develops during one epidemic rarely protects against the next one. This was evident in the 2017–2018 flu season in the United States, in which a record number of deaths of children (172) occurred for a single season (excluding pandemics)—80% of these children had not received flu vaccination.

 PATHOPHYSIOLOGY: Influenza spreads from person to person by virus-containing respiratory droplets and secretions. When it reaches the respiratory epithelial cell surface, the virus binds and enters the cell by fusion with the cell membrane, a process mediated by viral hemagglutinin glycoprotein, which binds sialic acid residues on respiratory epithelium. Once inside, the virus directs the cell to produce progeny viruses and causes cell death. Infection usually involves both the upper and the lower airways. Destruction of ciliated epithelium cripples the mucociliary blanket, predisposing to bacterial pneumonia, especially with *Staphylococcus aureus* and *Streptococcus pneumoniae.*

 PATHOLOGY: Influenza virus causes necrosis and desquamation of ciliated respiratory tract epithelium, associated with a predominantly lymphocytic inflammatory infiltrate. Extension of the infection to the lungs leads to necrosis and sloughing of alveolar lining cells and the histologic appearance of viral pneumonitis.

 CLINICAL FEATURES: Rapid onset of fever, chills, myalgia, headaches, weakness, and nonproductive cough are characteristic. Symptoms may be primarily those of an upper respiratory infection or those of tracheitis, bronchitis, and pneumonia. In epidemics there are deaths from influenza and its complications, particularly in the elderly and people with underlying cardiopulmonary disease. Killed viral vaccines specific to epidemic strains are 75% effective in preventing influenza.

Parainfluenza Virus Is Associated With Croup

The parainfluenza viruses cause acute upper and lower respiratory tract infections, particularly in young children. These are enveloped, single-stranded negative-sense RNA viruses with four distinct serotypes, of the paramyxovirus family. They are the most common cause of croup (laryngotracheobronchitis), which is characterized by stridor on inspiration and a "barking" cough.

 EPIDEMIOLOGY: Croup is common in children under 3 years worldwide, who have subglottic swelling, airway compression, and respiratory distress. These viruses spread through infectious respiratory aerosols and secretions. Infection is highly contagious. Parainfluenza viruses are isolated from 10% of young children with acute respiratory tract illnesses. Croup is the second leading cause of hospitalization for respiratory illness in children under 5 years.

PATHOLOGY: Parainfluenza viruses infect and kill ciliated respiratory epithelial cells and elicit an inflammatory response. In very young children, this process often involves the lower respiratory tract, causing bronchiolitis and pneumonitis. In young children, where the trachea is narrow and the larynx is small, the local edema of laryngotracheitis compresses the upper airway enough to obstruct breathing and cause croup. Parainfluenza infection is associated with fever, hoarseness, a barking cough, and inspiratory stridor. In older children and adults, symptoms are usually mild.

Respiratory Syncytial Virus (RSV) Causes Bronchiolitis in Infants

EPIDEMIOLOGY: Like parainfluenza virus, RSV belongs to the Paramyxoviridae family. It spreads rapidly from child to child in respiratory aerosols and secretions, and is common in daycare centers, hospitals, and other settings when small children are confined. RSV is worldwide and highly contagious. In the United States, 60% of infants are infected during their first RSV season, and nearly all will be infected by 2 to 3 years. RSV is the most common cause of bronchiolitis and pneumonia in children under 1 year.

PATHOLOGY: Viral surface proteins bind to specific receptors on host respiratory epithelium to cause fusion. The virus causes necrosis and sloughing of bronchial, bronchiolar, and alveolar epithelium, with a lymphocytic inflammatory infiltrate. Multinucleated syncytial cells are sometimes present.

 CLINICAL FEATURES: Infants and young children with RSV bronchiolitis or pneumonitis present with wheezing, cough and respiratory distress, sometimes accompanied by fever. The illness usually resolves in 1 to 2 weeks. In older children and adults, RSV produces much milder disease. Among otherwise healthy young children, mortality from RSV infection is very low, but it rises dramatically, up to 20% to 40%, among hospitalized children with congenital heart disease, chronic lung disease, prematurity, or immunosuppression.

Severe Acute Respiratory Syndrome (SARS) Is an Emergent Viral Disease Causing Outbreaks of Pneumonia

In early 2002 an epidemic of severe pneumonia was traced to Guangdong Province of China. As outbreaks occurred in Hong Kong, Viet Nam, and Singapore, the disease swept around the globe via routes of international air travel. This emerging clinical disease, SARS, eventually spread to North America and Europe. The causative agent is a novel coronavirus, the SARS-associated coronavirus (SARS-CoV), which is derived from a nonhuman host. In 2017, the source of the SARS virus was identified: a population of horseshoe bats in a remote cave in Yunnan province.

SARS is a potentially fatal viral respiratory illness with an incubation period of 2 to 7 days, with cases ranging up to 10 days. During the initial pandemic between November 2002 and July 2003, there were over 8,000 cases and 775 deaths—a case fatality rate of 9.6%. The last infected human case occurred in mid-2003, but SARS-CoV has not been eradicated and could reemerge.

 PATHOLOGY: Lungs of patients who died from SARS show diffuse alveolar damage (see Chapter 18). Multinucleated syncytial cells without viral inclusions have also been observed.

 CLINICAL FEATURES: SARS begins with fever and headache, followed shortly by cough and dyspnea. Coryza is often absent and diarrhea is common. Lymphopenia is common, and aminotransferase levels are modestly increased. Some patients develop adult respiratory distress syndrome (ARDS, see Chapter 18) and are at high risk of complications and death. Most patients recover, but mortality may reach 15% among the elderly and patients with other respiratory disorders. There are no controlled clinical trials, and no specific treatment is available.

Measles (Rubeola) Is a Highly Contagious Viral Exanthem That Can Be Fatal

Measles virus is an enveloped, single-stranded RNA paramyxovirus that causes an acute illness, characterized by upper respiratory tract symptoms, fever, and rash.

 EPIDEMIOLOGY: Measles virus is transmitted in respiratory aerosols and secretions. Among nonimmunized populations, it is primarily a disease of children. Current live, attenuated vaccines (measles is included in the 3-part MMR vaccine administered to infants and children) are highly effective in preventing measles and in eliminating its spread. Nationwide immunization has made measles uncommon in the United States. Similar efforts are under way worldwide to immunize all children.

In some settings, measles can be particularly severe with mortality rate of 10% to 25%. In immunocompromised and AIDS patients, the fatality rate may reach 30%. WHO estimates that there were 89,780 deaths worldwide in 2016 due to measles, and it remains a cause of major vaccine-preventable deaths. When measles was first introduced to previously unexposed populations (e.g., Native Americans, Pacific Islanders), resulting widespread infections had devastatingly high mortality rates.

Beginning in January 2019 an outbreak of measles occurred in the United States, mostly in non-vaccinated persons, with 626 cases confirmed in 15 states between January 1st and April 15th.

 PATHOPHYSIOLOGY: The initial site of infection is nasopharyngeal and bronchial mucous membranes. Two surface glycoproteins, "H" and "F" proteins, mediate viral attachment and fusion with respiratory epithelium. The virus then spreads to regional lymph nodes and the bloodstream, leading to widespread dissemination with prominent involvement of the skin and lymphoid tissues. T-cells attacking virally infected vascular endothelium cause the characteristic rash.

 PATHOLOGY: Measles virus produces necrosis of infected respiratory epithelium, with a predominantly lymphocytic inflammatory infiltrate. It causes vasculitis of small blood vessels in the skin. Lymphoid hyperplasia is often prominent in cervical and mesenteric lymph nodes, spleen, and appendix. In lymphoid tissues, measles virus sometimes causes fusion of infected cells, producing multinucleated giant cells containing up to 100 nuclei, with intracytoplasmic and intranuclear inclusions. These **Warthin–Finkeldey giant cells** (Fig. 9-2) are pathognomonic for measles.

 CLINICAL FEATURES: Measles first manifests with fever, rhinorrhea, cough, and conjunctivitis, progressing to characteristic mucosal and skin lesions. The mucosal lesions, or Koplik spots, are minute gray-white dots on a red base on the posterior buccal

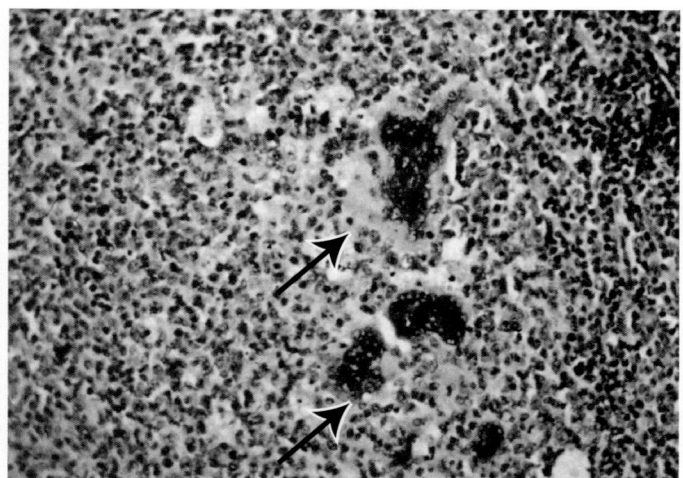

FIGURE 9-2. Warthin–Finkeldey giant cells in measles. A hyperplastic lymph node from a patient with measles shows several multinucleated giant cells (*arrows*).

mucosa. The skin lesions begin on the face as an erythematous maculopapular rash, which usually spreads to involve the trunk and extremities. The rash fades in 3 to 5 days, and symptoms gradually resolve.

The clinical course of measles may be much more severe in very young, malnourished, or immunocompromised patients. Measles often leads to secondary bacterial infections, especially otitis media and pneumonia. CNS invasion is probably common, as suggested by changes in electroencephalograph readings. Acute encephalitis is rare but does occur. Uncommonly, years after acute infection, patients can develop subacute sclerosing panencephalitis (SSPE), a slow, chronic neurodegenerative disorder. The pathophysiology of SSPE is unclear, but prophylactic vaccination against measles has greatly reduced the incidence of SSPE.

Rubella Infection *In Utero* Is Associated With Congenital Anomalies

Rubella virus is an enveloped, single-stranded RNA virus that causes a mild, self-limited systemic disease, usually associated with a rash (also known as "German measles"). Rubella virus is the only member of the genus of *Rubivirus*, in the family Togaviridae. Many infections are so mild that they go unnoticed. However, infection in a pregnant woman early in gestation can produce fetal death, premature delivery, and congenital anomalies, including deafness, cataracts, glaucoma, heart defects, and mental retardation.

EPIDEMIOLOGY: Rubella virus spreads primarily by the respiratory route. Infection occurs worldwide. Rubella is not highly contagious, and in unvaccinated populations, 10% to 15% of young women remain susceptible to infection into their reproductive years. The currently available live attenuated viral vaccine (part of MMR vaccine) prevents rubella and has largely eliminated the disease from developed countries. In the Americas, vaccination has interrupted transmission of the virus, and no endemic case has been observed since February 2009.

PATHOPHYSIOLOGY: Rubella infects respiratory epithelium, then disseminates through the bloodstream and lymphatics. Its rash is believed to result from an immunologic response to the disseminated virus. Fetal infection occurs through the placenta during the viremic phase of maternal illness. A congenitally infected fetus remains persistently infected and sheds large amounts of virus in body fluids, even after birth. Maternal infection after 20 weeks' gestation usually does not cause significant fetal disease.

PATHOLOGY: In the fetus, the heart, eye, and brain are the organs most frequently affected. Cardiac lesions include pulmonary valvular stenosis, pulmonary artery hypoplasia, ventricular septal defects, and patent ductus arteriosus (50% of patients). Cataracts, glaucoma, microphthalmia, and retinal defects may occur in 43% of patients. Severe brain involvement can produce microcephaly and mental retardation.

CLINICAL FEATURES: In most patients, rubella is a mild, acute febrile illness, with rhinorrhea, conjunctivitis, postauricular lymphadenopathy, and a rash that spreads from face to trunk and extremities. The rash resolves within 3 days; complications are rare. As many as 30% of infections are completely asymptomatic. Sensorineural deafness is a common (58%) complication of fetal rubella.

Zika Virus Is Profoundly Teratogenic if Exposure Occurs During Pregnancy

Zika virus is a flavivirus that is a newly emergent arbovirus that causes few or no symptoms in nonpregnant people. However, if it infects a pregnant woman, it can cause a fetal malformation syndrome that may include microcephaly and perinatal death.

EPIDEMIOLOGY: Zika virus is transmitted to humans via the bite of an infected *Aedes* mosquito—*A. aegyptii* or *A. albopictus*. Less frequently, Zika virus can be transmitted sexually from either gender. Like other mosquito-borne viruses, Zika virus occurs more often in low-income people in the warm regions of the world, where urban crowding favors breeding of the mosquito vectors and vector-borne transmission to humans. Following its initial recognition in the Western Hemisphere in Brazil in 2015, it became epidemic in South and Central America and the Caribbean from 2015 to 2016. It infected many hundreds of thousands of people, and possibly more. Its prevalence plummeted by 2017, probably because of an expanding population of immune people, or herd immunity.

PATHOPHYSIOLOGY: Zika virus infects cells of neuronal derivation. Following transplacental transmission from an infected mother to the fetus, it infects and kills primordial neural progenitor cells in the developing fetal brain. Virus RNA has been identified in several other maternal and fetal tissues including umbilical cord blood, several placental cell types including Hofbauer cells and trophoblast, decidual cells and amniotic fluid, as well as in the brain and placenta of human fetuses that were spontaneously aborted during the first and second trimesters.

 PATHOLOGY: Fetuses with congenital Zika syndrome show a spectrum of pathologic findings. Findings of fetal brain disruption sequence include severe microcephaly with partial collapse of the skull, overlapping cranial sutures, prominence of the occipital bone, and redundant scalp skin. Brain abnormalities are likely the result of direct cell injury by Zika virus, and include ventriculomegaly, microencephaly, hydrocephalus, agyria, cortical thinning, calcifications in the cortex and subcortical white matter and neuronal necrosis. Ocular abnormalities can include microphthalmia, cataracts, retinal findings such as chorioretinal atrophy, and optic nerve lesions. In some infected infants microcephaly begins following birth.

CLINICAL FEATURES: Most infected children and adults are asymptomatic. In the 20% of individuals with symptoms, most show fever, rash, conjunctivitis, joint and muscle pains, and headache. Fetuses with congenital infection can have contractual abnormalities including arthrogryposis or clubfoot in addition to CNS abnormalities. Zika virus infection is strongly associated with Guillain–Barré syndrome, but only a small number of infected people develop this disease.

Mumps Causes Acute Parotitis and Meningoencephalitis

Mumps virus is an enveloped, single-stranded RNA virus in the family Paramyxoviridae, that causes an acute, self-limited systemic illness.

EPIDEMIOLOGY: Mumps is mainly a disease of childhood, worldwide. It spreads via the respiratory route and is highly contagious: 90% of exposed, susceptible people become infected. Only 6% to 70% develop symptoms, however. A live attenuated mumps vaccine prevents mumps (part of MMR vaccine), and the disease has been largely eliminated from most developed countries.

PATHOPHYSIOLOGY: Mumps begins with viral infection of respiratory tract epithelium. The virus then disseminates through blood and lymphatic systems to other sites, most commonly the salivary glands (especially parotids), CNS, pancreas and testes. Over half of infections involve the CNS, with symptomatic disease in 10%. Epididymoorchitis occurs in 15% to 20% of males infected after puberty.

 PATHOLOGY: Mumps virus causes necrosis of infected cells, with a predominantly lymphocytic inflammatory infiltrate. Affected salivary glands are swollen, their ducts lined by necrotic epithelium and their interstitium infiltrated with lymphocytes. In mumps epididymoorchitis, testes can swell to three times normal size. As testes are confined by the tunica albuginea, focal infarcts may occur. Mumps orchitis is usually unilateral and so rarely causes sterility.

CLINICAL FEATURES: Mumps begins with fever and malaise, followed by painful salivary gland swelling, usually of one or both parotids. Symptomatic meningeal involvement most often manifests as headache, stiff neck, and vomiting. Before widespread vaccination, mumps was a leading cause of viral meningitis and encephalitis in the United States. Although severe disease of the pancreas is rare in mumps, most patients show elevated blood amylase.

Rotavirus Infection Is the Most Common Cause of Severe Diarrhea Worldwide

Rotavirus produces profuse watery diarrhea that can lead to dehydration and death if untreated. This double-stranded RNA virus, a member of the family Reoviridae, usually infects young children.

EPIDEMIOLOGY: Rotavirus infection spreads from person to person by the oral–fecal route. There are five species, termed Rotavirus A, B, C, D, and E. Rotavirus A, the most common to infect humans, causes >90% of cases. Infection is most common among children, who shed huge amounts of virus in the stool. Siblings, playmates, parents, as well as food, water, and environmental surfaces are readily contaminated with virus. The peak age of infection is 6 months to 2 years. Virtually all children have been infected by the age of 4 years. Rotavirus causes about 100 deaths annually in young children in the United States, and over 450,000 deaths worldwide among children under 5 years.

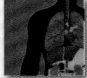 **PATHOPHYSIOLOGY:** Rotavirus infects enterocytes of the upper small intestine, disrupting absorption of sugars, fats, and various ions. Resulting osmotic load causes a net fluid loss into the bowel lumen, producing diarrhea and dehydration. Infected cells are shed from intestinal villi, and the regenerating epithelium initially lacks full absorptive capabilities.

 PATHOLOGY: Pathologic changes in rotavirus infection are largely confined to the duodenum and jejunum, with shortened villi and a mild infiltrate of neutrophils and lymphocytes.

CLINICAL FEATURES: Rotavirus infection manifests as vomiting, fever, abdominal pain and profuse, watery diarrhea. Vomiting usually lasts 2 to 3 days, but diarrhea continues for 5 to 8 days. Fluid replacement is critical: without adequate fluids, the diarrhea can cause fatal dehydration in young children.

Norwalk and Other Gastrointestinal Viruses Cause Outbreaks of Diarrhea

There are many viral causes of diarrhea. The best understood are the Norwalk family of nonenveloped RNA viruses, a group of caliciviruses whose names derive from the locations of particular outbreaks (e.g., Norwalk virus, Snow Mountain virus, Sapporo virus). Norwalk viruses are responsible for one-third of outbreaks of diarrheal disease. They produce gastroenteritis in children and adults, with self-limited vomiting and diarrhea, similar to that caused by rotavirus. Norwalk viruses infect cells of the upper small bowel and produce changes like those seen with rotavirus.

Viral Hemorrhagic Fevers Cause Hemorrhage, Shock, and Sometimes Death

There are many similar viral hemorrhagic fevers in different parts of the world, usually named for the area where they were first described. Members of five RNA virus families—Bunyaviridae, Flaviviridae, Arenaviridae, Filoviridae, and most recently, Rhabdoviridae—are responsible. Routes of transmission, vectors, and other epidemiologic characteristics divide these diseases into four epidemiologic groups (Table 9-1): mosquito-borne; tick-borne; zoonotic; and the filoviruses, Marburg and Ebola virus, in which the route of transmission is unknown.

Yellow Fever

Yellow fever is an acute hemorrhagic fever, sometimes associated with extensive hepatic necrosis and jaundice. It is caused by an insect-borne flavivirus, an enveloped, single-stranded RNA virus. Other pathogenic flaviviruses cause Omsk hemorrhagic fever and Kyasanur Forest disease.

EPIDEMIOLOGY: Yellow fever was first recognized in the 17th century. Today, the virus is restricted to parts of Africa and South America, including jungle and urban settings. The usual viral reservoir is tree-dwelling monkeys, for which the virus is not pathogenic, but among which it spreads in the forest canopy via mosquitoes. Humans acquire jungle yellow fever by entering the forest, after bites infected *Aedes mosquitoes.* Felling trees increases risk of infection, since mosquitoes are brought down with the tree. On returning to the village or city, the human victim becomes a reservoir for epidemic yellow fever in the urban setting, where *Aedes aegyptii* is the vector. Outbreaks of yellow fever continue to occur despite the availability of an effective vaccine. Beginning in 2017 a large multistate outbreak of yellow fever has been occurring in Brazil, including regions where the disease had not previously been a risk.

PATHOPHYSIOLOGY: On inoculation by the mosquito, the virus multiplies within tissue and vascular endothelium, then disseminates through the bloodstream. It has a tropism for liver cells, where it sometimes produces extensive acute hepatocellular destruction. Extensive damage to endothelium of small blood vessels may lead to loss of vascular integrity, hemorrhage, and shock.

PATHOLOGY: Yellow fever virus causes coagulative necrosis of hepatocytes, which characteristically begins in the middle of hepatic lobules and spreads toward central veins and portal tracts. Infection sometimes produces confluent areas of necrosis in the middle of the hepatic lobules (i.e., midzonal necrosis). In the most severe cases, an entire lobule may be necrotic. Virus-induced apoptosis may cause hepatocytes to become intensely eosinophilic and dislodge from adjacent cells, as Councilman bodies (see Chapter 1).

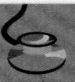

CLINICAL FEATURES: Yellow fever starts abruptly, with fever, chills, headache, myalgias, nausea, and vomiting. After 3 to 5 days, some patients develop signs of hepatic failure, with jaundice (hence the term "yellow" fever), deficiencies of clotting factors and diffuse hemorrhages. Vomiting of clotted blood ("black vomit") is a classic feature in severe cases. Patients with massive hepatic failure lapse into coma and die, usually within 10 days of onset of illness. Overall mortality is 5%, but among those with jaundice, it rises to 30%.

Ebola

Ebola virus is an RNA virus belonging to the Filoviridae family. It causes an acute febrile disease with a high mortality rate in humans in several regions of Africa. The only

TABLE 9-1
VIRAL HEMORRHAGIC FEVERS

Vector	Viral Fever
Mosquitoes	Yellow fever
	Rift valley fever
	Dengue hemorrhagic fever
	Chikungunya hemorrhagic fever
Ticks	Omsk hemorrhagic fever
	Crimean hemorrhagic fever
	Kyasanur Forest disease
Rodents	Lassa fever
	Bolivian hemorrhagic fever
	Argentine hemorrhagic fever
	Korean hemorrhagic fever
Fruit bats	Ebola virus disease

other filoviruses pathogenic to humans are the Marburg viruses, which produce Marburg virus disese.

 EPIDEMIOLOGY: Ebola virus first emerged in Africa with two major disease outbreaks that occurred almost simultaneously in Zaire and Sudan in 1976. Outbreaks of Ebola virus disease have occurred in Africa up to the present time, and are primarily caused by Zaire and Sudan strains. From 2000 to 2003, outbreaks caused by the Zaire strain of the virus occurred in Gabon, Republic of the Congo, and Uganda. Case fatality rates ranged from 53% to 89%. In January 2008, a new strain of Ebola virus, the Ebola Bundibugyo strain, emerged in Western Uganda, and reoccurred in 2012 in the Democratic Republic of the Congo. There are currently five viruses in the genus Ebola—Zaire ebolavirus (ZEBOV), Sudan ebolavirus (SEBOV), Reston ebolavirus (REBOV), Taï Forest virus (TAFV, formerly Côte d'Ivoire ebolavirus), and Bundibugyo ebolavirus (BEBOV). Beginning in late 2013 and lasting until 2016, the Ebola virus unexpectedly emerged in West Africa, where it rapidly became epidemic in Liberia, Sierra Leone, and Guinea, with over 28,000 suspected cases and more than 11,000 deaths. This was the first time that Ebola virus had infected urban areas. A post-Ebola syndrome was described from survivors of this epidemic. As a result of this epidemic, an effective vaccine was developed and tested, which was later successfully used to limit a subsequent outbreak of Ebola virus disease in DRC Congo in 2018.

In the wild, the virus infects humans, gorillas, chimpanzees, and monkeys. Recent field evidence from Gabon and the Republic of the Congo area of western Africa has implicated several species of fruit bats as the natural reservoir of Ebola virus. Healthcare workers and family members have become infected as a result of exposure while treating patients or during funerary preparation of bodies of deceased victims. Ebola virus can be transmitted via bodily secretions, blood and used needles, and it can persist in the semen.

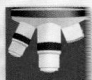 **PATHOPHYSIOLOGY, PATHOLOGY:** *Ebola virus results in the most widespread destructive tissue lesions of all viral hemorrhagic fever agents.* The virus replicates massively in endothelial cells, mononuclear phagocytes, and hepatocytes. Necrosis is most severe in the liver, kidneys, gonads, spleen, and lymph nodes. The liver characteristically shows hepatocellular necrosis, Kupffer cell hyperplasia, Councilman bodies, and microsteatosis. The lungs are usually hemorrhagic. Petechial hemorrhages are seen in the skin, mucous membranes, and internal organs. Injury to the microvasculature and increased endothelial permeability are important causes of shock.

CLINICAL FEATURES: Ebola virus disease incubates from 2 to 21 days, after which initial symptoms include headache, weakness and fever, followed by diarrhea, nausea, and vomiting. Some patients develop overt hemorrhage including bleeding from injection sites, petechiae, GI, and gingival hemorrhage. Ebola virus is especially lethal to unborn fetuses and newborns—of all Ebola virus epidemics since 1976, only two infants have survived, possibly due to the immediate administration of experimental therapy.

West Nile Virus (WNV)

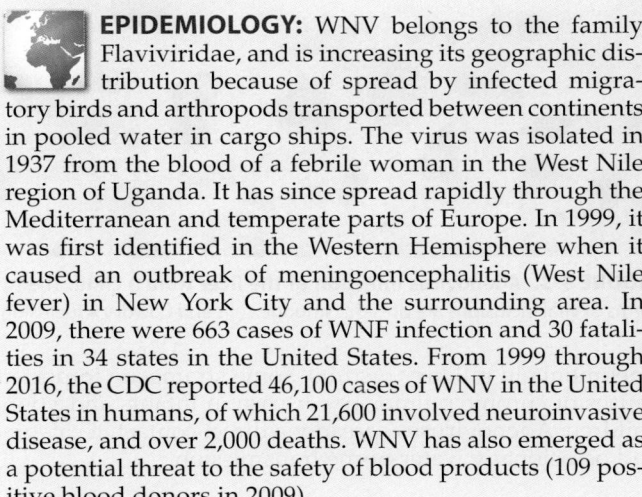 **EPIDEMIOLOGY:** WNV belongs to the family Flaviviridae, and is increasing its geographic distribution because of spread by infected migratory birds and arthropods transported between continents in pooled water in cargo ships. The virus was isolated in 1937 from the blood of a febrile woman in the West Nile region of Uganda. It has since spread rapidly through the Mediterranean and temperate parts of Europe. In 1999, it was first identified in the Western Hemisphere when it caused an outbreak of meningoencephalitis (West Nile fever) in New York City and the surrounding area. In 2009, there were 663 cases of WNF infection and 30 fatalities in 34 states in the United States. From 1999 through 2016, the CDC reported 46,100 cases of WNV in the United States in humans, of which 21,600 involved neuroinvasive disease, and over 2,000 deaths. WNV has also emerged as a potential threat to the safety of blood products (109 positive blood donors in 2009).

PATHOLOGY: WNV can be recovered from blood for up to 10 days in immunocompetent febrile patients, and longer in immunocompromised patients. Patients show slightly increased sedimentation rate and mild leukocytosis; cerebrospinal fluid in patients with CNS involvement is clear, with moderate pleocytosis and elevated protein. Brains show mononuclear meningoencephalitis or encephalitis. The brainstem, particularly the medulla, can be extensively involved, and in some cases cranial nerve roots had endoneural mononuclear inflammation. There are varying degrees of neuronal necrosis in gray matter, neuronal degeneration, and neuronophagia.

CLINICAL FEATURES: Most human WNV infections are subclinical, overt disease occurring in only 1 of 100 infections. Incubation periods range from 3 to 15 days. Symptoms, if they occur, are usually fever, often with rash, lymphadenopathy, and polyarthropathy. Patients with severe illness can develop acute aseptic meningitis or encephalitis, with convulsions and coma. Anterior myelitis, hepatosplenomegaly, hepatitis, pancreatitis, and myocarditis may develop. The probability of severe illness increases with increasing age. CNS infection is associated with a 4% to 13% mortality and is highest among elderly people.

DNA VIRUSES

Adenoviruses Cause Respiratory and Intestinal Diseases

Adenoviruses are nonenveloped DNA viruses. Certain serotypes commonly cause acute respiratory disease and

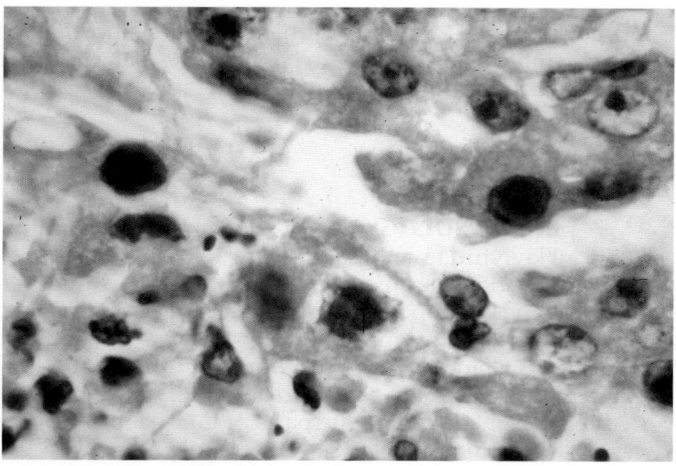

FIGURE 9-3. Adenovirus infection of the liver from a child. The two forms of viral inclusions are present: smudge cells and Cowdry A inclusions.

pneumonia in military recruits. Some strains are important causes of chronic pulmonary disease in infants and young children. Adenoviruses spread via direct contact, fecal–oral, and occasionally water-borne transmission.

PATHOLOGY: Pathologic changes include necrotizing bronchitis and bronchiolitis, in which sloughed epithelial cells and inflammatory infiltrate may fill the damaged bronchioles. Interstitial pneumonitis is characterized by areas of consolidation with extensive necrosis, hemorrhage, and a mononuclear inflammatory infiltrate. Two distinctive types of intranuclear inclusions (Fig. 9-3) involve bronchiolar epithelial cells and alveolar lining cells in areas of consolidation and among the necrotizing bronchiolar epithelial lesions. In early stages of adenovirus infection, cytopathic effects include granular, slightly enlarged nuclei with eosinophilic bodies intermixed with clumped basophilic chromatin. The eosinophilic bodies coalesce, forming large masses to end as a central, granular, ill-defined mass surrounded by a halo—a Cowdry A inclusion. The second type of inclusion, the "smudge cell," is more common and probably corresponds to a late-stage infected cell. Its nucleus is round or ovoid, large, and completely occupied by a granular amphophilic to deeply basophilic mass. There is no halo, and the nuclear membrane and nucleus are indistinct.

Adenoviruses types 40 and 41 infect colonic and small intestinal epithelial cells and may cause diarrhea in immunocompetent and immunocompromised hosts. AIDS patients are particularly susceptible to urinary tract infections caused by adenovirus type 35. In immunocompromised patients and transplant recipients, adenovirus can cause fulminant or disseminated disease such as colitis, pneumonitis, pancreatitis, nephritis, meningoencephalitis, and hepatitis.

Human Parvovirus B19 Causes Erythema Infectiosum in Children

This single-stranded DNA virus, now called erythrovirus, causes a benign self-limited febrile illness in children: **erythema infectiosum**. It also causes systemic infections characterized by rash, arthralgias, and transient interruption in erythrocyte production in nonimmune adults.

Erythrovirus spreads from person to person by the respiratory route. Infection is common and occurs in outbreaks, mostly among children. It is not known which cells, other than erythroid precursors, support virus replication, but the virus probably replicates in the respiratory tract before it spreads to erythropoietic cells.

PATHOLOGY: This virus gains entry to erythroid precursor cells via the P erythrocyte antigen, and produces characteristic cytopathic effects in those cells. Nuclei of affected cells are enlarged, with the chromatin is displaced peripherally by central glassy eosinophilic material nuclear inclusion bodies (giant pronormoblasts).

CLINICAL FEATURES: Erythema infectiosum is a mild exanthematous illness, accompanied by an asymptomatic interruption in erythropoiesis. In people with chronic hemolytic anemias, however, the pause in erythrocyte production may cause profound, potentially fatal anemia, known as **transient aplastic crisis** (see Chapter 26). When a fetus is infected by human parvovirus B19, transient cessation of erythropoiesis can lead to severe anemia and hydrops fetalis. Intrauterine death occurs in 10% of maternal infections.

Smallpox (Variola) Was a Highly Contagious, Often Lethal, Poxvirus Infection

EPIDEMIOLOGY: Smallpox is an ancient disease: a rash resembling smallpox was found in the mummified remains of Egyptian pharaoh Ramses V, who died in 1160 BC. In the 6th century, a Swiss bishop named the etiologic agent of smallpox "variola" from the Latin *varius*, meaning pimple or spot. The infection was common in Europe. It arrived in the New World with Spanish colonists, and often decimated native populations. In 1796, Edward Jenner performed the first successful vaccination when he inoculated a child with lymph from the hand of a milkmaid infected with cowpox. Once the cowpox pustule had regressed, Jenner challenged that child with smallpox and demonstrated that he was protected from the disease. In 1967, the WHO began its uniquely successful campaign to eradicate smallpox. The last occurrence of endemic smallpox was in Somalia in 1977, and the last reported human cases were laboratory-acquired infections in 1978. On May 8, 1980, the WHO declared that smallpox had been eradicated. Two known repositories of variola virus remain: one at the CDC in the United States, and one at the Institute for Virus Preparation in Russia. There has been considerable vigilance to its reemergence, either naturally or as a bioweapon.

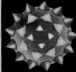 **ETIOLOGIC FACTORS:** Smallpox was transmitted between smallpox victims and susceptible people via droplets or aerosol of infected saliva. Viral titers in the saliva were highest in the first week of

infection. The virus is highly stable and remains infective for long periods outside its human host. Two types of smallpox have been recognized. *Variola major* was prevalent in Asia and parts of Africa and was the prototypical form of the infection. *Variola minor* was found in Africa, South America, and Europe. It was a milder disease, with smaller pox lesions.

PATHOLOGY: Skin vesicles of variola show reticular degeneration and scarce areas of ballooning degeneration. Eosinophilic, intracytoplasmic inclusion bodies (Guarnieri bodies) are seen, but are not specific for smallpox since they occur in most poxviral infections. Vesicles also occur in the palate, pharynx, trachea, and esophagus. In severe cases, there is gastric and intestinal involvement, hepatitis and interstitial nephritis.

CLINICAL FEATURES: Smallpox incubation period is about 12 days (range, 7 to 17 days) after exposure. After entering the respiratory tract, variola travels to regional lymph nodes, where it replicates and causes viremia. Clinical manifestations begin abruptly with malaise, fever, vomiting, and headache. The characteristic rash follows in 2 to 3 days. It is most prominent on the face but also involves the hands and forearms. After subsequent eruptions on the legs, the rash spreads centrally during the next week to the trunk. Lesions progress quickly from macules to papules, then to pustular vesicles (Fig. 9-4), and generally remain synchronous in their stage of development. By 8 to 14 days after onset, the pustules form scabs, which leave depressed scars on healing after 3 to 4 weeks. The case fatality rate is 30% in unvaccinated people.

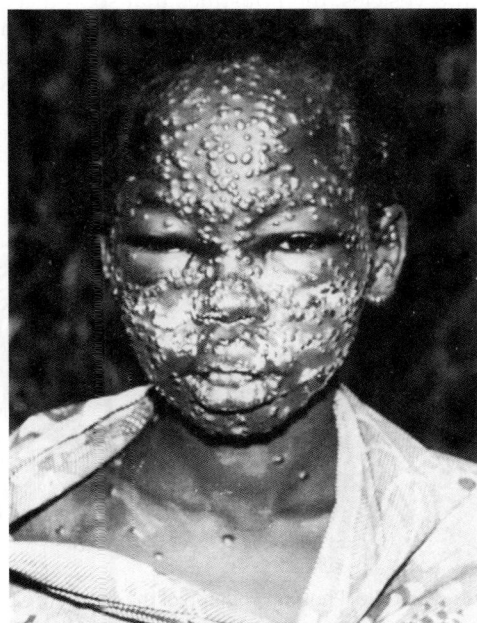

FIGURE 9-4. Child with smallpox, Bangladesh, 1973.

Monkeypox Is a Rare Poxviral Disease, Mainly in Central and West Africa

It is the only remaining potentially fatal poxvirus infection of humans. Since 2017, Nigeria has been experiencing the largest outbreak of monkeypox to occur in West Africa.

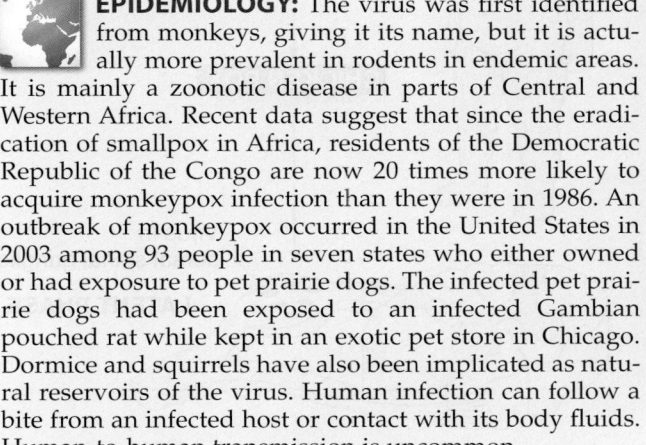

EPIDEMIOLOGY: The virus was first identified from monkeys, giving it its name, but it is actually more prevalent in rodents in endemic areas. It is mainly a zoonotic disease in parts of Central and Western Africa. Recent data suggest that since the eradication of smallpox in Africa, residents of the Democratic Republic of the Congo are now 20 times more likely to acquire monkeypox infection than they were in 1986. An outbreak of monkeypox occurred in the United States in 2003 among 93 people in seven states who either owned or had exposure to pet prairie dogs. The infected pet prairie dogs had been exposed to an infected Gambian pouched rat while kept in an exotic pet store in Chicago. Dormice and squirrels have also been implicated as natural reservoirs of the virus. Human infection can follow a bite from an infected host or contact with its body fluids. Human-to-human transmission is uncommon.

CLINICAL FEATURES: The incubation period in humans is about 12 days. It presents clinically like smallpox, but is milder. Illness begins with fever, headache, lymphadenopathy, malaise, muscle, and back ache, followed within 1 to 3 days by fever and a papular rash on the face or other body parts, which ultimately crusts and falls off. Illness typically lasts 2 weeks. In Africa, the case fatality is as high as 10%.

Herpesviruses Are Large, Enveloped Viruses, Many of Which Infect Humans

The virus family Herpesviridae includes a large number of enveloped, DNA viruses, many of which infect humans. Almost all herpesviruses express some common antigenic determinants, and many produce type A nuclear inclusions (acidophilic bodies surrounded by a halo). The most important pathogenic human herpesviruses are varicella-zoster (VZV or HHV-3), herpes simplex virus 1 and 2 (HHV-1 and HHV-2), Epstein–Barr virus (EBV or HHV-4), human herpesvirus 6 (HHV-6, the cause of roseola), cytomegalovirus (CMV or HHV-5), human herpesvirus 7 (HHV-7, a cause of exanthema subitum), and human herpesvirus 8 (KHSV or HHV-8, a human oncovirus causing Kaposi sarcoma, primary effusion lymphoma and some types of Castleman disease). *These viruses are distinguished by their capacity to remain latent for long periods of time.*

First Exposure to Varicella-Zoster Virus Causes Chickenpox

Chickenpox is an acute systemic illness characterized by a generalized vesicular skin eruption (Fig. 9-5). The virus then becomes latent. Its reactivation causes herpes zoster ("shingles"), a painful, localized vesicular skin eruption.

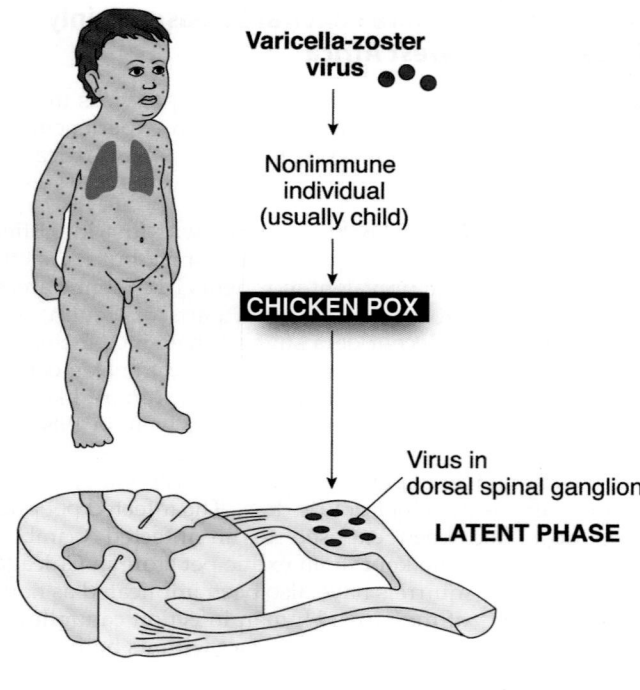

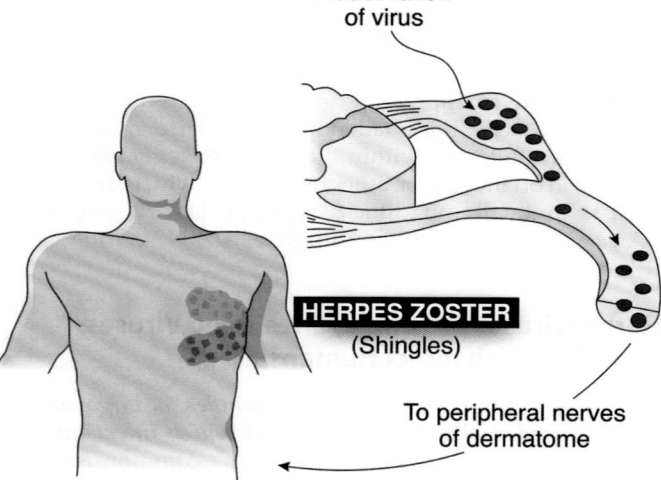

FIGURE 9-5. Varicella (chickenpox) and herpes zoster (shingles). Varicella-zoster virus (VZV) in droplets is inhaled by a nonimmune person (usually a child) and initially causes a "silent" infection of the nasopharynx. This progresses to viremia, seeding of fixed macrophages and dissemination of VZV to skin (chickenpox) and viscera. VZV resides in a dorsal spinal ganglion, where it remains dormant for many years. Latent VZV is reactivated and spreads from ganglia along the sensory nerves to the peripheral nerves of sensory dermatomes, causing shingles.

EPIDEMIOLOGY: VZV infects human hosts worldwide, is highly contagious, and spreads from person to person primarily by the respiratory route. It can also be spread by contact with secretions from skin lesions. Most children in the United States are infected by early school age, but an effective vaccine has reduced this incidence.

PATHOPHYSIOLOGY: VZV initially infects cells of the respiratory tract or conjunctival epithelium. There it reproduces and spreads through the blood and lymphatic systems. Many organs are infected during this viremic stage, but skin involvement usually dominates the clinical picture. VZV spreads from the capillary endothelium to the epidermis, where its replication destroys the basal cells. As a result, the upper layers of the epidermis separate from the basal layer to form vesicles.

During primary infection, VZV establishes latent infection in perineuronal satellite cells of the dorsal nerve root ganglia. Transcription of viral genes continues during latency, and viral DNA persists for years after the initial infection.

Shingles occurs when full virus replication occurs in ganglion cells and the agent travels down the sensory nerve from a single dermatome. It then infects the corresponding epidermis, producing a localized, painful vesicular eruption. The risk of shingles increases with age, and most cases occur among the elderly. Impaired cell-mediated immunity also increases the risk of herpes zoster reactivation.

PATHOLOGY: The skin lesions of chickenpox and shingles are identical to each other and also to the lesions of HSV. Vesicles fill with neutrophils and soon erode to become shallow ulcers. In infected cells, VZV produces a characteristic cytopathic effect, with nuclear homogenization, intranuclear inclusions (Cowdry type A). Inclusions are large and eosinophilic, and are separated from the nuclear membrane by a clear zone (halo). Multinucleated cells are common (Fig. 9-6). Over several days, vesicles become pustules, then rupture and heal.

CLINICAL FEATURES: Chickenpox causes fever, malaise, and a distinctive pruritic rash, that starts on the head and spreads to the trunk and extremities. Skin lesions begin as maculopapules that rapidly evolve into vesicles, then pustules that soon ulcerate and crust. Vesicles may also appear on mucous membranes, especially the mouth. Fever and systemic symptoms resolve in 3 to 5 days; skin lesions heal in several weeks.

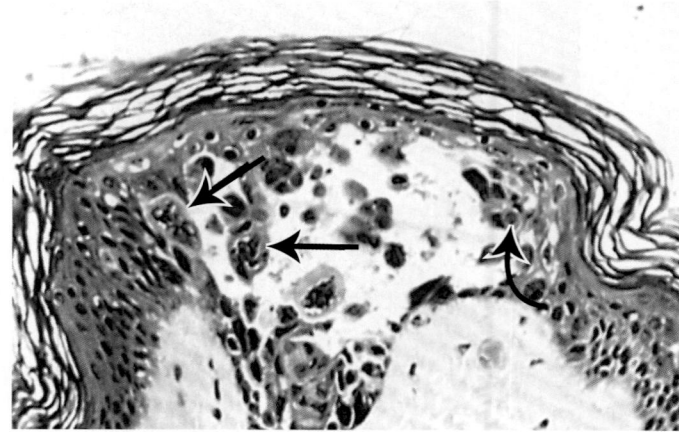

FIGURE 9-6. Varicella. Photomicrograph of the skin from a patient with chickenpox shows an intraepidermal vesicle. Multinucleated giant cells (*straight arrows*) and nuclear inclusions (*curved arrow*) are present.

TABLE 9-2
HERPES SIMPLEX VIRAL DISEASES

Viral Type	Common Presentations	Infrequent Presentations
HSV-1	Oral-labial herpes	Conjunctivitis, keratitis
		Encephalitis
		Herpetic whitlow
		Esophagitis[a]
		Pneumonia[a]
		Disseminated infection[a]
HSV-2	Genital herpes	Perinatal infection
		Disseminated infection[a]

[a]Usually occur in immunocompromised hosts.

Shingles presents with a unilateral, painful, vesicular eruption, similar in appearance to chickenpox, but in a dermatomal pattern, usually localized to a single dermatome. Pain can persist for months after resolution of the skin lesions.

Herpes Simplex Viruses (HSVs) 1 and 2 Are Transmitted in Oral and Genital Secretions, Respectively

HSVs are common human viral pathogens (Table 9-2). Two antigenically and epidemiologically distinct HSVs cause human disease (Fig. 9-7):

- **HSV-1** (also termed **HHV-1**) is transmitted in oral secretions and typically causes disease "above the waist," including oral, facial, and ocular lesions.
- **HSV-2** (also termed **HHV-2**) is transmitted in genital secretions and typically produces disease "below the waist," including genital ulcers and neonatal herpes infection.

EPIDEMIOLOGY: HSV spreads from person to person, primarily via direct contact with infected secretions or open lesions. HSV-1 spreads in oral secretions, and infection frequently occurs in childhood, most people (50% to 90%) being infected by adulthood. HSV-2 spreads by contact with genital lesions and is primarily a venereally transmitted pathogen. Neonatal herpes is acquired during birth, when a baby passes through an infected birth canal.

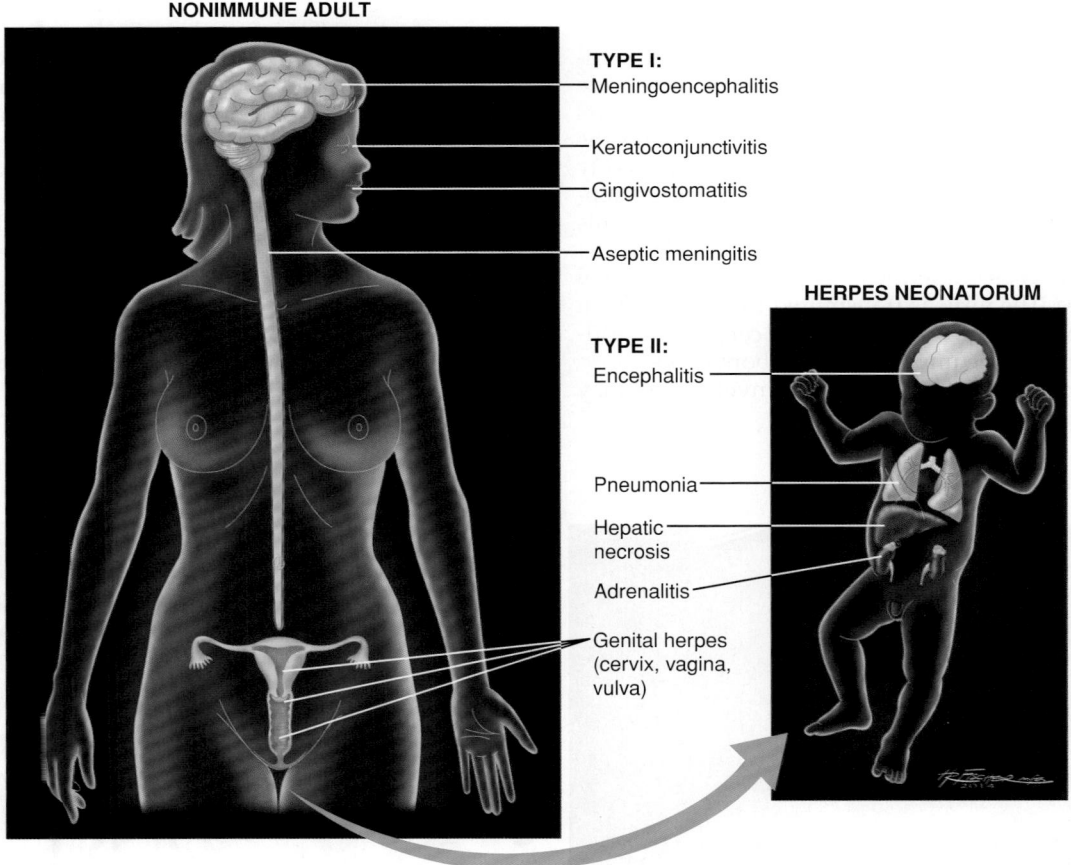

NONIMMUNE ADULT

TYPE I:
Meningoencephalitis
Keratoconjunctivitis
Gingivostomatitis
Aseptic meningitis

HERPES NEONATORUM

TYPE II:
Encephalitis
Pneumonia
Hepatic necrosis
Adrenalitis
Genital herpes (cervix, vagina, vulva)

FIGURE 9-7. Herpesvirus infections. Herpes simplex virus type 1 (HSV-1) infects a nonimmune adult, causing gingivostomatitis ("fever blister" or "cold sore"), keratoconjunctivitis, meningoencephalitis, and aseptic spinal meningitis. HSV-2 infects the genitalia of a nonimmune adult, involving the cervix, vagina, and vulva. HSV-2 infects the fetus as it passes through the birth canal of an infected mother. The infant's lack of a mature immune system results in disseminated infection with HSV-1. The infection is often fatal, involving lung, liver, adrenal glands, and central nervous system.

PATHOPHYSIOLOGY: Primary disease occurs at a site of initial viral inoculation, such as the oropharynx, genital mucosa, or skin. The virus infects epithelial cells, producing progeny viruses and destroying basal cells in the squamous epithelium, with resulting formation of vesicles. Cell necrosis also elicits an inflammatory response, initially mostly neutrophils, then followed by lymphocytes. Primary infection resolves when humoral and cell-mediated immunity to the virus develop.

Latent infection is established similarly to that of VZV. The virus invades sensory nerve endings in the oral or genital mucosa, ascends within axons and establishes a latent infection in sensory neurons within corresponding ganglia. From time to time, this latent infection reactivates, and HSV travels back down the nerve to the epithelial site served by the ganglion. There, it again infects epithelial cells. Sometimes this secondary infection produces ulcerating vesicular lesions. At other times, the secondary infection does not cause visible tissue destruction, but contagious progeny viruses are shed from the site of infection. Various factors, usually typical for a given person, can induce reactivation of latent HSV infection. These include intense sunlight, emotional stress, febrile illness and, in women, menstruation. Both HSV-1 and HSV-2 can cause severe protracted and disseminated disease in immunocompromised people.

Herpes encephalitis is a rare (1 in 100,000 HSV infections), but devastating, manifestation of HSV-1 infection. In some instances, it occurs when virus, latent in the trigeminal ganglion, is reactivated and travels retrograde to the brain. However, herpes encephalitis also occurs in people who have no history of "cold sores," and the pathogenesis of the encephalitis in these cases is poorly understood (see Chapter 32). Equally rare is **herpes hepatitis**, which may occur in immunocompromised patients but is also seen in previously healthy pregnant women.

Neonatal herpes is a serious complication of maternal genital herpes. The virus is transmitted to the fetus from the infected birth canal, often the uterine cervix, and readily disseminates in the unprotected newborn child.

Aseptic meningitis without genital involvement may be a manifestation of HSV-2 infection.

 PATHOLOGY: The skin and mucous membranes are the usual sites of HSV infection, but the disease sometimes involves the brain, eye, liver, lungs, and other organs. In any location, both HSV-1 and HSV-2 cause necrosis of infected cells, with a vigorous inflammatory response. Clusters of painful ulcerating vesicular lesions on the skin or mucous membranes are the most common manifestations (Fig. 9-8A). Lesions persist for 1 to 2 weeks and then resolve. The cellular alterations include (1) nuclear homogenization, (2) Cowdry type A intranuclear inclusions, and (3) multinucleated giant cells (Fig. 9-8B).

CLINICAL FEATURES: Clinical features of HSV infections vary according to host susceptibility (e.g., neonate, normal host, compromised host), viral type, and site of infection. A prodromal "tingling" sensation at the site often precedes the appearance of skin lesions. Recurrent lesions appear weeks, months or years later, at the initial site or at a site subserved by the same nerve ganglion. Recurrent herpetic lesions in the mouth or on the lip, commonly called "cold sores" or "fever blisters," may appear after sun exposure, trauma, or a febrile illness.

Immunocompromised patients are prone to develop herpes esophagitis. Early lesions consist of rounded 1- to 3-mm vesicles located mainly in the mid- to distal esophagus. As the HSV-infected squamous cells slough from these lesions, sharply demarcated ulcers with elevated margins form and coalesce. This process may result in denudation of the esophageal mucosa. Superimposed *Candida* infection is common at this stage. In immunocompromised patients, HSV may also infect the anal mucosa, where it causes painful blisters and ulcers.

Neonatal herpes begins 5 to 7 days after delivery, with irritability, lethargy, and a mucocutaneous vesicular eruption. Infection rapidly spreads to involve multiple organs, including the brain. The infected newborn develops jaundice, bleeding problems, respiratory distress, seizures, and coma. Treatment of severe HSV infections with acyclovir is often effective, but neonatal herpes still carries a high mortality.

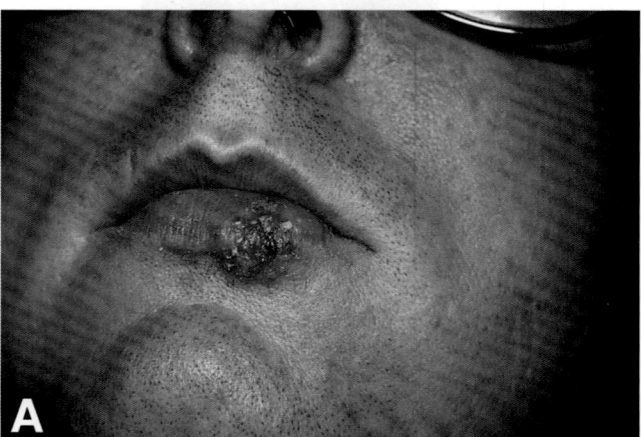
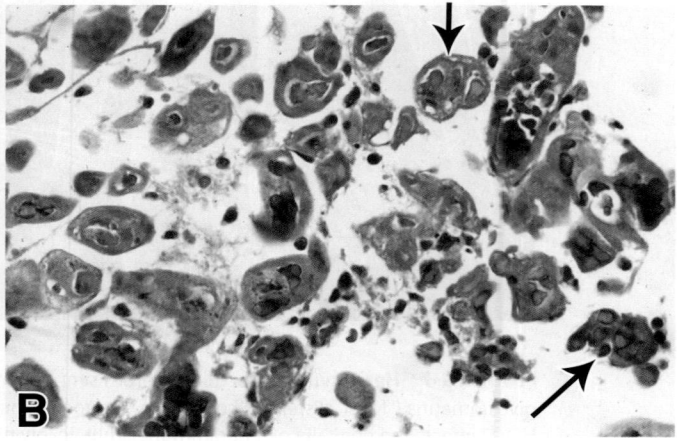

FIGURE 9-8. Herpes simplex virus type 1 (HSV-1). A. Herpetic vesicles are seen on the surface of the lower lip. **B.** Epithelial cells infected with HSV-1 demonstrate Cowdry type A intranuclear inclusions (*long arrow*) and multinucleated giant cells (*short arrow*).

Epstein–Barr Virus (EBV) Causes Infectious Mononucleosis and B-Cell Lymphomas

Infectious mononucleosis is a viral disease characterized by fever, pharyngitis, lymphadenopathy, and increased circulating atypical lymphocytes. By adulthood, most people have been infected with EBV. Most EBV infections are asymptomatic, but EBV may cause infectious mononucleosis. It is also associated with several cancers, including African Burkitt lymphoma, B-cell lymphoma in immunosuppressed patients, and nasopharyngeal carcinoma (Chapters 26 and 28).

 EPIDEMIOLOGY: In areas of the world where children often live in crowded conditions, infection with EBV usually occurs before 3 years of age, and infectious mononucleosis is not encountered. In developed countries, many people remain uninfected into adolescence or early adulthood. Two-thirds of those newly infected after childhood develop clinically evident infectious mononucleosis.

EBV spreads from person to person primarily through contact with infected oral secretions (Fig. 9-9). Once it enters the body, EBV remains for life, analogous to other latent herpesvirus infections. A few people (10% to 20%) shed the virus intermittently. Transmission requires close contact with infected people. Thus, EBV spreads readily among young children in crowded conditions, where there is considerable "sharing" of oral secretions. Kissing is also an effective mode of transmission, hence the term "kissing disease."

PATHOPHYSIOLOGY: The virus first binds to and infects nasopharyngeal cells and then B lymphocytes, which carry it throughout the body, producing a generalized infection of lymphoid tissues.

EBV is a polyclonal activator of B cells. These activated B cells stimulate proliferation of specific killer T lymphocytes and suppressor T cells. The former destroy virally infected B cells, while suppressor cells inhibit antibody production. The virus is also implicated in Burkitt lymphoma (see Chapters 5 and 26).

PATHOLOGY: The pathology of infectious mononucleosis involves the lymph nodes and spleen prominently. In most patients, lymphadenopathy is symmetric and most striking in the neck. The nodes are movable, discrete, and tender. Microscopically, nodal architecture is preserved. Germinal centers are enlarged and have indistinct margins, because of proliferation of immunoblasts. There are occasional large hyperchromatic cells with polylobular nuclei that resemble Reed–Sternberg cells of Hodgkin disease. Lymph node histology may be difficult to distinguish from Hodgkin disease or other lymphomas (see Chapter 26).

The spleen is large and soft, due to hyperplasia of the red pulp, and is susceptible to rupture. Immunoblasts are abundant, and infiltrate vessel walls, the trabeculae and the capsule. The liver is almost always involved, with sinusoids and portal tracts containing atypical lymphocytes.

Infectious mononucleosis is characterized by lymphocytosis with atypical lymphocytes. These are activated T cells with lobulated, eccentric nuclei and vacuolated cytoplasm, and are involved in suppression and killing of EBV-infected B lymphocytes. Patients with infectious mononucleosis develop a specific heterophile antibody—that is, an immunoglobulin produced in one species that reacts with antigens of another species—called Paul Bunnell antibody, identified by binding to sheep erythrocytes. This heterophile reaction is a standard diagnostic test for infectious mononucleosis. Specific serologic tests for antibodies against EBV and for EBV antigens are also available.

 CLINICAL FEATURES: Infectious mononucleosis manifests as fever, malaise, lymphadenopathy, pharyngitis, and splenomegaly. Patients usually have elevated leukocyte counts, predominantly lymphocytes and monocytes. Treatment is supportive; symptoms usually resolve in 3 to 4 weeks.

Cytomegalovirus (CMV) Is a Congenital and Opportunistic Pathogen

In normal people, CMV infection is usually asymptomatic, but it can be destructive in fetuses and immunocompromised patients. CMV infects 0.5% to 2.0% of fetuses and injures 10% to 20% of them, making it the most common congenital pathogen.

 EPIDEMIOLOGY: CMV spreads from person to person by contact with infected secretions and bodily fluids, and is transmitted to the fetus across the placenta. Children spread it in saliva or urine, while transmission among adolescents and adults is primarily through sexual contact.

 PATHOPHYSIOLOGY: CMV infects various human cells, including epithelial cells, lymphocytes, and monocytes, and establishes latency in white blood cells. Normal immune responses rapidly control infection and ill effects are rare. However, virus is shed periodically in body secretions. Like other herpesviruses, CMV may remain latent for life.

When an infected pregnant woman passes CMV to her fetus, the fetus is not protected by maternally derived antibodies and the virus invades fetal cells with little initial immunologic response, causing widespread necrosis and inflammation. CMV produces similar lesions in people with suppressed cell-mediated immunity.

CMV infection is often symptomatic in immunosuppressed people, such as organ transplant recipients. In that setting, the CMV infection usually represents reactivation of endogenous latent infection, whether the source is the graft or the recipient. Subsequent dissemination may lead to severe systemic disease.

 PATHOLOGY: CMV disease of the fetus most commonly involves the brain, inner ears, eyes, liver, and bone marrow. Severely affected fetuses

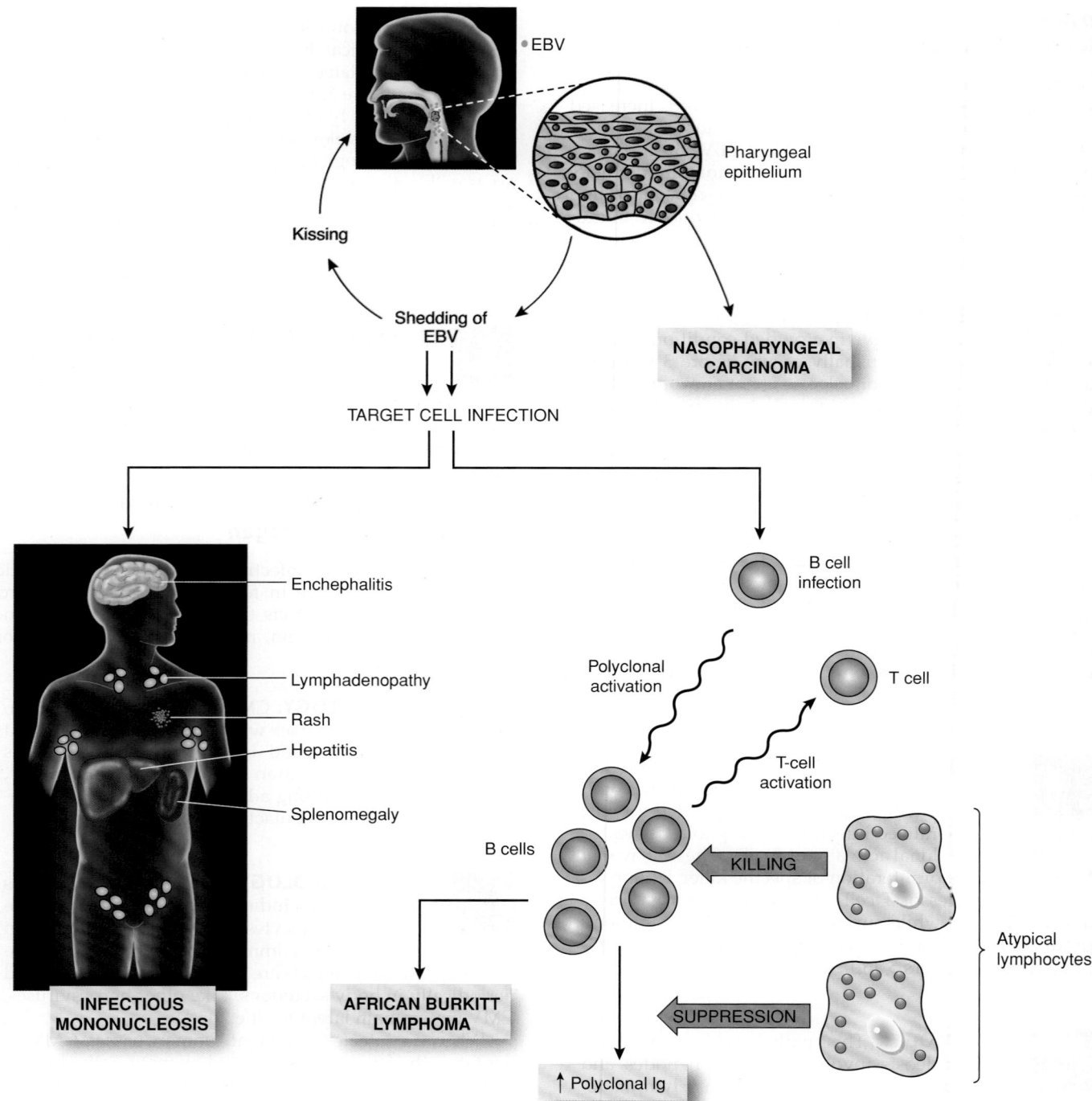

FIGURE 9-9. Role of Epstein–Barr virus (EBV) in infectious mononucleosis, nasopharyngeal carcinoma and Burkitt lymphoma. EBV invades and replicates within the salivary glands or pharyngeal epithelium and is shed into the saliva and respiratory secretions. In some people, the virus transforms pharyngeal epithelial cells, leading to nasopharyngeal carcinoma. In people who are not immune from childhood exposure, EBV causes infectious mononucleosis. EBV infects B lymphocytes, which undergo polyclonal activation. These B cells stimulate the production of atypical lymphocytes, which kill virally infected B cells and suppress the production of immunoglobulins. Some infected B cells are transformed into immature malignant lymphocytes of Burkitt lymphoma.

may have microcephaly, hydrocephalus, cerebral calcifications, hepatosplenomegaly, and jaundice. Lesions of fetal CMV disease show cellular necrosis and a characteristic cytopathic effect, with marked cellular and nuclear enlargement, with nuclear and cytoplasmic inclusions.

The giant nucleus, which is usually solitary, contains a large central inclusion surrounded by a clear zone. Smaller, granular intracytoplasmic CMV inclusions, which are not present in all infected cells, occur after the intranuclear inclusion (Fig. 9-10).

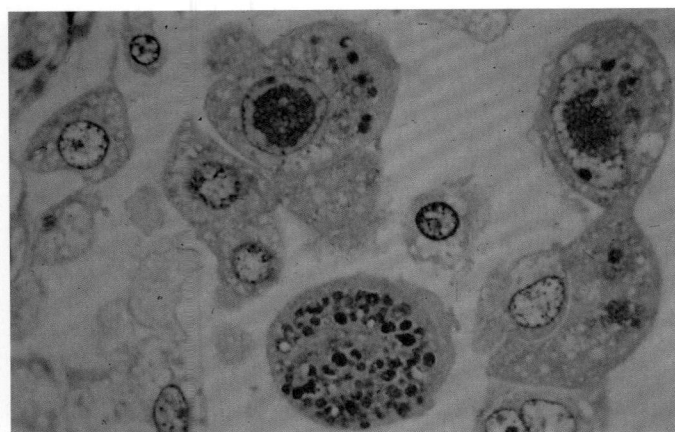

FIGURE 9-10. Cytomegalovirus (CMV) pneumonitis. Two type II pneumocytes display enlarged nuclei containing solitary CMV inclusions surrounded by a clear zone. The cell at the bottom shows abundant intracytoplasmic CMV inclusions.

CLINICAL FEATURES: Congenitally acquired CMV has diverse clinical presentations. Severe disease causes fetal death *in utero*, conspicuous CNS lesions, liver disease, and bleeding problems. However, most congenital CMV infections do not produce gross abnormalities, but manifest as subtle neurologic or hearing defects, which may not be detected until later in life.

CMV disease in immunosuppressed patients has a wide range of clinical presentations. It can manifest as decreased visual acuity (chorioretinitis), diarrhea or gastrointestinal hemorrhage (colonic ulcerations), change in mental status (encephalitis), shortness of breath (pneumonitis), or any number of other symptoms.

Human Papillomaviruses (HPVs) Cause Squamous Cell Proliferations

HPV-related lesions include common warts, flat warts, plantar warts, anogenital warts (condyloma acuminatum) as well as laryngeal papillomatosis. Some HPV serotypes cause squamous cell dysplasias and squamous cell carcinomas of the genital tract (see Chapter 18).

HPVs are nonenveloped, double-stranded DNA viruses. Over 100 serotypes of HPV are known, different ones being associated with different lesions. Thus, HPV types 1, 2, and 4 produce common warts and plantar warts. Types 6, 10, 11, and 40 through 45 cause anogenital warts. Types 16, 18, and 31 are associated with squamous carcinomas of the female genital tract (see Chapter 24) and elsewhere (see Chapters 19, 23, and 29).

HPV infection is widespread. It is transmitted by direct person to person contact. Most children develop common warts. The viruses that cause genital lesions are transmitted sexually.

PATHOPHYSIOLOGY: HPV infection begins with viral inoculation into a stratified squamous epithelium, where the virus enters the nuclei of basal cells. Infection stimulates epithelial proliferation, producing the various HPV-associated lesions. The rapidly growing squamous epithelium replicates innumerable progeny viruses, which are shed in the degenerating superficial cells. Many HPV lesions resolve spontaneously, but they may persist and spread in people with depressed cell-mediated immunity. HPV oncogenesis is discussed in Chapter 5.

PATHOLOGY: HPV-induced squamous proliferations vary in appearance and biologic behavior. Most show thickening of affected epithelium, due to enhanced squamous cell proliferation. Some HPV-infected cells show a characteristic cytopathic effect, **koilocytosis**, which features large squamous cells with shrunken nuclei enveloped in large cytoplasmic vacuoles (koilocytes).

CLINICAL FEATURES: Common warts (verruca vulgaris) are firm, circumscribed, raised, rough-surfaced lesions, usually on surfaces subject to trauma, especially the hands (see Chapter 24). **Plantar warts** are similar squamous proliferative lesions on the soles of the feet but are compressed inward by standing and walking.

Anogenital warts (condyloma acuminatum) are soft, raised, fleshy lesions on the penis, vulva, vaginal wall, cervix, or perianal region. Flat warts caused by certain HPV serotypes may evolve into malignant squamous cell proliferations (see Chapter 24).

ONCOVIRUSES

An oncovirus is a virus that causes cancer in its host. The International Agency for Research on Cancer of the WHO estimates that almost 18% of cancer in humans is caused by infection, and that 12% of cancers worldwide are caused by seven viruses (Table 9-3). Viral infection is believed to be the second most frequent risk factor for human cancer, exceeded only by tobacco. Oncoviruses can be DNA viruses such as EBV, or RNA viruses such as human thymus leukemia virus 1 (HTLV-1).

There are two major mechanisms by which a virus can cause cancer—direct oncogenesis (or acutely transforming) and indirect oncogenesis (or slowly transforming). In direct viral oncogenesis, a virus either insertions its own oncogene, or enhances endogenous cellular protooncogenes (see Chapter 5). Indirect oncogenesis involves virus-induced chronic inflammation persisting for decades of infection, as with chronic hepatitis C virus. Preliminary data link CMV infection and mucoepidermoid carcinoma. The development of effective vaccines to protect from two of the leading causes of viral-induced malignancies—hepatitis B and HPV—is of immense public health significance in preventing cancers caused by these viruses.

Prion Diseases

In the last several decades it has become clear that disease can be transmitted and propagated solely by proteins without nucleic acids. Despite considerable initial resistance to

TABLE 9-3
HUMAN ONCOVIRUSES

Virus	Cancer Types	% Cancers Worldwide
Human papillomaviruses (HPV-16, HPV-18, and others)	Cervical, vulvar, anal, vulva, vagina, penis, head and neck	5.2%
Hepatitis B and hepatitis C viruses	Hepatocellular carcinoma	4.9%
Human herpesvirus 8	Kaposi sarcoma, primary effusion lymphoma, Castleman disease	0.9%
Epstein–Barr virus	Hodgkin lymphoma, Burkitt lymphoma, nasopharyngeal carcinoma, post-transplant, lymphoproliferative disease	NA
Human T-lymphotropic virus	Adult T-cell leukemia and lymphoma	NA
Merkel cell polyoma virus	Merkel cell carcinoma	NA

this disease paradigm, it is clear that filterable particles that lack nucleic acids can transmit disease. To date, these particles, prions, are only known to cause CNS disease. Prions are essentially misfolded proteins that aggregate in CNS cells, are resistant to cellular proteostasis and cause progressive neurodegeneration that leads to death. **Prion protein (PrP)** exists in normal and pathogenic forms, the latter being transmissible. Pathogenic isoforms aggregate into prion rods which are characteristic of these rare disorders (see Chapter 32). Of particular importance is the uncommon persistence of these infectious agents that are highly resistant to normal methods of sterilization and may be transmitted via surgical instruments or electrodes when implanted in nervous tissue, unless special protocols are followed.

- **Kuru:** The prototypical human prion disease is Kuru, a progressive neurodegenerative disease that was only found in the South Fore tribe in the remote highlands of Papa New Guinea. Kuru, the Fore word for "trembling," was transmitted via cannibalism. Experimental transmission of Kuru has been accomplished using tissue from Kuru victims to pass the infection to nonhuman primates. Once funerary cannibalism among the Fore was eliminated, kuru disappeared within a generation.
- **Sporadic, Familial, and Iatrogenic Creutzfeldt–Jakob Disease (sCJD, fCJD, and iCJD):** CJD is a rapidly progressive neurodegenerative disorder characterized by myoclonus, behavior changes, and dementia (see Chapter 32). With a frequency of 1/1,000,000, sCJD is probably the most common human prion disease. Rarely, CJD resulted from transmission through transplanting such tissues as cornea and dura matter. Before the advent of recombinant protein therapeutics, CJD was also transmitted from human growth hormone isolated from human cadaver pituitaries.

- **New Variant Creutzfeldt–Jakob Disease (vCJD):** One of the more infamous emerging infectious diseases of the last few decades, both vCJD and the associated **bovine spongiform encephalopathy (BSE)**, also known as "mad cow" disease, underscore the interrelatedness of animal and human infectious agents. The use of certain animal products in feeds for domestic ungulates led to and amplified a prion disease epidemic in cattle herds of the United Kingdom. Nearly 150 people are known to have been infected with this relentless terminal disease. All patients to date have an uncommon genetic homozygosity: methionine–methionine at codon 129 of the gene (*PRNP*) that encodes the prion protein. Presentations differ from previously recognized forms of CJD in several ways, the age of onset being most notable. While CJD generally begins at about 65 years of age, vCJD affects younger adults, with a mean age of 26 years. Psychiatric signs and symptoms have also been predominant in vCJD. Pathologic changes in vCJD are strikingly similar to those seen in BSE and differ somewhat from changes seen in the sporadic form.
- **Fatal Familial Insomnia:** This is a rare inherited prion disorder that has as its hallmark progressive insomnia that worsens over time until the patient barely sleeps or is incapable of sleeping. There is also autonomic instability that usually appears as increased sympathetic tone. Altered sensorium may also be present, and signs of motor degeneration follow. Spongiform changes like those in other transmissible spongiform encephalopathies also develop later in the disease.
- **Gerstmann–Sträussler–Scheinker Syndrome:** This is another rare transmissible spongiform encephalopathy that is usually familial, although rare sporadic cases are described. Presentations vary, but signs and symptoms of cerebellar degeneration usually predominate. Dementia occurs late and often becomes a common feature.
- **Multiple System Atrophy (Shy Drager Syndrome):** In 2015, this rare neurodegenerative syndrome was identified as being transmissible. It is believed to be caused by a new prion—a misfolded form of the protein α-synuclein.

Bacterial Infections

Bacteria, at 0.1 to 10 μm, are the smallest living cells. They have three basic structural components: nuclear body, cytosol, and envelope. The **nuclear body** contains a single, coiled circular molecule of double-stranded DNA with associated RNA and proteins. It is not separated from the cytoplasm by a special membrane, which feature distinguishes bacteria, as prokaryotes, from eukaryotes. The **cytosol** is densely packed with ribosomes, proteins, and carbohydrates, and lacks the structured organelles, such as mitochondria and Golgi apparatus, of eukaryotic cells. The **bacterial envelope** is a permeability barrier and is also actively involved in transport, protein synthesis, energy generation, DNA synthesis, and cell division.

Bacteria are classified according to their envelope structure. The simplest envelope is a phospholipid–protein bilayer membrane. Mycoplasmas have such an envelope. Most bacteria also have a rigid cell wall that surrounds the cell membrane. Two types of bacterial cell walls are identified by their Gram staining properties:

- **Gram-positive bacteria** retain iodine-crystal violet when decolorized and appear dark blue. Their cell walls contain teichoic acids and a thick peptidoglycan layer.
- **Gram-negative bacteria** lose the iodine-crystal violet stain when decolorized and appear red with a counterstain. Outer membranes of gram-negative bacteria contain a lipopolysaccharide, called **endotoxin**, that is a potent mediator of the shock which complicates infections with these organisms.

Both gram-positive and gram-negative cell walls may be surrounded by an additional layer of polysaccharide or protein gel, a **capsule**. Capsules facilitate bacterial attachment and colonization, and may protect from phagocytosis. Because of this pathogenetic significance, bacteria may be classified as **encapsulated** or **unencapsulated**.

The cell wall confers rigidity to bacteria and allows them to be distinguished on the basis of shape and pattern of growth in cultures. Round or oval bacteria are **cocci**. Those that grow in clusters are called **staphylococci**, while those that grow in chains are called **streptococci**. Elongate bacteria are **rods**, or **bacilli**; curved ones are **vibrios**. Spiral-shaped bacteria are called **spirochetes**.

Most bacteria can be cultured on chemical media, and so may be described according to their growth requirements on these media. Bacteria that need high levels of oxygen are **aerobic**, those that grow best without oxygen are **anaerobic** and those that thrive with limited oxygen are **microaerophilic**. Bacteria that grow well with or without oxygen are **facultative anaerobes**.

BACTERIAL EXOTOXINS: Many bacteria secrete toxins (exotoxins) that damage human cells either at the site of bacterial growth or at distant sites. These toxins are often named for the site or mechanism of their activity. Thus, those that act on the nervous system are called **neurotoxins**; those that affect intestinal cells are **enterotoxins**. Some **cytotoxins** kill target cells, such as diphtheria toxin or some of the *Clostridium perfringens* toxins. Others may disturb normal functions of their target cells and damage or kill them, like the diarrheagenic toxin of *Vibrio cholerae* or the neurotoxin of *Clostridium botulinum*. *Clostridium perfringens* produces over 20 harmful toxins.

BACTERIAL ENDOTOXINS: As mentioned above, gram-negative bacteria contain structural **lipopolysaccharide**, or **endotoxin**, in their outer membranes. Lipopolysaccharide activates complement, coagulation, fibrinolysis, and bradykinin systems. It also causes release of primary inflammatory mediators, including TNFα, IL-1, and various colony-stimulating factors. Endotoxin may cause shock, complement depletion, and disseminated intravascular coagulation (DIC, see Chapters 7 and 26).

Many bacteria damage tissues by eliciting inflammatory or immune responses. The capsule of *Streptococcus pneumoniae* protects it from phagocytosis while activating a host's inflammatory response. Within the lung, the encapsulated organism causes fluid and cell exudation that fills alveoli. This inflammation impairs breathing but does not, at least initially, limit bacterial proliferation. *Treponema pallidum,* the spirochete that causes syphilis, persists in the body for years and elicits inflammatory and immune responses that continuously damage host tissues.

Many common bacterial infections (e.g., *Staphylococcus aureus* skin infections) are characterized by purulent exudates, but tissue responses to bacteria are highly variable. In some cases, such as cholera, botulism, and tetanus, there is no inflammatory response at critical sites of cellular injury. Other bacterial infections, including syphilis and Lyme disease, lead to a predominantly lymphocytic and plasma cellular response. Still others (e.g., brucellosis) are characterized by granuloma formation.

Many bacterial diseases are caused by organisms that normally inhabit the human body. The gut, upper respiratory tract, skin, and vagina are all home to diverse bacteria, which are normally commensal and cause no harm. However, if they gain access to usually sterile sites or if host defenses are impaired, they can cause extensive destruction. *Staphylococcus aureus, Streptococcus pneumoniae,* and *Escherichia coli* are normal flora that are also major human pathogens.

PYOGENIC GRAM-POSITIVE COCCI

Staphylococcus aureus Produces Suppurative Infections

S. aureus is a gram-positive coccus that typically grows in clusters and is among the most common bacterial pathogens. It normally resides on the skin, but can readily access deeper tissues, where it causes suppurative infections. *In fact, it is the most common cause of suppurative infections of skin, joints, and bones, and is a leading cause of infective endocarditis.* S. aureus is commonly distinguished from other, less virulent staphylococci by the coagulase test. *S. aureus* is coagulase-positive; the other staphylococci are coagulase-negative.

S. aureus spreads by direct contact with colonized surfaces or people. Most people are intermittently colonized with *S. aureus*, and carry it on the skin, nares, or clothing. The organism also survives on inanimate surfaces for long periods.

 PATHOPHYSIOLOGY: Many *S. aureus* infections begin as localized infections of skin and skin appendages, producing cellulites and abscesses. The organism, equipped with destructive enzymes and toxins, sometimes invades beyond the initial site, spreading by blood or lymphatics to almost any location in the body. Bones, joints, and heart valves are the most common sites of metastatic *S. aureus* infections. *S. aureus* also causes several distinct diseases by elaborating toxins that are carried to distant sites.

 PATHOLOGY: When *S. aureus* is introduced into a previously sterile site, infection usually produces suppuration and abscesses, ranging from microscopic foci to lesions several centimeters in diameter that are filled with pus and bacteria.

 CLINICAL FEATURES: Clinical manifestations of *S. aureus* disease vary according to the sites and types of infection.

- **Furuncles (boils) and styes:** Deep-seated *S. aureus* infections occur in and around hair follicles, often in a nasal carrier. They localize on hairy surfaces, such as

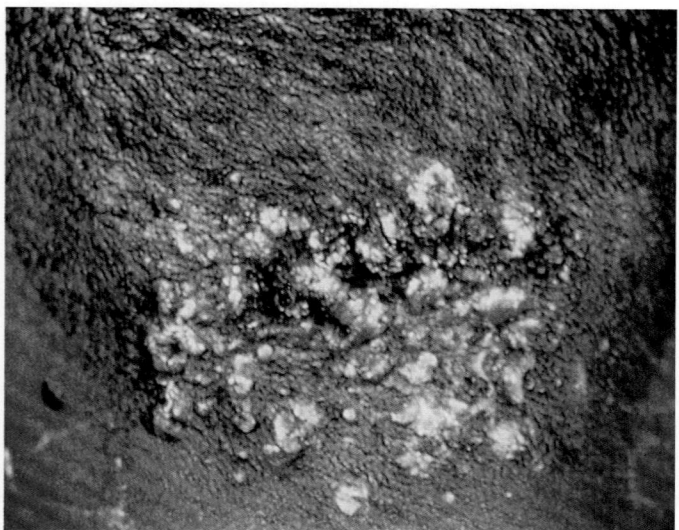

FIGURE 9-11. Staphylococcal carbuncle. The posterior neck is indurated and shows multiple follicular abscesses discharging purulent material.

the neck, thighs and buttocks of men, and the axillae, pubic area, and eyelids of both sexes. The boil begins as a nodule at the base of a hair follicle, followed by a pimple that remains painful and red for a few days. A yellow apex forms and the central core becomes necrotic and fluctuant. Rupture or incision of the boil relieves the pain. **Styes** are boils that involve the sebaceous glands around the eyelid. **Paronychia** are staphylococcal infections of nail beds and **felons** are the same infections on the palmar side of the fingertips.

- **Carbuncles:** These lesions, mostly on the neck, result from coalescing infections with *S. aureus* around hair follicles and produce draining sinuses (Fig. 9-11).
- **Scalded skin syndrome:** This disease affects infants and children under 3 years who present with a sunburnlike rash that begins on the face and spreads over the body. Bullae begin to form and even gentle rubbing causes skin to desquamate. The disease begins to resolve in 1 to 2 weeks, as the skin regenerates. Desquamation is due to systemic effects of a specific exotoxin. The site of *S. aureus* proliferation is often occult.
- **Osteomyelitis:** Acute staphylococcal osteomyelitis, usually in the bones of the legs, most commonly afflicts boys 3 to 10 years old. There is usually a history of infection or trauma. Osteomyelitis may become chronic if not properly treated. Adults over 50 may develop vertebral osteomyelitis after staphylococcal infections of the skin or urinary tract, prostatic surgery, or pinning of a fracture.
- **Infections of burns or surgical wounds:** These sites often become infected with *S. aureus* from the patient's own nasal carriage or from medical personnel. Newborns and elderly, malnourished, diabetic, and obese people are all highly susceptible.
- **Respiratory tract infections:** Staphylococcal respiratory tract infections occur mostly in infants under 2 years, and especially under 2 months. Infection is characterized by ulcers of the upper airway, scattered foci of pneumonia, pleural effusion, empyema, and pneumothorax. In adults, staphylococcal pneumonia may follow viral influenza, which destroys the ciliated surface epithelium and leaves the bronchial surface vulnerable to secondary infection.

- **Bacterial arthritis:** *S. aureus* causes half of all septic arthritis, mostly in patients 50 to 70 years old. Rheumatoid arthritis and corticosteroid therapy are common predisposing conditions.
- **Septicemia:** Septicemia with *S. aureus* afflicts patients with lowered resistance who are in the hospital for other diseases. Some have underlying staphylococcal infections (e.g., septic arthritis, osteomyelitis), some have had surgery (e.g., transurethral prostate resection) and some have infections from an indwelling intravenous catheter. Miliary abscesses and endocarditis are serious complications.
- **Bacterial endocarditis:** Bacterial endocarditis is a common complication of *S. aureus* septicemia. It may develop spontaneously on normal valves, on valves damaged by rheumatic fever or on prosthetic valves. Intravenous drug abuse predisposes to staphylococcal endocarditis.
- **Toxic shock syndrome:** This disorder most commonly afflicts menstruating women, who present with high fever, nausea, vomiting, diarrhea, and myalgias. They then develop shock and a sunburnlike rash within several days. Toxic shock syndrome is associated with use of tampons, particularly hyperabsorbent ones, which facilitate *S. aureus* replication and toxin elaboration. Toxic shock syndrome occurs rarely in children or men, and then is usually associated with occult *S. aureus* infection.
- **Staphylococcal food poisoning:** Staphylococcal food poisoning typically begins less than 6 hours after a meal. Nausea and vomiting start abruptly and usually resolve within 12 hours. This disease is caused by preformed toxin present in the food at the time it is eaten.
- **Antibiotic-resistant S. aureus.** Antibiotic-resistant *S. aureus* is a major clinical problem since penicillin was introduced in the early 1940s. *S. aureus* was one of the first important pathogens to become completely resistant to penicillin and, with time, to each subsequent generation of penicillin derivatives. **Methicillin-resistant S. aureus (MRSA)** infections are usually—but not exclusively—acquired in hospitals, where the environment selects for antibiotic-resistant bacteria. MRSA is one of the most dreaded of nosocomial infections. According to the CDC, between 1995 and 2004 in patients in intensive care units the percentage of *S. aureus* infections due to MRSA approximately doubled, to almost two-thirds. As of 2007, approximately 0.8% of the U.S. population were colonized with MRSA. MRSA infections are responsible for approximately 368,000 hospitalizations and 19,000 deaths annually in the United States. In 2010, a CDC study revealed that invasive and bloodstream MRSA infections occurring in healthcare settings were declining. The most worrisome feature of MRSA infection is the difficulty in treatment when it becomes invasive and imperils health. The recent increase in community-acquired MRSA (CA-MRSA) raises concerns of dissemination of antibiotic resistance among *Staphylococcus* and other bacteria. CA-MRSA appears to be a different strain of MRSA from that normally associated with hospital-acquired MRSA infections, with enhanced virulence and different antibiotic susceptibility profiles. It may spread in schools and gymnasiums, and mostly causes skin and soft tissue infections.

Coagulase-Negative Staphylococci Are Major Causes of Infections in Prosthetic Devices

Medical devices, including intravenous catheters, prosthetic heart valves, heart pacemakers, orthopedic prostheses, cerebrospinal fluid shunts, and peritoneal catheters are most affected.

The coagulase-negative staphylococci involved are usually from the normal bacterial flora. Of the more than 20 known species of coagulase-negative staphylococci, 10 reside normally on human skin and mucosal surfaces. Staphylococcus epidermidis *is the most frequent cause of infections associated with medical devices.* Another species, S. saprophyticus, causes 10% to 20% of acute urinary tract infections in young women.

PATHOPHYSIOLOGY: Coagulase-negative staphylococci readily contaminate foreign bodies, on which they proliferate slowly, inducing inflammatory responses that damage adjacent tissue. Bacteria present on an intravascular surface, such as the tip of an intravascular catheter, can spread through the bloodstream to cause metastatic infections. Unlike S. aureus, coagulase-negative staphylococci lack the enzymes and toxins to cause extensive local tissue destruction. Some strains of coagulase-negative staphylococci produce a polysaccharide gel biofilm which enhances their adherence to foreign objects and protects them from host antimicrobial defenses and from many antibiotics.

PATHOLOGY: Medical devices infected with coagulase-negative staphylococci are usually thinly coated with tan, fibrinous material. Coagulase-negative staphylococcal infections usually do not entail extensive local tissue necrosis or large quantities of pus. Microscopic examination of infected devices shows clusters of gram-positive bacteria embedded in fibrin and cellular debris, with an associated acute inflammatory infiltrate.

CLINICAL FEATURES: Coagulase-negative staphylococcal infections usually have subtle clinical presentations. The only symptom of infection may be persistent low-grade fever. Infection of orthopedic prostheses often causes progressive loosening and dysfunction of the devices. These infections are usually indolent, but may be fatal in compromised hosts. Treatment usually requires replacement of any infected foreign object and appropriate antibiotic therapy. Nosocomial strains of coagulase-negative Staphylococcus are often multi-drug resistant, with ≈80% carrying the mecA gene, which confers resistance to all classes of β-lactam antibiotics. Thus, treatment should be with non–β-lactam antibiotics.

Streptococcus pyogenes Causes Suppurative, Toxin-Related, and Immunologic Reactions

S. pyogenes, or group A streptococcus, is one of the most common human bacterial pathogens, causing many diseases of diverse organ systems, from acute self-limited pharyngitis to major illnesses such as rheumatic fever (Fig. 9-12). S. pyogenes, a gram-positive coccus, is frequently part of endogenous flora of the skin and oropharynx.

Diseases caused by S. pyogenes may be suppurative or nonsuppurative. The former occur at sites of bacterial invasion and consequent tissue necrosis, and usually involve acute inflammatory responses. Suppurative S. pyogenes infections include pharyngitis, impetigo, cellulitis, myositis, pneumonia, and puerperal sepsis. Nonsuppurative diseases caused by S. pyogenes are situated away from the site of bacterial invasion. The major nonsuppurative complications of S. pyogenes are rheumatic fever and acute poststreptococcal glomerulonephritis (see Chapters 17 and 22). These involve: (1) organs far from the sites of streptococcal invasion, (2) a time delay after the acute infection, and (3) immune reactions.

S. pyogenes elaborates several exotoxins, including erythrogenic toxins and cytolytic toxins (**streptolysins S and O**). Erythrogenic toxins cause the rash of scarlet fever. Streptolysin S lyses bacterial protoplasts (L forms) and probably destroys neutrophils after they ingest S. pyogenes. Streptolysin O induces persistently high antibody titers, and so is a useful marker for to diagnose S. pyogenes infections and their nonsuppurative complications.

Streptococcal Pharyngitis ("Strep Throat")

S. pyogenes, the common bacterial cause of pharyngitis, spreads from person to person by direct contact with oral or respiratory secretions. "Strep throat" occurs worldwide, mainly affecting children and adolescents.

 PATHOPHYSIOLOGY: S. pyogenes attaches to epithelial cells by binding to fibronectin on their surface. The bacterium produces hemolysins, DNAase, hyaluronidase, and streptokinase, which allow it to damage and invade human tissues. S. pyogenes also has cell wall components that protect it from the inflammatory response. One of these, **M protein**, protrudes from cell walls of virulent strains and protects bacteria from phagocytosis by preventing complement deposition. Another surface protein destroys C5a, blocking its opsonizing effect and inhibiting phagocytosis. The invading organism elicits acute inflammation, often producing an exudate of neutrophils in the tonsillar fossae.

 CLINICAL FEATURES: "Strep throat" is a sore throat, with fever, malaise, headache, and elevated leukocyte count. It usually lasts 3 to 5 days. *Streptococcal pharyngitis may lead to rheumatic fever or acute poststreptococcal glomerulonephritis.* Penicillin treatment shortens the course of strep throat and, more importantly, prevents nonsuppurative sequelae.

Scarlet Fever

Scarlet fever (**scarlatina**) is a punctate red rash on skin and mucous membranes in some suppurative S. pyogenes infections, mostly pharyngitis. It usually begins on the chest and spreads to the extremities. The tongue may develop a yellow-white coating, which sheds to reveal a "beefy-red" surface. Scarlet fever is caused by the erythrogenic toxin.

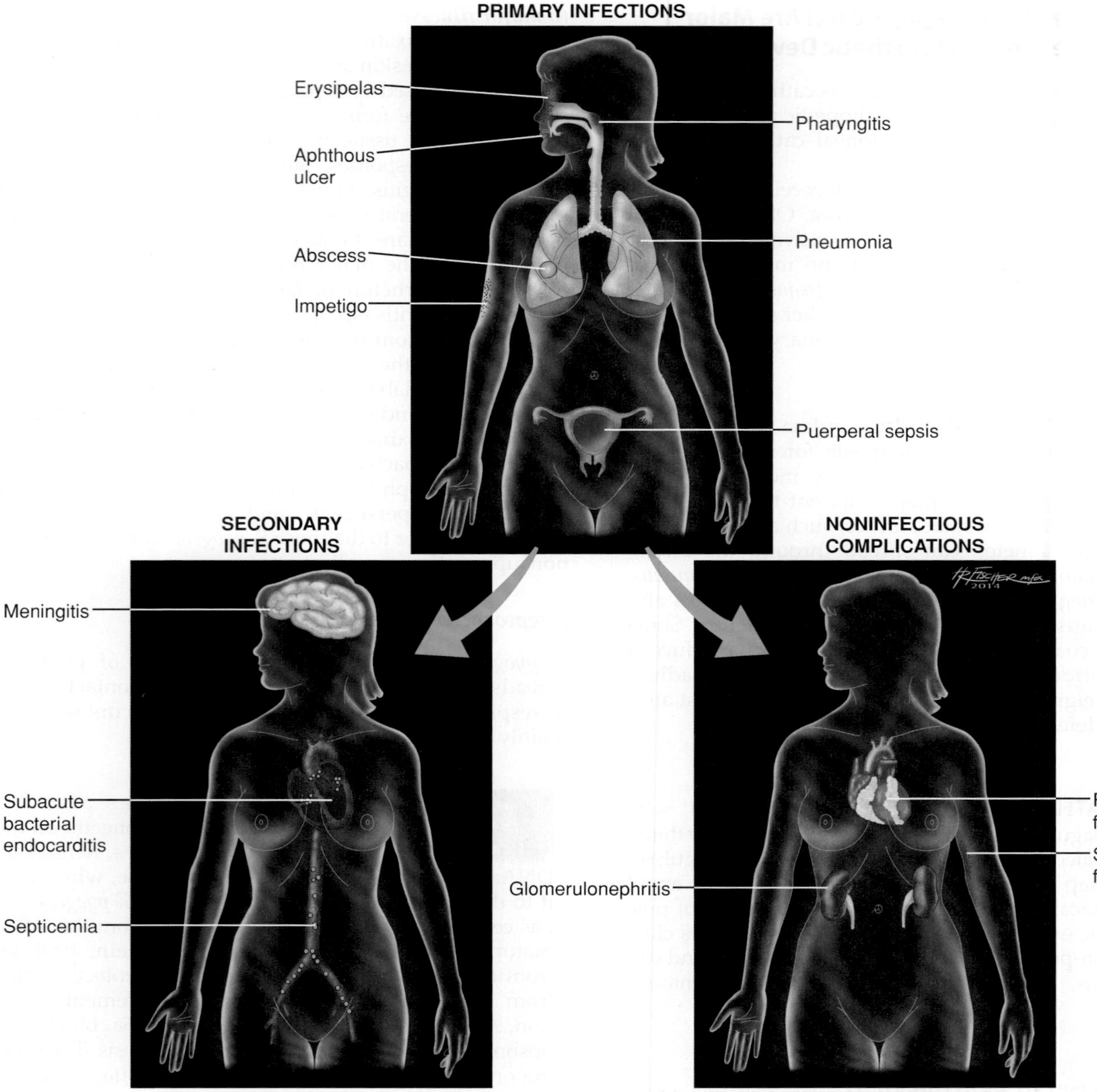

PRIMARY INFECTIONS

Erysipelas
Aphthous ulcer
Abscess
Impetigo
Pharyngitis
Pneumonia
Puerperal sepsis

SECONDARY INFECTIONS

Meningitis
Subacute bacterial endocarditis
Septicemia

NONINFECTIOUS COMPLICATIONS

Rheumatic fever
Scarlet fever
Glomerulonephritis

FIGURE 9-12. Streptococcal diseases.

Erysipelas

Erysipelas is erythematous swelling of the skin caused chiefly by *S. pyogenes* (Fig. 9-13). Erysipelas is common in warm climates, mostly in adults. It usually begins on the face and spreads rapidly. A diffuse, edematous, acute inflammatory reaction in the epidermis and dermis extends into subcutaneous tissues. The inflammatory infiltrate is mainly neutrophils and is most intense around cutaneous vessels and adnexa. Skin microabscesses and small foci of necrosis are common.

Impetigo

Impetigo (**pyoderma**) is a localized, intraepidermal infection caused by *S. pyogenes* or *S. aureus*. Strains of *S. pyogenes* that cause impetigo are antigenically and epidemiologically distinct from those that cause pharyngitis.

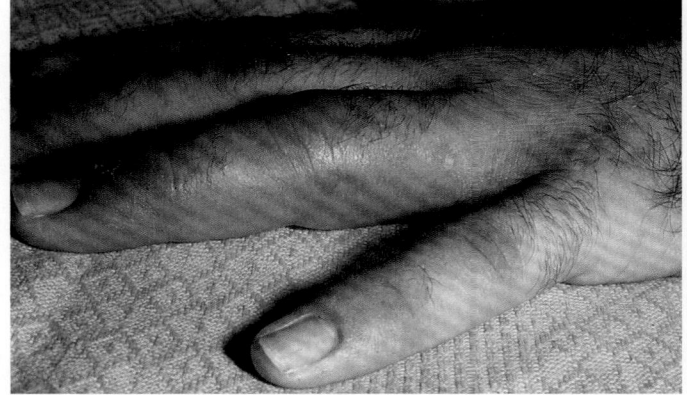

FIGURE 9-13. Erysipelas. Streptococcal infection of the skin has resulted in an erythematous and swollen finger.

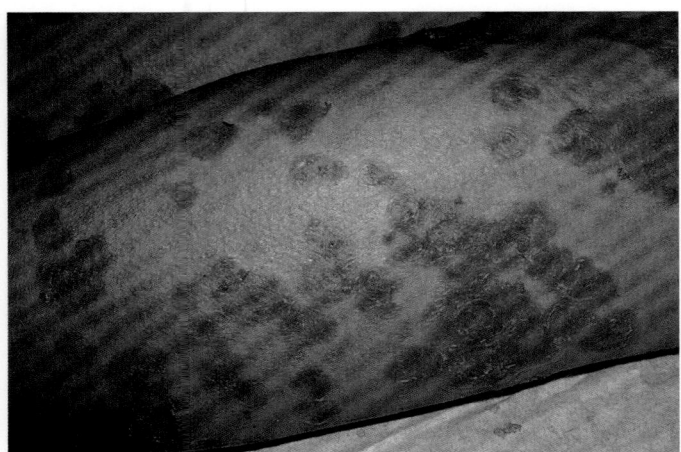

FIGURE 9-14. Streptococcal impetigo. The lower extremities contain many erythematous papules, with central ulceration and the formation of crusts.

Impetigo spreads from person to person by direct contact, and mostly affects children 2 to 5 years old. Infection begins with skin colonization with the causative organism. Minor trauma or an insect bite then inoculates the bacteria into the skin, where they form an intraepidermal pustule, which ruptures and leaks a purulent exudate.

Lesions begin on exposed body surfaces as localized erythematous papules (Fig. 9-14). These become pustules, which erode within a few days to form a thick honey-colored crust. Impetigo sometimes leads to poststreptococcal glomerulonephritis but it does not lead to rheumatic fever.

Streptococcal Cellulitis

S. pyogenes causes an acute spreading infection of the loose connective tissue of the deeper layers of the dermis. This suppurative infection results from traumatic inoculation of microorganisms into the skin and frequently occurs on the extremities in the context of impaired lymphatic drainage. Cellulitis usually begins at sites of unnoticed injury and appears as spreading areas of redness, warmth, and swelling.

Puerperal Sepsis

Puerperal sepsis is postpartum infection of the uterine cavity by *S. pyogenes*. The disease was once common, but is now rare in developed countries. It is spread by the contaminated hands of attendants at delivery.

Streptococcus pneumoniae Is a Major Cause of Lobar Pneumonia

S. pneumoniae, or simply **pneumococcus**, causes pyogenic infections, primarily of the lungs (**pneumonia**), middle ear (**otitis media**), sinuses (**sinusitis**), and meninges (**meningitis**). *It is one of the most common human bacterial pathogens. Most children in the world have had at least one episode of pneumococcal disease (usually otitis media) by age 5.*

S. pneumoniae is an aerobic, gram-positive diplococcus. Most strains that cause clinical disease have a capsule,

although nonserotypeable isolates are a known cause of epidemic conjunctivitis. There are over 80 antigenically distinct serotypes of pneumococcus; antibody to one does not protect from infection with another. *S. pneumoniae* is commensal in the oropharynx, and virtually everyone has been colonized at some time.

 PATHOPHYSIOLOGY: Pneumococcal disease begins when the organism gains access to sterile sites, usually those in proximity to its normal residence in the oropharynx. Pneumococcal sinusitis and otitis media are usually preceded by a viral illness, such as the common cold, which injures the protective ciliated epithelium and fills affected air spaces with fluid. Pneumococci then thrive in the nutrient-rich tissue fluid. Infection of the sinuses or middle ear can spread to the adjacent meninges.

Pneumococcal pneumonia arises similarly. The lower respiratory tract is protected by a mucociliary blanket and cough response, which normally expel organisms that reach the lower airways. Insults that interfere with respiratory clearance, including influenza, other viral respiratory illness, smoking and alcoholism, allow *S. pneumoniae* to reach alveoli. Once there, the organisms proliferate and elicit an acute inflammatory response. As the bacteria multiply and fill alveoli they spread to other alveoli. Their polysaccharide capsule prevents alternate complement pathway activation, and blocks production of the opsonin C3b. Consequently, the organism can proliferate and spread unimpeded by phagocytes until antibody is produced. In the lungs, *S. pneumoniae* spreads rapidly to involve an entire lobe or several lobes (lobar pneumonia).

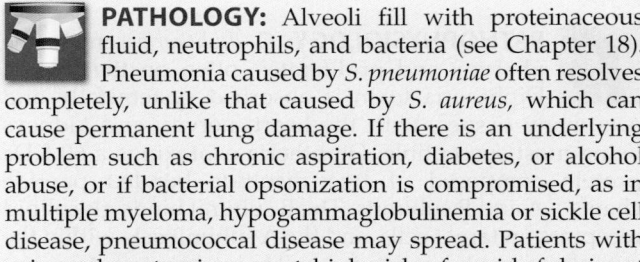 **PATHOLOGY:** Alveoli fill with proteinaceous fluid, neutrophils, and bacteria (see Chapter 18). Pneumonia caused by *S. pneumoniae* often resolves completely, unlike that caused by *S. aureus*, which can cause permanent lung damage. If there is an underlying problem such as chronic aspiration, diabetes, or alcohol abuse, or if bacterial opsonization is compromised, as in multiple myeloma, hypogammaglobulinemia or sickle cell disease, pneumococcal disease may spread. Patients with prior splenectomies are at high risk of rapid, fulminant septic shock and death.

Group B Streptococci Are the Leading Cause of Neonatal Pneumonia, Meningitis, and Sepsis

Group B streptococci are gram-positive bacteria that grow in short chains. They cause infrequent pyogenic infections in adults, but their main medical significance is the several thousand yearly neonatal infections with group B streptococci in the United States. About 30% of affected infants die. Group B streptococci are part of the normal vaginal flora in 10% to 30% of women. Most babies born to colonized women acquire the organisms as they pass through the birth canal.

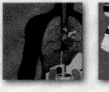 **PATHOPHYSIOLOGY AND PATHOLOGY:** Particular risk factors associated with development of neonatal group B streptococcal infections include premature delivery and

low levels of maternally derived IgG antibodies against the organism. Newborns have little functional reserve for granulocyte production, so once the bacterial infection is established, it rapidly overwhelms the body's defenses. Group B streptococcal infection may be limited to the lungs or CNS or may be widely disseminated. Involved tissues show a pyogenic response, often with overwhelming numbers of gram-positive cocci.

Diphtheria Is a Necrotizing Upper Respiratory Infection

Infection with *Corynebacterium diphtheriae*—an aerobic, pleomorphic, gram-positive rod—may lead to cardiac and neurologic disturbances due to toxin production. The disease is preventable by vaccination with inactivated *C. diphtheriae* toxin (toxoid).

EPIDEMIOLOGY: Humans are the only known reservoir for *C. diphtheriae,* and most people are asymptomatic carriers. The organism spreads from person to person in respiratory droplets or oral secretions. Diphtheria was once a leading cause of death in children 2 to 15 years of age. Immunization programs have largely eliminated the disease in the Western world, but diphtheria persists as a major health problem in less-developed countries. A recent outbreak occurred in 2011 in Kimba village, Nigeria affected over 100 nonimmunized people, mainly children, and had a case-fatality ratio of 22.4%.

PATHOPHYSIOLOGY: *C. diphtheriae* enters the pharynx and proliferates, often on the tonsils. Diphtheria toxin is absorbed systemically and acts many tissues, with the heart, nerves, and kidneys being most susceptible. Diphtheria exotoxin is a 60 KDa protein composed of two disulfide bonded peptide chains—A and B subunits. The B subunit binds glycolipid receptors on target cells, and the A subunit acts within the cytoplasm on elongation factor 2 to interrupt protein synthesis. Diphtheria toxin is one of the most potent known: one molecule suffices to kill a cell. Not all strains of *C. diphtheriae* produce exotoxin. The exotoxin is encoded by a lysogenic β-bacteriophage.

PATHOLOGY: The characteristic lesions of diphtheria are the thick, gray, leathery membranes composed of sloughed epithelium, necrotic debris, neutrophils, fibrin, and bacteria that line affected respiratory passages (from the Greek, *diphtheria*, "pair of leather scrolls"). The epithelial surface beneath the membranes is denuded, and the submucosa is acutely inflamed and hemorrhagic. The inflammation often causes swelling in surrounding soft tissues, which can be severe enough to cause respiratory compromise. When the heart is affected, the myocardium myocytes may show fat droplets and focal necrosis (Fig. 9-15). In the event of neural involvement, affected peripheral nerves show demyelination.

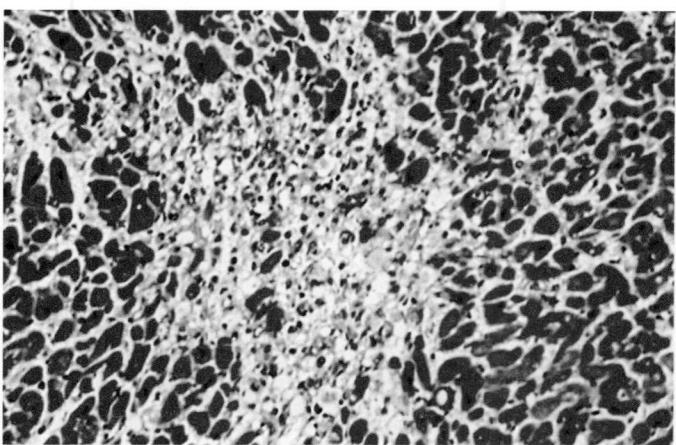

FIGURE 9-15. Diphtheritic myocarditis. Focal degeneration of cardiac myocytes is evident.

CLINICAL FEATURES: Diphtheria begins with fever, sore throat, and malaise. The dirty gray membrane usually develops first on the tonsils and may spread throughout the posterior oropharynx (Fig. 9-16). The membrane is firmly adherent, and an attempt to strip it from the underlying mucosa produces bleeding. Cardiac and neurologic symptoms develop in a minority of those infected, usually people with the most severe local disease.

Cutaneous diphtheria results from the organism entering via a break in the skin, and manifests as a pustule or ulcer; it rarely leads to cardiac or neurologic complications. Diphtheria is treated by prompt administration of antitoxin and antibiotics.

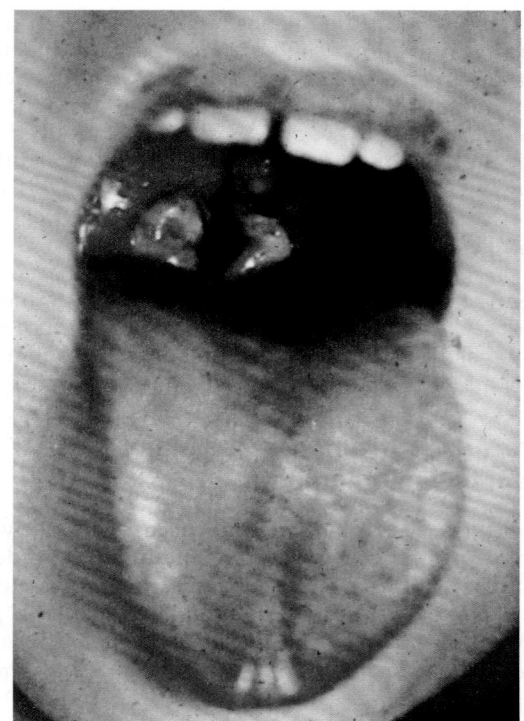

FIGURE 9-16. Characteristic diphtheric membrane in the oropharynx.

GRAM-NEGATIVE ORGANISMS

Pertussis Is Characterized by Debilitating Paroxysmal Coughing

The paroxysm is followed by a long, high-pitched inspiration, the "whoop," which gives the disease its name, "whooping cough." The causative organism is *Bordetella pertussis*, a small, gram-negative coccobacillus.

 EPIDEMIOLOGY: *B. pertussis* is highly contagious and spreads from person to person, primarily by respiratory aerosols. Humans are the only reservoir of infection. In susceptible populations, pertussis is mostly a disease of children under 5 years, but infection incidence is increasing among adults. Vaccination is protective, but there are some 50 million cases of pertussis each year worldwide, and almost 1 million deaths, particularly in infants. In 2012, the United States experienced the most severe outbreak of pertussis to occur in 50 years—exceeding 41,000 new cases—and highlighting a major public health problem in a vaccine-preventable disease.

PATHOPHYSIOLOGY: *B. pertussis* initiates infection by attaching to the cilia of respiratory epithelial cells. It then elaborates a cytotoxin that kills ciliated cells. The progressive destruction of ciliated respiratory epithelium and ensuing inflammatory response cause the local respiratory symptoms. Several other toxins include "pertussis toxin," which causes pronounced lymphocytosis that often accompanies whooping cough. Another toxin inhibits adenylyl cyclase, impeding bacterial phagocytosis.

PATHOLOGY: *B. pertussis* causes extensive tracheobronchitis, with necrosis of ciliated respiratory epithelium and an acute inflammatory response. Loss of the protective mucociliary blanket, increases risk of pneumonia from aspirated oral bacteria. Coughing paroxysms and vomiting make aspiration likely. Secondary bacterial pneumonia commonly causes death.

 CLINICAL FEATURES: **Whooping cough** is a prolonged upper respiratory tract illness, lasting 4 to 5 weeks and passing through three stages:

- The **catarrhal stage** resembles a common viral upper respiratory tract illness, with low-grade fever, runny nose, conjunctivitis, and cough.
- The **paroxysmal stage** occurs a week into the illness. Cough worsens and becomes paroxysmal, with 5 to 15 consecutive coughs, often followed by an inspiratory whoop. The patient develops a marked lymphocytosis: total leukocyte counts often exceed 40,000 cells/μL. The paroxysms persist for 2 to 3 weeks.
- The **convalescent phase** usually lasts for several weeks.

Haemophilus influenzae Causes Pyogenic Infections in Young Children

H. influenzae infections involve the middle ear, sinuses, facial skin, epiglottis, meninges, lungs, and joints. The organism is a major pediatric pathogen and a leading cause of bacterial meningitis worldwide. It is an aerobic, pleomorphic gram-negative coccobacillus that may be encapsulated or not. Nonencapsulated strains (type a) usually produce localized infections; encapsulated strains, type b, are more virulent and cause over 95% of the invasive bacteremic infections.

 EPIDEMIOLOGY: *H. influenzae* only infects humans, and spreads from person to person, mainly in respiratory droplets and secretions. It normally resides in the human nasopharynx of 20% to 50% of healthy adults. Most colonizing strains are nonencapsulated, but 3% to 5% are *H. influenzae* type b.

Most severe *H. influenzae* type b infections occur in children under 6 years. The incidence of serious disease peaks at 6 to 18 months of age, corresponding to the period between loss of maternally acquired immunity and acquisition of native immunity. *H. influenzae* type b (Hib) vaccine has greatly reduced the complications of invasive *H. influenzae* type b disease, particularly meningitis, in children. However, vaccination also reduces *H. influenzae* type b carriage and the repeated immunologic boosting that carriage provides, so continued vigilance is important.

 PATHOPHYSIOLOGY: Unencapsulated *H. influenzae* strains produce disease by spreading locally from their normal sites of residence to adjoining sterile locations, such as the sinuses or middle ear. This is facilitated by injury to normal defense mechanisms, as with a viral upper respiratory tract illness. At these previously sterile sites, unencapsulated organisms proliferate and elicit acute inflammatory responses, which injure local tissue but eventually contain the infection. Unencapsulated strains do not usually produce bacteremia.

In contrast, encapsulated H. influenzae type b is capable of tissue invasion. The capsular polysaccharide of type b organisms allows them to evade phagocytosis and bacteremic infections are common. Epiglottitis, facial cellulitis, septic arthritis, and meningitis result from invasive bacteremic infections. *H. influenzae* type b also elaborates an IgA protease, which facilitates local survival of the organism in the respiratory tract.

 PATHOLOGY: *H. influenzae* elicits strong acute inflammatory responses. Specific pathologic features vary according to the sites affected. *H. influenzae* meningitis resembles other acute bacterial meningitides, acute inflammatory leptomeningeal infiltration, sometimes involving the subarachnoid space.

H. influenzae pneumonia usually complicates chronic lung disease. In half of patients it follows a viral respiratory infection. Alveoli are filled with neutrophils, macrophages containing bacilli and fibrin. Bronchiolar epithelium is necrotic and infiltrated by macrophages.

Epiglottitis is swelling and acute inflammation of the epiglottis, aryepiglottic fold, and pyriform sinuses. It may sometimes completely obstruct the upper airway. In **facial cellulitis**, the site of infection and inflammation is the dermis, usually of the cheek or periorbital region. The first American president, George Washington, is believed to have died from acute epiglottitis.

 CLINICAL FEATURES: Most bacteremic *H. influenzae* infections afflict young children. **H. influenzae is the most common cause of meningitis in children under 2 years, although vaccination has reduced its frequency.** Onset is insidious and may follow an otherwise unremarkable upper respiratory tract infection or otitis media.

- **Bronchopneumonia or lobar pneumonia** is characterized by fever, cough, purulent sputum, and dyspnea.
- **Epiglottitis** affects primarily children 2 to 7 years old, but also occurs in adults. Upper respiratory obstruction may be fatal.
- **Septic arthritis** is secondary to bacteremic seeding of large weight-bearing joints. Symptoms include fever, heat, erythema, swelling, and pain on movement.
- **Facial cellulitis** or periorbital cellulitis is another severe bacteremic infection, mostly of young children. Patients present with fever, profound malaise, and a raised, hot, red-blue discolored area of the face, usually involving the cheek or an area about the eye. There is often concomitant meningitis or septic arthritis.

Neisseria meningitides Causes Pyogenic Meningitis and Overwhelming Shock

Neisseria meningitidis, or **meningococcus**, produces disseminated blood-borne infections, often accompanied by shock and profound disturbances in coagulation (Fig. 9-17). The organism is aerobic and appears as paired, bean-shaped, gram-negative cocci. There are eight major serogroups, A, B, and C being most important.

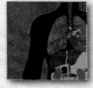 **EPIDEMIOLOGY:** Meningococci spread from person to person, largely in respiratory droplets. About 5% to 15% of the population carries them as commensals in the nasopharynx. Carriers develop antibodies to their colonizing strain of *N. meningitidis* and are not susceptible to disease caused by that strain.

Meningococcal diseases appear as sporadic cases, clusters of cases and epidemics. Most infections in industrialized countries are sporadic and afflict children under the age of 5. Epidemic disease occurs mostly in crowded quarters, such as among military recruits in barracks. There are over 6,000 cases of meningococcal meningitis each year in the United States, and over 600 deaths. Fatal meningococcal disease is more common in less-developed countries. There are several different vaccines against various strains of meningococcus, with efficacies generally in the range of 70% to 90%.

PATHOPHYSIOLOGY: Upon colonizing the upper respiratory tract, *N. meningitidis* attaches to nonciliated respiratory epithelium by means of

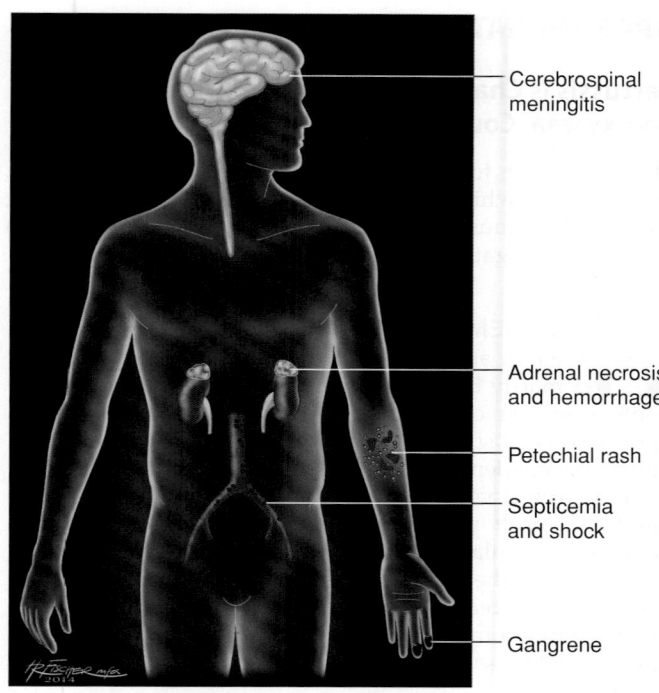

FIGURE 9-17. Meningococcemia. Meningococcal infections have a variety of clinical manifestations including meningitis, septicemia, shock, and associated complications.

its pili. Most exposed people then develop protective bactericidal antibodies over subsequent weeks, and some become carriers. If the organism spreads to the bloodstream before protective immunity develops, it can proliferate rapidly and cause fulminant meningococcal disease.

Many of the systemic effects of meningococcal disease are due to the endotoxin of the bacterial lipopolysaccharide. Endotoxin triggers increased TNFα production and simultaneous activation of complement and coagulation cascades. Disseminated intravascular coagulation, fibrinolysis, and shock follow.

 PATHOLOGY: Meningococcal disease can be confined to the CNS or may be disseminated throughout the body in the form of septicemia. In the former case, the leptomeninges and subarachnoid space are infiltrated with neutrophils and underlying brain parenchyma is swollen and congested. Meningococcal septicemia is characterized by diffuse damage to small vessel endothelium, with widespread petechiae and purpura in the skin and viscera.

Rarely (3% to 4% of cases), vasculitis and thrombosis produce hemorrhagic necrosis of both adrenals, called the **Waterhouse–Friderichsen syndrome.**

 CLINICAL FEATURES: Meningitis begins with rapid onset of fever, stiff neck, and headache. In meningococcal sepsis, fever, shock, and mucocutaneous hemorrhages appear abruptly. Patients may progress to shock within minutes, and treatment requires blood pressure support and antibiotics. Meningococcal disease was once almost invariably fatal, but antibiotic treatment has reduced mortality to less than 15%. Some patients who survive the early phase of meningococcemia develop late immunologic complications such as polyarthritis, cutaneous vasculitis, and pericarditis. Severe vasculitis may be associated with extensive cutaneous ulceration and even gangrene of the distal extremities.

Gonorrhea Is an Acute Suppurative Infection That May Cause Sterility

Neisseria gonorrhoeae, or **gonococcus**, causes gonorrhea, an acute suppurative genital tract infection, that presents with urethritis in men and endocervicitis in women. It is one of the oldest, and still one of the most common, sexually transmitted diseases. *N. gonorrhoeae* is an aerobic, bean-shaped, gram-negative diplococcus.

Gonococcal pharyngitis and proctitis are not uncommon, and are also sexually transmitted. In women, infection often ascends the genital tract, producing endometritis, salpingitis, and pelvic inflammatory disease. Ascending spread in men is less common, but if it occurs, epididymitis results. Gonococcal infection may rarely be bacteremic, in which case septic arthritis and skin lesions develop. Neonatal infections derived from the birth canal of a mother with gonorrhea usually manifest as conjunctivitis, although disseminated infections are occasionally seen. Neonatal gonococcal conjunctivitis remains a major cause of blindness in much of Africa and Asia but is largely prevented in developed countries by routine conjunctival instillation of antibiotics at birth.

EPIDEMIOLOGY: This common infection is spread directly from person to person. Except for perinatal transmission, spread is almost always by sexual contact. Infected people who are asymptomatic represent a significant reservoir of infection.

PATHOPHYSIOLOGY: Gonorrhea begins in the mucous membranes of the urogenital tract (Fig. 9-18). Bacteria attach to surface cells, after which they invade superficially and provoke acute inflammation. Gonococcus lacks a true polysaccharide capsule, but hairlike extensions, termed "pili," project from the cell wall. The pili contain a protease that digests IgA on the mucous membrane, thereby facilitating bacterial attachment to the columnar and transitional epithelium of the urogenital tract.

PATHOLOGY: Gonorrhea is a suppurative infection, eliciting a vigorous acute inflammatory response, with copious pus, and often forming submucosal abscesses. Stained smears of pus have many neutrophils, often containing phagocytosed bacteria. If untreated, the inflammation becomes chronic, with macrophages and lymphocytes predominant.

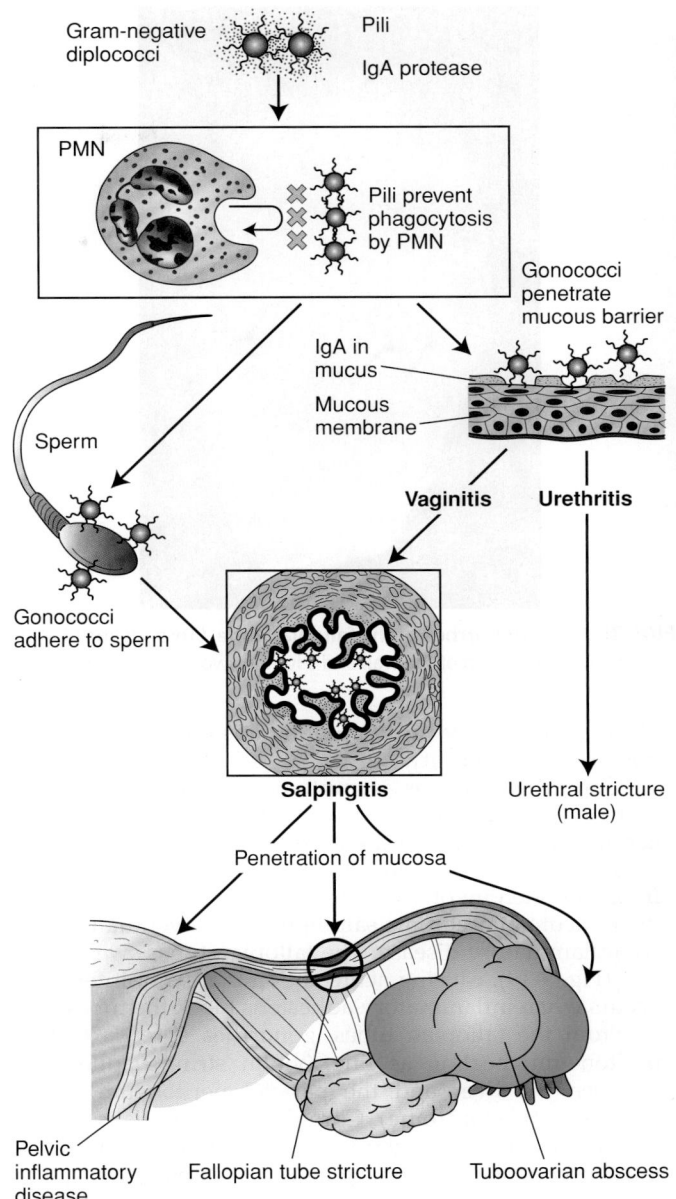

FIGURE 9-18. Pathogenesis of gonococcal infections. *Neisseria gonorrhoeae* is a gram-negative diplococcus whose surface pili form a barrier against phagocytosis by neutrophils. The pili contain an immunoglobulin A (IgA) protease that digests IgA on the luminal surface of the mucous membranes of the urethra, endocervix and fallopian tube, thereby facilitating attachment of gonococci. Gonococci cause endocervicitis, vaginitis, and salpingitis. In men, gonococci attached to the mucous membrane of the urethra cause urethritis and, sometimes, urethral stricture. Gonococci may also attach to sperm heads and be carried into the fallopian tube. Penetration of the mucous membrane by gonococci leads to stricture of the fallopian tube, pelvic inflammatory disease (PID), or tuboovarian abscess.

CLINICAL FEATURES: Men exposed to *N. gonorrhoeae* present with purulent urethral discharge and dysuria. If treatment is not instituted promptly, urethral stricture is a common complication. The organisms may also extend to the prostate, epididymis and accessory

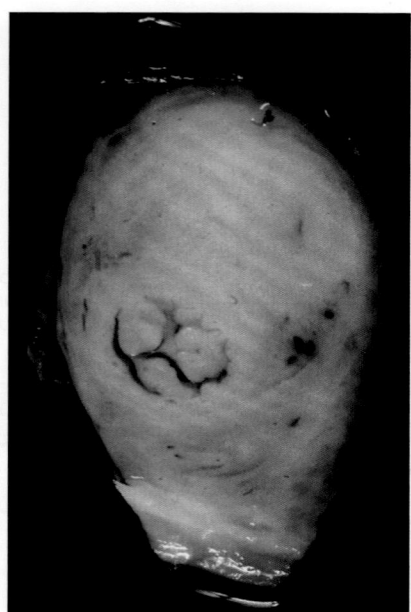

FIGURE 9-19. Gonorrhea of the fallopian tube. Cross-section of a "pus tube" shows thickening of the wall and a lumen swollen with pus.

glands, where they cause epididymitis and orchitis, and may result in infertility.

Gonorrhea remains asymptomatic in half of infected women. The other infected women initially show **endocervicitis**, with vaginal discharge or bleeding. Urethritis presents as dysuria rather than as a urethral discharge. Infection often involves the fallopian tubes, where it produces acute and chronic salpingitis and, eventually, pelvic inflammatory disease. The fallopian tubes swell with pus (Fig. 9-19), causing acute abdominal pain. Infertility occurs when inflammatory adhesions block the tubes.

From the fallopian tubes, gonorrhea spreads to the peritoneum, healing as fine "violin string" adhesions between the liver and the parietal peritoneum (**Fitz-Hugh–Curtis syndrome**). Chronic endometritis is a persistent complication of gonococcal infection and is usually the consequence of chronic gonococcal salpingitis.

Chancroid Causes Genital Ulcers, Usually in Tropical Regions

Chancroid is an acute sexually transmitted infection caused by *Haemophilus ducreyi*. The organism is a small, gram-negative bacillus, which appears in tissue as clusters of parallel bacilli and as chains, resembling schools of fish. Infections lead to painful genital ulceration and lymphadenopathy. *Chancroid is the leading cause of genital ulcers in many countries, especially in Africa and parts of Asia.* It has been suggested that these genital ulcers facilitate spread of HIV. In the United States, the incidence of chancroid is increasing, currently about 5,000 cases annually.

 PATHOLOGY: *H. ducreyi* enters through breaks in the skin, where it multiplies and produces a raised lesion, which then ulcerates. Ulcers vary from 0.1 to 2 cm in diameter. Organisms are carried within

macrophages to regional lymph nodes, which may suppurate. Seven to 10 days after the primary lesion appears, half of patients develop unilateral, painful, suppurative, inguinal lymphadenitis (**bubo**). Overlying skin becomes inflamed, breaks down and drains pus from the underlying node. The diagnosis is made by identifying the bacillus in tissue sections or gram-stained smears from the ulcers. Treatment with erythromycin is usually effective.

Granuloma Inguinale Is a Tropical Ulcerating Disease

Granuloma inguinale is a sexually transmitted, chronic, superficial ulceration of the genitalia and inguinal and perianal regions. It is caused by *Calymmatobacterium granulomatis*, a small, encapsulated, nonmotile, gram-negative bacillus.

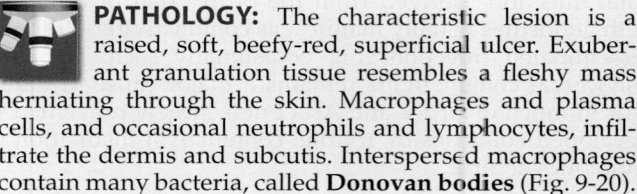 **EPIDEMIOLOGY:** Humans are the only hosts of *C. granulomatis*. Granuloma inguinale is rare in temperate climates but it is common in tropical and subtropical areas. New Guinea, central Australia, and India have the highest incidence. Most patients are 15 to 40 years of age.

PATHOLOGY: The characteristic lesion is a raised, soft, beefy-red, superficial ulcer. Exuberant granulation tissue resembles a fleshy mass herniating through the skin. Macrophages and plasma cells, and occasional neutrophils and lymphocytes, infiltrate the dermis and subcutis. Interspersed macrophages contain many bacteria, called **Donovan bodies** (Fig. 9-20).

CLINICAL FEATURES: Untreated granuloma inguinale follows an indolent, relapsing course, often healing with an atrophic scar. Secondary fusospirochetal infection may cause ulceration, mutilation, or amputation of the genitalia. Massive scarring of the dermis and subcutis may obstruct lymphatics and cause genital **elephantiasis**. Antibiotic therapy is effective in early cases.

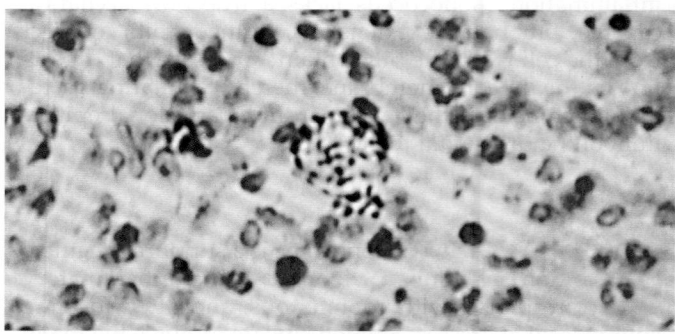

FIGURE 9-20. Granuloma inguinale. A skin lesion shows *Calymmatobacterium granulomatis* (Donovan bodies) clustered in a large macrophage. Intense silver staining by Warthin–Starry technique makes the organisms large, black, and easily seen.

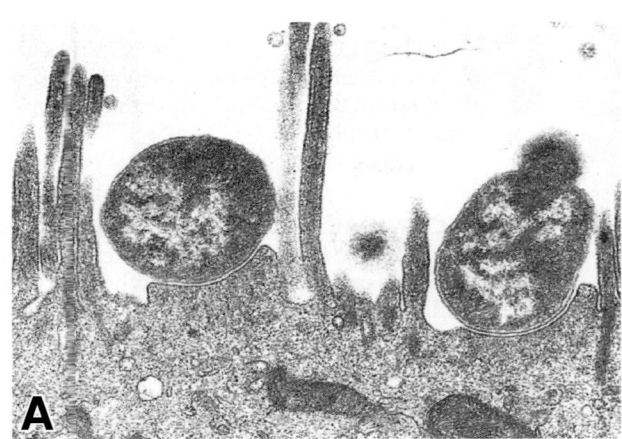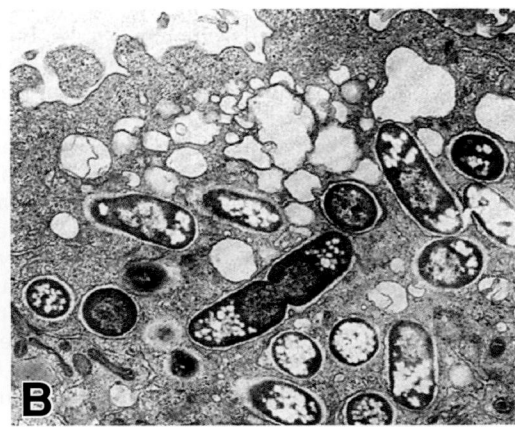

FIGURE 9-21. Enteric *Escherichia coli* infections. A. Enteropathogenic *E. coli* infection. An electron micrograph shows adherence of the bacteria to the intestinal mucosal cells and localized destruction of microvilli. **B.** Enteroinvasive *E. coli* infection. An electron micrograph shows organisms within a cell. (Reprinted from Farrar WE, Wood MJ, Innes JA, Tubbs H. *Infectious Diseases: Text and Color Atlas.* 2nd ed. New York: Gower Medical Publishing; 1992. Copyright © 1992 Elsevier. With permission.)

E. coli Is a Common Cause of Diarrhea and Urinary Tract Infections

E. coli is among the most frequent and important human bacterial pathogens. It causes over 90% of urinary tract infections and many cases of diarrheal illness worldwide. It is also a major opportunistic pathogen, frequently causing pneumonia and sepsis in immunocompromised hosts, and meningitis and sepsis in newborns.

E. coli are a group of antigenically and biologically diverse, aerobic (facultatively anaerobic), gram-negative bacteria. Most strains are intestinal commensals, well adapted to growth in the human colon without harming the host. However, *E. coli* can be aggressive when it gains access to usually sterile body sites, such as the urinary tract, meninges, or peritoneum. Strains of *E. coli* that produce diarrhea have specialized virulence properties, usually plasmid-mediated, that cause intestinal disease.

E. coli Diarrhea

There are four distinct strains of *E. coli* that cause diarrhea:

ENTEROTOXIGENIC E. coli: Enterotoxigenic E. coli are a major cause of diarrhea in poor tropical areas and probably cause most "traveler's diarrhea" among visitors to such regions. It is acquired from contaminated water and food. Many people in Latin America, Africa, and Asia are asymptomatic carriers.

PATHOPHYSIOLOGY: Nonimmune people (local children or travelers from abroad), develop diarrhea when they encounter the organism. Enterotoxigenic strains adhere to the intestinal mucosa and produce diarrhea by elaborating one or more of at least three enterotoxins that cause secretory dysfunction of the small bowel. One of the enterotoxins is structurally and functionally similar to cholera toxin, and another acts on guanylyl cyclase. Enterotoxigenic *E. coli* produces no distinctive macroscopic or light microscopic alterations in the intestine.

Enterotoxigenic *E. coli* causes an acute, self-limited diarrheal illness with watery stools lacking neutrophils and erythrocytes. In severe cases, fluid and electrolyte loss can cause extreme dehydration and even death.

ENTEROPATHOGENIC E. coli: This organism is a major cause of diarrheal illness in poor tropical areas, especially in infants and young children. It has virtually disappeared from developed countries, but still causes sporadic outbreaks of diarrhea, particularly among hospitalized infants younger than 2 years. Enteropathogenic *E. coli* is acquired by ingesting contaminated food or water. It is not invasive, and causes disease by adhering to and deforming the microvilli of intestinal epithelial cells (Fig. 9-21A). Enteropathogenic *E. coli* produces diarrhea, vomiting, fever, and malaise.

ENTEROHEMORRHAGIC E. coli: Enterohemorrhagic *E. coli* (serotype 0157:H7) causes a bloody diarrhea, which occasionally is followed by the **hemolytic–uremic syndrome** (see Chapter 22). Infection usually follows ingesting contaminated meat or milk. Enterohemorrhagic *E. coli* adheres to colonic mucosa and elaborates an enterotoxin, virtually identical to Shigatoxin (see below), that destroys epithelial cells. Patients infected with *E. coli* 0157:H7 present with cramping abdominal pain, low-grade fever and sometimes bloody diarrhea. Stool contains leukocytes and erythrocytes.

ENTEROINVASIVE E. coli: Enteroinvasive *E. coli* causes food-borne dysentery which is clinically and pathologically indistinguishable from that caused by *Shigella*, with which it shares extensive genetic, antigenic, and biochemical homology. It invades and destroys mucosal cells of the distal ileum and colon (Fig. 9-21B). As in shigellosis, the mucosae of the distal ileum and colon are acutely inflamed and focally eroded and are sometimes covered by an inflammatory pseudomembrane. Patients have abdominal pain, fever, tenesmus, and bloody diarrhea, usually for about a week. Antibiotic treatment is similar to that for shigellosis.

E. coli Urinary Tract Infection

EPIDEMIOLOGY: Urinary tract infections with *E. coli* are most common in sexually active women and in people of both sexes who have structural or functional abnormalities of the urinary tract. *Such infections are extremely common, afflicting more than 10% of the human population, often repeatedly.* *E. coli* in the urinary tract usually derive from resident flora of the perineum and periurethral—areas, reflecting fecal contamination of these regions.

PATHOPHYSIOLOGY: *E. coli* gains access to the sterile proximal urinary tract by ascending from the distal urethra. Women are much more prone to urinary tract infections because their shorter urethra provides a less effective mechanical barrier to infection. Sexual intercourse may propel organisms into the female urethra. Uropathogenic *E. coli* organisms have specialized adherence factors (Gal-Gal) on their pili, which enable them to bind to urothelial galactopyranosyl-galactopyranoside residues. Structural urinary tract abnormalities (e.g., congenital deformities, prostatic hyperplasia, strictures) and instrumentation (catheterization) overwhelm normal host defenses, predispose to urinary tract infections and account for most urinary tract infections in men.

 PATHOLOGY AND CLINICAL FEATURES: *E. coli* urinary tract infections initially produce acute inflammatory infiltrates at the site of infection, usually the bladder mucosa. Urinary tract infections involving the bladder or urethra present with urinary urgency, burning on urination (**dysuria**) and leukocytes in the urine. If infection ascends to the kidney (**pyelonephritis**), patients develop acute flank pain, fever, and leukocytosis. Neutrophils spill from the mucosa into the urine, and submucosal blood vessels are dilated and congested. Chronic infections show a mixed inflammatory infiltrate of neutrophils and mononuclear cells. Chronic renal infection may lead to chronic pyelonephritis and renal failure (see Chapter 22).

E. coli Pneumonia

Pneumonia caused by enteric gram-negative bacteria is considered opportunistic. It occurs mostly in debilitated people. *E. coli* is the most common cause, but other normal bowel flora, such as *Klebsiella, Serratia,* and *Enterobacter* species, produce similar disease. *The discussion below applies to all opportunistic gram-negative pneumonias.*

 PATHOPHYSIOLOGY: Enteric gram-negative bacteria are transiently introduced into the oral cavity of healthy people but cannot compete successfully with the dominant gram-positive flora, which adhere to the fibronectin that coats mucosal cell surfaces. Chronically ill or severely stressed people elaborate a salivary protease that degrades fibronectin, allowing gram-negative enteric bacteria to overcome the normal gram-positive flora and colonize the oropharynx.

Inevitably, droplets of resident oral flora are aspirated into the respiratory tract, where debilitated patients' often weak local defenses cannot destroy them. Decreased gag and cough reflexes, abnormal neutrophil chemotaxis, injured respiratory epithelium and foreign bodies, such as endotracheal tubes, all facilitate entry and survival of the aspirated organisms. *E. coli* pneumonia results from proliferation of aspirated organisms in terminal airways, usually at multiple sites in the lung.

 PATHOLOGY: There are multifocal areas of consolidation. Terminal airways and alveoli are filled with proteinaceous fluid, fibrin, neutrophils, and macrophages.

 CLINICAL FEATURES: Because pneumonia caused by *E. coli* and other enteric gram-negative organisms afflicts patients who are often already severely ill, symptoms of pneumonia may be less obvious than in healthy people. Increased malaise, fever, and labored breathing are often the first signs of pneumonia. If *E. coli* pneumonia remains untreated, the bacteria may invade the blood to produce fatal septicemia. Treatment requires parenteral antibiotics.

E. coli Sepsis (Gram-Negative Sepsis)

E. coli is the most common cause of enteric gram-negative sepsis, but other gram-negative rods, including *Pseudomonas, Klebsiella,* and *Enterobacter* species, produce identical disease. The discussion below applies to gram-negative sepsis in general.

 PATHOPHYSIOLOGY: *E. coli* sepsis is usually opportunistic. It occurs in people with predisposing conditions, for example, neutropenia, pyelonephritis, or cirrhosis, and in hospitalized patients. Together with other enteric gram-negative rods that normally reside in human colon, *E. coli* occasionally seeds the bloodstream. In healthy people, macrophages and circulating neutrophils ingest these bacteria. *E. coli* sepsis can develop in persons with normal immunity but who develop massive bacteremia (for example due to a ruptured abdominal organ), and in those patients who have an impaired ability to eliminate low-level bacteremia.

The presence of *E. coli* in the bloodstream causes septic shock through the effects of TNFα (among other factors), whose release from macrophages is stimulated by bacterial endotoxin (see Chapters 7 and 12).

Neonatal *E. coli* Meningitis and Sepsis

E. coli and group B streptococci are the main causes of meningitis and sepsis in the first month after birth. Both colonize the vagina, and newborns acquire them on passage through the birth canal. *E. coli* then colonize the infant's GI tract. It is postulated that the organisms spread to the bloodstream from the gut, then seed the meninges. Pathologically, *E. coli* meningitis resembles other bacterial meningitides. Although antibiotic treatment for neonatal *E. coli* meningitis and sepsis is often effective, mortality is still 15% to 50%. Almost half of survivors suffer neurologic sequelae.

Salmonella Cause Enterocolitis and Typhoid Fever

The bacterial genus *Salmonella* contains over 1,500 antigenically distinct but biochemically and genetically related gram-negative rods, which cause two important human diseases: *Salmonella* enterocolitis and typhoid fever.

Salmonella Enterocolitis

Salmonella enterocolitis is an acute self-limited (1 to 3 days) gastrointestinal illness that presents as nausea, vomiting, diarrhea, and fever. Infection is typically acquired by eating food containing nontyphoidal *Salmonella* strains, and is commonly called **Salmonella food poisoning.**

 EPIDEMIOLOGY: Nontyphoidal *Salmonella* infect many animal species, including amphibians, reptiles, birds, and mammals. They also readily contaminate foodstuffs derived from infected animals (e.g., meat, poultry, eggs, dairy products). If these foods are not cooked, pasteurized or irradiated, the bacteria persist and multiply, particularly at warm temperatures. Once a person is infected, the organism can spread from person to person by the fecal–oral route, which is infrequent among adults but common among small children in day-care settings or within families. *Salmonella* enterocolitis remains a major cause of childhood mortality in less-developed countries.

  PATHOPHYSIOLOGY AND PATHOLOGY: *Salmonella* proliferate in the small intestine and invade enterocytes in the distal small bowel and colon. Nontyphoidal *Salmonella* species elaborate several toxins that injure intestinal cells. Colonic and ileal mucosae are acutely inflamed and sometimes superficially ulcerated.

 CLINICAL FEATURES: *Salmonella* enterocolitis typically manifests as diarrhea, within 12 to 48 hours after consuming contaminated food. This contrasts with staphylococcal food poisoning, which is caused by a preformed toxin and begins 1 to 6 hours after eating. The diarrhea of *Salmonella* food poisoning is self-limited. It lasts 1 to 3 days and is often accompanied by nausea, vomiting, cramping abdominal pain, and fever. Treatment is supportive: antibiotics rarely improve the clinical course.

Typhoid Fever

Typhoid fever is an acute systemic illness caused by infection with *S. typhi*. **Paratyphoid fever** is a clinically similar but milder disease that results from infection with other species of *Salmonella*, including *S. paratyphi*. The term **enteric fever** includes both typhoid and paratyphoid fever.

 EPIDEMIOLOGY: Humans are the only natural reservoir for *S. typhi*, and typhoid fever is acquired from infected patients or chronic carriers. The latter tend to be older women with gallstones or biliary scarring: *S. typhi* colonizes their gallbladder or biliary tree. Infected food handlers and urine from patients with typhoid pyelonephritis can spread infection. Other sources include contaminated water and food, especially dairy products and shellfish, or, direct finger-to-mouth contact with feces, urine, or other secretions. Typhoid fever accounts for over 25,000 annual deaths worldwide but is uncommon in the United States.

 PATHOPHYSIOLOGY: *S. typhi* attaches to and invades small bowel mucosa without causing clinical enterocolitis. Invasion tends to be most prominent in the ileum, overlying Peyer patches. The bacteria are engulfed by macrophages, then block the respiratory burst of the phagocytes and multiply within these cells. Infected cells spread first to regional lymph nodes, then systemically via lymphatics and bloodstream, infecting mononuclear macrophages in lymph nodes, bone marrow, liver, and spleen. Infected macrophages produce IL-1 and TNFα, causing prolonged fever, malaise, and wasting characteristic of this disease.

 PATHOLOGY: The earliest pathologic change in typhoid fever is degeneration of the intestinal epithelium brush border. As bacteria invade, Peyer patches become hypertrophic. Intestinal lymphoid hyperplasia may progress to capillary thrombosis, causing necrosis of overlying mucosa and characteristic ulcers along the long axis of the bowel (Fig. 9-22). These ulcers frequently bleed and occasionally perforate, producing infectious peritonitis. Systemic bacterial spread leads to focal granulomas in the liver, spleen, and other organs, called **typhoid nodules**, containing aggregates of macrophages ("typhoid cells") with ingested bacteria, erythrocytes, and degenerated lymphocytes.

CLINICAL FEATURES: Untreated typhoid fever was classically divided into five stages (Fig. 9-23):

- **Incubation:** (10 to 14 days)
- **Active invasion/bacteremia:** Patients have about a week of nonspecific symptoms, including daily stepwise elevation in temperature (up to 41°C [105.8°F]), malaise, headache, arthralgias, and abdominal pain.
- **Fastigium:** Fever and malaise increase over several days to the point of prostration. Patients may become toxic from the release of endotoxins from dead bacteria. Hepatomegaly is accompanied by derangement in liver function. The spleen is conspicuously enlarged.
- **Lysis:** In patients destined to survive, fever and toxic symptoms gradually diminish. Gastrointestinal bleeding

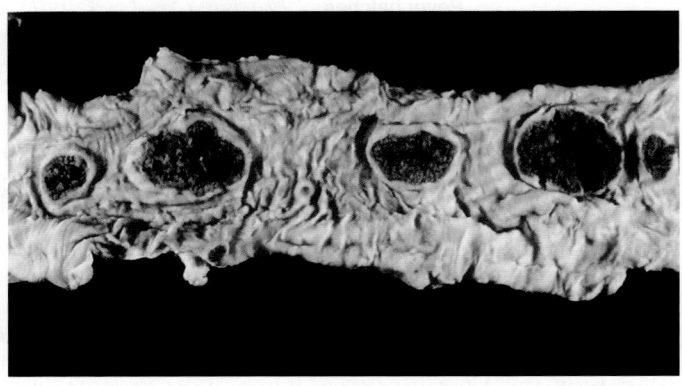

FIGURE 9-22. Ulcers of the terminal ileum in fatal typhoid fever. The ulcers have a longitudinal orientation because they are located over hyperplastic and necrotic Peyer patches.

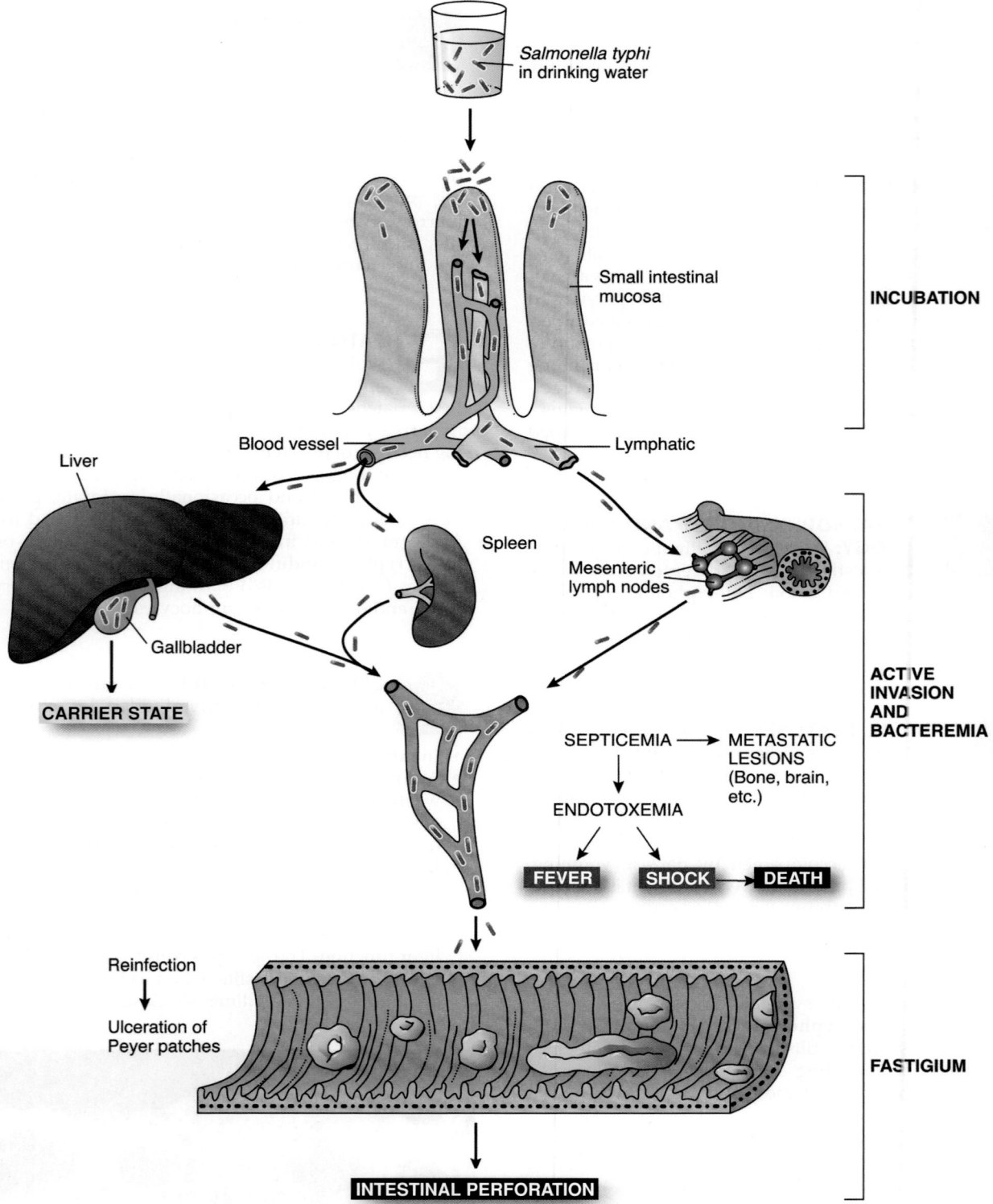

FIGURE 9-23. Stages of typhoid fever. Incubation (10 to 14 days). Water or food contaminated with *Salmonella typhi* is ingested. Bacilli attach to the villi in the small intestine, invade the mucosa and pass to the intestinal lymphoid follicles and draining mesenteric lymph nodes. The organisms proliferate further within mononuclear phagocytic cells of the lymphoid follicles, lymph nodes, liver, and spleen. Bacilli are sequestered intracellularly in the intestinal and mesenteric lymphatic system. **Active invasion/bacteremia** (1 week). Organisms are released and produce a transient bacteremia. The intestinal mucosa becomes enlarged and necrotic, forming characteristic mucosal lesions. The intestinal lymphoid tissues become hyperplastic and contain "typhoid nodules"—aggregates of macrophages ("typhoid cells") that phagocytose bacteria, erythrocytes, and degenerated lymphocytes. Bacilli proliferate in several organs, reappear in the intestine, are excreted in stool, and may invade through the intestinal wall. **Fastigium** (1 week). Dying bacilli release endotoxins that cause systemic toxemia. **Lysis** (1 week). Necrotic intestinal mucosa sloughs, producing ulcers, which hemorrhage or perforate into the peritoneal cavity.

and intestinal perforation at sites of ulceration may occur in any stage, but are most common during lysis, which commonly lasts a week.
- **Convalescence:** Fever abates and patients gradually recover over several weeks to months. Some relapse or have metastatic foci of infection.

Treatment of typhoid fever entails antibiotics and supportive care. Ten to 20% of untreated patients die, usually of secondary complications, such as pneumonia. However, treatment within 3 days of the onset of fever is generally curative.

Shigellosis Is a Necrotizing Infection of the Distal Small Bowel and Colon

It is caused by any of four species of *Shigella* (*S. boydii*, *S. dysenteriae, S. flexneri,* and *S. sonnei)*, which are aerobic, gram-negative rods. Of these, *S. dysenteriae* is the most virulent. Shigellosis is a self-limited disease that typically presents with abdominal pain and bloody, mucoid stools.

EPIDEMIOLOGY: *Shigella* organisms spread from person to person by the fecal–oral route. They have no animal reservoir and do not survive well outside the stool. Infection usually occurs through ingestion of fecally contaminated food or water, but can be acquired by oral contact with any contaminated surface (e.g., clothing, towels, or skin surfaces). As a result, endemic shigellosis is more common in areas with poor hygiene and sanitation. It is also spread in closed communities, such as hospitals, barracks, and households. In developed countries, *S. flexneri* and *S. sonnei* are more common, and infection tends to be sporadic.

In the United States, about 300,000 cases occur annually, but the incidence is much higher in countries lacking sanitary systems for human waste disposal. Like other diarrheal illnesses, shigellosis is a significant cause of childhood mortality in developing countries.

PATHOPHYSIOLOGY: Shigellae are among the most virulent enteropathogens. As few as 10 to 100 ingested bacteria can cause disease. There are few asymptomatic carriers. The agent proliferates rapidly in the small bowel and attaches to enterocytes, where it replicates within the cytoplasm. Endocytosis is essential for virulence and the virulence factor is encoded by a plasmid. Replicating shigellae kill infected cells then spread to adjacent cells and into the lamina propria.

Shigellae also produce a potent exotoxin, known as **Shiga toxin** that is like the verotoxin of *E. coli* O157:H7. Shiga toxin interferes with 60S ribosomal subunits and inhibits protein synthesis. It also causes watery diarrhea, probably by interfering with fluid absorption in the colon. Although shigellae damage the epithelium of the ileum and colon extensively, they rarely invade beyond the intestinal lamina propria, and bacteremia is uncommon.

PATHOLOGY: The distal colon is almost always affected, although the entire colon and distal ileum can be involved. The affected mucosa is edematous, acutely inflamed and focally eroded. Ulcers appear first on the edges of mucosal folds, perpendicular to the long axis of the colon. A patchy inflammatory **pseudomembrane** of neutrophils, fibrin, and necrotic epithelium is common in the most severely affected areas. Infected colonic epithelium regenerates rapidly, and healing is usually complete within 10 to 14 days.

CLINICAL FEATURES: Shigellosis often begins with watery diarrhea, which changes within 1 to 2 days to classic dysenteric stools. These are small-volume stools with gross blood, sloughed pseudomembranes, and mucus. Cramping abdominal pain, tenesmus, and urgency at stool typically accompany the diarrhea. Untreated, symptoms persist for 3 to 8 days. Antibiotic treatment shortens the course of the illness.

Cholera Is an Epidemic Enteritis Usually Acquired From Contaminated Water

Cholera is a severe diarrheal illness caused by the enterotoxin of Vibrio cholerae, *an aerobic, curved gram-negative rod. V. cholerae* proliferates in the lumen of the small intestine and causes profuse watery diarrhea, rapid dehydration and (if fluids are not restored) shock and death within 24 hours of the onset of symptoms.

EPIDEMIOLOGY: Cholera is common in most parts of the world, but it periodically "disappears" spontaneously. A major pandemic occurred between 1961 and 1974, throughout Asia, the Middle East, southern Russia, the Mediterranean basin, and parts of Africa. Cholera remains endemic in the river deltas of India and Bangladesh. It is a worldwide public health problem, affecting 3 to 5 million people, with 100,000 to 300,000 deaths per year. After the 2010 earthquake in Haiti, the largest outbreak of cholera in recent history killed 7,900 Haitians and hospitalized hundreds of thousands more while spreading to neighboring Cuba and Dominican Republic.

It is acquired by ingesting *V. cholerae*, mainly in contaminated food or water. Epidemics spread readily in areas where human feces pollute the water supply. Shellfish and plankton may serve as a natural reservoir for the organism. Shellfish ingestion accounts for most of the sporadic cases seen in the United States.

PATHOPHYSIOLOGY: Bacteria that survive passage through the stomach thrive and multiply in the mucous layer of the small bowel. They do not invade the mucosa but cause diarrhea by elaborating a potent exotoxin, **cholera toxin**, which has A and B subunits. The latter binds to GM_1 ganglioside in enterocyte cell membranes. The A subunit then enters the cell, where it activates adenylyl cyclase, increasing cAMP which

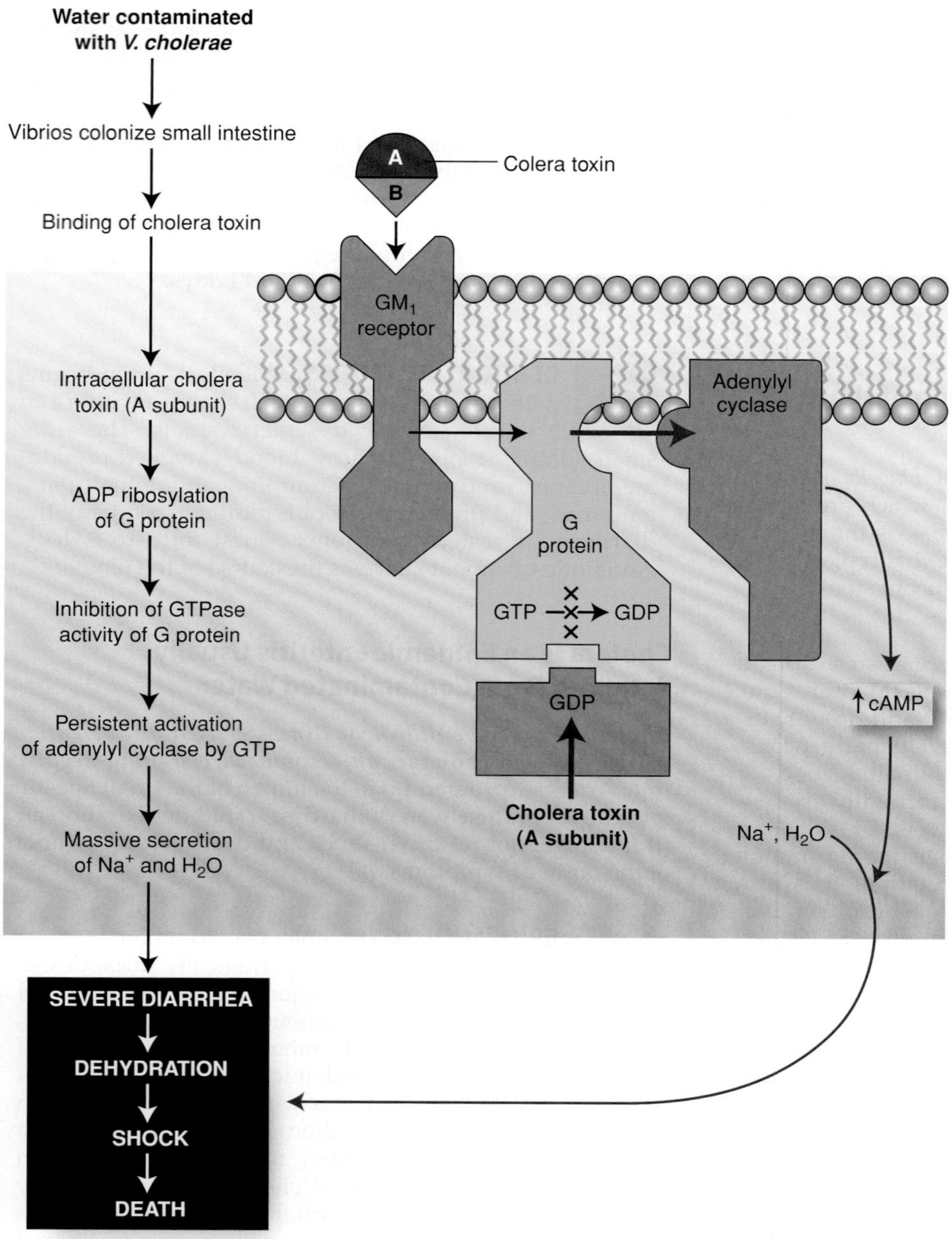

Water contaminated with *V. cholerae*

↓

Vibrios colonize small intestine

↓

Binding of cholera toxin

↓

Intracellular cholera toxin (A subunit)

↓

ADP ribosylation of G protein

↓

Inhibition of GTPase activity of G protein

↓

Persistent activation of adenylyl cyclase by GTP

↓

Massive secretion of Na^+ and H_2O

↓

SEVERE DIARRHEA
↓
DEHYDRATION
↓
SHOCK
↓
DEATH

A / B — Colera toxin

GM_1 receptor

Adenylyl cyclase

G protein

$GTP \longrightarrow GDP$

GDP

Cholera toxin (A subunit)

↑ cAMP

Na^+, H_2O

FIGURE 9-24. Cholera. Infection comes from water contaminated with *Vibrio cholerae* or food prepared with contaminated water. Vibrios traverse the stomach, enter the small intestine and propagate. Although they do not invade the intestinal mucosa, vibrios elaborate a potent toxin that induces a massive outpouring of water and electrolytes. Severe diarrhea ("rice water stool") leads to dehydration and hypovolemic shock.

causes massive secretion of sodium and water by the enterocyte into the intestinal lumen (Fig. 9-24). Most fluid secretion occurs in the small bowel, where there is a net loss of water and electrolytes.

PATHOLOGY: *V. cholerae* causes little visible alteration in the affected intestine, which appears grossly normal or only slightly hyperemic. Microscopically, the intestinal epithelium is intact but depleted of mucus.

CLINICAL FEATURES: Cholera begins with a few loose stools, usually evolving within hours into severe watery diarrhea. The stools are often flecked with mucus, imparting a "rice water" appearance. The volume of diarrhea is highly variable, but the rapidity and volume loss in severe cases can be staggering. With adequate volume replacement, infected adults can lose up to 20 L of fluid in a day. Fluid and electrolyte loss can lead to shock and death within hours if fluid volume is not replaced. Untreated cholera has a 50% mortality rate. Replacing lost salts and water is a simple, effective treatment, which can often be accomplished by oral rehydration with preparations of salt, glucose, and water. The illness subsides spontaneously in 3 to 6 days, which can be shortened by antibiotic therapy. Infection with *V. cholerae* confers long-term protection from recurrent illness. Available vaccines have limited effectiveness.

Vibrio parahaemolyticus

There are several "noncholera" vibrios, of which *V. parahaemolyticus* is the most common. This gram-negative bacillus is found in marine life and coastal waters around the world in temperate climates, and causes acute gastroenteritis in the summer. Its range may be expanding, perhaps due to global warming: confirmed cases have occurred in Alaska, over 1,000 miles north of any previous outbreaks. Gastroenteritis is associated with eating inadequately cooked or poorly refrigerated seafood. The clinical syndrome resembles *Salmonella* enteritis. No deaths have been reported.

Campylobacter jejuni Is the Most Common Cause of Bacterial Diarrhea in the Developed World

C. jejuni is the major human pathogen in the genus *Campylobacter*. It causes an acute, self-limited inflammatory diarrheal illness. *C. jejuni* is distributed worldwide and is responsible for over 2 million cases annually in the United States. It is a microaerophilic, curved gram-negative rod, morphologically similar to vibrios.

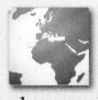 **EPIDEMIOLOGY:** *C. jejuni* infection is acquired through contaminated food or water. The bacteria inhabit GI tracts of many animals, including cows, sheep, chickens, and dogs, which are a significant animal reservoir for infection. In fact, *Campylobacter* infections cause abortions and infertility of infected cattle and sheep, and so serious economic losses. Raw milk and inadequately cooked poultry and meat are frequent sources of disease. *C. jejuni* can also spread from person to person by fecal–oral contact. It is a major cause of childhood mortality in developing countries and causes many cases of "travelers' diarrhea."

 PATHOPHYSIOLOGY: Ingested *C. jejuni* that survive gastric acidity multiply in the alkaline environment of the upper small intestine. The agent elaborates several toxic proteins that correlate with the severity of the symptoms.

 PATHOLOGY: *C. jejuni* causes a superficial enterocolitis, primarily involving the terminal ileum and colon, with focal necrosis of intestinal epithelium and acute inflammation. Severe cases progress to small ulcers and patchy inflammatory exudates (pseudomembranes) with necrotic cells, neutrophils, fibrin, and debris. Colon epithelial crypts often fill with neutrophils, forming the so-called crypt abscesses. These pathologic changes resolve in 7 to 14 days.

 CLINICAL FEATURES: Patients with *C. jejuni* usually produce more than 10 stools per day, varying from profuse watery stools to small-volume stools containing gross blood and mucus. Symptoms resolve in 5 to 7 days. Treatment with antibiotics is probably of marginal benefit. A few patients develop a more severe, protracted illness resembling acute ulcerative colitis. Gastrointestinal infections with *C. jejuni* have been associated with Guillain–Barré syndrome.

Yersinia Infections Produce Painful Diarrhea

Yersinia enterocolitica and *Y. pseudotuberculosis* are gram-negative coccoid or rod-shaped bacteria.

 EPIDEMIOLOGY: These organisms are facultative anaerobes found in feces of wild and domestic animals, including rodents, sheep, cattle, dogs, cats, and horses. *Y. pseudotuberculosis* also often occurs in domestic birds, including turkeys, ducks, geese, and canaries. Both organisms have been isolated from drinking water and milk. *Y. enterocolitica* is more likely acquired from contaminated meat, and *Y. pseudotuberculosis* from contact with infected animals.

 PATHOLOGY AND CLINICAL FEATURES: *Y. enterocolitica* proliferates in the ileum, invades the mucosa, causing ulceration and necrosis of Peyer patches. It migrates via lymphatics to mesenteric lymph nodes. Fever, diarrhea (sometimes bloody) and abdominal pain begin 4 to 10 days after mucosal penetration. Abdominal pain in the right lower quadrant may be mistaken for appendicitis. Arthralgia, arthritis, and erythema nodosum are complications. Septicemia is uncommon, but may be lethal in one-half of cases when it occurs.

Y. pseudotuberculosis penetrates ileal mucosa, localizes in ileal–cecal lymph nodes and produces abscesses and granulomas in the lymph nodes, spleen, and liver. Fever, diarrhea, and abdominal pain may also suggest appendicitis.

GRAM-NEGATIVE PNEUMONIAS

Klebsiella and *Enterobacter* Produce Nosocomial Infections That Cause Necrotizing Lobar Pneumonia

Klebsiella and *Enterobacter* species are short, encapsulated, gram-negative bacilli.

 EPIDEMIOLOGY: These organisms cause 10% of nosocomial infections, including pneumonia and infections of the urinary tract, biliary tract, and surgical wounds. Person-to-person transmission by hospital personnel is a special hazard. Predisposing factors are obstructive pulmonary disease in endotracheal tubes, indwelling catheters, debilitating conditions, and immunosuppression. Secondary pneumonia caused by these agents may complicate influenza or other respiratory viral infections.

 PATHOLOGY: *Klebsiella* and *Enterobacter* are inhaled and multiply in alveolar spaces. The lung parenchyma becomes consolidated, and a mucoid exudate of macrophages, fibrin, and edema fluid fills the alveoli. As the exudate accumulates, alveolar walls become compressed and then necrotic. Many small abscesses may coalesce and lead to cavitation.

CLINICAL FEATURES: The onset of pneumonia is sudden, with fever, pleuritic pain, cough, and a characteristic **thick mucoid sputum.** When infection is severe, these symptoms progress to dyspnea, cyanosis, and death in 2 to 3 days. *Klebsiella* and *Enterobacter* infections may be complicated by fulminating, often fatal, septicemia, and aggressive antibiotic therapy is required. Recently, a group of highly drug-resistant *Klebsiella* and *Enterobacter* have emerged and are spreading throughout the world. These organisms, termed carbapenem-resistant enterobacteriaceae (CRE), are resistant to carbapenem antibiotics, considered the "drugs of last resort" for such infections. Carbapenem-resistant *K. pneumoniae* (CRKP) produces carbapenamase, also called a β-metallo-lactamase 1 (NDM-1), so that these strains are resistant to almost all available antibiotics.

Legionella Cause Pneumonia That Ranges From Mild to Life-Threatening

Legionella pneumophila is a minute aerobic bacillus that has the cell wall structure of a gram-negative organism but stains poorly with Gram reagents. It was first identified 6 months after an outbreak of a severe respiratory disease of unknown cause at the 1976 American Legion convention in Philadelphia. Subsequently, retrospective studies showed antibodies in sera from previously unexplained epidemics, dating to 1957.

EPIDEMIOLOGY: *Legionella* are present in small numbers in natural bodies of fresh water. They survive chlorination and proliferate in devices such as cooling towers, water heaters, humidifiers, and evaporative condensers. Infection occurs when people inhale aerosols from contaminated sources. The disease is not contagious, and the organism is not normal human oropharyngeal flora. An estimated 8,000 to 18,000 cases of *Legionella* infection occur in the United States annually.

PATHOPHYSIOLOGY: *Legionella* causes two distinct diseases: **pneumonia** and **Pontiac fever**. The pathogenesis of *Legionella* pneumonia (Legionnaires disease) is understood in some detail, but that of Pontiac fever remains largely a mystery. *Legionella* pneumonia begins when the bacteria arrive in the terminal bronchioles or alveoli, where they are ingested by alveolar macrophages. There, they replicate within phagosomes, protecting themselves by blocking fusion of lysosomes with the phagosomes. The multiplying *Legionella* are released and infect freshly arriving macrophages. As immunity develops, macrophages become activated and cease to support intracellular growth.

Native respiratory tract defenses, such as the mucociliary airway blanket, provide a first line of defense against *Legionella* infection in the lower respiratory tract. Smoking, alcoholism, and chronic lung diseases, which interfere with respiratory defenses, also increase the risk of developing *Legionella* pneumonia.

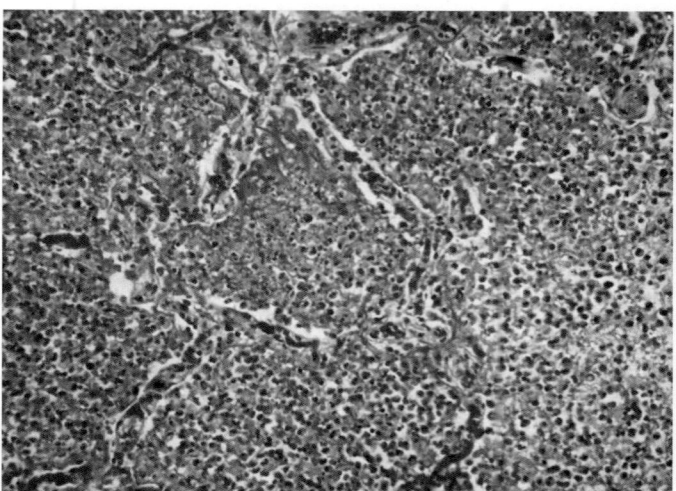

FIGURE 9-25. Legionnaires pneumonia. The alveoli are packed with an exudate composed of fibrin, macrophages, and neutrophils.

PATHOLOGY: Legionnaires disease is an acute bronchopneumonia. It is usually patchy but may show a lobar pattern of infiltration. Affected alveoli and bronchioles are filled with exudate containing proteinaceous fluid, fibrin, macrophages and neutrophils (Fig. 9-25), and microabscesses. Alveolar walls become necrotic and are destroyed. Many macrophages show eccentric nuclei, pushed aside by cytoplasmic vacuoles containing *L. pneumophila*. As the pneumonia resolves, the lungs heal with little permanent damage.

CLINICAL FEATURES: Clinical onset is rapid, following a 2- to 10-day incubation, with rapidly progressive pneumonia, fever, nonproductive cough, and myalgia. Chest radiographs show unilateral, diffuse, patchy consolidation, progressing to widespread nodular consolidation. Toxic symptoms, hypoxia, and obtundation may be prominent, and death may follow within a few days. In survivors, convalescence is prolonged. Mortality among hospitalized patients averages 15%, but is greater if there is a serious underlying illness. Macrolide antibiotics may be effective.

Pontiac fever is a self-limited, flulike illness with fever, malaise, myalgias, and headache. It differs from Legionnaires disease in showing no evidence of pulmonary consolidation. The disease resolves spontaneously in 3 to 5 days.

Pseudomonas aeruginosa Is a Highly Antibiotic-Resistant Opportunistic Pathogen

Pseudomonas only infrequently infects humans. In those cases where infections occur it commonly results in severe pneumonia, sepsis, and wound and urinary tract infections in hospital environments. Debilitated or immunosuppressed people are most at risk, with burns, catheterization, cystic fibrosis, diabetes, and neutropenia all being predisposing factors.

P. aeruginosa is a ubiquitous aerobic, gram-negative rod that requires moisture and only minimal nutrients. It thrives in soil and water, on animals and moist environmental surfaces.

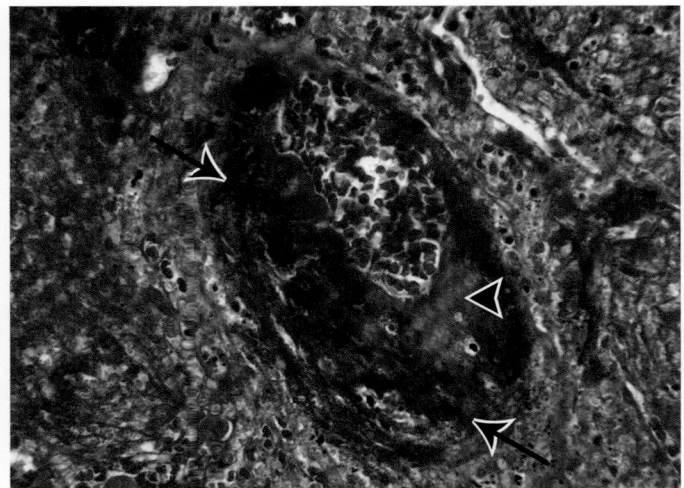

FIGURE 9-26. *Pseudomonas* vasoinvasiveness. A section of lung from a patient who died with *Pseudomonas* sepsis, showing a blood vessel, with masses of *Pseudomonas* (gram-negative rods) penetrating the vascular wall (*arrows*) and triggering thrombosis (*arrowhead*) in the vessel lumen. Surrounding lung is correspondingly infarcted.

Since it is resistant to most antibiotics, ongoing antibiotic treatment selects for it.

PATHOPHYSIOLOGY: Injury to epithelial cells uncovers surface molecules to which the bacteria's pili bind. Once attached, *P. aeruginosa* elaborates many proteins that allow it to invade and destroy host tissues, while evading host inflammatory and immune defenses. Many strains produce a proteoglycan that surrounds and protects the bacteria from mucociliary action, complement, and phagocytes. *Pseudomonas* releases extracellular enzymes—including an elastase, an alkaline protease and a cytotoxin—which facilitate tissue invasion and facilitate the characteristic necrotizing lesions. The elastase probably determines the distinctive ability of *P. aeruginosa* to invade blood vessel walls (Fig. 9-26). Systemic effects may be mediated by endotoxin and several systemically active exotoxins.

PATHOLOGY: *Pseudomonas* infection elicits an acute inflammatory response. The bacteria often invade small arteries and veins, causing thrombosis and hemorrhagic necrosis, particularly in the lungs and skin. Vascular invasion promotes dissemination and sepsis, and causes multiple nodular lesions in the lungs. Gram stains of necrotic tissue infected with *Pseudomonas* commonly show blood vessel walls densely infiltrated with organisms. Disseminated infections may include **ecthyma gangrenosum:** nodular, necrotic lesions represent sites where the organism spread to the skin, invaded blood vessels, and produced localized hemorrhagic infarcts.

CLINICAL FEATURES: *Pseudomonas* infections are among the most aggressive human bacterial diseases, often progressing rapidly to sepsis. They require immediate medical intervention and are associated with high mortality.

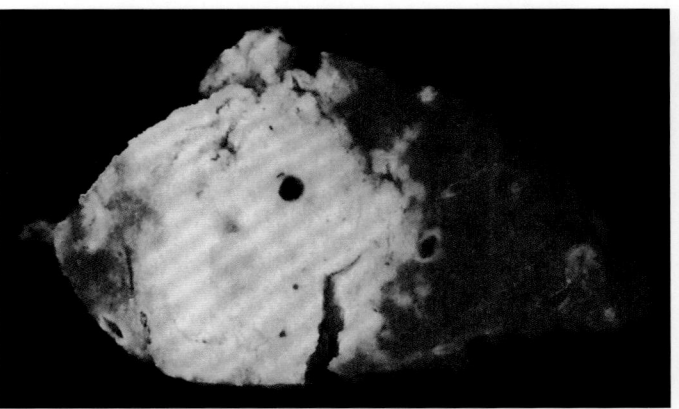

FIGURE 9-27. Acute melioidosis. The lung is consolidated and necrotic.

Melioidosis Is Characterized by Abscesses in Many Organs

Melioidosis (Rangoon beggars disease) is an uncommon disease caused by *Burkholderia* (formerly *Pseudomonas*) *pseudomallei*, a small gram-negative bacillus that inhabits the soil and surface water of Southeast Asia and other tropical areas. The bacteria flourish in wet environments, such as rice paddies and marshes. During the conflict in Vietnam, several hundred American servicemen acquired melioidosis. Bacteria enter the body through the skin, utilizing pre-existing lesions, including penetrating wounds and burns. Humans may also be infected by inhaling contaminated dust or aerosolized droplets. Incubation periods may be months to years. The clinical course is variable.

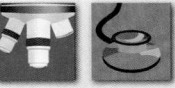

PATHOLOGY AND CLINICAL FEATURES: Acute melioidosis is a pulmonary infection, ranging from a mild tracheobronchitis to overwhelming cavitary pneumonia (Fig. 9-27). Patients with severe cases have sudden onset of high fever, constitutional symptoms and cough that may produce blood-stained sputum. Splenomegaly, hepatomegaly, and jaundice are sometimes present. Diarrhea may be as severe as in cholera. Fulminant septicemia, shock, coma, and death may develop despite antibiotic therapy. Acute septicemic melioidosis causes discrete abscesses throughout the body, especially in lungs, liver, spleen, and lymph nodes.

Chronic melioidosis is a persistent localized infection of the lungs, skin, bones, or other organs. Lesions may be suppurative or granulomatous abscesses, and in the lung they may be mistaken for tuberculosis. Chronic melioidosis may lie dormant for months or years, only to appear suddenly.

CLOSTRIDIA AND THEIR TOXINS

Clostridia are gram-positive, spore-forming, obligate anaerobic bacilli. The vegetative bacilli are found in the digestive tracts of herbivorous animals and humans. Anaerobic conditions promote vegetative division, while aerobic ones lead to sporulation. Spores pass in animal feces and contaminate soil and plants, where they survive well in unfavorable environments. Under anaerobic conditions, spores revert to vegetative cells, completing the cycle. During sporulation, vegetative cells degenerate. Plasmid-encoded toxins cause diverse diseases, depending on the species (Fig. 9-28).

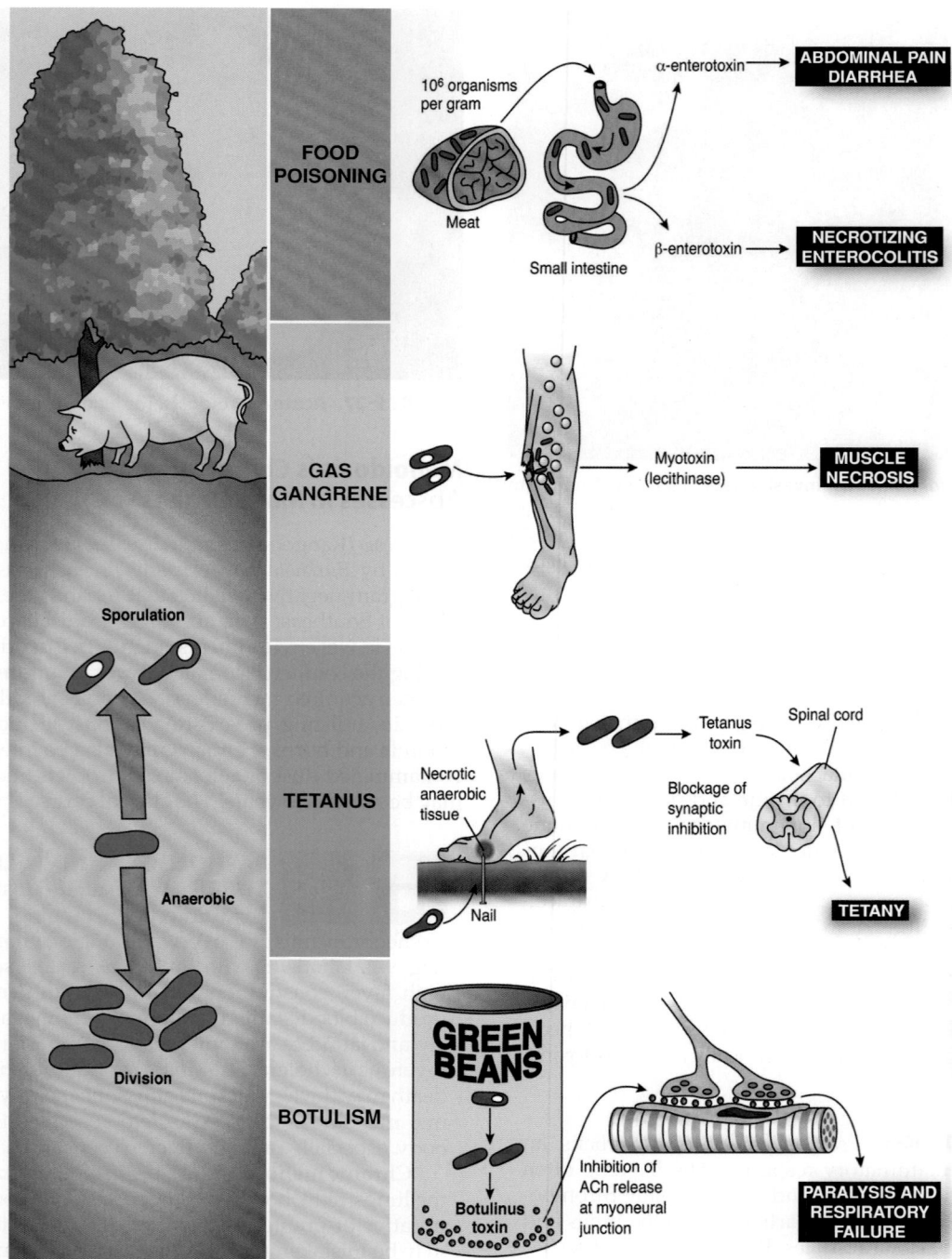

FIGURE 9-28. Clostridial diseases. Clostridia in the vegetative form (bacilli) inhabit the gastrointestinal tract of humans and animals. Spores pass in the feces, contaminate soil and plant materials and are ingested or enter sites of penetrating wounds. Under anaerobic conditions, they revert to vegetative forms. Plasmids in the vegetative forms elaborate toxins that cause several clostridial diseases. **Food poisoning and necrotizing enteritis.** Meat dishes left to cool at room temperature grow large numbers of clostridia (>10^6 organisms per gram). When contaminated meat is ingested, *Clostridium perfringens* types A and C produce α enterotoxin in the small intestine during sporulation, causing abdominal pain and diarrhea. Type C also produces β enterotoxin. **Gas gangrene.** Clostridia are widespread and may contaminate a traumatic wound or surgical operation. *C. perfringens* type A elaborates a myotoxin (α toxin), an α lecithinase that destroys cell membranes, alters capillary permeability, and causes severe hemolysis following intravenous injection. The toxin causes necrosis of previously healthy skeletal muscle. **Tetanus.** Spores of *Clostridium tetani* are in soil and enter the site of an accidental wound. Necrotic tissue at the wound site causes spores to revert to the vegetative form (bacilli). Autolysis of vegetative forms releases tetanus toxin. The toxin is transported in peripheral nerves and (retrograde) through axons to the anterior horn cells of the spinal cord. The toxin blocks synaptic inhibition, and the accumulation of acetylcholine in damaged synapses leads to rigidity and spasms of the skeletal musculature (tetany). **Botulism.** Improperly canned food is contaminated by the vegetative form of *Clostridium botulinum,* which proliferates under aerobic conditions and elaborates a neurotoxin. After the food is ingested, the neurotoxin is absorbed from the small intestine and eventually reaches the myoneural junction, where it inhibits the release of acetylcholine (ACh). The result is a symmetric descending paralysis of cranial nerves, trunk and limbs, with eventual respiratory paralysis and death.

- **Food poisoning and necrotizing enteritis (pigbel)** are caused by *C. perfringens* enterotoxins.
- **Gas gangrene** is produced by myotoxins of *C. perfringens, C. novyi, C. septicum, and* other species.
- **Tetanus** is due to *C. tetani* neurotoxin.
- **Botulism** results from neurotoxins of *C. botulinum.*
- **Pseudomembranous enterocolitis** is caused by exotoxins made by *C. difficile.*

Clostridia perfringens Toxins Cause Gastrointestinal and Wound Diseases

Food Poisoning due to C. perfringens

C. perfringens is one of the most common causes of bacterial food poisoning in the world, causing an acute, generally benign, diarrheal disease, usually lasting less than 24 hours. It is omnipresent in the environment, contaminating soil, water, air samples, clothing, dust, and meat.

Its spores survive cooking temperatures and germinate to yield vegetative forms, which proliferate when food is allowed to stand without refrigeration. Cooking drives out enough air to make the food anaerobic, which is conducive to growth but not sporulation. As a result, contaminated food contains vegetative clostridia but little preformed enterotoxin. Vegetative bacteria sporulate in the small bowel, where they make several exotoxins, which are cytotoxic to enterocytes and cause loss of intracellular ions and fluid. Certain types of food, including meats, gravies, and sauces, are ideal substrates for *C. perfringens.* Clostridial food poisoning presents as abdominal cramping and watery diarrhea, starting 8 to 24 hours after ingestion of contaminated food. It usually resolves within 24 hours.

C. perfringens Necrotizing Enteritis

C. perfringens type C also produces an enterotoxin that causes necrotizing enterocolitis. The illness is rare in the industrialized world but remains endemic in parts of New Guinea, especially in children who have participated in pig feasts (hence the pidgin term *pigbel*). Adults' circulating antibodies tend to protect them. Disease is segmental and may be restricted to a few centimeters, or may involve the entire small intestine. Green, necrotic pseudomembranes are seen in areas of necrosis and peritonitis. More advanced lesions perforate the bowel wall. Necrosis of intestinal mucosa, edema, hemorrhage, and a suppurative transmural infiltrate are characteristic.

Gas Gangrene

Gas gangrene (clostridial myonecrosis) is a necrotizing, gas-forming infection that begins in contaminated wounds and spreads rapidly to adjacent tissues. The disease can be fatal within hours of onset. *C. perfringens* is the most common cause of gas gangrene, but other clostridial species occasionally produce the disease.

 PATHOPHYSIOLOGY: Gas gangrene follows anaerobic deposition of *C. perfringens* into tissue. Clostridial growth requires extensive devitalized tissue, as in severe penetrating trauma, wartime injuries, and septic abortions. Clostridial myonecrosis is rare if wounds are débrided promptly.

Necrosis of previously healthy muscle is caused by myotoxins elaborated by a few species of clostridia. *C. perfringens* type A is the usual source of the myotoxin in 80% to 90% of cases, but *C. novyi* and *C. septicum* may also be responsible. The myotoxin is a phospholipase that attacks the membranes of myocytes, leukocytes, and erythrocytes.

 PATHOLOGY: Affected tissues rapidly become mottled, then frankly necrotic. Tissues such as muscle may even liquefy. Overlying skin becomes tense, as edema and gas expand underlying soft tissues. There is extensive tissue necrosis with dissolution of the cells. A striking feature is the paucity of neutrophils, which are apparently destroyed by the myotoxin. Affected tissues often show typical, lozenge-shaped, gram-positive rods.

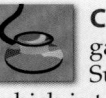 **CLINICAL FEATURES:** The incubation period of gas gangrene is commonly 2 to 4 days after injury. Sudden, severe pain occurs at the wound site, which is tender and edematous. Skin darkens, because of hemorrhage and cutaneous necrosis. The lesion develops a thick, serosanguineous discharge and an odor, and may contain gas bubbles. Hemolytic anemia, hypotension, and renal failure may develop; and in the terminal stages, coma, jaundice, and shock supervene.

Tetanus Is Spastic Skeletal Muscle Contractions Caused by *C. tetani* Neurotoxin

It is also known as "lockjaw" because of early involvement of the muscles of mastication.

 EPIDEMIOLOGY: *C. tetani* is present in the soil and lower intestine of many animals. Tetanus occurs when the organism contaminates wounds, proliferates in tissue, and releases its exotoxin. A vaccine made of inactivated tetanus toxin (**toxoid**) has largely eliminated the disease from developed countries. Tetanus remains a common and lethal disease in developing countries. Many deaths occur in newborns, where umbilical stumps are coated with dirt or dung to prevent bleeding.

 PATHOPHYSIOLOGY: Necrotic tissue and suppuration create a fertile anaerobic environment for the spores to revert to vegetative bacteria, which die and release their toxin. Although infection remains localized, the potent neurotoxin (**tetanospasmin**) is transported retrograde through the ventral roots of peripheral nerves to the anterior horn cells of the spinal cord. There, it crosses the synapse and binds to ganglioside receptors on presynaptic terminals of motor neurons. After it is internalized, its endopeptidase activity selectively cleaves a protein that mediates exocytosis of synaptic vesicles. Thus, release of inhibitory neurotransmitters is blocked, permitting unopposed neural stimulation and sustained contraction of skeletal muscles (**tetany**). The loss of inhibitory neurotransmitters also accelerates heart rate and leads to hypertension and cardiovascular instability.

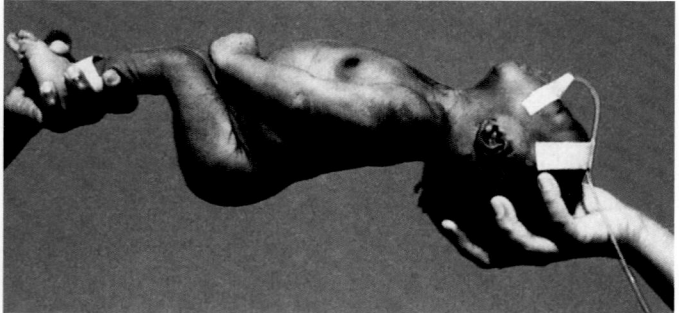

FIGURE 9-29. Tetanus. Opisthotonus (backward arching) in an infant due to intense contraction of the paravertebral muscles. (Reprinted from Farrar WE, Wood MJ, Innes JA, Tubbs H. *Infectious Diseases: Text and Color Atlas.* 2nd ed. New York: Gower Medical Publishing; 1992. Copyright © 1992 Elsevier. With permission.)

CLINICAL FEATURES: Tetanus incubates for 1 to 3 weeks, then begins subtly with fatigue, weakness, and muscle cramping that progresses to rigidity. Spastic rigidity often starts in the face, causing "lockjaw" and a fixed grin (**risus sardonicus**). Rigidity of the muscles of the back produces a backward arching (**opisthotonos**) (Fig. 9-29). Abrupt stimuli, including noise, light or touch, can precipitate painful generalized muscle spasms. Prolonged spasm of respiratory and laryngeal musculature may lead to death. Infants and people older than 50 years have the highest mortality.

Botulism Is a Paralyzing Disease Caused by *C. botulinum* Neurotoxin

The disease entails symmetric descending paralysis of cranial nerves, limbs, and trunk.

EPIDEMIOLOGY: *C. botulinum* spores are widely distributed and are especially resistant to drying and boiling. In the United States, the toxin occurs most often in foods that have been improperly home canned and stored without refrigeration. This setting provides suitable anaerobic conditions for growth of vegetative cells that elaborate the neurotoxin. Botulism can follow eating home-cured ham and other meats left unrefrigerated for several days, and from raw, smoked, and fermented fish products. It is also caused by absorption of toxin from organisms proliferating in infants' intestines (**infantile botulism**) or, rarely, by absorption of toxin from organisms growing in contaminated wounds (**wound botulism**).

PATHOPHYSIOLOGY: Ingested botulinum neurotoxin resists gastric digestion and is readily absorbed from the proximal small intestine. Circulating toxin reaches cholinergic nerve endings at the myoneural junction. There are 7 serotypes of neurotoxin (A–G), with diverse mechanisms of action. The most common serotype, A, binds gangliosides at presynaptic nerve terminals and inhibits acetylcholine release.

CLINICAL FEATURES: Botulism is characterized by a descending paralysis, first affecting cranial nerves and causing blurred vision, photophobia, dry mouth, and dysarthria. Weakness progresses to neck muscles, extremities, diaphragm, and accessory muscles of breathing. Respiratory weakness can progress rapidly to complete respiratory arrest and death. Untreated botulism is usually lethal, but treatment with antitoxin reduces mortality to 25%. Botulinum toxin is often used as treatment for many forms of dystonia, and has recently found popularity as a cosmetic vehicle to erase frown lines transiently (Botox).

Clostridium difficile Colitis May Complicate Antibiotic Treatment

C. difficile colitis is an acute necrotizing infection of the terminal small bowel and colon. It causes a large fraction (25% to 50%) of antibiotic-associated diarrheas and is potentially lethal.

EPIDEMIOLOGY: *C. difficile* resides in the colon in some healthy people. A change in intestinal flora, often due to antibiotic administration (e.g., clindamycin), allows it to flourish, produce toxin, and damage the colonic mucosa. Other precipitating insults to the colonic flora include bowel surgery, dietary changes, and chemotherapeutic agents. In hospitals where many patients receive antibiotics, fecal shedding of *C. difficile* results in person-to-person spread.

PATHOPHYSIOLOGY: Normal colonic bacteria ordinarily limit growth of *C. difficile*, but when normal flora are disturbed, *C. difficile* can proliferate, elaborate toxins, and destroy mucosal cells. It does this, not by invading the mucosa, but by elaborating two exotoxins. Toxin A causes fluid secretion; toxin B is directly cytopathic.

PATHOLOGY: *C. difficile* destroys colonic mucosal cells and incites an acute inflammatory infiltrate. Lesions range from focal colitis limited to a few crypts and only detectable on biopsy, to massive confluent mucosal ulceration (Fig. 9-30A). Inflammation initially involves only the mucosa, but if the disease progresses, it can extend into the submucosa and muscularis propria. An inflammatory exudate, or "pseudomembrane," of cell debris, neutrophils, and fibrin often forms over affected areas (Fig. 9-30B). Colitis caused by *C. difficile* is often called **pseudomembranous colitis**, even though that condition may have many etiologies.

CLINICAL FEATURES: *C. difficile* colitis may start with very mild symptoms, or with diarrhea, fever, and abdominal pain. Stools may be profuse and often contain neutrophils. Symptoms and signs are not specific and do not distinguish *C. difficile* colitis

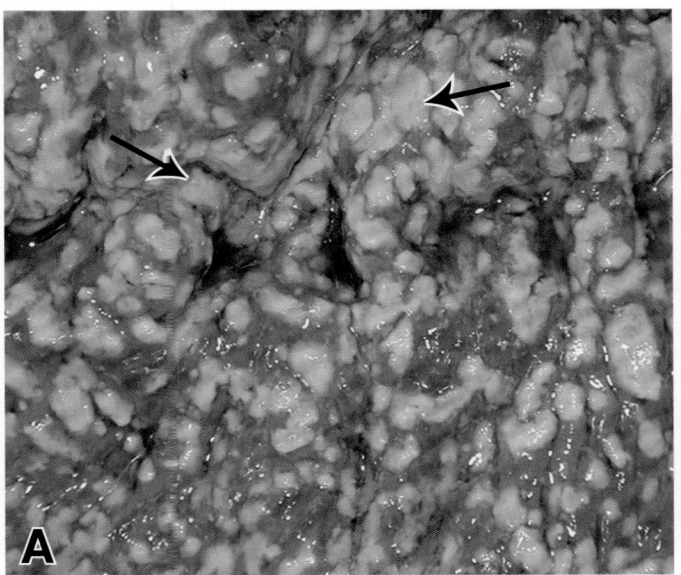 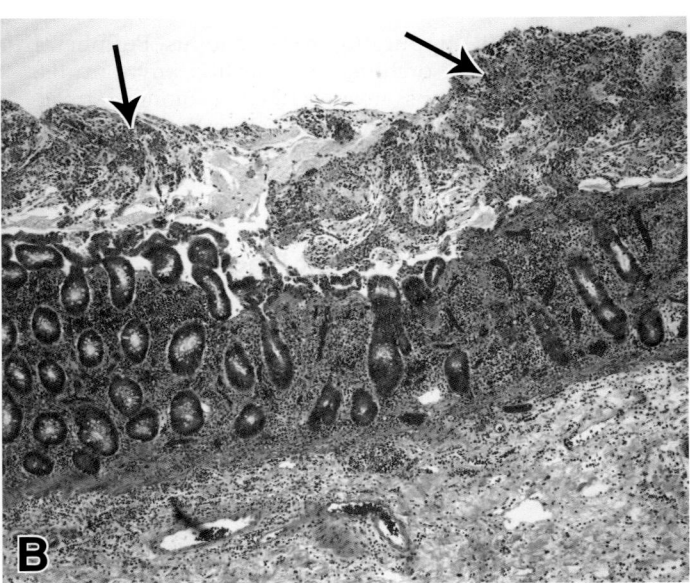

FIGURE 9-30. Pseudomembranous colitis. A. Gross appearance of pseudomembranous colitis. Representative areas of whitish pseudomembranes are highlighted by *arrows*. **B.** Pseudomembrane (*arrows*) with inflammation, debris, and fibrin at the mucosal surface, with partially denuded mucosal lining. (Photographs courtesy Dr. Jeffrey Baliff.)

from other acute inflammatory diarrheal illnesses. Mild cases can often be treated simply by discontinuing the precipitating antibiotic. More severe cases require an antibiotic effective against *C. difficile*.

BACTERIAL INFECTIONS WITH ANIMAL RESERVOIRS OR INSECT VECTORS

Brucellosis Is a Chronic Febrile Disease Acquired From Domestic Animals

Human brucellosis may be an acute systemic disease or a chronic infection with waxing and waning febrile episodes, weight loss, and fatigue. *Brucella* are small, aerobic, gram-negative rods. In humans they primarily infect monocytes/macrophages.

EPIDEMIOLOGY: Brucellosis is a zoonotic disease caused by one of four *Brucella* species, each with its own animal reservoir:

- *Brucella melitensis:* sheep and goats
- *Brucella abortus:* cattle
- *Brucella suis:* swine
- *Brucella canis:* dogs

Brucellosis is worldwide. Virtually every type of domesticated animal and many wild ones are affected. The bacteria reside in animals' genitourinary systems, are often endemic in herds. Humans acquire the bacteria by: (1) contact with infected blood or tissue, (2) ingesting contaminated meat or milk, or (3) inhaling contaminated aerosols. Brucellosis is an occupational hazard among ranchers, herders, veterinarians, and slaughterhouse workers.

Elimination of infected animals and vaccination of herds have reduced the incidence of brucellosis in many countries, including the United States, where only about

200 cases are reported annually. Yet, brucellosis persists in Central and South America, Africa, Asia, and Southern Europe. Unpasteurized milk and cheese remain a major source of infection in these areas. In arctic and subarctic regions, humans acquire brucellosis by eating raw bone marrow of infected reindeer.

PATHOLOGY: Bacteria enter the circulation through skin abrasions, lungs, conjunctiva, or oropharynx. They then spread in the bloodstream to the liver, spleen, lymph nodes, and bone marrow, where they multiply in macrophages. Generalized hyperplasia of these cells may ensue, causing lymphadenopathy and hepatosplenomegaly in 15% of patients infected with *B. melitensis,* and in 40% of those infected with *B. abortus.* Pathology varies with the *Brucella* species. *B. abortus* causes conspicuous noncaseating granulomas in the liver, spleen, lymph nodes, and bone marrow, while *B. melitensis* only elicits small aggregates of mononuclear cells in the liver and *B. suis* may cause liver abscesses. The bacteria are rarely seen histologically, but their periodic release from infected phagocytes may cause febrile episodes.

CLINICAL FEATURES: Brucellosis is a systemic infection that can involve any organ or organ system, with an insidious onset in half of cases. Systemic complaints include fever, sweats, anorexia, fatigue, weight loss, and depression. All patients are febrile at some time during the illness, but fevers can wax and wane (hence the term **undulant fever**) over a period of weeks to months if untreated. Mortality is rare (<1%), with death usually caused by endocarditis.

The most common complications of brucellosis involve bones and joints, and include spondylitis of the lumbar spine and suppuration in large joints. Peripheral neuritis, meningitis, orchitis, endocarditis, myocarditis, and pulmonary lesions are described. Prolonged treatment with tetracycline is usually effective; the relapse rate is dramatically reduced if rifampin or an aminoglycoside antibiotic is used.

Yersinia pestis Causes Bubonic Plague

Plague is a bacteremic, often fatal, infection that is usually accompanied by enlarged, painful regional lymph nodes (**buboes**). Historically, plague caused massive epidemics that killed many of the world's inhabitants. *Y. pestis* is a short gram-negative rod that stains more heavily at the ends (i.e., bipolar staining), particularly with Giemsa stains.

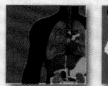 **EPIDEMIOLOGY:** *Y. pestis* infection is an endemic zoonosis in many parts of the world, including the Americas, Africa, and Asia, and affecting wild rodents, such as rats, squirrels, and prairie dogs. Fleas transmit it from animal to animal. Most human infections result from bites of infected fleas. People may develop plague pneumonia, and shed large numbers of organisms in aerosolized respiratory secretions, which allow person-to-person transmission.

Major plague epidemics have occurred when *Y. pestis* was introduced into large urban rat populations in crowded, squalid cities. Infection spread first among rats; then, as they died, infected fleas transmitted it to people, causing widespread disease. The Justinian plaque of 541–544 began in Ethiopia and spread throughout Europe, killing an estimated 25 million people. The Black Death pandemic in mid-14th century (1347–1350) Europe killed about a third of Europe's population, perhaps 34 million people. In the United States, 30 to 40 cases occur annually, mostly in the desert Southwest. Between 2,000 and 3,000 cases of plague are reported worldwide each year, but the likely number of infections is much higher. In 2017, an epidemic of both pneumonic and bubonic plague in Madagascar affected over 2,500 people and resulted in 221 deaths.

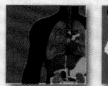 **PATHOPHYSIOLOGY AND PATHOLOGY:** After inoculation into the skin, *Y. pestis* is phagocytosed by neutrophils and macrophages. Bacteria ingested by neutrophils are killed, but those in macrophages survive, replicate intracellularly, and are carried to regional lymph nodes. There, they continue to multiply, producing extensive hemorrhagic necrosis. From regional lymph nodes, they disseminate via the bloodstream and lymphatics. In the lungs, *Y. pestis* produces a necrotizing pneumonitis that releases organisms into alveoli and airways. These are expelled by coughing, enabling pneumonic spread of the disease. Affected lymph nodes, "buboes," are enlarged and fluctuant, due to extensive hemorrhagic necrosis. Infected patients often develop necrotic, hemorrhagic skin lesions, hence the name "black death" for this disease.

 CLINICAL FEATURES: There are three clinical presentations of *Y. pestis* infection, although they often overlap.

- **Bubonic plague** begins within 2 to 8 days of the flea bite, with headache, fever, and myalgias. Painful enlargement of regional lymph nodes mostly affects the groin, as fleas usually bite in the legs. Disease progresses to septic shock within hours to days after buboes appear.
- **Septicemic plague** (10% of cases) occurs when bacteria are inoculated directly into the blood and do not produce buboes. Patients die of overwhelming bacterial growth in the bloodstream. Fever, prostration, and meningitis occur suddenly, with death within 48 hours. All blood vessels contain bacilli, and fibrin casts surround the organisms in renal glomeruli and dermal vessels.
- **Pneumonic plague** results from inhalation of airborne particles from carcasses of animals or the cough of infected people. Within 2 to 5 days, high fever, cough, and dyspnea begin suddenly. The sputum teems with bacilli. Respiratory insufficiency and endotoxic shock kill patients within 1 to 2 days.

All types of plague carry a high mortality rate (50% to 75%) if untreated. Tetracycline, combined with streptomycin, is the recommended therapy.

Tularemia Is an Acute Febrile, Disease Usually Acquired From Rabbits

Tularemia is caused by *Francisella tularensis*, a small, gram-negative coccobacillus.

 EPIDEMIOLOGY: Tularemia is a zoonosis whose most important reservoirs are rabbits and rodents, although other wild and domestic animals may harbor the organisms. Human infection results from contact with infected animals or from the bites of infected insects, including ticks, deerflies, and mosquitoes. Most human infections come from ticks and rabbits. Bacteria may enter the body when blood-sucking insects inoculate them through the skin, or via unnoticed breaks in the skin if there is direct contact with an infected animal. Inhaling infected aerosols, eating contaminated food and water, or spray into the eye may also cause tularemia. *F. tularensis* is found in temperate zones of the Northern Hemisphere. The incidence of tularemia has declined dramatically in the United States in the past 5 decades, to about 250 cases annually, presumably related to a decline in hunting and trapping.

 PATHOPHYSIOLOGY: *F. tularensis* multiplies at the site of inoculation, producing a focal ulcer there. The bacteria then spread to regional lymph nodes. Dissemination in the bloodstream leads to metastatic infections of mononuclear phagocytes, sometimes involving the lungs, heart, and kidneys. *F. tularensis* survives within macrophages until these cells are activated by a cell-mediated immune response to the infection.

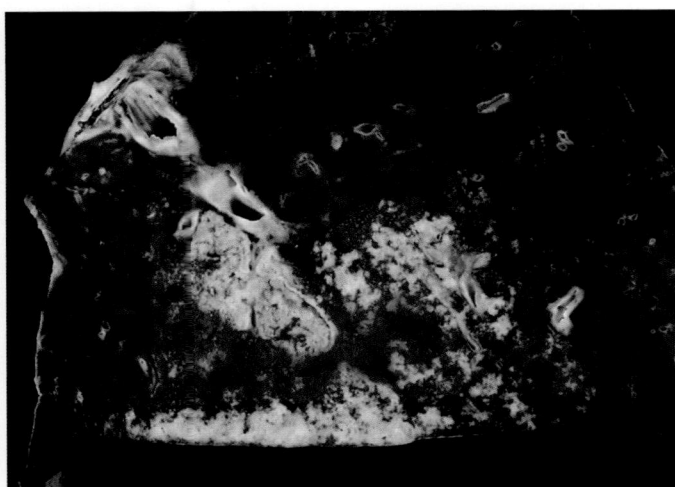

FIGURE 9-31. Tularemia. The lung shows firm, consolidated, and necrotic areas.

PATHOLOGY: Lesions of tularemia occur at the inoculation site and in lymph nodes, spleen, liver, bone marrow, lungs (Fig. 9-31), heart, and kidneys. Initial skin lesions are exudative, pyogenic ulcers. Later, disseminated lesions undergo central necrosis and are surrounded by a granulomatous reaction, like those of tuberculosis. Hyperemia and abundant macrophages in the sinuses make lymph nodes large and firm; they later soften as necrosis and suppuration develop. Pulmonary lesions resemble those of primary tuberculosis.

CLINICAL FEATURES: Tularemia incubation period is 1 to 14 days, depending on the dose and route of transmission, with a mean of 3 to 4 days. There are four distinct clinical presentations:

- **Ulceroglandular tularemia** is the most common presentation (80% to 90% of cases). It begins as a tender, erythematous papule at the site of inoculation, usually on a limb. This develops into a pustule, which then ulcerates. Regional lymph nodes become large and tender and may suppurate and drain through sinus tracts. Generalized lymphadenopathy **(glandular tularemia)** may be the first manifestation of infection.

    Initial bacteremia is accompanied by fever, headache, myalgias, and occasionally prostration. Within a week, generalized lymphadenopathy and splenomegaly develop. The most serious infections are complicated by secondary pneumonia and endotoxic shock, in which case the prognosis is grave. Some patients develop meningitis, endocarditis, pericarditis, or osteomyelitis.

- **Oculoglandular tularemia** is rare (<2% of cases) and is characterized by a primary conjunctival papule, which forms a pustule and ulcerates. Lymphadenopathy of the head and neck becomes prominent. Severe ulceration may cause blindness, if infection penetrates the sclera and reaches the optic nerve.

- **Typhoidal tularemia** is diagnosed when fever, hepatosplenomegaly, and toxemia are the presenting signs and symptoms.
- **Pneumonic tularemia**, in which pneumonia is a major feature, may complicate any of the other types.

    The illness lasts 1 week to 3 months, but this may be shortened by prompt treatment with streptomycin.

Anthrax Is Rapidly Fatal When It Disseminates

Anthrax is a necrotizing disease caused by *Bacillus anthracis*, which is a large spore-forming, gram-positive rod.

EPIDEMIOLOGY: Anthrax has been recognized for centuries, and descriptions of disease consistent with anthrax were reported in early Hebrew, Roman, and Greek records. The major reservoirs are goats, sheep, cattle, horses, pigs, and dogs. Spores form in the soil and dead animals, resisting heat, desiccation, and chemical disinfection for years. Humans are infected when spores enter the body via breaks in the skin, by inhalation or by ingestion. Human disease may also result from exposure to contaminated animal byproducts, such as hides, wool, brushes, or bone meal.

Anthrax has been a persistent problem in Iran, Turkey, Pakistan, and Sudan. One of the largest recorded naturally occurring outbreaks occurred in Zimbabwe, when 10,000 people became infected in 1978 to 1980. In North America, human infection is very rare (one case yearly) and usually results from exposure to imported animal products. However, increased vigilance for anthrax has increased after a bioterrorism episode involving transport of organisms by the postal system (see below).

PATHOPHYSIOLOGY: *B. anthracis* spores germinate in the human body to yield vegetative bacteria that multiply and release a potent necrotizing toxin. In 80% of cases of cutaneous anthrax, infection is localized, and host immune responses eliminate it. If infection disseminates, as occurs if the bacteria are inhaled or ingested, resulting widespread tissue destruction is usually fatal.

PATHOLOGY: *B. anthracis* produces extensive tissue necrosis at the sites of infection, associated with only a mild infiltrate of neutrophils. Cutaneous lesions are ulcerated, contain numerous organisms and are covered by a black scab. Lung infection produces a necrotizing, hemorrhagic pneumonia, with hemorrhagic necrosis of mediastinal lymph nodes and widespread dissemination of the organism.

CLINICAL FEATURES: Anthrax mode of presentation depends on the site of inoculation.

- **Malignant pustule** the cutaneous form, accounts for 95% of cases. Patients present with an elevated skin papule that enlarges and erodes into an ulcer. Bloody purulent exudate accumulates and gradually darkens to purple or black. The ulcer is often surrounded by a zone of brawny edema, which is disproportionately large for the size of the ulcer. Regional lymphadenitis portends a poor prognosis, since lymphatic invasion precedes septicemia. If infection does not disseminate, cutaneous lesions heal without sequelae.

- **Pulmonary, or inhalational, anthrax,** sometimes called **"woolsorters' disease,"** is a hazard of handling raw wool and develops after *B. anthracis* spores are inhaled. It begins as a flulike illness that rapidly progresses to respiratory failure and shock. Death often ensues within 24 to 48 hours. Only 18 cases of inhalational anthrax were reported in the United States from 1900 to 1980. The anthrax bioterror attack in the United States in 2001 caused 11 cases. Antibiotic therapy is the appropriate treatment.
- **Septicemic anthrax** follows pulmonary anthrax more than malignant pustules. Disseminated intravascular coagulation is a common complication. A bacterial toxin depresses the central respiratory center, which explains why death can occur even when antibiotic therapy has cured the infection.
- **Gastrointestinal anthrax** is rare and is acquired by eating contaminated meat. Stomach or bowel ulceration, and invasion of regional lymphatics, are common. Death is caused by fulminant diarrhea and massive ascites.

Listeriosis Is a Systemic Multiorgan Infection With a High Mortality

It is caused by *Listeria monocytogenes*, a small, motile, gram-positive coccobacillus.

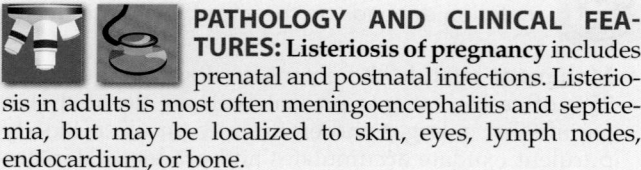 **EPIDEMIOLOGY:** Listeriosis is usually sporadic but may be epidemic. *L. monocytogenes* occurs worldwide in surface water, soil, vegetation, feces of healthy people, many species of wild and domestic mammals and several species of birds. However, spread of infection from animals to humans is rare. Most human infections occur in urban—not rural—environments, usually in the summer. *L. monocytogenes* grows at refrigerator temperatures, and outbreaks have been traced to unpasteurized milk, cheese, and dairy products.

PATHOPHYSIOLOGY: *L. monocytogenes* has an unusual life cycle, which allows it to evade host defenses. After phagocytosis by host cells, the bacteria enter phagolysosomes, where acidic pH activates *listeriolysin O*, an exotoxin that disrupts the vesicular membrane, so the bacteria escape into the cytosol. After replicating, they usurp host cytoskeleton contractile elements to form elongated protrusions that are engulfed by adjacent cells. Thus, *Listeria* spread from one cell to another without exposure to the extracellular environment.

PATHOLOGY AND CLINICAL FEATURES: Listeriosis of pregnancy includes prenatal and postnatal infections. Listeriosis in adults is most often meningoencephalitis and septicemia, but may be localized to skin, eyes, lymph nodes, endocardium, or bone.

Maternal infection early in pregnancy may lead to abortion or premature delivery. Infected infants rapidly develop respiratory distress, hepatosplenomegaly, cutaneous and mucosal papules, leukopenia, and thrombocytopenia. Intrauterine infections involve many organs and tissues, including amniotic fluid, placenta, and the umbilical cord. Abscesses are found in many organs. Foci of necrosis and suppuration contain many bacteria. Older lesions tend to be granulomatous. Neurologic sequelae are common, and the mortality of neonatal listeriosis is high even with prompt antibiotic therapy. Neonatal listeriosis may also be acquired during delivery, with the onset of clinical disease 3 days to 2 weeks after birth.

Chronic alcoholics, patients with cancer or who are immunosuppressed, are far more susceptible to infection than the general population. Meningitis is the most common form of the disease in adults and resembles other bacterial meningitides.

Septicemic listeriosis is a severe febrile illness most common in immunodeficient patients. It may cause shock and disseminated intravascular coagulation, leading to misdiagnosis as gram-negative sepsis. Prolonged treatment with antimicrobials is usually required because patients tend to relapse if therapy lasts less than 3 weeks. The mortality from systemic listeriosis remains at 25%.

Bartonella henselae Causes Cat-Scratch Disease

Cat-scratch disease is a self-limited infection usually caused by *Bartonella henselae* and more rarely by *B. quintana*. The bacteria are small (0.2 to 0.6 μm) gram-negative rods. They are difficult to culture but are easily seen in tissue sections of skin, lymph nodes, and conjunctiva, when stained with a silver impregnation technique (Fig. 9-32).

EPIDEMIOLOGY: The animal reservoir is thought to be cats; surveys have shown that up to 30% of cats are bacteremic. Infection begins when the bacillus is inoculated into the skin by the claws of cats (or rarely, other animals), or by thorns or splinters.

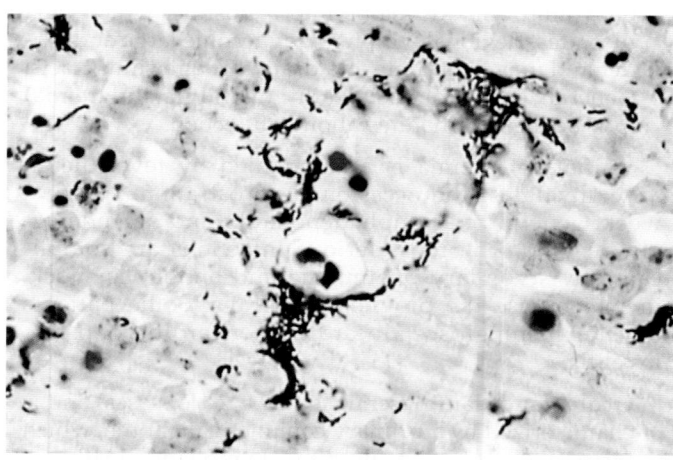

FIGURE 9-32. Cat-scratch disease. Section of a lymph node shows the bacilli, which are gram negative but difficult to visualize with tissue Gram stains. They are blackened by the Warthin–Starry silver impregnation technique.

Sometimes conjunctival contamination follows close contact, possibly by a cat licking around the eye. Infections are more common in children (80%) than adults.

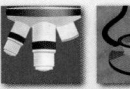 **PATHOLOGY AND CLINICAL FEATURES:** Bacteria multiply in small vessel walls and about collagen fibers at the site of inoculation, then are carried to regional lymph nodes, where they cause **suppurative** and **granulomatous lymphadenitis**. In early lesions, clusters of bacteria fill and expand lumina of small blood vessels. However, bacteria are rare in late lesions. A papule develops at the site of inoculation, followed by tenderness and enlargement of regional lymph nodes. Nodes remain enlarged for 3 to 4 months and may drain through the skin. About half of patients have other symptoms, including fever and malaise, rash, a brief encephalitis, and erythema nodosum.

Additional clinical manifestations include **Parinaud oculoglandular syndrome** (preauricular adenopathy secondary to conjunctival infection). **Bacillary angiomatosis** is a vascular skin disease that can extend to other organs—it is most common in immunocompromised people. **Bacillary peliosis** is affects the liver and spleen, causing blood-filled cystic spaces, and also mostly in severely immunocompromised patients. Antibiotics are not known to help.

Glanders Is a Granulomatous Infection Acquired From Horses

Glanders is an infection of equine species (horses, mules, donkeys) that is only rarely transmitted to humans, in whom it causes acute or chronic granulomatous disease. It is caused by *Pseudomonas mallei*, a small gram-negative, nonmotile bacillus. Although uncommon, glanders is endemic in South America, Asia, and Africa. Humans acquire the disease by contact with infected equines through broken skin or inhalation of contaminated aerosols.

- **Acute glanders** is characterized by bacteremia, severe prostration, and fever. Granulomatous abscesses form in subcutaneous tissues and other organs, including the lung, liver, spleen, muscles, and joints. Acute glanders is almost always fatal.
- **Chronic glanders** features low-grade fever, draining abscesses of the skin, lymphadenopathy, and hepatosplenomegaly. Granulomas in many organs mimic tuberculosis. The mortality in chronic glanders exceeds 50%.

Bartonellosis Causes Acute Anemia and Chronic Skin Disease

Bartonellosis is an infection by *Bartonella bacilliformis*, a small, multiflagellated, gram-negative coccobacillus.

 EPIDEMIOLOGY: Bartonellosis occurs only in Peru, Ecuador, and Colombia in river valleys of the Andes and is transmitted by sandflies. Humans are the only reservoir, and acquire infection at sunrise and sunset, when sandflies are most active. In endemic areas, 10% to 15% of the population have latent infections. Newcomers are susceptible, while indigenous populations tend to be resistant.

 PATHOLOGY AND CLINICAL FEATURES: Bartonellosis presents a biphasic pattern, in which acute hemolytic anemia (**Oroya fever**) is followed some months later by a chronic dermal phase (**verruga peruana**). Either phase may occur by itself.

The most severe consequence of bartonellosis is hemolytic anemia. After *B. bacilliformis* is inoculated into the skin by a sandfly, bacteria proliferate in the vascular endothelium and then invade erythrocytes, leading to profound hemolysis.

The **acute anemic phase** begins 3 weeks of incubation, with abrupt onset of fever, skeletal pains and severe, hemolytic anemia. If untreated, 40% of patients in the anemic phase die. Secondary *Salmonella* sepsis is frequent and contributes to the high mortality.

The **dermal eruptive phase** of bartonellosis may coexist with the anemic phase but is usually follows by 3 to 6 months. Many small hemangioma-like lesions stud the dermis, with bacteria in endothelial cells. Nodular lesions may be prominent on extensor surfaces of the arms and legs. Large deep-seated lesions, which tend to ulcerate, develop near joints and limit motion. The dermal eruptive phase is often prolonged but eventually heals spontaneously. Mortality in this phase is less than 5%.

BRANCHING FILAMENTOUS ORGANISMS

Actinomycosis Is Characterized by Abscesses and Sinus Tracts

Several anaerobic and microaerophilic *Actinomyces* species cause human disease, the most common being *Actinomyces israelii*. These are branching, filamentous, gram-positive rods that normally reside in the oropharynx, gastrointestinal tract, and vagina. Actinomycosis is a slowly progressive, suppurative, fibrosing infection affecting the jaw, thorax, or abdomen.

 PATHOPHYSIOLOGY: *Actinomyces* is not ordinarily virulent: the organisms reside as saprophytes in the body without producing disease. Two uncommon conditions must occur for *Actinomyces* to cause disease. First, it must be inoculated into deeper tissues, since it cannot invade. Second, it must have an anaerobic atmosphere. Trauma can produce tissue necrosis, which is an excellent anaerobic medium for *Actinomyces* growth, and can inoculate the organism into normally sterile tissue. Actinomycosis occurs at four distinct sites:

- **Cervicofacial actinomycosis** results from jaw injury, dental extraction, or dental manipulation.
- **Thoracic actinomycosis** is due to aspiration of organisms contaminating dental debris.

- **Abdominal actinomycosis** follows traumatic or surgical disruption of the bowel, especially the appendix.
- **Pelvic actinomycosis** is associated with prolonged use of intrauterine devices (IUDs).

Actinomycetes have a remarkable ability to burrow and create sinus tracts, irrespective of tissue boundaries and anatomic structures.

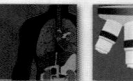

PATHOLOGY: Actinomycosis begins as a nidus of proliferating organisms that elicit an acute inflammatory infiltrate. The small abscess grows slowly, becoming a series of abscesses connected by sinus tracts. Tracts burrow across normal tissue boundaries and into adjacent organs. Eventually, a tract may reach an external surface or mucosal membrane, and produce a draining sinus. The walls of abscesses and tracts contain granulation tissue, often thick, densely fibrotic, and chronically inflamed. Within abscesses and sinuses are pus and colonies of organisms.

Actinomyces colonies within these lesions can grow to several millimeters in diameter and be visible to the naked eye. They appear as hard, yellow grains called **sulfur granules**, because they resemble elemental sulfur. These consist of tangled masses of narrow, branching filaments, embedded in a polysaccharide–protein matrix (**Splendore–Hoeppli material**). Histologically, the colonies are rounded, basophilic grains with scalloped eosinophilic borders (Fig. 9-33A). Individual filaments of *Actinomyces* cannot be discerned with hematoxylin and eosin stain, but are readily visible on Gram staining or silver impregnation (Fig. 9-33B).

CLINICAL FEATURES: The signs and symptoms of actinomycosis depend on the site of infection. If infection originates in a tooth socket or the tonsils, it is characterized by swelling of the jaw ("lumpy jaw"), face and neck, at first painless and fluctuant but later painful. In pulmonary infections, sinus tracts may penetrate from lobe to lobe, through the pleura and

into ribs and vertebrae. Abdominal or pelvic disease may present as an expanding mass, suggesting a locally spreading tumor. Actinomycosis responds to prolonged antibiotic therapy; penicillin is highly effective.

Nocardiosis Is a Suppurative Respiratory Infection in Immunocompromised Hosts

Nocardia are aerobic, gram-positive filamentous, branching bacteria. They are weakly acid-fast, which characteristic helps to distinguish them from the morphologically similar *Actinomycetes*. From the lungs, infection often spreads to the brain and skin.

EPIDEMIOLOGY: *Nocardia* species are widely distributed in soil. Human disease is caused by inhaling or inoculating soil-borne organisms, most often *N. asteroides*. It is not transmitted from person to person. Nocardiosis is most common in patients with impaired immunity, particularly cell-mediated immunity. Organ transplantation, long-term corticosteroid therapy, lymphomas, leukemias, and other debilitating diseases are predisposing factors.

Two other pathogenic species of *Nocardia*, *N. brasiliensis* and *N. caviae*, may cause pulmonary nocardiosis resembling that produced by *N. asteroides*. They are usually encountered in underdeveloped countries as a cause of mycetomas.

PATHOPHYSIOLOGY AND PATHOLOGY: *Nocardia* generally enter via the respiratory tract, where they elicit a brisk neutrophil response. Disease begins as a slowly progressive, pyogenic pneumonia. A vigorous cell-mediated immune response, may eliminate the infection, but immunocompromised patients may develop pulmonary abscesses, which are often multiple and confluent. Direct extension to the pleura, trachea and heart, and blood-borne metastases to the brain or skin carry a grave prognosis. Nocardial abscesses are filled with neutrophils, necrotic debris, and scattered

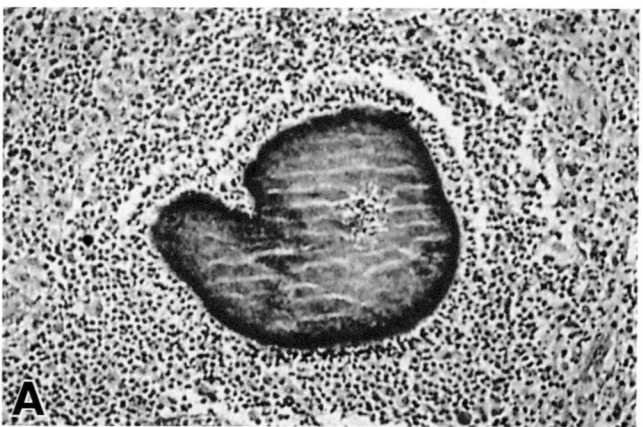

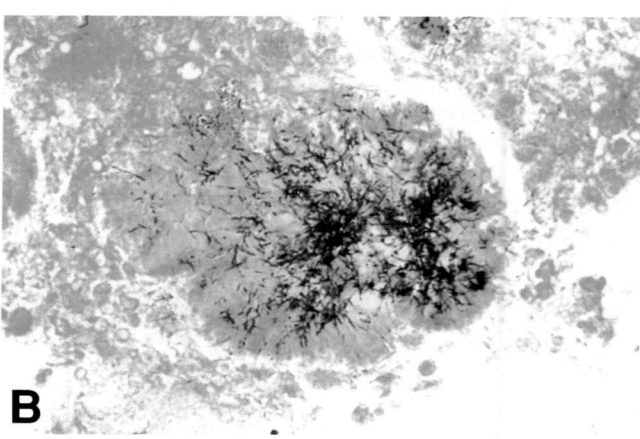

FIGURE 9-33. Actinomycosis. A. A typical sulfur granule lies within an abscess. **B.** The individual filaments of *Actinomyces israelii* are readily visible with the silver impregnation technique.

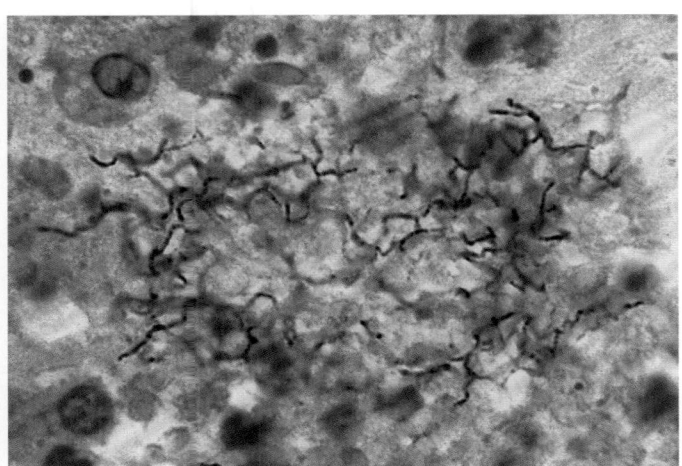

FIGURE 9-34. Nocardiosis. A silver stain of a necrotic exudate highlights the branching filamentous rods of *Nocardia asteroides*.

organisms. Bacteria can be demonstrated by silver impregnation (Fig. 9-34). With the Gram stain, *Nocardia* appear as beaded, filamentous, gram-positive rods. Untreated nocardiosis is usually fatal. Sulfonamides or related antibiotics for several months are often effective therapy.

SPIROCHETES

Spirochetes are long, slender, helical bacteria with specialized cell envelopes that permit them to move by flexion and rotation. They tend to be below the resolving power of routine light microscopy. Specialized techniques, such as darkfield microscopy or silver impregnation, are needed to visualize them. Although spirochetes have the basic cell wall structure of gram-negative bacteria, they stain poorly with the Gram stain.

Three genera of spirochetes cause human disease: *Treponema*, *Borrelia*, and *Leptospira*. Collectively, they are adept at evading host immune and inflammatory defenses, and generally cause chronic and relapsing disease (Table 9-4).

Syphilis Is a Sexually Transmitted Systemic Disease Caused by *T. pallidum*

Treponema pallidum is a thin, long spirochete (Fig. 9-35) that does not grow in artificial media. Syphilis was first recognized in Europe in the 1490s, possibly related to Columbus' return from the New World. Urbanization and mass movements of people caused by war contributed to its rapid spread. Originally, syphilis was an acute disease that caused destructive skin lesions and early death, but it has become milder, with a more protracted and insidious clinical course.

 EPIDEMIOLOGY: Syphilis is a worldwide disease that is transmitted almost exclusively by sexual contact. Infection may also spread from an infected mother to her fetus **(congenital syphilis)**. The incidence of primary and secondary syphilis has declined since the introduction of penicillin at the end of World War II.

 PATHOPHYSIOLOGY: *T. pallidum* is very fragile and is killed by soap, antiseptics, drying, and cold. Person-to-person transmission requires

TABLE 9-4
SPIROCHETE INFECTIONS

Disease	Organism	Clinical Manifestation	Distribution	Mode of Transmission
Treponemes				
Syphilis	*Treponema pallidum*	See text	Common worldwide	Sexual contact, congenital
Bejel	*Treponema endenicum (Treponema pallidum, subspecies endenicum)*	Mucosal, skin and bone lesions	Middle East	Mouth-to-mouth contact
Yaws	*Treponema pertenue (Treponema pallidum subspecies pertenue)*	Skin and bone	Tropics	Skin-to-skin contact
Pinta	*Treponema carateum*	Skin lesions	Latin America	Skin-to-skin contact
Borrelia				
Lyme disease	*Borrelia burgdorferi*	See text	North America, Europe, Russia, Asia, Africa, Australia	Tick bite
Relapsing fever	*Borrelia recurrentis*	Relapsing flulike illness	Worldwide	Tick bite, louse bite and related species
Leptospira				
Leptospirosis	*Leptospira interrogans*	Flulike illness, meningitis	Worldwide	Contact with animal urine

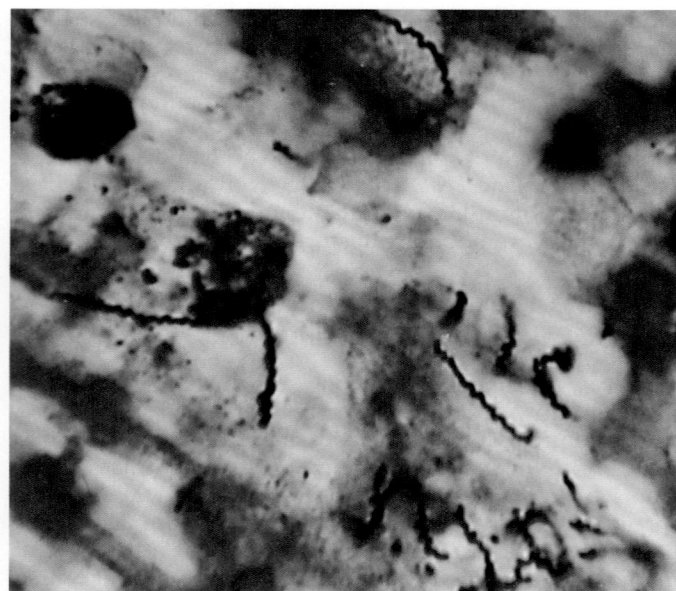

FIGURE 9-35. Syphilis. *Treponema pallidum* spirochetes, visualized by silver impregnation, in the eye of a child with congenital syphilis.

direct contact between a rich source of spirochetes (e.g., an open lesion) and mucous membranes or abraded skin of the genital organs, rectum, mouth, fingers, or nipples. The treponemes reproduce at the site of inoculation, then pass to regional lymph nodes, from which they spread to the blood and throughout the body. Although *T. pallidum* induces an inflammatory response and is taken up by phagocytes, it persists and proliferates. Chronic infection and inflammation cause tissue destruction, sometimes for decades.

The course of syphilis is classically divided into three stages (Fig. 9-36).

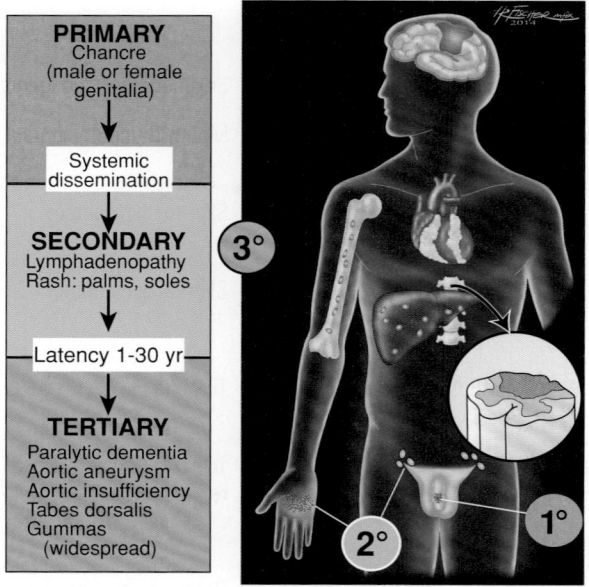

FIGURE 9-36. Clinical characteristics of the various stages of syphilis.

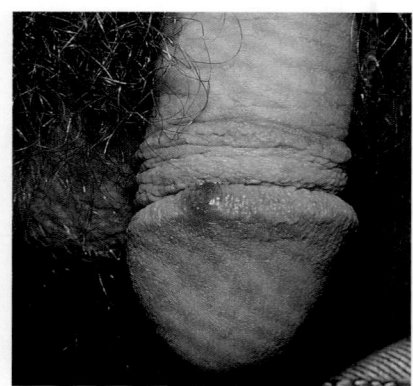

FIGURE 9-37. Syphilitic chancre. A patient with primary syphilis displays a raised, erythematous penile lesion.

The Classical Lesion of Primary Syphilis: The Chancre

Chancres (Fig. 9-37) are characteristic ulcers at sites of *T. pallidum* entry, usually the penis, vulva, anus, or mouth. They appear 1 week to 3 months after exposure, with an average of 3 weeks, and tend to be solitary, with firm, raised borders. Spirochetes tend to concentrate in vessel walls and in the epidermis around the ulcer. Chancres, like the lesions of all stages of syphilis, show **luetic vasculitis:** endothelial cell proliferation and swelling, and vessel walls becoming thickened by lymphocytes and fibrosis.

Chancres quickly erode to a characteristic ulcer. They are painless and can go unnoticed in some locations, such as the uterine cervix, anal canal, and mouth. They last 3 to 12 weeks, often elicit local lymphadenopathy and heal without scarring.

Secondary Syphilis

In secondary syphilis *T. pallidum* spreads systemically and proliferates to cause lesions in the skin, mucous membranes, lymph nodes, meninges, stomach, and liver. Lesions show perivascular lymphocytic infiltration and obliterative endarteritis.

- **Skin:** Secondary syphilis most often appears as an erythematous and maculopapular rash of the trunk and extremities, often including the palms (Fig. 9-38) and soles. A rash appears 2 weeks to 3 months after the chancre heals. Other skin lesions in secondary syphilis include **condylomata lata** (exudative plaques in the perineum, vulva or scrotum, full of spirochetes) (Fig. 9-39), **follicular syphilids** (small papular lesions around hair follicles that cause loss of hair) and **nummular syphilids** (coinlike lesions of the face and perineum).
- **Mucous membranes:** Lesions on mucosal surfaces of the mouth and genital organs, called **mucous patches**, teem with organisms and are highly infectious.
- **Lymph nodes:** Characteristic changes in lymph nodes, especially epitrochlear nodes, include a thickened capsule, follicular hyperplasia, increased plasma cells and macrophages, and luetic vasculitis. Spirochetes are numerous s in the lymph nodes of secondary syphilis.
- **Meninges:** Meninges are often seeded with *T. pallidum*, but meningeal involvement is generally asymptomatic.

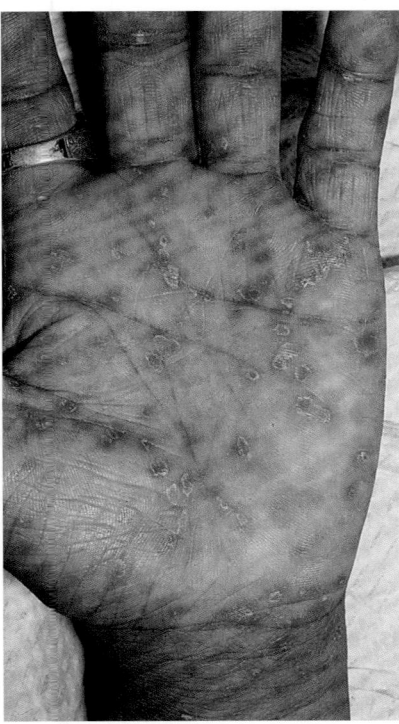

FIGURE 9-38. Secondary syphilis. A maculopapular rash is present on the palm.

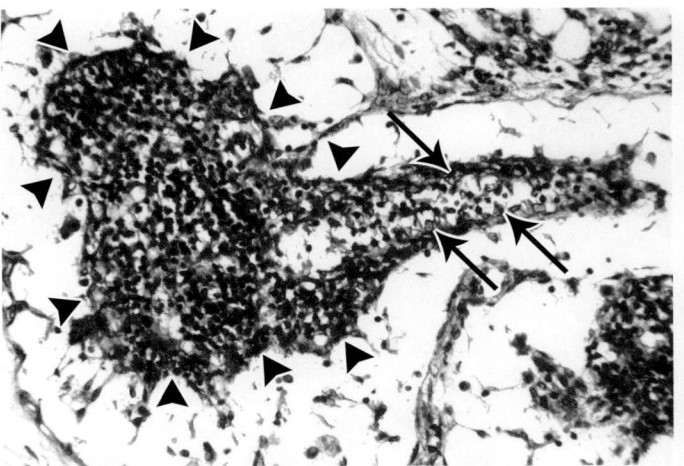

FIGURE 9-40. Obliterative endarteritis. Small vessel lesions of tertiary syphilis, with prominent endothelial cells (*arrows*) and exuberant perivascular mononuclear inflammatory infiltrate (*arrowheads*).

Tertiary Syphilis

After lesions of secondary syphilis subside, an asymptomatic period follows, lasting years to decades. During this time, spirochetes continue to multiply and the deep-seated lesions of tertiary syphilis gradually develop in one-third of untreated patients. *Focal ischemic necrosis secondary to obliterative endarteritis is the underlying mechanism for many of the processes associated with tertiary syphilis.* T. pallidum elicits mononuclear inflammation, mainly of lymphocytes and plasma cells. These cells infiltrate small arteries and arterioles, producing a characteristic obstructive vascular lesion (**endarteritis obliterans**) (Fig. 9-40). Small arteries are inflamed and their endothelial cells are swollen. They are surrounded by concentric layers of proliferating fibroblasts, giving the vascular lesions an "onion skin" appearance.

■ **Syphilitic aortitis:** This lesion results from a slowly progressive endarteritis obliterans of vasa vasorum, eventually causing necrosis of the aortic media, gradual weakening and stretching of the aortic wall, and aortic aneurysm. Syphilitic aneurysms are saccular and involve the ascending aorta, which is an unusual site for the much more common atherosclerotic aneurysms. On gross examination, the aortic intima is rough and pitted (**tree-bark appearance**) (Fig. 9-41) (see Chapter 16). The aortic media is gradually replaced by scar tissue, after which the aorta loses its strength and resilience. The aorta stretches, becoming progressively thinner to the point of rupture, massive hemorrhage, and sudden death. *Damage to, and scarring of, the ascending aorta may also lead to aortic ring dilation, separating the valve cusps and regurgitation through the aortic valve (aortic insufficiency).* Luetic vasculitis may narrow or occlude coronary arteries and cause myocardial infarction.

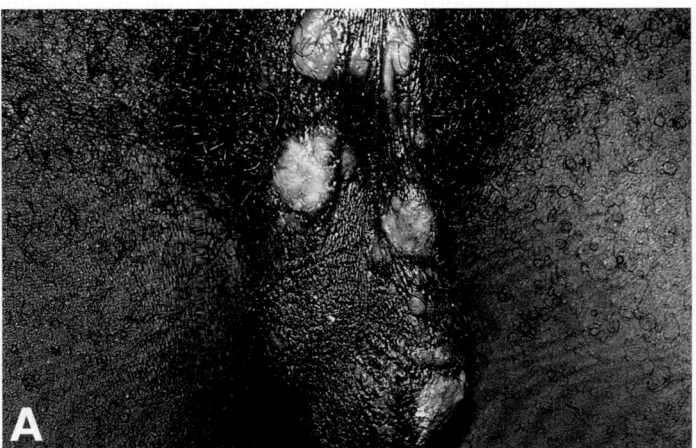

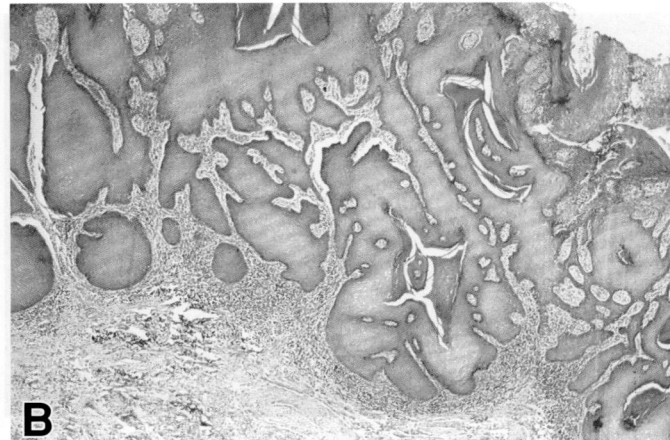

FIGURE 9-39. Condylomata lata in secondary syphilis. A. Whitish plaques are seen on the vulva and perineum. **B.** A photomicrograph shows papillomatous hyperplasia of the epidermis with underlying chronic inflammation.

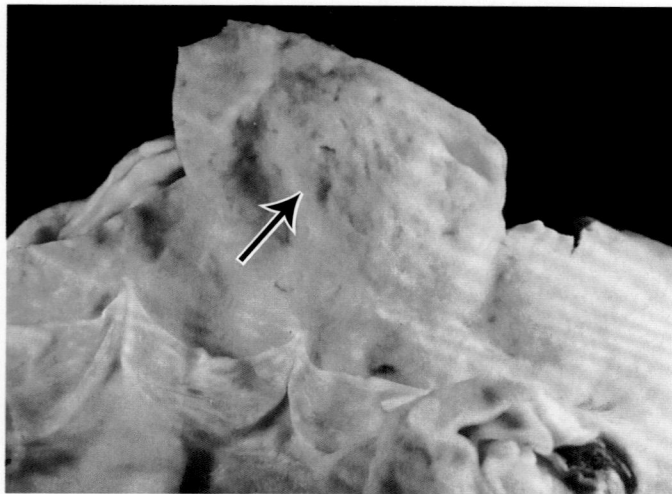

FIGURE 9-41. Syphilitic aortitis. The ascending aorta exhibits a roughened intima (*arrow,* "tree bark" appearance), owing to destruction of the media.

- **Neurosyphilis:** The slowly progressive infection damages the meninges, cerebral cortex, spinal cord, cranial nerves, or eyes. Tertiary CNS syphilis is subclassified according to the predominant pathology: **meningovascular syphilis** (meninges), **tabes dorsalis** (spinal cord), and **general paresis** (cerebral cortex) (see Chapter 32).
- **Benign tertiary syphilis:** The appearance of a gumma (Fig. 9-42) in any organ or tissue is the hallmark of benign tertiary syphilis. Gummas are most common in the skin, bone, and joints, although they can occur anywhere. These granulomatous lesions have a central area of coagulative necrosis, epithelioid macrophages, occasional giant cells, and peripheral fibrous tissue. Gummas are usually localized lesions that do not significantly damage the patient.

Congenital Syphilis

T. pallidum may cross the placenta and disseminate. Fetal tissues are injured by the proliferating bacteria and by accompanying inflammatory response. Fetal infection may cause stillbirth, neonatal illness or death, or progressive postnatal disease.

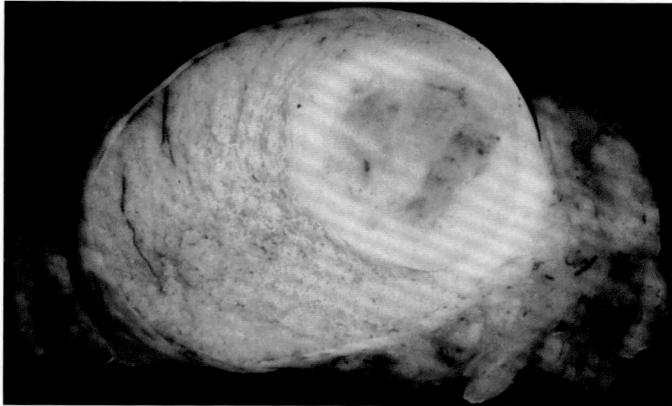

FIGURE 9-42. Syphilitic gumma. A patient with tertiary syphilis shows a sharply circumscribed gumma in the testis, characterized by a fibrogranulomatous wall and a necrotic center.

PATHOLOGY: Lesions of congenital syphilis are identical to those of adult disease. Infected tissues show a chronic inflammatory infiltrate of lymphocytes and plasma cells and endarteritis obliterans. Virtually any tissue can be affected, but skin, bones, teeth, joints, liver, and CNS are characteristically involved (see Chapter 6).

CLINICAL FEATURES: The presentation of congenital syphilis is variable; infected newborns are often asymptomatic. Early signs of infection include rhinitis (**snuffles**) and a desquamative rash. Infection of periosteum, bone, cartilage, and dental pulp produce deformities of bones and teeth, including **saddle nose,** anterior bowing of the legs (**saber shins**), **and** peg-shaped upper incisor teeth (**Hutchinson teeth**). Progression of congenital syphilis can be arrested by penicillin.

Nonvenereal Treponematoses Can Be Indistinguishable From Syphilis

These chronic diseases mostly occur in tropical and subtropical areas, and are caused by other treponemal species. Like syphilis, they result from inoculation into mucocutaneous surfaces. Clearly defined clinical and pathologic stages follow, including a primary lesion at the site of inoculation; secondary skin eruptions; a latent period; and a tertiary, late stage.

Yaws

Yaws is caused by *T. pertenue,* and occurs among poor rural populations in warm, humid areas of tropical Africa, South America, Southeast Asia, and Oceania. Children and adolescents are most at risk. Transmission is by skin-to-skin contact, facilitated by breaks or abrasions. Two to 5 weeks after exposure, a single "mother yaw" appears at the site of inoculation, usually on an exposed part. The lesion evolves from a papule to a 2- to 5-cm "raspberry-like" papilloma. The secondary or disseminated stage begins with similar, but smaller, yaws elsewhere on the skin. Lesions show hyperkeratosis, papillary acanthosis and intense neutrophilic infiltration of the epidermis. The epidermis at the apex of the papilloma lyses to form a shallow ulcer, and plasma cells invade the upper dermis. Spirochetes are abundant in the dermal papillae.

Painful papillomas on the soles of the feet lead patients to walk on the side of their feet like a crab, a condition called "**crab yaw.**" Treponemes are borne by the blood to bones, lymph nodes and skin, where they grow during a latent period of 5 or more years. Late-stage lesions include cutaneous gummas, which are destructive to the face and upper airways. Periostitis of the tibia causes "saber shins" or "boomerang legs." One dose of long-acting penicillin cures yaws.

Bejel

Bejel (also called "endemic syphilis," "frenga," and "belesh") is caused by *T. pallidum* subspecies *endemicum* and has a focal distribution in Africa, western Asia, and Australia. It is transmitted by nonvenereal routes, such as from an infected infant to the breast of the mother, from mouth to mouth, or from utensils to the mouth. The causative agent is morphologically and serologically indistinguishable from the causative agent of venereal syphilis, *Treponema pallidum.* Other than on the nursing breast, primary lesions are rare. Secondary lesions in the mouth are identical to the mucosal lesions of syphilis and may spread from the upper airway to the larynx. Lesions of the perineum and bone are encountered, and gummas of the breast occur.

Pinta

Pinta (from the Spanish for "painted" or "blemish") is caused by *T. carateum,* and features variably colored spots on the skin. It was first described in the 16th century in Aztec and Caribbean Amerindians. It is prevalent in remote, arid, inland regions and river valleys of the American tropics. Lesions of the three stages of pinta are limited to the skin and tend to merge. Transmission is by skin-to-skin inoculation, usually after long intimate contact with an infected person. Only a few hundred new cases are reported yearly from endemic areas, but this is probably an underestimate.

Lyme Disease Affects the Skin, Heart, Joints, and Nervous System

The causative agents are large, microaerophilic spirochetes belonging to the genus *Borrelia.*

EPIDEMIOLOGY: Lyme disease was first described in patients from Lyme, Connecticut, but has since been recognized in many other areas. *Borrelia burgdorferi* is the major cause of Lyme disease in the United States, while *B. afzelii* and *B. garinii* cause most cases in Europe. The spirochete is transmitted from its animal reservoir to humans by the tiny *Ixodes* tick. This pinhead-sized insect inhabits wooded areas, where it usually feeds on mice and deer. Transmission to humans is most likely from May through July, when nymph forms of the tick feed.

Lyme disease is an established public health problem in the United States, where it is the most common tickborne illness, annually causing 15,000 to 20,000 cases. It is concentrated along the eastern seaboard from Maryland to Massachusetts, in the Midwest in Minnesota and Wisconsin and in the West in California and Oregon. The disease also occurs in Europe, Australia, and Asia.

PATHOLOGY: *B. burgdorferi* reproduces locally at the site of inoculation, spreads to regional lymph nodes, and disseminates throughout the body via the bloodstream. Like other spirochetal diseases, Lyme disease is chronic and occurs in stages, with remissions and exacerbations. *B. burgdorferi* elicits a chronic inflammatory infiltrate of lymphocytes and plasma cells. In patients who died of the disease, organisms have been seen at autopsy in virtually every organ affected, including skin, myocardium, liver, CNS, and the musculoskeletal system.

CLINICAL FEATURES: Lyme disease is a prolonged illness in which three clinical stages are described:

- **Stage 1:** The characteristic skin lesion, **erythema chronicum migrans,** appears at the site of the tick bite, 3 to 35 days later, it is an erythematous macule or papule, which grows into an erythematous 3 to 7 cm patch. It often is intensely red at its periphery, with some central clearing, resembling a ring. It is accompanied by fever, fatigue, headache, arthralgias, and regional lymphadenopathy. Secondary annular skin lesions develop in about half of patients and may persist for long periods. During this phase, patients experience constant malaise and fatigue, headache, and fever. Intermittent manifestations may also include meningeal irritation, migratory myalgia, cough, generalized lymphadenopathy, and testicular swelling.
- **Stage 2:** The second stage begins several weeks to months after the skin lesion, with exacerbation of migratory musculoskeletal pains and cardiac and neurologic abnormalities. In 10% of cases, cardiac conduction abnormalities, particularly atrioventricular block, result from myocarditis. Neurologic abnormalities, most commonly meningitis and facial nerve palsies, occur in 15% of patients.
- **Stage 3:** The third stage of Lyme disease begins months to years later, with joint, skin, and neurologic abnormalities. Over half of these patients have arthralgia, with severe arthritis of the large joints, especially the knee. Affected joints are pathologically indistinguishable from rheumatoid arthritis, with villous hypertrophy and a conspicuous mononuclear infiltrate in the subsynovial lining area.

Neurologic manifestations may start months to years after the disease begins. They range from intermittent tingling paresthesias without demonstrable neurologic deficits to slowly progressive encephalomyelitis, transverse myelitis, organic brain syndromes, and dementia.

Distinctive late skin manifestations of Lyme disease include **acrodermatitis chronica atrophicans**. This occurs years after erythema chronicum migrans, and presents as patchy atrophy and sclerosis of the skin.

Culturing *B. burgdorferi* from infected patients can establish the diagnosis, but the sensitivity is low. Therefore, antibody titers (initially IgM and later IgG) the most practical way to establish the diagnosis. Treatment with tetracycline or erythromycin is effective in early Lyme disease. In later stages and when there are extensive extracutaneous manifestations, high doses of intravenous penicillin G or other combinations of antibiotic regimens for long periods are necessary.

Leptospirosis Is Usually a Mild, Self-Limited Febrile Disease

More severe infections may entail hepatic and renal failure, which may prove fatal.

EPIDEMIOLOGY: Leptospirosis is a worldwide zoonosis. Leptospires penetrate abraded skin or mucous membranes following contact with infected rats, contaminated water, or mud. Warm, moist environments favor survival of the spirochetes, so incidence is higher in the tropics. Between 30 and 100 cases are reported annually in the United States, some of them in slaughterhouse workers and trappers, but recently some cases were reported among destitute people in urban areas.

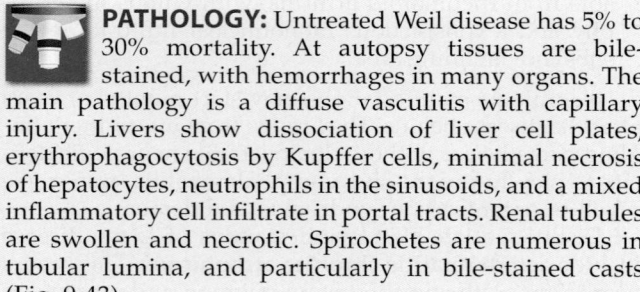

CLINICAL FEATURES: The symptoms of leptospirosis begin 4 days to 3 weeks after exposure to *Leptospira interrogans*. The disease usually resolves within a week without sequelae. In more severe cases, leptospirosis is a biphasic disease.

- In the **leptospiremic phase** leptospires are present in the blood and cerebrospinal fluid. Fever, shaking chills, headache, and myalgias begin abruptly. Symptoms abate within 1 to 2 weeks, as leptospires disappear from blood and bodily fluids.
- The **immune phase** begins within 3 days of the end of the leptospiremic phase, and is accompanied by IgM antibody production. The earlier symptoms recur, and signs of meningeal irritation become apparent. At this time, the CSF shows a prominent pleocytosis. In severe cases, jaundice appears. It may be followed by liver and renal failure, and widespread hemorrhages and shock. This severe form of leptospirosis has historically been called **Weil disease**.

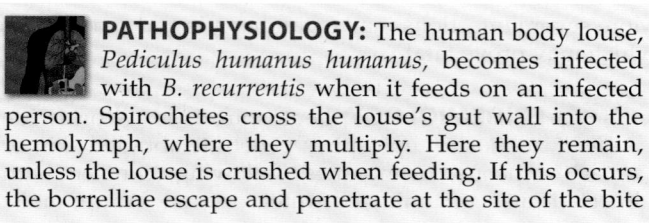

PATHOLOGY: Untreated Weil disease has 5% to 30% mortality. At autopsy tissues are bile-stained, with hemorrhages in many organs. The main pathology is a diffuse vasculitis with capillary injury. Livers show dissociation of liver cell plates, erythrophagocytosis by Kupffer cells, minimal necrosis of hepatocytes, neutrophils in the sinusoids, and a mixed inflammatory cell infiltrate in portal tracts. Renal tubules are swollen and necrotic. Spirochetes are numerous in tubular lumina, and particularly in bile-stained casts (Fig. 9-43).

Relapsing Fever Is an Acute, Febrile Illness Spread by Lice and Ticks

It is caused by spirochetes of the genus *Borrelia*. There are two main types of relapsing fever:

- **Epidemic relapsing fever** is caused by *Borrelia recurrentis* and is transmitted by the bite of an infected louse. Humans are the only reservoir.
- **Endemic relapsing fever** is produced by a number of *Borrelia* species and is transmitted from rodents and other animals by the bite of an infected tick.

PATHOPHYSIOLOGY: The human body louse, *Pediculus humanus humanus,* becomes infected with *B. recurrentis* when it feeds on an infected person. Spirochetes cross the louse's gut wall into the hemolymph, where they multiply. Here they remain, unless the louse is crushed when feeding. If this occurs, the borrelliae escape and penetrate at the site of the bite

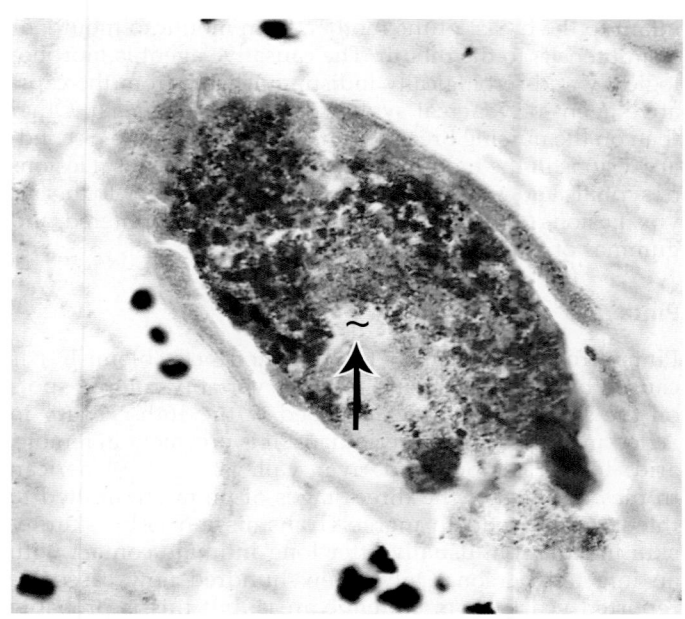

FIGURE 9-43. Leptospirosis. A distal renal tubule is obstructed by a bile-stained mass of hemoglobin and cellular debris. A leptospire (*arrow*) is in the center of this mass.

or even through the intact skin. War, crowded migrant worker camps, and heavy clothing during cold weather all favor mobilization of lice and disease spread. Also, lice dislike the higher temperatures of feverish victims and seek new hosts, another factor in the rapid spread of relapsing fever during epidemics. Louse-borne relapsing fever is mainly seen in several African countries, especially Ethiopia and Sudan and also in the South American Andes.

In endemic, tick-borne relapsing fever, ticks are infected while biting rats and other hosts. Borrelliae grow in ticks' hemocoeloms and invade other tissues, including the salivary glands. Humans are infected by saliva or coxal fluid of the tick. Ticks have a considerably longer life span than lice and may harbor spirochetes for 12 to 15 years without a blood meal. Tick-borne relapsing fever occurs sporadically worldwide.

PATHOLOGY: In fatal infections, the spleen is enlarged and contains miliary microabscesses. Spirochetes form tangled aggregates around necrotic centers. Lymphocytes and neutrophils infiltrate central and midzonal areas of the liver, where spirochetes lie free in the sinusoids. Focal hemorrhages involve many organs.

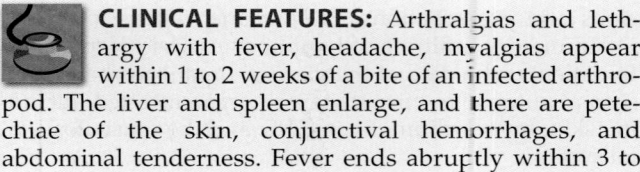

CLINICAL FEATURES: Arthralgias and lethargy with fever, headache, myalgias appear within 1 to 2 weeks of a bite of an infected arthropod. The liver and spleen enlarge, and there are petechiae of the skin, conjunctival hemorrhages, and abdominal tenderness. Fever ends abruptly within 3 to

9 days, only to begin again 7 to 10 days later. During the afebrile period, spirochetes disappear from the blood and change their antigenic coats. With each relapse, symptoms are milder and the illness shorter. In severe cases, the first episode may include a rash, meningitis, myocarditis, liver failure, and coma. Tetracycline is effective for both types of relapsing fever.

Tropical Phagedenic Ulcer Is a Painful Lesion of the Leg

Tropical phagedenic (rapid spreading and sloughing) ulcer, also called **tropical foot,** is a painful, necrotizing lesion of the skin and subcutaneous tissues of the leg that afflicts people in tropical climates. *Bacillus fusiformis* and *Treponema vincentii* are the responsible bacteria. Malnutrition may predispose to infection.

  PATHOLOGY AND CLINICAL FEATURES: The lesion usually starts on the skin at a point of trauma and develops rapidly. The surface sloughs to form an ulcer with raised borders and a cup-shaped crater, containing gray, putrid exudates (Fig. 9-44). The ulcer may be so deep that underlying bone and tendons are exposed. The margin becomes fibrotic, but complete healing may take years. In addition to secondary infection, tibial osteomyelitis and squamous carcinoma may be late complications. Antibiotics may be effective, but reconstructive plastic surgery is often necessary to close the defect.

Noma Is a Destructive Lesion of the Face

Noma (gangrenous stomatitis, cancrum oris) is a rapidly progressive necrosis of soft tissues and bones of the mouth and face and, less often, of other sites (chest, limbs, genitalia). It afflicts malnourished children in the tropics, many of whom are further debilitated by recent infections (e.g., measles, malaria, leishmaniasis). The main causes are *T. vincentii, B. fusiformis, Bacteroides* spp., and *Corynebacterium* spp.

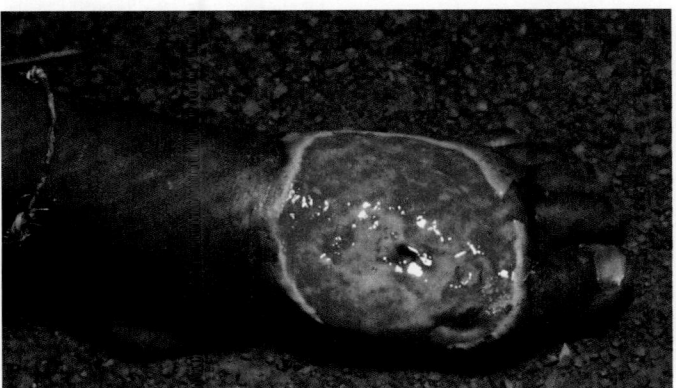

FIGURE 9-44. Tropical phagedenic ulcer caused by infection by fusospirochetal organisms, following penetrating trauma.

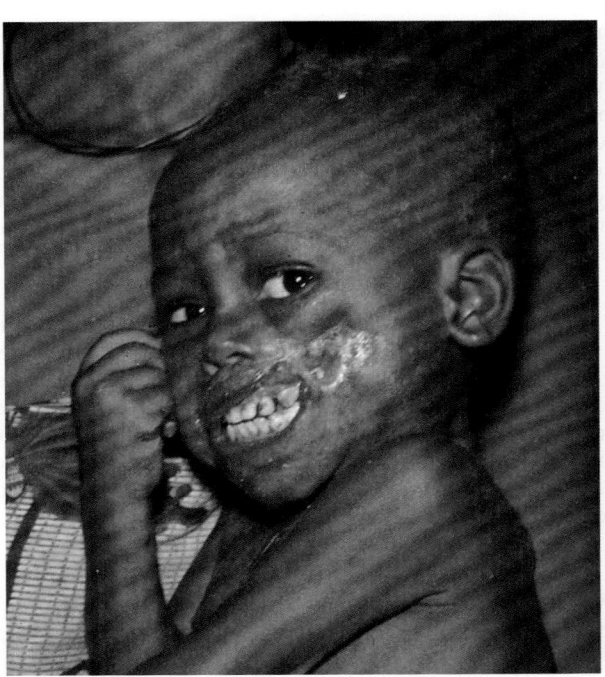

FIGURE 9-45. Noma. There is massive destruction of the soft tissues and bones of the mouth and cheek.

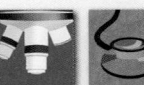 **PATHOLOGY AND CLINICAL FEATURES:** The ulcer is destructive, disfiguring, and usually unilateral (Fig. 9-45). Initially it is a small papule, often on the cheek opposite the molars or premolars. Large malodorous defects quickly develop. The lesions are painful and advance with necrosis of skin, muscle and adipose tissue, exposing underlying bone. Without treatment, patients usually die. Antibiotics are helpful, but reconstructive surgery is often required.

CHLAMYDIA

Chlamydiae are obligate intracellular parasites that are smaller than most other bacteria. They cannot make ATP, and so must parasitize host cell metabolic machinery. The chlamydial life cycle involves two morphologic forms. The **elementary body** is the smaller, metabolically inactive form, which survives extracellularly. It attaches to the appropriate host cell and induces endocytosis, forming a vacuole. It then transforms into the larger, metabolically active form, the **reticulate body,** which commandeers host cell metabolism to fuel chlamydial replication. The reticulate body divides repeatedly, forming daughter elementary bodies and destroying the host cell. Necrotic debris elicits inflammatory and immunologic responses that further damage infected tissue.

Chlamydial infections are widespread among birds and mammals, and perhaps 20% of humans are infected. Three species of chlamydiae (*C. trachomatis, C. psittaci,* and *C. pneumoniae*) cause human infection.

Infections With *C. trachomatis* Are Among the Most Common Sexually Transmitted Diseases

C. trachomatis serovars D through K cause genital epithelial infections that are the most common sexually contracted disease in North America. In men, they produce urethritis and sometimes epididymitis or proctitis. In women, infection usually starts as cervicitis and may progress to endometritis, salpingitis, and generalized infection of pelvic adnexal organs (pelvic inflammatory disease). Repeated episodes of salpingitis may cause scarring, and lead to infertility or ectopic pregnancy. Perinatal transmission of *C. trachomatis* causes neonatal conjunctivitis and pneumonia.

EPIDEMIOLOGY: *C. trachomatis* spreads in genital secretions. Infection is chronic and often asymptomatic, providing an enormous reservoir for transmission. As with all sexually transmitted diseases, risk of infection increases with the number of sexual partners. Newborns become infected upon contact with endocervical secretions during birth. Two-thirds of exposed newborns develop *C. trachomatis* conjunctivitis.

PATHOLOGY: Chlamydia elicit an infiltrate of neutrophils and lymphocytes. Lymphoid aggregates, with or without germinal centers, may appear at the site of infection. In newborns, conjunctival epithelium often contains vacuolar cytoplasmic inclusions, hence the name, **inclusion conjunctivitis**.

CLINICAL FEATURES: Most genital infections are asymptomatic. In men, clinically apparent infection presents as a purulent penile discharge, with dysuria and urinary urgency. Chlamydial cervicitis causes mucopurulent drainage from the cervical os. Chlamydial disease in newborns presents as reddened conjunctivae with a watery or purulent discharge. Untreated neonatal conjunctivitis is potentially serious, but may resolve without sequelae. Chlamydial pneumonia manifests in the second or third month with tachypnea and paroxysmal cough, usually without fever. Inclusion conjunctivitis is treated with systemic or topical antibiotics.

Lymphogranuloma Venereum (LGV) Is a Sexually Transmitted Disease That Causes Necrotizing Lymphadenitis

LGV starts as a genital ulcer, spreads to lymph nodes (Fig. 9-46A) and may cause local scarring. It is caused by *C. trachomatis* serovars L1 to L3.

EPIDEMIOLOGY: LGV is uncommon in developed countries, but is endemic in the tropics and subtropics. It accounts for 5% of sexually transmitted disease in Africa, India, parts of southeast Asia, South America, and the Caribbean. Since 2003, it has been increasingly reported from developed countries. Large outbreaks have been reported, mainly in men who have sex with men (MSM), with the biggest outbreaks in New York City and the United Kingdom, where proctitis was the main presentation.

PATHOLOGY: The spirochete enters through a break in the skin. After 4 to 21 days incubation, an ulcer appears, usually on the penis, vagina, or cervix, although lips, tongue, and fingers may also be primary sites. The organisms are carried by lymphatics to regional lymph nodes, where a **necrotizing lymphadenitis** erupts 1 to 3 weeks later. Abscesses develop within involved lymph nodes, often extending to adjacent lymph nodes. Over the next few weeks, the nodes become tender and fluctuant and frequently ulcerate and discharge pus. The intense inflammation may cause severe scarring and so produce chronic lymphatic obstruction, ischemic necrosis of overlying structures or strictures and adhesions. The necrotizing process produces enlarged and matted lymph nodes, containing multiple, coalescing abscesses, which often develop a stellate shape (Fig. 9-46B). Abscesses resemble granulomas, with neutrophils and necrotic debris in the center, surrounded by palisading epithelioid cells, macrophages, and occasional giant cells. There is a rim of lymphocytes, plasma cells, and fibrous tissue. Nodal architecture is eventually effaced by fibrosis.

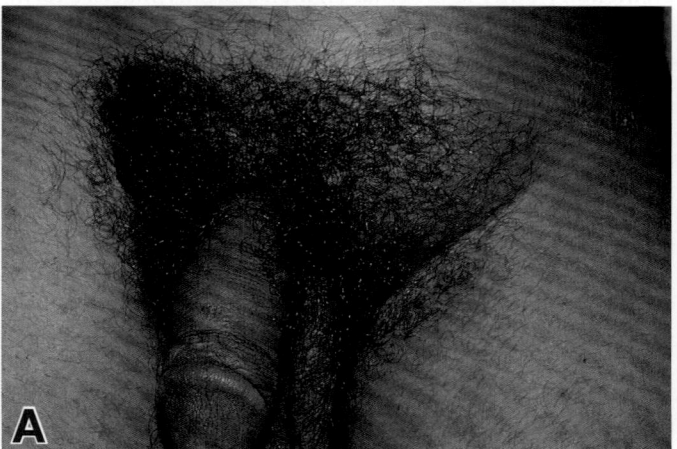
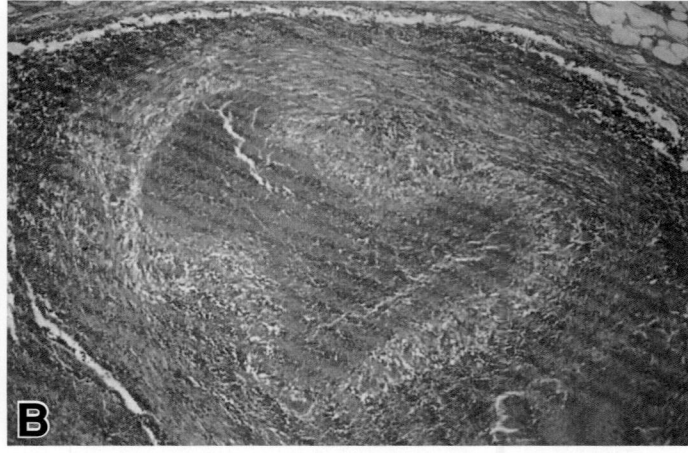

FIGURE 9-46. Lymphogranuloma venereum. A. Painful inguinal lymphadenopathy in a man infected with *Chlamydia trachomatis*. **B.** Microscopic section of a lymph node shows a necrotic central area surrounded by a granulomatous zone.

CLINICAL FEATURES: Patients with LGV present with lymphadenopathy. Most infections resolve completely, even without antibiotics. However, 5% of men develop progressive ulceration of the penis, urethra or scrotum, with fistulas and urethral stricture. Women and MSM often present with hemorrhagic proctitis, which may lead to rectal stricture, rectovaginal fistulas, and genital elephantiasis, occur in women.

Trachoma Is a Chronic Infection That Causes Ocular Scarring and Blindness

C. trachomatis serovars A, B, Ba, and C are responsible for the disease.

 EPIDEMIOLOGY: Trachoma is worldwide, associated with poverty and most prevalent in dry or sandy regions. Only humans are naturally infected, and poor personal hygiene and inadequate public sanitation are common factors. Trachoma remains a major problem in parts of Africa, India, and the Middle East. Infection is mostly spread by direct contact, but also by fomites, contaminated water and, probably, flies. Subclinical infections are an important reservoir. In endemic areas, infection starts early in childhood, becomes chronic and eventually progresses to blindness.

 PATHOLOGY: Once in the eye, *C. trachomatis* reproduces in conjunctival epithelium, inciting a mixed acute and chronic inflammatory infiltrate. Early lesions show chronic inflammation, lymphoid aggregates, focal degeneration, and chlamydial inclusions in the conjunctiva. As trachoma progresses, lymphoid aggregates enlarge and the conjunctiva becomes scarred and focally hypertrophic. Blood vessels and fibroblasts invade the cornea and form a scar reminiscent of a cloth ("pannus" in Latin), leading to corneal opacification (see Chapter 33).

 CLINICAL FEATURES: Palpebral and conjunctival inflammation begin abruptly, leading to tearing, purulent conjunctivitis, and photophobia. Lymphoid aggregates appear as small yellow grains beneath the palpebral conjunctivae within 3 to 4 weeks. After months to years, eyelid deformities eventually interfere with normal ocular function and secondary bacterial infections and corneal ulcers are common, leading to blindness.

Psittacosis Is a Self-Limited Pneumonia Transmitted by Birds

The causative agent, *C. psittaci,* is spread by infected birds. The resulting disease is called psittacosis (association with parrots) or ornithosis (contact with birds in general).

EPIDEMIOLOGY: *C. psittaci* is present in the blood, tissues, excreta, and feathers of infected birds. Humans inhale infectious excreta or dust from feathers. Although infection is endemic in tropical

birds, *C. psittaci* can infect almost any species and can spread to humans from many bird species, including parrots, parakeets, canaries, pigeons, sea gulls, ducks, chickens, and turkeys. Use of tetracycline-containing bird feeds and quarantine of imported tropical birds limits the spread of disease, and fewer than 50 cases are reported annually in the United States.

 PATHOLOGY: *C. psittaci* first infects pulmonary macrophages, which carry it to phagocytes in the liver and spleen, where it reproduces. It then spreads via the bloodstream to produce systemic infection, particularly diffusely in the lungs. *C. psittaci* reproduces in alveolar lining cells, whose destruction elicits inflammation. The pneumonia is predominantly an interstitial lymphocytic inflammatory infiltrate. There may be foci of necrosis in the liver and spleen and diffuse mononuclear cell infiltrates in the heart, kidneys, and brain.

 CLINICAL FEATURES: The spectrum of clinical illness varies widely. There is usually a persistent dry cough, with constitutional symptoms of high fever, headache, malaise, myalgias, and arthralgias. Untreated, fever persists for 2 to 3 weeks, then subsides as the pulmonary disease regresses. With tetracycline therapy, psittacosis is rarely fatal.

Chlamydia pneumoniae Causes Generally Mild Respiratory Infections

C. pneumoniae is transmitted from person to person, and infection appears to be very common. In the developed world, half of adults show evidence of past exposure, but only 10% of infections cause clinical pneumonia. Symptoms include fever, sore throat, and cough. Severe pneumonia occurs only if there is an underlying pulmonary condition. Untreated disease usually resolves in 2 to 4 weeks.

RICKETTSIAE

Rickettsiae are small, gram-negative coccobacilli. They are obligate intracellular pathogens and cannot replicate outside a host but, unlike chlamydiae, replicate by binary fission. They can synthesize their own ATP via a proton-translocating ATPase and can also obtain ATP from the host using ATP/ADP translocase. Rickettsiae induce endocytosis, and replicate in the cytoplasm of host cells. Their cell wall structures resemble gram-negative bacteria, but they do not stain well with Gram stain and are best demonstrated by the Gimenez method or with acridine orange.

Humans are accidental hosts for most species of *Rickettsia*, which normally reside in animals and insects. Human infection results from insect bites. Several species of *Rickettsia* cause different human diseases (Table 9-5), but these infections share many common features. ***In humans, rickettsiae target endothelial cells of capillaries and other small blood vessels***, in which they reproduce. They kill host cells in the process, producing a necrotizing vasculitis. Human rickettsial infections are traditionally divided into the "**spotted fever group**" and the "**typhus group**."

TABLE 9-5

RICKETTSIAL INFECTIONS

Disease	Organism	Distribution	Transmission
Spotted-fever Group (Genus *Rickettsia*)			
Rocky Mountain spotted fever	*R. rickettsii*	Americas	Ticks
Queensland tick fever	*R. australis*	Australia	Ticks
Boutonneuse fever, Kenya tick fever	*R. conorii*	Mediterranean, Africa, India	Ticks
Siberian tick fever	*R. sibirica*	Siberia, Mongolia	Ticks
Rickettsialpox	*R. akari*	United States, Russia, Central Asia, Korea, Africa	Mites
Flea-borne spotted fever	*R. felis*	North & South America, Europe, Australia	Ticks
Typhus Group			
Louse-borne typhus (epidemic typhus)	*R. prowazekii*	Latin America, Africa, Asia	Lice
Murine typhus (endemic typhus)	*R. typhi*	Worldwide	Fleas
Scrub typhus	*Orientia tsutsugamushi*	South Pacific, Asia	Mites
Q fever	*Coxiella burnetii*	Worldwide	Inhalation

Rocky Mountain Spotted Fever Is an Acute, Sometimes Fatal Vasculitis

It is usually attended by headache, fever, and rash. The causative organism, *Rickettsia rickettsii*, is transmitted to humans by tick bites.

EPIDEMIOLOGY: Rocky Mountain spotted fever is acquired by bites of infected ticks, which are the vectors for *R. rickettsii*. The organism passes from mother to progeny ticks without killing them, and so maintains a natural reservoir. Rocky Mountain spotted fever occurs in various areas throughout North, Central, and South America. About 500 cases occur annually in the United State, mostly from the eastern seaboard (Georgia to New York) westward to Texas, Oklahoma, and Kansas. Its name derives from its discovery in Idaho, but the disease is uncommon in the Rocky Mountain region.

PATHOPHYSIOLOGY: *R. rickettsii* in salivary glands of ticks enter the body as the ticks feed, then spread via lymphatics and small blood vessels to the circulation. They attach to vascular endothelial cells, are engulfed, reproduce in the cytoplasm and then are shed into the vascular and lymphatic systems. Further infection and destruction of vascular endothelium causes systemic vasculitis. The rash, produced by inflammatory damage to cutaneous vessels, is the most visible manifestation of the generalized vascular injury. Other rickettsiae infect only capillary endothelial cells, but *R. rickettsii* spreads to vascular smooth muscle and endothelium of larger vessels.

Extensive damage to blood vessel walls causes loss of vascular integrity, exudation of fluid, and disseminated intravascular coagulation. Fluid loss can be so extensive as to lead to shock. Damage to pulmonary capillaries can produce pulmonary edema and acute alveolar injury.

PATHOLOGY: The vascular lesions of Rocky Mountain spotted fever occur throughout the body, affecting capillaries, venules, arterioles, and sometimes larger vessels. Necrosis and reactive hyperplasia of vascular endothelium often lead to small vessel thrombosis. Vessel walls are infiltrated, initially with neutrophils and macrophages and later with lymphocytes and plasma cells. Microinfarcts with blood extravasation into surrounding tissues are common. The orientation of the intracellular bacilli in parallel rows and in an end-to-end pattern gives them the appearance of a "flotilla at anchor facing the wind."

CLINICAL FEATURES: Rocky Mountain spotted fever presents with fever, headache, myalgias, and then a rash. Skin lesions begin as a maculopapular eruption but rapidly become petechial, spreading centripetally from the distal extremities to the trunk (Fig. 9-47). Cutaneous lesions usually appear on the palms and soles, a distinctive feature of the disease. If untreated, 20% to 50% or more people die within 8 to 15 days. Prompt diagnosis and antibiotic treatment (chloramphenicol and tetracycline) is life saving: mortality in the United States is under 5%.

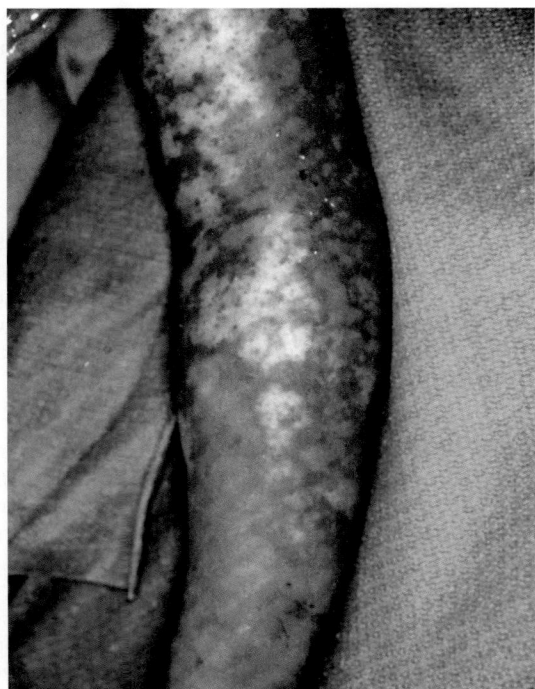

FIGURE 9-47. Rocky mountain spotted fever. A severe petechial and purpuric eruption occurred on the arm in this fatal case.

Epidemic Typhus Is Transmitted by Lice

It is caused by *Rickettsia prowazekii*, which has a human–louse–human life cycle (Fig. 9-48).

EPIDEMIOLOGY: Typhus is widely distributed in parts of Africa, Asia, Europe, and the Western Hemisphere. Devastating epidemics were associated with cold climates, poor sanitation and crowding during natural disasters, famine and, especially, war. Infrequent bathing and lack of changes of clothing lead to louse infestation of human populations and consequently epidemics of typhus. It is said that Napoleon's armies were not defeated in Russia by Russian armies, but by typhus. Mass displacements of populations in Eastern Europe in World War I led to epidemic typhus affecting over 30 million people and killing over 3 million. Epidemic louse-borne typhus last occurred in the United States in 1921.

PATHOPHYSIOLOGY: After a louse takes blood from an infected person, *R. prowazekii* enters the epithelial cells of the insect's midgut, multiplies there, and ruptures the cells within 3 to 5 days. Large numbers of rickettsiae flood the lumen of the louse intestine. Contaminated louse feces on the skin or clothing of a second host may remain infectious for over 3 months. Human infection begins when contaminated louse feces penetrate an abrasion or scratch, or when the person inhales airborne rickettsiae from clothing containing louse feces. Epidemic typhus begins as localized infection of capillary endothelium and progresses to

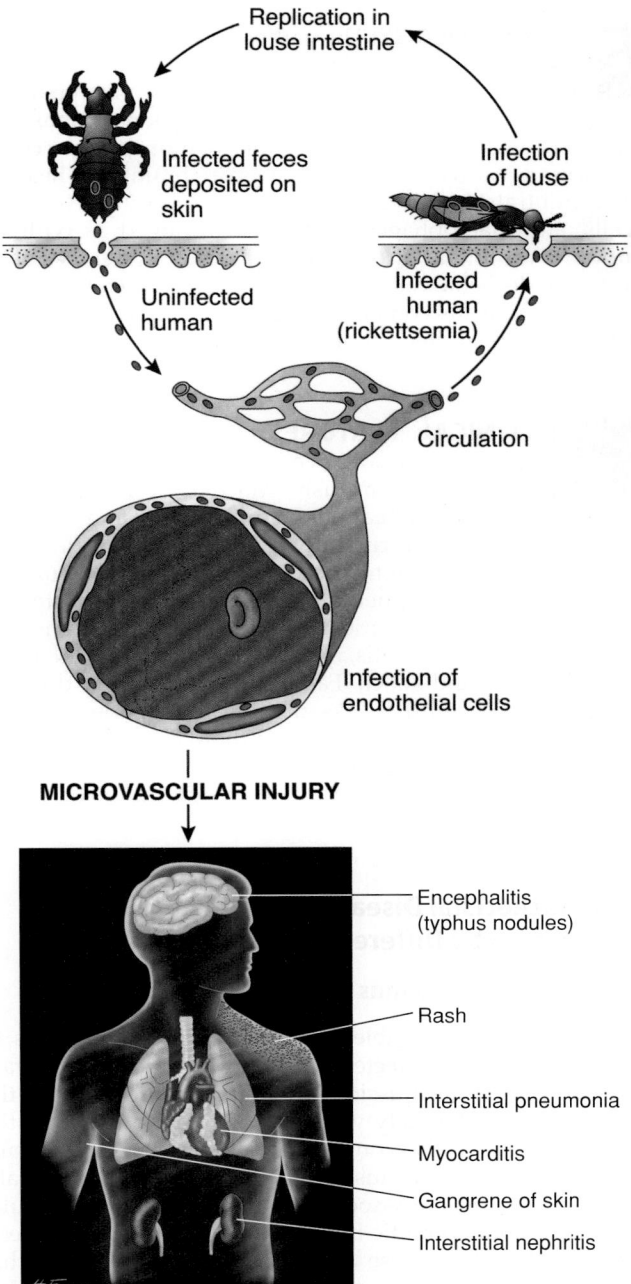

FIGURE 9-48. Epidemic typhus (louse-borne typhus). *Rickettsia prowazekii* has a man–louse–man life cycle. The organism multiplies in endothelial cells, which detach, rupture, and release organisms into the circulation (rickettsemia). A louse taking a blood meal becomes infected with rickettsiae, which enter the epithelial cells of its midgut, multiply and rupture the cells, thereby releasing rickettsiae into the lumen of the louse intestine. Contaminated feces are deposited on the skin or clothing of a second host, penetrate an abrasion or are inhaled. The rickettsiae then enter endothelial cells, multiply and rupture the cells, thus completing the cycle.

systemic vasculitis. Louse-borne typhus differs from other rickettsial diseases in that *R. prowazekii* can establish latent infection and produce recrudescent disease (Brill–Zinsser disease) many years after primary infection.

PATHOLOGY: The pathology of endemic typhus is similar to Rocky Mountain spotted fever and other rickettsial diseases. Gross examination mainly shows splenomegaly and occasional areas of necrosis. Microscopically, collections of mononuclear cells are found in various organs (e.g., skin, brain, and heart). The infiltrate includes mast cells, lymphocytes, plasma cells, and macrophages, frequently arranged as **typhus nodules** around arterioles and capillaries. Systemic small vessel endothelial cells are focally necrotic and hyperplastic, and the walls contain inflammatory cells. Rickettsiae can be demonstrated within the endothelial cells.

 CLINICAL FEATURES: Symptoms of louse-borne typhus are fever, headache, and myalgias, followed by a rash. Macular lesions, which become petechial, appear on the upper trunk and axillary folds and spread centrifugally to the extremities. In fatal cases, the rash commonly becomes confluent and purpuric. Mild rickettsial pneumonia may precede a bacterial pneumonia. Dying patients may show symptoms of encephalitis, myocarditis, interstitial pneumonia, interstitial nephritis, and shock. Fatalities usually occur during the second or third weeks of illness. In patients who recover, the symptoms abate after about 3 weeks.

Epidemic typhus can be controlled by large-scale delousing of the population, by steam sterilization of clothing and use of insecticides.

Other Rickettsial Diseases Are Transmitted by Different Vectors

Endemic (Murine) Typhus

Endemic typhus resembles epidemic typhus, but tends to be milder. Humans infected with *R. typhi,* interrupt the rat–flea–rat cycle of transmission. Contaminated flea feces on the skin may enter the body via the small wound made by the bite. *R. typhi* may also contaminate clothes and become airborne. If inhaled, they cause pulmonary infection. Outbreaks of murine typhus are associated with an exploding population of rats, but sporadic infections occur in the southwestern United States. These are associated with settings that bring humans into contact with rats, for example, handling and storage of grain.

Scrub Typhus

Scrub typhus **(Tsutsugamushi fever)** is an acute, febrile illness caused by *Orientia tsutsugamushi* (previously, *Rickettsia tsutsugamushi*), the only member of its genus. Rodents are the natural mammalian reservoir. Trombiculid mites (chiggers) transmit the infection to their larvae, which crawl to the tips of vegetation and attach to passers-by. While feeding, mites inoculate the Rickettsiae into the skin. Rickettsemia and lymphadenopathy follow. Scrub typhus is widely distributed in eastern and southern Asia and islands of the southern and western Pacific, including Japan. It is unknown in the Western world.

A multiloculated vesicle forms at the inoculation site and ulcerates, followed by an eschar. As the lesion heals,

headache and fever appear suddenly, then pneumonia, a macular rash, lymphadenopathy, and hepatosplenomegaly. Myocarditis, meningoencephalitis, and shock complicate severe cases, and mortality in untreated patients approach to 30%.

Q Fever Is a Self-Limited Systemic Infection

It usually presents as headache, fever, and myalgias. The disease is caused by *Coxiella burnetii,* a small pleomorphic coccobacillus with a gram-negative cell wall. Unlike true rickettsiae, *C. burnetii* enters cells passively, upon phagocytosis by macrophages. Infection does not produce a vasculitis, and thus there is no associated rash.

 EPIDEMIOLOGY: *C. burnetii* is endemic in many wild and domesticated animals, but exposure to cattle, sheep, and goats or their products usually causes human infection. These animals shed large numbers of organisms in urine, feces, milk, bodily fluids, and birth products. Q fever occurs most often after occupational exposure in herders, slaughterhouse workers, veterinarians, dairy workers, and others. Aerosol droplets may spread infection from person to person. Q fever is rare in the United States.

 PATHOPHYSIOLOGY: Q fever begins with inhalation of organisms, which are phagocytosed by alveolar macrophages and replicate in phagolysosomes. Recruitment of neutrophils and macrophages produces a focal bronchopneumonia. Nonactivated phagocytes fail to kill *C. burnetii*, and the organism disseminates through the body, primarily infecting monocytes and macrophages. Most infections resolve with the onset of specific cell-mediated immunity, but occasional cases persist as chronic infections.

 PATHOLOGY: The lungs and liver are most prominently involved in Q fever. The lungs show single or multiple irregular areas of consolidation, in which the pulmonary parenchyma is infiltrated by neutrophils and macrophages. Organisms may be demonstrated in macrophages by the Giemsa stain. In the liver, Q fever is usually characterized by multiple microscopic granulomas with a distinctive "fibrin ring." In these granulomas, epithelioid macrophages encircle a ring of fibrin, sometimes containing a lipid vacuole.

 CLINICAL FEATURES: Q fever is usually a self-limited mildly symptomatic febrile disease. More severe cases may present with headache, fever, fatigue, and myalgias, without rash. Pulmonary infection is virtually always present, but it may appear as an atypical pneumonia with dry cough, a rapidly progressive pneumonia or chest roentgenographic abnormalities without significant respiratory symptoms. Many patients have some hepatosplenomegaly. Q fever usually resolves spontaneously in 2 to 14 days.

TABLE 9-6
MYCOPLASMA INFECTIONS

Organism	Disease
Mycoplasma pneumoniae	Tracheobronchitis
	Pneumonia
	Pharyngitis
	Otitis media
Ureaplasma urealyticum	Urethritis
	Chorioamnionitis
	Postpartum fever
Mycoplasma hominis	Postpartum fever

MYCOPLASMA

At less than 0.3 μm in greatest dimension, mycoplasmas are the smallest free-living **prokaryotes**. They lack the rigid cell walls of more complex bacteria. Mycoplasmas are widespread, geographically and ecologically, as saprophytes and as parasites of many animals and plants. Many *Mycoplasma* species inhabit the human body, but only three are pathogenic: *M. pneumoniae, M. hominis,* and *Ureaplasma urealyticum* (Table 9-6).

M. pneumoniae Produces Acute, Self-limited Lower Respiratory Tract Infections, Mostly of Young People

It can also cause pharyngitis and otitis media.

 EPIDEMIOLOGY: Most infections are spread by aerosol from person to person. They occur worldwide, in small groups of people who have close contact (e.g., families, college fraternities, military units), with attack rates exceeding 50% within the group. *M. pneumoniae* causes 15% to 20% of pneumonias in developed countries.

 PATHOPHYSIOLOGY: *M. pneumoniae* initiates infection by attaching to a glycolipid on the surface of the respiratory epithelium. The organism remains outside the cells, where it reproduces and causes progressive dysfunction and eventual death of host cells. Because *M. pneumoniae* infection rarely produces symptomatic disease in children younger than the age of 5 years, it is thought that the host immune response plays a role in tissue injury.

PATHOLOGY: Pneumonia caused by *M. pneumoniae* usually shows patchy consolidation of a single segment of a lower lung lobe, although the process can be more widespread. The mucosa of affected airways is edematous and infiltrated by a mostly mononuclear inflammatory infiltrate. Alveoli show a largely interstitial process, with reactive alveolar lining cells and mononuclear infiltration. Pulmonary changes are often complicated by bacterial superinfection. The organism itself is too small to be seen by routine light microscopy.

 CLINICAL FEATURES: *Mycoplasma* pneumonia is sometimes called "walking pneumonia," as it tends to be milder than other bacterial pneumonias. Fever rarely lasts more than 2 weeks, but cough may linger for 6 weeks or more. Death from *M. pneumoniae* infection is rare. *However, life-threatening Stevens–Johnson syndrome may follow mycoplasma infection.*

MYCOBACTERIA

Mycobacteria are distinctive organisms, 2 to 10 μm in length. Their cell walls resemble gram-positive bacteria, but also contain large amounts of lipid. The high lipid content interferes with staining by aniline dyes, including crystal violet used in the Gram stain. Thus, although they are structurally gram-positive, routine staining does not demonstrate that. *Their waxy cell wall lipids make mycobacteria "acid fast" (i.e., they retain carbolfuchsin after rinsing with acid alcohol).*

Mycobacteria grow more slowly than other pathogenic bacteria, and their diseases are chronic, slowly progressive illnesses. They produce no known toxins. They damage human tissues by inducing inflammatory and immune responses. Most mycobacterial pathogens replicate within cells of the monocyte/macrophage lineage and elicit granulomatous inflammation. The outcome of mycobacterial infection largely reflects the host's capacity to contain the bacteria by mounting effective cell-mediated immune responses (see Chapter 4).

Mycobacterium tuberculosis and *M. leprae* only infect humans and have no environmental reservoir. Other pathogenic mycobacteria are environmental organisms that only occasionally cause human disease.

M. tuberculosis Elicits Necrotizing Granulomatous Inflammation

Tuberculosis is a chronic, communicable disease, primarily of the lungs, although any organ may be infected. Disease is mainly caused by **M. tuberculosis hominis** *(Koch bacillus) but occasionally by* **M. tuberculosis bovis.** *Characteristic lesions are spherical granulomas with central necrosis.*

M. tuberculosis is an obligate aerobe, a slender, beaded, nonmotile, acid-fast bacillus (Fig. 9-49). It grows slowly in culture, doubling every 24 hours, with 3 to 6 weeks commonly required to produce visible growth in culture.

 EPIDEMIOLOGY: Tuberculosis is worldwide and is one of the most important human diseases. It is now less common in developed countries, but HIV-infected, homeless, and malnourished people are highly susceptible, as are immigrants from areas where the disease is endemic. In the United States, annual incidence is 12 per 100,000, with mortality at 1–2 per 100,000. In some developing countries, incidence

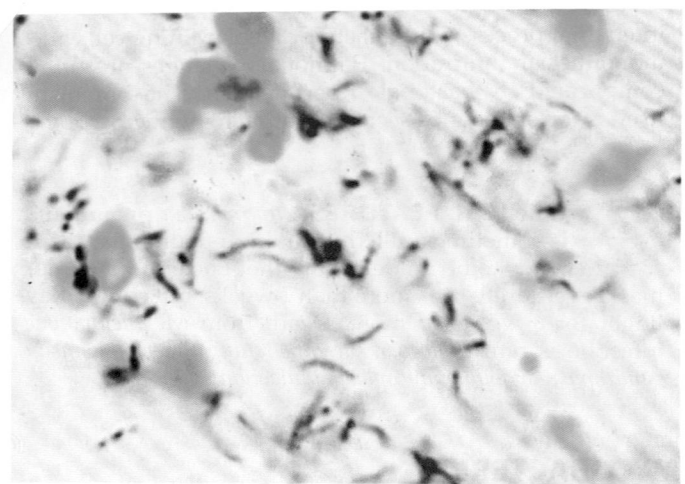

FIGURE 9-49. Mycobacterium tuberculosis. A smear of a pulmonary lesion shows slender, beaded, acid-fast bacilli.

reaches 450 per 100,000, with a high fatality rate. There are also racial and ethnic differences—African-Americans, and native populations are more susceptible than are white people. In the United States, tuberculosis is most common among the elderly, possibly reflecting reactivation of infections acquired early in life before its prevalence declined.

M. tuberculosis is transmitted from person to person by aerosolized droplets. Coughing, sneezing, and talking all create aerosolized respiratory droplets; usually, droplets evaporate, leaving an organism (droplet nucleus) that is readily carried in the air. Tuberculosis can also be caused by the closely related M. tuberculosis bovis, which is acquired by drinking nonpasteurized milk from infected cows.

The course of tuberculosis depends on age and immune competence, as well as total burden of organisms. Some patients have only an indolent, asymptomatic infection, while in others, tuberculosis is a destructive, disseminated disease. Many more people are infected than develop clinical symptoms. Thus, one must distinguish between infection and active tuberculosis. **Tuberculous infection** means that the organism is growing in a person, whether or not there is symptomatic disease. **Active tuberculosis** denotes the subset of tuberculous infections with destructive, symptomatic disease.

Primary tuberculosis occurs upon first exposure to M. tuberculosis, and may pursue an indolent or aggressive course (Fig. 9-50). **Secondary tuberculosis** develops long after primary infection, mostly by reactivation of primary infection. Secondary disease can also occur by exposure to exogenous organisms and is always an active disease.

Primary Tuberculosis

PATHOPHYSIOLOGY: Inhaled M. tuberculosis deposits in alveoli, usually in the lower segments of lower and middle lobes and anterior segments of upper lobes. The mycobacteria are phagocytosed by

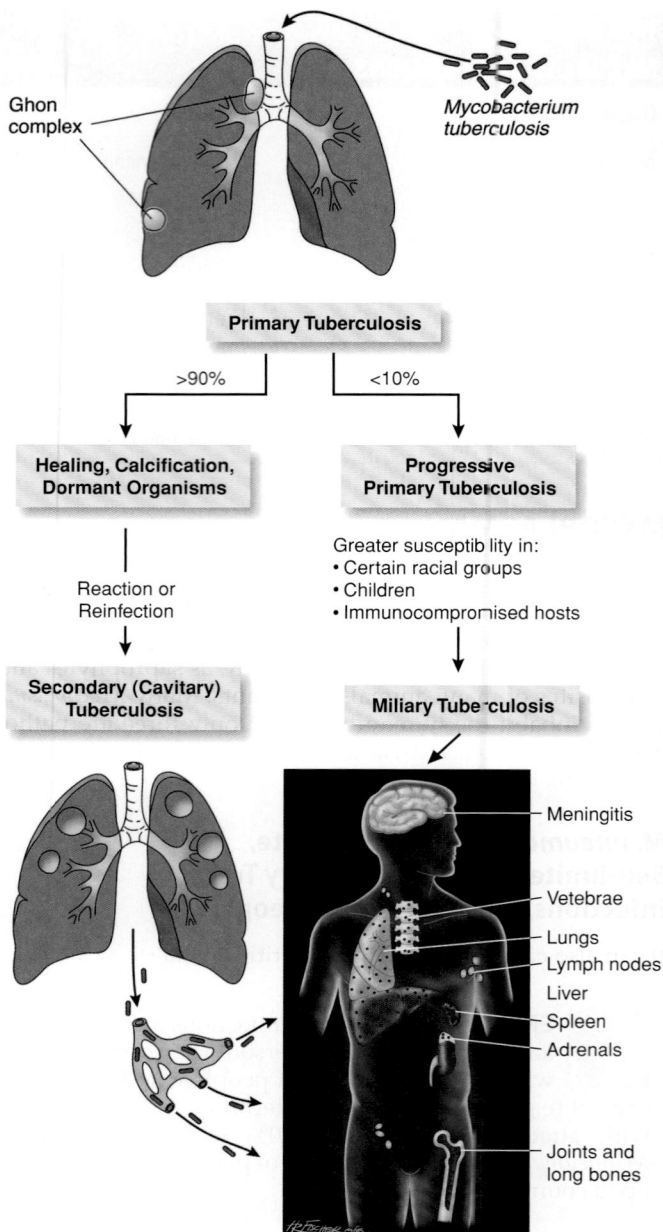

FIGURE 9-50. Stages of tuberculosis. Primary tuberculosis develops in a person lacking previous contact or immune responsiveness. **Progressive primary** tuberculosis develops in less than 10% of infected normal adults, but more frequently in children and immunosuppressed patients. **Secondary** (cavitary) tuberculosis results from reactivation of dormant endogenous bacilli or reinfection with exogenous bacilli. **Miliary** tuberculosis is caused by dissemination of tubercle bacilli to produce many, minute, yellow-white lesions (resembling millet seeds) in distant organs.

alveolar macrophages but resist killing; their cell wall lipids block fusion of phagosomes and lysosomes and allow them to proliferate within macrophages. As bacilli multiply, macrophages degrade some and present antigens to T lymphocytes (see below). Some macrophages carry organisms from the lung to regional (hilar and mediastinal) lymph nodes, from which they may disseminate by the bloodstream. Bacilli continue to proliferate at the primary site in the lungs, and elsewhere including lymph nodes, kidneys, meninges, epiphyseal plates of long bones and vertebrae, and apical areas of the lungs.

Although the macrophages that first ingest *M. tuberculosis* cannot kill it, they initiate hypersensitivity and cell-mediated immunologic responses that eventually contain the infection. Infected macrophages present mycobacterial antigens to T cells. Clones of sensitized T cells proliferate, produce IFNγ and activate macrophages, thus increasing their concentrations of lytic enzymes and augmenting their capacity to kill mycobacteria. The same lytic enzymes may, if released, also damage host tissues.

Development of activated lymphocytes responsive to M. tuberculosis antigen is the hypersensitivity response, leading to emergence of activated macrophages that can ingest and destroy the bacilli—the cell-mediated immune response. These responses together contain the infection, a process requiring 3 to 6 weeks to come into play.

If an infected person is immunologically competent and the burden of organisms is manageable, a vigorous granulomatous reaction is produced. Tubercle bacilli are ingested and killed by activated macrophages, surrounded by fibrous tissue, and successfully contained. If the number of bacilli is high, the hypersensitivity reaction produces significant tissue necrosis, with a consistency resembling cheese (caseous). *M. tuberculosis* does not always cause such necrosis, and is not the only agent that can elicit it, but caseous necrosis is so characteristic that it should raise suspicion of tuberculosis.

In young children or immunocompromised subjects, granulomas are poorly formed or not formed at all, and infection may progress at the primary site in the lung, in the regional lymph nodes or in multiple sites of dissemination. This process produces progressive primary tuberculosis.

PATHOLOGY: The lung lesion of primary tuberculosis is a **Ghon focus**. It occurs in the subpleural area of the upper segments of the lower lobes or in the lower segments of the upper lobes. It starts as a small, ill-defined area of inflammatory consolidation, which then drains to hilar lymph nodes. The combination of a peripheral Ghon focus and involved mediastinal or hilar lymph nodes is a **Ghon complex**. The classic histology of tuberculosis is a granuloma (Fig. 9-51), which has a soft, semisolid core of cheesy debris, surrounded by epithelioid macrophages, Langhans giant cells, lymphocytes, and peripheral fibrous tissue. If the host is immunocompromised, the granulomas may be less organized, with only aggregates of macrophages, without the architecture or Langhans giant cells of the classic granuloma.

In over 90% of normal adults, tuberculous infection is contained. In the lungs and lymph nodes, Ghon complexes heal and shrink, undergo scarring and calcification, the latter visible radiographically. Small numbers of organisms remain viable for years. There is evidence that the fibrosing process is directed by the bacilli, possibly to protect them from the effectiveness of otherwise mycobactericidal host immunity. Later, if immune mechanisms wane or fail, resting bacilli may proliferate and break out, causing serious secondary tuberculosis.

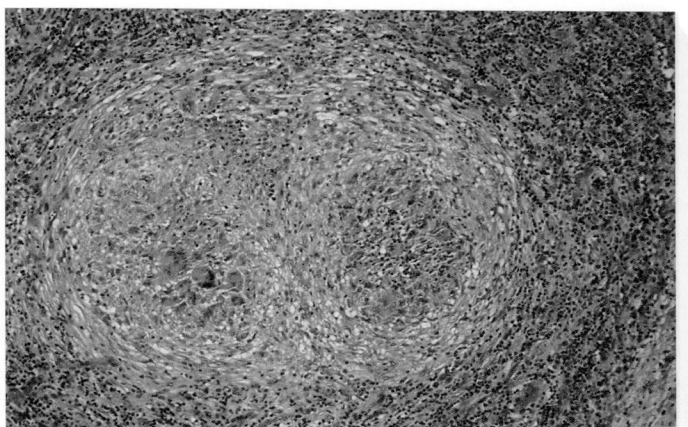

FIGURE 9-51. Primary tuberculosis. A hilar lymph node contains a tuberculous granuloma.

In <10% of normal adults, but more often in children and immunosuppressed patients, **progressive primary tuberculosis** develops. Then, host immune responses fail to control the bacilli. The Ghon focus enlarges and may erode into bronchi. Affected hilar and mediastinal lymph nodes enlarge, sometimes compressing right middle lobe bronchi to cause distal atelectasis (**middle lobe syndrome**). In some instances, the infected lymph nodes erode into an airway to spread organisms throughout the lungs.

Miliary tuberculosis (referring to the appearance of millet seeds) occurs when infection disseminates to produce multiple, small, yellow, nodular lesions in several organs (Fig. 9-52). Such lesions typically involve the lungs, lymph nodes, kidneys, adrenals, bone marrow, spleen, and liver. Progressive disease may affect the meninges, to cause tuberculous meningitis.

CLINICAL FEATURES: Most people contain primary infection successfully, and primary tuberculosis is generally asymptomatic. In those who develop progressive primary disease, symptoms are usually insidious and nonspecific, with fever, weight loss, fatigue, and night sweats. Sometimes onset of symptoms is abrupt, with high fever, pleurisy, pleural effusion, and lymphadenitis. Cough and hemoptysis develop only when active pulmonary disease is well established. In miliary tuberculosis, symptoms depend upon the organs affected and tend to occur late in the course of disease.

Secondary (Cavitary) Tuberculosis

The mycobacteria in secondary tuberculosis come from "dormant" old granulomas (usually) or, less often, newly acquired bacilli. Various conditions, including cancer, antineoplastic chemotherapy, immunosuppressive therapy, AIDS and old age, predispose to reemergence of endogenous hibernating *M. tuberculosis*. Secondary disease may develop even decades after primary infection.

PATHOLOGY: Any location may be involved but the lungs are by far the most common site. There, secondary tuberculosis usually begins in apical–posterior segments of the upper lobes, where organisms

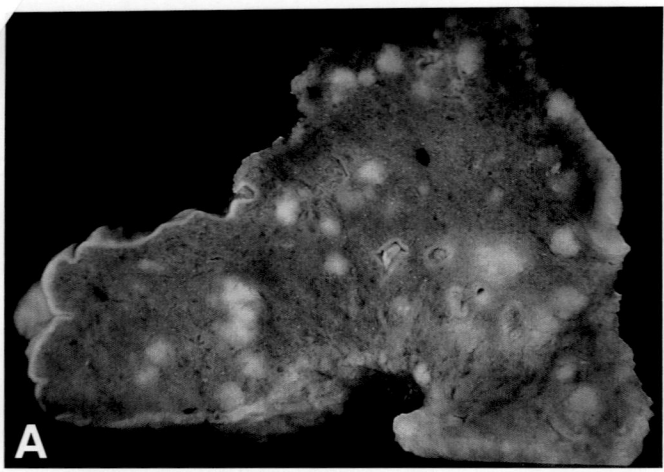
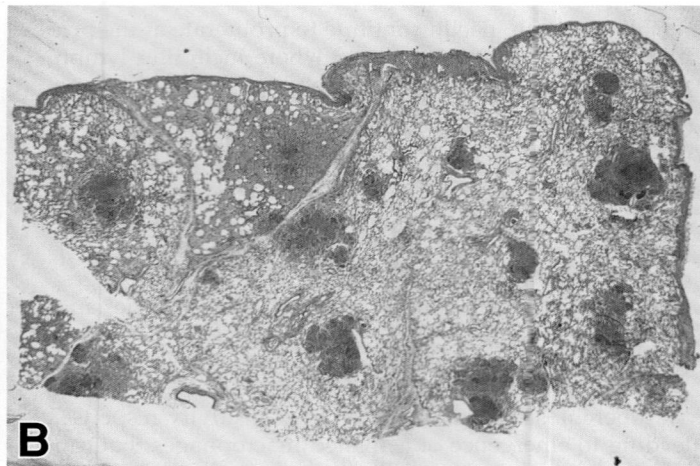

FIGURE 9-52. Miliary tuberculosis. A. The cut surface of the lung with abundant uniform, white nodules. **B.** A low-power photomicrograph discloses many foci of granulomatous inflammation.

are commonly seeded during primary infection. Bacilli proliferate, elicit inflammatory responses and cause localized consolidation. *Ensuing T cell–mediated immune responses to the now familiar tuberculous antigens lead to tissue necrosis and production of tuberculous cavities* (Fig. 9-53). Apical cavities are optimal for *M. tuberculosis* multiplication, and large numbers of organisms are produced in this environment. Cavities are typically 2 to 4 cm when first detected clinically but can exceed 10 cm. They contain necrotic material teeming with mycobacteria and are surrounded by a granulomatous response.

Lung lesions in secondary tuberculosis may be complicated by secondary effects:

- Scarring and calcification
- Spread to other areas
- Pleural fibrosis and adhesions
- Rupture of a caseous lesion, spilling bacilli into the pleural cavity
- Erosion into a bronchus, which seeds bronchioles, bronchi, and trachea
- Implantation of bacilli in the larynx, causing hoarseness and pain on swallowing

Tubercle bacilli may also spread throughout the body through the lymphatics and bloodstream to cause miliary tuberculosis.

 CLINICAL FEATURES: Cough (which may be mistakenly attributed to smoking or a cold), low-grade fever, general malaise, fatigue, anorexia, weight loss, and often night sweats are the usual manifestations. Tissue destruction may affect blood vessels and cause hemoptysis, which may be severe enough to cause exsanguination. Chest radiographs showing unilateral or bilateral apical cavities suggest secondary tuberculosis. If disease is disseminated, signs and symptoms reflect the organs involved.

Untreated secondary tuberculosis is a wasting disease that is eventually fatal. At one time, chronic cavitary tuberculosis was a most common cause of secondary amyloidosis (see Chapter 15). Tuberculosis is now treated with prolonged courses of antituberculous antibiotics, including isoniazid, pyrazinamide, rifampin, and ethambutol. Strains of *M. tuberculosis* resistant to all antibiotics have recently emerged, usually because of poor compliance with the full regimen of antibiotic therapy.

Leprosy Is a Slowly Progressive, Destructive Disease Affecting Skin, Nerves, and Mucous Membranes

It is caused by *Mycobacterium leprae*, a slender, weakly acid-fast rod which cannot be cultured.

EPIDEMIOLOGY: Leprosy is one of the oldest recognized human diseases. Lepers were isolated from the community in the Old Testament. For centuries, leprosy was widespread in Europe, including England. In 1873, Hansen first documented the causative agent (leprosy is also called "Hansen disease").

Lepra bacilli prefer temperatures lower than those in internal organs. Naturally acquired leprosy occurs in

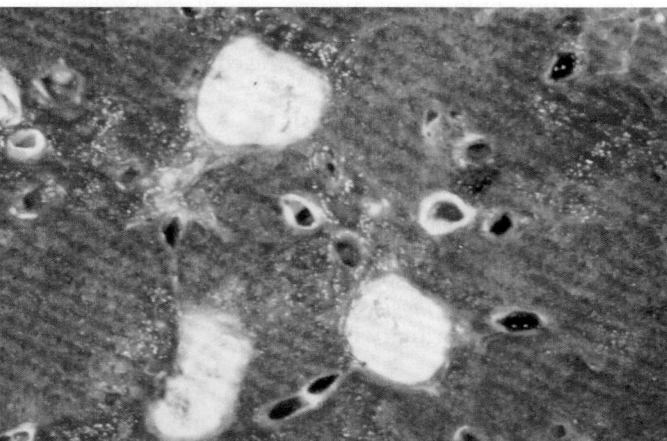

FIGURE 9-53. Secondary pulmonary tuberculosis. A cross-section of lung shows several tuberculous cavities filled with necrotic, caseous material.

armadillos in Louisiana and Texas whose susceptibility is related, at least in part, to their low body temperature (32° to 35°C [89.6° to 95°F]).

Leprosy is transmitted from person to person, after years of intimate contact. *M. leprae* is present in nasal secretions or ulcerated lesions of infected people. The mode of infection is unclear, but probably involves inoculation into the respiratory tract or open wounds. Leprosy is now rare in developed countries (<400 cases in the United States yearly), but worldwide 15 million people are infected, mainly in tropical areas. In total, there are about 6,500 people with leprosy in the United States, of whom 3,300 require active management.

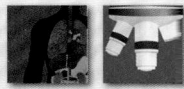 **PATHOPHYSIOLOGY AND PATHOLOGY:** *M. leprae* multiplies best at temperatures below core human body temperature so lesions tend to occur in cooler parts of the body (e.g., hands and face). Leprosy has a bewildering variety of clinical and pathologic features. Lesions vary from small, insignificant and self-healing macules of tuberculoid leprosy to the diffuse, disfiguring, and sometimes fatal lesions of lepromatous leprosy (Fig. 9-54). This extreme variation in disease presentation probably reflects differences in immune reactivity.

Most (95%) people have a natural protective immunity to *M. leprae* and are not infected, despite intimate and prolonged exposure. Susceptible individuals (5%) span a broad spectrum of immune function from anergy to hyperergy, and may develop symptomatic infection. At one end of the spectrum, anergic patients have little or no resistance and develop **lepromatous leprosy**, while hyperergic patients with high resistance contract **tuberculoid leprosy**. Most patients have **borderline leprosy**, in between these extremes.

TUBERCULOID LEPROSY: This is characterized by a single lesion or very few lesions of the skin, usually on the face, extremities, or trunk. Lesions show well-formed, circumscribed dermal granulomas with epithelioid macrophages, Langhans giant cells, and lymphocytes. Nerve fibers are almost invariably swollen and infiltrated with

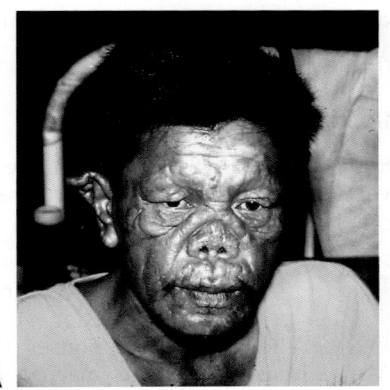 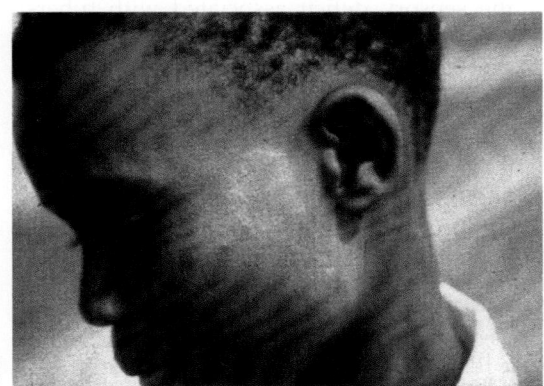
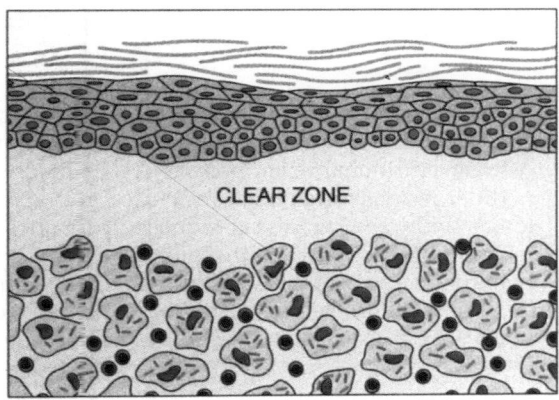 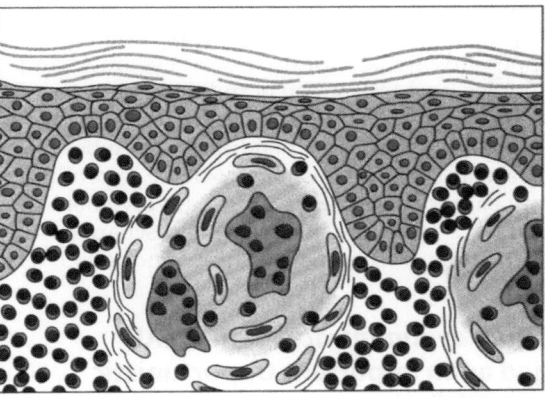

FIGURE 9-54. Leprosy A. (*Top*) **Leonine facies of lepromatous leprosy.** There is diffuse involvement, including a loss of eyebrows and eyelashes and nodular distortions of the face and ears, the exposed (cool) parts of the body. The septum and bone of the nose are damaged, producing "saddle nose" deformity. This Filipino patient also had deformities of the hands and feet. (*Bottom*) The nodular skin lesions of advanced lepromatous leprosy. Swelling has flattened the epidermis (loss of rete ridges). A characteristic "clear zone" of uninvolved dermis separates the epidermis from tumor-like accumulations of macrophages each full of lepra bacilli (*Mycobacterium leprae*). **B.** (*Top*) **Tuberculoid leprosy** on the cheek, showing a hypopigmented macule with a raised, infiltrated border. The central portion may be hypesthetic or anesthetic. (*Bottom*) Macular skin lesion of tuberculoid leprosy. Skin from the raised "infiltrated" margin of the plaque contains discrete granulomas that extend to the basal layer of the epidermis (without a clear zone). The granulomas are composed of epithelioid cells and Langhans giant cells and are associated with lymphocytes and plasma cells. Lepra bacilli are rare.

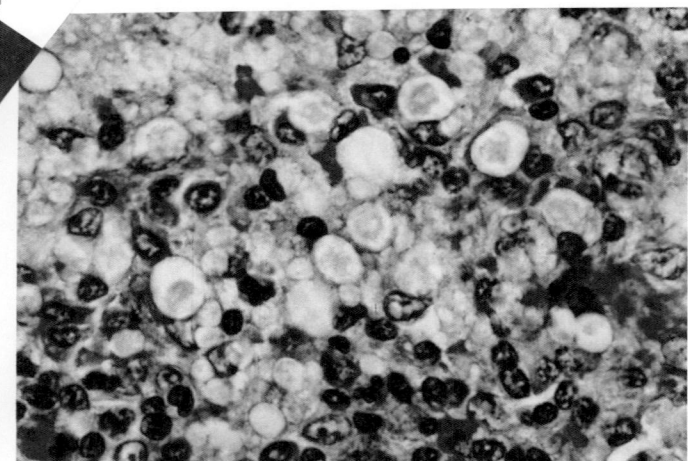

FIGURE 9-55. Lepromatous leprosy. Skin shows a tumor-like mass of foamy macrophages. Faint masses within the vacuolated macrophages are enormous numbers of lepra bacilli.

lymphocytes. Destruction of small dermal nerve twigs accounts for the sensory deficit associated with tuberculoid leprosy. Bacilli are rare and often not found with acid-fast stains. The term "tuberculoid leprosy" is used because the granulomas vaguely resemble those of tuberculosis, though they lack necrosis. The lesions of tuberculoid leprosy cause minimal disfigurement and are not infectious.

LEPROMATOUS LEPROSY: In this form, there are multiple, tumorlike lesions of the skin, eyes, testes, nerves, lymph nodes, and spleen. Nodular or diffuse infiltrates of foamy macrophages contain myriad bacilli (Fig. 9-55). The epidermis is stretched thinly over the nodules. Beneath it is a narrow, uninvolved "clear zone" of the dermis. Rather than destroying the bacilli, macrophages seem to be microincubators. With acid-fast staining, the many organisms inside the macrophages appear as aggregates of acid-fast material, called "globi." As dermal infiltrates expand slowly they distort and disfigure the face, ears and upper airways, and destroy eyes, eyebrows and eyelashes, nerves, and testes. The nodular skin lesions of lepromatous leprosy may ulcerate. Claw-shaped hands, hammertoes, saddle nose, and pendulous ear lobes are common. Nodular facial lesions may coalesce to produce a lionlike appearance ("leonine facies"). Involvement of the upper airways leads to chronic nasal discharge and voice change. Ocular infection may cause blindness.

Mycobacterium avium-intracellulare (MAI) Has Emerged as an Important Opportunistic Infection in AIDS Patients

Mycobacterium avium and *Mycobacterium intracellulare* are similar species that cause identical diseases and so are grouped as *M. avium-intracellulare* (MAI) complex, or simply MAI. They cause two types of disease: (1) a rare, slowly progressive granulomatous pulmonary disease in immunocompetent people, and (2) a progressive systemic disease in patients with AIDS. *MAI infection is the third most common opportunistic infection in AIDS patients in the United States.*

MAI occurs in soil, water, and foodstuffs worldwide. Humans probably acquire it from by inhaling aerosols from infected water. Colonization is common: as much as 70% of the population shows immunologic responsiveness to MAI, indicating prior exposure.

Granulomatous MAI Disease

Most immunocompetent people with granulomatous pulmonary disease caused by MAI are older (50 to 70 years), and have pre-existing pulmonary diseases. *Clinically and pathologically, MAI disease resembles tuberculosis but progresses much more slowly. It causes pulmonary nodules and cavities and necrotizing granulomas.*

CLINICAL FEATURES: Antecedent pulmonary illnesses predisposing to MAI infection in immunocompetent people include chronic obstructive pulmonary disease, treated tuberculosis, pneumoconiosis, and bronchiectasis. Cough is common, but tuberculosis-like symptoms are lacking. MAI lung disease is indolent or only slowly progressive, impairing lung function gradually over years to decades. MAI is resistant to first-line antituberculous drugs, and combination therapies often yield disappointing results.

MAI Infection in AIDS

One-third of AIDS patients in the United States develop overt MAI infection; and half may show evidence of infection at autopsy.

PATHOPHYSIOLOGY: In patients with AIDS, progressive depletion of helper T cells cripples the immune responses that normally prevent MAI disease. Although macrophages phagocytose the organisms, they cannot kill them. Bacilli replicate, fill cells, and spread—first to other macrophages and then throughout the body via the lymphatics and bloodstream.

PATHOLOGY: There are infected macrophages in many organs, and MAI proliferation recruits additional macrophages. As a result, expanding nodular lesions range from structured epithelioid granulomas with few organisms to loose aggregates of foamy macrophages packed with acid-fast bacilli (Fig. 9-56). Eventually, lymph nodes, spleen, and bone marrow may be almost completely replaced by aggregates of macrophages. Lesions in the bowel erode into the gut lumen.

CLINICAL FEATURES: Early, constitutional symptoms of MAI disease in AIDS resemble those of tuberculosis: fever, night sweats, fatigue, and weight loss. Progressive small bowel involvement produces malabsorption and diarrhea, often with abdominal pain. Pulmonary involvement is common but does not usually produce symptoms. Combinations of five or more antibiotics, including clarithromycin, may control, but rarely cure, widespread MAI infection in AIDS patients.

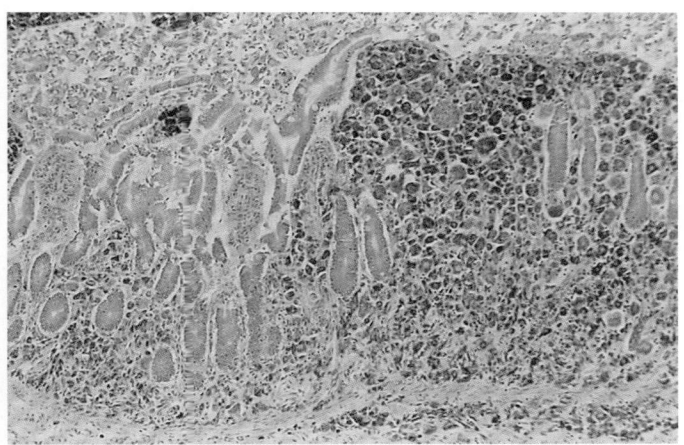

FIGURE 9-56. *Mycobacterium avium-intracellulare* **(MAI).** A section of small bowel from a patient with AIDS shows macrophages stuffed with acid-fast bacilli in the lamina propria.

Other Mycobacteria in Water, Dust, and Dirt May Cause Human Disease

Inhalation, inoculation, or ingestion of environmental material causes human infection.

These bacteria, including MAI, are often grouped as "atypical mycobacteria" (in contrast to the "typical" *M. tuberculosis*). These mycobacteria are biologically diverse and the uncommon diseases that they produce in humans differ (Table 9-7).

- *Mycobacterium kansasii* causes a chronic, slowly progressive granulomatous pulmonary disease in people over 50 years, like that produced by MAI in immunocompetent patients.

- *Mycobacterium scrofulaceum*, a common soil inhabitant, causes a draining, granulomatous, cervical lymphadenitis in young children (aged 1 to 5 years). It affects submandibular lymph nodes and probably results from inoculation or ingestion of organisms by toddlers playing in soil. Disease is localized, and surgical excision of affected lymph nodes is curative.

- *Mycobacterium marinum*, commonly found on underwater surfaces, produces a localized nodular skin lesion ("swimming pool granuloma"), sometimes with lymphatic involvement. Infection is acquired by traumatic inoculation, such as abrading an elbow on a swimming pool ladder or cutting a finger on a fish spine. Tissue reactions may be pyogenic or granulomatous.

- *Mycobacterium ulcerans* leads to a severe ulcerating skin disease in Australia, Africa, and New Guinea. Infection presents as a solitary, undermining, deep ulcer of the skin, and subcutaneous fat of the extremities.

- *Mycobacterium chelonae* and *Mycobacterium fortuitum* are closely related, ubiquitous, environmental organisms. Infection follows inoculation (usually traumatic) of contaminated material. Painless, fluctuant abscesses appear at the site of inoculation, ulcerate and gradually heal spontaneously. Tissue reactions can be pyogenic or granulomatous.

FUNGI

Pneumocystis jiroveci Causes Pneumonia in People With Impaired Immune Defenses

Pneumocystis jiroveci (formerly, carinii) *causes progressive, often fatal, pneumonia in people with impaired cell-mediated immunity.*

Pneumocystis has recently been reclassified as a fungus.

TABLE 9-7					
ATYPICAL MYCOBACTERIAL INFECTIONS					
Organism	**Disease**	**Ages Affected**	**Pathology**	**Source**	**Distribution**
Mycobacterium kansasii	Chronic granulomatous pulmonary disease (similar to that caused by *M. avium-intracellulare*)	50–70	Granulomatous inflammation	Inhaled organisms from soil, dust, or water	Worldwide
Mycobacterium scrofulaceum	Cervical lymphadenitis	1–5	Granulomatous inflammation	Probably ingested organisms from soil or dust	Worldwide
Mycobacterium marinum	Localized skin lesions	All	Granulomatous inflammation	Direct inoculation of organisms from fish or underwater surfaces (swimming pools, fish tanks)	Worldwide
Mycobacterium ulcerans	Large, solitary, severe ulcer of skin and subcutaneous tissue	Usually 5–25	Coagulative necrosis	Probably inoculation of environmental organisms	Australia, Africa
Mycobacterium fortuitum and *Mycobacterium chelonei*	Infections associated with traumatic or iatrogenic inoculations	All	Pyogenic inflammation	Inoculation of environmental organisms	Worldwide

EPIDEMIOLOGY: *P. jiroveci* occurs worldwide. Since 75% of people have antibodies by age 5, exposure is probably by inhalation. If cell-mediated immunity is intact, infection is rapidly contained without symptoms.

Until the 1980s, 100 to 200 cases of active *Pneumocystis* disease were reported annually in the United States, mainly in people with hematologic malignancies, transplant recipients, or those treated with corticosteroids or cytotoxic therapy. *Pneumocystis* became a common pathogen with the AIDS pandemic. Before the advent of effective antiretroviral therapy (see Chapter 4), 80% of AIDS patients developed *Pneumocystis* pneumonia.

PATHOPHYSIOLOGY: *P. jiroveci* reproduces in association with alveolar type 1 lining cells and active disease is confined to the lungs. Infection begins when *Pneumocystis* attaches to alveolar lining cells and feed on host cells. They enlarge and produce cysts that contain daughter organisms. Cysts rupture, releasing more *Pneumocystis*, and the process repeats. Unchecked by the host immune system or antibiotics, infected alveoli eventually fill with organisms and proteinaceous fluid. Progressive filling of alveoli impairs gas exchange and patients slowly suffocate.

It is assumed, but not proven, that most cases reflect reactivation of latent endogenous infection. Outbreaks of *Pneumocystis* pneumonia have also occurred among severely malnourished (and thus immunosuppressed) infants in nurseries; probably representing primary infection.

PATHOLOGY: *P. jiroveci* causes progressive consolidation of the lungs. Microscopically, alveoli contain a frothy eosinophilic material, composed of alveolar macrophages and cysts and *P. jiroveci* (Fig. 9-57A). There are hyaline membranes and prominent type 2 pneumocytes. In newborns, alveolar septa are thickened by lymphoid cells and macrophages. The prominent plasma cells in the infantile disease led to the now obsolete term *plasma cell pneumonia*.

The various forms of *P. jiroveci* are best visualized with methenamine silver stains. The cyst form measures about 60 μm in diameter (Fig. 9-57B); extracellular trophozoites and intracystic forms of the organism appear as irregularly shaped cells, 1 to 3 μm across, with punctate violet nuclei by Giemsa staining.

CLINICAL FEATURES: Patients with *P. jiroveci* pneumonia have fever, a nonproductive cough and progressive dyspnea, often exacerbated by exertion. The latter may start imperceptibly and progress slowly. Chest radiographs show a diffuse pulmonary process. Diagnosis requires recovery of alveolar material. The disease is fatal if untreated. Therapy is with trimethoprim-sulfamethoxazole or pentamidine.

Candida Species Are Common Opportunistic Pathogens

Many *Candida* species are endogenous human flora, well adapted to life on or in the human body, but they can cause disease if host defenses are impaired. *Candida* infections vary in severity, but most are localized and superficial, limited to a particular mucocutaneous site (Table 9-8).

Deep tissue **Candida** *infections are much less common than superficial ones but can be life-threatening.* The most common internal sites affected are the brain, eyes, kidney, and heart. Deep infections, candidal sepsis, and disseminated candidiasis, occur only in immunologically compromised people and are often fatal.

Most derive from endogenous flora. *C. albicans*, which lives in small numbers in the oropharynx, GI tract, and vagina, is most often the offender. It causes >95% of these infections.

PATHOPHYSIOLOGY: Mechanical barriers, inflammatory cells, humoral immunity, and cell-mediated immunity relegate *Candida* to superficial, nonsterile sites. Resident bacterial flora also limit numbers of fungi by: (1) blocking fungal attachment

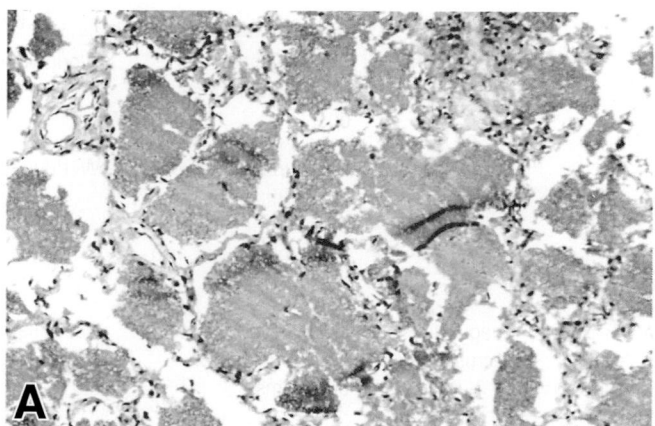
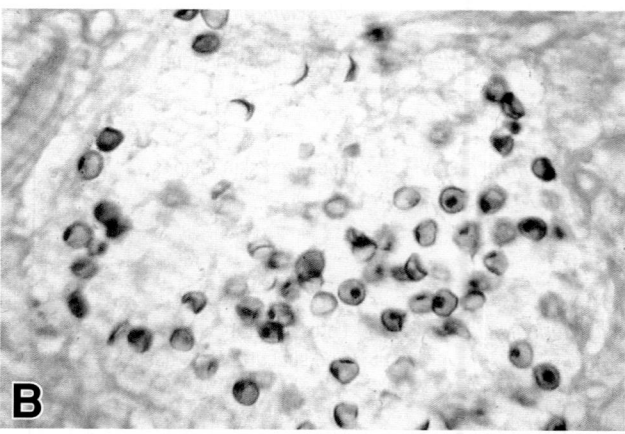

FIGURE 9-57. ***Pneumocystis jiroveci* pneumonia. A.** The alveoli contain a frothy eosinophilic material that is composed of alveolar macrophages and cysts and trophozoites of *P. jiroveci*. **B.** A silver stain shows crescent-shaped organisms, which are collapsed and degenerated. Some have a characteristic dark spot in their walls.

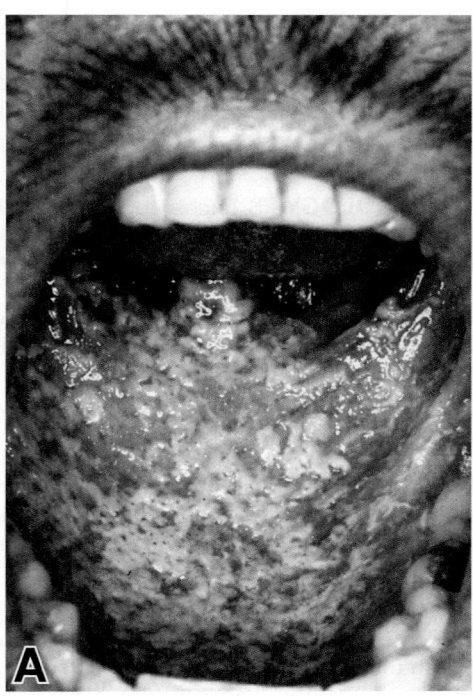

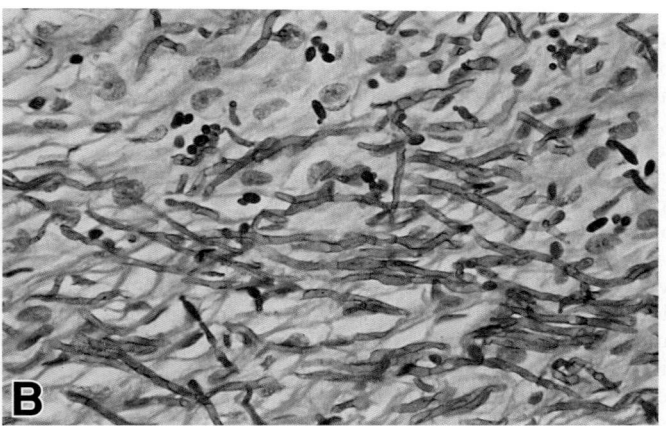

FIGURE 9-58. Candidiasis. A. The oral cavity of a patient with AIDS is covered by a white, curd-like exudate containing many fungal organisms. **B.** A periodic acid–Schiff (PAS) stain shows septate hyphae and yeast forms. 55A. (Reprinted from Farrar WE, Wood MJ, Innes JA, Tubbs H. *Infectious Diseases: Text and Color Atlas.* 2nd ed. New York: Gower Medical Publishing; 1992. Copyright © 1992 Elsevier. With permission.)

to epithelial cells; (2) competing with them for nutrients; and (3) preventing their conversion to tissue-invasive forms. When any of the above defenses is compromised, candidal infections can occur (Table 9-8). *Antibiotic use suppresses competing bacterial flora and is the most common precipitating factor for candidiasis.* Under conditions of unopposed growth, the yeast converts to its invasive form (hyphae or pseudohyphae), invades superficially and elicits inflammatory or immune responses.

Although *Candida* inhabits skin surfaces, it does not cause cutaneous disease without a predisposing skin lesion. The most common such factor is maceration, or softening and destruction of the skin. Chronically warm and moist areas, such as between fingers and toes, between skin folds and under diapers, are prone to maceration and superficial candidal disease.

The incidence of invasive candidal infections is increasing. Frequent use of potent broad-spectrum antibiotics eliminates bacteria that otherwise limit *Candida* colonization. Expanded use of medical devices, such as indwelling catheters, monitors, endotracheal tubes, and urinary catheters, provides access to sterile sites. Immune suppression renders patients less capable of defending themselves from even weak pathogens, such as *Candida*. Finally, IV drug users develop deep candidal infections because they inadvertently inoculate the fungi into the bloodstream.

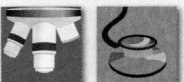 **PATHOLOGY AND CLINICAL FEATURES:** Superficial infections of the skin, oropharynx (Fig. 9-58A) and esophagus show invasive organisms in the most superficial epithelial layers and are associated with acute inflammatory infiltrates. Yeast, pseudohyphae, and hyphae are present (Fig. 9-58B). The yeasts are round and 3 to 4 µm in diameter; the hyphae are septate. In candidal vaginitis superficial fungal invasion of the squamous epithelium elicits scanty inflammation. Deep infections consist of multiple microabscesses with yeast, hyphae, necrotic debris, and neutrophils. Rarely, *Candida* elicit granulomatous responses.

The various superficial cutaneous infections present as tender, erythematous papules, which expand to form confluent erythematous areas.

TABLE 9-8
CANDIDAL INFECTIONS

Disease	Predisposing Conditions
Superficial Infections	
Intertrigo (opposed skin surfaces)	Maceration
Paronychia (nail beds)	Maceration
Diaper rash	Maceration
Vulvovaginitis	Alteration in normal flora
Thrush (oral)	Decreased cell-mediated immunity
Esophagitis	Decreased cell-mediated immunity
Deep Infections	
Urinary tract infections	Indwelling urinary catheters
Sepsis and disseminated infection	Neutropenia, indwelling vascular catheters and change in normal flora

hrush: This lesion involves the tongue and mucous membranes of the mouth. Early in life, it is the most common form of mucocutaneous candidiasis. Friable, white, curdlike membranes adhere to affected surfaces and patches contain fungi, necrotic debris, neutrophils, and bacteria. These can be dislodged by scraping, leaving a painful, bleeding surface.

- **Vulvovaginitis:** This condition causes a thick, white vaginal discharge with vaginal and vulvar itching. Involved vulvar areas are erythematous and tender. Candidal vaginitis is most intense when vaginal pH is low, and, during pregnancy, predisposes newborns to infection. Antibiotics, pregnancy, diabetes, and corticosteroids predispose to this form of vaginitis.
- **Sepsis and disseminated candidiasis:** Systemic candidiasis is rare, and is ordinarily a terminal event in someone with altered immunity or neutropenia. Several *Candida* species can produce such invasive disease. Organisms may enter through ulcerated skin or mucous membrane lesions or be introduced iatrogenically (e.g., intravenous lines, urinary catheters). The urinary tract is most commonly involved, and the incidence in women is four times that in men. Renal lesions may be bloodborne or may arise from ascending infection.
- **Endocarditis:** Large vegetations on the heart valves may lead to a high incidence of embolization to large arteries. Such patients are not usually immunosuppressed but have other vulnerabilities. Drug addicts who use unsterilized needles and people with pre-existing valvular disease who have had prolonged antibacterial therapy or indwelling vascular catheters are at risk for endocarditis. One of the most serious complications of invasive candidiasis is septic embolism to the brain.

Aspergillus Species Often Cause Opportunistic Lung Infections

These common environmental fungi usually cause three types of pulmonary disease: (1) **allergic bronchopulmonary aspergillosis**, (2) **colonization of a pre-existing pulmonary cavity** (**aspergilloma** or **fungus ball**), and (3) **invasive aspergillosis** (see Chapter 18). Of over 200 identified species of *Aspergillus*, about 20 cause human disease, *A. fumigatus* being by far the most frequent.

EPIDEMIOLOGY: *Aspergillus* is a saprophyte found worldwide in soil, decaying plant matter and dung. Pulmonary aspergillosis comes from inhaling small (2 to 3 μm) airborne spores, **conidia**, that are ubiquitous. The spores are small enough to reach alveoli when inhaled. Exposure is greatest when the fungus' habitat is disturbed, as during soil excavations or handling decaying organic matter.

In tissues, *Aspergillus* show septate hyphae, 2 to 7 μm, branching progressively at acute angles (*Aspergillus* from the Latin *aspergere*, "to sprinkle"). The aspergillum is used to sprinkle holy water during Catholic religious ceremonies.

Allergic Bronchopulmonary Aspergillosis

Inhaling *Aspergillus* spores delivers fungal antigens to airways and alveoli. Subsequent contact may trigger an allergic response in susceptible people. Spores that germinate and grow in airways may cause ongoing antigen exposure. Allergic bronchopulmonary aspergillosis is virtually restricted to asthmatics, 20% of whom eventually develop this disorder (see Chapter 18).

PATHOLOGY: Bronchi and bronchioles show infiltrates of lymphocytes, plasma cells, and variable numbers of eosinophils. Sometimes airways are impacted with mucus and fungal hyphae, which are not invasive. Patients experience exacerbations of asthma, often accompanied by pulmonary infiltrates and eosinophilia.

Aspergillomas

Inhaled spores germinate in the warm humid atmosphere provided by pre-existing cavities in the lungs, and fill them with masses of hyphae. The organisms do not invade (see Chapter 18).

PATHOLOGY: Aspergillomas are dense, roundish masses of tangled hyphae, 1 to 7 cm, within a fibrous cavity. The cavity wall is collagenous connective tissue, with lymphocytes and plasma cells. The hyphae do not invade adjacent tissues.

Aspergillomas occur most commonly in cavities left by previous tuberculous. Symptoms reflect the underlying disease. The radiologic appearance of a dense round ball in a cavity is characteristic. Aspergillomas are usually best left untreated, but surgical excision may be indicated in some cases.

Invasive Aspergillosis

Invasive aspergillosis may occur in immunocompromised people. The most common settings are high-dose steroid or cytotoxic therapy or acute leukemia. In profoundly neutropenic patients, inhaled spores germinate to produce hyphae. These invade through bronchi into lung parenchyma, from where the fungi may spread widely.

PATHOLOGY: *Aspergillus* readily invades blood vessels and produces thrombosis (Fig. 9-59). As a result, multiple nodular infarcts are seen throughout both lungs. Involvement of larger pulmonary arteries results in large, wedge-shaped, pleural-based infarcts. Vascular invasion also leads to fungus dissemination to other organs. Microscopically, *Aspergillus* hyphae are arranged radially around blood vessels and extend through their walls. Acute aspergillosis may also start in a nasal sinus and spread to the face, orbit, and brain.

CLINICAL FEATURES: Invasive aspergillosis presents as fever and multifocal pulmonary infiltrates in compromised patients. Frequent thrombosis and bloodstream dissemination portend a fatal outcome. Antifungal therapy with high-dose amphotericin B may be successful but if initiated early.

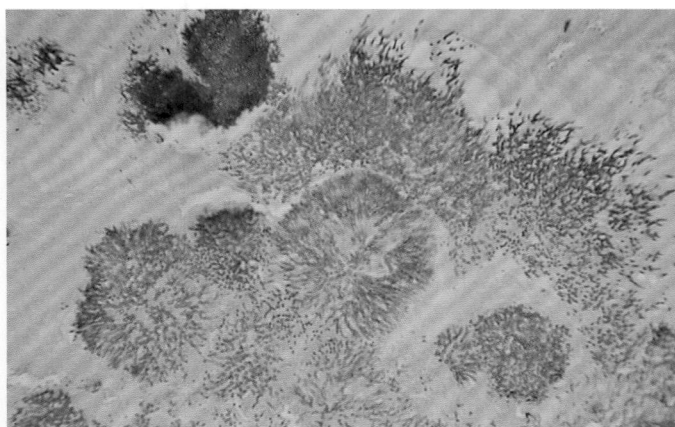

FIGURE 9-59. Invasive aspergillosis. A section of lung impregnated with silver shows branching fungal hyphae surrounding blood vessels and invading adjacent parenchyma.

Mucormycosis Is Usually a Necrotizing Opportunistic Infection

Several related environmental fungi of the class Zygomycetes—*Rhizopus, Mucor, Rhizomucor, and Absidia*—produce severe, invasive infections called **mucormycoses** or **zygomycoses** that begin in the nasal sinuses or lungs.

In tissues, zygomycetes have large (8 to 15 μm) hyphae that branch at right angles, have thin walls and lack septa. In tissue sections, they appear as hollow tubes. Lacking cross walls, their liquid contents flow, leaving long empty segments. They also may resemble "twisted ribbons," which represent collapsed hyphae.

EPIDEMIOLOGY: *Rhizopus, Rhizomucor, Mucor, and Absidia* are ubiquitous in soil, food, and decaying vegetable matter. Their spores are inhaled, and in susceptible people, disease begins in the respiratory system. Mucormycosis occurs almost exclusively in the setting of compromised defenses. Common causes include severe neutropenia (e.g., after treatment for leukemia), high-dose glucocorticoid therapy and, particularly, severe diabetes.

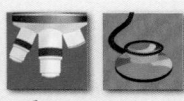

PATHOLOGY AND CLINI[...] TURES: The main forms of m[...] sis are rhinocerebral, pulmo[...] subcutaneous.

- **Rhinocerebral mucormycosis:** Fungi pro[...] in nasal sinuses, invade surrounding tissu[...] extend into facial soft tissues, nerves, blood v[...] and the brain. The palate or nasal turbinate[...] covered by a black crust and underlying tiss[...] friable and hemorrhagic. Fungal hyphae grow [...] the arteries and cause devastating, rapidly progr[...] sive, septic infarction of affected tissues. Extensi[...] into the brain causes fatal, necrotizing, hemorrhag[...] encephalitis. Involved tissues must be excise[...] amphotericin B given and the predisposing abnor[...] mality corrected.
- **Pulmonary mucormycosis:** This infection resembles invasive pulmonary aspergillosis, including vascular invasion and multiple areas of septic infarction (Fig. 9-60). Rhinocerebral and pulmonary mucormycosis are usually fatal.
- **Subcutaneous zygomycosis:** This infection is limited to the tropics and caused by *Basidiobolus haptosporus*, which grows slowly in the panniculus. It causes a slowly enlarging, hard inflammatory mass, usually on the shoulder, trunk, buttock, or thigh.

Cryptococcosis Mainly Affects Meninges and Lungs

Cryptococcosis is a systemic mycosis caused by *C. neoformans*, which mainly affects the meninges and lungs (Fig. 9-61). *C. neoformans* has a worldwide distribution. Its main reservoir is pigeon droppings, which are alkaline and hyperosmolar. These conditions keep cryptococci small, allowing inhaled organisms to reach the terminal bronchioles. *C. neoformans* is unique among pathogenic fungi in having a proteoglycan capsule, which is essential for pathogenicity. The organisms appear as faintly basophilic yeasts with a clear 3- to 5-μm thick mucinous capsule.

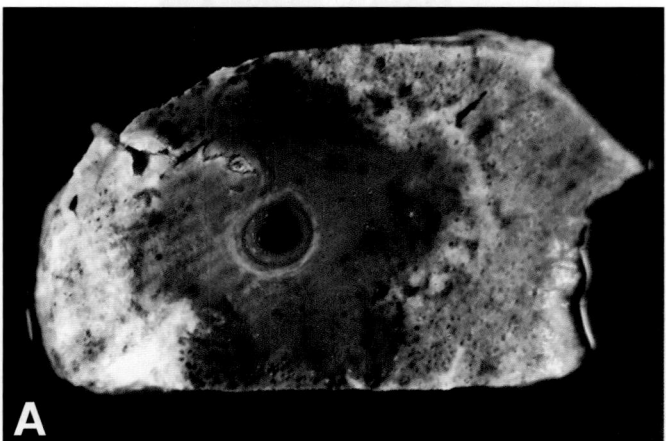

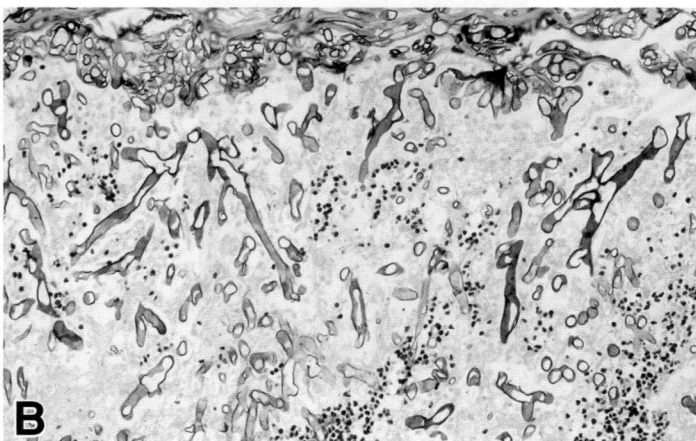

FIGURE 9-60. Pulmonary mucormycosis. A. A cross-section of the lung shows the vessel in the center of the field to be invaded by mucormycetes and occluded by a septic thrombus. The surrounding tissue is infarcted. **B.** Silver stained *Mucor*-infected lung, with broad, nonseptate hyphae of irregular caliber that branch at approximately 90-degree angles.

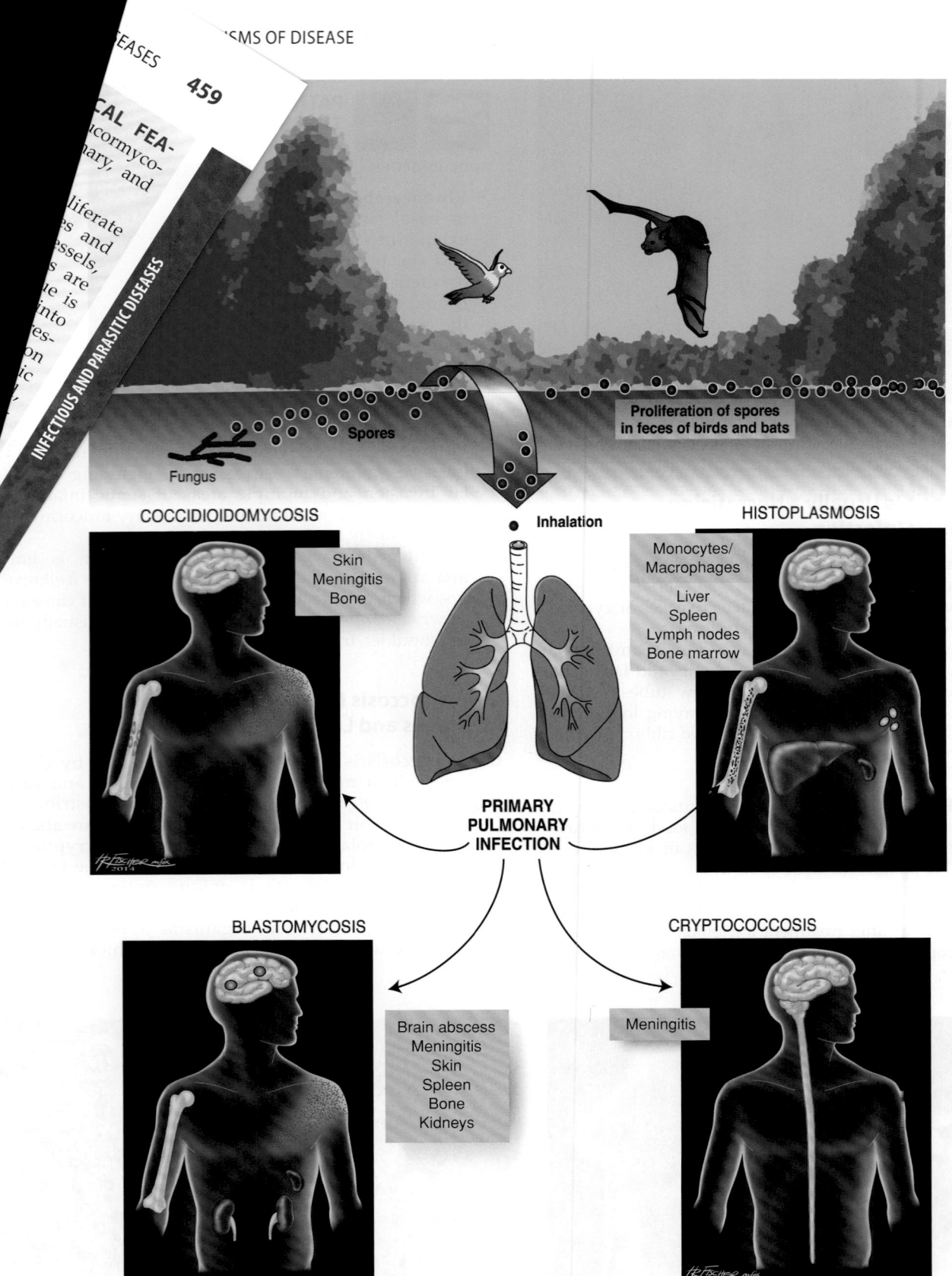

FIGURE 9-61. Pulmonary and disseminated fungal infection. Fungi grow in soil, air, and the feces of birds and bats; they produce spores, some of which are infectious. When inhaled, spores cause primary pulmonary infection. In a few patients, the infection disseminates. **Histoplasmosis.** Primary infection is in the lung. In susceptible patients, the fungus disseminates to target organs, namely, the monocyte/macrophage system (liver, spleen, lymph nodes, and bone marrow) and the tongue, mucous membranes of the mouth and the adrenals. **Cryptococcosis.** Primary infection of the lung disseminates to the meninges. **Blastomycosis.** Primary infection of the lung disseminates widely. The principal targets are the brain, meninges, skin, spleen, bone, and kidney. **Coccidioidomycosis.** Primary infection of the lung may disseminate widely. The skin, meninges, and bone are common targets.

EPIDEMIOLOGY: Cryptococcus *mainly affects people with impaired cell-mediated immunity.* Although the organism is ubiquitous and exposure is common, cryptococcosis is uncommon in the absence of predisposing illness. Disease is uncommon even among people such as pigeon fanciers, who are exposed to it in high concentrations. Cryptococcosis affects patients with AIDS, lymphomas (particularly Hodgkin disease), leukemias, sarcoidosis, and people on high doses of corticosteroids.

PATHOPHYSIOLOGY: In immunologically intact people, neutrophils and alveolar macrophages kill *C. neoformans* and no clinical disease develops. In patients with defective cell-mediated immunity, the fungi survive, reproduce locally, and then disseminate. Although the lung is the portal of entry, disease most often affects the CNS.

PATHOLOGY: Over 95% of cryptococcal infections involve the meninges and brain. Lesions in the lungs can be found in half of patients. In a small minority skin, liver, and other involvement occurs. In meningoencephalitis, the entire brain is swollen and soft. Leptomeninges are thickened and gelatinous due to the thickly encapsulated organisms. Inflammatory responses vary, but are often muted or minimal: large numbers of cryptococci infiltrate tissue with no inflammatory response. If present, inflammation may be neutrophilic, lymphocytic, or granulomatous.

Cryptococcosis in the lung may appear as diffuse disease or as isolated areas of consolidation. Affected alveoli are distended by clusters of organisms, usually with minimal inflammation.

Because of its thick capsule, *C. neoformans* stains poorly with routine H&E, and appears as bubbles or holes in tissue sections (Fig. 9-62A). Fungal stains (PAS and GMS) show the yeasts well but do not stain the polysaccharide capsule. The organism thus appears to be surrounded by a halo. The capsule can be highlighted by mucicarmine stain (Fig. 9-62B).

CLINICAL FEATURES: Cryptococc. ease often begins insidiously with symptoms, including headache, dizzin iness, and loss of coordination. Untreated cry meningitis is invariably fatal. Therapy requires p systemic administration of antifungal agents. Cry cal pneumonia presents as diffuse progressive puli disease.

Severity of Infection With *Histoplasma capsulatum* Varies Greatly

Histoplasmosis is caused by *H. capsulatum*. *Infection is ally self-limited but may cause systemic granulomate disease.* Most cases are asymptomatic, but progressive d seminated infections occur in people with impaired ce mediated immunity. *H. capsulatum* is a dimorphic fungu of worldwide distribution that grows as a mold at ambien temperatures and as a yeast in the body. The yeast cell is round and has a central basophilic body surrounded by a clear zone or halo, which in turn is encircled by a rigid 2- to 4-μm cell wall. In caseous lesions, silver impregnation identifies the remains of degenerating yeast forms.

EPIDEMIOLOGY: Histoplasmosis is acquired by inhaling infectious spores (Fig. 9-61). The reservoir for the fungus is bird droppings and soil. In the Americas, hyperendemic areas are the eastern and central United States, western Mexico, Central America, the northern countries of South America, and Argentina. In the tropics, bat nests, caves, and soil beneath trees are foci of exposure.

PATHOPHYSIOLOGY: Histoplasmosis resembles tuberculosis in many ways. Primary infection begins with phagocytosis of microconidia by alveolar macrophages. Like *M. tuberculosis*, *H. capsulatum* reproduces in immunologically naïve macrophages. As organisms grow, additional macrophages come to the site of infection, producing an area of pulmonary consolidation. A few macrophages carry organisms first to hilar and mediastinal

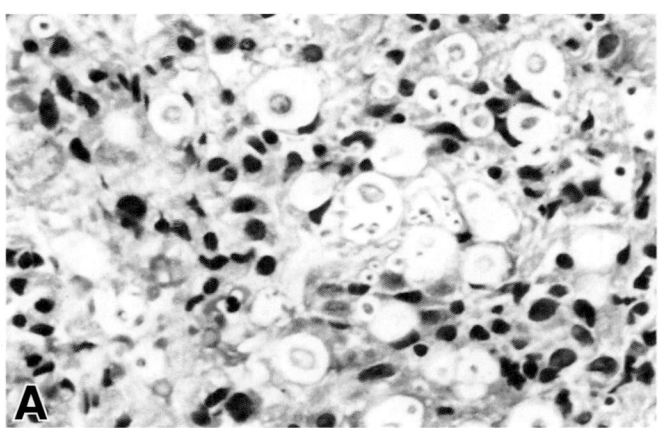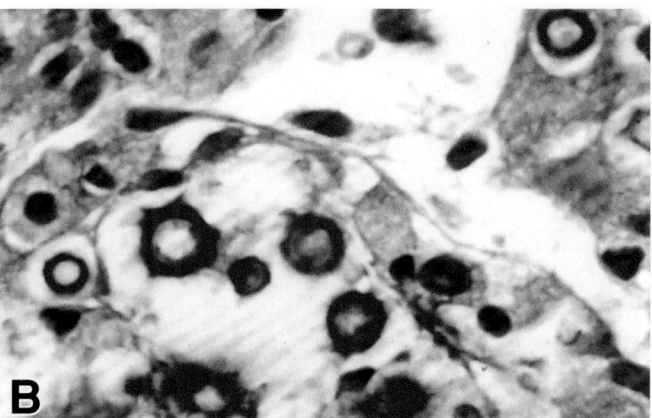

FIGURE 9-62. Cryptococcosis. A. In a section of the lung stained with hematoxylin and eosin, *Cryptococcus neoformans* appears as holes or bubbles. **B.** The same section stained with mucicarmine illustrates the capsule of the organism.

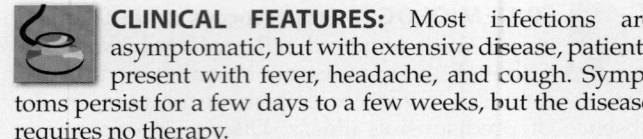

...ody, where fungi infect ... *capsulatum* proliferates ...sitivity and cell-mediated ...eeks later. Normal immune ... infection. Activated macro-...tosed yeasts, forming necrotiz-...nfection.

...n varies with the size of the infect-...e immunologic competence of the ...95%) involve small inocula of organ-...mpetent people. They affect small areas ...egional lymph nodes and remain unno-...er hand, exposure to a large inoculum, ...n excavated bird roost, may cause rapidly ...monary disease, large areas of consolidation, ...mediastinal and hilar nodal involvement and ...preading to the liver, spleen, and bone marrow. ...minated histoplasmosis develops in people who ...mount effective immune responses to *H. capsula-*...nfants, AIDS patients, and people treated with corti-...teroids are at particular risk. Some individuals with no ...own underlying illness may also develop disseminated ...istoplasmosis.

PATHOLOGY: In **acute self-limited histoplasmosis**, necrotizing granulomas occur in the lung, mediastinal and hilar lymph nodes, spleen, and liver. Early in infection, the caseous material is surrounded by macrophages, Langhans giant cells, lymphocytes, and plasma cells. Macrophages and the necrotic material contain yeast forms of *H. capsulatum*. Eventually, the cells in the granuloma largely disappear and the caseous material calcifies, forming a "fibrocaseous nodule" (Fig. 9-63A).

In **disseminated histoplasmosis** macrophages carrying *H. capsulatum* infiltrate many organs progressively (Fig. 9-63B). In mild cases, immune responses can control—but not eliminate—the organism. For long periods, disease remains limited to macrophages in infected organs. If a patient is immunocompromised, clusters of macrophages filled with *H. capsulatum* infiltrate the liver, spleen, lungs, intestine, adrenals, and meninges.

CLINICAL FEATURES: Most infections are asymptomatic, but with extensive disease, patients present with fever, headache, and cough. Symptoms persist for a few days to a few weeks, but the disease requires no therapy.

In disseminated histoplasmosis, weight loss, intermittent fever, and weakness occur. If the immunodeficiency is subtle, the disease may persist and progress for years, even decades. With more profound immunodeficiency, dissemination progresses rapidly, often with high fever, cough, pancytopenia, and changes in mental status. Disseminated histoplasmosis requires systemic antifungal agents.

Coccidioidomycosis Is a Chronic, Necrotizing Mycotic Infection

The disease, caused by *Coccidioides immitis*, resembles tuberculosis clinically and pathologically, and includes a spectrum of infections. They begin as focal pneumonitis. Most are mild and asymptomatic, and are limited to the lungs and local lymph nodes. Occasionally, *C. immitis* infections disseminate, to cause life-threatening disease.

EPIDEMIOLOGY: *C. immitis* is a dimorphic fungus that grows as a mold in the soil, where it forms spores. Inhaled spores reach the alveoli and terminal bronchioles (Fig. 9-61), enlarge into spherules and then mature to form **sporangia**, 30 to 60 μm across. These gradually fill with 1- to 5-μm **endospores**, which accumulate by endosporulation, a process unique among pathogenic fungi. The sporangia eventually rupture and release endospores, that then repeat the cycle.

C. immitis occurs in the soil in restricted climatic regions, particularly the Lower Sonoran life zones of the Western hemisphere. These are areas with sparse rainfall, hot summers, and mild winters. In the United States, large portions of California, Arizona, New Mexico, and Texas are natural habitats for *C. immitis*. The disease is particularly common in California's San Joaquin Valley, where it is called "**valley fever**." It also occurs in Mexico and parts of South America.

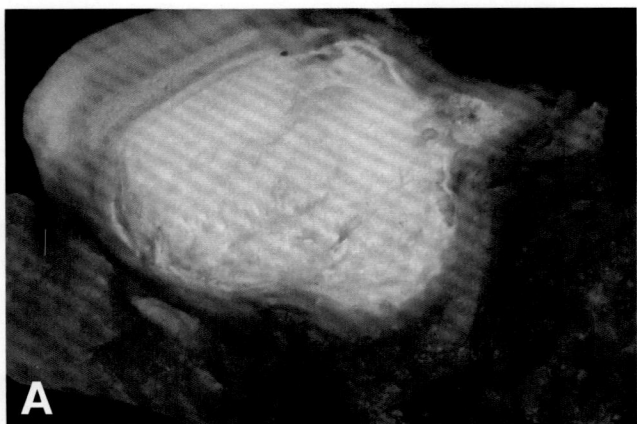

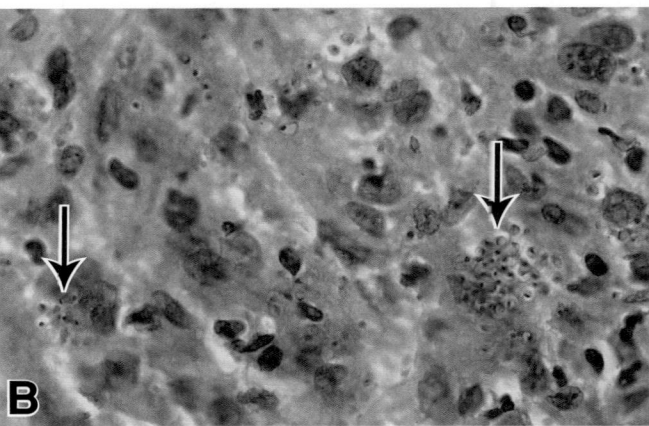

FIGURE 9-63. Histoplasmosis. A. A section of lung shows an encapsulated, subpleural, fibrocaseous nodule. **B.** Liver from a patient with disseminated histoplasmosis shows Kupffer cells containing yeasts of *Histoplasma capsulatum* (*arrows*) (periodic acid–Schiff [PAS] stain).

Long-term residents of endemic regions are almost always infected with *C. immitis*. Even brief visits to these areas can cause infection (usually asymptomatic). Dry, windy weather, which lifts spores into the air, favors infection. The disease is not contagious.

PATHOPHYSIOLOGY: Coccidioidomycosis begins with focal bronchopneumonia where the spores are deposited. These elicit mixed inflammatory infiltrates of neutrophils and macrophages, but the spores survive these. As in tuberculosis and histoplasmosis, the host controls *C. immitis* infection only when inflammatory cells become activated. Necrotizing granulomas form, coincident with specific hypersensitivity and cell-mediated immunity, which kills or contains the fungi.

The course of coccidioidomycosis varies from acute, self-limited disease to disseminated infection, depending on the infecting dose and immune status of the host. Coccidioidomycosis begins with focal bronchopneumonia. Most infections are caused by small inocula in immunocompetent hosts, and are acute and self-limited. Extensive pulmonary involvement and fulminant disease may occur when people from a nonendemic region are exposed to large numbers of organisms.

Disseminated coccidioidomycosis from a primary infection or reactivation of old disease. Immunologically compromised patients are at greatest risk. Certain racial groups, including Filipinos, other Asians, and African-Americans, are particularly susceptible to this form of infection, perhaps because of a specific immune deficit. The risk of dissemination among Filipinos is 175 times that in whites. Pregnant women are also unusually susceptible to disseminated disease if a primary infection occurs in the second half of pregnancy.

PATHOLOGY: Acute self-limited coccidioidomycosis causes solitary lesions or patchy pulmonary consolidation, in which affected alveoli are infiltrated by neutrophils and macrophages *C. immitis* spherules elicit an infiltrate of macrophages, but endospores mainly attract neutrophils. Once an immune response begins, necrotizing granulomas develop. Successful immune responses cause the granuloma to heal, sometimes leaving a fibrocaseous nodule, with a necrotic core, surrounded by residual macrophages and a thin capsule. Unlike histoplasmosis, old granulomas of coccidioidomycosis rarely calcify.

C. immitis spherules and endospores stain with H&E (Fig. 9-64). Spherules in various stages of development appear as basophilic rings. Mature spherules (sporangia) contain endospores that appear as smaller basophilic rings. As in other fungal infections, PAS and GMS stains help visualize *C. immitis*.

Disseminated coccidioidomycosis may involve almost any body site and may manifest as a single extrathoracic site or as widespread disease, involving the skin (Fig. 9-65), bones, meninges, liver, spleen, and genitourinary tract. Inflammatory responses at sites of dissemination are highly variable, ranging from infiltrates of neutrophils to granulomas.

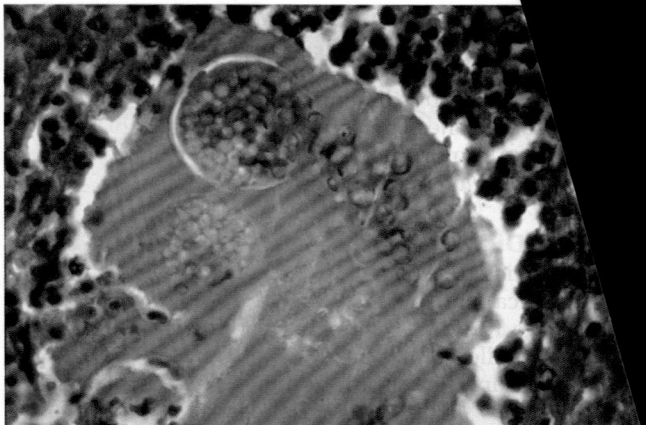

FIGURE 9-64. Coccidioidomycosis. Lung from a patient with ac coccidioidal pneumonia shows spherules containing endospores of *Coccidioides immitis*.

CLINICAL FEATURES: Coccidioidomycosis is a disease of protean manifestations, from a subclinical respiratory infection to one that disseminates and is rapidly fatal. Like syphilis and typhoid fever, it is a great imitator: almost any complaint or syndrome may be its initial presentation.

Most people with coccidioidomycosis (>60%) are asymptomatic. Others develop a flulike syndrome, with fever, cough, chest pain, and malaise, that resolves spontaneously. Cavitation, which may resemble that of tuberculosis, is the most common pulmonary complication, but it is fortunately uncommon (<5%). Such cavities are usually solitary and may persist for years. Progression or reactivation may lead to destructive lesions in the lungs, or more seriously, to disseminated lesions.

The signs and symptoms of disseminated coccidioidomycosis depend on the sites affected. Coccidioidal meningitis manifests with headache, fever, alteration in mental status or seizures and is fatal if untreated. Skin lesions in disseminated disease often have a warty appearance (Fig. 9-65). Even with prolonged amphotericin B therapy, the prognosis is poor in acute disseminated coccidioidomycosis but newer azole antifungal agents are promising.

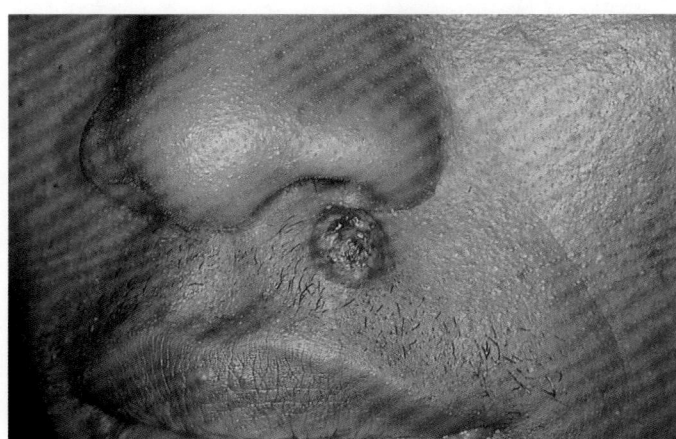

FIGURE 9-65. Disseminated coccidioidomycosis. A single raised, central ulcerated lesion is present on the face.

...ulomatous and ...se

...mation to other body sites, ...sative organism, *Blastomyces* ...ngus that grows as a mold in ...aying vegetable matter.

...GY: The infection occurs within ...ographic regions of the Americas, ... possibly the Middle East. In North ...us is endemic in the Mississippi and ...ys, the Great Lakes, and St. Lawrence ...ce of the soil, either by construction or by ...es such as hunting or camping, leads to for-...osols containing fungal spores.

PATHOPHYSIOLOGY: Blastomycosis is acquired ... by inhaling infectious spores of *B. dermatitidis* ... from the soil (Fig. 9-61). The spores germinate to ...n yeasts, which reproduce by budding. The host ...sponds to this challenge with neutrophils and macro-...phages, producing a focal bronchopneumonia. However, ...organisms persist until immunity starts and activated phagocytic cells kill the fungi.

PATHOLOGY: Blastomycosis is usually confined to the lungs, where it mostly produces small areas of consolidation. *B. dermatitidis* incites mixed suppurative and granulomatous inflammation. Even in the same patient, lesions may range from neutrophilic abscesses to epithelioid granulomas. Pulmonary disease usually resolves by scarring, but some patients develop progressive miliary lesions or cavities. The skin (>50%) and bones (>10%) are the most common sites of extrapulmonary involvement. Skin infection often elicits marked pseudoepitheliomatous hyperplasia, giving lesions a warty appearance.

Infected areas contain many yeast forms, which are spherical and 8 to 14 μm across, with broad-based buds and multiple nuclei in a central body (Fig. 9-66). With H&E

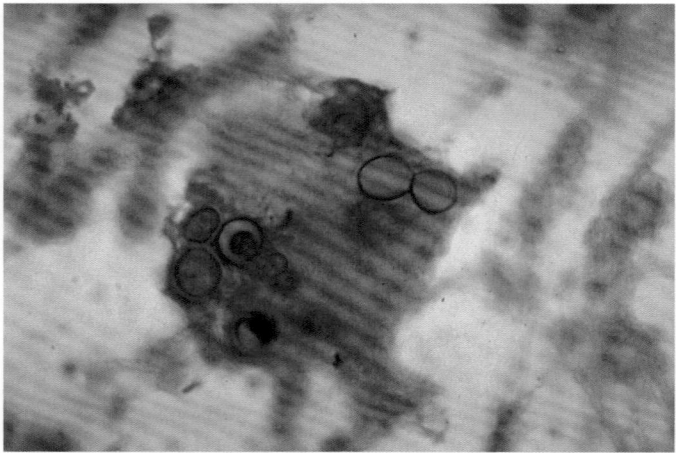

FIGURE 9-66. Blastomycosis. Yeasts of *Blastomyces dermatitidis* have a doubly contoured wall and nuclei in the central body. The buds have broad-based attachments.

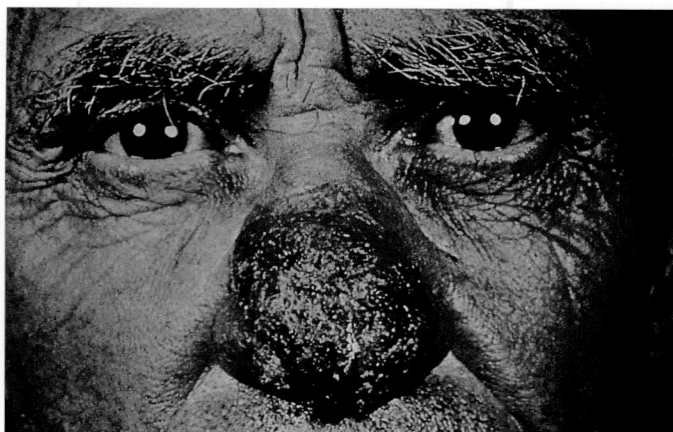

FIGURE 9-67. Cutaneous blastomycosis with ulceration.

stains, the yeasts are rings with thick, sharply defined cell walls. They may be in epithelioid cells, macrophages or giant cells, or they may lie free in microabscesses.

CLINICAL FEATURES: Pulmonary blastomycosis is self-limited in one-third of cases. Symptomatic acute infection begins as a flulike illness, with fever, arthralgias, and myalgias. In progressive pulmonary disease, low-grade fever, weight loss, cough, and mainly upper lobe infiltrates develop. Skin lesions are the most common signs of extrapulmonary dissemination, and resemble squamous cell carcinomas (Fig. 9-67). Although lung infections may appear to resolve totally, disease may reappear in some patients at distant sites months to years later.

Paracoccidioidomycosis Starts in Lungs and Disseminates Widely

Also called South American blastomycosis, paracoccidioidomycosis can involve skin, oropharynx, adrenals, and macrophages in the liver, spleen, and lymph nodes. *Paracoccidioides brasiliensis* is a dimorphic fungus, whose mold form is thought to live in soil.

EPIDEMIOLOGY: Infection begins by inhaling spores from the environment in limited regions of Central and South America. Most infections are asymptomatic. Reactivation of latent infection occurs and active disease can develop many years after someone leaves an endemic region. Men develop symptomatic infections 15 times more often than women.

PATHOLOGY: Paracoccidioidomycosis may only affect the lungs (Fig. 9-68), or involve extrapulmonary sites, like skin, mucosal surfaces, and lymph nodes. *P. brasiliensis* elicits a mixed suppurative and granulomatous response, with lesions like those in blastomycosis and coccidioidomycosis.

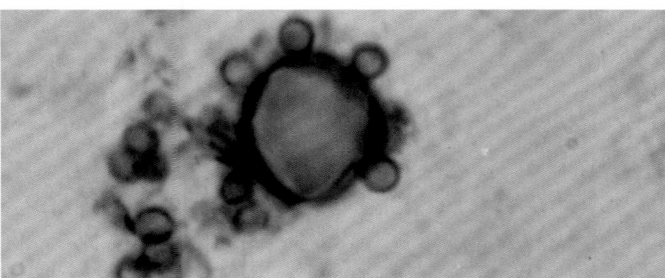

FIGURE 9-68. Paracoccidioidomycosis. The lung contains *Paracoccidioides braziliensis,* with many circumferential external buds arising from the mother organism.

 CLINICAL FEATURES: Disease is usually acute, self-limited and mild. Symptoms of progressive pulmonary involvement resemble those of tuberculosis. Chronic mucocutaneous ulcers are a frequent manifestation of extrapulmonary disease.

Sporotrichosis Is a Chronic Infection of Skin, Soft Tissues, and Lymph Nodes

It is caused by *Sporothrix schenckii.* This dimorphic fungus grows as a mold in soil and decaying plant matter and as yeast in the body.

 EPIDEMIOLOGY: Sporotrichosis is endemic in parts of the Americas and southern Africa. Most infections are cutaneous, from splinters, handling reeds or grasses, or minor puncture wounds. The fungus lives on thorns (particularly rose thorns). Cutaneous sporotrichosis is particularly common among gardeners, botanical nursery workers, and others who suffer abrasions while working with soil, moss, hay, or timbers. Infected animals, particularly cats, can also transmit the disease.

 PATHOLOGY: On entry into the skin, proliferates locally, eliciting an inf response that produces an ulceronodu Infection spreads along subcutaneous lympha nels, resulting in a chain of similar nodular ski (Fig. 9-69A). Disease is usually limited to the s may infrequently involve joints and bones, particu the wrist, elbow, or ankle.

The lesions of cutaneous sporotrichosis are usu the dermis or subcutaneous tissue, with a granulom edge and suppurative center. Surrounding skin shows berant pseudoepitheliomatous hyperplasia. Some ye are surrounded by an eosinophilic, spiculated zone, form "asteroid bodies" (Fig. 9-69B).

 CLINICAL FEATURES: Cutaneous sporotrichosis begins as a solitary nodular lesion at the site of inoculation, typically on a hand, arm, or leg. Weeks later, more nodules may appear along the path of lymphatic drainage from the primary lesion. Nodules often ulcerate and drain serosanguineous fluid. Joint involvement appears as pain and swelling of the affected joint, without involving overlying skin. Untreated cutaneous sporotrichosis continues to spread along the skin. The skin infection responds to systemic iodine therapy, but extracutaneous sporotrichosis requires systemic antifungal therapy.

Chromomycosis Is a Chronic Skin Infection

Several species of fungi from the soil and decaying vegetable matter are responsible. The fungi are brown, round, thick walled, 8 μm across, and resemble "copper pennies" (Fig. 9-70). The infection mostly occurs in barefooted agricultural workers in the tropics, in whom the fungus is implanted by trauma, usually below the knee. Lesions begin as papules and over

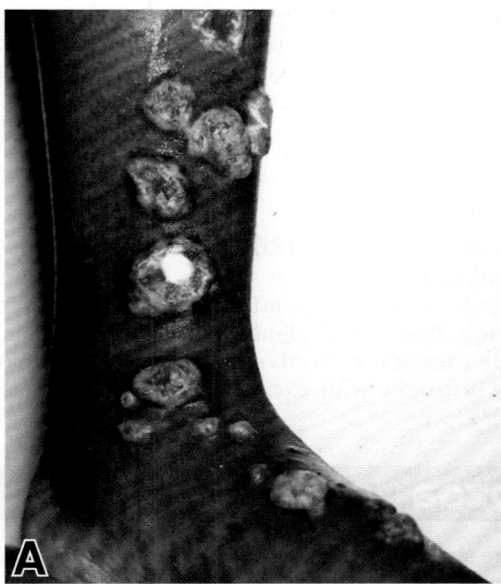

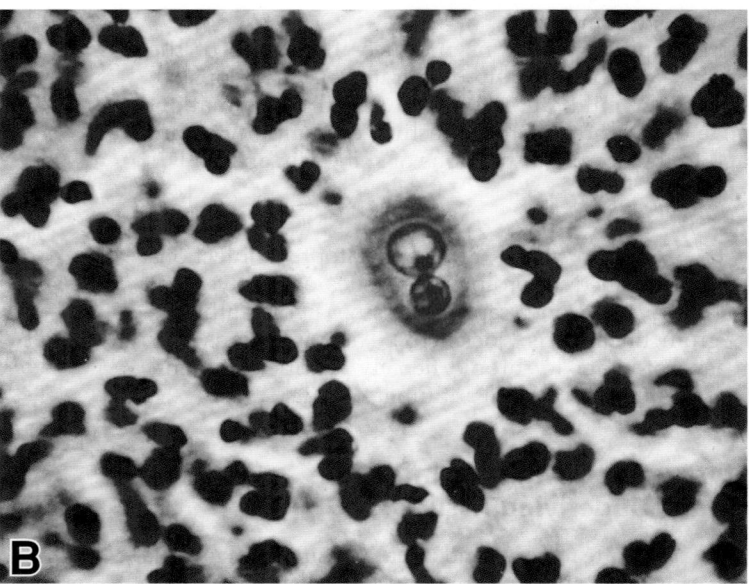

FIGURE 9-69. Sporotrichosis. A. The leg shows typical lymphocutaneous spread. **B.** A section of the lesion in (**A**) shows an asteroid body, composed of a pair of budding yeasts of *Sporothrix schenckii* surrounded by a layer of Splendore–Hoeppli substance, with radiating projections.

S. schenckii
ammatory
lar lesion.
tic chan-
n lesions
kin, but
larly of

lly in
atous
exu-
asts
to

Chromomycosis. A section of skin shows a giant cell in hich contains a thick-walled, brown, sclerotic body (copper w), representing the fungus.

ears become verrucous, crusted, and sometimes ulcer-. Infection spreads by contiguous growth and via lymatics. It may eventually involve an entire limb.

Dermatophyte Infections Affect Skin, Hair, and Nails

There are about 40 species of dermatophytes in 3 genera: *Trichophyton, Microsporum,* and *Epidermophyton.* They are resident in soil, on animals, and on humans. ***Dermatophyte infections are minor illnesses, but are very common.*** Most such infections in temperate countries are spread by direct contact, via infected hairs or skin scales.

PATHOLOGY: Dermatophytes proliferate in superficial keratinized tissues. They spread centrifugally from the initial site, producing round, expanding lesions with sharp margins that resemble worms, hence the names **ringworm** and **tinea** (from the Latin *tinea*, "worm").

Dermatophyte infections produce thickening of the squamous epithelium (hyperkeratosis). If biopsied, lesions show mild dermal lymphocytic inflammation. Hyphae and spores of the infecting dermatophytes are limited to the nonviable portions of skin, hair, and nails.

CLINICAL FEATURES: Dermatophyte infections are named according to the sites of involvement (e.g., scalp, tinea capitis; feet, tinea pedis, "athlete's foot"; groin, tinea cruris, "jock itch"). These infections vary from asymptomatic to chronic, fiercely pruritic eruptions, and are treated with topical antifungal agents.

Mycetomas Are Disfiguring Infections of Skin and Underlying Tissues

They may penetrate to bone, and usually result from inoculation of various soil-dwelling fungi and filamentous bacteria. Responsible organisms include *Madurella mycetomatis, Petrilidium boydii, Actinomadura madurae,* and *Nocardia brasiliensis.*

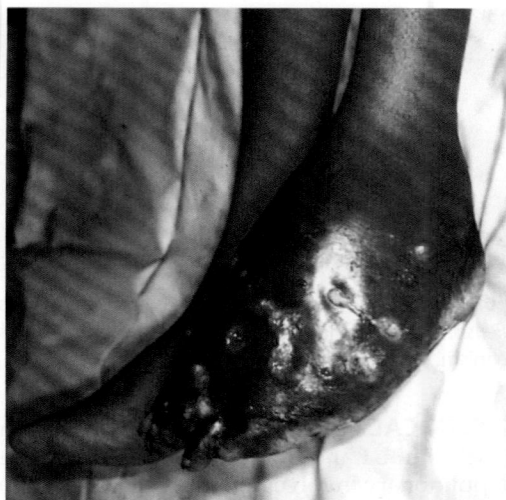

FIGURE 9-71. Mycetoma. The foot is swollen and painful and drains through the skin. The extremity was amputated.

EPIDEMIOLOGY: Mycetomas usually occur in the tropics among farmers and outdoor laborers whose skin is exposed to trauma. In places where people walk barefoot on soggy ground, feet are commonly infected. The disease is also called **Madura foot**. Frequent immersion of the foot macerates the skin and facilitates deep inoculation with soil organisms.

PATHOLOGY: The organisms proliferate in the subcutis, and spread to adjacent tissues, including bone. This incites a mixed suppurative and granulomatous inflammatory infiltrate which fails to eliminate the infecting organism. Surrounding granulation tissue and scarring produce progressive disfigurement of the affected sites.

Mycetomas begin as solitary subcutaneous abscesses, and slowly grow into multiple abscesses, interconnected by sinus tracts (Fig. 9-71). Sinus tracts eventually drain to the skin surface. Abscesses contain compact colonies of bacteria or fungi which resemble sulfur granules of actinomycosis. These are surrounded by neutrophils and an outer layer of granulomatous inflammation.

CLINICAL FEATURES: Mycetomas start as painless, swellings at sites of penetrating injury. Lesions slowly expand, and produce sinus tracts that tend to follow fascial planes, as they spread laterally and deeply through connective tissue, muscle, and bone. Treatment is usually wide excision of the affected area.

Protozoa

Protozoa are single-celled eukaryotes that fall into three general classes: **amebae, flagellates,** and **sporozoites**. Amebae move by projection of cytoplasmic extensions, or **pseudopods**. Flagellates use threadlike structures, flagella, which protrude from the cell membrane. Sporozoites do not have organelles of locomotion and also differ from amebae and flagellates in their mode of replication.

Protozoa cause human disease in several ways. Some, like *Entamoeba histolytica*, are extracellular parasites that digest and invade human tissues. Plasmodia are obligate intracellular parasites that replicate in and kill, human cells. Still others, for example, trypanosomes, do damage largely by eliciting inflammatory and immunologic responses. Some protozoa (e.g., *Toxoplasma gondii*) can establish latent infections that reactivate in immunocompromised hosts.

MALARIA

Malaria is a mosquito-borne, hemolytic, febrile illness. It affects over 200 million people and kills more than 1 million yearly. Four *Plasmodium* species cause malaria: *P. falciparum, P. vivax, P. ovale,* and *P. malariae.* All infect and destroy erythrocytes, producing chills, fever, anemia, and splenomegaly. Disease caused by *P. falciparum* is severe disease than the others, and accounts for most malarial deaths.

EPIDEMIOLOGY: Malaria has been eradicated in developed countries but continues to cause disease in tropical and subtropical areas. Rural poor, infants, children, malnourished people, and pregnant women are especially susceptible.

Malaria is transmitted by the bite of the female *Anopheles* mosquito. *P. falciparum* and *P. vivax* are the most common pathogens, but species distribution varies with geography. *P. vivax* is rare in Africa, where much of the population lacks the erythrocyte surface receptors required for infection. *P. falciparum* and *P. ovale* predominate in Africa. *P. malariae* has a broad distribution, is least common and causes the mildest form of malaria.

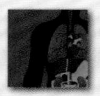

PATHOPHYSIOLOGY: The *Plasmodium* life cycle requires human and mosquito hosts (Fig. 9-72). Infected humans produce **gametocytes** that mosquitoes acquire when they feed. In mosquitoes, the plasmodium reproduces sexually to produce **sporozoites**. When the anopheline mosquito feeds, it inoculates the sporozoites into a human's bloodstream. There, they undergo asexual division "schizogony." Circulating sporozoites rapidly invade hepatocytes and reproduce in the liver to generate many daughter organisms "merozoites" (exoerythrocytic phase). Within 2 to 3 weeks, host hepatocytes rupture, merozoites enter the bloodstream and invade erythrocytes.

Merozoites feed on hemoglobin, grow, and reproduce inside erythrocytes. Within 2 to 4 days, mature progeny merozoites are produced. These daughter merozoites burst from infected erythrocytes, invade naive red cells, and initiate another cycle of erythrocytic parasitism. This cycle is repeated many times. Eventually, subpopulations of merozoites differentiate into sexual forms, **gametocytes**, which are ingested when a mosquito feeds on an infected host. This completes the parasite's life cycle.

When infected erythrocytes rupture, they release pyrogens, generating the characteristic fever and chills.

The fixed phagocytes of the liver and spleen asitized red blood cells, and cause hepatospl Thus, patients are anemic because of erythrocy sequestration of cells in the enlarging spleen.

P. falciparum causes a much more aggressive than other plasmodia. It differs from other mala sites in four ways:

- It has no secondary exoerythrocytic (hepatic) sta
- It parasitizes erythrocytes of any age (Fig. 9-73) ing marked parasitemia and anemia. In other ty malaria, only subpopulations of erythrocytes (e.g. young or old forms) are parasitized, so blood par levels are lower and anemia more mild.
- There may be several parasites in a single red cell.
- *P. falciparum* alters flow and adhesive properties infected erythrocytes, so they adhere to endotheli cells of small blood vessels. Obstruction of small ves sels may cause tissue ischemia, which contributes importantly to the organism's virulence.

PATHOLOGY: All forms of malaria have hepatosplenomegaly, as red blood cells are sequestered by fixed mononuclear phagocytes. Liver, spleen, and lymph nodes are darkened ("slate gray") by macrophages filled with hemosiderin and malarial pigment, the end-product of parasitic digestion of hemoglobin.

Infected red cells adhere to microvascular endothelium in falciparum malaria. Such parasitized erythrocytes attach to endothelial cells. Also, capillaries of deep organs, especially the brain, may become obstructed, causing ischemia affecting the brain, kidneys, and lungs. Brains of patients who die of cerebral malaria show congestion and thrombosis of small blood vessels in the white matter, which are rimmed with edema and hemorrhage ("ring hemorrhages") (Fig. 9-74). Obstruction of renal blood flow may cause acute renal failure. Intravascular hemolysis releases hemoglobin, leading to hemoglobinuric nephrosis (**blackwater fever**). Damage to alveolar capillaries produces pulmonary edema and acute alveolar damage.

CLINICAL FEATURES: Recurrent **paroxysms** of chills and high fever are typical. They begin with chills and sometimes headache, then, high, spiking fever, tachycardia, often with nausea, vomiting, and abdominal pain. The high fever causes marked vasodilation, leading to orthostatic hypotension. After several hours, patients are usually exhausted and drenched in sweat, and defervesce.

There follows a period of 2 to 3 days when patients feel well, only to repeat the experience. Paroxysms recur like this for weeks, eventually subsiding as an immune response is mounted. Each paroxysm reflects rupture of infected erythrocytes and release of daughter merozoites. As the mononuclear phagocytic system enlarges (see above), hepatosplenomegaly develops. Splenic enlargement can be dramatic: some of the largest spleens on record are due to chronic malaria. Hypersplenism can exacerbate the anemia of malarial infection. *P. falciparum* produces more severe disease than do other plasmodia.

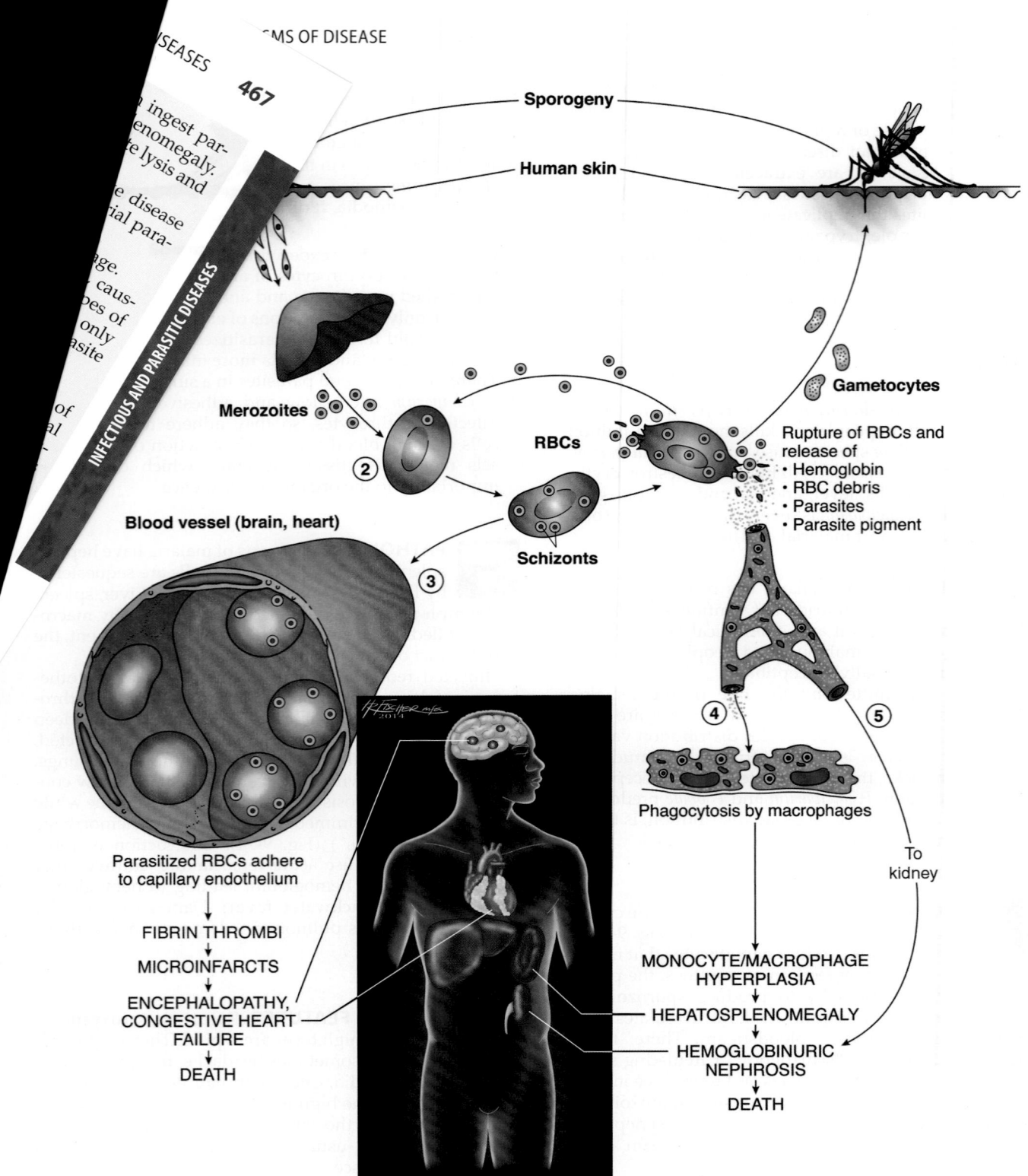

FIGURE 9-72. Life cycle of malaria. An *Anopheles* mosquito bites an infected person, taking blood that contains micro- and macrogametocytes (sexual forms). In the mosquito, sexual multiplication (sporogony) produces infective sporozoites in the salivary glands. **(1)** During the mosquito bite, sporozoites are inoculated into the bloodstream of the vertebrate host. Some sporozoites leave the blood and enter the hepatocytes, where they multiply asexually (exoerythrocytic schizogony) and form thousands of uninucleated merozoites. **(2)** Rupture of hepatocytes releases merozoites, which penetrate erythrocytes and become trophozoites, which then divide to form many schizonts (intraerythrocytic schizogony). Schizonts divide to form more merozoites, which are released on the rupture of erythrocytes and reenter other erythrocytes to begin a new cycle. After several cycles, subpopulations of merozoites develop into micro- and macrogametocytes, which are taken up by another mosquito to complete the cycle. **(3)** Parasitized erythrocytes obstruct capillaries of the brain, heart, kidney, and other deep organs. Adherence of parasitized erythrocytes to capillary endothelial cells causes fibrin thrombi, which produce microinfarcts. These result in encephalopathy, congestive heart failure, pulmonary edema, and frequently death. Ruptured erythrocytes release hemoglobin, erythrocyte debris, and malarial pigment. **(4)** Phagocytosis leads to monocyte/macrophage hyperplasia and hepatosplenomegaly. **(5)** Released hemoglobin produces hemoglobinuric nephrosis, which may be fatal. *RBCs* = red blood cells.

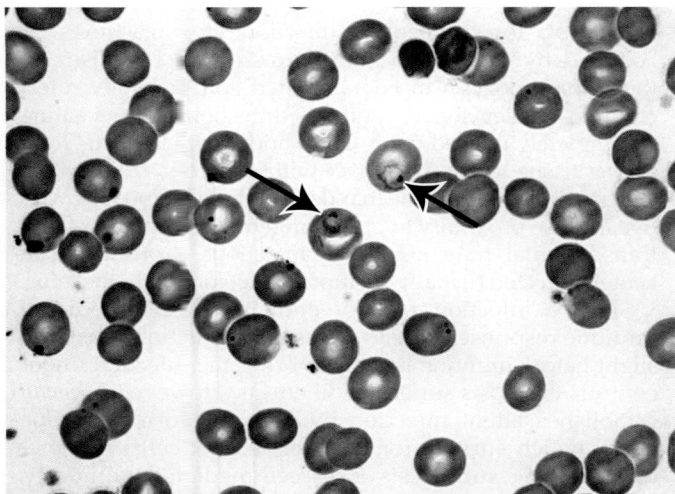

FIGURE 9-73. Plasmodia in erythrocytes. Red blood cells parasitized by malarial plasmodia (*arrows*), may circulate in the peripheral blood, which can help establish the diagnosis. (Photograph courtesy Dr. Gene Gulati.)

As levels of parasitemia increase, fever may be virtually continuous. Ischemic brain injury causes symptoms from somnolence, hallucinations and behavioral changes, to seizures and coma. CNS disease has a mortality of 20% to 50%.

Malaria is diagnosed by demonstrating the plasmodia on Giemsa-stained blood smears. The several species are distinguished by their appearance in infected erythrocytes. Nonfalciparum malarias are treated with oral chloroquine, sometimes with primaquine. Therapy for falciparum malaria varies, as widespread chloroquine resistance requires new treatments.

OTHER PROTOZOAL INFECTIONS

Babesiosis Is a Malaria-Like Infection Transmitted by Ticks

It is caused by protozoa of the genus *Babesia*.

 EPIDEMIOLOGY: *Babesia* infections are common in animals and in some locations may cause serious economic losses to the livestock industry. Human babesiosis is almost a medical curiosity, with the parasites infecting humans only when people intrude into the zoonotic cycle between the tick vector and its vertebrate host. Human babesiosis occurs only in Europe and North America. Infections in the United States have been concentrated in islands off the New England coast. The organisms invade and destroy erythrocytes, causing hemoglobinemia, hemoglobinuria, and renal failure. The disease is usually self-limited, but uncontrolled infections may be fatal (Fig. 9-75). *Babesia* spp. are resistant to most antiprotozoal drugs.

Toxoplasmosis Is Usually Mild But May Be Devastating *In Utero* or in Immunocompromised Hosts

Disease is caused by *Toxoplasma gondii*, and is worldwide.

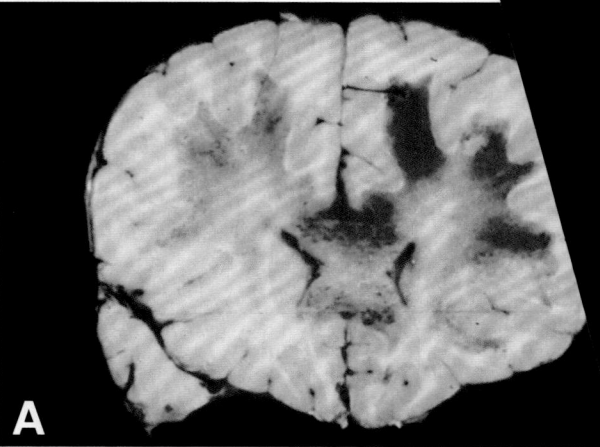

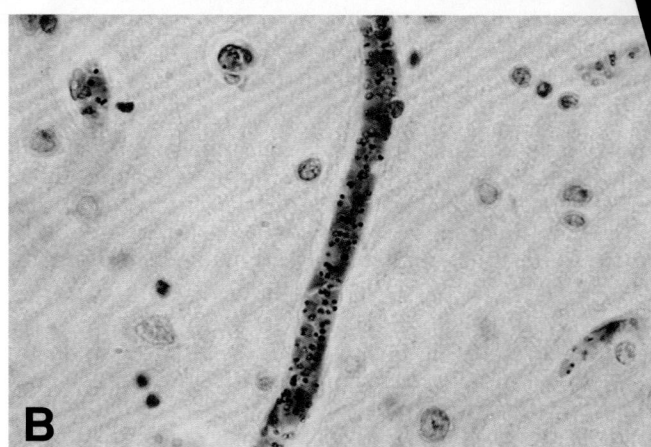

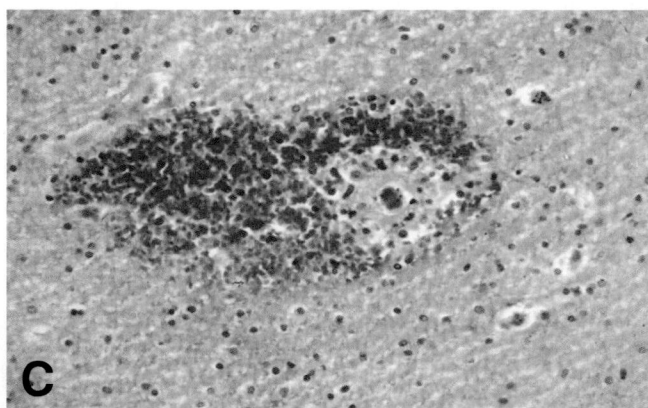

FIGURE 9-74. Acute falciparum malaria of the brain. A. There is severe diffuse congestion of the white matter and focal hemorrhages. **B.** A section of (**A**) shows a capillary packed with parasitized erythrocytes. **C.** Another section of (**A**) displays a ring hemorrhage around a thrombosed capillary, which contains parasitized erythrocytes in a fibrin thrombus.

EPIDEMIOLOGY: In some areas (e.g., France), prevalence of *T. gondii* infection exceeds 80% of adults; in other regions (e.g., the southwestern United States), it is uncommon. Many mammals and birds are intermediate hosts, but the only final hosts are cats, which become infected by ingesting toxoplasma cysts in tissues of an infected mouse or other intermediate

. Babesiosis. In the sinusoids of the liver, parasites appear
~~ar blue dots, in phagocytes and red blood cells (*arrows*).

In the cat's intestine, multiplicative stages end with
~~dding of **oocysts**. These sporulate in feces and soil and
~~fferentiate into **sporocysts** containing **sporozoites**.
These are ingested by intermediate hosts, such as birds,
mice, or humans, and complete the life cycle in them.

PATHOPHYSIOLOGY: *T. gondii* has two stages
in tissue, **tachyzoites** and **bradyzoites**, both
crescent-shaped and 2×6 μm. In acute infection,
tachyzoites multiply rapidly to form "groups" in intracellular vacuoles of parasitized cells. They eventually cause
the cells to rupture. Tachyzoites spread from the gut via
lymphatics to regional lymph nodes, then through the
blood to liver, lungs, heart, brain, and other organs.

During chronic infection, *Toxoplasma* bradyzoites multiply slowly. They store PAS-positive material and hundreds of organisms are tightly packed in "cysts," derived
from the intracellular vacuoles (see above), which enlarge
beyond the usual size of the cell and push the nucleus to
the periphery.

Except for congenital infection, toxoplasmosis is
acquired by eating infectious forms of the organism. In
the tropics, oocysts in contaminated soil generally infect
children. In developed countries, infection follows eating
incompletely cooked meat (lamb and pork) carrying *Toxoplasma* tissue cysts, or contact with cat feces, from which
oocysts contaminate the hands and food of people who
live in close proximity to cats. **Congenital infection** reflects
transplacental transmission of infectious forms from an
acutely infected (usually asymptomatic) mother to the fetus.

Active infection usually ends when cell-mediated
immune responses develop. Tissue destruction is usually
slight before immune responses bring the infection under
control, and hosts suffer few ill effects. However, *T. gondii*
establishes latent infection by forming dormant tissue
cysts, which survive for decades in host cells. If someone carrying such cysts loses cell-mediated immunity,
T. gondii can escape the cysts and reestablish a destructive infection.

Toxoplasma Lymphadenopathy

PATHOLOGY: The most common manifestation
of *T. gondii* infection in immunocompetent hosts
is lymphadenopathy (see Chapter 26). Any lymph
node group may be involved, but enlarged cervical nodes
are most readily apparent. The histology of affected lymph
nodes is distinctive: many epithelioid macrophages are
scattered, seemingly randomly, in the node. They may
even surround and encroach on reactive germinal centers.

CLINICAL FEATURES: In *Toxoplasma* lymphadenitis (Fig. 9-76A), patients present with nontender regional lymph node enlargement,
sometimes accompanied by fever, sore throat, hepatosplenomegaly, and circulating atypical lymphocytes.
Hepatitis, myocarditis (Fig. 9-76B), and myositis have
been documented. Lymphadenopathy usually resolves
spontaneously in weeks to months; therapy is seldom
required.

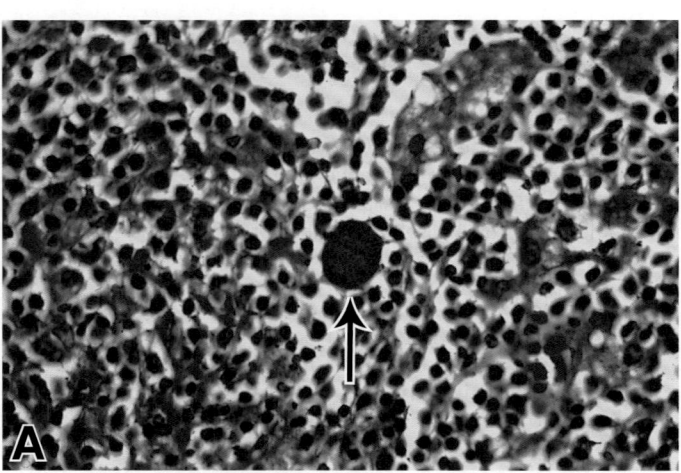

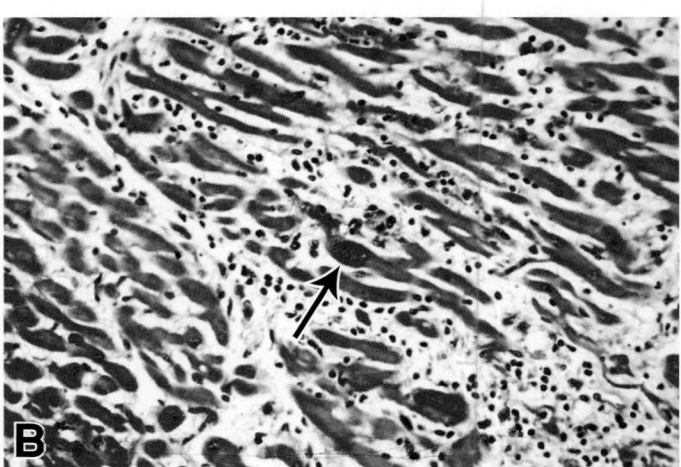

FIGURE 9-76. Toxoplasmosis. A. An enlarged lymph node contains bradyzoites of *Toxoplasma gondii* within a cyst (*arrow*). **B.** A section of heart shows
a cyst of bradyzoites of *T. gondii* within a myofiber (*arrow*), with edema and inflammatory cells in the adjacent tissue.

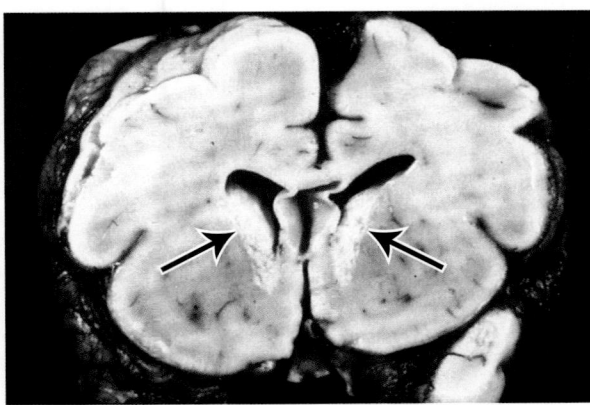

FIGURE 9-77. Congenital toxoplasmosis. The brain of a premature infant with subependymal necrosis with calcification appearing as bilaterally symmetric areas of whitish discoloration (*arrows*). (Reprinted from Farrar WE, Wood MJ, Innes JA, Tubbs H. *Infectious Diseases: Text and Color Atlas*. 2nd ed. New York: Gower Medical Publishing; 1992. Copyright © 1992 Elsevier. With permission.)

Congenital Toxoplasma Infection

T. gondii infection acquired *in utero* is highly destructive (see Chapter 6).

PATHOLOGY: If a pregnant woman contracts a primary *Toxoplasma* infection, the fetal immune system is too immature to contain the infection. The fetus' developing brain and eye are readily infected, leading to a necrotizing meningoencephalitis, which in the most severe cases leads to loss of brain parenchyma, cerebral calcifications (Fig. 9-77), and marked hydrocephalus. Ocular infection causes chorioretinitis (i.e., necrosis and inflammation of the choroid and retina).

CLINICAL FEATURES: Fetal disease is worst if infection occurs early in pregnancy, and spontaneous abortion may result. Brain involvement may vary from subtle psychomotor defects to severe mental retardation and seizures. Ocular involvement may cause congenital visual impairment. Latent ocular infection may be established *in utero* and recrudesce later in life to cause blindness. Some newborns have *Toxoplasma* hepatitis, with large areas of necrosis and giant cells. Occasionally, adrenal necrosis occurs. Congenital toxoplasmosis requires therapy with antiprotozoal agents.

Toxoplasmosis in Immunocompromised Hosts

Devastating *T. gondii* infections occur in people with impaired cell-mediated immunity, usually reflecting reactivation of latent infection. The brain is most commonly affected, with multifocal necrotizing encephalitis. Such patients present with paresis, seizures, alterations in visual acuity, and changes in mentation. *Toxoplasma* encephalitis in such patients is fatal if not treated with effective antiprotozoal agents.

Amebiasis Is Infection With *Entamoeba histolytica*

It mainly involves the colon, and occasionally the liver. *E. histolytica* is named for its ability to destroy tissue. Intestinal infection varies from asymptomatic colonization to severe invasive infection with bloody diarrhea. Sometimes, parasites invade through the colon, into other organs, most often the liver. There, *E. histolytica* causes slowly expanding, necrotizing abscesses.

EPIDEMIOLOGY: Humans are the only known reservoir for *E. histolytica*, which reproduces in the colon and passes in the feces. Amebiasis occurs worldwide, but is more common and more severe in tropical and subtropical areas. *Infection follows ingestion of materials contaminated with human feces.*

PATHOPHYSIOLOGY: *E. histolytica* lifecycle stages are: trophozoite, **precyst,** and cyst.

Amebic trophozoites, 10 to 60 μm across, are found in stools of patients with acute symptoms. They are spherical or oval, with a thin cell membrane, a single nucleus, condensed chromatin on the interior of the nuclear membrane and a central karyosome. The trophozoites may contain phagocytosed erythrocytes. PAS stains the cytoplasm of the trophozoites and makes them stand out in tissue sections. In the colon, trophozoites develop into cysts through an intermediate form, the **precyst**, during which process trophozoites stop feeding, become round and nonmotile, lose some digestive vacuoles and form glycogen masses and chromatoidal bodies.

Amebic cysts are the infecting stage, and are only in stool, as they do not invade tissue. They are spherical, have thick walls, measure 5 to 25 μm across and usually have four nuclei. Cysts in stool contaminate water, food, or fingers (Fig. 9-78). Once ingested, cysts traverse the stomach and excyst in the lower ileum. A metacystic ameba with four nuclei divides to form four small, immature trophozoites, which then grow to full size. These thrive in the colon and feed on bacteria and human cells. They may colonize any part of the large bowel, but the cecum is most affected. Patients with symptomatic amebic colitis pass both cysts and trophozoites. The latter survive only briefly outside the body and are also destroyed by gastric secretions. Host factors, such as nutritional status, coexistent colonic flora and immunologic status also affect the course of infection. Invasion begins when a trophozoite attaches to a colonic epithelial cell. The parasite kills target cells with a lytic protein that breaches the cell membrane. Progressive death of mucosal cells produces a superficial ulcer.

Intestinal Amebiasis

PATHOLOGY: Amebic lesions begin as small foci of necrosis that progress to ulcers (Fig. 9-79A). Undermining of the ulcer margin and confluence of expanding ulcers lead to irregular mucosal sloughing. The ulcer bed is gray and necrotic, with fibrin and cellular debris. The exudate raises the undermined mucosa, producing flask-shaped chronic amebic ulcers.

Trophozoites are present at the ulcer surface, and in the exudate and crater (Fig. 9-79B). They also occur in the submucosa, muscularis propria, serosa, and small

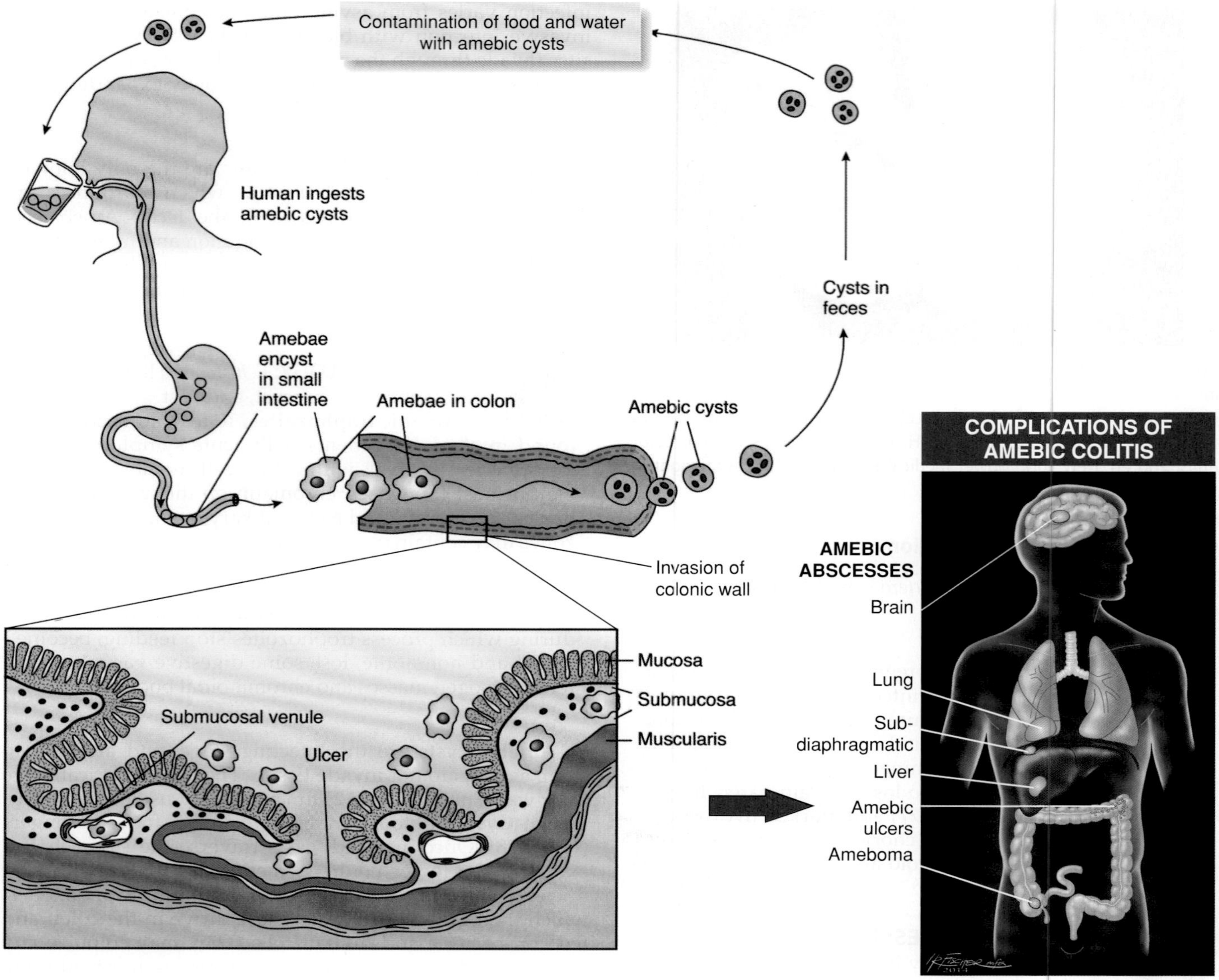

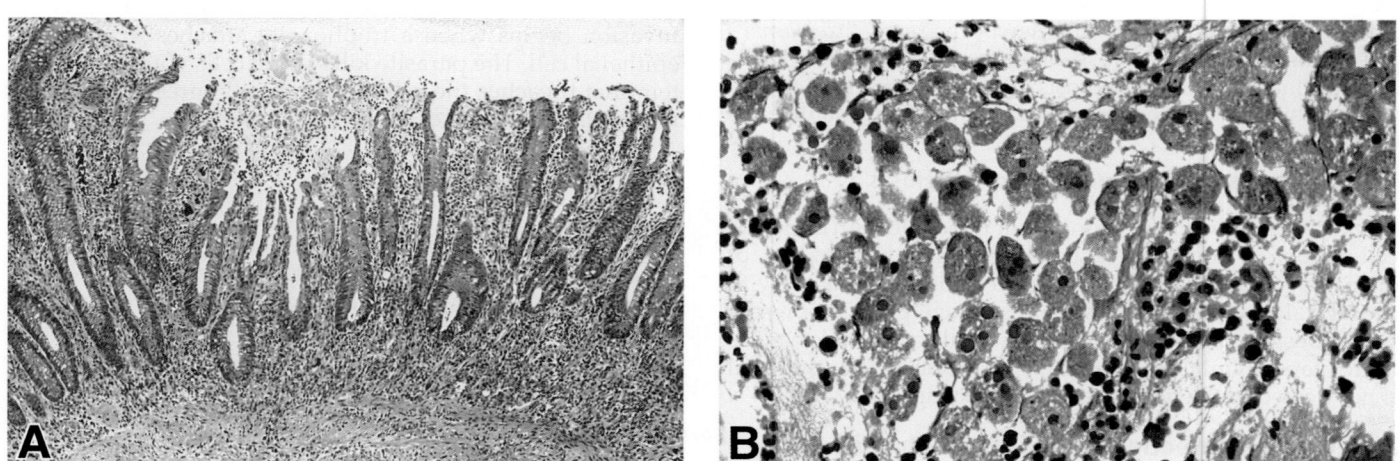

FIGURE 9-78. Amebic colitis and its complications. Amebiasis results from the ingestion of food or water contaminated with amebic cysts. In the colon, the amebae penetrate the mucosa and produce flask-shaped ulcers of the mucosa and submucosa. The organisms may invade submucosal venules, thereby disseminating the infection to the liver and other organs. The liver abscess can expand to involve adjacent structures.

FIGURE 9-79. Intestinal amebiasis. A. The colonic mucosa shows superficial ulceration beneath a cluster of trophozoites of *Entamoeba histolytica*. The lamina propria contains excess acute and chronic inflammatory cells, including eosinophils. **B.** Higher-power view shows trophozoites in the luminal exudate.

submucosal veins. There is little inflammatory response in early amebic ulcers, but as ulcers enlarge, acute and chronic inflammatory cells accumulate.

An ameboma may infrequently complicates amebiasis, if amebae invade through the intestinal wall. It is an inflammatory bowel wall thickening that resembles colon cancer and makes a "napkin-ring constriction." It consists of granulation tissue, fibrosis, and clusters of trophozoites.

CLINICAL FEATURES: Intestinal amebiasis varies from asymptomatic to severe dysentery. For acute disease, the incubation period is 8 to 10 days. Gradually increasing abdominal discomfort, tenderness, and cramps are accompanied by chills and fever, as well as nausea, vomiting, malodorous flatus, and intermittent constipation. Liquid stools (up to 25 a day) contain bloody mucus, but diarrhea is rarely prolonged enough to cause dehydration. Amebic colitis may persist for months to years. Patients may become emaciated and anemic. Clinically, its presentation can mimic appendicitis, cholecystitis, intestinal obstruction, or diverticulitis. In severe cases, massive destruction of colon mucosa may lead to fatal hemorrhage, perforation, or peritonitis. Therapy includes metronidazole, which acts against trophozoites and diloxanide, which is effective against cysts.

Amebic Liver Abscess

PATHOLOGY: *E. histolytica* trophozoites can invade submucosal veins, enter the portal circulation and reach the liver. There, they kill hepatocytes, to generate a slowly expanding necrotic cavity, filled with a dark brown, odorless, semisolid material, reported to resemble "anchovy paste" in color and consistency (Fig. 9-80). Neutrophils are rare within the cavity and trophozoites are found along the edges adjacent to hepatocytes.

Amebic liver abscesses may expand, rupture through the capsule and extend into the peritoneum,

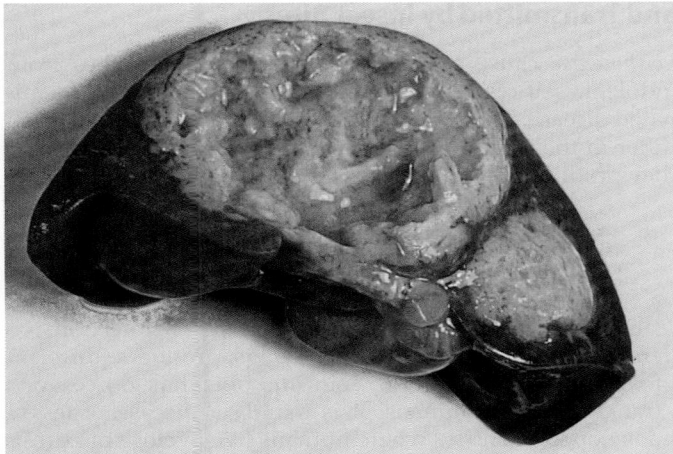
FIGURE 9-80. Amebic abscesses of the liver. The cut surface of the liver shows multiple abscesses containing "anchovy paste" material.

diaphragm, pleural cavity, lungs, or pericardium. Rarely, a liver abscess, or even a lesion in the colon, may traverse the diaphragm, into the pleural space, or spread to the brain by a hematogenous route to form large necrotic lesions.

CLINICAL FEATURES: Patients with amebic liver abscesses present with severe right upper quadrant pain, low-grade fever, and weight loss. Only a minority of patients give a history of an antecedent diarrheal illness and *E. histolytica* is demonstrable in the feces of under one-third of patients with extraintestinal disease. Radiography or ultrasound showing the abscess, plus serology showing antibodies to *E. histolytica*, make the diagnosis. Amebic abscesses are treated by percutaneous or surgical drainage and antiamebic drugs.

Cryptosporidiosis Causes Diarrhea in Immunosuppressed People

The severity of this infection varies from a self-limited to potentially life-threatening. Ingesting *Cryptosporidium* oocysts, present in feces of infected humans and animals, transmits the disease. Most infections probably reflect person-to-person transmission, but many domesticated animals harbor the parasite, and function as reservoirs.

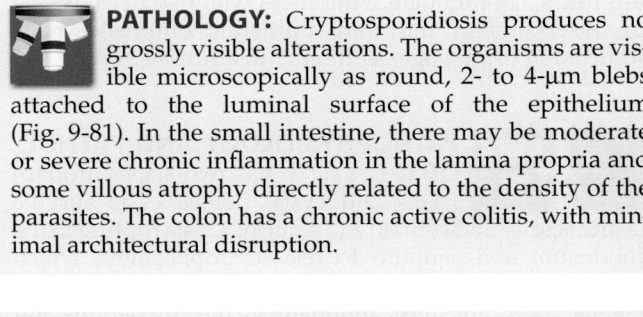**PATHOPHYSIOLOGY:** *Cryptosporidium* oocysts survive passage through the stomach and release forms that attach to small bowel microvilli, where they remain extracellular. They reproduce at the luminal surface of the gut, from stomach to rectum, forming progeny that also attach to the epithelium.

Immunocompetent people eliminate the infection by their immune responses. Patients with AIDS and other immunodeficiencies cannot contain the parasite and develop chronic infections, which may spread from the bowel to the gallbladder and intrahepatic bile ducts.

PATHOLOGY: Cryptosporidiosis produces no grossly visible alterations. The organisms are visible microscopically as round, 2- to 4-μm blebs attached to the luminal surface of the epithelium (Fig. 9-81). In the small intestine, there may be moderate or severe chronic inflammation in the lamina propria and some villous atrophy directly related to the density of the parasites. The colon has a chronic active colitis, with minimal architectural disruption.

CLINICAL FEATURES: Cryptosporidiosis presents as a profuse, watery diarrhea, sometimes with cramping abdominal pain or low-grade fever. Huge volumes of fluid can be lost as diarrhea and intensive fluid replacement is required. In immunocompetent patients, diarrhea resolves in 1 to 2 weeks. In immunocompromised patients, diarrhea may persist indefinitely and contribute to death.

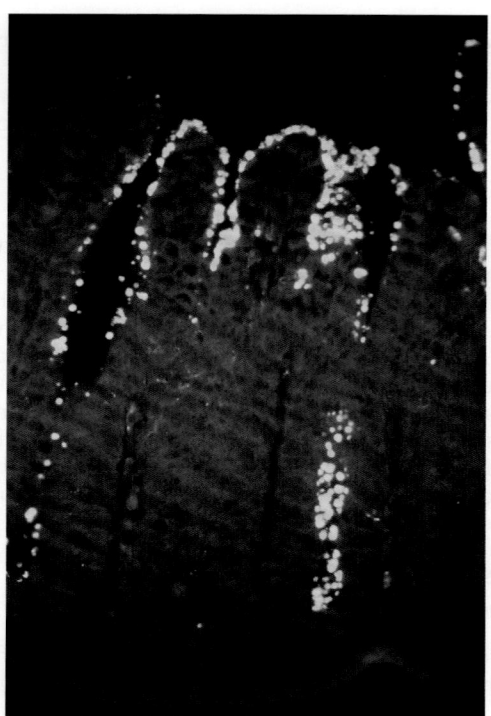

FIGURE 9-81. Cryptosporidiosis. A small intestinal biopsy stained with fluorescent antibody to *Cryptosporidium parvum* shows sporozoites covering the villi and lining the crypts.

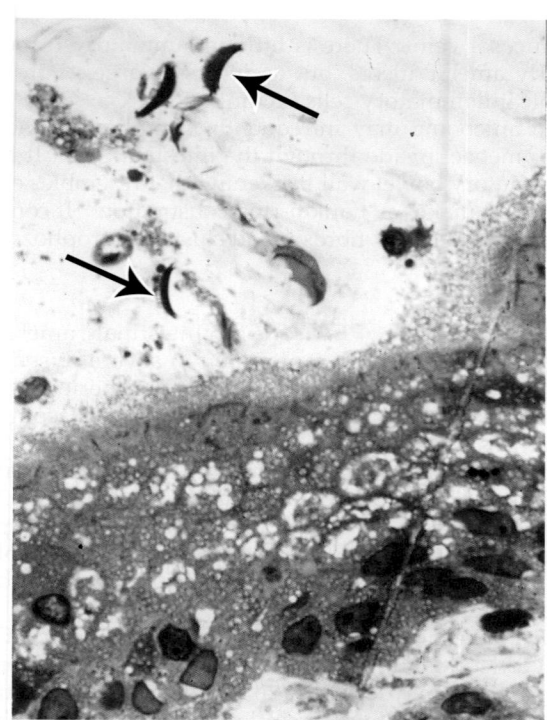

FIGURE 9-82. Giardiasis. Crescent-shaped trophozoites (*arrows*) of *Giardia lamblia* are present overlying the small intestinal mucosa.

Giardiasis Is an Intestinal Infection That Causes Diarrhea

EPIDEMIOLOGY: *Giardia lamblia* is a flagellated protozoan with worldwide distribution. The prevalence of infection varies from <1% to >25% in some warmer climates with crowded, unsanitary environments. Children are most at risk. People ingest infectious cyst forms of *Giardia*, which are shed in the feces of infected humans and animals. Infection may spread directly from person to person, and also via contaminated water or food. Feces from infected animals, like beavers and bears, contaminate wilderness water sources, which are reservoirs of infection. Epidemic outbreaks have occurred in orphanages and other institutions.

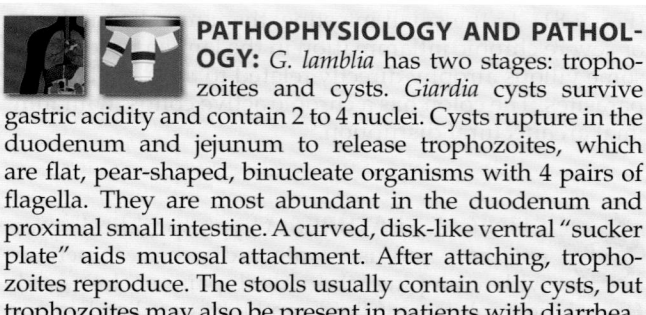

PATHOPHYSIOLOGY AND PATHOLOGY: *G. lamblia* has two stages: trophozoites and cysts. *Giardia* cysts survive gastric acidity and contain 2 to 4 nuclei. Cysts rupture in the duodenum and jejunum to release trophozoites, which are flat, pear-shaped, binucleate organisms with 4 pairs of flagella. They are most abundant in the duodenum and proximal small intestine. A curved, disk-like ventral "sucker plate" aids mucosal attachment. After attaching, trophozoites reproduce. The stools usually contain only cysts, but trophozoites may also be present in patients with diarrhea.

Giardiasis causes no grossly visible alterations. Microscopically, mucosal changes are minimal, with crescentic or semi-lunar–shaped *Giardia* trophozoites on villous surfaces and within crypts (Fig. 9-82).

CLINICAL FEATURES: *G. lamblia* is usually a harmless commensal, but can cause acute or chronic symptoms. Acute giardiasis starts abruptly, with abdominal cramping and frequent, foul-smelling stools. The course of infection varies greatly. Symptoms may resolve spontaneously in 1 to 4 weeks. Other patients have persistent abdominal cramping and poorly formed stools for months. In children, chronic giardiasis may cause malabsorption, weight loss, and retarded growth. The infection is treated effectively with various antibiotics, including metronidazole.

Leishmaniasis Is Caused by Protozoans and Transmitted by Insect Bites

Leishmaniae cause a spectrum of clinical syndromes from indolent, self-resolving cutaneous ulcers to fatal disseminated disease. There are numerous *Leishmania* species, which differ in their natural habitats and the types of disease that they produce.

EPIDEMIOLOGY: Leishmaniasis is transmitted by *Phlebotomus* sandflies, which acquire the infection by feeding on infected animals. In many subtropical and tropical areas, leishmanial infection is endemic in animal populations: dogs, ground squirrels, foxes, and jackals are reservoirs and potential sources for transmission to humans. It is mainly a disease of less-developed countries where humans live in close proximity to animal hosts and the fly vector. About 20 million people are infected worldwide.

PATHOPHYSIOLOGY: Infection begins when the organisms are inoculated into human skin by a sandfly bite. Leishmaniae are then phagocytosed by mononuclear phagocytes, transform into **amastigotes**, and reproduce within the macrophage. Daughter amastigotes eventually rupture from the cell, spread to other macrophages and continue the process at the site of inoculation.

From this humble beginning, the course of the infection depends on two factors: the host's immune status and the infecting species of *Leishmania*. There are three distinct clinical entities: (1) localized cutaneous leishmaniasis, (2) mucocutaneous leishmaniasis, and (3) visceral leishmaniasis.

Localized Cutaneous Leishmaniasis

Several *Leishmania* species in Central and South America, Northern Africa, the Middle East, India, and China cause localized skin disease, also called "tropical sore."

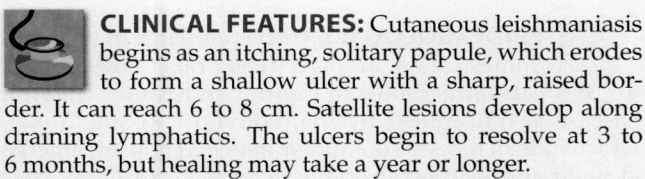 **PATHOLOGY:** Localized cutaneous leishmaniasis begins as a collection of amastigote-filled macrophages that ulcerates the overlying epidermis. In tissue sections, the 2-μm oval amastigotes a nucleus and a kinetoplast. Under low power, amastigotes in macrophages appear as multiple regular cytoplasmic dots, **Leishman-Donovan bodies.** As cell-mediated immunity develops, macrophages are activated and kill the intracellular parasites. The lesion slowly becomes a more mature granuloma, with epithelioid macrophages, Langhans giant cells, plasma cells, and lymphocytes. The ulcer heals spontaneously over the following months.

CLINICAL FEATURES: Cutaneous leishmaniasis begins as an itching, solitary papule, which erodes to form a shallow ulcer with a sharp, raised border. It can reach 6 to 8 cm. Satellite lesions develop along draining lymphatics. The ulcers begin to resolve at 3 to 6 months, but healing may take a year or longer.

Some patients have poor specific cell-mediated immune responses to leishmaniae, and may develop **diffuse cutaneous leishmaniasis**. This begins as a single nodule, but adjacent satellite nodules slowly form, and eventually involve much of the skin. These lesions resemble lepromatous leprosy so closely that some patients have been cared for in leprosaria. The nodule of anergic leishmaniasis contains enormous numbers of macrophages, replete with leishmaniae.

Mucocutaneous Leishmaniasis

Mucocutaneous leishmaniasis is caused by infection with *Leishmania braziliensis*. Most cases occur in Central and South America, where rodents and sloths are reservoirs.

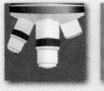 **PATHOLOGY AND CLINICAL FEATURES:** The early course and pathology of mucocutaneous leishmaniasis resemble localized cutaneous disease. A solitary ulcer appears,

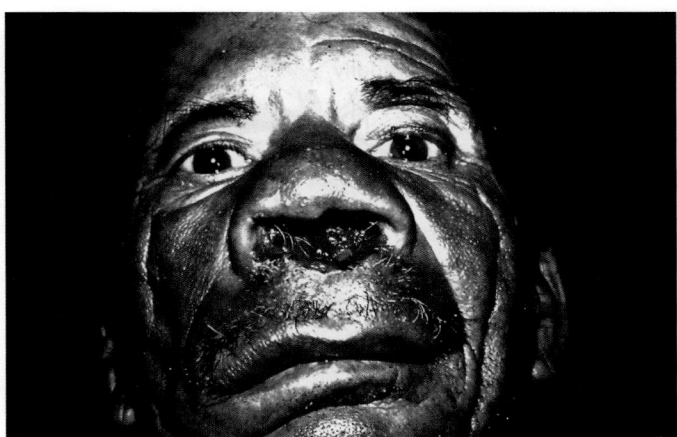

FIGURE 9-83. Mucocutaneous leishmaniasis. There is complete destruction of the basal septum and mucocutaneous ulceration.

expands, and resolves. Years afterwards, an ulcer develops at a mucocutaneous junction, such as the larynx, nasal septum, anus, or vulva. The mucosal lesion progresses slowly and is highly destructive and disfiguring. It erodes mucosal surfaces and cartilage (Fig. 9-83), and can destroy the nasal septum. Patients may die if ulcers obstruct the airways. Mucocutaneous leishmaniasis requires treatment with systemic antiprotozoal agents.

Visceral Leishmaniasis (Kala Azar)

 EPIDEMIOLOGY: Several subspecies of *Leishmania donovani* cause kala azar. Reservoirs of the agent and susceptible age groups vary in different parts of the world. Humans are the reservoir in India, and foxes in, for instance, southern France and central Italy. Other canine and rodent species are reservoirs elsewhere.

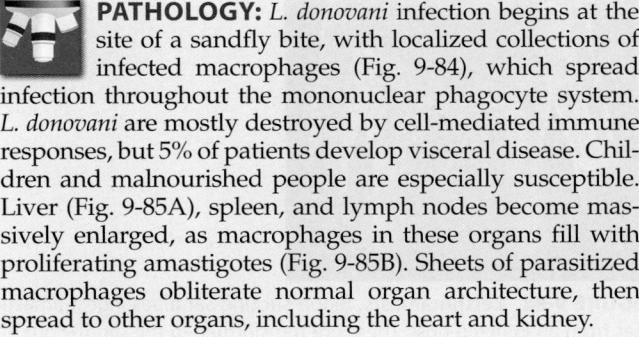 **PATHOLOGY:** *L. donovani* infection begins at the site of a sandfly bite, with localized collections of infected macrophages (Fig. 9-84), which spread infection throughout the mononuclear phagocyte system. *L. donovani* are mostly destroyed by cell-mediated immune responses, but 5% of patients develop visceral disease. Children and malnourished people are especially susceptible. Liver (Fig. 9-85A), spleen, and lymph nodes become massively enlarged, as macrophages in these organs fill with proliferating amastigotes (Fig. 9-85B). Sheets of parasitized macrophages obliterate normal organ architecture, then spread to other organs, including the heart and kidney.

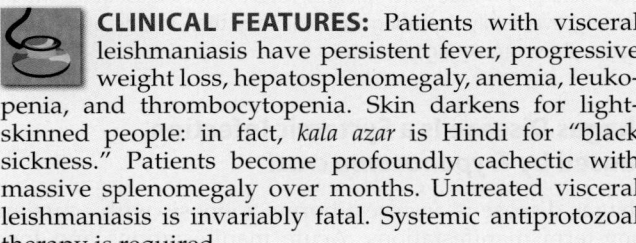 **CLINICAL FEATURES:** Patients with visceral leishmaniasis have persistent fever, progressive weight loss, hepatosplenomegaly, anemia, leukopenia, and thrombocytopenia. Skin darkens for light-skinned people: in fact, *kala azar* is Hindi for "black sickness." Patients become profoundly cachectic with massive splenomegaly over months. Untreated visceral leishmaniasis is invariably fatal. Systemic antiprotozoal therapy is required.

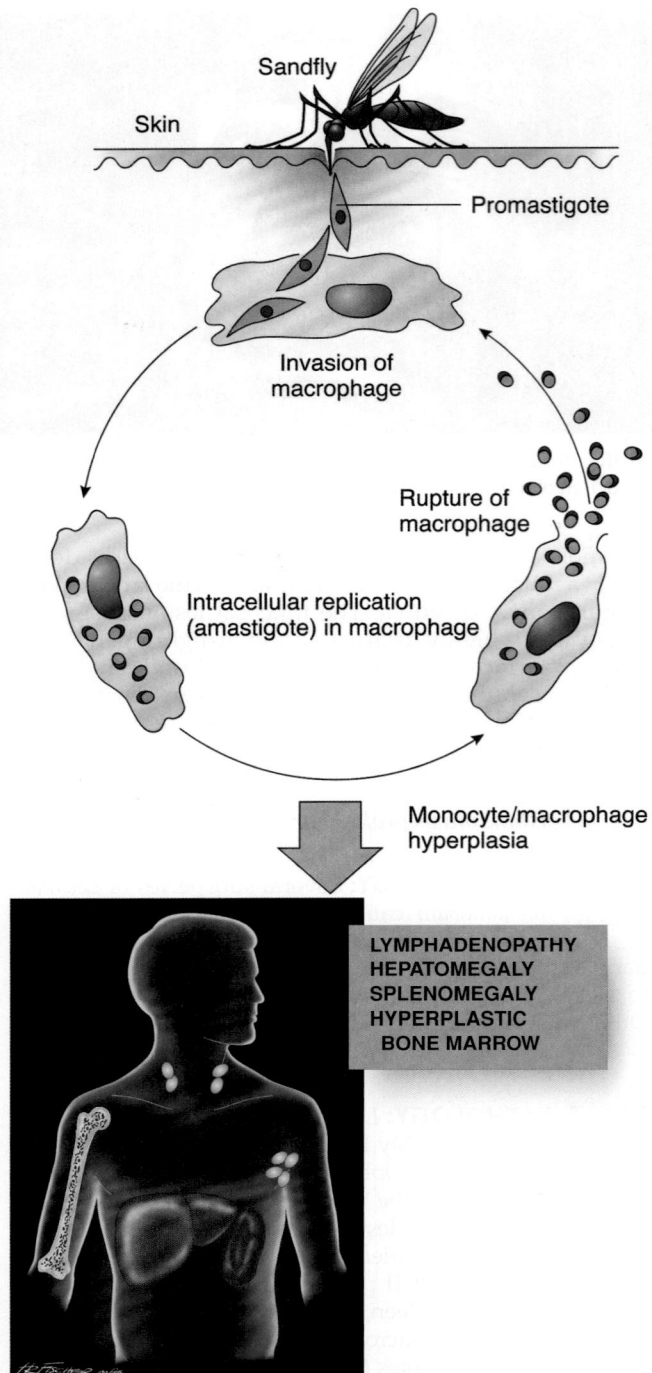

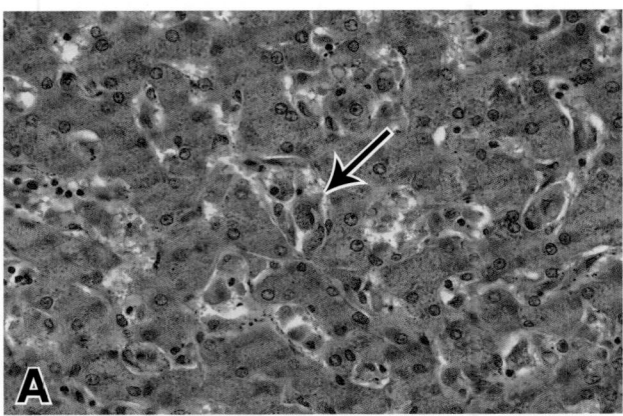

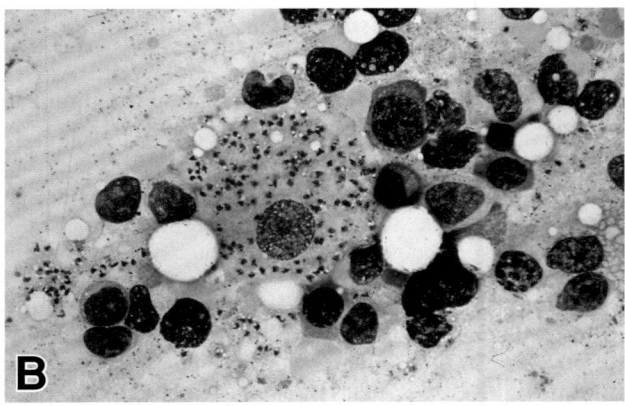

FIGURE 9-85. Visceral leishmaniasis. A. A photomicrograph of an enlarged liver shows prominent Kupffer cells distended by leishmanial amastigotes (*arrows*). **B.** A bone marrow aspirate from a patient with visceral leishmaniasis. Abundant leishmanial amastigotes are present, some of which are intracytoplasmic.

FIGURE 9-84. Leishmaniasis. Blood-sucking sandflies ingest amastigotes from an infected host. These are transformed in the sandfly gut into promastigotes, which multiply and are injected into the next vertebrate host. There they invade macrophages, revert to the amastigote form and multiply, eventually rupturing the cell. They then invade other macrophages, thus completing the cycle.

Chagas Disease Is a Systemic Infection Caused by *Trypanosoma cruzi*

Chagas disease is an insect-borne, zoonosis with acute and long-term manifestations. Acute manifestations and long-term sequelae occur in the heart and GI tract.

 EPIDEMIOLOGY: *T. cruzi* is endemic in wild and domesticated animals (e.g., rats, dogs, goats, cats, armadillos) in Central and South America. Disease is transmitted by the reduviid ("kissing") bug, which hide in recesses of mud or thatched houses, emerge at night and feed on sleeping victims. *T. cruzi* may pass from mother to fetus, to cause congenital infection. About 8 million people carry *T. cruzi*, mostly in Brazil. Chagas disease occurs in 18 nations in the Americas. It is an emerging public health concern in the United States, where about 300,000 people are infected. Between 10,000 and 50,000 people die from Chagas disease each year.

 PATHOPHYSIOLOGY: Infective forms of *T. cruzi* are discharged in the feces of the reduviid bug as it takes its blood meal. Itching and scratching promote contamination of the wound. The trypomastigotes penetrate at the site of the bite or at other abrasions, or may enter the mucosa of the eyes or lips. Once inside the body, they lose their flagella and undulating membranes and round up to become amastigotes.

T. cruzi infects and reproduces in macrophages at sites of inoculation, to form localized nodular inflammatory lesions, **chagomas**. The protozoa differentiate into trypomastigotes inside host cells, then break out and

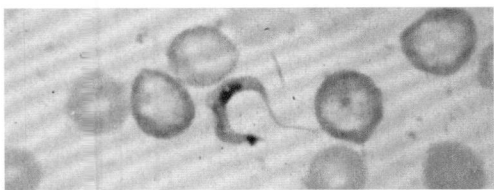

FIGURE 9-86. Chagas disease. A blood smear demonstrates a trypomastigote of *Trypanosoma cruzi* with its characteristic "C" shape, flagellum, nucleus, and terminal kinetoplast.

enter the blood (Fig. 9-86). It then disseminates throughout the body via the bloodstream. Different strains of *T. cruzi* target different cell types. Infections of cardiac myocytes, gastrointestinal ganglion cells and meninges cause the most severe disease. Parasitemia and widespread cellular infection are responsible for the systemic symptoms of acute Chagas disease. The onset of cell-mediated immunity eliminates the acute manifestations, but chronic tissue damage may continue. Progressive destruction of cells at sites of infection—particularly the heart, esophagus, and colon—causes organ dysfunction, manifested decades after the acute infection.

Ingested in a subsequent bite of a reduviid bug, trypomastigotes multiply in the insect's alimentary tract and differentiate into metacyclic trypomastigotes, which congregate in the rectum of the bug and are discharged in the feces, to repeat the cycle.

Acute Chagas Disease

 PATHOLOGY: *T. cruzi* circulates in the blood as a 20-µm long, curved, flagellate that is easily recognized on blood films. It reproduces in infected cells as a 2- to 4-µm nonflagellated amastigote. In fatal cases, the heart is enlarged and dilated, with a pale, focally hemorrhagic myocardium. Abundant parasites are visible in the heart, with amastigotes evident within pseudocysts in myofibers (Fig. 9-87). There is extensive chronic inflammation and phagocytosis of parasites is conspicuous.

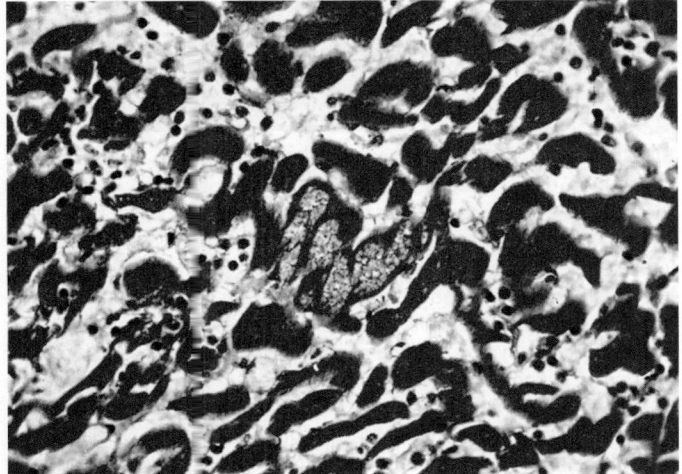

FIGURE 9-87. Acute Chagas myocarditis. Myofibers in the center contain amastigotes of *Trypanosoma cruzi* and are surrounded by edema and chronic inflammation.

 CLINICAL FEATURES: Acute symptoms develop 1 to 2 weeks after inoculation with *T. cruzi*. A chagoma (see above) develops at the site. Parasitemia appears within 2 to 3 weeks, usually with mild disease, including fever, malaise, lymphadenopathy, and hepatosplenomegaly. However, the disease can be lethal if there is extensive myocardial or meningeal involvement.

Chronic Chagas Disease

The most common and serious consequences of *T. cruzi* infection develop years or decades after acute infection. Up to 40% of those acutely infected eventually develop chronic disease. In this phase, *T. cruzi* is no longer evident in blood or tissue, but infected organs have been damaged by chronic, progressive inflammation.

 PATHOLOGY AND CLINICAL FEATURES: In chronic myocarditis, the heart is dilated, with prominent right ventricular outflow tract and dilated valve rings. The interventricular septum often deviates to the right and may immobilize the adjacent tricuspid leaflet. There are extensive interstitial fibrosis, hypertrophied myofibers, and focal lymphocytic inflammation, often involving the cardiac conduction system. Progressive cardiac fibrosis causes dysrhythmia or congestive heart failure. In endemic regions, chronic Chagas disease is a leading cause of heart failure in young adults.

Destruction of ganglion cells controlling gut motility may lead to esophageal and colonic dilatation (**megaesophagus** and **megacolon**). Impaired esophageal motility leads to difficulty in swallowing, which may be so severe that patients can consume only liquids. Progressive aganglionosis of the colon causes severe constipation.

In some pregnant women with parasitemia, infection may cross the placenta, involve the fetus and lead to spontaneous abortion. In the infrequent live births, infants die of encephalitis within a few days or weeks.

Antiprotozoal chemotherapy is effective for acute Chagas disease but not for its chronic sequelae. Cardiac transplantation has been effective in a number of patients.

African Trypanosomiasis, or Sleeping Sickness, Is Transmitted by Fly Bites

Infection with *Trypanosoma brucei gambiense* or *T. brucei rhodesiense* leads to life-threatening meningoencephalitis. Gambian trypanosomiasis is a chronic infection often lasting more than a year. East African (Rhodesian) trypanosomiasis is a rapidly progressive infection that kills patients in 3 to 6 months. Trypanosomes are curved, 15- to 30-µm flagellates, visible in blood or cerebrospinal fluid, but difficult to find in tissue.

 EPIDEMIOLOGY: *T. brucei gambiense* and *T. brucei rhodesiense* are hemoflagellate protozoa are transmitted by several species of blood-sucking tsetse flies of the genus *Glossina*. The patchy distribution of African trypanosomiasis is related to the habitats of these flies. In Gambian trypanosomiasis, *T. brucei gambiense* is transmitted by tsetse flies of the riverine bush, mainly in endemic pockets of West and Central Africa. *Humans are the only important reservoir for this trypanosome.*

In East African trypanosomiasis, *T. brucei rhodesiense* is spread by tsetse flies of the woodland savanna of East Africa. Antelope, other game animals, and domestic cattle are natural reservoirs of *T. brucei rhodesiense*. Infection of humans is an occupational hazard of game wardens, fishermen, and cattle herders.

 PATHOPHYSIOLOGY: While biting an infected animal or human, the tsetse fly ingests trypomastigotes with the blood (Fig. 9-88). These (1) lose their coat of surface antigen, (2) multiply in the fly's midgut, (3) migrate to the salivary gland, (4) develop for 3 weeks through the epimastigote stage, and (5) multiply in the fly's saliva as infective metacyclic trypomastigotes. During another bite, metacyclic trypomastigotes are injected into the lymphatics and blood vessels of a new host. They disseminate to the bone marrow and tissue fluids and some eventually invade the CNS. They replicate by binary fission in blood, lymph and spinal fluid, then are ingested by another fly to complete the cycle.

Immune complexes form, with variable trypanosomal antigens and antibodies. Autoantibodies to antigens of erythrocytes, brain, and heart may be present. Trypanosomes use a genetically encoded program to alter their glycoprotein antigen coats periodically, thus evading immune attack. As a result, each wave of circulating trypomastigotes carries different antigenic variants and the trypanosomes stay a step ahead of the host's immune response.

 PATHOLOGY: *T. brucei* multiplies at sites of inoculation, and may cause localized nodular lesions: "primary chancres." Generalized lymph node and spleen involvement is prominent early in the disease. Affected nodes and spleen show focal hyperplasia of lymphocytes and macrophages. Infection eventually localizes to small blood vessels of the CNS, where replicating organisms elicit a destructive vasculitis, producing the progressive decrease in mentation characteristic of sleeping sickness. With *T. brucei rhodesiense*, the organisms also localize to cardiac blood vessels, and may cause fulminant myocarditis.

Lesions in the lymph nodes, brain, heart, and various other sites (including the inoculation site) show small blood vessel vasculitis, with endothelial cell hyperplasia and dense perivascular infiltrates of lymphocytes, macrophages, and plasma cells. CNS vasculitis leads to neuron loss, demyelination, and gliosis. Perivascular infiltrates thicken the leptomeninges and involve the Virchow-Robin spaces (Fig. 9-89).

 CLINICAL FEATURES: African trypanosomiasis has three clinical stages:

1. **Primary chancre:** After 5 to 15 days, a 3- to 4-cm papillary swelling topped by a central red spot appears at the inoculation site. It subsides spontaneously within 3 weeks.

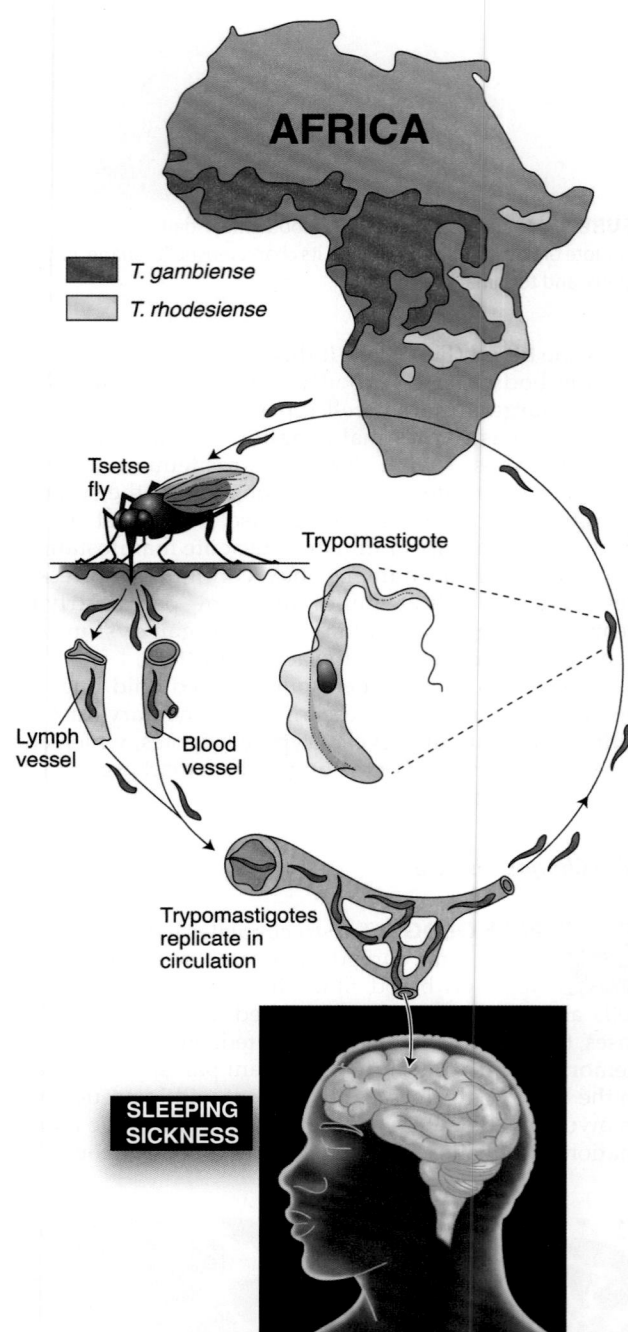

FIGURE 9-88. African trypanosomiasis (sleeping sickness). The distribution of Gambian and Rhodesian trypanosomiasis is related to the habitats of the vector tsetse flies (*Glossina* spp.). A tsetse fly bites an infected animal or human and ingests trypomastigotes, which multiply into infective, metacyclic trypomastigotes. During another fly bite, these are injected into lymphatic and blood vessels of a new host. A primary chancre develops at the site of the bite (stage 1a). Trypomastigotes replicate further in the blood and lymph, causing a systemic infection (stage 1b). Another fly ingests hypomastigotes to complete the cycle. In stage 2, invasion of the central nervous system by trypomastigotes leads to meningoencephalomyelitis and associated symptoms, including lethargy and daytime somnolence. Patients with Rhodesian trypanosomiasis may die within a few months. *T. gambiense = Trypanosoma brucei gambiense; T. rhodesiense = Trypanosoma brucei rhodesiense.*

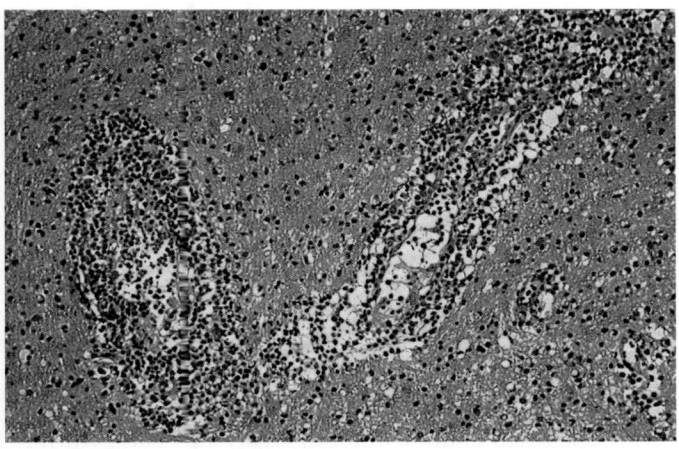

FIGURE 9-89. African trypanosomiasis. A section of brain from a patient who died from infection with *Trypanosoma brucei rhodesiense* shows a perivascular mononuclear cell infiltrate.

2. **Systemic infection:** Shortly after the chancre (if any) appears, and within 3 weeks of the bite, intermittent fever, for up to a week, often with splenomegaly and local and generalized lymphadenopathy herald bloodstream invasion. Enlarged posterior cervical lymph nodes, "Winterbottom sign," characterize Gambian trypanosomiasis. The evolving illness is marked by irregular remitting fevers, headache, joint pains, lethargy, and muscle wasting. Myocarditis may occur, more commonly and severely in Rhodesian trypanosomiasis. Dysfunction of lungs, kidneys, liver, and endocrine system occurs commonly in both forms of the disease.

3. **Brain invasion:** The two forms of sleeping sickness differ in the timing of CNS invasion. It occurs early (weeks to months) in Rhodesian trypanosomiasis and late (months to years) in the Gambian form. Brain invasion is marked by apathy, daytime somnolence, and sometimes coma. Diffuse meningoencephalitis causes tremors of the tongue and fingers; fasciculations of the muscles of the limbs, face, lips, and tongue; oscillatory movements of the arms, head, neck, and trunk; indistinct speech; and cerebellar ataxia, causing problems in walking.

Amebic Meningoencephalitis Is a Fatal Disease Caused by *Naegleria fowleri*

 EPIDEMIOLOGY: *N. fowleri* is a free-living, soil ameba that lives in ponds and lakes in tropical and subtropical regions. It also inhabits temperate areas, including the United States. Primary amebic meningoencephalitis is rare (fewer than 300 reported cases), and affects people who swim or bathe in these waters.

 PATHOPHYSIOLOGY: When someone swims in, or dives into, water with high concentrations of *N. fowleri*, it enters the nasal mucosa near the cribriform plate. Amebae invade the olfactory nerves, migrate into the olfactory bulbs, then proliferate in the meninges and brain.

 PATHOLOGY: Trophozoites are 8 to 15 μm, with sharply outlined nuclei that stain deeply with hematoxylin. The brain is swollen and soft, with vascular congestion and a purulent meningeal exudate, seen most over the lateral and basal areas, sometimes involving the length of the spinal cord. Amebae invade the brain along Virchow-Robin spaces, and cause massive tissue damage. Thrombosis and destruction of blood vessels lead to extensive hemorrhage. The olfactory tract and bulbs are enveloped and destroyed, and there is exudate between the bulb and the inferior surface of the temporal lobe. *Naegleria* proliferate in the brain and may produce solid masses of amebae (**amebomas**).

CLINICAL FEATURES: Primary amebic meningoencephalitis due to *N. fowleri* begins suddenly with fever, nausea, vomiting, and headache. Disease progresses rapidly. Within hours, patients suffer profound deterioration in mental status. CSF contains neutrophils, blood, and amebae. The disease is rapidly fatal.

Helminths

Helminths, or worms, are among the most common human pathogens. At any given time, a quarter to half of the world's population carries at least one helminth species. Although most do little harm, some cause significant disease. Schistosomiasis, for instance, is among the leading global causes of disease and death.

ETIOLOGIC AGENTS: Helminths are the largest (0.5 mm to 1 m) and most complex organisms that live within the human body. They are multicellular animals with the full range of body structures and complex life cycles, from eggs or larvae to adult worms, often with multiple morphologic transformations (molts). Some undergo these metamorphoses in different hosts before reaching adulthood, and human hosts may be only part of a series of hosts that support helminth maturation. Within the human body, helminths often migrate from the port of entry, through several organs, to a site of final infection.

PATHOPHYSIOLOGY: Most helminths that infect humans are well adapted to human parasitism, causing limited or no host tissue damage. They gain entry by ingestion, skin penetration or insect bites, and cause disease in various ways. A few compete with their human hosts for nutrients. Some grow to block vital structures, producing disease by mass effect. Most, however, cause dysfunction from the destructive inflammatory and immune responses that they elicit. For example, morbidity in schistosomiasis, the most destructive helminthic infection, results from granulomatous responses to schistosome eggs deposited in tissue.

Eosinophils' basic proteins are toxic to some helminths, and these cells are a major component of inflammatory responses to these organisms.

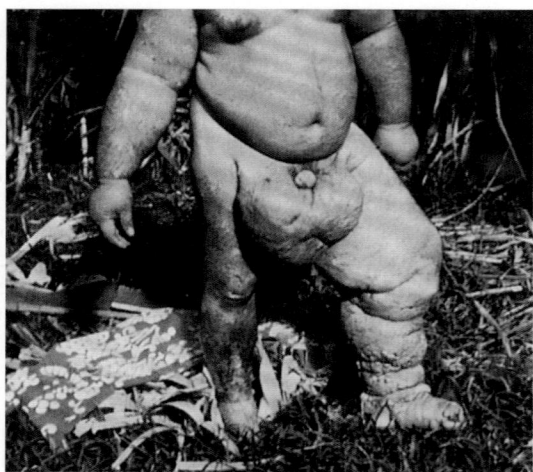

FIGURE 9-90. Bancroftian filariasis. Massive lymphedema (elephantiasis) of the scrotum and left lower extremity are present.

Parasitic helminths are grouped by overall morphology and digestive tissue structure:

- **Roundworms (nematodes)** are elongate and cylindrical, with tubular digestive tracts.
- **Flatworms (trematodes)** are flattened dorsoventrally, with digestive tracts that end in blind loops.
- **Tapeworms (cestodes)** are segmented, with separate head and body parts; they lack a digestive tract and absorb nutrients through their outer walls.

Lymphatic Filariasis Results in Massive Lymphedema (Elephantiasis)

Lymphatic filariasis (bancroftian and Malayan filariasis) is an inflammatory parasitic infection of lymphatic vessels caused by the roundworms *Wuchereria bancrofti* and *Brugia malayi*. Adult worms inhabit lymphatics, most often in inguinal, epitrochlear and axillary lymph nodes, testis, and epididymis. There they cause acute lymphangitis and, occasionally, obstruct lymphatics, causing severe lymphedema (Fig. 9-90). These filarial worms, are so called because they resemble threads (from Latin *filum*, meaning thread).

EPIDEMIOLOGY: Elephantiasis of lymphatic filariasis was familiar to Hindi and Persian physicians as early as 600 BC. Humans are the only definitive hosts, and acquire infection from bites of at least 80 species of *Culex, Aedes, Anopheles,* and *Mansonia* mosquitoes. *W. bancrofti* is widespread in southern Asia, the Pacific, Africa, and parts of South America. *B. malayi* is localized to coastal southern Asia and western Pacific islands. Worldwide, 100 to 200 million people are estimated to be infected.

PATHOPHYSIOLOGY: Mosquito bites transmit infectious larvae, which migrate to lymphatics and lymph nodes, where they mature over several months. Worms then mate and females release microfilariae into lymphatics and the bloodstream. Filariasis results from inflammatory responses to degenerating adult worms in the lymphatics. Repeated infections are common in endemic regions and cause bouts of lymphangitis (filarial fevers), that lead to extensive scarring and obstruct lymphatics over years. This blockage causes localized edema, mostly of legs, arms, genitalia, and breasts. In its most severe form (<5%), this is **elephantiasis**.

PATHOLOGY: Adult nematodes are white, threadlike very convoluted worms. Females are 80 to 100 mm long and 0.20 to 0.3 mm in width, twice the size of males. In Giemsa-stained blood films, microfilariae are curved, about 300 μm long.

Lymphatic vessels harboring adult worms are dilated, with thickened endothelium. In adjacent tissues, worms are surrounded by chronic inflammation, including eosinophils. Granulomatous reactions may develop and degenerating worms can provoke acute inflammation. Microfilariae in blood vessels and lymphatics, and degenerating microfilariae, also provoke a chronic inflammatory reaction. After repeated bouts of lymphangitis, lymph nodes and lymphatics become densely fibrotic, often containing calcified remnants of the worms.

CLINICAL FEATURES: In endemic areas, most of the infected population has antifilarial antibodies with no detectable infection, or asymptomatic microfilaremia. Some develop recurrent episodes of filarial fevers, with malaise, lymphadenopathy and lymphangitis, lasting 1 to 2 weeks, then resolving spontaneously. In a small subset of these, late manifestations of disease appear after 2 to 3 decades of recurrent bouts of filarial fevers. Lymphatic obstruction leads to chronic edema of dependent tissues. The overlying skin becomes thickened and warty. Identifying microfilariae in blood samples makes the diagnosis. Diethylcarbamazine and ivermectin are effective against lymphatic filariasis.

Occult filariasis, in patients who only have anti-filarial antibodies but no confirmed active disease, causes **tropical pulmonary eosinophilia**, which is only seen in southern India and some Pacific Islands. Patients have cough, wheezing, diffuse pulmonary infiltrates, and peripheral eosinophilia. Severity varies from mild to fatal.

Onchocerciasis Causes Blindness

Onchocerciasis ("**river blindness**") is a chronic inflammatory disease of the skin, eyes, and lymphatics caused by the filarial nematode *Onchocerca volvulus*.

EPIDEMIOLOGY: Onchocerciasis is one of the world's major endemic diseases. It afflicts about 40 million people, 2 million of whom are blind. It is transmitted by bites of *Simulium damnosum* blackflies, which inoculate infectious larvae into humans, who are the only definitive hosts. The flies require rapidly running water for breeding. Onchocerciasis is thus endemic along rivers and streams (hence, "river blindness") in parts of Africa, southern Mexico, and Central and South America.

PATHOPHYSIOLOGY: Adult worms live as coiled tangled masses in deep fasciae and subcutaneous tissues. Live worms cause no tissue damage and elicit no inflammatory response, but gravid females release millions of microfilariae, which migrate into the skin, eyes, lymph nodes and deep organs, and produce the onchocercal lesions. Ocular onchocerciasis results when microfilariae migrate throughout the eye, from the cornea to the optic nerve head.

When microfilariae die, they incite vigorous inflammatory and immune responses. Resulting damage to the cornea, choroids, or retina leads to partial or total loss of vision. Cutaneous inflammation causes microabscesses and chronic dermal and epidermal degeneration. In lymph nodes and lymphatics, responses to dying microfilariae cause chronic lymphatic obstruction and localized dependent edema.

 PATHOLOGY: *O. volvulus* is a thin, long nematode, the female is 400 × 0.3 mm and the male 30 × 0.2 mm. Massed adult worms become encapsulated by a fibrous scar, forming discrete, 1 to 3 cm, **onchocercal nodules** in the deep dermis and subcutis. Nodules form over bony prominences of the skull, scapula, ribs, iliac crest, trochanter, sacrum, and knee. These nodules show outer fibrosis, with inflammation, varying from suppurative to granulomatous inside. Active lesions in eyes and lymphatics show degenerating microfilariae surrounded by chronic inflammation, including eosinophils. Ocular involvement leads to sclerosing keratitis, iridocyclitis, chorioretinitis, and optic atrophy. Femoral inguinal nodes become enlarged, then fibrotic.

 CLINICAL FEATURES: Symptoms of onchocerciasis result from inflammatory responses to degenerating microfilariae. Skin manifestations begin with generalized pruritus that becomes so intense as to interfere with sleeping. Continuing damage produces patchy depigmentation, hypertrophy or atrophy of the skin. Progressive destruction of the cornea, choroid, or uvea causes loss of vision. Chronic lymphadenitis leads to localized edema that may cause chronic swelling (elephantiasis) of the legs, scrotum, or other dependent portions of the body. Systemic antihelminthic therapy, particularly with ivermectin, is effective.

Loiasis Principally Affects the Eyes and Skin

Loiasis is infection by the filarial nematode *Loa loa*, the African "eyeworm."

 EPIDEMIOLOGY AND PATHOPHYSIOLOGY: Loiasis is prevalent in the rain forests of Central and West Africa. Humans and baboons are the definitive hosts, and infection is transmitted by mango flies. Adult worms (4 cm long) migrate in the skin and occasionally cross the eye beneath the conjunctiva, making the patient acutely aware of this infection (Fig. 9-91). Gravid worms

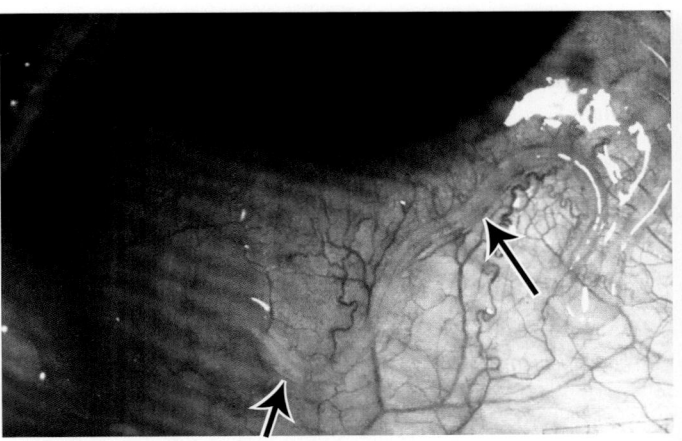

FIGURE 9-91. Loiasis. A thread-like *Loa loa* (*arrows*) is migrating in the subconjunctival tissues. (Reprinted from Farrar WE, Wood MJ, Innes JA, Tubbs H. *Infectious Diseases: Text and Color Atlas.* 2nd ed. New York: Gower Medical Publishing; 1992. Copyright © 1992 Elsevier. With permission.)

discharge microfilariae, which circulate in the blood during the day but reside in capillaries of the skin, lungs, and other organs at night.

 PATHOLOGY: Migrating worms cause no inflammation, but static ones are surrounded by eosinophils, other inflammatory cells and a foreign-body giant cell reaction. Rarely, acute generalized loiasis develops, with obstructive fibrin thrombi, containing degenerating microfilariae in small vessels of most organs. If such thrombi obstruct CNS vessels, lethal sudden and diffuse cerebral ischemia may result.

 CLINICAL FEATURES: Most infections are asymptomatic but persist for years. Some patients have pruritic, red, subcutaneous "Calabar" swellings, which may be reactions to migrating adult worms or microfilariae. Eyelids may swell, itch, and be painful. Worms may appear as they migrate beneath the conjunctiva. Systemic reactions include fever, pain, itching, urticaria, and eosinophilia. Dead worms in or near major nerves may cause paresthesia or paralysis. Microfilaricide therapy may cause massive death of microfilariae and provoke fever, meningoencephalitis, and death.

Patients With Symptomatic Nematode Infestations Generally Have Very Large Numbers of Parasites

Adult forms of several nematodes (Table 9-9) reside in the human bowel but rarely cause symptomatic disease. Clinical symptoms occur almost exclusively in patients with large infestations, or who are immunocompromised.

 EPIDEMIOLOGY: Humans are the only or primary host for all intestinal nematodes, and infection spreads from person to person via eggs or larvae passed in the stool or deposited in the perianal

TABLE 9-9
INTESTINAL NEMATODES

Species	Common Name	Site of Adult Worm	Clinical Manifestations
Ascaris lumbricoides	Roundworm	Small bowel	Allergic reactions to lung migration; intestinal obstruction
Ancylostoma duodenale	Hookworm	Small bowel	Allergic reactions to cutaneous inoculation and lung migration; intestinal blood loss
Necator americanus	Hookworm	Small bowel	Allergic reactions to cutaneous inoculation and lung migration; intestinal blood loss
Trichuris trichiura	Whipworm	Large bowel	Abdominal pain and diarrhea; rectal prolapse (rare)
Strongyloides stercoralis	Threadworm	Small bowel	Abdominal pain and diarrhea; dissemination to extraintestinal sites in immunocompromised people
Enterobius vermicularis	Pinworm	Cecum, appendix	Perianal and perineal itching

region. These diseases are most prevalent where hand washing and hygienic disposal of feces are lacking. Warm, moist climates are required for the infectious forms of many intestinal nematodes to survive outside the body. The worms are, thus, endemic in tropical and subtropical climates.

Ascariasis

Ascariasis is infection by the large roundworm *Ascaris lumbricoides*. It is the most common human helminthic infection, affecting at least one billion people, and is usually asymptomatic. Infection is worldwide, but is most common in areas with warm climates and poor sanitation.

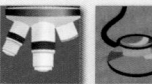 **PATHOPHYSIOLOGY:** Adult worms live in the small intestine, where gravid females discharge eggs that pass in the feces. These eggs hatch when ingested. *Ascaris* larvae emerge in the small intestine, penetrate the bowel wall, and reach the lungs through the venous circulation. They exit pulmonary capillaries, enter alveoli, then migrate up the trachea to the glottis. They are then swallowed, again reach the small bowel, to mature and reside in the lumen as adult worms for 1 to 2 years.

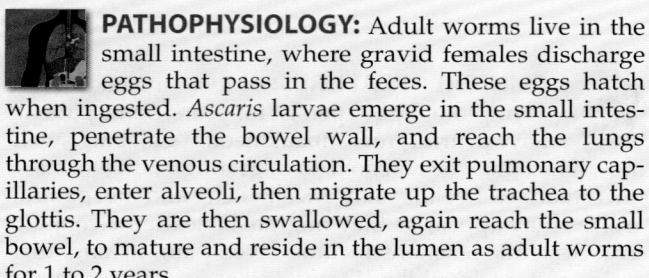 **PATHOLOGY AND CLINICAL FEATURES:** Adult worms (15 to 35 cm long) infrequently cause tissue reactions. Heavy infections may lead to vomiting, malnutrition, or intestinal obstruction (Fig. 9-92). Rarely, worms enter the pancreatic or biliary systems, and cause obstruction, acute pancreatitis, suppurative cholangitis, and liver abscesses. Eggs deposited in the liver or other tissues may produce necrosis, granulomatous inflammation, and fibrosis. *Ascaris* pneumonia, which may be fatal, develops when large numbers of larvae migrate within alveoli.

Ascariasis is diagnosed by identifying eggs in the feces. Adult worms may pass with the stools or even emerge from the nose or mouth. Ascaricidal drugs are effective.

Trichuriasis

Trichuriasis is caused by the intestinal nematode *Trichuris trichiura* ("**whipworm**").

 EPIDEMIOLOGY: Whipworm infection affects over 800 million people worldwide. Parasitism is most common in warm, moist places with poor sanitation, but over 2 million people in the United States are infected. Children are especially susceptible. Adult worms live in the cecum and upper colon, where females produce eggs that pass in the feces. Eggs embryonate in moist soil and become infective in 3 weeks. People are infected by ingesting eggs in contaminated soil, food, or drink.

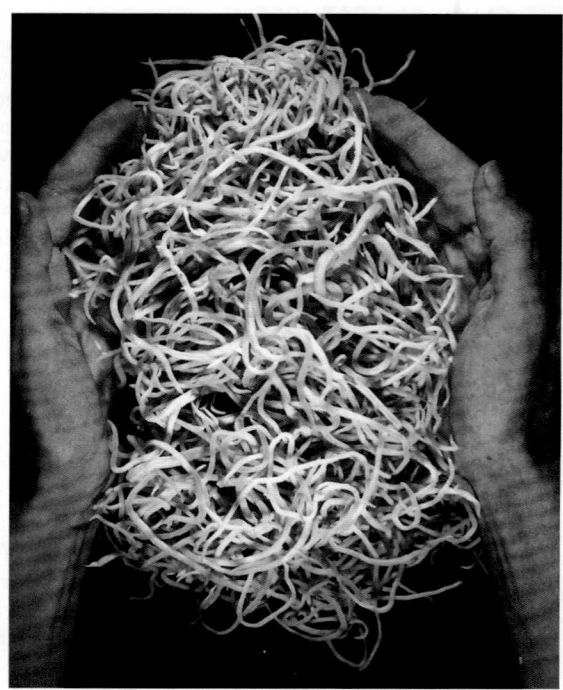

FIGURE 9-92. Ascariasis. This mass of over 800 worms of *Ascaris lumbricoides* obstructed and infarcted the ileum of a 2-year-old girl in South Africa.

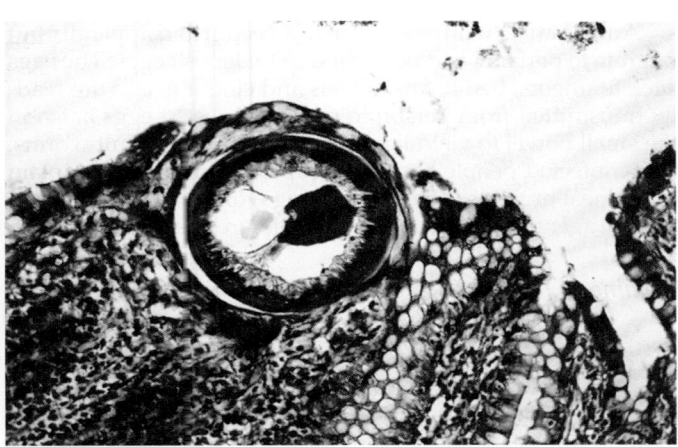

FIGURE 9-93. Trichuriasis. The anterior "whip" end of *Trichuris trichiura* is threaded into the mucosa of the colon.

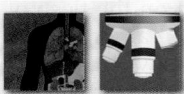 **PATHOPHYSIOLOGY AND PATHOLOGY:** Larvae emerge from ingested eggs in the small bowel and migrate to the cecum and colon, where adult worms attach to the superficial mucosa (Fig. 9-93). This causes small erosions, focal active inflammation and continuous loss of small quantities of blood. *T. trichiura* is 3 to 5 cm long, with a long, slender anterior and a short, blunt posterior.

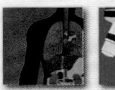 **CLINICAL FEATURES:** Most *T. trichiura* infections are asymptomatic. Heavy infestations may produce cramping abdominal pain, bloody diarrhea, weight loss, and anemia. The diagnosis is made by finding the characteristic eggs in the stool. Mebendazole is effective therapy.

Hookworm

Necator americanus and *Ancylostoma duodenale* ("hookworms") are intestinal nematodes that infect the human small bowel. They lacerate the bowel mucosa, causing intestinal blood loss, which can produce symptomatic disease in heavy infestations.

 EPIDEMIOLOGY: Hookworm infections are found in moist, warm, temperate, and tropical areas and cause serious public health problems worldwide. In fact, both *A. duodenale* ("Old World" hookworm) and *N. americanus* ("American" hookworm) both occur on most continents. Over 700 million people are infected with hookworms, including a half-million people in the United States.

PATHOPHYSIOLOGY AND PATHOLOGY: Filariform larvae directly penetrate the human epidermis on contact, enter the venous circulation and travel to the lungs. There, they lodge in alveolar capillaries, then rupture into alveoli, migrate up the trachea to the glottis and are swallowed. They molt in the duodenum, attach to its mucosal

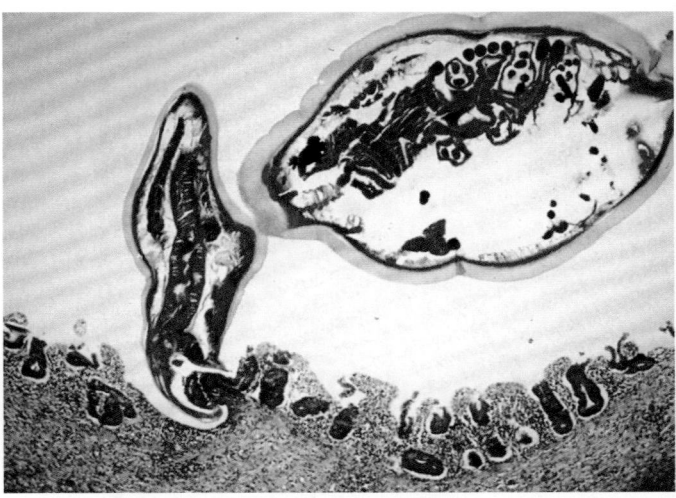

FIGURE 9-94. Ancylostomiasis. Section of the ileum shows two portions of a single adult worm, *Ancylostoma duodenale*. A plug of mucosa is in the buccal cavity of the hookworm.

wall with toothlike buckle plates and clamp off a section of a villus and ingest it (Fig. 9-94). In extensive infestations, particularly with *A. duodenale,* blood loss can be sufficient to cause anemia. Hookworms are about 1 cm long, grossly visible on the small bowel mucosa by punctate hemorrhages. There is no attendant inflammation.

 CLINICAL FEATURES: *Most people with infection have no symptoms, but hookworm is the most important cause of chronic anemia worldwide.* In people with heavy worm burdens and/or with inadequate iron intake (e.g., premenopausal women), chronic intestinal blood loss can produce severe iron deficiency anemia. Skin penetration may cause a pruritic eruption ("ground itch"), and larval migration through the lungs occasionally causes asthmalike symptoms.

Strongyloidiasis Is Disseminated in Immunocompromised Hosts

Strongyloidiasis is a small intestinal infection with a nematode, *Strongyloides stercoralis* ("threadworm"). *Most cases are asymptomatic, but infection can cause lethal disseminated disease in immunocompromised people.* Infection is most frequent in areas with warm, moist climates, and poor sanitation. Endemic pockets of strongyloidiasis exist in the United States, particularly in the Appalachian region and in institutions where personal hygiene may be poor.

  PATHOPHYSIOLOGY AND PATHOLOGY: *S. stercoralis* is the smallest intestinal nematode, 0.2 to 0.3 cm long. Adult females are buried in the crypts of the duodenum or jejunum but produce no visible reaction. The coiled females, their eggs and developing larvae, lie within the mucosa, usually with no associated inflammation (Fig. 9-95).

Parasitic females live in the mucosa of the small intestine, where they lay eggs that hatch quickly and release

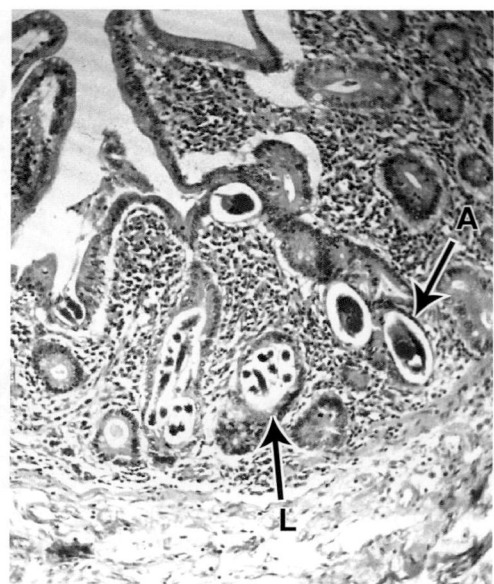

FIGURE 9-95. Strongyloidiasis. A section of jejunum shows adult worms, larvae and eggs of *Strongyloides stercoralis* in the mucosal crypts. The lamina propria is infiltrated with lymphocytes, plasma cells, and eosinophils. The patient had a hyperinfected syndrome and presented with malabsorption.

rhabditiform larvae. These pass into the feces, and become filariform in the soil. This infective stage penetrates human skin. Upon entry, *S. stercoralis* larvae invade the bloodstream, then travel to the lungs and subsequently to the small bowel, like hookworms. Worms mature in the small bowel. *S. stercoralis* may reproduce in human hosts by **autoinfection**. This occurs when rhabditiform larvae become infective (filariform) in a host's intestine, then repenetrate either the intestinal wall or the perianal skin, to start a new parasitic cycle within a single host.

CLINICAL FEATURES: Most infected people are asymptomatic, but moderate eosinophilia is common. Patients with impaired immunity, particularly if taking corticosteroids, may develop **disseminated strongyloidiasis** or **hyperinfection syndrome**. In them, internal autoinfection is greatly increased: huge numbers of filariform larvae penetrate intestinal walls and disseminate to distant organs. In disseminated strongyloidiasis, the gut may be ulcerated, edematous, and severely inflamed. Sepsis, usually with gram-negative organisms and infection of parenchymal organs follow. Untreated, disseminated strongyloidiasis is fatal; even with prompt treatment with thiabendazole or ivermectin, only one-third survive.

Pinworm

Enterobius vermicularis ("pinworm") is a worldwide intestinal nematode, most often encountered in temperate zones. People can be infected at any age, but parasitism is most common among young children. Over 200 million people carry *E. vermicularis* worldwide, including about 5 million school-age children in the United States.

Adult female worms reside in the cecum and appendix but migrate to perianal and perineal skin to deposit eggs. The eggs stick to fingers, bed linens, towels and clothing, and are readily transmitted from person to person. Ingested eggs hatch in the small bowel to yield larvae that mature into adult worms. Some infected people have no symptoms, but most complain of perineal pruritus, due to migrating worms depositing eggs. Several agents, including mebendazole, are effective treatment.

Trichinosis

EPIDEMIOLOGY: Humans worldwide acquire trichinosis by eating inadequately cooked meat with encysted *T. spiralis* larvae. Larvae are present in the skeletal muscles of various carnivorous or omnivorous wild and domesticated animals, including pigs, rats, bears, and walruses. Pork is the most common source of human trichinosis (Fig. 9-96).

Animals acquire trichinosis by feeding on the flesh of other infected animals. Infection is common among some wild animal populations and readily occurs when domesticated animals, such as pigs, they feed on garbage or uncooked meat. Meat inspection programs and restriction of feeding practices have largely eliminated *T. spiralis* from domesticated pigs in many developed countries. Only about 100 cases are reported in the United States annually, but these reflect only the most severely symptomatic cases and infection is probably much more common.

PATHOPHYSIOLOGY: In the small bowel, *T. spiralis* larvae emerge from ingested tissue cysts and burrow into the intestinal mucosa, where they develop into adult worms. The adults mate, and the female liberates larvae that invade the intestinal wall and enter the circulation. Production of larvae may continue for 1 to 4 months, until the worms are finally expelled from the intestine. Larvae can invade nearly any tissue but can survive only in striated skeletal muscle, where they encyst and remain viable for years. Resulting myositis is especially prominent in the diaphragm, extrinsic ocular muscles, tongue, intercostal muscles, gastrocnemius, and deltoids. CNS or cardiac involvement may cause meningoencephalitis or myocarditis.

PATHOLOGY: Skeletal muscle is the major site of tissue damage. When a larva infects a myocyte, the cell undergoes basophilic degeneration and swells. Early myocyte infection elicits an intense inflammatory infiltrate, rich in eosinophils and macrophages. Larvae grow to 10 times their initial size, fold on themselves and develop a capsule. With encapsulation, inflammation subsides. Several years later, larvae die and their cysts calcify. The small bowel is grossly normal but adult forms at the base of villi in heavy infestations may be associated with an inflammatory infiltrate.

CLINICAL FEATURES: Most human infections with *T. spiralis* involve small numbers of cysts and are asymptomatic. Symptomatic trichinosis is

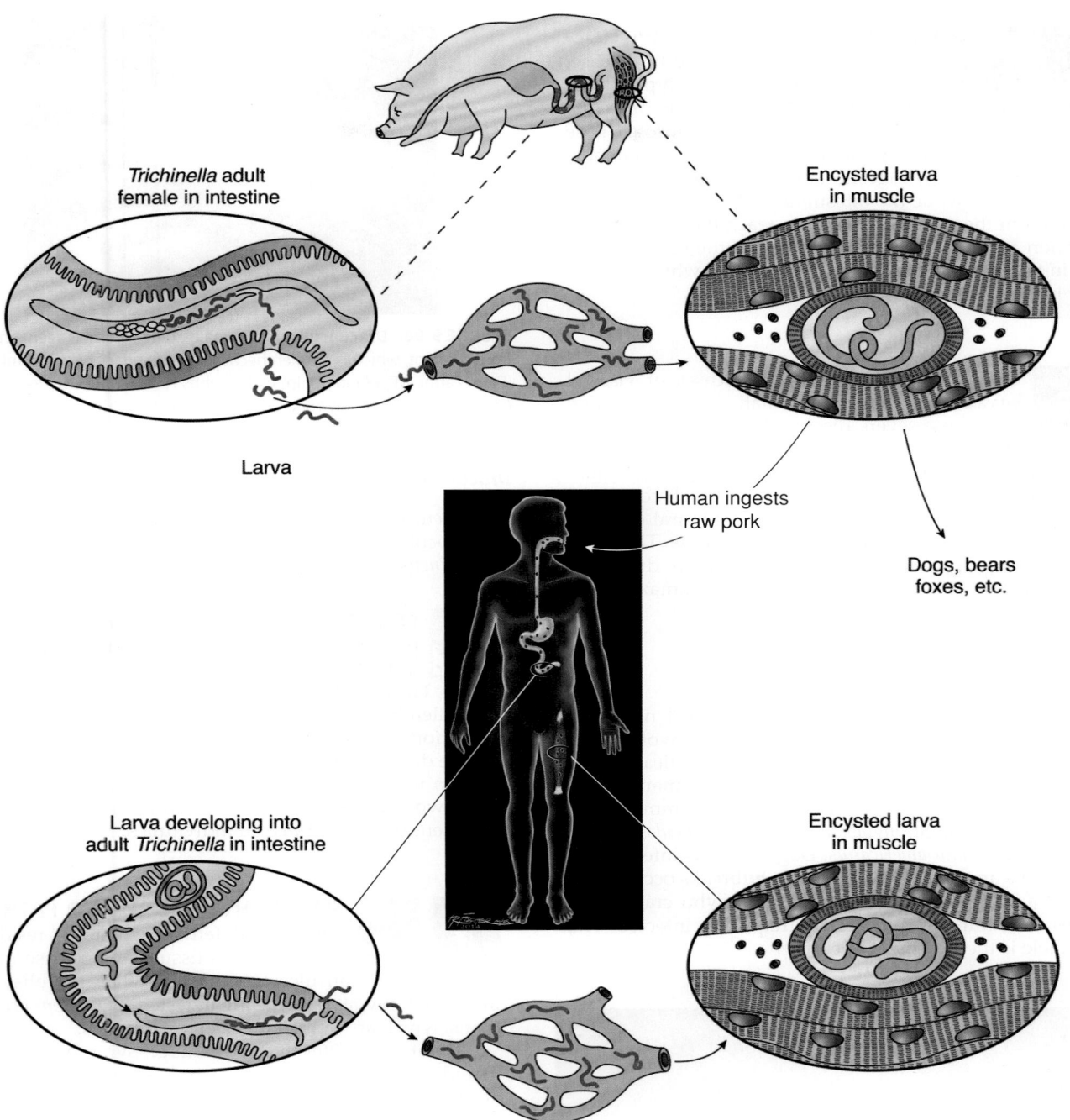

FIGURE 9-96. Trichinosis. After being ingested by the pig, cysts of *Trichinella* are digested in the gastrointestinal tract, liberating larvae that mature to adult worms. Female worms release larvae that penetrate the intestinal wall, enter the circulation and lodge in striated muscle, where they encyst. When humans ingest inadequately cooked pork, the cycle is repeated, resulting in the muscle disease characteristic of trichinosis.

usually self-limited and patients recover in a few months. If large numbers of cysts are eaten, abdominal pain and diarrhea may result when worms invade the small bowel. Major symptoms, like fever, weakness and severe pain and tenderness of affected muscles, usually develop several days later. **Eosinophilia may be extreme (>50% of blood leukocytes).** Extraocular muscle involvement may produce periorbital edema. Brain or heart infestation can

be fatal. Severe trichinosis requires corticosteroids to attenuate the inflammation. Antihelminthic drugs are needed to rid the intestine of adult worms.

Visceral Larva Migrans (Toxocariasis)

Toxocariasis is an infection of deep organs by helminthic larvae migrating in aberrant hosts.

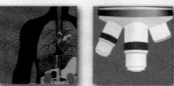 **PATHOPHYSIOLOGY AND PATHOLOGY:** Toxocariasis is a sporadic disease, mainly of young children, typically in overcrowded dwellings, with dogs and cats. *Toxocara canis* and *T. cati* are the most common causes. These roundworms live in dogs' and cats' intestines, and people acquire infection by ingestion of embryonated ova. Eggs hatch, larvae invade the intestinal wall, then travel to the liver. From there, a few emerge to reach the systemic circulation and are carried to any part of the body. Larvae die in tissues, and elicit small granulomas, which eventually heal by scarring.

CLINICAL FEATURES: Many cases of visceral larva migrans are asymptomatic, but any infection may cause severe disease. The typical symptomatic patient is a child with hypereosinophilia, pneumonitis, and hypergammaglobulinemia. In them, ocular manifestations are common, with the chief complaint often being loss of vision in one eye. Toxocaral endophthalmitis has been mistaken for retinoblastoma. The infection is generally self-limited, and symptoms disappear within a year. It is treated with diethylcarbamazine and thiabendazole.

Cutaneous Larva Migrans

Cutaneous larva migrans is caused by larval nematodes migrating through the skin, where they provoke severe inflammation that appears as serpiginous urticarial trails (Fig. 9-97). Cutaneous larva migrans goes by many names, and many organisms cause it. The more common larval nematodes include *Strongyloides stercoralis*, *Ancylostoma braziliensis* and *Necator americanus*. Dogs and cats infected with hookworms are the major reservoir. Outbreaks occur at subtropical and tropical beaches. Plumbers who crawl under houses and animal caretakers are frequently infected. Thiabendazole is the treatment of choice.

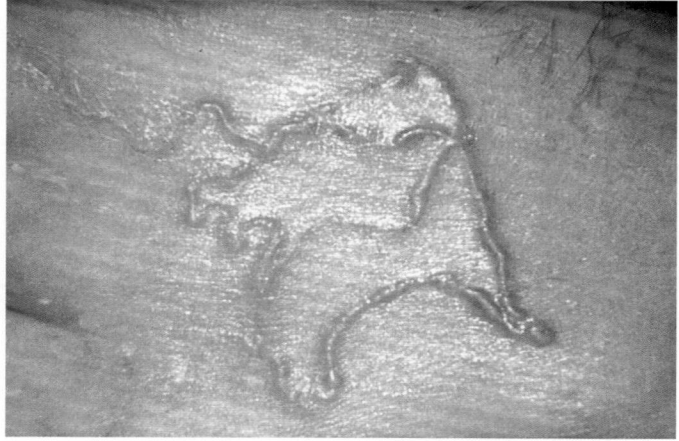

FIGURE 9-97. Cutaneous larva migrans. The skin shows a creeping eruption with the characteristic serpiginous, raised lesion. (Reprinted from Farrar WE, Wood MJ, Innes JA, Tubbs H. *Infectious Diseases: Text and Color Atlas.* 2nd ed. New York: Gower Medical Publishing; 1992. Copyright © 1992 Elsevier. With permission.)

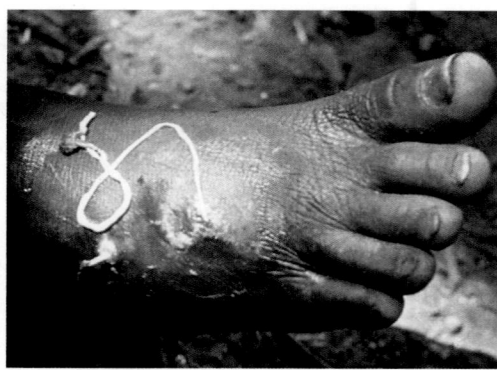

FIGURE 9-98. Dracunculiasis. A female guinea worm is seen emerging from the foot, which is swollen because of secondary bacterial infection. (From Farrar WE, Wood MJ, Innes JA, Tubbs H. *Infectious Diseases Text and Color Atlas.* 2nd ed. New York: Gower Medical Publishing; 1992.)

Dracunculiasis

Dracunculiasis (guinea worm) is an infection of connective and subcutaneous tissues with the guinea worm, *Dracunculus medinensis*.

 EPIDEMIOLOGY: Guinea worm infection was previously common in the rural areas of countries of the Middle East, South Asia and sub-Saharan Africa. However, the global prevalence of dracunculiasis has fallen by over 99 percent since the launch of eradication efforts in the 1980's, when 20 countries were endemic for the disease—in 1986 alone there were an estimated 3.5 million new cases. By 2018, new cases were confined to only two countries—Chad and South Sudan—and these represented only 28 infected individuals.

 PATHOPHYSIOLOGY AND PATHOLOGY: Adult female nematodes reside in subcutaneous tissues and release many larvae through an ulcerated blister. When the blister is immersed in water, larvae are ingested by *Cyclops* crustaceans, which are in turn ingested by humans.

About a year later, systemic allergic symptoms appear, including a pruritic urticarial rash. A reddish papule, often around the ankles, develops and vesiculates. Beneath this sterile blister is the anterior end of the female worm. The blister bursts upon contact with water and the worm, now measuring up to 120 cm and carrying 3 million larvae, partially emerges (Fig. 9-98). The worm then spews myriad larvae into the water. Secondary infection of the blister, often with spreading cellulitis, is common. Dead worms provoke intense inflammatory responses, which may be debilitating. The worm can be extracted by progressively twisting it onto a small stick. Treatment also includes anthelminthic drugs.

Schistosomiasis Causes Severe Inflammation in the Liver, Intestines, and Bladder

Schistosomiasis (bilharziasis) is the most important human helminthic disease. Intense inflammatory and immune responses cause tissue damage. Three species of schistosomes are responsible for the majority of infections: *Schistosoma mansoni, S. haematobium,* and *S. japonicum*.

EPIDEMIOLOGY: *Schistosomiasis affects about 10% of humanity and causes more morbidity and mortality than all other worm infections.* It is second only to malaria as a cause of disabling disease. In 2018, it is estimated that 779 million persons are at risk for infection, 207 million individuals in 74 countries were infected with schistosomiasis, and 120 million of them developed the disease. The three species affect distinct geographic regions, reflecting the distribution of their specific host snail species. *S. mansoni* occurs in much of tropical Africa, parts of southwest Asia, South America, and the Caribbean. *S. haematobium* is endemic in large regions of tropical Africa and parts of the Middle East. *S. japonicum* occurs in parts of China, the Philippines, Southeast Asia, and India.

PATHOPHYSIOLOGY: Schistosomes have complicated life cycles, alternating between asexual generations in their invertebrate host (snail) and sexual generations in vertebrate hosts (Fig. 9-99). A schistosome egg hatches in fresh water, liberating a motile **miracidium** that penetrates a snail, where it develops into the final larval stage, the **cercaria**. Cercariae escape into the water and penetrate human skin, during which process they lose their forked tails and become "schistosomula." These migrate through tissues, penetrate blood vessels, and migrate to the lungs and liver. In intestinal venules of the portal drainage, schistosomulae mature, forming pairs of male and female worms. Female *S. mansoni* and *S. japonicum* deposit eggs in intestinal venules; *S. haematobium* lays eggs in bladder venules. Embryos develop during as the eggs pass through these tissues. Larvae are mature when eggs pass through intestine or bladder walls, and are discharged in feces or urine. They hatch in fresh water, liberating miracidia and completing the life cycle.

PATHOLOGY: *The basic lesion is a circumscribed granuloma or a cellular infiltrate of eosinophils and neutrophils around an egg.* Adult schistosomes provoke no inflammation while alive in veins. Granulomas around the eggs may obstruct microvascular blood flow, cause ischemic damage to adjacent tissue and progressive scarring and dysfunction in affected organs.

Female worms deposit hundreds or thousands of eggs daily for 5 to 35 years. Most infected people harbor fewer than 10 adult females. However, if the worm burden is large, the granulomatous response to the enormous number of eggs can pose significant problems. Site of involvement reflects the tropisms of individual schistosome species.

- *S. mansoni* inhabits branches of the inferior mesenteric vein, affecting the distal colon and liver.
- *S. haematobium* winds its way to veins of the rectum, bladder, and pelvic organs.
- *S. japonicum* deposits its eggs mainly in the branches of the superior mesenteric vein, and so damages the small bowel, ascending colon, and liver.

Liver disease due to *S. mansoni* or *S. japonicum* begins as periportal granulomas (Fig. 9-100) and progresses to dense periportal fibrosis **(pipestem fibrosis)** (Fig. 9-101). In severe cases, this causes obstruction of portal blood flow and portal hypertension. *S. mansoni* and *S. japonicum* also damage the intestine, where granulomatous responses produce inflammatory polyps and foci of mucosal and submucosal fibroses.

In **urogenital schistosomiasis** with *S. haematobium*, eggs are most abundant in the bladder, ureter, and seminal vesicles, but may also reach lungs, colon, and appendix. Eggs in the bladder and ureters incite granulomatous inflammation, inflammatory protuberances, and patches of mucosal and mural fibrosis. These may obstruct urine flow, and so cause secondary inflammatory damage to the bladder, ureters, and kidneys. In the bladder, *S. haematobium* may cause **squamous cell carcinoma**. In areas where *S. haematobium* is prevalent, this is the most common malignancy.

The granulomas surround schistosome eggs. Eosinophils may predominate in early granulomas. In older granulomas, epithelioid macrophages and giant cells are prominent and the oldest granulomas are densely fibrotic. The eggs of the various schistosome species are identified on the basis of their size and shape.

CLINICAL FEATURES: When schistosome larvae penetrate skin, a self-limited, intensely pruritic rash may occur. However, chronic granulomatous tissue injury is the dominant problem. Liver involvement leads to portal hypertension, splenomegaly, ascites, and bleeding esophageal varices. Intestinal disease is usually minimally symptomatic, but some patients have abdominal pain and bloody stools. Bladder involvement causes hematuria, recurrent urinary infections. Progressive obstruction may occur and lead to renal failure. Identifying parasite eggs in the urine or feces establishes the diagnosis. Schistosomes are effectively killed by systemic antihelminthic agents, but structural changes due to extensive scarring are irreversible.

Other Fluke Infestations Mainly Affect GI, Respiratory, and Biliary Tracts

Clonorchiasis

Clonorchiasis is hepatobiliary infection caused by the Chinese liver fluke, *Clonorchis sinensis*. The fluke usually causes only mild symptoms, but is sometimes associated with bile duct stones, cholangitis, and bile duct cancer.

EPIDEMIOLOGY: Clonorchiasis is endemic in east Asia, from Vietnam to Korea, where people often eat uncooked freshwater fish and ingest fluke larvae. In parts of Vietnam, China, and Japan, over half of the adult population is infected.

Adult worms are flat and transparent, live in human bile ducts and pass eggs to the intestine and feces. After ingestion by a specific snail, the egg hatches into a miracidium. Cercariae escape from the snail and seek

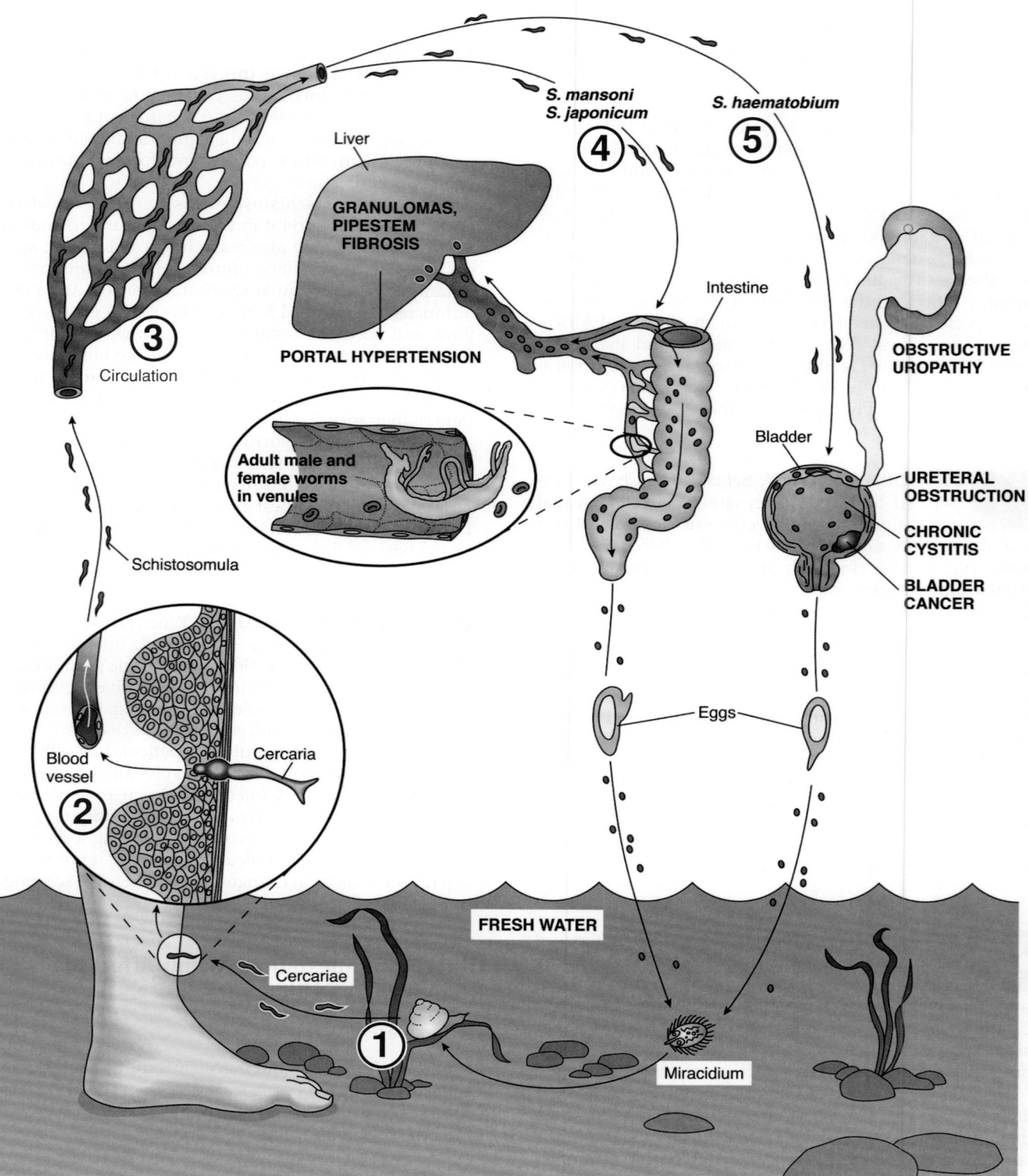

FIGURE 9-99. **Life cycle of *Schistosoma* and clinical features of schistosomiasis.** The schistosome egg hatches in water, liberates a miracidium that penetrates a snail and develops through two stages to a sporocyst to form the final larval stage, the cercaria. **(1)** The cercaria escapes from the snail into water, "swims" and penetrates the skin of a human host. **(2)** The cercaria loses its forked tail to become a schistosomulum, which migrates through tissues, penetrates a blood vessel and **(3)** is carried to the lung and later to the liver. In hepatic portal venules, the schistosomula become sexually mature and form pairs, each with a male and a female worm, the female worm lying in the gynecophoral canal of the male worm. The organism causes lesions in the liver, including granulomas, portal ("pipestem") fibrosis, and portal hypertension. **(4)** The female worm deposits immature eggs in small venules of the intestine and rectum (*Schistosoma mansoni* and *Schistosoma japonicum*) or **(5)** of the urinary bladder (*Schistosoma haematobium*). The bladder infestation leads to obstructive uropathy, ureteral obstruction, chronic cystitis, and bladder cancer. Embryos develop during passage of the eggs through tissues, and larvae are mature when eggs pass through the wall of the intestine or urinary bladder. Eggs hatch in water and liberate miracidia to complete the cycle.

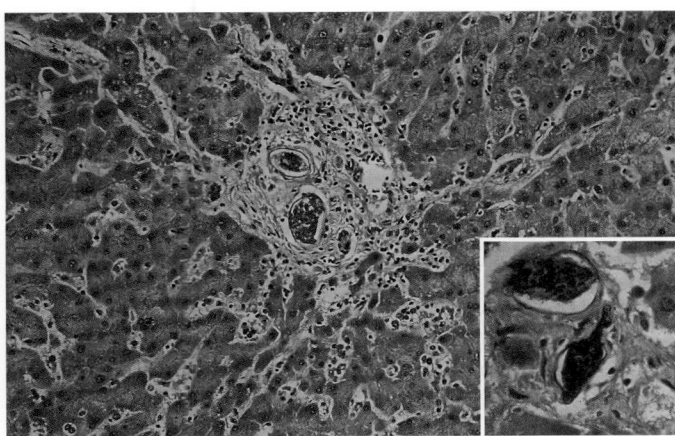

FIGURE 9-100. Hepatic schistosomiasis. A hepatic granuloma surrounds a degenerating egg of *Schistosoma mansoni*. A higher power of the organism is shown in the *inset*. (Reprinted from Farrar WE, Wood MJ, Innes JA, Tubbs H. *Infectious Diseases: Text and Color Atlas*. 2nd ed. New York: Gower Medical Publishing; 1992. Copyright © 1992 Elsevier. With permission.)

out certain fish, which they penetrate and in which they encyst. When humans eat uncooked fish, cercariae emerge in the duodenum, enter the common bile duct through the ampulla of Vater and mature in distal bile ducts to adult flukes.

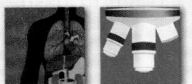 **PATHOPHYSIOLOGY AND PATHOLOGY:** The presence of *Clonorchis* in bile ducts elicits an inflammatory response that does not eliminate the worm, but causes ducts to dilate and scar. Sometimes the worms cause calculi in hepatic bile ducts, leading to obstruction. Adult *Clonorchis* persists in bile ducts for decades, and long-standing infection is associated with bile duct carcinoma (**cholangiocarcinoma**).

In heavy *Clonorchis* infestations, the liver may reach three times normal size. Dilated bile ducts are seen through the capsule, and the cut surface is punctuated with thick-walled dilated bile ducts (Fig. 9-102). Flukes (up to 2.5 cm), sometimes thousands, can be expressed from the bile ducts. Duct epithelium is initially hyperplastic, then metaplastic. Surrounding stroma is fibrotic. Secondary bacterial infection is common, with suppurative cholangitis. Eggs deposited in the liver parenchyma elicit fibrous

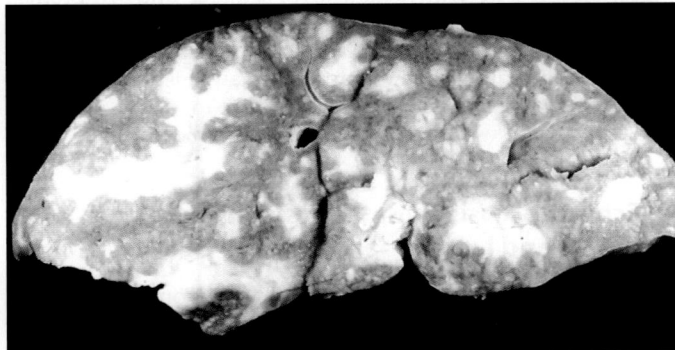

FIGURE 9-101. Hepatic schistosomiasis. Chronic infection of the liver with *Schistosoma japonicum* has led to the characteristic "pipestem" fibrosis.

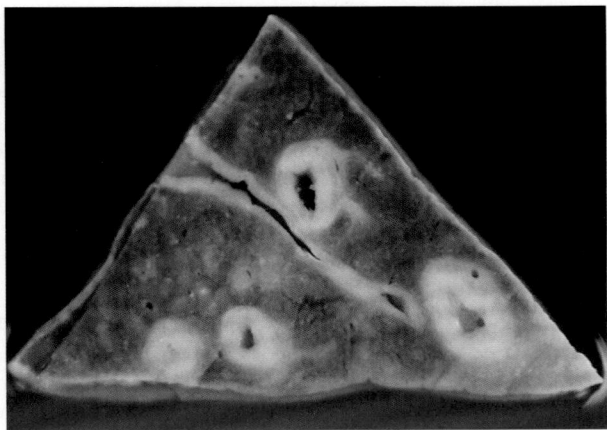

FIGURE 9-102. Clonorchiasis of the liver. The bile ducts are greatly thickened and dilated because of the presence of adult flukes (*Clonorchis sinensis*).

and granulomatous reactions. Masses of eggs lodged in bile ducts may cause cholangitis. If involved, pancreatic ducts may have metaplastic epithelium, and be dilated, thickened and eventually surrounded by fibrosis.

CLINICAL FEATURES: Transient fever and chills may occur when *C. sinensis* migrates into bile ducts, but most infected people are asymptomatic. A variety of complications may be fatal, including biliary obstruction, bacterial cholangitis, pancreatitis, and cholangiocarcinoma. Identifying *C. sinensis* eggs in stools or duodenal aspirates confirms the diagnosis. Systemic antihelminthic agents are effective.

Paragonimiasis

Paragonimiasis is a pulmonary infection by several species of the genus *Paragonimus,* the oriental lung fluke. The most common human pathogen is *P. westermani*, which is common in Asian countries (Korea, the Philippines, Taiwan, and China) where uncooked, lightly salted or wine-soaked fresh crabs are delicacies. Use of raw crab juices as medicines or seasonings may also cause the infection.

CLINICAL FEATURES: Pulmonary paragonimiasis is often mistaken for tuberculosis. It manifests as fever, malaise, night sweats, chest pain, and cough. However, unlike tuberculosis, peripheral eosinophilia is common. The sputum is sometimes blood-tinged and chest radiographs reveal transient diffuse pulmonary infiltrates. The prognosis is generally good, but ectopic lesions in the brain may be fatal. Finding eggs in the sputum or stools establishes the definitive diagnosis.

Fascioliasis

Fascioliasis is a liver infestation by the sheep liver fluke, *Fasciola hepatica*. Humans may acquire infection wherever sheep are raised, usually by eating vegetation, such as watercress, that is contaminated with the cysts passed by sheep.

PATHOPHYSIOLOGY: After reaching the duodenum, cysts liberate metacercariae that invade into the peritoneal cavity, penetrate the liver, then migrate through hepatic parenchyma into the bile ducts. Larvae mature to adults and live in both intrahepatic and extrahepatic bile ducts. Later, adult flukes penetrate bile duct walls, meander back into the liver, they feed on liver cells and deposit their eggs.

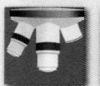 **PATHOLOGY AND CLINICAL FEATURES:** Eggs of *F. hepatica* cause hepatic abscesses and granulomas. The worms induce hyperplasia of bile duct epithelium, portal and periductal fibrosis, bile ductule proliferation and varying biliary obstruction. Eosinophilia, vomiting, and acute gastric pain are characteristic. Severe untreated infections may be fatal. Identifying eggs establishes the diagnosis.

Fasciolopsiasis

Fasciolopsiasis is common in the Orient, and is caused by the giant intestinal fluke, *Fasciolopsis buski*. Human acquire infection by eating aquatic vegetables contaminated with encysted cercariae. The worm is large (3 × 7 cm). It attaches to the duodenal or jejunal wall, which may ulcerate, become infected and cause pain like that of a peptic ulcer. Acute symptoms may also be due to intestinal obstruction or toxins released by large numbers of worms. Diagnosis is made by identifying *F. buski* eggs in the stool. Treatment is with systemic antihelminthic agents.

Taenia and *Diphyllobothrium* Species Cause Intestinal Tapeworm Infections

Taenia saginata, *T. solium*, and *Diphyllobothrium latum* infect humans, and grow to their adult forms within the intestine (Table 9-10). Presence of these adult worms rarely damages the human host.

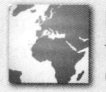 **EPIDEMIOLOGY:** People acquire intestinal tapeworm infections by eating poorly cooked beef (*T. saginata*), pork (*T. solium*), or fish (*D. latum*) containing larvae. Tapeworms have cystic larval stages in

TABLE 9-10
TAPEWORM INFECTIONS

Species	Human Disease	Source of Human Infection
Taenia saginata	Adult tapeworm in intestine	Beef
Taenia solium	Adult tapeworm in intestine; cysticercosis	Pork; human feces
Diphyllobothrium latum	Adult tapeworm in intestine	Fish
Echinococcus granulosus	Hydatid cyst disease	Dog feces

animals and worm stages in humans. Animals acquire beef and pork tapeworms by ingesting material tainted with infected human feces. The cystic larval forms develop in the animals' muscles. Modern cattle and pig farming practices, plus meat inspection, have largely eliminated beef and pork tapeworms in industrialized countries, but infection is still common elsewhere. Fish tapeworm infection occurs where raw, pickled, or partly cooked freshwater fish are common fare. Tapeworm infections are usually asymptomatic, but people may be distressed when passing parts of a worm in the stool. Fish tapeworm (*D. latum*) takes up vitamin B_{12} and a small number (<2%) of infected people develop pernicious anemia (see Chapter 26).

Cysticercosis

Adult *T. solium* is acquired by eating undercooked pork infected with cysticerci.

  PATHOPHYSIOLOGY AND EPIDEMIOLOGY: Pigs acquire cysticerci by ingesting eggs of *T. solium* in human feces. This cycle, although a public health concern, is essentially benign for both humans and pigs. However, when humans accidentally ingest tapeworm eggs from human feces and become infected with cysticerci, the consequences may be catastrophic. The eggs release oncospheres, which penetrate the gut wall, enter the bloodstream, lodge in tissue, encyst, and differentiate to cysticerci.

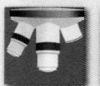 **PATHOLOGY:** *T. solium* causes a spherical, milky white 1 cm cyst containing fluid and an invaginated scolex (head of the worm) with birefringent hooklets. Cysts can remain viable indefinitely and provoke no inflammation; rather, as they grow they compress adjacent tissues. Degenerating cysts are what usually causes symptoms. They attach to tissue and are densely inflamed with eosinophils, neutrophils, lymphocytes, and plasma cells. Multiple cysticerci in the brain may impart a "Swiss cheese" appearance to the tissue (Fig. 9-103).

 CLINICAL FEATURES: Cerebral cysticercosis presents with headaches or seizures, and symptoms depend on the sites affected. Massive cerebral cysticercosis causes convulsions and death. Cysticerci in the retina blind the patient. In the heart, they may cause arrhythmias and sudden death. Depending on the site involved, cysticercosis is treated with surgery or antihelminthic therapy.

In Echinococcosis Hydatid Cysts Affect the Liver and Lungs

Echinococcosis (hydatid disease) is a zoonotic infection caused by larval cestodes of the genus *Echinococcus*. The most common offender is *Echinococcus granulosus*, which causes cystic hydatid disease. *E. multilocularis* and *E. vogeli* rarely infect humans.

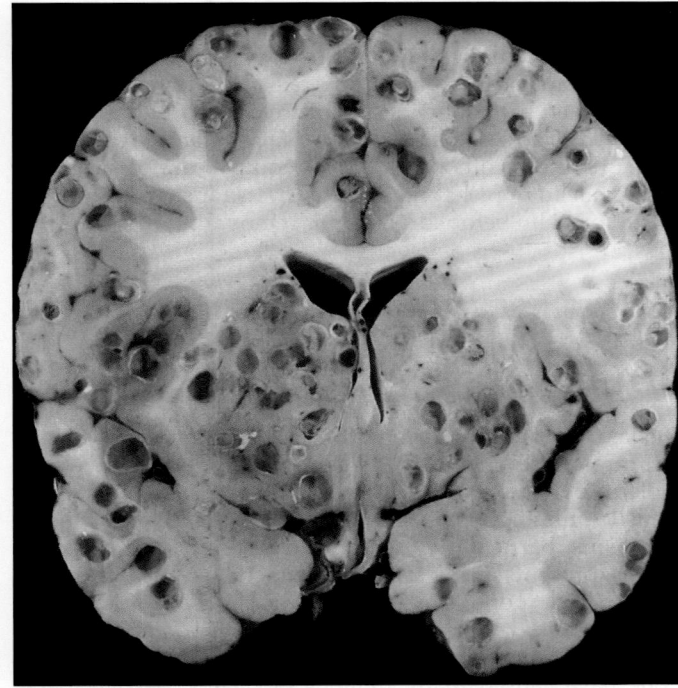

FIGURE 9-103. Cysticercosis. A cross-section of the brain from a patient infected with the larvae of *Taenia solium* shows many cysticerci in the gray matter, imparting a "Swiss cheese" appearance.

EPIDEMIOLOGY: Infestation with *E. granulosus* is endemic in sheep, goats, and cattle and their canine attendants. Dogs contaminate their habitats (and their human keepers) with infectious eggs. Humans become infected when they ingest tapeworm eggs inadvertently. Resulting hydatid disease occurs worldwide among herding populations who live in close proximity to dogs and herd animals, especially Australia, New Zealand, Argentina, Greece, and herding countries of Africa and the Middle East. In the United States, immigrants and indigenous sheep-herding populations of the southwest may be affected.

E. multilocularis causes rare alveolar hydatid disease in humans. Dogs and cats are domestic definitive hosts, house mice being intermediate hosts. Dogs are also definitive hosts for *E. vogeli*, with which people may become accidental intermediate hosts by ingesting eggs shed by domestic dogs.

PATHOPHYSIOLOGY: Adult tapeworms (2 to 6 mm long) live in the small intestines of carnivorous hosts, for example, wolves, foxes, etc. (Fig. 9-104). *E. granulosus* has a scolex with suckers and many hooklets that attach to intestinal mucosa. After a short neck are three segments (proglottids). The terminal gravid proglottid breaks off and releases eggs, which are eliminated in feces. Herbivorous intermediate hosts, like cattle and sheep, eat contaminated herbage. Humans who ingest plants contaminated by cestode eggs may also become infected. Larvae emerge from the eggs, penetrate the gut wall, enter the bloodstream, and disseminate to

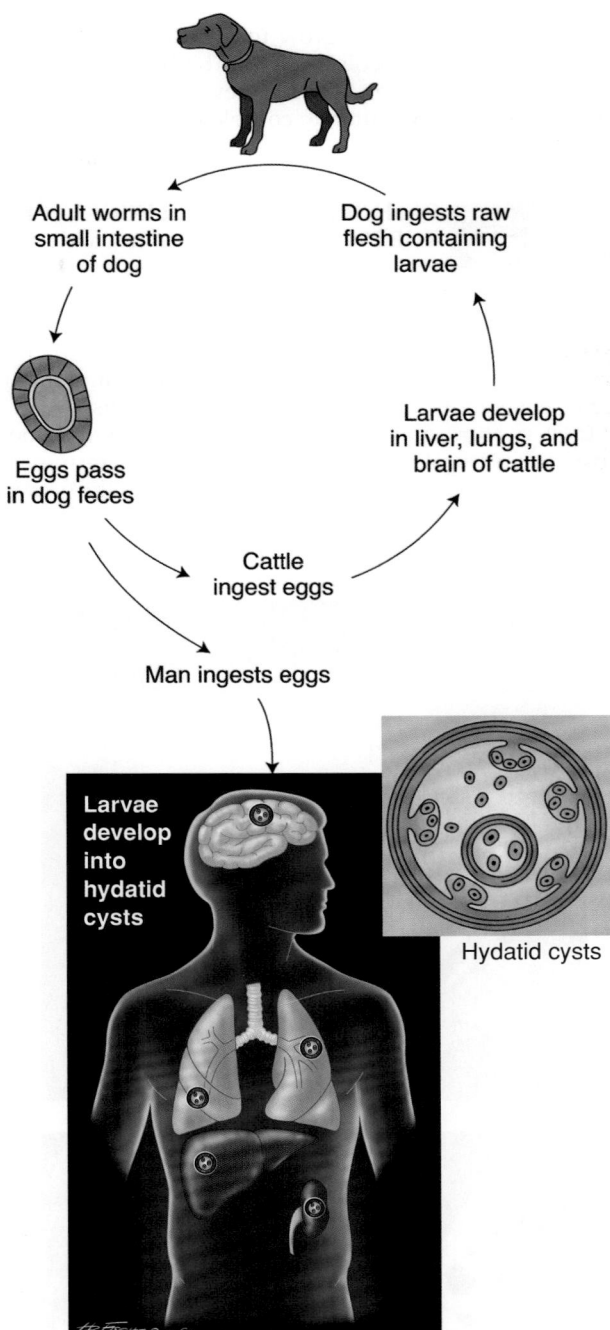

FIGURE 9-104. Life cycle of *Echinococcus granulosus* and cystic hydatid disease. The adult cestode lives in the small intestine of a dog (the definitive host). A gravid proglottid ruptures, releasing cestode eggs into the dog's feces. Cestode eggs are ingested by cattle or sheep (the intermediate hosts), hatch in the intestine and release oncospheres that penetrate the wall of the gut, enter the bloodstream, disseminate to various deep organs and grow to form hydatid cysts, containing brood capsules and scolices. When another dog ingests raw flesh from the cattle or sheep, the scolices are ingested and develop into mature worms in the dog's intestine to complete the cycle. A person who ingests cestode eggs in contaminated plant material becomes an accidental intermediate host. The larvae increase in size, but the parasite reaches a "dead end" without developing into an adult tapeworm. Hydatid cysts in humans occur predominantly in the liver but may also involve lung, kidney, brain, and other organs.

deep organs, where they grow to form large cysts with brood capsules and scolices. If the herbivore's flesh is eaten by a carnivore, scolices develop into sexually mature worms in the latter, to complete the cycle.

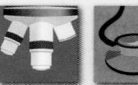 **PATHOLOGY AND CLINICAL FEATURES:** Slowly growing hydatid cysts are found by chance or when their size or position interferes with normal functions. A hepatic cyst may manifest as a palpable right upper quadrant mass. It may compress intrahepatic bile ducts to cause obstructive jaundice. Lung cysts (Fig. 9-105) are often asymptomatic and discovered incidentally on chest radiographs.

Cyst rupture may seed adjacent tissues with brood capsules and scolices. When these "seeds" germinate, they produce many additional cysts, each with the growth potential of the original cyst. Traumatic rupture of such a

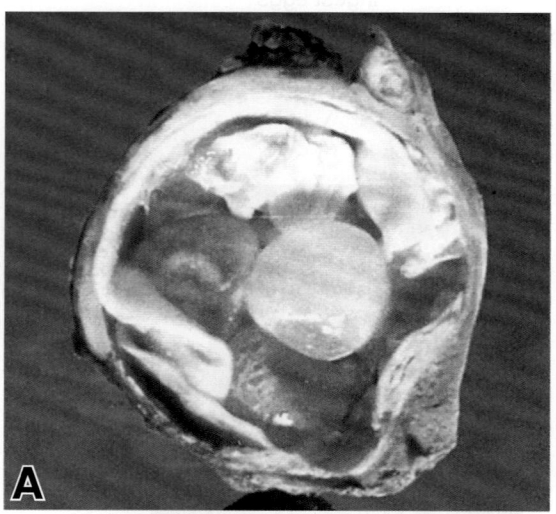

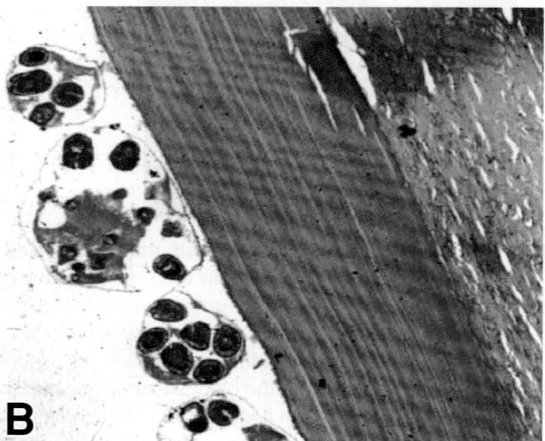

FIGURE 9-105. Echinococcal cyst. A. An echinococcal cyst showing daughter cysts was resected from the liver of a patient infected with *Echinococcus granulosus.* **B.** A photomicrograph of the cyst wall shows (*from right to left*) a laminated, nonnuclear layer, a nucleated germinal layer with brood capsules attached and many scolices in the cyst cavity. (Reprinted from Farrar WE, Wood MJ, Innes JA, Tubbs H. *Infectious Diseases: Text and Color Atlas.* 2nd ed. New York: Gower Medical Publishing; 1992. Copyright © 1992 Elsevier. With permission.)

hydatid cyst of the liver or abdominal organ causes severe diffuse pain, mimicking peritonitis. Rupture of a pulmonary cyst may cause pneumothorax and empyema. Moreover, when a hydatid cyst ruptures into a body cavity, released cyst contents can cause fatal allergic reactions. Treatment of echinococcal cysts requires careful surgical removal. To prevent anaphylaxis, cysts must be sterilized with formalin before drainage or removal.

Emerging and Reemerging Infections

The last few decades have witnessed reemergence of microbial threats that include resurgent well-known agents (e.g., cholera, dengue fever, influenza, anthrax), as well as previously unknown pathogens. Antibiotic-resistance among organisms, particularly communicable ones, such as tuberculosis, presents a new set of challenges.

Equally important has been the discovery of new pathogens belonging to all classes: viruses, bacteria, parasites, and fungi. AIDS and hepatitis C were unknown in the 1970s and alone have caused many millions of deaths, despite therapeutic advances. Frequent global influenza pandemics (e.g., H1N1, H5N1) underscore the resilience of influenza virus as a pathogen.

Table 9-11 is a partial list of newly recognized human infections. It should serve as a reminder that the equilibrium between us and our pathogens is a dynamic one: continuous vigilance is obligatory, and complacency invites disaster. The reader is referred to other sources for those infections not discussed above.

Agents of Biowarfare

Biologic agents have been used as weapons since ancient times. Biologic weapons are described in Hittite texts from 1500 to 2000 BCE, in which plague victims were driven into enemy lands. The great Carthaginian warrior, Hannibal, first delivered bioweapons in 184 BCE when, in preparing for a naval battle against King Eumenes of Pergamum, his army filled earthenware pots with serpents and hurled them to the decks of the Pergamene ships. In 1346, the Tatars lay siege to the Genoese-controlled seaport of Caffa (modern-day Feodosiya, Ukraine). During the siege, the Tatars were ravaged by plague. The Tatar leader catapulted his own dead soldiers, victims of the disease, into the besieged town to spread the epidemic, and forced the Genoese army to flee to Italy. Similar tactics were used at Karlstein in Bohemia in 1422 and by Russian troops in fighting Swedish forces in Reval in 1710.

Smallpox was used as a biologic weapon by Francisco Pizarro in his conquest of South America in the 15th century when he presented variola-contaminated clothing as gifts. The English used a similar tactic in the French-Indian War in 1763, when Sir Jeffrey Amherst presented smallpox-laden blankets to Delaware Indians loyal to the French. During the Revolutionary War, there were accusations of the potential use of smallpox as a weapon from both sides. There was a plan by the British and their colonial allies, the Loyalists, to spread smallpox among the American colonists (Fig. 9-106).

INFECTIOUS AND PARASITIC DISEASES

TABLE 9-11

SELECTED EXAMPLES OF NOTABLE PREVIOUSLY UNDESCRIBED OR EMERGING INFECTIONS IDENTIFIED SINCE THE YEAR 2000

Year	Agent	Human Disease/Association
2018	Human hepegivirus-1 (HHpgV-1) *Borrelia turicatae*	Tick-borne relapsing fever
2017	Maguari virus	Febrile illness
2017	Zika virus	Congenital syndrome including microcephaly and fetal malformations
2015	Bourbon virus	Tick-borne febrile disease
2014	Middle East Respiratory Syndrome Coronavirus (MERS Co-V)	SARS-like respiratory infection
2012	Bas Congo virus	Systemic disease
2012	*Exserohilum rostratum*	Fungal meningitis outbreak
2011	*Candidatus Neoehrlichia mikurensis*	Sepsis
2009	H1N1 "swine" influenza virus	Pneumonia
2008	Merkel cell polyomavirus (MC PyV)	Identified in Merkel cell carcinoma tissue
2007	Zika virus	Epidemic mosquito-borne viral syndrome
2005	Coronavirus HCoV-HKU-1	Pneumonia
2004	H5N1 "Avian" influenza	Pneumonia
2002	SARS-associated coronavirus	Severe atypical pneumonia (SARS-CoV)

Other previously unknown agents discovered within the 20 years earlier include human Herpes virus 8 (HHV-8, 1994), the causative agent of Kaposi sarcoma; *Bartonella henselae*, which causes cat-scratch disease (1992); hepatitis C virus (HCV, 1989), which causes hepatitis and hepatocellular carcinoma; HIV-1 (1983) and -2 (1986), which cause AIDS; *Helicobacter pylori*, which causes gastric and duodenal ulcers and malignancies (1983); hepatitis E virus (1983); and *Borrelia burgdorferi*, which causes Lyme disease (1983).

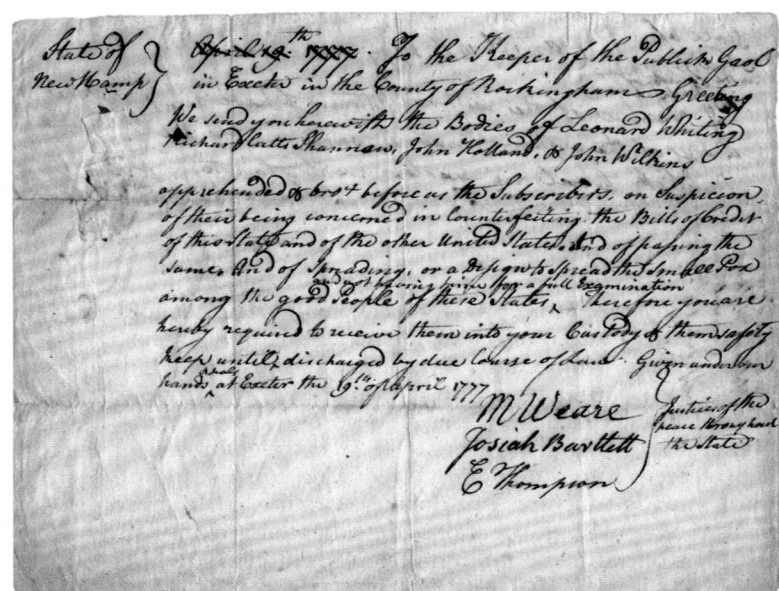

FIGURE 9-106. American Revolutionary War handwritten document describing the arrest and transport of three men "… on Suspicion of their being concerned in Counterfeiting the Bills of Credit of this State and of the other United States, and of passing the same and of Spreading or a Design to spread the Small Pox among the good People of these States…," dated April 19, 1777 and signed by Josiah Bartlett, a famed New Hampshire physician and signer of the Declaration of Independence. This letter describes the threat of deliberate biowarfare by British sympathizers (Loyalists) in the War of Independence, and led to General George Washington's order for smallpox inoculation of the Continental Army.

In addition, a smallpox outbreak was spreading through the Northern Continental Army. By 1777, General George Washington ordered mandatory smallpox inoculation of all military recruits who had not had the disease.

Allegations of biowarfare surfaced in World War I. The Germans were reported to have spread cholera to Italy, plague to St. Petersburg, and anthrax and glanders to the United States and elsewhere. Although the League of Nations after the war found no definite proof of any of these actions by Germany, the psychological impact of the potential use of biologic weaponry in inducing terror was firmly established in modern times. The United States established Camp Detrick in Maryland in 1942 to 1943 to investigate biologic weapons.

The 20th century has unfortunately witnessed many national bioweapons programs, mainly covert, and a few notorious for human experimentation. During the Sino-Japanese War, 1937 to 1945, Japanese Army Unit 731 conducted bioweapons experimentation on many thousands of Chinese civilians, as well as Russian and American prisoners of war. The Japanese Army used bioweapons during military campaigns against Chinese soldiers and civilians. In 1940, Japanese planes bombed Ningbo with ceramic bombs containing plague-infested fleas. It is estimated that 400,000 Chinese died as a direct result of this use of biologic weapons.

Accidental biologic contamination has also occurred. In 1942, Gruinard Island off the northwest coast of Scotland was rendered uninhabitable for almost 50 years after British field trials of anthrax. In 1979, accidental release of anthrax from a Sverdlovsk (now Yekaterinburg) military facility, Compound 19, was perhaps the largest biologic weapons accident known; sheep developed anthrax 200 km from the release point and over 60 people died.

There is legitimate fear in modern times over the use of bioweapons as a terrorist tool. In September 1984, an outbreak of salmonella gastroenteritis was caused by followers of the Indian guru Bagwan Shree Rajneesh in Oregon, infecting over 700 people. In 1993, an apocalyptic Japanese cult group sprayed anthrax spores from a high-rise building in Tokyo, but no one was injured. The same cult group was found to be preparing vast quantities of *Clostridium difficile* spores for terrorist use. In 1995, the American Type Culture Collection (ATCC), a nonprofit organization that supplies biologic specimens to scientists, shipped a package containing three vials of *Yersinia pestis* to the home of a political extremist in Ohio. A search of his home revealed a variety of explosive devices, detonating fuses and triggers. Most recently, dried anthrax was mailed in letters through the United States postal system, causing five deaths.

Only a few biologic agents have been considered or proven to be effective as weapons of biowarfare or bioterrorism (Table 9-12). Key factors that make an infectious agent suitable for large-scale biowarfare include: (1) ease of large-scale production; (2) ability to cause death or incapacity of humans at doses which are deliverable; (3) appropriate particle size as an aerosol; (4) ease of dissemination; (5) stability during storage, in the environment or placement into a delivery system; and (6) susceptibility of intended victims, but nonsusceptibility of friendly forces. Some biologic weapons are potentially extremely lethal: 1 g of purified botulinum toxin could kill 10 million people.

TABLE 9-12
POTENTIAL BIOLOGIC AGENTS OF WARFARE AND BIOTERROR

Bacteria

Bacillus anthracis

Brucella abortus, B. suis, B. melitensis

Listeria monocytogenes

Vibrio cholerae

Rickettsia prowazekii, R. rickettsii

Burkholderia mallei, B. pseudomallei

Coxiella burnetii, Francisella tularensis, Yersinia pestis

Clostridium botulinum and botulinum neurotoxin-producing species of *Clostridium*

Viruses

Arenaviruses— Lassa, Machupo, Sabia, Junin, Guanarito

Bunyaviruses—Rift Valley Fever virus, Congo-Crimean hemorrhagic fever virus

Filoviruses—Ebola virus, Marburg virus

Flaviviruses—Kyasanur Forest disease

Influenza

Kumlinge, Omsk hemorrhagic fever, Russian Spring-Summer encephalitis, Tick-borne encephalitis

Poxviruses—Smallpox (Variola) and Monkeypox

Togaviruses—Eastern Equine Encephalitis Virus

Venezuelan Equine Encephalitis Virus

Biologic Toxins

Botulinum, *Clostridium perfringens* epsilon toxin

Staphylococcal enterotoxin B

Shigatoxin

Conotoxins

Abrin

Ricin

Tetrodotoxin

Saxitoxin

T-2 toxin

Diacetoxyscirpenol

Microcystins

Aflatoxins

Satratoxin H

Palytoxin

Anatoxin A

Pathogenesis of Systemic Conditions

10 Aging

David B. Lombard

Harsh old age (Geras) will soon enshroud you—ruthless age which stands someday at the side of every man, deadly, wearying, dreaded even by the gods.

—**Homeric Hymn V to Aphrodite 243–224**

BIOLOGIC AGING

Questions related to aging and death have obsessed humanity since the dawn of recorded history. For example, after the debacle in the Garden of Eden, Adam and Eve were cursed with the certainty of mortality, that is, predestined aging. *Aging can be defined as a process of progressive dysfunction, frailty, and increasing mortality.* Biologic aging is distinct from disease: the latter represents an abnormal and unpredictable pathologic condition, whereas aging is both universal and inevitable. Yet, aging and disease are intimately related; aging represents a key risk factor—and often the dominant risk factor—for many diseases described elsewhere in this book.

The insidious effects of aging can be detected in otherwise healthy people. For example, in many sports, an athlete in his or her 30s is considered "old." Even in the absence of specific diseases or vascular abnormalities, beginning in the fourth decade of life, many physiologic functions decline progressively, including muscular strength, cardiac reserve, nerve conduction velocity, pulmonary vital capacity, glomerular filtration, and vascular elasticity (Fig. 10-1). Structural changes accompany this functional deterioration. Lean body mass decreases and the proportion of fat rises. Connective tissue matrix constituents are increasingly cross-linked and brittle. Lipofuscin ("aging")

pigment accumulates in organs such as the brain, heart, and liver. At the cellular level, the challenges imposed by aging on postmitotic cells such as neurons and cardiomyocytes are likely quite different from those faced by rapidly dividing cells, such as those of the gut or skin.

Life Span Is Subject to Environmental and Genetic Influences[1]

Considerable evidence shows that aging is subject to strong genetic and environmental influences. For example, it is now possible to achieve dramatic life span extension (up to 65%) in rodent models through single-gene mutations in specific signaling pathways, or even by administering certain small molecules. Reduced food intake without malnutrition (**dietary restriction [DR]**) promotes longevity in many species, from budding yeast to rodents and likely even nonhuman primates.

Those who live in advanced industrialized societies already benefit from a greatly increased life span, relative to our forebears. It is estimated that a typical age at death of Neolithic humans was 20 to 25 years, and the average life span today in some underdeveloped regions is often barely 10 years more. By contrast, female life expectancy at birth in industrialized countries over the past 160 years has risen

---

[1]In this chapter, we depart from our general promise to minimize discussion of animal and cell culture studies, and to avoid presenting hypotheses. Aging is central to the human condition. Throughout the ages, people have sought to prolong youth and to delay or evade death. Our current understanding of aging draws heavily on work done in experimental animals, and provocative but unproven hypotheses drawn from those experiments.

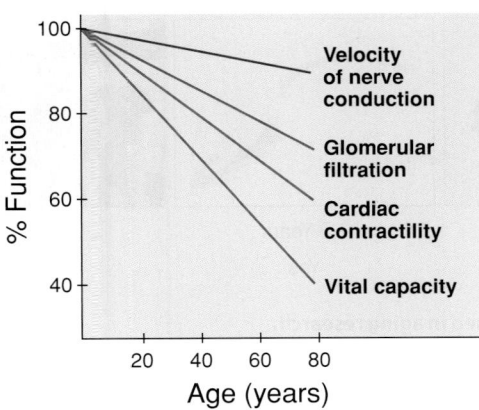

FIGURE 10-1. Decrease in human physiologic capacities as a function of age.

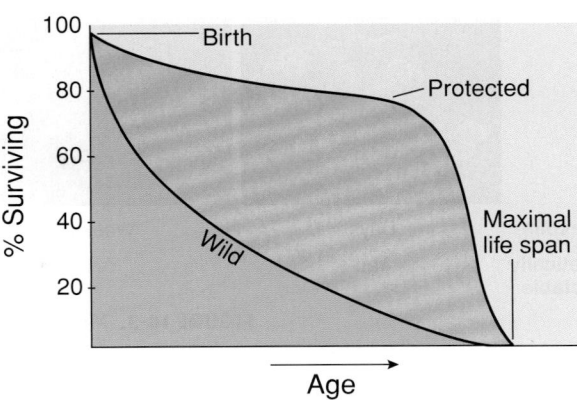

FIGURE 10-2. Life span of animals in their natural environment compared with that in a protected habitat. Note that both curves reach the same maximal life span.

linearly by nearly 3 months a year, from about 45 years in the mid-19th century to nearly 85 years in the present day (women live 5 to 6 years longer than men, on average). This dramatic increase in life span stems in part from reduced child mortality and improved public health measures, as well as advances in medical care. If current trends hold, life expectancy at birth in developed countries may reach 100 years by the mid-21st century. The **maximum** documented life span for any human is 122 years, and very few people live to be significantly older than 100.

Health Span

Health span is the *period of life spent free from major disease.* Remarkably, the prolongevity interventions described below not only extend life span but also delay or prevent many common diseases. For example, mice on a DR diet remain healthy into late old age, sometimes showing no evidence of clinically significant pathology at necropsy. By contrast, animals allowed to eat ad libitum typically show a diverse spectrum of advanced pathologies at the time of death.

An Evolutionary Perspective on Aging

Why do we age at all? Once development has ceased, why do we not remain young and in good health perpetually? The notion that aging is programmed is intuitively appealing: older individuals die to "make room" and free up resources for the next generation. However, from the standpoint of evolutionary biology, there are major conceptual problems with the notion of programmed aging. For example, mutations that speed aging would confer a selective disadvantage and so would not be maintained during evolution. So if aging is not a programmed process, akin to development, why does it occur? Evolutionary biology offers a conceptual answer, if not a biologic mechanism, to this question. We observe aging of organisms in the laboratory, or in other protected settings such as zoos. In this context, the maximal life span of animals in the wild differs little from the same animals in the zoo (Fig. 10-2).

In humans, aging is most evident in industrialized societies, where most people escape the ravages of infant mortality, infectious disease, trauma, starvation, and other causes of early death. Such protected environments differ greatly from those that occurred over the course of evolution. Most organisms evolved under conditions in which predation,

infectious disease, competition for resources, and environmental exposure eliminated much of the population early in life, independently of any effects of aging. For organisms evolving under such strong pressures, there was no evolutionary selective advantage in longevity, as most individuals died early from causes unrelated to age. Thus, processes underlying biologic aging persist, since there has been little evolutionary pressure to weed them out. This idea predicts that species that evolve in relatively protected environments will inherently live longer than those evolving in less forgiving circumstances. In fact, birds, bats, and flying squirrels, all of which can fly to escape from potential predators, live far longer than mice. Other rodents that have evolved inherent protection against would-be predators (e.g., porcupines) or that live in safe environments underground (the naked mole rat) also live longer than their less fortunate exposed kin.

Diverse Systems Exist to Study the Biology of Aging

Maximal life spans range from a few hours for adult forms of some insects, to a few weeks for the nematode *Caenorhabditis elegans* and fruit fly *Drosophila melanogaster,* to many decades for humans and other large mammals. At the upper end of longevity, there are clams that can live for centuries. A few species, such as hydra and lobster, may be entirely immune to aging. Key pathways that modulate longevity in invertebrates function similarly in rodents, and so potentially operate in the same way in humans.

Short-Lived Organisms and Mechanistic Insights into Aging

Model organisms have been invaluable tools to help elucidate aging biology (Fig. 10-3). Brewer's yeast (*Saccharomyces cerevisiae*) reproduces by budding. Individual yeast cells can bud only a finite number of times before ceasing to divide, a point known as *senescence.* Several genes (e.g., mammalian target of rapamycin [*mTOR*] [**see Chapter 1**] and *SIR2*) influence this process and also play key roles in modulating longevity in mammals. The roundworm (*C. elegans*) and the fruit fly (*D. melanogaster*) are more complex organisms that possess many tissue types seen in higher organisms, such as skeletal muscle and a nervous system. As they age, they show

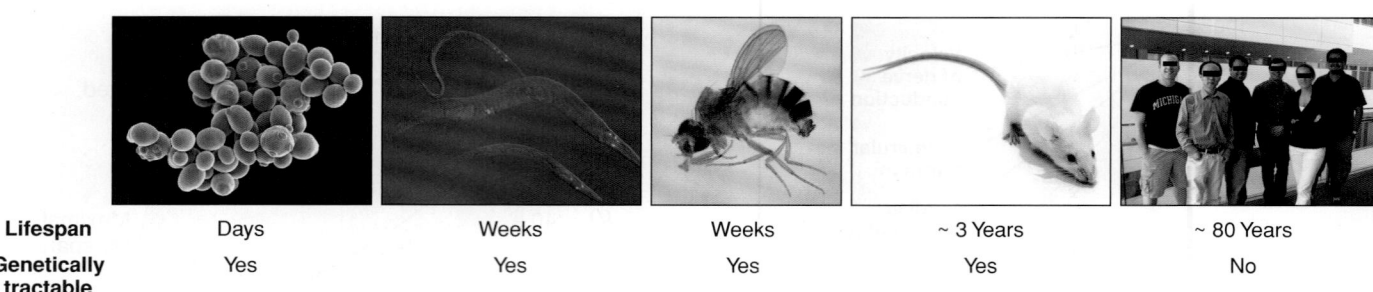

Lifespan	Days	Weeks	Weeks	~ 3 Years	~ 80 Years
Genetically tractable	Yes	Yes	Yes	Yes	No

FIGURE 10-3. **Model organisms commonly used in aging research.**

degenerative effects like those in higher organisms, including decreased movement and lipofuscin accumulation.

Among mammals, the laboratory mouse (*Mus musculus*) is the most popular system used to study life span. Aged mice show many of the same pathologies as older humans. Their small size, rapid generation time of roughly 12 weeks, and relatively short life span of 2 to 3 years, make mice the prime system for studying mammalian aging. The ease with which mouse strains with specific genomic alterations can be produced has greatly facilitated dissection of mechanisms of mammalian aging. Many diverse pathologies of old age in humans also afflict aged mice.

CELLULAR SENESCENCE AND ORGANISMAL AGING

Human fibroblasts passaged serially in culture do not replicate forever. Instead (like yeast), after many passages, they enter a nondividing state called **replicative senescence**. During this time, they remain postmitotic but are viable for an extended period. Senescent cells are characterized by specific markers, such as (1) an enlarged, flattened appearance; (2) absence of molecular markers of proliferation; (3) persistent foci of unrepaired DNA damage; and (4) expression of senescence-associated markers, such as β-galactosidase and p16^{Ink4a} protein.

Telomere Shortening Promotes Replicative Senescence

In human cells, replicative senescence occurs largely due to attrition of **telomeres**, a series of short repetitive nucleotide sequences (TTAGGG in vertebrates) at the ends of chromosomes (**see Chapters 1 and 5**). DNA polymerase, the enzyme that replicates DNA, begins at the 5' end, and works toward the 3' end. It cannot copy linear chromosomes right up to their distal ends, so telomeres shorten with each cell division. Telomeres protect DNA sequences that are near chromosomal termini from being lost with repeated cell divisions. Certain crucial cell types, such as stem cell populations, express an enzyme, **telomerase**, which restores sequences lost during replication and thus stabilizes their telomeres. Most human somatic cells, like fibroblasts, do not express significant levels of telomerase. Consequently, their telomeres shorten with each cell division, thus representing a "mitotic clock" that counts DNA replication events. Some types of cellular injury, such as oxidative stress, can directly damage telomeres, independent of replication.

Telomeres are normally protected by a protein complex, called **shelterin**. When telomeres shorten beyond a critical point, shelterin is released, triggering a DNA damage response that can cause irreversible cell cycle arrest or apoptosis (Fig. 10-4). Telomere attrition can also lead to end-to-end chromosomal fusions and other types of genomic instability via breakage–fusion–bridge cycles (**see Chapter 5**). Reintroducing telomerase into human fibroblasts enables them to bypass senescence, demonstrating that telomere attrition is limiting for their growth in culture.

In addition to telomere shortening, other types of injury also induce cellular senescence. These include many DNA-damaging agents, such as oxidative stress, excessive mitogenic stimulation associated with activated oncogenes (**see Chapter 5**), and chromatin disruption.

Senescence-Associated Secretory Phenotype

The link between cellular senescence and organismal aging is complex. There is solid evidence that senescence prevents cells with potentially oncogenic mutations from dividing (oncogene-induced senescence; **see Chapter 5**), and so helps prevent oncogenesis. Senescent cells also secrete proinflammatory cytokines, proteases, and other factors (**senescence-associated secretory phenotype,** or **SASP**). Via SASP, senescent cells likely contribute to diverse age-related pathologies, such

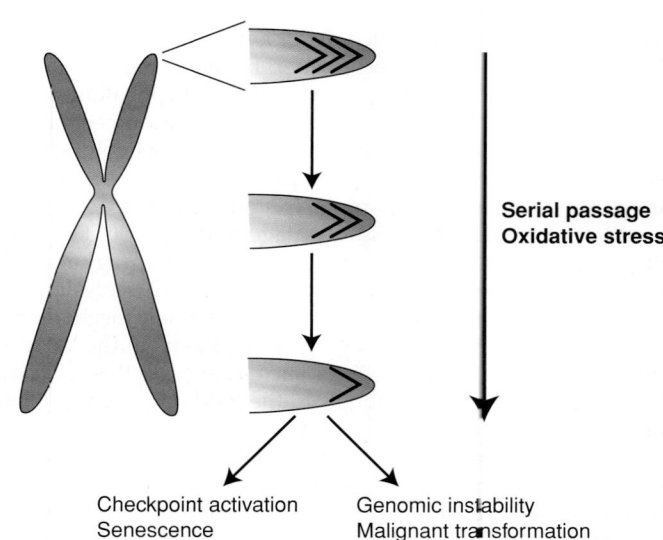

Serial passage
Oxidative stress

Checkpoint activation
Senescence

Genomic instability
Malignant transformation

FIGURE 10-4. **Deleterious consequences of telomere shortening in mammalian cells.**

as atherosclerosis, epidermal thinning, immune dysfunction, and degenerative joint disease. Senescent cells may also create a microenvironment that promotes growth of malignant cells, thus potentially contributing to increased rates of cancer as people age. Elimination of senescent cells with specific small molecules, termed **senolytics**, can extend mouse life span and delay age-associated pathologies.

Molecular Mechanisms of Aging Are Complex and Multifactorial

Macromolecular Damage in Aging

Many factors contribute to the degenerative manifestations of aging. Accumulated unrepaired macromolecular damage—to DNA, chromatin, proteins, and lipid—induces cellular dysfunction, manifesting at the organismal level as aging. To counter the effects of such damage, cells have evolved elaborate, well-regulated mechanisms to repair many macromolecular lesions. Cells with certain types of severe damage can also be removed by apoptosis or other forms of cell death (**see Chapter 1**). This damage-based model of aging predicts that mutant organisms with increased longevity should also show more robust resistance to damage-inducing stressors. This is in fact typically—though not always—observed. The model also predicts that cellular repair systems should be intimately related, genetically speaking, to prolongevity pathways. This is also observed empirically (see below).

Reactive Oxygen Species Contribute to Age-Associated Disease

A long-standing theory holds that macromolecular damage in the context of aging is caused by **reactive oxygen species (ROS)**, mostly generated endogenously in mitochondria (**see Chapter 1**). Important ROS include superoxide, peroxide, and nitric oxide. ROS can interact with and damage all cellular macromolecules, causing diverse lesions in nucleic acids, modifying and inactivating proteins, and damaging lipids. Most ROS generation occurs in mitochondria, due to "leakage" from electron transport chain. It is estimated that a single cell undergoes some 100,000 ROS attacks on DNA daily, and that at any time 10% of protein molecules in the cell are modified by oxidative carbonyl adducts.

Antioxidants

To counter these effects, cells possess a network of antioxidant defenses that detoxify ROS and repair ROS-related damage. These pathways include superoxide dismutases (SOD), catalase, glutathione peroxidase, thioredoxins, thioredoxin reductase, and many others. **Oxidative stress** occurs when ROS exceed cellular defenses.

ROS play important physiologic roles, besides potentially damaging macromolecules. For example, ROS modulate kinase signaling, defend against microbial pathogens and regulate vascular tone. Thus, it is neither possible nor desirable to eliminate cellular ROS entirely. Yet most long-lived invertebrate mutants have enhanced antioxidant defenses. DR induces increased antioxidant defenses, concomitant with diminished ROS levels and reduced macromolecular oxidation products.

However, current data strongly suggest that ROS are not a major driver of the rate of aging. In many invertebrate models, *elevated* ROS levels are paradoxically associated with *increased* longevity. Enhancing ROS defenses in mice by engineering overexpression of antioxidant enzymes generally does not extend longevity. Studies in hundreds of thousands of people given supraphysiologic doses of antioxidant dietary supplements have not found any significant benefit on life span, disease, or health; indeed, adding certain antioxidants is associated with *increased* mortality.

Telomere Maintenance in Longevity

The role of telomere erosion in aging is attributed to progressive cellular dysfunction and senescence, eventually leading to overall organismal aging. In humans, rare mutations in telomerase or shelterin components lead to shortened telomeres and aplastic anemia, skin and nail defects, infertility, pulmonary fibrosis, and cancer. Even in people without such defects, shortened telomeres are also found in association with cirrhosis, atherosclerosis, and ulcerative colitis, consistent with extended proliferative histories or high levels of oxidative stress in these conditions. Short telomere length in peripheral blood cells predicts susceptibility to coronary artery disease, neoplasia, and overall mortality in older people. Recent work has also revealed that short telomeres can lead to impairments in mitochondrial function. Genetically engineered mouse strains that cannot maintain telomeres show reduced longevity, as well as defects in tissues that require rapid cell proliferation and stem and progenitor cell activity, principally bone marrow, skin, gut, and testes. Conversely, improved telomere maintenance can extend longevity in mice.

Maintenance of Proteostasis Contributes to Longevity

Increasing evidence suggests that maintaining cellular protein homeostasis (**proteostasis**) is an important factor in longevity (**see Chapter 1**). All cellular proteins, collectively called the **proteome**, are constantly subject to diverse challenges. Translational errors, oxidative damage, mutations, and polymorphisms can lead to protein misfolding and aggregation, which can cause cellular injury. All of these mechanisms can be regulated by interventions that also promote longevity, implying an important relationship between proteostasis and life span. Moreover, older cells and organisms accumulate oxidatively damaged and cross-linked proteins. Studies of invertebrates suggest that diminished proteostasis is an early, and perhaps causative, event in organismal aging.

One proteostatic mechanism that is closely linked to aging is autophagy, a regulated process by which cells degrade damaged proteins, and even whole organelles, in lysosomes (**see Chapter 1**). In model organisms, autophagy is required for longevity induced by many environmental or genetic manipulations. Autophagic function declines with age in mammals and lower organisms, and restoring autophagy in older mice can improve tissue function.

Mitochondrial Function Declines With Aging

With age, mitochondria lose efficiency, and produce less ATP but more ROS. It is thought that this mitochondrial energetic decline contributes to major age-associated conditions such as sarcopenia, insulin resistance and type 2 diabetes, cardiac dysfunction, neurodegeneration, etc. The molecular basis for mitochondrial functional decline during aging is unclear; accumulation of damaged mitochondrial genomes may play a role. Since mitochondrial DNA lies in close proximity to components of the respiratory chain, it is highly susceptible to ROS-induced DNA damage. However, the role of mitochondria in longevity is not that straightforward. In *C. elegans, D. melanogaster*, and even rodents, certain mitochondrial defects present during development actually *extend* longevity. Mitochondria thus help determine organismal longevity, but via complex mechanisms.

Stem Cell Function Declines With Aging

Adult tissue stem cells are critical for proper organ function and for repair following injury. These stem cells lose functionality with age, thus impairing tissue homeostasis and contributing to degenerative disease. This notion is best illustrated by hematopoietic stem cells (HSCs), which give rise to all mature blood cell types. HSC function declines with age. Clinically, it has long been known that HSC transplants from young donors are more likely to succeed than those from older donors. In aged people, HSCs increasingly differentiate via myeloid, rather than lymphoid, lineages. There are progressive defects in HSC mobilization and homing. Aged HSCs also accumulate mutations in oncogenes and tumor suppressor genes, perhaps contributing to the increased incidence of blood cancers in the elderly.

The tumor suppressor p16^{Ink4a} (**see above and Chapter 5**) is upregulated in senescent cells. More generally, in aging tissues, p16^{Ink4a} and the related gene p19^{ARF} (the murine equivalent of human p14^{ARF}) are normally inhibited by Bmi-1, a protein required for renewal of all adult stem cell types. In aged mice, p16^{Ink4a} limits proliferative capacity in different types of stem cells. Increased p16^{Ink4a} in aging stem cells may defend against malignant transformation of these cells, at the expense of stem cell function, tissue repair, and overall organismal homeostasis. Interestingly, genetic studies in humans have linked polymorphisms near the p16^{Ink4a} locus to diverse age-associated pathologies (e.g., coronary atherosclerosis, type 2 diabetes, frailty). These data suggest that p16^{Ink4a} can regulate aging in humans via effects on stem cells or other cell types.

In recent years, it has become possible to convert somatic cells into induced pluripotent stem cells (iPSCs). Remarkably, this process reverses many effects of aging, including senescence, telomere erosion, and mitochondrial dysfunction, implying that iPSCs may be able to undo or prevent the ravages of aging in differentiated cells.

GENETIC DISEASES RESEMBLING PREMATURE AGING

There are rare diseases that resemble accelerated aging (**progerias**).

 MOLECULAR PATHOGENESIS: The two best-studied such conditions are **Werner syndrome (WS)** and **Hutchinson–Guilford progeria syndrome (HGPS)**.

- **WS** is caused by recessive mutations in the *WRN* gene, encoding a DNA helicase involved in DNA replication, repair, and telomere maintenance. Patients with mutations in *WRN* show poor growth in adolescence, premature hair graying, thinning of the skin, cataracts, diabetes, and atherosclerosis (Fig. 10-5). They also tend to develop cancer, specifically sarcomas, leukemias, and other malignancies. WS patients typically succumb to myocardial infarction or cancer by their 40s or 50s. Cultured WS fibroblasts show chromosomal instability, sensitivity to DNA cross-linking agents, and reduced replicative life span, further paralleling aging-associated changes.

  However, despite these similarities to normal aging, WS by no means mimics the aging process. For example, some disorders commonly associated with physiologic aging, such as Alzheimer disease, do not occur in WS patients. Thus, WS is an example of a **segmental progeria**, that is, a syndrome that recapitulates some, but not all, aspects of accelerated aging.

- **HGPS** is caused by autosomal dominant mutations in the *LMNA* gene, whose product is a protein, **lamin A**. Affected children show reduced growth, hair loss, scleroderma-like skin changes, and atherosclerosis (Fig. 10-6). Patients with HGPS typically die in their teens from myocardial infarction or stroke. The most common mutation associated with HGPS causes missplicing of the LMNA transcript, causing accumulation of **progerin**, a defective precursor of lamin A protein. Normally, lamin A is a key part of the nuclear lamina that provides structural integrity to nuclei in differentiated cells. By contrast, progerin accumulates in the nucleus, distorts nuclear outline, and causes nuclear blebbing. Progerin buildup interferes with chromatin organization, and impairs gene expression and DNA repair. HGPS is at the severe end of a spectrum of disorders associated with mutations in the *LMNA* gene,

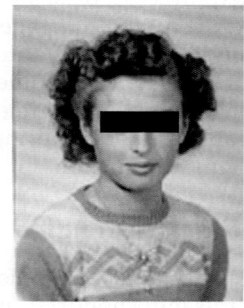 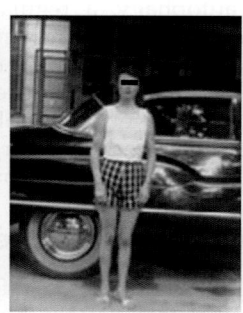 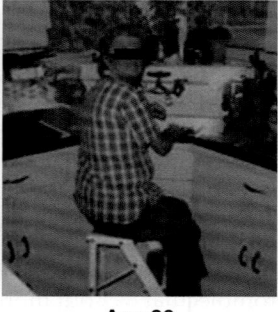 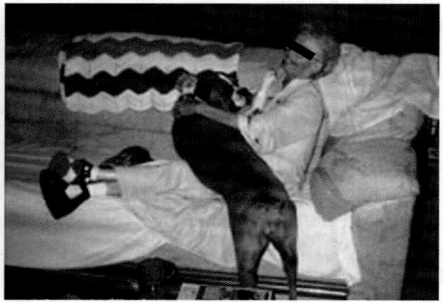

| Age 8 | Age 21 | Age 36 | Age 56 |

FIGURE 10-5. Werner syndrome. The premature appearance of aging phenotypes is evident. (Used with permission from Hisama FM, Bohr VA, Oshima J. WRN's tenth anniversary. *Sci Aging Knowledge Environ.* 2006;[10]:p. e18.)

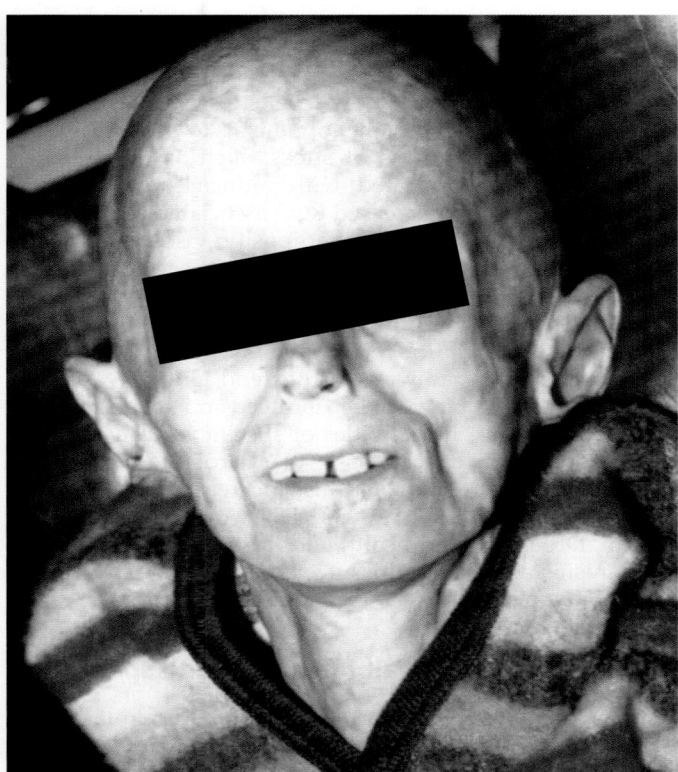

FIGURE 10-6. Hutchinson–Guilford progeria syndrome. A 10-year-old girl shows typical features of this disease.

collectively called "**laminopathies**." These diseases are associated with defects in muscle, adipose tissue, and peripheral nerves.

It is unclear whether and to what extent the study of WS, HGPS, and related disorders improves understanding of the biology of aging. These conditions may represent disease phenotypes whose pathogenesis is unrelated to physiologic aging. However, as non-HGPS cells may produce progerin as they age, HGPS may help provide insight into some aspects of normal aging.

Defects in DNA Repair Cause Degenerative Phenotypes

WS and HGPS are members of a larger group of syndromes that show accelerated degenerative, aging-like **(progeroid)** phenotypes. Many of these conditions have been produced in mice by inactivating genes involved in nuclear DNA repair. Thus, one model holds that DNA is an important target of age-associated damage. This is an intuitively appealing notion. Unlike other cellular macromolecules such as proteins and lipids, nuclear DNA cannot simply be replaced, but instead must be repaired once damaged. Consistent with this notion, increased levels of chromosomal aberrations, as well as more subtle mutations, occur in peripheral blood leukocytes and other tissues with advancing age.

Cells have evolved diverse systems to repair the different types of DNA lesions (**see Chapter 5**). Unrepaired DNA damage activates cellular checkpoint responses, causing cell cycle arrest, apoptosis, or senescence. Defects in DNA repair can cause dramatic harmful effects, but that does not prove

that DNA damage is the root of physiologic aging. Thus, a connection between DNA repair and aging remains an attractive, but unproven hypothesis.

A related model implicates **epigenetic** alterations in aging. Gene expression is regulated by many mechanisms affecting DNA, histones, chromatin-binding factors, protein alterations, and noncoding RNAs. DNA methylation and histone modifications change progressively with age, leading to less accurate regulation of gene expression. The methylation status of specific genomic CpG islands can predict biologic age accurately. In invertebrate systems, genetic manipulations involving the epigenome can prolong life span. Increased cell-to-cell variation in gene expression occurs in aging mammalian cardiomyocytes, further arguing that age-associated epigenetic dysregulation is harmful.

REDUCED CALORIC INTAKE AND LONGEVITY

As noted above, DR increases longevity in the vast majority of organisms in which it has been tested, from budding yeast to rodents. In mice, DR typically involves reducing caloric intake by 30% to 50%. This routinely extends life span by 25% to 40%. Perhaps even more striking than its prolongevity effects, DR delays or prevents many age-associated conditions, including cancers, cardiovascular disease, neurodegeneration, diabetes, sarcopenia, and many others. However, DR is not a "free ride"; in rodents, it impairs certain immune responses and delays wound healing. In humans, DR can reduce bone density and muscle mass, and has been associated with depression.

Prolonged Longevity With DR Is an Active Phenomenon

DR-related longevity DR is not simply a passive consequence of reduced caloric intake. Even reduction of specific dietary constituents can dramatically prolong longevity. Studies in mice identified protein as the most harmful dietary component. Similarly, in rodents, restriction of the amino acid, methionine, extends life span comparably to reduced overall caloric intake. Yet methionine-restricted animals actually consume *more* calories than do controls (Fig. 10-7).

In rodent models, DR initiated even in middle-aged adults has beneficial effects on longevity, although the

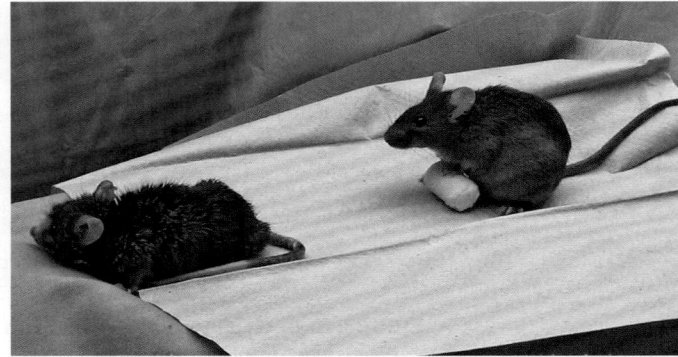

FIGURE 10-7. Methionine restriction extends mouse life span. Both mice are roughly 30 months old. The one in front is the last surviving member of a control group of mice fed regular chow. The one playing with the chalk was fed a low-methionine diet. (Courtesy of Dr. Richard Miller.)

magnitude of this effect diminishes the later in life that DR is started. Remarkably, in mice, DR imposed during the brief 3-week period from birth until weaning is sufficient to confer extended life span. This finding suggests that early DR may provoke long-lasting—possibly epigenetic—changes that favor longevity.

Can DR extend life span in humans? Studies of DR in our close cousins, rhesus monkeys, have so far yielded conflicting results as to its impact on longevity, though DR does exert consistent health benefits in these animals. Until recently, residents of the Japanese island of Okinawa ate on average substantially fewer calories than did those on the Japanese mainland or the United States. Okinawans had markedly reduced incidences of cardiac disease and cancer, and one of the world's largest populations of centenarians on a per capita basis. Certain people who voluntarily greatly limit their dietary intake show improved serum lipid parameters, increased insulin sensitivity, reduced blood pressure and protection against obesity, type 2 diabetes, inflammation, carotid artery intimal hyperplasia, and left ventricular diastolic dysfunction. Thus, DR in humans correlates with dramatic protection against cardiovascular risk factors. Yet the overall lowest mortality rate in humans is associated with a body mass index (BMI) of roughly 25, corresponding to a normal to slightly overweight status; both higher *and lower* BMIs are associated with increased risk of death. Thus, the low BMIs associated with DR in humans may have unforeseen negative consequences.

Hormesis

Conceptually, the longevity associated with DR represents an example of **hormesis**: a low-level stress such as reduced food intake may prime the organism to respond more effectively to other forms of stress, such as those linked to aging. DR is associated with reduced mitochondrial ROS production and decreased ROS-associated damage (see above). It also reduces overall adiposity; visceral adiposity in particular, exerts negative health effects (see Chapter 13). DR in rodents also increases insulin sensitivity in skeletal muscle and lowers serum levels of insulin and insulin-like growth factor-I (IGF-I, see Chapter 5). Genetic lesions in nutrient signaling pathways also extend longevity, providing a potential link between DR-induced and genetic longevity. DR modulates the activities of specific **sirtuin** proteins, NAD^+-dependent deacetylases that promote aspects of mammalian health span. DR also decreases inflammation and upregulates autophagy and DNA repair mechanisms. In sum, DR can extend health and life span. The molecular mechanisms underlying this effect are beginning to be elucidated, but are clearly complex and multifaceted.

Insulin and IGF-I Signaling Shorten Life Span

Insulin/IGF-I–like signaling (IIS) negatively regulates longevity. IIS is initiated when insulin or IGF family members bind their cognate cell surface receptor tyrosine kinases (Fig. 10-8). These interactions activate the kinase Akt, which

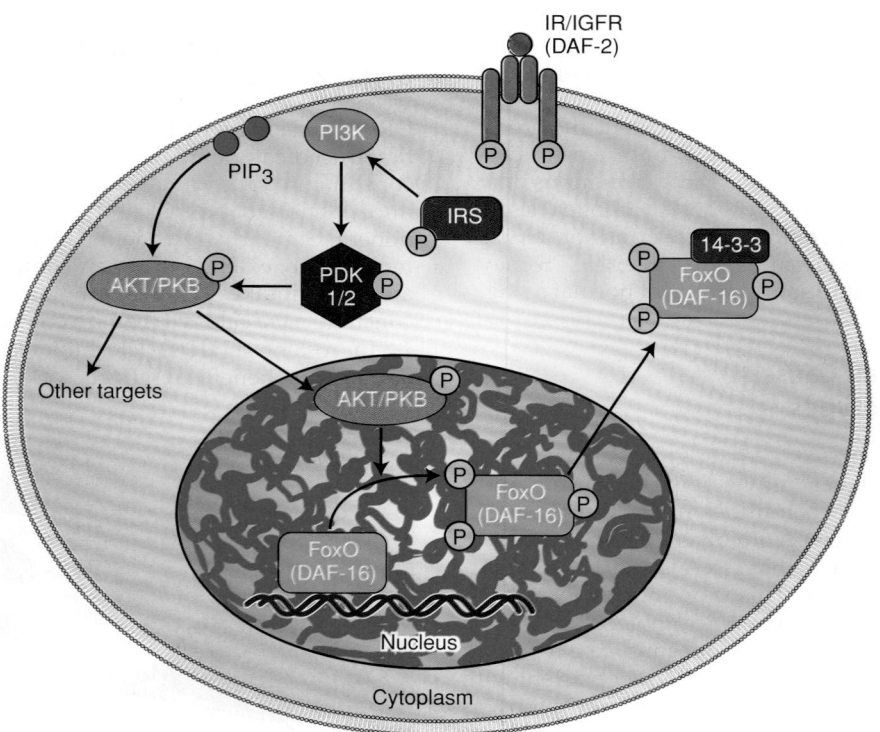

FIGURE 10-8. Insulin/insulin-like growth factor-I (IGF-I)–like signaling (IIS) pathway. IIS begins when insulin or IGF-I binds to its cell surface receptors, which are tyrosine kinases. This initiates an intracellular signaling cascade involving generation of phosphatidylinositol triphosphate by phosphatidylinositol 3-kinase (PI3K), in turn leading to activation of the downstream kinases PDK1 and Akt. FoxO transcription factors are key targets of this signaling pathway; in *C. elegans*, FoxO is termed DAF-16.

phosphorylates downstream proteins to regulate diverse processes, including cell survival, growth, cell cycle, metabolism, and stress resistance. FoxO transcription factors are key targets of Akt (**see Chapters 1 and 5**); when IIS is active, Akt phosphorylation sequesters FoxOs in the cytoplasm, where they are transcriptionally inert.

In 1993, it was shown that mutations in the *C. elegans* insulin receptor homolog *daf-2* more than doubled life span. This effect required that a FoxO homolog was active. Subsequent work showed that genetic lesions that impair several IIS components also extend life span. Increased FoxO activity is a key element in longevity related to reduced IIS. Interestingly, FoxO activity need only be increased in a subset of tissues to confer extended life span. These findings underscore the importance of neuroendocrine signaling in controlling overall life span.

Naturally occurring and genetically engineered mouse mutants with reduced growth hormone (GH) and IGF-I levels show extended longevity and delayed onset of age-associated disease. Remarkably, such mice also show preserved cognition in old age. In dogs and horses, small breeds show low serum IGF-I levels and longer life spans, compared to their larger cousins. Collectively, these data suggest a role for IIS in limiting mammalian life span.

How Does Reduced IIS Promote Longevity?

Experimental studies may be informative. In long-lived mouse strains, cells show increased resistance to oxidative and other stressors. Insulin sensitivity is a feature of mice with reduced GH signaling, an improved metabolic profile that may promote their longevity. Reduced IIS may contribute to the prolongevity effects of DR, but mechanisms of longevity underlying DR and reduced GH–IGF-I–IIS overlap only partially.

Could reduced IIS contribute to longevity in humans as well? Since insulin *resistance* in humans is typically a pathologic condition associated with disease states (obesity, atherosclerosis, dyslipidemia, etc.; **see Chapter 13**), the intuitive response to this question might be no. Yet genetic studies in humans support the notion that under some circumstances, reduced IIS may provide health and even longevity benefits. Congenital mutations in the GH receptor and consequent low serum IGF-I levels are the basis of **Laron dwarfism**. Affected individuals show very short stature and striking protection from cancer and type 2 diabetes. Centenarians in more typical populations show polymorphisms in genes for IGF-I receptor (IGFR), Akt, and FoxO. These IGFR polymorphisms correlate with reduced IGF-I signaling. Overall, there is solid evidence that chronically reduced IGF-I signaling in humans protects against disease and potentially promotes longevity.

mTOR Signaling

mTOR is a protein kinase (**see Chapters 1 and 5**) with conserved roles in limiting longevity seen in widely divergent species. Through complex signaling pathways, mTOR phosphorylates many cellular targets (Fig. 10-9). Genetic or pharmacologic inhibition of mTOR activity in invertebrates extends longevity. As with IIS, DR may work in part by reducing mTOR signaling. Genetic disruption of mTOR signaling components extends longevity in invertebrates

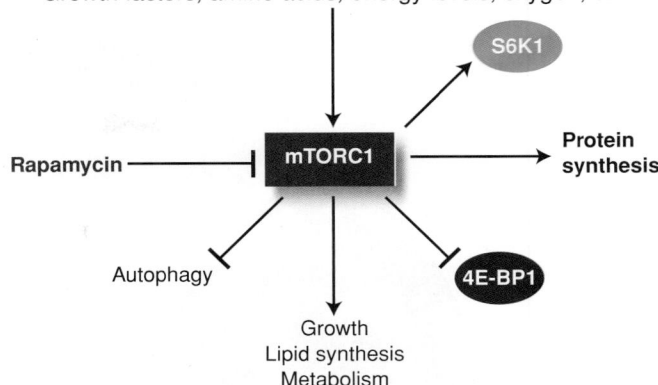

FIGURE 10-9. mTOR signaling. The mTOR kinase participates in two major complexes, termed mTORC1 and mTORC2. mTORC1 has been most closely linked to longevity. Multiple stimuli activate mTORC1. Two key downstream targets of mTORC1 are S6K1 and 4EBP1, through which mTORC1 promotes protein synthesis. Rapamycin acutely inhibits mTORC1 in a substrate-specific manner, but chronically can also inhibit mTORC2.

and in mice, and the mTOR inhibitor rapamycin robustly extends mouse life span, even when treatment is initiated in older adults. Rapamycin also suppresses neoplasia (**see Chapter 5**) and several other phenotypes of aging in treated animals. In humans, inhibition of mTOR activity enhances responses to influenza vaccination in healthy older individuals. Overall, these data indicate that mTOR signaling limits longevity in a manner that is conserved in many different organisms.

PERSPECTIVE: THE BIOLOGY OF AGING AND LONGEVITY

It seems likely that the protean effects of aging reflect multiple molecular causes, including diverse types of molecular damage and other phenomena, such as excess mTOR signaling. These effects may then converge to cause progressive dysfunction and eventual death. These phenomena have been codified in the form of nine "hallmarks" of aging, providing an initial conceptual framework for understanding major drivers of aging and potential points of therapeutic intervention (Fig. 10-10). There are now several means of extending life span experimentally, suggesting that such approaches can provide additional mechanistic insights into the aging process and, perhaps, means to extend healthy life spans in humans.

Although in some respects aging remains an enigma, we now have important molecular insights into its mechanisms, as well as environmental and genetic interventions that can dramatically slow the rate of aging in invertebrates and in mammals. Eventually, these efforts are likely to yield large dividends in medicine. In industrialized societies, most elderly people suffer from multiple diseases of old age. Consequently, disease-specific interventions, against heart disease or cancer for example, actually have fairly modest payoffs in terms of years of life gained. For example, based on demographic data, it has been estimated that for a 50-year-old woman, curing all forms of cancer would extend her life expectancy by less than 3 years. Even curing cancer,

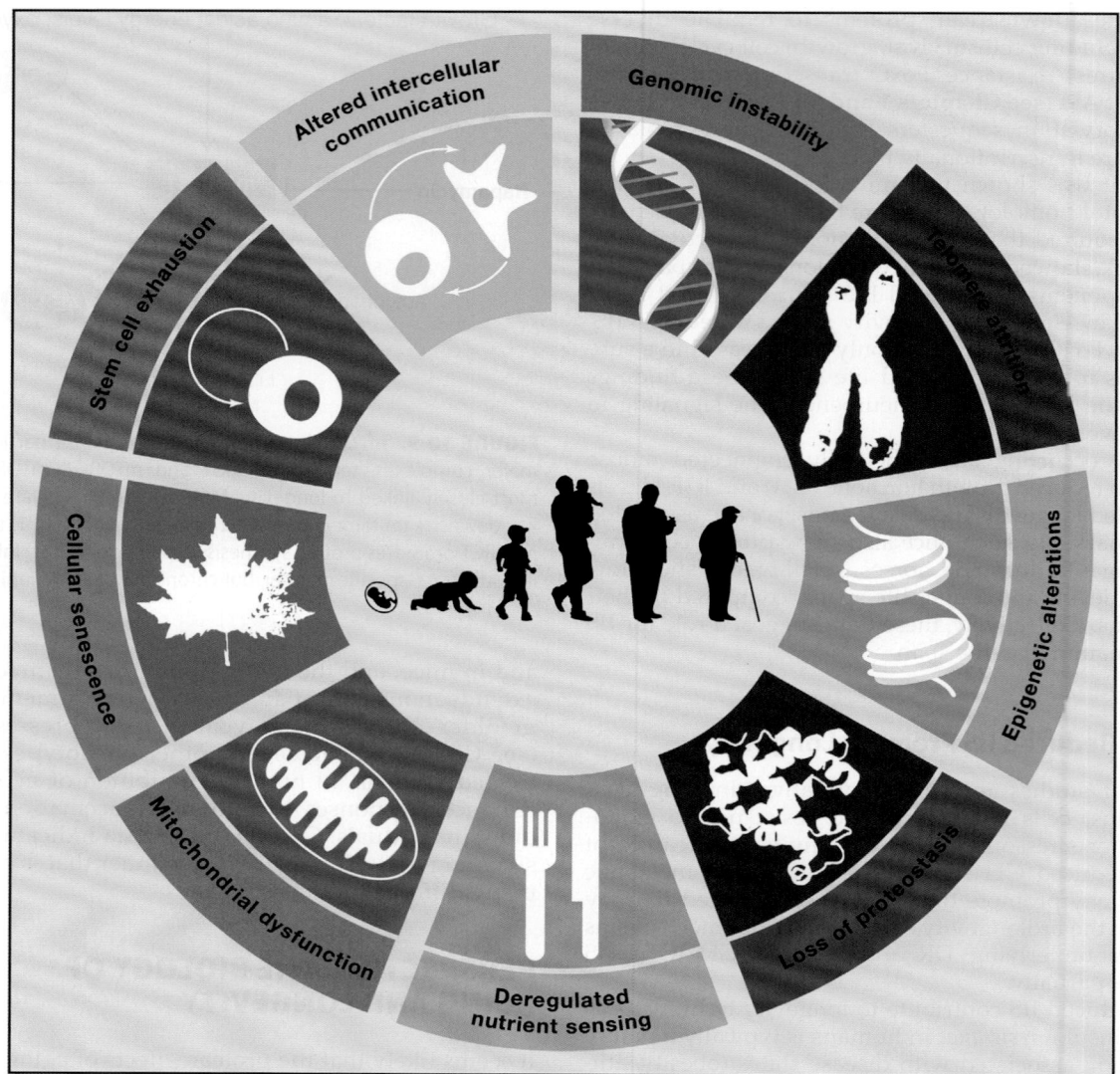

FIGURE 10-10. The nine proposed hallmarks of aging. (Reprinted from Lopez-Otin C, Blasco MA, Partridge L, Serrano M, Kroemer G. The hallmarks of aging. *Cell*. 2013;153[6]:1194–1217. Copyright © 2013 Elsevier. With permission.)

heart disease, stroke, and diabetes all simultaneously would add only 14 years of life, on average. These gains are fairly modest because deaths due to all causes of mortality rise exponentially with age. Thus, as she ages, our hypothetical 50-year-old woman will likely succumb to some other age-associated disease anyway (i.e., soon after she would have otherwise died from cancer, heart disease, stroke, or diabetes). On the other hand, life span extension proportional to that seen in rodent DR studies would increase her life expectancy by roughly 40%, from 80 to about 112 years. Moreover, if animal studies are any guide, most of those added years would likely be spent in good health. These figures illustrate how a deep, mechanistic understanding of the biology of aging may offer a powerful means to improve human well-being.

11 | Systemic Autoimmune Diseases

Philip L. Cohen, Jeffrey S. Warren, Sergio A. Jimenez

Mechanisms of Autoimmunity

Both the innate and adaptive immune systems have the capacity to injure host tissues, giving rise to a variety of human diseases, some entirely caused by self-reactivity, and others accompanied by self-reactivity. Autoimmune diseases can be divided into those affecting primarily one organ (e.g., myocarditis) and those involving multiple body systems (e.g., systemic lupus). More recently, a third group of autoimmune illnesses caused by inappropriate activation of the innate immune system has been recognized.

Autoimmunity Is Usually Defined as Specific Reactivity by the Adaptive Immune System Against Self-Tissue

This includes recognition of self-antigens by **autoantibodies** and self-reactive T cells. A broader definition of autoimmunity would include immune damage to tissues initiated by the innate immune system, for example, inflammation due to inappropriate activation of **inflammasomes** (see Chapter 2), key complexes of membrane-linked enzymes and adapter proteins that lead to generation of biologically active IL-1 or IL-18, with consequent inflammation. Similar activation of innate immunity affects the complement system due to faulty complement control proteins (e.g., factor H), which leads to hemolytic–uremic syndrome. Or, for example, inappropriately sensitive receptors may cause exaggerated responses to cytokines, as with TNF-α (causing TNF receptor-associated periodic syndrome [TRAPS]).

Self-recognition is woven into normal immune responses. For example, T cells normally recognize peptide antigens only when associated with self–MHC molecules (see Chapter 4). Autoantibodies are not always associated with disease. Certain autoantibodies are present even in normal individuals (e.g., rheumatoid factor; see below) and play a housekeeping role in removing superfluous antigens. In fact, B cells that make autoantibodies constitute a very large part of the fetal and neonatal antibody repertoire. Many, but not all of these cells are deleted by undergoing apoptosis, or are inactivated as the immune system matures (Fig. 11-1).

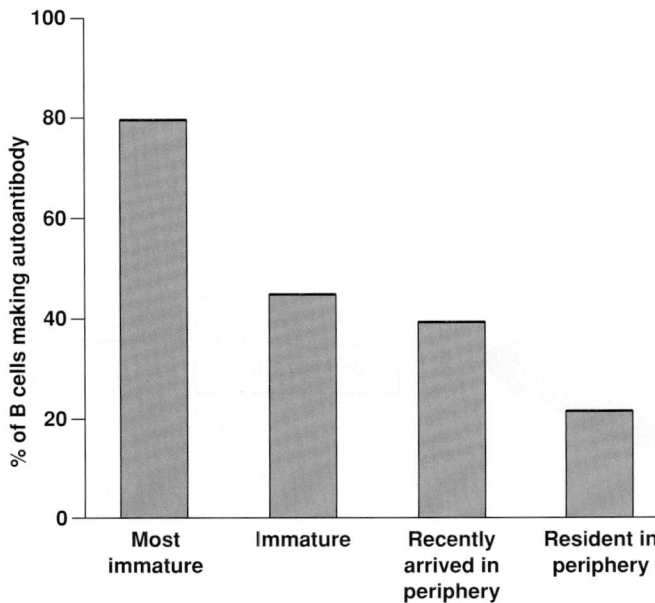

FIGURE 11-1. Autoantibody formation by normal B cells. Fractions of human B-cell lymphocytes produced autoantibodies, taken at different stages of development.

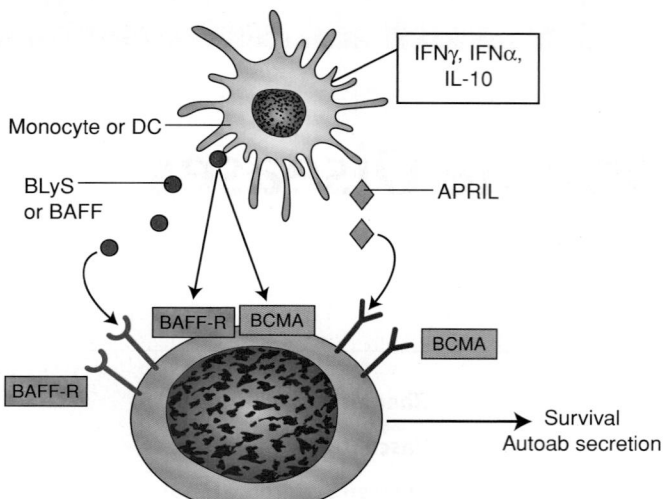

FIGURE 11-2.   BAFF and APRIL binding to B lymphocytes. Monocytes and dendritic cells produce BAFF (BLys) and APRIL when driven by certain cytokines. These bind to receptors on B cells, promoting their survival.

Humoral Autoimmunity

Like antibodies to pathogens or other exogenous antigens, autoantibodies are generated by rearrangement of VH and VL genes in B cells. B cells that by chance are autoreactive

must be eliminated or at least inactivated. Autoreactive B cells are vetted and deleted, or rendered inactive, at multiple checkpoints in normal B-cell development. Heavy (H) or light (L) chain Ig genes expressed by some autoreactive B cells may be replaced by different H or L chains, thus giving the B cell a new and nonautoreactive specificity. This process, called **receptor editing**, is an important mechanism of avoiding autoreactivity. **B-cell activating factor** (**BAFF**, also known as **BLyS**), a cytokine derived mainly from macrophages, regulates B-cell maturation (Fig. 11-2) and autoreactivity. Far more B cells are produced than will eventually survive. BAFF (and a related molecule, **A proliferation-inducing ligand**, or **APRIL**) control how many B cells reach maturity by rescuing immature B cells from apoptosis. Overproduction of BAFF causes hypergammaglobulinemia and humoral autoimmunity.

T-Cell–Mediated Autoimmunity

Acquisition of the mature T-cell repertoire is a complex process involving positive and negative selection in the thymus. The repertoire is further shaped by selection among peripheral T cells (i.e., mature T cells that have already exited the thymus). The **autoimmune regulator (AIRE)** thymic transcription factor plays a key role: it drives expression of many self-proteins in the thymus, so that potentially self-reactive T cells can be exposed to them and then eliminated (Fig. 11-3). Mutations in AIRE cause

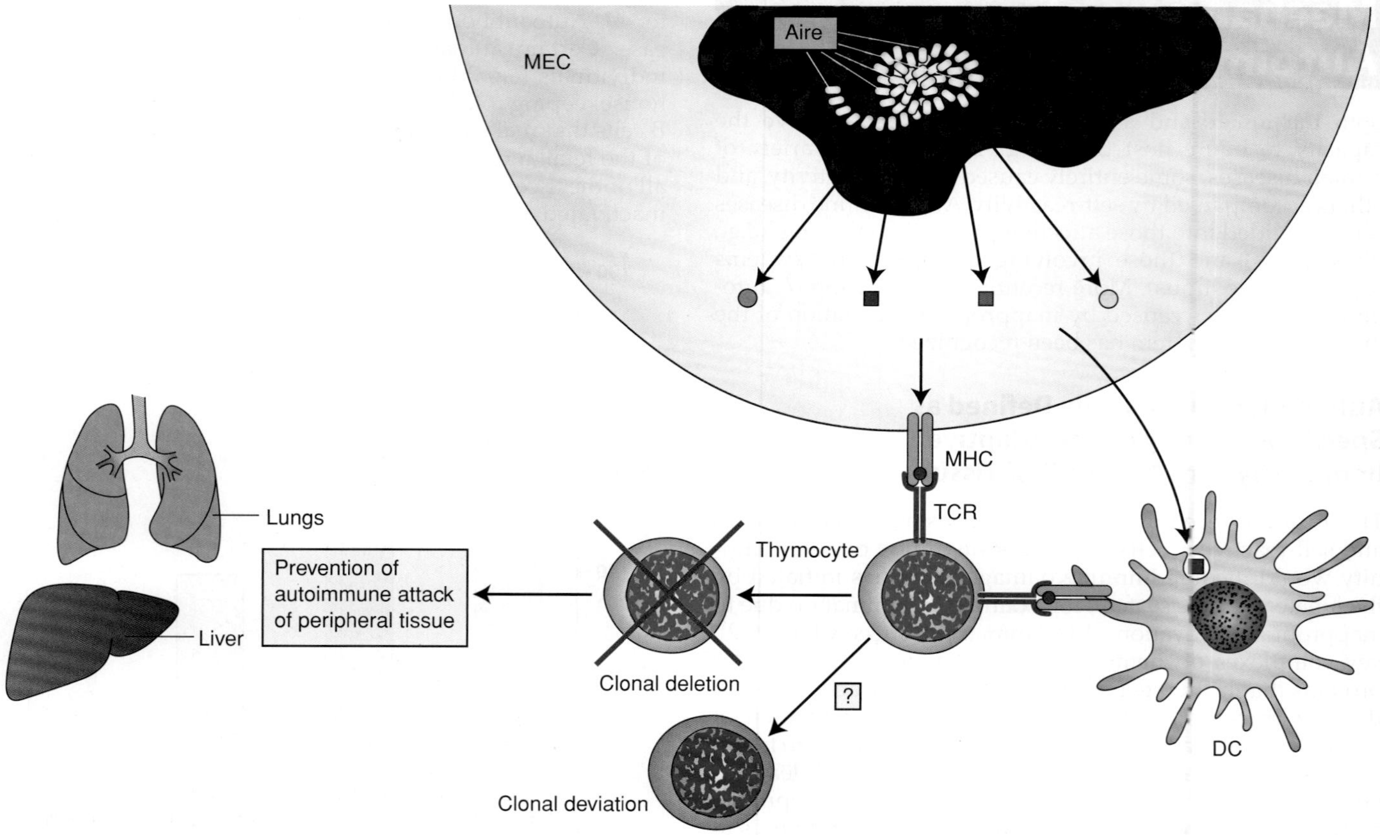

FIGURE 11-3.   T-lymphocyte clonal deletion in tolerance. AIRE transcription factor activates expression of antigens normally expressed in peripheral tissues, so that they are expressed in thymic medulla epithelial cells (MEC). Antigens so regulated may include those of any tissue, the liver, and lungs being shown here as representatives. Such self-antigens are presented to T lymphocytes developing in the thymus, directly by the MEC or by dendritic cells (DCs). The result is deletion of autoreactive T lymphocytes.

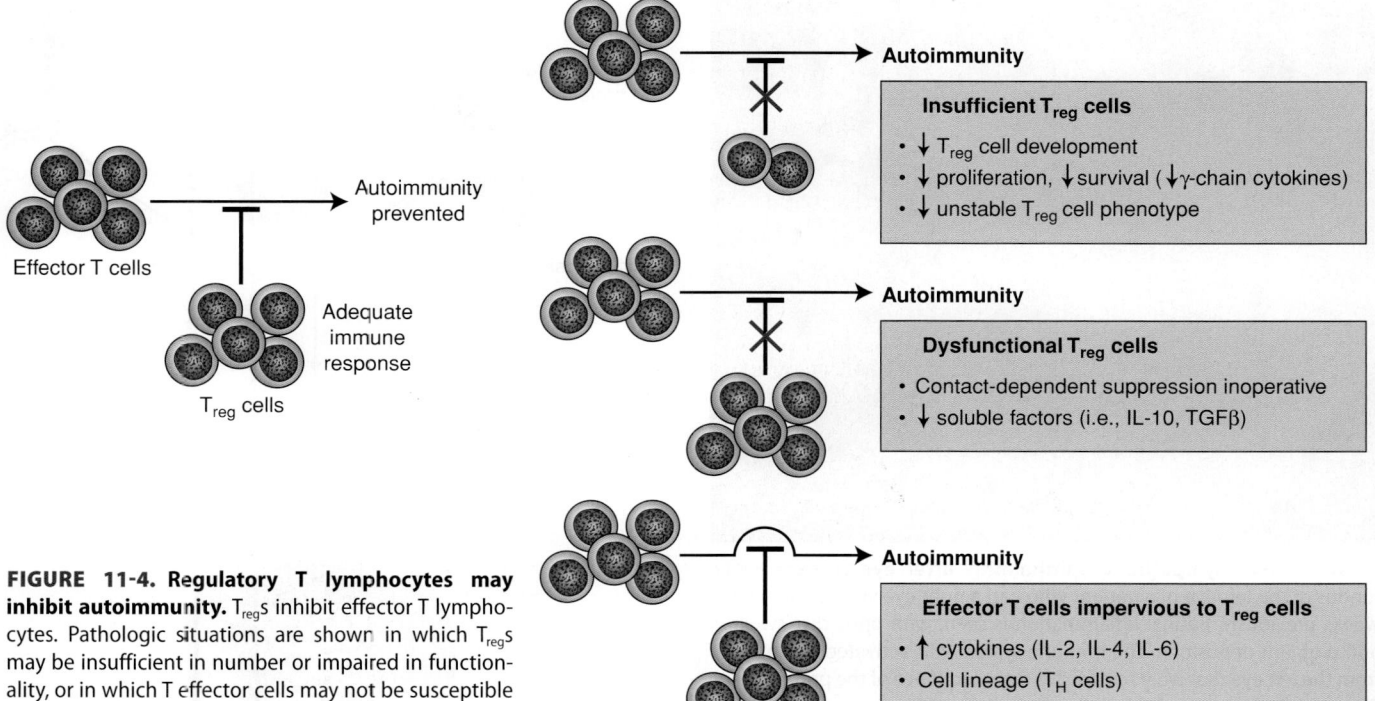

FIGURE 11-4. Regulatory T lymphocytes may inhibit autoimmunity. T_{reg}s inhibit effector T lymphocytes. Pathologic situations are shown in which T_{reg}s may be insufficient in number or impaired in functionality, or in which T effector cells may not be susceptible to the regulatory activities of T_{reg}s.

a serious systemic pediatric autoimmune disease (**autoimmune polyendocrinopathy–candidiasis–ectodermal dystrophy [APECED]**).

Regulatory T cells (T_{reg}) also control autoreactivity by limiting potentially harmful responses by other T cells. Mutations in **FoxP3**, a transcription factor for T_{reg}, lead to another serious autoimmune disease (**immunodysregulation, polyendocrinopathy and enteropathy, X-linked [IPEX]**) (Fig. 11-4).

Some Inflammatory Diseases Are Caused by Inappropriate Activation of the Innate Immune System

Thus, periodic fever syndromes, which are an important cause of morbidity in some parts of the world, are caused by genetic defects in control of **inflammasomes** (see above and Chapter 2) (Fig. 11-5). Other inherited "autoinflammatory" diseases entail widespread inflammation, for example, **neonatal-onset multisystem inflammatory disease (NOMID)**, in which a mutated **cryopyrin** protein (a key component of the inflammasome) is constitutively activated, causing unregulated IL-1 production and resulting in skin inflammation and arthritis. Likewise, mutations of **stimulator of interferon genes (STING)**, a key DNA sensing protein, lead to excessive interferon (INF) production and **systemic vasculitis (STING-associated vasculitis [SAV])**.

As noted above, inherited or acquired defects of complement regulatory proteins (factor H and others) can lead to severe microangiopathic disease (hemolytic–uremic syndrome). Similarly, defects in erythrocyte surface proteins that control complement activation can lead to paroxysmal nocturnal hemoglobinuria, a serious illness with anemia and hemolysis.

CAUSES OF AUTOIMMUNITY

Several mechanisms can lead to autoimmune disease. Despite considerable progress, our understanding of the pathophysiology of most autoimmune diseases is incomplete.

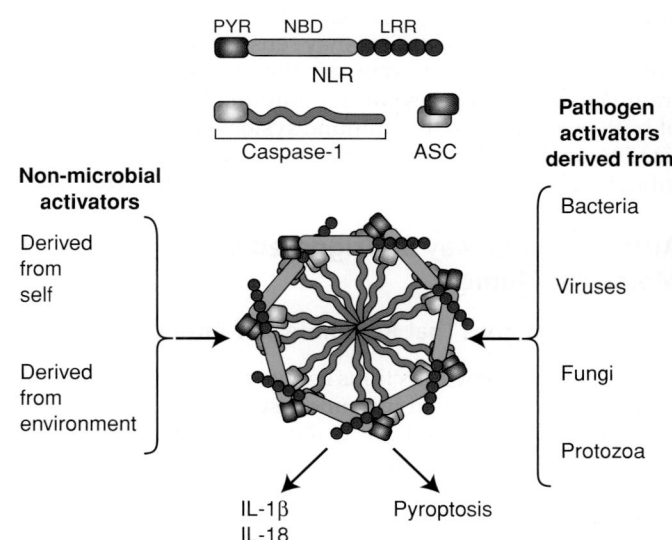

FIGURE 11-5. The inflammasome. The NLRP3 inflammasome, the best studied of these proinflammatory complexes, is a cluster of proteins (NLR, caspase 1, ASC) on macrophages and other innate immune cells. Several stimuli activate it to cause production of active interleukin-1 (IL-1) and IL-18 and to elicit cell death. *ASC* = apoptosis-associated speck-like protein containing a caspase recruitment domain; *CPPD* = calcium pyrophosphate dihydrate; *MDP* = muramyl dipeptide; *MSU* = monosodium urate; *NLR* = nucleotide-binding domain, leucine-rich repeat containing; *PAMP* = pathogen-associated molecule patterns.

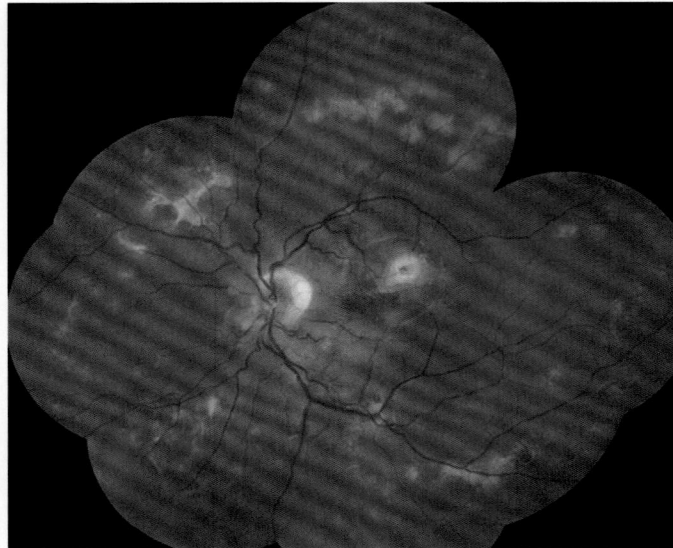

FIGURE 11-6. Sympathetic ophthalmitis after eye surgery. Optic fundus of the left eye of a patient who had a right eye vitrectomy several weeks previously. Retinal inflammation is seen, with optic disc swelling and pigment deposition. The immune system was activated by antigens from the left eye that were released as a consequence of the prior surgery. The result is damage in the previously normal right eye.

Breach of Immunologic Privilege

Certain body areas (e.g., the anterior chamber of the eye) are immunologically "privileged": the immune system has little or no contact with these areas. Neither immunity nor tolerance is established to their tissue-specific antigens. This is why transplanted corneas are not rejected. If the isolated antigens of privileged sites reach the immune system (e.g., via trauma), self-reactivity may ensue. This mechanism probably accounts for **sympathetic ophthalmitis,** where trauma to one eye causes chronic autoimmune inflammation of both eyes because the immune system has become sensitized to ocular antigens it normally ignores. Postmyocardial infarction pericarditis may have a similar etiology (Fig. 11-6).

Autoimmunity May Be Triggered by Molecular Mimicry

Microbial Antigens That Resemble Self-Antigens

Antigens from some infectious agents resemble human antigens structurally, so that immune responses to the pathogen may elicit antimicrobial antibodies or T cells which react with autologous tissues. Immunity against certain streptococcal antigens leads to antibodies that cross-react with antigens in the synovium, nervous system, and heart (see Chapter 17). This causes an acute febrile illness (**acute rheumatic fever)** with inflammation in and around the heart, in joints, and sometimes in the brain. It may lead to scarring in heart valves and may recur with reinfection. Why some people are susceptible and others are not remains unclear (see below).

    Guillain–Barré syndrome is a postviral autoimmune neuropathy apparently resulting from immunity originally directed against viral products, but now reactive against normal nervous system components. Some other viral diseases

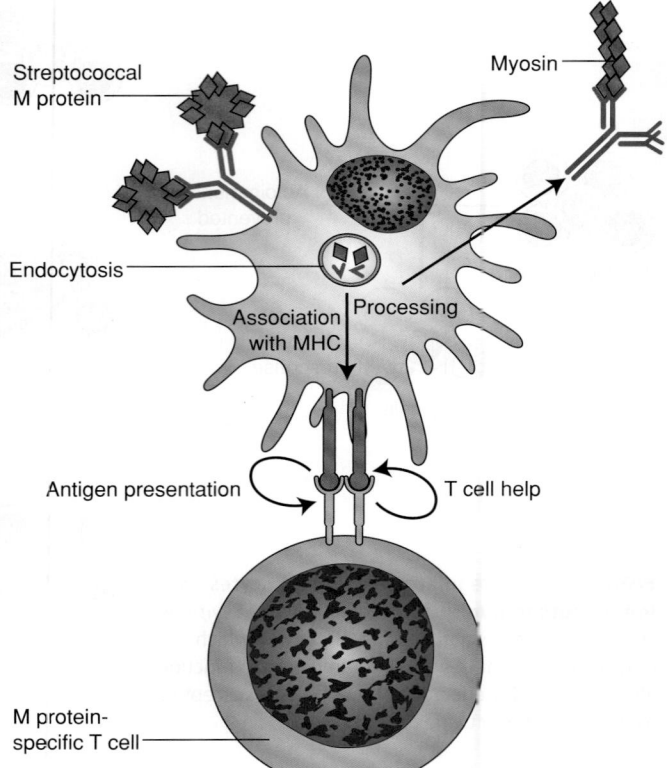

FIGURE 11-7. Molecular mimicry. In molecular mimicry, the immune system is sensitized by foreign proteins (here, *Streptococcus* M protein). M-protein–reactive T cells help B cells, which make antibody that cross-reacts with autologous cardiac myosin, to cause damage to the heart, as in rheumatic fever.

may also lead to autoimmunity—for example, postmeasles encephalomyelopathy (Fig. 11-7).

Polyclonal Activation and Autoimmunity

Certain environmental agents— for example, lipopolysaccharide (LPS) in gram-negative bacterial walls, but also many other substances—may diffusely activate the immune system. LPS binds toll-like receptor 4 ([TLR4]; see Chapter 2). Many other activators of the innate immune system can also activate toll-like receptors (TLRs). Because B cells have certain TLRs, they can be powerfully activated by ligands binding these receptors. For B cells, the result is that many different clones are activated simultaneously, causing a burst of antibody formation that represents all the specificities possessed by available B cells. This includes autoantibodies. Consequently, autoantibodies can be stimulated by particular viral or bacterial infections. For example, Epstein–Barr virus (EBV) binds to and activates B cells, and autoantibodies are often present during acute EBV infection. Chronic bacterial infections, such as endocarditis and osteomyelitis, are also often accompanied by autoantibodies. In most cases, these are not pathogenic, but occasionally they cause clinical disease.

Drugs and Toxins as Causes of Autoimmunity

Certain drugs can provoke autoantibodies, autoreactive T cells, and even clinical autoimmunity in ways that are still

ill-defined, leading to aberrations of tolerance. A systemic lupus-like syndrome, with antinuclear antibodies (ANAs), may occur in patients taking hydralazine, procainamide, and many other drugs. Methyldopa and some other drugs may cause antierythrocyte autoantibodies, and some patients given quinine and certain other medications may elicit antiplatelet antibodies.

Poisoning from environmental toxins, notably mercury and other heavy metals, is accompanied by autoimmune-mediated renal and nervous system disease. There have been outbreaks of inflammatory connective tissue disease traced to ingestion of contaminated tryptophan and other food supplements. Cocaine, especially when taken with the antihelminthic, levamisole, may induce granulomatous vasculitis.

 PATHOPHYSIOLOGY: Mechanisms that mediate such reactions are variably, and incompletely understood and documented:

1. A reactive exogenous compound (e.g., drug, microbial product) may bind covalently to an endogenous peptide, to form a hapten-carrier complex, thus creating a new antigen. This may elicit an antibody or cell-mediated response against the complex that could also recognize the noncomplexed endogenous carrier (Fig. 11-8[**A**]).
2. Similarly, an inert exogenous compound may be processed by the host (e.g., liver) to create an active derivative, which binds an endogenous peptide and repeats the process described in #1 above (Fig. 11-8[**B**]).

These two scenarios, which follow classical immunologic paradigms are not, however, sufficient to explain many autoimmune reactions triggered by exogenous substances. More recent data point to (at least) two additional mechanisms by which these situations arise:

3. An exogenous inert small peptide fits with high affinity into the binding site of either a T-cell receptor or a specific MHC molecule on an antigen-presenting cell. This may occur in a pre-existing setting of high levels of MHC and/or costimulatory molecule expression. The resulting complex strongly triggers T-cell signaling, associated with elevated concentrations of stimulatory cytokines (Fig. 11-8[**C**]).
4. In a parallel situation, an inert small peptide associates strongly with the peptide-binding pocket of a specific endogenous MHC molecule of target cell, to generate a new antigenic conformation. To the immune system, this altered MHC is no longer self-MHC, and so triggers an autoimmune response (Fig. 11-8[**D**]).

Genetics and Autoimmunity

Host genes profoundly affect susceptibility to autoimmunity triggers (see above) and autoimmune diseases. Concordance for SLE among identical twins is about 35%, and for RA about 15%. Autoimmune disease patients frequently report family members with the same or similar autoimmune disorders. Except for rare inherited conditions

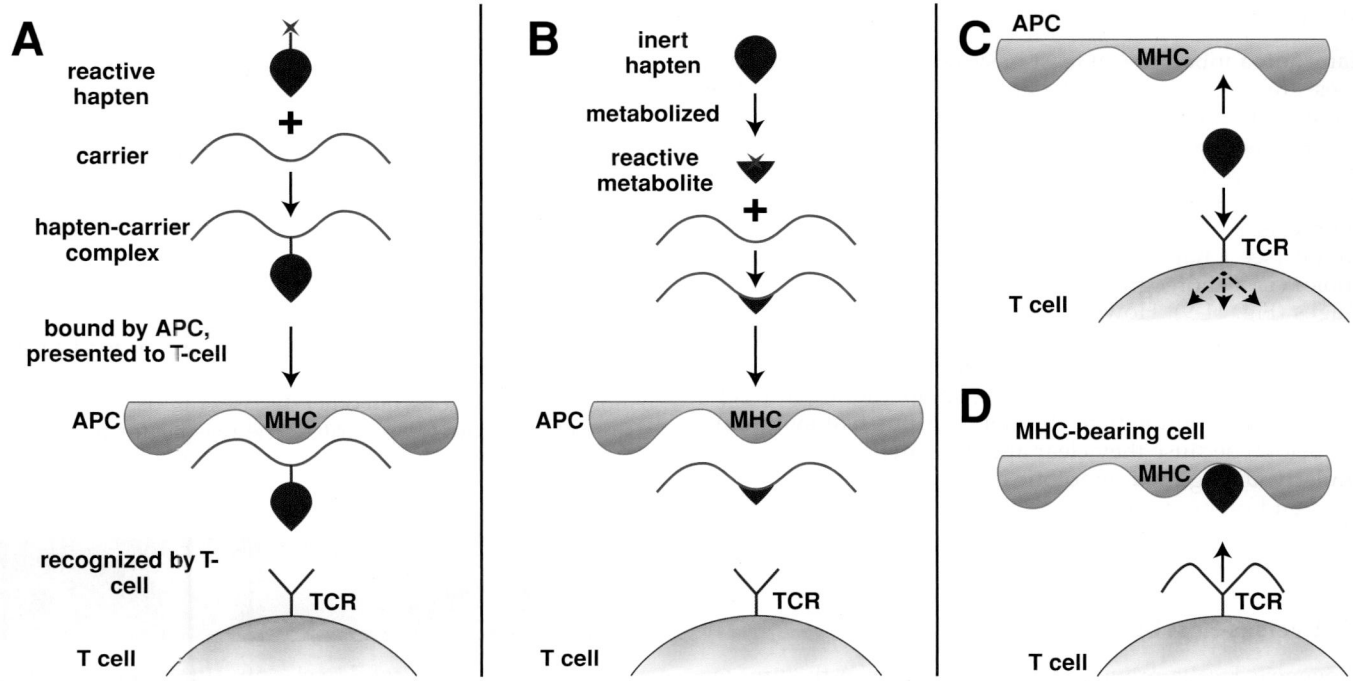

FIGURE 11-8. Mechanisms of small molecule–induced autoimmunity. A. A reactive small molecule binds a carrier protein, thereby creating a new antigen, which is the hapten-carrier complex, which can be presented to (here) T cells (or B cells) to elicit immunity that may cross-recognize the endogenous carrier. **B.** An inert small molecule is metabolized to a reactive derivative, and follows the same pathway as in **A**. **C.** An inert small molecule binds strongly to a *specific* self MHC molecule on an antigen-presenting cell (APC) and/or an antigen receptor, triggering extensive TCR-generated signaling and activating an immune response. **D.** An inert small molecule binds strongly to an endogenous MHC-bearing cell, to create an altered self MHC antigen, which now can be recognized by reactive (here) T cells as foreign, and generate an immune response that contains an element of antiself autoreactivity.

(e.g., APECED), inheritance is complex and multiple genes probably conspire with multiple environmental factors. Genetic links that influence development of autoimmune diseases include MHC alleles (mostly class II, but class I for spondyloarthropathies), and diverse genes involving immune signaling, such as IL-17, its receptor, and IL-23. TLR genes and genes for other cytokines, cytokine receptors, and tyrosine kinases involved in immune cell activation also participate in development of immune responses to self-antigens.

In addition, some of the mechanisms listed above are described specifically for certain HLA types.

Gender and Autoimmunity

Most autoimmune diseases occur more often in females. Female:male ratios range from up to 20:1 for autoimmune thyroiditis and lupus to 3:1 for rheumatoid arthritis (RA) and multiple sclerosis. Why women are more susceptible to autoimmunity is poorly understood. Sex hormones influence immune responses, and may contribute to increased female susceptibility, but other possibilities (e.g., X-chromosome gene dosage effects) are also possible.

Chance and Autoimmunity

Both B- and T-cell receptor formation involve random genetic recombination events. These are compounded by somatic mutation of receptors. The variability of autoimmunity—even in completely inbred susceptible animal strains—has led to the view that stochastic (random) events, probably in repertoire generation, may affect both the normal immune repertoire and development of autoimmunity.

Apoptosis and Autoimmunity

Many autoantibodies—at least in systemic autoimmune diseases—recognize intracellular antigens, especially those that reside normally in the nucleus. Such intracellular antigens may gain access to the immune system as cells die. Nuclear antigens appear on the surfaces of dying cells, where they may trigger self-immunization, leading to autoantibodies. Apoptosis is characterized by cell death without inflammation (see Chapter 1). Apoptotic cells are phagocytosed whole, via a choreographed set of interactions with macrophages (Fig. 11-9). However, abnormalities in the mononuclear phagocyte system may cause apoptotic cells to persist abnormally and can lead to autoimmunity in experimental systems. For example, mice lacking an apoptotic cell receptor-signaling intermediate develop a lupus-like syndrome (see below) because they clear apoptotic debris inefficiently. Similarly, unengulfed apoptotic debris is present in human lupus and other autoimmune diseases. Persistent apoptotic cell debris may progress to necrotic foci, which may provoke autoimmunity.

Graft-Versus-Host Disease

Allogeneic T cells provoke inflammation when they recognize histoincompatible tissue (as in recipients of allogeneic bone marrow; see Chapter 4). Autoantibodies may arise during chronic **graft-versus-host disease (GVHD)**. This is believed to result in abnormal interaction between donor T cells and recipient B cells, probably because those T cells have not been tolerized in the host thymus.

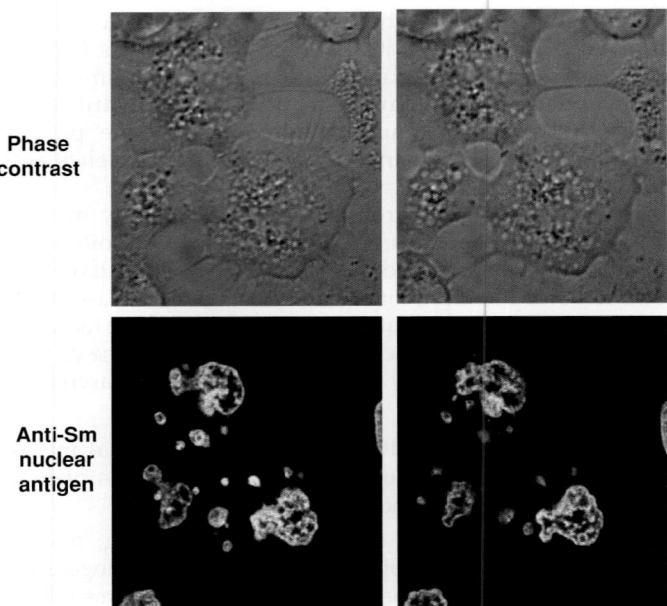

FIGURE 11-9. Expression and release of nuclear antigens by cells early (left) and late (right) in apoptosis. UV-irradiated skin cells became apoptotic, demonstrating the typical morphology (*upper panel*, phase contrast). Immunofluorescence staining was used to identify Sm nuclear antigen (*lower panel*). Sm was present on surface blebs. Such nuclear antigens may trigger autoimmune responses.

Marker Autoantibodies May Provide Clues About Autoimmunity

Marker autoantibodies are disease-specific autoantibodies that are so closely linked to certain diseases that their presence suffices to confirm the diagnosis. Some of these may be surprising; for instance, antibodies to transfer RNA (tRNA) synthetases (e.g., methionine tRNA synthetase) are virtually diagnostic of inflammatory myositis, and antibody to **topoisomerase I** (a DNA unwinding enzyme) is specific for scleroderma.

Remission–Exacerbation

Many autoimmune diseases, even if untreated, tend to flare and then remit. Multiple sclerosis is especially prone to exacerbations and remissions, but other diseases (lupus, RA, etc.) may also relent (usually temporarily). The reasons for this pattern of episodic peaks and valleys of disease activity are uncertain.

Systemic Autoimmune Diseases

As noted earlier, it is useful to classify autoimmune diseases as organ specific (affecting a single organ or organ system—for example, autoimmune thyroiditis—or as systemic, with multiple organs affected. Organ-specific autoimmunity can accompany systemic autoimmune disease. Manifestations of autoimmune diseases in individual organs (e.g., autoimmune hepatitis) are mainly described in the chapters that focus on organ-based pathology. We address below systemic autoimmune diseases, as they affect the whole patient. It should be emphasized that almost every organ can be afflicted with autoimmune disease.

AUTOANTIBODIES

Autoantibodies can be detected in normal people, and many do not cause disease. Some can cause disease when given to experimental animals, thus establishing a cause-and-effect relationship. Others may cross the placenta and harm the fetus, also supporting causality. For most autoimmune diseases, however, the inference that autoantibodies or autoreactive T cells cause the pathology is based on the presence of autoantibodies, often with complement components, or T cells in affected tissues.

Autoimmune Diseases May Reflect T- and B-Cell–Mediated Autoreactivity

Though many autoimmune diseases are largely caused by antibodies, others are mediated by T cells alone. Some (e.g., lupus; see below) seem to involve both autoreactive T and B cells. The sometimes surprising therapeutic effectiveness of B-cell depletion (using anti-CD20) has provoked a reevaluation of the relative role of T cells in certain autoimmune diseases, for example multiple sclerosis.

For some autoimmune diseases, target antigens are few, and well defined (e.g., α-gliadin in celiac disease). For others, it has been difficult to incriminate specific antigens, implying that more complex antigenic spectrum.

Immunity Is Usually Depressed in Patients With Autoimmune Diseases

People suffering from systemic autoimmune disorders have **reduced** immune responses to exogenous antigens (e.g., vaccines, infectious agents), independently of immunosuppressive treatments they may be receiving. It is almost as if an immune system that is preoccupied with responding to self cannot properly defend against infection. This disease-associated immune impairment can be clinically significant.

For the most part, the antibodies in systemic autoimmune disease patients have all of the characteristics of mature, high-affinity immune responses. Antibodies are against multiple epitopes on complex autoantigens, supporting the idea that the original autoantibody response was indeed antigen driven and not due to a fortuitous cross-reaction or aberrant immune regulation (Fig. 11-10).

Autoantibodies Predate Disease Onset

Studies using stored predisease serum samples have shown that detectable autoantibodies precede disease manifestations for systemic lupus and RA. Thus autoimmunity most likely leads to these illnesses, and autoantibodies are probably not secondary epiphenomena.

Autoantibody Specificities are Skewed

The specificities of disease-related autoantibodies are not easily predictable. Most antibodies in rheumatic disease

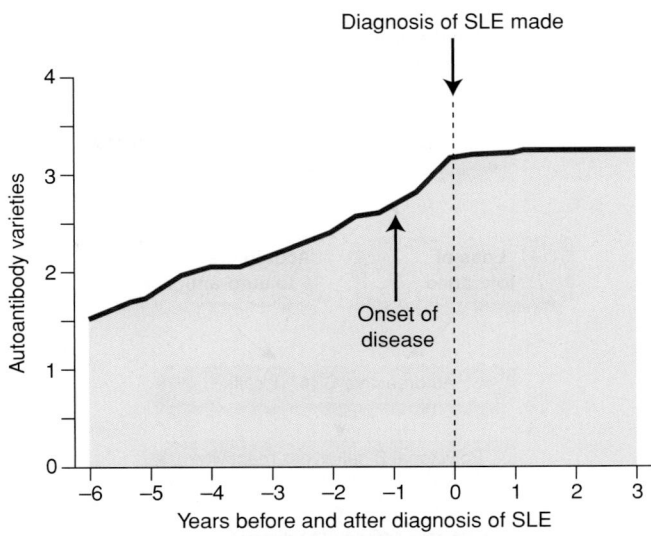

FIGURE 11-10. Time course of autoantibody formation in systemic lupus erythematosus (SLE). Average numbers of the different kinds of autoantibodies as a function of time of symptom onset and diagnosis in patients with SLE.

patients are directed against components of cell nuclei: **ANAs.** There are many proteins in the nucleus, but known autoantibodies only target some of them, and some are quite disease specific. For example, antibodies to **Smith (Sm) ribonuclear protein (RNP)** complex, which is crucial to splicing of premessenger RNA (pre-mRNA), are highly specific for lupus. Neither the amount nor the location of an individual self-protein clearly determines whether it will be a disease-related autoantigen. There is some evidence that the degree of molecular disorder and other structural characteristics of certain nuclear protein correlates with their autoantigenicity.

SYSTEMIC LUPUS ERYTHEMATOSUS

SLE Is a Multisystem Inflammatory Disease that May Involve Many Organs

It characteristically affects the skin, joints, serous membranes, CNS, and kidneys. Autoantibodies are directed against multiple self-antigens, including plasma proteins (complement components, clotting factors), protein–phospholipid complexes, cell surface antigens (lymphocytes, neutrophils, platelets, erythrocytes), intracellular cytoplasmic components (microfilaments, microtubules, lysosomes, ribosomes, RNA) and nuclear DNA, ribonucleoproteins, and histones. The spectrum of intracellular autoantigens includes the proteins and DNA that make up chromatin, proteins of the **spliceosome complex (small nuclear RNPs [snRNPs])** and the **Ro/La** small cytoplasmic ribonucleoprotein particle.

In SLE, antigen-antibody complexes deposit in tissues, provoking inflammation leading to characteristic vasculitis, synovitis, and glomerulonephritis. Although the role of T cells in provoking tissue damage in SLE is less well understood, it is clear that some damage is due to cell-mediated immune responses.

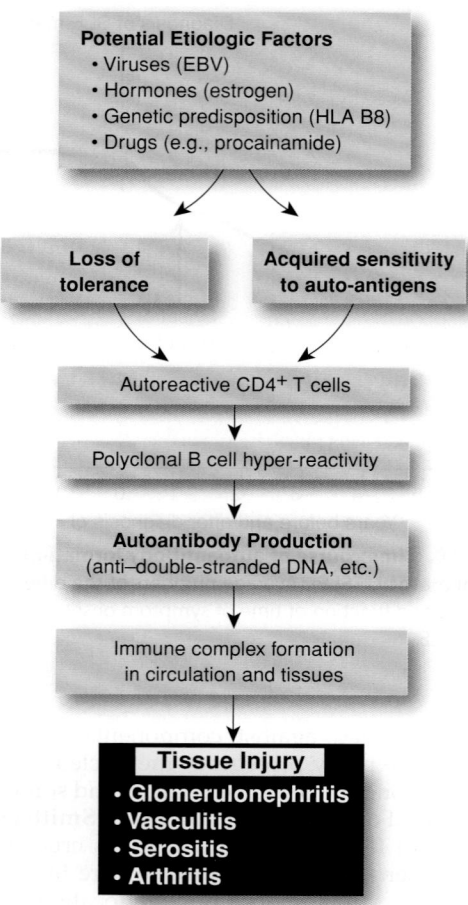

FIGURE 11-11. The pathogenesis of systemic lupus erythematosus is multifactorial. *EBV* = Epstein–Barr virus; *HLA* = human leukocyte antigen.

 PATHOPHYSIOLOGY: SLE patients have decreased cell membrane C3b receptors. Thus, Fc-receptor dependent phagocytosis of immune complexes is impaired, so ongoing autoimmunity may be exacerbated by persistent antigenic stimuli. Complement is important in clearing debris and apoptotic cells, and inherited deficiencies of certain complement components, particularly C2, C4, and C1q, are associated with an increased incidence of SLE and lupus-like disorders.

ENVIRONMENT. UV irradiation and viral infections can exacerbate pre-existing SLE disease. Lupus patients may experience disease flares after prolonged exposure to the sun or after a viral infection. Increased proinflammatory cell death accompanies these conditions, possibly serving to stimulate immunity against nucleic acids.

Silica exposure significantly increases the risk of developing lupus, perhaps because its toxicity for macrophages may impair clearance of apoptotic cells and so favor self-immunization.

HORMONES AND X-CHROMOSOME DOSAGE. SLE is predominantly a female disease. Onset of SLE before puberty and after menopause is uncommon. The female predilection becomes less pronounced outside the reproductive age range. These observations suggest a role for endogenous sex hormones in disease predisposition. Hormones can impact T cell and macrophage function, and estrogens increase B-cell differentiation and in vitro immunoglobulin (Ig) production including anti-dsDNA. There are other explanations for the female predominance in SLE, notably incomplete X chromosome inactivation, leading to increased dosage of genes affecting the immune system. In this regard, patients with Klinefelter's syndrome (XXY) are at increased risk for SLE.

EPIDEMIOLOGY: The prevalence of SLE varies worldwide. In North America and northern Europe, it is 40 in 100,000. In the United States, it appears to be more common and severe in African- and Hispanic-Americans, although socioeconomic factors may in part be responsible. Nearly 90% of cases are in women of childbearing age.

Genetic, immunologic, and environmental factors are all important (Fig. 11-11). However, many diagnostically helpful antinuclear autoantibodies are useful disease markers, but only a few directly cause inflammation.

MOLECULAR PATHOGENESIS: Susceptibility to lupus involves multiple genes. Close to 100 susceptibility genes contribute to disease, including Fc receptors (FcγRIIIA and FcγRIIA), PDCD1, and HLA-DR. Almost without exception, responsible genes encode proteins important in immune function, or are in regulatory regions that control expression of such proteins.

Immunologic Factors in the Pathogenesis of SLE

B Cells

Pathogenic autoantibodies produced by B cells are an important cause of tissue damage in SLE. B cells can also present self-antigens to T cells and are a significant source of cytokines. B-cell tolerance (specific unresponsiveness to self-antigens) is defective in SLE, causing autoreactive B cells to escape to the periphery. T cells are also important in the pathogenesis of lupus, both as helper cells for autoantibody production, and as cells directly involved in tissue injury.

CD4+ T cells may become autoreactive following DNA hypomethylation, and they overexpress the LFA (CD11a) cell adhesion molecules, which stabilize interactions between T cells and other cells. Follicular helper T cells have recently been shown to be especially important in providing help for autoreactive antibodies.

Dendritic Cells

Plasmacytoid dendritic cells contribute to lupus autoimmunity by producing IFN-α, which promotes inflammation and presentation of self-antigens to T cells. Leukocytes from SLE patients display what is called the "INF signature," namely activation of type I INF and of genes induced by this cytokine.

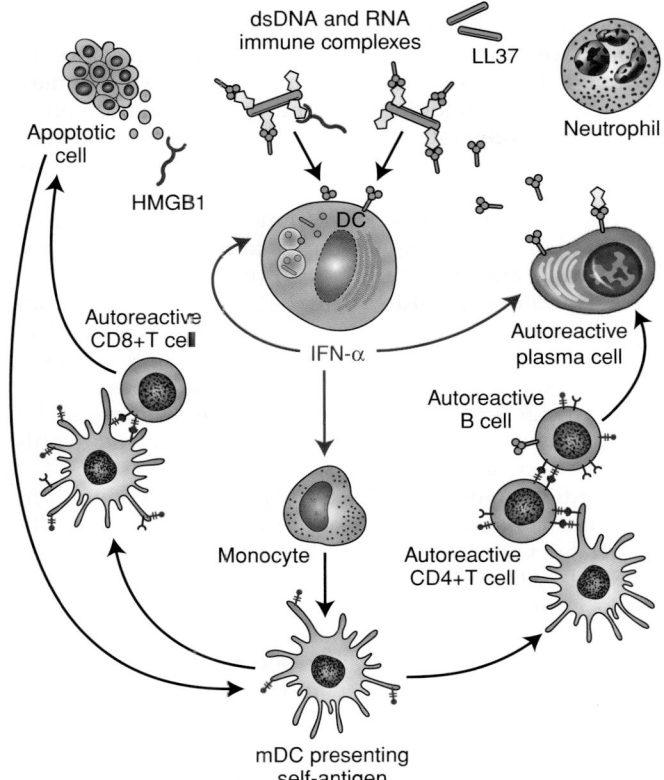

FIGURE 11-12. Immune pathogenesis of systemic lupus erythematosus (SLE). Nucleic acid complexes or toll-like receptor (TLR) agonists elicit interferon-α (IFN-α) by dendritic cells (DCs). This, in turn, triggers autoantigen presentation and autoantibody production by plasma cells.

Cytokines

Alterations in cytokine production in lupus reflect systemic inflammation and ongoing antigen-driven autoimmune responses. Some of these increased cytokines are IL-4, IL-6, IL-10, and IFN-α (Fig. 11-12).

Immune Complexes

A significant part of tissue injury in lupus reflects deposition of circulating immune complexes containing self-antigens, notably DNA. Immune complex formation may also occur *in situ*—Type II hypersensitivity reactions are also implicated in lupus, since cytotoxic antibodies against RBC and platelet membrane proteins can cause cytopenias (see Chapter 26).

Cell Death

Apoptosis (see Chapter 1) entails nuclear condensation, membrane blebbing, and subsequent cell shrinkage with preservation of an intact plasma membrane. As mentioned above, impaired apoptosis can cause an experimental disease like lupus, with lupus autoantibodies and glomerulonephritis.

Lupus patients have increased levels of circulating apoptotic debris and impaired capacity for uptake of dying cells. DNA/histones and RNA/proteins from apoptotic cells specifically bind to lupus autoantibodies and activate both DCs and autoreactive B cells via TLRs, serving to facilitate initiating or maintaining autoimmunity.

Toll-Like Receptors

TLRs pattern recognition receptors (PRRs) of the innate immune system (see Chapter 2), and recognize molecular patterns in microbial and other structures. Microbial TLR ligands include a wide range of molecules with strong adjuvant activity (such as LPS, lipopeptides, bacterial DNA, and viral RNA and DNA). These ligands are powerful activators of DCs, macrophages and other APCs, and allow effective presentation of microbial antigens to cells of the adaptive immune system. However, a substantial proportion of TLRs recognize endogenous ligands. In SLE, they bind circulating DNA/histone and RNA/protein complexes from apoptotic debris (see above), especially when complexed with autoantibodies. DNA/histone and RNA/protein, once taken up by DCs, engage TLR9 and TLR7, and stimulate DCs to produce large amounts of IFN-α. S100a and S100b proteins are abundant in neutrophil cytoplasm, and may bind to TLR 4 if released during inflammatory responses, leading to more inflammation and to chemotaxis of additional inflammatory cells.

IFN-α

There are two major types of IFNs: type I (IFN-α, β, ω) and type II (IFNγ, which is secreted only by T cells). IFN-α is secreted by virus-infected cells and plasmacytoid DCs; IFN-β is produced by many types of cells, such as myeloid DCs, following many—not necessarily infectious—stimuli. Type I IFNs share a ubiquitous heterodimeric receptor, mediate innate responses to viral infections, and are also required for full DC response to TLRs and their stimulation of T and B cells.

IFN-α strongly stimulates both innate and adaptive immune responses. In lupus in particular, circulating DNA/histone and RNA/protein complexes from apoptotic debris chronically stimulate its production via engagement and activation of TLR7 and TLR9. Most lupus patients have increased circulating levels of IFN-α. As noted above, levels of expression of many genes that are upregulated by IFN-α are higher in patients with SLE than in normal patients.

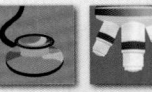 **CLINICAL FEATURES AND PATHOLOGY:** Because circulating immune complexes may accumulate in many tissues, virtually any organ may be affected (Fig. 11-13).

Joint disease is the most common manifestation of SLE; over 90% of patients have polyarthralgia. Inflammatory synovitis occurs, but unlike rheumatoid arthritis, joint destruction is unusual.

Skin involvement (see Chapter 28) is common, as a characteristic erythematous rash in sun-exposed sites, a malar "butterfly" rash. Perivascular lymphoid infiltrates and hydropic degeneration of keratinocytes (see Chapter 30) are seen. Immunofluorescence shows immunoglobulin and complement deposition along the dermal–epidermal junction ("lupus band"). An important role for T cells in these lesions is probable.

Renal disease, especially glomerulonephritis, affects over half of patients with SLE. Immune complexes, deposit in glomeruli, leading to glomerular inflammation (Fig. 11-14). These complexes contain IgG antibodies to double-stranded DNA, deposit in glomeruli in a

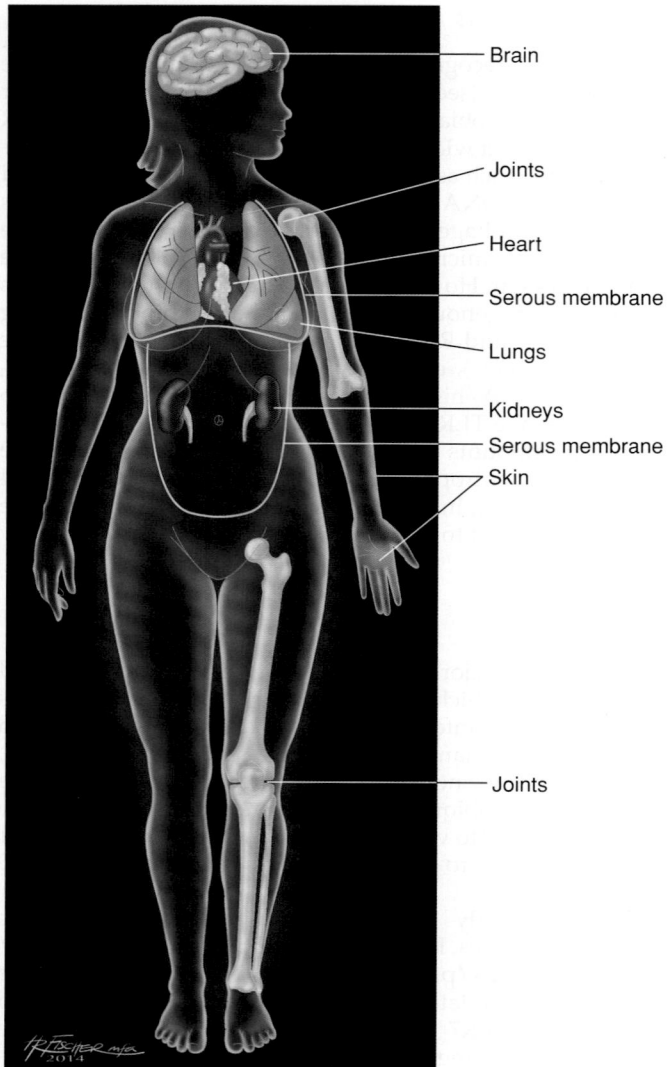

Brain

Joints

Heart

Serous membrane

Lungs

Kidneys

Serous membrane

Skin

Joints

FIGURE 11-13. Organ involvement in systemic lupus erythematosus.

membranous glomerulopathy (see Chapter 22). Glomerulonephritis is the most common renal manifestation of SLE, but interstitial nephritis or vasculitis (rarely) may also occur. Immunoglobulins and complement are often detectable in the interstitium and in renal blood vessels. There is T-lymphocyte infiltration and tissue injury as well.

Serous membranes are commonly involved. More than 1/3 of patients have pleuritis and pleural effusions. Pericarditis and peritonitis occur, but less frequently.

Respiratory disorders are common, ranging from pleural disease to upper airway and pulmonary parenchymal disease. Pneumonitis probably results from immune complex deposition in alveolar septa, and is associated with patchy acute inflammation. Progressive interstitial fibrosis develops in some patients, which may lead to pulmonary hypertension.

Cardiac involvement (see Chapter 17) is common in SLE, but congestive heart failure is rare and is usually associated with myocarditis. All layers of the heart may be affected, with pericarditis being most common. **Libman–Sacks endocarditis,** which is usually not clinically significant, is characterized by small nonbacterial vegetations on valve leaflets. These lesions should be differentiated from the larger, bulkier vegetations of bacterial endocarditis.

CNS disease can manifest as psychiatric disease or vasculitis, the latter a life-threatening complication. Vasculitis can lead to hemorrhage and infarction of the brain, which may be fatal.

Antiphospholipid antibodies and antibodies against related protein–phospholipid complexes circulate in 1/3 of SLE patients. They are associated with thromboembolic complications, including stroke, pulmonary embolism, deep venous thrombosis, portal vein thrombosis, and spontaneous abortions.

Other organ involvement is less common, and is often due to **vasculitis**. Lesions in the spleen include arterial thickening and concentric fibrosis, the so-called onion skin pattern.

The clinical course of SLE is extremely variable, with exacerbations and remissions. With immunosuppressive therapies, better recognition of mild forms of the disease and improved antihypertensive medication, overall 10-year survival approaches 90%. Patients with severe

"lumpy bumpy" pattern, and can be visualized using electron microscopy. They lead to various forms of glomerulonephritis including mesangial disease, focal proliferative nephritis, diffuse proliferative nephritis, and

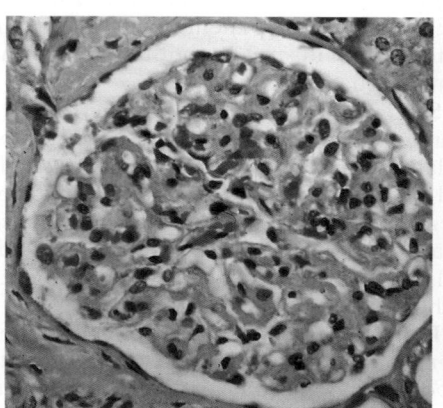
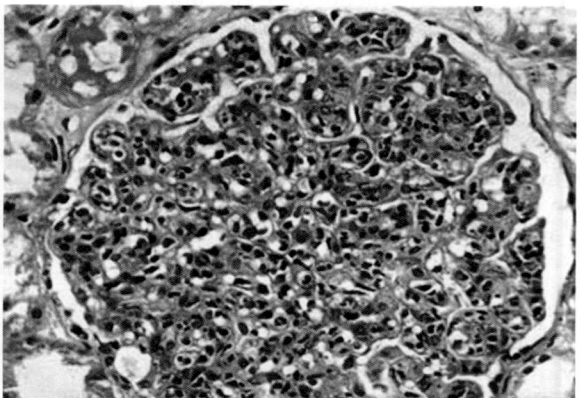

FIGURE 11-14.   Glomerulonephritis in systemic lupus erythematosus (SLE). A normal glomerulus is shown at left, highlighting the inflammatory hypercellularity of the glomerulus from a patient with lupus, shown at **right**.

renal or CNS disease, or with systolic hypertension, have a poorer prognosis.

There Are Several Variants of Lupus Erythematosus

Drug-Induced Lupus

As noted above, certain drugs may provoke a SLE-like syndrome. Patients typically have constitutional signs, polyarthritis, pleuritis, and ANAs. They may develop rheumatoid factor, false-positive tests for syphilis, and a positive direct antiglobulin (Coombs) test. Renal and CNS involvement rarely occur, and antibodies to double-stranded DNA and Sm antigen are distinctly uncommon. Autoantibodies to histones account for the positive ANA test result and are typical. As in idiopathic SLE, autoreactive CD4+ T cells have been implicated in polyclonal B-cell activation. The syndrome usually resolves when the offending drug is discontinued.

Chronic Discoid Lupus

Discoid lupus is a distinct clinical entity, with characteristic lesions limited to skin and no other pathology. Identical lesions may occur in some cases of SLE. Erythematous, depigmented, and telangiectatic plaques occur most commonly on the face and scalp. Lesional deposition of immunoglobulins and complement at the dermal–epidermal interface resembles that of SLE. However, unlike SLE, uninvolved skin contains no immune deposits. ANAs develop in about 1/3 of the patients, but antibodies against double-stranded DNA and Sm antigen are absent. Most patients with discoid lupus are not otherwise ill, but up to 10% eventually develop features of systemic disease.

Subacute Cutaneous Lupus

Subacute cutaneous lupus is characterized by papular and annular lesions, typically on the trunk. The disorder is aggravated by exposure to ultraviolet light, although lesions usually eventually resolve without scarring. Antibodies to SS-A (Ro antigen) (ribonucleoprotein complex) and an association with HLA-DR3 genotype are characteristic.

RHEUMATOID ARTHRITIS

RA is a systemic autoimmune disease, that may affect many organs, in addition to the joints. It has a particular predilection for the hands and wrists. Patients are usually (3:1) women, with a peak incidence in early middle age. They usually complain of symmetric stiffness and pain in the joints, and have associated swelling and warmth. Untreated, the disease destroys cartilage and bone, with loss of joint function and considerable disability.

MOLECULAR PATHOGENESIS: GENETIC FACTORS: The most important genetic loci that predispose to RA are a specific set of HLA-DR alleles (DR4, DR1, DR10, DR14). These alleles share a pentapeptide sequence motif (shared epitope) in a hypervariable segment of the HLA-DRB1 gene, which forms the peptide-binding pocket of the HLA molecule. It is likely that the binding properties of this pocket influence the type of peptides that can be bound by RA-associated HLA-DR molecules and so affect the immune response to these peptides. Interestingly, in seropositive RA (poor prognosis) there is often an arginine in the shared epitope, whereas in seronegative disease (good prognosis) lysine occupies the same position. This suggests that the physical characteristics of the rheumatoid pocket influence immune responses in RA. Several non-HLA loci have been linked to RA, including a region of chromosome 18q21 that encodes the receptor activator of NFκB, or RANK.

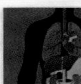

PATHOPHYSIOLOGY: HUMORAL IMMUNITY: Immunologic mechanisms are important in the pathogenesis of RA. Lymphocytes and plasma cells accumulate in the synovium, where they produce antibodies, mainly IgGs. In addition, immune complexes deposit in the articular cartilage and synovium.

Some 80% of patients with RA have elevated rheumatoid factor (RF) in their sera. RF is an autoantibody against the Fc fragment of IgG. Significant titers of RF also occur in patients with related collagen vascular diseases, such as systemic lupus, progressive systemic sclerosis, and dermatomyositis. RF is also present in many nonrheumatic disorders, including pulmonary fibrosis, cirrhosis, sarcoidosis, Waldenström macroglobulinemia, tuberculosis, kala-azar, lepromatous leprosy, and viral hepatitis. Even healthy elderly individuals, particularly women, occasionally test positive for RF.

Although patients with classic RA may be seronegative, the presence of RF in high titer often portends severe and unremitting disease, many systemic complications and a serious prognosis. The presence of IgG-type RF is sometimes associated with the development of systemic complications, such as necrotizing vasculitis.

Immune complexes (IgG RF + IgG) and complement components are found in the synovium, synovial fluid and extra-articular lesions of patients with RA. Furthermore, patients with seropositive RA have lower levels of complement in their synovial fluid than do those who are seronegative.

Anti-citrullinated protein antibodies (ACPA) are found in most RA patients and, unlike RF, may play a causative role in disease. Protein citrullination, a post-translational modification induced by tobacco smoke and other environmental agents, may such elicit ACPAs. In animal studies, these antibodies can induce or exacerbate disease.

CELLULAR IMMUNITY: It has also been postulated that cell-mediated immunity contributes to RA. Abundant T lymphocytes in rheumatoid synovium frequently express MHC class II, indicating activation, and most are CD4+. They are often in close contact with HLA-DR+ cells—either macrophages or dendritic Ia+ cells.

T cells may directly or indirectly interact with macrophages via production of cytokines that inhibit macrophage migration and proliferation. Such substances have been found in rheumatoid synovial fluid and in supernatants from rheumatoid tissue explants. These studies provide strong evidence that joint destruction in RA reflects local production of cytokines, especially TNF-α, IL-6, and IL-1.

INFECTIOUS AGENTS: Infectious bacteria and viruses are not present in joints of RA patients. Chronic oral infections with certain microorganisms, such as *Porphyromonas gingivalis*, can lead to periodontal disease and protein citrullination.

LOCAL FACTORS: Synovial cells cultured from rheumatic joints show decreased responsiveness to glucocorticoids and increased production of hyaluronate. They release a peptide (connective tissue-activating peptide) which may influence other cells' functions, increased production of prostaglandins, particularly PGE2.

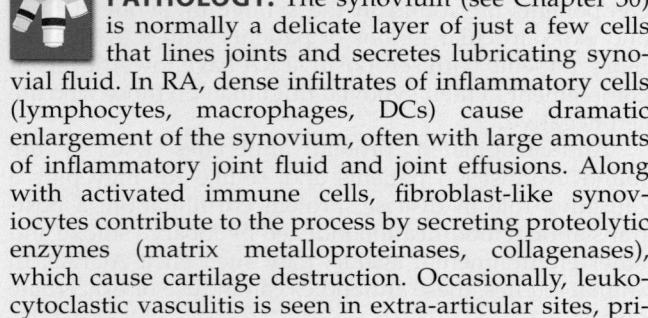 **CLINICAL FEATURES:** RA patients suffer from joint pain and stiffness. As the disease progresses, inflammation is accompanied by erosion of bone and cartilage, and progressive loss of motion and joint instability. Involvement of weight bearing joints like the hips and knees may cause difficulty walking and limit mobility. Patients note swelling and pain, together with stiffness, particularly upon arising.

RA inflammation outside the joints can cause:

- Subcutaneous nodules and occasionally nodules in the lungs
- Pericarditis and pleurisy
- Conjunctival and scleral inflammation—sometimes with diffuse eye inflammation
- Cutaneous vasculitis with troublesome ulcers
- Anemia and granulocytopenia
- Secondary Sjögren syndrome, with lymphocytic infiltration of salivary and lacrimal glands, leading to dry mouth and eyes (see primary Sjögren syndrome below) (Fig. 11-15).

PATHOLOGY: The synovium (see Chapter 30) is normally a delicate layer of just a few cells that lines joints and secretes lubricating synovial fluid. In RA, dense infiltrates of inflammatory cells (lymphocytes, macrophages, DCs) cause dramatic enlargement of the synovium, often with large amounts of inflammatory joint fluid and joint effusions. Along with activated immune cells, fibroblast-like synoviocytes contribute to the process by secreting proteolytic enzymes (matrix metalloproteinases, collagenases), which cause cartilage destruction. Occasionally, leukocytoclastic vasculitis is seen in extra-articular sites, primarily skin.

VASCULITIDES

Vasculitis is a term for a broad category of diseases characterized by inflammation of blood vessels of different types (see Chapter 16), causing disease because of impaired blood flow to tissues. This group of diseases is generally subdivided depending on the caliber of blood vessel involved and whether there is associated rheumatic disease. Thus, both SLE and RA can be associated with vasculitis, which

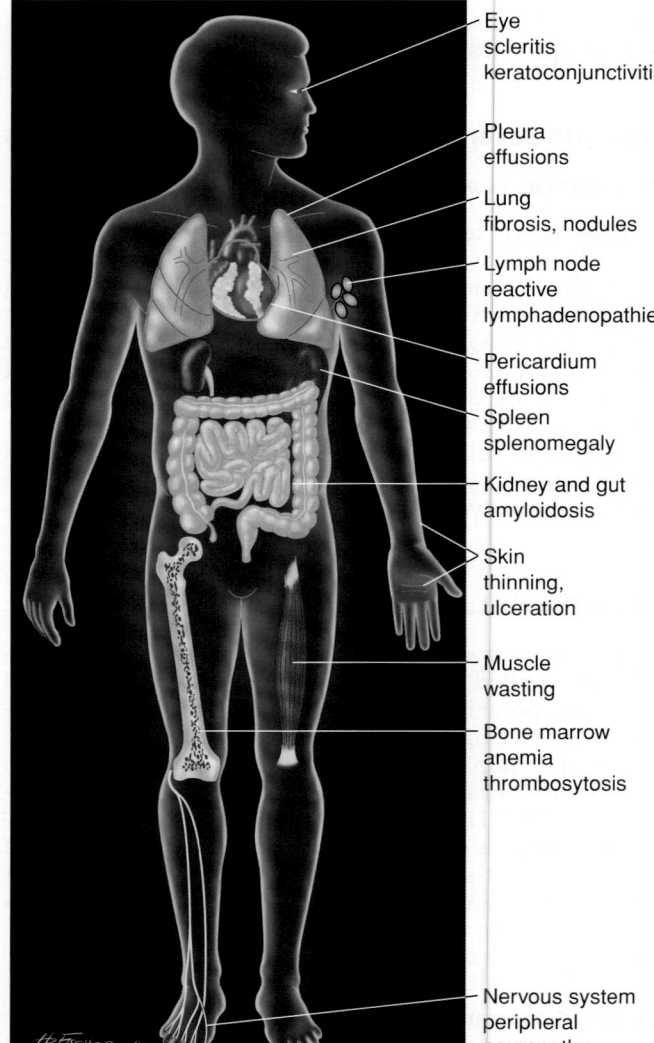

FIGURE 11-15. Organ involvement in rheumatoid arthritis.

is also seen in dermatomyositis (see below), especially in children. Vasculitis may accompany diverse infections, particularly viral infections, and result from taking certain drugs. Vasculitides not associated with systemic autoimmune diseases are discussed in Chapter 16, and those that accompany particular diseases are addressed with those specific diseases.

SJÖGREN SYNDROME

This disease is marked by lymphocytic infiltration of exocrine glands, primarily salivary and lacrimal glands, leading to dry mouth **(xerostomia)** and dry eyes **(xerophthalmia** or **keratoconjunctivitis sicca)**. It may be a single entity (primary Sjögren syndrome [SS]) or be part of other systemic autoimmune diseases such as SLE and RA. Primary SS may be associated with other organ involvement, affecting the thyroid, lungs, and kidneys (Fig. 11-16). The primary form of the disease most commonly begins in late middle age. Patients are overwhelmingly female.

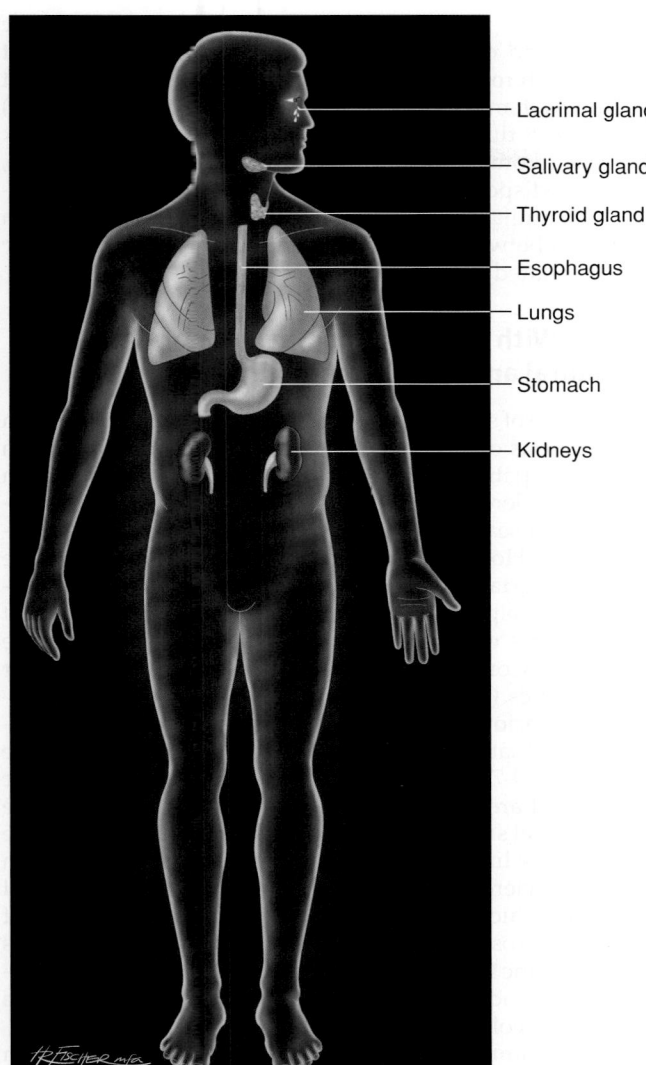

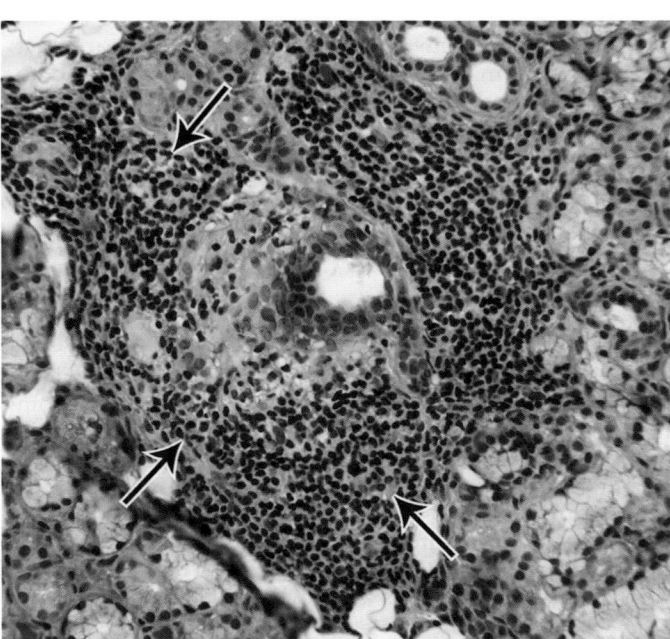

FIGURE 11-17. Histologic appearance of salivary glands in Sjögren syndrome. Note the infiltration of lymphocytes into the salivary gland tissue (*arrows*).

infiltrates destroy acini and ducts; the latter often become dilated and filled with cellular debris. Unlike lymphoma, which may supervene in SS, glandular stroma remains intact. The lymphocytic infiltrates are predominantly T cells, admixed with some B cells. Late in disease, affected glands atrophy and may be replaced by fibrosis. The salivary and lacrimal gland pathology is described in more detail in Chapter 29.

Involvement of extraglandular sites is also common in SS. Pulmonary disease occurs in many patients, particularly bronchial gland atrophy in association with lymphoid infiltration. Pulmonary SS is accompanied by thick tenacious secretions, focal atelectasis, bronchiectasis, and recurrent infections. The GI tract can be affected, and many patients have difficulty swallowing (dysphagia). Esophageal submucosal glands are infiltrated by lymphocytes. In addition, atrophic gastritis occurs secondary to lymphoid infiltration of the gastric mucosa. Liver disease, especially primary biliary cirrhosis, is present in 5% to 10% of patients with SS and is associated with nodular lymphoid infiltrates and destruction of intrahepatic bile ducts (see Chapter 20). Interstitial nephritis and chronic thyroiditis occasionally accompany SS. SS is associated with a 40-fold increased risk of lymphoma.

FIGURE 11-16. Organ involvement in Sjögren syndrome.

- Lacrimal glands
- Salivary glands
- Thyroid gland
- Esophagus
- Lungs
- Stomach
- Kidneys

PATHOPHYSIOLOGY: Lymphocytes infiltrate the salivary glandular tissue: mostly CD4$^+$ T cells, with a significant CD8$^+$ minority, plus B cells with occasional germinal centers. The genesis of this inflammation is unknown. It has been proposed that the primary abnormality is autoimmunity to salivary epithelial cells. Most patients with primary SS produce antibodies to the cytoplasmic RNA-associated proteins SS-A (Ro), and some of these also have antibodies to SS-B (La). ANAs are frequently present, as is rheumatoid factor.

Autoantibodies to DNA or histones are rare; their presence suggests secondary SS associated with lupus.

PATHOLOGY: Sjögren syndrome is characterized by intense lymphocytic infiltrates in salivary and lacrimal glands (see Chapter 29; Fig. 11-17). Lymphocytic infiltrates are initially periductal. Most lobules are affected, especially the centers. Well-defined germinal centers are rare. The lymphoid

CLINICAL FEATURES: Owing to insufficient and poor quality tears, patients with Sjögren syndrome complain of eye discomfort and can develop corneal and conjunctival ulcers and infections. Lack of saliva and its anti-bacterial proteins causes dry mouth, which may lead to increased dental caries and by thrush or other mouth infections, along with atrophy, inflammation, and cracking of the oral mucosa. Lymphocytic infiltration of other glands can lead to dry skin and dryness in the female reproductive tract. Respiratory tract involvement may impair mucus clearance and lead to interstitial lung disease. Hypergammaglobulinemia can lead to vasculitis, and some patients have renal dysfunction, or develop CNS involvement with transverse myelitis or cranial neuropathies.

SYSTEMIC SCLEROSIS (SCLERODERMA)

Systemic sclerosis is a systemic autoimmune disease of unknown etiology characterized by excessive deposition of collagen and other connective tissue macromolecules in the skin and multiple internal organs (Fig. 11-18), prominent and often severe alterations in the microvasculature and humoral and cellular immunologic abnormalities. It is a complex and heterogeneous disease with clinical forms ranging from limited skin involvement with minimal systemic alterations (**limited cutaneous systemic sclerosis,** previously called CREST syndrome; see below) to forms with diffuse skin sclerosis and severe and often progressive

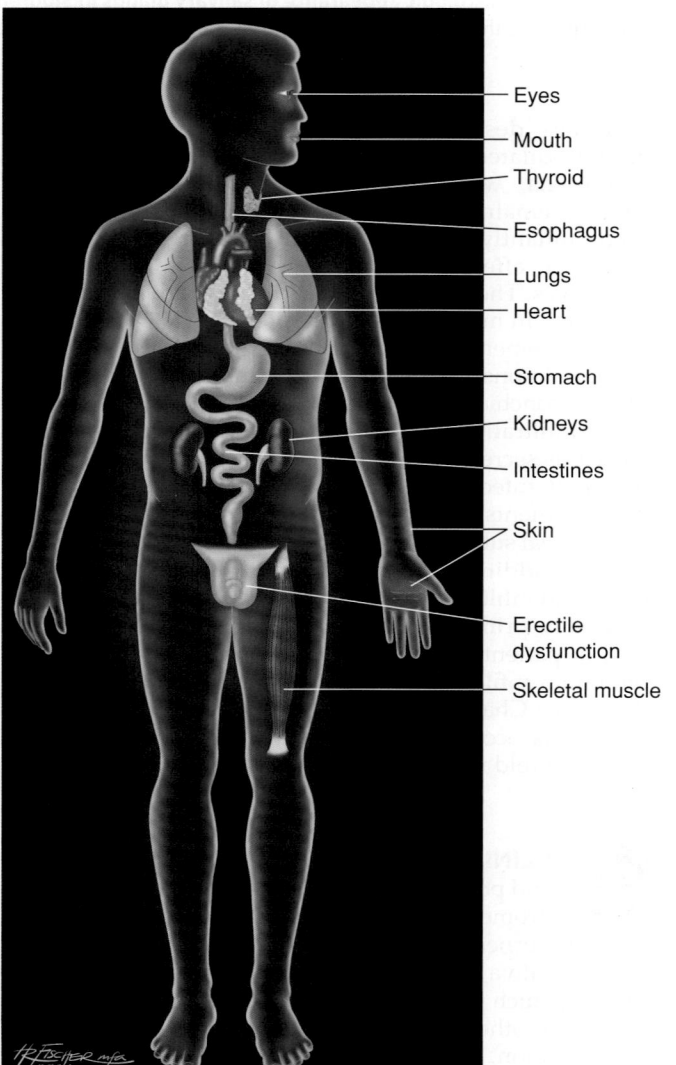

FIGURE 11-18. Organ involvement in systemic sclerosis.

internal organ involvement (**diffuse cutaneous systemic sclerosis**), and occasionally a fulminant course (**fulminant systemic sclerosis**). Systemic sclerosis is the third most common systemic autoimmune disease (after RA and SLE) and is 3 to 8 times more common in women, with a peak occurrence from 40 to 50 years. Although it is not inherited, genetic predisposition plays an important role in its development. Familial clusters have been reported, and there is an association between HLA-DQB1 and occurrence of systemic sclerosis-related autoantibodies.

Patients With Scleroderma Have Abnormalities in Humoral and Cellular Immunity

The presence of specific antibodies is one of the most common manifestations of systemic sclerosis, and they are present in over 90% of patients. Although autoantibodies are common in systemic sclerosis, they do not cause the clinical manifestations of the disease and their levels do not correlate with disease severity. However, because they occur commonly and are specific for certain clinical subsets of the disease, their presence is very helpful to establish the diagnosis and to predict likely patterns of organ involvement, severity, and disease progression. Commonly found antibodies include nucleolar autoantibodies (primarily against RNA polymerase I, fibrillarin, and various nucleolus-organizing proteins), antibodies to Scl-70 that target topoisomerase I, and anticentromere antibodies. Scl-70 antibodies are highly specific for systemic sclerosis and are present in 30% to 40% of patients with the diffuse clinical subset. Anticentromere antibodies occur more often with the limited cutaneous variant. A small proportion of systemic sclerosis patients harbor anti-RNA polymerase III antibodies, which are associated with increased incidence of systemic sclerosis–associated malignancies. Autoantibodies that are specific for certain tissues, for example, smooth muscle, thyroid, and salivary glands sometimes develop, as do antibodies to collagen types I and IV.

Cellular immune derangements are also present in patients with systemic sclerosis. Active disease often includes reduced circulating CD8+ T suppressor cells, evidence of T-cell activation, altered functions mediated by IL-1, and elevated IL-2 and soluble IL-2 receptor. Increased circulating IL-4 and IL-6 are also described. Systemic sclerosis-affected tissues have active mononuclear cell inflammation, which precedes development of the vasculopathy and fibrosis characteristic of this disease. The infiltrates contain increased CD4+ and γ/δ-T cells, and macrophages. Skin of scleroderma patients also contains degranulated mast cells. Incidence of other autoimmune disorders, such as autoimmune thyroiditis and primary biliary cirrhosis, is increased.

 PATHOPHYSIOLOGY: The pathogenesis of systemic sclerosis is extremely complex and not well understood. The clinical and pathologic manifestations of the disease result from three distinct processes: (1) fibroproliferative vascular lesions of small arteries and arterioles; (2) excessive and often progressive deposition of collagen and other fibrotic tissue extracellular matrix (ECM) macromolecules in skin and various internal organs; and (3) altered humoral and cellular immunity. Immunologic aberrations include innate immunity abnormalities, tissue infiltration with macrophages and T and B lymphocytes, production of numerous disease-specific autoantibodies and dysregulated cytokine, chemokine, and growth factor production. It is not clear which of these processes is of primary importance or how they are temporally related as the disease develops and progresses. However, because vascular alterations in affected tissues are universal and often cause clinical manifestations, the vasculopathy may be the primary event in the disease.

Unknown etiologic factors trigger a pathogenetic sequence in a genetically receptive host. These entail microvascular injury, characterized by structural and functional endothelial cell abnormalities. Endothelial cell abnormalities lead to either:

1. Increased production and release of many potent mediators including cytokines, chemokines, polypeptide growth factors and such other substances such as prostaglandins, reactive oxygen species (ROS), and thrombogenic and procoagulant activities, or
2. Reduced important compounds such as prostacyclin and nitric oxide.

Endothelial cell dysfunction allows chemokine- and cytokine-attracted inflammatory cells and fibroblast precursors to enter from the bloodstream and bone marrow. These cells transmigrate into the surrounding tissues to establish a chronic inflammatory process in which macrophages and T and B lymphocytes participate.

The tissue infiltrating inflammatory cells secrete additional cytokines and growth factors which activate resident fibroblasts, epithelial cells, endothelial cells, and pericytes. These cells then undergo phenotypic conversion into activated myofibroblasts (Fig. 11-19). This sequence of events causes severe, often progressive fibroproliferative vasculopathy, vessel rarefaction and exaggerated, widespread accumulation of fibrous tissue, the hallmark sclerosis that characterizes this disease.

Vascular Dysfunction Is One of the Earliest Manifestations of Systemic Sclerosis

Vascular alterations in systemic sclerosis are often heralded by Raynaud phenomenon. This episodic circulatory compromise mainly affects distal parts of the body, including the extremities, particularly the hands and toes, the tip of the nose, and the ear lobes. Raynaud phenomenon is often triggered by exposure to cold or tobacco smoke, and is accompanied by capillary microvascular alterations (observed by nailfold capillaroscopy) that often precede clinical evidence of tissue fibrosis. The initial events responsible for the vascular and endothelial cell injury and subsequent activation are not known. Many putative etiologies have been suggested, including vasculotropic viral pathogens, antiendothelial cell antibodies, cellular products from inflammatory cells or ROS generated during episodes of ischemia/reperfusion.

Endothelial cell activation induces expression of chemokines and cell adhesion molecules, causes trans-endothelial cellular migration, and leads to perivascular accumulation of immunologic/inflammatory cells. The latter include T and B lymphocytes and various macrophage populations. These inflammatory cells produce and secrete diverse cytokines and/or growth factors, including TGFβ and other profibrotic mediators such as endothelin-1, which stimulate smooth muscle cell proliferation and marked accumulation of subendothelial

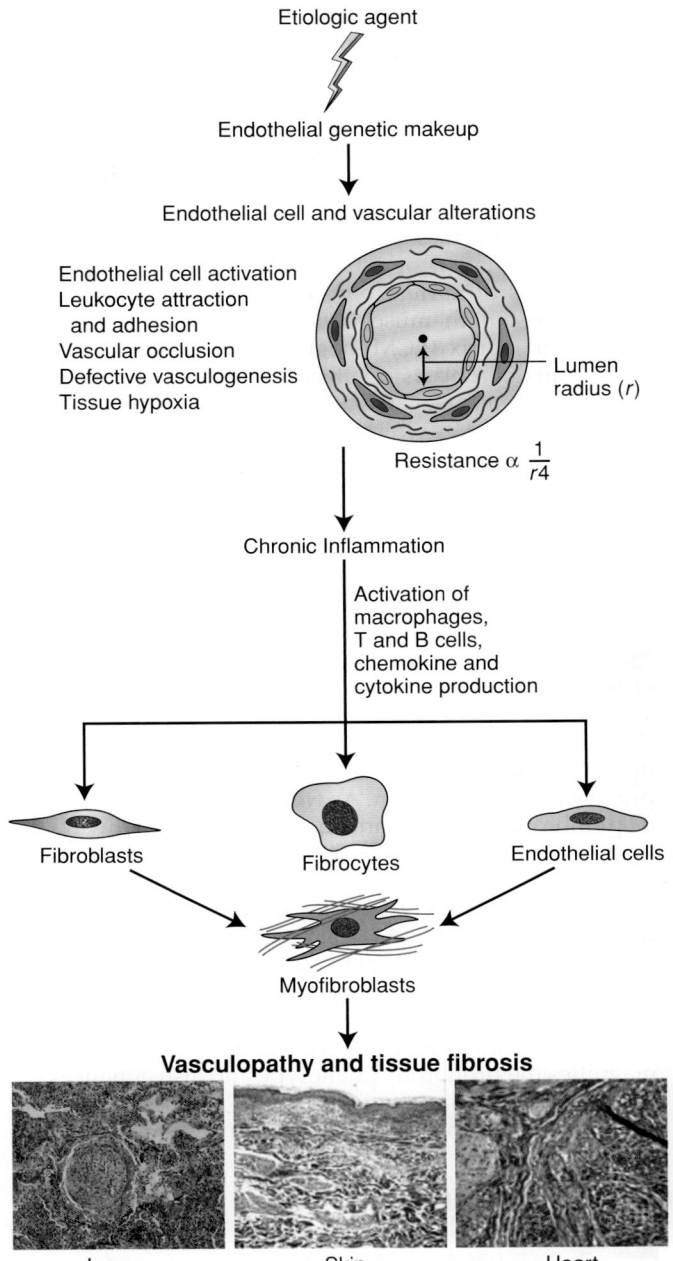

Resistance $\alpha \frac{1}{r4}$

FIGURE 11-19. Involvement of endothelial cells and vascular alterations in the pathogenesis of systemic sclerosis.

fibrotic tissue. They also trigger platelet aggregation, causing intravascular thrombosis and eventually microvascular occlusion. The effects of vascular dysfunction in patients with systemic sclerosis are most dramatic when they involve the renal and pulmonary arterioles, causing renal crisis and pulmonary arterial hypertension, respectively.

Myofibroblasts Are the Effector Cells in Systemic Sclerosis Tissue Fibrosis

The fibrotic process is the most notable characteristic of systemic sclerosis and causes most of its clinical manifestations (Fig. 11-18). It results from myofibroblast accumulation in skin and other affected tissues. These cells are ultimately responsible for the fibrosis, and originate from several sources: proliferation and activation of tissue fibroblasts or perivascular and vascular adventitial fibroblasts; chemokine-driven recruitment of fibroblast precursor cells from the bone marrow; transdifferentiation of epithelial cells to myofibroblasts (epithelial–mesenchymal transition [EMT; see Chapter 5]); and transition of endothelial cells to a mesenchymal phenotype (**endothelial–mesenchymal transition** or **EndMT**). The increased population of activated myofibroblasts produces large amounts of fibrillar type I and type III collagens and expresses α-smooth muscle actin. They also produce less extracellular matrix (ECM)-degradative enzymes. Accumulation of myofibroblasts in affected tissues and their uncontrolled, persistently elevated biosynthetic functions determine the extent and rate by which the fibrotic process progresses in systemic sclerosis, and presage the disease's clinical course, response to therapy, prognosis and mortality.

Role of TGFβ

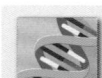 **MOLECULAR PATHOGENESIS:** TGFβ plays a crucial role in the fibrosis that accompanies systemic sclerosis. It strongly stimulates production of fibrotic tissue macromolecules resulting in severe tissue fibrosis. TGFβ also inhibits production of collagen-degrading metalloproteinases while simultaneously upregulating production of protease inhibitors, which prevent ECM breakdown. As well, it increases expression of profibrotic proteins, and uses autocrine pathways to upregulate its own expression. TGFβ binding to target cell surface receptors is the most important trigger for molecular pathways activating genes encoding fibrillar collagens and other ECM macromolecules (Fig. 11-20).

Connective tissue growth factor (CTGF) also plays a key role in systemic sclerosis–associated tissue fibrosis. TGFβ strongly stimulates CTGF synthesis in fibroblasts, vascular smooth muscle cells, and endothelial cells. CTGF magnifies the profibrotic phenotype and also enhances its own production via an autocrine loop. It thus maintains a continuous, prolonged cycle of excessive fibrosis.

Diffuse Systemic Sclerosis

PATHOLOGY: Sclerodermatous skin at first is edematous, then indurated. The thickened skin shows strikingly increased collagen fibers in the reticular dermis; epidermal thinning with loss of rete pegs; atrophy of dermal appendages (Fig. 11-21A); hyalinization and obliteration of arterioles; marked atrophy of subdermal adipose tissue; and variable mononuclear cell infiltrates, primarily of T cells and macrophages. The stage of induration may progress to atrophy or it may remain stable. Increased deposition of collagens and other fibrotic tissue ECM macromolecules can also occur in synovia, lungs, gut, heart, and kidneys.

ARTERIES: Lesions in arteries, arterioles, and capillaries are typical, and in some cases may be the first demonstrable pathology. Initial subintimal edema with fibrin deposition is followed by thickening and fibrosis of the vessel wall and reduplication or fraying of the internal elastic lamina. Involved vessels may become

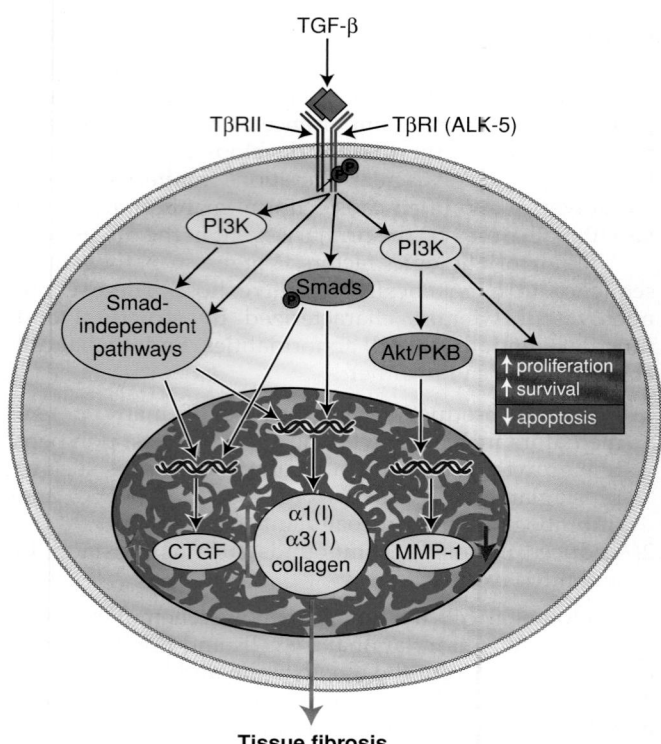

Tissue fibrosis

FIGURE 11-20. Involvement of transforming growth factor-β (TGF-β) in systemic sclerosis. Fibrogenic pathways are stimulated by TGF-β, and production of enzymes that degrade collagen is inhibited by TGF-β. Signaling pathways that are both independent of and that involve Smads mediate these effects. *PI3K* = phosphoinositol-3-kinase; *CTGF* = connective tissue growth factor; *MMP-1* = matrix metalloproteinase-1.

severely narrowed by fibrotic tissue or occluded by thrombi.

KIDNEYS: The kidneys are involved in more than half of patients, with severe vascular alterations, often with focal hemorrhages and cortical infarcts (see Chapter 22). The interlobular arteries and afferent arterioles tend to be most severely affected. Early subintimal fibromuscular thickening narrows vascular lumens, and is followed by fibrosis (Fig. 11-21B). Fibrinoid necrosis commonly occurs in afferent arterioles. Glomerular alterations are nonspecific, with focal changes ranging from necrosis extending from the afferent arterioles, to fibrosis. Early in disease, immunoglobulin, complement, and fibrin are diffusely deposited in affected vessels, probably caused by increased vascular permeability.

LUNGS: In the lung, vascular reactivity is increased ("pulmonary Raynaud phenomenon") with either pulmonary arterial hypertension or diffuse interstitial fibrosis. Pulmonary disease can progress to end-stage fibrosis (honeycomb lung; see Chapter 18).

HEART: Most patients with systemic sclerosis have patchy myocardial fibrosis. Over 10% of the myocardium is involved in about a quarter of patients. Cardiac fibrosis is among the most serious fibrotic complications, after pulmonary fibrosis.

GI TRACT: Systemic sclerosis can also involve any portion of the gastrointestinal tract. Esophageal dysfunction is most common and troublesome GI complication.

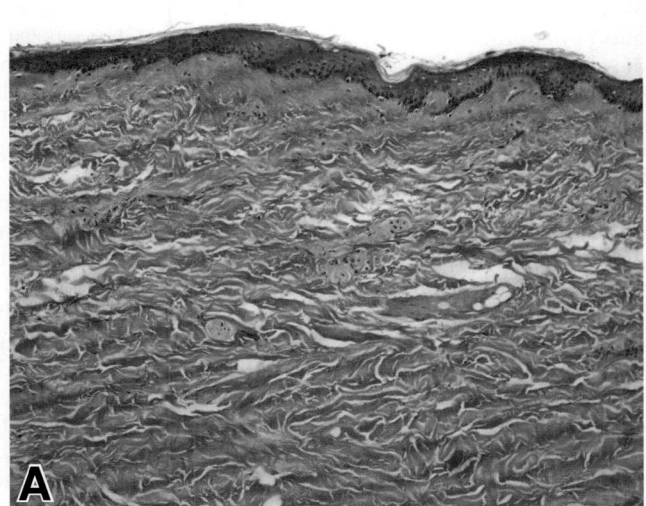
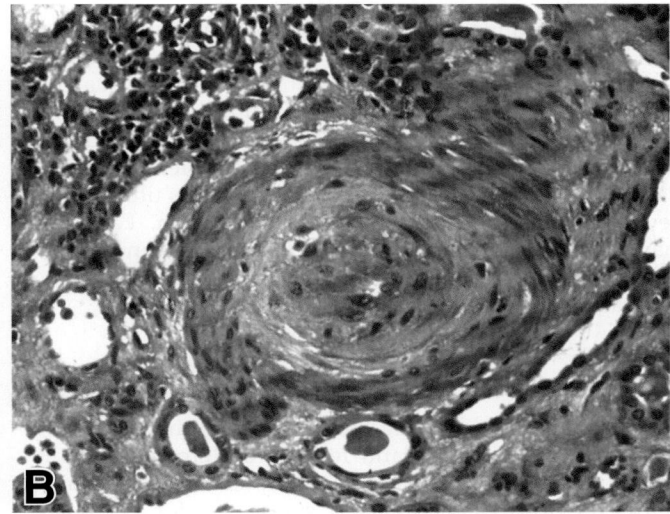

FIGURE 11-21. Histologic appearance of systemic sclerosis. A. Dermal fibrosis is characteristic of scleroderma. Dense collagen accumulation occurs beneath the epidermis. Note the absence of dermal appendages and the atrophy of subdermal adipose tissue. **B.** Scleroderma that affects the kidney is manifested by vascular involvement. Here, the interlobular artery exhibits marked luminal narrowing due to pronounced intimal thickening.

Atrophy and fibrous replacement of smooth muscle occur in the lower esophagus. The small bowel often has patchy fibrosis in the muscular layers. The colon is also frequently affected, with dilatation and characteristic "wide mouth" diverticulosis. Involvement of the anal sphincter may make it incompetent and cause rectal/anal incontinence.

CLINICAL FEATURES: The most apparent and almost universal clinical features of systemic sclerosis reflect progressive thickening and fibrosis of the skin. Scleroderma presents as two distinct clinical syndromes, a generalized or diffuse **(diffuse systemic)** form and a **limited variant** previously known as the CREST syndrome. Diffuse systemic sclerosis (diffuse scleroderma) includes severe, progressive skin disease and early onset of all or most of the associated abnormalities of visceral organs. Symptoms usually begin with Raynaud phenomenon (see above), with intermittent episodes of ischemia of the fingers, marked by triphasic color changes, paresthesias, and pain. This is accompanied, or followed, by edema of the fingers and hands, thickening and tightening of the skin, polyarthralgia, and involvement of specific internal organs. Affected skin is tight, indurated, and firmly bound to the subcutaneous tissue. The skin over the hands and face is most often involved. As the disease progresses, sclerotic changes extend and may affect the entire body.

The typical patient with generalized scleroderma has "stone facies," from tightening of facial skin, loss of facial wrinkles and restricted motion of the mouth. Progression of vascular lesions in the fingers may cause ischemic ulceration of the fingertips, with subsequent shortening and atrophy of the digits. Many patients suffer from painful tendonitis and joint pain.

OTHER ORGAN INVOLVEMENT. Musculoskeletal symptoms occur early in the disease. Severity may vary from mild to more severe polyarthralgias, but synovitis and frank arthritis are rare. As the disease advances, periarticular tissues become thickened and fibrotic, causing severe joint flexion contractures and distal phalangeal resorption—**acroosteolysis**. Muscle involvement may occasionally occur as a muscle inflammatory myopathy but frequently infiltration with fibrotic tissue results in a more indolent noninflammatory myopathy.

The gastrointestinal tract is the internal organ system most commonly involved. Esophageal involvement is almost universal, with symptoms of gastroesophageal reflux, heartburn, and dysphagia due to dysfunctional esophageal sphincter motility. In severe cases, stricture may result. Impaired gastric emptying and small intestine peristalsis may cause abdominal distention, bloating, nausea, and abdominal pain. Bacterial overgrowth may lead to secondary malabsorption and diarrhea.

Pulmonary involvement frequently causes severe respiratory disability, and may evolve as pulmonary arterial hypertension or as interstitial pulmonary fibrosis. The former is more closely associated with limited systemic sclerosis, while pulmonary fibrosis occurs more often and is more severe in diffuse systemic sclerosis. Patients develop progressively worsening tachypnea and exertional dyspnea, secondary to pulmonary fibrosis and/or pulmonary hypertension. Lung disease is the most common cause of death in systemic sclerosis.

Cardiac involvement is not uncommon and may manifest as chest pain, arrhythmias, and conduction defects. Infiltrative cardiomyopathy may cause left ventricular or biventricular failure. Cor pulmonale can develop in patients with pulmonary hypertension.

"Scleroderma renal crisis," as the renal disease may be known, typically begins abruptly, with malignant hypertension and rapidly progressive renal insufficiency. It is often heralded by severe headache, hypertensive retinopathy, seizures and other CNS symptoms, and/or myocardial ischemia, infarction or left ventricular failure. Prompt aggressive treatment can usually reverse this process, which otherwise is often fatal or may cause renal failure.

Functional thyroid abnormalities include elevated levels of antithyroid autoantibodies. Clinical and subclinical hypothyroidism are common. Impotence caused by erectile failure may be an early feature of systemic sclerosis, and many male systemic sclerosis patients ultimately develop some degree of erectile dysfunction. Patients may develop the **sicca syndrome** (**keratoconjunctivitis sicca** and **xerostomia**) caused by fibrosis and lymphocytic infiltration of salivary and lacrimal glands.

Limited Systemic Sclerosis

Cutaneous involvement may be confined to the digits and the dorsum of the hands and feet (**acrosclerosis**), and the sclerotic process may progress relatively slowly. This form of disease, previously called CREST syndrome (for calcinosis, Raynaud phenomenon, esophageal dysmotility, sclerodactyly and telangiectases) is now known as **limited systemic sclerosis** to differentiate this clinical presentation from its more severe cousin, diffuse systemic sclerosis. Other cutaneous manifestations include multiple telangiectasia, skin ulcers, usually localized to fingertips or knuckles and peculiar pigmentary changes with hyper- and hypopigmentation. Calcinosis is most commonly found in the fingertips and periarticular tissues.

MIXED CONNECTIVE TISSUE DISEASE

As suggested by the name, patients with mixed connective tissue disease (MCTD) combine features of several different autoimmune diseases including SLE, scleroderma, and polymyositis. The exact incidence of MCTD is unclear. From 80% to 90% of patients are female, and most are adults (mean age,

37 years). Findings reminiscent of SLE include rash, Raynaud phenomenon, arthralgias, and arthritis. Characteristics of scleroderma include swollen hands, esophageal hypomotility, and pulmonary interstitial disease. Some patients also develop symptoms suggestive of RA. Patients with MCTD reportedly respond well to corticosteroid therapy, although some studies have challenged this assertion.

The pathogenesis of MCTD is poorly understood. Patients often have evidence of B-cell activation with hypergammaglobulinemia and rheumatoid factor. ANAs are present but, unlike SLE, do not usually bind double-stranded DNA. The most distinctive ANA is directed against an extractable nuclear antigen. Specifically, patients with MCTD have high titers of antibody to uridine-rich ribonucleoprotein (anti-U1-RNP) in the absence of antibody to other extractable nuclear antigens, such as PM-1 and Jo-1. Most diagnostic criteria for MCTD include high-titer anti-U1-RNP ANA as a *sine qua non*. Anti-RNP antibodies may occur in SLE, but at much lower titers than in MCTD.

The cause of high titers of anti-U1-RNP antibody is unclear. However, there is an association with HLA-DR4 and HLA-DR2 genotypes, suggesting a role for T cells in autoantibody production. There is no direct evidence that these antibodies participate in the development of any of the characteristic lesions of MCTD.

There is controversy as to whether MCTD is a separate disease or a heterogeneous collection of patients with nonclassical presentations of SLE, scleroderma, or polymyositis. For example, in some patients, MCTD seems to evolve into typical scleroderma; other patients develop renal disease like that seen in SLE; still others develop features of RA. Thus, MCTD may be an intermediate stage in the progression to another recognized autoimmune disease. Patients whose disease remains undifferentiated may be a distinct subset. Thus, it is unclear whether MCTD represents a distinct entity or overlapping manifestations of other types of collagen vascular disease.

Sepsis

Daniel Remick

DEFINITIONS

In 2016, a consortium of physicians and investigators redefined sepsis as life-threatening organ dysfunction caused by a dysregulated host response to infection. A lay person's definition of sepsis was also provided: Sepsis is a life-threatening condition resulting from the body's response to an infection that damages its own organs and tissues. An important element is that there must be an infection, not just the presence of bacteria (see Box 12-1 for additional definitions). This new definition, called Sepsis-3, requires that three elements must be present in order to consider a patient septic. The first is the presence of an infection, the second is life-threatening organ injury, and the third is a dysregulated host response to the infection. Let us consider these elements separately.

First, there must be an infection, not just inflammation but invasion of the host by pathogens. It is not necessary to document the presence of pathogenic organisms, such as bacteria, to determine the presence of infection. In the correct clinical setting, other signs of infection would be considered sufficient, such as the presence of neutrophils in the sputum of a patient with pneumonia.

The second element is life-threatening organ dysfunction. There must be sufficient injury to the tissues or organs that the patient is at risk of dying. For example, coughing would not be considered a life-threatening organ injury in a patient with pneumonia, while being placed on a ventilator and requiring oxygen indicates that lung function is sufficiently compromised to be considered life threatening.

The third element is a dysregulated host response to the infection. Most infections elicit appropriate, regulated, host responses that eradicate the pathogen without causing organ injury. For example, about 30% of normal individuals will have detectable pathogenic bacteria in their bloodstream after brushing their teeth but they do not become septic, since the innate immune system quickly and efficiently eliminates these bacteria. Controlled inflammation is beneficial to the host.

The Sepsis-3 definition evolved from the concept that sepsis elicits the systemic inflammatory response syndrome (SIRS). SIRS criteria were developed so that septic patients could be quickly identified and treated. In order to make a diagnosis of SIRS, two of the four criteria need to be present (Box 12-2). These criteria can be quickly determined without sophisticated equipment, except for the white blood count. A major drawback to using SIRS to identify a septic patient is relative lack of specificity. Normal individuals who just finished exercising would manifest two of the criteria (tachycardia and tachypnea) but would not be considered septic.

BOX 12-1 BASIC DEFINITIONS FOR THE UNDERSTANDING OF SEPSIS

Bacteremia—bacteria in the bloodstream
Colonization—presence of bacteria without an inflammatory response, such as the bacteria in your mouth or colon
Infection—invasion of the host by disease-causing organisms such as bacteria, viruses, fungi, or parasites

---

BOX 12-2 CRITERIA FOR THE SYSTEMIC INFLAMMATORY RESPONSE SYNDROME (SIRS)

1. Temperature >38° or <36°C
2. Heart rate >90 beats/min
3. Respiratory rate >20 or $PaCO_2$ <32 mm Hg
4. White blood count >12,000 or <4,000/mm³, or >10% bands

Septic shock represents a subset of septic patients with circulatory and cellular abnormalities that are sufficiently severe to increase mortality substantially. These patients are identified by having persistent hypotension even when receiving appropriate therapy to increase their blood pressure. Sepsis may be considered as a continuum of disease, with septic shock representing the most severe form. The category of severe sepsis is no longer included in the newer sepsis definition.

Sepsis Has a Staggering Impact on Human Health

There are an estimated 31.5 million cases of sepsis worldwide yearly, causing 5.3 million deaths. Traditionally, sepsis mortality has been calculated as the survival rate after 28 days, in contrast to cancer mortality, which is typically determined on the basis of 5- or 10-year survival rates. In 2018, the expected mortality with optimal care was about 30%, although patients continued to die beyond the first month. Even among sepsis survivors, there is substantial morbidity, and many patients are not able to live independently 1 year after their initial sepsis diagnosis. Due to the high initial mortality, many scoring systems have evolved to determine prognosis.

EVOLUTION OF SEPSIS

No single pathophysiologic mechanism drives the septic response. The heterogeneity in the individual patients is an important element of sepsis and probably accounts for the failure of therapeutic interventions to be efficacious. Since multiple pathways may lead to the organ injury, individual patients will have individual immune aspects altered. These pathways change over time, so that appropriate therapy on one day may be inappropriate the following day. This resembles glucose control in a diabetic patient, which needs to be managed on a frequent basis and not just once a week.

Immune Cells Are Key to the Septic Response

Neutrophils

Virtually any cell may be involved during the host response to an infection but particular cells play an important role. Neutrophils, or polymorphonuclear leukocytes (PMNs; see Chapter 2), are phagocytic cells which engulf and eliminate bacteria and fungi. They are among the first cells recruited to the site of inflammation in response to host-produced chemotactic factors such as leukotriene B4, or such CXC chemokines as IL-8. As shown in Box 12-1, an increase in the number of circulating neutrophils is one component of the SIRS. Neutrophils are quickly released from the bone marrow in response to an infectious challenge to assist in the eradication of the pathogen. During the initial phase of this rapid release, immature neutrophil forms may be found in the circulation. Neutrophils are critical in the eradication of pathogens, which occurs via several mechanisms. Phagocytes, such as PMNs or macrophages, phagocytose, or engulf the pathogens into phagosomes (see Chapter 2), in which a portion of the cell membrane surrounds the pathogen. Within neutrophils' cytoplasm, lysosomes contain proteases such as lysozyme, and enzymes such as catalase that produce toxic reactive oxygen species (ROS) and nitric oxide synthase (NOS) to generate reactive nitrogen species (RNS). Phagosomes and lysosomes

fuse to create phagolysosomes, in which proteases, toxic ROS and RNS attack the ingested pathogen. Neutrophils may also form neutrophil extracellular traps (NETs, see Chapters 1 and 5) to help contain and kill the bacteria. NETs are strands of chromatin released from dying neutrophils which contain the DNA and proteases. Bacteria and other pathogens adhere to the strands of chromatin, such that the bacteria are in close contact with proteolytic enzymes such as elastase. While all of these mechanisms can protect the host from pathogens, in a septic patient, these normal eradication mechanisms may result in host damage.

It has been postulated that increased numbers of neutrophils may be responsible for the organ injury that lies at the heart of the sepsis-3 definitions. Specifically, these activated inflammatory cells may release proteases, ROS and RNS, which damage nearby normal tissues. Septic patients have delayed neutrophil apoptosis, which, when coupled with the release of neutrophils from the bone marrow, may result in increasing circulating numbers of the cells. In clinical studies, patients were given granulocyte colony stimulating factor (G-CSF, see Chapter 26) to increase production of neutrophils in septic patients. While numbers of circulating neutrophils increased, survival did not improve. Similar to so many other aspects of sepsis, the appropriate response at the appropriate time should provide the best outcome.

Lymphocytes

Lymphocytes assist phagocytic cells, such as neutrophils, to improve their function. Thus, B cells secrete antibodies which opsonize bacteria so that they are more effectively phagocytized by neutrophils. Natural killer (NK, see Chapter 4) cells secrete interferon gamma (IFNγ), which augments macrophage function including killing ingested bacteria. In septic patients, lymphocytes undergo extensive apoptosis. Those which are not apoptotic are often anergic, and fail to provide sufficient support to the immune system. These anergic lymphocytes have been called "zombie cells," not quite dead but unable to complete such normal functions as producing cytokines and antibodies. Checkpoint inhibitor therapies, currently successful for several different cancers, are in early clinical trials for treating septic patients. The concept is that a checkpoint inhibitor may reverse lymphocytes' anergy and restore their normal function.

Macrophages and Monocytes

Blood monocytes become macrophages once they exit the blood and move into tissues. There are fixed tissue macrophages such as Kupffer cells within the liver. Macrophages respond to septic insults by secreting proinflammatory mediators. Like neutrophils, macrophages are also important in phagocytosing and eradicating pathogens. Macrophage subsets exist, and classical or M1 macrophages secrete proinflammatory cytokines such as TNFα and IL-1β. Alternatively activated macrophages, also called M2 macrophages, are important in terminating inflammatory responses by secreting specific inhibitors.

Structural Elements Regulate the Host Response

Pathogen-Associated Molecular Patterns

These molecules are a specific feature of groups of pathogens. This is a structure of the pathogen typically recognized

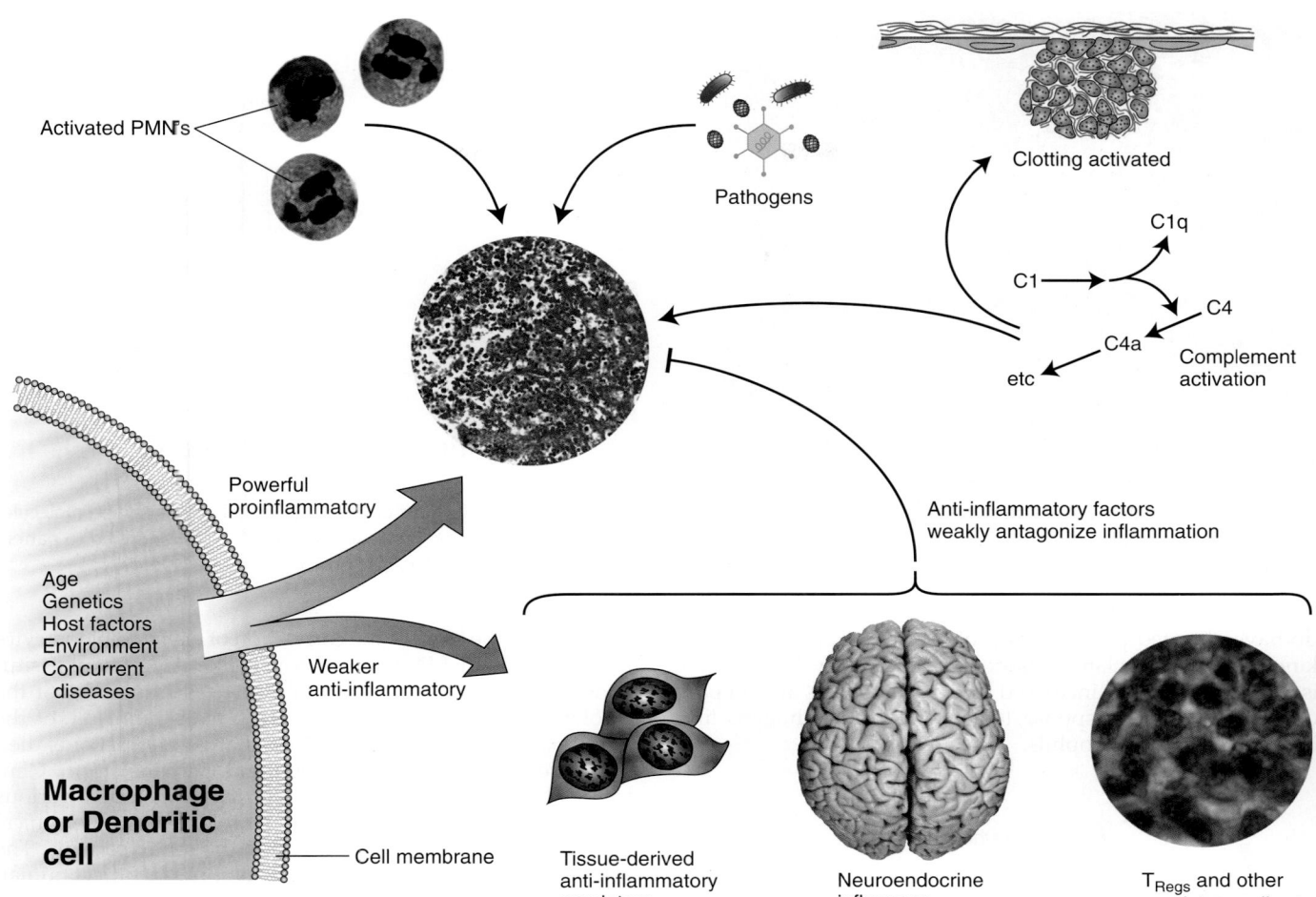

FIGURE 12-1. The elements of host responses favoring inflammatory activity during sepsis. Dendritic cell and macrophage responses are determined, both quantitatively and qualitatively, by a combination of genetics, environment, age, other concurrent illnesses, and other factors. When stimulated by an appropriate microbial trigger, whether bacterial, fungal, or viral, pro- and anti-inflammatory substances are secreted by these dendritic cells. Here, the former (**upper**) predominate and are involved in a series of reactions. These include activation of neutrophils, blood-clotting elements and complement, all of which lead to tissue necrosis. This, in turn, magnifies the proinflammatory response. Anti-inflammatory elements (**lower**) include tissue-derived anti-inflammatory regulators, neuroendocrine influences, and regulatory cells of different lineages, including T-regulatory cells (Tregs) and others.

by cells of the innate immune system. Many pathogen-associated molecular patterns (PAMPs) exist, one of the most studied being lipopolysaccharide (LPS) found in the cell wall of gram-negative bacteria. Other PAMPs include double-stranded RNA and lipoteichoic acid from gram-positive bacteria. Host elements that trigger inflammatory responses are shown in Figure 12-1.

Danger-Associated Molecular Patterns

Like PAMPs, there are molecules from the host that also stimulate innate immune cells. Similar inflammatory events may be initiated by either danger-associated molecular patterns (DAMPs) or PAMPs. Examples of DAMPs include ATP, uric acid, and heat shock proteins (Fig. 12-2).

Pattern Recognition Receptors

Either DAMPs or PAMPs bind to pattern recognition receptors (PRRs), and stimulate the innate immune system. PRRs

are found in different portions of the cell: at the cell membrane, in the cytoplasm, or within endosomes. Among the best studied PRRs are the toll-like receptors (TLRs), particularly TLR4, which is on the cell surface where it binds to LPS. Once TLR4 binds LPS, the cell triggers a sequence of events, culminating in acute inflammation (Fig. 12-3).

"Cytokine Storm" Provides a Key Lesson in Understanding Disease Pathogenesis

The concept of "Cytokine storm" postulated that there was massive and rapid production of cytokines in response to an infectious stimulus. This idea was based on experimental models in which LPS was injected into animals in an attempt to reproduce the septic phenotype. Extremely high levels of cytokines were measured within a few hours, and usually led to 100% mortality within 3 days. Unfortunately, this sequence does not reflect what happens in most septic patients; as well, under 5% of septic patients die within the first 3 days, and about 30% die over 28 days (see above). Human septic patients

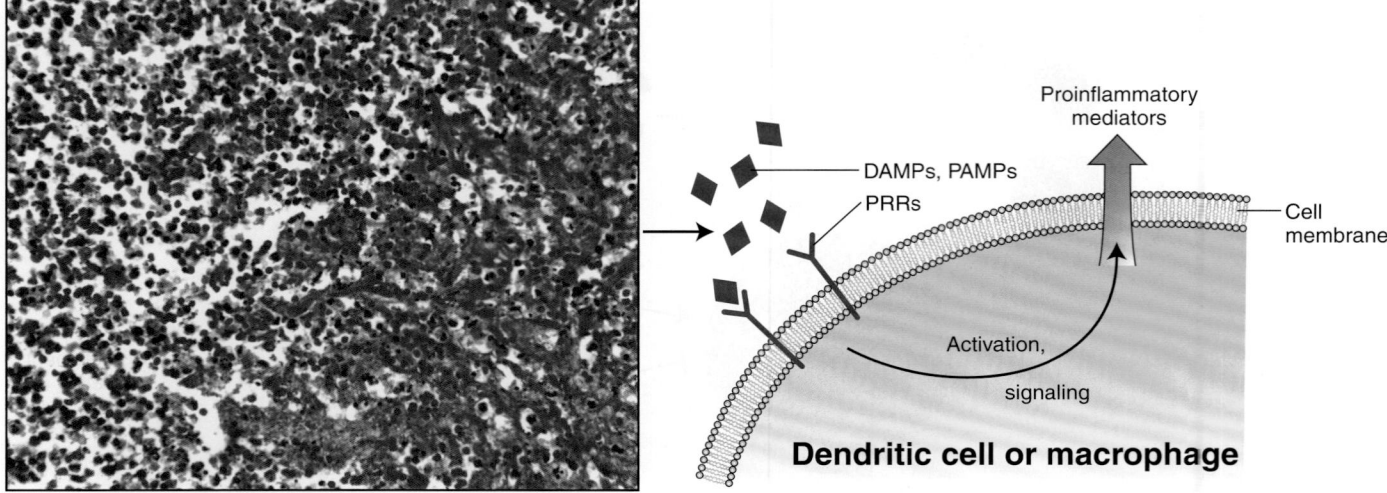

FIGURE 12-2. Tissue necrosis stimulates inflammation. Necrotic tissues, whether due to infections or other causes, release patterned molecules called damage-associated molecular patterns, or alarmins. These are similar to pathogen-associated molecular patterns (PAMPs) and bind to pattern recognition receptors (PRRs), in turn activating dendritic cells or macrophages to release proinflammatory cytokines.

do have elevated plasma levels of cytokines, and high cytokine levels do correlate with increased mortality. However, it is not clear that these increased levels of cytokines are not part of a host-protective response, to help eradicate pathogens, like increased blood neutrophils.

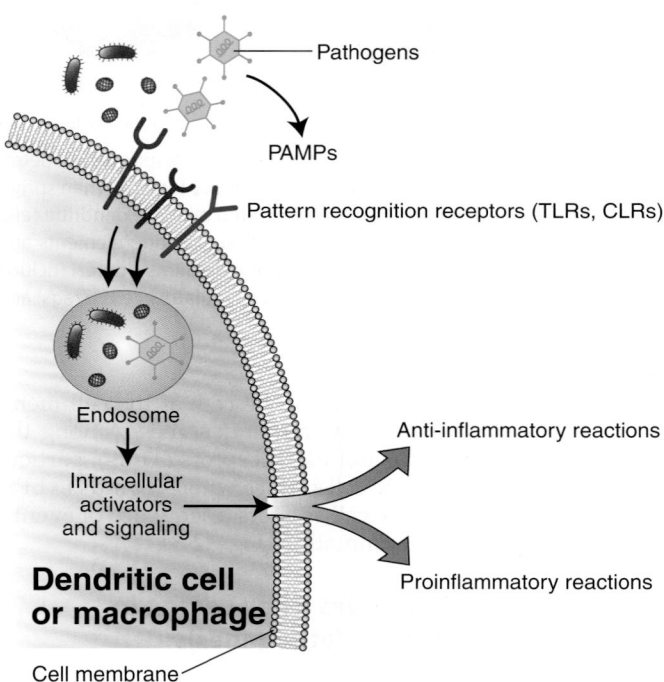

FIGURE 12-3. Mechanisms triggering soluble mediators in sepsis. Molecules containing pathogen-associated molecular patterns (PAMPs) are recognized by pattern recognition receptors (PRRs, mainly toll-like receptors [TLRs] and C-type lectin receptors [CLRs]) on cells of the innate immune system. Among other things, these interactions lead to phagocytosis of the pathogens, which is in turn followed by activation of intracellular response systems. As a consequence, dendritic cells and macrophages secrete a plethora of both proinflammatory and anti-inflammatory substances.

Thus, on the basis of the correlation of elevated blood cytokine levels with LPS-induced sepsis-like experimental situations and rapid, assured mortality, it was assumed that the cytokine levels were the cause, rather than the result, of the septic response and the mortality—that is, that patients died from overwhelming inflammation and cytokine storm. Clinical trials using cytokine inhibitors, have included various approaches to blocking TNFα and IL-1. None of these clinical trials demonstrated better survival in the septic patients. The inability of clinical trials of cytokine inhibitors to affect human mortality may reflect the inherent heterogeneity in patients' septic responses. (Parenthetically, though, agents developed for this purpose did prove helpful in chronic inflammatory conditions such as rheumatoid arthritis and Crohn disease.)

Other Attempted Therapies for Sepsis

Other treatment approaches have been tried for patients in sepsis, including:

- TLR4 antagonist. LPS activates cytokine secretion by binding TLR4, so that a TLR4 agonist might decrease production of inflammatory mediators.
- Antioxidants. As ROS produced during inflammation may damage tissues, antioxidant therapies, including free radical scavengers, could be protective.
- NOS inhibition. NO causes vasodilation and is cytotoxic, so that NOS inhibitors could protect from shock and tissue damage.
- NSAIDs. Inhibiting inflammation with nonsteroidal anti-inflammatory agents might mitigate overwhelming inflammatory responses.
- Glucocorticoids. In addition to their anti-inflammatory activity, glucocorticoids inhibit phospholipase, and so decrease release of inflammatory mediators, like leukotrienes and prostaglandins.
- IFNγ. This cytokine stimulates phagocytosis and disposal of pathogens, and so should help protect patients in sepsis.
- CSF. Increasing bone marrow production of leukocytes should improve the body's chances of defending itself against foreign invaders.

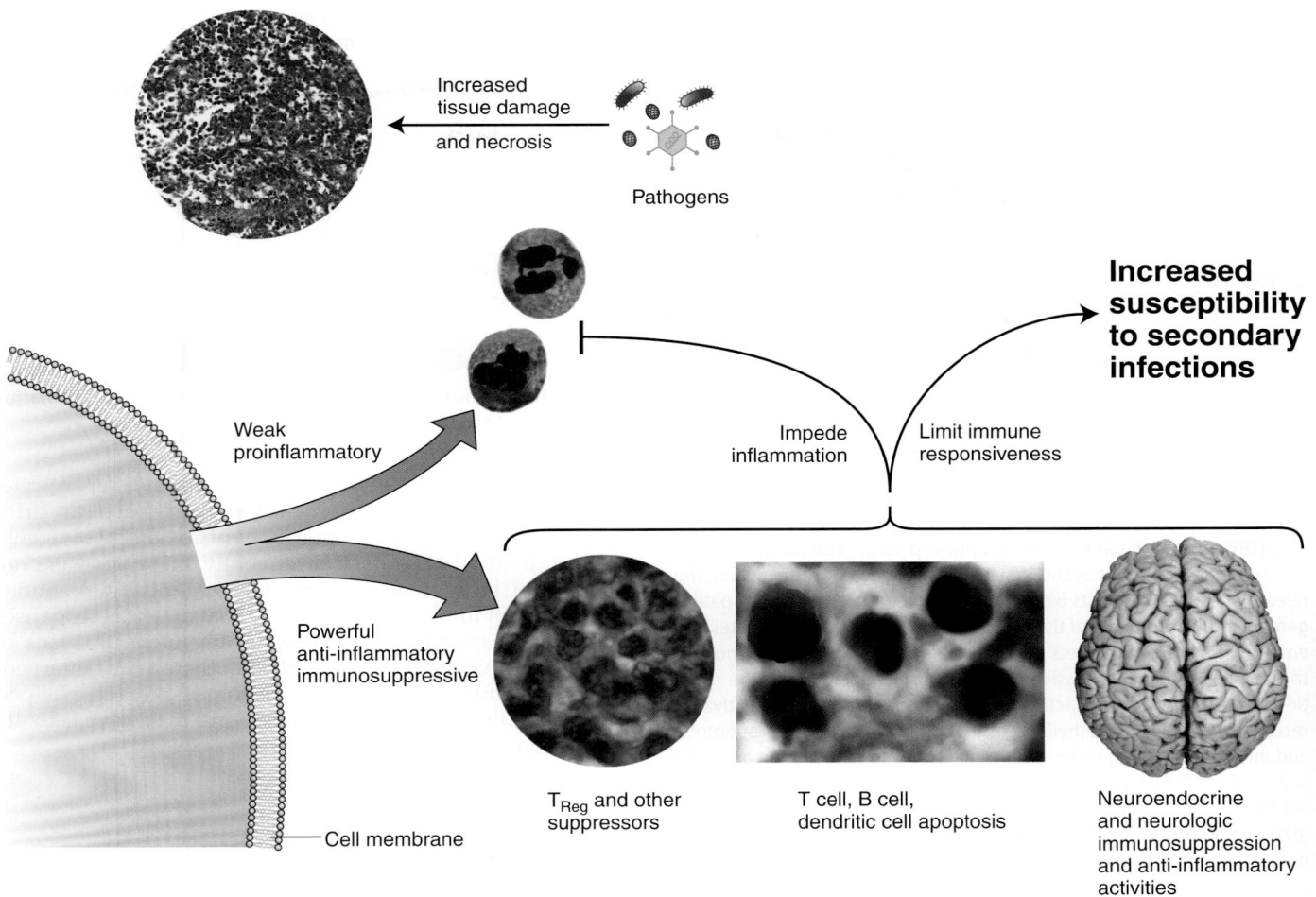

FIGURE 12-4. The host responses impeding inflammation and immune responsiveness during sepsis. The same dendritic cell and macrophage responses described in Figure 12-1 may be balanced differently, either because of genetics, environment, or as a function of timing following the initial infectious stimulus. In this setting, anti-inflammatory elements **(lower)** may predominate over proinflammatory agents **(upper)**. Depending on when such anti-inflammatory responses predominate during sepsis, they may impair immune responsiveness and limit inflammatory responses to secondarily invading pathogens. This may magnify the tissue damage that was initially due to exaggerated proinflammatory responses.

In clinical trials, none of these treatments proved efficacious in improving outcomes. That does not mean that some individual patients were not helped. Rather, as has been emphasized here, it is felt that sepsis progresses differently in each patient and over time, approaches to therapy should account for this pathogenetic diversity and plasticity.

Inflammatory Responses Are Tightly Regulated

After initial inflammatory responses, inhibitory pathways will become activated. There are several aspects to this inhibitory response. Macrophages may shift from M1, classically activated macrophages producing proinflammatory cytokines, to alternatively activated, M2 macrophages, producing cytokine inhibitors. These inhibitory responses include production of soluble TNF receptors, IL-10, and generation of T-regulatory cells (T_{reg}, see Chapter 4) (Fig. 12-4). Lymphocyte apoptosis may also be considered part of the inhibitory response. A recently described new class of lipid mediators, the resolvins, may actively resolve inflammatory responses. These would be different from inhibitors which block inflammation.

Adhesion Molecules

Traffic of inflammatory cells from blood into the tissues is complex and highly orchestrated. During inflammatory responses, specific molecules are upregulated on endothelial cells and on circulating leukocytes. These molecules, adhesion molecules, foster adhesion between inflammatory cells and vascular endothelium. There are many adhesion molecules with specificity for the different types of inflammatory cells. This specificity allows orchestrated recruitment of appropriate inflammatory cells to a site of inflammation.

There Is a Close Link Between Inflammation and Dysregulated Coagulation

Increased inflammation triggers the coagulation cascade, generating thrombi (Fig. 12-5). Under normal circumstances, once clotting starts, antagonistic mechanisms rapidly upregulate pathways to lyse newly formed thrombi (see Chapter 16). During sepsis, this process becomes dysregulated and patients develop disseminated intravascular coagulation (DIC). During DIC, thrombi form where they should not, and fail to form

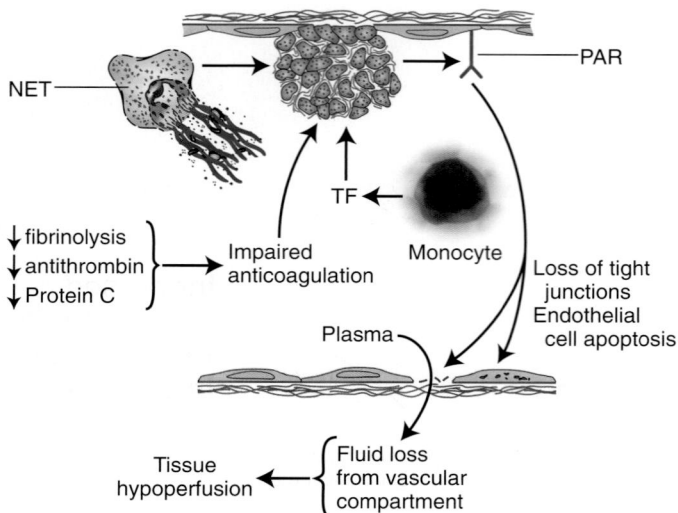

FIGURE 12-5. Pathogenesis of disseminated intravascular coagulation (DIC) and vascular insufficiency in sepsis. Several factors contribute to the development of DIC in patients with sepsis. These include the release of extracellular nets by neutrophils, trapping the microbial pathogens, and the production of tissue factor (TF) by activated monocytes and endothelial cells. TF both sets clotting in motion and inhibits fibrinolysis, the end result being excessive intravascular coagulation. At the same time, excessive thrombin activation in DIC triggers protease-activated receptors (PARs) on endothelial cells. Endothelium undergoes apoptosis and intercellular tight junctions loosen, leading to vasodilation and fluid leakage from the circulation into extravascular spaces. Activated endothelial cells produce nitric oxide (NO), which causes vasodilation and vascular leakiness. Impaired red blood cell deformability adds to these factors to decrease the effectiveness of oxygen delivery to tissues.

where they should. A consumptive coagulopathy occurs in DIC, with increased consumption of the elements of a normal thrombus including platelets and coagulation factors. Consequently, septic patients frequently have low platelet counts. There have been several attempts to treat the DIC that occurs in sepsis, but none of them have proven to be effective.

Current Understanding Suggests That Each Patient Has an Individualized Response to Pathogens

This response evolves over time and it is difficult to tell at any particular point in time where an individual patient lies in terms of her/his inflammation status. It is likely that the initial response in sepsis entails increased inflammation in an attempt to contain and eradicate the pathogen. It is this fact—that the evolution of sepsis appears to follow different routes in each individual patient—that makes interrupting the cascade described above so challenging.

First, it is difficult to ascertain when infection started. The subsequent trajectory is also difficult to predict: one patient may continue to increase the inflammatory response, another patient may have an elevated but appropriate level of inflammation, while a third quickly becomes immunosuppressed. There ought to be a balance between proinflammatory and anti-inflammatory reactions, but the lack of such balance results in dysregulated host responses (Fig. 12-6).

A diagnostic test for sepsis does not exist. As described in the scoring systems below, septic patients are identified on the basis of physiologic changes. Clinical trials have used

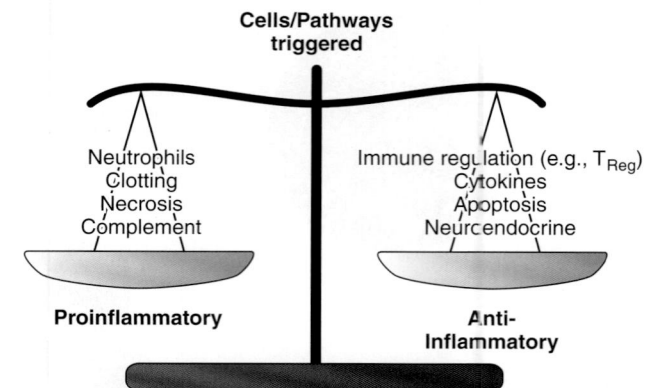

FIGURE 12-6. The balance of pro- and anti-inflammatory mediators that contribute to the heterogeneity in sepsis.

the approach of enrolling all patients who met sepsis criteria, regardless of their inflammatory status. Most of the prior failed sepsis therapies did not account for the heterogeneity of individual patients. Consequently, therapies were not tailored to individual patients. Therapeutic interventions also were not modified over time so that as septic responses evolved, the treatments remained static. Given this lack of tailored intervention, it is possible that therapeutic interventions to modulate inflammatory responses may have helped some patients, but been ineffective—and may have actually increased mortality—in others.

Biomarkers of Sepsis

The NIH defines a biomarker as "a characteristic that is objectively measured and evaluated as an indicator of normal biologic processes, pathogenic processes, or pharmacologic responses to a therapeutic intervention." Biomarkers have been used in sepsis studies in an attempt to identify those patients who have sepsis as well as those septic patients who will have a poor outcome. Elevated levels of cytokines have been used as biomarkers for sepsis, in addition to multiple other sophisticated measures of the inflammatory response. Some studies evaluated changes in biomarkers over time, reflecting the evolving inflammatory response to sepsis. Despite these prior studies, biomarkers have not often been used to direct therapy.

There may also be confusion between molecules that are considered biomarkers for septic inflammatory responses and molecules which are felt to be pathogenic mediators, driving the injurious septic response. In some settings, a biomarker may also be a mediator. For example, plasma TNFα is elevated in septic patients and TNFα may also be responsible for some aspects of cell and organ injury. However, in light of the heterogeneity of septic responses, it is not clear if every septic patient has elevated levels of TNFα which caused increased organ injury and mortality. There are several tests that are used to follow patients, such as lactate, WBC count, or blood gases, but a diagnostic laboratory test for sepsis does not yet exist.

METABOLIC AND PHYSIOLOGIC ABNORMALITIES DURING SEPSIS

The immunology, pathophysiology, and metabolic abnormalities of the septic response are all highly complex. A

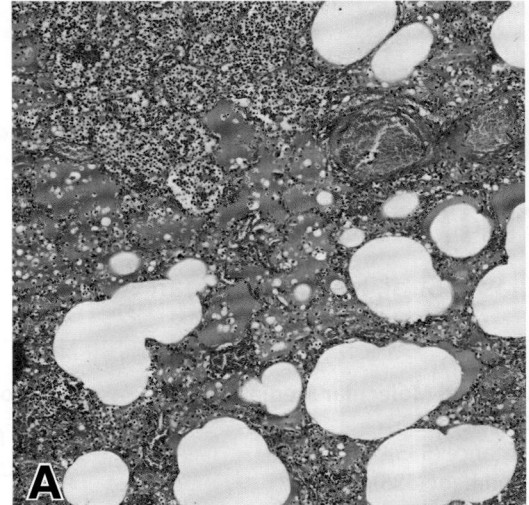 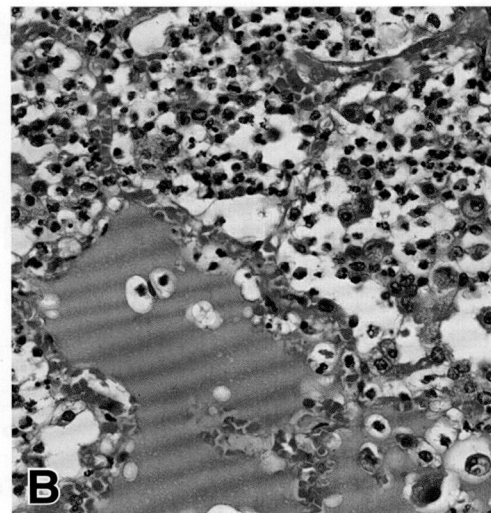

FIGURE 12-7. Histopathology of bacterial pneumonia. A. Some alveolar airspaces are filled with pink-stained protein-filled fluid. Numerous neutrophils have also infiltrated the alveolar space. The *white spaces* show alveoli where air was still exchanged through breathing. **B.** Higher power, showing intra-alveolar fluid, alveolar macrophages, and many neutrophils.

significant issue is what drives the physiologic abnormalities. Patients do not die from an elevated cytokine. Rather, organ injury or physiologic consequences of the elevated cytokine result in death. It is also important to differentiate systemic inflammation due to noninfectious causes from sepsis. Patients with sepsis respond to appropriate antibiotic therapy, while patients with systemic inflammation due to, for example, autoimmune disease will not.

Several Scoring Systems Help Predict Mortality in Septic Patients

Most such systems are based on a rapid assessment of specific physiologic parameters or clinical examination. For example, most scoring systems use respiratory rate as one component to predict outcome, demonstrating the importance of the pulmonary system in the septic response (Fig. 12-7). The fact that the respiratory rate is included in most scoring systems probably reflects the fact that pneumonia is the most frequent cause of sepsis. Other contributory physiologic parameters are heart rate, body temperature, and systolic blood pressure. Alterations in CNS status are typically included. Laboratory values are not included in these scoring systems, so that a rapid bedside assessment may be used to predict outcome. These scoring systems are also used to screen for the presence of sepsis. Such screens help to identify sepsis, but lack specificity, and do not identify underlying mechanisms driving an individual dysregulated host response that leads to organ injury.

Organ Injury Caused by Sepsis

The Sepsis-3 definition requires the presence of life-threatening organ dysfunction caused by dysregulated host response to infection. The urinary system is damaged in over 40% of septic patients and is the most frequently damaged organ/system during septic responses, followed by the respiratory. Organs may be damaged individually, or multisystem organ failure may develop. Mortality increases with the number of injured organs, such that a patient in whom a single organ is impaired has a 20% probability of dying, while if five organs are injured, likely mortality exceeds 60%. There may be end-organ damage in virtually any organ or system (Fig. 12-8).

CLINICAL FEATURES: Current treatment for sepsis. The surviving sepsis campaign includes a bundle of care for treating septic patient. This bundle of care calls for rapid identification of septic patients, controlling infection through appropriate means such as antibiotics, and treatment of physiologic abnormalities, for example, by providing fluids to support blood pressure. It is noteworthy that in the guidelines there are no recommendations for any specific immunologic therapy.

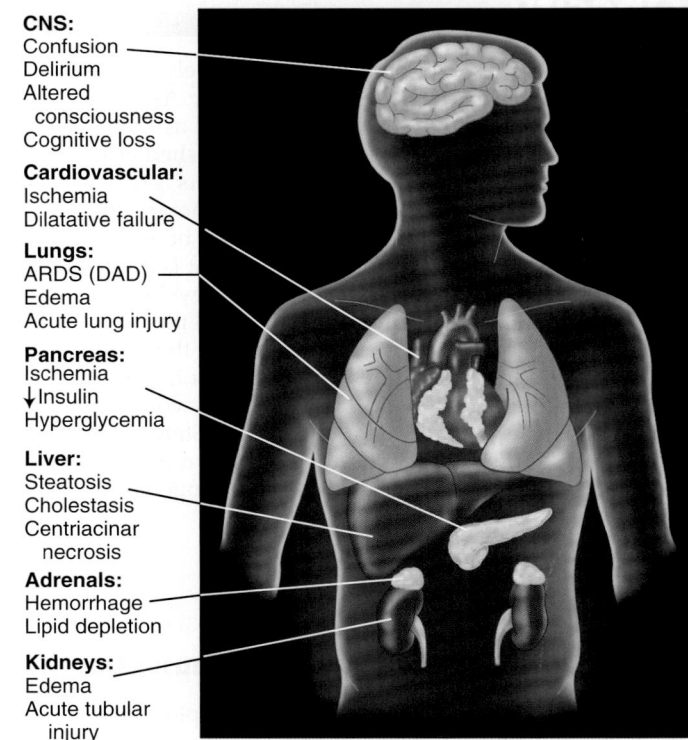

CNS:
Confusion
Delirium
Altered
 consciousness
Cognitive loss

Cardiovascular:
Ischemia
Dilatative failure

Lungs:
ARDS (DAD)
Edema
Acute lung injury

Pancreas:
Ischemia
↓Insulin
Hyperglycemia

Liver:
Steatosis
Cholestasis
Centriacinar
 necrosis

Adrenals:
Hemorrhage
Lipid depletion

Kidneys:
Edema
Acute tubular
 injury

FIGURE 12-8. End-organ damage in septic patients. Individual organ or multisystem organ failure may occur during the human response to sepsis.

13 Obesity, Diabetes Mellitus, and Their Harmful Sequelae

Kevin Jon Williams, Elias S. Siraj, Isaac E. Stillman

Obesity

Only three decades ago, obesity was relatively uncommon, but its prevalence has been increasing rapidly. Astonishingly, globally, 1 billion adults might be classified as overweight, and at least 400 million (4×10^8) meet established criteria for obesity. Approximately one-third of US adults is overweight and one-third obese. The rest are lean. Although the prevalence of obesity in the United States may be leveling off, rates of extreme obesity continue to rise, that is, individuals already obese are growing heavier. In the developed world, obesity is more common among women and the poor, while in developing countries, it mainly affects the well-to-do. This explosion in obesity rates indicates that the basic issue is environmental, not genetic. It is especially worrisome that at least one in seven children in the United States is obese; a recent study showed that childhood obesity more than doubles the risk of death before age 55 from endogenous causes.

CAUSATIVE AND UNDERLYING FACTORS IN OBESITY

Chronic, Positive Caloric Imbalance Causes Obesity

Nevertheless, underlying factors involve complex interactions of genetic, metabolic, physiologic, social, behavioral, technologic, governmental, and commercial influences that lead to overnutrition and underexertion. The magnitude of imbalance can be surprisingly small: thermodynamically correct models of human weight change indicate that the obesity epidemic in North America can be explained by only 220 kcal (Cal) average increased daily *intake* per person. Since maintaining and moving a larger body burn up 212.8 of this 220 additional kcal/day, the actual daily caloric *imbalance* per person that explains adult obesity is only +7.2 kcal, just over 7 kcal/person daily. This represents only 0.3% of a typical person's 2,500 kcal/day in the developed world, and translates into weight gain of about 1 g of tissue per day. Over 10,000 days (30 years), this represents approximately 10 kg (~22 lb) of adiposity, and matches the average adult weight gain from 1978 to 2005.

The daily caloric imbalance is the equivalent of mere cookie crumbs each day (one Oreo cookie has 53 kcal), or a few sips of a sugar-sweetened beverage (there are 150 kcal in a 12-ounce can of regular soda or two 6-ounce servings of fruit juice). Thus, a child who ingests a high-caloric snack going to and from school substantially increases his or her risk for obesity, unless other changes in intake or expenditure compensate for all that added energy load.

In considering the precision of energy balance required to defend body weight and prevent adiposity over the long run, consider that, in the West, each man consumes and expends roughly 1,000,000 kcal yearly, and, for Western women, 750,000 kcal per year. Proportionately small cumulative errors on this scale add up quickly. Severe clinical obesity may rarely have monogenic causes that impair satiety, described below, but most cases result from combined effects of lifestyle and environmental factors, superimposed on several partially heritable traits.

Societal and Other Factors Complicate Control of Body Weight

Traditionally, eating has been a highly social and cultural endeavor, and vigorous physical activity was a requirement for typical daily life. Several factors associated with rising rates of obesity in developed and developing countries disrupt long-standing patterns of dining and movement. Modern examples that alter eating include rising consumption of simple carbohydrate sweeteners, particularly sugary beverages; the invention of an evolutionarily unprecedented class of molecules—nonnutritive intense artificial sweeteners—that are widely sold without convincing evidence as "diet" aids for weight loss; recent breeding of domesticated crops and animals to enhance yield and shelf life but without adequate attention to flavor—common supermarket tomatoes are pre-eminent examples of a healthy food drained of taste and texture; replacement of regular, social meals with unscheduled snacking; agricultural and other subsidies that make carbohydrate calories cheaper—remarkably, the Food Stamp program in the United States spends an estimated nearly US\$15 × 10⁹ yearly to provide sweetened drinks, desserts, salty snacks, candy, and sugar to the poor, including children; over a half century of advice from cardiovascular and nutrition societies to avoid dietary fat, further shifting the public to carbohydrates that strongly associate with population-wide weight gain; and the growth of a sophisticated industry that has created a new class of food and drink that is low- or no-cost to the consumer, convenient, savory, calorically dense, yet conspicuously weak in its ability to satiate.

Diminished physical activity from labor-saving devices, such as washing machines and private cars; widespread use of television—with remote controls—and other electronic entertainment; and the growth of sedentary jobs—all now associate with worse health outcomes. Technologies that generate heat for buildings, vehicles, limited outdoor areas, and even some types of clothing cut down on normal, cold-induced expenditure of biologic energy stores.

However desirable these developments may be, when they are combined and used to excess, they disrupt normal mechanisms that defend body weight and limit adiposity. This leads to chronic positive caloric imbalance and increased obesity. Because performing long-term causal studies in humans is difficult, the contributions of many of these individual factors to human obesity have been inferred largely or entirely from associations, albeit strong ones.

Nevertheless, several points bear emphasis: Sustained reduction in energy intake, though difficult to achieve, reliably produces weight loss and improves metabolic status; bariatric surgery is currently the most effective clinical intervention to reduce energy intake, weight, the rate of type 2 diabetes mellitus (T2DM) and premature mortality in appropriately selected obese patients; regular exercise improves health even without weight loss; sufficient purposeful exercise aids long-term weight management; and obese and lean people in sedentary jobs exhibit huge differences in the daily amount of physical activity outside of purposeful exercise—such activity is also known as nonexercise activity thermogenesis or "NEAT" (see below).

Modern disruptions in caloric intake and expenditure that can contribute to metabolic disequilibrium (Fig. 13-1).

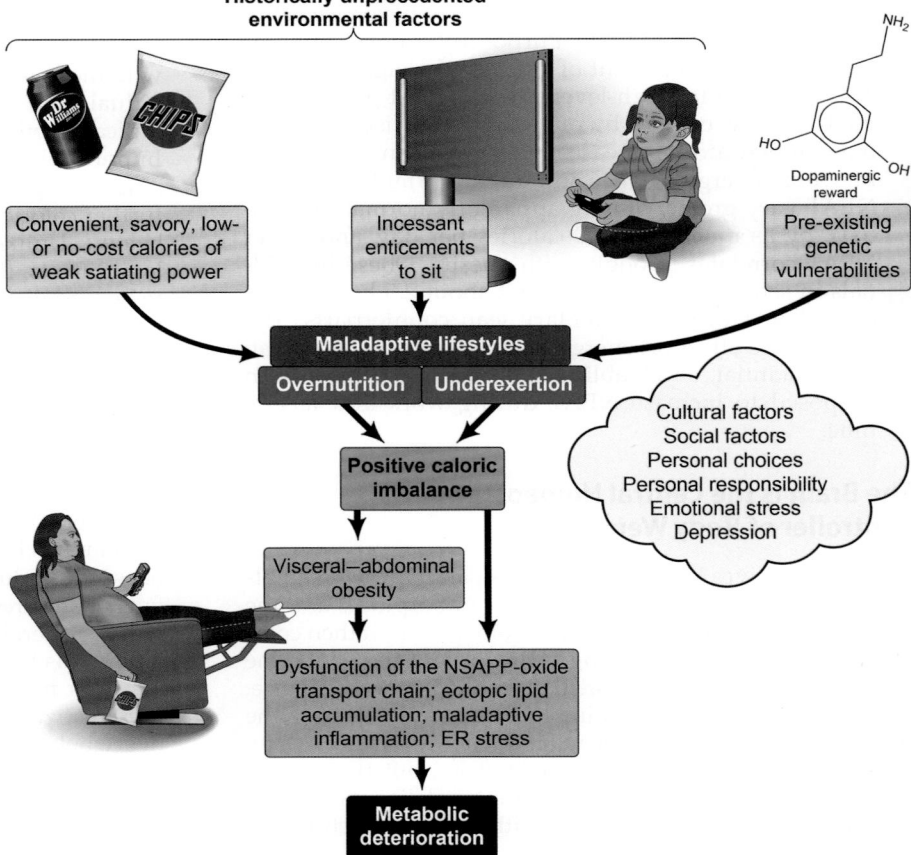

FIGURE 13-1. Causes and consequences of positive caloric imbalance. Historically unprecedented environmental factors combine with pre-existing vulnerabilities to promote maladaptive lifestyles that include overnutrition and underexertion. The main portion of the figure presents a causal chain, ending with metabolic deterioration. More complex factors of particular importance are listed in the cloud off to the right. *NSAPP* = an oxide transport chain from NOX4 to SOD3 to aquaporins to PTEN and PTPases that is required for balanced insulin signaling; *ER* = endoplasmic reticulum. (Adapted with permission from Williams K, Wu X. Imbalanced insulin action in chronic over nutrition: Clinical harm, molecular mechanisms, and a way forward. *Atherosclerosis* 2016;247:225–282.)

ENERGY INTAKE AND EXPENDITURE

Weight gain other than water occurs when energy intake exceeds expenditure: You are what you eat, minus what you burn, malabsorb, or excrete. Energy intake is conceptually straightforward: Many populations consume an overabundance of calories, and the normal human gut absorbs essentially all incoming simple fuels. Many behaviors related to caloric intake and expenditure are influenced by heredity. For example, offspring of mothers with high prepregnancy body weights tend to eat in the absence of hunger (EAH) and seek out foods of high energy density (kcal/g).

Total daily energy expenditure (TDEE) consists of several regulated components:

1. **Basal metabolic rate (BMR):** BMR is the energy expended at complete rest, lying down, in the postabsorptive state. It includes maintenance levels of breathing, circulation of blood and essential metabolic functions. For people with sedentary occupations, BMR is ~60% of TDEE. Over three-quarters of variations in BMR reflects differences in lean body mass. Minor differences in BMR are unlikely to explain human obesity. For example, extensive human data show no correlation between percent body fat and deviations from predicted BMRs.
2. **Calories spent to digest, absorb, and store ingested calories** (6% to 12% of TDEE). This is also known as the thermic effect of food.
3. **Energetic costs of emotion, medication, and adaptive thermogenesis in response to the environment** (e.g., changes in temperature, exposure to infectious agents).
4. **Activity thermogenesis** generated by physical movement during purposeful exercise and nonexercise activity thermogenesis (NEAT). Purposeful exercise remains an important component of successful weight-loss programs. Except for high-level athletes, most people burn relatively few calories by purposeful exercise, but without compensatory increases in intake, even small shifts in overall energy balance add up. Importantly, levels of NEAT vary greatly among apparently normal individuals, by as much as 2,000 calories per day, and lower NEAT correlates strongly with obesity. Obese individuals in sedentary occupations sit about 2.5 hours more each day than their sedentary lean counterparts. The cumulative effect on energy balance over the years can be substantial, and public health strategies have been proposed to increase NEAT during work and leisure time.

The Brain Is the Central Homeostatic Controller of Body Weight

The brain receives hormonal, neuronal, and nutrient signals from the periphery about food deficits or surpluses and the rate of fuel utilization. To maintain homeostasis, it then coordinates responses, modulating behavior and the endocrine and autonomic nervous systems to adjust energy balance. The **hypothalamus** is the main processor of signals from the periphery and is crucial to managing energy balance. Many hypothalamic nuclei regulate metabolism, but the arcuate nucleus is central to integrating peripheral signals via two distinct populations of neurons with opposing actions on food intake.

Anorexigenic Neuropeptides

One population produces **anorexigenic** (appetite-suppressing) neuropeptides including **proopiomelanocortin (POMC)** and **cocaine- and amphetamine-regulated transcript (CART)**. POMC is cleaved into α-**melanocyte stimulating hormone (αMSH)**, which binds melanocortin receptors MC3R and MC4R to decrease appetite.

Orexigenic Neuropeptides

The other group of neurons produces two **orexigenic** (appetite-stimulating) neuropeptides: **neuropeptide Y (NPY)** and a**gouti-related protein (AgRP)**. NPY is among the most abundant neuropeptides in the mammalian brain and is a potent stimulator of feeding. It may bind any of six G-protein–coupled NPY receptor subtypes (Y1 through Y6), but Y1 and Y2 NPY receptors seem to be most involved with feeding. AgRP antagonizes melanocortin receptors, thus blocking the anorexigenic effects of αMSH, stimulating food intake.

Multiple Hormones Stimulate and Suppress Appetite

Soluble mediators from many sources regulate hunger and satiety:

- **Leptin:** The discovery of **leptin** revealed a key link between neural and nonneural systems in controlling appetite and energy expenditure. Leptin (from the Greek λεπτός, meaning "thin") is produced mainly by adipocytes and is the protein product of the *LEP* gene, known historically as the *Ob* gene. Blood levels of leptin, like insulin, rise acutely after each meal and rise chronically with the mass of body fat (i.e., they are lower in lean individuals and rise with obesity). Thus, leptin and insulin indicate both short- and long-term energy availability. Importantly, each of these hormones enters the hypothalamus and provokes specific neuronal signals that inhibit further caloric intake (insulin in this context is discussed below). Unlike insulin, which has many other physiologic effects, the chief physiologic role of leptin appears to be signaling the brain that body energy stores are sufficient. Low serum leptin levels increase appetite. Normal leptin levels decrease appetite and increase energy expenditure.
- Leptin enters the brain and interacts with leptin receptors on POMC/CART and NPY/AgRP neurons, regulating them in opposite ways. Leptin directly activates (anorexigenic) POMC/CART neurons while inhibiting (orexigenic) NPY/AgRP neurons. The result is decreased food intake. Leptin blood levels are above normal in most obese individuals, but this increased leptin unfortunately fails to suppress appetite and halt excessive fat accumulation. Several explanations are possible, including that leptin fails to reach its neuronal targets, the leptin receptor does not signal normally despite binding to leptin (desensitization) and overwhelming cues to overeat may overwhelm physiologic restraints. Leptin injections to treat common forms of obesity have not been successful to date.
- **Circadian rhythms** affect, and are affected by, caloric flux. Mice with genetic disruption of the circadian system

develop obesity, hyperleptinemia, hyperlipidemia, and hyperglycemia. In humans, shift workers, who must alter their sleep rhythms, show increased prevalence of high body mass indexes (BMIs), the metabolic syndrome (see below), and cardiovascular events. Forced sleep restriction in humans disturbs appetite control and glucose tolerance, which is a particular concern given that obstructive sleep apnea often already disrupts sleep in obese individuals.

- **Endocannabinoids** are endogenous lipids that bind to cannabinoid receptors 1 and 2 (CB1, CB2). **CB1 receptors** are found in hypothalamic nuclei that are involved in control of energy balance and weight. CB1 receptors also occur in adipose tissue and the GI tract. When activated, they stimulate food intake and may play a role in the development and maintenance of obesity. Rimonabant, a synthetic blocker of the CB1 receptor, suppresses appetite, decreases weight, and improves metabolic parameters in obese subjects, but has prohibitive psychiatric side effects.

- The **gastrointestinal tract** is another major participant in energy homeostasis. Its multiple mechanoreceptors and chemosensitive receptors relay information via vagal afferent fibers to the brainstem nucleus tractus solitarii. For example, vagal activation by gastric distension causes satiety and meal termination. Taste receptors for bitter, sweet, and umami in the stomach, small intestine, and pancreas may act as nutrient sensors, and affect appetite and insulin release. In addition, several hormones produced by the gut signal to the CNS to regulate energy intake. **Glucagon-like peptide 1 (GLP1)** is produced by posttranslational processing of proglucagon by L-cells mainly in the mucosa of the distal ileum and colon. GLP1 binds GLP1 receptors, decreases food intake, slows gastric emptying, generates a feeling of satiety, augments postprandial glucose-stimulated insulin secretion and decreases secretion of glucagon, a hormone that opposes insulin action (see Chapter 21). These combined effects reduce caloric delivery into the intestines, and hence to the rest of the body, while enhancing insulin secretion and action. Liraglutide, semaglutide, and dulaglutide are long-acting GLP1 receptor agonists that are used to treat T2DM and also cause weight reduction and cardiovascular protection (discussed below).

- **Ghrelin** is produced primarily by gastric endocrine cells, but also to a lesser extent in the duodenum, ileum, and colon. It stimulates orexigenic NPY neurons in the hypothalamic arcuate nucleus. Circulating ghrelin levels increase during fasting, and its administration to normal subjects increases caloric intake. Patients with anorexia nervosa have high plasma concentrations of ghrelin, but administration of exogenous ghrelin to treat this condition has not been successful. Plasma ghrelin levels fall after gastric bypass, and may contribute to the continued weight loss after the procedure. Conversely, patients with the Prader–Willi syndrome exhibit hyperphagia and very high plasma ghrelin levels. *Moreover, serum ghrelin concentrations increase after diet-induced weight loss, which may contribute to poor long-term results of clinical weight loss programs.*

- **Cholecystokinin (CCK)** is mainly made by duodenal and jejunal mucosa. It is released in response to fat and protein intake and acts on two distinct receptors. CCK stimulates release of enzymes from the pancreas and gallbladder to aid digestion, slows gastric emptying, and reduces food intake. Regulation of food intake by CCK is mediated via vagal afferent signals to the brain.

- **Peptide YY (PYY)** is secreted along the entire GI tract, but is concentrated in the ileum and colon. PYY(3-36), the major circulating form, is released in response to food intake. Its numerous actions include delaying pancreatic and gastric secretions, gallbladder emptying, and gastric emptying. PYY(3-36) decreases appetite, duration of food intake, and total caloric intake.

- **Pancreatic polypeptide (PP)** is in the same peptide family as PYY. It is produced mainly in the pancreas, but also in the colon and rectum. Eating stimulates its release, and it acts to reduce appetite and decrease food intake.

- **Amylin** is a peptide mainly produced by pancreatic β-cells, but also found in gut endocrine cells, visceral sensory neurons, and the hypothalamus. It strongly inhibits gastric emptying and decreases food intake. An amylin analogue, pramlintide, is currently available for treatment of diabetes mellitus. Higher doses of pramlintide produced modest weight loss in clinical trials.

- **Insulin** is best known for its role in peripheral glucose uptake, but it also affects appetite. Injecting insulin into the third cerebral ventricle of rats decreases food intake via insulin receptors in the arcuate nucleus of the hypothalamus, where it increases messenger RNA (mRNA) for POMC (anorexigenic) and suppresses mRNA for NYP (orexigenic), similar to leptin. Clinically, however, peripheral administration of insulin often increases weight. Much of this effect has been attributed to control of glycosuria, thereby stopping caloric leakage via the urine that is not fully compensated by decreased appetite. A related effect, discussed below, occurs from SGLT2 inhibitors, which cause glycosuria and hence a caloric leak. The caloric leak from glycosuria is not fully compensated by increased appetite, and so promote modest weight loss. Exogenous insulin may also cause hypoglycemia, which may increase appetite.

- **Bile acids** and their receptors, such as the **farnesoid X-activated receptor (FXR**, also known as NR1H4), have been implicated in weight loss after bariatric surgery, in part because plasma concentrations of bile acids typically rise after these procedures. Definitive demonstrations that FXR ligands can produce weight loss, however, are still lacking.

- **Other substances** also regulate hunger, satiety, fat deposition, etc., in rodents, including galanin, adipocyte complement-related protein (ACRP), peroxisome proliferator-associated receptors (PPARs), and others.

- **Gut flora** affect body weight. Germ-free mice are protected from obesity induced by high-fat diets, and colonization of these mice with intestinal flora from conventionally raised mice enhances caloric uptake from complex dietary plant polysaccharides and modulates expression of specific host genes to increase caloric storage in adipose tissue. In humans, distal gut flora from obese individuals is different from flora in lean individuals. Gut bacteria from obese people may extract calories more effectively from complex dietary components than do microbiota from lean individuals. Nevertheless, modern foods of high-caloric density contain mostly simple carbohydrates and oils that are completely absorbed without any microbial assistance. Thus, research attention has focused instead on regulatory effects on the host from variations in gut flora.

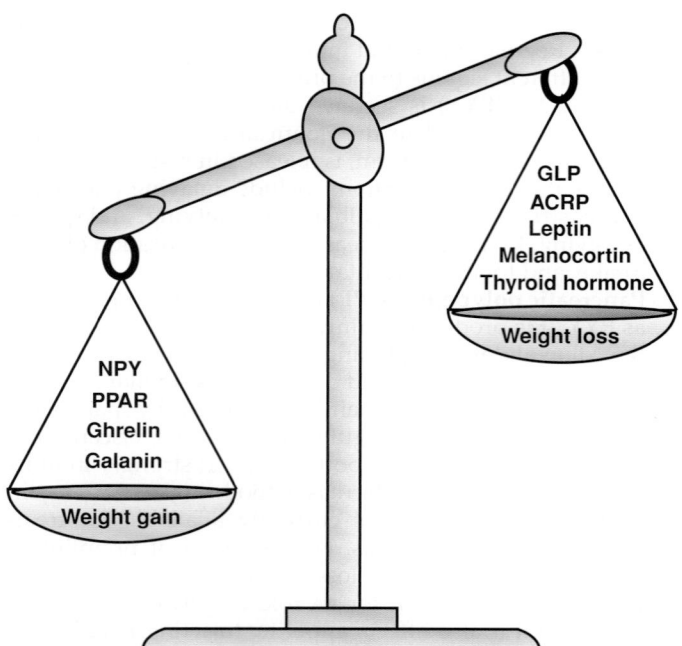

FIGURE 13-2. **The balance of chemical mediators that promote fat accumulation (weight gain) and those that promote fat loss (weight loss).** *ACRP* = adipocyte complement-related protein; *GLP* = glucagon-like peptide; *NPY* = neuropeptide Y; *PPAR* = peroxisome proliferator-activated receptor.

Gut flora "transplants" from lean to obese subjects have been attempted, but without clinically convincing results on weight or metabolic status.

Known orexigenic and anorexigenic factors are illustrated in Figure 13-2.

BODY MASS INDEX AND OBESITY

BMI is the standard most often used to define obesity:

$$BMI = [weight (kg)] \div [height (m)]^2$$

Although BMI is an excellent indicator of obesity, it does not distinguish between fat mass and lean mass. For example, a muscular person with little body fat could be misclassified as obese, and someone with excess adipose tissue and reduced muscle mass, who might be elderly or chronically ill, could have a normal BMI. In addition, there are racial/ethnic variations in adipose tissue volume, particularly visceral–abdominal adipose tissue, at a given BMI.

Obesity-Disease Correlations Often Vary With Ethnicity

Western Societies

Most health organizations define overweight as BMI between 25 and 29.9 kg/m². Someone whose BMI is 30 kg/m² or greater is considered obese, with 30 to 34.9 kg/m² being class I obesity; 35 to 39.9 kg/m², class II; and BMI >40 kg/m² being extreme (class III). These classifications are based on epidemiologic studies in Western countries showing that high BMI correlates with excess morbidity, mostly reflecting specific

metabolic abnormalities, particularly dyslipoproteinemia, hypertension, impaired glucose regulation, hypercoagulability, and risk of developing overt type 2 diabetes. Obesity correlates with shorter lifespan and a greater proportion of life lived with cardiovascular disease. People who are overweight have normal longevity, but spend a greater proportion of their lives with cardiovascular disease. Other work suggests that the association between obesity and mortality in Western countries may be weakening, perhaps because of improved public health and better treatment of cardiovascular risks.

Variation in Correlations Between BMI and Disease Susceptibility

There is substantial variation in susceptibilities of various populations worldwide to metabolic abnormalities at similar BMIs, perhaps due to diverse body composition, genetics, and lifestyle (e.g., cuisine, physical activity, tobacco use). A multiethnic cross-sectional study in Canada found that the same degree of impaired glucose control (dysglycemia) and dyslipoproteinemia seen on average in individuals of European descent with a BMI cutpoint of 30 kg/m²—the barely obese—occurred at much lower BMIs for people of different ethnicities (e.g., for dysglycemia—only 21.0 kg/m² with South Asian ancestry, 20.6 kg/m² with Chinese ancestry, and 21.8 kg/m² for Aboriginal Americans). Experience corroborates that overweight South Asians face a particular burden of dysglycemia and dyslipoproteinemia. Therefore, BMI values to define obesity and identify the need and intensity of intervention differ considerably among populations, and BMI cutpoints for people of European descent may understate cardiometabolic risks for other ethnic groups. Additional studies in other populations of non-European ancestry are ongoing.

The Role of Body Fat Distribution

Regional body fat distribution is an important correlate of health risk associated with obesity. Fat depots in different parts of the body play various roles including energy metabolism, secretion of circulating proteins and metabolites into the bloodstream and the physical cushioning and protection of internal organs. Visceral–abdominal obesity (also known as central adiposity or "apple-shaped") associates with a greater risk of dyslipoproteinemia, hypertension, heart disease, diabetes, and some forms of cancer than does gluteal–femoral obesity (termed lower-body obesity or "pear shaped" (Fig. 13-3).

As BMI does not account for fat distribution, abdominal obesity in many populations is better assessed by measuring the waist circumference. The waist:hip ratio once widely used, performs poorly in some sub-Saharan African populations. Adverse health outcomes are more likely with waist circumferences greater than 102 cm (40 in) in men, and 88 cm (35 in) in women. Thus, amounts of visceral fat and key, modifiable cardiovascular risk factors provide better guides to therapy than BMI. As noted in more detail below, surgical removal of adipose tissue produces no known metabolic benefits in obese humans, suggesting that adiposity is a marker, not a mediator, of their health problems. Liver fat (triglyceride) has been identified as a stronger marker of metabolic derangements than is visceral adiposity, but requires specialized magnetic resonance equipment.

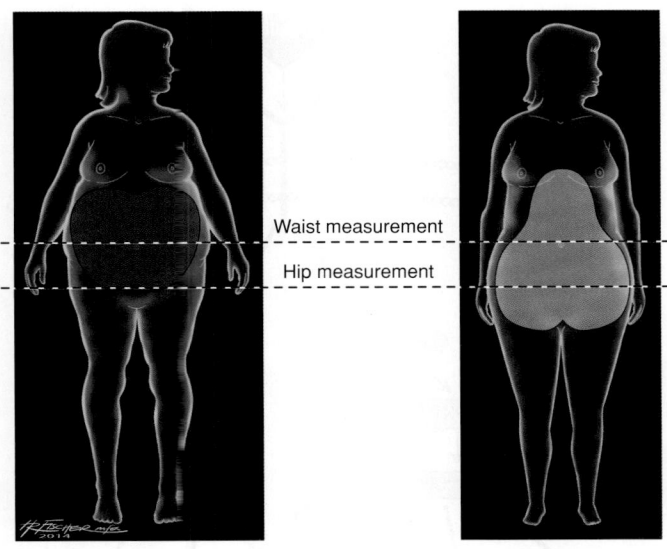

FIGURE 13-3. Regional adipose distribution and cardiometabolic risk. Individuals who accumulate adipose tissue in the abdomen ("apple-shaped") exhibit increased risk of insulin resistance for glucose, type 2 diabetes mellitus, and cardiovascular disease, compared to those with fat accumulation around the hips, buttocks, and thighs ("pear shaped"). Standard methods to assess abdominal obesity include waist circumference and the waist:hip ratio.

CAUSES AND MOLECULAR MEDIATORS OF OBESITY

Inheritance Is a Potent Factor in Predisposition to Obesity

Nearly everyone living in developed countries is exposed to a calorie-rich, sedentary environment, yet BMIs vary from extremely thin to morbidly obese. Inherited predisposition to obesity is clear: Twins (monozygotic and dizygotic), genetically full or half-siblings raised apart after adoption in infancy and in multigenerational kindreds have shown heritable BMI concordances from 20% to 80%. Most recently, a study of twins growing up *during* the obesity epidemic found 77% heritability in BMI and waist circumference. Behaviors linked to obesity (e.g., eating in the absence of hunger, impaired responses to internal signals of satiety but exaggerated responses to external food cues, rapid eating [increased bites/min], low levels of physical activity including low levels of NEAT) all showed substantial inherited tendencies.

 **MOLECULAR PATHOGENESIS:** Many genetic studies have identified specific gene variants that, when summed together, contribute only slightly to the population-wide development of obesity:

- Leptin gene mutations have been linked to rare monogenic syndromes of severe obesity in humans. Homozygotes have hyperphagia and severe, early-onset obesity. They die more readily from childhood infections and develop hypothalamic hypogonadism, insulin resistance for handling glucose and diabetes as adults. Heterozygotes have reduced blood levels of leptin and increased body weight compared with unaffected siblings. Unlike its ineffectiveness in people with ordinary obesity, leptin replacement therapy is effective in these individuals.
- Leptin receptor gene mutations occur in rare families with severe early-onset obesity. These people resemble patients with leptin gene mutations, except that patients with receptor mutations have markedly elevated serum leptin levels. They also have hypogonadotropic hypogonadism, failure of pubertal development, growth delay, and secondary hypothyroidism. As expected, leptin supplementation is ineffective in these individuals.
- Melanocortin-4 receptor gene (MC4R) mutations may be dominant or recessive, and are the leading cause of severe, monogenic childhood-onset obesity. Mutations in MC4R underlie an estimated ≈5% of cases of severe childhood-onset obesity. Because this syndrome is rare, MC4R mutations have a minor impact on population-wide prevalence of obesity. Patients tend to have no phenotype other than overeating, obesity, and the well-known cardiometabolic sequelae of obesity.
- Isolated cases of obesity have been linked to mutations or deficiencies in POMC/αMSH, αMSH, prohormone convertase 1, and hypothalamic transcription factor SIM1.
- The Human Genome Initiative has led to genome-wide association (GWA) studies of links between obesity and genomic polymorphisms. Several genes that encode brain/hypothalamic proteins are associated with variations in BMI. However, the sum of all the specific genetic polymorphisms identified to date reflects under 3% of BMI variations.
- Epigenetic programming during fetal or immediate postnatal life may influence adult physiology. Remarkably, large maternal weight loss from biliopancreatic bypass surgery before pregnancy seems to prevent transmission of obesity to subsequent children. In contrast, children born to the same mothers before weight loss surgery show high rates of obesity. It is not known if maternal weight loss from bariatric surgery has similar consequences.

Environmental Influences Are the Predominant Precipitants of Obesity

The impact of sociologic and psychological factors on development of positive caloric imbalance and obesity cannot be overstated. Genetic associations notwithstanding, the vast majority of obesity entails complex interactions of multiple genes with a person's environment. The marked increase in obesity in the past 30 years underscores how environmental influences drive obesity.

Striking examples of environmental influence on genetic predisposition include the Pima Native Americans in Arizona and the Aboriginal population of northern Australia. Pimas are now largely sedentary and eat a diet in which most of the energy derives from simple carbohydrates and fat, unlike their traditional low-fat diets that were rich in complex carbohydrates and fiber. The Pimas of Arizona have experienced dramatic increases in obesity and diabetes. In contrast, the genetically related Pimas in the Sierra Madre Mountains of Northern Mexico are more physically active, have maintained more traditional low-fat diets rich in complex carbohydrates and have much lower rates of obesity and T2DM.

Similarly, urbanized Aboriginal people in Australia have a high prevalence of diabetes and hypertriglyceridemia, compared with their nonurbanized counterparts. As little as a 7-week re-exposure of urbanized Aboriginals with T2DM and hypertriglyceridemia to the traditional lifestyle—eating less and moving more—led to weight loss, improved glucose tolerance, and lower blood glucose, insulin and triglycerides.

Regarding heritable predisposition, the risk of T2DM among members of the Pima Community is inversely related to a quantitative estimate of European genetic admixture in each individual, based on 18 genetic loci that are informative about ancestry. This finding is consistent with the three-fold difference in disease prevalence between the two parental populations.

Pathway-Selective Insulin Resistance and Responsiveness in Syndromes of Overnutrition

UNBALANCED INSULIN ACTION

Overnutrition and Obesity Cause Imbalances in Insulin Action

Consequences of overnutrition include harmful metabolic complications and T2DM. Appreciating the relationship of overnutrition and obesity to disturbed insulin action and type 2 diabetes requires understanding insulin receptor and its function.

PATHOPHYSIOLOGY: The insulin receptor is a tetrameric glycoprotein composed of two extracellular α-subunits that bind insulin and two transmembrane β-subunits with insulin-stimulated tyrosine kinase activity. Insulin binding activates the receptor kinase, leading to tyrosine phosphorylation of several docking proteins, such as insulin receptor substrate (IRS)-1, IRS2, and Src homologous and collagen-like protein (SHC) (Fig. 13-4). Newly phosphorylated sites on IRS1, IRS2, and SHC recruit other signal transduction molecules, such as downstream kinases or adaptor proteins which then activate still more downstream kinases. These phosphorylate lipid and protein substrates, causing glucose transport proteins to translocate from the cell's interior to the plasma membrane. This facilitates glucose entry, particularly into skeletal muscle and, to a lesser extent, adipocytes.

Insulin has several additional functions in normal physiology, unrelated to glucose transport. It:

- Suppresses hepatic glycogenolysis and gluconeogenesis, thus inhibiting hepatic glucose production in the postprandial state
- Induces hepatic fatty acid biosynthesis from carbohydrates (*de novo* lipogenesis), to package into triglycerides for export and storage in a compact, osmotically inactive form

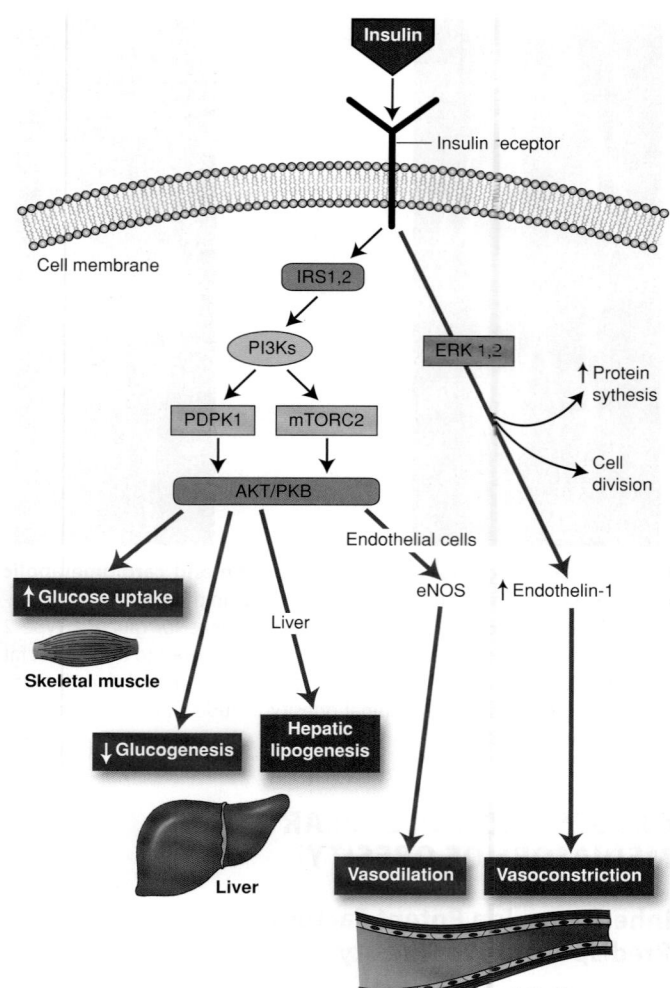

FIGURE 13-4. Key branches of insulin signaling and action. In normal physiology, insulin activates all pathways, but vasodilation produced by endothelial nitric oxide synthase (eNOS) dominates over vasoconstriction via ERK. Beneficial pathways when insulin is administered therapeutically are indicated in *blue* (glucose-lowering), while those that are potentially harmful are shown in *red* (hepatic lipogenesis and the ERK mitogen-activated protein [MAP] kinase). Strikingly, in obesity, type 2 diabetes and other conditions associated with pathway-selective insulin resistance and responsiveness (SEIRR), all pathways shown in blue become insulin resistant, while those in red remain insulin responsive. From the standpoint of human health, it is the worst possible combination of effects. *AKT/PKB* = protein kinase B; *ERK* = extracellular signal-regulated kinase; *Gluc* = glucose; *IRS1,2* = insulin receptor substrates 1 and 2; *mTORC2* = mammalian target of rapamycin complex-2; *PDPK1* = 3′-phosphoinositide-dependent protein kinase-1; *PI3Ks* = isoforms of phosphatidylinositol 3′-kinases; *SHC* = Src homologous and collagen-like protein. (Adapted with permission from Wu X, Williams KJ. NOX4 pathway as a source of selective insulin resistance and responsiveness. *Arterioscler Thromb Vasc Biol.* 2012;32[5]:1236–1245.)

- Activates endothelial nitric oxide synthase (eNOS). Resulting nitric oxide (NO) is a vasodilator that increases blood flow and hence glucose availability to skeletal muscle and
- Activates extracellular signal-regulated kinase (ERK), which then drives protein synthesis and cell division,

and increases endothelial production of endothelin-1, a vasoconstrictor that may moderate NO-mediated vasodilation.

All these effects are healthy responses to handle a normal meal's caloric content.

Insulin resistance has become a shorthand term for resistance to the *glucose-lowering* effects of insulin (or more simply, insulin resistance for handling glucose) (Figs. 13-4 and 13-5). Many other functions of insulin, however, remain fully active in obese subjects. Hence, obese people

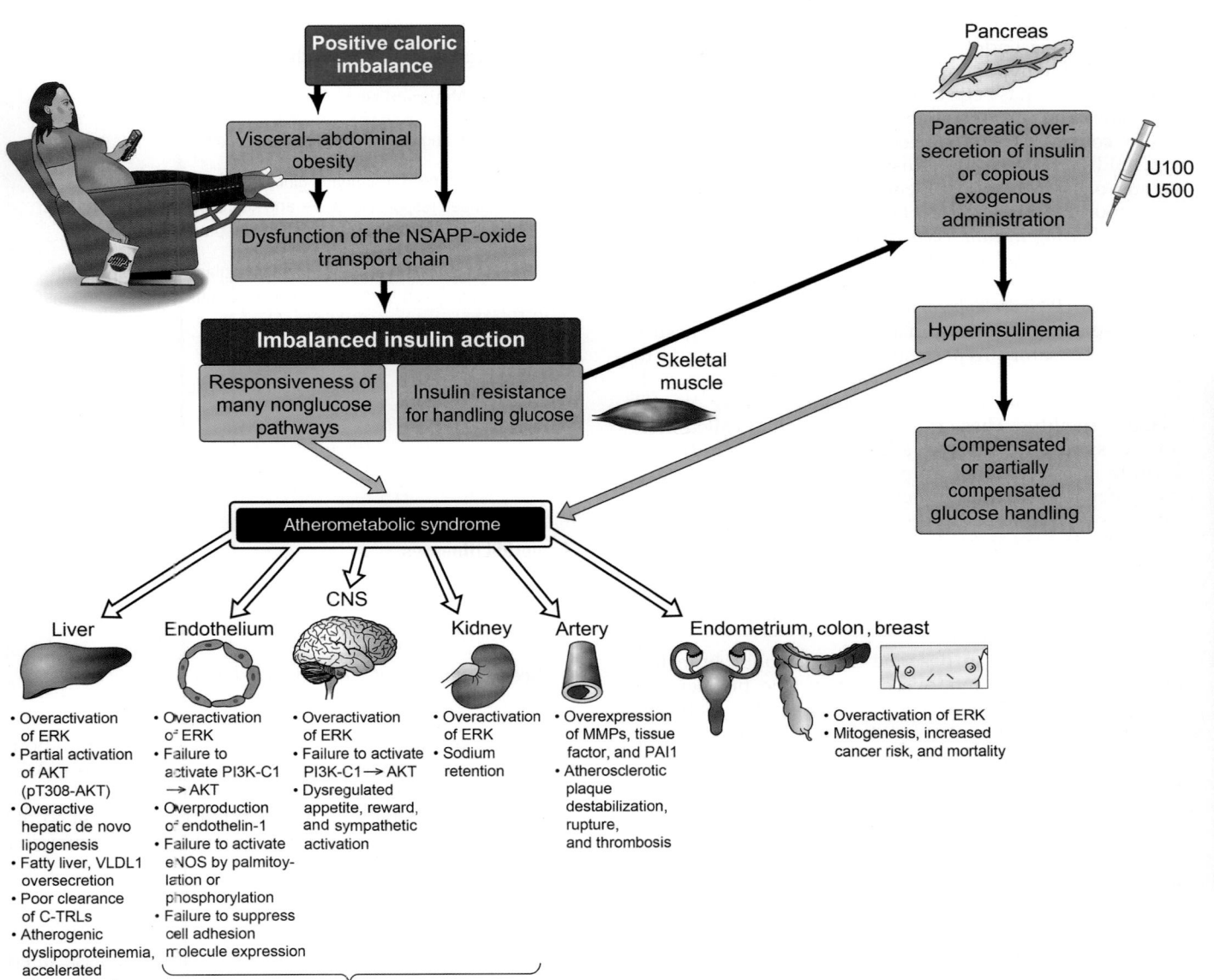

FIGURE 13-5. Imbalanced insulin action in the atherometabolic syndrome and T2DM. Imbalanced insulin action arises in association with overnutrition, underexertion, visceral–abdominal obesity, and dysfunction of molecular participants in insulin signaling. Because the atherometabolic syndrome and T2DM include insulin resistance for handling glucose, patients develop a significant compensatory hyperinsulinemia, either from endogenous oversecretion of this hormone by pancreatic β-cells or, if the β-cells cannot keep pace, from copious exogenous administration in the context of T2DM. The result is overdrive of those pathways that remain insulin-responsive, particularly ERK activation and hepatic de-novo lipogenesis (DNL). Importantly, raising insulin levels cannot make these individuals metabolically normal, even if they achieve normoglycemia, because hyperinsulinemia drives a number of processes unrelated to glucose control to become overactive. Harmful processes in liver, endothelium, the central nervous system (CNS), kidney, arterial wall, and other organs are illustrated. These effects drive fatty liver, atherogenic dyslipoproteinemia, vasoconstriction, failure to normally activate the endothelial nitric oxide synthase (eNOS), sympathetic overactivity, sodium retention, hypertension, accelerated atherosclerosis, plaque rupture and thrombosis, adverse cardiovascular events, and increased risk of specific cancers. In the CNS, imbalanced insulin action combined with hyperinsulinemia may also exacerbate the dysregulation of appetite and reward circuitry. *C-TRLs* = cholesterol- and triglyceride-rich apoB-containing remnant lipoproteins; *MMPs* = matrix metalloproteinases; *NSAPP* = a control node that regulates balanced insulin signaling and comprises N̲OX4, S̲OD3, A̲QP3, P̲TEN, and protein-tyrosine phosphatases; *PAI1* = plasminogen activator inhibitor-1; *VLDL1* = very-low density lipoprotein-1. (Adapted with permission from Williams KJ, Wu X. Imbalanced insulin action in chronic over nutrition: Clinical harm, molecular mechanisms, and a way forward. *Atherosclerosis* 2016;247:225–282.)

develop an imbalance amongst the actions of insulin. For example, overnutrition and obesity impair insulin's ability to increase blood flow into muscle, drive glucose uptake into skeletal myocytes, and block postprandial hepatic glucose production. However, insulin still stimulates hepatic lipogenesis, which contributes to development of fatty liver and hypertriglyceridemia. Insulin-induced activation of ERK continues unimpaired, and drives vasoconstriction via endothelin-1, mitogenesis, and possibly contributing to hypertension and cancer risk. This constellation of effects has been called **pathway-selective insulin resistance and responsiveness (SEIRR)**.

To control plasma glucose concentrations, patients with SEIRR become hyperinsulinemic, either from pancreatic overproduction of endogenous insulin or from therapeutic administration of large amounts of exogenous insulin. *Raising insulin levels cannot make these individuals metabolically normal,* **even if they achieve normoglycemia,** *because hyperinsulinemia drives lipid synthesis in the liver and the ERK MAP kinase to become overactive.*

These irregularities in insulin action in target tissues and compensatory hyperinsulinemia are closely tied to a diverse set of cardiovascular risk factors in obese, sedentary people, and patients with type 2 ("adult onset") diabetes mellitus. These risk factors, together called **metabolic syndrome** or **the atherometabolic syndrome**, include: (1) abdominal adiposity with increased waist circumference; (2) mild hypertension (perhaps related to failure of endothelium-dependent vascular relaxation, sympathetic overactivation, and renal salt retention); (3) high fasting plasma glucose levels; and (4) atherogenic dyslipoproteinemia with elevated fasting and nonfasting plasma triglycerides and low plasma HDL cholesterol (Fig. 13-5 and Table 13-1).

As well as we can describe the metabolic branches affected in obesity and overnutrition, the biochemical triggers remain elusive. There are several hypotheses which explain part of the equation but do not (at least, not yet) provide adequate overall understanding of how this all comes about. These hypotheses include:

- **Lipotoxicity**, which postulates that nonesterified fatty acids (NEFAs) activate PKC signaling and block insulin receptor signaling.
- **Maladaptive inflammation**, which suggests that elevated levels of proinflammatory cytokines induce insulin resistance.
- **ER stress**, in which the ER is activated by unfolded protein responses to impair insulin signaling.
- **NSAPP pathway** activation, that proposes that a recently discovered NADPH-related pathway that is triggered by insulin is impaired during SEIRR.

These pathways, or others as yet unknown, may participate in various aspects of the pathogenesis of SEIRR. But, to date, how obesity and excessive energy intake lead to metabolic syndrome is not clear.

Complications of Overnutrition and Obesity Affect Most Organ Systems

Many epidemiologic studies have shown that obesity and central adiposity correlate with increased morbidity and

TABLE 13-1
FREQUENTLY OBSERVED CONCOMITANTS OF THE METABOLIC SYNDROME
Clinical Signs
Central (visceral–abdominal) obesity with increased waist circumference
Acanthosis nigricans (hypertrophic, hyperpigmented skin changes)
Laboratory Abnormalities
Elevated fasting and/or postprandial glucose
Insulin resistance for handling glucose, with hyperinsulinemia, but continued responsiveness—and hence overactivity—of other pathways downstream of the insulin receptor
Dyslipidemia characterized by increased plasma concentrations of cholesterol- and triglyceride-rich apoB-containing lipoproteins (C-TRLs) and low concentrations of high-density lipoprotein cholesterol (HDLc)
Hypercoagulability and abnormal thrombolysis
Hyperuricemia
Endothelial and vascular smooth muscle dysfunction
Albuminuria
Comorbid Illnesses
Hypertension
Atherosclerosis
Hyperandrogenism with polycystic ovary syndrome

premature mortality (Fig. 13-6). Fat cells undergo both hyperplasia and hypertrophy. The surplus energy from kcal intake and kcal expenditure is stored in adipocytes that enlarge and/or increase in number: Extremely obese adults can have four times as many adipocytes, each containing twice as much lipid, as a lean adult.

Endocrine Complications

- **T2DM:** This disorder (see below) is strongly associated with obesity: Over 80% of cases of T2DM are attributed to obesity. Risk of diabetes increases linearly with BMI and with increments in abdominal fat mass or waist circumference at any given BMI. Conversely, weight loss and exercise decrease risk of T2DM and can prevent insulin resistance for handling glucose from progressing to frank diabetes. In a large American population with impaired glucose tolerance, simply walking briskly for 150 minutes per week and losing 7% of body weight reduced the progression to overt T2DM by 58%. More drastic measures for morbid obesity (e.g., decreased caloric intake, weight loss surgery) led to complete resolution of diabetes in 77% of patients. Thus, these harmful effects appear reversible in many patients.
- **Atherogenic dyslipidemia and dyslipoproteinemia:** By far, the major killer in obesity and diabetes is

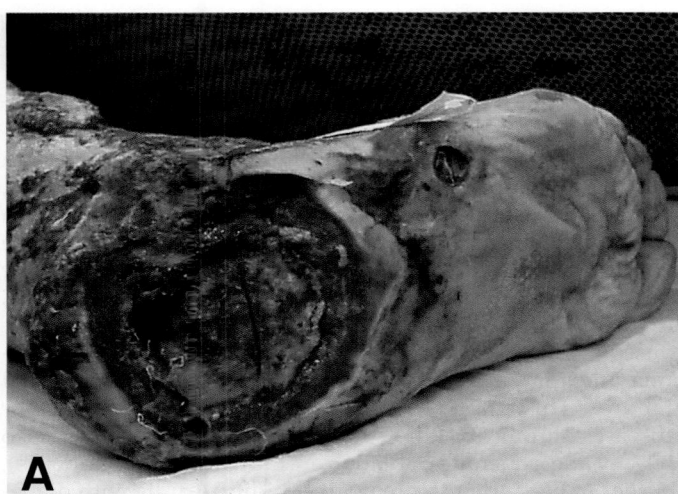
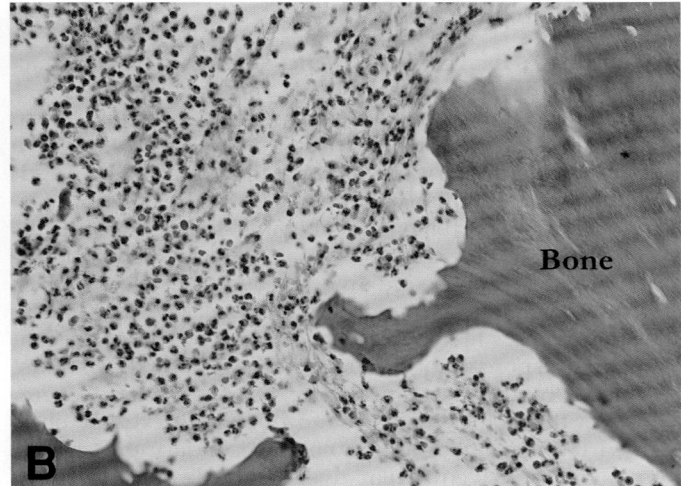

FIGURE 13-6. A: Most nontraumatic limb amputations in the United States are due to diabetes. Gangrene, secondary to ischemia resulting from diabetic macrovascular disease is the major factor, but diabetic neuropathies (leading to Charcot joint), as well as an enhanced susceptibility to infection, also play a role. **B:** Osteomyelitis secondary to bacterial infection, particularly in the lower extremities, is a major complication of diabetes. In the acute phase, the marrow space is filled with pus (neutrophils). With time, osteoclastic bone resorption creates "bitten (or scalloped) bone."

atherosclerotic cardiovascular disease (ASCVD). Several harmful plasma lipid and lipoprotein abnormalities often complicate obesity, including elevated fasting levels of cholesterol- and triglyceride-rich apolipoprotein-B (apoB)-containing lipoproteins (C-TRLs) and reduced high-density lipoprotein (HDL). These abnormalities are strongly associated with increased risk of cardiovascular disease, particularly in people with central adiposity. Although studies do not support a direct role for HDL in protecting people from ASCVD, low plasma HDL concentrations now appear to be a marker of elevated C-TRLs. In addition, nonfasting plasma triglyceride levels—which reflect persistence of a particular class of harmful C-TRLs, called remnants—independently predict subsequent heart attacks and strokes. Remnants circulate after each meal or snack. Like low-density lipoprotein (LDL), remnant particles contain apoB, can become trapped within arterial walls, and initiate and accelerate atherosclerotic vascular disease (see Chapter 16). As prevalence of obesity increases, dyslipoproteinemias other than simple elevations in plasma LDL cholesterol have become better recognized as contributors to population-wide cardiovascular risk. Clinically, plasma levels of non-HDL cholesterol (total cholesterol minus HDL cholesterol) and apoB predict ASCVD risk better than LDL cholesterol, because they capture LDL and C-TRLs together. Recent data show that lowering plasma triglycerides in statin-treated patients reduced ASCVD events. Ongoing clinical trials are testing agents to lower plasma concentrations of C-TRLs.

■ **Other endocrine complications:** Obesity is also associated with polycystic ovary syndrome, irregular menses, amenorrhea, infertility, and hypogonadism.

Cardiovascular Complications

■ **Hypertension:** Obesity entails a high risk of hypertension and is associated with heightened sympathetic activity. High insulin levels in obese patients with SEIRR act on pathways unrelated to glucose importation (see above),

including enhanced renal reabsorption of sodium, which contributes to hypertension, and endothelial production of endothelin-1, a vasoconstrictor mentioned above (Fig. 13-5). Obese adipose tissue also secretes substances that directly cause vasoconstriction and increase blood pressure, including angiotensin II and its precursors. Obesity therefore makes hypertension more difficult to control. Even a small reduction in weight may decrease blood pressure in this population.

■ **Coronary heart disease:** BMI has a graded association with myocardial infarction, but body fat distribution is a better indicator of risk. Dyslipoproteinemia and hypertension are the best predictors of ASCVD linked to obesity. Recent work shows that clinical control of five major factors (elevated glycated hemoglobin level, elevated plasma LDL cholesterol level, albuminuria, smoking, and elevated blood pressure) in patients with T2DM brings their risk of premature death, myocardial infarction, and stroke down to levels seen in the general nondiabetic population.

■ **Congestive heart failure:** Obesity and diabetes are associated with increased risk of heart failure. Heart failure with reduced ejection fraction occurs most often after a heart attack and loss of living myocardium. Heart failure with preserved ejection fraction may be related to cardiac fibrosis, diabetic intracardiac microvascular disease, and diabetic autonomic neuropathy. In addition, the combination of obesity and hypertension leads to ventricular wall thickening and larger heart volume. Obese patients are also at increased risk of atrial fibrillation and atrial flutter. Unfortunately, control of the same five factors mentioned above to manage ASCVD risk does not reduce heart failure in patients with T2DM. Major predictors of heart failure in diabetes include high BMI, sedentary lifestyle, and atrial fibrillation.

■ **Thromboembolic disease:** Deep venous thromboses and pulmonary embolism are more common in obese patients. Lower-extremity venous thromboembolic disease may be related to increased abdominal pressure, impaired fibrinolysis, and increased circulating cytokines, particularly with abdominal obesity.

Additional Complications of Obesity

- **Neurologic:** Increasing BMI increases risk of ischemic strokes.
- **Pulmonary:** Obesity may interfere mechanically with lung function. Obesity, especially abdominal obesity, decreases ventilatory drive, respiratory compliance, and ventilation, particularly at lung bases. It thus contributes to ventilation–perfusion mismatching. Obesity is a major risk factor for obstructive sleep apnea, in which patients are prone to apnea and hypopnea during sleep. Obesity hypoventilation syndrome is decreased ventilatory responsiveness to hypercapnia or hypoxia. This condition impairs responses to the increased ventilatory demands imposed by the mechanical effects of obesity. The severe form of this is Pickwickian syndrome, with extreme obesity, irregular breathing, cyanosis, secondary polycythemia, and right ventricular dysfunction leading to fixed pulmonary hypertension.
- **Hepatobiliary:** Obese people, particularly women, suffer from an increased incidence of gallstones. Interestingly, weight loss may also precipitate gallstones owing to increased cholesterol supersaturation in bile, enhanced cholesterol crystal nucleation, and decreased gallbladder contractility. Nonalcoholic fatty liver disease (NAFLD), with increased liver enzymes, hepatomegaly and altered liver histology, may also complicate obesity. Fat accumulates within hepatocytes (steatosis, see Chapter 20), and some patients progress to nonalcoholic steatohepatitis (NASH). Maladaptive inflammatory changes within the liver can lead to fibrosis, cirrhosis, and portal hypertension. NASH is the leading cause of the so-called "idiopathic" cirrhosis.
- **Gastrointestinal:** Gastroesophageal reflux is more common in obese individuals.
- **Cancer:** Certain cancers occur with greater frequency in people who are obese. Specifically, risks of esophageal, gallbladder, pancreatic, breast, renal, endometrial, cervical, and prostate cancers are all increased. Once a cancer is diagnosed, obesity is associated with a worse prognosis. It has been suggested that activation of ERK may provide a mitogenic stimulus that predisposes obese individuals to certain tumors (Fig. 13-5). Obesity has also been associated with overexpression of aromatase in adipose tissue within the breast, local production of estrogen, and increased breast cancer risk.
- **Musculoskeletal:** Hyperuricemia and gout are more common in obese people. Obesity increases the risk of osteoarthritis, particularly of weight-bearing joints such as the knees. However, non–weight-bearing joints may also be affected, suggesting mechanisms beyond increased mechanical load. Weight loss decreases the risk of osteoarthritis.
- **Skin:** Obesity causes striae—ribbon-like epidermal stretching and thinning. Acanthosis nigricans is a velvety, hypertrophic, hyperpigmented lesion, especially at skinfold areas (axillae, nape of the neck). It may be a response to high circulating insulin levels in obese individuals with insulin resistance for handling glucose. Excessive hair growth, hirsutism, can result from increases in circulating androgens in susceptible women.
- **Psychological and social:** Obesity has also been associated with worse quality of life, increased sick leave absences, and disability claims and depression (Fig. 13-1).

Diabetes Mellitus

Almost a century ago, the noted physician Sir William Osler defined diabetes mellitus as "a syndrome due to a disturbance in carbohydrate metabolism from various causes, in which sugar appears in the urine, associated with thirst, polyuria, wasting and imperfect oxidation of fats." With the advent of insulin and other therapeutic agents, these extreme features are unusual in properly managed diabetic patients. Long-term consequences persist, however. Hence, diabetes mellitus has become "a state of premature cardiovascular death that is associated with chronic hyperglycemia and may also be associated with blindness and renal failure." This emphasis reflects the fact that cardiovascular disease continues to kill ~70% of these patients (compared to 50% of the general population in industrialized countries), earlier in life and with greater morbidity. Adults with diabetes are two to four times more likely to have heart disease or a stroke than adults without diabetes.

TYPES OF DIABETES

The two major forms of diabetes have different underlying pathophysiologies. **Type 1 diabetes mellitus (T1DM)** (formerly, **insulin-dependent [IDDM]** or **juvenile-onset diabetes)** is caused by autoimmune destruction of insulin-producing pancreatic β-cells in the islets of Langerhans. In the United States, it affects about 5% of diabetic patients (5% to 10% globally).

T2DM (previously called **non–insulin-dependent [NIDDM]** or **maturity-onset diabetes**) is usually associated with obesity. It reflects target tissue resistance to insulin actions on glucose metabolism, but paradoxical responsiveness of the same tissues to other actions of insulin (see above). Oversecretion of insulin may, or may not, be sufficient to control plasma glucose concentrations. In other words, T1DM is a syndrome of frank insulin deficiency, while in T2DM, target tissues fail to respond normally to insulin, and oversecretion causes hyperinsulinemia (Table 13-2).

There are other forms of diabetes mellitus. **Gestational diabetes** develops in a percentage of pregnant women, because of resistance to the glucose-lowering actions of insulin in pregnancy, combined with a β-cell defect. It almost always abates after parturition.

Diabetes can also occur secondary to other endocrine conditions or drug therapy, especially in settings of glucocorticoid excess. Other rare genetic syndromes, such as **maturity-onset diabetes of the young (MODY)**, are associated with abnormal glucose metabolism or overt hyperglycemia, but the etiologies differ from the more common forms of diabetes, and so these syndromes are considered only briefly below (Table 13-3).

Ketosis-prone type 2 diabetes mellitus (KPD) was originally described in sub-Saharan African and in African-American patients, predominantly men, who presented with ketosis which resolved shortly after the acute episode. Glucotoxicity or lipotoxicity cause severe, acute, *reversible* insulin deficiency. The precise classification of KPD is controversial (Table 13-3).

Abnormal levels of blood glucose or glycated hemoglobin (hemoglobin A_{1c}) correlate with the chronic complications of diabetes. In particular, long-standing hyperglycemia

TABLE 13-2

COMPARISON OF TYPE 1 AND TYPE 2 DIABETES MELLITUS

	Type 1 Diabetes	Type 2 Diabetes
Age at onset	Half before age 30; half at age 30 or above	Usually after 30
Type of onset	Abrupt; symptomatic (polyuria, polydipsia, dehydration); often severe with ketoacidosis	Gradual; usually subtle; often asymptomatic
Usual body weight	Normal; recent weight loss is common	Overweight
Family history	<20%	>60%
Monozygotic twins	50% concordant	90% concordant
HLA associations	Yes	No
Antibodies to islet cell antigens (insulin, glutamic acid decarboxylase [GAD-65], IA-2, zinc transporter ZnT8)	Yes	No
Islet lesions	Early—inflammation Late—atrophy and fibrosis	Late—fibrosis, amyloid
β-cell mass	Markedly reduced	Normal or slightly reduced
Circulating insulin level	Markedly reduced	Early—elevated insulin concentrations from compensatory pancreatic oversecretion Late—decline in endogenous insulin concentration due to progressive β-cell dysfunction
Insulin resistance for handling glucose (Selective resistance to the glucose-lowering actions of insulin)	Absent	Present
Clinical management	Administration of exogenous insulin absolutely required	Exogenous insulin usually not needed initially; insulin supplementation may be needed at later stages; weight loss typically improves the condition; substantial weight loss such as after bariatric surgery often produces remission of T2DM, defined as normoglycemia off all anti-diabetes medications.

HLA = human leukocyte antigen; *IA-2* = islet cell antigen-512.

causes microvascular damage that leads to diabetic retinopathy, neuropathy, and renal glomerular damage. In a younger patient with abrupt onset of hyperglycemia, elevated plasma ketones or frank ketoacidosis, diagnosing T1DM due to absolute insulin deficiency is straightforward. In contrast, T2DM typically evolves gradually over years before it is recognized, most often in an overweight, middle-aged person with a genetic predisposition. Thus, patients with T1DM present early in their disease, long before microvascular complications have developed, while many T2DM patients are usually first recognized only after years of hyperglycemia, and may already have microvascular damage.

Recent American Diabetes Association recommendations suggest any of four diagnostic criteria (Table 13-4). One of these must be present for the diagnosis, but some criteria need confirmation by repeat testing. The ADA also recognizes three categories of increased risk for diabetes (Table 13-5). Some of these are often termed "prediabetes," but only half of such patients will ultimately develop diabetes.

TYPE 2 DIABETES MELLITUS

T2DM Entails Paradoxical Responsiveness and Unresponsiveness to Insulin

Tissues show reduced tissue sensitivity to insulin's glucose-lowering effects, but remain responsive to many other actions of insulin. Compensatory pancreatic oversecretion of insulin eventually becomes inadequate to control plasma glucose concentrations.

T2DM usually develops in adults, with an increased prevalence in obese and elderly people. Recently, it has been appearing increasingly in younger adults and adolescents, as obesity and inactivity among younger people increase. *Hyperglycemia in T2DM reflects the failure of the β-cells to overcome the body's increased resistance to insulin's glucose-lowering actions.* Compared to lean non-diabetics, however, patients with early T2DM are hyperinsulinemic, but their abnormally high insulin levels fail to control their

TABLE 13-3

ETIOLOGIC CLASSIFICATION OF DIABETES MELLITUS[a]

I. Type 1 diabetes (due to autoimmune β-cell destruction, usually leading to absolute insulin deficiency)
- A. Immune mediated
- B. Idiopathic

II. Type 2 diabetes (due to a progressive loss of β-cell insulin hypersecretion frequently on the background of insulin resistance for handling glucose)

III. Specific types of diabetes due to other causes
- Genetic defects of β-cell function (e.g., MODY)
- Genetic defects in insulin action (e.g., type A insulin resistance, which can be caused by mutations in the insulin receptor and typically impairs all downstream actions of insulin together, i.e., these individuals typically do not develop fatty liver owing to overactive hepatic de-novo lipogenesis)
- Diseases of the exocrine pancreas that cause collateral damage to the endocrine pancreas; also pancreatic surgery (e.g., Whipple procedure, also called pancreaticoduodenectomy)
- Endocrinopathies (e.g., Cushing disease, acromegaly, etc.)
- Drug or chemical induced (e.g., glucocorticoids)
- Infections (e.g., cytomegalovirus, rubella)
- Uncommon forms of immune-mediated diabetes (e.g., "stiff-man syndrome")
- Other genetic syndromes (e.g., Turner syndrome, Down syndrome)

IV. Gestational diabetes mellitus (diabetes diagnosed in the second or third trimester of pregnancy in a patient who did not have clear overt diabetes before gestation)

[a]Ketosis-prone type 2 diabetes (KPD) is a unique presentation with features of both T1DM and T2DM. Patients present in ketosis, but can stop exogenous insulin therapy shortly after the acute episode. It is most common in individuals of sub-Saharan African ancestry, but occurs in many other racial/ethnic groups as well. Whether KPD deserves a separate category is still being actively debated. See the text for further details.

Adapted from Classification and Diagnosis of Diabetes. Standards of Medical Care in Diabetes—2018. *Diabetes Care.* 2018;41(Supplement 1):S13.

blood sugar. When they receive exogenous insulin, their daily doses are much higher than in lean T1DM (insulin-deficient) patients. Because a number of insulin actions in obesity, prediabetes and T2DM still remain responsive, such as ERK activation and hepatic *de novo* lipogenesis, the hyperinsulinemia that occurs in these patients may be harmful (Fig. 13-5).

 EPIDEMIOLOGY: As of 2017, there were about 30.3 million Americans with T2DM (12.2% of those older than 18), about a quarter of whom are undiagnosed. About 25% of people older than 65 have diabetes. An additional 84 million Americans above 18 (33.9%) are estimated to have prediabetes. In the United States, obesity and T2DM are most prevalent in women, lower socioeconomic strata, and all nonwhite ethnic groups.

Diabetes is also increasing worldwide. The International Diabetes Federation, estimated in 2017 that ≈425 million people have diabetes (5.7% of total world population). For people 20 to 79 years old, T2DM prevalence rates vary: 10.9% in China, 5.2% in Ethiopia, 18% in Saudi Arabia, 8.9% in Mexico, and 8.7% in Brazil. In China,

TABLE 13-4

CRITERIA FOR THE DIAGNOSIS OF DIABETES

1. Fasting plasma glucose (FPG) ≥126 mg/dL (7.0 mmol/L). Fasting is defined as no caloric intake for at least 8 hours.[a]

OR

2. 2-hour plasma glucose ≥200 mg/dL (11.1 mmol/L) during oral glucose tolerance test (OGTT). The OGTT should be performed as described by the WHO, using a glucose load containing the equivalent of 75-g anhydrous glucose dissolved in water.[a]

OR

3. Hemoglobin A$_{1c}$ (HbA$_{1c}$) ≥6.5% (48 mmol/mol). The test should be performed in a laboratory using a method that is NGSP certified and standardized to the DCCT assay.[a]

OR

4. In a patient with classic symptoms of hyperglycemia or hyperglycemic crisis, a random plasma glucose ≥200 mg/dL (11.1 mmol/L)

[a]In the absence of unequivocal hyperglycemia, criteria 1–3 should be confirmed by repeat testing.

Modified from American Diabetes Association. Classification and diagnosis of diabetes: Standards of Medical Care in Diabetes—2018. *Diabetes Care.* 2018;41(Suppl 1):S13–S27. Copyright and all rights reserved. Material from this publication has been used with the permission of American Diabetes Association.

India, and Africa, unlike North America, obesity and T2DM are most prevalent among the wealthy.

Diabetes is the leading cause of kidney failure, non-traumatic lower limb amputations, and a common cause of osteomyelitis (Fig. 13-6A,B) and new cases of blindness among adults in the United States. It is also a major contributor to heart disease and stroke, as well as the seventh leading cause of death in the United States. Prevalence of diabetes in the United States has increased dramatically between 1994 and 2010, mostly related to obesity (Fig. 13-7).

T2DM Is a Two-Hit Disease

T2DM parallels obesity and metabolic syndrome for much of its evolution. Therefore, the discussion below necessarily overlaps in part the prior section.

TABLE 13-5

CATEGORIES OF INCREASED RISK FOR DIABETES (ALSO CALLED "PREDIABETES")[a]

Fasting plasma glucose (FPG) of 100 mg/dL (5.6 mmol/L) to 125 mg/dL (6.9 mmol/L) (also called impaired fasting glucose or IFG)

2-h plasma glucose in the 75-g OGTT of 140 mg/dL (7.8 mmol/L) to 199 mg/dL (11.0 mmol/L) (also called impaired glucose tolerance, IGT)

HbA$_{1c}$ of 5.7%–6.4%

[a]For all three tests, risk is continuous, extending below the lower limit of the range and becoming disproportionately greater at the higher ends of the range.

Modified from American Diabetes Association. Classification and diagnosis of diabetes: Standards of Medical Care in Diabetes—2018. *Diabetes Care.* 2018;41(Suppl 1):S13–S27. Copyright and all rights reserved. Material from this publication has been used with the permission of American Diabetes Association.

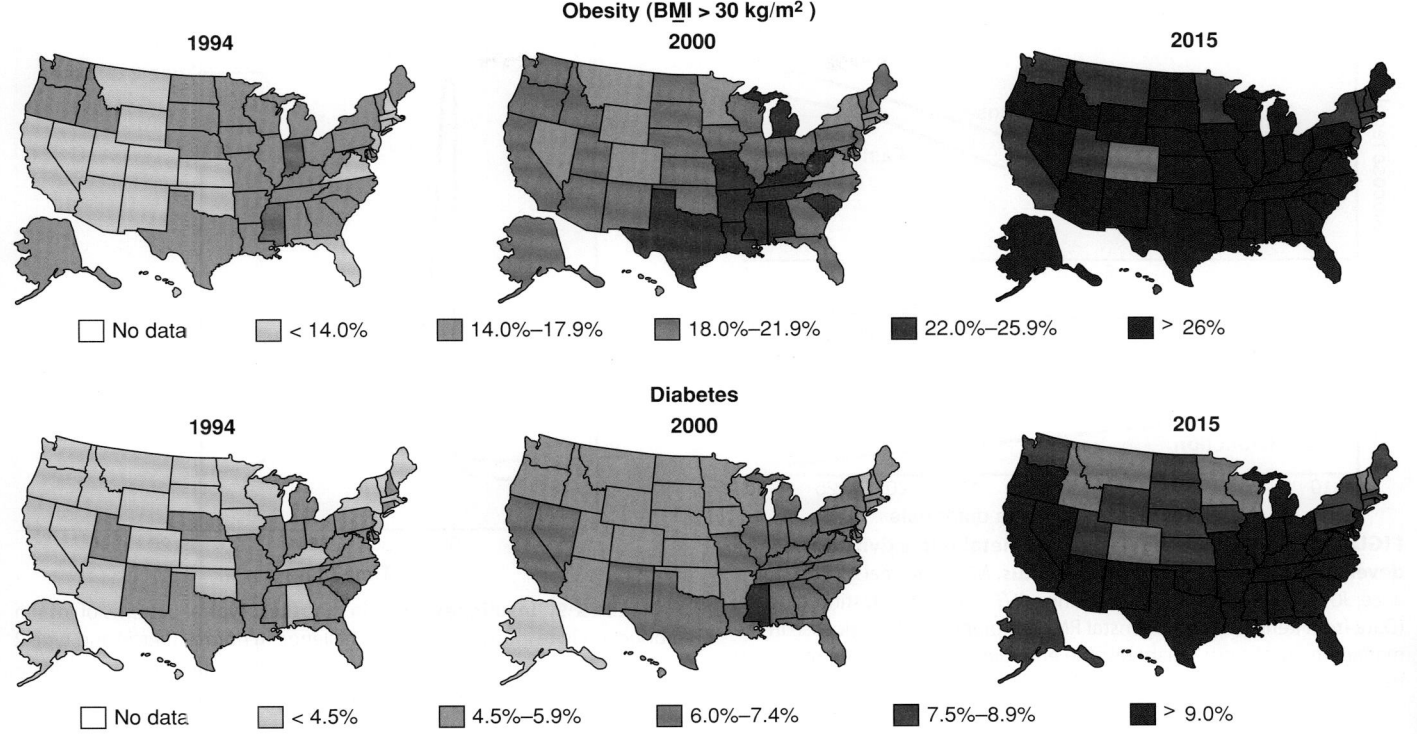

FIGURE 13-7. **Prevalence of diabetes and obesity in the United States.** (Data from the Centers for Disease Control and Prevention, 2017.)

PATHOPHYSIOLOGY: The first "hit" is resistance to glucose-lowering actions of insulin in its metabolic target tissues (liver, skeletal muscle, adipose tissue, and others). This defect alone evokes increased total pancreatic output of insulin, causing hyperinsulinemia. Because many other actions of insulin remain fully active, as noted above, this pattern reflects unbalanced (or imbalanced) insulin action (see Fig. 13-5). Through the ERK signaling pathway, which remains responsive to insulin, hyperinsulinemia may increase cell proliferation and cancer risk; sodium retention by the kidney; sympathetic activation; and abnormal vasoconstriction to contribute to hypertension (see above). By stimulating hepatic *de novo* lipogenesis, hyperinsulinemia contributes to NAFLD and an atherogenic dyslipoproteinemia, steatohepatitis (NASH) and cirrhosis. This constellation is "metabolic" or "atherometabolic" syndrome (see above), which occurs often in overt T2DM and also in prediabetes (see Fig. 13-5).

The second "hit" in T2DM occurs when the pancreas can no longer compensate for the highly increased demand for insulin to control blood sugar levels. Degenerative changes in the pancreatic islet occur often in these patients. Prediabetes and overt T2DM evolve most often in patients with both of these hits (see Fig. 13-5).

As described above, insulin resistance for glucose in states of chronic overnutrition, underexertion, and obesity, normal insulin control of glucose metabolism is impaired. Initially, this impairment is subclinical. In time, fasting glucose and/or glucose tolerance become abnormal. When frank hyperglycemia sets in, T2DM can be diagnosed (Fig. 13-8). Hepatic glucose production

increases, but glucose uptake by peripheral tissues, primarily muscles and adipose tissue decreases.

By itself, insulin resistance for handling glucose rarely causes T2DM, because increased insulin secretion (hyperinsulinism) by β-cells compensates for defects in insulin action and prevents blood glucose levels from rising. It is only when the β-cells can no longer keep up with this high demand that blood glucose levels start to increase (Fig. 13-8). In many patients with obesity and prediabetes, subclinical β-cell dysfunction can appear before overt diabetes.

β-CELL DYSFUNCTION: In the first phase, which may precede overt glucose intolerance, insulin secretion after glucose stimulation is diminished (Fig. 13-9). In the second phase, release of newly synthesized insulin is impaired, due to paradoxical inhibition of insulin release by glucose, and sometimes occurs with high blood glucose levels ("glucose toxicity"). In some patients, this can be reversed by restoring normoglycemia.

THE ROLE OF INCRETINS: An oral glucose load stimulates significantly more insulin secretion than does a comparable intravenous glucose infusion. This discrepancy (Fig. 13-10A) is due to peptides (incretins) secreted by the gut in response to meals. Incretins, mainly **glucose-dependent insulinotropic peptide (GIP)** and **glucagon-like peptide-1 (GLP1)**, act to: (1) enhance glucose-dependent stimulation of insulin secretion by β-cells; (2) inhibit glucagon secretion by α-cells; (3) inhibit appetite; and (4) slow gastric emptying. Incretins are rapidly inactivated in the circulation by dipeptidyl peptidase 4 (DPP4).

In patients with T2DM, the incretin effect is markedly reduced (Fig. 13-10B), which has been attributed to

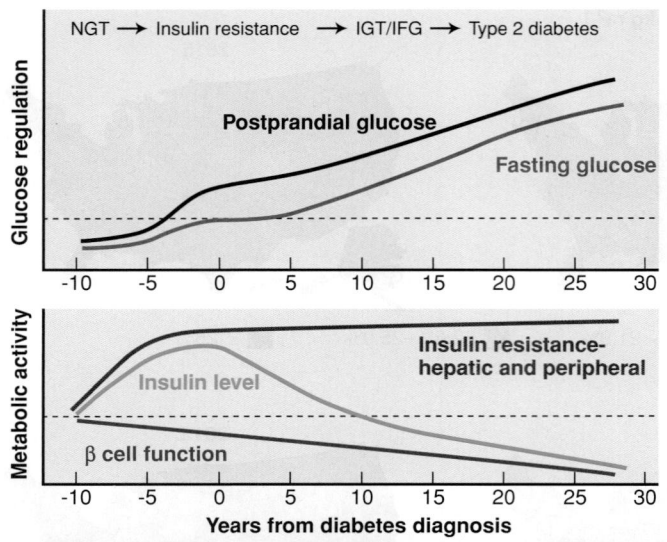

FIGURE 13-8. Glucose regulation and metabolic activity during the development of type 2 diabetes mellitus. *NGT* = normal glucose tolerance; *IGT* = impaired glucose tolerance; *IFG* = impaired fasting glucose. (Data from Kendall DM, Bergenstal RM. Postprandial blood glucose in the management of type 2 diabetes: the emerging role of incretin mimetics: the role of PPG in type 2 diabetes. *Medscape Diabetes*. 2005;7[2].)

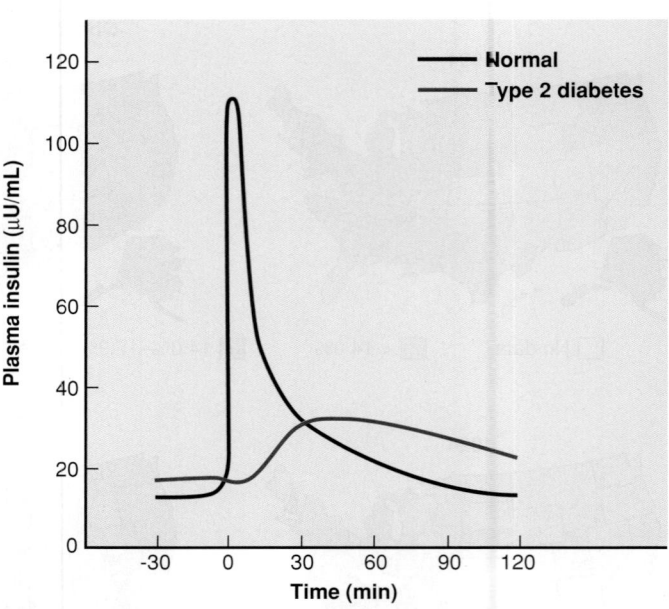

FIGURE 13-9. Insulin response in diabetes. Typical patterns of insulin production in response to glucose challenge in normal (*black*) and type 2 diabetic (*red*) patients. (Redrawn from Pfeifer MA, Halter JB, Porte D. Insulin secretion in diabetes mellitus. *Am J Med*. 1981;70:579–588.)

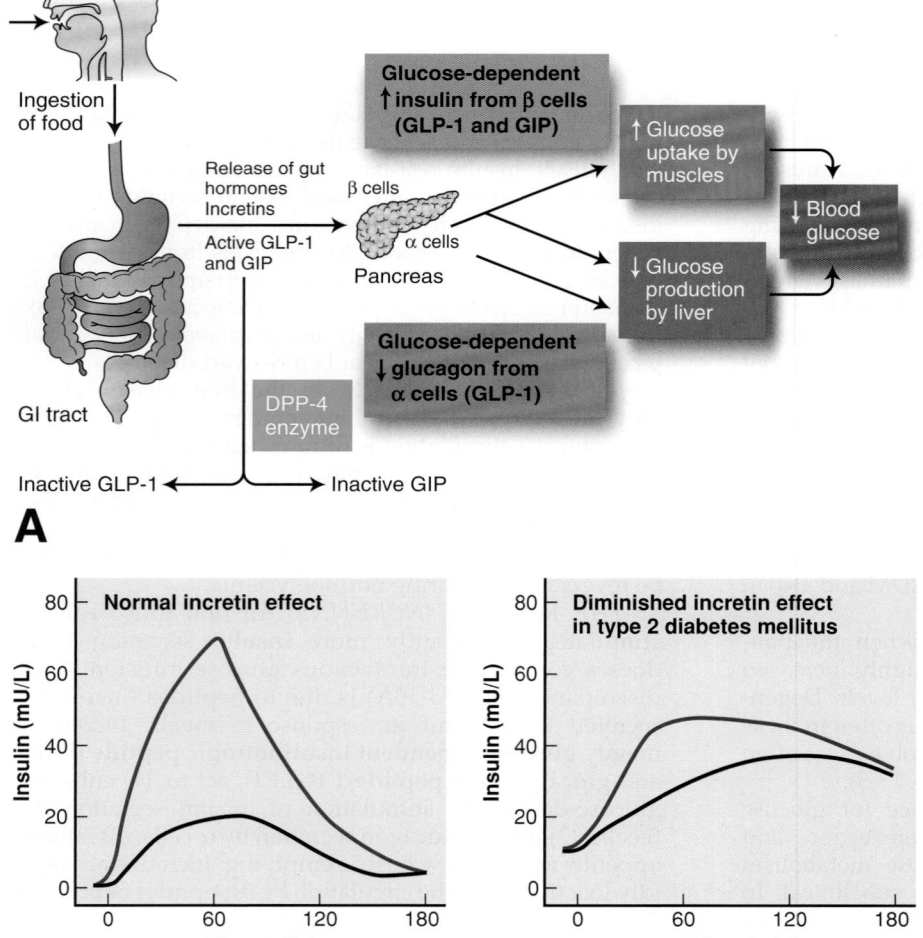

FIGURE 13-10. Incretins. A: Physiologic roles of incretins in glucose metabolism. Involvement of incretins in regulating the responses of the body to a caloric load. *GIP* = glucose-dependent insulinotropic peptide; *GLP-1* = glucagon-like peptide-1. **B:** Diminished incretin responsiveness in type 2 diabetes mellitus.

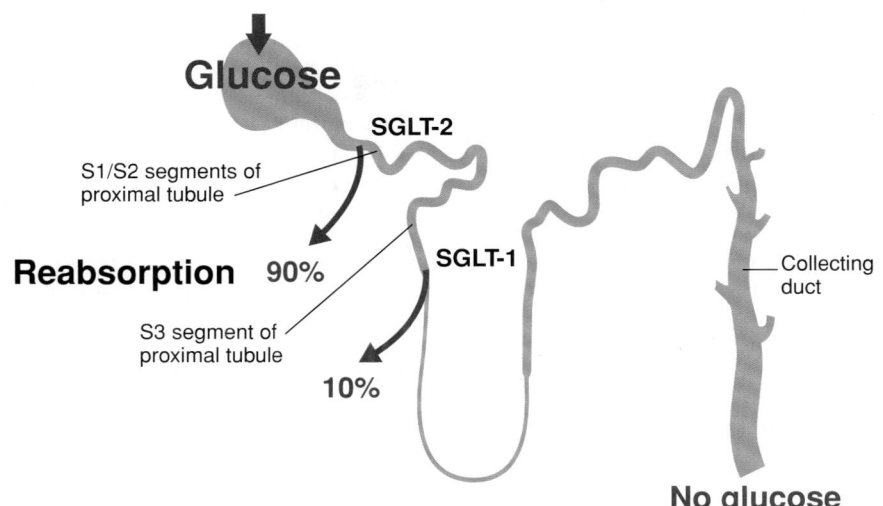

FIGURE 13-11.　Renal glucose handling.

impaired GLP-1 and GIP secretion. How these changes in incretins affect the pathogenesis of T2DM has not yet been clarified.

THE KIDNEY AND GLUCOSE HOMEOSTASIS: In spite of the daily fluctuations in the supply of glucose and the body's need for it, homeostatic mechanisms maintain plasma glucose levels within a narrow range of about 90–100 mg/dL. Besides the liver, the kidney supplies glucose during fasting. The renal-contribution to gluconeogenesis is about 15 to 55 g/day (20% to 25% of the glucose released into the circulation after an overnight fast).

The kidney mainly influences glucose homeostasis by reabsorbing glucose from the glomerular filtrate. In healthy individuals, renal proximal convoluted tubules (PCT) reabsorb essentially all of the (about) 180 g of glucose that it filters daily via two isoforms of the renal sodium-glucose cotransporter (SGLT). SGLT2, in S1 and S2 segments of the PCT, has a high capacity but low affinity for glucose transport, and normally reabsorbs ≈90% of filtered glucose (Fig. 13-11). SGLT1 is a low-capacity, high-affinity glucose transporter in the S3 segment and reabsorbs the remaining 10% of filtered glucose. This active glucose transport is coupled to the downhill sodium transport, which, in turn, requires active sodium extrusion across the basolateral surface into the intracellular fluid (Fig. 13-12). Facilitated glucose transporters

(GLUTs) carry glucose across the basolateral membrane by facilitated diffusion.

This SGLT2 mechanism is a therapeutic target: Its inhibition increases glucosuria and so improves blood glucose levels. SGLT2 inhibitors can also facilitate small amounts of weight loss through the renal caloric leak, which is only partially compensated by increased appetite.

Risk Factors

Risk factors clearly associated with T2DM include **over-nutrition, low levels of physical activity, and obesity.** As noted above, risk of T2DM increases linearly with BMI. Most cases of T2DM can be attributed to obesity. Visceral–abdominal obesity ("apple shaped") is more associated with insulin resistance for glucose and with T2DM than is gluteal–femoral obesity ("pear shaped"). Accordingly, weight loss through dieting, exercise, and medications like metformin lowers the risk of T2DM and can prevent high-risk individuals from progressing to frank diabetes. Surgical removal of subcutaneous adipose tissue through liposuction or visceral–abdominal adiposity through omentectomy produces no known metabolic benefits.

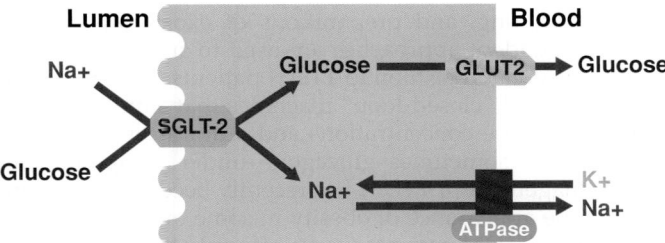

FIGURE 13-12.　SGLT2 normally mediates glucose reabsorption in the kidney. SGLT2 catalyzes the active transport of glucose (against a concentration gradient) across the luminal membrane by coupling it with the downhill transport of Na+. (Modified from Chao EC. SGLT-2 inhibitors: A new mechanism for glycemic control. *Clin Diabetes.* 2014;32[1]:4–11. Copyright and all rights reserved. Material from this publication has been used with the permission of American Diabetes Association.)

MOLECULAR PATHOGENESIS: *Polygenic inheritance is a key contributor to the development of T2DM:*

- More than one-third of patients with T2DM have at least one parent with T2DM.
- Among monozygotic twins, concordance for T2DM approaches 100%
- T2DM prevalence among different ethnic groups who live in similar environments varies tremendously
- First-degree relatives of patients with T2DM have significantly higher lifetime risk of T2DM compared with matched subjects without family history.

Despite its high familial prevalence, inheritance of T2DM is complex and probably involves multiple interacting susceptibility genes. As with obesity, monogenic causes of T2DM represent only a small fraction of cases, and commonly inherited polymorphisms individually contribute only small degrees of risk for, or protection from, T2DM. Moreover, all genetic polymorphism identified to date by genome-wide scans of T2DM patients account for only 10% to 18% of inherited risk for T2DM, despite the high heritability of the disorder. Factors such as obesity (which itself has strong genetic determinants, see above), hypertension, and exercise influence T2DM phenotypic expression and complicate genetic analysis

A rare autosomal dominant form of inherited diabetes, MODY, is associated with several gene defects affecting β-cell function, including the gene for glucokinase, which senses glucose metabolism within β-cells, and several mutations in genes that control β-cell development and function. Mutations in these genes, however, do not account for the typical T2DM.

CLINICAL FEATURES: Early in T2DM, insulin resistance for handling glucose and hyperinsulinemia are the predominant presentations. Both can dramatically improve with even modest weight loss and exercise, and lifestyle interventions remain at the center of clinical management. In addition, medication with insulin sensitizing effects are useful in those patients. Metformin is considered an "insulin sensitizer," because it improves glucose uptake by muscle and inhibits hepatic glucose production, although its molecular mechanism of action remains controversial. Thiazolidinediones, a class of PPARγ agonists, also classified as insulin sensitizers, lower insulin requirements and improve fatty liver. Water retention, increased appetite, and other side-effects have led to declines in their use.

Later in the course of diabetes, as β-cell dysfunction sets in, insulin sensitizers alone cannot control T2DM. Other agents such as secretagogues (e.g., sulfonylureas), incretin-based agents (GLP1 receptor agonists, DPP4 inhibitors), SGLT2 inhibitors and, ultimately, exogenous insulin, are needed.

Cardiovascular disease is a major cause of morbidity, and the leading cause of death, in patients with diabetes. Recently, some SGLT2 inhibitors (empagliflozin, canagliflozin, and dapagliflozin) and GLP1 receptor agonists (liraglutide, semaglutide, and dulaglutide) have reportedly reduced the occurrence of major adverse cardiovascular events, though by as yet unclear mechanisms. The former appear mostly to mitigate the effects of heart failure, and the latter help prevent atherosclerosis-related events, though the mechanisms by which both achiever these effects remain unclear.

PATHOLOGY: Microscopic lesions may be found in the islets of Langerhans of many, but not all, patients with T2DM. Unlike T1DM, β-cells are not consistently reduced in T2DM, and no morphologic lesions of these cells have been found by light or electron microscopy.

In some islets, fibrous tissue accumulates, sometimes to such a degree that the islets are obliterated. Islet amyloid is often present (Fig. 13-13), particularly in patients over 60 years old. This type of amyloid is composed of

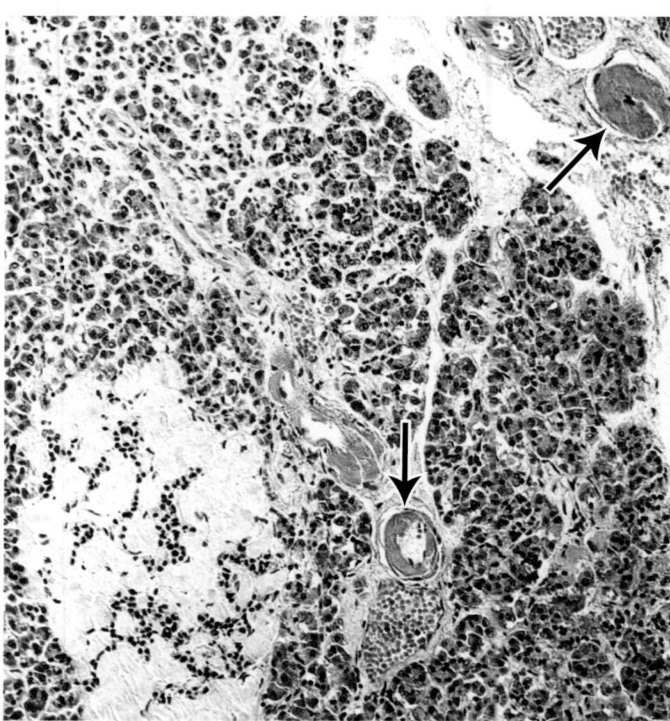

FIGURE 13-13. Amyloid deposition (hyalinization) of an islet in the pancreas of a patient with type 2 diabetes mellitus (*lower left*). Blood vessels adjacent to the islet show the advanced hyaline arteriolosclerosis (*arrows*) characteristic of diabetes.

the polypeptide, amylin, which is secreted with insulin by β-cells. As many as 20% of aged nondiabetics also have amyloid deposits in their pancreas, which finding has been attributed to aging itself (see Chapter 10).

TYPE 1 DIABETES MELLITUS

Unlike T2DM, T1DM Is One-Hit Disease Caused by Autoimmune Destruction of β-Cells

Triggers for this autoimmune reaction are unknown (see below). Because T1DM arises from a deficiency of insulin, rather than complex defects in insulin action, these patients can approach metabolic normalcy by close control of the amounts, timing, and preparations of exogenous insulin. Two independent approaches are used to supply insulin in a highly regulated fashion to T1DM patients: Islet cell transplantation and "closed-loop" machines that simultaneously monitor glucose concentrations and administer exogenous insulin—and sometimes glucagon—under computer control. Management of T1DM has recently become more complex by the appearance of obesity in some of these patients; historically, T1DM patients were uniformly lean.

In T1DM there are few, if any, functional β-cells, and extremely limited or nonexistent insulin secretion. Without insulin, the body switches energy use to a pattern that resembles starvation, regardless of the availability of food. Thus, adipose stores, rather than exogenous glucose, are preferentially metabolized for energy. Oxidation of fat overproduces **ketone bodies** (acetoacetic acid, β-hydroxybutyric

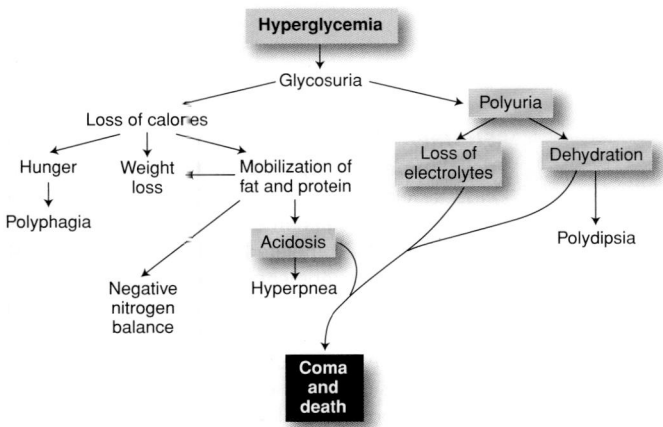

FIGURE 13-14. Symptoms and signs of uncontrolled hyperglycemia in diabetes mellitus.

acid), which are released into the blood from the liver and cause metabolic ketoacidosis. Hyperglycemia results from unsuppressed hepatic glucose output and reduced glucose uptake into skeletal muscle and adipose tissue, and leads to glucosuria and dehydration from loss of body water into glucose-rich urine. If uncorrected, progressive acidosis and dehydration ultimately lead to coma and death (Fig. 13-14).

EPIDEMIOLOGY: Over 1.25 million people in the United States are afflicted with T1DM. Most patients develop T1DM within the first two decades of life, but increasingly, cases are being recognized in older people. Some older patients may present with autoimmune β-cell destruction that developed slowly over many years, which is termed, **latent autoimmune diabetes in adults (LADA)**.

T1DM is most common among northern Europeans and their descendants and occurs less often among Asians, Asian Americans, African Americans, and Native Americans. For example, in Finland T1DM occurs 20 to 40 times more often than in Japan. It can develop at any age, but peak age of onset coincides with puberty. Its incidence increases in late fall and early winter, suggesting a role for seasonal infectious agents as autoimmune triggers (see below).

PATHOPHYSIOLOGY: *AUTOIMMUNITY:* The concept of an autoimmune pathogenesis for T1DM is supported by the observation that pancreatic islets from patients who die shortly after the onset of the disease often shows mild mononuclear infiltration–insulitis (Fig. 13-15). Among the inflammatory cells, CD8+ T-lymphocytes predominate, with some CD4+ cells also present. The infiltrating inflammatory cells also elaborate cytokines like IL-1, IL-6, interferon-α, and NO, which may compound β-cell injury.

Autoantibodies against β-cell components (including insulin) occur in most children newly diagnosed with T1DM. Many patients develop anti-islet cell antibodies months or years *before* insulin production decreases or symptoms appear, a situation called "pre-type 1 diabetes"

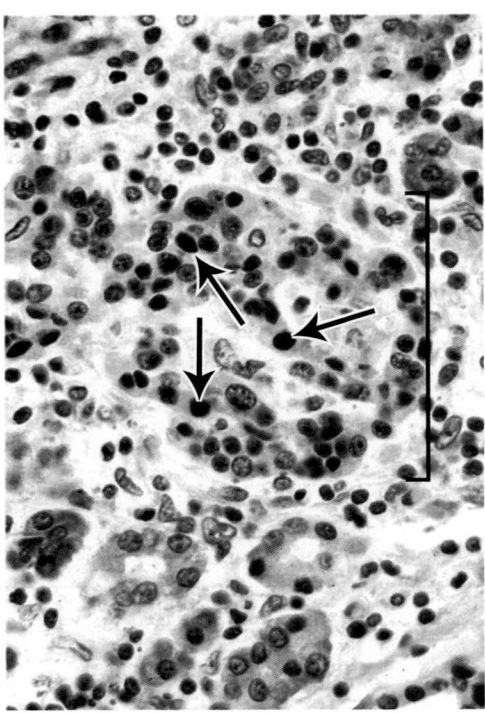

FIGURE 13-15. Insulitis in type 1 diabetes mellitus. A lymphocytic inflammatory infiltrate (*arrows*) is seen in and around the islet (*left of bracket*).

(Fig. 13-16). These autoantibodies are interpreted as responses to antigens released as cell-mediated immune mechanisms destroy β-cells, rather as causing β-cell depletion. Nevertheless, detection of such antibodies is useful—especially in obese patients—for differentiating T1DM, which has an autoimmune basis, from T2DM, which does not.

CELL-MEDIATED IMMUNE MECHANISMS ARE FUNDAMENTAL TO THE PATHOGENESIS OF T1DM: Cytotoxic T-lymphocytes sensitized to β-cells in T1DM persist indefinitely, possibly for a lifetime. Patients transplanted with a donor pancreas or a preparation of purified islets must be treated with immunosuppressive drugs. Of patients with T1DM, 10% show at least one other organ-specific autoimmune disease, including Hashimoto thyroiditis, Graves disease, myasthenia gravis, Addison disease, or pernicious anemia. Interestingly, most patients with polyendocrine immune syndromes (see Chapter 21) are also HLA-DR3 and -DR4 positive.

β-cell destruction in T1DM generally develops slowly over years, and specific stages of the disease have been described (Fig. 13-16). First-degree relatives of patients with T1DM show that antibodies against islet cells are present several years before the disease starts. T1DM with hyperglycemia or ketoacidosis is clinically evident only when ~80% or more of insulin-secreting cells are lost and insulin deprivation is severe.

There are three distinct stages: Stage 1, characterized by autoimmunity and normoglycemia; stage 2 in which there is autoimmunity and mild dysglycemia; and the final stage with new onset symptomatic hyperglycemia establishing the diagnosis of diabetes (Table 13-6).

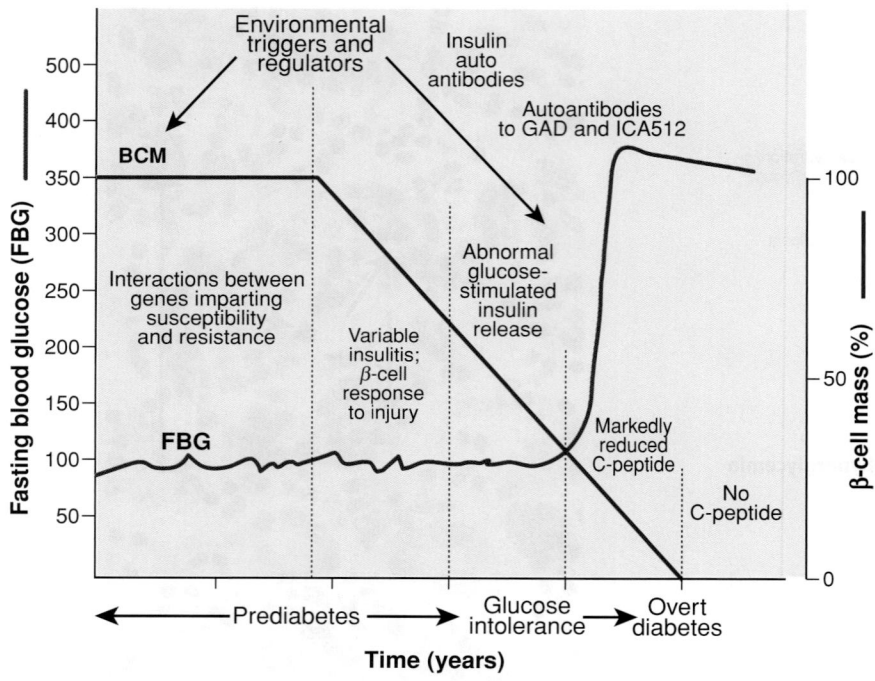

FIGURE 13-16. Pathogenetic stages in the development of type 1 diabetes (T1DM). The disease develops from an initial genetic susceptibility to defective recognition of β-cell epitopes and ends with essentially complete β-cell destruction in most patients. An environmental event is believed to trigger the immune attack, and people with certain genetic markers (human leukocyte antigen [HLA]-DR3 and -DR4) are particularly susceptible to the autoimmune disease. Patients with islet cell antibodies and normal blood glucose levels are considered to have a state of "pre–type 1 diabetes." The rate of decline in β-cell mass (*blue line*) determines the length of time between onset of β-cell destruction and eventual hyperglycemia (*red line*, fasting blood glucose) owing to loss of greater than 90% of functioning β-cells. In the serum, autoantibodies to insulin appear early, followed by antibodies to the β-cell antigen glutamic acid decarboxylase (GAD-65) and the islet cell antigen (ICA-512). *BCM* = β-cell mass.

 MOLECULAR PATHOGENESIS: Evidence for the role of genetic factors in the pathogenesis of T1DM includes:

1. Relatives of people with T1DM have increased risk for development of T1DM. The lifetime risk of T1DM in the US general population is 0.4%, but for first-degree relatives of people with T1DM, it is 3% to 8%. An identical twin has a 30% to 50% risk of developing T1DM once the other twin develops it. Interestingly, children of fathers with T1DM are three times more likely to develop the disease than are children of mothers with T1DM, suggesting genetic imprinting involving paternal susceptibility genes or protective intrauterine or other maternal influences.

2. There are differences in risk among different ethnic groups who live in similar environments, with the highest burden among Caucasians.

3. There is a strong linkage of T1DM to the highly polymorphic HLA class II antigens—DR and DQ—on chromosome 6. There are many high- and low-risk HLA alleles. For example, only 45% of the US population expresses DR3 or DR4, but 95% of those who develop T1DM carry these haplotypes. Because HLA molecules participate in antigen presentation, such HLA linkage and association is consistent with an autoimmune component in T1DM.

4. Many other independent chromosomal regions (several of them non-HLA) have been associated with susceptibility to T1DM.

TABLE 13-6
STAGING OF TYPE 1 DIABETES

	Stage 1	Stage 2	Stage 3
Characteristics	• Autoimmunity • Normoglycemia • Presymptomatic	• Autoimmunity • Dysglycemia • Presymptomatic	• New-onset hyperglycemia • Symptomatic
Diagnostic criteria	• Multiple autoantibodies • No IGT or IFG	• Multiple autoantibodies • Dysglycemia: IFG and/or IGT • FPG 100–125 mg/dL (5.6–6.9 mmol/L) • 2-h PG 140–199 mg/dL (7.8–11.0 mmol/L) • A1C 5.7–6.4% (39–47 mmol/mol) or ≥10% increase in A1C	• Clinical symptoms • Diabetes by standard criteria

ETIOLOGIC FACTORS: *ENVIRONMENTAL FACTORS:* Evidence for a role of environmental factors in the pathogenesis of T1DM includes:

- Only 33% to 50% of monozygotic twins of T1DM patients develop T1DM.
- Recent increases in T1DM incidence in some populations suggest an etiologic role for environmental factors.
- About 80% to 90% of T1DM patients have no family history of the disease.
- There are seasonal differences in the incidence of T1DM.

Viruses have been implicated in triggering at least some cases of T1DM. Thus, the disease occasionally develops after infection with Coxsackie B and, less often, mumps viruses. Certain viral proteins appear to share antigenic epitopes with human cell-surface proteins and may trigger autoreactivity by molecular mimicry. For example, a Coxsackie B virus protein has close similarity to the human GAD-65 islet protein.

It has been suggested that some early dietary exposures may also be associated with T1DM, but these associations have not been established.

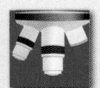 **PATHOLOGY:** As noted above, the most characteristic early lesion in the pancreas of T1DM is a mononuclear infiltrate in the islets (insulitis), chiefly lymphocytes, sometimes accompanied by a few macrophages and neutrophils (see Fig. 13-15). As the disease becomes chronic, islet β-cells become progressively depleted; eventually insulin-producing cells are no longer discernible. Loss of β-cells results in variably sized islets, many resembling ribbon-like cords that may be indistinguishable from the surrounding acinar tissue. Fibrosis of the islets is uncommon. Unlike T2DM, amyloid does not deposit in pancreatic islets in T1DM. The exocrine pancreas in chronic T1DM often shows diffuse interlobular and interacinar fibrosis, accompanied by atrophy of the acinar cells.

 CLINICAL FEATURES: The clinical presentation of T1DM results from lack of insulin, which has a unique role in energy metabolism. Patients classically present with acute metabolic decompensation characterized by hyperglycemia and ketoacidosis. Depending on the degree of absolute insulin deficiency, severe ketoacidosis may be preceded by weeks to months of increased urine output (**polyuria**) and increased thirst (**polydipsia**). Excessive diuresis results from the osmotic load from glucose in the urine. Weight loss in spite of increased appetite (**polyphagia**) reflects inefficient energy use with unregulated catabolism of body fat stores, protein, and carbohydrate. Often the clinical onset of T1DM coincides with another acute illness, such as a febrile viral or bacterial infection (Fig. 13-14).

COMPLICATIONS OF DIABETES

The discovery of insulin in the early 20th century promised to cure diabetes, but as diabetic patients lived longer, they developed diverse complications. *The severity and chronicity of hyperglycemia in both T2DM and T1DM are the major pathogenetic factors leading to the "microvascular" complications of diabetes including retinopathy, nephropathy, and neuropathy. Control of blood glucose therefore remains the major approach to preventing microvascular diabetic complications.* It has been more difficult to demonstrate that glucose control can prevent "macrovascular" (large-vessel) complications, meaning atherosclerosis and its sequelae (coronary artery, peripheral vascular, and cerebrovascular disease). These macrovascular complications are especially common in patients with T2DM, because the patients tend to be older and frequently have additional cardiovascular risk factors, particularly dyslipoproteinemia, hypertension, and hypercoagulability.

 PATHOPHYSIOLOGY: Several biochemical mechanisms have been proposed to account for the development of pathologic changes in diabetes:

ADVERSE EFFECTS ON KNOWN CARDIOVASCULAR RISK FACTORS: In T2DM, pathway-selective insulin resistance and responsiveness:

- Promote fatty liver
- Lead to overproduction of triglyceride-rich apoB-lipoproteins
- Impair hepatic removal of circulating atherogenic postprandial lipoproteins
- Cause vasoconstriction
- Lead to overexpression of tissue factor and possibly salt retention.

Enhanced production or action of angiotensin II may also play a role. Many prospective clinical trials have demonstrated benefit from lipid-lowering agents (statins), treatment of hypertension, and particularly with ACE inhibitors or ARBs. Inhibition of platelet activation by low-dose aspirin helps prevent thrombosis-related arterial narrowing when an atherosclerotic plaque ruptures, which helps limit ASCVD.

In T1DM, significant hypertriglyceridemia may develop due to poor glycemic control. However, this usually corrects quickly once insulin doses and diet are properly managed.

REACTIVE OXYGEN SPECIES (ROS): ROS are implicated in many types of cellular injury (see **Chapter 1**). In cultured cells, hyperglycemia increases ROS production from oxidative phosphorylation. Although there are several candidate mediators of glucose-induced oxidative damage, there is no evidence in humans that excessive ROS contribute to diabetes or its complications.

PROTEIN GLYCATION: Nonenzymatic covalent glucose binding to many proteins (**glycation**, or **nonenzymatic glycosylation**) roughly reflects blood glucose levels. Proteins modified in this manner include hemoglobin, components of the crystalline lens, and cellular basement membrane proteins. Nonenzymatic hemoglobin glycation is irreversible, so glycated hemoglobin levels in circulating erythrocytes (hemoglobin A_{1c}) reflect the overall degree of hyperglycemia during the prior 6 to 12 weeks, and help assess glycemic control.

Initial glycation products (which are Schiff bases) are labile and can dissociate rapidly. However, over time, they undergo chemical rearrangements to form stable **advanced glycosylation end-products (AGEs),** in which a glucose derivative covalently binds protein amino groups. This permanently alters protein structure and possibly, function. For example, albumin and IgG do not normally bind to collagen, but they adhere to glycated collagen. AGEs can cause modified proteins to undergo cross-linking with nearby proteins, possibly contributing to the characteristic thickening of vascular basement membranes in diabetes. Importantly, unlike their labile glycated predecessors, AGEs can continue to cross-link proteins even if blood glucose returns to normal. Patients with diabetic retinopathy have higher levels of AGEs than do diabetics without this complication. However, the role of AGEs in diabetic microvascular disease is uncertain, and studies preventing their formation been disappointing.

THE ALDOSE REDUCTASE PATHWAY: By mass action, hyperglycemia also increases glucose uptake into tissues that do not depend on insulin. Some of the increased intracellular glucose is metabolized to sorbitol by aldose reductase:

$$Glucose + NADPH \rightarrow Sorbitol + NADP$$

While this reaction lowers intracellular reducing equivalents, clinical trials of aldolase reductase inhibition have shown no benefit. Thus, the role of aldose reductase and sorbitol in the complications of diabetes is unclear.

Atherosclerosis Is a Common and Deadly Complication of T1DM and T2DM

Cardiovascular disease, including atherosclerotic heart disease and ischemic stroke, accounts for about 70% of deaths among adults with diabetes. The extent and severity of atherosclerotic lesions in medium-sized and large arteries are increased in patients with long-standing diabetes. Diabetes eliminates the usual protective effect of being female, and coronary artery disease develops at a younger age than in nondiabetic people. Moreover, mortality from myocardial infarction is higher in patients with diabetes than in those without. As indicated above, patients with T2DM often have risk factors related to the metabolic syndrome that contribute to atherogenesis.

Atherosclerotic peripheral vascular disease, particularly of the legs, is a common complication of diabetes. Vascular insufficiency leads to ulcers and gangrene of the toes and feet, complications that ultimately necessitate amputation. *Indeed, diabetes is the leading cause of nontraumatic limb amputations in the United States.*

Although levels of chronic hyperglycemia correlate with higher rates of cardiovascular disease, glucose levels *per se* may not be culpable. In most randomized clinical trials in T2DM, improving HbA$_{1c}$ levels does not improve macrovascular outcomes.

 PATHOPHYSIOLOGY: There are at least three general schools of thought as to how diabetes promotes atherosclerosis:

1. **Direct effects of diabetes or hyperglycemia on the arterial wall.** Gene polymorphisms associated with just small increases in plasma glucose—below the threshold for diagnosing diabetes—increase atherosclerotic cardiovascular risk. As noted above, however, no clinical therapies based on this idea have reduced this type of complication of T2DM.

2. **Side effects of diabetic therapy,** such as high insulin concentrations associated with certain forms of treatment.

3. **Exacerbation of general risk factors for atherosclerosis** (e.g., hypertension, dyslipoproteinemia, hypercoagulability). Dyslipoproteinemia in T2DM in part reflects hepatic and intestinal overproduction of cholesterol- and triglyceride-rich apoB-lipoproteins, defective lipoprotein lipase that impairs clearance of chylomicrons and leads to postprandial hypertriglyceridemia and impaired hepatic uptake of atherogenic postprandial remnant lipoprotein particles. Current successful strategies to reduce cardiovascular events in T2DM include managing these risk factors (e.g., LDL-lowering therapies [statins, ezetimibe, and PCSK9 inhibitors], antihypertensive agents and, in secondary prevention, low-dose aspirin), plus new agents recently shown to confer cardiovascular protection (some GLP1 receptor agonists and SGLT2 inhibitors, see above). Gastric bypass surgery for weight loss substantially reduces cardiovascular deaths in properly selected obese patients.

 PATHOLOGY: The pathology of diabetes-related macrovascular disease reflects the accelerated atherogenesis described above. Arteries show intimal thickening and fibrosis (Fig. 13-17).

Diabetic Microvascular Disease Causes Many of the Complications of Diabetes, Including Renal Failure, Blindness, and Neuropathy

Arteriolosclerosis and capillary basement membrane thickening are characteristic vascular changes in diabetes

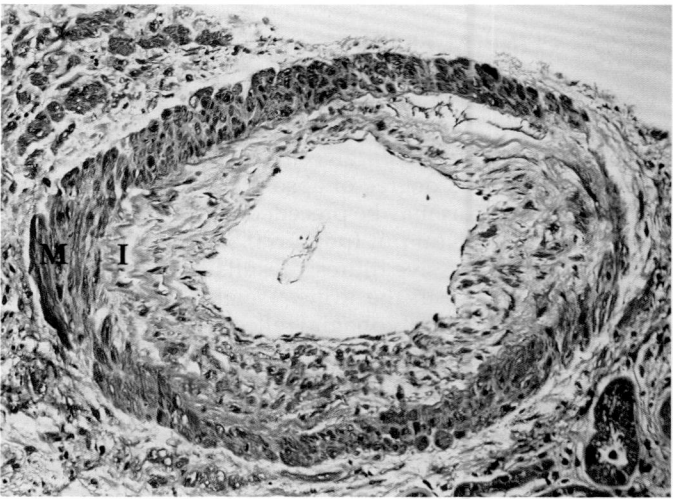

FIGURE 13-17. The Arcuate artery of a diabetic kidney displays macrovascular disease. Endothelial dysfunction due to hyperglycemia leads to accelerated atherosclerosis with intimal fibroplasia and thickening (*I*) and medial fibrosis (*M*) as demonstrated on this Trichrome stain.

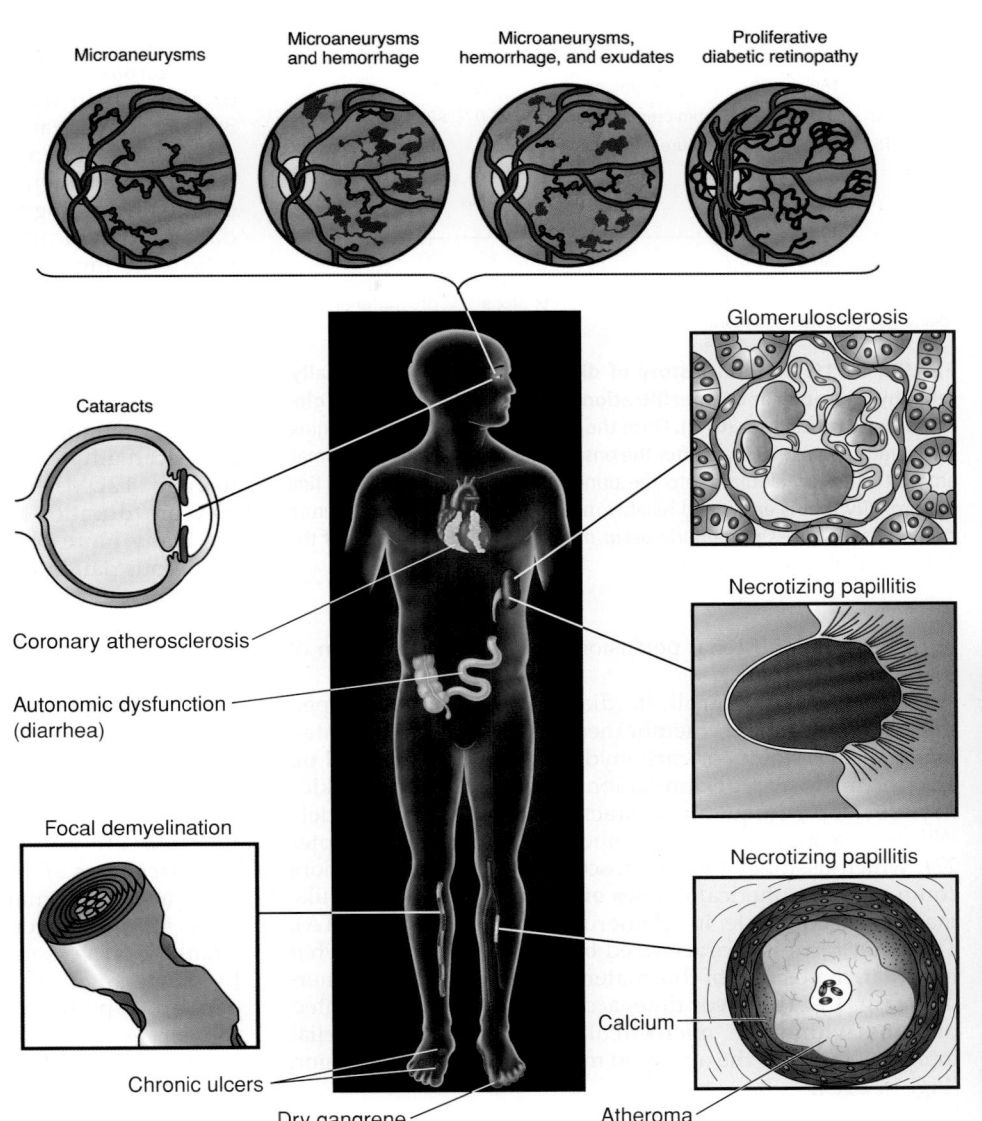

FIGURE 13-18. Secondary complications of diabetes. The effects of diabetes on a number of vital organs result in complications that may be incapacitating (cerebral and peripheral vascular disease), painful (neuropathy) or life-threatening (coronary artery disease, pyelonephritis with necrotizing papillitis).

(see Chapter 10). Hypertension contributes to these arteriolar lesions. Deposition of basement membrane proteins, which may also be glycated, increases in diabetes. Platelet aggregation in smaller blood vessels and impaired fibrinolytic mechanisms may also contribute to diabetic microvascular disease.

Whatever its pathogenesis, diabetic microvascular disease affects tissue perfusion and wound healing profoundly. Blood flow to the heart, already compromised by large-vessel disease (see above), is further reduced by small-vessel disease. Poor sensation from neuropathy predisposes diabetic patients to trauma, leading to infection and chronic ulcers, particularly in the feet. In part due to microvascular disease, these tend to heal poorly. The major complications of diabetic microvascular disease involve the kidney, the retina, and peripheral nerves (Fig. 13-18).

Diabetic Nephropathy

Diabetes is the leading cause of renal failure in the United States, accounting for nearly half of new cases and occurring in 30% to 40% of patients with T1DM. Up to 20% of patients with T2DM are similarly affected. Although some patients with T1DM die from uremia, most patients who develop nephropathy succumb to cardiovascular disease, the risk of which is much higher in T1DM patients who have end-stage renal disease. The prevalence of diabetic nephropathy increases with the severity and duration of hyperglycemia. *Diabetic kidney disease is the most common reason for renal transplantation in adults.*

Initially, hyperglycemia leads to glomerular hypertension and renal hyperperfusion (Fig. 13-19). Increased glomerular pressure favors deposition of protein in the mesangium, resulting in glomerulosclerosis and, eventually, renal failure. AGEs and lipoprotein abnormalities may contribute to changes in the glomerular basement membrane chemical composition. In addition, growth factors, particularly TGFβ, that are increased in diabetic kidneys, have been implicated in some of the cellular abnormalities in diabetic nephropathy. Inhibition of TGFβ in some animal models of diabetes attenuates renal disease. Regardless of the underlying mechanism, strict control of blood glucose levels and blood pressure retards development of diabetic nephropathy. Antihypertensive treatment targeting angiotensin or its receptor reduces systemic blood pressure, glomerular

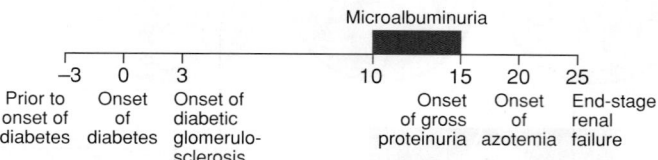

	−3	0	3	Time (years)		15	20	25
	120	150	150	GFR (mL/min)		120	60	<10
	1.0	0.8	0.8	Serum creatinine (mg/dL)		1.0	>2.0	>10.0
	15	10	10	Serum urea nitrogen (mg/dL)		15	>30	>100

Microalbuminuria

−3	0	3		10	15	20	25
Prior to onset of diabetes	Onset of diabetes	Onset of diabetic glomerulo-sclerosis		Onset of gross proteinuria		Onset of azotemia	End-stage renal failure

FIGURE 13-19. Natural history of diabetic nephropathy. Initially, renal hypertrophy and hyperfiltration lead to an increase in the glomerular filtration rate (GFR). Once the decline in renal function begins, on average at least 10 years after the onset of diabetes, leakage of a small amount of serum albumin into the urine (microalbuminuria) is the first abnormality that is easily and reliably measured. The elevation in serum creatinine and gross proteinuria occur much later. (Data courtesy of the American Diabetes Association.)

hypertension, and renal perfusion, and slow progression of diabetic nephropathy.

Eventually, glomeruli in diabetic kidneys developed thickened basement membranes, which are highlighted using special stains for carbohydrates (Fig. 13-20A) and on electron microscopic examination (Fig. 13-20B). Diabetic kidneys develop a unique and characteristic lesion: Kimmelstiel–Wilson disease or nodular glomerulosclerosis (see Chapter 22), which assumes two microscopic patterns. In the more common one, spherical masses of basement membrane–like material accumulate in glomerular lobules (Fig. 13-21A). The other form is characterized by more diffuse, somewhat irregular, deposition of this material throughout the glomerulus (Fig. 13-21B). Over time, accumulation of glycosylated proteins within the microcirculation impairs endothelial integrity and thus the ability to maintain effective perfusion (Fig. 13-21C).

Onset of glomerular disease is heralded clinically by the **microalbuminuria**, the appearance of small amounts of albumin in the urine. Formally, this represents 30 to 300 mg/day or an albumin-to-creatinine ratio between 30 and 300 mg/g in a spot urine sample. Proteinuria increases with time and with progressive decline in renal function, eventually leading to **macroalbuminuria**, defined as ≥300 mg daily, and typically assessed by an albumin-to-creatinine ratio ≥300 mg/g. Both microalbuminuria and macroalbuminuria indicate deteriorating renal function and worsening cardiovascular risk.

Diabetic Retinopathy

Diabetic retinopathy is the leading cause of blindness in American adults under age 74. The risk is higher in T1DM than in T2DM. In fact, 10% of patients with T1DM of 30 years' duration become legally blind. Nevertheless, there are many more patients with T2DM, so they are the most numerous patients with diabetic retinopathy. Retinopathy is the most devastating ophthalmic complication of diabetes, although glaucoma, cataracts, and corneal disease are also increased. Like nephropathy, the prevalence of diabetic retinopathy reflects the duration and degree of glycemic control (also see **Chapter 33**).

Diabetic Neuropathy

Peripheral sensory impairment and autonomic nerve dysfunction are among the most common and distressing complications of diabetes. Changes in the nerves are complex, and abnormalities in axons, myelin, and Schwann cells all may occur. Microvasculopathy involving the small blood vessels of nerves contributes to the disorder. Evidence suggests that hyperglycemia increases the perception of pain, independent of any structural lesions in the nerves.

Peripheral neuropathy is initially characterized by pain and abnormal sensations in the extremities. However, fine

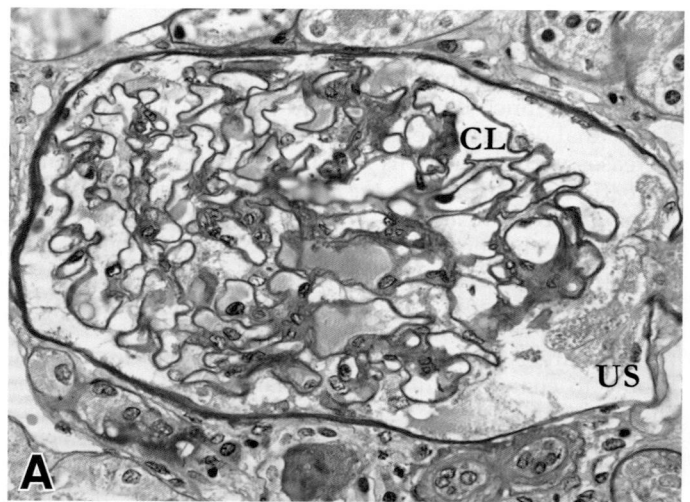

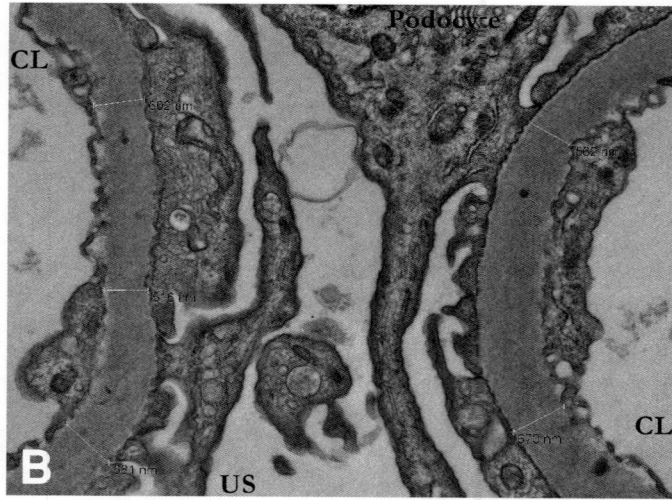

FIGURE 13-20. Diabetes leads to basement membrane thickening throughout the body. A: This glomerulus displays the earliest stage of diabetic glomerulosclerosis, glomerular basement membrane thickening (best seen on PAS stain), prior to the development of mesangial matrical increase. *CL* = capillary lumen; *US* = urinary space. **B:** Electron micrograph of diabetic glomerular basement membrane thickening. Early thickening can only be detected on EM, which is the only way to accurately measure thickness (upper limit of normal ~450 nm). Despite the thickening, the capillaries are leakier to plasma proteins, and lead to proteinuria. *CL* = capillary lumen; *US* = urinary space.

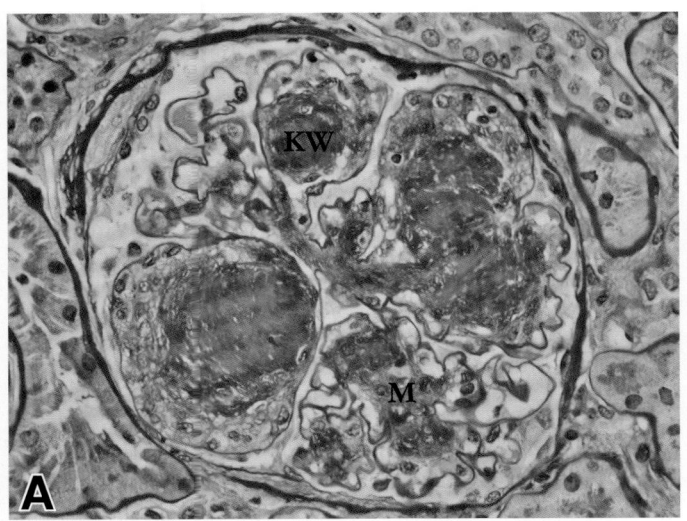

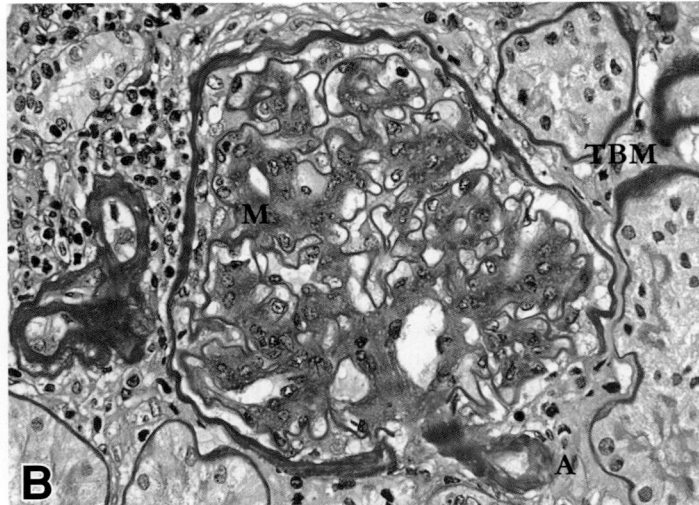

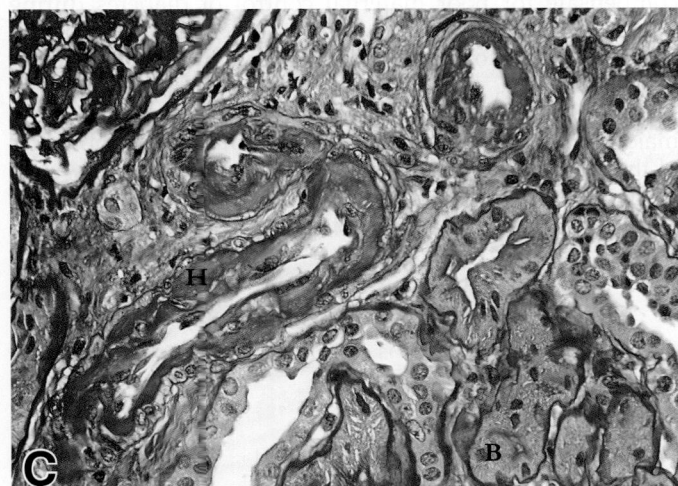

FIGURE 13-21. Diabetic glomerulopathy. A: Nodular diabetic glomerulosclerosis is superimposed on the diffuse form of mesangial expansion, and is the most specific form of diabetic glomerulosclerosis. The PAS-positive nodules, often laminated and centrally acellular, may be associated with loss of mesangial integrity (mesangiolysis) and capillary dilation, as seen here. *M* = diffusely expanded mesangium; *KW* = Kimmelstiel–Wilson mesangial nodules. **B:** As diabetic glomerulosclerosis progresses, the mesangial matrix (*M*) also expands, initially and most commonly in a diffuse (nonnodular) pattern, as seen on this PAS stain. Adjacent nonatrophic tubules also show thickening of their tubular basement membranes (*TBM*). The arteriole (*A*) shows mural hyalinosis. **C:** Hyaline arteriosclerosis may be seen in aging and hypertension but is significantly worse in diabetes where it is part of diabetic microvascular disease. Chronic endothelial dysfunction leads to the accumulation of glassy plasma proteins (*H*), compromising the microvascular circulation, and leading to tubulo-interstitial scarring. Glomeruli may also show hyaline deposition in the capillaries or Bowman capsule. Adjacent proximal tubules show an intact PAS positive brush border (*B*).

touch, pain detection, and proprioception are ultimately lost. As a result, patients with diabetes tend to ignore irritation and minor trauma to feet, joints, and legs. Peripheral neuropathy can thus lead to foot ulcers, which often plague patients with severe diabetes. It also plays a role in the painless destructive joint disease that occasionally occurs (Charcot joint, Fig. 13-22).

Although autonomic nerve dysfunction is subtle, abnormalities in neurogenic regulation of cardiovascular and gastrointestinal functions frequently lead to postural hypotension and problems of gut motility, such as gastroparesis and diarrhea. Erectile dysfunction and retrograde ejaculation also complicate autonomic dysfunction, although vascular disease also contributes. Hypotonic urinary bladder

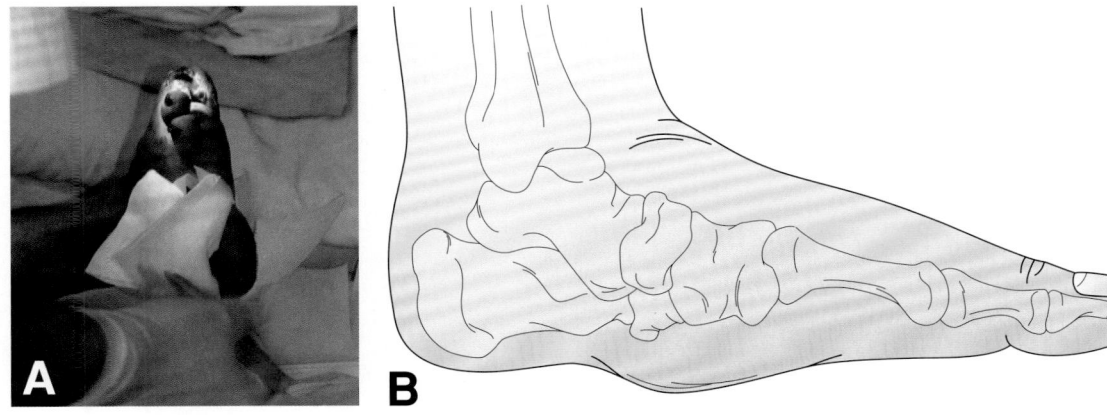

FIGURE 13-22. Foot complications of diabetes mellitus. A: Foot ulcer. **B:** Charcot foot.

develops occasionally, results in urinary retention, which predisposes to infection.

Bacterial and Fungal Infections Occur in Diabetic Patients Whose Hyperglycemia Is Poorly Controlled

Abnormal host responses to microbial pathogens occur in patients with poorly controlled diabetes. Leukocyte function is compromised and immune responses are blunted. Before the use of insulin, tuberculosis and purulent infections were often life-threatening. Now, patients with well-controlled diabetes are much less susceptible to infections. However, **urinary tract infections** continue to be problematic because glucose in the urine provides an enriched culture medium. A new class of medications, SGLT2 inhibitors, discussed above, aids glycemic control and weight management by inhibiting renal reabsorption of glucose. This causes glucosuria and increases risk for genitourinary infections. Any urinary tract infection can become further complicated in patients with autonomic neuropathy, which impairs bladder emptying and causes urinary retention. Infection ascending from the bladder to the kidney (i.e., **pyelonephritis**) is thus a constant concern. **Renal papillary necrosis** may be a devastating complication of bladder infection.

Mucormycosis is a dreaded infectious complication of poorly controlled diabetes. It tends to originate in the nasopharynx or paranasal sinuses and spreads rapidly to the orbit and brain, and is often fatal (see Chapter 9).

Diabetes Occurring During Pregnancy (Gestational Diabetes) May Put Both Mother and Fetus at Risk

Gestational diabetes develops during pregnancy in only a few percent of seemingly healthy women, in a small percentage of whom it continues after parturition. Pregnancy is a state of insulin resistance for handling glucose, but only pregnant women with impaired β-cell insulin secretion become diabetic. These women show abnormalities in the amount and timing of insulin secretion, making them highly susceptible to overt T2DM later in life when not pregnant.

Poor control of diabetes in pregnancy (either gestational diabetes or pre-existing diabetes) may lead to the birth of large infants, complicating labor and delivery, and necessitating cesarean section. The fetal pancreas may try to compensate for poor maternal control of diabetes during gestation. Such fetuses may develop β-cell hyperplasia, which may lead to transient hypoglycemia at birth and early in postnatal life.

About 5% to 10% of infants of diabetic mothers show major developmental abnormalities, including anomalies of the heart and great vessels, and neural tube defects, such as anencephaly and spina bifida. These lesions often reflect poor control of maternal diabetes during early gestation.

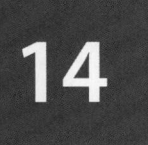

14 The Pathology of Pregnancy

David A. Schwartz

Obstetric and Placental Pathology and the Pathology of Pregnancy

In normal pregnancies, almost every maternal organ system changes profoundly to accommodate the needs of the fetoplacental unit. The placenta, with its two separate vascular supplies from two genetically distinct individuals, is an important part of obstetric pathology. It normally invades its host, but it can also cause potentially fatal cancer.

PLACENTA

The placenta includes a **placental disc, umbilical cord**, and **extraplacental membranes** (Fig. 14-1). It is a flattened discoid organ with two surfaces. The fetus faces one aspect **(fetal or chorionic surface)**, which is covered by membranes, the **amnion** and **chorion**. These contain the **amniotic fluid** that surrounds the fetus. Opposite, is the **maternal** (or **decidual**) **surface** which abuts a decidualized endometrium.

Fetal blood enters the placenta through two umbilical arteries that spiral around an umbilical vein. Each artery supplies half of the placenta. The umbilical cord inserts into the chorionic surface on the placenta. The major branches of the umbilical arteries and vein (chorionic plate blood vessels) then branch along the surface of the disc and penetrate the placental disc to form the chorionic villous tree. Primary stem villi originate at the chorionic plate and contain the major umbilical arterial and venous branches. These villous trunks progressively subdivide into smaller branches, ending in the terminal (or, tertiary) villi, where oxygen and nutrient transport occurs. At term, the terminal villi constitute 40% of villous volume and 60% of villous cross-sections.

The **decidua** forms the border between fetal tissue composing the villous trees and the underlying uterus. The decidua contains 80 to 100 small **spiral arterioles**, which are branches of myometrial arteries, and supply the placenta with maternal blood (Fig. 14-2). These arteries undergo

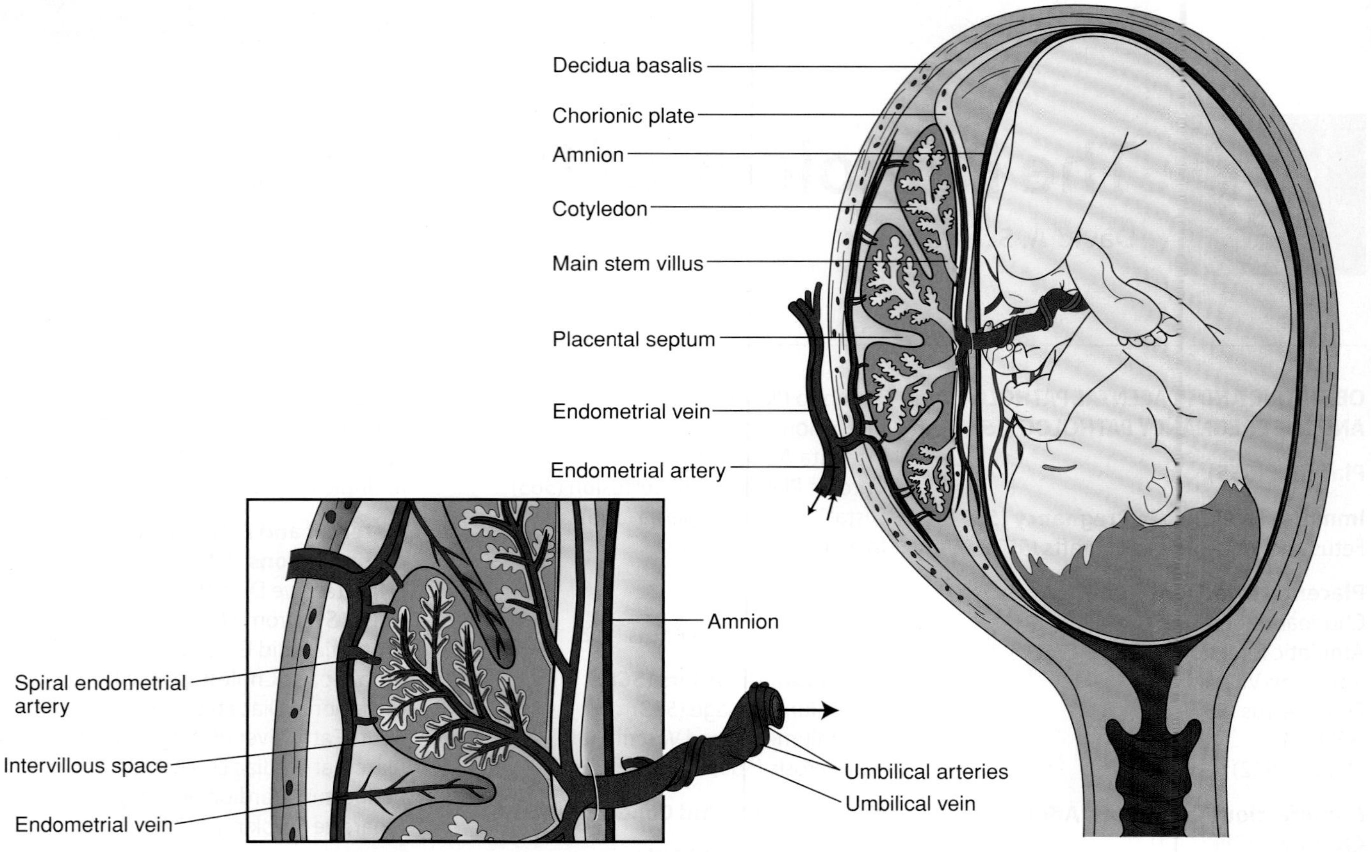

Decidua basalis

Chorionic plate

Amnion

Cotyledon

Main stem villus

Placental septum

Endometrial vein

Endometrial artery

Amnion

Spiral endometrial artery

Intervillous space

Endometrial vein

Umbilical arteries
Umbilical vein

FIGURE 14-1. Pregnant uterus including fetus, placenta, and circulation.

remodeling changes that decrease their resistance to uterine blood flow and support the developing placenta and fetus. Each spiral arteriole delivers maternal blood to the center of an anatomic subunit of the placenta, the **cotyledon**. Maternal blood entering the placental disc is not confined to a vessel, but instead occupies a cavity, the **intervillous space**, where it exchanges oxygen and nutrients. Maternal

and fetal circulations in the placenta are entirely separate (Fig. 14-2).

The terminal villus is the placenta's functional unit of exchange. The trophoblastic layer covers the chorionic villous tree. It contains an inner **cytotrophoblast (Langhans cells)**, a middle layer of **intermediate trophoblast** and an outer layer of **syncytiotrophoblast**. The villous stroma is

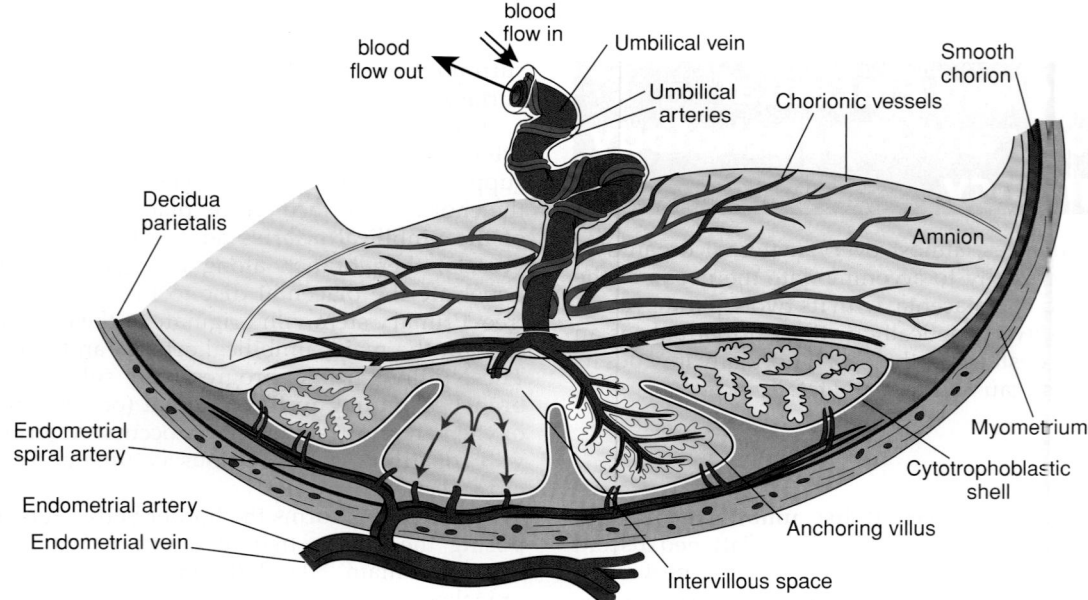

blood flow in

blood flow out

Umbilical vein

Umbilical arteries

Chorionic vessels

Smooth chorion

Amnion

Decidua parietalis

Endometrial spiral artery

Endometrial artery

Endometrial vein

Intervillous space

Myometrium

Cytotrophoblastic shell

Anchoring villus

FIGURE 14-2. Cross-section of the placenta and its circulation.

loose mesenchyme containing embryonal macrophages—**Hofbauer cells.** In the third trimester, syncytiotrophoblast nuclei aggregate to form multinuclear protrusions **(syncytial knots)**. Syncytium between the knots along the villous surface becomes markedly attenuated. At these points, trophoblastic cytoplasm comes into direct contact with fetal capillary endothelium, to form the **vasculosyncytial membrane**. These specialized zones facilitate gas and nutrient transfer across the placenta.

In addition to releasing waste and absorbing oxygen and nutrients, the villi are hormonally active. The syncytiotrophoblast secretes **human chorionic gonadotropin (hCG)**, which maintains the corpus luteum. It also secretes **progesterone** to assure the integrity of the decidua, and **human placental lactogen (HPL)**, which raises maternal glucose levels and so assists in adequate fetal nutrition.

Placental Size

Placental size increases as gestation progresses—for example, mean placental weight at 30 weeks' gestation is 316 g; at 35 weeks, 434 g; and at term (40 weeks), 537 g. An abnormally small placenta (≤10th percentile for gestational age) is associated with maternal hypertensive disease of pregnancy and low birth weight. It can cause poor fetal outcomes, including neurologic abnormalities and perinatal death. Abnormally large placentas (≥90th percentile) may reflect villous edema, fetal hydrops, placental hemorrhage, syphilis, placental tumors, and maternal diabetes. At term, 1 g of placenta can oxygenate 7 g of fetal tissue. This relationship, called the **fetal–placental weight ratio**, helps to determine the "placental reserve" and how placental insufficiency can occur. A fetus too large for its placenta (i.e., increased fetal:placental weight ratio) can lead to a poor obstetric outcome, as can abnormally thin placentas (<2 cm thickness at term).

Placental Shape

A typical placental disc is round or ovoid.

- **Bilobed placenta** (2% to 8%) appears as two equal-sized discs, separated by membranes.
- **Succenturiate placenta** (5%) is bilobed, with one lobe smaller than the other. Bilobed and succenturiate placentas have membranous blood vessels connecting each lobe, which may be damaged by compression, thrombosis, or rupture.
- In **vasa previa** (1 in 2,500), membranous vessels are between the fetus and the internal cervical os. These vessels may rupture before or during delivery, causing fetal bleeding that may rapidly lead to fetal exsanguination.
- **Circumvallate placentas** (1% to 6%) have membranes that extend away from the margin toward the center of the placental disc. The margin has fibrin and clotted blood. It is thought to result from either marginal hemorrhage early in development or a deep implantation of the fetus into the decidua.
- **Circummarginate placenta** (4%) differs from circumvallate placenta by not having reflected membranes fold back.

Placental Implantation

Placentas normally implant in the uterine wall above the internal cervical os. Implantation lower in the uterus, may partially or completely cover the internal os (**placenta previa**, 0.3% to 1%

of pregnancies). Risk factors include smoking, increased age, multiple prior pregnancies, previous cesarean sections, and prior abortions. Placenta previa must be recognized before delivery to avoid a fetus being delivered through its own placenta, risking life-threatening hemorrhage. Placenta previa is one of the most common causes of third-trimester bleeding and entails a high risk of abruption, postpartum hemorrhage, prolapsed umbilical cord, fetal malpresentation, intrauterine growth restriction (IUGR), and fetal and perinatal mortality. Placenta previa is often associated with another abnormal condition, **placenta accreta** (see below), in which case it is **placenta previa accreta**.

Placenta implantation outside the uterine cavity, that is, **ectopic pregnancy**, usually involves the fallopian tube. But 2% of ectopic pregnancies occur in the ovary, cervix, or abdomen. Unless removed surgically, abdominal pregnancy carries a high maternal mortality.

Umbilical Cord Abnormalities

At term, umbilical cords normally measure 35 to 100 cm. Abnormally short cords predispose to perinatal mortality, intrauterine fetal distress, and IUGR. The cord normally inserts at or near the center of the placental disc, but 7% insert at the placenta's edge (**marginal insertion**) and 1% insert into the membranes—**velamentous** or **membranous insertion**, which may cause **vasa previa** (see above). Velamentous and marginal cord insertions are common in spontaneous abortions and fetuses with congenital anomalies.

IMMUNE TOLERANCE IN PREGNANCY

The Mother Tolerates the Fetus and Placenta as Allografts

The conceptus differs genetically from the mother and so represents an allograft. Why, then, does the mother not reject her fetus as foreign like other genetically foreign tissues? **Immune tolerance in pregnancy** describes the absence of a maternal immune response against the fetus and its placenta.

 PATHOPHYSIOLOGY: The placenta is the major immunologic barrier between mother and conceptus, and creates an immunologically privileged site.

- Placental trophoblast does not express class I HLA-A and -B MHC antigens, helping protect the fetus from recognition as foreign.
- Trophoblast-expressed atypical MHC class I isotypes HLA-E and HLA-G may prevent attack by maternal natural killer (NK) cells.
- The trophoblast syncytium, lacks intercellular spaces or connections between cells, thus restricting migratory immune cells from passing between the maternal and fetal bloodstreams.
- The placenta permits some maternal IgG to cross the vasculosyncytial barrier and enter the fetal circulation, helping protect from infectious diseases.
- Fetal cells that enter maternal circulation elicit antibodies targeting fetal antigens. ABO blood group differences between mother and fetus could trigger maternal

antibodies against fetal antigens, potentially destroying fetal erythrocytes. This develops rarely, however, because maternal anti-A and anti-B antibodies are IgM, which does not cross the placenta.

- The placenta secretes **neurokinin B**, a peptide that binds the immune-cloaking molecule **phosphocholine**.
- Regulatory T lymphocytes (T_{reg}; see Chapters 4 and 11) and NK cells may help avoid maternal immunologic rejection by fetal tissues, but the mechanisms are uncertain.

PLACENTAL INFECTIONS

Chorioamnionitis Reflects Ascending Infection

Infectious organisms, almost exclusively bacteria, can ascend from the maternal birth canal, pass through the cervical os and infect the decidua and placental tissues, the amniotic fluid and, potentially, the fetus.

 ETIOLOGIC FACTORS: Acute chorioamnionitis is usually caused by bacteria normally present in the maternal cervicovaginal canal. The most common offenders are group B and other *Streptococcus* species, *Escherichia coli*, *Enterococcus*, *Staphylococcus* sp., gram-negative bacilli, *Bacteroides*, *Mycoplasma hominis*, and *Ureaplasma*.

PATHOLOGY: Upon reaching the uterine cavity, bacteria initially elicit a maternal inflammatory response (MIR). Maternal neutrophils circulating in the intervillous space migrate upward toward the fetal surface, or chorionic plate, causing **acute subchorionitis**. They then migrate upward, into the chorion. Maternal neutrophils recruited from the decidual blood vessels enter the chorion (Fig. 14-3A), to cause **acute chorioamnionitis**. Maternal inflammatory cells can also migrate from decidual and spiral arteries into the decidua underlying the extraplacental membranes or the placental disc, to cause **acute deciduitis**. Severe deciduitis may cause necrosis of the decidua **(necrotizing deciduitis)** (Fig. 14-3B), or it can form focal **decidual microabscesses**. Since maternal spiral arteries in the decidua supply the placenta with oxygenated maternal blood, decidual infection can threaten the pregnancy.

A fetal inflammatory response (FIR) may also develop. **Acute chorionic vasculitis**, a component of FIR, occurs when fetal neutrophils migrate from the fetal bloodstream into the walls of the large chorionic plate vessels (branches of the umbilical cord vessels) at the surface of the placental disc (Fig. 14-4A). Fetal neutrophils also migrate from umbilical blood vessel lumens into the muscular vessel walls, causing umbilical vasculitis, or **acute funisitis** (Fig. 14-4B). Fetal neutrophils can migrate completely through umbilical vessel walls and infiltrate the mesenchyme (Wharton jelly). Cerebral palsy is statistically associated with severe—but not mild or moderate—FIR (see below) in term infants.

CLINICAL FEATURES: Acute chorioamnionitis (10% of placentas) can cause preterm labor, premature rupture of membranes, fetal and neonatal infections, and intrauterine hypoxia. The mother may have fever, uterine tenderness, and foul-smelling or cloudy amniotic fluid. Major risks are postpartum endometritis and pelvic sepsis with venous thrombosis.

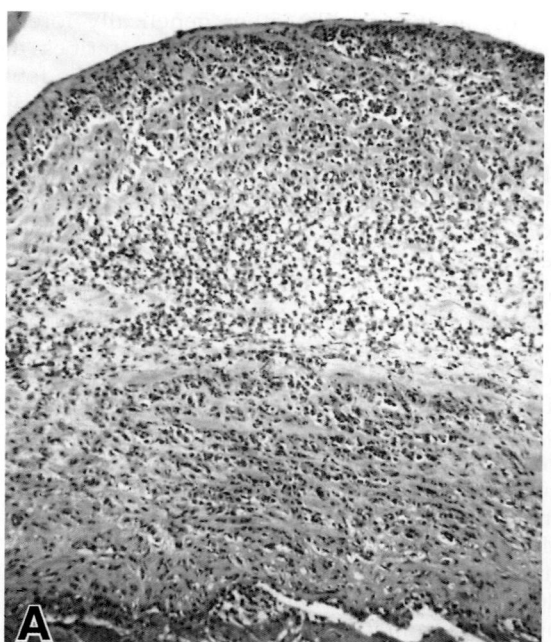
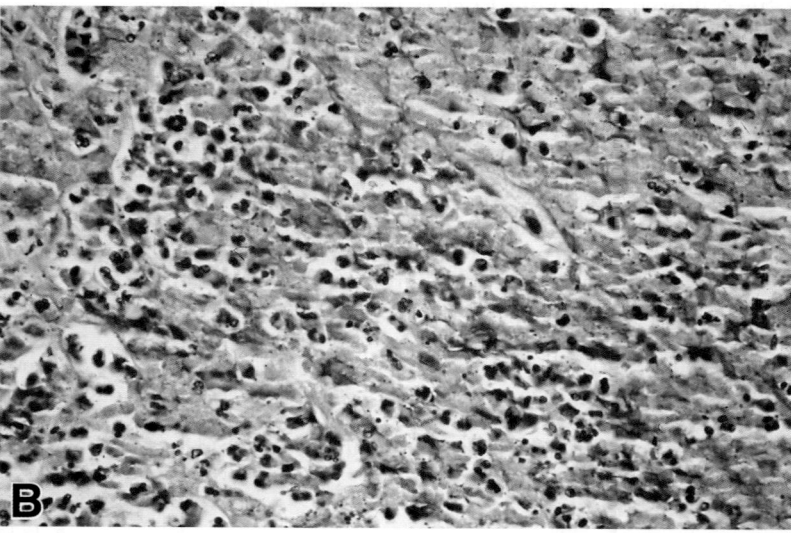

FIGURE 14-3. Maternal inflammatory responses to ascending infection. A. Acute chorioamnionitis (maternal inflammatory response [MIR]). The chorion contains many acute inflammatory cells, recruited from the maternal intervillous space. **B. Acute necrotizing deciduitis (MIR).** The decidua contains abundant inflammatory cells of maternal origin and is necrotic.

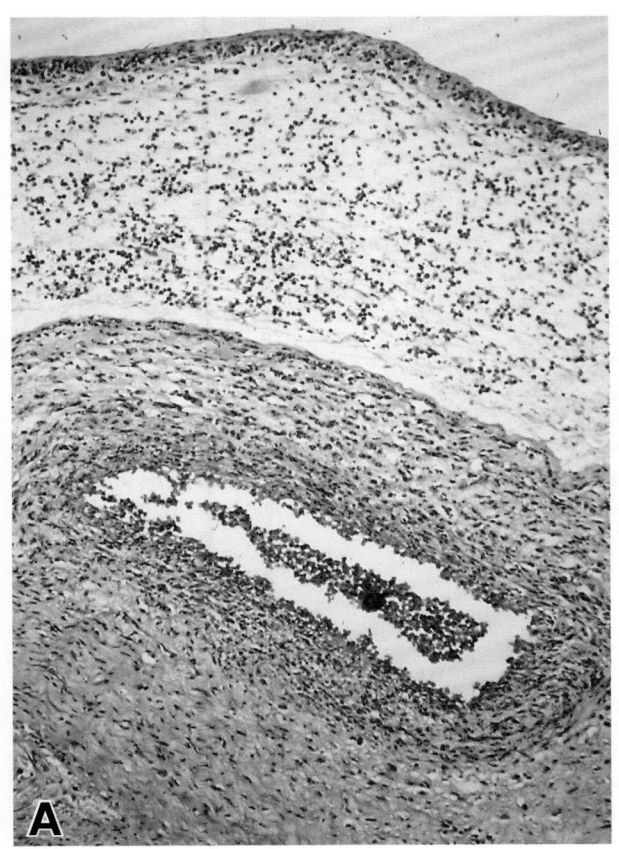

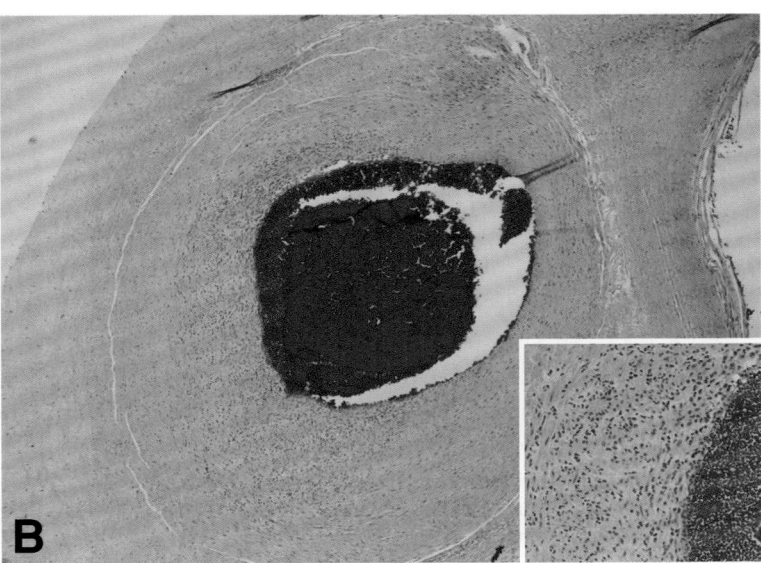

FIGURE 14-4. Fetal inflammatory responses to ascending infection. A. Acute chorionic vasculitis (fetal inflammatory response [FIR]). The wall of this large chorionic plate blood vessel is infiltrated by fetal neutrophils. The overlying chorion shows acute chorioamnionitis. **B. Acute funisitis (FIR).** The muscular wall of this umbilical vessel contains numerous fetal inflammatory cells (*Inset:* higher magnification).

In preterm, low–birth-weight (LBW) (<2,500 g) infants, especially those with very low birth weight (VLBW) (<1,500 g), acute chorioamnionitis often leads to severe neurologic disease, stillbirth, neonatal sepsis, and death. However, it can also cause morbidity and mortality in full-term infants. The risks of chorioamnionitis to the fetus include (1) pneumonia after inhalation of infected amniotic fluid; (2) skin or eye infections from direct contact with organisms in the fluid; (3) neonatal gastritis, enteritis, or peritonitis from ingesting infected fluid; (4) neonatal sepsis; and (5) neurologic injury including cerebral palsy.

Amniotic Infection Syndrome Can Cause Intrauterine Fetal Infection

Amniotic Fluid

At first, amniotic fluid is a transudate of maternal fluids, but later the amnion, fetal lungs, and kidneys also contribute. The fetus inhales and exhales amniotic fluid during breathing movements before birth.

Intra-Amniotic Infection

Amniotic fluid is normally sterile, but sometimes contains bacteria. Amniotic fluid infection gives microorganisms a portal of entry into the fetus, especially the respiratory tract, from where infection can enter the bloodstream and spread to other fetal organs. These infants can be born with "congenital" or

early-onset neonatal infections, including pneumonia, sepsis, and meningitis. Placentas of these infants typically show acute chorioamnionitis, often with FIR. Amniotic infections can portend serious or fatal outcomes for the neonate.

Villitis Can Indicate a Maternal Infection

Villitis—inflammation of chorionic villi—may reflect infection spreading from the maternal circulation to the placenta. It may also be of unknown etiology. Causative agents include (1) most commonly, viruses (rubella, CMV, Herpes); (2) bacteria (*Listeria, Treponema pallidum, Mycobacterium tuberculosis, Mycoplasma, Chlamydia*); (3) parasites and protozoa (*Toxoplasma, Trypanosoma cruzi*); and (4) fungi (*Candida*). Villitis can impair oxygen transport to the fetus. The etiologic agent can also traverse the villi and infect the fetus. If villitis from any cause is extensive or causes tissue necrosis (necrotizing villitis), perinatal morbidity, including brain damage, and mortality may result.

Maternal blood-borne infections do not always cause villitis. Notable exceptions are HIV and Zika virus.

Cytomegalovirus

Cytomegalovirus (CMV) is one of the TORCH agents (see Chapter 6) that can cause congenital infections. The most serious fetal complications occur when a mother becomes infected for the first time while pregnant. Reactivation of latent maternal CMV infection during pregnancy is less dangerous. In Western nations, 8% of women develop primary infection during pregnancy, and half will transmit the virus

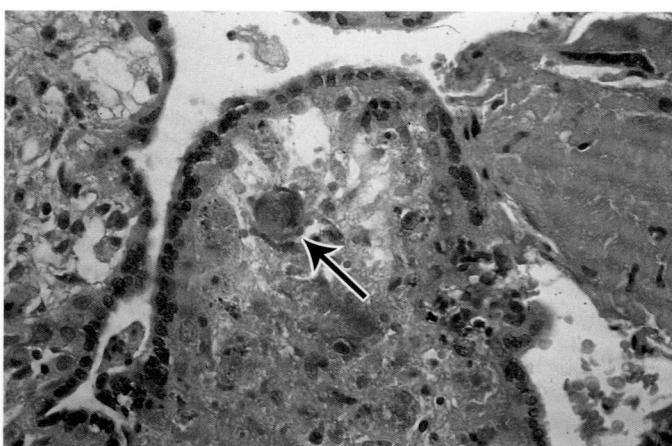

FIGURE 14-5. Chronic villitis caused by cytomegalovirus (CMV). The villi are infiltrated by chronic inflammatory cells. An enlarged cell with a CMV inclusion is present (*arrow*).

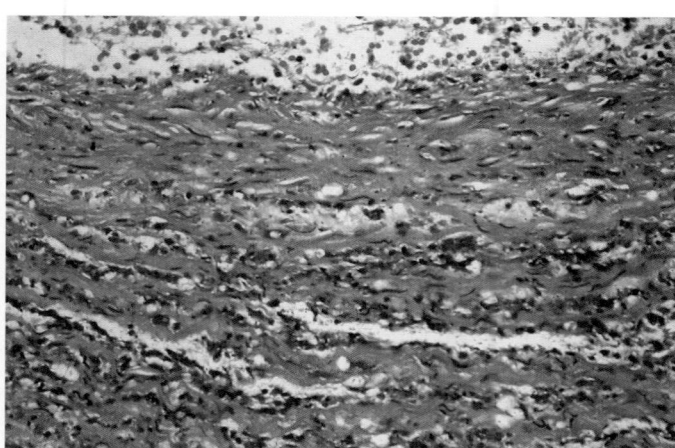

FIGURE 14-6. Necrotizing funisitis due to syphilis. The smooth muscle cells of the umbilical vessels are necrotic, and "smudgy" chronic inflammatory cells are causing a funisitis.

to their fetus. In less affluent settings, congenital CMV infections are less common, because primary CMV exposure likely occurred previously.

PATHOLOGY: CMV entering the placenta from maternal blood causes endothelial infection with cellular swelling, luminal occlusion, endothelial necrosis, and vascular destruction. Thrombosis, ischemic villous necrosis and, eventually, avascular villi with villous scarring (fibrosis) result. Villous stromal macrophages (Hofbauer cells) may be increased. Remote CMV infection can cause villous microcalcifications. Intranuclear and intracytoplasmic inclusions may be visible if CMV infection occurs near the time of delivery (Fig. 14-5), but rarely if infection is remote.

CLINICAL FEATURES: Among fetuses infected with CMV, 1/4 are born with clinical symptoms. Some 5% to 10% of neonates will not have symptoms at birth but will later develop hearing loss, visual impairment, and mental retardation. In more severe cases, generalized neonatal infections may entail low birth weight, microcephaly, seizures, and skin manifestations. With multiorgan dissemination, infants may show cerebral abnormalities, splenomegaly, and hepatitis. Occasionally, congenital CMV may be lethal.

Syphilis

Treponema pallidum (see Chapter 9) can pass from the maternal circulation to the fetal circulation through chorionic villi, mostly during the secondary phase.

PATHOLOGY: Placentas in infants with congenital syphilis are large—1 kg or more. Villi appear hypercellular and enlarged, usually with Hofbauer cell hyperplasia and stromal fibrosis. Chronic villitis is usually present and decidual plasma cells may be abundant. The umbilical cord can show **necrotizing**

funisitis, which grossly resembles a "barber pole" and microscopically shows necrosis of umbilical vessel walls, perivascular concentric rings of smudgy-appearing chronic inflammatory cells, necrotic debris, or calcium deposits (Fig. 14-6). Spirochetes in placental tissues are visualized using Warthin–Starry silver stain or fluorescent antibodies (Fig. 14-7).

CLINICAL FEATURES: Syphilis is an important cause of stillbirth, and liveborn infants with early congenital syphilis may be premature. Nevertheless, most newborns with congenital syphilis are asymptomatic. Symptomatic infants suffer hepatosplenomegaly, snuffles, lymphadenopathy, mucocutaneous lesions, pneumonia, edema, rash, hemolytic anemia, or thrombocytopenia at birth or within the first 4 to 8 weeks. Children with late congenital syphilis show facial and other defects (see Chapter 6).

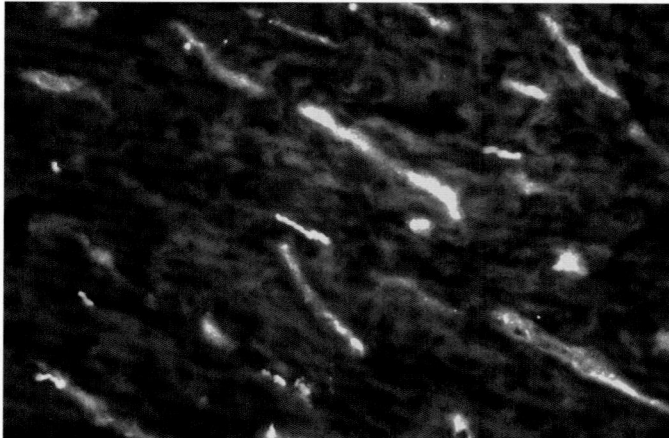

FIGURE 14-7. Spirochetes of *Treponema pallidum* in the wall of an umbilical cord blood vessel with necrotizing funisitis. The organisms are visible using a fluorescent antibody stain.

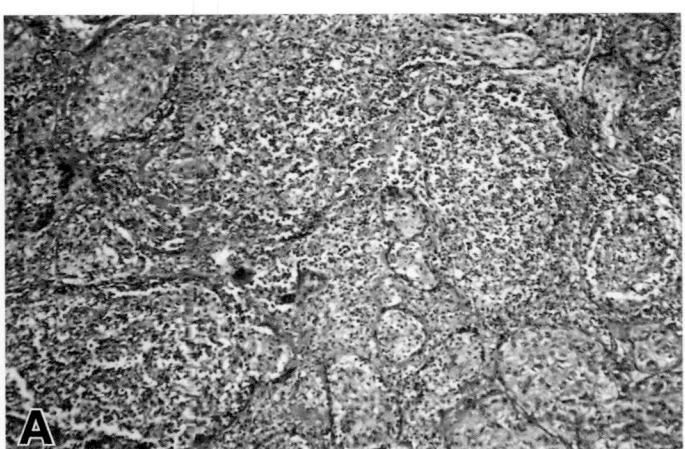 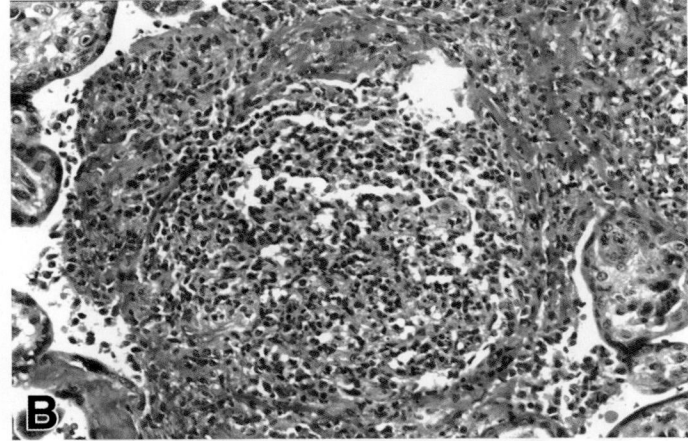

FIGURE 14-8. *Listeria* infection. A. Necrotizing villitis and intervillositis with microabscesses caused by *Listeria monocytogenes*. B. Higher magnification of acute villitis caused *by L. monocytogenes.* Acute inflammation has destroyed the central villus, which has become a microabscess. Neutrophils extend from the inflamed villus into the intervillous space and adjacent villi.

Listeria

Listeriosis is a potentially serious infection that occurs most commonly when pregnant women eat food contaminated with *Listeria monocytogenes*. The bacteria can circulate in maternal blood and infect the placenta and fetus. This may cause miscarriage, stillbirth, and premature delivery. Infants with *Listeria* infection show granulomatous rash and pyogenic granulomas throughout the body. *Listeria* also causes 5% of cases of neonatal meningitis.

PATHOLOGY: Placentas infected with *Listeria* contain abundant microabscesses that destroy villi and produce an acute intervillositis (Fig. 14-8). Necrotizing chorioamnionitis and severe funisitis are frequent.

Toxoplasma

T. gondii, a protozoan parasite in cats, is a potentially severe hazard. Fetal infections acquired early in pregnancy are more likely to be severe than those acquired later.

PATHOLOGY: Characteristic cysts of *Toxoplasma* can be present in subamnionic connective tissue, chorionic villi, trophoblast, and umbilical cord. Like syphilis and CMV, Hofbauer cell hyperplasia can also occur. Placental vascular thrombosis may occur, with or without calcification.

CLINICAL FEATURES: The classical triad of congenital toxoplasmosis, namely, hydrocephalus, intracranial calcifications, and chorioretinitis, is well known but does not occur in most infants infected *in utero.* Severe manifestations include encephalitis, multiple organ infection, epilepsy, mental retardation, blindness, and stillbirth.

Erythrovirus (Parvovirus B19) Causes Fetal Hydrops and Stillbirth

Erythrovirus, formerly called parvovirus B19, is a DNA virus that causes erythema infectiosum, a benign disease with fever and rash in children. When a pregnant woman becomes infected, the risk for stillbirth rises, especially if infection occurs in the first and second trimester. About 30% of acutely infected mothers transmit the virus to their fetus. Erythrovirus produces distinctive ground-glass intranuclear inclusions, called "lantern cells," which are most evident in nucleated fetal red blood (Fig. 14-9). Placentas are typically enlarged and villi are edematous. Newborns tend to be hydropic (Fig. 14-10) and anemic, and may have cardiac involvement.

HIV Can Be Transmitted From Mother to Fetus

When a woman infected with HIV becomes pregnant, her infant can become infected via three major routes. The virus can cross the placenta; it can infect the newborn at the time

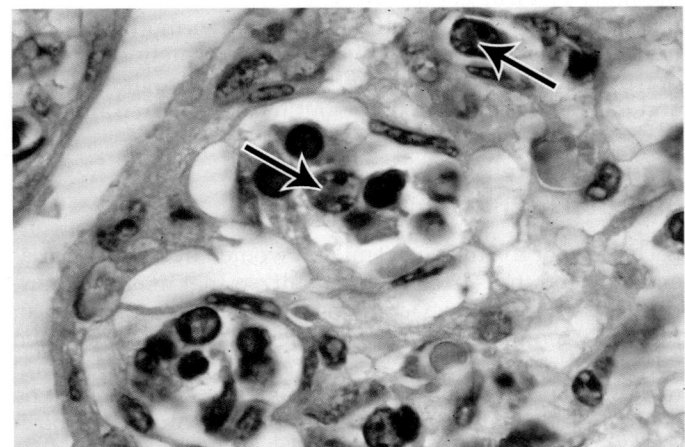

FIGURE 14-9. Intranuclear inclusions ("lantern cells," *arrows*) of erythrovirus (parvovirus) in nucleated fetal red blood cells in the placenta.

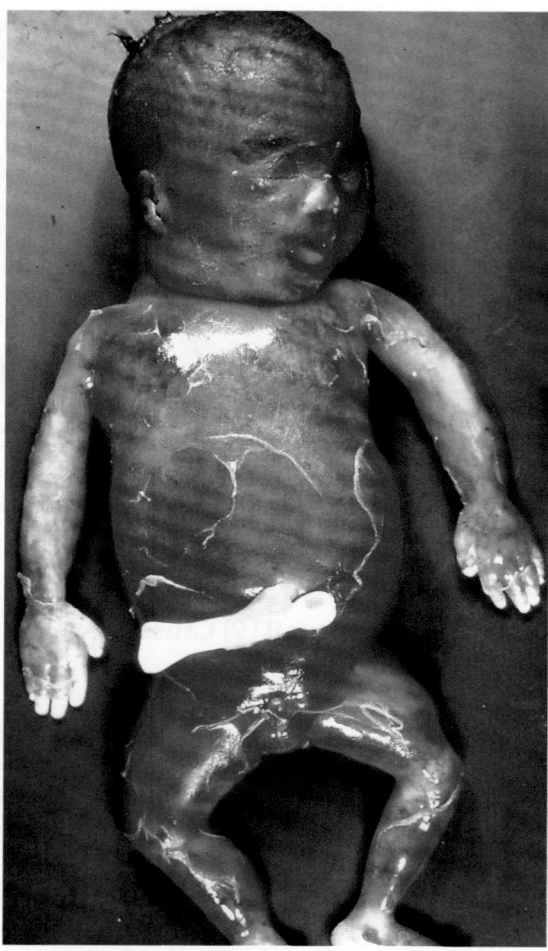

FIGURE 14-10. Stillbirth due to erythrovirus (parvovirus). The infant is hydropic (edematous).

of delivery; or infection can be transmitted through breast-feeding. Table 14-1 shows risk factors for maternal–fetal HIV transmission. Because HIV does not cause discernible abnormalities in the placenta, examining the placenta does not help establish that route of intrauterine transmission. Prenatal antiretroviral medication, education, and barrier methods of birth control have greatly reduced maternal–fetal HIV transmission. Without intervention, mother-to-child transmission rates are 15% to 45%. Unfortunately, one-fourth of women who are HIV+ do not receive antiretroviral therapy, and transmit HIV infection to about 160,000 children annually.

Malaria Remains a Perinatal Infection in Endemic Areas

Each year approximately 50 million women living in malaria-endemic countries become pregnant, so that malaria occurring during pregnancy remains an important problem in places where *Plasmodium* is endemic. Pregnant women who lack pre-existing immunity are at high risk for cerebral malaria, hypoglycemia, pulmonary edema, severe hemolytic anemia, and death. Malaria infection can cause low birth weight, and possibly abortion and stillbirth. In malaria-endemic African countries, 15% of infant deaths can be attributed to low birth weight.

TABLE 14-1

RISK FACTORS FOR PERINATAL TRANSMISSION OF HIV

Maternal Factors

Low CD4+ lymphocyte counts (T cells)

High HIV-1 RNA levels (viral load)

Acute retroviral syndrome during pregnancy

Presence of coinfections (hepatitis C, bacterial vaginosis, CMV)

Injection drug use

Absence of antiretroviral therapy or prophylaxis

Absence of prenatal care

Obstetric Factors

Duration of placental membrane rupture and/or chorioamnionitis

Invasive procedures

Vaginal delivery

Infant Factors

Premature delivery

Breastfeeding

CMV = cytomegalovirus.

 PATHOLOGY: Placentas of mothers with malaria may show maternal red blood cells infected with *Plasmodium* in the intervillous space. Malarial pigment may be abundant in intervillous spaces, villous stroma, and fibrin deposits (Fig. 14-11). Chronic intervillositis is common.

NONINFECTIOUS CONDITIONS AFFECTING CHORIONIC VILLI

Villitis of Unknown Etiology (VUE) Causes Reproductive Loss and Brain Damage, and Recurs in Subsequent Pregnancy

VUE is abnormal inflammation in chorionic villi, for which no infectious agent is found. Severe cases are associated with

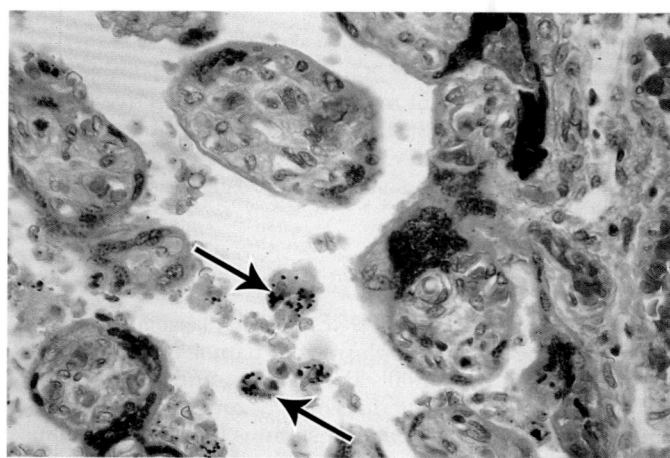

FIGURE 14-11. Placenta from mother with malaria. There is abundant intracellular brown pigment (hemosiderin, *arrows*) in the intervillous space.

significant rates of recurrence and with poor obstetric outcomes. Pregnancy failures occur in about 60% of pregnancies with recurrent VUE. Mild forms of VUE occur in 5% to 10% of pregnancies. They involve a single villus or very few villi, are not diffuse or necrotizing, and do not result in placental insufficiency.

 PATHOLOGY: VUE may be focal or diffuse. If it destroys chorionic villi, it is called necrotizing villitis of unknown etiology. This has an ominous prognosis for the fetus. Chronic uteroplacental malperfusion and insufficiency often coexist with other pathologic findings, including fetal thrombotic vasculopathy, distal villous hypoplasia, increased fibrin, and avascular chorionic villi.

Villous Edema Results From Fetal Stress

Villous edema, derived from the fetal chorionic circulation, is one of the most frequent causes of an enlarged placenta, especially in preterm deliveries.

ETIOLOGIC FACTORS: Villous edema has many causes. If it accompanies immunologic reactions and certain infections, it is **villous hydrops** and is often associated with **hydrops fetalis** (see Chapter 6), for example, in maternal–fetal Rh incompatibility and intrauterine erythrovirus infection (see above). However, villous edema can also occur without an edematous fetus, with intrauterine fetal stress usually the trigger. Other causes of villous edema include abruptio placentae, chorioamnionitis, umbilical cord accidents, fetal malformations, and genetic disorders. If edema is severe, it can compress fetal villous vessels, causing fetal hypoxia and stillbirth.

PATHOLOGY: Terminal villi are enlarged and edematous (Fig. 14-12). Edema fluid may be phagocytized by villous Hofbauer cells, where it appears as intracellular microdroplets. As edema accumulates in villi, it can cause clefts, or lacunae, in the villous interstitium, imparting a "bubbly" appearance. Villous edema tends to be most severe in immature placentas and preterm infants.

VASCULAR DISORDERS OF THE PLACENTA

Fetal Thrombotic Vasculopathy (FTV) Reflects Clotting in Placental Vessels

Thrombosis anywhere in the circulation of the placenta is called FTV, or fetal vascular malperfusion (FVM). It indicates an unfavorable intrauterine environment for the fetus. Clots can develop in arterial or venous circulations of the placenta and umbilical cord, although the venous circulation is most often affected. Risk factors for development of FTV include villitis and disorders of coagulation, particularly hypercoagulable syndromes (see Chapter 26). Clots forming in the placental circulation can cause terrible placental insufficiency by obstructing blood flow and thus perfusion in parts of the villous trees. Poor outcomes are associated with FTV, include stillbirth, neonatal death, IUGR and, in surviving infants, neurologic injury. FTV may occur with similar clots in fetal organs.

PATHOLOGY: Thrombi of varying ages are present in chorionic villous blood vessels. In acute FTV, large thrombi may occur in umbilical vessels or in the large vessels of the chorionic plate. Acute thrombi may affect smaller fetal vessels, including secondary and tertiary villi. In chronic FTV, chorionic villi downstream from thrombosed vessels undergo progressive fibrosis, giving a distinctive appearance to clusters of scarred, **avascular villi** (Fig. 14-13). Thrombi can be incorporated into vessel walls as mural thrombi, or **cushion defects**. In addition to the placenta, clots may also occur in fetal internal organs in FTV, e.g., brain, lungs, heart.

FTV in umbilical cord vessels (Fig. 14-14) can be catastrophic, and can complicate abnormally long or excessively twisted cords, velamentous cord insertion, or cord entanglement and knots.

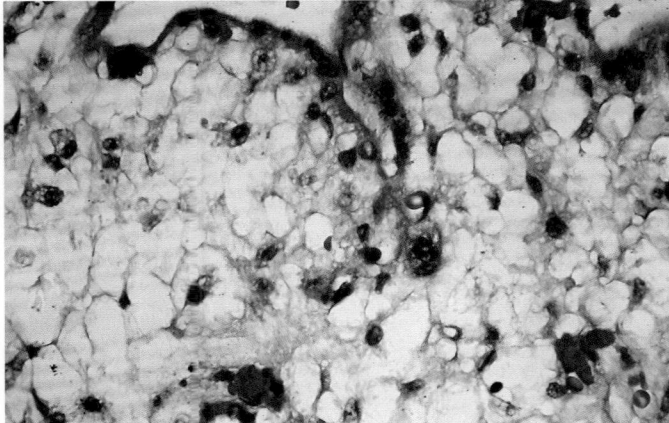
FIGURE 14-12. Villous edema. This villus is enlarged and hydropic, and the fetal capillaries appear compressed. Especially in premature infants, the stromal edema can inhibit oxygen transfer from maternal to fetal circulations.

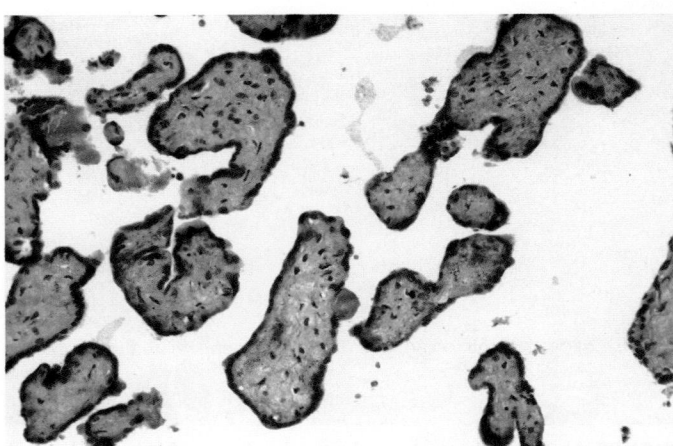
FIGURE 14-13. Avascular villi. The villous capillaries have been replaced by fibrous tissue as a result of a chronic thrombus in a larger upstream stem villus.

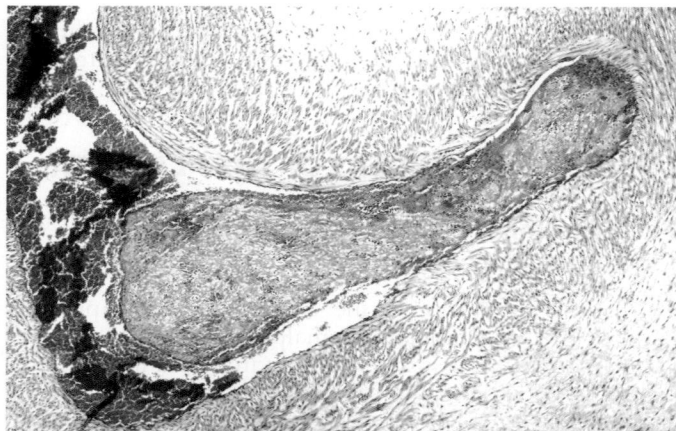

FIGURE 14-14.   Thrombus within an umbilical cord blood vessel.

Villous Stromal-Vascular Karyorrhexis Is Caused by Ischemic Injury to Chorionic Blood Vessels

Villous stromal-vascular karyorrhexis (previously, "hemorrhagic endovasculopathy") results from irreversible injury to endothelial cells lining fetal blood vessels in chorionic villi. It is associated with increased perinatal morbidity and mortality, neurologic impairment, and impaired fetal growth and development. This abnormality often accompanies other placental abnormalities, like fetal vascular malperfusion, VUE, villous fibrosis, infarcts, erythroblastosis, and meconium staining. Hypertensive disease of pregnancy is the only known risk factor.

PATHOLOGY: It can affect any vessel in the chorionic villous tree. Extravasated fetal red blood cells extend from the lumen through the intimal lining and into the surrounding blood vessel wall or stroma (Fig. 14-15). The vessel wall may be necrotic. Red blood cells can be fragmented, and karyorrhexis of endothelial and nucleated red blood cells is common.

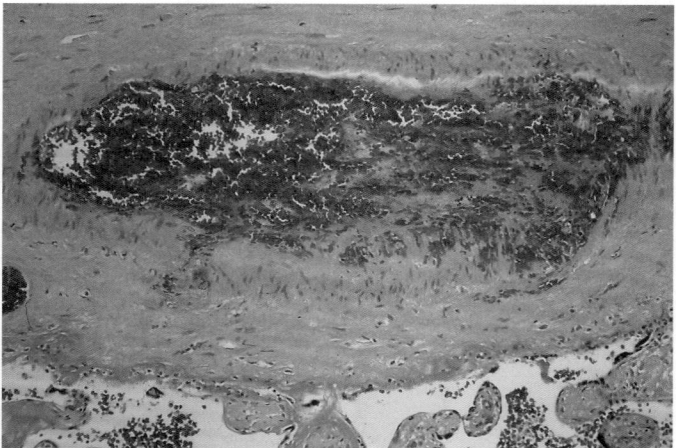

FIGURE 14-15. Villous stromal-vascular karyorrhexis (or hemorrhagic endovasculopathy). Fetal red blood cells in a large chorionic villus vessel extend from the lumen, through the ischemic endothelium and into the surrounding villous stroma.

Abruptio Placentae Causes Retroplacental Hematoma

Retroplacental hematoma occurs between the basal plate of the placenta and the uterine wall, and accounts for 8% of perinatal deaths. Hemorrhage derives from a ruptured maternal (spiral) artery or premature placental separation. Retroplacental hemorrhage can be due to placental abruption **(abruptio placentae)**. However, in 1/3 of cases it occurs without clinical abruption, and the reverse is also true. Abruptio placentae is often the final dramatic consequence of a chronic placental disorder, mostly maternal vascular disease that affects decidual blood vessels. Key risk factors for retroplacental hematoma include maternal smoking, hypertensive disease of pregnancy, late maternal age, acute chorioamnionitis, uterine malformation, placenta previa, history of previous abruption, short umbilical cord, thrombophilia, multiparity, and cocaine use. Abruption may occasionally be due to trauma.

PATHOLOGY: Premature placental detachment or rupture of a uterine blood vessel causes blood to accumulate between the placenta and the decidua basalis, forming a hematoma (Fig. 14-16). When a retroplacental hematoma is present for some time, overlying villous tissue may show ischemic infarction. Abruption can result from trauma (a fall or motor vehicle accident), but is usually nontraumatic—the culmination of a long-standing disorder of the mother's decidual blood vessels.

CLINICAL FEATURES: Abruptio placentae complicates 1% of pregnancies worldwide. Presentations depend upon the extent of abruption and include vaginal bleeding, uterine tenderness, abdominal or back pain, uterine tetanic contractions, fetal distress,

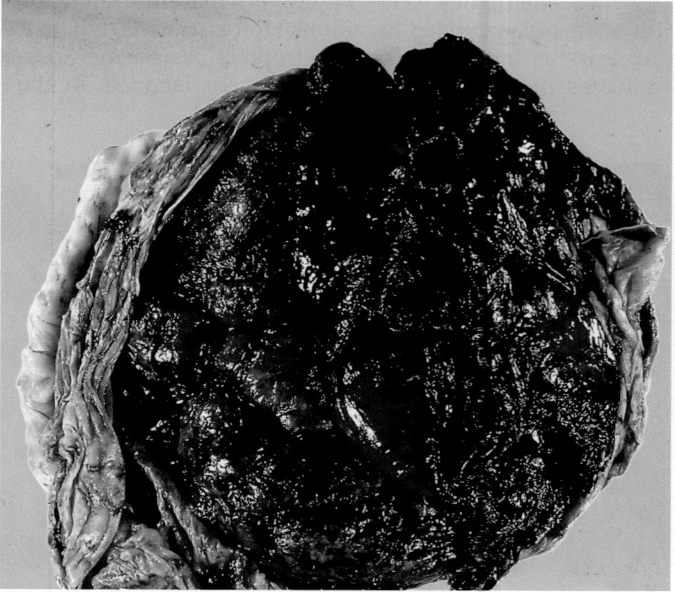

FIGURE 14-16.   Retroplacental hematoma. The occurrence of a retroplacental hemorrhage such as this large hematoma may correlate with the presence of a clinical abruption.

maternal shock, hypofibrinogenemia, coagulopathy, and maternal or fetal death.

In the half of placental abruptions that are mild, neither the fetus nor the mother suffers ill consequences. However, many abruptions result in poor fetal outcomes, including neonatal shock from hypoxia and anemia, irreversible neurologic injury, and perinatal death.

In some cases, blood forces its way into the underlying myometrium, resulting in a **"Couvelaire uterus."** In such cases, mothers may develop anemia, coagulopathy, disseminated intravascular coagulation (DIC), acute respiratory distress syndrome (ARDS), shock, and death. Maternal death due to abruptio placentae is rare in developed nations (0.4 per thousand cases of abruption), but is an important cause of maternal death in the resource-poor regions of the world.

Intervillous Thrombi Represent Fetomaternal Hemorrhage

When a chorionic villous blood vessel ruptures, blood accumulates in the placenta and forms an intervillous thrombus, or hematoma. Since the pressure of the fetal circulation in the placenta exceeds that of the maternal circulation, this represents **fetomaternal hemorrhage**, and fetal blood entering the maternal circulation can have clinical implications if fetal and maternal blood groups are not compatible.

Small, usually clinically insignificant, intervillous thrombi occur in up to 20% of full-term placentas. A larger thrombus or multiple thrombi can cause fetal blood loss or hypoxia. Intervillous thrombi can develop as a result of preeclampsia or maternal thrombophilias, and when there is thrombosis in the maternal circulation.

PATHOLOGY: Intervillous thrombi appear as well-demarcated red firm areas, much different from the surrounding spongy placental parenchyma. Hemorrhage compresses nearby villi (Fig. 14-17). When intervillous thrombi occur remotely from the time of delivery, the rim of surrounding compressed villi show infarction or avascular scarring.

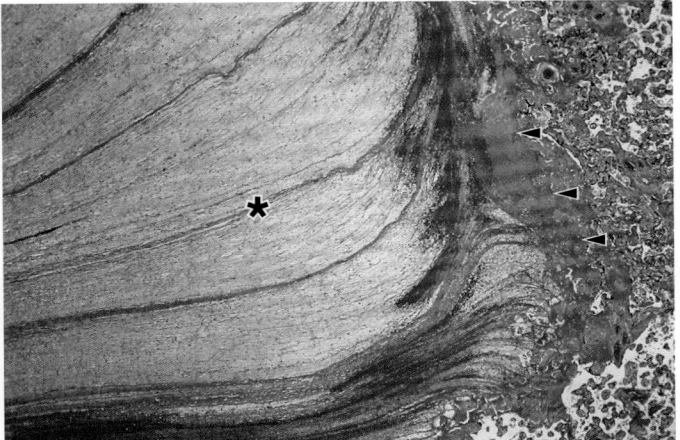

FIGURE 14-17. Intervillous thrombus (hematoma). This intraplacental hematoma (*) represents an area of fetal–maternal hemorrhage. It is surrounded by a zone of fibrin (*arrowheads*) and ischemic villi.

If significant amounts of fetal blood enter the maternal bloodstream from an intervillous thrombus, the fetal red blood cells may be detected using the **Kleihauer–Betke (KB)** test, which utilizes the differing sensitivity of fetal and adult hemoglobin to acid.

Placenta Accreta Is Abnormal Placental Adherence to the Uterus

Placenta accreta is caused by failure to form decidua. Normally, decidual endometrium separates the base of the placenta from underlying uterine muscle. Placenta accreta occurs when the decidual layer is partially or totally absent, so the villi contact the underlying decidua or uterine muscle directly. In that case, the placenta does not separate normally from the uterine wall at the time of delivery, which may lead to life-threatening maternal hemorrhage. Risk factors for placenta accreta include placenta previa, prior cesarean sections, advanced maternal age, high parity, and endometrial defects.

 PATHOLOGY: Placenta accreta is classified by the depth of myometrial invasion by the villi:

- In **placenta accreta**, villi attach to the surface of the uterine wall without further invasion (Fig. 14-18A).
- **Placenta increta** occurs when villi invade underlying myometrium, penetrating either superficially, or deep into the myometrium (Fig. 14-18B).
- In **placenta percreta**, villi traverse the entire uterine wall thickness. Sometimes, placenta percreta goes through the uterine serosa and invades adjacent organs such as the colon or urinary bladder; it can also result in uterine rupture.

CLINICAL FEATURES: Patients with placenta accreta can have a normal pregnancy and delivery. However, complications may occur during pregnancy, during delivery, or especially in the immediate postpartum period. Third-trimester bleeding is the most common presenting sign; substantial fragments of placenta may remain adherent after delivery and cause hemorrhage, endometritis, and DIC. Bleeding may threaten the lives of both mother and baby and necessitate emergency hysterectomy.

Chronic Placental Malperfusion Can Cause Poor Obstetric Outcomes

Adequate fetal oxygenation requires that both fetal and maternal circulations between the uteroplacental and fetal structures operate properly. Chronic placental malperfusion and insufficiency are important causes of perinatal morbidity and mortality. They can result in stillbirth, neonatal death, preterm birth, IUGR and, if the infant survives, neurologic damage. Chronic placental malperfusion can result from **maternal vascular malperfusion (MVM)**, where the placenta is not adequately perfused by maternal blood, or from fetal vascular malperfusion where there is suboptimal placental perfusion arising from disease of the fetal vessels. Some of the most frequent causes include distal villous hypoplasia,

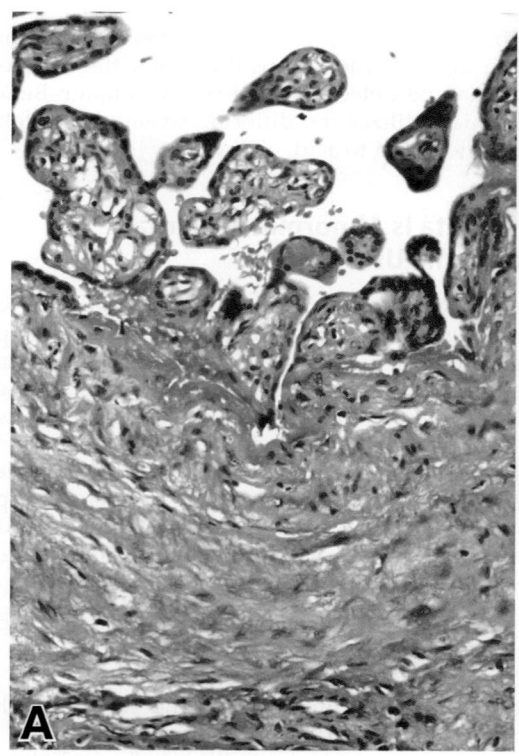

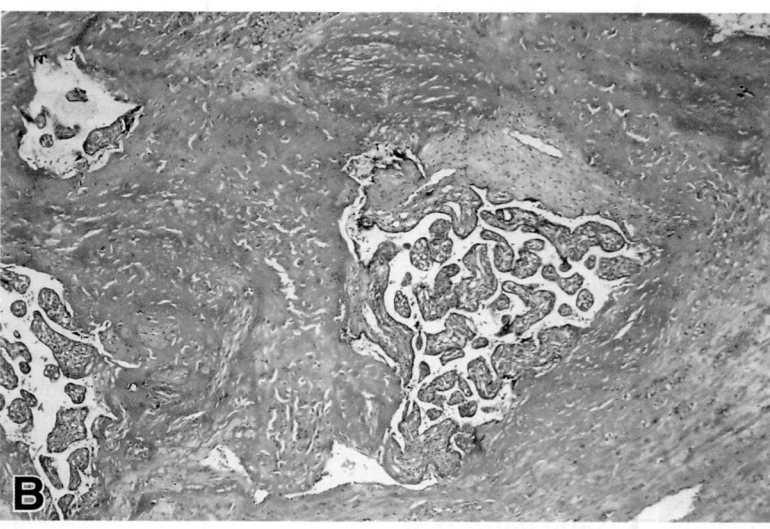

FIGURE 14-18. A. Placenta accreta. Some of the chorionic villi (*top*) are in contact with the underlying muscle. The decidua is absent. **B. Placenta increta.** The chorionic villi have invaded deeply into the uterine wall.

maternal floor infarction, massive perivillous fibrin deposition, diabetes, hypertension, cigarette smoking, autoimmune diseases, villitis, placental infarcts, chronic abruption, FVM, abnormally small or thin placentas, large chorangiomas, multiple or large remote intervillous thrombi and chronic umbilical cord abnormalities.

Distal Villous Hypoplasia Is Caused by Insufficient Maternal Blood Flow to the Placenta

Distal villous hypoplasia (or, uneven accelerated maturation) results from chronic underlying disease of spiral arterioles, including stenosis, fluctuating vasoconstriction or, as occurs with preeclampsia, defective remodeling (see below). It is an important cause of chronic maternal vascular malperfusion. Decreased maternal perfusion of the placental intervillous space leads to ischemic degeneration of chorionic villi (Fig. 14-19A,B). Resulting fetal hypoxia can produce stillbirth, neonatal death, IUGR, preterm birth, and neurologic injury in infants who survive.

Increased Fibrin Results in a Spectrum of Placental Disorders

Small amounts of fibrin from the maternal circulation deposit in the placenta under normal conditions. Fibrin occurs

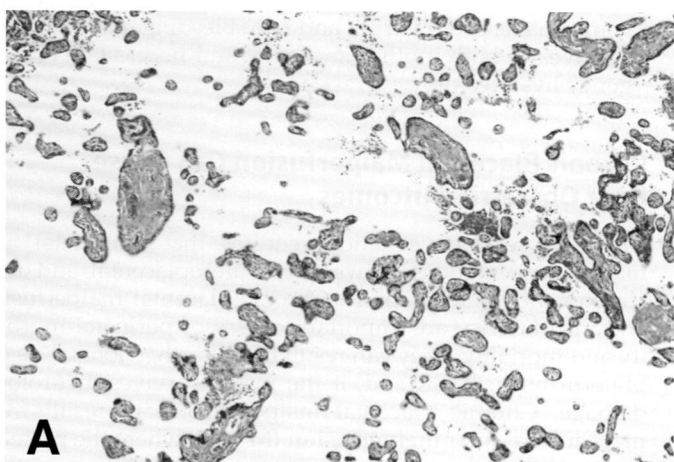

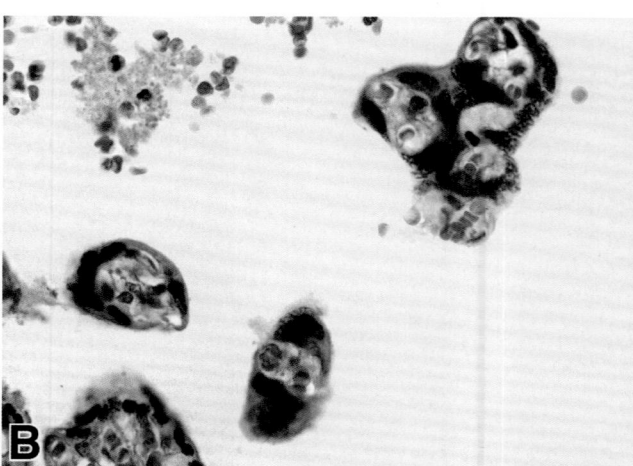

FIGURE 14-19. Distal villous hypoplasia. A. The diameter of the villi is decreased, resulting in an apparent increase in the intervillous space between villi. **B. High magnification of distal villous hypoplasia.** The characteristic features of chronic ischemia are present including small, ischemic, and shrunken villi with stromal fibrosis and clumped trophoblast.

normally under the fetal surface (chorionic plate) of the placenta where it is called **subchorionic fibrin** or **Langhans stria**, and results from eddying of maternal blood and, potentially, from fetal movement. **Rohr fibrin** is a necessary component of the basal plate of the placenta, where it faces the intervillous plate. **Nitabuch fibrin** deposits in the deep part of the basal plate. *Deficiency of Nitabuch fibrin causes placenta accreta.* Several chronic pathologic conditions are caused by fibrin abnormal deposition in the placenta.

Increased Perivillous Fibrin

Excess deposition of fibrin around villi can cause placental insufficiency. Pathologically increased fibrin deposited in intervillous spaces and around chorionic villi interferes with perfusion of the villi. It impairs oxygen delivery to the fetus by blocking oxygen-bearing maternal blood flow through the intervillous space and eventually causes ischemic necrosis of the villi (Fig. 14-20). This can result in chronic placental malperfusion and insufficency. Increased fibrin is also associated with infant brain injury.

Massive perivillous fibrin deposition (MPFD) can cause perinatal death. The cause of MPFD is unknown. The fibrin extends from the basal (decidual) part of the placenta up to the fetal (chorionic) surface. Dense fibrin fills the intervillous space, causing villous ischemic necrosis (Fig. 14-21). MPFD often leads to poor pregnancy outcomes including IUGR, perinatal death, and in infants who survive, neurologic injury.

Maternal Floor Infarction (MFI)

MFI is not a true infarct but shares some morphologic features with MPFD. Excessive fibrin extends confluently across the width of the placenta, mainly affecting the basal surface and decidua, and extending upward to involve the villi. The placental floor is firm, thickened and often discolored tan-yellow. Like MPFD, villi involved with MFI are embedded in dense fibrin and are necrotic. MFI has the same perinatal outcomes as does MPFD. It recurs in a subsequent pregnancy in up to 30% of women.

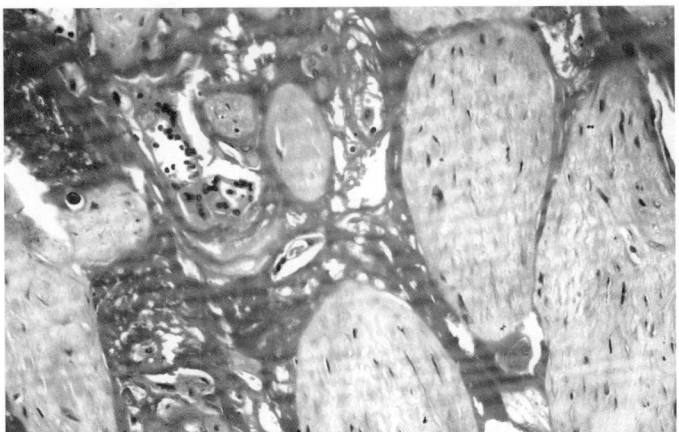

FIGURE 14-20. Increased villous fibrin. The fibrin has covered the chorionic villi, obstructed the intervillous space, and resulted in villous necrosis.

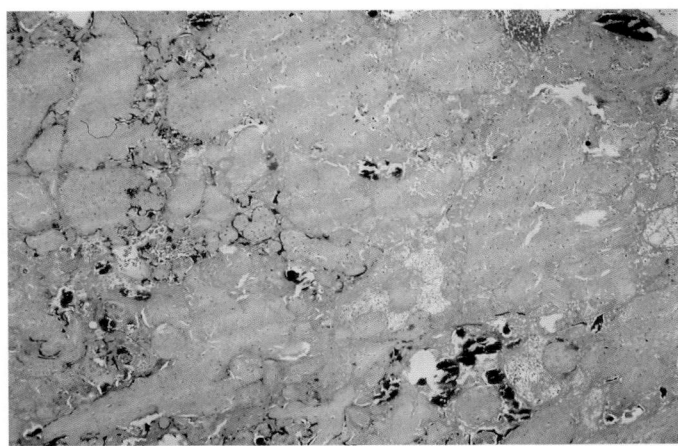

FIGURE 14-21. Massive perivillous fibrin deposition (MPFD). Low magnification showing confluent villous necrosis and fibrin deposition in the intervillous space. The small, dark purple microcalcifications attest to the chronicity of this process.

Infarcts Are the Most Frequently Diagnosed Vascular Condition of the Placenta

Complete interruption of maternal vascular supply causes placental infarction. The most common causes of placental infarction are hemorrhage between the base of the placenta and the uterine wall (retroplacental hemorrhage and abruptio placentae) and occlusion or thrombosis of the uterine spiral artery.

Placental infarcts often accompany hypertensive diseases of pregnancy including preeclampsia, maternal thrombophilia, and cigarette smoking. Small infarcts in placentas of full-term infants are common, and usually harmless. Multiple infarcts, especially if they are large or in the central part of the placenta, can result in placental insufficiency, leading to IUGR, neurologic injury, and perinatal death. Infarcts in any part of the placenta are never normal in the first two trimesters, and may signal a poor outcome.

PATHOLOGY: Infarcts are dark red areas that are firmer than surrounding placental tissue. As they age, infarcts become firmer, change from dark red to yellow and then to tan. They finally become white and sharply delineated from adjacent tissue.

Chorangiosis Is Abnormally Increased Chorionic Vasculature

Normal terminal chorionic villi contain five to six or fewer fetal blood vessels. In chorangiosis, terminal chorionic villi show marked increased numbers of vessels, due to capillary (endothelial) proliferation. This benign endothelial proliferation increases villous capillary surface area in the face of chronic intrauterine hypoxia. Chorangiosis takes many weeks to develop fully. It does not cause fetal damage but is a microscopic marker of significant uteroplacental insufficiency and fetal hypoxia that may arise from diverse causes.

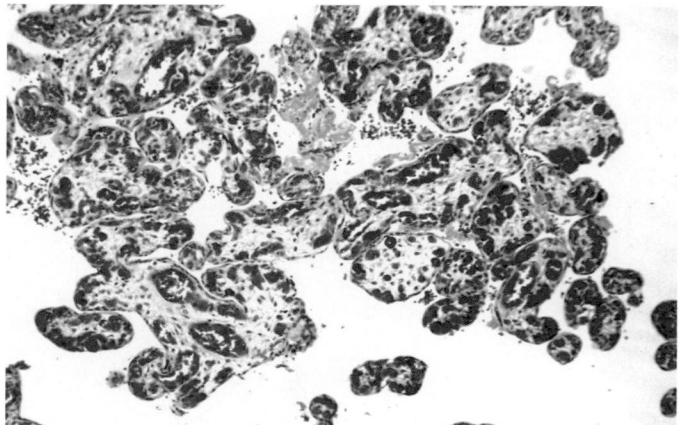

FIGURE 14-22. Chorangiosis. Chorangiosis results from chronic fetal hypoxia. The chorionic villi in these villi are hypervascular—most contain greater than 10 capillary cross-sections, and a few villi contain 20 or more vessels.

PATHOLOGY: Chorangiotic villi contain 10 or more vessels, affecting numerous villi. The increased vascularity may be so marked that some villi have 30 to 40 or more fetal vessels (Fig. 14-22).

Increased Syncytial Knots Indicate Uteroplacental Malperfusion

Chorionic villi are covered by a layer of multinucleated syncytiotrophoblast cells (see above). During chronic uteroplacental malperfusion, the syncytiotrophoblast forms prominent bulbous knots or folds, often bridging intervillous spaces and touching the trophoblast of adjacent villi (Fig. 14-23). Such **increased syncytial knots** (or syncytiotrophoblastic hyperplasia and Tenney–Parker changes) often reflects chronic malperfusion from all causes.

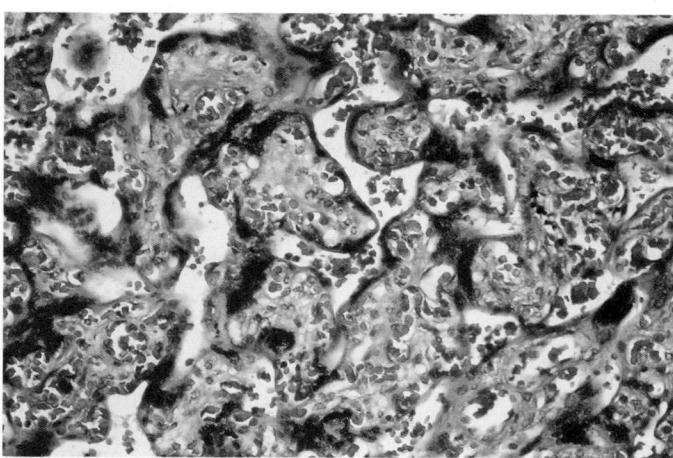

FIGURE 14-23. Increased syncytial knots (syncytiotrophoblastic hyperplasia or Tenney–Parker change). The syncytiotrophoblast is knotted and hyperbasophilic and bridges the intervillous space to connect to adjacent villi. This is caused by chronic uteroplacental malperfusion of either maternal or fetal origin.

MECONIUM DISORDERS

Meconium (Greek *me-ko-n,* or "poppy") is the earliest stools of the fetus or newborn. It is present in the intestine of the fetus until it is discharged, which may be before birth, during labor and delivery or following birth. Its composition is different from feces formed later in life: meconium is composed of materials ingested by the fetus while *in utero.* It includes water (80%), amniotic fluid, mucopolysaccharides, intestinal enzymes, bile, lanugo, and epithelial cells from the skin and intestines. Typically, meconium is sticky and tarry, dark olive green, and usually odorless.

Meconium Passage by the Fetus May Indicate Fetal Stress

Physiologic passage of meconium can be facilitated in full-term fetuses because of the maturity of the fetal gut. It can also be released when a term fetus experiences hypoxia or distress. Chorioamnionitis and amniotic infection syndrome, compression of the fetal head or umbilical cord, fetal asphyxia and acidosis and gestational cholestasis in the mother may all trigger meconium release. Meconium passage in preterm infants (<37 weeks) is always abnormal.

PATHOLOGY: Following delivery, the fetal surfaces of the placenta, membranes or umbilical cord appear discolored, varying from brown to green to golden yellow. Within 1 to 3 hours after meconium passage, the amnion will be stained. Beyond 3 to 4 hours before delivery, intracellular meconium is evident within the resident macrophages in the membranes or chorionic surface of the placenta (Fig. 14-24). When meconium has been present more than 24 hours, it may be seen in the umbilical cord mesenchyme (Wharton jelly) or in the trophoblast or decidual layers of the extraplacental membranes. In remote meconium passage, the amnionic epithelium is thickened or thrown up into finger-like projections owing to irritation, which is called **amnionic papillary hyperplasia**.

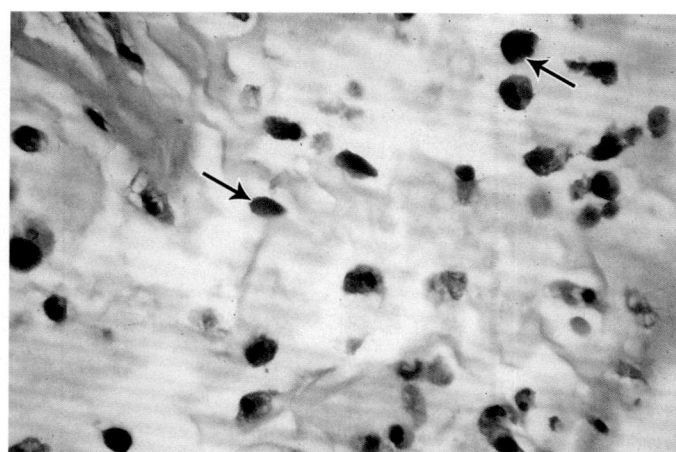

FIGURE 14-24. Abundant meconium in chorionic macrophages in a premature infant (*arrows*). It takes a minimum of 3 to 4 hours for meconium to be absorbed into the chorion and macrophages from the amniotic fluid following its passage by the fetus.

Meconium-Induced Vascular Necrosis (MIVN) Can Threaten the Life of the Fetus or Cause Brain Damage

MIVN is an important potential complication of meconium discharge. Meconium passed by the fetus long before delivery has sufficient time to penetrate the connective tissue (Wharton jelly) of the umbilical cord or through the chorionic plate, to reach and permeate the muscular walls of the umbilical cord or large chorionic plate blood vessels. A toxic reaction ensues, leading to apoptotic degeneration and necrosis of the smooth muscle cells over a period of several days or greater. Once blood vessels undergo MIVN-induced smooth muscle necrosis, they cannot regulate fetal blood flow adequately. Poor obstetric outcomes including brain injury (e.g., cerebral palsy) and death may result.

PATHOLOGY: Umbilical cord vessels and large chorionic plate blood vessels can be involved in MIVN (Fig. 14-25). In affected blood vessels, only eosinophilic remnants of the cytoplasm remain visible. In remote cases of MIVN, muscular walls of affected vessel are thinned. Meconium is often visible within connective tissues near the injured vessels.

MULTIPLE COMORBID CONDITIONS

Sometimes in a pregnancy, two or more abnormal conditions or diseases occur in the mother, placenta, fetus, or all three.

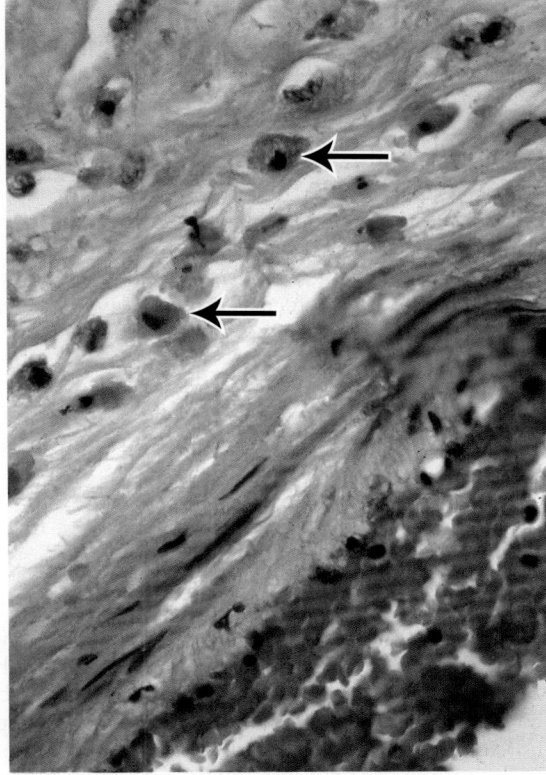

FIGURE 14-25. Meconium-induced vascular necrosis (MIVN). Smooth muscle cells of the fetal blood vessel have undergone degeneration and necrosis, and appear rounded and hyperchromatic (*arrows*).

Multiple simultaneous abnormalities, or comorbid conditions, may vary in etiologies, severity, timing, and duration, and are not necessarily causally linked. If multiple adverse uteroplacental conditions coexist, the risk of poor obstetrical outcomes—e.g., growth restriction, birth depression, stillbirth, neonatal death, brain injury and neurobehavioral abnormalities—are **synergistic, exponential** or **multiplicative**. Disorders of differing durations are particularly dangerous combinations. Chronic uteroplacental placental problems can reduce the threshold needed for later abnormalities to cause brain damage or perinatal death. Thus, evaluating placental size, fetal weight and placental and fetal reserve is particularly important in understanding poor obstetrical and neonatal outcomes.

ABNORMALITIES OF BIRTH WEIGHT

IUGR is an abnormality of fetal growth and development that affects 3% to 10% of deliveries. IUGR can be asymmetric (60% to 70%) or symmetric (20% to 30%), or have a combined or mixed pattern in 5% to 10% of cases.

Asymmetric IUGR Usually Reflects Chronic Uteroplacental Insufficiency

Asymmetric IUGR occurs when the placenta cannot provide adequate oxygen and nutrition to the fetus for a long period of time. Fetal soft tissues of the extremities (skeletal muscle mass) and body (subcutaneous fat, especially at the abdomen) undergo gradual wasting. The liver also becomes smaller due to decreased hepatic fat and glycogen. Infants with asymmetrical IUGR often have normal body weight, length, and head circumference for gestational age and gender. Because the head usually continues to grow despite soft-tissue wasting, this is often termed *"head-sparing IUGR."* Diagnosis of asymmetrical IUGR can be definitively made at birth using the **Ponderal Index**, which utilizes the relationship between birth weight and length. If under the 10th percentile for gestational age, the Ponderal Index is diagnostic of asymmetric IUGR. This index requires either ultrasonography or measurement after delivery, so many cases of asymmetrical IUGR are only appreciated after birth.

Asymmetric IUGR can become a mixed pattern of IUGR if uteroplacental insufficiency is sufficiently long-lasting or severe. Resulting newborns have 5 to 10 times increased risk for perinatal mortality and morbidity than those who are not growth restricted. Placentas with asymmetric IUGR may be small and thin, and typically show distal villous hypoplasia, FTV and avascular villi, increased fibrin, infarcts and other pathologies.

 ETIOLOGIC FACTORS: Placentas from neonates with asymmetrical IUGR are almost always abnormal and typically show lesions of chronic fetal or maternal vascular malperfusion, or chronic maternal disease. *Maternal cigarette smoking is the most important preventable cause of asymmetric IUGR.*

Symmetrical IUGR Develops Early in Pregnancy

Symmetrical IUGR generally results from intrinsic fetal diseases that develop early in pregnancy. It is less common than asymmetrical IUGR, accounting for 20% to 30% of growth-restricted newborns. Unlike asymmetrical IUGR, in symmetrical IUGR most of the baby's size parameters are abnormally small—infants typically have low birth weights, small head circumference, short body length, etc.

 ETIOLOGIC FACTORS: Causes of symmetrical IUGR include genetic disorders of the fetus such as chromosome aberrations, metabolic disorders and inborn errors of metabolism, malformation syndromes, maternal malnutrition, maternal substance abuse (e.g., alcohol), infections early in pregnancy (e.g., toxoplasmosis, rubella, CMV), anemia, and some drugs. Similar to asymmetrical IUGR, symmetrical IUGR has a 5 to 10 times increased risk for perinatal mortality and morbidity.

Abnormal Weights for Gestational Age May Reflect Intrauterine Exposures

Small-for-gestational-age (**SGA**) infants weigh below the 10th percentile for their gestational age and gender. Similarly, **large-for-gestational-age** (**LGA**) infants weigh above the 90th percentile. Average birth weights vary with geography, ethnicity, and socioeconomic status. However, SGA or LGA infants may be products of intrauterine diseases or toxicities. Related terms for infant birth weight are:

- **Low birth weight (LBW):** a newborn weighing <2,500 g regardless of gestational age
- **Very low birth weight (VLBW):** infants weighing <1,500 g
- **Extremely low birth weight (ELBW):** newborns weighing <1,000 g

LBW Is Associated With Increased Neonatal Morbidity and Mortality

LBW infants are 20-fold more likely to die than are normal–birth-weight infants. They tend to remain malnourished, with intellectual and cognitive disabilities. More than 95% of such babies are born in developing countries. LBW in developing countries mostly reflects IUGR, while in the developing world most LBW is due to prematurity.

Most ELBW Infants Are Born at Under 27 Weeks

Such infants represent <1% of live births in Western nations. Only 14% of infants weighing less than 500 g at birth survive their first year; between 500 and 749 g, 51% live to be 1 year old; 85% of infants between 750 and 1,000 g at birth are alive at 1 year. In the resource-poor nations, data for ELBW infants are scarce, and survival is most likely rare.

Macrosomia Can Be Constitutional or Caused by Intrauterine Disease

Depending on the criteria used, macrosomic newborns weigh >4,000 g (8 lb, 13 oz) or >4,500 g (9 lb, 15 oz), regardless of gestational age or gender. Macrosomia differs from LGA because the latter is based on birth weight exceeding the 90th percentile.

Fetal macrosomia presents problems for both mother and infant. Potential maternal complications include difficulty

in labor, genital tract lacerations, postpartum bleeding, and uterine rupture. Macrosomic fetuses have more body mass and so require more oxygen. Poor outcomes may result if uteroplacental unit cannot satisfy this demand. Stillbirth is twice as common for macrosomic infants as for normal-sized infants, regardless of maternal diabetes.

 ETIOLOGIC FACTORS: The most frequent cause of neonatal macrosomia is maternal diabetes. Gestational diabetes increases maternal serum glucose levels. The infant responds to this stimulus by increasing its insulin secretion, which in turn stimulates fetal growth. Male infants are at greater risk than females. Other risk factors for macrosomia include maternal obesity, excessive maternal weight gain, prior history of macrosomic infants, prolonged pregnancy (>41 weeks) and advanced maternal age.

VARIATIONS IN CARRYING PREGNANCIES

Spontaneous Abortion, or Miscarriage Occurs When a Pregnancy Ends Before the 20th Week

About 10% to 15% of recognized pregnancies miscarry, that is, abort spontaneously. An additional 30% of women abort without being aware that they were pregnant. Thus, almost half of pregnancies miscarry, making it the most common complication of early pregnancy. The most common symptom of spontaneous abortion is bleeding.

 ETIOLOGIC FACTORS: Most spontaneous abortions occur before 12 weeks of gestation. Karyotypic anomalies are present in 50% of spontaneous abortions, and in up to 70% of those occurring before the 7th week of gestation. The main factors responsible for spontaneous abortion are:

- Infection early in pregnancy (e.g., *Listeria*, CMV, *Toxoplasma*, coxsackievirus)
- Mechanical factors (e.g., uterine leiomyoma, septate uteri, cervical incompetence)
- Endocrine factors (e.g., maternal diabetes, polycystic ovary, luteal phase defects, progesterone deficiency, hypothyroidism)
- Immunologic factors
- Cigarette smoking
- Cocaine use
- Congenital fetal malformations (e.g., neural tube defects)
- Chromosomal abnormalities
- Increasing maternal age
- Multiple gestation (e.g., twins, triplets, etc.)

 PATHOLOGY: An empty gestational sac with hydropic swelling of the chorionic villi (blighted ovum) suggests early fetal demise. The embryo may be grossly disorganized or show defects such as spina bifida, anencephaly, or cleft palate. Chorionic villi may be histologically normal or show intravillous fibrosis or hydropic change. If infection preceded miscarriage, there is often microscopic evidence of the infectious agent (see Chapter 9).

Recurrent Pregnancy Loss

For most fertile couples miscarriage is a sporadic event, but 1% to 5% of fertile couples experience **recurrent pregnancy loss** (RPL; also termed **habitual abortion**).

 ETIOLOGIC FACTORS: The **antiphospholipid syndrome** accounts for 3% to 15% of RPL. Another important cause is **thrombophilia**, mostly **factor V Leiden** and **prothrombin G20210A** (factor II) mutations. Chromosomal aberrations in one or both partners occur in 4% of couples with RPL. Diverse endocrine factors—hypothyroidism, polycystic ovary disease, diabetes, and inadequate production of progesterone—can cause RPL. Anatomic conditions, such as cervical incompetence and uterine malformations, or immune factors including antithyroid autoantibodies and maternal immunization against male-specific minor histocompatibility (H-Y) antigens are also involved in some cases. Certain ovarian factors increase risk for RPL, including luteal phase defects and advanced maternal age, with decreased ovarian reserve and decreased egg quality.

Multiple Gestations May Be Dizygotic or Monozygotic

Slightly under 1% of normal pregnancies are dizygotic or monozygotic twins (Fig. 14-26).

DIZYGOTIC TWINS: Fertilization of two separate ova yields genetically different twins, of the same or opposite sex. Dizygotic twinning has a strong hereditary component, only on the maternal side. Dizygotic twinning and multiple gestations occur more often in women who used hormones to induce ovulation artificially or who underwent *in vitro* fertilization.

Separate placentas develop when two fertilized ova implant apart from one another. If they implant near each other, the two placentas may show varying degrees of fusion, and even appear to be one. If the ova implant apart, there are discrete conceptuses, each placenta having its own amniotic sac. When two placentas fuse, the membranes between the two fetuses show two amnions and two chorions (diamnionic, dichorionic gestation).

MONOZYGOTIC TWINS: Early division of a single fertilized ovum results in genetically identical twins of the same sex. If a fertilized ovum divides within 2 days of fertilization, before the trophoblast has differentiated, two separate embryos develop, each with its own placenta and amniotic sac (dichorionic, diamniotic twinning). Hence, dichorionic placentas may be either monozygotic or dizygotic, while monochorionic placentas are always monozygous. If division occurs from the third to eighth days after conception, the trophoblast (but not the amniotic cavity) has already differentiated. A single placenta with two amniotic sacs develops (monochorionic, diamniotic twinning). A monochorionic, monoamniotic placenta is formed if division occurs between the 8th and 13th day postconception, because the amniotic cavity has already developed. Incomplete separation of monozygous twins results in **conjoint (formerly Siamese) twins** within a monoamniotic, monochorionic placenta.

MATERNAL AND FETAL OBSTETRICAL COMPLICATIONS

Preeclampsia and Eclampsia Are Hypertensive Disorders of Pregnancy

Together, they define a syndrome of hypertension, protein-uria and, most severely, CNS complications. Preeclampsia occurs in 2% to 8% of pregnancies, most often in primagravidas. It usually occurs in the third trimester, but earlier onset often portends worse outcomes. If seizures occur, the syndrome is eclampsia. Preeclampsia causes about 50,000 maternal deaths worldwide yearly.

 ETIOLOGIC FACTORS: Preeclampsia probably arises because of faulty remodeling of uterine spiral arteries that supply maternal blood to the placenta. Immunologic and genetic factors, as well as altered vascular reactivity, endothelial injury and coagulation abnormalities, may also contribute. The characteristics of preeclampsia are (Fig. 14-27):

- Maternal blood flow to the placenta is markedly reduced because of ineffective remodeling of maternal spiral arteries of the decidua.

THE PATHOLOGY OF PREGNANCY

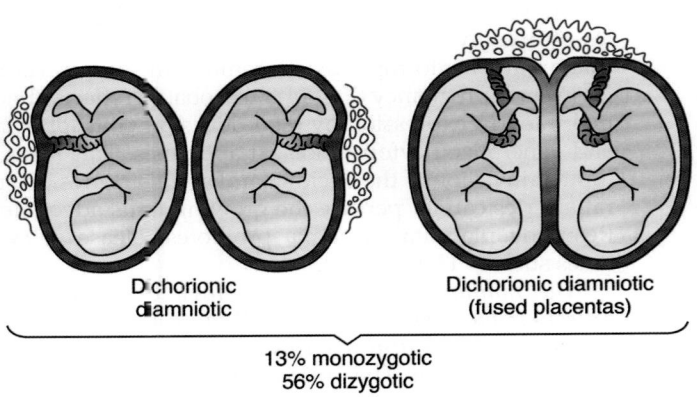
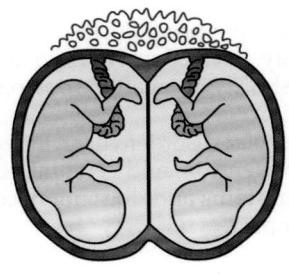
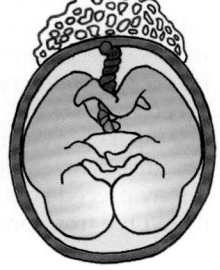

Dichorionic diamniotic

Dichorionic diamniotic (fused placentas)

13% monozygotic
56% dizygotic

Monochorionic diamniotic

30% monozygotic

Conjoint twins monochorionic monoamniotic

<<1% monozygotic

FIGURE 14-26. Placental structure in twin pregnancies. The percentages in the figure refer to the proportion of total twin pregnancies (100%) accounted for by each variant.

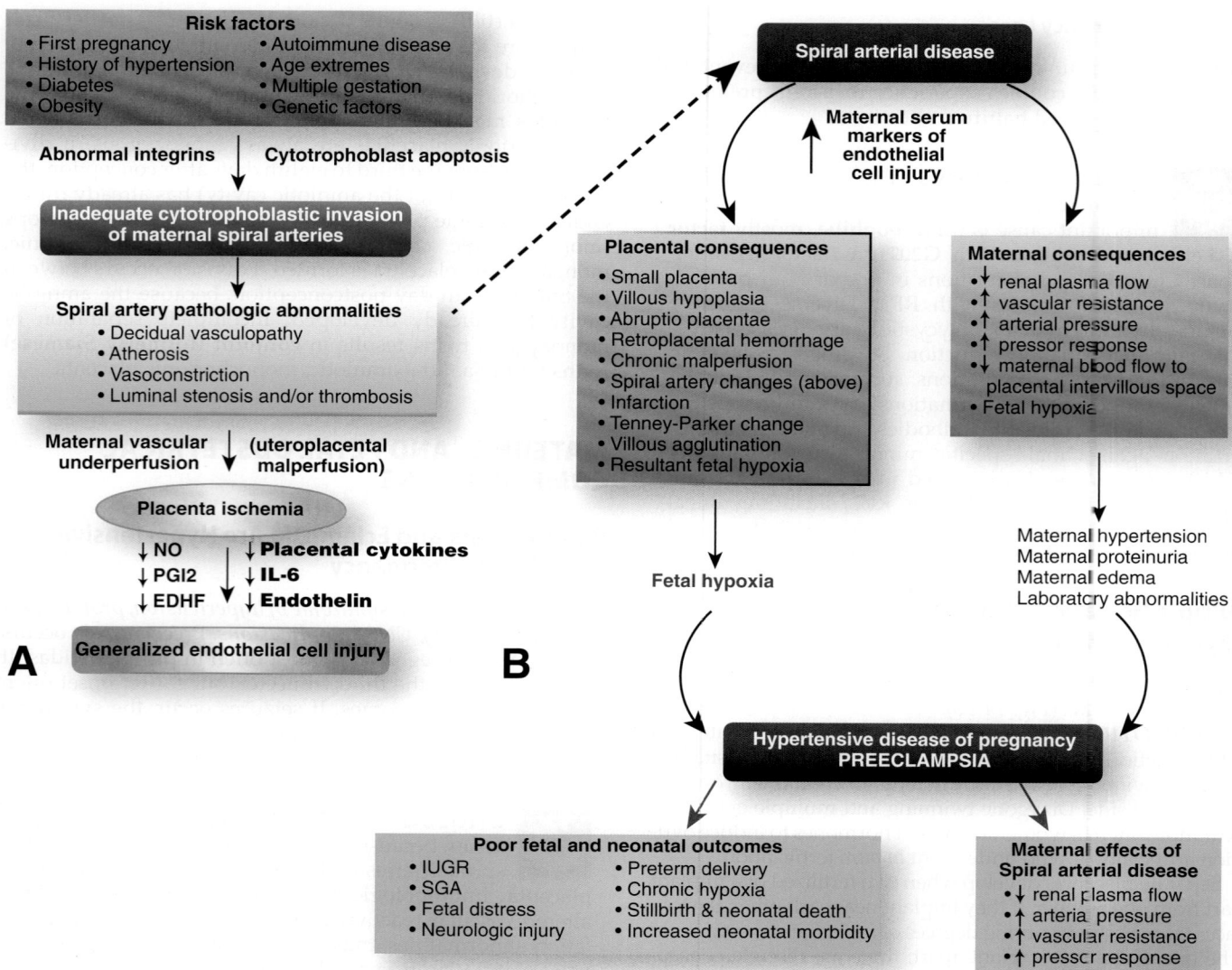

FIGURE 14-27. **Pathogenesis of preeclampsia.** *EDHF* = endothelium-derived hyperpolarizing factor; *IUGR* = intrauterine growth retardation.

- Renal involvement contributes to hypertension and proteinuria.
- Disseminated intravascular coagulation (DIC) may occur in preeclampsia.
- The risk of preeclampsia in a first pregnancy is many-fold higher than in subsequent pregnancies.
- Rarely, preeclampsia may not occur until the time of labor and delivery, or shortly thereafter (postpartum preeclampsia).
- Eclampsia is a cerebrovascular disorder characterized by seizures, worsening hypertension, and cerebral edema. It may precede other symptoms and does not necessarily evolve from preeclampsia.

PATHOPHYSIOLOGY: Early in a normal pregnancy, fetal cytotrophoblast cells extend downward into the decidua and uterus. They invade the uterine spiral arteries and progressively replace the maternal-derived endothelium, medial elastic tissue, smooth muscle and neural tissue. By the end of the second trimester, the normally narrow spiral arteries are dilated tubes lined by fetal-derived cytotrophoblast. This low-resistance arterial circuit supplies the increasing oxygen and nutrient demands of the developing fetus.

In preeclampsia, many maternal uterine (spiral) arteries escape invasion by trophoblastic tissue and so never dilate. Faulty cytotrophoblastic remodeling of spiral arteries in early pregnancy (Fig. 14-27) probably reflects abnormal integrin expression by fetal-derived cytotrophoblast and generalized cytotrophoblast apoptosis. This leads to limited invasion of the decidua and spiral arteries, so spiral arteries cannot perfuse the growing fetus adequately. Resulting placental ischemia promotes release of cytokines such as TNFα and IL-6.

The fundamental pathophysiology of preeclampsia reflects reduced maternal blood flow to the uteroplacental unit, as the spiral arteries of the uteroplacental bed never fully dilate. The combination of vasoconstriction and structural changes in spiral arteries contributes to inadequate blood flow, placental ischemia, villous hypoplasia, and fetal hypoxia. The effectiveness of vasodilators in treating preeclampsia, including nitric oxide (NO•), prostacyclin (PGI₂), and endothelium-derived hyperpolarizing factor (EDHF), is further evidence for endothelial dysfunction in preeclampsia.

Upregulation of placental antiangiogenic factors (e.g., VEGF, see Chapter 5) and soluble endoglin may play a role in the onset of the clinical features of preeclampsia, including hypertension and proteinuria. Roles, if any, of other factors are unclear.

PATHOLOGY: *Placental pathology usually precedes the clinical onset of maternal hypertension.* Extensive placental infarction is seen in 1/3 of women with severe preeclampsia, although it is often negligible in mild preeclampsia. Retroplacental hemorrhage or abruptio placentae occurs in 15% and abnormally small placentas (<10th percentile) in 10% of cases (Fig. 14-16). Chorionic villi show signs of chronic maternal underperfusion, consisting of ischemically degenerated chorionic villi (villous hypoplasia; Fig. 14-19), fibrin (Fig. 14-20), increased placental site giant cells, syncytiotrophoblastic hyperplasia (Tenney–Parker change) (Fig. 14-23) and mural hypertrophy of membrane arterioles. The spiral arteries commonly show fibrinoid necrosis, clusters of lipid-rich macrophages, and a perivascular infiltrate of mononuclear cells; collectively called **acute atherosis** (Fig. 14-28). These vessels are often thrombosed, causing focal placental infarcts.

Maternal kidneys always show glomerular changes. Glomeruli are enlarged and endothelial cells are swollen, forming classic "bloodless" glomeruli of preeclampsia (glomerular endotheliosis) (Fig. 14-29). Fibrin deposits between endothelial cells and the glomerular capillary basement membrane. Mesangial cell hyperplasia is the rule. These maternal renal changes are reversible with therapy or after delivery.

Fatal cases of eclampsia often show cerebral hemorrhages, ranging from petechiae to large hematomas. *Liver abnormalities occur in 60% of women dying from preeclampsia,* including periportal fibrin deposits and necrosis (Fig. 14-30), lobular hemorrhage, and hepatic infarction.

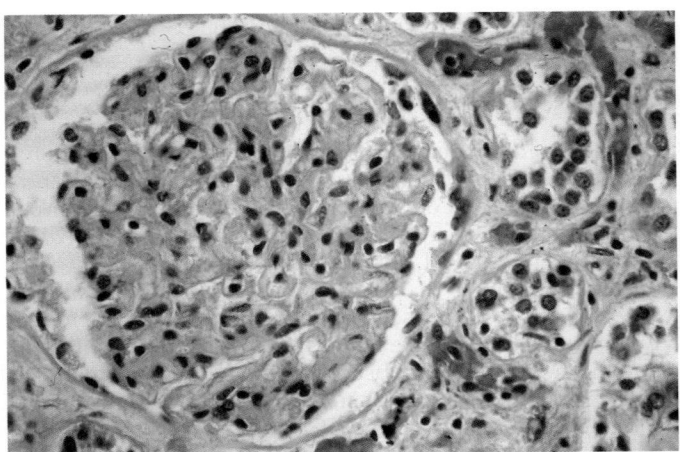

FIGURE 14-29. Glomerular endotheliosis. This is the "bloodless glomerulus" from a woman dying from preeclampsia.

CLINICAL FEATURES: Preeclampsia usually begins insidiously after the 20th week of pregnancy, with excessive weight gain due to fluid retention, increased maternal blood pressure, and proteinuria. As preeclampsia progresses from mild to severe, diastolic pressure persistently exceeds 110 mm Hg, proteinuria reaches over 3 g/day and renal function declines. DIC often supervenes. Preeclampsia is treated with antihypertensive and antiplatelet drugs, but definitive therapy requires removing the placenta. Eclampsia is treated with magnesium sulfate, which reduces cerebrovascular tone.

Preeclampsia Predisposes to HELLP Syndrome

HELLP syndrome—hemolytic anemia, elevated liver enzymes, and low platelet count—is a potentially fatal condition of pregnant women and their infants that most often follows third trimester preeclampsia. It occurs in 0.2% to 0.6% of pregnancies, and in 4% to 12% of women with preeclampsia or eclampsia. It may occur before (70%) or after (30%) delivery.

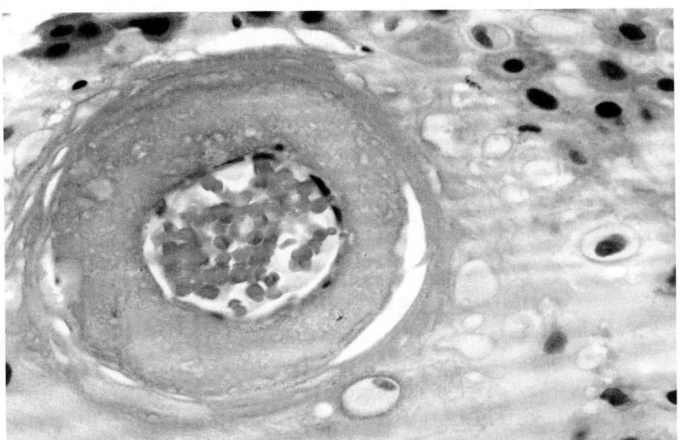

FIGURE 14-28. Decidual atherosis in preeclampsia. A small decidual artery shows fibrinoid thickening of the vessel wall.

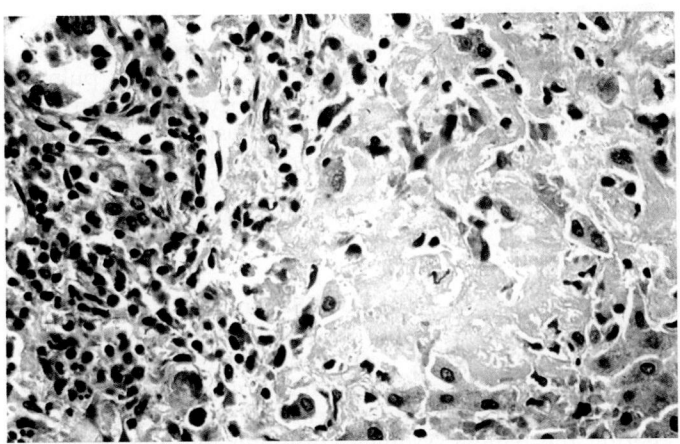

FIGURE 14-30. Liver of a woman with preeclampsia. The periportal area (zone 1) demonstrates fibrin deposition.

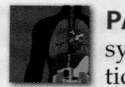 **PATHOPHYSIOLOGY:** The trigger for HELLP syndrome is unknown, but generalized activation of coagulation is thought to be the major problem. The syndrome evolves from microvascular endothelial damage and intravascular platelet activation. The latter causes vasospasm, platelet agglutination, and further endothelial damage. Excessive platelet consumption results in DIC and microangiopathic anemia in 20% of women with HELLP syndrome.

Fibrin deposits in hepatic sinusoids obstructs blood flow, causing liver ischemia and periportal necrosis. Liver enzyme levels are increased. In severe cases, intrahepatic hemorrhage, subcapsular hematoma formation, or hepatic rupture may occur. Additional complications include hemorrhage from DIC, pulmonary edema, placental abruption, ARDS, acute hepatorenal failure, and fetal death. The maternal mortality rate is 1%. Infant morbidity and mortality vary from 10% to 60%, depending on the severity of maternal disease.

Amniotic Fluid Embolism (AFE) Is a Obstetrical Emergency

AFE is a rare, life-threatening event that results in an anaphylaxis-like syndrome. It occurs when amniotic fluid, fetal squamous cells, hair, vernix, and other amniotic materials enter the maternal circulation through the uterine veins in the decidual bed at the base of the placenta. Maternal mortality has declined to 25%, but it still accounts for 5% to 10% of maternal deaths in the United States. About 20% of infants die after their mothers develop AFE.

 PATHOPHYSIOLOGY: Amniotic fluid constituents entering the maternal bloodstream are thought to trigger the acute onset of symptoms of AFE (Fig. 14-31). Many pathogenetic aspects of AFE resemble those of preeclampsia (see above).

However, amniotic fluid cellular elements are not always identified in women who die with AFE. If amniotic fluid materials enter the maternal bloodstream during labor and delivery, they trigger anaphylaxis, complement activation or both.

PATHOLOGY: In fatal cases of AFE, the lungs show diffuse alveolar damage (see Chapter 18). Platelet–fibrin aggregates are present in pulmonary vessels, and increased megakaryocytes are often seen in alveoli, heralding the onset of DIC. Distinctive fetal squamous epithelial cells are often present in both alveolar capillaries and larger blood vessels (Fig. 14-32A). Rarely, other fetal elements are present, including fetal hair (Fig. 14-32B).

CLINICAL FEATURES: Initially, pulmonary arterial vasospasm, pulmonary hypertension, and elevated right ventricular pressure cause hypoxia. Myocardial and pulmonary capillary damage follow, with ARDS and left heart failure, further endangering the patient. Women surviving the first phase of AFE may develop a second phase, including uterine

atony, hemorrhage and DIC. A fatal consumptive coagulopathy may be the initial presentation.

Intrahepatic Cholestasis of Pregnancy (ICP) Is a Leading Cause of Gestational Jaundice

ICP occurs in 1 to 2 women per 1,000 pregnancies, typically presenting as intense pruritus. It usually begins in the third trimester, but may occur any time during pregnancy. It can endanger a fetus' health, and may cause fetal distress, spontaneous premature delivery, meconium aspiration syndrome, intrauterine fetal demise, and neonatal death.

 ETIOLOGIC FACTORS: The cause of ICP is not known, but pregnancy hormones and genetic factors are probably involved. ICP most commonly occurs in the third trimester, when maternal pregnancy hormone levels are at their highest, and it occurs more often in multifetal pregnancies, which are associated with higher hormone levels. Estrogens and glucuronides can cause cholestasis, and high-dose estrogen oral contraceptives can trigger features of ICP in nonpregnant women.

 CLINICAL FEATURES: The most common maternal complaint is intense itching without a rash, most often involving the palms and soles. Circulating liver enzymes and bile acids can be elevated. Jaundice, dark urine, right upper quadrant pain, and lighter stools occur less often. Risks of recurrence may be 90% in subsequent pregnancies.

In Gestational Diabetes a Previously Normal Woman Develops Abnormally High Blood Glucose Levels During Pregnancy

Gestational diabetes develops in 3% to 10% of pregnancies. It usually reverses after delivery, butt recurs in 20% to 80% of future pregnancies. Half of such women will develop diabetes within 6 years of delivering. This risk is highest among women who required insulin, developed autoantibodies, had multiple prior pregnancies and are obese. Children of women with gestational diabetes have 4- to 8-fold greater risk of developing type II diabetes.

 PATHOPHYSIOLOGY: The hallmark of gestational diabetes is resistance to maternal insulin (Fig. 14-33). Pregnancy hormones and other factors interfere with insulin binding to its receptor, leading to hyperglycemia.

 CLINICAL FEATURES: As mentioned above, infants of women with gestational diabetes may be abnormally large (macrosomia), unusually small or growth restricted. Congenital fetal malformations are increased with gestational diabetes, as are fetal and placental thrombosis. Neonates are at risk for hypoglycemia, jaundice, polycythemia, hypocalcemia, and hypomagnesemia.

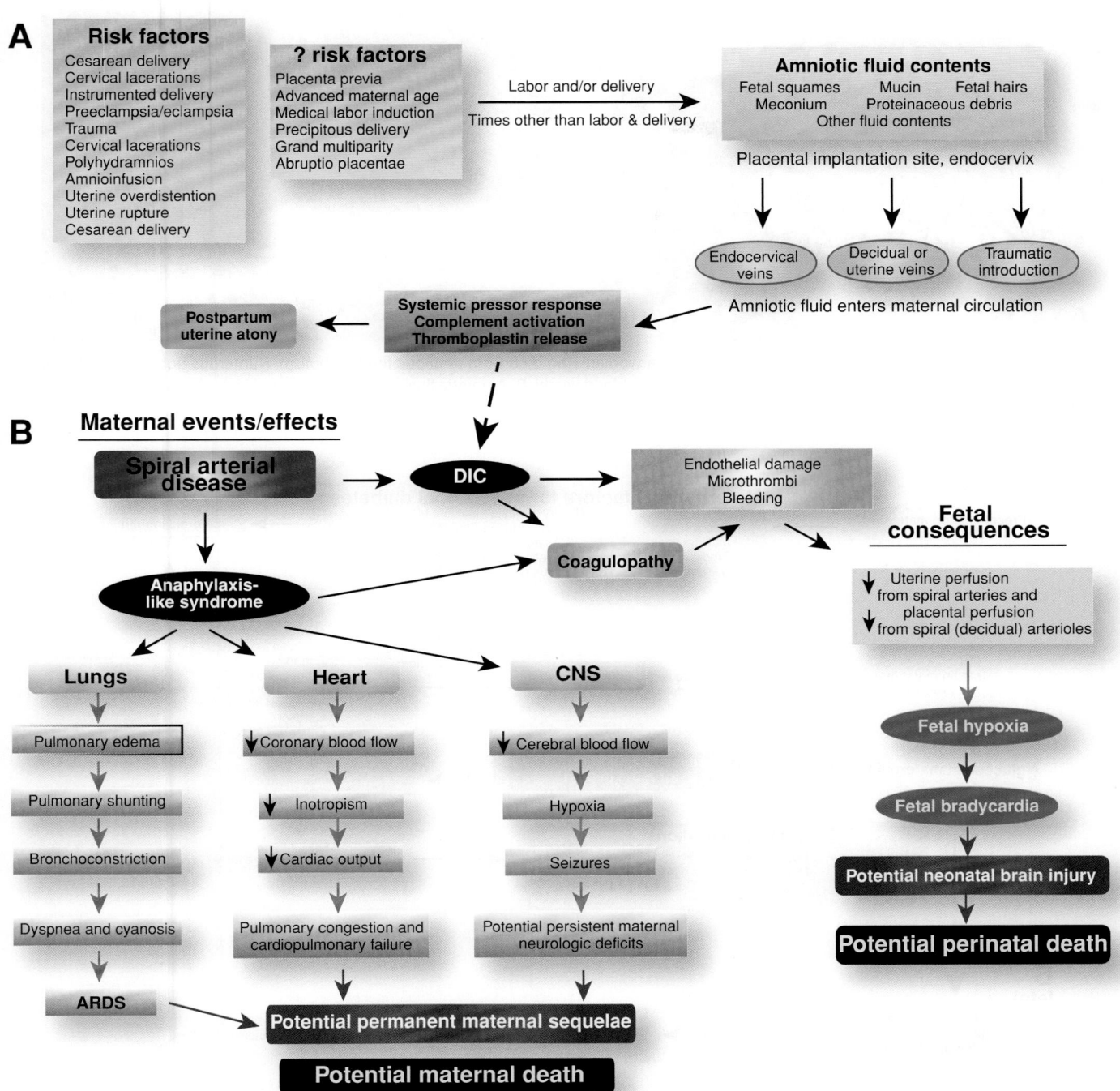

FIGURE 14-31. Current concepts of the pathophysiology of amniotic fluid embolism (anaphylactoid syndrome of pregnancy).

Acute Fatty Liver of Pregnancy (AFLP) Reflects Disordered Mitochondrial Fatty Acid Metabolism

AFLP is a rare, life-threatening complication of pregnancy, usually associated with preeclampsia. It can recur in subsequent pregnancies. AFLP occurs almost exclusively in the third trimester and is characterized by the onset of abdominal pain, jaundice, and anorexia, with elevated levels of liver enzymes and bilirubin. DIC may occur in severe cases. Additional complications include pancreatitis and encephalopathy. AFLP is associated with 18% maternal mortality and 23% fetal mortality.

MOLECULAR PATHOGENESIS: Acute fatty liver of pregnancy is caused by a mitochondrial dysfunction, generally thought to be a deficiency in long-chain 3-hydroxyacyl-coenzyme A dehydrogenase (LCHAD). When fatty acid oxidation is deficient in the fetus, unmetabolized fatty acids reenter maternal circulation through the placenta, overwhelming maternal β-oxidation enzymes. Microvesicular steatosis in the mothers' liver occurs as a result.

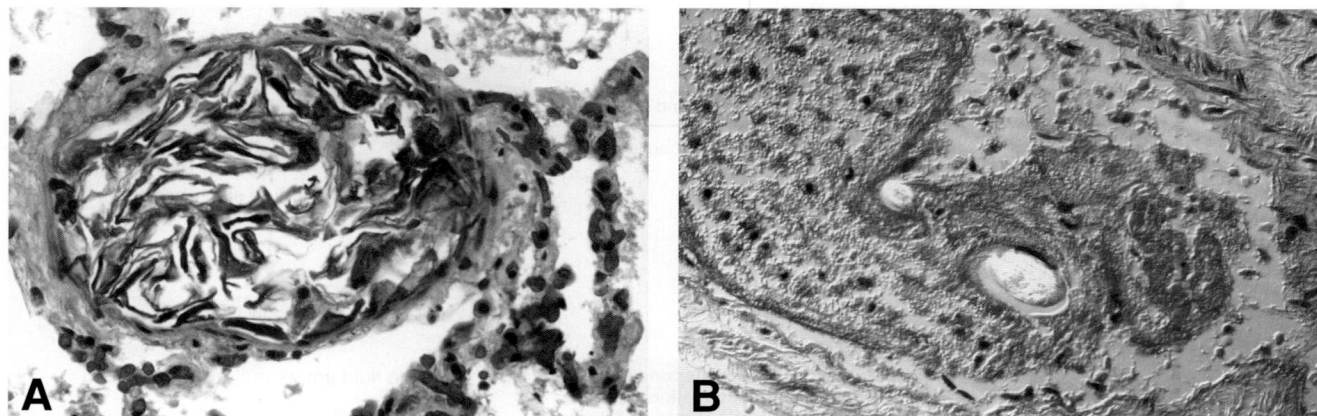

FIGURE 14-32. Amniotic fluid embolism. A. Lung from a woman who died from amniotic fluid embolism. Numerous tightly packed fetal squamous epithelial cells obstruct the lumen of this pulmonary blood vessel. **B.** Amniotic fluid embolism: Nomarski interference contrast highlights two golden brown cross-sections of a fetal hair in the maternal pulmonary circulation.

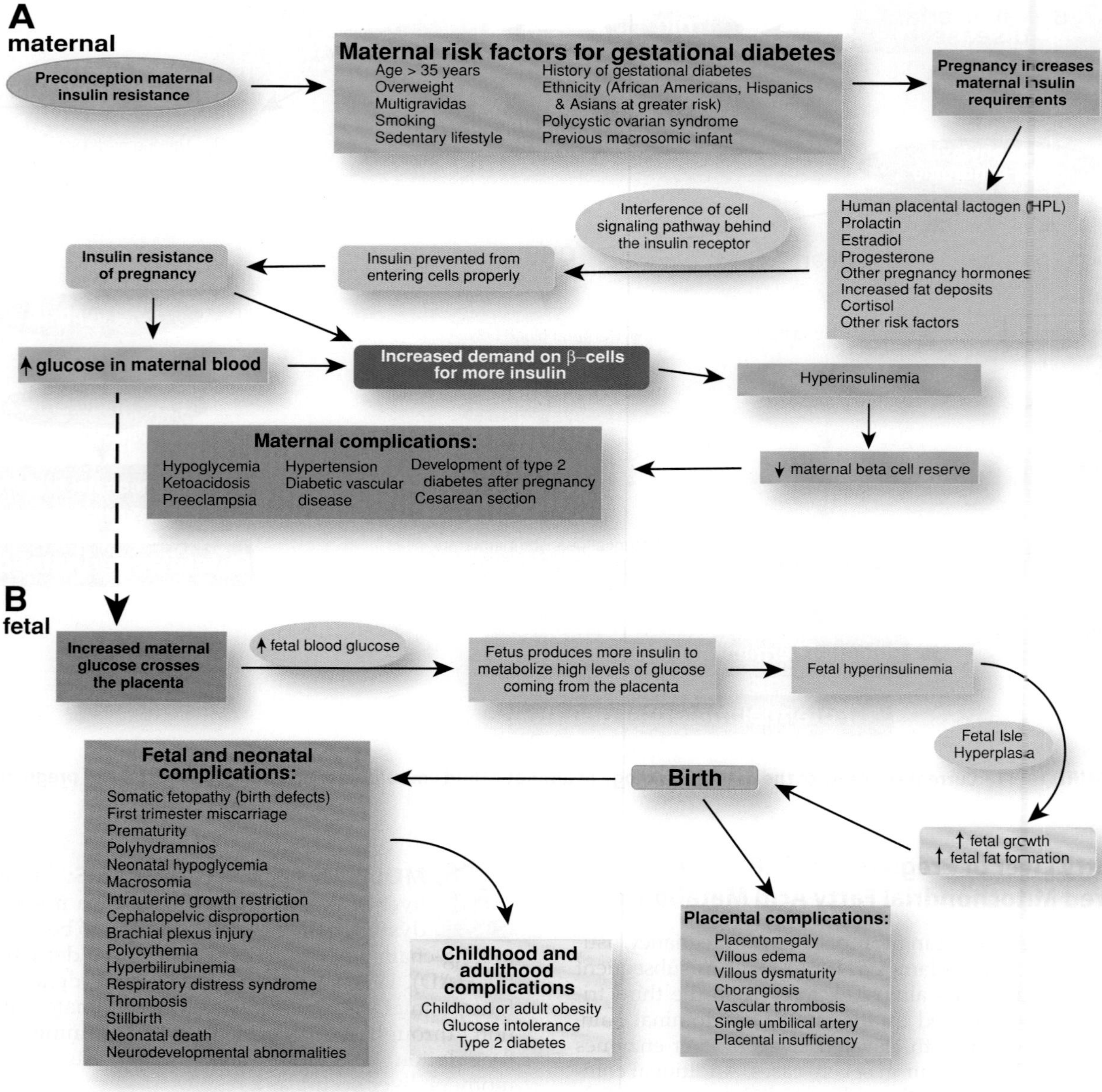

A
maternal

Preconception maternal insulin resistance

Maternal risk factors for gestational diabetes
Age > 35 years   History of gestational diabetes
Overweight   Ethnicity (African Americans, Hispanics
Multigravidas   & Asians at greater risk)
Smoking   Polycystic ovarian syndrome
Sedentary lifestyle   Previous macrosomic infant

Pregnancy increases maternal insulin requirements

Human placental lactogen (HPL)
Prolactin
Estradiol
Progesterone
Other pregnancy hormones
Increased fat deposits
Cortisol
Other risk factors

Interference of cell signaling pathway behind the insulin receptor

Insulin prevented from entering cells properly

Insulin resistance of pregnancy

↑ glucose in maternal blood

Increased demand on β–cells for more insulin

Hyperinsulinemia

↓ maternal beta cell reserve

Maternal complications:
Hypoglycemia   Hypertension   Development of type 2
Ketoacidosis   Diabetic vascular   diabetes after pregnancy
Preeclampsia   disease   Cesarean section

B
fetal

Increased maternal glucose crosses the placenta

↑ fetal blood glucose

Fetus produces more insulin to metabolize high levels of glucose coming from the placenta

Fetal hyperinsulinemia

Fetal Isle Hyperplasia

Fetal and neonatal complications:
Somatic fetopathy (birth defects)
First trimester miscarriage
Prematurity
Polyhydramnios
Neonatal hypoglycemia
Macrosomia
Intrauterine growth restriction
Cephalopelvic disproportion
Brachial plexus injury
Polycythemia
Hyperbilirubinemia
Respiratory distress syndrome
Thrombosis
Stillbirth
Neonatal death
Neurodevelopmental abnormalities

Birth

↑ fetal growth
↑ fetal fat formation

Childhood and adulthood complications
Childhood or adult obesity
Glucose intolerance
Type 2 diabetes

Placental complications:
Placentomegaly
Villous edema
Villous dysmaturity
Chorangiosis
Vascular thrombosis
Single umbilical artery
Placental insufficiency

FIGURE 14-33. Current concepts of the pathophysiology of gestational diabetes and its consequences.

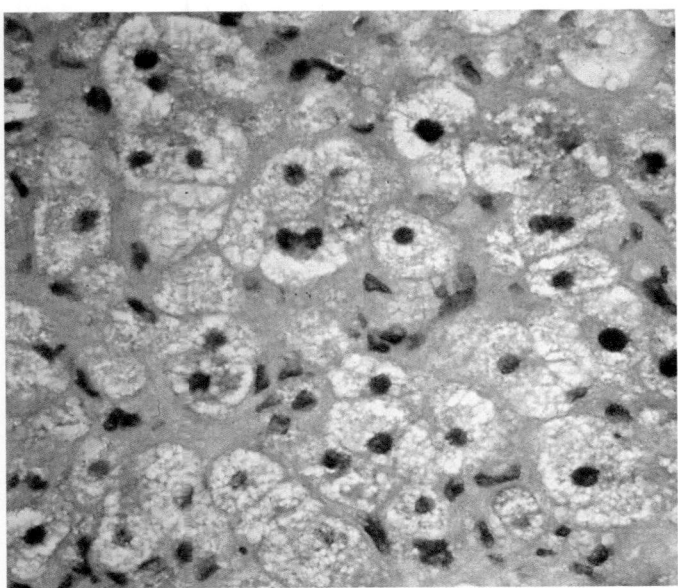

FIGURE 14-34. Acute fatty liver of pregnancy (AFLP). The hepatocytes contain microvesicular fat droplets.

PATHOLOGY: Livers in AFLP show characteristic microvesicular fat droplets in the cytoplasm of enlarged hepatocytes (see Chapter 20) (Fig. 14-34). Hepatocellular necrosis is usually absent, but severe cases may show hepatocyte dropout, collapse of reticulin fibers, and portal tract inflammation.

Maternal Cardiac Disease Endangers Both Mother and Fetus

In developed nations, maternal cardiac disease is a frequent cause of maternal morbidity and death. A woman with pre-existing cardiac disease who become pregnant has a 1% probability of dying. Pre-existing maternal cardiac disease also increases the risk of death of the infant 10-fold. Among women with severe cardiac conditions, pregnancy carries a 25% to 50% likelihood of maternal death.

Peripartum Cardiomyopathy Is Rarely Diagnosed Before Delivery

This type of cardiomyopathy accounts for only 1% of cardiac events during pregnancy, but it is the cause of an increasing number of pregnancy-related maternal deaths. Only 10% of cases are diagnosed prior to delivery, with 75% detected in the postpartum period. Although the exact cause of peripartum cardiomyopathy is unknown, it is associated with increased maternal age, obesity, hypertension, multiparity, tocolysis with β-agonists, preeclampsia, low socioeconomic status, and black race. Mortality is 25% to 50%.

The large majority (65%) of pregnant women who die from pre-existing heart conditions have congenital cardiac disease. The second leading cause of death is vascular heart disease (25%); 6% have cardiomyopathy.

Cigarette Smoking is the Leading Avoidable Cause of Morbidity and Mortality in Pregnant Women and Their Infants

Maternal Cigarette Smoking

About 13% of women report smoking during the last 3 weeks of pregnancy. Even more pregnant adolescents smoke (27% to 37%). Cigarette smoking during pregnancy is associated with diverse poor obstetric and infant outcomes. However, if mothers stop smoking in the first trimester, their offspring are protected from most smoking-related excess morbidity and mortality.

 ETIOLOGIC FACTORS: The key factors in cigarette smoke that contribute include carbon monoxide (CO) and nicotine. CO in cigarette smoke displaces oxygen from hemoglobin, reducing oxygen delivery to the fetus, and causing fetal hypoxia. In heavy smokers, CO may reduce fetal oxygen-carrying capacity by up to 25%. Nicotine, a potent vasoconstrictor, reduces uterine and placental blood flow in the blood vessels of all anatomic components of the uteroplacental unit. Uterine spiral arteries that deliver maternal blood to the placenta, placental villous vessels that transport oxygen and nutrients, and umbilical vessels carrying placental blood to and from the fetus are all affected. Placentas of women who smoke may show features of chronic uteroplacental malperfusion (see below).

 PATHOPHYSIOLOGY AND PATHOLOGY: Effects of cigarette smoking on the placenta and fetus reflect damage to placental and uterine blood vessels, impaired fetal physiology, genetic damage, placental dysfunction, and poor pregnancy outcomes. These include damage to:
  Umbilical and placental vessels: intimal degeneration, vasoconstriction, decreased blood flow, impaired vasodilatation, and anticoagulation.
  Uterine spiral arteries: increased fragility, vasoconstriction, and decreased blood flow.
  Fetal physiology: acidosis, hypoxia, nicotine accumulation, increased toxins (e.g., CO, cyanide, nicotine).
  DNA: increased trophoblast double-strand breaks and DNA adducts, altered mitochondrial DNA, and abnormal placental DNA methylation.
  Placental structure: villous hypoplasia, atrophic and fibrotic villi, trophoblast hyperplasia (Tenney--Parker change), infarcts, chorangiosis, villous agglutination, increased fibrin, evidence of malperfusion.

Cigarette smokers are at increased risk of spontaneous abortion early in gestation and other placental abnormalities later in pregnancy (see Chapter 8). Nicotine also crosses the placenta readily, and may reach higher levels in fetal tissues and amniotic fluid than in the mother. This may lead to postnatal neurobehavioral and other CNS abnormalities (see Chapter 8).

Environmental Tobacco Smoke (ETS)

Unfortunately, even if pregnant women do not smoke, ETS contains many toxic and carcinogenic chemicals that may still reach the fetus. Such exposures correlate with neurobehavioral disorders, as well as adverse pregnancy and neonatal outcomes (see Chapters 6 and 8). Damage to the infant's DNA due to ETS can be as severe as that caused by maternal smoking. Pregnant women exposed to second-hand smoke have greater risk of miscarriages: if a housemate smokes >20 cigarettes daily risk of early pregnancy loss may increase by 81%.

GESTATIONAL TROPHOBLASTIC DISEASE

Gestational trophoblastic disease reflects abnormal trophoblast proliferation and maturation, including neoplasms derived from trophoblast (Fig. 14-35).

Complete Hydatidiform Moles Contain No Embryo

A complete hydatidiform mole is a placenta with grossly swollen chorionic villi, resembling bunches of grapes, with varying degrees of trophoblastic proliferation. Villi are enlarged, often exceeding 5 mm in diameter (Fig. 14-36).

 MOLECULAR PATHOGENESIS: *Complete mole results from fertilization of an empty ovum that lacks functional maternal DNA.* Most commonly, a haploid (23,X) set of paternal chromosomes introduced by monospermy duplicates to 46,XX, but dispermic 46,XX and 46,XY moles also occur. *Moles characteristically lack maternal chromosomes.* Paternally imprinted genes, such as *p57*, in which only the maternal allele is expressed, are not expressed in villous trophoblasts of androgenetic-derived complete moles. Embryos die before placental circulation has developed, so few chorionic villi contain blood vessels. Fetal parts are absent.

EPIDEMIOLOGY: The risk of hydatidiform mole relates to maternal age and has two peaks. Girls under 15 years of age have 20-fold higher risk than do women 20 to 35 years old. Risk increases progressively for women over 40, and 50+ year old women have 200-fold greater risk than those between 20 and 40. The incidence is many-fold higher in Asian women than in white women. In Taiwan, risk is 25 times that in the United States. Women with a prior hydatidiform mole are 20-fold more susceptible to subsequent molar pregnancy than the general population.

PATHOLOGY: Molar tissue is voluminous and consists of obviously swollen, grossly visible villi (Fig. 14-36). Many individual villi have cisternae, which are central, acellular, fluid-filled spaces lacking mesenchymal cells. Trophoblast is hyperplastic with syncytiotrophoblast, cytotrophoblast, and intermediate trophoblast. Considerable cellular atypia is present.

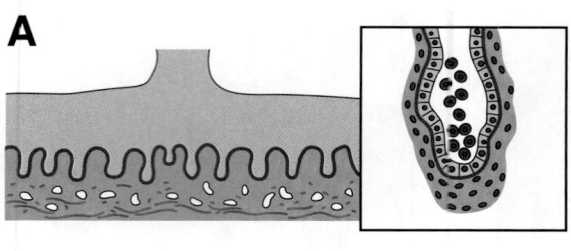
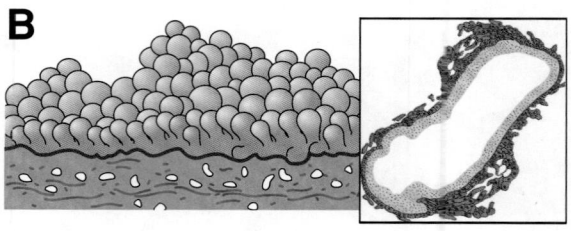
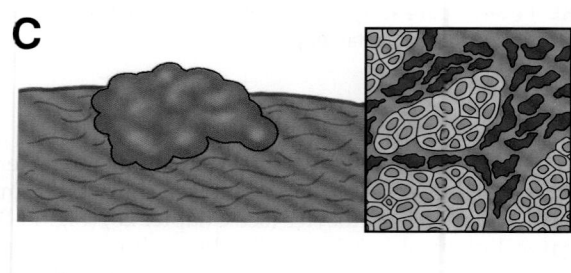
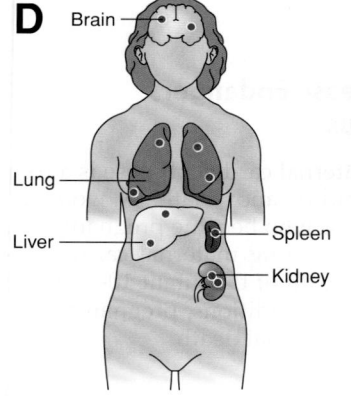
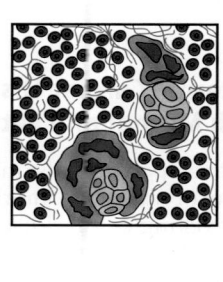

FIGURE 14-35. Proliferative disorders of the trophoblast. A. Normal chorionic villus of 8-week fetus, with blood vessel containing nucleated red blood cells. **B.** Complete hydatidiform mole with hydropic villi (also see Fig. 14-38). The villi are enlarged by an edematous stroma devoid of blood vessels. The trophoblastic epithelium is hyperplastic and exhibits variable atypia. **C.** Choriocarcinoma that has arisen in a molar pregnancy invades the myometrium and consists of admixed syncytiotrophoblastic and cytotrophoblastic elements. **D.** Common sites of metastasis from choriocarcinoma.

CLINICAL FEATURES: Patients with complete moles commonly present at 11 to 25 weeks of pregnancy with excessive uterine enlargement and often uterine bleeding. They often pass tissue fragments resembling small, grape-like masses. Serum hCG levels are markedly elevated and increase rapidly.

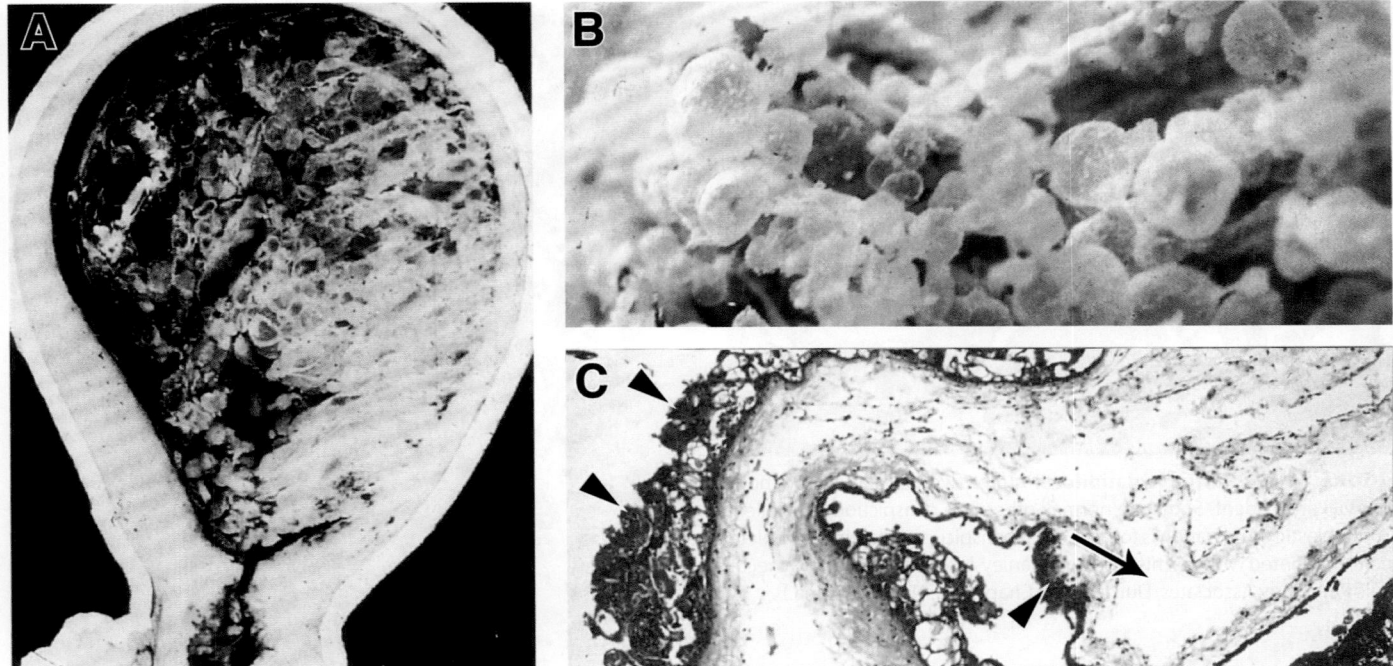

FIGURE 14-36. Complete hydatidiform mole. A. Complete mole in which the entire uterine cavity is filled with swollen villi. **B.** The villi are each 1 to 3 mm in diameter and appear grape-like. **C.** Individual molar villi, many of which have cavitated central cisterns (*arrow*), show considerable trophoblastic hyperplasia (*arrowheads*) and atypia. Villous blood vessels have atrophied and disappeared.

Complications of complete mole include uterine hemorrhage, DIC, uterine perforation, trophoblastic embolism, and infection. Choriocarcinoma (see below) occurs in 2% of patients whose moles were evacuated.

Treatment is suction curettage of the uterus and subsequent monitoring of serum hCG levels. Up to 20% of patients show stable or rising hCG levels requiring adjuvant chemotherapy for persistent disease, and survival approaches 100%.

Partial Hydatidiform Moles Have Triploid Genomes

Partial hydatidiform mole is a distinct entity that almost never evolves into choriocarcinoma (Table 14-2). Partial moles have 69 chromosomes (triploidy): one haploid maternal set—and two haploid paternal—and results when two spermatozoa fertilize a normal ovum (23,X). Sometimes, a single spermatozoon that failed meiotic reduction, and so has 46 chromosomes, is involved. Fetuses associated with a partial mole usually die after 10 weeks of gestation. Moles are aborted shortly thereafter. Thus, fetal parts may be present.

PATHOLOGY: Partial moles have two populations of chorionic villi. Some are normal; others are enlarged by hydropic swelling and show central cavitation, resulting from tangential histologic sections of invaginated surface epithelium ("fjord-like") (Fig. 14-37). Trophoblastic proliferation is focal and less pronounced than in complete moles. Chorionic villi contain blood vessels with fetal (nucleated) erythrocytes.

TABLE 14-2

COMPARATIVE FEATURES OF COMPLETE AND PARTIAL HYDATIDIFORM MOLE

Features	Complete Mole	Partial Mole
Karyotype	46,XX	47,XXY or 47,XXX
Parental origin of haploid genome sets	Both paternal	1 maternal, 2 paternal
Preoperative diagnosis	Mole	Missed abortion
Marked vaginal bleeding	3+	1+
Uterus	Large	Small
Serum hCG	High	Less elevated
Hydropic villi	All	Some
Trophoblastic proliferation	Diffuse	Focal
Atypia	Diffuse	Minimal
hCG in tissue	3+	1+
Embryo present	No	Some
Blood vessels	No	Common
Nucleated erythrocytes	No	Sometimes
Persists after initial therapy	20%	7%
Choriocarcinoma	2% after mole	No choriocarcinoma

hCG = human chorionic gonadotropin.

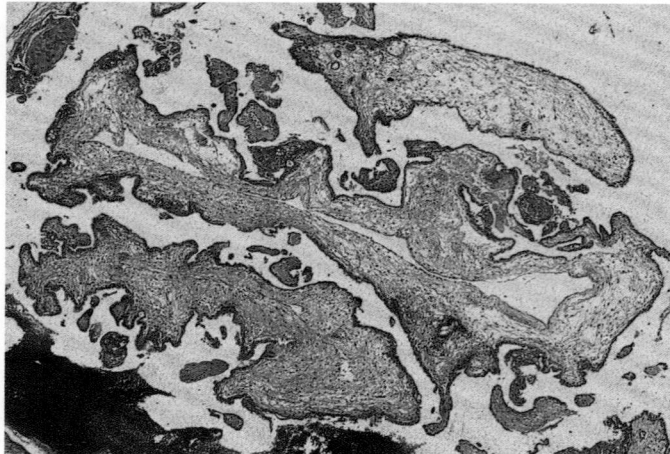

FIGURE 14-37. Partial hydatidiform mole. Two populations of chorionic villi are evident. Some are normal; others are conspicuously swollen. Trophoblastic proliferation is focal and less conspicuous than in a complete mole. (Reprinted with permission from Stanley J. Robboy, MD, and Gynecologic Pathology Associates, Durham and Chapel Hill, North Carolina.)

Invasive Moles Penetrate Underlying Myometrium

PATHOLOGY: The villi of a hydatidiform mole may be limited to the superficial myometrium, or they may invade the uterus and even the broad ligament. They tend to enter myometrial venous channels. One-third spread to distant sites, mostly the lungs. Unlike choriocarcinoma (see below), distant deposits of an invasive mole remain within blood vessels in which they lodge, and rarely cause death. Clinical distinction between invasive mole and choriocarcinoma may be difficult.

Histologically, invasive moles show less hydropic change than do complete moles. Trophoblastic proliferation is usually prominent. Uterine perforation is a major complication, but only occurs in a minority of cases. Theca lutein cysts (see Chapter 24), which may occur with any form of trophoblastic disease as a result of hCG stimulation, are prominent with invasive moles.

Gestational Choriocarcinoma Derives From Trophoblast

EPIDEMIOLOGY: Choriocarcinoma occurs once in 30,000 pregnancies in the United States; in eastern Asia, the frequency is far greater. The incidence seems related to abnormalities of pregnancy. In whites, 25% arise from term deliveries, 25% from spontaneous abortions and 50% from complete hydatidiform moles. Although the risk of a complete hydatidiform mole becoming choriocarcinoma is ≈2%, it is still several orders of magnitude higher than if the pregnancy were normal.

PATHOLOGY: Uterine lesions of choriocarcinoma vary from microscopic foci to huge necrotic and hemorrhagic tumors. Viable tumor is usually confined to the rim of the neoplasm because, unlike most

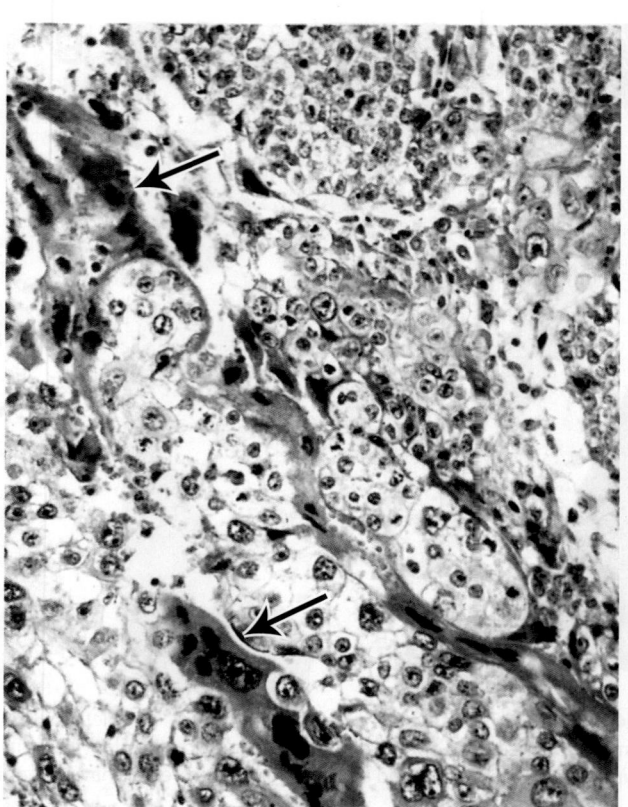

FIGURE 14-38. Choriocarcinoma. Malignant cytotrophoblast and syncytiotrophoblast (*arrows*) are present.

other cancers, choriocarcinomas lack intrinsic tumor vasculature. They contain both cytotrophoblast and syncytiotrophoblast, with varying degrees of intermediate trophoblast (Fig. 14-38). The tumor resembles the trophoblast of an early implanting blastocyst. Rims of syncytiotrophoblast surround central cytotrophoblastic cores, in addition to being arranged around maternal blood spaces, which resemble the intervillous space of normal placentation. hCG is localized to the syncytiotrophoblastic element. *By definition, tumors containing any villous structures, even if metastatic, are hydatidiform moles and not choriocarcinomas.*

Choriocarcinomas invade mainly via venous sinuses in the myometrium. They metastasize widely hematogenously, especially to lungs (>90%), brain, GI tract, liver, and vagina (Table 14-3).

CLINICAL FEATURES: Abnormal uterine bleeding is the most common first symptom of choriocarcinoma. Occasionally, a tumor first presents with metastases to lungs or brain. In some cases, it may only become evident 10 or more years after the last pregnancy.

With current chemotherapy, survival rates exceed 70%, even when tumors have metastasized. Virtually 100% remission is expected if a tumor is localized. Serial serum hCG levels are used to monitor the effectiveness of treatment.

TABLE 14-3	
CLINICAL STAGING OF GESTATIONAL TROPHOBLASTIC TUMORS	
I	Confined to the uterus
Ia	0 risk factors
Ib	1 risk factor
Ic	2 risk factors
II	Extends outside of the uterus but limited to genital structures
III	Extends to lungs
IV	All other metastatic sites

Risk factors affecting stage include (1) human chorionic gonadotropin (hCG) >100,000 mIU/mL and (2) duration of disease >6 months from termination of antecedent pregnancy.

Placental Site Trophoblastic Tumor Outcomes Are Unpredictable

Placental site trophoblastic tumors are the least common trophoblastic tumors. They are mainly composed of intermediate trophoblastic cells.

 PATHOLOGY: Placental site trophoblastic tumors are grossly more variable than are choriocarcinomas. Often, the myometrium shows an ill-defined, yellowish tumor without conspicuous hemorrhage. The extent of myometrial invasion varies, and patterns of infiltration resemble normal trophoblast in the placental bed. Since intermediate trophoblast in a normal pregnancy anchors the pregnancy to the superficial myometrium, these tumors appear microscopically like exaggerated placental sites. Mononuclear and multinuclear trophoblast may be single cells or cords, islands and sheets of cells interspersed among myometrial cells. Neither necrosis nor villi are present. Placental site trophoblastic tumor is also distinguished from choriocarcinoma by its monomorphic (intermediate) trophoblastic proliferation, unlike the dimorphic pattern of trophoblast in choriocarcinoma. Most trophoblastic cells express human placental lactogen (hPL), but a few express hCG.

 CLINICAL FEATURES: The age and parity of patients with placental site trophoblastic tumor are like those of patients with choriocarcinoma. Half report amenorrhea, while vaginal bleeding usually occurs with choriocarcinoma. Past history of molar pregnancy is much less common (5%) than with choriocarcinoma (50%).

Placental site trophoblastic tumors must be excised completely (hysterectomy) to prevent local recurrence. They sometimes metastasize and may be fatal. Large tumors and high mitotic indices carry a worse prognosis. Because hPL has a short half-life, serum levels of hCG are more useful in monitoring response to treatment. Conservative management usually suffices. If hCG persists, even at low levels, or mitotic count is elevated, aggressive treatment with hysterectomy or chemotherapy is indicated.

15 Systemic Amyloidosis

Vaishali Sanchorawala, John L. Berk

INTRODUCTION

The term, *amyloidosis*, covers a group of protein-misfolding disorders involving extracellular deposition of insoluble fibrillar proteins in tissues and organs. These diseases are a subset of a growing group of disorders recognized to be caused by misfolding of proteins; these include Alzheimer and other neurodegenerative diseases, prion diseases, some cases of cystic fibrosis, and others. All amyloidoses show a common unparalleled β-pleated sheet structural conformation that confers unique staining properties. The pathologist Rudolf Virchow (1821 to 1902) coined the term "amyloid" in 1854, because their peculiar staining reaction with iodine and sulfuric acid convinced him that such deposits in autopsy livers were starch-like. One hundred years later, "amyloid" was found to be a proteinaceous fibrillar deposit in tissues.

Biochemical characterization of the fibril proteins from clinical cases showed that "amyloidoses" are a spectrum of diseases, often with a fatal outcome due to progressive amyloid fibril deposition in major organs. Different types of amyloid appear indistinguishable by hematoxylin/eosin and Congo red staining (Fig. 15-1), but >30 proteins misfold, aggregate, and form amyloid. Each different amyloidogenic protein confers specific organ tropisms, defining clinical course and potential therapeutic interventions. Thus, a diagnosis of amyloidosis requires that the misfolded protein be identified.

CLASSIFICATION AND EPIDEMIOLOGY

Historically, amyloidoses were classified by the clinical or pathologic features of their associated diseases. Secondary

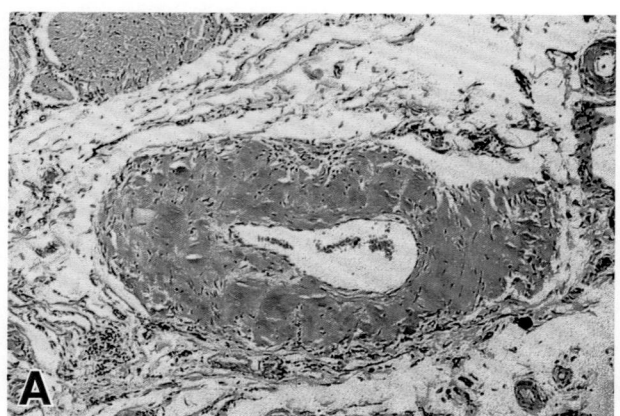
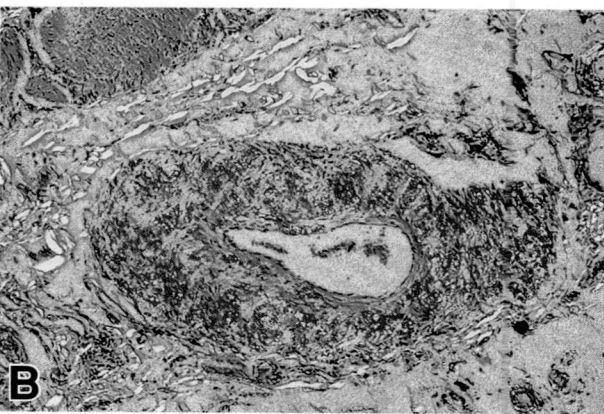

FIGURE 15-1. **AL amyloid** involving the wall of an artery stained with Congo red is shown under **(A)** ordinary light and **(B)** polarized light. Note the red-green birefringence of the amyloid. Collagen has a silvery appearance.

TABLE 15-1
AMYLOID PRECURSOR PROTEINS AND THEIR CLINICAL SYNDROMES

Designation	Precursor	Clinical Syndrome	Clinical Involvement
Systemic Amyloidoses			
AL	Immunoglobulin light chain	Primary or myeloma-associated[a]	Any
AH	Immunoglobulin heavy chain	Rare variant of primary or myeloma-associated	Any
AA	Serum amyloid A protein	Secondary; reactive[b]	Renal, heart, other
$A\beta_2M$	β_2-microglobulin	Hemodialysis-associated	Synovial tissue, bone
ATTR	Transthyretin	Familial (mutant) Age-related (wild type)	Cardiac, peripheral, and autonomic nerves
AApoAI	Apolipoprotein AI	Familial	Hepatic, renal
AApoAII	Apolipoprotein AII	Familial	Renal
AGel	Gelsolin	Familial	Cornea, cranial nerves, skin, renal
AFib	Fibrinogen Aα	Familial	Renal
ALys	Lysozyme	Familial	Renal, hepatic
ALECT2	Leukocyte chemotactic factor 2	Undefined	Renal
Localized Amyloidoses			
Aβ	Amyloid β protein	Alzheimer disease; Down syndrome	Central nervous system
ACys	Cystatin C	Cerebral amyloid angiopathy	Central nervous system, vascular
APrP	Prion protein	Spongiform encephalopathies	Central nervous system
AIAPP	Islet amyloid polypeptide (amylin)	Diabetes-associated	Pancreas
ACal	Calcitonin	Medullary carcinoma of the thyroid	Thyroid
AANF	Atrial natriuretic factor	Atrial fibrillation	Cardiac atria
APro	Prolactin	Endocrinopathy	Pituitary
ASgI	Semenogelin I	Age-related; incidental autopsy or biopsy finding	Seminal vesicles

[a]Localized AL deposits can occur in skin, conjunctiva, urinary bladder, and the tracheobronchial tree.
[b]Secondary to chronic inflammation or infection or to a hereditary periodic fever syndrome such as familial Mediterranean fever.

(AA) amyloidosis accompanied chronic inflammatory processes. Familial (AF) amyloidosis caused distinctive clinical manifestations within kindreds. All other types, except that associated with myeloma, were termed *primary*, in the sense that they were idiopathic. Development of methods for characterizing amyloid fibrils extracted from tissues permits us to identify 30 different amyloid precursor proteins so far (Table 15-1). Current classification now rests on the chemical nature of the fibrils that constitute the deposits, for example, immunoglobulin light chains in AL amyloidosis. These etiologically and chemically based terms have replaced older ones, such as *primary, secondary, senile, dialysis-associated,* and *myeloma-associated* amyloidoses.

In localized forms of amyloidosis, deposits occur at the site where the precursor protein is synthesized. In systemic amyloidoses, deposits form in organs at a distance from the precursor-producing cells.

 EPIDEMIOLOGY: Data on the epidemiology of amyloidosis are limited. One study based on data from the National Center for Health Statistics estimated incidence of AL as 4.5 per 100,000. AL amyloidosis, like other plasma cell dyscrasias, usually begins after age 40 and progresses rapidly, with multisystem involvement and short survival. AA amyloidosis is increasingly rare in the Western world, occurring in less than 1% of people with chronic inflammatory diseases. However, it is more common in Turkey and the Middle East, where it may complicate familial Mediterranean fever. It may begin within a year after onset of the underlying inflammatory disease or many years later. It is the only type of amyloidosis that occurs in children. $A\beta_2M$ amyloidosis occurs in patients on long-term dialysis and usually manifests as deposits in joint synovia. Its incidence is declining as dialysis techniques change.

Inherited amyloidoses have an estimated incidence of less than 1 per 100,000. They are autosomal dominant diseases in which a variant plasma protein forms amyloid deposits, generally beginning in midlife, however, rarely before childhood. The most common form is caused by variant transthyretin (TTR), of which there are nearly 100 associated with amyloidosis. Carrier frequency for one variant, V122I, may be as high as 4% of the African-American population. This variant is associated with late-onset cardiac amyloidosis. There are also regions with high incidence of particular ATTR mutations such as V30M in Portugal, Sweden, Japan, and other countries. Even wild-type TTR can form fibrils, leading to age-related systemic amyloidosis, which predominantly affects the heart, in older patients. Other familial amyloidoses, caused by variant apolipoprotein A-I, A-II, gelsolin, fibrinogen Aα, or lysozyme, are reported.

 PATHOPHYSIOLOGY: The mechanism by which amyloid deposits impair organ function is actively debated. Amyloid deposits can significantly alter cardiac geometry, affect kidney size, and alter glomerular appearance. In extreme cases, it may threaten spontaneous rupture of the liver and spleen. These observations suggest that the volume of infiltrated extracellular amyloid can damage organs overwhelmingly and disrupt their function. In other cases, however, demonstrable amyloid deposits (e.g., in nerves) or anticipated amyloid burden (heart) do not cause extensive organ dysfunction. Tissues from patients with severe sensorimotor peripheral neuropathy typically show extensive axonal degeneration that are consistent with the length-dependent deficits detected clinically, but no or limited amyloid deposits. Similarly, AL amyloidosis patients with advanced congestive heart failure often have only minor infiltrative echocardiographic changes.

Alternatively, misfolded proteins may disrupt organ function because of apparent tissue toxicity of prefibrillary forms of the amyloid cascade, specifically oligomers and protein aggregates of misfolding proteins. *Ex vivo* studies show that perfusing rodent hearts with amyloidogenic light chains immediately alter myocardial calcium fluxes and impair cardiac contractility—even without amyloid fibril deposition. Mounting clinical evidence supports the toxicity of circulating amyloidogenic oligomers, explaining the dissociation of organ dysfunction and identifiable amyloid deposits.

ETIOLOGIC FACTORS: Mechanisms of amyloid fibril formation. The exact mechanism of fibril formation is unknown and may be different among the various types of amyloid. However, studies suggest there may be a common underlying mechanism in which a partially unfolded protein intermediate forms oligomers and then higher-order polymers. Some factors which contribute to fibrillogenesis may include: variant or unstable protein structure, extensive β-conformation of the precursor protein, proteolytic processing of the precursor protein, association with serum or extracellular matrix components (e.g., amyloid P-component, amyloid-enhancing

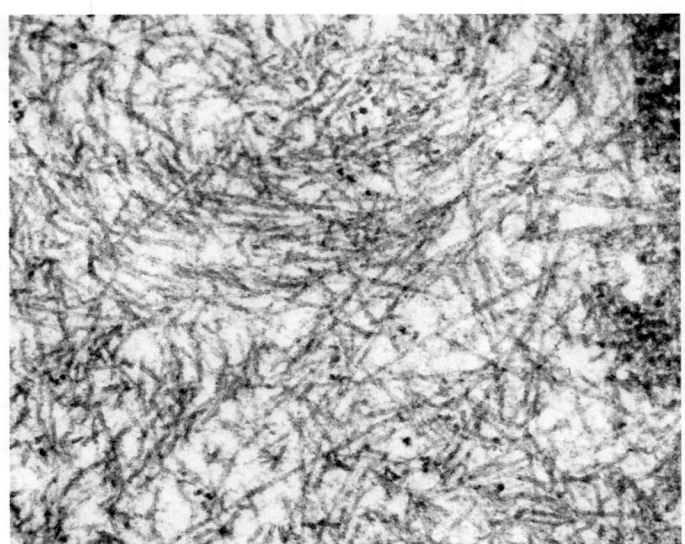

FIGURE 15-2. Amyloid deposits in tissue. Parallel and interlacing arrays of fibrils are evident in this electron micrograph.

factor, apolipoprotein E, or glycosaminoglycans), and physical properties including pH at the tissue site.

Amyloid Precursor Proteins. Amyloid precursor proteins are usually small, with molecular weights between 4 and 25 kDa. They lack any discernible amino acid sequence homology, but the secondary structures of many of amyloid proteins have substantial β-pleated sheet structure and comparable ultrastructural appearance (Fig. 15-2). Clinical amyloidoses are disorders of protein structure in which cells secrete soluble precursor protein that become insoluble at some tissue site, ultimately compromising organ function. They represent a part of the total spectrum of protein deposition disorders.

MOLECULAR PATHOGENESIS: In some cases, the aberrant secondary structure seen in amyloid reflects a hereditary alteration in sequence that predisposes to fibril formation, as in the proteins transthyretin (TTR), lysozyme, fibrinogen, cystatin c, gelsolin, amyloid-β protein precursor (AβPP), and apolipoprotein A1 (ApoA1). In other cases, wild-type molecules are the fibril precursors (TTR, β_2-microglobulin [β_2M], ApoA1).

Accessory Molecules. The role of *P component* and of the other accessory molecules in amyloid deposition is not clear. Although they do not appear to be required for fibril formation, they may stabilize the fibril, protecting it from proteolysis once it is formed, or enhance the transition from protofibril to fibril. In experimental systems, amyloid deposition is slower in the absence of P component. Intravenously injected purified P component preferentially binds to amyloid deposits. This property has been exploited clinically, using radiolabeled P component to localize and quantify total body burden of amyloid in the so-called "SAPscan." The scan has been particularly useful in evaluating liver, spleen, and endocrine deposits, but less so when disease involves the heart because of "signal-to-noise" issues.

Apolipoprotein E (ApoE) is found in all types of amyloid deposits. One ApoE allele (ApoE4) is strongly associated with Alzheimer disease. ApoE4 has been suggested to also be a risk factor for other forms of amyloidosis, but its association with other amyloidoses is less well supported by the epidemiologic evidence. The mechanism of ApoE involvement is not known.

The heparan sulfate proteoglycan **perlecan** is a basement membrane component intimately associated with all types of tissue amyloid deposits. As with P component and ApoE, its role in amyloidogenesis is undefined. Compounds that bind heparan sulfate proteoglycans, such as anionic sulfonates, decrease fibril deposition in murine models of AA disease and have been suggested as potential therapeutic agents.

Role of Proteolysis. In some cases, amyloid precursors undergo proteolysis, which may hasten folding into prefibrillar structural intermediates. In, for example, Aβ or AA amyloidoses, a normal proteolytic process may be disturbed, yielding excessive concentrations of a prefibrillar molecule. Whether tissue deposition is purely physicochemical or depends on an interaction like that between ligands and receptors, where some component of tissue ground substance is the binding target, is not known. If proteolysis does occur, its timing, relative to deposition, also is not known.

ORIGINS OF AMYLOID PROTEINS

AL Amyloidosis Is Usually due to a Plasma Cell Dyscrasia

It may occur in isolation, or along with multiple myeloma. Similar cytogenetic changes have been identified in both cases, suggesting they may have a common molecular pathogenesis. Electrophoretic and mass spectrographic analyses show that these amyloid fibril deposits are intact 23-kD monoclonal immunoglobulin light chains, as well as C-terminal truncated fragments. Although all kappa (κ) and lambda (λ) light-chain subtypes have been identified in amyloid fibrils, λ subtypes predominate. The λ VI subtype appears to have unique structural properties that predispose it to fibril formation, often in the kidney. AL amyloidosis is usually rapidly progressive with amyloid deposits in multiple tissues. It can also occur in other B-lymphoproliferative disorders including Waldenström macroglobulinemia and non-Hodgkin lymphoma.

Secondary (AA) Amyloidosis May Complicate Severe, Long-Standing Inflammation

Most often, this occurs in rheumatic diseases or in chronic infections such as tuberculosis. AA amyloid fibrils are usually composed of an 8 kDa, 76-residue NH2-terminal portion of the 12-kDa precursor, serum amyloid A (SAA). SAAs are a group of related proteins, encoded by a family of SAA genes. SAAs are acute phase apoproteins made in the liver and transported by the plasma high-density lipoprotein, HDL3, in the plasma.

Usually, several years of an underlying inflammatory disease that causes elevated SAA precedes fibril formation, although AA amyloidosis associated with infections may develop more quickly. Several factors may accelerate AA fibril formation, such as an amyloid-enhancing factor present at high concentrations in the spleen, basement membrane heparan sulfate proteoglycan, or seeding with AA or heterologous fibrils.

Other Forms of Amyloidosis Reflect Diverse Pathogenetic Mechanisms

β_2M

Factors related to β_2M fibril formation, which used to occur in patients on long-term hemodialysis, are not clear. Possible explanations include dialysis membrane permeability, with 11.8-kDa β_2-microglobulin exceeding the porosity of standard membranes. As well, dialysis membranes may induce proinflammatory mediators that stimulate or modify β_2-microglobulin and contribute to fibril formation.

Familial Amyloidosis and Aging

In variant **ATTR amyloidosis** (also called familial amyloidotic polyneuropathy or cardiomyopathy), and all other forms of familial amyloidosis, inherited mutations or polymorphisms in genes encoding large serum proteins produce amyloid-prone variants. This is best understood for TTR, in which variant TTR molecules appear to be prone to dissociate from stable tetramers and then unfold, leading to misfolding, polymerization, and fibril formation. Since patients possess variant TTRs since birth, but do not have clinically apparent disease in childhood, age plays a role in this form of the disease. An age-related "trigger" activates cardiac amyloidosis, which occurs exclusively in the elderly, with deposits of wild-type TTR fibrils.

DIAGNOSIS

PATHOLOGY: A tissue biopsy demonstrating amyloid fibrils is necessary to diagnose amyloidosis. The least invasive biopsy is an abdominal fat aspirate, which is positive in 80% of patients with AL or ATTR amyloidosis and in 60% to 70% of patients with AA amyloidosis. If the aspirate is negative but clinical suspicion remains high, more invasive biopsies should be done. Sampling a clinically involved organ is recommended, but almost any tissue biopsy is likely to be positive if the patient has systemic disease. Once the diagnosis of amyloidosis is made, careful clinical evaluation, including presentation, organ system involvement, underlying diseases, and family history should suggest the type of amyloid. However, diagnosis and treatment require accurate typing of amyloid deposits to identify the specific precursor protein.

The presence of a plasma cell dyscrasia (**see Chapter 26**) distinguishes AL from other types of amyloidosis. Over 90% of AL patients have a monoclonal immunoglobulin protein or free light chain in their serum or urine, assayed by immunofixation electrophoresis or using a recently available nephelometric assay for free light chains. In addition, bone marrow biopsy often shows increased monoclonal plasma cells. A monoclonal serum protein alone is not diagnostic of

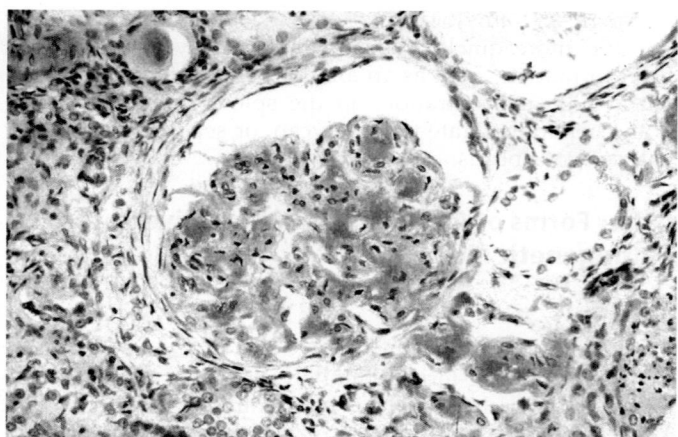

FIGURE 15-3. Microscopic appearance of AA amyloid in a glomerulus. Note the lobular pattern of the amyloid deposit and the involvement of the afferent arteriole.

amyloidosis, since monoclonal gammopathy of uncertain significance (**MGUS, see Chapter 26**) is common in older patients. However, if "MGUS" is present in someone with biopsy-proven amyloidosis, the AL type should be strongly suspected. Laboratories establish clonality by various techniques, including immunochemistry, in situ hybridization, and mass spectrometry–based microsequencing of protein extracted from fibril deposits.

One should suspect AA amyloidosis in patients with renal amyloidosis (Fig. 15-3) and a chronic inflammatory condition or infection. AL and ATTR amyloidosis must be ruled out, and AA amyloidosis confirmed, by immunostaining for AA protein.

If a patient does not have a plasma cell dyscrasia or AA amyloidosis, one must exclude possible familial amyloidosis. Although the disease has a dominant inheritance, family history may not be apparent if amyloidosis occurs later in life; also, some cases arise through new mutations. Isoelectric focusing (IEF) can usually detect variant TTR proteins, and an abnormal IEF should lead to sequencing of TTR exons to determine the precise mutation. If AF is suspected and TTR IEF is negative, exon sequencing may detect mutations in fibrinogen, lysozyme, and apolipoproteins.

CLINICAL FEATURES

AL Amyloidosis Most Often Affects the Kidneys and Heart

However, virtually any tissue other than the brain can be involved. Renal involvement usually presents as nephrotic syndrome with progressive worsening of renal function. In a small proportion of patients (~10%), amyloid deposits are in the renal vasculature or tubulointerstitium, causing renal dysfunction without significant proteinuria. Amyloid deposition in the heart results in rapidly progressive heart failure from restrictive cardiomyopathy (**see Chapter 17**). Ventricular walls are concentrically thickened with normal or reduced cavity size. Ventricular ejection fraction may be normal or only slightly decreased, but impaired ventricular filling limits cardiac output. EKG shows low voltage in many patients, often with a pseudoinfarct pattern.

Hepatomegaly is common and can result from either congestion due to right heart failure or amyloid infiltrating the liver. Hepatomegaly from amyloid infiltration can be massive and on physical examination, the liver is typically "rock-hard" and nontender. Since amyloid infiltrates the sinusoids, alkaline phosphatase may be severely elevated, with only mildly increased transaminases.

Autonomic nervous system involvement by AL amyloidosis can cause orthostatic hypotension, early satiety due to delayed gastric emptying, erectile dysfunction, and impaired intestinal motility. Painful, bilateral, symmetric, distal sensory neuropathy that progresses to motor neuropathy is the usual manifestation of peripheral nervous system involvement. Macroglossia, carpal tunnel syndrome, skin nodules, arthropathy, alopecia, nail dystrophy, submandibular gland enlargement, periorbital purpura, and hoarseness all characterize soft tissue involvement. Although macroglossia is present in a minority of patients, it is a hallmark of AL amyloidosis.

Endocrinopathies such as hypothyroidism and hypoadrenalism are rare, but may occur if AL amyloid infiltrates the glands. Many clotting abnormalities have been described in AL. Amyloid fibrils may bind factor X, and cause its rapid clearance from the blood, with consequent prolongation of prothrombin and partial thromboplastin times. Elevated levels of tissue and urine plasminogen activators and decreased tissue plasminogen activator inhibitor, may lead to hyperfibrinolytic states.

Secondary (AA) Amyloidosis May Occur at Any Age

Its primary clinical manifestation is proteinuria and/or renal insufficiency. Hepatomegaly, splenomegaly, and autonomic neuropathy often develop often as the disease progresses; cardiomyopathy is rare. When it complicates chronic inflammatory diseases, AA amyloid progression is slow and patients survive 10 years or more, particularly with treatment for renal failure. In contrast, when it occurs with untreated infections like osteomyelitis or tuberculosis, a more rapidly progressive amyloid syndrome may develop, which can remit with effective treatment of the infection.

Aβ_2M Amyloidosis May Manifest With Bone and Joint Complaints

Commonly observed conditions include carpal tunnel syndrome, persistent joint effusions, spondyloarthropathy, and cystic bone lesions. Carpal tunnel syndrome is usually the first symptom of disease. Persistent joint effusions accompanied by mild discomfort occur in up to 50% of patients on dialysis for more than 12 years. Involvement is bilateral and large joints (shoulders, knees, wrists, and hips) are most affected. Synovial fluid is noninflammatory, and its sediment contains β_2-microglobulin amyloid deposits on Congo red staining. β_2-microglobulin amyloid deposits may cause spondyloarthropathy with destructive changes of intervertebral discs and paravertebral erosions. Cystic bone lesions, sometimes leading to pathologic fractures, may occur in the femoral head, acetabulum, humerus, tibial plateau, vertebral bodies, and carpal bones. Although less common, visceral β_2-microglobulin amyloid deposits occasionally occur in the gut, heart, tendons, and subcutaneous tissues.

Clinically, ATTR Familial Amyloidosis Resembles AL Amyloidosis

In fact, the diseases are virtually indistinguishable on clinical grounds alone. A family history makes ATTR more likely, but many patients present with no such history, due to new TTR mutations or lack of ascertainment in parents. Within a family, disease symptoms tend to be similar. For ATTR V30M, peripheral neuropathy begins in the extremities as sensory neuropathy and progresses to motor neuropathy. This pattern varies with different TTR variants. Autonomic neuropathy causes GI symptoms: diarrhea with weight loss and orthostatic hypotension. Patients with TTR T60A and several other mutations have myocardial thickening, like that seen in AL amyloidosis, but heart failure is less common and the prognosis is better. Vitreous opacities due to amyloid deposits are pathognomonic of ATTR amyloidosis.

The TTR variant, V122I, is a common allele among the African-American population and is associated with cardiomyopathy. About 25% of black patients with amyloidosis have this TTR variant. This disease is probably underdiagnosed because of a lack of physician awareness and difficulties distinguishing amyloid and hypertensive cardiomyopathy without an endomyocardial biopsy.

Other Amyloidoses Reflect Deposits of Diverse Proteins and Have Variable Clinical Presentations

Hereditary Renal Amyloidoses

Hereditary renal amyloidoses (amyloidosis ApoAI [AApoAI], ApoAII [AApoAII], amyloidosis fibrinogen α-chain [AFib], amyloidosis lysozyme [ALys]) can resemble AL with renal involvement and should be considered when kidney biopsies show amyloid. Family history and immunoglobulin studies may help distinguish hereditary renal amyloidoses from AL with a dominant renal presentation. Immunohistochemical analysis of biopsy material to detect the various candidate amyloid proteins, establishes the diagnosis definitively.

Amyloidoses Localized to the CNS

AL amyloid may occur in cerebral vasculature, but it rarely accumulates in the CNS. Thus, it is easily distinguished clinically from the primarily CNS amyloidoses. The latter include amyloidosis cystatin C (ACys); hereditary cerebral hemorrhage with amyloidosis–Icelandic type, in which the precursor is the protease inhibitor cystatin c; the Aβ amyloidoses, including Dutch-type hereditary cerebral hemorrhage with amyloidosis, Alzheimer disease (Fig. 15-4), and Down syndrome; amyloidosis PrP (APrP), prionoses including Creutzfeldt–Jakob disease (CJD), Gerstmann–Sträussler–Scheinker (GSS) disease, fatal familial insomnia (FFI), bovine spongiform encephalopathy, kuru, and scrapie; and ABri/ADan, familial British/Danish dementia (**see Chapter 32**).

Localized Light-Chain Amyloidosis

Localized amyloid deposits, including amyloid masses called *amyloidomas*, may develop in various sites, even without systemic disease. Sometimes, plasma cells surround the deposits. DNA sequencing may show that the local plasma cells are producing the deposited light chains. For unknown reasons, the tracheobronchial tree is the most common site

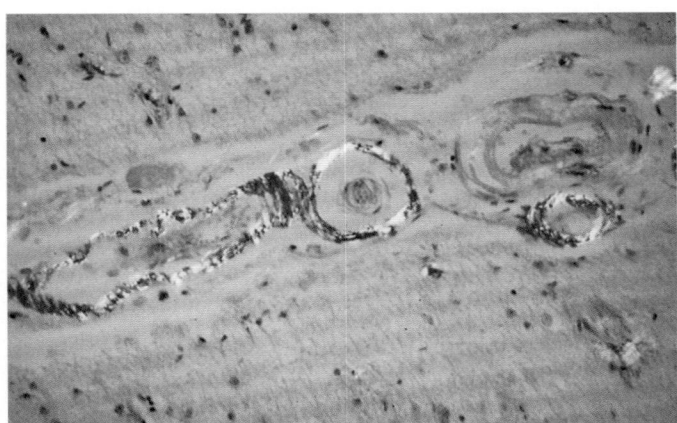

FIGURE 15-4. Cerebrovascular amyloid in a case of Alzheimer disease. The section was stained with Congo red and examined under polarized light.

of localized AL. It does not progress to systemic disease. Other localized AL deposits may involve the urinary tract, mediastinum, retroperitoneum, breast, and skin (as plaques or nodules).

TREATMENT AND PROGNOSIS OF SYSTEMIC AMYLOIDOSIS

Multiple Approaches May Be Used to Treat Systemic Amyloidosis

Modulating Overproduction

AL amyloid deposits reflect overproduction of immunoglobulin paraproteins. Median survival without treatment is usually only ~1 to 2 years from the time of diagnosis. Historically, treatment strategies have largely targeted production of the amyloidogenic protein. In AL amyloidosis, this has generally meant targeting plasma cells that make the immunoglobulin L chain that forms the amyloid fibrils (**see Chapter 26** for discussion). This approach, which may include stem cell transplants, has led to considerable success among selected patients.

However, for patients with myocardial involvement in AL amyloidosis, and impaired cardiac function or arrhythmias, median survival is ~6 months without treatment. In these patients, combined cardiac and stem cell transplantation can be performed. For this and other specific organ involvement, supportive therapies to address individual problems are used.

Stabilization

Without intervention, survival after ATTR disease onset is 5 to 15 years. Orthotopic liver transplantation, which removes the major source of variant TTR and replaces it with normal TTR, is the major treatment. Liver transplantation arrests disease progression and some improvement in autonomic and peripheral neuropathy can occur.

In this form of amyloidosis, the target, TTR, is structurally uniform among affected patients. Thyroxine binds and stabilizes circulating TTR tetramers. Thyroxine mimetics can prevent monomer release and amyloid fibril formation from variant-destabilized tetramers, and so block progression of neurologic disease.

Addressing Underlying Inflammatory and Infectious Diseases

The major focus in treating AA amyloidosis is the underlying inflammatory or infectious disease. Anti-inflammatory or anti-microbial treatment decreases SAA protein. New strategies include interfering with AA protein interaction with tissue gly-cosaminoglycans to prevent fibril formation and deposition.

Preventing Amyloid Protein Production

In cases where variant and wild-type TTR misfolding leads to amyloidosis, specific molecular suppressants may target the TTR in question. These have been shown to suppress blood TTR levels by 75% to 85%.

Cellular Proteostasis Pathways

Cellular proteostasis mechanisms are discussed in detail in Chapter 1. These cytoprotective pathways include autoph-agy relating to the endoplasmic reticulum (ER-associated degradation, or ERAD), autophagy, and related signaling pathways. Stimulating these pathways (or inhibiting their inhibitors) may protect from protein misfolding.

Disrupting Amyloid Deposits

Amyloid deposits encompass fibrils and ground substance, with SAP, ApoAIV, ApoE, and glycosaminoglycans. Anti-bodies against specific amyloidogenic proteins or targeting a ubiquitous component of amyloid ground substance, SAP, may allow removal of deposits and promote remodeling of major end organs.

Altering Dialysis in Aβ_2M Amyloidosis

In this disease, the 11-kD β_2-microglobulin molecule can-not pass through dialysis membranes. However, copper is thought to initiate Aβ_2M fibrillogenesis, and copper-free dialysis membranes appear to reduce the incidence of disease. Peritoneal dialysis, which is associated with lower plasma levels of β_2-microglobulin than hemodialy-sis, may slow amyloid development. Kidney transplanta-tion may mitigate symptoms in patients who developed Aβ_2M.

Diseases of Individual Organ Systems

16 Blood Vessels

Avrum I. Gotlieb, Myron I. Cybulsky

ANATOMY OF BLOOD VESSELS

Arteries Include Conducting and Resistance Vessels

The circulatory system includes several types of blood vessels that are categorized by size, structure, and function. These include arteries, which are conducting and resistance vessels; capillaries; and veins (Fig. 16-1).

Elastic Arteries

The largest blood vessels, the aorta and the elastic arteries, are conduits for blood flow to smaller arterial branches and are composed of three layers:

- Intima: This contains a single layer of endothelial cells, a subendothelial compartment with a few smooth muscle cells, and an extracellular matrix (ECM) reaching the luminal side of the internal elastic lamina. The aortic intima is thicker than that of other elastic arteries and its matrix proteins include collagen, proteoglycans, and small amounts of elastin. Occasional resident lymphocytes, macrophages, dendritic cells, and other blood-derived inflammatory cells are also present.

- Media: The next layer outward is the tunica media, the thickest tunica. It is bounded by internal and external elastic laminae and itself has many elastic laminae and smooth muscle cells within an extracellular connective tissue matrix. The aortic media is organized into lamellar units, each consisting of two concentric elastic laminae, with smooth muscle cells and their associated matrix in between the laminae. The media of the thoracic aorta contains more elastin; that of the abdominal aorta has more collagen. In elastic arteries, elastic fibers are interposed between smooth muscle cells and serve to minimize energy loss as pressure changes between systole and diastole.

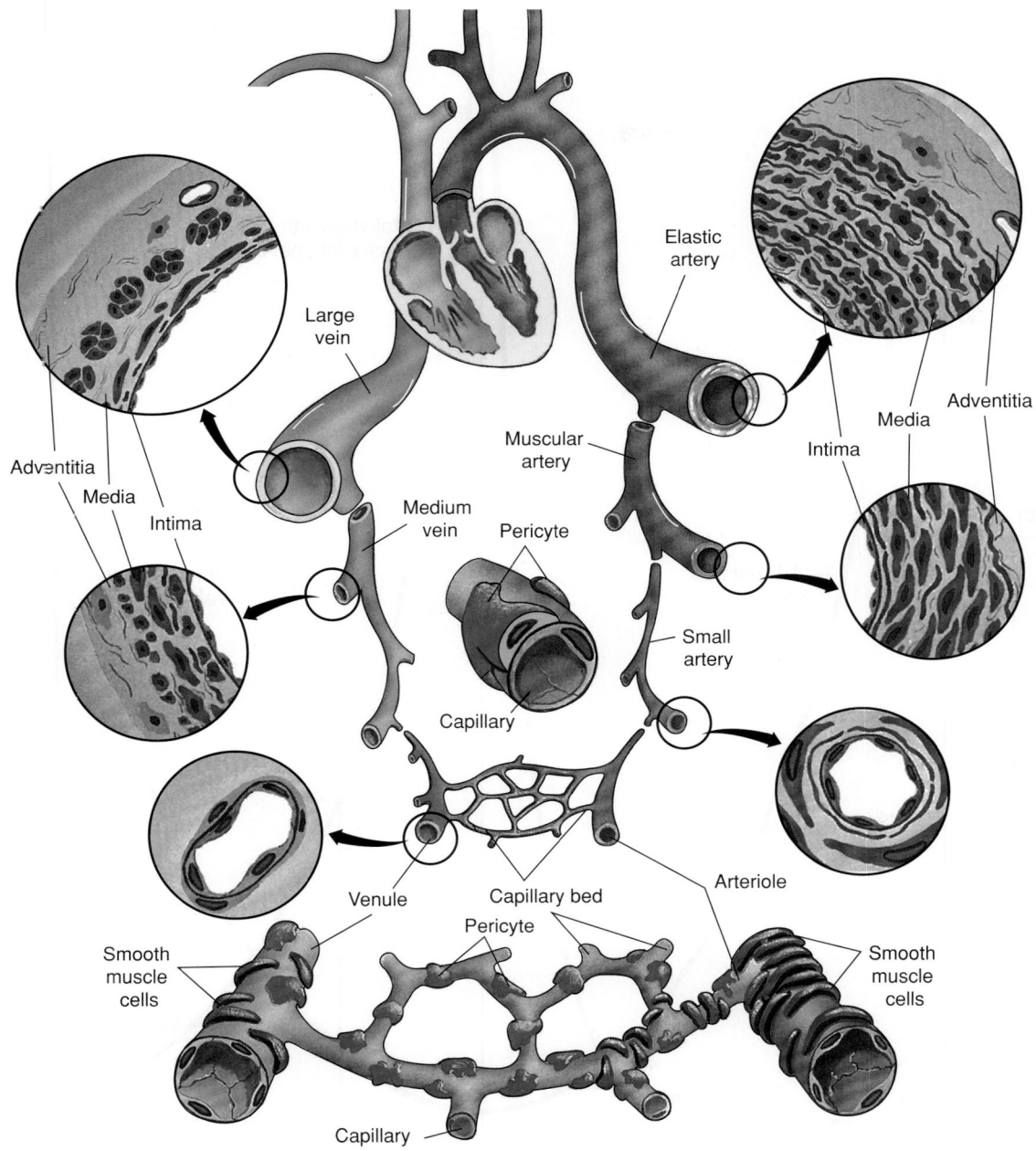

FIGURE 16-1. Subdivisions and histologic structure of the vascular system. Each subdivision is subject to a set of pathologic changes conditioned by the structure–function relationship of that part of the system. For example, the aorta, an elastic artery subject to great pressure, frequently shows a pathologic dilation (aneurysm) if the supporting elastic media is damaged. Muscular arteries are the most significant sites of atherosclerosis. Small arteries, particularly arterioles, are sites of hypertensive changes. Capillary beds, venules, and veins each display their own types of pathologic changes.

In smaller elastic arteries, the media is nourished by diffusion from the blood vessel lumen through the endothelium and the layers of smooth muscle. However, blood vessels with more than 28 layers of smooth muscle cells have a vasculature of their own, the *vasa vasorum*. These small vessels arise from the visceral and parietal branches of the aorta, and both form a superficial plexus at the adventitia–media border, when they penetrate into the outer 2/3 of the media. The media also contains autonomic nerve fibers that influence vascular contractility.

■ Adventitia: The outermost vessel wall layer contains fibroblasts, connective tissue, nerves, and small vessels

that give rise to the vasa vasorum. Occasional inflammatory cells, including collections of lymphocytes, may also be present.

Muscular Arteries

Blood conducted by elastic arteries is distributed to individual organs through large muscular arteries (Figs. 16-1 and 16-2). The media of muscular arteries contains layers of smooth muscle cells lacking prominent elastin bands, but with conspicuous internal and usually external elastic laminae. Fenestrae

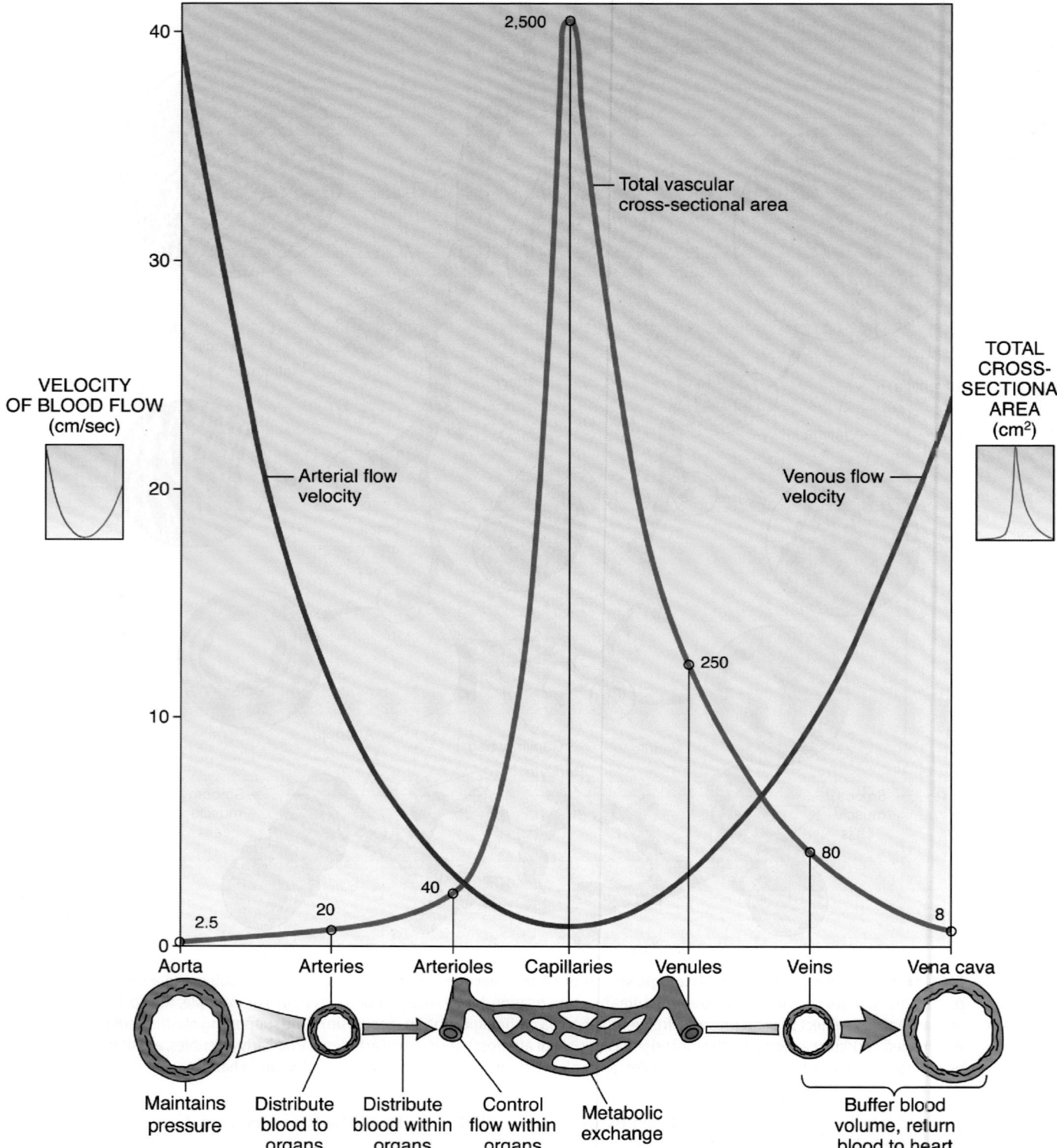

FIGURE 16-2. Relationship between velocity of blood flow and cross-sectional area in the vasculature. The vascular tree is a circuit that conducts blood from the heart through large-diameter, low-resistance conducting vessels to small arteries and arterioles, which lower blood pressure and protect the capillaries. The capillaries are thin walled and allow the exchange of nutrients and waste products between tissue and blood, a process that requires a very large surface area. The circuit back to the heart is completed by the veins, which are distensible and provide a volume buffer that acts as a capacitance for the vascular circuit.

interrupt the continuity of the internal elastic lamina, permitting smooth muscle cells to migrate from the media into the intima. Without heavy elastin layers, muscular arteries contract more efficiently. The intima of muscular arteries, like that of the aorta, also contains some smooth muscle cells, connective tissue, and occasional inflammatory cells. Vasa vasorum nourish the outer walls of thicker muscular arteries, but not smaller ones. As the vascular tree branches further, the media thins, and except for the endothelium, the intima disappears.

Small muscular arteries are important regulators of blood flow. Their narrow lumens increase resistance, and reduce blood pressure to levels appropriate to exchange water and plasma constituents across downstream thin-walled capillaries. Small muscular arteries, also called resistance vessels, help to maintain systemic pressure by regulating total peripheral resistance.

Arterioles

Arterioles are the smallest parts of the arterial system. They have an endothelial lining surrounded by one or two layers of smooth muscle cells, without elastic layers. The smallest arterioles regulate blood flow by vasomotion (change in an artery's caliber), thus controlling blood distribution through the capillary tree.

Capillaries Permit Transport From the Blood to the Interstitium

In capillaries, the smallest blood vessels, the endothelium is supported only by sparse smooth muscle cells. Capillary endothelium allows exchange of solutes and cells between blood and extracellular fluid. A necessary feature of this exchange is a marked decrease in pressure, which prevents intravascular fluid from shifting into the extracellular space.

The capillary endothelium is a semipermeable membrane, in which molecular size and charge determine exchange of plasma solutes with extracellular fluid. Capillary permeability depends on their endothelial cells. Brain capillaries, where junctions between endothelial cells are tightly sealed, are highly impermeable. Proteins do not traverse their walls. Transport in other capillary beds is mediated by passage of molecules through incomplete cell junctions or by transcytosis, in which vesicles transport molecules across the cytoplasm, possibly with continuity between vesicles, forming a continuous channel. In some capillaries, there may be permanent channels through discontinuous gaps between endothelial cells. Fenestrated renal glomerular capillaries are specifically adapted to filter plasma. Fenestrated endothelium also lines liver sinusoids, which are not true capillaries, facilitating access of plasma to hepatocytes.

Veins Return Blood to the Heart

Venules are the first vessels to collect blood from capillaries. They do not face high intraluminal pressures, and so have thin media. Venules merge into small and medium-sized veins, eventually emptying into large veins. Large veins do not contain elastic lamellae; even the internal elastic lamina is well developed only in the largest veins. The media is thin and is virtually absent in smaller tributaries. Many veins, particularly in the extremities, have valves made of endothelial-lined folds of the intima. These prevent backflow and facilitate blood movement in the low-pressure venous circulation. Postcapillary venules are where leukocytes transmigrate into tissue in inflammatory reactions (see Chapter 2).

Lymphatics Drain Interstitial Fluid

In lymphatic circulation, blind-ended lymphatic capillaries with endothelium but not pericytes, empty into precollecting lymphatics, which in turn drain into collecting lymphatics that pump lymph toward lymph nodes, lymphatic trunks, and finally thoracic and right lymphatic ducts. These return lymph back to the blood. Filtrate from capillaries and venules enters lymphatics, which are pathways to regional lymph nodes for cells, foreign material, and microorganisms. Collecting lymphatics have a contractile layer of smooth muscle cells to propel lymph forward. As in veins, intraluminal valves prevent backflow.

CELLS OF THE BLOOD VESSEL WALL

The vascular wall cells have unique properties that contribute to normal physiology, and to the pathogenesis of vascular diseases.

A Single Endothelial Cell Layer Forms a Thromboresistant Barrier

Endothelial cells are metabolically active and are intimately involved in several biologic functions, including vascular permeability, coagulation, platelet regulation, fibrinolysis, inflammation, immune regulation, and repair. They also modulate vascular smooth muscle cell function through paracrine pathways. Endothelial cells are unique mechanotransduction structures that mitigate the effects of luminal hemodynamic shear stress on the vessel wall. Endothelial cell membranes may deform in response to mechanical forces, which induce expression of vasoactive compounds, growth factors, coagulation/fibrinolytic/complement factors, matrix degradation enzymes, inflammatory mediators, and adhesion molecules.

Endothelial integrity depends on several types of adhesion complexes that promote cell–substratum and cell–cell adhesions (see Chapter 2).

- Cell-substrate adhesion molecules attach endothelial cells to their substratum (e.g., basal lamina). These molecules complex with intracellular cytoskeleton that participates in intracellular signal transduction. Integrins are transmembrane molecules that bind endothelial cells to ECM adhesive molecules, including laminin, fibronectin, fibrinogen, von Willebrand factor, and thrombospondin. Integrins' cytoplasmic tails bind the complex of proteins that regulate adhesion at focal contact sites and associate with actin microfilaments and microtubules of the cytoskeleton (Fig. 16-3).
- Cell–cell adhesion molecules link endothelial cells to their neighbors: cadherin at intercellular adhesion junctions and occludin, claudins, and junctional adhesion molecules (JAMs) at tight junctions. These connect to the actin cytoskeleton. Platelet endothelial cell adhesion molecule-1 (PECAM-1) and VEGFR-2 in adherens junctions help sense shear stress. Gap junctions, made of connexins, regulate ion passage between adjacent cells.

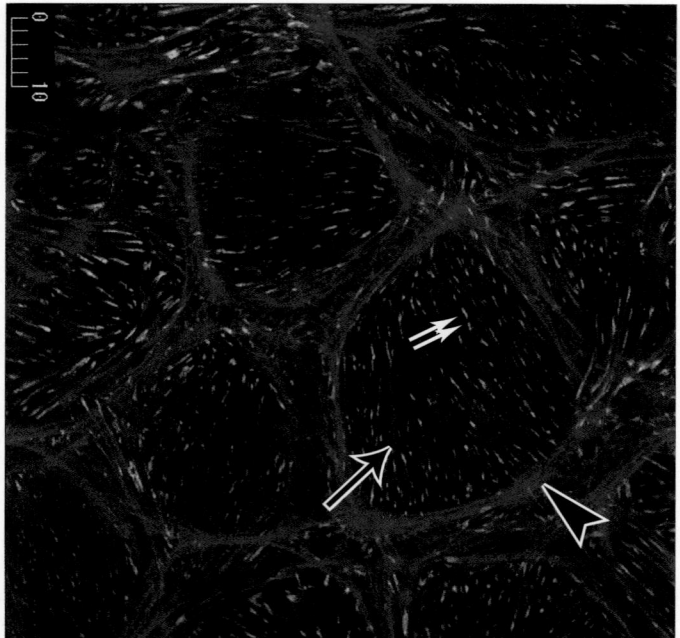

FIGURE 16-3. Focal adhesion protein, vinculin. Porcine aortic endo-thelial cells were grown to confluency and double-stained for actin/vincu-lin. Endothelial cells in confluent monolayers contain a dense peripheral band of actin microfilament bundles (*arrowhead*) and central microfila-ment or "stress fibers" (*single arrow*). Vinculin in confluent monolayer localizes to the tips of stress fibers (*double arrow*).

Endothelial cells subserve many important metabolic functions (Table 16-1), often regulated by serum and hemo-dynamic factors that activate surface receptors and signal transduction pathways or regulate gene transcription. Endo-thelial cells do not usually proliferate, but after vascular injury with loss of endothelium, they spread, migrate, and proliferate rapidly to reestablish endothelial structural integ-rity and so protect the wall (Fig. 16-4).

TABLE 16-1

FUNCTIONS OF ENDOTHELIAL CELLS OF THE BLOOD VESSELS

Semipermeable barrier (adherens junctions)

Thromboresistant surface

Mechanotransducer (shear stress response elements)

Vasoactive factors: Nitric oxide (endothelium-derived relaxing factor), prostacyclin (PGI$_2$), endothelin

Antithrombotic agent production: Adenine metabolites

Antiplatelet agent production: Prostacyclin (PGI$_2$)

Anticoagulant production: Thrombomodulin, other proteins; tissue factor pathway inhibitor

Fibrinolytic agent production: Tissue plasminogen activator, urokinase-like activator

Procoagulant production: Tissue factor, factor V, factor VIIIa (von Willebrand factor), receptors for factor IX, factor X, plasminogen activator inhibitor

Inflammatory mediator production: Cytokines, chemokines, interleukin-1, cell adhesion molecules, tumor necrosis factor

Growth factor production: Blood cell colony-stimulating factors, insulin-like growth factors, fibroblast growth factor, platelet-derived growth factor

Growth inhibitor of smooth muscle cells (heparin)

Lipid metabolism, low-density lipoproteins, modified low-density lipoproteins

Proliferation and migration in response to injury

Matrix secretion and remodeling

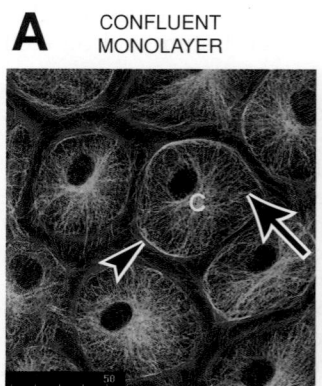 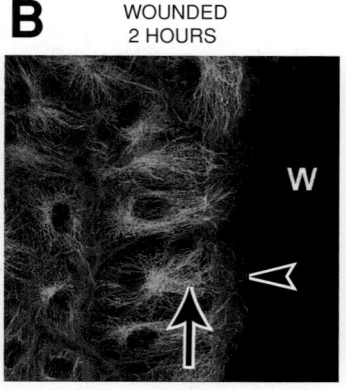 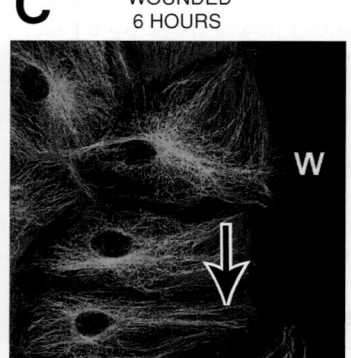 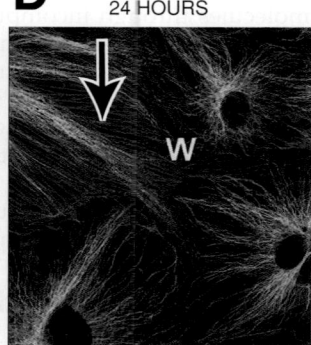

A CONFLUENT MONOLAYER **B** WOUNDED 2 HOURS **C** WOUNDED 6 HOURS **D** WOUNDED 24 HOURS

FIGURE 16-4. Remodeling in response to loss of endothelial integrity. Porcine aortic endothelial cells were grown to confluency, and a 1-mm wound was created using a scraper. Cells were fixed and double-stained for actin/tubulin at 2, 6, and 24 hours after wounding. **A.** Endothelial cells in confluent monolayers contain a dense peripheral band (DPB) of actin microfilament bundles (*arrowhead*) and centrosomes (C) (*arrow*) toward the cell periphery. **B.** Two hours after wounding, there is formation of lamellipodia (*arrowhead*), and stress fibers (*arrow*) rearrange to become parallel to the wound edge (*W*). Centrosomes migrate around the nucleus toward the wound edge, and the microtubules begin emanating toward the wound (*W*). **C.** By 6 hours, changes in microtubules and microfilaments are more prominent and the microtubule–microfilament networks (*arrow*) begin to reorganize perpendicu-lar to the wound edge (*W*) as the cells begin to spread. **D.** Twenty-four hours after wounding, the microtubule–microfilament networks (*arrow*) are aligned perpendicular to the wound edge (*W*) as the cells migrate into the wound.

Endothelial cells release a number of biologically potent factors when they are activated. Some of these bioactive molecules are released locally, act at short distances, and are rapidly inactivated. For example, prostacyclin (PGI$_2$), derived from the cyclooxygenase (COX) pathway, relaxes smooth muscle and inhibits platelet aggregation. Endothelial nitric oxide synthase (NOS) converts L-arginine and O$_2$ to L-citrulline and nitric oxide (NO•) (see below). It also modulates vascular tone and vascular smooth muscle cell proliferation by increasing cyclic guanosine monophosphate (cGMP), in turn activating cGMP-dependent protein kinase. NO• also helps to control the muscular tone of large arteries and resistance vessels. After agonists stimulate endothelial cell receptors, prostacyclin and NO• are released and together inhibit platelet aggregation. Compounds that promote NO• release include acetylcholine, bradykinin, and adenosine diphosphate (ADP). NO• is even more labile than prostacyclin, with a half-life of 6 seconds.

Several bioactive peptides also alter vascular tone. **Endothelins** are a family of potent vasoconstrictive proteins made by endothelial cells. They bind two receptors: both occur on smooth muscle cells, but only one on endothelial cells. **Angiotensin-converting enzyme (ACE)**, an endothelial product, converts angiotensin I to angiotensin II, a potent vasoconstrictor that is important in the pathogenesis of hypertension.

Endothelial cell–derived factors also control some immune responses. Like macrophages, when stimulated, endothelial cells express class II histocompatibility antigens. They may thus work with monocytes—or even replace them—in activating lymphocytes. Immune responses against endothelium are a key part of organ rejection after transplantation, and in the pathogenesis of graft arteriosclerosis.

Smooth Muscle Cells Maintain Blood Vessel Integrity

Vascular smooth muscle cells are derived from local mesoderm after endothelial tubes are formed (Fig. 16-5). However, the smooth muscle cells of major upper body arteries derive instead from neural crest.

Smooth muscle cells, in association with ECM, maintain blood vessel integrity and provide support for endothelium. They control blood flow by contracting or dilating in response to specific stimuli. They also synthesize the vessel's connective tissue matrix, including elastin; collagen, especially type I and III collagen; and proteoglycan. These cells produce proteolytic enzymes and their inhibitors, which regulate tissue remodeling and repair. In normal arteries, smooth muscle cells rarely divide. Rather, like endothelial cells, they proliferate in response to injury and are important in atherogenesis. In the latter case, they differentiate to a synthetic phenotype, expressing genes regulating secretion, migration, and proliferation. PDGF, microRNAs (miRNAs), and oxidized **low-density lipoprotein (LDL)** are important drivers of the switch of smooth muscle cells from contractile to synthetic phenotype. Smooth muscle cells are major producers of growth factors, cytokines, and chemokines involved in atherogenesis. They may also alter phenotype, to assume phagocytic or osteogenic characteristics, as part of arterial calcification.

Pericytes Are Modified Smooth Muscle Cells Around Capillaries

Pericytes regulate endothelial functions in angiogenesis and capillary stability. Endothelial tip cells (see Chapter 5)

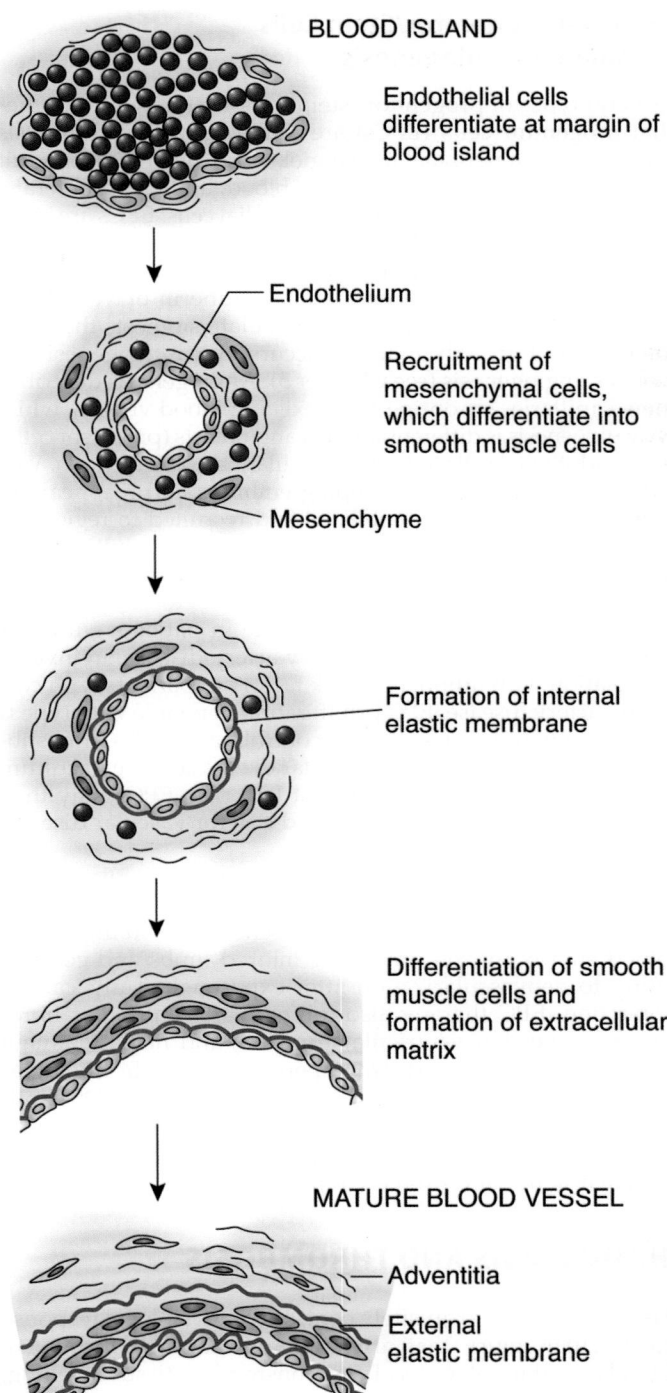

BLOOD ISLAND

Endothelial cells differentiate at margin of blood island

Endothelium

Recruitment of mesenchymal cells, which differentiate into smooth muscle cells

Mesenchyme

Formation of internal elastic membrane

Differentiation of smooth muscle cells and formation of extracellular matrix

MATURE BLOOD VESSEL

Adventitia

External elastic membrane

FIGURE 16-5. Differentiation of vessels in early embryos. The course of events from the development of blood islands on the chorioallantoic membrane starts with differentiation of endothelium and proceeds to fully developed arteries and veins.

activate pericyte migration and proliferation via platelet-derived growth factor-β (PDGFβ). Pericytes may act as stem or precursor cells, differentiating into myofibroblasts and smooth muscle cells. They may also regulate endothelial cell activities and proliferation.

Vascular Progenitor/Stem Cells Regulate Vasculogenesis

Several types of progenitor/stem cells are known. **Endothelial progenitor cells (EPCs)** are multipotent immature cells that arise from perinatal hemangioblasts. They reside in adult bone marrow and circulate in the blood, and can proliferate, migrate, and differentiate into endothelial cells. EPCs are identified by their expression of CD133, CD34, c-kit, VEGFR-2, CD144, and Sca-1. Unlike mature endothelial cells, they express CD133, but not endothelial cadherin or von Willebrand factor. The fact that EPCs circulate suggests that new blood vessel growth in adults occurs by vasculogenesis, as well as angiogenesis (see Chapter 5). Angiogenesis describes new capillaries sprouting from existing blood vessels, while vasculogenesis is differentiation of angioblasts (precursor cells) into endothelial cells to form a vascular network de novo. Vasculogenesis occurs in developing embryos and reappears in adults when EPCs are mobilized and recruited to regions of new blood vessel formation. As embryonic and adult vasculogenesis are similar, initiating stimuli and regulatory pathways for both are probably comparable.

Fewer EPCs circulate and migrate in patients with diabetes mellitus and stable coronary artery disease, in inverse correlation with numbers of risk factors in patients with coronary artery disease. EPC proliferation in people with type II diabetes mellitus is less than in controls, and EPCs from subjects at high risk for cardiovascular events senesce in culture faster than do cells from those at low risk. EPCs may thus be sensitive indicators of increased risk for vascular disease, especially atherosclerosis.

EPCs may have therapeutic potential in vascular regeneration, for example, transplanted EPCs may promote collateral circulation and treat tissue ischemia, as in improving blood supply in experimentally injured limbs and contributing to neovascularization after experimental myocardial infarction. EPC therapy also inhibits left ventricular fibrosis, preserves left ventricular function, and helps maintain blood vessel patency after therapeutic stenting. Technologies to capture EPCs, for example, incorporating anti-CD34 antibody into stents, have shown promise in keeping implanted stents patent. Adult circulating EPCs may thus help treat vascular injury and promote repair.

HEMOSTASIS AND THROMBOSIS

Hemostasis is an exquisitely controlled physiologic response to vascular injury that arrests hemorrhage by forming a blood clot. It involves local vasoconstriction, tissue swelling, and platelet adhesion, aggregation, and activation. Coagulation and fibrin formation follow, producing a hemostatic plug at sites of injury.

Thrombosis is the process that promotes formation of a blood clot, or thrombus, within the circulation. A thrombus is an aggregate of coagulated blood that contains platelets, fibrin, leukocytes, and red blood cells. It forms when the balance of factors favor clotting, as compared to inhibiting it—that is, when prothrombotic processes overcome antithrombotic ones. Thrombosis involves (1) activation of platelets, (2) activation of coagulation pathways, (3) participation of the monocyte/macrophage system, (4) active involvement of the endothelial cells of the vessel wall and, under certain conditions, extrusion of neutrophil DNA (NETosis, see Chapter 1).

TABLE 16-2	
COAGULATION FACTOR DESIGNATIONS	
Factor	**Standard Name**
I	Fibrinogen
II	Prothrombin
III	Tissue factor
IV	Calcium ions
V	Proaccelerin
VII	Proconvertin
VIII	Antihemophilic factor (AHF)
IX	Plasma thromboplastin component (PTC)
X	Stuart factor
XI	Plasma thromboplastin antecedent (PTA)
XII	Hageman factor
XIII	Fibrin-stabilizing factor (FSF)
–	Prekallikrein
–	High–molecular-weight kininogen

Hemostasis (see Chapters 7 and 26) involves the coagulation network of activating and inactivating enzymes, and cofactors derived from different cells and tissues, some circulating and some locally produced (Table 16-2).

Blood Coagulates When Fibrinogen Is Converted to Fibrin

The endpoint of blood coagulation is conversion of soluble plasma fibrinogen to an insoluble fibrillar polymer—fibrin. This reaction is catalyzed by the protease, thrombin. A series of finely tuned steps is mediated by several coagulation factors (Table 16-2). To prevent extensive clotting throughout the entire circulation, many of these factors are restricted by specific inhibitors. The coagulation cascade amplifies an initial signal into eventual generation of thrombin, production of which is key to clot progression and stabilization. For example, one molecule of an upstream coagulation factor, factor Xa, generates about 1,000 molecules of thrombin.

The coagulation cascade was once divided into "intrinsic" and "extrinsic" pathways, now called the contact activation pathway and the tissue factor (TF) pathway, respectively. However, this dichotomy does not accurately reflect the main mechanisms of clotting, in which the contact activation pathway actually plays a minor role.

Current views of coagulation (Fig. 16-6) highlight the centrality of TF, a membrane-bound glycoprotein. The dynamic association of factor VIIa–TF complexes with TF pathway inhibitor (TFPI) is crucial to thrombosis. TFPI inhibits initiation of coagulation by binding TF–FXa–FVIIa complex. A major pool of TFPI on endothelial cell surfaces thus probably regulates coagulation. Hemostasis starts when activated

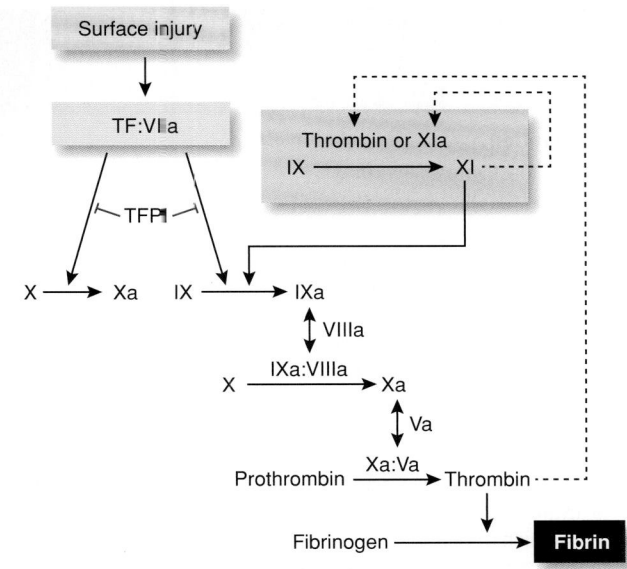

FIGURE 16-6. Coagulation cascade. The coagulation cascade is initiated by endothelial injury, which releases tissue factor (*TF*). The latter combines with activated factor VII (VIIa) to form a complex that activates small amounts of X to Xa and IX to IXa. The complex of IXa with VIIIa further activates X. The complex of Xa with Va then catalyzes the conversion of prothrombin to thrombin, after which fibrin is formed from fibrinogen. *TFPI* = tissue factor pathway inhibitor. Positive feed back loops are indicated by dashed lines.

factor VII (VIIa) encounters TF at a site of injury, forming the TF–VIIa complex. This complex activates small amounts of factors IX and X to IXa and Xa. Factors VIIIa and IXa convert greater amounts of X to Xa.

Xa converts small amounts of prothrombin to thrombin, which activates factor XI to XIa. XIa increases its own generation from XI (positive feedback) and increases factor IX conversion to IXa. The IXa and VIIIa complex generates more factor Xa from X. This Xa and Va form the prothrombinase complex, which activates prothrombin to thrombin. Thrombin converts fibrinogen to fibrin monomers, which then polymerize. Thrombin also activates factor XIII to XIIIa, cross-linking fibrin strands to stabilize the clot.

Besides its important role in coagulation and platelet aggregation, thrombin participates in production of fibrinolytic molecules and regulation of growth factors and leukocyte adhesion molecules. It also mediates the protein C anticoagulant pathway by binding thrombomodulin at the surface of endothelial cells. Factor V, an essential protein coagulation cofactor, also has anticoagulant activity by exerting a cofactor function in the activated protein C system, which then downregulates factor VIIIa activity. Thrombin also increases vessel permeability via G protein-coupled receptors (PARs), by promoting alterations in endothelial cell shape and disrupting endothelial cell–cell adhesion junctions.

Blood Vessel Injury Causes Platelet Adhesion and Aggregation

Normally, circulating platelets do not adhere to each other or to the surface of the vessel wall. However, injury upregulates platelet adhesiveness, after which platelets interact with one another to form a platelet thrombus, that is, an aggregate of activated platelets (Fig. 16-7). This process

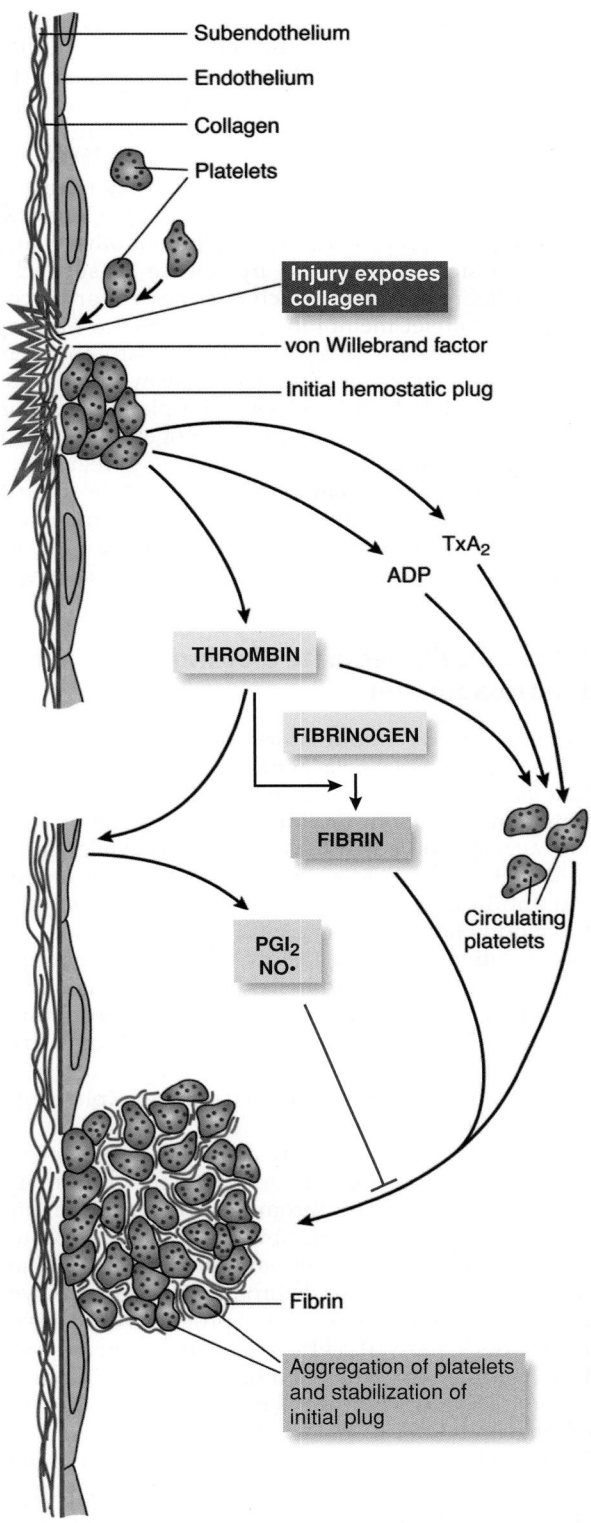

FIGURE 16-7. The role of platelets in thrombosis. Following vessel wall injury and alteration in flow, platelets adhere and then aggregate. Adenosine diphosphate (*ADP*) and thromboxane A_2 (*TxA₂*) are released and, along with locally generated thrombin, recruit additional platelets, causing the mass to enlarge. The growing platelet thrombus is stabilized by fibrin. Other elements, including leukocytes and red blood cells, are also incorporated into the thrombus. The release of prostacyclin (*PGI₂*) and nitric oxide (*NO•*) by endothelial cells regulates the process by inhibiting platelet aggregation.

requires that platelets change shape, requiring reorganization of actin microfilaments. Thrombin, collagen, ADP, epinephrine, thromboxane A_2, platelet-activating factor (PAF), and vasopressin promote platelet aggregation. Platelet aggregates occlude injured small vessels and prevent leakage of blood.

Once platelets adhere to a vessel wall, they release their granular contents, in part by contraction of platelet cytoskeleton. These granules promote aggregation of other platelets. Platelet adhesion is enhanced by release of subendothelial von Willebrand factor, which is adhesive for glycoprotein (Gp) Ib platelet membrane protein and for fibrinogen. Activated platelets also release ADP and thromboxane A_2, a product of arachidonic acid metabolism, which recruit additional platelets to the process. The platelet membrane protein complex GpIIb–IIIa binds fibrinogen to form fibrinogen bridges between platelets, enhance aggregation, and stabilize the nascent thrombus. Activated platelets in turn release factors that initiate coagulation, thus forming a complex thrombus on the surface of the vessel wall. Thrombin itself stimulates further release of platelet granules and subsequent recruitment of new platelets.

Endothelial Cells Regulate Clotting and Anticoagulation

Endothelium-derived modulators of coagulation are listed in Table 16-3. Endothelial cells synthesize a number of anticoagulant factors. They produce and secrete PGI_2, which inhibits platelet aggregation. Endothelial NO• strongly inhibits platelet aggregation and adhesion to vessel walls. Endothelial cells metabolize ADP, a strong promoter of thrombogenesis, to antithrombogenic metabolites. The luminal surface of the endothelium is coated with heparan sulfate, which binds a number of clotting factors, including the antiprotease β_2-macroglobulin. Endothelial heparan sulfate activates antithrombin, which binds to several coagulation factors, IIa, IXa, Xa, XIa, and XIIa, which are free and not bound in complexes or in the clot. Endothelial cells may also lyse some clots as they form through the plasminogen/plasminogen activator/plasmin system.

Among other anticoagulant activities, endothelial cell surfaces have a cofactor which inactivates thrombin, by forming a complex with thrombin and antithrombin III (a plasma antiprotease). Thrombin itself activates protein C by binding its receptor, thrombomodulin, at endothelial cell surfaces. Both protein C and thrombomodulin are synthesized by endothelial cells. Activated protein C destroys coagulation factors V and VIII. TFPI generated during coagulation binds to endothelium, where it inhibits the TF–VIIa complex (Fig. 16-6). TF and TFPI are synthesized and secreted by endothelial and other vascular cells.

The endothelium is also intimately involved in initiating and propagating thrombosis. The event that triggers most thrombosis is endothelial injury, which imparts a prothrombotic property to endothelium (Fig. 16-7). Endothelial cells synthesize **von Willebrand factor,** which promotes platelet adherence and activates clotting factor V. Endothelial cells also bind factors IX and X, which favors coagulation at endothelial surfaces. Finally, inflammatory agents, including cytokines released from monocytes, activate procoagulants on the surface of intact endothelium. IL-1 and TNF-α cause endothelial cells to present thromboplastin to the plasma, thereby potentially triggering the TF pathway.

TABLE 16-3

REGULATION OF COAGULATION AT THE ENDOTHELIAL CELL SURFACE

Downregulation

1. Thrombin inactivators
   a. Antithrombin III
   b. Thrombomodulin
2. Activated protein C pathway
   a. Synthesis and expression of thrombomodulin
   b. Synthesis and expression of protein S
   c. Thrombomodulin-mediated activation of protein C
   d. Inactivation of factor V_a and factor VIII_a by APC–protein S complex
3. Tissue factor pathway inhibition
4. Antithrombin III inactivates factors IX, X, XI, XII
5. Fibrinolysis
   a. Synthesis of tissue plasminogen activator, urokinase plasminogen activator, and plasminogen activator inhibitor-1
   b. Conversion of Glu-plasminogen to Lys-plasminogen
   c. Antithrombin III
   d. APC-mediated potentiation
6. Synthesis of unsaturated fatty acid metabolites
   a. Lipoxygenase metabolites—13-HODE
   b. Cyclooxygenase metabolites—PGI_2 and PGE_2

Procoagulant Pathways

1. Synthesis and expression of:
   a. Tissue factor (thromboplastin)
   b. Factor V
   c. Thrombin activatable fibrinolysis inhibitor (TAFI)
   d. Platelet-activating factor (PAF)
2. Binding of clotting factors IX/IX_a, X (prothrombinase complex)
3. Downregulation of APC pathway
4. Increased synthesis of plasminogen activator inhibitor
5. Synthesis of 15-HPETE

APC = adenomatous polyposis coli; 13-HODE = 13-hydroxyoctadecadienoic acid; 15-HPETE = 15-hydroperoxyeicosatetraenoic acid; PGE_2 = prostaglandin E_2; PGI_2 = prostacyclin.

Thus, thrombi may form when endothelial function is altered, endothelial continuity is lost, or blood flow in a vessel becomes abnormal, such as turbulent or static. Simple endothelial cell loss, or injury to a vessel with good flow, causes platelet pavementing but not thrombosis (Fig. 16-8).

Endothelial Cells Repair Defects in Damaged Areas

The most common denuding injury to endothelium is progressive disruption by atherosclerotic plaque. Denuding endothelial damage also occurs in homocystinuria, hypoxia, and endotoxemia, and during invasive procedures like harvesting and implanting saphenous vein bypass grafts, angioplasty, inserting intravascular stents, and atherectomy. Interactions of a thrombus with subjacent endothelial cells may further disturb endothelial integrity. Both fibrin and thrombin affect endothelial cell cytoskeleton and initiate endothelial shape changes to form intercellular gaps that disrupt endothelial integrity.

In that setting, endothelial cells can spread rapidly and migrate into the denuded area to reestablish a thrombo-resistant barrier (Fig. 16-4). The cells then proliferate to restore normal cell density. These mechanisms may become

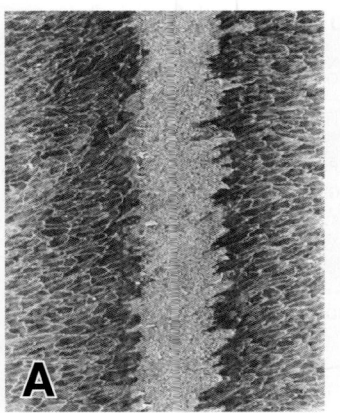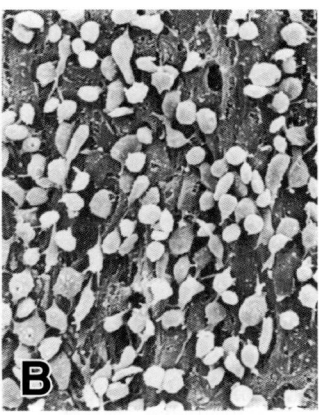

FIGURE 16-8. Scanning electron micrograph of the endothelial surface of a rat aorta 1 hour after the endothelial cells were removed by scraping with a nylon filament. A. Intact endothelium and scratched portion. **B.** Higher-power view of the scratched area shows a pavement of intact platelets that adheres to the underlying connective tissue in the high-velocity arterial stream.

dysfunctional at sites of persistent endothelial cell damage, causing focal erosions, ulcers, and fissures.

In addition, marrow-derived EPCs may proliferate after vascular injury and physiologic stress. They then are released into the peripheral circulation, where they attach to denuded vessel wall surfaces and differentiate, to reestablish endothelial integrity.

Clot Lysis Is a Regulatory Mechanism

Thrombi may undergo several fates: (1) lysis, (2) growth and propagation, (3) embolization, and (4) organization and canalization. The combination of aggregated platelets and clotted blood is made unstable by activation of the fibrinolytic enzyme plasmin (Fig. 16-9). During clot formation, plasminogen binds to fibrin and therefore is an integral part of the forming platelet mass. Endothelial cells make plasminogen activator, but in larger thrombi, circulating plasminogen may also be converted to plasmin by products of the coagulation cascade. Plasminogen activator bound to fibrin activates plasmin. Plasmin digests fibrin strands into

smaller fragments, lysing and disrupting the thrombus. These smaller fragments inhibit thrombin and fibrin formation. Clearance of fibrin also limits its accumulation in atherosclerotic plaques, where it can promote plaque growth and attract inflammatory cells. Endothelial cells also synthesize plasminogen activator inhibitor-1 (PAI-1), and plasmin is inhibited by α_2-antiplasmin. Thus, a regional fibrinolytic state reflects the balance between plasminogen and plasmin activation and inhibition.

Thrombi may undergo organization and become incorporated into vessel walls. The fibrin meshwork contracts to reduce thrombus size. Arterial smooth muscle cells, endothelium, and venous fibroblasts migrate into the cross-linked fibrin and produce ECM and contribute to canalization.

Proteolytic enzymes and their inhibitors secreted by smooth muscle cells and macrophages remodel, digest, and then recanalize the clot with its own new blood vessels, elicited by angiogenic factors in the thrombus. However, blood flow through canalized thrombi is usually limited.

ATHEROSCLEROSIS

The Classic Atherosclerotic Lesion Is a Fibroinflammatory Lipid Plaque

Atherosclerosis is characterized by progressive accumulation of inflammatory, immune, and smooth muscle cells, lipids, and connective tissue in the intima of large and medium-sized elastic and muscular arteries. These fibroinflammatory plaques (atheromas) develop over several decades (Tables 16-4 and 16-5). Their continued growth encroaches on arterial wall media and narrows vessel lumens. Atherosclerotic lesions are also called plaques, atheromas, fibrous plaques, or fibrofatty lesions.

EPIDEMIOLOGY: The major complications of atherosclerosis include ischemic heart disease (coronary artery disease), myocardial infarction, stroke, and gangrene of the extremities. These, together, cause over half of annual mortality in the Western world. Deaths from ischemic heart disease in Western countries peaked in the late 1960s, then declined dramatically, but

FIGURE 16-9. Mechanisms of fibrinolysis. Plasmin formed from plasminogen lyses fibrin. The conversion of plasminogen to plasmin and the activity of plasmin itself are suppressed by specific inhibitors.

```
Tissue-Type Plasminogen Activator
Urokinase-Type Plasminogen
        |
        v
   Plasminogen Activator Inhibitors
        |
Plasminogen -------> Plasmin
                       |
                       |--- α₂-Antiplasmin
                       v
Fibrin -------> Fibrin Degradation Products
```

TABLE 16-4
ATHEROGENESIS
• Initiation and growth of fibroinflammatory lipid atheroma is a slowly evolving dynamic process with superimposed acute events.
• Reversible and nonreversible risk factors promote initiation and accelerate progression of plaques.
• The pathogenesis is multifactorial and thus the relative importance of specific genetic and environmental factors may vary in individuals.
• Interactions between cellular and matrix components of the vessel wall and serum constituents, leukocytes, platelets, and physical forces regulate the formation of the fibroinflammatory lipid atheroma.
• The genetic effect in atherosclerosis is polygenic: There is no single genetic determinant.

TABLE 16-5

IMPORTANT COMPONENTS OF FIBROINFLAMMATORY LIPID ATHEROMA

Cells		
	• Endothelial cells	• Lipids and lipoproteins
	• Smooth muscle cells	• Serum proteins
	• Foam cells	• Platelet products
	• Giant cells	• Leukocyte products: cytokines, chemokines
	• Lymphocytes	• Necrotic debris, cholesterol crystals
	• Dendritic cells	
	• Mast cells	• New microvessels
	• Macrophages	• Hydroxyapatite crystals
Matrix		
	• Collagen	• Growth factors
	• Elastin	• Oxidants/antioxidants
	• Glycoproteins	• Proteolytic enzymes
	• Proteoglycans	• Procoagulant factors

are still the leading cause of death. There are wide geographic and racial variations in the incidence of ischemic heart disease. Important risk factors include hyperlipidemia, hypertension, diabetes mellitus, smoking, microparticle pollutants, obesity, advanced age, and a strong family history.

 MOLECULAR PATHOGENESIS: Except for rare monogenic disorders of lipid metabolism, there is no single molecular trigger causing atherosclerosis. Instead, over 60 single nucleotide polymorphisms (SNPs) are known to contribute. As well, certain miRNAs are enriched in atherosclerotic vessels, some of which are known to be flow sensitive, regulating inflammation, endothelial proliferation, NO• signaling, and apoptosis. Circulating microvesicles containing miRNAs may transport these functions from one endothelial cell to another.

 PATHOPHYSIOLOGY: Even as plaque formation, growth, and clinical presentation vary from patient to patient, the pathogenesis of atherosclerosis is reasonably well understood. The seeds of atherogenesis (Figs. 16-10 to 16-13) may begin in fetal or early postnatal life, with the formation of intimal cell masses, or when fatty streaks begin to evolve. However, typical atherosclerotic lesions, which are clinically insignificant at first, form over 20 to 30 years. (An exception is homozygous familial hypercholesterolemia, in which lesions develop in the first decade of life.)

The life of a plaque has three stages: (1) initiation and formation, (2) adaptation, and (3) clinical. In this process, biologically active molecules regulate several dynamic cellular functions, and multiple gene polymorphisms most likely interact with the environmental factors, and with each other.

Initiation and Formation Stage

1. Uniform laminar flow with normal shear stress helps maintain normal endothelial thromboresistance and integrity. Proinflammatory cytokines and tissue factor

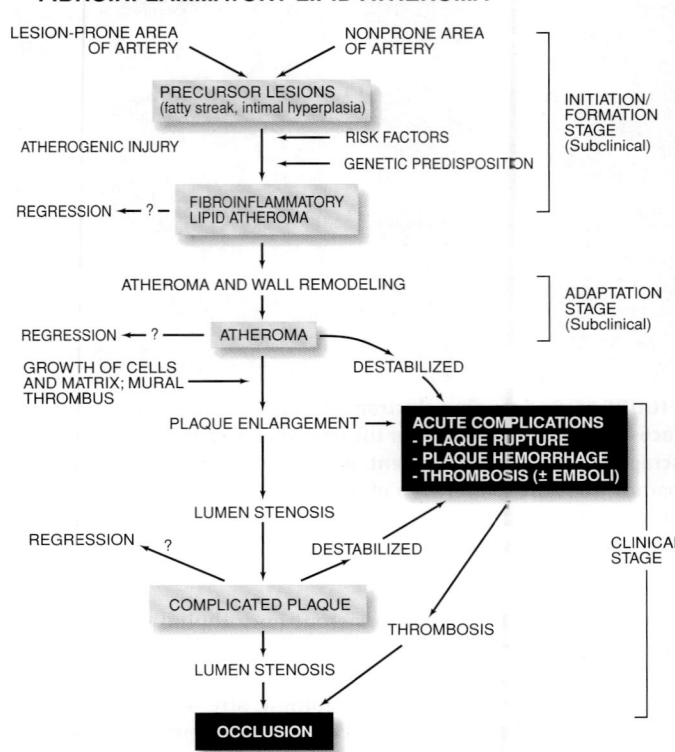

FIGURE 16-10. A unifying hypothesis for the pathogenesis of atherosclerosis.

(TF) are suppressed. Endothelial dysfunction may also reflect hemodynamic shear stress or may be constitutive, in association with vessel wall structure. Intimal lesions initially occur at structurally predisposed sites with intimal cell mass, bifurcations, branch points, and arterial curvatures, including where shear stresses are low but fluctuate rapidly. At such points, subendothelial smooth muscle cells accumulate in intimal cell masses, which predispose to plaque formation, especially in coronary arteries. Inflammatory cells, including macrophages and dendritic cells, arrive in the intima of these atherosclerosis-prone areas.

At such sites, expression of proinflammatory genes, **vascular cell adhesion molecule-1 (VCAM-1)** and **intercellular adhesion molecule-1 (ICAM-1),** by endothelial cells increases. These molecules recruit monocytes into vessel walls, as one of the early events in atherogenesis that is orchestrated through a multistep process involving adhesion and transmigration. Adhesion is regulated by cell surface adhesion molecules including P-selectin, E-selectin, VCAM-1, ICAM-1, and several chemokines. Transmigration involves **platelet endothelial cell adhesion molecule-1 (PECAM-1).**

The preference of atherosclerotic lesions for large vessels and particular vascular beds, as well as the fact that hypertension enhances the severity of atherosclerosis, all underscore the importance of hemodynamic factors. Hemodynamic forces induce expression of several factors in endothelial cells that are likely to promote atherosclerosis, for example,

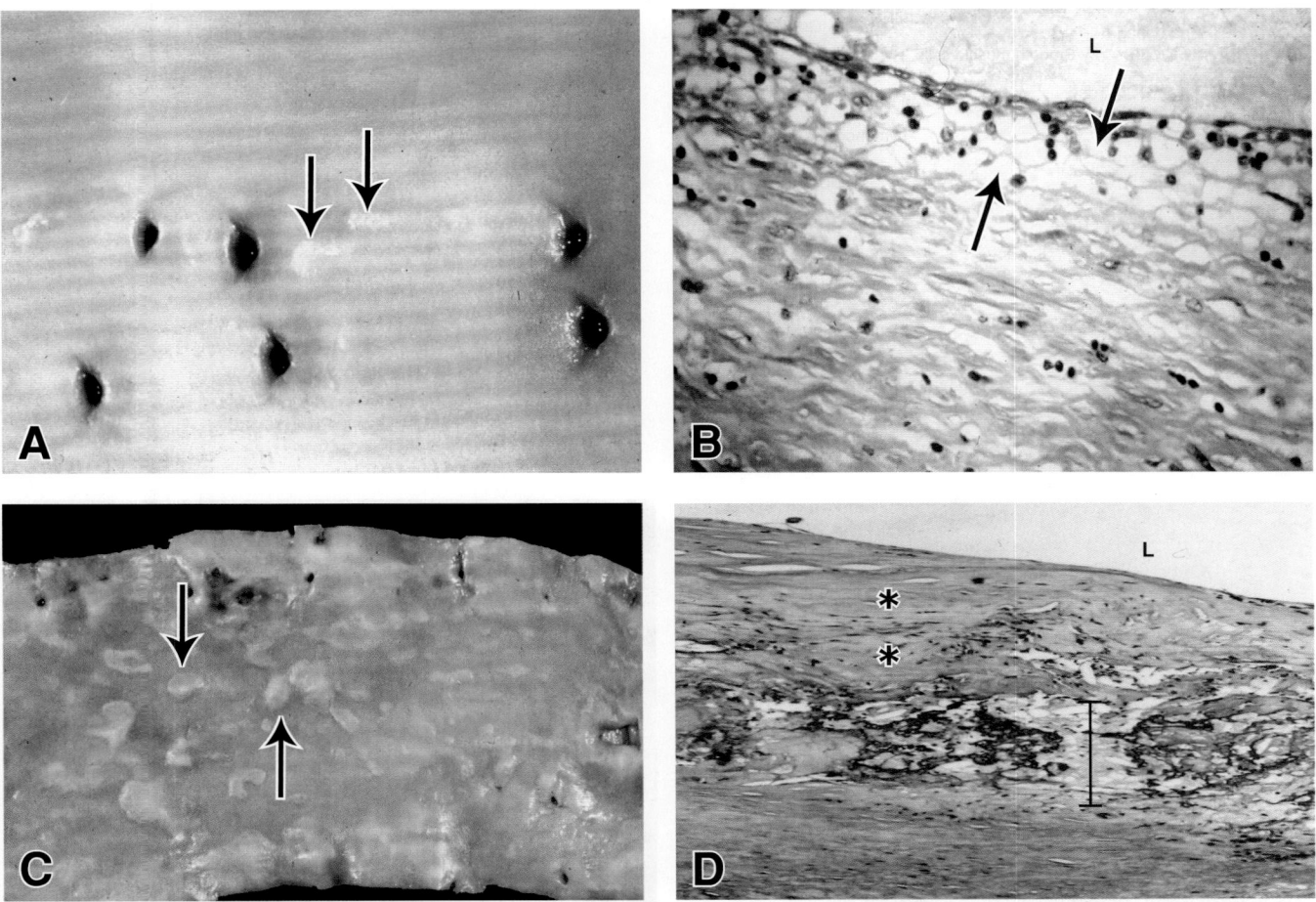

FIGURE 16-11. Fatty streak and atherosclerosis. A. Fatty streak. Gross photo of yellow fatty streaks (*arrows*) in the thoracic aorta. **B.** Fatty streak. Microscopic features of fatty streak in artery wall with intimal foam cells (*arrows*). *L* = lumen. **C.** Fibroinflammatory lipid plaques. Focal elevated plaques in thoracic aorta (*arrows*). **D.** Fibroinflammatory lipid plaques. Fibrous cap (*asterisks*) separating lumen (*L*) from central necrotic core (*bracket*).

FGF-2, TF, plasminogen activator, endothelin, and PECAM. However, shear stress also induces expression of genes that may be antiatherogenic, including NOS and PAI-1. In people at increased risk for atherosclerosis, lesions also occur in areas that are not usually affected.

2. Lipid accumulation requires disruption of the integrity of the endothelium, through gaps between cells, cell loss, or endothelial cell dysfunction. This injury may be due to high blood cholesterol or homocysteine, abnormal laminar flow, ROS, cytokine-induced inflammation, or advanced glycation end-products in diabetes. Hypertension also promotes endothelial dysfunction. Oxidative stress in endothelial cells and macrophages leads to cellular dysfunction and damage. LDLs carry lipids into the intima. Since oxidized LDL activates cell adhesion molecules, macrophages adhere to activated endothelial cells, then transmigrate between endothelial cells into the intima, bringing lipids with them. Some of these "foamy" macrophages die and release lipids. Alterations in types of matrix proteoglycans synthesized by intimal smooth muscle cells also predispose these sites to accumulate lipids by binding and trapping them in the intima. Reduced

egress of lipids out of the artery wall also promotes lipid accumulation.

3. Macrophages, in addition to bringing in fats, release growth factors that stimulate further accumulation of smooth muscle cells. Oxidized LDLs induce tissue damage and recruit macrophages. They also promote endothelial and smooth muscle cell release of chemokines, which regulate immune cell recruitment into the plaque. The NFκB pathway contributes to several stages of plaque growth and progression. It activates recruitment of leukocytes by endothelial cells, cytokine expression, and extracellular matrix remodeling. Monocytes/macrophages synthesize PDGF, FGF, TNF, IL-1, interferon (IFN)-α, and TGFβ, each of which can stimulate or inhibit growth of smooth muscle or endothelial cells. For example, IFN and TGF limit cell proliferation or inhibit growth-stimulatory peptides, which could explain how endothelial cells fail to maintain continuity over the lesion. IL-1 and TNF stimulate endothelial cells to produce PAF, TF, and PAI. Thus, macrophages and endothelial cells together may transform the normal anticoagulant vascular surface to a procoagulant one.

4. As a lesion progresses, mural thrombi often form on the damaged intimal surface. This stimulates PDGF

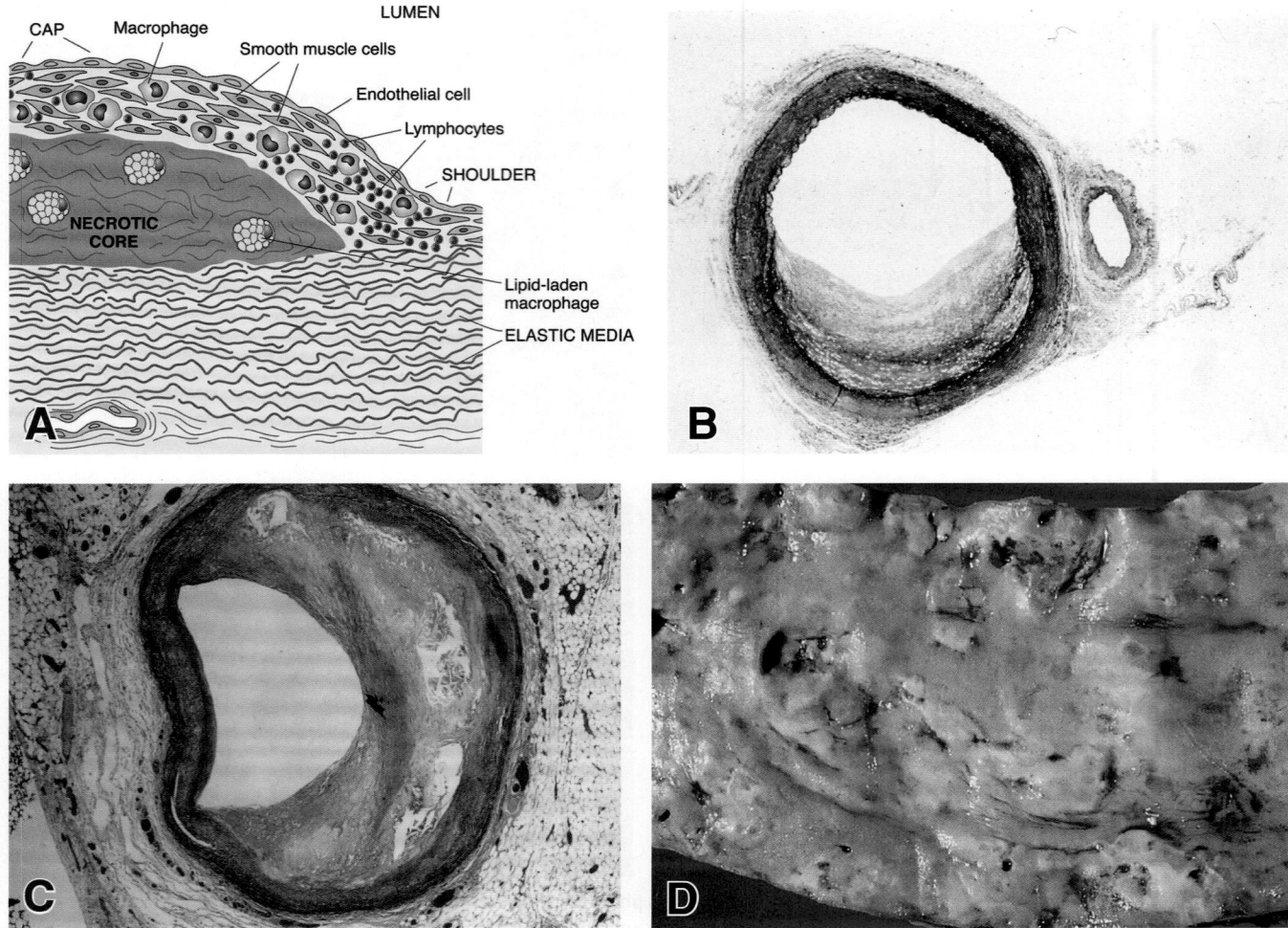

FIGURE 16-12. Fibrofatty plaque of atherosclerosis. A. In this fully developed fibrous plaque, the core contains lipid-filled macrophages and necrotic smooth muscle cell debris. The "fibrous" cap is composed largely of smooth muscle cells, which produce collagen, small amounts of elastin, and glycosaminoglycans. Also shown are infiltrating macrophages and lymphocytes. Note that the endothelium over the surface of the fibrous cap frequently appears intact. **B.** Adaptive stage with atherosclerotic plaque and vessel wall dilatation to maintain the normal size of the lumen. Normal artery wall is at the top. **C.** Stenotic coronary artery with atherosclerotic plaque. **D.** The aorta shows discrete, raised, tan plaques. Focal plaque ulcerations are also evident.

release, accelerating smooth muscle proliferation and secretion of matrix components. The thrombus may grow, lyse, or become organized and incorporated into the plaque.

5. The deeper parts of the now-thickened intima are poorly nourished because their increased distance limits diffusion. This tissue undergoes ischemic necrosis, which is augmented by proteolytic enzymes released by macrophages (i.e., cathepsins) and tissue damage caused by oxidized LDLs, ROS, and other agents, generating a central necrotic core. This necrotic core, together with platelet- and macrophage-derived angiogenic factors, stimulates angiogenesis, and new vasa vasorum form in the plaque.

6. The fibroinflammatory lipid plaque develops with a central necrotic core and a fibrous cap, which separates the core from the blood in the lumen. The core contains highly thrombogenic tissue debris, dead cells, necrotic foam cells, cholesterol crystals, and focal calcification. A fibrous cap contains contractile smooth muscle cells, which produce ECM, proteinases, and proteinase inhibitors, separating the thrombogenic necrotic plaque core from the vessel lumen. Cholesterol clefts stimulate more inflammation. Inflammatory and immune cells infiltrate, mingling with smooth muscle cells, deposited lipids and variably organized matrix. TGFβ regulates ECM deposition, stimulates deposition of several types of collagen, fibronectin, and proteoglycans, and limits matrix degradation by inhibiting proteolytic enzymes. TGFβ also has anti-inflammatory properties and promotes growth of smooth muscle cells. Its effects are context dependent, so that TGFβ may be both atherogenic and antiatherogenic.

7. The immune system participates in atherogenesis. Dendritic cells are present in early lesions, and T lymphocytes also increase in the plaque. HLA-DR antigen expression on endothelial and smooth muscle cells in plaques suggests that these cells have undergone immunologic activation, perhaps in response to IFN

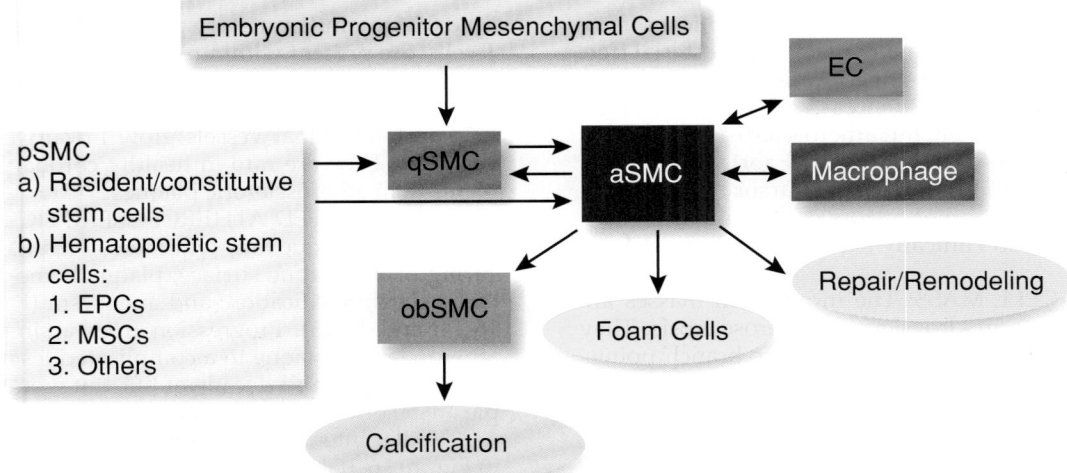

FIGURE 16-13. The hypothesized roles of smooth muscle cells (SMCs) in the pathogenesis of atherosclerosis. SMCs are quiescent (*qSMC*) in the normal artery wall and are derived embryonically from progenitor mesenchymal cells and neural crest cells. SMCs become activated (*aSMC*) by lipids and a variety of cytokines, chemokines, other mediators secreted by macrophages and endothelial cells through paracrine pathways in the lesion, and function in repair and remodeling of the lesion. aSMCs migrate, proliferate, and secrete prominent extracellular matrix, while qSMCs exhibit a differentiated and contractile phenotype. aSMCs can accumulate lipids and become foam cells in the lesion. aSMCs can also undergo a change in phenotype to show osteoblastic functions (*obSMC*) promoting calcification in the atherosclerotic lesion. Progenitor SMCs (*pSMCs*) such as resident stem cells, bone marrow–derived hematopoietic stem cells, endothelial progenitor cells (*EPCs*), and bone marrow–derived mesenchymal stem cells (*MSCs*) may replenish SMCs in the vasculature, especially during a response to injury. aSMCs interact with endothelial cells (*ECs*) and macrophages directly or indirectly to regulate atherosclerotic plaque growth.

released by activated T cells in the plaque. Thus, the presence of T cells in plaques reflects an autoimmune response (against, e.g., oxidized LDLs).

Adaptation Stage

As plaque protrudes into the lumen (e.g., in coronary arteries), the arterial wall remodels to maintain lumen size. However, when plaque occupies about half of the lumen, such remodeling can no longer compensate, and the arterial lumen narrows (stenosis). Hemodynamic shear stress, which regulates vessel wall remodeling, acts via the mechanotransduction properties of endothelial cells. These include the cell cytoskeleton, cell membrane ion channels, and the cell coat. Smooth muscle cell turnover, proliferation, apoptosis and matrix synthesis and degradation modulate remodeling of the vessel and the atherosclerotic plaque. MMPs and their inhibitors (TIMPs) are important in this process (see Chapter 3). Just as remodeling maintains vessel patency, it also allows a plaque to remain clinically silent. Even a small plaque at this stage can rupture, with catastrophic results, as noted below.

Clinical Stage

1. As a plaque grows into the lumen, fragile new vessels are formed within the plaque, and may bleed into it. The plaque may thus increase its size without rupture. Macrophages clean up resulting debris.
2. Complications—surface ulceration, calcification, and fissure or aneurysm formation—develop in the plaque. Activated mast cells at sites of erosion may release proinflammatory mediators and cytokines. Continued

plaque growth leads to severe stenosis or occludes the lumen.

3. Pressurized circulating blood may undermine and raise the plaque. Hemorrhage and thrombosis combine to obstruct the vessel. Plaque rupture, involving the fibrous cap, with ensuing thrombosis and occlusion, may precipitate catastrophic events in these advanced plaques (e.g., acute myocardial infarction). Even plaques causing less than 50% stenosis may suddenly rupture. There are several conditions that appear to favor rupture, as noted in Figure 16-10. These include hemodynamic shear stress, fissure formation, a thin fibrous cap, reduced number of smooth muscle cells, increased matrix metalloproteinase activity, inflammation, foam cell accumulation, and focal nodular calcification.

Figure 16-10 shows how these mechanisms may operate in atherogenesis.

Initial Lesions of Atherosclerosis

PATHOLOGY: Two distinct lesions precede atherosclerotic plaques.
FATTY STREAK: Fatty streaks are flat or slightly elevated lesions in the intima in which intra- and extracellular lipids accumulate. They are seen in young children as well as in adults. Cells filled with lipid droplets ("foam cells") congregate (Fig. 16-11). Macrophages contain the most lipid, but smooth muscle cells contain fat as well.

In children who die accidentally, significant fatty streaks may be evident in many parts of the arterial tree, but not necessarily in the same locations as atherosclerotic lesions in adults. Fatty streaks are common in the thoracic aorta in children, but atherosclerosis in adults is far more prominent in the abdominal aorta. Still, many believe that fatty infiltration is a precursor lesion of atherosclerosis and that other factors control the transition from fatty streak to clinically significant atherosclerotic plaque.

INTIMAL CELL MASS: The intimal cell masses are also candidate precursor lesions of atherosclerosis. They are white, thickened areas at arterial tree branch points, and contain smooth muscle cells and connective tissue but no lipid. Their situation at branch sites correlates well with locations of later atherosclerotic lesions.

CHARACTERISTIC LESIONS OF ATHEROSCLEROSIS: Atherosclerotic lesions are characteristically fibroinflammatory lipid plaques. Simple plaques are focal, elevated, pale yellow, smooth-surfaced lesions, irregularly shaped, but with well-defined borders. Fibrofatty plaques (Fig. 16-12) represent more-advanced lesions. They tend to be oval and up to 12 cm in diameter. In smaller vessels, such as coronary or cerebral arteries, plaques are often eccentric—occupying only part of the circumference of the lumen. In later stages, plaques in muscular arteries fuse to produce larger lesions, which occupy several square centimeters.

Atherosclerotic plaques are initially covered by endothelium and tend to involve the intima and very little of the upper media (Fig. 16-12B). The area between the lumen and the necrotic core—the fibrous cap—contains smooth muscle cells, macrophages, lymphocytes, lipid-laden cells (foam cells), and connective tissue components. The central core contains necrotic debris. Cholesterol crystals and foreign body giant cells may be present within the fibrous tissue and necrotic areas. Foam cells are both macrophages and smooth muscle cells that have taken up

lipids. Many inflammatory and immune cells, especially T cells, are present within plaques.

Neovascularization is an important contributor to plaque growth and its subsequent complications (Fig. 16-13). It is postulated that vessels grow inward from the vasa vasorum. They are rare in healthy coronary arteries but plentiful in atherosclerotic plaques.

COMPLICATED ATHEROSCLEROTIC PLAQUES: A complicated plaque may reflect erosion, ulceration, or fissuring of the plaque surface; plaque hemorrhage; mural thrombosis; calcification; and aneurysm (Figs. 16-12C,D; 16-14; and 16-15). Progression from a simple fibrofatty atherosclerotic plaque to a complicated lesion may occur as early as the third decade of life, but most affected people are 50 or 60 years old.

Cellular interactions in atherogenesis are summarized in Figure 16-16.

- Calcification involving osteochondrocytic differentiation occurs in areas of necrosis and elsewhere in the plaque. Oxidized lipids and inflammatory cytokines promote vascular calcification. Arterial calcification thought to depend on mineral deposition and resorption, which are regulated by osteoblast-like and osteoclast-like cells in the vessel wall. These cells are considered to be rare precursor cells in the artery wall, derived from smooth muscle-type cells that have transformed phenotypically, or possibly bone marrow–derived circulating stem/precursor cells. Several transcription factors, as well as oxidized LDL (Ox-LDL), promote cell osteoblast development. Calcification may also reflect changes in physical–chemical properties of a diseased vessel wall that provoke formation of hydroxyapatite crystals.
- Where the plaque protrudes into the lumen, it creates turbulence, reduced luminal flow, or stasis, leading to mural thrombosis. The flow disturbances also damage the endothelial lining, which may become dysfunctional or locally denuded, and so no longer presents a

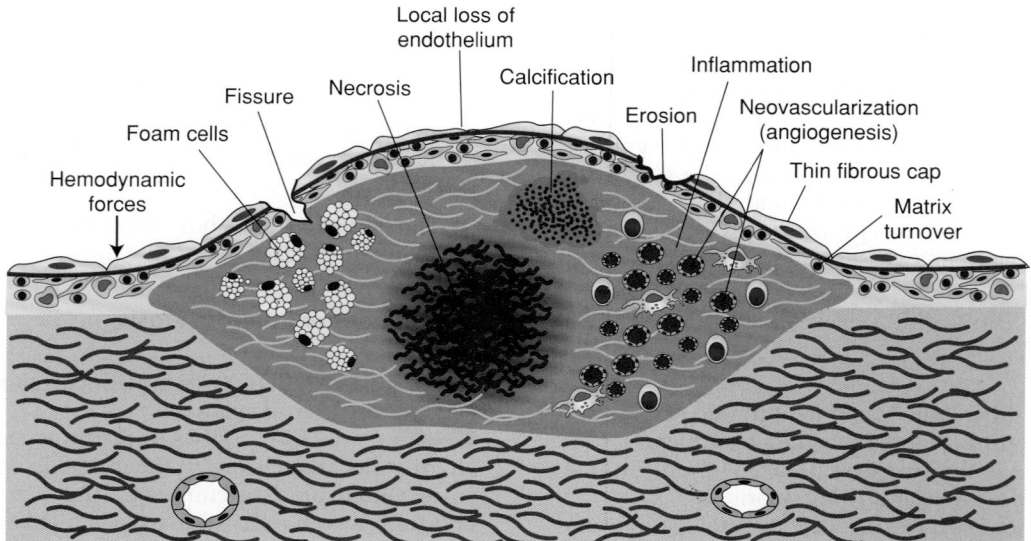

FIGURE 16-14. Complicated atherosclerotic plaque. The surface shows endothelial denudation, erosion, and fissure formation. The plaque shows a thin fibrous cap, a central necrotic core, inflammation, lipids, calcification, and neovascularization.

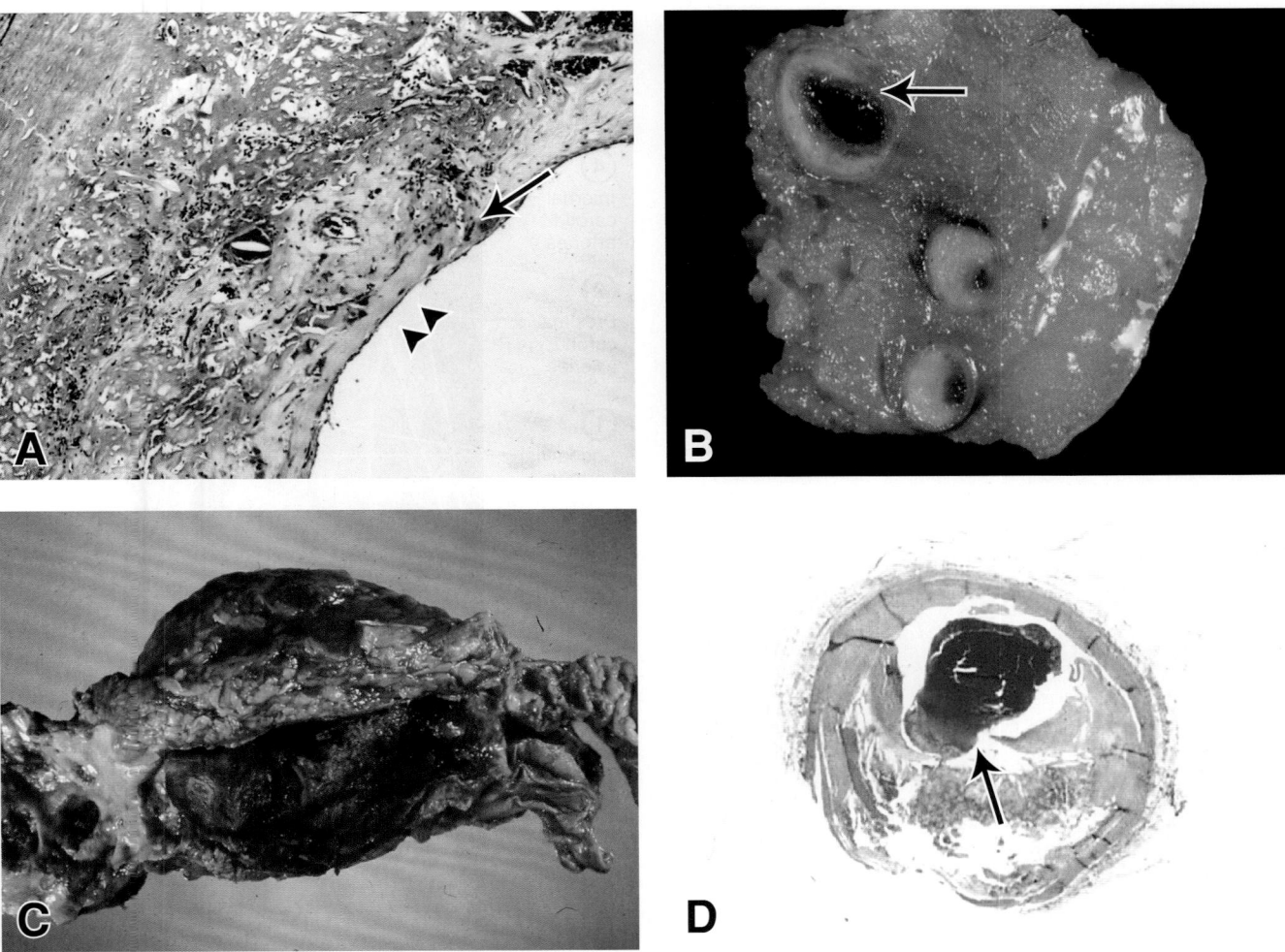

FIGURE 16-15. Complications of atherosclerosis. A. Fibroinflammatory lipid plaque. Microscopic features of plaque erosion (*arrowheads*) and fissure formation (*arrow*). **B. Fibroinflammatory lipid plaque** with occlusive luminal thrombosis (*arrow*). **C. Abdominal aortic aneurysm with thrombus. D.** Rupture of fibrous cap and occlusive luminal thrombosis (*arrow*) in atherosclerotic coronary artery.

thromboresistant surface. Thrombi often form at sites of erosion and fissuring on the surface of the fibrous cap. Mural thrombi in the proximal region of a coronary artery may embolize to more distal sites in the vessel. At this point, the atheromatous plaque has developed destabilizing structural and functional alterations.

- Atheroma destabilization may occur whenever the dynamic balance of opposing biologic and physical processes is disrupted. Plaque hemorrhage due to rupture of thin, newly formed vessels may occur within a plaque, with or without a subsequent rupture of the fibrous cap. In a ruptured plaque, the necrotic material that comes in contact with blood contains TF and is highly thrombogenic. This leads to mural thrombosis, fibrous cap rupture, or more intraplaque hemorrhage. Adjacent endothelium has reduced inhibitor (TFPI) levels and lower antiplatelet and fibrinolytic activities, all favoring coagulation. Exposed thrombogenic material promotes clot formation in the lumen, causing an occlusive thrombus, and hemorrhage may expand the plaque and further narrow the lumen.

- Elevated circulating markers of inflammation, like C-reactive protein (CRP), fibrinogen, soluble VCAM, IL-1, IL-6, and TNF, suggest that procoagulant inflammatory mediators may also participate, and increase plaque burden.
- The hemorrhage will be resorbed over time within the plaque, leaving telltale residual hemosiderin-laden macrophages.

Most plaques that rupture show less than 50% luminal stenosis, and over 95% are less than 70% stenosed. Plaque rupture often occurs at the shoulder of the plaque, suggesting that hemodynamic shear stress weakens and tears the fibrous cap. If not repaired, endothelial loss leads to plaque erosion, weakening the fibrous cap and exposing the plaque to blood constituents. Plaque rupture has been associated with (1) areas of inflammation, (2) large lipid core size, (3) thin fibrous cap, (4) decreased smooth muscle cells owing to apoptosis, (5) imbalance of proteolytic enzymes and their inhibitors in the fibrous cap, (6) calcification in the plaque, and (7) intraplaque hemorrhage, leading to inside-out rupture of the fibrous cap.

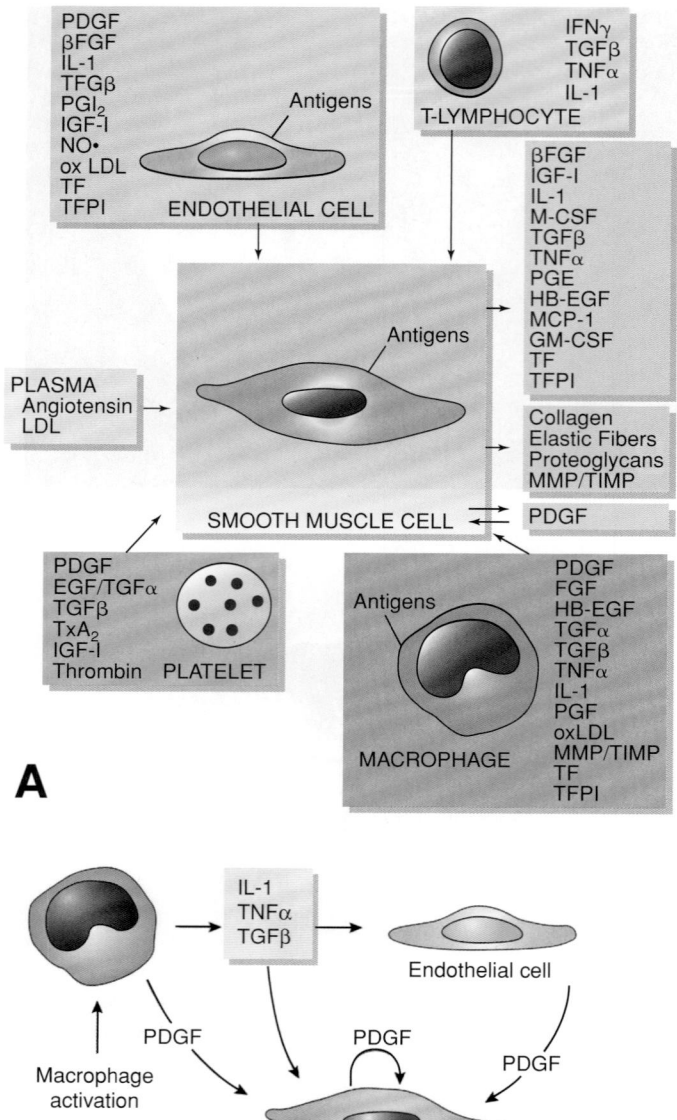

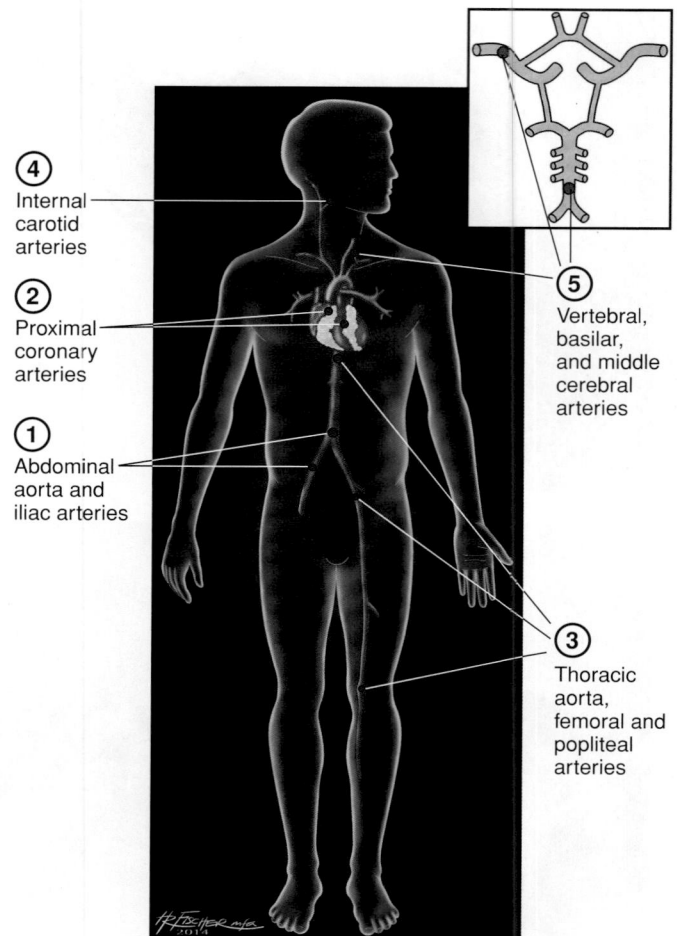

FIGURE 16-17. Sites of severe atherosclerosis in order of frequency.

■ **Acute occlusion:** Thrombosis on an atherosclerotic plaque may abruptly occlude a muscular artery (Fig. 16-18). The result is ischemic necrosis (infarction) of the tissue supplied by that vessel, manifested clinically as myocardial infarction, stroke, or gangrene of the intestine or lower

FIGURE 16-16. Cellular interactions in the progression of the athero-sclerotic plaque. A. Endothelium, platelets, macrophages, T lymphocytes, and smooth muscle cells elaborate a variety of cytokines, growth factors, and other substances. The scheme illustrated here emphasizes their influence on smooth muscle cells. **B.** The cellular interactions that promote the proliferation of smooth cells. *EGF* = endothelial growth factor; *FGF* = fibroblast growth factor; *HB-EGF* = heparin-binding epidermal growth factor; *IFN* = interferon; *IGF-I* = insulin-like growth factor I; *IL* = interleukin; *MCP-1* = monocyte chemotactic protein-1; *M-CSF* = macrophage colony-stimulating factor; *MMP* = matrix metalloproteinase; *NO•* = nitric oxide; *oxLDL* = oxidated low-density lipoprotein; *PDGF* = platelet-derived growth factor; *PGE* = prostaglandin; PGI_2 = prostacyclin; *TF* = tissue factor; *TGF* = tumor growth factor; *TFPI* = tissue factor pathway inhibitor; *TNF* = tumor necrosis factor; *TIMP* = inhibitors of MMPs; TxA_2 = thromboxane A_2.

Complications of Atherosclerosis

The complications of atherosclerosis depend on the location and size of the affected vessel (Fig. 16-17) and the chronicity of the process.

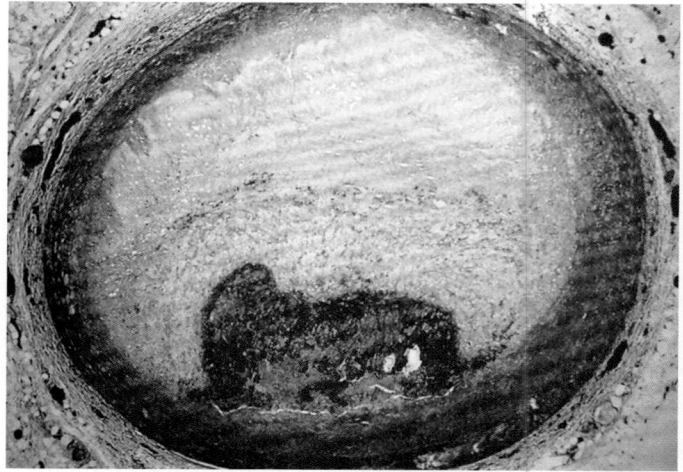

FIGURE 16-18. Coronary artery thrombosis. A microscopic section of a coronary artery shows severe atherosclerosis and a recent thrombus in the narrowed lumen.

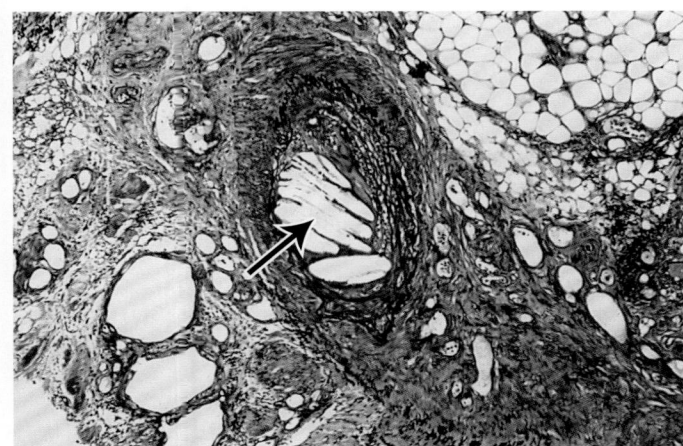

FIGURE 16-19. Cholesterol crystal embolus. Needle-shaped clefts (*arrow*) are seen in an atherosclerotic embolus that has occluded a small artery.

extremities. Some occlusive thrombi can be dissolved therapeutically by enzymes that activate plasma fibrinolysis, including streptokinase and tissue plasminogen activator.

- **Chronic narrowing of a vessel lumen:** As an atherosclerotic plaque grows, it may narrow the lumen, progressively reducing blood flow to tissue served by that artery. Chronic ischemia of the affected tissue causes atrophy of the organ, for example, unilateral renal artery stenosis causing renal atrophy, mesenteric artery atherosclerosis producing intestinal stricture, or cutaneous atrophy in a diabetic with severe peripheral vascular disease.
- **Aneurysm formation:** Complicated atherosclerotic lesions may extend into the media of elastic arteries and weaken their walls, so as to allow aneurysm formation, typically in the abdominal aorta. Reduced elastin causes the wall to thin and balloon outward. Simultaneously, MMPs secreted by smooth muscle cells and macrophages break down collagen. Such aneurysms often contain thrombi, which may embolize. Or, they may rupture catastrophically, especially in the aorta and cerebrum.
- **Embolism:** A thrombus formed over an atherosclerotic plaque may detach and lodge in a distal vessel. Thus, embolization from a thrombus in an abdominal aortic aneurysm (AAA) may acutely occlude the popliteal artery, causing gangrene of the leg.
- **A plaque may ulcerate,** dislodging atheromatous debris that embolizes to produce so-called cholesterol crystal emboli. These appear as needle-shaped spaces in affected tissues (Fig. 16-19), most often the kidney.

Restenosis May Complicate Repair of Stenotic Vessels

Percutaneous transluminal coronary angioplasty (PTCA) is an important treatment for stenotic atherosclerotic vascular disease, especially for the epicardial coronary arteries. Using a catheter to insert and then dilate a balloon catheter, a stenotic portion of the artery can be reopened. However, the balloon causes endothelial damage and tears in the plaque and the media. In 30% to 40% of cases with successful dilatation, the artery restenoses within 3 to 6 months.

Intimal hyperplasia due to smooth muscle cell proliferation and matrix deposition leads to restenosis. An organized mural thrombus on the luminal surface may or may not be involved. Vascular wall remodeling, induced in part by trauma to the vessel wall and involving the adventitia, may contract the vessel wall and narrow the lumen.

Stenting

A stent, a tubular scaffold device deployed via catheter, keeps the diseased atherosclerotic artery open. Stents are now coated with biocompatible polymers and biologically active agents, greatly reducing restenosis. For example, drug-eluting stents with antiproliferative agents block cell cycle progression and thus inhibit overgrowth of smooth muscle cells in the vessel wall. Although long-term complications are not fully known, especially as they relate to thrombosis, drug-eluting stents are used extensively.

Coronary Artery Bypasses

Transplanted saphenous vein autografts used in coronary artery bypass operations undergo adaptive and reparative changes. These include (1) intimal thickening associated with phlebosclerosis, (2) occasional medial calcification, (3) focal muscle cell hypertrophy, and, eventually, (4) adventitial scarring. Venous grafts in place for a few years develop atherosclerotic plaques indistinguishable from those in native coronary arteries (Fig. 16-20). Half of such bypass grafts occlude within 5 to 10 years from neointimal hyperplasia and atherosclerosis.

Many Factors Increase Risk for Atherosclerosis

 CLINICAL FEATURES: Factors associated that increase risk of ischemic heart disease by twofold or more include:

- **Hypertension:** High blood pressure increases the risk of myocardial infarction. Both diastolic and systolic hypertension contributes equally to this increased risk. Men with systolic blood pressures over 160 mm Hg have almost triple the incidence of myocardial infarction compared to those with systolic pressures under 120 mm Hg. Use of antihypertensive drugs has significantly reduced myocardial infarction and stroke.
- **Blood cholesterol:** Serum cholesterol levels correlate with development of ischemic heart disease and account for much of the geographic variation in its incidence. Absent of the presence of genetic disorders of lipid metabolism (see below), blood cholesterol correlates strongly with dietary intake of saturated fat. Cholesterol-lowering drugs lower the risk of myocardial infarction. Total serum cholesterol does not necessarily predict risk of ischemic heart disease, since cholesterol is transported by atherogenic and antiatherogenic lipoproteins. Thus, therapeutic decisions are mainly based on LDL cholesterol levels.
- **Cigarette smoking:** Coronary and aortic atheroscleroses are more severe and extensive in cigarette smokers than in nonsmokers, and the effect is dose related (see Chapter 8). Thus, smoking markedly increases the risk of myocardial infarction, ischemic stroke, and abdominal aortic aneurysms.

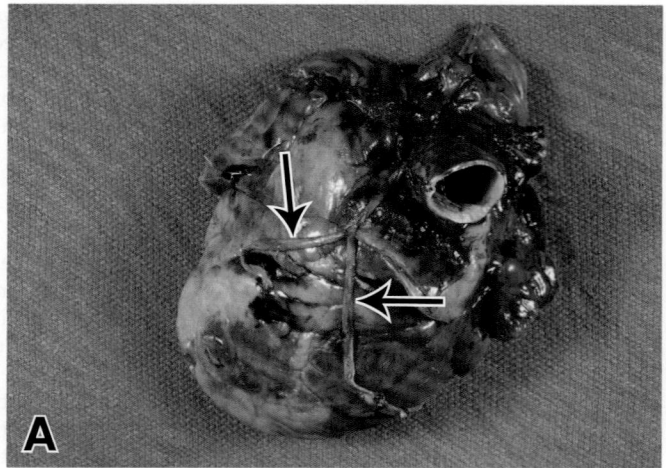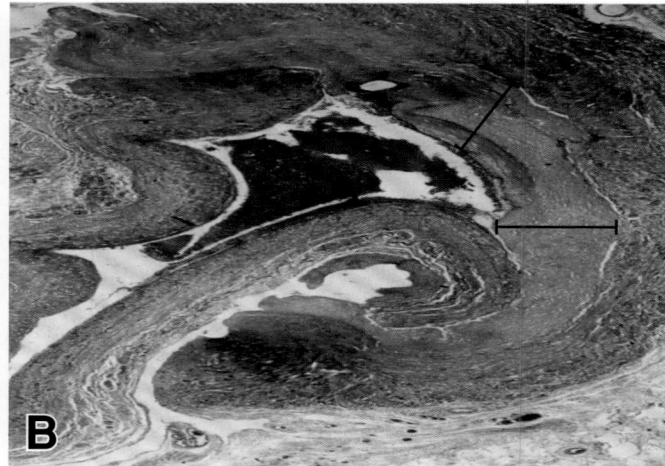

FIGURE 16-20. Saphenous vein aortocoronary bypass. A. Saphenous vein aortocoronary bypass on the surface of the heart (epicardium) (*arrows*). **B.** Distal anastomosis site with atherosclerotic coronary artery (*brackets*).

- **Diabetes:** Diabetics are at increased risk for occlusive atherosclerotic vascular disease in many organs. However, the relative contributions of carbohydrate intolerance alone, as opposed to the hypertension and hyperlipidemias common in diabetics, are not well defined (see Chapter 13).
- **Increasing age** and **male sex:** Both correlate strongly with the risk of myocardial infarction, but probably as reflections of accumulated effects of other risk factors.
- **Physical inactivity** and **stressful life patterns:** These factors correlate with increased risk of ischemic heart disease, but their role in atherosclerogenesis is not clear.
- **Obesity:** Obesity is a risk factor for atherosclerotic coronary artery disease, hypertension, and type II diabetes, and so increases risk in several ways.
- **Homocysteine:** Homocystinuria, a rare autosomal recessive disease caused by mutations in the gene encoding cystathionine synthase, causes premature and severe atherosclerosis. Mildly elevated plasma homocysteine in people without homocystinuria are common, and are an independent risk factor for coronary and other atherosclerosis. The increased risk is comparable to smoking and hyperlipidemia. Homocysteine is toxic to endothelial cells. It also impairs their anticoagulant mechanisms by inhibiting thrombomodulin at endothelial cell surfaces, antithrombin III–binding activity of heparan sulfate proteoglycan, binding of tissue plasminogen activator, and ecto-ADPase activity on endothelial cell surfaces. The latter promotes platelet aggregation. Oxidative interactions between homocysteine, lipoproteins, and cholesterol further complicate the situation. Low dietary folate may aggravate genetic predisposition to hyperhomocysteinemia, but whether folic acid treatment protects from atherosclerosis is unknown.
- **C-reactive protein** (**CRP**): CRP is an acute phase reactant mainly made by hepatocytes. It is a serum marker for systemic inflammation and has been linked to increased risk of myocardial infarction and ischemic stroke. This fact, together with the presence of CRP in atherosclerotic plaques, suggests that systemic inflammation may contribute to atherogenesis.

- **Lipoproteins:** Elevated Lp(a) increases risk for myocardial infarction and ischemic heart disease. An Lp(a) component (apolipoprotein[a]) stimulates inflammation and lipid peroxidation. Lp(a) also increases cholesterol deposition and smooth muscle proliferation in injured vessels, and suppresses thrombolysis. Pharmacologic PCSK9 inhibition aims to decrease Lp(a).
- **Metabolic syndrome:** People with metabolic syndrome (see Chapter 13) have greater risk for cardiovascular disease. They have elevated triglycerides, reduced HDL-C, hypertension, and elevated blood glucose and waist circumference.

Infection and Atherosclerosis

Some infectious agents may stimulate atherosclerosis. *Chlamydia pneumoniae* and cytomegalovirus have been studied most, but *Helicobacter pylori*, herpesvirus, and others may also contribute. Some atheromas may contain DNA from these agents, but the nature of this association is obscure.

Lipid Metabolism

We have learned a lot since Rudolf Virchow first identified cholesterol crystals in atherosclerotic lesions. Lipoprotein particles transport cholesterol and other lipids (mainly triglycerides) (Table 16-6; Fig. 16-21). These particles differ in protein and lipid composition, size, and density, and are categorized by density:

- Chylomicrons
- Very–low-density lipoproteins (VLDLs)
- Intermediate-density lipoproteins (IDLs)
- Low-density lipoproteins (LDLs)
- High-density lipoproteins (HDLs)

Apolipoproteins are amphipathic structural proteins in outer membranes of lipoproteins, which regulate (up/down) receptor-mediated endocytosis and plasma enzymes that metabolize lipids. **B apolipoproteins** (apoB100, apoB48) accompany the particles from synthesis to breakdown, while other apolipoproteins may be exchanged among lipoproteins.

TABLE 16-6

LIPOPROTEINS

Features			Composition (%)				Apolipoproteins	
Lipoprotein Class	Density (g/mL)	Particle Diameter (nm)	Prot	Chol	PL	TG and CE	Non-Ex	Ex
Chylomicron	<0.950	80–1,200	<2	1–3	6–12	80–90*	B48	A, C, E
VLDL	0.950–1.006	30–80	4–10	22	18	45–60	B100	C
IDL	1.006–1.019	25–50	15	29	22	30–35	B100	C, E
LDL	1.019–1.063	18–28	25	50	21	8–10	B100	
HDL	>1.063	5–15	33	30	29	4–8	A	C, E

Functions	
Lipoprotein	Key Function
Chylomicron	Transport of dietary TG
VLDL	Transport of endogenous lipids
IDL	Transport of endogenous lipids
LDL	Transport of endogenous cholesterol
HDL	Reverse cholesterol transport, exchange of apolipoproteins

VLDL = very–low-density lipoproteins; IDL = intermediate-density lipoproteins; LDL = low-density lipoproteins; HDL = high-density lipoproteins; Prot = protein; Chol = cholesterol; PL = phospholipid; TG = triglyceride (triacylglycerol); CE = cholesteryl ester; Ex = exchangeable; * = mostly TG.

The liver is central to regulating cholesterol distribution (Fig. 16-22). Lipoproteins made there and in the small intestine deliver cholesterol and free fatty acids (FFAs) to tissues. Cholesterol is a key component of membranes, steroids, and vitamin D. HDLs transport cholesterol from tissues back to the liver (reverse transport). The liver controls circulating lipid levels by removing lipoproteins from the blood by endocytosis, via apolipoprotein-binding receptors LDL receptor (LDLR) and a related protein (LRP1). Bile made in the liver (see Chapter 20) mediates lipid absorption from the gut.

MOLECULAR PATHOGENESIS: EXOGENOUS PATHWAY: Chylomicrons produced by small intestinal epithelium contain apoB48, and transport lipid from intestine to liver. ApoB48 is produced by the action of an mRNA editing enzyme, **APOBEC**. Chylomicrons are absorbed into gut lymphatics, and enter the blood, where **lipoprotein lipase (LPL)** on the capillary endothelial cell surface hydrolyzes them to FFAs. Inactivating mutations of (GP1HBP1) prevent transport of LPL made by adipocytes and muscle cells to the surface of endothelial cells, and thus cause severe hypertriglyceridemia. Once triglycerides are hydrolyzed and FFAs removed, the liver endocytoses the remnant particles.

ENDOGENOUS PATHWAY: Hepatocytes make and secrete VLDL particles, which acquire apoCII and apoE in the blood and are first converted to IDLs, then, by plasma hepatic lipase, to LDLs. Inactive hepatic lipase is released

and activated by HDL. Hepatocytes take up and catabolize IDL and LDL (Fig. 16-23).

Endothelial cells facilitate LDL entry into tissues by transcytosing it from the plasma to tissue fluid, where tissue cells take it up via LDLR. Interaction of LDL with its receptor initiates receptor-mediated endocytosis, leading to catabolism of LDL. Arterial endothelial cells transcytose IDL and LDL into the intima, where they bind ECM molecules, leading to oxidative and other lipoprotein modifications. Elevated plasma LDL magnifies this process.

REVERSE CHOLESTEROL TRANSPORT: HDLs made by the liver and intestinal cells contain apoAI and apoAII. These include direct HDL secretion by intestine and liver, and transfer of lipid and apolipoprotein constituents released during lipolysis of apoB-containing lipoproteins. HDLs: (1) are reservoirs for apolipoproteins, mainly apoCII and apoE, and (2) transport extrahepatic cholesterol, including that in arterial walls, to the liver for elimination (reverse cholesterol transport). Low HDL states may occur with diets high in polyunsaturated fats or low in fats, truncal obesity, diabetes, smoking, and excess androgens. Vigorous exercise, moderate alcohol consumption, and estrogens increase HDL.

In tissues, cholesterol removed from cells is principally free cholesterol, which is rapidly esterified by **lecithin cholesterol acyl transferase (LCAT)** to **cholesteryl esters**. The latter are transferred to the cores of lipoprotein particles or are exchanged to VLDL and LDL. Specific transfer proteins (e.g., cholesterol ester transfer protein

A

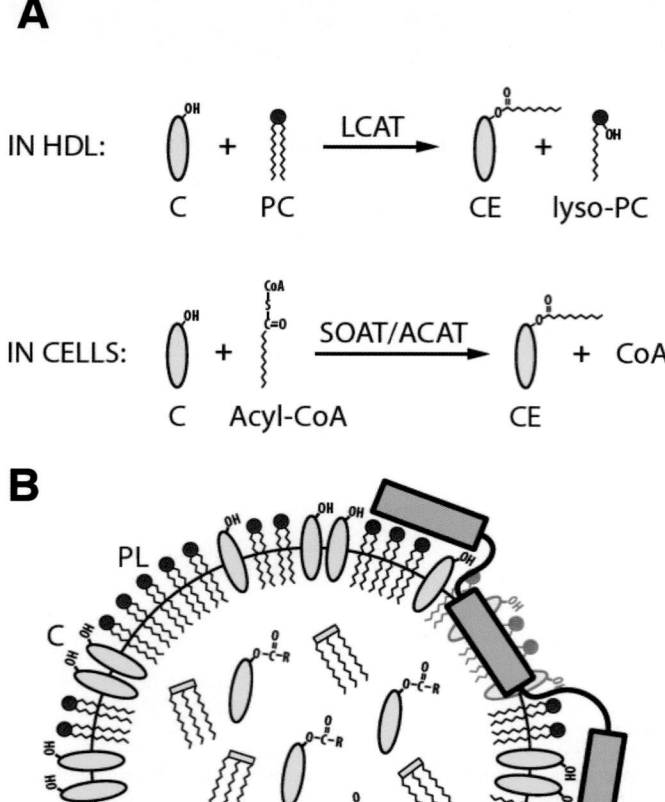

B

FIGURE 16-21. Cholesterol, cholesterol esters and lipoproteins. A. Conversion of cholesterol (*C*) to cholesterol ester (*CE*) in HDL and cells. *PC* = phosphatidylcholine; *CoA* = coenzyme A; *LCAT* = lecithin cholesterol acyl transferase; *SOAT* = Sterol O-acyltransferase; *ACAT* = Acyl-CoA cholesterol acyltransferase. **B.** Schematic of a lipoprotein particle, with a phospholipid (*PL*) membrane that contains *C* and apolipoproteins, and a core of neutral lipids, predominately *CE* and triglycerides (*TG*).

[CETP]) mediate these transfers. Defective cholesteryl ester transfer and exchange lead to dyslipoproteinemia, increased intracellular cholesteryl esters, and accelerated atherosclerosis.

CHOLESTEROL HOMEOSTASIS: Cells bind LDL apoB100 via LDLR, internalize LDLs, then recycle LDLR to their surfaces. The LDL particle moves to lysosomes, which hydrolyze cholesteryl esters to release cholesterol (Fig. 16-23). Hepatocytes secrete proprotein convertase subtilisin kexin type 9 (PCSK9) into the blood, where it has two functions that raise LDL: it binds LDLR and causes its degradation; and it binds LDL and prevents LDLR-mediated endocytosis.

Cholesterol levels also reflect de novo synthesis, which is regulated by ER enzymes. Its biosynthesis is complex, and starts with acetyl-CoA, which is modified by

the enzyme HMG-CoA synthase. The modified product (hydroxymethylglutaryl-CoA, or HMG-CoA), is then reduced by the rate-limiting enzyme, HMG-CoA reductase (HMGCR). High ER cholesterol levels lead to HMGCR polyubiquitination and degradation (Fig. 16-24A). In addition, production of these enzymes is highly regulated by sterol response regulatory elements (SRE, Fig. 16-24B).

Familial Hypercholesterolemias (FHs)

Familial clustering of ischemic heart diseases is well documented (Table 16-7).

MOLECULAR PATHOGENESIS: Hepatocytes clear LDL exclusively via LDLR, and mutations in this gene cause familial hypercholesterolemia (FH), inherited as an autosomal dominant disease. About 1 in 500 people are heterozygotes and 1 in a million are homozygotes (see Chapter 6). More than 400 mutant alleles are known, including point mutations, insertions, and deletions.

Mutations in other genes may also cause hypercholesterolemia. Thus, mutations in apoB100 may decrease LDL binding to LDLR. Gain of function mutations in PCSK9 (see above) may alter LDLR availability for binding, and impede LDL binding to remaining LDLR. Mutations in genes for apoE proteins may alter clearance of chylomicron remnants and IDLs. Hypertriglyceridemia may result from deficiencies in apoAI. Lipoprotein(a) (Lp[a]) enhances cholesterol delivery to injured blood vessels, suppresses plasmin, and promotes smooth muscle proliferation. Inherited predispositions to high blood Lp(a) levels increase risk of coronary and cerebral artery atherosclerosis.

CLINICAL FEATURES: Most untreated homozygotes have 6- to 10-fold higher plasma LDL than normal, and die from coronary artery disease before they reach 20. Among people under 60 who have had myocardial infarction, 5% are heterozygous for familial hypercholesterolemia. Their plasma LDL levels are twice normal, and they tend to suffer myocardial infarction earlier than usual, but later than do homozygotes (40 to 45 years old in men). In addition to premature atherosclerosis, LDL cholesterol also deposits in skin and tendons to form xanthomas (Fig. 16-25). In some cases (before age 10 in homozygotes), an arcus lipoides is present in the cornea.

HYPERTENSIVE VASCULAR DISEASE

Blood pressure fluctuates over the course of the day, in response to exercise, emotion, sleep, etc. Average systolic blood pressure increases with age, as arteries become stiffer. Recent guidelines define hypertension as sustained ambulatory systolic blood pressure ≥ 130 mm Hg. It may be asymptomatic, but therapies should be initiated in order to minimize complications (Fig. 16-26).

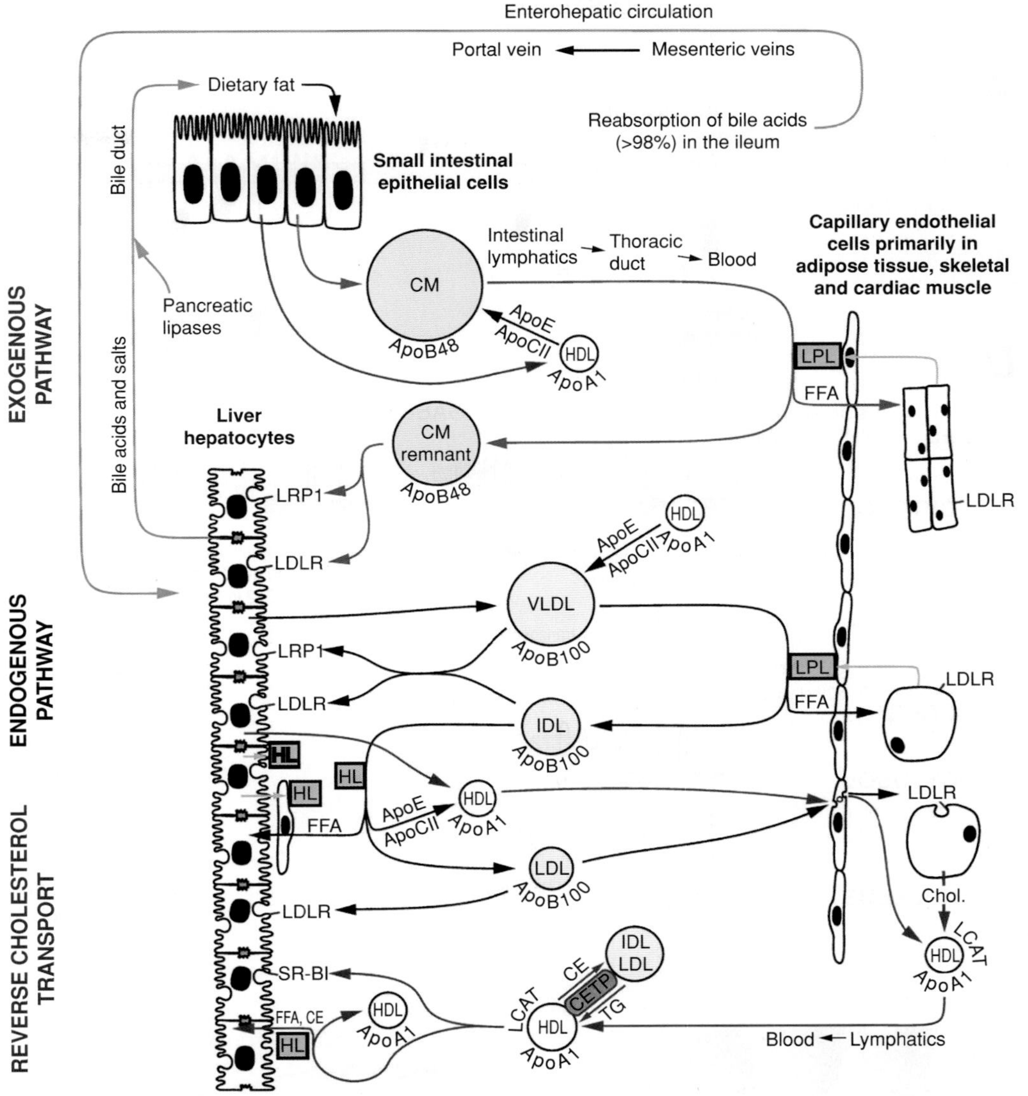

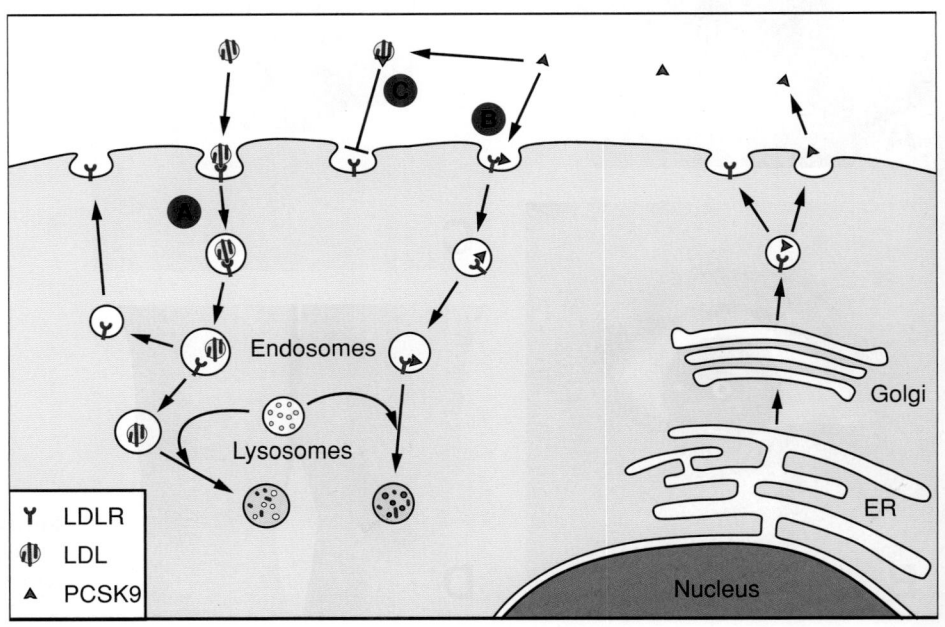

FIGURE 16-22. Cholesterol distribution pathways.

FIGURE 16-23. Effects of PCSK9 on LDL endocytosis in hepatocytes through binding to LDLR. A. Endocytosis of LDL in the absence of PCSK9 leads to recycling of LDLR. **B.** Binding of PCSK9 to LDLR leads to endocytosis and degradation of the receptor. **C.** Binding of PCSK9 to apoB100 inhibits LDL binding to LDLR.

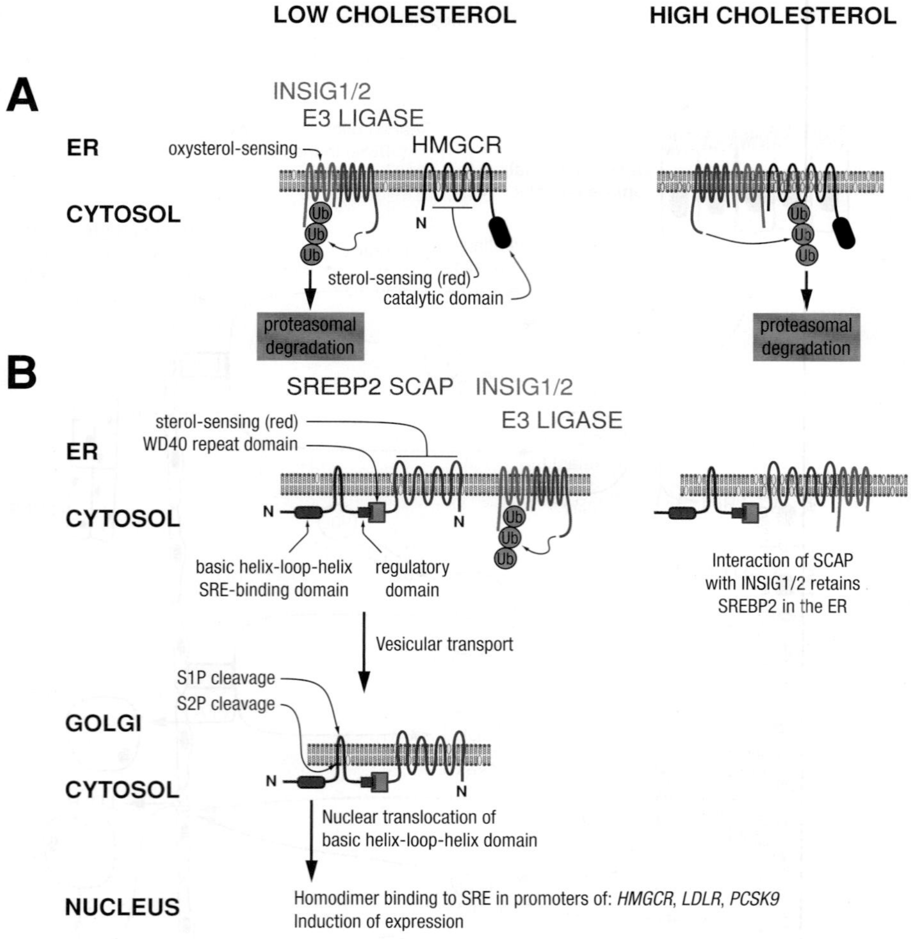

LOW CHOLESTEROL   HIGH CHOLESTEROL

A

INSIG1/2
E3 LIGASE

ER   oxysterol-sensing   HMGCR

CYTOSOL

Ub
Ub
Ub

sterol-sensing (red)
catalytic domain

N

proteasomal
degradation

proteasomal
degradation

B

SREBP2 SCAP   INSIG1/2
E3 LIGASE

sterol-sensing (red)
WD40 repeat domain

ER

CYTOSOL

N   N

basic helix-loop-helix   regulatory
SRE-binding domain   domain

Ub
Ub
Ub

Interaction of SCAP
with INSIG1/2 retains
SREBP2 in the ER

Vesicular transport

S1P cleavage
S2P cleavage

GOLGI

CYTOSOL

N   N

Nuclear translocation of
basic helix-loop-helix domain

NUCLEUS

Homodimer binding to SRE in promoters of: *HMGCR, LDLR, PCSK9*
Induction of expression

FIGURE 16-24. Regulation of cell cholesterol homeostasis. A. High-cholesterol levels in the endoplasmic reticulum (*ER*) membrane leads to polyubiquitination and degradation of HMGCR, resulting in a reduction in cholesterol biosynthesis. *Ub* = ubiquitin. **B.** *SREBP2* regulates the transcription of genes involved in cholesterol metabolism.

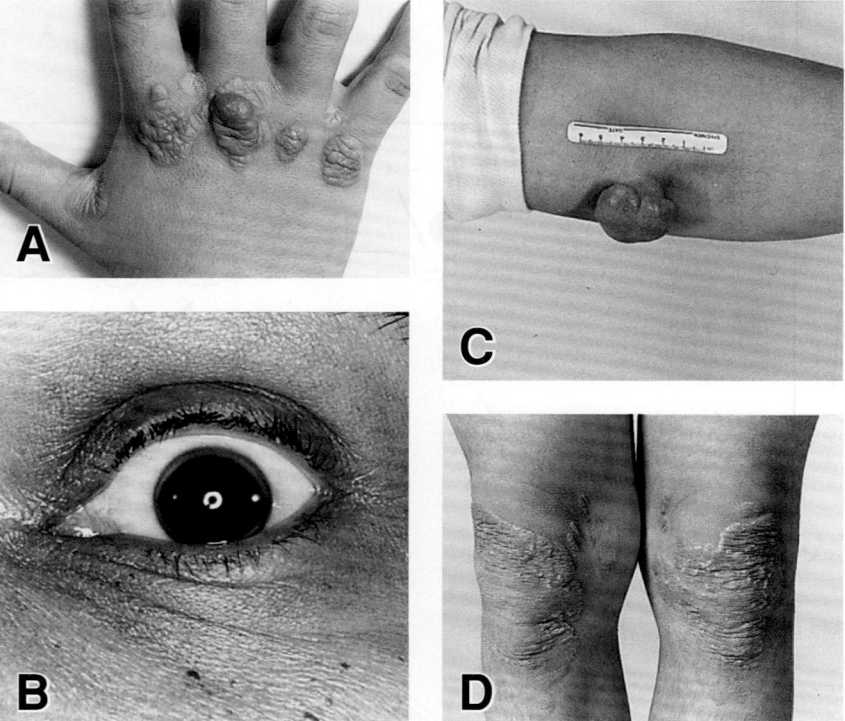

FIGURE 16-25. Xanthomas in familial hypercholesterolemia. A. Dorsum of the hand. **B.** Arcus lipoides represents the deposition of lipids in the peripheral cornea. **C.** Extensor surface of the elbow. **D.** Knees.

TABLE 16-7

MOLECULAR DEFECTS IN DYSLIPOPROTEINEMIAS

Defect/Condition	Gene Mutation(s)	Clinical Features
Abetalipoproteinemia (absence of VLDL and chylomicrons)		
Defective lipid-loading of apoB48 and apoB100 by microsomal triglyceride transfer protein (MTTP)	*MTTP* (4q23)	Malabsorption of lipids and fat-soluble vitamins; ataxia; hemolytic anemia; visual defects; reduced incidence of atherosclerosis
ApoB48 and apoB100 deficiency	*ApoB* (2p24.1)	
Familial α-lipoprotein deficiency (low or absent HDL)		
ApoAI deficiency	*ApoA1* (11q23.3)	Hypertriglyceridemia; corneal opacities; xanthomas; high risk of early-onset atherosclerosis
Lecithin:cholesterol acyltransferase (LCAT) deficiency complete and partial (fish-eye disease)	*LCAT* (16q22.1)	Mild hypertriglyceridemia, reduced HDL; corneal opacities; kidney disease; variable atherosclerosis
ATP-binding cassette A1 defect inhibiting transport of cholesterol and phospholipid to apoAI (Tangier disease)	*ABCA1* (9q31.1)	Mild hypertriglyceridemia, reduced HDL; neuropathy; corneal opacities; risk of atherosclerosis is inversely related to HDL levels
Enzyme defects causing hypertriglyceridemia (type I hyperlipidemia)		
Lipoprotein lipase inactivating mutations	*LPL* (8p21.3)	Elevated chylomicrons, cholesterol, and TG (type Ia hyperlipidemia); pancreatitis; hepatosplenomegaly; xanthomas, minimal atherosclerosis
ApoCII deficiency, inability to activate lipoprotein lipase	*APOC2* (19q13.32)	
Enzyme defects causing hyperlipoproteinemia		
Hepatic lipase deficiency	*LIPC* (15q21.3)	Elevations of IDL, HDL, TG, and cholesterol; severe atherosclerosis
GPIHBP1 inactivating mutations; inability to transport LPL to the capillary endothelial cell surface	*GPIHBP1* (8q24.3)	Elevated chylomicrons and TG (type Id hyperlipidemia); autosomal recessive
Defects in LDL receptor (LDLR) biology		

Apo = apolipoprotein; HDL = high-density lipoprotein; IDL = intermediate-density lipoprotein; LDL = low-density lipoprotein; TG = triglyceride (triacylglycerol).

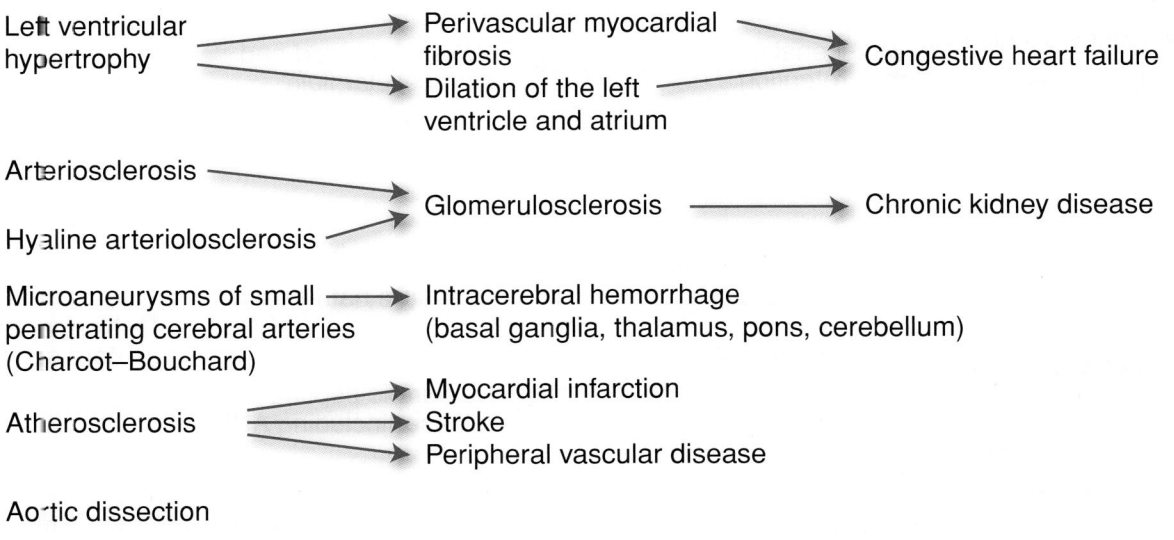

FIGURE 16-26. Conditions associated with chronic system hypertension.

Essential Hypertension, the Most Common Form, Is Idiopathic

EPIDEMIOLOGY: Incidence of hypertension has increased to the point where it affects over 30% of the American population, and is present in most cases of myocardial infarction, stroke, and chronic renal disease and the vast majority of dissecting aortic aneurysm, intracerebral hemorrhage, myocardial wall rupture, and ascending aortic dissections and rupture. It is part of metabolic syndrome (see Chapter 13). African-Americans are particularly plagued by hypertension and are more likely than are whites to experience severe complications.

ETIOLOGIC FACTORS: Essential or **primary hypertension** affects over 90% of patients with hypertension. The remaining minority develop **secondary hypertension** caused by renal, metabolic, endocrine diseases, sleep apnea, cardiovascular conditions, rare neoplasms and monogenic disorders (see below). The etiology of essential hypertension is complex and dependent on polygenic, environmental, demographic and epigenetic factors, such as sodium versus potassium ingestion, gender, age, body mass index, birth weight, low number of nephrons in the kidney, etc. Genome-wide association studies (GWAS) have reported multiple loci that are associated with essential hypertension, supporting a polygenic etiology, i.e., many genes contribute small effects that collectively elevate blood pressure.

Many factors, both environmental and genetic, contribute to the development of hypertension. Genetic associations, except for genes affecting renal sodium handling, tend to contribute only slightly.

PATHOPHYSIOLOGY: Mean arterial blood pressure is the product of cardiac output and total peripheral resistance to blood flow. Neuroendocrine and renal systems, plus multiple feedback loops, regulate blood pressure. Key mediators include sympathetic activity, the renin–angiotensin system, and whole-body sodium homeostasis, the latter being a critical determinant of blood volume. Hypertension results when the relationship between cardiac output and peripheral resistance is altered (Fig. 16-27). The pathophysiology of most forms of secondary hypertension is understood, but in primary hypertension, the imbalance is complex and multifactorial. Irrespective of the initial perturbation, increased total peripheral resistance ultimately occurs. Initially, changes in vascular reactivity are reversible, but with time, structural changes in renal vasculature reduce kidney function and lead to sodium retention.

Arteriolar dilatation and constriction regulate peripheral resistance, relying on systemic, local, and neural factors, and autoregulation. Nitric oxide, PGE_2, kinins, and

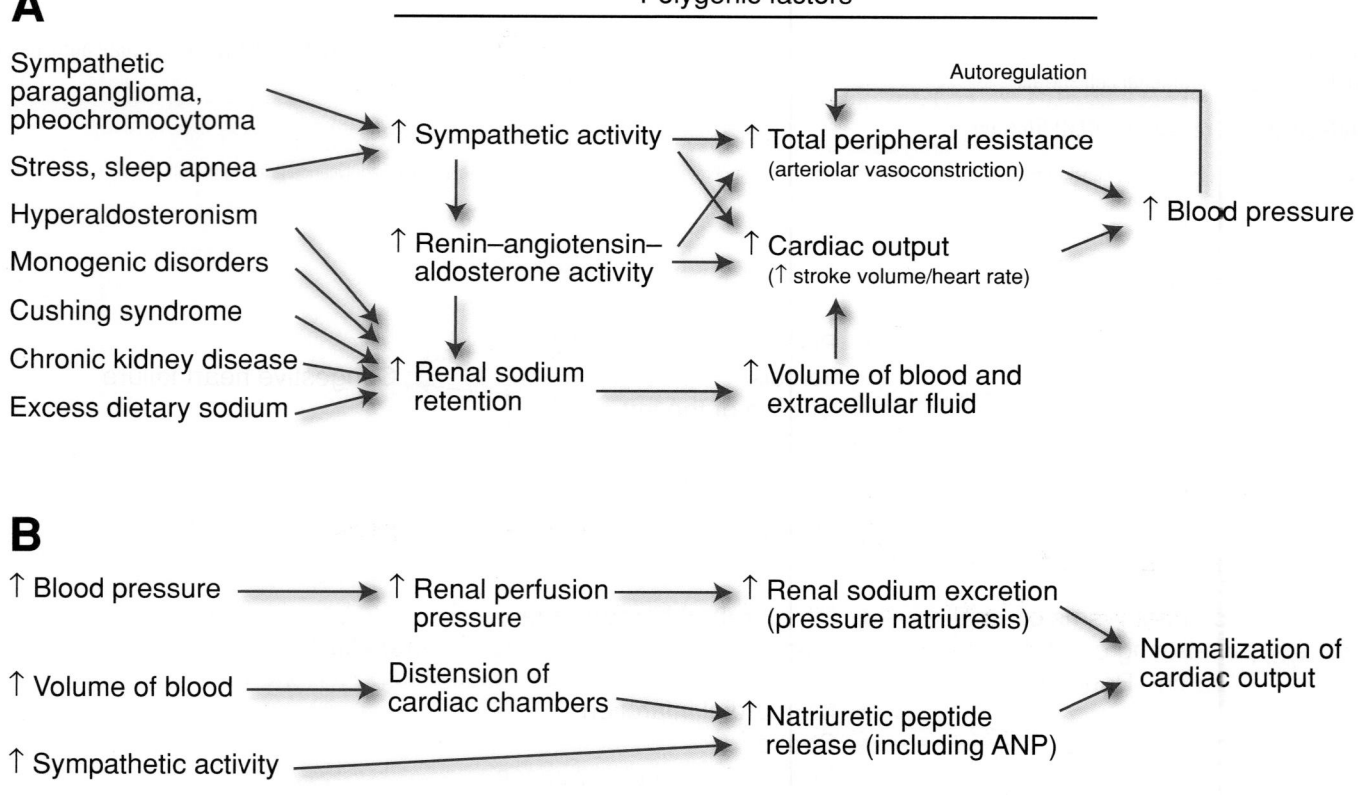

FIGURE 16-27. Relationships between cardiac output, total peripheral resistance, and hypertension. A. Pathogenic mechanisms of hypertension dependent on known causes and polygenic factors in essential hypertension that influence cardiac output and total peripheral resistance. **B.** Physiologic responses attempt to normalize blood pressure by increasing renal sodium excretion and normalizing cardiac output.

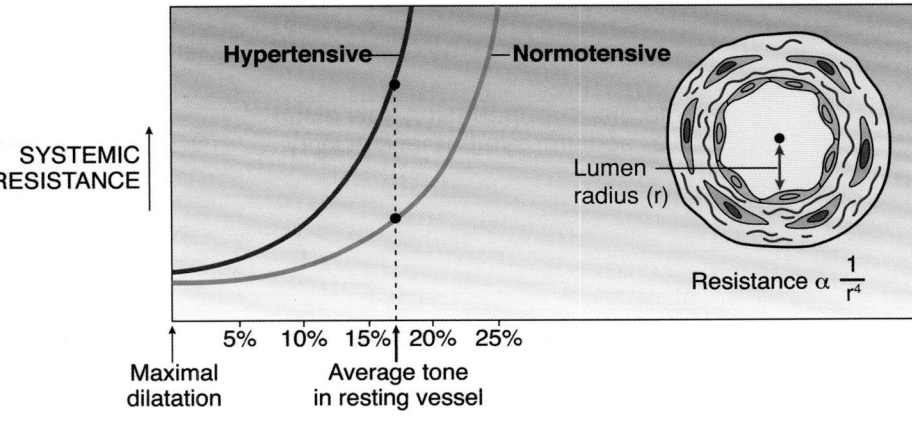

FIGURE 16-28. Autoregulation of blood pressure. Hypertension, regardless of its primary cause, increases the ability of the resistance vessel walls to respond to vasoactive stimuli. Resistance is increased even in maximally dilated vessels because the lumen size is decreased in the hypertensive vascular bed. As the smooth muscle cells contract, the increase in vessel wall thickness increases the resistance, which is inversely proportional to the fourth power of the radius of the lumen. Note that at the average resting muscular tone, the resistance in hypertensive patients is considerably higher than normal.

hypoxia stimulate dilatation. Endothelin-1, TxA$_2$, leukotrienes, angiotensin II, vasopressin, and catecholamines do the opposite. Balanced dilatory and constricting factors regulate arteriolar tone and provide adequate tissue perfusion and oxygenation, and protect organ microvascular beds from hyperperfusion and pressure injury. Autoregulation of small arteries and arterioles through local myogenic responses to altered perfusion pressure normalizes organ blood flow (Fig. 16-28).

Renal function is fundamental to blood pressure regulation, reflecting the centrality of sodium (and, consequently, water) retention. The **renin–angiotensin system** (RAS, Fig. 16-29) reflects contributions from many organ systems, and RAS dysregulation is implicated in over 2/3 of patients with hypertension. Renal artery occlusion or dietary salt restriction increases renal secretion of renin. Renin is a protease that cleaves **angiotensinogen** to a decapeptide, **angiotensin I**. In turn, angiotensin I is converted to **angiotensin II** by **angiotensin-converting enzyme (ACE)** on endothelial surfaces. Common polymorphisms of the angiotensinogen gene may contribute to primary hypertension. Angiotensin II causes vasoconstriction and affects centers in the brain that control sympathetic outflow and stimulate adrenal aldosterone release. Aldosterone increases renal tubular sodium reabsorption. The net effect of all these actions is increased total body fluid.

This axis is antagonized by **atrial natriuretic peptide (ANP),** a polypeptide hormone secreted by specialized cells in the cardiac atria. ANP binds specific receptors in the kidney and increases urinary sodium excretion, and so opposes angiotensin II–induced vasoconstriction. ANP secretion may be controlled by stretch–secretion coupling after atrial distention, due to increased volume, or by as-yet undefined endocrine interactions, possibly involving endothelin-1.

The importance of this hormonal axis in regulating blood pressure in hypertension is demonstrated by the therapeutic success of sympathetic antagonists (β-adrenergic blockers), diuretics, and ACE inhibitors. Nonetheless, no central defect in the RAS has been identified, in part because the vasculature responds quickly to hemodynamic changes by autoregulation (Fig. 16-28).

Thus, the renin–angiotensin system elevates blood pressure by three mechanisms:

- Increased sympathetic output
- Increased mineralocorticoid secretion
- Direct vasoconstriction

PATHOLOGY: Chronic hypertension has multiple consequences (Fig. 16-26), which involve left ventricular myocardium, atherosclerosis in conduit arteries, and aortic dissection. Vascular changes mostly involve small arteries and arterioles, especially in the kidney. Initially, smooth muscle cell hypertrophy in resistance arterioles may contribute to hyperreactivity to vasoactive stimuli (Fig. 16-28). **Arteriosclerosis** of small muscular arteries in chronic hypertension presents as fibromuscular intimal thickening by new layers of elastin, with reduplication of the intimal elastic lamina and increased connective tissue (Fig. 16-30A). Arteriosclerosis is not diagnostic of hypertension, since similar pathologies are associated with aging. In hyaline arteriolosclerosis arteriole walls have a glassy appearance by light microscopy. Thickened arteriolar walls show deposition of basement membrane material and accumulated plasma proteins (Fig. 16-30B). Hyaline arteriosclerosis may also be present in diabetes. Kidneys affected with chronic hypertension may be contracted, have a granular surface, and microscopically often show **glomerulosclerosis** and interstitial fibrosis.

Monogenic and Acquired Hypertensive Disorders

Single gene mutations that may cause childhood hypertension include defects in:

- Mineralocorticoid synthesis, metabolism, and signaling
- Sodium channels and cotransporters

Disordered Aldosterone

Aldosterone release from the adrenal zona glomerulosa is stimulated by angiotensin II and hyperkalemia (Fig. 16-29). In autosomal dominant **glucocorticoid-remediable aldosteronism (GRA)** (also called **familial hyperaldosteronism**

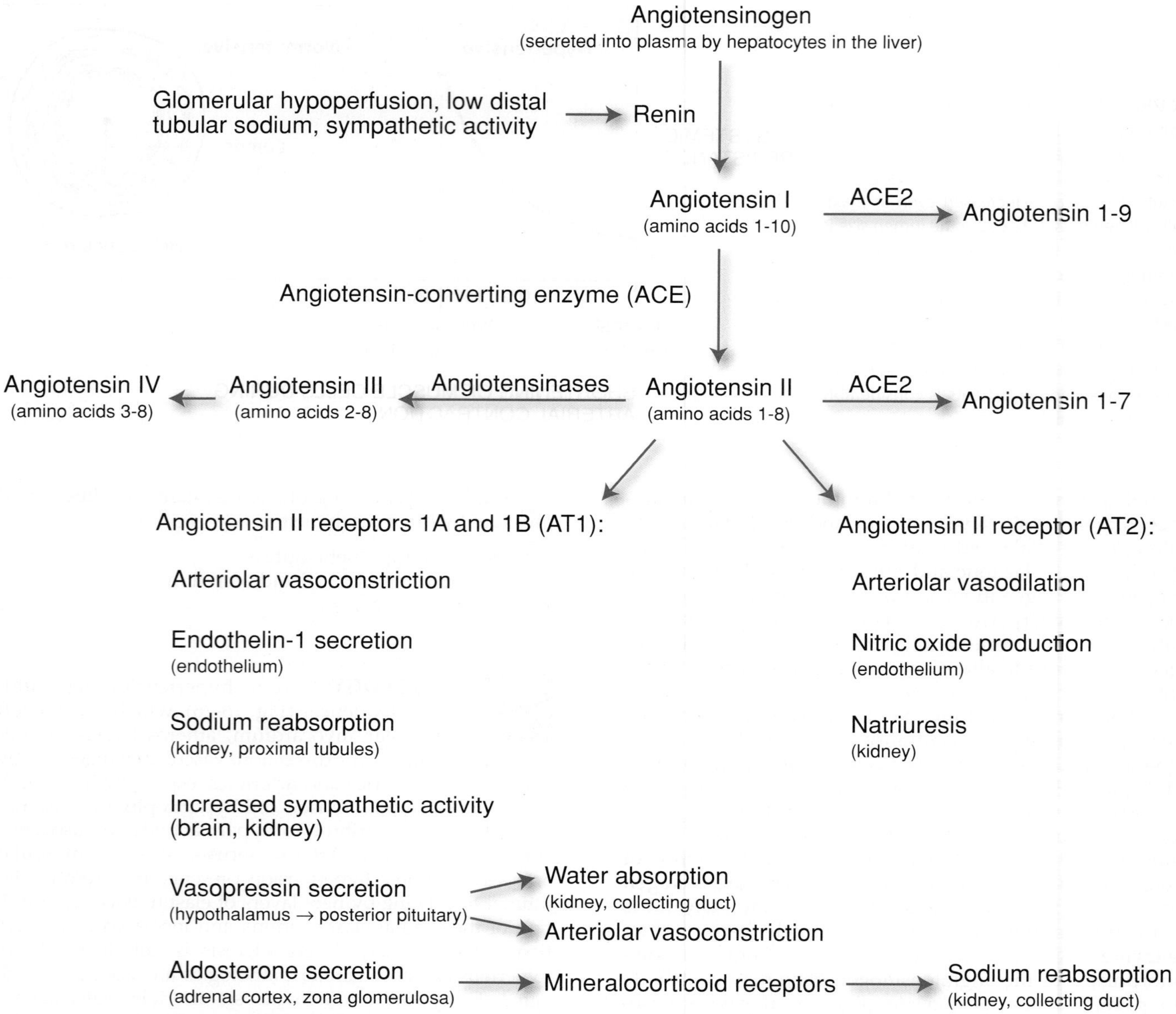

Angiotensinogen
(secreted into plasma by hepatocytes in the liver)

Glomerular hypoperfusion, low distal tubular sodium, sympathetic activity → Renin

Angiotensin I
(amino acids 1-10) → ACE2 → Angiotensin 1-9

Angiotensin-converting enzyme (ACE)

Angiotensin IV
(amino acids 3-8) ← Angiotensin III
(amino acids 2-8) ← Angiotensinases ← Angiotensin II
(amino acids 1-8) → ACE2 → Angiotensin 1-7

Angiotensin II receptors 1A and 1B (AT1):

Arteriolar vasoconstriction

Endothelin-1 secretion
(endothelium)

Sodium reabsorption
(kidney, proximal tubules)

Increased sympathetic activity
(brain, kidney)

Vasopressin secretion
(hypothalamus → posterior pituitary) → Water absorption
(kidney, collecting duct)
→ Arteriolar vasoconstriction

Aldosterone secretion
(adrenal cortex, zona glomerulosa) → Mineralocorticoid receptors → Sodium reabsorption
(kidney, collecting duct)

Angiotensin II receptor (AT2):

Arteriolar vasodilation

Nitric oxide production
(endothelium)

Natriuresis
(kidney)

FIGURE 16-29. The renin–angiotensin system and its role in fluid and sodium homeostasis.

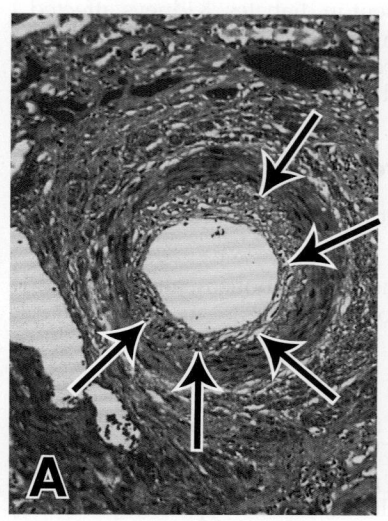
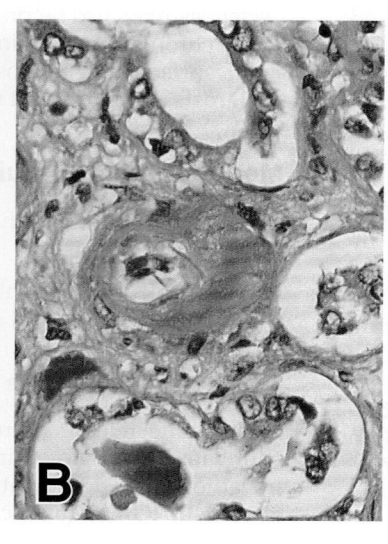

FIGURE 16-30. Arteriosclerosis and arteriolosclerosis. A. A cross-section of a renal intralobular artery shows irregular thickening of the intima (*arrows*). **B.** A renal arteriole exhibits hyaline arteriolosclerosis (*center*).

type 1 [FH-II], a crossover on chromosome 8 puts the regulatory region for an enzyme needed to synthesize all steroids (11β-hydroxylase) in control of aldosterone synthase, leading to ACTH-stimulated hyperaldosteronism. In another form of genetically increased aldosteronism, **FH-III**, a potassium channel mutation causes the zona glomerulosa to secrete excessive aldosterone.

Other morogenic disorders include **syndrome of apparent mineralocorticoid excess (AME)**. Normally, the slight mineralocorticoid activity of cortisol is inactivated by an enzyme in the collecting ducts. In AME, this enzyme is deficient, causing cortisol to mimic aldosterone. Collecting duct hyperresponsiveness also occurs in **Liddle syndrome**, in which a mutation in its polyubiquitination site leads to abnormal persistence of the sodium resorption channel.

Of course, some monogenic diseases lead to the opposite phenomenon: excessive sodium wastage and hypotension.

Acquired Forms of Hypertension

These include renal artery stenosis, most forms of chronic renal disease, diabetes mellitus, primary elevation of aldosterone levels (Conn syndrome), Cushing syndrome, pheochromocytoma, hyperthyroidism, coarctation of the aorta, and renin-secreting tumors. In addition, people with severe atherosclerosis may have high systolic pressures because a sclerotic aorta cannot properly absorb the pulsatile kinetic energy of systole, and because they often have renovascular hypertension.

Prothrombotic Paradox of Hypertension

Hypertension exposes the arterial tree to increased pulsatile stress and is an important risk factor for atherosclerosis. Paradoxically, most major complications of chronic hypertension, such as myocardial infarction and stroke, are thrombotic, rather than hemorrhagic. This is known as the prothrombotic paradox of hypertension. Hypertension also increases the load on the myocardium, which impairs coronary blood flow, gives rise to left ventricular hypertrophy and eventually leads to congestive heart failure and associated arrhythmias.

Malignant Hypertension

A very small fraction of hypertensive patients have **malignant hypertension**, with rapid and severe increases in systolic (≥180 mm Hg) and diastolic (≥120 mm Hg) pressures, which causes symptoms of organ injury (headache, nausea, retinal hemorrhage, papilledema, proteinuria) and can be fatal via CNS, myocardial and renal infarction. Causes include discontinuation of antihypertensive medications, cerebrovascular accidents, stimulants such as cocaine and amphetamines that cause autonomic hyperactivity, preeclampsia and eclampsia (see Chapter 14), autoimmune diseases, glomerulonephritis, etc. As with ordinary hypertension, malignant hypertension occurs more often in patients of African descent.

 PATHOLOGY: Malignant hypertension produces dramatic pathologic changes in small vessels. Segmental constriction and dilation of retinal

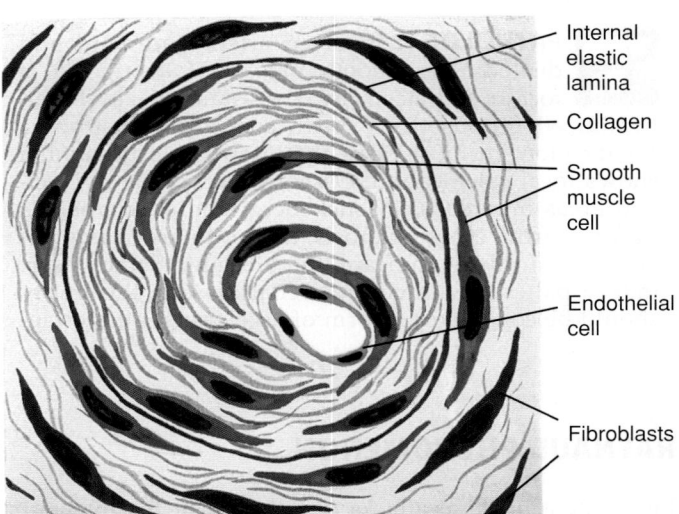

FIGURE 16-31. Hyperplastic arteriosclerosis. In cases of malignant hypertension, the arterioles exhibit smooth muscle cell proliferation and increased amounts of intercellular collagen and glycosaminoglycans, resulting in an "onion-skin" appearance. The mass of smooth muscle and associated elements tend to fix the size of the lumen and restrict the arteriole's capacity to dilate.

arterioles in severely hypertensive patients are sufficiently prominent to allow one to make the diagnosis by ophthalmoscopy (see Chapter 33). If blood pressure rises rapidly, retinal arterioles show microaneurysms, focal hemorrhages, and retinal scarring. Ischemic necrosis and edema of the retina appear as "cotton wool spots" with the ophthalmoscope. These retinal changes are typical of those in other resistance vessels when pressure rises rapidly.

In malignant hypertension, necrosis of smooth muscle cells in small muscular arteries causes segmental dilation. In those regions, vessels lose endothelial integrity, which increases vascular permeability and causes plasma proteins to seep into the vessel wall. Fibrin deposits, creating **fibrinoid necrosis** (see Chapter 1). Acute injury is rapidly followed by smooth muscle proliferation and a striking concentric increase in the number of layers of smooth muscle cells, producing an "onion-skin" appearance (Fig. 16-31). This form of smooth muscle proliferation may be a response to release of growth factors from platelets and other cells at sites of vascular injury. Together, these changes comprise malignant arteriosclerosis or arteriolosclerosis, depending on the size of the vessels affected. In the kidney, such lesions are called **malignant nephrosclerosis**.

MÖNCKEBERG MEDIAL SCLEROSIS

Mönckeberg medial sclerosis entails degenerative calcification of the media of large and medium-sized muscular arteries. It occurs mainly in older people and mostly involves arteries of the arms and legs. It is also common in advanced chronic renal disease and type II diabetes.

PATHOLOGY: Involved arteries are hard and dilated. The smooth muscle of the media is focally replaced by pale-staining, acellular, hyalinized fibrous tissue, with concentric dystrophic calcification. In most cases the internal elastic lamina shows focal calcification. Osseous metaplasia in calcified areas may occur. Mönckeberg medial sclerosis is different from atherosclerosis, and ordinarily does not entail clinically significant impairment. Some assert that in patients with chronic renal disease, this entity should be considered a form of accelerated atherosclerosis.

RAYNAUD PHENOMENON

Intermittent bilateral attacks of ischemia of the fingers or toes, and sometimes the ears or nose, are called Raynaud phenomenon.

CLINICAL FEATURES: It is characterized by severe pallor (Fig. 16-32), often accompanied by paresthesias and pain. Symptoms are precipitated by cold or emotional stimuli and relieved by heat. Primary cold sensitivity of the Raynaud type is more common in women, and it often starts in the late teens. It is bilateral and symmetric. Rarely, it may lead to ulcers or gangrene of the tips of digits. The hands are more commonly affected than feet.

Raynaud phenomenon may occur as an isolated disorder or as part of systemic autoimmune diseases (see Chapter 11), particularly scleroderma and systemic lupus erythematosus. It includes primary and secondary cold sensitivity, livedo reticularis, and acrocyanosis. Whatever its associations, Raynaud phenomenon reflects vasospasm of arteries and arterioles in the skin. Dysregulation of vascular tone by sympathetic nerve activity and neurohumoral factors may play a role. Phosphodiesterase type 5 inhibitors induce vasodilation and have some therapeutic value.

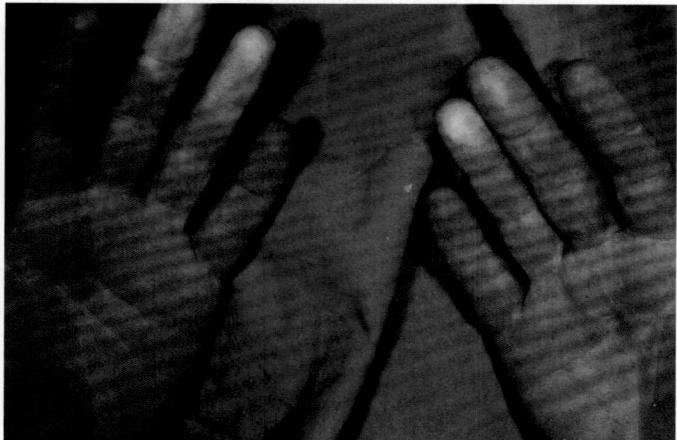

FIGURE 16-32. Raynaud phenomenon. The tips of the fingers show marked pallor.

FIBROMUSCULAR DYSPLASIA

Fibromuscular dysplasia is a rare noninflammatory thickening of large and medium-sized muscular arteries, distinct from atherosclerosis and arteriosclerosis. The cause is unknown; however, it may be developmental in nature. Renal artery stenosis due to this condition is an important cause of renovascular hypertension, but fibromuscular dysplasia may affect almost any vessel, including carotid, vertebral, and splanchnic arteries. It is typically a disease of women during their reproductive years but may appear at any age, even in childhood.

PATHOLOGY: In most cases, the distal 2/3 of the renal artery and its primary branches have several segmental stenoses, which represent fibrous and muscular ridges that project into the lumen. In these segments arrangement and proliferation of the cellular elements of the vessel wall is disorderly, without necrosis or inflammation. Fibrous tissue and myofibroblasts replace smooth muscle, and the media may be thinned. In some cases, intimal fibroplasia predominates, and in unusual instances, connective tissue encircles the adventitia. Other than renal hypertension, the major complication of fibromuscular dysplasia is dissecting aneurysm due to thinning of the media of affected arteries.

VASCULITIS

Vasculitis is inflammation and necrosis of blood vessels. It may affect arteries, veins, and capillaries (Table 16-8). Vessels may be damaged by immune mechanisms (see Chapter 4), infectious agents, mechanical trauma, radiation, or toxins. However, in many cases, no specific cause is determined.

PATHOPHYSIOLOGY: Vasculitic syndromes are thought to involve immune mechanisms, including (1) deposition of immune complexes, (2) direct attack by circulating antibodies on vessels, and (3) various forms of cell-mediated immunity. Agents that incite these reactions are largely unknown, but vasculitis may be associated with viral infection.

Serum sickness was one of the first human immunologic disorders to be linked with vasculitis. In animal models of serum sickness, immune complexes and complement deposit in local tissue reactions (see Chapter 4). In human cases, immune complexes are only sometimes present, and firm evidence for them in most cases of vasculitis is lacking.

Viral antigens may cause vasculitis. Thus, chronic infection with hepatitis B virus is associated with some cases of **polyarteritis nodosa** (see below and Chapter 11). In this case, viral antigen–antibody complexes circulate and are deposited in the vascular lesions. Human vasculitis has also been associated with other infections, including herpes simplex, CMV, and parvovirus, as well as with several bacterial antigens.

Small vessel vasculitides (e.g., polyangiitis with granulomatosis; see below) are associated with circulating antineutrophil cytoplasmic antibodies (ANCAs), but why these autoantibodies appear and how they lead to

TABLE 16-8

INFLAMMATORY DISORDERS OF BLOOD VESSELS

Polyarteritis Nodosa Group of Systemic Necrotizing Vasculitis

Classic polyarteritis nodosa

Allergic angiitis and granulomatosis (Churg–Strauss variant)

"Overlap syndrome" of systemic angiitis

Hypersensitivity Vasculitis

Serum sickness and similar reactions

Henoch–Schönlein purpura

Vasculitis associated with connective tissue disorders

Vasculitis in cases of essential mixed cryoglobulinemia

Vasculitis associated with other primary disorders

Wegener Granulomatosis

Lymphomatoid Granulomatosis

Giant Cell Arteritis

Temporal arteritis

Takayasu arteritis

Central Nervous System Vasculitis

Vasculitis Associated With Cancer

Mucocutaneous Lymph Node Syndrome (Kawasaki Disease)

Thromboangiitis Obliterans (Buerger Disease)

Behçet Disease

Miscellaneous Vasculitis Syndromes

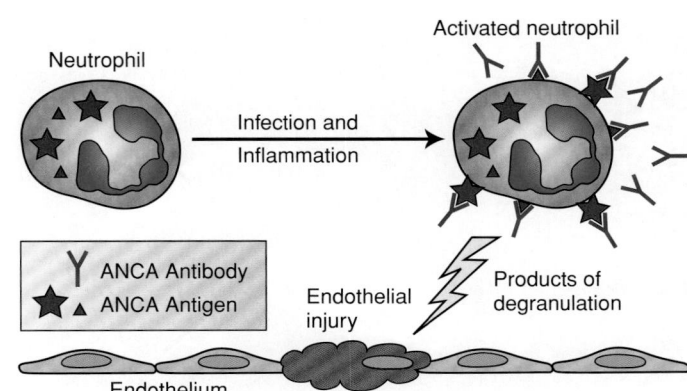

FIGURE 16-33. Model of the pathogenesis of antineutrophil cytoplasmic antibody (ANCA) vasculitis. ANCA antigens are normally found in the neutrophil cytoplasm with very little surface expression. In inflammation and infection, increased cell surface expression of ANCA antigens is induced in the neutrophils. ANCA present in the circulation owing to previous formation through unknown mechanisms binds to these ANCA antigens on the surface, leading to neutrophil activation and interaction with endothelial cells. Neutrophil degranulation releases toxic factors including reactive oxygen species, proteinase 3 (PR3), and myeloperoxidase, and other granule enzymes cause endothelial cell apoptosis and necrosis, leading to endothelial injury.

vasculitis are not known. Infection may play a role in the development of ANCAs. ANCA may cause endothelial damage by activating neutrophils, and antibody titers correlate with disease activity in some cases. Perinuclear antigenic targets (P-ANCA) are mostly directed against myeloperoxidase; more general cytoplasmic immunofluorescence (C-ANCA), mainly targets proteinase 3.

When neutrophils are activated (e.g., by TNF-α) and degranulate, myeloperoxidase and proteinase 3 are present at their surfaces. ANCA, which may be part of a response to infection, can then bind and activate the neutrophils. Other autoantibodies that activate neutrophils and injure endothelial cells also occur in vasculitides (Fig. 16-33).

Polyarteritis Nodosa Is an Acute, Necrotizing Vasculitis

Polyarteritis nodosa affects medium-sized and smaller muscular arteries and, occasionally, larger arteries. It is more common in men than in women. The disease was rare until the 1940s, when there was a striking rise in its incidence. The increased frequency of polyarteritis nodosa at that time seemed to be associated with the widespread use of antisera to bacteria and toxins produced in animals, and with use of sulfonamides. The incidence of polyarteritis nodosa now seems to be subsiding.

PATHOLOGY: Characteristically, lesions of polyarteritis nodosa are <1-mm long areas of fibrinoid necrosis, and occur patchily in small to medium-sized muscular arteries—although they may occasionally involve larger arteries, such as renal, splenic, or coronary arteries. They may involve all or part of a vessel's circumference. Medial muscle and adjacent tissues are fused into a featureless eosinophilic mass that stains for fibrin. Vigorous acute inflammation envelops the area of necrosis, usually involving the entire adventitia (periarteritis), and extends through the other coats of the vessel (Fig. 16-34). Neutrophils, lymphocytes, plasma cells, and macrophages are present in varying proportions, and eosinophils may be conspicuous.

Thrombosis in affected segments of arteries commonly causes infarcts in involved organs. Injury to larger arteries may cause small aneurysms (<0.5 cm), especially in renal, coronary, and cerebral artery branches. An aneurysm may rupture and, if located in a critical area, may cause fatal hemorrhage.

Over time, many vascular lesions start to heal, especially if corticosteroids have been given. Necrotic tissue and inflammatory exudate are resorbed, and the vessel is left with fibrosis of the media and conspicuous gaps in the elastic laminae.

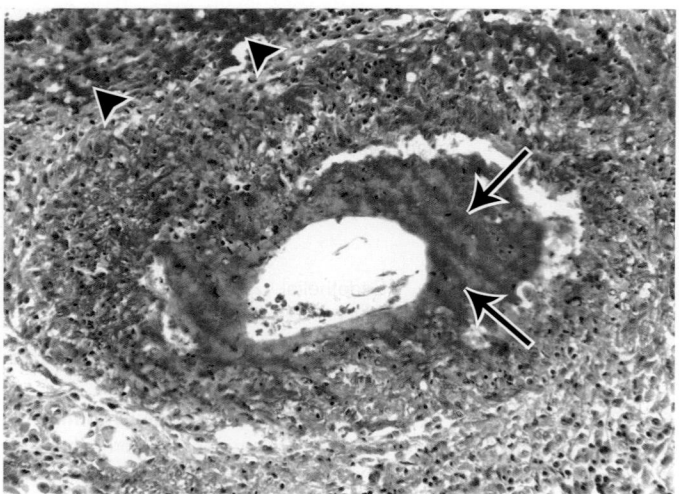

FIGURE 16-34. Polyarteritis nodosa. The intense inflammatory cell infiltrate in the arterial wall and surrounding connective tissue is associated with fibrinoid necrosis (*arrows*) and disruption of the vessel wall with hemorrhage into surrounding tissues (*arrowheads*).

CLINICAL FEATURES: Clinical manifestations of polyarteritis nodosa are variable and depend on the organs affected by the lesions. Kidneys, heart, skeletal muscle, skin, and mesentery are most often involved, but lesions may occur almost anywhere, including the bowel, pancreas, lungs, liver, and brain. Constitutional symptoms such as fever and weight loss are common. Polyarteritis nodosa-like lesions may complicate infections with hepatitis B and C viruses, and HIV.

Untreated polyarteritis nodosa was usually fatal, but anti-inflammatory and immunosuppressive therapies, for example, corticosteroids, cyclophosphamide, usually induce remissions or cures.

Hypersensitivity Angiitis Is a Response to Foreign Substances

Hypersensitivity angiitis is a broad category of inflammatory vascular lesions considered to represent a reaction to foreign materials (e.g., bacterial products or drugs). For lesions mainly confined to skin, the terms **leukocytoclastic vasculitis** (i.e., with debris from disintegrating neutrophils), **cutaneous vasculitis,** or **cutaneous necrotizing venulitis** (reflecting the predominant involvement of venules) are used. **Systemic hypersensitivity angiitis,** or **microscopic polyangiitis,** affects many of the same organs as polyarteritis nodosa but is restricted to the smallest arteries and arterioles.

CLINICAL FEATURES AND PATHOLOGY: Cutaneous vasculitis may follow administration of many drugs, including aspirin, penicillin, and thiazide diuretics. It is also commonly related to streptococcal and staphylococcal infections, viral hepatitis, tuberculosis, and bacterial endocarditis. The disease typically presents as palpable purpura, largely on the legs. Microscopically, superficial cutaneous venules show fibrinoid necrosis with acute inflammation. Cutaneous vasculitis is generally self-limited (see Chapter 28).

Systemic hypersensitivity angiitis may be an isolated entity or a part of other conditions, such as collagen vascular diseases (lupus erythematosus, rheumatoid arthritis, Sjögren syndrome), Henoch–Schönlein purpura, dysproteinemias, and several malignancies. Patients with systemic hypersensitivity angiitis may also have cutaneous purpuric lesions. The most feared complication of microscopic polyangiitis is renal involvement, with rapidly progressive glomerulonephritis and renal failure (see Chapter 22). *Microscopic polyarteritis is strongly associated with P-ANCA.*

Giant Cell Arteritis Mainly Affects Temporal Arteries

Granulomatous arteritis (temporal arteritis) most often affects the temporal artery, but may also involve other cranial arteries, the aorta (giant cell aortitis) and its branches, and occasionally other arteries. Aortic aneurysms and dissection occur. The average age at onset is 70 years; it is rare before age 50. Giant cell arteritis is the most common vasculitis; its incidence rises with age and may reach 1% by age 80. Women are affected slightly more often than men. The age at onset helps differentiate it from other vasculitides that may involve the same vessels in younger people, such as Takayasu disease.

PATHOPHYSIOLOGY: The etiology of giant cell arteritis is obscure. Its association with HLA-DR4 and its occurrence in first-degree relatives support a genetic component in its pathogenesis. Immunologic features, including activated CD4+ T-helper cells and macrophages, and the association of the disease with a specific polymorphism of ICAM-1 suggest an immune reaction. B lymphocytes are lacking. Macrophages at the border of the intima and media produce MMPs that digest ECM. ANCA is absent in giant cell arteritis. Generalized symptoms of muscle aching and the widespread distribution of its manifestations are consistent with a relationship to rheumatoid diseases.

PATHOLOGY: Affected vessels are cord-like, with nodular thickening. Lumens are reduced to slits or may be obliterated by a thrombus (Fig. 16-35A). Microscopically, the media and intima show granulomatous inflammation; aggregates of macrophages, lymphocytes, and plasma cells are admixed with variable numbers of eosinophils and neutrophils. Giant cells tend to be distributed at the internal elastic lamina (Fig. 16-35B) but vary widely in number. Both foreign body and Langhans giant cells are seen. There are foci of necrosis, with changes in the internal elastica, which become swollen, irregular, and fragmented. In advanced lesions, it may completely disappear. Fragments of the elastica occasionally appear in the giant cells. In late stages, the intima is conspicuously thickened and the media is fibrotic. Thrombi may obliterate the lumen, after which organization and canalization occur.

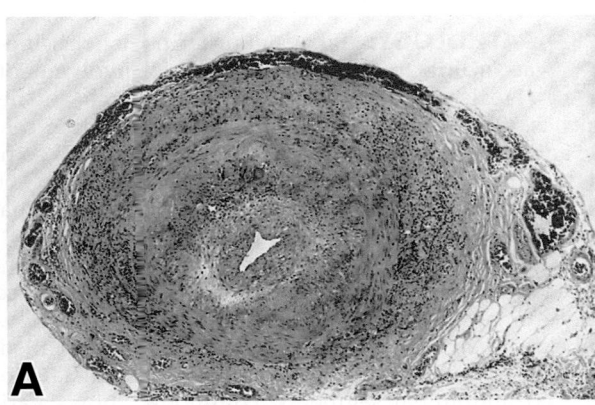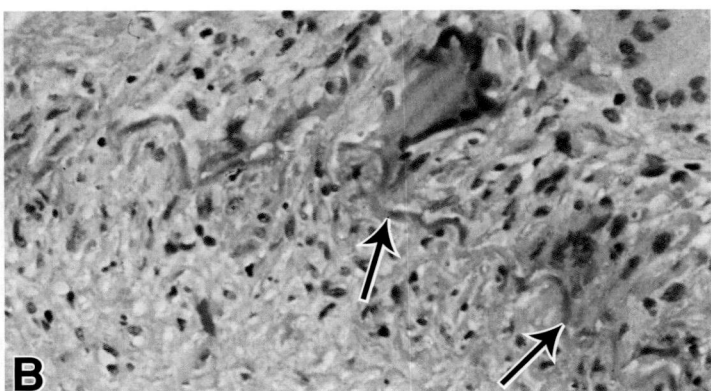

FIGURE 16-35. Temporal arteritis. A. A photomicrograph of a temporal artery shows chronic inflammation throughout the wall and a lumen severely narrowed by intimal thickening. **B.** A high-power view shows giant cells adjacent to the fragmented internal elastic lamina (*arrows*).

CLINICAL FEATURES: Giant cell arteritis tends to be benign and self-limited, and symptoms subside in 6 to 12 months. Patients present with headache and throbbing temporal pain. Sometimes there are early constitutional symptoms, including malaise, fever, weight loss, and generalized muscular aching or stiffness in the shoulders and hips. Throbbing and pain over the temporal artery are accompanied by swelling, tenderness, and redness in overlying skin. Almost half of patients have visual symptoms, which may progress from transient to permanent blindness in one or both eyes, sometimes rapidly. Occasionally, the disease causes myocardial, CNS, or gastrointestinal infarcts, which may be fatal. Because the inflammatory process is patchy, temporal artery biopsy may not be diagnostic in up to 40% of patients with otherwise classic manifestations. Response to corticosteroids is usually dramatic, and symptoms subside within days.

Granulomatosis With Polyangiitis Affects the Respiratory Tract and Kidney

Granulomatosis with polyangiitis (GPA) (formerly Wegener granulomatosis) is a systemic necrotizing vasculitis of unknown etiology, with granulomatous lesions of the nose, sinuses, and lungs and renal glomerular disease. Men are affected more than women, usually in their fifth and sixth decades. Over 90% of patients with GPA are positive for ANCA, of whom 75% have C-ANCA. Possibly, antibodies activate circulating neutrophils to attack blood vessels. The response to immunosuppressive therapy supports an immunologic basis for the disease.

PATHOLOGY: Lesions of GPA feature parenchymal necrosis, vasculitis, and granulomatous inflammation composed of neutrophils, lymphocytes, plasma cells, macrophages, and eosinophils. Individual lesions in the lung may reach 5 cm, and must be distinguished from tuberculosis. Vasculitis involving small arteries and veins may occur anywhere but most affects the respiratory tract (Fig. 16-36), kidney, and spleen. Inflammation in arteries is mainly mononuclear, although acute inflammation, necrotizing and nonnecrotizing granulomas, and fibrinoid necrosis are often present. Medial thickening and intimal proliferation are common and often narrow or obliterate the lumen.

In the lungs, persistent bilateral pneumonitis, with nodular infiltrates that undergo cavitation, resembles tuberculous lesions. Chronic sinusitis and nasopharyngeal mucosal ulcers are frequent. The kidney at first shows focal necrotizing glomerulonephritis, which progresses to crescentic glomerulonephritis (see Chapter 23).

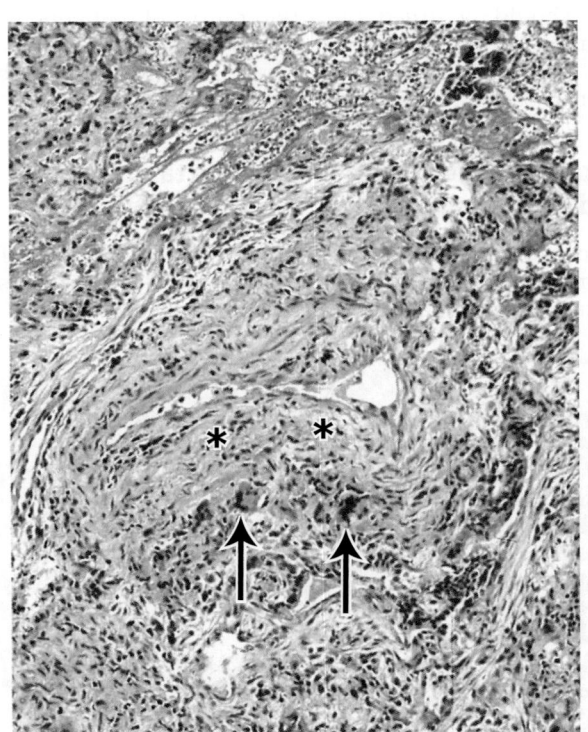

FIGURE 16-36. Granulomatosis with polyangiitis (GPA). A photomicrograph of the lung shows vasculitis of a pulmonary artery. There are chronic inflammatory cells and Langerhans giant cells (*arrows*) in the wall, together with thickening of the intima (*asterisks*).

CLINICAL FEATURES: Most patients present with respiratory symptoms, particularly pneumonitis and sinusitis. The lung is eventually involved in over 90% of patients, with multiple—often cavitary—pulmonary infiltrates. Hematuria and proteinuria are common, and glomerular disease can progress to renal failure. Rash, muscular pains, joint involvement, and neurologic symptoms occur. Without treatment, GPA is rapidly fatal, with a mean survival of 5 to 6 months. However, cyclophosphamide produces both complete remissions and substantial disease-free intervals in most patients. Interestingly, antimicrobial sulfa drugs significantly reduce the incidence of relapses, suggesting a relationship of the disease to bacterial infection.

Allergic Granulomatosis and Angiitis (Churg–Strauss Syndrome) Occurs in Young People With Asthma

PATHOLOGY: Tissues show widespread necrotizing granulomatous lesions and intense eosinophilic infiltrates in and around blood vessels of small and medium-sized arteries (Fig. 16-37), arterioles, and veins in the lungs, spleen, kidney, heart, liver, CNS, and other organs. Although Churg–Strauss syndrome seems to be a distinct entity, it may resemble other diseases: fibrinoid necrosis, thrombosis, and aneurysm formation may simulate polyarteritis nodosa, and other eosinophilic syndromes, such as parasitic and fungal infestations, polyangiitis with granulomatosis, eosinophilic pneumonia (Loeffler syndrome), and drug vasculitis should be ruled out. Two-thirds of patients with Churg–Strauss syndrome have P-ANCA.

Untreated, these patients have a poor prognosis, but corticosteroid therapy is almost always effective.

Takayasu Arteritis Affects the Aorta and Its Branches

Takayasu arteritis is seen worldwide. It mainly affects women (90%), usually under 30 years of age. Its cause is unknown, but an autoimmune basis has been proposed.

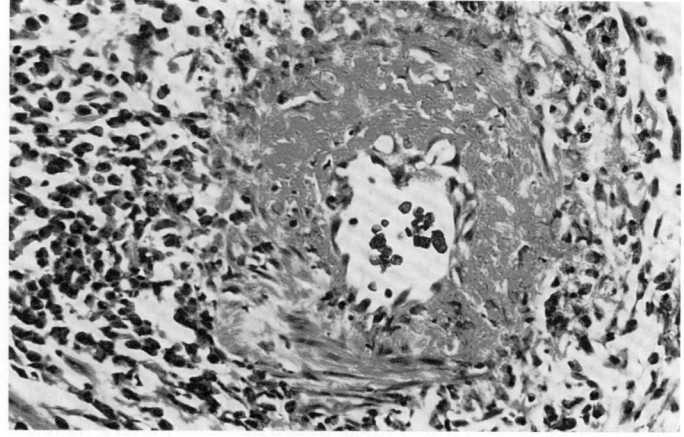

FIGURE 16-37. Churg–Strauss syndrome. A medium-sized artery shows fibrinoid necrosis and a surrounding eosinophilic infiltrate.

PATHOLOGY: Takayasu arteritis is classified according to the extent of aortic involvement: (1) disease restricted to the aortic arch and its branches, (2) arteritis only affecting the descending thoracic and abdominal aorta and its branches, and (3) combined involvement of the arch and descending aorta. The pulmonary artery is occasionally affected and the retinal vasculature is frequently involved.

The aorta wall is thickened, with focal, raised intimal plaques. Branches of the aorta often have localized stenosis or occlusion, which interferes with blood flow. If subclavian arteries are affected, it is sometimes called, "pulseless disease." The aorta, particularly the distal thoracic and abdominal segments, commonly shows variably sized aneurysms. Early lesions of the aorta and its main branches show acute panarteritis, with infiltrates of neutrophils, mononuclear cells, and occasional Langhans giant cells. Inflammation of vasa vasorum in Takayasu arteritis resembles that in syphilitic aortitis. Late lesions show fibrosis and severe intimal proliferation. Secondary atherosclerosis may obscure the basic disease.

CLINICAL FEATURES: Patients with early Takayasu arteritis complain of constitutional symptoms, dizziness, visual disturbances, dyspnea, and, occasionally, syncope. As the disease progresses, cardiac symptoms become more severe, with intermittent claudication of the arms or legs. Asymmetric differences in blood pressure may develop and pulses in one extremity may sometimes actually disappear. Hypertension may reflect coarctation of the aorta or renal artery stenosis. Most patients eventually develop congestive heart failure. Loss of visual acuity ranges from field defects to total blindness. Early Takayasu arteritis responds to corticosteroids, but the later lesions require surgical reconstruction.

Kawasaki Disease Mainly Targets Coronary Arteries in Children

Kawasaki disease (mucocutaneous lymph node syndrome) is an acute necrotizing vasculitis of infancy and early childhood, with high fever, rash, conjunctival and oral lesions, and lymphadenitis. In 70% of patients, coronary artery vasculitis causes aneurysms (Fig. 16-38), 1% to 2% of which are lethal.

ETIOLOGIC FACTORS: Kawasaki disease is usually self-limited. Despite high suspicion and considerable effort, no infectious cause has been identified. *Parvovirus B19* or *New Haven coronavirus* has been implicated in some cases, as have various bacteria, including *Staphylococcus, Streptococcus,* and *Chlamydia* in others. The common theme seems to be viral or bacterial production of superantigens. These are molecules that bind to major histocompatibility complex (MHC) class II receptors and the Vβ region of the T-cell receptor, massively activating immune responses. IL-1β and IL-18 processing and secretion contribute to excess proinflammatory cytokines in coronary arterial walls. Some patients show autoantibodies to endothelial and smooth muscle cells.

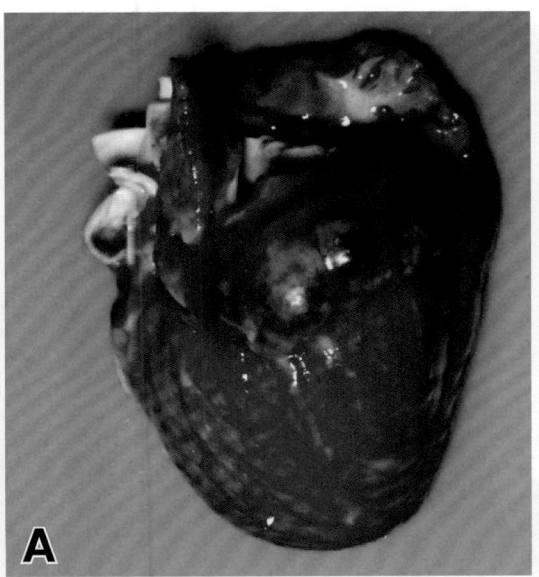
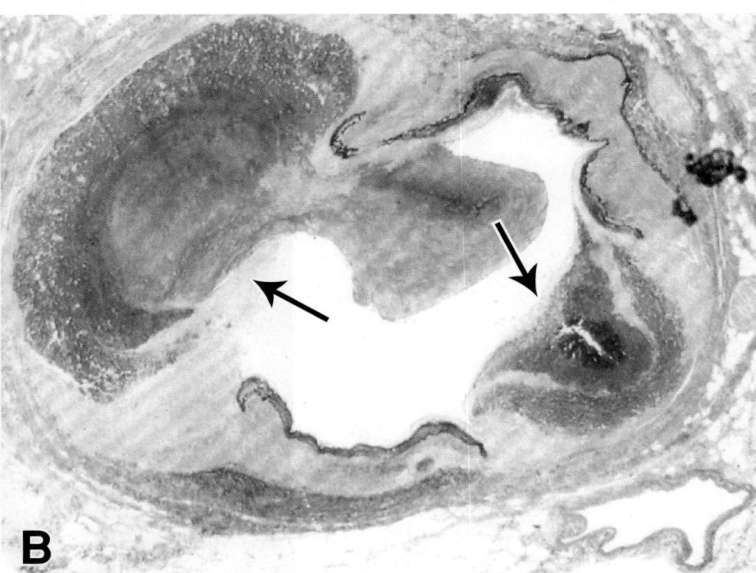

FIGURE 16-38. Kawasaki disease. A. The heart of a child who died from Kawasaki disease shows conspicuous coronary artery aneurysms. **B.** A microscopic section of a coronary artery from the same patient shows two large defects (*arrows*) in the internal elastic lamina, with two small aneurysms filled with thrombus.

Buerger Disease Is a Peripheral Vascular Disease of Smokers

Buerger disease (thromboangiitis obliterans) is an occlusive inflammatory disease of medium and small arteries in the distal arms and legs. It once occurred almost only in young and middle-aged men who smoked heavily, but it is now also described in women. It is more common in the Mediterranean area, Middle East, and Asia.

 ETIOLOGIC FACTORS: The role of smoking in Buerger disease is underscored by the fact that stopping smoking may lead to remission, and resuming it to exacerbation. Yet, how tobacco smoke acts here is obscure. Certain polyphenols from tobacco elicit antibodies and can induce inflammation. Smokers show a higher incidence of such sensitivity to tobacco than do nonsmokers. Cell-mediated hypersensitivity to collagen types II and III has also been observed. Endothelium-dependent vasodilatory responses in disease-free blood vessels are dysfunctional in some patients, suggesting a generalized impairment of endothelial function. HLA-A9 and HLA-B5 haplotypes are more common among Buerger patients, further suggesting that a genetically controlled hypersensitivity to tobacco is involved. In some patients, endothelial vasodilatory responses, even in seemingly normal vessels, are dysfunctional, suggesting a generalized impairment in endothelial function.

PATHOLOGY: The earliest change in Buerger disease is acute inflammation of medium-sized and small arteries. Neutrophilic infiltrates extend to involve neighboring veins and nerves. Endothelial involvement leads to thrombosis and obliteration of the lumen (Fig. 16-39A). Small microabscesses of the vessel wall, with a central area of neutrophils surrounded by fibroblasts and Langhans giant cells, distinguish this process from thrombosis associated with atherosclerosis. Early lesions often are severe enough to cause gangrene of the extremity, leading to amputation. Late in the course of the disease, thrombi are completely organized and partly canalized.

CLINICAL FEATURES: Symptoms of Buerger disease usually start between the ages of 25 and 40 years as intermittent claudication (cramping pains in muscles after exercise, quickly relieved by rest). Patients often present with painful ulceration of a digit, which progresses to destruction of the tips of the involved digits (Fig. 16-39B). Those who continue to smoke may slowly lose both hands and feet.

Behçet Disease Is a Vasculitis of Many Mucous Membranes

Behçet disease is a systemic vasculitis characterized by oral aphthous ulcers, genital ulcers, ocular inflammation, and occasional CNS, GI, and cardiovascular lesions. Both large and small vessels show vasculitis. The mucocutaneous lesions show nonspecific vasculitis involving arterioles, capillaries, and venules, with infiltration of vessel walls and perivascular tissue by lymphocytes and plasma cells. Occasional endothelial cells are proliferated and swollen. Medium and large arteries show destructive arteritis, with fibrinoid necrosis, mononuclear infiltration, thrombosis, aneurysms, and hemorrhage. The cause is unknown, but the effectiveness of corticosteroid treatment and an association with specific HLA subtypes suggest an immune basis.

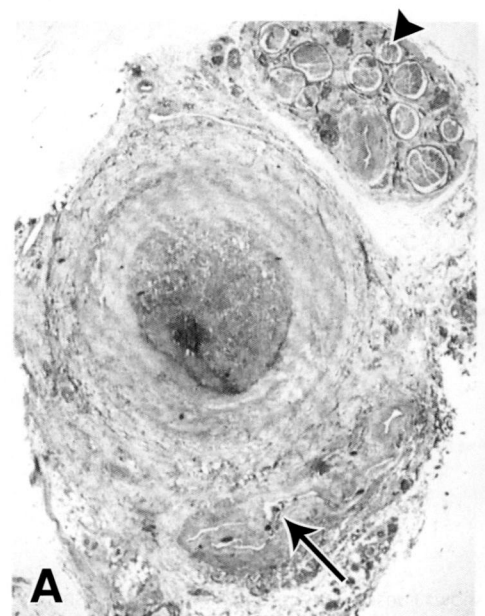
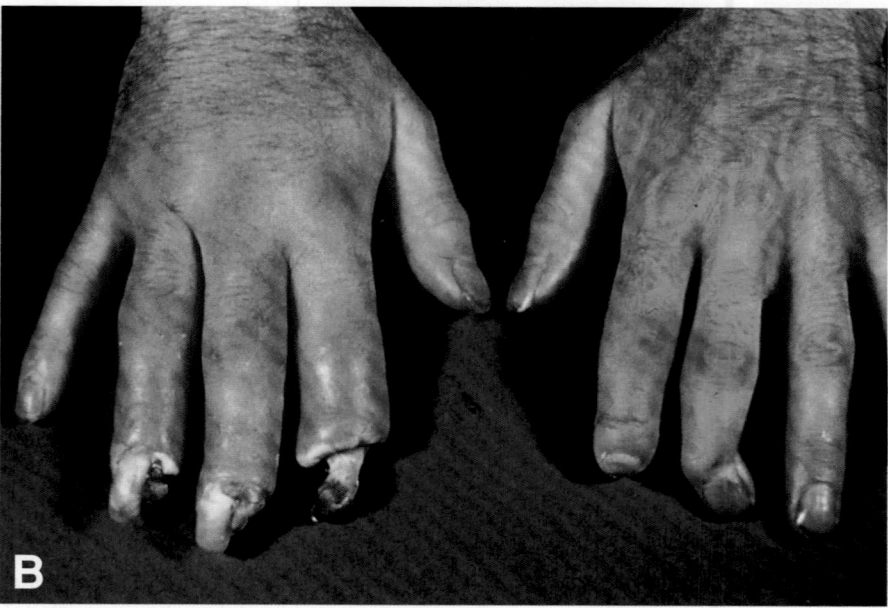

FIGURE 16-39. Buerger disease. A. Section of the upper extremity shows an organized arterial thrombus that has occluded the lumen. Some inflammatory cells are evident in the adventitial fat. In this instance, the vein (*arrow*) and the adjacent nerve (*arrowhead*) show foci of chronic inflammation. **B.** The hand shows necrosis of the tips of the fingers.

Radiation Vasculitis Has Acute and Chronic Phases

Acute radiation vasculitis shows endothelial injury and denudation, ballooning degeneration of intimal smooth muscle cells, and macrophages and smooth muscle cell necrosis in the media, which may appear fibrinoid. Thrombi occur in small arteries and arterioles. In the chronic phase, intimal hyperplasia and vessel wall fibrosis are prominent. Vessels may be completely scarred and occluded. Radiation damage predisposes to accelerated atherosclerosis.

Rickettsial Vasculitis Is Caused by Intracellular Parasites

Rickettsiae are obligate intracellular parasites that produce a characteristic vasculitis (see Chapter 9). Each rickettsial disease affects different types of small vessels, and to variable extent and severity. The organisms usually disseminate from the entry site into the blood and invade endothelial cells, smooth muscle cells of the media of small vessels and capillaries.

ANEURYSMS

Arterial aneurysms are localized vascular dilations due to congenital or acquired weakness of the media. They are not rare, and their incidence tends to rise with age. Aneurysms of the aorta and other arteries are found in as many as 10% of unselected autopsies. Aneurysm walls are formed by stretched arterial wall remnants.

Aneurysms are classified by location (which artery or vein, e.g., aorta or popliteal vein), configuration, and etiology (Fig. 16-40). There are several categories of aneurysms:

- **Fusiform aneurysms** are ovoid swellings parallel to the long axis of the vessel.

- **Saccular aneurysms** are bubble-like arterial wall outpouchings at a site of weakened media.
- **Dissecting aneurysms** are actually dissecting hematomas, in which blood from hemorrhage into the media separates the layers of the vascular wall.
- **Arteriovenous aneurysms** are direct conduits between an artery and a vein.

Abdominal Aortic Aneurysms Complicate Atherosclerosis

AAAs are dilations that increase vessel wall diameter by at least 50%. They are the most common aneurysms, usually develop after age 50, and are associated with severe atherosclerosis of the artery. The prevalence rises to 6% after age 80. They occur much more often in men than in women, and half of patients are hypertensive. Occasionally, aneurysms may be found in all parts of the thoracic aorta and in iliac and popliteal arteries.

 PATHOPHYSIOLOGY: AAAs invariably occur in the context of atherosclerosis. However, the disease is probably multifactorial, with inflammation and dysregulation of matrix remodeling and repair. The growth of the aneurysm is regulated in part by hemodynamic forces that occur in the aneurysm; as the radius of the vessel increases, so does circumferential wall stress. Enzymes important in proteolysis of medial and adventitial type I/III fibrillar collagen promote the growth of abdominal aneurysms. These include MMPs; cysteine protease cathepsins K, L, and S; and osteoclastic proton pump vH$^+$-ATPase. Proinflammatory cytokines, such as IL-1β, TNF-α, monocyte chemotactin protein-1 (MCP-1), and IL-8, have also been linked to the pathogenesis of abdominal aneurysms. The walls of AAAs contain

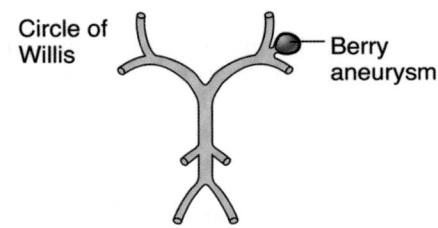

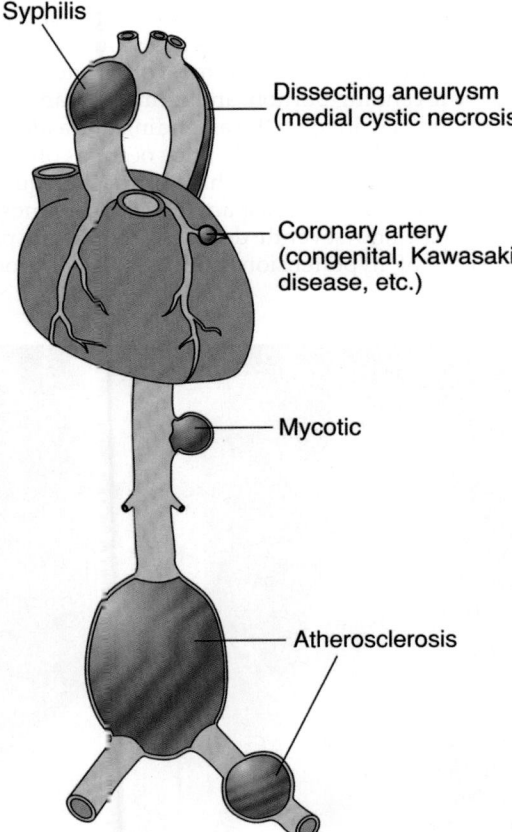

FIGURE 16-40. The locations of aneurysms. Syphilitic aneurysms are the common variety in the ascending aorta, which is usually spared by the atherosclerotic process. Atherosclerotic aneurysms can occur in the abdominal aorta or muscular arteries, including the coronary and popliteal arteries and other vessels. Berry aneurysms are seen in the circle of Willis, mainly at branch points; their rupture leads to subarachnoid hemorrhage. Mycotic aneurysms occur almost anywhere that bacteria can deposit on vessel walls.

chemokines and growth factors that regulate remodeling—for example, granulocyte colony-stimulating factor (G-CSF), macrophage colony-stimulating factor (M-CSF), IL-13, IGF-1, TGFβ, and macrophage inflammatory proteins (MIP)-1α and -1β. Familial clustering suggests a genetic predisposition, but this is poorly understood.

 PATHOLOGY: Most AAAs occur distal to the renal arteries and proximal to the aortic bifurcation (Fig. 16-41). They are usually fusiform, but saccular varieties do occur. Any sized aneurysm may be

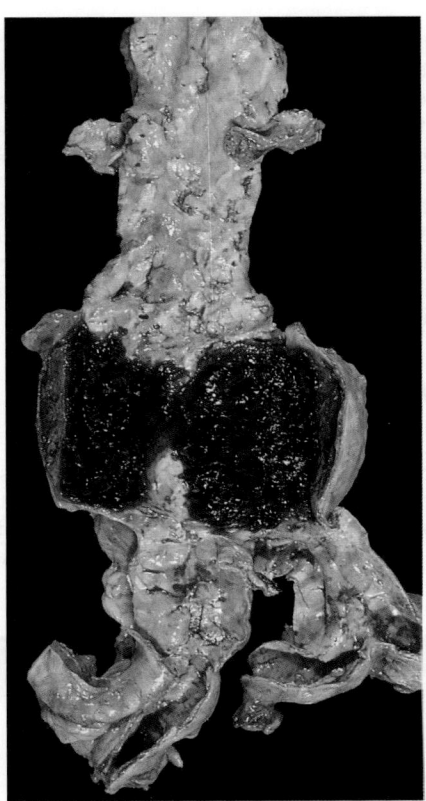

FIGURE 16-41. Atherosclerotic aneurysm of the abdominal aorta. The aneurysm has been opened longitudinally to reveal a large mural thrombus in the lumen. The aorta and common iliac arteries display complicated lesions of atherosclerosis.

symptomatic, but most symptomatic lesions are >5–6 cm. Some extend into the iliac arteries, which occasionally have additional aneurysms, beyond to the one in the aorta. Aneurysms that extend above the renal arteries may occlude the origin of the superior mesenteric artery and the celiac axis.

Most of these aneurysms are lined by raised, ulcerated, and calcified (complicated) atherosclerotic lesions. Most also contain variably organized mural thrombi, portions of which may embolize to peripheral arteries. Infrequently, a thrombus itself enlarges enough to compromise aortic blood flow.

Walls of AAAs complicated by atherosclerotic lesions are destroyed and replaced by fibrous tissue. There are focal remnants of normal media, with atheromatous lesions extending to variable depths. The adventitia is thickened and focally inflamed in response to severe atherosclerosis.

CLINICAL FEATURES: Many AAAs are asymptomatic and are discovered only when a mass in the abdomen is palpated or appears on radiologic examination done for some other reason. Patients may complain of abdominal pain, which often reflects the aneurysm's expansion. Abrupt occlusion of a peripheral artery by an embolus from a mural thrombus may present suddenly with ischemic symptoms. Rupture and exsangui-nation into the retroperitoneum (or chest) are the most dreaded complications, in which case patients present emer-gently with pain, shock, and a pulsatile abdominal mass. Half of such patients die, even with prompt surgical inter-vention. Therefore, even asymptomatic large aneurysms are often replaced by or bypassed with prosthetic grafts.

The risk of rupture of an abdominal aortic aneurysm depends on its size. Aneurysms <4 cm rarely rupture (2%); 25% to 40% of those >5 cm rupture within 5 years of their discovery.

Cerebral Arterial Aneurysms Cause Subarachnoid Hemorrhage

The most common type of cerebral aneurysm is a saccular structure known as **berry aneurysm,** because it resembles a berry attached to a twig of the arterial tree. Berry aneu-rysms reflect congenital defects in arterial walls and tend to

arise at branches in the circle of Willis or at arterial junctions (see Chapter 32). The most common sites are between the anterior cerebral and anterior communicating arteries; the internal carotid and posterior communicating arteries; and the first main divisions of the middle cerebral artery and the bifurcation of the internal carotid artery.

In Dissecting Aneurysms Blood Tunnels Into the Arterial Wall

The dissection occurs on a path along the length of the vessel (Fig. 16-42) and essentially represents a false lumen within the arterial wall. Dissecting aneurysms most often affect the aorta, especially the ascending portion, and its major branches. Tho-racic dissections may involve the ascending aorta alone (type A) or only the distal aorta (type B). They occur as often as 1 in 400 autopsies, with men affected three times as frequently as women. They may affect almost any age, but are most com-mon in the sixth and seventh decades. Almost all patients have a history of hypertension, and associated conditions

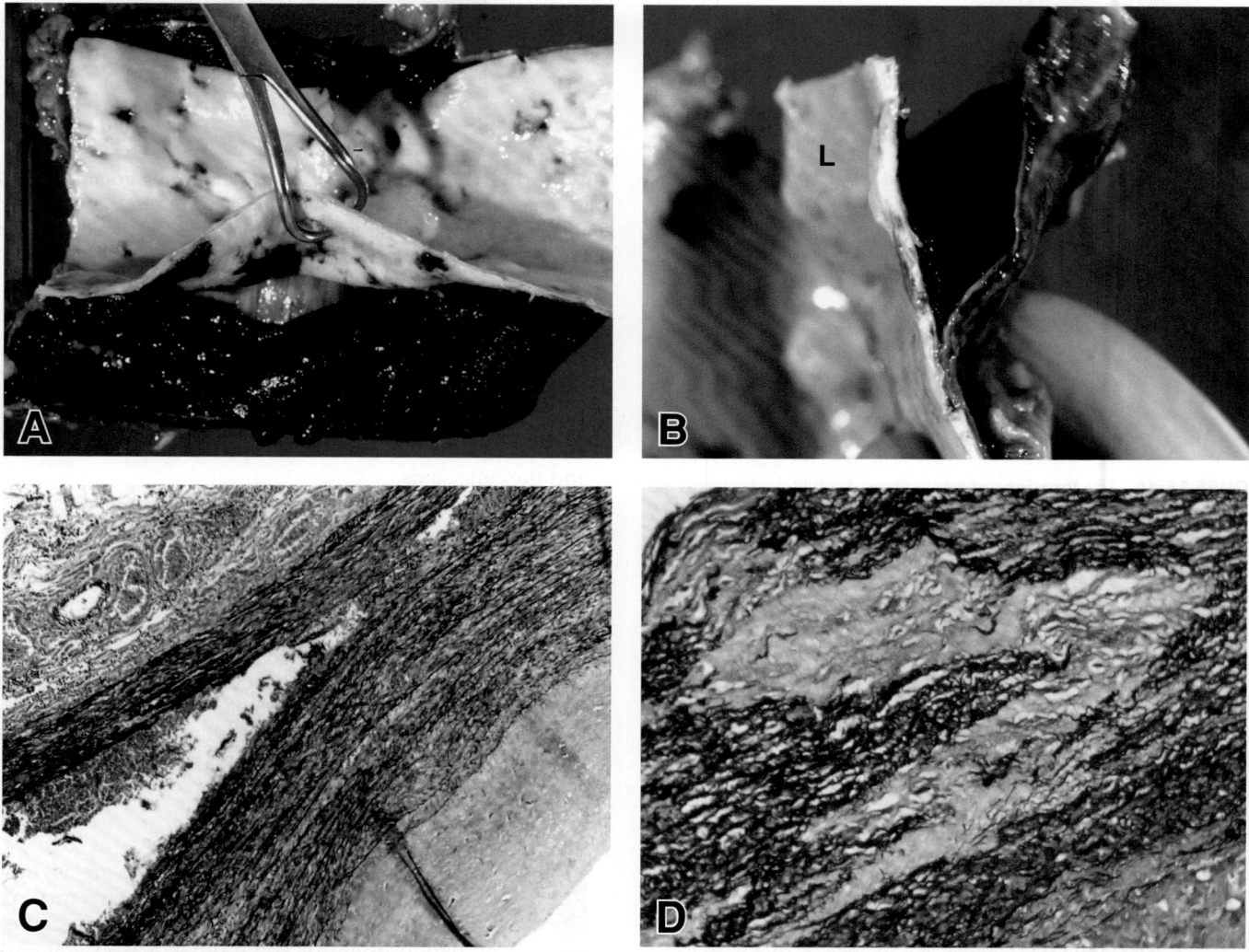

FIGURE 16-42. Dissecting aortic aneurysm. A. Thoracic aorta with metal clamps revealing the dissection and hematoma in the wall with old blood clot. **B.** The thoracic aorta has been opened longitudinally and reveals clotted blood dissecting the media of the vessel. *L* = lumen. **C.** Athero-sclerotic aorta with dissection along the outer third of the media (elastic stain). **D.** A section of the aortic wall stained with aldehyde fuchsin shows pools of metachromatic material characteristic of the degenerative process known as cystic medial necrosis.

include atherosclerosis, bicuspid aortic valve, and idiopathic aortic root dilation.

 PATHOPHYSIOLOGY: Dissecting aneurysms usually reflect weakened aortic media. The changes were originally described as **cystic medial necrosis (of Erdheim)**, because focal loss of elastic and muscle fibers in the media leads to "cystic" spaces filled with a metachromatic myxoid material. These spaces are not true cysts but are rather pools of matrix collected between the cells and tissues of the media. The mechanisms of medial degeneration are not well understood. However, some cases occur with specific disorders—Marfan, Ehlers–Danlos, and Loeys–Dietz syndromes, and with filamin mutations. In Marfan syndrome, a systemic connective tissue abnormality, specific mutations in the gene encoding fibrillin (an extracellular matrix protein) have been identified (see Chapter 6). Some patients have mutations in other genes, including TGFβ receptors 1 and 2, smooth muscle cell–specific β–myosin (MYH11), and α–actin (ACTA2). Aging also causes mild degenerative changes in the aorta, with focal elastin loss and medial fibrosis. Patients with thoracic aorta dissections show decreased expression of fibulin-5, an extracellular protein that regulates elastic fiber assembly. Abnormal release of MMP-2 and its inhibitor by smooth muscle cells has also been implicated. In animals, defective cross-linking of collagen induced by a copper-deficient diet (lysyl oxidase is a copper-dependent enzyme) causes dissecting aneurysm of the aorta. The same lesion is produced by feeding β–aminopropionitrile, an inhibitor of lysyl oxidase. People with Wilson disease who are treated with penicillamine, a copper chelator, also may develop medial necrosis of the aorta. Taken together, these data suggest that the common factor in these several situations is a molecular defect that brings on weakness of aortic connective tissue.

PATHOLOGY: The triggering event for medial dissection is controversial. Over 95% of cases have a transverse tear in the intima and internal media. The spontaneous laceration in the intima allows blood from the lumen to enter and dissect the media. Alternatively, hemorrhage from vasa vasorum into a media weakened by cystic medial necrosis may initiate stress on the intima, in turn causing the ubiquitous intimal tear.

Most intimal tears are in the ascending aorta, 1 to 2 cm above the aortic ring. Dissection in the media occurs within seconds and separates the inner 2/3 of the aorta from the outer third. It can also involve coronary arteries, great vessels of the neck, and renal, mesenteric, or iliac arteries. Since the outer wall of the false channel of the dissecting aneurysm is thin, hemorrhage into the extravascular space—including the pericardium, mediastinum, pleural space, and retroperitoneum—frequently causes death. In 5% to 10% of cases, the blood within the dissection reenters the lumen via a second distal tear to form a "double-barreled aorta." In a comparable proportion, a reentry site produces communication of the aorta with a major artery, most often the iliac artery.

CLINICAL FEATURES: Patients typically present with acute onset of severe, "tearing" pain in the anterior chest, which may be misdiagnosed as myocardial infarction. Loss of one or more arterial pulses is common, as is a murmur of aortic regurgitation. Hypertension is a frequent finding in patients with dissecting aneurysms, but hypotension ominously suggests aortic rupture. Cardiac tamponade or congestive heart failure is diagnosed by the usual criteria.

Before antihypertensive and surgical treatments were available, mortality was very high, with 80% of patients dying within 2 weeks, and half of the rest within 3 months. Now, prompt surgical intervention and control of hypertension have reduced overall mortality to under 20%.

Syphilitic Aneurysms Reflect Inflammation of Aortic Vasa Vasorum

Syphilis was once the most common cause of aortic aneurysms, but as the infection has become less common, so has syphilitic vascular disease, including aortitis and aneurysms. Syphilitic aneurysms mainly affect the vasa vasorum of the ascending aorta, which show periarteritis and obliterative endarteritis. Vasa vasorum ramify in the adventitia and penetrate the outer and middle thirds of the aorta. There, they become encircled by lymphocytes, plasma cells, and macrophages, with lumenal obliteration causing focal aortic wall medial necrosis and scarring, disrupting elastic lamellae. The depressed medial scars create a roughened intimal surface, a "tree-bark" appearance (Fig. 16-43). The relentless pressure of the blood eventually forces the weakened wall of the ascending aorta and aortic arch to form a fusiform aneurysm, which may rupture.

Mycotic Aneurysms Are Microbial Infections of Vessel Walls

Mycotic (infectious) aneurysms tend to rupture and bleed. They may develop in the aortic wall or in cerebral vessels during septicemia, most commonly due to bacterial endocarditis. Mesenteric, splenic, or renal arteries are also commonly affected. Mycotic aneurysms may also occur adjacent to a focus of tuberculous or a bacterial abscess.

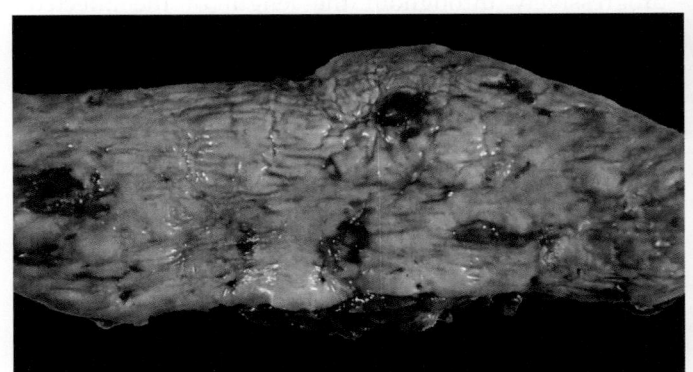

FIGURE 16-43. Syphilitic aortitis. The thoracic aorta is dilated, and its inner surface shows the typical "tree-bark" appearance.

VEINS

Varicose Veins Are Enlarged and Tortuous

Superficial varicosities of leg veins, usually in the saphenous system, are very common. They vary from a trivial knot of dilated veins to painful and disabling distention of the whole venous system of the leg, with secondary trophic disturbances. Up to 10% to 20% of the population has some varicosities in leg veins, of which only a fraction develop symptoms.

 ETIOLOGIC FACTORS: There are several risk factors for varicose veins:

- **Age:** Varicose veins increase in frequency with age and may reach 50% in people over 50 years. This increased incidence may reflect age-related degenerative changes in venous wall connective tissue, loss of supporting fat and connective tissues, more flaccid muscle tone, and inactivity.
- **Gender:** Among 30 to 50 year olds, women are more often affected by varicose veins than men, particularly those who have experienced increased venous pressure on the iliac veins from a pregnant uterus.
- **Heredity:** There is a strong familial predisposition to varicose veins, possibly due to inherited configurations or structural weaknesses of the venous walls or valves.
- **Posture:** Leg vein pressure is 5 to 10 times higher when a person is erect rather than when recumbent. Thus, varicose veins and their complications are more common in people whose occupations require them to stand for long periods.
- **Obesity:** Excessive body weight predisposes to varicose veins, possibly because of increased intra-abdominal pressure or poor external support provided by subcutaneous fat.

Other factors that raise venous pressure in the legs can cause varicose veins, including pelvic tumors, congestive heart failure, and thrombotic obstruction of the main venous trunks of the thigh or pelvis.

In the pathogenesis of varicose veins, it is not clear which comes first: valvular incompetence or venous dilation. Whatever the case, the two reinforce each other. As the vein increases in length and diameter, tortuosities develop. Once the process begins, the varicosity extends progressively throughout the length of the affected vein. As each valve becomes incompetent, increasing strain is put on the vessel and valve below. The role of inflammation is unclear, but affected veins may show elevated expression of leukocyte–endothelial adhesion molecules.

PATHOLOGY: Varicose veins show variations in wall thickness. Some areas are thin and dilated, while others are thickened by smooth muscle hypertrophy, subintimal fibrosis, and incorporation of mural thrombi into the wall. Patchy calcification is common. Valve deformities include thickening, shortening, and rolling of the cusps.

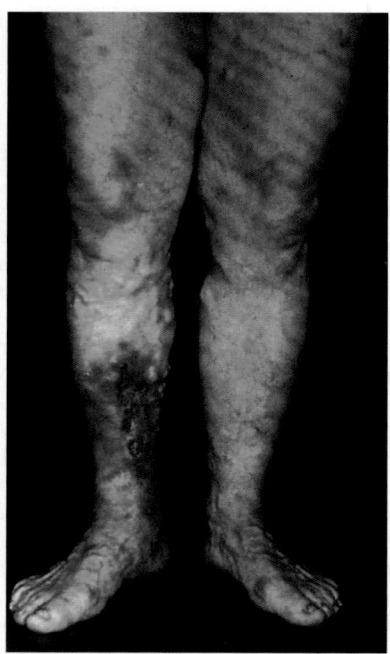

FIGURE 16-44. Varicose veins of the legs. Severe varicosities of the superficial leg veins have led to stasis dermatitis and secondary ulcerations.

CLINICAL FEATURES: Visual inspection makes the diagnosis of varicose veins of the leg. Most affected vessels and veins have little clinical effect and are mainly cosmetic problems. The principal symptoms are aching in the legs, aggravated by standing and relieved by elevation. Severe varicosities (Fig. 16-44) may give rise to trophic changes in the skin drained by the affected veins, called **stasis dermatitis**. Surgery is required if the overlying skin has ulcerated or if spontaneous bleeding or extensive thrombosis (which may lead to pulmonary embolism) occurs.

Varicose Veins Also Occur at Other Sites

HEMORRHOIDS: These are dilations of the veins of the rectum and anal canal and may occur inside or outside the anal sphincter (see Chapter 19). There may be a hereditary predisposition, but factors that increase intra-abdominal pressure contribute strongly. These include constipation, pregnancy, and venous obstruction by rectal tumors. Hemorrhoids often bleed, an occurrence that may be confused with bleeding rectal cancers. Thrombosed hemorrhoids are exquisitely painful.

ESOPHAGEAL VARICES: This complication of portal hypertension is caused mainly by hepatic cirrhosis (see Chapter 20). High portal pressure distends anastomoses between portal and systemic venous circulations at the lower end of the esophagus. Although they may be prominent radiologically, esophageal varices are usually unimpressive at autopsy. They collapse at death, leaving bluish streaks in the esophageal mucosa. Hemorrhage from esophageal varices can be lethal in patients with cirrhosis.

VARICOCELE: Varicosities of the pampiniform plexus (see Chapter 23) may cause a palpable scrotal mass.

Deep Venous Thrombosis Mainly Affects Leg Veins

- **Thrombophlebitis** is inflammation and secondary thrombosis of small veins and sometimes larger ones, commonly as part of a local reaction to bacterial infection.
- **Phlebothrombosis** describes venous thrombosis that occurs without an initiating infection or inflammation.
- **Deep venous thrombosis (DVT)** (see Chapter 7) encompasses phlebothrombosis and thrombophlebitis. Since most cases of venous thrombosis are not associated with inflammation or infection, this condition is usually associated with prolonged bed rest or reduced cardiac output. It is most common in deep leg veins and can be a major threat to life because of pulmonary embolization (exemplified by sudden death with ambulation after surgery). Deficiencies of anticoagulants, such as protein C and antithrombin, increase the incidence of venous thromboembolism.

LYMPHATIC VESSELS

Lymphatic vessels are thin-walled low-pressure channels. They maintain normal tissue fluid balance, and provide drainage of plasma filtrates, cells, and foreign material from tissue interstitial spaces. They are also important in fat digestion, through lacteals in intestinal villi, and in immune surveillance. Lymphatic vessels have few tight junctions, and so are more permeable than blood vessels. NO• may act as a mediator of several growth factors that are lymphangiogenic and may be important in lymphatic function. For example, NO• may inhibit pumping in collecting lymphatics. Inflammation and tumors frequently spread via lymphatics.

MOLECULAR PATHOGENESIS: Fox2, the forkhead transcription factor, regulates lymphatic valve morphogenesis and maintains the lymphatic capillary phenotype late in development. The VEGF-C/VEGFR-3 pathway (see Chapter 5) mediates lymphatic endothelial cell migration, proliferation, and survival. Missense mutations in VEGFR-3 result in lymphedema and lymphatic hypoplasia. PROX-1 is essential for early steps in lymphatic formation, like budding from the anterior cardinal vein and forming lymph sacs. Along with podoplanin, VEGFR-3 and neuropilin-2, it also contributes to primary lymphatic plexus development. In inflammatory conditions, VEGF-C is upregulated by cytokines, and macrophages express VEGFR-3 and secrete VEGF-C. Experimentally, tumor metastasis and lymphangiogenesis can be blocked by inhibiting VEGF-C/VEGFR-3. In some patients, primary lymphedema is associated with mutations in VEGFR-3, FOXC2, SOX18, and germline GATA2.

Lymphangitis Reflects Infection in Lymphatic Vessels

Transport of infectious material to regional lymph nodes incites **lymphadenitis**. At the edges of inflammatory foci dilated lymphatics are filled with fluid exudate, cells, cellular debris, and bacteria. If tissues are expanded by exudate, there is comparable distention of lymphatic channels and an opening of intercellular channels between endothelial cells.

Almost any pathogen can cause acute lymphangitis, but β-hemolytic *Streptococci* (*S. pyogenes*) are particular offenders. Inflammation and infection may extend beyond lymphatic channels into surrounding tissues, and draining lymph nodes are regularly enlarged and inflamed. Painful subcutaneous red streaks, often with similarly painful regional lymph nodes, characterize acute lymphangitis.

Lymphatic Obstruction Causes Lymphedema

Scar tissue, intraluminal tumor cells, pressure from surrounding tumor, or plugging with parasites may all obstruct lymphatics. As collateral lymphatic channels are abundant, lymphedema (distention of tissue by lymph) usually occurs only when major trunks are obstructed, especially in the axilla or groin. For example, when radical mastectomy for breast cancer was routine, axillary lymph node dissection frequently disrupted lymphatic channels and led to lymphedema of the arm. Prolonged lymphatic obstruction causes progressive dilation of lymphatic vessels, or **lymphangiectasia,** and overgrowth of fibrous tissue. In **elephantiasis**, a lymphedematous limb becomes grossly enlarged. In tropical filariasis, a parasitic worm invades lymphatics, and commonly causes elephantiasis (see Chapter 9).

Milroy disease is an inherited type of lymphedema that is present at birth. It is associated with mutations in VEGF3 receptor, which is normally activated by VEGF-C and VEGF-D in lymphatic embryogenesis. It usually affects only one limb, but it may be more extensive and involve the eyelids and lips. Affected tissues show hugely dilated lymphatic channels, and the entire area appears honeycombed or spongy. This lesion is more properly considered lymphangiectasia rather than simply lymphedema.

BENIGN TUMORS OF BLOOD VESSELS

Tumors of the vascular system are common. Many are hamartomas, rather than true neoplasms. Some mutations have been linked to vascular anomalies. For example, endoglin and ALK-1 mutations have been identified in hereditary hemorrhagic telangiectasia, as have several gene mutations causing familial cerebral cavernous malformation.

Hemangiomas Are Common Benign Tumors of Vascular Channels

Hemangiomas usually occur in the skin but may also be found in internal organs.

 PATHOLOGY: *CAPILLARY HEMANGIOMA: This lesion contains vascular channels with the size and structure of normal capillaries.* Capillary hemangiomas may occur anywhere. The most common sites are skin; subcutaneous tissues; mucous membranes of the lips and mouth; and internal viscera, including spleen, kidneys, and liver. The lesions vary from a few millimeters to several centimeters. They are bright red to blue, depending on the degree of oxygenation of the blood. In the skin, capillary hemangiomas are called **birthmarks** or **ruby spots**. The only disability is cosmetic disfiguration.

JUVENILE HEMANGIOMA: Also called **strawberry hemangiomas,** these lesions occur on the skin of newborns. They grow rapidly in the first months of life, begin to fade at 1 to 3 years of age, and 80% completely regress by 5 years. Juvenile hemangiomas contain packed masses of capillaries separated by connective tissue stroma (Fig. 16-45). Endothelial-lined channels are usually filled with blood. Thromboses, sometimes organized, are common. Occasionally, the vascular channels rupture, causing scarring and accumulation of hemosiderin. Juvenile hemangiomas are usually well demarcated despite lacking capsules. Although finger-like projections of the vascular tissue may give the impression of invasion, these are benign; they do not invade or metastasize.

CAVERNOUS HEMANGIOMA: These lesions contain large vascular channels, often interspersed with small, capillary-type vessels. When they occur in the skin (Fig. 16-46), they are called **port wine stains**. They also appear on mucosal surfaces and visceral organs, including the spleen, liver, and pancreas. If they occur in the brain, they may enlarge slowly and cause neurologic symptoms after long quiescent periods.

Cavernous hemangiomas are red-blue, soft, spongy masses, up to several centimeters in diameter. Unlike capillary hemangiomas, these do not regress spontaneously. They are demarcated by sharp borders, but

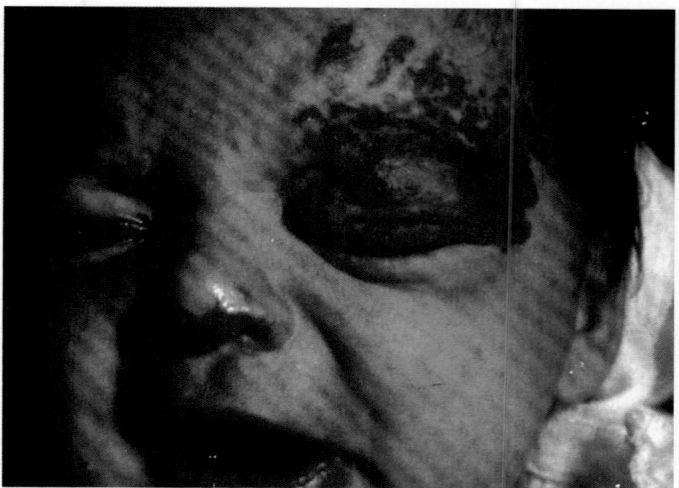

FIGURE 16-46. Congenital cavernous hemangioma of the skin.

are not encapsulated. Large endothelial-lined, blood-containing spaces are separated by sparse connective tissue. Cavernous hemangiomas can undergo a variety of changes, including thrombosis, fibrosis, cystic cavitation, and intracystic hemorrhage.

MULTIPLE HEMANGIOMATOUS SYNDROMES: More than one hemangioma may occur in a single tissue. Two or more tissues may be involved, such as skin and nervous system or spleen and liver. In **von Hippel–Lindau syndrome** (see Chapters 5 and 6), cavernous hemangiomas occur in the cerebellum or brainstem and the retina. **Sturge–Weber syndrome** involves a developmental disturbance of blood vessels in the brain and skin. Other closely related lesions are plexiform or racemose angiomas, cirsoid aneurysms, and angiomatous dilation of vessels of the brain and elsewhere.

 ETIOLOGIC FACTORS: Although hemangiomas are clearly benign, their origin is uncertain; they may be true neoplasms or they may be hamartomas. Evidence favoring the latter includes (1) the lesion is present at birth; (2) it grows only as the rest of the body grows and remains limited in size; and (3) after growth ceases, it usually remains unchanged indefinitely absent of trauma, thrombosis or hemorrhage.

The development of these vascular malformations recapitulates vascular embryology. A network of endothelial channels undergoes remodeling, acquiring a muscular coat and adventitia. In this view, vascular malformations reflect persistence of the original or modified channels and mixtures of connective tissue elements derived from the mesenchyme. Hemangiomas are classified by histologic type and location. Molecular characterization will likely provide new classifications and better understanding of these lesions.

Glomus Tumors Are Painful Tumors of the Glomus Body

Glomus bodies are normal neuromyoarterial receptors that are sensitive to temperature and regulate arteriolar flow.

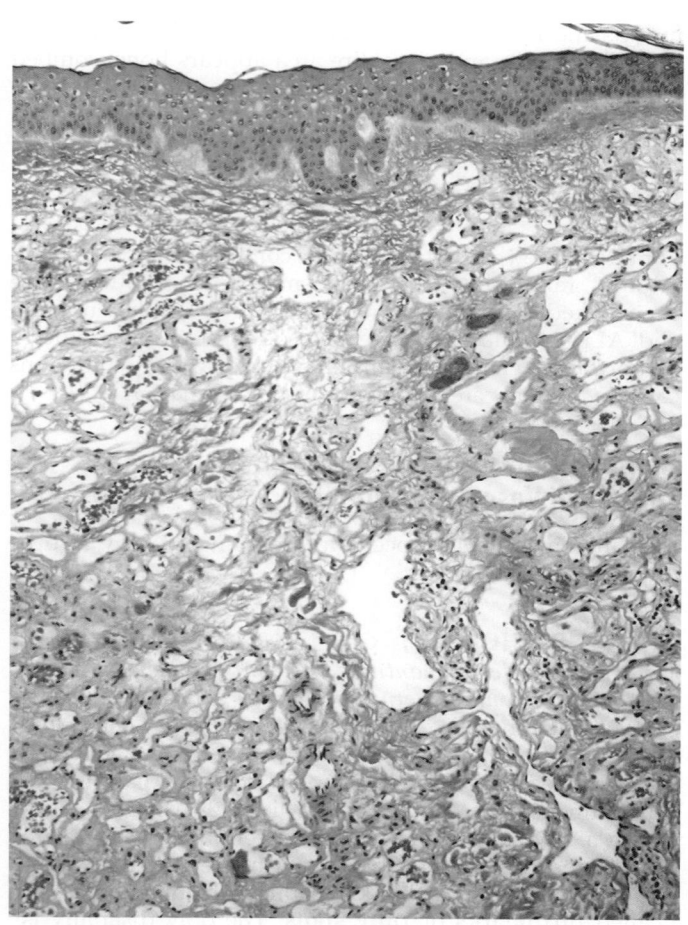

FIGURE 16-45. Juvenile hemangioma. A network of delicate, anastomosing vessels is present subcutaneously.

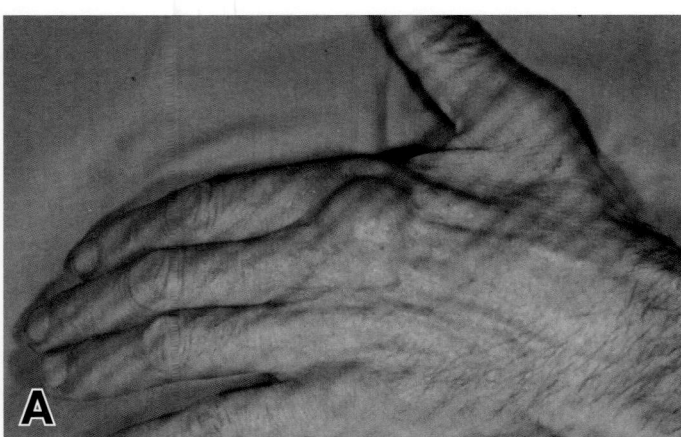
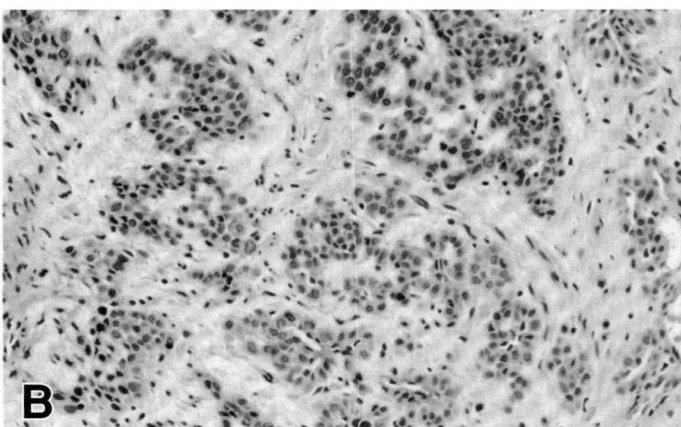

FIGURE 16-47. Glomus tumor. A. The dorsal surface of the hand displays a prominent tumor nodule on the proximal third finger. **B.** A photomicrograph of (**A**) reveals nests of glomus tumor cells embedded in a fibrovascular stroma.

They occur widely in the skin, mostly in the distal fingers and toes. This parallels the sites of glomus tumors (glomangiomas), typically under the nails. The lesions tend to be unusually painful.

PATHOLOGY: Glomus tumors are small, usually <1 cm; many are smaller than a few millimeters. In the skin, they are slightly elevated, rounded, red-blue, and firm (Fig. 16-47). The main histologic components are branching vascular channels in a connective tissue stroma and aggregates or nests of specialized glomus cells. The latter are regular, round to cuboidal cells that resemble smooth muscle cell ultrastructurally.

Hemangioendotheliomas Are Intermediate Between Hemangiomas and Angiosarcomas

Epithelioid or histiocytoid hemangioendotheliomas have endothelial cells with abundant eosinophilic, often vacuolated, cytoplasm. Vascular lumina are evident, as are a few mitoses. These tumors occur in almost all locations. They may recur locally, and about 1/5 develop metastases, but surgical removal is generally curative.

Spindle cell hemangioendotheliomas occur mostly in males of any age, usually in the dermis and subcutaneous tissue of distal extremities. They contain vascular, endothelial-lined spaces into which papillary projections extend.

MALIGNANT TUMORS OF BLOOD VESSELS

Malignant vascular neoplasms are rare. They rarely arise in preexisting benign tumors.

Angiosarcoma Is a Rare Malignant Tumor of Endothelial Cells

These tumors occur in either sex and at any age. They begin as small, painless, sharply demarcated, red nodules, most commonly in the skin, soft tissue, breast, bone, liver, and spleen. Eventually, most enlarge to become pale gray, fleshy masses without a capsule. Angiosarcomas often undergo central necrosis, with softening and hemorrhage.

PATHOLOGY: Angiosarcomas show variable differentiation, from those composed mainly of distinct vascular elements to undifferentiated tumors with few recognizable blood channels (Fig. 16-48). The latter have frequent mitoses, pleomorphism, and giant cells, and tend to be more aggressive. Almost half of patients with angiosarcoma die of the disease.

Hepatic angiosarcomas have been associated with environmental carcinogens, particularly arsenic (in pesticides) and vinyl chloride (used in production of plastics). They occurred in patients given thorium dioxide, a radioactive contrast medium (Thorotrast) used by radiologists before 1950. Thorotrast, engulfed by macrophages in liver sinusoids, remained there for life.

There is a long latent period between exposure to the chemicals or radionuclide and development of hepatic angiosarcoma. The earliest detectable changes are atypia and diffuse hyperplasia of the cells lining the hepatic sinusoids. The tumors are frequently multicentric and may arise in the spleen as well. Hepatic angiosarcomas are highly malignant and spread by both local invasion and metastasis.

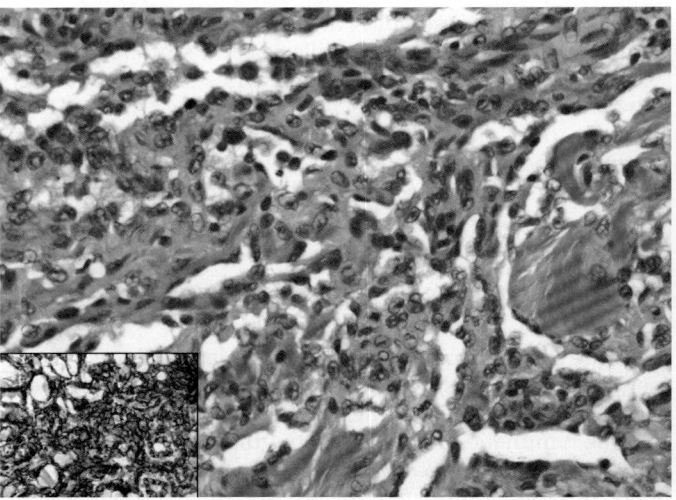

FIGURE 16-48. Angiosarcoma. Malignant spindly cells line vague channels. *Inset.* Immunostain for CD31, an endothelial marker.

Hemangiopericytomas Are Rare Tumors of Pericytes

Pericytes, which are modified smooth muscle cells, lie outside capillary and arteriolar walls. However, it is not clear that these tumors actually derive from these cells. Hemangiopericytomas present as masses of capillary-like channels surrounded by, and frequently enclosed within, nests and masses of round to spindle-shaped cells. Tumor cells are characteristically invested by a basement membrane.

These tumors can occur anywhere but are most common in the retroperitoneum and legs. Most are removed surgically without having invaded or metastasized. Malignant hemangiopericytomas metastasize to lungs, bone, liver, and lymph nodes.

Kaposi Sarcoma Is Caused by Human Herpesvirus 8

Kaposi sarcoma is a malignant angioproliferative tumor derived from endothelial cells.

EPIDEMIOLOGY: Kaposi sarcoma was originally described in the 19th century by Moritz Kaposi in Vienna. It also occurred as a sporadic tumor endemic in parts of central Africa, but was otherwise an oddity that mainly afflicted older men. It is now seen in epidemic form in immunosuppressed patients, especially those with AIDS. Human herpesvirus 8 (HHV8), also called Kaposi sarcoma–associated herpes virus (KSHV), is responsible for this tumor, which arises in endothelial cells. About 10% of the US population is HHV8 positive, but only a small fraction of them develop Kaposi sarcoma. VEGF and hypoxia-inducible factor (HIF) seem to play important roles in pathogenesis of the tumor, as does the PI3K/Akt/mTOR pathway (see Chapters 1 and 5). What determines whether Kaposi sarcoma develops in HHV8+ individuals is unclear.

PATHOLOGY: Kaposi sarcomas start as painful purple or brown 1-mm to 1-cm cutaneous nodules. They appear most often on the hands or feet but may occur anywhere. Their histology is highly variable. One form resembles a simple hemangioma, with tightly packed clusters of capillaries and scattered hemosiderin-laden macrophages. Other types are highly cellular with less prominent vascular spaces (Fig. 16-49). They may be difficult to distinguish from fibrosarcomas, but immunochemistry identifies their endothelial origin. Kaposi sarcomas are considered malignant, and may be widely distributed in the body, but they rarely cause death.

TUMORS OF THE LYMPHATIC SYSTEM

There are many histologic and clinical variants of local enlargements of lymphatics, but it is difficult to distinguish among anomalies, proliferations due to stasis and true neoplasms. In general, lymphatic tumors are distinguished by their size and location. The spaces may be small, as in capillary lymphangiomas, or large and dilated, as in cystic or cavernous lesions. Lymphangiomatous lesions can arise at almost any site, including skin, mediastinum, retroperitoneum, and spleen.

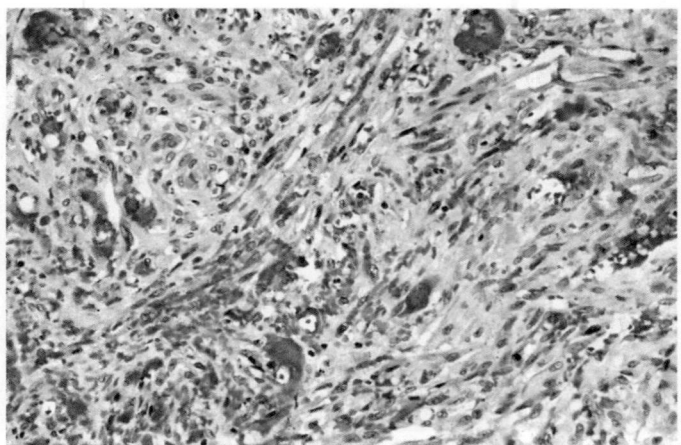

FIGURE 16-49. Kaposi sarcoma. A photomicrograph of a vascular lesion from a patient with acquired immune deficiency syndrome shows numerous poorly differentiated, spindle-shaped neoplastic cells and a vascular lesion filled with red blood cells.

Capillary Lymphangiomas May Be Single or Multiple

These small, benign tumors are circumscribed, grayish-pink, fleshy nodules. They are subcutaneous and occur on the skin of the face, lips, chest, genitalia, or extremities. Capillary lymphangiomas contain variably sized, thin-walled spaces lined by endothelial cells, with lymph and occasional leukocytes.

Cystic Lymphangiomas Are Often Congenital Lesions

These benign lesions (also called **cystic hygromas,** see Chapter 6) are most common in the neck and axilla but also may occur in the mediastinum and retroperitoneum. They may reach 10 to 15 cm or more, and fill the axilla or distort the neck.

PATHOLOGY: Cystic lymphangiomas are soft, spongy, and pink. Watery fluid exudes from their cut surfaces. They contain endothelial-lined spaces filled with protein-rich fluid. These spaces differ from blood vessels because they lack erythrocytes and leukocytes. Abundant irregularly distributed smooth muscle and connective tissue cells may be present.

Lymphangiosarcoma May Occur After Lymphedema or Radiation

These rare malignant tumors develop in 0.1% to 0.5% of patients with lymphedema of the arm after radical mastectomy. Distinction between this tumor and angiosarcoma is difficult, and some authors equate the two. Lymphangiosarcoma may also occur in other regions, for example, in the leg after radiation therapy for uterine cervical carcinoma.

PATHOLOGY: Lymphangiosarcomas are purplish, frequently multiple, nodules in edematous skin. Their cells resemble capillary endothelial cells and show intercellular zonulae adherentes. The walls of tumor vessels have a rudimentary form of basal basement membrane. Lymphangiosarcomas are highly aggressive. Even with radical surgery, their prognosis is poor.

17 The Heart

Jeffrey E. Saffitz

INTRODUCTION

The heart is a fist-sized muscular pump that has the remarkable capacity to work unceasingly for the 90 or more years of a human lifetime. On average, it pumps 8,000 L of blood each day. As demand requires, it can increase its output many fold, in part because the coronary circulation can augment its blood flow to 5× normal. It also responds to short-term increases in workload by increasing heart rate and contractility, the latter in accordance with the Frank–Starling law of the heart. If it must increase workload for longer periods (e.g., systemic hypertension), the left ventricle hypertrophies, an adaptation that increases its work capacity. However, this compensatory mechanism has its limits: The heart reaches a point where it can no longer supply blood adequately to peripheral tissues; the result is heart failure. Damage to the myocardium, caused most commonly by coronary artery disease, also limits the left ventricle's ability to pump blood and similarly results in heart failure.

CARDIAC ANATOMY

The heart of a normal adult man weighs 280 to 340 g; that of a normal adult woman, 230 to 280 g. It is a two-sided pump. Blood enters each side through a thin-walled **atrium**, from which it is propelled forward by thicker muscular **ventricles**. The right ventricle is considerably thinner (<0.5 cm) than the left ventricle (1.3 to 1.5 cm) because the right side has low venous filling pressure and relatively low afterload.

Blood enters the ventricles across atrioventricular valves, the mitral valve on the left and the tricuspid valve on the right. The leaflets of these valves are tethered by chordae tendineae, strong fibrous cords attached to the inner ventricular wall surface by papillary muscles. The entrances to the aorta and pulmonary arteries are guarded, respectively by the aortic and pulmonary valves, each with three semilunar cusps.

The heart wall has three layers: outer epicardium, middle myocardium, and inner endocardium. Visceral and parietal pericardia, separated by the pericardial cavity, surround the heart.

Cardiac Myocytes Generate Contractile Force

The myocardium is a network of individual myocytes linked by intercalated disks containing cell–cell adhesion and electrical junctions. Electron microscopy reveals the structure and distribution of the sarcolemma, **sarcoplasmic reticulum** (SR), T tubules, nucleus, and *many* mitochondria (a normal heart consumes >15 times its weight in ATP daily) (Fig. 17-1A). Myocyte contractile elements, called **myofilaments**, are arranged in bundles called **myofibrils**. These are separated by

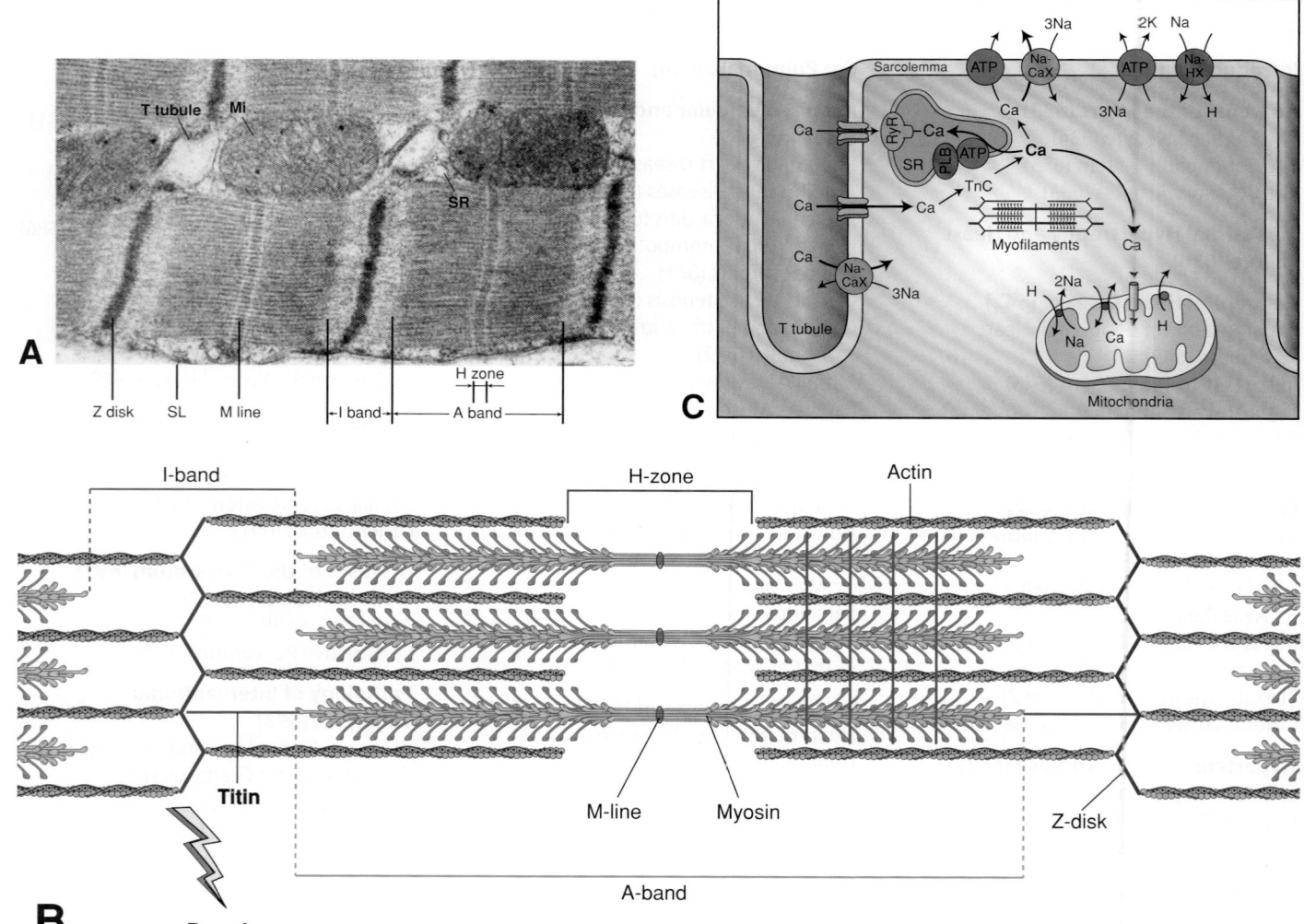

FIGURE 17-1. Ultrastructure of the myocardium. A. Electron micrograph of a ventricular myocyte sectioned longitudinally, showing the sarcolemma (SL) and sarcomeres composed of myofibrils. Sarcomeres are delimited by Z disks and include M lines, H zones, A bands, and I bands. Also present are mitochondria (Mi), sarcoplasmic reticulum (SR) and T tubules. I bands and H zones are absent when myofibrils are contracted. **B.** The molecular basis for the banding seen in the electron micrograph. In each sarcomere, thick filaments composed of myosin extend from the M line toward Z disks. Myosin head-domains form the cross-bridges that generate force by interacting with the thin actin filaments, which are connected to Z disks. The amount of force that can be generated is proportional to the extent to which myosin and actin filaments overlap and is maximal when sarcomeres are between 2 and 2.2 µm long. When sarcomeres are less than 2 µm, the thin filaments slide across each other and overlap, decreasing the potential for force-generating cross-links; similarly, when the sarcomeres are stretched beyond 2.2 µm, force is decreased proportionately to the widening of the H zone. This mechanism can be invoked as the basis for the Frank–Starling law of the heart. The giant sarcomeric protein titin spans the full distance between the Z disk and the M line within each sarcomere and contributes to the viscoelastic properties of the myocyte. The intermediate filament protein desmin extends across the full length of the myocyte and binds to Z disks of each sarcomere, thus helping to maintain sarcomeres in register. **C.** Pathways regulating Ca^{2+} homeostasis and excitation–contraction coupling in cardiac myocytes. The cardiac action potential brings depolarizing current into T tubules where voltage-gated L-type Ca^{2+} channels reside in high concentrations (green channel structures). Influx of Ca^{2+} through these channels stimulates Ca^{2+} release from the SR (located in immediate proximity to the T tubule) via the ryanodine receptor, RyR2. The transient increase in cytosolic Ca^{2+} concentration promotes contraction through interactions with cardiac troponin T (TnC). Resting diastolic Ca^{2+} levels are restored by reuptake into the SR and extrusion via sodium–calcium exchange (Na-CaX) and an ATP pump.

mitochondria and SR. Myofibrils are organized into repeating units called **sarcomeres**.

The sarcomere is the basic functional unit of the contractile apparatus. It contains a Z disk on each end and interdigitated thick and thin filaments, oriented perpendicular to the Z disk (Fig. 17-1B). The thick filaments contain myosin heavy chains, myosin-binding protein C, and myosin light chains. The thick filaments are limited to the A band and interact with the giant sarcomeric protein, **titin** (~27,000 amino acids), which spans from the Z disk to the M line, to form a third sarcomere filament system. Titin helps maintain precise assembly of myofibrillar proteins and contributes to the viscoelastic properties of cardiac muscle. The thin filaments contain actin and regulatory proteins, including α-**tropomyosin-1** and the **troponin complex** (cardiac troponins I, C, T), and extend from the Z disk through the I band and into the A band. Interaction of these myofilaments generates the force for contraction. The force that can be produced is proportional to the overlap between adjoining thick and thin filaments, and is maximal when sarcomeres are 2.0 to 2.2 μm.

When sarcomere length is under 2 μm, the thin filaments slide across each other and overlap, decreasing the potential for force-generating cross-links. If it is stretched beyond 2.2 μm, force decreases in proportion to the widening of the H zone. *This is the basis for the Frank–Starling law of the heart, which states that cardiac contractile force is a function of fiber length during diastole.* Average sarcomere length is about 2.2 μm when left ventricular end-diastolic pressure is at the upper limit of normal.

Increased cytosolic free calcium initiates cardiac muscle contraction. In a normal myocyte, an action potential triggers calcium ion entry into the myocyte through voltage-gated L-type Ca^{2+} channels in T tubules. These invaginations of the sarcolemma bring depolarizing current and resultant voltage-gated Ca^{2+} entry into intimate proximity to intracellular organelles regulating calcium homeostasis (lateral cisterns of the SR) and the contractile apparatus itself (Fig. 17-1C). Entering calcium stimulates release of Ca^{2+} sequestered in the SR (Ca^{2+}-induced Ca^{2+} release) via cardiac ryanodine receptors (RyR2) Increased cytosolic Ca^{2+} produces a conformational change in regulatory myofilament proteins, in particular troponin, allowing cross-bridges between actin and myosin to break and reform repeatedly. As a result, the filaments slide over one another, causing myocardial contraction. *The number of contractile sites activated and the resulting force generated are directly proportional to the concentration of Ca^{2+} near the myofibrils.*

The myocardium relaxes when cytosolic Ca^{2+} returns to its normal low (diastolic) concentration of 10^{-7} M. This process depends on calcium adenosine triphosphatase (ATPase) of the SR, which pumps Ca^{2+} from the cytosol into the SR. Outward Ca^{2+} transport by Na^+–Ca^{2+} exchange and sarcolemmal calcium pumps returns cytosolic Ca^{2+} also to normal resting diastolic concentration (Fig. 17-1C). *Thus, myocardial relaxation is an active, energy-requiring event.*

The Conduction System Consists of Specialized Myocytes

These myocytes have two major functions: (1) they initiate heartbeats by generating electrical current through their automatic rhythmicity, which is more rapid in the sinoatrial (SA) node than more distally in the system; and (2) they distribute this current to activate atrial and ventricular myocardium in an appropriate temporal–spatial pattern. Fibers of the atrioventricular (AV) conduction system generally conduct impulses faster (~1 to 2 m/sec) than do working (contractile) atrial and ventricular fibers (~0.5 to 1 m/sec). Conduction through the atrioventricular node is exceptionally slow (~0.1 m/sec). Slow conduction at the AV junction delays ventricular activation and facilitates ventricular filling.

Heartbeats normally originate in the SA node, near the junction of the superior vena cava and the roof of the right atrium. If the node is diseased or otherwise prevented from functioning as the pacemaker, a condition known as sick sinus syndrome, more distal components of the conduction system or even ventricular muscle itself assume the role of pacemaker. *As a rule, the more distal the pacemaker site, the slower the heart rate.* On leaving the SA node, an electrical impulse activates the atria. Atrial wavefronts converge on the AV node, which conducts the impulse through the common bundle (bundle of His) to the left and right bundle branches of the Purkinje system. Purkinje fibers run within the endocardium on both sides of the interventricular septum and distribute current to overlying ventricular muscles. Each cycle, ventricular contraction begins along the interventricular septum and at the apex. It progresses from apex to base, allowing smooth and efficient ejection of blood into the great vessels.

The His bundle in normal adult hearts is the only electrical connection between atria and ventricles. Additional abnormal connections may occasionally arise during development as small bundles or tracts of cardiac myocytes. Such "bypass tracts" can activate ventricular muscle before the normal impulse arrives via the conduction system (ventricular pre-excitation). They are found in patients with **Wolff–Parkinson–White syndrome** and can establish circuits that promote **supraventricular tachycardia**. Congenital conduction system discontinuities may result from placentally transmitted autoantibodies in mothers with diseases such as systemic lupus erythematosus (SLE). Acquired defects may arise due to infarction, inflammation or infiltrative disease, or as a complication of cardiac surgery or cardiac catheterization.

Coronary Arteries Supply Blood to the Heart

The right and left main coronary arteries originate in, or immediately above, the sinuses of Valsalva of the aortic valve. The left main coronary artery bifurcates within 1 cm of its origin into the left anterior descending (LAD) and left circumflex coronary arteries. The latter rests in the left atrioventricular groove and supplies the lateral wall of the left ventricle (Fig. 17-2). The LAD coronary artery lies in the anterior interventricular groove and provides blood to the (1) anterior left ventricle, (2) adjacent anterior right ventricle, and (3) anterior 1/2 to 2/3 of the interventricular septum. In the apical region, the LAD artery supplies the ventricles circumferentially (Fig. 17-2).

The right coronary artery travels along the right atrioventricular groove and feeds most of the right ventricle and posteroseptal left ventricle (Fig. 17-2), including the posterior third to half of the interventricular septum at the base of the heart (also called the "inferior" or "diaphragmatic" wall). Thus, one can predict locations of infarcts that result from occlusion of any of these major epicardial coronary arteries.

The epicardial coronary arteries are usually arranged in a so-called right coronary–dominant distribution. In this pattern of dominance the coronary artery contributes the most

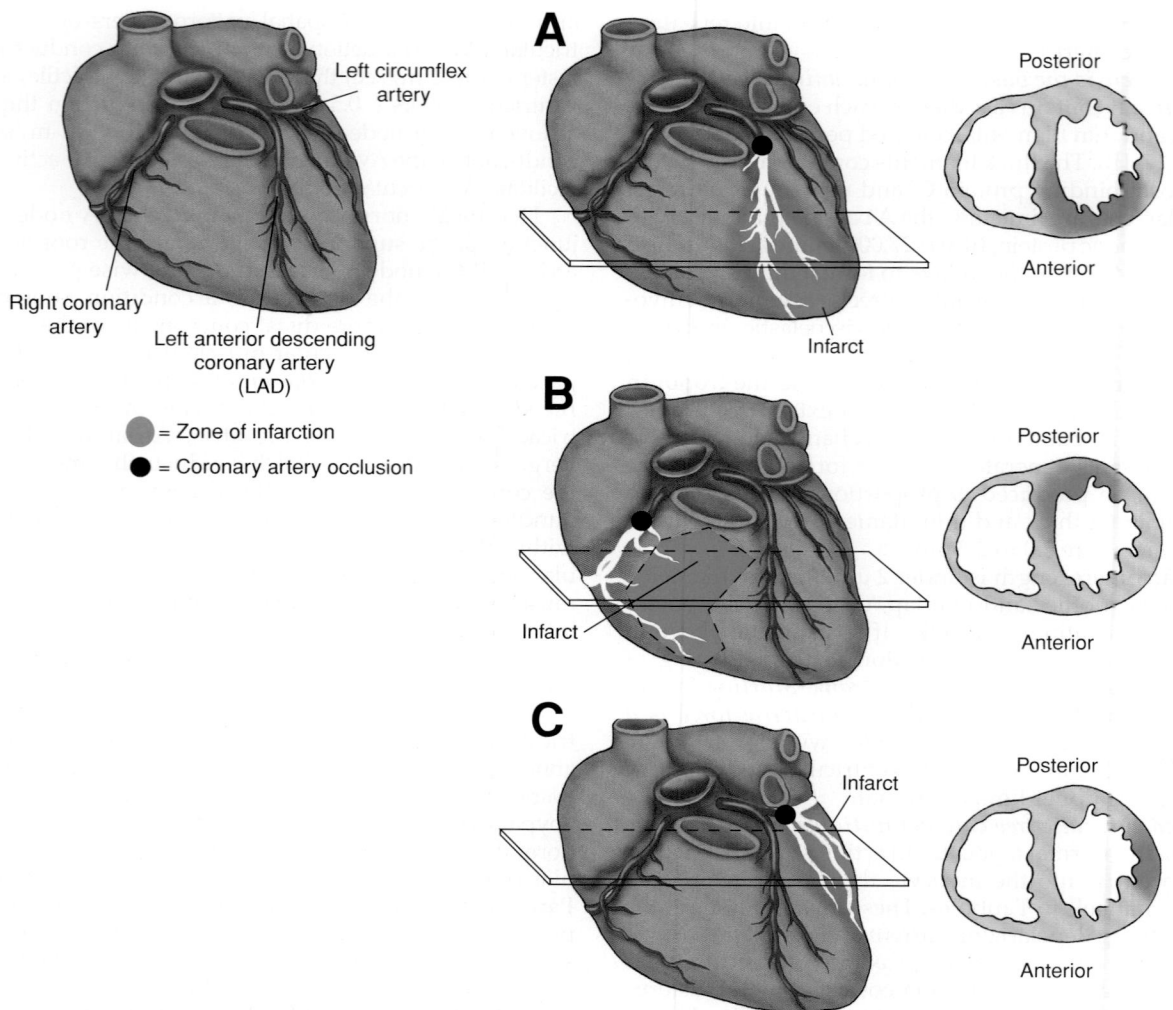

FIGURE 17-2. Location of left ventricular infarcts caused by occlusion of each of the main coronary arteries. A. Anterior infarct follows occlusion of the anterior descending branch (left anterior descending, LAD) of the left main coronary artery. The infarct is in the anterior free wall and adjacent two-thirds of the septum. It involves the entire wall circumference near the apex. **B. A posterior ("inferior" or "diaphragmatic") infarct** results from right coronary artery occlusion and involves the posterior wall, including the posterior one-third of the interventricular septum, and the posteromedial papillary muscle in the basal half of the ventricle. **C. Lateral infarct** in the posterolateral wall, which follows occlusion of the left circumflex artery.

blood to the posterior descending coronary artery. In 5% to 10% of people, the left circumflex coronary artery contributes the most (left dominant).

Blood flows in the myocardium inward from epicardium to endocardium. Thus, endocardium is generally most vulnerable to ischemia when flow through a major epicardial coronary artery is compromised. Some of the small intramyocardial coronary arteries branch as they traverse the ventricular wall; others maintain a large diameter and pass to the endocardial surface without branching (Fig. 17-3). Because capillary networks arising from penetrating arteries do not interconnect, the borders between viable and infarcted myocardium after coronary artery occlusion are distinct.

The epicardial portion of each coronary artery fills and expands during systole and empties and narrows during diastole. Intramyocardial arteries are compressed by systolic muscular pressure and do the opposite. Thus, blood flow in the myocardium, especially in subendocardial ventricular

regions, is lower or absent in systole. Autoregulation of blood flow roughly equalizes myocardial supply, however.

MYOCARDIAL HYPERTROPHY AND HEART FAILURE

Normally, ventricles are compliant, and diastolic filling occurs at low atrial pressures. During systole, ventricles contract vigorously and eject about 60% of the blood that is in them at the end of diastole **(ejection fraction)**. In an injured heart, the clinical consequences are similar, regardless of the cause of cardiac dysfunction. *If initial impairment is severe, cardiac output may not be sustainable despite compensatory changes, causing acute, life-threatening* **cardiogenic shock.** For lesser impairment, compensatory mechanisms (see below) maintain output by increasing diastolic ventricular filling pressure and end-diastolic volume. This results

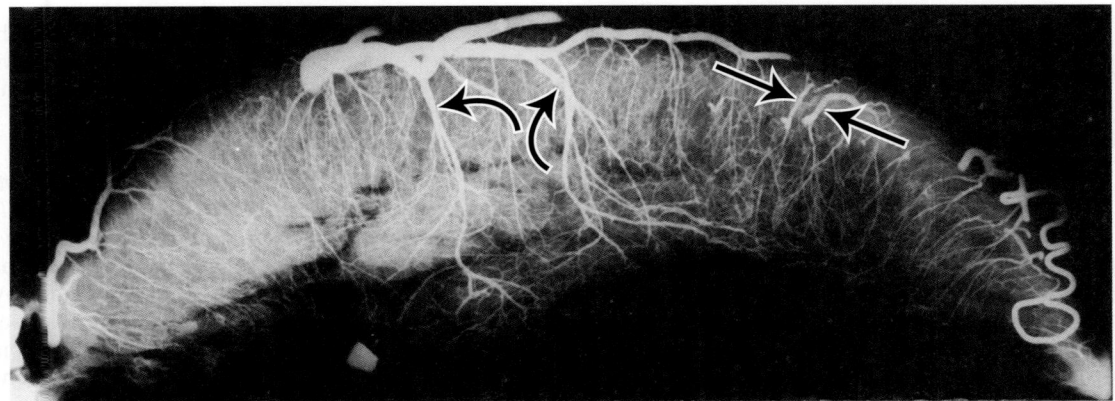

FIGURE 17-3. **Arteriogram of a longitudinal segment of the left ventricle posterior wall, including the postero-medial papillary muscle.** Note the two types of branches passing into the myocardium at right angles to the epicardial artery (*top*): class A, which quickly divide into a fine network (*straight arrows*), and class B, which maintain a large diameter and pass with little branching into the subendocardial region and the papillary muscle (*curved arrows*).

in the characteristic signs and symptoms of heart failure. Because of the heart's capacity to compensate, heart failure is often tolerated for years.

The heart's ability to adapt to injury depends on the same mechanisms that allow cardiac output to rise in response to stress. *Compensation reflects the Frank–Starling law: cardiac stroke volume is a function of diastolic fiber length; within certain limits, a normal heart will pump whatever volume the venous circulation brings to it* (Fig. 17-4). Stroke volume, a measure of ventricular function, increases with greater ventricular end-diastolic volume due to increased atrial filling pressure.

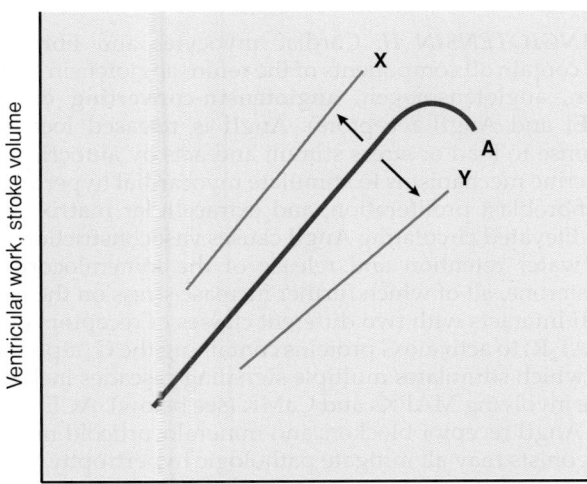

FIGURE 17-4. **Relation between cardiac work (or stroke volume) and the level of venous inflow, as measured by atrial pressure, ventricular end-diastolic volume (EDV) or end-diastolic pressure (EDP).** *Curve A* indicates that as ventricular EDV, EDP or left atrial pressure increase, the amount of work done by the heart increases linearly up to a point. Beyond this point, the work done decreases, and the heart fails. However, the downslope of this curve is reached only at very high left atrial pressures. The curve may shift upward to position *X* or downward to position *Y*, depending on whether contractility has increased (e.g., due to the action of norepinephrine) or decreased (i.e., in failure), respectively. A failing heart usually functions on the ascending limb of a depressed curve.

Increased contractile force in response to ventricular dilation reflects myofibrillar organization: stretching of sarcomeres allows thick and thin filaments to overlap more during contraction. This permits enhanced force generation, as long as the sarcomere does not stretch beyond 2.2 μm. When there is a sudden need to increase cardiac output in a normal heart, as during exercise, catecholamine stimulation increases heart rate and contractility. The latter is mainly mediated by modulating activities of key proteins that regulate Ca^{2+} transients during excitation–contraction coupling. Thus, the normal relationship between end-diastolic volume and stroke volume is shifted upward (from curve A to curve X in Fig. 17-4). End-diastolic volume may also increase, greatly increasing cardiac output.

In injured hearts, overall basal cardiac function tends to be depressed. Higher than normal filling pressures are then needed to maintain cardiac output (curve Y in Fig. 17-4). In heart failure, the basal state requires catecholamine stimulation. Comparable increases in cardiac output thus require greater increases in atrial pressure in failing hearts than in normal ones. *The most prominent feature of heart failure is abnormally high atrial filling pressure relative to stroke volume.* However, absolute values of stroke volume and cardiac output are generally well maintained.

PATHOPHYSIOLOGY: Myocardial hypertrophy is an adaptive response that augments myocyte contractile strength and mitigates increases in ventricular wall stress. **Physiologic hypertrophy**, which develops in highly trained athletes, differs from **pathologic hypertrophy** due to injury or disease. While there is some overlap in molecular mechanisms leading to these different forms of hypertrophy, there are also important differences: an athlete's enlarged heart is highly efficient while a diseased heart of similar mass is structurally and functionally impaired.

Physiologic hypertrophy follows activation of signaling cascades that antagonize cardiac myocyte death and stimulate production of new myocytes and produces growth that increases ventricular chamber size and wall thickness proportionately, associated with increases in cardiac myocyte length and width (Fig. 17-5).

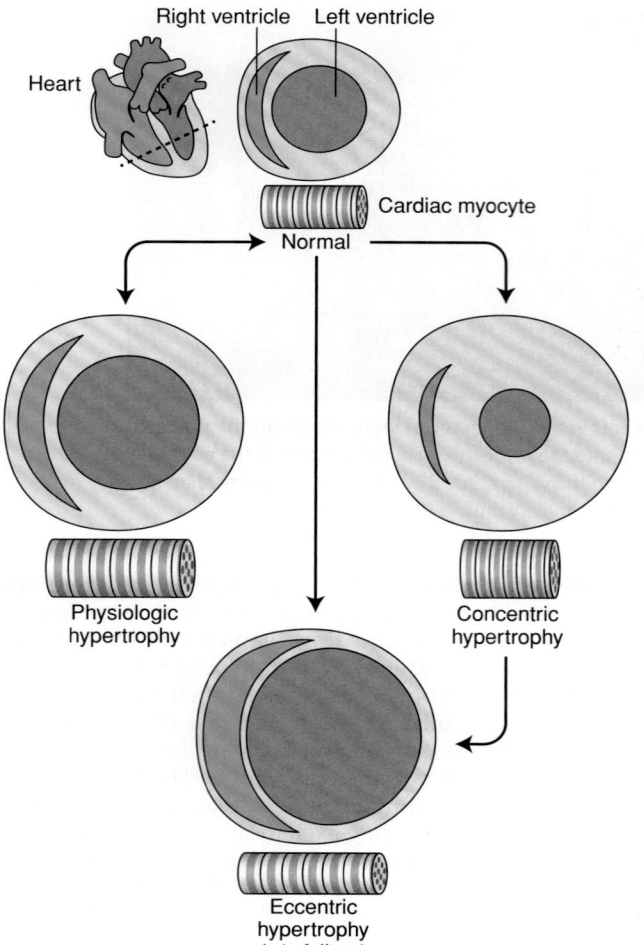

FIGURE 17-5. Different types of cardiac hypertrophy. In physiologic hypertrophy, the ventricular walls and chambers grow proportionately, because myocytes increase in both length and width. In pathologic hypertrophy, the ventricle thickens without an increase in chamber size, giving rise to "concentric" hypertrophy, associated with increased caliber but not length of cardiac myocytes. When pathologic hypertrophy becomes decompensated, the ventricle dilates and hypertrophied cardiac myocytes lengthen, giving rise to "eccentric" hypertrophy, which is often associated with a clinical picture of heart failure. (Reprinted with permission from van Berlo JH, Maillet M, Molkentin JD. Signaling effectors underlying pathologic growth and remodeling of the heart. *J Clin Invest.* 2013;123[1]:37–45.)

Pathologic hypertrophy thickens the ventricular wall without a proportionate increase in chamber size (the so-called ***concentric hypertrophy****)* (Fig. 17-5) *and reflects signaling pathways activated by neuroendocrine factors or incompletely understood sensors of abnormal wall stress.* Pathologic hypertrophy is a compensatory response to hemodynamic overload, which occurs in association with chronic hypertension or valvular stenosis **(pressure overload)**, myocardial injury, valvular insufficiency **(volume overload)** and other stresses that persistently increase cardiac workload. It also develops with primary injury of cardiac myocytes as in cardiomyopathies (see below). At first, pathologic hypertrophy maintains pump function and normalizes wall stress. However, with ongoing injury, further remodeling causes chamber dilatation and increased myocyte

length (**eccentric hypertrophy**) (Fig. 17-5). This type of hypertrophic remodeling is often associated with clinical heart failure with reduced ventricular function.

MOLECULAR PATHOGENESIS: *Receptor-mediated myocardial events triggered by a stimulus promote hypertrophic responses by autocrine and paracrine mechanisms.* Contractile cells respond to mechanical stimuli, such as stretching or pressure overload, by releasing ligands that activate receptor-mediated signaling pathways to produce hypertrophy (Fig. 17-6). Key among these ligands are (1) **angiotensin II** (AngII), (2) **endothelin-1** (ET-1), (3) **norepinephrine** (NE), and (4) various growth factors, including **insulin-like growth factor-I (IGF-I)** and **transforming growth factor β (TGFβ)**. Some of these, especially AngII and TGFβ, transform cardiac fibroblasts into proliferative myofibroblasts that synthesize and deposit extracellular matrix. Ligands that promote hypertrophy bind to and activate **G-protein–coupled receptors** and receptor tyrosine kinases to activate intracellular signaling, the most important of which include (1) **mitogen-activated protein kinases (MAPKs), phosphoinositide-3-kinases (PI3Ks)**, and β-adrenergic (**protein kinase A**) and **protein kinase C (PKC)** pathways, which are all activated by G-protein–coupled receptors; and (2) **Ca^{2+}/calmodulin-dependent protein kinase (CaMK)** pathways, which are regulated by Ca^{2+}. Events mediated by β-adrenergic receptors are implicated in the transition from compensatory hypertrophy to heart failure. Ligands, signaling cascades, downstream targets, and mechanisms mediating the hypertrophic response are described below (**see Chapter 1**).

ANGIOTENSIN II: Cardiac myocytes and fibroblasts both contain all components of the renin–angiotensin system (renin, angiotensinogen, **angiotensin-converting enzyme [ACE]** and AngII receptors). AngII is released locally in response to load or stress stimuli and acts by autocrine and paracrine mechanisms to stimulate myocardial hypertrophy, myofibroblast proliferation, and extracellular matrix secretion. Elevated circulating AngII causes vasoconstriction, Na$^+$ and water retention and release of the mineralocorticoid aldosterone, all of which further increase stress on the heart. AngII interacts with two different classes of receptors (AT$_1$R and AT$_2$R) to activate G proteins containing the G$_q$ alpha subunit which stimulates multiple signaling cascades including those involving MAPKs and CaMK (see below). ACE inhibitors, AngII receptor blockers and mineralocorticoid receptor antagonists may all mitigate pathologic hypertrophy.

β-ADRENERGIC SIGNALING AND DESENSITIZATION: Stimulation of β-adrenergic receptors by norepinephrine (NE) turns on the stimulatory G protein G$_s$ and activates adenylyl cyclase. This produces the **cyclic adenosine monophosphate (cAMP)** second messenger to activate PKA. PKA then phosphorylates Ca^{2+} regulatory and sarcomeric proteins to enhance myocardial contractility in the acute "fight-or-flight" response in a normal heart. Persistent β-adrenergic receptor stimulation, as in hypertension and heart failure, produces hypertrophy and desensitizes β-adrenergic receptors. Treatment with β-adrenergic receptor blockers is among the most effective therapies to reduce mortality and improve cardiac function in patients with advanced heart

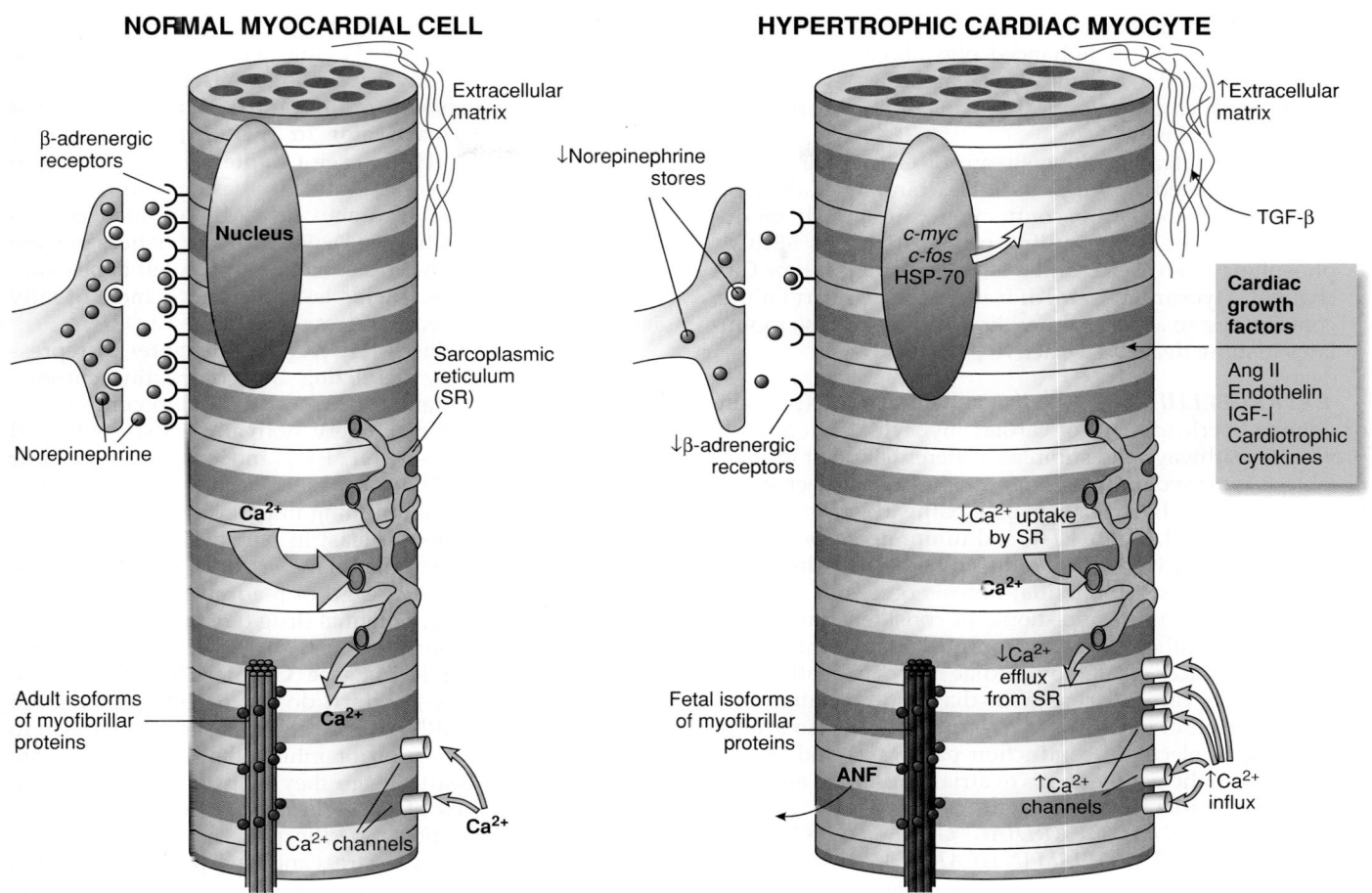

FIGURE 17-6. **Biochemical characteristics of myocardial hypertrophy and congestive heart failure.** *ANF* = atrial natriuretic factor; *Ang II* = angiotensin II; *HSP-70* = heat shock protein 70; *IGF* = insulin-like growth factor; *TGF* = transforming growth factor.

failure. Seemingly paradoxically, this response is consistent with abundant evidence that β_1-adrenergic receptors mediate cardiotoxic effects of NE in failing hearts, including maladaptive cardiac myocyte hypertrophy and apoptosis, interstitial fibrosis, contractile dysfunction, and sudden death. Desensitization of β-adrenergic receptors is mediated by specific G-protein–coupled receptor kinases (GRKs). Inhibition of GRK2 ameliorates heart failure in experimental models and is under investigation as a potential therapeutic strategy in patients.

IGF-1 and PHOSPHOINOSITIDE-3-KINASE (PI3K) PATHWAYS: IGF-1 binds its tyrosine kinase receptor to activate the p100α isoform of PI3K, causing phosphorylation of membrane lipids and generating second messengers like phosphatidylinositol-3,4,5-trisphosphate. This signaling cascade plays an important role in physiologic hypertrophy induced by exercise. PI3K activates **protein kinase B (Akt)** and downstream mediators such as **CCAAT/enhancer-binding protein β (CEBP/β)** which promote adaptive cardiac myocyte growth, improve myocyte survival, and stimulate angiogenesis and changes in ion channel proteins that reduce risk of arrhythmias. They also counteract fibrosis and myocyte cell death mechanisms.

MITOGEN-ACTIVATED PROTEIN KINASE PATHWAYS: The MAPK cascade has 3 main branches. **ERK1/2 (extracellular receptor kinase 1/2)** signaling stimulates growth and survival of cardiac myocytes. Activation of **JNK (c-Jun N-terminal kinase)** and p38 MAPK cascades leads to pathologic remodeling and apoptosis of cardiac myocytes.

ENDOTHELIN-1: ET-1 is a powerful vasoconstrictor produced by many cells, including endothelial cells and cardiac myocytes. It is also a potent growth factor for cardiac myocytes. Like AngII, ET-1 activates a G_q-protein–coupled receptor to stimulate MAPK cascades (mainly JNK pathways) that promote maladaptive cardiac hypertrophy.

CALCIUM HOMEOSTASIS: Defects in Ca^{2+} homeostasis occur in pathologic hypertrophy and heart failure. Expression and function of key Ca^{2+}-regulating proteins in cardiac myocytes are altered (see Fig. 17-1C):

- **Ryanodine receptor-2 (RyR2)**, the major Ca^{2+} release channel in the SR, is activated during action potential by influx of extracellular Ca^{2+} via voltage-gated channels in T tubules. Decreased numbers and/or abnormal regulation of RyR2 channels impair contractility by reducing Ca^{2+} release from SR in excitation–contraction coupling.
- **Sarco/endoplasmic reticulum Ca^{2+}-ATPase (SERCA)** is the pump responsible for Ca^{2+} reuptake into SR after contraction. Abnormal expression or regulation of SERCA lowers SR Ca^{2+} uptake. Resultant elevated diastolic Ca^{2+} impairs relaxation, depletes SR Ca^{2+} stores needed for optimal contractile function and promotes arrhythmias via afterdepolarizations that can cause ectopic ventricular activation.

- **Phospholamban** is a key regulator of cardiac contractility that inhibits SERCA. Enhanced phospholamban–SERCA interactions lead to chronically elevated Ca^{2+} levels during diastole, which play a critical role in chronic heart failure and arrhythmias.

- **CaMKII** is activated downstream of G_q signaling pathways stimulated by AngII and ET-1 binding. CaMKII is important in excitation–contraction coupling. It modulates actions of Ca^{2+}-handling proteins such as SERCA, phospholamban, RyR2, and the voltage-gated L-type Ca^{2+} channel. Myocardial CaMKII is increased in heart failure, contributing to abnormal Ca^{2+} homeostasis. It also modulates **histone deacetylase** activity (see below).

EXTRACELLULAR MATRIX: Mechanical stress (pressure or volume overload) and/or cardiac myocyte death activate profibrotic pathways and stimulate differentiation of resident fibroblasts into myofibroblasts that synthesize and secrete collagenous matrix. The major signaling pathways include those mediated by AngII, TGFβ, ET-1, and **tumor necrosis factor α (TNFα)** all of which may be produced by both cardiac myocytes and fibroblasts. Interstitial fibrosis occurs in virtually all forms of heart failure and should be considered an obligatory feature of pathologic hypertrophy. Replacement fibrosis occurs to fill spaces created by cardiac myocyte death. Myocardial fibrosis can interfere with diastolic relaxation and impair diffusion of oxygen and nutrients. It can also lead to remodeling of electrical conduction pathways, and so is a major factor in the pathogenesis of atrial fibrillation and ventricular tachycardia.

CHANGES IN MYOCARDIAL GENE EXPRESSION AND ENERGY METABOLISM IN HEART FAILURE: Cardiac myocytes respond to acute pressure overload by expressing **proto-oncogenes** such as c-*jun* and c-*fos* and heat shock protein 70 (Hsp70, **see Chapter 1**). These effects are mediated by AngII and other G_q signaling pathways. In pathologic hypertrophy, proto-oncogene activation directs myocardial gene expression to favor **re-expression of fetal protein isoforms** (Fig. 17-6). For example, **atrial natriuretic factor (ANF)** is made in fetal hearts, but, after birth, is only made in atria. In hypertrophic ventricles, however, ANF and brain natriuretic protein (now called **B-type natriuretic protein or BNP**) are re-expressed and reduce hemodynamic overload by altering salt and water metabolism (**see Chapter 7**). Blood BNP levels are a useful clinical biomarker of the severity of heart failure.

Fetal isoforms of contractile proteins also reemerge during cardiac hypertrophy. There are two forms of β-myosin: a more slowly contracting fetal form with less ATPase activity, and an adult form that is faster and has greater ATPase activity. Normal ventricles contain only slow myosin, but in hypertrophied hearts, atria change from fast to slow β-myosin. This impairs contractility but is also adaptive, as it conserves energy by increasing the tension generated during systole and improving contraction efficiency. Fetal isoforms of other myofibrillar proteins, including actin and tropomyosin, appear in hypertrophic ventricular myocardium. Hypertrophied hearts also contain abnormal varieties of lactic dehydrogenase (LDH), creatine kinase (CK), and the sarcolemmal Na^+ pump.

Energy metabolism differs in failing, compared to normal, hearts. Fetal hearts rely largely on maternally derived glucose for ATP production. After birth, hearts downregulate glycolytic enzymes and increase expression of genes that encode proteins mediating β-oxidation of fatty acids derived from breast milk. Failing hearts revert to glucose as an energy source, by expressing transcriptional regulators such as **peroxisome proliferator-activated receptor α (PPARα)**, **PPARγ co-activator 1α (PGC1α)**, and hypoxia-inducible factor 1α (HIF1α, **see Chapter 1**) increasing glucose uptake and glycolysis, and decreasing fatty acid oxidation. Failing hearts also activate AMP-activated protein kinase (AMPK, **see Chapter 1**), which also enhances glucose uptake and utilization. This substrate shift is felt to be adaptive: a mole of glucose yields less ATP than a mole of fatty acid, but glycolysis requires less oxygen.

Histone deacetylases (HDACs, **see Chapter 5**) repress gene transcription by stabilizing and compacting chromatin structure, thus making it less accessible to components of the transcriptional machinery. Activation of stress-related G_q signaling pathways by NE, ET-1, and AngII alters nuclear shuttling of specific HDACs which is thought to be responsible for genetic reprogramming in pathologic hypertrophy. This effect is mediated at least in part by CaMKII. HDAC inhibitors reduce experimental hypertrophy caused by pressure overload or chronic AngII or β-adrenergic stimulation. HDACs are, therefore, potential drug targets in patients.

An emerging regulatory network in cardiac myocytes involves **noncoding RNAs** (**see Chapter 5**). Hundreds of microRNAs (miRNAs)—which do not encode proteins but rather bind target mRNAs in a sequence-specific manner, to promote their degradation or inhibit their translation—are expressed in the heart, where they help to regulate expression of large groups of genes in cardiac development and phenotypic specification. Specific patterns of miRNAs are upregulated in response to stress and have been implicated in mediating the hypertrophic response. Long noncoding RNAs (lncRNAs, **see Chapter 5**), non–protein-coding RNA transcripts of >200 nucleotides, are also expressed in the heart. LncRNAs modulate mRNA expression and regulate chromatin structure. Such lncRNAs also appear to participate in molecular mechanisms in hypertrophy and heart failure. Circulating miRNAs and lncRNAs may become useful prognostic and therapeutic biomarkers in patients with heart failure.

APOPTOSIS AND AUTOPHAGY IN HEART FAILURE: Pathologic hypertrophy is associated with increased cardiac myocyte apoptosis, which may contribute to the transition from compensated hypertrophy to heart failure. Signaling by agonists such as AngII and ET-1 increases expression of pro-apoptotic genes via JNK and p38 MAPK pathways and signaling by adrenergic agonists increases cardiac myocyte sensitivity to apoptotic stimuli. Signaling via p110α PI3K, triggered by the IGF-1 receptor enhances survival. Thus, diverse signaling pathways in cardiac hypertrophy may exert pro- or anti-apoptotic influences, the final outcome depending on the balance between them.

Autophagy is an intracellular mechanism to degrade and recycle aged proteins and organelles (**see Chapter 1**). Because cardiac myocytes are so long-lived and have such high metabolic activity, autophagy helps them maintain normal function. Enhanced autophagy in times of stress helps protect cardiac myocytes that would other accumulate defective proteins and senescent organelles. However, excessive autophagy may promote cell injury and death. This is a developing topic in heart failure research.

CARDIAC STEM CELLS AND MYOCARDIAL REGENERATION: Lower vertebrates, such as zebrafish and salamanders, can regenerate new myocardium by division of existing cardiac myocytes after removal of a portion of the heart. Fetal and neonatal mice show a similar capability but lose it in early postnatal life. Thereafter, cardiac growth occurs almost exclusively by nuclear division (karyokinesis) without cell division (mitosis), and by hypertrophy enlarging cardiac myocytes. Humans undergo a similar transition but with less karyokinesis. Nevertheless, more than half of cardiac myocytes in normal adult human hearts are polyploid, even though they remain mononuclear. Hypertrophy stimulates DNA synthesis and karyokinesis, which explains the marked enlargement and hyperchromatic staining of nuclei (see, e.g., Fig. 17-26) and the greater proportion of binucleated myocytes in pathologic hypertrophy. Resident cardiac progenitor (stem) cells exist but are rare. Their capacity to replace myocardium lost to disease is minimal. The total number of cardiac myocytes in normal, uninjured adult hearts is essentially stable. The best estimates are that 0.5% to 2.0% of human cardiac myocytes turn over per year. Cardiac injury is associated with both increased myocyte loss through apoptosis and/or necrosis, and increased myocyte renewal. However, myocyte loss greatly exceeds the gain in common chronic heart diseases. Redressing this imbalance is an active area of research.

 PATHOLOGY: Anything that increases cardiac workload for a prolonged period or produces structural damage may lead to heart failure. *Coronary artery disease is by far the most common cause of heart failure.* Other important causes are hypertension, valvular disease, nonischemic heart muscle disease (cardiomyopathies) and persistent atrial fibrillation. Increasingly, heart failure is being seen in patients with congenital heart disease (CHD) who survive into adulthood. Virtually all body organs suffer when the heart fails (see Chapter 7).

Other than changes characteristic of specific diseases (e.g., ischemic heart disease, cardiac amyloidosis, congenital malformations), the morphology of failing hearts is nonspecific. *Ventricular hypertrophy is seen in virtually all conditions associated with chronic heart failure.* Initially, only the left ventricle may be affected, as in compensated hypertensive heart disease. But when the left ventricle fails, increased workload is imposed on the right ventricle, so some right ventricular hypertrophy usually follows. *In most cases of clinically severe systolic heart failure, ventricles are conspicuously dilated.* The distribution of end-organ involvement depends on whether the heart failure is predominantly left sided or right sided.

Left-sided heart failure is more common, as the most common causes of cardiac injury (e.g., ischemic heart disease and hypertension) primarily affect the left ventricle. To compensate for left ventricular failure, left atrial and pulmonary venous pressures rise, causing passive pulmonary congestion. Alveolar septal capillaries fill with blood and small ruptures spill erythrocytes into alveoli, which may therefore contain many hemosiderin-laden macrophages (heart failure cells). If capillary hydrostatic pressure exceeds plasma osmotic pressure, fluid leaks from capillaries into alveoli, causing **pulmonary edema** (see Chapters 16 and 18), with alveoli being variably filled by the transudate. Interstitial pulmonary fibrosis results if congestion persists for an extended period.

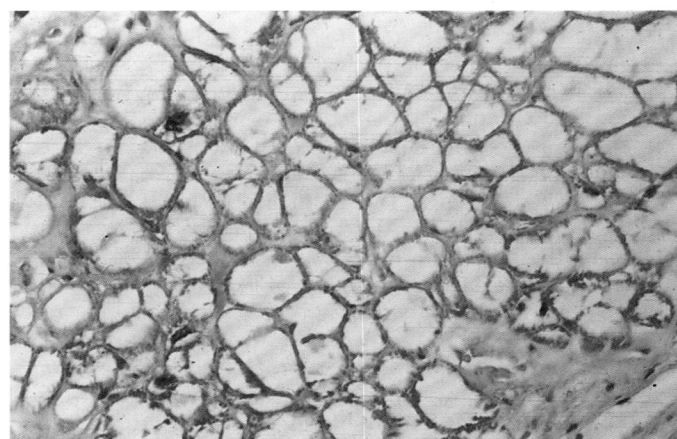

FIGURE 17-7. Severe myocytolysis in a patient with end-stage heart failure. Chronically injured myocytes show dramatic loss of myofibrils, giving cells a marked vacuolated appearance. Only a thin rim of contractile cytoplasm (stained red) is present, immediately beneath the sarcolemma.

Right-sided heart failure occurs most commonly as a complication of left-sided failure but can develop independently due to intrinsic lung disease or pulmonary hypertension. The latter creates resistance to blood flow through the lung, causing right atrial pressure and systemic venous pressure to increase. Jugular veins become distended, edema accumulates in the legs, and the liver and spleen become congested. Hepatic congestion in heart failure is characterized by distended central veins, which stand out on the cut surface of the liver as dark red foci against the yellow of cells in the lobular periphery. This gross appearance has been compared to the cut surface of a nutmeg ("nutmeg liver"; see Chapter 20).

Chronically injured cardiac myocytes lose myofibrils. Regardless of the type of injury, dysfunctional myocytes lose sarcomeres and correspondingly increase cytosol and glycogen. This process **(myocytolysis)** makes cells appear vacuolated (Fig. 17-7 shows a dramatic example). These changes likely result from reversible perturbations in myocyte protein metabolism and turnover. Myocytolysis may be an adaptive response to keep myocytes alive during chronic injury. It occurs in "hibernating myocardium," in which contractile function is impaired at rest because of chronically reduced coronary blood flow.

CLINICAL FEATURES: Symptoms of left-sided failure include respiratory distress with exercise **(dyspnea on exertion), orthopnea** (dyspnea when lying down) and **paroxysmal nocturnal dyspnea** (dyspnea that awakens patients from sleep). Dyspnea on exertion reflects increasing pulmonary congestion that accompanies higher end-diastolic pressure in the left atrium and ventricle. Orthopnea and paroxysmal nocturnal dyspnea result when lung blood volume increases, due to reduced blood volume in the legs during recumbency.

The clinical presentation of heart failure can largely be explained by venous congestion **(backward failure)**, but congestive failure also involves inadequate perfusion of vital organs **(forward failure)**. Most patients with left-sided heart failure retain sodium and water (edema) because of poor renal perfusion, decreased glomerular filtration and renin–angiotensin–aldosterone system activation (**see Chapter 7**). Inadequate cerebral perfusion can lead to confusion, memory loss and disorientation. Reduced skeletal muscle perfusion causes fatigue and weakness.

HEART FAILURE WITH PRESERVED EJECTION FRACTION (HFpEF): Almost one-half of patients with heart failure have a normal ejection fraction (≥50%). Once called diastolic heart failure, HFpEF typically occurs in older, hypertensive patients, especially women. Other risk factors include obesity, metabolic syndrome, and renal dysfunction. The heart may be normal in size or show concentric hypertrophy. Increased myocardial collagen content augments ventricular stiffness and helps explain the greater filling (diastolic) pressures seen in HFpEF. However, diastolic dysfunction occurs with aging and increasing evidence suggests that systolic dysfunction, which can occur even if ejection fraction is in the normal range, may play a role in HFpEF. Reduced myocardial capillary density may also contribute to the pathophysiology of HFpEF. Not surprisingly, high left atrial pressure and pulmonary hypertension are common. HFpEF entails greater risk of right ventricular dysfunction and atrial fibrillation. Molecular mechanisms underlying HFpEF are poorly understood, but suggested causes include hypophosphorylation of sarcomeric titin, reduced cGMP levels and increased expression of wildtype transthyretin amyloid.

CONGENITAL HEART DISEASE (CHD)

CHD is defined as a structural malformation of the heart and/or great vessels that is present at birth. It results from faulty embryonic development, expressed either as misplaced structures (e.g., transposition of the great vessels) or arrested progression of a normal structure from an early stage to a more advanced one (e.g., atrial septal defect [ASD] or tricuspid atresia). Significant CHD occurs in ~0.8% of live births.

It does not include certain common defects that are not functionally important, such as an anatomically patent foramen ovale that is functionally closed by the left atrial flap that covers it. In this case, the foramen ovale remains closed as long as left atrial pressure exceeds that in the right atrium. Bicuspid aortic valves are also common and are usually asymptomatic until adulthood. Estimates of the incidence of specific cardiovascular anomalies depend on many factors. A range derived from several sources is shown in Table 17-1. Medical and surgical advances have greatly improved outcomes for CHD patients. For example, the prevalence of *severe* CHD requiring surgical intervention in the first year of life (e.g., univentricular hearts, heterotaxy [left–right asymmetry defects], conotruncal abnormalities, ventricular outflow obstructions, atrioventricular canal defects) increased substantially between 2000 and 2010, such that two-thirds of the CHD population was 18 years or older in 2010.

 ETIOLOGIC FACTORS: Genetic, epigenetic and environmental factors all may play significant roles. Environmental factors are estimated to be responsible for 10% of CHD, for example, maternal infection with rubella virus during the first trimester, especially

TABLE 17-1
RELATIVE INCIDENCE OF SPECIFIC ANOMALIES IN PATIENTS WITH CONGENITAL HEART DISEASE
Ventricular septal defects: 25–30%
Atrial septal defects: 10–15%
Patent ductus arteriosus: 10–20%
Tetralogy of Fallot: 4–9%
Pulmonary stenosis: 5–7%
Coarctation of the aorta: 5–7%
Aortic stenosis: 4–6%
Complete transposition of the great arteries: 4–10%
Truncus arteriosus: 2%
Tricuspid atresia: 1%

during the first 4 weeks of gestation. Associations with other viral infections are suspected but are not as well documented. Maternal use of certain drugs in early pregnancy may also lead to cardiac defects in offspring: 10% of babies with thalidomide syndrome (phocomelia) had CHD (**see Chapter 6**). Other drugs implicated in CHD include alcohol, amphetamines, phenytoin, lithium, and estrogens. Maternal diabetes is also associated with increased incidence of CHD.

 EPIDEMIOLOGY: The causes of CHD are unknown in most cases, but epidemiologic studies have documented that heredity is critical. For example, CHD concordance is greater in monozygotic than dizygotic twins. Risk of CHD is greater among siblings of an affected child: CHD occurs in 1% of the general population but becomes 2% to 15% for pregnancies that follow the birth of a child with a heart defect. Risk of a third affected child may reach 30%. Infants born to mothers with CHD also have increased risk for CHD. Still, most cases of CHD, especially severe forms, occur in families with no history of CHD. It is estimated that de novo mutations in 400 genes could explain 10% of sporadic CHD. Many of these affect epigenetic mechanisms involving histone methylation.

 MOLECULAR PATHOGENESIS: The most important genetic contributions to CHD are aneuploidies, copy number variations and point mutations.

ANEUPLOIDIES were the first genetic defects to be linked to CHD. Cardiac malformations, often severe, occur in 40% to 50% of live-born infants with trisomy 21 (Down syndrome, **see Chapter 6**), in >60% with trisomy 13 and trisomy 18, and in a third with monosomy X. Given the large number of dysregulated genes involved in such chromosome abnormalities, extracardiac malformations occur in the vast majority CHD cases associated with aneuploidies.

COPY NUMBER VARIATIONS, arising from deletions or duplications from 1 kilobase to several megabases, may be responsible for up to 10% of cases of CHD. Del22q11 causes DiGeorge syndrome which includes CHD (usually conotruncal malformations) and extracardiac features such as immune deficiencies related to thymic aplasia, and facial abnormalities. This deletion includes the T-box transcription factor *TBX1* in which point mutations have been implicated in malformations of **outflow septation** such as **tetralogy of Fallot (TOF)** and persistent truncus arteriosus. **Del8p23** includes the transcription factor *GATA4* and has been linked to atrial and ventricular **septal defects**. Del7q11 causes **William syndrome** involving supravalvular aortic and pulmonary stenosis related to haploinsufficiency for elastin.

INHERITED POINT MUTATIONS in genes encoding a core group of cardiac transcription factors including *NKX2.5*, the **GATA** family of zinc finger proteins, **T-box factors** (*TBX5* and *TBX1*) and **MEF2** factors, have been implicated in CHD. The best studied is *NKX2.5*, deletion of which leads to failure of cardiac myocyte fate specification and lack of formation of a heart. Cardiac myocytes develop without *NKX2.5*, but certain features of morphogenesis are arrested and growth of the heart tube is retarded. Expression of several cardiac genes is also lower, including genes encoding myosin light chain 2v, ANF and cardiac ankyrin repeat protein and others that regulate right and left ventricle development. Point mutations in human *NKX2.5* may lead to several types of CHD, including atrial and ventricular septal defects, TOF, double-outlet right ventricle, tricuspid valve abnormalities and hypoplastic left heart syndrome (HLHS). Mutations in *TBX5* have been linked to **Holt–Oram syndrome**, with defects in cardiac septation and conduction, and upper limb malformations. Mutations in *NOTCH1* (**see Chapter 5**) may cause severe malformations, like HLHS, but may also be linked to ~5% of cases of bicuspid aortic valve, which affects up to 2% of adults. Recently mutations in genes that control the structure and function of cilia have been identified in humans with CHD. Cilia play an important role in establishing left–right asymmetry by determining the direction of looping of the embryonic heart. Accordingly, mutations affecting ciliary motility may result in heterotaxy.

Classifications of Congenital Heart Disease Reflect Cyanosis and Shunting

There are several ways to categorize congenital heart defects. One clinically useful approach, based on the presence or absence of cyanosis, puts cases into three groups:

- **The acyanotic group** does not have an abnormal communication between systemic and pulmonary circuits. Examples include coarctation of the aorta, right-sided aortic arch, and Ebstein malformation.
- **The cyanose tardive group** is defined as an initial left-to-right shunt with late reversal of flow, including patent ductus arteriosus (PDA), patent foramen ovale, and ventricular septal defect. In patients with these anomalies, cyanosis supervenes later (i.e., tardive). The shunt is initially left to right, but later becomes right to left

TABLE 17-2
CLASSIFICATION OF CONGENITAL HEART DISEASE
Initial Left-to-Right Shunt
Ventricular septal defect
Atrial septal defect
Patent ductus arteriosus
Persistent truncus arteriosus
Anomalous pulmonary venous drainage
Hypoplastic left heart syndrome
Right-to-Left Shunt
Tetralogy of Fallot
Tricuspid atresia
No Shunt
Complete transposition of the great vessels
Coarctation of the aorta
Pulmonary stenosis
Aortic stenosis
Coronary artery origin from pulmonary artery
Ebstein malformation
Complete heart block

(**Eisenmenger complex**) because progressively increasing pulmonary vascular resistance causes right ventricular pressure to increase and eventually exceed that in the left ventricle (see below).

- **The cyanotic group** entails a permanent right-to-left shunt. These include TOF, truncus arteriosus, tricuspid atresia, and complete transposition of the great vessels.

Additional classification schemes may provide the detail necessary to meet clinical requirements, especially for a cardiac surgeon. **A more contemporary classification divides cases is in** Table 17-2.

Early Left-to-Right Shunt Reflects the Higher Pressure on the Left Side of the Heart

Ventricular Septal Defect (VSD)

VSDs are among the most common congenital heart lesions (Table 17-1). They occur as isolated lesions or in combination with other malformations.

 ETIOLOGIC FACTORS: The fetal heart has a single chamber until the fifth week of gestation, after which development of interatrial and interventricular septa and formation of atrioventricular valves from endocardial cushions divide it. A muscular interventricular

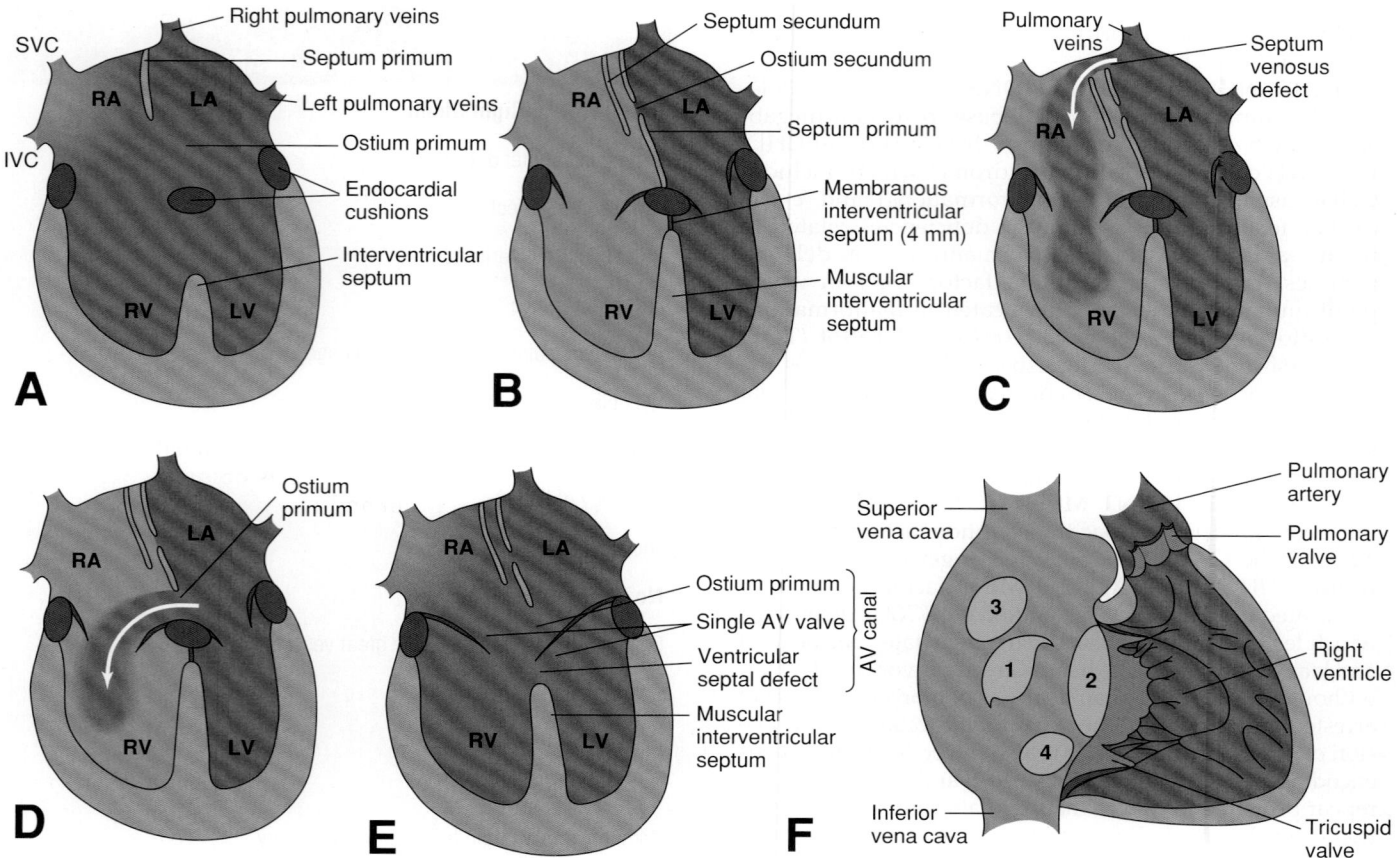

FIGURE 17-8. Pathogenesis of ventricular and atrial septal defects. Shunts are illustrated by varying shades depicting mixtures of red oxygenated and blue venous blood. **A.** The common atrial chamber is being separated into the right and left atria (RA and LA) by the septum primum. Because the septum primum has not yet joined the endocardial cushions, there is an open ostium primum. The ventricular cavity is being divided by a muscular interventricular septum into right and left chambers (right and left ventricles, RV and LV). *IVC* = inferior vena cava; *SVC* = superior vena cava. **B.** The septum primum has joined the endocardial cushions but at the same time has developed an opening in its midportion (the ostium secundum). This is partly overlaid by the septum secundum, which has grown down to cover, in part, the foramen ovale. Simultaneously, the membranous septum joins the muscular interventricular septum to the base of the heart, completely separating the ventricles. **C.** The **sinus venosus type of atrial septal** defect is in the most cephalad region and is adjacent to the inflow of the right pulmonary veins, which thus tend to open into the RA. **D.** The **ostium primum defect** occurs just above the atrioventricular (AV) valve ring, sometimes in the presence of an intact valve ring. It may also, in conjunction with a defect of the valve ring and ventricular septum, form an AV canal, as shown in panel. **E.** This common opening allows free communication between atria and ventricles. **F. Location of atrial septal defects.** In decreasing order of frequency: 1. Ostium secundum. 2. Ostium primum. 3. Sinus venosus. 4. Coronary sinus type.

septum grows upward from the apex toward the base of the heart (Fig. 17-8). It is eventually joined by the downward-growing membranous septum, separating right and left ventricles. *The most common VSD is related to partial or incomplete formation of the membranous portion of the septum.*

PATHOLOGY: VSDs occur as: (1) a small hole in the membranous septum; (2) a large defect involving more than the membranous region (perimembranous defects); (3) defects in the muscular portion, which are more common anteriorly but can occur anywhere in the muscular septum and are often multiple; or (4) complete absence of the muscular septum (single ventricle).

VSDs are most common in the superior portion of the septum below the pulmonary artery outflow tract (below the crista supraventricularis, i.e., infracristal) and behind the septal leaflet of the tricuspid valve. The common bundle (bundle of His) is immediately below the defect (inlet type). Less often, the defect is above the crista supraventricularis (supracristal) and just below the pulmonary valve (infra-arterial). The supracristal variety of septal defect is often associated with other defects, such as an overriding pulmonary artery (the **Taussig–Bing** type of double-outlet right ventricle), transposition of the great vessels, or persistent truncus arteriosus.

CLINICAL FEATURES: *A small septal defect may have little functional significance and may close spontaneously as the child matures.* Either hypertrophy of adjacent muscle or adherence of tricuspid valve leaflets to the margins of the hole may close the defect. In infants with large septal defects, higher left ventricular pressure creates initially a left-to-right shunt. Left ventricular dilation and heart failure (eccentric hypertrophy) are common complications of such shunts. If a defect is small enough to permit prolonged survival, augmented pulmonary blood flow caused by shunting of blood into the right ventricle eventually causes pulmonary arterial thickening and increases pulmonary vascular resistance. The latter may be so great that the direction of the shunt reverses and goes from right to left (**Eisenmenger complex**). Such patients develop late-onset cyanosis (i.e., tardive cyanosis), right ventricular hypertrophy, and right-sided heart failure.

Additional complications include (1) infective endocarditis at the lesion site, (2) paradoxical emboli, and (3) prolapse of an aortic valve cusp (causing aortic insufficiency). Large VSDs are repaired surgically, usually in infancy.

Atrial Septal Defect (ASD)

ASDs arise from defects in embryologic atrial septum formation, and range in severity from clinically insignificant and asymptomatic to life-threatening. Atrial septa develop embryologically in a sequence that allows continued passage of oxygenated placental blood from the right to the left atrium through the patent foramen, which process continues until birth. Beginning at the fifth week of intrauterine life, the septum primum extends downward from the roof of the common atrium to join to the endocardial cushions, thus closing the incomplete segment, or "ostium primum" (Fig. 17-8A). Before this closure is complete, the midportion of the septum primum develops a defect, or "ostium secundum," allowing right-to-left flow to continue. During the sixth week, a second septum (septum secundum) develops to the right of the septum primum, passing from the roof of the atrium toward the endocardial cushions (Fig. 17-8B). This process leaves a patent foramen, the **foramen ovale**, where the original ostium secundum was. The defect persists until it is sealed after birth by fusion of the septum primum and septum secundum, whereupon it becomes the **fossa ovalis**.

MOLECULAR PATHOGENESIS: The cause of most ASDs is not known, but a minority of them are parts of certain genetic syndromes. Mutations in genes encoding cardiac transcription factors may be involved (see above). Thus, about 15% of familial ASDs and 3% of sporadic ASDs are associated with coding errors in *NKX2.5*, and other genes are implicated in other ASD-containing syndromes, for example, *TBX1* deletion in DiGeorge syndrome (del22q11), *TBX5*, in large secundum-type ASDs in Holt–Oram syndrome and both ASDs and VSDs with *GATA4* mutations.

PATHOLOGY: ASDs occur at several sites (Fig. 17-8).

- **Patent foramen ovale:** Tissue derived from the septum primum situated on the left side of the foramen ovale functions as a flap valve that normally fuses with the margins of the foramen ovale, thereby sealing the opening. An incomplete seal allows a probe to pass through it (**probe patent foramen ovale**) and occurs without clinical problems in 25% of normal adults. However, if right atrial pressure increases (e.g., with recurrent pulmonary emboli) it may allow a right-to-left shunt to develop. Then, emboli from the right-sided circulation may pass directly into the systemic circuit. Such **paradoxical emboli** may cause infarcts in parts of the arterial circulation, most significantly in the brain, heart, spleen, intestines, kidneys, and legs. A widely patent foramen ovale, which occurs occasionally, is actually an acquired ASD that is caused by a disproportion between the size of the foramen ovale and the length of the valve covering it.

- **Ostium secundum-type ASD:** This defect accounts for 90% of ASDs. It is a true deficiency of the atrial septum and should not be confused with a patent foramen ovale. Ostium secundum defects occur in the middle portion of the septum and vary from trivial openings to large defects of the entire fossa ovalis region. Small defects are usually not problematic, but larger ones may allow sufficient blood to shunt from left to right to cause dilation and hypertrophy of the right atrium and ventricle. In this setting, pulmonary artery diameter may exceed that of the aorta.

  Lutembacher syndrome, a variant of the ostium secundum ASD, combines mitral stenosis and an ostium secundum defect. The mitral stenosis may be congenital or acquired (see below). Increased left atrial pressure due to mitral valve obstruction keeps the atrial septum patent.

- **Sinus venosus defect:** This anomaly accounts for 5% of ASDs. It occurs in the upper portion of the atrial septum, above the fossa ovalis, near the entry of the superior vena cava (Fig. 17-8C). It is usually accompanied by drainage of right pulmonary veins into the right atrium or superior vena cava.

- **ASD, ostium primum type:** This condition involves the region adjacent to the endocardial cushions (Fig. 17-8D) and makes up 7% of ASDs. There are usually clefts in the anterior mitral valve leaflet and the septal leaflet of the tricuspid valve, which may be accompanied by a defect in the adjacent interventricular septum.

- **Atrioventricular (AV) canal:**
  - **Persistent common AV canal** represents fully developed combined atrial and ventricular septal defects (Fig. 17-8E). Although uncommon, this defect occurs often in patients with Down syndrome.
  - **Complete AV canal** occurs when atrioventricular endocardial cushions fail to fuse. As a result, the defect includes (1) an enlarged ostium primum ASD, (2) an inlet ventricular septal defect, and (3) a single (common) atrioventricular valve with clefts in the mitral valve anterior leaflet and the tricuspid valve septal leaflet.
  - **Incomplete (partial) AV canal** is a situation in which an ostium primum ASD is adjacent to the atrioventricular valves, which are often abnormal.

- **Coronary sinus ASD:** This is the rarest ASD and is in the posteroinferior part of the interatrial septum, by the coronary sinus ostium. It is associated with a persistent left superior vena cava, which drains into the roof of the left atrium (Fig. 17-8F).

THE HEART

CLINICAL FEATURES: Young children with ASDs usually are asymptomatic, although they may complain of easy fatigability and dyspnea on exertion. Later in life, usually in adulthood, changes in the pulmonary vasculature may reverse blood flow through the defect and create a right-to-left shunt. This may cause cyanosis and clubbing of the fingers. Complications of ASDs include atrial arrhythmias, pulmonary hypertension, right ventricular hypertrophy, heart failure, paradoxical emboli, and bacterial endocarditis. Symptomatic cases are treated surgically or with new closure devices, which can be delivered and deployed percutaneously.

Patent Ductus Arteriosus (PDA)

In early embryos, six pairs of aortic arches connect ventral and dorsal aortas as part of the branchial cleft system (Fig. 17-9A). The left sixth aortic arch is partly preserved as the pulmonary arteries, and the arterial continuation on the left to the descending thoracic aorta becomes the **ductus arteriosus**. The ductus conveys most of the pulmonary outflow into the aorta. It constricts after birth due to increased arterial oxygen content and becomes occluded by fibrosis (**ligamentum arteriosus**) (Fig. 17-9B).

ETIOLOGIC FACTORS: Persistent PDA is among the most common congenital cardiac defects, especially in infants whose mothers were infected with rubella virus early in pregnancy. It is also common in premature infants, in whom prematurity precluded closure. In these patients, the ductus usually closes spontaneously. In full-term infants with PDA, however, the ductus has an abnormal endothelium and media, and only rarely closes spontaneously. PDAs occur in some patients with Down and DiGeorge syndromes.

CLINICAL FEATURES: Luminal diameters of PDAs vary greatly. A small shunt has little effect on the heart, although it serves as a nidus for infective endarteritis. A large shunt may divert blood from the aorta to the low-pressure pulmonary artery. In severe cases, more than one-half of left ventricular output may be shunted into the pulmonary circuit. Resulting increased demand for cardiac output may cause left ventricular hypertrophy and heart failure. In patients with large PDAs, the increased pulmonary blood volume and pressure eventually lead to pulmonary hypertension and its cardiac complications. Infective endarteritis involving the pulmonary artery side of the ductus is a frequent complication of untreated PDA.

PDAs can be corrected surgically or by interventional cardiac catheterization or caused to contract and then closed by instilling prostaglandin synthesis inhibitors (e.g., indomethacin). Conversely, a patient born with a cardiac defect may require a left-to-right or right-to-left shunt for survival, in which case PDAs can be kept open after birth by administering prostaglandins (PGE$_2$). Such patients may have isolated pulmonary stenosis, complete transposition of the great vessels or HLHS.

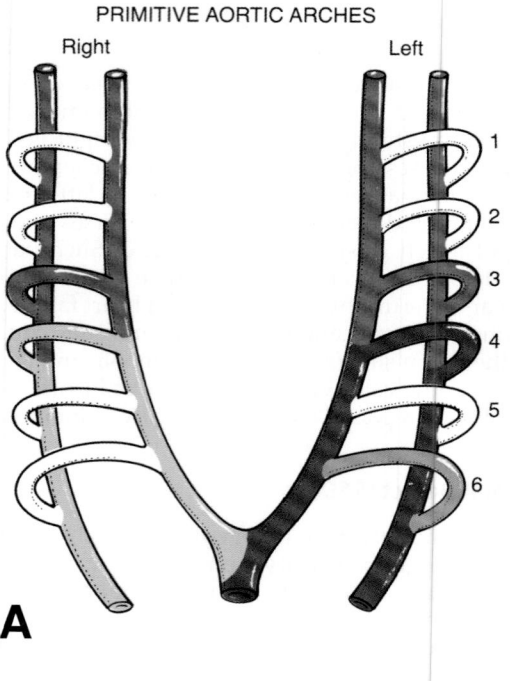

PRIMITIVE AORTIC ARCHES

Right   Left

1
2
3
4
5
6

A

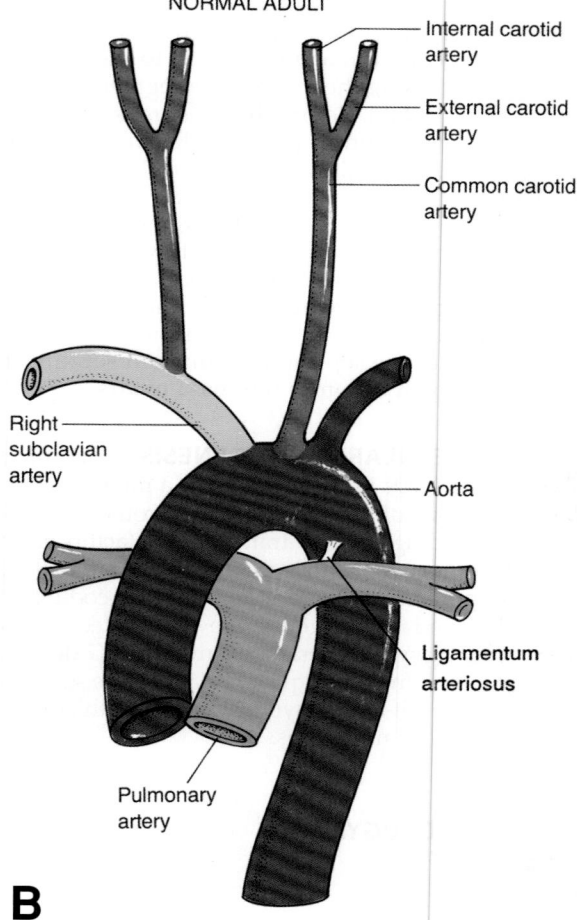

NORMAL ADULT

Internal carotid artery

External carotid artery

Common carotid artery

Right subclavian artery

Aorta

Ligamentum arteriosus

Pulmonary artery

B

FIGURE 17-9. Derivatives of the aortic arches. Colors identify corresponding structures in each panel. **A.** Complete primitive aortic arch system. **B.** In normal adults, the left fourth aortic arch is preserved as the arch of the adult aorta, and the left sixth arch gives rise to the pulmonary artery and ligamentum arteriosus (closed ductus arteriosus).

Aortopulmonary window is a rare defect between the base of the aorta and the pulmonary artery. It resembles PDA functionally and may be difficult to differentiate from it clinically.

Other abnormalities of the aortic arches can be understood as that may occur if the complete aortic arch system develops incorrectly (Fig. 17-9). Thus, if right arch system, rather than the left, is retained, a **right aortic arch** results. This occurs in about 25% of patients with TOF and 50% of those with truncus arteriosus. A right aortic arch is innocuous unless it creates a vascular ring that compresses the esophagus and trachea.

Persistent Truncus Arteriosus

The truncus arteriosus is the embryonic arterial trunk that initially opens from both ventricles and is later separated into the aorta and pulmonary trunk by the spiral septum. *In persistent truncus arteriosus, absent or incomplete partitioning of the truncus arteriosus by the spiral septum leads to a common trunk for the aorta, pulmonary, and coronary arteries. The truncus arteriosus always overrides a VSD and receives blood from both ventricles.* The valve of the truncus has from 2 to 6 semilunar cusps, but usually 3 or 4. Coronary arteries arise from the base of the valve.

 PATHOLOGY: There are several variants of truncus arteriosus:

- **Type 1** is most common, with a single trunk giving rise to a common pulmonary artery and ascending aorta.
- **Type 2** has right and left pulmonary arteries arising from a common site in the posterior midline of the truncus.
- **Type 3** features separate pulmonary arteries arising laterally from a common trunk.
- **Type 4** covers other rare variants, lacking any pulmonary trunk, with pulmonary circulation derived from the aorta via enlarged bronchial arteries. This type is difficult to differentiate from TOF with pulmonary artery atresia.

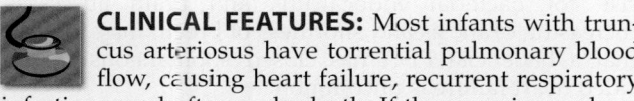 **CLINICAL FEATURES:** Most infants with truncus arteriosus have torrential pulmonary blood flow, causing heart failure, recurrent respiratory infections, and often early death. If they survive, pulmonary vascular disease develops, with cyanosis, polycythemia, and clubbing of the fingers. Corrective surgery before significant pulmonary vascular changes develop is effective treatment.

Hypoplastic Left Heart Syndrome (HLHS)

PATHOLOGY: In this usually profound malformation, the left ventricle and ascending aorta are hypoplastic, and left-sided valves are hypoplastic or atretic. Severe aortic valvular stenosis or aortic atresia is often the main defect. Some mitral valve structures are usually present, but the mitral valve may also be atretic. If the mitral valve is atretic rather than hypoplastic, the left ventricle may only be a thin slit lined by endocardium.

 MOLECULAR PATHOGENESIS: Genetic factors likely play a role in this complex malformation, since there is a 2% to 4% risk of recurrence in future pregnancies (in families with two affected children, the risk increases to 25%). However, the sporadic occurrence of HLHS suggests a complex genetic landscape. Maternal copy number variations occur in about 10% of cases, the most common being del11q24-25 (**Jacobsen syndrome**), in which 10% of children have HLHS. Other copy number variations, inherited and de novo, are rare.

 CLINICAL FEATURES: Aortic valve atresia precludes left ventricular outflow into the aorta. There is an obligate left-to-right shunt through a patent foramen ovale. Cardiac output is entirely via the right ventricle and pulmonary artery. Systemic blood flow depends on flow from the pulmonary trunk to the aorta through a PDA. Coronary blood flow depends on retrograde flow from a hypoplastic ascending aorta to the sinuses of Valsalva. Because pulmonary vascular resistance is high at birth and both the foramen ovale and ductus arteriosus are patent, newborns with HLHS may appear well initially. As pulmonary vascular resistance falls and systemic (and especially coronary) blood flow decreases, infants become symptomatic. Without surgical correction or transplantation, over 95% die within their first month.

Anomalous Pulmonary Vein Drainage

Developing pulmonary veins form a network in the dorsal mesoderm. A bud from the region of the atrium joins the pulmonary venous confluence, and eventually all four pulmonary veins drain into the left atrium. If these tissues fail to join correctly, various venous anomalies result.

PATHOLOGY: Total anomalous pulmonary vein drainage may occur as an isolated defect, or as part of the asplenia syndrome (a heterotaxy syndrome including splenic agenesis, congenital heart defects and situs inversus of abdominal organs). Most often, the pulmonary veins drain into a common pulmonary venous chamber and then via a persistent left superior vena cava (persistent left pericardial vein) into the innominate vein or right superior vena cava. Or, a common pulmonary vein may drain into the coronary sinus or persistent posterior and subcardinal veins. The latter form a middorsal trunk that crosses the diaphragm and enters the portal vein or ductus venosus and may be associated with some pulmonary venous obstruction.

 CLINICAL FEATURES: In total anomalous pulmonary drainage, there is no direct pulmonary venous return to the left side of the heart, and only an ASD or patent foramen ovale sustains life. Heart failure, severe hypoxemia, and pulmonary venous obstruction result from total anomalous pulmonary vein drainage. Surgery often provides good correction.

Partial anomalous pulmonary venous drainage may result from less severe circulatory impairment. This anomaly may involve one or two pulmonary veins, especially with a sinus venosus type of ASD. Prognosis is excellent, like that for ASDs.

Right-to-Left Shunt Is the Most Common Cyanotic Congenital Heart Disease

Tetralogy of Fallot (TOF)

TOF represents 10% of CHD. Adults with this malformation represent the largest group of survivors with surgically repaired cyanotic CHD.

 PATHOLOGY: Four congenital cardiac anomalies define TOF (Fig. 17-10):

- **Pulmonary stenosis**
- **Ventricular septal defect**
- **Dextroposition of the aorta so that it overrides the ventricular septal defect**
- **Right ventricular hypertrophy**

The VSD, which may be as large as the aortic orifice, results from incomplete closure of the membranous septum and affects both the muscular septum and the endocardial cushions. In addition, the spiral septum, which normally divides the common truncus region into an aorta and a pulmonary artery, does not develop normally. As a result, the aorta is displaced to the right and overlies the septal defect. The VSD is just below the overriding

aorta. Pulmonary stenosis is often due to subpulmonary muscular hypertrophy, with an enlarged infundibular muscle obstructing blood flow into the pulmonary artery. In about one-third of cases, the valve itself is the main cause of stenosis, and the valve will usually be funnel shaped, with the narrow part more distal.

The heart is hypertrophied so as to give it a boot shape. Almost half of patients with TOF have other cardiac anomalies, including ostium secundum ASDs, PDA, left superior vena cava, and endocardial cushion defects. The aortic arch is on the right side in one-fourth of cases. The surgeon must remember that a large branch of the right coronary artery may cross the pulmonary conus region, which is the site of the cardiotomy made to enlarge the outflow tract. The PDA is actually protective, because it provides a source of blood to an otherwise deprived pulmonary vascular bed.

 MOLECULAR PATHOGENESIS: TOF has a familial recurrence rate of 2% to 3%, but genetic determinants are complex. It occurs in some patients with Down and DiGeorge syndromes. Mutations in *NOTCH1* are implicated in some affected families, and mutations in the NOTCH ligand *JAG1* occur in ~90% of patients with **Alagille syndrome**, a rare autosomal dominant condition that includes cholestatic liver disease, kidney involvement, and CHD, most commonly TOF. Rare inherited and de novo copy number variations have also been linked to this malformation.

 CLINICAL FEATURES: In the face of severe pulmonary stenosis, right ventricular blood is shunted through the VSD into the aorta, causing arterial desaturation and cyanosis. Corrective surgery is usually performed in the first 2 years of life. Otherwise, affected children develop slowly physically, complain of dyspnea on exertion and often assume a squatting position to relieve the shortness of breath. Cerebral thromboses may occur, due to marked polycythemia. Patients are also at risk for bacterial endocarditis and brain abscesses. Increasing cyanosis and shortness of breath may indicate that a beneficial PDA has closed spontaneously. Left-sided heart failure is uncommon.

Without treatment, the prognosis of TOF is dismal. However, total correction is possible with surgery, which has less than 10% mortality. After successful surgery, patients become asymptomatic and have excellent long-term prognoses.

Tricuspid Atresia

 PATHOLOGY: *Tricuspid atresia, a congenital absence of the tricuspid valve, causes obligate right-to-left shunting through A patent foramen ovale.* The defect usually occurs with a VSD through which blood gains access to the pulmonary artery. In **type I** tricuspid atresia (75% of patients), the great arteries are normal, while in **type II** D-transposition of the great arteries (TGA) occurs. A rare **type III** has L-malposition (see below).

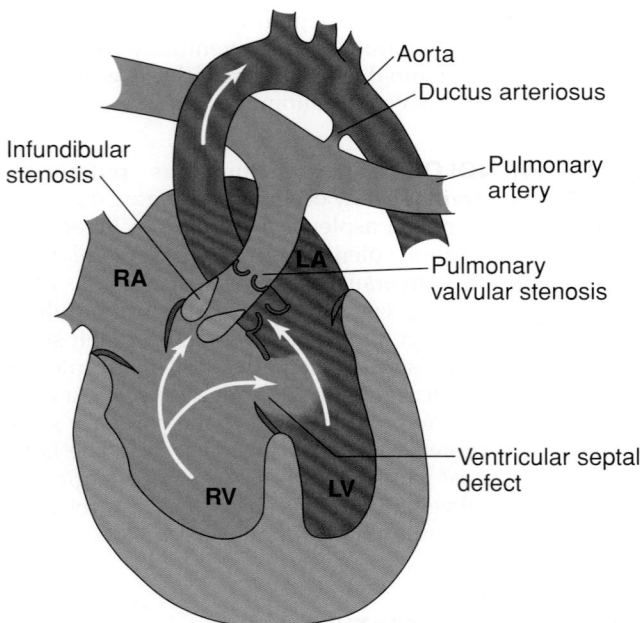

FIGURE 17-10. Tetralogy of Fallot. Note the pulmonary stenosis, due to infundibular hypertrophy *and* pulmonary valvular stenosis. The ventricular septal defect involves the membranous septum region. Dextroposition of the aorta and right ventricular hypertrophy are shown. Because of pulmonary obstruction, the shunt is from right to left, and the patient is cyanotic. *LA* = left atrium; *LV* = left ventricle; *RA* = right atrium; *RV* = right ventricle.

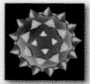 **CLINICAL FEATURES:** Infants with tricuspid atresia have cyanosis due to atrial right-to-left shunt. If the VSD is small, pulmonary blood flow is limited, which can result in even worse cyanosis. In that case, a cardiac murmur is prominent. Surgical intervention tries to bypass the atretic tricuspid valve and small right ventricle. Staged surgical palliation is the goal of current therapy.

Congenital Heart Diseases May Occur Without Shunting of Blood

Transposition of the Great Arteries (TGA)

In TGA, the aorta arises from the right ventricle and the pulmonary artery from the left ventricle. TGA has a male predominance and is more common if mothers are diabetic. It causes over half of deaths from cyanotic heart disease in the first year of life.

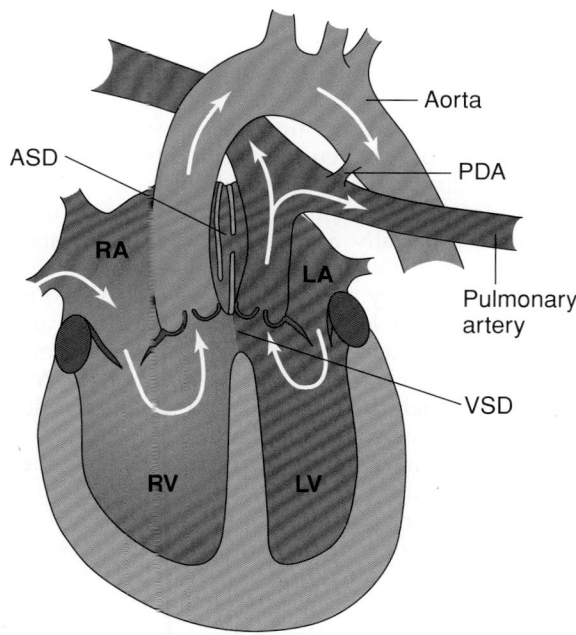 **ETIOLOGIC FACTORS:** Abnormal development of the spiral septum can produce aberrant positioning of the great arteries, such that the aorta is anterior to the pulmonary artery and connects to the right ventricle. Then, the pulmonary artery receives the left ventricular outflow (Fig. 17-11). Venous blood from the right side of the heart flows to the aorta and oxygenated blood from the lungs returns to the pulmonary artery. Thus, there

FIGURE 17-11. Complete transposition of great arteries, regular type. The aorta arises from the right ventricle, and is anterior to, and to the right of, the pulmonary artery ("D-transposition"). Without interatrial or interventricular connections or patent ductus arteriosus, this anomaly is incompatible with life. The volume and direction of blood flow through intracardiac communications and patent ductus arteriosus, if present, depend on pressure gradients across the communications, which vary during early stages of extrauterine life. *ASD* = atrial septal defect; *LA* = left atrium; *LV* = left ventricle; *RA* = right atrium; *RV* = right ventricle; *PDA* = patent ductus arteriosus; *VSD* = ventricular septal defect.

are in effect two independent and parallel circuits, for systemic and pulmonary circulations. Survival requires that these circuits communicate, so virtually all such infants have an ASD, one-half have a VSD and two-thirds have a PDA.

 PATHOLOGY: Normally, the aorta arises posterior to, and left of, the pulmonary artery, then ascends behind and right of it. In all forms of TGA, the aorta is anterior to the pulmonary artery. In **"D" or dextrotransposition**, the aorta arises from the right ventricle and to the right of the pulmonary artery, which arises from the left ventricle.

 CLINICAL FEATURES: It is possible to correct TGA within the first 2 weeks of life using an arterial-switch operation. Overall survival is 90%.

In **congenitally corrected transposition**, the aorta is anterior to, but passes to the left of, the pulmonary artery (**"L" transposition**). Although the great arteries are thus abnormally related to each other, they arise from discordant ventricles. Thus, the circulatory pattern is functionally corrected because of transposition of both the ventricles and the great vessels, and the discordant relationship between the atria and ventricles. Patients in whom corrected TGA is the only malformation are clinically normal but there are often other anomalies that require their own interventions.

Taussig–Bing malformation is a double-outlet right ventricle (both great vessels arise from the right ventricle) in which a VSD is above the crista supraventricularis and directly beneath an overriding pulmonary artery. This condition is functionally and clinically similar to TGA with a VSD and pulmonary hypertension.

 MOLECULAR PATHOGENESIS: Various types of double-outlet right ventricle occur in patients with autosomal trisomies (13, 18, 21) and des22q11. Mutations in *NKX2.5* and maternal exposure to teratogens that influence neural crest development have also been implicated in a few cases.

Coarctation of the Aorta

Coarctation of the aorta is a local constriction, almost always immediately below the origin of the left subclavian artery, at the site of the ductus arteriosus. Rare aortic coarctations may occur at any point from the arch to the abdominal bifurcation. The condition is two to five times more common in men than in women and is associated with bicuspid aortic valves in two-thirds of cases. Mitral valve malformations, VSDs and subaortic stenosis may also be present. Turner syndrome, in particular, is associated with coarctation, as are berry aneurysms in the brain (**see Chapter 16**).

  ETIOLOGIC FACTORS AND PATHOPHYSIOLOGY: The pathogenesis of aortic coarctation reflects the pattern of flow in the ductus arteriosus in fetal life (Fig. 17-12). In utero, much more blood flows through the ductus than

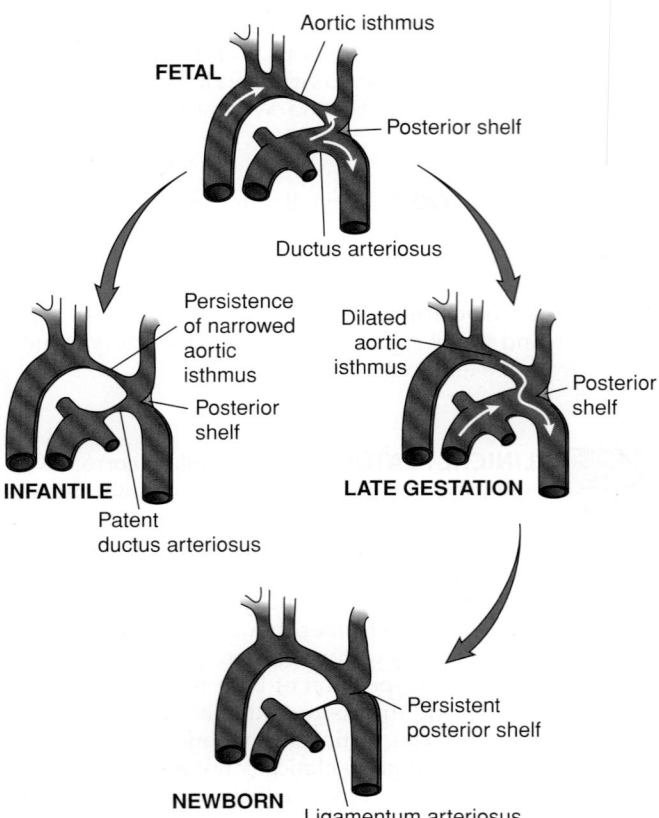

FIGURE 17-12. Pathogenesis of coarctation of the aorta. In the fetus, ductal blood is diverted into cephalad and descending streams by the posterior aortic shelf. In late fetal life, the isthmus dilates and the increased descending blood flow is accommodated by the ductal orifice. After birth, if the shelf does not undergo the normal involution, obliteration of the ductal orifice does not permit free flow around the persistent posterior shelf, creating a juxtaductal obstruction of blood flow to the distal aorta. If the aortic isthmus does not dilate during late fetal life, it remains narrow, resulting in an infantile or preductal coarctation. Then, the ductus arteriosus usually remains patent.

across the aortic valve. Blood leaving the ductus is diverted into two streams by a posterior aortic shelf opposite the orifice of the ductus. One stream passes cephalad into a relatively hypoplastic aortic isthmus to supply the head and arms; the other enters the descending thoracic aorta. In late fetal life, increasing left ventricular output dilates the isthmus and bypasses the obstruction (represented by the posterior shelf) through the wide ductal orifice. After birth, the ductal orifice is obliterated and the posterior shelf normally involutes, removing the obstruction. The shelf may not involute, as anomalies that limit left ventricular output (e.g., bicuspid aortic valve) may generate inadequate antegrade flow in the aortic arch in utero. The obstructing shelf may fail to involute for unknown reasons. In any event, the result is the most common aortic coarctation, a **juxtaductal constriction**.

The **infantile (preductal) type of coarctation** occurs when the aortic isthmus remains narrow (hypoplastic) into late fetal life and after birth. This is usually accompanied by a PDA and a right-to-left shunt through a VSD.

 CLINICAL FEATURES: *The clinical hallmark of coarctation of the aorta is a discrepancy in blood pressure between the upper and lower extremities.* The pressure gradient from the coarctation causes hypertension proximal to the narrowed segment, occasionally with dilation of that part of the aorta.

Hypertension in the upper part of the body results in left ventricular hypertrophy and may produce dizziness, headaches, and nosebleeds. The elevated pressure may also increase the risk of rupture of a berry aneurysm and consequent subarachnoid hemorrhage (**see Chapter 32**). Hypotension downstream of the coarctation leads to weakness, pallor, and coldness of the legs. In an attempt to bridge the obstruction between the upper and lower aortic segments, collateral vessels enlarge. Chest radiography shows notching of the inner surfaces of the ribs, caused by increased pressure in markedly dilated intercostal arteries.

Untreated, most patients with coarctation of the aorta die by age 40. Complications include (1) heart failure, (2) rupture of a dissecting aneurysm (due to medial degeneration in the aorta), (3) infective endarteritis at the point of narrowing or at the site of jet-stream impingement on the wall immediately distal to the coarctation, (4) cerebral hemorrhage, and (5) stenosis or infective endocarditis of a bicuspid aortic valve if one accompanies the coarctation. For asymptomatic patients, preferably between 1 and 2 years old, surgically removing the narrowed segment is effective treatment. Balloon dilation of the narrowed area by cardiac catheterization has also been performed.

Pulmonary Stenosis

Pulmonary stenosis results from (1) developmental deformities in the endocardial cushion region (with involvement of the pulmonary valves), (2) an abnormality of the right ventricular infundibular muscle (subvalvular or infundibular stenosis, especially as part of TOF), or (3) abnormal development of distal parts of the pulmonary artery tree (peripheral pulmonary stenosis). Peripheral (distal) pulmonary stenosis is much less common than the others and may cause pulmonary artery "coarctation" at one or more sites. This anomaly is more common in newborns with **Williams syndrome**, in which there are deletion mutations (del7q11) that include the gene encoding elastin.

Isolated pulmonary stenosis ordinarily involves the valve cusps, which are fused to form a constrictive inverted cone or funnel. The artery distal to the valve may develop post-stenotic dilation after several years. In severe cases, infants have right ventricular and atrial hypertrophy. If the foramen ovale is patent, there is a right-to-left shunt producing cyanosis, secondary polycythemia, and clubbing of the fingers. Balloon dilation of the stenotic valve by cardiac catheterization can be effective.

Congenital Aortic Stenosis

Congenital aortic stenosis may be valvular, subvalvular, or supravalvular.

VALVULAR AORTIC STENOSIS: The most common form of congenital aortic stenosis, bicuspid valve, arises through abnormal development of the endocardial cushions. A congenitally bicuspid aortic valve is much more common (4:1) in males than females and is associated with other cardiac anomalies (e.g., coarctation of the aorta) in 20% of cases. Typically, two of the three semilunar cusps (the right coronary cusp with one of the adjacent two cusps) are fused.

 CLINICAL FEATURES: Many children with bicuspid aortic stenosis are asymptomatic. Over years, the bicuspid valve tends to become thickened and calcified, generally causing symptoms in adulthood. More severe forms of congenital aortic stenosis cause a unicommissural valve or one without any commissures (acommissural). These malformations cause symptoms in early life, such as exertional dyspnea and angina pectoris. Sudden death, mainly due to ventricular arrhythmias, is a danger for patients with severe obstruction. Bacterial endocarditis may complicate the disease. Valve replacement may be indicated.

SUBVALVULAR AORTIC STENOSIS: This defect accounts for roughly 1% of CHD and 15% to 20% of congenital obstructive left ventricular outflow tract anomalies. It is caused by abnormal development of a band of subvalvular fibroelastic tissue or a muscular ridge. Stenosis results from a membranous diaphragm or fibrous ring that encircles the left ventricular outflow tract immediately below the aortic valve. It is two to three times more common in males than females.

Many people with subvalvular aortic stenosis develop thickening and immobility of the aortic cusps, with mild aortic regurgitation. Bacterial endocarditis carries its own risks and may also aggravate the regurgitation. Surgical treatment of subvalvular aortic stenosis involves excising the membrane or fibrous ridge.

SUPRAVALVULAR AORTIC STENOSIS: This type of stenosis is the least common and is often associated with idiopathic infantile hypercalcemia **(Williams syndrome)**, with mental retardation and multiple system disorders.

Origin of a Coronary Artery From the Pulmonary Artery

One coronary artery—or, rarely, both—may originate from the pulmonary artery rather than the aorta. When one coronary artery has an anomalous origin (most often the left coronary), anastomoses develop between right and left coronary arteries. This produces an arterial–arterial shunt, with blood flowing from the artery originating from the aorta to the one arising from the pulmonary artery. The myocardium supplied by the anomalous artery is vulnerable to episodic ischemia, causing possible myocardial infarction, with fibrosis and calcification. Anomalous origin of a coronary artery is seen in about 15% to 20% of young (under age 35) victims of sudden cardiac death.

Ebstein Malformation

Ebstein malformation results from downward displacement of an abnormal tricuspid valve into an underdeveloped right ventricle. One or more tricuspid valve leaflets are plastered to the right ventricular wall for a variable distance below the right atrioventricular annulus.

 PATHOLOGY: Septal and posterior tricuspid valve leaflets are usually affected. They are irregularly elongated and adherent to the right ventricular wall, so that the upper part of the right ventricular cavity (inflow region) functions separately from the distal chamber. The anterior leaflet is usually the least involved and may be normal. The valve ring may or may not be displaced downward from its usual position. In any event, the effective tricuspid valve orifice is displaced downward into the ventricle, thus dividing it into two separate parts: an "atrialized" (proximal) ventricle and a functional right (distal) ventricle. In two-thirds of cases, conspicuous dilation of the functional ventricle limits its ability to pump blood well to the pulmonary arteries. The degree of tricuspid insufficiency reflects the severity and configuration of the defect in the leaflets.

 CLINICAL FEATURES: Ebstein malformation leads to heart failure, massive right atrial dilation, arrhythmias with palpitations, and tachycardia and sudden death. Surgical treatment has met with variable success.

Congenital Heart Block

ETIOLOGIC FACTORS: Congenital complete heart block is usually associated with other cardiac anomalies, with the accompanying cardiac abnormality causing conduction system discontinuities. However, isolated complete heart block is believed to result from failure of atrioventricular conduction, due to lack of regression of the sulcus tissue that encloses the conducting tissue during early development. Congenital heart block without structural heart disease has been linked to maternal connective tissue disease, especially systemic lupus. If maternal SS-A/Ro or SS-B/La autoantibodies are transmitted to the fetus transplacentally, incidence of congenital complete heart block approaches 100%.

  PATHOLOGY AND CLINICAL FEATURES: Hearts of patients with congenital heart block tend to show a discontinuity between the atrial myocardium and the AV node. Alternatively, the defect may be a fibrous separation of the AV node from the ventricular conducting tissue. The heart rate is abnormally slow, but patients with isolated heart block rarely have functional difficulty. Later in life, cardiac hypertrophy, attacks of Stokes–Adams syncope (dizziness, unexpected fainting), arrhythmias, and heart failure may develop.

Dextrocardia

Dextrocardia is rightward orientation of the base–apex axis of the heart. It is often associated with a mirror image of the normal left-sided location and configuration. The position of the ventricles is determined by the direction of the embryonic cardiac loop. If the loop protrudes to the right, the future right ventricle develops on the right, and the left ventricle comes to occupy its proper position. If the loop protrudes to the left, the opposite occurs.

PATHOLOGY: Dextrocardia without abnormal positioning of the visceral organs (**situs inversus**) is invariably associated with severe cardiovascular anomalies: TGA, various atrial and ventricular septal defects, anomalous pulmonary venous drainage, and others. If dextrocardia occurs with situs inversus, the heart is functionally normal, but minor anomalies may be seen.

ISCHEMIC HEART DISEASE

Ischemic heart disease develops when blood flow is inadequate to meet the heart's oxygen needs and is usually due to coronary artery atherosclerosis. Ischemic heart disease is by far the most common type of heart disease in industrialized nations, where it is the leading cause of death and is responsible for ≥80% of deaths from heart disease. Atherosclerotic heart disease is less common in developing countries. Ischemic heart disease causes angina pectoris, myocardial infarction, chronic heart failure, and sudden death. Acute clinical events such as myocardial infarction and sudden death are caused by **acute coronary syndromes** which include any process that abruptly reduces coronary blood flow in one or more epicardial coronary arteries.

ANGINA PECTORIS: This is the pain of myocardial ischemia. It typically feels like severe substernal crushing or burning, which may radiate to the left arm, jaw, or epigastrium. It is the most common symptom of ischemic heart disease. Coronary atherosclerosis becomes symptomatic only when severe luminal narrowing compromises blood flow through one or more of the large epicardial coronary arteries. A patient with stable angina pectoris typically has recurrent episodic chest pain, usually brought on by physical or emotional stress. The pain usually lasts 1 to 10 minutes and is relieved by rest or treatment with sublingual nitroglycerin (a potent vasodilator).

Although the most common cause of angina pectoris is severe coronary atherosclerosis, decreased coronary blood flow can result from other conditions, including coronary vasospasm, aortic stenosis, or aortic insufficiency. Stable angina pectoris is not an acute coronary syndrome and is not, therefore, associated with myocardial pathology as long as its duration and severity do not cause myocardial necrosis. However, repetitive bouts of angina may eventually contribute to myocytolytic degeneration of the myocardium (Fig. 17-7).

Prinzmetal angina (variant angina) *is an atypical form of angina that occurs at rest and is caused by coronary artery spasm.* The mechanisms responsible are not fully understood, but endothelial dysfunction plays a major role. Patients typically show vasoconstrictor responses to acetylcholine, reflecting abnormal nitric oxide production. Thromboxane, derived from platelet activation, may also be involved. While spasm in structurally normal coronary arteries may be part of a systemic syndrome of abnormal arterial vasomotor reactivity that includes migraine headaches and Raynaud phenomenon, it usually develops in near a plaque in atherosclerotic coronary arteries. In this case, coronary artery spasm may contribute to acute myocardial infarction or affect the size of an infarct but is generally not the principal cause of infarction.

In **unstable angina,** *chest pain has a less predictable relationship to exercise than does stable angina, may occur during rest or sleep and is often associated with nonocclusive thrombi over atherosclerotic plaques.* In some cases of unstable angina, episodes of chest pain become progressively more frequent and longer over 3 to 4 days. Electrocardiographic (ECG) changes are not characteristic of infarction and serum levels of cardiac-specific intracellular proteins, such as the MB isoform of CK (MB-CK) or cardiac troponins T or I (evidence of myocardial necrosis), remain normal. Unstable angina is also called **preinfarction angina, accelerated angina,** or **"crescendo" angina**. Without pharmacologic or mechanical intervention to treat the coronary narrowing, many such patients progress to myocardial infarction.

MYOCARDIAL INFARCTION: Acute myocardial infarct is a discrete focus of myocardial necrosis in the heart caused by an acute coronary syndrome. This definition excludes patchy necrosis caused by drugs, toxins, or viruses. Development of an infarct is related to the duration of ischemia and the metabolic demands of the ischemic tissue. In experimental coronary artery ligation, foci of necrosis form after 20 minutes of ischemia and become more extensive as the period of ischemia lengthens.

CHRONIC HEART FAILURE: Early mortality associated with acute myocardial infarction is now less than 5%. Many patients with ischemic heart disease survive longer and develop chronic heart failure. Coronary artery disease is responsible for over 75% of heart failure. Contractile impairment is due to previous infarcts, with irreversible myocardial loss, and hypoperfusion of surviving muscle. These lead to chronic ventricular dysfunction ("hibernating" myocardium; Fig. 17-7). Some patients die suddenly, especially those in whom contractile impairment is not severe. However, sudden death in people with heart failure has declined steadily in the past 20 years, and most patients develop progressive pump failure and die of multiorgan failure. Because their coronary artery disease is often so extensive and many have already had coronary artery bypass surgery or one or more stents, the only treatments available for end-stage disease in these patients are heart transplantation or the use of artificial pumps (ventricular assist devices).

SUDDEN DEATH: In some patients, the first and only clinical manifestation of an acute coronary syndrome is sudden death due to spontaneous ventricular tachycardia that degenerates into ventricular fibrillation. Definitions of sudden death vary. Some authorities require that death occurs within 1 hour of the onset of symptoms, or that sudden death be unexpected. Others consider death within 24 hours of the onset of symptoms to be sudden. *In any event, coronary atherosclerosis underlies most cases of cardiac death that occur within an hour of the onset of symptoms.*

Experimental acute coronary occlusion causes a high incidence of ventricular fibrillation within 1 hour. Sudden cardiac death due to ventricular fibrillation also occurs in people as a result of acute coronary artery thrombosis. On the other hand, such an arrhythmia may appear in patients with marked coronary artery disease but no apparent thrombotic occlusion of a major epicardial coronary artery. Many patients who have been defibrillated and survived an arrhythmia have not suffered acute myocardial infarction: serum markers and ECG changes characteristic of infarction do not develop. *Thus, in many cases, lethal arrhythmia is likely triggered by acute ischemia (acute coronary syndrome) without overt myocardial infarction.* The presence of a healed infarct or ventricular hypertrophy increases the risk that an episode of acute ischemia will initiate life-threatening ventricular arrhythmia.

EPIDEMIOLOGY: *Major risk factors predisposing to coronary artery disease are (1) systemic hypertension, (2) cigarette smoking, (3) diabetes mellitus, and (4) elevated blood cholesterol.* The presence of any one of these factors significantly increases risk of myocardial infarction; a combination of multiple factors increases that risk by >7-fold (**see Chapter 8**).

During the 20th century, the United States first experienced a dramatic increase and then a marked decrease in mortality from ischemic heart disease. In 1950, the age-adjusted death rate from myocardial infarction was 226 per 100,000 people; 40 years later it was 108. This shift reflects reduced smoking, lower dietary saturated fat and new drugs that control hypertension, reduce cholesterol and dissolve coronary thrombi. Important medical advances include construction of coronary care units, coronary revascularization procedures, and use of defibrillators and ventricular assist devices. Concurrently, the role of hyperlipidemia in the pathogenesis of coronary artery atherosclerosis attracted much more attention. This was driven initially by epidemiologic evidence showing that populations in which men have high mean serum cholesterol values had higher rates of coronary artery disease. Since then, multiple studies established that elevated serum low-density lipoproteins (LDLs) are associated with increased risk of myocardial infarction, and high levels of high-density lipoproteins (HDLs) are associated with decreased risk. The total cholesterol–to–HDL cholesterol ratio appears to be a better predictor of coronary artery disease than is serum cholesterol level alone. Reducing LDL cholesterol in the blood clearly reduces risk of major adverse cardiac events. This relationship has been strongly confirmed in recent clinical studies with inhibitors of **proprotein convertase subtilisin/kexin type 9 (PCSK9)**, an enzyme that degrades LDL receptors in the liver, and thereby reduces the number of receptors on the cell surface. However, little if any evidence shows that raising HDL cholesterol levels provides benefit. Thus, low levels of HDL cholesterol may be a marker of risk but not a cause of disease.

Blood lipid profiles are important indicators of risk of atherogenesis, but other factors exert powerful independent effects. Someone whose blood pressure is 160/95 mm Hg has twice the risk of ischemic heart disease as someone whose blood pressure is 140/75. Reducing systolic blood pressure from 140 to 120 mm Hg further decreases risk of major adverse cardiac events (defined as a composite of myocardial infarction, acute coronary syndrome without myocardial infarction, stroke, acute decompensated heart failure, and cardiovascular death). Risk of ischemic heart disease increases in proportion to numbers of cigarettes smoked. Serum factors involved in thrombosis or thrombolysis or that contribute to endothelial injury have also been implicated in atherogenesis. For example, plasma fibrinogen levels directly correlate with risk of ischemic heart disease, presumably because of fibrinogen's role in atherogenesis and coronary artery thrombosis. Other factors that increase risk of myocardial infarction include factor VII, plasminogen activator inhibitor-1 (PAI-1), homocysteine, and low fibrinolytic activity. Levels of selected serum markers of inflammation such as C-reactive protein (CRP) and IL-6 also predict greater ischemic heart disease risk.

Recent years have seen a huge increase in the incidence of type 2 diabetes in the United States, reflecting a similar increase in obesity (**see Chapter 13**). Ischemic heart disease complicates type 1 and type 2 diabetes and occurs two- to threefold more than in nondiabetic people. Conversely, atherosclerotic cardiovascular disease (myocardial infarction, stroke, peripheral vascular disease) accounts for 80% of deaths in diabetics.

Other risk factors for ischemic heart disease include:

- **Obesity:** In a major, longitudinal study of one population (Framingham Heart Study), obesity was identified as an independent risk factor for cardiovascular disease, with an increased risk for obese people over lean ones of 2.0 to 2.5.
- **Age:** Risk of infarction increases with increasing age, up to 80 years. Age emerges as a powerful independent predictor of cardiovascular risk even after being adjusted for age-related increases in blood pressure or blood lipids. The responsible mechanisms are not well understood.
- **Sex:** Most (60%) coronary events occur in men. Angina pectoris is more common in men than women; the ratio at ages under 50 years is 4:1 and is 2:1 after age 60.
- **Family history:** In one study that controlled for other risk factors, relatives of patients with ischemic heart disease had two- to fourfold higher risk for coronary artery disease. Genetics of familial risk may interact with other risk factors. Genome-wide association studies identified several single nucleotide polymorphisms in patients with myocardial infarction, but specific genes involved and underlying mechanisms are not yet known.
- **Use of oral contraceptives:** Women over 35 years of age who smoke cigarettes and use oral contraceptives have modestly increased risk of myocardial infarction.
- **Sedentary life:** Regular exercise lowers myocardial infarction risk, via mechanisms that are likely complex and multifactorial. In one study, people in the least-fit quartile had 6× greater risk than did those in the fittest quartile.
- **Personality:** Early studies suggested that aggressive, time-conscious, executive-type ("type A") individuals have more heart disease than do easygoing, relaxed people ("type B"). "Coronary-prone" subjects, with type A behaviors have higher plasma triglycerides and cholesterol, and greater urinary catecholamines. Yet, the link between coronary artery disease and personality is controversial. Recent studies have not shown as strong an association as had previously been reported.

Many Conditions Limit Blood Supply to the Heart

The heart is an aerobic organ, using oxidative phosphorylation to generate energy for contraction. Skeletal muscle switches to anaerobic glycolysis under conditions of extreme physical exertion, but that cannot sustain the heart. Ischemic heart disease represents an imbalance between the heart's oxygen needs and its supply (Table 17-3).

Atherosclerosis and Thrombosis

The pathogenesis of atherosclerosis is detailed in Chapter 16. Here we discuss only briefly the features of special importance to ischemic heart disease. Coronary arteries are conductance

TABLE 17-3

CAUSES OF ISCHEMIC HEART DISEASE

Decreased Supply of Oxygen

Conditions that influence the supply of blood

Atherosclerosis and thrombosis

Thromboemboli

Coronary artery spasm

Collateral blood vessels

Blood pressure, cardiac output, and heart rate

Miscellaneous: arteritis (e.g., periarteritis nodosa), dissecting aneurysm, luetic aortitis, anomalous origin of coronary artery, muscular bridging of coronary artery

Conditions that influence the availability of oxygen in the blood

Anemia

Shift in the hemoglobin–oxygen dissociation curve

Carbon monoxide

Cyanide

Increased Oxygen Demand (i.e., Increased Cardiac Work)

Hypertension

Valvular stenosis or insufficiency

Hyperthyroidism

Fever

Thiamine deficiency

Catecholamines

vessels—small muscular arteries with a prominent internal elastic lamina. Their main role is to deliver blood to the regulatory vasculature (small intramural arteries and arterioles) that controls nutritive myocardial blood flow.

A healthy person has substantial coronary flow reserve and myocardial perfusion can increase to five times resting levels with intense exercise. In a normal heart, the large coronary arteries provide almost no resistance to blood flow: myocardial circulation is mainly controlled by constriction and dilation of small, intramyocardial branches less than 400 μm in diameter. In advanced atherosclerosis of the main epicardial coronary arteries, luminal stenosis decreases blood pressure distal to the narrowed zone. To compensate for reduced perfusion pressure, microvessels dilate, thus maintaining normal resting blood flow. Thus, most patients with coronary atherosclerosis do not have ischemia or angina at rest. However, the microcirculation can only dilate so much, so when exercise increases myocardial oxygen need in excess of supply, ischemia, and angina result.

Maximal blood flow to the myocardium is not impaired until about 75% of the cross-sectional area of an epicardial

coronary artery (~50% of diameter, as assessed by coronary angiography) is compromised by atherosclerosis. Resting blood flow is not reduced until >90% of the lumen is occluded. Moreover, coronary arteries remodel and enlarge their lumens as atherosclerosis develops. In patients with long-standing angina pectoris, the extent and distribution of collateral circulation exerts an important influence on the risk of acute myocardial infarction. In some settings (e.g., hypotension or tachycardia) demand for oxygen and perfusion pressure may be so out of balance that myocardial infarction ensues even when a coronary artery is not ordinarily sufficiently narrowed to produce ischemia.

Although myocardial infarction often occurs during physically demanding activities such as running or shoveling snow, many infarcts occur at rest or even while asleep. Thus, for most people, conversion of clinically silent coronary atherosclerosis to catastrophic myocardial infarction involves a sudden, marked decrease in myocardial blood flow, accompanied, or not, by increased myocardial oxygen demand. *Coronary artery thrombosis is the event that usually precipitates acute myocardial infarction. Thrombosis typically results from spontaneous rupture or erosion of a "vulnerable" atherosclerotic plaque, usually one with a lipid-rich necrotic core, many inflammatory cells and a thin fibrous cap.* Hemorrhage into or under the plaque may be the trigger.

Thromboemboli

Thromboembolism is a rare cause of myocardial infarction. Coronary emboli often come from the heart itself, usually valvular vegetations due to infective or nonbacterial endocarditis, or in patients with atrial fibrillation and mitral valve disease who have mural thrombi in the left atrial appendage. Thromboembolic occlusion of a coronary artery also happens in patients with left ventricular mural thrombi due to prior infarction, aneurysm, or dilated cardiomyopathy.

Coronary Collateral Circulation

Normal coronary arteries act as functional endarteries. Most normal hearts have anastomoses 20 to 200 μm in diameter between coronary vessels, but such collateral vessels do not function under normal circumstances as there is no pressure gradient between the arteries that they connect. However, a pressure gradient due to abrupt occlusion of a coronary artery allows blood to flow from a patent artery to the ischemic area. Extensive collateral connections develop in hearts with severe coronary atherosclerosis and may provide enough arterial flow to prevent infarction completely or to limit infarct size when a major epicardial coronary artery is acutely occluded.

Well-developed coronary collaterals can explain certain unusual situations, such as anterior infarction after recent thrombotic occlusion of the right coronary artery (the so-called *infarction at a distance*). This reflects opening of collaterals between the LAD and right coronary arteries (formed, e.g., in response to gradual atherosclerotic narrowing of the LAD). As a result, myocardium normally supplied by the LAD distal to the occlusion now depends on blood flow from the right coronary artery via collaterals. Acute thrombosis of the right coronary artery may thus cause paradoxical infarction of the anterior left ventricular wall.

Other Conditions That Limit Coronary Blood Flow

- **Coronary arteritis** occurs in various vasculitides, such as polyarteritis nodosa or Kawasaki disease (**see Chapter 16**). It may cause luminal narrowing from vessel wall thickening or create local aneurysms that may become occluded by thrombus.
- **Dissecting aortic aneurysms** may involve and obstruct coronary arteries. Rarely, medial necrosis and dissecting aneurysms are limited to a coronary artery.
- **Syphilitic aortitis** characteristically affects the ascending aorta, where it may obliterate a coronary artery orifice.
- **Congenital anomalous origin of a coronary artery** (origin of a coronary artery from the pulmonary trunk or passage of an anomalous coronary artery between the aorta and pulmonary artery) may cause sudden death in young, otherwise healthy people.
- **An intramural course of the LAD artery** may cause myocardial ischemia and sudden death. The artery normally runs in epicardial fat, but in some hearts, it dips into the myocardium for a short distance. This muscular digression may compress the artery during systole or predispose it to coronary spasm.

If Oxygen Supply Is Inadequate, the Myocardium Is at Risk for Ischemia

Anemia is a common cause of decreased myocardial oxygen delivery. A heart with normal circulation can survive severe anemia, but severe atherosclerosis may so limit the effectiveness of compensatory increases in coronary blood flow that infarction results. Anemia also increases cardiac workload because increased output is required to oxygenate vital organs adequately.

Carbon monoxide (CO) **poisoning** (**see Chapter 8**) decreases oxygen delivery to tissues. The high affinity of hemoglobin for CO displaces oxygen, thus depriving tissues of oxygen. It should be noted that cigarette smoking generates significant levels of carboxyhemoglobin (a measure of CO) in the blood.

Increased Oxygen Demand May Cause Cardiac Ischemia

Any increase in cardiac workload increases the heart's need for oxygen. Conditions that raise blood pressure or cardiac output, such as exercise, stress or pregnancy, increase myocardial demand, which may lead to angina pectoris or infarction. Disorders in this category include valvular disease (mitral or aortic insufficiency, aortic stenosis), infection and conditions such as hypertension, coarctation of the aorta, and hypertrophic cardiomyopathy (Table 17-3).

Hyperthyroid patients have increased metabolic rates and tachycardia, which increase oxygen demand and cardiac workload. Treatment of the underlying thyroid disease is the best therapy for a hyperthyroid patient with symptoms of cardiac ischemia. Fever also increases basal metabolic rate, cardiac output, and heart rate.

Myocardial Infarcts Are Classified on the Basis of Clinical and Pathologic Features

Acute myocardial infarcts are generally classified into those associated with ST elevation in the ECG (**STEMI** or ST elevation myocardial infarcts) and those without ST elevation (non–ST elevation MI: **NON-STEMI** or NSTEMI). Most patients with STEMIs go on to develop stable Q waves in their ECG (Fig. 17-13).

Myocardial infarction is also classified into six separate categories based on clinical and pathogenic mechanisms. **Type 1 myocardial infarcts** occur spontaneously, usually as a result coronary thrombosis. These infarcts are often STEMIs (Fig. 17-13). **Type 2 myocardial infarcts** result from ischemia produced by severe, prolonged imbalance between myocardial oxygen demand and blood flow. This occurs, for example, in coronary artery spasm, tachy- or bradyarrhythmias, anemia, or hypotension. In most cases, type 2 infarcts are non-STEMIs (Fig. 17-13). Other types involve those in which symptoms of myocardial ischemia precede death, but in which serum biomarkers were not obtained (**type 3**), acute infarcts arising as complications of percutaneous coronary interventions (**type 4a**), stent thrombosis (**type 4b**), or coronary artery bypass grafting (**type 5**).

Location of Infarcts

PATHOLOGY: In general, type 1 infarcts produce discrete, transmural myocardial necrosis, while type 2 infarcts are typically subendocardial and often patchy. There are important differences between these two types of infarcts (Table 17-4).

A **subendocardial infarct** affects the inner 1/3 to 1/2 of the left ventricle. It may arise within the territory of one of the major epicardial coronary arteries or it may be circumferential, involving subendocardial distributions of multiple coronary arteries. It may be due to atherothrombosis in one coronary artery (type 1 infarct) or related to conditions that limit myocardial blood flow globally, such as aortic stenosis, hemorrhagic shock or hypoperfusion during cardiopulmonary bypass (type 2 infarct). Circumferential subendocardial infarction caused by global hypoperfusion of the myocardium does not require that

TABLE 17-4

DIFFERENCES BETWEEN SUBENDOCARDIAL AND TRANSMURAL INFARCTS

Subendocardial Infarcts	Transmural Infarcts
Multifocal	Unifocal
Patchy	Solid
May be circumferential	In distribution of a specific coronary artery
Coronary thrombosis less common (mainly type 2 infarcts; usually non-STEMI)	Coronary thrombosis common (type 1 infarcts; often STEMI)
Often result from hypotension or shock	Often cause shock
No epicarditis	Epicarditis common
Do not form aneurysms or lead to ventricular rupture	May result in aneurysm or ventricular rupture

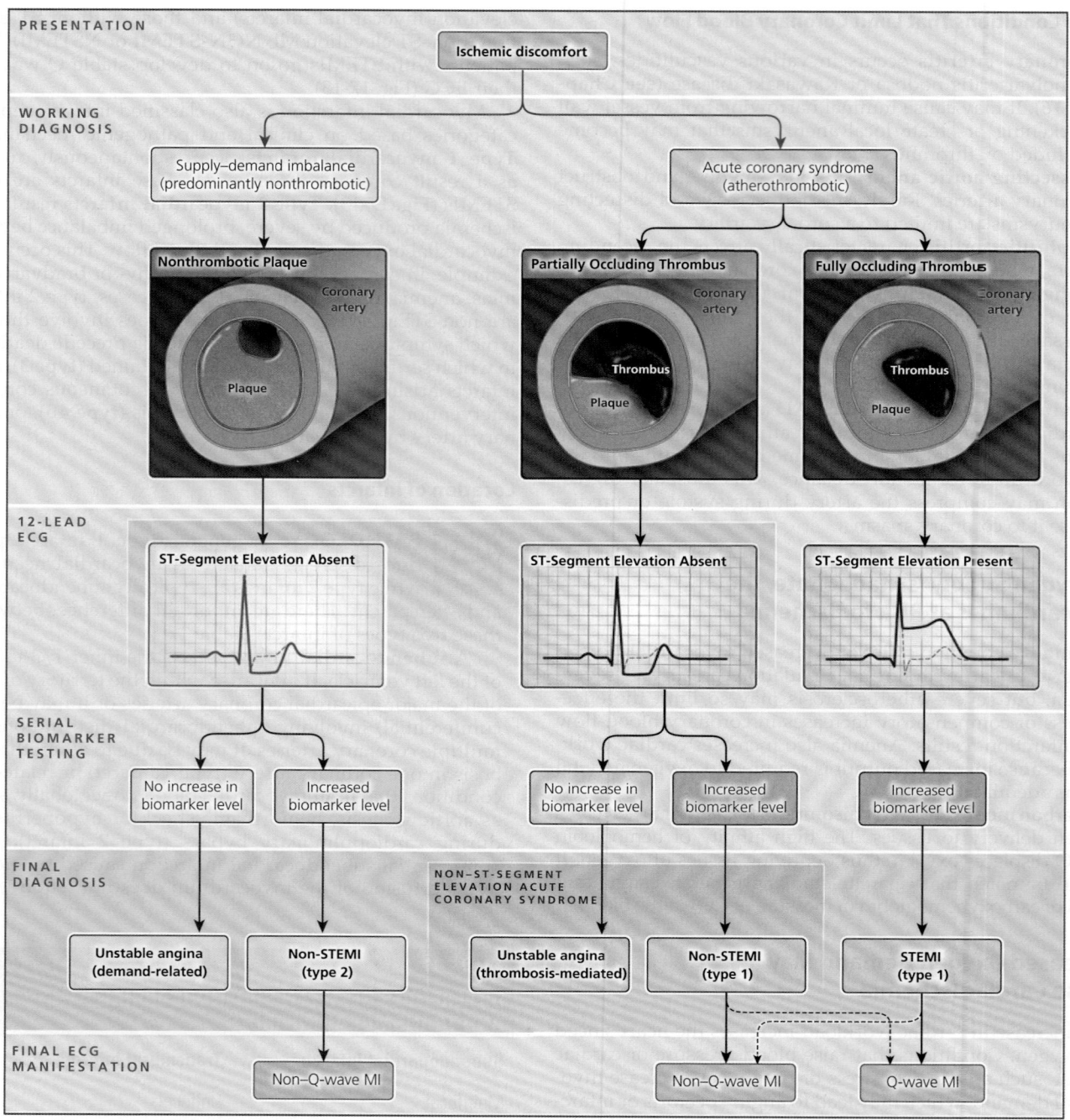

FIGURE 17-13. Clinical and pathologic features of ST elevation and non-ST elevation myocardial infarcts (STEMI and non-STEMI). (From Anderson JL, Morrow DA. Acute myocardial infarction. *N Engl J Med*. 2017; 376[21]:2053–2064. Copyright © 2017 Massachusetts Medical Society. Reprinted with permission from Massachusetts Medical Society.)

coronary artery stenosis be present. Because necrosis is limited to the inner layers of the heart, complications arising in transmural infarcts (e.g., pericarditis and ventricular rupture) do not follow subendocardial infarction.

A **transmural infarct** usually follows coronary artery occlusion and involves the full left ventricular wall thickness (type 1 infarct, usually STEMI). These infarcts thus tend to conform to the distribution of one of the major coronary arteries (Fig. 17-2):

■ **Right coronary artery:** Proximal occlusion of this vessel causes an infarct of the posterior basal left ventricle and the posterior 1/3 to 1/2 of the interventricular septum ("inferior" infarct).
■ **LAD coronary artery:** LAD blockage produces apical, anterior, and anteroseptal wall left ventricle infarcts.
■ **Left circumflex coronary artery:** Obstruction of this vessel is the least common cause of myocardial infarction, causing infarcts of the lateral left ventricle wall.

Myocardial infarction does not occur instantaneously. Rather, it begins in the subendocardium and progresses outward as a wavefront of necrosis to subepicardium over several hours. Transient coronary occlusion may cause only focal subendocardial necrosis, but persistent occlusion eventually leads to transmural necrosis. The goal of acute coronary interventions (pharmacologic or mechanical thrombolysis) is to interrupt this wavefront and limit the amount of myocardial necrosis.

The volume of arterial collateral flow is the chief determinant of transmural progression of an infarct. In chronic cardiac hypoperfusion, extensive collaterals, which preferentially supply the outer or subepicardial layer, often limit infarction to the subendocardial myocardium. However, in fatal cases, acute transmural infarcts are more common than those restricted to the subendocardium.

Infarcts involve the left ventricle much more often and extensively than the right ventricle. This difference is largely due to the greater workload imposed on the left ventricle by systemic vascular resistance and the greater thickness of the left ventricular wall. Right ventricular hypertrophy (e.g., in pulmonary hypertension) increases the incidence of right ventricular infarction. Infarction of the posterior right ventricle may occur in about 1/3 of left ventricular posteroseptal infarcts (right coronary artery territory), but infarcts limited to the right ventricle are rare.

Macroscopic Characteristics of Myocardial Infarcts

The early stages of myocardial infarction have been characterized most thoroughly in experimental animals. Within 10 seconds after ligation of a coronary artery, affected myocardium becomes cyanotic and, rather than contracting, bulges outward during systole. If the obstruction is promptly relieved, myocardial contractions resume and there is no anatomic damage, but contractility may be depressed in the affected area for hours (**stunned myocardium**) due to the effects of reactive oxygen radicals formed by reperfusion of acutely ischemic myocardium (see below). This reversible stage lasts for 20 to 30 minutes of total ischemia. Then, damaged myocytes progressively die.

Acute myocardial infarcts are not grossly discernable within the first 12 hours. By 24 hours, they are recognized by pallor on cut surfaces of the involved ventricle. After 3 to 5 days, they become mottled and more sharply outlined, with a central pale, yellowish, necrotic region bordered by a hyperemic zone (Fig. 17-14). By 2 to 3 weeks, the infarcted region is depressed and soft, with a refractile, gelatinous appearance. Older, healed infarcts are firm and contracted, with pale gray scar tissue (Fig. 17-15).

Microscopic Characteristics of Myocardial Infarcts

THE FIRST 24 HOURS: Electron microscopy is required to see the earliest morphologic features of ischemic injury (Fig. 17-16). Reversibly injured myocytes show subtle changes of sarcoplasmic edema, mild mitochondrial swelling, and loss of glycogen (the ultrastructural correlates of stunned myocardium). After 30 to 60 minutes of ischemia myocyte injury has become irreversible: mitochondria are greatly swollen with disorganized cristae and amorphous matrix densities containing lipid material. Nuclei show clumping and margination of chromatin and the sarcolemma is focally disrupted.

Loss of sarcolemmal integrity leads to release of intracellular proteins, such as myoglobin, LDH, CK, and troponins

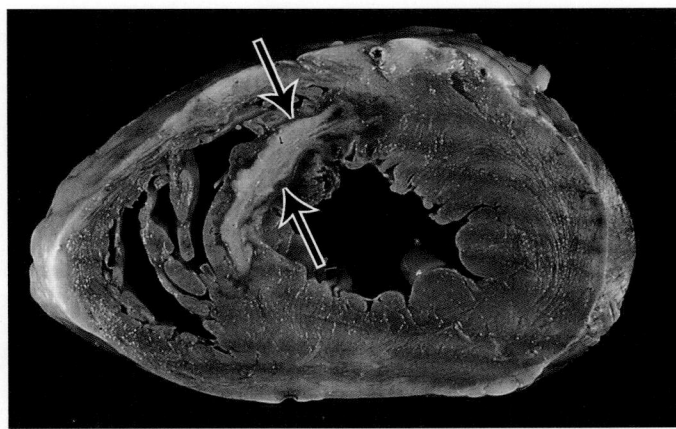

FIGURE 17-14. Acute myocardial infarct. A transverse section of the heart of a patient who died a few days after the onset of severe chest pain shows a transmural infarct in the anteroseptal region of the left ventricle (left anterior descending coronary artery territory). The necrotic myocardium is soft, yellowish and sharply demarcated (*arrows*).

I and T. Ion gradients are also dissipated, and tissue potassium decreases as sodium, chloride, and calcium increase.

The noncontractile ischemic myocytes are stretched with each systole and become **"wavy fibers."** By 24 hours, they are deeply eosinophilic (Fig. 17-17) with changes characteristic of coagulative necrosis (**see Chapter 1**). However, it takes several days for myocyte nuclei to disappear totally.

TWO TO 3 DAYS: Polymorphonuclear leukocytes are attracted to necrotic myocytes, but only gain access at the edge of the infarct, where blood still flows. They accumulate at infarct borders and reach peak concentrations at 2 to 3 days (Figs. 17-17 and 17-18). Interstitial edema and microscopic areas of hemorrhage may also appear. By 2 to 3 days, muscle cells are more clearly necrotic, nuclei disappear and striations become less prominent. Some of the neutrophils begin to undergo karyorrhexis.

FIVE TO 7 DAYS: By this time few, if any, intact neutrophils remain. At the periphery of the infarct, macrophages phagocytose dead muscle. Myofibroblasts begin to proliferate. New collagen is deposited. Lymphocytes and pigment-laden macrophages are prominent. The process of replacing

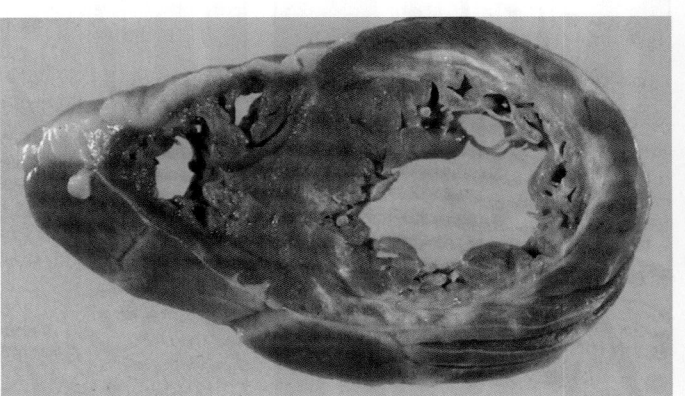

FIGURE 17-15. Healed myocardial infarct. A cross-section of the heart from a man who died after a long history of angina pectoris and several myocardial infarctions shows near-circumferential scarring of the left ventricle.

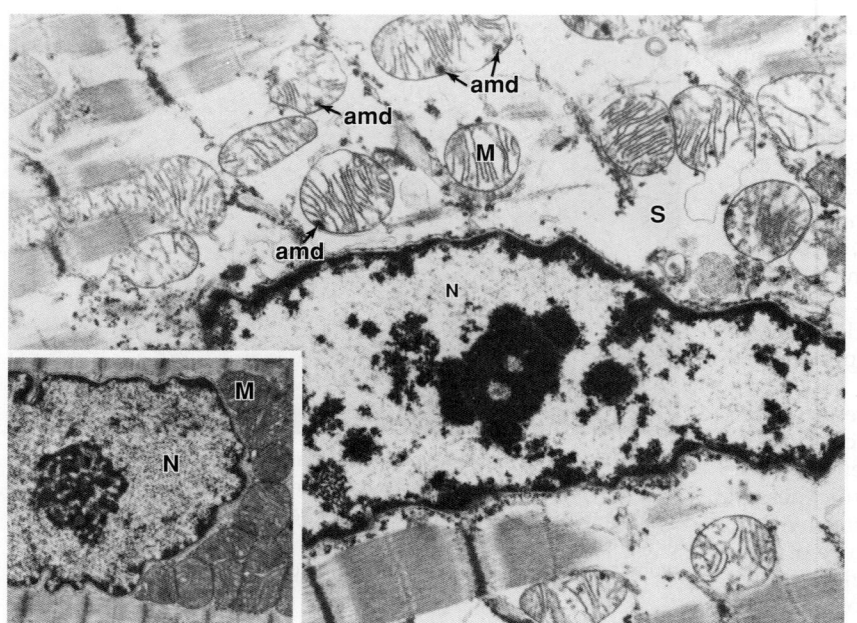

FIGURE 17-16. Ultrastructure of myocardial ischemia. Electron micrograph of an irreversibly injured myocyte from a canine heart subjected to 40 minutes of ischemia induced by proximal occlusion of the circumflex branch of the left coronary artery. (*Inset* shows a nonischemic control myocyte from the same heart. *N* = nucleus.) The affected myocyte is swollen and has abundant clear sarcoplasm (*S*). The mitochondria (*M*) are also swollen and contain amorphous matrix densities (*amd*), which are characteristic of lethal cell injury. The sarcolemma of this myocyte (*not shown*) showed small areas of disruption. Nuclear chromatin (*N*) is aggregated peripherally, in contrast to uniformly distributed chromatin in normal tissue.

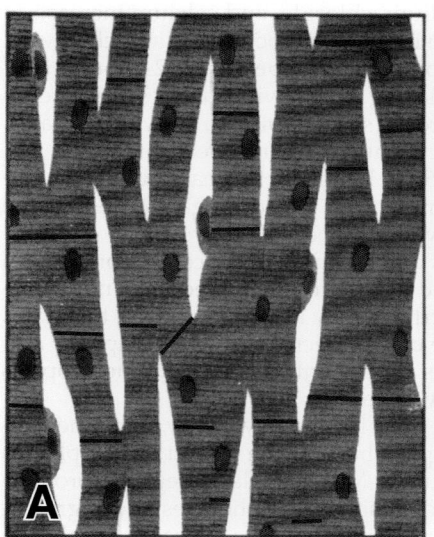
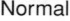

Normal

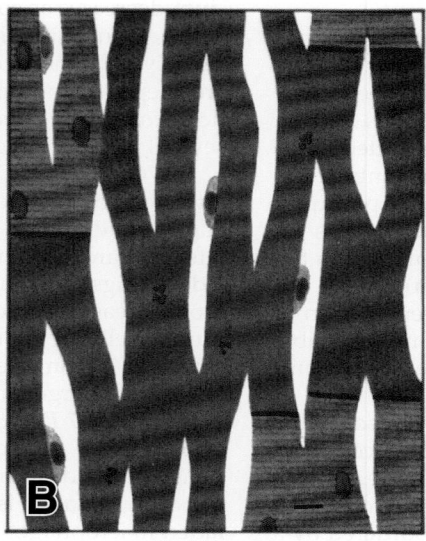

12–18 hours

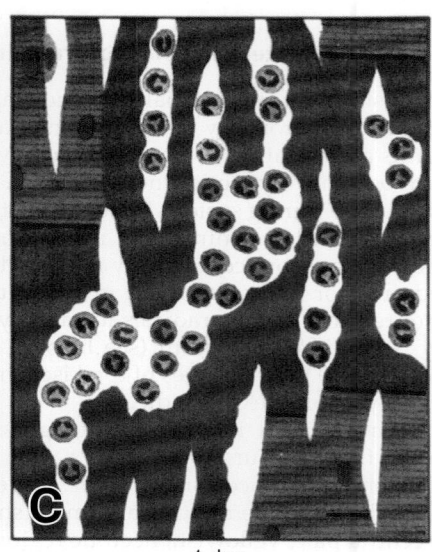

1 day

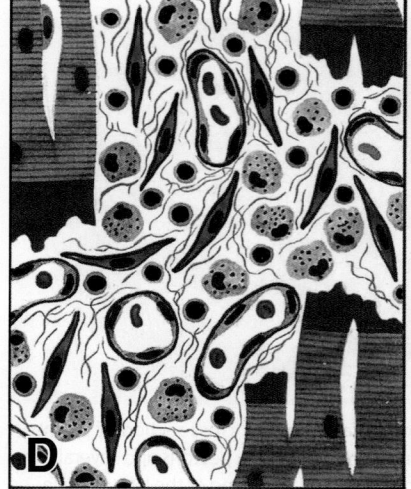

3 weeks

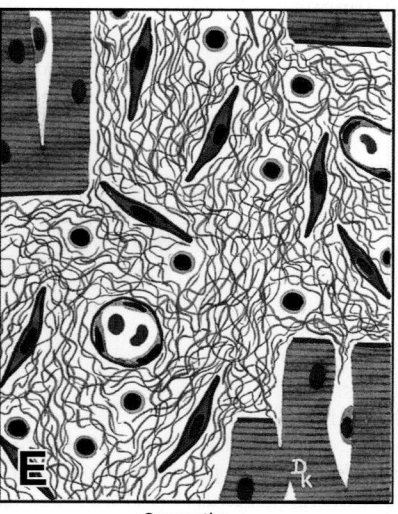

3 months

FIGURE 17-17. Development of a myocardial infarct. A. Normal myocardium. **B.** After about 12 to 18 hours, infarcted myocardium is eosinophilic (*red staining*) in hematoxylin and eosin-stained sections. **C.** About 24 hours after the onset of infarction, neutrophils infiltrate spaces between necrotic myocytes at the periphery of the infarct. **D.** After about 3 weeks, peripheral portions of the infarct contain granulation tissue with prominent capillaries, myofibroblasts, lymphoid cells, and macrophages. Necrotic debris has been largely removed, and a small amount of collagen has been laid down. **E.** After 3 months or more, the infarcted region has been replaced by scar tissue.

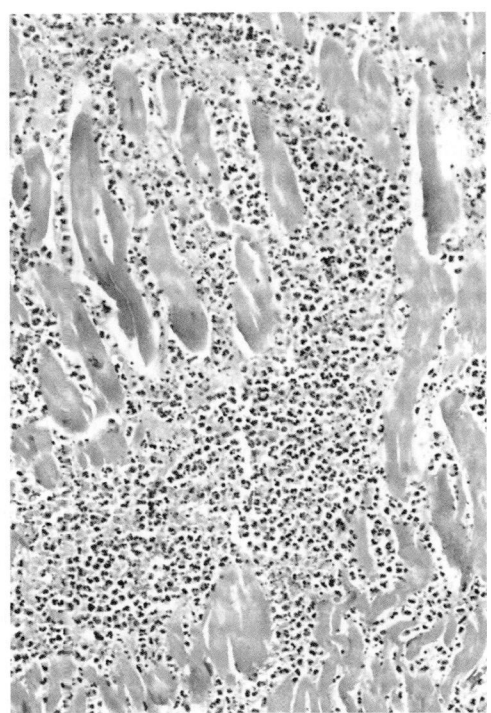

FIGURE 17-18. Acute myocardial infarct. Necrotic myocardial fibers, which are eosinophilic and lack cross-striations and nuclei, are immersed in a sea of acute inflammatory cells.

necrotic muscle with scar tissue begins at about 5 days, first at the infarct's edge, gradually moving inward.

ONE TO 3 WEEKS: Collagen deposition proceeds, inflammation gradually recedes, and the newly sprouted capillaries are progressively obliterated.

MORE THAN 4 WEEKS: Considerable dense fibrous tissue is present. Debris is slowly removed, and the scar is more solid and less cellular as it matures (Fig. 17-19).

This sequence of inflammatory and reparative events can be altered by local or systemic factors. For example, immediate extension of an infarct into a region that previously had patchy necrosis may not show expected changes. Large infarcts tend not to mature at centrally as rapidly as do smaller ones. In estimating the age of a large infarct, it is more accurate to base interpretation on the outer border where repair begins, rather than on the central region. In fact, in some large infarcts, dead myocytes are not removed but rather remain indefinitely "mummified."

Reperfusion and Ischemic Myocardium

The above descriptions pertain to healing of infarcts caused by persistent coronary occlusion, such as those arising from thrombotic occlusion of an epicardial coronary artery. However, blood flow may be restored to regions of evolving infarcts by spontaneous thrombolysis or through coronary intervention to open an occluded artery. When that happens, an infarct's appearance changes. Reperfused infarcts are typically hemorrhagic, from blood flow through damaged microvasculature. Thus, infarcts due to persistent occlusion are only apparent grossly after about 12 hours and are pale, but hemorrhage immediately highlights reperfused infarcts. Reperfusion also accelerates acute inflammation: neutrophils permeate the infarct, rather than only the periphery. They accumulate more rapidly, and then disappear more rapidly. Replacement of necrotic muscle by fibrous scar is also faster, at least where perfusion persists.

A characteristic feature of reperfused acute infarcts is **contraction band necrosis**. Contraction bands are thick, irregular, transverse eosinophilic bands in necrotic myocytes (Fig. 17-20). These bands are small groups of hypercontracted and disorganized sarcomeres with thickened Z disks. The sarcolemma is disrupted. Mitochondria located between the contraction bands are swollen and may contain calcium phosphate deposits in the matrix and amorphous matrix densities. Contraction bands occur whenever there is a massive influx of Ca^{2+} into cardiac myocytes. Reperfusion of ischemic myocardium causes extensive sarcolemmal damage mediated largely by reactive oxygen species (ROS), which permits unrestrained entry of extracellular Ca^{2+} into

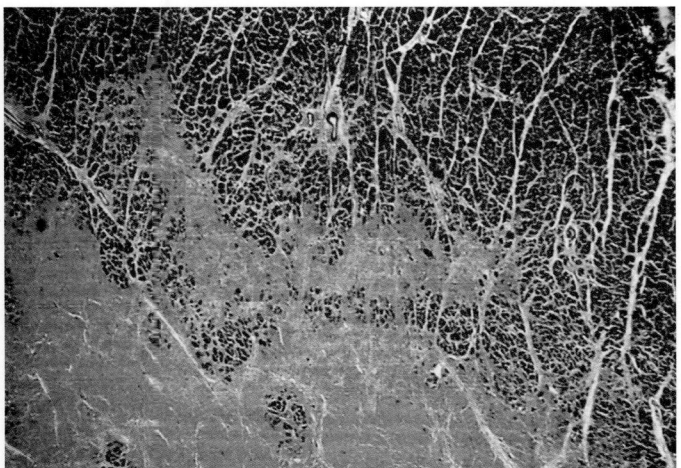

FIGURE 17-19. Healed myocardial infarct (trichrome stain for collagen). At the edge of a healed infarct, dense, acellular regions of collagenous matrix (blue-green here) are sharply demarcated from adjacent viable myocardium.

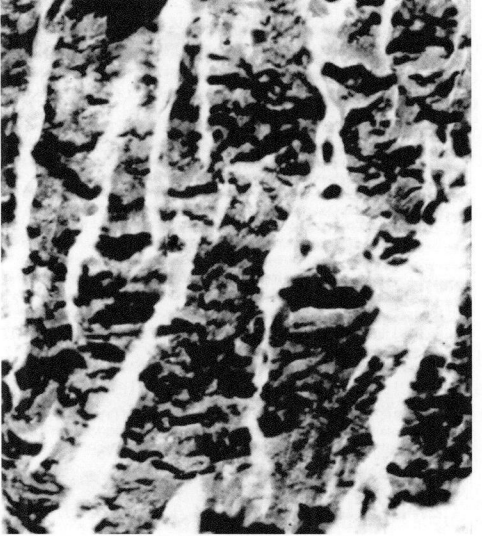

FIGURE 17-20. Contraction band necrosis. Infarcted myocardium shows prominent, thick, wavy, transverse bands in myofibers.

myocytes. This massive Ca^{2+} influx leads to hypercontraction in cells still able to contract. Contraction band necrosis is most extensive when acutely ischemic myocardium is reperfused (e.g., after thrombolytic therapy or with prolonged cardiopulmonary bypass during which myocardium has sustained irreversible injury). In infarcts arising from persistent coronary occlusion, microscopic foci of contraction band necrosis may be limited to the margins of the infarct, where dynamic ebb and flow of blood favor Ca^{2+} influx. Other conditions promoting abnormal Ca^{2+} influx leading to contraction bands include massive catecholamine release in patients with head injuries or pheochromocytoma, or patients in shock treated with large doses of pressors.

Clinical Diagnosis

CLINICAL FEATURES: *The onset of acute myocardial infarction is often sudden, with severe, crushing substernal or precordial pain.* The pain may be reported as epigastric burning (simulating indigestion) or it may extend into the jaw or down the inside of either arm. It is often accompanied by sweating, nausea, vomiting, and shortness of breath. In some cases, acute myocardial infarction is preceded by several days of unstable angina. *Up to a third of nonfatal Q-wave myocardial infarctions occur without symptoms and are identified only later by ECG changes or at autopsy.* These "clinically silent" infarcts are particularly common among diabetics with autonomic dysfunction and in cardiac transplant patients whose hearts are denervated.

Diagnosis of acute myocardial infarction is confirmed by ECG changes and by increased serum levels of certain enzymes or proteins. The ECG shows ST depression in non-STEMI and ST elevation in STEMI. Q waves typically develop in the latter (Fig. 17-13). The pathologic distinction of transmural versus subendocardial infarcts correlates reasonably well with ECG distinction of STEMI versus non-STEMI events.

Elevation in serum of cardiac proteins such as MB-CK or cardiac troponins is evidence of myocardial necrosis. The most widely assayed biomarker is cardiac troponin (I or T) which is highly specific for cardiac muscle and can be measured with high clinical sensitivity. Diagnosis of myocardial infarction requires a rise and/or fall in the level of the biomarker within the time frame of clinical events. Although clinical symptoms of myocardial ischemia and acute ST depression may reflect unstable (demand-associated) angina or non-STEMI (Fig. 17-13), elevated biomarker levels are seen only in the latter. An increase in biomarker level is invariable in STEMI.

Complications of Myocardial Infarction

Early (<30 days) mortality in acute myocardial infarction has dropped from 30% in the 1950s to less than 5% now. Nevertheless, the clinical course after acute infarction may be dominated by electrical or mechanical complications of the infarct.

CLINICAL FEATURES: *ARRHYTHMIAS:* Virtually all patients who have a myocardial infarct have abnormal cardiac rhythm at some time

during their illness. Arrhythmias still account for half of deaths caused by ischemic heart disease, but the advent of coronary care units and defibrillators has greatly reduced early mortality. Premature ventricular beats, sinus bradycardia, ventricular tachycardia, ventricular fibrillation, paroxysmal atrial tachycardia, and partial or complete heart block may occur. The causes of these arrhythmias are often multifactorial. Acute ischemia alters conduction, increases automaticity and promotes triggered activity related to afterdepolarizations driven by abnormal myocyte Ca^{2+} homeostasis. Enhanced sympathetic activity mediated by increased levels of local or circulating catecholamines plays an important role.

LEFT VENTRICULAR FAILURE AND CARDIO-GENIC SHOCK: Development of left ventricular failure soon after myocardial infarction is an ominous sign that generally indicates massive muscle loss. Thanks to coronary interventions that limit the extent of infarction (thrombolytic therapy, angioplasty) or assist damaged myocardium (intra-aortic balloon pump), cardiogenic shock occurs in under 5% of cases. Cardiogenic shock tends to develop early after infarction when 40% or more of the left ventricle has been lost; mortality may reach 90%.

REINFARCTION: This is defined as acute myocardial infarction that occurs within 28 days of a previous infarction. In many cases, it involves extension or enlargement of the antecedent infarct. In the current era, reinfarction is often caused by stent thrombosis. In up to 10% of patients, reinfarction typically occurs in the first 1 to 2 weeks. In careful echocardiographic studies, half of patients with anterior myocardial infarction showed some infarct extension in the first 2 weeks, suggesting that many episodes of infarct extension are not recognized. Clinically significant infarct extension doubles mortality.

RUPTURE OF THE FREE WALL OF THE MYOCAR-DIUM: Myocardial rupture (Fig. 17-21) may occur at almost any point in the 3 weeks after acute infarction, but is most common between days 2 and 7, when the infarcted wall is weakest. During this vulnerable period, infarcted tissue is soft and necrotic. Its extracellular matrix has

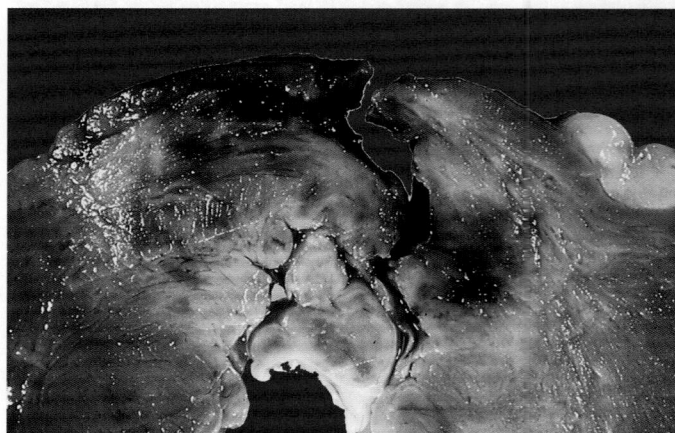

FIGURE 17-21. Rupture of an acute myocardial infarct. An elderly woman with a recent myocardial infarct died of cardiac tamponade. The pericardium was filled with blood. The cut surface of the left ventricle shows a linear rupture of the necrotic myocardium.

been degraded by proteases from inflammatory cells, but significant new matrix has not yet been deposited. Once scars begin to form, rupture is less likely. Rupture of the free wall is a complication of transmural infarcts; surviving muscle overlying subendocardial infarcts prevents rupture. However, rupture usually occurs in relatively small transmural infarcts. The remaining viable, contractile myocardium produces mechanical forces that may initiate and propagate tearing along the infarct's edge, where neutrophils accumulate.

Rupture of the left ventricular free wall most often leads to hemopericardium and death from pericardial tamponade. Myocardial rupture accounts for 10% to 20% of deaths after acute myocardial infarction among hospitalized patients. It occurs in less than 1% of patients undergoing acute coronary interventions. It is more common among elderly people, mostly women, having a first infarct, usually anterior in location. Treating with β-adrenergic blockers, which are negative inotropes, or concurrent heart failure, both reduce risk of myocardial rupture because they decrease contractile forces. Rarely, a ruptured ventricle may be walled off and the patient survives with a false aneurysm (Fig. 17-22).

OTHER FORMS OF MYOCARDIAL RUPTURE: A few patients in whom a myocardial infarct involves the interventricular septum develop **septal perforations**, 1 cm or longer. The magnitude of the resulting left-to-right shunt and, therefore, the prognosis depend on the size of the rupture.

Rupture of a portion of a papillary muscle results in mitral regurgitation. In some cases, an entire papillary muscle is transected, in which case, massive sudden mitral valve incompetence may be fatal.

ANEURYSMS: Left ventricular aneurysms complicate 10% to 15% of transmural infarcts. After acute transmural infarction, the affected ventricular wall tends to bulge outward during systole in one-third of patients. As the infarct heals, newly deposited collagenous matrix is susceptible to further stretching, although eventually the scar becomes nondistensible. Localized thinning and stretching of the ventricular wall in the region of a healing infarct is called "infarct expansion" but is actually an early aneurysm. Such an aneurysm is composed of a thin layer of necrotic myocardium and collagenous tissue, which expands with each cardiac contraction. As evolving aneurysms become more fibrotic, their tensile strength increases. However, aneurysms continue to dilate with each beat, thus "stealing" some left ventricular output and increasing the heart's workload. Left ventricular aneurysms predispose patients to ventricular tachycardia, due to increased opportunities for electrical current reentry at the edge of the aneurysm. Mural thrombi can develop within aneurysms and be sources of systemic emboli.

A distinction should be made between "**true**" and "**false**" **aneurysms** (Fig. 17-22). True aneurysms are much more common, and are caused by bulging of an intact, but weakened, left ventricular wall (Fig. 17-23). False aneurysms form when a left ventricle rupture is walled off by pericardial scar tissue. Thus, the wall of a false aneurysm contains pericardium and scar tissue, not left ventricular myocardium.

MURAL THROMBOSIS AND EMBOLISM: From 1/3 to 1/2 of patients who die after myocardial infarction have mural thrombi overlying the infarct at autopsy (Fig. 17-24). This occurs particularly often when the infarct involves the apex of the heart. Half of these patients have some evidence of systemic embolization. Inflammation of the endocardium lining an infarct promotes platelet adhesion and fibrin deposition. Also, poor contractile function of the underlying myocardium allows fibrin–platelet mural thrombi to grow. Fragments of thrombus can embolize, to cause strokes or myocardial or visceral infarcts. Documented mural thrombosis justifies anticoagulant and antiplatelet therapy.

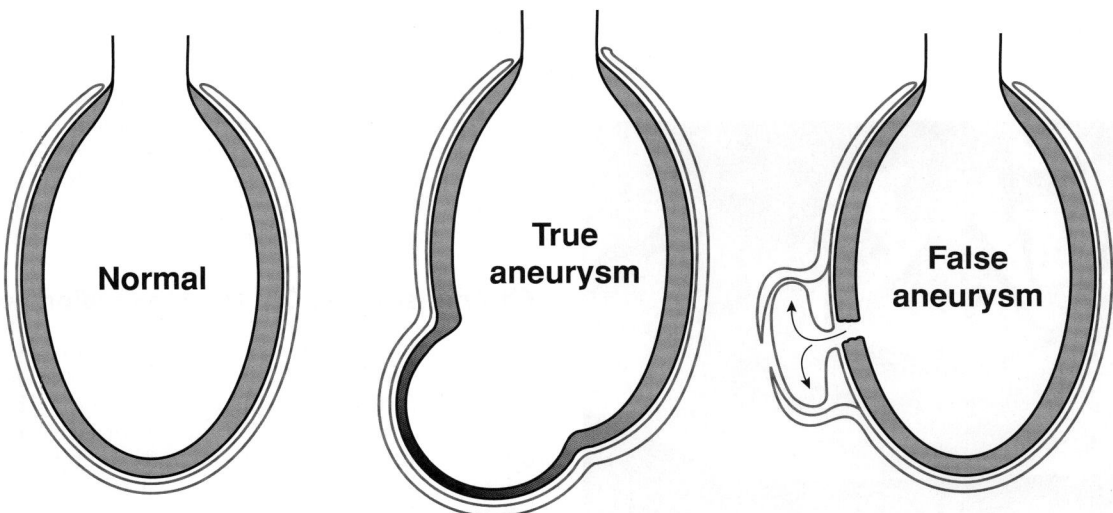

FIGURE 17-22. True and false aneurysms of the left ventricle. Left. Normal heart. The left ventricular wall (*shaded*) is enclosed by the pericardial sac. **Center.** True aneurysm shows an intact wall (*black*), which bulges outward. **Right.** False aneurysm shows a ruptured infarct, walled off externally by adherent pericardium. Note that the mouth of the true aneurysm is wider than that of the false aneurysm.

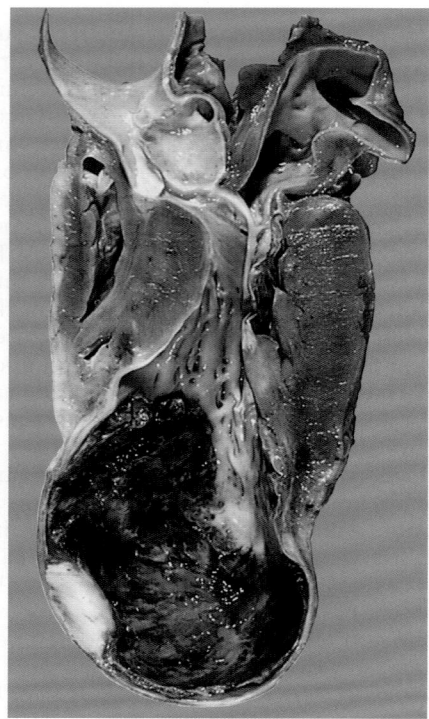

FIGURE 17-23. Ventricular aneurysm. The heart of a patient with a history of an anteroapical myocardial infarct who developed a massive ventricular aneurysm. The apex of the heart shows marked thinning and aneurysmal dilation.

PERICARDITIS: A transmural myocardial infarct involves the epicardium and leads to pericardial inflammation in 10% to 20% of patients. Pericarditis manifests clinically as chest pain and may produce a pericardial friction rub. One-quarter of patients with acute myocardial infarction, particularly those with larger infarcts and heart failure, develop pericardial effusions, with or without pericarditis. Less often, anticoagulant therapy may lead to hemorrhagic pericardial effusions and even cardiac tamponade.

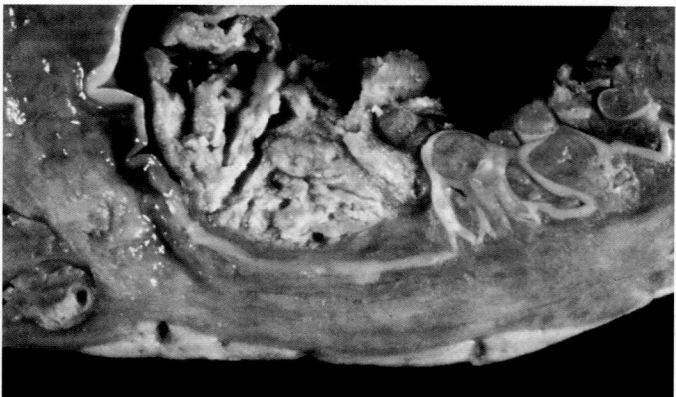

FIGURE 17-24. Mural thrombus overlying a healed myocardial infarct. In this cross-section of a fixed heart, an organized, friable, grayish white mural thrombus overlies a thickened endocardium situated over scarred myocardium.

Postmyocardial infarction syndrome (Dressler syndrome) is a delayed form of pericarditis that develops 2 to 10 weeks after infarction. A similar disorder may occur after cardiac surgery. Patients develop antibodies to heart muscle and improve with corticosteroid therapy, suggesting that the syndrome has an autoimmune basis.

Therapeutic Interventions Can Limit Infarct Size

Because the amount of myocardium that undergoes necrosis is an important prognostic predictor, any therapy that limits infarct size should be beneficial. Such therapy is directed at preventing reversibly injured, ischemic myocytes from dying and limiting infarct extension. Damaged myocytes can be salvaged for some time after the onset of ischemia if arterial blood flow resumes.

- **Restoring arterial blood flow**, often in association with reduction in myocardial oxygen demand via β-adrenergic blockers, is the only effective way to salvage ischemic myocytes permanently. Other interventions can slow ischemic injury, most notably hypothermia, which is used to minimize myocardial damage during cardiopulmonary bypass. Several methods have been developed to restore blood flow to myocardium supplied by an obstructed coronary artery.
- **Thrombolytic enzymes** such as tissue plasminogen activator or streptokinase can be infused intravenously to dissolve a clot causing vascular obstruction.
- **Percutaneous coronary intervention (PCI)** is dilation of a narrowed coronary artery by inflating a balloon catheter. PCI is useful as a primary procedure, immediately after the onset of ischemia or as a rescue procedure if thrombolytic agents fail to restore arterial blood flow. It nearly always includes placing a drug-eluting stent in the coronary artery to maintain its patency. Slow release of drugs such as paclitaxel, an anti-mitotic that interferes with microtubule (spindle) formation, or everolimus and related drugs that inhibit mTOR (**see Chapters 1 and 5**) signaling, limits subsequent restenosis by blocking smooth muscle cell proliferative responses to local injury caused by inflating the balloon catheter and deploying the stent.
- **Coronary artery bypass grafting** can restore blood flow to the coronary artery segment beyond a proximal occlusion.

Time is of the essence: interventions to restore blood flow must be done as soon as possible, preferably within the first few hours after symptoms begin. After 12 hours, it is unlikely that much salvageable ischemic myocardium remains, although reperfusion at this point may aid infarct healing and limit maladaptive postinfarct remodeling.

Chronic Ischemia Can Lead to Cardiomyopathy

In a minority of patients with severe coronary atherosclerosis, myocardial contractility is impaired globally without discrete infarcts, as in dilated cardiomyopathy. This situation usually reflects a combination of ischemic myocardial dysfunction, diffuse fibrosis and multiple small healed microinfarcts. However, there is a group of patients with left ventricular failure in whom cardiac dysfunction occurs without obvious infarction. These patients are said to have **ischemic cardiomyopathy**. In some, the dysfunctional myocardium has experienced repetitive episodes of ischemic injury, which causes degenerative changes in myocytes, with loss of myofibrils (hibernating myocardium) (Fig. 17-7). Contractile function of hibernating myocardium is restored when affected tissue is revascularized. Thus, to the extent that hibernation plays a role in ischemic cardiomyopathy, surgical revascularization may be beneficial.

HYPERTENSIVE HEART DISEASE

The World Health Organization has traditionally defined normal blood pressure as 120 mm Hg systolic and 80 mm Hg diastolic, and hypertension as persistent systemic blood pressure >140 mm Hg systolic and or >90 mm Hg diastolic (**see Chapter 16**). As reflected by the gap between normal and elevated blood pressures in these definitions, physicians have struggled to identify target blood pressure goals for patients with hypertension. Recent evidence shows that reducing systolic pressure from 140 to 120 mm Hg substantially reduces risk for adverse cardiovascular events. And although hypertension is a well-established risk factor for cardiovascular disease, most cardiovascular disease events occur in people with blood pressures below 140/90 mm Hg. In 2017, new guidelines issued by the American College of Cardiology and American Heart Association defined normal blood pressure <120/80 mm Hg, and *elevated blood pressure* as 120 to 129 systolic *and* >80 diastolic. **Stage 1 hypertension** was defined as 130 to 139 systolic *or* 80 to 89 diastolic, and **stage 2 hypertension** was defined as ≥140 systolic *or* ≥90 diastolic. Using these criteria, it was estimated that nearly half (46%) of the U.S. adult population has high blood pressure.

Chronic Hypertension Is a Common Cause of Heart Disease

It leads to pressure overload leading first to compensatory left ventricular hypertrophy and, eventually, cardiac failure. In **hypertensive heart disease**, there is no cause for a heart to be enlarged other than hypertension.

PATHOLOGY: The increased workload caused by hypertension leads to concentric left ventricular hypertrophy. *Left ventricular free walls and interventricular septum become thickened uniformly, but with no corresponding increase in chamber size* (Figs. 17-5 and 17-25). Heart weight increases, exceeding 375 g in men and 350 g in women. Hypertrophic myocardial cells are thicker, with enlarged, hyperchromatic, and rectangular ("boxcar") nuclei (Figs. 17-5 and 17-26).

CLINICAL FEATURES: Myocardial hypertrophy allows the heart to handle increased workload and normalize elevated wall stress caused by increased systemic vascular resistance. However, there is a limit beyond which additional hypertrophy no longer compensates. This upper limit to useful hypertrophy may reflect increasing diffusion distance between the interstitium and the center of each myofiber; if that distance is too great, oxygen supply to the myofiber will be impaired. Untreated hypertensive heart disease typically progresses to eccentric hypertrophy (Fig. 17-5) associated with heart failure.

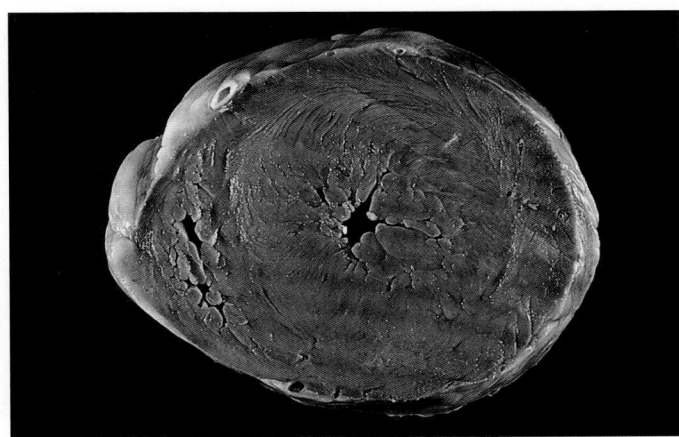

FIGURE 17-25. Hypertensive heart disease. A transverse section of the heart shows marked left ventricular myocardial hypertrophy, without dilation of the chamber (concentric hypertrophy). The right ventricle is normal size.

Diastolic dysfunction is the most common operative abnormality caused by hypertension and by itself can lead to heart failure. Hypertrophy causes some interstitial fibrosis, which makes the left ventricle stiffer. Hypertension also is associated with more severe coronary artery atherosclerosis. *The combination of greater cardiac workload (systolic dysfunction), diastolic dysfunction, and narrowed coronary arteries increases risk of myocardial ischemia, infarction, and heart failure.*

Heart Failure Is the Major Cause of Death in Patients With Untreated Hypertension

Fatal intracerebral hemorrhage, coronary atherosclerosis and myocardial infarction, dissecting aortic aneurysm or ruptured cerebral berry aneurysm are common as well. If hypertension becomes severe, nephrosclerosis may lead to renal failure.

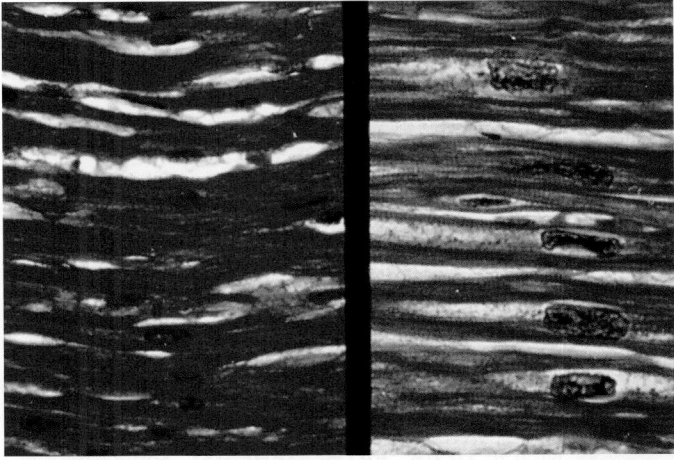

FIGURE 17-26. Hypertensive heart disease with myocardial hypertrophy. Left. Normal myocardium. Right. Hypertrophic myocardium (same magnification) shows thicker fibers and enlarged, hyperchromatic, rectangular nuclei.

COR PULMONALE

Cor pulmonale is right ventricular hypertrophy and dilation due to pulmonary hypertension. Increased pulmonary arterial pressure may reflect a disorder of lung parenchyma or, more rarely, a primary pulmonary vascular disease (e.g., primary pulmonary hypertension, recurrent small pulmonary emboli). It may also develop in response to alveolar hypoxia caused by abnormal breathing.

Acute cor pulmonale is an abrupt onset pulmonary hypertension, most often due to sudden, massive pulmonary embolization. This condition causes acute right-sided heart failure and is a medical emergency. At autopsy, the only cardiac findings are severe right ventricular, and sometimes right atrial, dilation.

CLINICAL FEATURES: Chronic cor pulmonale occurs to some extent in 30% to 40% of people with heart failure, reflecting the prevalence of lung disease—especially chronic bronchitis and emphysema—in such patients. Cor pulmonale is a component of heart failure with preserved ejection fraction (HFpEF) which is often associated with pulmonary hypertension. In chronic lung disease, the degree of pulmonary hypertension often correlates more closely with survival than other variables: <10% of patients with pulmonary artery pressures over 45 mm Hg survive 5 years.

Chronic cor pulmonale may be caused by any lung disease that impairs ventilatory mechanics or gas exchange or obstructs the pulmonary vasculature (Table 17-5). *The most common causes are obstructive sleep apnea, chronic obstructive pulmonary disease, and pulmonary fibrosis* (see Chapter 18). Severe kyphoscoliosis may deform the chest wall, impede its function as a bellows and so cause hypoxemia and pulmonary vasoconstriction. **Primary pulmonary hypertension** may also cause cor pulmonale. Some congenital heart diseases associated with increased pulmonary blood flow (see above) are complicated by pulmonary hypertension and cor pulmonale.

PATHOPHYSIOLOGY: The pathogenesis of pulmonary hypertension due to recurrent pulmonary emboli is related clearly to progressive mechanical obstruction of blood flow. However, mechanisms of pulmonary hypertension in chronic parenchymal diseases of the lungs are more complicated. In addition to obliteration of blood vessels in the lung, these disorders lead to pulmonary arteriolar vasoconstriction, which reduces the effective cross-sectional area of the pulmonary vascular bed without destroying vessels. Hypoxia, acidosis, and hypercapnia directly cause pulmonary vasoconstriction. Hypoxia also indirectly raises pulmonary vascular resistance by inducing polycythemia, which increases blood viscosity. People living at very high altitude often develop cor pulmonale because of the effects of chronic hypoxemia.

MOLECULAR PATHOGENESIS: Some people with pulmonary arterial hypertension have a familial disease with dominant inheritance and incomplete penetrance. Many of them have mutations in the gene

TABLE 17-5
CAUSES OF COR PULMONALE

Parenchymal Diseases of the Lung

Chronic bronchitis and emphysema

Pulmonary fibrosis (from any cause)

Cystic fibrosis

Pulmonary Vascular Diseases

Recurrent pulmonary emboli

Primary pulmonary hypertension

Peripheral pulmonary stenosis

Intravenous drug abuse

Residence at high altitude

Schistosomiasis

Congenital Heart Diseases

Impaired Movement of the Thoracic Cage

Kyphoscoliosis

Pickwickian syndrome and other causes of obstructive sleep apnea

Pleural fibrosis

Neuromuscular disorders

Idiopathic hypoventilation

encoding bone morphogenic protein receptor type 2 (*BMPR2*), a member of the TGFβ superfamily. BMPR2 helps regulate gene expression and intersects with other signaling cascades (e.g., MAPK pathways). A consequence of this aberrant signaling is endothelial dysfunction with insufficient production of vasodilators such as NO and prostacyclin, and overexpression of vasoconstrictors such as thromboxane. Resulting imbalances between vasoconstrictive and vasodilatory forces favor the former, which leads to smooth muscle hyperplasia and thickening of small pulmonary arteries, as is typically seen in pulmonary arterial hypertension. Genomic analysis has also identified variants other TGFβ superfamily members and rare recessive variants in other genes including *CAV1*, which encodes caveolin1; *KCNK3*, a K+ channel in pulmonary artery smooth muscle cells that regulates proliferation; and *EIF2AK4*, a translation initiation factor.

PATHOLOGY: Right ventricular hypertrophy (Fig. 17-27), which may exceed 1.0 cm in thickness (normal, 0.3 to 0.5 cm), is characteristic of chronic cor pulmonale. The right ventricle and right atrium are often dilated. Normally, the interventricular septum is curved to the left (i.e., it is part of the left ventricle), but may straighten or even curve to the right (Fig. 17-27) if right ventricular hypertrophy is severe.

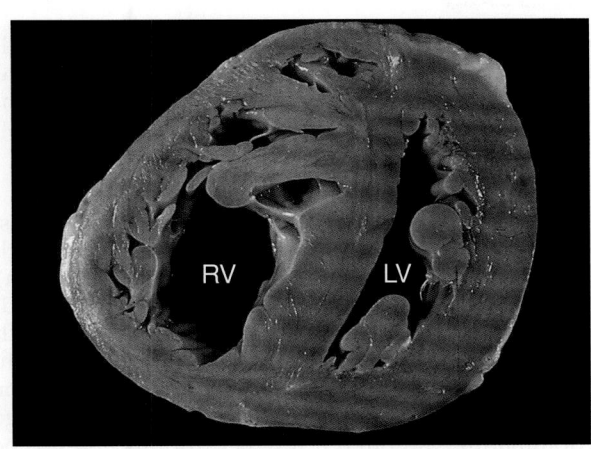

FIGURE 17-27. Cor pulmonale. A transverse section of the heart from a patient with primary (idiopathic) pulmonary hypertension shows a markedly hypertrophied right ventricle (on the left in this image). The right ventricular free wall thickness nearly equals the left ventricular wall. The right ventricle is dilated. The straightened interventricular septum has lost its normal curvature toward the left ventricle, due to remodeling in cor pulmonale.

ACQUIRED VALVULAR AND ENDOCARDIAL DISEASES

Many inflammatory, infectious and degenerative diseases damage and impair heart valves. Valves are normally thin flexible membranes that close tightly to prevent backward blood flow. The semilunar valves are structurally and functionally simple compared with atrioventricular valves, which consist of valve leaflets, fibrous and muscular valve annuli and a subvalvular apparatus (chordae tendineae and papillary muscles). Valvular stenosis usually involves pathologic changes of leaflets themselves, but regurgitation can be caused by abnormalities of valve leaflets, annulus, and/or subvalvular apparatus.

Damaged leaflets or cusps may be thickened and fused sufficiently to narrow the aperture and obstruct blood flow. This is **valvular stenosis**. Diseases that destroy valve tissue may also allow retrograde blood flow into atria during systole—**valvular regurgitation** or **insufficiency**. Diseases of cardiac valves may produce both stenosis and insufficiency, but one or the other generally predominates.

Cardiac valve stenosis causes **pressure overload** (concentric) hypertrophy of heart muscle upstream of the obstruction. Once compensatory mechanisms are exhausted, dilation and failure of the proximal chamber eventually occur (eccentric hypertrophy; see Fig. 17-5). Thus, mitral stenosis leads to left atrial hypertrophy and dilation. As the left atrium decompensates and can no longer propel pulmonary venous return through the stenotic mitral valve, blood backs up into the pulmonary venous circuit and signs of pulmonary congestion develop. This is followed by right ventricular hypertrophy and may lead to cor pulmonale (see above). Similarly, aortic stenosis causes left ventricular hypertrophy and eventually left heart failure.

Valve regurgitation or insufficiency causes **volume overload** with hypertrophy and dilation of the chamber proximal to the valve. In aortic insufficiency, the left ventricle first hypertrophies, and then dilates, when it can no longer handle

the regurgitant volume and maintain adequate cardiac output. An incompetent mitral valve volume overloads both the left atrium and ventricle, causing hypertrophy and dilation.

Marked left ventricular dilation from any cause that limits cardiac contractility (e.g., heart failure after a large myocardial infarct) may also widen the mitral valve ring and splay the left ventricular papillary muscles. These effects may be so severe that the valve leaflets do not close properly, leading to mitral regurgitation.

Rheumatic Heart Disease Encompasses Acute Myocarditis and Residual Valvular Deformities

Acute Rheumatic Fever

Rheumatic fever (RF) is a multisystem childhood disease that follows streptococcal infection. It entails an inflammatory reaction involving the heart, joints, and central nervous system.

EPIDEMIOLOGY: RF is a complication of acute streptococcal infection, almost always pharyngitis (i.e., "strep" throat; **see Chapter 9**). The cause is *Streptococcus pyogenes,* or group A β-hemolytic *Streptococcus.* In some epidemics of streptococcal pharyngitis, incidence of RF may be as high as 3%. RF is mainly a disease of children, with peak age incidence at 5 to 15 years. It may occur in adults but is rare after age 30.

In the first half of the 20th century, RF reached almost epidemic proportions in the United States, but its incidence has decreased dramatically. Between 1950 and 1972, the death rate fell from 14.5 to 6.8 per 100,000 and is now rarely fatal in the United States. Widespread antibiotic treatment explains part of this decrease, but the death rate from RF had begun declining well before antibiotics were generally available. Better socioeconomic conditions, particularly less crowded living circumstances, probably also contributed. *RF is still an important cause of cardiac deaths in young people in parts of Africa, Asia, the Middle East, and Latin America.*

 MOLECULAR PATHOGENESIS: For acute RF to develop, there must be a genetically susceptible host, a rheumatogenic strain of group A *Streptococcus* and an abnormal host immune response. It is unknown why only relatively few people infected with the offending *Streptococcus* develop RF. Autoimmunity and molecular mimicry are most likely involved (Fig. 17-28). For example, streptococcal antigens may resemble specific human leukocyte antigen (HLA) class II molecules, leading to aberrant cytokine production, and eliciting antibodies against proteins on valves and other host tissues.

Streptococcal M protein contains a coiled α-helical domain that structurally resembles domains in myosin and other cardiac proteins. Antibodies from acute RF patients can recognize both the M protein and epitopes within the myocardium. The levels of these antibodies correlate with disease severity and fall after replacement of diseased valves in RF patients. Some streptococcal M proteins contain a PARF domain (peptide associated with rheumatic fever) that can bind type IV collagen and

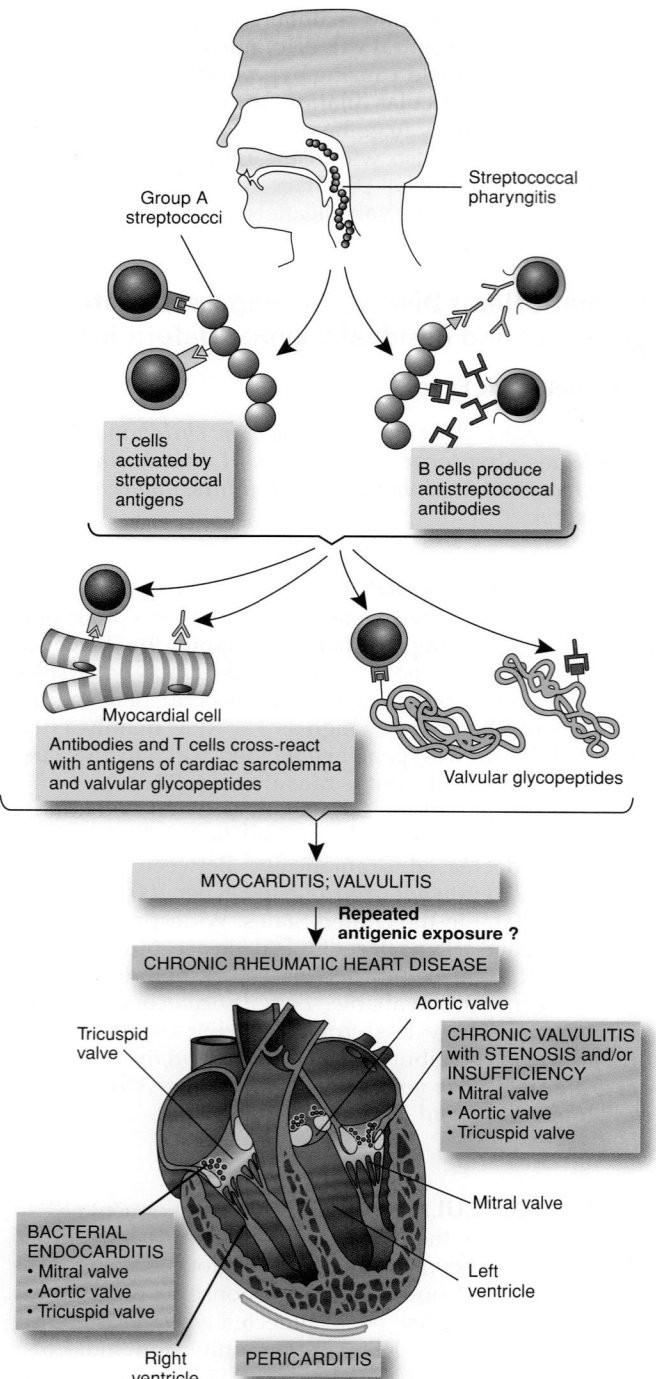

FIGURE 17-28. Biologic factors in rheumatic heart disease. The upper portion shows the trigger, β-hemolytic streptococcal pharyngitis, introducing streptococcal antigens into the body, eliciting antibodies and activating cytotoxic T cells. Resulting immune responses can cross-react with certain cardiac antigens, including those from myocyte sarcolemma and valvular glycoproteins. This may lead to inflammation of the heart in acute rheumatic fever, which involves all cardiac layers (endocarditis, myocarditis, pericarditis). This inflammation becomes apparent after 2- to 3 weeks. Active inflammation of the valves may eventually lead to chronic valvular stenosis or insufficiency. These lesions involve mitral, aortic, and tricuspid valves, in that order of frequency.

thereby stimulate an antibody response against collagen. Additional autoimmune mechanisms, not yet well defined, also probably contribute to the acute inflammatory response in RF.

PATHOLOGY: Acute rheumatic heart disease is a pancarditis; that is, it affects all three layers of the heart (endocardium, myocardium, pericardium).
MYOCARDITIS: In severe RF, some patients may die during the earliest acute phase of the illness before the typical granulomatous inflammation develops. At this early stage, the heart tends to be dilated and shows a nonspecific myocarditis, with lymphocytes and macrophages predominating, although a few neutrophils and eosinophils may be present. Fibrinoid degeneration of collagen, in which fibers become swollen, fragmented and eosinophilic, is characteristic of this early phase.

The **Aschoff body** is the characteristic granulomatous lesion of rheumatic myocarditis (Fig. 17-29). It develops several weeks after symptoms start. At first, it is a perivascular focus of swollen eosinophilic collagen surrounded by lymphocytes, plasma cells, and macrophages. With time, the Aschoff body assumes a granulomatous appearance, with a fibrinoid center and a perimeter of lymphocytes, plasma cells, macrophages, and giant cells. In time, it is replaced by a nodular scar.

Anitschkow cells are unusual cells within Aschoff bodies, whose nuclei contain a central band of chromatin. These nuclei have an "owl eye" appearance in cross-section and resemble a caterpillar when cut longitudinally

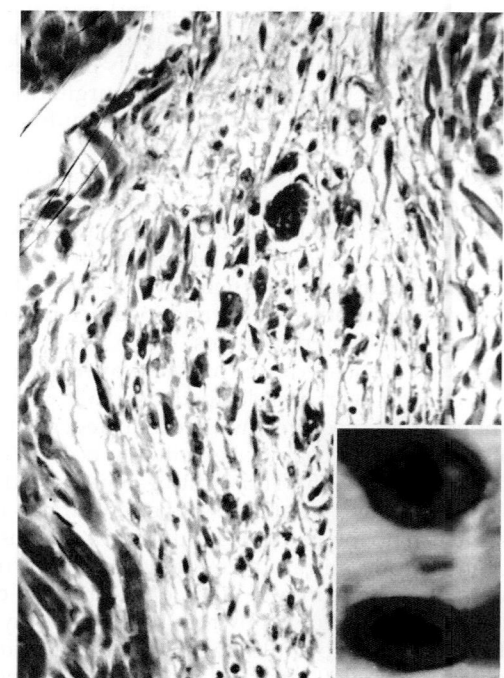

FIGURE 17-29. Acute rheumatic heart disease. An Aschoff body in the myocardial interstitium. Note collagen degeneration, lymphocytes and a multinucleated Aschoff giant cell. *Inset.* Nuclei of Anitschkow myocytes, showing "owl-eye" appearance in cross-section and "caterpillar" shape longitudinally.

(Fig. 17-29). Anitschkow cells are macrophages that are normally present in small numbers but accumulate and become prominent in certain types of inflammatory diseases of the heart. They may become multinucleated, in which case they are called **Aschoff giant cells**.

PERICARDITIS: Tenacious irregular fibrin deposits on visceral and parietal pericardial surfaces develop during the acute inflammatory phase of RF. These exudates resemble the shaggy surfaces of two slices of buttered bread that have been pulled apart ("bread-and-butter pericarditis"). This pericarditis may manifest clinically as a friction rub, but it is functionally minor and only infrequently leads to constrictive pericarditis.

ENDOCARDITIS: During the acute stage of rheumatic carditis, valve leaflets become inflamed and edematous. All four valves are affected, but left-sided valves sustain the worst injury, because they close under much higher pressures than right-sided valves. The result is damage and focal loss of endothelium along valve leaflet closure lines. This leads to deposition of tiny nodules of fibrin, recognized grossly as "verrucae" along the leaflets (the so-called verrucous endocarditis of acute RF).

 CLINICAL FEATURES: There is no specific test for RF. Clinically, the diagnosis is made if two major—or one major and two minor—criteria **(Jones criteria)** are met. Evidence of recent streptococcal infection increases the probability of RF.

Major criteria of acute RF include carditis (murmurs, cardiomegaly, pericarditis, congestive heart failure), polyarthritis, chorea, erythema marginatum, and subcutaneous nodules.

Minor criteria are previous history of RF, arthralgia, fever, certain laboratory tests indicating an inflammatory process (e.g., increased sedimentation rate, positive test result for C-reactive protein, leukocytosis) and ECG changes.

Symptoms of RF begin 2 to 3 weeks after an infection with *S. pyogenes.* By then, throat cultures are usually negative. Rising serum antibody titers to group A streptococcal antigens, such as antistreptolysin O, anti-DNase B, and antihyaluronidase, provide concrete evidence of a recent infection with group A *Streptococcus.* Acute symptoms of RF usually subside within 3 months, but with severe carditis, clinical activity may go on for 6 months or more. Mortality in acute rheumatic carditis is low. The main cause of death is heart failure due to myocarditis, but valvular dysfunction may also play a role.

Recurrent attacks of RF are associated with types of group A β-hemolytic streptococci to which the patient has not been exposed previously and, thus, to which immunity has not developed. RF recurrence rates reflect the time between the first episode and a later streptococcal infection. Recurrence rates may reach 65% if there had been a recent attack of RF; recurrence after 10 years affects only 5% of patients.

Prompt treatment of streptococcal pharyngitis with antibiotics prevents a first attack of RF and, less often, recurrences. There is no specific treatment for acute RF, but corticosteroids and salicylates help to manage the symptoms.

Chronic Rheumatic Heart Disease

 PATHOLOGY: Myocardial and pericardial components of RF typically resolve without permanent sequelae. By contrast, rheumatic valvulitis often causes long-term structural and functional changes. During the healing phase, diffuse fibrosis develops, and valve leaflets eventually become thickened, shrunken, and less pliable. At the same time, the verrucous lesions along the lines of closure often "heal" with fibrous "adhesions" that develop between leaflets, especially at the commissures (commissural fusion). The result is a stenotic valve that does not open freely because its leaflets are rigid and partially fused. Blood flow across such valves is turbulent, causing chronic hemodynamic "wear and tear" and eventuating in even more scarring and deformation of leaflets. Severe valvular scarring may develop months or years after a single bout of acute RF. On the other hand, recurrent episodes of acute RF can lead to repeated and progressively increasing damage to the heart valves.

The mitral valve is most commonly and severely affected valve in chronic rheumatic disease. It snaps shut under systolic pressure and so bears the greatest mechanical burden of all the valves. In chronic mitral valvulitis, valve leaflets are thickened and calcified, often with fused commissures and chordae tendineae (Fig. 17-30). In severe chronic rheumatic mitral valvular disease, valve orifices become reduced to a fixed narrow slit resembling a "fish mouth" when viewed from the ventricular aspect (Fig. 17-31). Stenosis may dominate functionally, but such valves are also regurgitant. Chronic regurgitation produces a "jet" of blood directed at the posterior aspect of the left atrium, damaging atrial endocardium and producing focal rough, wrinkled endocardium called "**MacCallum plaque.**"

Aortic valves, which snap shut under diastolic pressure, are second most often affected valve in rheumatic heart disease. Aortic stenosis occurs because cusps undergo diffuse fibrous thickening, with fusion of the commissures. Stenosis may at first be mild, but it progresses because of the chronic effects of turbulent blood flow across the valve. Often, cusps become rigidly calcified as patients age, causing varying degrees of stenosis and insufficiency (Fig. 17-32). The lower right heart pressures usually protect

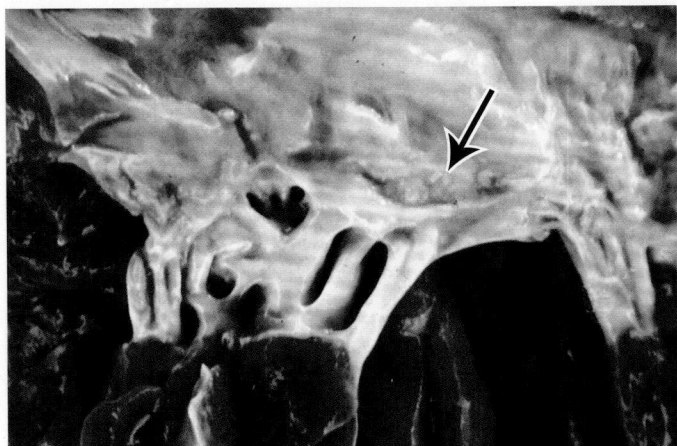

FIGURE 17-30. Chronic rheumatic valvulitis. The mitral valve leaflets are thickened and focally calcified (*arrow*), and the commissures are partially fused. The chordae tendineae are also short, thick, and fused.

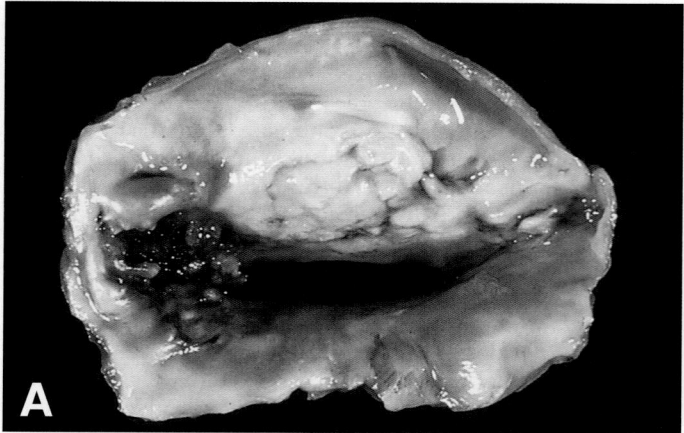
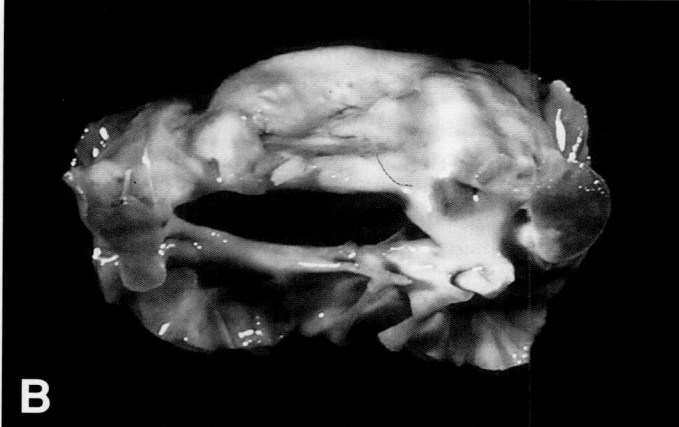

FIGURE 17-31. Chronic rheumatic valvulitis. A surgically excised rheumatic mitral valve, viewed from the left atrium (**A**) and left ventricle (**B**), shows rigid, thickened, and fused leaflets with a narrow orifice, creating the characteristic "fish mouth" appearance of rheumatic mitral stenosis. Note that the tips of the papillary muscles (in **B**) attach directly to the underside of the valve leaflets, reflecting marked shortening and fusion of chordae tendineae.

right-sided valves. Recurrent RF may, however, deform the tricuspid valve, virtually always together with mitral and aortic lesions. The pulmonic valve is rarely affected.

Complications of Chronic Rheumatic Heart Disease

- **Bacterial endocarditis** follows episodes of bacteremia (e.g., during dental procedures). The scarred valves of rheumatic heart disease are an attractive environment for bacteria that would bypass a normal valve.
- **Mural thrombi** form in atria or ventricles in 40% of patients with rheumatic valve disease. They give rise to thromboemboli, which can produce infarcts in various organs. Rarely, a large thrombus in the left atrial appendage develops a stalk and acts as a ball valve to obstruct the mitral valve orifice.
- **Heart failure** complicates rheumatic disease of both mitral and aortic valves.
- **Adhesive pericarditis** often follows the fibrinous pericarditis of acute attacks, but rarely causes constrictive pericarditis.

Autoimmune Diseases Affect Cardiac Valves and Myocardium

Systemic Lupus Erythematosus

SLE often involves the heart, but cardiac symptoms are usually less prominent than other manifestations of the disease.

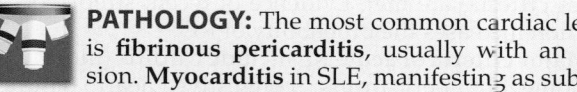

PATHOLOGY: The most common cardiac lesion is **fibrinous pericarditis**, usually with an effusion. **Myocarditis** in SLE, manifesting as subclinical left ventricular dysfunction, is also common and reflects the severity of the disease in other organs. Fibrinoid necrosis of small vessels and focal degeneration of interstitial tissue are seen.

Endocarditis is the most striking cardiac lesion of SLE. Verrucous vegetations, up to 4 mm, occur on endocardial surfaces and are called **Libman–Sacks endocarditis**. They occur most often on the mitral valve (Fig. 17-33), usually on atrial surfaces, close to the origin of the leaflets from the valve ring. They may also extend onto chordae tendineae

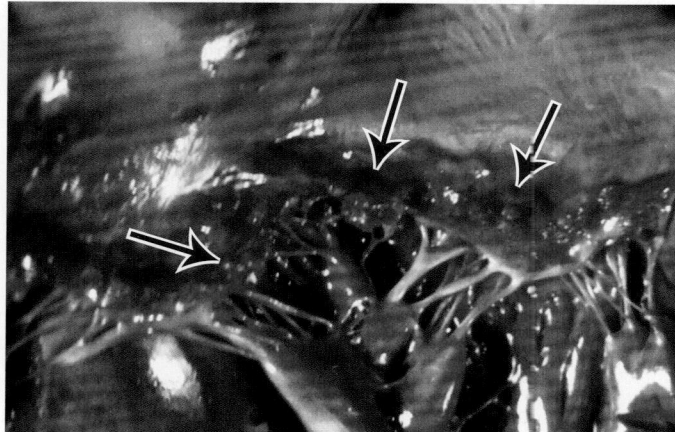

FIGURE 17-32. Chronic rheumatic aortic valvulitis with severe rheumatic aortic stenosis. Three sinuses of Valsalva are recognizable, but the cusps are rigidly fibrotic and calcified, and extensive fusion of the commissures has narrowed the orifice into a fixed slit-like configuration that does not change during the cardiac cycle.

FIGURE 17-33. Libman–Sacks endocarditis. The heart of a patient who died of complications of systemic lupus erythematosus has verrucous vegetations (*arrows*) on the leaflets of the mitral valve.

and papillary muscles. Aortic valve involvement is rare. *Libman–Sacks endocarditis usually heals without scarring and does not cause a functional deficit.*

Rheumatoid Arthritis

The heart is rarely compromised in patients with rheumatoid arthritis. Characteristic rheumatoid granulomatous inflammation, with fibrinoid necrosis and palisaded lymphocytes and macrophages, may occur in the pericardium, myocardium or valves, but heart function remains intact.

Ankylosing Spondylitis

A characteristic aortic valve lesion develops in up to 10% of patients with long-standing ankylosing spondylitis. The valve ring is dilated and its cusps are scarred and shortened. Focal inflammatory lesions occur in all layers of the aortic wall, particularly near the valve ring. Aortic regurgitation is the principal functional consequence.

Scleroderma (Progressive Systemic Sclerosis [PSS])

Scleroderma affects the heart mainly by causing intimal sclerosis in small arteries, with consequent cardiac ischemia, small infarcts, and fibrosis. Heart failure and arrhythmias are common. In fact, ECGs show ventricular ectopy in up to 2/3 of patients with PSS, and serious arrhythmias in 1/4. Only renal disease exceeds cardiac involvement as a cause of death in scleroderma. Cor pulmonale (due to pulmonary interstitial fibrosis) and hypertensive heart disease (caused by renal involvement) also occur.

Polyarteritis Nodosa

The heart is affected in up to 75% of patients with polyarteritis nodosa. Necrotizing lesions in branches of the coronary arteries cause myocardial infarction, arrhythmias or heart block. Cardiac hypertrophy and failure due to renal vascular hypertension are common.

Bacteria Cause Most Infectious Endocarditis

Other organisms, like fungi, chlamydia and rickettsiae are less commonly responsible.

Before the antibiotic era, bacterial endocarditis was untreatable and almost invariably fatal. Infections were classified by their course as acute or subacute, with **acute bacterial endocarditis** generally reflecting infection of normal cardiac valves with highly virulent organisms, like *Staphylococcus aureus* and *S. pyogenes* causes. **Subacute bacterial endocarditis** was generally due to colonization of structurally abnormal valves, often deformed by prior rheumatic heart disease, with less virulent organisms (e.g., *Streptococcus viridans* or *Staphylococcus epidermidis*).

Infectious endocarditis is now classified according to anatomic location and the offending organism (Table 17-6).

EPIDEMIOLOGY: Most children with bacterial endocarditis have an underlying cardiac lesion. While rheumatic heart disease accounted for one-third of such cases, it is rarely responsible for childhood bacterial endocarditis in the United States. *The most*

TABLE 17-6
ETIOLOGIC FACTORS IN BACTERIAL ENDOCARDITIS

	Children (%)		Adults (%)	
	Newborns	<15 Years	15–60 Years	>60 Years
Underlying Disease				
Congenital heart disease	30	80	10	2
Rheumatic heart disease	—	5	25	8
Mitral valve prolapse	—	10	10	10
Valvular calcification	—	—	5	30
Intravenous drug abuse	—	—	15	10
Other	—	—	10	10
None	70	5	25	30
Microorganisms[a]				
Staphylococcus aureus	45	25	35	30
Coagulase-negative staphylococci	10	5	5	10
Streptococci	15	45	45	35
Enterococci	—	5	5	15
Gram-negative bacteria	10	5	5	5
Fungi	10	Rare	Rare	Rare
Negative culture	5	10	5	5

[a]Five percent of neonatal infections are polymicrobial.

common predisposing condition for bacterial endocarditis in children currently is congenital cardiac malformations.

In adults, where rheumatic heart disease once counted for 75% of cases, it is now uncommon. Most adults with bacterial endocarditis have no known predisposing cardiac lesion. *Mitral valve prolapse (MVP) and CHD are now the most frequent bases for bacterial endocarditis in adults.*

- When bacterial endocarditis is superimposed on **rheumatic heart disease**, the mitral valve is affected in over 85%, and the aortic valve in 50%. Lone mitral valve endocarditis occurs more often in women (2:1), but the ratio is reversed, 4:1, in isolated aortic valve endocarditis.
- **Intravenous drug abusers** inject pathogenic organisms along with illicit drugs, and bacterial endocarditis is a notorious complication. In such patients, 80% have no underlying cardiac lesion, and the tricuspid valve is involved in half of cases. The most common source of bacteria in IV drug abusers is the skin, with *S. aureus* causing over half of the infections.
- **Prosthetic valves** are sites of infection in 20% of cases of endocarditis in adults, and 4% of patients with prosthetic valves have this complication. Risk of infection is greater in patients with bioprosthetic valves than with

mechanical valves. Staphylococci are again responsible for half of these infections. Most of the rest are caused by gram-negative aerobic organisms, streptococci, enterococci, and fungi. Indwelling vascular catheters are another source of iatrogenic endocarditis.

- **Transient bacteremia** from any source may lead to infective endocarditis. Dental procedures, urinary catheterization, gastrointestinal endoscopy, and obstetric procedures may all be responsible. Antibiotic prophylaxis is recommended for patients (e.g., with histories of RF or a cardiac murmur) who are at increased risk for bacterial endocarditis.
- **The elderly** are increasingly susceptible to endocarditis, due to age-related changes in heart valves, including calcific aortic stenosis and calcification of mitral annuli.
- **Diabetes** and **pregnancy** may also increase the incidence of bacterial endocarditis.

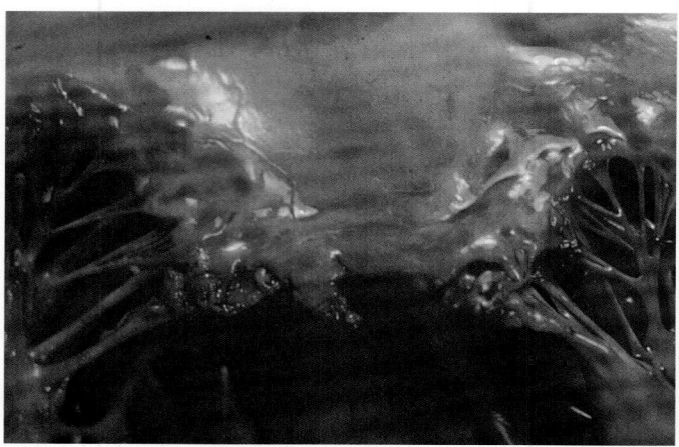

FIGURE 17-34. Bacterial endocarditis. The mitral valve shows destructive vegetations, which eroded through the free margins of the valve leaflets.

 ETIOLOGIC FACTORS: Virulent organisms, such as *S. aureus,* can infect apparently normal valves, but how this happens is poorly understood. Infection of previously damaged valves by less virulent organisms has been tied to (1) hemodynamic factors, (2) formation of an initially sterile platelet–fibrin thrombus, and (3) adherence properties of the microorganisms.

 PATHOPHYSIOLOGY: A key feature is abnormal blood flow across a damaged valve. Lesions form on the inflow portions of valves, where high pulsatile shear stresses occur. The pressure gradient across a narrow orifice (valve or congenital defect) produces turbulent flow at the periphery and a high-velocity jet at the center, both of which tend to denude valve endothelial surfaces. This leads to focal deposition of platelets and fibrin, creating small sterile vegetations that are hospitable sites for bacterial colonization and growth. Indeed, platelet adhesion is enhanced at high shear rates, which occur at leaflet free edges. Surrounding endothelium becomes activated by the presence of platelet–fibrin thrombi and upregulates expression of adhesion molecules (vascular cell adhesion molecule-1 [VCAM-1], intracellular adhesion molecule-1 [ICAM-1], and E-selectin). These, in turn, attract inflammatory cells. Microorganisms that gain access to the circulation, as a result of dental manipulation, for example, can deposit within the vegetations. In this protected environment, there may be 10^{10} organisms per gram of tissue. Matrix metalloproteinases made by bacteria begin to destroy valves, facilitating formation of adjacent vegetations.

Factors that promote bacterial adherence to sterile vegetations are believed to be important in the pathogenesis of endocarditis. Cell-associated and circulating fibronectin both bind to surface molecules of the bacteria, facilitating adhesion of fibrin, collagen, and cells. Some microorganisms produce extracellular polysaccharides, which also function as adhesion factors.

PATHOLOGY: Bacterial endocarditis most commonly involves left-sided heart valves (mitral, aortic, or both). The most common congenital heart lesions that predispose to bacterial endocarditis are PDA, TOF, VSD, and bicuspid aortic valve, which is an increasingly recognized risk factor, especially in men over 60. *As a rule, vegetations form on the upstream sides of the valves (i.e., the atrial side of AV valves and the ventricular side of semilunar valves), often at points where leaflets or cusps close* (Fig. 17-34). Vegetations consist of platelets, fibrin, cell debris, and masses of organisms. Underlying valve tissue is edematous and inflamed and may eventually become so damaged that a leaflet perforates, causing regurgitation. Lesions vary from small, superficial deposits to bulky, exuberant vegetations. The infective process may spread locally to involve valve rings or adjacent mural endocardium and chordae tendineae.

Infected thromboemboli travel to multiple systemic sites, causing infarcts or abscesses in many organs, including the brain, kidneys, intestine, and spleen.

Focal segmental glomerulonephritis may complicate infective endocarditis (**see Chapter 22**). It results from immune complex deposition in glomeruli, producing a patchy hemorrhagic appearance—the so-called flea-bitten kidneys.

 CLINICAL FEATURES: Many patients show early symptoms of bacterial endocarditis within a week of the bacteremic episode, and almost all are symptomatic within 2 weeks. Nonspecific symptoms—low-grade fever, fatigue, anorexia, weight loss—predominate at first. Heart murmurs develop almost invariably and often change during the course of the disease. In cases lasting over 6 weeks, splenomegaly, petechiae, and clubbing of the fingers are common. Systemic emboli are recognized at some point in one-third of cases. Mycotic aneurysms of cerebral vessels, brain abscesses, and intracerebral bleeding may occur. Cerebral emboli cause neurologic dysfunction in one-third of patients. Tricuspid valve endocarditis in drug addicts may cause septic pulmonary emboli.

Antibacterial therapy is effective in limiting morbidity and mortality of bacterial endocarditis. Most patients defervesce within a week of instituting such therapy. However, prognosis depends to some extent on the offending organism and the stage at which infection is treated. *A quarter of cases of S. aureus endocarditis are fatal.* Surgical replacement of a valve destroyed by endocarditis is risky and carries high surgical mortality as long as infection is active. *The most common serious complication of bacterial endocarditis is heart failure, which is usually due to valve destruction, and portends a grim prognosis.* Myocardial abscesses and infarction from coronary artery emboli may contribute to heart failure.

Nonbacterial Thrombotic Endocarditis (NBTE) May Complicate Some Cancers and Wasting Diseases

NBTE, also called marantic endocarditis, entails sterile vegetations on apparently normal cardiac valves, almost always in association with cancer or some other wasting disease. It affects mitral (Fig. 17-35) and aortic valves equally often. NBTE grossly resembles infective endocarditis but does not destroy affected valves and lacks both inflammation and microorganisms.

The cause of NBTE is poorly understood. It is seen commonly as a paraneoplastic condition, usually complicating adenocarcinomas (particularly of pancreas and lung) and hematologic malignancies. NBTE may also accompany disseminated intravascular coagulation or debilitating nonneoplastic diseases, accounting for the term "marantic endocarditis" (from the Greek, *marantikos*, "wasting away"). It may reflect increased blood coagulability or immune complex deposition. NBTE is often an incidental finding at autopsy; and vegetations remain small and do not destroy valves. The main danger, which is uncommon, is distant embolization, with infarcts of many organs.

Calcific Aortic Stenosis Reflects Chronic Valve Damage

In calcific aortic stenosis the aortic valve orifice narrows from calcium deposition in valve cusps.

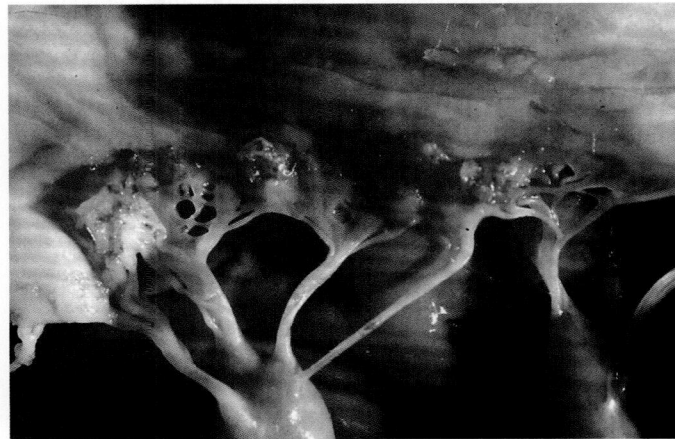

FIGURE 17-35. Marantic endocarditis. Sterile platelet–fibrin vegetations are seen on the mitral valve leaflets.

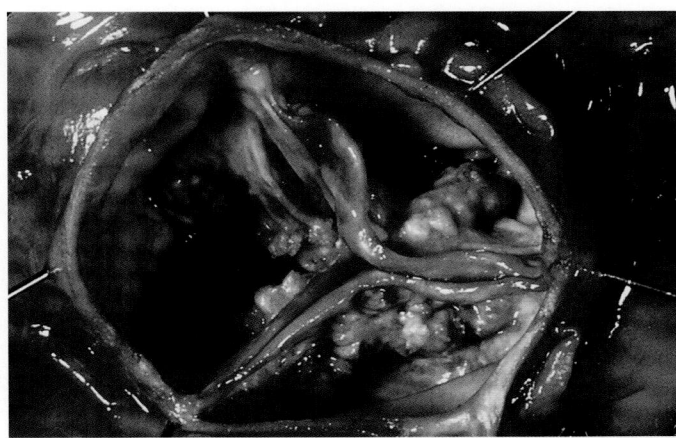

FIGURE 17-36. Calcific aortic stenosis in a three-cuspid aortic valve in an elderly person. Leaflets are heavily calcified, but there is no commissural fusion (compare to Fig. 17-32).

  ETIOLOGIC FACTORS, PATHOLOGY: Calcific aortic stenosis has 3 main causes.

- **Rheumatic aortic valve disease** is characterized by diffuse fibrous thickening and scarring of the cusps, commissural fusion and calcium deposition, all of which shrink the valve orifice and limit valve mobility (Fig. 17-32). Rheumatic aortic stenosis almost never occurs in isolation; it usually accompanies rheumatic mitral valve disease. As RF is now so rare in the United States, and as most rheumatic valves have been replaced surgically, calcific aortic stenosis is usually attributed to other causes.
- **Degenerative (senile) calcific stenosis** develops in the elderly as a degenerative process in a tricuspid aortic valve. Valve cusps become rigidly calcified, but commissural fusion (Fig. 17-36), which is a hallmark of rheumatic aortic valves, is not seen. The mitral valve is usually normal in patients with senile calcific aortic stenosis, although the mitral annulus may also be calcified.
- **Congenital bicuspid aortic stenosis** often develops with age (Fig. 17-37).

PATHOPHYSIOLOGY: Calcific aortic stenosis in damaged, malformed, and structurally normal valves is related to cumulative effects of years of turbulent blood flow across the valve. Bicuspid valves are not inherently stenotic, but flow across their elliptical orifice is more turbulent than with a tricuspid aortic valve. Increasing cusp rigidity eventually produces functional derangements, typically in patients over age 60. In all forms of calcific aortic stenosis, calcific nodules are restricted to the base and lower half of the cusps within the sinuses of Valsalva (see Figs. 17-36 and 17-37), and rarely involve the free margins. Without rheumatic scarring, commissures are not fused and 3 distinct cusps (or 2 in bicuspid valves) are evident.

Aortic valve calcification is not a purely passive process in which devitalized tissue becomes mineralized. In fact, valvular calcification is an active process involving modulation of valvular interstitial cells to

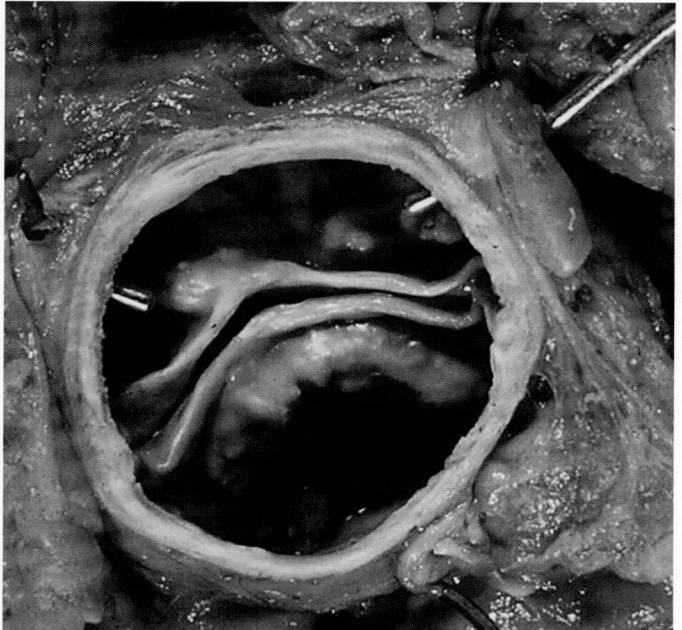

FIGURE 17-37. Calcific aortic stenosis of a congenitally bicuspid aortic valve. The two leaflets are heavily calcified, but there is no commissural fusion. Probes show the openings of the coronary ostia.

an osteoblastic phenotype and new gene expression resulting in cell-mediated mineralization of the extracellular matrix. Circulating osteoprogenitor cells may also migrate to the valve interstitium and contribute to mineralization. Many of the mechanisms and risk factors associated with valvular calcification are like those for atherosclerosis. For example, elevated LDL levels are associated with increased risk of aortic valve disease. Mechanical forces promote accumulation of LDL particles which become oxidized and stimulate inflammation with production of IL-1β, TNFα, and TGFβ. These inflammatory mediators activate matrix metalloproteinases which degrade valve extracellular matrix. In this milieu, fibroblasts are stimulated to differentiate into myofibroblasts with an osteoblast-like phenotype which, under the influence of oxidized LDL, TGFβ, and osteopontin, promote calcification of matrix proteins, mainly collagen. Despite these similarities between atherosclerosis and aortic valve calcification, however, drugs such as statins which reduce atherosclerosis, do not prevent calcific aortic stenosis.

CLINICAL FEATURES: Severe aortic stenosis causes striking concentric left ventricular hypertrophy. Eventually, the ventricle dilates and fails (eccentric hypertrophy). Surgical valve replacement is highly successful (5-year survival rate, 85%), if done before ventricular dysfunction is irreversible. The hypertrophic left ventricle then returns toward normal size. Transcatheter aortic valve replacement (TAVR) is being used increasingly in elderly patients with aortic stenosis who are poor candidates for open-chest valve replacement procedures.

Mitral Valve Annulus Calcification Is Usually Asymptomatic

Calcification of the mitral valve annulus is common among the elderly and usually carries no functional significance, although it often produces a murmur. Mitral regurgitation may occur if the process is severe enough to interfere with posterior mitral leaflet excursion during systole. Unlike calcification in RF-damaged valves, valve leaflets are not deformed in this entity, and calcification mainly affects the annulus, rather than the leaflets. About 40% of women over 90 have this lesion, compared to 15% of men. Mitral annulus calcification is aggravated if the patient has aortic stenosis, hypertension, or diabetes.

Calcific deposits transform the mitral ring into a rigid, curved bar up to 2 cm in diameter, which may be seen radiologically. Amorphous masses of calcified material first develop in the connective tissue of the valve ring, but, with time, extend into the base of the leaflets and eventually to the ventricular septum.

Mitral Valve Prolapse (MVP) Is the Most Common Indication for Valve Repair or Replacement

In MVP, also called "floppy mitral valve syndrome," mitral valve leaflets become enlarged and redundant. Chordae tendineae are thinned and elongated, so that the leaflets billow and prolapse into the left atrium during systole (Fig. 17-38A). Up to 3% of adults may show echocardiographic evidence of MVP, but regurgitation in most will not be severe enough to require surgery. MVP may be primary (nonsyndromic) or secondary (syndromic). The latter are associated with inborn errors of matrix proteins such as Ehlers–Danlos syndrome, osteogenesis imperfecta, or pseudoxanthoma elasticum. Over 90% of patients with Marfan syndrome have MVP.

MOLECULAR PATHOGENESIS: There is a heritable component in nonsyndromic MVP transmitted as an autosomal dominant trait with variable penetrance related to age and sex. Loci have been mapped to chromosomes 16, 11, and 13, but responsible alleles are not known. Recently, a missense mutation in *DCHS1*, at 11p15.4 and encodes a protein in the cadherin superfamily, has been implicated in a large family with nonsyndromic MVP.

Because MVP is so prevalent in Marfan syndrome, it was thought that variants in *FBN1* (the fibrillin-1 gene that is mutated in Marfan syndrome) might play a role in nonsyndromic MVP but this has not been observed. Dysregulated TGFβ signaling occurs in surgically excised valves from patients with primary MVP. TGFβ activates valve interstitial cells and promotes extracellular matrix remodeling. It also reduces expression of metallothioneins involved in response to oxidative stress, and downregulates expression of genes in the ADAMTS family that degrade proteoglycans. Abnormal TGFβ signaling has also been implicated in syndromic MVP. For example, Marfan syndrome may be caused by mutations in the TGFβ receptor-2 gene, *TGFBR2*. Loeys–Dietz syndrome, a connective tissue disorder associated with a high prevalence of MVP, is also caused by heterozygous mutations in either *TGFBR1* or *TGFBR2*. AngII receptor blockers can block abnormal TGFβ, and clinical trials testing effects on aortic root dilatation and MVP have shown encouraging initial results.

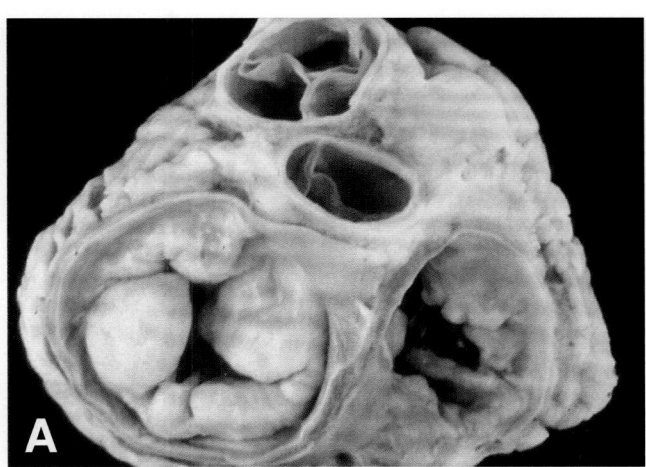
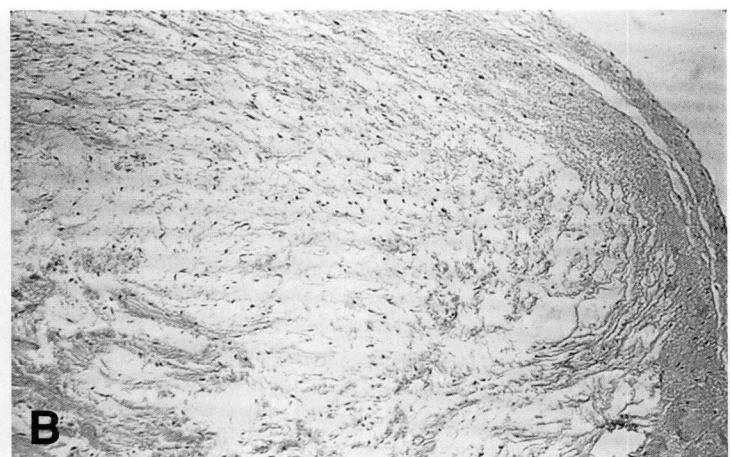

FIGURE 17-38. Mitral valve prolapse. A. A view of the mitral valve (*left*) from the left atrium shows redundant and deformed leaflets, which billow into the left atrial cavity. **B.** A microscopic section of one of the mitral valve leaflets shows conspicuous myxomatous connective tissue in the center of the leaflet.

 PATHOLOGY: Prolapsed mitral valve leaflets are redundant and deformed (Fig. 17-38A), with striking amounts of myxomatous connective tissue in the spongiosa, the middle layer of the valve leaflet (Fig. 17-38B). Accumulation of proteoglycans (acid mucopolysaccharides) imparts a gelatinous appearance and slippery texture to valve cut surfaces. Collagen fibrils are fragmented. Myxomatous degeneration also affects the valve annulus and chordae tendineae, increasing prolapse and regurgitation. Damage to chordae may be so severe that they break. Rupture of multiple chordae can yield a "flail mitral valve" that is totally incompetent. The mitral valve is usually the only valve affected, but myxomatous degeneration can occur in other valves, especially in patients with Marfan syndrome, in whom the tricuspid valve is often abnormal.

CLINICAL FEATURES: Most patients with MVP are asymptomatic. Clinical suspicion of MVP is based on classical auscultatory findings: a mid- to late-systolic click, caused by redundant leaflets snapping as they prolapse into the left atrium. A late-systolic murmur is present if regurgitation is significant. Endocarditis is a potentially serious complication (see above). Significant mitral regurgitation develops in 15% of patients after 10 to 15 years of MVP, after which mitral valve repair or replacement is indicated.

Risk of sudden death, presumably due to ventricular tachyarrhythmias, is twice that in the general population. The mechanisms are not well understood, but risk appears mainly to reflect the degree of regurgitation, perhaps related to ventricular remodeling associated with volume overload. Repair of regurgitant floppy valves lowers this risk.

Papillary Muscle Dysfunction May Cause Mitral Regurgitation

Left ventricular papillary muscle dysfunction is usually due to ischemia. Papillary are supplied by terminal branches of intramyocardial coronary arteries muscles, and so are especially vulnerable to ischemic injury. Any reduction in blood flow preferentially interferes with papillary muscle function. Brief periods of ischemia (e.g., during episodes of angina pectoris) can cause transient papillary muscle dysfunction (stunning) and temporary mitral regurgitation. Permanent mitral regurgitation may be due to infarction and subsequent scarring of papillary muscles. One-third of patients being evaluated for coronary artery bypass surgery show evidence of "ischemic mitral regurgitation." Papillary muscle dysfunction may also be associated with healed myocardial infarct, in which impaired myocardial contractility at the base of a papillary muscle impedes its function. Rarely, patients may suddenly develop life-threatening mitral regurgitation when an acutely infarcted papillary muscle ruptures.

Carcinoid Heart Disease Affects Right-Sided Valves

Carcinoid heart disease occurs in people with carcinoid tumors and may lead to tricuspid regurgitation and pulmonic stenosis.

PATHOPHYSIOLOGY: Carcinoid heart disease is not fully understood, but valve and endocardial lesions are thought to reflect high concentrations of serotonin and/or other vasoactive substances secreted by carcinoid tumors that have metastasized to the liver. These chemicals are metabolized in the liver and lung, so carcinoid heart disease affects the right side of the heart almost exclusively, and only after liver metastases. Rarely, patients with ASDs and right-to-left shunts may show left-sided involvement.

During the 1990s, reports surfaced of mitral and aortic valve disease in patients taking the appetite-suppressing drugs fenfluramine-phentermine ("fen-phen"). Affected valves had pathologic features strikingly like those in carcinoid heart disease, except on left-sided valves. Other anorexigenic drugs and ergot alkaloid drugs, for example, ergotamine and methysergide used to treat migraine headaches have also been linked to this type of valve disease.

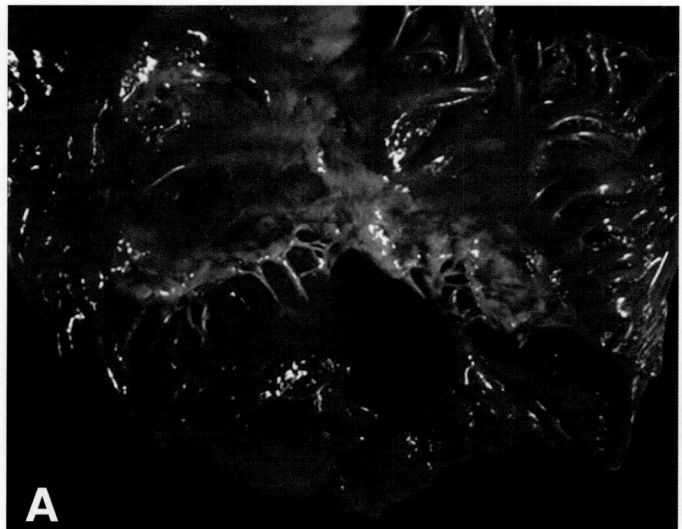
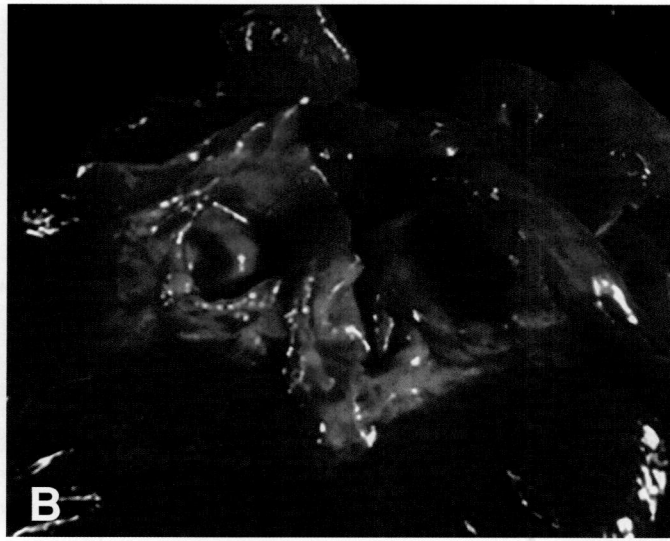

FIGURE 17-39. Carcinoid heart disease. A. Tricuspid valve leaflets are thickened by plaque-like fibrous deposits; chordae are thickened and fused. The deformed valve is unable to close normally and causes tricuspid regurgitation. The right atrium is greatly enlarged as a result of volume overload. **B.** Pulmonic valve leaflets are thickened by fibrosis and show reduced surface area. The deformed valve cannot open fully, thus producing pulmonic stenosis and pressure overload of the right ventricle.

These drugs interfere with serotonin metabolism and signaling, so the pathogenesis of drug-related and carcinoid valve disease is similar.

PATHOPHYSIOLOGY: The cardiac lesions are plaque-like deposits of dense, pearly gray, fibrous tissue on tricuspid (Fig. 17-39) and pulmonary valves and on the endocardial surface of the right ventricle. These patches look "tacked on" to valve leaflets, with no associated inflammation or apparent damage to underlying valve structures. However, leaflets become deformed, with reduced surface area, so tricuspid leaflets appear stuck onto adjacent right ventricular mural endocardium. Tricuspid insufficiency or stenosis results. Shrinkage of the pulmonic valve and its annulus leads to stenosis.

MYOCARDITIS

Myocarditis is myocardial inflammation with myocyte necrosis. This definition specifically excludes ischemic heart disease. The true incidence of myocarditis is hard to establish, as many cases are asymptomatic. It occurs at any age but is most common in children 1 to 10 years old. It is one of the few heart diseases that can cause acute heart failure in previously healthy children, adolescents, or young adults. Severe myocarditis can cause extensive myocardial necrosis, arrhythmias, and sudden cardiac death.

Most Cases of Myocarditis Are Caused by Viruses

Viral etiology is generally suspected, but unless special studies identify viral genomes in heart biopsies, evidence is usually circumstantial. During the second half of the 20th century, enteroviruses, especially coxsackie virus, were most commonly identified in the western world. Since then, sensitive methods to detect viral genomes have identified H1N1 strain influenza, adenovirus, cytomegalovirus, parvovirus B-19, and others in viral myocarditis. Etiologies of myocarditis are listed in Table 17-7.

PATHOPHYSIOLOGY: Viral myocarditis develops in phases. Virus first enters myocytes and activates innate immune responses. Coxsackie and adenoviruses gain entry by binding the coxsackie-adenovirus receptor (CAR). CAR belongs to the family of intercellular adhesion molecules. It is especially abundant in children, which may explain why viral myocarditis so

---

TABLE 17-7

CAUSES OF MYOCARDITIS

Idiopathic

Infectious

- Viral: Coxsackievirus, adenovirus, echovirus, influenza virus, human immunodeficiency virus, and many others
- Rickettsial: Typhus, Rocky Mountain spotted fever
- Bacterial: Diphtheria, staphylococcal, streptococcal, meningococcal, *Borrelia* (Lyme disease), and leptospiral infection
- Fungi and protozoan parasites: Chagas disease, toxoplasmosis, aspergillosis, cryptococcal and candidal infection
- Metazoan parasites: *Echinococcus, Trichina*

Noninfectious

- Hypersensitivity and immunologically related diseases: Rheumatic fever, systemic lupus erythematosus, scleroderma, drug reaction (e.g., to penicillin or sulfonamide) and rheumatoid arthritis
- Radiation
- Miscellaneous: Sarcoidosis, uremia

often afflicts them. Intracellular coxsackie viruses produce proteases 2A and 3C which are crucial for viral replication but may also impair myocardial function. Protease 2A cleaves myocyte proteins such as dystrophin, which increases cell permeability and diminishes contractile function. Viral proteases may also activate myocyte apoptosis pathways by cleaving caspases. During active viral replication, myocytes produce type 1 (i.e., virus-induced) interferons. Antibodies to viral and cardiac proteins, the latter probably arising via molecular mimicry, further contribute to tissue damage and contractile dysfunction. At this point, myocytes undergo degeneration and apoptosis, with minimal inflammation.

A second phase, develops over days to weeks, with activation of acquired immunity. Infected myocytes produce and release cytokines including TNFα, IL-1, IL-2, and IFNγ. NK cells, macrophages, and T lymphocytes accumulate at sites of infection producing the classic pathology of viral myocarditis (Fig. 17-40). T cells eventually clear viruses resolving inflammation, healing by fibrosis in areas of myocyte necrosis and restored contractile function. Sometimes, impaired viral clearance and/or persistent immune activation may lead to dilated cardiomyopathy.

The above sequence describes common forms of myocarditis caused by viruses that infect cardiac myocytes. Other viruses can cause myocarditis by infecting cardiac endothelial cells. For example, parvovirus B-19, a frequent cardiac pathogen, stimulates production of IL-6 and TNFα and upregulates adhesion molecules, like E-selectin, in endothelial cells. Resulting endothelial injury, and accumulation of intravascular T cells, may cause enough microvascular damage to produce local ischemia and further impair cardiac function.

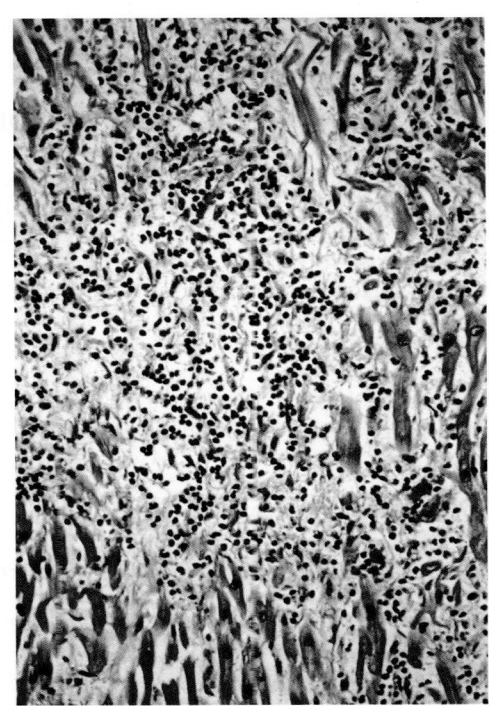

FIGURE 17-40. Viral myocarditis. Myocardial fibers are disrupted by a prominent interstitial infiltrate of lymphocytes and macrophages.

PATHOLOGY: Histologic features of viral myocarditis vary with the clinical disease, but with few exceptions, microscopic features are nonspecific and indistinguishable from toxic myocarditis. The classical picture during the phase of active acquired immunity, shows patchy or diffuse interstitial T-cell and macrophage infiltrates (Fig. 17-40). Multinucleated giant cells may also be present. Inflammatory cells often surround individual myocytes. Focal myocyte necrosis is seen. During the resolving phase, fibroblasts proliferate and deposit interstitial collagen. Neutrophils are uncommon, but if necrosis is extensive, the histology may resemble an acute infarct—a neutrophilic infiltrate followed by organization and repair. Most viruses that cause myocarditis also cause pericarditis.

CLINICAL FEATURES: Many people with viral myocarditis have no symptoms. When symptoms do occur, they usually start a few weeks after infection, coincident with acquired immune responses. Most patients recover from acute myocarditis, though some may die suddenly during the acute inflammatory phase. In the United States, for example, myocarditis is seen in a few percent of young adults (younger than age 35) autopsies for sudden, unexpected deaths. Others may progress to chronic heart failure, with features of dilated cardiomyopathy. Randomized clinical trials of immune suppression in active (biopsy-proven) viral myocarditis have been disappointing, but immunosuppression may be effective, at least in the short term, in a subset of patients with "virus-negative" (no viral genomes detected in heart biopsies) and "inflammation-positive" (ongoing production of cardiac-specific autoantibodies) myocarditis.

MYOCARDITIS IN AIDS: A significant number of AIDS patients have clinical or pathologic evidence of cardiac disease (pericardial effusions, myocarditis, endocarditis, or cardiomyopathy). They are unusually susceptible to viral myocarditis, largely due to cardiotropic viruses, like coxsackievirus and adenovirus. HIV-1 infection of cardiac myocytes appears to play a minor role.

Nonviral Infectious Agents Can Cause Myocarditis

Other blood-borne microorganisms can infect the heart. Among these, brucellosis, meningococcemia, and psittacosis (**see Chapter 9**) often lead to infectious myocarditis. Some bacteria (e.g., diphtheria) make cardiotoxins, which may cause fatal myocarditis. Myocarditis in South America is often Chagas disease, caused by the protozoan, *Trypanosoma cruzi* (**see below, Chapter 9**).

- **Bacterial infection** of the myocardium is characterized by multiple foci of a mixed inflammatory infiltrate, mainly polymorphonuclear. Microabscesses occur if septic emboli lodge in the coronary circulation, often because of infective endocarditis.
- **Rickettsia** often causes widespread vasculitis, affecting small coronary blood vessels.
- **Fungal myocarditis** mostly affects immunocompromised patients, although the heart is relatively resistant to fungal infection.

- **Toxoplasmosis** can involve the myocardium in immunosuppressed patients or be acquired transplacentally; the intracellular parasites proliferate in cardiac myocytes and elicit focal mixed inflammation, with neutrophils and eosinophils.

- **Chagas disease** is an insect-borne protozoal myocarditis, endemic to Latin America, caused by *Trypanosoma cruzi*. The acute stage may be asymptomatic or associated with mild systemic features of infection. Parasites proliferate in cardiac myocytes and stimulate inflammation, mainly of lymphocytes, plasma cells, and macrophages. A third to half of patients develop chronic Chagasic cardiomyopathy with heart failure, ventricular tachyarrhythmias, and thromboembolism.

Granulomatous Myocarditis May Be Caused by Microorganisms or Immunologically Mediated Injury

Microorganisms associated with granulomatous myocarditis include *Mycobacteria* and some types of fungi. Immune-mediated myocardial injury, for example, rheumatic myocarditis (Fig. 17-29) and sarcoidosis, may also cause granulomatous myocarditis.

Sarcoidosis Granulomatous Myocarditis Is Highly Arrhythmogenic

Sarcoidosis is a generalized granulomatous disease that may involve the heart (**see Chapter 18**). Although its cause remains enigmatic, considerable evidence implicates immune dysregulation. Attempts to identify an infectious source using the most sensitive methods have consistently failed. Sarcoidosis most often involves the lungs and mediastinal lymph nodes, but cardiac involvement is common and, in some cases, may be isolated. One-quarter of cases show some granulomas in the heart at autopsy, but <5% of patients with sarcoidosis have cardiac symptoms. Sarcoid granulomas may cause extensive myocardial damage, especially the base of the interventricular septum. Since this region contains major components of the AV conduction system, bundle branch blocks or complete heart block is common, as well as serious life-threatening ventricular tachyarrhythmias and sudden death. Microscopically, the heart in cases of severe sarcoid heart disease shows noncaseating granulomas infiltrating the myocardium, massive myocyte destruction, and interstitial fibrosis (Fig. 17-41).

Hypersensitivity Myocarditis Is a Reaction to Drugs

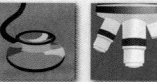 **PATHOLOGY:** In hypersensitivity myocarditis, inflammation is interstitial and perivascular. It is often confined to the myocardium and does not affect other organs. The inflammation in hypersensitivity myocarditis resembles that in viral myocarditis but with numerous eosinophils, in addition to lymphocytes and plasma cells. Myocyte necrosis is typically absent, even with intense inflammation.

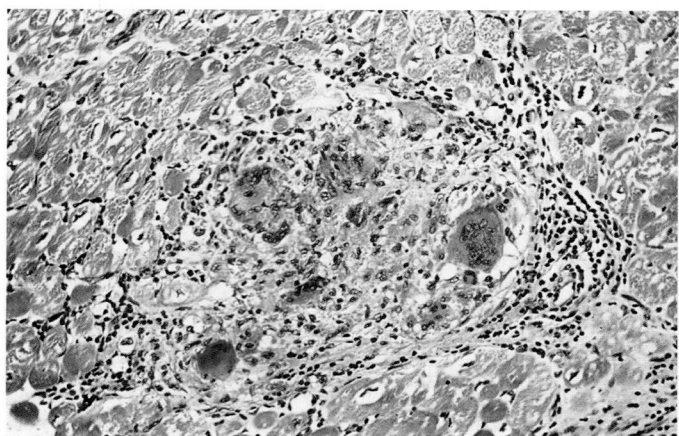

FIGURE 17-41. Cardiac sarcoidosis. The myocardium is infiltrated by nonnecrotizing granulomas, with prominent giant cells. There is considerable destruction of cardiac myocytes with fibrosis.

CLINICAL FEATURES: Hypersensitivity myocarditis is usually clinically silent and is often diagnosed incidentally at autopsy. However, it may produce chest pain and ECG changes resembling acute myocardial ischemia, or, occasionally, fatal ventricular arrhythmias. If there are symptoms, the offending drug should be discontinued and corticosteroids or immunosuppressive agents given.

Giant Cell Myocarditis Is Usually Fatal

Giant cell myocarditis is a rare, idiopathic, highly aggressive disease with intense inflammation, extensive myocyte necrosis and many multinucleated giant cells derived from macrophages. It sometimes occurs in patients with SLE, hyperthyroidism, or thymoma. Autoimmune etiology, with dysregulated T lymphocytes, has been suggested.

CLINICAL FEATURES, PATHOLOGY: Giant cell myocarditis usually affects adults in the third to fifth decades and is rapidly fatal. Patients die of heart failure or suddenly from arrhythmias. At autopsy, hearts are flabby and dilated, possibly with mural thrombi. Prominent giant cells, lymphocytes, and macrophages cluster at the margins of serpiginous areas of myocardial necrosis. There are many giant cells, but no granulomas. Long-term immunosuppression can benefit some patients. For others, cardiac transplantation may be needed. However, in 25% of cases giant cell myocarditis recurs in transplanted hearts.

METABOLIC DISEASES OF THE HEART

Hyperthyroidism Causes High-Output Failure

Thyroid hormone has direct inotropic and chronotropic effects on the heart by: (1) increasing activity of the sarcolemmal sodium-potassium pump (Na^+/K^+-adenosine triphosphatase [ATPase]); (2) enhancing synthesis of a myosin isoform with rapid ATPase activity and reducing production of a slower isoform; and (3) upregulating SERCA and exerting direct effects on voltage-gated Ca^{2+} channels in the sarcolemma, to augment contractility. Hyperthyroidism thus causes tachycardia. It increases cardiac workload by decreasing peripheral resistance and increasing cardiac output. It may eventually cause angina pectoris, high-output failure, and/or arrhythmias (atrial fibrillation, most commonly).

Hypothyroidism Lowers Cardiac Output

Patients with severe hypothyroidism (**myxedema**) have low cardiac output, reduced heart rate, and poor myocardial contractility—the opposite of hyperthyroidism. A pericardial effusion may result from increased capillary permeability, with leakage of fluid and protein into the pericardial cavity. Pulse pressure is low because of higher peripheral resistance and lower blood volume.

Hearts from patients with myxedema are flabby and dilated, with myofiber swelling. Basophilic (mucinous) degeneration and interstitial fibrosis may be present. Still, myxedema alone does not cause heart failure.

Thiamine Deficiency (Beriberi) Heart Disease Resembles Hyperthyroidism

Heart disease develops in people with insufficient dietary vitamin B_1 (thiamine) intake for at least 3 months (**see Chapter 8**). In the United States, thiamine deficiency sometimes occurs in alcoholics or neglected people. It was once common in parts of Asia where vitamin-rich bran had been removed from rice, but this is rare today. Beriberi heart disease resembles hyperthyroidism: peripheral vascular resistance decreases and cardiac output increases, causing high-output failure. Heart failure may develop so abruptly that patients die within 2 days of the onset of symptoms. Hearts are dilated and show only nonspecific microscopic changes.

CARDIOMYOPATHY

Cardiomyopathies are primary diseases of the myocardium. Most common heart diseases damage coronary arteries, peripheral vasculature or cardiac valves, and affect the myocardium secondarily. Cardiomyopathies, however, target cardiac myocytes.

The American Heart Association defines cardiomyopathies as "a heterogeneous group of diseases of the myocardium associated with mechanical and/or electrical dysfunction" and "inappropriate ventricular hypertrophy or dilatation." Primary cardiomyopathies are: **dilated cardiomyopathy (DCM)**, **hypertrophic cardiomyopathy (HCM)**, **arrhythmogenic cardiomyopathy (ACM)**, **restrictive cardiomyopathy (RCM)**, and **left ventricular noncompaction (LVNC)**. These are mostly familial diseases. Many are monogenic, with thousands of mutations in over 100 genes implicated. They are often autosomal dominant traits, but autosomal recessive, X-linked recessive, and mitochondrial inheritance have all been described. Table 17-8 lists some of these genes, and Figure 17-42 shows major proteins and organelles in which pathogenic variants have been identified. Defects in virtually every major cardiac myocyte organizational unit can cause cardiomyopathy: myocyte cytoskeleton and the dystrophin/sarcoglycan complex which links internal cell structures to the extracellular matrix; the contractile apparatus; proteins regulating nuclear-cytoplasmic interactions; and intercalated disk proteins which mechanically and electrically couple cardiac myocytes to one another. These protein/organelle units are structurally and functionally highly integrated within cardiac myocytes. It should be no surprise, then, that *different variants within a single gene may yield highly variable clinical and pathologic phenotypes depending on the specific nature of the defect.* For example, actin has both cytoskeletal and contractile functions. Gain-of-function mutations that enhance actin–myosin interaction in sarcomeres thus can cause HCM phenotype, while loss-of-function mutations that disrupt actin binding to the dystrophin/sarcoglycan complex may lead to DCM (see Fig. 17-42). Table 17-8 lists pleotropic features of many cardiomyopathy disease genes.

HCM and ACM have a strong genetic basis, and pathogenic variants can usually be identified in patients with clinical and pathologic features of these cardiomyopathies. DCM is seen as more of a "mixed" cardiomyopathy in which both genetic and environmental factors play important causal roles. In most cases, however, *familial cardiomyopathies are characterized by highly variable genetic penetrance and disease expression.* It is not unusual for first-degree relatives of a proband with a fully expressed clinical phenotype to harbor the same mutant allele but show no apparent disease. Development of clinical and pathologic features in cardiomyopathies depends on complex interactions between mutant alleles and "modifiers"—genetic, epigenetic, and environmental—which ultimately determine disease expression. Relatively little is known about specific genetic and epigenetic modifiers but the ensemble effects of each individual's unique genetic makeup may enhance or mitigate the pathogenic influence of a disease allele. Other modifiers that affect disease expression include gender, presence of hypertension or other cardiovascular diseases, exercise (particularly important in ACM), and diet.

Contractility Is Impaired in Dilated Cardiomyopathy

DCM is most common cardiomyopathy, and a leading indication for heart transplantation. It is characterized clinically by biventricular dilation, impaired contractility, and heart failure. DCM can develop after a large number of known insults that directly injure cardiac myocytes (**secondary DCM**), or it may mainly be driven by genetic determinants in cardiac myocytes (**primary DCM**). The fact that so many diverse agents (infectious, toxic, immune, genetic) can injure cardiac myocytes explains the frequency of this clinical/pathologic form of cardiomyopathy

MOLECULAR PATHOGENESIS: Most cases of DCM likely develop through complex interactions between genetic, epigenetic, and environmental factors. At least one-third of DCM patients inherit the disease as a Mendelian single-gene disorder. The proportion may actually be even greater, as incomplete penetrance often makes it difficult to identify early or latent disease in family members. Most familial cases seem to be autosomal dominant traits, but autosomal recessive (e.g., mutations in *TNNC1* or *TAZ*), X-linked recessive (e.g., cardiomyopathies associated with mutations in *RVDMD* causing muscular dystrophies), and mitochondrial inheritance have all been described (see Table 17-8).

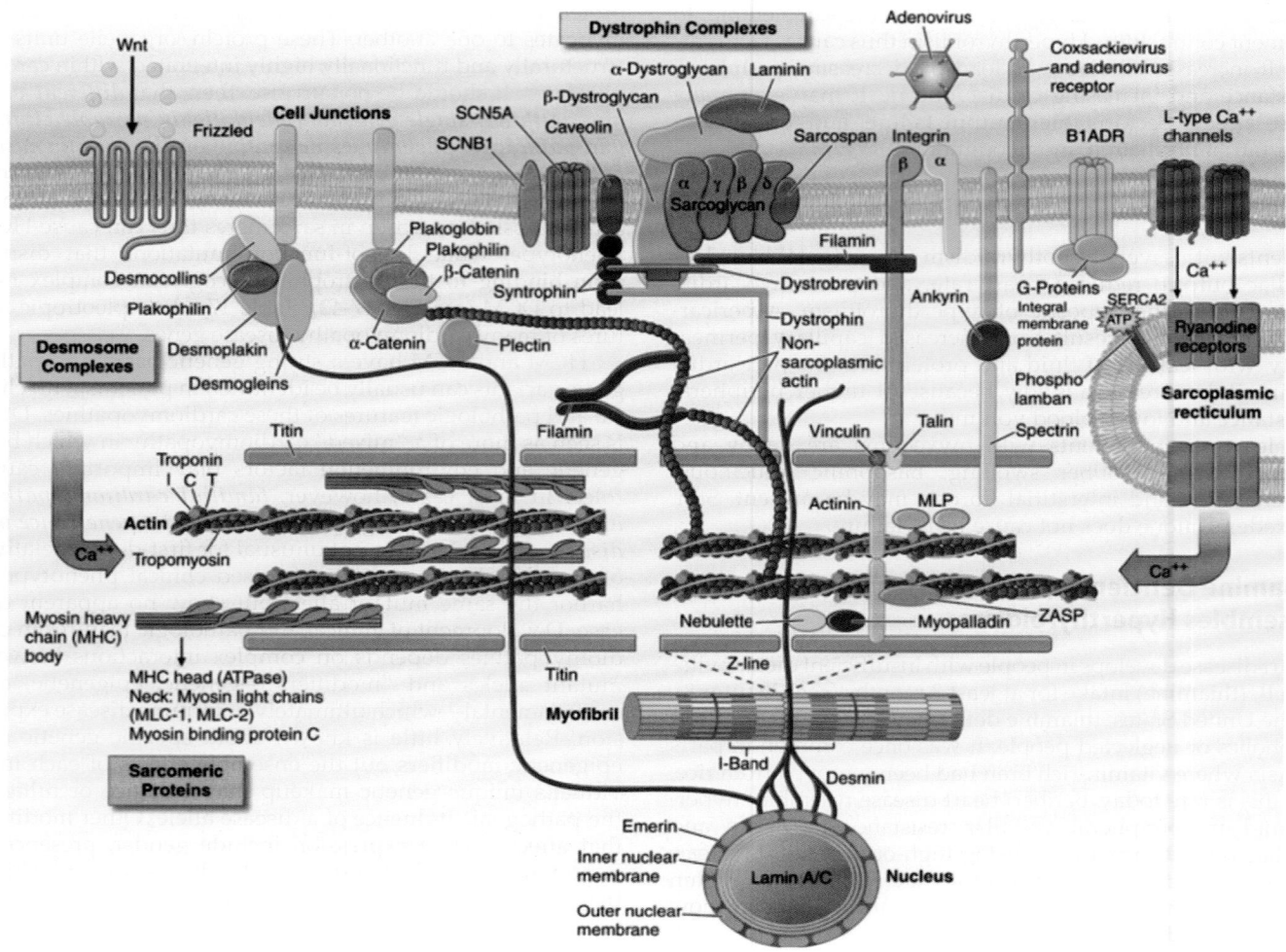

FIGURE 17-42. Subcellular distribution and molecular interactions of mutant proteins implicated in the pathogenesis of the familial non-ischemic cardiomyopathies. Genes in which variants have been linked to these heart muscle diseases are listed in Table 17-8. (Republished with permission of McGraw-Hill Education from Jameson JL, Fauci AS, Kasper DL, Hauser SL, Longo DL, Loscalzo J. *Harrison's Principles of Internal Medicine.* 20th ed. McGraw-Hill Education; 2018; Fig. 254-1. Permission conveyed through Copyright Clearance Center, Inc.)

Mutations in more than 50 genes have been linked to DCM. Several occur in genes encoding such cytoskeletal filament and anchor proteins as actin, desmin, vinculin, lamin A/C, and emerin. Others occur in genes encoding δ-sarcoglycan and dystrophin, proteins involved in anchoring the cytoskeleton and the sarcolemma to the extracellular matrix (Table 17-8, Fig. 17-42). These tend to be loss-of-function mutations and may cause defective force transmission. Other mechanisms are also undoubtedly related to other mutations. For example, 35% to 45% of genetic causes of DCM may be related to mutations in genes encoding sarcomeric proteins such as tropomyosin 1, troponins C, I, or T, and myosin heavy or light chains. Mutations (mainly truncations) in the giant sarcomeric protein titin, which has 35,000 amino acids, may alone account for up to 20% of genetic causes of DCM.

Some mutations that cause DCM have also been linked to a variety of other heart muscle diseases. Thus, mutations in *DES*, which encodes the intermediate filament protein desmin, can cause DCM, ACM, or RCM. Mutations in *PLN*, the gene for the Ca²⁺ regulatory protein phospholamban, can cause DCM, HCM, or ACM. Mutations in the *SCN5A*, which encodes the cardiac Na⁺ channel, can cause DCM or the long-QT syndrome. How specific variants give rise to such diverse clinical/pathologic phenotypes is poorly understood. At the same time, distinctions among traditional clinical/pathologic subtypes among cardiomyopathies have become blurred. A subset of DCM patients who have a particularly arrhythmogenic phenotype often have mutations in genes encoding desmosomal proteins or Ca²⁺ regulatory proteins, which are implicated in both DCM and ACM. As the list of genetic factors expands, so does our insight into potential molecular mechanisms and genotype–phenotype relationships.

VIRAL MYOCARDITIS may eventually lead to DCM. In most patients, innate and acquired immune mechanisms clear the virus, after which active inflammation ebbs. In some people, however, viral genomes persist in

TABLE 17-8

CARDIOMYOPATHY GENES AND THEIR RELATIONSHIP TO CLINICAL PHENOTYPES

Cardiomyopathy Genes (thousands of variants in >100 genes)

Gene	Gene Name	Cardiomyopathy Subtype(s)
ABCC9	ATP-binding cassette, sub-family C, member 9	DCM
ACTC1	Actin cardiac muscle 1	DCM, HCM, LVNC
ACTN2	Actinin, 2	DCM, HCM
ANKRD1	Ankyrin repeat domain 1 (cardiac muscle)	DCM, HCM
BAG3	BCL2-associated athanogene 3	DCM
CASQ2	Calsequestrin 2 (cardiac muscle)	LVNC
CAV3	Caveolin 3	HCM
COX15	COX15 homolog, cytochrome c oxidase assembly protein	HCM
CRYAB	Crystallin αB	HCM
CSRP3	Cysteine and glycine-rich protein 3	DCM, HCM
CTF1	Cardiotrophin 1	DCM
DES	Desmin	DCM, ACM, RCM
RVDMD	Dystrophin	DCM
DNAJC19	DnaJ (Hsp40) homolog, subfamily C, member 19	DCM
DSC2	Desmocollin 2	DCM, ACM
DSG2	Desmoglein 2	ACM
DSP	Desmoplakin	DCM, ACM
DTNA	Dystrobrevin	LVNC
EMD	Emerin	DCM
EYA4	Eyes absent homolog 4	DCM
FHL2	Four-and-a half LIM domains 2	DCM
FKTN	Fukutin	DCM
FOXD4	Forkhead box D4	DCM
GLA	Galactosidase	HCM
JUP	Junctional plakoglobin	ACM
LAMA4	Laminin, α4	DCM
LAMP2	Lysosomal-associated membrane protein 2	DCM, HCM
LDB3	LIM domain binding 3	DCM, LVNC
LMNA	Lamin A/C	DCM, LVNC
MYBPC3	Myosin-binding protein C, cardiac	DCM, HCM, LVNC
MYH6	Myosin, heavy chain 6, cardiac muscle	DCM, HCM

(continued)

TABLE 17-8

CARDIOMYOPATHY GENES AND THEIR RELATIONSHIP TO CLINICAL PHENOTYPES (*CONTINUED*)

Cardiomyopathy Genes (thousands of variants in >100 genes)

Gene	Gene Name	Cardiomyopathy Subtype(s)
MYH7	Myosin, heavy chain 7, cardiac muscle	DCM, HCM, RCM, LVNC
MYL2	Myosin, light chain 2, regulatory, cardiac, slow	HCM
MYL3	Myosin, light chain 3, alkali; ventricular, skeletal, slow	HCM
MYLK2	Myosin light chain kinase 2	HCM
MYOZ2	Myozenin 2	HCM
MYPN	Myopalladin	DCM, HCM, RCM
NEXN	Nexilin (F actin-binding protein)	DCM, HCM
PKP2	Plakophilin 2	ACM
PLN	Phospholamban	DCM, HCM, ACM
PRKAG2	Protein kinase, AMP-activated, gamma 2, noncatalytic subunit	HCM
PSEN1	Presenilin 1	DCM
PSEN2	Presenilin 2	DCM
RBM20	RNA-binding motif protein 20	DCM
RYR2	Ryanodine receptor 2 (cardiac)	CPVT
SCN5A	Sodium channel, voltage-gated, type V, α subunit	DCM
SDHA	Succinate dehydrogenase complex, subunit A, flavoprotein	DCM
SGCD	Sarcoglycan	DCM
SYNE1	Spectrin repeat containing, nuclear envelope 1	DCM
SYNE2	Spectrin repeat containing, nuclear envelope 2	DCM
TAZ	Tafazzin	DCM, LVNC
TCAP	Titin-cap (telethonin)	DCM
TMEM43	Transmembrane protein 43	ACM
TMPO	Thymopoietin	DCM
TNNC1	Troponin C type 1 (slow)	DCM, HCM
TNNI3	Troponin I type 3 (cardiac)	DCM, HCM, RCM
TNNT2	Troponin T type 2 (cardiac)	DCM, HCM, LVNC
TPM1	Tropomyosin 1	DCM, HCM
TTN	Titin	DCM, HCM, ACM
TTR	Transthyretin	HCM
VCL	Vinculin	DCM, HCM

the heart and stimulate ongoing immune mechanisms. In addition, impaired T-cell tolerance to cardiac self-antigens may cause chronic autoantigen-driven myocardial inflammation, which, eventually may progress to clinical DCM and end-stage heart failure. This may persist in the absence of virus and be asymptomatic until heart failure ensues. Subsequent noninfectious cardiotoxic agents may stimulate this process. Why some patients with acute myocarditis ultimately develop DCM is not well understood. Genetic factors, both host and viral, molecular mimicry between cardiac proteins and infectious agents, and environment factors likely all contribute. *Finally, one should understand that the meaning of circulating autoantibodies versus cardiac antigens (e.g., mitochondrial, sarcomeric, and G-protein–coupled receptor proteins) seen in diverse heart diseases is unclear. They may cause cardiac injury, or they may reflect nonimmune injury and have no pathogenic significance.*

PATHOLOGY: The gross and microscopic pathology of DCM is generally nonspecific and is similar whatever its genesis. The heart is invariably enlarged, with conspicuous left and right ventricular hypertrophy. In extreme cases, heart weight may be tripled (>900 g). All chambers are usually dilated, with ventricles more severely affected than atria (Fig. 17-43). At end-stage, left ventricular dilation is usually so severe that its free wall appears to be of normal thickness or even thinned, masking the considerable amount of hypertrophy that invariably develops in DCM. The myocardium is flabby and pale, sometimes with small subendocardial scars. Left ventricle endocardium tends to be thickened, especially at the apex, where adherent mural thrombi are common.

DCM is characterized by atrophic and hypertrophic myocardial fibers. Cardiac myocytes, especially in the subendocardium, often show advanced degenerative changes, with myofibrillar loss (myocytolysis) giving cells a vacant, vacuolated look. Interstitial and perivascular myocardial fibrosis is also most prominently in the subendocardial zone. Scattered chronic inflammatory cells may be present but are not conspicuous. Electron microscopy typically shows loss of sarcomeres and apparently increased mitochondria. Occasionally, insights into etiology may be gleaned from special microscopic features. For example, in DCM due to mutations in desmin cardiac myocytes may contain intracellular aggregates of misfolded intermediate filaments.

CLINICAL FEATURES: The clinical courses of primary and secondary DCM are comparable. Both begin insidiously with compensatory ventricular hypertrophy and asymptomatic left ventricular dilation. Exercise intolerance usually progresses relentlessly to overt heart failure, and nearly half of patients die or undergo transplantation within 5 years of onset of symptoms. Roughly 25% of deaths in DCM patients are sudden, attributed to ventricular arrhythmias. Abnormal signaling cascades in heart failure lead to altered activity and/or distribution of various intracellular Ca^{2+} homeostasis proteins and selected repolarizing (K^+) currents. These changes tend to prolong QT intervals on the surface ECG and create intracellular conditions that increase risk of arrhythmias initiated by triggered activity. Despite advances in treating heart failure, many DCM patients eventually need ventricular assist devices or heart transplants.

Over 100 Injurious Agents May Cause Secondary DCM

Secondary DCM is best viewed as a final common pathway for virtually any toxic, metabolic, or pathophysiologic disorder that injures cardiac myocytes. In this context, alcohol abuse, various drugs and pregnancy may all lead to secondary DCM. Diabetes mellitus and cigarette smoking are also associated with increased incidence of DCM. Even lacking a known pathogenetic mutation, these agents interact with host genetic factors to determine disease susceptibility and severity.

Toxic Cardiomyopathy

Many chemicals and drugs cause myocardial injury, but only a few of the more important ones are discussed here.

ETHANOL: Alcohol is the single most common identifiable cause of DCM in the United States and Europe. Although moderate alcohol consumption is associated with reduced risk of major adverse cardiac events, ethanol abuse can lead to chronic, progressive cardiac dysfunction, which may be fatal. The disorder is more common in men, because alcoholism is more frequent in men. Typical patients are 30 to 55 years old and have been drinking heavily for at least 10 years. Clinically and pathologically, alcoholic cardiomyopathy looks like DCM: the diagnosis is largely based on excluding other potential causes of DCM and documenting a history of excessive alcohol consumption.

 PATHOPHYSIOLOGY: The pathogenesis of alcoholic cardiomyopathy is complex and multifactorial. Increasing evidence implicates harmful effects of alcohol on cardiac mitochondrial structure and function. Exposing cardiac myocytes to alcohol leads to

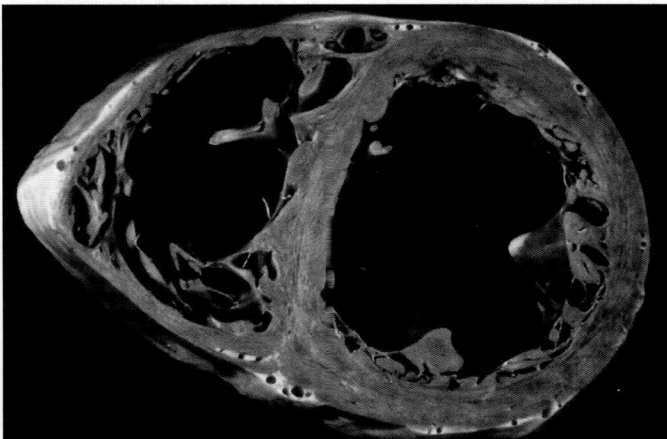

FIGURE 17-43. Idiopathic dilated cardiomyopathy. A transverse section of the enlarged heart reveals conspicuous biventricular dilatation. Although the ventricular wall appears thinned, the increased mass of the heart indicates considerable hypertrophy.

degenerative changes in the mitochondrial inner membrane and depolarization of the mitochondrial membrane potential, which is a robust indicator of mitochondrial dysfunction. Alcohol also reduces expression and activities of enzymes in the tricarboxylic acid cycle and electron transport chain in cardiac myocytes. This increases generation of ROS and reduces expression and/or activity of enzymes that detoxify ROS. Alcohol also impairs mitochondrial biogenesis and damages mtDNA. Chronic alcohol abuse increases the rate of apoptosis in human cardiac myocytes and exerts inhibitory effects on certain types of progenitor cells. This is associated with increased expression of pro-apoptotic proteins such as caspase 3 and Bax. These changes are related, at least in part, to the complex derangements in mitochondria produced by alcohol.

COBALT: The cardiac toxicity of cobalt is discussed in Chapter 8.

CATECHOLAMINES: In high concentrations, catecholamines can cause focal myocyte necrosis (contraction band necrosis, see Fig. 17-20). This type of myocardial injury may occur in patients with pheochromocytomas or who require high doses of inotropic drugs to maintain blood pressure, and in accident victims who sustain massive head trauma. Multiple mechanisms contribute to myocardial injury, but the most important is enhanced Ca^{2+} flux into myocytes. Focal ischemia caused by platelet aggregation and microvascular constriction may also contribute. Catecholamine toxicity has been implicated in **Takotsubo cardiomyopathy**, also called apical ballooning- or stress-induced cardiomyopathy, with abrupt onset of transient left ventricular dysfunction with apical dilation, often triggered by severe emotional or physical stress.

CARDIOTOXICITY OF CANCER THERAPY: With increasing numbers of cancer survivors and an ever-expanding armamentarium of anti-cancer drugs, a new field of *oncocardiology* has emerged to address cardiotoxic effects of cancer therapy. Multiple drugs have been linked to cardiac damage via "off-target" effects that are independent of their primary anti-tumor mechanisms. Widely used cancer drugs that can injure the heart include anthracyclines such as doxorubicin, HER2/neu receptor blockers such as trastuzumab, alkylating agents such as cyclophosphamide, antimetabolites such as 5-fluorouracil, tyrosine kinase inhibitors such as imatinib, and more recently, checkpoint inhibitors such as pembrolizumab. Many are directly toxic to cardiac myocytes while others can cause hypertension, coronary vasospasm, thromboembolism, or arrhythmias. Affected patients may develop heart failure resembling secondary DCM.

PATHOPHYSIOLOGY: The prototypical cardiotoxic cancer drugs are anthracyclines. Doxorubicin (Adriamycin) and other anthracycline drugs are potent chemotherapeutic agents whose usefulness is limited by cumulative, dose-dependent, cardiac toxicity. DCM begins to appear in patients who receive a cumulative dose of more than 450-mg doxorubicin per m^2. Risk is higher in females older than age 65 who have pre-existing cardiovascular diseases including hypertension and receive concomitant mediastinal radiation and/or other cardiotoxic drugs such as cyclophosphamide. It is now recognized that anthracyclines injure cardiac myocytes through off-target effects that alter activity of topoisomerase II. This causes double-strand DNA breaks and marked changes in the myocyte transcriptome, with profoundly affecting mitochondria and increasing ROS generation. HER2/neu receptor blockers such as trastuzumab and tyrosine kinase inhibitors such as imatinib have off-target effects that disrupt signaling by vascular endothelial growth factor and, thereby, limit stress-induced angiogenesis in the heart. The alkylating agent cyclophosphamide does not cause classical DCM but can cause pericarditis and occasionally massive hemorrhagic myocarditis. The latter is thought to reflect endothelial injury and thrombocytopenia. Assays of cardiac myocyte biomarkers and sensitive imaging are now being used to detect early cardiotoxicity and implement emerging strategies, such as topoisomerase II inhibitors in the case of anthracycline therapy, to limit long-term damage to the heart in cancer patients.

COCAINE: Cocaine use is often associated with chest pain and palpitations. True DCM is an unusual complication of cocaine abuse, but myocarditis, focal necrosis and thickening of intramyocardial coronary arteries have been reported. Myocardial ischemia or infarction associated with cocaine use has been attributed to coronary vasoconstriction in the face of increased myocardial oxygen demand. Sudden death due to spontaneous ventricular tachyarrhythmias is well documented. Cocaine-induced arrhythmias may be due to drug-related vasoconstriction, sympathomimetic activity, hypersensitivity responses, and direct toxicity.

Peripartum Cardiomyopathy (PPCM)

A unique form of DCM develops in the last trimester of pregnancy or the first 6 months after delivery. PPCM is relatively uncommon in the United States (~1 in 1,000 to 4,000 live births), but in some areas in Africa, it affects as many as 1% of pregnant women. Risk of cardiomyopathy of pregnancy is greatest in black, multiparous women older than 30 years. Preeclampsia and hypertension are strong predisposing factors. Unlike most other varieties of DCM, half of women with PPCM spontaneously recover normal cardiac function. In the other half, left ventricular dysfunction persists. It may progress to overt heart failure, leading to early death. In patients who survive, subsequent pregnancies pose a high risk of recurrence and maternal mortality, especially if baseline left ventricular function remains reduced.

PATHOPHYSIOLOGY: PPCM is caused by toxic effects of late-gestational hormones on maternal vasculature. Genetic factors also appear to play an important role and likely explain wide variations in incidence in different populations. Ten to 15% of women with PPCM carry a pathogenic DCM mutation, with variants in *DMD* and *TTN* most commonly identified. Early development of the placenta involves extensive vasculogenesis (new blood vessel formation) and angiogenesis (sprouting of new vessels from existing blood vessels), driven largely by vascular endothelial growth factor (VEGF, **see Chapter 5**) and related hormones. After

25 weeks of gestation, such growth is regulated by anti-angiogenic factors including soluble **Fms-like tyrosine kinase 1 (sFlt1)**, which neutralizes much of the free VEGF in the maternal circulation. Abnormally high sFlt1 levels occur in preeclampsia and PPCM. This creates a problem for the heart, which must produce more VEGF locally to counteract sFlt1 anti-angiogenic effects, and thereby to meet the circulatory demands of late pregnancy. Insufficient myocardial production of VEGF, especially in concert with pathogenic alleles, can lead to a clinical and pathologic picture of secondary DCM.

In Hypertrophic Cardiomyopathy, Cardiac Hypertrophy Is Out of Proportion to Hemodynamic Load

The hallmark of HCM is unexplained left ventricular hypertrophy. Secondary causes of hypertrophy such as hypertension, aortic stenosis, or physiologic hypertrophy in highly trained athletes must thus be excluded to diagnose HCM.

MOLECULAR PATHOGENESIS: Most cases of HCM are due to dominant mutations in single genes that encode sarcomeric proteins (Table 17-8). Most cases involve pathogenic variants in 8 genes: *MYH7* (β-myosin H-chain), *TPM1* (α-tropomyosin), *TNNT2* (cardiac troponin T), *MYBPC3* (cardiac myosin-binding protein C), *MYL2* (myosin regulatory light chain), *MYL3* (myosin essential light chain), *TNNI3* (cardiac troponin I), and *ACTC1* (cardiac α-actin). Mutations in *MYH7* and *MYBPC3* account for 50% of HCM cases. Disease-causing mutations in these genes occur in ~60% of probands with the highest detection rate seen in those with early onset, more severe hypertrophy, and a family history of HCM. *TTN* (titin) mutations, so common in DCM, are unusual in HCM.

The prevalence of clinically identified unexplained hypertrophy in the general population is 1 in 500, which greatly exceeds the prevalence of pathogenic mutations. Modern sequencing studies have identified variants in sarcomeric genes in people with clinically silent, unexplained hypertrophy. Working individually or collectively, these variants can apparently produce left ventricular hypertrophy without causing overt HCM.

PATHOPHYSIOLOGY: How these mutations cause HCM is only now being elucidated. Mutations in the myosin head domain enhance contraction and impair relaxation, both of which are pathophysiologic hallmarks of HCM. As mentioned above, different mutations in the same gene can lead to disparate phenotypes. Those causing HCM tend to be gain-of-function mutations while those causing DCM lead to loss-of-function. Thus, HCM-causing mutations in *MYH7* produce a hypercontractile phenotype with increased force and velocity of contraction, while DCM-causing mutations in the same gene reduce contractile power and speed. HCM mutations in *TNNT2* enhance the Ca²⁺ sensitivity of actin-activated myosin ATPase activity, but DCM mutations in the same gene desensitize myosin ATPase.

Perturbed myocardial energetics appears to play a role in HCM. Some nonsarcomere gene mutations linked to HCM affect glucose metabolism and clearance. These include variants in *PRKAB2* (AMP-activated protein kinase noncatalytic subunit), *LAMP2* (lysosomal-associated membrane protein 2), and *GLA* (galactosidase). How the complex clinical phenotype of HCM results from these mutations is poorly understood, and there is debate as to how classical the resultant HCV is. Nevertheless, abundant evidence implicates abnormal myocardial energetics in HCM: ratios of phosphorylated creatinine to ATP are reduced, ATPase activity is abnormal and there is increased energetic flux in actin–myosin cross-bridge cycling.

By increasing contractile force and velocity, and enhancing ATP hydrolysis and Ca²⁺ sensitivity, HCM mutations activate signaling pathways that promote hypertrophic growth in cardiac myocytes and also affect vascular and interstitial cells in the myocardium. Augmented Ca²⁺ signaling and profibrotic mediators such as TGFβ, elaborated and secreted by cardiac myocytes, stimulate vascular smooth muscle cell and interstitial fibroblast proliferation, and expand the extracellular matrix via paracrine mechanisms. This explains how mutations in genes expressed only in cardiac myocytes can cause changes in nonmyocyte components of the myocardium (see Fig. 17-44). It also accounts, at least partly, for the abnormal left ventricle diastolic properties in HCM.

As in the other cardiomyopathies, age-related penetrance of common disease alleles is variable in HCM. *MYH7* mutations are highly penetrant. Over 90% of carriers develop HCM by their second decade. Carriers of *MYBPC3* mutations, however, may not develop disease until their 50s or 60s. Patients with some forms of HCM are at high risk of sudden death. However, except for some *TNNT2* mutations, which carry particular risk, meaningful molecular predictors have been elusive.

PATHOLOGY: Hearts in HCM patients are always enlarged, but how much so vary among different genetic forms. The left ventricular free wall is thick, and its cavity is small, sometimes only a slit. Papillary muscles and trabeculae carneae are prominent and encroach on the lumen. More than half of cases show asymmetric interventricular septal hypertrophy, with a ratio of septum to left ventricular free wall thickness >1.5 (Fig. 17-44A). In some uncommon genetic forms of HCM, only the apical portion of the left ventricle or the papillary muscles may be selectively hypertrophied. The thickened, hypertrophied interventricular septum may bulge into the left ventricular outflow tract early in ventricular systole, obstructing aortic outflow. In this situation, a fibrous endocardial mural plaque is typically seen in the outflow tract, corresponding to the contact point where the anterior mitral valve leaflet impinges on the septal wall of the outflow tract during systole. Both atria are commonly dilated.

***The most notable histologic feature of HCM is* myofiber disarray**, most markedly in the interventricular septum. Instead of the usual parallel arrangement of myocytes into muscle bundles, there are oblique and often perpendicular orientations of adjacent hypertrophic

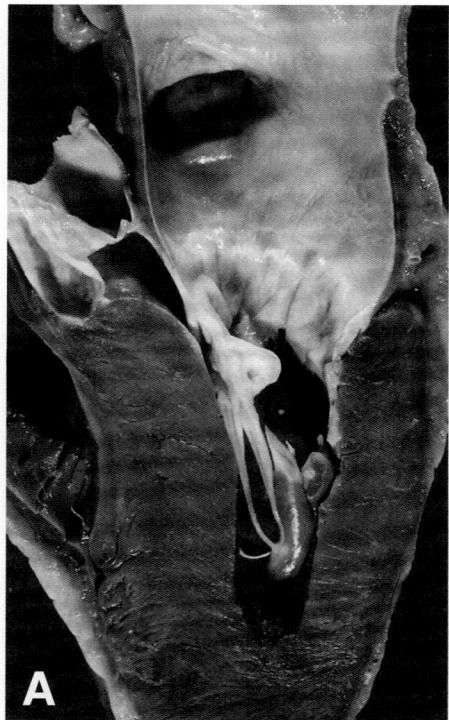
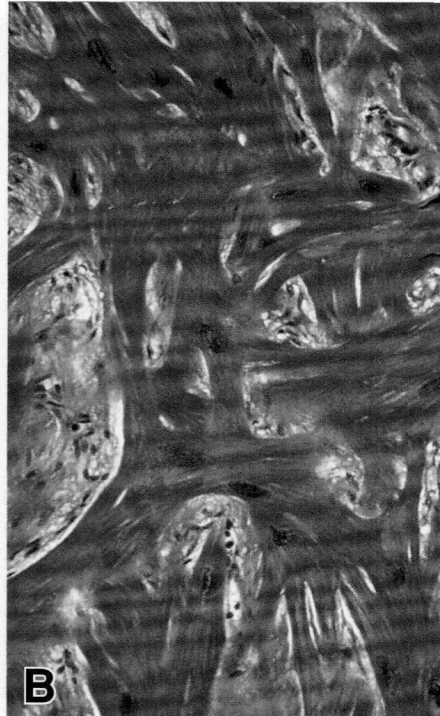
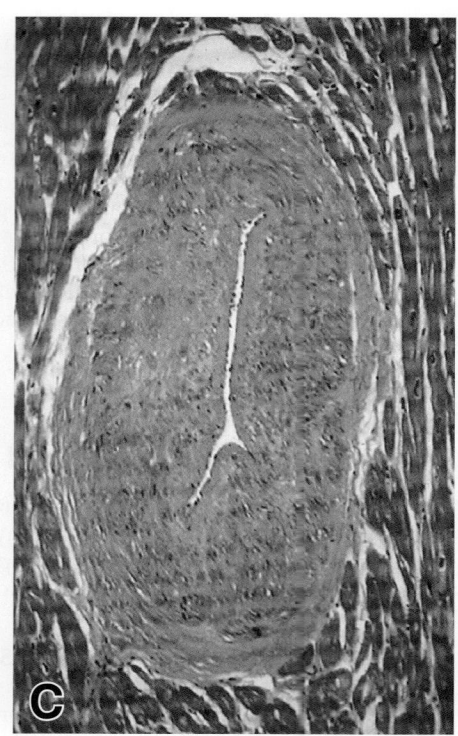

FIGURE 17-44. Hypertrophic cardiomyopathy (HCM). A. The heart has been opened to show striking asymmetric left ventricular hypertrophy. The interventricular septum is thicker than the free wall of the left ventricle and impinges on the outflow tract such that it contacts the underside of the anterior mitral valve leaflet. The left atrium is markedly enlarged. **B.** A section of the myocardium shows characteristic myofiber disarray and hyperplasia of interstitial cells. **C.** A small intramural coronary artery shows a thickened, hypercellular media. This type of remodeling of coronary vessels could contribute to development of angina-like symptoms in some patients with HCM.

myocytes (Fig. 17-44B). Myofibrils and myofilaments within individual myocytes are also disorganized. Similar structural disarrangements may occur in infants with congenital heart defects and in other settings, but in HCM they are always extensive. There are also more interstitial cells, and extracellular matrix is expanded (Fig. 17-44B). Intramural coronary arteries may be thick and cellular (Fig. 17-44C).

CLINICAL FEATURES: Many patients with HCM have few, if any, symptoms, and the diagnosis is commonly made during family screening if there is an affected member. Risk of death is ~1% per year. About 60% of deaths are sudden. Even without symptoms, such people may be at risk for sudden death. In fact, unsuspected HCM is found at autopsy in roughly one-half of young athletes who die suddenly (see Fig. 17-48). HCM may become clinically apparent at any age, often in the third to fifth decades, but it also is first found in the elderly (mainly with *MYBPC3* mutations). Some patients are incapacitated by dyspnea, angina pectoris, and syncope. These symptoms stem from dynamic outflow tract obstruction by asymmetric septal hypertrophy, and local ischemia due to abnormal myocardial energetics and thickening of intramural coronary arteries. Its clinical course tends to be stable for years, but HCM may lead to heart failure with impaired systolic function. In 10% of patients, a DCM-like picture supervenes.

Contractile function in HCM tends to be hyperdynamic. Ejection fractions are typically very high and with of the stroke volume is ejected during early systole. The remodeled left ventricle in HCM is stiff and noncompliant, resulting in impaired diastolic relaxation and increased end-diastolic pressure. Mitral regurgitation is common, especially in patients with dynamic outflow tract obstruction. This contributes to the atrial dilatation often seen in HCM (note the enlarged left atrium in Fig. 17-44A). It also predisposes to atrial fibrillation, which greatly impairs filling of the stiff, noncompliant left ventricle, and exacerbates symptoms.

HCM is treated with negative inotropes, like β-adrenergic blockers and Ca^{2+} channel blockers, which reduce contractility, decrease outflow tract obstruction, and may improve diastolic left ventricular relaxation. Surgically excising part of a hypertrophic septum or injecting ethanol into a septal artery to cause localized infarction may relieve symptoms of outflow tract obstruction, but the risk of sudden death remains.

Arrhythmogenic Cardiomyopathy (ACM) Is a Disease of the Desmosome With a High Risk of Sudden Death

ACM is a primary heart muscle disease with a high incidence of early-onset ventricular tachyarrhythmias. It affects roughly 1 in 5,000 individuals and is most common in Mediterranean countries, where it is a leading cause of sudden death in young people (<35 years). Overall risk of death is about ~1% per year but >80% of deaths in ACM are sudden. Although originally described as a right ventricular disease (arrhythmogenic right ventricular cardiomyopathy, or ARVC), it is now known to have biventricular and left dominant forms, which may be misdiagnosed as DCM. That said, there is considerable overlap in clinical and pathologic phenotypes in ACM and DCM and their genetic causes. Although sudden death is much more common in ACM as in DCM, a subset of DCM patients follow a highly arrhythmogenic clinical course, with genotypes that can cause either DCM or ACM phenotypes (see Table 17-8).

PATHOLOGY: ACM is associated with serious arrhythmias and/or sudden death, which may occur early in the disease, before significant structural remodeling and contractile dysfunction develop. The classical form (ARVC) affects the right ventricular free wall but some left ventricular free wall involvement, especially in posterolateral segments, is present in most cases. Characteristic pathology includes degeneration of epicardial cardiac myocytes and replacement by fat and fibrous tissue (Fig. 17-45). The extent of this change can be quite variable and is not necessarily conspicuous in patients who die suddenly.

MOLECULAR PATHOGENESIS: ACM is a familial disease, usually inherited as an autosomal dominant. Its true frequency is probably underestimated because of variable penetrance, age-related progression and large phenotypic variation. Diagnosis can be difficult, and requires analysis of various clinical criteria, which, although relatively specific, are not highly sensitive. Mutations in genes encoding proteins in desmosomes, cell–cell adhesion organelles, can be identified in more than half of individuals who fulfill these criteria. These include genes for desmosomal adhesion molecules (desmoglein-2, desmocollin-2), and intracellular desmosomal linker proteins (plakoglobin, desmoplakin, plakophilin-2), which form a complex that connects the adhesion molecules to the intermediate filament (desmin) cytoskeleton in cardiac myocytes (Table 17-8). Mutations in *PKP2*, the gene for plakophilin-2, are seen most commonly in classical ARVC; mutations in *DSP*, the gene for desmoplakin, are often associated with biventricular or left-sided forms of ACM. Desmosomes are particularly abundant in heart and skin, two organs that experience the greatest mechanical burden, and mutations in desmosomal genes generally cause cutaneous and/or cardiac disease depending on the mutant isoform's tissue-specific expression patterns. The mechanism by which desmosome mutations cause ACM is not fully understood, but increasing evidence implicates deranged Wnt signaling pathways and abnormal responses to mechanical stimulation of the heart during exercise.

Restrictive Cardiomyopathy (RCM) Impairs Diastolic Function

RCM is a group of diseases with restrictive ventricular filling, reduced diastolic volume in one or both ventricles, and normal or near-normal ventricular systolic function and wall thickness. It is the least common cardiomyopathy, comprising 2% to 5% of pediatric cardiomyopathies, but it carries a high mortality rate with death and disability due mainly to heart failure. **Primary restrictive cardiomyopathy** (also called "idiopathic") is caused by genetic mutations and/or other derangements in that alter cardiac myocyte biophysical properties and account for the characteristic diastolic dysfunction. Unlike other familial cardiomyopathies in which structural ventricular remodeling correlates with functional derangements (e.g., dilatation in DCM, hypertrophy and myofiber disarray in HCM, fibrofatty infiltration in ACM), the myocardium in primary RCM shows few if any pathologic changes to explain the abnormal diastolic properties. Biopsies of affected ventricle(s) may be normal or show some interstitial fibrosis.

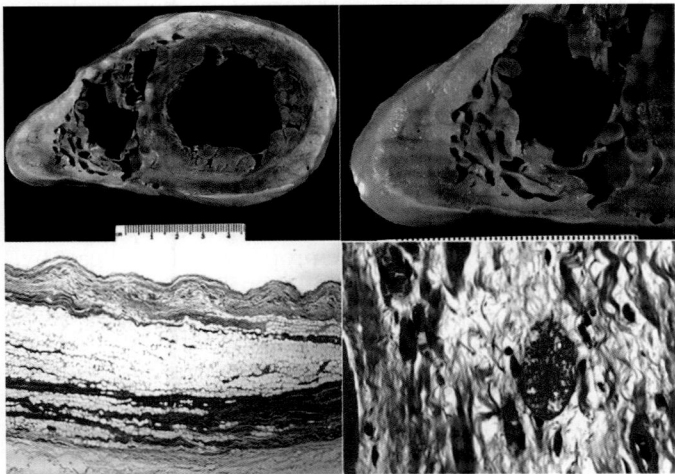

FIGURE 17-45. Arrhythmogenic cardiomyopathy. Upper panels show the typical gross features in which epicardial muscle of the right ventricular free wall has been replaced by fatty tissue and only subendocardial trabeculae remain. As is often the case, the left ventricular wall, especially lateral and posterolateral segments, is also affected. **Lower panels** show microscopic features of fibrofatty replacement of cardiac muscle and myocyte degeneration (shown in the higher magnification image). In these trichrome-stained sections, fibrous tissue is blue and cardiac myocytes are brick-red.

MOLECULAR PATHOGENESIS: The genetic bases of RCM are less well understood as in HCM or ACM. Still, dominant mutations in several genes have been implicated in RCM (Table 17-8). The most frequently identified mutations in RCM involve sarcomeric genes *MYH7* (myosin heavy chain) and *TNNI3* (cardiac troponin I), which may often be mutated in HCM and DCM. In fact, clinical and pathologic phenotypes in RCM may overlap HCM, and patients with features of both tend to have worse outcomes. Mutations in *MYPN*, which encodes the Z-disk protein myopalladin, have also been linked to RCM (and DCM and HCM). Mutations and variants in *TTN* (titin) have been reported in patients with idiopathic RCM. Thus, it appears that a significant proportion of patients with primary RCM have pathogenic variants in sarcomeric genes that presumably alter diastolic function of the contractile apparatus without affecting systolic function. Increased Ca²⁺ sensitivity and altered conformation of the cardiac troponin complex have been suggested, but exactly how such changes would alter diastolic versus systolic function of the contractile apparatus is unclear.

Secondary Restrictive Cardiomyopathies Have Diverse Causes

In **secondary RCM**, abnormal ventricular filling is caused by changes in the myocardial interstitium (e.g., accumulation of amyloid or metastatic carcinoma), or diseases causing the endocardium to become thickened and stiffened by fibrosis. Restrictive pathophysiology also occurs in hemochromatosis and desmin-related cardiomyopathies in which cardiac myocytes accumulate intracellular iron or aggregates of misfolded intermediate filaments. Cardiac sarcoidosis (see above) can also impair diastolic function. Thus, restrictive pathophysiology in secondary RCM does not reflect genetic changes in the contractile apparatus *per se* but rather in other components of the myocardium. The result is a preload-dependent state with defective diastolic compliance, restricted ventricular filling, increased end-diastolic pressure, atrial dilation, and venous congestion. These hemodynamics resemble those of constrictive pericarditis, which may be difficult to distinguish from restrictive myocardial disease.

Amyloidosis

Amyloid accumulation in the heart causes an RCM. Many proteins can form amyloid fibrils (**see Chapter 15**) but the vast majority of patients with cardiac amyloidosis have accumulated immunoglobulin light chains amyloid (**AL** or **primary amyloidosis**), or amyloid transthyretin (**ATTR**). Transthyretin, produced primarily in the liver, transports retinol (vitamin A) and thyroxine. Cardiac ATTR is caused by myocardial accumulation of either wildtype transthyretin (ATTRwt) or variant forms encoded by relatively frequent variant alleles in the transthyretin gene, *TTR*.

PATHOLOGY: Amyloid infiltration in the heart results in cardiac enlargement without ventricular dilation. Grossly, the heart may resemble that seen in HCM. Ventricular walls are typically thickened, firm, and rubbery. Amyloid accumulation is most prominent in interstitial, perivascular, and endocardial regions (Fig. 17-46). Endocardial involvement is common in atria, where nodular deposits often impart a granular appearance and gritty texture to the endocardial surface. Amyloid deposits also can thicken cardiac valves. Amyloid accumulation in walls of intramural coronary arteries and arterioles is also common. Occasionally, vascular amyloid can narrow lumens to the point of causing ischemic injury. AL and ATTR have a similar histologic appearance but they can be distinguished in heart biopsies by mass spectrometry.

CLINICAL FEATURES: AL and ATTR cardiac amyloidosis usually present in people aged 60 to 80 years. Patterns of systemic involvement vary (**see Chapter 15**), but when the heart is affected, the clinical

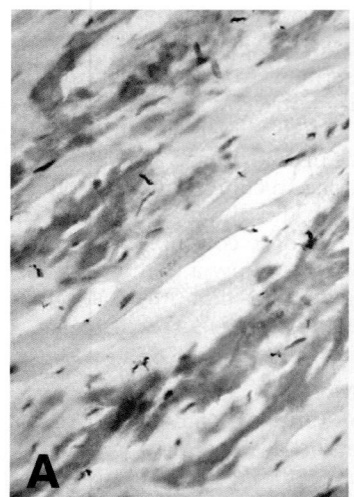

FIGURE 17-46. Cardiac amyloidosis. A. A section of myocardium stained with Congo red shows interstitial, red-staining amyloid deposits. **B.** Under polarized light, the characteristic green birefringence of amyloid fibrils is evident.

picture initially resembles RCM with progressive diastolic and, eventually, systolic dysfunction. Some cases of heart failure with preserved ejection fraction (HFpEF) may be due to ATTR. ATTRwt is often seen in the heart and blood vessels in elderly people at autopsy. Such "senile" cardiac amyloidosis is usually clinically silent, but it can produce restrictive pathophysiology. Indeed, ATTRwt may be responsible for up to 10% of cases of heart failure in elderly people. Extensive conduction system infiltration by amyloid can cause heart block and contribute to arrhythmias. In symptomatic patients, echocardiography typically shows concentric left ventricular thickening and, at least in early stages, near-normal ejection fractions. Atrial enlargement, due to the noncompliant ventricular walls, is common. Low-voltage QRS complexes on ECG are characteristic. Once it is symptomatic, cardiac amyloidosis has a poor prognosis although recent advances have improved the outlook considerably.

In AL amyloidosis, Ig light chains are made by monoclonal plasma cell proliferations. This is an acquired condition without an apparent heritable component. In addition to altering diastolic properties of the heart by filling the interstitium, amyloidogenic free lights chains can cause lysosomal abnormalities in cardiac myocytes resulting in production of ROS and cell death. ATTR cardiac amyloidosis is caused by myocardial accumulation of ATTRwt or variants, the latter encoded by *TTR* variants. In the United States, the most common isoforms causing cardiac ATTR are ATTRwt, Val122Ile, and Thr60Ala. Val122Ile is the most prevalent variant in the United States and occurs mainly in patients of African descent. Over 80% of patients with ATTR cardiac amyloidosis are male. Efforts to treat AL amyloidosis depend on eliminating the underlying plasma cell disorder. Newer treatments for ATTR include gene silencing to decrease hepatic production of pathologic transthyretin, and pharmacologic transthyretin stabilization (**see Chapter 15**).

Desmin-Related Cardiomyopathies

Desmin is the intermediate filament protein in cardiac, striated, and smooth muscle. It binds to desmosomes at intercalated disks and spans the length of the cardiac myocyte by binding to sarcomere Z-disks and other intracellular organelles (see Fig. 17-42).

 MOLECULAR PATHOGENESIS, PATHOLOGY: Restrictive cardiac pathophysiology is the most common clinical phenotype associated with mutations in *DES*. Because desmin is also expressed in skeletal and smooth muscle, **desminopathies** may include distal and proximal muscle weakness, and respiratory and gastrointestinal problems related to smooth muscle dysfunction, as well as cardiomyopathy. Restrictive cardiac pathophysiology is often associated with accumulated aggregates of misfolded desmin filaments in ventricular myocytes. These aggregates presumably affect the biophysical properties of the myocardium and impair relaxation. Mutations in *DES* are also linked to ACM and DCM, perhaps due to abnormal molecular interactions between desmin and components of desmosomes, Z-disk, and the cardiac myocyte cytoskeleton.

Endomyocardial Disease (EMD)

EMD causes fibrous thickening of the ventricular endocardial lining, which interferes with ventricular filling and produces restrictive pathophysiology. EMD consists of two geographically separate groups of disorders.

ENDOMYOCARDIAL FIBROSIS: This disorder is particularly common in equatorial Africa, where it accounts for 10% to 20% of deaths from heart disease. It also occurs occasionally in other tropical and subtropical regions of the world. While it is most common in children and young adults, endomyocardial fibrosis may occur in people up to age 70. Its etiology and pathogenesis are poorly understood, but parasitic infection, especially with helminths that cause eosinophilia, likely plays an important role. It produces restrictive pathophysiology leading to heart failure and arrhythmias.

EOSINOPHILIC ENDOMYOCARDIAL DISEASE (LÖFFLER ENDOCARDITIS): This is a cardiac disorder of temperate regions characterized by hypereosinophilia (up to 50,000/μL). It usually occurs in men in the fifth decade, often accompanied by rash. Löffler endocarditis typically progresses to heart failure and death, although corticosteroids may improve survival.

 ETIOLOGIC FACTORS: Endomyocardial fibrosis and Löffler endocarditis are probably variants of the same pathophysiology. *They may reflect myocardial injury by cardiotoxic components of eosinophil granules.* In the tropics, parasitic infestations may trigger transient high blood eosinophilia; in temperate climates, idiopathic hypereosinophilia is often persistent. EMD can be divided into three stages:

1. The necrotic stage occurs within the first few months of the illness, with intense eosinophilic infiltration of inner myocardial layers, usually in both ventricles. The infiltrate is perivascular and interstitial, with evidence of vascular injury and myocyte necrosis. This stage lasts for several months, usually without significant functional impairment.
2. The thrombotic stage develops about a year later. Mural thrombi attach to injured, slightly thickened endocardium. The myocardium is no longer inflamed but shows early hypertrophy. Emboli may occur at this time.
3. The fibrotic stage is the chronic phase of EMD, with conspicuous fibrotic endocardial thickening and marked fibrosis. This decreases compliance and causes diastolic dysfunction. Mitral and tricuspid leaflets and subvalvular apparatus may also become fibrotic and regurgitant, further compromising ventricular function and enlarging the atria.

 PATHOLOGY: Grossly, a thickened grayish-white endocardium extends from the left ventricle apex, over the posterior papillary muscle and chordae, to the posterior leaflet of the mitral valve, and then for a short distance into the left outflow tract. Interstitial and replacement fibrosis involves the inner 1/3 to 1/2 of the ventricle wall. Mural thrombi in various stages of organization may be present. When the right ventricle is involved, the entire cavity may show endocardial thickening with tricuspid valve and chorda involved. The fibrotic endocardium has only a few elastic fibers. Myofibers trapped within the collagenous tissue show nonspecific degenerative changes.

In Left Ventricular Noncompaction (LVNC) Trabeculae Are Prominent in the Ventricular Apex

In LVNC, the endocardium shows thick trabeculations and deep intratrabecular recesses, especially in the apex, encroaching into what is normally the compact portion of the ventricular wall (Fig. 17-47). LVNC occurs in the course of some congenital heart diseases including septal defects, pulmonic stenosis, and HLHS. It also occurs as an isolated disease, often considered a cardiomyopathy. It may be

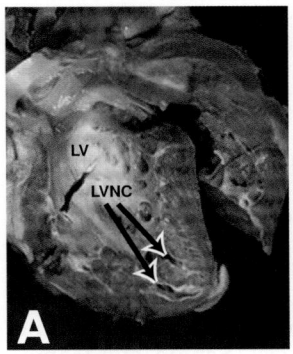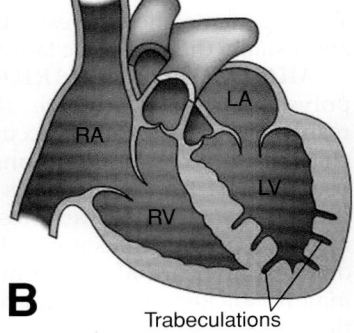

FIGURE 17-47. Left ventricular noncompaction. A. Gross appearance of a heart in LVNC with accentuated trabeculae and deep intertrabecular grooves in the apex of the left ventricle. **B.** Diagram showing the usual distribution of myocardial noncompaction. (Reprinted by permission from Towbin JA, Bowles NE. The failing heart. *Nature.* 2002;415:227–233; Fig 4. Copyright © 2002 Springer Nature.)

accompanied by ventricular hypertrophy or dilatation, and clinical features of heart failure, ventricular tachyarrhythmias, and complete heart block. Echocardiography in otherwise asymptomatic people may identify LVNC, suggesting that it may be more common than originally suspected, and raising questions about the relationship between structural and functional abnormalities in LVNC.

 MOLECULAR PATHOGENESIS: Known mutations cause LVNC in 30% to 50% of symptomatic patients (Table 17-8). Some males with isolated LVNC show X-linked inheritance of mutations in *TAZ*, which encodes tafazzin, a highly expressed cardiac and skeletal muscle phospholipid transacylase involved in cardiolipin metabolism. Other autosomal dominant mutations involve many of the same sarcomeric protein genes as are linked to HCM (Table 17-8). How mutations in these genes cause such diverse clinical and pathologic phenotypes is unknown.

Storage Diseases Can Mimic Primary Cardiomyopathies

Mutations in genes that regulate cardiac metabolism and clearance of cellular byproducts can cause left ventricular hypertrophy that mimics diverse primary cardiomyopathies (Table 17-8). For example, mutations in *LAMP2* (lysosomal-associated membrane protein 2) may cause a DCM or HCM phenotype. Diseases caused by mutations in *GLA* (galactosidase) and *PRKAG2* (AMP-activated protein kinase) may resemble HCM. The presence of vacuoles in cardiac myocytes containing lipid (*GLA* mutations), lysosomal remnants (*LAMP2* mutations), or glycogen (*PRKAG2* mutations) helps distinguish these diseases from true primary cardiomyopathies. Classical lysosomal diseases (**see Chapter 6**) may also mimic primary cardiomyopathies. Only cardiac manifestations of storage diseases are reviewed here.

GLYCOGEN STORAGE DISEASES: Of the various forms of glycogen storage disease, types II (Pompe disease), III (Cori disease), and IV (Andersen disease) affect the heart. Pompe disease is the most common and severe. Infants with this condition have markedly enlarged hearts (up to 7x normal), and 20% have endocardial fibroelastosis. Myocytes are vacuolated because they store large amounts of glycogen. These patients show a restrictive type of cardiomyopathy and usually die of cardiac failure.

MUCOPOLYSACCHARIDOSES: Several of the mucopolysaccharidoses involve the heart. Cardiac disease results from lysosomal accumulation of mucopolysaccharides (glycosaminoglycans). In general, ventricular pseudohypertrophy develops and contractility gradually diminishes. Coronary arteries may be narrowed by intimal and medial thickening. In **Hurler** and **Hunter** syndromes, myocardial infarction is common. Valve leaflets may be thickened, causing progressive valvular dysfunction, manifested as aortic stenosis (**Scheie syndrome**), or mitral regurgitation (Hurler, **Morquio** syndromes). Hypoxic pulmonary vasoconstriction due to narrowing of the airways causes pulmonary hypertension, which leads to cor pulmonale.

SPHINGOLIPIDOSES: In **Fabry disease**, glycosphingolipid accumulation in the heart may cause functional and pathologic changes like those in the mucopolysaccharidoses. Fabry disease produces gross and microscopic changes resembling HCM. However, the characteristic vacuolated cardiac myocytes denote an underlying storage disease. **Gaucher disease** rarely involves the heart but may feature left ventricular interstitial infiltration by cerebroside-laden macrophages, impaired left ventricular compliance, and cardiac output.

HEMOCHROMATOSIS: This multiorgan disease is associated with excessive iron deposition in many tissues (**see Chapter 20**). The extent of cardiac iron deposition varies, and correlates only roughly with that in other organs. Cardiac involvement has features of DCM and RCM, with systolic and diastolic impairment. Heart failure occurs in up to one-third of patients.

Hearts are dilated, with thickened ventricular walls. The myocardium reflects iron deposition in cardiac myocytes. Interstitial fibrosis is always present, but the amount does not correlate with levels of iron accumulation. The severity of myocardial dysfunction seems to reflect the quantity of iron deposited.

SUDDEN CARDIAC DEATH

Over 300,000 people in the United States die suddenly each year. Most of these deaths are caused by spontaneous lethal ventricular tachyarrhythmias—ventricular tachycardia and ventricular fibrillation—in patients with some type of heart disease. Many sudden deaths occur out of the hospital in apparently healthy individuals who have coronary artery disease at autopsy but may have shown little clinical evidence of it during life.

Common causes of sudden cardiac death differ in young and old individuals. This has been studied best in competitive athletes (Fig. 17-48). In subjects under 35, HCM, idiopathic left ventricular hypertrophy (presumably reflecting genetic forms of heart muscle disease in at least some), and congenital coronary anomalies account for over 75% of sudden deaths. In Italy and other Mediterranean countries, ACM is a leading cause of sudden death in young people. *However, in developed nations, coronary artery disease is responsible for most sudden deaths in middle-aged and older adults.*

PATHOLOGY: The surface ECG may occasionally indicate a specific pathologic structure that can be implicated in causing sudden death, such as an accessory atrioventricular connection in Wolff–Parkinson–White syndrome or a lesion that disrupts a discrete component of the ventricular conduction system causing new bundle branch block. *However, lethal arrhythmias usually arise from complex functional and structural changes in the working ventricular myocardium that lead to ectopic beats (triggered activity) and/or abnormal conduction (reentry).* Grossly, hearts of sudden death victims typically exhibit myocardial alterations that create "anatomic substrates of arrhythmias." These changes may be localized (e.g., healed myocardial infarcts or left ventricular aneurysms) or diffuse (e.g., variable degrees of cardiac myocyte hypertrophy and interstitial fibrosis). Spontaneous lethal cardiac arrhythmia may be seen as a stochastic event arising from complex

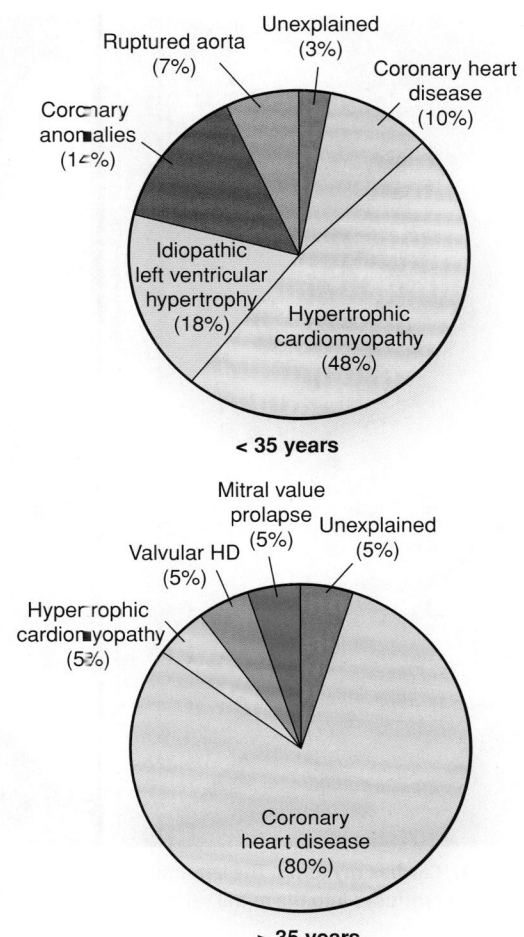

FIGURE 17-48. Different causes of sudden cardiac death in young and older adult competitive athletes. *HD* = heart disease.

interactions between relatively fixed anatomic substrates and acute, transient triggering events such as acute ischemia, neurohormonal activation, changes in electrolytes or other stresses. Many patients have potential arrhythmia substrates in their hearts. In most cases, they may be necessary but they are not sufficient for arrhythmogenesis. Arrhythmias are most likely when acute electrophysiologic changes (triggers) are superimposed on an existing substrate of remodeled myocardium with characteristic conduction abnormalities. Indeed, most often sudden death involves acute ischemia (a transient triggering event) in an area of the heart containing a healed infarct (a common anatomic substrate).

Sudden Cardiac Death Occurs in Patients With Structurally Normal Hearts but Is Rare

Some (perhaps many) of such patients have "channelopathies," genetic diseases in which mutations in genes for Na⁺, K⁺, and Ca²⁺ channel proteins or proteins important in their intracellular trafficking and turnover are responsible for sudden death syndromes (see Chapter 1). These syndromes are rare but have provided valuable insights into molecular mechanisms of lethal arrhythmias.

 MOLECULAR PATHOGENESIS: *LONG QT SYNDROME:* This inherited condition is defined by prolonged QT interval and T-wave abnormalities on the surface ECG and a history of syncope, ventricular arrhythmias or sudden, unexpected death. More than 15 different types of congenital long QT syndrome are defined, based on the specific gene in which mutations have been linked to the long QT phenotype. Most are caused by loss-of-function mutations in genes encoding proteins that form K⁺ channels. The loss of function prolongs repolarization of cardiac action potentials (thus increasing QT intervals on surface ECGs) and promotes arrhythmias by increasing the likelihood of afterdepolarizations. Long QT syndrome can also be caused by gain-of-function mutations in *SCN5A*, the gene for the α-subunit of the cardiac Na⁺ channel, or *CACNA1C*, which encodes the pore-forming protein of the cardiac L-type Ca²⁺ channel. These mutations prolong QT intervals by allowing leakage of depolarizing current during repolarization. Mutations in ankyrin B and caveolin-3, which mediate ion channel protein trafficking or scaffolding, also cause long QT syndrome. Arrhythmias occur in long QT syndrome because the mutated ion channels are normally distributed in the heart in a spatially heterogeneous fashion. The functional defect caused by the mutation creates ionic gradients that promote abnormal electrical impulse formation (afterdepolarizations) and abnormal impulse conduction, conditions conducive to development of ventricular tachycardias. QT prolongation also occurs in heart failure and likely contributes to increased risk of arrhythmias and sudden death. It arises as a result of acquired rather than genetic "electrophysiologic remodeling" that accompanies changes in signaling pathways and protein expression patterns in failing hearts. Many commonly prescribed drugs including antibiotics, antihistamines, and various psychotropic drugs prolong QT intervals as off-target effects. Drug-induced QT prolongation increases risk of serious arrhythmia, especially in people with genetic predisposition and/or acquired conditions that also prolong repolarization. The U.S. Food and Drug Administration requires that all new nonantiarrhythmic drugs undergo clinical electrocardiographic trial to evaluate effects on cardiac repolarization.

BRUGADA SYNDROME: This is an autosomal dominant disease with characteristic ST-segment elevation in right precordial leads, right bundle branch block, and susceptibility to life-threatening arrhythmias. Approximately 25% of cases have loss-of-function mutations in *SCN5A*. Many Brugada syndrome hearts are structurally normal, but some patients' hearts may have varying amounts of fibrosis. There may also be phenotypic overlap between Brugada syndrome and ACM.

CATECHOLAMINERGIC POLYMORPHIC VENTRICULAR TACHYCARDIA: In this condition, arrhythmias and sudden death occur in response to catecholamine surges associated with exercise or emotional stress. Mutations in genes encoding proteins that regulate intracellular Ca²⁺ homeostasis and excitation–contraction coupling, such as RyR2 and calsequestrin, are typical. These mutations promote leakage of Ca²⁺ from the SR and resultant arrhythmias triggered by afterdepolarizations.

THE HEART

CARDIAC TUMORS

Cardiac tumors are rare but can cause serious problems when they occur. Metastatic tumors to the heart are 100 times more common than primary tumors, and roughly 90% of primary cardiac tumors are benign. Most are myxomas.

Myxomas Are the Most Common Primary Cardiac Tumors

These benign tumors account for 50% to 80% of primary cardiac tumors.

MOLECULAR PATHOGENESIS: Most cardiac myxomas are sporadic, but about 5% to 10% are part of an autosomal dominant syndrome, the Carney complex, that also includes myxomatous tumors of other tissues, cutaneous hyperpigmentation and increased endocrine activity. It has been linked to inactivating germline mutations in *PRKAR1A*, which encodes the α-regulatory subunit of cAMP-dependent protein kinase type 1. This tumor suppressor gene controls cell proliferation. The cell of origin is still not fully resolved but most authorities agree that cardiac myxomas arise from multipotent mesenchymal stem cells in the fossa ovalis and elsewhere in the endocardium. These cells and many of the tumors they give rise to express markers characteristic of both primitive cardiac myocytes and endothelial cell precursors. They also produce α-smooth muscle actin which is expressed by cardiac myocytes early in development.

PATHOLOGY: Myxomas can occur in any cardiac chamber or on a valve, but most (75%) arise in the left atrium. They are glistening, gelatinous, polypoid masses, 5 to 6 cm, with a short stalk (Fig. 17-49), and may be sufficiently mobile to obstruct the mitral valve orifice. Their loose myxoid stroma contains abundant proteoglycans, and polygonal stellate cells, singly or in small clusters.

CLINICAL FEATURES: Over half of patients with left atrial myxomas have clinical evidence of mitral valve dysfunction. The tumor does not metastasize in the usual sense, but it may fragment and embolize. Some patients with myxomas of the left heart die of strokes because of tumor emboli to the brain. Surgical tumor removal is usually curative.

Rhabdomyomas Are the Most Common Primary Childhood Cardiac Tumors

They form nodular myocardial masses. Rhabdomyomas may really be hamartomas (see below) and not true neoplasms, but this question is not settled. Almost all are multiple and involve both ventricles and, in one-third of cases, atria as well. In half of cases, the tumors project into a cardiac chamber and obstruct a lumen or valve orifice.

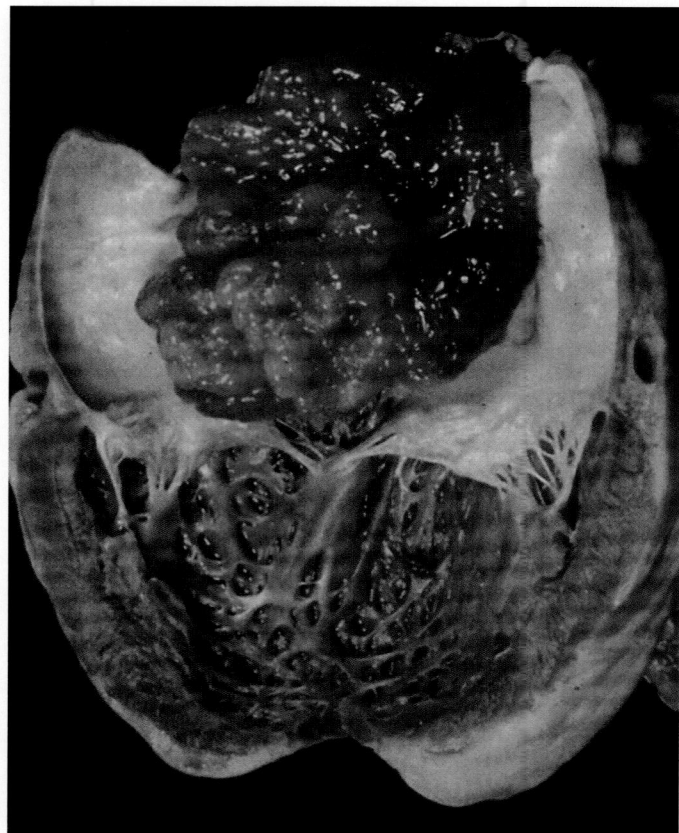

FIGURE 17-49. Cardiac myxoma. The left atrium contains a large, polypoid tumor that protrudes into the mitral valve orifice.

MOLECULAR PATHOGENESIS: Rhabdomyomas occur in one-third of patients with tuberous sclerosis, the familial form of which is caused by mutations in *TSC1* and *TSC2*, which encode hamartin and tuberin, respectively. Both are tumor suppressors (**see Chapter 5**) and regulate embryonic and neonatal growth and differentiation of cardiac myocytes.

PATHOLOGY: Cardiac rhabdomyomas are pale, 1 mm to several centimeter masses. Tumor cells show small central nuclei and abundant glycogen-rich clear cytoplasm, in which fibrillar processes containing sarcomeres radiate to the margin of the cell ("spider cell"). About one-third to one-half of these tumors occur in association with tuberous sclerosis. A few cardiac rhabdomyomas have been successfully excised.

Papillary Fibroelastoma Involves the Valves

Papillary fronds resembling a sea anemone and measuring up to 3 to 4 cm may grow on heart valves. These are not true neoplasms, but rather **hamartomas**. The fronds have central dense cores of collagen and elastic fibers surrounded by looser connective tissue. They are covered by a continuation of valvular endothelium on which the tumor originates. In most instances, papillary fibroelastomas are not clinical problems, but they can fragment and embolize to distant

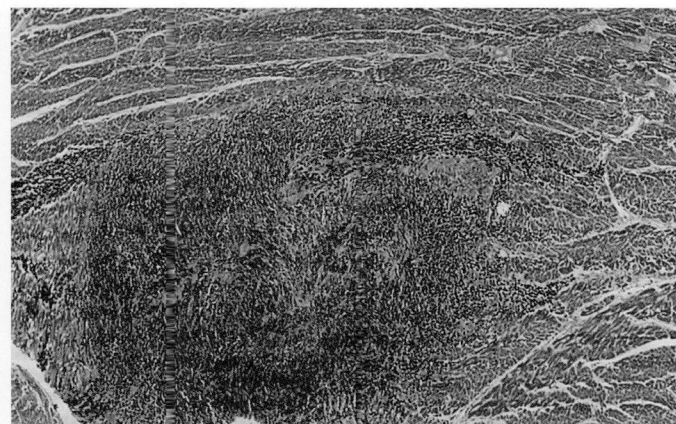

FIGURE 17-50. Malignant melanoma metastatic to the heart. The myocardium contains a heavily pigmented tumor metastasis.

organs, or occlude a coronary artery orifice and cause myocardial ischemia.

Other Cardiac Tumors Are Rare

Other primary tumors of the heart include angiomas, fibromas, lymphangiomas, neurofibromas, and their sarcomatous counterparts. Lipomatous hypertrophy of the interatrial septum and encapsulated lipomas have been reported.

Metastatic tumors to the heart are seen most often in patients with the most common carcinomas—that is, lung, breast, and gastrointestinal tract. Still, only a minority of patients with these tumors develop cardiac metastases. Lymphomas and leukemia also may involve the heart. The tumor most likely to metastasize to the heart is malignant melanoma (Fig. 17-50). Metastatic cancer involving the myocardium can result in clinical manifestations of RCM, particularly if the cardiac tumors are associated with extensive fibrosis. Occasionally, metastatic tumors may disrupt the AV conduction system, and cause heart block or bundle branch block patterns on the surface electrocardiogram.

DISEASES OF THE PERICARDIUM

Pericardial Effusions Can Cause Cardiac Tamponade

Pericardial effusions are accumulations of excess fluid within the pericardial cavity, as either a transudate or an exudate. The pericardial sac normally contains no more than 50 mL of lubricating fluid. If the pericardium is slowly distended, it can accommodate up to 2 L of fluid without serious hemodynamic consequences. However, rapid accumulation of as little as 150 to 200 mL of pericardial fluid or blood may significantly increase intrapericardial pressure and restrict diastolic filling, especially of the right atrium and ventricle.

- **Serous pericardial effusion** often complicates an increase in extracellular fluid volume, as occurs in heart failure or nephrotic syndrome. The fluid has low-protein content and few cellular elements.
- **Chylous effusion** (fluid containing chylomicrons) results when the thoracic duct communicates with the pericardial space, due to lymphatic obstruction by tumor or infection.

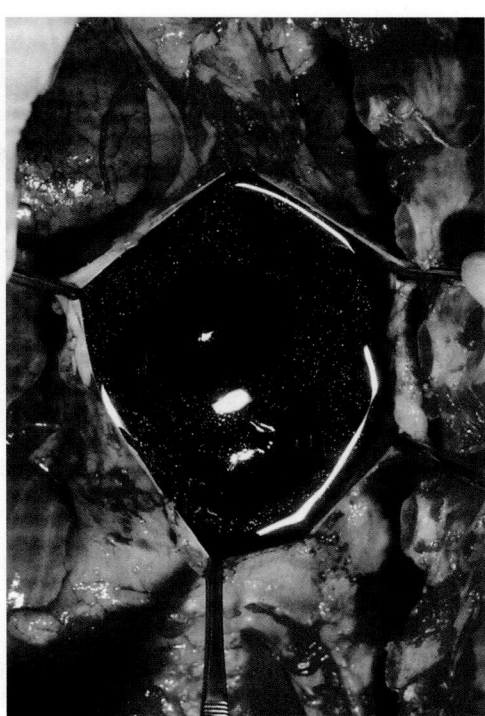

FIGURE 17-51. Hemopericardium. The parietal pericardium has been opened to reveal the pericardial cavity distended with fresh blood. The patient sustained a ruptured myocardial infarct.

- **Serosanguineous pericardial effusion** may develop after chest trauma, either accidentally or after cardiopulmonary resuscitation.
- **Hemopericardium** is bleeding directly into the pericardial cavity (Fig. 17-51). The most common cause is ventricular free wall rupture at a myocardial infarct. Less frequent causes are penetrating cardiac trauma, rupture of a dissecting aneurysm of the aorta, infiltration of a vessel by tumor or a bleeding diathesis.

Cardiac tamponade *occurs when pericardial fluid accumulates rapidly, restricting the filling of the heart.* Hemodynamic consequences range from a minimally symptomatic condition to abrupt cardiovascular collapse and death. As pericardial pressure increases, it reaches and then exceeds central venous pressure, thus limiting blood return to the heart. Cardiac output and blood pressure decrease, and **pulsus paradoxus** (an abnormal decrease in systolic pressure with inspiration) occurs in almost all patients. Acute cardiac tamponade is almost always fatal unless the pressure is relieved by removing pericardial fluid, via needle pericardiocentesis or surgery.

Acute Pericarditis May Follow Viral Infections

Pericarditis is inflammation of the visceral or parietal pericardium.

 ETIOLOGIC FEATURES: The causes of pericarditis are similar to those for myocarditis (Table 17-7). It may complicate myocardial infarction or rheumatic fever (see above), but most cases of pericarditis are

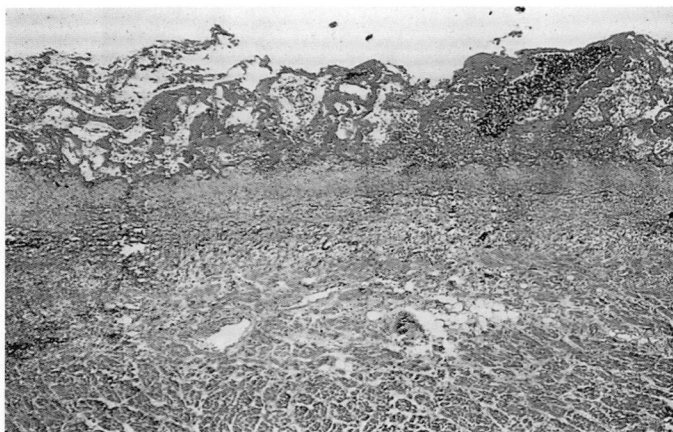

FIGURE 17-52. Fibrinous pericardial exudate. The epicardial surface is edematous, inflamed, and covered with tentacles of fibrin.

idiopathic, and are generally attributed to undiagnosed viral infections. Bacterial pericarditis is unusual in the antibiotic era.

Metastatic tumors that involve the pericardium may induce serofibrinous or hemorrhagic exudative and inflammatory reactions. Breast and lung cancers most often involve the pericardium and cause malignant pericardial effusions.

PATHOLOGY: Acute pericarditis can be **fibrinous, purulent**, or **hemorrhagic**, depending on gross and microscopic characteristics of the pericardial surfaces and fluid. Fibrinous pericarditis is most common: normally smooth, glistening pericardial surfaces are replaced by a dull, granular fibrin-rich exudate (Fig. 17-52). The rough texture of inflamed pericardial surfaces causes a typical friction rub on auscultation. Effusion fluid in fibrinous pericarditis is usually rich in protein, and the pericardium contains mainly mononuclear inflammatory cells. Pericarditis is most commonly due to viral infection and myocardial infarction. Uremia can cause fibrinous pericarditis (Fig. 17-53), but with ubiquitous renal dialysis, uremic pericarditis is rare in the United States.

Bacterial infection may cause purulent pericarditis, in which the pericardial exudate resembles pus and is full of neutrophils. Bleeding into the pericardial space caused by aggressive infectious or neoplastic processes or coagulation defects leads to hemorrhagic pericarditis.

CLINICAL FEATURES: Initial manifestations of acute pericarditis are sudden, severe, substernal chest pain, sometimes referred to the back, shoulder, or neck. Unlike the pain of angina pectoris or myocardial infarction pericarditis pain does not radiate down the left arm. A characteristic pericardial friction rub is easily audible. Electrocardiographic changes reflect repolarization abnormalities of the myocardium.

Idiopathic or viral pericarditis is self-limited but may infrequently lead to constrictive pericarditis. Corticosteroids are the treatment of choice. Therapy for other specific forms of acute pericarditis varies with the cause.

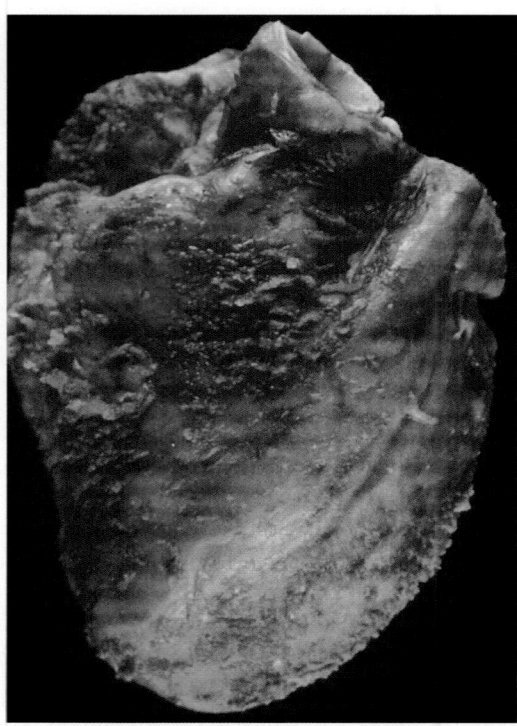

FIGURE 17-53. Fibrinous pericarditis. The heart of a patient who died in uremia displays a shaggy, fibrinous exudate covering the visceral pericardium.

Constrictive Pericarditis May Mimic Right Heart Failure

Constrictive pericarditis is a chronic fibrotic disease of the pericardium that compresses the heart and restricts inflow.

  ETIOLOGIC FACTORS, PATHOLOGY: Constrictive pericarditis is not an active inflammatory condition. Rather, it reflects exuberant healing after acute pericardial injury. The pericardial space becomes obliterated, and visceral and parietal layers become fused in a dense, rigid mass of fibrous tissue. The scarred pericardium may be so thick (up to 3 cm) that it narrows the orifices of the venae cavae (Fig. 17-54). The fibrous envelope may contain calcium. This condition is uncommon today and, in developed countries, is mostly idiopathic. Prior radiation therapy to the mediastinum and cardiac surgery account for more than one-third of cases. In others, it follows a purulent or tuberculous infection. Tuberculosis today accounts for <15% of cases of constrictive pericarditis in industrialized countries but is still the major cause elsewhere.

CLINICAL FEATURES: Patients with constrictive pericarditis have small, quiet hearts in which venous inflow is restricted, since the rigid pericardium limits diastolic filling of the heart. These patients have high venous pressure, low cardiac output, small pulse pressure, and fluid retention with ascites and peripheral edema. Total pericardiectomy is the treatment of choice.

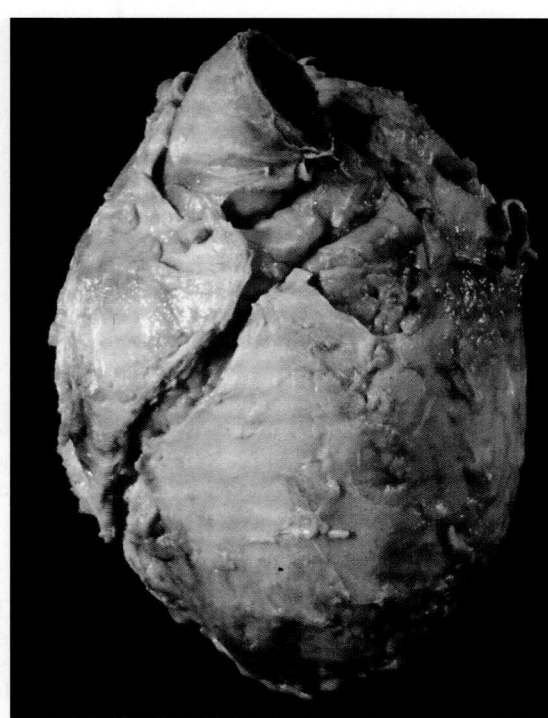

FIGURE 17-54. Constrictive pericarditis. The pericardial space has been obliterated, and the heart is encased in a fibrotic, thickened pericardium.

Adhesive pericarditis is a much milder form of healing of an inflamed pericardium. Commonly seen as an incidental finding at autopsy, it is the outcome of many different types of pericarditis that have healed and left only minor fibrous adhesions between the visceral and parietal surfaces.

PATHOLOGY OF INTERVENTIONAL THERAPIES

Percutaneous Coronary Interventions (PCI) Are Used to Treat Atherosclerotic Coronary Artery Disease

PCI is used to dilate mechanically an artery narrowed by atherosclerosis and keep its lumen open. A catheter with a deflated balloon covered by a collapsed cylindrical metallic mesh **(stent)** is positioned in the stenotic segment. Inflating the balloon fractures the plaque and stretches the vessel wall. As the stent deploys, it holds the fragmented wall open and keeps the vessel lumen patent. Acute complications of PCI such as coronary artery dissection, acute thrombotic occlusion and perforation are uncommon. Most patients receive drug-eluting stents, which slowly release antiproliferative agents such as everolimus or paclitaxel. Their use has dramatically reduced the incidence of restenosis. Stents with bioabsorbable scaffolds are under study but have not been shown to be superior to second-generation drug-eluting stents.

Coronary Bypass Grafts Circumvent Obstructed Segments

Coronary bypasses use saphenous vein or left internal mammary artery grafts to circumvent proximal coronary artery

stenosis. Operative mortality is low and most patients experience early symptomatic relief, but several complications limit long-term improvement in myocardial perfusion: (1) early thrombosis, (2) intimal hyperplasia, and (3) atherosclerosis developing in vein grafts. Progressive atherosclerosis of native coronary arteries is not affected by such grafting. Nevertheless, in patients with severe left main coronary artery or diffuse epicardial coronary disease, coronary bypasses are still considered the "gold standard" and are superior to PCI in long-term outcomes.

Internal mammary artery grafts are less problematic than vein grafts, and so last longer. Unavoidable surgical manipulation of excised saphenous vein segments, and endothelial cell damage due to brief ischemia during harvesting injure the grafted veins. Exposure to arterial pressures far exceeds those native venous pressures. Finally, the vein is expanded by high arterial blood pressures, to become much larger than the distal coronary artery at the graft anastomosis. This mismatch promotes blood stasis. Immediately postoperatively, these factors enhance the chance of thrombosis and probably eventually lead to **intimal hyperplasia**. Intimal hyperplasia is a concentric increase of smooth muscle cells, fibroblasts, and collagen in the intima of the vein. After several years, lipids accumulate. Atherosclerotic plaques that form in the thickened intima of vein grafts represent the most frequent cause of vein graft failure in patients who have had several years of good graft function. Over 50% of saphenous vein grafts become totally or partly occluded within 10 to 15 years.

Since arteries are better aortocoronary bypass conduits than veins, some surgeons have advocated total arterial bypass procedures that use internal mammary, radial and selected abdominal arteries that can be taken without end-organ damage.

Bioprosthetic and Mechanical Valves Are Used to Replace Damaged Cardiac Valves

Many patients with mitral regurgitation undergo valve repair procedures that mitigate regurgitant flow by reducing leaflet redundancy, shortening stretched chordae, and tightening annular circumference. However, patients with severe valve dysfunction require replacement with a prosthetic valve for long-term symptomatic improvement. Operative mortality is low, especially for patients with good preoperative myocardial function. Half of patients with prosthetic valves are free of complications after 10 years. Recent advances have made TAVR a viable option in elderly patients with severe aortic valve disease who are poor candidates for open-chest valve replacement operations. Catheter-deployed mitral valve prostheses are also in early clinical use.

BIOPROSTHETIC VALVES: The most commonly used bioprosthetic valves are made from glutaraldehyde-fixed porcine valve cusps or pieces of bovine pericardium attached to a frame or stent covered with fabric that serves as a sewing ring. Stentless bioprosthetic valves offer larger valve orifice areas. All transcatheter aortic and mitral valves are made of trileaflet porcine or bovine tissues on an expandable metal frame.

Bioprosthetic valves have good hemodynamic characteristics, cause little obstruction and resist thromboembolic complications. Unfortunately, they are not very durable. The most common reason these prostheses fail is tissue degeneration with calcification and fragmentation of prosthetic

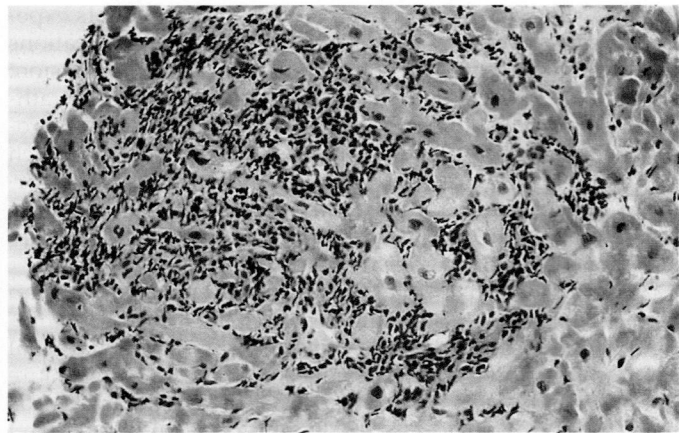

FIGURE 17-55. Cardiac transplant rejection. An endomyocardial biopsy shows lymphocytes surrounding individual myocytes and expanding the interstitium.

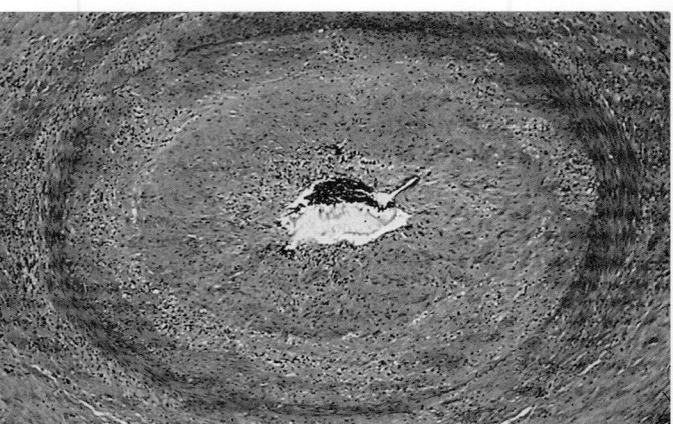

FIGURE 17-56. Chronic cardiac transplant rejection. An intramyocardial branch of a coronary artery shows prominent intimal proliferation and inflammation with concentric narrowing of the lumen.

valve cusps. This affected virtually all early-generation porcine aortic valves and caused valve failure in 20% to 30% within 10 years. Tissue-valve calcification mainly affects residual cells killed by glutaraldehyde treatment. Preventing or delaying such calcification improved valve longevity and performance.

MECHANICAL VALVES: The most widely used mechanical prostheses involve single or bileaflet tilting disk designs that do not obstruct blood flow across the valve and are highly durable. However, risk of thromboembolism makes long-term anticoagulant therapy imperative.

Heart Transplantation Extends Life in Patients With End-Stage Heart Diseases but Is Subject to Host Rejection Processes

Development of effective immune suppressive regimens and endomyocardial biopsy protocols has made cardiac transplantation an effective treatment for end-stage heart disease. Allograft rejection (**see Chapter 4**), however, is a major complication of cardiac transplantation.

Hyperacute rejection usually reflects blood-group incompatibility or major histocompatibility differences. Preformed host antibodies cause immediate vascular injury to the donor heart: diffuse hemorrhage, edema, intracapillary platelet–fibrin thrombi, vascular necrosis, and infiltration of neutrophils. This complication is rare.

In **acute humoral rejection**, antibody and complement deposit in graft vasculature, with endothelial cell swelling and edema. This form of rejection has a worse prognosis than acute cellular rejection.

Acute cellular rejection, the most common form of allograft rejection, usually occurs in the first few months

after transplantation. It begins as focal perivascular T-cell infiltration, not associated with acute myocyte necrosis. It often resolves spontaneously and so does not necessitate changing the immunosuppressive regimen. In moderate cellular rejection, T cells infiltrate into adjacent interstitial spaces, surround individual myocytes and expand the interstitium (Fig. 17-55). In this instance, focal acute myocyte necrosis also occurs. Moderate cellular rejection usually does not impair function detectably, and usually resolves within a few days to a week after treatment. However, because moderate cellular rejection can progress to severe rejection, additional immunosuppression is applied. Severe rejection is characterized by vascular damage, widespread myocyte necrosis, neutrophil infiltration, interstitial hemorrhage, and functional impairment, which is difficult to reverse.

The early stage of cellular allograft rejection is often asymptomatic. Once symptoms develop, rejection is usually advanced and has caused irrecoverable loss of cardiac myocytes. The most reliable screening procedure is endomyocardial biopsy of the right side of the interventricular septum.

Chronic vascular rejection, also called **accelerated coronary artery disease**, is the most common cause of death in heart transplant patients beyond the first year after transplantation. It affects proximal and distal epicardial coronary arteries, penetrating coronary artery branches, and arterioles. Accelerated coronary artery disease is characterized by concentric intimal proliferation (Fig. 17-56), which can lead to vascular occlusion. Resulting myocardial infarction is painless, because transplanted hearts are denervated. Thus, extensive myocardial damage can develop before a transplant patient is aware that ischemic injury has occurred.

18

The Respiratory System

Mary Beth Beasley, William D. Travis

The Normal Respiratory System

EMBRYOLOGY

The respiratory system includes the larynx, trachea, bronchi, bronchioles, and alveoli. During the fourth week of gestation, the laryngotracheal groove develops as a ventral outpouching of the foregut.

1. **Embryonic period:** Between 4 and 6 weeks of gestation, the tracheobronchial bud divides to form proximal airways to the level of segmental bronchi.
2. **Pseudoglandular period:** From 6 to 16 weeks of gestation, the distal airways are formed to the level of the terminal bronchioles.

3. **Acinar or canalicular development:** During weeks 17 to 28, (a) the framework of the gas-exchanging unit of the lung develops, (b) acini are formed, (c) the vascular system develops, (d) capillaries reach the epithelium, and (e) gas exchange can occur. At this point extrauterine life becomes possible.

4. **Saccular period:** At 28 to 34 weeks of gestation, primary saccules become subdivided by secondary crests, resulting in greater complexity of the gas-exchanging surface and thinning of airspace walls.

5. **Alveolar period:** The last step is alveolar development during weeks 34 to 36. At birth, the number of alveoli is highly variable, ranging from 20 to 150 million. Most alveoli develop in the first 2 years of life.

ANATOMY

TRACHEA AND BRONCHI: The trachea is a hollow tube up to 25 cm in length and 2.5 cm in diameter. The right bronchus diverges at a lesser angle from the trachea than does the left, which is why foreign material is more frequently aspirated on the right side. On entering the lung, the main bronchi divide into lobar bronchi, then into segmental bronchi, which supply the 19 lung segments. Since segments are individual units with their own bronchovascular supply, they can be resected individually.

The tracheobronchial tree contains cartilage and submucosal mucus glands in their walls (Fig. 18-1). The latter are compound tubular glands, which contain **mucus cells** (pale) and **serous cells** (granular, more basophilic). The pseudostratified epithelium appears as layers, but all cells reach the basement membrane. Most cells are ciliated, but there are also mucus-secreting **(goblet)** cells and basal cells. The **basal cells,** which do not reach the surface, are precursors that differentiate into more specialized tracheobronchial epithelial cells. There are also nonciliated columnar cells, or **club cells** (formerly **Clara cells),** which sequester and detoxify inhaled toxic agents (e.g., nitrogen dioxide [NO_2]). **Neuroendocrine cells**, scattered within the tracheobronchial mucosa, produce a variety of hormonally active polypeptides and vasoactive amines.

BRONCHIOLES: Distal to the bronchi are the bronchioles, which differ from bronchi in that they lack cartilage and mucus-secreting glands (Fig. 18-1). Bronchiolar epithelium becomes thinner with progressive branching, until only a single cell layer is present. The last purely conducting structure free of alveoli is the **terminal bronchiole,** which exhibits pseudostratified ciliated respiratory epithelium and a smooth muscle wall. Individual mucus cells gradually disappear from the lining of the bronchioles until they are replaced entirely in the small bronchioles by nonciliated, columnar club cells (formerly Clara cells). Terminal bronchioles divide into **respiratory bronchioles,** which merge into **alveolar ducts** and **alveoli.** The gas exchange units of the lung are called **acini** and consist of respiratory bronchioles, alveolar ducts, and alveoli.

ALVEOLI: Alveoli are lined by two types of epithelial cells (Fig. 18-1). **Type I cells** cover 95% of the alveolar surface but constitute only 40% of alveolar epithelial cells. They are thin and have a large surface area, a combination that facilitates gas exchange. **Type II cells** produce surfactant and make up 60% of the alveolar lining cells. As they are more cuboidal than type I cells, they cover only 5% of the alveolar surface. Type I cells are highly vulnerable to injury. When they are lost, type II pneumocytes multiply and differentiate to form new type I cells, restoring the integrity of the alveolar surface.

Alveolar epithelial and endothelial cells are ideally arranged for gas exchange. The cytoplasm of epithelial and endothelial cells is spread very thinly on either side of a fused basement membrane, allowing efficient exchange of oxygen and carbon dioxide. An extensive capillary network supplies 85% to 95% of the alveolar surface. Away from the site of gas exchange, interstitial connective tissue is more abundant, consisting of collagen, elastin, and proteoglycans. Fibroblasts and myofibroblasts may also be present. This expanded region forms the interstitial space of the alveolar wall, where significant fluid and molecular exchange occurs.

PULMONARY VASCULATURE: The lung has a **dual blood supply** from the pulmonary and the bronchial systems. Pulmonary arteries accompany airways in a sheath of connective tissue, the **bronchovascular bundle.** The more proximal arteries are elastic and are succeeded by muscular arteries, pulmonary arterioles, and eventually pulmonary capillaries.

The smallest veins, which resemble the smallest arteries, join other veins and drain into lobular septa, connective tissue partitions that subdivide the lung into small respiratory units. In these septa, the veins form a network separate from the bronchovascular bundles.

Bronchial arteries arise from the thoracic aorta and nourish the bronchial tree as far as the respiratory bronchioles. These arteries are accompanied by their respective veins, which drain into the azygos or hemiazygos veins.

There are no lymphatics in most alveolar walls. These vessels begin in alveoli at the periphery of acini, which lie along lobular septa, bronchovascular bundles, or the pleura. The lymphatics of the lobular septa and bronchovascular bundle accompany these structures, and the pleural lymphatics drain toward the hilus through the bronchovascular lymphatics.

DEFENSE MECHANISMS

The respiratory system has effective defense mechanisms to cope with the numerous particulates and infectious agents inhaled on inspiration.

The **nose and trachea** warm and humidify air entering the lung. The nose traps almost all particles over 10 μm in diameter and about half of all particles of 3 μm aerodynamic diameter (Fig. 18-2, see also Chapter 8). (Aerodynamic diameter refers to the way particles behave in air rather than to their actual size.)

The **mucociliary blanket** of the airway epithelium disposes of particles 2 to 10 μm in diameter. The ciliary beat drives the mucus blanket toward the trachea. Particles that land on it are thus removed from the lungs and swallowed or coughed up.

Alveolar macrophages protect the alveolar space. These cells are derived from the bone marrow, probably undergo a maturation division in the interstitium of the lung and then enter the alveolar space. They are particularly effective in dealing with particles with aerodynamic diameters under 2 μm. Very small particles are not phagocytosed and are exhaled.

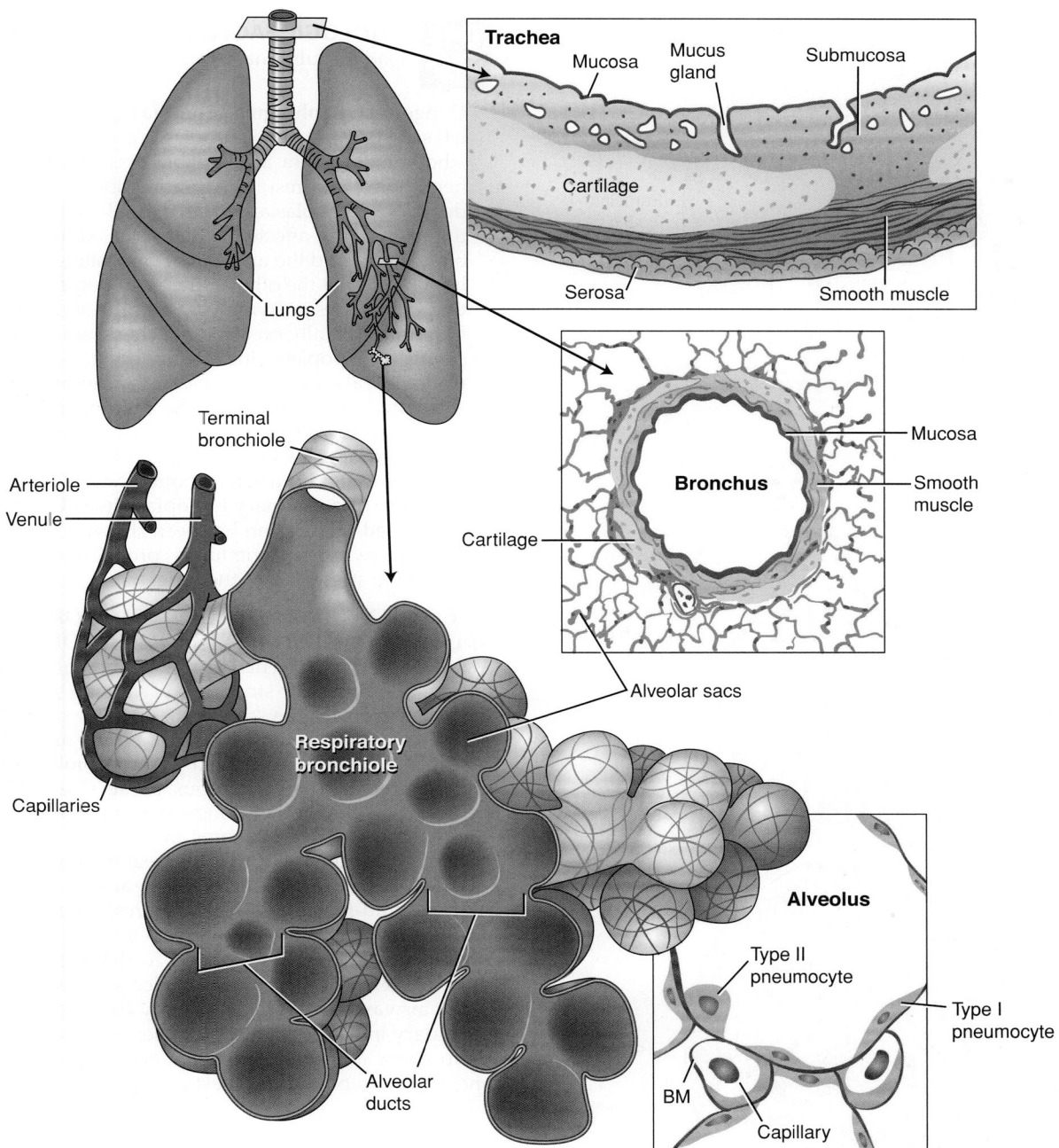

FIGURE 18-1. Anatomy of the lung. The conducting structures of the lung include (1) the trachea, which has horseshoe-shaped cartilages; (2) the bronchi, which have plates of cartilage in their walls (both the trachea and bronchi have mucus-secreting glands in their walls); and (3) the bronchioles, which do not have cartilage in their walls and terminate in the terminal bronchioles. The gas-exchanging components compose the acinus, the unit distal to the terminal bronchiole. Alveoli are lined by type I cells, which are large, flat cells that cover most of the alveolar wall, and by type II cells, which secrete surfactant and are the progenitor cells of the alveolar epithelium. Gas exchange occurs at the level of the alveolar wall.

The Lungs

CONGENITAL ANOMALIES

BRONCHIAL ATRESIA: This abnormality most often involves the bronchus to the apical posterior segment of the left upper lobe. In infants, the lesion may result in an overexpanded part of the lung. In later life, the over-expanded lobe may become emphysematous. Bronchial mucous accumulating distal to the atretic region may appear on radiologic examination as a mass.

PULMONARY HYPOPLASIA: This condition reflects incomplete or defective lung development. The lung is smaller than normal, with fewer and smaller acini. This is the most common congenital lesion of the lung, found in 10% of

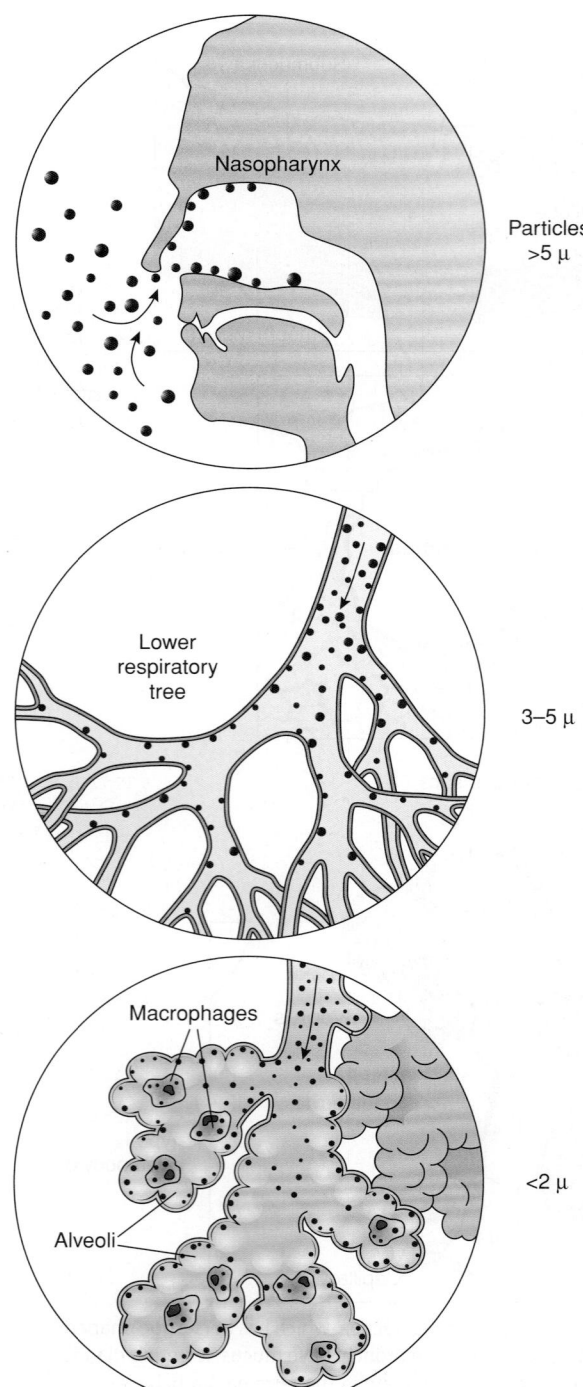

FIGURE 18-2. Deposition of particles in the respiratory tract. Large particles are trapped in the nose. Intermediate-sized particles deposit on the bronchi and bronchioles and are removed by the mucociliary blanket. Smaller particles terminate in the airspaces and are removed by macrophages. Very small particles behave as a gas and are breathed out.

neonatal autopsies. In most cases (90%), it occurs in association with other congenital anomalies, most of which involve the thorax. The lesion may be accompanied by hypoplasia of bronchi and pulmonary vessels if the insult occurs early in gestation, as in congenital diaphragmatic hernia. Pulmonary hypoplasia is also seen in trisomies 13, 18, and 21.

 ETIOLOGIC FACTORS: Three major factors may lead to pulmonary hypoplasia:

- **Congenital diaphragmatic hernia** typically occurs on the left side, because the pleuroperitoneal canal fails to close. Abdominal viscera are variably present in the affected hemithorax and result in compression of the lung. The degree of hypoplasia is thus variable. At one extreme, the lung on the affected side is reduced to a small nubbin of tissue and the lung on the opposite side is severely hypoplastic. At the other extreme, hypoplasia is so slight that it produces no symptoms and the abnormalities are found incidentally on a routine chest radiograph. Other causes of hypoplasia include abnormalities of the chest wall, pleural effusions, and ascites, as in hydrops fetalis. Abnormal development of the pulmonary vasculature often leads to persistent pulmonary hypertension.
- **Oligohydramnios** (low amniotic fluid volume) is usually due to genitourinary anomalies and is an important cause of pulmonary hypoplasia (see Chapter 6).
- **Decreased respiration** has been shown experimentally to produce hypoplastic lungs, probably due to lack of repetitive stretching of the lung.

CONGENITAL CYSTIC ADENOMATOID MALFORMATION (CONGENITAL PULMONARY ADENOMATOID MALFORMATION): This common anomaly consists of abnormal bronchiolar structures of varying sizes or distribution. Most cases are seen in the first 2 years of life. The lesion usually affects one lobe of the lung and consists of multiple cyst-like spaces lined by bronchiolar epithelium and separated by loose fibrous tissue (Fig. 18-3). Some patients will have other congenital anomalies. The most common presenting symptoms are respiratory distress and cyanosis. Surgical resection is the treatment of choice.

BRONCHOGENIC CYSTS: These are discrete, extrapulmonary, fluid-filled masses lined by respiratory epithelium and limited by walls that contain muscle and cartilage. They are most commonly found in the middle mediastinum. In newborns, a bronchogenic cyst may compress a major airway and cause respiratory distress. Later in life, secondary infections of cysts may lead to hemorrhage and perforation. Many bronchogenic cysts are asymptomatic and are found on routine chest radiographs.

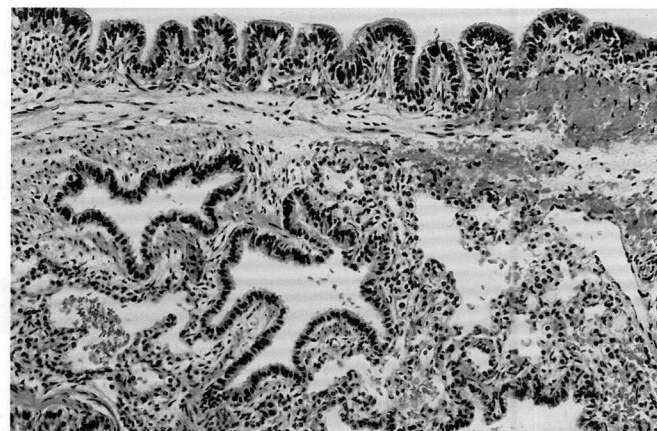

FIGURE 18-3. Congenital cystic adenomatoid malformation. Multiple gland-like spaces are lined by bronchiolar epithelium.

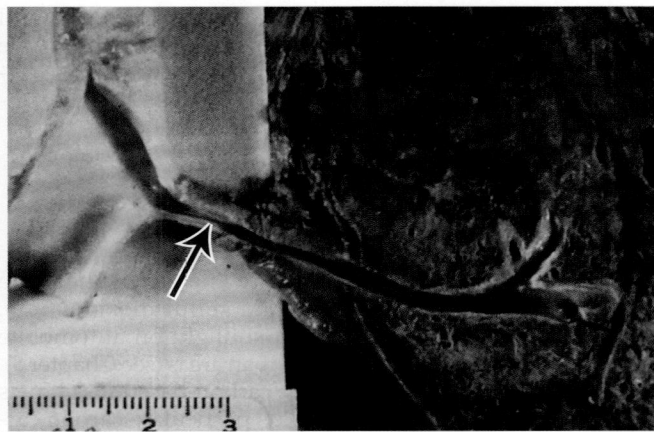

FIGURE 18-4. Extralobar sequestration. The sequestered pulmonary tissue is situated outside the lung parenchyma. It is supplied by an aberrant artery (*arrow*) from the aorta and is not connected to the bronchial tree.

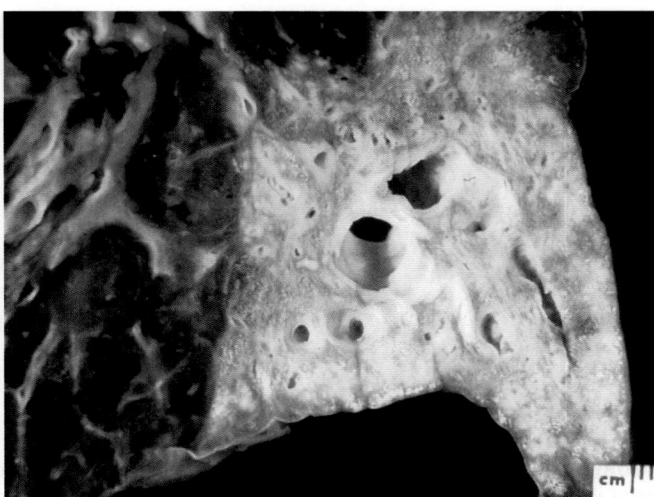

FIGURE 18-5. Intralobar sequestration. The sequestered tissue lies within the visceral pleura and exhibits cystic change and dense fibrosis. It was supplied by an aberrant pulmonary artery (not shown).

EXTRALOBAR SEQUESTRATION: Extralobar sequestration is a mass of lung tissue that is not connected to the bronchial tree and is covered by its own visceral pleura independent from the main lung. An abnormal artery, usually arising from the aorta, supplies the sequestered tissue (Fig. 18-4).

 ETIOLOGIC FACTORS: This lesion is thought to originate from an outpouching of the foregut, distinct from the pulmonary anlage, that later loses its connection to the original foregut. It occurs three to four times more often in males than in females and is associated with other anomalies in two-thirds of patients.

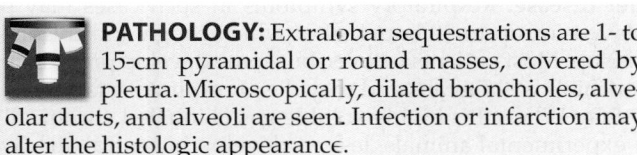 **PATHOLOGY:** Extralobar sequestrations are 1- to 15-cm pyramidal or round masses, covered by pleura. Microscopically, dilated bronchioles, alveolar ducts, and alveoli are seen. Infection or infarction may alter the histologic appearance.

CLINICAL FEATURES: In half of cases, extralobar sequestration is detected before 1 month of age, and is recognized by 2 years of age in 75% of patients. The condition is often associated with congenital cystic adenomatoid malformation. In the neonatal period, extralobar sequestration may cause dyspnea and cyanosis, often in the first day of life. In older children, recurrent bronchopulmonary infections may bring it to medical attention. Surgical excision is curative.

INTRALOBAR SEQUESTRATION: Intralobar sequestrations are masses of lung tissue located within the visceral pleura of the lung but isolated from the tracheobronchial tree and supplied by a systemic artery (Fig. 18-5). These are felt to be acquired abnormalities.

 PATHOLOGY: Intralobar sequestrations are almost always found in a lower lobe. Bilateral involvement is distinctly unusual. On gross examination, the sequestered tissue shows the result of chronic recurrent pneumonia, with end-stage fibrosis and honeycomb cystic changes. These cysts range up to 5 cm in diameter and lie in a dense fibrous stroma. Microscopically, the cystic spaces are lined mostly by cuboidal or columnar epithelium and the lumen contains foamy macrophages and eosinophilic material. Interstitial chronic inflammation and follicular lymphoid hyperplasia are often prominent. Acute and organizing pneumonia may be seen.

CLINICAL FEATURES: Cough, sputum production, and recurrent pneumonia are seen in almost all patients. Most cases are discovered in adolescents or young adults. Only one-fourth of patients are in the first decade of life, and the lesion is rarely identified in infants. Surgical resection is often indicated.

DISEASES OF THE BRONCHI AND BRONCHIOLES

Most bronchial and bronchiolar diseases are acute conditions and their sequelae. Chronic bronchitis is discussed later.

Airway Infections Are Caused by Diverse Organisms

Here, we distinguish between airway and parenchyma infections for convenience and for reasons of classification, but this division should not be thought of as rigid. Causative agents are discussed in Chapter 9.

Many infectious agents that involve the intrapulmonary airways tend to affect the peripheral airways **(bronchiolitis)**. Examples include adenovirus, respiratory syncytial virus (RSV), and measles. All are more serious in malnourished children and in populations not ordinarily exposed to these agents. Severe symptomatic infections occur more often in infants and children, and recovery is the rule. Symptoms include cough, a feeling of tightness in the chest and, in extreme cases, shortness of breath and even cyanosis.

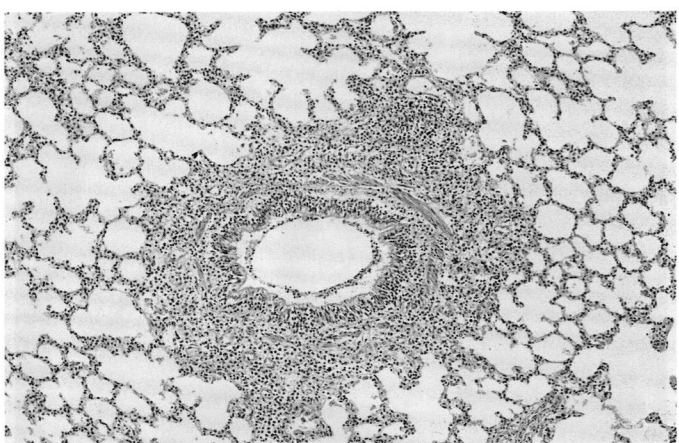

FIGURE 18-6. Bronchiolitis due to adenovirus. The wall of this bronchiole shows an intense chronic inflammatory infiltrate with local extension into the surrounding peribronchial tissue.

INFLUENZA: This is a characteristic example of tracheobronchitis, and in the occasional patient who dies with this infection, the appearance of the bronchi is dramatic. The surface of the airway is fiery red, reflecting acute inflammation and congestion of the mucosa.

ADENOVIRUS: Infection with adenovirus causes the most serious sequelae, with extensive bronchiolitis (Fig. 18-6) and then healing by fibrosis. Bronchioles may become obliterated or occluded by loose fibrous tissue (**constrictive bronchiolitis**).

RESPIRATORY SYNCYTIAL VIRUS (RSV): RSV infection often occurs in epidemics in nurseries. It is usually self-limited, but rare fatal cases do occur. It can cause nosocomial infection in children and (rarely) in adults. Histologically, peribronchiolar inflammation and disorganization of the epithelium are evident. Severe overdistention may be found without obvious bronchiolar obstruction, possibly due to displacement of surfactant from the bronchiolar surface.

MEASLES: At one time a major cause of bronchiolitis, measles is rarely a problem in developed countries since the advent of the measles vaccine. However, measles-induced bronchiolitis remains a serious problem particularly in populations seldom exposed to the virus. Similar to adenovirus, it may cause bronchiolar obliteration and bronchiectasis.

BORDETELLA PERTUSSIS: This bacterium commonly infects the airways and is the cause of whooping cough. With widespread use of a pertussis vaccine, the disease became rare in the United States. Unfortunately, vaccination is no longer compulsory in England, and the incidence of pertussis is rising. Clinically, whooping cough is typified by fever and prolonged severe bouts of coughing, followed by a characteristic deep whooping inspiration. Severe bronchial and bronchiolar inflammation are found in fatal cases. Before immunization was available, whooping cough commonly led to the development of bronchiectasis.

HAEMOPHILUS INFLUENZAE AND STREPTOCOCCUS PNEUMONIAE: In addition to causing pneumonia, these organisms have been implicated in exacerbations of chronic bronchitis. Such episodes contribute to the morbidity of chronic bronchitis and are treated with antibiotics.

CANDIDA ALBICANS: This fungus is a normal commensal organism in the oral cavity, gut, and vagina and is best known for causing infections in those regions. It may also affect the lungs, usually as a noninvasive growth on airway surface epithelium, where it may produce mucosal ulceration. Predisposing factors for invasive growth include trauma, burns, gastrointestinal surgery, indwelling catheters, and neutropenia, such as may be associated with cytotoxic chemotherapy for acute leukemia.

Respiratory Irritants Derive From Air Pollution and Industrial Accidents

The most important irritant gases in the atmosphere are oxidants (ozone, nitrogen oxides) and sulfur dioxide (SO_2). Oxidants derive from the action of sunlight on automobile exhaust and are important in major urban areas (see Chapter 8). SO_2 is produced mainly by burning carbon-based fossil fuels that contain sulfur. These gases, plus particulate carbon carrying toxins from diesel exhaust, may compound adverse effects of tobacco smoke. Indeed, inhabitants of urban areas and environments with greater air pollution have worse pulmonary function (e.g., reduced expiratory flow rates) than do those who reside in cleaner environments. Respiratory infections are also more common in young children who live in regions of high pollution. These effects are small in the healthy population, but in people with chronic pulmonary disease, the situation is different. For example, ozone makes airways more reactive, an effect related to airway inflammation. *Thus, air pollution can exacerbate symptoms in asthmatic people and in those with established respiratory disease. In high concentrations, irritant gases produce serious morphologic and functional effects.*

NO$_2$: NO_2 is often encountered in industrial settings, including welding, electroplating, metal cleaning, and blasting. It is also produced by decaying grain stored in silos. As NO_2 is heavier than air, it accumulates immediately above the surface of the grain. A worker entering the silo inhales it in high concentrations, resulting in lung injury known as **silo-filler disease.** Respiratory symptoms in such cases may be delayed for up to 30 hours, after which cough and dyspnea develop. Most patients recover, but some develop progressive bronchiolitis obliterans and may die of respiratory failure.

SO$_2$: When this highly soluble gas is inhaled chronically by experimental animals, lesions develop in central airways that resemble chronic bronchitis and may progress to squamous metaplasia. In humans, exposure to high concentrations of SO_2 has been associated with severe inflammation and bronchiolitis.

CHLORINE AND AMMONIA: These gases may be released in high concentrations in industrial accidents. If inhaled, they cause extensive bronchial and bronchiolar mucosal injury. Secondary inflammation may lead to bronchiectasis, owing partly to bronchiolar obliteration and partly to direct bronchial damage.

Bronchocentric Granulomatosis Is Usually a Response to Infection

Bronchocentric granulomatosis is a nonspecific granulomatous inflammation centered on bronchi or bronchioles (Fig. 18-7). *This histologic pattern can be seen in a number of clinical settings and is not a distinct clinical entity.*

Asthmatic patients, for the most part, have allergic bronchopulmonary aspergillosis (see below). In addition to having bronchocentric granulomatosis, they have bronchial mucus plugs, bronchiectasis and bronchiolectasis, and

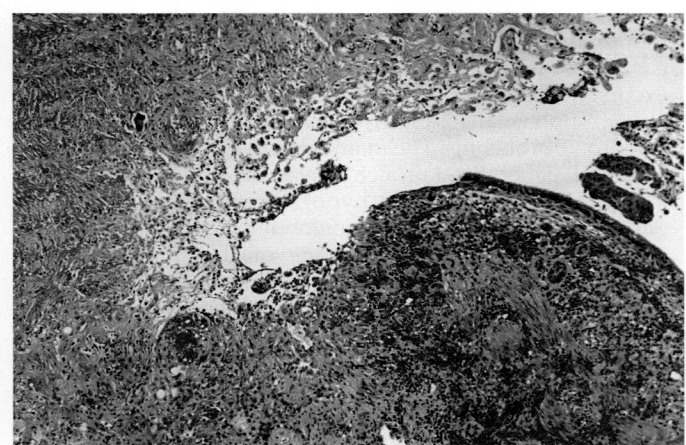

FIGURE 18-7. Bronchocentric granulomatosis. This bronchiole shows ulceration and necrosis of the mucosa and submucosa with granulomatous inflammation. The patient had granulomatosis with polyangiitis (formerly Wegener granulomatosis) with lung involvement in the pattern of bronchocentric granulomatosis.

eosinophilic pneumonia. Irregular, fragmented *Aspergillus* hyphae may be seen in the mucus plugs. A nonspecific secondary vasculitis is centered on airways rather than vessels.

Nonasthmatic patients with bronchocentric granulomatosis are likely to have an infection, especially tuberculosis or fungi such as *Histoplasma capsulatum*. The disorder can also be a manifestation of immune problems, such as rheumatoid arthritis, ankylosing spondylitis, and granulomatosis with polyangiitis (formerly Wegener granulomatosis). Patients with bronchocentric granulomatosis of either allergic or nonallergic type generally respond well to corticosteroid therapy.

Constrictive Bronchiolitis May Obliterate Bronchioles

In constrictive bronchiolitis, an initial inflammatory bronchiolitis is followed by bronchiolar scarring and fibrosis, with progressive narrowing and, eventually, complete destruction of the airway lumen (Fig. 18-8). **Obliterative bronchiolitis** is a synonym.

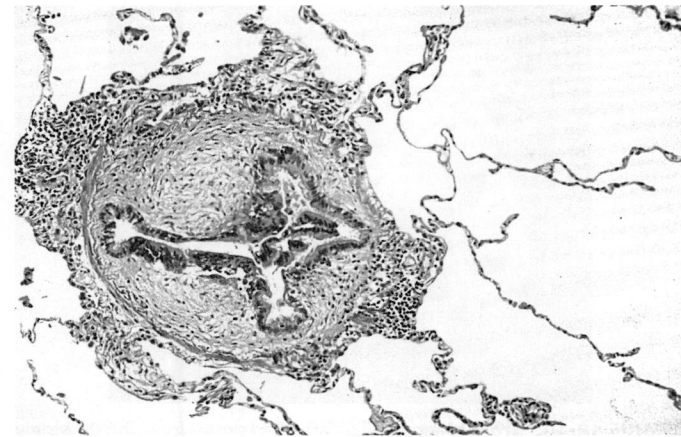

FIGURE 18-8. Constrictive bronchiolitis. The lumen of a bronchiole is markedly narrowed, owing to marked submucosal fibrosis.

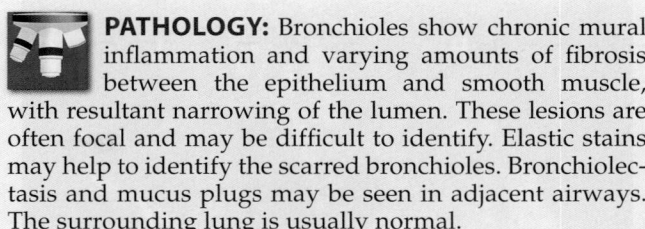

PATHOLOGY: Bronchioles show chronic mural inflammation and varying amounts of fibrosis between the epithelium and smooth muscle, with resultant narrowing of the lumen. These lesions are often focal and may be difficult to identify. Elastic stains may help to identify the scarred bronchioles. Bronchiolectasis and mucus plugs may be seen in adjacent airways. The surrounding lung is usually normal.

CLINICAL FEATURES: Patients may have dyspnea and wheezing due to severe obstructive pulmonary function. Chest radiographs and computed tomography (CT) scans may be normal or show overinflation caused by air trapping distal to the obliterated bronchioles. Constrictive bronchiolitis may be idiopathic; however, this pattern of fibrosis is seen in several situations, including (1) bone marrow transplantation (graft-versus-host disease), (2) lung transplantation (chronic rejection), (3) collagen vascular diseases (especially rheumatoid arthritis), (4) postinfectious disorders (especially viral infections), (5) after inhalation of toxins (SO_2, ammonia, phosgene), and (6) ingestion of certain drugs (penicillamine). Additionally, constrictive bronchiolitis has been associated with exposure to diacetyl and 2,3-pentanedione which are used as flavoring substances. This has been most widely reported in workers involved in the manufacture of butter flavoring in microwave popcorn. These substances are found in other flavoring compounds, including those used in electronic cigarettes raising concerns about exposures in e-cigarette users. Most patients have a relentless progressive clinical course. Although many patients are treated with steroids, no therapy is effective for this disease.

Bronchial Obstruction Leads to Atelectasis

Bronchial obstruction in adults occurs mostly because of endobronchial extension of primary lung tumors. Mucus plugs, aspirated gastric contents, or foreign bodies may also be responsible, especially in children. If obstruction is partial, trapped air may cause overdistention of the distal affected segment; complete obstruction results in atelectasis. Areas distal to the obstruction may develop pneumonia, abscesses, and bronchiectasis (see below).

Atelectasis is the collapse of expanded lung tissue (Fig. 18-9). If the air supply is obstructed, gas transfers from alveoli to the blood, causing the affected region to collapse. Atelectasis is an important postoperative complication of abdominal surgery, because of mucus obstruction of a bronchus and/or diminished respiratory movement resulting from postoperative pain. It is often asymptomatic, but when severe, it can cause hypoxemia and a shift of the mediastinum *toward* the affected side.

Atelectasis is usually caused by bronchial obstruction but may also result from direct compression of the lung (e.g., hydrothorax or pneumothorax). If the compression is severe enough, the function of the affected lung may be jeopardized and the mediastinum may shift *away* from the affected side.

In long-standing atelectasis, the area of collapsed lung becomes fibrotic and bronchi dilate, in part owing to infection distal to the obstruction. Permanent bronchial dilation (bronchiectasis) results.

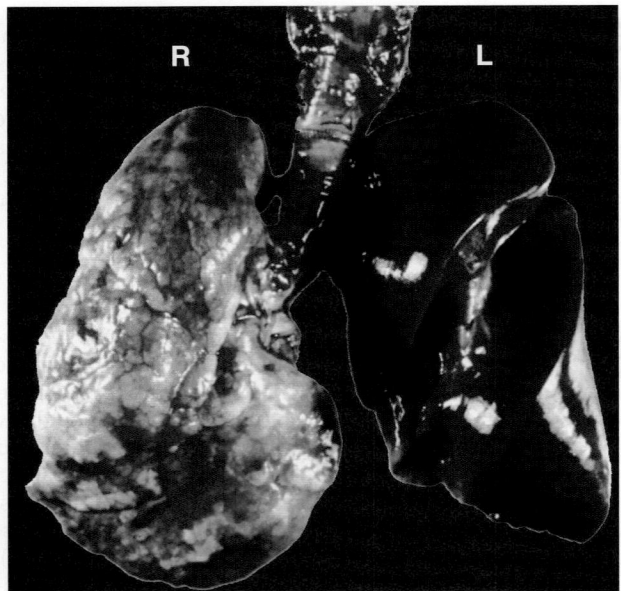

FIGURE 18-9. Atelectasis. The right lung (**R**) of an infant is pale and expanded by air; the left lung (**L**) is collapsed (i.e., atelectatic).

Right middle lobe syndrome refers to atelectasis due to obstruction of the bronchus to the right middle lobe, usually from external compression by hilar lymph nodes. This bronchus is particularly susceptible to external compression because it is long and slender and surrounded by lymph nodes. Histologically, the lung shows bronchiectasis, chronic bronchitis and bronchiolitis, lymphoid hyperplasia, abscess formation, and dense fibrosis. Acute and organizing pneumonia may both be present. Tuberculous lymphadenitis or metastatic lung cancer may cause the lymph node enlargement, but the cause of the obstruction is often undetermined.

Bronchiectasis Is Irreversible Bronchial Dilation Caused by Destruction of Bronchial Wall Muscle and Elastic Elements

ETIOLOGIC FACTORS: Bronchiectasis may be obstructive or nonobstructive.

Obstructive bronchiectasis is localized and occurs distal to a mechanical obstruction of a central bronchus by, for example, tumors, inhaled foreign bodies, mucus plugs in asthma, or lymph node enlargement. **Nonobstructive bronchiectasis** usually follows respiratory infections or defects in airway defenses from infection. It may be localized or generalized.

Localized nonobstructive bronchiectasis was once common, usually after childhood bronchopulmonary infections with measles, pertussis, or other bacteria. Vaccines and antibiotics have reduced the incidence of bronchiectasis, but most cases still follow bronchopulmonary infection, usually with adenovirus or RSV. Childhood respiratory infections continue to cause bronchiectasis in less developed parts of the world.

Generalized bronchiectasis is, for the most part, secondary to inherited impairment in host defense mechanisms or acquired conditions that permit introduction of infectious organisms into the airways. Acquired disorders

that predispose to bronchiectasis include (1) neurologic diseases that impair consciousness, swallowing, respiratory excursions, and the cough reflex; (2) incompetence of the lower esophageal sphincter; (3) nasogastric intubation; and (4) chronic bronchitis. The main **inherited conditions** associated with generalized bronchiectasis are cystic fibrosis, dyskinetic ciliary syndromes, hypogammaglobulinemia, and deficiencies of specific immunoglobulin (Ig) G subclasses.

Kartagener syndrome is one of the immotile cilia syndromes (ciliary dyskinesia). It consists of the triad of dextrocardia (with or without situs inversus), bronchiectasis, and sinusitis. It is caused by defects in the outer or inner dynein arms of cilia, which generate or regulate cilia beats, respectively. Other dyskinetic ciliary syndromes include **radial spoke deficiency** ("Sturgess syndrome") and absence of the central doublet of cilia. In these diseases, cilia are deficient throughout the body. Both men and women are sterile, because of impaired ciliary mobility in the vas deferens and the fallopian tube. In the respiratory tract, ciliary defects lead to repeated upper and lower respiratory tract infections and, thus, to bronchiectasis.

Immunodeficiencies may also predispose to repeated pulmonary infection and bronchiectasis. In hypogammaglobulinemia, lack of IgAs or IgGs that protect against viruses or bacteria can lead to recurrent lung infections. Acquired and inherited defects of neutrophils also increase the risk of respiratory infections and bronchiectasis.

PATHOLOGY: Bronchial dilation may be described as saccular, varicose, or cylindrical depending on the level of bronchial branch involved (Fig. 18-10). This designation is not as critical as the severity and extent of disease.

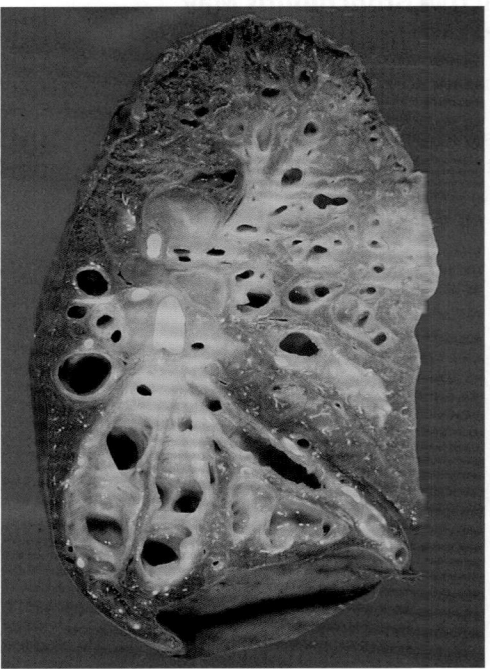

FIGURE 18-10. Bronchiectasis. The resected upper lobe shows widely dilated bronchi, with thickening of the bronchial walls and collapse and fibrosis of the pulmonary parenchyma.

Generalized bronchiectasis is usually bilateral and is most common in the lower lobes, the left more than the right. Localized bronchiectasis may occur wherever there was prior obstruction or infection. Bronchi are dilated, with thick, white or yellow walls. Bronchial lumens often contain dense, mucopurulent secretions. Severe inflammation of bronchi and bronchioles results in destruction of all components of the bronchial wall. Collapse of distal lung parenchyma causes damaged bronchi to dilate. Inflammation of central airways leads to mucus hypersecretion and abnormalities of the surface epithelium, including squamous metaplasia and increased goblet cells. Lymphoid follicles are often seen in bronchial walls, and distal bronchi and bronchioles are scarred and often obliterated. Bronchial arteries enlarge to supply the inflamed bronchial wall and fibrous tissue. A vicious cycle may be established in which pools of mucous become infected, which further promotes destruction of the bronchial walls.

 CLINICAL FEATURES: Patients with bronchiectasis have chronic cough, often producing several hundred milliliters of mucopurulent sputum a day. Hemoptysis is common, as bronchial inflammation erodes the walls of adjacent bronchial arteries. Dyspnea and wheezing are variable, depending on the extent of the disease. Pneumonia is common, and patients with long-standing cases are at risk of chronic hypoxia and pulmonary hypertension. Radiographically, the bronchi appear dilated and have thickened walls. Definitive diagnosis is made by CT scan of the lung. Surgical resection of localized bronchiectasis may be necessary, especially if complications such as severe hemoptysis or pneumonia arise. However, in the generalized disease, surgical resection is more palliative than curative.

Acute, reversible bronchial dilation may follow bacterial or viral respiratory infections, but it may take months before the bronchi return to normal size.

INFECTIONS

Pulmonary infections are discussed in detail in Chapter 9. The major pulmonary entities are described below, with particular emphasis on pathologic features.

Bacterial Pneumonia Is Inflammation and Consolidation of Lung Parenchyma

Bacterial pneumonia has historically been divided into lobar pneumonia or bronchopneumonia, but these terms have little clinical relevance today. In **lobar pneumonia,** an entire lobe is consolidated (Fig. 18-11), whereas **bronchopneumonia** refers to scattered solid foci in the same or several lobes, generally surrounding an airway (Fig. 18-12).

ETIOLOGIC FACTORS: *Streptococcus pneumoniae* (pneumococcus) was the classic cause of lobar pneumonia, but with antibiotic therapy, involvement of a lobe tends to be incomplete, and more than one lobe is usually affected. By contrast, bronchopneumonia is still a common cause of death. It typically develops in terminally ill patients, usually in dependent and posterior

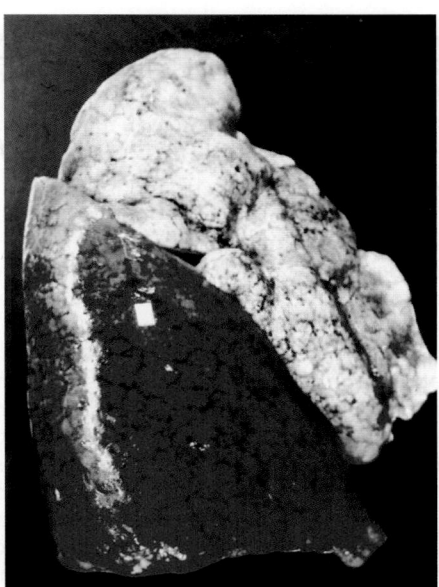
FIGURE 18-11. Lobar pneumonia. The entire left lower lobe is consolidated and in the stage of red hepatization. The upper lobe is normally expanded.

portions of the lung. Scattered irregular foci of pneumonia are centered on terminal bronchioles and respiratory bronchioles. Bronchiolitis is seen, with polymorphonuclear exudates in adjacent alveoli. Large contiguous areas of alveolar involvement do not occur in bronchopneumonia.

Bacterial pneumonias occur in three settings:

- **Community-acquired pneumonia** arises outside the hospital in people with no primary disorder of the immune system. The term is also used loosely to denote lobar pneumonia.

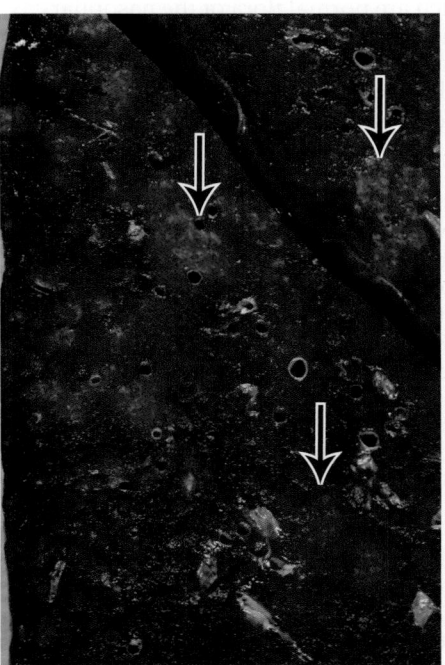
FIGURE 18-12. Bronchopneumonia. Scattered foci of consolidation (*arrows*) are centered on bronchi and bronchioles.

- **Nosocomial pneumonia** is infection that develops in hospital environments. It tends to affect compromised patients.
- **Opportunistic pneumonia** afflicts people whose immune status is defective.

Bacterial pneumonias are best classified by etiologic agent, as clinical and morphologic features, and thus therapies, often vary with the causative organism.

Most bacteria that cause pneumonia are normal inhabitants of the oropharynx and nasopharynx that reach alveoli by aspiration of secretions. Other routes of infection include inhalation from the environment, hematogenous dissemination from an infectious focus elsewhere, and (rarely) spread of bacteria from an adjacent site. Emergence of a virulent organism in the oropharyngeal flora often precedes the development of pneumonia. Predisposing conditions usually entail depressed host defenses related to cigarette smoking, chronic bronchitis, alcoholism, severe malnutrition, wasting diseases, and poorly controlled diabetes. Debilitated or immunosuppressed patients in the hospital often have altered oropharyngeal flora, and as many as 25% may develop nosocomial pneumonia.

Pneumococcal Pneumonia

Antibiotic therapy notwithstanding, *S. pneumoniae* (pneumococcus) pneumonia remains a significant problem. It is mainly a disease of young to middle-aged adults. It is rare in infants, less common in the elderly, and much more frequent in men than women.

ETIOLOGIC FACTORS: Pneumococcal pneumonia is mostly a result of altered respiratory tract defenses. For example, an upper respiratory viral infection (e.g., influenza) stimulates bronchial secretions. These provide a hospitable environment for *S. pneumoniae,* which are normal flora of the nasopharynx, to proliferate. The thin, watery secretions carry the organisms into the alveoli, thus initiating an inflammatory response. The remarkably severe acute inflammation with spreading edema reflects a vigorous immune response. Aspiration of pneumococci may also follow impaired epiglottic reflexes, as occurs with exposure to cold, anesthesia, and alcohol intoxication. Lung injury caused, for example, by congestive heart failure or irritant gases also increases susceptibility to pneumococcal pneumonia.

The pneumococcal capsule protects the bacteria against phagocytosis by alveolar macrophages. The organisms must therefore be opsonized before they can be ingested and killed. In an immune-competent person, antipneumococcal antibodies act as opsonins, but a host not previously exposed to the specific infecting strain of *S. pneumoniae* must use the alternative complement pathway to opsonize the bacteria.

PATHOLOGY: In the earliest stage of pneumococcal pneumonia, protein-rich edema fluid with abundant organisms fills the alveoli (Fig. 18-13). Marked capillary congestion leads to massive outpouring of polymorphonuclear leukocytes and intra-alveolar hemorrhage (Fig. 18-14). Because the color and firm consistency of the affected lung are reminiscent of the liver, this stage has been aptly named **"red hepatization"** (Fig. 18-13).

The next phase, 2 or more days later (depending on the success of treatment), involves lysis of neutrophils and appearance of macrophages, which phagocytose the fragmented leukocytes and other inflammatory debris. At this stage, congestion has diminished, but the lung is still firm (**"gray hepatization"**) (Fig. 18-13). The alveolar exudate is then removed and the lung gradually returns to normal.

A number of complications can follow pneumococcal pneumonia:

- **Pleuritis (inflammation of the pleura)**, often painful, is common, because the pneumonia readily extends to the pleura.
- **Pleural effusion (fluid in the pleural space)** is also common but usually resolves.
- Empyema/**pyothorax (pus in the pleural space)** results from infection of a pleural effusion and may heal with extensive fibrosis.
- **Bacteremia** occurs during the early stages of pneumococcal pneumonia in more than 25% of patients and may lead to endocarditis or meningitis. Patients whose spleens have been removed often die of this bacteremia.
- **Pulmonary fibrosis** is a rare complication of pneumococcal pneumonia. The intra-alveolar exudate organizes to form intra-alveolar plugs of granulation tissue, known as **organizing pneumonia.** Gradually, increasing alveolar fibrosis leads to a shrunken and firm lobe, a rare complication known as **carnification.**
- **Lung abscess (localized collection of pus)** is an unusual complication of pneumococcal pneumonia.

CLINICAL FEATURES: Pneumococcal pneumonia begins abruptly, with fever and chills. Chest pain due to pleural involvement is common. Sputum is characteristically "rusty," because it is derived from altered blood in alveolar spaces. Radiographic studies show alveolar filling in large areas of lung, producing a solid appearance that extends to entire lobes or segments. Before antibiotic therapy, severe fever, dyspnea, debility, and even loss of consciousness were common. Such symptoms were followed by **"crisis"** after 5 to 10 days, when a moribund patient would suddenly become afebrile and return from death's door. Satisfactory resolution of a crisis reflected effective immune responses to the infection. Nevertheless, about one-third of patients died. Current treatment for pneumococcal pneumonia is effective, and although symptoms resolve rapidly, radiographic lesions still take several days to clear.

Klebsiella Pneumonia

Other than *S. pneumoniae, Klebsiella pneumoniae* is the only organism that causes lobar pneumonia with any frequency. However, *K. pneumoniae* accounts for only about 1% of community-acquired pneumonias. *K. pneumonia* occurs mostly in middle-aged, often alcoholic, men. Diabetes and chronic lung disease also increase the risk.

PATHOLOGY: The pathologic stages of *Klebsiella* pneumonia are not as distinctly defined as those in pneumococcal pneumonia, but acute phase

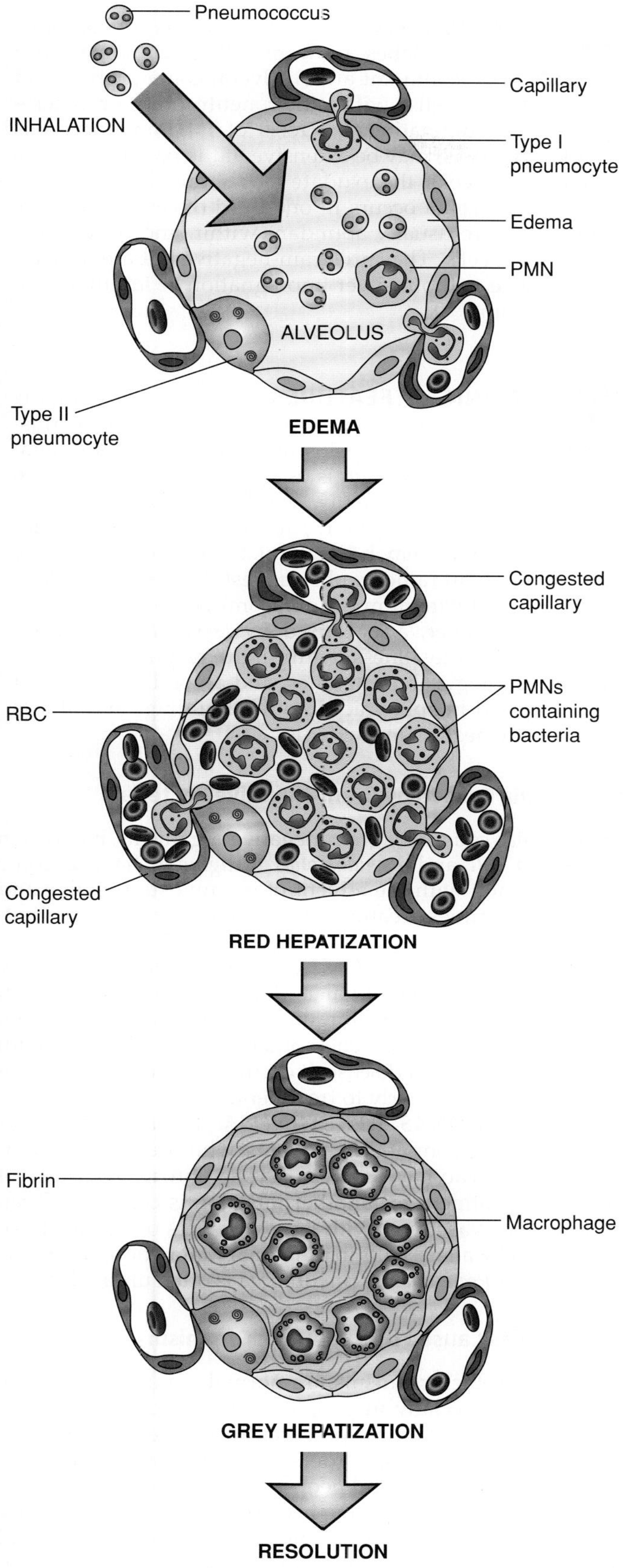

Pneumococcus

INHALATION

Capillary

Type I
pneumocyte

Edema

PMN

ALVEOLUS

Type II
pneumocyte

EDEMA

Congested
capillary

PMNs
containing
bacteria

RBC

Congested
capillary

RED HEPATIZATION

Fibrin

Macrophage

GREY HEPATIZATION

RESOLUTION

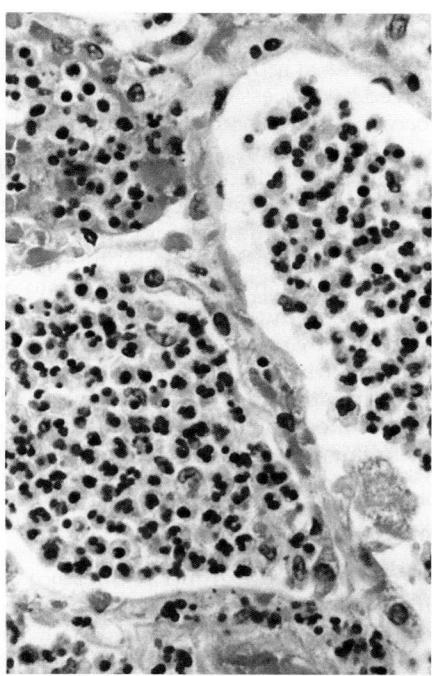

FIGURE 18-14. Pneumococcal pneumonia. Alveoli are packed with an exudate composed of polymorphonuclear leukocytes and occasional macrophages.

congestion and hemorrhage are less pronounced. *K. pneumoniae* has a thick, gelatinous capsule, giving the cut lung surface a characteristic mucoid appearance. Another distinctive feature of *Klebsiella* pneumonia is increased size of the affected lobe, causing the fissure to "bulge" toward the unaffected region. There is a tendency toward tissue necrosis and abscess formation. A serious complication is **bronchopleural fistula** (i.e., a communication between the bronchial airway and the pleural space).

The onset of *Klebsiella* pneumonia is less dramatic than that of pneumococcal pneumonia, but the disease may be more dangerous. Before antibiotics, mortality from *Klebsiella* pneumonia was 50% to 80%. Even with prompt antibiotic treatment, mortality remains considerable.

Staphylococcal Pneumonia

Staphylococci account for only 1% of community-acquired bacterial pneumonias. However, *Staphylococcus aureus* is a common pulmonary superinfection after influenza and other viral respiratory tract infections. Repeated episodes of staphylococcal pneumonia are seen in patients with cystic fibrosis, owing to colonization of bronchiectatic airways. Nosocomial staphylococcal pneumonia typically occurs in chronically ill people who are prone to aspiration and in intubated patients.

FIGURE 18-13. Pathogenesis of pneumococcal lobar pneumonia. Pneumococci, characteristically in pairs (diplococci), multiply rapidly in alveolar spaces and induce extensive edema. They also incite an acute inflammatory response in which polymorphonuclear leukocytes and congestion are prominent (red hepatization). As the inflammatory process progresses, macrophages replace the polymorphonuclear leukocytes and ingest debris (gray hepatization). The process usually resolves, but complications may ensue. *PMN* = polymorphonuclear neutrophil; *RBC* = red blood cell.

PATHOLOGY: Like staphylococcal infections elsewhere, staphylococcal pneumonia is characterized by abscess development. Multiple foci of staphylococcal pneumonia produce many small abscesses. In infants and, less often, in adults, these may lead to **pneumatoceles**, thin-walled cystic spaces lined primarily by respiratory tissue. Pneumatoceles may enlarge rapidly and compress surrounding lung or rupture into the pleural cavity and cause a tension pneumothorax. A pneumatocele develops when an abscess breaks into an airway, allowing drainage of purulent material and expansion of the former abscess by the pressure of inspired air. Cavitation and pleural effusions are common complications of staphylococcal pneumonia, but empyema is infrequent. Staphylococcal pneumonia requires aggressive therapy, particularly because *S. aureus* is often antibiotic resistant.

Other Streptococcal Pneumonias

Pulmonary infections with group A *Streptococcus pyogenes* were identified among soldiers during the 19th century. Its features were described during World War I. Streptococcal pneumonia typically follows viral respiratory tract infections. It is distinctly unusual in a community setting but is occasionally encountered in debilitated patients.

PATHOLOGY: On gross examination, the lungs of patients who die of streptococcal pneumonia are heavy, with bloody edema. Dry consolidation (hepatization) is not a feature of this disease. Microscopically, alveoli are filled with fibrin-containing fluid, but neutrophils are few. Alveolar necrosis may follow prolonged pneumonia. Empyema is a common complication.

CLINICAL FEATURES: Patients with streptococcal pneumonia have abrupt fever, dyspnea, cough, chest pain, hemoptysis, and often cyanosis. Radiographically, a bronchopneumonia pattern is observed; lobar consolidation is not seen. Intensive antibiotic therapy is indicated.

Streptococcal pneumonia in the newborn is usually caused by group B streptococci (*Streptococcus agalactiae*), a normal resident of the female genital tract. Symptoms are similar to those of the infantile respiratory distress syndrome. The infants, however, are often full term, have severe toxemia, and may die within a few hours.

Legionella Pneumonia

In 1976, a mysterious respiratory disease with high mortality broke out at an American Legion convention in Philadelphia. The responsible organism, *Legionella pneumophila*, is a fastidious bacterium that is difficult to grow in culture. Serologic and histologic studies showed that several previously unrecognized epidemics of the same disease had occurred. *Legionella* organisms thrive in aquatic environments, and outbreaks of pneumonia have been traced to contaminated water in air-conditioning cooling towers, evaporative condensers, and construction sites. Person-to-person spread does not occur, and there is no animal or human reservoir.

PATHOLOGY: In fatal *Legionella* pneumonia, multiple lobes show bronchopneumonia, with large confluent areas. Alveoli contain fibrin and inflammatory cells, with either neutrophils or macrophages predominating. Necrosis of inflammatory cells (leukocytoclasis) may be extensive. If the patient survives for several weeks, the exudate may show fibrous organization. Empyema occurs in one-third of cases. *Legionella* organisms are usually abundant within and outside the phagocytic cells. They are gram-negative but are difficult to visualize without silver impregnation or immunofluorescent stains.

CLINICAL FEATURES: *Legionella* pneumonia tends to begin abruptly, with malaise, fever, muscle aches and pains and, curiously, abdominal pain. A productive cough is usual, and chest pain due to pleuritis occurs occasionally. The chest radiograph is variable, but the most common pattern shows focal alveolar infiltrates, which may be bilateral. Symptoms are usually less severe than radiographs suggest. Mortality is 10% to 20%, especially in immunocompromised patients.

Pontiac fever, also caused by *Legionella* species, is mainly a febrile illness with slight respiratory symptoms, radiologic abnormalities, and a good prognosis. It has occurred in epidemics in office buildings and affects apparently healthy individuals.

Pneumonia Caused by Gram-Negative Bacteria

Pneumonias caused by gram-negative organisms, most often *Escherichia coli* and *Pseudomonas aeruginosa,* have become more common with the advent of immunosuppressive and cytotoxic therapies, treatment with broad-spectrum antibiotics and AIDS.

ESCHERICHIA COLI: E. coli pneumonia may follow bacteremia after abdominal and urogenital surgery, even in patients who are not immunosuppressed. It also is seen in cancer patients given chemotherapy and in people with chronic lung or heart disease. It occurs as a bronchopneumonia and responds poorly to treatment.

PSEUDOMONAS AERUGINOSA: Pseudomonas pneumonia is most common in patients who are immunocompromised or who have burns or cystic fibrosis. A history of antibiotic treatment for another infection is common. Often an infectious vasculitis, with large numbers of organisms in blood vessel walls, results in pulmonary infarction. Antibiotic treatment of *Pseudomonas* pneumonia is often unsatisfactory.

Pneumonias Caused by Anaerobic Organisms

Many anaerobic organisms are normal commensals of the oral cavity, especially in people with poor dental hygiene. These include certain streptococci, fusobacteria, and *Bacteroides* sp. Swallowing disorders, as in stuporous alcoholics, anesthetized patients, and people subject to seizures, predispose to aspirating anaerobic bacteria. Resulting pulmonary infections cause necrotizing pneumonias, which often lead to lung abscesses. The most dramatic complication is gangrene of the lung, a result of thrombosis of a branch of the pulmonary artery and consequent infarction. This is a medical emergency and requires resection of the affected lung.

Psittacosis

Psittacosis is a lung infection due to inhalation of *Chlamydia psittaci* in dust contaminated with excreta from birds, usually pets and often parrots. It is characterized by severe systemic symptoms, with fever, malaise, and muscle aches, but surprisingly few respiratory symptoms other than cough. Chest radiographs may be negative, and when abnormal, they show irregular consolidation and an interstitial pattern. The morphologic patterns in most cases are unknown, but the disease is likely to be an interstitial pneumonia. In fatal cases, varying degrees of diffuse alveolar damage (DAD) (a pattern of injury described in more detail in a later section) are present, together with edema, intra-alveolar pneumonia, and necrosis.

Anthrax Pneumonia and Pneumonic Plague

Recent world events have focused attention on infectious agents that could be used as weapons of bioterrorism. Chief among these are *Bacillus anthracis* and *Yersinia pestis.*

B. anthracis, a gram-positive, spore-forming bacillus, is the causative agent of anthrax. Anthrax occurs in many species of domestic animals, but human infection occurs rarely, or in sporadic outbreaks. Transmission is via direct contact with the spores; person-to-person transmission is uncommon. Cutaneous anthrax is rarely fatal, but inhalational anthrax has a high mortality. Anthrax spores are extremely resistant to drying. When inhaled, they are transported to mediastinal lymph nodes where bacilli emerge and disseminate rapidly through the bloodstream to other organs, including the lungs. Hemorrhagic necrosis of infected organs ensues along with severe hemorrhagic mediastinitis related to local lymphadenopathy. In the lungs, the disease is manifested by hemorrhagic bronchitis and confluent areas of hemorrhagic pneumonia.

Y. pestis, the causative agent of **plague**, produces two main forms of infection, a bubonic form and a pneumonic form. In pneumonic plague, the organisms are inhaled directly without an intermediary arthropod vector, and disease may be spread from person to person. The lungs typically show extensive hemorrhagic bronchopneumonia, pleuritis, and mediastinal lymph node enlargement. Untreated disease progresses rapidly and is highly fatal.

Mycoplasma Pneumoniae Causes "Atypical Pneumonia"

Unlike lobar pneumonia, atypical pneumonia begins insidiously. Leukocytosis is absent or slight and the course is prolonged. Respiratory symptoms may be minimal or severe, and chest radiographs shows patchy intra-alveolar pneumonia or interstitial infiltrates. Infection characteristically causes a bronchiolitis with a neutrophilic intraluminal exudate and intense lymphoplasmacytic infiltration in bronchiolar walls (Fig. 18-15). *Mycoplasma* lack rigid cell walls that most bacteria possess. They grow slowly and are difficult to culture by traditional methods. Diagnosis is usually established by serologic detection of *Mycoplasma pneumoniae* antibodies or cold agglutinins. Erythromycin is effective, and the infection is only rarely fatal.

Tuberculosis Is the Classic Granulomatous Infection

Known since ancient Egypt, tuberculosis was the scourge of the industrialized world in the 19th and early 20th centuries. It declined quickly as living and working conditions improved

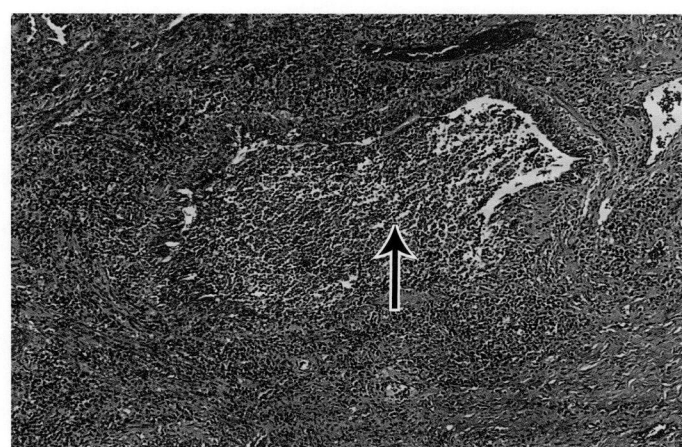

FIGURE 18-15. Mycoplasma pneumonia. The lung shows chronic bronchiolitis with a neutrophilic luminal exudate (*arrow*).

during the 20th century, and the introduction of antituberculosis drugs further decreased its impact. However, tuberculosis has recently reemerged, particularly drug-resistant strains and among patients with AIDS (see Chapter 9).

Tuberculosis mostly represents infection with *Mycobacterium tuberculosis,* although atypical mycobacterial infections may cause similar manifestations. The disease is divided into primary and secondary (or reactivation) tuberculosis.

PRIMARY TUBERCULOSIS: The disease is acquired after initial exposure to *M. tuberculosis,* most commonly from inhaling infected aerosols generated when a person with cavitary tuberculosis coughs. Inhaled organisms multiply in the alveoli because alveolar macrophages cannot readily kill them.

PATHOLOGY: The **Ghon lesion** is the first lesion of primary tuberculosis and consists of a peripheral parenchymal granuloma, often in the upper lobes. When this lesion is associated with an enlarged mediastinal lymph node, a **Ghon complex** is formed (Fig. 18-16). On gross examination, the healed, subpleural Ghon nodule is 1 to 2 cm in diameter, well circumscribed and centrally necrotic. In later stages, it is fibrotic and calcified. Microscopically, a granuloma with central caseous necrosis (Fig. 18-17) shows varying degrees of fibrosis. The microscopic features of draining hilar lymph nodes are similar to those of the peripheral parenchymal lesion.

Most (>90%) primary tuberculous infections are asymptomatic; lesions remain localized and heal. Sometimes there is self-limited extension to the pleura, with secondary pleural effusion. Less often, primary tuberculosis is not limited but spreads to other parts of the lung (**progressive primary tuberculosis**). This usually occurs in young children or immunosuppressed adults. In this situation, the initial lesion enlarges, producing necrotic areas up to 6 cm. Central liquefaction results in cavities, which may expand to occupy most of the lower lobe. At the same time, draining lymph nodes display similar histologic changes. Erosion of a bronchus by the necrotizing process leads to further pulmonary dissemination of the disease.

SECONDARY TUBERCULOSIS: This stage represents reactivation of primary pulmonary tuberculosis or new infection in someone previously sensitized by primary tuberculosis.

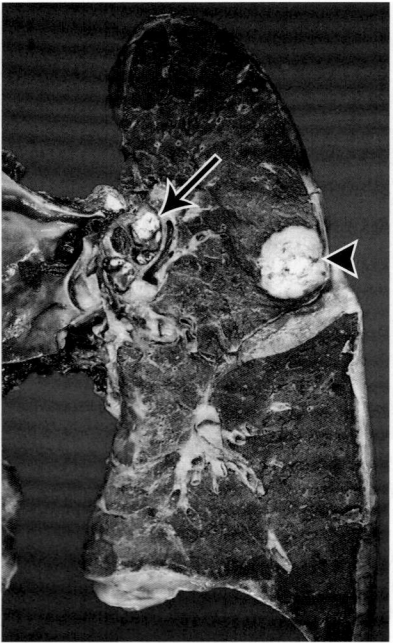

FIGURE 18-16. Primary tuberculosis. A healed Ghon complex is comprised of a subpleural nodule (*arrowhead*) and an involved draining hilar lymph nodes (*arrow*).

PATHOLOGY: The initial reaction to *M. tuberculosis* is different in secondary tuberculosis. A cellular immune response occurs after a latent interval and leads to formation of many granulomas and extensive tissue necrosis. Apical and posterior segments

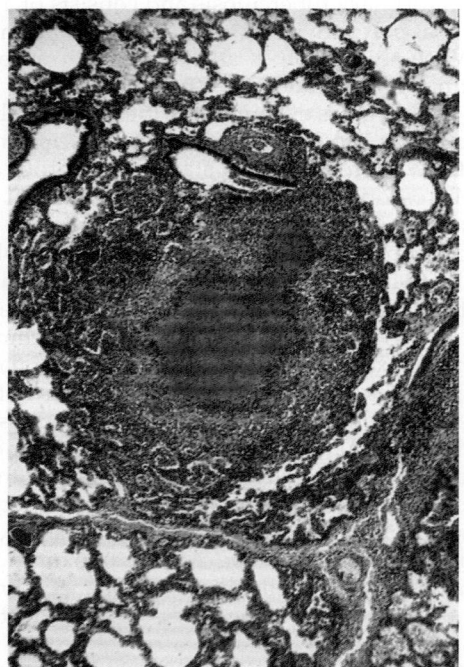

FIGURE 18-17. Necrotizing granuloma due to *Mycobacterium tuberculosis*. A small tuberculous granuloma with conspicuous central caseation is present in the pulmonary parenchyma. The necrotic center is surrounded by histiocytes, giant cells, and fibrous tissue.

of the upper lobes are most commonly involved, but the superior segment of the lower lobe is also often affected, and no part of the lung can be excluded. A diffuse, fibrotic, poorly defined lesion develops, with focal areas of caseous necrosis. Often these foci heal and calcify, but some may erode into bronchi, after which drainage of infectious material creates a tuberculous cavity.

Tuberculous cavities range from under 1 cm to large, cystic areas occupying almost the entire lung. Most measure 3 to 10 cm. They prefer the apices of the upper lobes (Fig. 18-18) but may occur anywhere in the lung. The cavity wall is composed of an inner, thin, gray membrane encompassing soft necrotic nodules; a middle zone of granulation tissue; and an outer collagenous border. The lumen is filled with caseous material containing acid-fast bacilli. Cavities often communicate with a bronchus, and the release of infectious material into airways spreads infection within the lung. The walls of healed tuberculous cavities eventually become fibrotic and calcified.

Secondary tuberculosis is associated with a number of complications:

- **Miliary tuberculosis** is the presence of multiple, small (size of millet seeds), tuberculous granulomas (Fig. 18-19) in many organs. The organisms disseminate from the lung or other sites via the blood, usually during secondary tuberculosis, but occasionally in primary disease.
- **Hemoptysis** is caused by erosion into small pulmonary arteries adjacent to the cavity wall. It may be severe enough to drown patients in their own blood.
- **Bronchopleural fistula** occurs when a subpleural cavity ruptures into the pleural space. In turn, tuberculous empyema and pneumothorax result.
- **Tuberculous laryngitis** is a consequence of coughing up infectious material.
- **Intestinal tuberculosis** may follow swallowing of the same tuberculous material.
- **Aspergilloma** is a fungal mass arising by superinfection of a persistent open cavity with *Aspergillus*; fungi may fill the entire cavity.

MYCOBACTERIUM AVIUM-INTRACELLULARE (MAI): In immunodeficient patients, whose ability to mount a granulomatous reaction may be impaired, MAI

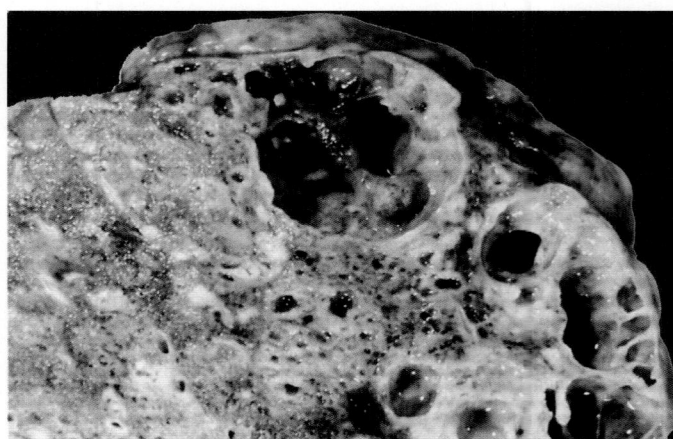

FIGURE 18-18. Cavitary tuberculosis. The apex of the left upper lobe shows tuberculous cavities surrounded by consolidated and fibrotic pulmonary parenchyma that contains small tubercles.

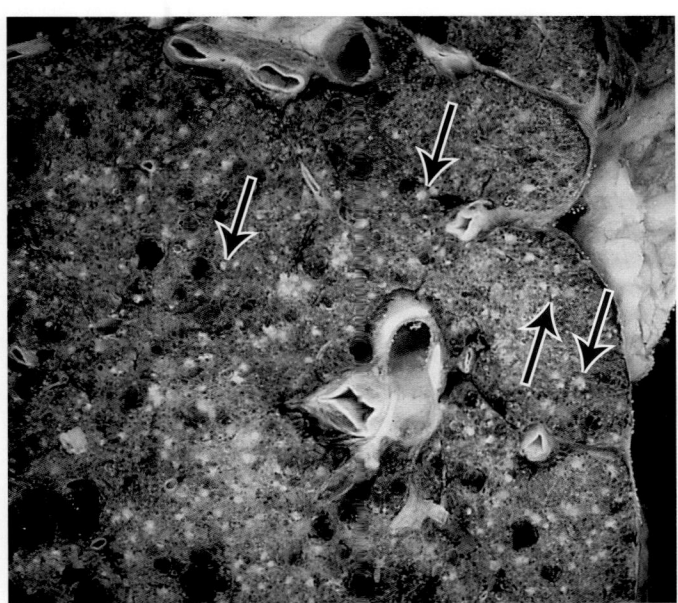

lung by aspiration of oropharyngeal contents or by extension from an actinomycotic subdiaphragmatic abscess or liver abscess.

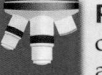 **PATHOLOGY:** Lung lesions of actinomycosis consist of multiple, interconnecting, small lung abscesses. The abscess margins are granulomatous, but central necrotic areas are purulent and contain colonies of thin, branching, filamentous, gram-positive bacteria. Clubbed basophilic filaments, noted at the colony margins, are visible to the naked eye as small yellow particles (**"sulfur granules"**). The abscesses may extend to the pleura and produce bronchopulmonary fistulas and empyema. They may also invade the chest wall.

Nocardia Is Usually an Opportunistic Organism

Nocardia is a gram-positive filamentous bacterium that causes an acute progressive or chronic bacterial pneumonia. Infection is mostly seen in immunocompromised patients, particularly those with lymphomas, neutropenia, chronic granulomatous disease of childhood, and pulmonary alveolar proteinosis. *Nocardia asteroides* is the most common *Nocardia* sp. to cause pneumonia.

 PATHOLOGY: Histologically, lungs show abscesses (Fig. 18-21A), which may have granulomatous features in chronic infections. The organisms are delicate, beaded, thin filaments, which branch mostly at right angles (Fig. 18-21B). They are best seen with Gram or Gomori methenamine silver stains (Fig. 18-21B). They are also weakly acid fast.

Fungal Infections May Be Geographic or Opportunistic

Histoplasmosis

Histoplasmosis is a disease of the midwestern and southeastern United States, particularly the Mississippi and Ohio river valleys. It is caused by inhalation of *H. capsulatum* in infected dust, commonly from bird droppings.

FIGURE 18-19. Miliary tuberculosis. Multiple millimeter-sized nodules (*arrows*) are scattered throughout the lung parenchyma.

pneumonia is characterized by an extensive infiltrate of macrophages and innumerable acid-fast organisms (Fig. 18-20). MAI may colonize airways of older, immunocompetent individuals with underlying pulmonary disorders such as bronchiectasis, or it may produce granulomatous inflammation with or without cavitation. *Mycobacterium kansasii* produces a spectrum of disease similar to that of MAI but is not as frequently encountered, owing to a more restricted geographic distribution.

Actinomycosis Features Multiple Lung Abscesses

Actinomycosis is caused by infection with actinomycetes, and the usual pulmonary organism is *Actinomyces israelii*. Although actinomycetes resemble fungi in appearance, they are anaerobic, gram-positive, filamentous bacteria. They normally inhabit the mouth and nose and infect the

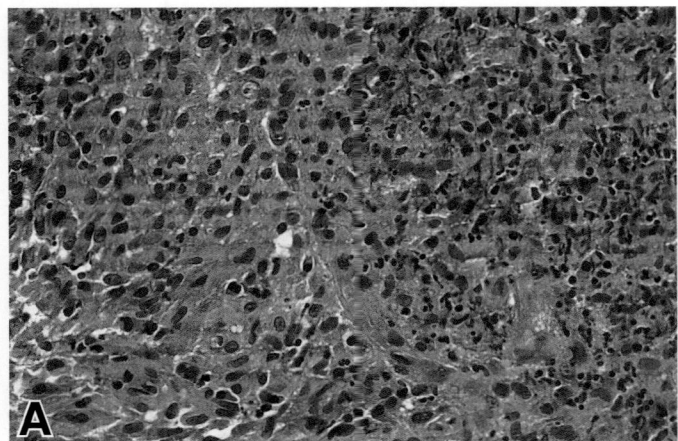
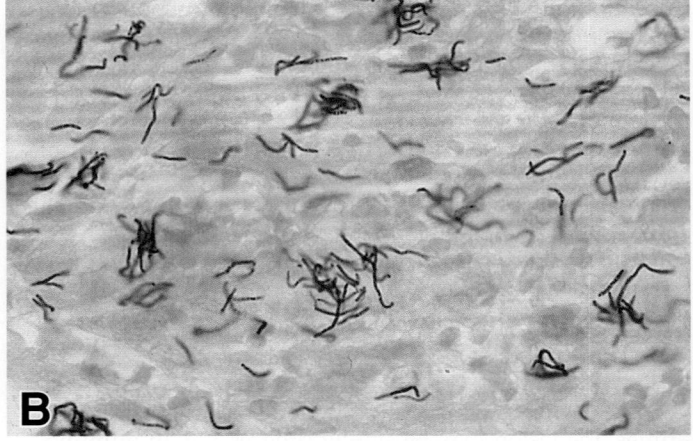

FIGURE 18-20. *Mycobacterium avium-intracellulare* pneumonia in AIDS. **A.** The pneumonia is characterized by an extensive infiltrate of macrophages. **B.** The Ziehl–Neelsen stain shows numerous acid-fast organisms.

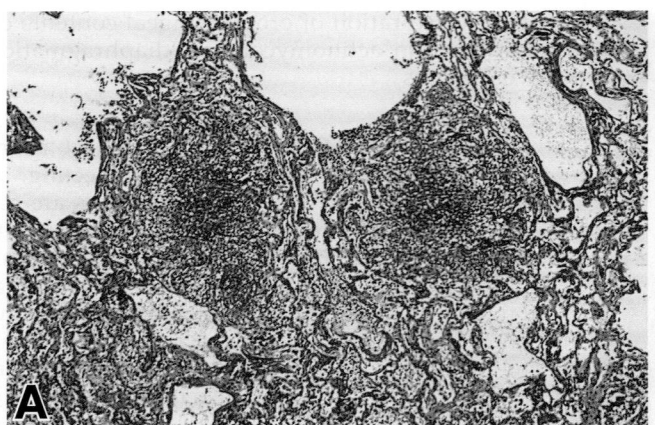
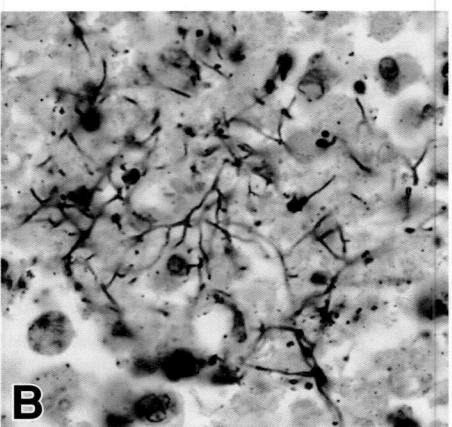

FIGURE 18-21. Nocardiosis. A. This lung contains abscesses consisting of focal collections of acute inflammation. **B.** The organisms are thin, filamentous, branching bacteria (Gomori methenamine silver stain).

PATHOLOGY: Histoplasmosis resembles tuberculosis clinically and pathologically. Most infections are asymptomatic and result in lesions like Ghon complexes, including a parenchymal granuloma and similar lesions in the draining lymph nodes. The granulomas are particularly prone to calcify, often with a concentric laminar pattern. In the acute phase, numerous organisms are seen within macrophages. Granulomatous inflammation follows, often with central areas of necrosis. The granulomas heal by fibrosis and calcification, but central necrotic areas may persist. The spherical organisms are best seen with a silver stain as 2 to 4 μm in diameter with narrow-based budding.

In a few cases, pulmonary lesions progress or reactivate, leading to a progressive fibrotic and necrotic lesion that closely resembles that of reactivation tuberculosis. However, histoplasmosis lesions are more fibrotic than those of tuberculosis, and cavitation is less common. The reason for progression is not known, although large infective doses and poor host responses are usually considered to be responsible. Immunocompromised patients are at particular risk for dissemination of *Histoplasma* within the lungs and spread to other organs.

Coccidioidomycosis

Coccidioidomycosis, caused by inhalation of spores of *Coccidioides immitis,* was originally known as San Joaquin Valley fever, after the location where the disease has been endemic for many years. However, the infection is widespread throughout the southwestern part of the United States and shares many of the clinical and pathologic features of histoplasmosis and tuberculosis. In histologic sections, the organism is a spherule, 30 to 100 μm, with a thick refractile wall. Spherules contain many 2- to 5-μm endospores. Empty spherules or endospores that have been released into the tissue may also be visible.

PATHOLOGY: In most instances, lesions are limited to a peripheral parenchymal granuloma, with or without lymph node granulomas. Sometimes, the lesion may be slowly progressive. In immunocompromised hosts, the disease may progress rapidly, with release of endospores into the lung, in which case the tissue reaction may be purulent as well as granulomatous.

Cryptococcosis

Cryptococcosis results from the inhalation of spores of *Cryptococcus neoformans*, which are often found in pigeon droppings. Lung lesions range from small parenchymal granulomas to several large granulomatous nodules, pneumonic consolidation, and even cavitation. Most serious cases of pulmonary cryptococcosis occur in immunocompromised patients, in whom the organisms proliferate extensively within alveolar spaces, with little tissue reaction. The organisms are 4 to 6 μm, but may be larger, with narrow-based budding and a thick mucoid capsule.

North American Blastomycosis

Blastomycosis is an uncommon condition caused by *Blastomyces dermatitidis*. It is concentrated in the Missouri, Mississippi, and Ohio river basins in the United States, and in southern Manitoba and northwestern Ontario in Canada. Clinical and pathologic features resemble those of the fungi mentioned above. Initial infection produces a lesion resembling a Ghon complex or progressive pneumonitis. Unlike tuberculous Ghon complexes, the focal lesions of blastomycosis show central necrosis with a purulent reaction, surrounded by granulomatous inflammation. The organisms are 8 to 15 μm, have a thick refractile wall, and exhibit broad-based budding.

Aspergillosis

Lung infections by *Aspergillus* spp., usually *Aspergillus niger* or *Aspergillus fumigatus,* may occur as:

- **Invasive aspergillosis:** This is the most serious form of *Aspergillus* infection, occurring almost exclusively as an opportunistic infection in people with compromised immunity, usually due to cytotoxic therapy or AIDS. The lungs show patchy, multifocal consolidation and, occasionally, cavities. Extensive blood vessel invasion (usually arterial [Fig. 18-22]) causes occlusion, thrombosis, and infarction of lung tissue. Invasive aspergillosis is a fulminant pulmonary infection that is not amenable to therapy.

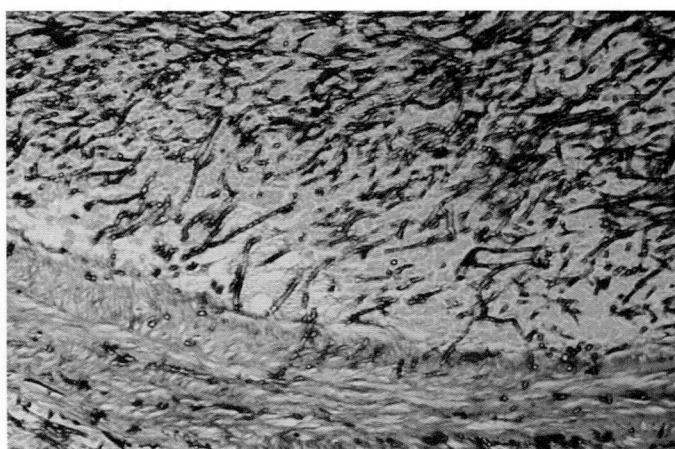

FIGURE 18-22. Invasive pulmonary aspergillosis. A branch of the pulmonary artery shows fungal hyphae (*dark filamentous structures*) in the wall and within the lumen (Gomori methenamine silver stain).

■ **Aspergilloma ("fungus ball" or mycetoma):** *Aspergillus* spp. may grow in preexisting cavities, such as those caused by tuberculosis or bronchiectasis, where they proliferate to form fungus balls (Fig. 18-23). Radiographs show a large mass within an air-filled cavity. Fungus balls are usually clinically silent and merely represent incidental radiographic findings. However, if they become clinically evident, they most often cause hemoptysis, arising either from the underlying condition or, less commonly, fungal infection of the cavity wall.

■ **Allergic bronchopulmonary aspergillosis (ABPA):** Some asthmatics have an unusual immunologic reaction to *Aspergillus* characterized by (1) transient pulmonary infiltrates on chest radiographs, (2) eosinophilia of blood and sputum, (3) skin sensitivity and serum precipitins to *A. fumigatus* antigens, and (4) increased serum IgE. CT scans shows thickened bronchial walls and mucus plugs in bronchi.

> **PATHOLOGY:** ABPA is invariably associated with proximal (central) bronchiectasis, involving segmental bronchi and the next 2 to 4 orders of subsegmental bronchi. Bronchial and bronchiolar mucus

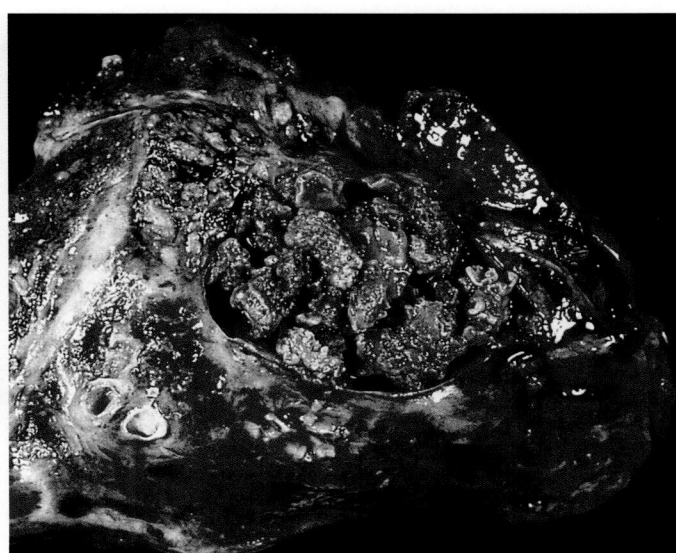

FIGURE 18-23. *Aspergillus* **fungus ball.** The lung contains a cavity filled with a fungus ball.

plugs, eosinophilic infiltrates, and Charcot-Leyden crystals are all seen (Fig. 18-24A,B). Bronchocentric granulomatosis and eosinophilic pneumonia may also be present. Bronchial mucous may contain septate, fungal hyphae, with 45-degree branching. Interestingly, the peripheral bronchial tree is spared.

> **CLINICAL FEATURES:** Patients with ABPA wheeze, with chest pain and cough, and often have thick mucus plugs. Systemic corticosteroids usually control acute episodes.

Pneumocystis jiroveci

First described as "plasma cell pneumonia" in malnourished infants at the end of World War II, pulmonary infections with *Pneumocystis jiroveci* (formerly *Pneumocystis carinii*) most often cause pneumonia in immunosuppressed patients or those with immunodeficiencies such as HIV/AIDS. Patients

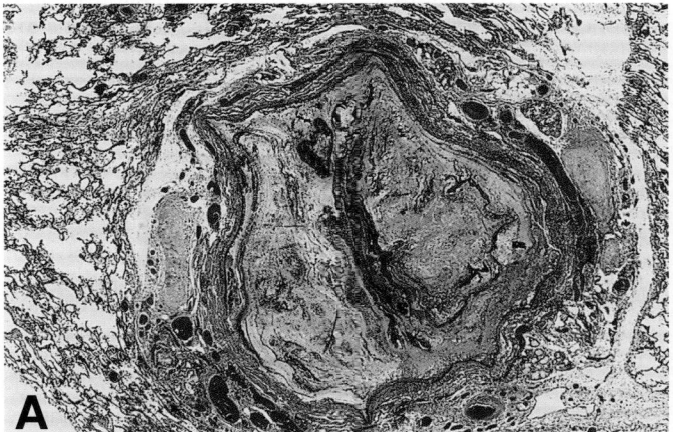
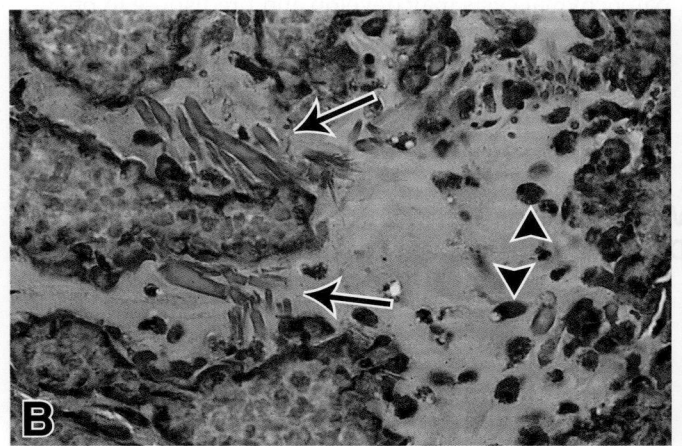

FIGURE 18-24. Allergic bronchopulmonary aspergillosis. A. A dilated bronchus is filled with a mucus plug that has dense layers of eosinophilic infiltrates. **B.** Higher magnification shows numerous eosinophils (*arrowheads*) and Charcot-Leyden crystals (*arrows*).

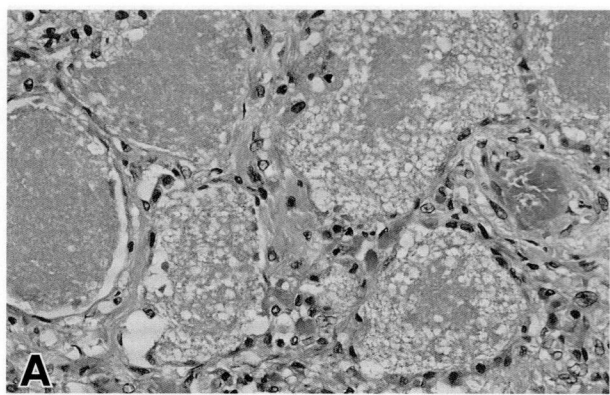
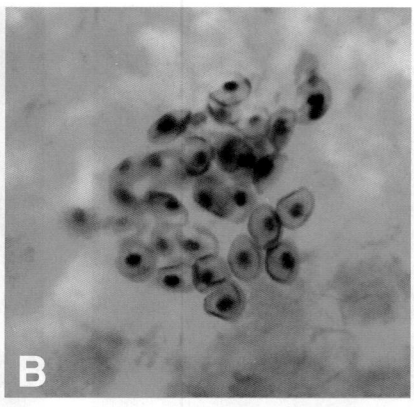

FIGURE 18-25. *Pneumocystis jiroveci* pneumonia. A. Alveoli are filled with a foamy exudate, and the interstitium is thickened and contains a chronic inflammatory infiltrate. **B.** A centrifuged bronchoalveolar lavage specimen impregnated with silver shows a cluster of *Pneumocystis* cysts.

receiving immunosuppressive drugs after organ transplantation or chemotherapy for malignant disease are particularly at risk. Once considered a protozoan, *Pneumocystis* is now recognized as a fungus.

PATHOLOGY: The classic lesions of *Pneumocystis* pneumonia are interstitial infiltrates of plasma cells and lymphocytes and hyperplasia of type II pneumocytes. Alveoli are filled with a characteristic foamy exudate, in which the organisms appear as small bubbles in a background of proteinaceous exudate (Fig. 18-25A). With silver impregnation, cysts appear as round or indented ("crescent moon") bodies, 5 μm in diameter (Fig. 18-25B). After sporozoites develop within the cyst, it ruptures and assumes an indented shape. Sporozoites develop into trophozoites, which may be seen with stains such as Giemsa in cytology specimens but are difficult to see in routine histologic sections. Granulomatous inflammation in *Pneumocystis* pneumonia is rare but occurs in up to 5% of lung biopsies from HIV-infected patients. In some cases, *Pneumocystis* also produces DAD (see below).

CLINICAL FEATURES: Clinically and radiographically, *Pneumocystis* pneumonia presents a variable picture. At one extreme, symptoms may be minimal, while at the other, there is rapidly progressive respiratory failure. In AIDS patients, thin-walled parenchymal cysts may develop and predispose to pneumothorax. The diagnosis is made by identifying the organism by sputum examination, bronchoalveolar lavage, transbronchial biopsy, needle aspiration of the lung, or open lung biopsy. Treatment is with trimethoprim–sulfamethoxazole or pentamidine.

Viral Pneumonitides Cause Diffuse Alveolar Damage or Interstitial Pneumonia

PATHOLOGY: Viral infections initially affect the alveolar epithelium and elicit interstitial mononuclear infiltrates (Fig. 18-26). Hyaline membranes and necrosis of type I epithelial cells lead to an appearance indistinguishable from DAD from other causes. Sometimes, alveolar damage is indolent, and disease is characterized by type II pneumocyte hyperplasia

and chronic interstitial inflammation. This is unlike most bacterial infections, in which intra-alveolar neutrophilic exudates predominate and the interstitium is only incidentally involved (Fig. 18-27).

Cytomegalovirus (CMV) pneumonia entails intense interstitial lymphocytic infiltration. Alveoli are lined by type II cells that have regenerated to cover the epithelial defect left by necrosis of type I cells. The infected alveolar cells are very large (cytomegaly) with a single, dark, basophilic nuclear inclusion with a peripheral halo and multiple, indistinct cytoplasmic, basophilic inclusions (Fig. 18-28).

Measles infection involves both the airways and the parenchyma. It is characterized by large (100 μm across) multinucleated giant cells with nuclear inclusions and large eosinophilic cytoplasmic inclusions (Fig. 18-29). Interstitial pneumonia, a well-characterized complication of measles, is rarely fatal, except in immunocompromised, previously unexposed individuals.

Varicella infection (chickenpox and herpes zoster) produces disseminated, focally necrotic lung lesions and interstitial pneumonia. Pulmonary involvement is usually asymptomatic, except in immunocompromised hosts, in whom it may be fatal. The viral inclusions are nuclear, eosinophilic, and refractile and are surrounded by a clear halo. Multinucleation can occur.

Herpes simplex can cause a necrotizing tracheobronchitis as well as DAD. Viral inclusions are identical to those seen in varicella infection.

Adenovirus causes necrotizing bronchiolitis and bronchopneumonia. Two types of nuclear inclusions are seen: eosinophilic nuclear inclusions surrounded by a clear halo and "smudge cells," with indistinct, basophilic, nuclear inclusions that fill the entire nucleus and are surrounded by only a thin rim of chromatin (Fig. 18-30).

Influenza virus typically produces interstitial pneumonitis and bronchiolitis similar to those seen in other viral pneumonias. It does not produce characteristic viral cytopathic changes in histologic sections. A recent pandemic of H1N1 influenza drew attention to the pathology of influenza pneumonia. Most cases of H1N1 infection are fortunately mild and self-limited. But in some patients, mainly those with underlying health problems, fatal disease may occur. Pathologies vary from interstitial pneumonia and bronchiolitis to DAD. In some cases, extensive hemorrhage is present. With most strains of influenza, bacterial superinfection is not uncommon.

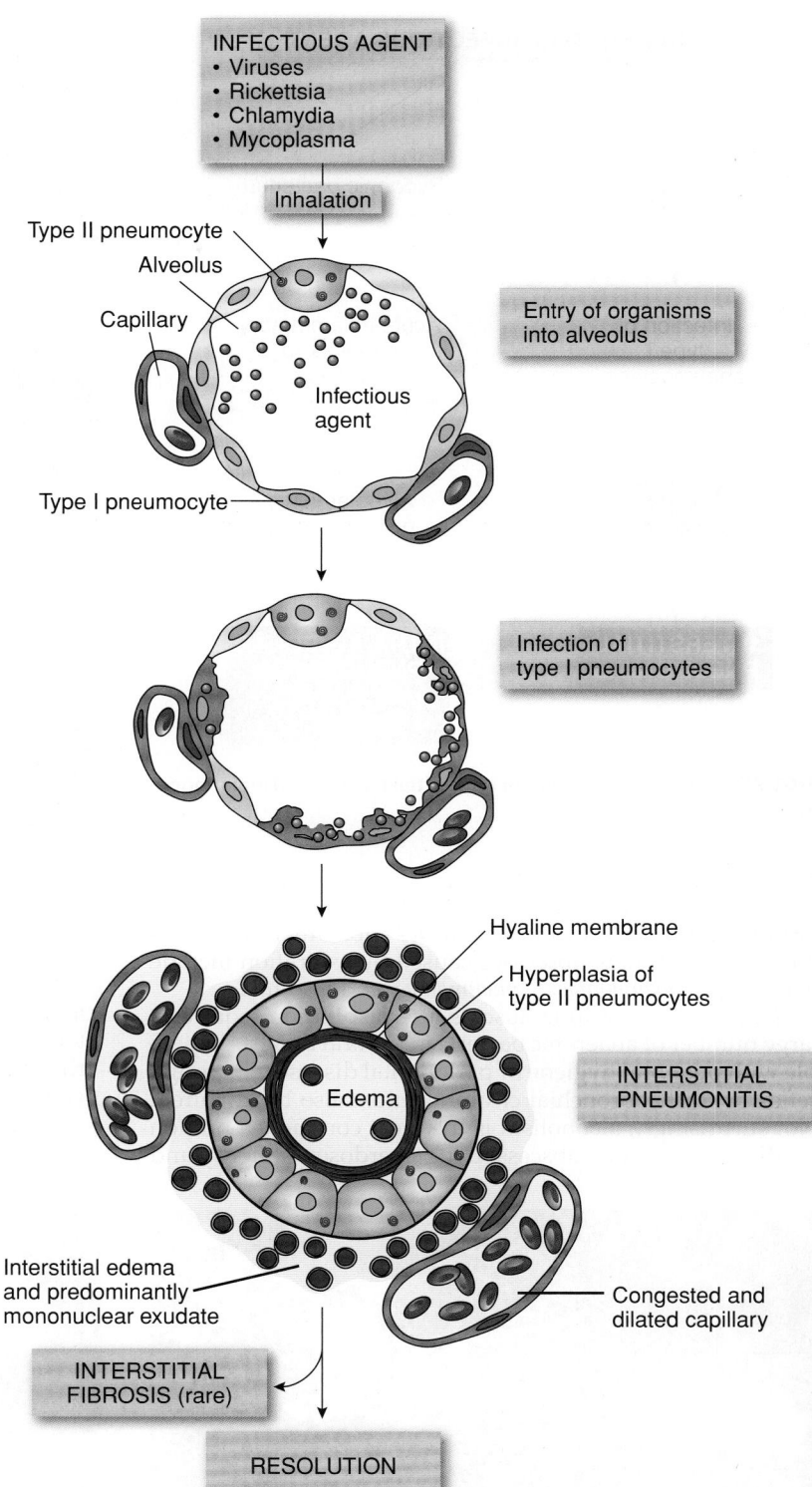

FIGURE 18-26. Pathogenesis of interstitial pneumonia. Although interstitial pneumonia is usually caused by viruses, other organisms also may cause significant interstitial inflammation. Type I cells are the most sensitive to damage. Once infected, injured type I cells degenerate, which leads to intra-alveolar edema. The proteinaceous exudate and cell debris form hyaline membranes, and type II cells multiply to line the alveoli. Interstitial inflammation is characterized mainly by mononuclear cells. The disease usually resolves completely but occasionally progresses to interstitial fibrosis.

Coronavirus family members, *Coronaviridae*, have been responsible for outbreaks of severe acute respiratory syndrome (SARS), primarily in China and Southeast Asia and Middle East Respiratory Syndrome (MERS), primarily in the Arabian Peninsula. Pathology is primarily DAD lacking characteristic viral cytopathic changes.

The Most Common Cause of Lung Abscess Is Aspiration

Lung abscesses are localized accumulations of pus, with destruction of pulmonary parenchyma, including alveoli, airways, and blood vessels.

States of depressed consciousness often predispose to the aspiration that causes lung abscesses, and aspirated

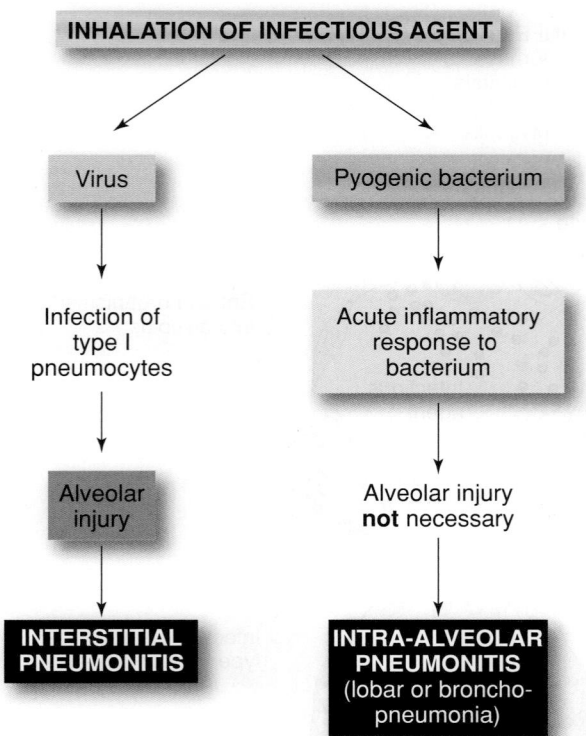

FIGURE 18-27. Pathogenesis of interstitial and intra-alveolar pneumonitis.

oropharyngeal anaerobic bacteria are responsible in over 90% of cases. Infections are typically polymicrobial, often with fusiform bacteria and *Bacteroides* spp. Other organisms encountered in lung abscesses caused by aspiration include *S. aureus, K. pneumoniae, S. pneumoniae,* and *Nocardia.*

Development of lung abscess after aspiration requires a large number of anaerobic bacteria in the oral flora, as in people with poor oral hygiene or periodontal disease. The cough reflex or tracheobronchial clearance must also be impaired. Not surprisingly, alcoholism is the most common condition predisposing to lung abscess. Drug overdoses, epilepsy and

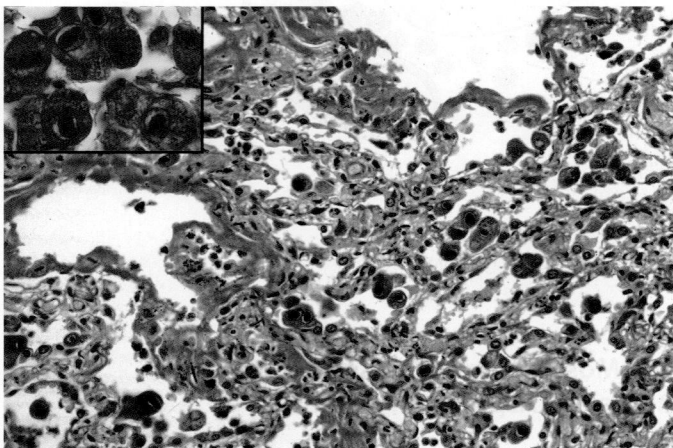

FIGURE 18-28. Cytomegalovirus pneumonitis. Infected alveolar cells are enlarged. A higher-power view shows infected alveolar cells that display a single basophilic nuclear inclusion with a perinuclear halo and multiple, indistinct, basophilic, cytoplasmic inclusions (*inset*).

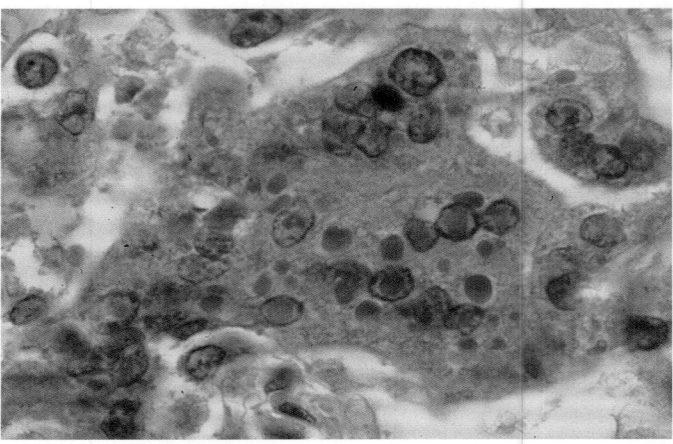

FIGURE 18-29. Measles pneumonitis. This multinucleated giant cell shows single, refractile, eosinophilic inclusions within each of the nuclei, as well as multiple, irregular, eosinophilic, cytoplasmic inclusions.

neurologic impairment also increase the risk. Other causes of lung abscess include necrotizing pneumonias, bronchial obstruction, infected pulmonary emboli, penetrating trauma, and extension of infection from adjacent tissues.

PATHOLOGY: Lung abscesses typically range from 2 to 6 cm in diameter; 10% to 20% have multiple cavities, usually arising after a necrotizing pneumonia or a shower of septic pulmonary emboli. The right side of the lung is more often involved than the left, because the right main bronchus follows the direction of the trachea more closely at its bifurcation. Acute lung abscesses are not distinctly separated from the surrounding lung parenchyma. They contain abundant polymorphonuclear leukocytes and, depending on the age of the lesion, variable numbers of macrophages and necrotic tissue debris. Initially, they are surrounded by hemorrhage, fibrin, and inflammation, but as they age, a fibrous wall forms around the margin. Lung abscesses differ from

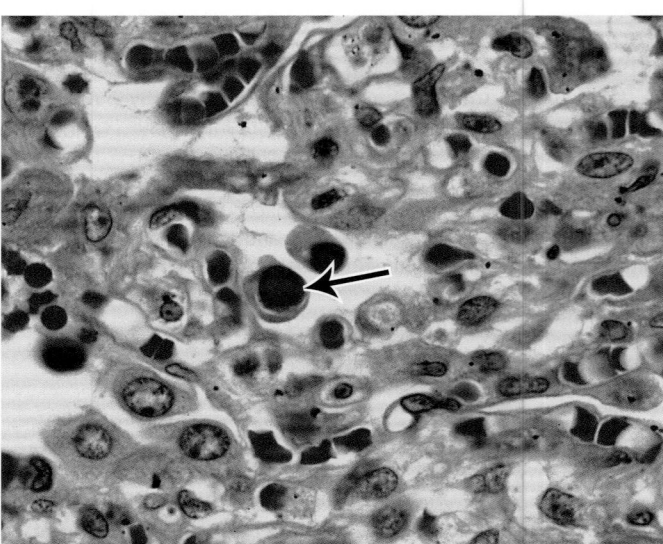

FIGURE 18-30. Adenovirus pneumonia. The "smudge" cell in the center (*arrow*) contains a smudgy basophilic nuclear inclusion.

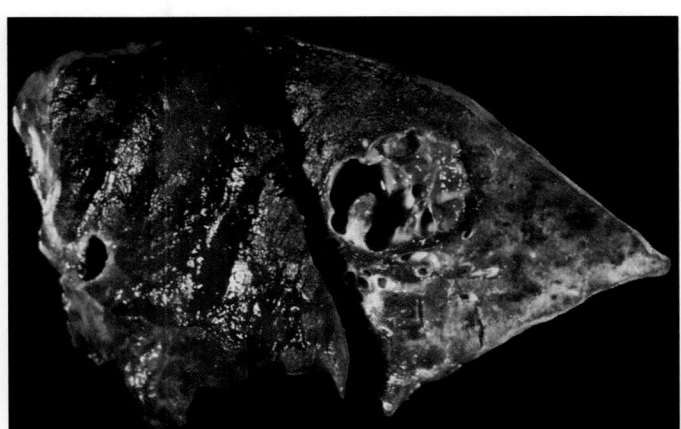

FIGURE 18-31. Pulmonary abscess. A large cystic abscess contains purulent exudate and is lined by a fibrous wall. Pneumonia is present in the surrounding pulmonary parenchyma.

abscesses elsewhere in that they may drain spontaneously into an airway. The cavity thus formed contains air, necrotic debris, and inflammatory exudate (Fig. 18-31), creating an air-fluid level that is easily seen radiographically. The cavity lining eventually becomes covered with regenerating squamous epithelium. Walls of old abscesses may be lined by ciliated respiratory epithelium, making them difficult to distinguish from bronchiectasis.

CLINICAL FEATURES: Almost all patients with lung abscess present with fever and cough, characteristically producing large amounts of foul-smelling sputum. Many patients complain of pleuritic chest pain, and 20% develop hemoptysis.

The differential diagnosis of lung abscess includes lung cancer and cavitary tuberculosis. Indeed, cancer is a more common cause of cavitation than lung abscess. Cavitation due to cancer arises from tumor necrosis half the time, with the other half following bronchial obstruction with subsequent infection. Tuberculous cavities only rarely show the air-fluid levels characteristic of lung abscesses.

Complications of lung abscess include rupture into the pleural space, which causes empyema, and severe hemoptysis. Abscess drainage into a bronchus may spread infection to other parts of the lung. Despite vigorous antimicrobial therapy, principally directed against anaerobic bacteria, the mortality of lung abscess remains 5% to 10%.

DIFFUSE ALVEOLAR DAMAGE

DAD is a pattern of reaction of alveolar epithelial and endothelial cells to a variety of acute insults (Table 18-1). The clinical expression of severe DAD is **acute respiratory distress syndrome** (ARDS). In ARDS, apparently normal lungs sustain damage that progresses rapidly to respiratory failure. Lung compliance is impaired (usually requiring mechanical ventilation), with hypoxemia and extensive bilateral radiographic opacities ("white-out"). ARDS mortality exceeds 50%, and in patients over 60, it is as high as 90%.

 ETIOLOGIC FACTORS: DAD is a final common pathologic pathway triggered by a large variety of insults (Table 18-1), including infections, sepsis, shock, aspiration of gastric contents, inhalation of toxic gases, near-drowning, radiation pneumonitis, and many drugs and other chemicals. The common pathogenic link is acute alveolar epithelial and endothelial cell injury, thus producing DAD. *Unless a specific infectious agent is identified, the trigger for DAD is not evident from the lung histology alone.* In some patients, no cause is found. Such idiopathic DAD, referred to clinically as **acute interstitial pneumonia** (AIP), also includes cases historically called **Hamman–Rich disease (see below).**

MOLECULAR PATHOGENESIS: Endothelial cell injury allows protein-rich fluid to leak from alveolar capillaries into the interstitial space (Fig. 18-32). Loss of type I pneumocytes permits fluid to enter alveolar spaces, where plasma proteins form fibrin-containing precipitates (hyaline membranes) on the injured alveolar walls (Fig. 18-33). In response to cell injury in DAD, inflammatory cells accumulate in the interstitium. Although lacking type I pneumocytes, alveolar basement membranes remain intact and act as scaffolds for type II pneumocytes, which proliferate to replace the normal alveolar epithelial lining.

If the patient survives the acute phase of ARDS, fibroblasts proliferate in the interstitial space and deposit collagen in the alveolar walls (Fig. 18-34). With complete recovery, the alveolar exudate and hyaline membranes are resorbed and normal alveolar epithelium is restored. Fibroblast proliferation ceases, the extra collagen is metabolized, and patients regain normal lung function. In patients who do not recover, DAD can progress to end-stage fibrosis:

TABLE 18-1			
IMPORTANT CAUSES OF ACUTE RESPIRATORY DISTRESS SYNDROME			
Nonthoracic Trauma	**Infection**	**Aspiration**	**Drugs and Therapeutic Agents**
Shock due to any cause	Gram-negative septicemia	Near-drowning	Heroin
Fat embolism	Other bacterial infections	Aspiration of gastric contents	Oxygen
	Viral infections		Radiation
			Paraquat
			Cytotoxic drugs

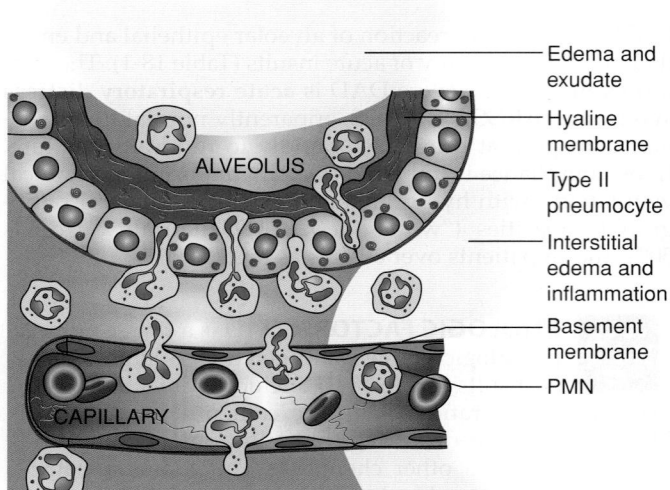

FIGURE 18-32. Diffuse alveolar damage (acute respiratory distress syndrome [ARDS]). In ARDS, type I cells die as a result of diffuse alveolar damage. This is followed by intra-alveolar edema and formation of hyaline membranes composed of proteinaceous exudate and cell debris. In the acute phase, the lungs are markedly congested and heavy. Type II cells multiply to line the alveolar surface. Interstitial inflammation is characteristic. The lesion may heal completely or progress to interstitial fibrosis. *PMN* = polymorphonuclear neutrophil.

remodeling of lung architecture produces many cyst-like spaces throughout the lung (**honeycomb lung**). These spaces are separated by thick fibrous walls lined by type II pneumocytes, bronchiolar epithelium, or squamous cells.

Mechanisms of acute injury in DAD are not entirely clear. It is thought that activation of complement (e.g., by endotoxin in the case of gram-negative septicemia) leads to sequestration of neutrophils in the marginating pool. Only a small proportion, perhaps one-third, of neutrophils actively circulate in the blood; most of the rest are in the lung. Normally, they cause no damage there, but upon activation by complement, they release oxygen

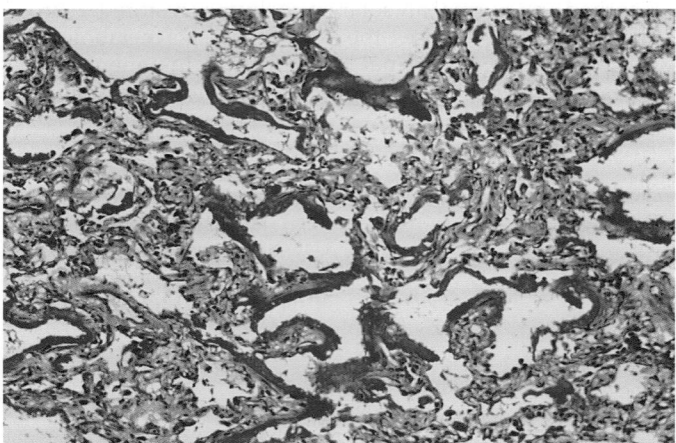

FIGURE 18-33. Diffuse alveolar damage, acute (exudative) phase. Alveolar septa are thickened by edema and a sparse inflammatory infiltrate. Alveoli are lined by eosinophilic hyaline membranes.

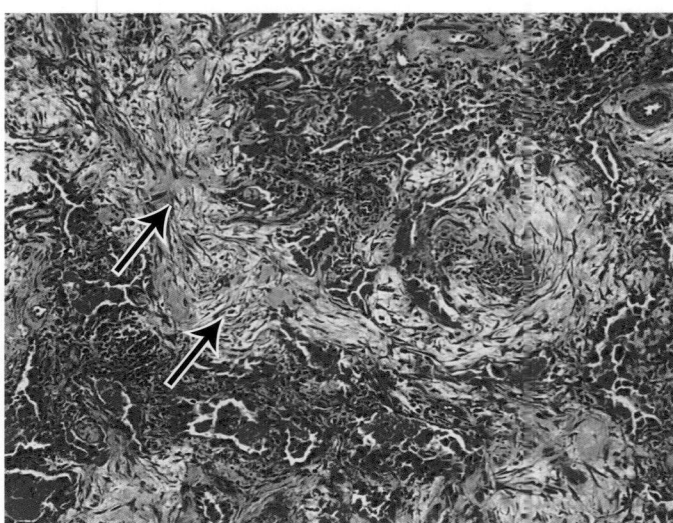

FIGURE 18-34. Diffuse alveolar damage, acute and organizing phase. Alveolar walls are thickened by fibroblasts and loose connective tissue (*arrows*).

radicals and hydrolytic enzymes, which damage pulmonary capillary endothelium. However, neutrophils cannot be obligatory for DAD, because ARDS can develop in severely neutropenic patients.

In DAD following toxic gas inhalation or near-drowning, the damage is mostly at the alveolar epithelial surface. Normal alveolar epithelial junctions are very tight, but epithelial injury disrupts these junctions, permitting exudation of fluid and proteins from the interstitium into alveolar spaces.

PATHOLOGY: The first step is the **exudative phase of DAD,** which develops within a week after pulmonary insult. Edema, hyaline membranes, and leakage of plasma proteins are evident, as is accumulation of inflammatory cells (Fig. 18-33). The earliest evidence of alveolar injury is seen by electron microscopy as degenerative changes in endothelial cells and type I pneumocytes. This is followed by sloughing of type I cells, thus denuding basement membranes. Interstitial and alveolar edema is prominent by the first day but soon recedes. "**Hyaline membranes**" appear by the second day and are the most conspicuous morphologic feature of the exudative phase after 4 to 5 days. They are eosinophilic and glassy, consisting of precipitated plasma proteins and cytoplasmic and nuclear debris from sloughed epithelial cells. Interstitial inflammation, with lymphocytes, plasma cells, and macrophages, develops early and peaks in about a week. Toward the end of the first week and persisting during the subsequent **organizing stage,** regularly spaced, cuboidal type II pneumocytes become arrayed along the denuded alveolar septa. Alveolar capillaries and pulmonary arterioles may contain fibrin thrombi. When DAD is fatal, the lungs are heavy, edematous, and virtually airless.

The organizing phase of DAD starts about a week after the initial injury and is marked by fibroblast proliferation within alveolar walls (Fig. 18-34). Interstitial inflammation and proliferated type II pneumocytes persist, but no additional hyaline membranes are formed. Alveolar macrophages digest the remnants of hyaline membranes and other debris, and are thought to release cytokines such as transforming growth factor beta (TGF-β) and platelet derived growth factor (PDGF), which stimulate fibroblast growth. Loose fibrosis expands alveolar septa but resolves in mild cases. In severe DAD, fibrosis progresses to restructuring of the pulmonary parenchyma.

CLINICAL FEATURES: Patients destined to develop ARDS are symptom-free for a few hours after the initial insult, but then tachypnea and dyspnea mark the onset of clinical manifestations. Blood gas analyses show arterial hypoxemia and decreased pCO_2. As ARDS progresses, dyspnea worsens and the patient becomes cyanotic. Diffuse, bilateral, interstitial, and alveolar infiltrates are noted radiographically. Increasing the concentration of inspired oxygen alone does not restore adequate blood oxygenation, necessitating mechanical ventilation. In fatal cases, the combination of increasing tachypnea and decreasing tidal volume causes alveolar hypoventilation, progressive hypoxemia, and increasing pCO_2.

Patients who survive ARDS may recover normal pulmonary function, but in severe cases, they are left with scarred lungs, respiratory dysfunction and, in some instances, pulmonary hypertension.

Diffuse Alveolar Damage Has Diverse Causes

Oxygen Toxicity

Patients who receive high oxygen levels for respiratory problems can develop DAD. Lung lesions may rarely follow long-term exposure to as little as 28% oxygen, but it is usually safe to breathe 40% to 60% oxygen for long periods. Oxygen toxicity is thought to be caused by increased production of reactive oxygen species in the lung (see Chapter 1).

Shock

ARDS often follows shock from any cause, including sepsis (see Chapter 12), trauma, or blood loss. The pulmonary consequences are often called "shock lung." The pathogenesis of DAD associated with shock is poorly understood but is likely multifactorial. Tissue necrosis in organs damaged by trauma or ischemia may lead to release of vasoactive peptides into the circulation. These enhance vascular permeability in the lung. Disseminated intravascular coagulation may damage alveolar capillaries, and fat emboli from bone fractures may obstruct the distal capillary bed of the lung. The pathogenesis of endothelial cell injury in endotoxic shock is discussed in Chapter 7.

Aspiration

Aspiration of gastric contents introduces material with a pH less than 3.0 into the alveoli. The severe chemical injury to the alveolar lining cells leads to DAD. In near-drowning, aspiration of water produces pulmonary injury and ARDS.

Drug-Induced DAD

Many drugs cause DAD, especially cytotoxic chemotherapeutic agents. The best known is bleomycin, but others

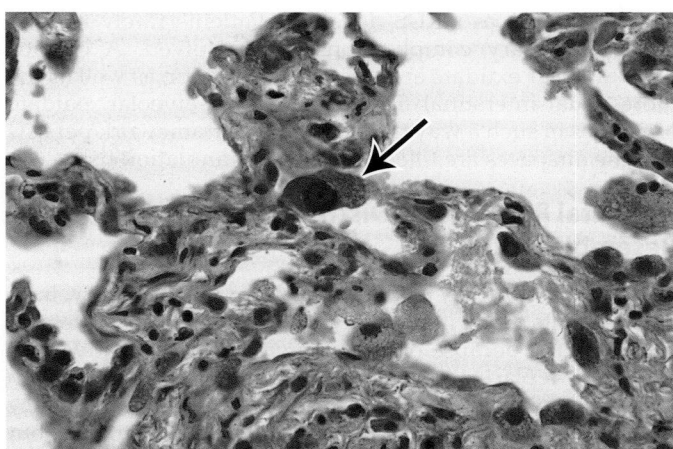

FIGURE 18-35. Diffuse alveolar damage (DAD) associated with busulfan treatment. An atypical pneumocyte (*arrow*) is seen in a case of organizing DAD associated with busulfan therapy.

include 1,3-bis-(2-chloroethyl)-1-nitrosourea (BCNU), methotrexate, 5-fluorouracil, busulfan, and cyclophosphamide. With bleomycin, an imprecise dose-dependent relation has been demonstrated, but such an effect is not apparent with most other drugs.

Bizarre, atypical, hyperchromatic nuclei in type II cells are particularly common when alveolar damage is due to chemotherapy (Fig. 18-35). Damage progresses even when the offending agent is discontinued, but corticosteroid treatment may be helpful. Progressive interstitial fibrosis occurs, usually with retention of lung structure. Methotrexate differs from other chemotherapeutic agents in that it may sometimes cause a hypersensitivity reaction in the lung, in which case the DAD is reversible after the drug is discontinued. Hypersensitivity lesions are characterized by granulomatous inflammation and occasionally vasculitis. Drugs other than chemotherapeutic agents that may cause DAD include nitrofurantoin, amiodarone, and penicillamine.

Radiation Pneumonitis

There are two forms of radiation pneumonitis: acute DAD and chronic pulmonary fibrosis. Alveolar injury is believed to be caused by oxygen radicals generated by the radiolysis of water (see Chapter 1).

Acute radiation pneumonitis occurs in as many as 10% of patients irradiated for lung or breast cancer or for mediastinal lymphoma. DAD caused by radiation is mostly dose related and appears 1 to 6 months after radiation therapy, when patients develop fever, cough, and dyspnea. Pathologically, the lungs show atypical alveolar lining cells, with enlarged hyperchromatic nuclei and multinucleated cells. Most patients recover from acute radiation pneumonitis.

In **chronic radiation pneumonitis,** interstitial fibrosis may follow acute DAD or develop insidiously. Lung biopsy demonstrates interstitial fibrosis, radiation-induced vascular changes, and atypical type II pneumocytes. The disease is asymptomatic unless it affects a substantial volume of the lung.

Paraquat

Exposure to paraquat, a common herbicide, may cause DAD. Pulmonary disease becomes apparent 4 to 7 days after ingestion, as ARDS develops. Patients rarely recover once pulmonary complications have evolved. A curious intra-alveolar exudate and organization occur, as well as the more usual interstitial fibrosis. The intra-alveolar exudate organizes in such a way that the alveolar framework persists and the airspaces are filled with loose granulation tissue.

Neonatal Respiratory Distress Syndrome Resembles ARDS

Neonatal respiratory distress syndrome (NRDS) (see Chapter 6) results from immaturity of the surfactant system at birth, usually because of severe prematurity. The advent of surfactant replacement therapy and better ventilatory techniques have increased survival and decreased the frequency of complications of NRDS in older premature infants, but very premature infants may still develop **bronchopulmonary dysplasia (BPD)**. Previously, BPD reflected damage to lung acini and subsequent repair, which led to atelectasis, fibrosis, and destruction of clusters of acini. With the advent of surfactant replacement therapy, the necrotizing bronchiolitis and alveolar septal fibrosis of BPD have largely disappeared, and decreased alveolarization is the main finding now. NRDS and BPD are discussed in further detail in Chapter 6.

RARE ALVEOLAR DISEASES

Alveolar Proteinosis Features Excess Intra-Alveolar Lipid-Rich Material

Alveolar proteinosis, also called **lipoproteinosis**, is a rare condition in which alveoli are filled with a granular eosinophilic material rich in surfactant. Initially considered idiopathic, alveolar proteinosis is now known to be associated with compromised immunity; various cancers, particularly leukemia and lymphoma; respiratory infections; and exposure to environmental inorganic dusts. There is also a rare congenital form caused by a point mutation in *CSF2RA*, the gene for the granulocyte-macrophage colony-stimulating factor (GM-CSF) receptor.

PATHOPHYSIOLOGY: Alveolar proteinosis is thought to be related to defective surfactant clearance by macrophages. It has recently been attributed to defective activity, or deficiency, of GM-CSF. Anti–GM-CSF autoantibodies are detected in most patients with the idiopathic form of the disease, suggesting an autoimmune etiology. The pathogenesis of secondary alveolar proteinosis is less clear, but appears related to defective macrophage function via altered GM-CSF activity.

PATHOLOGY: The lungs are heavy and viscid, yellow fluid leaks from cut surfaces. They contain scattered, firm, yellow-white nodules that vary in diameter from a few millimeters to 2 cm. Granular material composed of surfactant, cell debris, foamy macrophages, and detached type II pneumocytes is seen in alveoli, respiratory bronchioles, and alveolar ducts (Fig. 18-36). Electron microscopy shows characteristic tubular myelin structures of surfactant. Importantly, the interstitial architecture of the lung is intact, and little inflammation is present.

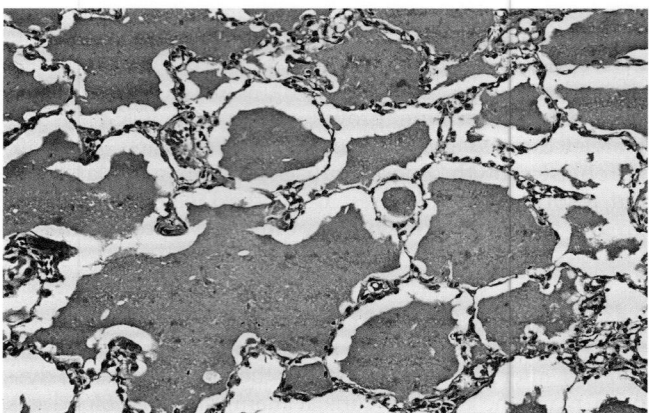

FIGURE 18-36.   Alveolar proteinosis. Alveoli and alveolar ducts contain abundant granular, eosinophilic material.

CLINICAL FEATURES: A few cases have been reported in infants and children, but alveolar proteinosis is a disease of adults. Patients have fever, productive cough, and dyspnea. Chest radiographs show diffuse, bilateral, symmetric, alveolar infiltrates, which may radiate from the hilar regions. Repeated respiratory tract infections, often with fungi or *Nocardia*, are common, perhaps due to altered neutrophil and macrophage activity. Infections occur at both pulmonary and extrapulmonary sites, suggesting a systemic predisposition to infections. Before treatment became available, alveolar proteinosis often progressed gradually to respiratory failure. Today, bronchoalveolar lavage can remove the alveolar material, and repeated lavage (sometimes for years) cures or arrests the disease. GM-CSF reconstitution is being investigated.

Diffuse Pulmonary Hemorrhage Syndromes Are Immunologic Disorders

Diffuse alveolar hemorrhage can occur in diverse clinical settings (Table 18-2). These diseases are characterized by acute hemorrhage (numerous intra-alveolar red blood cells) or chronic hemorrhage (hemosiderosis). In virtually all of these disorders, neutrophils infiltrate the alveolar capillary walls (**neutrophilic capillaritis**), reminiscent of leukocytoclastic vasculitis seen in other organs such as the skin. This finding tends to be most prominent in hemorrhagic syndromes associated with polyangiitis with granulomatosis (formerly Wegener granulomatosis) or systemic lupus erythematosus.

Some diffuse pulmonary hemorrhage syndromes are associated with characteristic immunofluorescence patterns. Linear fluorescence along alveolar walls is seen in antibasement membrane antibody disease, or Goodpasture syndrome. A granular pattern occurs in immune complex–associated diseases, such as systemic lupus erythematosus. Pauci-immune disorders consist of antineutrophil cytoplasm antibody (ANCA)-associated diseases (e.g., polyangiitis with granulomatosis, microscopic polyangiitis, or idiopathic pulmonary hemorrhage syndromes), in which no etiology or immunologic mechanism can be determined (Table 18-2).

Goodpasture Syndrome

Goodpasture syndrome (Antiglomerular basement membrane antibody disease) entails a triad: diffuse alveolar hemorrhage,

TABLE 18-2

CONDITIONS ASSOCIATED WITH PULMONARY HEMORRHAGE

Disease	Immunologic Mechanism	Immunofluorescence Pattern
Goodpasture syndrome	Antibasement membrane antibody	Linear
Microscopic polyangiitis	Antineutrophilic cytoplasmic antibody (ANCA)	Negative/pauci-immune
Systemic lupus erythematosus	Immune complexes	Granular
Mixed cryoglobulinemia		
Henoch–Schönlein purpura		
Immunoglobulin A (IgA) disease		
Granulomatosis with polyangiitis (formerly Wegener granulomatosis)	ANCA	Negative or pauci-immune
Idiopathic glomerulonephritis		
Idiopathic pulmonary hemorrhage	No immunologic marker	

glomerulonephritis, and circulating cytotoxic autoantibody to a component of basement membranes. Cross-reactivity between alveolar and glomerular basement membranes accounts for the simultaneous attack on the lung and kidney (see Chapter 22 for details about the pathogenic mechanism).

PATHOLOGY: Patients with Goodpasture syndrome have extensive intra-alveolar hemorrhage (Fig. 18-37A). Their lungs are dark red and heavy in the acute phase and rusty brown later, when extravasated erythrocytes have been phagocytosed. Red blood cells and hemosiderin-laden macrophages fill airspaces. The presence of neutrophils in and around alveolar capillaries may suggest an "alveolitis," but this reaction may be transient. Alveolar septa are mildly thickened by interstitial fibrosis and type II pneumocyte hyperplasia is seen. Immunofluorescence studies show deposition of IgG and complement in the basement membranes of alveoli and glomeruli (Fig. 18-37B).

CLINICAL FEATURES: Goodpasture syndrome may affect adults of either sex and any age, but it occurs mostly in young men. Most (95%) patients present with hemoptysis, often accompanied by dyspnea, weakness, and mild anemia. Evidence of glomerulonephritis follows pulmonary manifestations within about 3 months (1 week to 1 year), although some patients do not develop renal disease. Radiographic imaging reveals diffuse, bilateral alveolar infiltrates, which may resolve rapidly in a matter of days as erythrocytes lyse and are phagocytosed. Hypoxemia and respiratory alkalosis are common, but respiratory function returns to normal as the hemorrhage resolves. The diagnosis is made on the basis of a renal or pulmonary biopsy with characteristic immunofluorescence findings.

Goodpasture syndrome is treated with corticosteroids, cytotoxic drugs, and plasmapheresis. Before such aggressive treatment was used, mortality was 80%. Even with current therapy, 2-year survival is now only 50%, and the outlook is worse if renal failure develops.

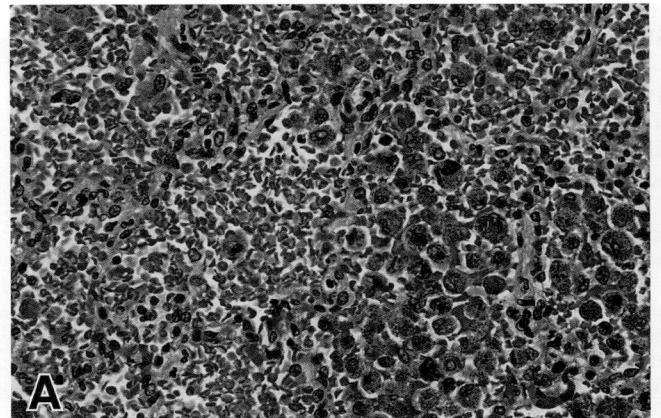 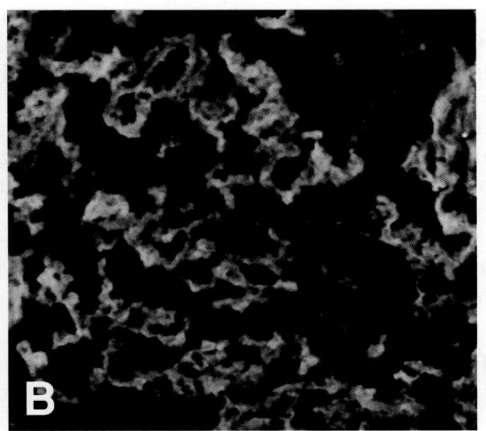

FIGURE 18-37. Goodpasture syndrome. A. A section of lung shows extensive intra-alveolar hemorrhage (*left*) and collections of hemosiderin-laden macrophages (*right*). Alveolar septa are thickened, and alveoli are lined by hyperplastic type II pneumocytes. **B.** Linear deposition of immunoglobulin G (IgG) within the alveolar septa is demonstrated by immunofluorescence.

Idiopathic Pulmonary Hemorrhage

This rare disease (also called **idiopathic pulmonary hemosiderosis**) is characterized by diffuse alveolar bleeding similar to that of Goodpasture syndrome but without renal involvement or antibasement membrane antibodies. It is microscopically indistinguishable from the lung of Goodpasture syndrome.

 CLINICAL FEATURES: Idiopathic pulmonary hemosiderosis affects mainly children, but 20% of patients are adults, usually younger than 30. Males predominate, 2:1, among adults, but sex distribution is equal in children. Patients complain of cough (with or without hemoptysis), dyspnea, substernal chest pain, fatigue, and iron-deficiency anemia. Pulmonary hemorrhages are recurrent and intermittent. The course is more protracted than that of Goodpasture syndrome.

The response to corticosteroids is variable, and mean survival is 3 to 5 years. One-fourth of patients die rapidly of massive hemorrhage. Another 25% have persistent, active disease; repeated episodes of hemoptysis result in interstitial fibrosis and cor pulmonale. In another one-fourth of patients, the disease remains inactive, but dyspnea and anemia may persist. The remaining patients recover completely without recurrence.

Eosinophilic Pneumonia

Eosinophilic pneumonia entails accumulation of eosinophils in alveolar spaces. The disease is classified as **idiopathic** or **secondary** to an underlying illness (Table 18-3).

Idiopathic Eosinophilic Pneumonia

SIMPLE EOSINOPHILIC PNEUMONIA: Simple eosinophilic pneumonia (also called Löffler syndrome) is a mild condition characterized by fleeting pulmonary infiltrates, which usually resolve within a month. Patients typically have peripheral blood eosinophilia but are often asymptomatic. Histologically, the lung shows eosinophilic pneumonia, but the diagnosis is usually established clinically, and lung biopsy is rarely performed.

ACUTE EOSINOPHILIC PNEUMONIA: Patients present with acute (<7 days) symptoms, including fever, hypoxemia, and diffuse interstitial and alveolar infiltrates on chest radiograph. The etiology is not known but is thought to be a hypersensitivity reaction. Peripheral blood eosinophilia is often absent, but bronchoalveolar lavage consistently contains increased eosinophils. Histologically, the lung shows eosinophilic pneumonia accompanied by features of DAD (i.e., hyaline membranes). Patients respond dramatically to corticosteroids, and unlike chronic eosinophilic pneumonia, acute eosinophilic pneumonia does not recur.

CHRONIC EOSINOPHILIC PNEUMONIA: The etiology of chronic eosinophilic pneumonia is unknown, but an allergic diathesis is noted in some patients.

 PATHOLOGY: Alveolar spaces contain eosinophils, alveolar macrophages, and a proteinaceous exudate (Fig. 18-38). Some cases may also show an eosinophilic interstitial pneumonia. Hyperplasia of type II pneumocytes may be prominent. Eosinophilic abscesses, with central masses of necrotic eosinophils surrounded by palisaded macrophages, are sometimes found. A mild

TABLE 18-3
TYPES OF EOSINOPHILIC PNEUMONIA

Idiopathic

  Chronic eosinophilic pneumonia

  Acute eosinophilic pneumonia

  Simple eosinophilic pneumonia (Löffler syndrome)

Secondary Eosinophilic Pneumonia

  Infection

    Parasitic

      Tropical eosinophilic pneumonia

      Ascaris lumbricoides, Toxocara canis, filarial

      Dirofilaria

    Fungal

      Aspergillus

  Drug induced

    Antibiotics

    Cytotoxic drugs

    Anti-inflammatory agents

    Antihypertensive drugs

    L-Tryptophan (eosinophilic fasciitis)

  Immunologic or systemic diseases

    Allergic bronchopulmonary aspergillosis

    Eosinophilic granulomatosis with polyangiitis (formerly Churg–Strauss syndrome)

    Hypereosinophilic syndrome

eosinophilic vasculitis may be seen. An organizing pneumonia pattern is also occasionally described (see below).

 CLINICAL FEATURES: Patients have fever, night sweats, weight loss, cough productive of eosinophils, and dyspnea. Asthma is present in many patients, and circulating eosinophilia may be conspicuous. The chest radiograph is diagnostic and has been

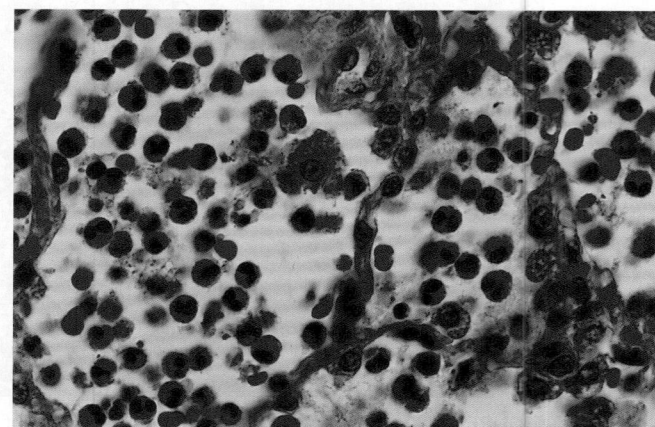

FIGURE 18-38. Eosinophilic pneumonia. Alveolar spaces are filled with an inflammatory exudate composed of eosinophils and macrophages. Alveolar septa are thickened by the presence of numerous eosinophils.

described as "the photographic negative of pulmonary edema," characterized by peripheral alveolar infiltrates with sparing of the hilum. The response to corticosteroids is dramatic and helps confirm the diagnosis.

Secondary Eosinophilic Pneumonia

Eosinophilic pneumonia can occur in a variety of clinical settings, including parasitic or fungal infection, drug toxicity, and systemic disorders such as Churg–Strauss syndrome (Table 18-3). In industrialized countries, the most frequent cause of eosinophilic pneumonia is drug hypersensitivity, including reactions to antibiotics, anti-inflammatory agents, cytotoxic drugs, and antihypertensive agents. The pulmonary disease resolves without long-term sequelae. The clinical presentations and histologic findings are the same as described above.

The classic form of **infectious eosinophilic pneumonia** associated with parasitic infection is **tropical eosinophilic pneumonia**. Migration of parasites through the lung elicits an acute, self-limited, respiratory illness characterized clinically by fever, a cough productive of sputum containing eosinophils, and transient pulmonary infiltrates.

In temperate zones, the roundworm *Ascaris lumbricoides* is the usual culprit, but the dog roundworm, *Toxocara canis,* is also occasionally involved. However, the most distinctive infection associated with eosinophilic pneumonia is allergic bronchopulmonary aspergillosis (see above).

In tropical regions, eosinophilic pneumonia is most commonly a response to infestation with the filarial nematodes *Wuchereria bancrofti* and *Brugia malayi,* although other parasites may also be responsible.

Endogenous Lipid Pneumonia Reflects Bronchial Obstruction

This disease, also called "golden pneumonia," is a localized condition distal to an obstructed airway, which is characterized by lipid-laden macrophages in alveolar spaces. The size of the affected area corresponds to the caliber of the involved bronchus. Bronchial obstruction leads to retention of secretions and breakdown products of inflammatory and epithelial cells. Although the protein component is readily digested, lipids are phagocytosed by macrophages, which fill alveoli distal to the obstruction.

 PATHOLOGY: Endogenous lipid pneumonia has a characteristic golden-yellow color, from lipid accumulation within alveolar macrophages. Alveoli are flooded by foamy macrophages with needle-shaped clefts characteristic of cholesterol crystals, with mild chronic inflammation and fibrosis. Alveolar walls are intact. If the obstruction is relieved, the affected lung can return to its normal state unless bronchiectasis and chronic recurrent bronchopneumonia have caused irreversible damage.

Exogenous Lipid Pneumonia Is a Response to Aspirated Oils

Causes of exogenous pneumonia include mineral oil (a laxative and a carrier for medications in nose drops), vegetable oils used in cooking, and animal oils ingested in the form of cod-liver oil and other vitamin preparations. Oil-based contrast media used for radiologic bronchography have also been

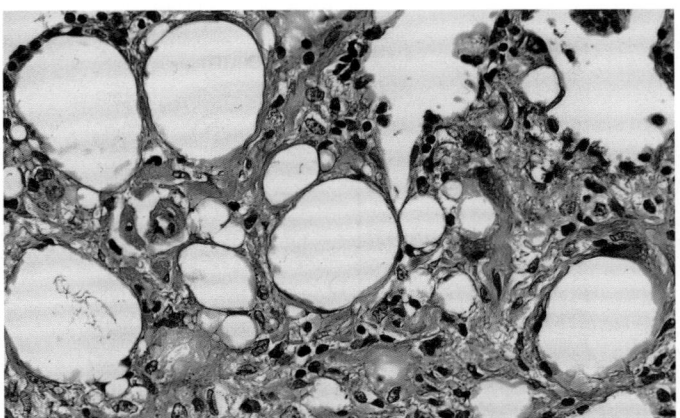

FIGURE 18-39. Exogenous lipoid pneumonia (mineral oil aspiration). The cystic spaces are empty because the lipid was dissolved during tissue processing. A giant cell reaction is present.

associated with the disorder. Exogenous lipid pneumonia is most common in older individuals, who take nose drops or laxatives at bedtime and aspirate during sleep. Computed tomography may reveal a spiculated mass that appears worrisome for malignancy. Children may aspirate oily medications while vigorously resisting attempted administration.

PATHOLOGY: Exogenous lipid pneumonia is gray, greasy, and poorly demarcated. Foamy macrophages are seen in alveolar and interstitial spaces (Fig. 18-39). Large oil droplets in both locations are surrounded by foreign body granulomas. As processing for paraffin embedding removes most of the oil, empty vacuolar spaces are seen in histologic sections. In chronic cases, affected areas may become densely fibrotic.

Patients with exogenous lipid pneumonia are usually asymptomatic; the condition comes to medical attention when a mass simulating an infection or a tumor is seen on a chest radiograph.

OBSTRUCTIVE PULMONARY DISEASES

Several diseases, including chronic bronchitis, emphysema, asthma, and in some classifications bronchiectasis and cystic fibrosis, are grouped together because they all entail obstruction to airflow in the lungs.

Chronic obstructive pulmonary disease (COPD) includes chronic bronchitis and emphysema, in which forced expiratory volume, measured by spirometry, is decreased.

Airflow can be reduced by increasing resistance to airflow or by reducing outflow pressure. In the lung, narrowed airways produce increased resistance, whereas loss of elastic recoil results in diminished pressure. Airway narrowing occurs in chronic bronchitis or asthma, and emphysema causes loss of recoil.

In Chronic Bronchitis, Patients Have a Chronic Productive Cough Without a Discernible Cause for 50% or More Days During 2 or More Years

The pathologic definition of the disease is less satisfactory, as its morphologic alterations are a continuum; mild chronic bronchitis may show normal histology.

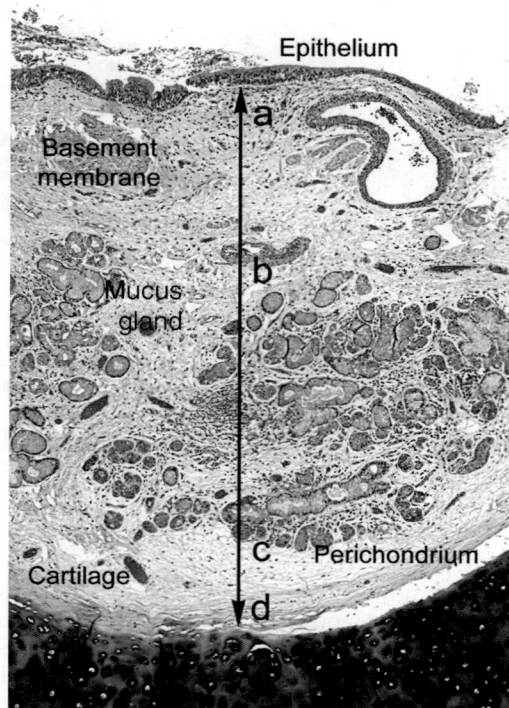

FIGURE 18-40. Chronic bronchitis. The bronchial submucosa is greatly expanded by hyperplastic submucosal glands that compose more than 50% of the thickness of the bronchial wall. The Reid index equals the maximum thickness of the bronchial mucus glands internal to the cartilage (*b* to *c*) divided by the bronchial wall thickness (*a* to *d*). (From Travis WB, Colby TV, Koss MN, et al. *Non-neoplastic Disorders of the Lower Respiratory Tract.* Washington, DC: American Registry of Pathology; 2002.)

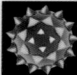 **ETIOLOGIC FACTORS:** *Since 90% of chronic bronchitis cases are smokers, the disease mainly reflects the consequences of cigarette smoke* (see Chapter 8). Chronic bronchitis occurs in less than 5% of nonsmokers, but it is seen in 10% to 15% of moderate smokers and over 25% of heavy smokers. The frequency and severity of acute respiratory tract infections are increased in patients with chronic bronchitis; conversely, infections have been incriminated in its etiology and progression. Chronic bronchitis occurs more often in people in areas of substantial air pollution and in workers exposed to toxic industrial inhalants, but the effects of cigarette smoking far outweigh other contributing factors.

How cigarette smoke and other pollutants injure bronchi is not well understood. Experimentally, rodents that inhale cigarette smoke or SO_2, or are given dilute acids by instillation, exhibit squamous metaplasia of the bronchial epithelium. A similar change occurs when certain proteases are introduced into the bronchi, and this effect can be prevented by pretreating with antiproteases. Bronchial epithelial metaplasia also occurs in rodents given adrenergic and cholinergic agonists, suggesting that autonomic stimulation may play a role in the pathogenesis of chronic bronchitis.

PATHOLOGY: The main pathology in chronic bronchitis is increased bronchial mucus-secreting tissue (Fig. 18-40). Two types of cells line bronchial mucus glands: the more abundant pale mucus cells, and basophilic, granular serous cells. **In *chronic bronchitis, mucus cells undergo hyperplasia and hypertrophy and are increased relative to serous cells.*** Thus, both individual acini and glands enlarge (Fig. 18-41).

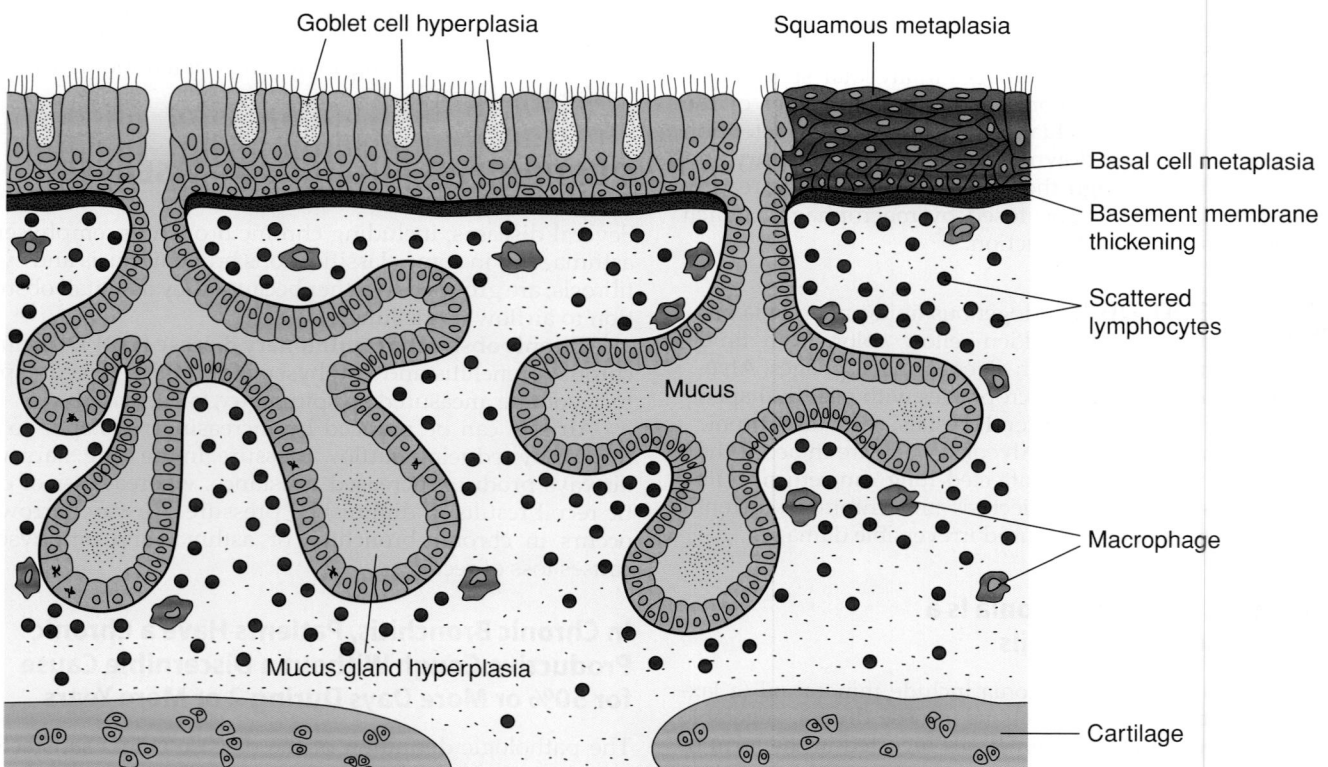

FIGURE 18-41. Morphologic changes in chronic bronchitis.

The **Reid index** measures the size of the mucus glands (Fig. 18-40): the area occupied by the glands in the plane vertical to the epithelium as a proportion of the thickness of the entire bronchial wall (basement membrane to inner perichondrium). A normal Reid index is 0.4 or less; in chronic bronchitis, it is more than 0.5.

Other morphologic changes in chronic bronchitis are variable and include:

- Excess mucous in central and peripheral airways
- "Pits" on the surface of the bronchial epithelium, which represent dilated ducts into which several bronchial glands open
- Thickening of the bronchial wall by mucus gland enlargement and edema, encroaching on the bronchial lumen
- Increased numbers of goblet cells (hyperplasia) in the bronchial epithelium
- Increased smooth muscle, which may underlie bronchial hyperreactivity
- Squamous metaplasia of the bronchial epithelium, reflecting epithelial damage from tobacco smoke, an effect that is probably independent of the other changes seen in chronic bronchitis

 CLINICAL FEATURES: Chronic bronchitis is often accompanied by emphysema (see below), and separating the clinical contributions of each in an individual patient may be difficult. In general, patients with mainly chronic bronchitis have had a productive cough for many years. Cough and sputum production are initially more severe in the winter but progress over time from hibernal to perennial. Exertional dyspnea and cyanosis supervene, and cor pulmonale may ensue. The combination of cyanosis and edema due to cor pulmonale has led to the label "blue bloater" for such patients.

In patients with advanced chronic bronchitis, multiple factors such as pulmonary infections, thromboembolism, left ventricular failure, and major episodes of air pollution may precipitate acute respiratory failure, with progressive hypoxemia and hypercapnia. Because of retained mucus secretions, people with chronic bronchitis are prone to bacterial lung infections, particularly with *Haemophilus influenzae* and *S. pneumoniae*.

People with chronic bronchitis must be warned to stop smoking. Prompt antibiotic treatment of pulmonary infections, use of bronchodilator drugs, and occasionally bronchopulmonary drainage are mainstays of treatment.

Emphysema Causes Overinflation of the Lungs in Smokers

Emphysema is a chronic lung disease in which airspaces distal to terminal bronchioles are enlarged owing to destruction of their walls, without fibrosis. Although it is classified in anatomic terms, the severity of emphysema is more important than the anatomic type. In practical terms, as emphysema becomes more severe, it becomes more difficult to classify. Moreover, several anatomic patterns may be present in the same lung.

 ETIOLOGIC FACTORS AND PATHOPHYSIOLOGY: The major cause of emphysema is cigarette smoking. Moderate to severe emphysema is rare in nonsmokers (see Chapter 8). In considering the pathogenesis of emphysema, it is thought that a balance exists between elastin synthesis and catabolism in the normal lung. Emphysema results when elastolytic activity increases and/or antielastolytic activity is reduced (Fig. 18-42).

Increased numbers of neutrophils, which contain serine elastase and other proteases, are found in the bronchoalveolar lavage fluid of smokers. Smoking also interferes with α_1-antitrypsin (α_1-AT) activity, by oxidizing methionine residues in α_1-antitrypsin. In this way, unopposed and increased elastolytic activity leads to destruction of elastic tissue in the walls of distal airways, impairing elastic recoil and, as discussed above, contributing to airflow obstruction. At the same time, other cellular proteases may be involved in injury to the airspace walls. This theory, although attractive, awaits further confirmation.

α_1**-ANTITRYPSIN (α_1-AT) DEFICIENCY:** Genetic deficiency of α_1-AT accounts for about 1% of patients with COPD and is much more common in young people with severe emphysema. α_1-AT is a circulating inhibitor of serine proteases, including elastase, trypsin, chymotrypsin, thrombin, and bacterial proteases. Made in the liver, it accounts for 90% of blood antiproteinase activity. In the lung, it inhibits neutrophil elastase, an enzyme that digests elastin and other alveolar wall components.

 MOLECULAR PATHOGENESIS: The amount and type of α_1-AT is determined by a pair of codominant alleles for the *SERPINA1* gene, also known as *Pi* (protease inhibitor). The most common allele is *PiM and the most common genotype is PiMM*, but more than 100 variants are known. The amount of α_1-AT in the blood depends on the genotype. Some mutant forms fail to fold properly and are thus targeted for proteasomal degradation in liver cells. Other mutant forms polymerize and accumulate within hepatocytes. The most serious abnormality involves the *PiZ* allele, which occurs in 5% of the population. It is more common in people of Scandinavian origin and is rare in Jews, blacks, and Japanese. Because the abnormal protein is poorly secreted by the liver, plasma α_1-AT in *PiZZ* homozygotes is only 15% to 20% of normal. These people are at risk for cirrhosis of the liver (see Chapter 20) and emphysema. **Most patients with clinically diagnosed emphysema under age 40 have genetic α_1-AT deficiency (PiZ).** In *PiZZ* homozygotes who do not smoke, emphysema begins between ages 45 and 50; those who smoke develop it 5 to 10 years earlier. However, most nonsmoking *PiZZ* homozygotes show no evidence of emphysema. The association of α_1-AT deficiency with emphysema supports the concept that cigarette smoking by itself causes emphysema by altering the balance of proteases and antiproteases in the lung.

PATHOLOGY: Emphysema is morphologically classified according to the location of the lesions within the pulmonary acinus (Fig. 18-43). Only the proximal acinus (the respiratory bronchiole) is affected in centrilobular emphysema, whereas the entire acinus is destroyed in panacinar emphysema.

CENTRILOBULAR EMPHYSEMA: This form of emphysema is most common. It usually accompanies

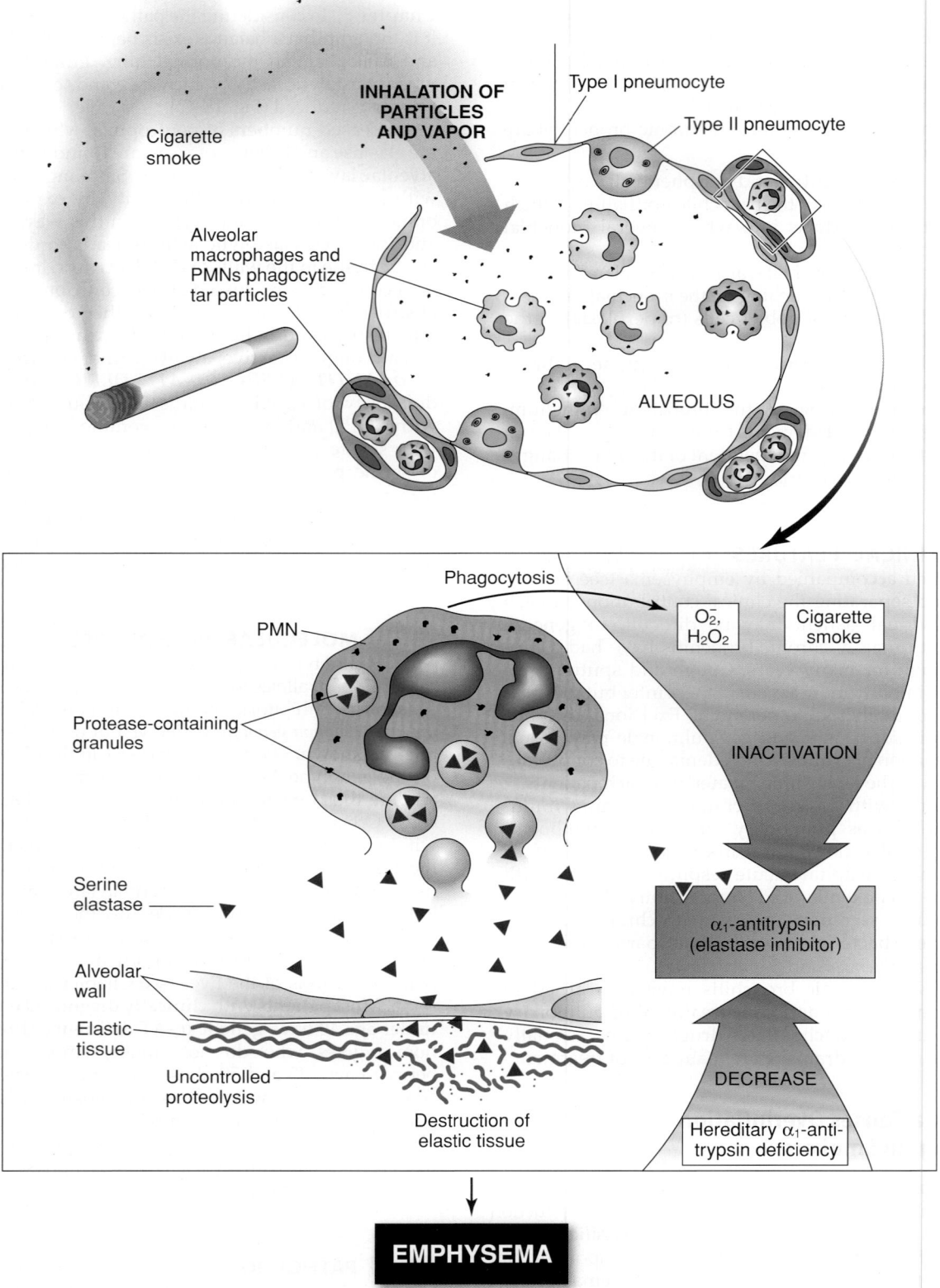

FIGURE 18-42. The proteolysis–antiproteolysis theory of the pathogenesis of emphysema. Cigarette (tobacco) smoking is closely related to the development of emphysema. Some products in tobacco smoke induce an inflammatory reaction. The serine elastase in polymorphonuclear leukocytes, a particularly potent elastolytic agent, injures the elastic tissue of the lung. Normally, this enzyme activity is inhibited by α_1-antitrypsin, but tobacco smoke, directly or through the generation of free radicals, inactivates α_1-antitrypsin (protease inhibitor). H_2O_2 = hydrogen peroxide; O_2^- = superoxide ion; PMN = polymorphonuclear neutrophil.

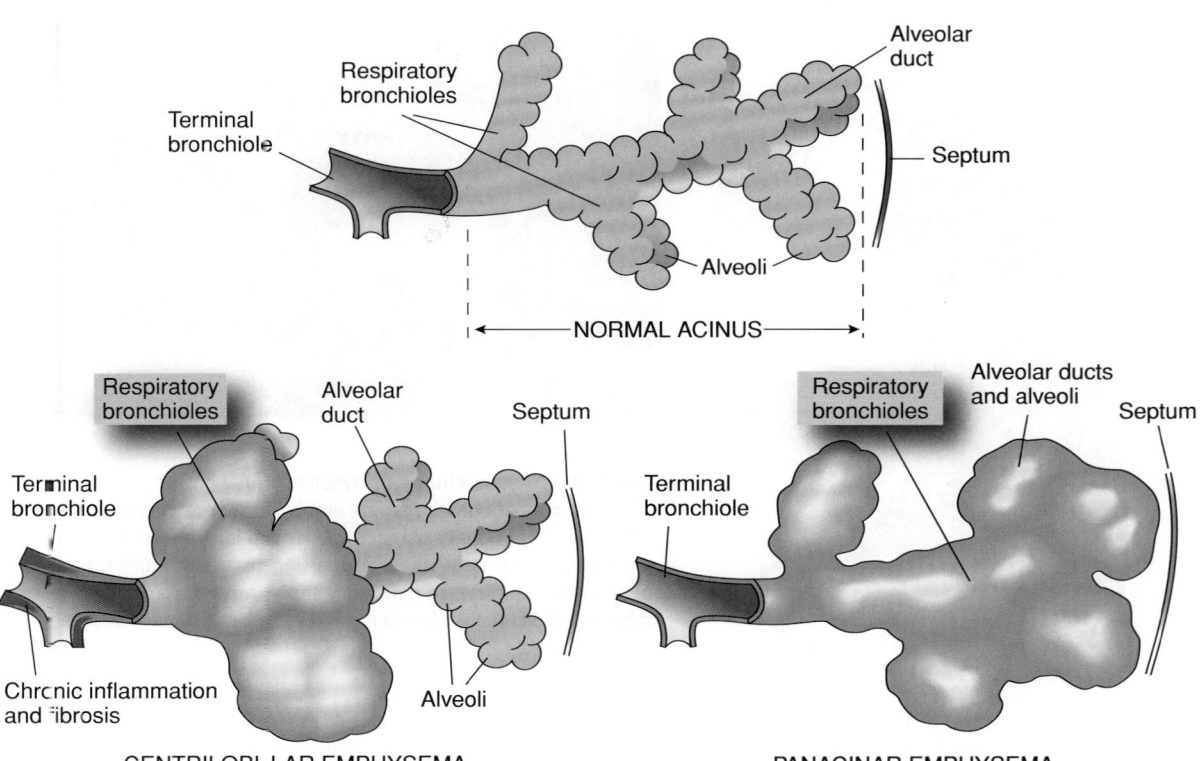

FIGURE 18-43. Types of emphysema. The acinus is the gas-exchanging structural unit of the lung distal to the terminal bronchiole. It consists of (from proximal to distal) respiratory bronchioles, alveolar ducts, and alveoli. In centrilobular (proximal acinar) emphysema, the respiratory bronchioles are predominantly involved. In paraseptal (distal acinar) emphysema, the alveolar ducts are particularly affected. In panacinar (panlobular) emphysema, the acinus is uniformly damaged.

cigarette smoking and is symptomatic. The clusters of terminal bronchioles near the end of the bronchiolar tree in the central part of the pulmonary lobule are destroyed (Fig. 18-44A). These are the smallest portion of the lung bounded by septa and include several acini. Dilated respiratory bronchioles form enlarged airspaces separated from

each other and from lobular septa by normal alveolar ducts and alveoli. As centrilobular emphysema progresses, these distal structures may also be involved (Fig. 18-44B). Bronchioles proximal to emphysematous spaces are inflamed and narrowed. Centrilobular emphysema is most severe in the upper lobes and in superior segments of the lower lobes.

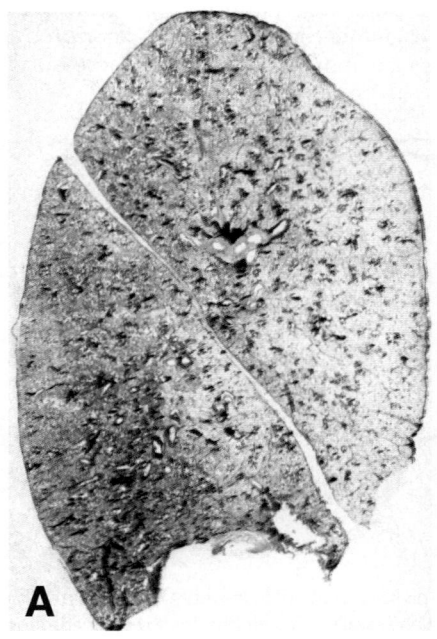

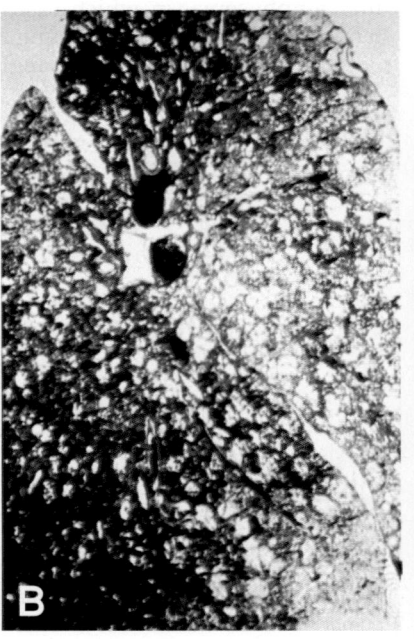

FIGURE 18-44. Centrilobular emphysema. A. A whole mount slice of the left lung of a smoker with mild emphysema shows enlarged airspaces scattered throughout both lobes, which represent destruction of terminal bronchioles in the central part of the pulmonary lobule. These abnormal spaces are surrounded by intact pulmonary parenchyma. **B.** In a more advanced case of centrilobular emphysema, destruction of the lung has progressed to produce large, irregular airspaces.

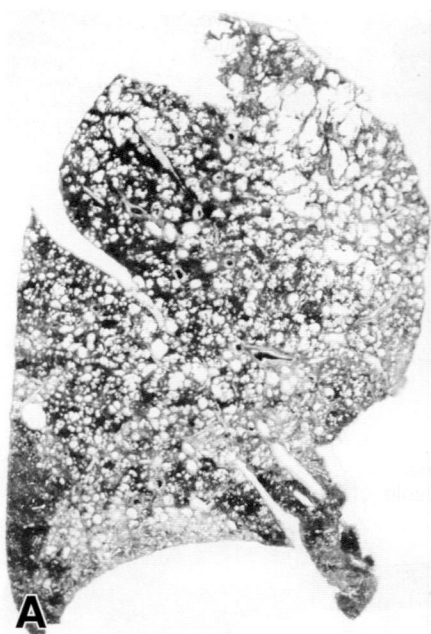

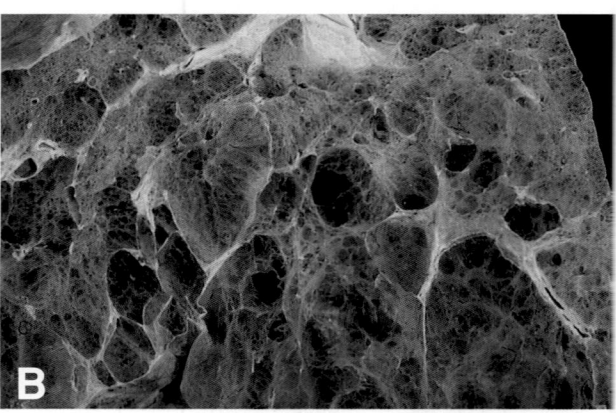

FIGURE 18-45. Panacinar emphysema. A. A whole mount of the left lung from a patient with severe emphysema reveals widespread destruction of pulmonary parenchyma, which in some areas leaves behind only a lacy network of supporting tissue. **B.** Lung from a patient with α_1-antitrypsin deficiency shows a panacinar pattern of emphysema. Loss of alveolar walls has resulted in markedly enlarged airspaces.

Focal dust emphysema, a disease of coal miners, resembles centrilobular emphysema but differs in that affected spaces are smaller and more regular and lack inflammation of the bronchioles. The lesions mainly distend, rather than destroy, alveolar walls. This disease is discussed below with coal workers' pneumoconiosis.

PANACINAR EMPHYSEMA: In panacinar emphysema, acini are uniformly involved, with destruction of alveolar septa from the center to the periphery of acini (Fig. 18-45). Loss of alveolar septa is illustrated by histologic comparison of normal lungs with those affected by α_1-AT deficiency (Fig. 18-46). In its final stage, panacinar emphysema leaves behind a lacy network of supporting tissue ("cotton-candy lung"). This type of emphysema is typically associated with α_1-AT deficiency. But it may also occur in cigarette smokers in association with centrilobular emphysema, in which cases the panacinar pattern tends to occur in more basal lung zones, while centrilobular emphysema prefers upper regions (see above).

LOCALIZED EMPHYSEMA: This disease, also called distal acinar or "paraseptal emphysema," entails alveolar destruction and leads to emphysema at only one or at most a few locations. The remainder of the lungs is normal. The lesion is usually found at the apex of an upper lobe in a subpleural location but may occur anywhere (Fig. 18-47). It is not clinically significant itself, but a focus of localized emphysema may rupture and cause spontaneous pneumothorax, particularly in younger individuals (see below). Localized emphysema can also progress to large areas of destruction, or **bullae**, which can be as small as 2 cm or can occupy an entire hemithorax.

CLINICAL FEATURES: Most patients with emphysema present at age 60 or older, with long histories of exertional dyspnea but minimal, nonproductive cough. They have lost weight and use accessory muscles of respiration to breathe. Weight loss is

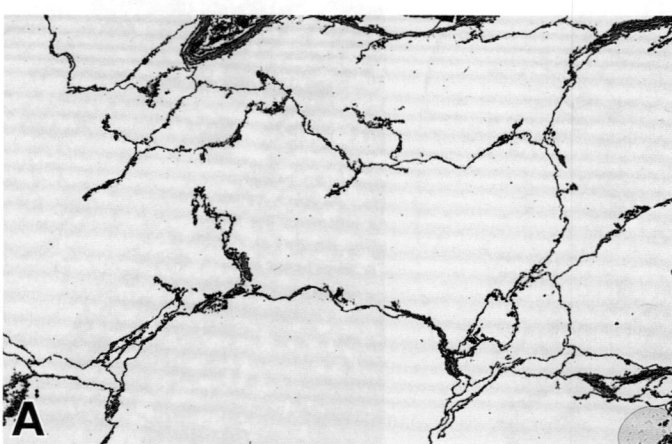

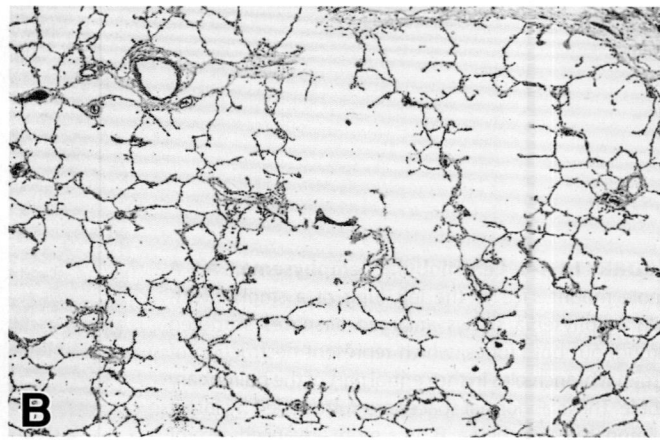

FIGURE 18-46. Panacinar emphysema. A. This lung, from a patient with α_1-antitrypsin deficiency, shows large, irregular airspaces and a markedly reduced number of alveolar walls. **B.** Extensive loss of alveolar walls in **A** is emphasized by comparison with this section of normal lung at the same magnification.

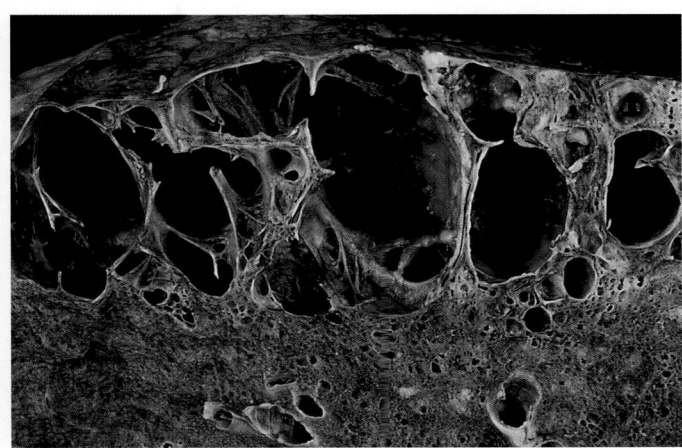

FIGURE 18-47. Localized emphysema. The subpleural parenchyma shows markedly enlarged airspaces owing to the loss of alveolar tissue.

probably due less to lack of calories than to the increased work of breathing. Tachypnea and a prolonged expiratory phase are typical. Radiographically, the lungs are overinflated: they are enlarged, diaphragms are depressed, and the posteroanterior diameter is increased (barrel chest). Bronchovascular markings do not reach the peripheral lung fields. Since these patients have increased respiratory rates and minute volumes, they can maintain arterial hemoglobin saturation at near-normal levels and so are called "pink puffers." Unlike patients with predominantly chronic bronchitis, those with emphysema are not at higher risk for recurrent pulmonary infections and are not so prone to develop cor pulmonale. Emphysema entails an inexorable decline in respiratory function and progressive dyspnea, for which no treatment other than lung transplantation is adequate.

In Asthma a Number of Stimuli Trigger Episodic Airflow Obstruction

Asthmatic patients typically have paroxysms of wheezing, dyspnea, and cough. Attacks may alternate with asymptomatic periods or be superimposed on a background of chronic airway obstruction. Severe acute asthma that is unresponsive to therapy is **status asthmaticus.** Most asthmatic patients, even when apparently well, have some persistent airflow obstruction and morphologic lesions.

In the United States, bronchial asthma affects up to 10% of children and 5% of adults. The prevalence of asthma in the United States has doubled since 1980. Initial asthma attacks may occur at any age, but half of cases begin in patients under age 10, and they are twice as common in boys as in girls. By age 30, both sexes are affected equally.

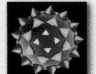 **ETIOLOGIC FACTORS:** Asthma was once divided into **extrinsic (allergic)** and **intrinsic (idiosyncratic)** forms, depending on inciting factors. It is now described in terms of the different inciting factors and the common effector pathways.

Bronchial hyperresponsiveness in asthma generally reflects inflammatory reactions to diverse stimuli. After exposure to an inciting factor (e.g., allergens, drugs, cold, exercise), inflammatory mediators released by activated macrophages, mast cells, eosinophils, and basophils trigger bronchoconstriction, increased vascular permeability, and mucus secretion. Resident inflammatory cells release chemotactic factors, which in turn recruit more effector cells and amplify the response of the airways. Inflammation of bronchial walls also may injure the epithelium, stimulating nerve endings and initiating neural reflexes that further aggravate and propagate the bronchospasm.

Many inflammatory mediators and chemotactic factors may participate in the bronchospasm and mucus hypersecretion of asthma. The relative contributions of the different substances probably vary with the inciting stimulus. The best-studied situation associated with the induction of asthma is inhaled allergens.

In a sensitized person, an inhaled allergen interacts with $T_H 2$ cells and IgE antibody bound to the surface of mast cells, which are interspersed among the bronchial epithelial cells (Fig. 18-48). The $T_H 2$ cells and mast cells release mediators of type I (immediate) hypersensitivity, including histamine, bradykinin, leukotrienes, prostaglandins, thromboxane A_2, and platelet-activating factor (PAF), as well as cytokines such as interleukin (IL)-4 and IL-5. These inflammatory mediators promote (1) **smooth muscle contraction,** (2) **mucus secretion,** and (3) **increased vascular permeability and edema.** Each of these effects is a potent, albeit reversible, cause of airway obstruction. IL-5 also stimulates terminal differentiation of eosinophils in the bone marrow. Chemotactic factors, including leukotriene B_4 and neutrophil and eosinophil chemotactic factors, attract neutrophils, eosinophils, and platelets to the bronchial wall. Eosinophils then release leukotriene B_4 and PAF, aggravating bronchoconstriction and edema. Discharge of eosinophil granules containing eosinophil cationic protein and major basic protein into the bronchial lumen further impairs mucociliary function and damages epithelial cells. Epithelial cell injury is suspected to stimulate nerve endings in the mucosa, initiating autonomic discharge that contributes to airway narrowing and mucus secretion. Leukotriene B_4 and PAF recruit more eosinophils and other effector cells, and thus act to prolong and amplify the attack.

Bronchial epithelial dysfunction also plays a role in the pathogenesis of various asthma phenotypes. The inflammatory response disrupts tight junctions in bronchial epithelium and so impairs barrier function and increases permeability. The mucosal epithelium itself also secretes various cytokines and chemokines that participate in regulating cells of the immune system. Since the bronchial mucosa is the first structure to come into contact with inhaled allergens and infectious agents, the importance of epithelial cells in the pathogenesis of asthma has recently been emphasized.

ALLERGIC ASTHMA: This is the most common form of asthma and is usually seen in children. One-third to one-half of all patients with asthma have known or suspected reactions to such allergens as pollens, animal hair or fur, and house dust contaminated with mites. Allergic asthma correlates strongly with skin-test reactivity. Half of children with asthma have substantial or complete remission of symptoms by age 20, but in many, asthma may recur after age 30.

INFECTIOUS ASTHMA: A common precipitating factor in childhood asthma is a viral respiratory tract infection rather than an allergic stimulus. In children under 2 years of age, RSV is the usual agent; in older children, rhinovirus,

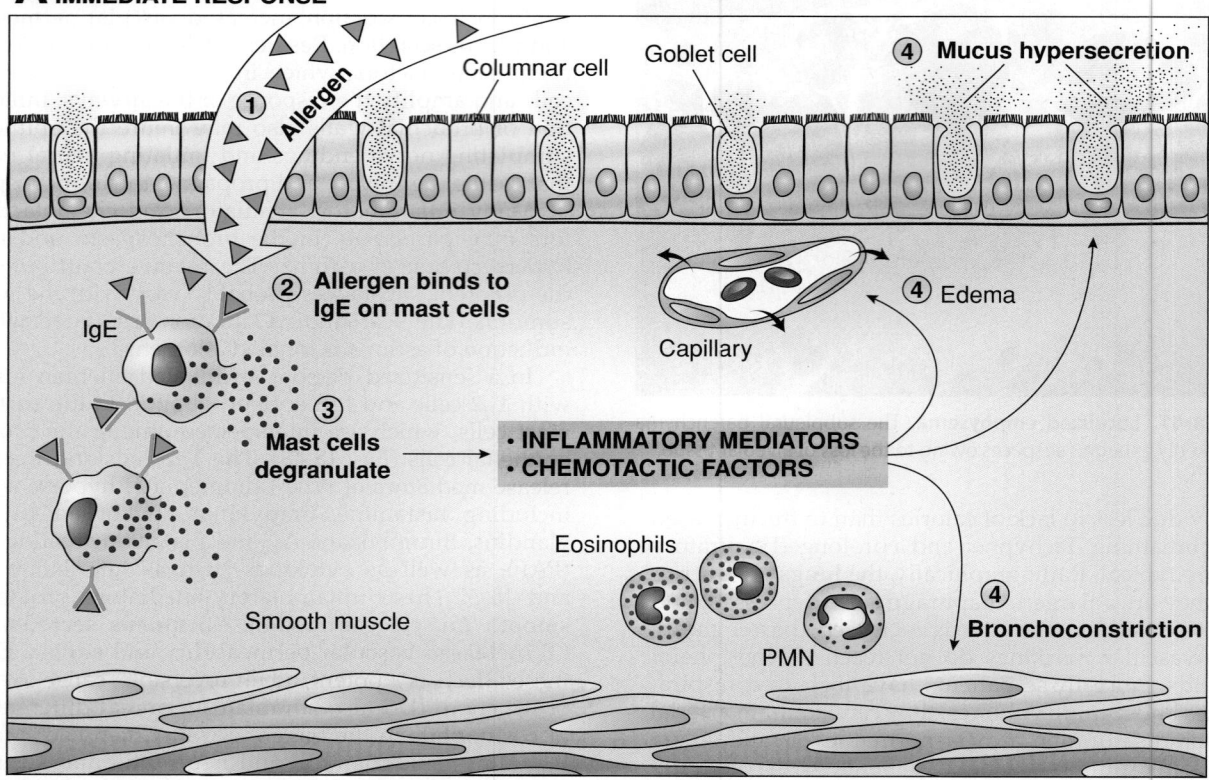

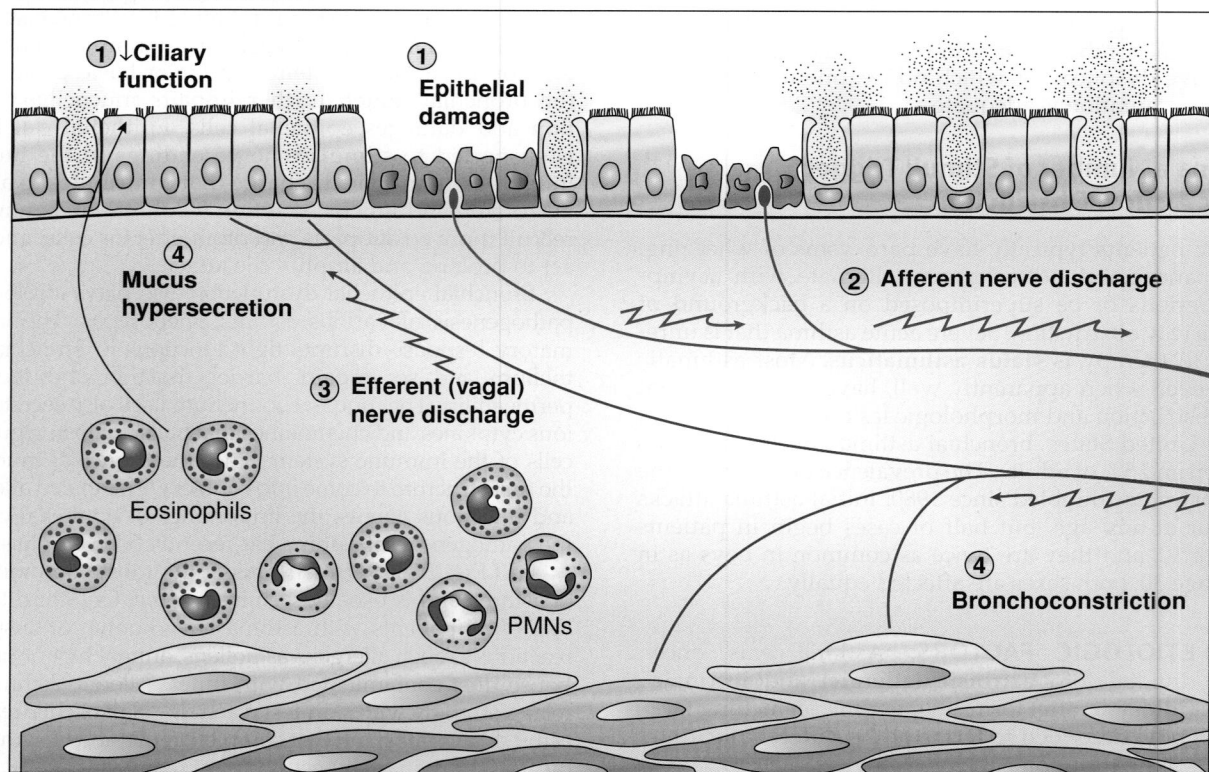

FIGURE 18-48. Pathogenesis of asthma. A. Immunologically mediated asthma. Allergens interact with immunoglobulin E (IgE) on mast cells, either on the surface of the epithelium or, when there is abnormal permeability of the epithelium, in the submucosa. Released mediators may react locally or by vagal reflexes. **B.** Discharge of eosinophilic granules further damages epithelial cells and impairs mucociliary function. Epithelial cell injury stimulates nerve endings (*in red*) in the mucosa, initiating an autonomic discharge that contributes to airway narrowing and mucus secretion. *PMNs* = polymorphonuclear neutrophils.

influenza, and parainfluenza are common inciting organisms. Inflammatory responses to viral infection in susceptible people may trigger the episode of bronchoconstriction. In support of this hypothesis, bronchial hyperreactivity may persist for as long as 2 months after a viral infection in nonasthmatics.

EXERCISE-INDUCED ASTHMA: Exercise can precipitate bronchospasm in more than half of all asthmatics. In some patients, it may be the only inciting factor. Exercise-induced asthma is related to the magnitude of heat or water loss from airway epithelium. The more rapid the ventilation (intensity of exercise) and the colder and drier the air breathed, the more likely is an attack of asthma. Thus, an asthmatic playing hockey on an outdoor rink in Canada in winter is more likely to have an attack than one swimming slowly in Texas during the summer. Mechanisms underlying exercise-induced asthma are unclear. They may be related to mediator release or vascular congestion secondary to rewarming of bronchi after the exertion.

OCCUPATIONAL ASTHMA: More than 80 different occupational exposures have been linked to asthma. Some substances may provoke allergic asthma via IgE-related hypersensitivity (e.g., in animal handlers, bakers, and workers exposed to wood and vegetable dusts, metal salts, pharmaceutical agents, and industrial chemicals). Occupational asthma may also result from direct release of mediators of smooth muscle contraction after contact with an offending agent, as is postulated in byssinosis ("brown lung"), an occupational lung disease of cotton workers. Some occupational exposures affect the autonomic nervous system directly. For instance, organic phosphorus insecticides act as anticholinesterases and produce overactivity of the parasympathetic nervous system. Substances such as toluene diisocyanate and western red cedar dust are thought to operate through hypersensitivity mechanisms, although specific IgE antibodies to these substances have not been identified.

DRUG-INDUCED ASTHMA: Drug-induced bronchospasm occurs mostly in patients with known asthma. The best-known offender is aspirin, but other nonsteroidal anti-inflammatory agents also have been implicated. Up to 10% of adult asthmatics may be sensitive to aspirin. Immediate hypersensitivity does not seem to be involved, and these patients can be desensitized by daily administrations of small doses of aspirin. Rhinitis and nasal polyps are also common in these individuals. β-Adrenergic antagonists consistently induce bronchoconstriction in asthmatics and are contraindicated in such patients.

AIR POLLUTION: Massive air pollution, usually occurring during temperature inversions, may cause bronchospasm in patients with asthma and other preexisting lung diseases. Gasses such as SO_2, nitrogen oxides, and ozone are commonly implicated, but particulate carbon, carrying toxic chemicals in diesel exhaust, may also contribute.

EMOTIONAL FACTORS: Psychological stress can aggravate or precipitate attacks of bronchospasm in as many as half of asthmatics. Vagal efferent stimulation is thought to be the underlying mechanism.

PATHOLOGY: The pathology of asthma has been studied in autopsies of patients who died in status asthmaticus, where the most severe lesions are described. Grossly, the lungs are highly distended with air, and airways are filled with thick, tenacious, adherent mucus plugs. Microscopically, these plugs (Fig. 18-49A) contain strips of epithelium and many eosinophils. Charcot-Leyden crystals, derived from phospholipids of the

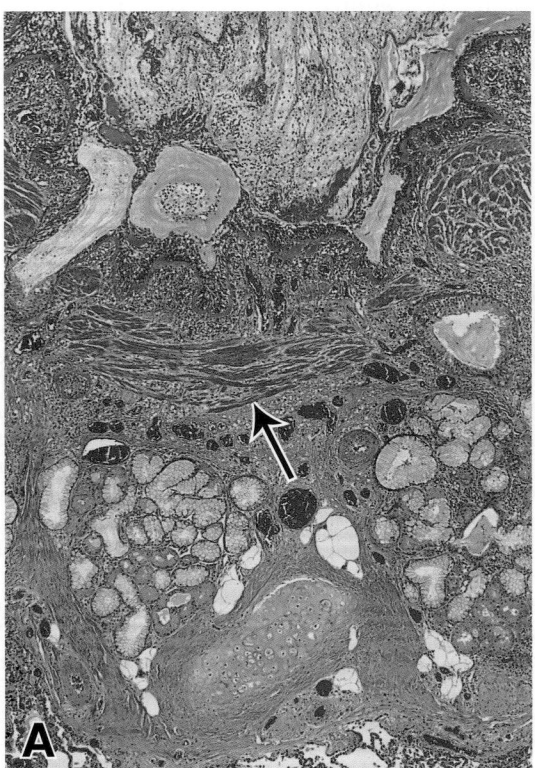

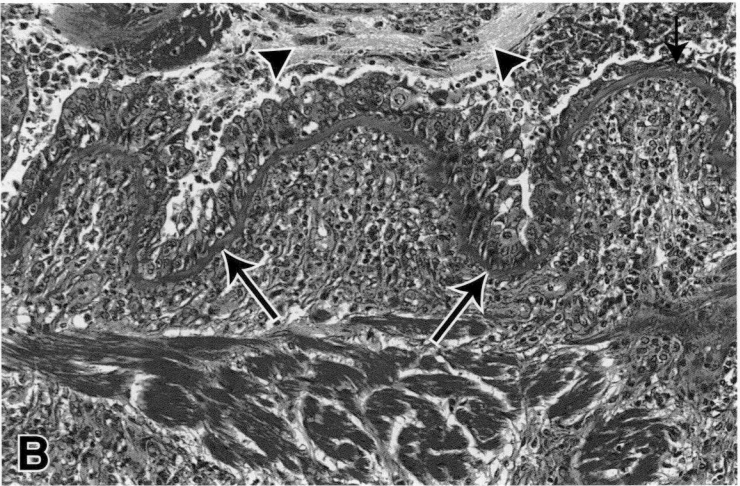

FIGURE 18-49. Asthma. A. A section of lung from a patient who died in status asthmaticus reveals a bronchus containing a luminal mucus plug (*top*), submucosal gland hyperplasia, and smooth muscle hyperplasia (*arrow*). **B.** Higher magnification shows hyaline thickening of the subepithelial basement membrane (*long arrows*) and marked inflammation of the bronchiolar wall, with numerous eosinophils. The mucosa exhibits an inflamed and metaplastic epithelium (*arrowheads*). The epithelium is focally denuded (*short arrow*).

eosinophil cell membrane, are also seen (Fig. 18-24B). In some cases, mucoid casts of the airways (Curschmann spirals) may be expelled with coughing, as may compact clusters of epithelial cells (Creola bodies).

One of the most characteristic features of status asthmaticus is hyperplasia of bronchial smooth muscle. Bronchial submucosal mucus glands are also hyperplastic (Fig. 18-49A). The submucosa is edematous, with a mixed inflammatory infiltrate containing variable numbers of eosinophils. The epithelium does not show the normal pseudostratified appearance and may be denuded, with only basal cells remaining (Fig. 18-49B). The basal cells are hyperplastic, and squamous metaplasia and goblet cell hyperplasia are seen. Bronchial epithelial basement membranes are thickened, owing to an increase in collagen deep to the true basal lamina.

 CLINICAL FEATURES: A typical attack of asthma begins with tightness in the chest and nonproductive cough. Inspiratory and expiratory wheezes appear, respiratory rate increases, and the patient becomes dyspneic. The expiratory phase is particularly prolonged. The attack often ends with fits of severe coughing and expectoration of thick mucous containing Curschmann spirals, eosinophils, and Charcot-Leyden crystals.

Status asthmaticus is severe bronchoconstriction unresponsive to drugs that usually abort the acute attack. It is serious and requires hospitalization. Patients in status asthmaticus have hypoxemia and often hypercapnia. They require oxygen and other pharmacologic interventions. Severe episodes may be fatal. The cornerstone of asthma treatment includes administration of β-adrenergic agonists, inhaled corticosteroids, cromolyn sodium (which stabilizes mast cells and limits release of mediators), methylxanthines, and anticholinergic agents. Systemic corticosteroids are reserved for status asthmaticus or resistant chronic asthma. The inhalation of bronchodilators often provides dramatic relief.

PNEUMOCONIOSES

Pneumoconioses are pulmonary diseases caused by mineral dust inhalation. Over 40 inhaled minerals cause lung lesions and radiographic abnormalities. Most, like tin, barium, and iron, are innocuous and simply accumulate in the lung. However, some lead to crippling lung diseases. The specific types of pneumoconioses are named by the substance inhaled (e.g., silicosis, asbestosis, talcosis). Sometimes, the offending agent is uncertain, and the occupation is simply cited (e.g., "arc welder's lung"), as before etiologies were identified, some occupations were known to predispose to lung disease. Thus, "knife grinder's lung" was used before the disease was recognized as silicosis.

 ETIOLOGIC FACTORS: *The key factor in the genesis of symptomatic pneumoconioses is the capacity of inhaled dusts to stimulate fibrosis* (Fig. 18-50). Thus, small amounts of silica produce extensive fibrosis, whereas coal and iron are only weakly fibrogenic.

In general, lung lesions produced by inorganic dusts reflect the dose and size of inhaled particles. The dose is a function of the concentration of dust in the air and the duration of exposure. As inhaled particles are often irregular, their size should be expressed as aerodynamic particle diameter, a parameter that describes the particle's motion in inspired air and that determines where inhaled dusts deposit in the lung (Fig. 18-2, Chapter 8). The most dangerous particles are those that reach the farthest periphery (i.e., the smallest bronchioles and acini). Particles 2.5 to 10 μm in diameter deposit on bronchi and bronchioles and are removed by mucociliary action. Smaller particles (<2.5 μm) reach acini, and the tiniest ones (<100 nm) may penetrate alveolar walls and enter the bloodstream.

Alveolar macrophages ingest inhaled particles and are the main defenders of the alveolar space. Most phagocytosed particles ascend to the mucociliary carpet, to be coughed up or swallowed. Others migrate into the lung interstitium, and thence into lymphatics. Many ingested particles accumulate in and about respiratory bronchioles and terminal bronchioles. Others are not phagocytosed but migrate through epithelial cells into the interstitium.

Silicosis Is Caused by Inhaled Silicon Dioxide (Silica)

The earth's crust is composed largely of silicon and its oxides, and silicosis is one of the oldest recorded diseases, possibly having begun in the Paleolithic period when humans began to fashion flint instruments. Dyspnea in metal diggers was reported by Hippocrates, and early Dutch pathologists wrote that the lungs of stone cutters sectioned like a mass of sand. The 19th-century English literature provided numerous descriptions of silicosis, and the disease remained the major cause of death in workers exposed to silica dust for the first half of the 20th century.

Silicosis was first described as a disease of sandblasters, but exposure to silica occurs in many occupations, including mining, stone cutting, polishing and sharpening of metals, ceramic manufacturing, foundry work, and cleaning of boilers. The use of air-handling equipment and face masks has substantially reduced the incidence of silicosis. Nevertheless, its incidence has increased lately in coal miners who must cut through more quartz to reach ever diminishing seams of coal.

 ETIOLOGIC FACTORS: The biologic effects of silica particles depend on a number of factors, some involving the particle itself and others related to the host response. Crystalline silica (quartz) is more toxic than amorphous forms, and its biologic activity is related to its surface properties. Particles of 0.2 to 2.0 μm are the most dangerous. Removal of the soluble surface layer by acid washing or creation of new surfaces by sandblasting enhances the biologic activity of silica particles.

After their inhalation, silica particles are ingested by alveolar macrophages. Silicon hydroxide groups on the particles' surface form hydrogen bonds with phospholipids and proteins. This interaction damages cellular membranes and so kills the macrophages. The dead cells release free silica particles and fibrogenic factors. The released silica is then reingested by macrophages and the process is amplified.

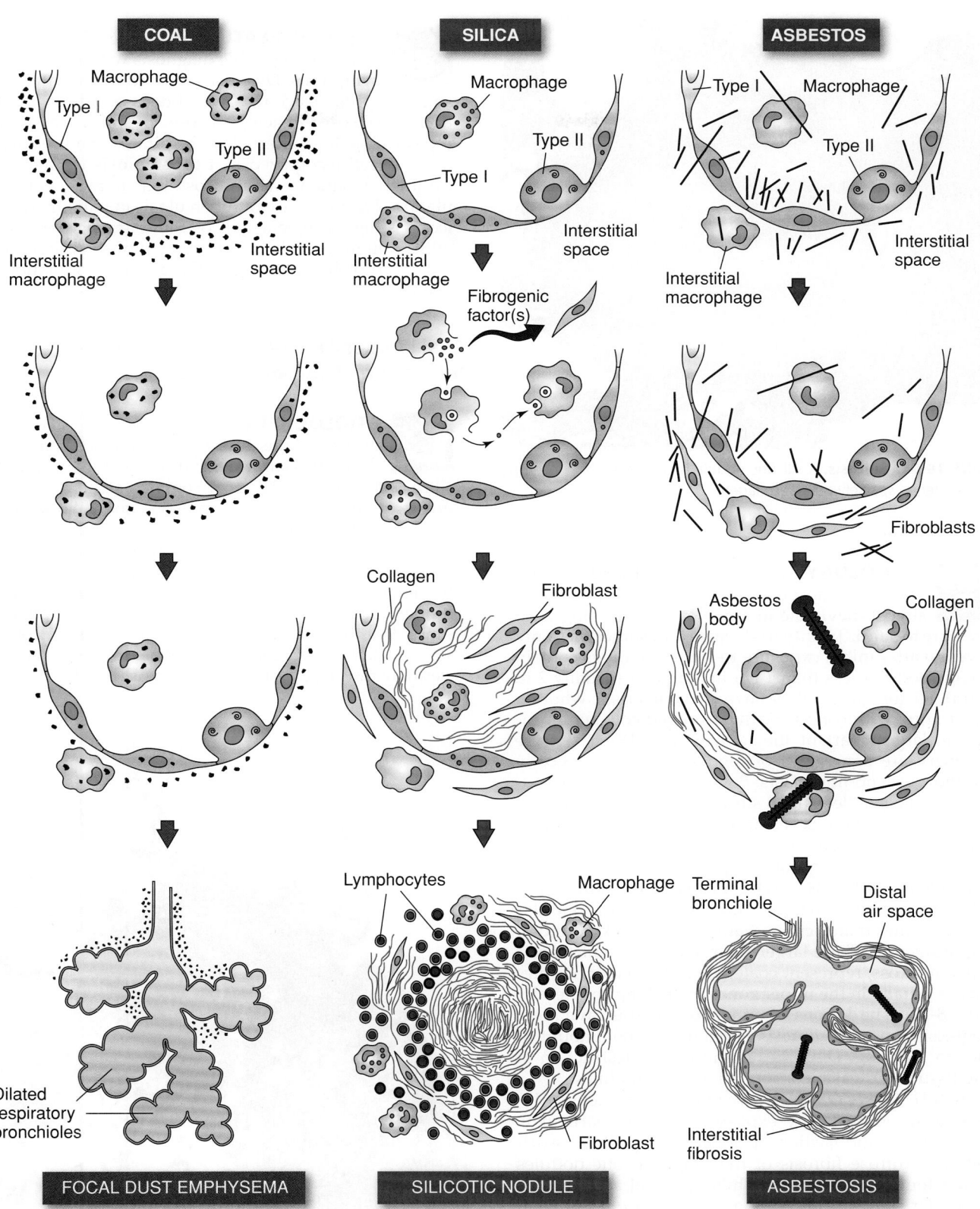

FIGURE 18-50. Pathogenesis of pneumoconioses. The three most important pneumoconioses are illustrated. In simple coal workers' pneumoconiosis, massive amounts of dust are inhaled and engulfed by macrophages. The macrophages pass into the interstitium of the lung and aggregate around respiratory bronchioles, which subsequently dilate. In silicosis, silica particles are toxic to macrophages, causing them to die and release fibrogenic factors. In turn, the released silica is again phagocytosed by other macrophages. The result is a dense fibrotic nodule, the silicotic nodule. Asbestosis is characterized by considerable interstitial fibrosis. Asbestos bodies are the classic features.

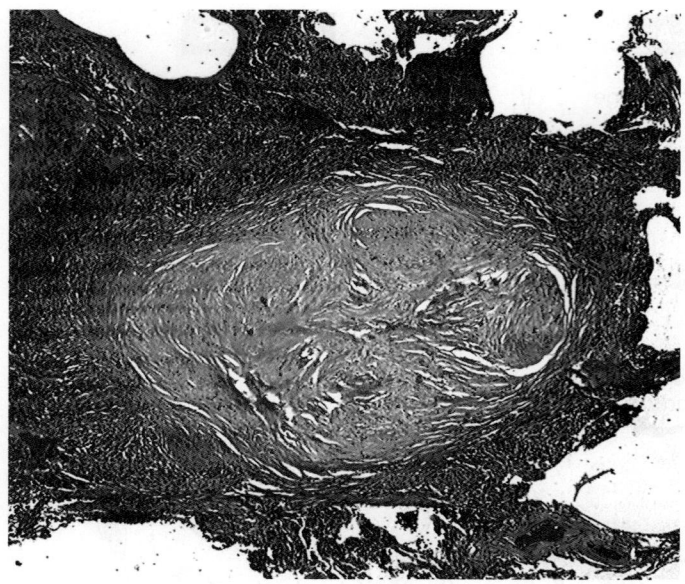

FIGURE 18-51. Silicosis. A silicotic nodule is composed of concentric whorls of dense, sparsely cellular collagen.

 PATHOLOGY: *SIMPLE NODULAR SILICOSIS:* This is the most common form of silicosis and is almost inevitable in any worker with long-term exposure to silica. Twenty to 40 years (but sometimes only 10 years) after initial exposure to silica, the lungs contain silicotic nodules less than 1 cm in diameter (usually 2 to 4 mm). Histologically, they have a characteristic whorled appearance, with concentrically arranged collagen forming the largest part of the nodule (Fig. 18-51). At the periphery are aggregates of mononuclear cells, mostly lymphocytes and fibroblasts. Polarized light reveals doubly refractile needle-shaped silicates within the nodule.

Hilar nodes may be enlarged and calcified, often at their edges ("eggshell calcification"). Simple silicosis does not usually impair respiration significantly.

PROGRESSIVE MASSIVE FIBROSIS: Radiographically, progressive massive fibrosis signifies nodular masses greater than 2 cm in diameter, in a background of simple silicosis. These larger lesions, most of which are 5 to 10 cm across, represent coalescence of smaller nodules and are usually in the upper zones of the lungs bilaterally (Fig. 18-52). The lesions often exhibit central cavitation. Progressive massive fibrosis is related to the amount of silica in the lung. Disability is caused by destruction of lung tissue that was incorporated into the nodules.

ACUTE SILICOSIS: Now uncommon, acute silicosis results from heavy exposure to finely particulate silica during sandblasting or boiler scaling. It is associated with diffuse fibrosis of the lung. Silicotic nodules are not found. Dense eosinophilic material accumulates in alveolar spaces to produce an appearance resembling alveolar lipoproteinosis **(silicoproteinosis).** The disease progresses rapidly over a few years, unlike other forms of silicosis in which progression is measured in decades. Radiographically, acute silicosis shows diffuse linear fibrosis and reduced lung volume. Clinically, there is a severe restrictive defect.

CLINICAL FEATURES: Simple silicosis is usually a radiographic diagnosis without significant symptoms. Dyspnea on exertion and later at rest suggests progressive massive fibrosis or other complications of silicosis. In acute silicosis, dyspnea may become rapidly disabling, after which respiratory failure ensues.

It is well recognized that **tuberculosis** is much more common in patients with silicosis than in the general population. The incidence of tuberculosis in patients with silicosis is higher in acute silicosis and among populations with a high prevalence of tuberculosis. Although the incidence of tuberculosis in the general population has declined, the association with silicosis persists.

Coal Workers' Pneumoconiosis Is due to Inhalation of Carbon Particles

ETIOLOGIC FACTORS: Coal dust is composed of amorphous carbon and other constituents of the earth's surface, including variable amounts of silica. Anthracite (hard) coal contains significantly more quartz than does bituminous (soft) coal. Workers who inhale large amounts of quartz particles, such as those who work within mines, are at greater risk than those working above ground or loading coal for transport. In this context, amorphous carbon by itself is not fibrogenic. It does not kill alveolar macrophages, but is simply a nuisance dust that causes innocuous anthracosis. By contrast, silica is highly fibrogenic, and inhaled anthracotic particles may thus lead to **anthracosilicosis** (Fig. 18-53).

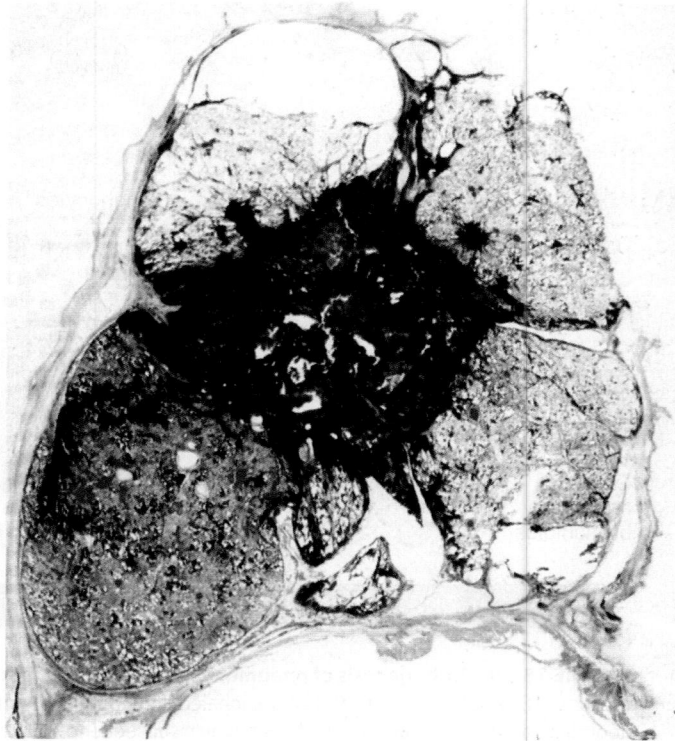

FIGURE 18-52. Progressive massive fibrosis. A whole mount of a silicotic lung from a coal miner shows a large area of dense fibrosis containing entrapped carbon particles.

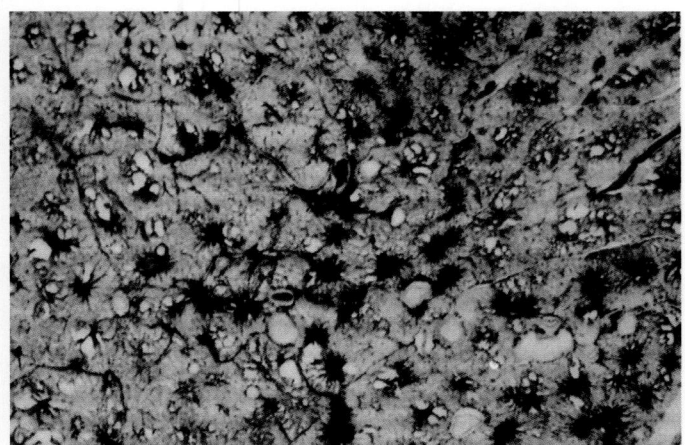

FIGURE 18-53. Anthracosilicosis. A whole mount of the lung of a coal miner demonstrates scattered, irregular, pigmented nodules throughout the parenchyma.

 PATHOLOGY: Coal workers' pneumoconiosis (CWP) is typically divided into **simple CWP** and **complicated CWP** (a.k.a. progressive massive fibrosis). The typical lung lesions of simple CWP include nonpalpable **coal-dust macules** and palpable **coal-dust nodules,** both of which are multiple and scattered throughout the lung as 1- to 4-mm black foci. Microscopically, coal-dust macules contain many carbon-laden macrophages, which surround distal respiratory bronchioles, extend to fill adjacent alveolar spaces and infiltrate peribronchiolar interstitial spaces. Respiratory bronchioles may be mildly dilated (focal dust emphysema), probably owing to atrophy of smooth muscle.

Nodules are round or irregular, and may or may not be associated with bronchioles. They consist of dust-laden macrophages associated with a fibrotic stroma. They occur when coal is admixed with fibrogenic dusts such as silica, and are more properly classified as anthracosilicosis (Fig. 18-53). Coal-dust macules and nodules appear on chest radiographs as small nodular densities. Simple CWP was once thought to cause severe disability, but it is now clear that at worst it causes minor impairment of lung function. If coal miners have severe airflow obstruction, it is usually due to smoking. **Complicated CWP** occurs on a background of simple CWP and is defined by the presence of a lesion 2.0 cm or greater in size. It may cause significant respiratory impairment.

Caplan syndrome was first described as rheumatoid nodules (**Caplan nodules**) in the lungs of coal miners with rheumatoid arthritis. However, it now also refers to the association of pulmonary rheumatoid nodules with other pneumoconioses, such as silicosis or asbestosis. The nodular lesions are large (1 to 10 cm), multiple, bilateral, and usually peripheral. Microscopically, they resemble rheumatoid nodules associated with inhaled dust deposits. True rheumatoid nodules have large, central necrotic areas with a border of chronic inflammation and palisading macrophages (see Chapters 11 and 30). Caplan nodules are not identical to rheumatoid nodules and may represent a combination of silicotic and rheumatoid nodules.

Asbestos-Related Diseases May Be Reactive or Neoplastic

Asbestos (Greek, "unquenchable") includes a group of fibrous silicate minerals that occur as thin fibers. It has been used for diverse purposes for over 4,000 years, since early Finns fashioned pottery from it. Roman vestal virgins used it to manufacture oil-lamp wicks, and Marco Polo remarked that asbestos-containing Chinese cloth resisted fire. More recently, asbestos has been used in insulation, construction materials, and automotive brake linings. Asbestos mining proceeded exponentially in the 20th century until its deleterious effects eventually elicited alarm.

There are six natural types of asbestos, which can be divided into two mineralogic groups. **Chrysotile** accounts for the bulk of commercially used asbestos. The other group called **amphiboles** include amosite, crocidolite, tremolite, actinolite, and anthophyllite. Of the amphiboles, only amosite and crocidolite have been used commercially to any significant extent. Erionite, a fibrous zeolite found in Turkey and adjacent areas, has pathogenic properties similar to the amphiboles. Exposure to asbestos can cause *asbestosis, benign pleural effusion, pleural plaques, diffuse pleural fibrosis, rounded atelectasis,* and *mesothelioma* (Table 18-4). All commercially used forms of asbestos are associated with lung diseases, but the amphiboles, and crocidolite in particular, have a much greater propensity to produce disease than does chrysotile.

ASBESTOSIS: Asbestosis is diffuse interstitial fibrosis resulting from inhalation of asbestos fibers. Development of asbestosis requires heavy exposure to asbestos of the type historically seen in asbestos miners, millers, and insulators.

ETIOLOGIC FACTORS: Although asbestos fibers may be long (up to 100 μm), they are thin (0.5 to 1 μm) so their aerodynamic particle diameter is small. They deposit in distal airways and alveoli, particularly at bifurcations of alveolar ducts. The smallest particles are engulfed by macrophages, but many larger fibers penetrate into the interstitial space. They first cause an alveolitis that is directly related to asbestos exposure. Subsequent release of inflammatory mediators by activated macrophages and the fibrogenic character of the free asbestos fibers in the interstitium promote interstitial pulmonary fibrosis.

TABLE 18-4
ASBESTOS-RELATED LUNG DISEASE

Pleural Lesions
   Benign pleural effusion
   Parietal pleural plaques
   Diffuse pleural fibrosis
   Rounded atelectasis

Interstitial Lung Disease
   Asbestosis

Malignant Mesothelioma
   Carcinoma of the lung (in smokers)

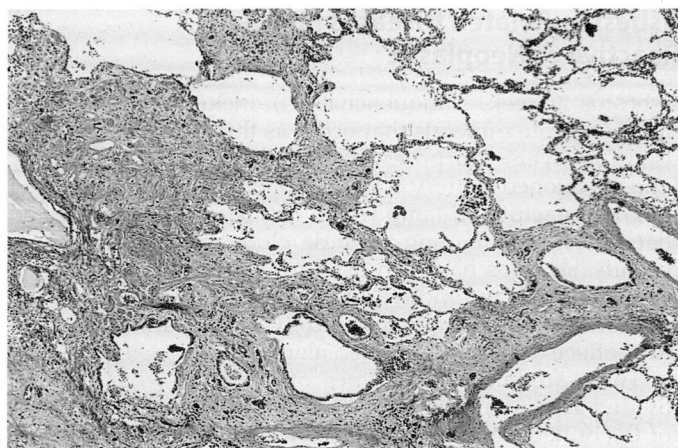

FIGURE 18-54. Asbestosis. The lung shows patchy, dense, interstitial fibrosis.

PATHOLOGY: Asbestosis is characterized by bilateral, diffuse interstitial fibrosis and asbestos bodies in the lung (Figs. 18-54 and 18-55). In early stages, fibrosis occurs in and around alveolar ducts and respiratory bronchioles, and in the periphery of the acinus. When the fibers deposit in bronchioles and respiratory bronchioles, they incite a fibrogenic response that leads to mild chronic airflow obstruction. Thus, asbestos may produce obstructive as well as restrictive defects. As the disease progresses, fibrosis spreads beyond the peribronchiolar location and eventually results in an end-stage or "honeycomb" lung. Asbestosis is usually more severe in the lower zones of the lung.

Asbestos bodies are found in the walls of bronchioles or within alveolar spaces, often engulfed by alveolar macrophages. The particles have a distinctive morphology, consisting of a clear, thin asbestos fiber (10 to 50 µm long) surrounded by a beaded iron–protein coat. By light microscopy, they are golden brown (Fig. 18-55) and react strongly with the Prussian blue stain for iron. The fibers are only partly engulfed by macrophages because they are too large for a single cell. The macrophages coat the asbestos fiber with protein, proteoglycans, and ferritin.

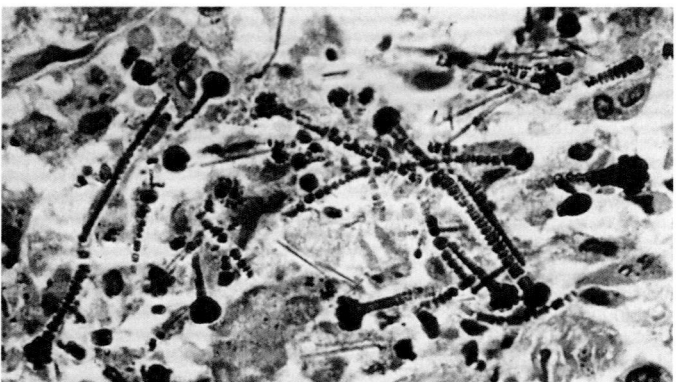

FIGURE 18-55. Asbestos bodies. These ferruginous bodies contain central, colorless, nonbirefringent core asbestos fibers. They are encrusted with protein and iron, which gives them their characteristic golden brown color and beaded appearance. (Courtesy of the Armed Forces Institute of Pathology.)

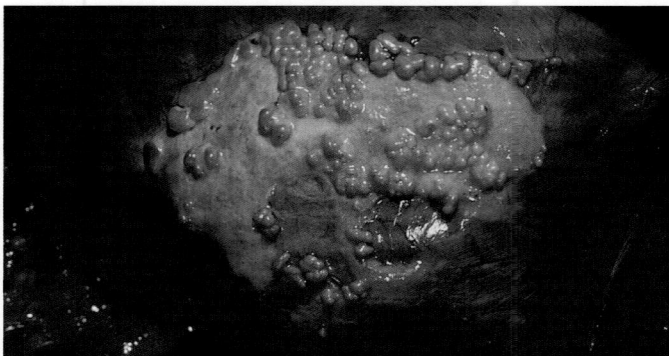

FIGURE 18-56. Pleural plaque. The dome of the diaphragm is covered by a pearly white, nodular plaque.

Finding asbestos bodies incidentally at autopsy does not warrant a diagnosis of asbestosis; the lungs must also show diffuse interstitial fibrosis. Digests and concentrates of autopsy lungs demonstrate asbestos bodies to varying degrees in the lungs of virtually all adults.

BENIGN PLEURAL EFFUSION: Benign pleural effusion associated with asbestos inhalation is diagnosed by (1) a history of asbestos exposure, (2) identification of a pleural effusion with radiographs or thoracentesis, (3) absence of other diseases that could cause effusion, and (4) no malignant tumor after 3 years of follow-up. Pleural effusions often occur within 10 years of initial exposure and are seen in about 3% of workers exposed to asbestos.

PLEURAL PLAQUES: Pleural plaques, mainly on parietal and diaphragmatic pleura, occur 10 to 20 years after exposure to asbestos. They presumably arise in response to asbestos fibers that have gained access to the pleural space, possibly via lymphatics. They may be found in up to 15% of the general population, and half of all patients with plaques at autopsy may not have a known history of asbestos exposure. Plaques occur most often on the parietal pleura, in the posterolateral regions of the lower thorax and on the domes of the diaphragm.

Grossly, pleural plaques are pearly white and have a smooth or nodular surface (Fig. 18-56). They are usually bilateral, but not necessarily symmetric. Plaques may measure over 10 cm in diameter and become calcified. Histologically, they consist of dense, acellular hyalinized fibrous tissue, with numerous slit-like spaces in a parallel fashion ("basket-weave pattern"). Pleural plaques are not predictors of asbestosis, nor do they evolve into mesotheliomas.

DIFFUSE PLEURAL FIBROSIS: Fibrosis limited to the pleura is usually detected at least 10 years after the initial exposure and should be distinguished from asbestosis, in which fibrosis affects the interstitium of the underlying lung diffusely.

ROUNDED ATELECTASIS: Asbestosis exposure occasionally leads to pleural fibrosis and adhesions associated with atelectasis, which has a rounded appearance on chest radiograph. Radiographically, rounded atelectasis is characterized by a pleural-based, rounded or oval, 2.5- to 5-cm shadow, which usually lies along the posterior surface of a lower lobe. Pathologically, the lung shows pleural fibrosis or plaques, with curved pleural invaginations extending several centimeters into the underlying parenchyma. The condition is clinically benign.

MESOTHELIOMA: The relation between asbestos exposure and malignant mesothelioma is firmly established. Sometimes exposure is indirect (e.g., wives of asbestos workers who wash their husbands' clothes). More often, mesothelioma is seen in workers with significant occupational exposure to asbestos, mainly crocidolite and amosite. This malignancy is discussed below with diseases of the pleura.

CARCINOMA OF THE LUNG: There are reports that lung cancer is more common in nonsmoking asbestos workers than in similar workers not exposed to asbestos, but data are limited and no firm conclusion is possible at this point. However, in asbestos workers who smoke, the incidence of carcinoma of the lung is vastly increased: up to 40 to 60 times that of the general nonsmoking population. The link between asbestos and lung cancer is most convincingly supported in the presence of asbestosis (diffuse interstitial fibrosis).

Berylliosis Is Characterized by Noncaseating Granulomas

Berylliosis refers to the pulmonary disease that follows the inhalation of beryllium. Today this metal is used principally in structural materials in aerospace, industrial ceramics, and nuclear industries. Exposure to beryllium may also occur in those who mine and extract beryllium ores.

PATHOLOGY: Berylliosis may occur as an acute chemical pneumonitis or a chronic pneumoconiosis. In the acute form, symptoms begin within hours or days after inhalation of metal particles and manifest pathologically as DAD. Of all patients with acute beryllium pneumonitis, 10% progress to chronic disease, although chronic berylliosis is often observed in workers without a history of an acute illness.

Chronic berylliosis differs from other pneumoconioses in that the inciting exposure may be brief and minimal. The lesion is thus suspected to be a hypersensitivity reaction. Pulmonary lesions are indistinguishable from those of sarcoidosis (see below). Multiple noncaseating granulomas are distributed along the pleura, septa, and bronchovascular bundles (Fig. 18-57). The beryllium lymphocyte

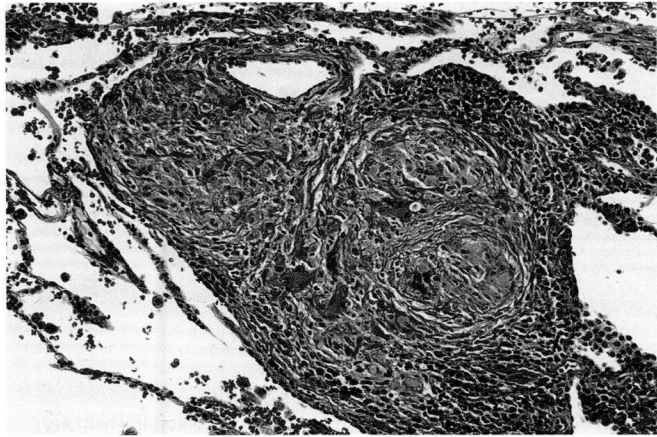

FIGURE 18-57. Berylliosis. A noncaseating granuloma consists of a nodular collection of epithelioid macrophages and multinucleated giant cells.

proliferation test (demonstration of beryllium sensitization by proliferation of isolated peripheral blood lymphocytes incubated with beryllium) may aid in separating these two entities. The disease may progress to end-stage fibrosis and **honeycomb lung** (see below). Patients with chronic berylliosis experience insidious onset of dyspnea 15 or more years after the initial exposure. The disease appears to be associated with an increased risk of lung cancer.

Talcosis Results From Prolonged and Heavy Exposure to Talc Dust

Talc consists of magnesium silicates that are used in several industries as lubricants, and in cosmetics and pharmaceuticals. Occupational exposure to talc occurs among workers engaged in mining and milling the mineral and in the leather, rubber, paper, and textile industries. Industrial talcs may include other minerals such as tremolite asbestos or silica. Cosmetic talc is more than 90% pure and rarely causes lung disease.

PATHOLOGY: Talcosis lesions vary from tiny nodules to severe fibrosis. Foreign body granulomas associated with birefringent plate-like talc particles are scattered throughout the parenchyma, which displays fibrotic nodules and interstitial fibrosis. Associated minerals such as silica may contribute to the fibrotic changes.

People who inject illicit drugs that include talc as a carrier may develop vascular and interstitial granulomas in the lung and variable fibrosis. Arterial changes of pulmonary hypertension are common and may be associated with cor pulmonale.

INTERSTITIAL LUNG DISEASE

Many pulmonary disorders are characterized by interstitial inflammatory infiltrates and have similar clinical and radiographic presentations, and so are grouped as interstitial, infiltrative, or restrictive diseases. These may be acute or chronic and of known or unknown etiology. They vary from minimally symptomatic to severely incapacitating and lethal interstitial fibrosis. Restrictive lung diseases are characterized by decreased lung volume and decreased oxygen-diffusing capacity on pulmonary function studies.

Hypersensitivity Pneumonitis Is a Response to Inhaled Antigens

Inhalation of many antigens leads to hypersensitivity pneumonitis (also called extrinsic allergic alveolitis), with acute or chronic interstitial inflammation in the lung. Most such antigens are encountered in occupational settings, and resulting diseases are labeled accordingly: **farmer's lung** occurs in people exposed to *Micropolyspora faeni* from moldy hay; **bagassosis** results from exposure to *Thermoactinomyces sacchari* in moldy sugar cane; **maple bark–stripper's disease** follows exposure to the fungus *Cryptostroma corticale* in moldy maple bark; and **bird fancier's lung** affects bird keepers with long-term exposure to proteins from bird feathers, blood, and excrement. Other causes of hypersensitivity pneumonitis include inhalation of pituitary snuff (**pituitary snuff taker's disease**), moldy cork (**suberosis**), and moldy

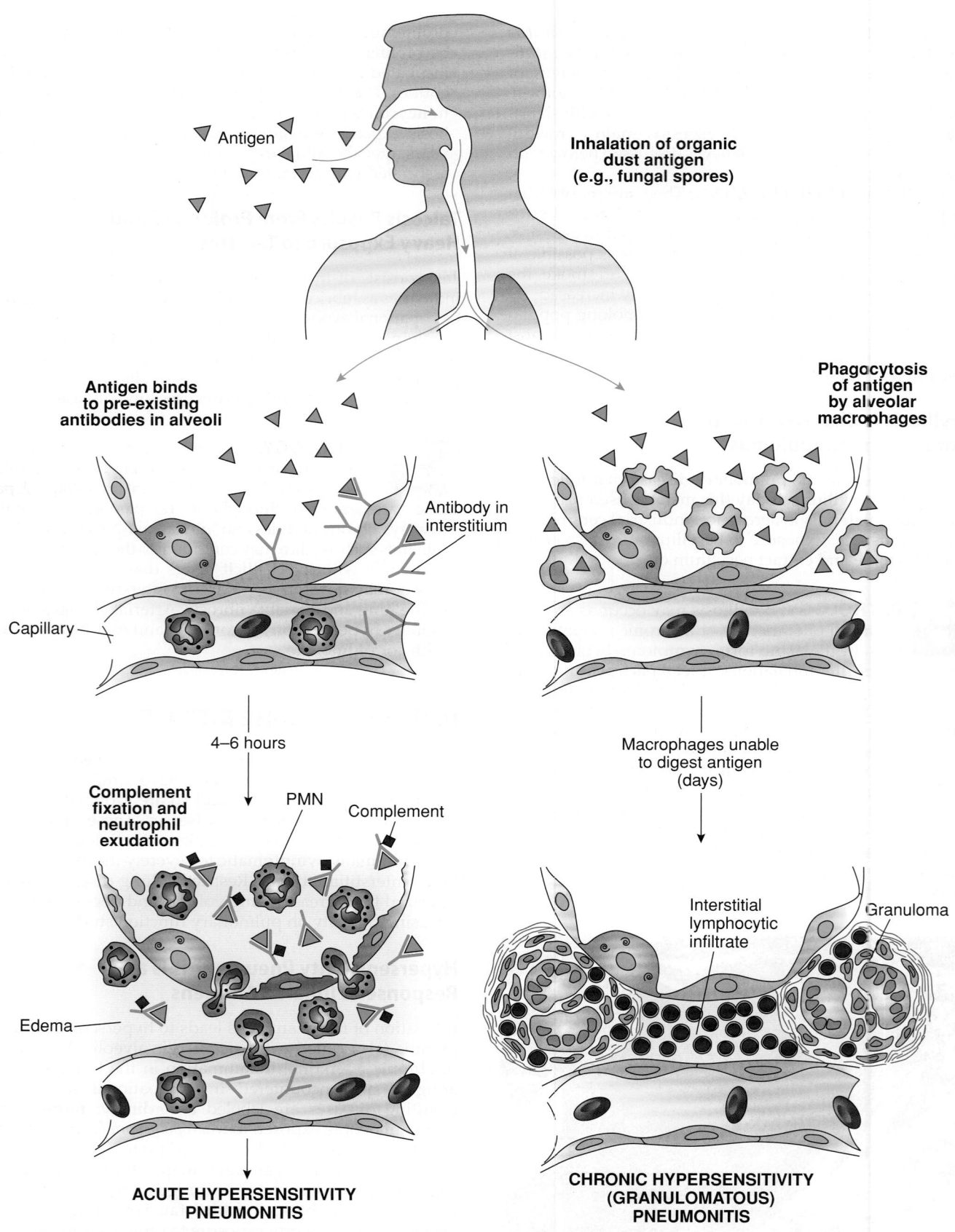

FIGURE 18-58. Hypersensitivity pneumonitis. An antigen–antibody reaction occurs in the acute phase and leads to acute hypersensitivity pneumonitis. Continued exposure is followed by a cellular or subacute phase, with formation of granulomas and chronic interstitial pneumonitis. *PMN* = polymorphonuclear neutrophil.

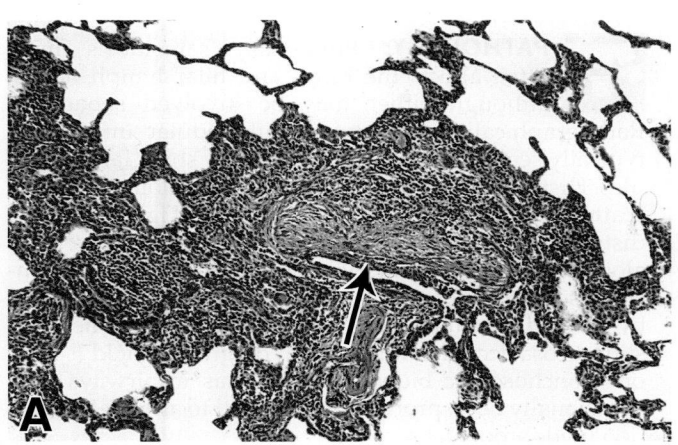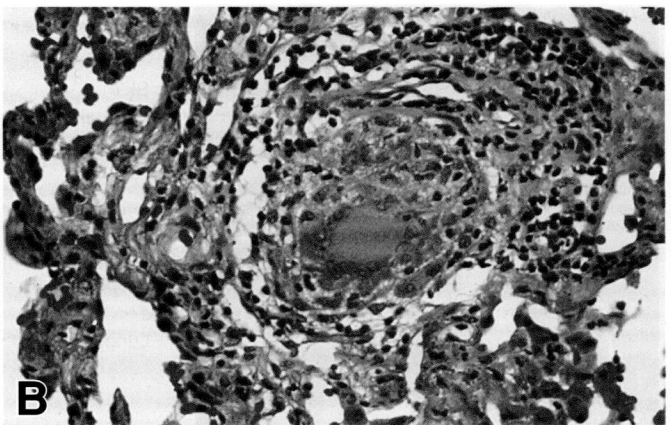

FIGURE 18-59. Hypersensitivity pneumonitis. A. A lung biopsy shows a mild peribronchiolar chronic inflammatory interstitial infiltrate, with a focus of intraluminal organizing fibrosis (*arrow*). **B.** Focal poorly formed granulomas were scattered in the lung biopsy specimen.

compost (**mushroom worker's disease**). Hypersensitivity pneumonitis may also be caused by fungi that grow in stagnant water in air conditioners, swimming pools, hot tubs, and central heating units. Skin tests and serum precipitating antibodies are used to confirm the diagnosis. Often, however, an inciting antigen is never identified, especially in chronic hypersensitivity pneumonitis. In acute cases, the diagnosis is usually established clinically, so lung biopsies are performed only in chronic cases.

PATHOPHYSIOLOGY: Acute hypersensitivity pneumonitis is characterized by neutrophilic infiltrates in alveoli and respiratory bronchioles; chronic lesions show mononuclear cells and granulomas, typical of delayed hypersensitivity. Most cases have serum IgG precipitating antibodies against the offending agent. Hypersensitivity pneumonitis represents a combination of immune complex–mediated (type III) and cell-mediated (type IV) hypersensitivity reactions, although the precise contribution of each is still debated (Fig. 18-58). Importantly, most people who have serum precipitins to inhaled antigens do not develop hypersensitivity pneumonitis, suggesting a genetic component in host susceptibility.

PATHOLOGY: The histology in florid cases of chronic hypersensitivity pneumonitis is virtually diagnostic. However, in subtle cases, the diagnosis may require careful clinical and radiographic correlation, and even then it may remain tentative. Microscopic features of chronic hypersensitivity pneumonitis are bronchiolocentric cellular interstitial pneumonia, noncaseating granulomas, and organizing pneumonia (Fig. 18-59A,B). The bronchiolocentric cellular interstitial infiltrate consists of lymphocytes, plasma cells, and macrophages and varies from severe to subtle; eosinophils are uncommon. Poorly formed noncaseating granulomas are seen in two-thirds of cases (Fig. 18-59B), as is organizing pneumonia (Fig. 18-59A). In the end stage, interstitial inflammation recedes, leaving pulmonary fibrosis, which may resemble usual interstitial pneumonia.

CLINICAL FEATURES: Hypersensitivity pneumonitis may present as acute, subacute, or chronic pulmonary disease, depending on the frequency and intensity of exposure to the offending antigen. Farmer's lung, the prototype of hypersensitivity pneumonitis, is caused by inhaling thermophilic actinomycetes from moldy hay. Typically, a farm worker enters a barn where hay has been stored for winter feeding. After a lag period of 4 to 6 hours, he or she rapidly develops dyspnea, cough, and mild fever. Symptoms remit within 24 to 48 hours but return on reexposure; with time, the disorder becomes chronic. Patients with chronic hypersensitivity pneumonitis have a more nonspecific presentation, with a gradual onset of dyspnea and cor pulmonale.

Pulmonary function studies show a restrictive pattern, with decreased compliance, reduced diffusion capacity, and hypoxemia. In the chronic stage, airway obstruction may be troublesome. Bronchoalveolar fluid contains increased T lymphocytes, mostly CD8+ suppressor/cytotoxic cells. Removing the offending antigen is the only adequate treatment for hypersensitivity pneumonitis. Steroid therapy may be effective in acute forms and for some chronically affected patients.

Sarcoidosis Is a Granulomatous Disease of Unknown Etiology

The lung is the organ most often involved, but lymph nodes, skin, eye, heart, and other organs are also common targets (Fig. 18-60).

EPIDEMIOLOGY: Sarcoidosis occurs worldwide and affects all races and both sexes, but with strong racial and ethnic predilections. In North America, it is much more common among blacks than whites (15:1), but it is uncommon in tropical Africa. In Scandinavian countries, its prevalence is 64 in 100,000, but is 10 in 100,000 in France and 3 in 100,000 in Poland; among Irish women in London, its prevalence is an astonishing 200 in 100,000. Sarcoidosis is distinctly uncommon in China.

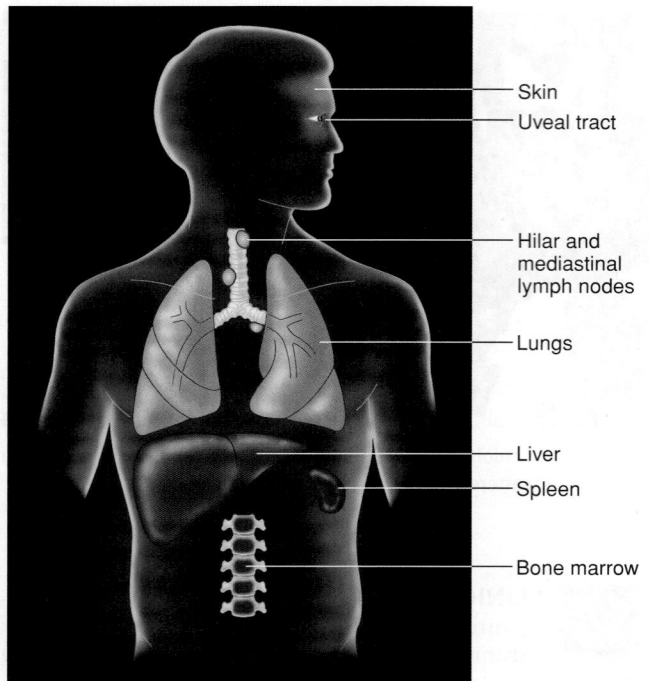

FIGURE 18-60. Organs commonly affected by sarcoidosis. Sarcoidosis involves many organs, most commonly the lymph nodes and lung.

PATHOPHYSIOLOGY: The pathogenesis of sarcoidosis remains obscure, but there is a consensus that helper/inducer T-lymphocyte responses to exogenous or autologous antigens are exaggerated. These cells accumulate in affected organs, where they secrete lymphokines and recruit macrophages, which help form noncaseating granulomas. CD4+:CD8+ T-cell ratios are 10:1 in organs with sarcoid granulomas, but are 2:1 in uninvolved tissues. Why helper/inducer T lymphocytes accumulate is unclear. A defect in suppressor cell function may permit unopposed helper cell proliferation. Inherited or acquired differences in immune response genes may favor one type of T-cell response over another. Nonspecific polyclonal activation of B cells by T-helper cells leads to hyperglobulinemia, a characteristic feature of active sarcoidosis.

PATHOLOGY: Pulmonary sarcoidosis most often affects the lungs and hilar lymph nodes, although either may be involved separately. Radiographically, a diffuse reticulonodular infiltrate is typically seen, but occasional cases may show larger nodules. Histologically, multiple sarcoid granulomas are seen scattered in the interstitium of the lung (Fig. 18-61). The distribution is distinctive with preferential involvement along the pleura and interlobular septa and around bronchovascular bundles (Fig. 18-61A). Frequent infiltration by sarcoid granulomas of the bronchial or bronchiolar submucosa accounts for the high diagnostic yield (~90%) on bronchoscopic biopsy. Granulomas in airways may occasionally be so prominent as to lead to airway obstruction (endobronchial sarcoid).

The granulomatous phase of sarcoidosis can progress to a fibrotic phase. Fibrosis often begins at the periphery of a granuloma and may show an onion-skin pattern of lamellar fibrosis around the giant cells. Significant necrosis is uncommon, but one-third of open lung biopsies show small foci of necrosis. Interstitial chronic inflammation tends to be inconspicuous. Granulomatous vasculitis is seen in two-thirds of open lung biopsies from patients with sarcoidosis. Although **asteroid bodies** (star-shaped crystals) (Fig. 18-61B) and **Schaumann bodies** (small lamellar calcifications) are commonly encountered, they are not specific for sarcoidosis and may be seen in most granulomatous processes.

Interstitial fibrosis is not prominent in pulmonary sarcoidosis. However, progressive pulmonary fibrosis leads to honeycomb lung, respiratory insufficiency, and cor pulmonale.

CLINICAL FEATURES: Sarcoidosis is most common in young adults of both sexes. **Acute sarcoidosis** has an abrupt onset, usually followed by spontaneous remission within 2 years and an excellent response to steroids. **Chronic sarcoidosis** begins insidiously, and patients are more likely to have persistent or progressive disease. Sarcoidosis causes several chest radiographic patterns, the most classic of which is bilateral hilar adenopathy, with or without interstitial pulmonary

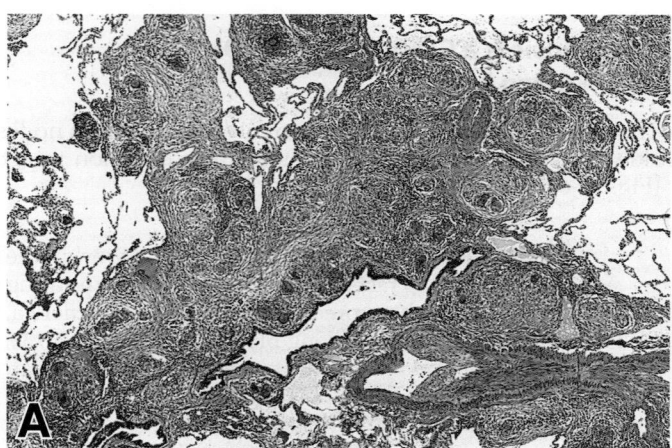
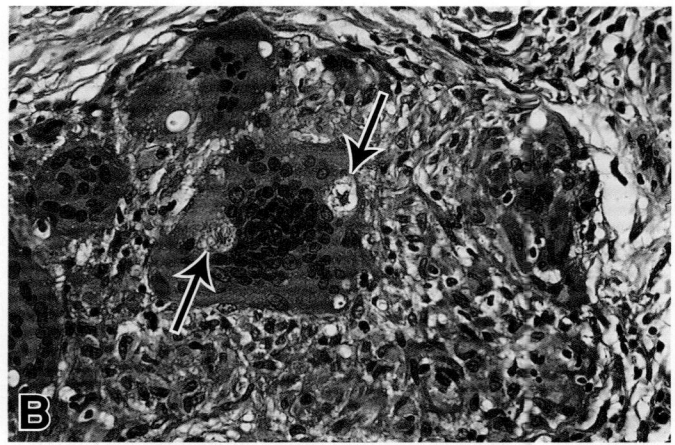

FIGURE 18-61. Sarcoidosis. A. Multiple noncaseating granulomas are present along the bronchovascular interstitium. **B.** Noncaseating granulomas consist of tight clusters of epithelioid macrophages and multinucleated giant cells. Several asteroid bodies are present (*arrows*).

infiltrates. It may also affect the skin (erythema nodosum), mostly in women. Black patients tend to have more severe uveitis, skin disease, and lacrimal gland involvement. Cough and dyspnea are the major respiratory complaints. However, the disease can be mild and may be discovered as an incidental finding on a chest radiograph in an asymptomatic patient.

No laboratory test is specific for the diagnosis of sarcoidosis. Transbronchial lung biopsy via a fiberoptic bronchoscope often reveals granulomas. Occasionally, the diagnosis is made by mediastinoscopy, identifying multiple noncaseating granulomas in a mediastinal lymph node. Bronchoalveolar lavage often shows an increase in the proportion of CD4+ T lymphocytes. Increased uptake of gallium-67, a material phagocytosed by activated macrophages, can demonstrate granulomatous areas. Serum angiotensin-converting enzyme (ACE) levels are elevated in two-thirds of patients with active sarcoidosis, and 24-hour urine calcium is frequently increased. These laboratory data, together with supportive clinical and radiologic findings, allow the diagnosis of sarcoidosis to be made with a high probability.

Other organs commonly involved include the skin, eye (uveal tract), heart (where it is associated with arrhythmias), central nervous system, extrathoracic lymph nodes, spleen, and liver (Fig. 18-60). These are discussed separately in individual chapters.

The prognosis in pulmonary sarcoidosis is favorable and most patients do not develop clinically significant sequelae. In 60% of patients, pulmonary sarcoidosis resolves, but this is less likely in older patients and those with extrathoracic disease, particularly in the bone and skin. In up to 20% of cases, sarcoidosis does not remit or recurs at intervals, but it leads to death in only 10% of cases. Corticosteroid therapy is effective for active sarcoidosis.

Usual Interstitial Pneumonia Is the Histologic Finding in Clinical Idiopathic Pulmonary Fibrosis

Usual interstitial pneumonia (UIP) is one of the most common types of interstitial pneumonia, with an annual incidence of 6 to 14 cases per 100,000 people. It has a slight male predominance and a mean age at onset of 50 to 60 years. UIP is the histologic pattern present on biopsy, and the clinical term **idiopathic pulmonary fibrosis** (IPF) is applied when the disease is determined to be of unknown origin.

ETIOLOGIC FACTORS: The etiology of IPF is unknown, but immunologic, viral, and genetic factors probably contribute. Some patients have histories of flu-like illnesses, suggesting viral involvement. Familial clusters of IPF, and association of UIP-like diseases in patients with inherited disorders such as neurofibromatosis and Hermansky–Pudlak syndrome, indicate that genetic factors contribute. Mutations in genes encoding telomerase reverse transcriptase (*TERT*), surfactant protein C and MUC5B are common in familial IPF but are implicated in less than one-third of cases. The genetic abnormality in most patients is unknown.

UIP histology accompanies autoimmune diseases, including rheumatoid arthritis, systemic lupus erythematosus, and progressive systemic sclerosis, in 20% of cases, suggesting impaired immunity. It also occurs with autoimmune disorders like Hashimoto thyroiditis, primary biliary cirrhosis, autoimmune hepatitis, idiopathic thrombocytopenic purpura, and myasthenia gravis. Autoantibodies (e.g., antinuclear antibodies and rheumatoid factor) and immune complexes are often found in blood, inflamed alveolar walls, and bronchoalveolar lavage fluids. No antigen has yet been identified. Activated alveolar macrophages may release cytokines, which recruit neutrophils. These in turn damage alveolar walls, stimulating a series of events that culminates in interstitial fibrosis.

PATHOLOGY: As emphasized above, UIP is a histologic pattern that occurs in several clinical settings (e.g., collagen vascular disease, chronic hypersensitivity pneumonitis, drug toxicity, and asbestosis). Many cases have no identifiable etiology and are so considered idiopathic (IPF). The lungs are small in UIP, and fibrosis tends to be worse in the lower lobes, in subpleural regions and along interlobular septa. Retraction of the scars, especially of lobular septa, gives the pleural surface of the lung a hobnail or cobblestone appearance, reminiscent of cirrhosis of the liver. Fibrosis is often patchy, with areas of dense scarring and honeycomb cystic change (Fig. 18-62A).

The histologic hallmark of UIP is patchy interstitial fibrosis, with areas of normal lung adjacent to fibrotic areas (Fig. 18-62B). The fibrosis is of different ages, which has been called "**temporal heterogeneity**." Areas of loose fibroblastic tissue (**fibroblast foci**) may be adjacent to dense collagen (Fig. 18-62C). The fibrosis is most pronounced beneath the pleura and adjacent to interlobular septa (Fig. 18-62B).

Bronchiolar epithelium grows into the dilated airspaces, which may be damaged but unrecognizable proximal respiratory bronchioles (Fig. 18-63). The areas of dense scarring fibrosis cause remodeling of the lung architecture, leading to alveolar wall collapse and formation of cystic spaces (Fig. 18-62A). These spaces are typically lined by bronchiolar or cuboidal epithelium and contain mucous, macrophages, or neutrophils. If such changes are extensive, the term "**honeycomb lung**" may be used to describe the gross cystic changes. Interstitial chronic inflammation is mild or moderate. Lymphoid aggregates, sometimes containing germinal centers, are occasionally noted, particularly in UIP associated with a collagen vascular disease such as rheumatoid arthritis. Extensive vascular changes of intimal fibrosis and medial thickening may be associated with pulmonary hypertension.

CLINICAL FEATURES: UIP begins insidiously, with gradual onset of dyspnea on exertion and dry cough, usually for 1 to 3 years. Patients have restrictive lung disease by pulmonary function testing. Finger clubbing is common, especially late in the disease. In half of patients, CT scans show distinctive peripheral, subpleural reticular opacities, traction bronchiectasis, and honeycombing, mostly in posterior lower lobes. These patients do not require surgical lung biopsy.

The classic auscultatory finding is late inspiratory crackles and fine ("Velcro") rales at the lung bases. Tachypnea at

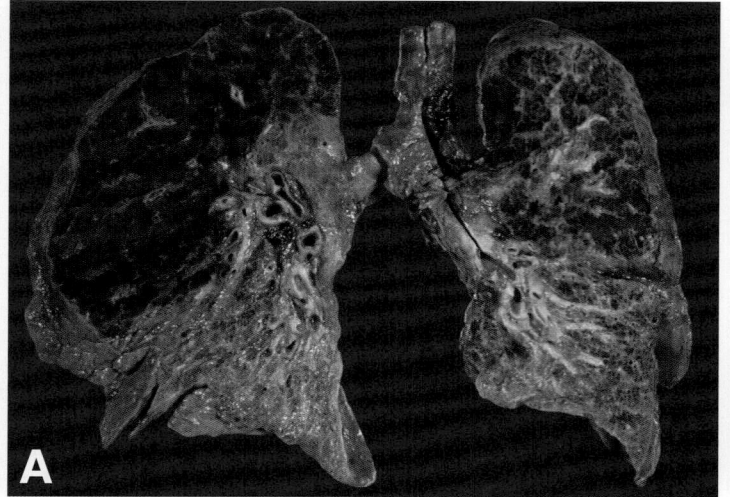

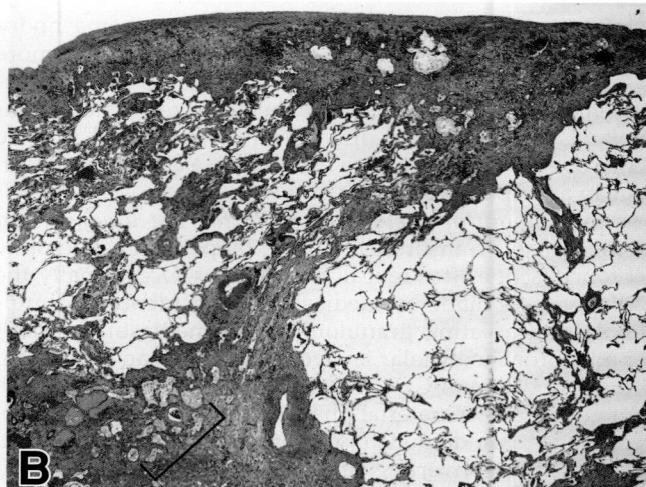

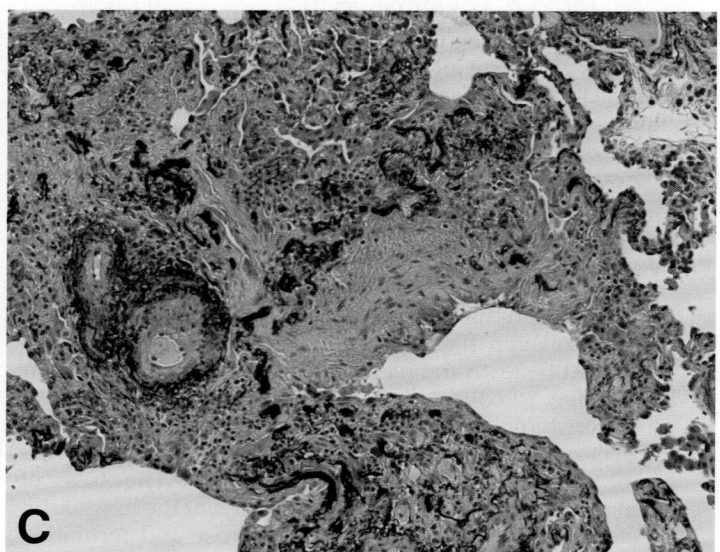

FIGURE 18-62. Usual interstitial pneumonitis. A. Grossly, the lungs show patchy dense scarring with extensive areas of honeycomb cystic change, predominantly affecting the lower lobes. This patient also had polymyositis. **B.** A microscopic view shows patchy subpleural fibrosis with microscopic honeycomb fibrosis (*bracket*). The areas of dense fibrosis display remodeling, with loss of the normal lung architecture. **C.** Elastin stain highlights the fibroblastic focus in green, which contrasts with the adjacent area of yellow staining of dense collagen and black staining of collapsed elastic fibers.

rest, cyanosis, and cor pulmonale eventually follow. The prognosis is bleak, with a mean survival of 4 to 6 years. Patients are treated with corticosteroids and sometimes cyclophosphamide, but lung transplantation generally offers the only hope of survival. Antifibrotic drugs pirfenidone and nintedanib that block signaling by TGF-β, fibroblast growth factor (FGF), and PDGF are FDA approved for slowing progression of disease.

Nonspecific Interstitial Pneumonia Has Multiple Etiologies

Nonspecific interstitial pneumonia (NSIP) is a histologic pattern that reflects diverse potential etiologies (infection, collagen vascular disease, hypersensitivity pneumonitis, drug reaction) or it may be idiopathic.

PATHOLOGY: NSIP shows a spectrum of **cellular** and **fibrosing patterns.** Unlike the patchy distribution and temporal heterogeneity of UIP, lung changes in NSIP are diffuse and uniform. In the

cellular form, alveolar septa are diffusely involved by a mild to moderate lymphocytic infiltrate. In the **fibrosing form,** septa show diffuse fibrosis, with or without significant associated inflammation. Honeycombing and fibroblastic foci are inconspicuous or absent.

CLINICAL FEATURES: In idiopathic NSIP, shortness of breath and cough develop over months to years. Computed tomography features are variable but mostly show bilateral lower lobe "ground glass" changes or reticulation with traction bronchiectasis. The prognosis of idiopathic NSIP is favorable compared to IPF; 5-year survival is 80%.

Desquamative Interstitial Pneumonia Is a Diffuse Lung Disease Seen Mostly in Smokers

Interstitial fibrosis is minimal in desquamative interstitial pneumonia (DIP) (Fig. 18-64A,B). The term "desquamative" is a misnomer based on the original idea that the intra-alveolar cells were desquamated epithelial cells. They are now

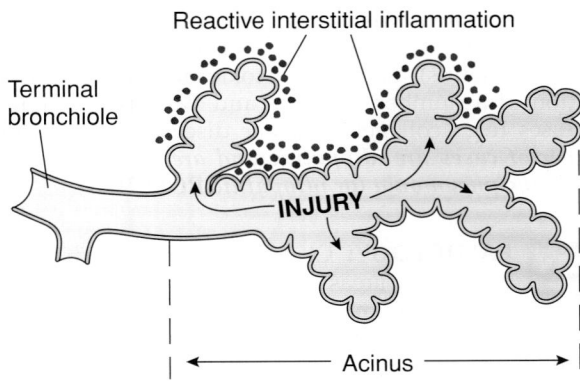

Reactive interstitial inflammation

Terminal bronchiole

INJURY

Acinus

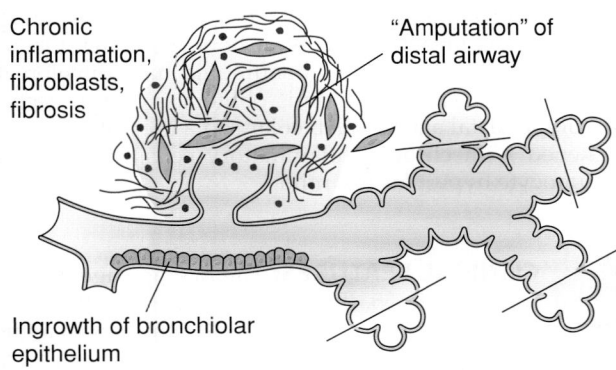

Chronic inflammation, fibroblasts, fibrosis

"Amputation" of distal airway

Ingrowth of bronchiolar epithelium

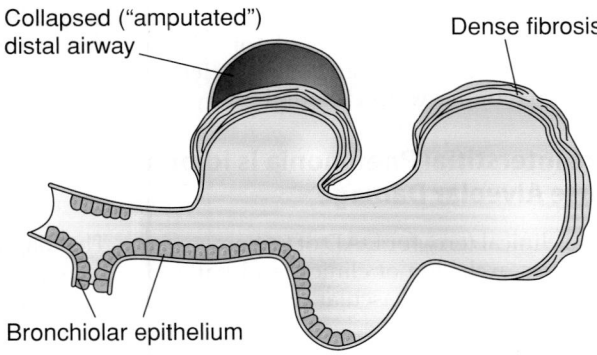

Collapsed ("amputated") distal airway

Dense fibrosis

Bronchiolar epithelium

FIGURE 18-63. Pathogenesis of honeycomb lung. Honeycomb lung is the result of a variety of injuries. Interstitial and alveolar inflammation destroys ("amputates") the distal part of the acinus. The proximal parts dilate and become lined by bronchiolar epithelium, and their walls become fibrotic.

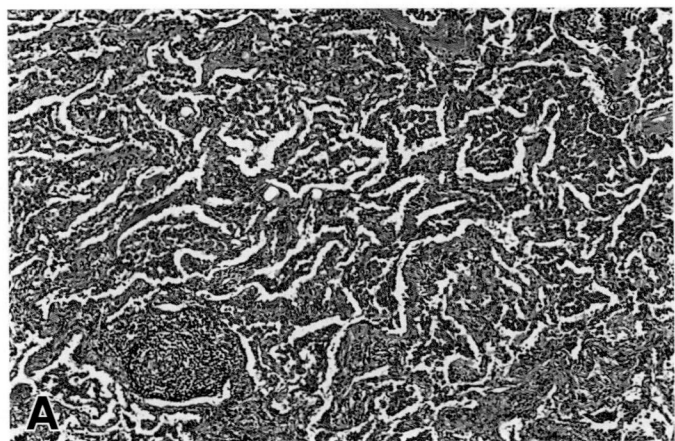

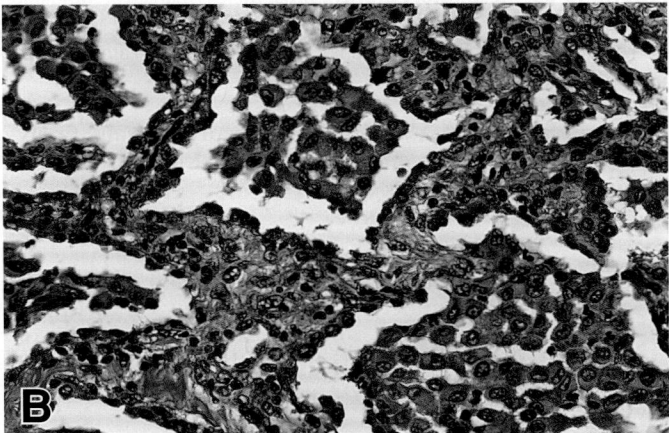

FIGURE 18-64. Desquamative interstitial pneumonia (DIP). A. This diffuse process in the lungs is characterized by accumulation of alveolar macrophages, preservation of alveolar architecture, and formation of lymphoid aggregates. **B.** There is also mild alveolar septal fibrosis, type II pneumocyte hyperplasia, and mild interstitial chronic inflammation.

recognized to be macrophages. In DIP, unlike UIP, alveolar architecture is preserved, and the disorder lacks the patchy scarring and remodeling of lung parenchyma seen in UIP. Alveolar walls in DIP may, however, be mildly thickened by chronic inflammation and interstitial fibrosis (Fig. 18-64B). Intra-alveolar macrophages contain a fine golden-brown pigment. Scattered lymphoid aggregates also may be present. Hyperplasia of type II pneumocytes is often prominent.

DIP occurs almost exclusively in cigarette smokers, typically in the fourth or fifth decade, and is twice as common in men as in women. Probably, DIP and respiratory bronchiolitis–interstitial lung disease (ILD) (see below) are a spectrum of disease related to cigarette smoking, although the

mechanism is unclear. The radiographic picture of DIP is not specific but most often shows bilateral lower lobe ground glass infiltrates. DIP has a much better prognosis than UIP, with an overall 10-year survival between 70% and 100%. Most patients respond well to steroid therapy and smoking cessation.

Respiratory Bronchiolitis–Interstitial Lung Disease Occurs in Smokers

Respiratory bronchiolitis (RB) is a histologic lesion that occurs in cigarette smokers. It is most often an incidental histologic finding, but it may rarely be the sole cause of ILD, and the clinical term **respiratory bronchiolitis–interstitial lung disease** (RB-ILD) is appropriate in this setting.

PATHOLOGY: RB is a patchy accumulation of pigmented macrophages in airspaces, centered on bronchioles (Fig. 18-65). These macrophages are present in bronchiolar lumens and adjacent alveoli. Bronchiolar walls show mild chronic inflammation and fibrosis, but interstitial fibrosis does not extend into the

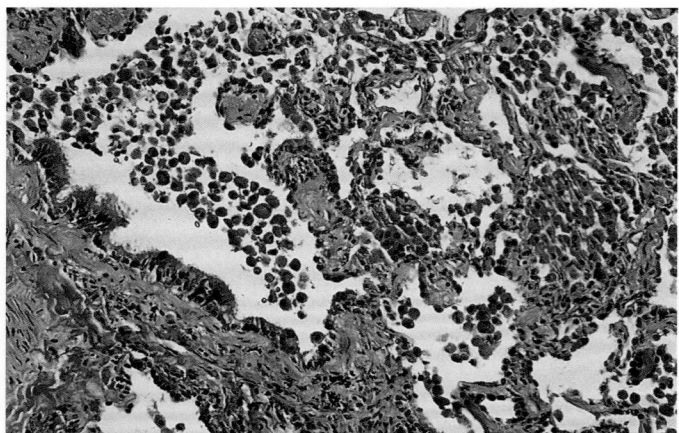

FIGURE 18-65. Respiratory bronchiolitis. There is marked accumulation of macrophages within bronchioles and surrounding airspaces. Mild fibrotic thickening and chronic inflammation of the bronchiolar wall are present.

surrounding lung. Macrophages usually contain finely granular, brown pigment. The lesions in RB are bronchiolocentric and patchy.

CLINICAL FEATURES: Patients have mild respiratory dysfunction. Imaging shows that upper lobes are most affected, with thickening of peripheral bronchioles. Patients with RB-ILD have an excellent prognosis, and symptoms usually resolve after smoking cessation.

In Organizing Pneumonia Pattern (Cryptogenic Organizing Pneumonia) Polypoid Plugs of Tissue Fill Alveolar Spaces, Alveolar Ducts, and Bronchiolar Lumens

Organizing pneumonia pattern, previously called "bronchiolitis obliterans–organizing pneumonia" (BOOP), is not specific for any etiologic agent, and its cause cannot be determined from the histopathology. Thus, it is seen in many settings, including respiratory tract infections (particularly viral bronchiolitis), inhalation of toxic materials, after administration of a number of drugs and various inflammatory processes (e.g., collagen vascular diseases). *A substantial number of cases are idiopathic and are called cryptogenic organizing pneumonia (or idiopathic BOOP).*

PATHOLOGY: Organizing pneumonia pattern has patchy areas of loose organizing fibrosis and chronic inflammatory cells in distal airways, adjacent to normal lung. Plugs of organizing fibroblastic tissue occlude bronchioles (bronchiolitis obliterans), alveolar ducts, and surrounding alveoli (organizing pneumonia; Fig. 18-66). Alveolar organizing pneumonia predominates; bronchiolitis obliterans may not be seen in all cases. Lung architecture is preserved, without honeycombing. Obstructive or endogenous lipid pneumonia may develop if there is significant bronchiolitis obliterans due to occlusion of the distal airways. Alveolar septa are only slightly thickened with chronic inflammatory cells, and type II pneumocyte hyperplasia is mild.

CLINICAL FEATURES: The average age at presentation is 55. The onset is acute, with fever, cough, and dyspnea, often with a history of a flu-like illness 4 to 6 weeks previously. Some patients may have predisposing conditions. Chest radiographs reveal localized opacities or bilateral interstitial infiltrates, which may migrate over time. Pulmonary function studies demonstrate a restrictive ventilatory pattern. Corticosteroid therapy is effective, and some patients recover within weeks to months even without therapy.

Acute Interstitial Pneumonia Is Idiopathic Diffuse Alveolar Damage

AIP is a clinical term for DAD of unknown cause. The diagnosis requires exclusion of clinical and pathologic causes such as infection, collagen vascular diseases, and drug toxicity.

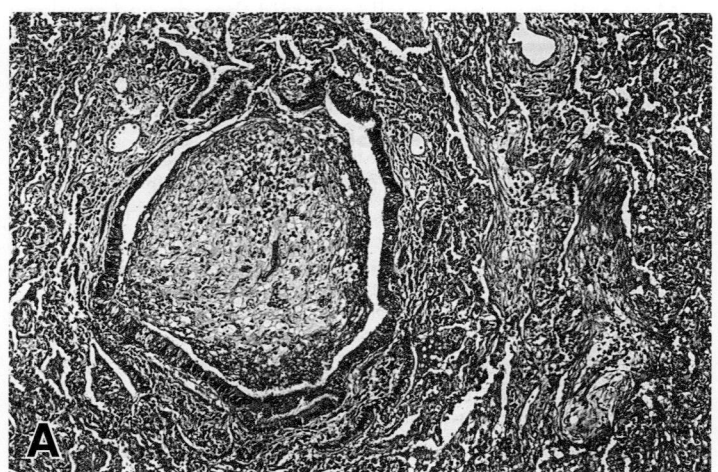
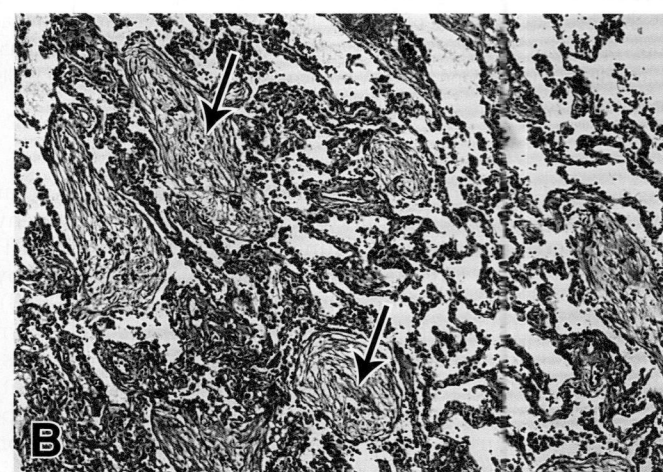

FIGURE 18-66. Organizing pneumonia pattern. A. Polypoid plugs of loose fibrous tissue are present in a bronchiole and adjacent alveolar ducts and alveoli. **B.** Alveolar spaces contain similar plugs of loose organizing connective tissue (*arrows*).

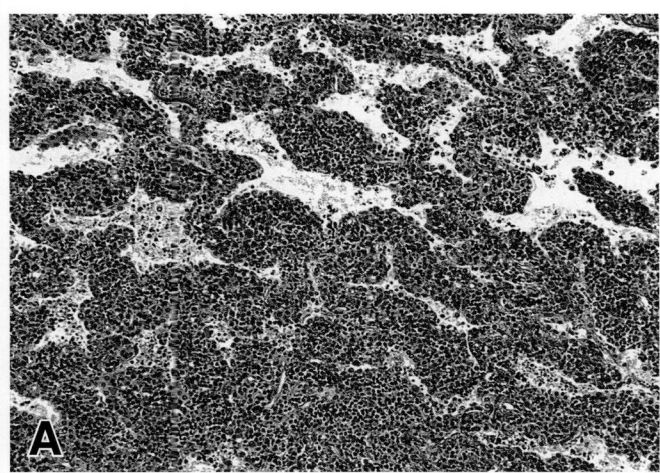
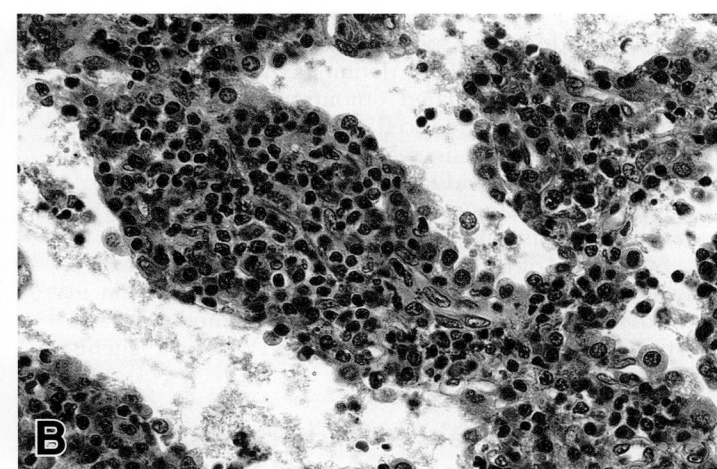

FIGURE 18-67. Lymphocytic interstitial pneumonia (LIP). A. The walls of the alveolar septa are diffusely infiltrated by chronic inflammatory cells. **B.** The inflammatory infiltrate is composed of lymphocytes and plasma cells.

PATHOLOGY: The pathology is identical to DAD associated with known causes (see above), but histologic features such as necrosis, acute pneumonia, eosinophilia, vasculitis, or hemorrhage, all of which suggest specific etiologies, must be excluded. In AIP, the pattern is usually of organizing DAD, so hyaline membranes may be inconspicuous and it consists mainly of organizing loose connective tissue causes thickening of alveolar walls.

CLINICAL FEATURES: AIP has a mean age at onset of 50 with a wide range and no sex predominance. It usually begins after an illness that resembles an upper respiratory tract infection with myalgias, arthralgias, fever, chills, and malaise. Patients develop severe exertional dyspnea over several days and usually present less than 3 weeks after experiencing the first symptoms. CT scan shows widespread consolidation. Mortality is approximately 50%, and those who survive may either recover completely or follow a course with recurrences and progressive ILD.

Lymphoid Interstitial Pneumonia Often Accompanies Autoimmune Diseases

Lymphoid interstitial pneumonia (LIP) is a rare disease with lymphoid infiltrates distributed diffusely in interstitial spaces.

PATHOLOGY: The hallmark of LIP is diffuse lymphocytic infiltration of alveolar septa and peribronchiolar spaces, with plasma cells and macrophages (Fig. 18-67). Alveolar architecture is preserved without scarring or remodeling. Marked type II pneumocyte hyperplasia may be seen, and inconspicuous foci of organizing interstitial fibrosis are occasionally present. Noncaseating sarcoid-like granulomas are often seen. Alveolar spaces tend to contain a proteinaceous exudate. Occasionally, scattered lymphoid aggregates are present, some containing germinal centers. Hyperplasia of peribronchiolar lymphoid tissue may be prominent.

CLINICAL FEATURES: LIP may be idiopathic but often occurs in patients with collagen vascular diseases (especially Sjögren syndrome), dysproteinemia, or HIV infection (Table 18-5). It is largely a

TABLE 18-5

CONDITIONS ASSOCIATED WITH LYMPHOCYTIC INTERSTITIAL PNEUMONIA

Idiopathic

Dysproteinemia
  Polyclonal gammopathy
  Macroglobulinemia
  Hypogammaglobulinemia
  Pernicious anemia

Collagen Vascular Disease
  Sjögren syndrome
  Systemic lupus erythematosus
  Rheumatoid arthritis

Immunodeficiency
HIV infection
Severe combined immunodeficiency syndrome

Infection
  Pneumocystis jiroveci pneumonia
  Epstein–Barr virus (lymphoproliferative disorder)
  Chronic hepatitis

Iatrogenic
  Bone marrow transplantation
  Phenytoin (Dilantin)

disease of adults, but pediatric cases have been documented. In children, LIP is a defining criterion for the diagnosis of AIDS. Associated autoimmune manifestations include increased or reduced serum γ-globulins, various dysproteinemias, and increased circulating autoantibodies, such as rheumatoid factor and antinuclear antibodies. Lymphoma may rarely develop in patients with LIP, particularly in patients with Sjögren syndrome and AIDS.

Symptoms of LIP include cough and progressive dyspnea. The disease varies from an indolent condition to one that progresses to end-stage lung remodeling and respiratory failure. Corticosteroids and cytotoxic agents have been of some benefit.

Pulmonary Langerhans Cell Histiocytosis Entails a Bronchiolocentric Proliferation of Langerhans Cells

Different presentations of Langerhans cell histiocytosis (LCH) have been called **eosinophilic granuloma, Hand–Schüller–Christian disease** and **Letterer–Siwe disease** (see Chapter 26). LCH can affect the lung as a distinctive form of ILD. In adults, LCH is *primarily seen in cigarette smokers*. It may occur as an isolated lesion (previously **pulmonary eosinophilic granuloma**) or as diffuse cystic lung disease. Extrapulmonary manifestations such as bone lesions or diabetes insipidus occur in 10% to 15% of cases. In children, lung involvement may occur in association with the multiorgan Letterer–Siwe disease or Hand–Schüller–Christian disease.

PATHOLOGY: Histologically, pulmonary LCH appears as scattered nodular infiltrates with a stellate border extending into the surrounding interstitium (Fig. 18-68A). These lesions are frequently subpleural or centered on bronchioles. They contain varying proportions of Langerhans cells admixed with lymphocytes, eosinophils, and macrophages. Langerhans cells are round to oval, with a moderate amount of eosinophilic cytoplasm and prominently grooved nuclei with small inconspicuous nucleoli (Fig. 18-68B). As the disease progresses, lesions cavitate and become fibrotic, and honeycomb fibrosis may result. Parenchyma adjacent to the nodular lesions may show marked accumulation of

intra-alveolar macrophages, owing to respiratory bronchiolitis caused by smoking.

Langerhans cells are distinctive: they show cytoplasmic Birbeck granules (on electron microscopy), C3, IgG-F$_c$ receptors, CD1a, and human leukocyte antigen (HLA)-DR and S-100 protein expression. Whether pulmonary LCH is a neoplastic proliferation or an abnormal immunologic response to antigens within cigarette smoke is unclear. Recently, *BRAF* mutations have been reported in a subset of pulmonary LCH.

CLINICAL FEATURES: Pulmonary LCH usually affects patients in their third and fourth decades. The most common presenting symptoms are nonproductive cough, dyspnea on exertion, and spontaneous pneumothorax, but 25% of patients are asymptomatic at the time of diagnosis. Chest radiographs show diffuse, bilateral, reticulonodular lesions, usually in the upper lobes. The lesions frequently undergo cavitation. Although most patients have a good prognosis, some develop chronic pulmonary dysfunction. In a few cases, progressive pulmonary fibrosis can lead to death. Cessation of smoking is beneficial in early stages of the disease.

In Lymphangioleiomyomatosis Abnormal Smooth Muscle Proliferates in the Lung and Lymphatics

Lymphangioleiomyomatosis (LAM) is a rare ILD that occurs almost exclusively in women of child-bearing age. It is characterized by widespread abnormal proliferation of smooth muscle in the lung, mediastinal and retroperitoneal lymph nodes, and major lymphatic ducts. Its etiology is unknown, but clinical responses to oophorectomy and progesterone therapy suggest that the smooth muscle proliferation is under hormonal control. Its occurrence in patients with tuberous sclerosis and its association with renal angiomyolipomas suggest that LAM may be a forme fruste of **tuberous sclerosis.** LAM is also associated with tuberous sclerosis gene complex (*TSC*) mutations, whether or not fully developed tuberous sclerosis is present. LAM cells are thought to be derived from perivascular epithelioid cells similar to

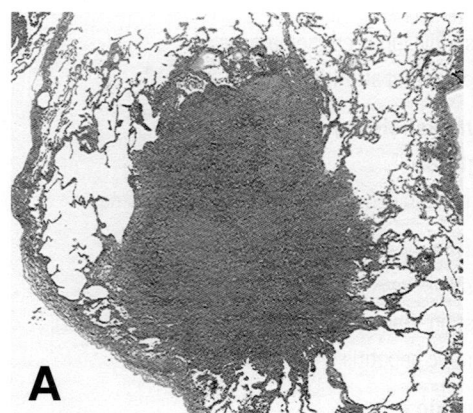
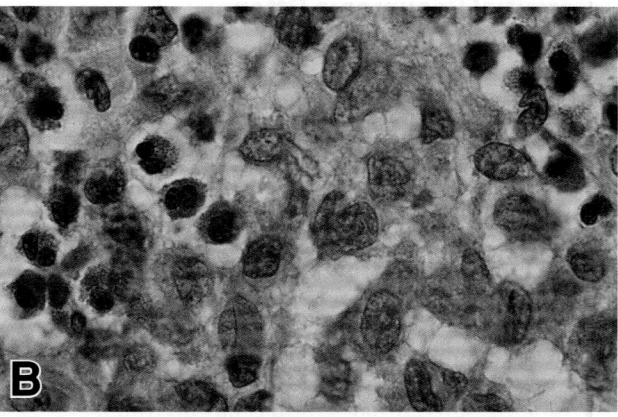

FIGURE 18-68. Langerhans cell histiocytosis. A. The nodular interstitial infiltrate has a stellate shape, with extension of cells into adjacent alveolar septa. **B.** Higher-power view shows Langerhans cells with a moderate amount of eosinophilic cytoplasm and prominently grooved nuclei. Eosinophils are also present.

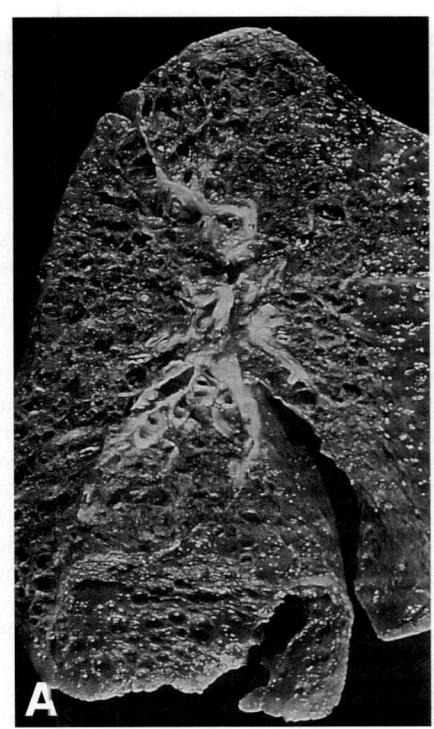

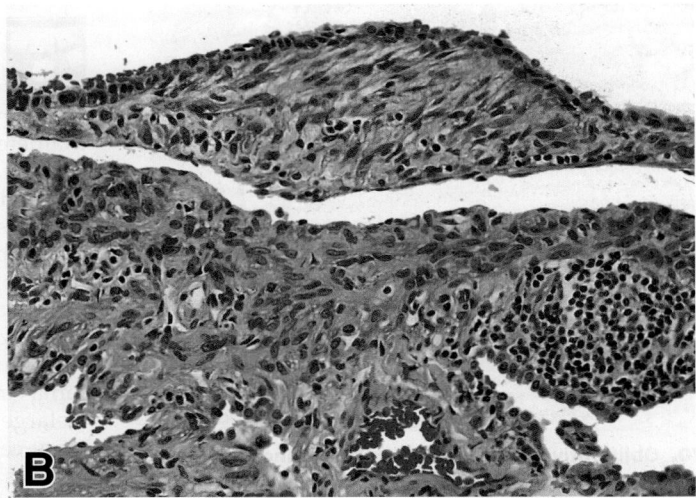

FIGURE 18-69. Lymphangioleiomyomatosis. A. The cut surface of the lung displays extensive cystic change. **B.** Abnormal cystic spaces are lined by smooth muscle bundles in which myocytes are haphazardly arranged.

other lesions associated with tuberous sclerosis, such as angiomyolipoma and clear cell tumor.

PATHOLOGY: The lungs show bilateral, diffuse enlargement, with extensive cystic changes associated with proliferation of abnormal smooth muscle or LAM cells (Fig. 18-69A). Many cystic spaces are lined by focal nodules or bundles of LAM cells. These round or spindle-shaped cells resemble immature smooth muscle cells but lack the parallel orientation of normal smooth muscle around airways and blood vessels (Fig. 18-69B). This proliferation typically follows a lymphatic distribution in the lung, around blood vessels and bronchioles, and along pleura and interlobular septa. Blood vessel walls, especially in small pulmonary veins, may also be infiltrated, causing microscopic hemorrhages and hemosiderin accumulation in alveolar macrophages. Immunostaining for HMB-45 (a melanoma antigen) specifically identifies LAM cells and distinguishes them from other lung smooth muscle cells. LAM cells usually also express estrogen or progesterone receptors.

CLINICAL FEATURES: Patients with LAM have shortness of breath, spontaneous pneumothorax, hemoptysis, cough, and chylous effusions. In early stages, the chest radiograph may be normal, but then shows a diffuse interstitial reticular or cystic pattern as the disease progresses. Pleural effusions, marked hyperinflation of the lungs and pneumothorax may ensue. Pulmonary function tests show markedly increased total lung capacity, decreased diffusing capacity, and obstructive or restrictive features. Some patients have an indolent clinical course, but many die of progressive respiratory failure. Hormonal ablation through oophorectomy, as well as antiestrogen (tamoxifen) and progesterone therapy, showed initial promise but has not proven to be effective over time. Mutations of the *TSC* genes lead to activation of the mammalian target of rapamycin (mTOR) pathway; thus, sirolimus is currently under investigation as a potential therapy.

LUNG TRANSPLANTATION

Patients who undergo lung transplantation are prone to acute and chronic rejection and infection. The histology of acute rejection includes perivascular infiltrates of small round lymphocytes, plasmacytoid lymphocytes, macrophages, and eosinophils. In severe cases, inflammation may involve adjacent alveoli, and hyaline membranes may be seen. The major pattern of chronic rejection is bronchiolitis obliterans, characterized by bronchiolar inflammation and varying degrees of fibrosis. The latter can take the form of polypoid plugs of intraluminal granulation tissue or concentric mural fibrosis, with the pattern of constrictive bronchiolitis (Fig. 18-70). Bronchiectasis is common in long-term survivors of lung transplants, perhaps related to poor perfusion of the airways, denervation, and/or recurrent airway infection.

Opportunistic infections, including those caused by bacteria, fungi, viruses, and *Pneumocystis*, are common in transplant patients. The most common fungal pathogens are *Candida* and *Aspergillus* spp. CMV is the most common cause of viral pneumonia. Of lung transplant patients who survive more than 30 days, 3% to 8% develop **lymphoproliferative disorders**, owing to uncontrolled proliferation of Epstein–Barr virus (EBV)–infected B lymphocytes as a result of immunosuppression by cyclosporine.

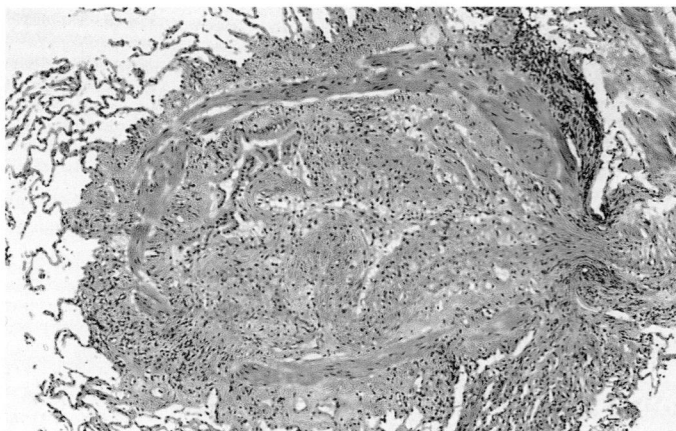

FIGURE 18-70. Obliterative bronchiolitis in the setting of chronic rejection in lung transplantation. The lumen of this bronchiole is virtually obliterated by concentric fibrosis. (The authors would like to gratefully acknowledge Dr. Anthony Gal for the contribution of Figure 18-70.)

VASCULITIS AND GRANULOMATOSIS

Many pulmonary conditions result in vasculitis, most of which are secondary to other inflammatory processes, such as necrotizing granulomatous infections. Only a few primary idiopathic vasculitis syndromes affect the lung, the most important of which are granulomatosis with polyangiitis (GPA, formerly called Wegener granulomatosis), microscopic polyangiitis, eosinophilic granulomatosis with polyangiitis (EGPA, formerly called Churg–Strauss granulomatosis), and necrotizing sarcoid granulomatosis.

Granulomatosis With Polyangiitis Has Aseptic, Necrotizing Granulomas and Vasculitis

GPA (formerly called Wegener granulomatosis) is a disease of unknown cause. It affects small and medium-sized blood vessels. It occurs mainly in the upper and lower respiratory tracts and the kidneys (see Chapters 16, 22, and 29), but many cases also involve the eyes, joints, skin, and peripheral nerves. Here, we deal only with pulmonary manifestations of GPA.

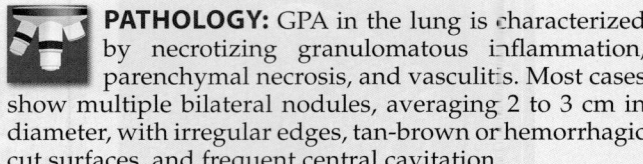

PATHOLOGY: GPA in the lung is characterized by necrotizing granulomatous inflammation, parenchymal necrosis, and vasculitis. Most cases show multiple bilateral nodules, averaging 2 to 3 cm in diameter, with irregular edges, tan-brown or hemorrhagic cut surfaces, and frequent central cavitation.

Nodules of parenchymal consolidation show (1) tissue necrosis; (2) granulomatous inflammation with a mixture of lymphocytes, plasma cells, neutrophils, eosinophils, macrophages, and giant cells; and (3) fibrosis. Necrosis may feature neutrophilic microabscesses or large basophilic zones of "geographical" necrosis with irregular serpiginous borders (Fig. 18-71A). Patterns of GPA granulomas include palisading macrophages along the borders of large necrotic zones, loosely clustered multinucleated giant cells, and scattered giant cells. Vasculitis may affect arteries (Fig. 18-71B), veins, or capillaries and may show acute, chronic, or granulomatous inflammation. Organizing pneumonia is common at the edges of the nodules of inflammatory consolidation. The lungs often show acute or chronic alveolar hemorrhage. "Neutrophilic capillaritis," with neutrophils in alveolar walls, is common.

CLINICAL FEATURES: GPA mostly affects the head and neck, then the lung, kidney, and eye. Respiratory manifestations include cough, hemoptysis, and pleuritis. Chest radiographs often show multiple intrapulmonary nodules, although single nodules may also be seen. Head and neck manifestations include sinusitis, nasal disease, otitis media, hearing loss, subglottic stenosis, ear pain, cough, and oral lesions. Systemic symptoms include arthralgias, fever, skin lesions, weight loss, peripheral neuropathy, central nervous system abnormalities, and pericarditis.

Diffuse pulmonary hemorrhage, an important complication of GPA, is a fulminant life-threatening crisis that produces severe respiratory failure. It is also usually accompanied by acute renal failure.

It is currently thought that antineutrophil cytoplasmic antibodies (ANCAs) are responsible for the inflammation in GPA. Serum ANCAs are a useful marker for

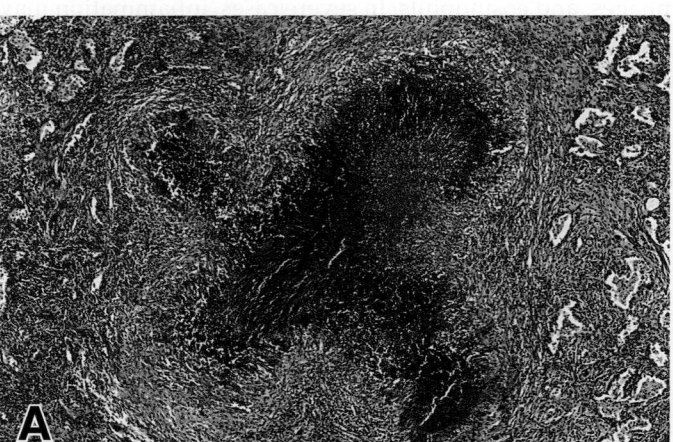
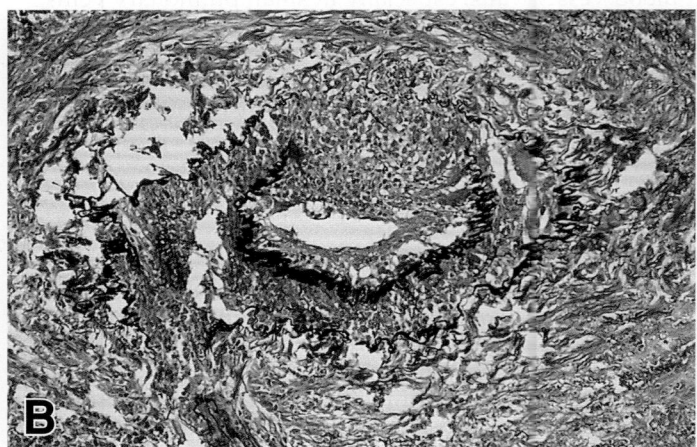

FIGURE 18-71. Granulomatosis with polyangiitis (formerly Wegener granulomatosis). A. This large area of necrosis has a "geographical" pattern with serpiginous borders and a basophilic center. **B.** Vasculitis in this artery is characterized by a focal, eccentric, transmural chronic inflammatory infiltrate that has destroyed the inner and outer elastic laminae (elastic stain).

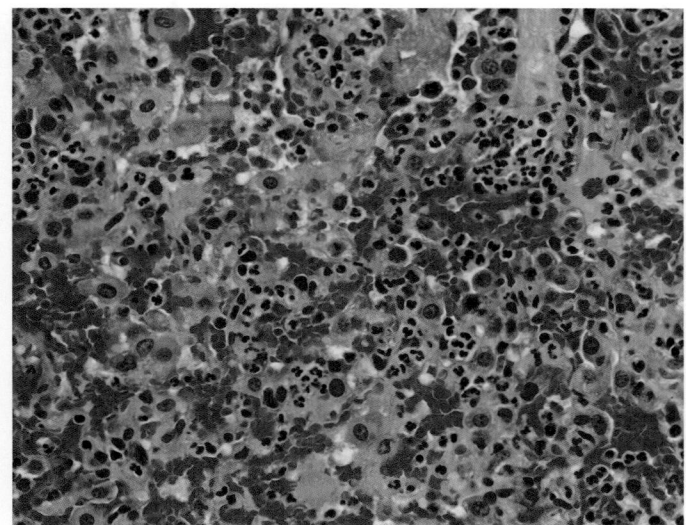

FIGURE 18-72. Microscopic polyangiitis. Alveolar walls are thickened owing to prominent infiltration by neutrophils.

GPA and other vasculitis syndromes. Patient serum yields two major immunofluorescence patterns when applied to neutrophils: cytoplasmic (C-ANCA) and perinuclear (P-ANCA). C-ANCAs reacting with neutrophil proteinase 3 occur in more than 85% of patients with active generalized GPA. Most P-ANCAs are specific for myeloperoxidase and are also seen with idiopathic necrotizing and crescentic glomerulonephritis, polyarteritis nodosa, or Churg–Strauss syndrome.

Most patients with GPA are treated effectively with corticosteroids and cyclophosphamide, and 5-year survival is now almost 90%.

Microscopic Polyangiitis

Microscopic polyangiitis is a pauci-immune vasculitis involving arterioles, venules, and capillaries. Almost all patients also show evidence of glomerulonephritis, and microscopic polyangiitis has emerged as one of the more common causes of "pulmonary-renal syndrome." Joints and muscles, upper respiratory tract, and skin may also be involved. Over 80% of patients have a positive ANCA, most often of the "perinuclear" type (P-ANCA), directed against myeloperoxidase. Microscopic polyangiitis may occur at any age and is of equal incidence in males and females. Lung biopsies show alveolar hemorrhage with neutrophilic capillaritis (Fig. 18-72). Immunoglobulin deposition is not seen.

Eosinophilic Granulomatosis With Polyangiitis Is a Disorder of Unknown Etiology, Defined by Asthma, Eosinophilia, and Vasculitis

 PATHOLOGY: The lungs of patients with EGPA (formerly called Churg–Strauss syndrome or allergic angiitis and granulomatosis) show changes of asthmatic bronchitis or bronchiolitis (see above), including eosinophilic pneumonia, vasculitis (Fig. 18-73A), parenchymal necrosis (Fig. 18-73B), and granulomatous inflammation. Infiltrates of eosinophils may be seen in any anatomic compartment of the lung. Involvement of blood vessel walls causes vasculitis and damage to airway walls and results in bronchitis or bronchiolitis. The vasculitis includes eosinophils, lymphocytes, plasma cells, macrophages, giant cells, and neutrophils (Fig. 18-73A). Necrotic foci have eosinophilic centers owing to accumulation of dead eosinophils (Fig. 18-73B).

CLINICAL FEATURES: EGPA has three clinical phases.

- **Prodrome:** Patients have one or more of the following: allergic rhinitis, asthma, peripheral eosinophilia, and eosinophilic infiltrative disease (eosinophilic pneumonia or eosinophilic enteritis).
- **Systemic vasculitic phase:** Extrapulmonary vasculitic manifestations are present, such as cutaneous leukocytoclastic vasculitis or peripheral neuropathy.
- **Postvasculitic phase:** Asthma, allergic rhinitis, and complications of neuropathy and hypertension may persist. Cardiovascular manifestations are common and include pericarditis, hypertension, and heart failure.

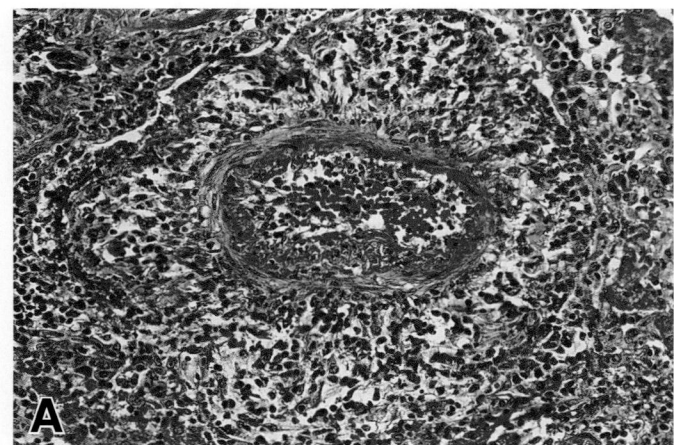

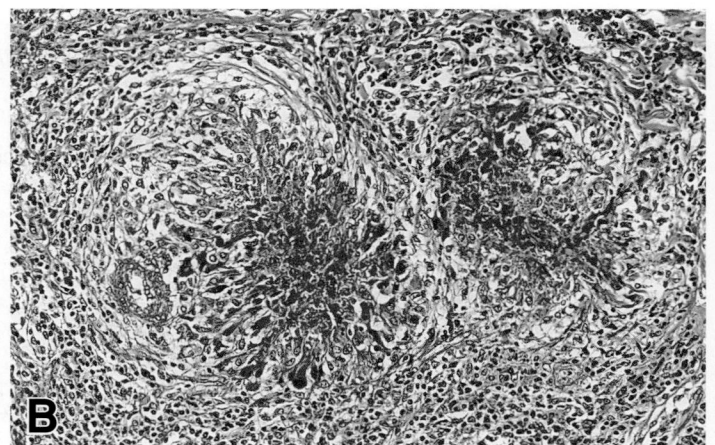

FIGURE 18-73. Allergic granulomatosis with polyangiitis (formerly Churg–Strauss syndrome). A. An artery shows severe vasculitis consisting of a dense infiltrate of chronic inflammatory cells and eosinophils. **B.** A necrotic ("allergic") granuloma has a central eosinophilic area of necrosis surrounded by palisading macrophages and giant cells.

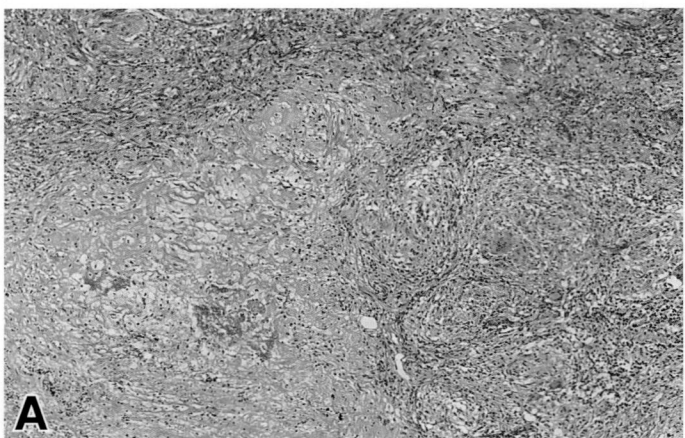
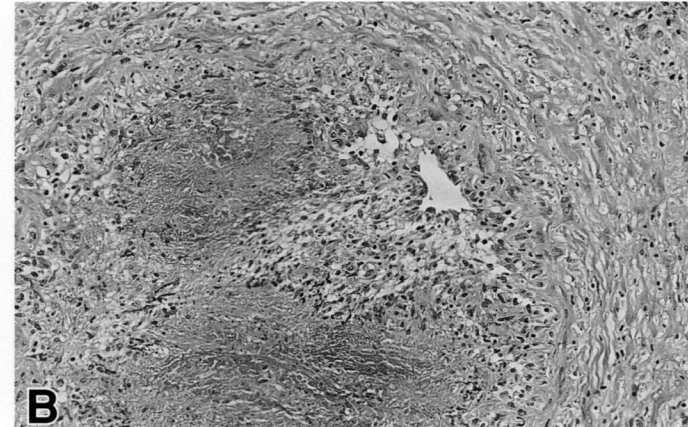

FIGURE 18-74. Necrotizing sarcoid granulomatosis. A. A large area of necrosis is surrounded by confluent sarcoid granulomas. **B.** The vasculitis consists of a necrotizing granuloma in the wall of an artery.

Renal disease and sinus involvement are usually less severe than those in GPA.

The cause of EGPA is obscure. An autoimmune mechanism is likely, in view of the presence of hypergammaglobulinemia, increased IgE, rheumatoid factor, and ANCAs.

Patients with EGPA usually are positive for P-ANCA in the vasculitic phase. Most patients respond to corticosteroid therapy, but cyclophosphamide may be needed in severe cases. With treatment, the 5-year survival is 60%.

Necrotizing Sarcoid Granulomatosis Shows Large Zones of Necrosis and Vasculitis

Necrotizing sarcoid granulomatosis is a rare condition featuring nodular confluent sarcoidal granulomas (Fig. 18-74). It is not a systemic vasculitis, but is usually limited to the lung. Giant cells and necrotizing granulomas (Fig. 18-74B) are seen, as is chronic inflammation with lymphocytes and plasma cells. Most patients are asymptomatic, and chest radiographs typically show multiple, well-circumscribed, pulmonary nodules. Extrapulmonary disease is uncommon, and localized lesions may be treated effectively by surgical removal. Corticosteroids are usually effective for patients with multiple lesions. The prognosis is excellent.

PULMONARY HYPERTENSION

In fetal life, pulmonary arterial walls are thick, as pulmonary arterial pressure is high. Blood is oxygenated through the placenta, not the lungs, and high fetal pulmonary arterial resistance helps shunt right ventricular output through the ductus arteriosus into the systemic circulation. After birth, the ductus arteriosus closes and the lungs must oxygenate venous blood. The lungs must therefore adapt to accept the entire cardiac output, which demands the high-volume and low-pressure system of the mature lung. By the third day of life, pulmonary arteries dilate, their walls become thin, and pulmonary arterial pressure declines.

Elevated pulmonary arterial pressure is defined as a mean pressure over 25 mm Hg at rest. Increased pulmonary blood flow or vascular resistance may lead to higher pulmonary arterial pressure. Whatever the cause, increased pulmonary artery pressure alters pulmonary artery structure (Fig. 18-75). The Heath and Edwards grading system describes a spectrum of structural changes seen in pulmonary hypertension and

SMALL PULMONARY ARTERIES

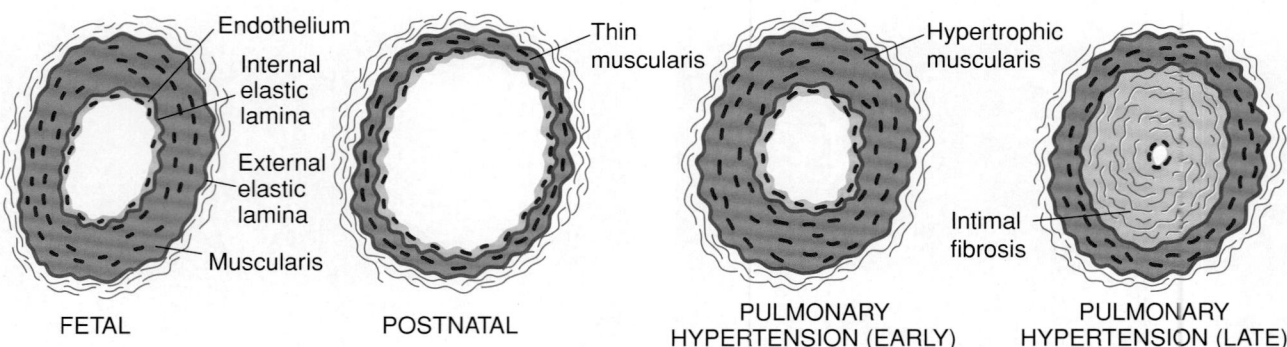

FIGURE 18-75. Histopathology of pulmonary hypertension. In late gestation, the pulmonary arteries have thick walls. After birth, the vessels dilate, and the walls become thin. Mild pulmonary hypertension is characterized by thickening of the media. As pulmonary hypertension becomes more severe, there is extensive intimal fibrosis and muscle thickening.

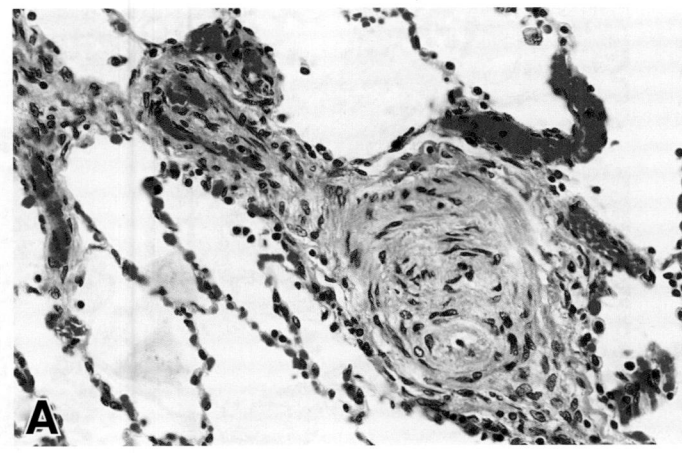

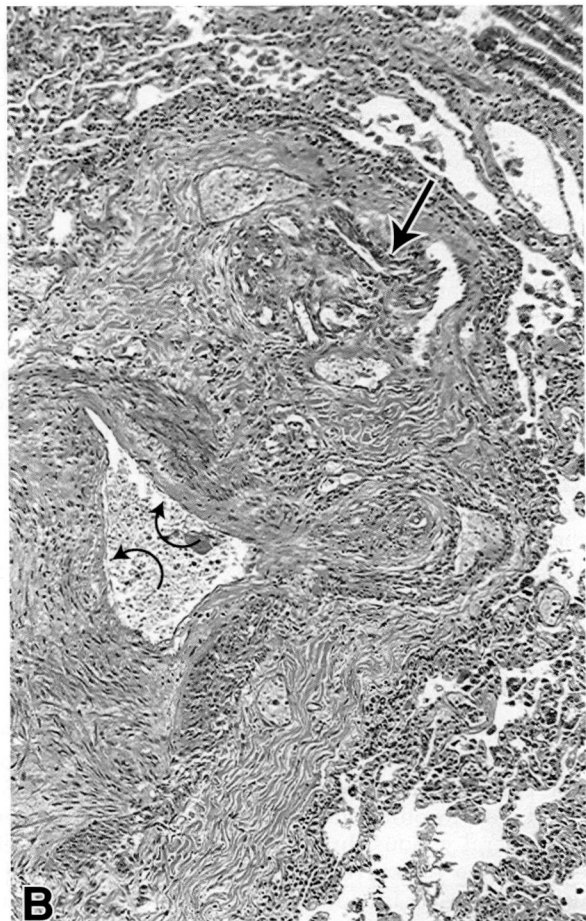

FIGURE 18-76. Pulmonary arterial hypertension. A. A small pulmonary artery is virtually occluded by concentric intimal fibrosis and thickening of the media. **B.** A plexiform lesion (*arrow*) is characterized by a glomeruloid proliferation of thin-walled vessels adjacent to a parent artery, which shows marked hypertensive changes of intimal fibrosis and medial thickening (*curved arrows*).

correlates the potential for reversibility following corrective cardiac surgery to relieve pulmonary hypertension. Grades 1, 2, and 3 are generally reversible; grades 4 and above are generally not.

- **Grade 1:** Medial hypertrophy of muscular pulmonary arteries and appearance of smooth muscle in pulmonary arterioles.
- **Grade 2:** Intimal proliferation with increasing medial hypertrophy.
- **Grade 3:** Intimal fibrosis of muscular pulmonary arteries and arterioles, which may be occlusive (Fig. 18-76A).
- **Grade 4:** Plexiform lesions, dilation and thinning of pulmonary arteries. These nodular lesions are composed of irregular interlacing blood channels and further obstruct pulmonary blood flow (Fig. 18-76B).
- **Grade 5:** Plexiform lesions in combination with dilation or angiomatoid lesions. Rupture of dilated thin-walled vessel, with parenchymal hemorrhage and hemosiderosis, is also present.
- **Grade 6:** Fibrinoid necrosis of arteries and arterioles.

Even mild pulmonary atherosclerosis is uncommon if pulmonary arterial pressure is normal. However, atherosclerosis, typically in the form of intimal lipid plaques, is seen in the largest pulmonary arteries with all grades of pulmonary hypertension. Increased pressure in the lesser circulation leads to hypertrophy of the right ventricle **(cor pulmonale).**

Pulmonary Hypertension May Be Precapillary or Postcapillary in Origin

Whether the primary source of increased flow or resistance is proximal or distal to the pulmonary capillary bed may be used to understand the pathophysiology of pulmonary hypertension. Precapillary hypertension includes left-to-right cardiac shunts, primary pulmonary hypertension, thromboembolic pulmonary hypertension, and hypertension due to fibrotic lung disease and hypoxia. Postcapillary hypertension includes pulmonary veno-occlusive disease (PVOD) and hypertension secondary to left-sided cardiac disorders, such as mitral stenosis and coarctation of the aorta.

Left-to-Right Shunts

Shunts from the systemic to the pulmonary circuit increase blood flow to the lungs. Most cases represent congenital cardiac malformations causing left-to-right shunts (see Chapter 17). At birth, the pulmonary artery and the aorta have about the same number of elastic lamellae in their media. Normally, elastic lamellae in the pulmonary artery are lost after birth, but if pulmonary hypertension is present, the fetal pattern of elastic lamellation persists.

Primary Pulmonary Hypertension

Primary pulmonary hypertension is a rare precapillary disorder caused by increased pulmonary arterial tone. The condition may be idiopathic, but some cases are hereditary and have been linked to mutations in *BMPR2*, which encodes bone morphogenetic protein receptor type 2; *ALK1*, which makes activin receptor-like kinase 1; and *ENG*, which encodes endoglin. Together, these genetic defects implicate a role for altered TGF-β signaling in pulmonary arterial hypertension. Recent advances have also focused attention on altered patterns of gene expression mediated by microRNAs. Pulmonary arterial hypertension may also be encountered in association with underlying collagen vascular diseases or induced by drugs or toxins (an example being the diet drug "fen-phen"). Pulmonary arterial hypertension occurs at all ages but is most common in young women in their 20s and 30s. It presents with insidious onset of dyspnea. Physical signs and radiologic abnormalities are initially slight but become more apparent with time. Severe pulmonary hypertension, typically associated with plexiform lesions histologically, eventually ensues, and patients die of cor pulmonale. Although medical treatment is mostly ineffective, recent use of prostacyclin analogs, endothelin receptor antagonists, and phosphodiesterase-5 inhibitors have led to a 5-year survival of about 30%. Lung transplantation, or heart and lung transplantation if there is an irreversible cardiac defect, is often indicated.

Recurrent Pulmonary Emboli

Multiple thromboemboli in smaller pulmonary vessels often result from asymptomatic, episodic showers of small emboli from the periphery. They gradually limit pulmonary circulation and lead to pulmonary hypertension. Some patients have peripheral venous thromboses, usually in deep veins in the legs, or a history of circumstances predisposing to venous thrombosis. In addition to causing the vascular lesions of pulmonary hypertension, organized thromboemboli can produce fibrous bands ("webs") that extend across the lumens of small pulmonary arteries. If the condition is diagnosed during life, placement of a filter in the inferior vena cava reduces risk of further embolization.

Any Disorder That Produces Alveolar Hypoxia Can Constrict Small Pulmonary Arteries and Lead to Pulmonary Hypertension

Low alveolar oxygen tension in a portion of the lung promotes constriction in vessels perfusing that area. This basic mechanism is designed to match ventilation and perfusion for optimal gas exchange. Thus, any condition that produces alveolar hypoxia can promote pulmonary hypertension. These include chronic airflow obstruction (chronic bronchitis), ILD, and living at high altitude. Severe kyphoscoliosis or extreme obesity (**Pickwickian syndrome**) may also impede ventilation and lead to hypoxemia and pulmonary hypertension.

Left Ventricular Failure Increases Pulmonary Venous Pressure and Secondarily Pulmonary Arterial Pressure

Both mitral stenosis and regurgitation can produce severe pulmonary venous hypertension and thus significant pulmonary artery hypertension. In such cases, the lungs exhibit lesions of both pulmonary hypertension and chronic passive congestion (see Chapter 7).

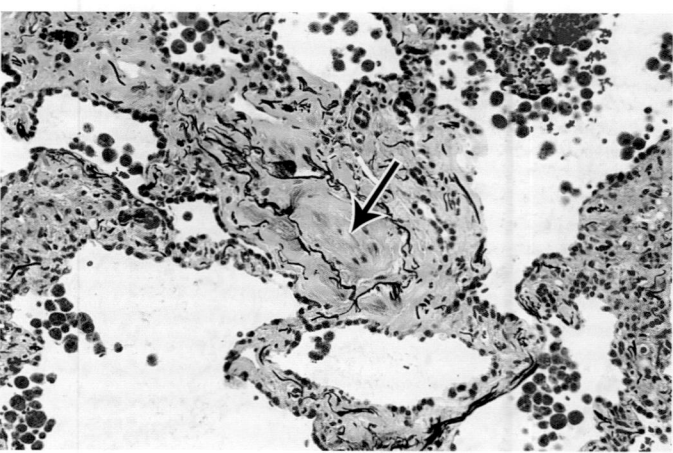

FIGURE 18-77. Veno-occlusive disease of the lung. This pulmonary vein is occluded by intimal fibrosis (*arrow*; Movat stain).

Pulmonary Veno-Occlusive Disease Involves Fibrotic Obstruction of Small Veins

PVOD is a rare condition of uncertain etiology in which small pulmonary veins and venules become occluded by loose, sparsely cellular, intimal fibrosis (Fig. 18-77). Some large veins may also be involved, and in half of cases, similar but less severe lesions affect pulmonary arteries. The obstructive lesions may canalize, and so could represent organized thrombi, possibly due to endothelial damage. PVOD may follow viral infections, exposure to toxic agents, and chemotherapy. More than half of cases occur in the first three decades of life. In children, girls and boys are affected similarly, but after age 15, it is more common in men.

PATHOLOGY: PVOD produces severe pulmonary hypertension. Grossly, the lung shows brown induration and atherosclerosis of large pulmonary arteries. Microscopically, small veins and venules are partly or totally occluded and larger veins show eccentric intimal thickening. Moderate alveolar wall fibrosis and foci of hemosiderosis are common. Pulmonary arteries show recent thrombi and lesions of severe pulmonary hypertension.

CLINICAL FEATURES: The clinical presentation of progressive dyspnea is similar to that of primary pulmonary hypertension, but PVOD has a more fulminant course. Radiographic examination reveals scattered infiltrates in the lung, representing hemorrhage and hemosiderosis, which increase as the disease progresses. There is no effective therapy, and lung transplantation should be contemplated.

Pulmonary Neoplasms

PULMONARY HAMARTOMA

The term "hamartoma" implies a malformation, but hamartomas are true tumors that consist of a benign proliferation of

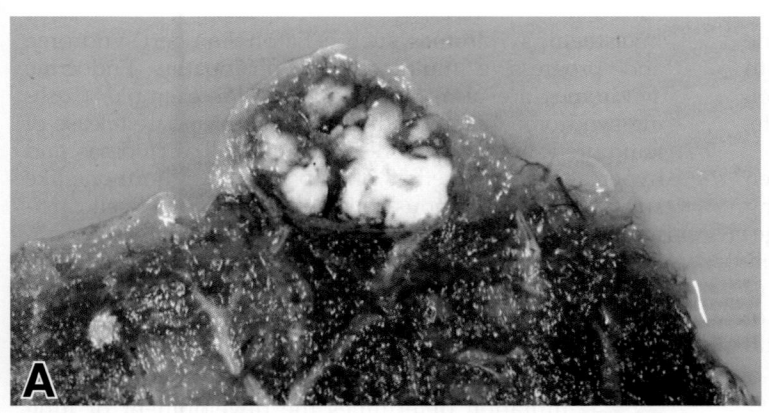
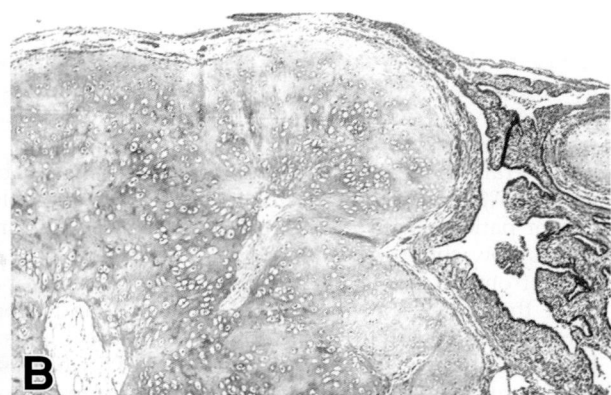

FIGURE 18-78. Pulmonary hamartoma. A. The cut surface of a sharply circumscribed, peripheral pulmonary nodule shows a lobulated structure. **B.** Microscopy reveals nodules of hyaline cartilage separated by connective tissue lined by respiratory epithelium.

cells that normally occur in the involved organ. Pulmonary hamartomas typically occur in adults, with a peak in the sixth decade of life. They account for 10% of "coin" lesions discovered incidentally on chest radiographs. A characteristic ("popcorn") pattern of calcification is often seen by x-ray.

PATHOLOGY: Grossly, pulmonary hamartomas are solitary, circumscribed, lobulated masses, averaging 2 cm in diameter, with a white or gray, cartilaginous cut surface (Fig. 18-78A). The tumor has elements usually present in the lung: cartilage, fibromyxoid connective tissue, fat, bone, and occasionally smooth muscle (Fig. 18-78B), interspersed with clefts lined by respiratory epithelium. Hamartomas are benign and well circumscribed and shell out from the surrounding lung parenchyma. Most are seen in the periphery, but 10% occur in a central endobronchial location. The latter may cause symptoms due to bronchial obstruction.

CARCINOMA OF THE LUNG

EPIDEMIOLOGY: Regarded as a rare tumor as recently as 1945, lung cancer is the most common cause of cancer mortality worldwide. In the United States, where it is the leading cause of cancer death in both men and women, 85% to 90% of lung cancers occur in cigarette smokers (see Chapter 8); conversely, the lifetime risk of developing lung cancer in smokers is 12% to 17%. Smokers are at risk for both "non–small cell lung carcinomas" (NSCLCs)—encompassing squamous cell carcinoma, adenocarcinoma, and large cell carcinoma (see also Pathology paragraph below)—and small cell lung carcinoma (SCLC). Most of the never-smokers who develop lung cancer have an adenocarcinoma. In general, 80% of lung cancers are NSCLC and 17% are SCLC. The distribution of histologic subtypes of NSCLC according to gender is shown in Table 18-6. The peak age for lung cancer is between 60 and 70 years, with most patients between 50 and 80 years. The former male predominance is decreasing as smoking increases among women.

General Features of Lung Cancer

CLINICAL FEATURES: Lung cancer presents in early stages in 30% of patients where the primary treatment approach is surgical resection and pathologic assessment is based on evaluation of the entire tumor. However, the remaining 70% of lung cancers present as advanced, unresectable disease. Then, diagnosis is based on nonresection specimens (small biopsies and cytology) and treatment is mostly chemotherapy and/or radiation.

Lung cancers historically have been categorized as SCLCs and NSCLCs, with the latter encompassing squamous cell carcinoma, adenocarcinoma, and large cell carcinoma. The reason for this was that small cell carcinomas responded to specific chemotherapies, but non–small cell tumors did not. Now, some NSCLCs can be treated with chemotherapy: lung adenocarcinoma patients whose tumors express endothelial growth factor receptor (*EGFR*) mutations or rearrangements involving the anaplastic lymphoma kinase gene (*ALK*) or the *ROS1* gene show

TABLE 18-6

FREQUENCY OF LUNG CARCINOMA HISTOLOGIC TYPES (%) BY GENDER (NCI SEER DATA, HISTOLOGICALLY CONFIRMED, 2006–2010)

Subtype	Males	Females	Males and Females
Adenocarcinoma	32.9	40.5	36.4
Squamous cell carcinoma	23.8	15.6	20
Small cell carcinoma	13.0	14.7	13.8
Large cell carcinoma	3.6	2.9	3.3
Other carcinomas	23.7	21.8	22.8
Carcinoid	2.0	3.5	2.7
Adenosquamous carcinoma	1.0	1.0	1.0

better progression-free survival if treated with tyrosine kinase inhibitors or crizotinib, respectively. Patients with advanced-stage adenocarcinoma—but not squamous cell carcinoma—may respond to the folate antimetabolite, pemetrexed.

Overall survival for all patients with NSCLC has been about 15% for the past few decades, but advanced lung cancer patients with *EGFR* mutations or *ALK* rearrangements now show improved 2-year progression-free survival, from 20% to 60%, with tyrosine kinase inhibitor and ALK therapy, respectively. The molecular landscape of lung cancer is evolving rapidly. Small cell carcinomas still have a dismal prognosis: 5-year survival of 5% or less.

Tumor stage is the single most important predictor of prognosis. The staging system for lung carcinoma uses the TNM scoring approach. This system is based on specific parameters regarding tumor size and extent of local and/or regional spread in the lung and chest (the T component); spread of tumor to specific groups of regional or distant lymph nodes (the N component); and the presence of distant metastases or malignancy involving the pleural fluid (the M component). Tumor stage is determined by the combination of the various T, N, and M categories. Stage I requires small tumor size and absence of lymph node involvement and metastases. Stages II and III are determined largely by the extent of regional lymph node involvement, and Stage IV applies to any tumor with distant metastasis.

LOCAL EFFECTS: Lung cancer can produce cough, dyspnea, hemoptysis, chest pain, obstructive pneumonia, and pleural effusion. A lung cancer (usually squamous) in the apex of the lung (**Pancoast tumor**) may extend to involve the eighth cervical and first and second thoracic nerves, leading to shoulder pain that radiates down the arm in an ulnar distribution (**Pancoast syndrome**). A Pancoast tumor also may paralyze cervical sympathetic nerves and cause **Horner syndrome** on the affected side with (1) depression of the eyeball (enophthalmos), (2) ptosis of the upper eyelid, (3) constriction of the pupil (miosis), and (4) absence of sweating (anhidrosis).

Most central endobronchial tumors produce symptoms related to bronchial obstruction: persistent cough, hemoptysis, and obstructive pneumonia, or atelectasis. Effusions can result from tumor extension into the pleura or pericardium. Lymphangitic spread of the tumor within the lung may interfere with oxygenation. Tumors arising peripherally are more likely to be discovered on routine chest radiographs or after they have become advanced. The latter circumstance features invasion of the chest wall with resulting chest pain, superior vena cava syndrome, and nerve entrapment syndromes.

MEDIASTINAL SPREAD: Tumor growth within the mediastinum can cause superior vena cava syndrome (owing to tumorous obstruction of this vein) and nerve entrapment syndromes.

METASTASES: Lung cancers metastasize most often to regional lymph nodes, particularly hilar and mediastinal nodes, and to the brain, bone, and liver. Extranodal metastases often involve the adrenal gland, but adrenal insufficiency is uncommon.

PARANEOPLASTIC SYNDROMES: Disorders associated with lung cancer include acanthosis nigricans, dermatomyositis/polymyositis, clubbing of the fingers, and myasthenic syndromes, such as Eaton–Lambert syndrome and progressive multifocal encephalopathy. Endocrine syndromes are also seen including, for example, Cushing syndrome or the syndrome of inappropriate release of antidiuretic hormone (SIADH) in small cell carcinomas, and hypercalcemia (secretion of a parathyroid hormone-like substance) in squamous cell carcinomas. Small cell carcinomas may also be associated with a syndrome of paraneoplastic encephalomyelitis and sensory neuropathy associated with circulating anti-Hu antibodies.

 MOLECULAR PATHOGENESIS: No single mutation determines the development of lung cancer, but some are common and may allow for targeted chemotherapy.

- *EGFR:* Activating mutations in the tyrosine kinase domain of this gene are of particular interest in lung adenocarcinomas, owing to the responsiveness of mutated tumors to tyrosine kinase inhibitor drugs targeted against this receptor, such as erlotinib and gefitinib. *EGFR* mutations are more common in adenocarcinomas in nonsmokers, Asians, and women. These mutations occur in 10% to 15% of lung adenocarcinomas in the United States, with higher percentages in nonsmokers and women, but 40% to 60% of East Asians have *EGFR* mutations.

- *KRAS:* Mutations in this oncogene, particularly in codons 12 and 13, occur in 25% of adenocarcinomas, 20% of large cell carcinomas, and 5% of squamous carcinomas, but rarely in SCLCs. These mutations correlate with cigarette smoking and with a poor prognosis in patients with adenocarcinoma. No effective targeted molecular therapy is available for *K-ras* mutations.

- **EML4-ALK translocations:** Fusion between the genes for echinoderm microtubule-associated protein-like 4 (*EML4*) and anaplastic lymphoma kinase (*ALK*) is encountered in approximately 5% of advanced pulmonary adenocarcinomas, most frequently in nonsmokers. Adenocarcinomas harboring this translocation are responsive to targeted therapy with crizotinib.

- *ROS1 translocations:* Fusions between *ROS1* and a variety of fusions partners (*FIG*, *TPM3*, *SLC34A2*, numerous others) occur in approximately 2% of all lung cancers but retain the tyrosine kinase domain which allows for response to targeted therapy agents such as crizotinib.

- *MYC:* Overexpression of this oncogene occurs in 10% to 40% of small cell carcinomas but is rare in other types.

- *TP53:* Mutations in *TP53* are identified in more than 80% of small cell carcinomas and 50% of non–small cell tumors.

- *RB:* Mutations in the retinoblastoma (*RB*) gene occur in over 80% of small cell cancers and 25% of non–small cell carcinomas.

- **Chromosome 3 (3p):** Deletions in the short arm of this chromosome are frequently found in all types of lung cancers.

- *BCL2:* This protooncogene encodes Bcl-2, a protein that inhibits apoptosis (see Chapter 1). It is expressed in 25% of squamous cell carcinomas and 10% of adenocarcinomas.

- **PTEN:** This tumor suppressor gene regulates cell survival signaling and is deficient by one of a number of mechanisms (loss of heterozygosity, mutation, promoter methylation, etc.) in many non–small cell lung cancers. Loss of PTEN is associated with poor prognosis and drug resistance.
- **FGFR1** (fibroblast growth factor receptor 1): Amplification of *FGFR1* has been reported in 20% of squamous cell carcinoma, and FGFR inhibitors are currently the subject of clinical testing.
- **Other mutations:** Abnormalities of *BRAF, PIK3CA, ERBB2, RET, c-MET* and others have been reported in small percentages of lung carcinoma and are the focus of ongoing efforts to identify effective targeted therapies.

PATHOLOGY: Squamous cell carcinoma, adenocarcinoma, large cell carcinoma, and small cell carcinoma are the major forms of lung cancer. Although the term **bronchogenic** carcinoma was once used, about one-fourth of primary lung cancers do not have an obvious bronchial origin, so this term is no longer recommended. Squamous cell carcinoma, adenocarcinoma, and large cell carcinoma have traditionally been lumped together from a clinical standpoint as "non–small cell carcinoma" because of historically similar treatment; however, advances in chemotherapy and targeted therapies in particular have made subtyping of critical importance, and the usage of "non–small cell carcinoma" is discouraged.

Histologic subtyping of lung cancer is based on the best-differentiated component, unless an area of small cell carcinoma is present. However, the degree of differentiation is graded according to the worst-differentiated component. Thus, if a tumor is mostly poorly differentiated large cells but has foci of squamous cells or adenocarcinoma, it is classified as a poorly differentiated squamous cell carcinoma or adenocarcinoma, respectively. Any cancer with a component of small cell carcinoma is regarded as a subtype of that tumor (see below).

Histologic Subtypes of Lung Carcinoma

Squamous Cell Carcinoma

Squamous cell carcinoma is the second most common histologic type of lung cancer, accounting for 20% of all lung cancers in the United States. It is more common in men than in women (Table 18-6). In response to injury of the bronchial epithelium, such as occurs with cigarette smoking, regeneration from the pluripotent basal layer commonly entails squamous metaplasia. The metaplastic squamous mucosa follows the same sequence of dysplasia, carcinoma in situ, and invasive tumor seen in other sites normally lined by squamous epithelium, such as the cervix or skin.

Most squamous cell carcinomas arise centrally in the lung, from major or segmental bronchi, although 10% originate in the periphery. They tend to be firm, gray-white, 3- to 5-cm ulcerated lesions that extend through the bronchial wall into the adjacent lung parenchyma (Fig. 18-79A). Central cavitation is frequent. On occasion, a central squamous carcinoma occurs as an endobronchial tumor.

These tumors vary widely in degrees of squamous differentiation. There are three histologic subtypes: keratinizing, nonkeratinizing, and basaloid. Many show overt keratinization or intercellular bridges. Well-differentiated tumors have keratin "pearls," small round nests of brightly eosinophilic aggregates of keratin surrounded by concentric ("onion skin") layers of squamous cells (Fig. 18-79B). Individual cell keratinization also occurs, in which the cytoplasm becomes glassy and intensely eosinophilic. Intercellular bridges (representing desmosomes) in some well-differentiated squamous cancers are slender gaps between adjacent cells, traversed by fine strands of cytoplasm. By contrast, some squamous tumors are very poorly differentiated. They lack keratinization and are difficult to distinguish from large cell, small cell, or spindle cell carcinomas. Basaloid tumors have small tumor cells with moderate eosinophilic cytoplasm and peripheral palisading. Focal abrupt keratinization may be present. Diffuse expression of immunohistochemical squamous markers such as p40 is helpful in making the diagnosis of nonkeratinizing and basaloid squamous cell carcinomas.

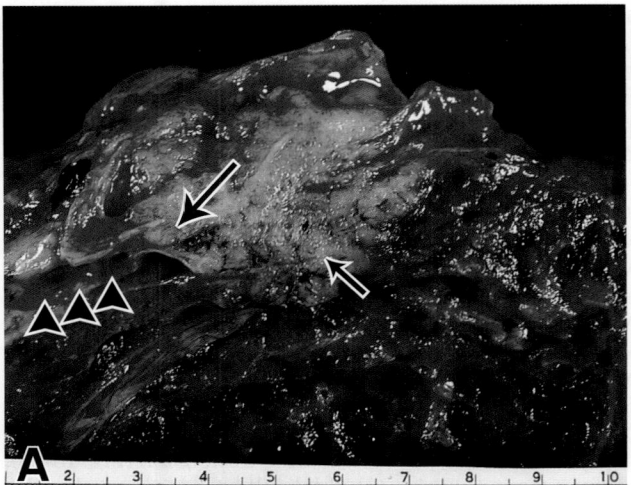
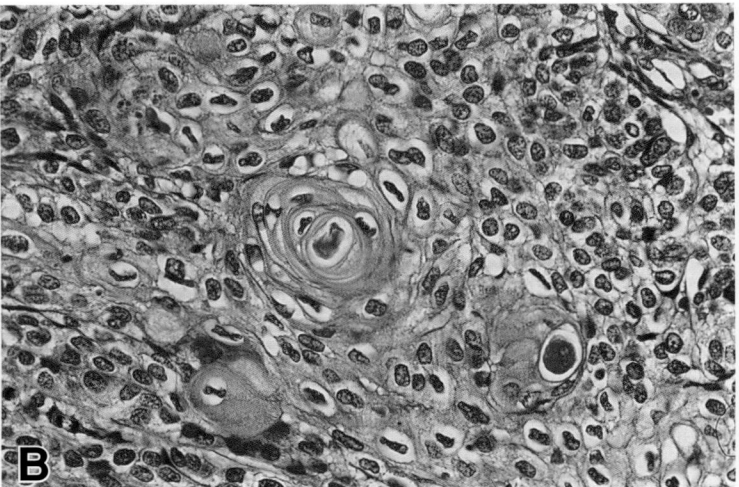

FIGURE 18-79. Squamous cell carcinoma of the lung. A. The tumor (*large arrow*) grows within the lumen of a bronchus (*arrowheads* highlight the course of the bronchus) and invades adjacent intrapulmonary lymph nodes (*small arrow*). **B.** Microscopy reveals well-differentiated squamous cell carcinoma composed of cells with brightly eosinophilic cytoplasm and keratin pearls (one shown in *center*).

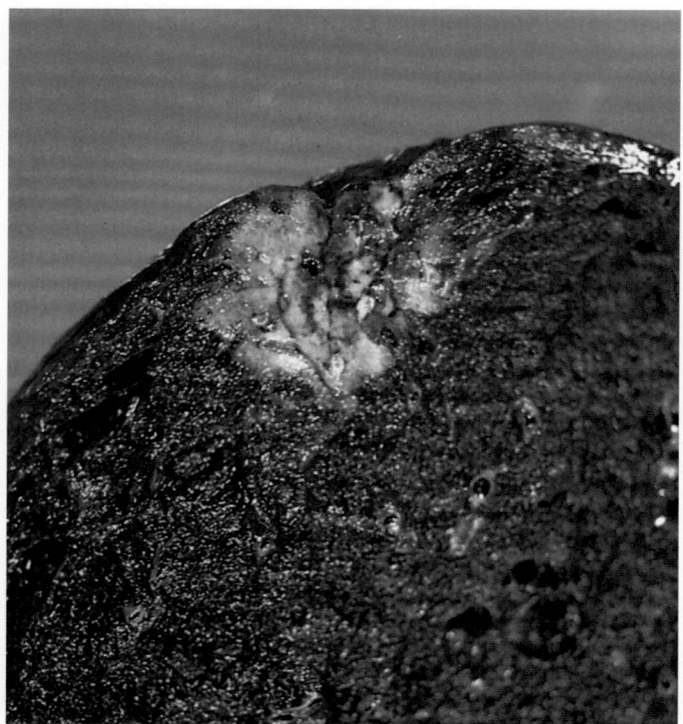

FIGURE 18-80. Invasive adenocarcinoma of the lung. A peripheral tumor in the right upper lobe has an irregular border and a tan or gray cut surface. It causes puckering of the overlying pleura.

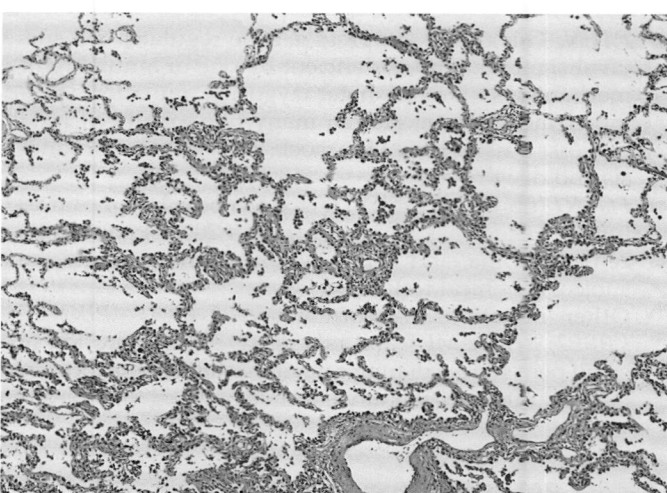

FIGURE 18-81. Atypical adenomatous hyperplasia. This millimeter-sized bronchioloalveolar proliferation is ill-defined with mild thickening of alveolar walls lined by hyperplastic pneumocytes showing minimal atypia.

Adenocarcinoma

Worldwide, adenocarcinoma has overtaken squamous cell carcinoma as the most common subtype of lung cancer in most countries, and it is the most common type in nonsmokers. In the United States, it accounts for 36% of all invasive lung malignancies and is more common in women (41% of all lung cancers) than in men (33% of all lung cancers) (Table 18-6). It tends to arise in the periphery of the lung and is often associated with pleural fibrosis and subpleural scars, which can lead to pleural puckering (Fig. 18-80). These cancers were once thought to arise in scars left by old tuberculosis or healed infarcts, but it is now recognized that such scars represent a desmoplastic response to the tumor. Adenocarcinoma classification has recently been revised. The term "bronchioloalveolar carcinoma" has been dropped because it was found to represent five different entities. Also, the term "mixed subtype adenocarcinoma" is no longer used.

Atypical adenomatous hyperplasia (AAH) is recognized as a putative precursor lesion for adenocarcinomas. AAH is a well-demarcated lesion, usually less than 5 mm in greatest dimension, with atypical proliferation of epithelial cells along alveolar septa (Fig. 18-81). In a sequence similar to the "adenoma–carcinoma" sequence in colon cancers, lung adenocarcinomas are thought to originate as AAH, progress to adenocarcinoma in situ (AIS), and then to more aggressive invasive adenocarcinomas. The progressive accumulation of mutations as the lesions advance supports this hypothesis, but it remains unclear whether all foci of AAH will progress to carcinoma or if all adenocarcinomas arise via this sequence of events.

Adenocarcinoma In Situ

AIS, once called bronchioloalveolar carcinoma, is a preinvasive form of adenocarcinoma in which tumor cells grow only along preexisting alveolar walls (lepidic growth). It accounts for 1% to 5% of lung adenocarcinomas. Patients with tumors meeting criteria for AIS have a 100% 5-year survival rate after resection.

Minimally Invasive Adenocarcinoma

For adenocarcinomas, a small amount of invasion in a tumor otherwise showing lepidic growth does not adversely affect prognosis. This has led to the introduction of a category of adenocarcinoma called minimally invasive adenocarcinoma (MIA, formerly bronchioloalveolar carcinoma), which has the same favorable prognosis as AIS. MIA is defined as a tumor with lepidic growth as seen in AIS, but with foci of invasive tumor measuring 5 mm or less in maximal diameter and lacking pleural or lymphovascular invasion and necrosis.

Both AIS and MIA may be seen radiographically as single peripheral nodules with a "ground glass" appearance or as multiple nodules. AIS shows pure ground glass changes radiographically, while MIA may show a small solid component. Grossly, both tumors should measure less than or equal to 3 cm and typically appear as ill-defined tan lesions, which may be difficult to distinguish from surrounding normal tissue.

Most AIS and MIA are nonmucinous, and contain club cells (formerly Clara cells) and/or type II pneumocytes. Only rarely are they mucinous. AIS has a pure lepidic pattern without invasion (Fig. 18-82A,B). MIA is lepidic-predominant adenocarcinoma with an invasive component less than or equal to 5 mm in maximal dimension (Fig. 18-83). In nonmucinous tumors, cuboidal cells grow along alveolar walls. Mucinous tumors contain columnar cells with abundant apical cytoplasm filled with mucous, sometimes with a goblet cell appearance. Particularly for mucinous tumors,

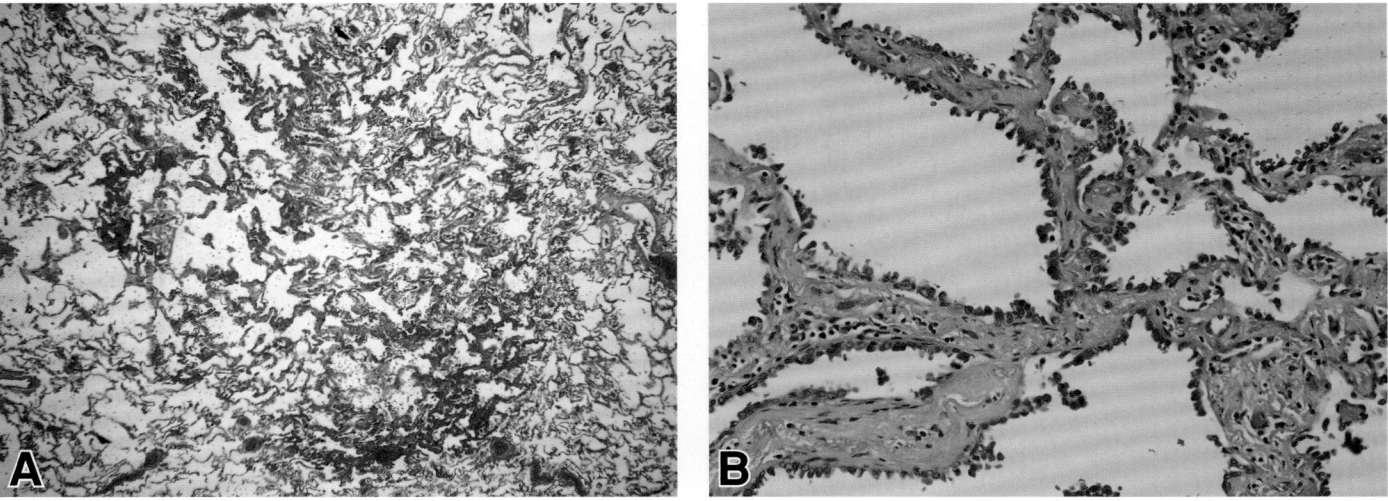

FIGURE 18-82. Adenocarcinoma in situ. A. This circumscribed nonmucinous tumor grows purely with a lepidic pattern. No foci of invasion or scarring are seen. **B.** A layer of atypical pneumocytes lines alveolar walls.

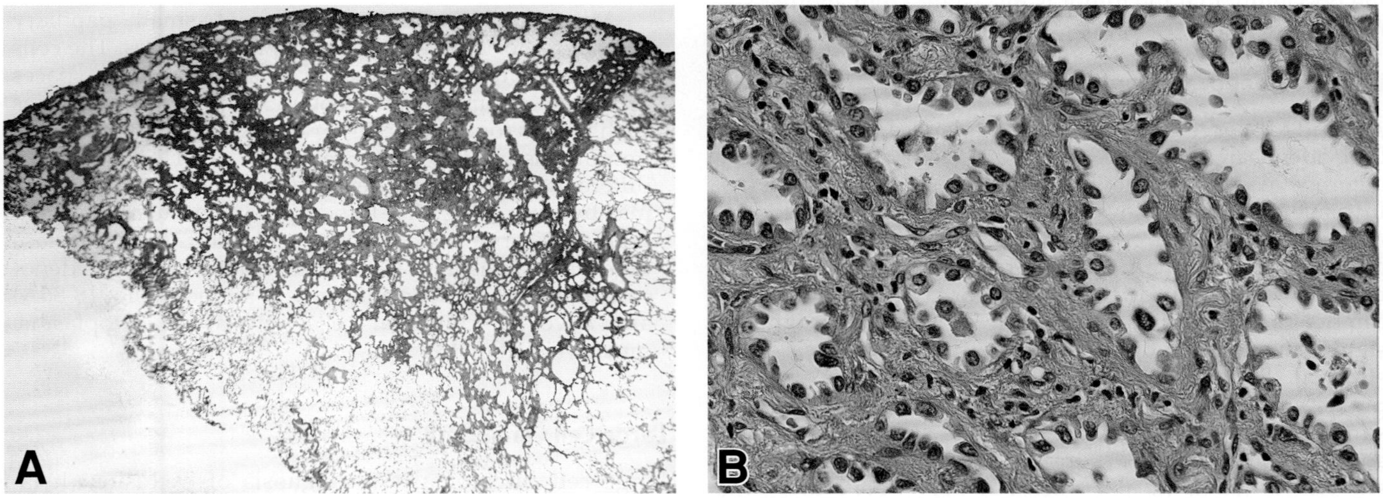

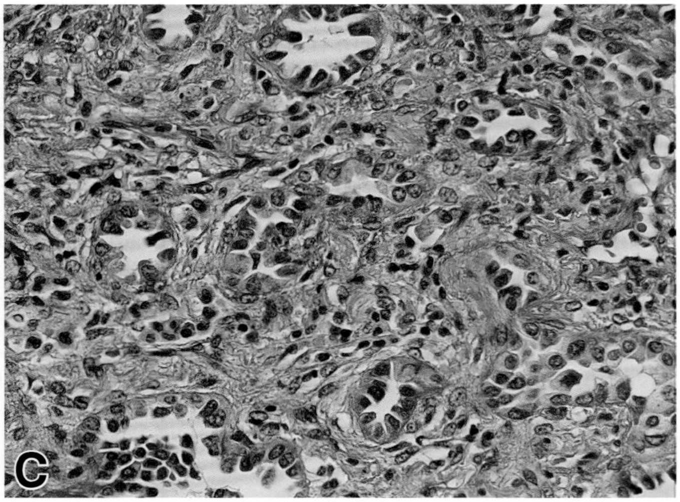

FIGURE 18-83. Minimally invasive adenocarcinoma. A. This nonmucinous adenocarcinoma consists primarily of lepidic growth with a small (<0.5 cm) area of invasion. **B.** The lepidic component shows alveolar walls lined by atypical pneumocytes. **C.** The invasive area shows acinar glands within a fibrous stroma.

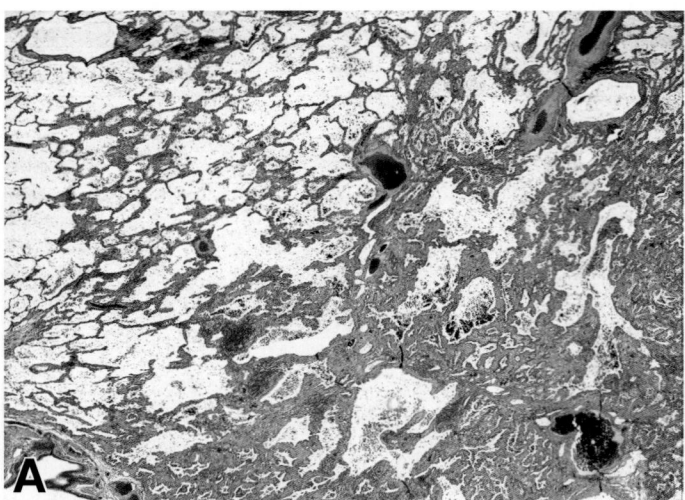
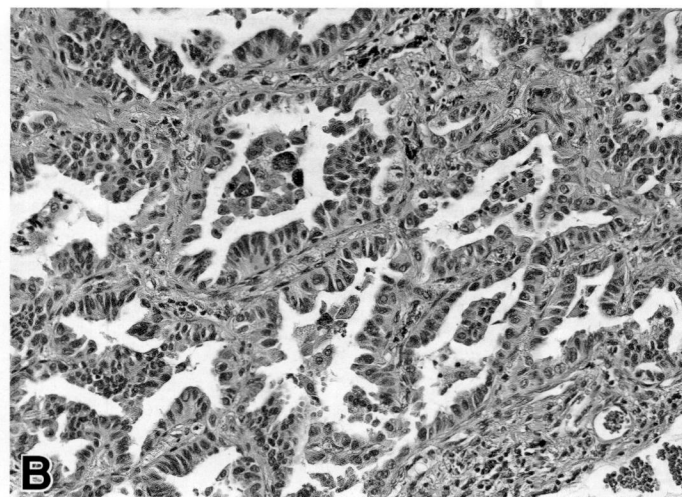

FIGURE 18-84. Adenocarcinoma with lepidic-predominant pattern. A. The tumor shows mostly lepidic growth (*upper left*) and an area of invasive acinar adenocarcinoma (*lower right*). **B.** Lepidic pattern consists of a proliferation of type II pneumocytes and Clara cells along the surface of alveolar walls.

the possibility that the tumor is metastatic from another site must be excluded.

Invasive Adenocarcinomas

AIS and MIA account for only 5% of adenocarcinomas. Most lung adenocarcinomas are more invasive. They are typically heterogeneous and show a mixture of growth patterns. Invasive tumors are now classified based on the predominant growth pattern. Such patterns include lepidic, acinar, papillary, solid, and micropapillary. Rarely, tumors will contain only a single growth pattern. For completely resected tumors, the predominant histologic subtype has prognostic significance. AIS and MIA have 100% 5-year disease-free survival. For stage I invasive adenocarcinomas, lepidic-predominant adenocarcinoma has excellent 5-year disease-free survival (>90%), with an intermediate survival for acinar and papillary types (80% to 90%). The worst disease-free survival is for solid and micropapillary adenocarcinoma (60% to 80%).

PATHOLOGY: Invasive lung adenocarcinomas appear mostly as irregular 2- to 5-cm masses but may be so large as to replace an entire lobe. On cut section, nonmucinous tumors are grayish white. Mucinous tumors may be glistening or gelatinous depending on the amount of mucin production. Central adenocarcinomas may grow mainly endobronchially and invade bronchial cartilage.

Most invasive adenocarcinomas contain heterogeneous mixtures of lepidic, acinar, papillary, micropapillary, and solid patterns. Lepidic-predominant tumors are invasive lung adenocarcinomas in which lepidic growth is the most prominent pattern (Fig. 18-84). The acinar pattern is distinguished by regular glands lined by cuboidal or columnar cells (Fig. 18-85A). Acinar-predominant adenocarcinomas are the most common category of invasive adenocarcinomas. Papillary adenocarcinomas exhibit a single cell layer on a core of fibrovascular connective tissue (Fig. 18-85B).

Micropapillary carcinomas show small papillary tufts of tumor cells with no fibrovascular cores. The cells may appear to float in alveolar spaces, glands, or spaces in fibrous stroma (Fig. 18-85C). Solid adenocarcinomas with mucus formation and/or expression of pneumocyte immunohistochemical markers such as TTF-1 are poorly differentiated tumors. They differ from large cell carcinomas by expressing TTF-1 and/or having mucin detected with mucicarmine or periodic acid–Schiff (with diastase digestion) stains (Fig. 18-85D). Invasive mucinous adenocarcinomas show solid mucoid cut surfaces (Fig. 18-86A) and have tall columnar cells with apical cytoplasmic mucin (Fig. 18-86B).

Large Cell Carcinoma

Large cell carcinoma is a diagnosis of exclusion: it is a poorly differentiated non–small cell carcinoma lacking squamous or glandular morphology and lacking expression of p40, TTF-1, or mucin (Fig. 18-87). This tumor type accounts for 3% of invasive lung tumors in the United States (Table 18-6). The cells are large and exhibit ample cytoplasm. Nuclei frequently show prominent nucleoli and vesicular chromatin.

Large cell neuroendocrine carcinoma is a rare high-grade neuroendocrine carcinoma with a growth pattern similar to carcinoid tumors (see below), with an organoid pattern, trabecular growth, peripheral palisading of cells, and rosette formation. It shows neuroendocrine differentiation by immunohistochemistry or ultrastructure. Mitotic rates are high and necrosis is common. These are aggressive tumors with 5-year survival rates similar to small cell carcinoma.

Small Cell Carcinoma

Small cell carcinoma (formerly "oat cell" carcinoma) is a highly malignant epithelial tumor of the lung with neuroendocrine features. It accounts for 14% of all lung cancers

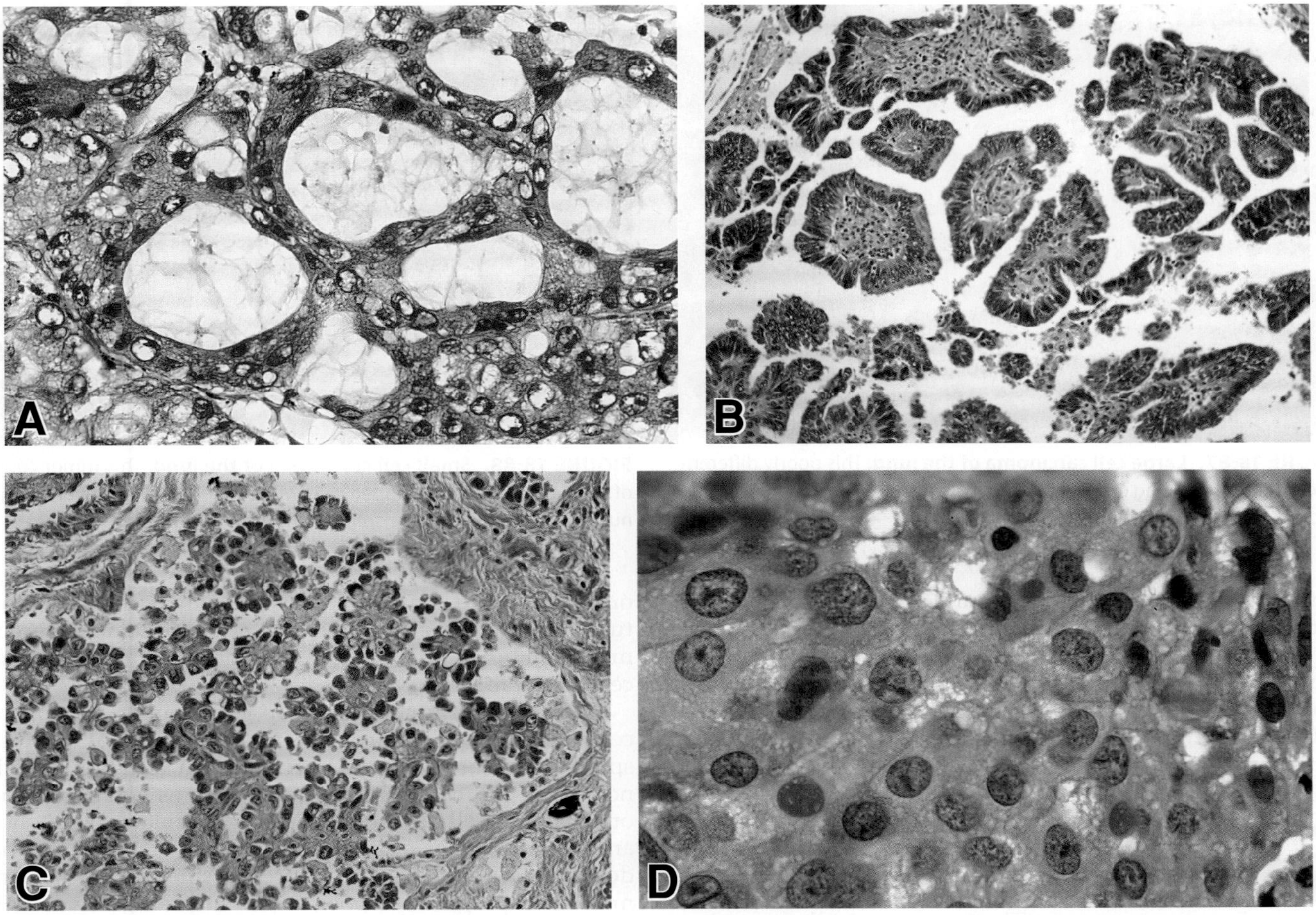

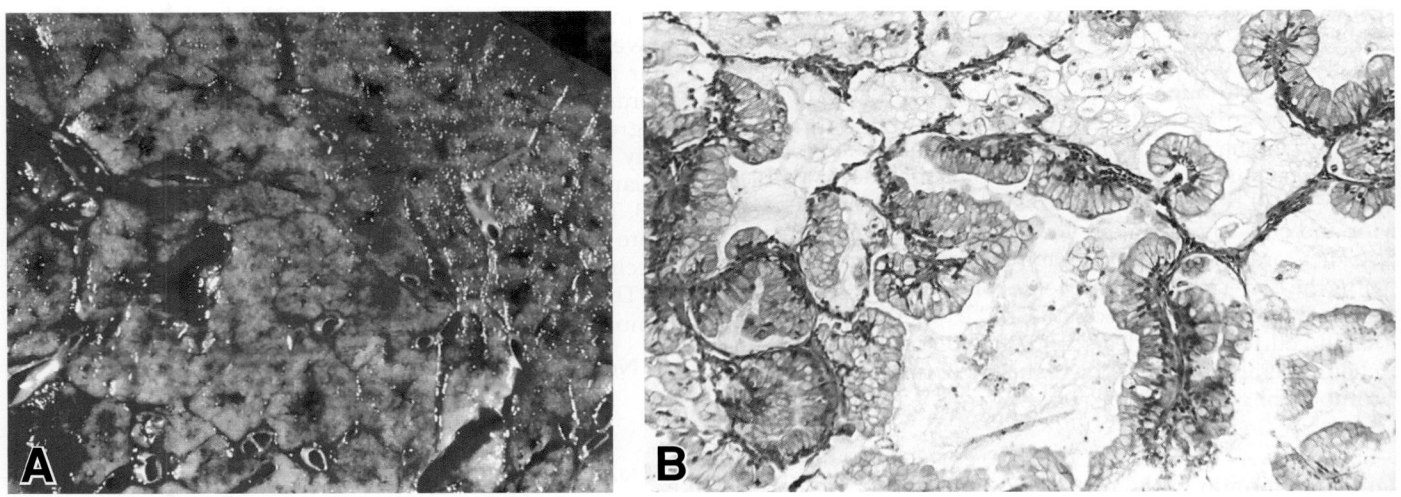

FIGURE 18-85. Invasive adenocarcinoma of the lung. A. Acinar adenocarcinoma is composed of round to oval-shaped malignant glands. **B. Papillary adenocarcinoma** consists of malignant cuboidal to columnar tumor cells growing on the surface of fibrovascular cores. **C. Micropapillary adenocarcinoma** consists of small papillary clusters of glandular cells growing within this airspace, most of which do not contain fibrovascular cores. **D. Solid adenocarcinoma** with mucin formation consists of solid sheets of tumor cells with red intracytoplasmic mucin droplets that stain positively with the mucicarmine stain.

FIGURE 18-86. Invasive mucinous adenocarcinoma. A. The cut surface of the lung is solid, glistening, and mucoid, an appearance that reflects a diffusely infiltrating tumor. **B.** Mucinous bronchioloalveolar carcinoma consists of tall columnar cells, filled with apical cytoplasmic mucin, that grow along existing alveolar walls.

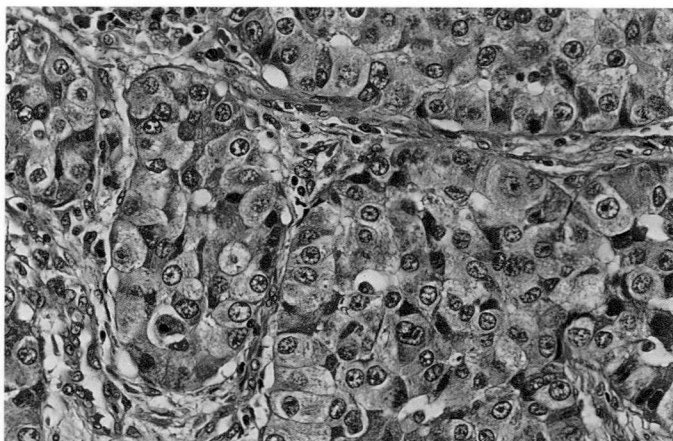

FIGURE 18-87. Large cell carcinoma of the lung. This poorly differentiated tumor is growing in sheets. Tumor cells are large and contain ample cytoplasm and prominent nucleoli.

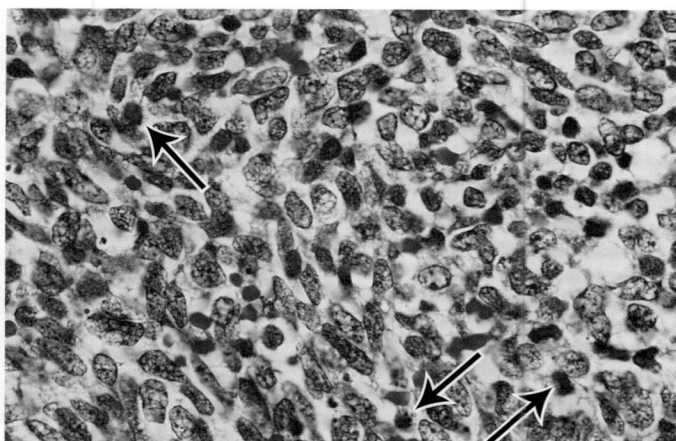

FIGURE 18-88. Small cell carcinoma of the lung. This tumor consists of small oval to spindle-shaped cells with scant cytoplasm, finely granular nuclear chromatin, and conspicuous mitoses (*arrows*).

in the United States (Table 18-6) and is strongly associated with cigarette smoking. SCLCs grow and metastasize rapidly: 70% of patients are first seen at advanced stages. These tumors often cause paraneoplastic syndromes, including **diabetes insipidus, ectopic adrenocorticotropic hormone (ACTH; corticotropin) syndrome**, and **Eaton–Lambert syndrome**.

PATHOLOGY: SCLCs are usually perihilar masses, with extensive lymph node metastases. They are soft and white, often with extensive hemorrhage and necrosis. The tumor typically spreads along bronchi in a submucosal and circumferential fashion.

Small cell carcinomas have sheets of small, round, oval, or spindle-shaped cells with scant cytoplasm. Their nuclei are distinctive, with finely granular nuclear chromatin and absent or inconspicuous nucleoli (Fig. 18-88). Most tumors express detectable neuroendocrine markers such as CD56, chromogranin, or synaptophysin. Mitotic rates are very high, with 60 to 70 mitoses per 2-mm^2 area of tumor (10 high-power fields). Necrosis is frequent and extensive. Although there is no absolute measure for the size of the tumor cells, a useful rule of thumb in small cell carcinoma is the diameter of three small resting lymphocytes. Rarely, a small cell carcinoma may occur with a "non–small cell carcinoma." In such cases, tumor behavior and clinical outcome reflect the small cell component, so they are classified as combined small cell carcinoma plus the non–small cell type (e.g., combined small cell carcinoma and adenocarcinoma). Unlike other lung cancers, small cell tumors, at least initially, are very sensitive to chemotherapy, which is the mainstay of treatment for this tumor type.

Lung Carcinomas With Combined Histology

Lung carcinomas may contain a combination of histologic subtypes within one tumor: small cell carcinomas may occur in combination with components of non–small cell carcinomas (known as "combined small cell carcinoma"),

or different non–small cell subtypes may occur in the same tumor, primarily exemplified by adenosquamous carcinomas. Combined small cell carcinomas are treated as small cell carcinomas.

Sarcomatoid tumors make up less than 1% of lung cancers. Most are pleomorphic carcinomas with at least 10% spindle and/or giant cell carcinoma in addition to other non–small cell carcinoma patterns such as adenocarcinoma or squamous cell carcinoma. If true sarcomatous components are present such as osteosarcoma, chondrosarcoma, or rhabdomyosarcoma, these tumors are classified as carcinosarcomas. Their prognosis is poor, with a median survival of 9 to 12 months.

DIAGNOSIS OF LUNG CANCER IN SMALL BIOPSIES AND CYTOLOGY SPECIMENS: The initial diagnosis of lung cancer is frequently made by analyzing a small biopsy or cytology specimen, which in patients with advanced disease, may be the only specimens available. Subtyping of NSCLC on small biopsies may be difficult as histologic features of differentiation may be lacking. Historically, classifying such tumors merely as NSCLC was sufficient. Now, however, subtyping is critical due to the need for molecular testing to identify genetic abnormalities for targeted therapy, especially in adenocarcinomas. Immunostains are of great utility in this regard. Adenocarcinomas are typically positive for markers such as TTF-1 and Napsin, and squamous cell carcinomas are usually positive for p40 or p63. This approach makes it possible to accurately subtype more than 95% of lung cancers in small biopsies or cytology specimens.

The recommended terminology and criteria for these tumors are summarized below:

Non–small cell carcinoma, favor adenocarcinoma: An NSCC-NOS by light microscopy that is positive for adenocarcinoma markers (TTF-1 or mucin) and negative for squamous markers (p63 or p40) (Fig. 18-89)

Non–small cell carcinoma, favor squamous carcinoma: An NSCC-NOS by light microscopy that is positive for squamous markers (p40 or p63) but negative for adenocarcinoma markers (Fig. 18-90)

Non–small cell carcinoma, not otherwise specified: An NSCC-NOS by light microscopy either that is negative

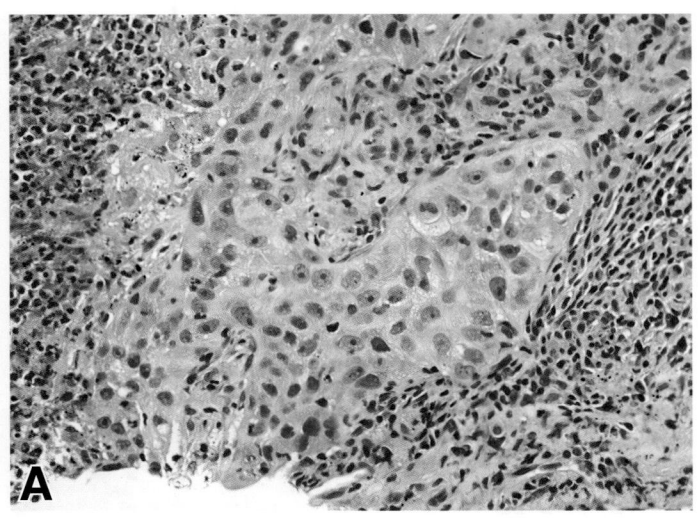

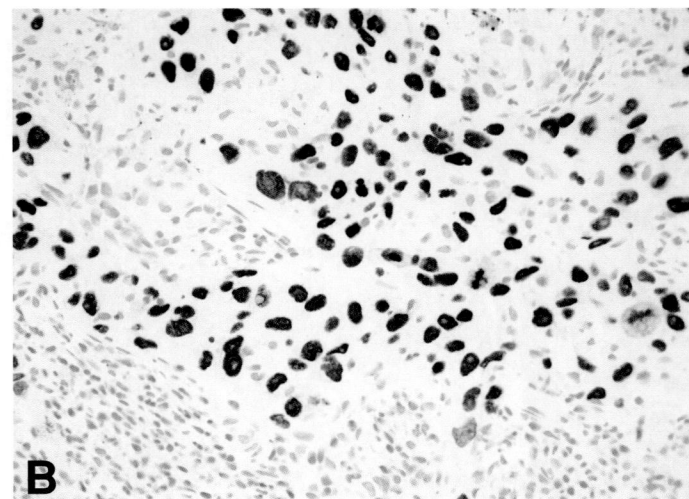

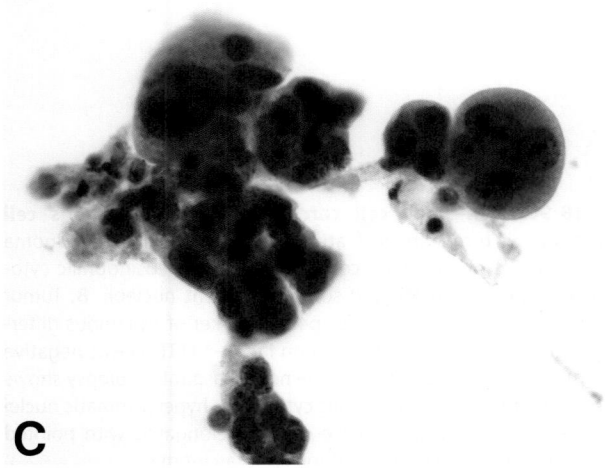

FIGURE 18-89. Non–small cell carcinoma, favor adenocarcinoma. A. This tumor shows features of a non–small cell carcinoma with large cell size, abundant cytoplasm, and prominent nucleoli. **B.** Tumor cells show strong nuclear staining for the immunohistochemical marker thyroid transcription factor-1 (TTF-1), a marker not only for adenocarcinoma differentiation but also for lung origin. Staining for p40 was negative (not shown). **C.** Papanicolaou stain of fine needle aspiration shows malignant cells in clusters with glandular structures and large hyperchromatic nuclei with some nucleoli.

for adenocarcinoma and squamous markers or one in which the staining pattern is not clear (Fig. 18-91)

All tumors classified as adenocarcinoma and NSCC-NOS must be tested for *EGFR* mutation and *ALK* or *ROS* rearrangement at a minimum. Chemotherapy, if needed, is often determined based on the presence or absence of specific mutations.

Evidence-based molecular targeted therapies are not yet established for squamous cell carcinomas. Thus, routine molecular testing for squamous cell carcinomas is not currently recommended.

Carcinoid Tumors

Two subtypes of carcinoid tumors of the lung (**typical carcinoid** and **atypical carcinoid**) are thought to arise from resident neuroendocrine cells in the normal bronchial epithelium. Carcinoid tumors account for 2% to 3% of all primary lung cancers in the United States (Table 18-6), show no sex predilection, and are not related to cigarette smoking. Although neuropeptides are readily demonstrated in the tumor cells, most are endocrinologically silent. A small subset of cases is associated with an endocrinopathy, such as

Cushing syndrome with ectopic ACTH production by tumor cells. The carcinoid syndrome (see Chapter 19) occurs in 1% of cases, usually in the setting of hepatic metastases. Nodular neuroendocrine proliferations less than 0.5 cm are called tumorlets. They may arise in the setting of interstitial fibrosis or small airway disorders and usually represent incidental findings of no clinical significance.

 PATHOLOGY: One-third of carcinoid tumors are central, one-third are peripheral (subpleural) and one-third arise in the midportion of the lung. Central carcinoid tumors tend to have a large endobronchial component, with fleshy, smooth, polypoid masses protruding into bronchial lumens (Fig. 18-92A). The tumors average 3.0 cm in diameter, but range from 0.5 to 10 cm.

Carcinoid tumors are characterized by organoid growth patterns and uniform cytologic features: eosinophilic, finely granular cytoplasm and nuclei with finely granular chromatin (Fig. 18-92B). A variety of neuroendocrine patterns may be seen, including trabecular growth, peripheral palisading, and rosettes.

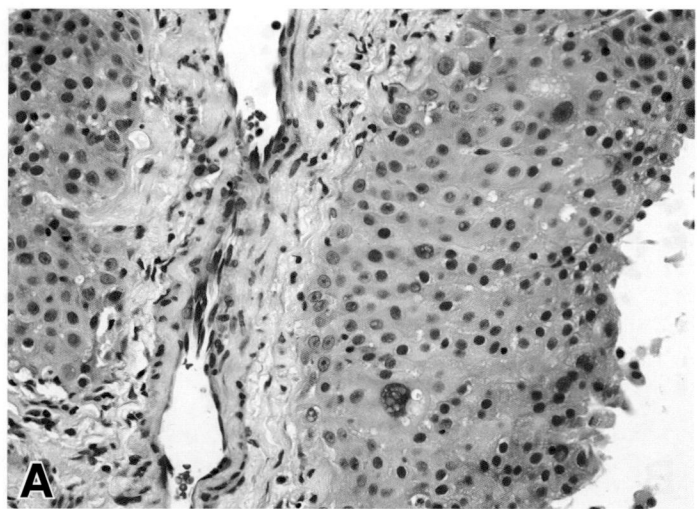

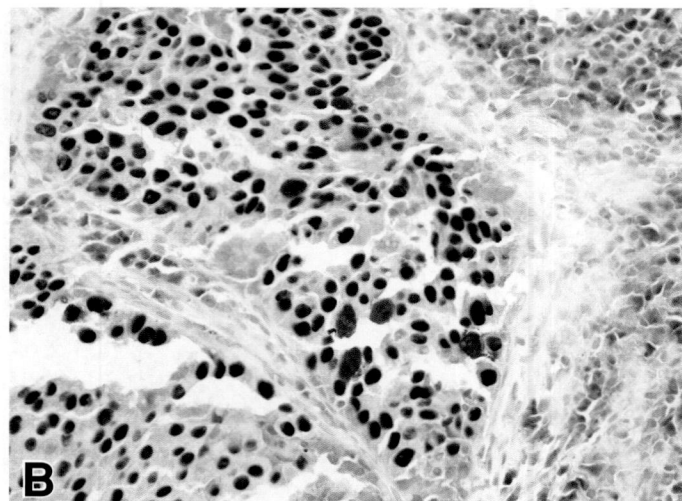

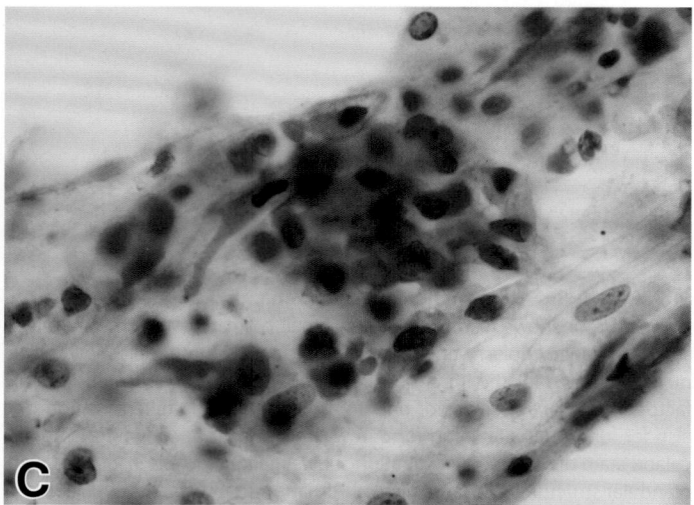

FIGURE 18-90. Non–small cell carcinoma, favor squamous cell carcinoma. A. This tumor shows features of a non–small cell carcinoma consisting of sheets of malignant cells with abundant eosinophilic cytoplasm, hyperchromatic nuclei, and some prominent nucleoli. **B.** Tumor cells show strong nuclear staining for p40, a marker of squamous differentiation. Staining for thyroid transcription factor-1 (TTF-1) was negative (not shown). **C.** Papanicolaou stain of fine needle aspiration biopsy shows clusters of cells with dense eosinophilic cytoplasm, hyperchromatic nuclei with sharply angulated shapes. Some cells are elongated with pointed ends. All of these are features of squamous cell carcinoma.

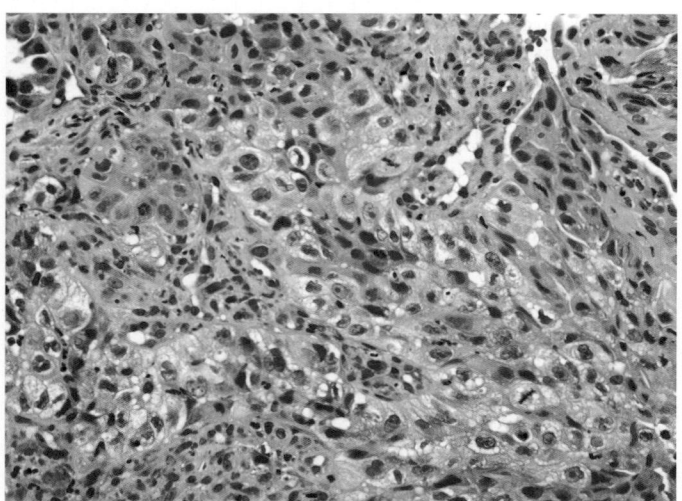

FIGURE 18-91. Non–small cell carcinoma, not otherwise specified. This tumor consists of sheets of large malignant cells with abundant eosinophilic cytoplasm and hyperchromatic and vesicular nuclei, many of which show prominent nucleoli.

Atypical carcinoid tumors are distinguished from typical carcinoid tumors by the presence of 2 to 10 mitoses per 2 mm² or by necrosis (Fig. 18-93).

CLINICAL FEATURES: Carcinoid tumors grow slowly, so half of patients are asymptomatic at presentation. They are often discovered incidentally as a mass in a chest radiograph. If a patient is symptomatic, the most common pulmonary manifestations are hemoptysis, postobstructive pneumonitis, and dyspnea. There is a slight female predominance. The mean age at diagnosis is 55, but these tumors can occur at any age. In fact, bronchial carcinoids are the most common lung tumors in childhood. Atypical carcinoid tumors tend to be more aggressive than typical ones. Regional lymph node metastases occur in 15% of patients with typical carcinoids and 50% of those with atypical carcinoids. Patients with typical carcinoids have 90% 5-year survival after surgery, compared with 60% for atypical carcinoids.

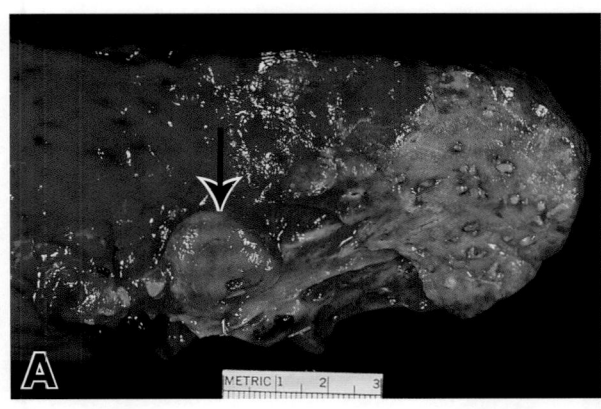

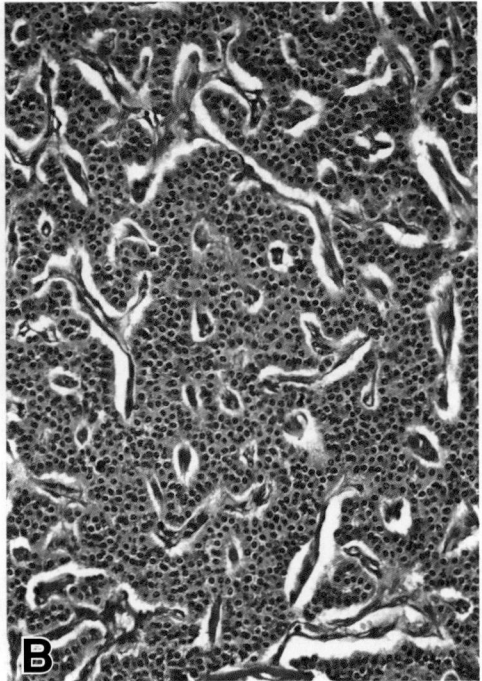

FIGURE 18-92. Carcinoid tumor of the lung. A. A circumscribed central carcinoid tumor (*arrow*) protrudes into the lumen of a main bronchus. Compression of the bronchus by the tumor caused the postobstructive pneumonia seen in the distal lung parenchyma (*right*). **B.** Microscopy shows ribbons of tumor cells embedded in a vascular stroma.

Rare Pulmonary Tumors

Inflammatory Myofibroblastic Tumor/Inflammatory Pseudotumor: Inflammatory myofibroblastic tumor of the lung is an uncommon lesion that consists of variable amounts of inflammatory cells, foamy macrophages, and fibroblasts. Most of these masses grow within the lung, although the pleura may be involved. In 5% of cases, tumors invade structures outside the lung, such as the esophagus, mediastinum, chest wall, diaphragm, or pericardium.

Inflammatory myofibroblastic tumors encompass a spectrum of lesions with a range of histologic findings as described below. As knowledge advances, some of these lesions may be reclassified as other entities. Some originally thought to be a nonneoplastic inflammatory process are now known to be inflammatory myofibroblastic tumors, a lesion originally described in soft tissue. Identification of *ALK* gene mutations provides additional evidence that at least some are true neoplasms. Other lesions previously categorized as so-called plasma cell granuloma variants of inflammatory myofibroblastic tumor may be pulmonary manifestations of immune-related processes such as IgG4-related systemic sclerosing disease.

PATHOLOGY: The tumors are solitary circumscribed, with a mean size of 4 cm. The tumor cells consist of spindle-shaped myofibroblasts. The stroma can be composed of varying amounts of inflammatory cells, including lymphocytes, plasma cells, macrophages, giant cells, mast cells, and eosinophils. Inflammatory myofibroblastic tumor causes consolidation of the lung parenchyma and loss of architecture. Two major histologic patterns are fibrohistiocytic (Fig. 18-94) and plasma cell granuloma, depending on the predominant component. In some cases, foamy macrophages impart a xanthomatous picture.

CLINICAL FEATURES: Most patients are under 40, but inflammatory myofibroblastic tumors can occur at any age and are among the most common lung tumors of childhood. Half of patients are asymptomatic at presentation. A previous history of a pulmonary infection is present in one-third of patients. Most inflammatory myofibroblastic tumors are cured by surgical excision, but 5% recur within the chest.

Pulmonary Epithelioid Hemangioendothelioma: Pulmonary epithelioid hemangioendotheliomas are rare low- to intermediate-grade vascular sarcomas. Most patients are young adults; 80% are women. Half are asymptomatic.

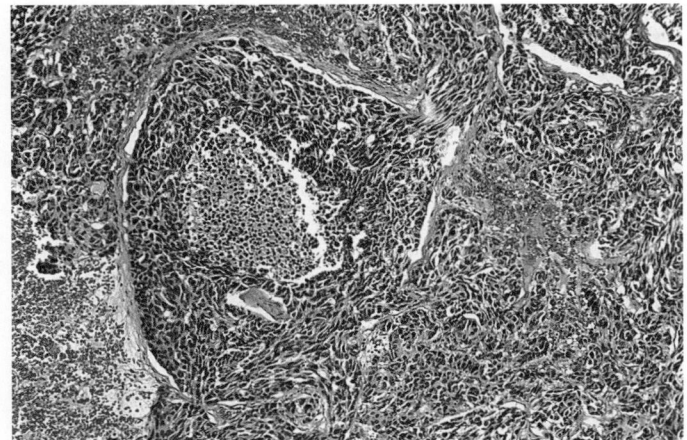

FIGURE 18-93. Atypical carcinoid tumor of the lung. A cellular tumor shows central necrosis and a disorganized architecture.

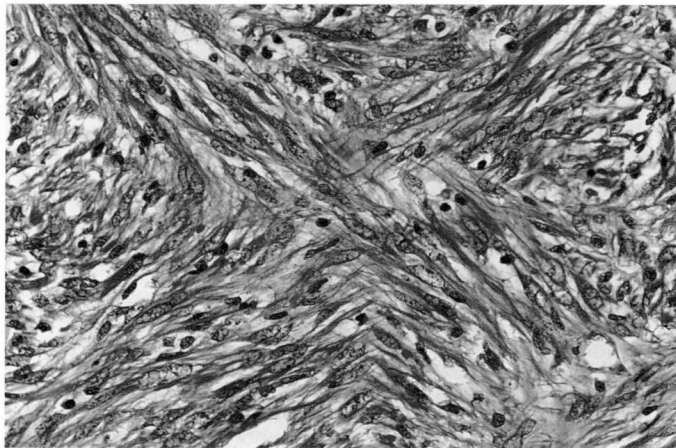

FIGURE 18-94. Inflammatory pseudotumor. Microscopy shows intersecting spindle cells with scattered lymphocytes and macrophages.

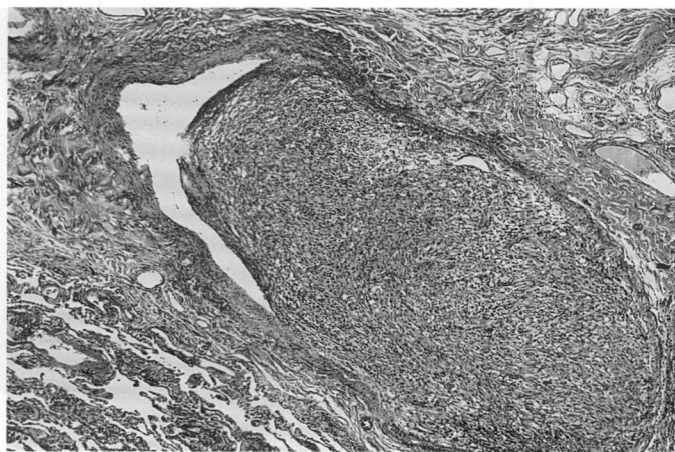

FIGURE 18-96. Pulmonary artery sarcoma. A polypoid mass of malignant spindle cells is spreading within the lumen of this pulmonary artery.

PATHOLOGY: Most patients are first seen with multiple pulmonary nodules. Histologically, these tumors consist of oval-shaped nodules with central, sclerotic, hypocellular zones and cellular peripheral zones. They spread within alveolar spaces (Fig. 18-95). Tumor cells have abundant cytoplasm, with frequent intracytoplasmic vascular lumens, which may contain red blood cells. The tumor matrix is abundant and eosinophilic. The tumors express vascular markers, such as factor VIII, CD34 or CD31. Additionally, most tumors are characterized by a *WWTR1-CAMTA1* gene fusion although some variants have been associated with a *YAP-TFE3* gene fusion. Both of these gene fusions result in dysregulation of the Hippo signaling pathway and promote anchorage-independent cell proliferation. Epithelioid hemangioendotheliomas with a histologic pattern similar to that seen in the lung may occur in the liver, bone, and soft tissue. Pulmonary epithelioid hemangioendothelioma has a variable clinical course, with a mean survival of 5 years.

Pulmonary Blastoma: This malignant tumor resembles embryonal lung, with a glandular component of poorly differentiated columnar cells in tubules, lacking

mucus secretion. The intervening tumor contains spindle cells that resemble embryonal mesoderm. There is histologic overlap between pulmonary blastoma and carcinosarcoma, including heterologous elements. The clinical features are also similar.

Despite its embryonal appearance, pulmonary blastomas occur mainly in adults (median age range, 35 to 43), and most patients are cigarette smokers. The prognosis for patients with biphasic tumors is poor and comparable to that for carcinoma of the lung. Pulmonary blastomas are often associated with mutations in *CTNNB*, which encodes β-catenin.

Mucoepidermoid Carcinoma and Adenoid Cystic Carcinoma: These neoplasms resemble their namesakes in the salivary glands. They are derived from tracheobronchial mucus glands and are seen in the trachea or proximal bronchus as a luminal mass, often associated with obstructive symptoms. Adenoid cystic carcinomas are difficult to resect locally and often metastasize.

Pulmonary Artery Intimal Sarcoma: Pulmonary artery intimal sarcoma is a rare tumor of connective tissue (Fig. 18-96), which has a broad histologic spectrum, including fibrosarcoma, leiomyosarcoma, osteosarcoma, rhabdomyosarcoma, angiosarcoma, or unclassifiable sarcoma. These tumors are rarely diagnosed during life, but may be discovered because of pulmonary hypertension. They often grow in an intraluminal fashion, within proximal arteries, and may extend, worm-like, to peripheral pulmonary artery branches, causing peripheral infarcts.

Pulmonary Lymphomas

All lymphomas, both Hodgkin and non-Hodgkin types, may involve the lung (see also Chapter 26). Most lymphomas involving the lung are metastatic. Primary pulmonary lymphomas are rare, the most common being **extranodal marginal zone B-cell lymphoma.** These tumors are thought to arise from *mucosa-associated lymphoid tissue* of the lung and are sometimes designated "MALT" lymphomas. They are low-grade tumors, generally with a favorable prognosis.

Diffuse large B-cell lymphoma may also arise as a primary pulmonary lymphoma (see Chapter 26). **Lymphomatoid granulomatosis,** a subtype of diffuse large B-cell

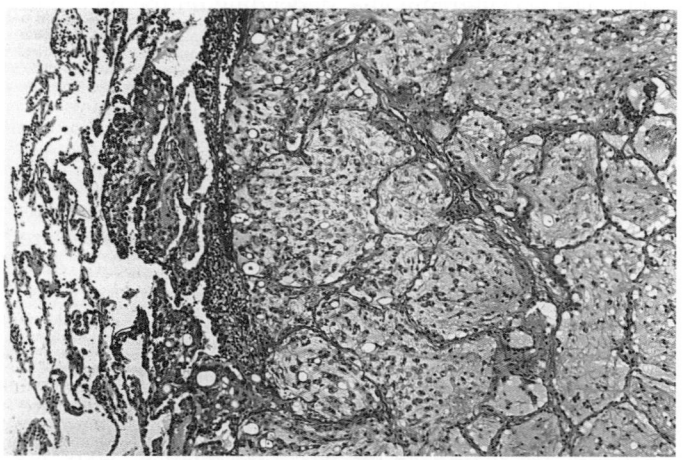

FIGURE 18-95. Epithelioid hemangioendothelioma. A nodule of tumor has spread within alveolar spaces.

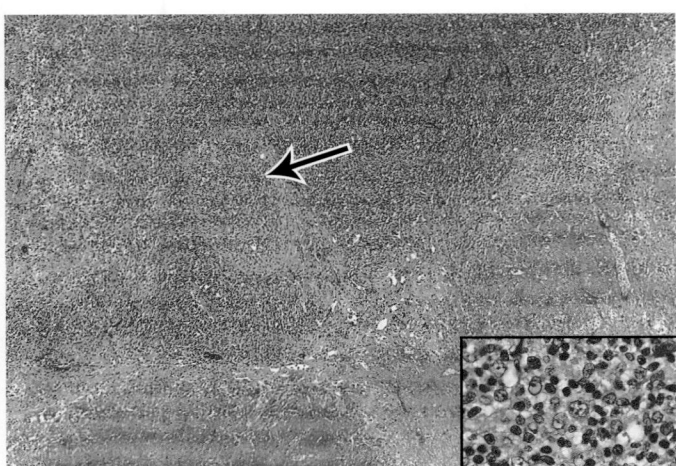

FIGURE 18-97. Lymphomatoid granulomatosis. This extensively necrotic nodular mass consists of a lymphoid infiltrate that penetrates a blood vessel (*arrow*) at the edge of the lesion. The lymphoid infiltrate is composed of a polymorphous population of small, medium-sized, and large atypical lymphoid cells (*inset*).

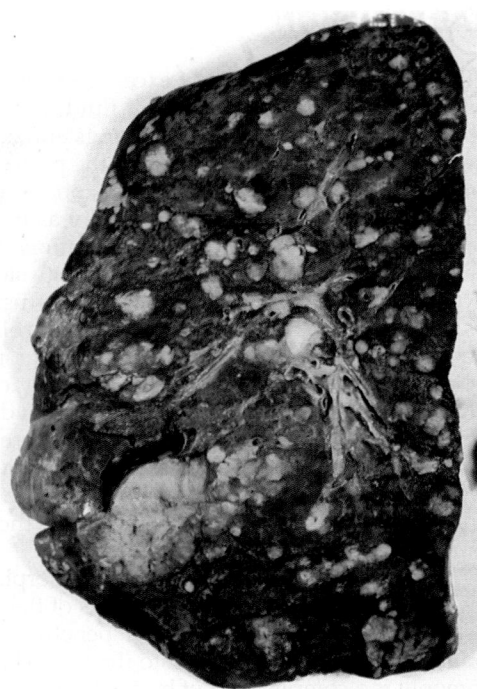

FIGURE 18-98. Metastatic carcinoma of the lung. A section through the lung shows numerous nodules of metastatic carcinoma corresponding to the "cannon ball" pattern of metastases seen radiographically.

lymphoma, is characterized by nodular pulmonary lymphoid infiltrates with frequent central necrosis and vascular permeation (Fig. 18-97). It affects middle-aged people and is more common in immunosuppressed individuals. The lung is the major location, but the kidney, skin, and upper respiratory tract may also be involved. The lymphoid infiltrate is angiocentric and angioinvasive, with polymorphous, small to medium-sized lymphocytes, mainly T cells, admixed with variable numbers of large atypical B cells. The latter typically express EBV, which is thought to drive the proliferation. Lymphomatoid granulomatosis is typically divided into grades depending on the percentage of atypical B cells present. Previously, only the highest grade was considered a "true" lymphoma, and the lower grades were thought to be less aggressive; however, all grades are now considered to be subtypes of diffuse large B-cell lymphoma for treatment purposes. Despite remissions with chemotherapy, half of all patients eventually develop large cell lymphoma.

Extrapulmonary Tumors Often Metastasize to the Lung

In one-third of all fatal cancers, lung metastases are found at autopsy. In fact, metastatic tumors are the most common malignancies in the lung. They are typically multiple and circumscribed. Large metastatic nodules in the lungs seen radiologically are called "cannon ball" metastases (Fig. 18-98). Most metastases resemble their primary tumors. Rarely, metastatic tumors show lepidic growth, particularly mucinous types, in which cases the usual primary site is the pancreas or stomach.

In **lymphangitic carcinoma**, metastatic tumor spreads widely through pulmonary lymphatic channels to form a sheath of tumor around the bronchovascular tree and veins. Clinically, patients suffer from cough and shortness of breath and display a diffuse reticulonodular pattern on the chest radiograph. The common primary sites are the breast, stomach, pancreas, and colon.

The Pleura

PNEUMOTHORAX

Pneumothorax is the presence of air in the pleural cavity. It may occur with traumatic perforation of the pleura or may be "spontaneous." Traumatic causes include penetrating wounds of the chest wall (e.g., a stab wound or a rib fracture). Traumatic pneumothorax is most commonly iatrogenic and is seen after therapeutic aspiration of fluid from the pleura (thoracentesis), pleural or lung biopsies, transbronchial biopsies, and positive pressure–assisted ventilation.

Spontaneous pneumothorax is typically seen in young adults. For example, a young man may develop acute chest pain and shortness of breath during vigorous exercise. A chest radiograph shows collapse of the lung on the side of the pain and a large collection of air in the pleural space. The cause is rupture, usually of a subpleural emphysematous bleb. In most cases, spontaneous pneumothorax resolves by itself, but some patients require withdrawal of the air.

Tension pneumothorax refers to unilateral pneumothorax extensive enough to shift the mediastinum to the opposite side, with compression of the opposite lung. The condition may be life-threatening and must be relieved by immediate drainage.

Bronchopleural fistula is a serious condition involving free communication between an airway and the pleura. It is usually iatrogenic, caused by the interruption of bronchial continuity during biopsy or surgery. It may also be due to extensive infection and necrosis of lung tissue, in which case the infection is more important than the air.

PLEURAL EFFUSION

Pleural effusion is accumulation of excess fluid in the pleural cavity. Normally, a small amount of fluid in the pleural cavity lubricates the space between the lungs and chest wall. Fluid is secreted into the pleural space by the parietal pleura and absorbed by the visceral pleura. Effusions vary from a few milliliters, detectable only radiologically as blunting of the costophrenic angle, to massive accumulations that shift the mediastinum and the trachea to the opposite side.

HYDROTHORAX: Hydrothorax is an effusion that resembles water and would be regarded as edema elsewhere. It may be due to increased capillary hydrostatic pressure, as occurs in patients with heart failure or in any condition that produces systemic or pulmonary edema. Hydrothorax also occurs in patients with low serum oncotic pressure, as in nephrotic syndrome, cirrhosis of the liver, or severe starvation. Other important causes of hydrothorax are collagen vascular diseases (notably systemic lupus erythematosus and rheumatoid arthritis) and asbestos exposure.

PYOTHORAX: A turbid effusion full of polymorphonuclear leukocytes (pyothorax) results from infections of the pleura. It may occasionally be caused by an external penetrating wound that introduces pyogenic organisms into the pleural space but more commonly is a complication of bacterial pneumonia that extends to the pleural surface, the classic example of which is pneumococcal pneumonia. Pyothorax is a rare complication of medical procedures involving the pleural cavity.

EMPYEMA: This disorder is a variant of pyothorax in which thick pus accumulates within the pleural cavity, often with loculation and fibrosis.

HEMOTHORAX: Blood in the pleural cavity as a result of trauma or rupture of a vessel (e.g., dissecting aneurysm of the aorta) is hemothorax. A pleural effusion may be blood stained in tuberculosis, cancers involving the pleura, and pulmonary infarction.

CHYLOTHORAX: Chylothorax is accumulation of milky, lipid-rich fluid (chyle) in the pleural cavity due to lymphatic obstruction. It has an ominous portent, because lymphatic obstruction suggests disease of the lymph nodes in the posterior mediastinum. Chylothorax is thus a rare complication of mediastinal tumors, such as lymphoma. In tropical countries, it may result from nematode infestations. It can also be seen in pulmonary LAM.

PLEURITIS

Pleuritis, or inflammation of the pleura, may result from extension of any pulmonary infection to the visceral pleura, bacterial infections within the pleural cavity, viral infections, collagen vascular disease, or pulmonary infarction that involves the lung surface. The most striking symptom is sharp, stabbing chest pain on inspiration. It is often associated with pleural effusions.

TUMORS OF THE PLEURA

Localized (Solitary) Fibrous Tumors of the Pleura Are Usually Benign

Solitary fibrous tumor of the pleura is an uncommon localized neoplasm arising in the pleura. Most are benign, but a few are malignant. Some 80% arise on the visceral pleura, the remainder being from the parietal pleura. Similar tumors can develop on any mesothelial surface, including the mediastinum, peritoneum, pericardium, liver, and tunica vaginalis. They arise from submesothelial connective tissue, not mesothelium, and are unrelated to asbestos exposure.

PATHOLOGY: The tumors are usually pedunculated. More than 60% are greater than 10 cm in diameter and some reach 40 cm and may weigh up to 3,800 g. The cut surface is gray-white, with a nodular, whorled, or lobulated appearance (Fig. 18-99A). Cysts are occasionally present, especially at the base near the pleural attachment.

The most common histologic appearance is the "patternless pattern" of disorderly or randomly arranged mixtures of fibroblast-like cells and connective tissue. Other arrangements include hemangiopericytoma-like, storiform (star-like, or spiral), herringbone, leiomyoma-like, or neurofibroma-like arrangements (Fig. 18-99B). The tumor cells are spindle to oval shaped, often with a fibroblast-like appearance. Collagen is compressed between the cells in a lacy network or it may form dense, wire-like bands. Histologic features suggesting malignancy include increased cellularity, pleomorphism, necrosis, and more

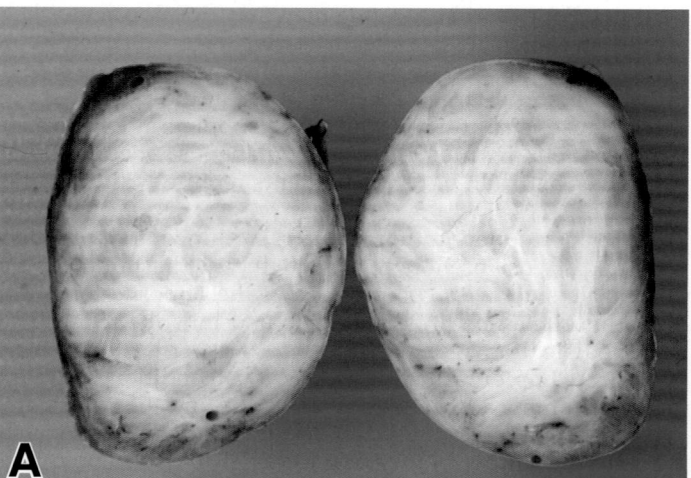
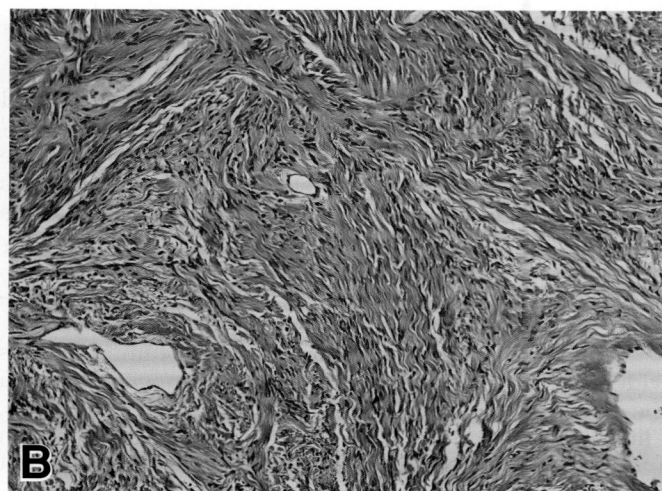

FIGURE 18-99. Pleural localized (solitary) fibrous tumor. A. The tumor is circumscribed with a whorled, tan cut surface. **B.** Tumor cells are round to oval and spindle shaped, with a dense eosinophilic or "ropy" collagen stroma and slit-like blood vessels.

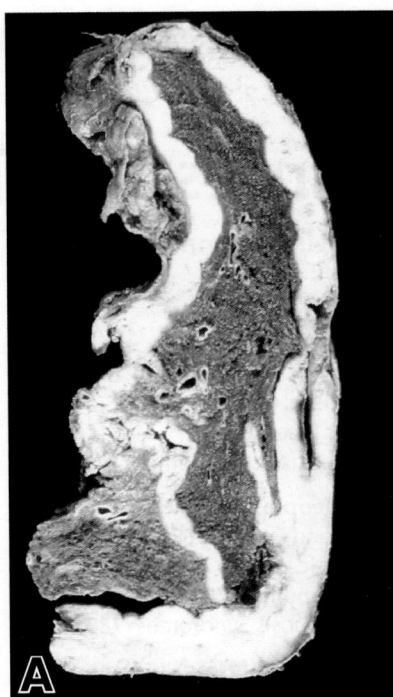
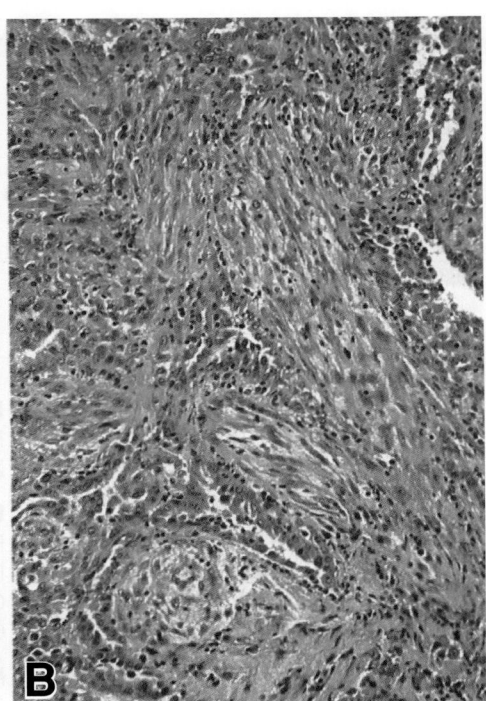

FIGURE 18-100. Pleural malignant mesothelioma. A. The lung is encased by a dense pleural tumor that extends along interlobar fissures but does not invade the underlying lung parenchyma. **B.** This mesothelioma is composed of a biphasic pattern of epithelial and sarcomatous elements.

than four mitoses per 10 high-power fields. Most tumors are immunopositive for CD34 and Bcl-2. The majority of cases also harbor a *NAB2-STAT6* gene fusion which results in positive immunostaining for STAT-6.

 CLINICAL FEATURES: The median age of patients diagnosed with localized fibrous tumor of the pleura is 55 years (range, 9 to 86 years) without a sex predominance. They present most often with chest pain, followed by shortness of breath, cough, hypoglycemia, weight loss, hemoptysis, fever, and night sweats. Patients with benign fibrous tumors of pleura have an excellent prognosis. Half of histologically malignant tumors are cured if resected completely.

Malignant Mesothelioma Usually Reflects Asbestos Exposure

Malignant mesothelioma is a neoplasm of mesothelial cells. It is most common in the pleura but also occurs in the peritoneum, pericardium, and tunica vaginalis of the testis.

EPIDEMIOLOGY: Some 2,000 new cases of malignant mesothelioma develop yearly in the United States. In the United States, Great Britain, and South Africa, 80% of patients report exposure to asbestos. Mesothelioma typically develops after a long latency period, which averages 30 to 40 years.

PATHOLOGY: Grossly, pleural mesotheliomas often encase and compress the lung, extending into fissures and interlobar septa, a distribution often referred to as a "pleural rind" (Fig. 18-100A). Invasion of pulmonary parenchyma is generally limited to the periphery adjacent to the tumor. Lymph nodes tend to be spared. Microscopically, classic mesotheliomas show both epithelial and sarcomatous patterns (Fig. 18-100B). Glands and tubules that resemble adenocarcinoma are admixed with sheets of spindle cells similar in appearance to a fibrosarcoma. In some instances, only one or the other component is present. If it is epithelial, the tumor may be difficult to distinguish from adenocarcinoma. Less commonly, only a sarcomatous component is present.

Immunohistochemistry is essential for differentiating mesothelioma from adenocarcinoma (see Chapter 5). Both are positive for cytokeratins; however, adenocarcinomas often, but not always, express carcinoembryonic antigen, claudin-4, Leu-M1, B72.3, and Ber-EP4, but mesotheliomas are negative for these markers. In contrast, mesotheliomas are typically positive for calretinin, WT-1, and D2-40 (podoplanin), for which adenocarcinomas are typically negative. Other criteria supportive of a diagnosis of mesothelioma include absence of mucin, presence of hyaluronic acid (positive Alcian blue staining) and long, slender microvilli seen by electron microscopy.

CLINICAL FEATURES: The average age of patients with mesothelioma is 60 years. Patients first present with a pleural effusion or a pleural mass, chest pain, and nonspecific symptoms, such as weight loss and malaise. Pleural mesotheliomas tend to spread locally within the chest cavity, invading and compressing major structures. Metastases can occur to the lung parenchyma and mediastinal lymph nodes, as well as to extrathoracic sites such as liver, bones, peritoneum, and adrenals. Treatment is largely ineffective and prognosis is poor. Few patients survive longer than 18 months after diagnosis.

THE RESPIRATORY SYSTEM

19 The Gastrointestinal Tract

Jeffrey P. Baliff, Jonathan N. Glickman

The Esophagus

ANATOMY

The gut and respiratory tract arise embryologically from the foregut, which then divides into two separate tubes, the dorsal esophagus and the ventral trachea. The adult esophagus is a conduit for food and liquid into the stomach. As measured during upper endoscopy, its length is 38 to 43 cm (average 40) from the incisor teeth to the gastroesophageal junction. It contains striated and smooth muscle in its upper portion and smooth muscle only in its lower portion. It is fixed superiorly by the cricopharyngeal and inferior pharyngeal constrictor muscles, which together form the upper esophageal sphincter. It courses inferiorly through the posterior mediastinum behind the trachea and heart and exits the thorax through the diaphragm. Tonic muscular contraction at its lower end creates the **lower esophageal sphincter**, which is a functional sphincter, rather than a true anatomic one.

The esophagus has a mucosa, muscularis mucosae, submucosa, muscularis propria, and adventitia. The mucosa is lined by nonkeratinizing, stratified squamous epithelium. A transition to gastric mucosa at the **gastroesophageal (GE) junction** occurs abruptly at the level of the diaphragm. The esophageal submucosa contains mucous glands, a rich lymphatic plexus and nerve fibers. Lymphatics of the upper third of the esophagus drain to cervical lymph nodes, those of the middle third to mediastinal nodes and those of the lower third to celiac and gastric lymph nodes. These anatomic features are significant in the spread of esophageal cancer.

Venous drainage of the esophagus is important, because the veins can form varices if there is portal hypertension. Varices occur only in the lower third of the esophagus, as the veins of the upper third drain into the superior vena cava and those of the middle third drain into the azygous system. Only the veins of the lower third drain into the portal vein via the gastric veins.

CONGENITAL DISORDERS

Tracheoesophageal Fistula Leads to Aspiration Pneumonia

Congenital **atresias** and **stenoses** may occur at any site in the gastrointestinal tract. Esophageal atresia occurs in 1 in 3,500 births and stenosis in 1 in 50,000 births. Atresias are a complete interruption of the lumen, whereas a fistula is an abnormal connection between two normally separated structures. Stenoses, or narrowings, are mainly acquired but can be congenital. They usually occur in the distal esophagus and reflect abnormal wall architecture.

Esophageal atresia with or without tracheoesophageal fistula is the most common congenital esophageal anomaly (Fig. 19-1), with an increased frequency in preterm babies of male gender. Atresia results from a failure of the primitive forgut to recanalize, whereas tracheoesophageal fistula results from incomplete separation of the primitive foregut into two completely separate tubes. Half of patients have other congenital anomalies. One-fifth have VACTERL

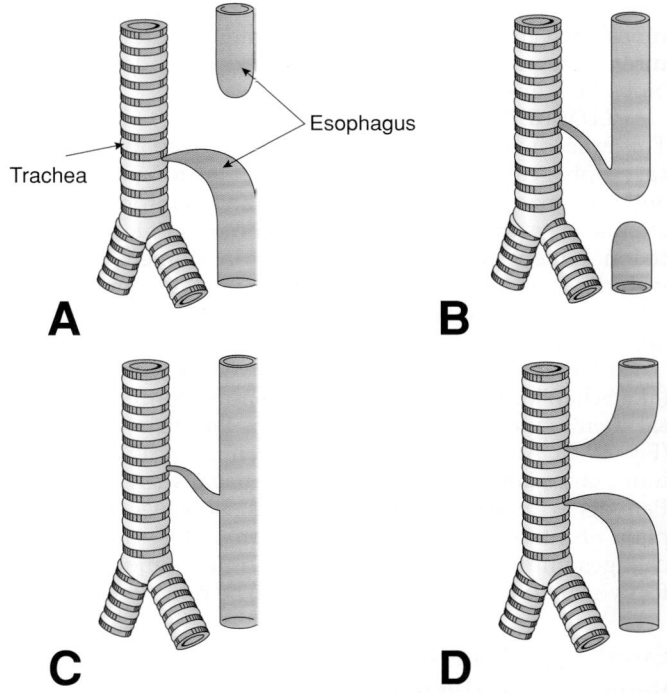

FIGURE 19-1. Congenital tracheoesophageal fistulas. A. The most common type (85% of cases) is a communication between the trachea and the lower portion of the esophagus. The upper segment of the esophagus ends in a blind sac. **B.** In a few cases, the proximal esophagus communicates with the trachea. **C.** H-type fistula without esophageal atresia. **D.** Tracheal fistulas to both a proximal esophageal pouch and distal esophagus.

syndrome (vertebral defects, anal atresia, cardiac defects, tracheoesophageal fistula, renal dysplasia, and limb abnormalities). The etiology of esophageal atresias and fistulas is unknown, but genetic and environmental factors are thought to contribute. Prenatal diagnosis is suggested by polyhydramnios, as amniotic fluid cannot reach the stomach in the case of an upper esophageal atresia.

PATHOLOGY: In about 85% of tracheoesophageal fistulas, the upper portion of the esophagus ends in a blind pouch and the superior end of the lower segment communicates with the trachea (Fig. 19-1A). *In this type of atresia, the upper blind sac fills with mucus, which the infant aspirates.* Another type of fistula is a communication between the proximal esophagus and the trachea; the lower esophageal pouch communicates with the stomach (Fig. 19-1B). *Infants with this condition aspirate shortly after birth.* In an **H-type fistula,** there is a communication between an intact esophagus and an intact trachea (Fig. 19-1C). This lesion may not become symptomatic until adulthood, presenting with repeated pulmonary infections.

Rings and Webs Cause Dysphagia

ESOPHAGEAL WEBS: Occasionally, a mucosal membrane projects into the esophageal lumen. Webs are usually thin (<2 mm), eccentric, and occur in the proximal esophagus. They have a core of fibrovascular tissue lined by normal mucosa and submucosa. Middle-aged women are most affected and present with difficulty swallowing (dysphagia). They are typically treated with rubber bougies, cylindrical tubes used to dilate constricted segments of tubular structures. If necessary, webs can be excised via endoscopy with biopsy forceps.

PLUMMER–VINSON (PATERSON–KELLY) SYNDROME: This exceedingly rare disorder is characterized by (1) a cervical esophageal web, (2) inflammation of the tongue (glossitis) and corners of the mouth (cheilitis), and (3) iron-deficiency anemia. Dysphagia is the most common clinical manifestation. Ninety percent of cases occur in women. Treatment includes iron supplementation and, if necessary, mechanical dilation of the esophagus. *Carcinoma of the oropharynx and upper esophagus is a possible complication.*

SCHATZKI RING: In contrast to webs, esophageal rings (aka Schatzki ring) are thicker (2 to 5 mm), concentric mucosal membranes that usually occur in the distal esophagus (Fig. 19-2). Although they may be seen in up to 14% of barium examinations, Schatzki rings are usually asymptomatic. Patients with narrow Schatzki rings, however, may complain of intermittent dysphagia. Often dietary and lifestyle changes improve symptoms. If these interventions are ineffective, dilation with bougies can also be done.

Esophageal Diverticula Often Reflect Motor Dysfunction

A **true diverticulum** is an outpouching of the tubular gastrointestinal tract that contains all layers—mucosa, submucosa, and muscularis propria. An outpouching of mucosa and submucosa through the muscularis propria is a **false diverticulum**. Esophageal diverticula occur in the hypopharyngeal area above the upper esophageal sphincter, in the

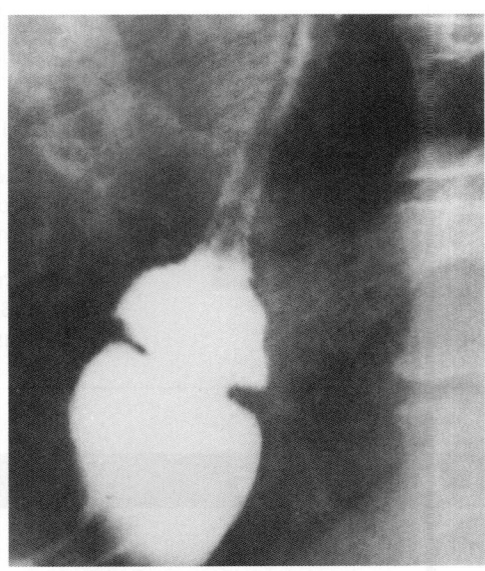

FIGURE 19-2. Schatzki mucosal ring. A contrast radiograph illustrates the lower esophageal narrowing.

middle esophagus, and just proximal to the lower esophageal sphincter.

ZENKER DIVERTICULUM: The most common type of esophageal diverticulum, Zenker diverticula appear in the proximal esophagus in elderly patients, men more than women. These acquired false diverticula probably reflect disordered function of cricopharyngeal musculature.

These diverticula can enlarge conspicuously and accumulate a large amount of food. Symptoms include halitosis (bad breath), regurgitation of undigested food, cough, choking, and possibly aspiration pneumonia. Long-standing inflammation caused by stasis of food contents within the diverticulum may lead to squamous cell carcinoma in up to 7% of patients. When symptomatic, these lesions are surgically removed or treated endoscopically.

MIDESOPHAGEAL (TRACTION) DIVERTICULA: Diverticula in the middle of the esophagus are often due to periesophageal inflammation and/or scarring that pulls the esophageal wall outward (thus the term traction diverticula). These true diverticula may be caused by a lung mass or necroinflammation in mediastinal lymph nodes caused by tuberculosis, histoplasmosis, or sarcoidosis, for example. Less commonly, motility disorders like achalasia may be the cause. These diverticula do not retain food or secretions and remain asymptomatic, with only rare complications.

EPIPHRENIC DIVERTICULA: These diverticula are located in the distal esophagus, usually immediately above the diaphragm. Motor disturbances of the esophagus (e.g., achalasia, diffuse esophageal spasm) are found in two-thirds of patients with this false diverticulum. Abnormalities of the lower esophageal sphincter may also lead to an epiphrenic diverticula. When symptomatic, surgery to correct the underlying motor abnormality (e.g., myotomy) is appropriate.

MOTOR DISORDERS

Autonomic coordination of muscular movement during swallowing is a **motor function** and results in free passage of food through the esophagus. The hallmark of motor disorders is difficulty in swallowing, or **dysphagia**. Dysphagia is often an awareness that food is not moving downward and in itself is not painful. Pain on swallowing is **odynophagia**. Motor disorders can be caused by:

- **Systemic diseases of skeletal muscle** (in the upper esophagus) such as myasthenia gravis, dermatomyositis, amyloidosis, hypothyroidism, and myxedema
- **Neurologic diseases** affecting nerves to skeletal or smooth muscle (e.g., cerebrovascular accidents, amyotrophic lateral sclerosis)
- **Peripheral neuropathy** associated with diabetes or alcoholism

In Achalasia, Lower Esophageal Sphincter Function Is Abnormal

Achalasia involves failure of the lower esophageal sphincter to relax with swallowing and poor peristalsis in the body of the esophagus. As a result of these defects in both the outflow tract and esophageal pumping mechanisms, food is retained in the esophagus with consequent proximal dilation (Fig. 19-3).

Primary achalasia is an inflammatory disease that causes loss of inhibitory neurons in the esophageal myenteric plexus. Chronic inflammation (mainly T cells) in the myenteric plexus leads to neuritis and ganglionitis, and eventually to ganglion cell loss and fibrosis. The cause of the inflammation is unknown, but genetic, viral, and autoimmune factors have been suggested. Degenerative changes in the dorsal motor nucleus of the vagus and extraesophageal vagus nerves may also contribute. In Latin America, secondary achalasia is a common complication of **Chagas disease** (see Chapter 9), in which ganglion cells are destroyed by the protozoan *Trypanosoma cruzi*. The term pseudoachalasia refers to damage to myenteric plexus nerves by infiltrative disorders, such as amyloidosis, sarcoidosis, or invasive tumors.

Symptoms of achalasia include dysphagia (to both solids and liquids) and occasionally odynophagia and regurgitation of material retained in the esophagus. Squamous cell carcinoma may develop in long-standing cases. Radiography may show a "bird-beak" gastroesophageal junction, but manometry is the standard diagnostic test for confirming achalasia. Treatment may include endoscopic balloon dilation, botulinum toxin injection of the lower esophageal sphincter, endoscopic myotomy, or surgical myotomy of the lower esophageal sphincter. Patients may develop gastroesophageal reflux after treatment.

Systemic Sclerosis Causes Fibrosis of the Esophageal Wall

Systemic sclerosis (scleroderma) causes fibrosis in many organs and involves the gastrointestinal tract 80% of the time (see Chapter 11). Any segment of the tubal gut may be affected. The esophagus is most frequently impacted, often with severely abnormal esophageal muscle function. The lower esophageal sphincter may be so impaired that the lower esophagus and upper stomach no longer form distinct functional entities and are visualized as a common cavity. Peristalsis may be impaired throughout the esophagus.

 PATHOLOGY: Fibrosis is present in the esophageal smooth muscle (especially the inner muscularis propria). Nonspecific inflammation is also evident. Small arteries and arterioles show intimal fibrosis, which may contribute to the fibrosis.

CLINICAL FEATURES: Patients have dysphagia, regurgitation, and heartburn caused by peptic esophagitis, owing to reflux of acid from the stomach. Severe reflux changes may occur (see below).

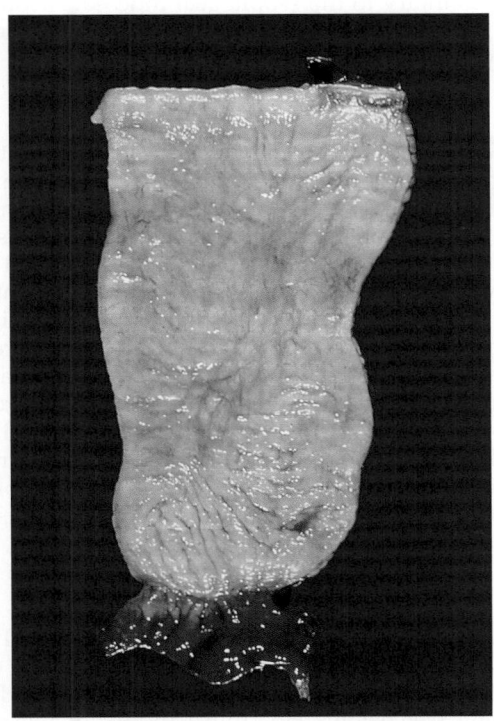

FIGURE 19-3. Esophagus and upper stomach of a patient with advanced achalasia. The esophagus is markedly dilated above the esophagogastric junction, where the lower esophageal sphincter is located. The esophageal mucosa is redundant and has hyperplastic squamous epithelium.

HIATAL HERNIA

Hiatal hernia is a protrusion of the stomach into the chest, through an enlarged diaphragmatic opening. There are two basic types of hiatal hernia (Fig. 19-4).

SLIDING HERNIA: Enlargement of the diaphragmatic hiatus and laxity of the circumferential connective tissue allow a cap of gastric mucosa to move upward, above the diaphragm. This common condition accounts for 85% of hiatal hernias and is usually asymptomatic. The most commonly associated symptom is GE reflux, although it is unclear whether hernias are the cause or the result of reflux.

PARAESOPHAGEAL HERNIA: In this uncommon form of hiatal hernia, a portion of gastric fundus herniates through a defect in the diaphragmatic connective tissue that normally forms the esophageal hiatus. The hernia progressively enlarges and the hiatus grows increasingly wide. This

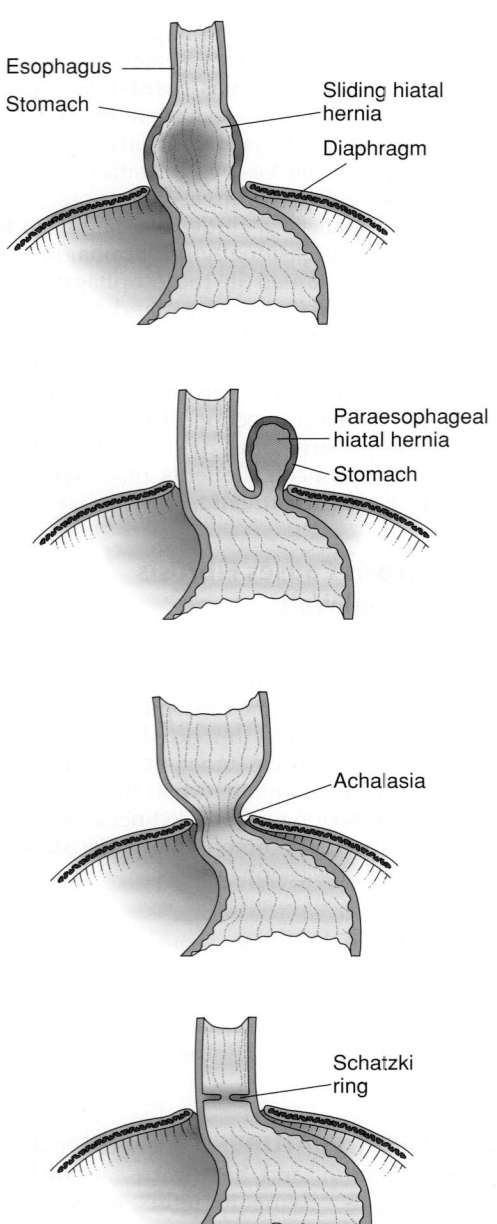

FIGURE 19-4. Disorders of the esophageal outlet.

can compress the esophagus, leading to a decrease in reflux of gastric contents. In extreme cases, the entire stomach and other abdominal organs can herniate into the thorax.

CLINICAL FEATURES: Symptoms of sliding hiatal hernia, mostly heartburn and regurgitation, result from reflux of gastric contents into the esophagus, primarily due to incompetence of the lower esophageal sphincter. Classically, symptoms are worse when subjects recline, as this position facilitates acid reflux. Dysphagia, fullness after meals, shortness of breath, painful swallowing, and occasionally bleeding peptic ulcers may be seen in paraesophageal hernias. Large hernias carry a risk of gastric volvulus or intrathoracic gastric dilation.

Sliding hiatal hernias generally do not require surgery and are treated medically. An enlarging paraesophageal hernia should be corrected surgically, even if it is asymptomatic.

ESOPHAGITIS

Reflux Esophagitis Is Caused by Reflux of Gastric Contents (Gastroesophageal Reflux Disease)

This is by far the most common type of esophagitis. It often occurs together with sliding hiatal hernias but may develop because of an incompetent lower esophageal sphincter with no anatomic lesion.

 ETIOLOGIC FACTORS: The main barrier to reflux of gastric contents into the esophagus is the lower esophageal sphincter. Episodic reflux is normal, particularly after a meal. The mucosa is partially protected by the alkaline secretions of submucosal glands. Esophagitis results when episodes are frequent and prolonged. Agents that decrease lower esophageal sphincter pressure (e.g., alcohol, chocolate, fatty foods, cigarette smoking) also cause reflux, as may certain central nervous system (CNS) depressants (e.g., morphine, diazepam), abdominal obesity, pregnancy, estrogen therapy, and the presence of a nasogastric tube. Acid damages the esophageal mucosa, but the combination of acid plus pepsin is particularly injurious. Moreover, gastric fluid often contains refluxed bile from the duodenum, which magnifies injury to the esophageal mucosa. Alcohol, hot beverages, and spicy foods may also injure the mucosa directly.

PATHOLOGY: The first grossly apparent effect of GE reflux is hyperemia. Affected areas are susceptible to superficial mucosal erosions and ulcers, which often appear as vertical linear streaks. Mild injury to the squamous epithelium appears as cell swelling (hydropic change; see Chapter 1). With continued injury, hyperplasia develops: the basal epithelium is thickened and the papillae of the lamina propria are elongated and approach the surface (Fig. 19-5). Capillaries in the papillae are often dilated. Lymphocytes, neutrophils, and eosinophils infiltrate the epithelium. Mucosal ulceration develops in severe cases. Esophageal stricture may occur if the ulcer persists and damages the esophageal wall deep to the lamina propria. In this circumstance, reactive fibrosis can narrow the esophageal lumen.

CLINICAL FEATURES: Gastroesophageal reflux disease (GERD) can occur at any age and can be nonerosive, erosive, or involved by Barrett esophagus (see below). Heartburn and dysphagia are the usual presenting symptoms and generally respond to agents that reduce gastric acidity, in particular proton pump inhibitors (PPIs). In cases of erosive GERD, ulceration, hematemesis, and stricture may occur.

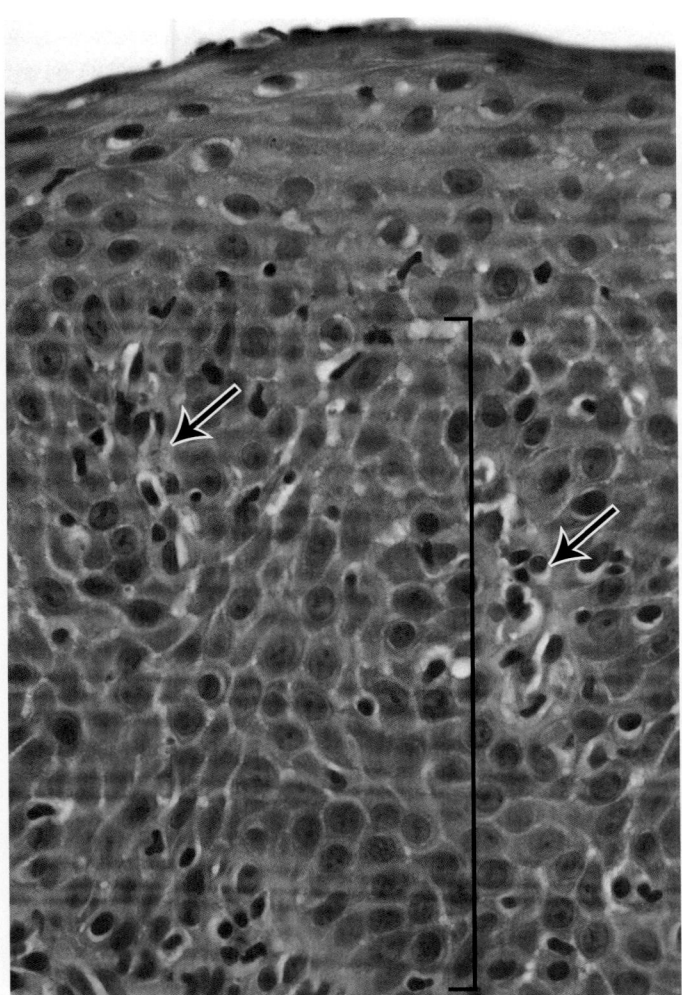

FIGURE 19-5. Reflux esophagitis. Biopsy from a patient with long-standing heartburn. Note the basal hyperplasia (*bracket*) and papillae, squamous hyperplasia and inflammation (*arrows*).

Barrett Esophagus Is Replacement of Esophageal Squamous Epithelium by Columnar Epithelium With Goblet Cells (Intestinal Metaplasia)

Barrett esophagus is a result of chronic GERD. For reasons unknown, its incidence has been increasing in recent years, particularly among white men. This disorder occurs in the lower third of the esophagus but may extend higher.

PATHOLOGY: Metaplastic Barrett epithelium may partially involve the circumference of short segments or may line the entire lower esophagus (Fig. 19-6A). The sine qua non of Barrett esophagus is a distinctive "specialized epithelium." By endoscopy, it has a typical salmon-pink color and, histologically, the normal squamous epithelium is replaced by an admixture of intestine-like epithelium with well-formed goblet cells and gastric foveolar cells (Fig. 19-6B). Dysplasia develops in this epithelium in a minority of patients (Fig. 19-6C) and, if left untreated, may progress to adenocarcinoma (Fig. 19-6D). *The risk of Barrett esophagus transforming*

into adenocarcinoma correlates with the length of esophagus involved and the degree of dysplasia.

CLINICAL FEATURES: The diagnosis of Barrett esophagus is established by endoscopy with biopsy, usually after complaints of GERD, although many do not report reflux symptoms. Males predominate (3:1). Prevalence increases with age, and most patients are diagnosed after age 50. Smokers have twice the risk of Barrett esophagus as nonsmokers. Obesity and white race are other risk factors.

While Barrett esophagus is common with a prevalence of 5% to 15% of adults with GERD, the estimated annual risk of adenocarcinoma in patients with Barrett esophagus is low at 0.1% to 0.3%. To prevent the development of adenocarcinoma, patients with Barrett esophagus are followed closely to detect early microscopic evidence of dysplastic mucosa, with surveillance endoscopies at 3- to 5-year intervals if no dysplasia is detected. According to the American College of Gastroenterology 2016 guidelines, patients with low-grade dysplasia should undergo radiofrequency ablation of the Barrett segment with possible endomucosal resection for nodular areas, although annual surveillance biopsies only are acceptable (but not preferred). Patients with high-grade dysplasia should undergo radiofrequency ablation of the Barrett segment combined with endomucosal resection for visible (nodular) lesions.

Eosinophilic Esophagitis Is an Immune-Mediated Disorder Common in Patients With Allergies and Asthma

A diagnosis of eosinophilic esophagitis requires clinical–pathologic correlation. While the pathogenesis is not completely understood, allergies to ingested food and environmental allergens likely play a prominent role. Patients often complain of dysphagia or feeling food "sticking" upon swallowing, which they may relate to specific foodstuffs. Affected individuals are often first identified after they fail to improve on standard antireflux therapy. It is important to rule out GERD either by pH monitoring or after several weeks of PPI therapy.

PATHOLOGY: On endoscopy, eosinophilic esophagitis shows concentric mucosal rings (described as trachealization or felinization because it resembles the trachea or a cat esophagus), vertical linear furrows, strictures, and small white plaques/exudates (Fig. 19-7A). Some patients have a normal-appearing esophagus at endoscopy. Since the disease can be quite patchy, multiple biopsies from various levels of esophagus should be assessed. The epithelium shows hyperplasia (papillary and basal layer hyperplasia), intercellular edema, increased intraepithelial eosinophils (≥15 per high-power field), superficial layering of eosinophils, eosinophilic microabscesses, and prominent degranulation of eosinophils (Fig. 19-7B). Importantly, GERD may also show increased eosinophils, but these should subside after antireflux therapy and are usually located in the distal esophagus.

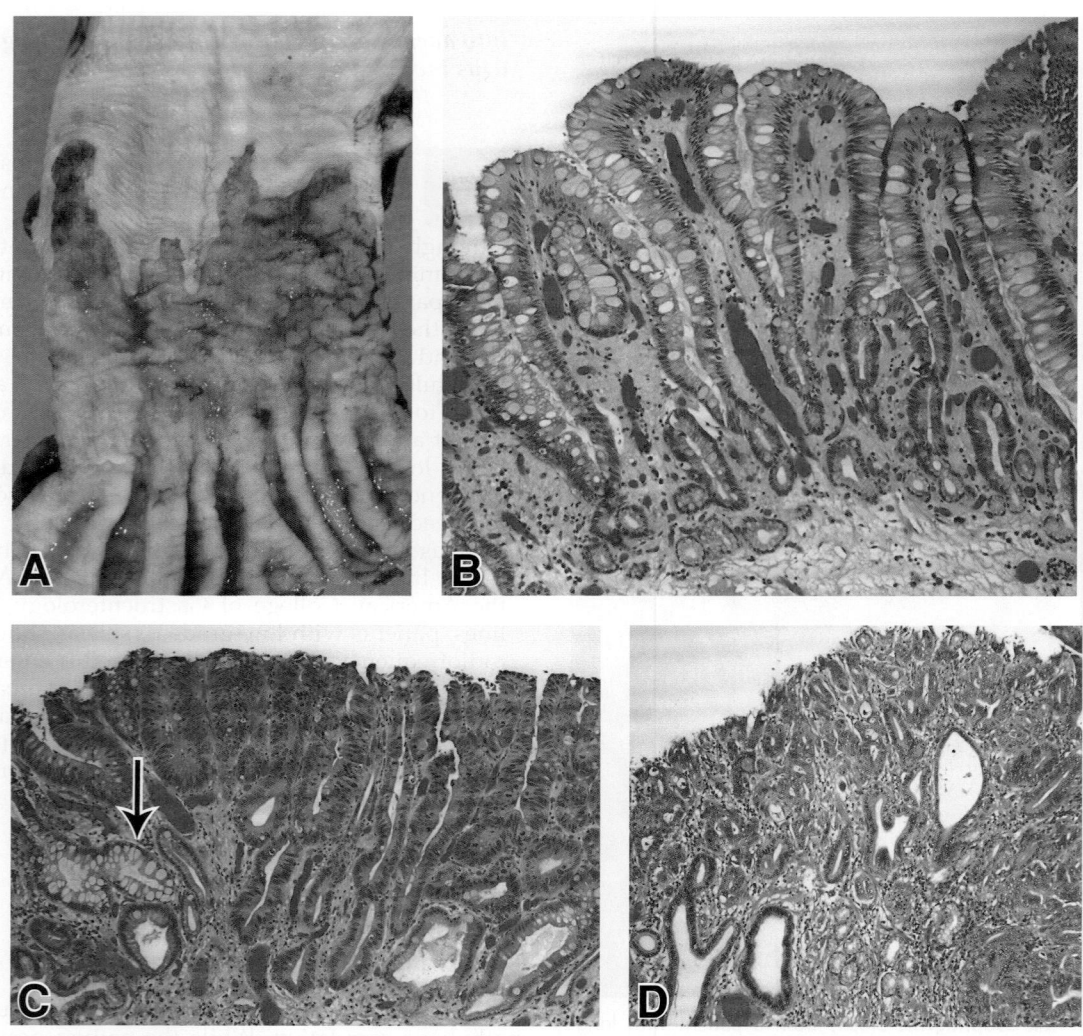

FIGURE 19-6. Barrett esophagus. A. The presence of the tan tongues of epithelium interdigitating with the more proximal squamous epithelium is typical of Barrett esophagus. **B.** The specialized epithelium has a villiform architecture and is lined by cells that are foveolar gastric-type cells and intestinal goblet-type cells. **C. High-grade dysplasia.** Markedly dysplastic glands predominate with hyperchromatic nuclei and early architectural distortion. Intestinalized, nondysplastic glands persist (*arrow*). **D. Intramucosal adenocarcinoma.** Malignant glands (*left*) are restricted to the mucosa.

In eosinophilic esophagitis, by contrast, eosinophils do not respond to antireflux therapy and are usually located in the proximal and/or mid esophagus.

CLINICAL FEATURES: Eosinophilic esophagitis can present at any age and is more common in males. Adults typically complain of dysphagia to solids or food impaction, while young children may show food intolerance, vomiting, feeding difficulties, or failure to thrive. Many patients have a personal or family history of atopy (asthma, allergic rhinitis, eczema, atopic dermatitis), and some may have mildly increased blood eosinophils. Eliminating inciting food from the diet can lead to remission in many patients. Swallowed corticosteroids, leukotriene inhibitors, and other immunomodulators are also used to treat eosinophilic esophagitis.

Infective Esophagitis Is Associated With Immunosuppression

CANDIDA ESOPHAGITIS: This fungal infection is the most common infection of the esophagus because of the increasing numbers of immunocompromised patients with HIV/AIDS, chemotherapy for malignant disease, or immunosuppression after organ transplantation. Esophageal candidiasis also occurs in patients with diabetes, in those receiving antibiotic or acid-suppressive therapy, or in people using inhaled or swallowed corticosteroids. It is uncommon in the absence of known predisposing factors. Dysphagia and severe pain on swallowing are the usual symptoms.

PATHOLOGY: White mucosal plaques on the esophageal mucosa are characteristic. Microscopically, neutrophils are typically seen within the squamous epithelium, although they may be absent in

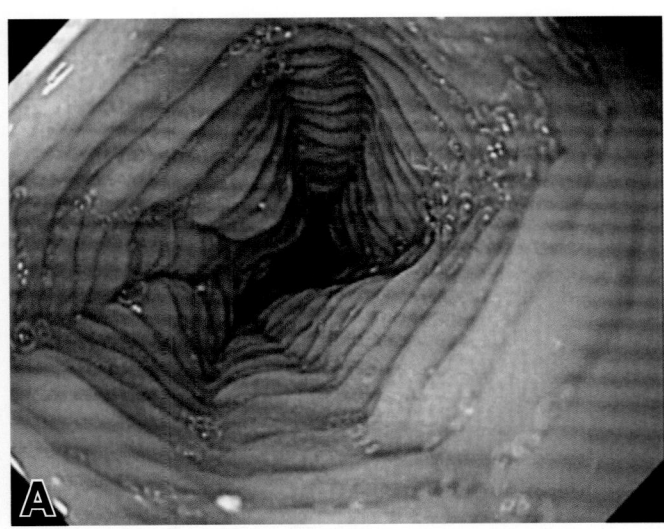
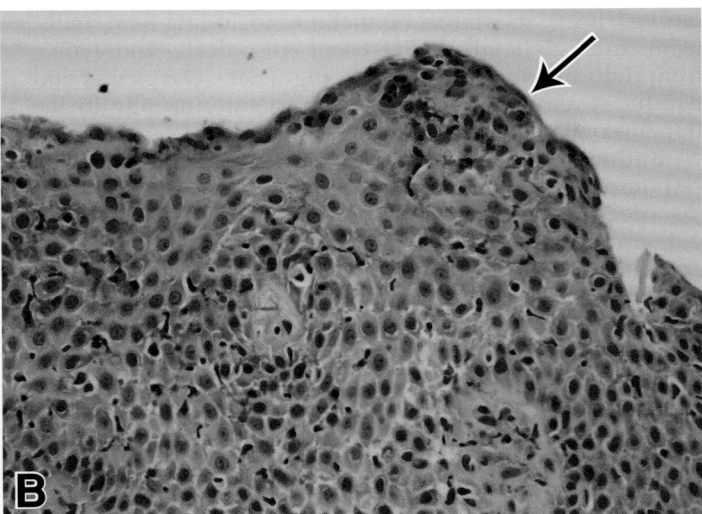

FIGURE 19-7. Eosinophilic esophagitis. A. Endoscopic view of an esophagus from a patient with eosinophilic esophagitis showing concentric mucosal rings (called trachealization or felinization because of its resemblance to the trachea or cat esophagus). **B.** Microscopic image showing increased intraepithelial eosinophils (intensely red staining cells) (≥15 per high-power field), superficial layering of eosinophils, eosinophilic microabscesses, and prominent degranulation of eosinophils (*arrow*).

severely immunosuppressed patients. Yeast and pseudo-hyphal fungal organisms are best seen within necrotic squamous debris by silver or PAS stains.

HERPETIC ESOPHAGITIS: Esophageal infection with herpesvirus type I most commonly follows solid-organ or bone marrow transplantation. Patients complain of odynophagia. Herpetic esophagitis may occur on occasion in otherwise healthy people.

PATHOLOGY: Early cases show vesicles, small erosions or plaques; as infection progresses, sharply demarcated ulcers are characteristic. Epithelial cells at the ulcer edges show typical nuclear herpetic inclusions, either Cowdry A type (eosinophilic inclusion with surrounding clear halo) or Cowdry B type (groundglass intranuclear inclusion) with occasional multinucleation and nuclear molding.

CYTOMEGALOVIRUS (CMV) ESOPHAGITIS: Involvement of the esophagus, or other segments of the gastrointestinal tract, with CMV usually reflects systemic viral disease in severely immunosuppressed patients (e.g., those with AIDS, transplant recipients, etc.). Mucosal ulceration, as in herpetic esophagitis, is common.

PATHOLOGY: CMV preferentially infects endothelial cells and stromal cells, whereas herpes simplex virus (HSV) usually affects epithelial cells. CMV differs from HSV in other ways. For example, CMV virus is usually located at the ulcer base, whereas HSV is found at the ulcer edge. And, a cell infected with CMV shows both nuclear and cytoplasmic enlargement with a single large "owl's eye" Cowdry-A type intranuclear inclusion and smaller intracytoplasmic inclusions, whereas HSV has intranuclear inclusions only.

Chemical Esophagitis Results From Ingestion of Corrosive Agents

Chemical injury to the esophagus usually follows accidental poisoning in children, attempted suicide in adults or contact with medication ("pill esophagitis"). Strong alkaline agents (e.g., lye) or strong acids (e.g., sulfuric or hydrochloric acid), which are used in various cleaning solutions, can produce chemical esophagitis. The former are particularly insidious, since they are generally odorless and tasteless and are easily swallowed before protective reflexes come into play. Those who survive ingestion of caustic substances are at a greatly increased lifelong risk for squamous cell carcinoma.

PATHOLOGY: Alkaline agents cause liquefactive necrosis with conspicuous inflammation and saponification of membrane lipids of all layers of the esophagus and stomach. Small vessel thrombosis adds ischemic necrosis to the injury. Severe damage is the rule with liquid alkali, but fewer than 25% of those who ingest granular preparations suffer severe complications.

Strong acids produce immediate coagulative necrosis. Resultant protective eschars limit injury and penetration. Still, half of patients who ingest concentrated hydrochloric or sulfuric acid develop severe esophageal injury.

Drug-related esophagitis is most often caused by direct chemical effects on the squamous mucosa, especially with capsules; esophageal dysmotility and cardiac enlargement (which impinges on the esophagus) may be contributing factors.

Esophagitis May Complicate Systemic Illnesses

Esophageal squamous mucosa resembles, and shares some reactions with, the skin.

The **dermolytic (dystrophic) form of epidermolysis bullosa** (see Chapter 28) involves all organs lined by, or derived from, squamous epithelium, including skin, nails, teeth, and esophagus. Bullae occur episodically and evolve from fluid-filled vesicles to weeping ulcers. Dysphagia and painful swallowing are common. Stricture, usually in the upper esophagus, may occur.

Bullous pemphigoid causes subepithelial bullae in the skin and esophagus without scarring. Other dermatologic disorders associated with esophagitis include pemphigus vulgaris, dermatitis herpetiformis, Behçet syndrome, and erythema multiforme.

Graft-versus-host disease (GVHD; see Chapter 4) in recipients of bone marrow transplants can cause esophageal lesions and dysphagia, odynophagia, and GE reflux.

Esophagitis May Be Iatrogenic

External irradiation for treatment of thoracic cancers may affect parts of the esophagus and lead to esophagitis and stricture. **Nasogastric tubes** may cause pressure ulcers if left in place for prolonged periods, but acid reflux also plays a role in these cases.

ESOPHAGEAL VARICES

Esophageal varices are dilated veins just beneath the mucosa (Fig. 19-8) *that are prone to rupture and hemorrhage* (also see Chapter 20). They arise in the lower third of the esophagus, virtually always in patients with hepatic cirrhosis and portal hypertension. GE anastomoses link lower esophageal veins to the portal system. If portal pressure exceeds a critical level, these anastomoses dilate in the upper stomach and lower esophagus. Without treatment, varices rupture in approximately one-third of patients, leading to life-threatening hemorrhage. Reflux injury or infective esophagitis can contribute to variceal bleeding. Esophageal banding and β-adrenergic blockers to reduce portal hypertension are used to prevent esophageal varices from rupturing.

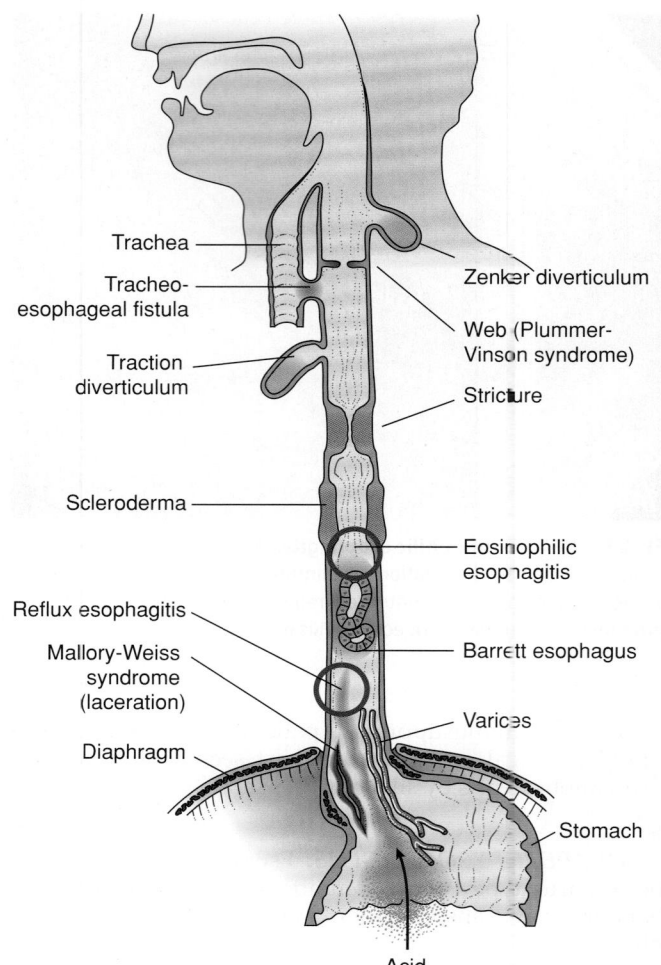

FIGURE 19-9. Nonneoplastic disorders of the esophagus.

LACERATIONS AND PERFORATIONS

Lacerations of the esophagus result from external trauma, such as automobile accidents, medical instrumentation, or severe vomiting, during which intraesophageal pressure may reach 300 mm Hg. Forceful retching may cause mucosal tears, first in the gastric epithelium and then extending into the esophagus.

Mallory–Weiss syndrome refers to severe retching, often associated with alcoholism. It leads to mucosal lacerations of the upper stomach and lower esophagus. These tears cause patients to vomit bright red blood. Bleeding may be so severe as to require transfusion of many units of blood. Perforation into the mediastinum, called **Boerhaave syndrome**, may result.

The major nonneoplastic esophageal disorders are summarized in Figure 19-9.

NEOPLASMS OF THE ESOPHAGUS

Benign Tumors of the Esophagus Are Uncommon

Unlike other parts of the gastrointestinal tract, most spindle cell submucosal tumors of the esophagus derive from

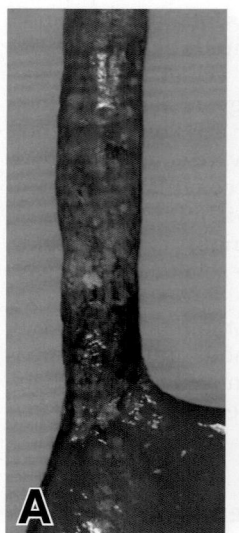 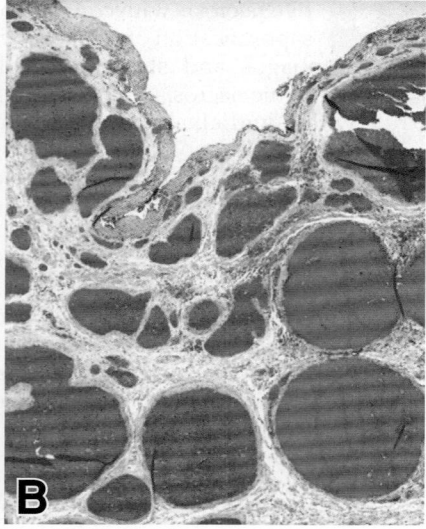

FIGURE 19-8. Esophageal varices. A. Numerous prominent blue venous channels are seen beneath the mucosa of the everted esophagus, particularly above the gastroesophageal junction. **B.** Section of the esophagus reveals numerous dilated submucosal veins.

smooth muscle (**leiomyoma**) rather than from interstitial cells of Cajal (gastrointestinal stromal tumors [GISTs]; see below). They are almost always benign. **Squamous papillomas** of the esophagus are uncommon and may be related to human papillomavirus (HPV) infection.

Esophageal Squamous Carcinomas Vary Geographically and Histologically

EPIDEMIOLOGY: Esophageal cancer is the eighth most common cancer globally. Worldwide, most esophageal cancers are squamous cell carcinomas. In the United States, adenocarcinoma is now more common (see below).

Global geographic variations in the incidence of esophageal squamous carcinomas are striking: areas of high incidence often abut areas of low incidence. The greatest frequency is in China, Iran, South America, and South Africa. In the United States, black men have a much higher incidence than whites, and American urban dwellers are at greater risk than those in rural areas. Esophageal squamous cell carcinoma is more common in older males.

ETIOLOGIC FACTORS: The variable distribution of esophageal squamous carcinomas, even among relatively homogeneous populations, suggests that environmental factors strongly affect its development. The most common factors are smoking and alcohol, which have a synergistic rather than additive effect. Other contributors include diet, consuming large amounts of hot beverages, HPV, radiation exposure, dietary nitrates and nitrosamines, vitamin deficiencies, genetic factors, Plummer–Vinson syndrome, achalasia, and prior caustic injury.

PATHOLOGY: About half of esophageal squamous cell carcinomas involve the middle and upper thirds of the esophagus (in contrast to esophageal adenocarcinoma, see below). Tumors may be endophytic or exophytic (Fig. 19-10). They can also be infiltrating, growing mainly in the wall. Bulky polypoid tumors tend to obstruct early, but ulcerated ones are more likely to bleed. Infiltrating tumors gradually narrow the lumen by circumferential compression. Extension of tumor into mediastinal structures is often a major problem.

Neoplastic squamous cells range in microscopic appearance from well differentiated, with keratin "pearls," to poorly differentiated, without evident squamous differentiation. Some tumors have a predominant spindle cell population of tumor cells.

The rich lymphatic drainage of the esophagus provides a route for most metastases. Tumors of the upper third spread to cervical, internal jugular, and supraclavicular nodes. Those of the middle third metastasize to paratracheal and hilar lymph nodes and to nodes in the aortic, cardiac, and paraesophageal regions. Since the lower third of the esophagus is supplied by the left gastric artery, lower esophageal tumors spread via accompanying lymphatics to retroperitoneal, celiac, and left gastric nodes. Metastases to liver and lung are common, but almost any organ may be affected.

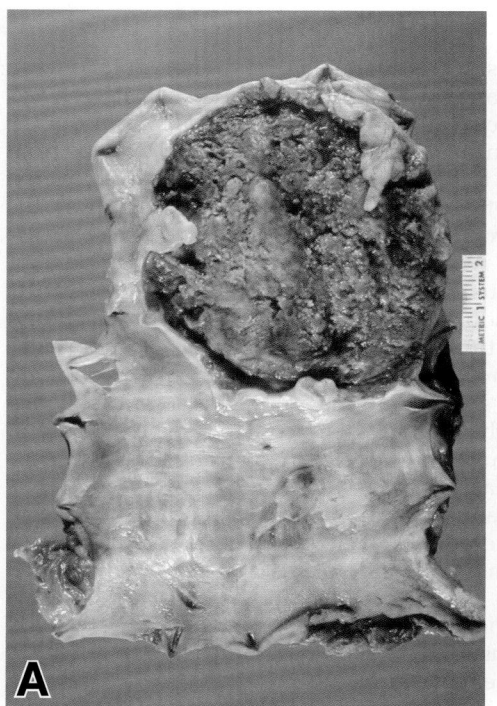
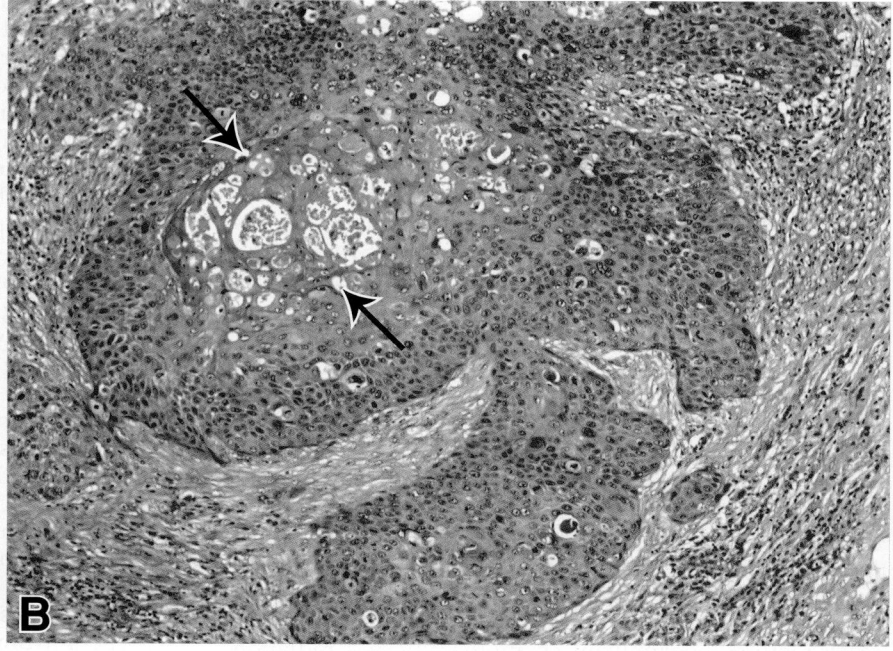

FIGURE 19-10. Esophageal squamous cell carcinoma. A. A large ulcerated mass is present in the squamous mucosa with normal squamous mucosa intervening between the carcinoma and the stomach. **B.** Nests of malignant squamous cells with abnormal keratin production in the center of one nest (*arrows*).

CLINICAL FEATURES: Dysphagia is the most common presenting complaint, but by the time this occurs, most tumors are inoperable. Patients may become cachectic from anorexia, difficulty in swallowing, and the systemic catabolic effects of cancer. Odynophagia occurs in half of patients. Persistent pain suggests extension to the mediastinum or to spinal nerves. Compression of the recurrent laryngeal nerve causes hoarseness, and tracheoesophageal fistula presents clinically as a chronic cough. Treatment is similar to esophageal adenocarcinoma (see below).

Adenocarcinoma of the Esophagus Often Arises in a Background of Barrett Esophagus

EPIDEMIOLOGY: In North America, Western Europe, and Australia, esophageal adenocarcinoma is far more common than squamous cancer. Incidence of esophageal adenocarcinoma is increasing faster than any solid tumor: it has increased sevenfold in the United States in the last 30 years. Men are affected more often than women.

ETIOLOGIC FACTORS: Most esophageal adenocarcinomas arise from dysplasia in Barrett esophagus and so have similar underlying risk factors. These include white race, male gender, obesity, GERD, diet, tobacco use, and genetic factors. Other risk factors that lead to increased gastric acid production or reflux include lower esophageal sphincter dilation or myotomy, scleroderma, Zollinger–Ellison syndrome (see below), or use of medications that relax the lower esophageal sphincter.

PATHOLOGY: The majority of esophageal adenocarcinomas involve the distal esophagus or GE junction, and can extend into the proximal stomach. Tumors may be flat, ulcerated, polypoid, or fungating. Often there is surrounding nonneoplastic Barrett mucosa that can be seen grossly or microscopically (Fig. 19-11).

These tumors may be well differentiated, with well-developed glands, ranging to poorly differentiated tumors with essentially no glandular differentiation. Some poorly differentiated adenocarcinomas have signet ring cellular morphology.

CLINICAL FEATURES: The symptoms and clinical course of esophageal adenocarcinoma are like those of squamous carcinoma. Symptoms generally appear in white, obese men with histories of GERD. Diagnosis and staging are typically done using endoscopy with ultrasound. Early invasive cancers (T1) can be treated with endoscopic mucosal resection. Patients with T2 cancers (invading into the submucosa) usually undergo primary esophagectomy. More advanced disease requires neoadjuvant chemotherapy and radiation treatment, which may be followed by surgical resection in patients who show a good clinical response.

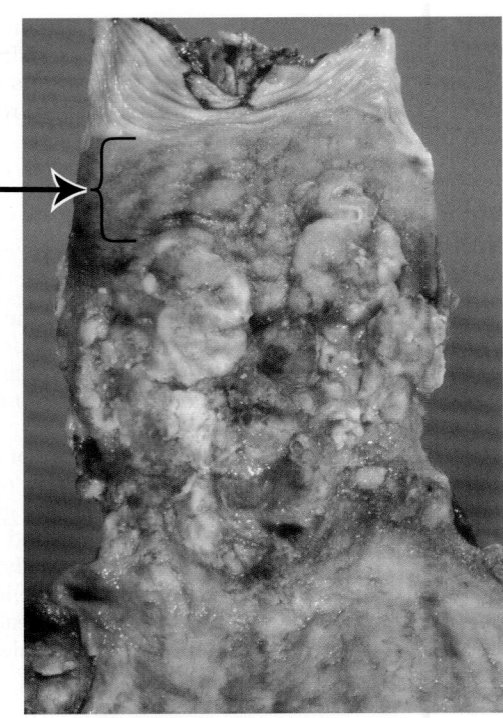

FIGURE 19-11. Esophageal adenocarcinoma. A large exophytic ulcerated mass lesion is seen just proximal to the gastroesophageal junction. This well-differentiated adenocarcinoma was separated from the most proximal squamous epithelium by a tan area representing Barrett esophagus (*arrow and bracket*).

The Stomach

ANATOMY

The stomach arises as a dilatation of the embryonic foregut. In adult life, it assumes a J configuration with its convexity (the greater curvature) extending leftward from the GE junction. The concave aspect (lesser curvature) extends from the GE junction to the right. The entire stomach is covered by peritoneum; the omentum extends downward from the greater curvature.

The stomach is divided into four regions: the cardia, fundus, body (corpus), and antrum (Fig. 19-12A,B). The **cardia** separates the esophagus from the rest of the stomach and it begins where the rugal folds begin. This is of importance in determining where the GE junction lies. While columnar metaplasia may ascend into the esophagus for variable distances, causing the esophageal mucosa to resemble the stomach, the gastric rugal folds do not change, and thus define the start of the stomach.

The **fundus** and **body** are basically identical except that the fundus is the portion of the stomach that bulges above the GE junction. Acid and intrinsic factor are produced in these regions, as these are the only parts of the stomach that contain parietal cells. The boundary between the body and antrum is usually taken to be the incisura angularis, a notch in the lesser curvature.

The **antrum** is the distal stomach, ending in the duodenum, from which it is separated by the pyloric sphincter. The hormone gastrin, produced in the antrum, stimulates acid production in the gastric body.

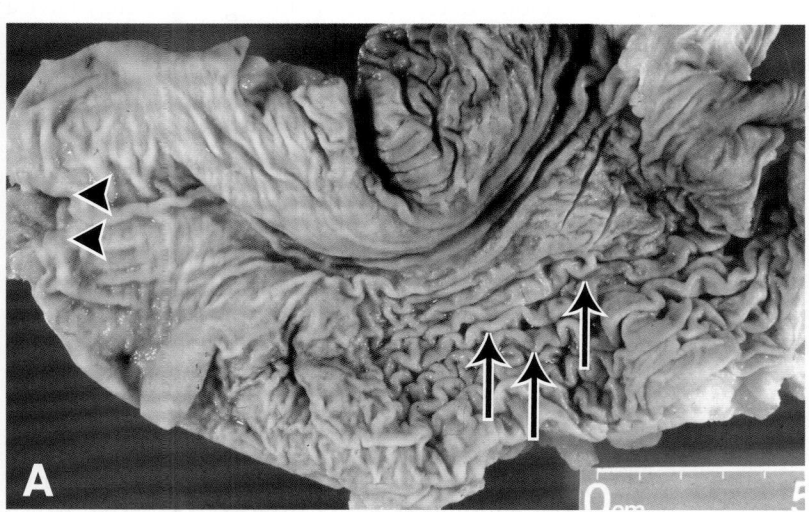

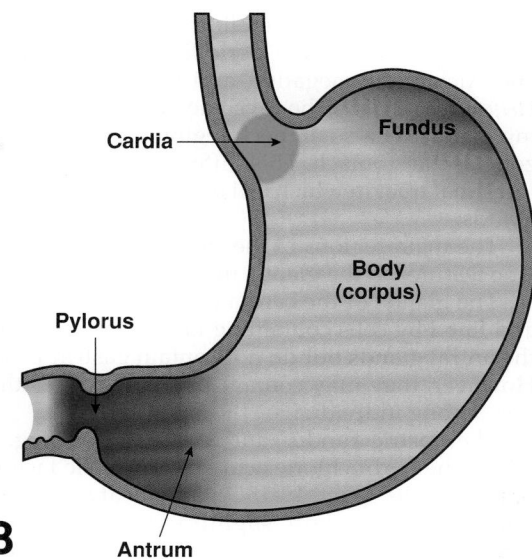

FIGURE 19-12. A. A **normal stomach** from an autopsy. The rugal folds are readily seen in the body (*arrows*). The sweep of the lesser curvature leads into the V-shaped antrum (*arrowheads*). **B.** Anatomic regions of the stomach.

In addition to the inner circular and outer longitudinal layers of the muscularis propria seen elsewhere in the gut, there is an oblique layer that aids in mixing gastric contents to promote early phases of digestion.

Although the cardia, fundus/body, and antrum each have distinct histologic features, the mucosal surface of the entire stomach is composed of a characteristic "foveolar" epithelium (Fig. 19-13A), a term that refers to the shallow

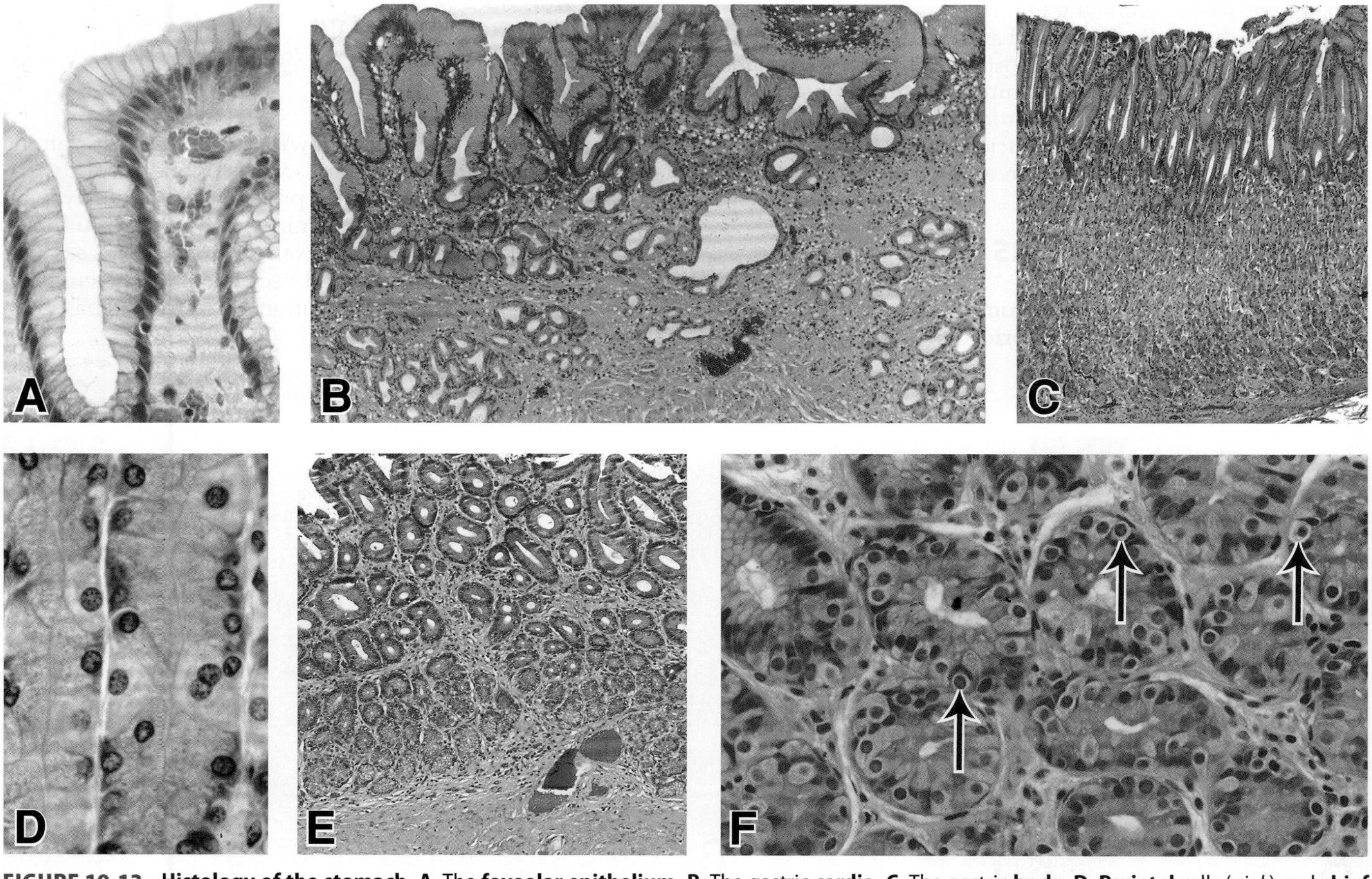

FIGURE 19-13. Histology of the stomach. A. The **foveolar epithelium. B.** The gastric **cardia. C.** The gastric **body. D. Parietal** cells (*pink*) and **chief cells** (*granular blue*). **E.** The gastric **antrum. F. Gastrin**-producing cells in antrum; they resemble fried eggs (*arrows*). See text for further description.

pits formed by this epithelium. The neutral pink mucin in these epithelial cells is periodic acid–Schiff (PAS) positive and Alcian blue negative, and it provides a safe haven for *Helicobacter pylori*. The foveolae are separated from underlying glands by a small neck region which is the proliferative zone in the stomach. This differs from the rest of the gastrointestinal tract in which cell division occurs in the base of the glands.

The main regions of the stomach take on their characteristic features in the glands underlying the foveolae.

The glands of the cardia (Fig. 19-13B) are loosely packed and lined by cells containing neutral mucus. They resemble the antral glands but do not contain gastrin-producing cells. However, they may contain parietal cells, as there is variation among individuals.

The gastric fundus and body glands (Fig. 19-13C) are where the hydrochloric acid- and intrinsic factor–producing parietal cells (Fig. 19-13D) are located. These are large polygonal cells with slightly granular pink cytoplasm. Deep in these glands, chief cells predominate. They have granular blue cytoplasm, a histologic feature reflecting production of the protein zymogen pepsinogen. The deepest aspect of the glands is also home to neuroendocrine cells—the enterochromaffin-like (ECL) cells.

The antral (or pyloric) mucosa (Fig. 19-13E) also contains loosely packed glands lined by cells that make neutral mucus. However, it is the presence of neuroendocrine cells that distinguishes the antrum from the cardia. Gastrin-producing G cells (Fig. 19-13F) are numerous here. There are also enterochromaffin cells (ECs) that produce serotonin, and somatostatin-producing D cells.

Because the cardia, body, and antrum are distinct in their anatomy and function, it is important to keep track of landmarks during endoscopic examination and biopsy of the stomach. However, transitions from one part to another are not very sharp, and their characteristic histologic features may intermingle somewhat in areas of transition.

CONGENITAL DISORDERS

Congenital disorders of the stomach are uncommon. Of these, most are **congenital pyloric stenosis**. This condition presents with **projectile vomiting** during the first 6 months of life. It is more common in boys than girls and may have a genetic basis.

ACUTE GASTRITIS

Acute Gastritis Results From an Imbalance Between Mucosal Protective Mechanisms and Damaging Agents or Processes

In thinking about conditions may lead to acute gastritis, it is helpful to conceptualize gastritis as a losing battle by mucosal protective mechanisms against injurious agents or mechanisms. Mucosal protective mechanisms include mucosal blood flow, mucus production, and cellular tight junctions. Injurious agents or mechanisms include ischemia (from many causes such as hypotension, hypovolemia, or cocaine), inhibition of prostaglandin synthesis (e.g., from nonsteroidal anti-inflammatory drugs or NSAIDs), which helps maintain the mucus layer, and direct mucosal damage by alkali, acid, or alcohol. If the losing battle is relatively brief, then acute gastritis ensues and may result in formation of gastric ulcers. These ulcers are typically shallow and multiple. They occur in the acid-producing mucosa of the body (Fig. 19-14A,B). The gastritis itself (Fig. 19-15) is usually hemorrhagic (acute hemorrhagic gastritis) but can show a significant fibro-inflammatory reaction (acute erosive gastritis). These processes can be life-threatening and patients with predisposing conditions may be treated prophylactically.

CHRONIC GASTRITIS

Chronic gastritis is associated with an increase in lamina propria inflammatory cells and is very common worldwide. It may be asymptomatic, or may present with vague dyspeptic symptoms. Endoscopic examination is less accurate in assessing gastritis than similar examinations are for esophagitis and colitis. As a result, and because of the heterogeneity of this disorder, the classification of gastritis is based on highly variable nomenclature.

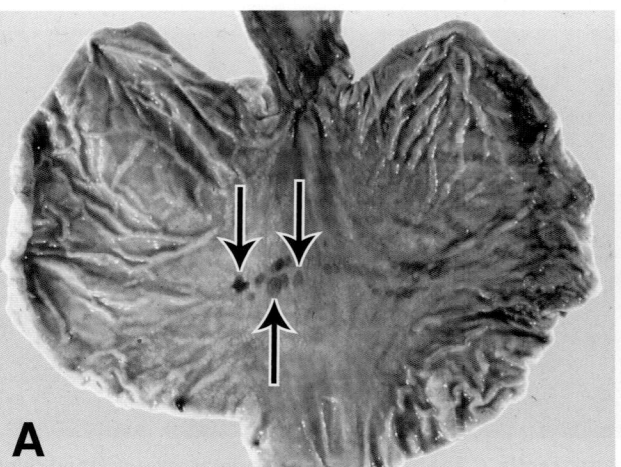
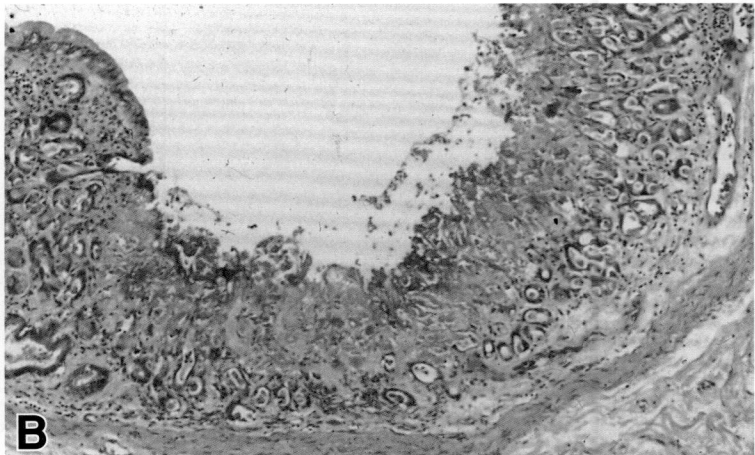

FIGURE 19-14.   A. Several shallow erosions/ulcers are scattered in the gastric body (*arrows*). **B.** There is an area of erosion with hemorrhage.

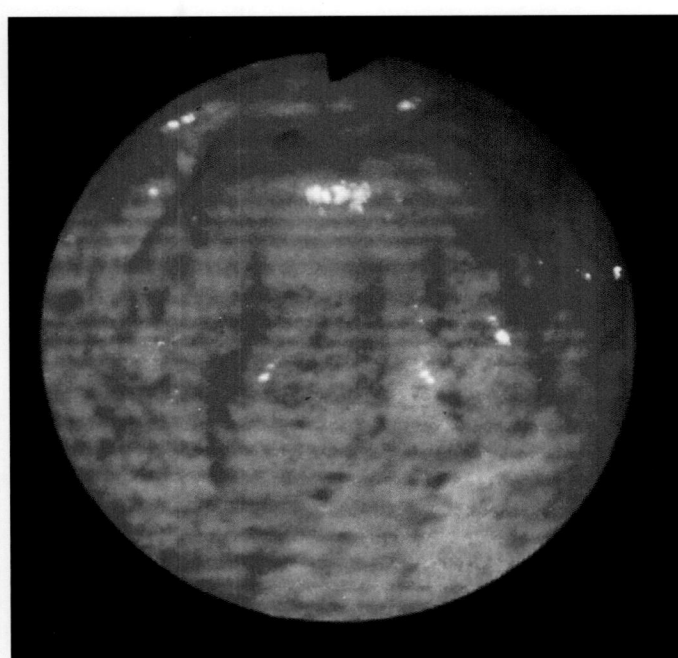

FIGURE 19-15. Endoscopic view of erosive gastritis from a patient who had ingested NSAIDs. Note the hemorrhagic mucosal lesions. (Courtesy of Dr. Cecilia M. Fenoglio-Preiser.)

Helicobacter pylori Infection Is the Major Cause of Gastritis and Gastric Cancer Worldwide

Helicobacter are short rod-shaped bacteria with a unique habitat: the surface of foveolar epithelial cells. The presence and significance of these bacteria went unnoticed for many years, until the astute observations of Warren and Marshall in 1984, for which they were awarded the Nobel Prize, explained the mystery of chronic gastritis. In some countries, over 80% of people are affected. It is most prevalent in developing countries and among low socioeconomic populations. In the United States, it is estimated that 4% to 30% of people are affected, but over the past 30 years, increased recognition and treatment of *Helicobacter pylori* gastritis has significantly reduced these percentages. Treatment consists of triple drug therapy with a proton-pump inhibitor, clarithromycin, and either amoxicillin or metronidazole.

PATHOLOGY: *Helicobacter* gastritis tends to be localized. In most cases, the antrum is affected but with prolonged infection or chronic use of PPIs, the more proximal stomach may become involved. Inflammation starts in the superficial lamina propria (Fig. 19-16A), since the organisms reside in a thin layer of mucus adherent to the surface foveolar cells. In fact, what adapts *Helicobacter* so well to this mucus layer niche is its ability to produce the enzyme urease, which converts urea to ammonia. As a base, ammonia acts to neutralize gastric acid and thereby help the bacteria to survive in what would otherwise be an inhospitable acidic environment. *Helicobacter* do not invade. Rather, they cause damage by releasing cytotoxins (vacA and cagA) that are directly injurious to the mucosal epithelium and/or induce

inflammation. Lymphoid aggregates are often present in *Helicobacter* gastritis (Fig. 19-16B). The inflammatory infiltrate is largely a mixture of lymphocytes and plasma cells. Neutrophils are often present and may accumulate in foveolae to form "pit abscesses" (Fig. 19-16C). The presence of such neutrophils does not denote acute gastritis, which is an entirely different process (see above). Rather, they indicate flares of inflammation in an underlying chronic gastritis.

Helicobacter (Fig. 19-16D) are small curvilinear bacilli found in the mucin-covered surface of foveolar cells. With a trained eye (and mind), they are usually visible with hematoxylin and eosin stains, but special stains enhance their recognition: silver impregnation, as in the Warthin–Starry stain, is used most often. Immunostaining is also effective.

Gastritis Caused by Non–*Helicobacter pylori* *Helicobacter* Species

Other species of *Helicobacter*, often collectively called *Helicobacter heilmannii*, can cause human disease. These species are commonly found in the stomachs of domestic animals such as cats, dogs, and pigs. They are longer and thicker than *H. pylori* and have several tight spirals. Gastritis caused by these organisms is similar to that seen with *H. pylori* and like *H. pylori*, these species produce urease and respond to the same treatment regimens.

Significance of *Helicobacter* Infections

The most common problem caused by chronic *Helicobacter* gastritis is peptic ulcer disease. Duodenal ulcers occur in 5% to 10% of patients with antral-predominant gastritis. More ominously, however, is the increased risk for gastric cancer, with 70% of distal gastric cancers attributable to chronic *Helicobacter* infection. Cancers are thought to arise through the sequence of inflammation leading to intestinal metaplasia, dysplasia, and finally adenocarcinoma. Countries with a high incidence of *H. pylori* gastritis also have high rates if gastric cancer.

In addition to adenocarcinoma, patients with *Helicobacter* infection are at risk for gastric lymphoma of mucosa-associated lymphoid tissue (MALT). Interestingly, lasting remission is achieved in about 75% of patients through eradication of the infection alone.

Multifocal Atrophic Gastritis May Be due to Factors Other Than Helicobacter and Increase Cancer Risk

The term multifocal atrophic gastritis is applied when mucosal atrophy (loss of glands) with intestinal metaplasia affects the antrum, body, and/or fundus (Fig. 19-17).

While *Helicobacter* is the leading cause (75% of cases), other factors such as a diet rich in smoked and salted foods may contribute when infection is absent. Thus, this entity is also called "environmental" multifocal atrophic gastritis because it encompasses infectious as well as noninfectious etiologies (with the exclusion of autoimmune atrophic gastritis as explained next). As mentioned, atrophic gastritis leads to intestinal metaplasia, which then predisposes to dysplasia and increases the risk for gastric adenocarcinoma.

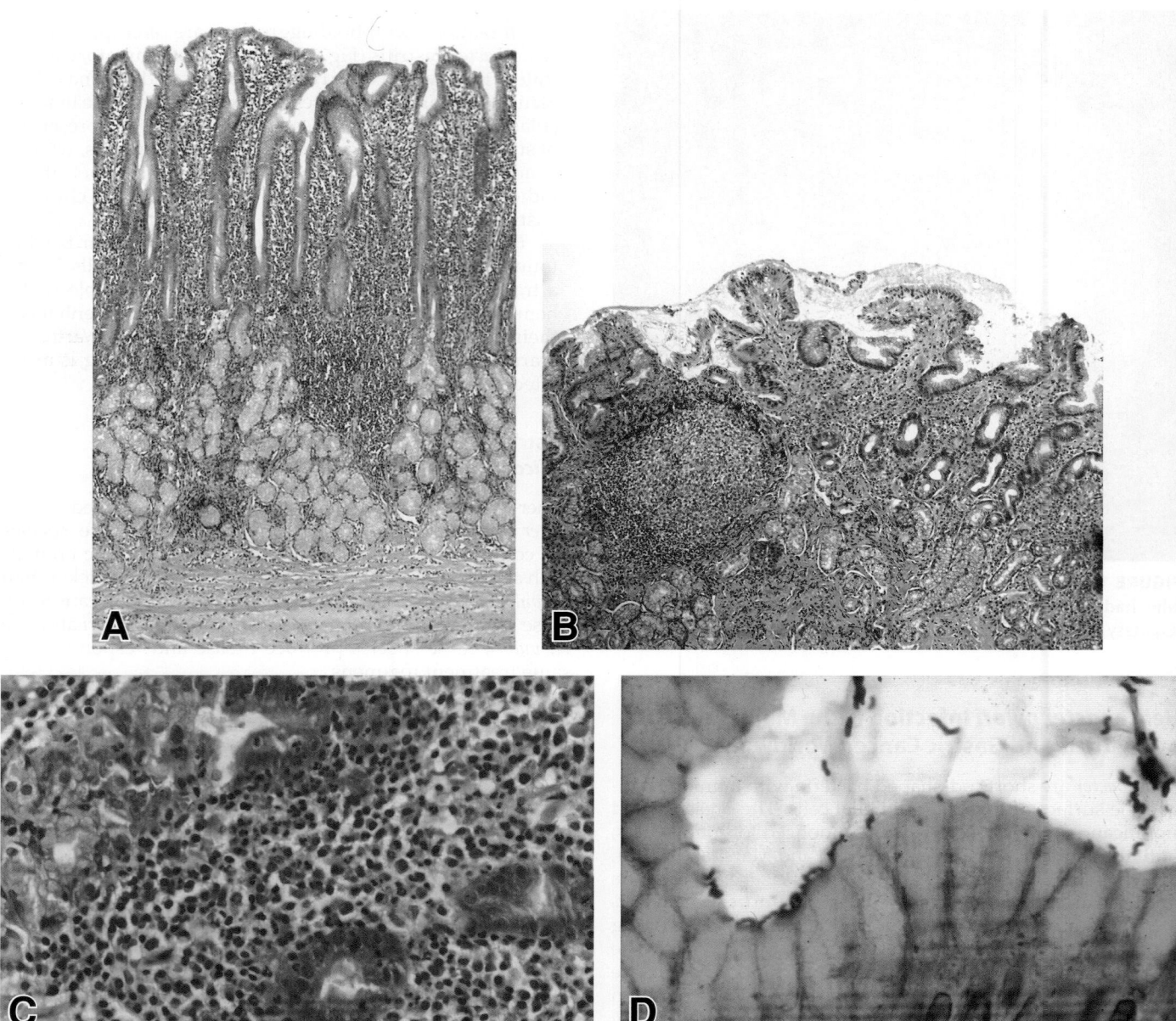

FIGURE 19-16. **A.** A superficial dense lymphoplasmacytic infiltrate is present in the lamina propria. **B.** A lymphoid aggregate; when present, these are highly suggestive of *Helicobacter*. **C.** A higher magnification view of the infiltrate shows lymphocytes and plasma cells in the lamina propria. Neutrophils are scattered in the lamina propria and infiltrating the glandular epithelium. **D.** The Warthin–Starry stain highlights the small curvilinear organisms at the foveolar surface.

Autoimmune Gastritis Is Limited to the Gastric Body and Fundus and Is Caused by Anti-Parietal and Anti-Intrinsic Factor Antibodies, Leading to Pernicious Anemia

Autoimmune gastritis has a 1% to 2% prevalence rate among older adults; it is female predominant. The target of the autoimmune reaction is gastric parietal cells, specifically the H^+/K^+ ATPase and intrinsic factor. This explains why it is limited to the gastric body and fundus, the only regions of the stomach in which parietal cells are found.

Loss of parietal cells leads to predictable clinical and laboratory abnormalities. Reduced gastric acid production leads to clinical hypo- or achlorhydria. Responding to the loss of acid, antral G cells increase gastrin production which induces corpus ECL cells to produce histamine to stimulate any remaining parietal cells to secrete acid. Thus, hypergastrinemia ensues. Loss of intrinsic factor leads to vitamin B_{12} deficiency, as intrinsic factor mediates absorption of vitamin B_{12} from the ileum. This is called pernicious anemia because a megaloblastic anemia results from vitamin B_{12} deficiency (see Chapter 26). Thus, hypo- or achlorhydria, hypergastrinemia, and vitamin B_{12} deficiency are all expected in a patient with anti-parietal cell and/or anti-intrinsic factor antibodies with mucosal atrophy and intestinal metaplasia limited to the gastric body and fundus.

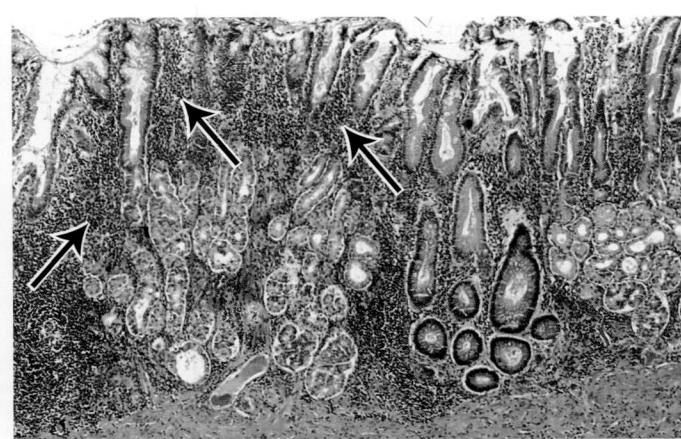

FIGURE 19-17. Atrophic gastritis. Inflammatory infiltrate fills the lamina propria (*arrows*). There is loss of gland volume (atrophy), with a striking loss of parietal cells as compared to the normal gastric body (see Fig. 19-13C).

TABLE 19-1		
COMPARISON OF AUTOIMMUNE AND ENVIRONMENTAL ATROPHIC GASTRITIS		
	Autoimmune Atrophic Gastritis	**Environmental Multifocal Atrophic Gastritis**
Etiology	Immune mediated	*H. pylori* infection, diet
Sex	Female predominate	No sex predilection
Location	Body and fundus	Antral predominant with extension to body, multifocal
H. pylori colonization	<20%	90–100%
Anti-parietal cell antibodies	+	–
Anti-intrinsic factor antibodies	+	–
Vitamin B$_{12}$ level	Low	Normal
Serum gastrin	High	Normal/high

PATHOLOGY: These conditions lead to the characteristic histology of autoimmune gastritis (Fig. 19-18A,B). Parietal cells are absent and there is significant mononuclear inflammation and intestinal and pseudopyloric metaplasia. In time, neuroendocrine hyperplasia may become prominent. Patients with autoimmune gastritis and their family members have a significant predisposition to other autoimmune diseases (see Chapter 11). These diseases include type I diabetes, hypothyroidism, and Addison disease.

Features seen in autoimmune versus environmental atrophic gastritis are compared in Table 19-1.

Lymphocytic Gastritis

As the name suggests, this process is characterized by increased numbers of mature intraepithelial lymphocytes in the surface epithelium (Fig. 19-19). Several clinical associations underscore the importance of this entity. The most important is its relationship to celiac disease. Some 40% of patients with lymphocytic gastritis have celiac disease, while 20% have *Helicobacter* infection. Other less common etiologies include allergy, drug reaction, and Crohn disease.

Portal Hypertensive Gastropathy

This lesion is seen in patients with portal hypertension, typically due to cirrhosis. The characteristic endoscopic appearance ("mosaic" or "snakeskin") is due to abnormal dilatation of lamina propria capillaries and submucosal vasculature.

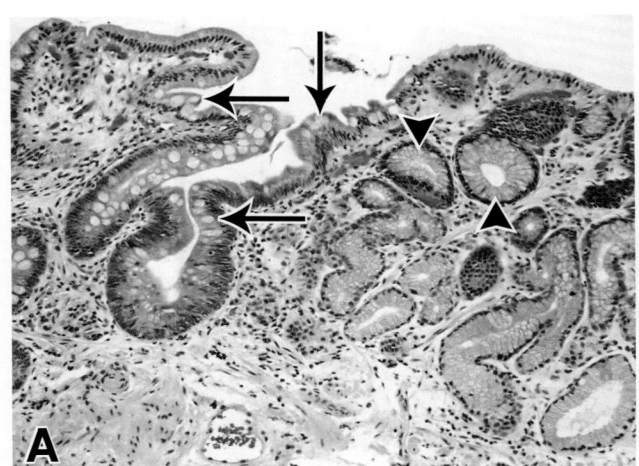
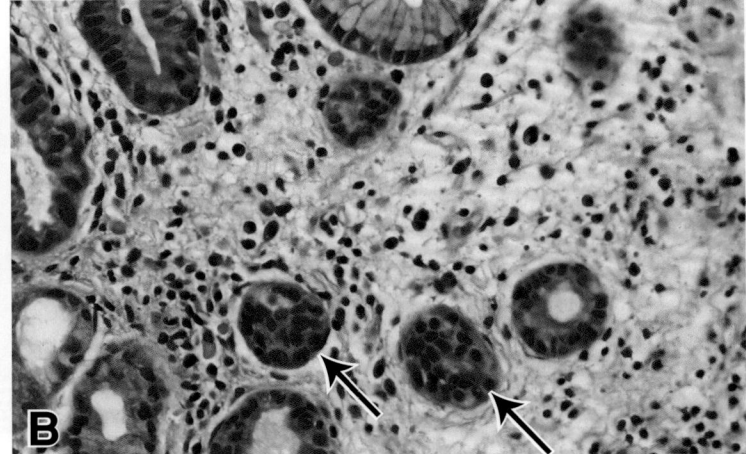

FIGURE 19-18. A. The gastric body is atrophic and devoid of parietal cells. There is intestinal metaplasia (goblet cells, *arrows*) and pseudopyloric metaplasia (*arrowheads*). **B.** Elsewhere in the body there are micronodules composed of enterochromaffin-like (ECL) cells (*arrows*).

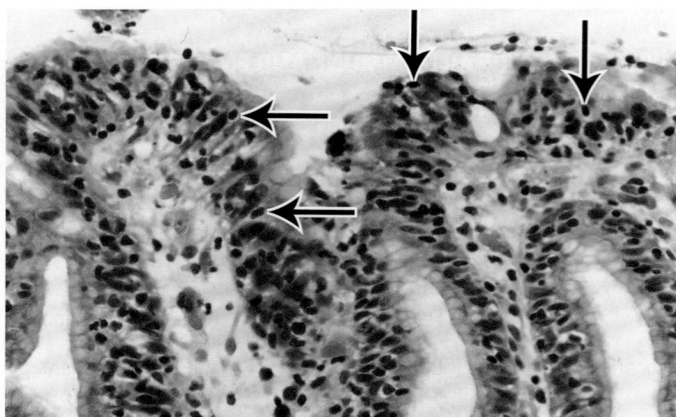

FIGURE 19-19. Lymphocytic gastritis. A dense infiltrate of lymphocytes (*arrows*) is seen in the surface epithelium and extending into the rest of the gland.

Granulomas in Gastric Mucosa

There are multiple causes of gastric granulomas, otherwise known as granulomatous gastritis. The presence of granulomas in the gastric mucosa should prompt a search for responsible processes (e.g., sarcoidosis or Crohn disease). Associated findings elsewhere (lung, ileum, etc.) are necessary to establish such diagnoses. Infections (fungal and mycobacterial) must also be excluded.

Reactive (Chemical) Gastropathy Is Most Often due to NSAIDs

Reactive gastropathy is defined as a hyperplastic mucosal response to a variety of irritants, most commonly NSAIDs. In fact, up to 40% of chronic NSAID users manifest reactive gastropathy. Other causes include bile reflux, radiation, and excess alcohol consumption. These injurious agents induce hyperplasia of foveolar cells, which may cause gastric pits to become irregular, resulting in a "corkscrew" appearance (Fig. 19-20A). Additional changes may include proliferation of lamina propria smooth muscle (Fig. 19-20B). Inflammation

is infrequent unless an ulcer or mucosal erosion elicits a localized inflammatory response. Withdrawal of the offending agent is the treatment of choice.

PEPTIC ULCER DISEASE

"Peptic ulcer disease" is focal destruction of the mucosa of the stomach and small intestine, mainly the proximal duodenum where it is caused by gastric secretions. Duodenal ulcers have declined greatly in frequency over the past 30 years.

Peptic ulceration may occur as far proximally as the esophagus and as far distally as a Meckel diverticulum with gastric heterotopia (see below), but the disease mostly affects the distal stomach and proximal duodenum. Many clinical and epidemiologic features distinguish gastric from duodenal ulcers; the common factors that unite them are gastric hydrochloric acid secretion and *H. pylori* infection.

 EPIDEMIOLOGY: Peptic ulcers may occur at any age (including infancy), but the peak incidence has progressively changed, so that it is now between 30 and 60 years of age. Gastric ulcers usually afflict the middle-aged and elderly and affect both sexes equally. Duodenal ulcers are more common in males.

Racial differences have been studied, but most data suggest that all ethnic groups are susceptible in an urban Western setting. Surveys in the United States and Great Britain show a modest inverse relation between duodenal ulcers and socioeconomic status and education.

ETIOLOGIC FACTORS: No single agent appears to be responsible, although many etiologies have been proffered.

H. PYLORI: H. pylori can be isolated from the gastric antrum of virtually all patients with duodenal ulcers. The converse is not true, however. Only a small minority of those carrying the bacterium have duodenal ulcer disease. Thus, *H. pylori* infection may be necessary, but is

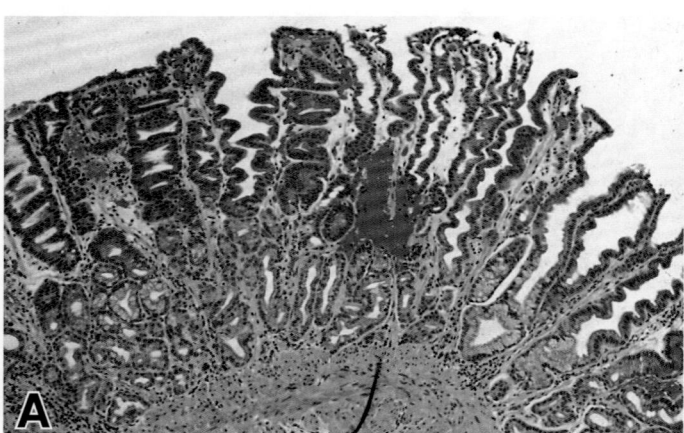

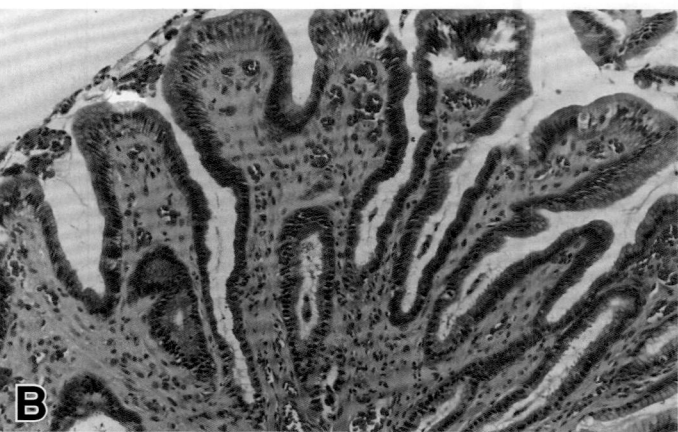

FIGURE 19-20. Examples of reactive gastropathy. A. The corkscrew contour of the antral glands deviates from normal architecture in this patient with bile reflux. **B.** There is increased smooth muscle in the villiform structures in the antrum of a patient with chronic use of nonsteroidal anti-inflammatory drugs (NSAIDs).

not sufficient, for development of peptic duodenal ulcers. Nevertheless, such ulcers heal more quickly and recur less frequently after treatment for *H. pylori* infection.

How *H. pylori* infection predisposes to duodenal ulcers is not completely clear, but several mechanisms have been proposed. Cytokines produced by inflammatory cells in response to the infection stimulate gastrin release and suppress somatostatin secretion. These effects, plus release of histamine metabolites from the organism itself, **may stimulate basal gastric acid secretion**. In addition, luminal cytokines from the stomach may gain access to and injure duodenal epithelium.

H. pylori infection may also block inhibitory signals from the antrum to G cells and the parietal cell region, thus increasing gastrin release and impairing inhibition of gastric acid secretion. Such an effect might **increase acid load in the duodenum**, contributing to duodenal ulceration. Acidification of the duodenal bulb induces islands of metaplastic gastric mucosa in the duodenum in many patients with peptic ulcers. Such gastric epithelium in the duodenum is sometimes colonized with *H. pylori*, like the gastric mucosa, and infection of the metaplastic epithelium by *H. pylori* may render the mucosa more susceptible to peptic injury (Fig. 19-21).

H. pylori infection is probably also important in the pathogenesis of gastric ulcers, because the organism causes most of the chronic gastritis that underlies this disease. About 75% of patients with gastric ulcers harbor *H. pylori*. The other 25% likely have other types of chronic gastritis. The gastric and duodenal factors implicated as possible mechanisms in the pathogenesis of duodenal ulcers are summarized in Figure 19-22.

HCl SECRETION: Hyperacidity due to increased hydrochloric acid secretion is necessary for peptic ulcers to form and persist in the stomach and duodenum. This mechanism is supported by the following observations: (1) all patients with duodenal ulcers and nearly all with gastric ulcers are gastric acid secretors; (2) experimental ulcer production in animals requires acid; (3) hypersecretion of acid is present in many, but not all, patients with duodenal ulcers (there is no evidence that acid overproduction alone explains duodenal ulceration); and (4) surgical and medical treatments that reduce acid production promote healing of peptic ulcers. Gastric secretion of pepsin, which may also play a role in peptic ulceration, parallels that of hydrochloric acid.

DIET: Despite the folk wisdom that spicy food and caffeine are ulcerogenic, there is little evidence that any food or beverage, including coffee and alcohol, leads to the development or persistence of peptic ulcers.

DRUGS: Aspirin is an important contributor to duodenal, and especially gastric, ulcers. Other NSAIDs and analgesics have been incriminated in peptic ulcerogenesis. Prolonged treatment with high doses of corticosteroids also slightly increases risk of peptic ulceration.

CIGARETTE SMOKING: Smoking is a definite risk factor for duodenal and gastric ulcers, particularly gastric ulcers.

GENETIC FACTORS: First-degree relatives of people with duodenal or gastric ulcers have a threefold higher risk of developing an ulcer—but only at the same site. Monozygotic twins show much higher (50%) concordance for these ulcers than do dizygotic twins, but this figure also indicates that environmental factors must also be involved.

The role of genetic factors is further supported by the fact that blood-group antigens correlate with peptic ulcer disease. Duodenal ulcers occur 30% more often in people with type O blood than in those with other types. This does not hold for gastric ulcers. People who do not secrete blood-group antigens in saliva or gastric juice have 50% higher risk of duodenal ulcers. Those who are both type O and nonsecretors (10% of white people) have a 2.5-fold increase in duodenal ulcers.

Pepsinogen I is secreted by gastric chief and mucous neck cells and appears in gastric juice, blood, and urine. Serum levels of this proenzyme correlate with the capacity for gastric acid secretion and reflect parietal cell mass. Someone with high blood pepsinogen I levels has five times the normal risk of developing a duodenal ulcer. Hyperpepsinogenemia has been attributed to autosomal dominant inheritance and may reflect an inherited tendency to increased parietal cell mass. Half of children of ulcer patients with hyperpepsinogenemia have hyperpepsinogenemia themselves.

Familial tendencies for other features are reported in ulcer patients. Many such patients have normal pepsinogen I levels but still show familial aggregation. Family clustering of duodenal ulcers and rapid gastric emptying has been noted, as has familial hyperfunction of antral G cells. Patients with a childhood duodenal ulcer are much more likely to have a family history of ulcers than people in whom the disease begins in adulthood.

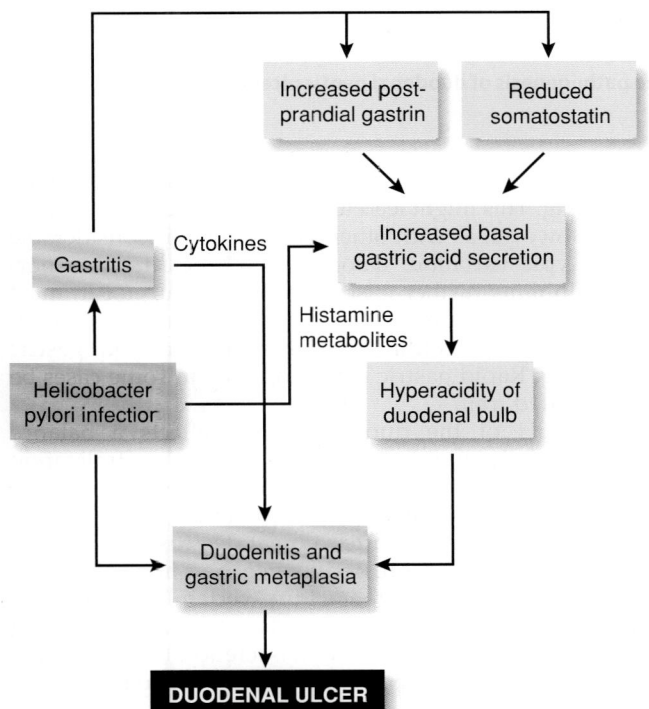

FIGURE 19-21. Possible mechanisms in the pathogenesis of duodenal ulcer disease associated with *Helicobacter pylori* infection.

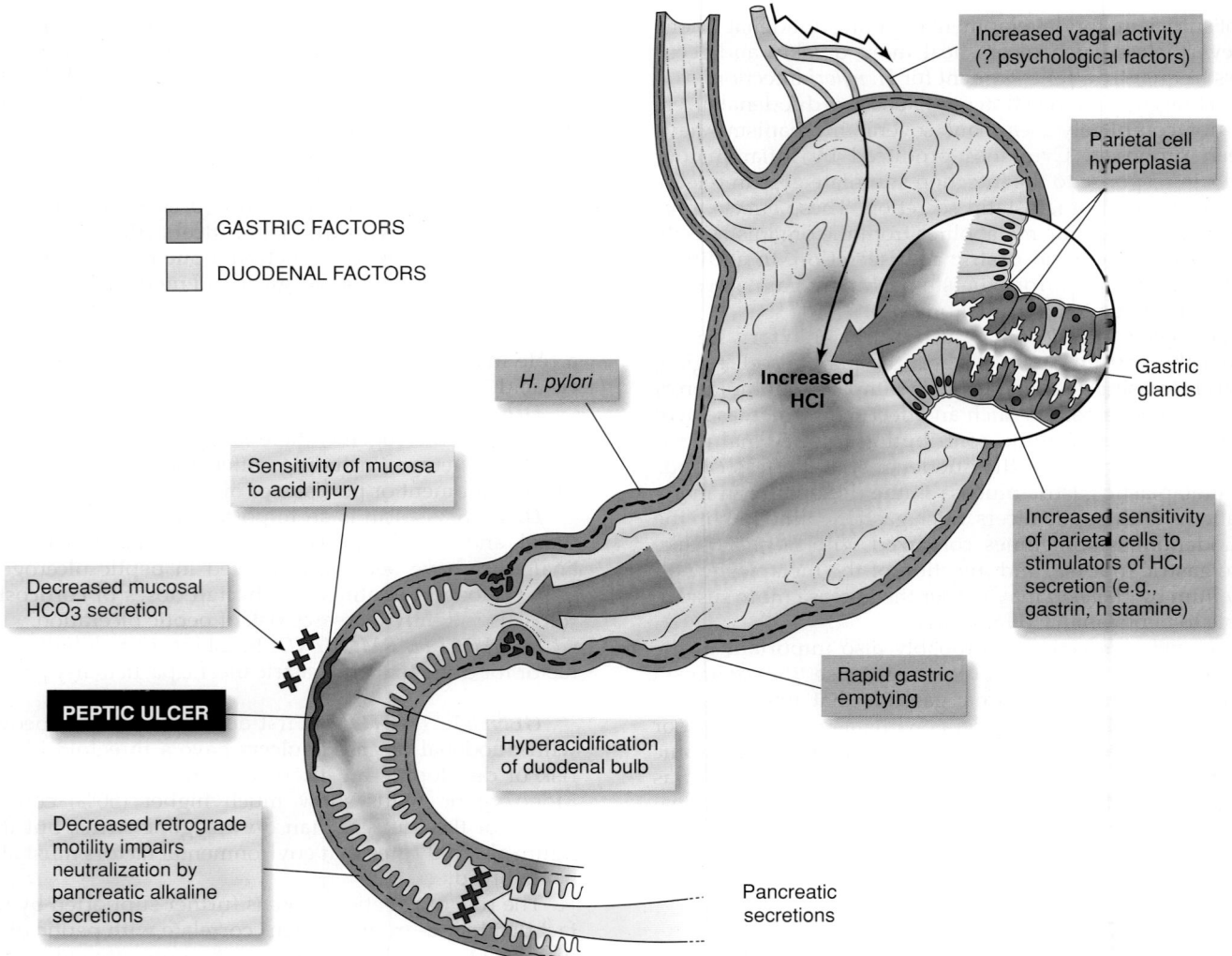

FIGURE 19-22. Gastric and duodenal factors in the pathogenesis of duodenal peptic ulcers.

PATHOPHYSIOLOGY: *DUODENAL ULCERS:* Maximal capacity for gastric acid production is a function of total parietal cell mass. Patients with duodenal ulcers may have up to double the normal parietal cell mass and maximal acid secretion. However, there is a wide variation, and only a third of ulcer patients secrete excess acid. Increased chief cell mass often accompanies increased parietal cells, reflecting the prevalence of hyperpepsinogenemia in patients with ulcers.

Food-stimulated gastric acid secretion is increased in magnitude and duration in people with duodenal ulcers, but here, too, there is significant overlap with normal values. This may involve, at least in part, altered G-cell responses to meals. Such patients show postprandial hypergastrinemia and increased antral G cells. Most people with duodenal ulcers, however, do not show G-cell hyperfunction. Acid secretion in people with duodenal ulcers may also be more sensitive than normal to gastric secretagogues such as gastrin, possibly owing to increased vagal tone or increased affinity of parietal cells for gastrin. Brisk secretion of acid after a meal may reflect increased vagal tone.

Patients with duodenal ulcers show accelerated gastric emptying. This might lead to excessive duodenal acidification. However, as with other factors, there is considerable phenotypic variation. Duodenal bulb acidification normally inhibits further gastric emptying, but not in most people with duodenal ulcers. In them, duodenal acidification leads to continued, rather than delayed, gastric emptying. Rapid gastric emptying may in some cases be an inherited trait.

The pH of the duodenal bulb reflects a balance between delivery of gastric juice and its neutralization by biliary, pancreatic, and duodenal secretions. Duodenal ulceration requires an acidic pH in the bulb. In ulcer patients, duodenal pH after a meal decreases to a lower level and remains depressed longer than in normal people. Such duodenal hyperacidity certainly reflects the gastric factors discussed above. The role of neutralizing factors, particularly bicarbonate secretion by the duodenal mucosa or by the pancreas in response to secretin, is uncertain.

Impaired mucosal defenses may also contribute to peptic ulceration. Factors such as prostaglandins may or may not protect the duodenum as they do the gastric mucosa (see above).

GASTRIC ULCERS: Gastric ulcers almost invariably arise in the setting of epithelial injury by *H. pylori* or chemical gastritis, but how chronic gastritis predisposes to gastric ulceration remains unclear. Most patients with gastric ulcers secrete less acid than do those with duodenal ulcers and even less than normal people. Factors implicated in gastric ulceration include (1) back-diffusion of acid into the mucosa, (2) decreased parietal cell mass, and (3) abnormalities of parietal cells themselves. A few gastric ulcer patients produce excess acid. Their ulcers are usually near the pylorus and are considered variants of duodenal ulcers. Interestingly, intense gastric hypersecretion such as occurs in the Zollinger–Ellison syndrome (see below) is associated with severe ulceration of the duodenum and even the jejunum, but rarely of the stomach.

The concurrence of gastric ulcers and gastric hyposecretion in gastric ulcer patients implies that (1) their gastric mucosa may in some way be abnormally sensitive to low concentrations of acid; (2) agents other than acid may damage the mucosa (e.g., NSAIDs); or (3) the gastric mucosa may be exposed to potentially injurious agents for unusually long periods. As discussed above, the mucosal barrier to acid and perhaps to other contents within the stomach may be impaired in some patients with gastric ulcers, although the evidence is not conclusive. Reflux of bile constituents (especially deoxycholic acid and lysolecithin) and pancreatic secretions may also contribute to the development of gastric ulcers.

PATHOLOGY: Most peptic ulcers arise in the lesser gastric curvature in the antral and prepyloric regions and in the first part of the duodenum.

Gastric ulcers are usually single and less than 2 cm in diameter. Ulcers on the lesser curvature are often associated with chronic gastritis; those on the greater curvature are commonly related to NSAIDs. Edges tend to be sharply punched out, with overhanging margins. Deeply penetrating ulcers produce a serosal exudate that may cause the stomach to adhere to adjacent structures. Scarring in healed ulcers in the prepyloric region may be severe enough to cause pyloric stenosis. Grossly, chronic peptic ulcers may resemble ulcerated gastric carcinomas. They differ from the latter by their tendency to produce radiating folds in the surrounding mucosa, their lack of a raised border and a "clean" (fibrin-covered)-appearing base (Fig. 19-23). Endoscopists must biopsy the edges and bed of gastric ulcers, as ulcer centers tend to show only necrotic tissue.

Duodenal ulcers (Fig. 19-24) are ordinarily on the anterior or posterior wall of the first part of the duodenum, near the pylorus. They are usually solitary, but paired ulcers on both walls, the so-called "kissing ulcers" are not uncommon.

Gastric and duodenal ulcers are histologically similar (Fig. 19-25A,B). From the lumen inward, they are composed of several layers: (1) a superficial zone of fibrinopurulent exudate, (2) necrotic tissue, (3) granulation tissue, and (4) fibrotic tissue with variable amounts of chronic inflammation at the depth of the ulcer's base. Ulceration

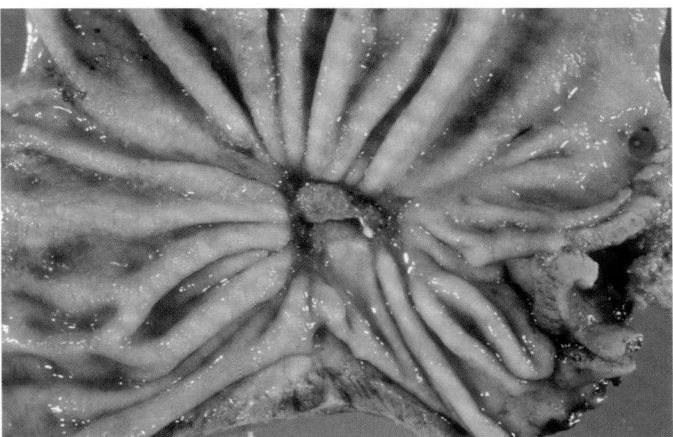

FIGURE 19-23. Gastric ulcer. There is a characteristic sharp demarcation from the surrounding mucosa, which has prominent radiating folds. The base of the ulcer is covered with fibrin, giving it a gray color.

may penetrate muscle layers, interrupting them with scar tissue after healing. Blood vessels at the margins of the ulcer are often thrombosed. Mucosal margins tend to be slightly hyperplastic. With healing, mucosa grows over ulcerated areas as a single epithelial layer. Duodenal ulcers are usually accompanied by peptic duodenitis, with Brunner gland hyperplasia and gastric mucin cell metaplasia.

CLINICAL FEATURES: The symptoms of gastric and duodenal ulcers are generally not distinguishable by history or physical examination. Classic duodenal ulcers cause epigastric pain 1 to 3 hours after a meal or that awakens a patient at night. Alkali and food relieve these symptoms. Dyspeptic symptoms associated with gallbladder disease, such as fatty food intolerance, distention, and belching, occur in half of patients with peptic ulcers.

The major complications of peptic ulcer disease are hemorrhage, obstruction, and perforation with peritonitis.

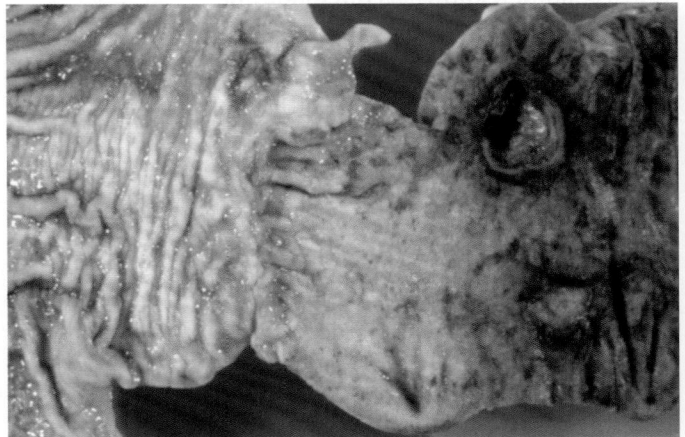

FIGURE 19-24. Duodenal ulcers. Two sharply demarcated duodenal ulcers are surrounded by inflamed duodenal mucosa. The gastroduodenal junction can be seen in the midportion of the photograph.

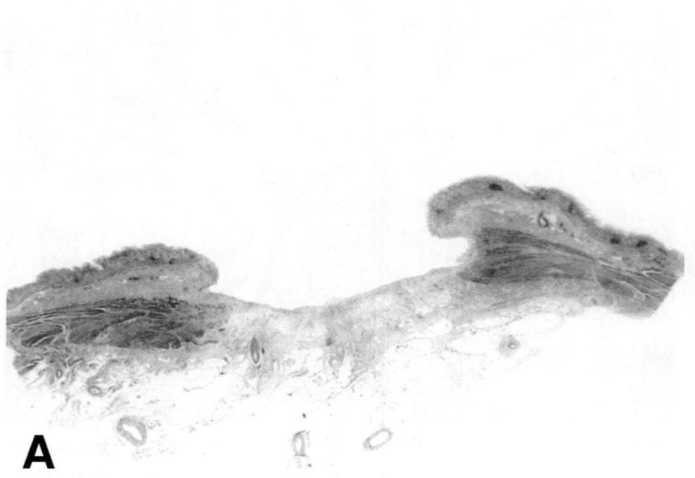
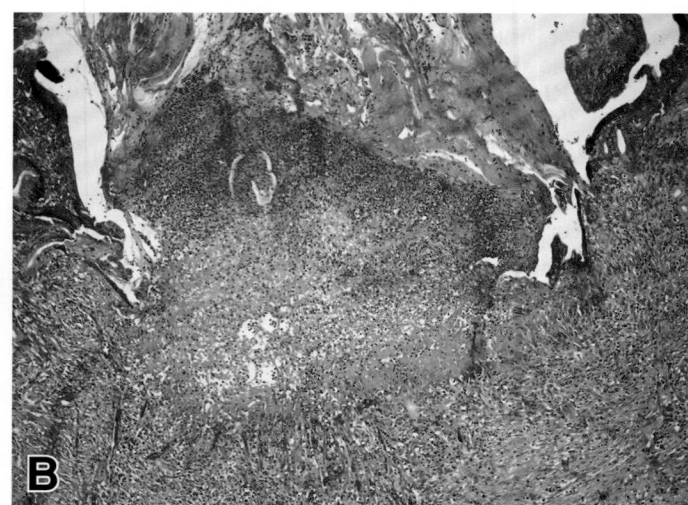

FIGURE 19-25. A. Gastric ulcer: The destructive nature of this lesion is shown by the loss of the underlying muscle in the muscularis propria with replacement by fibrous tissue. **B.** Classic appearance of peptic ulcer with superficial fibrin exudate over necrosis, followed by granulation tissue and fibrosis in the deep aspect.

Of these, the most common is bleeding, which occurs in up to 20% of patients. It is often occult. If there are no other symptoms, it may be manifest clinically as iron-deficiency anemia or occult blood in stools. Massive life-threatening bleeding is a well-known complication of active peptic ulcers.

Perforation is a serious complication that occurs in 5% of patients. In one-third of these, there are no antecedent symptoms of a peptic ulcer. Duodenal ulcers perforate more often than do gastric ulcers, mostly on the anterior wall of the duodenum. As the anterior gastric and duodenal walls are undefended by contiguous tissue, perforations there are more likely to lead to generalized peritonitis and air in the abdominal cavity, called **pneumoperitoneum**. Posterior gastric ulcers perforate into the lesser peritoneal sac, where inflammation may be contained. An ulcer that penetrates the pancreas, liver or greater omentum can cause severe intractable pain. Ulcers may also penetrate the biliary tract and fill it with air, a condition known as **pneumobilia**.

Perforation carries a high mortality rate of 10% to 40% for gastric ulcers, two to four times more than for duodenal ulcers. Perforations may lead to significant hemorrhage. Shock, abdominal distention, and pain are common symptoms. Occasionally, perforations are diagnosed for the first time at autopsy, particularly in institutionalized, elderly patients.

Pyloric obstruction occurs in up to 10% of ulcer patients, and peptic ulcer disease is its most common cause in adults. Narrowing with eventual obstruction of the pyloric lumen by an adjacent peptic ulcer may be caused by muscular spasm, edema, muscular hypertrophy, or contraction of scar tissue, or, most commonly, a combination of these.

Gastric and duodenal ulcers occur together in the same patient far more often than can be accounted for by chance alone. Patients with either one have a much greater risk of later developing the other.

HYPERPLASTIC GASTROPATHIES

Two entities comprise the hyperplastic gastropathies, but the same cellular component undergoes abnormal hyperplasia in both. Only the gastric body/fundus is affected, while the antrum is spared. Thus, both entities have a similar gross appearance but differ microscopically and clinically.

Ménétrier Disease Includes Foveolar Hyperplasia With Excess Mucus Production, Leading to Hypoalbuminemia and an Increased Risk for Gastric Carcinoma

In Ménétrier disease, endoscopy shows **markedly thickened gastric folds with mucus production limited to the body/ fundus with antral sparing** (Fig. 19-26). Microscopically, the thickened folds are attributable to massive foveolar

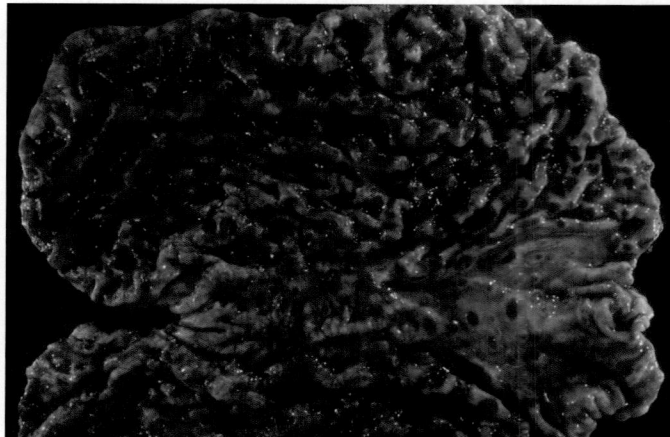

FIGURE 19-26. Ménétrier disease. The rugal folds are diffusely enlarged. They appear to be hemorrhagic because of the accompanying lymphocytic gastritis. Note the relative antral sparing (right of photograph).

hyperplasia with cystic glandular dilatation and loss of parietal and chief cells. These changes occur in response to overexpression of transforming growth factor α (TGFα), an activator of the EGFR signaling cascade, which may be idiopathic, genetic, or related to infection by CMV, HSV, or *Helicobacter*. Ménétrier disease is more common in men in the fifth and sixth decades and develops insidiously. Patients present with abdominal pain and, in severe cases, peripheral edema. Laboratory findings show **hypoproteinemia and hypoalbuminemia**, the latter of which results from mucosal protein loss. Treatment options include gastrectomy, cetuximab (an EGFR inhibitor), octreotide, and, if related to infection, antibacterial or antiviral therapy. Patients with Ménétrier disease have a predisposition to develop gastric carcinoma.

Zollinger–Ellison Syndrome Involves Parietal Cell Hyperplasia due to a Gastrinoma, Leading to Refractory Peptic Ulcers

Zollinger–Ellison (Z–E) syndrome also causes enlarged rugal folds with antral sparing, but this is due to a proliferation of parietal cells rather than foveolar cells. The cause is dysregulated gastrin production by a neuroendocrine tumor (gastrinoma). Most of these tumors are sporadic, in which case they are more commonly duodenal than pancreatic. Up to 25% of cases are related to multiple endocrine neoplasia syndrome type 1 (MEN1). Gastrinomas in Z–E patients may occur in the duodenum, pancreas, or gastric antrum, and they may be exceedingly small. Rugal folds are enlarged owing to the autonomous hypergastrinemia causing parietal cell hyperplasia; the rugae thus have a characteristic bumpy appearance (Fig. 19-27). Z–E patients have intractable peptic ulcer disease, often with multiple ulcers in unusual locations. Treatment involves acid suppression and surgical resection of the primary gastrinoma if it is a solitary mass and has not metastasized.

BENIGN NEOPLASMS

Gastric polyps, as seen endoscopically or at autopsy, are grossly identifiable elevations of the mucosa. In the stomach, unlike the colon, the vast majority are not true neoplasms.

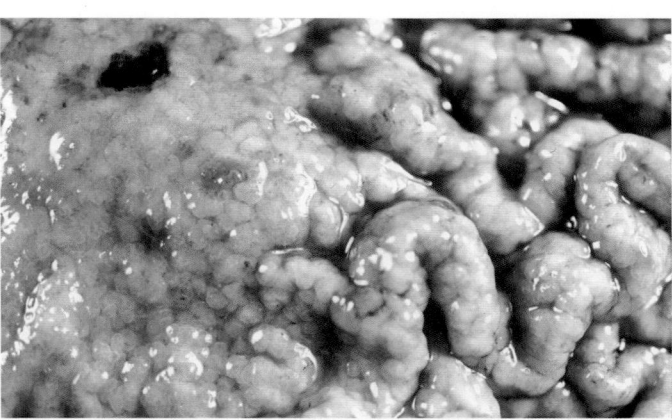

FIGURE 19-27. Zollinger–Ellison syndrome. The rugal folds are convoluted and thickened. They appear bumpy owing to hyperplasia of the parietal cells occurring in groups.

Fundic Gland Polyps Occur Only in the Body and Fundus

These are mucosal elevations composed of cystically dilated glands lined by a mixture of parietal cells, chief cells, and neutral mucous cells (Fig. 19-28A,B). They were first described in patients with familial adenomatous polyposis (FAP; see below). Such patients have a myriad of polyps carpeting the proximal gastric mucosa. Rarely, fundic gland polyps in these patients show focal dysplasia. Far more common are isolated or small numbers of fundic polyps in patients taking PPIs.

The mechanism responsible for formation of polyps involves alterations in the Wnt/β-catenin signaling pathway in both sporadic and syndromic (FAP) polyps. Polyps related to use of PPIs appear to be innocuous. Because of the ever-increasing use of PPIs in recent years, fundic gland polyps are now the most common form of polyp seen in the stomach.

Hyperplastic Polyps Often Occur in the Setting of Chronic Gastritis or Mucosal Injury

This term is somewhat of a misnomer, and these polyps have nothing in common with polyps of the colon that

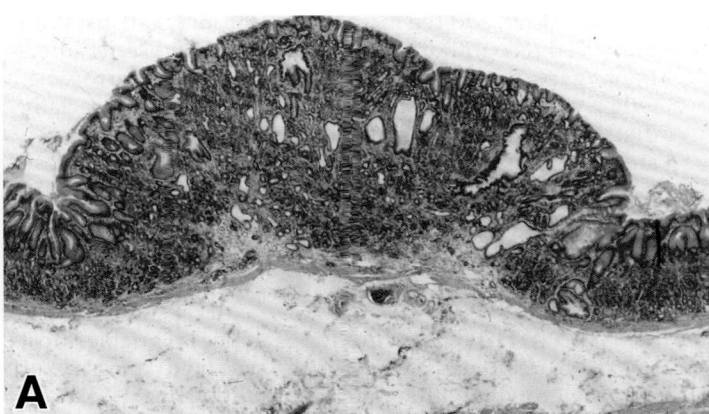

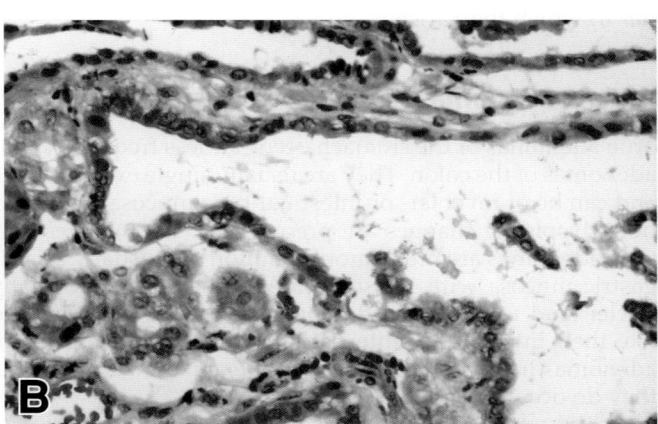

FIGURE 19-28. Fundic gland polyp. A. Low-power view shows the polyp as a slight elevation above the surrounding body-type mucosa. **B.** The cystically dilated glands contain parietal and chief cells.

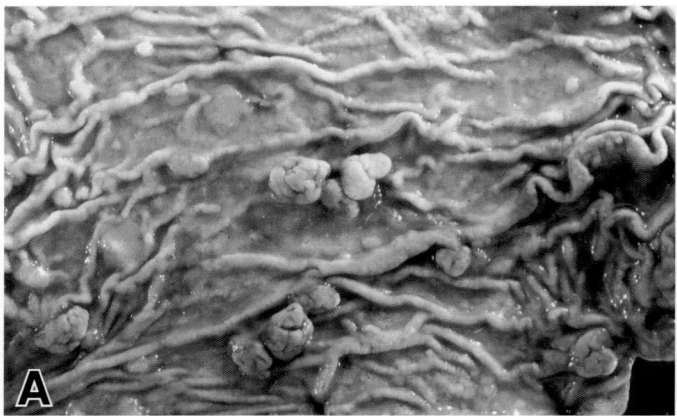

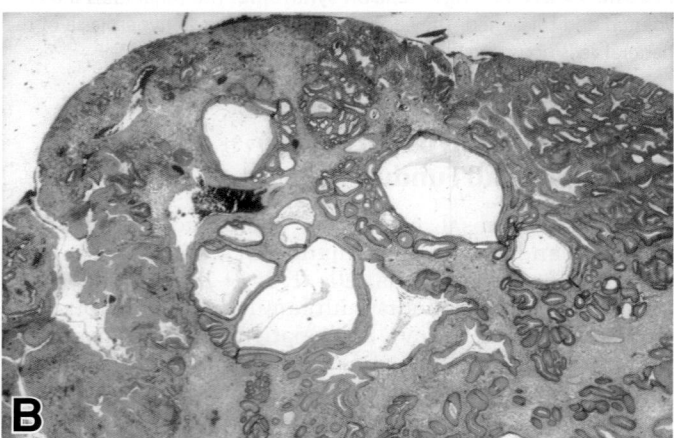

FIGURE 19-29. Hyperplastic polyp. A. Multiple mucosal elevations are seen in this resected stomach. **B.** The polyp is a mound of inflamed lamina propria. The cystically dilated glands are lined by foveolar epithelium.

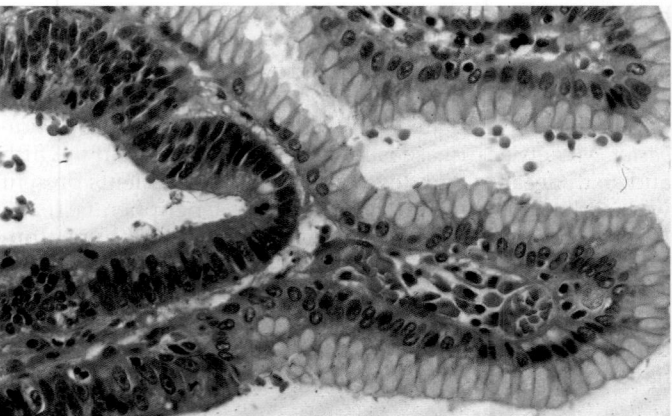

FIGURE 19-30. Gastric adenoma. There is sharp demarcation between the glandular epithelium with enlarged, hyperchromatic pencil-shaped nuclei in the adenoma (*left*) and adjacent normal foveolar epithelium (*right*).

Gastric Polyposis Syndromes

Multiple gastric polyps can be seen in FAP and in several other distinct syndromes. These include generalized familial juvenile polyposis (Fig. 19-31A–C), and Peutz–Jeghers, Cronkhite–Canada, and Cowden syndromes. The polyps in these syndromes are usually bland in appearance, often resembling large hyperplastic polyps. Their true nature is established by identifying the characteristic features of the respective underlying syndrome.

MALIGNANT NEOPLASMS

Adenocarcinoma Is the Most Common Gastric Malignancy

EPIDEMIOLOGY: There are striking geographical differences in its incidence. Gastric adenocarcinoma has declined markedly in incidence in Western countries over the past century. Many Eastern countries have a far higher incidence. Multiple factors play a role, but the most important appears to reflect differences in the prevalence of *Helicobacter*, different strains of *Helicobacter*, and the incidence of chronic gastritis. With improved recognition and treatment of *Helicobacter* infections, gaps between the West and East are narrowing. Other environmental factors also contribute, especially diet. Consumption of smoked or pickled foods is associated with a higher cancer rate, while a diet rich in fresh vegetables and leafy greens has the opposite effect. Genetic factors also play a significant role, particularly with some types of gastric cancer.

PATHOLOGY: Gross appearance is variable. Most carcinomas form large polypoid masses or growths with significant ulceration (Fig. 19-32A,B). Malignant ulcers differ from benign peptic ulcers by their large size, raised firm irregular borders and ragged ulcer

bear the same name (see below). They are exaggerated focal responses to mucosal injury in the setting of chronic gastritis or reactive gastropathy. They may be single or multiple and consist of hyperplastic foveolar cells sometimes forming small cysts with an inflamed lamina propria (Fig. 19-29A,B). Reactive atypia may be present, particularly if surface erosions occur. They are sometimes called "hyperplastic/inflammatory" polyps, reflecting the manner in which they arise.

Gastric Adenomas Are Relatively Uncommon

True adenomas of the stomach occur far less frequently than adenomas of the colon. They are usually single except in FAP, and can be of foveolar- or intestinal-type mucosa. By definition, dysplastic changes are present (Fig. 19-30). Intestinal-type adenomas are much more common and usually arise in gastric mucosa with intestinal metaplasia. Microscopically, nuclei tend to be enlarged, elongated and hyperchromatic, like their intestinal counterparts. In contrast, foveolar-type adenomas have no relationship to intestinal metaplasia, but they do occur in FAP.

Although gastric adenomas may be related to gastric carcinoma, the close relationship of adenoma to carcinoma seen in the colon is not present.

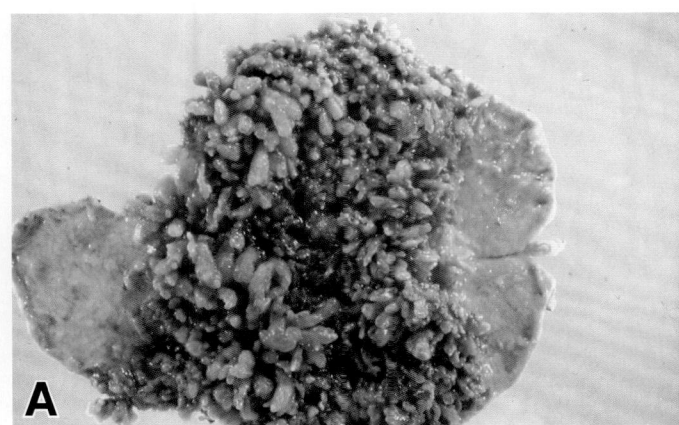

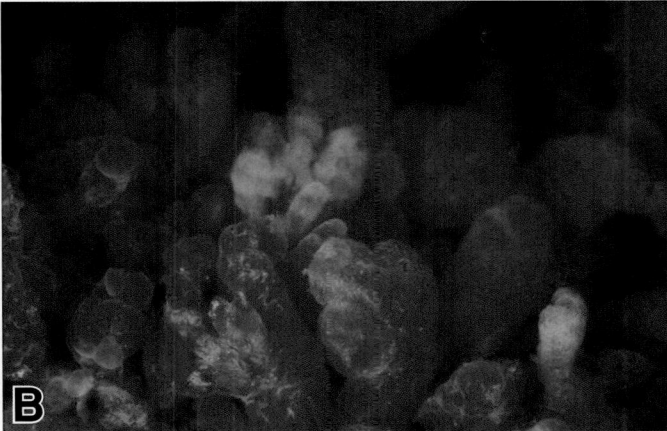

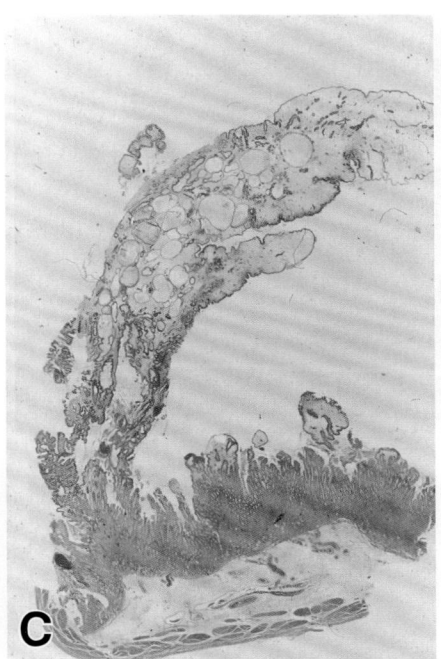

FIGURE 19-31. Familial juvenile polyposis. A, B. While the colon is the main target organ in this syndrome, the stomach can be involved and carpeted by polyps. **C.** Histologically, they are innocuous and somewhat resemble hyperplastic polyps.

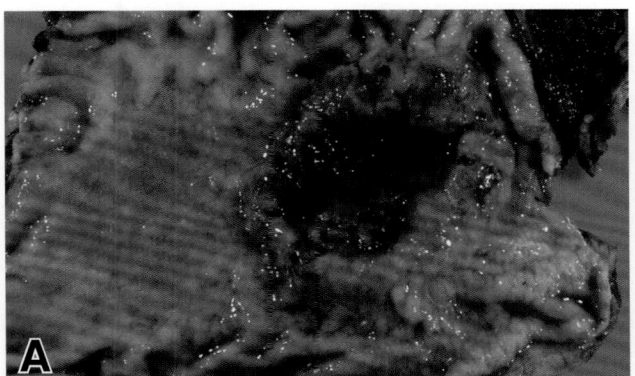

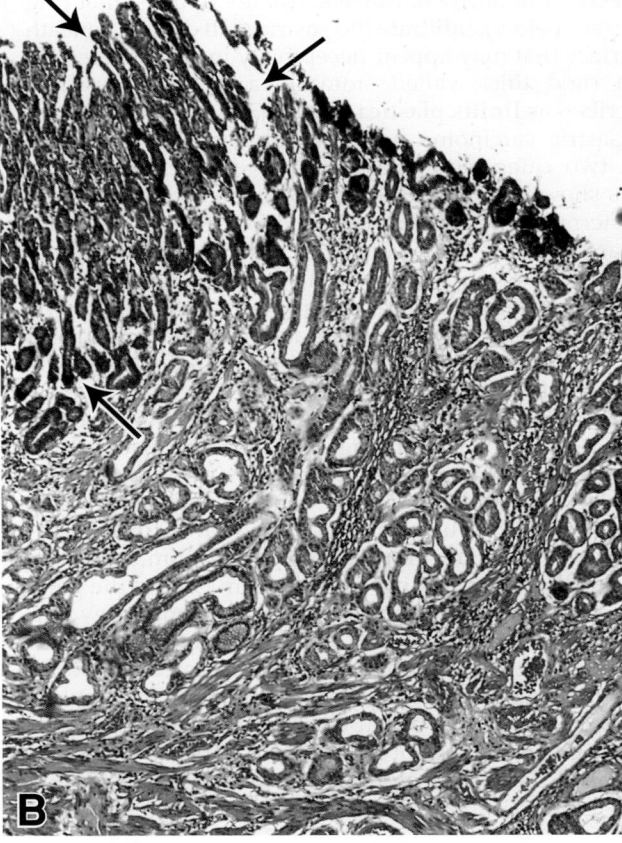

FIGURE 19-32. Gastric carcinoma. A. This large antral lesion is clearly distinguished from a benign ulcer by its raised firm edges and necrotic base. **B.** Microscopically, innumerable poorly formed glands (*arrows*) replace the mucosa in this intestinal-type carcinoma.

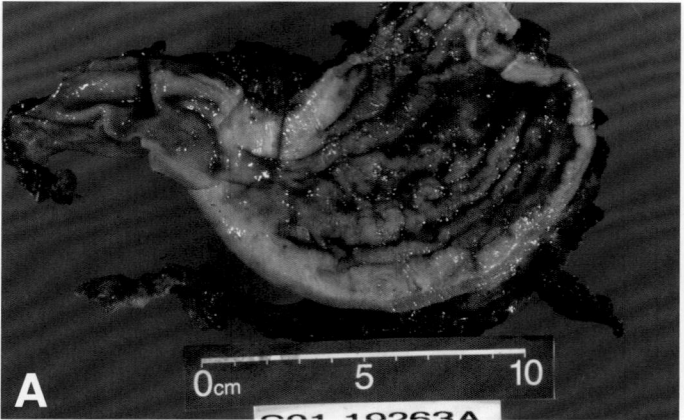

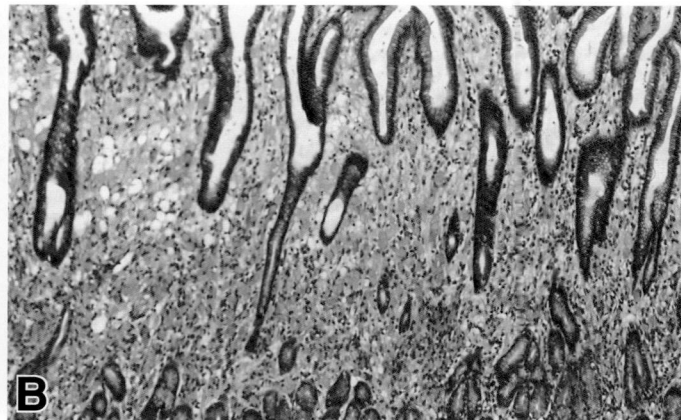

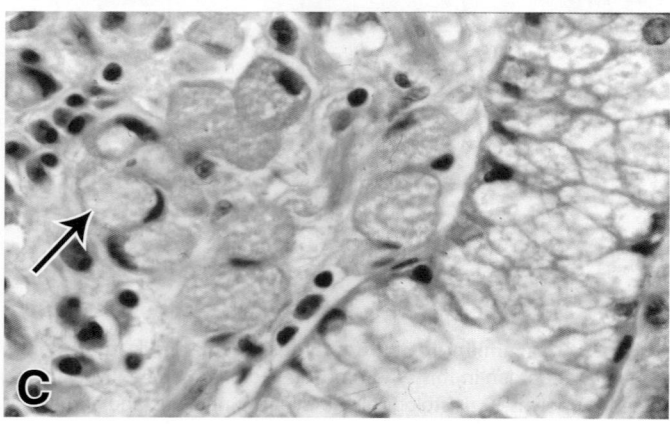

FIGURE 19-33. Gastric carcinoma. A. The wall is white and thickened owing to the diffuse infiltrate of tumor cells. The mucosal surface is deceptively free of mass lesions. **B.** The infiltrate fills and expands the lamina propria but leaves glands and surface epithelium intact. **C.** The tumor cells in this diffuse-type cancer are present next to an intact gland. Note the signet ring appearance (*arrow*).

surfaces. A minority of cancers, usually of the signet ring type (see below), infiltrate the gastric wall deeply, beneath a surface that may appear deceptively intact. This results in a rigid thick-walled stomach, a feature classically described as **linitis plastica** (Fig. 19-33A–C).

Gastric carcinoma has traditionally been separated into two categories, intestinal and diffuse, with some cases showing overlap (this is the Lauren classification). The term "intestinal" in this context mainly describes the architecture, rather than the cell type. Such tumors form glands or papillae, as well as some solid areas. The intestinal type is the more common pattern and is the one associated with chronic gastritis and intestinal metaplasia as a precursor. It is declining in incidence because of its relationship to *Helicobacter*.

Diffuse-type carcinoma contains poorly cohesive cells, usually of signet-ring type, that diffusely infiltrate the gastric wall. The incidence of this tumor has been relatively stable in all countries. It also has a clearer genetic cause. Indeed, hereditary diffuse gastric cancer is an uncommon autosomal dominant condition linked to germline mutations in *CDH1*, the gene that encodes E-cadherin. Such patients may develop cancer at an early age and often have multiple small foci of signet ring carcinoma in situ detectable only by thorough microscopic examination. Prophylactic gastrectomy is a therapeutic option. As one might expect given the loss of E-cadherin, patients also have increased risk of developing lobular carcinoma of the

breast. E-cadherin inactivation also occurs in sporadic diffuse gastric carcinomas.

Early Versus Advanced Gastric Adenocarcinoma

Complex systems are used to describe the character and depth of gastric carcinomas, but there is one simple fact of paramount importance: *patients with early gastric cancer (i.e., tumors confined to the mucosa and submucosa) have a much better prognosis (80% to 90% survival at 5 years) than patients with advanced adenocarcinomas (i.e., lesions that extend into the muscularis propria and beyond) who have only 16% to 80% survival at 5 years. Prognosis is even worse if invasion is deeper.*

The Stomach Is a Common Site of Extranodal Lymphomas Related to *Helicobacter* Infection

The gastrointestinal tract is the most common location for extranodal lymphomas, and the stomach is the most common portion of the gastrointestinal tract affected. Most gastric lymphomas are either extranodal marginal zone lymphomas of mucosa-associated lymphoid tissue (MALT lymphoma; see Chapter 26) or diffuse large B-cell lymphomas. Both are associated with *Helicobacter* infection; **eradication of the organisms leads to remission** in a striking majority (up to 80%) of cases. However, some lymphomas acquire an (11;18)(q21;q21) translocation in which case the tumor is no longer responsive to *H. pylori*

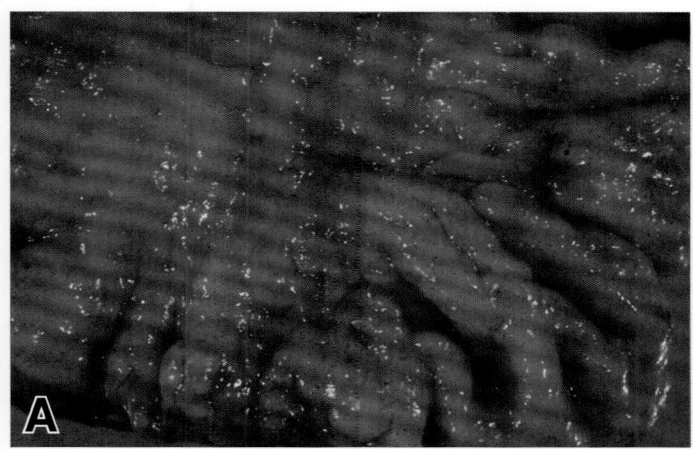

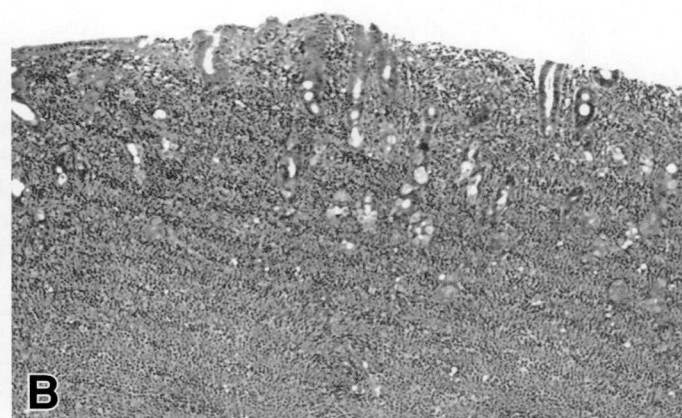

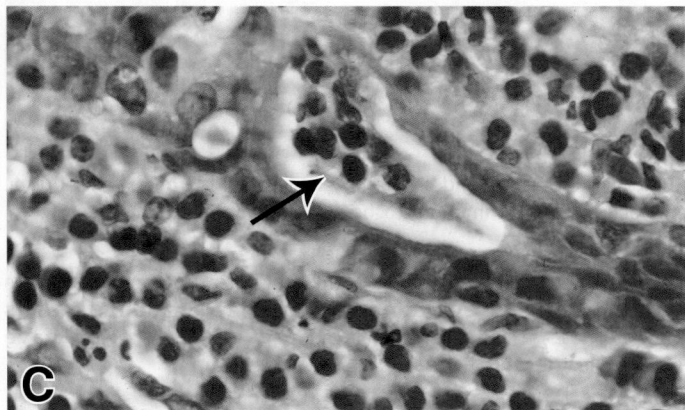

FIGURE 19-34. Gastric lymphoma, mucosa-associated lymphoid tissue (MALT) type. A. There is loss of detail within the gastric mucosa as a MALT lymphoma infiltrates the mucosa over a large surface area, although a discrete mass was not formed. **B.** Microscopically, a monotonous population of lymphoid cells greatly expands the lamina propria. **C.** A **lymphoepithelial lesion,** with tumor lymphocytes penetrating into a gland (*arrow*).

eradication therapy. MALT lymphoma is difficult to distinguish from chronic gastritis with lymphoid hyperplasia. The presence of gastric glands infiltrated by lymphocytes (lymphoepithelial lesions) and uniform monocytoid morphology of cells infiltrating the lamina propria are distinguishing features (Fig. 19-34). Diffuse large B-cell lymphomas are more readily recognized because of their pleomorphic appearance.

Gastrointestinal Stromal Tumors (GISTs) Derive From the Interstitial Cells of Cajal

Interstitial cells of Cajal, from which these tumors derive, normally reside in the muscularis propria and are pacemaker cells, transducing signals between the enteric nervous system and the smooth muscle of the gastrointestinal tract to ensure coordinated peristalsis.

GIST tumors are usually large and bulky (Fig. 19-35A). They arise in the muscularis propria but may show central ulceration of the overlying mucosa, and thus present with bleeding. They are comprised of a solid proliferation of tumor cells with a spindled or epithelioid morphology (Fig. 19-35B). These tumors are most commonly driven by mutations in *KIT,* which encodes a receptor tyrosine kinase. Accordingly, most GISTs stain positively for CD117, an immunohistochemical stain targeting the C-Kit tyrosine kinase. A minority are linked to mutations in *PDGFRα,* another receptor tyrosine kinase, or in the succinate dehydrogenase complex of genes.

GISTs occur throughout the gastrointestinal tract but are most common in the stomach followed by the small bowel. The best pathologic predictors of behavior include tumor site, size, and mitotic count. Treatment includes surgical resection and drug therapy, with the drug of choice determined by the specific mutations present. As most GISTs are related to mutations in *KIT,* imatinib mesylate (Gleevec) is used to inhibit the tyrosine kinase. The same drug is used in chronic myelogenous leukemia to block the kinase activity of the BCR-ABL1 fusion protein.

Neuroendocrine Tumors of the Stomach Behave Differently, Depending Upon the Background Conditions in Which They Arise

These tumors were once called "carcinoids," but that term has been replaced by "well-differentiated neuroendocrine tumor" (NET). As for GISTs, the site of origin is the major determinant of biologic behavior. Additional predictive features at a given site are tumor size and mitotic rate (proliferative activity may be assessed immunohistochemically by the percentage of tumor cells expressing the cell cycle marker Ki-67).

Behavior of gastric NETs depends on the conditions in which the neoplasms arise. These tumors are found in three major clinical settings. The first is autoimmune gastritis. As described previously, profound activation of antral G cells results in hypergastrinemia and proliferation of ECL cells in the body and fundus. The

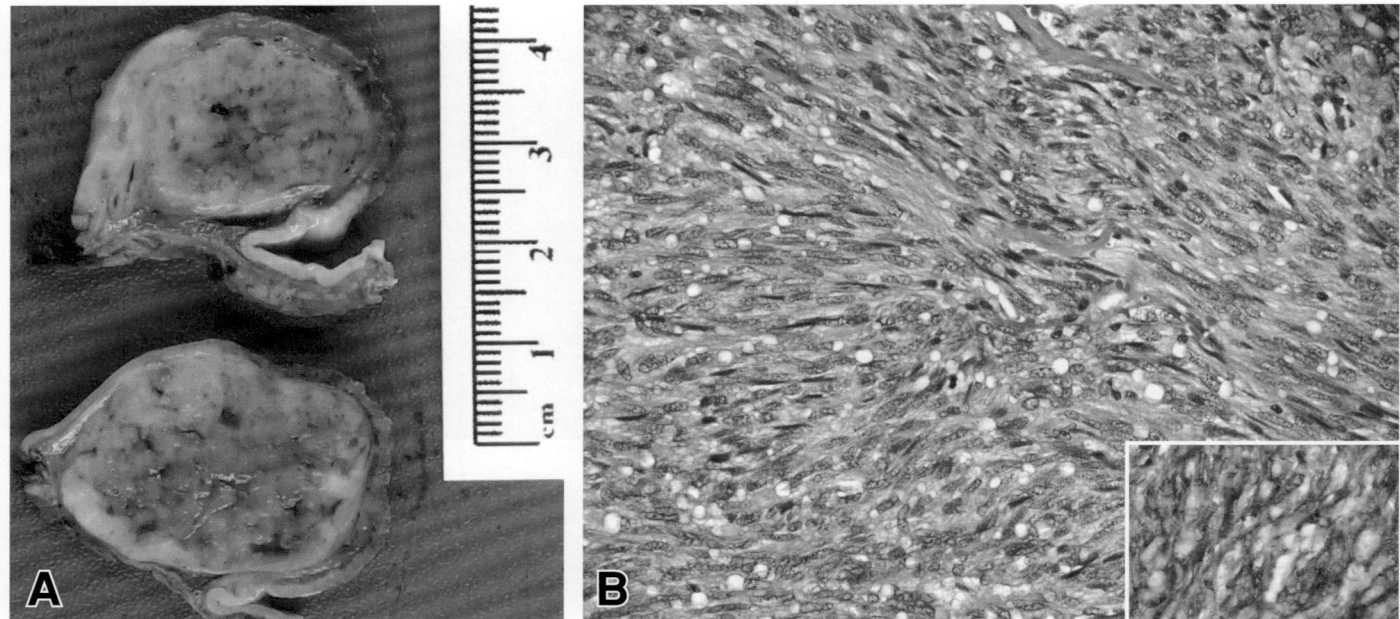

FIGURE 19-35. Gastrointestinal stromal tumor (GIST). A. The resected tumor is submucosal and covered by mucosa with a deep central ulcer. **B.** Microscopic appearance of tumor cells that are spindled and have cytoplasmic vacuoles. *Inset:* Immunohistochemical stain positive for c-kit.

initial response is ECL-cell hyperplasia but then strings of cells form linear arrays, which later coalesce to form micronodules that separate from the bases of gastric glands. Propelled by prominent hypergastrinemia, these micronodules eventually coalesce into larger structures until a clinically evident neoplasm is formed. Patients with NETs arising in autoimmune gastritis often have multiple visible tumors (Fig. 19-36).

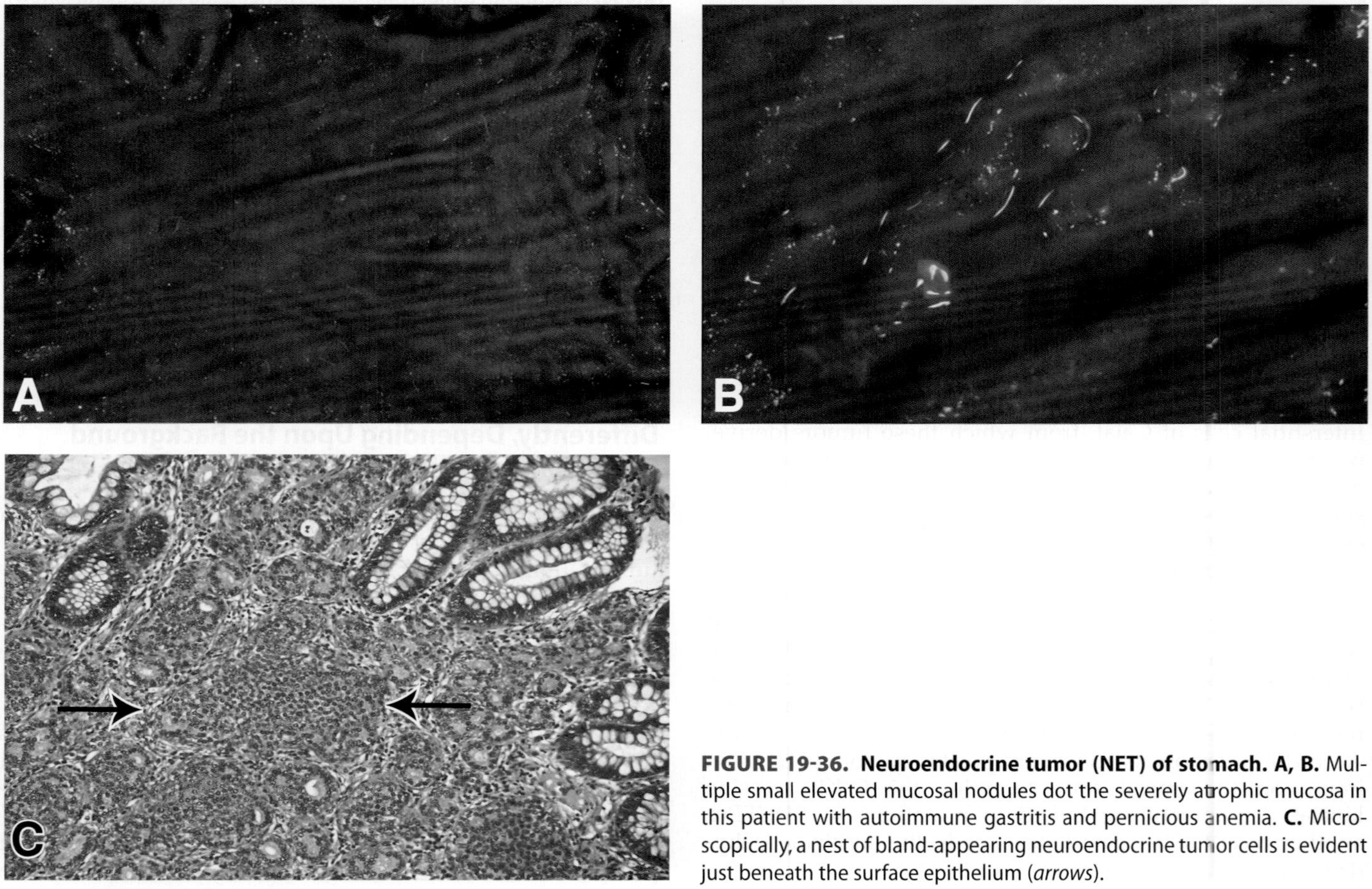

FIGURE 19-36. Neuroendocrine tumor (NET) of stomach. A, B. Multiple small elevated mucosal nodules dot the severely atrophic mucosa in this patient with autoimmune gastritis and pernicious anemia. **C.** Microscopically, a nest of bland-appearing neuroendocrine tumor cells is evident just beneath the surface epithelium (*arrows*).

A second clinical setting in which gastric neuroendocrine tumors arise is the hypergastrinemic state associated with Z–E syndrome (see above). Finally, gastric NETs can occur sporadically in which case they are more frequently antral. Of interest, tumors arising in autoimmune gastritis are rarely aggressive, whereas sporadic NETs have a worse prognosis. Those arising in association with Z–E syndrome are intermediate in behavior.

The Small and Large Intestine

ANATOMY

Embryologically, the intestinal tract develops as a tube that elongates progressively from the stomach to the cloaca. Its cephalic portion becomes the segment that extends from the distal duodenum to the proximal ileum. The more caudal portion develops into distal ileum and the proximal 2/3 of transverse colon. The vitelline duct, which connects the primitive duct to the yolk sac, may persist as a Meckel diverticulum (see below). To reach its final disposition, the fetal gut undergoes a complex series of rotations.

The small intestine extends from the pylorus to the ileocecal valve and, depending on its muscle tone, is from 3.5 to 6.5 m long, on average. It is divided into three regions:

1. **The duodenum** extends to the ligament of Treitz.
2. **The jejunum** is the proximal 40% of the remainder of the small intestine.
3. **The ileum** is the distal 60%.

The C-shaped duodenum is almost entirely retroperitoneal and thus fixed. It surrounds the head of the pancreas, and receives biliary drainage from the liver and pancreatic secretions through the common bile duct at the ampulla of Vater. The remainder of small intestine, which is disposed in redundant loops, is movable.

In most individuals, the common bile duct and the main pancreatic duct (duct of Wirsung) meet to form a common chamber, the **ampulla**, which projects into the duodenal lumen through the major **papilla of Vater**. The terminal parts of both ducts and ampulla are surrounded by a circular muscle, the **sphincter of Oddi**. In some people, an accessory pancreatic duct, the duct of Santorini, may branch off the main pancreatic duct and separately drain the pancreatic head, entering the duodenum at the **minor duodenal papilla**.

The distal duodenum becomes invested by mesentery and merges with the jejunum at the **ligament of Treitz**. There is no demarcation between jejunum and ileum, which merge gradually.

The **large intestine** is that portion of the gut from the ileocecal valve to the anus. It is 90 to 125 cm long in adults and has six regions, distally from the ileocecal valve: (1) cecum, (2) ascending colon, (3) transverse colon, (4) descending colon, (5) sigmoid colon, and (6) rectum. The bend between the ascending and transverse colon in the right upper quadrant is the **hepatic flexure**, and that between the transverse and descending segments in the left upper quadrant is the **splenic flexure**. The lumen narrows progressively from the cecum to the sigmoid colon.

The arterial blood supply of the small and large intestine is provided by three major vessels. The duodenum is served by the pancreaticoduodenal branch of the hepatic artery, which arises from the celiac artery. The jejunum, ileum, and colon up to the splenic flexure are supplied by the superior mesenteric artery (a branch of the aorta), which is arranged in arcades in the mesentery, thus providing abundant collateral circulation in its distal reaches. The left colon is supplied by the inferior mesenteric artery. Venous flow and lymphatic drainage from the small intestine and colon empty into the portal circulation.

Differences in the histology of the small and large intestines reflect the major functions of these two gastrointestinal tract segments—nutrient absorption in the small intestine and storage of feces with water and salt absorption in the large intestine.

The small intestine is notable for its extensive surface area. The surface area is not only maximized by its overall length (average of 3 to 5 m), but by its mucosal folds, the **plicae circulares**. Lining the plicae are even more folds, **the villi**, finger-like projections of mucosa which are covered by the enterocytes and goblet cells (Fig. 19-37). The luminal surfaces of the enterocytes are covered with **microvilli**, colloquially

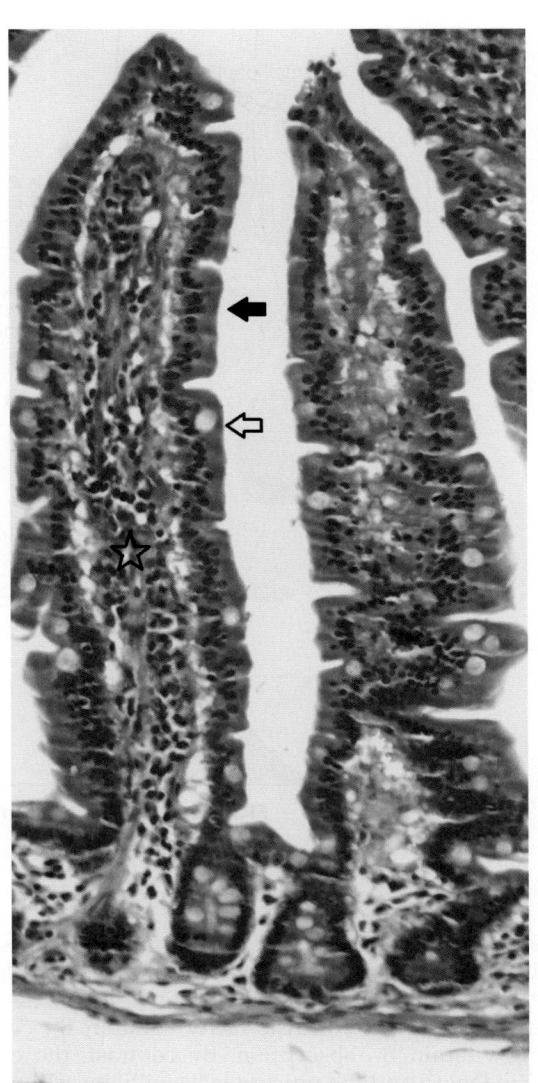

FIGURE 19-37. Intestinal villi from the jejunum. The villi are several times longer than the crypts that gave rise to them. The lamina propria (*star*) normally contains a mixture of lymphocytes and plasma cells with some scattered eosinophils. The villous epithelium is comprised of a mixture of absorptive enterocytes (*filled arrow*) and goblet cells (*open arrow*).

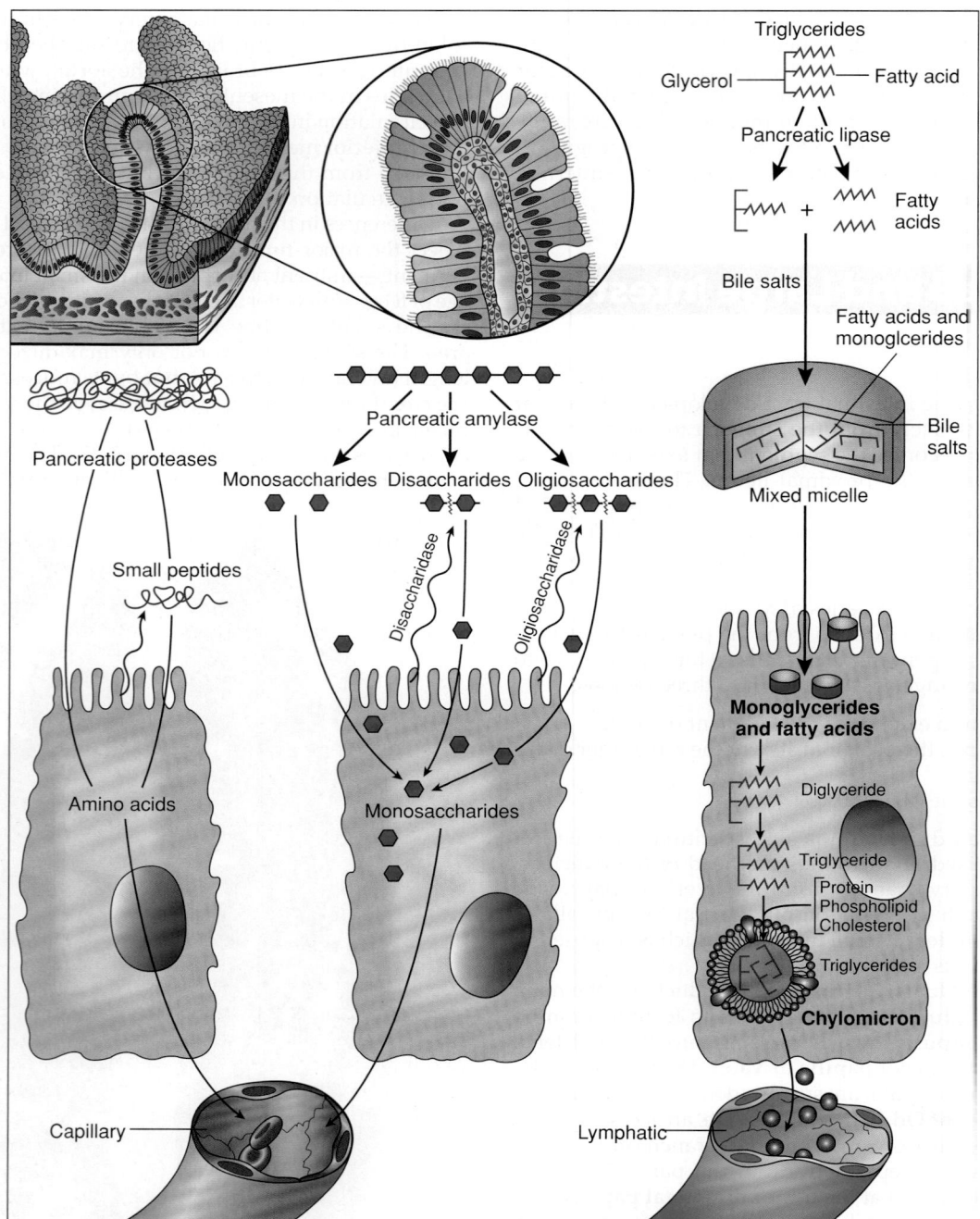

FIGURE 19-38. Mechanisms of nutrient absorption in the small intestine.

referred to as the brush border, further maximizing surface area. It is here where most digestive enzymes are located (Fig. 19-38). Enterocytes in the terminal ileum also contain receptors for the intrinsic factor–vitamin B_{12} complex, enabling vitamin B_{12} absorption. By contrast, the colon is shorter in length and the mucosa lacks villi; instead of being specialized to absorb nutrients from food intake, it is lined by crypts and a surface epithelium whose more limited function is to absorb water and store feces.

A closer look reveals additional differences in the small and large intestinal mucosa with a greater degree of

complexity in the small intestine. Four cell types occur in the small intestinal crypts:

- **Paneth cells** at crypt bases resemble pancreatic or salivary zymogen cells and are active in exocrine secretion. Their basophilic cytoplasm is filled with eosinophilic secretory granules. Paneth cells also function in mucosal defense, as mediated by lysozyme; antimicrobial products, including peptides called crypt defensins (cryptdins); and CD95 ligand, a member of the tumor necrosis factor (TNF) family of cytokines.

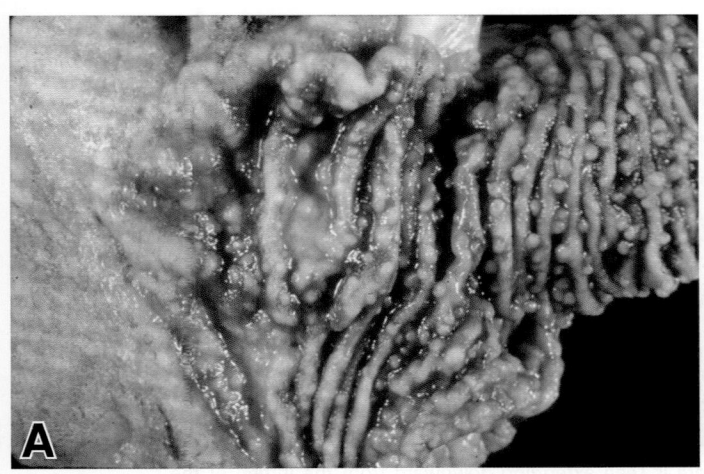
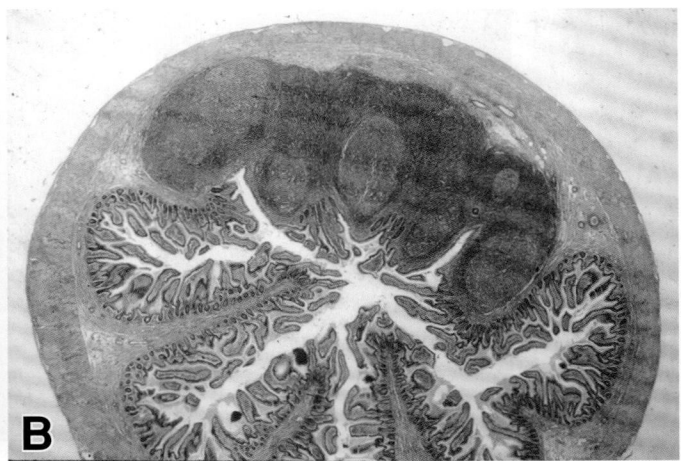

FIGURE 19-39. A. Peyer patches are particularly prominent in the terminal ileum and are seen as small come-shaped mucosal mounds. **B.** They are composed of lymphoid tissue, often with prominent germinal centers, displacing the epithelial structures.

- **Goblet cells** of the crypts are flask shaped and filled with mucous granules. They resemble goblet cells elsewhere both structurally and functionally, and contain neutral and acid mucins.
- **Endocrine cells** have apical nuclei and basal eosinophilic granules. They produce several gastrointestinal hormones and peptides, including gastrin, secretin, cholecystokinin, glucagon, vasoactive intestinal peptide (VIP), and serotonin. These hormones regulate many gastrointestinal functions, and tumors derived from these cells often exhibit striking hormone secretion.
- **Undifferentiated cells** reside in the lateral crypt walls and are interspersed between Paneth cells at crypt bases. They are the most abundant cells in the crypts and act as mitotically active reserve cells, from which all other mucosal cell populations are renewed.

The colonic mucosa, by contrast, is composed primarily of two cell types, simple columnar cells and goblet cells. The crypts mostly contain goblet cells, except at their bases, where a few undifferentiated cells and a variety of neuroendocrine cells are located.

The submucosa of the small intestine has two unique regions. In the proximal duodenum, **Brunner glands** secrete mucus and bicarbonate, which protect the duodenal mucosa from peptic ulceration. The other specialized region, in the terminal ileum, is notable for its collection of lymphoid tissue known as **Peyer patches** (Fig. 19-39A,B). Having a structure analogous to that of lymph nodes, Peyer patches are important components of the adaptive immune system, in which B or T lymphocyte activation occurs in response to luminal antigens.

Finally, the muscular layers of the small and large intestine are relatively similar. Both have two layers: an outer longitudinal and inner circular layer, which act together to propel intestinal contents by peristalsis. Parasympathetic and sympathetic innervations terminate in the submucosal Meissner plexus and the muscular Auerbach plexus to coordinate this peristalsis. The colon, however, is unique in that the longitudinal muscle layer is aggregated into three separate bundles, the **taeniae coli**. Evaginations of the colonic wall between taeniae, the **haustra**, appear as external sacculations. The **appendices epiploicae** are small serosal masses of fat, invested by peritoneum.

Cell renewal in the small and large intestine occurs only in the crypts, where undifferentiated cells divide. New cells migrate up the crypt and into the villus, where they differentiate into goblet cells and absorptive cells, and eventually slough into the lumen at the tip of the villus. Their absorptive capacity is maximal in the upper 1/3 of villi. The mucosal epithelium of the small intestine is replaced every 4 to 7 days. Intestinal epithelium is therefore very sensitive to radiation and chemotherapeutic agents.

CONGENITAL AND NEONATAL DISORDERS

Meckel Diverticulum Is Present in About 2% of the Population and Is the Most Common Cause of Gastrointestinal Tract Bleeding Before Age 2

This is the most commonly encountered clinically significant congenital disorder of the small intestine. It is solitary true diverticulum, containing all layers of the intestinal wall (Fig. 19-40A,B). It arises as a remnant of the vitelline duct, which fails to involute, and so extends from the antimesenteric side of the distal ileum. Meckel diverticula occur more often in males than females. Most are asymptomatic, but bleeding, perforation, or obstruction due to intussusception may occur. Bleeding and perforation may result from peptic ulceration due to the presence of heterotopic gastric tissue with acid-producing parietal cells. Rarely, neoplasms develop in this location, usually neuroendocrine tumors.

Necrotizing Enterocolitis, a Complication of Prematurity, Is the Most Serious Acquired Neonatal Gastrointestinal Disorder

Neonatal necrotizing enterocolitis, commonly known as NEC, is, unfortunately, one of the most common acquired surgical emergencies in newborns. It is more common and severe in premature and low–birth-weight infants. Onset usually follows the start of enteral feeding. As the name suggests, NEC may result in full-thickness coagulative necrosis of the bowel with perforation (Fig. 19-41); less severe cases may involve mucosal ischemia that later heals with strictures. Pneumatosis cystoides intestinalis, the

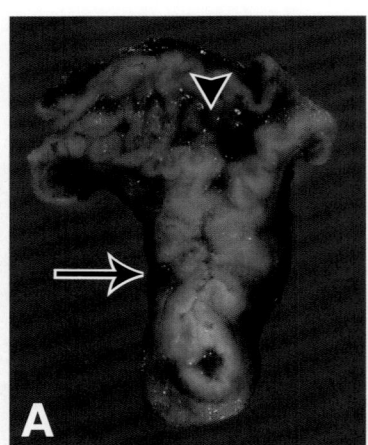
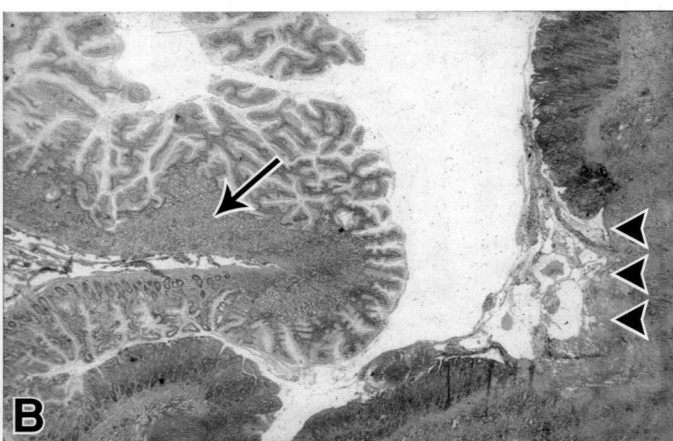

FIGURE 19-40. A. The **Meckel diverticulum** (*arrow*) here is seen extending downward from the lumen of the ileum (*arrowhead*). **B.** Low-power microscopic view shows heterotopic gastric mucosa (*arrow*) and mucosal ulceration (*arrowheads*).

classic radiologic finding in NEC (see below), is frequent. While its exact pathogenesis is not known, NEC is thought to be related to bowel immaturity, an imbalance in the normal microbiome, and solute loading, in that hyperosmolar feedings increase the risk of disease. Surgical resection of the affected segment may lead to a phenomenon known as short gut syndrome. This is an iatrogenic malabsorption disorder caused by a critical reduction in the amount of functional small bowel. Perforation is associated with 20% to 40% overall mortality from sepsis, with lower weight infants doing worse.

Meconium Ileus May Be an Early Complication of Cystic Fibrosis

In the neonatal period, infants with cystic fibrosis may develop intestinal obstruction caused by plugging of the lumen of the distal ileum by thick viscid mucus characteristic of that condition. Perforation and peritonitis due to the meconium may occur.

Hirschsprung Disease Is Caused by Segmental Absence of Ganglion Cells

In Hirschsprung disease, colon dilation (Fig. 19-42) results from absence of ganglion cells beginning in the internal anal sphincter and extending proximally for variable lengths

(Fig. 19-43). Most commonly the rectum and left colon are affected, but in about 10% of cases, the entire colon is aganglionic. Rarely, the small intestine is also involved. Hirschsprung disease affects 1 in 5,000 live births; 80% of patients are male except in long segment disease where the male:female ratio is equal.

The incidence of Hirschsprung disease is 1 in 300 in infants with Down syndrome, and Down syndrome is found in approximately 4% of all patients with Hirschsprung disease. Most cases are solitary lesions, but congenital anomalies of the kidneys and lower urinary tract, as well as imperforate anus and cardiac malformations, have also been reported.

Interestingly, like achalasia, which is caused by destruction of esophageal ganglion cells, Chagas disease may cause aganglionic megacolon. In fact, the most common cause of megacolon in Central and South America in Chagas disease in which the responsible parasite destroys cells of the autonomic nervous system.

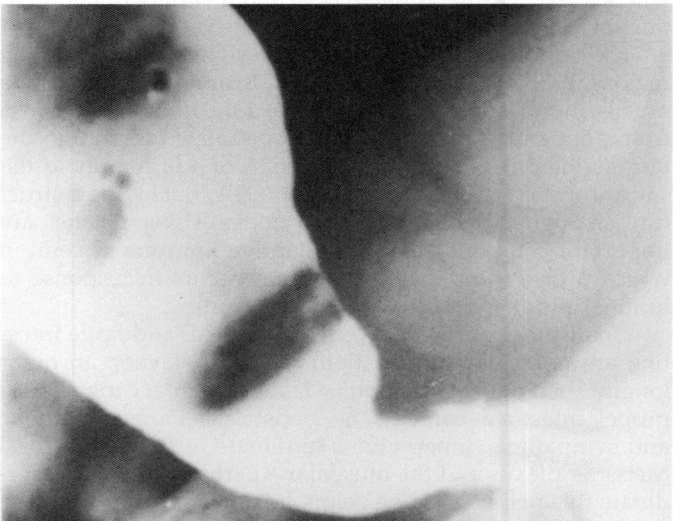

FIGURE 19-42. Hirschsprung disease. A contrast radiograph shows marked dilation of the rectosigmoid colon proximal to the narrowed rectum. (From Mitros FA. *Atlas of Gastrointestinal Pathology*. New York: Gower Medical Publishing; 1988. Copyright Lippincott Williams & Wilkins.)

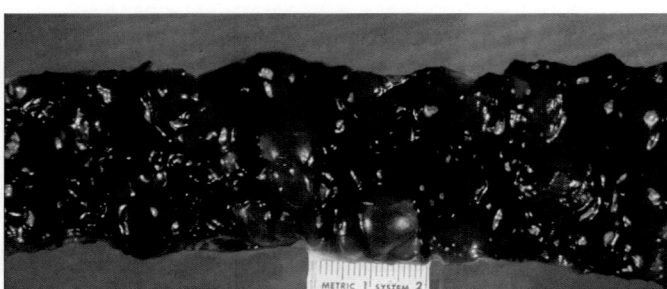

FIGURE 19-41. A segment of necrotic ileum with hemorrhage and pneumatosis from a premature infant with **neonatal necrotizing enterocolitis (NEC).**

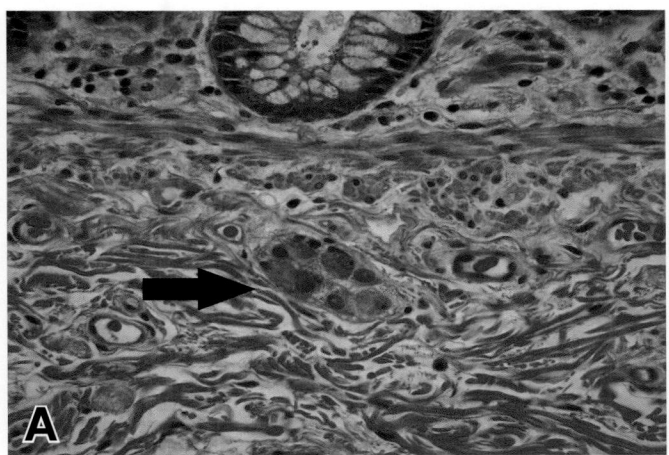
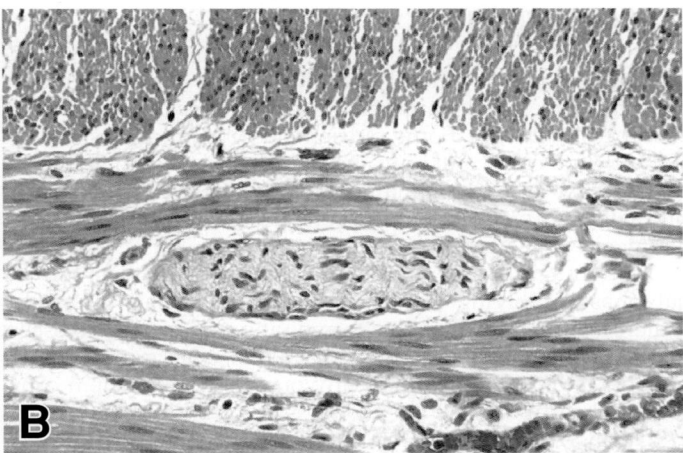

FIGURE 19-43. Hirschsprung disease. A. A photomicrograph of ganglion cells in the submucosa of a normal rectum (*arrow*). **B.** A rectal biopsy specimen from a patient with Hirschsprung disease shows a nonmyelinated nerve in the mesenteric plexus and an absence of ganglion cells.

PATHOGENESIS: In Hirschsprung disease, the normal cranial to caudal migration of neuroblasts from the neural crest to the distal aspect of the rectum during embryogenesis fails to occur. Consequently, ganglion cells will be absent from the submucosal and myenteric plexuses starting where this neuroblast migration halts, with aganglionosis extending distally to the internal anal sphincter. This aganglionic segment is permanently contracted because of the absence of tonic relaxation neural stimuli. As a result, fecal contents cannot readily enter the contracted area.

Most cases of Hirschsprung disease are sporadic, but 10% are familial. Half of familial cases, and 15% of sporadic ones, have been linked to loss-of-function mutations of the RET receptor tyrosine kinase gene on chromosome 10q (see MEN2 syndrome, Chapter 27). Some cases involve mutations in the endothelin-B receptor or genes that encode ligands of these two receptors.

PATHOLOGY: The aganglionic segment of the large intestine in Hirschsprung disease is constricted and spastic. Proximal to this, the bowel is very dilated. Definitive diagnosis requires demonstrating the absence of ganglion cells on rectal biopsy (Fig. 19-43B). Because it is difficult to prove a negative, the diagnosis requires careful and comprehensive analysis of an adequate amount of tissue. There is also a striking increase in nonmyelinated cholinergic nerve fibers in the submucosa and between muscle coats (neural hyperplasia). The lack of ganglion cells leads to accumulation of acetylcholine and acetylcholinesterase, which are evident using histochemical staining. Immunohistochemistry of calretinin, a calcium-binding protein expressed in enteric neurons, has also been used in diagnosing Hirschsprung disease in rectal suction biopsies.

CLINICAL FEATURES: *Hirschsprung disease is the most common cause of congenital intestinal obstruction.* Typically, newborns show delayed passage of meconium and vomiting in the first few days of life. In some cases, complete intestinal obstruction may require immediate surgical relief. Children whose involved rectal segments are short may experience only partial obstruction, constipation, abdominal distention, and recurrent fecal impactions.

The most serious complication is enterocolitis, in which the dilated proximal segment of the colon becomes ulcerated and necrotic. This process may extend proximally into the small intestine. Hirschsprung disease is treated by surgical removal of the aganglionic segment and reconstruction.

Acquired Megacolon Is Any Cause of Constipation With Colonic Dilatation

Acquired megacolon sometimes occurs in children and often has a psychogenic component. In adults, acquired megacolon can result from disorders that interfere with bowel innervation or smooth muscle function, such as Chagas disease, diabetic neuropathy, Parkinsonism, myotonic dystrophy, scleroderma, amyloidosis, and hypothyroidism.

Anorectal Malformations Often Accompany Other Developmental Defects

These malformations vary from minor narrowings to serious and complex defects. They result from arrested development of the caudal region of the gut in the first 6 months of fetal life. These anomalies are now categorized by their precise anatomy:

- **Anorectal agenesis and rectal atresia.**
- **Anal agenesis and anorectal stenosis.**
- **Imperforate anus** is a deformity in which the anal opening is covered by a cutaneous membrane behind which meconium is visible. **Anal stenosis** is a variant of imperforate anus.
- **Fistulas** between the rectum and perineum, bladder, urethra, or vagina may occur alone or in association with other anorectal anomalies.

MALABSORPTION

Malabsorption is a general term that covers diverse clinical conditions in which important nutrients are inadequately absorbed by the gut. Some nutrient absorption occurs in the stomach and colon, but only absorption from the small intestine, mainly in the proximal portion, is clinically important. Bile salts and vitamin B_{12} are preferentially absorbed by the ileum.

Nutrient absorption in the intestine proceeds via a luminal phase involving processes within the small intestine lumen, and an intestinal phase involving transport processes in cells of the intestinal mucosa. Each phase has critical components and derangement in any one or more of them can impair absorption.

During the luminal phase, the physicochemical state of nutrients is altered to allow them to be taken up by absorptive cells. Pancreatic enzymes and bile acids secreted into the duodenum facilitate digestion of lipids. Normal, regulated flow of gastric contents into the duodenum and a sufficiently high duodenal pH are also needed. And, normal pancreatic enzyme delivery to the duodenum requires adequate pancreatic exocrine function and unobstructed flow of pancreatic juice.

Supplying bile in normal quantity and quality to the duodenum requires (1) adequate liver function, (2) unobstructed bile flow, and (3) intact enterohepatic bile salt circulation. This enterohepatic circulation begins with absorption of most intestinal bile salts from the distal ileum and ends with their excretion into the duodenum through the bile ducts. Normally, 95% of intestinal bile salts are recycled via this circuit; 5% are excreted in the stool. Normal enterohepatic circulation requires (1) normal intestinal microflora, (2) normal ileal absorptive function, and (3) an unobstructed biliary system.

While the luminal phase depends on contributions from multiple organs and segments of the gastrointestinal tract, the intestinal phase, discussed next, involves several specific cellular mechanisms in the intestinal mucosa.

Intestinal-Phase Malabsorption Frequently Reflects Specific Enzyme Defects, Microvillus Damage, or Impaired Transport

Abnormalities in any of the four parts of the intestinal phase may cause malabsorption, but some diseases affect more than one of these components. A brief description of these four parts with their corresponding diseases is helpful, followed by a more in-depth discussion of each disease.

 ETIOLOGIC FACTORS: *MICROVILLI:* Intestinal disaccharidases and oligopeptidases are present at the surface of the microvilli. Disaccharidases are essential for sugar absorption, since only monosaccharides can be absorbed by intestinal epithelial cells. Oligopeptides and dipeptides may be absorbed by alternate routes that do not require peptidases. Abnormal microvillus function may be primary—as in primary disaccharidase deficiencies—or secondary, if there is damage to villi, as in celiac disease (see below). Enzyme deficiencies lead to intolerance to the respective disaccharides (e.g., lactose intolerance in lactase deficiency).

ABSORPTIVE AREA: As already discussed, the considerable length of the small bowel and the amplification of its surface by intestinal folds and villi provide a large absorptive surface. Severe diminution in this area may cause malabsorption. Surface area may be decreased by (1) small bowel resection (short gut syndrome), (2) gastrocolic fistula (bypassing the small intestine), or (3) mucosal damage due to small intestinal diseases such as celiac disease, tropical sprue, or Whipple disease.

METABOLIC FUNCTION OF ABSORPTIVE CELLS: Before they can be transported to the circulation, nutrients must first be metabolized within absorptive cells. For example, monoglycerides and free fatty acids are reassembled into triglycerides and coated with proteins (apoproteins) to make chylomicrons and lipoprotein particles. Genetic defects in synthesis of apoproteins required for assembly of lipoproteins and chylomicrons may cause specific metabolic syndromes such as abetalipoproteinemia (associated with erythrocyte acanthocytosis; see Chapter 26). Nonspecific damage to small intestinal epithelial cells occurs in celiac disease, tropical sprue, Whipple disease, and hyperacidity due to a gastrinoma.

TRANSPORT: Nutrients are moved from the intestinal epithelium through the intestinal wall via blood capillaries and lymphatic vessels. Impaired transport of nutrients through these conduits is probably important in malabsorption due to Whipple disease, as explained below.

 CLINICAL FEATURES: Malabsorption may be specific or generalized:

- **Specific or isolated malabsorption** reflects an identifiable molecular defect that causes malabsorption of a single nutrient. Examples include disaccharidase deficiencies (e.g., lactase deficiency) and vitamin B_{12} insufficiency (pernicious anemia) from lack of intrinsic factor due to autoimmune gastritis. Anemias may be caused by deficiencies of iron, folic acid, vitamin B_{12}, or a combination of these. A bleeding diathesis may be due to vitamin K deficiency; malabsorption of vitamin D and calcium may lead to tetany, osteomalacia (in adults), or rickets (in children) (also see Chapter 8).
- **Generalized malabsorption** refers to impaired absorption of several or all major nutrient classes. It leads to generalized malnutrition. In adults, this appears as weight loss and sometimes cachexia; children show "failure to thrive" with poor growth and weight gain.

Diverse Laboratory Studies May Detect Specific Forms of Malabsorption

Absorption of dietary fat is almost always impaired in generalized malabsorption, resulting in **steatorrhea** (fat in the stools). Quantitative fecal fat analysis is the most reliable and sensitive test of overall digestive and absorptive function and is a standard for all other tests for malabsorption.

Other clinical tests may be used to assess causes of malabsorption.

- **D-xylose absorption:** Absorption of xylose, a 5-carbon sugar, does not require any component of the luminal phase. Thus, measurements of blood levels and urinary excretion after eating a defined load of xylose are useful tests of the intestinal phase of absorption.

- **$^{14}CO_2$-cholyl-glycine breath test:** Measuring $^{14}CO_2$ in exhaled air after ingestion of $^{14}CO_2$-cholylglycine tests bile salt absorption by the ileum. It is used to diagnose blind- or stagnant-loop syndrome (due to bacterial overgrowth) and to assess ileal absorptive function.

Lactase Deficiency Causes Intolerance to Milk Products

Lactose is abundant in milk and other dairy products and is one of the most common disaccharides in the diet. It cannot be absorbed unless hydrolyzed to glucose and galactose by lactase, a disaccharidase present in the intestinal brush border. Before domestication of milk-producing animals about 9,000 years ago, human milk was probably the only milk consumed by babies and young children. Otherwise, dairy products were not part of the normal human diet. The recent (evolutionarily speaking) availability of nonhuman milk in the diet favored lactase production, perhaps explaining why cattle-herding societies (e.g., Europeans) tend to be lactose tolerant, while non–cattle herders (e.g., Native Americans, Asians) are lactose intolerant.

Acquired lactase deficiency is common. Symptoms typically begin in adolescence, and include abdominal distention, flatulence, and diarrhea after consuming dairy products. Removing milk and dairy products from the diet provides relief. Diseases that injure the intestinal mucosa (e.g., celiac disease) may also cause acquired lactase deficiency. Congenital lactase deficiency is rare but may be lethal if not recognized.

Celiac Disease Is Caused by Sensitivity to Gluten

PATHOPHYSIOLOGY: Gluten-sensitive enteropathy (GSE) is an immunologic malabsorption disorder that occurs in genetically susceptible individuals in response to ingestion of gluten found in wheat, rye, and barley. Gluten is actually a complex of two proteins, glutenin and gliadin. The main culprit of GSE appears to be **gliadin**. The genetic nature was first established by family studies; the fact that a significant percentage of people with type 1 diabetes, another immunologic disorder (see Chapter 13), have GSE is further confirmation. It appears that specific alleles in the major histocompatibility complex, namely, class II HLA-DQ2 and DQ8, are present in nearly all patients (Fig. 19-44). While the presence of these alleles does not inevitably lead to celiac disease, their absence virtually excludes the diagnosis. Other environmental factors may also be operative.

Both cellular immunity and antibodies are involved. Modified peptides derived from gliadin are presented on HLA DQ2- or DQ8-positive antigen presenting cells, which then activate T lymphocytes. Activated mucosal T lymphocytes cause mucosal injury via release of cytokines; antigen–antibody complex deposition with complement activation may also lead to injury. Activated T cells also provide help to B lymphocytes which secrete circulating antibodies, which form the basis of serologic tests that are useful in diagnosing GSE. The most

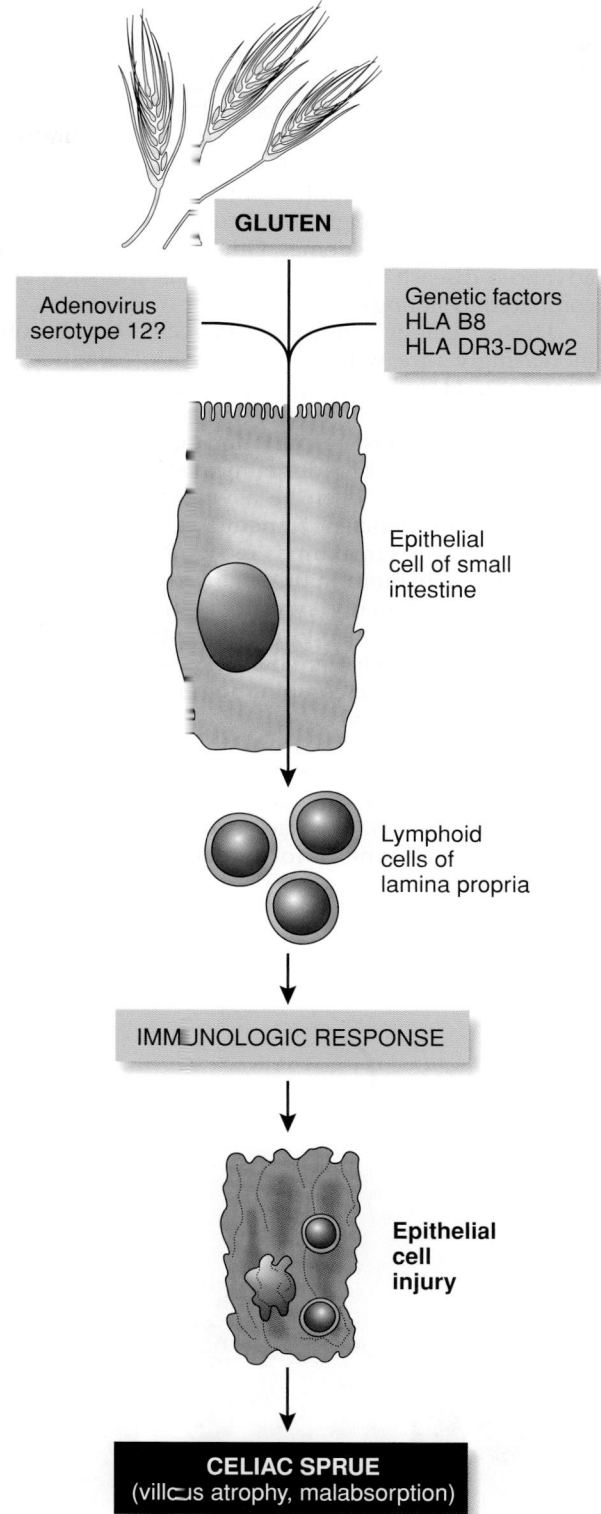

FIGURE 19-44. Proposed mechanism of the pathogenesis of celiac disease. *HLA* = human leukocyte antigen.

important of these are **tissue transglutaminase (tTG)** and **antiendomysial antibody;** the former is now the test of choice. Testing for antigliadin antibody has a much lower sensitivity and specificity than these two tests.

CLINICAL FEATURES: The classic symptoms are abdominal discomfort and diarrhea. With more advanced disease and consequent increased difficulty in absorbing fat, steatorrhea develops. Because of its high fat content, the stool tends to float and develops a particularly offensive odor owing to the action of intestinal bacteria on lipid. Eventually there can be severe malnutrition with weight loss, muscle wasting and hypoalbuminemia with edema. Other clinical sequelae of advanced disease include osteoporosis and short stature compared to siblings.

These "classic" findings in GSE are becoming increasingly rare with better means of diagnosis and treatment. However, improved understanding of the pathogenesis of GSE and better means of recognizing the process serologically and morphologically has uncovered a much broader clinical spectrum of the disease. Patients may even be asymptomatic, or present only with iron-deficiency anemia resistant to oral iron therapy. At the same time, recognition that GSE can manifest much more subtly than previously believed has also caused many symptoms or conditions to be attributed to GSE, or to gluten ingestion, without clear supporting evidence. Care must be taken, as the diagnosis of GSE requires a combination of clinical, serologic, and histologic evidence.

Exclusion of gluten from the diet is usually an effective treatment. However, gluten is ubiquitous and adhering to the diet can be difficult. As well, diet change has been known to lead to a placebo effect, underscoring the need for concrete evidence before diagnosing GSE.

PATHOLOGY: The histologic hallmarks of GSE are (1) increased mucosal inflammation, including an **increase in intraepithelial lymphocytes (IELs)**, and (2) variable architectural derangement in the small intestinal villi. In it most marked form, the mucosa shows total or near-total atrophy of villi, accompanied by crypt hyperplasia.

T lymphocytes normally reside in small numbers in the surface epithelium (Fig. 19-45A,B), but in GSE their density increases significantly. As an isolated finding, increased intraepithelial T cells are not specific for GSE (they may be seen in NSAID exposure and *H. pylori* gastritis), but IELs are essentially always increased in patients with GSE. As a result, the diagnosis of GSE requires correlation with clinical symptoms and laboratory data such as serology, as well as characteristic histology.

Surface epithelial cells are damaged and lose their brush border. This damage shortens their life span, so that mitotic activity in the crypts increases to compensate for the increased cell loss. As a result, there is hyperplasia of the crypts. This leads to deeper crypts, even as villi decrease in height (Fig. 19-46). Eventually a flat mucosa may result, but often a spectrum of changes is seen, ranging between total loss of villi to normal villi showing an increase in IELs, particularly at their tips. The mucosal changes are most prominent in the proximal small intestine where the most intense gluten exposure occurs; the distal ileum is only rarely involved.

There is evidence that patients with chronic GSE have increased risk for primary intestinal T-cell lymphoma (called enteropathy-associated T-cell lymphoma) and small intestinal adenocarcinoma, but the exact magnitude of this risk is unclear.

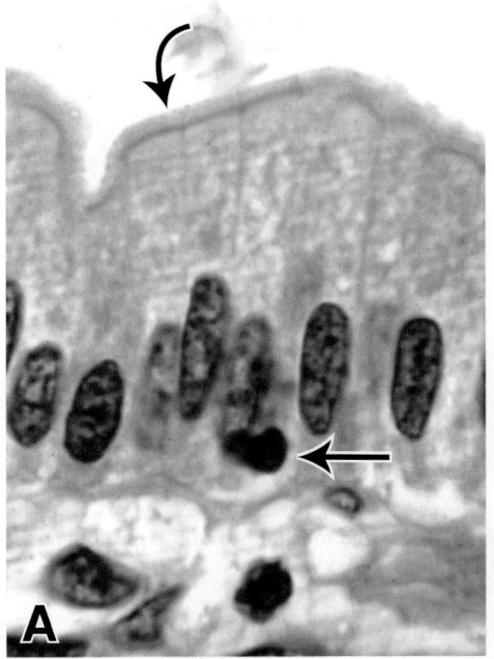

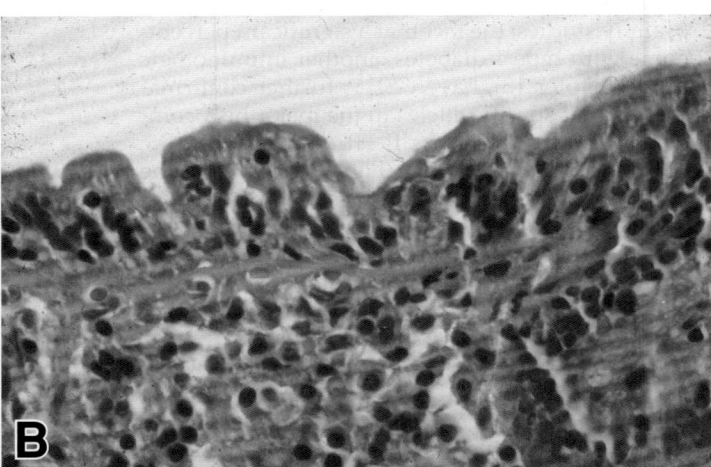

FIGURE 19-45. A. High-power view of small intestine surface epithelium; note the **brush border** (*curved arrow*) and rare intraepithelial lymphocyte (*arrow*). **B.** The surface epithelium in **celiac disease:** the epithelial height is reduced, the brush border is damaged and intraepithelial lymphocytes are numerous.

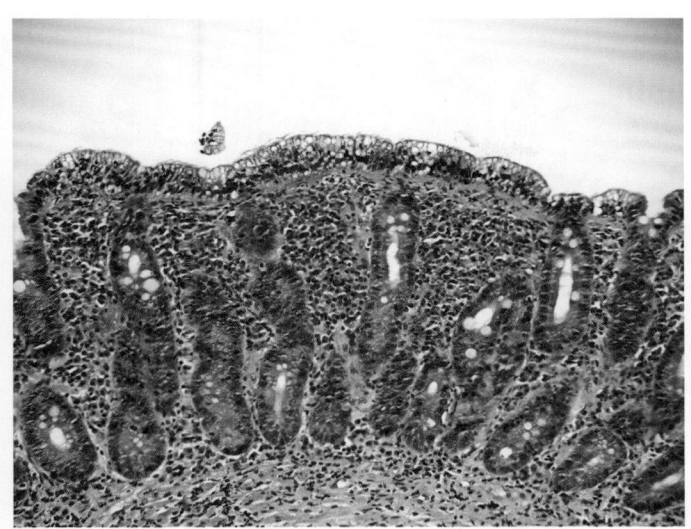

FIGURE 19-46. Classic advanced celiac disease: villi are blunted, crypts are taller than normal and a lymphoplasmacytic infiltrate expands the lamina propria. Damage to the surface epithelium is evident.

Tropical Sprue Is Chronic Malabsorption That Is Restricted Geographically

Affected locations are the Indian subcontinent, portions of Southeast Asia, Central America, and the Caribbean. Tropical sprue can develop both in residents and in visitors to the area. The term "sprue" is from a Dutch term meaning diarrhea and has also been applied to GSE at times ("nontropical sprue"). Evidence supports a complex bacterial etiology as antibiotics are effective in alleviating the condition. However, the exact nature of the causative agent(s) is uncertain.

In contrast to GSE, histologic changes in tropical sprue often involve the entire small intestine including ileum (rather than being limited to the duodenum). IELs are more prominent in the crypts than in the villus tips, and completely flat mucosa is less common than in GSE.

Severe folate and B_{12} deficiency may occur, the latter reflecting ileal involvement; this may lead to megaloblastic change.

Autoimmune Enteropathy Is a Rare Disease but Is Increasing in Frequency

Patients with this disorder present with severe diarrhea and have circulating antibodies directed against the intestinal epithelial cells themselves (**anti-enterocyte antibodies**). Severe villous atrophy may be present, but IELs are not as prominent as in GSE. Also, there is usually loss of goblet and Paneth cells, with epithelial apoptosis consistent with the immune-mediated nature of the injury. Importantly, the stomach and colon are often involved in addition to the small intestine. Likewise, extraintestinal sites, such as the pancreas and lung, may also be involved. Treatment differs radically from that for GSE; immunosuppressant medication is required and gluten restriction has no effect.

Whipple Disease Is Caused by *Tropheryma whippelii*

Whipple disease is a multiorgan infectious disorder. Only recently was it shown to be caused by an actinobacterium, many years after it was first described. These bacteria accumulate within macrophages which are unable to degrade them. This results in build-up of masses of bacteria-laden macrophages in multiple organs, including small bowel villi and extraintestinal sites such as the heart, joints, lymph nodes, and brain. Villi become enlarged and bulbous owing to large numbers of affected macrophages, which appear histologically to have "foamy" cytoplasm (Fig. 19-47A–D). Because of their polysaccharide content, the bacteria impart striking PAS-staining positivity to the foamy macrophages. This time-honored method of establishing the diagnosis is being replaced by specific polymerase chain reaction (PCR) identification of the causative organism. Malabsorption is thought to result from compression of villous lymphatics due to massive macrophage accumulation, thereby affecting the transport component of the intestinal phase discussed earlier. Because of CNS involvement, these patients may first present with neuropsychiatric symptoms. Whipple disease responds dramatically to antibiotic therapy.

Small Bowel Bacterial Overgrowth Usually Results From Disordered Motility

In this condition, overgrowth of colonic-type anaerobic bacteria in the small bowel causes bloating and diarrhea. Conditions interfering with overall gut motility, such as diabetes, scleroderma, and pseudo-obstruction, can lead to the syndrome. The term "blind loop syndrome" is used if stasis is due to an anatomic defect such as small bowel diverticula or prior surgery such as a Billroth II. The mucosa may appear to be normal or show varying degrees of patchy nonspecific inflammation. It is thought that deconjugation of bile salts by the bacteria or their use of micronutrients is the major contributing pathogenic factor. Diagnosis is by breath test to measure hydrogen and methane gas, both products of bacterial fermentation in the small bowel that are transported to the lungs and exhaled. Cultures of intestinal fluid may also be performed. Antibiotic therapy usually results in symptomatic improvement. This and the other multiple causes of malabsorption are depicted in Figure 19-48.

OBSTRUCTION

Mechanical obstruction can affect any segment of the gastrointestinal tract; the small bowel is frequently involved. The common causes include entrapment of bowel in hernias, intussusception (see below), adhesions from prior surgery or peritoneal infection, and volvulus. In volvulus, a segment of the intestinal tract twists on its mesentery, causing obstruction and ischemic damage. Neoplasms can also cause luminal obstruction with or without intussusception.

In Intussusception, a Segment of Bowel Is Drawn Into a Distal Segment

In this setting, peristalsis pushes a part of bowel distally into an adjacent segment, causing it to telescope (Fig. 19-49A,B). The mesentery and blood vessels accompany the bowel and can become compressed, leading to edema, ischemic damage, and entrapment. Intussusception can reverse spontaneously, or sometimes a barium enema may reduce it. Surgical removal may be necessary. In children, there is

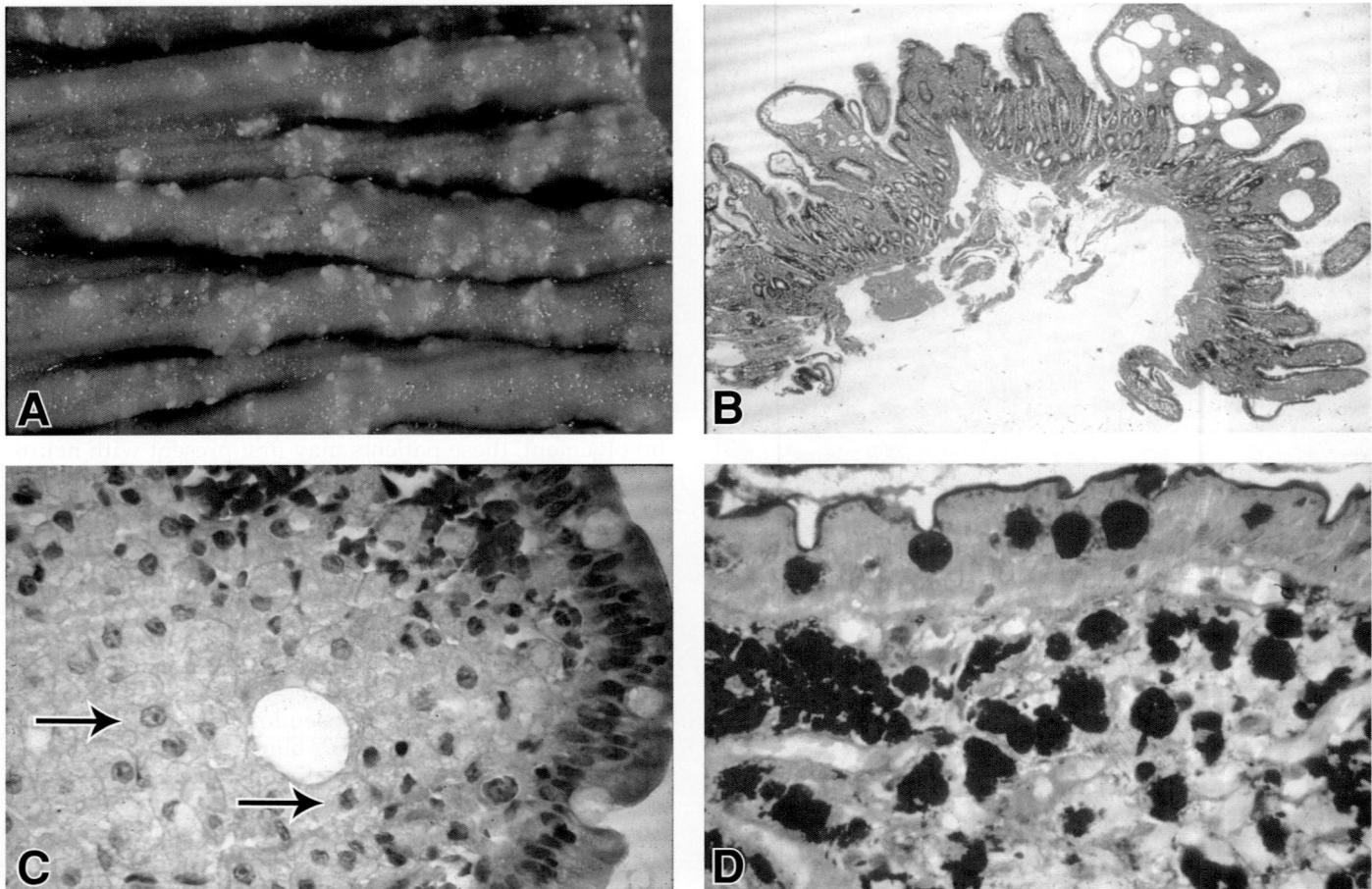

FIGURE 19-47.　Whipple disease. A. The gross specimen shows elevated white areas due to lymphatic fluid collecting in the damaged mucosa. **B.** At low-power villi are short and club shaped; large cystic-appearing areas represent dilated lymphatics (lymphangiectasia) owing to compression of mucosal lymphatic vessels by macrophage accumulation. **C.** The lamina propria contains abundant foamy macrophages (*arrows*). **D.** The partially digested bacteria in these macrophages impart strong periodic acid–Schiff (PAS) positivity.

usually no causative anatomic defect other than lymphoid hyperplasia. This may be physiologic for age, but in some, rotavirus or adenovirus may be responsible for the hyperplasia. In adults, a neoplastic luminal process is often the cause of intussusception, with the mass serving as a point of traction that prevents reduction.

Pseudo-Obstruction

In pseudo-obstruction, symptoms and signs of obstruction occur, but without any of the mechanical lesions previously discussed. There are both primary and secondary causes; they all impair gut motility by affecting smooth muscle cells and/or their neural inputs. In primary pseudo-obstruction, smooth muscle may become replaced by fibrous tissue leading to profoundly altered motility. This may occur as a familial condition. Muscular abnormalities are more common than neural defects, which are often difficult to identify morphologically. Secondary pseudo-obstruction may arise as a complication of well-defined systemic diseases. Chief among these is scleroderma which interferes with normal smooth muscle function. Amyloidosis and endometriosis may similarly affect the muscularis and cause secondary pseudo-obstruction.

INTESTINAL ISCHEMIA

Impaired intestinal blood flow for any reason can cause ischemic bowel disease. Manifestations of intestinal ischemia are diverse. The most common type of ischemic bowel disease is acute intestinal ischemia, which causes injury ranging from mucosal necrosis to transmural bowel infarction. Chronic intestinal ischemia syndromes, caused by repetitive bouts of ischemia, are less common and generally require severe compromise of two or more major arteries, usually by atherosclerosis.

Mesenteric Arterial Occlusion Causes Segmental Ischemia

This is the most common cause of acute intestinal ischemia. Sudden occlusion of a large artery by thrombosis or embolization leads to infarction before collateral circulation can compensate. A lesser frequent cause is vasculitis, which often involves small arteries. In addition to intrinsic vascular lesions, volvulus, intussusception, and incarceration of the intestine in a hernia sac may lead to arterial as well as venous occlusion. Thrombophilic states, several prescription medications and the

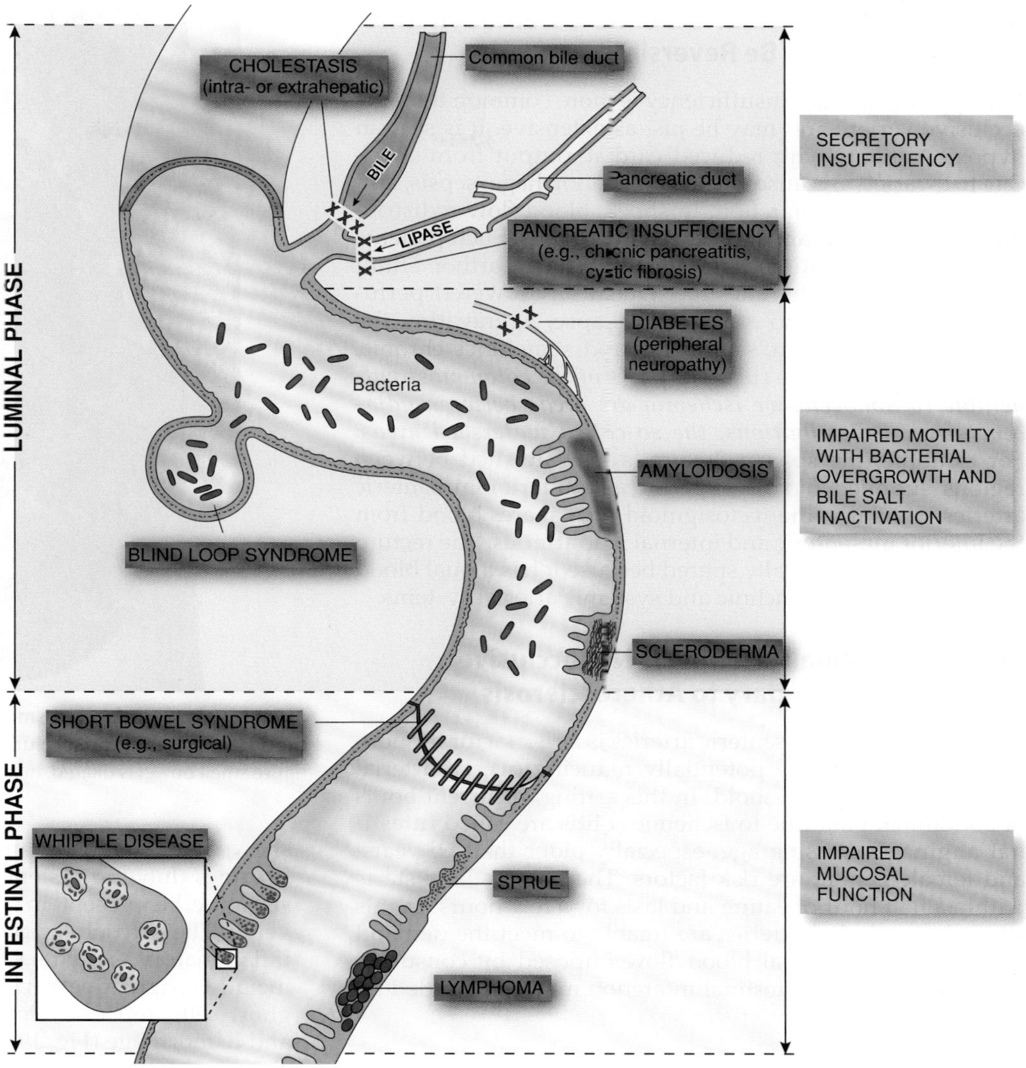

CHOLESTASIS
(intra- or extrahepatic)
Common bile duct
BILE
SECRETORY
INSUFFICIENCY
Pancreatic duct
LIPASE
PANCREATIC INSUFFICIENCY
(e.g., chronic pancreatitis,
cystic fibrosis)
LUMINAL PHASE
DIABETES
(peripheral
neuropathy)
Bacteria
IMPAIRED MOTILITY
WITH BACTERIAL
OVERGROWTH AND
BILE SALT
INACTIVATION
AMYLOIDOSIS
BLIND LOOP SYNDROME
SCLERODERMA
SHORT BOWEL SYNDROME
(e.g., surgical)
INTESTINAL PHASE
WHIPPLE DISEASE
IMPAIRED
MUCOSAL
FUNCTION
SPRUE
LYMPHOMA

FIGURE 19-48. The causes of malabsorption.

illicit drug cocaine also increase the risk of ischemic bowel disease by causing microvacular occlusion and/or constriction. Depending on the size of the occluded artery, infarction may be segmental or cause gangrene of virtually the entire small bowel.

Occlusive ischemia may also be associated with infections by *E. coli* O157:H7 and *Shigella* spp., in which bacterial toxins damage vascular endothelium (see below), and vasculitic syndromes such as polyarteritis nodosa and Henoch–Schönlein purpura.

A
0cm
5
10

B

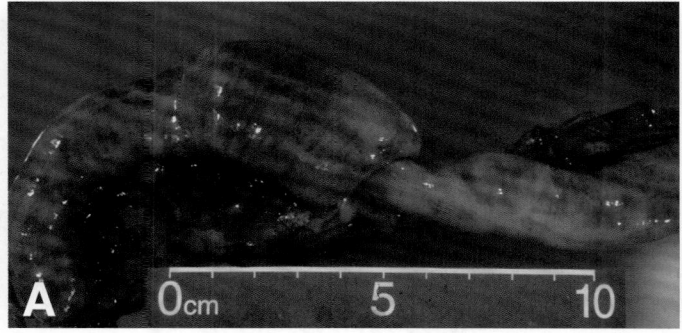

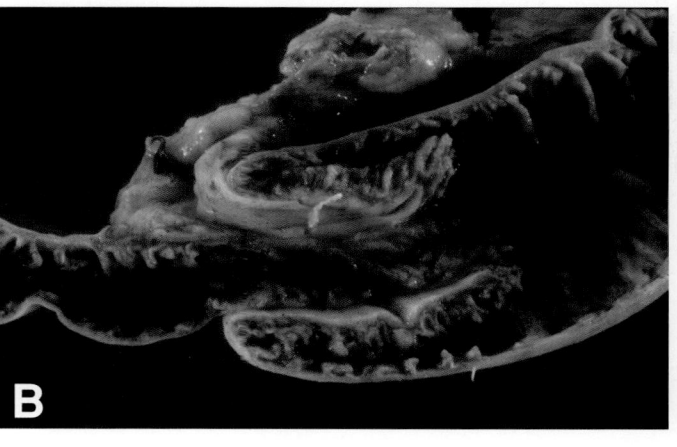

FIGURE 19-49. Intussusception. A, B. The proximal ileum has telescoped into the distal ileum in this case of **intussusception;** the anatomy is well seen in the cut section.

THE GASTROINTESTINAL TRACT

Nonocclusive Intestinal Ischemia Is Hemodynamic in Nature and May Be Reversible

This type of vascular insufficiency is more common than the occlusive variety and may be just as extensive. It is seen in hypoxic patients with reduced cardiac output from shock due to a variety of causes including hemorrhage, sepsis, and acute myocardial infarction. In shock, blood flow redistributes to favor the brain and other vital organs. Such patients often received α-adrenergic agents, which further shunt blood away from the intestine. Drastically lowered perfusion pressure leads to arteriolar collapse, aggravating the ischemia. In the colon, segmental, and sometimes chronic, ischemic disease is the rule. *The parts of the colon most vulnerable to nonocclusive ischemia are areas between adjacent arterial distributions, the so-called watershed areas.* For example, the splenic flexure is in watershed between regions supplied by the superior and inferior mesenteric arteries. Similarly, the rectosigmoid area shares blood from the inferior mesenteric and internal iliac arteries. The rectum itself, however, is usually spared because it has a dual blood supply, from the splanchnic and systemic arterial systems.

Chronic Intestinal Ischemia Is Nonocclusive and Usually Secondary to Atherosclerosis

Atherosclerosis of mesenteric arteries is a risk factor for nonocclusive ischemia by potentially reducing overall arterial blood to a critical threshold. In this setting, recurrent bouts of abdominal pain due to ischemic colitis are called **intestinal angina**. Increasing age, especially older than 65 years, and female gender are risk factors. The pain usually starts within a half hour of eating and lasts for a few hours. In this situation, occluded arteries are unable to meet the demand for increased intestinal blood flow imposed by consumption of food. Frank intestinal infarction may be heralded by abdominal angina.

Mesenteric Vein Thrombosis Causes Venous Outflow Obstruction

Mesenteric vein thrombosis is also a common cause of ischemic damage. Causes of mesenteric vein thrombosis include hypercoagulable states, stasis, and inflammation (pylephlebitis). Almost all thromboses affect the superior mesenteric vein; only 5% involve the inferior mesenteric vein. Collateral flow in the distribution of the superior mesenteric vein is usually sufficient to prevent infarction of the intestine. As result of the blockage to venous outflow, blood and fluid builds up in the affected segment, compromising arterial perfusion and leading to ischemia. Treatment is to correct the underlying cause.

PATHOLOGY: On endoscopy, multiple ulcers, hemorrhagic nodular lesions or a pseudomembrane may be seen. Infarcted bowel is edematous and diffusely purple (Fig. 19-50). The demarcation between the infarcted bowel and normal tissue is usually sharp, although venous occlusion may lead to a more diffuse border. Hemorrhage is prominent in the infarcted mucosa and submucosa, especially in venous occlusion (e.g., mesenteric vein thrombosis). The mucosal surface

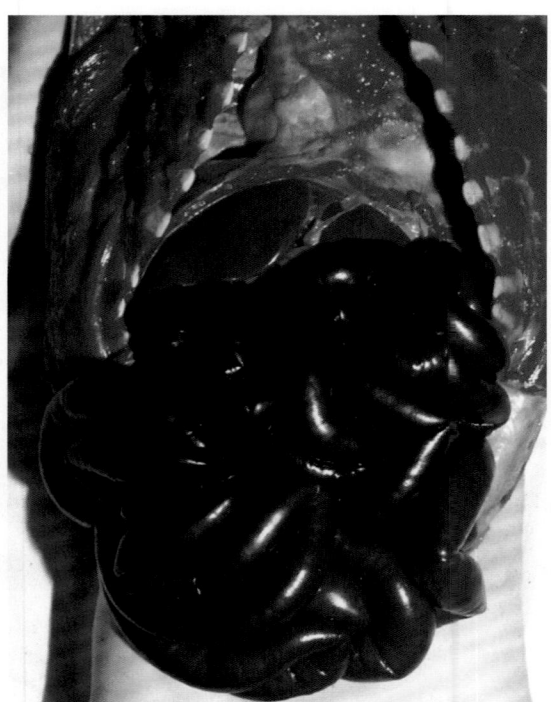

FIGURE 19-50. Infarcted small bowel at autopsy of an infant who died after volvulus had occluded the superior mesenteric artery. The entire small bowel is dilated, hemorrhagic, and necrotic.

shows irregular wide areas of sloughing, and the wall becomes thin and distended. Bubbles of gas (pneumatosis) may be present in the bowel wall and mesenteric veins. The serosal surface is cloudy and covered by an inflammatory exudate. Characteristic histologic changes include coagulative necrosis of surface epithelium with ghost cells, mucosal ulceration, crypt abscesses, edema, and hemorrhage (Fig. 19-51). In more severe cases, necrosis affects deeper layers of bowel and can evolve to full-thickness necrosis.

Chronic vascular insufficiency of the small intestine may lead to fibrosis and stricture formation. Ischemic strictures of the small bowel may be single or multiple and produce intestinal obstruction or, occasionally,

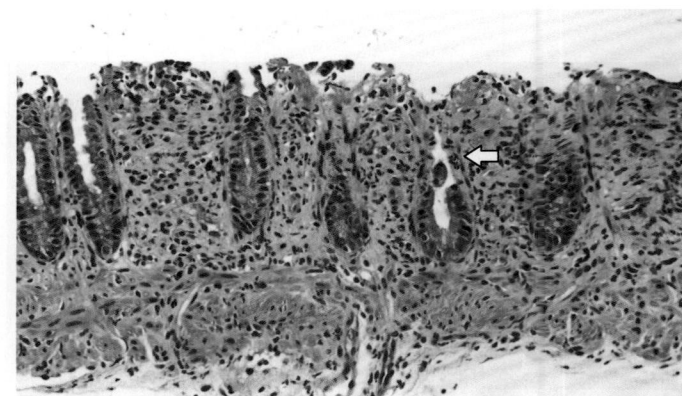

FIGURE 19-51. Ischemic colitis. A mucosal biopsy shows coagulative necrosis with "ghostly" outlines of the pre-existing crypts (*arrow*). Only a small portion of the base of several crypts remains.

malabsorption owing to stasis and bacterial overgrowth. These strictures are concentric, and the mucosa of this region is atrophic, often with one or more small ulcers. The submucosa is thickened and fibrotic with granulation tissue, which may involve the muscular layers. Hemosiderin deposition may be seen, particularly near the muscularis mucosae.

CLINICAL FEATURES: Symptoms of acute ischemia include abdominal pain, which begins abruptly, often with bloody diarrhea, bright red blood in stools or with maroon stools, depending on the location of the bleeding. Patients without bleeding may have a worse prognosis. In untreated cases, perforation is frequent and shock may ensue. As infarction progresses, systemic symptoms become more severe (multiple organ dysfunction syndrome). In extensive infarction that is a result of occlusion in the proximal superior mesenteric artery, nearly the entire small bowel must be surgically resected, a situation not compatible with ultimate survival. In the colon, ischemic colitis may be indistinguishable clinically from other forms of colitis (infectious, IBD). Prognosis and treatment depend on the primary cause and extent of involvement. The goal is to improve blood supply to the colon by treating patients' overall cardiovascular status and providing bowel rest. There may also be a role for antibiotics. In severe cases, mortality exceeds 50%, and urgent surgical removal of the involved bowel may be necessary. Patients may recover completely or develop a stricture, in which case surgical removal of the obstructed segment may be necessary.

Angiodysplasia (Vascular Ectasia) May Cause Intestinal Bleeding

Angiodysplasia (vascular ectasia) is the historical term for localized colonic arteriovenous malformations, arising most commonly in the cecum and ascending colon. These may cause lower intestinal bleeding, especially in people over 60 years of age. Younger people may have lesions at other sites, including the rectum, stomach, and small bowel. Aortic valvular disease may be associated in some cases.

It has been suggested that angiodysplasia results from chronic intestinal circulatory insufficiency, intestinal muscle hypertrophy and consequent venous obstruction. Patients complain of multiple bleeding episodes, but chronic bleeding may also be occult. Radiologic studies and examination at laparotomy are usually negative. Thus, the diagnosis is difficult and often requires selective mesenteric arteriography or colonoscopy. Colonoscopic interventions are usually sufficient to stop the bleeding, but surgical removal of the affected segment may be necessary in some cases.

PATHOLOGY: The resected specimen has one or more collections of closely spaced vascular channels, which viewed from the mucosal aspect appear as erythematous patches less than 0.5 cm in diameter. Submucosal veins and capillaries are tortuous, thin walled, and dilated. These vessels have attenuated walls, presumably accounting for their propensity to bleed.

RADIATION ENTEROCOLITIS

Radiation therapy for malignancies in the pelvis or abdomen may injure the small intestine (radiation enteritis) and colon (radiation colitis).

PATHOLOGY: Clinically significant radiation colitis occurs most often in the rectum (radiation proctitis). Lesions vary from reversible intestinal mucosal injury to chronic inflammation, ulceration, and fibrosis of the intestine. In the short term, radiation damages epithelium and endothelium, impairs normal bowel mucosal renewal and, in the small bowel, leads to villous shortening. Mucosal inflammation is conspicuous and abscesses may be seen in colonic crypts. Failure of epithelial renewal may lead to ulceration. Chronic changes occur 9 to 14 months after radiation therapy, after the mucosa has healed. Damage to submucosal vessels leads to thrombosis, lumenal occlusion, and chronic mucosal ischemia. The submucosa becomes fibrotic and often contains bizarre-appearing fibroblasts.

Complications of radiation enterocolitis include perforation and subsequent development of internal fistulas, fibrous adhesions, and strictures. These may be severe enough to obstruct the intestines and require surgical resection.

INTESTINAL INFECTIONS AND TOXINS

Infectious diarrhea is particularly lethal in underdeveloped countries. Infants are especially vulnerable. In countries with poor sanitation, the death toll from childhood diarrhea is staggering: 1.5 million children under 5 years die annually of diarrhea, over 80% of them in Africa and south Asia.

The small bowel normally contains few bacteria (usually $<10^4$/mL), most of which are lactobacilli and other organisms that travel in the food stream and ordinarily do not colonize the small intestine. Infectious diarrhea is caused by bacterial colonization (e.g., with toxigenic strains of *Escherichia coli* and *Vibrio cholerae*). The most significant factor in infectious diarrhea is increased intestinal secretion. Bacterial toxins impair mucosal ion channels and pumps resulting in unrestrained secretion of ions and water. Decreased absorption and increased peristaltic activity contribute less to the diarrhea.

The colon harbors abundant bacteria, at concentrations seven orders of magnitude greater than in the small intestine. Anaerobic bacteria in the colon (e.g., *Bacteroides* and *Clostridium* species) outnumber aerobic organisms by 1,000-fold. With the more rapid transit of intestinal contents during diarrhea, the colon may become overpopulated by more aerobic species, including *E. coli*, *Klebsiella*, and *Proteus*. Moreover, offending organisms themselves become conspicuous and pathogens of the small intestine such as *V. cholerae* may be the major isolate in the stool.

Several factors limit the numbers of bacteria in the stomach and small bowel: (1) gastric acid inhibits bacterial growth, which explains bacterial overgrowth in the stomach in achlorhydria; (2) bile has an antimicrobial activity; (3) peristalsis propels intestinal contents, limiting bacterial accumulation; (4) normal flora secrete their own antimicrobial

TABLE 19-2

HISTOLOGIC PATTERNS OF BACTERIAL INFECTIONS OF THE GASTROINTESTINAL TRACT

Minimal inflammatory changes	*Vibrio cholerae*
	Toxigenic *Escherichia coli*
	Neisseria sp.
Acute self-limited colitis	*Shigella*
	Campylobacter jejuni
	Aeromonas
	Salmonella
	Clostridium difficile
Pseudomembranous pattern	*C. difficile*
	Shigella
	Enterohemorrhagic *E. coli*
Granulomas	*Yersinia* sp.
	Mycobacterium bovis
	Mycobacterium avium-intracellulare
	Actinomycosis
Histiocytic	Whipple disease (*Tropheryma whippelii*)
	M. avium-intracellulare
Lymphohistiocytic	*Lymphogranuloma venereum*
Architectural distortion	*Salmonella typhimurium*
	Shigella

substances to maintain an ecologic balance (indeed, treatment with broad-spectrum antibiotics alters the natural flora and allows overgrowth of ordinarily harmless organisms); and (5) plasma cells of the lamina propria secrete IgA into the intestinal lumen.

Individual agents responsible for infectious diarrhea are discussed in Chapter 9. Here we review the major entities only briefly. Agents of infectious diarrhea are classified into **toxigenic** (i.e., producing diarrhea by elaborating toxins) or as adherent or invasive bacteria (Table 19-2 lists reaction patterns).

Toxigenic Diarrhea Is Most Often due to *Escherichia coli*

The prototypical organisms that cause diarrhea by secreting toxins are *V. cholerae* and toxigenic strains of *E. coli*.

The characteristics of toxigenic diarrhea are:

- Damage to the intestinal mucosal is minimal or absent.
- The organism remains on the mucosal surface, where it secretes its toxin.
- Fluid secreted into the small intestine causes watery diarrhea, which can lead to dehydration, which in the case of cholera can be lethal.

Many organisms have been isolated in the so-called traveler's diarrhea, but toxigenic *E. coli* is the most common in almost all studies.

Invasive Bacteria Cause Diarrhea by Direct Mucosal Injury

Among these invasive organisms, *Shigella, Salmonella,* certain strains of *E. coli, Yersinia,* and *Campylobacter* are the most widely recognized. Invasive organisms tend to infect the distal ileum and colon, while toxigenic bacteria mainly involve the upper intestinal tract. The mechanisms by which invasive bacteria produce diarrhea are uncertain. Enterotoxins have been identified, but their role in causing diarrhea is not established. Mucosal invasion by bacteria increases synthesis of prostaglandins in affected tissues, and inhibitors of prostaglandin synthesis seem to block fluid secretion. It also may be that damaged mucosa cannot absorb fluid from the lumen.

Shigella

Shigellosis, caused by any of the four species of the genus *Shigella,* mainly affects the colon, but the terminal ileum is occasionally involved. A granular and hemorrhagic mucosa has many shallow serpiginous ulcers. Inflammation is especially severe in the sigmoid colon and rectum, but is usually superficial. In the early stage, neutrophils accumulate in damaged crypts (crypt abscesses), and the lymphoid follicles of the mucosa break down to form ulcers. Unlike ulcerative colitis (see below), histologic features of chronicity such as crypt branching or dense lymphoplasmacytic infiltrate in the lamina propria are absent. As infection recedes, ulcers heal and the mucosa returns to normal.

Typhoid Fever

Typhoid fever (*Salmonella typhi* enteritis) is uncommon in the industrialized world but is still a problem in underdeveloped countries. Infection of Peyer patches causes necrosis of lymphoid tissue, mainly in the terminal ileum but occasionally in the appendix or colon, and this leads to scattered ulcers. The base of the ulcer contains black necrotic tissue mixed with fibrin.

Histologically, early lesions of typhoid fever contain erythrocytes, necrotic debris, and large basophilic macrophages filled with typhoid bacilli. Similar lymphoid hyperplasia and necrosis are seen in regional lymph nodes. Within a week of onset of acute symptoms, ulcers heal completely, leaving little fibrosis or other sequelae. Intestinal hemorrhage and perforation, principally in the ileum, are the most feared complications of typhoid fever and tend to occur in the third week and during convalescence.

Nontyphoidal Salmonellosis

Formerly known as **paratyphoid fever**, enteritis caused by *Salmonella* strains other than *S. typhi* is generally far less serious than typhoid fever. The principal target is the ileum, but minor involvement of the colon may also occur. Organisms invade the mucosa, which shows mild ulceration, edema, and infiltration with neutrophils. Hematogenous dissemination from the intestine may carry infection to bones, joints, and meninges. People with sickle cell disease tend to develop *Salmonella* osteomyelitis, possibly because phagocytosis of products of hemolysis interferes with cellular ingestion of the organisms and allows their dissemination through the bloodstream.

Escherichia coli

Enteroinvasive, enteroadherent, and enterohemorrhagic strains of *E. coli* may uncommonly cause bloody diarrhea similar to shigellosis and are a prominent cause of traveler's diarrhea. Certain strains of *E. coli*, particularly serotype 0157:H7, produce *Shigella*-like toxins, but the role of these proteins in the pathogenesis of the enterocolitis is not understood. Serotype 0157:H7 has also been implicated in the hemolytic–uremic syndrome in children.

Yersinia

Yersinia enterocolitica and *Yersinia pseudotuberculosis* are transmitted by pets or contaminated food. Infection is most common in young children and lasts 1 to 3 weeks. *Yersinia* infection causes diarrhea, cramps, and fever. Peyer patches are hyperplastic, with acute ulceration of overlying mucosa. A fibrinopurulent exudate covering the ulcers often contains many organisms.

In addition to causing enterocolitis, *Yersinia* causes acute mesenteric adenitis and right lower quadrant pain. It may so resemble appendicitis that infected children have mistakenly been taken to laparotomy for appendectomy. Lymph nodes show epithelioid granulomas with central necrosis in the case of *Y. pseudotuberculosis*. The ileum and appendix may contain similar granulomas, imparting an appearance that resembles that of Crohn disease.

Adults, who are less susceptible to *Yersinia* infection than are children, have acute diarrhea, often followed within a few weeks by erythema nodosum, erythema multiforme, or polyarthritis. Patients with underlying chronic debilitating diseases may develop *Yersinia* bacteremia, resistant to antibiotic treatment. Interestingly, people with thalassemia are particularly susceptible to *Y. enterocolitica* infection. Although the mechanism is not fully understood, iron overload in thalassemia is thought to play a role in *Yersinia* infection perhaps by impairing macrophage function. Identification of *Yersinia* by culture can be difficult, but PCR analysis is effective.

Campylobacter jejuni

Campylobacter jejuni is one of the most common causes of bacterial diarrhea, with a higher incidence than nontyphoidal *Salmonella* and *Shigella* in some U.S. studies. In a report from Great Britain, *Campylobacter* caused half of bacterial diarrhea. Humans contract the disease mainly by contact with infected domestic animals or by eating poorly cooked or contaminated food. The histology is similar to that of *Shigella*. Adults usually recover in less than 1 week.

Food Poisoning Reflects Bacterial Toxins in Contaminated Food

STAPHYLOCOCCUS AUREUS: Symptoms result from eating food contaminated with *Staphylococcus* strains that produce an exotoxin that damages gastrointestinal epithelium. Severe vomiting and abdominal cramps occur within 6 hours, often followed by diarrhea. Most patients recover in 1 to 2 days.

CLOSTRIDIUM PERFRINGENS: This bacterium produces an enterotoxin that causes vomiting and diarrhea. The organism is anaerobic but tolerates exposure to air for up to 3 days. Enterotoxin activity is maximal in the ileum. In most cases, watery diarrhea and severe abdominal pain begin 8 to 24 hours after ingestion of contaminated food and last about 1 day.

Rotavirus and Norwalk Virus Are the Most Common Causes of Viral Gastroenteritis in the United States

ROTAVIRUS: Rotavirus infection is a common cause of infantile diarrhea. It accounts for about half of acute diarrhea in hospitalized children younger than 2 years. Rotavirus has been demonstrated in duodenal biopsy specimens. It is associated with injury to the surface epithelium and impaired intestinal absorption for periods of up to 2 months.

NOROVIRUSES: These highly infectious agents account for one-third of the epidemics of viral gastroenteritis in the United States. The virus targets the upper small intestine, causing patchy mucosal lesions and malabsorption. Vomiting and diarrhea are usual, but symptoms typically resolve within 2 days.

Other viruses implicated as etiologic agents of infective diarrhea include echovirus, coxsackievirus, cytomegalovirus, adenovirus and coronavirus.

Intestinal Tuberculosis Is Mostly Caused by Ingesting Bacteria in Food or Swallowing Infectious Sputum

The tubercle bacillus (either *Mycobacterium tuberculosis* or *Mycobacterium bovis*) is protected from gastric acid by its cell wall. Once it passes into the small bowel, it establishes a locus of infection, usually (90% of patients) in the ileocecal region, where lymphoid tissue is abundant. Infection also occurs in the colon, jejunum, appendix, rectum, and duodenum, in that order of frequency.

 PATHOLOGY: Intestinal tuberculosis may present with ulcers of varying size in the transverse plane of the bowel. As these ulcers heal, reactive fibrosis may cause localized circumferential ("napkin ring") stricture of the bowel lumen. Mesenteric lymph nodes are typically enlarged, and show caseous necrosis.

Necrotizing granulomas containing small numbers of organisms may occur throughout the bowel wall, particularly in Peyer patches and lymphoid follicles. Tuberculous strictures are difficult to distinguish from other causes of stricture, such as ischemic enterocolitis or Crohn disease.

 CLINICAL FEATURES: Almost all patients with intestinal tuberculosis complain of chronic abdominal pain and many have a palpable abdominal mass, usually in the right lower quadrant. Malnutrition, weight loss, fever, and weakness are common. Complications include obstruction, fistulas, perforation, and abscess.

Giardiasis Is the Leading Gastrointestinal Protozoal Infection in the United States

The causative agent is *Giardia lamblia*. *Giardia* spores are extremely hardy; infections can be acquired by person-to-person transmission or after drinking from unprotected water sources. The trophozoites can be identified in duodenal fluid

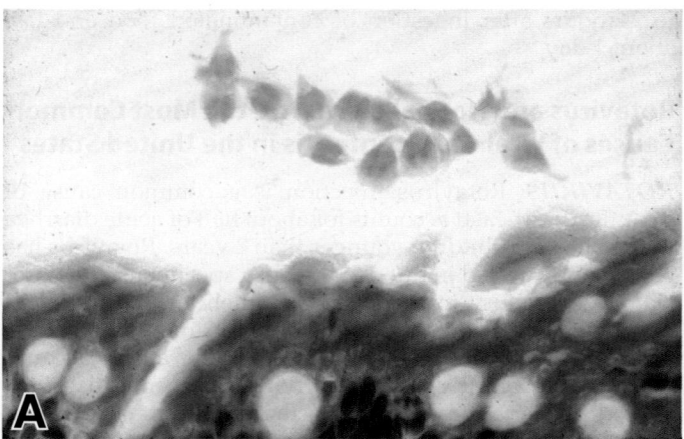
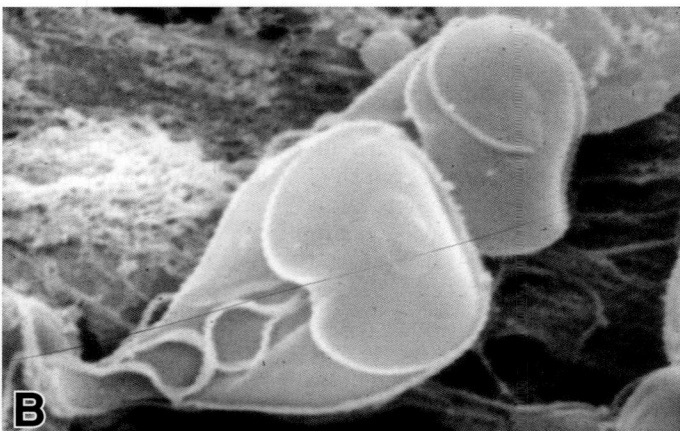

FIGURE 19-52. **A.** A group of *Giardia* is seen just above the surface epithelium in this jejunal biopsy. **B.** A trophozoite from this area is seen here by scanning electron microscopy.

or stool, but are often first identified in a duodenal biopsy. While they have a characteristic pear shape when seen in fluids, they tend to be seen in profile as sickle or triangular shapes in biopsies (Fig. 19-52A,B). They are usually very numerous, adhere to the epithelial surface, and do not invade. The underlying mucosa is often completely normal or may show mild nonspecific inflammatory changes including a slight increase in IELs. *Giardia* are among the most common infections in common variable immunodeficiency which is characterized by low levels of immunoglobulins. In such cases, lamina propria plasma cells are sparse to absent and lymphoid aggregate may be present. Identifying *Giardia* in a biopsy should trigger a search for plasma cells to exclude this possibility.

Symptoms may include severe watery diarrhea as well as abdominal discomfort with nausea and vomiting. Malabsorption can occur.

OTHER INFECTIONS OF THE LARGE INTESTINE

A number of sexually transmitted infections involve the anorectal region. These include gonorrhea, syphilis, lymphogranuloma venereum, anorectal herpes, and HPV infections (venereal warts or condylomata acuminata). Immunosuppressed people have a high incidence of colonic infections (e.g., amebiasis, shigellosis).

Pseudomembranous Colitis Usually Follows Antibiotic Treatment

Pseudomembranous colitis is a generic term for an inflammatory disease of the colon that is characterized by **exudative mucosal plaques**. It is most often caused by *C. difficile*.

ETIOLOGIC FACTORS: The major risk factor for developing *C. difficile* infection is antibiotic therapy. Virtually all antibiotics have been implicated, although some are associated with a higher risk. Hospitalization is another major risk factor. About 1% to 5% of adults are *C. difficile* carriers, but 30% of hospitalized patients become carriers. In elderly hospitalized

patients, *C. difficile* carriage may approach 70%. Immunosuppression and underlying inflammatory bowel disease are also risk factors.

C. difficile is transmitted via the fecal–oral route and is ingested in vegetative form or as spores. When normal protective gut flora are killed by antibiotics, the more resistant *C. difficile* can gain a foothold and begin producing its toxins: toxins A and B. Toxin A activates and recruits inflammatory mediators, and toxin B is directly cytotoxic. *It is important to note that C. difficile is not invasive and mediates damage via production of toxins.*

Other conditions that can produce pseudomembranes include ischemic colitis and other enteric infections, most notably verotoxin-producing *E. coli*.

PATHOLOGY: The entire colon is often involved and sometimes the small intestine is as well. The characteristic gross feature is raised yellowish plaques up to 2 cm that adhere to the underlying mucosa (Fig. 19-53). The intervening mucosa is congested and edematous, but not ulcerated. In severe cases, plaques coalesce into extensive pseudomembranes, consisting of debris from necrotic epithelial cells, mucus, fibrin, and neutrophils. Superficial epithelial necrosis is believed to be the initial pathologic event. Colonic crypts then become disrupted and expanded by mucin and neutrophils. In milder cases, well-formed pseudomembranes may be absent and the pathology is more subtle, showing only focal damage to the surface epithelium.

CLINICAL FEATURES: Antibiotic-associated *C. difficile* infections are virtually always accompanied by mild to moderate watery diarrhea, but the disorder does not usually progress to colitis. In patients with pseudomembranous colitis, fever, leukocytosis, and abdominal cramps are superimposed on a severe diarrhea that can be bloody. In some cases, the disease can progress to fulminant colitis, which can lead to serious complications such as colonic perforation, toxic megacolon, and death.

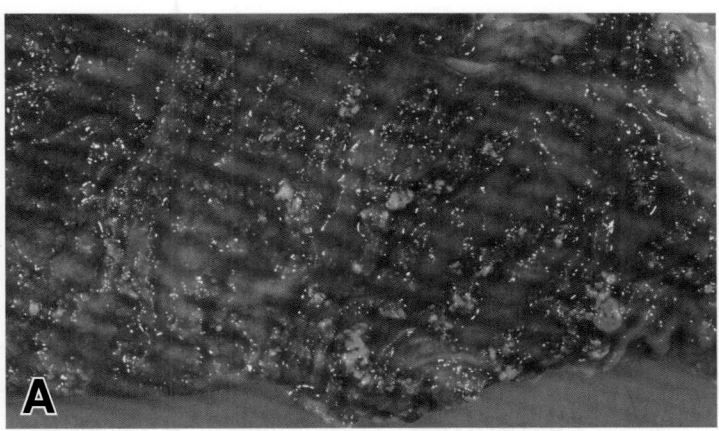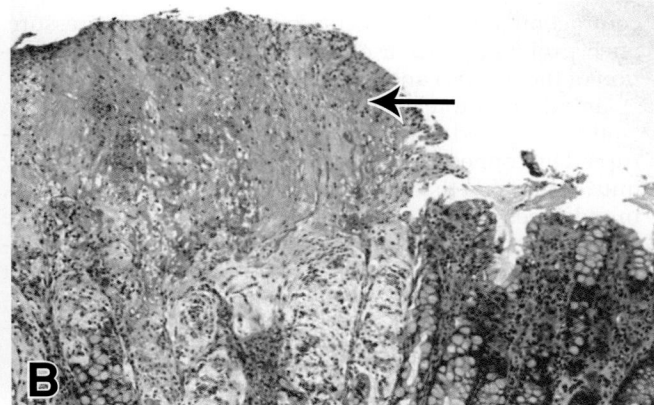

FIGURE 19-53. Pseudomembranous colitis. A. The colon shows variable involvement ranging from erythema to yellow-green areas of pseudomembrane. **B.** Microscopically, the pseudomembrane (*arrow*) consists of fibrin, mucin, and inflammatory cells (largely neutrophils).

The diagnosis is usually made by identifying toxins in stool by cytotoxin assay, enzyme-linked immunosorbent assay (ELISA) or molecular methods. *C. difficile* infections are treated with antibiotics (metronidazole or vancomycin) and supportive fluid and electrolyte therapy. It is important to withdraw the inciting antibiotic as soon as possible. In cases of fulminant colitis, colectomy may be necessary. *C. difficile* infection recurs in one-fifth of patients. Treatment for patients with multiple recurrences is replenishment of normal gut flora with a **"fecal transplant."** Preventing *C. difficile* transmission in hospitals is critically important in reducing the incidence of the disease.

Opportunistic Infections Are Common Complications of AIDS and Other Causes of Immunosuppression

The AIDS epidemic that began in the 1980s resulted in many gastrointestinal infections that had previously been considered rare. Most AIDS patients have chronic diarrhea. Virtually all forms of infectious agents—bacteria, fungi, protozoa, and viruses—afflict these patients (Table 19-3). The risk of contracting such infections increases with reductions in CD4 count, indicating the crucial role of normal host immunity in suppressing these potential pathogens. Similarly, patients who have undergone bone marrow transplantation or who receive immunosuppressive medications are at increased risk for contracting opportunistic infections. Cytomegalovirus infection, usually by reactivation of latent infection and involving endothelial and other mesenchymal cells, is a frequent example.

DIVERTICULAR DISEASE

Diverticular disease covers two entities: **diverticulosis** and its inflammatory complication, **diverticulitis**.

Diverticulosis Reflects Environmental and Structural Factors

Diverticulosis entails acquired herniation of the mucosa and submucosa through the muscularis propria.

ETIOLOGY: Diverticulosis is common in Western societies but not in Asia, Africa, and underdeveloped countries. Because of this striking geographic variability, diet and lifestyle factors are thought to play a prominent role in the development of diverticulosis. For example, people who consume a vegetarian diet and/or a diet rich in fiber are at lower risk for diverticular disease than those whose diet is rich in refined carbohydrates and meat. According to the fiber theory, Western diets lack dietary residue, leading to sustained bowel

TABLE 19-3
GASTROINTESTINAL PATHOGENS ASSOCIATED WITH AIDS

Bacteria
Mycobacterium avium-intracellulare
Shigella
Salmonella
Clostridium difficile

Viruses
Cytomegalovirus
Herpes simplex

Fungi
Candida
Aspergillus

Protozoa
Cryptosporidium
Toxoplasma
Giardia
Entameba histolytica
Microsporidia
Isospora belli

Helminths
Strongyloides
Enterobius

contraction and thus increased intraluminal pressure. Such prolonged increased pressure may lead to herniation of the mucosa and submucosa of the colon.

In addition to elevated pressure, defects in the colon wall are required. The circular muscle of the colon is interrupted by connective tissue clefts at sites of penetration by nutrient vessels that supply the submucosa and mucosa. In older people, this connective tissue loses its resilience and thus its resistance to the effects of increased intraluminal pressure. This concept is supported by the fact that people with heritable connective tissue disorders (e.g., Marfan syndrome, Ehlers–Danlos syndrome) acquire precocious diverticulosis, primarily of the small bowel.

PATHOLOGY: In diverticulosis, the structures are actually pseudodiverticula, in which only the mucosa and submucosa are herniated through the muscle layers. By contrast, true diverticula involve all layers of the intestinal wall. The sigmoid colon is affected in 95% of cases, but diverticulosis can affect any segment of the colon, including the cecum. Diverticula vary in number from a few to hundreds.

Diverticula are characteristically seen as flask-like structures that extend from the lumen through the muscle layers (Fig. 19-54). They measure up to 1 cm and are connected to the intestinal lumen by necks of varying length and caliber. Their walls are continuous with the surface mucosa and thus have epithelium *and* submucosa. The muscularis propria of the affected colon is often thickened.

CLINICAL FEATURES: *At least 80% of affected individuals are symptom free.* Symptomatic patients complain of episodic colicky abdominal pain. Both constipation and diarrhea, sometimes alternating, may occur, and flatulence is common. Sudden, painless, and severe bleeding from colonic diverticula is a cause of serious lower gastrointestinal hemorrhage in the elderly, occurring in as many as 5% of patients with diverticulosis. Chronic blood loss may lead to anemia.

Diverticulitis Is Inflammation at the Base of a Diverticulum

Of patients with diverticulosis, 10% to 20% will develop diverticulitis at some point. Acute diverticulitis is believed to be precipitated by irritation due to retained fecal material. This irritation and obstruction lead to inflammation of the diverticulum, which can eventually rupture. Beyond this acute episode, chronic diverticular disease may develop from a combination of abnormal colonic motility, visceral hypersensitivity, imbalance among intestinal flora (called dysbiosis), and chronic inflammation leading to an irritable bowel–like syndrome.

PATHOLOGY: Diverticulitis produces inflammation of the wall of the diverticulum, which may lead to perforation and release of fecal bacteria into peridiverticular tissues. The resulting abscess is usually contained by the appendices epiploicae and pericolonic adipose tissue. Infrequently, perforation leads to generalized peritonitis. Fibrosis in response to repeated episodes of diverticulitis may constrict the bowel lumen, causing obstruction. Fistulas may form between the colon and adjacent organs, including the bladder, vagina, small intestine, and skin of the abdomen. Additional complications include pylephlebitis and liver abscesses.

CLINICAL FEATURES: The most common symptoms of acute diverticulitis, which usually occur after perforation, are persistent lower abdominal pain and fever. Changes in bowel habits, from diarrhea to constipation, are frequent. Most patients have left lower quadrant tenderness and, often, a palpable mass in that area. Leukocytosis is the rule. Antibiotics and supportive measures usually alleviate acute diverticulitis, but about 20% of patients eventually require surgery. Medical management to prevent subsequent attacks and chronic diverticular disease includes high-fiber diet; long-term, cyclical antibiotic therapy; anti-inflammatory medication (mesalamine); and, potentially, probiotics.

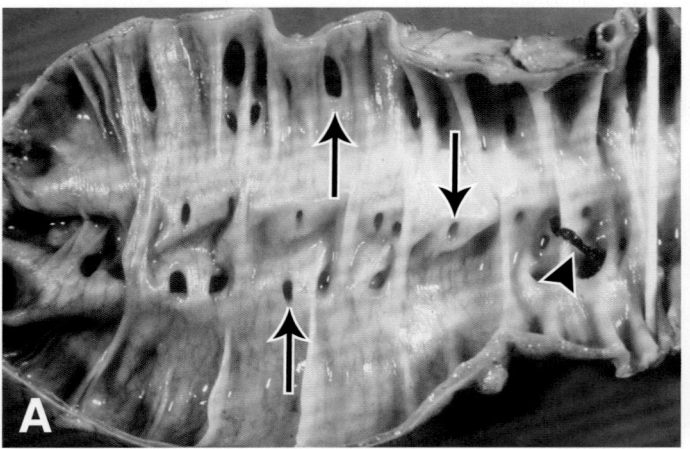
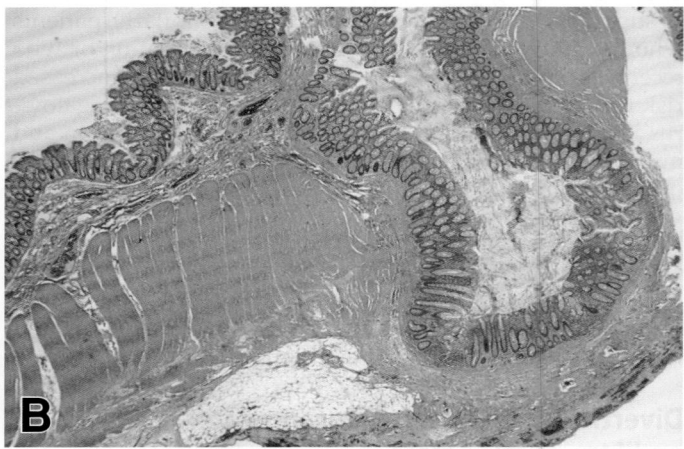

FIGURE 19-54. Diverticulosis of the colon. A. The mouths of numerous diverticula are seen between the taenia (*arrows*). There is a blood clot seen protruding from the mouth of one of the diverticula (*arrowhead*). This was the source of massive gastrointestinal bleeding. **B.** The histologic section shows mucosa including muscularis mucosa and submucosa, which has herniated through a defect in the bowel wall, producing a diverticulum.

SOLITARY RECTAL ULCER SYNDROME

Internal rectal mucosal prolapse can cause mucosal changes that are easily mistaken clinically and pathologically for chronic inflammatory disease or a tumor. Patients often have a history of severe straining during defecation. Despite the name, some patients have no ulcers, while others have multiple erosions, ulcers, or even polypoid lesions/masses that can simulate a neoplasm. While often found in the rectum, other regions of the colon can be affected. The hallmark of solitary rectal ulcer syndrome is smooth muscle proliferation from the muscularis mucosae into the lamina propria often with accompanying mucosal hyperplastic changes. Dilated glands can be trapped in the rectal wall, a condition called **colitis cystica profunda**.

IDIOPATHIC INFLAMMATORY BOWEL DISEASE

The term **inflammatory bowel disease** (IBD) encompasses **Crohn disease** and **ulcerative colitis**, both of which are chronic immune-mediated disorders of the gastrointestinal tract and other organs. These two disorders share certain common features but usually differ enough to be clearly distinguishable. Patients with IBD that cannot be classified with certainty are referred to as having **indeterminate colitis**.

Extraintestinal manifestations of IBD are more common with Crohn disease but also occur in ulcerative colitis (Fig. 19-55). While their precise causes are unknown, epidemiologic, clinical, and animal studies suggest that mucosal injury accrues from altered immune responses and abnormal interactions of bacteria with intestinal epithelia. The differences between the two diseases are described below.

PATHOGENESIS: The causes of Crohn disease and ulcerative colitis are not fully understood. The current leading theories involve a combination of a genetically susceptible host, defective mucosal barrier, intestinal dysbiosis (altered intestinal flora), and dysregulated immune response, leading to bowel inflammation. Genome-wide association studies have identified more than 50 loci that confer susceptibility for Crohn disease, ulcerative colitis, or both, although these account for a minority of cases. Some genetic associations involve genes controlling innate and adaptive immunity. Polymorphisms identified in the innate system occur in *NOD2 (CARD15)* and in two genes related to autophagy (*ATG16L1, IRGM*). These variants implicate problems in recognition and handling of intracellular bacteria. Others encode proteins involved in epithelial cell adhesion and so perhaps contribute to mucosal barrier dysfunction. The T-cell response (adaptive immune system) in Crohn disease involves T_H1 (see Chapter 4), which is mediated by interleukin-12, interferon γ (IFNγ), and TNF, whereas the T-cell response in ulcerative colitis is T_H2 dominant and mediated by natural killer T cells. This combination of factors leads to mucosal hyperresponsiveness to commensal bacteria and an exaggerated immune response causing chronic inflammation and damage.

Crohn Disease Is Chronic Segmental Transmural Intestinal Inflammation

Crohn disease mainly affects the distal small intestine but may involve any part of the digestive tract and even extraintestinal tissues. The colon, particularly the right colon, is often affected.

EPIDEMIOLOGY: Crohn disease has a worldwide incidence of 0.7 to 14.6 per 100,000 but is more common in developed countries. Its incidence has increased dramatically in the past 30 years, probably owing to a combination of factors related to adoption of a "Western lifestyle." Age distribution is bimodal, with a peak in adolescents or young adults and a second smaller peak in the 50s and 60s. It is most common in people of European origin, with a considerably higher frequency among Ashkenazi Jews. Males predominate among children, but in adults there is a slight female predominance. Smokers are at an increased risk of developing Crohn disease and of having more severe disease, compared with nonsmokers.

PATHOLOGY: Two key features of Crohn disease differentiate it from other gastrointestinal inflammatory diseases. First, inflammation usually involves all layers of the bowel wall and is thus referred to as **transmural**. Second, intestinal involvement is discontinuous: areas of inflammation are separated by apparently normal intestine.

Crohn disease may involve different parts of the bowel singly or in combination. It affects the ileum and cecum in half of cases, only the small intestine in 30% and only the colon in 20%. Ileal and cecal disease is more common in younger patients; colitis is common among older patients. Crohn disease sometimes affects the duodenum, stomach, and esophagus as focal acute inflammation with or without granulomas. In women with anorectal disease, inflammation may spread to the external genitalia.

The pathology of Crohn disease is highly variable. The bowel and adjacent mesentery are thickened and edematous. Mesenteric fat often surrounds the bowel (the so-called "fat wrapping," Fig. 19-56A), a favorite sign of the disease for surgeons that is best seen in the small intestine; it is a result of transmural disease. Nodular swelling, fibrosis, and linear mucosal ulceration lead to a "cobblestone" appearance, particularly in the small intestine (Figs. 19-56B and 19-57). In early cases, ulcers have either an aphthous or a serpiginous appearance; later they become deeper and appear as linear clefts or fissures (Fig. 19-57B). The transmural involvement with subsequent luminal narrowing often produces obstructive symptoms related to the small intestine, one of the major debilitating symptoms of Crohn disease.

The appearance of the bowel wall underscores the fact that the process affects the entire thickness of the bowel wall: all layers show thickening, edema, and fibrosis. The serosal surfaces of involved loops of bowel are often adherent. Fistulas may form between such segments (Fig. 19-58A–C). These are late results of deep mural ulcers and may also penetrate from the bowel into,

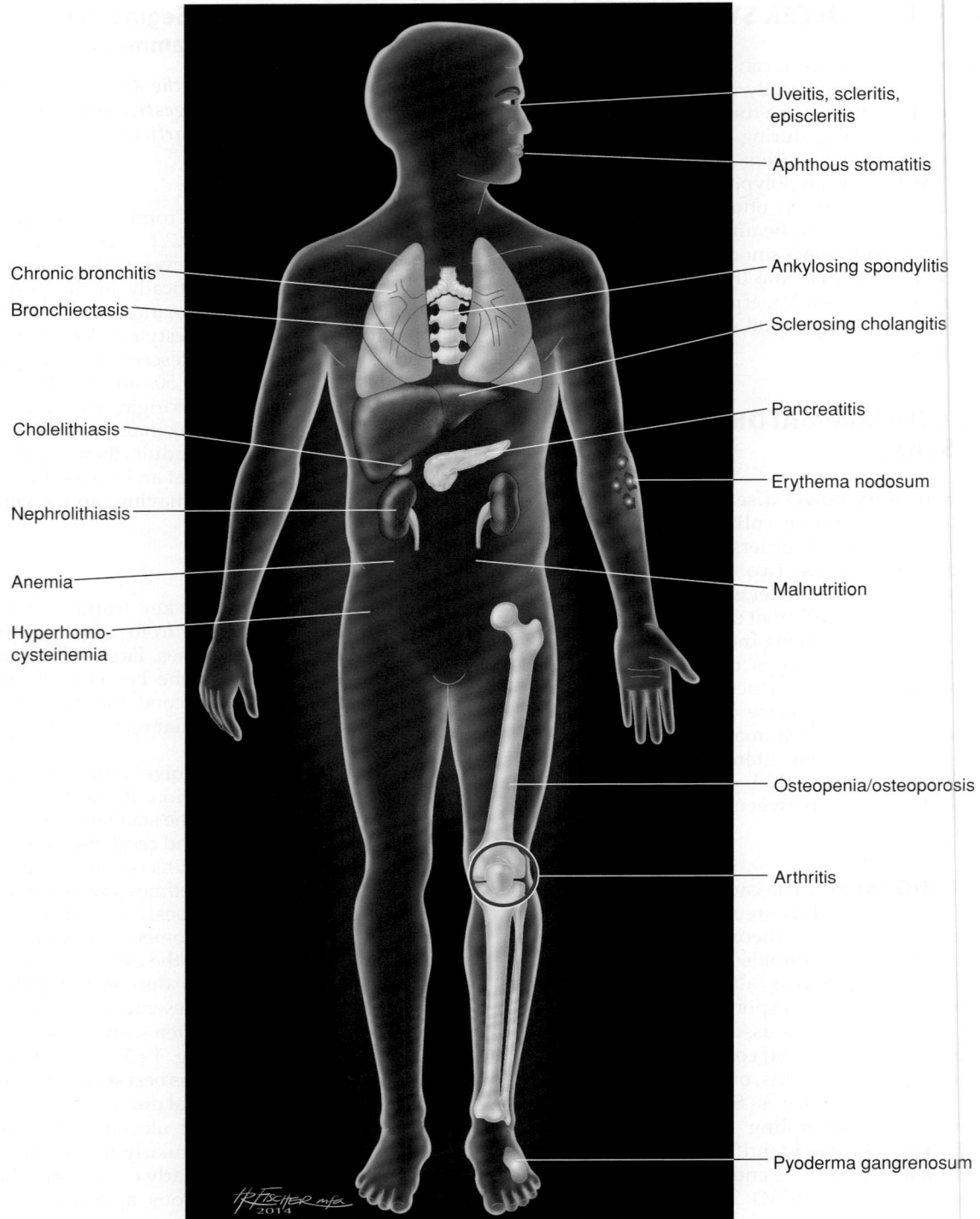

FIGURE 19-55. Systemic complications of inflammatory bowel disease. These conditions are more common with Crohn disease but may also be seen in ulcerative colitis.

for example, the bladder, uterus, vagina, and skin. Most fistulas end blindly, to form abscess cavities in the peritoneum, mesentery, or retroperitoneal structures. Lesions in the distal rectum and anus may create perianal fistulas, a well-known presenting feature.

Early in the disease, histologic inflammation may be confined to the mucosa and submucosa. Small, superficial mucosal ulcers (aphthous ulcers) are seen, as are mucosal and submucosal edema and infiltrates of lymphocytes, plasma cells, eosinophils, and macrophages. Crypt regenerative changes and villous distortion also occur. With prolonged disease, histologic features of chronicity including architectural glandular distortion, increased chronic inflammation with or without active neutrophilic

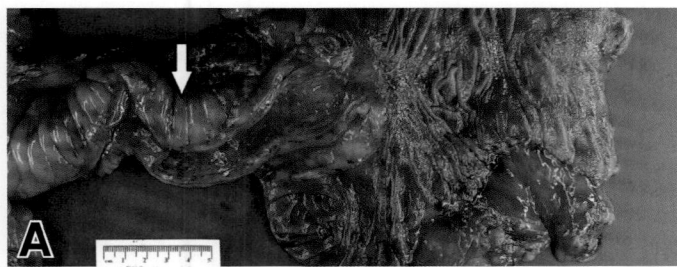

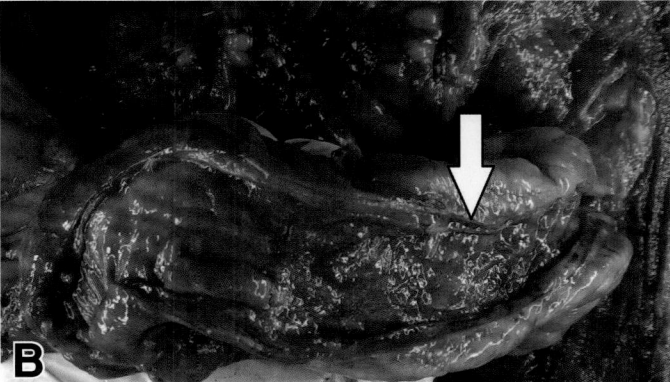

FIGURE 19-56. A. Mesenteric fat wrapping (*arrow*), seen in this resection of a diseased terminal ileum, is a manifestation of transmural involvement in Crohn disease, but is not always evident. **B.** Close up of inflamed ileal mucosa, showing erythema granularity and cobblestoning (*arrow*). See also Figure 19-57 for a linear ulcer.

inflammation, pyloric metaplasia, and Paneth cell metaplasia are common in the small and large intestines. Later, long, deep, fissure-like ulcers, vascular hyalinization, and fibrosis appear.

Discrete, noncaseating granulomas may be present, mostly in the submucosa (Fig. 19-59). These resemble those of sarcoidosis, with focal aggregates of epithelioid cells, surrounded by a rim of lymphocytes. Multinucleated giant cells may be present. The centers of the granulomas usually have hyaline material but only very rarely necrosis.

Such discrete granulomas strongly suggest Crohn disease. However, their absence does not exclude the diagnosis, as they are present in less than half of cases. The pathologic features of Crohn disease are summarized in Figure 19-60.

CLINICAL FEATURES: The clinical manifestations and natural history of Crohn disease are highly variable and reflect the diversity of anatomic sites affected. The most common symptoms are abdominal pain and diarrhea, with passage of blood and/or mucus. Recurrent fever is frequent. If it mainly involves the ileum and cecum, its sudden onset may mimic appendicitis, with right lower quadrant pain, intermittent diarrhea, fever, and a tender right lower quadrant mass. When the small intestine is diffusely involved, malabsorption and malnutrition may be major features. Lipid malabsorption may also result from interruption of the enterohepatic cycle of bile salts secondary to ileal disease. Colonic involvement leads to **diarrhea** and sometimes **colonic bleeding**. In a few patients, the major site of involvement may be the anorectal region and recurrent anorectal fistulas may be the presenting sign.

The transmural involvement with subsequent luminal narrowing often produces obstructive symptoms and fistula tract formation, one of the major debilitating complications of Crohn disease. Occasionally, free perforation of the bowel occurs. When it begins in childhood, it may slow growth and physical development.

There are many extraintestinal manifestations and associated disorders (Fig. 19-55). Small bowel cancer occurs at least threefold more commonly in patients with Crohn disease. Risk of colorectal cancer is also higher, more so in patients with more extensive involvement of the colon, a family history of colorectal cancer and/or sclerosing cholangitis.

There is no known cure. Corticosteroids, sulfasalazine, metronidazole, azathioprine, 6-mercaptopurine, methotrexate, and anti–TNF-α antibodies such as infliximab may suppress the inflammatory reaction. However, these

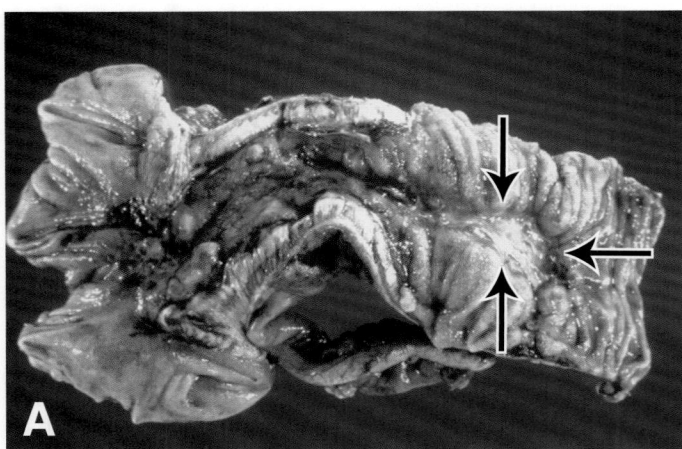

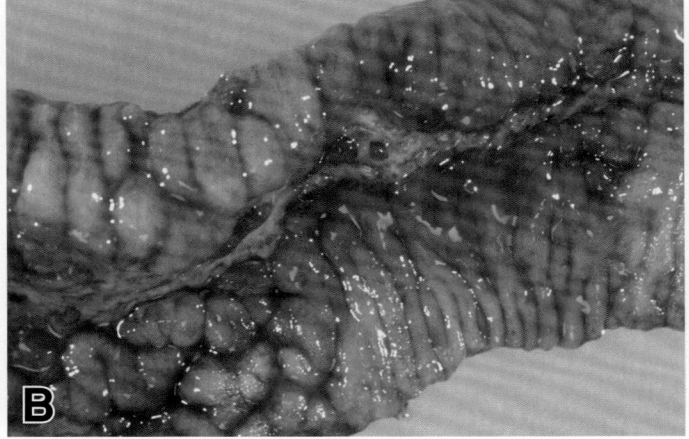

FIGURE 19-57. Crohn disease. A. The terminal ileum shows striking thickening of the wall of the distal portion with distortion of the ileocecal valve. A longitudinal ulcer is present (*arrows*). **B.** Another longitudinal ulcer is seen in this segment of ileum. The large rounded areas of edematous damaged mucosa give a "cobblestone" appearance to the involved mucosa. A portion of the mucosa seen at the lower right is uninvolved.

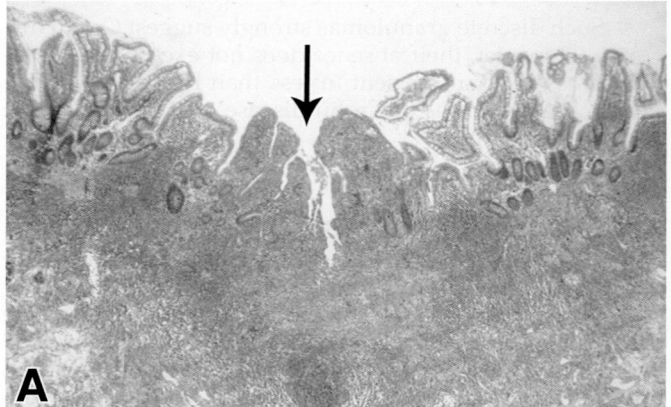

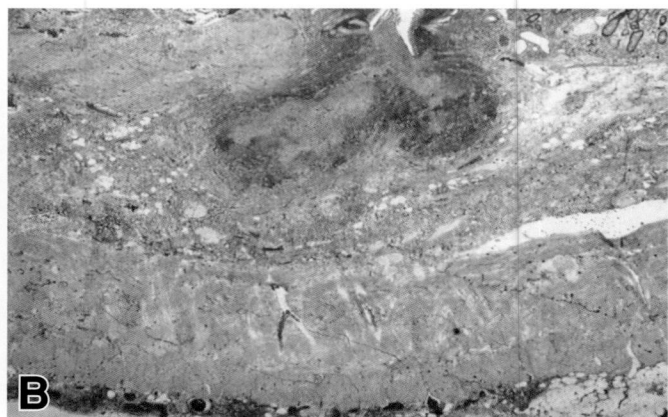

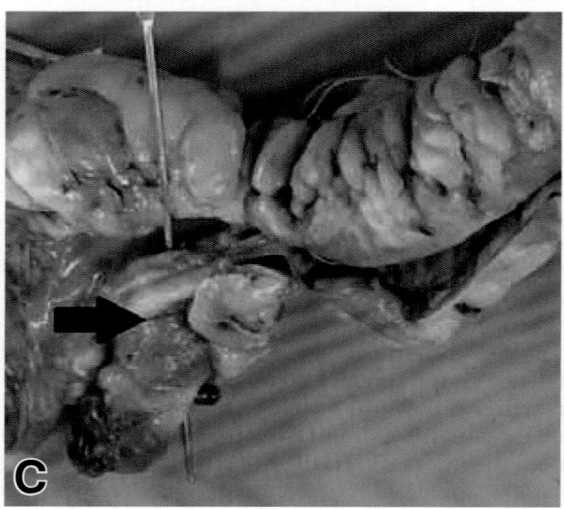

FIGURE 19-58. Crohn disease. A. A small **fissuring ulcer,** here knife-like (*arrow*), often starts over a lymphoid aggregate. **B.** The process continues, causing a fissure extending into the submucosa and beyond, ultimately penetrating the bowel wall. **C.** A **fistula** may result from such transmural involvement. In this resection a probe has been inserted through the fistula (*arrow*).

medications put patients at increased risk for opportunistic infections.

Surgical resection of obstructed or severely involved portions of intestine and drainage of abscesses caused by fistulas are required in some cases. Unfortunately,

preanastomotic or prestomal recurrences after an enterostomy is constructed occur often and make clinical management difficult. The need for repeated resections can lead to short-bowel syndrome in some patients.

Additional adjunct therapies that show possible benefit in small series include dietary modifications, antibiotics, probiotics, and fecal transplant.

Ulcerative Colitis Is Chronic, Superficial Inflammation of the Colon and Rectum

EPIDEMIOLOGY: Worldwide, the incidence of ulcerative colitis ranges from 1.5 to 24.5 per 100,000. It occurs more often in developed countries. Like Crohn disease, its incidence is increasing in countries that adopt "Western" lifestyles, suggesting that environmental factors may contribute to the pathogenesis of the disease. It also has a bimodal age distribution, with a peak from 15 to 30 years and another between 50 and 70. In the United States, whites are affected more than blacks. Smoking seems to inhibit development of ulcerative colitis, but ex-smokers are at an increased risk. People with a family history of IBD have a higher risk of developing ulcerative colitis, although this relationship is not as strong as that in Crohn disease.

FIGURE 19-59. Crohn disease. This mucosal biopsy in Crohn disease shows small noncaseating epithelioid granulomas (*arrows*) between two intact crypts.

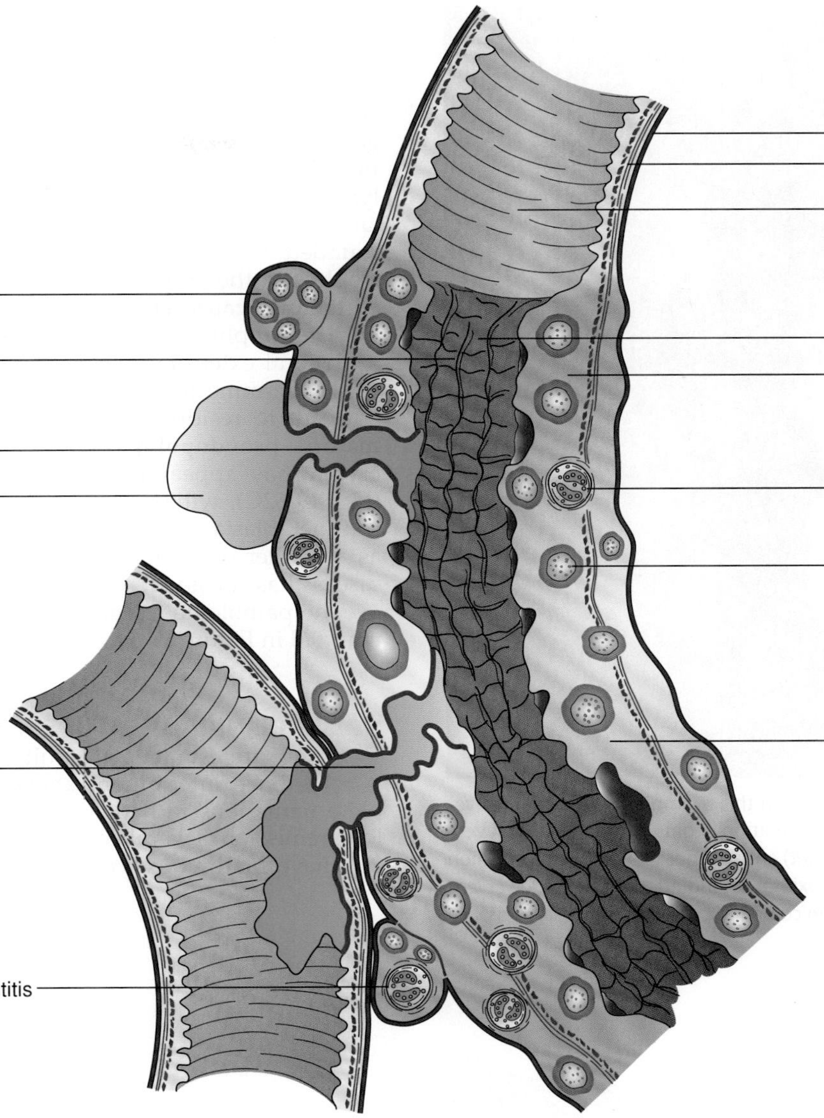

Hyperplastic lymph node

Linear ulceration

Perforation

Abscess

Fistula into loop
of small bowel

Granulomatous lymphadentitis

Serosa

Muscularis

Uninvolved (skipped) area

Narrow lumen

Thickened wall

Granuloma

Lymphoid follicle

Transmural chronic
inflammation

FIGURE 19-60. A schematic representation of the major features of Crohn disease in the small intestine.

PATHOLOGY: Major pathologic features of ulcerative colitis that help to differentiate it from other inflammatory conditions, particularly Crohn disease, are:

- **Ulcerative colitis diffusely involves the rectum and a variable portion of the colon.** Isolated rectal involvement is referred to as **ulcerative proctitis**, while extension to the splenic flexure is called **proctosigmoiditis** or **left-sided colitis**. If the entire colon is involved, it is called **pancolitis**. If untreated, the disease is confluent without skip lesions (Fig. 19-61). The exception to this rule is the occasional patient with left-sided colitis and an area of cecal involvement, a so-called "cecal patch." Sparing of the rectum is possible but should raise the possibility of Crohn disease.
- **Inflammation in ulcerative colitis is limited to the colon and rectum.** If the cecum is affected, the disease ends at the ileocecal valve, although minor inflammation of the adjacent ileum (**backwash ileitis**) may sometimes occur.
- **Ulcerative colitis is a mucosa only disease.** Deeper layers are involved only in infrequent fulminant cases and this is usually associated with toxic megacolon.

This morphologic sequence may develop rapidly or it may take years.

Gross findings: Early in the disease, the mucosal surface is raw, red, and granular. It is frequently covered with a yellowish exudate and bleeds easily. Later, small superficial ulcers or erosions may appear. These occasionally coalesce into irregular, shallow, ulcerated areas that seem to surround islands of intact mucosa. Importantly, the strictures and fistula tracts characteristic of Crohn disease are absent because such complications require involvement of the muscularis and serosal structures. In long-standing cases, the large bowel may become shortened, especially on

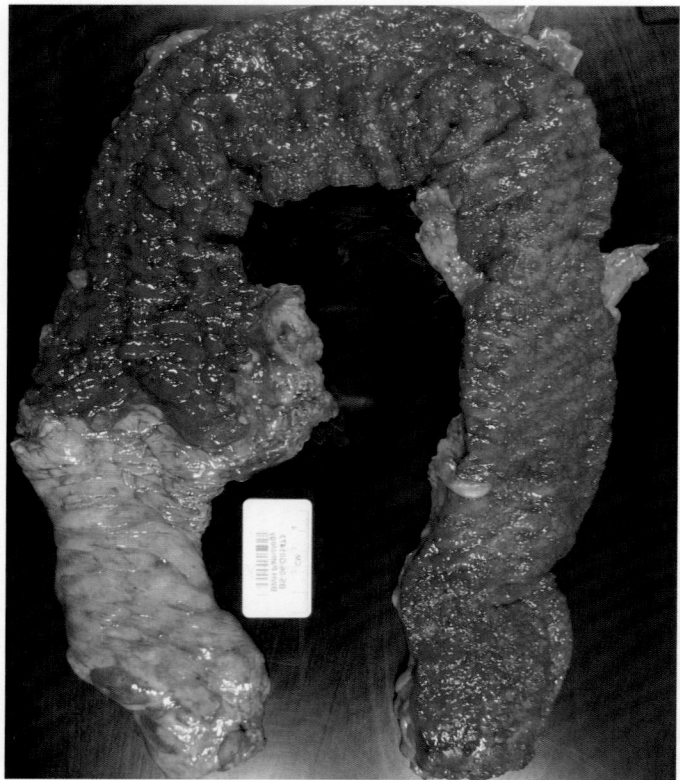

FIGURE 19-61. Ulcerative colitis. In this example of subtotal involvement of the colon, erythema and ulceration begins in and are most severe in the rectosigmoid area (*lower right*) and extends in a continuous fashion into the ascending colon. The proximal ascending and cecum (*lower left*) are spared, as indicated by the tan color and preserved mucosal folds.

the left side. Mucosal folds are indistinct and are replaced by a granular or smooth mucosal pattern.

The histology of early ulcerative colitis correlates with colonoscopic appearances and includes (1) mucosal congestion, edema, and tiny hemorrhages; (2) diffuse mixed inflammation in the lamina propria, including prominent lymphocytes and plasma cells (Fig. 19-62A); and (3) damage and distortion of colorectal crypts, which are often surrounded and infiltrated by neutrophils (**cryptitis**). Neutrophils in the crypts and suppurative necrosis of crypt epithelium cause **crypt abscesses** (dilated crypts filled with neutrophils) (Fig. 19-62B).

Lateral extension and coalescence of crypt abscesses can undermine the mucosa, leaving areas of ulceration adjacent to residual islands of mucosa termed **inflammatory pseudopolyps** (Fig. 19-63). At later stages, crypts may appear tortuous, branched, and shortened (Fig. 19-62C), with diffuse mucosal atrophy and Paneth cell metaplasia. This crypt distortion frequently persists as a marker of chronic mucosal injury, even after active disease has subsided.

The pathologic features of ulcerative colitis are summarized in Figure 19-64.

CLINICAL FEATURES: The clinical course and manifestations are quite variable. Most patients have intermittent attacks, with partial or complete remissions in between. A few (<10%) have a very long remission (several years) after their first attack. About 20% have continuous symptoms without remission.

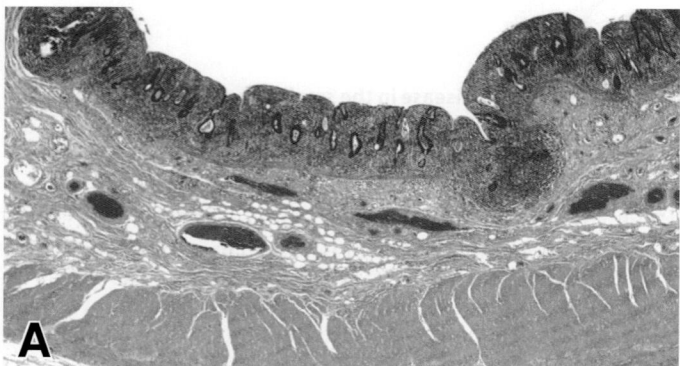

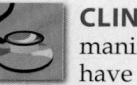

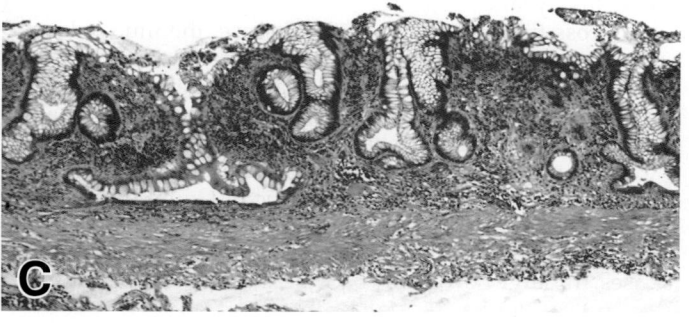

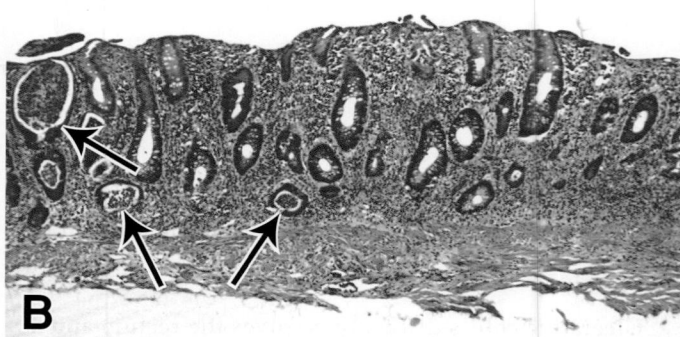

FIGURE 19-62. Ulcerative colitis. A. A full-thickness section of colon resected for ulcerative colitis shows inflammation affecting the mucosa with sparing of the submucosa and muscularis propria. **B.** A higher magnification view of the mucosa in active ulcerative colitis shows expansion of the lamina propria by inflammatory cells and several neutrophilic crypt abscesses (*arrows*). **C.** Chronic ulcerative colitis shows significant crypt distortion and atrophy.

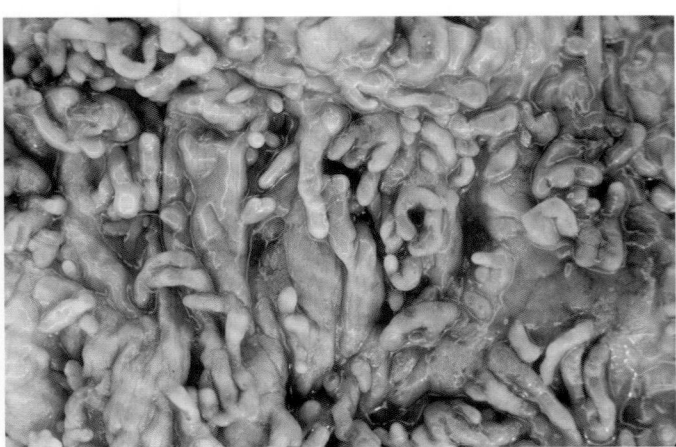

FIGURE 19-63. Inflammatory pseudopolyps of the colon in ulcerative colitis. Nodules of regenerative mucosa and inflammation surrounded by denuded areas provide a diffuse polypoid appearance of the mucosa.

Half of patients with ulcerative colitis have mild disease limited to the rectum or distal sigmoid colon. Their major symptom is rectal bleeding, sometimes with **tenesmus** (rectal pressure and discomfort). Extraintestinal complications are uncommon. Most patients in this category experience mild disease throughout their lives.

About 40% of patients have moderate disease, often corresponding to left-sided colitis. They usually have episodic loose bloody stools, crampy abdominal pain, and often low-grade fever, lasting days or weeks. Anemia is commonly due to chronic fecal blood loss.

About 10% of patients have severe or fulminant disease, with subtotal or complete involvement of the colon (pancolitis). The disease may start out this way, but more often severe colitis supervenes during a flare of activity. These patients have many (sometimes >20) bloody bowel movements daily, often with fever and other systemic symptoms. Blood and fluid loss rapidly lead to anemia, dehydration, and electrolyte depletion. Massive hemorrhage may be life-threatening. *Toxic megacolon*—extreme dilation of the colon that carries a high risk for perforation—is particularly dangerous. Fulminant ulcerative colitis is a medical emergency. It requires immediate, intensive medical therapy and, sometimes, prompt colectomy. Despite aggressive management, some patients with fulminant disease die.

Medical treatment of ulcerative colitis depends on the sites involved and the severity of the inflammation. The 5-aminosalicylate–based compounds (e.g., mesalamine) are mainstays of treatment for patients with mild to moderate disease. Corticosteroids and immunosuppressive/immunoregulatory agents (azathioprine, cyclosporine, or anti–TNFα agents) are used in patients with severe and refractory disease. Because infection with C. *difficile* or CMV can precipitate or exacerbate an attack of ulcerative colitis, these should be ruled out and treated if identified. Fecal transplant may be of some benefit in patients with refractory disease.

Differential Diagnosis

The most important conditions to be distinguished from inflammatory bowel disease are other forms of colitis or enteritis due to specifically treatable causes, including NSAID-related damage, infection, and radiation-related strictures, all of which can mimic Crohn disease. NSAIDs are known to cause solitary ulcers and diaphragm-like strictures, usually more proximally in the small intestine. More subtle changes, including erosive and shallow ulcers with associated inflammation in the distal ileum, can occur even with low-dose NSAIDs. These can cause great diagnostic difficulty in terminal ileal biopsies.

Other conditions in the differential diagnosis of ulcerative colitis are bacterial infections and amebic colitis, especially in areas where it is endemic. If inflammation is limited to the rectum, other infectious agents, including viruses, chlamydia, fungi, and other parasites, merit consideration. Other conditions that may mimic ulcerative colitis are ischemic colitis, antibiotic-associated colitis, radiation injury, and solitary rectal ulcer syndrome.

Distinguishing between ulcerative colitis and Crohn colitis is important because (1) surgical approaches are different (Crohn disease often recurs, so continent ileostomy and ileoanal pouches may be contraindicated), (2) ulcerative colitis carries a higher risk of cancer, and (3) medical treatments differ. The distinction between ulcerative colitis and Crohn colitis is based on different anatomic localization and histopathology (summarized in Table 19-4). Ulcerative colitis is a diffuse process, usually more severe distally, while Crohn colitis is patchy or segmental and often spares the rectum. Inflammation in ulcerative colitis is superficial (i.e., usually limited to the mucosa), but that in Crohn colitis is transmural and involves all layers, with granulomas in some of the specimens.

In 10% of cases, definitive discrimination is impossible and the disease is denoted as indeterminate colitis. This occurs mostly in fulminant colitis.

LOCAL COMPLICATIONS

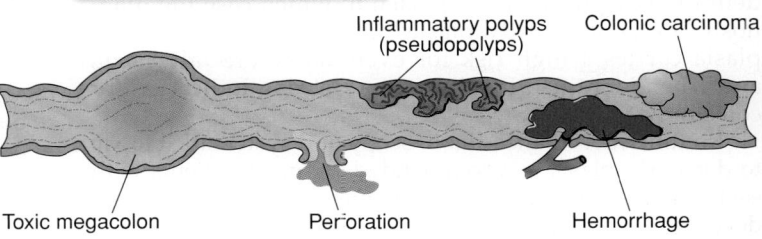

Inflammatory polyps (pseudopolyps)

Colonic carcinoma

Toxic megacolon

Perforation

Hemorrhage

FIGURE 19-64. Ulcerative colitis. A schematic representation of the major features of ulcerative colitis in the colon.

TABLE 19-4

COMPARISON OF THE PATHOLOGIC FEATURES IN THE COLON OF CROHN DISEASE AND ULCERATIVE COLITIS

Lesion	Crohn Disease	Ulcerative Colitis
Macroscopic		
Thickened bowel wall	Typical	Uncommon
Luminal narrowing	Typical	Uncommon
"Skip" lesions	Common	Absent
Right colon predominance	Typical	Absent
Fissures and fistulas	Common	Absent
Circumscribed ulcers	Common	Absent
Confluent linear ulcers	Common	Absent
Inflammatory polyps	Absent	Common
Microscopic		
Transmural inflammation	Typical	Rare
Submucosal fibrosis	Typical	Absent
Fissures	Typical	Rare
Granulomas	Common	Absent
Crypt abscesses	Typical	Typical

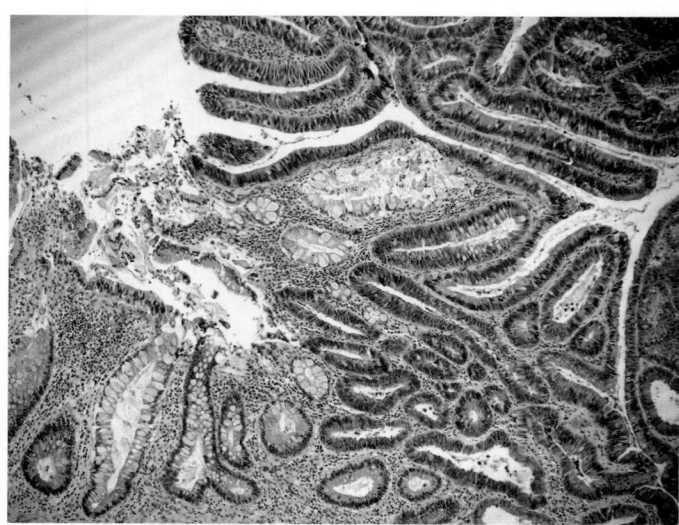

FIGURE 19-65. Dysplasia in ulcerative colitis. The colonic mucosa shows the chronic changes of ulcerative colitis. The crypts on the righthand side of the image show low-grade dysplasia, with increased nuclear cytoplasmic ratio, hyperchromatic nuclei, and lack of surface maturation.

Inflammatory Bowel Disease and Colorectal Cancer

Patients with long-standing ulcerative colitis and Crohn colitis have a higher risk of colorectal cancer than the general population. The magnitude of this increased risk is related to the extent and duration of the disease (elevated risk with >10 years disease). If inflammation is limited to the rectum, the risk of colorectal cancer is similar to that of the general population. Patients with ulcerative colitis who develop primary sclerosing cholangitis are at a higher risk of dysplasia and colorectal cancer.

Colorectal epithelial dysplasia is a neoplastic epithelial proliferation and precursor to colorectal carcinoma (Fig. 19-65). The dysplasia can occur in flat mucosa or in a polypoid lesion, sometimes called dysplasia-associated lesion or mass (DALM), based on its endoscopic appearance. Epithelial dysplasia is characterized by increased nuclear cytoplasmic ratio, nuclear atypia, and failure of maturation. It may be classified as low grade or high grade, depending on the degree of cytologic and architectural changes. Marked inflammation may preclude a definitive diagnosis of dysplasia, in which case the diagnosis "indefinite for dysplasia" is used. High-grade dysplasia carries a high risk for eventual colorectal cancer, and when identified in a biopsy is a strong indication for colectomy.

Routine surveillance colonoscopy and systematic biopsy to detect dysplasia is recommended for most patients with established IBD. Newer technologies such as chromoendoscopy (applying a topical dye to the mucosa during endoscopy) or confocal laser endomicroscopy (enhancing magnification of the endoscopic picture down to the cellular level) may increase biopsy yields of dysplastic lesions. With surveillance endoscopy with routine biopsies and medical therapy to reduce inflammation, dysplasia, and cancer risk can be reduced.

COLLAGENOUS AND LYMPHOCYTIC COLITIS CAUSE CHRONIC DIARRHEA

These entities are collectively referred to as microscopic colitis, so named because the colon appears grossly normal and only microscopic evaluation reveals an abnormality. The incidence of microscopic colitis has been increasing over the past 20 years. At least part of this increase reflects greater awareness of the disease. The main presenting symptom is chronic watery diarrhea. Patients may also have abdominal pain and weight loss, which are typically mild.

The disease increases with age, is more common in women and is associated with some medications, autoimmune diseases, and smoking. Treatment involves removing potentially offending medications, smoking cessation, antidiarrheal medications, and immune suppressants/modulators.

ETIOLOGY: The causes of collagenous colitis and lymphocytic colitis are unknown. Autoimmunity has been suggested, based on occasional association with autoimmune diseases such as rheumatoid arthritis, thyroid dysfunction, and psoriasis. Microscopic colitis is also frequently associated with celiac disease. Several medications have been implicated in both diseases; most are NSAIDs, but whether this association is causal or incidental is unclear, as many of these patients use NSAIDs for arthralgias.

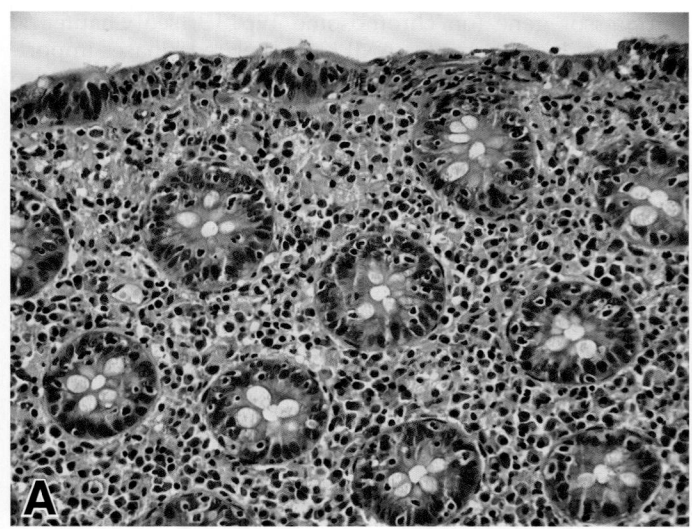 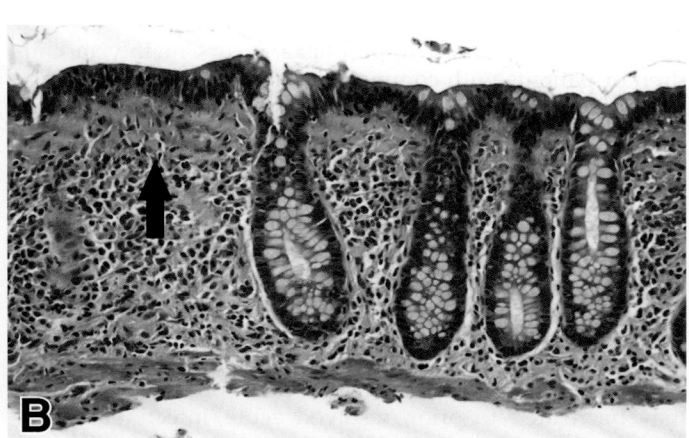

FIGURE 19-66. A. Lymphocytic colitis also shows increased intraepithelial lymphocytes but has a normal subepithelial collagen table. **B.** Collagenous colitis. Characteristic thickening of the collagen table (*arrow*) causes entrapment of capillaries. The intercryptal surface epithelium is flattened and contains an increased number of intraepithelial lymphocytes.

PATHOLOGY: Lymphocytic colitis has surface damage with increased intraepithelial lymphocytes (>20 per 100 epithelial cells) (Fig. 19-66A). Chronic inflammation of the lamina propria is increased, and typically more prominent superficially. Mild active inflammation may also be present. Gland architecture is normal, unlike in IBD. Changes may be more pronounced in the right colon, so random biopsies of the whole colon are useful in evaluating microscopic colitis.

Collagenous colitis typically shows similar changes to the colonic mucosa as lymphocytic colitis (normal architecture, surface damage, increased lamina propria inflammation, intraepithelial lymphocytosis), plus an irregularly thickened subepithelial collagen band, usually greater than 10 µm, which entraps capillaries (Fig. 19-66B). The collagen table is usually thickened irregularly, and thus multiple biopsies may be needed to make this diagnosis.

Pneumatosis Cystoides Intestinalis Is Gas Bubbles in the Bowel Wall

The small intestine and colon are most commonly affected (Fig. 19-67). Pneumatosis almost always complicates another condition, such as NEC (see above). In adults, it may be seen in pulmonary disease as a complication of emphysema or complicating such processes as endoscopic polypectomy, ischemia, *Clostridium difficile* colitis, or AIDS. Entrapped gas may cause a mass effect that can be mistaken for a neoplastic process.

Gas may enter the bowel wall by several routes. In pulmonary disease, air from ruptured blebs may track through the retroperitoneum and follow vascular adventitia into the bowel wall. Increased intra-abdominal pressure may force luminal gas through minute mucosal defects. Finally, some cases result from gas formed by luminal anaerobic organisms. Prognosis is related to the underlying condition.

POLYPS AND NEOPLASMS OF THE SMALL AND LARGE INTESTINE

A gastrointestinal polyp is a mass that protrudes into the gut lumen. Polyps are classified by their attachment to the bowel wall (e.g., sessile, or pedunculated with a discrete stalk), their histology (e.g., hyperplastic or adenomatous) and their neoplastic potential (i.e., benign or malignant). By themselves, polyps are not usually symptomatic and their clinical importance lies in the potential of some polyp types for malignant transformation. Despite the length and large surface area of the small intestine, primary small intestinal neoplasms occur less commonly than do those in the esophagus, stomach, or colon.

Lymphoid Polyps Are Solitary Submucosal Lymphoid Accumulations

They are normally present in the colorectal mucosa and vary in size from pinpoint to 5 cm. On occasion, multiple lesions

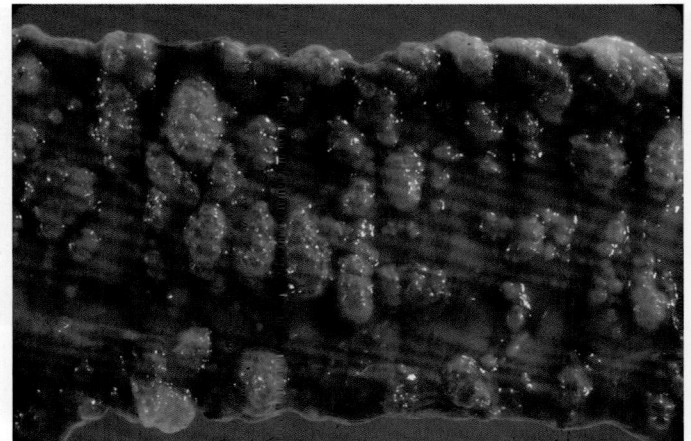

FIGURE 19-67. Multiple gas-filled blebs protrude into the lumen in this **case of pneumatosis cystoides intestinales.**

impart a cobblestone appearance to the mucosa. They are covered by intact mucosa and contain prominent lymphoid follicles with germinal centers. Lymphoid polyps are benign and usually asymptomatic.

Nodular lymphoid hyperplasia occurs mainly in children or patients with **common variable immunodeficiency syndrome** (see Chapter 4) and is characterized by excessive accumulation of normal colonic lymphoid follicles. The condition is rarely related to malignant lymphoma, but its radiologic appearance can be mistaken for FAP.

Inflammatory Polyps Are Elevated Areas of Inflamed, Regenerating Epithelium

They are commonly found in patients with ulcerative colitis and Crohn disease but may result from any cause of colitis. They also occur without demonstrable colonic disease and may be related to prior, resolved acute/infectious colitis. These polyps have variable components of distorted and inflamed mucosal glands, often intermixed with granulation tissue. By definition, these polyps do not show dysplasia, and as such have no malignant potential.

Hamartomatous Polyps Typically Have Both Stromal and Epithelial Elements

They are composed of a disorganized overgrowth of cells and tissue native to the anatomic location. They occur sporadically and may also be associated with a variety of heritable syndromes.

Peutz–Jeghers Polyps

Polyps in this syndrome may occur anywhere in the gastrointestinal tract but are most common in the small intestine. They have a characteristic gross and microscopic (Fig. 19-68A,B) appearance. The surface of the polyp is composed of bland-appearing small intestinal epithelium, often with an unusual architectural arrangement, overlying a core of large arborizing branches of smooth muscle. This autosomal dominant disorder is characterized by buccal pigmentation and macular lesions on the lips, hands, feet, and genitals. Most patients have loss-of-function mutations in the *LKB1* tumor

suppressor gene (on chromosome 19p13.3; see Chapter 5) which normally activates AMPK and related kinases important in regulating growth and energy metabolism. There is also an increased risk for cancer, largely outside the gastrointestinal tract, involving the testis, ovary, uterus, or pancreas.

Juvenile Polyps (Retention Polyps)

Juvenile polyps occur most commonly in children younger than 10 years, although up to 30% may arise in adults. They develop sporadically or may be part of a polyposis syndrome. When sporadic, they typically arise in the rectum and present with rectal bleeding or with the polyp prolapsing through the rectum.

A juvenile polyposis syndrome can be diagnosed if there are:

1. Five or more juvenile polyps in the colorectum
2. Juvenile polyps occurring outside the colon
3. Any number of juvenile polyps, plus a family history of juvenile polyposis

 MOLECULAR PATHOGENESIS: Mutations of *SMAD4* or *BMPR1A*, which affect control of cell proliferation by the TGFβ pathway, have been identified in some families with this syndrome. However, 30% to 40% of patients do not have an identified mutation. Patients with juvenile polyposis syndrome have an increased risk for gastrointestinal and pancreatic carcinomas. By contrast, people who present with sporadic juvenile polyps do not have an increased risk of malignancy.

 PATHOLOGY: Juvenile polyps are single or (rarely) multiple. They occur mostly in the rectum but may be anywhere in the small or large bowel. Most are pedunculated lesions up to 2 cm, with smooth, rounded surfaces. Dilated and cystic epithelial tubules are filled with mucus and inflammatory cells and are embedded in a fibrovascular lamina propria (Fig. 19-69). Surface epithelial erosion with underlying granulation tissue is common, as is reactive epithelial proliferation. Dysplasia is rare.

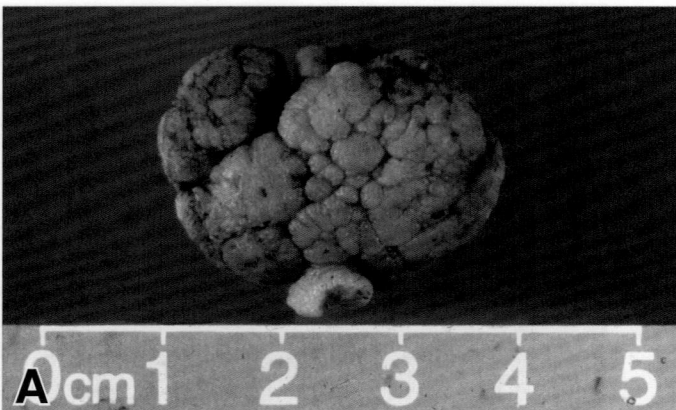
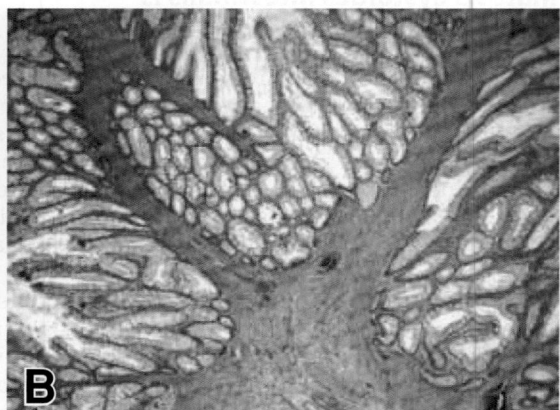

FIGURE 19-68. A. This **Peutz–Jeghers polyp** has a characteristic striking bosselated appearance. **B.** The histology is characterized by arborizing bundles of smooth muscle. The epithelium and glands between closely resemble the bland appearance of their normal counterparts but form an unusual architectural configuration.

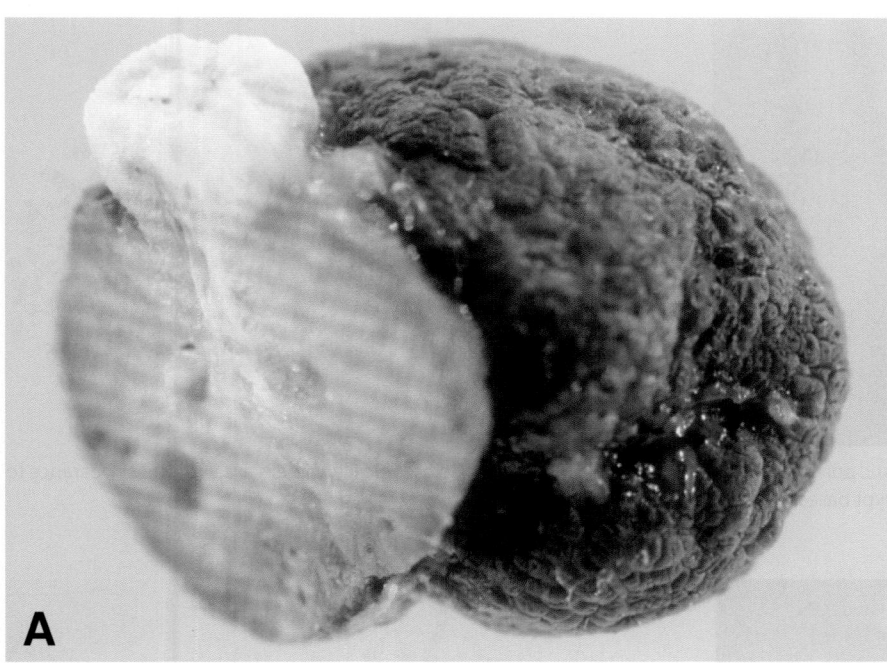
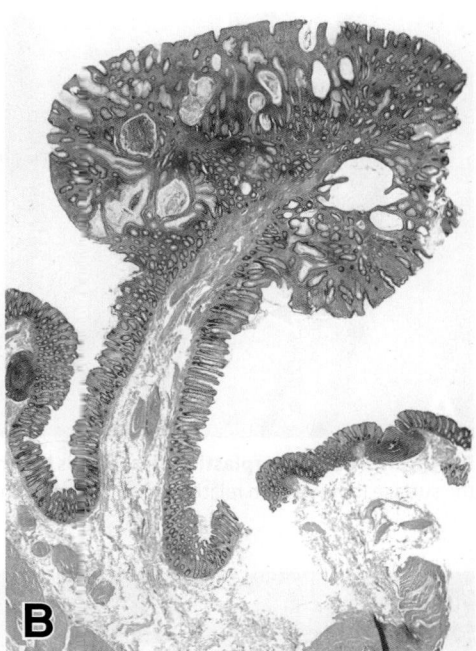

FIGURE 19-69. Juvenile polyp. A. The resected specimen shows a rounded surface. The cut surface (*left*) is cystic. **B.** Microscopically, the polyp displays cystically dilated glands.

PTEN Hamartomatous Tumor Syndromes

These rare autosomal dominant syndromes (Cowden syndrome and Bannayan–Ruvalcaba–Riley syndrome) are associated with germline *PTEN* mutations (see Chapter 5) and inherited with near-complete penetrance. These patients develop hamartomas of the skin, intestine, breast, and thyroid gland. Gastrointestinal polyps in these patients are often indistinguishable in appearance from juvenile polyps, although some may contain a prominent component of neurons and ganglion cells. Thus, the diagnosis of Cowden syndrome is made clinically and by identifying extraintestinal manifestations. Patients with Cowden syndrome are at increased risk of developing breast, thyroid, ovarian, cervical, uterine, and bladder cancers as well as meningiomas (see Chapter 32). They do not appear to be at increased risk of gastrointestinal cancers.

Cronkhite–Canada Syndrome

Cronkhite–Canada syndrome is characterized by hamartomatous polyps of the gastrointestinal tract, indistinguishable from juvenile polyps. However, unlike juvenile polyposis or Cowden syndrome, this is not an inherited disorder. Such patients can develop a protein-losing enteropathy, anemia, and electrolyte disturbances. They also present with scalp and body alopecia, nail dystrophy and skin hyperpigmentation. It is not entirely clear, but these patients may be at an increased risk for gastric and colorectal cancers.

Hyperplastic Polyps Are Benign Serrated Lesions

Hyperplastic polyps are small, sessile mucosal protrusions with exaggerated crypt architecture. They are the most common polyps of the colon, especially in the rectum. Hyperplastic polyps are present in 40% of rectal specimens in people younger than 40 years and in 75% of older people. They are more common in colons with adenomatous polyps

and in populations with higher rates of colorectal cancer. Hyperplastic polyps are felt to be due to defective proliferation and maturation of normal epithelium. In this setting, cell proliferation occurs at the base of the crypt, and upward migration of the cells is slowed. The epithelial cells differentiate and acquire absorptive characteristics lower in the crypts and persist at the surface longer than do normal cells.

PATHOLOGY: Hyperplastic polyps are small, sessile, raised mucosal nodules, up to 0.5 cm, but occasionally larger (Fig. 19-70A). They are almost always multiple. The crypts of hyperplastic polyps are elongated and show relatively normal crypt bases. The epithelium in the upper third of the crypts contains hyperplastic goblet and mucinous cells and absorptive cells, with no dysplasia, giving them a serrated contour and tufted surface (Fig. 19-70B).

Sessile Serrated Adenomas Resemble Hyperplastic Polyps but Have Malignant Potential

Also called sessile serrated polyps, these lesions typically arise in the right colon and show hypermethylation of the promoter for the mismatch-repair enzyme, *MLH1*; mutations in *BRAF*; and a high incidence of microsatellite instability. **Unlike hyperplastic polyps, sessile serrated adenomas are an important precursor lesion for colorectal carcinoma. Because of their malignant potential, these polyps should be entirely resected.**

PATHOLOGY: These lesions are sessile or flat. They may appear as misshapen, abnormal mucosal folds, and often have abundant adherent mucin (Fig. 19-71A). They are typically larger than 1 cm. They show irregular, asymmetric cell proliferation in which

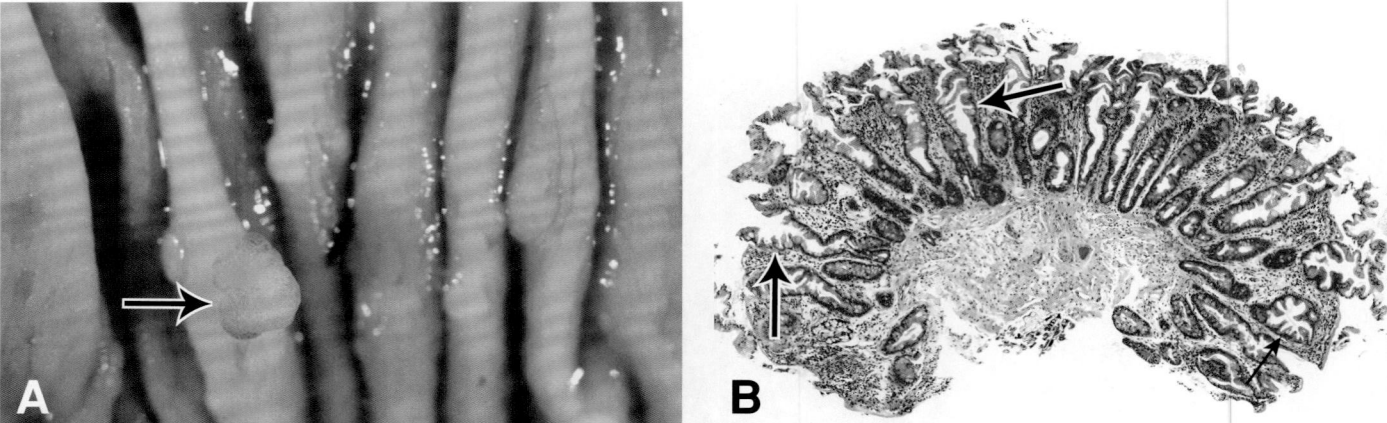

FIGURE 19-70.   Hyperplastic polyp. A. This hyperplastic polyp is small, sessile, and pale (*arrow*). **B.** Microscopically, there is a "sawtooth" appearance to the surface (*arrows*) with relatively normal-appearing crypt bases.

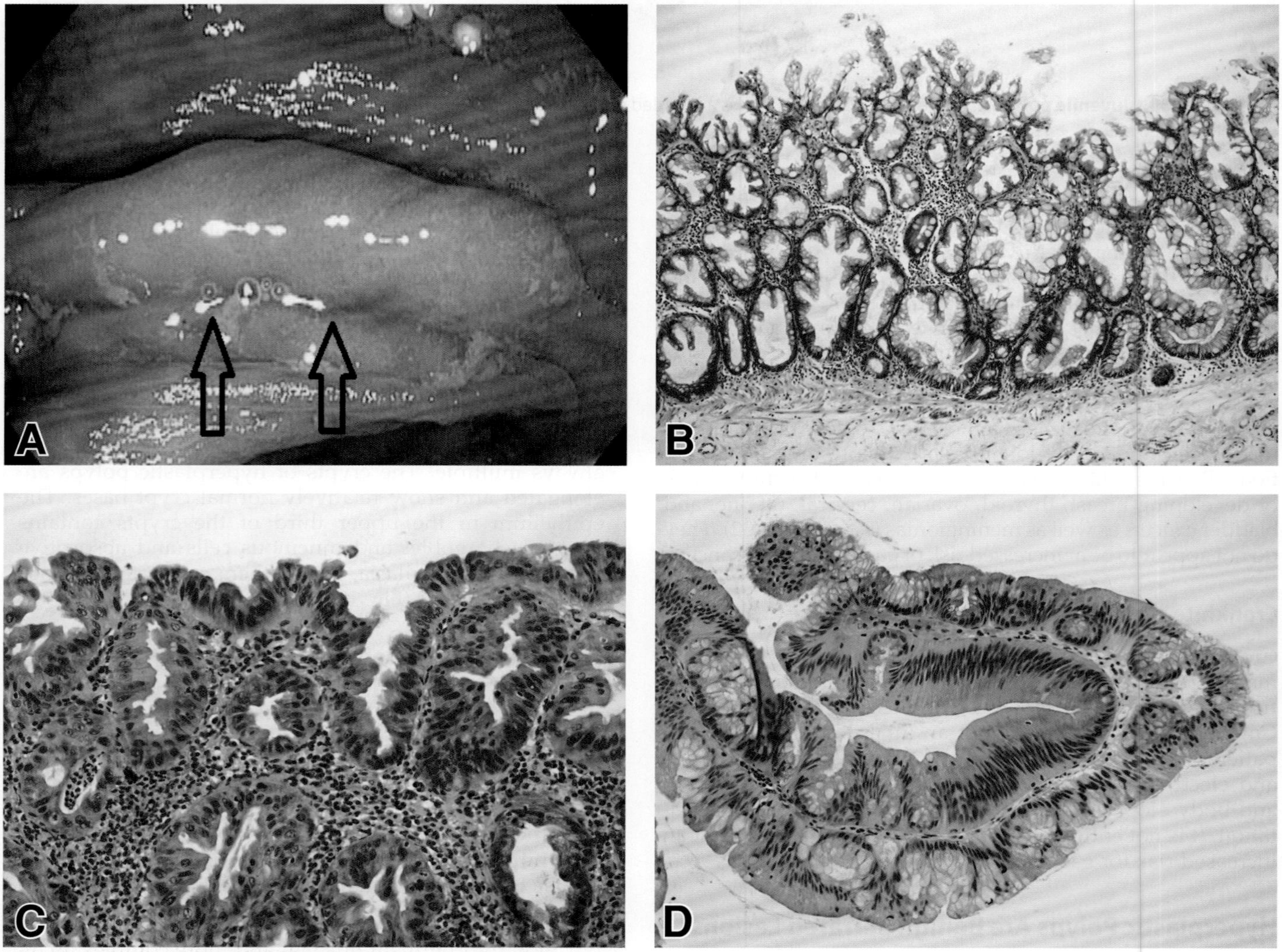

FIGURE 19-71.   Premalignant serrated polyps. A. Sessile serrated adenoma. The gross appearance is often that of an enlarged flattened mucosal fold, as seen in this endoscopic photograph (*arrows*). **B. Sessile serrated adenoma.** Microscopically, the abnormal proliferation of goblet cells gives the crypts a serrated appearance down to the bases, causing the bases to become dilated with abundant mucin and the characteristic formation of boot-, "L"-, or inverted "T"-shaped crypts. **C. Sessile serrated adenoma** with cytologic high-grade dysplasia. **D. Traditional serrated adenoma.** The most characteristic feature of this polyp type is formation of ectopic crypts, often with a villous architecture and lining epithelial cells with abundant eosinophilic cytoplasm.

cells may divide anywhere along the crypt. Intermixed goblet and mucin cells extend to the base. Some crypt bases are dilated with abundant mucin, while others show boot-, "L"-, or inverted "T"-shaped crypts (Fig. 19-71B). Although these crypt architectural features are useful in distinguishing sessile serrated adenomas from hyperplastic polyps, this differential diagnosis can be challenging in individual cases if the histologic features are subtle. These lesions may develop low- to high-grade dysplasia (Fig. 19-71C) and eventually invasive carcinoma.

Traditional Serrated Adenomas Occur Mainly in the Distal Colon and May Be Premalignant

These polyps are much less common than hyperplastic polyps or sessile serrated adenomas. They show diverse molecular abnormalities: some have *ERAF* mutations, some have *KRAS* mutations, and some show a CpG island methylator phenotype that involves methylation of the promoter for *MGMT* (see Chapter 5). Like sessile serrated adenomas, these polyps should be entirely removed.

 PATHOLOGY: Traditional serrated adenomas typically show tubulovillous or villous architecture. Lining epithelial cells have a serrated architecture, abundant eosinophilic cytoplasm with elongated nuclei and open or hyperchromatic chromatin, indicative of low-grade dysplasia (Fig. 19-71D).

Serrated Polyposis Syndrome Is Characterized by Multiple Serrated Polyps

Also called hyperplastic polyposis syndrome, this rare disorder is characterized by multiple serrated colorectal polyps, usually hyperplastic polyps and sessile serrated adenomas. Risk factors include European descent and increased age, although younger people are sometimes affected. There is no gender preference. No specific mutations have yet been identified, although the disease shows familial clustering. People are diagnosed with this syndrome if there are:

1. At least 5 serrated polyps proximal to the sigmoid colon, and 2 or more are >1 cm
2. Any number of serrated polyps proximal to the sigmoid colon in an individual with a first-degree relative with serrated polyposis syndrome
3. More than 20 serrated polyps of any size, distributed throughout the colon

Because of their increased risk of colorectal cancer, patients with a first-degree relative with serrated polyposis syndrome should begin screening colonoscopy at age 40, or 10 years younger than age at diagnosis of the youngest affected relative. All lesions greater than 5 mm, especially if right sided, should be removed.

Adenomatous Polyps Are Dysplastic Premalignant Lesions

These polyps are the usual precursors to colon carcinoma (see below), and their epithelium is by definition dysplastic.

 PATHOGENESIS: The pathogenesis of adenomas involves neoplastic alteration of crypt epithelium with (1) diminished apoptosis, (2) persistent cell replication, and (3) failure of epithelial cells to mature and differentiate as they migrate toward crypt surfaces. Normally, DNA synthesis stops when cells reach the upper 1/3 of crypts, after which they mature, migrate to the surface, and are then sloughed into the lumen. Adenomas represent focal disruption of this orderly sequence, in that epithelial cells may proliferate throughout the entire depth of the crypt. As the lesion evolves, the proliferation rate exceeds that of sloughing, and cells accumulate in upper crypts and on the surface.

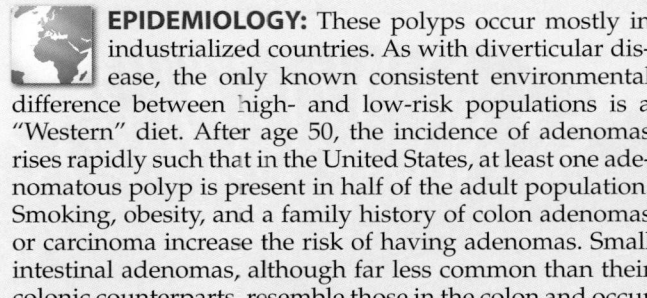 **EPIDEMIOLOGY:** These polyps occur mostly in industrialized countries. As with diverticular disease, the only known consistent environmental difference between high- and low-risk populations is a "Western" diet. After age 50, the incidence of adenomas rises rapidly such that in the United States, at least one adenomatous polyp is present in half of the adult population. Smoking, obesity, and a family history of colon adenomas or carcinoma increase the risk of having adenomas. Small intestinal adenomas, although far less common than their colonic counterparts, resemble those in the colon and occur both sporadically and in the setting of FAP (see below).

PATHOLOGY: Almost half of adenomatous polyps of the colon in the United States are in the rectosigmoid. The remaining half are evenly distributed throughout the rest of the colon. Adenomas vary from barely visible nodules or small, pedunculated adenomas to large, sessile (flat) lesions. They are classified by architecture into **tubular**, **villous**, and **tubulovillous** types, depending on the proportion of the lesion comprised of villi (thin, tall, finger-like processes that resemble the villi of the small intestine).

Tubular Adenomas represent 2/3 of large bowel adenomas. They are typically smooth-surfaced lesions, less than 2 cm, often with a stalk (Fig. 19-72). Some tubular adenomas, particularly the smaller ones, may be sessile. Tubular adenomas show closely packed epithelial tubules, which may be uniform or irregular and excessively branched (Fig. 19-72C). Polyps with 25% to 75% villous architecture are termed "**tubulovillous.**" Villous adenomas are the least common type and are found mainly in the rectosigmoid region. They are typically large (>2 cm) sessile lesions with shaggy, cauliflower-like surfaces (Fig. 19-73A), but they can be small and pedunculated. They are lined externally by neoplastic epithelial cells and are supported by a core of lamina propria (Fig. 19-73B).

By definition, adenomas show at least low-grade epithelial dysplasia, with enlarged "cigar-shaped" hyperchromatic nuclei showing slight stratification. High-grade dysplasia is characterized by increased nuclear pleomorphism with prominent nucleoli and more complex architecture, including cribriform glandular arrangements. As long as dysplasia is confined to the mucosa, the lesion is cured by complete polypectomy.

High-grade dysplasia can progress to invasive adenocarcinoma, the diagnosis of which requires neoplastic

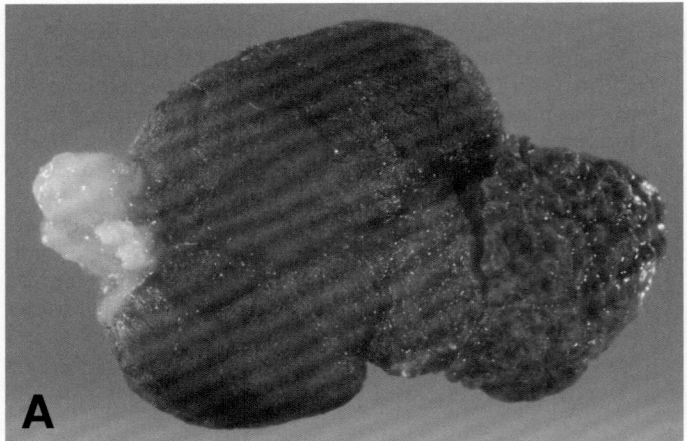

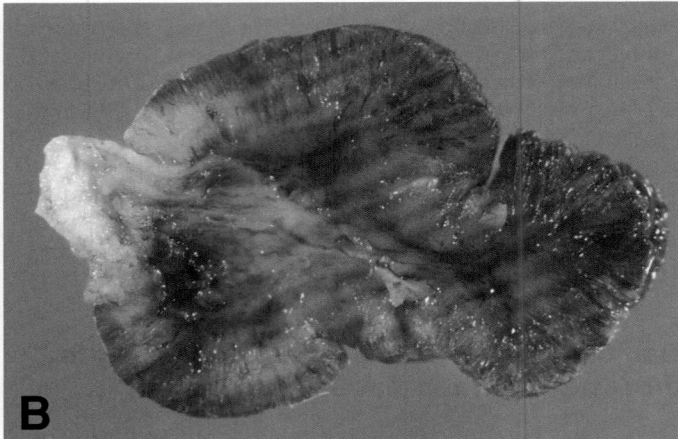

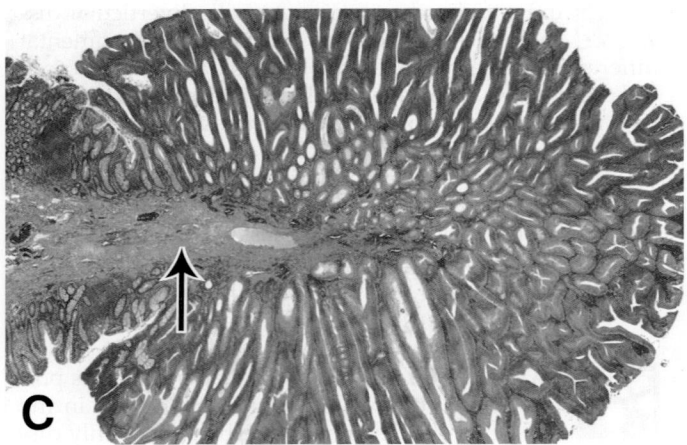

FIGURE 19-72. Tubular adenoma of the colon. A. The adenoma shows a characteristic stalk (*white area*) and bosselated surface. **B.** The bisected adenoma shows the stalk covered by the adenomatous epithelium. The *ashen white color* is due to cautery at the resection margin from the polypectomy. **C.** Microscopically, the adenoma shows a repetitive pattern that is largely tubular. The stalk (*arrow*), which is in continuity with the submucosa of the colon, is not involved and is lined by normal colonic epithelium.

glands below the muscularis mucosae (Fig. 19-74). The risk of invasive carcinoma correlates with the size of the adenoma, with the presence of high-grade dysplasia, and with the presence of villous morphology. For example, only 1% of tubular adenomas less than 1 cm have invasive cancer at the time of resection. Of those 1 to 2 cm, 10% harbor malignancy, and of those greater than 2 cm, 35%

are malignant. In villous adenomas under 1 cm, the risk of cancer is 10 times higher than that for tubular adenomas of comparable size, and up to 50% of villous adenomas greater than 2-cm harbor invasive carcinoma. Invasive adenocarcinoma may be cured by polypectomy alone if the tumor shows low-risk features and there is an adequate margin of resection at the base.

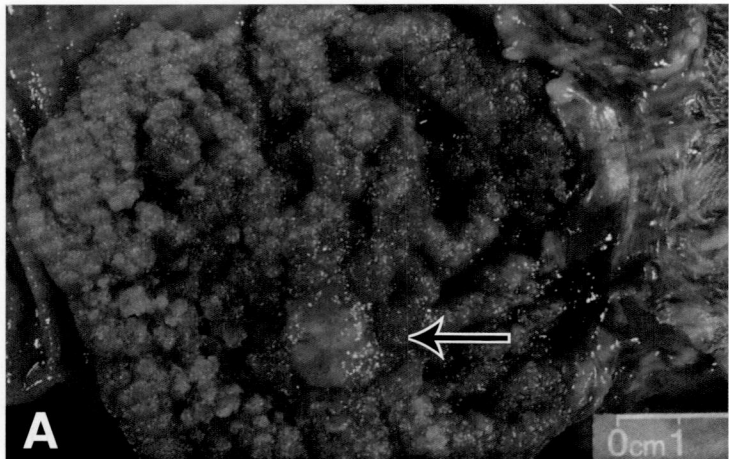

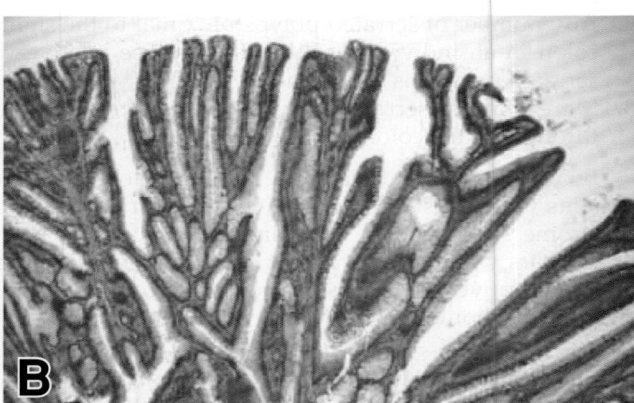

FIGURE 19-73. Villous adenoma of the colon. A. The colon contains a large, broad-based, elevated lesion that has a cauliflower-like surface. A firm area near the center of the lesion (*arrow*) proved on histologic examination to be an adenocarcinoma. **B.** Microscopic examination shows finger-like processes with fibrovascular cores lined by low-grade dysplastic epithelium.

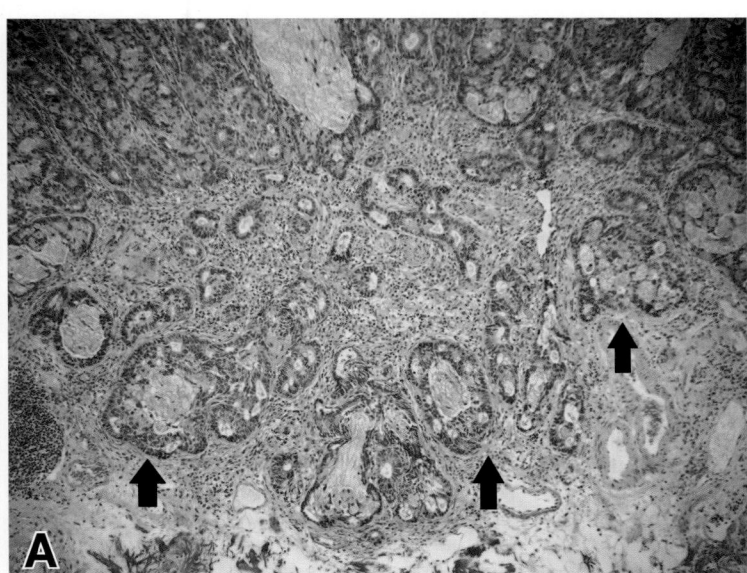
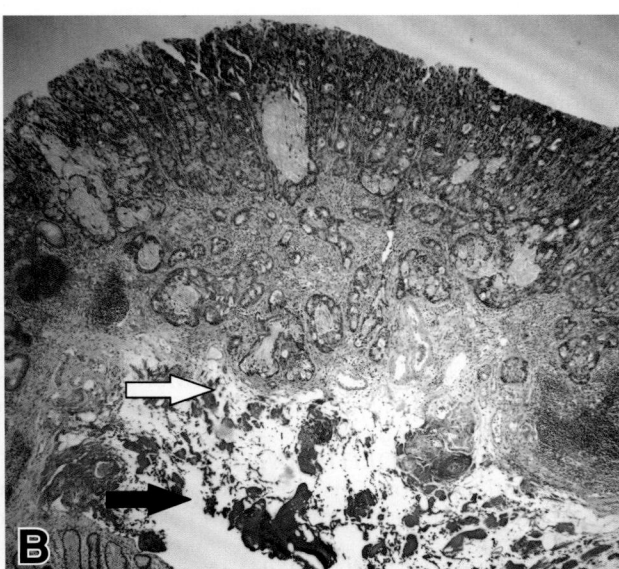

FIGURE 19-74. Adenocarcinoma arising in a pedunculated adenomatous polyp. A. The invasive component consists of infiltrating glands with high-grade dysplastic epithelium, characterized by a cribriform pattern and increased nuclear pleomorphism (*arrows*). **B.** Low-power shot of adenocarcinoma invading the polyp stalk. Since the invasive tumor (*white arrow*) is less than 1 mm from the cauterized deep margin of resection (*black arrow*), additional resection should be considered.

Familial Adenomatous Polyposis Is an Autosomal Dominant Trait That Invariably Leads to Cancer

FAP accounts for less than 1% of colorectal cancers. It is caused by a heritable, germline loss-of-function mutation in the *APC* gene on the long arm of chromosome 5 (5q21-22) (see below). As detailed below, this gene normally acts as a tumor suppressor. It participates in the Wnt/β-catenin signaling pathway which, among other functions, regulates proliferation of colonic mucosa cells. Most cases are familial, but 30% to 50% reflect new mutations. In FAP, there are hundreds to thousands of adenomas carpeting the colorectal mucosa, sometimes throughout its entire length, but particularly in the rectosigmoid region (Fig. 19-75). These are mostly tubular adenomas, but tubulovillous and villous adenomas may also be present. Microscopic adenomas, sometimes involving a single crypt, are numerous. A few polyps are usually already present by age 10, but symptoms usually begin by age 36. Carcinoma of the colon and rectum is inevitable in FAP patients, with the mean age of onset at 40 years.

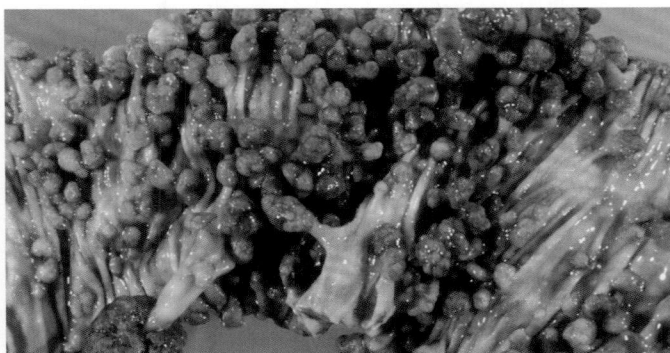

FIGURE 19-75. Familial adenomatous polyposis. The colon contains thousands of adenomatous polyps with several exceeding 1 cm in diameter.

Total colectomy before the onset of cancer is curative, but some patients may also have tubular adenomas in the small intestine and stomach, and these have the same malignant potential as those in the colon.

APC mutations are found in only three-fourths of familial cases. Some APC mutation-negative patients have homozygous mutations in *MYH* which encodes a DNA repair enzyme. This causes a distinct, rare, autosomal recessive polyposis syndrome that clinically overlaps FAP. Subtypes of FAP (which may be associated with particular APC mutations) include:

■ **Attenuated FAP:** In this condition there are fewer than 100 adenomas in the colon. Colorectal cancer develops an average of 15 years later than in classical FAP and carries a 70% risk of invasive cancer by age 80.

■ **Gardner syndrome:** In this variant, extracolonic lesions include osteomas of the skull, mandible, and long bones; epidermoid cysts; desmoid tumors; and congenital hypertrophy of retinal pigment epithelium. *APC* mutations do not predict this phenotype.

■ **Turcot syndrome:** This rare disorder combines FAP with malignant CNS tumors. Many cases, especially those with medulloblastoma, are due to germline mutations of the *APC* gene.

Most Colorectal Adenocarcinomas Arise in Adenomatous Polyps

In Western societies, colorectal cancer is the third most common cause of cancer and the second leading cause of cancer death. The term "colorectal" is used because cancers of the colon and rectum share certain biologic features, but there are also differences between colonic and rectal cancers. For instance, colon cancer rates are about equal between men and women, but rectal cancer shows a slight male predominance. The two tumors are also treated differently.

Risk Factors for Colorectal Carcinoma

Most colorectal cancers arise in adenomatous polyps. Thus, factors that lead to the development of such polyps favor colorectal cancer as well.

AGE: Increasing age is probably the single most important risk factor for colorectal cancer in the general population. The risk is low (but not zero) before age 40 in the absence of a polyposis syndrome. It then increases steadily to age 50, after which it doubles each decade.

PRIOR COLORECTAL CANCER: Patients with one colorectal cancer are at increased risk for a subsequent tumor. In fact, 5% to 10% of patients treated for colorectal cancer develop a second such malignancy. Moreover, 2% to 5% of those with a new colorectal cancer have a simultaneous (synchronous) second cancer.

ULCERATIVE COLITIS AND CROHN DISEASE: These chronic inflammatory diseases increase colorectal cancer risk in proportion to their duration and extent of large bowel involvement.

GENETIC FACTORS: Risk of colorectal cancer is increased in relatives of patients with the disease, suggesting a genetic contribution to tumorigenesis. People with two or more first- or second-degree relatives with colorectal cancer constitute 20% of all patients with this tumor. Some 5% to 10% of colorectal cancers are inherited as autosomal dominant traits, the most common syndrome being hereditary nonpolyposis colorectal carcinoma (HNPCC, Lynch syndrome [see below]), in addition to FAP.

DIET: Consumption of animal products including fat, cholesterol, and protein parallels incidence of colorectal cancer. This is one of the key factors underlying the marked geographic variation in the incidence of this cancer, with rates differing by 10-fold between developing and developed countries. Possibly, ingestion of animal products favors bacterial flora that degrade bile salts to N-nitroso compounds, which may contribute to tumorigenesis.

Diets low in fruits, vegetables, and whole grains (fiber) have also been implicated in colorectal carcinogenesis. Reasons for this are not entirely clear but may be related to an effect on gut flora and stool transit time.

PHYSICAL ACTIVITY AND OBESITY: These factors combined are thought to account for up to one-third of colorectal cancers. While not well understood, physical inactivity decreases gut motility. Obesity increases circulating estrogens and decreases insulin sensitivity, factors that are believed to influence cancer risk.

CIGARETTE SMOKING AND ALCOHOL: Cigarette smoking and heavy alcohol consumption are independent risk factors for colon cancer. If present together, they may act synergistically. DNA mutations induced by smoking are repaired less efficiently in the presence of alcohol. Nutritional deficiencies may also play a role in heavy alcohol users.

MOLECULAR PATHOGENESIS: In 85% of cases of colorectal carcinoma, it is estimated that at least 8 to 10 mutational events must accumulate before an invasive cancer with metastatic potential develops. This process is initiated in histologically normal mucosa, proceeds through a precursor stage and ends as invasive adenocarcinoma (see Chapter 5).

The most important mutational events involve (Fig. 19-76A):

- *APC* **gene:** As noted above, germline mutations in the *APC* (adenomatous polyposis coli) tumor suppressor gene are responsible for FAP. The APC gene product negatively regulates β-catenin by stimulating its phosphorylation, followed by ubiquitination and proteasomal degradation. Mutant APC allows β-catenin to accumulate in the nucleus, where it is a transcriptional activator of key proliferation genes (e.g., *cyclin D1* and *MYC*). *APC* mutations in normal colonic mucosa precede development of sporadic adenomas, highlighting the "gatekeeper" role of this gene preventing the early development of dysplasia. This relationship also explains how FAP patients develop large numbers of adenomas, since one APC allele is already mutated. *APC* **mutations are found in 70% to 80% of sporadic colorectal cancers.** Some tumors with normal *APC* have mutations in the **β-catenin gene** itself. A specific *APC* mutation (isoleucine → lysine at codon 1307) occurring in 6% of Ashkenazi Jews, renders surrounding regions of the gene susceptible to inactivating frame-shift mutations and increases risk of colon cancer.
- *KRAS:* Activating mutations of the *KRAS* protooncogene occur early in tubular adenomas of the colon.
- *TP53:* Mutations in p53 facilitate the transition from adenoma to the most common type of adenocarcinoma and are late events in colon carcinogenesis.

In 15% of colorectal cancers, the process of **DNA mismatch repair** (MMR; see Chapter 5) is impaired, leading to deficient repair of spontaneous replication errors and increased mutations in coding and noncoding regions of multiple genes, and in regions with simple repetitive sequences (microsatellites). MMR deficiency occurs via two mechanisms. In a hereditary form (HNPCC; see below), a germline mutation in one of the MMR genes is followed by somatic mutation of the other allele ("second hit"; see Chapter 5) later in life. In sporadic tumors, hypermethylation of an MMR promoter, usually for the *MLH1* gene, inactivates transcription of the gene (Fig. 19-76B).

PATHOLOGY: Grossly, colorectal cancers resemble adenocarcinomas elsewhere in the gut. They tend to be polypoid and ulcerating or infiltrative, and may be annular and constrictive (Fig. 19-77). Polypoid cancers are more common in the right colon, particularly the cecum, where the large lumen allows unimpeded intraluminal growth. Annular constricting tumors occur more often in the distal colon. Tumors often ulcerate, regardless of growth pattern.

The vast majority of colorectal cancers are adenocarcinomas comprised of infiltrating glands and tubules, similar to their counterparts elsewhere in the digestive tract (Fig. 19-77B). About 15% secrete abundant mucin and are called **mucinous** adenocarcinomas. Other tumors (particularly MMR deficient tumors) are poorly differentiated and consist of sheets of malignant cells.

Colon cancers spread by direct extension or lymphovascular invasion. The former is common in resected specimens. Serosal connective tissue offers little resistance to tumor spread, and cancer cells are often seen in the pericolonic

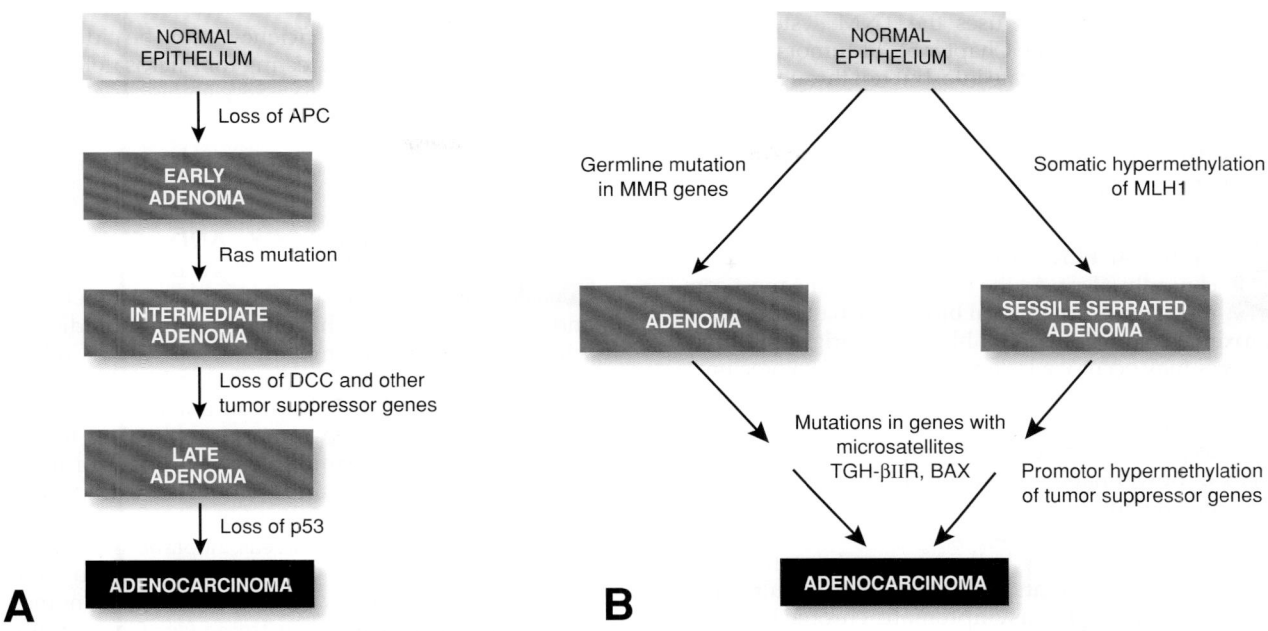

FIGURE 19-76. Model of genetic alterations involved in colonic carcinogenesis. A. The tumor suppressor pathway. **B.** The mismatch repair (MMR) defect pathway. *APC* = adenomatous polyposis coli; *DCC* = deleted in colon cancer; *MLH1* = MutL homolog 1; *TGF-βIIR* = transforming growth factor-β2 receptor; *BAX* = BCL2-associated X protein.

fat far from the primary site. The peritoneum is occasionally involved, in which case there may be multiple deposits throughout the abdomen.

Colorectal cancer invades lymphatic channels and initially involves lymph nodes in the vicinity of the tumor. The liver is the most common distant metastatic site, but the tumor may spread more widely. The prognosis of colorectal cancer is more closely related to tumor extension through the large bowel wall than to its size or histopathology.

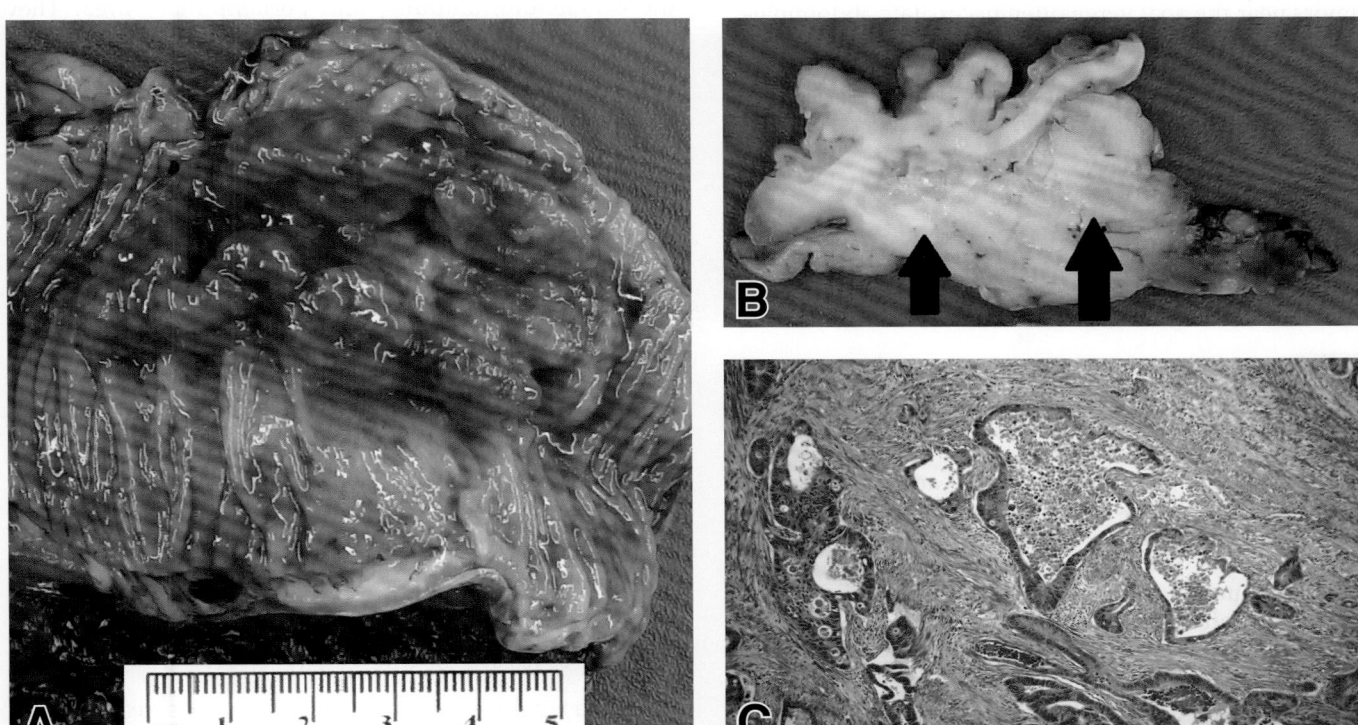

FIGURE 19-77. Adenocarcinoma of the colon. A. A resected colon shows an ulcerated mass with enlarged, firm, rolled borders. **B.** Cut section shows the tumor extending through the muscularis propria into the pericolonic adipose tissue (*left arrow*). A pericolonic lymph node replaced by tumor is also visible (*right arrow*). **C.** Microscopically, this colon adenocarcinoma consists of moderately differentiated glands with a prominent cribriform pattern and frequent central necrosis.

Staging of these tumors uses the TNM system (tumor, lymph nodes, metastasis; see Chapter 5). T1 tumors invade the submucosa; T2 tumors infiltrate into, but not through, the muscularis propria; T3 tumors invade pericolorectal soft tissue; and T4 tumors penetrate the serosa (T4a) or involve adjacent organs (T4b). N reflects the presence or absence of lymph node metastases, and M the presence or absence of distant metastases.

 CLINICAL FEATURES: Initially, colorectal cancer is clinically silent. As the tumor grows, the most common sign is **occult fecal blood** when the tumor is in the proximal colon. Both occult blood and **bright red blood** in the feces may occur if a lesion is in the distal colorectum.

Cancers on the left side of the colon, where the lumen is narrow and feces are more solid, often constrict the lumen and produce **obstructive symptoms**. These include changes in bowel habits and abdominal pain. Colorectal cancers may **perforate** early and cause peritonitis. By contrast, right-sided cancers may grow large without causing obstruction, especially in the cecum where the lumen is large and fecal contents are liquid. As a result, right-sided tumors can lead to asymptomatic chronic bleeding. **Iron-deficiency anemia** may be the first indication of colorectal cancer. A tumor that spreads beyond the colorectum may cause enterocutaneous and rectovaginal **fistulas**, tumor masses in the abdominal wall, bladder symptoms and sciatic nerve pain. Spread within the abdomen may cause **small intestinal obstruction** and malignant **ascites**.

Resection is the primary curative treatment for colorectal cancer, sometimes followed by adjuvant chemotherapy or radiotherapy. Small polyps are easily removed endoscopically; large lesions require segmental resection. Tumors near the anal verge often necessitate abdominal–perineal resection and colostomy, although newer surgical techniques may preserve sphincter function. Preoperative (neoadjuvant) chemotherapy and radiotherapy are typically used in all but very early rectal cancers.

Hereditary Nonpolyposis Colorectal Cancer (Lynch Syndrome)

Lynch Syndrome is an autosomal dominant inherited disease that accounts for 3% to 5% of colorectal cancers.

 MOLECULAR PATHOGENESIS: Lynch syndrome (LS) is caused by germline mutations in a DNA MMR gene. Usually, *hMSH2* (human MutS homolog 2) on chromosome 2p and *hMLH1* (human MutL homolog 1) on chromosome 3p are affected. Less common mutations involve *hMSH6* (human MutS homolog 6) or *hPMS2* (human postmeiotic segregation 2) on chromosomes 2p and 7p, respectively. In LS, there is a germline mutation in one allele of one MMR gene. The fact that one allele is mutated hinders repair of any second sporadic mutation in the other (formerly) wild-type allele: a somatic "second hit" (see Chapter 5). Thereafter, repair of spontaneous replication errors is ineffective. Widespread genomic instability results, particularly in simple repetitive sequences (microsatellites), which are particularly prone to replication errors. Thus, genes that regulate growth and differentiation, and other mismatch repair genes, are disabled by unrepaired mutations.

Mismatch repair deficiency can be identified by sequencing MMR genes, testing for microsatellite instability and immunostaining to assess levels of MMR proteins in a tumor. A specific mutation can be used to evaluate other family members.

 PATHOLOGY AND CLINICAL FEATURES: Lynch syndrome tumors more often show mucinous, signet ring cell and solid (medullary) histologies than sporadic tumors, with many intratumor lymphocytes and Crohn's-like lymphocytic reactions. LS patients tend to (1) present with cancer at a young age; (2) have few adenomas (hence "nonpolyposis"); (3) develop tumors proximal to the splenic flexure (70%); (4) have multiple synchronous or metachronous colorectal cancers; and (5) develop extracolonic cancers, especially of the endometrium, ovary, stomach, small intestine, urinary tract, pancreas, hepatobiliary tract, skin, and CNS. Patients with Lynch syndrome who have skin involvement (sebaceous adenomas and carcinomas) are said to have **Muir–Torre syndrome** (see Chapter 28). Specific criteria for the diagnosis of Lynch syndrome are listed in Table 19-5.

Small Intestinal Adenocarcinomas Are Far Less Common Than in the Colon

These tumors resemble their colonic counterparts and also arise from adenomatous precursors, but are much less frequent. They occur more often proximally, particularly in the duodenum, ampulla, and periampullary area. They can be polypoid or ulcerated or have a peculiar constricted napkin ring appearance (Fig. 19-78A,B). There is a much greater (80-fold) risk of small bowel adenocarcinoma in patients with Crohn disease or celiac disease. In the former, tumors arise distally, in inflamed intestine. These tumors are also increased in FAP and Peutz–Jeghers syndrome.

Because of their crucial anatomic location, ampullary tumors may present clinically with jaundice even when relatively small. Tumors may have an intestinal or a pancreaticobiliary phenotype. The former tend to have a somewhat better prognosis.

TABLE 19-5

CLINICAL SITUATIONS WHICH RAISE THE POSSIBILITY OF LYNCH SYNDROME

Revised Bethesda Guidelines (only one criterion needs to be met)

Diagnosed with colorectal cancer (CRC) before the age of 50 years
Individuals with more than one CRC or other LS-related tumor
CRC with high-microsatellite instability morphology, diagnosed before the age of 60 years
CRC and a first-degree relative with CRC or other LS-related tumor. One cancer must have been diagnosed at younger than age 50 years or one adenoma at younger than age 40 years
CRC with at least two relatives with CRC or other LS-related tumor, regardless of age

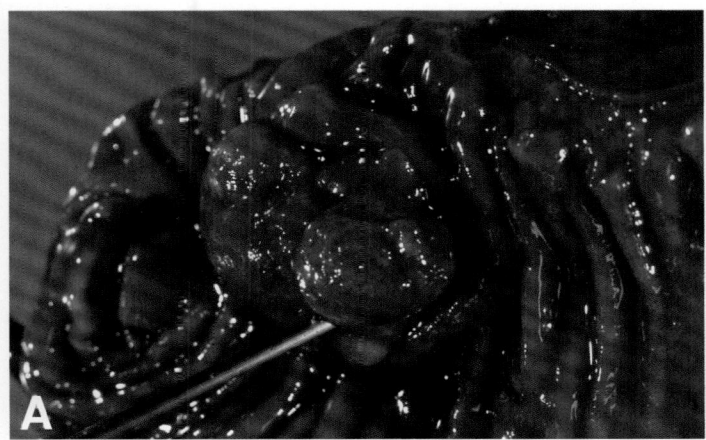
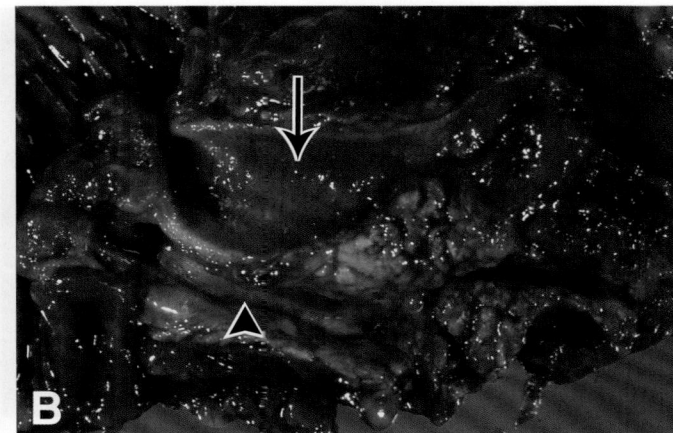

FIGURE 19-78. A. A probe was placed into the ampulla and common bile duct in this carcinoma of the ampulla. **B.** Upon dissection, both the common bile duct (*arrow*) and the pancreatic duct (*arrowhead*) are dilated owing to obstruction by the tumor.

OTHER TUMORS OF THE INTESTINES

Intestinal Neuroendocrine Tumors Vary in Their Biologic Behavior

As noted above in the section on the stomach, the term **well-differentiated neuroendocrine tumor** has replaced "carcinoid" in designating these tumors. In addition to the site of origin, the size, depth of invasion, hormonal responsiveness, and presence or absence of function are major indicators of likely aggressiveness. The appendix is the most common gastrointestinal site of origin, followed by the rectum; tumors in these sites are usually indolent. By contrast, NETs of the ileum are usually small but are often more aggressive. NETs may also arise in the ampullary region. Some develop as part of neurofibromatosis, produce somatostatin and are known as somatostatinomas.

PATHOLOGY: Small NETs usually present as submucosal nodules covered by intact mucosa. Larger tumors may grow in polypoid, intramural or annular patterns and often undergo secondary ulceration. Cut surfaces are firm and white to yellow. As they enlarge, the tumors invade the muscular coat and penetrate the serosa, often causing a conspicuous fibrosis reaction (desmoplasia), which can lead to peritoneal adhesions, kinking of the bowel and possible intestinal obstruction. Ileal NETs are multiple in about 40% of cases (Fig. 19-79A,B).

Small, round cells in NETs form nests, cords, and rosettes. Nuclei are remarkably regular and mitoses are rare. The abundant eosinophilic cytoplasm contains neurosecretory-type granules (Fig. 19-79C).

When these tumors metastasize to regional lymph nodes, they may produce a bulky mass far larger than the primary tumor. Subsequent hematogenous spread causes metastases at distant sites, particularly the liver.

CLINICAL FEATURES: Carcinoid syndrome occurs in a small percentage of patients with NETs. It is a unique but uncommon clinical condition caused by release of active tumor products. Most NETs are somewhat functional, but carcinoid syndrome mainly occurs in patients with extensive hepatic metastases. *Classic symptoms include diarrhea (often the most distressing symptom), episodic flushing, bronchospasm, cyanosis, telangiectasia, and skin lesions.* Half of patients also have right-sided cardiac valvular disease (see Chapter 17). Diarrhea is thought to be caused by serotonin.

After its release into the blood, serotonin is metabolized to 5-hydroxyindoleacetic acid (5-HIAA) by monoamine oxidase (MAO) in the liver or other tissues. Urine 5-HIAA is a diagnostic test for carcinoid syndrome. Liver, lung, and brain all have high levels of MAO activity, but the right side of the heart is affected mainly when there are metastases in the liver, allowing secreted serotonin to bypass hepatic detoxification. Fibrous plaques form on tricuspid and pulmonic valves, the endocardium of the right-sided cardiac chambers, the vena cava, the coronary sinus and the pulmonary artery. Valvular distortion leads to pulmonic stenosis and tricuspid regurgitation. The left heart is not involved because of high levels of MAO in the lungs.

Intestinal Mesenchymal Tumors Encompass the Range of Benign and Malignant Soft Tissue Tumors

Gastrointestinal stromal tumors are the most common mesenchymal tumor of the small intestine. The small intestine is the second most common site for GISTs after the stomach. Like their gastric counterparts, they arise in deeper layers of the bowel wall but may be associated with mucosal ulceration, which can cause severe bleeding (Fig. 19-35A). Small intestinal GISTs are usually composed of spindled cells (see Fig. 19-35B), and are more likely to behave aggressively than gastric GISTs. By contrast, the most frequently encountered colonic mesenchymal tumors are benign submucosal lipomas and leiomyomas derived from the muscularis mucosae, with GISTs being significantly less common.

An assortment of other soft tissue tumors such as liposarcoma, neurofibroma, ganglioneuroma, peripheral nerve sheath tumors, leiomyosarcoma, and vascular tumors are all seen rarely.

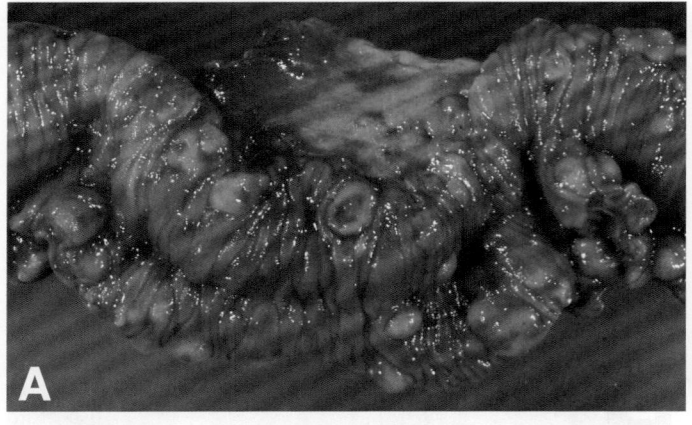

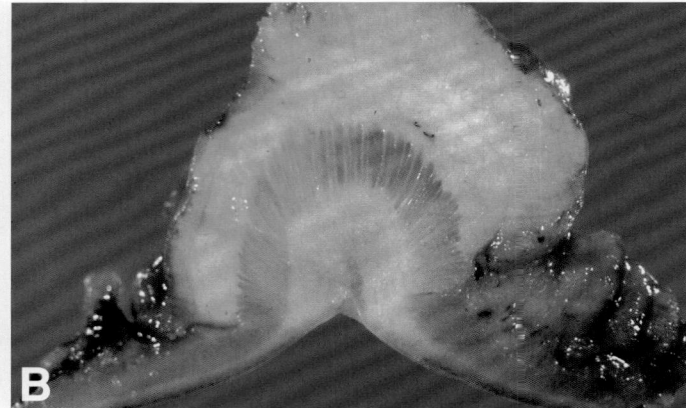

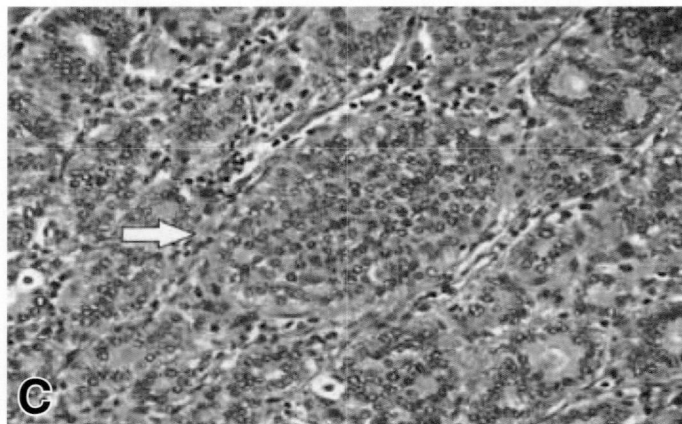

FIGURE 19-79. A. Ileal neuroendocrine tumors (NETs) are frequently multiple, here producing several mucosal-covered pa e yellow tumors. **B.** The characteristic "knuckling" of the intestinal wall i; due to the brisk fibrous response to the invading tumor. **C.** Most neuroendocrine tumors are well differentiated and are comprised of nests of tumor cells with round nuclei, finely granular "salt and pepper" chromatin, and moderate amounts of cytoplasm (*arrow*).

Intestinal Lymphomas Are Diverse

Four major types of lymphoma arise in the small intestine (see Chapter 26): Burkitt lymphoma, immunoproliferative small intestinal disease ([IPSID], Mediterranean lymphoma), diffuse large B-cell lymphoma, and enteropathy-associated T-cell lymphoma (EATL).

Burkitt lymphoma develops mainly in the terminal ileum in children, with males predominating. The tumors form bulky masses. The B cells composing the tumor may have a plasmacytoid appearance. Many cases are EBV positive. The process can be seen in young adults who have immunodeficiency; some are HIV positive.

Patients with IPSID are most commonly young adults of lower socioeconomic status living in the Middle East. This appears to be a distinctive type of extranodal marginal B-cell lymphoma. Environmental factors are thought to play a role, and there is evidence implicating *Campylobacter jejuni*. Abdominal pain, malabsorption, diarrhea, and weight loss dominate the clinical picture. Diffuse mural thickening with luminal dilatation is often present. Free immunoglobulin α-heavy chains are often found in the serum. An extensive mucosal lymphoid infiltrate may distort small intestinal villi.

Diffuse large B-cell lymphoma often presents as a large luminal mass in an older adult. It tends to be quite aggressive.

EATL complicates celiac disease, which may be long-standing but can be of short duration (Fig. 19-80A–C). Severe malnutrition despite adherence to a gluten-free diet often heralds its onset. It has the worst prognosis of the intestinal lymphomas.

Primary lymphoma of the colorectum is uncommon. It may be seen with (1) segmental mucosal involvement, (2) diffuse polypoid lesions, or (3) a mass extending beyond the colorectum. Symptoms are like those of other intestinal cancers, but the diffuse polypoid form may resemble inflammatory or adenomatous polyps. Most colonic lymphomas are B-cell non-Hodgkin lymphomas such as mantle cell lymphoma or large cell lymphoma.

Finally, the small and large intestines may be secondarily involved by many types of lymphoma originating in lymph nodes or other sites.

Metastases

Secondary carcinomas are about as common as are primary adenocarcinomas in the small intestine. The primary tumor may be of any origin, but melanomas and tumors of the lung, breast, colon, and kidney are the most common. In the colon, metastases are outnumbered by primary malignancies, but patients with carcinomas of the pancreas, urinary female genital tracts, among others, can show large intestinal involvement. Careful attention to historical and histologic detail is necessary to establish the diagnosis.

Endometriosis Involving the Colon Can Mimic Colorectal Cancer

Colorectal endometriosis is mostly asymptomatic and may be discovered incidentally during laparotomy for other reasons. If symptoms occur (abdominal pain, constipation,

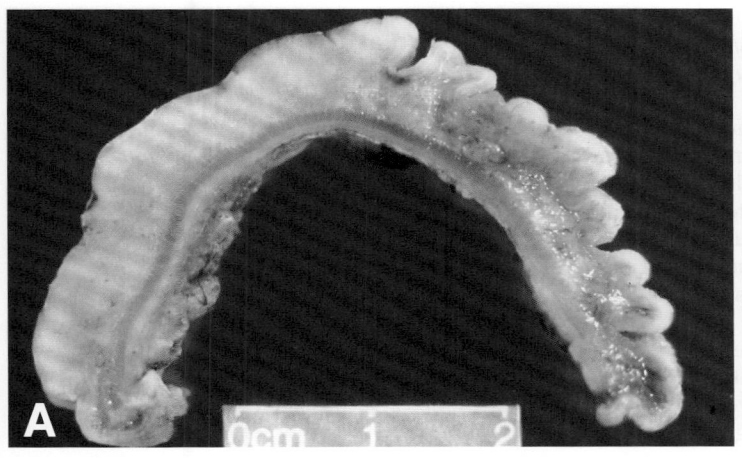

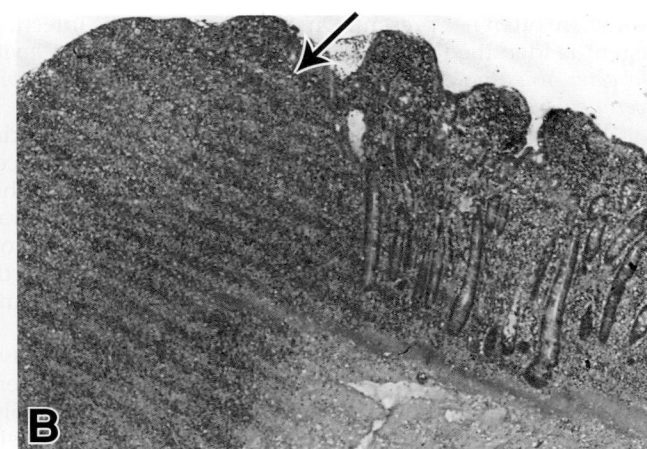

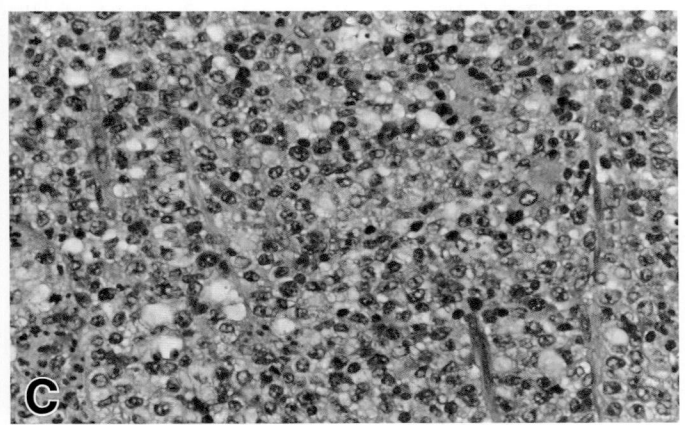

FIGURE 19-80. A. A **lymphoma** diffusely penetrating the bowel wall has given it a peculiar pale white color often referred to as "fish flesh." **B.** The infiltrate in this enteropathy-associated T-cell lymphoma (EATL) (*arrow*) is adjacent to the flat mucosa in this patient with celiac disease. **C.** The lymphomatous infiltrate pushes aside the epithelial and muscular structures.

intestinal obstruction), they may be mistaken for those of colorectal cancer. As a result of repeated hemorrhage, the lesions are surrounded by reactive fibrosis, which, when severe, can lead to a classic "apple core" appearance to the colon or rectum and grossly mimic a primary colorectal carcinoma (see Chapter 24).

The Appendix

The appendix is a true diverticulum of the cecum. Its histology is the same as that of the colon from which it arises, although the submucosal lymphoid tissue is particularly robust, especially in childhood.

APPENDICITIS

The most important disease of the appendix is acute appendicitis (Fig. 19-81). This may occur at any age, but children and adults over 60 are most affected. The familiar presenting sign is right lower quadrant pain, which, if not treated, is followed by signs of peritoneal inflammation. Treatment is surgical removal. Despite its common occurrence, the genesis of appendicitis remains largely mysterious. In many there appears to be some component of luminal obstruction by lumps of fecal concretions known as fecaliths. However,

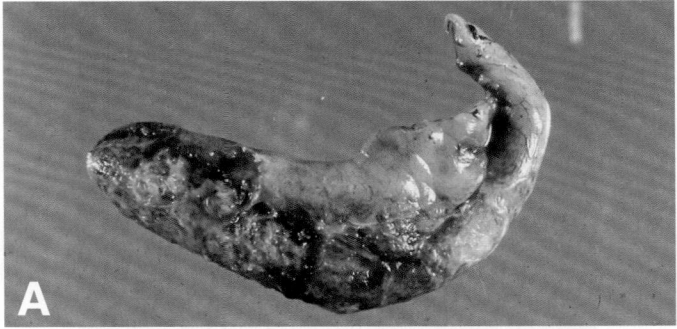

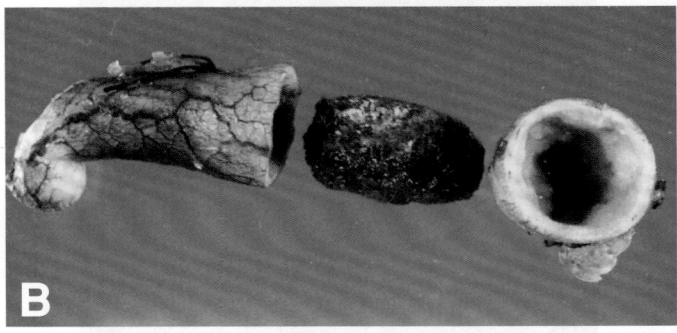

FIGURE 19-81. Acute appendicitis. A. The distal appendix is dilated, congested and partly covered by fibrin in this case of **appendicitis**. **B.** The lumen in this case of appendicitis was dilated owing to a large **fecalith**.

these are often not present. On occasion, a specific infectious agent is identified, such as *Yersinia, Actinomyces,* or *Campylobacter.* In some children, a tangle of pinworms (*Enterobius vermicularis*) may contribute to luminal obstruction.

However, in most cases, there is no apparent-specific infectious agent. There is often a mucosal erosion or ulceration, followed by a transmural infiltrate of neutrophils which can extend into the periappendiceal fat or penetrate the serosa and cause perforation. Periappendicitis without appendicitis can also reflect secondary involvement of the appendix from an external source, such as pelvic inflammatory disease involving the ovary or fallopian tube.

Granulomatous appendicitis may represent involvement by Crohn disease (see above) or an infectious agent. However, most granulomas involving the appendix involve neither of these entities and are of unknown cause and significance.

A **mucocele** is a distended appendix filled with mucinous material. Rarely these are due to inflammation causing focal luminal obstruction; these lesions rarely exceed 2 cm in diameter. More commonly, a dilated mucin-filled appendix reflects a neoplastic process (see below).

APPENDICEAL NEOPLASMS

Appendiceal NETs Are Generally Benign

Neuroendocrine tumors are common in the appendix. Most such tumors are quite small and benign and are found incidentally at the time of appendectomy. Abundant empirical data show that small (<1.5 cm) NETs of the appendix are of no clinical significance.

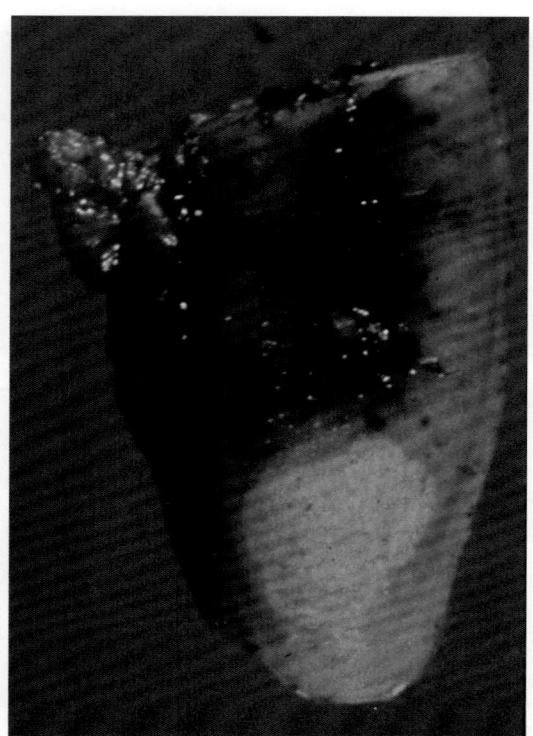

FIGURE 19-82. An oval yellow 1.1-cm **neuroendocrine tumor** was found incidentally in this appendix removed for appendicitis.

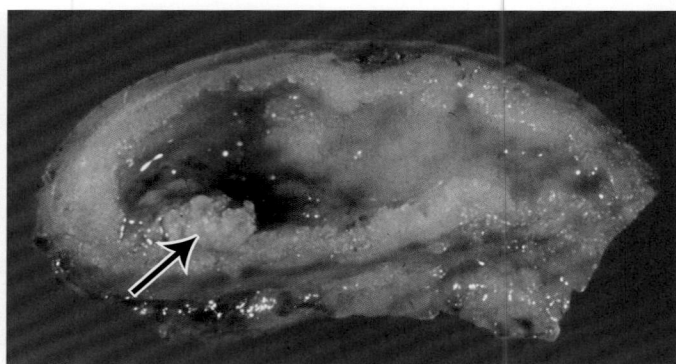

FIGURE 19-83. This appendiceal **mucinous neoplasm** (*arrow*) has led to the dilatation of the appendix by massive mucin production.

Most NETs of the appendix arise from endocrine cells. These tumors are almost always under 1 cm in diameter. At this size, the behavior of these tumors is invariably clinically benign. They tend to be oval and located at the tip of the appendix (Fig. 19-82). Tumors between 1 and 2 cm in diameter show a low rate of metastasis (about 1%). Larger lesions are increasingly aggressive.

Epithelial Tumors Are the Most Clinically Important Appendiceal Neoplasms

A variety of benign and malignant epithelial polyps and neoplasms affect the appendix. Some lesions resemble adenomas, hyperplastic polyps, and sessile serrated adenomas of the colon.

Appendiceal mucinous neoplasms may arise from progressive growth of adenomatous lesions which dilate the lumen as mucin accumulates (Fig. 19-83). The neoplastic epithelial lining of these lesions is that of low-grade adenomatous dysplasia (Fig. 19-84A,B). Mucin can infiltrate the wall of the appendix and eventually lead to appendiceal perforation. When this happens, abundant mucin admixed with dysplastic tumor cells may fill the peritoneal cavity, causing a lesion known as **pseudomyxoma peritonei** (Fig. 19-85). Some consider ovarian mucinous tumors to be another potential origin for pseudomyxoma, but experience has shown that most patients have an appendiceal primary.

Conventional appendiceal adenocarcinomas histologically resembling their colonic counterparts are less common but have been described.

The Anus

The anal canal extends from the level of the pelvic floor to the proximal margin of the anal verge. It is about 4 cm long and is divided into three parts, based on its lining epithelium: the colorectal zone (lined by glandular mucosa), the transition zone (varying, transitional mucosa) and the distal, squamous zone (lined by squamous mucosa). The dentate (pectinate) line (formed by the anal valves, roughly midway through the anal canal) is easily identified, and the superior border of the anal canal may be defined as 2 cm above this line. The internal sphincter of the anal canal is continuous with the muscularis of the rectum. The external anal sphincter is the major mechanism by which bowel continence is maintained. It surrounds the anal canal with a layer of skeletal muscle.

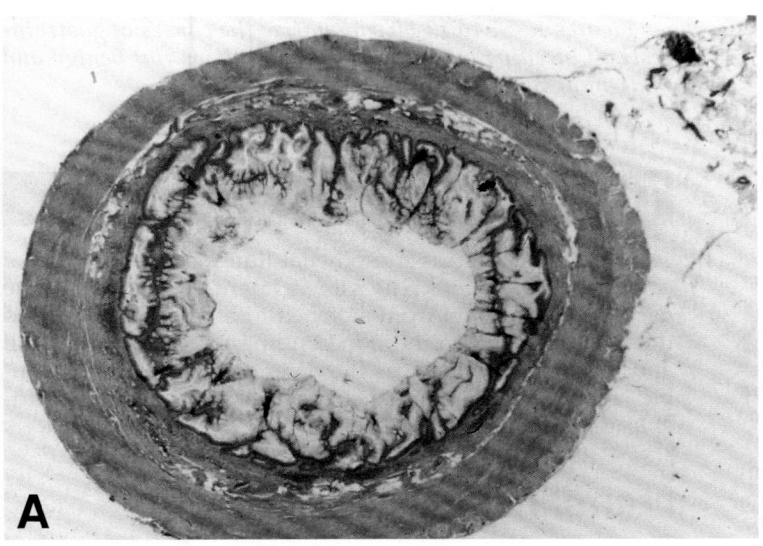 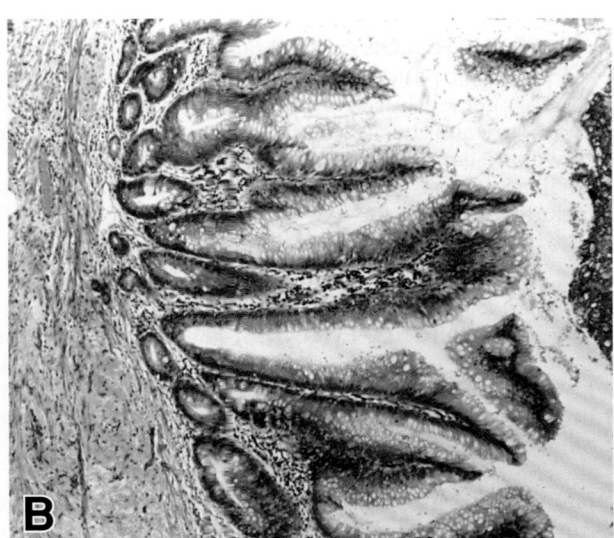

FIGURE 19-84. A. The mucinous neoplasm here encircles the entire lumen. **B.** At higher power its peculiar villous configuration is appreciated.

BENIGN LESIONS OF THE ANAL CANAL

Hemorrhoids Are Dilated Venous Channels of the Hemorrhoidal Plexuses

They result from downward displacement of the anal cushions. Internal hemorrhoids arise from the superior hemorrhoidal plexus above the dentate (pectinate) line. They are covered by rectal or transitional mucosa. External hemorrhoids originate from the inferior hemorrhoidal plexus, below that line, and are covered by squamous mucosa. *Hemorrhoids affect at least 5% of people in Western countries (likely a gross underestimate since most people treat themselves for this condition).* They are most common in whites between 45 and 65 years old. Pregnancy is another risk factor, presumably related to increased abdominal pressure.

 PATHOLOGY: Hemorrhoids are dilated vascular spaces with excess smooth muscle in their walls. Hemorrhage and thrombosis are common.

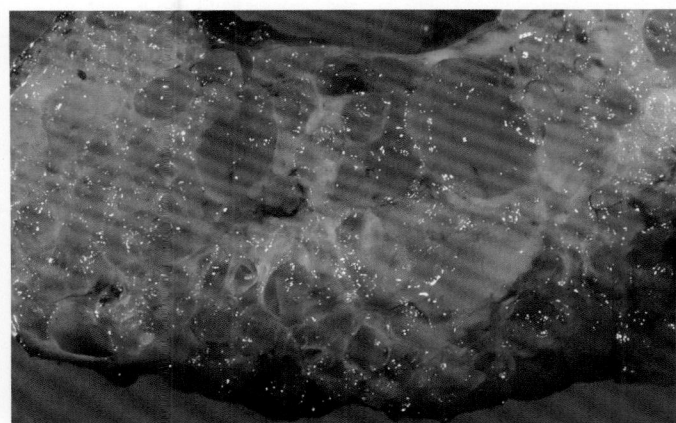

FIGURE 19-85. This large mass of mucin was removed from the abdomen of a patient with **pseudomyxoma peritonei** due to a mucinous tumor of the appendix.

 CLINICAL FEATURES: Hemorrhoids cause painless rectal bleeding associated with bowel movements. While chronic blood loss may lead to **iron-deficiency anemia,** other causes must be ruled out before it is attributed to hemorrhoidal bleeding. **Rectal prolapse** is common and may cause perineal irritation or anal itching. Prolapsed hemorrhoids may become irreducible and lead to painful, strangulated hemorrhoids. **Thrombosed** external hemorrhoids are exquisitely painful and require evacuation of the offending clots. Hemorrhoids are treated with dietary and lifestyle modifications aimed at improving the quality of stools and reducing straining on the toilet. Medical and surgical interventions are also available.

Anal Condylomata Acuminata (Anal Warts) Are Related to HPV Infection

These lesions are typically benign but may potentially develop into squamous cancers.

PATHOLOGY: Condylomas have a cauliflower-like growth pattern of papillary excrescences lined by squamous epithelium that is often hyperkeratotic. The squamous cells show characteristic koilocytic change, with enlarged nuclei, irregular nuclear contours, and perinuclear cytoplasmic clearing. Condylomas can develop dysplasia—graded mild, moderate, or severe, similar to the grading scheme in the cervix (see Chapter 24).

MALIGNANT TUMORS OF THE ANAL CANAL

Anal Canal Cancers Are Mostly Squamous Cell Carcinomas

These cancers, while increasing in frequency, are relatively uncommon; their incidence is 1.4 per 100,000. They are more common in women than in men. In the highest-risk group, people who practice anal-receptive intercourse, incidence approaches 35 per 100,000.

PATHOLOGY: Anal cancers have various histologic patterns (e.g., squamous or basaloid [cloacogenic]). But all tumor types tend to behave similarly and so are simply classified as **squamous cell carcinomas. Bowen disease of the anus** is squamous carcinoma in situ. Anal carcinomas spread directly into surrounding tissues, including internal and external sphincters, perianal soft tissues, the prostate, and the vagina.

 CLINICAL FEATURES: The major risk factor for anal squamous cell carcinoma is infection with HPV. Other risk factors include HIV infection, immunosuppression in organ transplantation, presence of an immune disorder, and smoking.

The usual symptom of anal cancers is bleeding, but pain and/or a palpable mass are also possible. Often a tumor is not first recognized as malignant and may be discovered only in a hemorrhoidectomy specimen. Combined chemotherapy and radiation therapy is the customary treatment, although abdominal–perineal resection is sometimes used. The 5-year survival rate averages 75%, but patients with more advanced tumors (greater size, lymph, node and/or distant metastases) do worse.

Extramammary Paget Disease May Involve the Anus

Paget disease is classically described in the breast (Chapter 25) but also occurs elsewhere, including the anogenital region. It can be primary when it arises from the epidermis or secondary if it is associated with an underlying adenocarcinoma.

 PATHOLOGY: Grossly involved areas may appear normal or be erythematous, scaly or ulcerated. The epidermis often shows reactive changes including hyperplasia and hyperkeratosis. The hallmark finding is malignant cells with pale, granular, or vacuolated cytoplasm scattered throughout the epidermis (Fig. 19-86).

Figures 19-87 to 19-90 summarize the causes of gastrointestinal bleeding and obstruction and the major benign and malignant tumors of the gastrointestinal tract.

The Peritoneum

The peritoneum is the mesothelial lining of the abdominal cavity and its viscera. The visceral peritoneum invests the gastrointestinal tract from stomach to rectum and encircles the liver. The parietal peritoneum lines the abdominal wall and retroperitoneal space. The omentum, which has a double layer of peritoneum, encloses blood vessels and a variable amount of fat.

PERITONITIS

Bacterial Peritonitis Is Usually Caused by Intestinal Organisms

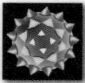 **ETIOLOGIC FACTORS:** *PERFORATION: The most common cause of bacterial peritonitis is perforation of an abdominal viscus* (e.g., an inflamed appendix, peptic ulcer, or colonic diverticulum). Peritonitis results in an acute abdomen, with severe abdominal pain and tenderness. Nausea, vomiting, and a high fever are usual. In severe cases, paralytic ileus and septic shock (see Chapter 12) ensue. Often the perforation is "walled off," in which case a peritoneal abscess results.

Bacteria released into the peritoneal cavity from the gastrointestinal tract vary according to the site of perforation and the duration of the peritonitis. Diverse aerobic and anaerobic species usually participate, including *E. coli, Bacteroides* sp., various *Streptococcus* sp., and *Clostridium*. Despite antibiotic treatment, surgical drainage and supportive measures, generalized peritonitis still carries substantial mortality and is especially dangerous in the elderly.

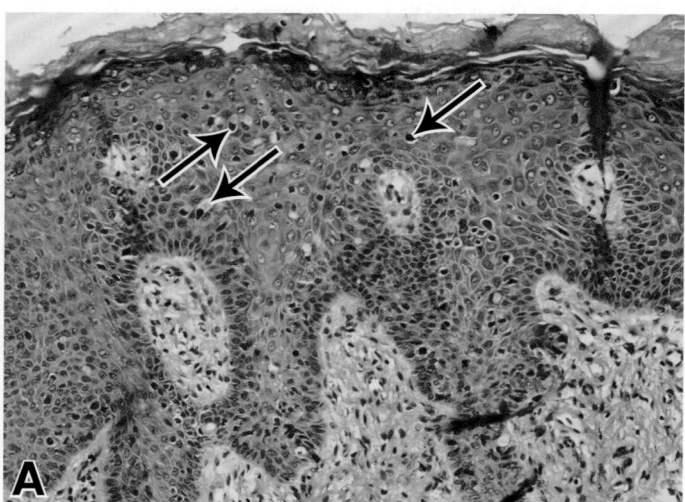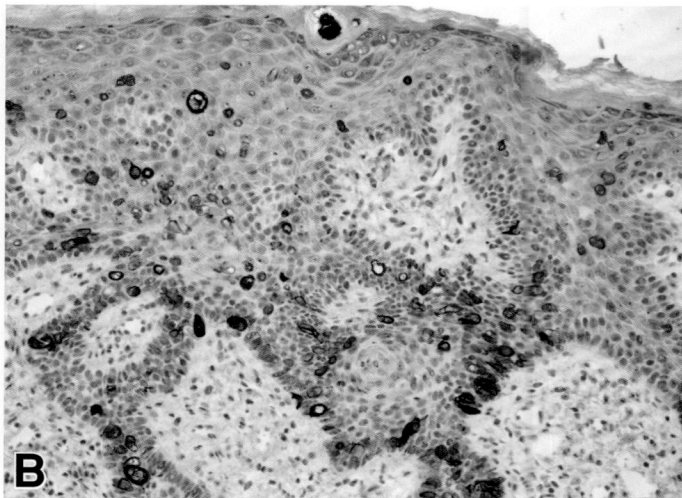

FIGURE 19-86. Paget disease of the anal canal. A. Microscopic image showing squamous epithelium with scattered malignant cells with pale or vacuolated cytoplasm seen throughout the epidermis (*arrows*). **B.** Immunohistochemical stain for CK20 highlights the malignant cells.

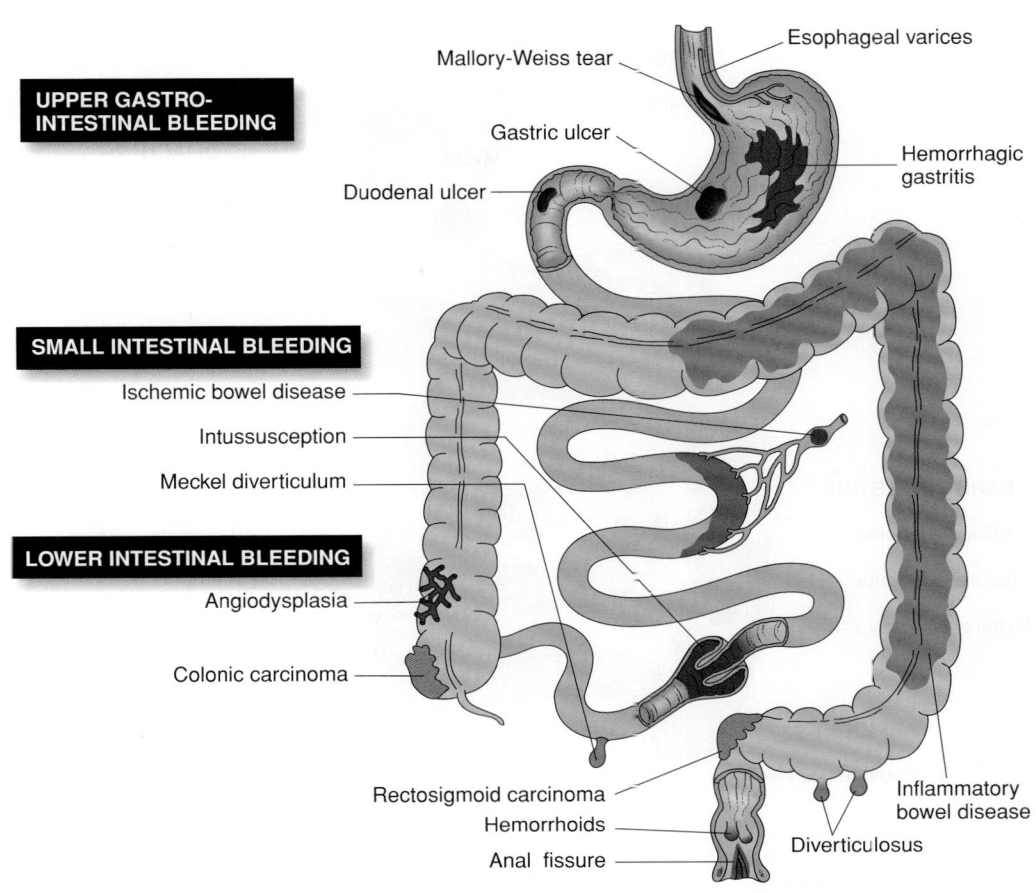

FIGURE 19-87. Causes of gastrointestinal bleeding.

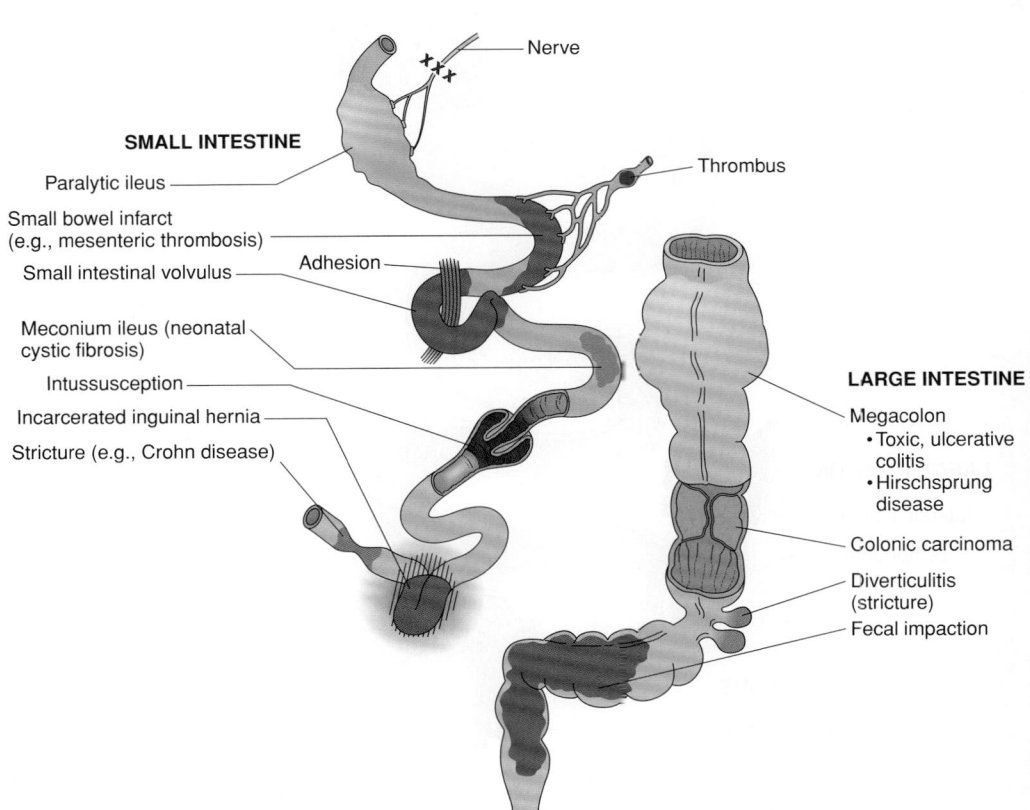

FIGURE 19-88. Causes of gastrointestinal obstruction.

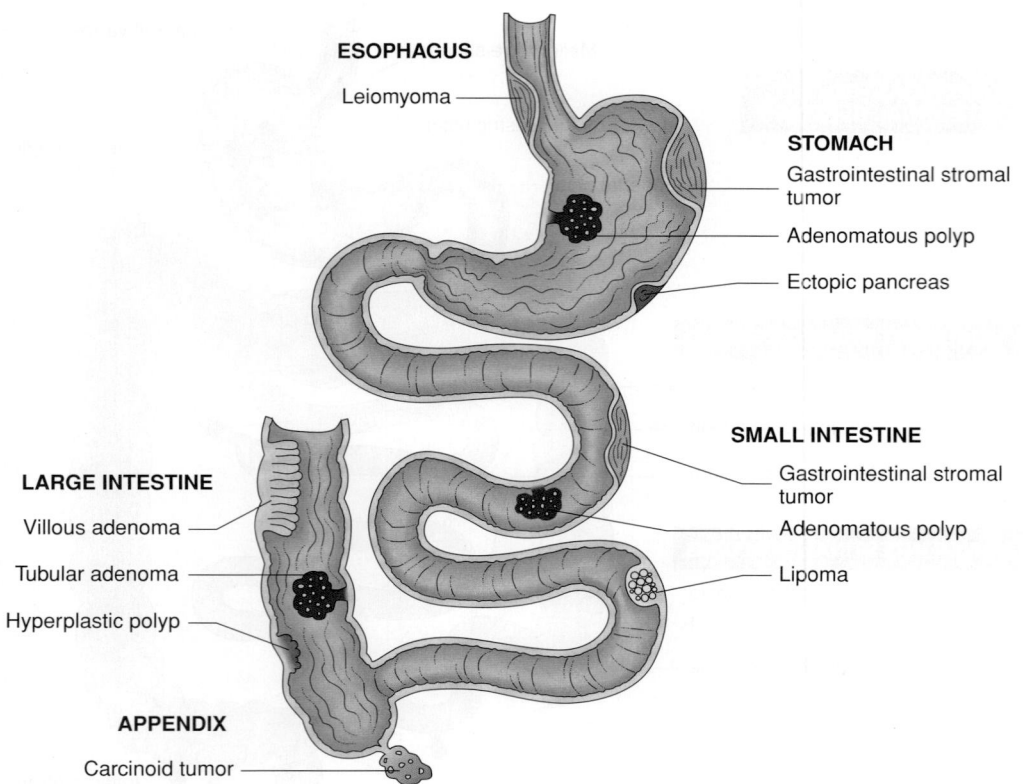

FIGURE 19-89. Major benign tumors of the gastrointestinal tract.

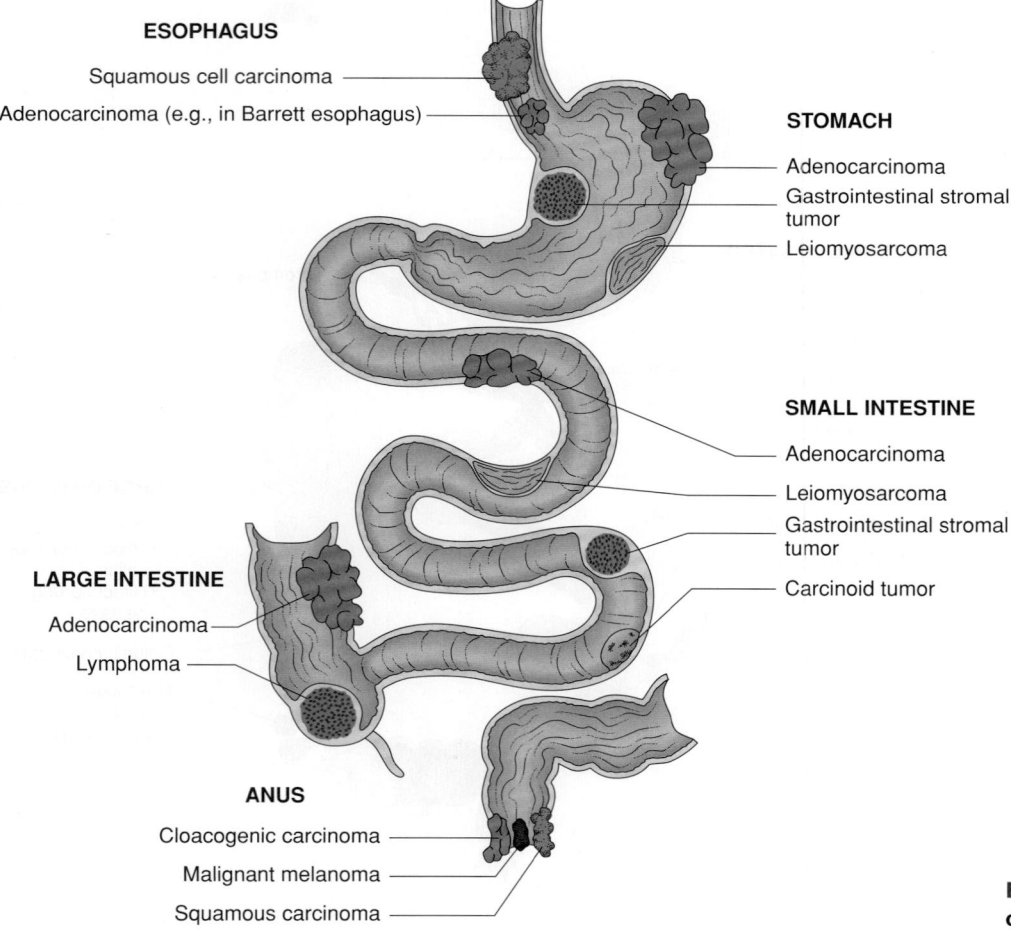

FIGURE 19-90. Major malignant tumors of the gastrointestinal tract.

PERITONEAL DIALYSIS: Chronic peritoneal dialysis is a frequent cause of bacterial peritonitis, due to contamination of instruments or dialysate. The clinical course is usually milder than with a perforated viscus; *Staphylococcus* and *Streptococcus* spp. are most often responsible. Chronic dialysis can also cause aseptic peritonitis, presumably due to a chemical in the dialysate to which the peritoneum is sensitive.

SPONTANEOUS BACTERIAL PERITONITIS: Sometimes, peritoneal infection lacks a clear cause. *Such spontaneous bacterial peritonitis occurs most often in adults with cirrhosis complicated by portal hypertension and ascites* (see Chapter 20). Enteric organisms, mainly gram-negative bacilli, appear to move from the gut to mesenteric lymph nodes. From there, they seed the ascitic fluid, where phagocytic and antibacterial activities are low.

In children, spontaneous bacterial peritonitis can complicate the **nephrotic syndrome** (see Chapter 22). Spontaneous peritonitis in children is mostly due to gram-negative organisms, usually from urinary tract infections. The disease causes symptoms of an acute abdomen and usually leads to surgical intervention, unless the child is known to have nephrotic syndrome. Even with antibiotic treatment, mortality is 5% to 10%.

TUBERCULOUS PERITONITIS: Tuberculous peritonitis is rare in industrialized countries, but it may occur in developing countries. Many patients with tuberculous peritonitis do not have apparent pulmonary or miliary disease, which suggests that it represents activation of latent tuberculous foci in the peritoneum derived from previous hematogenous dissemination.

PATHOLOGY: Grossly, bacterial peritonitis resembles purulent infection elsewhere. A fibrinopurulent exudate rich in neutrophils covers the surface of the intestines. When it organizes, fibrinous and fibrous adhesions form between loops of bowel, which then adhere to each other. Such adhesions may eventually be lysed, or they may lead to **volvulus** and **intestinal obstruction**.

Chemical Peritonitis Usually Results From Endogenous Sources

- **Bile peritonitis** occurs when bile enters the peritoneum, usually from a perforated gallbladder but sometimes from needle biopsy of the liver. This abrupt insult may lead to shock.
- **Hydrochloric acid or hemorrhage** from a perforated peptic ulcer of the stomach or duodenum may elicit an inflammatory reaction in the peritoneum.
- In **acute pancreatitis**, activated lipolytic and proteolytic enzymes are released into the peritoneum, where they cause severe peritonitis with fat necrosis. Shock is common and may be lethal unless it is adequately treated.
- **Foreign materials** introduced by surgery (e.g., talc) or by trauma are unusual causes of chemical peritonitis.
- **Leakage of urine** can produce ascites.

NEOPLASMS OF THE PERITONEUM

Mesenteric and Omental Cysts Are Usually of Lymphatic Origin

They may also derive from other embryonic tissues. Usually a slowly enlarging, painless mass is discovered in a child older than 10 years. The cyst may come to medical attention because of rupture, bleeding, torsion, or intestinal obstruction. Surgical excision is curative.

Malignant Peritoneal Mesotheliomas Are Rare, Aggressive Tumors

One-quarter of mesotheliomas arise in the peritoneum. *Like pleural mesotheliomas, most of these malignant tumors are associated with exposure to asbestos.* Pathologic characteristics of peritoneal mesotheliomas are identical to those of their pleural counterparts (see Chapter 18).

Primary Peritoneal Carcinomas Resemble Ovarian Carcinoma

Primary peritoneal carcinomas present as tumor masses involving the omentum and peritoneum. They are morphologically identical to serous carcinomas of the ovary, except that in primary peritoneal carcinomas, the ovaries are normal (see Chapter 24).

The Most Common Malignancies of the Peritoneum are Metastatic Carcinomas

Ovarian, gastric, and pancreatic carcinomas are particularly likely to seed the peritoneum, but any intra-abdominal malignancy can spread to the peritoneum.

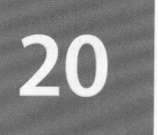

20 The Liver and Biliary System

Arief A. Suriawinata, Swan N. Thung

The Liver

ANATOMY

The liver arises from the embryonic foregut as an endodermal bud that differentiates into the hepatic diverticulum. Strands of endodermal cells mingle with proliferating mesenchymal cells to form the adult liver, gallbladder, and extrahepatic bile ducts.

The liver weighs about 1,500 g in an average adult man and is in the right upper quadrant of the abdomen, just below the diaphragm. It has two lobes, a larger **right lobe** and a smaller **left lobe,** which meet at the level of the gallbladder bed. Inferiorly, the right lobe has lesser segments, the **caudate** and **quadrate lobes.** The **gallbladder** lies inferiorly, in a fossa of the right hepatic lobe, and extends a little below the inferior margin of the liver.

The liver has a dual blood supply: (1) the **hepatic artery,** a branch of the celiac axis, and (2) the **hepatic portal vein,** formed when the splenic and superior mesenteric veins join. The **hepatic veins** empty into the inferior vena cava, which is partly surrounded by the posterior surface of the liver. Hepatic lymphatics drain mainly into porta hepatis and celiac lymph nodes.

The right and left hepatic ducts merge to form the **hepatic duct,** which joins the cystic duct from the gallbladder to make the **common bile duct.** The latter meets the pancreatic duct just before emptying into the duodenum. It terminates in the ampulla of Vater, where its lumen is guarded by the sphincter of Oddi.

The Lobule Is the Basic Unit of the Liver

Liver lobules are polyhedral (Figs. 20-1 and 20-2), classically depicted as hexagons. **Portal triads** (or portal tracts) are

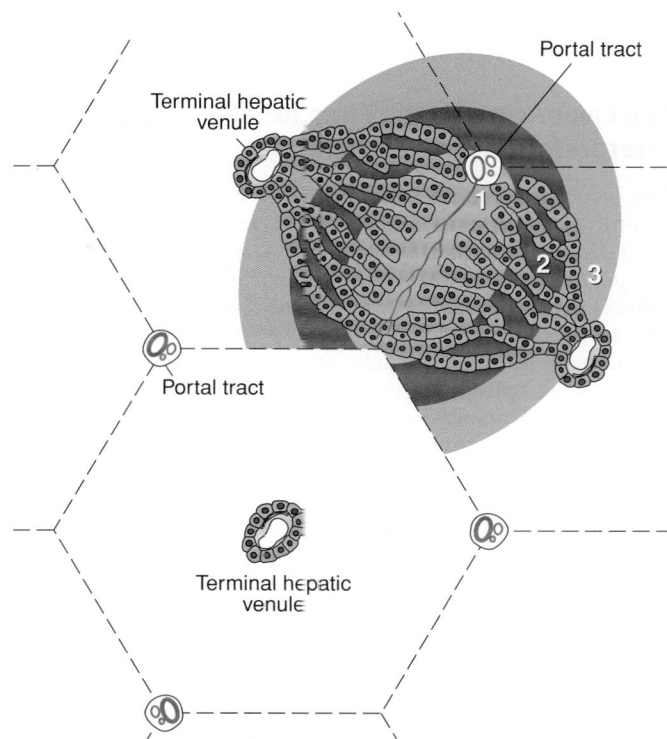

FIGURE 20-2. Morphologic and functional concepts of the liver lobule. In the classic *morphologic* liver lobule, the periphery of the hexagonal lobule is anchored in the portal tracts, and the terminal hepatic venule is in the center. The *functional* liver lobule is an acinus derived from the gradients of oxygen and nutrients in the sinusoidal blood. In this scheme, the portal tract, with the richest content of oxygen and nutrients, is in the center (zone 1). The region most distant from the portal tract (zone 3) is poor in oxygen and nutrients and surrounds the terminal hepatic venule. The white numbers identify the locations of these zones.

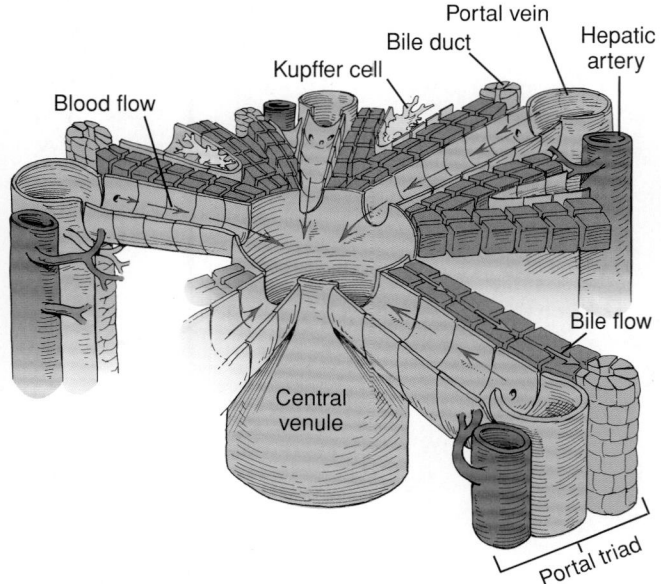

FIGURE 20-1. Microanatomy of the liver. The classic lobule is composed of portal triads, hepatic sinuses, a terminal hepatic venule (central venule) and associated plates of hepatocytes. *Red arrows* indicate the direction of sinusoidal blood flow. *Green arrows* show the direction of bile flow. (From Ross MH, Pawlina W. *Histology: A Text and Atlas.* 6th ed. Philadelphia, PA: Lippincott Williams & Wilkins, 2011: 636.)

peripheral, at the angles of the polygon, and contain intrahepatic branches of the (1) **bile ducts,** (2) **hepatic artery,** and (3) **portal vein.** Portal tracts are invested by the **limiting plate,** a layer of adjacent hepatocytes. The **central venule** (or, **terminal hepatic venule**) is at the center of the lobule. Radiating from it are **one-cell-thick plates of hepatocytes,** which extend to the edge of the lobule, where they are continuous with plates of other lobules. Between plates of hepatocytes are **hepatic sinusoids,** which are lined by endothelial cells, Kupffer cells, and stellate cells.

The hepatic artery and portal vein enter the liver at the porta hepatis and eventually divide into the small interlobular branches in the portal triads. From there, interlobular vessels distribute blood into hepatic sinusoids, where it flows centripetally toward the central venule. Central venules coalesce into sublobular veins, which eventually merge into the hepatic veins.

Bile is secreted by hepatocytes into **bile canaliculi.** These are formed by apposed lateral surfaces of contiguous hepatocytes. Bile flows in a direction opposite to that of the blood. Contraction of the bile canaliculus by the hepatocyte pericanalicular cytoskeleton propels bile toward the portal tract. From canaliculi, bile flows into canals of Hering, to **bile ductules,** or **cholangioles,** at the border of portal tracts. It then enters a branch of the **intrahepatic bile ducts.** Within each liver lobe, smaller bile ducts progressively merge, eventually forming right and left hepatic ducts.

The Liver Acinus Is the Functional Interpretation of the Lobule

The structural lobule described above is arranged around a central venule and reflects the liver's histologic appearance. *However, a functional unit can be conceptualized with the portal tract at the center* (Fig. 20-2). Such a construct reflects the functional gradients within lobules. That is, oxygen, nutrients, etc., delivered by the blood are most concentrated near the portal tracts, then progressively decline as hepatocytes extract these materials from the blood going through the sinusoids toward the central venule. Such a construct allows for concentric functional zones. **Zone 1** is the most highly oxygenated zone, around portal tracts. **Zone 3** surrounds central venules and is oxygen-poor. **Zone 2** is intermediate and midlobular. Ischemic injury usually affects zone 3 first. Differences between hepatocytes are not limited to blood flow. The acinus is also heterogeneous with respect to metabolism, independent of oxygenation. In particular,

toxic injury is often prominent in zone 3, which is enriched in hepatocyte enzymes that perform drug detoxification and biotransformation. For convenience, pathologic changes in the liver are usually designated in relation to the classic histologic lobule. For example, centrilobular necrosis describes a lesion around central venules, and periportal fibrosis occurs at the periphery of the classic lobule.

Hepatocytes Carry Out the Major Functions of the Liver

Hepatocytes comprise 60% of liver cells and about 90% of the organ's volume. They are roughly 30 μm across and have three specialized surfaces: **sinusoidal, lateral,** and **canalicular**. Each cell has two sinusoidal surfaces, with numerous slender microvilli. Hepatocyte sinusoidal surfaces are separated from the endothelial cells that line sinusoids by the **space of Disse** (Fig. 20-3). Canalicular surfaces of adjacent hepatocytes form the **bile canaliculus,** which is actually an intercellular space without a separate wall. Along this surface, microvilli extend into the lumen. Tight junctions between adjacent hepatocytes prevent bile leakage from

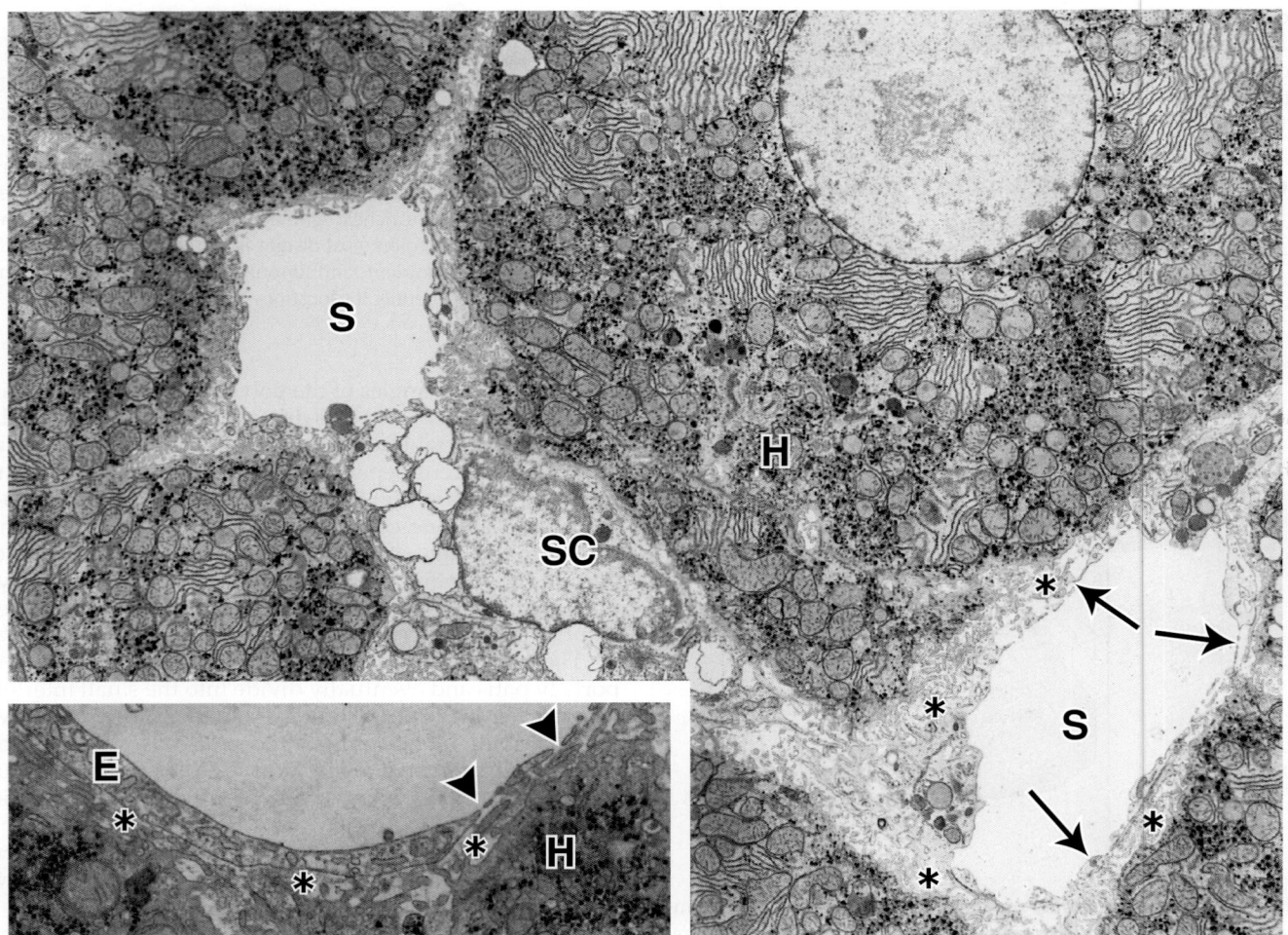

FIGURE 20-3. Hepatic sinusoids and space of Disse. An electron micrograph illustrates the relationship between hepatocytes (*H*), sinusoids (*S*), the space of Disse (indicate by *asterisks)* and hepatic stellate cells (*SC*). The *arrows* indicate endothelial cells lining the space of Disse. *Inset.* The relationship between hepatocytes (*H*) and endothelial cells (*E*). The *arrowheads* indicate fenestrae in endothelial cells; the *asterisks* are in the space of Disse.

canaliculi. Lateral, or intercellular, surfaces of adjacent hepatocytes are in close contact and contain gap junctions composed mainly of connexin32 (Cx32).

Centrally placed, occasionally multiple, hepatocyte nuclei are spherical, with one or more nucleoli. Most are diploid, but tetraploid and octaploid nuclei are common. The cytoplasm is rich in organelles, with prominent rough and smooth endoplasmic reticulum (SER), Golgi complexes, mitochondria, lysosomes, and peroxisomes. In addition, in the fed state, abundant glycogen and occasional fat droplets are evident.

Blood Traverses the Liver Through Hepatic Sinusoids

Sinusoids contain three cell types: endothelial, Kupffer, and stellate cells.

ENDOTHELIAL CELLS: Endothelial cells line sinusoids and are penetrated by many holes, or **fenestrae** (Fig. 20-3). Adjacent endothelial cells do not form junctions in the liver, and there are many gaps between them. The result is a sieve-like structure that provides free communication between the sinusoidal lumen and the space of Disse. There is no basement membrane between endothelial cells and hepatocytes, further facilitating access of sinusoidal plasma to hepatocytes.

KUPFFER CELLS: Kupffer cells are macrophages, found in gaps between adjacent endothelial cells or on their surfaces (Fig. 20-1). Because they derive from bone marrow, the Kupffer cells that repopulate transplanted livers are from the recipient, not the donor. Like other macrophages, they protect against infection and circulating toxins (e.g., endotoxin), but with higher efficiency. Activated Kupffer cells also release cytokines, such as TNFα, interleukins, interferons, and TGFs α and β.

STELLATE CELLS: Stellate cells (also known as Ito cells) are occasionally seen beneath endothelial cells in the space of Disse and have specialized storage capacities. They contain fat, vitamin A, and other lipid-soluble vitamins. Stellate cells also secrete extracellular matrix components, including collagens, laminin, and proteoglycans. In some diseases, they make these matrix molecules in great excess, leading to hepatic fibrosis and eventually cirrhosis.

The most abundant extracellular matrix component in the space of Disse is fibronectin. Bundles of type I collagen fibers provide a scaffold for liver lobules.

FUNCTIONS OF THE LIVER

Hepatocytes Serve Myriad Functions

Hepatocytes perform metabolic, synthetic, storage, catabolic, and excretory functions.

METABOLIC FUNCTIONS: The liver is a center of **glucose homeostasis** and responds rapidly to fluctuations in blood glucose levels. After feeding, excess blood glucose is shunted to the liver to be stored as glycogen. During fasting, blood glucose levels are stabilized by hepatic **glycogenolysis** and **gluconeogenesis**. For the latter, the liver uses amino acids, lactate, and glycerol. Amino acid nitrogen is converted to urea. Free fatty acids are taken up by the liver and oxidized to produce energy, or are converted to triglycerides and secreted as **lipoproteins** to be used elsewhere.

SYNTHETIC FUNCTIONS: Most serum proteins are synthesized in the liver. **Albumin** is the main source of plasma osmotic pressure; in chronic liver disease, decreased albumin causes edema and ascites. Blood **clotting factors,** including prothrombin and fibrinogen, are produced by hepatocytes. Severe and often life-threatening bleeding may thus complicate liver failure. Hepatic endothelial cells manufacture **factors V and VIII;** thus, hemophilia can be treated by liver transplantation. **Complement** and other "acute-phase reactants" (e.g., ferritin, C-reactive protein, serum amyloid A) are also secreted by the liver. Numerous specific **binding proteins** (such as those for iron, copper, and vitamin A) are also made by the liver.

STORAGE FUNCTIONS: The liver stores glycogen, triglycerides, iron, copper, and lipid-soluble vitamins. Severe liver disease can result from excessive storage—for example, abnormal glycogen deposition in type IV glycogenosis, excess iron in hemochromatosis, and copper in Wilson disease (WD).

CATABOLIC FUNCTIONS: The liver catabolizes many endogenous substances, such as hormones and serum proteins. As a result, in chronic liver disease, impaired elimination of estrogens causes feminization in men. The liver is also the principal **detoxifier of foreign compounds** such as drugs, industrial chemicals, environmental contaminants and, perhaps, products of intestinal bacterial metabolism

Ammonia from amino acid metabolism is mainly removed by the liver. Serum ammonia increases in liver failure and is used as a marker for this condition.

EXCRETORY FUNCTIONS: The principal excretory product of the liver is **bile,** an aqueous mixture of conjugated bilirubin, bile acids, phospholipids, cholesterol, and electrolytes. Bile is a repository for the products of heme catabolism and is vital for fat absorption in the small intestine. Normal bile production is critical for eliminating environmental toxins, carcinogens and drugs and their metabolites.

Regeneration Is a Unique Characteristic of the Liver

Liver size is normally maintained within narrow limits, relative to body size. If there is substantial loss of liver tissue (e.g., after mechanical, toxic, or viral insult), the organ regrows from the undamaged tissue, a process called **liver regeneration**. Hepatocytes, which are normally in a fully differentiated, quiescent state (G₀), reenter the cell cycle for as many synchronized rounds of replication as are needed to recover the organ's original size. Uniquely, the liver maintains its differentiated functions during this process. Little is known about how this process is triggered or how the liver recognizes when it has reattained its normal size and architecture. *Conditions that interfere with regeneration may cause permanent liver dysfunction and may bring about liver failure.*

Several phases are distinguished in liver regeneration:

- **Priming:** Liver tissue recognizes that damage has occurred and that remaining functional parenchymal cells must transition from their peaceful G₀ state to enter the cell cycle. This process, called *priming,* entails expression of many genes, especially transcription factors which are required to drive cell cycling (see Chapter 5). Priming also requires the release of TNFα, IL-6, and other cytokines.
- **Progression to mitosis:** In the next phase, the cell progresses through G₁ into S phase, where DNA synthesis occurs. This is followed by G₂ and M phases, where cell division occurs. Several growth factors drive this part of the process, including hepatocyte growth factor

(HGF/SF), epidermal growth factor (EGF), TGFα, and others. Several growth factors (e.g., HGF, IL-6) promote protection of the liver and survival in various models of hepatic injury. After one or two rounds (depending on need) of mitosis, hepatocytes become quiescent again and resume normal function.

- **Nonparenchymal and progenitor cells:** In the final phase, nonparenchymal cells (sinusoidal endothelium, Kupffer cells, stellate cells, and biliary epithelium) replicate. The tissue remodels to recover the original structure of liver cell plates.

Hepatic progenitor cells ("oval cells"), which lie within the terminal branches of bile ductules and canals of Hering, contribute to ductular proliferation after extensive hepatic necrosis. However, the role of these cells in hepatic regeneration is unclear, as is any involvement of bone marrow–derived stem cells (see Chapter 3).

BILIRUBIN METABOLISM AND MECHANISMS OF JAUNDICE

Bilirubin Is the End-Product of Heme Catabolism

About 80% of this heme comes from senescent erythrocytes, removed by mononuclear phagocytes of the spleen, bone marrow, and liver from the circulation. The remainder of the heme comes from other sources, including cytochrome P450 isoenzymes, myoglobin, and premature breakdown of erythroid progenitors in the bone marrow. Beyond this, no specific physiologic role for bilirubin is known.

Bilirubin dissolves poorly in water but is quite miscible with fat. Thus, in the circulation, it is transported bound to albumin. The albumin in the blood and extracellular space is a large reservoir for binding bilirubin, ensuring a low extracellular concentration of free (unbound) bilirubin. Bilirubin that is not bound to albumin or conjugated to glucuronic acid easily enters the lipid-rich brain. There, it is very toxic, and high concentrations of it in newborns causes irreversible brain injury, **kernicterus**.

Transfer of bilirubin from blood to the bile involves four steps:

1. **Uptake:** The albumin–bilirubin complex is dissociated when it reaches hepatocytes, and the bilirubin is transported across the plasma membrane. Transporter proteins facilitate mostly passive uptake by hepatocytes.
2. **Binding:** Once inside hepatocytes, bilirubin binds to cytosolic proteins, known collectively as **glutathione S-transferases** (also termed *ligandin*).
3. **Conjugation:** Bilirubin is converted to a water-soluble glucuronic acid conjugate for excretion. This is done in the endoplasmic reticulum (ER), where the uridine diphosphate-glucuronyl transferase (UGT) system attaches glucuronic acid to bilirubin. The process yields mostly water-soluble bilirubin diglucuronide and a small amount (<10%) of monoglucuronide.
4. **Excretion:** Conjugated bilirubin diffuses through the cytosol to bile canaliculi and is excreted into the bile by an energy-dependent carrier-mediated process. This is the rate-limiting step in the transhepatic transport of bilirubin.

Conjugated bilirubin enters the small intestine as part of mixed micelles but is not absorbed there. It remains intact until

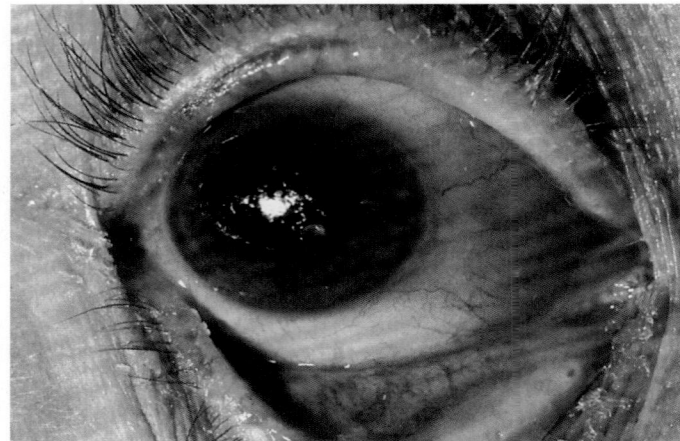

FIGURE 20-4. Jaundice. A patient in hepatic failure displays yellow sclerae.

it reaches the distal small bowel and colon, where it is hydrolyzed by bacterial flora into free (unconjugated) bilirubin, which is reduced to a mixture of pyrroles, collectively called **urobilinogen**. Most urobilinogen is excreted in feces, but a small amount is absorbed in the terminal ileum and colon, returned to the liver and reexcreted into the bile. Bile acids are also reabsorbed in the terminal ileum and salvaged by the liver. This recycling process is the **enterohepatic circulation of bile**. Some urobilinogen escapes reabsorption by the liver, reaches the systemic circulation and is excreted in the urine.

- **Hyperbilirubinemia** means increased blood levels of bilirubin (>1.0 mg/dL).
- **Jaundice** or **icterus** is yellow skin and sclerae (Fig. 20-4), the color becoming apparent when circulating bilirubin concentrations exceed 2.5 to 3.0 mg/dL.
- **Cholestasis** is pathologic plugging of dilated bile canaliculi by inspissated bile. Bile pigment, which is normally invisible, is seen in hepatocytes.
- **Cholestatic jaundice** is histologic cholestasis and hyperbilirubinemia. Many conditions are associated with hyperbilirubinemia (Fig. 20-5).

Overproduction of bilirubin, interference with its hepatic uptake or intracellular metabolism and impaired bile excretion and flow may all cause jaundice (Fig. 20-5).

Bilirubin Overproduction Can Lead to Unconjugated Hyperbilirubinemia

Increased production of free bilirubin results from enhanced destruction of erythrocytes (e.g., hemolytic anemia) or ineffective erythropoiesis. Rarely, erythrocyte breakdown in a large hematoma (e.g., after trauma) may also generate excess unconjugated bilirubin.

In adults, even severe hemolytic anemia does not lead to sustained increases in serum bilirubin above 4.0 mg/dL as long as hepatic bilirubin clearance is normal. However, prolonged hemolysis, as in sickle cell anemia, in the context of intrinsic liver disease, such as viral hepatitis, may cause extremely high blood bilirubin levels (up to 100 mg/dL) and pronounced jaundice.

Hyperbilirubinemia from uncomplicated hemolysis is mainly unconjugated bilirubin, whereas parenchymal liver disease causes elevation of both conjugated and

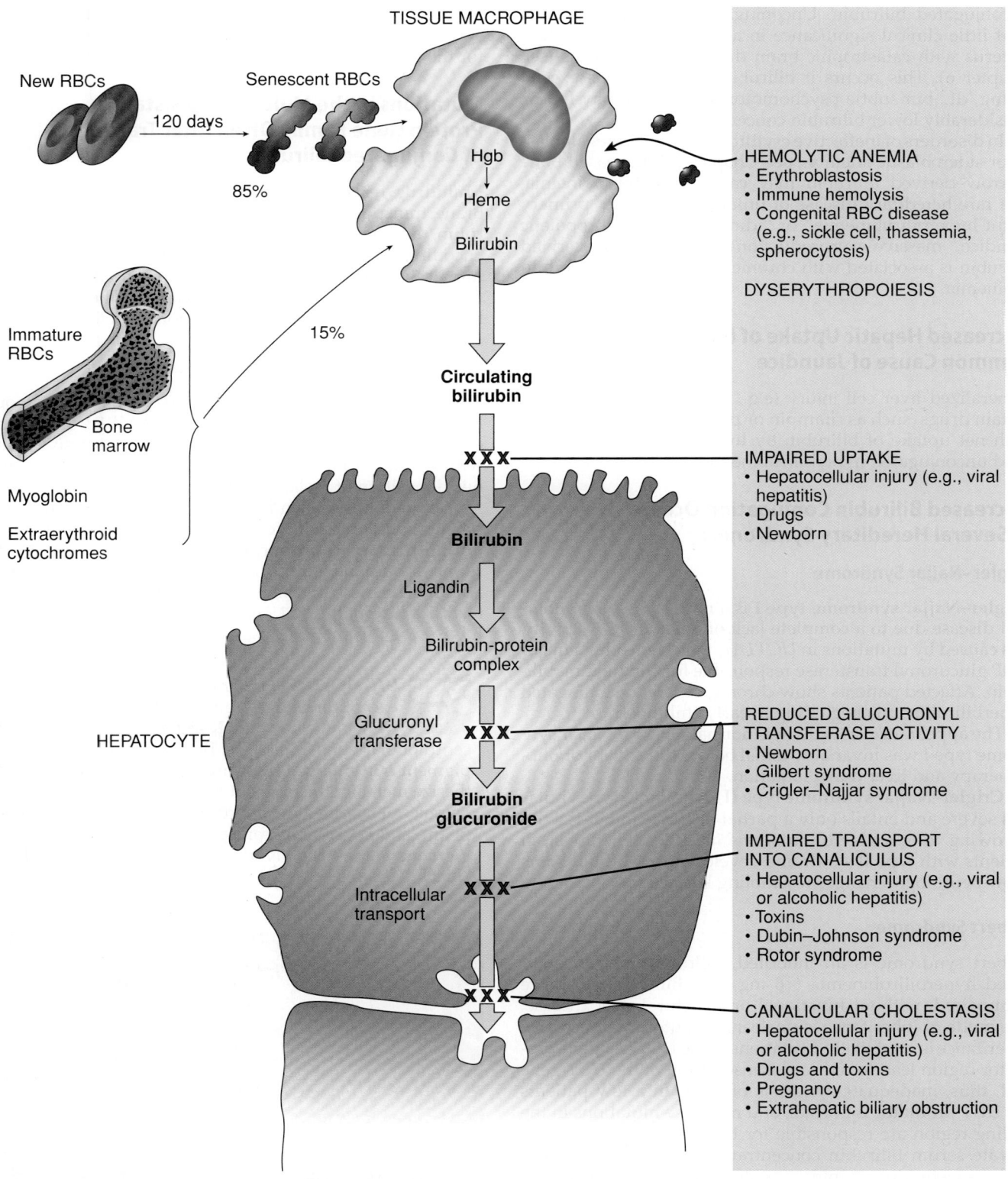

FIGURE 20-5. Mechanisms of hyperbilirubinemia at the level of the hepatocyte. Bilirubin is derived principally from catabolism of heme in senescent circulating red blood cells (RBCs), with a smaller contribution from the degradation of erythropoietic elements in the bone marrow, myoglobin, and extraerythroid cytochromes. Hyperbilirubinemia and jaundice result from overproduction of bilirubin (e.g., in hemolytic anemia), dyserythropoiesis, impaired bilirubin uptake or defects in its hepatic metabolism. The locations of specific blocks in the metabolic pathway of bilirubin in the hepatocyte are illustrated. *Hgb* = hemoglobin.

unconjugated bilirubin. Unconjugated hyperbilirubinemia is of little clinical significance in adults but can cause kernicterus with catastrophic brain damage in newborns (see Chapter 6). This occurs if bilirubin concentrations exceed 20 mg/dL, but subtle psychomotor retardation may follow considerably lower bilirubin concentrations.

In disorders of ineffective erythropoiesis (e.g., megaloblastic or sideroblastic anemias; see Chapter 20), increased bone marrow–derived bilirubin may cause hyperbilirubinemia. In a rare hereditary disease of unknown etiology, "primary shunt hyperbilirubinemia" or "idiopathic dyserythropoietic jaundice," massive overproduction of bone marrow–derived bilirubin is associated with chronic unconjugated hyperbilirubinemia.

Decreased Hepatic Uptake of Bilirubin Is a Common Cause of Jaundice

Generalized liver cell injury (e.g., due to viral hepatitis or certain drugs, such as rifampin or probenecid) may interfere with net uptake of bilirubin by liver cells. This can cause mild unconjugated hyperbilirubinemia.

Decreased Bilirubin Conjugation Occurs in Several Hereditary Syndromes

Crigler–Najjar Syndrome

Crigler–Najjar syndrome type I is a rare, recessively inherited disease due to a complete lack of hepatic UGT activity. It is caused by mutations in *UGT1A1*, which encodes a major UDP glucuronyl transferase responsible for conjugating bilirubin. Affected patients show chronic, severe, unconjugated hyperbilirubinemia beginning in early childhood.

The appearance of the liver is normal. Crigler–Najjar syndrome type I was invariably lethal before the advent of phototherapy and liver transplantation.

Crigler–Najjar syndrome type II is similar to type I but is less severe and entails only a partial decrease in UGT activity owing to less severe mutations in *UGT1A1*. Almost all patients with type II syndrome develop normally, but some show neurologic changes resembling kernicterus.

Gilbert Syndrome

Gilbert syndrome is an inherited, mild, chronic unconjugated hyperbilirubinemia (<6 mg/dL). Bilirubin clearance is impaired, without functional or structural liver disease. The mode of inheritance is unclear, but autosomal recessive inheritance is most likely. Mutations in the *UGT1A1* gene promotor region lead to reduced transcription of the *UGT* gene and, thus, inadequate synthesis of UGT. In a few patients the *UGT* promotor is normal, and missense mutations in the coding region are responsible for the disorder. Factors that elevate serum bilirubin concentrations in normal persons, such as fasting or an intercurrent illness, produce exaggerated increases in people with Gilbert syndrome. Mild hemolysis, which also tends to increase bilirubin levels, occurs in more than 1/2 of persons with Gilbert syndrome, but the mechanism is unclear.

Gilbert syndrome is exceptionally common, occurring in 5% to 10% of the population. It occurs more often in men than in women and is usually recognized after puberty. Differences and the age at onset and patient gender suggest that

hormones influence hepatic bilirubin metabolism. Gilbert syndrome is generally without clinical significance, except for the possibility that drug metabolism may be altered.

Mutations in the Multidrug Resistance Protein Gene Family Often Alter Transport of Conjugated Bilirubin

Multidrug resistance proteins (MRPs) mediate transmembrane transport of organic ions, including conjugated bilirubin, bile acids, and phospholipids. Mutations in genes encoding these proteins, or in other canalicular transporters, impair hepatocellular secretion of bilirubin glucuronides and other organic anions into canaliculi. The clinical spectrum of diseases varies from innocuous to lethal.

Dubin–Johnson Syndrome

This syndrome is caused by homozygous or compound heterozygous mutations in the *ABCC2/MRP2* gene, which encodes an MRP. It is a benign, autosomal recessive disease with chronic conjugated hyperbilirubinemia and conspicuous deposition of melanin-like pigment in the liver.

Dubin–Johnson syndrome can be distinguished from other conditions with conjugated hyperbilirubinemia by testing **urinary coproporphyrin excretion**. There are two forms of human coproporphyrins, **isomer I** and **isomer III**. A shift in the ratio of urinary coproporphyrin isomer I and III from 1:3 (normal) to 4:1 (abnormal) is diagnostic of Dubin–Johnson syndrome.

PATHOLOGY: Liver histology is entirely normal, except for coarse, iron-free, **dark-brown granules** in hepatocytes and Kupffer cells, mainly in the centrilobular zone (Fig. 20-6). By electron microscopy, the pigment is in enlarged lysosomes. As liver cells do not synthesize melanin, the pigment may reflect auto-oxidation of anionic metabolites (e.g., tyrosine, phenylalanine, tryptophan), and possibly of epinephrine. Accumulation of this pigment causes the liver to be grossly pigmented, or "black."

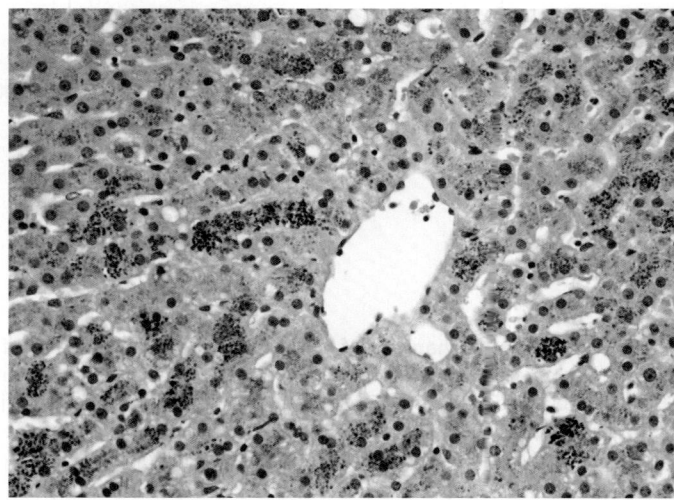

FIGURE 20-6. Dubin–Johnson syndrome. Hepatocytes contain coarse, iron-free, dark-brown granules.

> **CLINICAL FEATURES:** Symptoms are mild: slight intermittent jaundice and vague nonspecific complaints. Dark urine is present in 1/2 of those affected. In women, the disease may be diagnosed when jaundice appears with use of oral contraceptives or during pregnancy. Serum bilirubin is 2 to 5 mg/dL but may transiently be much higher.

Rotor Syndrome

Rotor syndrome is an autosomal recessive, familial conjugated hyperbilirubinemia, clinically similar to Dubin–Johnson syndrome but without liver pigmentation. Defective hepatic uptake or intracellular binding of organic ions has been blamed. The pattern of urinary coproporphyrins is like that of most hepatobiliary disorders with conjugated hyperbilirubinemia (i.e., increased total urinary coproporphyrins, 65% of which are isomer I). Patients with Rotor syndrome have few symptoms and lead normal lives.

Progressive Familial Intrahepatic Cholestasis

Progressive familial intrahepatic cholestases (PFICs) are a heterogeneous group of rare, inherited, autosomal recessive disorders of infancy or early childhood in which intrahepatic cholestasis progresses relentlessly to cirrhosis. PFIC1, PFIC2, and PFIC3, now called FIC1 deficiency, BSEP deficiency, and MDR3 deficiency, respectively, are due to mutations of different genes. In FIC1 deficiency, mutant *ATP8B1* causes deficiency in FIC1 protein, an ATPase in bile canalicular membranes that functions as an aminophospholipid transporter. BSEP deficiency is a defect in a bile salt export pump (BSEP) encoded by the *ABCB11* gene. MDR3 deficiency is caused by multidrug resistant 3 (MDR3) protein deficiency, encoded by the *ABCB4* gene. Both benign recurrent intrahepatic cholestasis and intrahepatic cholestasis of pregnancy (ICP; see below) are milder forms of PFIC that do not progress to cirrhosis.

The first patients with FIC1 deficiency were descendants of an Amish man, Jacob Byler (Byler syndrome), but PFIC is not limited to that ethnic group. There is an associated high incidence of retinitis pigmentosa. The children are often mentally retarded. Most affected children die within the first 2 years of life.

Benign Recurrent Intrahepatic Cholestasis

In benign recurrent intrahepatic cholestasis, self-limited, episodic intrahepatic cholestasis may be preceded by malaise and itching. The occurrence of familial cases suggests a genetic origin. Symptoms tend to last several weeks to several months. Patients usually have three to five episodes in their lives, but some may have as many as 10. Recurrences may be separated by weeks to years. Serum bilirubin during the acute episodes ranges from 10 to 20 mg/dL, mostly conjugated.

The liver shows centrilobular cholestasis (bile plugs in bile canaliculi) and a few mononuclear inflammatory cells in portal tracts. All structural and functional alterations disappear during remissions. No permanent sequelae have been reported.

Intrahepatic Cholestasis of Pregnancy

ICP is a rare disease marked by pruritus and cholestasis, usually in the last trimester of each pregnancy. These promptly disappear after delivery. Women with ICP fare well, but fetal morbidity and mortality are increased, as are premature labor, fetal distress, and placental insufficiency. Mutations in the ATP-cassette transporter B4 (*ABCB4*) and the multidrug resistance protein-3 (MDR3) have been described in women with ICP. Increased gonadal and placental hormones during pregnancy most likely cause cholestasis in susceptible women. Mothers' livers show mainly centrilobular cholestasis. The diagnosis is generally made by clinical observation and confirmed by the markedly increased maternal total bile acid levels. Therapy with ursodeoxycholic acid (UDCA) provides some relief of pruritus.

Sepsis Can Cause Jaundice

Severe conjugated hyperbilirubinemia may occur in sepsis involving either gram-positive or gram-negative bacteria. In such situations, serum alkaline phosphatase and cholesterol levels are usually low, suggesting a defect in excretion of conjugated bilirubin. Liver pathology is nonspecific and includes mild canalicular cholestasis and slight fat accumulation. Portal tracts may contain excess inflammatory cells and show variable ductular reaction (bile ductile proliferation). Occasionally, dilated ductules are filled with inspissated bile.

Neonatal (Physiologic) Jaundice Occurs in Most Newborns

Neonatal hyperbilirubinemia occurs in the absence of any specific disorder. Hepatic clearance of bilirubin in the fetus is minimal; hepatic uptake, conjugation and biliary excretion are all much lower than in children and adults. Liver UGT activity is less than 1% of that in adults, and ligandin levels are low. Fetal bilirubin levels are low because bilirubin crosses the placenta and is conjugated and excreted by the mother's liver.

The livers of newborns thus become responsible for clearing bilirubin before the conjugation and excretion are fully developed. Moreover, increased erythrocyte destruction in the postnatal period adds to the liver's duties in the newborn. ***Thus, 70% of normal infants have transient unconjugated hyperbilirubinemia.*** Such physiologic jaundice is more pronounced in premature infants, because liver clearance of bilirubin is less developed and red blood cell turnover is greater than in term infants. When hepatic bilirubin-conjugating capacity reaches adult levels, about 2 weeks after birth (ligandin takes somewhat longer), serum bilirubin levels rapidly decline to normal adult values. Absorption of light by unconjugated bilirubin generates water-soluble bilirubin isomers. ***Thus, phototherapy is now routinely used to treat neonatal jaundice.***

Maternal–fetal blood group incompatibilities may lead to **erythroblastosis fetalis** (see Chapter 6), in which striking bilirubin overproduction in the fetus is due to immune-mediated hemolysis. Newborns with erythroblastosis fetalis show increased cord blood bilirubin. However, jaundice becomes severe only after birth, since the mother's liver no longer compensates for the immaturity of the neonatal liver.

Cholestasis Reflects Extra- or Intrahepatic Biliary Obstruction

Functionally, cholestasis represents decreased bile flow through the canaliculus and reduced secretion of water,

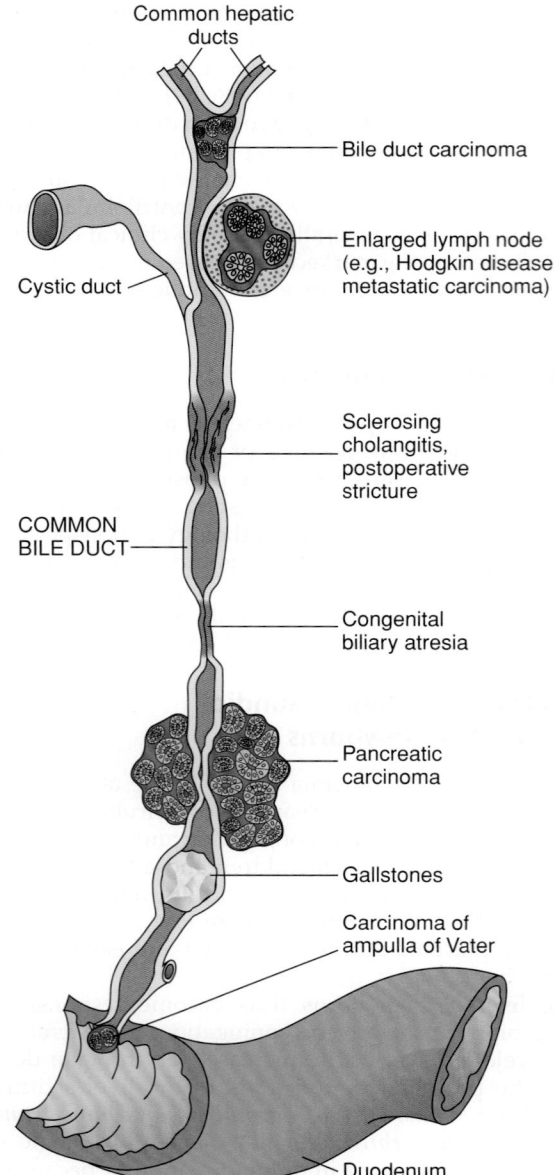

FIGURE 20-7. Major causes of extrahepatic biliary obstruction.

The extrahepatic biliary system may be obstructed by gallstones lodged in the common bile duct, cancers of the bile duct, or surrounding tissues (pancreas or ampulla of Vater), external compression by enlarged neoplastic lymph nodes in the porta hepatis (as in Hodgkin lymphoma), benign strictures (postoperative scarring or primary sclerosing cholangitis [PSC]), and biliary atresia (BA) (Fig. 20-7).

PATHOPHYSIOLOGY: Bile secretion into canaliculi and passage into the biliary collecting system depend on (1) functional and structural characteristics of canalicular microvilli, (2) permeability of canalicular plasma membranes, (3) intracellular contractile systems around canaliculi (microfilaments, microtubules), and (4) interactions of bile acids with the secretory apparatus.

The biochemical basis of cholestasis is unclear, but several abnormalities in bile formation and movement of bile have been described. For extrahepatic biliary obstruction, the effects clearly begin with increased pressure within bile ducts. However, in the early stages, the biochemistry and morphology at the canalicular level resemble those in intrahepatic cholestasis, including initial centrilobular canalicular bile plugs (Fig. 20-8).

The invariable presence of bile constituents in the blood of people with cholestasis implies regurgitation of conjugated bilirubin from hepatocytes into the blood. Hepatic clearance of unconjugated bilirubin in cholestasis is normal. Even if bile duct obstruction is complete, serum bilirubin levels only reach 30–35 mg/dL because renal excretion of bilirubin prevents further accumulation.

In both intra- and extrahepatic cholestasis, bile pigment initially is centrilobular. Fluid secretion into the canalicular bile has two components: one that is dependent on bile acid secretion and the other that is not. Since periportal hepatocytes secrete most of the bile acids, the fluid content in the periportal zone of the canaliculus exceeds that in the central zone, thus keeping bilirubin in solution.

bilirubin, and bile acids by hepatocytes. Clinical diagnosis depends on the accumulation in the blood of materials that are normally transferred to the bile, including bilirubin, cholesterol and bile acids, and elevated blood activities of certain enzymes, typically alkaline phosphatase. Cholestasis due to intrinsic liver disease is **intrahepatic cholestasis** (Fig. 20-5), whereas that caused by obstruction of large bile ducts is **extrahepatic cholestasis.** *In any event, it reflects a defect in bile transport across the canalicular membrane.*

The inability to excrete bile acids into canaliculi raises serum and hepatocellular bile acid levels. As detergents, bile acids injure cells by both detergent action and direct activation of apoptosis. They are thus potent hepatotoxins, and their accumulation within hepatocytes causes much of the hepatic injury and progression to cirrhosis associated with cholestasis. Elevation of serum bile acids is the likely cause of severe itching **(pruritus)**.

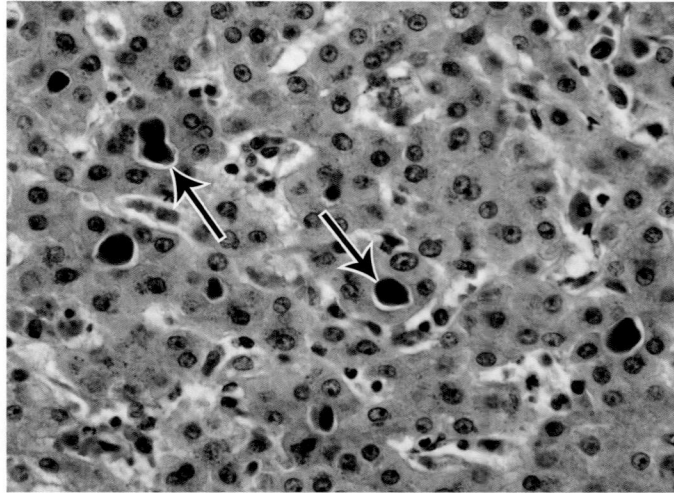

FIGURE 20-8. Bile stasis. The liver from a patient with drug-induced cholestasis shows prominent bile plugs in dilated bile canaliculi *(arrows)*. In the absence of inflammation (as seen here), this lesion may be termed *pure cholestasis.*

In addition, the bile acids themselves act as detergents in the intestine and solubilize aggregates of bilirubin in the periportal areas. As well, the higher activity of microsomal mixed-function oxidases in the central zone predisposes central hepatocytes to injury by a variety of drugs and toxins. Such an effect may favor bile deposition in centrilobular areas in cholestasis.

Several mechanisms of cholestasis have been proposed. *DAMAGE TO CANALICULAR PLASMA MEMBRANES:* The canalicular plasma membrane is the site of sodium (and therefore fluid) secretion into the bile. This membrane also participates in bile acid and bilirubin secretion. Fluid secretion is controlled by the Na$^+$/K$^+$-ATPase of the canalicular membrane. Alterations in the canalicular membrane by drugs and other agents that can perturb its structure inhibit the Na$^+$/K$^+$-ATPase, decrease bile flow or produce morphologic alterations.

ALTERED CONTRACTILE PROPERTIES OF THE CANALICULUS: Bile is propelled along the canaliculus by peristalsis-like contractile activity of hepatocytes. Agents that perturb pericanalicular actin microfilaments (e.g., cytochalasin and phalloidin) inhibit this peristalsis and may cause cholestasis.

ALTERATIONS IN CANALICULAR MEMBRANE PERMEABILITY: Agents that cause cholestasis, including estrogens and taurolithocholate, may allow back-diffusion of bile components by making canalicular membranes more permeable, or "leaky."

PATHOLOGY: *Cholestasis is characterized by the presence of brownish bile pigment within dilated canaliculi and in hepatocytes* (Figs. 20-8 to 20-10). Canaliculi are enlarged. By electron microscopy, microvilli are blunted and fewer in number or even absent. Bile accumulates in hepatocytes in large, bile-laden lysosomes.

When cholestasis persists, secondary morphologic abnormalities develop. Scattered necrotic hepatocytes probably reflect the toxicity of excess intracellular bile. Intrasinusoidal macrophages and Kupffer cells contain bile pigment and cellular debris. Whereas early cholestasis is limited almost entirely to the central zone, chronic cholestasis is also marked by bile plugs at the periphery of lobules.

In **extrahepatic biliary obstruction,** the liver is swollen and bile stained. Prolonged obstruction suppresses bile secretion, causing the bile to become almost colorless ("white bile"). The liver, however, remains green. At first, edema in portal tracts accompanies centrilobular cholestasis, progressing to portal mononuclear infiltrates as obstruction persists. Tortuous and distended bile ductules proliferate and attract neutrophils (Fig. 20-9). Damaged hepatocytes swollen with bile show (1) hydropic swelling, (2) diffuse impregnation with bile pigment, and (3) a reticulated appearance. This triad is called **feathery degeneration** (Fig. 20-10). Cholestasis eventually reaches the periphery of the lobule. Dilated bile ducts or ductules may rupture, leading to **bile lakes** (Fig. 20-11)—focal, golden-yellow deposits surrounded by degenerating hepatocytes. Infection of obstructed biliary passages often leads to superimposed suppurative cholangitis, intraluminal pus,

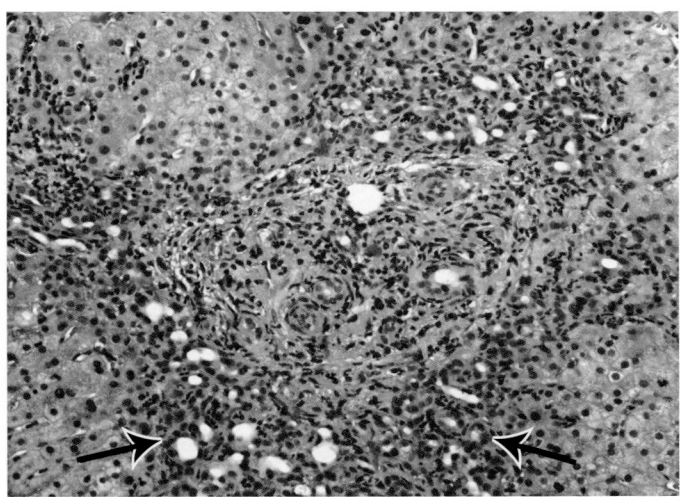

FIGURE 20-9. Extrahepatic biliary obstruction. A portal tract is expanded by ductular reaction (*arrows*) and acute and chronic inflammation.

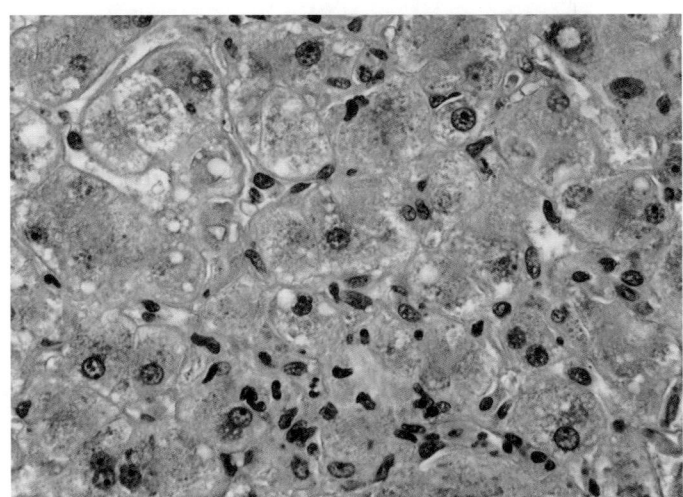

FIGURE 20-10. Cholestasis. Hepatocytes are swollen and bile stained (feathery degeneration).

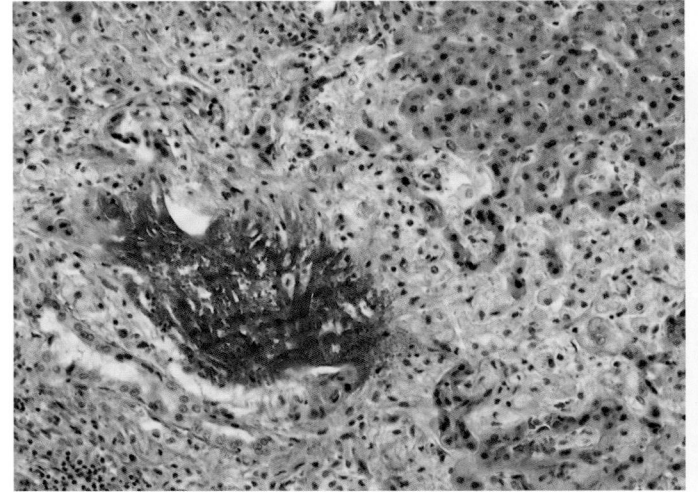

FIGURE 20-11. Bile infarct (bile lake). The liver in a patient with extrahepatic biliary obstruction, showing an area of necrosis (pale-appearing hepatocytes) and accumulation of extravasated bile.

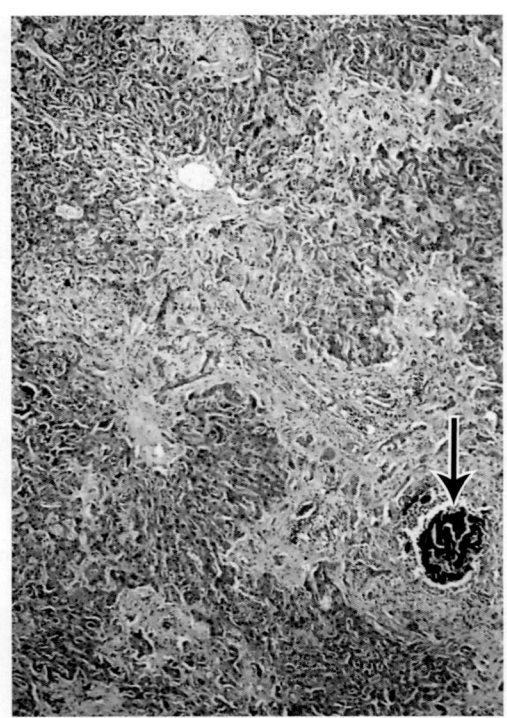

FIGURE 20-12. Secondary biliary cirrhosis. Liver from a patient with a carcinoma of the pancreas that obstructed the common bile duct. Irregular fibrous septa extend from enlarged portal tracts containing a dilated interlobular bile duct that encloses a dense bile concretion (*arrow*). Proliferating bile ducts (ductular reaction) are seen within the septa.

and even intrahepatic abscesses. Within bile ducts and ductules, biliary concretions may be conspicuous.

In time, portal tracts become enlarged and fibrotic (Fig. 20-12). If extrahepatic biliary obstruction is untreated, septa eventually extend between portal tracts of contiguous lobules to form **biliary cirrhosis** (see below).

CLINICAL FEATURES: Whatever the cause, cholestasis usually presents with jaundice. **Pruritus** (itching) is common and can be severe and intractable. It may be caused by deposition of bile acids in the skin, but other bile components may play a role. Cholesterol accumulates in the skin to form **xanthomas. Malabsorption** may develop in cases of protracted cholestasis (see Chapter 13).

CIRRHOSIS

Cirrhosis is destruction of normal liver architecture by fibrous bands around regenerative nodules of hepatocytes. This pattern invariably results from persistent liver cell necrosis. Advanced cases of cirrhosis all tend to have a similar appearance, and the cause often can no longer be ascertained by morphologic examination alone. In earlier stages, on the other hand, features characteristic of an inciting pathogenic insult may be evident. For example, the presence of fat and Mallory–Denk hyalins is typical of alcoholic liver injury, whereas chronic inflammation and interface hepatitis

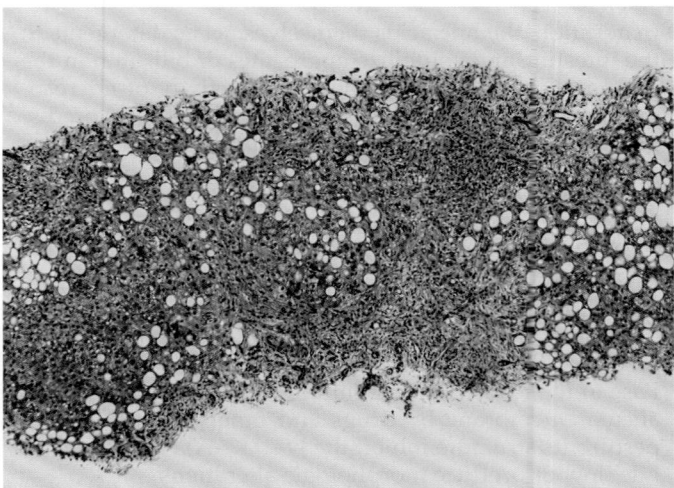

FIGURE 20-13. Micronodular cirrhosis. Cirrhotic liver from a chronic alcoholic. Note the small, regenerative nodules of parenchyma and fatty change surrounded by blue staining fibrous tissue.

(inflammation and necrosis of hepatocytes at limiting plates adjacent to portal tracts) are prominent in chronic hepatitis.

The pathogenesis of cirrhosis involves death and regeneration of hepatocytes, extracellular matrix deposition by activated hepatic stellate cells and resulting alterations in hepatic vascular architecture.

Many terms are applied to the different forms of cirrhosis, rivaling the number of etiologies incriminated in chronic liver disease, but some patterns emerge. At one end of this spectrum, usually early in the evolution of cirrhosis, is the **micronodular** type (Fig. 20-13), characterized by small, uniform nodules separated by fibrous septa. At the other end, ordinarily seen late in the disease or in postnecrotic liver diseases such as autoimmune and viral hepatitis, is **macronodular cirrhosis** (Fig. 20-14), with grossly visible, coarse, irregular nodules, mirrored histologically by large nodules that vary in size and shape and are encircled by similarly variably broad bands of connective tissue from extensive parenchymal damage. *Between these extremes are many cases with features of both. In practice, the different appearances of cirrhosis are less important than their etiologies.*

Once considered to be irreversible, cirrhotic livers may undergo collagen resorption, hepatic regeneration, and remodeling over years to decades—if the underlying cause of cirrhosis is removed. However, even as functional and structural improvement may occur, complete regression is unlikely and portal hypertension may persist.

MICRONODULAR CIRRHOSIS: This form of liver disease was previously termed **Laennec cirrhosis,** to honor the early 19th-century French physician who first described it accurately. (He also invented the stethoscope.) Nodules in micronodular cirrhosis are usually less than 3 mm, scarcely larger than a lobule (Fig. 20-13). They show no landmarks of lobular architecture, such as portal tracts or central venules. Fibrous septa separating nodules are usually thin, but irregular focal collapse of necrotic parenchyma may lead to wider septa. In its active stages, mononuclear inflammatory cells and ductular reaction inhabit the septa. *The prototypical cause of micronodular cirrhosis is alcoholic injury, but other etiologies may also be responsible.*

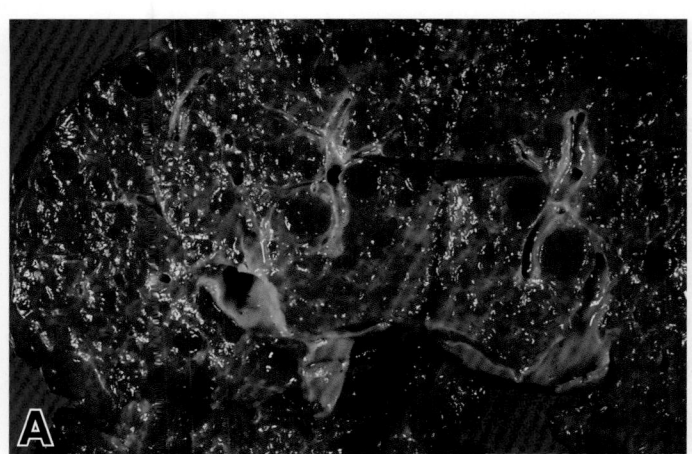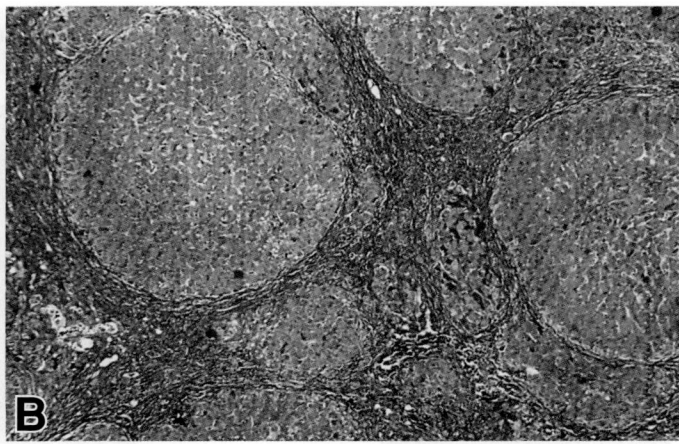

FIGURE 20-14. Macronodular cirrhosis. A. The liver is misshapen, and the cut surface reveals irregular nodules and connective tissue septa of varying width. **B.** Nodules of varying size and irregular fibrous septa.

MACRONODULAR CIRRHOSIS: Macronodular cirrhosis is classically due to chronic hepatitis. Broad connective tissue septa (Fig. 20-14) show elements of pre-existing portal tracts, mononuclear inflammatory cells, interface hepatitis, and ductular reaction. Micronodular cirrhosis can become macronodular with continued regeneration and expansion of existing nodules, especially in alcoholics who stop drinking.

The diseases associated with cirrhosis are listed in Table 20-1. They have little in common except that they all entail ongoing liver cell necrosis. Most cases of cirrhosis are attributable to alcoholism and chronic viral hepatitis. But for 15% of cases, etiologies remain unknown. These are labeled **cryptogenic cirrhosis**. Nonalcoholic steatohepatitis (NASH) is now felt to account for a significant proportion of cryptogenic cirrhosis.

TABLE 20-1
MAJOR CAUSES OF CIRRHOSIS

Alcoholic Liver Disease

Nonalcoholic Fatty Liver Disease

Chronic Hepatitis
Chronic viral hepatitis
Autoimmune hepatitis
Drugs

Biliary Disease
Extrahepatic biliary obstruction
Primary biliary cholangitis
Primary sclerosing cholangitis

Metabolic Disease

Hemochromatosis	Glycogen storage disease
Wilson disease	Hereditary fructose intolerance
α_1-Antitrypsin deficiency	Hereditary storage diseases
Tyrosinemia	Galactosemia

Cryptogenic

HEPATIC FAILURE

Hepatic failure is the clinical syndrome that occurs when the liver cannot sustain its vital activities. It may develop acutely, mostly due to viral hepatitis, autoimmune hepatitis, or toxic exposure. Chronic liver diseases, such as chronic viral hepatitis or cirrhosis, may lead to insidious onset of hepatic failure. Advances in supportive care have improved survival in acute hepatic failure or acute-on-chronic liver failure, but mortality for this condition without liver transplantation exceeds 50%. The consequences of hepatic failure are depicted in Figure 20-15.

Jaundice Reflects Inadequate Clearance of Bilirubin by the Liver

Hyperbilirubinemia in hepatic failure is mostly conjugated, although unconjugated bilirubin levels also tend to increase. On occasion, increased erythrocyte turnover may add to unconjugated hyperbilirubinemia, thus aggravating the jaundice.

The Effect of Liver Failure on the CNS Is Hepatic Encephalopathy

Altered mental status is common in patients with acute liver failure and portal hypertension (see below).

PATHOPHYSIOLOGY: No one factor explains the clinical syndrome of hepatic encephalopathy. Because of hepatocyte dysfunction and/or structural or functional vascular shunts, harmful compounds absorbed from the intestine escape hepatic detoxification. This is particularly evident after surgical construction of a portal–systemic anastomosis (portal vein to inferior vena cava or its equivalent) to relieve portal hypertension (see below). Hence, the term **portal–systemic encephalopathy** is used to describe post-shunt encephalopathy.

AMMONIA: Ammonia levels are usually increased in the blood and brain of patients with hepatic encephalopathy. Most of the body's ammonia is derived from ingestion of ammonia in foods, digestion of proteins in

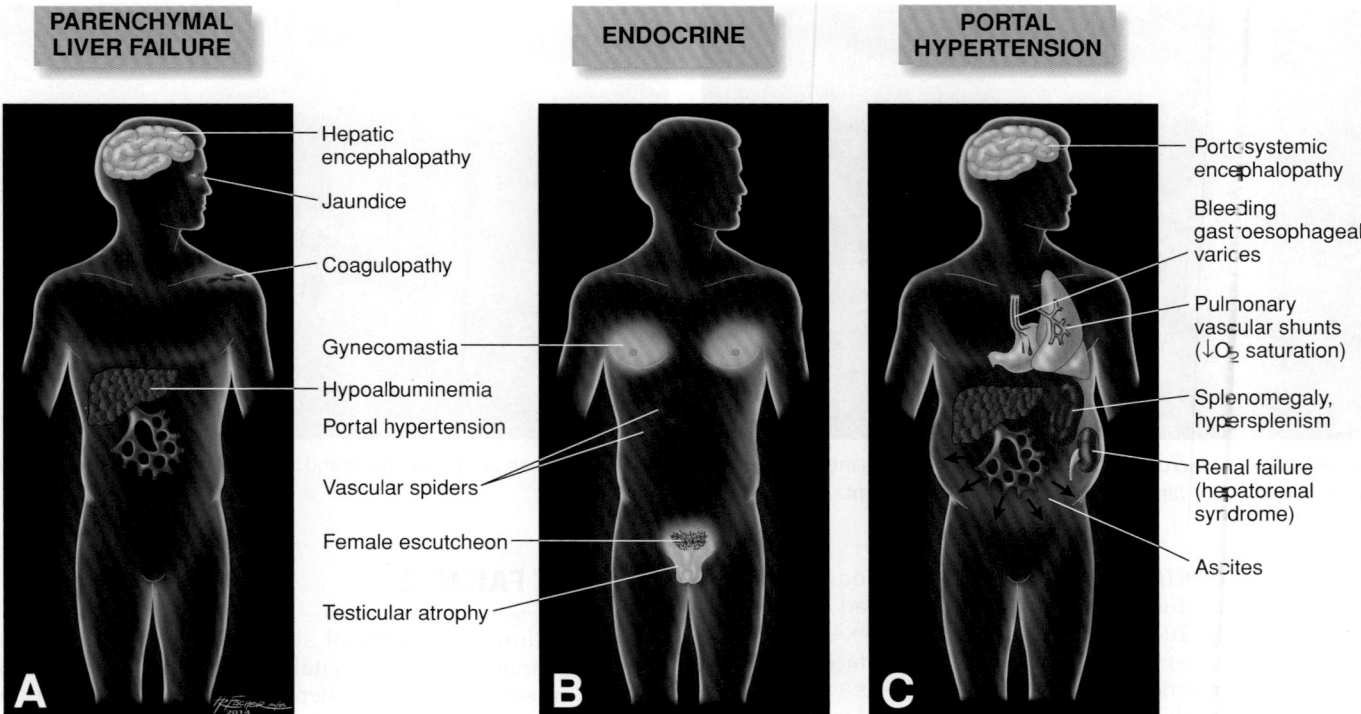

FIGURE 20-15. Complications of cirrhosis and hepatic failure. Clinical features are related to (**A**) **parenchymal liver failure,** (**B**) **endocrine disturbances,** and (**C**) **portal hypertension.** There is considerable overlap of these clinical features with regard to their pathogeneses.

the small intestine and bacterial catabolism of dietary protein and urea secreted into the intestine. Ammonia is produced in the small bowel when glutamine is deaminated by glutaminase, an enzyme that is more active in cirrhosis than normally. Ammonia is detoxified by the liver. However, in patients with acute liver failure or cirrhosis, reduced hepatocyte mass or portal–systemic shunts, respectively, an excess of ammonia escapes into the systemic circulation.

Ammonia has several harmful effects. The brain detoxifies ammonia by using it as a substrate to synthesize glutamate and glutamine. Excess levels of these molecules may alter neurotransmission and brain osmolality. However, correlation between blood ammonia levels and the severity of hepatic encephalopathy is inexact, and thus the neurotoxicity of ammonia remains only partly understood.

γ-AMINOBUTYRIC ACID: Neural inhibition, mediated by the γ-aminobutyric acid (GABA)–benzodiazepine receptor complex, is accentuated in hepatic encephalopathy by increased levels of benzodiazepine-like molecules.

OTHER SUBSTANCES: Other compounds that may contribute to hepatic encephalopathy include **mercaptans** from the breakdown of sulfur-containing amino acids in the colon. A characteristic breath odor of patients with hepatic failure, **fetor hepaticus,** is due to these mercaptans in saliva. Blood levels of aromatic amino acids are also increased in hepatic failure. They impair synthesis of normal neurotransmitters such as norepinephrine but increase production of **false neurotransmitters** (e.g., octopamine). Toxicity of **phenols** and **short-chain fatty acids** on the brain has also been postulated in hepatic encepha-

lopathy. Finally, the blood–brain barrier may be impaired in patients with hepatic failure.

 PATHOLOGY: Cerebral edema is the major cause of death in most patients with acute hepatic failure. It often coincides with uncal and cerebellar herniation. This edema is a specific lesion associated with hepatic coma, although the precise mechanism is obscure.

The brains of patients who died with chronic liver disease and hepatic coma show striking changes in astrocytes. Termed **Alzheimer type II astrocytes** (see Chapter 28), these cells are swollen, increased in number and size and show nuclear enlargement and nuclear inclusions. Deep layers of the cerebral cortex and subcortical white matter, the basal ganglia and the cerebellum show laminar necrosis and a spongiform appearance.

 CLINICAL FEATURES: Hepatic encephalopathy traverses four stages:

- **Stage I:** Sleep disturbance, irritability, and personality changes
- **Stage II:** Lethargy and disorientation
- **Stage III:** Deep somnolence
- **Stage IV:** Coma

This sequence may require many months, or it may evolve in days or weeks in cases of acute liver failure. Associated neurologic symptoms include (1) a flapping tremor of the hands, or **asterixis,** and hyperactive reflexes in the early stages; (2) extensor toe responses (Babinski reflex) later; and (3) decerebrate posture in terminal stages. Intensive supportive measures may be beneficial early in hepatic encephalopathy, but patients with stages III and IV encephalopathy usually require liver transplantation.

Treatment of hepatic encephalopathy hinges on reversal of the underlying hepatic disease and reduction in ammonia levels. The latter requires purgatives (to rid the bowel of protein, the substrate for ammonia formation), nonabsorbable antibiotics (to reduce urease-producing bacteria that make ammonia) and correction of other sources of ammonia production, including infections and electrolyte disturbances.

Defects of Coagulation Often Cause Bleeding

In liver failure, impaired synthesis of coagulation factors and thrombocytopenia lead to poor hemostasis. The clotting factors—fibrinogen, prothrombin, and factors V, VII, IX, and X—are reduced, reflecting generalized impairment of hepatic protein synthesis.

Thrombocytopenia (<80,000/μL) is common in hepatic failure, as are qualitative defects in platelet function. Hypersplenism, bone marrow depression, and platelet loss due to **disseminated intravascular coagulation** (DIC) decrease circulating platelets.

DIC occurs frequently in liver failure. It may be stimulated by liver cell necrosis, activation of factor XII (Hageman factor; see Chapter 4) by endotoxin or inadequate hepatic clearance of activated clotting factors from the circulation.

Hypoalbuminemia Complicates Hepatic Failure

Impaired hepatic albumin synthesis causes hypoalbuminemia. This is an important factor in the pathogenesis of edema that often complicates chronic liver disease.

Liver Failure Causes Imbalances in Steroid Hormones

Hyperestrogenism in chronic liver failure in men leads to **gynecomastia,** a female body habitus and female distribution of pubic hair (female escutcheon). Vascular effects of hyperestrogenism are common and include **spider angiomas** in the drainage territory of the superior vena cava (upper trunk and face) and **palmar erythema**.

Feminization reflects reduced catabolism of estrogens and weak androgens by a dysfunctional liver. Weak androgens (androstenedione and dehydroepiandrosterone) are converted to estrogens in peripheral tissues, thus increasing circulating estrogen levels. Extrahepatic portal–systemic shunts due to portal hypertension in cirrhosis (see below) permit these hormones to bypass the liver.

Men with alcoholic liver disease are more likely to be feminized than those with liver disease from other causes, and the feminization is usually more severe. Chronic alcoholics also suffer hypogonadism, with testicular atrophy, impotence, and loss of libido. Alcoholic women also have gonadal failure, which presents as oligomenorrhea, amenorrhea, infertility, ovarian atrophy, and loss of secondary sex characteristics. These effects in both sexes reflect a direct toxic action of alcohol on gonadal function and are independent of chronic liver disease.

PORTAL HYPERTENSION

The superior mesenteric and splenic veins meet to make the hepatic portal vein. This vessel carries the major venous drainage from the gastrointestinal tract, pancreas, and spleen to the liver. It accounts for 2/3 of the liver's blood flow but provides less than half of its total oxygen supply. The remainder is supplied by the hepatic artery. *Portal hypertension is either an absolute increase in portal venous pressure, usually above 8 mm Hg, or an increase in the pressure gradient between the portal vein and the hepatic vein of 5 mm Hg or more.* Obstruction to blood flow somewhere in the portal circuit is responsible. Increased portal pressure causes opening of **portal–systemic collateral channels,** bleeding from gastroesophageal varices, ascites, splenomegaly, and renal and pulmonary disease (Fig. 20-15).

Portal hypertension is most accurately assessed by directly measuring hepatic vein pressure: a balloon-tipped catheter inserted into the internal jugular vein is advanced to a terminal hepatic vein to obtain the **free hepatic vein pressure** (FHVP). The **wedged hepatic vein pressure** (WHVP), determined after balloon inflation, is an indirect measure of portal vein pressure. The difference between WHVP and FHVP is the **hepatic vein pressure gradient** (HVPG); that is, WHVP – FHVP = HVPG.

Increased resistance to portal blood outflow is the basis for diagnosing portal hypertension (Fig. 20-16). This increase in resistance can originate in one of three areas:

1. **Sinusoidal (intrahepatic):** Injury to sinusoids leads to sinusoidal, or intrahepatic, portal hypertension. In the Western world, cirrhosis is the most common cause of all forms of portal hypertension. In cirrhosis, fibrosis leads to obstruction of intrahepatic sinusoids. This, in turn, impedes the inflow of portal blood. The result is increased pressure in the portal vein, relative to the hepatic vein. In sinusoidal portal hypertension, the pressure difference between the WHVP and FHVP (HVPG) is usually 5 mm Hg or more.
2. **Presinusoidal:** Resistance to blood flow in the extrahepatic portal vein or intrahepatic portal veins or venules (e.g., caused by thrombotic occlusion) is known as **presinusoidal portal hypertension**. If the point of resistance is within portal venules (i.e., within the liver), the HVPG may be increased. However, if the point of resistance is more distal, allowing for a zone of normal pressure in the portal vein between the occlusion and the sinusoids, the HVPG can be normal.
3. **Postsinusoidal:** If the point of resistance is in the hepatic veins, venules, or cardiac circulation, **postsinusoidal portal hypertension** may result. This can occur if blood flow in the hepatic veins is impeded, as in Budd–Chiari syndrome or congestive heart failure. The HVPG is usually normal in this situation. That is, if the hepatic vein pressure is measured distal to the point of postsinusoidal obstruction, the FHVP will be increased, and the HVPG can be expected to be normal, as the sinusoids are normal and pose no significant resistance to the flow of blood into the liver. However, if high pressure due to outflow resistance is constant, the sinusoids may become progressively injured, leading to eventual elevation in the HVPG.

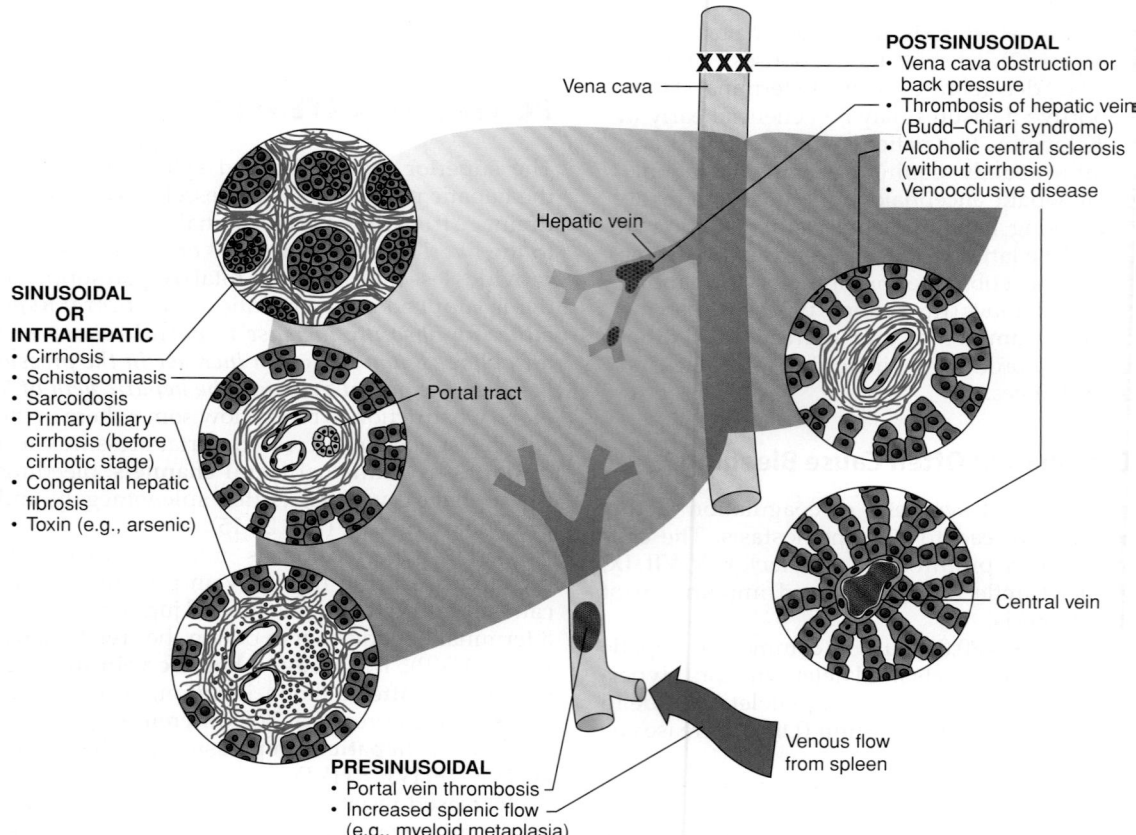

FIGURE 20-16. Causes of portal hypertension.

Intrahepatic Portal Hypertension Is Usually Caused by Cirrhosis

PATHOPHYSIOLOGY: Intrahepatic portal hypertension, such as occurs in cirrhosis, offers the best paradigm for understanding the pathogenesis of portal hypertension. Even before fibrosis distorts sinusoidal architecture, active contraction of vascular smooth muscle and stellate cells initiates resistance to the flow of blood into the liver from the portal vein. The trigger for this is not clear but is probably related to factors that incite inflammation, such as alcoholic hepatitis and viral hepatitis. As fibrosis develops, sinusoids become increasingly disordered. Regenerative nodules in the cirrhotic liver impinge on hepatic veins, obstructing blood flow beyond the lobules. Small portal veins and venules are trapped, narrowed, and often obliterated by scarring of the portal tracts. Blood flow through the hepatic artery is increased and small arteriovenous communications open. In this way, arterial blood flow increases and adds to portal hypertension due to obstruction of blood flow distal to the sinusoid.

In cirrhosis, **endothelial cell dysfunction** occurs both in the liver and in the systemic circulation. Hepatic vascular tone increases, and intrahepatic vessels constrict. Impaired phosphorylation of endothelial nitric oxide synthase (eNOS), reduced nitric oxide (NO) availability due to oxidative stress and excess vasoconstrictive factors (e.g., angiotensinogen, endothelin, and eicosanoids) all reduce eNOS activity. This decreases hepatic NO production.

Ensuing vasoconstriction increases resistance to portal blood flow into the liver.

Progressive portal hypertension parallels mesenteric arterial vasodilation. That is, to make matters worse, **mesenteric arterial vasodilation** increases blood flow into the portal vein just when portal vein resistance is going up. Mesenteric arterial vasodilation is driven by increased NO production in response to greater shear forces upon the mesenteric vessels (owing to increased resistance to portal blood flow into the liver), and by other vasodilating factors including increased vascular endothelial growth factor (VEGF) and inflammatory mediators such as TNFα. *Mesenteric artery vasodilation provokes systemic circulatory dysfunction, systemic arterial vasodilation, and reduced effective arterial blood volume.*

This decrease in effective arterial blood volume causes the clinical syndrome of advanced portal hypertension: **ascites,** and **hepatorenal syndrome (HRS)** and **hepatopulmonary syndrome (HPS)**. The increase in portal pressure also opens vascular shunts that decompress the portal circuit. Although this may be regarded as an adaptive compensatory mechanism, these shunts are a mixed blessing, as they may cause such complications as bleeding varices and encephalopathy (see above).

Worldwide, hepatic schistosomiasis is a major cause of intrahepatic portal hypertension (see Chapter 9). Ova released from intestinal veins traverse the portal system and lodge in intrahepatic portal venules, where they elicit a granulomatous reaction that heals by scarring.

Because the obstruction within the liver occurs mainly before portal blood enters the hepatic sinusoids, hepatic schistosomiasis is functionally akin to prehepatic portal hypertension. Liver function is well maintained, but the intrahepatic presinusoidal vascular obstruction leads to severe portal hypertension.

Idiopathic portal hypertension, also called **noncirrhotic portal hypertension, hepatoportal sclerosis** or **obliterative portal venopathy,** refers to occasional cases of intrahepatic portal hypertension with splenomegaly in the absence of demonstrable intra- or extrahepatic disease. Known causes of idiopathic portal hypertension are chronic exposure to copper, arsenic, and vinyl chloride. In some countries (England, Japan), idiopathic portal hypertension accounts for 15% to 35% of all cases that require surgery to decompress the portal circulation.

Intrahepatic portal hypertension can be caused by other conditions that interfere with blood flow through the liver, including cystic disease of the liver (see Chapter 16), partial nodular transformation of the liver in the region of the porta hepatis, nodular regenerative hyperplasia (small regenerative nodules without fibrosis that compress the intervening hepatic parenchyma), immune-mediated diseases, hypercoagulable states, recurrent infections, and exposure to toxins/medications.

Portal Vein Thrombosis Often Causes Presinusoidal Portal Hypertension

 ETIOLOGIC FACTORS: Portal vein thrombosis occurs most often in the setting of cirrhosis. Other causes include tumors, infections, hypercoagulability states, pancreatitis, and surgical trauma. Some cases are of unknown etiology. Primary hepatocellular carcinoma (HCC) may invade branches of the portal vein and occlude the main portal vein. When the portal vein is obstructed by a septic thrombus, bacteria may seed intrahepatic branches of the portal vein (suppurative pylephlebitis) and cause multiple hepatic abscesses.

Portal vein occlusion (Fig. 20-17) may occur in the neonatal period or in early childhood. Umbilical sepsis

is an important cause in some cases, but other local and systemic infections may also play a role. Sometimes the thrombosed portal or splenic vein is replaced by a fibrous cord or interlacing vascular channels, a condition termed **cavernous transformation**.

The liver normally offers little resistance to blood flow through the sinusoids and it can accommodate substantial increases in blood volume without a secondary increase in pressure. However, increased portal venous blood flow can occasionally lead to prehepatic portal hypertension. Arteriovenous fistulas (abnormal communications between an artery and the portal vein) may cause prehepatic portal hypertension. These generally arise from trauma or rupture of an aneurysm of the splenic or hepatic artery. They may also develop in patients with hereditary hemorrhagic telangiectasia (Osler–Weber–Rendu syndrome). Splenomegaly due, for example, to myeloproliferative neoplasms (see Chapter 20) may result in portal hypertension. The splenomegaly that accompanies cirrhosis tends to aggravate portal hypertension.

Postsinusoidal Portal Hypertension Is Obstruction to Blood Flow Beyond Liver Lobules

Budd–Chiari Syndrome

Budd–Chiari syndrome is a congestive disease of the liver caused by occlusion of the hepatic veins and their tributaries.

 ETIOLOGIC FACTORS: Hepatic vein thrombosis is the main cause of Budd–Chiari syndrome, and it may occur in such diverse diseases as myeloproliferative neoplasms (especially polycythemia vera), hypercoagulable states associated with malignancies, use of oral contraceptives, pregnancy, bacterial infections, paroxysmal nocturnal hemoglobinuria, metastatic and primary tumors in the liver, and surgical trauma. In 20% of cases, there is no clear cause. Thrombi form most often in the large hepatic veins, near their exit from the liver, and in the intrahepatic portion of the inferior vena cava. In parts of Africa and Asia, membranous webs of unknown cause can compromise the vena cava above the orifices of the hepatic veins and lead to Budd–Chiari syndrome. Increased venous back-pressure from severe congestive heart failure, tricuspid stenosis or regurgitation, or constrictive pericarditis may mimic the syndrome.

Hepatic veno-occlusive disease is a variant of Budd–Chiari syndrome, caused by hepatic sinusoidal injury resulting in occlusion of the centrilobular hepatic sinusoids, central venules, and small branches of the hepatic veins. This disorder is most often traced to ingestion of toxic pyrrolizidine alkaloids in plants of the *Crotalaria* and *Senecio* genera, which are used in "bush teas." It is also seen in patients given certain antineoplastic agents, after hepatic irradiation and after bone marrow transplantation, possibly as a manifestation of graft-versus-host disease.

PATHOLOGY: In the acute stage of **hepatic vein thrombosis,** the liver is swollen and tense. Its cut surface is mottled and oozes blood (Fig. 20-18A). In the chronic stage, the cut surface is paler, and the liver

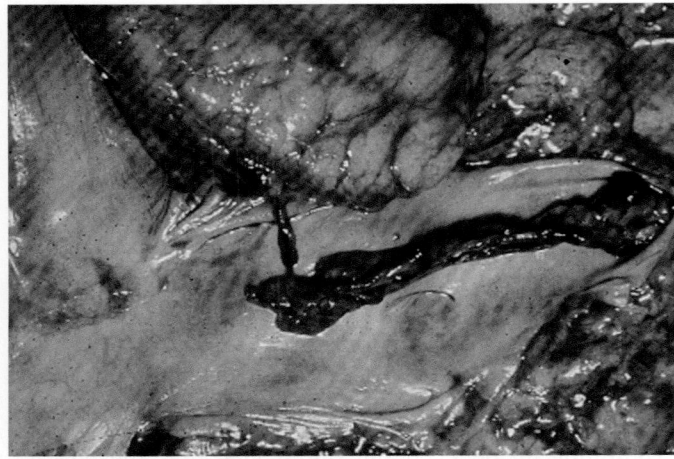

FIGURE 20-17. Portal vein thrombosis.

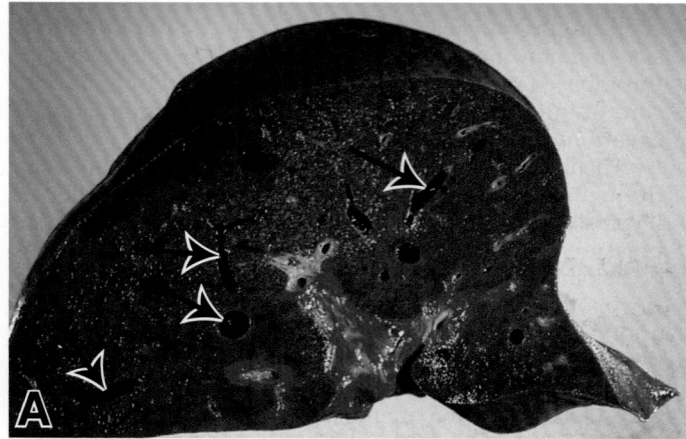

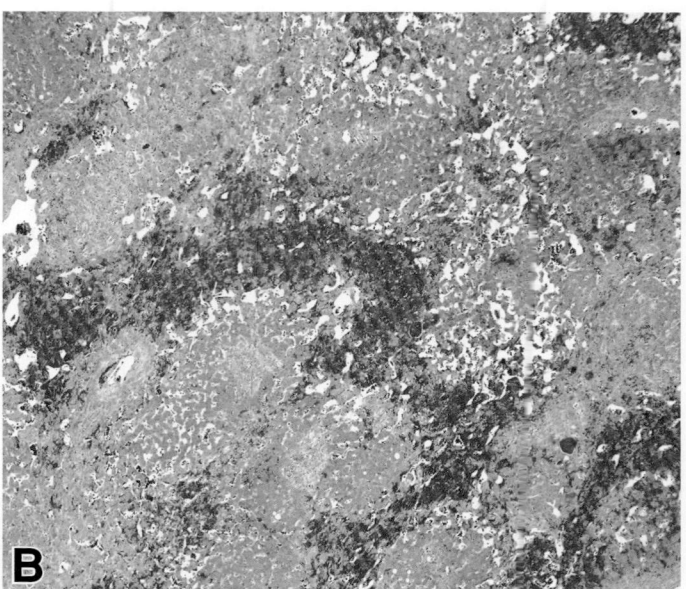

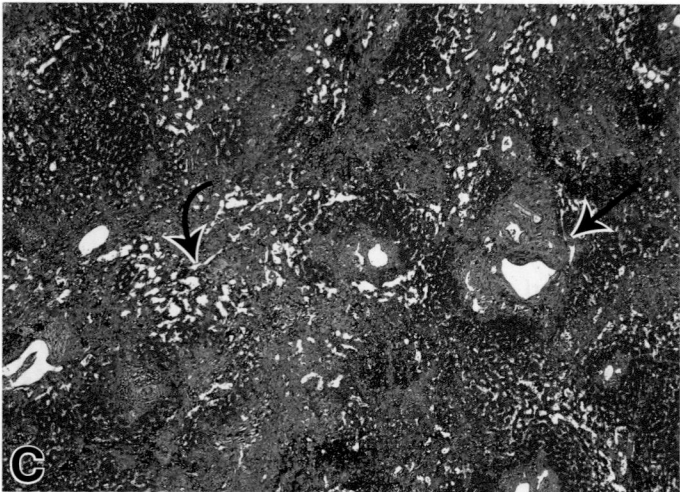

FIGURE 20-18. Budd–Chiari syndrome. A. The cut surface of the liver from a patient who died of Budd–Chiari syndrome shows thrombosis of the hepatic veins (*arrows*) and diffuse congestion of the parenchyma. **B.** Liver parenchyma from a patient with **acute Budd–Chiari syndrome** reveals centrilobular necrosis (pale pink staining regions) and hemorrhage. **C. Chronic Budd–Chiari syndrome**. Cirrhosis has developed with bridging fibrosis emanating from the central venules rather than the portal tracts. Note the dilated sinusoids (*curved arrow*) and intact portal tract (*arrow*).

is firm, owing to an increase in connective tissue. Hepatic veins contain thrombi in varying stages of evolution, from recent clots to well-organized thrombi that have been recanalized.

In the acute stage of both Budd–Chiari syndrome and veno-occlusive disease, the sinusoids of the central zone are dilated and packed with erythrocytes (Fig. 20-18B). Liver cell plates are compressed, with hemorrhage and necrosis of centrilobular hepatocytes. In long-standing venous congestion, fibrosis of the central zone may radiate to more peripheral portions of the lobules (Fig. 20-18C). Sinusoids are dilated, and central-to-midzonal hepatocytes show pressure atrophy. Eventually, **reverse lobulation** occurs, with connective tissue septa linking adjacent central zones to form nodules with a single central portal tract. This fibrosis is usually not severe enough to justify a label of cirrhosis.

 CLINICAL FEATURES: Complete thrombosis of the hepatic veins presents as an acute illness with abdominal pain, enlargement of the liver, ascites, and mild jaundice. Acute hepatic failure and death often follow quickly. Most often, the obstruction of the hepatic venous circulation is incomplete, and similar symptoms

persist for periods from a month to a few years. More than 90% of patients with Budd–Chiari syndrome develop ascites, usually severe, and splenomegaly is common. Typically, serum bilirubin levels and aminotransferase activities increase only modestly. Most patients eventually die in hepatic failure or from complications of portal hypertension. Liver transplantation may be curative.

Portal Hypertension Affects Many Organ Systems

Esophageal Varices

Esophageal varices are the most important complication of portal hypertension. They arise when collateral portal–systemic vascular channels open to relieve pressure in the portal circuit. A common cause of death in patients with disorders associated with portal hypertension is exsanguinating upper gastrointestinal hemorrhage from **bleeding esophageal varices** (see Chapter 13).

PATHOPHYSIOLOGY: The collaterals of greatest clinical significance are in the submucosa of the lower esophagus and upper stomach, where they communicate between the portal vein and the gastric coronary vein. Normally, these collaterals are closed. However, when the portal circulation sustains increased blood flow and higher pressures that follow, they open. They are submucosal veins near the esophagogastric junction, and they become dilated and protrude into the lumen. There is no simple correlation between the magnitude of the portal venous pressure and the risk of variceal bleeding, but that risk does rise with increasing size of the varices.

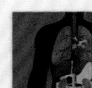 **CLINICAL FEATURES:** Bleeding esophageal varices portend a poor prognosis; acute mortality may be as high as 40%. In patients with cirrhosis who have survived one episode of variceal bleeding, long-term survival is unlikely because the chances of recurrent bleeding or worsening liver failure are high. By contrast, patients in whom portal hypertension is caused by a presinusoidal block without underlying hepatic dysfunction, as in schistosomiasis, have a much better prognosis than those with cirrhosis. Death from bleeding esophageal varices is usually due to hepatic failure precipitated by stress, ischemic necrosis of the liver, and the encephalopathy caused by the nitrogenous load imposed by blood in the intestinal tract. Exsanguination and shock are only infrequently the direct causes of death.

Initial treatment of acute variceal hemorrhage focuses on stopping the bleeding by endoscopic variceal ligation, injection of a sclerosing agent during endoscopy or direct tamponade with an inflatable balloon. In addition, intravenous administration of a somatostatin analog, octreotide, inhibits splanchnic vasodilation. This, in turn, reduces splanchnic blood flow and portal venous pressure. If these measures fail and varices rebleed, permanent portal circulation decompression may be needed. Angiographically a small stent or shunt is placed in the liver to join the portal and systemic circulations (transjugular intrahepatic portal–systemic shunt [TIPS]). This procedure, in addition to surgically constructed portal–systemic shunts, diverts blood from the high-pressure portal circulation to the lower-pressure systemic venous circulation. In some cases, liver transplantation is an alternative to shunt surgery.

Back-pressure in the portal vein also dilates its tributaries, including the inferior hemorrhoidal veins, which become dilated and tortuous (**anorectal varices**). Collateral veins radiating about the umbilicus produce a pattern known as **caput medusae**.

Splenomegaly

The spleen in portal hypertension enlarges progressively and often causes **hypersplenism** (hyperactive splenic function), leading to decreased life spans (i.e., increased rates of removal) and consequent reduced levels in the circulation of all formed elements of the blood (pancytopenia). Hypersplenism is attributed to a prolonged transit time through the hyperplastic spleen.

The spleen is firm and weighs up to 1,000 g (normal, <180 g). Its cut surface is uniformly deep red, and white pulp is inconspicuous. Sinusoids are dilated and lined by hyperplastic endothelium and macrophages. Their walls are thickened by fibrous tissue. Focal hemorrhages cause fibrotic, iron-laden nodules known as **Gamna-Gandy bodies**.

Ascites

Ascites is accumulation of fluid in the peritoneal cavity. It often accompanies portal hypertension, and the amount of fluid may be so great (often many liters) that it distends the abdomen and interferes with breathing. The onset of ascites in cirrhosis portends a poor prognosis.

 PATHOPHYSIOLOGY: Reduced effective arterial blood volume and mean arterial pressure lead to predictable homeostatic responses. Early in portal hypertension, heart rate and cardiac output increase, thus preserving arterial pressure. However, as peripheral arterial vasodilation worsens, circulatory dysfunction worsens; cardiac output cannot keep pace with homeostatic demand, and endogenous vasoactive mechanisms become engaged. To preserve arterial pressure, activities of the renin–angiotensin system and sympathetic nervous system increase. These effects raise renal sodium and water resorption. Vasodilation also activates antidiuretic hormone secretion, promoting additional water retention and dilutional hyponatremia.

Increased liver sinusoidal pressure results in hydrostatic movement of fluid and lymph from the sinusoids into the space of Disse. This compounds the effects of greater sodium and water retention. These fluids spill into the peritoneal cavity and accumulate as ascites. Decreased albumin synthesis lowers intravascular oncotic pressure and further facilitates movement of fluid into the peritoneal space.

Progressive deposition of fibrous tissue compromises endothelial permeability which, in turn, reduces the amounts of protein and albumin that spill into the ascites fluid. This increases the serum:ascites albumin gradient (SAAG). A SAAG exceeding 1.1 is associated with ascites due to portal hypertension from cirrhosis.

The pathogenesis of ascites is illustrated in Figure 20-19.

Spontaneous Bacterial Peritonitis

Spontaneous bacterial peritonitis (SBP) is an important complication in patients with both cirrhosis and ascites.

 ETIOLOGIC FACTORS: SBP is due to translocation of intestinal bacteria into the systemic circulation, with secondary infection of ascitic fluid. The most common bacteria are the gram negatives of the gut (*Escherichia coli, Klebsiella*); *Streptococcus pneumoniae* is also a common cause of SBP. Patients with low complement levels in ascitic fluid, reflected as low protein levels (<1 g/dL), are at particular risk for SBP.

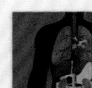 **CLINICAL FEATURES:** Patients with SBP typically present with ascites and abdominal pain, or other signs of infection such as fever or leukocytosis. Up to 20% of patients are asymptomatic. A finding of more than 250 neutrophils/μL in ascitic fluid establishes the diagnosis. *Without appropriate therapy, SBP mortality exceeds 80%.* Even if the acute infection is treated and resolved, an episode of SBP is associated with a 70% 1-year mortality. Therefore, SBP is often an indication for liver transplantation.

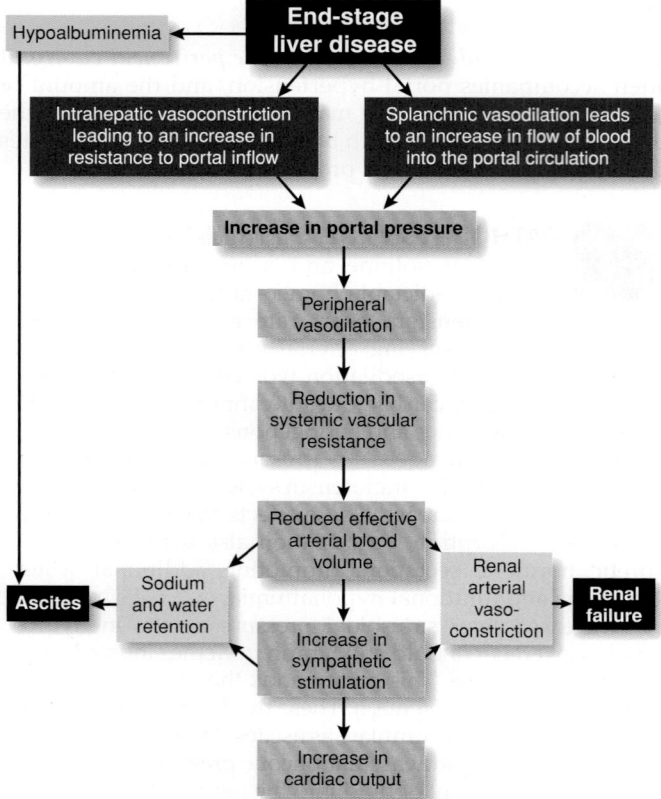

FIGURE 20-19. Pathogenesis of ascites.

Hepatorenal Syndrome

HRS is characterized by renal hypoperfusion, with oliguria, azotemia, and increased plasma creatinine. It usually occurs in the setting of cirrhosis and indicates a poor prognosis. Renal dysfunction in HRS is reversible. Kidneys from patients who died with HRS function normally when transplanted into recipients with chronic renal failure. Similarly, renal function is restored after liver transplantation in patients with HRS.

 PATHOPHYSIOLOGY: In the early stages of portal hypertension, glomerular filtration pressure is protected from systemic arteriolar vasodilation by intrarenal prostaglandins. As vasodilation worsens, these compensatory intrarenal mechanisms become ineffective, and renal vasoconstriction intensifies and glomerular perfusion and filtration decline. Eventually, this leads to clinically evident renal dysfunction, or HRS. The diagnosis of HRS also requires that serum creatinine exceeds 1.5 mg/dL and does not improve after diuretic withdrawal and volume expansion.

There are two types of HRS. Type I HRS is rapidly and inexorably progressive. Liver transplantation is the only definitive therapy. Type II HRS progresses more slowly and usually occurs in the setting of severe ascites unresponsive to conventional therapies with salt restriction and diuretics. This form of HRS may be mitigated by volume expansion or diuretic withdrawal. However, type II ultimately progresses to type I HRS if portal hypertension is not reversed.

Pulmonary Complications of Portal Hypertension

Cirrhosis and portal hypertension can lead to HPS, **portopulmonary hypertension** (PPHTN), and **hepatic hydrothorax**. Directly or indirectly, these are due to the circulatory and vascular disturbances of advanced liver disease.

Up to a third of patients with cirrhosis show signs of HPS, which results from shunts in the pulmonary vascular bed due to portal hypertension. They present with progressive shortness of breath, although chest radiography and pulmonary hemodynamics are typically normal. Treatment with supplemental oxygen may be useful, but liver transplantation is the only effective therapy because it reverses the intrapulmonary shunting. HPS is associated with reduced survival, particularly if arterial oxygen is less than 50 mm Hg.

PPHTN is increased pulmonary vascular resistance in the setting of portal hypertension. Usually, it is associated with increased mean pulmonary arterial pressure, to more than 25 mm Hg, and occurs in 2% of those with portal hypertension. The pathophysiology of the disorder is unclear. It may reflect consequences of the hyperdynamic circulation of portal hypertension including increased shear stress, endothelial injury, vasoconstriction, and liberation of vasoactive factors. Proliferative pulmonary arteriopathy develops such that PPHTN is inexorably progressive and usually does not reverse following liver transplantation. In fact, severe PPHTN it is a risk factor for intraoperative death due to acute heart failure and represents a contraindication to liver transplantation.

Hepatic hydrothorax is a pleural effusion attributed to portal hypertension. Most such effusions occur in the right chest and arise by movement of ascitic fluid through the diaphragm into the pleural space. Thus, the fluid has the same composition and protein content as ascites and, like ascites, is prone to spontaneous infection.

VIRAL HEPATITIS

Viral hepatitis is infection of hepatocytes that causes liver necrosis and inflammation. It was known as "epidemic jaundice" for millennia. Worldwide, more than 500 million people are infected with hepatotropic viruses and, as a result, are at great risk for HCC. Many viruses and other infectious agents can produce hepatitis and jaundice (Table 20-2), but in the industrialized world, more than 95% of cases of viral

TABLE 20-2	
INFECTIOUS AGENTS THAT CAUSE HEPATITIS	
Hepatitis A virus (HAV)	Herpes simplex virus
Hepatitis B virus (HBV)+/− HDV	Cytomegalovirus
Hepatitis C virus (HCV)	Enteroviruses other than HAV
Hepatitis E virus (HEV) Yellow fever virus	Leptospires (leptospirosis)
Epstein–Barr virus (infectious mononucleosis)	*Entamoeba histolytica* (amebic hepatitis)
Lassa, Marburg, and Ebola viruses	

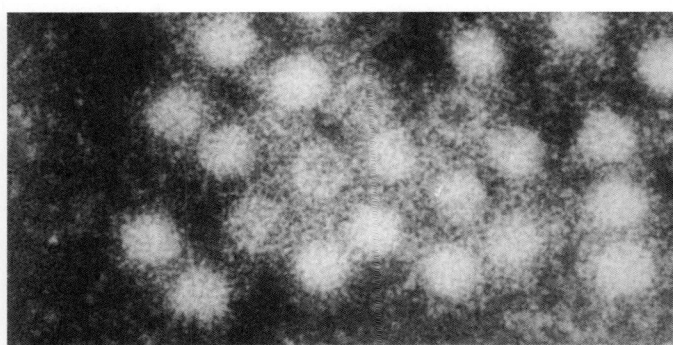

FIGURE 20-20. Electron micrograph of hepatitis A virus (HAV). A fecal extract was treated with convalescent serum containing anti-HAV to aggregate the viral particles.

hepatitis are caused by hepatitis A, B, C, D, and E viruses (HAV, HBV, etc.).

The following discussion emphasizes the illnesses commonly termed **viral hepatitis**. The reader is referred to Chapter 9 for consideration of the other agents.

Hepatitis A Virus Is the Most Common Cause of Acute Hepatitis

Hepatitis A virus (HAV) is a small RNA-containing enterovirus of the picornavirus family (which includes polio virus) (Fig. 20-20). It mainly replicates in hepatocytes, but gastrointestinal epithelial cells may also be infected. Infectious virus progeny are shed into the bile and excreted in feces. HAV is not directly cytopathic; rather, hepatic injury is mediated by the immunologic reaction against virally infected hepatocytes.

 EPIDEMIOLOGY: The only reservoir for HAV is acutely infected people, so transmission is mostly from person to person by the fecal–oral route. Epidemics of hepatitis A occur in crowded and unsanitary conditions, such as exist in warfare, or by fecal contamination of water and food. Edible shellfish in contaminated waters concentrate the virus and may transmit infection if not adequately cooked.

In industrialized countries with low rates of infection, most cases of hepatitis A are seen in older children and adults. By contrast, in less developed regions, where the disease is endemic, most of the population is infected before 10 years of age.

In the United States, about 10% of the population younger than 20 years show serologic evidence of previous HAV infection. Thus, *most HAV infections are anicteric.* Hepatitis A is common in day care centers and among international travelers and men who have sex with men. However, no source is identified in about 1/2 of cases. Hepatitis A vaccination confers long-term protection from the disease. Universal vaccination programs have significantly reduced the incidence of acute hepatitis A in the United States.

 CLINICAL FEATURES: After an incubation period of 3 to 6 weeks (mean, about 4 weeks), HAV-infected patients develop nonspecific symptoms,

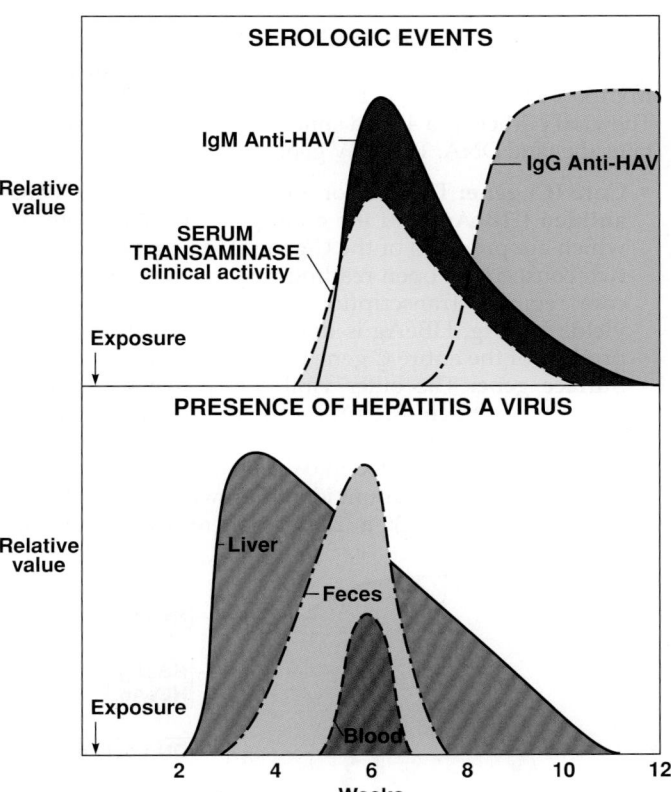

FIGURE 20-21. Typical serologic events associated with hepatitis A (HAV).

including fever, malaise, and anorexia. Liver injury is evidenced by a rise in serum aminotransferases (Fig. 20-21). Aminotransferase levels begin to decline, usually 5 to 10 days later. Jaundice may then appear. It remains evident for an average of 10 days but may persist for more than a month. Aminotransferase levels generally return to normal by the time jaundice has disappeared. *Hepatitis A never becomes chronic. There is no carrier state, and infection provides lifelong immunity.* Fulminant hepatitis is rarely seen, and virtually all patients recover without sequelae.

HAV is detectable in the liver about 2 weeks after infection, peaks in another 2 weeks and disappears shortly thereafter (Fig. 20-21). Fecal shedding of HAV follows its appearance in the liver by about a week and is brief. The period of viremia is also short, occurring early in the disease.

Anti-HAV IgM is the first detectable immune response to HAV. It appears in the blood during the acute illness. IgM titers begin to decline within a few weeks and are undetectable by 3 to 5 months. Anti-HAV IgM appears as patients recover and persists for life. Serum IgM anti-HAV in a patient with acute hepatitis confirms HAV as the cause.

Hepatitis B Is a Major Cause of Acute and Chronic Liver Disease

 ETIOLOGIC FACTORS: Hepatitis B virus (HBV) is a hepatotropic DNA virus of the **hepadnavirus** group, whose genomes are among the smallest of all known viruses. The HBV genome is circular and predominantly double-stranded DNA with the entire genome, plus a shorter complementary strand that varies from 50% to 85% of the length of the longer strand (Fig. 20-22). The viral particle is a 42-nm sphere (*Dane particle*) that contains the viral DNA. The HBV genome has four genes:

- **Core (C) gene:** The core of the virus contains the **core antigen (HBcAg)** and the **e antigen (HBeAg),** both of which are products of the *C* gene. The *C* gene includes two consecutive open reading frames, the precore and core regions. Transcription of the core frame alone yields HBcAg. HBeAg is derived from the translation product of the entire *C* gene by proteolysis.
- **Surface gene:** The outer viral coat contains **hepatitis B surface antigen (HBsAg).** HBsAg is synthesized by infected hepatocytes independently of the viral core, and vast amounts are secreted into the blood. Electron microscopy of centrifuged serum identifies two distinct HBsAg particles (Fig. 20-22): a 22-nm sphere and a tubular

structure 22 nm in diameter and 40 to 400 nm in length. These particles are immunogenic but not infectious.
- **Polymerase gene:** The *P* gene encodes viral DNA polymerase.
- **X gene:** The small X protein activates viral transcription and probably plays a role in HBV-related hepatocarcinogenesis associated with chronic HBV infection.

HBV attaches to host hepatocytes and then enters the cell, where it uncoats. Its genome then goes into the nucleus, where it is converted into a covalently closed circular DNA (cccDNA) that is the template for transcription of viral mRNA. Persistence of cccDNA prevents HBV clearance from the host, even with potent antiviral pharmacotherapy.

There are six distinct HBV serotypes (A through F). Mutations are common, both in unmolested infection and under the influence of pharmacotherapy. *Precore mutant HBV DNA-containing viruses do not express HBeAg,* and their function is unclear. Antiviral treatment selects for HBV mutants at high (50%) rates after years of therapy. Newer nucleoside and nucleotide analogs cause lower rates of HBV mutation.

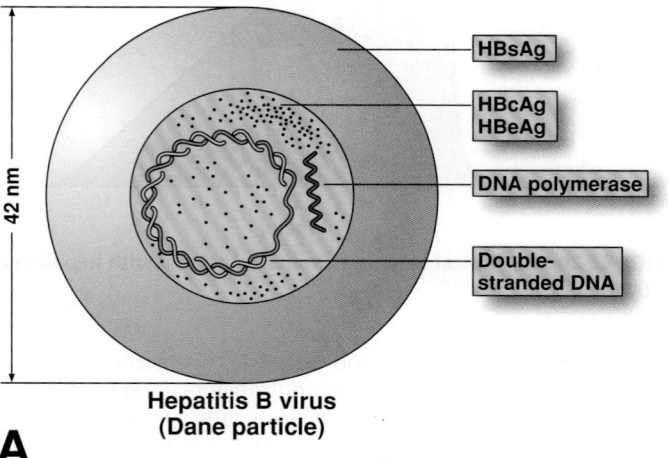

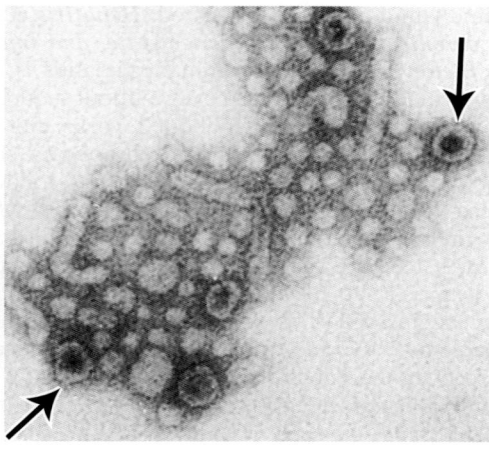

FIGURE 20-22. Hepatitis B virus (HBV). A. Schematic representation of HBV and serum particles associated with HBV infection. (Antigens [Ag] for hepatitis B are indicated by their letters: c = core; e is located between the core and the lipid envelop that forms the surface; and s = surface.) **B.** Electron micrograph of particles from centrifuged serum from a patient with hepatitis B. Rod-like and spherical particles containing HBsAg are evident. The complete virion, composed of the viral core and its surrounding envelope, is represented by Dane particles (*arrows*).

EPIDEMIOLOGY: It is estimated that there are more than 350 million chronic carriers of HBV in the world, constituting an enormous reservoir of infection (Fig. 20-23). Depending on the rate of primary infection with HBV, carrier rates of chronic infection vary from 0.3% (United States, Western Europe) to 20% (Southeast Asia, sub-Saharan Africa, Oceania, and the Pacific and Amazon basins). In endemic areas, high carrier rates are sustained by vertical transmission from carrier mothers to newborns.

In the United States, between 500,000 and 1.5 million people are chronically infected HBV carriers. Between 200,000 and 300,000 new cases of HBV occur annually. The use of a protective vaccine lowered the incidence of HBV in the United States from 10.7/100,000 in 1983 to 1.6/100,000 in 2006. Only 1/4 of new cases present with jaundice. Fulminant hepatitis B causes 250 to 300 deaths annually in the United States. Posttransfusion hepatitis, once common, is now a memory due to routine blood screening for HBsAg.

The incidence of HBV chronicity is inversely proportional to the age at viral acquisition. In countries with high endemicity, the high chronicity rate is due to vertical transmission and unsafe injection practices. In areas with lower rates of infection, HBV transmission is most frequently horizontal. No more than 10% of people infected with HBV as adults become carriers, but neonatal hepatitis B generally leads to persistent infection. Males become carriers more often than females. In the United States, chronic HBV carriers are common among male homosexuals and IV drug users.

Humans are the only significant reservoir of HBV. Unlike hepatitis A, HBV is not transmitted by the fecal–oral route, nor does it contaminate food and water supplies. *HBsAg is found in most secretions, but infectious virus is only present in blood, saliva, and semen.* Most cases of hepatitis B are now transmitted by intimate contact. Such contact transmission largely involves direct

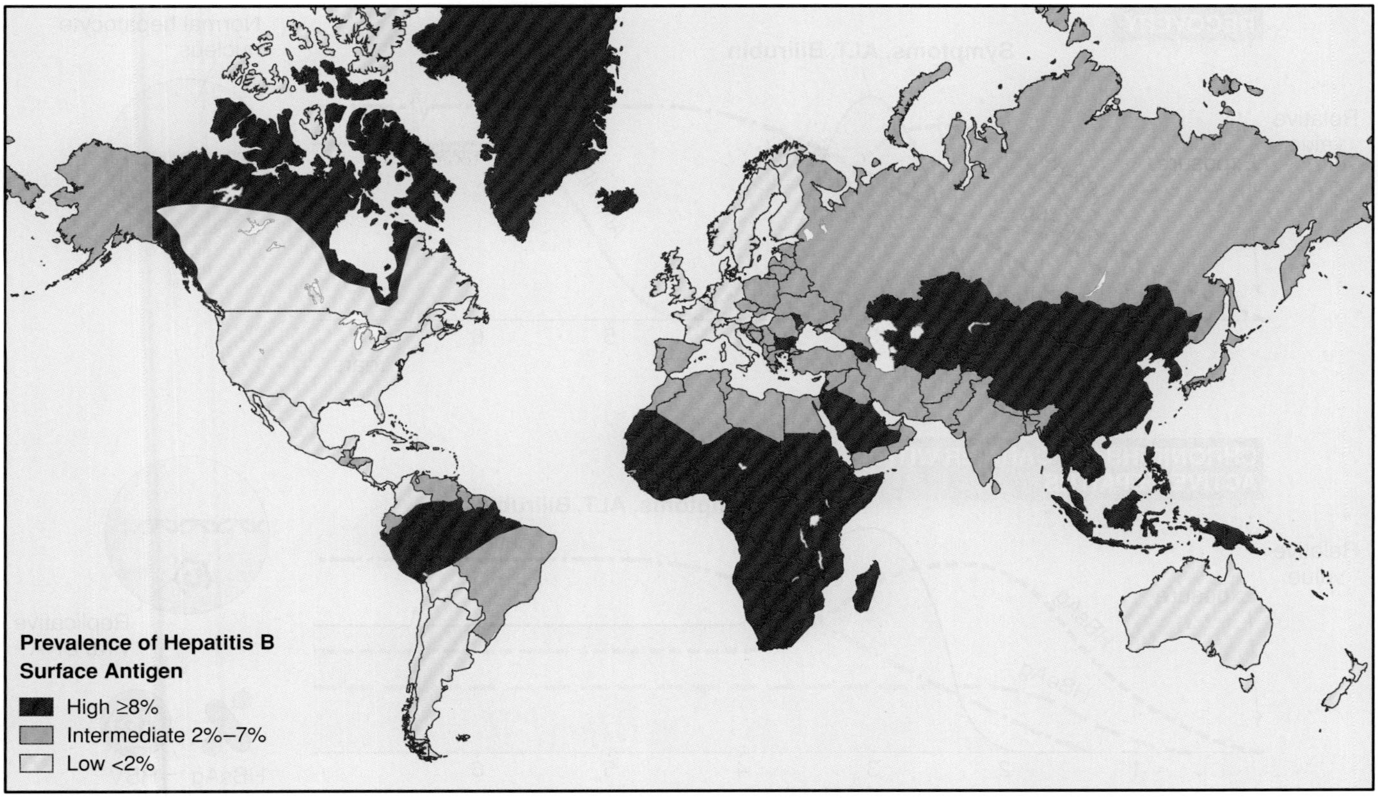

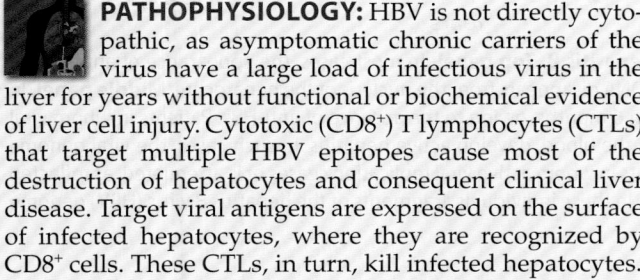

Prevalence of Hepatitis B Surface Antigen

■ High ≥8%
■ Intermediate 2%–7%
□ Low <2%

FIGURE 20-23. Geographic prevalence of hepatitis B infection.

transfer of virus through breaks in the skin or mucous membranes. Anal sexual contact is thus an important mode of transmission.

Synthetic hepatitis B vaccines, containing recombinant HBsAg or its immunogenic epitopes, are highly effective and confer lifelong immunity. In some regions where hepatitis B is endemic, vaccination has significantly reduced the prevalence of the disease. In the United States, it is now routine to administer the vaccine. Vaccination of infants is common in most nations (currently 177 of 193 countries).

PATHOPHYSIOLOGY: HBV is not directly cytopathic, as asymptomatic chronic carriers of the virus have a large load of infectious virus in the liver for years without functional or biochemical evidence of liver cell injury. Cytotoxic (CD8⁺) T lymphocytes (CTLs) that target multiple HBV epitopes cause most of the destruction of hepatocytes and consequent clinical liver disease. Target viral antigens are expressed on the surface of infected hepatocytes, where they are recognized by CD8⁺ cells. These CTLs, in turn, kill infected hepatocytes.

The infectivity of blood from patients with chronic hepatitis B declines with the duration of the disease. This is largely due to decreased episomal (extrachromosomal) replication of infectious virions. The intact viral genome does not integrate into host DNA. However, genomic fragments are progressively integrated, after which they produce several viral antigens, contributing to viral persistence.

CLINICAL FEATURES: Hepatitis B may follow three courses (Fig. 20-24):

- Acute hepatitis
- Fulminant hepatitis
- Chronic hepatitis

ACUTE HEPATITIS B: Most adult patients have acute, self-limited hepatitis B, similar to that produced by HAV, usually followed by complete recovery and lifelong immunity. Symptoms of hepatitis B are largely similar to those of hepatitis A, but acute hepatitis B tends to be somewhat more severe, and its incubation period is much longer. Typically, symptoms appear 2 to 3 months after exposure, but incubation periods may vary from under 6 weeks to 6 months. As in hepatitis A, many cases, including virtually all infections in infants and children, are anicteric and thus not clinically apparent.

HBsAg is the first marker to appear in the serum of patients with acute hepatitis B. It appears 1 to 8 weeks after exposure (Fig. 20-24) and disappears from the blood during convalescence in those patients who recover rapidly. Simultaneously with, or shortly after, HBsAg disappears, serum antibody to HBsAg (anti-HBs) is detectable. Its appearance heralds complete recovery, and it provides lifelong immunity.

HBcAg (core antigen) is not seen in blood of persons with acute hepatitis B, but antibody to HBcAg (anti-HBc) appears shortly after HBsAg. Antibody to HBcAg is a marker of a prior HBV infection but it does not clear the virus or protect from reinfection.

THE LIVER AND BILIARY SYSTEM

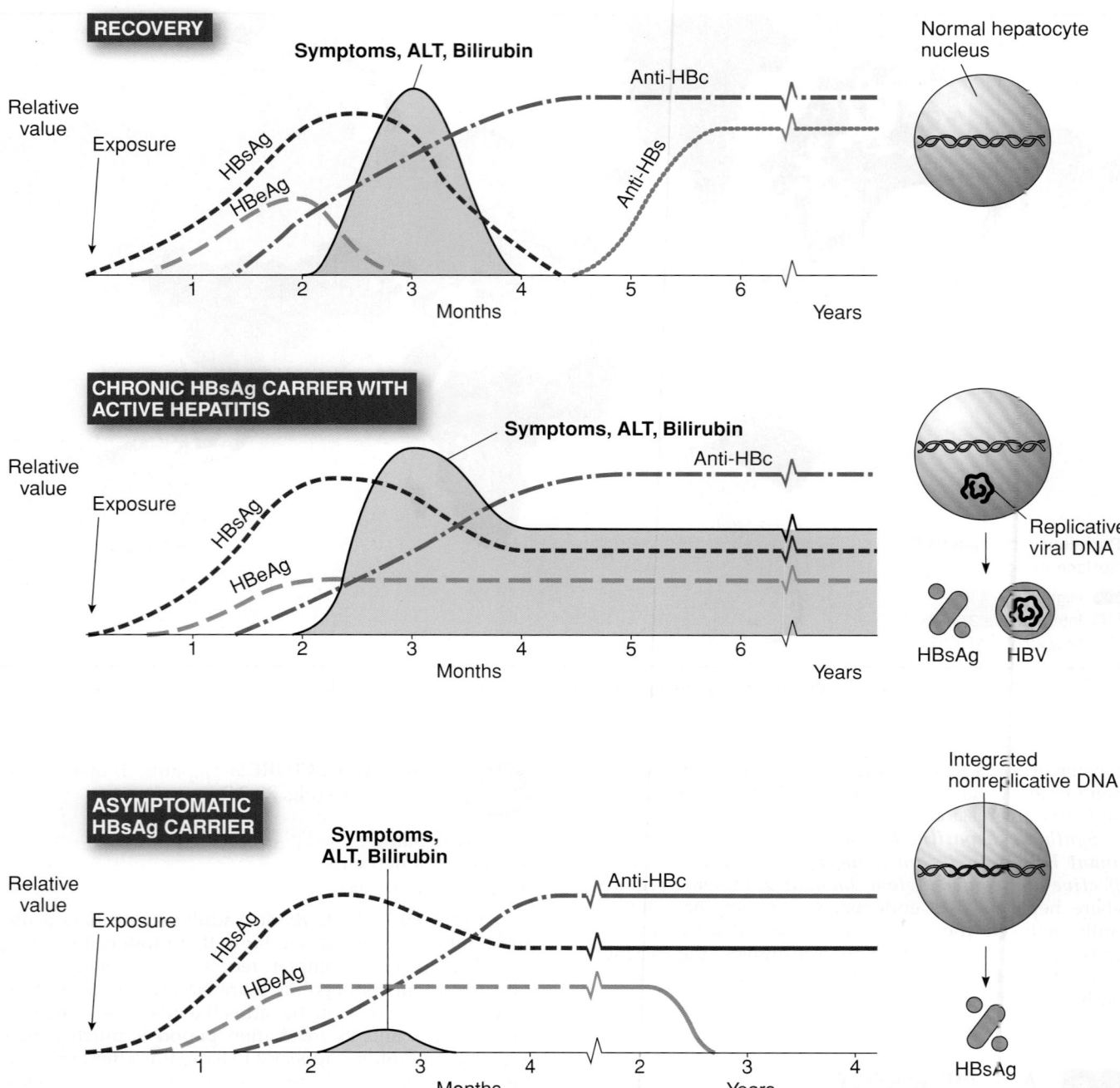

FIGURE 20-24. Typical serologic events in three distinct outcomes of hepatitis B. Top panel. In most cases, the appearance of antibody to hepatitis B surface antigen (HBsAg; anti-HBs) ensures complete recovery. Viral DNA disappears from the nucleus of the hepatocyte. **Middle panel.** In about 10% of cases of hepatitis B, HBs antigenemia is sustained for longer than 6 months, owing to the absence of anti-HBs. Patients in whom viral replication remains active, as evidenced by sustained high levels of HBeAg in the blood, develop active hepatitis. In such cases, the viral genome persists in the nucleus but is not integrated into host DNA. **Lower panel.** Patients in whom active viral replication ceases or is attenuated, as reflected in the disappearance of HBeAg from the blood, become asymptomatic carriers. In these individuals, fragments of the hepatitis B virus (HBV) genome are integrated into the host DNA, but episomal DNA is absent.

HBeAg circulates before the onset of clinical disease and after the appearance of HBsAg. It generally disappears within about 2 weeks, whereas HBsAg is still present. Serum HBeAg correlates with a period of intense viral replication and, hence, maximal infectivity of the patient. Anti-HBe antibody appears shortly after the antigen disappears and is detectable up to 2 or more years after the hepatitis resolves. A minor subset of patients who seroconvert to anti-HBe antibody and lose serum HBeAg have persistent HBV replication. HBV viruses in these cases are replication competent but do not produce HBeAg because of mutations in the HBV genome.

FULMINANT HEPATITIS B: More often than hepatitis A, but still only rarely, acute hepatitis B can be a fulminant disease, with massive liver cell necrosis, hepatic failure, and high mortality. Treatment with nucleoside and nucleotide analogs has improved outcomes for patients with fulminant hepatitis B compared to historical controls. Patients with fulminant acute hepatitis B can decompensate rapidly. Death is primarily caused by cerebral edema, cardiopulmonary collapse, or sepsis. Liver transplantation, when available, gives excellent patient survival.

CHRONIC HEPATITIS B: Chronic hepatitis is characterized by continued necrosis and inflammation in the liver for more than 6 months. People with chronic HBV infection are at increased risk for cirrhosis and HCC. Men are more susceptible than women. Other risk factors include age greater than 40 years, high levels of HBV viremia, viral genotypes C and F, or a precore promoter mutation.

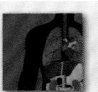 **PATHOPHYSIOLOGY:** Three phases of chronic hepatitis B are recognized: (1) immune tolerant phase, (2) immune active phase, and (3) inactive phase. A fourth phase, recovery, is not yet generally accepted. People chronically infected with HBV often progress temporally through these phases but can also revert backward.

1. **Immune tolerant phase:** Patients in this phase are HBeAg positive, with very high HBV DNA levels (>20,000 IU/mL). There is little significant hepatocellular inflammation or necrosis, and serum aminotransferase levels are normal. This phase may last for decades and is common among those who acquired HBV by vertical transmission. Since HBV DNA integrates into cellular DNA, even patients in this phase are at increased risk for HCC.
2. **Immune active phase:** This phase is characterized by HBV viremia and liver cell necrosis (i.e., elevated serum aminotransferases). Portal-based inflammatory infiltrates and hepatocyte necrosis are seen. Patients with detectable HBe tend to have greater viremia than those who are HBe negative/anti-HBe positive. Significant liver injury, cirrhosis, and HCC tend to develop in this phase. Antiviral therapy is often initiated in the immune active phase.
3. **Inactive phase:** In the inactive phase, anti-HBe antibody circulates but HBeAg does not, and serum aminotransferases are normal and blood HBV DNA is low (<2,000 IU/mL). These people are "asymptomatic carriers" and are at very low risk of progression to cirrhosis or HCC. However, they may revert to the immune active disease phase and thus require long-term follow-up.

In some chronic HBV carriers, HBsAg–anti-HBs complexes circulate in the blood. Thus, these patients produce antibody but do not clear the virus antigen from the circulation. Such circulating immune complexes may lead to **extrahepatic** complications, including a serum sickness–like syndrome (fever, rash, urticaria, acute arthritis), polyarteritis, glomerulonephritis, and cryoglobulinemia. In fact, 1/3 to 1/2 of patients with polyarteritis nodosa are HBV carriers. Chronic hepatitis B is associated with a significant risk of liver cancer (see below). *The possible outcomes of infection with HBV are summarized in Figures 20-24 and 20-25.*

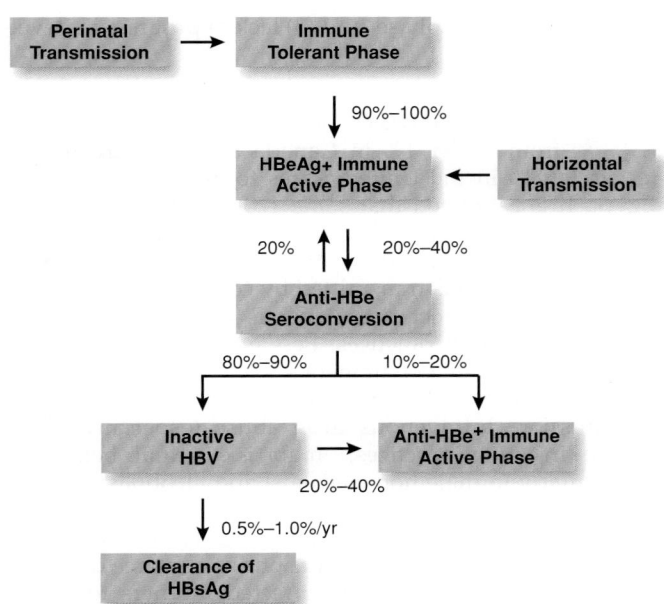

FIGURE 20-25. Outcomes of infection with the hepatitis B virus (HBV).

Hepatitis D Virus Is a Defective RNA Virus

Assembly of hepatitis D virus (HDV) in the liver requires HBsAg to be present. Therefore, infection with HDV is limited to people who are also infected with HBV. The two infections may be simultaneous (coinfection), or HDV infection may follow HBV infection (superinfection). HDV and HBsAg are cleared together, and the clinical course is usually similar to that for the usual acute hepatitis B. However, in some patients, coinfection with HDV leads to severe, fulminant and often fatal hepatitis, particularly in intravenous drug abusers. *Superinfection of an HBV carrier with HDV typically increases the severity of an existing chronic hepatitis.* In fact, 70% to 80% of HBsAg carriers superinfected with HDV develop chronic hepatitis. Since the discovery of HDV in 1979, recognition of its natural history has led to a significant drop in HDV transmission. The virus remains a clinical problem especially in developing nations endemic for HBV.

Hepatitis C Virus Commonly Causes Chronic Hepatitis and Cirrhosis

Hepatitis C virus (HCV) is an enveloped flavivirus. Its single-stranded RNA genome of 9,600 bases encodes one transcript. This mRNA is translated into a polyprotein of about 3,000 amino acids, which is cleaved into three structural proteins (one core and two envelope proteins) and six nonstructural proteins. Short untranslated regions at the end of the genome are required for replication.

The virus is genetically unstable, which accounts for the presence of multiple genotypes and subtypes. Six different but related HCV genotypes are known. Types 1, 2, and 3 are most common (about 75% in the United States and Western Europe). Genotypes 2 and 3 respond better to antiviral therapy than does type 1. In an individual patient, many mutant HCVs arise, which likely explains several features of infection, including (1) the inability of anti-HCV antibodies to clear the infection, (2) persistent and relapsing infection in the chronic hepatitis phase, and (3) lack of progress in developing a vaccine.

EPIDEMIOLOGY: The prevalence of HCV ranges from under 1% in Canada and Scandinavia to 1.8% in the United States to as high as 22% in Egypt. It is estimated that some 170 million people (3% overall prevalence) are infected worldwide. HCV accounts for the majority of patients waiting for liver transplants.

HCV infection is transmitted by contact with infected blood through direct percutaneous exposure to blood or unsafe injection practices. Less efficient transmission occurs via smaller percutaneous exposures (needlestick injuries) or mucosal routes such as vertical and sexual transmission. Intravenous drug abuse (especially with unsafe injection practices), high-risk sexual behavior (particularly in male homosexuals) and alcoholism place individuals at high risk for contracting HCV infection. Screening of the blood supply for anti-HCV antibodies has virtually eliminated transfusions as a source of HCV infection. Transmission from infected mothers to newborn babies is infrequent (2.7% to 8.4%) but is four to five times more common in women coinfected with HIV. In a minority of cases, there are no known risk factors. The incidence of new cases of acute HCV infection in the United States has fallen from 230,000 annually in the 1980s to 16,000 now, a drop of 93%. Much of this decrease probably reflects declining use of injectable illicit drugs. Mortality due to hepatitis C is increasing, as people infected long ago are aging. This aging population will likely be increasingly susceptible to decompensated cirrhosis and HCC over the next 20 years.

PATHOPHYSIOLOGY: HCV is not directly cytopathic, and many chronic HCV carriers have no liver cell injury. Despite active humoral and cellular immune responses against all viral proteins, most patients have persistent viremia. *Liver cell injury probably reflects CTL killing of virus-infected hepatocytes.* HCV persistence is not well understood. The high level of virus genome mutation (see above) and defects in HCV-specific cellular immunity probably contribute.

CLINICAL FEATURES: The incubation period of hepatitis C is similar to that of hepatitis B. Serum aminotransferases (Fig. 20-26) usually rise 4 to 12 weeks after exposure (range, 2 to 26 weeks). Within 1 to 3 weeks of infection, HCV RNA circulates in the blood. Anti-HCV antibodies usually appear 7 to 8 weeks after infection and persist during the chronic phase. Acute hepatitis C is quite mild, or asymptomatic, in most people; only 10% to 20% develop jaundice. About 20% of HCV patients spontaneously clear the virus. Persistent viremia is milder in patients who develop jaundice and greater in those who acquire HCV via IV drug use. Fulminant hepatitis, if it occurs at all, is rare.

The most important consequences of HCV infection relate to chronic disease. Despite complete recovery from clinical and biochemical acute liver disease, 85% of patients develop chronic disease (Fig. 20-27). Cirrhosis

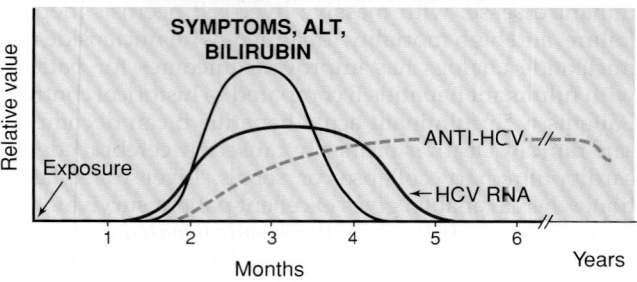

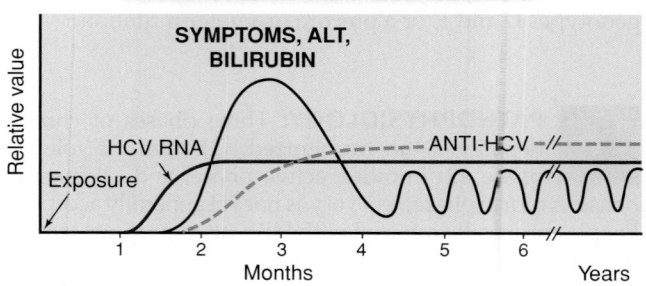

FIGURE 20-26. Clinical course of hepatitis C virus (HCV). Typical serologic events in two distinct outcomes. **Top panel.** About 20% of the patients with acute hepatitis C have a self-limited infection that resolves in a few months. Anti-HCV appears at the end of the clinical course and persists. **Bottom panel.** The remaining patients with hepatitis C develop chronic illness, with exacerbations and remissions of clinical symptoms. The development of anti-HCV does not affect the clinical outcome. Chronic hepatitis often leads to cirrhosis. *ALT* = alanine aminotransferase.

develops in 15% to 20% of people chronically infected with HCV for 10 to 30 years. The risk of cirrhosis is greater in men, the elderly, alcoholics, and those who are also infected with HIV or HBV. Even in the absence of elevated aminotransferases or significant risk factors for progression, patients can present with significant fibrosis and even cirrhosis. Liver biopsy is vital to estimating the risk of clinical progression.

Chronic hepatitis is mild in most patients for at least 10 years and often for 20 or more years. Some 20% of patients with chronic hepatitis C eventually develop cirrhosis. *Of patients with cirrhosis, up to 5% per year develop HCC.*

Liver disease in patients with chronic HCV infection tends to be more severe in the face of concurrent hepatitis B, alcoholic liver disease, hemochromatosis, or α_1-antitrypsin (α_1-AT) deficiency. About 25% of patients with advanced alcoholic liver disease have antibodies to HCV, although rates vary in different locales. The relationship is unexplained, and some cases classified as alcoholic cirrhosis may actually be due to HCV.

Extrahepatic manifestations of hepatitis C are common and include mixed cryoglobulinemia (see Chapter 20), a systemic vasculitis due to deposition of circulating immune complexes in the microvasculature. The skin (leukocytoclastic vasculitis), salivary glands (sicca syndrome), nervous system (mononeuritis multiplex), and

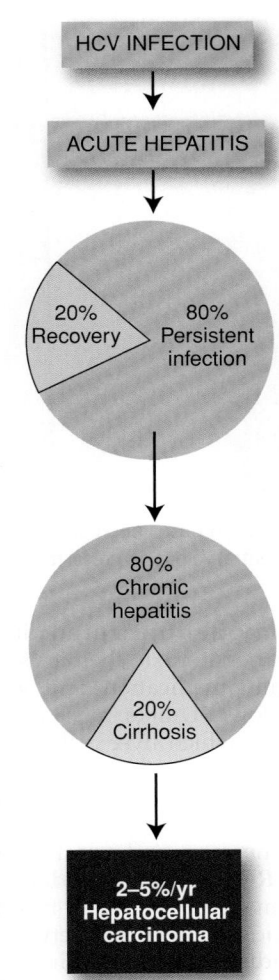

FIGURE 20-27. Outcomes of infection with hepatitis C virus (HCV).

TABLE 20-3			
COMPARATIVE FEATURES OF THE COMMON FORMS OF VIRAL HEPATITIS			
	Hepatitis A	**Hepatitis B**	**Hepatitis C**
Genome	RNA	DNA	RNA
Incubation period	3–6 weeks	6 weeks–6 months	7–8 weeks
Transmission	Oral	Parenteral	Parenteral
Blood	No	Yes	Yes
Feces	Yes	No	No
Vertical	No	Yes	5%
Fulminant	Very rare	Yes	Rare hepatic necrosis
Chronic hepatitis	No	10%	80%
Carrier state	No	Yes	Yes
Liver cancer	No	Yes	Yes

kidney (membranoproliferative glomerulonephritis) may be affected. Non-Hodgkin B-cell lymphomas are more common in patients with chronic hepatitis C.

Since it is largely asymptomatic, acute HCV rarely comes to medical attention. For patients who are treated for acute HCV, success rates are higher than in chronic cases. Chronic hepatitis C was previously treated with a combination of injected interferon-α and oral ribavirin. New therapies combining sofosbuvir and ledipasvir act synergistically to impair viral replication. This enables the immune system to clear the virus and results in a cure rate of ~99%. A sustained virologic response (i.e., no detectable HCV RNA) is associated with a conspicuous decrease in the risk of HCC.

Table 20-3 compares the major features of the common forms of viral hepatitis.

Hepatitis E Virus Is a Major Cause of Epidemic Hepatitis

Hepatitis E is a self-limited, acute, icteric disease similar to hepatitis A. Hepatitis E virus (HEV) is an enteric RNA virus of the Hepeviridae family, five species of which are now known. It accounts for more than 1/2 of cases of acute viral

hepatitis in young to middle-aged people in poorer regions of the world. Large outbreaks have been reported in India, Nepal, Burma, Pakistan, the former Soviet Union, Africa, and Mexico. Most of these epidemics have followed heavy rains in areas with inadequate sewage disposal. HEV infection may be transmitted via several routes: waterborne, zoonotic (especially eating raw or undercooked meat of infected wild animals such as pig, boar, or deer) and parenteral and vertical transmission. HEV closely resembles a swine virus, suggesting that the latter may represent a reservoir of infection.

The incubation period for HEV is 35 to 40 days. Jaundice, hepatomegaly, fever, and arthralgias are common and usually resolve within 6 weeks, with 1% to 12% mortality. Like hepatitis A, clinical illness from hepatitis E is far more common in adults than in children; in the latter, infection may often be subclinical. The disease is very dangerous in pregnant women, in whom mortality may reach 20% to 40%. Chronic disease and carrier states are unknown in immunocompetent patients, but immunocompromised people may develop chronic hepatitis E. A successful vaccine against HEV infection has been developed and tested in Nepal but is not yet licensed in the United States.

PATHOLOGY OF VIRAL HEPATITIS

All Forms of Acute Viral Hepatitis Are Pathologically Similar

 PATHOLOGY: The hallmark of acute viral hepatitis is liver cell death (Fig. 20-28). Within the hepatic lobule, scattered single cell necrosis or death of small clusters of hepatocytes is seen. A few apoptotic liver cells appear as small, deeply eosinophilic bodies **(acidophilic bodies),** sometimes with pyknotic nuclei. Acidophilic bodies are characteristic of viral hepatitis but are also

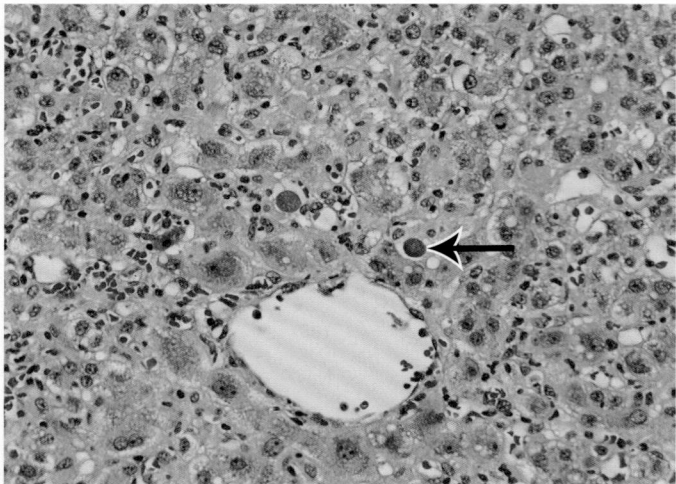

FIGURE 20-28. Acute viral hepatitis. Disarray of liver cell plates, swollen (ballooned) hepatocytes and an infiltrate of lymphocytes and scattered mononuclear inflammatory cells are typical features. Remnants of apoptotic hepatocytes have been extruded into sinusoids, where they appear as acidophilic bodies (*arrow*).

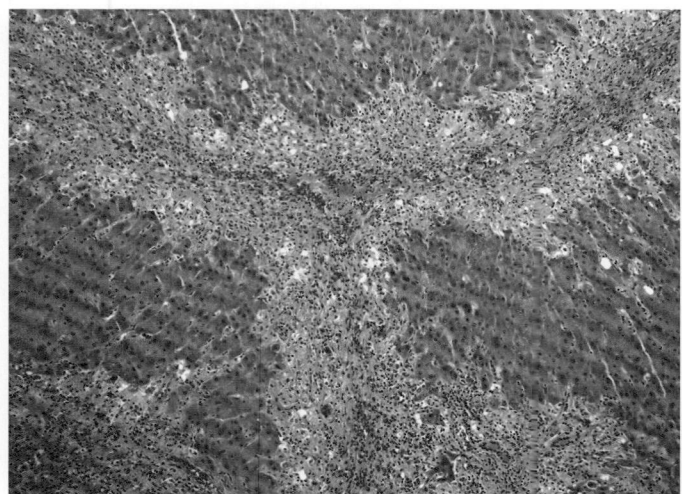

FIGURE 20-29. Confluent hepatic necrosis. Hemorrhagic zones of necrosis bridge adjacent central veins and portal tracts (bridging necrosis).

seen in many other liver diseases. In acute viral hepatitis, many liver cells show varying degrees of hydropic swelling and differences in size, shape, and staining properties. Concomitantly, regenerative liver cells may have larger nuclei and basophilic cytoplasm. Resulting irregular liver cell plates are described as **lobular disarray**.

Mononuclear cells, mostly lymphocytes, infiltrate lobules diffusely, surround individual necrotic liver cells and accumulate in areas of focal necrosis. Macrophages may be prominent, whereas eosinophils and polymorphonuclear leukocytes are less common. Characteristically, lymphocytes infiltrate between the wall of the central vein and the liver cell plates, an appearance termed **central phlebitis**. Swelling and proliferation of the endothelium of central veins (**endophlebitis**) may develop. Kupffer cells are enlarged, project into sinusoid lumens and contain lipofuscin pigment and phagocytosed debris. Cholestasis is common. If severe, it is called **cholestatic hepatitis**, in which many liver cells are arrayed around dilated bile canaliculi, giving an acinar or glandular appearance. Lumens of dilated canaliculi may contain bile plugs.

Mononuclear inflammatory cells accumulate within portal tracts. Lymphocytes in portal tracts may form follicles, particularly in hepatitis C. The limiting plate of hepatocytes around the portal tracts is usually intact. These changes are gradually reversed during recovery, and normal hepatic architecture is completely restored.

Confluent Hepatic Necrosis Affects Whole Regions of the Lobule

Confluent hepatic necrosis reflects particularly severe forms of acute viral hepatitis, characterized by death of many hepatocytes in a geographical distribution. In extreme cases, nearly all liver cells in a lobule die (**massive hepatic necrosis**). The most common viral cause is acute hepatitis B; only rarely does confluent hepatic necrosis result from infection with other hepatotropic viruses. The lesions are not unique

to viral hepatitis but may also occur in autoimmune hepatitis and after exposure to hepatotoxic chemicals or drugs, which include over-the-counter medications and herbal and dietary supplements (see below). Unlike most common forms of acute viral hepatitis, in which liver cell necrosis appears to be random and patchy, confluent hepatic necrosis typically affects whole regions of lobules. The lesions of confluent hepatic necrosis, in order of increasing severity, are bridging necrosis, submassive necrosis, and massive necrosis.

BRIDGING NECROSIS: At the milder end of the spectrum of lesions that make up confluent hepatic necrosis are bands of necrosis (bridging necrosis) between adjacent portal tracts, between adjacent central veins and from portal tracts to central veins (Fig. 20-29). Adjacent plates of hepatocytes die, causing collapse of the collagenous stroma to form bands of connective tissue. These are best seen with a reticulin stain. If such bands encircle an area of liver cells, they may impart a nodular appearance, as in cirrhosis.

SUBMASSIVE HEPATIC NECROSIS: This form of acute hepatitis defines an even more severe injury in which entire lobules or groups of adjacent lobules die. Clinically, these patients manifest as severe hepatitis, which may rapidly progress to hepatic failure, in which case the disease is classified as **fulminant hepatitis**.

MASSIVE HEPATIC NECROSIS (ACUTE YELLOW ATROPHY): This is the most feared form of acute viral hepatitis, but fortunately it is rare. It is almost invariably fatal. Grossly, the liver becomes shrunken to as little as 500 g (1/3 of normal weight). The capsule is wrinkled, with mottled, soft, and flabby red-tan parenchyma. Nearly all hepatocytes are dead (Fig. 20-30), and only the collagenous frameworks remain as epitaphs of liver lobules that collapsed and perished. Macrophages, erythrocytes and necrotic debris fill sinusoids. For unknown reasons, the massive necrosis does not elicit a vigorous inflammatory response in either the parenchyma or portal tracts. Liver transplantation is a mainstay of therapy.

Chronic Hepatitis May Complicate Hepatitis B and C, Metabolic Diseases, and Immune Disorders

The morphologic spectrum of chronic hepatitis ranges from mild portal inflammation with little or no liver cell necrosis

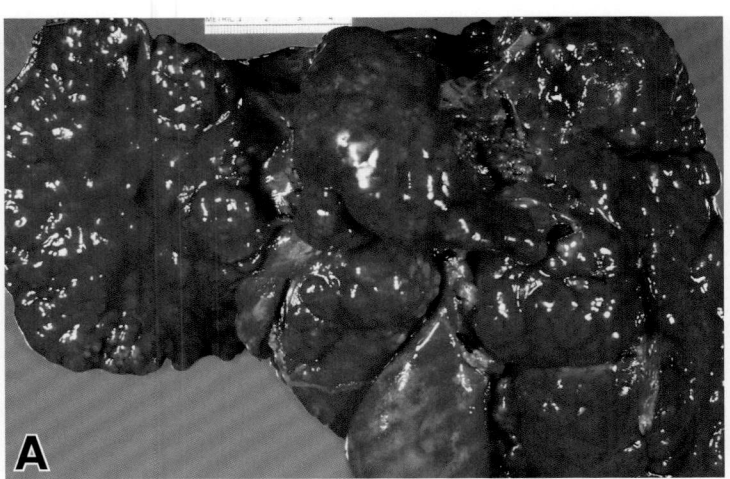
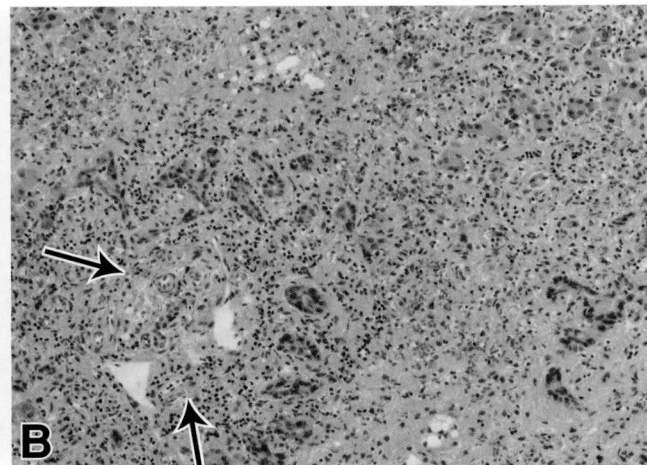

FIGURE 20-30. Massive hepatic necrosis. A. The liver is soft and reduced in size and grossly shows a mottled, yellowish surface ("acute yellow atrophy"). **B.** Microscopic examination shows complete loss of hepatocytes. The framework of the lobule has collapsed. The portal tracts (*arrows*) are expanded and contain ductular reaction.

(Fig. 20-31) to widespread inflammation, necrosis, and fibrosis eventuating in cirrhosis (Fig. 20-32).

PORTAL TRACT LESIONS: In chronic hepatitis, portal tracts are variably infiltrated by lymphocytes, plasma cells, and macrophages (Figs. 20-31 and 20-32). These expanded portal tracts often show mild to severe proliferation of bile ductules, which is a nonspecific response to chronic liver injury. In the case of chronic hepatitis C, lymphoid aggregates or follicles with reactive centers are often present. Eosinophils may be seen in autoimmune hepatitis.

INTERFACE HEPATITIS: This is focal inflammatory destruction of the limiting plate of hepatocytes. A periportal chronic inflammatory infiltrate creates an irregular border between portal tracts and the lobular parenchyma (Fig. 20-32A).

INTRALOBULAR LESIONS: Focal necrosis and parenchymal inflammation typify chronic hepatitis. Scattered acidophilic bodies and enlarged Kupffer cells are common (Fig. 20-28). In chronic hepatitis B, scattered hepatocytes may have enlarged pale light pink cytoplasm containing abundant HBsAg in SER **(ground-glass hepatocytes)** (Fig. 20-33).

PERIPORTAL FIBROSIS: Progressive loss of periportal hepatocytes by interface hepatitis leads to deposition of collagen, giving portal tracts a stellate (star-shaped) appearance. In time, fibrosis may extend to join adjacent portal tracts or approach the central vein, ultimately developing into cirrhosis (Fig. 20-32B).

AUTOIMMUNE HEPATITIS

Autoimmune hepatitis is a severe type of chronic hepatitis associated with circulating autoantibodies and elevated serum immunoglobulins. It may appear at any age; 70% of cases occur in women. In the United States, autoimmune hepatitis affects up to 200,000 people and accounts for 6% of liver transplants.

PATHOPHYSIOLOGY: There are two types of autoimmune hepatitis:

- **Type I** disease is more common (80% of cases). It features antinuclear and anti–smooth muscle antibodies. Some 70% of cases occur in women younger than 40 years, among whom 1/3 have other autoimmune diseases, including thyroiditis, rheumatoid arthritis, and ulcerative colitis. Of those patients with type I autoimmune hepatitis, 1/4 present with cirrhosis, indicating that the disease usually has a prolonged asymptomatic course. Antibodies against many cytosolic enzymes may be detected, but the hepatocyte membrane asialoglycoprotein receptor is the main candidate target for antibody-dependent cell-mediated cytotoxicity (ADCC). The HLA-*DRB1* gene confers particular susceptibility to type I autoimmune hepatitis. Some patients may present with a poorly characterized "overlap syndrome" with mixed clinical and histologic features of autoimmune hepatitis and either primary biliary cholangitis (PBC) or PSC.
- **Type II** autoimmune hepatitis occurs mainly in children who are 2 to 14 years old. Antibodies against liver and kidney microsomes (anti-LKM) are characteristic.

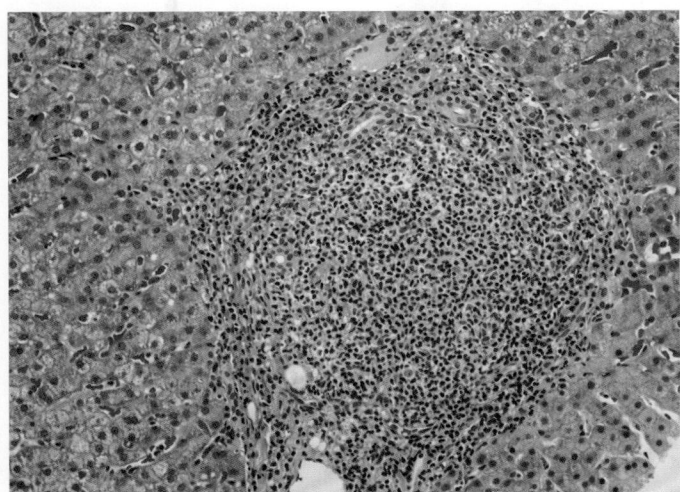

FIGURE 20-31. Mild chronic hepatitis. A portal tract has become infiltrated by mononuclear inflammatory cells. The lobular parenchyma is intact.

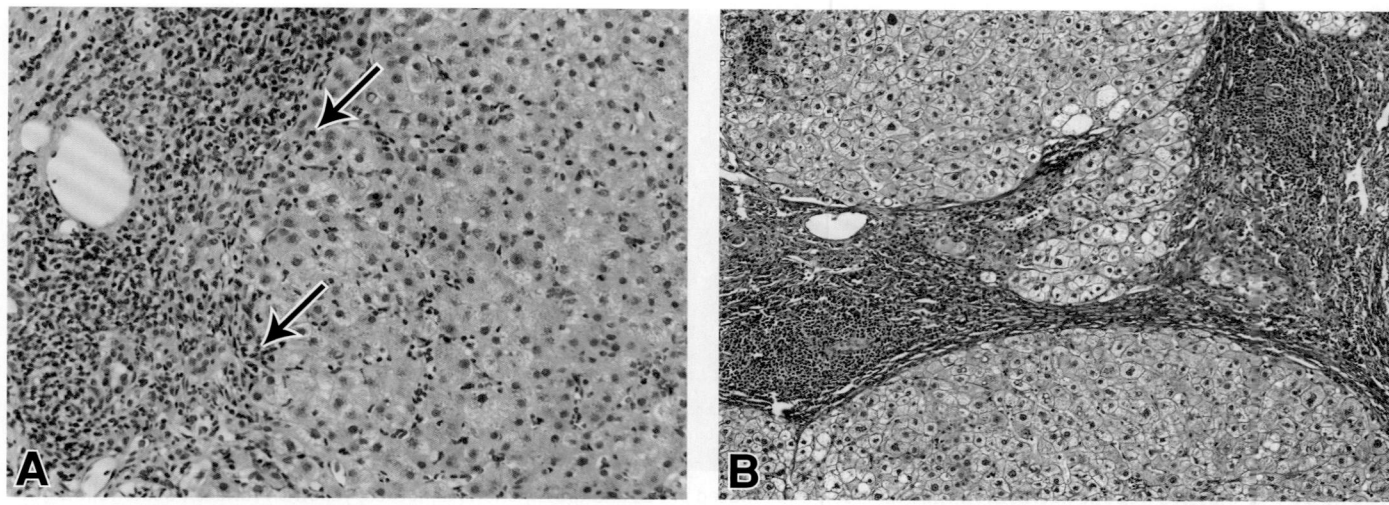

FIGURE 20-32. Severe chronic hepatitis. A. Mononuclear inflammatory infiltrate has accumulated in an expanded portal tract (*left*). Interface hepatitis is penetration of inflammation to the limiting plate where it surrounds groups of hepatocytes at the border of the portal tract (*arrows*). **B. Chronic hepatitis with cirrhosis.** Liver from a patient with long-standing chronic hepatitis C shows lymphocytic aggregates, bridging fibrosis, and nodular transformation.

However, the key autoantigen is a P450-type drug-metabolizing enzyme (CYP 2D6). These patients often have other autoimmune diseases (i.e., type I diabetes and thyroiditis). Genetic determinants of type II disease are not defined.

PATHOLOGY: Autoimmune hepatitis basically resembles acute and chronic viral hepatitis histologically, but lobular inflammation and necrosis, and interface hepatitis are more pronounced. The inflammatory infiltrate is rich in plasma cells, an important diagnostic feature (Fig. 20-34). Confluent hepatic necrosis may be seen in severe cases.

CLINICAL FEATURES: Autoimmune hepatitis can arise insidiously, with fatigue and mild right upper quadrant discomfort. Often, there is a personal or family history of autoimmunity. With time, aminotransferase levels rise markedly and may exceed 1,000 IU/mL. Marked hyperglobulinemia is common. In severe cases, jaundice, hepatic synthetic dysfunction and even liver failure ensue, but it rarely presents as fulminant disease. Untreated, autoimmune hepatitis often progresses to cirrhosis.

Autoimmune hepatitis usually responds to combinations of corticosteroids and immunosuppressants such as azathioprine. Patients whose disease progresses to cirrhosis may receive liver transplants. Autoimmune hepatitis recurs in up to 20% of patients after liver transplantation.

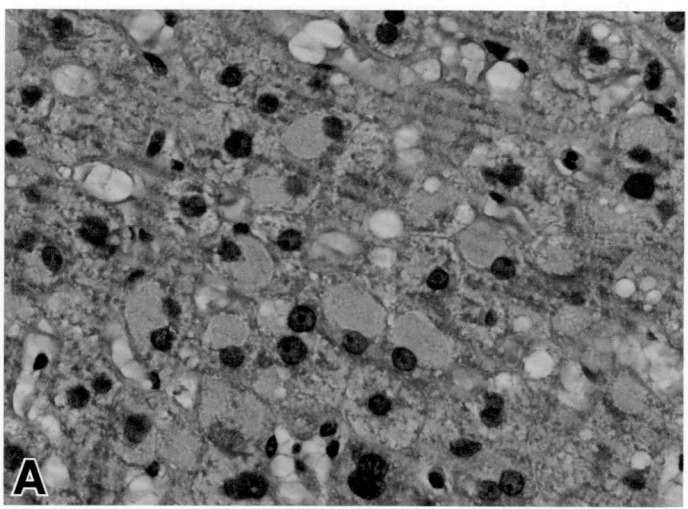
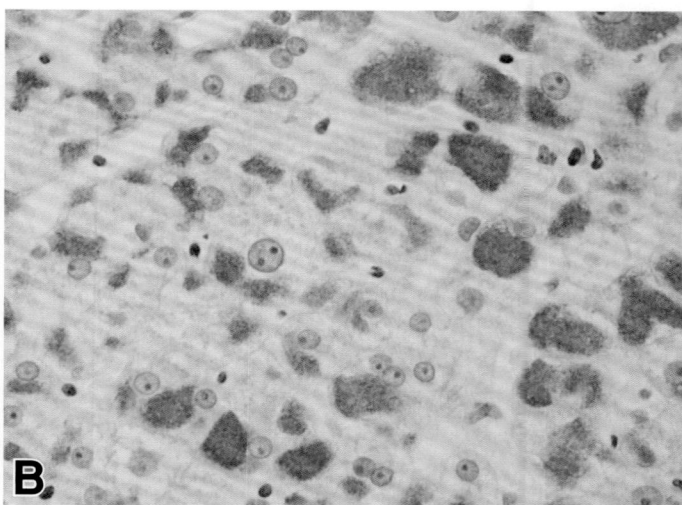

FIGURE 20-33. "Ground-glass" hepatocytes. A. Liver from a patient with chronic hepatitis B shows scattered hepatocytes with an abundant light pink cytoplasm containing hepatitis B surface antigen (HBsAg). **B.** The same specimen has been stained for HBsAg by the immunoperoxidase method. The abundant cytoplasmic HBsAg appears brown.

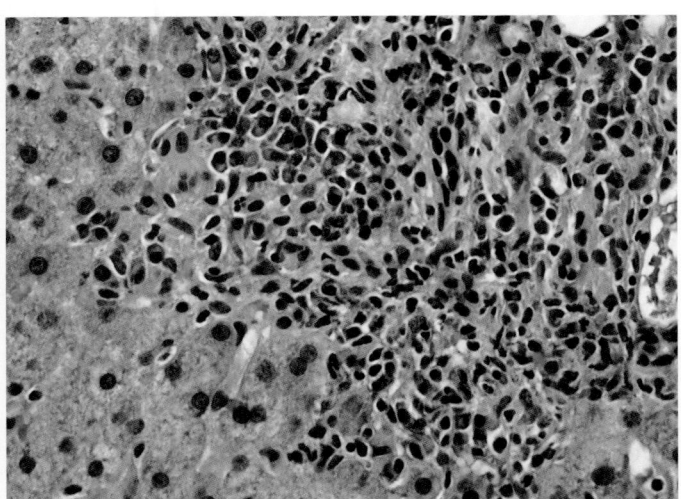

FIGURE 20-34. Autoimmune hepatitis. The inflammatory infiltrate is rich in plasma cells.

ALCOHOLIC LIVER DISEASE

The harmful effects of excess alcohol (ethanol, ethyl alcohol) consumption have been recognized almost since the dawn of recorded history. The prophet Isaiah warned, "Woe to him that is mighty to drink wine." Ethanol is now seen as a hepatotoxin that acts both directly and indirectly.

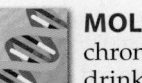 **EPIDEMIOLOGY:** *Alcoholic cirrhosis is most common in countries where people consume the most alcohol,* regardless of the specific alcoholic beverage (e.g., wine in France, beer in Australia, spirits in Scandinavia). Only a minority of chronic alcoholics develop cirrhosis, but there is a dose–response relationship between lifetime dose of alcohol (duration of exposure and daily amount of alcohol consumed) and the appearance of cirrhosis.

About 10% of men and 5% of women in the United States abuse alcohol. In some other countries, this figure is much higher. *Some 15% of alcoholics develop cirrhosis; many of them die in hepatic failure or from extrahepatic complications of cirrhosis.* In many urban areas of the United States with high alcoholism rates, cirrhosis of the liver is the third or fourth leading cause of death in men younger than 45 years.

The amount of alcohol required to produce chronic liver disease depends on body size, age, gender, and ethnicity, but the lower range seems to be about 20 g/day (about 2 oz of 86 proof [43%] whiskey, two glasses of wine or two 12-oz bottles of beer daily) for women and 40 g/day in men. In general, more than 10 years of alcohol use at this level is needed to produce cirrhosis, although a few cirrhotic patients give shorter histories of heavy alcohol use.

Women are more predisposed to the harmful effects of alcohol, for unknown reasons. However, women metabolize alcohol differently and have lower body masses.

The epidemiology of alcoholic liver disease is complicated by its association with the hepatotropic viruses. HBV seropositivity is two- to fourfold more common in alcoholics than in control populations. The prevalence of anti-HCV antibodies is up to 10% among alcoholics and even higher among alcoholics with chronic liver disease. As noted above, people who abuse alcohol and also have hepatitis C are more likely to develop liver disease than their counterparts not so infected.

Ethanol Is Mainly Metabolized in the Liver

Ethanol is absorbed rapidly from the stomach and eventually distributed in body water space. Between 5% and 10% is excreted unchanged, mostly in the urine and expired breath. The remaining 90% is metabolized by the liver to acetaldehyde and acetate, largely by cytosolic **alcohol dehydrogenase (ADH)**. The mixed-function oxidases in the **microsomal ethanol-oxidizing system** in the SER are a minor metabolic pathway for alcohol. Clearance of alcohol from the body, unlike most drugs, is linear—that is, a fixed quantity is metabolized per unit time. Roughly, for the average man, 7 to 10 g of alcohol is eliminated per hour. However, since the microsomal pathway (see above) is upregulated in chronic alcoholics, they metabolize ethanol more rapidly, as long as they do not suffer from active liver disease.

Alcohol Consumption Causes a Spectrum of Liver Diseases

Alcoholic liver disease spans three major morphologic and clinical entities: **fatty liver, acute alcoholic hepatitis,** and **cirrhosis**. These lesions usually occur in sequence, but they may coexist in any combination and may actually be independent entities.

Fatty Liver

MOLECULAR PATHOGENESIS: Virtually all chronic alcoholics, regardless of their pattern of drinking, accumulate fat in hepatocytes (**steatosis**). The relative contributions of different metabolic pathways to steatosis may depend on the amount of alcohol consumed, dietary lipid content, body stores of fat, hormonal status, and other variables. *Still, accumulation of fat clearly depends on alcohol intake, as it is fully and rapidly reversible if alcohol ingestion stops.*

Dietary fat, as chylomicrons and free fatty acids, is transported to the liver, where it is taken up by hepatocytes. Triglycerides are then hydrolyzed to free fatty acids. These, in turn, undergo β-oxidation in mitochondria or are converted by the ER to triglycerides. These newly synthesized triglycerides are secreted within lipoprotein particles (mainly chylomicrons and very low density lipoprotein or VLDL) or are retained for storage.

Most of the fat deposited in the liver after chronic alcohol consumption is from the diet. Ethanol increases lipolysis and thus delivery of free fatty acids to the liver. Within hepatocytes, ethanol (1) increases fatty acid synthesis, (2) decreases mitochondrial oxidation of fatty acids, (3) raises triglyceride production, and (4) impairs release of lipoproteins. Collectively, these metabolic consequences produce a fatty liver.

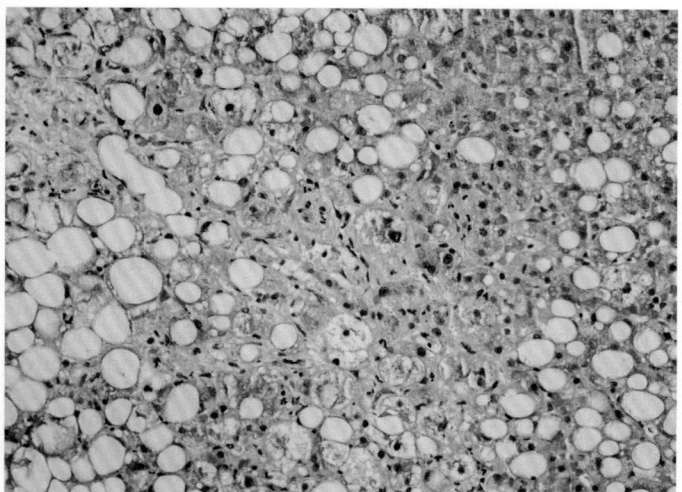

FIGURE 20-35. Alcoholic fatty liver. The cytoplasm of nearly all of the hepatocytes is distended by fat which displaces the nucleus to the periphery.

PATHOLOGY: In the setting of high alcohol intake, the liver becomes yellow and enlarged, sometimes to as much as three times its normal weight. This increased weight reflects not only fat accumulation; protein and water content are also increased. The extent of visible fat accumulation varies from minute droplets scattered in the cytoplasm of a few hepatocytes to distention of the entire cytoplasm of most cells by coalesced droplets (Fig. 20-35). In the latter case, liver cells may be barely recognizable as such and resemble adipocytes, with their cytoplasm distended by a clear area and their nuclei flattened and displaced to the periphery of the cell.

Ultrastructurally, hepatocytes in alcohol-induced fatty livers reflect the cytotoxicity of ethanol rather than any direct effect of fat. Mitochondria are enlarged, with occasional bizarre giant forms. The smooth ER is hyperplastic, resembling that produced by other inducers of microsomal drug-metabolizing enzymes (see Chapter 1).

Chronic ethanol ingestion elicits pronounced hepatic functional alterations. Liver mitochondria show decreased rates of substrate oxidation (e.g., of fatty acids) and impaired ATP formation. Smooth ER hyperplasia is accompanied by increased activity of the cytochrome P450–dependent mixed-function oxidases. Not only is the microsomal ethanol-oxidizing system induced, but metabolism of a variety of drugs is also enhanced. *This increased microsomal function also augments metabolism of hepatic toxins, thus exaggerating the danger of agents such as acetaminophen, in which it is the drug's metabolic products that are most toxic.* Whereas chronic alcohol consumption promotes microsomal functions, acute alcohol ingestion inhibits mixed-function oxidases and acutely reduces the rate of clearance of drugs from the body.

CLINICAL FEATURES: Patients with uncomplicated alcoholic fatty liver have surprisingly few symptoms of liver disease. Despite the striking morphologic change in the liver, alcoholic fatty liver is fully reversible and does not by itself progress to more severe disease. The best treatment for fatty liver due to alcohol is

abstinence. Fatty liver, although characteristic of alcoholism, is not limited to it. Fatty liver may also be seen in nonalcoholic fatty liver disease (NAFLD; see below), hepatitis C, after certain drugs and in many other conditions.

Alcoholic Hepatitis

Alcoholic hepatitis is characterized by (1) hepatocyte necrosis, mainly in the central zone; (2) cytoplasmic hyalin inclusions within hepatocytes (Mallory-Denk hyalins); (3) an acute inflammatory infiltrate in the lobule; and (4) pericellular fibrosis (Fig. 20-36). **The pathogenesis of alcoholic hepatitis is a mystery.** Alcoholics may have mild fatty liver for many years and, without any change in drinking habits, suddenly develop acute alcoholic hepatitis. It may be that long-standing, subclinical alcoholic hepatitis precedes clinically overt hepatitis. Nevertheless, the often explosive presentation of alcoholic hepatitis suggests that some environmental or physiologic cofactor is involved, although none has been identified.

PATHOLOGY: Typically, hepatic architecture is intact. Hepatocytes show variable hydropic swelling, giving them a heterogeneous appearance. Isolated necrotic liver cells or clusters of them have pyknotic nuclei and show karyorrhexis. Scattered hepatocytes contain **Mallory–Denk hyalins** (Fig. 20-36). These cytoplasmic inclusions are more common in visibly damaged, swollen hepatocytes and appear as irregular skeins of eosinophilic material or as solid eosinophilic masses, often in a perinuclear location. They are aggregates of intermediate (cytokeratin) filaments (Fig. 20-36C). The damaged, ballooned hepatocytes, particularly those containing Mallory–Denk hyalins, are surrounded by neutrophils (satellitosis). A more diffuse, intralobular inflammatory infiltrate is also present. Mallory–Denk hyalins are characteristic of, but not specific for, alcoholic liver disease, as they may also be present in nonalcoholic steatohepatitis (NASH), chronic cholestatic syndromes, WD and HCC. Mild to severe cholestasis is seen in up to 1/3 of cases. Alcoholic hepatitis is usually superimposed on an existing fatty liver, but there is no evidence that fat accumulation per se predisposes or contributes to development of alcoholic hepatitis.

Collagen deposition is always seen in alcoholic hepatitis, especially around central veins (terminal hepatic venules). Chronic alcohol exposure activates hepatic stellate cells to deposit intrasinusoidal collagen. In severe cases, venules and perivenular sinusoids become obliterated and surrounded by dense fibrous tissue to yield **central hyaline sclerosis** (Figs. 20-36 and 20-37). This condition is often associated with noncirrhotic portal hypertension.

The appearance of portal tracts in alcoholic hepatitis is highly variable. Some are virtually normal, whereas others are enlarged, with mononuclear infiltrate and ductular reaction. Altered portal tracts often show spurs of fibrous tissue that penetrate the lobules.

CLINICAL FEATURES: Patients with alcoholic hepatitis have malaise and anorexia, fever, right upper quadrant abdominal pain, and jaundice. Leukocytosis is common. Serum aminotransferase activities,

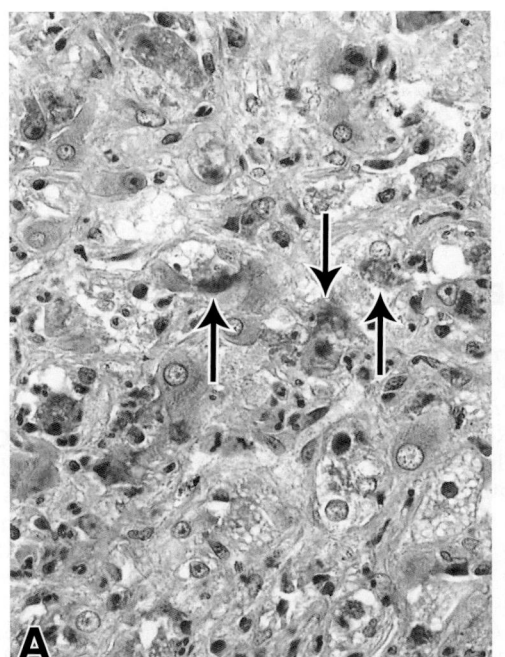

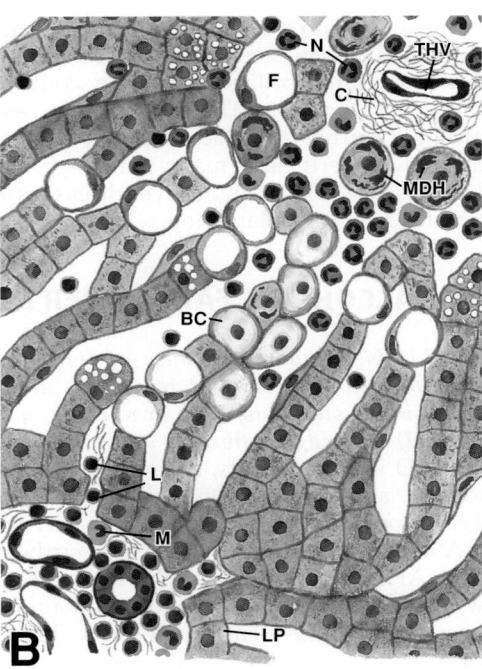

FIGURE 20-36. Alcoholic hepatitis. A. Necrosis and degeneration of hepatocytes, with Mallory–Denk hyalins in the cytoplasm of injured hepatocytes (*arrows*) and infiltration by neutrophils. **B. Schematic representation of the major pathologic features of alcoholic hepatitis.** The lesions are predominantly centrilobular and include necrosis and loss of hepatocytes, ballooned cells (*BC*) and Mallory–Denk hyalins (*MDH*) in the cytoplasm of damaged hepatocytes. The inflammatory infiltrate consists predominantly of neutrophils (*N*), although a few lymphocytes (*L*) and macrophages (*M*) are also present. The central venule, or terminal hepatic venule (*THV*), is encased in connective tissue (*C*) (central hyaline sclerosis; also see Fig. 14-36). Fat-laden hepatocytes (*F*) are evident in the lobule. The portal tract displays moderate chronic inflammation, and the limiting plate (*LP*) is focally breached. **C. Ultrastructure of Mallory–Denk hyalins.** These are composed of dense, interwoven bundles of cytokeratin filaments in the cytoplasm of hepatocytes.

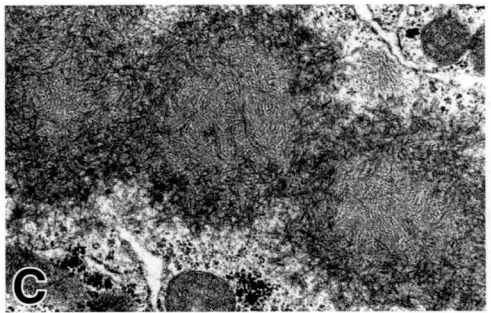

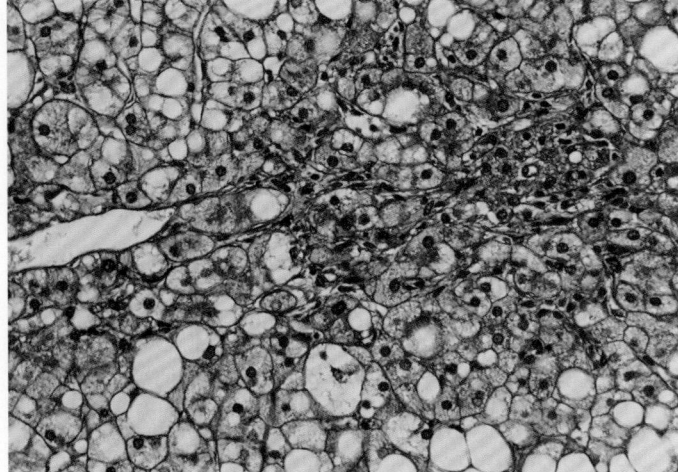

FIGURE 20-37. Pericellular fibrosis in nonalcoholic steatohepatitis (NASH). This trichrome-stained liver from a patient with NASH shows pericellular fibrosis around the central venule (*blue*). Note the macrovesicular fat. This lesion mimics that seen in alcoholic liver disease.

particularly AST, are moderately elevated but not as high as in viral hepatitis: AST usually remains under 400. The AST:ALT ratio is typically 2:1. Serum alkaline phosphatase activity is usually increased. In severe cases, a prolonged prothrombin time often portends an ominous prognosis.

The outlook in patients with alcoholic hepatitis reflects the severity of liver cell injury. In some patients, the disease progresses rapidly to hepatic failure and death. Mortality in the acute stage of alcoholic hepatitis is about 10%. Most of those who abstain from alcohol after recovery from acute alcoholic hepatitis recover. However, of those who continue to drink, up to 70% ultimately develop cirrhosis.

There is no specific treatment for acute alcoholic hepatitis. Corticosteroids improve short-term mortality and thus are often given if there is no infection or renal failure. Nutritional therapy can be beneficial.

Alcoholic Cirrhosis

In about 15% of alcoholics, hepatocellular necrosis, fibrosis, and regeneration eventually lead to formation of fibrous septa around hepatocellular nodules (Fig. 20-13). The other lesions of alcoholic liver disease—fatty liver and acute or persistent alcoholic hepatitis—are often seen in conjunction with cirrhosis. Some assert that progression to alcoholic cirrhosis requires at least subclinical alcoholic hepatitis. Activated hepatic stellate cells, which produce sinusoidal and pericellular collagen, probably contribute to the development of cirrhosis. The prognosis in cases of established alcoholic cirrhosis is much better in those who abstain from alcohol. Nevertheless, many patients progress to end-stage liver disease, and alcoholic liver disease is a common indication for liver transplantation.

NONALCOHOLIC FATTY LIVER DISEASE

NAFLD is so named because of its close resemblance to alcoholic liver disease. It represents diverse liver injuries from simple steatosis, with or without associated hepatitis (NASH) to bridging fibrosis and cirrhosis. Risk factors for NAFLD include obesity, type 2 diabetes mellitus, hyperlipidemia, and metabolic syndrome (see Chapter 22). About 1/2 of people with both severe obesity and diabetes have NASH, of whom up to 1/5 develop cirrhosis.

NAFLD overlaps alcoholic liver disease histologically, with steatosis, lobular and portal inflammation, hepatocyte necrosis, Mallory–Denk hyalins and fibrosis. As in alcoholic liver disease, centrilobular fibrosis is common (Fig. 20-37). If cirrhosis develops, steatosis often disappears. *Thus, NAFLD is the likely cause of many cases of the so-called cryptogenic cirrhosis.*

PATHOPHYSIOLOGY: The pathogenesis of NAFLD and NASH may overlap that of alcoholic hepatitis. Insulin resistance is associated with increased hepatic mitochondrial oxidation of free fatty acids, increased oxidative stress and lipid peroxidation, and it appears to be the strongest risk factor for NAFLD and NASH. Progression to cirrhosis in NAFLD is often insidious, and many patients remain asymptomatic, with only moderate increases in serum liver enzyme activities.

NAFLD is considered the hepatic manifestation of the metabolic syndrome, which consists of abdominal obesity, dyslipidemia, insulin resistance, and hypertension (see Chapter 13). Weight reduction, including that via bariatric surgery, tends to improve NAFLD and NASH, but no definitive treatment is yet available.

PRIMARY BILIARY CHOLANGITIS

PBC is an immune-mediated, chronic, progressive cholestatic disease in which intrahepatic bile ducts are destroyed **(non-suppurative destructive cholangitis)**. Loss of bile ducts leads to impaired bile secretion, cholestasis, and hepatic damage. PBC occurs mainly in middle-aged women (10:1 female predominance).

It accounts for up to 2% of deaths from cirrhosis. Cases are sporadic, although the prevalence of PBC in families of patients with PBC is considerably higher than that in the general population, suggesting a genetic predisposition.

MOLECULAR PATHOGENESIS: PBC is associated with many immune abnormalities and thus is widely held to be an autoimmune disease. Most (85%) patients have at least one other autoimmune

disease (chronic thyroiditis, rheumatoid arthritis, scleroderma, Sjögren syndrome, systemic lupus erythematosus), and almost 1/2 (40%) have two or more such diseases.

The *DRB1*008* family of major histocompatibility complex–encoded genes is associated with PBC, whereas the disease is less common in people carrying *DRB1*11* and *DRB1*13*. Polymorphisms of key immune regulatory genes, such as those encoding TNFα and the CTL antigen 4 (CTLA4), are reported in patients with several autoimmune diseases, including PBC. Increased X chromosome monosomy may explain the strong female predominance of PBC.

PATHOPHYSIOLOGY: Humoral and cellular immunity are both impaired. Serum immunoglobulin levels are increased, especially IgM. *More than 95% of patients have circulating antimitochondrial antibodies (AMAs), a finding of which is commonly used to diagnose PBC.* Autoantibodies bind epitopes associated with the mitochondrial pyruvate dehydrogenase complex. Despite their specificity, AMAs do not affect mitochondrial function and play no known role in the pathogenesis or progression of the disease. Thus, they are markers but not effectors of disease. Other circulating autoantibodies include antinuclear, antithyroid, antiplatelet, antiacetylcholine receptor, and antiribonucleoprotein antibodies. The complement system is also chronically activated.

The cells surrounding and infiltrating sites of bile duct damage are mostly suppressor/cytotoxic (CD8⁺) lymphocytes, suggesting that they mediate the destruction of the ductal epithelium.

PATHOLOGY: Pathologic stages of PBC are portal stage, periportal stage, septal stage, and biliary cirrhosis.

- *STAGE 1: FLORID DUCT LESION OR PORTAL STAGE:* Early PBC features a unique lesion, a **chronic destructive cholangitis** involving small and medium-sized intrahepatic bile ducts. Injury to the ducts is segmental and thus appears focal in tissue sections. Lymphocytes, plasma cells, and macrophages surround the ducts, disrupting the basement membrane (Fig. 20-38). Bile duct epithelium is irregular and hyperplastic, with stratification and occasional papillary ingrowths of epithelial cells. Epithelioid granulomas often occur in portal tracts and may impinge on the bile ducts.
- *STAGE 2: PERIPORTAL STAGE:* In this stage, bile ducts are reduced in number and ductular proliferation is evident in periportal areas. Inflammation is less than in stage 1.
- *STAGE 3: SEPTAL STAGE:* As a result of the destructive inflammation in stages 1 and 2 PBC, small bile ducts virtually disappear during the septal stage. Scarring of medium-sized bile ducts is common. Collagenous septa extend from the portal tracts into the lobular parenchyma and begin to encircle some lobules.
- *STAGE 4: CIRRHOSIS:* The end stage of PBC is cirrhosis, producing a dark-green bile-stained nodular liver with

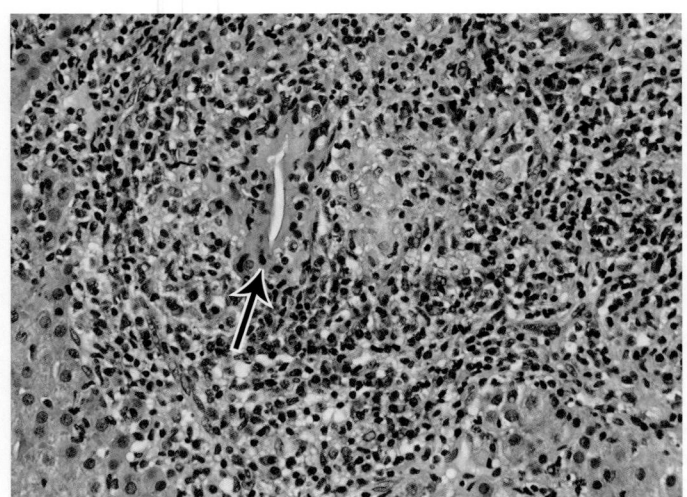

FIGURE 20-38. Florid duct lesion in primary biliary cholangitis (PBC), stage I. A portal tract is expanded by an inflammatory infiltrate consisting of lymphocytes, plasma cells, eosinophils, and macrophages. Florid duct lesion represents a damaged bile duct (*arrow*) by the inflammation.

mainly portal-to-portal bridging fibrous septa. This fibrosis gives a "jigsaw puzzle" appearance to the cirrhotic parenchyma and the chronic cholestasis give a "halo" appearance to the cirrhotic nodules. Small bile ducts are scarce, and medium-sized ducts are conspicuously fewer in number. There is little inflammation within either the fibrous septa or the parenchymal nodules.

CLINICAL FEATURES: *Some 90% to 95% of those afflicted with PBC are women, usually those who are 30 to 65 years old.* Fatigue and pruritus are the most common initial symptoms, but many patients have no symptoms during the early stage of PBC. Some remain asymptomatic and appear to have an excellent prognosis; others ultimately develop advanced cirrhosis and its complications. The diagnosis of PBC is confirmed when a patient meets two of three criteria: (1) AMA titer of 1:40 or higher; (2) biochemical cholestasis, as indicated by elevated serum alkaline phosphatase activity for at least 6 months; and (3) typical liver histology seen in a biopsy. The unusual diagnosis of the so-called AMA-negative PBC rests on characteristic histologic and clinical findings (criteria 2 and 3).

Early in PBC, serum alkaline phosphatase activity is usually high, but bilirubin is normal or slightly elevated. The patient may complain of severe pruritus. As the disease advances, serum bilirubin progressively increases in most patients. Serum AST and ALT are only moderately elevated. Blood cholesterol levels increase strikingly, and an abnormal lipoprotein (lipoprotein-X) appears, a finding in many forms of chronic cholestasis. Cholesterol-laden macrophages accumulate in subcutaneous tissues, where they form localized lesions termed **xanthomas.** Impaired bile excretion into the intestine often leads to severe **steatorrhea** due to fat malabsorption. Associated malabsorption of vitamin D and calcium leads to **osteomalacia** and **osteoporosis,** two important complications of PBC. About 1/3 of patients develop gallstones. Those patients

who eventually develop cirrhosis die of liver failure or complications of portal hypertension.

PBC is treated with ursodeoxycholic acid (UDCA), which improves bile transport in the liver. It does not treat the underlying causes of PBC but it does, increase transplant-free survival and leads to biochemical remission in about 40% of patients. The course of PBC is usually indolent and may last as long as 20 to 30 years. Liver transplantation is highly effective in end-stage PBC.

PRIMARY SCLEROSING CHOLANGITIS

PSC is a chronic cholestatic liver disease of unknown etiology, in which inflammation and fibrosis narrow and then obstruct intrahepatic and extrahepatic bile ducts. It usually occurs in men (70%), with a mean age of 40 years. PSC prevalence is 14 cases per 100,000 population. Progressive biliary obstruction typically leads to persistent obstructive jaundice, recurrent cholangitis, and eventually to secondary biliary cirrhosis.

PATHOPHYSIOLOGY: *The cause of PSC is unknown, but 2/3 of patients also have ulcerative colitis.* A few cases have been described in patients with Crohn disease of the colon. Associations with retroperitoneal fibrosis, lymphoma, and the fibrosing variant of chronic thyroiditis (Riedel struma) are also reported. In 1/4 of cases, no other disease is present. Increased colonic permeability to bacteria has been suggested as a factor, but this possibility remains speculative.

Genetic and immunologic factors are implicated in the pathogenesis of PSC. It can occur in families, and is sometimes associated with certain HLA haplotypes, including HLA B8. Hypergammaglobulinemia is common, as are circulating immune complexes and antineutrophil cytoplasmic antibodies (perinuclear or P-ANCAs), and complement activation by the classic pathway. Portal tracts contain increased numbers of T cells.

PATHOLOGY: As in PBC, the pathology of PSC liver disease has four stages:

- *STAGE 1: PORTAL STAGE:* At first, there is periductal inflammation and "concentric, onion skin" fibrosis in the portal tracts (Fig. 20-39A).
- *STAGE 2: PERIPORTAL STAGE:* Many bile ducts become obliterated (Fig. 20-39B), portal fibrosis with fibrous septa extends into the parenchyma.
- *STAGE 3: SEPTAL STAGE:* Bridging fibrosis.
- *STAGE 4: CIRRHOSIS:* Secondary biliary cirrhosis eventuates.

Similar inflammatory and fibrotic changes may be seen in large intra- and extrahepatic bile ducts, and these changes can obstruct both. The disease tends to be segmental; thus, the intrahepatic biliary tree shows a characteristic beaded appearance seen by contrast radiography. The same inflammatory process affects the gallbladder wall. Some patients with typical clinical features of PSC have normal-appearing bile ducts on cholangiography, in which case the condition is termed *small duct PSC.*

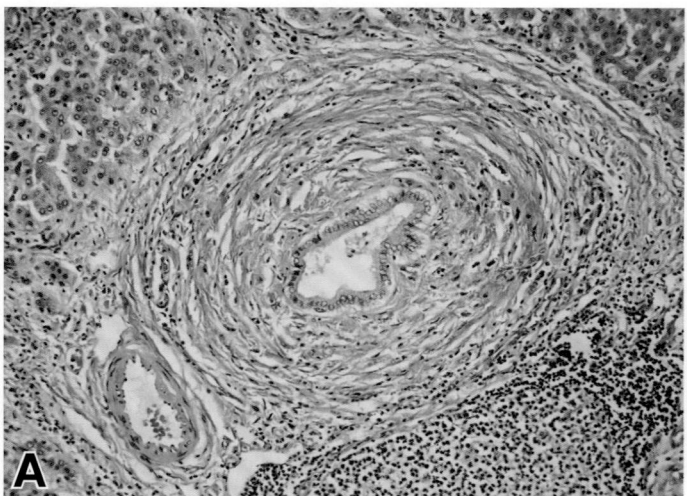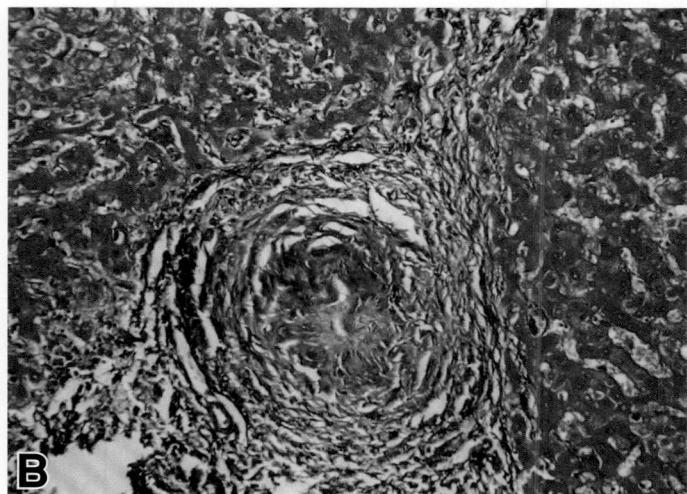

FIGURE 20-39. Primary sclerosing cholangitis (PSC). A. A mildly inflamed portal tract with "onion skin" periductal fibrosis. **B.** A bile duct scar represents a destroyed bile duct in PSC (trichrome stain).

CLINICAL FEATURES: The median survival in symptomatic patients with PSC is 8 to 9 years. Asymptomatic patients have a better prognosis. Clinical presentations vary from asymptomatic elevations in cholestatic liver tests to symptoms of biliary obstruction, recurrent cholangitis and evidence of end-stage liver disease. Infection may lead to abscess formation. *Cholangiocarcinoma develops in up to 20% of patients with PSC.* Liver transplantation may be curative; however, PSC often recurs in the transplanted liver.

IRON OVERLOAD SYNDROMES

Excessive iron accumulates in the body (*siderosis*) in several conditions. There are two major groups of iron overload syndromes, divided on the basis of etiology. **Hereditary hemochromatosis (HH)** is caused by a common genetic alteration in control of intestinal iron absorption. **Secondary iron overload** complicates certain hematologic disorders. It entails parenteral iron overload, in which the iron accrues due to multiple blood transfusions or parenteral administration of iron itself, or is caused by huge dietary intake of iron. Secondary iron overload alone rarely causes liver disease.

Body Iron Stores Are Tightly Regulated

An understanding of normal iron metabolism is central to an appreciation of the pathophysiology of diseases of iron overload, such as HH. The normal total body content of iron is 3 to 4 g. Most of this (about 2.5 g) is bound up in hemoglobin. Iron normally enters the body by being absorbed through the duodenal mucosa. There is no mechanism for iron excretion: men and postmenopausal women eliminate 1 to 2 mg daily in desquamated cells. Therefore, maintaining body iron within acceptable limits requires strict control of intestinal iron uptake (Fig. 20-40).

Several principal proteins control this process:

- **Hepcidin:** This 25 amino acid peptide is manufactured and exported by the liver and is the key to iron regulation.

Hepcidin blocks transit of iron through enterocytes to the blood and inhibits its secretion from stores in hepatocytes and macrophages. It does this by binding the main iron export channel in these cells, **ferroportin,** and promoting its degradation.

- Regulation of hepcidin levels is thus central to iron homeostasis. Hepcidin synthesis is stimulated when body iron stores are sufficient and it is downregulated when the body needs more iron. Several important proteins—transferrin receptor 2 (TfR2), hemojuvelin, and the human hemochromatosis protein HFE—are all necessary to stimulate hepcidin production. Interestingly, hepcidin is also an acute phase reactant and is upregulated by the pro-inflammatory cytokine, IL-6 (see below). Other factors, such as bone morphogenesis proteins, increase hepcidin levels in ways that are not well understood. In addition, hepcidin, as a small peptide, passes through glomeruli. It is degraded in proximal tubules. As a consequence, in renal failure, hepcidin is not eliminated efficiently and its levels are generally elevated.

- **Ferroportin:** This protein is the obligatory iron channel in cells. It is required for cells (mainly enterocytes, hepatocytes, and macrophages) to export iron or to transport it through the cell. Hepcidin inhibits ferroportin function by displacing iron from it, then causing the hepcidin–ferroportin complex to be internalized and degraded.

- **Transferrin (Tf):** There is more than one isoform of this molecule. However, the principal isoform of the Tf molecule is the main iron carrier in the blood. One Tf molecule binds two Fe^{3+} ions. Tf also mediates iron uptake by cells via its main receptor (TfR1). Normal plasma iron levels range from 80 to 100 mg/dL, and Tf is ordinarily about 33% saturated. A small amount of free iron—not bound by Tf—also circulates normally. In times of huge iron excess, free iron may be the predominant form of iron in the blood.

- **Ferritin:** This multimeric protein is responsible for storing iron within cells and is present in every cell type. It binds the ferric (Fe^{3+}) form of iron to form a complex called **hemosiderin,** and in so doing prevents the stored iron from generating free radical species via the Fenton

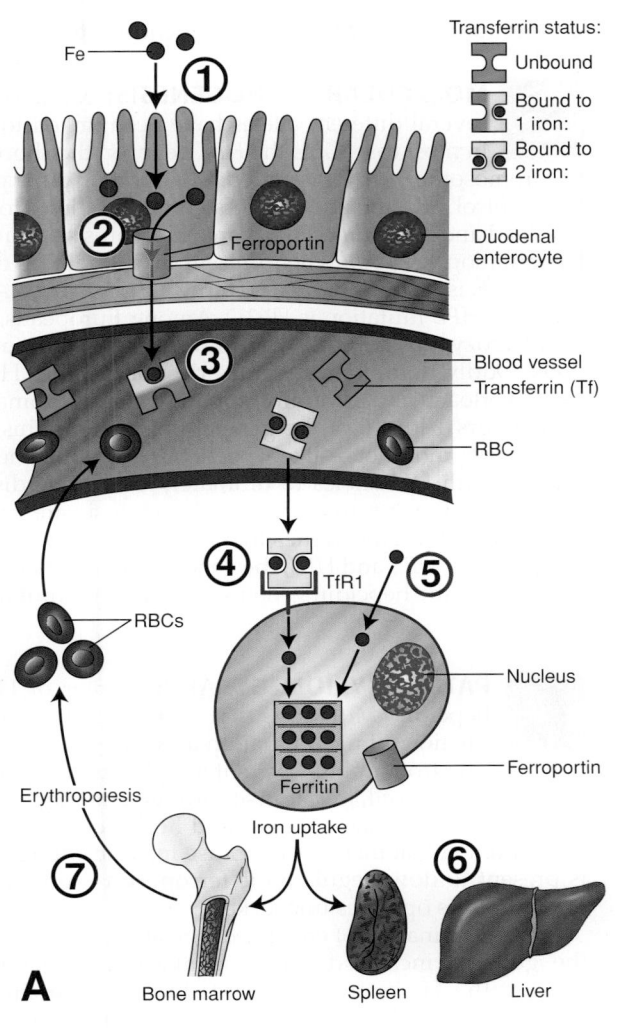

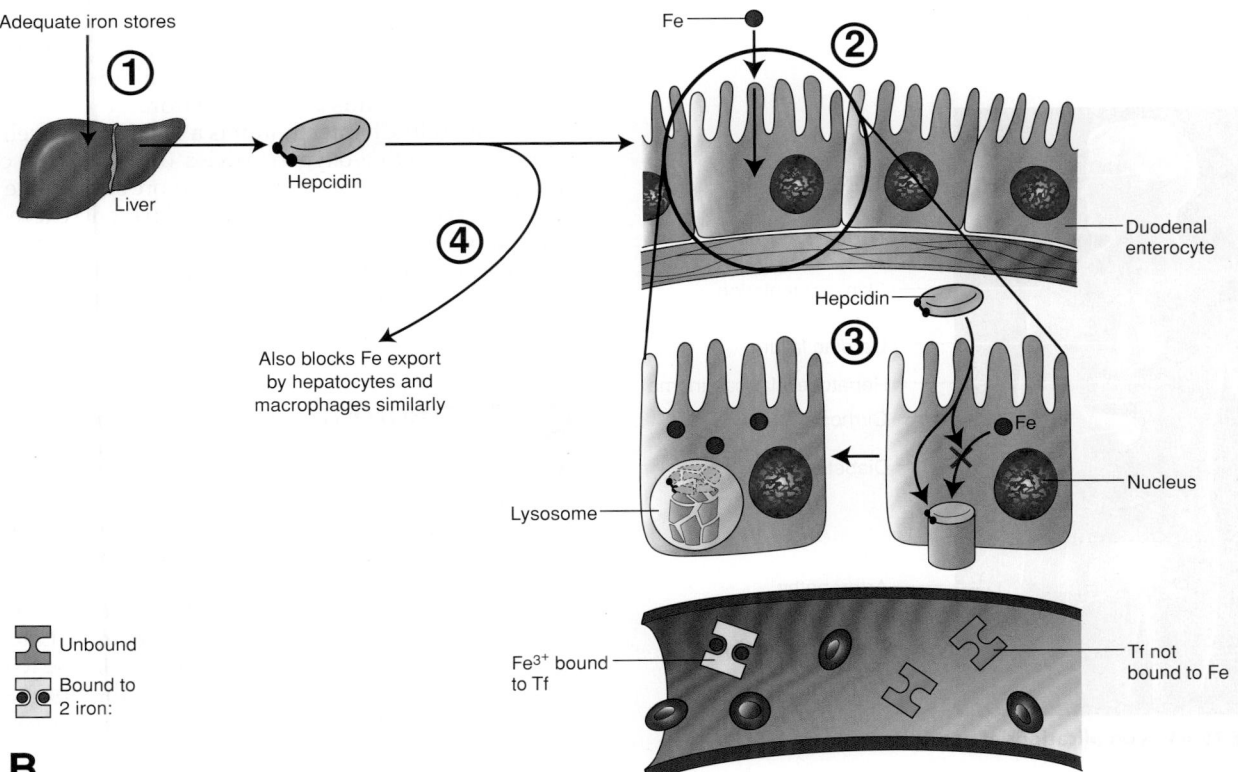

FIGURE 20-40. Normal iron metabolism and the role of hepcidin in its regulation. A. Iron absorption and utilization. 1. Iron enters duodenal enterocytes. These cells have a specific transporter that mediates iron entry. 2. Iron traverses enterocytes on its way to the circulation. Once in enterocyte cytosol, iron is exported by a specific channel, ferroportin, which mediates iron export in enterocytes and other cells. 3. Having traversed the enterocytes, Fe^{3+} binds to Tf, the principal means by which iron circulates. (Some free iron, i.e., iron not bound to Tf, circulates in normal circumstances.) 4. Tf is recognized by a receptor (TfR1) on cells that are engaged in iron uptake. It is stored bound to ferritin. 5. A small amount of iron enters cells as free iron, unbound to Tf. It, too, is stored as ferritin. 6. Excess iron supplies are stored in macrophages and hepatocytes. 7. Cells in the bone marrow incorporate iron into hemoglobin for use in erythrocytes. **B.** Hepcidin regulation of iron uptake. 1. Hepcidin is produced by hepatocytes and exported into the circulation. 2. The duodenum, the principal portal of iron entry into the body, is a key site of hepcidin action. 3. If hepcidin is present, it binds ferroportin. This has two consequences. First, iron is denied access to ferroportin and thus cannot be exported. Second, hepcidin binding causes the hepcidin–ferroportin complex to be internalized and degraded. 4. The sequence is illustrated here for enterocytes but applies comparably to other cells that store and export iron, such as macrophages and hepatocytes.

reaction (see Chapter 1). Each ferritin complex (molecular size, 450 kDa) can store up to 4,500 Fe^{3+} ions. Blood ferritin levels generally reflect the status of the body's iron stores: low serum ferritin generally reflects iron deficiency. High ferritin levels occur when the body has large amounts of stored iron or, as well, during acute inflammatory reactions.

Iron Entry Into Cells

Under normal circumstances, the main portal of iron entry into enterocytes is a cell membrane channel referred to as divalent metal transporter 1 (DMT-1). Other cells generally admit iron via a different receptor-mediated pathway in which Tf-bound iron is recognized by TfR1 and internalized. Free iron (not bound by Tf) enters cells differently, via poorly understood mechanisms. It is this pathway, by which unbound iron enters cells, that allows intracellular iron accumulation when regulatory mechanisms malfunction (see below). Normally, iron is stored mainly in hepatocytes and is bound to **ferritin**. Some is also stored in macrophages. In iron overload states, however, it can accumulate in many cell types.

Hereditary Hemochromatosis Is a Systemic Disease Caused by Excessive Iron Absorption

Toxic iron accumulation in HH is harmful to parenchymal cells, particularly of the liver, heart, and pancreas. Up to 20 to 40 g of iron may accumulate, only within body storage compartments. *The clinical hallmarks of advanced HH are cirrhosis, diabetes, skin pigmentation, and cardiac dysfunction* (Fig. 20-41). HH is the most common inherited metabolic disorder in whites. It manifests most often in patients 40 to 60 years of age. Men are affected 10 times as often as women, probably because women lose iron by menstruation. However, postmenopausal women may also develop HH. As maximum daily iron absorption is about 4 mg, hemochromatosis develops over years.

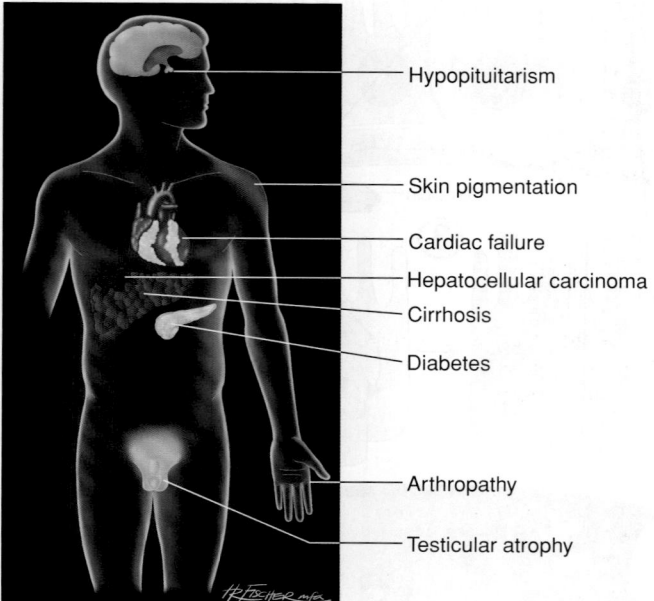

FIGURE 20-41. Complications of hemochromatosis.

Iron Metabolism in Hereditary Hemochromatosis

 MOLECULAR PATHOGENESIS: Mutations in several different alleles have been linked to HH. In most cases, it is the *HFE* gene, on the short arm of chromosome 6, that is mutated. Mutations in other genes that control iron metabolism less commonly lead to iron overload and syndromes like hemochromatosis. A particular mutation (C282Y), when present in both alleles of the *HFE* gene, is responsible for HH in 90% of patients. A less common *HFE* mutation is H63D. Among Europeans, 10% are heterozygous for C282Y, and 1 of 200 to 400 is homozygous. Oddly, some homozygotes do not develop HH or iron overload, and clinically apparent hemochromatosis only occurs 1 in 400 of the general population. This suggests that modifiers—likely genetic and epigenetic—interact with HH alleles to ultimately determine disease expression. Rarer forms of hemochromatosis are caused by mutations in other genes that control hepcidin expression, such as *TfR2* and *HJV*, the gene that makes hemojuvelin. Rarely, the hepcidin gene itself (*HAMP*) is mutated.

 PATHOPHYSIOLOGY: At the center of HH is hepcidin. Mutations that decrease hepcidin production mimic a situation in which there is insufficient iron. Iron uptake by enterocytes thus increases (Fig. 20-42). As well, iron transit through enterocytes, and iron export from macrophages and hepatocytes, into the circulation are all increased because insufficient hepcidin is present to downregulate the ferroportin exporter. The exporter thus operates unchecked.

The combination of enhanced iron absorption through the gut and increased export from storage sites overwhelms the Tf system and results in very high circulating free iron levels. Massive influx of iron into many cells ensues. In hepatocytes, this flood of free iron exceeds even the accelerated iron export (see above) that occurs in the absence of hepcidin-mediated inhibition of ferroportin. Hepatocytes thus accumulate iron.

As noted in Chapter 1, iron is a key factor in cell injury caused by reactive oxygen species (ROS). Excess cellular iron probably renders HH patients more susceptible to oxidative injury. Serum iron levels in HH patients exceed twice normal, with 100% saturation of Tf. Blood ferritin, which parallels the amount of stored iron, is greatly increased.

The causes of iron overload are summarized in Table 20-4.

 PATHOLOGY: In HH, large amounts of iron accumulate in parenchymal cells of a variety of organs and tissues.

LIVER: The liver is always affected in HH and contains more than 0.5-g iron per 100 g wet weight in the late stages. It is enlarged and red-brown with micronodular cirrhosis. Hepatocytes and bile duct epithelium are filled with iron granules (Fig. 20-43). Excess cellular iron is mostly stored in lysosomes as ferric iron. Late in the disease, iron is conspicuous in Kupffer cells due to phagocytosis of necrotic hepatocytes. Within the fibrous septa, iron is prominent in bile ductules and macrophages.

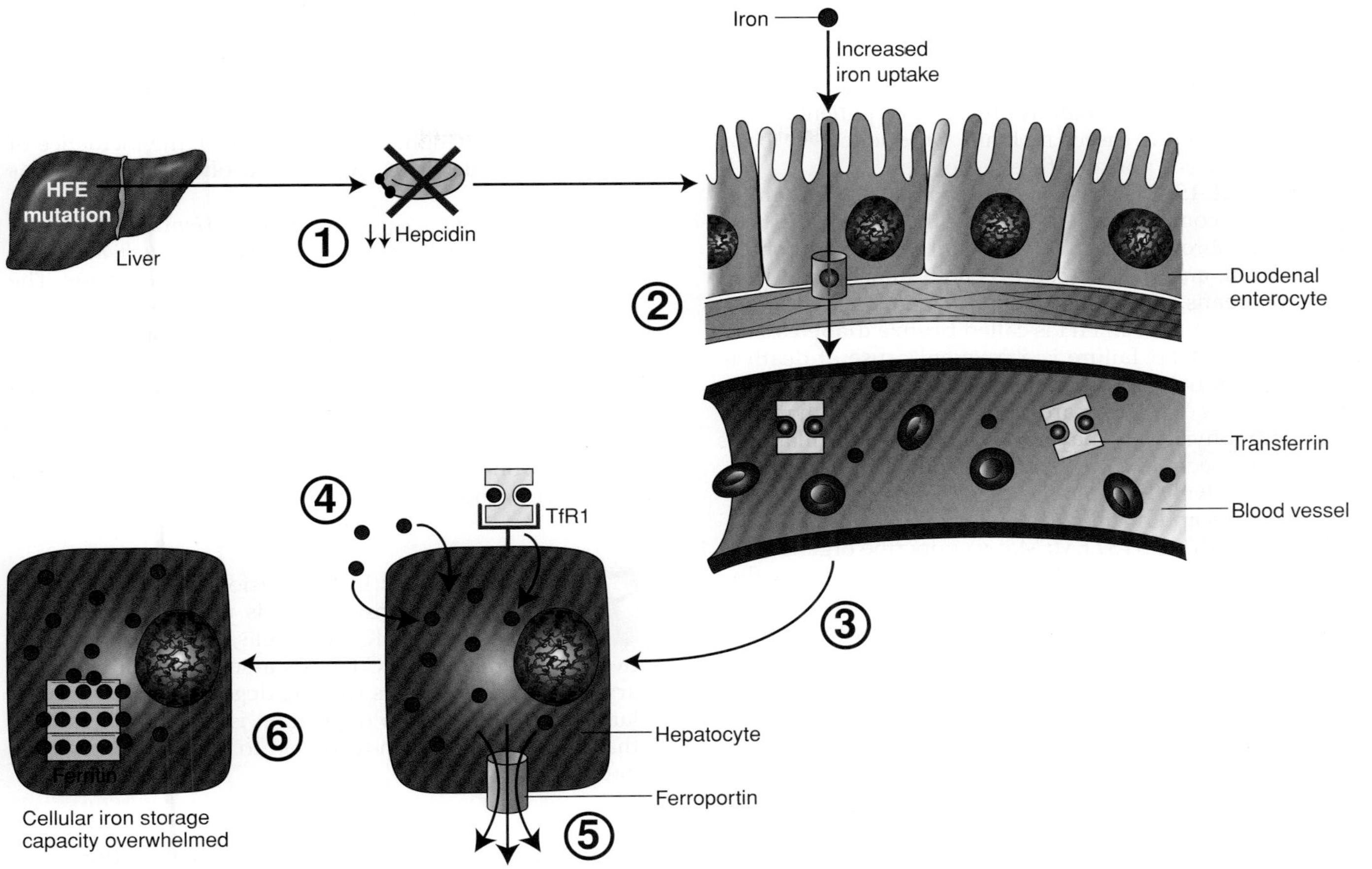

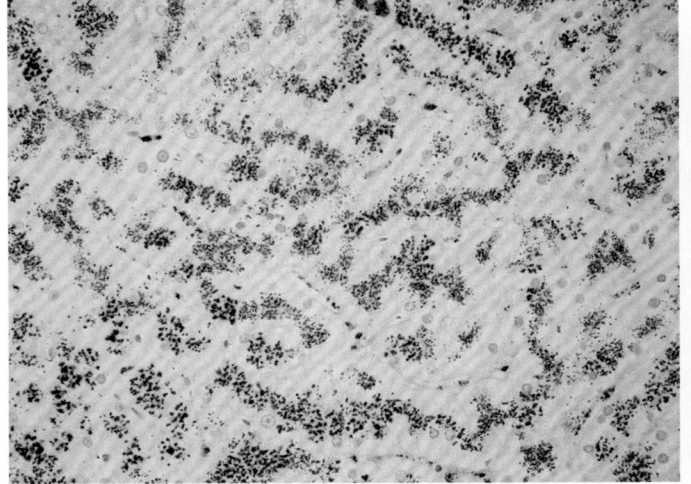

FIGURE 20-42. The fate of iron in the absence of hepcidin in hereditary hemochromatosis (HH). 1. The genetic defect in HH leads to decreased hepatic production of hepcidin. 2. As a consequence, when iron in the duodenal lumen enters enterocytes, its export through ferroportin is not regulated appropriately. The situation mimics that which occurs in iron deficiency (when hepcidin production is suppressed because of the need for increased iron uptake), even though there is abundant iron. Too much iron is absorbed and transported through the enterocytes into the blood. 3. Normally, iron is transported in the blood bound to Tf, and Tf is usually about 1/3 saturated with iron. In HH, not only is Tf iron-carrying capacity saturated (100%), but free iron (i.e., unbound to Tf) is also abundant in the blood. 4. Iron enters hepatocytes both as Tf-bound iron and as free iron. Tf-bound iron enters via the TfR1 pathway. Free iron enters via a different, poorly understood pathway. 5. Lacking inhibition by hepcidin, ferroportin export of iron is very active. 6. However, probably because of massive entry of free iron into hepatocytes, iron storage, and export capacities are overwhelmed. Therefore, the excess iron accumulates.

TABLE 20-4

CAUSES OF IRON OVERLOAD

Increased Iron Absorption

    Hereditary hemochromatosis

        HFE associated: C282Y and H63D homozygotes and C282/H63D heterozygotes

        Hemochromatosis associated with mutations in transferrin receptor 2 (TfR2) and ferroportin

        Juvenile hemochromatosis: mutations in hemojuvelin and hepcidin

    Chronic liver disease (e.g., alcoholic liver disease)

    Iron-loading anemias

    Porphyria cutanea tarda

    Dietary iron overload; excess medicinal iron

Parenteral Iron Overload

    Multiple blood transfusions

    Injectable medicinal iron

FIGURE 20-43. Hemochromatosis. Perl iron stain demonstrates marked iron (*blue*) in hepatocytes along the bile canaliculi.

Eventually, as with other forms of micronodular cirrhosis, macronodular cirrhosis supervenes.

SKIN: In HH, the skin is pigmented, but marked iron deposits occur in the skin in only 1/2 of patients. Most patients have increased melanin production in basal melanocytes as a nonspecific effect of iron.

PANCREAS: Diabetes due to deposition of iron in the pancreas is common in HH. Grossly, the organ is rust colored and fibrotic. Exocrine and endocrine cells contain excess iron, and there is cell loss both in acini and islets of Langerhans. The combination of pigmented skin and glucose intolerance in HH is called **bronze diabetes**.

HEART: Heart failure is a frequent cause of death in HH. This is usually associated with clinical and pathologic features of dilated cardiomyopathy although restrictive pathophysiology may also occur. Atrial fibrillation is commonly seen. Myocardial fibers contain iron pigment, more extensively in ventricles than in atria. Cardiac myocyte necrosis and resulting fibrosis are common.

ENDOCRINE SYSTEM: Many endocrine organs accumulate iron in HH, including the pituitary, adrenal, thyroid, and parathyroid glands. Except for the pituitary, in which release of gonadotropins is impaired, tissue damage does not occur in these organs. As a result, testicular atrophy is seen in 1/4 of male patients, even without iron deposition in the testes. Altered pituitary–gonadal axis function presents as loss of libido and amenorrhea in women, and impotence and sparse body hair in men.

JOINTS: About 1/2 of patients with HH show arthropathy, which is most severe in the fingers and hands. HH arthritis affecting larger joints, like the knee, can be disabling.

CLINICAL FEATURES: HH generally becomes symptomatic in midlife. The liver disease usually progresses slowly, but 1/4 of untreated patients eventually die in hepatic coma or from gastrointestinal hemorrhage. Cirrhosis may lead to HCC; the 10-year cumulative chance of developing liver cancer may reach 30%.

Treatment of HH involves removal of iron from the body, most effectively by repeated phlebotomy. Weekly phlebotomies for 2 to 3 years can remove 20 to 40 g of iron, after which phlebotomies every 2 to 3 months maintain iron balance. In homozygotes without cirrhosis or diabetes, iron depletion allows a life expectancy identical to that of the general population. Without treatment, 10-year survival with HH is only 6%.

Secondary Iron Overload Occurs in People Without HH Mutations

PATHOPHYSIOLOGY: Within certain limits, the amount of iron absorbed is a function of the amount ingested. For example, hemochromatosis is unlikely to develop in someone with a diet low in iron. Many patients (up to 40%) with secondary iron overload have a long history of alcohol abuse; it is thought that alcohol increases both iron storage and associated cell injury.

Iron accumulation among blacks of sub-Saharan Africa, commonly misnamed "Bantu siderosis," is an example of secondary iron overload. This disorder occurs because these populations consume large amounts of iron-containing alcoholic beverages. As "home-brewed" beverages (low alcohol, high iron) have been replaced by Western spirits (high alcohol, low iron), the incidence of siderosis has declined, whereas alcoholic cirrhosis has increased.

Massive iron overload occurs in patients with certain diseases with ineffective erythropoiesis, such as sickle cell anemia, thalassemia major, and other anemias. The excess iron derives from hemolysis or transfused blood. Increased iron absorption also occurs despite Tf saturation. Multiple blood transfusions alone are generally insufficient to produce secondary iron overload, even in patients with hypoplastic anemia who receive many transfusions (250-mg iron/500 mL unit of blood). In these patients, iron is concentrated principally in mononuclear phagocytes, and cirrhosis is rare.

PATHOLOGY: In transfusion-related and other types of siderosis, there is uniform, initial iron deposition in Kupffer cells, eventually spilling over into hepatocytes. Cirrhosis associated with secondary iron overload shows varying degrees of iron accumulation, but hepatic iron deposition is generally less than that in HH and is often restricted to the periphery of the nodules.

A Footnote to Hepcidin-Regulated Iron Metabolism

The centrality of hepcidin to iron metabolism has implications far beyond hereditary iron storage disorders. As mentioned above, in chronic renal failure, the inability of the kidneys to eliminate hepcidin may lead to its accumulation. Excess hepcidin production, such as is stimulated by IL-6 in settings of chronic infection and inflammation, and in some malignancies, may also lead to excessively high levels of hepcidin.

In this setting, elevated hepcidin concentrations may severely restrict ferroportin function. This could impair iron absorption in the gut and lead to excessive iron retention in stores due to inadequate release from macrophages and hepatocytes. If hepcidin remains elevated for prolonged periods of time, iron-deficiency anemia may develop. Thus, anemia in some chronic inflammatory diseases, such as Crohn disease and rheumatoid arthritis, or in some tumors, such as certain lymphomas, may be associated with high circulating hepcidin levels. Such anemias, although they show low blood iron levels, are not amenable to treatment with dietary iron, as high hepcidin levels impede enteric iron absorption.

HERITABLE DISORDERS ASSOCIATED WITH CIRRHOSIS

Wilson Disease Is an Inherited Disorder of Copper Metabolism

WD is an autosomal recessive disease in which excess copper is deposited in the liver and brain (Fig. 20-44). One in 150 to 180 people is a carrier, and 1 in 30,000 children develop clinical disease.

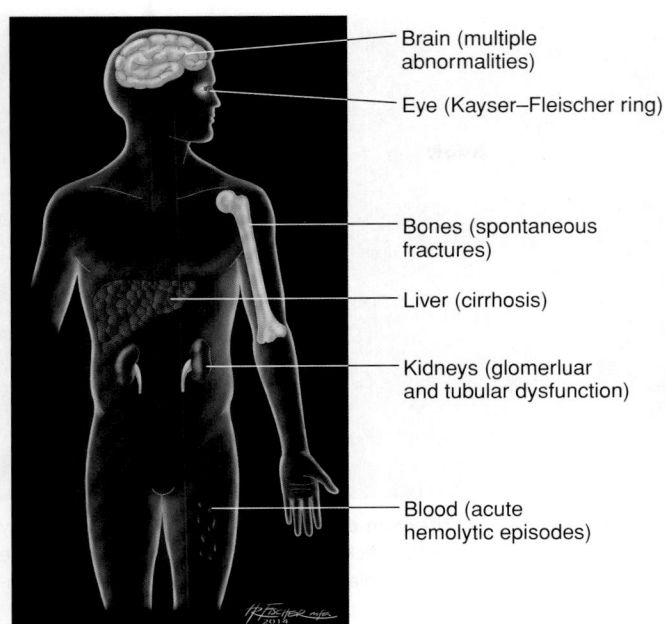

FIGURE 20-44. Organs principally affected in Wilson disease.

- Brain (multiple abnormalities)
- Eye (Kayser–Fleischer ring)
- Bones (spontaneous fractures)
- Liver (cirrhosis)
- Kidneys (glomerluar and tubular dysfunction)
- Blood (acute hemolytic episodes)

MOLECULAR PATHOGENESIS: Dietary copper intake usually exceeds the body's needs. The excess is excreted by the liver into the bile. Copper is normally bound to ceruloplasmin in hepatocytes and then secreted into the blood. The gene for WD, namely *ATP7B* on chromosome 13, encodes an ATP-dependent, transmembrane cation channel, which transports copper within hepatocytes before it is excreted. *Mutations in ATP7B impair copper transport. Both biliary copper excretion and incorporation into ceruloplasmin are deficient.* Some 200 different mutations in the WD gene are known. In European and North American populations, a single variant, H1069Q, accounts for 70% of WD, but this mutation is rare in India and Asia. Most patients are compound heterozygotes and possess two different mutant alleles.

In WD, serum ceruloplasmin levels are very low, a deficiency thought to be due to hepatic copper overload. Excess copper is toxic to hepatocytes, which die and release their copper into the blood, to then deposit in extrahepatic tissues. The central role of the liver in WD is underscored by the fact that liver transplantation is curative.

Just how excess copper injures cells is unclear. Copper can replace iron in the Fenton reaction to convert hydrogen peroxide into hydroxyl radicals (see Chapter 1).

PATHOLOGY: *In WD, the liver progresses from mild to severe chronic hepatitis. Cirrhosis may develop rapidly, even in childhood (Fig. 20-45).* Features of severe hepatocyte injury and steatosis may be seen. Hepatocytes often contain Mallory–Denk hyalins, and cholestasis is common. Initially, cirrhosis is micronodular, but in time, it becomes macronodular. Chemical measurement of liver copper in unfixed tissue or uncut paraffin blocks from livers of patients with WD reveals more than 250 μg of copper per gram of dry weight.

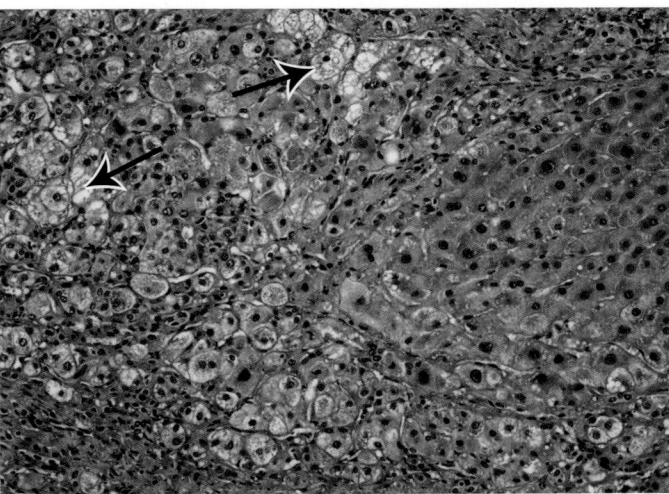

FIGURE 20-45. Wilson disease. The liver shows cirrhosis, with severe hepatocyte injury and hydropic change (*arrows*).

CLINICAL FEATURES: In 1/2 of patients with WD, some symptoms are shown by adolescence. The rest usually become ill early in adulthood, but WD can present later. Initial symptoms reflect chronic liver disease in about 1/2 of patients, 1/3 are first seen with neurologic complaints, and about 1/10 have psychiatric illnesses.

LIVER: Liver-related symptoms are nonspecific at first and may progress to chronic liver disease indistinguishable from that of other forms of chronic hepatitis. Eventually, chronic hepatitis and cirrhosis result in jaundice, portal hypertension and hepatic failure. WD may present as acute liver failure. There is increased risk of liver cancer in WD, although not as great as that in HH.

BRAIN: Neurologic disease begins with mild incoordination and tremors. If untreated, dysarthria and dysphagia appear, then disabling dystonia and spasticity.

EYE: Ocular manifestations invariably accompany neurologic disease. **Kayser–Fleischer rings** are golden-brown, bilateral corneal discolorations around the edge of the iris that obscure its muscular pattern (Fig. 20-46). They

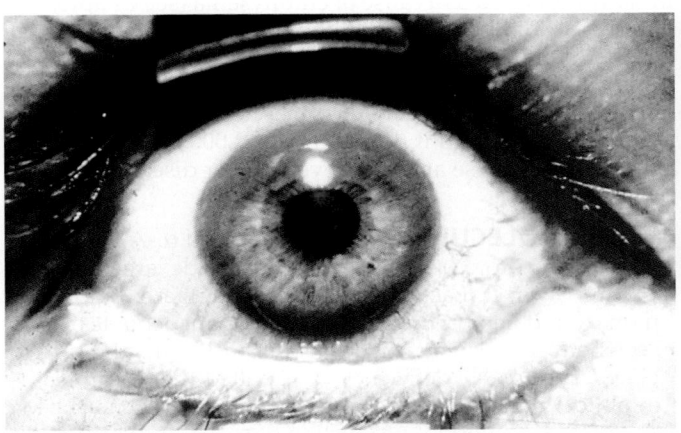

FIGURE 20-46. Kayser–Fleischer ring. Deposition of copper in the Descemet membrane produces a peripheral brown color, which obstructs the view of the underlying iris.

represent copper deposited in Descemet membrane. In some patients, these rings are accompanied by "sunflower cataracts," which are green copper discs in the anterior capsule of the lens.

BONES: Skeletal lesions are common and include osteomalacia, osteoporosis, spontaneous fractures, and various arthropathies.

KIDNEY: Renal glomerular and tubular dysfunction is common in WD and is manifested by proteinuria, lowered glomerular filtration, aminoaciduria, and phosphaturia. These abnormalities are due to copper deposition in renal tubules.

BLOOD: Transient acute hemolytic episodes, presumably related to a sudden release of free copper from the liver, occur in 15% of patients with WD.

Treatment of WD is designed to prevent copper accumulation in tissues and remove copper already deposited. Copper-chelating agents, trientine and D-penicillamine, augment urinary copper excretion. Treatment often reverses central nervous system (CNS) dysfunction and liver disease. Presymptomatic patients are given supplemental dietary zinc, which blocks intestinal absorption of copper. Liver transplantation is curative for WD.

Cystic Fibrosis May Cause Biliary Obstruction

The cystic fibrosis transmembrane regulator (CFTR; see Chapter 6) is expressed in biliary epithelial cells. In cystic fibrosis (CF), tenacious mucus plugs obstruct intrahepatic biliary channels, sometimes as early as in the first few weeks of life. Some infants die in hepatic failure. The most common hepatic lesion is focal or diffuse biliary cirrhosis. In patients who survive to adolescence, liver involvement becomes clinically symptomatic in 15%. Secondary biliary cirrhosis occurs in 10% of those who survive beyond 25 years. Liver disease accounts for 2.5% of deaths in CF, making it the most common nonpulmonary cause of death in this disease. UDCA therapy, also used in treating PBC, improves liver function, chemistry and histology in CF, but not survival.

α_1-Antitrypsin Deficiency Leads to Cirrhosis

α_1-AT deficiency is an autosomal recessive disease that was initially described as a cause of emphysema (see Chapter 12). Later, cases of liver disease without lung involvement were reported, and disease involving both organs is recognized. α_1-AT deficiency is the most common genetic liver disease and the most common genetic disease treated by liver transplantation. Although it occurs in 1 of 2,000 live births, only 10% to 15% of those affected develop liver disease.

 MOLECULAR PATHOGENESIS: α_1-AT is a serine protease inhibitor (serpin) made largely in the liver. It inactivates neutrophil elastase. Both pulmonary and hepatic disorders are due to inadequate α_1-AT secretion by the liver. Mutations in *SERPINA1*, the α_1-AT gene, cause α_1-AT deficiency. Also called the *PI* (protease inhibitor) gene, the most common allele of this gene, the M allele, leads to normal production of α_1-AT and most people in the general population have two copies of this allele (MM). The S allele and especially the Z allele produce

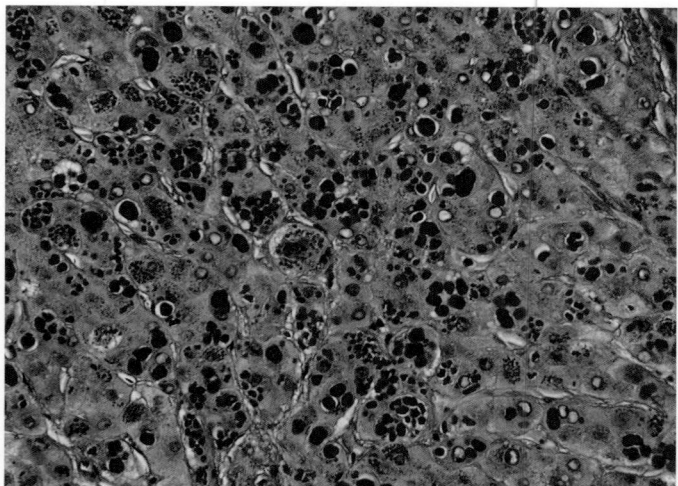

FIGURE 20-47. α_1-Antitrypsin deficiency. A cirrhotic liver stained by the periodic acid–Schiff (PAS) reaction with diastase digestion to remove glycogen reveals numerous cytoplasmic globules in the hepatocytes composed of misfolded α_1-antitrypsin protein.

lower amount of α_1-AT such that people homozygous for Z likely have α_1-AT deficiency. More than 75 variants have been identified in *SERPINA1* that account for loss of function in the S and Z alleles. The most common (95% of cases), called PiZ, causes a lysine for glutamate substitution at position 342. The resultant mutant protein folds abnormally and is retained within the hepatocyte ER. Insoluble aggregates of the mutant protein cannot be exported and accumulate, thereby damaging the cell.

PATHOLOGY: Hepatocytes in patients with α_1-AT deficiency contain faintly eosinophilic, PAS-positive cytoplasmic droplets (Fig. 20-47), which contain amorphous material (i.e., the misfolded mutant protein) within dilated ER cisternae. The disease often presents with chronic hepatitis, which terminates in cirrhosis.

α_1-AT deficiency may cause hepatitis in the newborn (see below). Micronodular cirrhosis develops by the ages of 2 to 3 years in these children and may ultimately become macronodular.

CLINICAL FEATURES: Liver disease in α_1-AT deficiency varies from rapidly fatal neonatal hepatitis to no hepatic dysfunction at all. *Of infants with the ZZ genotype—who are susceptible to development of clinical disease—10% have neonatal cholestatic jaundice (conjugated hyperbilirubinemia).* In fact, α_1-AT deficiency accounts for 30% of cases of neonatal conjugated hyperbilirubinemia. Most infants recover within 6 months, but 10% to 20% develop permanent liver disease. Children with cirrhosis usually die before 10 years of age from hepatic failure or other complications of the disease. However, liver transplantation is curative.

Some patients are asymptomatic until early adulthood, when symptoms of cirrhosis may be the initial complaint. *Cirrhosis in α_1-AT deficiency is prone to a high incidence of HCC.*

Inborn Errors of Carbohydrate Metabolism Affect the Liver

Glycogen Storage Diseases

The biochemical basis of glycogen storage diseases is discussed in Chapter 6. *Only glycogenosis type IV (brancher deficiency, Andersen disease) is usually complicated by cirrhosis.* Slowly developing cirrhosis may also occur in glycogenosis type III (debrancher deficiency, Cori disease) but is not inevitable. Glycogenosis type I (glucose-6-phosphatase deficiency, von Gierke disease) is associated with striking hepatomegaly, and type II (acid-glucosidase deficiency, Pompe disease) features mild hepatomegaly. Neither type I nor type II is complicated by cirrhosis.

GLYCOGENOSIS TYPE I: Hepatocytes are distended by large amounts of glycogen, which appears pale in sections stained with hematoxylin and eosin and red with PAS. Fat accumulation varies from mild to severe, but fibrosis is usually absent. Hepatic adenomas often develop in adolescence but regress with dietary therapy designed to avoid hypoglycemia and limit intake of fructose and galactose neither of which are properly metabolized in type I disease.

GLYCOGENOSIS TYPE II: Infants with Pompe disease typically present with muscle weakness (myopathy), poor muscle tone (hypotonia), hepatomegaly, and cardiomegaly. The hepatocyte appearance with abundant glycogen is similar to glycogenosis type I.

GLYCOGENOSIS TYPE III: Infants with Cori disease show severe hepatomegaly, and the liver morphologically resembles that seen in type I. Fat is less conspicuous, but fibrosis is present and may progress to cirrhosis.

GLYCOGENOSIS TYPE IV: Infants present with severe hepatomegaly and usually succumb to cirrhosis by 4 years of age. Sharply circumscribed, PAS-positive inclusions are seen in enlarged hepatocytes. These inclusions are fibrillar and represent abnormal glycogen. Deposits of mutant glycogen are also found in the heart, skeletal muscle, and brain. Liver transplantation is curative for glycogenosis type IV.

Galactosemia

This autosomal recessive trait is caused by deficiency in galactose-1-phosphate uridyl transferase. This enzyme catalyzes the second step in the conversion of galactose to glucose. Thus, galactose and its metabolites accumulate in the liver and other organs. Affected infants who are fed milk rapidly develop hepatosplenomegaly, jaundice, and hypoglycemia. Cataracts and mental retardation are common.

Within 2 weeks of birth, the liver shows extensive and uniform fat accumulation and striking bile ductule proliferation in and around portal tracts. Cholestasis is often seen in canaliculi and bile ductules. Bile plugs fill many of these pseudoacini. By about 6 weeks of age, fibrosis begins to extend from portal tracts into the lobules and progresses to cirrhosis by 6 months. A galactose-free diet improves the disease and reverses many of the morphologic alterations.

Hereditary Fructose Intolerance

This is an autosomal recessive deficiency of fructose-1-phosphate aldolase. Fructose feeding early in infancy causes hepatomegaly, jaundice, and ascites. However, if initial exposure to fructose occurs after 6 months, resulting disease is far milder; the only clinical impairment is spontaneous hypoglycemia. Infants with liver disease show changes of neonatal hepatitis. Fat accumulation may be marked, resembling that in galactosemia. If left untreated, progressive fibrosis culminates in cirrhosis.

Tyrosinemia

This autosomal recessive trait is caused by impaired tyrosine catabolism to fumarate and acetoacetate. The missing enzyme is fumarylacetoacetate hydrolase (FAH). More than 30 different mutations in the *FAH* gene are known. Succinyl acetone and succinyl acetoacetate accumulate. Both are potent electrophiles that can react with the sulfhydryl groups of glutathione and proteins, and damage the liver and kidneys.

Acute tyrosinemia begins within a few weeks or months of birth with hepatosplenomegaly. Liver failure and death are usual before 1 year of age. The liver pathology is remarkably like that in galactosemia, and progression to cirrhosis is the rule.

Chronic tyrosinemia begins in the first year of life, manifesting as growth retardation, renal disease, and hepatic failure. Death usually supervenes before 10 years of age. Tyrosinemia is treated by liver transplantation. *The incidence of HCC in untreated chronic tyrosinemia is extremely high.*

Miscellaneous Inherited Causes of Cirrhosis

Several inborn errors of metabolism are associated with cirrhosis, including storage diseases such as Gaucher disease, Niemann–Pick disease, mucopolysaccharidoses, neonatal adrenoleukodystrophy, Wolman disease and Zellweger syndrome.

INDIAN CHILDHOOD CIRRHOSIS

Indian childhood cirrhosis (ICC) is a fatal disorder affecting mainly, but not only, preschool children in India. It predominantly affects boys 1 to 4 years old. The liver shows micronodular cirrhosis and many Mallory–Denk hyalins, as in alcoholic liver disease.

The etiology and pathogenesis of ICC are not well understood. Familial cases are reported, but no hereditary pattern has been established nor have potential disease alleles been identified. Interestingly, children with this disease have a marked excess of copper and copper-binding protein in the liver, but the significance of these findings in terms of disease pathogenesis remains obscure.

DRUG-INDUCED LIVER INJURY

Drug-induced liver injury can mimic nearly any type of liver disease, with severity ranging from asymptomatic elevations of transaminases to acute liver failure. *In fact, drugs are the most common cause of acute liver failure in the United States.* Chapter 1 includes a discussion of mechanisms by which toxins may produce liver necrosis. Chapter 4 reviews immune-mediated mechanisms of injury.

Drugs cause injury in either **predictable** or **unpredictable** **patterns.** The former refers to drugs that cause liver injury in a dose-dependent manner (e.g., carbon tetrachloride, the mushroom poison phalloidin, the analgesic acetaminophen). The latter reflects injury that occurs with low frequency, independent of dose and without apparent predisposition (**idiosyncratic reaction**).

The defining characteristics of predictable drug-induced hepatoxicity are:

- The agent, in sufficiently high doses, always produces liver cell damage.
- The extent of hepatic injury is dose dependent.
- Liver necrosis is zonal and often, but not always, centrilobular.
- The time between exposure and development of liver cell necrosis is short.

Most drug reactions are unpredictable and seem to represent idiosyncratic events. This type of hepatotoxicity occurs in people with metabolic or genetic predispositions. It usually reflects unusual sensitivity to a dose-related off-target side effect. Thus, individuals may be predisposed to idiosyncratic reactions because their metabolic pathways differ from those of the general population (*metabolic idiosyncrasy*) or because they possess genetic variations in systems of biotransformation or detoxification of reactive metabolites. As well, some drugs or their metabolites may trigger immunologic reactions in the liver (autoimmune hepatitis).

There is no specific test to predict or diagnose drug-induced hepatotoxicity. A detailed history of medications, drugs, and dietary supplements must be elicited from patients with elevated liver enzymes or jaundice. Other liver diseases must be ruled out (e.g., viral hepatitis, genetic disease, autoimmune hepatitis, alcoholic hepatitis). Liver biopsy is often of limited value in diagnosing drug injury, as histologic patterns of acute or chronic drug-induced liver disease overlap with non–drug-related diseases.

Histologic Patterns of Drug-Induced Liver Disease Are Diverse

Drug toxicities can cause nearly the entire gamut of pathologies seen in non–drug-induced liver diseases. However, individual drugs usually have characteristic patterns of liver toxicity.

Zonal Hepatocellular Necrosis

Toxic doses of acetaminophen *predictably* cause centrilobular necrosis (Fig. 20-48A), but very high doses can cause panlobular necrosis (see Chapter 1). A metabolite of acetaminophen depletes glutathione and thus impairs the ability of hepatocytes to detoxify peroxides. This zonal pattern probably reflects the greater activity of drug-metabolizing enzymes in the central zones. Classic agents that produce this pattern of injury are carbon tetrachloride and the toxin of the mushroom *Amanita phalloides*. In affected zones, hepatocytes show coagulative necrosis, hydropic swelling, and variable small fat droplets. Inflammation is sparse. Patients either die in acute hepatic failure or recover without sequelae. *Acetaminophen-induced hepatotoxicity is the most common cause of acute liver failure in the United States and is frequently seen in suicidal gestures. Patients usually present soon after drug ingestion.*

Chronic exposure to various hepatotoxins that cause zonal necrosis (e.g., carbon tetrachloride) is not generally a problem: once acute toxic injury is recognized, reexposure to the offending agent is rare.

Cholestasis

Injury to intralobular and interlobular bile ducts is a common but unpredictable reaction to drugs. When it occurs, bile accumulates in hepatocytes and canaliculi. It is called *pure cholestasis* (Fig. 20-8) if there is no inflammation. Drugs that cause pure cholestasis include estrogens, androgens, and several antibiotics (e.g., sulfamethoxazole). If cholestasis is accompanied by inflammation, the term **cholestatic hepatitis** is used.

Acute and Chronic Hepatitis

Inflammation is common in many *unpredictable* hepatotoxic drug reactions. All of the features of acute viral hepatitis can occur after exposure to a wide variety of drugs (e.g., isoniazid, antibiotics). The inflammation is a general response to cell injury and necrosis, such as in viral or autoimmune hepatitis (Fig. 20-48B). *The entire range of acute liver injury, from mild anicteric hepatitis to rapidly fatal massive hepatic necrosis, is encountered.* Typically, drug-induced hepatitis and associated liver enzyme elevations resolve when the offending drug is withdrawn. If exposure continues, chronic hepatitis and even cirrhosis may develop. Sometimes inflammation may reflect **drug-induced autoimmune hepatitis** (e.g., as with nitrofurantoin) either as an immune response to the drug or by unmasking classical autoimmune hepatitis. The presence of eosinophils in the inflammatory infiltrate suggests such a drug reaction (Fig. 20-48C). *An inflammatory infiltrate, regardless of its composition, is not specific for drug-associated hepatotoxicity.* Granulomatous hepatitis is also a rare reaction to drugs.

Fatty Liver

Accumulation of triglycerides within hepatocytes (i.e., hepatic steatosis or fatty liver) generally occurs in a predictable fashion. Although there may be substantial overlap, two morphologic patterns are recognized: macrovesicular and microvesicular steatosis.

Macrovesicular Steatosis

In addition to its association with chronic ethanol ingestion, accumulation of macrovesicular fat within hepatocytes results from accidental exposure to direct hepatotoxins, such as carbon tetrachloride. Corticosteroids and some antimetabolites, such as methotrexate, may also cause macrovesicular steatosis. Fat per se does not injure hepatocytes (see above). A variant of toxic macrovesicular steatosis that resembles alcoholic hepatitis (**steatohepatitis**) occurs after administration of certain drugs (e.g., the antiarrhythmic agent amiodarone). Both hepatocytes and Kupffer cells are enlarged, with foamy cytoplasm that reflects accumulation of **phospholipids**. Mallory–Denk hyalins are abundant (Fig. 20-48D). Macrovesicular steatosis is itself clinically inconsequential.

Microvesicular Steatosis

Unlike macrovesicular steatosis, microvesicular fatty liver is often associated with severe, and sometimes fatal, liver disease. Small fat vacuoles are dispersed throughout the cytoplasm of hepatocytes, and the nucleus retains its central position (Fig. 20-48E). The microvesicular fat is important, not in and of itself but as a manifestation of metabolic severe injury to subcellular structures, mainly mitochondria.

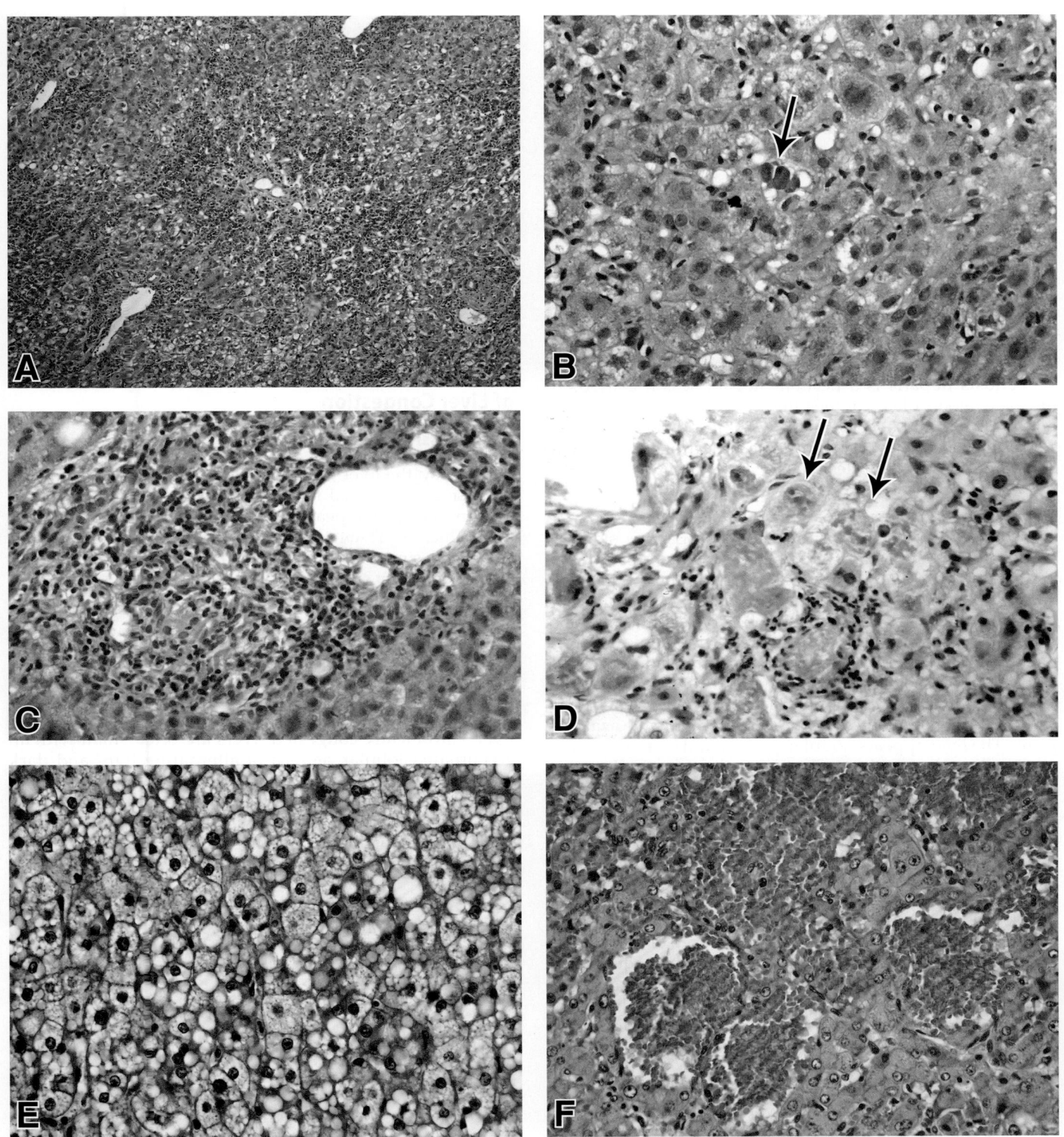

FIGURE 20-48. Drug-induced hepatotoxicity. A. Toxic centrilobular necrosis. This liver biopsy was from a 20-year-old man who attempted suicide with an overdose of acetaminophen. It shows centrilobular hemorrhagic necrosis. Note that the surviving hepatocytes are markedly swollen. **B. Acute hepatitis.** This patient was started on isoniazid for treatment of tuberculosis. After 3 weeks, the aspartate aminotransferase (AST) and alanine aminotransferase (ALT) were elevated. The liver biopsy shows features of acute hepatitis including lobular disarray, inflammation, acidophilic bodies (*arrow*), and focal necrosis. **C. Eosinophilic portal inflammatory infiltrate.** A 33-year-old woman developed fatigue 2 weeks after initiating therapy with a nonsteroidal anti-inflammatory agent. The AST was 250 U/L. Portal tracts show expansion by acute and chronic inflammation with eosinophils. **D. Phospholipidosis.** This liver biopsy is from a patient treated with the anti-arrhythmic drug amiodarone. Hepatocytes are swollen and display ample Mallory–Denk hyalins (*arrows*). **E. Reye syndrome.** A liver biopsy shows small-droplet fat in hepatocytes and centrally located nuclei. **F. Peliosis hepatis.** The patient was a 44-year-old weight lifter who used anabolic steroids. The liver contains numerous large, irregular, blood-filled spaces.

REYE SYNDROME: This rare acute disease of children is characterized by microvesicular steatosis, hepatic failure, and encephalopathy. Edema and fat accumulation can also occur in the brain. Symptoms usually begin after a febrile illness, such as influenza or varicella infection, and may correlate with aspirin administration. However, retrospective review of some cases has shown that the doses of aspirin involved were far too low to cause liver injury, and it is now recognized that Reye syndrome is more complex than simple aspirin toxicity. In any event, as the use of aspirin and the incidence of influenza have declined in children, Reye syndrome has fortunately become uncommon.

Vascular Lesions
Occlusion of hepatic veins **(Budd–Chiari syndrome;** Fig. 20-18) may follow use of oral contraceptives, perhaps because they induce hypercoagulability in some people.

Peliosis hepatis is a peculiar hepatic lesion composed of cystic, blood-filled cavities that are lined by hepatocytes and not by endothelial cells (Fig. 20-48F). Anabolic sex steroids, contraceptive steroids, and the antiestrogen tamoxifen sometimes produce this lesion.

Mass Lesions and Altered Hepatic Morphology
Hepatocellular adenoma, induced by exogenous steroids (estrogens and anabolic steroids), and **hemangiosarcoma,** caused by intravenous administration of the radioactive contrast agent thorium dioxide (Thorotrast; see Chapter 8) dye (no longer used), are among the very few mass lesions caused by drugs. Chronic exposure to inorganic arsenic, usually in insecticides, and occupational inhalation of vinyl chloride have also been linked to hepatic angiosarcomas.

Nodular regenerative hyperplasia may occur after therapy with antimetabolites (e.g., 6-thioguanine) and azathioprine. The liver appears nodular, grossly and on microscopic examination, but without fibrosis. Patients typically present with portal hypertension as the architectural distortion impairs portal blood flow into the liver.

THE PORPHYRIAS

Porphyrias are caused by deficiencies in heme biosynthesis and are characterized by accumulation of porphyrin intermediates (see Chapter 20). They may be acquired or inherited. They are divided into hepatic and erythropoietic types, based on where the defective heme metabolism and the accumulation of porphyrins and their precursors occur. Genetic porphyrias are heterogeneous, and usually involve unique mutations in individual families.

Hepatic porphyrias are inherited as autosomal dominant traits and are often precipitated by administration of drugs, sex hormones, starvation, hepatitis C, HIV infection, and alcohol. The liver shows variable steatosis, hemosiderosis, fibrosis, and cirrhosis. Needle-shaped cytoplasmic inclusions composed of crystals of porphyrinogens, porphyrins, and uroporphyrins may be present.

ACUTE INTERMITTENT PORPHYRIA: This is the most common genetic porphyria. It is caused by a deficiency in porphobilinogen deaminase activity in the liver. Only 10% of gene carriers show clinical symptoms, which generally affect young adults. Colicky abdominal pain and neuropsychiatric symptoms predominate.

PORPHYRIA CUTANEA TARDA: This chronic hepatic porphyria is the most frequent porphyria. It may be acquired or inherited as an autosomal dominant trait and is characterized by deficient uroporphyrinogen decarboxylase activity. Typical patients are of middle age or elderly, with cutaneous photosensitivity and liver disease with hepatic iron overload.

Other inherited porphyrias, termed **erythropoietic porphyrias** and **congenital erythropoietic porphyrias,** are caused by enzyme deficiencies in erythrocytes. They are characterized by cutaneous photosensitivity and occasionally liver disease.

VASCULAR DISORDERS

Heart Failure Is the Major Cause of Liver Congestion

Acute Passive Congestion

At autopsy, the liver is often acutely congested, presumably because of a terminal failing heart (see Chapter 7). On cut section, the liver appears diffusely speckled with small red foci, which represent centrilobular zones with dilated and congested sinusoids and terminal venules. These changes are not clinically significant.

Chronic Passive Congestion

Chronic passive liver congestion occurs when long-standing heart failure increases the back-pressure in the peripheral venous circulation, impeding venous outflow from the liver. Chronically congested livers are often small with an accentuated lobular pattern of alternating light and dark areas (Fig. 20-49A), called **nutmeg liver** because it resembles the appearance of the interior of a nutmeg. In severe cases, centrilobular terminal venules and adjacent sinusoids are greatly dilated and filled with blood (Fig. 20-49B). Liver cell plates in this zone are thinned by pressure atrophy.

If **right-sided heart failure** is severe and long-standing (e.g., tricuspid valvular disease or constrictive pericarditis), chronic passive congestion may progress to hepatic fibrosis (Fig. 20-49C). Delicate fibrous strands envelop terminal venules, and septa radiate from centrilobular zones. Fibrous septa may link adjacent central veins, producing a "reverse lobulation." Pressure atrophy of centrilobular hepatocytes is prominent. This is not "cardiac cirrhosis," however. Complete septa and regenerative nodules, as are seen in true cirrhosis, are rarely encountered.

Chronic passive liver congestion rarely affects hepatic function. Infrequently, features of portal hypertension, such as splenomegaly and ascites, may develop.

Shock Results in Decreased Liver Perfusion

Shock from any cause may cause ischemic necrosis of centrilobular hepatocytes and hemorrhage. The centrilobular zone—that is, zone 3 (Fig. 20-2)—is farthest from the blood that originates in the portal tracts and thus is the area most vulnerable to ischemic insult.

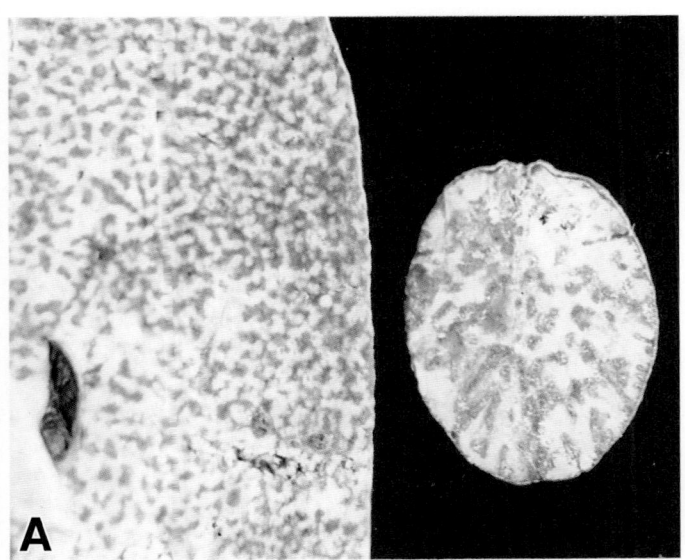

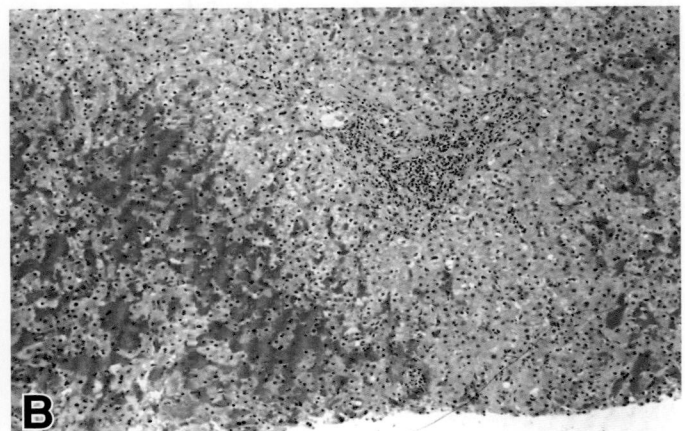

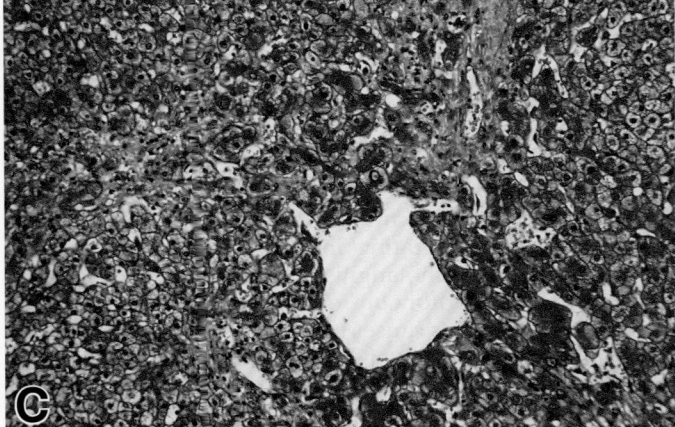

FIGURE 20-49. Chronic passive congestion of the liver. A. The cut surface of this fixed liver exhibits an accentuated lobular pattern, an appearance resembling that of a nutmeg (*right*). **B.** Microscopic examination shows congestion and widening of central sinusoids. **C.** A Masson-trichrome stain shows fibrosis (*blue*) emanating out of central veins.

Liver Infarction Is Uncommon Because of Its Dual Blood Supply

Acute occlusion of the hepatic artery or its branches is rare. When it occurs, it is usually due to embolism, polyarteritis nodosa, or accidental ligation during surgery. In such an event, irregular pale areas, often surrounded by a hyperemic zone, reflect the ischemic necrosis.

Acute occlusion of intrahepatic branches of the portal vein, generally in the setting of elevated hepatic venous pressure, classically produces a **Zahn infarct,** a discrete dark-red, triangular area with its base at the liver surface. Only sinusoidal dilation and congestion are present, not necrosis. Thus, the term *infarct* is actually a misnomer.

BACTERIAL INFECTIONS

Bacterial infections rarely cause liver disease in industrialized countries and are mostly complications of infections elsewhere. Granulomas, abscesses, and diffuse inflammation are the most common pathologic features. Infections associated with granulomatous inflammation elsewhere (e.g., tuberculosis, tularemia, brucellosis) also cause granulomatous hepatitis.

Pyogenic liver abscesses are usually caused by staphylococci, streptococci, and gram-negative enterobacteria. Gut anaerobes, mostly *Bacteroides* and microaerophilic streptococci, commonly cause liver abscesses. These resemble abscesses in other sites. Organisms reach the liver in arterial or portal blood, or via the biliary tract. In sepsis, the liver is seeded with organisms from distant sites through the arterial blood.

Pylephlebitic abscesses (Fig. 20-50) result from intraabdominal suppuration, as in peritonitis or diverticulitis, with microorganisms entering the liver in the portal blood. Pylephlebitis was once the most common cause of hepatic abscesses, but with antibiotic control of abdominal sepsis, this has become an uncommon route of infection.

Cholangitic abscesses in the liver are the most common form of hepatic abscess in Western countries today. Biliary obstruction from any cause is often complicated by bacterial

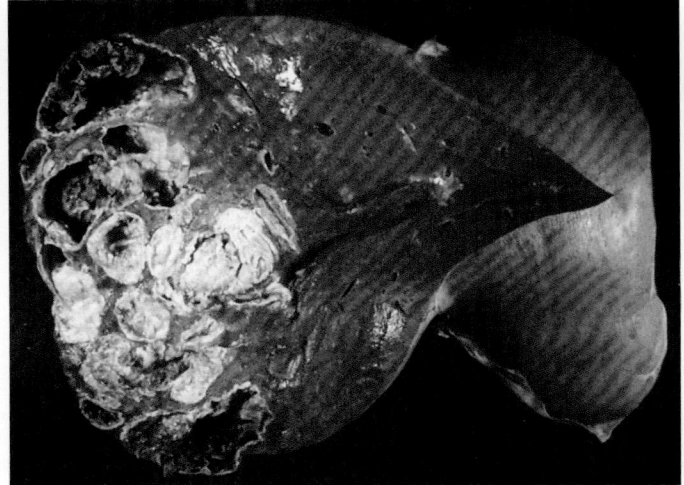

FIGURE 20-50. Pylephlebitic abscesses of the liver. The cut surface of the liver shows large, confluent, irregular abscess cavities.

infection of the biliary tree, called **ascending cholangitis**. Retrograde biliary dissemination of organisms (usually *E. coli*) then leads to cholangitic abscesses.

Hepatic abscesses occur more commonly in the right lobe of the liver. Diffuse inflammation of the liver from bacterial infection is distinctly uncommon today but may be encountered in septicemia, particularly in immunocompromised patients. The source of infection is unknown in about 1/2 of cases.

CLINICAL FEATURES: A patient with a hepatic abscess typically presents with high fever, rapid weight loss, right upper quadrant abdominal pain, and hepatomegaly. Jaundice occurs in 1/4 of cases; serum alkaline phosphatase is almost always elevated. Solitary abscesses are treated with percutaneous or surgical drainage and antibiotics, but with multiple abscesses, treatment is more problematic. The main complications are rupture and direct spread of infection. Pleuropulmonary fistulas, from rupture of an abscess through the diaphragm, and peritonitis, from leakage into the abdominal cavity, may occur. Dissemination of organisms in the blood may promote septicemia and metastatic abscesses elsewhere in the body. Mortality from hepatic abscess, even when treated, is high, ranging from 40% to 80%.

PARASITIC INFESTATIONS

Parasitic disease in the liver is a serious public health problem worldwide but is rare in industrialized countries (for details, see Chapter 9). The major parasitic diseases are summarized here.

Protozoal Diseases Frequently Involve the Liver

AMEBIASIS: In the United States, the carrier rate for *Entamoeba histolytica* in the colon is probably less than 5%, but rates approaching 35% are reported in homosexual men. Amebiasis of the liver, the most common extraintestinal site, causes amebic abscesses, which are multiple in about 1/2 of cases (Fig. 20-51). Amebic abscesses are typically 8 to 12 cm in diameter, well circumscribed and filled with thick, dark pasty material. Trophozoites are usually seen at the edges of the necrotic debris.

Symptoms associated with amebic abscesses are similar to those of pyogenic abscesses. With appropriate treatment (tissue amebicides), the abscess may heal with only a residual scar remaining. Percutaneous or surgical drainage of large abscesses is important. If an amebic abscess continues to grow, it may rupture into the peritoneum and produce peritonitis, which carries a mortality rate as high as 40%. Amebae may also invade the blood and cause abscesses of the brain and lung.

MALARIA: Hepatic involvement in malaria is a common cause of hepatomegaly in endemic areas (see Chapter 9). It reflects Kupffer cell hypertrophy and hyperplasia owing to phagocytosis of debris from rupture of parasitized erythrocytes. Liver function remains intact.

VISCERAL LEISHMANIASIS (KALA-AZAR): As in malaria, chronic visceral leishmaniasis causes hyperplasia of mononuclear phagocytes in the liver. Unlike malaria, however, the Kupffer cells ingest the parasitic organisms

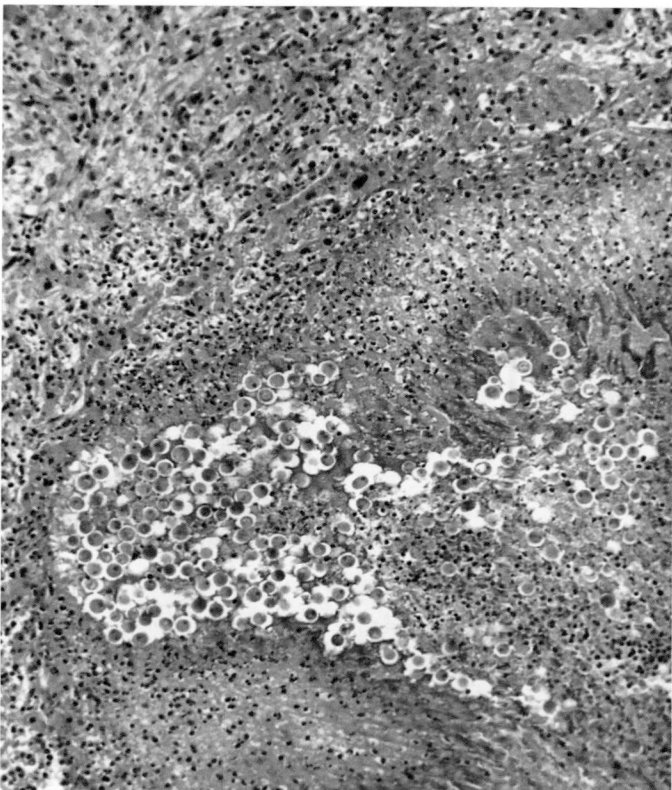

FIGURE 20-51. Amebic abscess of the liver. An amebic abscess shows fibroblastic proliferation surrounding the cavity and amebic trophozoites in the lumen.

themselves, which appear as **Donovan bodies**. Clinically, there is little evidence of hepatic dysfunction.

Helminthic Diseases Are Problems of Underdeveloped Areas

Diseases caused by helminths are described in Chapter 9, and **hepatic schistosomiasis** is discussed above in the context of portal hypertension.

ASCARIASIS: From the duodenum, *Ascaris lumbricoides* worms enter the biliary tree, where they may cause acute biliary colic. They lodge in intrahepatic biliary passages, where they disintegrate, liberating innumerable eggs that cause severe, suppurative cholangitis. Cholangitic abscesses may rupture into the peritoneum or pleural space. Spread into hepatic or portal veins causes pylephlebitis, a highly dangerous complication. The liver is enlarged and contains many irregular cavities full of foul-smelling material composed of degenerated parasites.

LIVER FLUKES: The major parasitic flukes of the human liver are *Clonorchis sinensis* and *Fasciola hepatica*. Humans are the definitive host for *C. sinensis*, whereas sheep and cattle are the main reservoir of *F. hepatica*. Both parasites lodge in the intrahepatic biliary tree, where they provoke hyperplasia of the biliary epithelium, which is particularly severe in clonorchiasis (Fig. 20-52). In high-grade infestations with *C. sinensis*, degenerated worms, parasite eggs and viscid mucus (secreted by metaplastic goblet cells in the biliary epithelium) accumulate and obstruct intrahepatic bile flow. This typically leads to intrahepatic pigment gallstones. Secondary

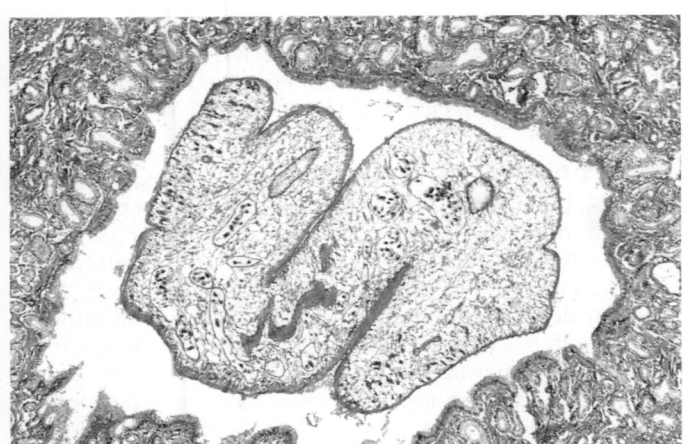

FIGURE 20-52. Infection of the liver by *Clonorchis sinensis.* The lumen of a bile duct contains an adult liver fluke, and the mucosa is hyperplastic.

infection of the bile with *E. coli* may cause cholangitis and cholangitic abscesses, which are frequent surgical emergencies in some Asian countries. *Biliary* **C. sinensis** *infestation is associated with development of cholangiocarcinoma.*

ECHINOCOCCOSIS (CYSTIC HYDATID DISEASE): Hepatic infection with tapeworms of the genus *Echinococcus,* principally *E. granulosus,* is an important zoonosis affecting humans. Echinococcal cysts expand slowly and produce symptoms only after many years. They behave as space-occupying lesions. Systemic manifestations reflect toxic or allergic reactions to the absorption of constituents of the organisms.

Leptospirosis Is an Accidental Human Infection From a Zoonosis

Leptospira spirochetes infect many animal species. Despite the large animal reservoir, fewer than 1/5 of patients who develop leptospirosis give a history of direct contact with animals. **Weil syndrome** is leptospirosis that is complicated by prolonged fever and jaundice, and, in severe cases, azotemia, hemorrhages, and altered consciousness. Weil syndrome occurs in only 1% to 6% of cases of leptospirosis. Liver pathology in fatal cases is nonspecific and includes focal necrosis, enlarged Kupffer cells and centrilobular cholestasis. Organisms are generally not demonstrable in the liver.

Liver Lesions May Occur in Congenital or Tertiary Syphilis

Congenital syphilis causes neonatal hepatitis, with diffuse fibrosis in portal tracts and around individual liver cells or groups of hepatocytes. In **tertiary syphilis,** hepatic gummas (i.e., focal lesions resembling granulomas) develop and eventually heal with dense scars. Scar retraction produces deep clefts and leads to gross pseudolobation of the liver called **hepar lobatum,** a condition that should not be confused with cirrhosis.

CHOLESTATIC SYNDROMES OF INFANCY

Diseases characterized by prolonged cholestasis and jaundice in infants either primarily affect hepatocytes or cause biliary obstruction.

Neonatal Hepatitis Entails Prolonged Cholestasis, Inflammation, and Liver Cell Injury

 ETIOLOGIC FACTORS: A specific cause can be identified in about 1/2 of cases of neonatal hepatitis (Table 20-5). About 30% are due to α_1-AT deficiency. Most other cases of known etiology are due to congenital infections with HBV, toxoplasma, rubella, cytomegalovirus, herpes simplex virus, or other agents. Hepatic injury caused by metabolic defects (e.g., galactosemia or fructose intolerance) account for some cases, and neonatal hepatitis occurs occasionally in patients with

TABLE 20-5

CAUSES OF NEONATAL HEPATITIS

Idiopathic
  Idiopathic neonatal hepatitis
  Prolonged intrahepatic cholestasis
    Arteriohepatic dysplasia (Alagille syndrome)
    Paucity of intrahepatic bile ducts not associated with specific syndromes
    Zellweger syndrome (cerebrohepatorenal syndrome)
    Byler disease

Mechanical Obstruction of the Intrahepatic Bile Ducts
  Congenital hepatic fibrosis
  Caroli disease (cystic dilation of intrahepatic ducts)

Metabolic Disorders
  Defects of carbohydrate metabolism
    Galactosemia
    Hereditary fructose intolerance
    Glycogenosis type IV
  Defects in lipid metabolism
    Gaucher disease
    Niemann-Pick disease
    Wolman disease
  Tyrosinemia (defect of amino acid metabolism)
  α_1-Antitrypsin deficiency
  Cystic fibrosis
  Parenteral nutrition

Hepatitis
  Hepatitis B
  TORCH agents (toxoplasmosis, "other," rubella, cytomegalovirus, and herpes simplex)
  Varicella
  Syphilis
  ECHO (enteric cytopathic human orphan) viruses
  Neonatal sepsis

Chromosomal Abnormalities
  Down syndrome
  Trisomy 18

Extrahepatic Biliary Obstruction

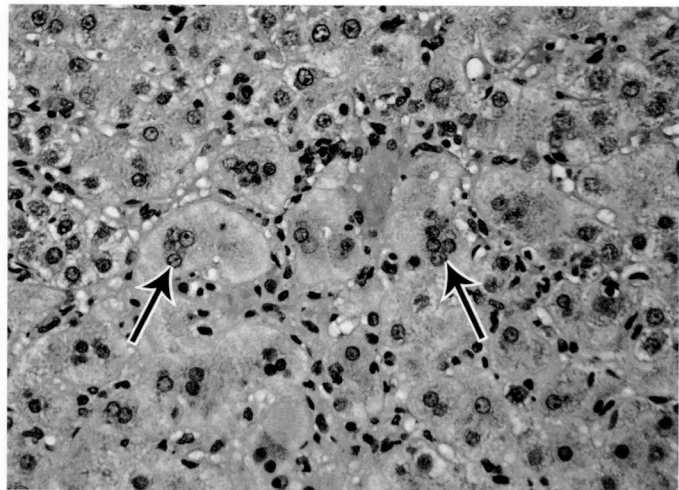

FIGURE 20-53. Neonatal hepatitis. Characteristic features include severe hepatocyte swelling (hydropic change), multinucleated giant hepatocytes (*arrows*), mild chronic inflammatory infiltrate and fibrosis.

Down syndrome and other chromosomal disorders. The other 1/2 of cases of neonatal hepatitis are unexplained.

PATHOLOGY: The characteristic lesion of neonatal hepatitis is giant cell transformation of hepatocytes, hence the older term **giant cell hepatitis** (Fig. 20-53). These giant cells may contain up to 40 nuclei and may appear detached from other cells in the liver plate. Their pale, distended cytoplasm contains large amounts of glycogen and iron. Their numbers decline with time, and they are rare in children older than 1 year. Bile pigment is prominent within canaliculi and hepatocytes. Ballooned hepatocytes, acinar transformation of hepatocytes, and acidophilic bodies are also typical of neonatal hepatitis. Extramedullary hematopoiesis is often conspicuous. Chronic inflammatory infiltrates are seen in portal tracts and in the lobular parenchyma. Pericellular fibrosis around degenerating hepatocytes, singly or in groups, is common, and fibrous tissue septa extend from the portal tracts.

Part of the Biliary Tree Has No Lumen in Biliary Atresia

Extra- and intrahepatic biliary atresias may resemble neonatal hepatitis pathologically.

Biliary Atresia

BA is a cholestatic disease in which inflammation obliterates the lumen of all or part of the biliary tree, in the absence of calculi, tumor, or rupture. BA is rare. Its estimated incidence is 1 in 5000–19,000 live births, with a higher frequency in East Asia. Biliary atresia is the most common indication for liver transplantation in children. It is thought to represent the end result of heterogeneous conditions during gestational and perinatal development. Other organs, including the heart, intestine and spleen, show anomalies in 20% of cases. BA may be associated with known causes of neonatal

hepatitis, such as various viral infections and chromosomal abnormalities (e.g., trisomy 18 and 21). Cholangiograms in BA show no bile flow into the duodenum or liver, depending on the site of the affected segment of the biliary tract.

PATHOLOGY: BA may involve all extrahepatic bile ducts or be limited to parts of the proximal or distal biliary tree. The gallbladder is often atretic. At one extreme, acute and chronic periluminal inflammation is prominent, with epithelial necrosis, and cellular debris within the obstructed or narrowed lumen. At the other extreme, the original lumen is completely replaced by mature connective tissue, and little or no inflammation. Histologically, cholestasis and periportal marginal bile ductular proliferation in the liver are evident. Some cases have multinucleated giant hepatocytes, like those seen in neonatal hepatitis. Although intrahepatic bile ducts may initially appear normal, they are gradually obliterated with the persistent cholestasis. Eventually, secondary biliary cirrhosis supervenes.

Paucity of Intrahepatic Bile Ducts

In paucity of intrahepatic bile ducts, there are few bile ducts within the liver. This occurs under three circumstances:

- In association with known causes of neonatal hepatitis (e.g., α_1-AT deficiency, various chromosomal anomalies, and metabolic derangements).
- **Alagille syndrome** (syndromic bile duct paucity), an autosomal dominant disease, also characterized by congenital abnormalities of the heart, eye, skeleton, kidneys, and CNS. This syndrome involves mutations in the Notch signaling pathway. Affected patients show five major features: chronic cholestasis, peripheral pulmonary artery stenosis, butterfly-like vertebral arch, hypertelic facies, and an eye abnormality involving the iris and cornea known as posterior embryotoxon. The liver pathology is characterized by the absence of bile ducts in portal tracts.
- Unassociated with other conditions (idiopathic).

Neonatal hepatitis, paucity of intrahepatic bile ducts, BA, and possibly choledochal cyst all probably result from infantile obstructive cholangiopathy, a common inflammatory process.

PATHOLOGY: With paucity of intrahepatic bile ducts, very few bile ducts are seen in the liver. Giant cell transformation, cholestasis, and ductular reaction are common; cirrhosis is not.

CLINICAL FEATURES: Most patients with uncomplicated neonatal hepatitis recover without sequelae, but the prognosis is poor if it is associated with paucity of intrahepatic bile ducts. Many such children develop biliary cirrhosis. By contrast, the outlook in Alagille syndrome is good. If uncorrected, BA invariably leads to progressive secondary biliary cirrhosis and death. Surgical correction (by hepatoportojenunostomy) may be curative in some anatomically favorable cases, but transplantation is the best treatment for biliary atresia.

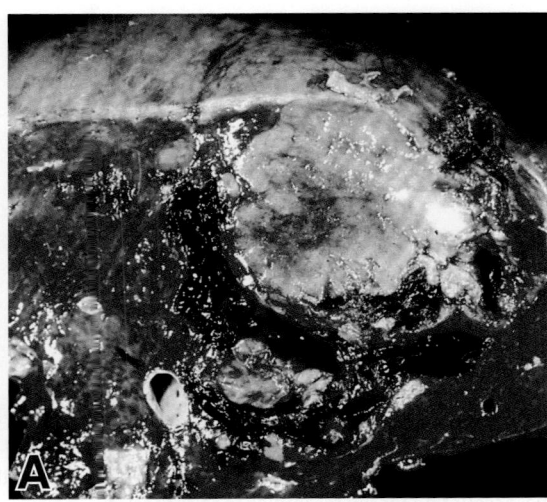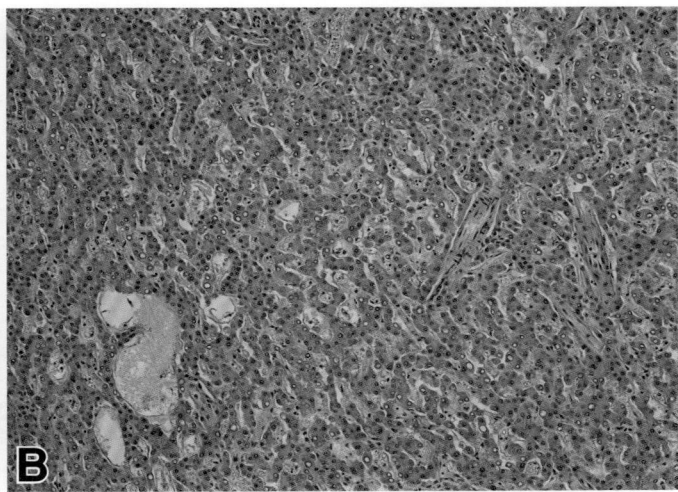

FIGURE 20-54. Hepatocellular adenoma. A. A surgically resected portion of liver shows a tan, lobulated mass beneath the liver capsule. The tumor has ruptured, resulting in intraparenchymal and intraperitoneal hemorrhage. The patient was a woman who had taken birth control pills for a number of years and presented with sudden intraperitoneal bleeding. **B.** The adenomatous hepatocytes do not differ from normal hepatocytes and are arranged without discernible lobular architecture. Note the absence of portal tracts.

BENIGN TUMORS AND TUMOR-LIKE LESIONS

Liver Adenomas Are Benign Tumors That Occur Mainly in Women

Once rare, these tumors became more common with oral contraceptive use. Lower-dose estrogen and progesterone combinations have reduced the incidence of liver adenomas.

PATHOLOGY: Hepatocellular adenomas are usually solitary, sharply demarcated masses measuring up to 40 cm in diameter and weighing up to 3 kg (Fig. 20-54A). Multiple smaller adenomas are present in 1/4 of cases. The diagnosis of hepatocellular adenomatosis is applied if more than 10 adenomas are present. These tumors are encapsulated and paler than nearby liver parenchyma. *The neoplastic hepatocytes resemble normal hepatocytes but are not arrayed in a lobular architecture.* Portal tracts and central venules are absent (Fig. 20-54B). The cells of adenomas may be very and eosinophilic, or filled with glycogen or fat, which makes the cytoplasm appear clear or vacuolated. The presence of small arteries within the parenchyma suggests an adenoma as opposed to normal liver.

CLINICAL FEATURES: In about 1/3 of patients with hepatic adenomas (particularly pregnant women who have used oral contraceptives), these tumors bleed into the peritoneal cavity and require immediate surgery. However, even large adenomas may disappear if oral contraceptives are discontinued. Occasional liver adenomas have been reported in men who use anabolic steroids.

Hepatocellular adenomas are subclassified into HNF1-alpha–inactivated adenomas, inflammatory adenomas, beta-catenin–activated adenomas, and unclassified adenomas. HNF1-alpha–inactivated adenomas make up 35% of all adenomas. They exhibit macrovesicular steatosis and are often associated with adenomatosis. Inflammatory adenomas make up 45% of all adenomas. They demonstrate lymphocytic inflammation and sinusoidal dilatation/congestion, and are associated with fatty liver disease. Inflammatory adenomas were historically referred to as telangiectatic focal nodular hyperplasia (FNH). Beta-catenin–activated adenomas make up 10% of all adenomas and are associated with increased risk of malignant transformation. Unclassified adenomas make up <10% of all adenomas and have no specific pathologic features.

Focal Nodular Hyperplasia Resembles Cirrhosis

FNH is characterized by multiple fibrous septa and regenerative nodules (Fig. 20-55A). It measures up to 15 cm in diameter and weighs as much as 700 g. On occasion, FNH protrudes from the surface of the liver, and may even be pedunculated. The cut surface has a central scar from which fibrous septa radiate. Hepatocytic nodules are circumscribed by fibrous septa (Fig. 20-55B), with many tortuous bile ductules and mononuclear inflammatory cells. Lobular architecture is absent within nodules. Septa contain large dystrophic arteries and veins, but show little hemorrhage. These abnormal vessels suggest that FNH forms as a result of localized vascular malformation.

FNH occurs in both sexes and at all ages. It is not a neoplasm nor it is associated with use of oral contraceptives, and only rarely bleeds.

Nodular Regenerative Hyperplasia Causes Portal Hypertension

Nodular regenerative hyperplasia, also called *nodular transformation of the liver* or *partial nodular transformation*, is neither neoplastic nor preneoplastic. It is characterized by small, hyperplastic nodules without fibrosis in an otherwise normal liver. It may be isolated and located predominantly in the perihilar region, or occur diffusely throughout the liver.

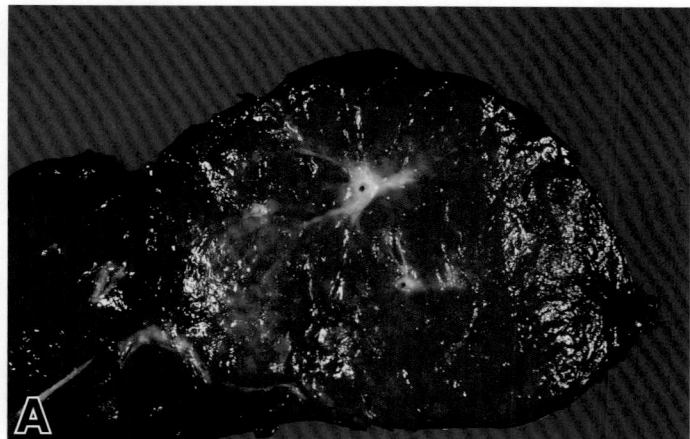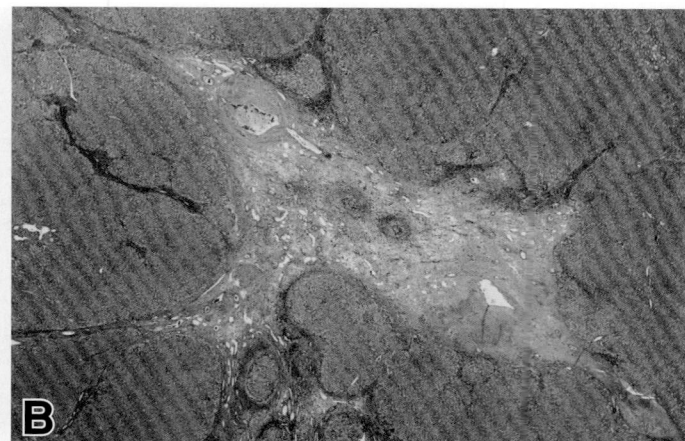

FIGURE 20-55. Focal nodular hyperplasia. A. A resected mass shows nodules with central scarring. **B.** This surgically resected mass from the liver shows a vascular central scar and irregular fibrous septa dissecting hepatic parenchyma, accounting for the resemblance to cirrhosis.

Nodules are composed of liver cells in plates two and three cells thick, compressing the surrounding parenchyma.

Nodular regenerative hyperplasia is associated with portal hypertension. Once called **noncirrhotic portal hypertension,** its etiology is unknown, but it has been linked to use of oral contraceptives or anabolic steroids, extrahepatic infections, tumors, and chronic inflammatory and autoimmune diseases.

Hemangiomas Are the Most Common Tumors of the Liver

Benign hemangiomas in the liver occur at all ages and in both sexes. They are common, being present in up to 7% of autopsy livers (Fig. 20-56). They are normally small and asymptomatic, although larger tumors may cause abdominal symptoms and even hemorrhage into the peritoneum. Grossly, hemangiomas are usually solitary and under 5 cm, but multiple hemangiomas and giant forms (>15 cm) have been described. They resemble cavernous hemangiomas found elsewhere (see Chapter 10).

Cystic Diseases of the Liver Represents a Spectrum of Lesions

BILE DUCT MICROHAMARTOMAS: These clinically inapparent lesions (also called *von Meyenburg complexes*) are composed of anomalous, small cystic bile ducts in a fibrous stroma. They are usually multiple and vary from pinpoint grayish white foci to nodules up to 1 cm. Cysts are lined by bile duct epithelium and may contain inspissated bile (Fig. 20-57).

SOLITARY AND MULTIPLE SIMPLE CYSTS: Simple liver cysts are lined by cuboidal to columnar epithelium and may be associated with adult polycystic kidney disease (see Chapter 16). They may be seen in livers with von Meyenburg complexes.

CONGENITAL HEPATIC FIBROSIS: This recessively inherited disorder is marked by enlarged portal tracts with extensive fibrosis and many well-formed bile ductules (Fig. 20-58). It is seen mainly in children and adolescents. Bile ducts may become so dilated that they resemble microcysts, but they still communicate with the biliary

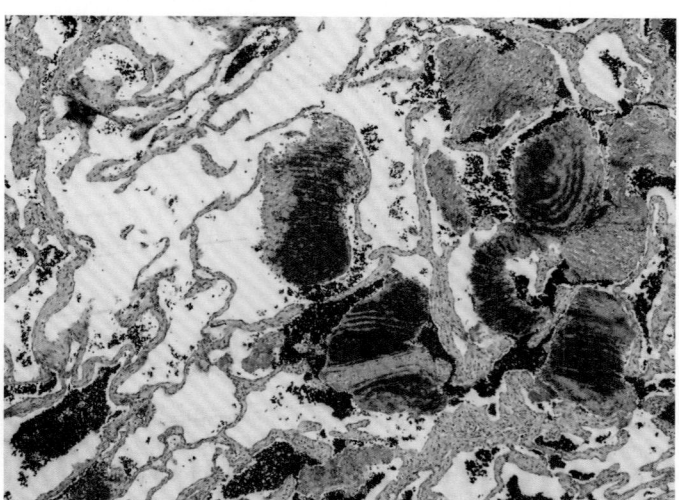

FIGURE 20-56. Cavernous hemangioma. This is benign vascular tumor composed of blood-filled cavernous spaces.

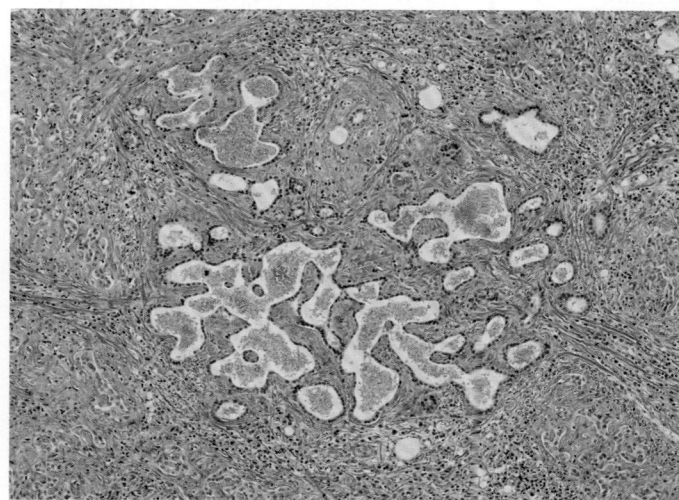

FIGURE 20-57. Bile duct microhamartoma (von Meyenburg complex). A bile duct microhamartoma is composed of cystically dilated spaces lined by a single layer of duct epithelium and containing inspissated bile.

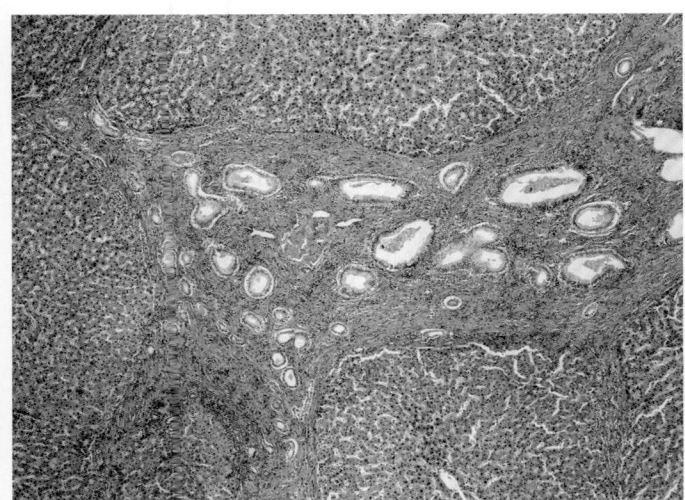

FIGURE 20-58. Congenital hepatic fibrosis. An enlarged and fibrotic portal tract contains ductal plate remnant microcysts.

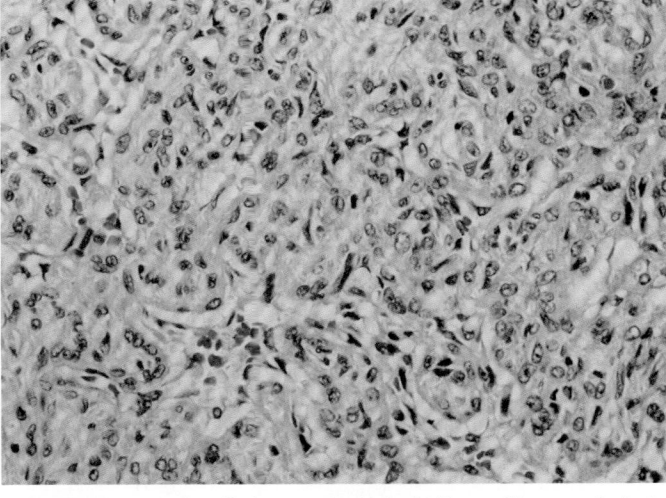

FIGURE 20-60. Infantile hemangioendothelioma. Plump endothelial cells line anastomosing slit-like vascular spaces.

system. Regenerative nodules are absent, thus distinguishing this condition from cirrhosis. The origin of the lesion is unknown. The main complication of congenital hepatic fibrosis is severe portal hypertension with recurrent bleeding from esophageal varices. **Infantile polycystic disease** of the liver resembles congenital hepatic fibrosis. It is also inherited as an autosomal recessive trait.

Angiomyolipoma Is a Benign Tumor of Stromal Elements

Angiomyolipoma is a rare tumor composed of varying proportions of blood vessels, smooth muscle, and mature fatty tissue (Fig. 20-59). It is derived from perivascular epithelial cells (PECs) and thus belongs to a group of tumors usually associated with tuberous sclerosis, referred to as PEC-omas. Hepatic angiomyolipomas resemble the more common angiomyolipoma of the kidney (see Chapter 16).

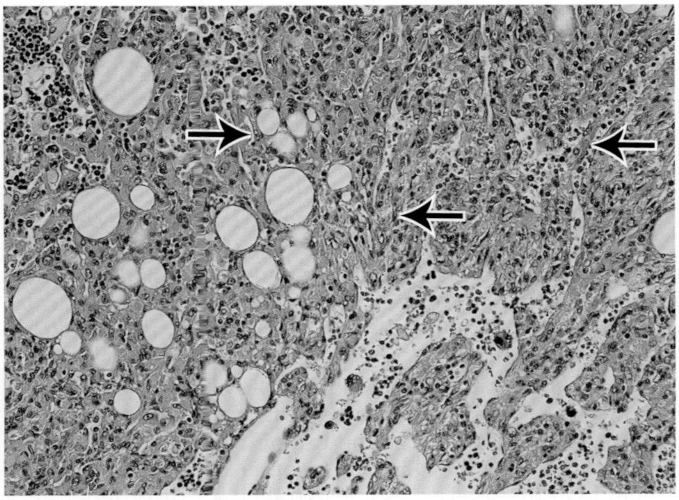

Infantile Hemangioendothelioma Is a Type of Hemangioma That Occurs in Infants

Infantile hemangioendothelioma is a benign vascular tumor of intercommunicating vascular channels lined by a single layer of plump endothelial cells in a fibrous stroma (Fig. 20-60). It is found mostly in infants, usually females. Spontaneous involution is common. However, a large tumor may cause high-output cardiac or liver failure.

Mesenchymal Hamartoma Is a Developmental Malformation

Mesenchymal hamartoma is a benign liver tumor formed as a developmental malformation of liver mesenchyme. It is composed of large, serous fluid cysts surrounded by loose mesenchyme containing a mixture of bile ducts, hepatocyte cords, and clusters of vessels (Fig. 20-61). The mesenchymal tissue consists of scattered stellate-shaped cells in a loose matrix. Complete surgical excision is curative.

FIGURE 20-59. Angiomyolipoma. An angiomyolipoma is composed of a mixture of epithelioid and spindle-shaped smooth muscle (*arrows*), vascular spaces, and round fat cells.

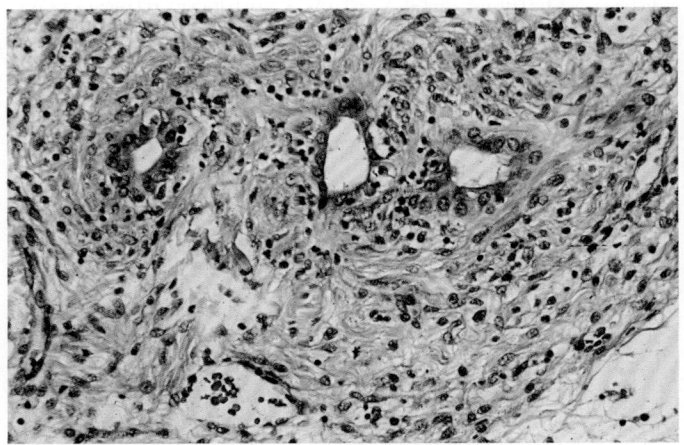

FIGURE 20-61. Mesenchymal hamartoma. These consist of bile ducts in loose mesenchymal tissue stroma.

THE LIVER AND BILIARY SYSTEM

MALIGNANT TUMORS OF THE LIVER

Hepatocellular Carcinoma Is a Malignant Tumor of Hepatocytes

EPIDEMIOLOGY: HCC is the most common primary liver malignancy and is a leading cause of cancer-related death. It occurs worldwide but with striking geographic variability. In industrialized Western countries, HCC is uncommon, although its incidence has nearly doubled in the past 20 years, mostly in patients with chronic hepatitis C. In sub-Saharan Africa and Southeast Asia, HCC may occur up to 50 times more often. For example, in Mozambique, which has the highest incidence in the world, 2/3 of all cancers in men and 1/3 in women are HCC.

PATHOPHYSIOLOGY: *HEPATITIS B:* More than 85% of cases of HCC occur in countries with a high prevalence of chronic HBV infection. Most patients have had chronic hepatitis B for years, often after vertical or perinatal transmission from an infected mother to her newborn child. Individuals with persistent HBV infection have up to 200-fold increased risk for HCC. When chronic hepatitis B is acquired at or near birth, 1/4 will ultimately develop HCC. Risk of this cancer in men who are positive for HBsAg and HBeAg is four times higher than those with HBsAg alone. Most (>80%) cases of HCC associated with HBV infection occur in patients with cirrhosis.

Cirrhosis has been blamed for the development of HCC in HBV-infected livers, but many HBV-associated HCCs occur in patients without cirrhosis. It is likely that integration of the HBV genome into the host DNA and expression of HBV genes are the key factors. For example, the viral protein HBxAg, encoded by the *X* gene of HBV, inactivates tumor suppressor proteins and transactivates certain oncogenes.

HEPATITIS C: HCV is less common than HBV worldwide, but most cases of HCC in Europe, North America, and Japan are associated with hepatitis C. In the United States, HCV infection is present in about 50% of HCC. As with HCC in hepatitis B, most patients with HCV who develop HCC have underlying cirrhosis, and the cumulative occurrence of HCC in HCV-induced cirrhosis is as high as 70% after 15 years.

Coinfection with HBV and HCV increases the risk of liver cancer threefold, relative to infection with either virus alone. Carcinogenesis by HCV is poorly understood, but interactions between virus proteins and cellular constituents are likely involved.

OTHER CAUSES OF HEPATOCELLULAR CARCINOMA: **Alcoholic cirrhosis** predisposes to HCC, but the risk is not large, and the mechanism is unknown. Because many alcoholics are infected with HBV and HCV, the role of alcohol alone in HCC is difficult to determine. Alcoholics with chronic hepatitis C have double the risk for HCC compared with HCV infection alone.

Hemochromatosis and α_1-**AT deficiency** carry a substantial risk of HCC. About 10% of patients with hemochromatosis may be expected to develop the tumor. On the other hand, a lower risk of HCC is seen in patients with autoimmune hepatitis, WD or PBC with cirrhosis. *As with HCC in patients with chronic hepatitis B without cirrhosis, this suggests that cirrhosis itself is not sufficient to cause liver cancer but it may magnify HCC risk due to other etiologies.*

Aflatoxin B$_1$ is a fungal contaminant of many foods, found mostly in developing tropical countries. It causes HCC in a number of animal species. The incidence of liver cancer in humans correlates roughly with dietary intake of aflatoxin. The presence of urinary aflatoxin B$_1$ metabolites is associated with a threefold increased risk of HCC. Aflatoxin and HBV infection are synergistic; combined exposure increases the risk of HCC 60-fold.

Mutations in the *TP53* gene are present in 1/2 of DNA samples from HCCs occurring in areas endemic for aflatoxin. Most of these mutations are G-to-T substitutions at codon 249, a change that is produced experimentally by aflatoxin B$_1$.

PATHOLOGY: HCCs are solitary or multiple soft, hemorrhagic tan masses (Fig. 20-62A). Occasionally, a green color indicates bile production. They tend to grow into portal and hepatic veins, and may extend from the latter into the vena cava and even the right atrium. The tumor may spread widely, but metastases favor the lungs and portal lymph nodes.

HCCs range from well differentiated and difficult to distinguish from normal liver to anaplastic or undifferentiated neoplasms. In most, tumor cells are arranged in trabeculae or plates as in normal liver ("trabecular pattern"). These plates are separated by endothelium-lined sinusoids. In a "pseudoglandular (adenoid, acinar) pattern," malignant hepatocytes are arranged around a lumen, which may contain bile (Fig. 20-62B). Despite their resemblance to glands, these are not true glands, and the lesion should not be confused with cholangiocarcinoma or other adenocarcinomas. Neither histologic pattern carries a particular prognostic significance.

Fibrolamellar carcinoma is an uncommon variant of HCC with a distinctive histology. It arises in noncirrhotic livers, mostly in adolescents and young adults, and is composed of clusters of large, eosinophilic, neoplastic hepatocytes with cytoplasmic pale bodies containing fibrinogen. The cells are surrounded by thick collagen fibers (Fig. 20-63). The prognosis of fibrolamellar HCC is similar to that of other types of HCC in noncirrhotic livers.

CLINICAL FEATURES: HCC usually presents as a painful, enlarging mass. If discovered at an advanced stage, the prognosis is dismal. Patients die of malignant cachexia, rupture of the tumor with catastrophic bleeding into the peritoneal cavity or complications of cirrhosis.

HCC may cause paraneoplastic syndromes (e.g., polycythemia, hypoglycemia, hypercalcemia) due to ectopic hormone production by the tumor. α-Fetoprotein (AFP) levels are often elevated, as in other benign and malignant liver diseases and some extrahepatic disorders.

Surveillance of patients with increased risk for HCC has led to early detection.

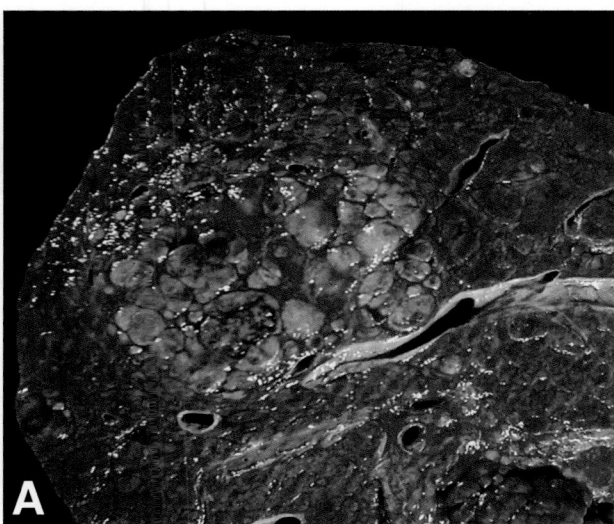
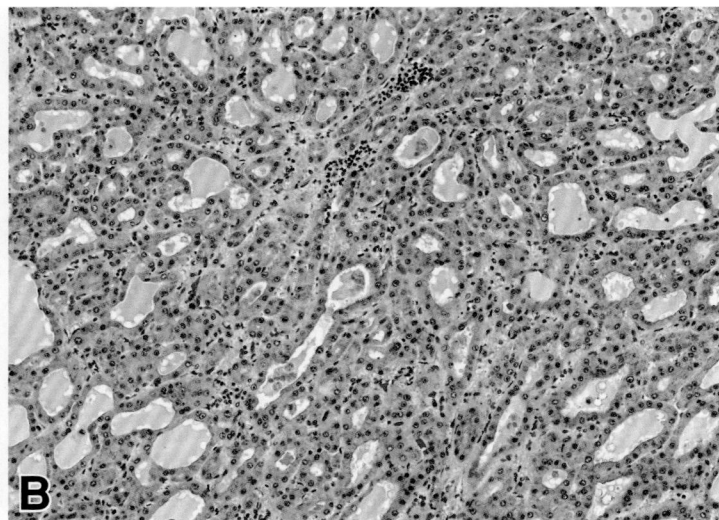

FIGURE 20-62. Hepatocellular carcinoma (HCC). A. Cut surface of a cirrhotic liver shows a poorly circumscribed, nodular area of yellow, partially hemorrhagic HCC. **B.** In this moderately differentiated tumor, HCC cells are arranged in an acinar pattern and surround concretions of inspissated bile.

If a small tumor is confined to one hepatic lobe, segmental resection can provide acceptable tumor-free survival rates. Ablative therapies (e.g., ethanol injection, radiofrequency ablation, cryotherapy, and transarterial embolization) can slow tumor progression. In patients with cirrhosis and limited tumor burden, liver transplantation gives the best tumor-free survival.

Cholangiocarcinomas Arise From Biliary Epithelium

Intrahepatic cholangiocarcinoma is a bile duct carcinoma that originates anywhere in the biliary tree, from large intrahepatic bile ducts to the smallest ducts at the edges of hepatic lobules, and peribiliary glands. It occurs mainly in older people of both sexes, with an average age at presentation of 60 years. It may occur anywhere but is particularly common in parts of Asia where the liver fluke *C. sinensis* (see above) is endemic. In fact, the incidence of intrahepatic cholangiocarcinoma is also increasing in association with chronic liver diseases, such as hepatitis C, hepatitis B, and alcoholic cirrhosis. PSC predisposes strongly to cholangiocarcinoma. Of livers with PSC removed for transplantation, 1/4 are found to have cholangiocarcinoma. Choledochal cysts and Caroli disease (see below) are also risk factors.

PATHOLOGY: Intrahepatic cholangiocarcinomas form small cuboidal cells in ductular or glandular patterns (Fig. 20-64). They often show substantial fibrosis and thus may be confused with metastatic breast or pancreas carcinomas on liver biopsy. Tumors with both HCC and intrahepatic cholangiocarcinoma morphologies are **combined hepatocellular–cholangiocarcinomas**.

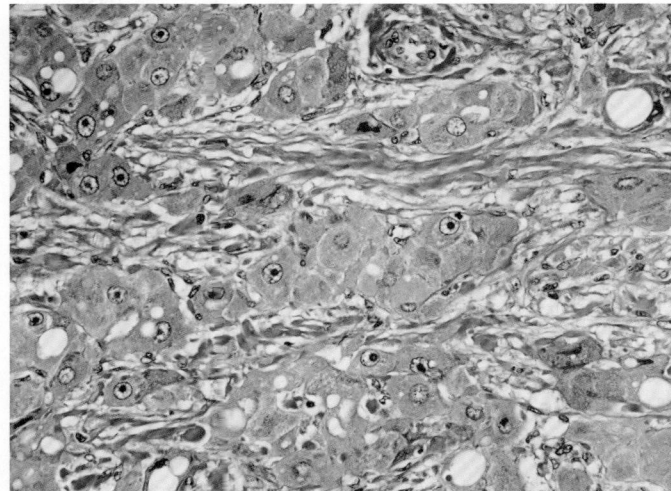

FIGURE 20-63. Fibrolamellar hepatocellular carcinoma. Clusters of eosinophilic tumor cells with abundant cytoplasm are separated by lamellated fibrous bands.

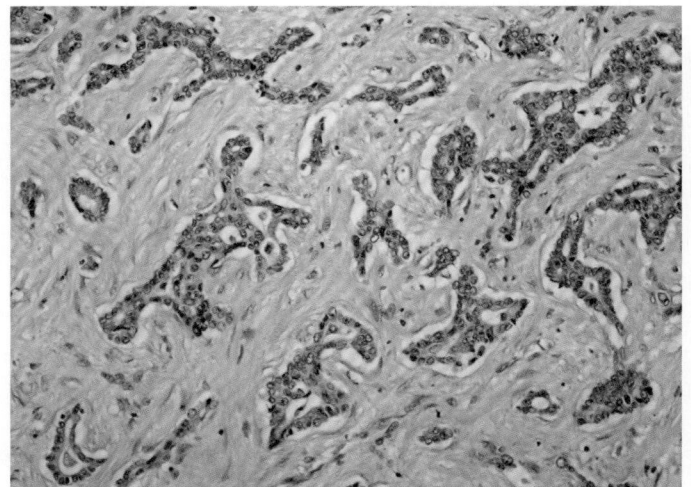

FIGURE 20-64. Cholangiocarcinoma. Well-differentiated neoplastic glands are embedded in a dense fibrous stroma.

Perihilar cholangiocarcinomas are bile duct carcinomas that arise around the convergence of the right and left hepatic ducts. They present as (1) small sclerosing tumors that obliterate the duct, (2) tumors that spread within the duct wall, or (3) a rare intraductal papillary variant. They may grow to "mass-forming" tumors. All produce symptoms of extrahepatic biliary obstruction.

Cholangiocarcinomas invade portal and hepatic veins less aggressively than do HCCs, but they spread locally along nerves and metastasize throughout the body, particularly to portal lymph nodes. Liver transplantation is rarely successful in eradicating the tumor.

Hepatoblastoma Is a Rare Malignant Tumor of Children

Hepatoblastomas are usually discovered at birth or before the age of 3 years.

 PATHOLOGY: Hepatoblastomas are circumscribed masses up to 25 cm in diameter. Typically, they are partially necrotic and hemorrhagic, and composed of both epithelial- and mesenchymal-appearing cells. Occasionally, the latter are not seen. The epithelial component resembles embryonic and fetal cells. The "embryonal" cells are small and fusiform, arranged in ribbons or rosettes. The "fetal" cells resemble hepatocytes, contain glycogen and fat and form trabeculae with intervening sinusoids. The mesenchymal elements include connective tissue, cartilage, and osteoid. Foci of squamous epithelium are occasionally encountered.

 CLINICAL FEATURES: Abdominal enlargement, vomiting, and failure to thrive are common presenting symptoms. Serum AFP is almost always elevated, and occasionally secretion of ectopic gonadotropin leads to sexual precocity. Congenital anomalies, including cardiac and renal malformations, hemihypertrophy and macroglossia, may be present. Untreated, these tumors are fatal, but liver transplantation or partial hepatectomy is often curative.

Epithelioid Hemangioendothelioma Is a Low-Grade Malignancy

This type of vascular tumor occurs predominantly in middle-aged women.

 PATHOLOGY: Epithelioid hemangioendotheliomas may be single or multiple firm, gray tumors. They have a zonal pattern of cellularity with a hypocellular central area and a hypercellular periphery, the latter corresponding to its advancing front. The central zone is often sclerotic or calcified. Tumor cells, which are endothelial in origin, are spindle shaped, dendritic patterned, or epithelioid (Fig. 20-65). The latter commonly form lumens, which may contain red blood cells.

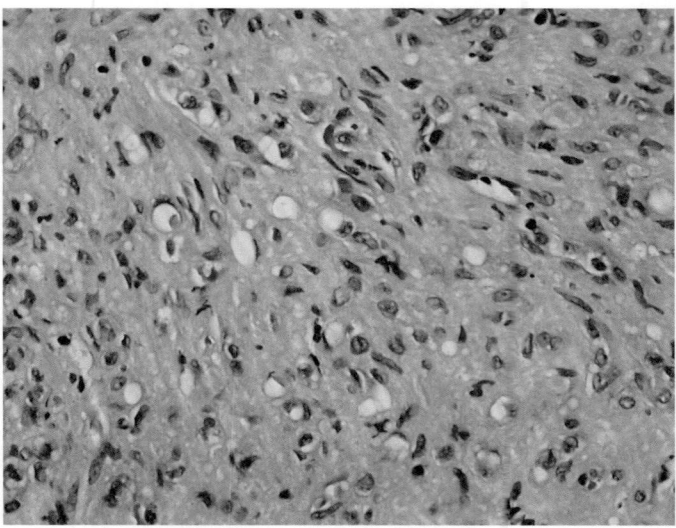

FIGURE 20-65. Epithelioid hemangioendothelioma. Tumor cells are scattered in a fibrous stroma. Some resemble signet rings with intracellular lumens containing red blood cells.

 CLINICAL FEATURES: Patients present with abdominal pain, enlarging mass, weight loss, or malaise. Imaging studies show single or multiple avascular or calcified tumors. Treatment includes surgical resection for localized lesions or liver transplantation for patients with multiple tumors.

Hemangiosarcoma May Result From Chemical Exposures

This is the only significant sarcoma of the liver. It is linked to exposure to thorium dioxide, vinyl chloride, or inorganic arsenic and is now distinctly uncommon.

 PATHOLOGY: These are mostly multicentric tumors, starting as multiple hemorrhagic nodules that may coalesce. Spindle-shaped, neoplastic, endothelial cells line sinusoids, and compress liver cell plates (Fig. 20-66). Cavernous blood spaces and solid masses of neoplastic cells are common. Widespread metastases are usual.

 CLINICAL FEATURES: Patients present with hepatomegaly, jaundice, and ascites. Hematologic abnormalities, including pancytopenia and hemolytic anemia, are often prominent and in many cases due to splenomegaly from noncirrhotic portal hypertension. Tumor rupture with vigorous intra-abdominal hemorrhage is common. The prognosis is dismal.

Metastatic Cancer Is the Most Common Malignancy in the Liver

Of all metastatic cancers, 1/3 affect the liver, including 1/2 of cancers of the gastrointestinal tract, breast, and lung. Pancreatic carcinoma, malignant melanoma, and hematologic malignancies also often metastasize to liver, but any tumor may do so.

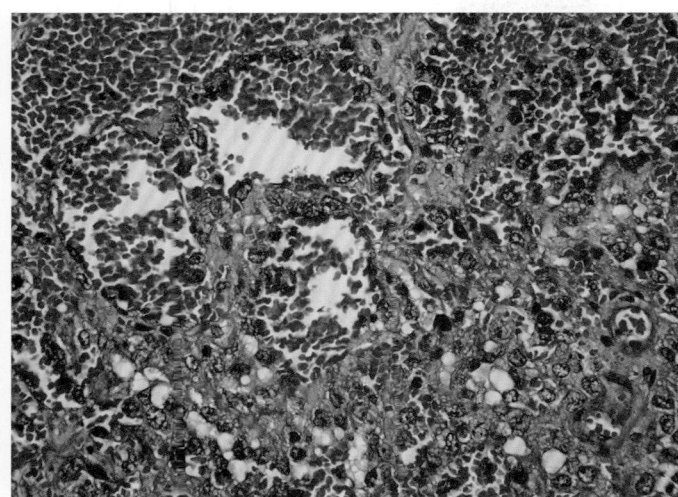

FIGURE 20-66. Hemangiosarcoma. Tumor cells with bizarre nuclei line vascular spaces.

PATHOLOGY: The liver may have a single metastatic nodule or become virtually replaced by metastases (Fig. 20-67), in which case it may weigh more than 5 kg. *Such metastases are the most common cause of massive hepatomegaly.* Metastatic tumors can appear on the liver surface as umbilicated masses. Hepatic metastases tend to resemble their primary tumors but may be so poorly differentiated that a primary site cannot be determined.

CLINICAL FEATURES: Metastatic cancers to the liver often lead to weight loss as a presenting symptom. Portal hypertension and its complications may occur. Bile duct obstruction or replacement of most of the liver parenchyma may cause jaundice. If the patient lives long enough, hepatic failure may ensue. Often the first indication of a metastatic tumor is an unexplained increase in serum alkaline phosphatase. Most patients die within a year of diagnosis, but surgical resection of a solitary metastasis may be curative.

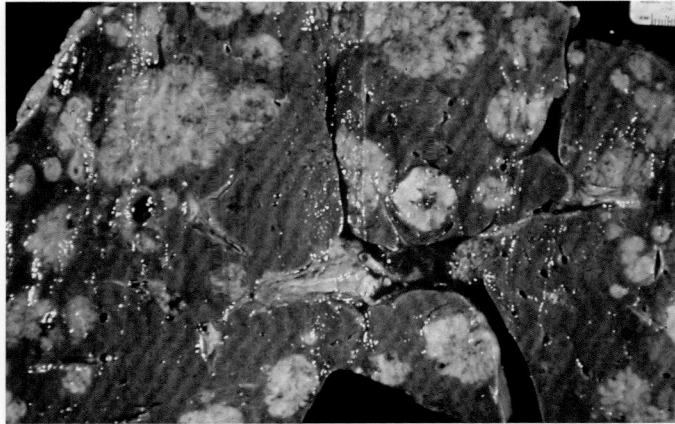

FIGURE 20-67. Metastatic carcinoma in the liver. The cut surface of the liver shows many firm, pale masses of metastatic colon cancer.

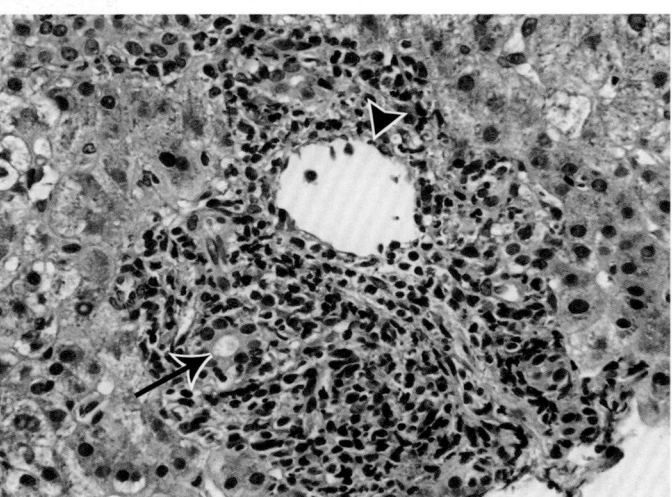

FIGURE 20-68. Acute rejection in a liver allograft. A portal tract is expanded by a polymorphous inflammatory infiltrate consisting of large and small lymphocytes, plasma cells, macrophages, neutrophils, and eosinophils. The bile ducts (*arrow*) are damaged. A vein (*arrowhead*) is also inflamed (endophlebitis).

LIVER TRANSPLANTATION

With increasing use of hepatic transplantation, the pathologic diagnosis of allograft rejection requires useful criteria by which outcome can be assessed and therapy recommended.

PATHOLOGY: In acute rejection, bile ducts are distorted by mixed cellular portal inflammation that may involve the ductal epithelium itself. Eosinophils are almost always present. Epithelial atypia may be seen (Fig. 20-68). Lymphocytes often adhere to the endothelium of terminal venules and small branches of the portal veins, with or without subendothelial inflammation (endothelialitis).

In allograft rejection lasting more than 2 months, interlobular bile ducts become damaged. These small bile ducts are progressively destroyed, causing persistent cholestasis, the end stage of which is **chronic ductopenic rejection** or **vanishing bile duct syndrome** (Fig. 20-69).

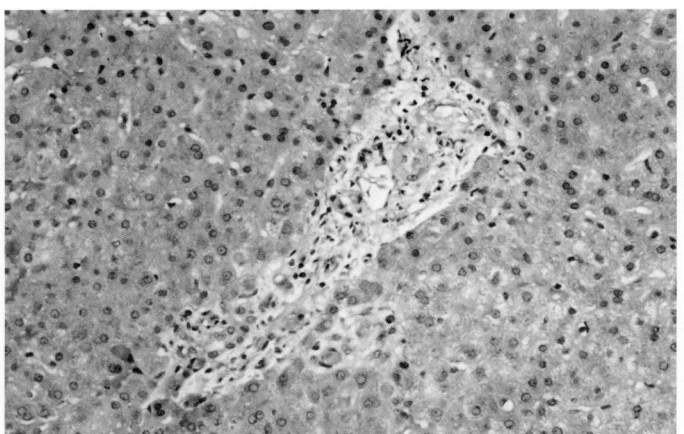

FIGURE 20-69. Chronic ductopenic rejection (vanishing bile duct syndrome). A portal tract shows mild chronic inflammation and absence of the bile duct.

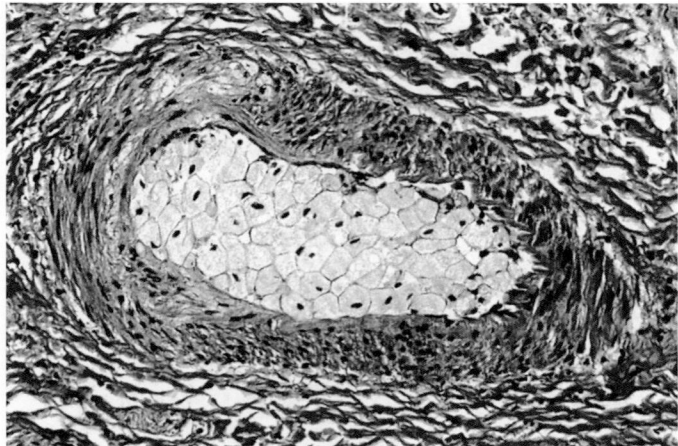

FIGURE 20-70. Arterial lesions in chronic rejection in a liver transplant. Subintimal foam cells, intimal sclerosis, and myointimal hyperplasia virtually obliterate the lumen of a hepatic artery. These changes reflect chronic immune-mediated injury of allograft blood vessels.

Subintimal foam cells, intimal sclerosis and myointimal hyperplasia, that is, rejection arteriopathy, may cause arterial narrowing or occlusion (Fig. 20-70).

The Gallbladder and Extrahepatic Bile Ducts

ANATOMY

The gallbladder is a thin, elongated sac about 8 cm long and about 50 mL in volume, which occupies a fossa on the inferior surface of the liver between the right and quadrate lobes. It originates from the same foregut diverticulum that gives rise to the liver. Its primary function is storage, concentration, and release of bile. The cystic duct is about 3 cm long and drains the gallbladder into the hepatic duct. It conducts dilute bile from the hepatic duct into the gallbladder, where it is concentrated and subsequently discharged into the common bile duct.

The gallbladder wall is composed of a mucous membrane, a muscularis, and an adventitia. It is covered by a reflection of visceral peritoneum. The mucosa is thrown into folds and consists of columnar epithelium and a lamina propria of loose connective tissue. **Rokitansky–Aschoff sinuses** are mucosal diverticula that dip into the gallbladder wall.

CONGENITAL ANOMALIES

Developmental anomalies of the gallbladder are rare and of little clinical significance except for surgeons. Bile duct anomalies include **duplications** and **accessory bile ducts**. Congenital bile duct dilations include **choledochal cysts** (85% of all cases), **choledochal diverticula**, or **choledochoceles** (Fig. 20-71). Multiple cysts may occur as segmental dilations in the entire extrahepatic biliary tree. Similar multiple dilations in the intrahepatic biliary tree, called **Caroli disease**, predispose to bacterial cholangitis.

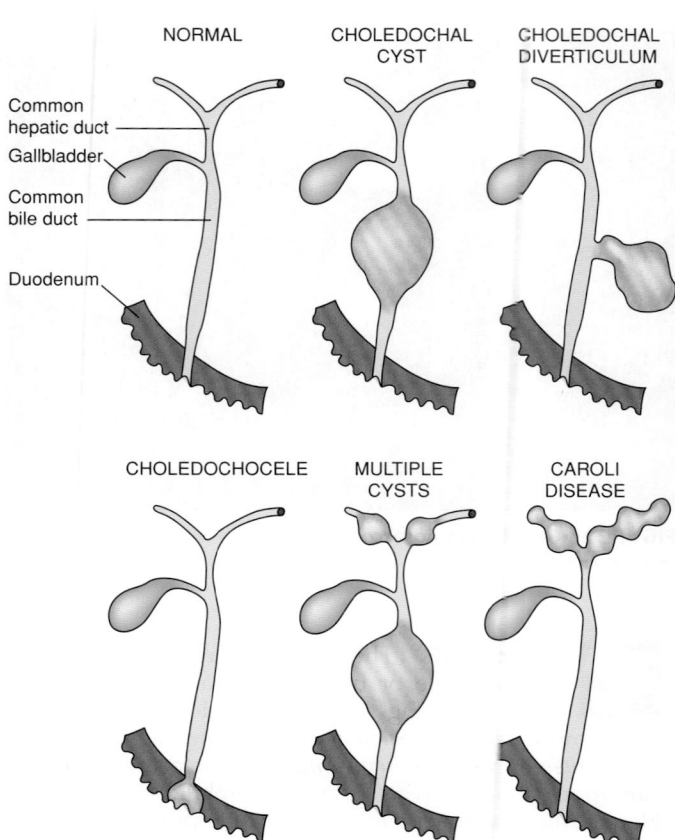

FIGURE 20-71. Congenital dilations of the bile ducts.

CHOLELITHIASIS

This is one or more stones in the gallbladder lumen or the extrahepatic biliary tree. In the industrialized countries, 3/4 of gallstones are composed mainly of **cholesterol**; the rest are made of **calcium bilirubinate** and **other calcium salts (pigment gallstones)**. Pigment stones are more common in the tropics and Asia. Most gallstones are not radiopaque but are readily detected by ultrasonography. They are often asymptomatic but cause mild to severe pain **(biliary colic)** if they become lodged in the cystic or common bile ducts.

Cholesterol Stones Are the Most Common Gallstones

Cholesterol stones measure up to 4 cm in diameter and may be round or faceted, yellow to tan, single or multiple (Fig. 20-72). They are mostly cholesterol, plus some calcium salts and mucin.

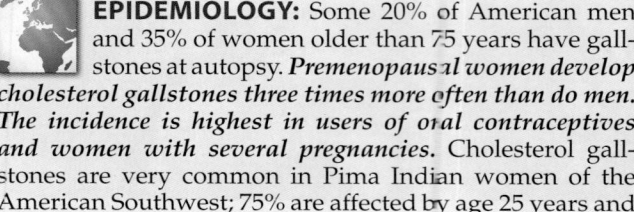
EPIDEMIOLOGY: Some 20% of American men and 35% of women older than 75 years have gallstones at autopsy. *Premenopausal women develop cholesterol gallstones three times more often than do men. The incidence is highest in users of oral contraceptives and women with several pregnancies.* Cholesterol gallstones are very common in Pima Indian women of the American Southwest; 75% are affected by age 25 years and 90% by age 60.

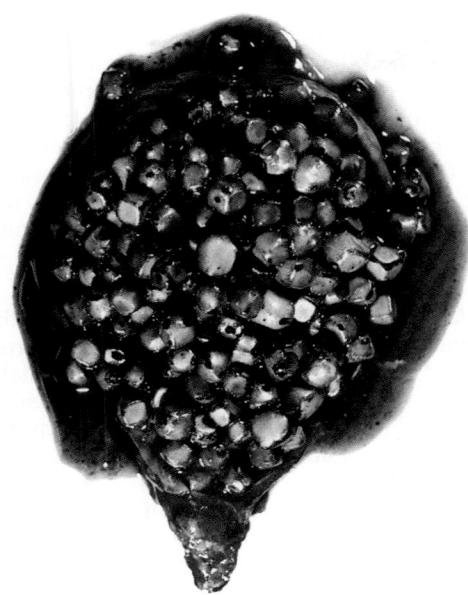

FIGURE 20-72. Cholesterol gallstones. The gallbladder has been opened to reveal numerous yellow cholesterol gallstones.

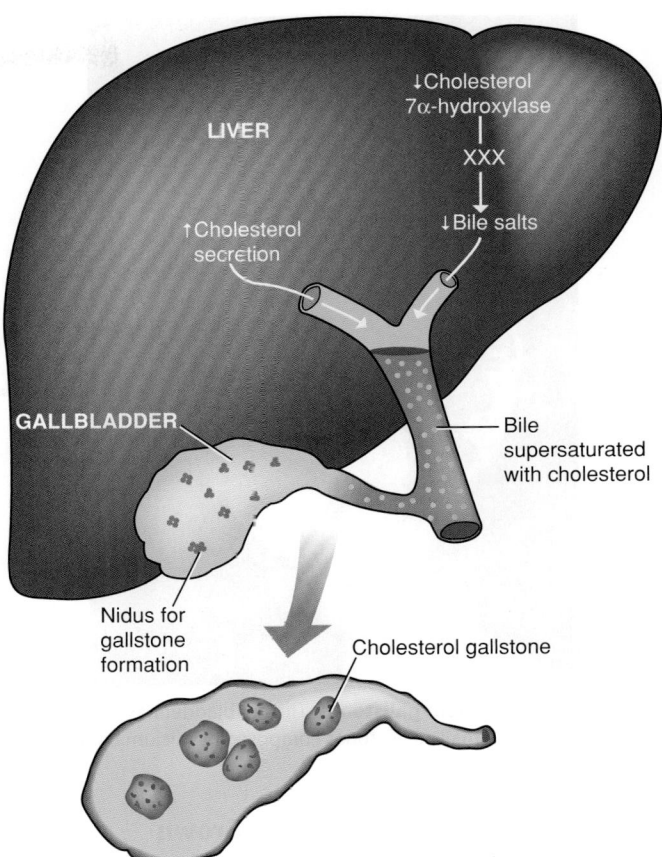

FIGURE 20-73. Pathogenesis of cholesterol gallstones.

 PATHOPHYSIOLOGY: Formation of cholesterol gallstones reflects the physicochemical qualities of bile and local factors in the gallbladder (Fig. 20-73):

- **Bile formation in the liver:** Cholesterol is insoluble in water. When secreted by hepatocytes into the bile, it is held in solution by the combined action of bile acids and lecithin and is carried as mixed lipid micelles. Bile containing too much cholesterol or that is deficient in bile acids becomes supersaturated in cholesterol, which then precipitates as solid crystals to form stones **(lithogenic bile)**. Bile from people who have cholesterol gallstones contains more cholesterol and less bile salts as it leaves the liver than does bile of normal people. Obesity increases hepatic cholesterol secretion even more, further supersaturating the bile with cholesterol.
- **Local factors in the gallbladder:** Bile components in the gallbladder from patients with gallstones crystallize more easily than normal. Biliary proteins can function as nuclei of crystallization, and hypersecretion of gallbladder mucus accelerates cholesterol precipitation from gallbladder bile.
- **Gallbladder motility:** Impaired gallbladder motor function leads to stasis causing bile sludging, which progresses to macroscopic stones.

Estrogens increase hepatic secretion of cholesterol and decrease secretion of bile acids, perhaps explaining why women form cholesterol gallstones more often. Pregnancy magnifies these effects. Progesterone, the main hormone of pregnancy, inhibits discharge of bile from the gallbladder. The gallbladder empties more slowly, and the resulting stasis increases the opportunity for precipitation of cholesterol crystals. Similar mechanisms may also explain the increase in gallstones with oral contraceptive use.

Other major risk factors for cholesterol gallstones include increased biliary cholesterol secretion, decreased secretion of bile salts and lecithin or both.

Factors associated with **increased biliary cholesterol secretion** include:

- Increasing age
- Obesity
- Ethnicity (e.g., Native Americans, Chilean women, some northern Europeans)
- Familial predisposition
- Diet high in calories and cholesterol
- Certain metabolic abnormalities associated with high blood cholesterol levels (e.g., diabetes, some genetic hyperlipoproteinemias, PBC)

The risk of symptomatic gallstones is a direct function of body weight. In obese people, the relative risk of gallstones may be fivefold above normal. Hepatic cholesterol synthesis is stimulated by insulin, and the hyperinsulinism that accompanies increased body fat may explain why biliary excretion of cholesterol increases with obesity.

Decreased secretion of bile salts and lecithin occurs in nonobese whites who develop gallstones. Disorders that interfere with enterohepatic circulation of bile acids (e.g., pancreatic insufficiency in CF or Crohn disease) also decrease bile acid secretion and favor gallstone formation.

Cholesterol synthesis is elevated and bile salts and lecithin are lower in Pima Indians and in people taking certain drugs (e.g., clofibrate). Moderate alcohol intake lowers biliary cholesterol concentration and decreases the risk of gallstones.

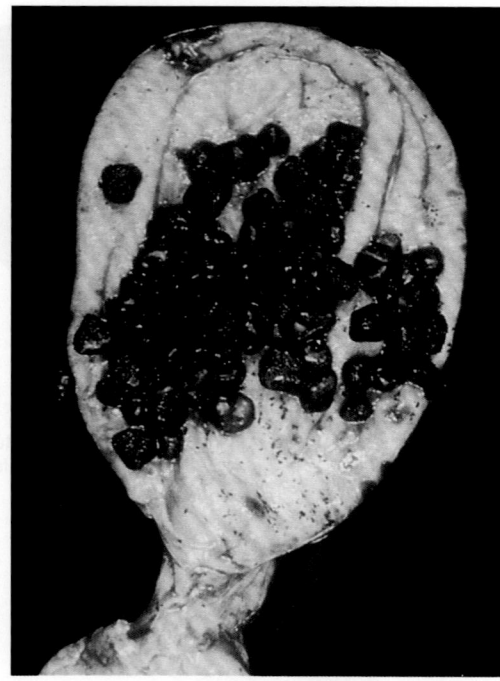

FIGURE 20-74. Pigment gallstones. The gallbladder has been opened to reveal numerous small, dark stones composed of calcium bilirubinate.

Pigment Stones May Be Black or Brown

Black Pigment Stones

Black pigment stones measure less than 1 cm and are irregular and glassy (Fig. 20-74). They contain calcium bilirubinate, bilirubin polymers, calcium salts, and mucin.

Black stones are more common in older or undernourished people. Chronic hemolysis, as in hemoglobinopathies, predisposes to development of black pigment stones, either because it increases hemolysis or because of damage to liver cells. Cirrhosis is also associated with a high incidence of black stones. However, usually no cause for formation of black pigment stones is found.

Unconjugated bilirubin is insoluble in bile and is normally present in only trace amounts. If increased unconjugated bilirubin is secreted by hepatocytes, it precipitates as calcium bilirubinate, probably around a nidus of mucinous glycoproteins. Patients without known predisposing factors who develop black pigment stones have increased concentrations of unconjugated bilirubin in the bile for unknown reasons.

Brown Pigment Stones

Brown pigment stones are spongy and laminated. They contain calcium bilirubinate, cholesterol, and calcium soaps of fatty acids. Unlike other types of gallstones, they are more common in intra- and extrahepatic bile ducts than in the gallbladder.

 ETIOLOGIC FACTORS: *Brown stones are almost always associated with bacterial cholangitis—E. coli is the main cause.* They are uncommon in Western countries but are not infrequent in Asia, where they are almost entirely seen in people infested with *A. lumbricoides* or *C. sinensis,* helminths that may invade the biliary tract. The rare cases in Western countries are seen in patients with chronic mechanical obstruction to bile flow, as in sclerosing cholangitis, or the presence of a catheter in the common bile duct after common bile duct surgery. Bacterial β-glucuronidase or other enzymes hydrolyze conjugated bilirubin to its unconjugated form, which favors formation of brown stones.

 CLINICAL FEATURES: Gallstones within the gallbladder may remain "silent" for many years, and few patients die as a result of cholelithiasis itself. The 15-year cumulative probability that asymptomatic stones will lead to biliary pain or other complications is less than 20%. Laparoscopic cholecystectomy is the treatment of choice.

Most complications of cholelithiasis relate to gallstones obstructing the cystic or common bile ducts. Passage of a stone into the cystic duct often, but not always, causes severe biliary colic and may lead to acute cholecystitis. Repeated bouts of acute cholecystitis give rise to chronic cholecystitis, which may also result from the presence of stones alone. Gallstones entering the common duct **(choledocholithiasis)** may cause obstructive jaundice, cholangitis, and pancreatitis. They are the most common cause of acute pancreatitis in people who do not drink alcohol. Passage of a large gallstone into the small intestine can even cause intestinal obstruction, known as **gallstone ileus.** In cystic duct obstruction with or without acute cholecystitis, bile in the gallbladder is reabsorbed and replaced by a clear mucinous fluid secreted by gallbladder epithelium. **Hydrops of the gallbladder (mucocele)** (Fig. 20-75) refers to a distended and palpable gallbladder, which may become secondarily infected.

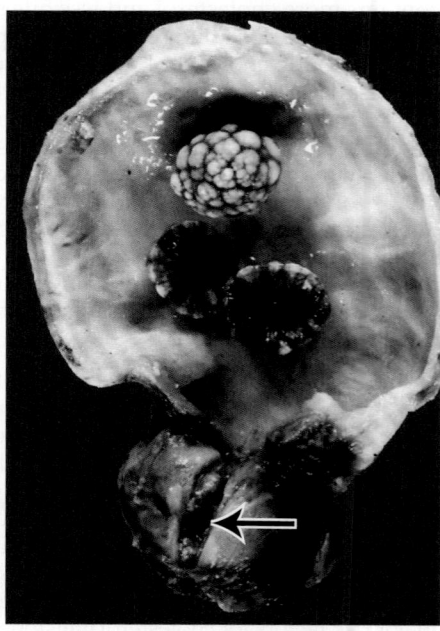

FIGURE 20-75. Hydrops of the gallbladder. The lumen of the dilated gallbladder is filled with clear mucus and contains cholesterol stones. Note the stone (*arrow*) obstructing the cystic duct.

ACUTE CHOLECYSTITIS

Acute cholecystitis is diffuse inflammation of the gallbladder, usually secondary to obstruction of the gallbladder outlet.

 PATHOPHYSIOLOGY: *People with gallstones account for 90% of cases of acute cholecystitis.* The remaining cases **(acalculous cholecystitis)** are linked to sepsis, severe trauma, infection of the gallbladder with *Salmonella typhosa* and polyarteritis nodosa. Bacterial infection is usually a consequence of biliary obstruction rather than a primary event.

Obstruction of the cystic duct by a gallstone may cause release of phospholipase by the gallbladder epithelium. This enzyme hydrolyzes lecithin to lysolecithin, a membrane-active toxin. The mucous coat of the epithelium is disrupted, exposing mucosal cells to the detergent action of concentrated bile salts. Bile supersaturated with cholesterol may be toxic to the epithelium.

PATHOLOGY: In acute cholecystitis, the external surface of the gallbladder is congested and layered with fibrinous exudate. The wall is thickened by edema, and the mucosa appears fiery red or purple. Gallstones are usually found in the lumen, and one is often seen obstructing the cystic duct. Rarely, in **empyema of the gallbladder,** the cystic duct is completely obstructed, allowing bacteria to invade the gallbladder and distending the organ with cloudy, purulent fluid.

Edema and hemorrhage of the gall bladder wall are striking, with accompanying acute and chronic inflammation (Fig. 20-76). Suppuration in the wall often follows bacterial invasion. The mucosa shows focal ulcers or, in severe cases, widespread necrosis **(gangrenous cholecystitis).**

Perforation is a dreaded complication of bacterial infection. Bile leakage into the peritoneum can cause **bile peritonitis.** More often, inflammatory adhesions create a **pericholecystic abscess** and limit spread of gallbladder

contents after perforation. Erosion of gallbladder contents into a viscus may create a **cholecystenteric fistula**.

CLINICAL FEATURES: Right upper quadrant abdominal pain is usually the presenting symptom. Most patients have had prior episodes of biliary colic. Mild jaundice, caused by stones in, or edema of, the common bile duct, is seen in 20% of patients. The acute illness generally subsides within a week, but persistent pain, fever, leukocytosis, and shaking chills herald progression of the disease and the need for cholecystectomy. As inflammation resolves, the gallbladder wall becomes fibrotic and the mucosa heals. However, the function of the gallbladder remains impaired.

CHRONIC CHOLECYSTITIS

Chronic cholecystitis (i.e., persistent chronic inflammation) is the most common disease of the gallbladder. It is almost always associated with gallstones but may also result from repeated attacks of acute cholecystitis. In the latter case, the pathogenesis probably relates to chronic irritation and chemical injury to the gallbladder epithelium.

PATHOLOGY: The wall of a chronically inflamed gallbladder is thickened and firm (Fig. 20-77A), and its serosal surface commonly shows fibrous adhesions to surrounding structures, which are residues of previous episodes of acute cholecystitis. Gallstones are usually found within the lumen. The bile frequently contains gravel or sludge (i.e., fine precipitates of calculous material) with coliform organisms in about 1/2 of cases. The mucosa tends to be focally ulcerated and atrophic but may be intact. The fibrotic wall is chronically inflamed throughout and penetrated by Rokitansky–Aschoff sinuses (Fig. 20-77B). Long-standing inflammation may lead to calcification of the gallbladder wall **(porcelain gallbladder)**.

CLINICAL FEATURES: Many patients with chronic cholecystitis complain of nonspecific abdominal symptoms, but it is not at all clear that these are related to the gallbladder disease. On the other hand, pain in the right hypochondrium is typical and often episodic. The diagnosis is best made by ultrasound examination, which shows gallstones in a thick, contracted gallbladder. Cholecystectomy is the final treatment.

CHOLESTEROLOSIS

Cholesterolosis of the gallbladder is accumulation of cholesterol-laden macrophages in the submucosa. It reflects supersaturation of bile with cholesterol and does not ordinarily cause symptoms. The mucosa shows scattered, yellow flecks (strawberry gallbladder), and mucosal folds are swollen with large, foamy macrophages, in which small nuclei are displaced to the periphery.

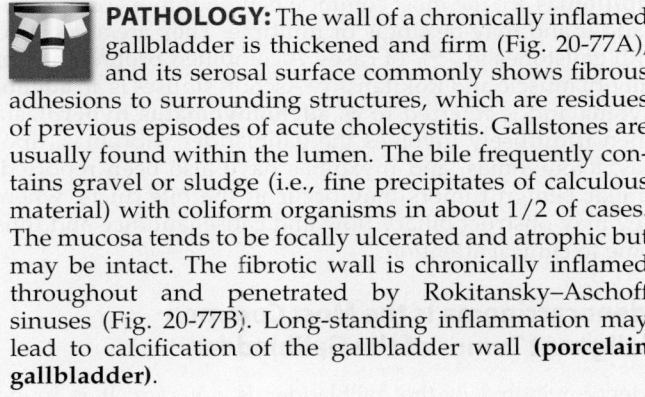

FIGURE 20-76. Acute cholecystitis. The gallbladder removed from a patient with acute cholecystitis shows ulceration of the mucosa (*left*) and acute and chronic inflammation.

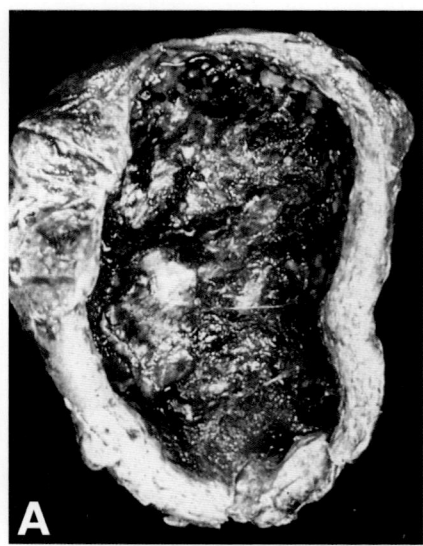

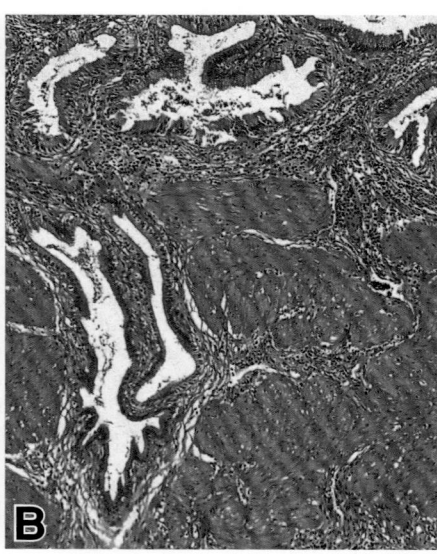

FIGURE 20-77. Chronic cholecystitis. A. The gallbladder is thickened and fibrotic. The lumen had previously contained several gallstones. **B.** Microscopic examination of the same specimen as in A shows chronic inflammation of the gallbladder and a sinus of Rokitansky–Aschoff extending into the muscularis.

TUMORS

Benign Tumors of the Gallbladder and Extrahepatic Biliary Ducts Are Rare

Papillomas are the most common benign tumors of the gallbladder and may be single or multiple. They are associated with gallstones in 75% of cases. A combined proliferation of smooth muscle and Rokitansky–Aschoff sinuses is an **adenomyoma** and is referred to as **adenomyomatus hyperplasia** when it diffusely involves the gallbladder. Fibromas, lipomas, leiomyomas, and myxomas have also been reported. Similar benign tumors may occur in the bile ducts, where they may obstruct biliary flow and cause jaundice and thus come to clinical attention.

Adenocarcinoma Is the Most Common Malignant Tumor of the Gallbladder

Adenocarcinoma of the gallbladder is not rare. It is found incidentally in 2% of patients who undergo cholecystectomy.

Because this cancer is usually associated with cholelithiasis and chronic cholecystitis, it is much more common in women and in populations with a high incidence of cholelithiasis, such as Native Americans. Calcified (porcelain) gallbladders (see above) are particularly prone to developing gallbladder cancer.

 PATHOLOGY: Gallbladder carcinoma may occur anywhere in the gallbladder but most often involves the fundus. The tumor is usually an infiltrative, well-differentiated adenocarcinoma. It is usually desmoplastic, and thus the gallbladder wall becomes thickened and leathery (Fig. 20-78). Anaplastic, giant cell and spindle cell forms, as well as adenosquamous carcinoma of the gallbladder, have been reported. Metastases occur via both lymphatic spread and direct extension into the liver, contiguous structures, and peritoneum.

CLINICAL FEATURES: The symptoms of gallbladder carcinoma are like those of gallstone disease. However, by the time these tumors become

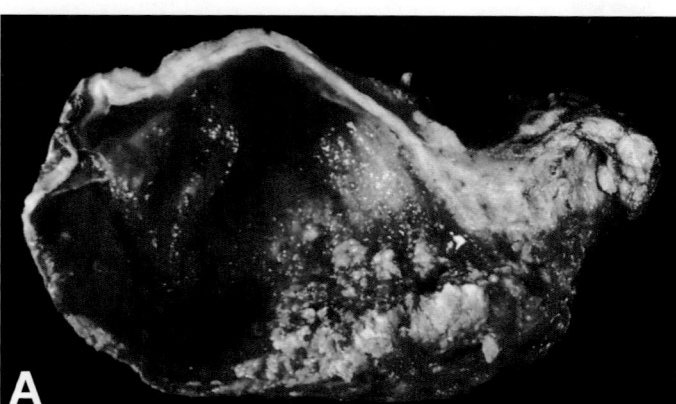

FIGURE 20-78. Carcinoma of the gallbladder. A. A surgically resected gallbladder has been opened to reveal a thickened wall infiltrated by adenocarcinoma, which also demonstrates exophytic growth into the lumen. **B.** The gallbladder wall is infiltrated by adenocarcinoma.

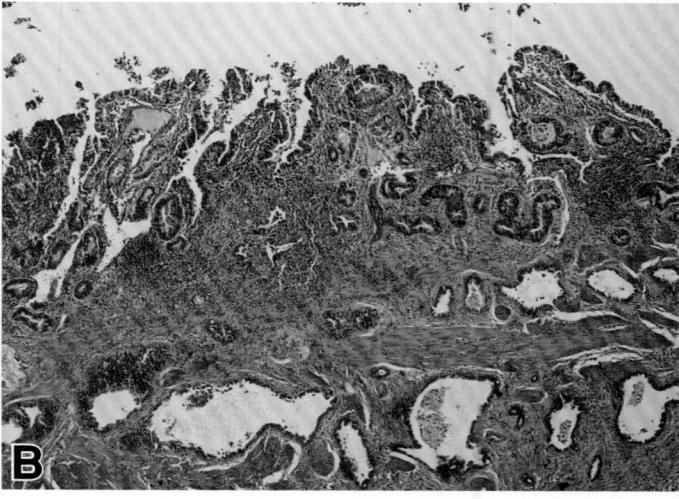

symptomatic, they are almost always incurable; 5-year survival is less than 3%. For practical purposes, only those patients whose tumors are discovered incidentally during cholecystectomy are cured.

Carcinomas of the Bile Duct and Ampulla of Vater Present as Obstructive Jaundice

Cancer of the extrahepatic bile ducts (extrahepatic cholangiocarcinoma; see above) is almost always adenocarcinoma. It may occur anywhere along the duct, including the point where the right and left hepatic ducts join to form the common hepatic duct (hilar cholangiocarcinoma).

These tumors are less common than gallbladder cancer and affect both sexes comparably. Gallstones are often found in those affected, and there is an association with inflammatory diseases of the colon. The tumor may occur in choledochal cysts and in Caroli disease. In Asia, bile duct carcinoma is associated with biliary infestation by the fluke *C. sinensis*. As in carcinoma of the gallbladder, growth may be endophytic (into the lumen) or diffusely infiltrative. The prognosis is poor, but as symptoms arise early in the disease, the outcome is somewhat better than for gallbladder carcinoma.

SUGGESTED READINGS

Books

Arias IM, Wolkoff AW, Boyer JL, et al., eds. *The Liver: Biology and Pathobiology*. Chichester: Wiley Blackwell; 2009.

Burt AD, Ferrell L Hubscher S, eds. *MacSween's Pathology of the Liver*. Elsevier; 2017.

Dooley JS, Lok ASF, Garcia-Tsao G, et al., eds. *Sherlock's Diseases of the Liver and Biliary System*. Chichester: Wiley Blackwell; 2011.

Kaplowitz N, DeLeve LD, eds. *Drug-Induced Liver Disease*. Academic Press; 2013.

Schiff ER, Maddrey WC, Reddy KR, eds. *Schiff's Diseases of the Liver*. Chichester: Wiley Blackwell; 2017.

Suriawinata A, Thung SN, eds. *Liver Pathology: An Atlas and Concise Guide*. New York: Demos Medical; 2011.

Journal Articles

Adams PC. The natural history of untreated HFE-related hemochromatosis. *Acta Haematol*. 2009;122(2–3):134–139.

Alexander J, Kowdley KV. HFE-associated hereditary hemochromatosis. *Genet Med*. 2009;11(5):307–313.

Alter MJ. Epidemiology of hepatitis C virus infection. *World J Gastroenterol*. 2007;13(17):2436–2341.

Banff schema for grading liver allograft rejection: an international consensus document. *Hepatology*. 1997;25(3):658–663.

Bioulac-Sage P, Sempoux C, Balabaud C. Hepatocellular adenomas: morphology and genomics. *Gastroenterol Clin North Am*. 2017;46(2):253–272.

Bogdanos DP, Mieli-Vergani G, Vergani D. Autoantibodies and their antigens in autoimmune hepatitis. *Semin Liver Dis*. 2009;29(3):241–253.

Bosma PJ. Inherited disorders of bilirubin metabolism. *J Hepatol*. 2003;38(1):107–117.

Brunt E, Aishima S, Clavien PA, et al. cHCC-CCA: Consensus terminology for primary liver carcinomas with both hepatocytic and cholangiocytic differentiation. *Hepatology*. 2018;68(1):113–126.

Chang TT, Lai CL, Chien RN, et al. Four years of lamivudine treatment in Chinese patients with chronic hepatitis B. *J Gastroenterol Hepatol*. 2004;19(11):1276–1282.

Colombo C. Liver disease in cystic fibrosis. *Curr Opin Pulm Med*. 2007;13(6):529–536.

Demetris A, Adams D, Bellamy C, et al. Update of the International Banff Schema for Liver Allograft Rejection: working recommendations for the histopathologic staging and reporting of chronic rejection. An International Panel. *Hepatology*. 2000;31(3):792–799.

Fairbanks KD, Tavill AS. Liver disease in alpha 1-antitrypsin deficiency: a review. *Am J Gastroenterol*. 2008;103(8):2136–2141; quiz 2142.

Feldstein AE. Novel insights into the pathophysiology of nonalcoholic fatty liver disease. *Semin Liver Dis*. 2010;30(4):391–401.

Garcia-Tsao G, Bosch J. Management of varices and variceal hemorrhage in cirrhosis. *N Engl J Med*. 2010;362(9):823–832.

Ge D, Fellay J, Thompson AJ, et al. Genetic variation in IL28B predicts hepatitis C treatment-induced viral clearance. *Nature*. 2009;461(7262):399–401.

Gong Y, Huang ZB, Christensen E, et al. Ursodeoxycholic acid for primary biliary cirrhosis. *Cochrane Database Syst Rev*. 2008;(3):CD000551.

Hay JE. Liver disease in pregnancy. *Hepatology*. 2008;47(3):1067–1076.

Heathcote EJ. Demography and presentation of chronic hepatitis B virus infection. *Am J Med*. 2008;121(12 Suppl):S3–S11.

Hennes EM, Zeniya M, Czaja AJ, et al; International Autoimmune Hepatitis Group. Simplified criteria for the diagnosis of autoimmune hepatitis. *Hepatology*. 2008;48(1):169–176.

Henriksen JH, Møller S. Cardiac and systemic haemodynamic complications of liver cirrhosis. *Scand Cardiovasc J*. 2009;43(4):218–225.

Hohenester S, Oude-Elferink RP, Beuers U. Primary biliary cirrhosis. *Semin Immunopathol*. 2009;31(3):283–307.

Hoofnagle JH, Seeff LB. Peginterferon and ribavirin for chronic hepatitis C. *N Engl J Med*. 2006;355(23):2444–2451.

Hui DK, Leung N, Yuen ST, et al. Natural history and disease progression in Chinese chronic hepatitis B patients in immune tolerant phase. *Hepatology*. 2007;46(2):395–401.

Hytiroglou P, Snover DC, Alves V, et al. Beyond "cirrhosis": a proposal from the International Liver Pathology Study Group. *Am J Clin Pathol*. 2012;137(1):5–9.

Hytiroglou P, Theise ND. Regression of human cirrhosis: an update, 18 years after the pioneering article by Wanless et al. *Virchows Arch*. 2018;473(1):15–22.

Kamar N, Selves J, Mansuy JM, et al. Hepatitis E virus and chronic hepatitis in organ-transplant recipients. *N Engl J Med*. 2008;358(8):811–817.

Khuroo MS, Khuroo MS. Hepatitis E virus. *Curr Opin Infect Dis*. 2008;21(5):539–543.

Kim WR. Epidemiology of hepatitis B in the United States. *Hepatology*. 2009;49(5 Suppl):S28–S34.

Kleiner DE, Brunt EM, Van Natta M, et al; Nonalcoholic Steatohepatitis Clinical Research Network. Design and validation of a histological scoring system for nonalcoholic fatty liver disease. *Hepatology*. 2005;41(6):1313–1321.

Kondrackiene J, Kupcinskas L. Intrahepatic cholestasis of pregnancy-current achievements and unsolved problems. *World J Gastroenterol*. 2008;14(38):5781–5788.

Krawitt EL. Autoimmune hepatitis. *N Engl J Med*. 2006;354(1):54–66.

Lee NM, Brady CW. Liver disease in pregnancy. *World J Gastroenterol*. 2009;15(8):897–906.

Leemans WF, Ter Borg MJ, de Man RA. Success and failure of nucleoside and nucleotide analogues in chronic hepatitis B. *Aliment Pharmacol Ther*. 2007;26 Suppl 2:171–182.

Maheshwari A, Ray S, Thuluvath PJ. Acute hepatitis C. *Lancet*. 2008;372(9635):321–332.

Manns MP, Vogel A. Autoimmune hepatitis, from mechanisms to therapy. *Hepatology*. 2006;43(2 Suppl 1):S132–S144.

Mazzaferro V, Chun YS, Poon RT, et al. Liver transplantation for hepatocellular carcinoma. *Ann Surg Oncol*. 2008;15(4):1001–1007.

McMahon BJ. The natural history of chronic hepatitis B virus infection. *Hepatology*. 2009;49(5 Suppl):S45–S55.

Mendes F, Lindor KD. Primary sclerosing cholangitis: overview and update. *Nat Rev Gastroenterol Hepatol*. 2010;7(11):611–619.

Mieli-Vergani G, Vergani D. De novo autoimmune hepatitis after liver transplantation. *J Hepatol*. 2004;40(1):3–7.

Moon DB, Lee SG. Liver transplantation. *Gut Liver*. 2009;3(3): 145–165.

Morotti RA, Suchy FJ, Magid MS. Progressive familial intrahepatic cholestasis (PFIC) type 1, 2, and 3: a review of the liver pathology findings. *Semin Liver Dis*. 2011;31(1):3–10.

Nemeth E, Ganz T. The role of hepcidin in iron metabolism. *Acta Haematol*. 2009;122(2-3):78–86.

Olynyk JK, Trinder D, Ramm GA, et al. Hereditary hemochromatosis in the post-HFE era. *Hepatology*. 2008;48(3):991–1001.

Poupon R. Primary biliary cirrhosis: a 2010 update. *J Hepatol*. 2010;52(5):745–758.

Rizzetto M. Hepatitis D: thirty years after. *J Hepatol*. 2009;50(5): 1043–1050.

Roberts EA, Yeung L. Maternal-infant transmission of hepatitis C virus infection. *Hepatology*. 2002;36(5 Suppl 1):S106–S113.

Runyon BA; AASLD Practice Guidelines Committee. Management of adult patients with ascites due to cirrhosis: an update. *Hepatology*. 2009;49(6):2087–2107.

Schilsky ML. Wilson disease: new insights into pathogenesis, diagnosis, and future therapy. *Curr Gastroenterol Rep*. 2005;7(1):26–31.

Sempoux C, Jibara G, Ward SC, et al. Intrahepatic cholangiocarcinoma: new insights in pathology. *Semin Liver Dis*. 2011;31(1): 49–60.

Shepard CW, Finelli L, Alter MJ. Global epidemiology of hepatitis C virus infection. *Lancet Infect Dis*. 2005;5(9):558–567.

Shrestha MP, Scott RM, Joshi DM, et al. Safety and efficacy of a recombinant hepatitis E vaccine. *N Engl J Med*. 2007;356(9):895–903.

Strassburg CP. Pharmacogenetics of Gilbert's syndrome. *Pharmacogenomics*. 2008;9(6):703–715.

Suriawinata AA, Thung SN. Acute and chronic hepatitis. *Semin Diagn Pathol*. 2006;23(3-4):132–148.

Terrault NA, Shiffman ML, Lok AS, et al; A2ALL Study Group. Outcomes in hepatitis C virus-infected recipients of living donor vs. deceased donor liver transplantation. *Liver Transpl*. 2007;13(1):122–129.

Yang JD, Roberts LR. Hepatocellular carcinoma: a global view. *Nat Rev Gastroenterol Hepatol*. 2010;7(8):448–458.

Yugo DM, Meng XJ. Hepatitis E virus: foodborne, waterborne and zoonotic transmission. *Int J Environ Res Public Health*. 2013;10(10):4507–4533.

Zignego AL, Craxì A. Extrahepatic manifestations of hepatitis C virus infection. *Clin Liver Dis*. 2008;12(3):611–636, ix.

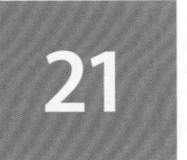

21 The Pancreas

David S. Klimstra, Edward B. Stelow

ANATOMY AND PHYSIOLOGY

Pancreatic development begins at 4 weeks' post-fertilization as two endodermal outpouchings on the dorsal and ventral sides of the embryonic duodenal tube. The ventral pancreas along with the common bile duct migrates posteriorly around the duodenum, and the ductal systems of the two embryonic pancreatic anlagen merge at 7 weeks, giving rise to a main pancreatic duct (**duct of Wirsung**) composed of the ventral pancreatic duct that extends from the ampulla of Vater at the duodenum into the distal portion of the dorsal pancreatic duct. The proximal remnant of the dorsal duct becomes the **duct of Santorini**, which may remain patent through the minor papilla into the duodenum, but this connection usually obliterates. The ducts branch progressively into smaller ducts and ductules that extend into the pancreatic lobules. Acinar cells arise from the ductules and acquire their distinctive zymogen granules. The enzymatic secretions of the acinar cells drain into the smallest ductules between the centroacinar cells, which bridge the acinar lumina into the ductal system. Islet cells are also derived from the ducts and acquire small, dense, neurosecretory granules of different types, each characteristic of the specific peptide cells types of the endocrine pancreas.

The pancreas is a mixed exocrine and endocrine gland that lies transversely in the upper abdomen, cradled between the loop of the duodenum and the hilum of the spleen. It is retroperitoneal, behind the lesser omental sac and the stomach, although the anterior surface is covered by peritoneum. This location renders it inaccessible to physical examination. The adult pancreas is 10 to 15 cm long and weighs 60 to 150 g. It is divided into three anatomical subdivisions: (1) **the head** lies in the concavity of the duodenum and extends to the superior mesenteric vessels, which pass through a groove immediately behind the organ, (2) **the neck** connects the head to the distal portion of the gland, and (3) **the tail** constitutes the distal two-thirds of the pancreas and extends to the hilum of the spleen.

Exocrine pancreatic secretions drain into the major ducts of Wirsung and Santorini, which empty along with the common bile duct into the duodenum through the papilla of Vater. These pancreatic and biliary ducts usually merge a variable distance (1 to 5 mm) below the duodenal mucosa in a common channel that constitutes the prototypical ampulla of Vater, although in a significant minority of individuals, the ducts remain separated by a septum and enter the duodenum independently. The ampulla is surrounded by a circular complex of smooth muscle fibers, the sphincter of Oddi, that controls the passage of pancreatic juice and bile into the duodenum.

Exocrine tissue makes up 80% to 85% of the pancreas and consists of acinar cells composed of a single layer of pyramidal cells, whose basal cytoplasm is basophilic due to abundant rough endoplasmic reticulum. The apical cytoplasm is filled with eosinophilic zymogen granules. Acinar cells synthesize some 20 different digestive enzymes, mostly in the form of inactive proenzymes. Following neural and hormonal stimulation, pancreatic enzymes including trypsin, chymotrypsin, amylase, lipase, and elastase are secreted and subsequently activated in the duodenum. Amylase and lipase are secreted in their active forms. The daily secretion of 1.5 to 3 L of pancreatic juice attests to the remarkable synthetic and secretory capacity of the exocrine pancreas.

The endocrine pancreas is organized into islets of Langerhans distributed throughout the organ but comprising only 1% to 2% of the total pancreatic mass. Most of the islets consist of circumscribed lobules of cells that are derived from the dorsal embryonic pancreas. These compact islets contain several cell types, including predominantly alpha and beta cells that synthesize glucagon and insulin, respectively; somatostatin producing delta cells and pancreatic polypeptide cells are present in small numbers. The islets derived from the ventral embryonic pancreas contain predominantly beta and pancreatic polypeptide cells. These diffuse islets are arranged in cords interspersed between acinar cells. Each islet cell synthesizes only one peptide hormone, which is secreted directly into the blood (see below). The major endocrine disease of the pancreas, diabetes mellitus, is discussed in Chapter 13.

CONGENITAL ANOMALIES

Numerous anatomic variations can occur in the configuration of the major pancreatic ducts and their relationship to the common bile duct. Most of these variations are regarded to be normal and are rarely of clinical significance. Other developmental variations have clinical consequences and are therefore regarded as developmental defects.

PANCREAS DIVISUM: Pancreas divisum, the most common congenital anomaly, results from failure of the two embryonic pancreatic ducts to fuse. This leads to the formation of two separate ductal systems, each draining into the duodenum through the major and minor papillae, respectively. Consequently, the major portion of the pancreas is drained by the duct of Santorini through the minor papilla. Chronic pancreatitis develops in up to 25% of persons with pancreas divisum.

HETEROTOPIC PANCREAS: In this anomaly, pancreatic tissue develops outside its normal location, most commonly in the wall of the duodenum, stomach, and jejunum, and in Meckel diverticula. It is an incidental finding in 2% to 15% of autopsies. The heterotopic tissue may contain all components of normal pancreas, but some cases contain only ducts without acini and islets. Smooth muscle fibers are usually abundant in pancreatic heterotopia involving the tubular gastrointestinal tract. Different type of pancreatic neoplasms can arise in heterotopic tissue, the most common being infiltrating ductal adenocarcinoma.

ANNULAR PANCREAS: In this uncommon condition, the pancreatic head surrounds the second portion of the duodenum; encirclement may be complete or partial. Infants with annular pancreas frequently have other congenital anomalies, including trisomy 21 (Down syndrome). Some affected patients also have duodenal atresia, an anomaly that requires surgery immediately after birth. About half of patients with annular pancreas do not require surgery in early life but develop symptoms by 60 or 70 years of age.

CYSTS: True cysts of the pancreas are believed to arise from faulty development of pancreatic ducts. There is an association with other anatomic anomalies, including renal tubular dysplasia, anorectal malformations, polydactyly, and thoracic dystrophy.

PARTIAL AND COMPLETE PANCREATIC AGENESIS: Homozygous germline mutations in the transcription factor *PDX1*, the pancreatic and duodenal homeobox 1 gene (formerly known as *IPF1* or insulin promoter factor 1), have been reported in these rare conditions.

ACUTE PANCREATITIS

Acute Pancreatitis results from the aberrant release of pancreatic exocrine enzymes. It is not truly an inflammatory condition, but instead encompasses the myriad of locoregional and systemic changes seen with the release of these enzymes. The devastation of acute pancreatitis was justly described by Lord Moynihan in 1925 as the "most terrible of all calamities [of] the abdominal viscera. The suddenness of its onset,

the illimitable agony which accompanies it and the mortality attendant upon it render it a formidable disease." For unknown reasons, the incidence of acute pancreatitis has increased 10-fold in the past few decades.

The clinical and anatomic severity of acute pancreatitis varies greatly from case to case. At one end of the spectrum is a mild, self-limited disease, associated with acute inflammation and stromal edema, and little or no acinar cell necrosis. This is usually not associated with systemic manifestations of disease. At the other extreme is a severe, sometimes fatal, acute hemorrhagic pancreatitis with massive necrosis. With this severe injury, systemic manifestations such as shock, acute respiratory distress, acute renal failure, and disseminated intravascular coagulation may develop.

Repeated episodes of acute pancreatitis may lead to chronic pancreatitis, which is characterized clinically by recurrent attacks of severe abdominal pain and pathologically by progressive fibrosis, ultimately leading to pancreatic insufficiency. However, no acute episodes are recognized clinically in about half of the cases of chronic pancreatitis.

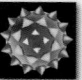 **PATHOGENESIS:** Acinar cell injury and duct obstruction are the major causes of acute pancreatitis. These processes lead to inappropriate extracellular leakage of activated digestive enzymes and consequent autodigestion of pancreatic and extrapancreatic tissues. A number of factors have been implicated in acute pancreatitis. Genetic determinants appear to contribute to the development of acute pancreatitis but because the same molecular and genetic factors are also associated with the pathogenesis of chronic pancreatitis they are discussed in that section below.

ETIOLOGIC FACTORS: *ACTIVATED PANCREATIC ENZYMES:* Inappropriate activation of pancreatic proenzymes occurs in all forms of pancreatitis. Acinar cells are shielded from the potentially destructive action of their digestive enzymes (proteases, nucleases, amylase, lipase, and phospholipase A) by three mechanisms.

1. Various enzymes are physically isolated from cytoplasmic components by an intricate, intracellular, cavitary system of endoplasmic reticulum, Golgi complex, and zymogen granule membranes.
2. Many of the digestive enzymes are synthesized and secreted as inactive forms (e.g., chymotrypsinogen, proelastase, prophospholipase, and trypsinogen).
3. Specific enzyme inhibitors tend to protect the pancreas.

The various inhibitors of proteolytic enzymes present in many body fluids and tissues constitute a defense against inappropriate activation of pancreatic proenzymes. Four potent protease inhibitors have been identified in human plasma: α1-antitrypsin, α2-macroglobulin, C1 esterase inhibitor, and pancreatic secretory trypsin inhibitor. Despite the variety of trypsin inhibitors in different body compartments, the protection they render is clearly incomplete. Trypsin activation is central to the pathogenesis of acute pancreatitis. By itself, trypsin does not produce cell necrosis, but it activates other pancreatic proenzymes, including prophospholipase A2 and proelastase.

SECRETION AGAINST OBSTRUCTION AND DUCT INSUFFICIENCY: Most enzymes secreted by acinar cells are discharged into the ductal system and enter the duodenum. A small amount diffuses back into periductular extracellular fluid and eventually into plasma. Any condition that narrows the lumens of pancreatic ducts or impairs the easy outflow of exocrine secretions can raise intraductal pressure and exacerbate back-diffusion across the ducts. This phenomenon is suspected to cause inappropriate activation of digestive proenzymes. Heavy meals may lead to release of pancreatic secretagogues, and so augment production of pancreatic enzymes.

Gallstones sometimes cause pancreatic duct obstruction. Some 45% of all patients with acute pancreatitis also have cholelithiasis. *Conversely, about 5% of patients with gallstones develop acute pancreatitis and the risk of developing acute pancreatitis in patients with gallstones is 25 times higher than in the general population.* Also, unless gallstones are eliminated after the first attack, recurrent acute pancreatitis occurs in half the cases. However, fewer than 5% of patients with acute pancreatitis have impacted stones at the ampulla of Vater, and the reason for the association between pancreatitis and cholelithiasis remains obscure. Neither ligation of the pancreatic duct nor its occlusion by tumor generally causes severe acute pancreatitis. It has been suggested that the reflux of bile or duodenal contents into the pancreatic duct may lead to pancreatitis, but there is little evidence to support this theory.

Anatomic anomalies (e.g., pancreas divisum) and **neoplasms** (ampullary and pancreatic neoplasms, including intraductal processes) can also lead to acute pancreatitis due to duct insufficiency or obstruction, respectively.

ETHANOL: Chronic alcohol abuse accounts for one-third of cases of acute pancreatitis, although only 5% to 10% of chronic alcoholics develop this complication. Ethanol is well recognized as a chemical toxin, but a significant injurious effect on pancreatic acinar or duct cells has yet to be demonstrated. The pathogenesis of ethanol-induced pancreatitis (acute and chronic) is not well understood. The mechanism of ethanol-induced chronic pancreatitis is discussed below.

Ethanol consumption may adversely affect the pancreas by causing spasm or acute edema of the sphincter of Oddi, especially after an alcoholic binge. It also stimulates secretion from the small intestine, which triggers the exocrine pancreas to release pancreatic juice.

OTHER CAUSES OF ACUTE PANCREATITIS:

- **Viruses,** such as mumps, coxsackievirus, and cytomegalovirus, can cause pancreatitis. The incidence of acute pancreatitis is particularly high in patients with acquired immunodeficiency syndrome (AIDS) owing to human immunodeficiency virus (HIV) itself, or, more commonly, cytomegalovirus infection.
- **Therapeutic drugs** have been reported to cause acute pancreatitis. These include immunosuppressive drugs (e.g., azathioprine), antineoplastic agents, estrogens, sulfonamides, and diuretics. The mechanisms of pancreatic injury by these compounds are unclear.
- **Blunt trauma** to the upper abdomen can cause contusive injury to the pancreas, with leakage of digestive enzymes into the pancreas and peripancreatic tissues. Patients undergoing endoscopic retrograde

cholangiopancreatography (ERCP), fine needle aspiration biopsy, and surgical manipulation occasionally develop acute pancreatitis.

- **Acute ischemia** due to shock, vasculitis, and thrombosis may injure the pancreas.
- **Hyperlipidemia** can induce acute pancreatitis. The mechanism is thought to involve hydrolysis of triglycerides in the extracellular space by inappropriate leakage of lipase by pancreatic cells. Released free fatty acids are cytotoxic.
- **Hypercalcemia**, regardless of its cause, is associated with acute pancreatitis. Mechanisms include secretory block, intracellular zymogen accumulation, and activation of proteases. **Obesity** is a risk factor for pancreatitis, especially for severe disease. Increased deposition of peripancreatic fat may predispose obese people to more extensive fat necrosis after local release of pancreatic lipase.
- **Idiopathic pancreatitis** is still the third most common form of the disease, accounting for 10% to 20% of all cases.
- **Parasites** (e.g., Ascariasis), **bacteria** (e.g., Mycoplasma species), and **pregnancy** are rare causes of acute pancreatitis.

Factors involved in the pathogenesis of acute hemorrhagic pancreatitis are shown in Figure 21-1.

PATHOLOGY: In acute hemorrhagic pancreatitis, the pancreas is initially edematous and hyperemic. Within a day, pale, gray foci appear, rapidly becoming friable and hemorrhagic (Fig. 21-2A). *In severe cases, these foci enlarge and become so numerous that most of the pancreas is converted into a large retroperitoneal hematoma, in which pancreatic tissue is barely recognizable.* Yellow-white areas of fat necrosis appear around the pancreas, including the adjacent mesentery (Fig. 21-2B). These nodules of necrotic fat have a pasty consistency that becomes firmer and chalklike as more calcium and magnesium soaps of fatty acids are produced. Saponification reflects the interaction of cations with free fatty acids released by the action of activated lipase on triglycerides in fat cells. As a result, the level of blood calcium may be depressed, sometimes to the point of causing neuromuscular irritability.

The most prominent microscopic findings in acute pancreatitis are acinar cell and fat necrosis, often associated with some degree of acute inflammation (Fig. 21-3). Necrosis is usually patchy, rarely involving the entire gland. Irregular fibrosis of the pancreas and occasionally calcification (i.e., chronic pancreatitis) result from healed acute pancreatitis.

PANCREATIC PSEUDOCYST: As many as half of patients who survive acute pancreatitis are at risk for developing pancreatic pseudocysts (Fig. 21-4). These are delimited by connective tissue and contain degraded blood, inflammatory cells, debris, and fluid rich in pancreatic enzymes. Pseudocysts may enlarge to compress and even obstruct the duodenum or other structures. They may become secondarily infected and form an abscess. Rupture of a pseudocyst is a rare complication that leads to chemical or septic peritonitis or both.

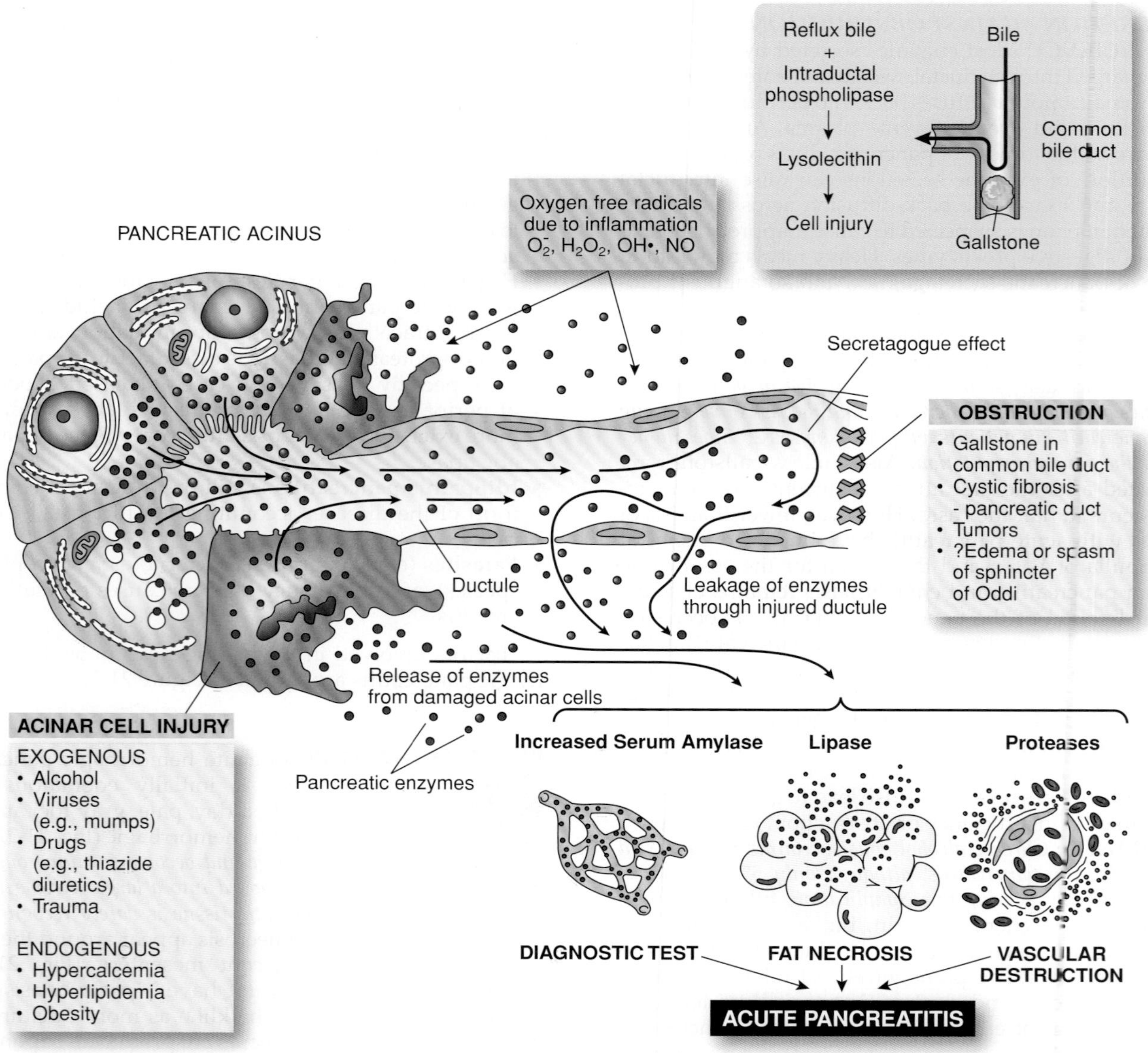

Reflux bile
+
Intraductal
phospholipase
↓
Lysolecithin
↓
Cell injury

Bile

Common
bile duct

Gallstone

PANCREATIC ACINUS

Oxygen free radicals
due to inflammation
O_2^-, H_2O_2, OH•, NO

Secretagogue effect

OBSTRUCTION

• Gallstone in
  common bile duct
• Cystic fibrosis
  - pancreatic duct
• Tumors
• ?Edema or spasm
  of sphincter
  of Oddi

Ductule

Leakage of enzymes
through injured ductule

Release of enzymes
from damaged acinar cells

ACINAR CELL INJURY

EXOGENOUS
• Alcohol
• Viruses
  (e.g., mumps)
• Drugs
  (e.g., thiazide
  diuretics)
• Trauma

ENDOGENOUS
• Hypercalcemia
• Hyperlipidemia
• Obesity

Pancreatic enzymes

Increased Serum Amylase   **Lipase**   **Proteases**

DIAGNOSTIC TEST   **FAT NECROSIS**   **VASCULAR DESTRUCTION**

ACUTE PANCREATITIS

FIGURE 21-1. The pathogenesis of acute pancreatitis. Injury to ductules or acinar cells leads to the release of pancreatic enzymes. Lipase and proteases destroy tissue, thereby causing acute pancreatitis. The release of amylase and its accumulation in the blood is the basis of a laboratory test for acute pancreatitis. H_2O_2 = hydrogen peroxide; NO• = nitric acid; O_2^- = superoxide ion; •OH = hydroxyl radical.

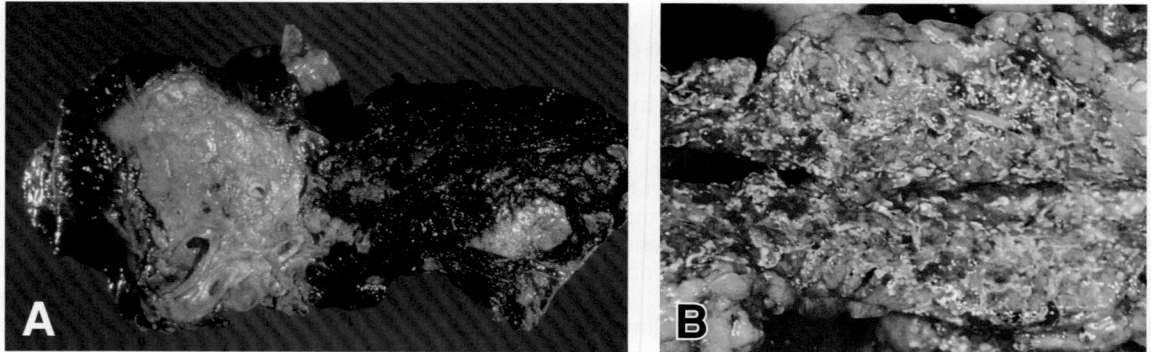

FIGURE 21-2. Acute hemorrhagic pancreatitis. A. Large areas of the pancreas are intensely hemorrhagic. **B.** The cut surface of the pancreas in a less severe case of acute pancreatitis, and at a later stage than in **A**, shows numerous yellow-white foci of fat necrosis.

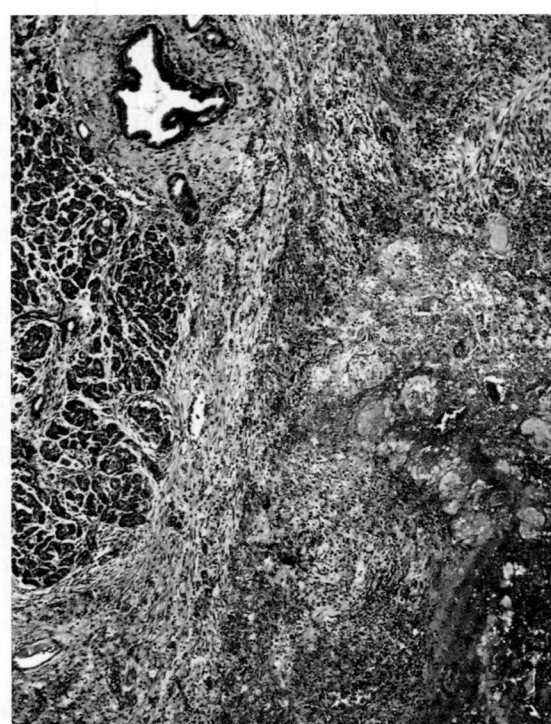

FIGURE 21-3. Acute hemorrhagic pancreatitis. A photomicrograph of the pancreas shows areas of acinar cell necrosis (*right*), hemorrhage, and fat necrosis (*lower right*). An intact lobule is seen on the *left*.

CLINICAL FEATURES: Patients with acute pancreatitis present with severe epigastric pain that is referred to the upper back and is accompanied by nausea and vomiting. Catastrophic peripheral vascular collapse and shock may ensue within hours. If shock is sustained and profound, adult respiratory distress syndrome and acute renal failure may occur within the first week. Early in the disease, pancreatic digestive enzymes are released from injured acinar cells into the blood and retroperitoneal cavity. *Documentation of elevated serum amylase and lipase within 24 to 72 hours is diagnostic for acute pancreatitis.* The necrotic pancreas sometimes becomes infected with gram-negative bacteria from the intestinal tract which greatly increases mortality.

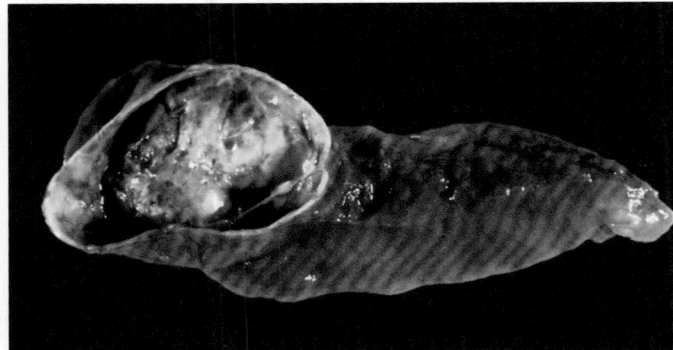

FIGURE 21-4. Pancreatic pseudocyst. A cystic cavity arising in the head of the pancreas.

CHRONIC PANCREATITIS

Chronic pancreatitis results from the progressive destruction of pancreatic parenchyma and its replacement with fibrosis. Despite its original description and association with stones two centuries ago, the pathogenesis, clinical course and treatment of chronic pancreatitis remain enigmatic. Clinically, it can manifest as recurrent or persistent abdominal pain, or only with signs and symptoms of pancreatic exocrine or endocrine insufficiency.

PATHOGENESIS: Most factors that cause acute pancreatitis also cause chronic pancreatitis. The fact that chronic pancreatitis is often characterized by intermittent "acute" attacks followed by periods of quiescence suggests that it may evolve from repeated bouts of acute pancreatitis, followed by scarring. However, about half of patients present without a clinical history of acute pancreatitis.

ETIOLOGIC FACTORS:
- **Alcoholism** of long standing duration is the major cause of chronic pancreatitis, being responsible for nearly 80% of adult cases. Almost half of alcoholics who had no symptoms of chronic pancreatitis during life show evidence of the disease at autopsy. A comparable proportion of asymptomatic alcoholics manifest abnormal pancreatic exocrine function tests. The role of alcohol is undisputed, but the mechanism by which it causes chronic pancreatitis is still debated.

  The most widely accepted theory is based on the fact that alcohol is a pancreatic secretagogue. Hypersecretion of enzyme proteins by acinar cells, without a concomitant increase in fluid volume results in precipitation of "protein plugs" in small branches of the pancreatic ducts. These deposits can cause obstruction, that, at first, may produce only mild acute pancreatitis. The development of fibrosis (chronic pancreatitis) and additional plugs (that grow and promote formation of calcium carbonate stones) increase the risk of developing new, more severe bouts of acute pancreatitis. This process continues in a viscous cycle. As only a minority of severe alcoholics develop clinical chronic pancreatitis, other factors may also play a role. For example, anatomic abnormalities (e.g., pancreatic divisum) or genetic predisposition (e.g., variants in the cystic fibrosis gene, *CFTR*) may predispose some alcoholics to developing chronic pancreatitis.
- **Obstruction or insufficiency of the pancreatic duct** sometimes leads to chronic pancreatitis. It is interesting to note, however, that acute obstruction by gallstones causes acute pancreatitis that does not seem to progress to chronic pancreatitis.

  Paraduodenal or "groove" pancreatitis is a particular form of chronic pancreatitis that develops within the "groove" region between the head of the pancreas, the common bile duct, and the duodenum. Its etiology is not entirely clear, but it usually develops in alcoholics and certain anatomic variations in the region of the minor papilla may predispose these people to develop disease here. Because of the location of the disease, patients frequently develop jaundice (secondary to bile duct obstruction) or duodenal obstruction. Cystic changes in the pancreas are also common in this condition. Thus patients are often brought to surgery for expected pancreatic ductal adenocarcinoma or cystic neoplasm.

- **Chronic injury to acinar cells** (e.g., in hemochromatosis) is associated with pancreatic fibrosis and atrophy.
- **Chronic renal failure** is linked to increased incidence of acute and chronic pancreatitis.

PATHOGENESIS:

- **Autoimmune chronic pancreatitis** (also termed **lymphoplasmacytic sclerosing pancreatitis, duct-destructive chronic pancreatitis,** etc.) frequently occurs in association with other autoimmune and sclerosing disorders such as chronic sclerosing sialadenitis, retroperitoneal fibrosis, or inflammatory bowel disease. It affects both sexes, often in early adulthood. Symptoms vary from abdominal discomfort to painless jaundice. Imaging studies can be particularly worrisome, ranging from a mass-like lesion (mimicking an adenocarcinoma) to irregular beading of the pancreatic or bile ducts.

  The pathogenesis of autoimmune pancreatitis is unclear and multiple forms of the disease exist. In one form (type 1), serum immunoglobulin IgG4 is elevated and numerous IgG4-positive plasma cells (>50 per high-power microscopic field) of are seen in the pancreatic parenchyma. Immunoglobulin deposits within basement membranes have also been described. An autoimmune etiology is further suggested by the presence of hypergammaglobulinemia and serum autoantibodies, including antinuclear antibody (ANA), rheumatoid factor, antilactoferrin, and anticarbonic anhydrase. Type 2 autoimmune pancreatitis lacks IgG4-positive plasma cells and is more closely associated with inflammatory bowel disease. Both types of autoimmune pancreatitis may respond to steroid therapy.
- **Cystic fibrosis** (CF; see Chapter 6) is briefly reviewed here because it can manifest as chronic pancreatitis. In patients with CF, intraductal pancreatic secretions are abnormally viscid, accounting for the older name, **mucoviscidosis**. Plugs of inspissated mucus obstruct cystically distended pancreatic ducts, leading to chronic pancreatitis and exocrine pancreatic insufficiency. In its late stages, the entire parenchyma is replaced by adipose tissue. By then, malabsorption is a common feature of CF in children, who may have bulky, fatty stools (steatorrhea). Death, however, usually results from the pulmonary complications of the disease.
- **Hereditary pancreatitis** is a rare autosomal dominant disease with 80% penetrance. It is characterized by recurrent episodes of severe abdominal pain that often manifests in childhood. Disease develops because of genetic point mutations that result in increased trypsin levels within the pancreas, often associated with autoactivation of trypsinogen. Most cases are caused by one of three point mutations in the **cationic trypsinogen gene** (**protease serine 1**, *PRSS1*; chromosome 7q). Point mutations in the **serine protease inhibitor gene** (*SPINK 1*) have also been associated with the disease.

Hereditary pancreatitis is occasionally accompanied by aminoaciduria, although the two conditions are not necessarily linked etiologically. Some patients exhibit hypercalcemia secondary to parathyroid hyperplasia or adenomas. *About 40% of patients with hereditary pancreatitis subsequently develop pancreatic ductal adenocarcinoma.* The clinicopathologic features of hereditary pancreatitis are indistinguishable from those of other forms of chronic pancreatitis, including ductal stones and the late complications.

- **Idiopathic chronic pancreatitis** has a bimodal distribution: a juvenile form with a mean age of 25 years, and a second form that occurs in older patients with a peak at age 60. Variants in the cystic fibrosis transmembrane conductance regulator (*CFTR*) gene are seen in 10% to 30% of patients with idiopathic chronic pancreatitis. Somatic mutations in the gene for pancreatic secretory trypsin inhibitor (*SPINK1*) have also been associated with chronic pancreatitis. Thus although considered "idiopathic," many cases may actually result from cystic fibrosis or represent hereditary pancreatitis that lacks other clinical signs of the diseases.

PATHOLOGY:

By the time chronic pancreatitis becomes clinically evident, the disease process is usually at an advanced stage of development. Its pathologic features vary somewhat based on the etiology. Chronic calcifying pancreatitis, the most common type of the disease, is associated with chronic alcoholism in over 90% of cases. The pancreas can be affected in a focal, segmental, or diffuse distribution. The parenchyma is firm, and the cut surface lacks the usual lobular architecture (Fig. 21-5A). The main pancreatic duct and its tributaries are commonly dilated, owing to obstruction by thick proteinaceous plugs, intraductal stones, or strictures. Pseudocysts or abscess formation are common.

Microscopically, large regions of the pancreas show irregular areas of fibrosis with loss of acinar cells, and, eventually the endocrine parenchyma (Fig 21-5B). As the disease progresses, islets of Langerhans become embedded in sclerotic fibrous tissue, and may appear fused and enlarged until they, too, disappear. Fibrotic areas contain myofibroblasts and variable numbers of lymphocytes, plasma cells, and macrophages. Pancreatic ducts of all sizes contain variably calcified proteinaceous material, a finding more commonly associated with alcoholism. Ductal epithelium may be atrophic or hyperplastic, and may show squamous metaplasia. Microscopically, autoimmune pancreatitis is characterized by fibrosis of the parenchyma with a dense lymphoplasmacytic inflammatory infiltrate surrounding the ductal epithelium (Fig. 21-6). Type 2 autoimmune pancreatitis is associated with intraepithelial acute inflammation. Obliterative venulitis is seen with both type 1 and type 2 forms of the disease.

CLINICAL FEATURES:

Half of patients with chronic pancreatitis have suffered repeated antecedent episodes of acute pancreatitis. One-third of cases experience the gradual onset of continuous or intermittent pain, without any acute attacks (Fig. 21-7).

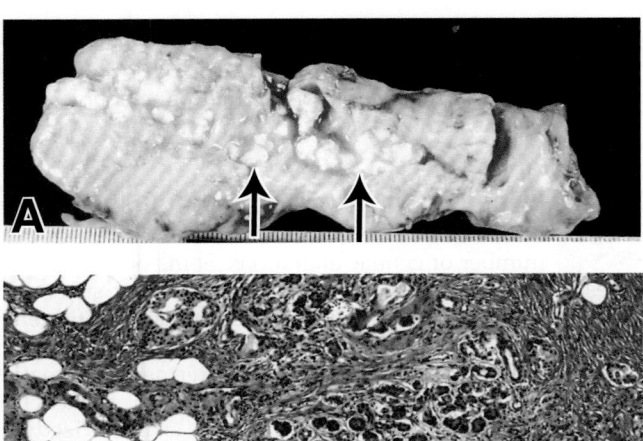

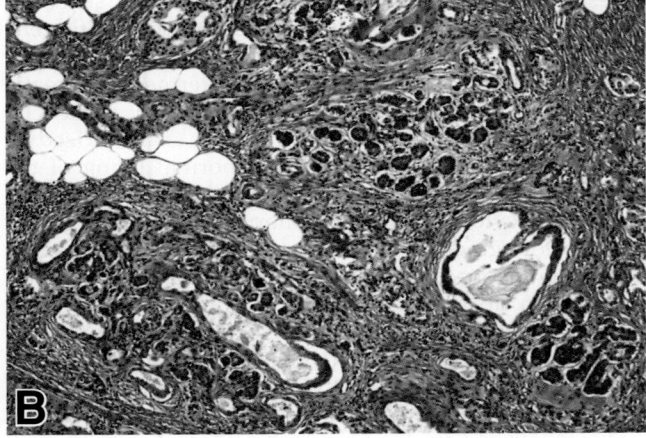

FIGURE 21-5. Chronic calcifying pancreatitis. A. The pancreas is shrunken and fibrotic, and the dilated duct contains numerous stones (*arrows*). **B.** Atrophic lobules of acinar cells are surrounded by dense fibrous tissue infiltrated by lymphocytes. The pancreatic ducts are dilated and contain inspissated proteinaceous material.

In a few patients, chronic pancreatitis is initially painless but presents with diabetes or malabsorption. Once pancreatic calcifications are detectable radiographically, most patients will have developed diabetes, malabsorption, or both. Conspicuous weight loss is common, and unrelenting epigastric pain, radiating to the back, may cripple the patient. The mortality rate is 3% to 4% per year, and approaches 50% within 20 to 25 years. One-fifth of patients

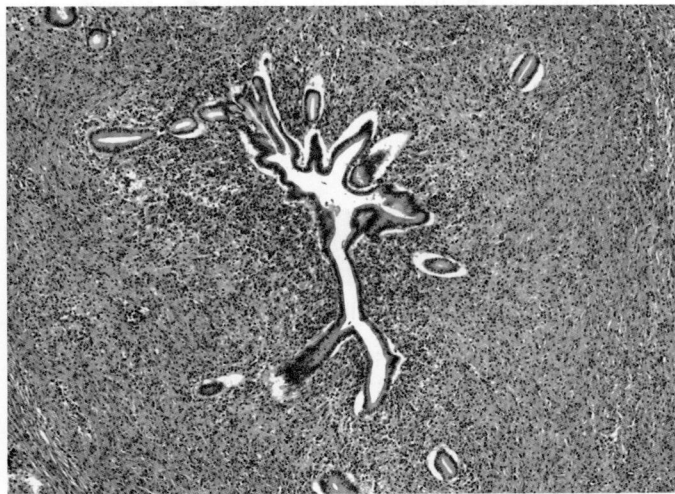

FIGURE 21-6. Autoimmune pancreatitis. There is a loss of acinar tissue and the pancreatic duct is surrounded by dense lymphoplasmacytic inflammatory infiltrate.

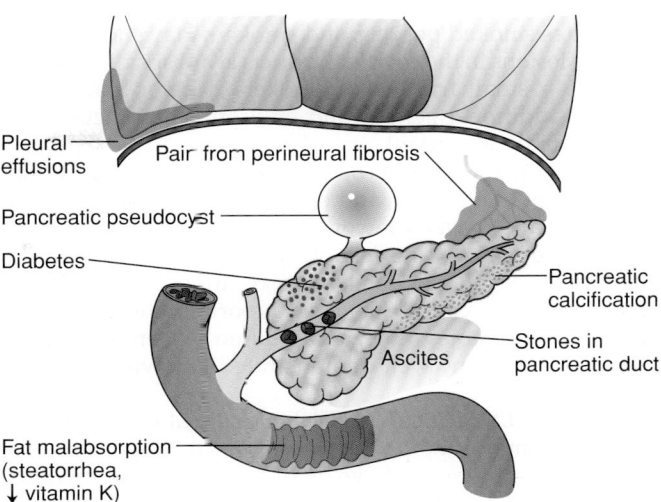

FIGURE 21-7. Complications of chronic pancreatitis.

die of complications associated with attacks of acute pancreatitis. The remaining deaths are attributable to other causes, mainly alcohol-related disorders.

PANCREATIC EXOCRINE NEOPLASIA

The Vast Majority (~85%) of Pancreatic Tumors in Adults Are Infiltrating Ductal Adenocarcinomas

Because of this, this neoplasm is commonly referred to simply as "pancreatic cancer." In the United States, pancreatic cancer is the fourth most common cause of cancer death in both women and men. The prognosis is dismal: the 5-year survival is less than 3%. The incidence of pancreatic cancer seems to be increasing in all countries studied, and it has tripled in the United States over the past 50 years.

 EPIDEMIOLOGY: Pancreatic cancer is seen worldwide. The highest incidence (twice that in the United States) is among male Maoris, Polynesian aborigines of New Zealand, and female natives of Hawaii. Over 55,000 new cases occur each year in the United States, where the incidence in Native Americans and African-Americans is about 50% higher than in whites. Although it can arise in people in their 20s or 30s, pancreatic cancer is a disease of late life, with the greatest incidence in those more than 60 years of age. It shows a significant male predominance (up to 3:1) in younger age groups but almost equal sex distribution in old age.

ETIOLOGIC FACTORS: The factors responsible for the development of pancreatic cancer are not rigorously established. Epidemiologic studies have implicated both host and environmental factors as being of possible etiologic significance.

SMOKING: About 25% of pancreatic cancers are attributable to cigarette smoking, and there is a two- to threefold increased risk of pancreatic cancer in cigarette smokers. There is an apparent relationship with the number of

cigarettes smoked per day, and smokers may show proliferative lesions in the pancreatic ducts at autopsy. However,
as only a small fraction of smokers develop pancreatic
cancer, additional genetic and environmental factors are
undoubtedly important.

BODY MASS INDEX (BMI) AND DIETARY FACTORS:
A diet high in meat, fat, and nitrates may increase the risk
of pancreatic cancer. However, confounding factors such
as methods of cooking (e.g., frying, boiling, barbecuing)
may play a role. A positive association between BMI
and pancreatic cancer has been reported, and diets rich
in fruits, vegetables, fiber, and vitamin C seem to be protective. There is no well-demonstrated link with coffee or
alcohol consumption.

DIABETES MELLITUS: Diabetics are at increased risk
for carcinoma of the pancreas, and up to 80% of patients
with pancreatic cancer have evidence of diabetes mellitus
at the time of cancer diagnosis. In some patients, however,
diabetes may be the result, rather than the cause, of pancreatic cancer. In any event, patients with diabetes mellitus for
5 or more years have double the risk for pancreatic cancer.

CHRONIC PANCREATITIS: Chronic pancreatitis is
a risk factor for pancreatic cancer, although conventional
types (such as alcoholic pancreatitis) likely account for
few cases. Hereditary pancreatitis and tropical calcifying pancreatitis are more clearly linked to cancer. Since
chronic pancreatitis may occasionally be mild and clinically silent, its role in the development of pancreatic
carcinoma may be underestimated. On the other hand,
pancreatic cancers commonly cause obstructive chronic
pancreatitis because they invade the pancreatic ducts and
obstruct the distal gland. Thus, the relationship of pancreatitis and cancer has proven difficult to unravel.

ADDITIONAL FACTORS: Some environmental factors are suggested by increased risk linked to specific
occupations. Workers exposed to coal gas, metallurgi-
cal chemicals, dry cleaning agents, and leather tanning
chemicals have a higher incidence of pancreatic cancer.

FAMILIAL PANCREATIC CANCER: Hereditary factors play a role in pancreatic cancer risk, and a number of
defined cancer-associated hereditary diseases have been
linked to pancreatic cancer (Table 21-1; also see Chapter 5).
In such cases, the underlying gene defect plays a role in
the development of the neoplasm (see below). However,
cases due to known germline mutations comprise only a
small fraction of all pancreatic cancers, and families that
have multiple affected members usually do not suffer from
one of these defined syndromes. Increased risk has recently
been linked to specific ABO blood group types, but the
genetic causes of most cases of familial pancreatic cancer
remain to be determined.

MOLECULAR PATHOGENESIS: Pancreatic
infiltrating ductal adenocarcinomas exhibit a
number of genetic alterations. Some occur in most
cases whereas others are only found in a minor subset. A
proposed tumor progression model, based on specific gene
mutations, is supported by the morphologic finding of
neoplastic ductal proliferative lesions, termed **pancreatic
intraductal neoplasia** (PanIN), the more recent nomenclature for dysplasia of the ducts. PanINs are characterized by
mucinous epithelium replacing the normal lining of the
ducts. They are categorized into two grades that reflect
increasing cytoarchitectural abnormalities. Early events
occur in low-grade PanIN and include telomere shortening
and mutational activation of the *KRAS* oncogene, which is
mutated in up to 95% of ductal adenocarcinomas. Later
events in the sequence of neoplastic progression involve
mutational inactivation or deletion of tumor suppressor
genes, including *p53* (50% to 75%), *p16/CDKN2A* (which
encodes cyclin-dependent kinase inhibitor 2A) (95%), and
SMAD4/DPC-4 (involved in transforming growth factor-β
[TGF-β] signaling) (55%). Interestingly, deletions in chromosome 18 are present in 90% of pancreatic cancers.
Although *DPC-4* (named for "deleted in pancreatic cancer
locus 4") is located on chromosome 18, only half of all pancreatic cancers show loss or inactivation of this gene, suggesting that another nearby tumor suppressor gene
contributes to the development of the remaining 40%.
Overactivity or inappropriate expression of several growth
factors and their receptors has been described, including
epidermal growth factor (EGF) and its receptor, TGF-β,
fibroblast growth factor (FGF) and its receptor, and HER2/
neu. Up to 7% of pancreatic carcinomas have inactivating
mutations of *BRCA2* and a similar fraction have loss of
DNA mismatch repair genes. Many other genes involved
in ductal adenocarcinoma are being identified now that the
pancreatic cancer genome has been sequenced, but most
are implicated in only a small proportion of cases. The
sequential development of morphological abnormalities
and acquisition of the most common genetic defects in the
progression of PanIN to invasive carcinoma are shown in
Figure 21-8.

TABLE 21-1

FAMILIAL CANCER SYNDROMES AND RELATIVE RISK FOR PANCREATIC CANCER

Syndrome	Chromosome	Gene Mutation	Relative Risk of Pancreatic Cancer
Peutz–Jegher syndrome	19p13	*STK11/LKB1*	132-fold
Hereditary pancreatitis	7q35	*PRSS1*	50- to 80-fold
Familial atypical multiple mole melanoma	9p21	*P16 (CDKN2A)*	9- to 38-fold syndrome (FAMM)
Hereditary breast-ovarian cancer syndrome (HBOC)	13q12–13	*BRCA2*	3.5- to 10-fold
Hereditary nonpolyposis cancer syndrome (HNPCC)	3p21, 2p22	*hMLH1, hMSH2*	Unknown

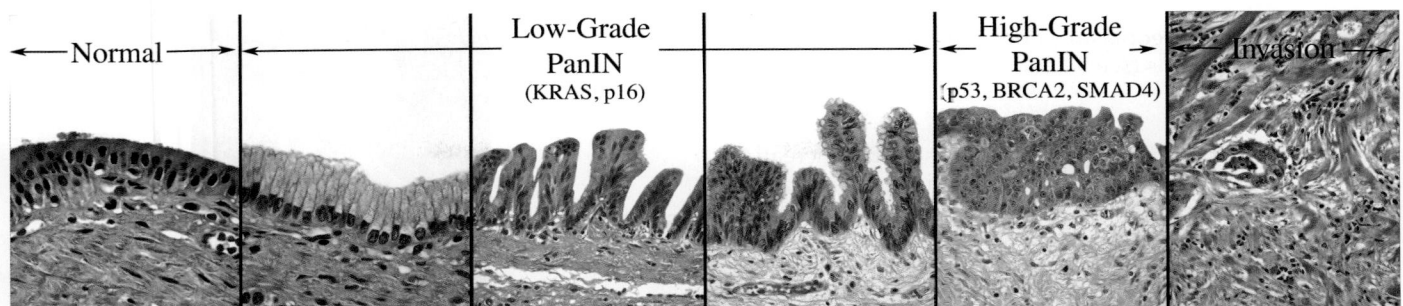

FIGURE 21-8. Pancreatic intraepithelial neoplasia (PanIN). The sequence proceeds left to right from normal ductal epithelium to invasive carcinoma. Common gene mutations are acquired during the progression from normal to invasive cancer.

PATHOLOGY: Ductal adenocarcinoma may arise anywhere in the pancreas, the most frequent location being in the head (60% to 70%), followed by the body (10%), and tail (10% to 15%). In some cases, the pancreas is diffusely involved. Carcinomas of the head of the pancreas may cause biliary obstruction by compressing the intrapancreatic common bile duct or ampulla of Vater. Classically, both the bile duct and the pancreatic duct become dilated. Because they tend to cause signs and symptoms earlier, carcinomas arising in the head are often smaller at the time of diagnosis than those of the body and tail and show more limited spread to regional lymph nodes and distant sites.

On gross examination, ductal adenocarcinomas are usually a very firm, gray, poorly demarcated masses (Fig. 21-9A) that can be difficult to distinguish from surrounding areas of fibrosing chronic pancreatitis. Invasion of peripancreatic tissues and other local structures is common. Tumors of the head of the pancreas may invade the common bile duct and duodenal wall. They may also obstruct the main pancreatic duct and cause atrophy of the body and tail. Carcinomas of the tail of the gland may extend into the spleen, transverse colon, or stomach. Metastases are commonly found in regional lymph nodes and liver. Other frequent metastatic locations include peritoneum, lungs, adrenals, and bones; involvement of distant sites renders most cases unresectable.

Microscopically, more than 75% of infiltrating ductal adenocarcinomas are well- to moderately-differentiated (Fig. 21-9B). They are characterized by well-formed individual tubular glands containing mucin-producing epithelial cells. Nuclear atypia may be marked, but in some cases the malignant glands are so bland as they are difficult to distinguish from nonneoplastic ducts. Typically there is a striking desmoplastic stromal component surrounding the neoplastic glands. Ductal carcinomas are highly infiltrative and poorly circumscribed, and microscopic extension well beyond the grossly apparent limits of the tumor is common. Perineural invasion is characteristic of ductal adenocarcinoma and accounts for the early and persistent pain associated with this disease. The remaining 25% of ductal adenocarcinomas are poorly differentiated. They may be composed of sheets of cells or individual cells, or represent variants of ductal adenocarcinoma such as colloid carcinoma, medullary carcinoma, adenosquamous carcinoma, and various types of undifferentiated carcinoma, including undifferentiated carcinoma with osteoclast-like giant cells.

Some ductal adenocarcinomas and their variants arise in association with preinvasive neoplasms such as

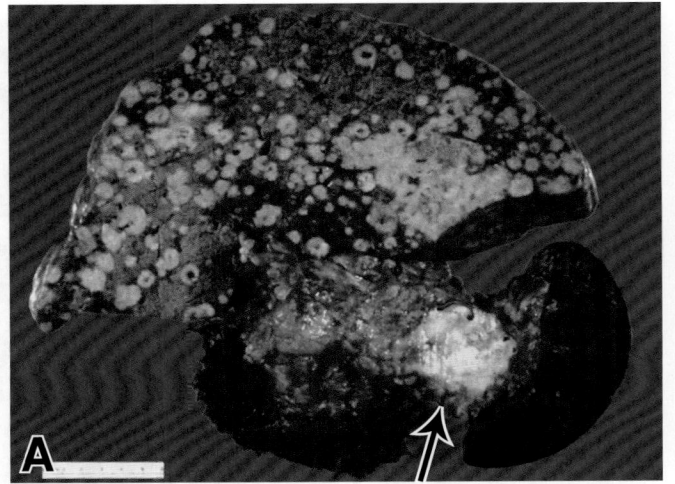

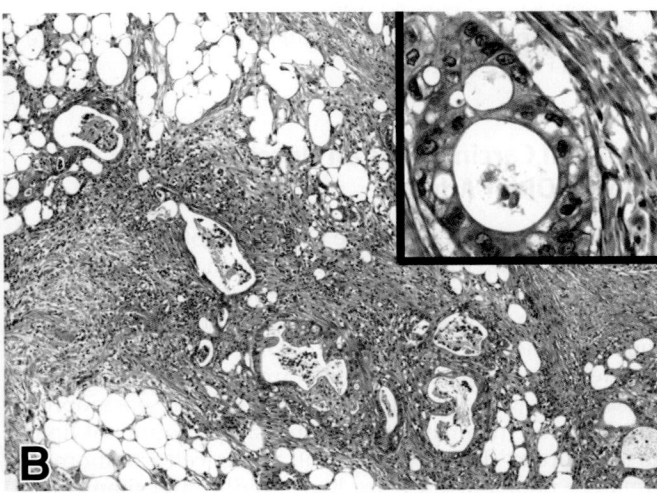

FIGURE 21-9. Infiltrating ductal adenocarcinoma of the pancreas. A. An autopsy specimen shows a large tumor in the tail of the pancreas (*arrow*) and extensive metastases in the liver. **B.** A section of the tumor reveals malignant glands infiltrating into adipose tissue with surrounding fibrous stroma. (Inset shows high power image of a malignant gland.)

mucinous cystic neoplasms and intraductal papillary mucinous neoplasms (see below).

CLINICAL FEATURES: Patients with pancreatic cancer present with anorexia, conspicuous weight loss, and a gnawing pain in the epigastrium, which often radiates to the back. Painless jaundice is seen in about half of all patients with cancer localized to the head of the pancreas, but in less than 10% of tumors of the body or tail. Serum levels of cancer antigen (CA)19-9, a Lewis blood group antigen, are usually increased, but this finding is not specific. Early diagnosis of pancreatic cancer is unusual because the tumor is not ordinarily symptomatic until it is well advanced. Most have already metastasized or invaded local major vessels by the time of diagnosis, and curative surgery is uncommon. Progressive deterioration almost invariably ensues, with intractable pain, cachexia, and death. Half of patients die within 6 months of diagnosis, and the overall 5-year survival rate is less than 8%.

Courvoisier sign is acute, painless gallbladder dilation accompanied by jaundice, owing to common bile duct obstruction by tumor. In about one-third of patients, it may be the first sign of pancreatic cancer but it does not identify potentially curable tumors.

Migratory thrombophlebitis (deep venous thrombosis) develops in 10% of patients with pancreatic cancer, especially when the tumor involves the body and tail of the pancreas. It is not uncommon for migratory thrombophlebitis, also known as **Trousseau syndrome**, to be the first evidence of an underlying pancreatic malignancy, although it may be seen with other cancers as well. Unexplained thrombophlebitis in an otherwise healthy person demands a careful search for occult malignancy. Mechanisms responsible for the hypercoagulable state that leads to migratory thrombophlebitis are not completely understood, but several factors have been implicated: (1) a serine protease synthesized and released by malignant tumor cells directly activates plasma factor X; (2) tumor cells spontaneously shed plasma membrane vesicles, which exhibit procoagulant activity; and (3) intracellular tissue thromboplastin is released from necrotic tumor.

The complications of pancreatic ductal carcinoma are shown in Figure 21-10.

Acinar Cell Carcinoma Is an Uncommon Tumor of Older Adults

Acinar cell carcinomas are rare (1% to 2% of pancreatic carcinomas) tumors that recapitulate the normal pancreatic acini, including the production of exocrine enzymes by the tumor cells. They usually occur in the seventh decade of life, although some occur in children. Some patients develop a characteristic paraneoplastic syndrome of subcutaneous fat necrosis, polyarthralgia, and peripheral eosinophilia attributable to hypersecretion of massive amounts of lipase into the serum. The prognosis of acinar cell carcinoma is ultimately poor but they are less rapidly fatal than ductal adenocarcinomas. Acinar cell carcinomas are large and circumscribed and lack the desmoplastic stroma of ductal adenocarcinomas. Microscopically they are composed of

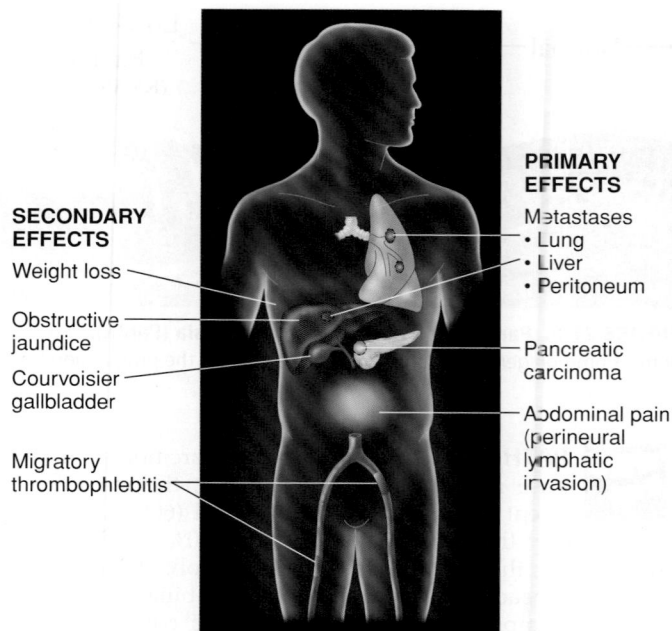

FIGURE 21-10. Complications of pancreatic ductal adenocarcinoma.

uniform cells arranged in small acini and nests (Fig. 21-11), and the production of exocrine enzymes can be demonstrated with immunohistochemistry. The molecular pathogenesis of acinar cell carcinoma is very different from that of ductal adenocarcinoma. Some cases have abnormalities in the APC/beta-catenin pathway or fusions involving *BRAF*, but the genetic defects typically observed in ductal adenocarcinoma are not seen in acinar cell cancers.

Pancreatoblastoma Is a Tumor of Childhood

Usually detected in the first decade of life, pancreatoblastoma is closely related to acinar cell carcinoma. It may occur in the setting of Beckwith–Wiedemann syndrome, an overgrowth syndrome that affects multiple organs and is associated with an increased risk of developing several types

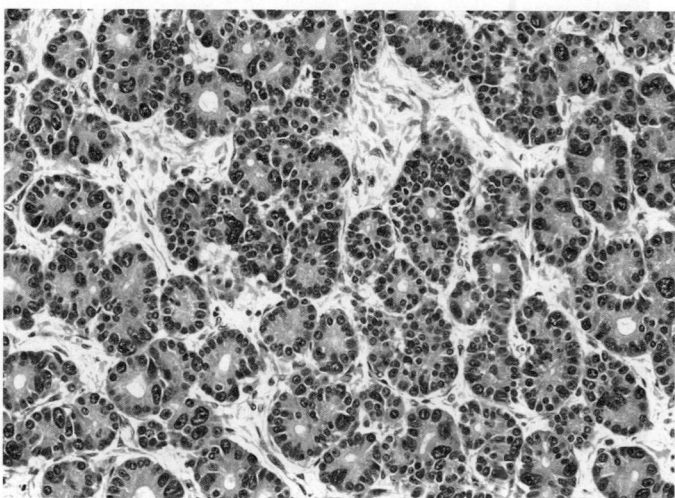

FIGURE 21-11. Acinar cell carcinoma. This malignant tumor is characterized by acinar formations reminiscent of normal pancreatic parenchyma.

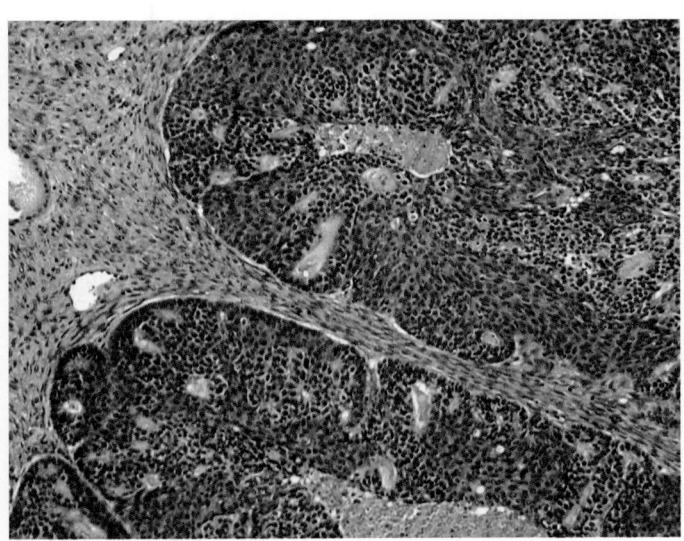

FIGURE 21-12. Pancreatoblastoma. Sarcomatoid features with spindle cells are interspersed with scattered acinar structures.

of benign and malignant neoplasms. Serum α-fetoprotein levels may be elevated. Microscopically, the tumor is composed of polygonal cells arrayed in solid islands and acinar structures, with interspersed squamoid nests (Fig. 21-12). Acinar differentiation, with production of exocrine enzymes, is consistently present, and some cases also show ductal or endocrine differentiation. Lymph node or hepatic metastases occur in a third of patients, and are associated with a poor prognosis. Surgery and chemotherapy can be curative in patients without metastatic disease.

Serous Cystic Neoplasms of the Pancreas Are Nearly Always Benign

Serous cystic neoplasms are almost always benign tumors composed of cystic structures lined by glycogen-rich cuboidal epithelium (Fig. 21-13). They usually arise in the pancreatic body or tail in adults, with a 3:1 female predominance.

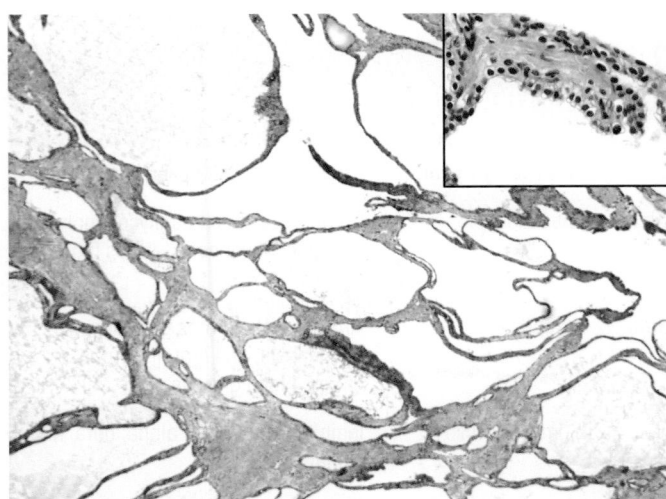

FIGURE 21-13. Serous cystadenoma. Cysts are embedded in a dense, fibrous stroma. The epithelial lining is composed of a single layer of glycogen-rich clear cells (*inset*).

Patients with von Hippel–Lindau syndrome are at increased risk for its development. Inactivation of the tumor suppressor *VHL* gene in von Hippel–Lindau syndrome results in defective degradation of various growth factors and thereby promote development of multiple neoplasms including, among others, cystic tumors of the pancreas and kidneys. Serous cystadenomas range from 1 to 25 cm in diameter. They often contain a large, stellate central scar, sometimes with microcalcifications, giving a "sunburst" pattern on imaging studies. Most patients present with nonspecific symptoms related to local mass effects, but many are asymptomatic. These tumors are sometimes excised surgically because of clinical concern for malignancy or because of symptoms.

Intraductal Papillary Mucinous Neoplasms Are Sometimes Associated With Invasive Carcinoma

Intraductal papillary mucin-producing neoplasms (IPMNs) are composed of dilated pancreatic ducts (>5 mm) lined by neoplastic mucinous epithelium and filled with mucus. Frequently, numerous papillary proliferations extend into the duct lumen (Fig. 21-14). The tumors are usually diagnosed in late adulthood, after being found incidentally or in patients with chronic pancreatitis. Most IPMNs arise in the head of the pancreas. Duct involvement may be unifocal, multifocal, or diffuse. Some IPMNs involve the main pancreatic ducts whereas others are localized to the peripheral (branch) ducts and mimic cystic lesions on imaging studies. IPMNs exhibit a varying degrees of epithelial atypia, and are classified accordingly. They may show either low-grade or high-grade dysplasia, categorized in a similar fashion to PanINs. A focus of invasive adenocarcinoma is found in up to one-third of

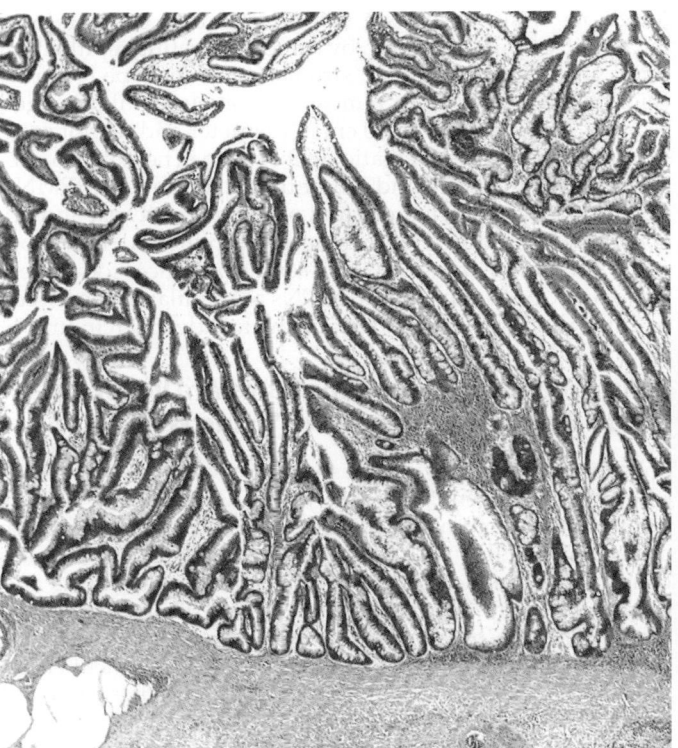

FIGURE 21-14. Intraductal papillary mucinous neoplasm. An exuberant papillary proliferation of tall mucin-secreting epithelium fills the pancreatic duct.

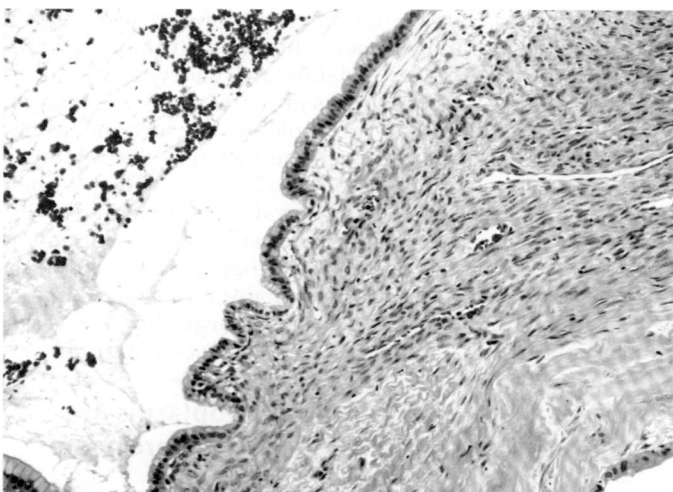

FIGURE 21-15. Mucinous cystic neoplasm. A mucin-rich epithelial lining of this cystic lesion rests on an ovarian type stroma.

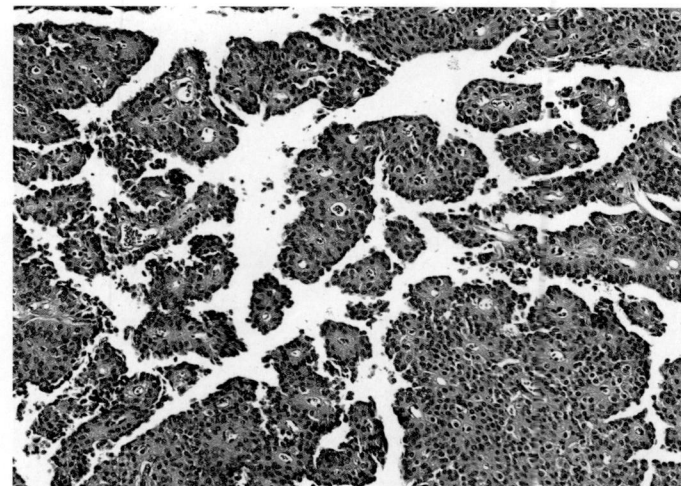

FIGURE 21-16. Solid pseudopapillary neoplasm. The tumor is composed of pseudopapillae with vascular cores.

cases. Because of their risk for harboring invasive carcinomas, clinically concerning lesions, such as larger tumors or those with atypical radiographic features, are often resected. The molecular pathogenesis of many of these tumors is similar to that of PanIN and pancreatic ductal adenocarcinoma. Some IPMNs, however, develop via alternative molecular pathways, likely explaining why some exhibit different phenotypes when compared to PanIN.

Mucinous Cystic Neoplasms Are Most Often Found in the Pancreatic Tails of Middle-Aged Women

Mucinous cystic neoplasm (MCN) is a uni- or multilocular cystic neoplasm lined by mucin-secreting epithelium with underlying cellular stroma (ovarian-type stroma) (Fig. 21-15). MCNs occur almost exclusively in middle-aged women. They may reach 10 cm in diameter and do not communicate with the pancreatic duct system. They have a predilection for the body and tail of the pancreas. Like IPMNs, they may show varying degrees of epithelial atypia and are sometimes associated with invasive carcinoma. The prognosis for noninvasive MCN is excellent once completely removed. Genetic changes in MCNs are similar to those seen in PanIN and invasive pancreatic ductal adenocarcinoma.

Solid Pseudopapillary Neoplasms Are Very Low–Grade Malignancies Found in Young Women

Solid pseudopapillary neoplasm (SPN) occurs almost exclusively in adolescent girls and young women. The tumors are solid and circumscribed, often with large areas of cystic degeneration filled with blood and necrotic debris. They are composed of monomorphic cells forming loose sheets and pseudopapillary structures (Fig. 21-16). That vast majority of SPNs are indolent and curable by complete surgical resection, although metastases occur in about 10% of cases, usually to the liver. Even these patients usually live for many years, emphasizing the slow-growing nature of this neoplasm. Clinically, SPNs may mimic other malignant neoplasms of the pancreas. Most have mutations in *CTNNB1*, the β-catenin gene, and show abnormal nuclear localization of the corresponding protein.

THE ENDOCRINE PANCREAS

The Islets of Langerhans Form the Endocrine Pancreas

These islets are scattered irregularly throughout the pancreas and consist of richly vascularized spherical or lobulated aggregates of endocrine cells. Four major distinct cell types are present in the islets, and each cell produces only one specific peptide hormone (Table 21-2).

- **Alpha cells** synthesize glucagon and are located at the peripheral of the islet lobules. They constitute 15% to 20% of the total islet cell population (Fig. 21-17A). Glucagon induces glycogenolysis and gluconeogenesis in the liver, thereby raising blood glucose. Its secretion is stimulated by hypoglycemia and by ingestion of a low-carbohydrate, high-protein meal. By virtue of these responses, glucagon, together with insulin, serves to maintain glucose homeostasis.
- **Beta cells** make up 60% to 70% of all islet cells and produce insulin (Fig. 21-17B). They are found in central

TABLE 21-2		
SECRETORY PRODUCTS OF ISLET CELLS AND THEIR PHYSIOLOGICAL ACTIONS		
Cell	**Secretory Product**	**Physiological Actions**
Alpha	Glucagon	Catabolic, stimulates glycogenolysis and gluconeogenesis, raises blood glucose
Beta	Insulin	Anabolic, stimulates glycogenesis, lipogenesis, and protein synthesis, lowers blood glucose
Delta	Somatostatin	Inhibits secretion of alpha, beta, and acinar cells
PP	Human pancreatic polypeptide (HPP)	Stimulates gastric enzyme secretion, inhibits intestinal motility and bile secretion

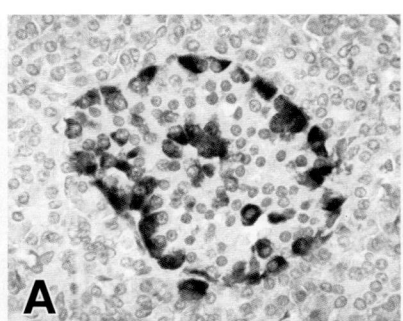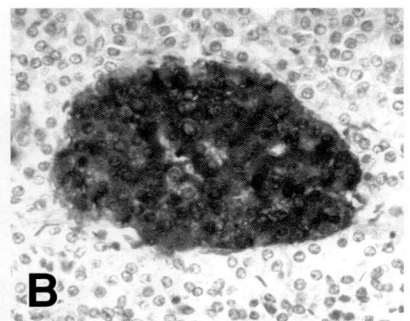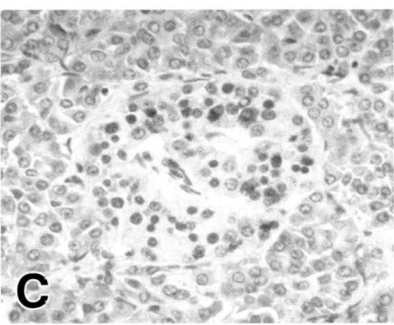

FIGURE 21-17. Localization of hormones of the pancreatic islet by specific antibodies. The immunoperoxidase technique reveals (**A**) glucagon in alpha cells at the periphery of the islet, (**B**) insulin in beta cells distributed throughout the islet, and (**C**) somatostatin in sparsely distributed delta cells.

regions of the islets. By electron microscopy, beta cells contain characteristic polygonal and rhomboidal crystals enclosed in secretory vesicles. The major obligatory stimulus for insulin secretion is the binding of glucose to receptors on the beta cell surface.

- **Delta cells** secrete somatostatin. They are fewer in number (5% to 10%) and, like alpha cells, tend to be at the periphery of the islets (Fig. 21-17C). Pancreatic somatostatin inhibits pituitary release of growth hormone, secretion by alpha, beta, and acinar cells of the pancreas, and certain hormone-secreting cells in the gastrointestinal tract. These hormonal interactions suggest that somatostatin plays a regulatory role in glucose homeostasis.
- **Pancreatic polypeptide-secreting cells** are located primarily in the diffuse islets of the portion of the head of the pancreas derived from the embryonic ventral pancreas. They synthesize a polypeptide that appears to have variable and opposing functions. For example, pancreatic polypeptide stimulates secretion of enzymes from the gastric mucosa, and inhibiting a number of functions including smooth muscle contraction in intestine and gallbladder, production of gastric acid, and secretion by the exocrine pancreas and biliary system.

Pancreatic Neuroendocrine Tumors Comprise About 5% of Pancreatic Neoplasms

Pancreatic neuroendocrine tumors (PanNETs) have distinctive morphologic features resembling those of normal islet cells and other well-differentiated neuroendocrine tumors of the body, such as pulmonary carcinoid tumors. Previously known as "islet cell tumors," PanNETs may secrete hormones that cause dramatic paraneoplastic syndromes or may be nonfunctioning. Functioning PanNETs include insulinoma, glucagonoma, somatostatinoma, gastrinoma, VIPoma, and other rare types. Of the functioning tumors, insulinomas are the most common. More than half of PanNETs are nonfunctioning. PanNETs exhibit a range of clinical aggressiveness; when small, they are easily cured by surgical resection, but larger tumors may develop incurable metastases. Prediction of the likely clinical course of PanNETs is difficult, although features such as large size, a relatively high rate of tumor cell proliferation, and more extensive invasion increase the likelihood of recurrence. Even when they give rise to distant metastases, PanNETs may grow relatively slowly, and survival for years or even decades can occur. When functioning PanNETs cannot be completely removed by surgery,

complications of the hormonal syndromes may be highly morbid. Very small PanNETs (less than 0.5 cm) are common incidental findings and are designated pancreatic neuroendocrine microadenomas.

PanNETs can occur at any age but are most common between 40 and 60 years. Men and women are equally affected. Nonfunctioning tumors are detected incidentally by imaging studies or come to attention due to local mass effects or because of metastatic disease, which occur most commonly in the liver.

PanNETs are a component of the multiple endocrine neoplasia syndrome, type 1 (MEN1), which also involves adenomas of the pituitary and parathyroid glands, and less commonly neuroendocrine tumors of other organs. Affected patients usually have multiple pancreatic neuroendocrine microadenomas and PanNETs, at least one of which is functioning. Patients with von Hippel–Lindau syndrome also develop nonfunctioning PanNETs.

Patients with hereditary PanNETs can show biallelic inactivation of *MEN1* or *VHL*, genes linked to the MEN1 and von Hippel–Lindau syndromes, respectively. *MEN1* encodes a protein called menin which acts as a tumor suppressor by regulating DNA repair and apoptosis. As discussed above, *VHL* regulates timely degradation of various growth factors and thus its inactivation promotes unrestrained proliferation. The genes most commonly involved in the development of PanNETs include *MEN1*, *DAXX* (which encodes a death domain protein critical in apoptosis), and *ATRX* (which makes a chromatin remodeling protein). Genes in which defects have been implicated in the development of ductal adenocarcinoma are usually normal in PanNETs.

Functioning PanNETs Produce Dramatic Paraneoplastic Syndromes

- **Insulinomas**, the most frequent functioning PanNET, secrete sufficient insulin to cause hypoglycemia. The neoplastic cells are not regulated by low blood glucose levels, so the tumors continue to secrete insulin. Although the tumors are usually small (75% are less than 2 cm), the symptoms are profound and include both the direct central nervous system effects of hypoglycemia as well as the secondary effects of the resulting catecholamine response. Patients suffer from sweating, visual changes, confusion, nervousness, and hunger, which may progress to confusion, lethargy, and even seizures or coma. Abnormal behavior may falsely suggest a psychiatric disorder.

Insulinomas are somewhat more common in the tail of the pancreas. Although 30% of the functioning PanNETs in patients with MEN1 are insulinomas, only 5% of insulinomas arise in the setting of MEN1. Compared to other PanNETs, insulinomas have a benign clinical course, perhaps because they are usually very small when detected. Surgical removal, even by enucleation, is usually curative.

■ **Glucagonomas** are associated with a syndrome of (1) mild diabetes; (2) a necrotizing, migratory, erythematous rash; (3) anemia; (4) diarrhea; and (5) deep vein thromboses. Psychiatric disturbances also occur. Glucagonomas constitute 8% to 13% of functioning PanNETs and occur between the ages of 40 and 70 years, with a slight female predominance. In patients with alpha cell tumors, plasma glucagon levels are elevated up to 30 times above normal. Like other functioning PanNETs (other than insulinomas) and nonfunctioning PanNETs, glucagonomas exhibit malignant behavior in 50% to 70% of cases.

■ **Somatostatinomas** are rare. They produce a syndrome consisting of mild diabetes, gallstones, steatorrhea, hypochlorhydria, anemia, and weight loss. These effects result from the inhibitory actions of somatostatin on other cells of the pancreatic islets and on neuroendocrine cells of the gastrointestinal tract. Consequently, levels of insulin and glucagon in blood are low.

■ **Pancreatic gastrinoma** is a functioning PanNET composed of so-called G cells, which produce gastrin, a potent hormonal stimulus for gastric acid secretion. The location of this tumor in the pancreas is curious, because gastrin-producing cells do not normally occur in the islets. Pancreatic gastrinoma causes Zollinger–Ellison syndrome, a disorder characterized by (1) intractable gastric hypersecretion, (2) severe peptic ulceration of the duodenum and jejunum, and (3) high blood gastrin levels. Among functioning PanNETs, gastrinomas are second in frequency to insulinomas, and they are the most common functioning tumor in MEN1 patients. However, the pancreas has proven to be a less common location for gastrinomas than the duodenum, especially in cases not associated with MEN1. Gastrinomas of the pancreas are usually relatively large (over 2 cm), whereas duodenal gastrinomas can measure only a few millimeters. In some cases, only lymph node metastases are found, with no detectable evidence of a primary gastrinoma. Gastrinomas occur most commonly between the ages of 30 and 50, with a slight male predominance. Most pancreatic gastrinomas arise in the head of the gland. Pancreatic

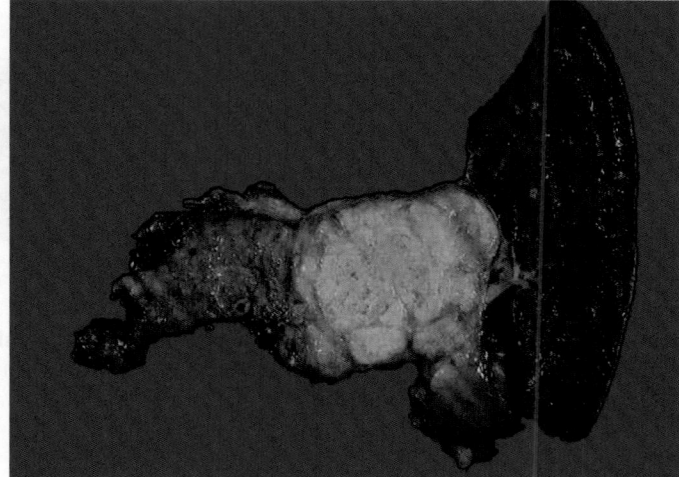

FIGURE 21-18. Pancreatic neuroendocrine tumor. This well-circumscribed somewhat nodular tumor arose in the tail of the pancreas near the spleen.

gastrinomas are locally aggressive, although those arising in the duodenum are usually less so, even when lymph node metastases are present.

■ **VIPomas** are functioning PanNETs that produce vasoactive intestinal polypeptide (VIP), another hormone not normally found in nonneoplastic islet cells but rather in ganglion cells and nerve fibers of pancreas, gut, and brain. VIP induces glycogenolysis and hyperglycemia and regulates ion and water secretion by epithelial cells of the gastrointestinal tract. VIPomas induce Verner–Morrison syndrome, which is characterized by explosive and profuse watery diarrhea, accompanied by hypokalemia and achlorhydria (also known as WDHA syndrome or pancreatic cholera). VIPomas are rare tumors (3% to 8% of all PanNETs and 10% of functioning PanNETs) and are usually large and solitary.

■ PanNETs may rarely secrete other hormones not ordinarily produced in the pancreas (ectopic hormones), including ACTH, parathyroid hormone, calcitonin, and vasopressin. These ectopic hormones may be produced either alone or in combination with normally occurring pancreatic hormones. Pancreatic polypeptide can also be secreted by some PanNETs, dubbed "PPomas," but no specific clinical syndrome is attributable to this hormone, so technically PPomas are clinically nonfunctioning.

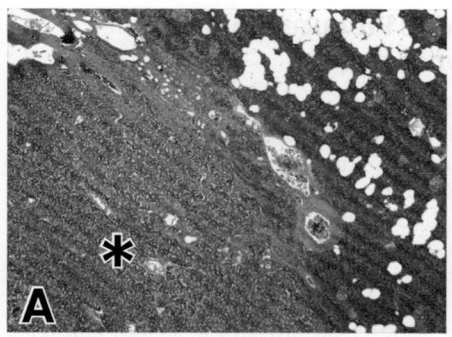
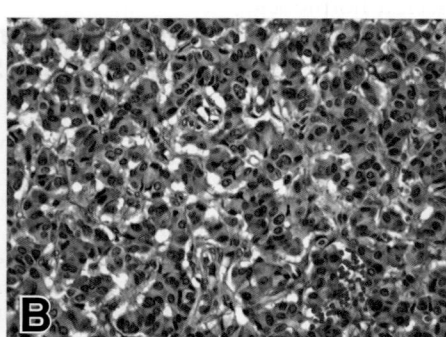
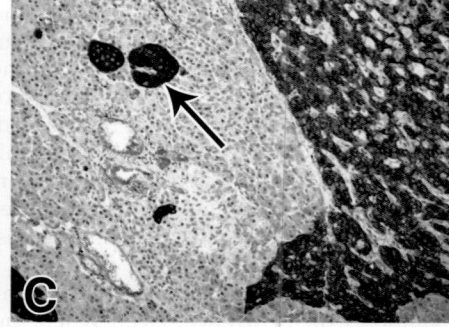

FIGURE 21-19. Pancreatic neuroendocrine tumor. A. The well-circumscribed nature of the tumor (*) can be appreciated at low power. **B.** A higher power image shows uniform neoplastic epithelioid cells arranged in cords. **C.** An immunohistochemical stain for chromogranin, a neuroendocrine antigen, highlights tumor cells and islets (*arrow*) within the adjacent pancreas.

PATHOLOGY: Other than the smaller size characteristic of insulinomas, functioning and nonfunctioning PanNETs are grossly similar. They are usually solitary, circumscribed masses of pink to tan, soft tissue (Fig. 21-18). Larger tumors can be multinodular and contain areas of hemorrhage. Cystic degeneration can occur, or some cases can appear firm and fibrotic. Microscopically, PanNETs are composed of uniform cells arranged in so-called organoid patterns, including nests, ribbons, and festoons (Fig. 21-19). Gland formation can also occur. Nuclei are uniform and have a coarsely stippled chromatin pattern, and the proliferative rate is low. Sometimes the stroma contains amyloid, or it may be sclerotic. Certain histologic patterns have previously been attributed to various functioning types of PanNETs, but such relationships are loose at best and cannot be used to identify the cell type of the PanNET. The neuroendocrine nature of the tumor can be demonstrated using immunohistochemistry with antibodies against chromogranin A and synaptophysin. Functioning PanNETs can often be shown by immunohistochemistry to produce the hormone responsible for the clinical syndrome but production of a number of different hormones in minor cell populations is not uncommon, even in clinically nonfunctioning PanNETs. Electron microscopy can demonstrate characteristic neurosecretory granules, and in some functioning PanNETs, the granule morphology matches that of the specific granules in the nonneoplastic islet cell counterparts.

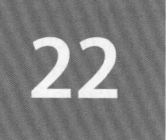

22 | The Kidney

J. Charles Jennette, Harsharan K. Singh

Anatomy

The kidneys are paired, bean-shaped organs located on both sides of the vertebral column in the retroperitoneal space. Adult kidneys average 150 g and are approximately 11-cm long, 6-cm wide, and 3-cm thick. Each kidney consists of an outer cortex and an inner medulla (Fig. 22-1). When a kidney is bisected, the medulla has approximately 12 pyramids, with their bases at the corticomedullary junction. A medullary pyramid and its overlying cortex constitute a renal lobe. A pyramid has an inner and an outer zone. The inner zone, the **papilla,** empties into a calyx, a funnel-shaped structure that conducts urine into the renal pelvis, which empties into the ureter.

BLOOD VESSELS

The kidneys are among the most vascular organs in the body and they receive 20% to 25% of systemic cardiac output.

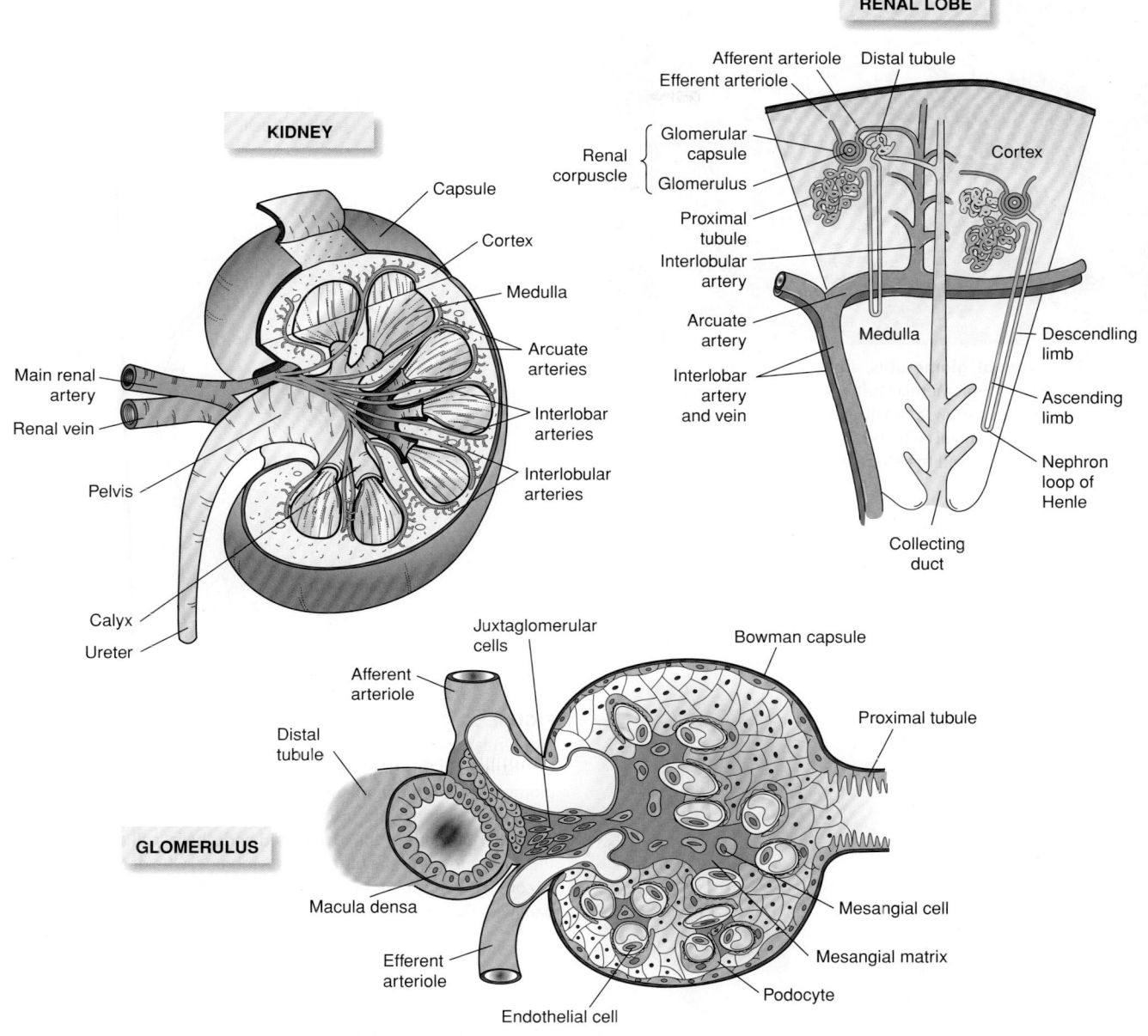

FIGURE 22-1. The gross and microscopic anatomy of the kidney.

The blood supply to each kidney usually derives from a single main renal artery, although 1/4 of kidneys have one or more accessory renal arteries. Before entering the renal parenchyma, the renal artery divides into anterior and posterior branches, which in turn give rise to interlobar arteries (Fig. 22-1). The latter branch into arcuate arteries, which run parallel to the renal surface near the corticomedullary junction. Interlobular arteries arise from the arcuate arteries and extend toward the renal surface, giving off afferent arterioles, each of which supplies a single glomerulus. Efferent arterioles drain the glomeruli and then branch into peritubular capillaries. Those in the outer cortex give rise to capillaries that supply blood to the cortical parenchyma, and those in the deep cortex, adjacent to the medulla, provide vessels that extend into the medulla to become the medullary peritubular vessels, the **vasa recta**.

The Glomerulus Is the Renal Filter

The **nephron** is the functional unit of the kidney; it includes the glomerulus and its tubule, which terminates at a common collecting system (Fig. 22-1). The glomerulus is a specialized network of capillaries covered by epithelial cells called **podocytes** and supported by modified smooth muscle cells called **mesangial cells** (Figs. 22-1 to 22-4). As it enters the glomerulus, the afferent arteriole branches into capillaries, which form the convoluted glomerular tuft and eventually coalesce into the efferent arteriole that exits the glomerulus. Glomerular capillaries are lined by fenestrated endothelial cells lying on a basement membrane. The outer surface of this basement membrane is covered by podocytes. The Bowman space lies between the podocytes and the epithelial cells that line the Bowman capsule.

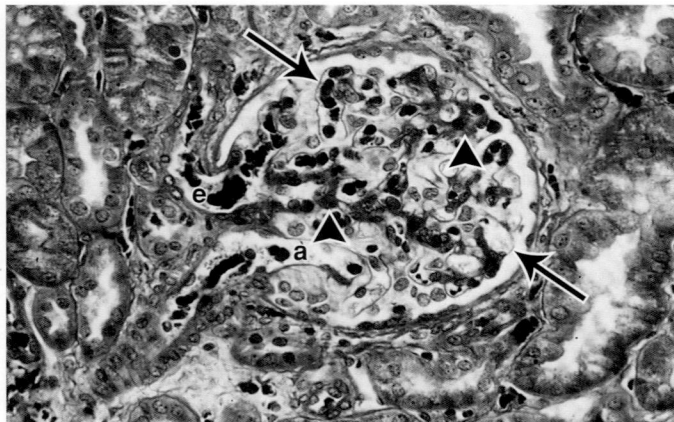

FIGURE 22-2. Normal glomerulus, light microscopy. The Masson trichrome stain shows a glomerular tuft with delicate blue capillary wall basement membranes (*arrows*), small amounts of blue matrix (*arrowheads*) surrounding mesangial cells and the hilum on the left. The afferent arteriole (*a*) enters below, and the efferent arteriole (*e*) exits above.

Glomerular Basement Membrane

The glomerular basement membrane (GBM) (Figs. 22-3 to 22-5) separates endothelial cells from podocytes in peripheral capillary walls and also podocytes from the mesangium. Since the GBM does not completely surround each capillary lumen, but rather splays out over the mesangium as the

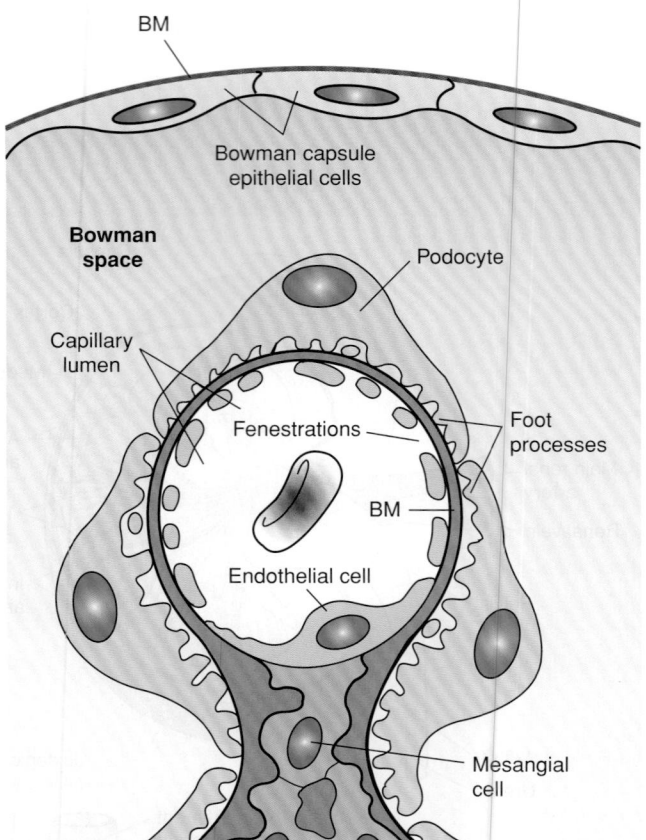

FIGURE 22-4. Normal glomerulus. The relationship of the different glomerular cell types to the basement membrane and mesangial matrix is illustrated in this single glomerular loop. The entire outer aspect of the glomerular basement membrane (peripheral loop and stalk shown in *orange*) is covered by the visceral epithelial cell (podocyte) foot processes. The outer portions of the fenestrated endothelial cell are in contact with the inner surface of the basement membrane, whereas the central part is in contact with the mesangial cell and adjacent mesangial matrix. Compare with Figure 22-3.

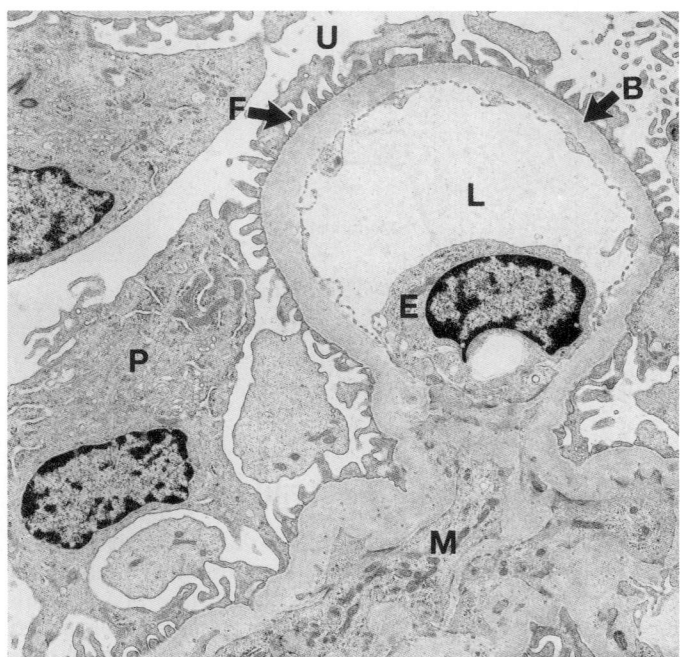

FIGURE 22-3. Normal glomerular capillary. In this electron micrograph of a single capillary loop and adjacent mesangium, the capillary wall portion of the lumen (*L*) is lined by a thin layer of fenestrated endothelial cytoplasm (shown at higher magnification in Fig. 22-5) that extends out from the endothelial cell body (*E*). The endothelial cell body is in direct contact with the mesangium, which includes the mesangial cell (*M*) and adjacent matrix. The outer aspect of the basement membrane (*B*) is covered by foot processes (*F*) from podocytes (*P*) that line the urinary space (*U*). Compare this figure with Figures 22-4 and 22-5.

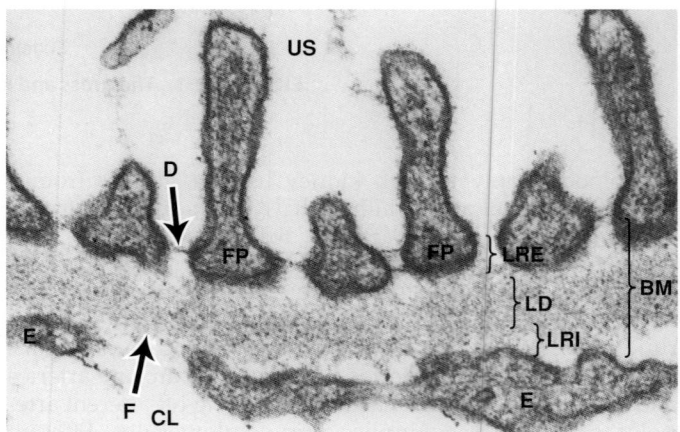

FIGURE 22-5. The glomerular filter. This electron micrograph illustrates the structures of the glomerular filter. Molecules that pass from the capillary lumen (*CL*) to the urinary space (*US*) traverse the fenestrations (*F*) of the endothelial cell (*E*), the trilaminar basement membrane (*BM*) (lamina rara interna [*LRI*], lamina densa [*LD*] and lamina rara externa [*LRE*]) and the slit pore diaphragms (*D*) that connect podocyte foot processes (*FP*).

paramesangial GBM, substances in the blood may potentially enter the mesangium without crossing the GBM.

Although morphologically similar to many other basement membranes, the GBM is functionally and structurally distinct. It is approximately 350 nm thick and has three ultrastructurally definable layers (Fig. 22-5):

- **Lamina densa:** A central electron-dense zone
- **Lamina rara interna:** A thin inner electron-lucent zone
- **Lamina rara externa:** A thin outer electron-lucent zone

The GBM is composed mainly of type IV collagen, which provides its major scaffolding. Genetic abnormalities in type IV collagen and autoantibodies directed against type IV collagen cause glomerular disease. Other constituents include glycosaminoglycans, laminin, entactin, and fibronectin. The polyanionic glycosaminoglycans, which are rich in heparan sulfate, impart a strong negative charge to the GBM. This allows selective filtration of electrically neutral and cationic molecules and relative exclusion of negatively charged molecules such as albumin. The GBM also discriminates among molecules on the basis of size.

Glomerular Endothelial Cells

The glomerular endothelial cell layer is 50-nm thick and contains numerous 60- to 100-nm pores or fenestrations (Fig. 22-5) that are not spanned by diaphragms. Thus, they permit passage of fluid, ions, and proteins (Fig. 22-4). Endothelial surface membrane proteins (e.g., adhesion molecules) and endothelial secretory products (e.g., prostaglandins and nitric oxide) play important roles in the pathogenesis of inflammatory and thrombotic glomerular diseases (Figs. 22-4 and 22-5).

Podocytes

Podocytes rest on the outer aspect of the GBM and send cytoplasmic projections, called **foot processes,** onto the lamina rara externa of the GBM (Fig. 22-5). Between adjacent foot processes is a thin membrane called the **slit diaphragm,** which is a modified adherens junction. Podocytes are the major glomerular barrier to protein loss in the urine. Mutations in genes encoding proteins in podocytes and the slit diaphragm (e.g., **nephrin, podocin, α-actinin-4** and **transient receptor potential cation channel 6 [TRPC6]**) can result in abnormal protein loss into the urine (proteinuria).

Mesangium

The mesangium is a cellular and matrix network that supports the glomerulus. Mesangial cells are modified smooth muscle cells situated in the center of the glomerular tuft between capillary loops. Important functions of the mesangium are:

- Mechanical support for the glomerulus
- Endocytosis and processing of plasma proteins, including immune complexes
- Maintenance of mesangial extracellular matrix
- Modulation of glomerular blood flow and filtration by mesangial cell contractility
- Generation of molecular mediators (e.g., prostaglandins and cytokines)

Tubules Comprise Most of the Nephron

The major segments of the tubule that arise from each glomerulus are the proximal tubule, loop of Henle and distal tubule, which empties into the collecting duct. At the origin of the proximal tubule from the glomerulus, the flat epithelium of the Bowman capsule abruptly transforms into tall columnar cells of the **proximal tubule,** which have numerous tall microvilli that form a brush border. The initial segment, called the **proximal convoluted tubule**, is very tortuous. As it descends into the medulla, the proximal tubule straightens into the thick **descending limb of the loop of Henle**. Further into the medulla, the thick descending limb thins into the **thin limb of the loop of Henle,** which eventually loops back toward the cortex.

Approaching the cortex, the thin limb becomes the **thick ascending limb**. This abuts the glomerulus from which it arose, contributes to that glomerulus' juxtaglomerular apparatus and then becomes the **distal convoluted tubule**. Several distal tubules unite to form a **collecting duct,** which ultimately empties into the ducts of Bellini, which discharge urine through the papillae into the calyces.

The Juxtaglomerular Apparatus Secretes Renin and Angiotensin

The juxtaglomerular apparatus is situated at the hilus of the glomerulus and it consists of:

- **Macula densa,** a region of the thick ascending limb of the loop of Henle that has closely packed nuclei
- **Extraglomerular mesangial cells,** between the macula densa and the hilar arterioles
- **Terminal afferent arteriole** and **proximal efferent arteriole**

The wall of the afferent arteriole contains characteristic granular cells involved in the synthesis and secretion of renin and angiotensin.

The Interstitium Provides Structural Support

The renal interstitium is composed of interstitial cells that resemble fibroblasts and surrounding collagenous matrix. The interstitium occupies only 10% of cortical volume but constitutes 20% to 30% of medullary volume. In addition to providing structural support, some cortical interstitial cells secrete erythropoietin and some medullary cells elaborate prostaglandins.

Congenital and Inherited Renal Diseases

CONGENITAL ANOMALIES OF THE KIDNEY AND URINARY TRACT

Potter Sequence Results From Insufficient Amniotic Fluid

Potter sequence (oligohydramnios sequence) is a syndrome of pathologic abnormalities that are caused by markedly reduced intrauterine urine production (also see Chapter 6). Reduced urine production due, for example, to bilateral

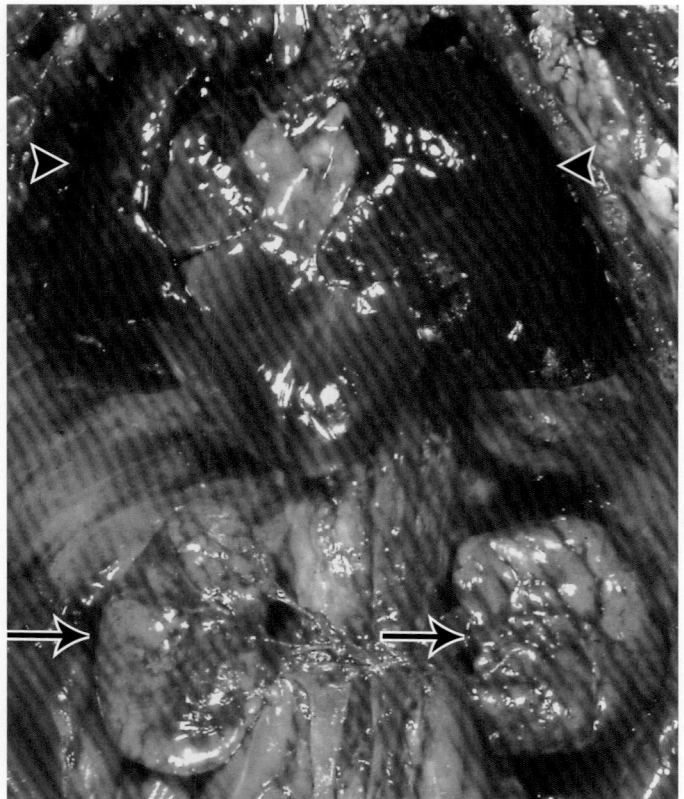

FIGURE 22-6. Bilateral renal agenesis. The Potter sequence includes congenitally nonfunctional kidneys, pulmonary hypoplasia and other anomalies. In this case, there was bilateral renal agenesis, with only mesenchymal elements in the renal rudiments (*arrows*). Consequently, the lungs were hypoplastic (*arrowheads*). This infant was stillborn.

renal agenesis (Fig. 22-6) results in less amniotic fluid (oligohydramnios). The amniotic fluid normally cushions the fetus. With less fluid, the fetus is compressed by the uterus. This compression causes flattening of the face with low-set ears, a small receding chin and a flattened beak-like nose; it also restricts movement of the arms and legs, often leading to abnormally bent lower extremities. The most life-threatening component of Potter sequence is pulmonary hypoplasia (Fig. 22-6), which is caused by inadequate maturational stimuli from amniotic fluid and by compression of the chest wall by the uterus. Because even neonates can be dialyzed to accommodate renal failure, severe respiratory insufficiency due to Potter sequence (rather than renal failure) may be the cause of death in infants with severe congenital renal anomalies.

Renal Agenesis Is the Complete Absence of Renal Tissue

Most infants born with bilateral renal agenesis (Fig. 22-6) are stillborn and have Potter sequence. Bilateral agenesis is often associated with other anomalies, especially elsewhere in the urinary tract or lower extremities. Unilateral renal agenesis is not serious if there are no other associated anomalies, as the contralateral kidney hypertrophies sufficiently to maintain normal renal function. If unilateral renal agenesis is accompanied by hypoplasia of the contralateral kidney, there is an increased risk for developing progressive glomerular sclerosis (secondary focal segmental glomerulosclerosis [FSGS]) due to overwork of nephrons.

In Renal Hypoplasia, Kidneys Are Histologically Normal but Smaller

Congenital hypoplastic kidneys are formed by six or fewer renal lobes (medullary pyramids with overlying cortex) and have reduced numbers of nephrons. Hypoplastic kidneys usually weigh less than 50% of normal. Hypoplasia must be differentiated from small kidneys due to atrophy or scarring. A frequent variant of hypoplasia features enlargement of the too few glomeruli and thus is called **oligomeganephronia**. This enlargement indicates overwork of too few nephrons and predisposes to developing FSGS.

Renal Ectopia Is a Normal Kidney in an Abnormal Location

The misplaced kidney is usually in the pelvis, due to failure of the fetal kidney to migrate from the pelvis to the flank. One or both kidneys may be affected. In **simple ectopia,** the ureters drain into the appropriate side of the bladder. In **crossed ectopia,** the ectopic kidney is on the same side as its normal mate; the ectopic ureter crosses the midline and drains into the contralateral side of the bladder.

Horseshoe Kidney Is a Single, Large, Midline Organ

The kidneys are fused, usually at the lower poles (Fig. 22-7). This anomaly increases the risk for obstruction and renal infection (pyelonephritis) because the ureters are compressed as they cross over the junction between the two kidneys when the organ is fused at the lower pole.

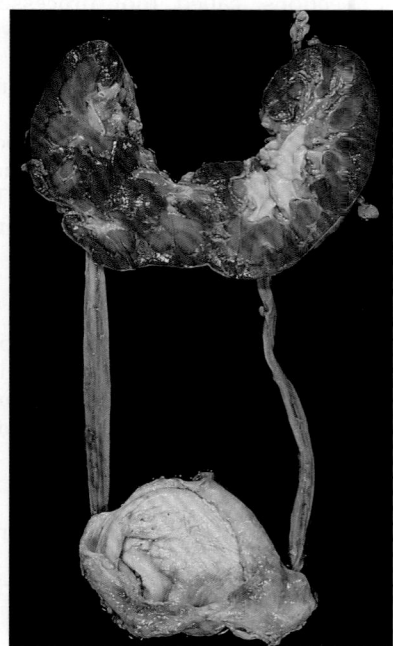

FIGURE 22-7. Horseshoe kidney. The kidneys are fused at the lower pole.

In Renal Dysplasia, Primitive Mesenchyme Surrounds Undifferentiated Tubules

This mesenchyme sometimes contains heterotopic tissue such as cartilage. Cysts often form from the abnormal tubules.

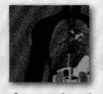 **PATHOPHYSIOLOGY:** Renal dysplasia results from abnormal metanephric differentiation and has multiple genetic and somatic causes. Some familial forms of dysplasia result from abnormal differentiation signals that affect the inductive interactions between the ureteric bud and the metanephric blastema. Many forms of dysplasia are accompanied by other urinary tract abnormalities, especially ones that cause obstruction of urine flow. This association suggests that obstruction to urine flow in utero can cause dysplasia. Frequent associated anomalies include:

- Ureteral agenesis
- Ureteral atresia
- Ureteropelvic junction obstruction
- Ureterovesical stenosis or posterior urethral valves

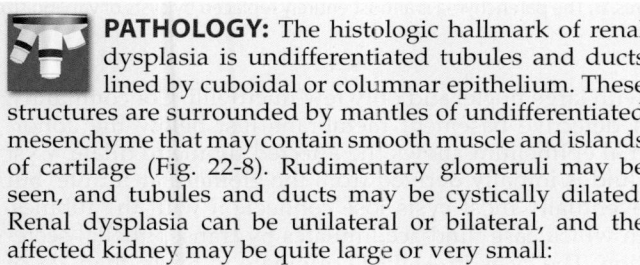 **PATHOLOGY:** The histologic hallmark of renal dysplasia is undifferentiated tubules and ducts lined by cuboidal or columnar epithelium. These structures are surrounded by mantles of undifferentiated mesenchyme that may contain smooth muscle and islands of cartilage (Fig. 22-8). Rudimentary glomeruli may be seen, and tubules and ducts may be cystically dilated. Renal dysplasia can be unilateral or bilateral, and the affected kidney may be quite large or very small:

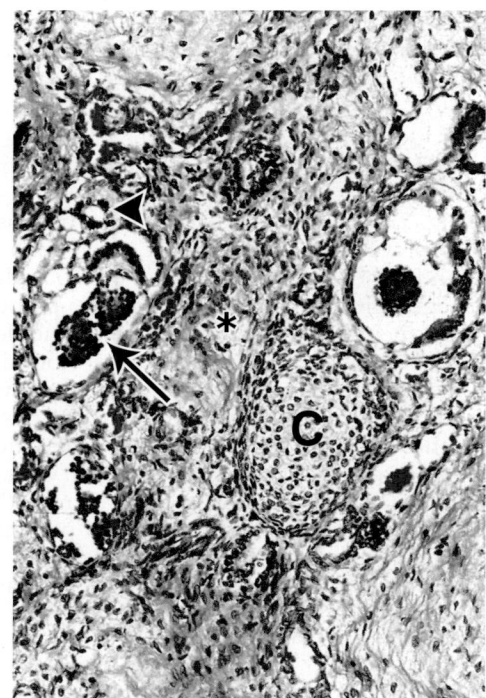

FIGURE 22-8. Renal dysplasia. Immature glomeruli (*arrow*), tubules (*arrowhead*) and cartilage (*C*) are surrounded by loose, undifferentiated mesenchymal tissue (***).

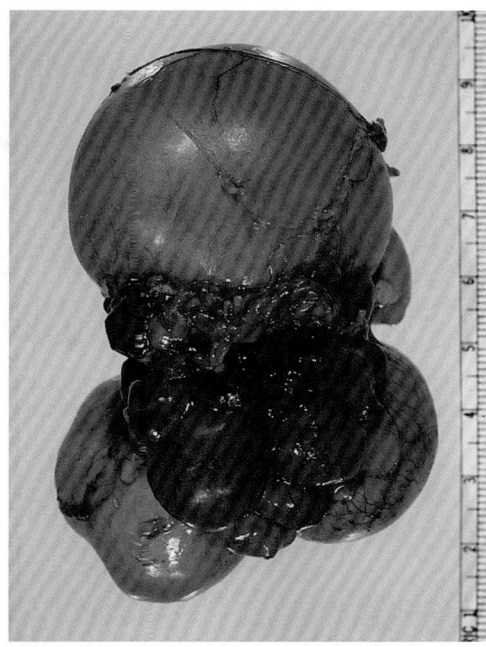

FIGURE 22-9. Multicystic renal dysplasia. This irregular mass of variably sized cysts does not have a reniform shape.

- **Aplastic renal dysplasia** results in very small misshapen dysplastic kidneys, which may be difficult to identify by gross examination.
- **Multicystic renal dysplasia** is usually unilateral and is characterized by renal enlargement by multiple cysts, ranging from microscopic to several centimeters in diameter. The kidney does not have the usual kidney shape but is rather an irregular mass of cysts (Fig. 22-9).
- **Diffuse cystic renal dysplasia** features more uniformly sized cysts and preservation of a kidney shape.
- **Obstructive renal dysplasia,** focal or diffuse, unilateral or bilateral, is caused by intrauterine obstruction to urine flow, such as posterior urethral valves or ureteropelvic junction stenosis.

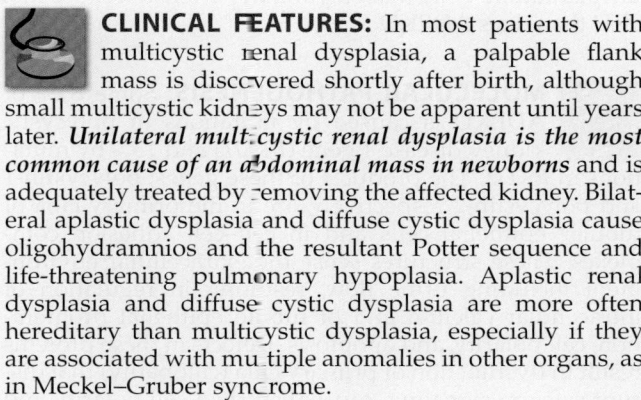 **CLINICAL FEATURES:** In most patients with multicystic renal dysplasia, a palpable flank mass is discovered shortly after birth, although small multicystic kidneys may not be apparent until years later. *Unilateral multicystic renal dysplasia is the most common cause of an abdominal mass in newborns* and is adequately treated by removing the affected kidney. Bilateral aplastic dysplasia and diffuse cystic dysplasia cause oligohydramnios and the resultant Potter sequence and life-threatening pulmonary hypoplasia. Aplastic renal dysplasia and diffuse cystic dysplasia are more often hereditary than multicystic dysplasia, especially if they are associated with multiple anomalies in other organs, as in Meckel–Gruber syndrome.

In Autosomal Dominant Polycystic Kidney Disease, Kidneys Are Enlarged and Multicystic

Autosomal dominant polycystic kidney disease (ADPKD) is the most common of a group of congenital diseases in which

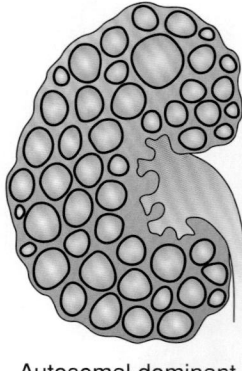
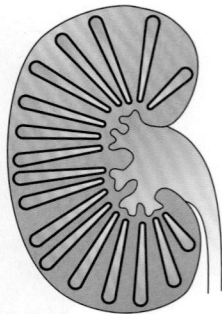

Autosomal dominant polycystic disease

Autosomal recessive polycystic disease

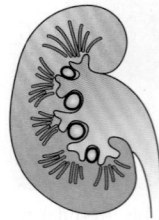
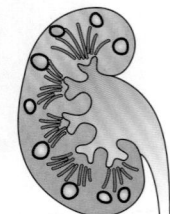

Medullary sponge kidney

Medullary cystic disease

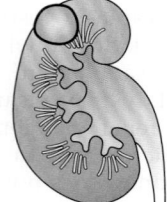

Simple cyst

FIGURE 22-10. Cystic diseases of the kidney.

the renal parenchyma contains many cysts (Fig. 22-10). It affects 1:400 to 1:1,000 people in the United States, 1/2 of whom eventually develop end-stage renal disease (ESRD). ADPKD is responsible for 5% of ESRD requiring dialysis or transplantation. Only diabetes and hypertension cause more ESRD than does ADPKD.

 MOLECULAR PATHOGENESIS: Some 85% of ADPKD is caused by mutations in polycystic kidney disease 1 gene (*PKD1*) and 15% by mutations in *PKD2*. The products of these genes, polycystin-1 and polycystin-2 respectively, are in the primary cilia of tubular epithelial cells and in cell–cell adhesion complexes. These structures sense the extracellular environment including urine flow, resulting in regulation of intracellular calcium and of tubule epithelial proliferation, cell polarity, and apoptosis. Defects in these proteins result in dysfunction of primary cilia (ciliopathy) that disrupt calcium signaling, cause disturbed cell polarity and induce tubular epithelial cell proliferation.

Although the precise pathogenesis of ADPKD remains unclear, it is thought that cysts arise in segments of renal tubules from a few cells that proliferate abnormally. The tubule wall becomes covered by undifferentiated cells

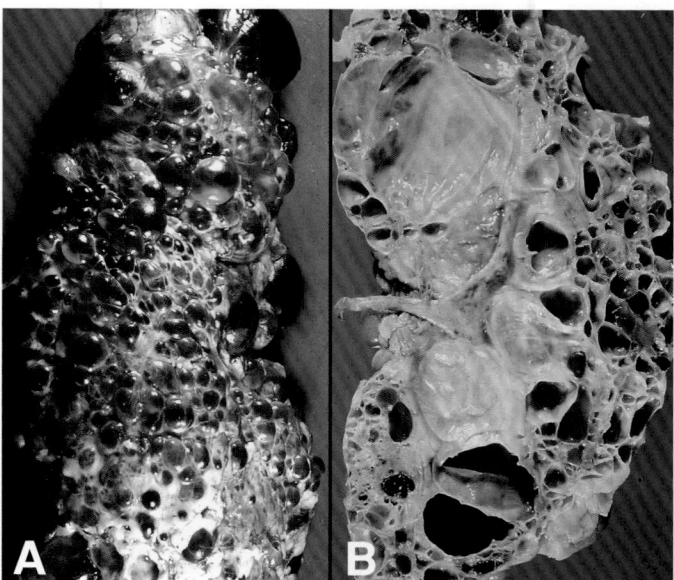

FIGURE 22-11. Autosomal dominant polycystic kidney disease. A. The kidneys are enlarged and studded with multiple fluid-filled structures. **B.** The parenchyma is almost entirely replaced by cysts of varying size.

with large nuclei and only few microvilli. Concomitantly, a defective basement membrane just below the abnormal epithelium allows the affected tubule to dilate. Cyst fluid is initially derived from the glomerular filtrate, but eventually most cysts lose connection with the tubules, in which case fluid accumulates by transepithelial secretion. The cysts in ADPKD originate in fewer than 2% of nephrons. Thus, factors other than crowding of normal tissue by expanding cysts likely impair functional renal tissue. Apoptotic loss of renal tubules and accumulation of inflammatory mediators have been implicated in the destruction of normal renal mass.

 PATHOLOGY: The kidneys in ADPKD are both markedly enlarged and can weigh up to 4,500 g (Fig. 22-11). The external contours are distorted by numerous cysts, as large as 5 cm, filled with straw-colored fluid. These cysts are lined by cuboidal and columnar epithelium. Cysts arise from any point along the nephron, including glomeruli, proximal tubules, distal tubules, and collecting ducts. Areas of normal renal parenchyma between the cysts undergo progressive atrophy and fibrosis as the disease advances with age.

Of patients with ADPKD, 1/3 also have **hepatic cysts,** whose lining resembles bile duct epithelium. Cysts occur in the spleen (10% of patients) and pancreas (5%) as well. **Cerebral aneurysms** occur in 1/5 of patients, and intracranial hemorrhage is the cause of death in 15% of patients with ADPKD. Interestingly, many patients with ADPKD also develop colonic diverticula.

 CLINICAL FEATURES: Most patients with ADPKD do not manifest clinically until the fourth decade of life, which is why this condition was once called *adult* polycystic kidney disease. A small minority of patients develop symptoms during childhood, and only rarely do signs and symptoms occur at birth. Symptoms include a sense of heaviness in the loins, bilateral flank and abdominal pain, and abdominal masses. Hypertension is one of the earliest and most common manifestations. Eventually, hematuria, low-level proteinuria and progressive renal insufficiency develop.

Collecting Ducts Are Cystically Dilated in Infants With Autosomal Recessive Polycystic Kidney Disease

Compared with ADPKD, autosomal recessive polycystic kidney disease (ARPKD) is rare, occurring in about 1 in 6,000 to 140,000 live births. In the neonatal period, 1/4 of these infants die, often because of pulmonary hypoplasia caused by oligohydramnios (Potter sequence) and because the large size of the kidneys impairs lung development and function. Children who survive the neonatal period have varying onset and rate of progression of renal insufficiency as well as hepatic fibrosis with portal hypertension.

MOLECULAR PATHOGENESIS: ARPKD is caused by mutations in *PKHD1*. This gene encodes **fibrocystin,** which is found in the primary cilia of the collecting ducts of the kidney, biliary ducts of the liver, and exocrine ducts of the pancreas. It is involved in regulation of cell differentiation, proliferation, and adhesion. Mutations of *PKHD1* also cause pancreatic cysts and hepatic biliary dysgenesis and fibrosis.

PATHOLOGY: Unlike ADPKD, the external kidney surface in ARPKD is smooth. The disease is invariably bilateral. The kidneys are often so large that delivery of the infant is impeded. The cysts are fusiform dilations of cortical and medullary collecting ducts and have a striking radial arrangement, perpendicular to the renal capsule (Fig. 22-12). Interstitial fibrosis and tubular atrophy are common, particularly in children

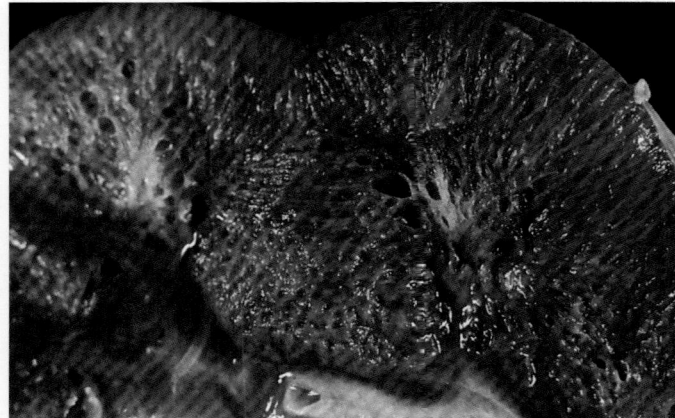

FIGURE 22-12. Autosomal recessive polycystic kidney disease. The dilated cortical and medullary collecting ducts are arranged radially, and the external surface is smooth.

in whom disease presents later. As in ADPKD, the calyceal system is normal. The liver is usually affected by **congenital hepatic fibrosis,** with fibrous expansion of portal tracts with bile duct proliferation (see Chapter 20).

Bowman Capsule Is Dilated in Many Glomeruli in Glomerulocystic Disease

Glomerulocystic kidney disease may be an isolated process or a component of other cystic disease, such as ADPKD, nephronophthisis–medullary cystic disease complex, and diffuse cystic dysplasia. Thus, glomerulocystic disease has multiple causes. Familial forms are caused by mutations in the gene for hepatocyte nuclear factor-1β (*HNF-1β*). Also known as *TCF2*, this gene encodes a transcription factor that plays fundamental roles in hepatic and renal development.

PATHOLOGY: The kidneys may be large or small. The cut surface reveals numerous small round cysts rarely more than 1 cm in diameter. Light microscopy shows dilation of the Bowman capsule in many glomeruli. The residual glomerular tuft is often distorted or appears immature.

Nephronophthisis and Medullary Cystic Disease Cause Tubulointerstitial Injury and Medullary Cysts

MOLECULAR PATHOGENESIS: Nephronophthisis and medullary cystic disease both cause pathologically similar progressive medullary tubulointerstitial disease. However, they have different genetic causes and inheritance patterns. Nephronophthisis is autosomal recessive, with onset in infancy, childhood, or adolescence. It is caused by mutations in many genes that encode proteins expressed in centrosomes and primary cilia, including *NPHP* genes (*NPHP1* through *10* identified to date). Their gene products, nephrocystins, link primary cilia to the *PKD* and *PKHD* gene products, also in primary cilia. Medullary cystic kidney disease (MCKD) is autosomal dominant with onset in adolescence and renal failure in adulthood. It has two main forms. MCKD1 is caused by mutations in *MUC1*, which encodes a protein called mucin 1. In addition to its role as a component of mucus, mucin 1 regulates cell growth and adhesion in the kidney. MCKD2 is caused by mutations in *UMOD*, the gene that encodes a protein called uromodulin. This protein regulates excretion of uric acid, and it is normally secreted in the urine. When mutated, it can accumulate in cells and apparently induce apoptosis.

PATHOLOGY: The kidneys often, but not always, have multiple, variably sized cysts (up to 1 cm) at the corticomedullary junction (Fig. 22-10). These cysts arise from distal portions of the nephron. Atrophic tubules with markedly thickened and laminated basement membranes and loss of tubules out of proportion to glomerular loss are early histologic features of the disease. Eventually, corticomedullary cysts may develop, and the

THE KIDNEY

rest of the parenchyma becomes increasingly atrophic. Secondary glomerular sclerosis, interstitial fibrosis, and nonspecific inflammatory infiltrates dominate the late histologic picture.

CLINICAL FEATURES: Patients present initially with deteriorating tubular function, such as impaired concentrating ability and sodium wasting, manifested as polyuria, polydipsia, and enuresis (bed-wetting). Progressive azotemia and renal failure follow. Nephronophthisis is seen in three clinical variants: infantile, juvenile, and adolescent. The juvenile form is most common and accounts for 5% to 10% of ESRD in children. Symptoms begin between 4 and 6 years, and ESRD usually develops within 10 years. The onset and progression to ESRD of adolescent nephronophthisis overlap with the juvenile form, but the adolescent form results from defects in *NEPH3* and more often causes ESRD at 10 to 20 years. Defects in *NPHP2* are most common in the infantile form, which progresses to ESRD before 2 years. Among all patients with nephronophthisis, the *NEPH1* mutation is most common.

Medullary cystic disease is characterized by onset of renal failure after the fourth decade and usually presents with polyuria. Hyperuricemia and gout, related to defects in uromodulin, may be accompanying findings.

Medullary Sponge Kidney Is Distinguished by Cysts in the Papillae

The papillary cysts are multiple and small (<5 mm in diameter) (Fig. 22-10). They arise from collecting ducts in the renal papillae and are lined by cuboidal or columnar epithelium. The disease is bilateral in 75% of patients. It is usually sporadic but a few familial cases have been described.

Medullary sponge kidney is asymptomatic in young adults. Symptomatic cases are usually discovered between the ages of 30 and 60 years, presenting with flank pain, dysuria, hematuria, or "gravel" in the urine caused by stone formation in the cysts. Although the disease itself does not pose a threat to health, the cysts may predispose to secondary pyelonephritis.

ACQUIRED CYSTIC KIDNEY DISEASE

Simple Renal Cysts Occur in Half of People Older Than 50 Years

Simple cysts are usually incidental findings at autopsy and are rarely clinically symptomatic unless they become very large. They may be solitary or multiple and are usually found in the outer cortex, where they bulge the capsule. Simple cysts occur less commonly in the medulla. Microscopically, they are lined by flat epithelium.

Long-Term Dialysis Leads to Acquired Cystic Disease

Multiple cortical and medullary cysts may form in kidneys of patients with ESRD who are maintained on dialysis. After 5 years of dialysis, more than 75% of patients show bilateral cystic kidneys. The cysts are initially lined by flat-to-cuboidal epithelium, but hyperplastic and neoplastic epithelial proliferation may develop within 10 years of initiating dialysis. **Renal cell carcinoma (RCC)** develops in approximately 5% of patients with acquired cystic disease.

Acquired Nonneoplastic Diseases of the Kidney

GLOMERULAR DISEASES

Many renal disorders are caused by injury to the glomerulus that can produce acute kidney injury (AKI) or chronic kidney disease (CKD). Glomeruli may be the only major site of disease (primary glomerular disease; e.g., immunoglobulin [Ig]A nephropathy) or part of a systemic disease affecting several organs (secondary glomerular disease; e.g., lupus glomerulonephritis). Signs and symptoms of glomerular disease fall into one of the following categories:

- Asymptomatic proteinuria
- Nephrotic syndrome
- Asymptomatic hematuria
- Nephritic syndrome
- Rapidly progressive nephritic syndrome
- CKD
- ESRD

Proteinuria Exceeds 3.5 g/day in Nephrotic Syndrome

It is also characterized by hypoalbuminemia, edema, hyperlipidemia, and lipiduria. Increased glomerular capillary wall permeability allows loss of protein from plasma into the urine (proteinuria). Proteinuria is caused by many different glomerular diseases and by a variety of mechanisms.

Severe proteinuria causes the nephrotic syndrome (Fig. 22-13), but lower levels of proteinuria may be asymptomatic. Nephrotic syndrome results from **primary** glomerular diseases unrelated to a systemic disease, or they may be **secondary** to a systemic disease that affects other organs as well as the kidneys. Diabetic glomerulosclerosis is the most common cause of secondary nephrotic syndrome in adults. Table 22-1 lists the major causes and approximate frequency of the primary nephrotic syndromes in adults and children. Table 22-2 details selected pathologic features of some of these diseases (discussed below).

The incidence of specific glomerular diseases that cause nephrotic syndrome varies considerably in adults and children. For example, minimal-change disease is responsible for most (70%) cases of primary nephrotic syndrome in children, but only 15% in adults. The primary glomerular diseases that most often cause nephrotic syndrome in adults are membranous nephropathy and FSGS. The most common cause of secondary nephrotic syndrome in adults is diabetes. Membranous nephropathy is the most frequent cause in whites and Asians, whereas FSGS is the most common etiology in American blacks. The incidence of FSGS has been increasing over the past decade. Systemic diseases that involve the kidney, such as diabetes, amyloidosis, and

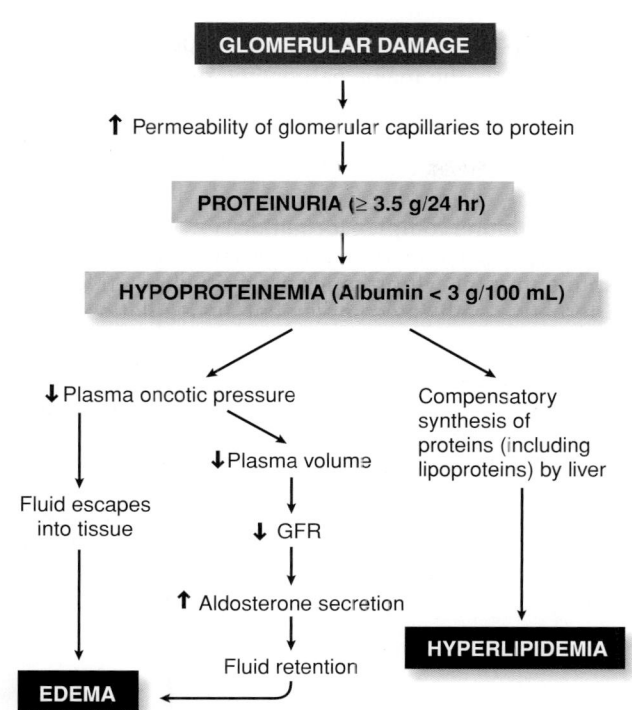

FIGURE 22-13. Pathophysiology of the nephrotic syndrome. *GFR* = glomerular filtration rate.

systemic lupus erythematosus (SLE), account for many of the remaining cases of nephrotic syndrome in adults. In third world countries, where chronic infectious diseases are common, infection-induced immune complex-mediated glomerulonephritis is a frequent cause of nephrotic syndrome.

Nephritic (Glomerulonephritis) Syndrome Is an Inflammatory Disease With Hematuria, Proteinuria, and Decreased Glomerular Filtration Rate

Hematuria may be microscopic or grossly visible, and proteinuria varies. Decreased GFR causes elevated blood urea nitrogen and serum creatinine, oliguria, salt and water retention, hypertension, and edema. Glomerular diseases associated with the nephritic syndrome are caused by inflammatory changes in glomeruli (e.g., infiltration by leukocytes, hyperplasia of glomerular cells and, in severe

Cause	Children (%)	Adults (%)
Minimal-change disease	75	10
Membranous nephropathy	5	30
Focal segmental glomerulosclerosis	10	35
Membranoproliferative glomerulo-nephritis	5	5
Other glomerular diseases[a]	5	20

TABLE 22-1

FREQUENCY OF CAUSES OF THE NEPHROTIC SYNDROME INDUCED BY PRIMARY GLOMERULAR DISEASES IN CHILDREN AND ADULTS

[a]Includes many forms of mesangioproliferative and proliferative glomerulonephritis, such as immunoglobulin A nephropathy, which may cause nephritic and nephrotic features.

lesions, necrosis). Injury to glomerular capillaries results in spillage of protein and blood cells into the urine (proteinuria and hematuria). The inflammatory damage may also impair glomerular flow and filtration, resulting in renal insufficiency, fluid retention, and hypertension. Nephritic manifestations may: (1) develop rapidly and result in reversible renal insufficiency (acute glomerulonephritis); (2) progress rapidly, with renal failure that resolves only with aggressive treatment (rapidly progressive glomerulonephritis); or (3) persist for years continuously or intermittently and proceed slowly to renal failure (chronic glomerulonephritis).

Some glomerular diseases tend to cause the nephrotic syndrome, while others lead to the nephritic syndrome (Table 22-3). However, except for minimal-change disease (which almost always causes nephrotic syndrome), all glomerular diseases may occasionally cause mixed nephritic and nephrotic manifestations that confound clinical diagnosis. *Renal biopsy evaluation is the only means of definitive diagnosis for most glomerular diseases, although clinical and laboratory data may provide presumptive evidence for a specific disease.*

 PATHOPHYSIOLOGY: Glomerulonephritis is often caused by immunologic mechanisms. Antibody- and cell-mediated immunity may both lead to glomerular inflammation, but three types of

TABLE 22-2

PATHOLOGIC FEATURES OF IMPORTANT CAUSES OF THE NEPHROTIC SYNDROME

	Minimal-Change Disease	Focal Segmental Glomerulosclerosis	Membranous Nephropathy	Membranoproliferative Glomerulonephritis
Light microscopy	No lesion	Focal and segmental glomerular consolidation	Diffuse global capillary wall thickening	Capillary wall thickening and endocapillary hypercellularity
Immunofluorescence microscopy	No immune deposits	No immune deposits	Diffuse capillary wall immunoglobulin	Diffuse capillary wall complement with or without immunoglobulin
Electron microscopy	No immune deposits	No immune deposits	Diffuse subepithelial deposits	Subendothelial dense deposits; intramembranous dense deposits (dense deposit disease)

TABLE 22-3

TENDENCIES OF GLOMERULAR DISEASES TO MANIFEST NEPHROTIC AND NEPHRITIC FEATURES

Disease	Nephrotic	Nephritic
Minimal-change disease	++++	–
Membranous nephropathy	+++	++
Focal segmental glomerulosclerosis	+++	++
Mesangioproliferative glomerulonephritis[a]	++	++
Membranoproliferative glomerulonephritis	++	++
Proliferative glomerulonephritis[a]	+	+++
Crescentic glomerulonephritis[a]	+	++++

[a]These histologic phenotypes can be caused by many categories of glomerular disease, including immunoglobulin A nephropathy, postinfectious glomerulonephritis, lupus glomerulonephritis, antineutrophil cytoplasmic autoantibody glomerulonephritis, anti–glomerular basement membrane glomerulonephritis, and C3 glomerulopathy.

antibody-induced inflammatory mechanisms have been incriminated as the major pathogenic processes in most forms of glomerulonephritis (Fig. 22-14). A fourth less frequent cause of glomerulonephritis is dysregulation and uncontrolled activation of the alternative complement pathway.

- *In situ* immune complex formation
- Deposition of circulating immune complexes
- Antineutrophil cytoplasmic autoantibodies (ANCAs)
- Alternative pathway complement dysregulation

Immune complex formation *in situ* involves binding by circulating antibodies to intrinsic antigens or foreign antigens within glomeruli. For example, circulating anti-GBM autoantibodies bind a specific epitope on the α4 chain of type IV collagen in GBMs. Resultant immune complexes in glomerular capillary walls attract leukocytes and activate complement and other humoral inflammatory mediators, resulting in inflammatory injury. In the most common form of primary membranous nephropathy, immune complexes form *in situ* between an antigen

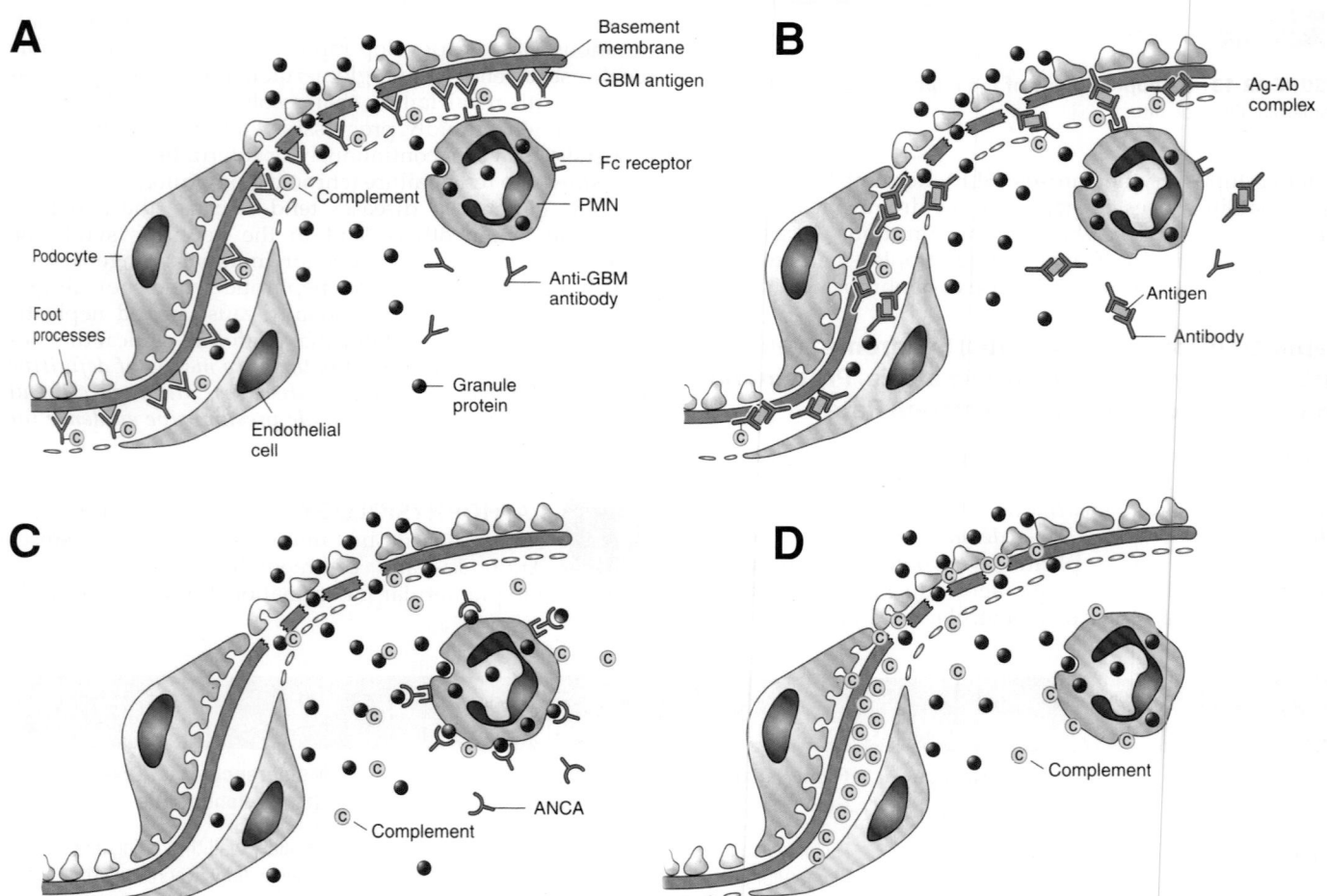

FIGURE 22-14. Pathogenesis of immune-mediated glomerulonephritis. A. Anti–glomerular basement membrane (GBM) antibodies cause glomerulonephritis by binding *in situ* to basement membrane antigens. This activates complement and recruits inflammatory cells. *PMN* = polymorphonuclear neutrophil. **B.** Immune complexes that deposit from the circulation also activate complement and recruit inflammatory cells. Ag-Ab complex = antigen–antibody complex. **C.** Antineutrophil cytoplasmic antibodies (ANCAs) cause inflammation by activating leukocytes via direct binding of the antibodies to the leukocytes and by Fc receptor engagement of ANCA bound to antigen. **D.** As in A, B, and C, complement is activated and deposits in glomeruli to cause inflammation; however, this results primarily from dysregulation of complement activation in the absence of substantial immunoglobulin deposits.

produced by podocytes, phospholipase A₂ receptor (PLA₂R) and anti-PLA₂R antibodies in the circulation.

Circulating immune complexes may deposit in glomeruli and incite inflammation like that produced when immune complexes form *in situ*. For example, circulating antibodies can bind to antigens released into the blood by bacterial or viral infection to produce immune complexes. If these complexes escape phagocytosis, they can deposit in glomeruli and incite inflammation. Immunofluorescence microscopy detects such immune complexes in glomeruli. Anti-GBM antibodies produce linear staining of GBMs, but other immune complexes produce granular staining in capillary walls, mesangium, or both.

ANCAs cause severe glomerulonephritis with little or no glomerular immunoglobulin deposition. Such patients often have circulating autoantibodies specific for antigens in the cytoplasm of neutrophils, which activate them and thereby mediate glomerular inflammation. Most ANCAs are directed against myeloperoxidase (MPO-ANCA) or proteinase-3 (PR3-ANCA). Even minor stimulation of neutrophils and monocytes, such as by increased circulating levels of cytokines during viral infection, causes them to express surface MPO and PR3, which then can interact with ANCAs. This interaction activates neutrophils and causes them to adhere to microvascular endothelial cells, especially glomerular capillaries. There, they release products that promote vascular inflammation, including glomerulonephritis, arteritis, and venulitis. This inflammation is amplified by release of factors from ANCA-activated neutrophils that activate the alternative complement pathway.

Formation of glomerular immune complexes *in situ*, deposition of immune complexes and interaction of ANCAs with leukocytes all initiate glomerular inflammatory injury, with attraction and activation of leukocytes (Fig. 22-14).

A fourth immunopathology category of glomerulonephritis **(C3 glomerulopathy)** is mediated by dysregulation of the alternative complement pathway caused either by the genetic absence or dysfunction of complement regulatory proteins (e.g., complement factor H, complement factor I), autoantibodies that inhibit complement regulatory proteins or autoantibodies that stabilize the alternative pathway C3 convertase (C3 nephritis factor).

 PATHOLOGY: Specific glomerular diseases have distinctive pathologic features, as well as different natural histories and appropriate treatments. *Accurate pathologic diagnosis of glomerular diseases requires examination of renal tissue by light, immunofluorescence and electron microscopy, and integration of these findings with clinical information.* Table 22-4 lists pathologic features used in diagnosing glomerular diseases (see Table 22-2 for a summary of pathologic features of important causes of the nephrotic syndrome). The algorithm in Figure 22-15 shows how pathologic and clinical data mesh to diagnose specific glomerular diseases.

In general, pathologic features of acute inflammation, such as leukocyte infiltration and necrosis, and crescent formation, are more common in patients with nephritic rather than nephrotic clinical signs and symptoms. **Glomerular crescent formation** (extracapillary hypercellularity in Bowman space) correlates with a more

---

TABLE 22-4

DIAGNOSTIC FEATURES OF GLOMERULAR DISEASES

I. Light microscopic features
A. Increased cellularity
   Hyperplasia of mesangial cells and endothelial cells
   Accumulation of leukocytes (e.g., neutrophils, monocytes, macrophages) in capillary lumens and mesangium
   Increased cells in Bowman space (crescent formation) caused by epithelial proliferation and influx of leukocytes.
B. Increased extracellular material
   Localization of immune complexes
   Thickening or reduplication of GBM
   Increases in collagenous matrix (sclerosis)
   Insudation of plasma proteins (hyalinosis)
   Fibrinoid necrosis
   Deposition of amyloid

II. Immunofluorescence features
A. Linear staining of GBM
   Anti-GBM antibodies
   Multiple plasma proteins (e.g., diabetic glomerulosclerosis)
   Monoclonal immunoglobulin heavy and light chains
B. Granular immune complex staining or complement staining alone
   Mesangium (e.g., IgA nephropathy)
   Capillary wall (e.g., membranous nephropathy)
   Mesangium and capillary wall (e.g., lupus glomerulonephritis, C3 glomerulopathy)
C. Irregular amorphous staining
   Monoclonal light chains (AL amyloidosis)
   AA protein (AA amyloidosis)
   IgG, C3, and DnaJ heat shock protein B9 (DNAJB9) (fibrillary glomerulonephritis)

III. Electron microscopic features
A. Electron-dense immune complex deposits or complement deposits
   Mesangial (e.g., IgA nephropathy)
   Subendothelial (e.g., lupus glomerulonephritis)
   Subepithelial (e.g., membranous nephropathy)
B. GBM thickening (e.g., diabetic glomerulosclerosis)
C. GBM remodeling (e.g., membranoproliferative glomerulonephritis)
D. Collagenous matrix expansion (e.g., focal segmental glomerulosclerosis)
E. Fibrillar deposits (e.g., amyloidosis, fibrillary glomerulonephritis)

GBM = glomerular basement membrane; IgA = immunoglobulin A.

---

rapidly progressive course. Crescents are not specific for a particular cause of glomerular inflammation. They are, rather, markers of severe injury causing extensive rupture of capillary walls, which allows inflammatory mediators to enter the Bowman space, where they stimulate macrophage infiltration and epithelial proliferation.

Minimal-Change Disease Causes Nephrotic Syndrome

Pathologically, this disease entails global effacement of podocyte foot processes.

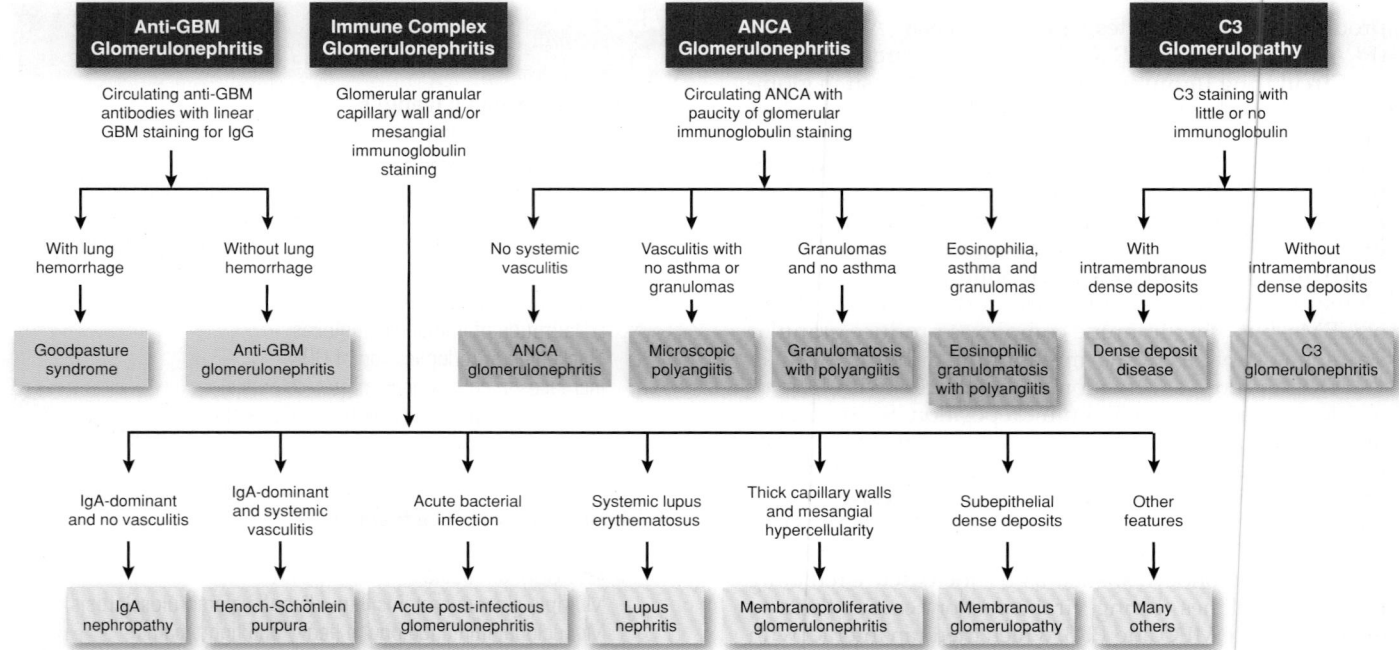

FIGURE 22-15. Algorithm demonstrating the integration of pathologic findings with clinical data to diagnose specific forms of primary or secondary glomerulonephritis. The important initial categorization includes anti–glomerular basement membrane glomerulonephritis (anti-GBM), immune complex glomerulonephritis, antineutrophil cytoplasmic autoantibody (ANCA) glomerulonephritis, or C3 glomerulopathy. Once this determination is made, a more specific diagnosis depends on additional clinical or pathologic observations.

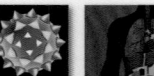 **ETIOLOGY AND PATHOPHYSIOLOGY:** Minimal-change disease occurs as a primary (idiopathic) form especially in children and as a secondary form especially in adults due to infection (e.g., HIV, mononucleosis), allergy (e.g., drugs especially nonsteroidal anti-inflammatory drugs, immunization, bee venom), and lymphomas (e.g., Hodgkin, mantle-cell). The pathogenesis of idiopathic (primary) minimal-change disease is unknown. The immune system may be involved: the disease may remit with corticosteroid treatment, and it may occur in association with an allergic disease or a lymphoid neoplasm. Occasional associations with Hodgkin disease (in which there is T-cell dysfunction) and with thymomas and T-cell lymphomas has led to speculation that minimal-change disease may reflect a disorder of T lymphocytes, possibly involving production of a cytokine(s) that increases glomerular permeability via effects on podocytes. The heavy proteinuria of minimal-change disease is accompanied by loss of GBM and podocyte polyanionic sites. This allows anionic proteins, especially albumin, to pass more readily across capillary walls. There may be a pathogenic relationship between minimal-change disease and some forms of FSGS, with the potential for the former to evolve into the latter in some patients, but this has not been confirmed.

PATHOLOGY: *Glomeruli in minimal-change disease appear essentially normal on light microscopy* (Fig. 22-16). Proteinuria leads to hypoalbuminemia, and a compensatory increase in lipoprotein secretion by the liver results in hyperlipidemia.

Loss of lipoproteins through glomeruli causes lipids to accumulate in proximal tubular cells, reflected histologically as glassy (hyaline) droplets in tubular epithelial cytoplasm. Such droplets are not specific for minimal-change disease but can also be seen in any glomerular disease causing nephrotic syndrome.

Electron microscopy shows extensive (>75%)/global **fusion of podocyte cell foot processes** (Figs. 22-17 and 22-18). This occurs in almost all cases of nephrotic range proteinuria; it is not specific for minimal-change disease. Immunofluorescence studies for immunoglobulin and complement deposition are most often negative, but there

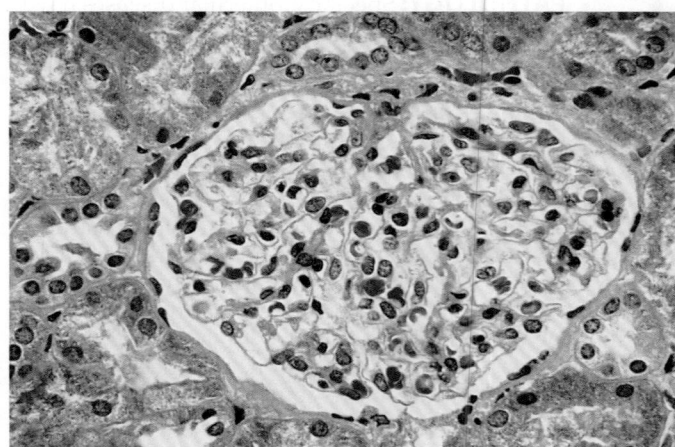

FIGURE 22-16. Minimal-change disease. A light micrograph shows no abnormality.

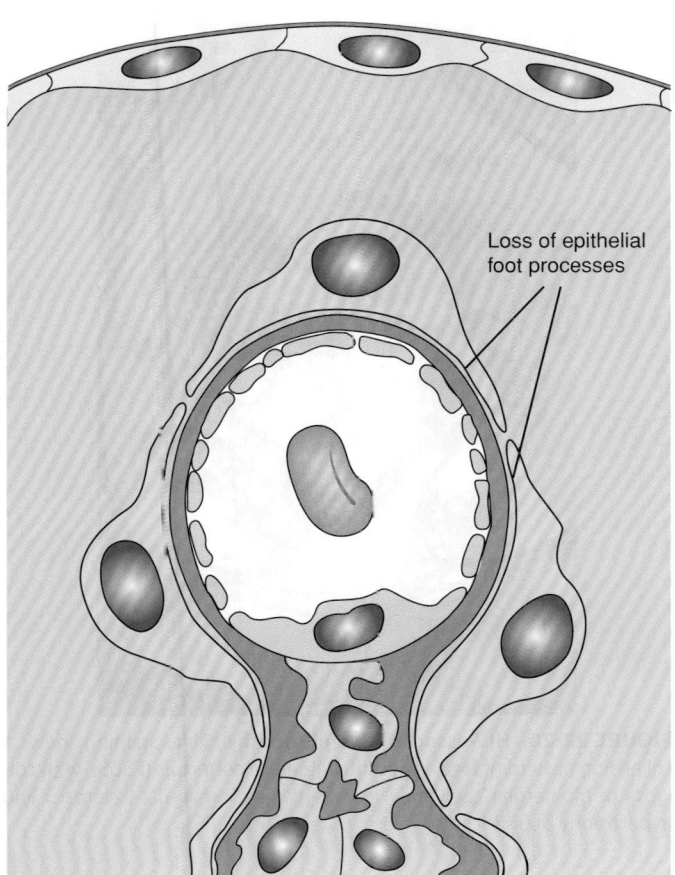

FIGURE 22-17. **Minimal-change disease.** This condition is characterized mainly by epithelial cell changes, particularly effacement of foot processes. All other glomerular structures appear intact.

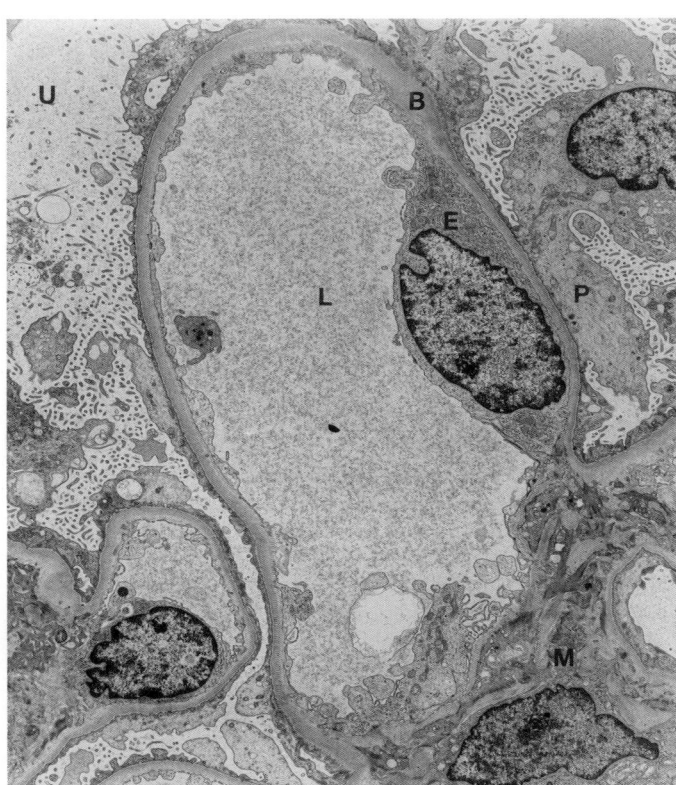

FIGURE 22-18. **Minimal-change disease.** In this electron micrograph, the podocyte (*P*) displays extensive effacement of foot processes and has numerous microvilli projecting into the urinary space (*U*). *B* = basement membrane; *E* = endothelial cell; *L* = lumen; *M* = mesangial cell. Compare with Figure 22-3.

is occasional weak mesangial staining for IgM and the complement component C3.

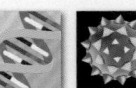

CLINICAL FEATURES: *Minimal-change disease causes 90% of primary nephrotic syndrome cases in children younger than 5, 50% in older children, and 15% in adults.* Proteinuria is generally more selective (albumin > globulins) than in the nephrotic syndrome caused by other diseases, but there is too much overlap for this to be a useful diagnostic criterion. In more than 90% of children and in fewer adults with minimal-change disease, proteinuria remits completely within 8 weeks of initiating corticosteroid therapy. Adults often require a longer course of steroids for remission. If corticosteroids are withdrawn, most patients experience intermittent relapses for up to 10 years. A small subgroup of patients has only partial remission with corticosteroid therapy and continues to lose protein in the urine. An even smaller group is totally resistant to corticosteroid therapy. In such cases, the diagnosis of minimal-change disease may not be correct, and FSGS not sampled in the initial biopsy specimen may be present.

In the absence of complications, the long-term outlook for patients with minimal-change disease is no different from that of the general population. Development of azotemia in a patient previously diagnosed as having minimal-change disease should suggest failure to sample FSGS in the original biopsy. It may also reflect evolution into FSGS or perhaps a complication such as drug-induced interstitial nephritis.

Focal Segmental Glomerulosclerosis May Reflect Diverse Etiologies and Pathogenic Mechanisms

In FSGS, glomerular consolidation affects some (focal), but not all, glomeruli and initially involves only part of an affected glomerular tuft (segmental). Consolidated segments often show increased collagenous matrix (sclerosis; Fig. 22-19). There are primary (idiopathic) and secondary forms of FSGS.

MOLECULAR PATHOGENESIS AND ETIOLOGIC FACTORS: The term **FSGS** is a pattern of injury rather than a specific disease and it has many different etiologies, pathogenic mechanisms, responses to treatment, and outcomes. It may be idiopathic (primary) or secondary to a diverse group of conditions (Table 22-5). Multiple factors lead to a final common pathway of injury. Pathologic features and genetic evidence suggest that injury to podocytes may be common to all types of FSGS.

Some forms of FSGS are caused by genetic abnormalities in podocyte proteins (e.g., podocin, nephrin, α-actinin-4,

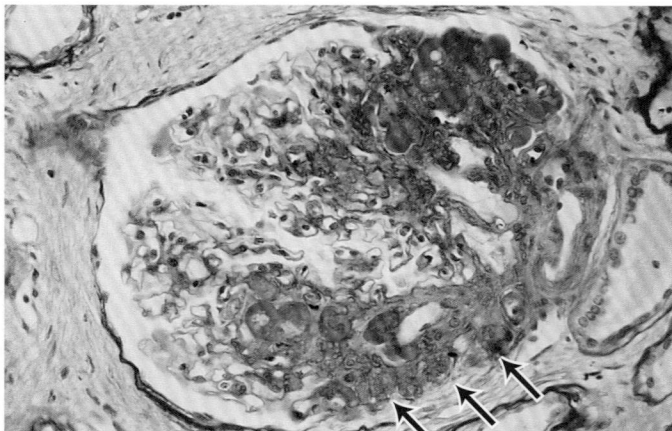

FIGURE 22-19. Focal segmental glomerulosclerosis. Periodic acid–Schiff (PAS) staining shows perihilar areas of segmental sclerosis and adjacent adhesions to the Bowman capsule (*arrows*).

TRPC6, collagen 4). This implicates injury to, or dysfunction of, podocytes in FSGS.

Congenital (e.g., unilateral agenesis with contralateral hypoplasia) and acquired (e.g., reflux nephropathy) reductions in renal mass place adaptive stress on the reduced number of nephrons. In turn, this strain appears to cause FSGS from overwork, with increased glomerular capillary pressure and filtration, and glomerular enlargement. A normal amount of renal tissue can also be stressed by excessive body mass (obesity), resulting in FSGS. Reduced blood oxygen (e.g., as in sickle cell disease or cyanotic congenital heart disease) also causes a similar pattern of glomerular injury. In all of these settings, glomerular enlargement reflects functional overwork, placing undue stress on podocytes because of their limited proliferative capacity.

Viruses, drugs, and serum factors are implicated as causes of FSGS. Infection with HIV, especially in blacks, is associated with a specific variant of FSGS with a collapsing pattern of sclerosis (Fig. 22-20). Such an appearance may also occur in an idiopathic form of FSGS. Collapsing FSGS may also be caused by viral infection of podocytes.

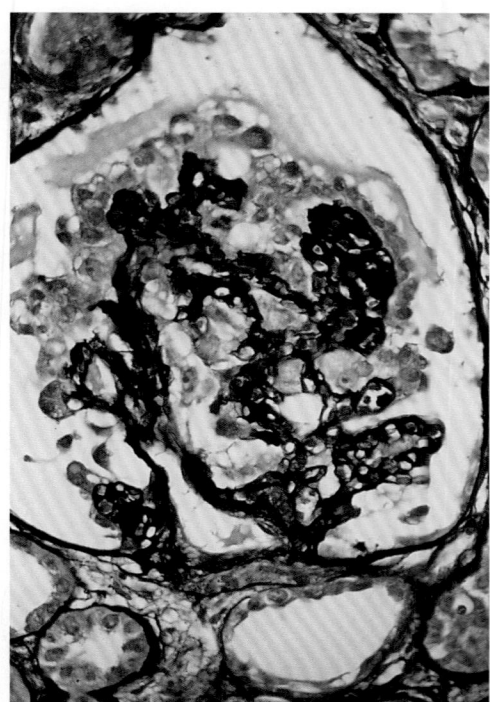

FIGURE 22-20. HIV-associated nephropathy. Silver staining shows a collapsing pattern of focal segmental glomerulosclerosis (FSGS), with collapse of glomerular capillaries, increased matrix material (sclerosis) and hypertrophy of podocytes.

Pamidronate, a drug used to treat osteolytic bone disease in patients with cancer, causes collapsing FSGS in some patients. The drug probably causes FSGS by injuring podocytes.

A serum permeability factor has been detected in some patients with FSGS, which suggests a systemic cause for the glomerular injury. This is further supported by the recurrence of FSGS in renal transplants, especially in patients who have the permeability factor. Sequence variants in the gene encoding apolipoprotein 1 (*APOL1*) have been linked to FSGS in blacks, who are known to have a high incidence of FSGS and hypertension-related ESRD. Apparently, these variants provide protection against African sleeping sickness (trypanosomiasis), which may explain their prevalence in blacks. As in sickle cell disease, this is an example of how a genetic variant can cause a common disease while providing protection against a major infectious disease.

TABLE 22-5

CATEGORIES OF FOCAL SEGMENTAL GLOMERULOSCLEROSIS (A PATTERN OF INJURY)

Primary (idiopathic) focal segmental glomerulosclerosis (FSGS)

Secondary FSGS

  Hereditary/genetic (e.g., mutations in podocyte genes)

  Obesity (perihilar variant)

  Reduced renal mass (perihilar variant)

  Cyanotic congenital heart disease (usually perihilar variant)

  Sickle cell nephropathy (usually perihilar variant)

  Infection induced (e.g., HIV; collapsing variant)

  Drug induced (e.g., pamidronate; collapsing variant)

Note: Primary and secondary FSGS can have various histologic patterns of injury: perihilar, tip lesion, cellular, collapsing, not otherwise specified (NOS).

PATHOLOGY: Varying numbers of glomeruli show segmental obliteration of capillary loops by increased matrix or accumulation of cells, or both. Insudation of plasma proteins and lipid gives lesions a glassy appearance, called **hyalinosis**. Adhesions to the Bowman capsule occur adjacent to sclerotic lesions. Uninvolved glomeruli may look entirely normal, although mild mesangial hypercellularity is occasionally present. Because uninvolved glomeruli usually appear normal, FSGS can be mistaken for minimal-change disease in small biopsy specimens that contain only nonsclerotic glomeruli.

Several histologic variants of FSGS are recognized. Particularly in patients with reduced renal mass or obesity, the sclerosis localizes in **perihilar** segments within glomeruli and in deep cortical (juxtamedullary) glomeruli (Fig. 22-19). A **collapsing** pattern of sclerosis with hypertrophied and hyperplastic podocytes adjacent to sclerotic segments is typical of HIV-associated nephropathy and also occurs with intravenous drug abuse, with pamidronate-induced disease and as an idiopathic process. This collapsing variant has a poor prognosis, and 1/2 of patients reach end-stage disease within 2 years. Sclerosis limited to glomerular segments adjacent to the origin of the proximal tubule has been designated **tip lesion** and is more likely to respond to steroid therapy than other forms of FSGS. A **cellular variant** of FSGS has prominent lipid-laden cells within the sites of glomerular consolidation.

By electron microscopy, epithelial cell foot processes are diffusely effaced in FSGS, with occasional focal detachment or loss of podocytes from the GBM. Sclerotic segments show increased matrix material, wrinkling and thickening of basement membranes, and capillary collapse. Accumulation of electron-dense material in sclerotic segments represents insudative trapping of plasma proteins and corresponds to hyalinosis seen by light microscopy. *Immune complexes are absent.*

Immunofluorescence microscopy shows irregular trapping of IgM and C3 in the segmental areas of sclerosis and hyalinosis. IgG, C4, and C1q are less often found in sclerotic segments. Nonsclerotic segments do not stain or do so weakly, usually for IgM and C3 in the mesangium.

 CLINICAL FEATURES: FSGS causes 1/3 of primary nephrotic syndrome in adults and 10% in children. It is more common in blacks than in whites and is the leading cause of primary nephrotic syndrome in blacks. Its frequency has been increasing over the past few decades for unknown reasons. Clinical presentations and outcomes vary among the different patterns of injury. Most often, asymptomatic proteinuria begins insidiously and progresses to the nephrotic syndrome. Many patients are hypertensive. Microscopic hematuria is frequent.

Most people with FSGS show persistent proteinuria and progressive decline in renal function. Many progress to ESRD after 5 to 20 years. Some, but not all, patients improve with corticosteroid therapy. Although renal transplantation is the preferred treatment for ESRD, FSGS recurs in 1/2 of transplanted kidneys.

Patients with FSGS due to obesity or reduced renal mass usually have a more indolent course with lower levels of proteinuria that benefits from treatment with angiotensin-converting enzyme (ACE) inhibitors or angiotensin receptor blockers (ARBs). People with the tip lesion variant often present with severe nephrotic syndrome. This variant resembles minimal-change disease and responds better to corticosteroids than do other forms of FSGS. HIV-associated and idiopathic collapsing FSGS have the worst prognoses. They are typically associated with severe nephrotic syndrome and renal failure, often progressing to ESRD within a year.

HIV-1–Associated Nephropathy Is a Severe, Rapidly Progressive Collapsing Form of FSGS

 ETIOLOGIC FACTORS: Nephropathy in patients with HIV-1 infection could be caused by HIV-1 within the renal parenchyma. An alternative hypothesis proposes that the nephropathy is caused by another virus that has infected the kidney of an immunocompromised person.

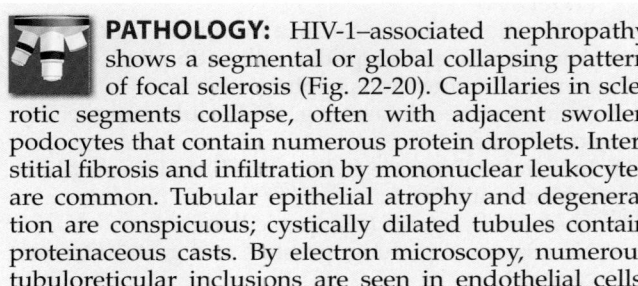 **PATHOLOGY:** HIV-1–associated nephropathy shows a segmental or global collapsing pattern of focal sclerosis (Fig. 22-20). Capillaries in sclerotic segments collapse, often with adjacent swollen podocytes that contain numerous protein droplets. Interstitial fibrosis and infiltration by mononuclear leukocytes are common. Tubular epithelial atrophy and degeneration are conspicuous; cystically dilated tubules contain proteinaceous casts. By electron microscopy, numerous tubuloreticular inclusions are seen in endothelial cells, similar to those in lupus nephritis.

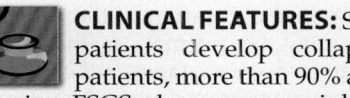 **CLINICAL FEATURES:** Some 5% of HIV-positive patients develop collapsing FSGS. Of these patients, more than 90% are black. Idiopathic collapsing FSGS also occurs mainly in blacks. It presents with severe proteinuria (often >10 g/day) and renal insufficiency. More than 1/2 of patients progress to ESRD in less than 2 years.

Membranous Nephropathy Is a Disease of Immune Complex Deposition

Membranous nephropathy is a common cause of nephrotic syndrome in adults. It reflects subepithelial immune complex accumulation in glomerular capillaries.

PATHOPHYSIOLOGY: Immune complexes localize in the **subepithelial zone** (in the outer aspect of the GBM below the podocytes) either as a result of immune complex formation *in situ* or deposition of circulating immune complexes. Formation *in situ* occurs in an animal model of membranous nephropathy called **Heymann nephritis,** in which rats are immunized with a renal epithelial antigen and develop autoantibodies. The antibodies cross GBMs and bind antigens on podocytes. Resultant immune complexes are shed into the adjacent subepithelial zone to cause membranous nephropathy. A rare form of neonatal membranous nephropathy is caused by transplacental passage of antibodies that react with an alloantigen on neonatal podocytes (neutral endopeptidase) that is not shared by the mother. Approximately 75% of patients with primary membranous nephropathy have circulating autoantibodies against PLA$_2$R, a podocyte transmembrane receptor. Both PLA$_2$R and anti-PLA$_2$R can be isolated from the immune complexes, supporting *in situ* subepithelial immune complex formation.

Repeated experimental exposure to foreign proteins elicits antibodies, which form circulating immune complexes. A subpopulation of these complexes deposits in glomerular capillary walls. Sometimes, free antigens and antibodies cross the GBM independently and form subepithelial immune complexes *in situ*.

General causes of nephropathy glomerulonephritis are:

- Primary membranous nephropathy
  - Anti-PLA$_2$R autoantibodies
  - Anti-thrombospondin type-1 domain-containing 7A (THSD7A)
  - Anti-cationic bovine serum albumin (in children)
  - Anti–neutral endopeptidase alloantibodies
- Secondary membranous nephropathy
  - Autoimmune disease (e.g., SLE, autoimmune thyroid disease)
  - Infectious disease (e.g., hepatitis B, malaria, syphilis, schistosomiasis)
  - Therapeutic agents (e.g., penicillamine)
  - Neoplasms (e.g., lung, prostate and gastrointestinal cancers)

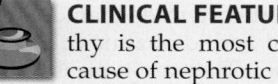 **PATHOLOGY:** Glomeruli are usually normocellular. Depending on the duration of the disease, capillary walls may be normal or thickened (Fig. 22-21). In intermediate disease stages, silver stains (which highlight basement membranes) reveal multiple "spikes" of argyrophilic material on the epithelial side of the basement membrane (Fig. 22-22). These spikes are projections of basement membrane material around subepithelial immune complexes (which do not stain with silver). As disease progresses, capillary lumens narrow, and glomerular sclerosis eventually ensues. Advanced membranous nephropathy cannot be distinguished from other forms of chronic glomerular disease. Atrophy of tubules and interstitial fibrosis parallel the degree of glomerular sclerosis.

By electron microscopy, immune complexes appear in capillary walls as electron-dense deposits (Figs. 22-23 and 22-24). The progressive ultrastructural changes caused by subepithelial immune complexes are divided into stages:

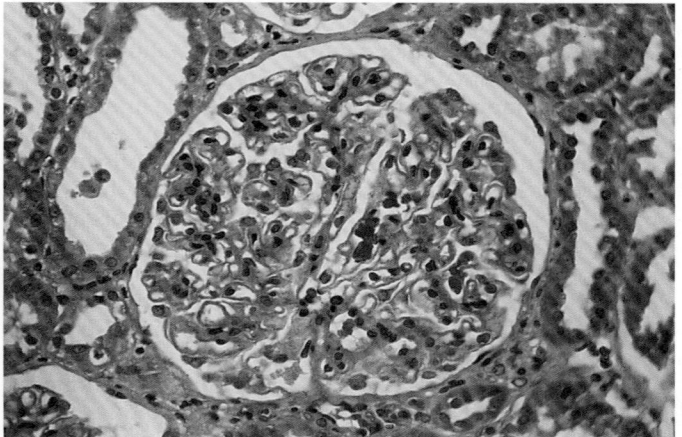

FIGURE 22-21. Membranous nephropathy. This glomerulus is slightly enlarged and shows diffuse thickening of capillary walls. There is no hypercellularity. Compare capillary walls to those shown in Figures 22-2 and 22-16.

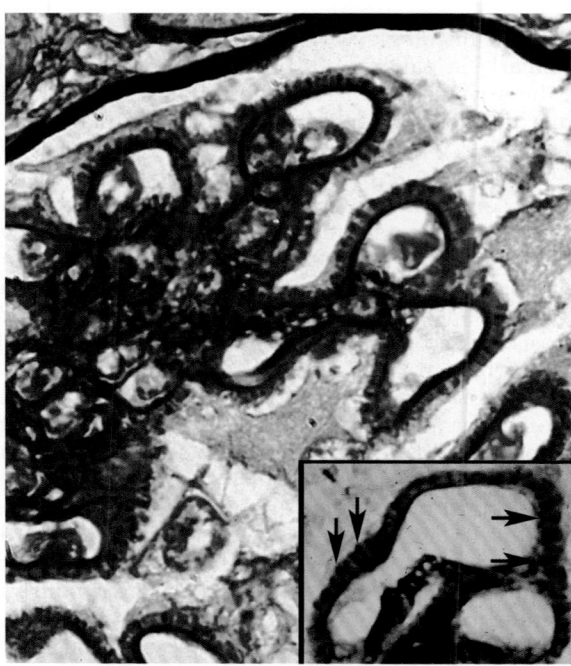

FIGURE 22-22. Membranous nephropathy. Silver staining reveals multiple "spikes" diffusely distributed in the glomerular capillary basement membranes (identified by *arrows* in the higher magnification *inset*). This pattern corresponds to the stage II lesion illustrated in Figures 22-23 and 22-24. The appearance is produced by deposition of silver-positive basement membrane material around silver-negative immune complex deposits.

- **Stage I:** Subepithelial dense deposits without adjacent projections of GBM material
- **Stage II:** Projections of GBM material adjacent to dense deposits (Fig. 22-24)
- **Stage III:** Enclosure of dense deposits within GBM material
- **Stage IV:** Rarefaction of deposits within a thickened GBM

Mesangial electron-dense deposits are rare in primary membranous nephropathy but are more common in secondary disease (e.g., in lupus nephropathy). This difference may reflect the fact that primary disease is caused by antigens normally present in the subepithelial zone (e.g., podocyte PLA$_2$R and neutral endopeptidase), but the secondary type is produced by circulating antigens (e.g., hepatitis B virus antigens) in complexes with circulating antibodies that can accumulate in mesangial as well as subepithelial locations.

Immunofluorescence reveals diffuse granular staining of capillary walls for IgG and C3 (Fig. 22-25). There is intense staining for terminal complement components, including the membrane attack complex, which participate in inducing glomerular injury, especially affecting podocytes.

CLINICAL FEATURES: Membranous nephropathy is the most common primary glomerular cause of nephrotic syndrome in white and Asian adults in the United States (the most common secondary glomerular cause is diabetic glomerulosclerosis). The

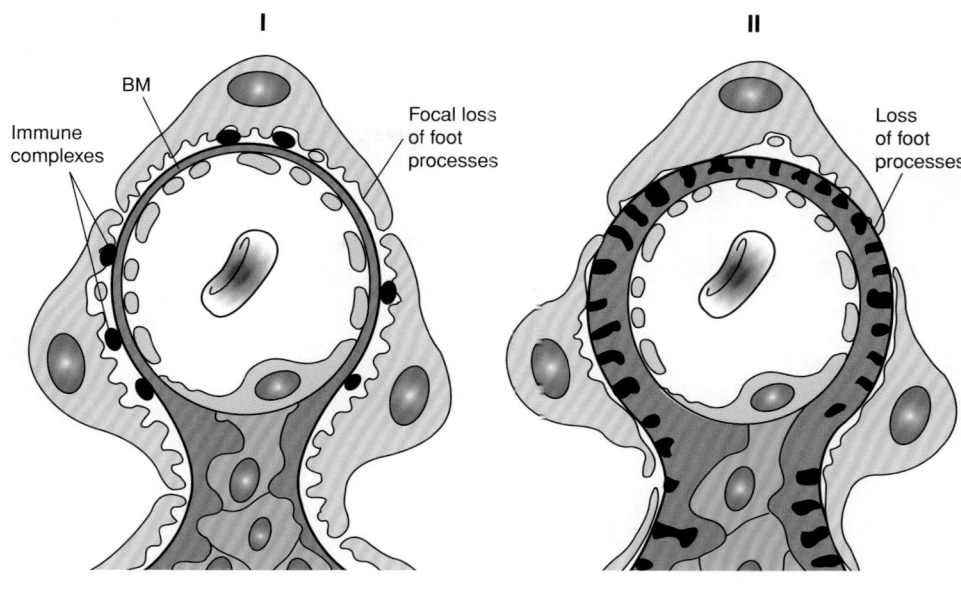

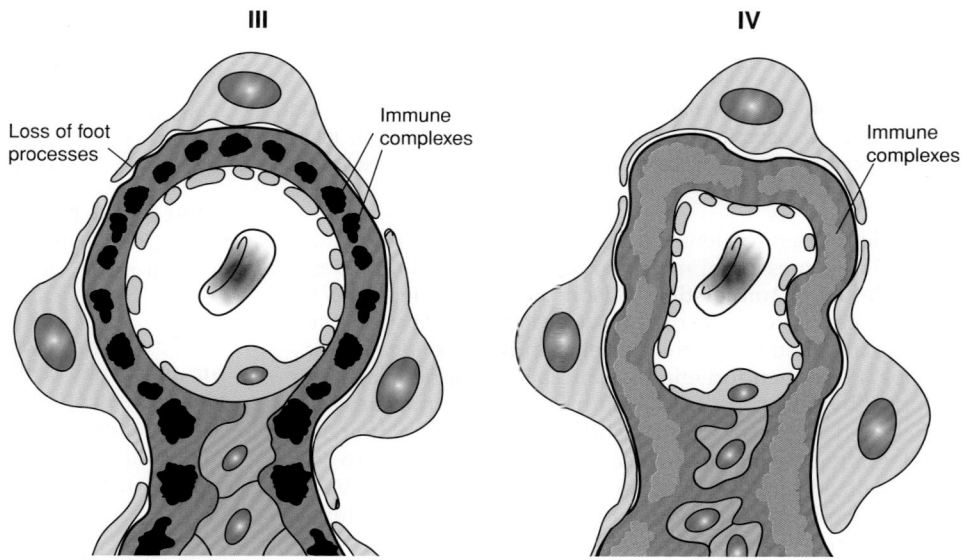

FIGURE 22-23. Membranous nephropathy. This disease is caused by the subepithelial accumulation of immune complexes and the accompanying changes in the basement membrane (BM). Stage I exhibits scattered subepithelial deposits. The outer contour of the basement membrane remains smooth. Stage II disease has projections (spikes) of basement membrane material adjacent to the deposits. In stage III disease, newly formed basement membrane has surrounded the deposits. With stage IV disease, the immune complex deposits lose their electron density, resulting in an irregularly thickened basement membrane with irregular electron-lucent areas.

course of membranous nephropathy is highly variable. Spontaneous remission occurs in 1/4 of patients within 20 years, and 10-year renal survival rate is greater than 65%. Lower survival correlates with male gender, age above 50, proteinuria of more than 6 g/day, extensive glomerular sclerosis, and chronic tubulointerstitial disease. Patients with progressive renal failure receive corticosteroids and/or immunosuppressive drugs. The prognosis is better in children because of a higher rate of permanent spontaneous remission.

Diabetic Glomerulosclerosis Causes Proteinuria and Progressive Renal Failure

 PATHOPHYSIOLOGY: Glomerulosclerosis is part of a vasculopathy that affects small vessels throughout the body in diabetic patients (see

Chapter 13). The abnormal metabolic state leads to a general increase in synthesis of basement membrane material in the microvasculature. One hypothesis proposes that increased **oxidative injury** and abnormal **nonenzymatic glycosylation** of plasma proteins (e.g., immunoglobulins) and matrix proteins (including those of the GBM and mesangial matrix) induce excessive matrix production and podocyte injury.

PATHOLOGY: The earliest lesions of diabetic glomerulosclerosis are glomerular enlargement, GBM thickening, and mesangial matrix expansion (Fig. 22-26). Numbers of podocytes decline. Mild mesangial hypercellularity may develop along with the increase in mesangial matrix. In patients with symptomatic disease, GBM thickening and especially mesangial matrix expansion are visible on light microscopy. In

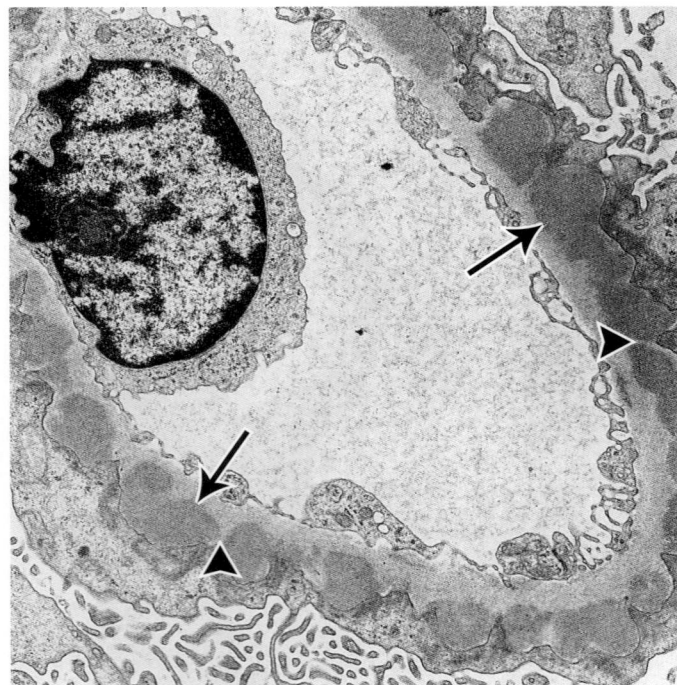

FIGURE 22-24. Stage II membranous nephropathy. This electron micrograph shows deposits of electron-dense material (*arrows*), with intervening delicate projections of basement membrane material (*arrowheads*).

diabetic glomerulosclerosis, diffuse global GBM thickening and diffuse mesangial matrix expansion are accompanied by sclerotic **Kimmelstiel–Wilson nodules** (Fig. 22-27). Insudated proteins form rounded nodules between the Bowman capsule and the parietal epithelium ("capsular drops") or subendothelial accumulations along capillary loops ("hyaline caps"). Tubular basement membranes are thickened. Sclerosing and insudative changes in afferent and efferent arterioles cause hyaline arteriolosclerosis. Generalized renal arteriosclerosis is usually present. Vascular narrowing and reduced blood flow to the medulla predispose to papillary necrosis and pyelonephritis.

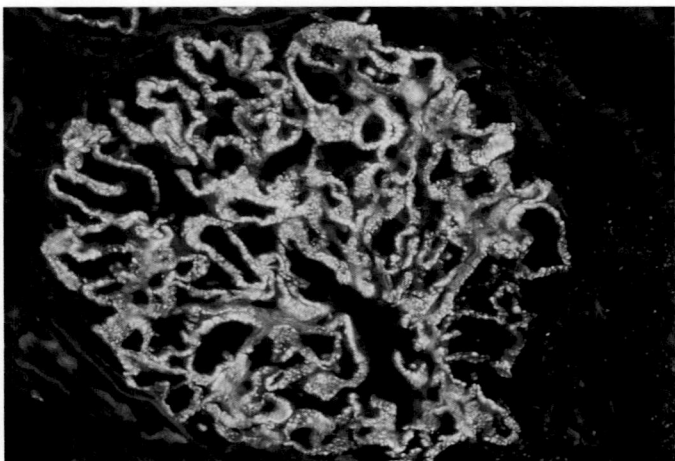

FIGURE 22-25. Membranous glomerulonephritis. Immunofluorescence microscopy shows granular deposits of immunoglobulin G (IgG) outlining the glomerular capillary loops.

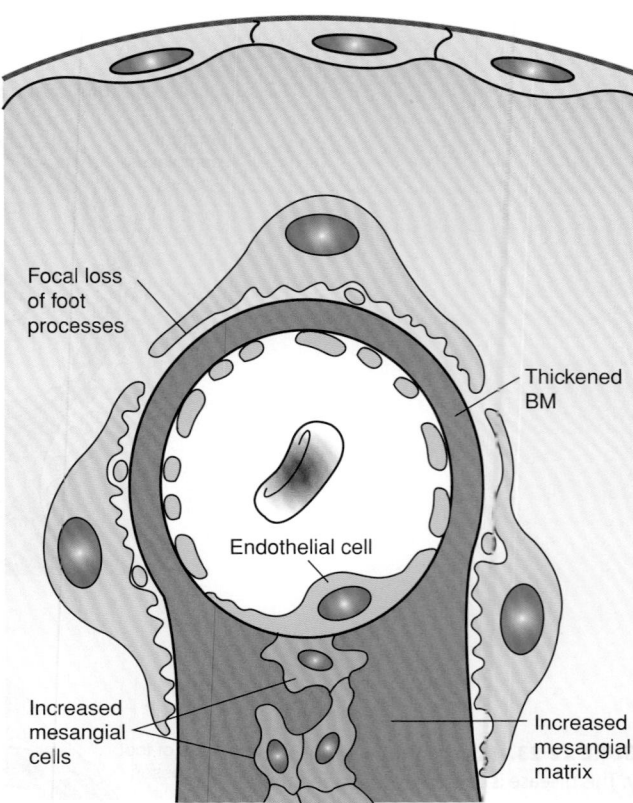

FIGURE 22-26. Diabetic glomerulosclerosis. The lamina densa of the glomerular basement membrane is thickened, and there is an increase in mesangial matrix material.

By electron microscopy, the basement membrane lamina densa may be thicker by 5- to 10-fold. Mesangial matrix is increased, particularly in nodular lesions (Fig. 22-28). The hyaline insudative lesions appear as electron-dense masses that contain lipid debris. By immunofluorescence, there is diffuse linear trapping of IgG, albumin, fibrinogen,

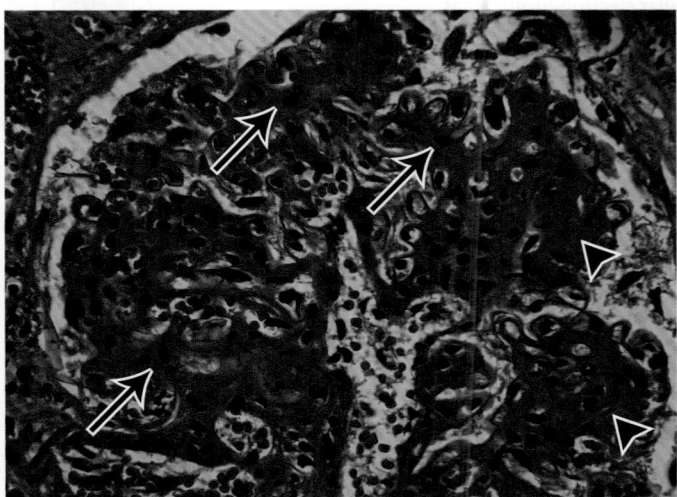

FIGURE 22-27. Diabetic glomerulosclerosis. A prominent increase in the mesangial matrix (*arrows*) forms several nodular lesions (*arrowheads*). Dilation of glomerular capillaries is evident, and some capillary basement membranes are thickened.

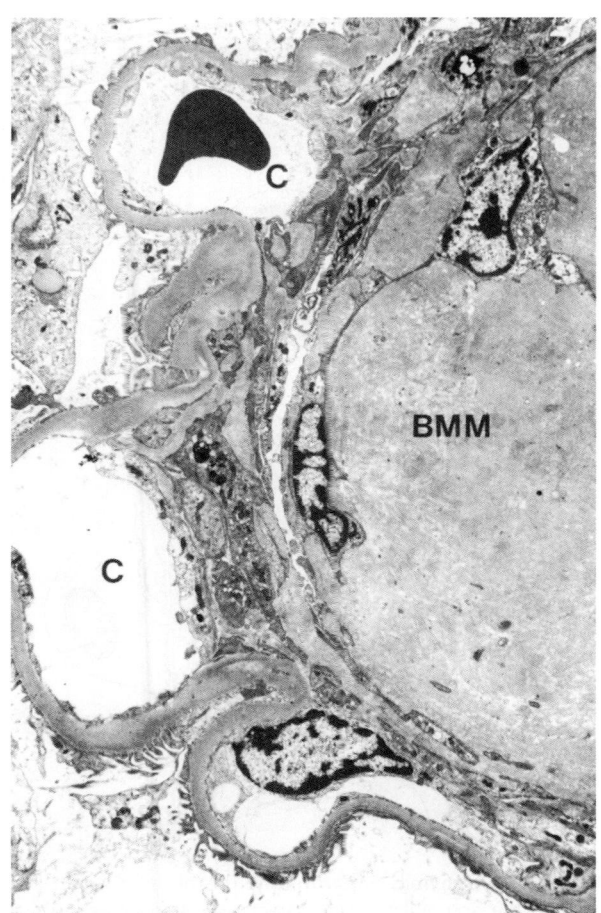

FIGURE 22-28. Advanced diabetic glomerulosclerosis. This electron micrograph shows a nodular aggregate of basement membrane–like material (*BMM*). Peripheral capillaries (*C*) demonstrate diffuse basement membrane widening but with a normal texture.

and other plasma proteins in the GBM. This reflects non-specific adsorption of these proteins to the thickened GBM, possibly due to nonenzymatic glycosylation of GBM and plasma proteins.

CLINICAL FEATURES: *Diabetic glomerulosclerosis accounts for 40% of ESRD and thus is the leading cause of ESRD in the United States.* It occurs in type 1 and type 2 diabetes mellitus. There is a higher risk of diabetic glomerulosclerosis in blacks and native Americans with type 2 diabetes mellitus. Approximately 25% of patients with diabetes develop diabetic glomerulosclerosis. The earliest manifestation is microalbuminuria (slightly increased proteinuria). Overt proteinuria occurs 10 to 15 years after the onset of diabetes and often becomes severe enough to cause the nephrotic syndrome. In time, diabetic glomerulosclerosis progresses to renal failure. Strict control of blood glucose reduces the incidence of diabetic glomerulosclerosis and retards progression once it develops. Control of hypertension and dietary protein restriction also slow progression of the disease.

Amyloidosis Leads to Nephrotic Syndrome and Renal Failure

Renal disease is a frequent complication of AA and AL amyloidosis (see Chapter 15).

 MOLECULAR PATHOGENESIS: Amyloid may be formed from >30 different precursor proteins. In North America, AL amyloidosis accounts for 80% of renal amyloidosis; AA amyloidosis accounts for 10% and the remaining 10% is due to other types of amyloidosis (e.g., composed of fibrinogen, leukocyte chemotactic factor 2, apolipoprotein). AA is more common is areas with high rates of endemic infections. All forms of amyloidosis appear similar histologically and ultrastructurally. Immunohistochemical tests are required to differentiate among the different types. Mass spectrometry may be useful in typing cases of amyloidosis as some are due to genetic mutations (e.g., transthyretin and gelsolin). **AA amyloid** is derived from serum amyloid A (SAA) protein, which increases markedly during inflammation. Thus, AA amyloid is often associated with chronic inflammatory disorders (e.g., rheumatoid arthritis, chronic infections, familial Mediterranean fever). **AL amyloid** is derived from immunoglobulin light chains made by neoplastic clones of B cells or plasma cells. Thus, it often occurs in, or presages, multiple myeloma. **ALECT2 amyloidosis** (leukocyte chemotactic factor 2 amyloidosis) is a renal-limited form that occurs most commonly in the United States in elderly patients of Mexican ancestry.

PATHOLOGY: Amyloid appears by light microscopy as an eosinophilic, amorphous material (Fig. 22-29) with a characteristic apple-green color under polarized light in sections stained with Congo red (Fig. 22-30). Acidophilic deposits are initially most apparent in the mesangium but later extend into capillary walls and may obliterate capillary lumens (Figs. 22-29 and 22-31). Glomerular structure is completely obliterated in advanced amyloidosis, and glomeruli appear as amorphous eosinophilic spheres.

Amyloid is composed of nonbranching fibrils, about 10 nm in diameter. These are initially most abundant in the mesangium but often extend into capillary walls, especially in advanced cases (Figs. 22-31 and 22-32). Podocyte foot processes overlying the GBM are effaced.

CLINICAL FEATURES: Renal involvement is prominent in most cases of systemic AL and AA amyloidosis. Proteinuria is often the initial manifestation. Proteinuria is nonselective (both albumin and globulins are in the urine) and nephrotic syndrome occurs in 60% of patients. Eventually, severe infiltration of glomeruli and blood vessels by amyloid results in renal failure. AL amyloidosis is treated with chemotherapy for multiple myeloma. AA amyloidosis, especially when caused by familial Mediterranean fever, is ameliorated by colchicine therapy. New therapies designed to block protein misfolding appear promising.

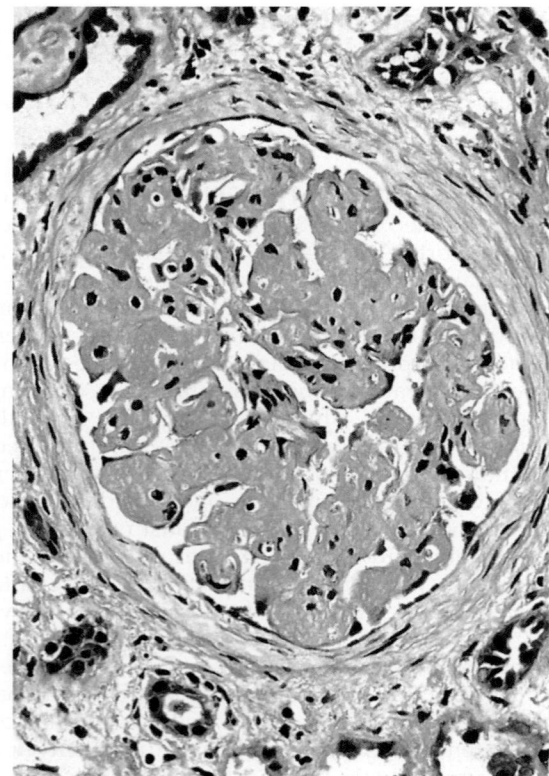

FIGURE 22-29. Amyloid nephropathy. Amorphous acellular material expands mesangial areas and obstructs glomerular capillaries. The deposits of amyloid may take on a nodular appearance, somewhat resembling those of diabetic glomerulosclerosis (see Fig. 22-27). However, amyloid deposits are not periodic acid–Schiff positive and are identifiable by Congo red staining as shown in Figure 22-30.

Nonfibrillary Monoclonal Immunoglobulin Deposition in Kidneys Can Cause Disease

Such deposition may be in GBMs, glomerular mesangial matrix, capillary walls, and tubular basement membranes.

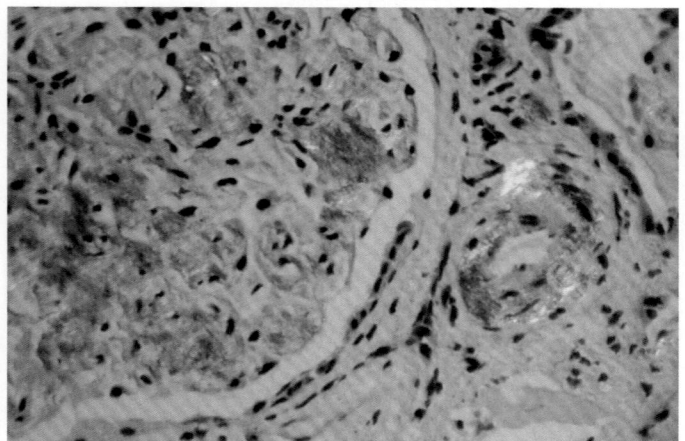

FIGURE 22-30. Amyloid nephropathy. This section stained with Congo red and examined under polarized light shows amyloid deposits in a glomerulus and adjacent arteriole which exhibit characteristic apple-green birefringence.

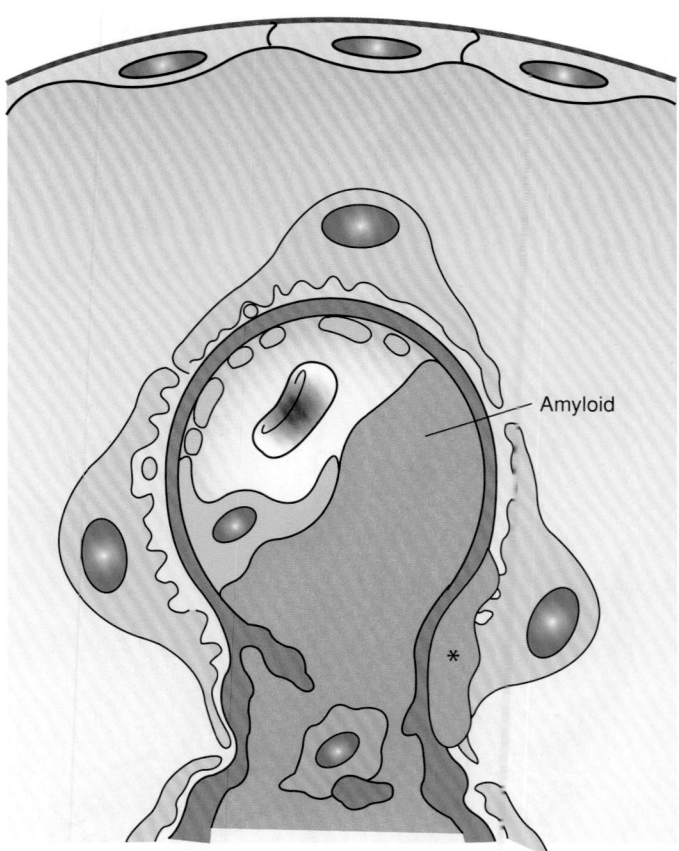

FIGURE 22-31. Amyloid nephropathy. This disorder is initially associated with the accumulation of characteristic fibrillar deposits in the mesangium. These inert masses, which are fibrillar by electron microscopy, extend along the inner surface of the basement membrane, frequently obstructing the capillary lumen. Focal extension of amyloid through the basement membrane (*) may elevate the epithelial cell.

Unlike the deposits of AL amyloid, these do not form fibrils. The two major phenotypes are nodular sclerosing glomerular disease with granular deposits by electron microscopy and proliferative (or membranoproliferative) glomerulonephritis with homogeneous dense deposits by electron microscopy.

PATHOLOGY: The underlying B-cell dyscrasia may be occult, or there may be overt multiple myeloma or lymphoma. Monoclonal immunoglobulin deposition stimulates increased glomerular matrix production and/or mesangial hyperplasia. Nodular expansion of mesangial regions resembles diabetic glomerulosclerosis. The increased extracellular material does not stain with Congo red, which distinguishes monoclonal immunoglobulin deposition disease from amyloidosis. Immunofluorescence microscopy demonstrates staining for monoclonal immunoglobulin chains. Monoclonal immunoglobulin deposition disease with nodular sclerosis usually manifests clinically as nephrotic syndrome, whereas proliferative glomerulonephritis with monoclonal immunoglobulin deposits often manifests as mixed nephritic and nephrotic syndrome.

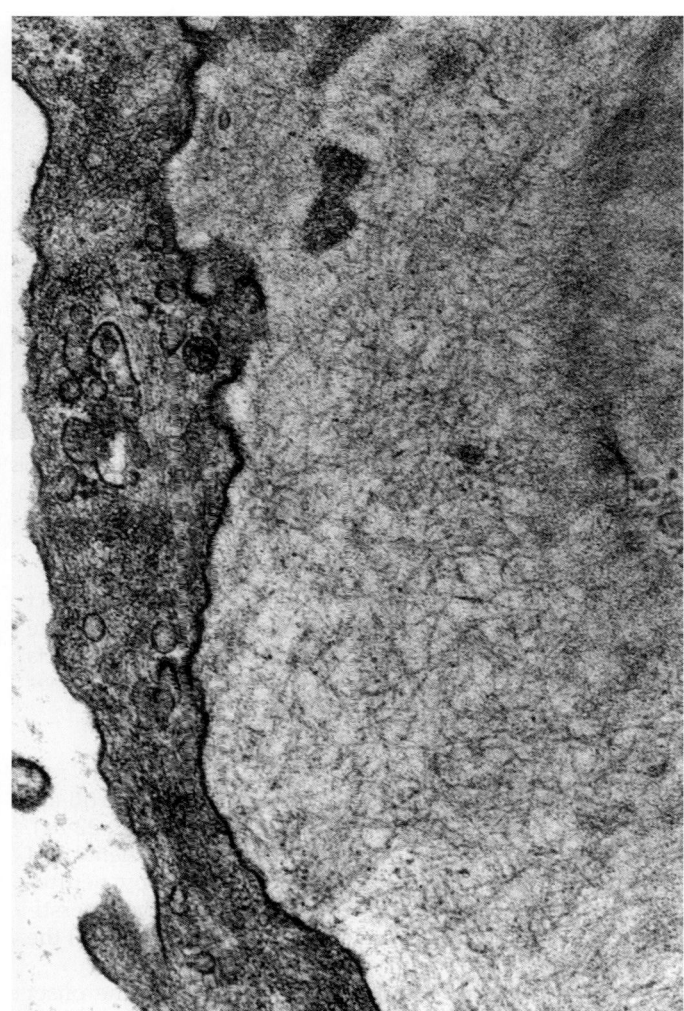

FIGURE 22-32. Amyloid nephropathy. Masses of fibrils (10 nm in diameter) in a glomerulus are adjacent to a podocyte (seen on the *left*) with effaced foot processes.

Hereditary Nephritis (Alport Syndrome) Reflects Abnormal Glomerular Basement Membrane Type IV Collagen

Hereditary nephritis is a proliferative and sclerosing glomerular disease, often accompanied by defects of the ears or eyes. It is caused by genetic defects in type IV collagen. In Alport syndrome, a hereditary hearing deficit accompanies nephritis.

MOLECULAR PATHOGENESIS: Several genetic mutations cause molecular defects in the GBM that lead to the renal lesions of hereditary nephritis. The most common, accounting for 85% of hereditary nephritis, is X-linked and is caused by a mutation in the gene for the α5 chain of type IV collagen (*COL4A5*). A deletion at the 5′ end of *COL4A5* that extends into the *COL4A6* gene, which codes for the α6 chain of type IV collagen, causes hereditary nephritis and multiple leiomyomas in the gastrointestinal and genital tracts. An autosomal recessive form of hereditary nephritis is caused by mutations in *COL4A3* and *COL4A4*.

As basement membrane structure is disturbed in hereditary nephritis, serum from patients with anti-GBM disease (e.g., Goodpasture syndrome) fails to react with GBMs from patients with hereditary nephritis. Conversely, patients with hereditary nephritis who have renal transplants are at risk for developing antibodies to allograft GBMs.

PATHOLOGY: Early glomerular lesions of hereditary nephritis show mild mesangial hypercellularity and matrix expansion. Renal disease progression is associated with increasing focal and eventually diffuse glomerular sclerosis. Tubular atrophy, interstitial fibrosis and foam cells in tubules and interstitium accompany advanced glomerular lesions. Electron microscopy makes the diagnosis, demonstrating an irregularly thickened GBM with splitting of the lamina densa into interlacing lamellae that surround electron-lucent areas (Fig. 22-33).

CLINICAL FEATURES: Hematuria develops early in boys with X-linked hereditary nephritis, and proteinuria and progressive renal failure usually follow in the second to fourth decades of life. In females, the X-linked disease is generally milder, with the

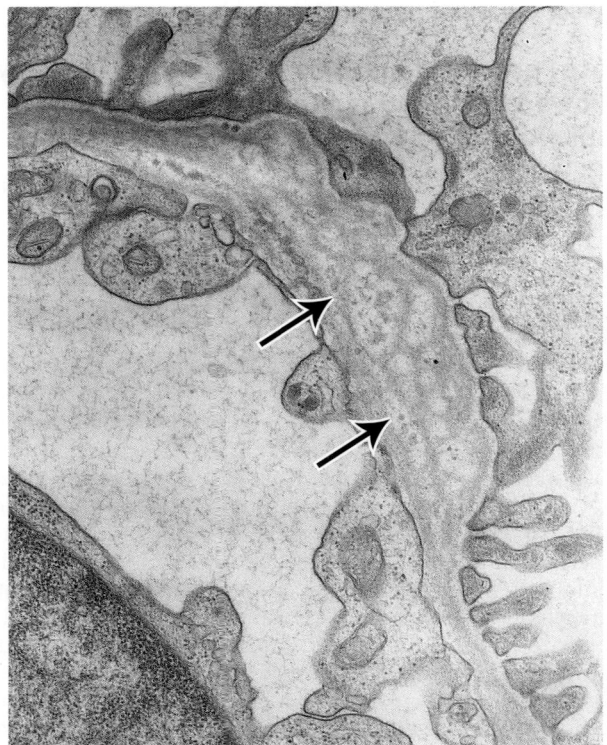

FIGURE 22-33. Hereditary nephritis (Alport syndrome). The lamina densa of the glomerular basement membrane is laminated (*arrows*) rather than forming a single dense band (compare this electron micrograph with Fig. 22-5).

rate of progression varying substantially among patients, possibly due to the degree of random inactivation (lyonization) of the mutated X chromosome. Autosomal recessive hereditary nephritis resembles X-linked disease except that males and females are affected equally. Autosomal dominant hereditary nephritis with progressive renal failure is rare and difficult to distinguish from severe thin basement membrane disease (see below). Sensorineural, high-frequency hearing loss affects 1/2 of males with X-linked disease and a higher proportion of males and females with autosomal disease. Ocular defects, largely of the lens, occur in 1/4 to 1/3 of patients.

Thin Glomerular Basement Membrane Nephropathy Is a Common Cause of Hereditary Benign Hematuria

This nephropathy, also called **benign familial hematuria,** often presents as asymptomatic microscopic hematuria, with occasional intermittent gross hematuria. This disease and IgA nephropathy are common diagnostic considerations in patients with asymptomatic glomerular hematuria. Patients with thin basement membrane nephropathy usually do not develop renal failure or substantial proteinuria. By light microscopy, glomeruli are unremarkable. Electron microscopy shows reduced thickness of the GBM (150 to 300 nm; normal is 350 to 450 nm). The most common mode of inheritance is autosomal dominant. Heterozygous mutations in *COL4A3* and *COL4A4* lead to thin basement membrane disease, and homozygous variants lead to Alport syndrome. Variants in *COL4A3* and *COL4A4* are also detected in adult patients with sporadic and familial FSGS.

Acute Postinfectious Glomerulonephritis Usually Follows Acute β-Hemolytic Streptococcal or Staphylococcal Infection

Complement-rich immune complex deposits in glomeruli cause this disease.

PATHOPHYSIOLOGY: Nephritogenic strains of group A streptococci or staphylococci usually cause acute postinfectious glomerulonephritis. Rare cases result from viral (e.g., hepatitis B) or parasitic (e.g., malaria) infections. Poststreptococcal glomerulonephritis has a 9- to 14-day latent period between onset of infection and glomerulonephritis. As described below, postinfectious glomerulonephritis involves extensive glomerular localization of immunoglobulin and complement, or complement alone. One possible pathogenic mechanism is immune complex formation in glomeruli-containing pathogen antigen and antibodies that activate complement and induce inflammation. Alternatively, nephritogenic bacteria could release factors that activate complement without requiring immune complex formation. This would explain why complement, but not immunoglobulin, is sometimes present in glomerular deposits.

Complement activation, as well as activation of other humoral and cellular inflammatory mediators, causes glomerular inflammation. Complement activation is so extensive that more than 90% of patients develop

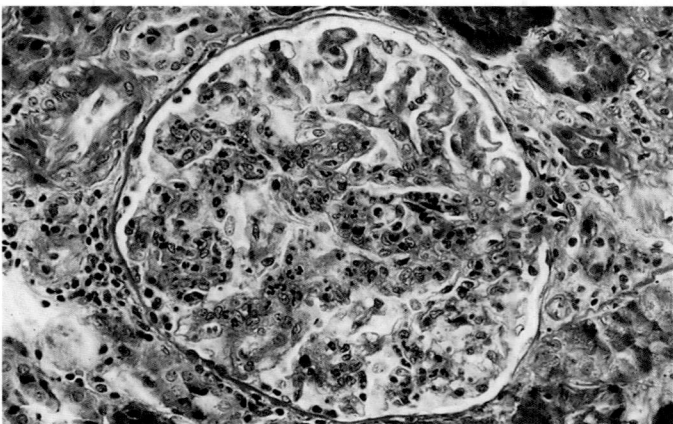

FIGURE 22-34. Acute poststreptococcal glomerulonephritis. This glomerulus from a patient who developed glomerulonephritis after a streptococcal infection contains many neutrophils (Masson trichrome stain).

hypocomplementemia. The inflammatory mediators attract and activate neutrophils and monocytes, and stimulate mesangial and endothelial cell proliferation. These effects result in marked glomerular hypercellularity which defines acute diffuse proliferative glomerulonephritis.

PATHOLOGY: In the acute phase, glomeruli are diffusely enlarged and hypercellular (Fig. 22-34). The latter reflects proliferation of endothelial and mesangial cells (Fig. 22-35), and infiltration by neutrophils and monocytes. Crescents are uncommon. Interstitial edema and mild mononuclear infiltration parallel the glomerular changes.

The acute phase begins 1 to 2 weeks after the onset of the nephritogenic infection and resolves in more than 90% of patients after several weeks. Neutrophils and endothelial hypercellularity disappear first. Mesangial hypercellularity and matrix expansion remain, but all of these changes resolve completely in most patients after several months.

Ultrastructurally, acute postinfectious glomerulonephritis shows distinctive **subepithelial dense deposits** shaped like **"humps"** (Figs. 22-35 and 22-36). These are invariably accompanied by mesangial and subendothelial deposits, which may be more difficult to detect but are probably more important in pathogenesis by virtue of their proximity to inflammatory mediator systems in the blood. The variably sized, dome-shaped humps are on the epithelial side of the GBM. They are not as widely distributed as the deposits of membranous nephropathy (compare Figs. 22-23 and 22-35). Granular deposits of C3 with or without immunoglobulin are observed by immunofluorescence microscopy in capillary walls, corresponding to the humps (Fig. 22-37). A rare variant of postinfectious glomerulonephritis, usually caused by methicillin-resistant staphylococcus, has conspicuous IgA in the immune deposits.

CLINICAL FEATURES: The incidence of acute postinfectious glomerulonephritis is declining in most developed countries but remains high

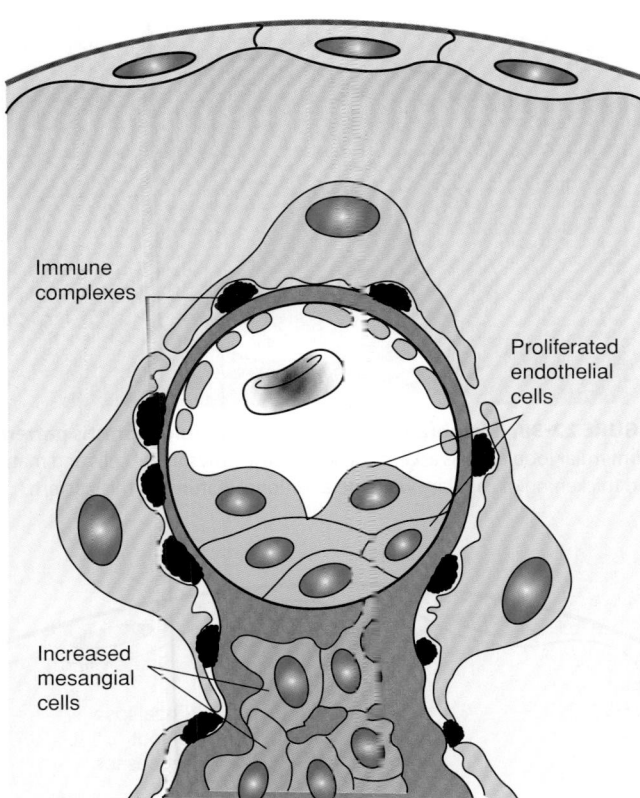

FIGURE 22-35. Postinfectious glomerulonephritis. Accumulation of numerous subepithelial immune complexes as hump-like structures is a characteristic feature. Less prominent subendothelial immune complexes are associated with endothelial cell proliferation and are related to increased capillary permeability and narrowing of the lumen. Frequently, proliferation of mesangial cells and a thickened mesangial matrix result in widening of the stalk and conspicuous trapping of immune complexes.

because of higher rates of nephritogenic infections. It is still one of the most common childhood renal diseases. Primary infection involves the pharynx (pharyngitis, often "Strep throat") or, especially in hot and humid environments, the skin (pyoderma). In recent years, the proportion of cases following staphylococcal infection has been increasing. Because organisms may not be present at the time nephritis develops, the diagnosis may depend on serologic evidence of increasing antibody titers to streptococcal antigens. The nephritic syndrome begins abruptly with oliguria, hematuria, facial edema, and hypertension. Serum C3 levels are lower during the acute syndrome but return to normal within 1 to 2 weeks. Overt nephritis resolves after several weeks, but hematuria and especially proteinuria may persist for several months. A few patients have abnormal urinary sediment for years after the acute episode, and rare patients (particularly adults) develop progressive renal failure.

Immune Complex Membranoproliferative Glomerulonephritis Has Multiple Causes

MPGN is a pattern of glomerular inflammation with hypercellularity and capillary wall thickening caused by multiple different etiologies and pathogenic mechanisms.

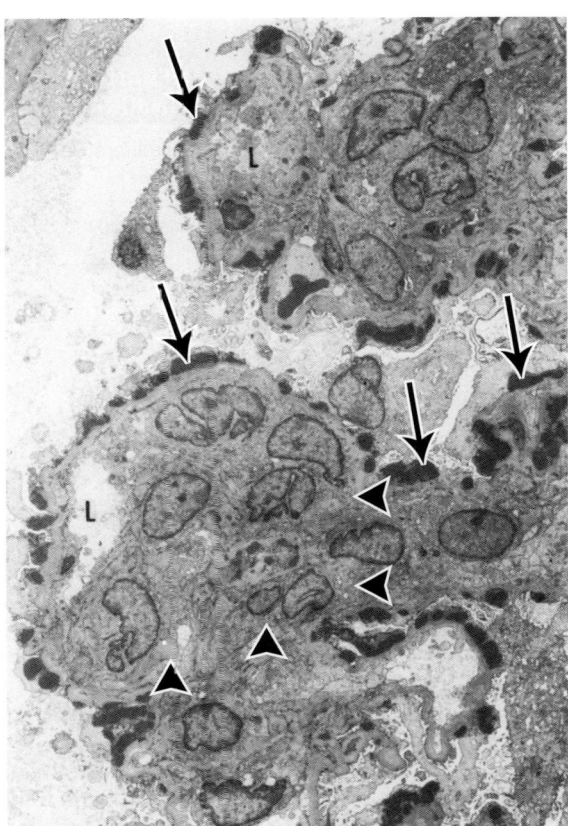

FIGURE 22-36. Acute postinfectious glomerulonephritis. This electron micrograph demonstrates numerous subepithelial humps (*arrows*) and mesangial hypercellularity (*arrowheads*). Capillary lumens (*L*) are markedly narrowed.

PATHOPHYSIOLOGY: MPGN is caused by deposits in the mesangium and capillary walls containing immune complexes or activated complement without immunoglobulin. Subepithelial deposits may also occur. The two major immunopathologic

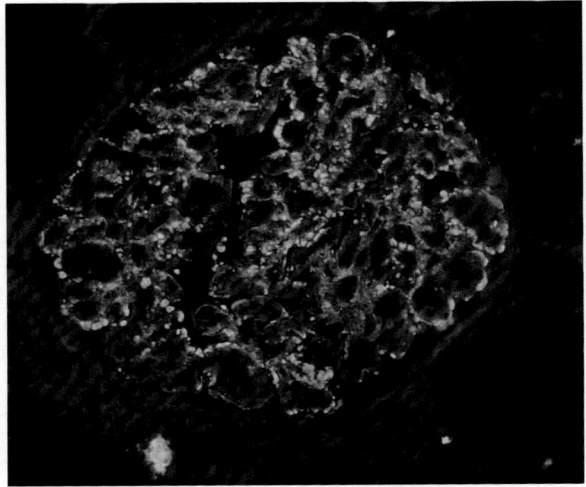

FIGURE 22-37. Acute postinfectious glomerulonephritis. This immunofluorescence micrograph demonstrates granular staining for C3 in capillary walls and the mesangium.

TABLE 22-6

CLASSIFICATION OF MEMBRANOPROLIFERATIVE GLOMERULONEPHRITIS (A PATTERN OF INJURY)

Primary Immune Complex–Mediated Membranoproliferative Glomerulonephritis (MPGN)

Secondary Immune Complex–Mediated MPGN caused by:

    Subacute bacterial endocarditis

    Infected ventriculoatrial shunt

    Osteomyelitis

    Hepatitis C virus infection

    Cryoglobulinemia

    Monoclonal immunoglobulins

    Neoplasia

C3 glomerulopathy

    Dense deposit disease

    C3 glomerulonephritis

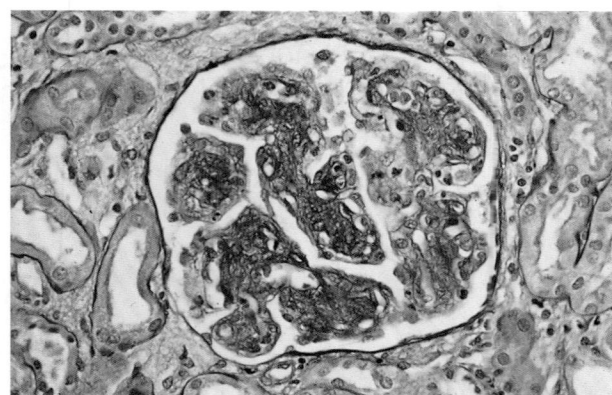

FIGURE 22-38. Membranoproliferative glomerulonephritis pattern. Glomerular lobulation is accentuated. Increased mesangial cells and matrix and thickening of capillary walls are additional features of this pattern.

categories are immune complex–mediated MPGN and C3 glomerulopathy (Table 22-6). The nephritogenic antigens in immune complex–mediated MPGN are usually unknown. However, the sources of the antigens may be infectious or autoimmune conditions (Table 22-6). A rare MPGN variant is caused by monoclonal immunoglobulin. C3 glomerulopathy is caused by genetic or autoimmune disruption of regulatory mechanisms that normally hold the alternative complement pathway in check. C3 glomerulopathy, which can cause patterns of glomerulonephritis in addition to MPGN, is discussed in the next section.

Eliminating the associated condition (e.g., bacterial endocarditis or osteomyelitis) may be followed by resolution of immune complex–mediated MPGN, thus suggesting a causal relationship between the two. Unlike the pathogens of acute postinfectious glomerulonephritis, those associated with immune complex–mediated MPGN cause persistent, indolent infections with chronic antigenemia. This condition leads to chronic localization of immune complexes in glomeruli and resultant hypercellularity and matrix remodeling.

PATHOLOGY: Glomeruli in MPGN are diffusely enlarged, with florid mesangial cell proliferation and infiltration of monocytes/macrophages. The resultant glomerular lobular accentuation ("hypersegmentation"; Fig. 22-38) was once called **lobular glomerulonephritis**. Of these patients, 20% have crescents, usually involving only a minority of glomeruli. Capillary walls are thickened, and silver stains show a doubling or complex replication of GBMs.

Electron microscopy reveals thickening and replication of GBMs probably caused by endothelial cell activation as well as extension of mesangial cytoplasm into the subendothelial zone and deposition of new basement membrane material between the mesangial cytoplasm and endothelial cell (Figs. 22-39 and 22-40). Subendothelial

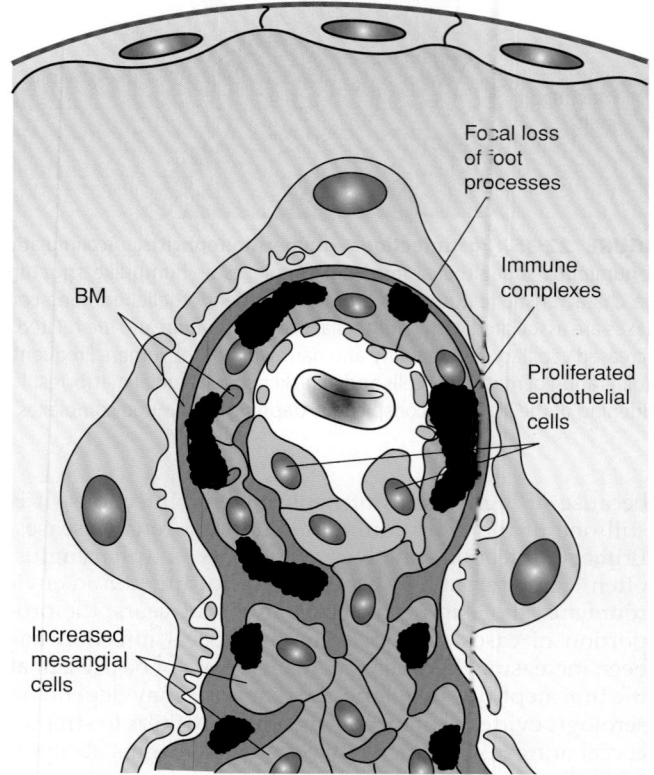

FIGURE 22-39. Membranoproliferative glomerulonephritis. In this pattern of injury, glomeruli are enlarged. Hypercellular tufts and narrowing or obstruction of capillary lumens are seen. Large subendothelial deposits of immune complexes or complement extend along the inner border of the basement membrane (*BM*). Mesangial cells proliferate and migrate peripherally into the capillary. Basement membrane material accumulates in a linear fashion parallel to the basement membrane in a subendothelial position. The interposition of mesangial cells and basement membrane between the endothelial cells and the original basement membrane creates a double-contour effect. Accumulation of mesangial cells and stroma in the tufts narrows the capillary lumen. Proliferation of mesangial cells and accumulation of basement membrane material also widens the mesangium. The entire process leads to progressive lobulation of the glomerulus. Note the proliferation of endothelial cells and focal effacement of foot processes.

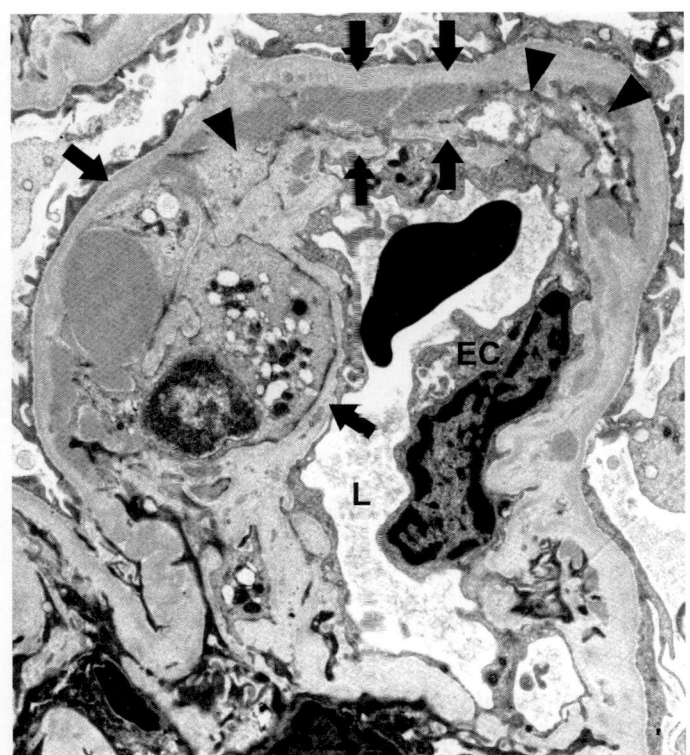

FIGURE 22-40. Membranoproliferative glomerulonephritis. This electron micrograph demonstrates a double-contour basement membrane (*arrows*), with mesangial interposition (*arrowhead*) and prominent subendothelial deposits. *EC* = endothelial cell; *L* = capillary lumen.

and mesangial electron-dense deposits, corresponding to immune complexes or complement deposits, are the likely stimuli for the endothelial and mesangial response. Variable numbers of subepithelial dense deposits may also be seen. Immunofluorescence microscopy shows granular deposition of immunoglobulins and complement in glomerular capillary loops and mesangium in immune complex MPGN and complement alone in C3 glomerulopathy (Fig. 22-41).

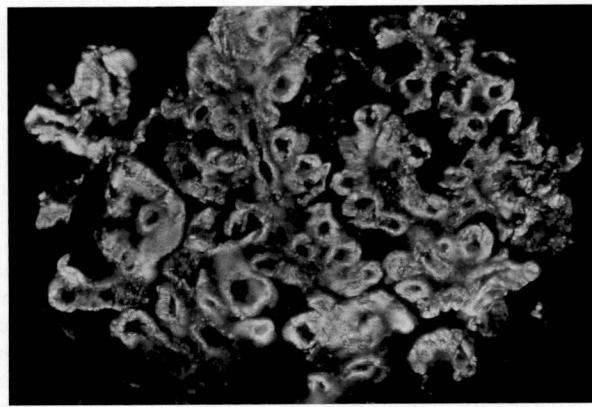

FIGURE 22-41. Membranoproliferative glomerulonephritis. This immunofluorescence micrograph shows granular to band-like staining for C3 in the capillary walls and mesangium.

CLINICAL FEATURES: Immune complex–mediated MPGN can occur at any age but is most frequent in older children and young adults. It may manifest as nephrotic or nephritic syndromes, or a combination of both. MPGN accounts for 5% of primary nephrotic syndrome in children and adults in the United States. Immune complex–mediated MPGN occurs much more commonly in countries where chronic infections are more prevalent. Patients often have low C3 levels. The differential diagnosis includes acute postinfectious glomerulonephritis and lupus glomerulonephritis, both of which can cause nephritis with hypocomplementemia. MPGN is usually a persistent, slowly progressive disease. After 10 years, 1/2 of patients reach ESRD.

C3 Glomerulopathy Is Caused by Dysregulation of the Alternative Complement Pathway

C3 glomerulopathy is caused by complement dysregulation that includes **dense deposit disease** (formerly called *type II MPGN*) and **C3 glomerulonephritis** (including a variant with an MPGN pattern).

PATHOPHYSIOLOGY: Extensive glomerular localization of complement *with* minimal to absent immunoglobulin indicates that complement activation is a major mediator of the structural and functional abnormalities. Deficient or ineffective alternative pathway complement regulatory factors (e.g., complement factor H, complement factor I) cause C3 glomerulopathy. Complement activation abnormality results from genetic defects or autoantibodies that impair alternative pathway regulatory mechanisms. Some patients have a serum IgG autoantibody, **C3 nephritic factor,** which stabilizes activated C3 convertase (C3bBb) of the alternative complement pathway and prolongs C3 activation. C3 glomerulopathy often recurs in renal transplants because the defect in complement regulation is in the recipient.

PATHOLOGY: The two pathologic subtypes of C3 glomerulopathy are dense deposit disease and C3 glomerulonephritis. C3 glomerulopathy may resemble immune complex–mediated MPGN histologically, with capillary wall thickening and increased cellularity (Fig. 22-42). However, in many patients, the glomerular injury does not show a MPGN pattern. The distinctive pathologic feature of dense deposit disease is a ribbon-like zone of increased density in the center of a thickened GBM and in the mesangial matrix seen by electron microscopy (Fig. 22-43). There are also areas of density in peritubular capillary basement membranes and arteriolar walls. C3 deposits linearly in capillary walls, with little or no antibody (Fig. 22-44). C3 glomerulonephritis, on the other hand, lacks intramembranous dense deposits. It has deposits similar to those of immune complex–mediated glomerulonephritis, except there is little to no immunoglobulin.

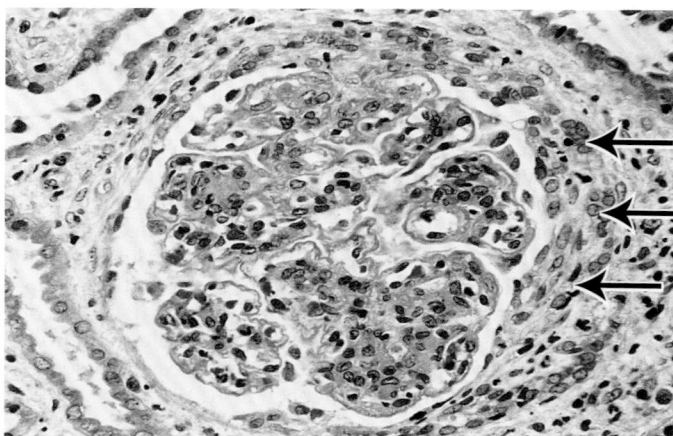

FIGURE 22-42. Dense deposit disease variant of C3 glomerulopathy. Capillary wall thickening, hypercellularity and a small crescent (*arrows*) are evident.

CLINICAL FEATURES: C3 glomerulopathy is rare, and 80% of patients are children. Patients usually present with proteinuria (often nephrotic range), hematuria, hypertension, and impaired renal function. Hypocomplementemia with low C3 and normal

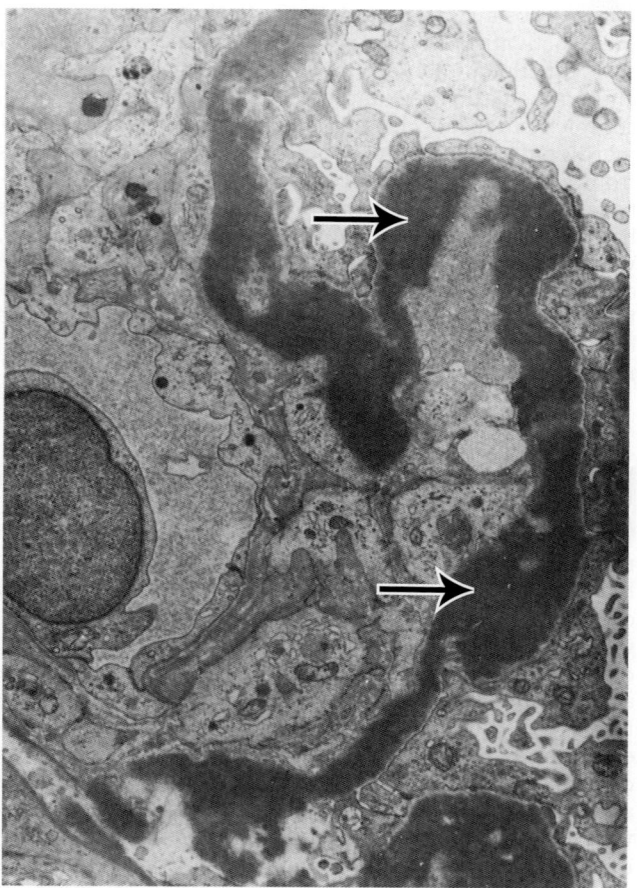

FIGURE 22-43. C3 glomerulopathy (dense deposit disease). This electron micrograph shows thickening of the basement membrane with intramembranous dense deposits (*arrows*).

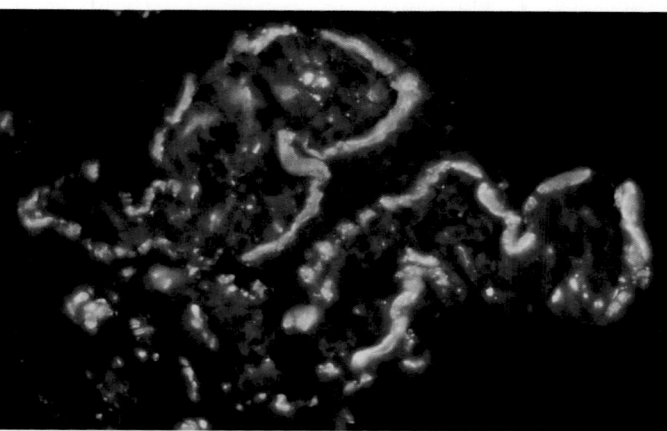

FIGURE 22-44. C3 glomerulopathy (dense deposit disease). This immunofluorescence micrograph shows bands of capillary wall staining and coarsely granular mesangial staining for C3.

C4 is common. Prognosis is sobering, as 40% reach ESRD within 10 years.

Lupus Glomerulonephritis Includes Diverse Patterns of Immune Complex Deposition

SLE (see Chapter 11) is an autoimmune disease with generalized B-cell dysregulation and hyperactivity, and production of autoantibodies to many nuclear and nonnuclear antigens, including DNA, RNA, nucleoproteins, and phospholipids. SLE is most common in women, especially of child-bearing age. Blacks, Asians, and Hispanics generally have more severe disease than do whites. Nephritis is one of the most common complications of SLE.

Immune complexes in the mesangium cause less inflammation than subendothelial immune complexes. The latter are more accessible to cellular and humoral inflammatory mediator systems in blood and are, therefore, more likely to initiate inflammation. Subepithelial localization of immune complexes causes proteinuria but does not stimulate overt glomerular inflammation.

PATHOPHYSIOLOGY: Defective apoptosis and impaired clearance of chromatin fragments may contribute to antinuclear autoimmune responses and provide target antigens for nephritogenic immune complex formation. Immune complexes may localize in glomeruli by deposition from the circulation, formation *in situ* or both. Circulating immune complexes formed by high-avidity antibodies deposit in subendothelial and mesangial zones; low-affinity antibodies form immune complexes *in situ* in the subepithelial zone. Immune complexes formed *in situ* may involve antigens such as double-stranded DNA and nucleosomes that accumulate on GBMs or in mesangial matrix due to charge interactions. Glomerular immune complexes activate complement and initiate inflammation. Complement activation often causes hypocomplementemia. Immune complexes also localize in the renal interstitium, walls of interstitial vessels, and tubular basement membranes, where they may activate the tubulointerstitial inflammation seen in patients with lupus nephritis.

TABLE 22-7

PATHOLOGIC AND CLINICAL FEATURES OF LUPUS NEPHRITIS

Location of Immune Lupus Nephritis Class	Location of Immune Clinical Complexes	Clinical Manifestations
I: Minimal mesangial	Mesangial	Mild hematuria and proteinuria
II: Mesangial proliferative	Mesangial	Mild hematuria and proteinuria
III: Focal	Mesangial and subendothelial	Moderate nephritis
IV: Diffuse	Mesangial and subendothelial	Severe nephritis
V: Membranous	Subepithelial and mesangial	Nephrotic syndrome
VI: Chronic sclerosing	Variable	Chronic renal failure

PATHOLOGY: The pathologic and clinical manifestations of lupus nephritis vary with the diverse patterns of immune complex accumulation in different patients (Table 22-7) and in the same patient over time.

- **Class I (minimal mesangial lupus glomerulonephritis):** Immune complexes are confined to mesangium and produce no changes by light microscopy.
- **Class II (mesangial proliferative lupus glomerulonephritis):** Immune complexes are confined to mesangium and induce varying degrees of mesangial hypercellularity and matrix expansion (Fig. 22-45).
- **Class III (focal lupus glomerulonephritis):** Subendothelial immune complexes accumulate, together with mesangial immune complexes. These trigger mesangial and endothelial cell proliferation, inflammation and influx of neutrophils and monocytes. This overt glomerular inflammation is called **focal proliferative lupus glomerulonephritis** if it involves less than 50% of glomeruli.
- **Class IV (diffuse lupus glomerulonephritis):** This type is similar to class III but involves more than 50% of glomeruli. Glomerular involvement may be predominantly global (IV-G) or predominantly segmental (IV-S).
- **Class V (membranous lupus glomerulonephritis):** Immune complexes are mostly in the subepithelial zone. Some patients show a background of class V injury with concurrent class III or IV injury. Even pure class V lupus nephritis has mesangial immune complexes that can be detected by electron microscopy.
- **Class VI (advanced sclerosing lupus glomerulonephritis):** Advanced chronic disease.

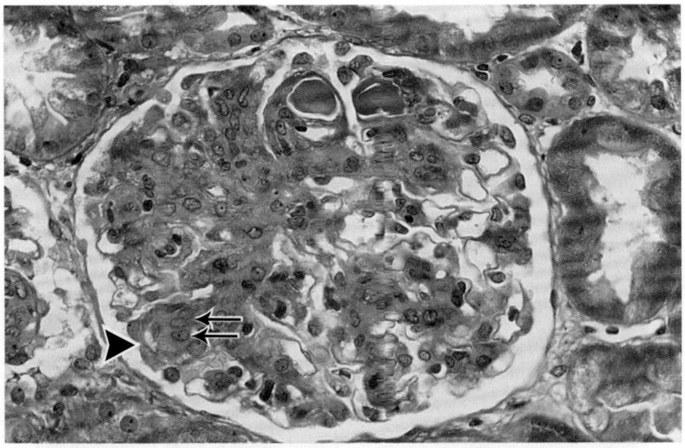

Immune complex dense deposits occur in mesangial, subendothelial, and subepithelial locations. Class I and II lesions have mainly mesangial deposits. Classes III and IV-G have mesangial and subendothelial deposits, and usually scattered subepithelial deposits (Fig. 22-46). Class IV-S tends to show fewer glomerular immune complexes and more segmental necrosis. Class V lesions contain many subepithelial dense deposits. In 80% of cases, endothelial cells have cytoplasmic **tubuloreticular inclusions** detected by electron microscopy (Fig. 22-46). These reflect high levels of interferon. Lupus nephritis and HIV-associated nephropathy are the major renal diseases that feature such inclusions.

By immunofluorescence, subepithelial complexes are granular; subendothelial deposits may be granular or band like (Fig. 22-47). The immune complexes often stain most intensely for IgG, but IgA and IgM are also almost always present, as are C3, C1q, and other complement components. Granular staining along tubular basement membranes and interstitial vessels occurs in more than 1/2 of patients.

FIGURE 22-45. Proliferative lupus glomerulonephritis. Segmental endocapillary hypercellularity (*arrows*) and thickening of capillary walls (*arrowhead*) are present.

CLINICAL FEATURES: Renal disease develops in 70% of patients with SLE and is often the major cause of morbidity and mortality. Clinical manifestations and prognosis of renal dysfunction vary (Table 22-7), depending on the pathology of the underlying renal disease. *Renal biopsy specimens from patients with lupus are used to assess disease category, activity and chronicity, as well as to diagnose lupus glomerulonephritis.* Class III and class IV lupus nephritis have the poorest prognosis and are treated most aggressively, usually with

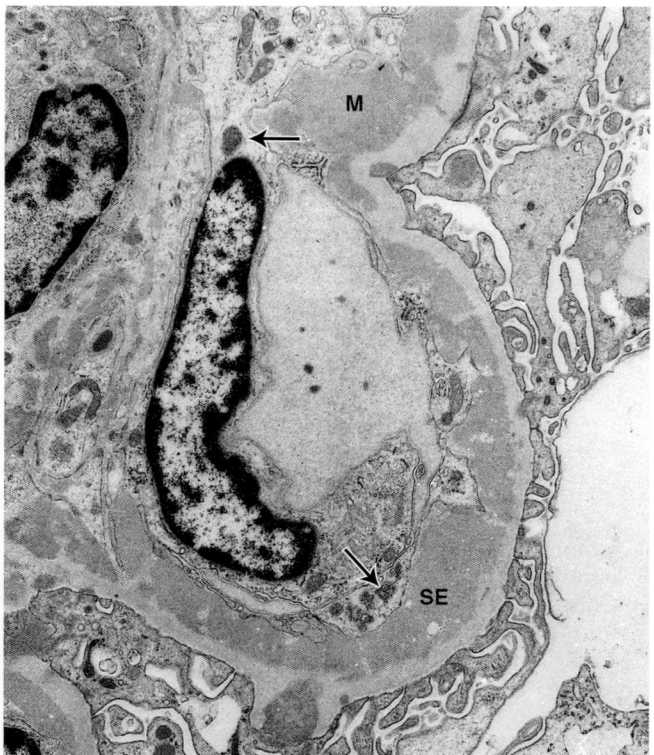

FIGURE 22-46. Diffuse proliferative class IV lupus glomerulonephritis. This electron micrograph reveals large subendothelial and mesangial dense deposits (*M*) and a few subepithelial (*SE*) deposits. Endothelial tubuloreticular inclusions (*arrows*) are present.

high doses of corticosteroids and immunosuppressive drugs. Over time, sometimes due to treatment, lupus nephritis may change from one type to another, with parallel changes in clinical manifestations. Fewer than 20% of patients with class IV disease reach ESRD within 5 years.

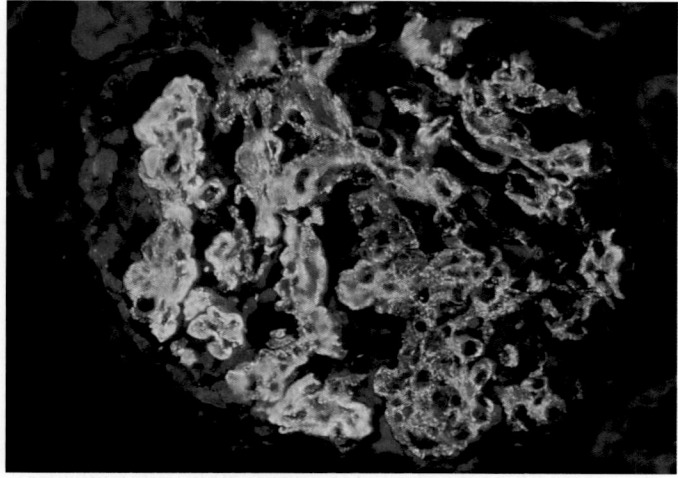

FIGURE 22-47. Diffuse proliferative lupus glomerulonephritis. This immunofluorescence micrograph shows segmental staining for immunoglobulin G in capillary walls and the mesangium.

IgA Nephropathy Is Caused by IgA1 Immune Complexes

PATHOPHYSIOLOGY: Deposition of IgA-dominant immune complexes is the cause of IgA nephropathy, but what the constituent antigens are and how they accumulate (deposition vs. formation *in situ*) are uncertain. Patients with IgA nephropathy often have aberrant IgA1 molecules, elevated blood levels of IgA1, and circulating IgA1-containing immune complexes or aggregated IgA1. Mesangial accumulation of IgA-dominant immune complexes may entail several mechanisms.

Respiratory or gastrointestinal infections often trigger exacerbations of IgA nephropathy. Mucosal exposure to viral, bacterial, or dietary antigens stimulates IgA-dominant immune responses, leading to glomerular immune complex accumulation. Abnormal glycosylation of the IgA1 hinge region appears to be an important factor in many patients with IgA nephropathy. The immune deposits contain mainly IgA1 rather than IgA2. IgA1, but not IgA2, has a hinge region with O-linked glycan chains. In IgA nephropathy, serum IgA1 has less terminal galactosylation and sialylation of these chains. Autoantibodies against these abnormal chains may develop.

As well, the abnormal IgA1 galactosylation may impair receptor engagement of the abnormal IgA1, reducing clearance of immune complexes containing IgA1 from the blood. As a result, IgA forms aggregates in the circulation. The mesangium traps these aggregates. Immune complexes form between the abnormal IgA1 and IgG antibodies against the abnormal IgA1.

IgA-containing immune complexes in the mesangium most likely activate complement by the alternative pathway. The demonstration of C3 and properdin, but not C1q and C4, in the IgA deposits supports this hypothesis.

PATHOLOGY: Immunofluorescence microscopy is essential for diagnosis of IgA nephropathy. The diagnostic finding is mesangial immunostaining for IgA more intense than, or equivalent to, staining for IgG or IgM (Fig. 22-48). This is almost always accompanied

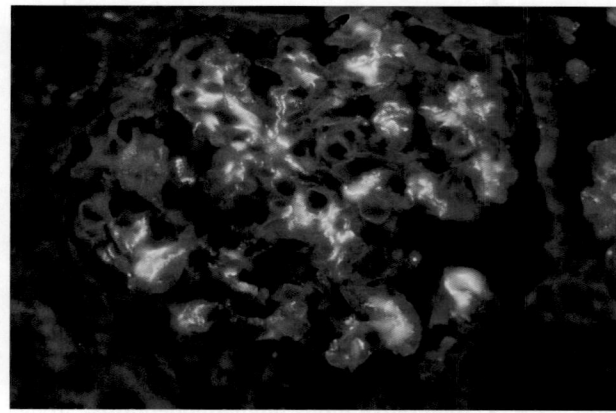

FIGURE 22-48. Immunoglobulin A (IgA) nephropathy. This immunofluorescence micrograph shows deposits of IgA in mesangial areas.

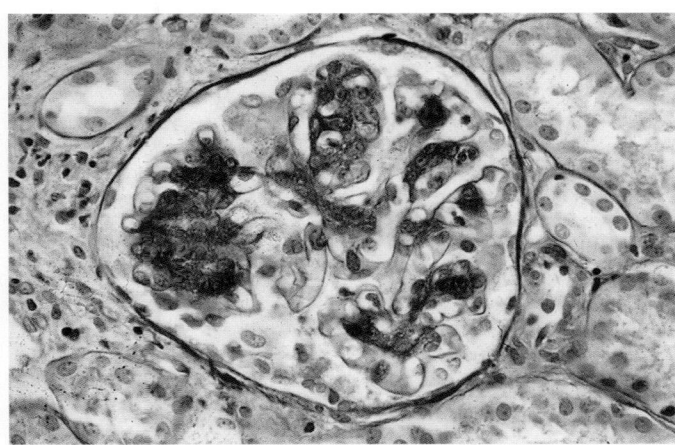

FIGURE 22-49. Immunoglobulin A nephropathy. Mesangial immune deposits (periodic acid–Schiff stain) cause segmental mesangial hypercellularity and matrix expansion.

by staining for C3. IgA deposited in the glomerular capillary wall (in addition to the mesangium) may be present in more severe cases and suggests a less favorable prognosis.

Depending on the severity and duration of the disease, a continuum of histologic findings is seen in IgA nephropathy, from: (1) no discernible light microscopic changes; to (2) focal or diffuse mesangial hypercellularity; to (3) focal or diffuse proliferative glomerulonephritis (Fig. 22-49); and to (4) chronic sclerosing glomerulonephritis. Focal proliferative glomerulonephritis is the most frequent manifestation seen at the time of initial renal biopsy diagnosis. Crescents are not common, except in unusually severe cases. This spectrum of pathologic changes is analogous to that seen with lupus nephritis but tends to be less severe.

Ultrastructural examination reveals mesangial electron-dense deposits (Figs. 22-50 and 22-51). Capillary wall immune complex deposition is usually seen in patients with severe disease.

CLINICAL FEATURES: *IgA nephropathy is the most common form of glomerulonephritis in developed countries.* It accounts for 10% of cases in the United States, 20% in Europe, and 40% in Asia. IgA nephropathy is common in Native Americans and rare in blacks. It occurs most often in young men, with a peak age of 15 to 30 years at diagnosis. Clinical presentations vary, which reflects the varied pathologic severity: 40% of patients have asymptomatic microscopic hematuria, 40% have intermittent gross hematuria, 10% have nephrotic syndrome, and 10% have renal failure. The disease rarely resolves completely but may follow an episodic course, with exacerbations often coinciding with upper respiratory tract infections. IgA nephropathy is slowly progressive, with 20% of patients reaching end-stage renal failure after 10 years. In systemic IgA vasculitis (Henoch–Schönlein purpura), deposits of IgA and resultant inflammation affect small vessels throughout the body including the skin (causing purpura) and gut (causing abdominal pain). When patients with IgA

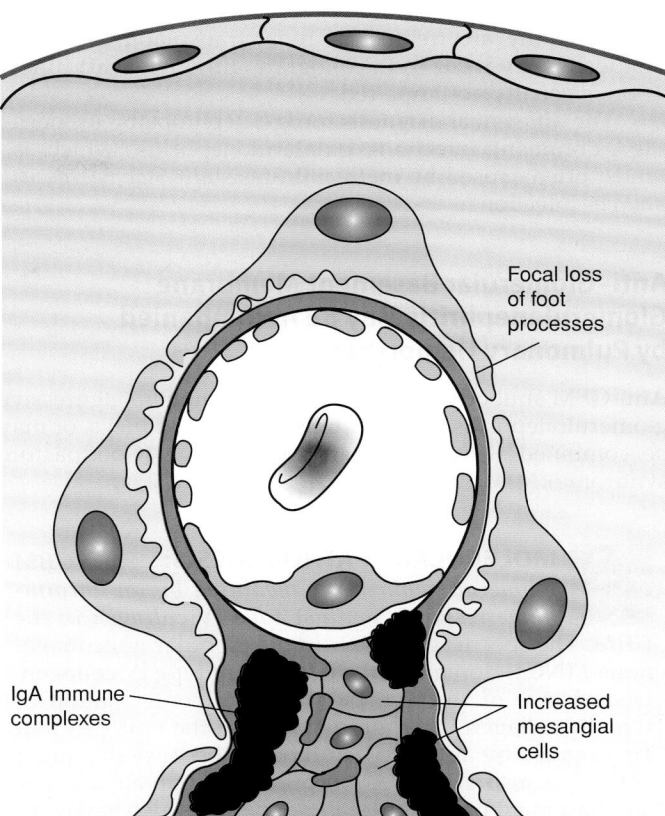

FIGURE 22-50. Immunoglobulin A (IgA) nephropathy. Significant accumulation of IgA is seen in the mesangium, most commonly between mesangial cells and the basement membrane.

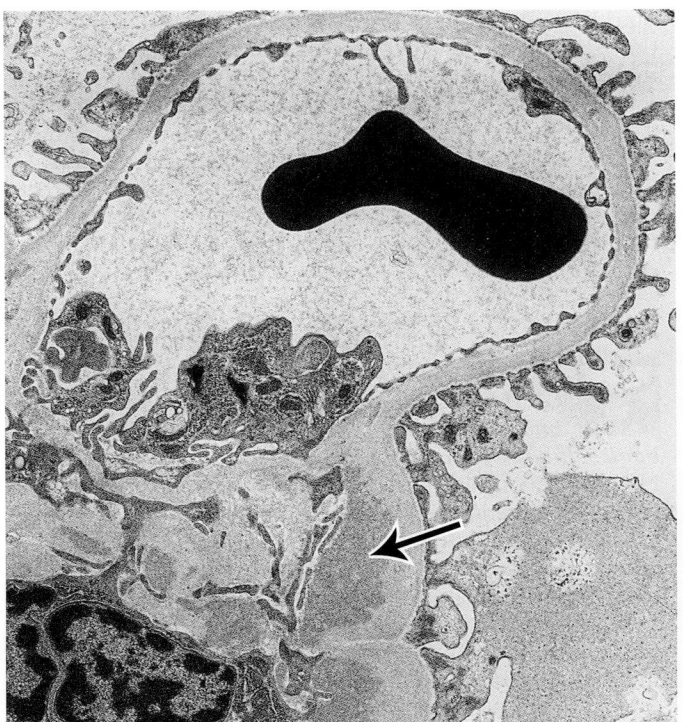

FIGURE 22-51. Immunoglobulin A nephropathy. This electron micrograph demonstrates prominent dense deposits in the mesangial matrix (*arrow*).

nephropathy are treated by renal transplantation, IgA deposits may recur in the allograft, although graft function is usually not impaired.

The differential diagnosis for IgA nephropathy includes IgA-dominant infectious glomerulonephritis, which is most often caused by methicillin-resistant *Staphylococcus aureus* infection.

Anti–Glomerular Basement Membrane Glomerulonephritis May Be Accompanied by Pulmonary Hemorrhage

Anti-GBM antibody disease is an uncommon but aggressive glomerulonephritis that may only affect the kidneys, or may be combined with pulmonary hemorrhage (Goodpasture syndrome).

 MOLECULAR PATHOGENESIS: *Anti-GBM glomerulonephritis is mediated by an autoimmune response against type IV collagen in the GBM.* The specific epitope is in the globular noncollagenous 1 (NC1) domain of the α3 chain of type IV collagen. Disturbance of the tertiary structural conformation of type IV collagen is required to expose the epitopes that are targeted by anti-GBM antibodies. Because the target antigen is also expressed on pulmonary alveolar capillary basement membranes, 1/2 of patients also have pulmonary hemorrhages and hemoptysis, sometimes severe enough to be life-threatening. If lungs and kidneys are both involved, the eponym **Goodpasture syndrome** is used (Fig. 22-15). Anti-GBM antibodies, anti-GBM T cells, or both may mediate the injury. The antibodies bind the autoantigens *in situ*, initiating acute inflammation by activating mediator systems, such as complement. Experimental studies suggest that T cells specific for GBM antigens may also mediate vascular injury. Genetic susceptibility to anti-GBM disease is strongly associated with human leukocyte antigen (HLA)-DRB1. Disease onset often follows viral upper respiratory tract infections, and pulmonary involvement appears to require synergistic injurious agents, such as cigarette smoke.

 PATHOLOGY: *The pathologic hallmark of anti-GBM glomerulonephritis is diffuse linear GBM immunostaining for IgG, indicating autoantibodies bound to the basement membrane* (Fig. 22-52). However, this finding is not entirely specific. Binding of IgG to basement membranes also occurs in diabetic glomerulosclerosis and monoclonal immunoglobulin deposition disease via mechanisms other than antigen recognition. More than 90% of patients with anti-GBM glomerulonephritis have glomerular crescents **(crescentic glomerulonephritis)** (Figs. 22-53 and 22-54), usually involving more than 50% of glomeruli. Focal glomerular fibrinoid necrosis is common. Involved lungs have marked intra-alveolar hemorrhage. By electron microscopy, GBMs show focal breaks, but no immune complex–type electron-dense deposits.

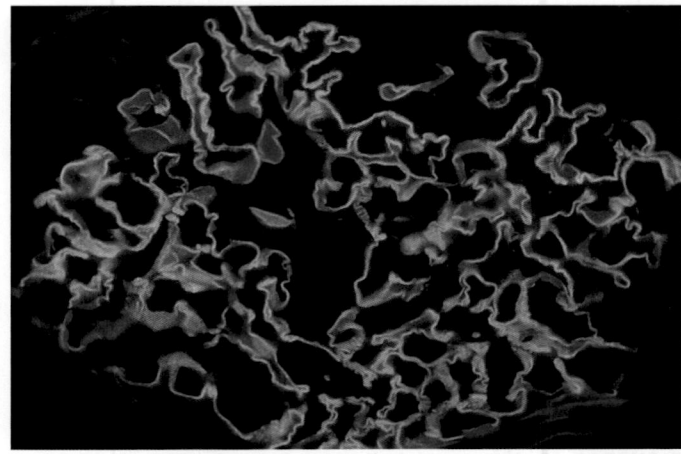

FIGURE 22-52. Anti–glomerular basement membrane (GBM) glomerulonephritis. Linear immunofluorescence for immunoglobulin G is seen along the GBM. Contrast this linear pattern of staining with the granular pattern of immunofluorescence typical for most types of immune complex deposition within capillary walls (see Fig. 22-36).

 CLINICAL FEATURES: Anti-GBM glomerulonephritis typically presents with rapidly progressive renal failure and nephritic signs and symptoms. *It accounts for 10% to 20% of rapidly progressive (crescentic) glomerulonephritis* (Table 22-8). Anti-GBM antibodies are detectable in approximately 90% of patients. Treatment consists of high-dose immunosuppressive therapy and plasma exchange, which are most effective at an early stage of the disease, before severe renal failure supervenes. If ESRD develops, renal transplantation is successful with little risk of losing the allograft to recurrent glomerulonephritis if transplantation occurs after anti-GBM antibodies have disappeared.

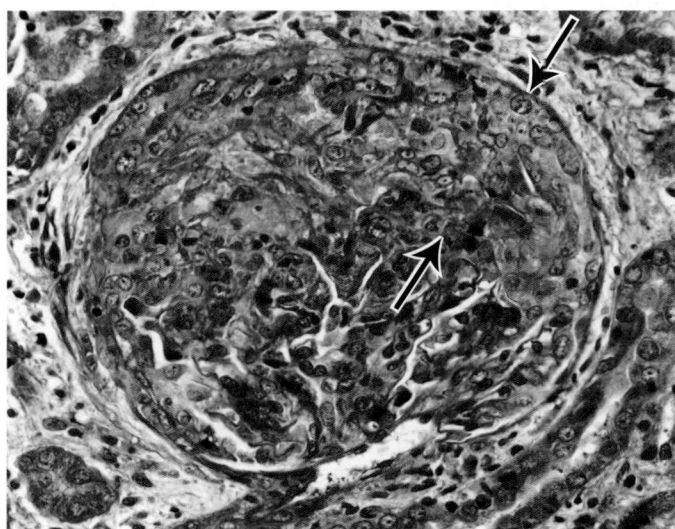

FIGURE 22-53. Crescentic anti–glomerular basement membrane glomerulonephritis. Bowman space is filled by a cellular crescent (*between arrows*). The injured glomerular tuft is at the bottom (Masson trichrome stain).

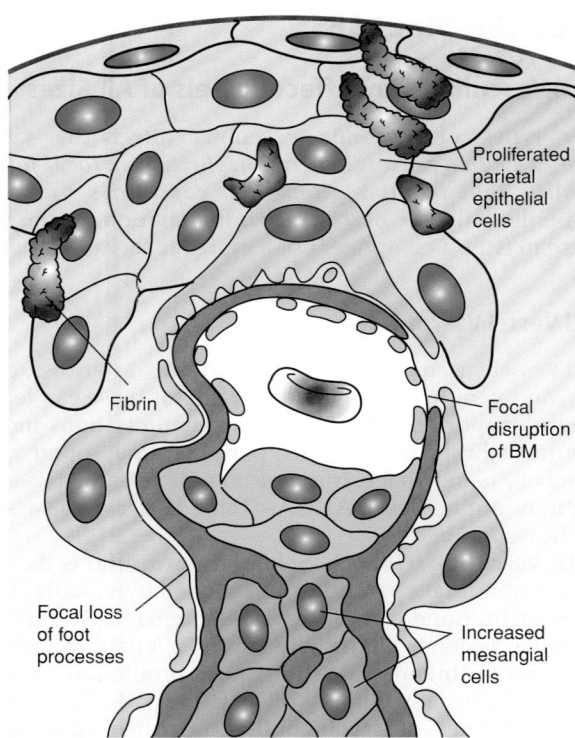

FIGURE 22-54. Crescentic (rapidly progressive) glomerulonephritis. Different pathogenic mechanisms cause crescent formation by disrupting glomerular capillary walls. This allows plasma constituents, including coagulation factors and inflammatory mediators, access to the Bowman space. Fibrin forms, and proliferation of parietal epithelial cells and influx of macrophages (not shown) results in crescent formation.

Antineutrophil Cytoplasmic Autoantibody Glomerulonephritis Is an Aggressive Disease Mediated by Neutrophils

ANCA glomerulonephritis is characterized by glomerular necrosis and crescents.

 PATHOPHYSIOLOGY: ANCA glomerulonephritis was once called *idiopathic crescentic glomerulonephritis* because there was no evidence of

TABLE 22-8

FREQUENCY (%) OF IMMUNOPATHOLOGIC CATEGORIES OF CRESCENTIC GLOMERULONEPHRITIS^a IN DIFFERENT AGE GROUPS

Category	Age (years)		
	<20	20–64	>65
Anti–glomerular basement membrane	10	10	10
Immune complex	55	40	10
Antineutrophil cytoplasmic autoantibody	30	45	75
No evidence for the three categories above	5	5	5

^{a}Glomerulonephritis with crescents in more than 50% of glomeruli.

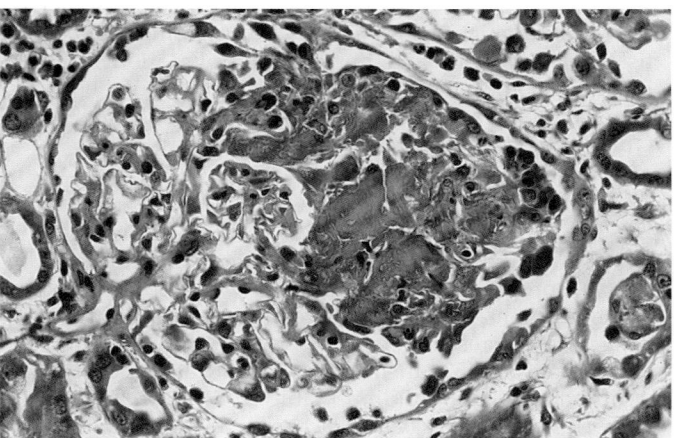

FIGURE 22-55. Antineutrophil cytoplasmic autoantibody glomerulonephritis. Segmental fibrinoid necrosis is seen on the *right side* of this glomerulus. In time, this lesion stimulates crescent formation.

glomerular deposition of anti-GBM antibodies or immune complexes. The discovery that 90% of patients with this pattern of glomerular injury have circulating ANCAs led to the demonstration that these autoantibodies cause the disease. *ANCAs are specific for cytoplasmic proteins in neutrophils and monocytes, usually myeloperoxidase (MPO-ANCA) or proteinase 3 (PR3-ANCA).* These autoantibodies activate neutrophils to adhere to endothelial cells, release toxic oxygen metabolites, degranulate and kill endothelial cells. Neutrophils activated by ANCAs also stimulate the alternative complement pathway and kinin system, which further amplifies the inflammation.

PATHOLOGY: More than 90% of patients with ANCA glomerulonephritis have glomerular necrosis (Fig. 22-55) and crescent formation (Fig. 22-56), often in more than 50% of glomeruli. Nonnecrotic segments may appear normal or have slight neutrophil infiltration or mild endocapillary hypercellularity. There is little or no immunoglobulin or complement

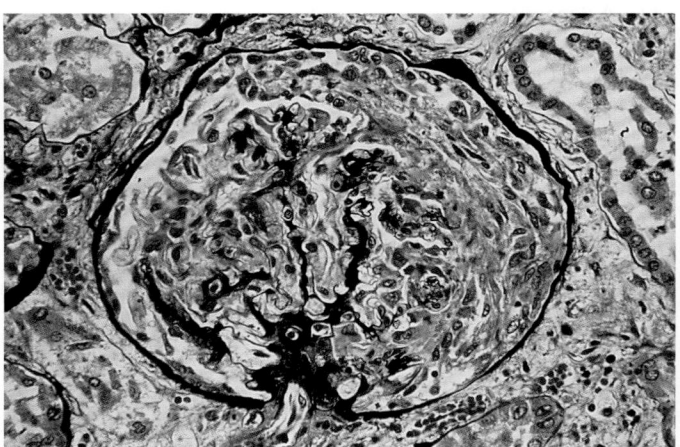

FIGURE 22-56. Antineutrophil cytoplasmic autoantibody glomerulonephritis. Silver staining shows focal disruption of glomerular basement membranes and crescent formation within the Bowman space.

deposition, which distinguishes ANCA glomerulonephritis from anti-GBM and immune complex glomerulonephritides. Some patients with crescentic glomerulonephritis have serologic and pathologic evidence of ANCAs, anti-GBM antibodies, and/or immune complexes.

CLINICAL FEATURES: ANCA glomerulonephritis most commonly presents with rapidly progressive renal failure, with nephritic signs and symptoms. The disease accounts for 75% of rapidly progressive (crescentic) glomerulonephritis in patients older than 60, 45% in middle-aged adults, and 30% in young adults and children (Table 22-8). *Systemic small vessel vasculitis (see below) occurs in 3/4 of patients with ANCA glomerulonephritis and this has many systemic manifestations, including pulmonary hemorrhage.* ANCA glomerulonephritis with pulmonary vasculitis causing **pulmonary–renal vasculitic syndrome** is far more frequent than Goodpasture syndrome. More than 80% of patients with ANCA glomerulonephritis develop ESRD within 5 years if left untreated. Immunosuppressive therapy reduces this to less than 20%. Once remission is induced with high-dose immunosuppression, patients are at risk for recurrent disease. The disease recurs in 15% of renal transplant recipients.

VASCULAR DISEASES

Renal Vasculitis May Affect Vessels of All Sizes

Many types of systemic vasculitis affect the kidney (Table 22-9). *In a sense, glomerulonephritis is a local form of vasculitis that involves glomerular capillaries.* Glomeruli may be the only site of vascular inflammation, or the renal disease may be a component of a systemic vasculitis.

Small Vessel Vasculitides

Small vessel vasculitis affects small arteries, arterioles, capillaries, and venules. Involvement of any of these can lead to glomerulonephritis. Other common manifestations include purpura, arthralgias, myalgias, peripheral neuropathy, and pulmonary hemorrhage. Immune complexes, anti–basement membrane antibodies or ANCAs (Table 22-9) can cause small vessel vasculitides.

IgA vasculitis (Henoch–Schönlein purpura) is the most common childhood vasculitis. It is caused by vascular localization of immune complexes containing mostly IgA. The glomerular lesion is identical to that of IgA nephropathy.

Cryoglobulinemic vasculitis causes proliferative glomerulonephritis, usually with a MPGN pattern. By light microscopy, aggregates of cryoglobulins are often seen within capillary lumens ("hyaline thrombi") (Fig. 22-57).

TABLE 22-9

TYPES OF VASCULITIS THAT INVOLVE THE KIDNEYS

Type of Vasculitis	Major Target Vessels in Kidney	Major Renal Manifestations
Small Vessel Vasculitis		
Immune Complex Vasculitis		
IgA vasculitis (Henoch–Schönlein purpura)	Glomeruli	Nephritis
Cryoglobulinemic vasculitis	Glomeruli	Nephritis
Anti-GBM vasculitis		
Goodpasture syndrome	Glomeruli	Nephritis
ANCA Vasculitis		
Granulomatosis with polyangiitis (Wegener granulomatosis)	Glomeruli, arterioles, interlobular arteries	Nephritis
Microscopic polyangiitis	Glomeruli, arterioles, interlobular arteries	Nephritis
Eosinophilic granulomatosis with polyangiitis (Churg-Strauss syndrome)	Glomeruli, arterioles, interlobular arteries	Nephritis
Medium-Sized Vessel Vasculitis		
Polyarteritis nodosa	Interlobar and arcuate arteries	Infarcts and hemorrhage
Kawasaki disease	Interlobar and arcuate arteries	Infarcts and hemorrhage
Large Vessel Vasculitis		
Giant cell arteritis	Main renal artery	Renovascular hypertension
Takayasu arteritis	Main renal artery	Renovascular hypertension

ANCA = antineutrophil cytoplasmic autoantibody; GBM = glomerular basement membrane.

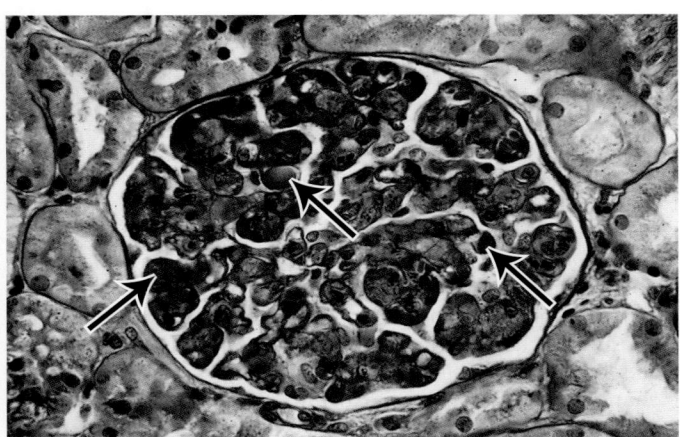

FIGURE 22-57. Cryoglobulinemic glomerulonephritis. This pattern of glomerular inflammation is similar to that of type I membranoproliferative glomerulonephritis. However, as in this example, conspicuous glassy aggregates ("hyaline thrombi," *arrows*) typically occur in capillary lumens and subendothelial spaces. These are not true thrombi but instead are aggregates of cryoglobulins (periodic acid–Schiff stain).

ANCA vasculitis involves vessels outside the kidneys in 75% of patients with ANCA glomerulonephritis. Based on clinical and pathologic features, patients with systemic ANCA vasculitis are classified as follows (Fig. 22-15):

- **Microscopic polyangiitis,** if there is pauci-immune vasculitis with no asthma or granulomatous inflammation
- **Granulomatosis with polyangiitis (formerly Wegener granulomatosis),** if there is necrotizing granulomatous inflammation, usually in the respiratory tract
- **Eosinophilic granulomatosis with polyangiitis (Churg–Strauss syndrome),** if there is eosinophilia and asthma

In addition to causing necrotizing and crescentic glomerulonephritis, ANCA vasculitides often entail necrotizing inflammation in other renal vessels, such as arteries (Fig. 22-58), arterioles, and medullary peritubular capillaries.

Medium-Sized Vessel Vasculitis

Medium-sized vessel vasculitides affect arteries, but not arterioles, capillaries or venules (see Chapter 16). The necrotizing

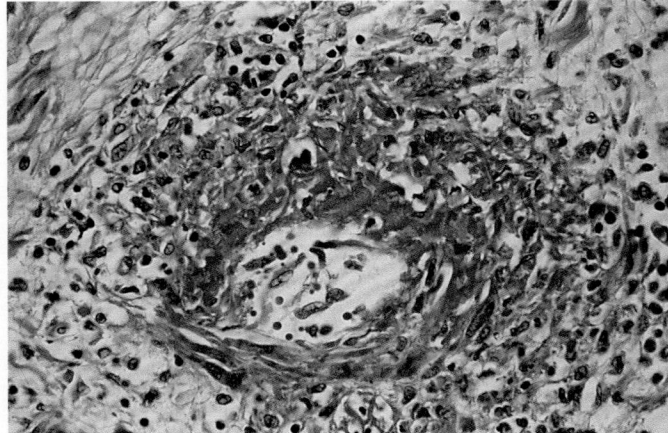

FIGURE 22-58. Antineutrophil cytoplasmic autoantibody necrotizing arteritis. Fibrinoid necrosis and inflammation involve an interlobular artery in the renal cortex.

arteritides, such as **polyarteritis nodosa,** which occurs mainly in adults, and **Kawasaki disease,** which principally afflicts young children, rarely cause renal dysfunction. However, they may involve renal arteries and cause pseudoaneurysm formation and renal thrombosis, infarction, and hemorrhage.

Large Vessel Vasculitis

Large vessel vasculitides, such as **giant cell arteritis** and **Takayasu arteritis,** affect the aorta and its major branches. These disorders may cause renovascular hypertension by involving the main renal arteries or the aorta at the origins of the renal arteries (see Chapter 16). Narrowing or obstruction of these vessels results in renal ischemia, which stimulates increased renin production and consequent hypertension (Table 22-9).

Hypertensive Nephrosclerosis May Obliterate Glomeruli

 ETIOLOGIC FACTORS: Sustained systolic pressures greater than 140 mm Hg and diastolic pressures higher than 90 mm Hg define hypertension, although these cutoffs are changing in light of recent clinical studies (see Chapter 16). Mild to moderate hypertension causes typical hypertensive nephrosclerosis, thus belying the previous term, *benign nephrosclerosis.* In fact, hypertensive nephrosclerosis is identified in about 15% of patients with "benign hypertension" and we recognize that there is nothing benign about hypertension. Changes like those in hypertensive nephrosclerosis may occur in older individuals who have never had hypertension and are attributed to aging itself.

Hypertensive nephrosclerosis is most prevalent and aggressive in blacks, among whom hypertension is the leading cause of ESRD. Black patients have an approximate eightfold elevation in the risk of hypertension-induced end-stage renal disease (ESRD) and this increase in risk may persist even with "adequate" blood pressure control. The recent recognition of an association between two independent sequence variants in the apolipoprotein 1 (*APOL1*) gene on chromosome 22 and renal disease in blacks, including focal segmental glomerular sclerosis and hypertension-related ESRD, provides a likely pathophysiologic mechanism and suggests that hypertensive nephrosclerosis in blacks and whites may arise by diverse mechanisms.

PATHOLOGY: The kidneys are smaller than normal (atrophic) and are usually affected bilaterally. Renal cortical surfaces are finely granular (Fig. 22-59), but coarser scars are occasionally present. On cut section, the cortex is thinned. Many glomeruli appear normal; others show varying degrees of ischemic change. Initially, glomerular capillaries are broader because of thickening, wrinkling, and collapse of GBMs. Cells of the glomerular tuft are progressively lost, and collagen and matrix material are deposited within the Bowman space. Eventually, glomerular tufts are obliterated by a dense, eosinophilic globular scar, all inside the Bowman capsule. Tubular atrophy, due to glomerular obsolescence, is associated with interstitial fibrosis and chronic inflammation.

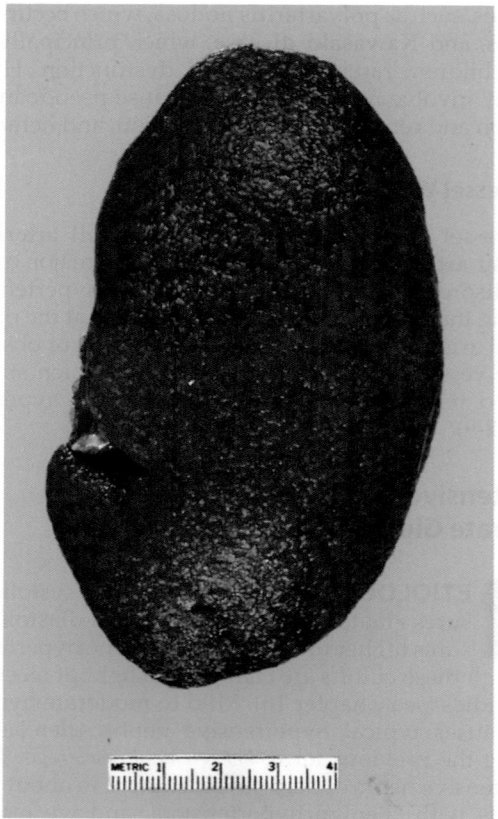

FIGURE 22-59. Hypertensive nephrosclerosis. The kidney is reduced in size, and the cortical surface exhibits fine granularity.

Globally, sclerotic glomeruli and surrounding atrophic tubules are often clustered in focal subcapsular zones, with adjacent areas of preserved glomeruli and tubules (Fig. 22-60), which accounts for the granular surfaces of nephrosclerotic kidneys.

The pattern of change in renal blood vessels depends on vessel size. Intimas of arteries as small as arcuate arteries show fibrotic thickening, replication of the elastica-like lamina, and partial replacement of the muscularis with fibrous tissue. Interlobular arteries and arterioles may develop medial hyperplasia. Arterioles show concentric hyaline thickening of the wall, often with smooth muscle cell loss or displacement to the periphery. This arteriolar change is called **hyaline arteriolosclerosis**.

CLINICAL FEATURES: Although hypertensive nephrosclerosis does not usually impair renal function, some people with hypertension develop progressive renal failure, which may lead to ESRD. Since hypertension is so common, the relatively small percentage of hypertensive patients who develop renal insufficiency still amounts to 1/3 of patients with ESRD.

Malignant Hypertensive Nephropathy Causes Rapid Loss of Renal Function

ETIOLOGIC FACTORS: No specific blood pressure defines malignant hypertension, but diastolic pressures greater than 130 mm Hg, retinal

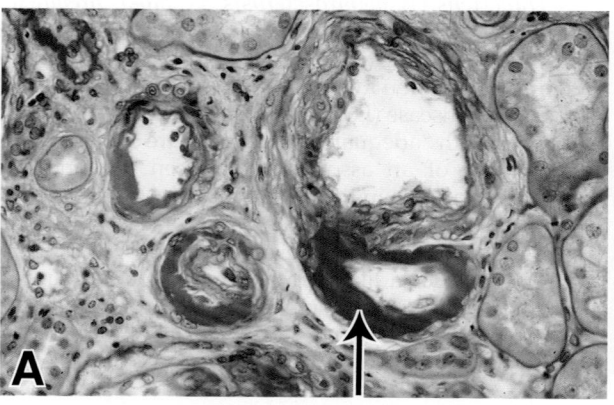

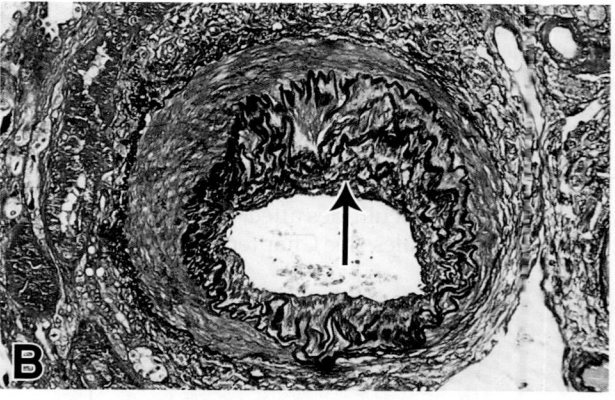

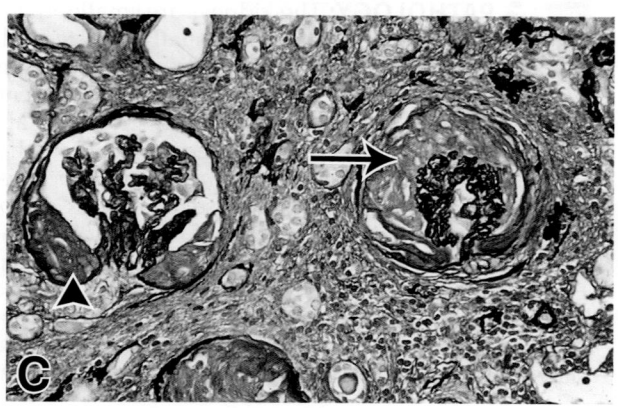

FIGURE 22-60. Features of hypertensive nephrosclerosis. A. Arterioles show hyaline sclerosis (*arrow*) (periodic acid–Schiff stain). **B.** This arcuate artery shows fibroelastotic intimal thickening causing narrowing of the lumen (*arrow*) (silver stain). **C.** One glomerulus exhibits global sclerosis (*arrow*) and another shows segmental sclerosis (*arrowhead*). Note also tubular atrophy, interstitial fibrosis, and chronic inflammation (silver stain).

vascular changes, papilledema, and renal functional impairment are usual criteria. There is a prior history of benign hypertension in 1/2 of patients, and many others have a background of chronic renal injury caused by many different diseases. Occasionally, malignant hypertension arises *de novo* in apparently healthy people, particularly young black men. The pathogenesis of the vascular injury in malignant hypertension is not entirely clear. One hypothesis proposes that very high blood pressure, combined with microvascular vasoconstriction, causes endothelial injury as blood slams into narrowed small vessels. At such sites, plasma constituents leak into injured arteriolar walls (causing fibrinoid necrosis), into arterial intimas (inducing edematous intimal thickening), and into the subendothelial zone of glomerular capillaries (consolidating glomeruli). At these sites of vascular injury, thrombosis can result in focal renal cortical necrosis (infarcts).

PATHOLOGY: Kidneys in malignant hypertensive nephropathy vary in size from small to enlarged, depending on the duration of pre-existing benign hypertension. The cut surface is mottled red and yellow, with occasional small cortical infarcts. Malignant hypertensive nephropathy is often superimposed on hypertensive nephrosclerosis, with edematous (myxoid, mucoid) intimal expansion in arteries and fibrinoid necrosis of arterioles. Glomerular changes vary from capillary congestion to consolidation to necrosis (Fig. 22-61). Severe cases show thrombosis and focal ischemic cortical necrosis (infarction). Electron microscopy shows electron-lucent material expanding glomerular subendothelial zones. There may be focal insudation of plasma proteins into injured vessel walls. These changes are identical to those seen in other forms of thrombotic microangiopathy (see below).

CLINICAL FEATURES: Malignant hypertension is more common in men than in women, typically presenting around the age of 40. Patients suffer headache, dizziness, and visual disturbances and

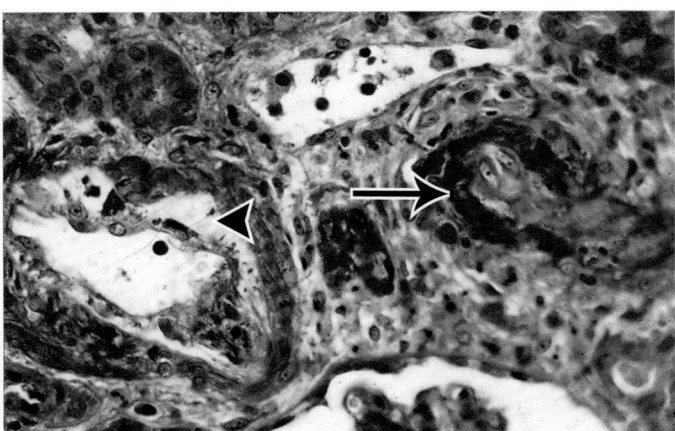

FIGURE 22-61. Malignant hypertensive nephropathy. Characteristic features include red fibrinoid necrosis (*arrow*) in the wall of the arteriole on the right and clear edematous expansion (*arrowhead*) in the intima of the interlobular artery on the left (Masson trichrome stain).

may develop overt encephalopathy. Hematuria and proteinuria are frequent. Progressive renal deterioration develops if the condition persists. Aggressive antihypertensive therapy often controls the disease.

Renovascular Hypertension Follows Narrowing of a Major Renal Artery

 PATHOPHYSIOLOGY: Stenosis or total occlusion of a main renal artery produces hypertension that is potentially curable if the arterial lumen is restored. Harry Goldblatt, an experimental pathologist, pioneered the initial studies of this syndrome in dogs in 1934. Since then, a kidney deprived of vascular supply has been known as a **Goldblatt kidney**. In patients with renal artery stenosis, hypertension is caused by increased production of renin, angiotensin II, and aldosterone all of which are released in response to hypoperfusion of the affected kidney. The level of renin in the venous drainage from an ischemic kidney is elevated, but it is normal in the contralateral kidney. Most (95%) cases are caused by atherosclerosis, which explains why this disorder is twice as common in men as in women, and occurs mainly at older ages (average age, 55). Fibromuscular dysplasia and vasculitis are less common causes overall but are the most frequent causes in children.

 PATHOLOGY: Regardless of the cause of renal artery stenosis, renal parenchymal changes are the same. The size of the involved kidney is reduced. Glomeruli appear normal but are closer to each other than normal, because intervening tubules show marked ischemic atrophy without extensive interstitial fibrosis. Many glomeruli lose their attachments to proximal tubules. Juxtaglomerular apparati are prominent, hyperplastic, and more granular than usual, due to greater renin production.

When atherosclerotic plaques cause the vascular stenosis, they impinge on the aortic ostium or narrow the renal artery lumen, more often on the left than on the right. Occasionally, an abdominal aortic aneurysm affects the origin of the renal arteries. Takayasu arteritis and giant cell arteritis cause renal artery stenosis by inflammatory and sclerotic thickening of the artery wall with resultant narrowing of the lumen.

In **fibromuscular dysplasia,** the renal artery becomes fibrous and shows stenosis due to muscular hyperplasia. Several patterns of renal artery involvement can occur: intimal fibroplasia, medial fibroplasia, perimedial fibroplasia, and periarterial fibroplasia. As the names imply, these disorders affect different layers of the artery, from the intima to the adventitia. Medial fibroplasia is the most common and accounts for 2/3 of cases. This process creates areas of medial thickening alternating with areas of atrophy, producing a "string of beads" pattern in angiograms.

CLINICAL FEATURES: Renovascular hypertension is characterized by mild to moderate blood pressure elevations. A bruit may be heard over

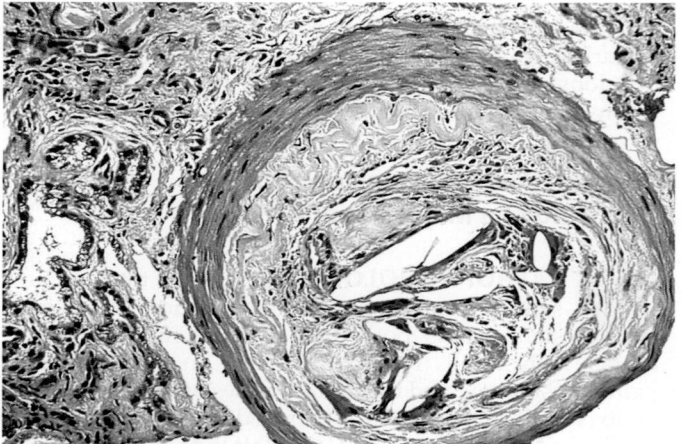

FIGURE 22-62. Atheroembolus. An atheroembolus obstructs an arcuate artery. Note the cholesterol clefts.

the renal artery. Diagnosis requires imaging studies, such as angiography. In more than 1/2 of patients, surgical revascularization, angioplasty, or nephrectomy cures the hypertension. If renovascular hypertension is long standing, the uninvolved kidney may develop hypertensive nephrosclerosis.

Renal Atheroembolism May Complicate Aortic Atherosclerosis

In patients with severe aortic atherosclerosis, atheromatous debris may embolize into the renal arteries, progress into the vascular tree as far as glomerular capillaries and cause acute renal failure. This may occur spontaneously or be initiated by trauma, such as angiographic procedures. **Cholesterol clefts** are seen in vessel lumens (Fig. 22-62). Early lesions are surrounded by atheromatous material or thrombus. They may later elicit a foreign body reaction and stimulate fibrosis in the adjacent vessel wall.

Thrombotic Microangiopathies Cause Microangiopathic Hemolytic Anemia and Renal Failure

PATHOPHYSIOLOGY: Thrombotic microangiopathy has a variety of causes and at least two distinct pathogenic pathways. One pathogenic pathway causes typical and atypical **hemolytic–uremic syndrome (HUS)** by producing endothelial damage. This allows plasma constituents to enter the intima of arteries, walls of arterioles, and subendothelial zone of glomerular capillaries, narrowing vessel lumens and causing ischemia. The injured endothelial surfaces promote thrombosis, which worsens ischemia and may cause focal ischemic necrosis. **Typical HUS** follows diarrhea due to toxin-producing bacteria, most often *Escherichia coli* (usually the O157:H7 strain), in contaminated food. The toxin injures glomerular endothelial cells, initiating the sequence described above. **Atypical HUS** is unrelated to diarrhea

and is caused by different mechanisms, including genetic abnormalities in complement regulatory proteins (mostly factor H but also factor I and membrane cofactor protein), autoantibodies to complement regulatory proteins (anti–factor H), or both.

A second pathogenic pathway causes **thrombotic thrombocytopenic purpura (TTP)**. This is related to genetic or acquired deficiency of a protease, ADAMTS 13, which cleaves multimers of von Willebrand factor on the surface of endothelial cells (see Chapter 26). As a result, large uncleaved multimers accumulate on endothelial cell surfaces and promote platelet aggregation and microvascular thrombosis. Passage of blood through vessels injured by HUS or TTP leads to a nonimmune (Coombs-negative) hemolytic anemia, with misshapen and disrupted erythrocytes (schistocytes) along with thrombocytopenia. This syndrome is **microangiopathic hemolytic anemia (MAHA)**. Because both HUS and TTP present with MAHA, they can be difficult to distinguish clinically. Thrombotic microangiopathies that resemble HUS and TTP can also be due to drugs, autoimmune diseases, and malignant hypertension (Table 22-10).

TABLE 22-10
CATEGORIES OF THROMBOTIC MICROANGIOPATHY
Thrombotic Thrombocytopenic Purpura
Autoantibodies against ADAMTS13
Inherited deficiency in ADAMTS13
Typical Hemolytic–Uremic Syndrome
Escherichia coli
Shigella spp.
Pseudomonas spp.
Atypical Hemolytic–Uremic Syndrome
Genetic mutation (e.g., factor H, factor I, membrane cofactor protein)
Autoantibodies to complement regulatory proteins (e.g., anti–factor H)
Drug-Induced Thrombotic Microangiopathies
Mitomycin
Cisplatin
Cyclosporine
Tacrolimus
Anti-VEGF therapy
Autoimmune Diseases
Systemic sclerosis (scleroderma)
Systemic lupus erythematosus
Antiphospholipid antibody syndrome
Malignant Hypertension
Pregnancy and Postpartum Factors

VEGF = vascular endothelial growth factor.

PATHOLOGY: The renal pathology of HUS is like that of malignant hypertensive nephropathy (see above), which is a form of thrombotic microangiopathy. The basic renal lesions are:

- Arteriolar fibrinoid necrosis
- Arterial edematous intimal expansion
- Glomerular consolidation, necrosis, or congestion
- Vascular fibrin-rich thrombosis

Electron microscopy of glomeruli shows electron-lucent expansion of the subendothelial zone (Figs. 22-63 and 22-64), due to insudation of plasma proteins under injured endothelial cells. Fluorescence microscopy reveals fibrin and insudated plasma proteins in injured vessel walls.

TTP may produce vascular lesions that resemble HUS, but TTP is characterized by more numerous platelet-rich thrombi in glomerular capillaries as well as in capillaries, arterioles, and small arteries in many tissues of the body.

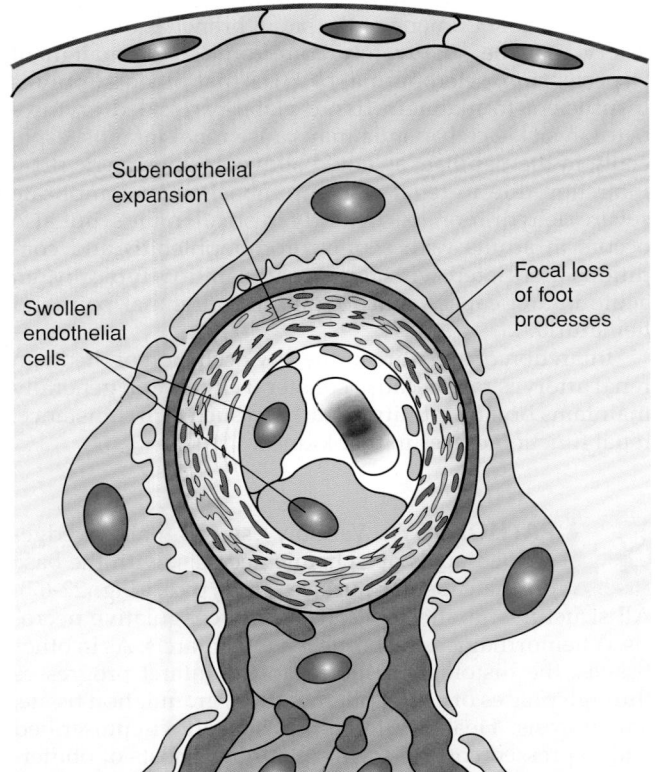 **CLINICAL FEATURES:** Their clinical presentations and causes allow discrimination among the different categories of thrombotic microangiopathy. The MAHAs all have in common microangiopathic hemolytic anemia, thrombocytopenia, hypertension, and renal failure, but to different degrees. An accompanying disease process in a patient with thrombotic microangiopathy (e.g., bloody diarrhea, SLE, systemic sclerosis) or a history of a specific treatment (e.g., mitomycin, cisplatin,

FIGURE 22-63. Hemolytic–uremic syndrome. Subendothelial expansion caused by insudation of plasma proteins narrows the capillary lumen. Endothelial cell swelling further contributes to narrowing of the lumen.

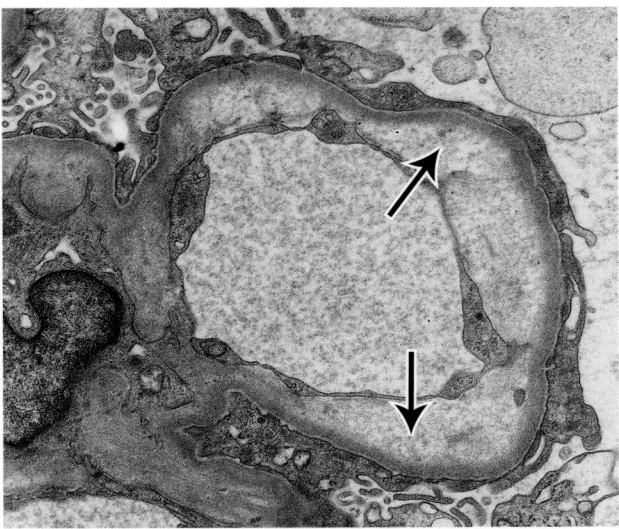

FIGURE 22-64. Thrombotic microangiopathy. This electron micrograph shows a band of lucent material in the subendothelial zone (*arrows*) which narrows the capillary lumen. This is an example of subendothelial expansion depicted in Figure 22-63.

vascular endothelial growth factor [VEGF] inhibitor) may help pinpoint the cause of the MAHA.

Hemolytic–Uremic Syndrome

Typical postdiarrheal HUS features MAHA and acute renal failure, with little or no significant vascular disease outside the kidneys. *Typical HUS is among the most common causes of acute renal failure in children.* It is less common in adults. HUS occurs as isolated cases or in epidemics caused by food contaminated with enterohemorrhagic *Escherichia coli*. Patients present with hemorrhagic diarrhea and rapidly progressive renal failure. Even when dialysis is required, normal renal function usually returns within several weeks. However, impaired renal function may eventually reemerge after 15 to 25 years in more than 1/2 of patients. Atypical HUS is more frequent in adults and is not preceded by diarrhea. Its prognosis is worse than that for typical HUS, often with multiple recurrences and a greater chance of progression to ESRD.

Thrombotic Thrombocytopenic Purpura

In TTP, systemic microvascular thrombosis is characterized clinically by thrombocytopenia, purpura, fever and changes in mental status. Unlike HUS, renal involvement is often absent or less prominent than disease in other organs (e.g., CNS involvement). Bleeding, caused by the consumptive thrombocytopenia, is also more severe in TTP than it is in HUS. TTP is more common in adults than children. Treatment involves plasmapheresis to remove the anti-ADAMTS13 antibody and/or plasma infusion to replace genetically deficient ADAMTS13 (see Chapter 26).

Hypertension, Proteinuria, and Edema Occur in the Third Trimester of Pregnancy in Preeclampsia

If these features are complicated by **convulsions,** the process is called **eclampsia** (see Chapter 14). Glomeruli in

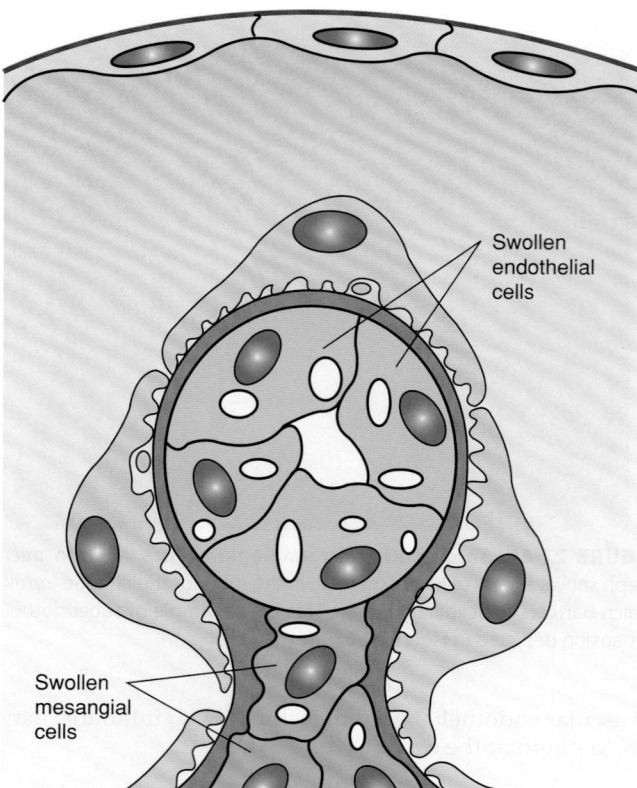

FIGURE 22-65. Preeclamptic nephropathy. Also known as pregnancy-induced nephropathy, preeclamptic nephropathy exhibits marked swelling of endothelial cells and narrowing of the lumens. Both endothelial and mesangial cells are enlarged and have multiple vacuoles and vesicular structures.

preeclampsia are uniformly enlarged and endothelial cells are swollen, resulting in apparently bloodless glomerular tufts (Figs. 22-65 and 22-66). Elevated levels in the maternal circulation of antiangiogenic factors released by the placenta may trigger these endothelial changes. By electron microscopy, the swollen endothelial cells contain large, irregular vacuoles. Vacuoles are also present in podocytes. Bed rest and antihypertensive agents suffice to control mild to moderate disease. More severe cases may require induction of

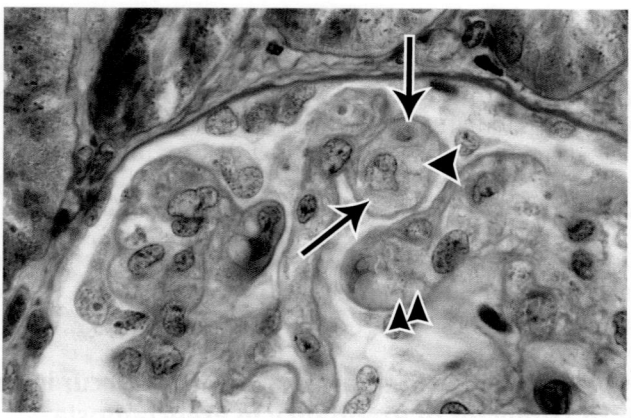

FIGURE 22-66. Preeclampsia. Capillary lumens (*large arrowhead*) are obliterated by swollen endothelial cells (*arrows*). Mesangial vacuolization is also present (*small double arrowheads*) (Masson trichrome stain).

delivery. Hypertension and proteinuria typically disappear by 1 to 2 weeks after delivery.

Nephropathy Is the Most Common Organ Manifestation of Sickle Cell Disease

The interstitial tissue in which the vasa recta course is hypertonic and has a low oxygen tension. As a result, in sickle cell patients, erythrocytes tend to sickle as they go through the vasa recta. In so doing, they occlude the vascular lumens and cause infarcts in the medulla and papilla. The latter may be severe enough to cause grossly apparent papillary necrosis. Ischemic scarring of the medulla leads to focal tubular loss and atrophy. Glomeruli are conspicuously congested with sickled cells. FSGS or, less often, MPGN occurs in a minority of patients and may cause nephrotic syndrome.

Renal Infarcts Are Mostly due to Embolic Arterial Obstruction

Such emboli most often involve interlobar or arcuate arteries.

 ETIOLOGIC FACTORS: The size of the infarct varies with the size of the occluded vessel. Common sources of emboli include:

- **Mural thrombi** overlying myocardial infarcts or related to atrial fibrillation
- **Infected valves** in bacterial endocarditis
- **Complex ulcerated atherosclerotic plaques** in the aorta

Occasionally, a branch of the renal artery is occluded by thrombosis superimposed on underlying atherosclerosis or arteritis. Lumens of the small branches of the renal artery may be so severely compromised in malignant hypertension, scleroderma, or HUS that blood supply is insufficient to maintain tissue viability. Sickled erythrocytes in sickle cell anemia may cause renal infarcts, especially in the papillae, as noted above. Hemorrhagic renal infarction due to renal vein thrombosis may complicate severe dehydration, particularly in small infants, but also occurs in adults with septic thrombophlebitis and conditions associated with hypercoagulability. Typically, an acute infarct causes sharp flank or abdominal pain and hematuria.

Infarction of an entire kidney by occlusion of the main renal artery is rare because collateral circulation generally maintains organ viability. Clearly, in such a circumstance, renal function ceases in that kidney.

 PATHOLOGY: Variably sized, pale wedge-shaped areas of ischemic necrosis, with the base on the capsular surface, are typical (Fig. 22-67). All structures in affected zones show coagulative necrosis. A hemorrhagic zone borders acute infarcts. As in other tissues, the histologic response to the infarct progresses through phases of acute inflammation, granulation tissue, and fibrosis. Healed infarcts are sharply circumscribed and depressed cortical scars containing ghosts of obliterated glomeruli, atrophic tubules, interstitial fibrosis, and a mild chronic inflammatory infiltrate. Old infarcts may undergo dystrophic calcification. At the margins of a

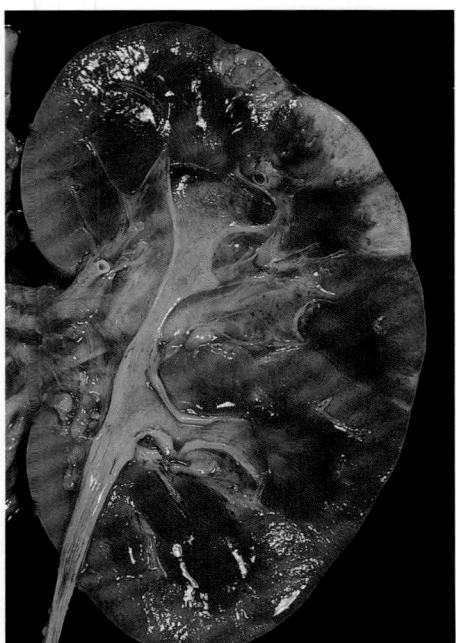

FIGURE 22-67. Renal infarcts. A bisected kidney shows three discrete areas of recent infarction characterized by marked pallor, which extends to the subcapsular surface.

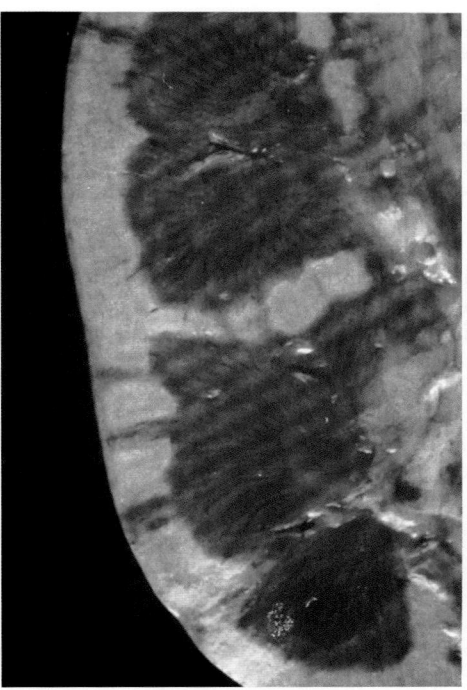

FIGURE 22-68. Renal cortical necrosis. The cortex of the kidney is pale yellow and soft owing to diffuse cortical necrosis.

healed infarct, the viable tissue may show changes attributable to recurrent episodes of sublethal ischemia, including tubular atrophy, interstitial fibrosis, and infiltration by chronic inflammatory cells.

Cortical Necrosis Is due to Severe Ischemia

Cortical necrosis affects all or part of the renal cortex. The term **infarct** applies if there is one area (or only a few areas) of necrosis caused by arterial occlusion, but **cortical necrosis** implies more-widespread (geographic) ischemic necrosis.

 ETIOLOGIC FACTORS: Renal cortical necrosis can complicate any condition associated with hypovolemic or endotoxic shock, the classical situation being premature placental separation late in pregnancy (see Chapter 12). All forms of shock can result in either reversible prerenal or intrarenal ischemia, which precedes irreversible cortical necrosis.

Vasa recta that supply arterial blood to the medulla arise from juxtamedullary efferent arterioles, proximal to vessels supplying the outer cortex. Thus, occlusion of outer cortical vessels (e.g., by vasospasm, thrombi or thrombotic microangiopathy) leads to cortical necrosis and spares the medulla. Experimentally, renal cortical necrosis may be caused by vasoconstrictors such as vasopressin and serotonin, or by eliciting disseminated intravascular coagulation (DIC) (see Chapter 26).

 PATHOLOGY: Cortical necrosis may vary from patchy to confluent (Fig. 22-68). In the most severely involved areas, all parenchymal elements exhibit coagulative necrosis. The proximal convoluted tubules are invariably necrotic, as are most of the distal tubules. In adjacent viable portions of the cortex, glomeruli and distal convoluted tubules are usually unaffected, but many proximal convoluted tubules may show ischemic injury, such as epithelial flattening or necrosis.

With extensive necrosis, the cortex is pale and diffusely necrotic, except for thin rims of viable tissue just beneath the capsule and at the corticomedullary junction. These areas are supplied by capsular and medullary collateral blood vessels, respectively. In patients who survive cortical necrosis, dystrophic calcification may develop in the necrotic areas.

 CLINICAL FEATURES: Severe cortical necrosis manifests as acute renal failure, which initially may be indistinguishable from that produced by acute tubular injury (ATI). However, the former is more often irreversible. A renal arteriogram or biopsy may be required for diagnosis. Recovery is determined by the extent of the disease, but hypertension is common among survivors.

DISEASES OF TUBULES AND INTERSTITIUM

AKI is defined clinically an acute rise in serum creatinine. It is classified as **prerenal** if caused by reduced blood flow to the kidneys, **intrarenal** if due to injury to the renal parenchyma, and **postrenal** if caused by urinary tract obstruction. Intrarenal AKI is further categorized by the portion of the kidney that is mainly injured: **glomeruli** (e.g., acute glomerulonephritis), **vessels** (e.g., thrombotic microangiopathy), **tubules** (e.g., ischemic acute tubular injury), or **interstitium** (acute tubulointerstitial nephritis). *The most common cause of intrarenal AKI is ischemic acute tubular injury*.

Acute Ischemic and Nephrotoxic Acute Tubular Injury Commonly Cause AKI

Ischemic AKI is severe, but potentially reversible, renal failure due to impaired tubular epithelial function caused by ischemia or toxic injury. By definition, ischemic prerenal AKI is reversible pathophysiologic AKI with no structural tubular epithelial changes. *If ischemia is severe enough to cause histologic tubular epithelial injury, it is considered intrarenal ischemic AKI.* Extensive ischemia can cause overt necrosis of tubular epithelium, or **ATN**. However, most ischemic acute tubular injury does not produce widespread tubular epithelial necrosis, and thus in this setting, the term *acute tubular necrosis (ATN)* is a misnomer.

 PATHOPHYSIOLOGY AND ETIOLOGIC FACTORS: Table 22-11 lists some causes of AKI due to acute tubular injury. **Ischemic acute tubular injury** results from reduced renal perfusion, usually associated with hypotension. Tubular epithelial cells have a high metabolic rate and thus are particularly vulnerable to oxygen deprivation, which rapidly depletes intracellular ATP. The most frequent histologic abnormality is flattening (simplification) of tubular epithelial cells due to sloughing of the apical cytoplasm into the urine. This generates granular pigmented casts that can be seen in the urine and detected by urinalysis. Tubular epithelial cells may be simplified (flattened) but not necrotic in some patients with typical ischemic AKI. Overt necrosis is uncommon.

TABLE 22-11
CAUSES OF ACUTE TUBULAR INJURY

Ischemic Prerenal Acute Renal Failure or Ischemic Acute Kidney Injury

    Massive hemorrhage

    Septic shock

    Severe burns

    Dehydration

    Prolonged diarrhea

    Congestive heart failure

    Volume redistribution (e.g., pancreatitis, peritonitis)

Nephrotoxin Acute Tubular Injury

    Antibiotics (e.g., aminoglycosides, amphotericin B)

    Radiographic contrast agents

    Heavy metals (e.g., mercury, lead, cisplatin)

    Organic solvents (e.g., ethylene glycol, carbon tetrachloride)

    Poisons (e.g., paraquat)

Hemeprotein Cast Nephropathies

    Myoglobin (from rhabdomyolysis, e.g., with crush injury)

    Hemoglobin (from hemolysis, e.g., with transfusion reaction)

Nephrotoxic acute tubular injury is caused by some form of chemical injury to epithelial cells. In addition to their sensitivity to ischemia, their active metabolic state makes tubular epithelial cells susceptible to injury by toxins that perturb oxidative or other metabolic pathways. At the same time, these cells also absorb and concentrate toxins. Hemoglobin and myoglobin act as endogenous toxins that can induce acute tubular injury **(pigment nephropathy)** if they are present at high concentrations in the urine.

The pathophysiology of ischemic AKI involves decreased glomerular filtration and tubular epithelial dysfunction due to some or all of the following (Fig. 22-69):

- Intrarenal vasoconstriction
- Alteration of arteriolar tone by tubuloglomerular feedback
- Decreased glomerular hydrostatic pressure
- Decreased glomerular capillary permeability (K_f)
- Tubular obstruction by cellular debris, with increased hydrostatic pressure
- Back leakage of glomerular filtrate into the interstitium through damaged tubular epithelium

 PATHOLOGY: In ischemic AKI, the kidneys are swollen. The cortex appears pale and the medulla is congested. Glomeruli and blood vessels are normal. Tubule injury is focal in distribution and is most pronounced in the proximal tubules and thick ascending limb of the loop of Henle of the outer medulla. The tubular epithelium is flattened, lumens are dilated and brush borders are lost (epithelial simplification), due in part to sloughing of apical cytoplasm, which appears in distal tubular lumens and urine as brown granular casts ("muddy casts"; the color reflects renal cytochrome pigments). Electron microscopy shows decreased basolateral membrane infoldings of proximal tubular epithelial cells. Widespread necrosis of tubular epithelial cells is uncommon, but simplification may be more evident. Instead, "necrosis" is subtle and appears as individual necrotic cells in some proximal or distal tubules. These single necrotic cells, plus a few viable cells, are shed into the tubular lumen, thus focally denuding the tubular basement membrane (Fig. 22-70). Interstitial edema is common. The vasa recta of the outer medulla are congested and often contain nucleated cells, which are predominantly mononuclear leukocytes.

Toxic acute tubular injury shows more-extensive tubular epithelial cell necrosis than is typically seen in the setting of ischemic acute tubular injury (compare Figs. 22-70 and 22-71). However, toxic necrosis is limited largely to tubular segments that are most sensitive to a particular toxin, usually the proximal tubule. In acute tubular injury due to hemoglobinuria or myoglobinuria, there are, as well, many red-brown tubular casts ("pigment casts") that are colored by heme pigments.

During the recovery phase of acute tubular injury, tubular epithelial cells regenerate, with mitoses, increased size of cells and nuclei, and cell crowding. Surviving cells eventually display complete restoration of normal renal architecture.

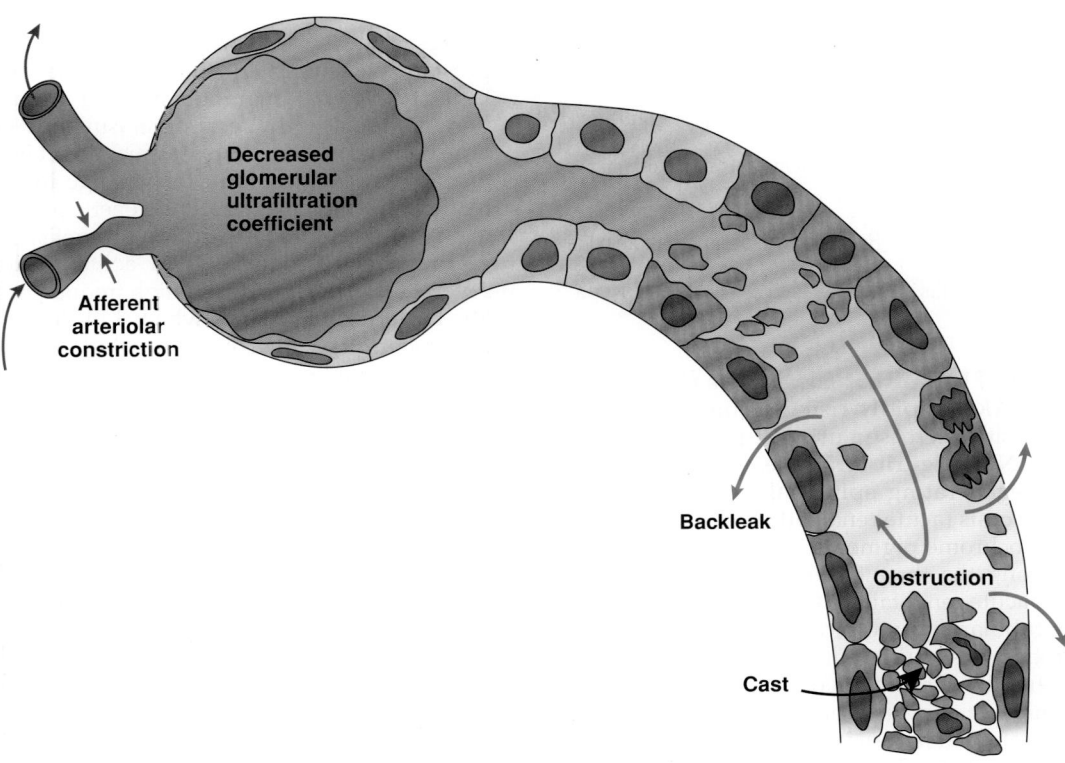

FIGURE 22-69. Pathogenesis of acute renal failure caused by acute tubular injury (ATI). Sloughing and necrosis of epithelial cells result in cast formation. Casts cause tubular obstruction and increased intraluminal pressure, which reduces glomerular filtration. Afferent arteriolar vasoconstriction, caused in part by tubuloglomerular feedback, further decreases glomerular capillary filtration pressure. Tubular injury and increased intraluminal pressure cause leakage of fluid from the tubular lumen into the interstitium.

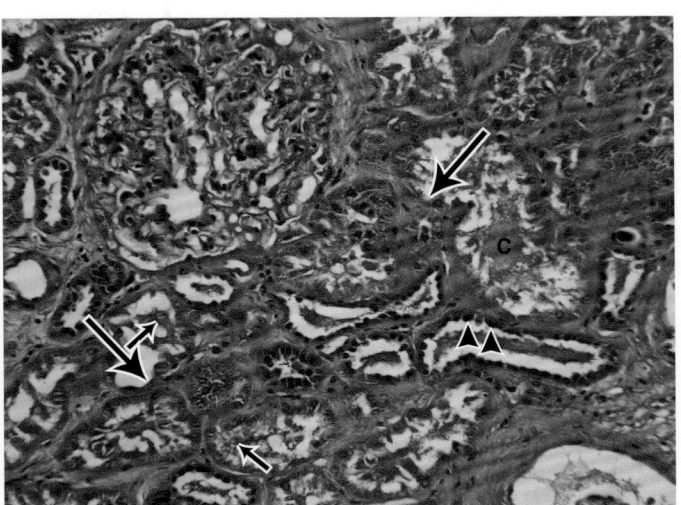

FIGURE 22-70. Ischemic acute tubular injury (ischemic ATI). Necrosis of individual tubular epithelial cells is evident both from focal denudation of the tubular basement membrane (*thick arrows*) and from individual necrotic epithelial cells (*thin arrows*) in some tubular lumens. Casts, the debris of dead tubular epithelium, fill many tubules (*C*). Some enlarged, regenerative-appearing epithelial cells are also present (*arrowheads*). Note the lack of significant glomerular or interstitial inflammation.

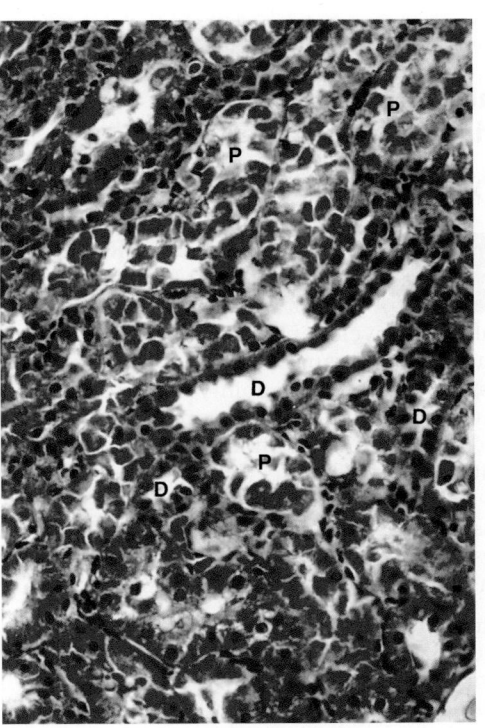

FIGURE 22-71. Toxic acute tubular injury (ATI) due to mercury poisoning. There is widespread necrosis of proximal tubular (*P*) epithelial cells, with sparing of distal and collecting tubules (*D*). Interstitial inflammation is minimal.

THE KIDNEY

TABLE 22-12

URINALYSIS IN ACUTE KIDNEY INJURY

Causes of Acute Kidney Injury	Urinalysis Sediment Findings
Acute tubular injury	Dirty brown casts and epithelial cells
Acute glomerulonephritis	Red blood cell casts and proteinuria
Acute tubulointerstitial nephritis	White blood cell casts and pyuria

 CLINICAL FEATURES: *Ischemia is the leading cause of AKI.* Rapidly rising serum creatinine, usually with decreased urine output **(oliguria),** is characteristic. **Nonoliguric** AKI is less common. Urinalysis shows degenerating epithelial cells and **"dirty brown" granular casts** (acute renal failure casts) with cell debris rich in cytochrome pigments. Urinalysis may help differentiate among the three major intrinsic renal diseases that cause acute renal failure (Table 22-12). Prerenal ischemic acute tubular injury typically has a less than 1% fractional excretion of sodium, but intrarenal acute tubular injury has a fractional excretion of sodium greater than 2%, which is a marker of overt tubular epithelial damage.

The duration of renal failure in patients with ischemic acute tubular injury depends on many factors, especially the nature and reversibility of the cause. Many patients develop at least transient uremia (azotemia, fluid retention, metabolic acidosis, hyperkalemia), and may require dialysis. If the insult is removed right after injury begins, renal function may return within 1 to 2 weeks. However, recovery may take months. Increased urine output and decreased serum creatinine herald the recovery phase.

Pyelonephritis Usually Reflects Bacterial Infection of the Kidney

Acute Pyelonephritis

 ETIOLOGIC FACTORS AND PATHOPHYSIOLOGY: Gram-negative bacteria from feces, mostly *Escherichia coli,* cause 80% of acute pyelonephritis. *E. coli* that cause urinary tract infections **(uropathogenic E. coli)** have virulence factors that enhance their ability to cause not only urinary tract infections but also pyelonephritis. Of these, the best studied are adhesins on fimbria (pili) encoded by pyelonephritis-associated pili (*PAP*) genes. Uropathogenic *E. coli* pili attach to adhesin-binding sites on urothelial cells as well as epithelial cells of the kidney. Infection reaches the kidney by ascending through the urinary tract, a process that depends on several factors:

- Bacterial urinary infection
- Reflux of infected urine up the ureters into the renal pelvis and calyces
- Bacterial entry through the papillae into the renal parenchyma

Bladder infections (cystitis) usually precede acute pyelonephritis. These occur more commonly in females because they have short urethras and lack antibacterial prostatic secretions. In addition, sexual intercourse can facilitate bacterial migration. Normal urethral commensal flora are replaced by fecal organisms in women who are unusually prone to recurrent urinary tract infections. Many factors may contribute to this change in flora, including hygiene, hormonal effects, and genetic predisposition (e.g., increased receptors for *E. coli* on urothelial cells).

Pregnancy predisposes to acute pyelonephritis for several reasons, including a high frequency of asymptomatic bacteriuria (10%), of which 1/4 develops into acute pyelonephritis. Other causes include increased residual urine volume because high levels of progesterone make bladder musculature flaccid and less able to expel urine.

The bladder normally empties all but 2 to 3 mL of residual urine. Subsequent addition of sterile urine from the kidneys dilutes any bacteria that may have gained access to the bladder. However, if residual urine volume is increased (e.g., with prostatic obstruction or bladder atony due to neurogenic disorders such as paraplegia or diabetic neuropathy), sterile urine from the kidneys may be insufficient to dilute residual bladder urine and prevent bacterial accumulation. Diabetic glycosuria also facilitates infection by providing a rich bacterial growth medium.

Bacteria in bladder urine usually do not ascend to infect the kidneys. The ureter commonly inserts into the bladder wall at a steep angle (Fig. 22-72), and its most distal portion courses parallel to the bladder wall, between the mucosa and muscularis. Increased intravesicular pressure during micturition occludes the distal ureteral lumen and prevents urinary reflux. An anatomic abnormality, a short passage of the ureter within the bladder wall, causes the ureter to insert more perpendicularly to the bladder mucosal surface. As a result, rather than occluding the lumen, micturition increases intravesicular pressure and pushes urine into the patent ureter. This reflux can force the urine into the renal pelvis and calyces.

Even if reflux pressure delivers bacteria to the calyces, the renal parenchyma is not necessarily contaminated. The convexity of the simple papillae of central calyces blocks reflux urine from entering (Fig. 22-72), but the concavity of peripheral compound papillae allows easier access to the collecting system. *However, if pressure is prolonged, as in obstructive uropathy, even simple papillae eventually become vulnerable to retrograde entry of urine.* From the collecting tubules, bacteria access the renal interstitium and tubules.

In addition to ascending through urine, bacteria and other pathogens can gain access to renal parenchyma through the bloodstream, causing **hematogenous pyelonephritis**. In bacterial endocarditis, for example, gram-positive organisms, such as staphylococci, can spread from an infected valve and establish infection in the kidney. The kidney is commonly involved in miliary tuberculosis. Fungi, such as *Aspergillus,* can seed kidneys in immunosuppressed hosts. Hematogenous infections preferentially affect the cortex, which receives abundant blood flow.

PATHOLOGY: The kidneys in acute pyelonephritis are swollen and may contain medullary abscesses, if the infection is ascending. Abscesses are present in the cortex when the infection is

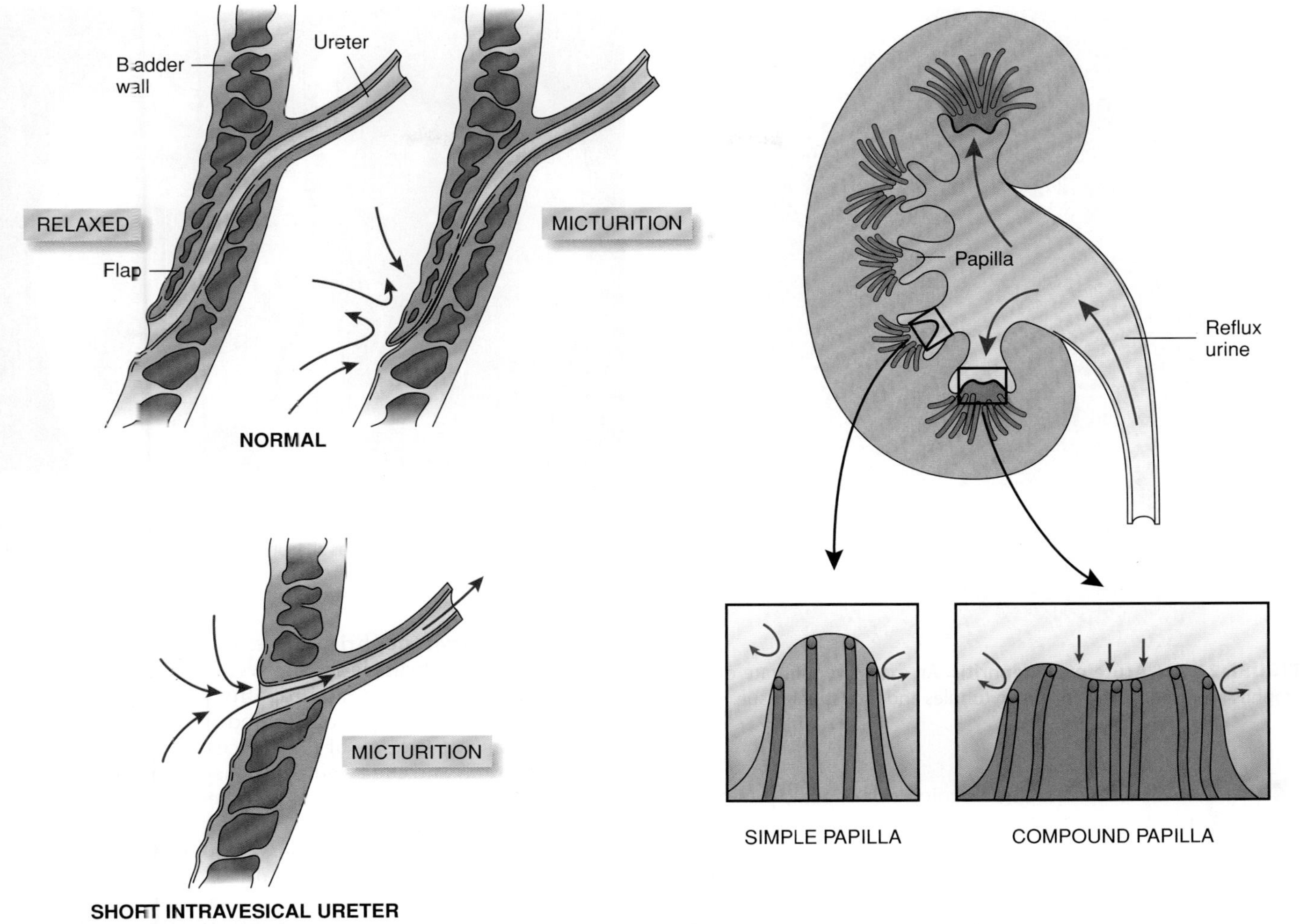

Bladder wall

Ureter

RELAXED

Flap

MICTURITION

NORMAL

MICTURITION

SHORT INTRAVESICAL URETER

Papilla

Reflux urine

SIMPLE PAPILLA

COMPOUND PAPILLA

FIGURE 22-72. Anatomic features of the bladder and kidney in pyelonephritis caused by ureterovesical reflux. In the normal bladder, the distal portion of the intravesical ureter courses between the mucosa and the muscularis, forming a mucosal flap. On micturition, the elevated intravesicular pressure compresses the flap against the bladder wall, occluding the lumen. People with a congenitally short intravesical ureter have no mucosal flap, because the angle of entry of the ureter into the bladder approaches a right angle. Thus, micturition forces urine into the ureter. In the renal pelvis, simple papillae of the central calyces are convex and do not readily allow reflux of urine. By contrast, peripheral compound papillae are concave and permit entry of refluxed urine.

hematogenous. Pelvic and calyceal urothelium may be hyperemic and covered by purulent exudate. The disease is often focal, and much of the kidney may be normal.

Most infections involve only a few papillary systems. Renal parenchyma, particularly the cortex, typically shows extensive focal destruction by inflammation, although vessels and glomeruli are often preferentially preserved. Infiltrates mainly contain neutrophils, which often fill tubules and especially collecting ducts (Fig. 22-73). In severe cases of acute pyelonephritis, necrosis of the papillary tips may occur (Fig. 22-74) or infection may extend beyond the renal capsule to cause a perinephric abscess.

CLINICAL FEATURES: Symptoms of acute pyelonephritis include fever, chills, sweats, malaise, flank pain, and costovertebral angle tenderness. Blood neutrophilia is common. Clinical differentiation of upper from lower urinary tract infections is often

difficult, but **leukocyte casts** in the urine suggest a pyelonephritis.

Chronic Pyelonephritis

ETIOLOGIC FACTORS: Chronic pyelonephritis is caused by recurrent and persistent bacterial infection due to urinary tract obstruction, urine reflux, or both (Fig. 22-75). Whether reflux without infection can produce chronic pyelonephritis is controversial.

In chronic pyelonephritis caused by reflux or obstruction, medullary tissue and overlying cortex are preferentially injured by recurrent acute and chronic inflammation. Progressive atrophy and scarring ensue, leading to contraction of involved papillary tips (or sloughing if there is papillary necrosis) and thinning of the overlying cortex. This process causes a distinctive gross appearance of broad depressed areas of cortical fibrosis and atrophy overlying a dilated calyx **(caliectasis)** (Fig. 22-76).

THE KIDNEY

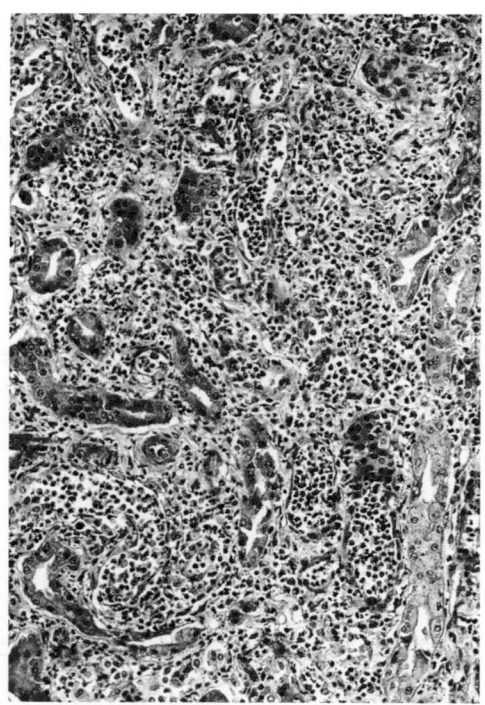

FIGURE 22-73. Acute pyelonephritis. An extensive infiltrate of neutrophils is present in the collecting tubules and interstitial tissue.

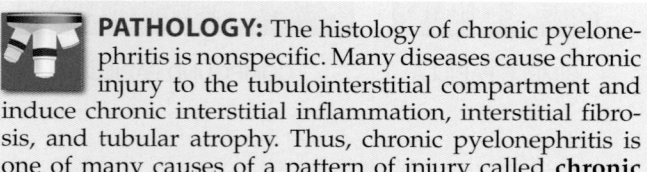

PATHOLOGY: The histology of chronic pyelonephritis is nonspecific. Many diseases cause chronic injury to the tubulointerstitial compartment and induce chronic interstitial inflammation, interstitial fibrosis, and tubular atrophy. Thus, chronic pyelonephritis is one of many causes of a pattern of injury called **chronic**

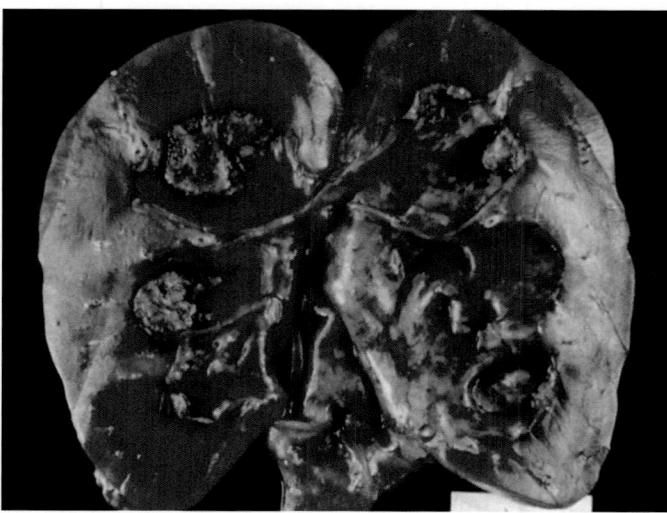

FIGURE 22-74. Papillary necrosis. The bisected kidney shows a dilated renal pelvis and dilated calyces secondary to urinary tract obstruction. The papillae are necrotic and appear as sharply demarcated, ragged, yellowish areas.

tubulointerstitial nephritis. The gross appearance of chronic pyelonephritis is distinctive. Only chronic pyelonephritis and analgesic nephropathy produce both caliectasis and overlying corticomedullary scarring. In obstructive uropathy, all of the calyces and the renal pelvis are dilated, and the parenchyma is uniformly thinned (Fig. 22-76). In cases associated with vesicoureteral reflux, the calyces at the poles of the kidney are preferentially expanded and are associated with overlying discrete, coarse scars that indent the renal surface. The scars are composed of atrophic dilated tubules surrounded by interstitial fibrosis and chronic inflammatory infiltrates

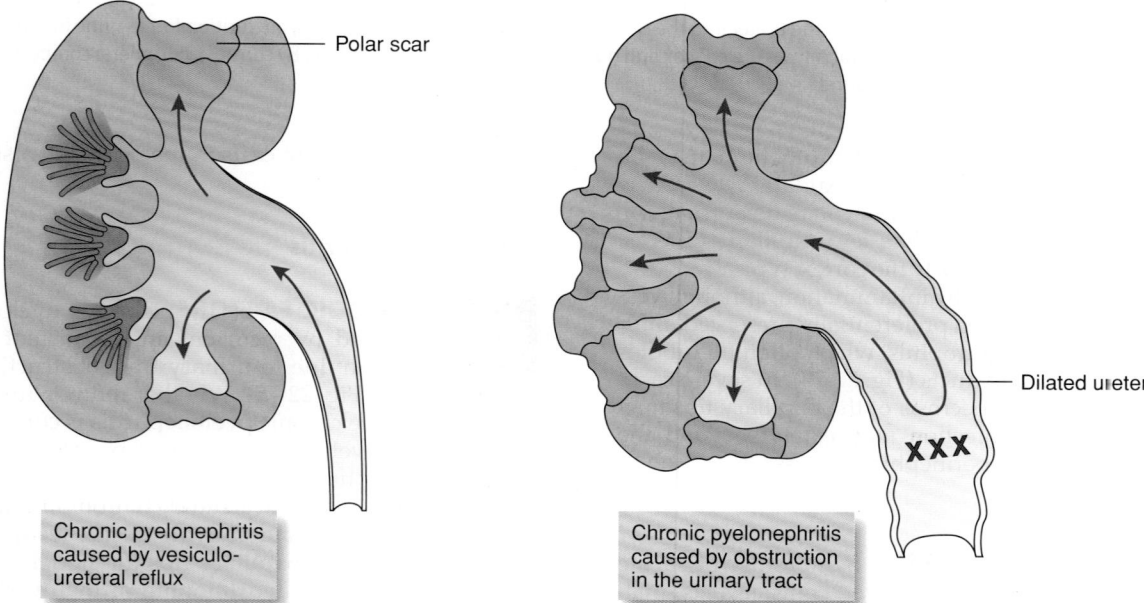

Polar scar

Chronic pyelonephritis caused by vesiculoureteral reflux

Dilated ureter

Chronic pyelonephritis caused by obstruction in the urinary tract

FIGURE 22-75. The two major types of chronic pyelonephritis. Left. Vesicoureteral reflux causes infection of the peripheral compound papillae and, therefore, scars in the poles of the kidney. **Right.** Obstruction of the urinary tract leads to high-pressure backflow of urine, which causes infection of all papillae, diffuse scarring of the kidney and thinning of the cortex.

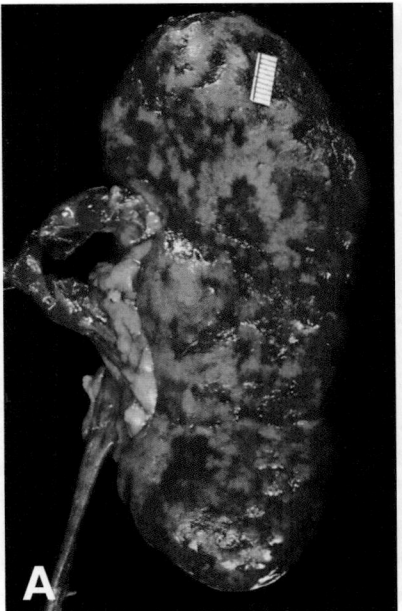
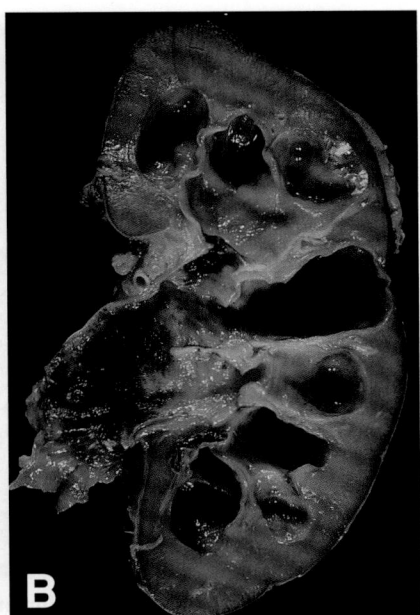

FIGURE 22-76. Chronic pyelonephritis. A. The cortical surface contains many irregular, depressed scars (reddish areas). **B.** There is marked dilation of calyces (caliectasis) caused by inflammatory destruction of papillae, with atrophy and scarring of the overlying cortex.

(Fig. 22-77). The most characteristic (but not specific) tubular change is severe epithelial atrophy, with diffuse, eosinophilic, hyaline casts. Such tubules are "pinched-off" spherical segments, resembling colloid-containing thyroid follicles. This pattern, called **thyroidization,** results from breakup of tubules and residual segments forming spherules. Glomeruli may be uninvolved, show periglomerular fibrosis or glomerulosclerosis. Loss of most functioning nephrons may lead to secondary FSGS. Fibrosis in arterial and arteriolar walls is common. There is marked scarring and chronic inflammation of the calyceal mucosa.

Xanthogranulomatous pyelonephritis is an uncommon form of chronic pyelonephritis that is often caused by diverse pathogens, such as *Proteus, Escherichia coli, Klebsiella,* and *Pseudomonas.* Its name derives from the yellow gross appearance of nodular renal lesions, caused by numerous lipid-laden foamy macrophages **(xanthoma cells)** (Fig. 22-78A). The disease is usually unilateral. Because this form of inflammation often presents as a mass lesion (Fig. 22-78B), it can be confused with renal cell carcinoma (RCC).

CLINICAL FEATURES: Most patients with chronic pyelonephritis have episodic symptoms of urinary tract infection or acute pyelonephritis, such as recurrent fever and flank pain. Some have a silent course until ESRD develops. Urinalysis shows leukocytes, and imaging studies reveal caliectasis and cortical scarring.

Analgesic Nephropathy Results From Chronic Overconsumption of Phenacetin

Patients with analgesic nephropathy typically have taken more than 2 kg of analgesics, often in combinations, such as aspirin and phenacetin, or aspirin and acetaminophen. Phenacetin most often leads to nephropathy and is banned in many countries, including the United States. The pathogenesis of analgesic nephropathy is not clear. Possibilities include direct nephrotoxicity, ischemic damage due to drug-induced vascular changes or both. Analgesic nephropathy is distinct from AKI caused by analgesic-induced acute tubulointerstitial nephritis (e.g., caused by NSAIDs).

PATHOLOGY: Medullary injury with papillary necrosis occurs early in analgesic nephropathy. Atrophy, chronic inflammation, and scarring of the overlying cortex follow. The earliest histologic abnormality is a distinctive homogeneous thickening of capillary walls just beneath the transitional epithelium of the urinary tract. Early parenchymal changes are confined to papillae and the inner medulla, and they consist of focal basement membrane thickening of tubules and capillaries,

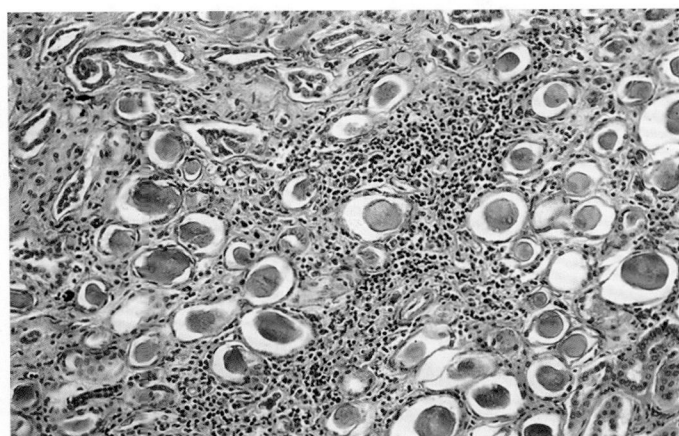

FIGURE 22-77. Tubular dilation and atrophy. Many tubules contain eosinophilic hyaline casts resembling the colloid of thyroid follicles (so-called thyroidization). The interstitium is scarred and contains a chronic inflammatory cell infiltrate.

THE KIDNEY

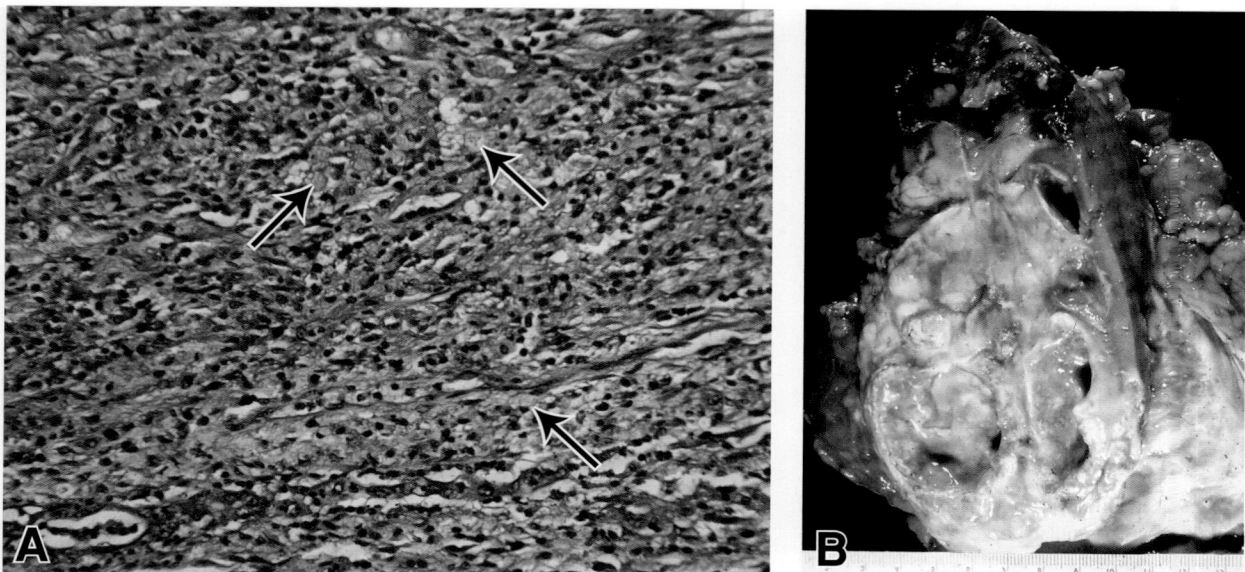

FIGURE 22-78. Xanthogranulomatous pyelonephritis. A. This lesion is characterized by a granulomatous reaction, with foamy histiocytes (*arrows*) admixed with other types of inflammatory cells. **B.** This type of pyelonephritis can present as a mass lesion, simulating a tumor.

interstitial fibrosis, and focal coagulative necrosis. Necrotic areas eventually become confluent, first affecting the corticomedullary junction and then the collecting ducts. The necrotic foci contain few inflammatory cells. Eventually, the entire papilla becomes necrotic **(papillary necrosis),** often remaining in place as an amorphous mass. Dystrophic calcification of such necrotic papillae is common. Papillae may remain partly attached at the demarcation zone or be completely sloughed. Secondary tubular atrophy, interstitial fibrosis, and chronic inflammation develop in the overlying cortex.

CLINICAL FEATURES: Signs and symptoms occur only late in analgesic nephropathy and include an inability to concentrate the urine, distal tubular acidosis, hematuria, hypertension, and anemia. Sloughing of necrotic papillary tips into the renal pelvis may result in colic as they pass through the ureters. Progressive renal failure often develops and leads to ESRD.

Drug-Induced (Hypersensitivity) Acute Tubulointerstitial Nephritis Is a Cell-Mediated Immune Response

PATHOPHYSIOLOGY: Acute drug-induced tubulointerstitial nephritis causes AKI. It entails infiltration by activated T cells and eosinophils, indicating a type IV cell-mediated immune reaction. The immunogen could be the drug itself, the drug bound to certain tissue components, a drug metabolite, or a tissue component altered by the drug. Drugs most commonly implicated include NSAIDs, diuretics, and certain antibiotics, especially β-lactam antibiotics (e.g., synthetic penicillins, cephalosporins).

PATHOLOGY: There is patchy cortical infiltration by lymphocytes and occasional eosinophils (5% to 10% of the total leukocytes in the tissue) (Fig. 22-79). The medulla is usually less involved. Eosinophils tend to cluster, especially in tubular lumens and in the urine. Neutrophils are rare; their presence should raise suspicion of pyelonephritis or hematogenous bacterial

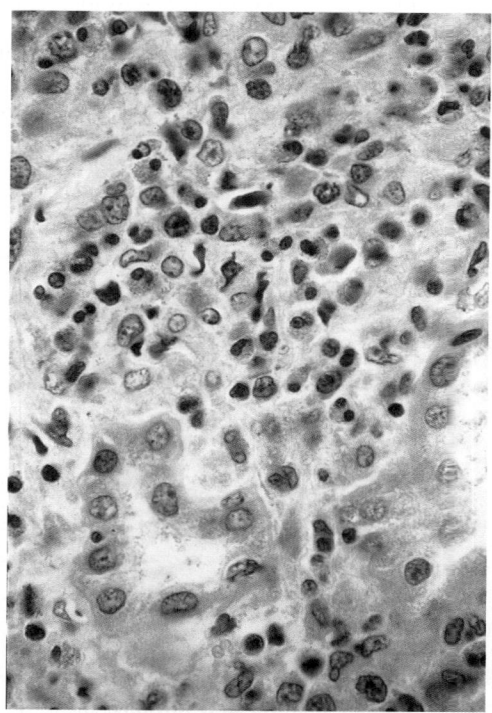

FIGURE 22-79. Hypersensitivity tubulointerstitial nephritis. There is interstitial edema and infiltration by mononuclear leukocytes, with admixed eosinophils.

infection. There may be small granulomatous foci, especially later in the disease. Proximal and distal tubular epithelial cells are focally invaded by white blood cells ("tubulitis"). Glomeruli and vessels are not inflamed, but features of minimal-change disease may occur in drug-induced tubulointerstitial nephritis caused by NSAIDs.

CLINICAL FEATURES: Acute tubulointerstitial nephritis usually presents as AKI, typically about 2 weeks after a drug is started. Urinalysis shows erythrocytes, leukocytes (including eosinophils) and sometimes leukocyte casts. Tubular defects are common, including sodium wasting, glucosuria, aminoaciduria, and renal tubular acidosis. Systemic allergic symptoms, such as fever and rash, may also be present. Most patients recover fully within several weeks or months if the offending drug is discontinued.

Light-Chain Cast Nephropathy May Complicate Multiple Myeloma

Light-chain cast nephropathy is caused by monoclonal Ig light chains in the urine. These cause tubular epithelial injury and tubular casts.

PATHOPHYSIOLOGY: As discussed above, multiple myeloma may produce AL amyloidosis, light-chain deposition disease, heavy-chain deposition disease and light-chain cast nephropathy. The latter is the most common kidney disease in patients with multiple myeloma. Glomeruli filter circulating light chains. However, at the acidic pH typical of urine, these light chains form casts by binding to Tamm–Horsfall glycoproteins secreted by distal tubular epithelial cells. Renal dysfunction results from both the toxicity of free light chains for tubular epithelium and obstruction by the casts. Light chain structure determines whether they produce light-chain cast nephropathy, AL amyloidosis, or light-chain deposition disease. Occasional patients can show several of these renal diseases concomitantly.

PATHOLOGY: Many dense, brightly eosinophilic and glassy (hyaline) casts may be seen in distal renal tubules and collecting ducts (Fig. 22-80). Casts appear crystalline, often with fractures and sharp angular borders. They may elicit foreign body reactions, with macrophages and multinucleated giant cells. Interstitial chronic inflammation and edema typically accompany the tubular lesions. More chronic lesions show interstitial fibrosis and tubular atrophy. Focal calcium deposits **(nephrocalcinosis)** often occur in the fibrotic tubular interstitium. Immunostaining visualizes antibody light chains and Tamm–Horsfall proteins.

CLINICAL FEATURES: Light-chain cast nephropathy may manifest as acute or chronic renal failure. Proteinuria, predominantly of immunoglobulin light chains, is usually present, although not necessarily in

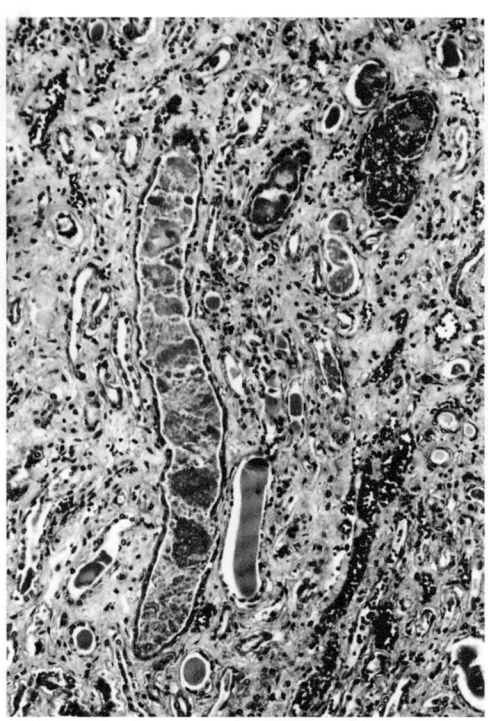

FIGURE 22-80. Light-chain cast nephropathy. This light micrograph shows numerous casts within tubular lumina.

the nephrotic range. Nephrotic-range proteinuria in patients with multiple myeloma suggests AL amyloidosis or light-chain deposition disease rather than light-chain cast nephropathy.

Urate Crystals Deposit in the Tubules and Interstitium in Urate Nephropathy

Any condition with elevated blood levels of uric acid may cause urate nephropathy. The classic chronic disease in this category is primary gout (see Chapter 30).

PATHOPHYSIOLOGY: In **chronic urate nephropathy** due to gout, crystalline monosodium urate deposits in the tubules and interstitium. **Acute urate nephropathy** can be due to increased cell turnover. For example, chemotherapy for malignant neoplasms may cause extensive tumor cell death. In **tumor lysis syndrome,** blood uric acid levels suddenly increase as massive numbers of tumor cells die. Catabolism of huge amounts of purines from DNA released by dying tumor cells leads to hyperuricemia. Uric acid crystals precipitate in the acidic pH of collecting ducts, obstructing them and causing AKI. Interference with uric acid excretion (e.g., chronic intake of certain diuretics) can also cause hyperuricemia. Chronic lead intoxication interferes with uric acid secretion by proximal tubules and leads to **saturnine gout.**

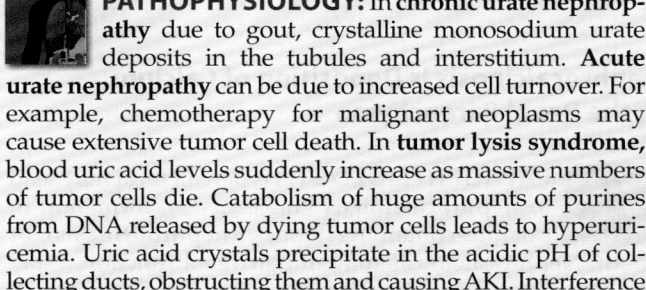 **PATHOLOGY:** In acute urate nephropathy, uric acid precipitated in collecting ducts appears as yellow streaks in the papillae (Fig. 22-81A). The

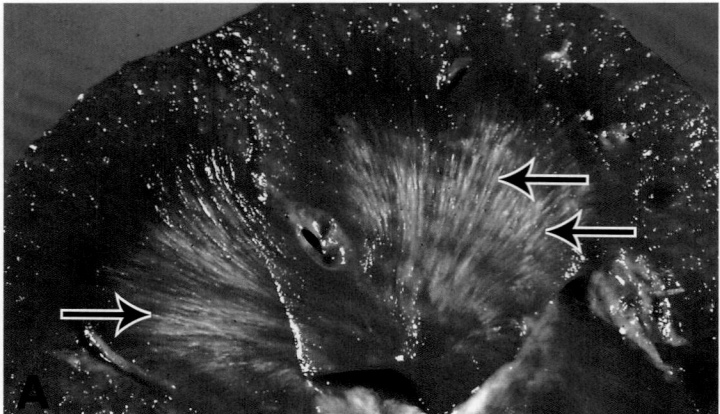
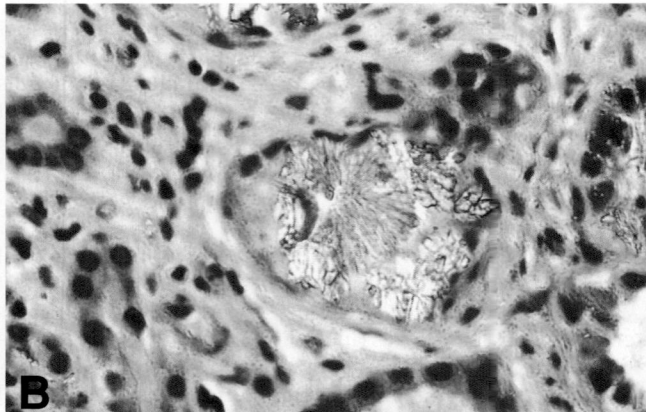

FIGURE 22-81. Urate nephropathy. A. Urate deposits appear as golden streaks in the medulla (*arrows*). **B.** A frozen section shows deposits of uric acid crystals in tubules.

tubular deposits are amorphous after tissue processing, but birefringent crystals are visible in frozen sections (Fig. 22-81B). Tubules are dilated upstream of the obstruction. Uric acid crystals in collecting ducts may also elicit foreign body reactions.

The pathogenesis of chronic urate nephropathy is similar to that of the acute form, but because the course is prolonged, more urate accumulates in the interstitium, causing interstitial fibrosis and cortical atrophy. The **gouty tophus** is diagnostic. It is a focal accumulation of urate crystals surrounded by inflammatory cells, which may appear granulomatous and include multinucleated giant cells. Uric acid stones account for 10% of **urolithiasis** and occur in 20% of patients with chronic gout and 40% of those with acute hyperuricemia.

CLINICAL FEATURES: Acute urate nephropathy presents as AKI; chronic urate nephropathy causes chronic renal tubular defects. Although histologically apparent renal lesions occur in most patients with chronic gout, less than 1/2 exhibit significant renal dysfunction.

Nephrocalcinosis Is Deposition of Calcium in the Renal Parenchyma

PATHOPHYSIOLOGY: Hypercalciuria may lead to **nephrocalcinosis** (Table 22-13), formation of calcium-containing stones **(nephrolithiasis)** or both. Nephrocalcinosis may impair renal function, especially by causing tubular defects such as poor concentrating ability, salt wasting, and renal tubular acidosis. Nephrocalcinosis caused by hypercalcemia is an example of **metastatic calcification,** whereas calcification at sites of renal parenchymal injury (e.g., infarcts or cortical necrosis) is representative of **dystrophic calcification**.

Acute phosphate nephropathy is a form of nephrocalcinosis that is an uncommon complication of phosphate bowel-cleansing preparations used in patients about to undergo colonoscopy. Risk factors for this complication include older age, renal insufficiency, and use of ACE inhibitors or ARBs. Risk is reduced by avoiding excessive dehydration during bowel cleansing. In acute phosphate nephropathy, AKI occurs several weeks after use of phosphate bowel-cleansing preparations. Pathologically, calcium phosphate deposits in injured distal tubules and collecting ducts, usually accompanied by interstitial fibrosis and chronic inflammation.

PATHOLOGY: At autopsy, 20% of kidneys have small calcium deposits that have no functional significance or recognized association with hypercalcemia. In patients with nephrocalcinosis caused by hypercalcemia, calcification varies from tiny deposits to grossly and radiologically visible calcium aggregates. If hypercalcemia is severe (e.g., as in primary hyperparathyroidism), kidneys may contain wedge-shaped scars interspersed with relatively normal renal tissue. These scars reflect parenchymal atrophy and interstitial fibrosis caused by the calcification. Renal tubular basement membrane calcification may be striking, particularly in proximal convoluted tubules. Interstitial tissues also contain calcium precipitates. Such deposits also accumulate in the

TABLE 22-13
CAUSES OF HYPERCALCEMIA THAT LEAD TO NEPHROCALCINOSIS

Increased Resorption of Calcium from Bone

Renal osteodystrophy

Primary hyperparathyroidism

Neoplasms producing parathormone or parathormone-like protein

Osteolytic neoplasms and metastases

Increased Intestinal Absorption of Calcium

Idiopathic hypercalcemia

Vitamin D excess

Milk–alkali syndrome

Sarcoidosis

cytoplasm of tubular epithelial cells, which eventually degenerate and are sloughed into the lumens to aggregate as calcified casts. Scattered glomeruli show calcification of the Bowman capsule. Intrarenal arteries may also be calcified. Calcium deposits stain deeply blue with hematoxylin. They are black with the more specific von Kossa stain. Electron microscopy shows abundant calcium deposits in mitochondria of renal tubular epithelial cells.

RENAL STONES (NEPHROLITHIASIS AND UROLITHIASIS)

Nephrolithiasis refers to stones within the renal collecting system and **urolithiasis** is stones elsewhere in the collecting system of the urinary tract. Calculi often form and accumulate in the renal pelvis and calyces. Stones vary in composition, depending on geography, metabolic alterations, and the presence of infection.

For unknown reasons, renal stones are more common in men than in women. They vary in size from gravel (<1 mm) to large stones that dilate the entire renal pelvis. Although they may be well tolerated, in some cases they lead to severe hydronephrosis and pyelonephritis. They can also erode the mucosa and cause hematuria. Passage of a stone into the ureter causes excruciating flank pain, **renal colic**. Larger kidney stones required open surgical removal in the past, but ultrasonic disintegration (lithotripsy) and endoscopic removal are now effective.

A urinary stone is usually associated with increased blood levels and urinary excretion of its principal component. This is the case with uric acid and cystine stones. However, many patients with calcium stones have hypercalciuria without hypercalcemia. Mixed urate and calcium stones are common with hyperuricemia, as urate crystals act as a nidus for calcium salts to precipitate.

- **Calcium stones:** Most (75%) renal stones are calcium complexed with oxalate or phosphate, or a mixture of these anions. Calcium oxalate is more common in the United States, whereas in England, calcium phosphate predominates. Calcium oxalate stones are hard and occasionally dark, because they are covered by hemorrhage from the mucosa of the renal pelvis injured by the sharp calcium oxalate crystals. Calcium phosphate stones tend to be softer and paler.
- **Infection stones:** Infection, often with urea-splitting bacteria like *Proteus* or *Providencia* spp., causes 15% of stones. Resulting alkaline urine favors magnesium ammonium phosphate (**struvite**) and calcium phosphate (**apatite**) precipitation. Such stones may be hard, or soft and friable. Infection stones occasionally fill the pelvis and calyces to form a cast of these spaces, a **staghorn calculus** (Fig. 22-82). This name refers to the shape of the calculus which resembles a deer horn. Infection stones cause frequent complications, such as intractable urinary tract infection, pain, bleeding, perinephric abscess, and urosepsis.
- **Uric acid stones:** These stones occur in 25% of patients with hyperuricemia and gout, although most patients with uric acid stones have neither (**idiopathic urate lithiasis**). Urate stones are smooth, hard, and yellow, and are usually less than 2 cm. Unlike calcium-containing stones, pure uric acid stones are radiolucent.

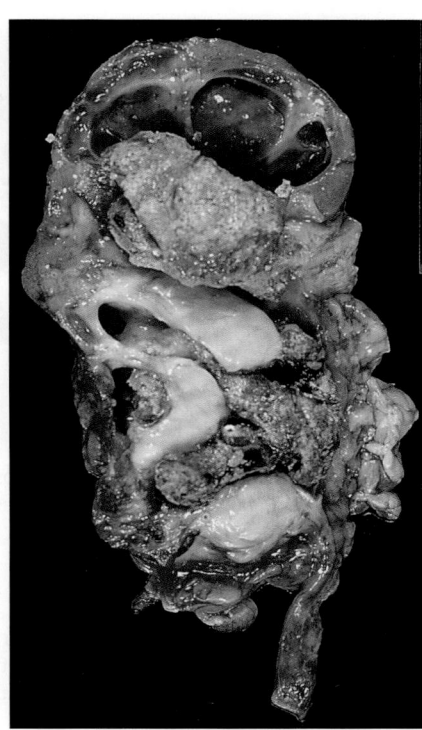

FIGURE 22-82. Staghorn calculi. The kidney shows hydronephrosis and stones that are casts of the dilated calyces. The shape of the calculi resembles deer horns.

- **Cystine stones:** These account for only 1% of renal stones overall but are a significant fraction of childhood calculi. They occur only in hereditary cystinuria. Although composed only of cystine, they may be enveloped by a layer of calcium phosphate.

OBSTRUCTIVE UROPATHY AND HYDRONEPHROSIS

Obstructive uropathy is caused by structural or functional abnormalities in the urinary tract that impede urine flow, which may cause renal dysfunction (obstructive nephropathy) and dilation of the collecting system (hydronephrosis). Urinary tract obstruction is detailed in Chapter 23.

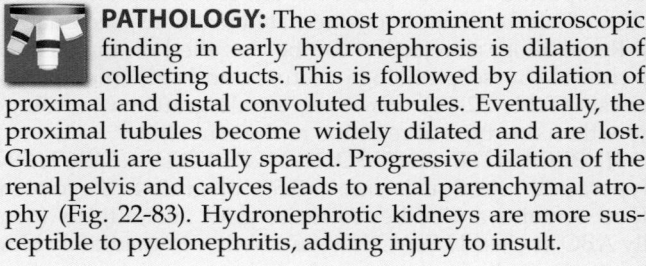 **PATHOLOGY:** The most prominent microscopic finding in early hydronephrosis is dilation of collecting ducts. This is followed by dilation of proximal and distal convoluted tubules. Eventually, the proximal tubules become widely dilated and are lost. Glomeruli are usually spared. Progressive dilation of the renal pelvis and calyces leads to renal parenchymal atrophy (Fig. 22-83). Hydronephrotic kidneys are more susceptible to pyelonephritis, adding injury to insult.

 CLINICAL FEATURES: Bilateral acute urinary tract obstruction causes acute renal failure (**postrenal acute renal failure**). Unilateral obstruction is often asymptomatic. Many causes of acute obstruction

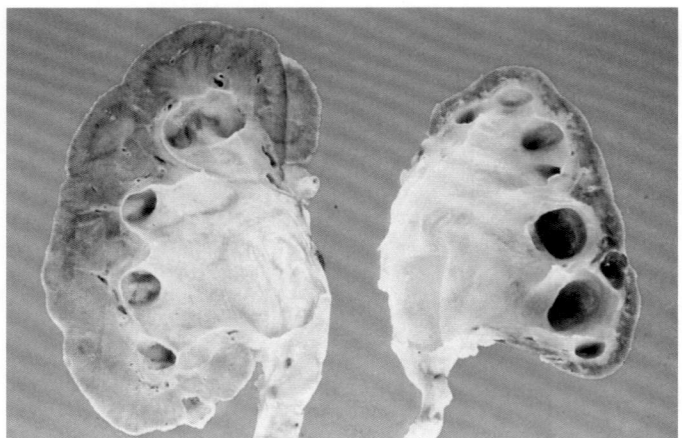

FIGURE 22-83. Hydronephrosis. Bilateral urinary tract obstruction has led to conspicuous dilation of the ureters, pelves, and calyces. The kidney on the right shows severe parenchymal atrophy.

are reversible; thus, prompt recognition is important. Left untreated, an obstructed kidney undergoes atrophy. If obstruction is bilateral, chronic renal failure ensues.

RENAL TRANSPLANTATION

Kidney transplantation is the treatment of choice for most patients with ESRD. The major obstacle is allograft rejection. However, the transplanted organ is also susceptible to recurrence of the disease that destroyed the native kidneys and to nephrotoxicity from immunosuppressive drugs. Table 22-14 lists distinct, but often coexisting, patterns of antibody-mediated and cellular renal allograft rejection.

ABO blood group antigens and **HLA antigens** are the main antigenic targets on transplanted kidneys. ABO antigens are expressed on endothelial cells and red blood cells, and are the most problematic barriers to transplantation. Because anti-ABO antibodies are preformed, they bind to graft endothelial cells and cause immediate (hyperacute) rejection (see below). *More common (and more gradual) patterns of acute and chronic rejection are due mainly to recipient reactivity against donor HLA antigens (see Chapter 4).* HLA antigens are expressed on most cells, including endothelial cells, but not erythrocytes. Development of donor-specific HLA immunity in allograft recipients causes cell-mediated and antibody-mediated reactions (see Chapter 4). Renal allograft rejection can be classified on the basis of its clinical course, pathologic features, and presumed pathogenesis (Table 22-14). However, an allograft may undergo more than one type of rejection at the same time.

HYPERACUTE ANTIBODY-MEDIATED REJECTION: Hyperacute rejection is rare (<0.5% of grafts). If recipient blood contains antibodies to major graft alloantigens (usually ABO or class I HLA), those antibodies immediately bind endothelial cells in the transplanted organ and cause irreversible injury within minutes. The graft may become mottled, cyanotic, and flaccid intraoperatively. Antibody binds endothelial cell antigens, activates complement and thus attracts neutrophils. The cytotoxic effects of complement and neutrophils cause endothelial cells to swell, become vacuolated and lyse. Accumulation of neutrophils in glomerular

TABLE 22-14
CATEGORIES OF RENAL ALLOGRAFT REJECTION

Category	Most Characteristic Lesion
Antibody-Mediated Rejection	
Hyperacute antibody-mediated rejection	Neutrophils in peritubular capillaries (peritubular capillaritis), hemorrhage, and necrosis
Acute antibody-mediated rejection	Neutrophils in peritubular capillaries (peritubular capillaritis), complement degradation factor C4d deposition along peritubular capillaries by immunofluorescence or immunohistochemistry
Acute necrotizing transplant arteritis	Arterial fibrinoid necrosis
T-cell–Mediated Rejection	
Acute tubulointerstitial cellular rejection	Tubulitis (infiltrating mononuclear leukocytes between epithelial cells of tubules) and interstitial activated lymphocytes
Acute endarteritis	Mononuclear leukocytes infiltrating into arterial intima
Acute transplant glomerulitis	Mononuclear leukocytes filling glomerular capillaries lumens (most often focal/segmental distribution)
Acute transplant necrotizing arteritis	Acute transmural inflammation or necrosis
Chronic Rejection	
Interstitial fibrosis and tubular atrophy	Tubular atrophy, interstitial fibrosis, interstitial chronic inflammatory cells
Chronic transplant vasculopathy	Arterial fibrotic intimal thickening containing myofibroblasts and no duplication of elastica
Chronic transplant glomerulopathy	Glomerular capillary wall thickening with glomerular basement membrane duplication/remodeling

capillaries portends impending rejection. Endothelial cell changes are followed by formation of platelet thrombi and then fibrin thrombi (Fig. 22-84). Interstitial edema, hemorrhage (Fig. 22-84), and cortical necrosis develop over the ensuing 12 to 24 hours.

ACUTE ANTIBODY-MEDIATED REJECTION: The most common type of acute antibody-mediated rejection is directed primarily at capillaries and may cause only subtle or no pathologic changes by light microscopy. Neutrophils or mononuclear leukocytes are increased in peritubular and glomerular capillaries, and in tubules. Complement activation products, especially C4d, localize consistently to the walls of peritubular

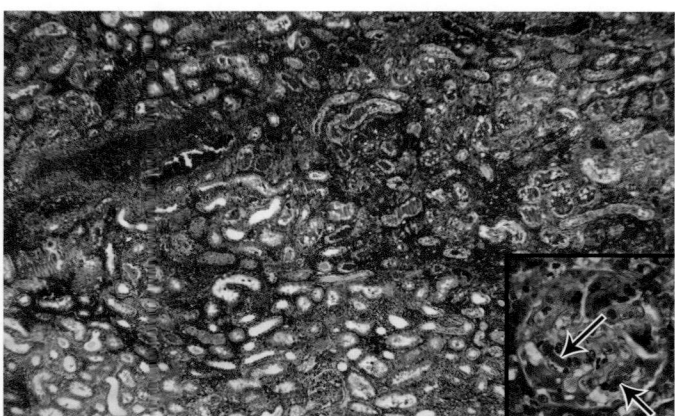

FIGURE 22-84. Hyperacute rejection. Preformed antibody against recipient antigens causes an immediate *in situ* reaction, with hemorrhage due to vascular necrosis. Fibrin thrombi (*arrows*) are abundant in glomeruli (*inset*).

and glomerular capillaries (Fig. 22-85A). The most severe, but least common, pattern of acute antibody-mediated rejection involves **necrotizing arteritis** with fibrinoid necrosis of the media (Fig. 22-85B). It occurs in less than 1% of allografts in patients whose immunosuppression includes a calcineurin inhibitor, although before these agents were introduced it occurred in 5% of renal allografts. If necrotizing arteritis develops, fewer than 30% of grafts survive 1 year, even with aggressive immunosuppression.

ACUTE CELLULAR REJECTION: This is the most common form of acute rejection. It is characterized by infiltration of the interstitium, tubules, arteries, arterioles, or glomeruli by T lymphocytes and macrophages. Nuclei of infiltrating lymphocytes vary in size and shape because the cells are at various stages of activation and include immunoblasts (see Chapter 26). Usually, interstitial infiltrates are patchy rather than diffuse. Involvement of tubules **(tubulitis)** includes movement of lymphocytes across tubular basement membranes to lie between tubular epithelial cells (Fig. 22-86A). Arterial involvement by cellular rejection involves T lymphocytes and monocytes traversing the endothelium, expanding the intima with mononuclear leukocytes **(endarteritis)** (Fig. 22-86B). Arterioles may be similarly affected. Glomerular infiltration by mononuclear

leukocytes with dilatation and filling/obliteration of capillary lumens causes **acute transplant glomerulitis**. Renal transplants with tubulitis but not endarteritis have an 80% chance of 1-year graft survival, compared with 60% for allografts with endarteritis.

CHRONIC REJECTION: Chronic rejection features interstitial fibrosis and tubular atrophy, interstitial mononuclear infiltrates, thickening (multilamination) of peritubular capillary basement membranes, **chronic transplant arteriopathy,** and **chronic transplant glomerulopathy** (see below) (Table 22-14).

Chronic transplant arteriopathy affects arteries of all sizes, including the main renal artery. The intima is thickened by stromal cell proliferation and matrix deposition (Fig. 22-87), but without the dense fibrosis and elastic lamination seen in nonspecific arteriosclerosis. Inflammation is absent (inactive phase), or is much less prominent (chronic active transplant arteriopathy) than in active acute cell-mediated intimal arteritis (compare to Fig. 22-83). Foam cells may be conspicuous, and the internal elastic lamina may be disrupted. Peritubular capillaries show basement membrane thickening and multilayering.

In chronic transplant glomerulopathy, glomerular capillary walls become thickened, due to expansion of the glomerular capillary subendothelial zone and formation of new lamina densa material (GBM replication). The mesangium is widened. Ischemia due to arterial and capillary narrowing may lead to tubular atrophy and interstitial fibrosis. Tubulointerstitial injury may also result from indolent tubulitis.

RECURRENCE OF KIDNEY DISEASE: The same disease that caused the native kidneys to fail may recur in a transplanted kidney. The frequency and significance of recurrence vary among different types of glomerular disease (Table 22-15).

CALCINEURIN INHIBITOR NEPHROTOXICITY OF CYCLOSPORINE AND TACROLIMUS: Cyclosporine and tacrolimus are immunosuppressive inhibitors of calcineurin that have dramatically improved allograft survival for kidneys and other organs (e.g., liver, heart, lungs). Unfortunately, both drugs are nephrotoxic and can injure both kidney allografts and native kidneys of patients taking these drugs for other reasons. Acute or chronic renal failure can result.

The most characteristic renal lesion is an **arteriolopathy** that begins with smooth muscle cell degeneration and necrosis. The destroyed arteriolar muscle cells are replaced

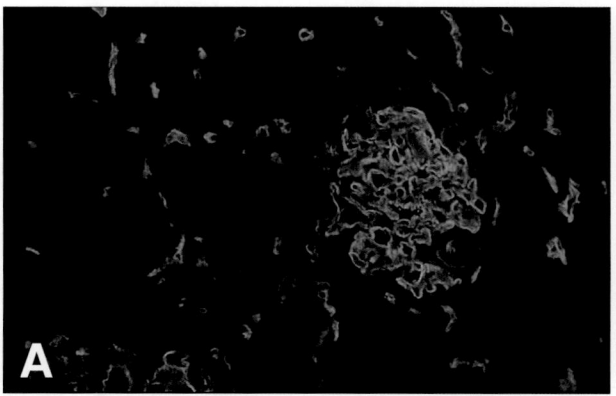

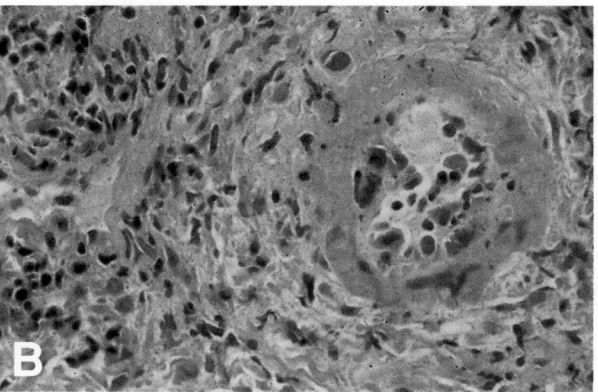

FIGURE 22-85. Acute antibody-mediated allograft rejection. A. Staining of peritubular and glomerular capillaries with an anti-C4d antibody provides evidence of complement activation by antibodies directed against donor antigens on endothelial cells. **B.** Acute antibody-mediated necrotizing acute vasculitis in an interlobular artery shows extensive fibrinoid necrosis of the muscularis. The vascular and interstitial infiltrates of mononuclear leukocytes indicate concurrent acute cellular rejection.

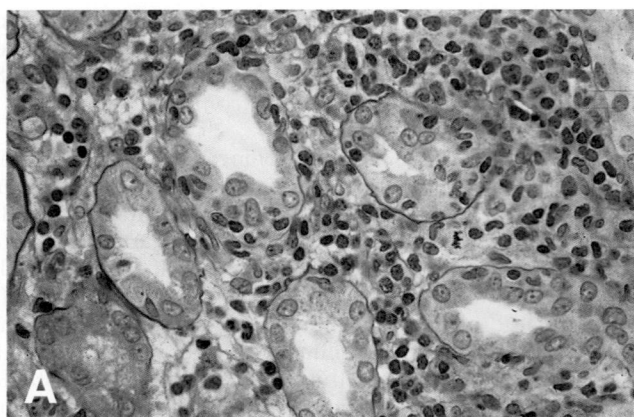

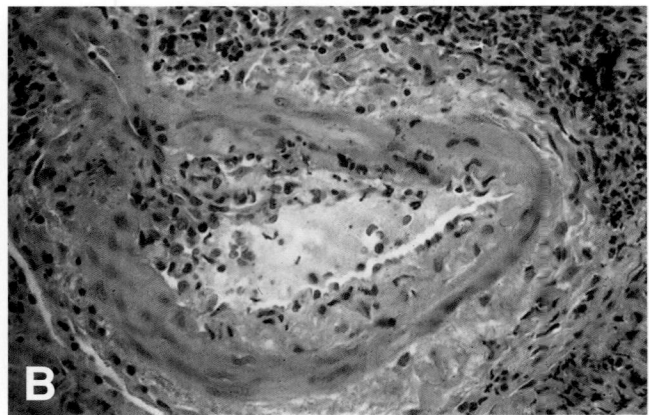

FIGURE 22-86. Acute cellular allograft rejection. A. Acute tubulointerstitial cellular rejection with tubulitis indicated by lymphocytes on the epithelial side of the basement membrane (periodic acid–Schiff stain). **B.** Acute cellular vascular rejection with endarteritis indicated by mononuclear leukocytes infiltrating the intima of an arcuate artery.

by acidophilic hyaline material (Fig. 22-88). In fulminant cases, vascular lesions resemble full-blown thrombotic microangiopathy, with circumferential fibrinoid arteriolar necrosis. In chronic toxicity, there are zones of interstitial fibrosis and tubular atrophy ("striped fibrosis").

BK POLYOMAVIRUS INFECTION: Immunosuppression can reactivate latent BK virus infection in a transplanted kidney and can lead to acute tubular injury and tubulointerstitial nephritis. Intranuclear viral inclusions in proximal tubular epithelial cells may suggest this possibility, and immunochemical staining for the SV40 large T antigen can confirm the diagnosis.

TABLE 22-15

RECURRENCE OF DISEASE IN RENAL ALLOGRAFTS

Disease	Recurrence Rate (%)	Rate of Graft Loss (%)
C3 glomerulopathy (e.g., dense deposit disease)	>90	15
Diabetic glomerulosclerosis	>90	<5
IgA nephropathy	40	<10
Focal segmental glomerulosclerosis	35	30
Membranous nephropathy	20	<5
ANCA glomerulonephritis	15	<5
Anti-GBM glomerulonephritis	5	<5
Lupus glomerulonephritis	5	<5

ANCA = antineutrophil cytoplasmic autoantibody; GBM = glomerular basement membrane; IgA = immunoglobulin A.

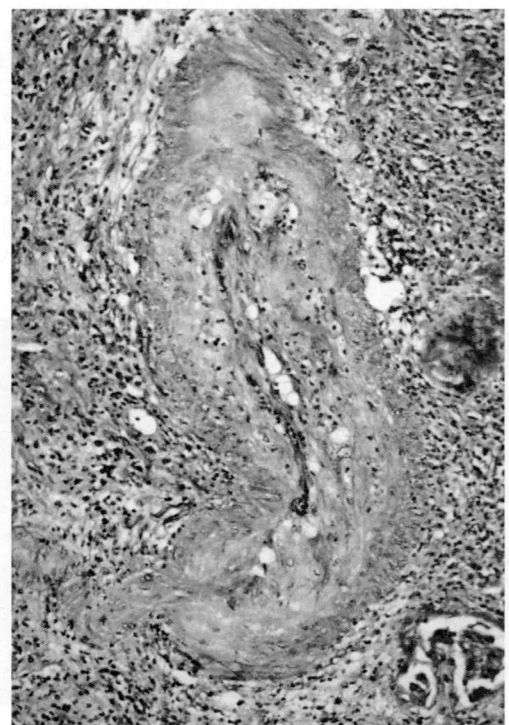

FIGURE 22-87. Chronic allograft rejection. The lumen of this medium-sized artery is occluded by a thickened intima, which contains a few inflammatory cells.

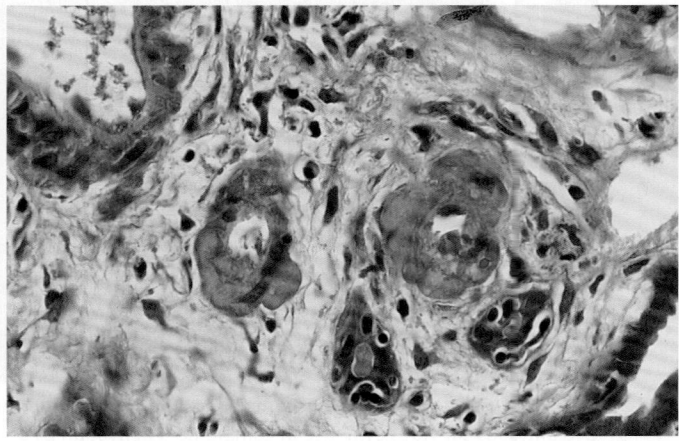

FIGURE 22-88. Cyclosporine nephrotoxicity with arteriolopathy. Marked destructive hyalinosis of arterioles is present.

Renal Tumors

BENIGN RENAL TUMORS

PAPILLARY RENAL ADENOMA: Whether any epithelial renal cell tumor should be considered benign remains controversial. Tumor size, which has been used to separate adenomas from carcinomas, is problematic because all carcinomas start out as small lesions. Renal epithelial neoplasms smaller than 3 cm rarely metastasize, but "rarely" is not "never." Tumors composed of cells resembling clear cell, chromophobe or collecting duct RCCs should not be referred to as adenomas even if they are small. Neoplasms smaller than 5 mm with papillary or tubulopapillary growth patterns can be considered adenomas. Papillary renal adenomas occur more often with advancing age and are incidental autopsy findings in 40% of patients older than 70.

RENAL ONCOCYTOMA: This benign neoplasm accounts for 5% to 10% of primary renal tumors removed surgically. It derives from collecting duct intercalated cells. The neoplastic cells are plump, with abundant, finely granular, acidophilic cytoplasm, and round nuclei that lack atypia. The distinctive appearance of the tumor cells is due to abundant mitochondria in the cytoplasm. Oncocytomas are typically mahogany-brown due to mitochondrial lipochrome pigments. These tumors rarely metastasize.

MEDULLARY FIBROMA: Medullary fibromas (renomedullary interstitial cell tumors) are typically small (<0.5 cm in diameter), pale gray, well-circumscribed tumors, usually in the midportion of medullary pyramids. They are composed of small stellate to polygonal cells in a loose stroma. Renal medullary fibromas are incidental findings in as many as 1/2 of all adult autopsies (Fig. 22-89).

ANGIOMYOLIPOMA: These tumors are strongly associated with tuberous sclerosis. Of patients with tuberous sclerosis, 80% have angiomyolipomas, but most patients with angiomyolipomas do not have tuberous sclerosis.

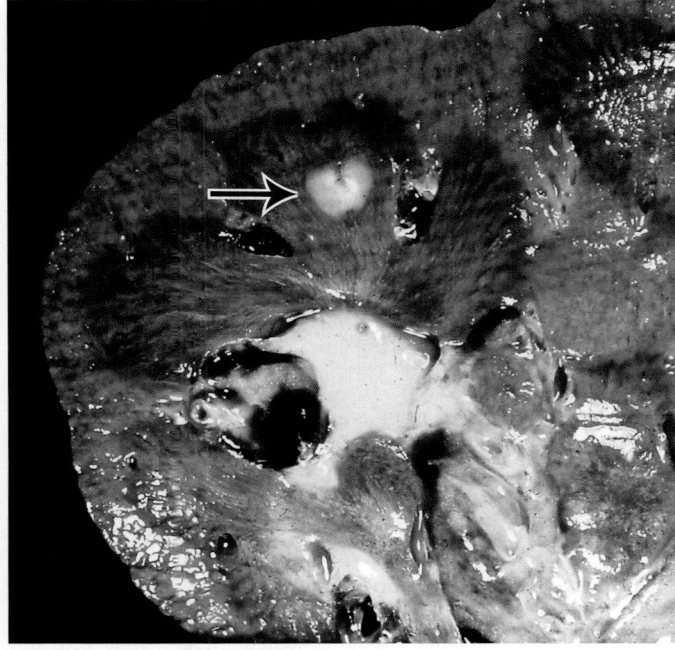

FIGURE 22-89. Medullary fibroma (*arrow*).

These lesions are mixtures of well-differentiated adipose tissue, smooth muscle and thick-walled vessels. Grossly, they are yellow and bosselated, and may resemble RCCs. However, they are always well encapsulated and lack necrosis.

MESOBLASTIC NEPHROMA: Mesoblastic nephromas are benign congenital neoplasms or hamartomas usually found in the first 3 months of life. They must be differentiated from Wilms tumors. The lesions range from smaller than 1 cm to larger than 15 cm and are composed of spindle cells of fibroblastic or myofibroblastic lineage. Tumor margins are usually irregular, with bands of cells interdigitating with adjacent renal parenchyma. Mesoblastic nephromas may recur if some of these tongues of tumor tissue are left behind after surgical resection.

MALIGNANT TUMORS OF THE KIDNEY

Wilms Tumor (Nephroblastoma) Is a Malignancy of Embryonal Renal Elements

Component nephrogenic elements in Wilms tumors include admixed blastema, stroma, and epithelium. Its incidence is 1 in 10,000, making it the most common abdominal solid tumor in children.

MOLECULAR PATHOGENESIS: In most (90%) cases, Wilms tumors are sporadic and unilateral. In 5% of cases, however, they arise as part of three different congenital syndromes, all of which increase the risk of developing Wilms tumors at an early age and often bilaterally:

- **WAGR syndrome: W**ilms tumor, **a**niridia, **g**enitourinary anomalies, mental **r**etardation
- **Denys–Drash syndrome (DDS):** Wilms tumor, intersexual disorders, glomerular mesangial sclerosis
- **Beckwith–Wiedemann syndrome (BWS):** Wilms tumor, overgrowth ranging from gigantism to hemihypertrophy, visceromegaly and macroglossia

Approximately 6% of Wilms tumors are familial. These have an early onset and are bilateral but are not associated with other syndromes.

WAGR syndrome is caused by a deletion in the short arm of chromosome 11 (11p13). Affected genes include the aniridia gene (*PAX6*) and **Wilms tumor gene 1 (*WT1*).** WT1 protein (see below) is expressed in kidneys, thymus, spleen, and gonads. Loss or mutation of one *WT1* allele leads to genitourinary anomalies. A defect in *PAX6* causes aniridia. Of children with WAGR syndrome, 1/3 develop Wilms tumors. The presence of a germline mutation in one *WT1* allele and loss of heterozygosity (LOH) at this locus in the tumors of WAGR syndrome implies that acquired somatic mutation in the remaining *WT1* allele is required for Wilms tumor to occur (as in retinoblastomas; see Chapter 5). Unlike deletions in WAGR syndrome, mutations in *WT1* in DDS are considered dominant negative mutations, possibly accounting for the fact that the DDS phenotype is far more severe than that of WAGR syndrome. *WT1* mutations also occur in Frasier syndrome, but affected patients develop gonadoblastomas, rather than Wilms tumors.

WT1 is a tumor-suppressor protein that regulates transcription of several other genes, including insulin-like growth factor-II (*IGF-II*), snail (*SNAI1*), E-cadherin (*CDH1*), and platelet-derived growth factor (*PDGF*). Wilms tumors arising in the context of WAGR syndrome all have *WT1* mutations, but only 10% to 20% of sporadic Wilms tumors do. Thus, genes other than *WT1* must contribute to the genesis of sporadic Wilms tumors. Among sporadic Wilms tumors, 10% have a gain-of-function mutation in the gene for β-catenin (*CTNNB1*), a key component of the developmentally important Wnt signaling pathway. An additional 5% have mutations in the p53 gene (*TP53*; see Chapter 5).

Approximately 70% of Wilms tumors show LOH or loss of imprinting (LOI) at a second locus on chromosome 11 (11p15.5). This site, also linked to BWS, is distinct from, but close to, the *WT1* gene. Interestingly, LOH at this locus in sporadic Wilms tumors invariably results in loss of the maternal allele. In addition, some BWS patients have germline duplications of the paternal locus, whereas others have two copies of chromosome 11 with the same imprinting pattern at this locus as the father (*paternal uniparental isodisomy*). Because *IGF-II 2* maps to chromosome 11p15 and has paternal imprinting, an increased dose of *IGF-II 2* might contribute to BWS and to tumorigenesis. Another possibility is that a closely linked gene, such as *H19* (a long noncoding RNA gene), expressed only by the maternal allele, is a tumor suppressor or regulates imprinting in the region.

The *WTX* gene on the X chromosome is mutated in 20% to 30% of Wilms tumors with about 2/3 of these carrying deletions of the entire gene. *WTX* may act as a tumor suppressor by downregulating Wnt/β-catenin signaling by promoting degradation of β-catenin. Mutations in *CTNNB1* that increase Wnt/β-catenin stability occur in approximately 15% of Wilms tumors. Thus, constitutive activation of Wnt/β-catenin signaling may be important in Wilms tumorigenesis. About 3/4 of Wilms tumors with mutant *WT1* also have *CTNNB1* mutations, suggesting that *WT1* loss does not fully activate Wnt/β-catenin signaling.

Nephrogenic rests (small foci of persistent primitive blastemal cells) are found in the kidneys of all children with syndromic Wilms tumors and in 1/3 of sporadic cases. Given that such rests in the nontumorous kidney have the same somatic *WT1* mutations as are present in the tumors, these rests may represent clonal precursor lesions that are one or more steps along the pathway to tumor formation.

PATHOLOGY: Most Wilms tumors are solitary lesions. Wilms tumors tend to be large when detected, with bulging, pale tan, cut surfaces enclosed by a thin rim of renal cortex and capsule (Fig. 22-90). Wilms tumors resemble normal fetal renal tissue (Fig. 22-91), including metanephric blastema, immature stroma (mesenchymal tissue), and immature epithelial elements.

Most Wilms tumors contain all three elements in varying proportions, but only two elements or even only one may be present on occasion. The blastema-like component contains small ovoid cells with scanty cytoplasm,

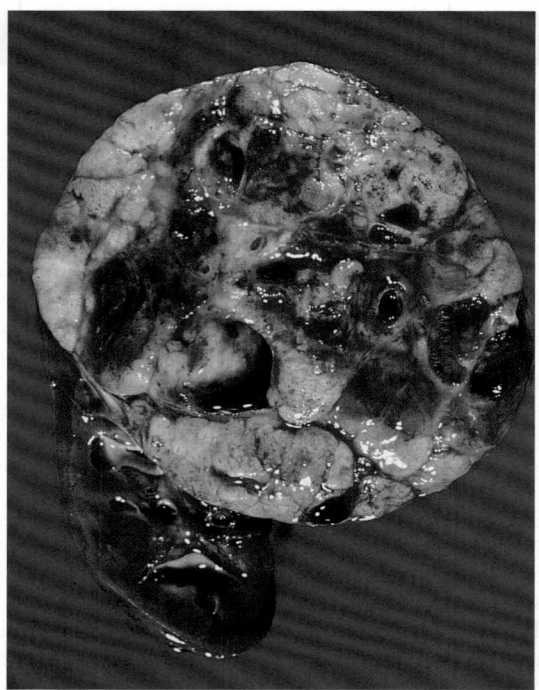

FIGURE 22-90. Wilms tumor. A cross-section shows a pale tan neoplasm attached to a residual portion of the kidney.

arranged in nests, and trabeculae. The epithelial component appears as small tubular structures. Structures resembling immature glomeruli may sometimes be seen. The tumor stroma contains spindle cells, which are mostly

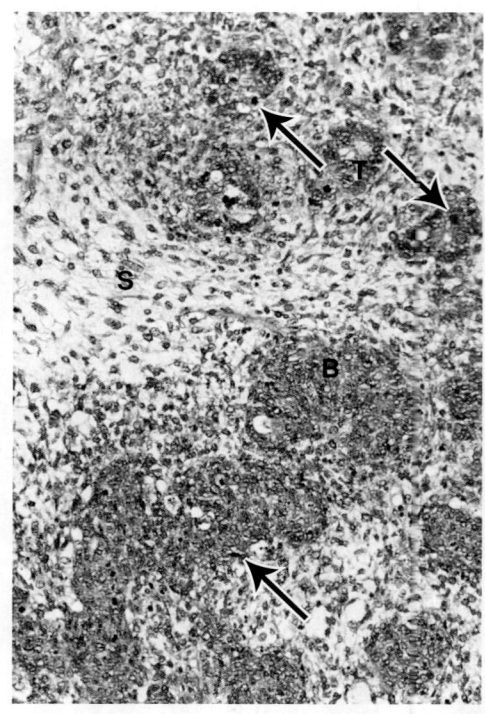

FIGURE 22-91. Wilms tumor (nephroblastoma). This Wilms tumor shows highly cellular areas composed of undifferentiated blastema (*B*), loose stroma (*S*) containing undifferentiated mesenchymal cells and immature tubules (*T*). Note the many mitotic figures (*arrows*).

undifferentiated but may show smooth muscle or fibroblast differentiation. Skeletal muscle is the most common heterotopic stromal element, although bone, cartilage, fat or neural tissue may rarely be encountered.

 CLINICAL FEATURES: Wilms tumors account for 85% of pediatric renal neoplasms. They occur in 1 in 10,000 children, usually 1 to 3 years old, and 98% present before age 10. Familial cases usually show autosomal dominant inheritance. Only 5% of sporadic cases are bilateral, in contrast to 20% of familial cases. The diagnosis is usually made after recognition of an abdominal mass. Additional manifestations include abdominal pain, intestinal obstruction, hypertension, hematuria, and symptoms of traumatic tumor rupture.

Several histologic and clinical parameters are used to predict the behavior of Wilms tumors, with varying success. Patients younger than 2 years tend to fare better. Presence of tumor outside the renal capsule at the time of surgery is a negative prognostic sign. Anaplasia (large, hyperchromatic nuclei, and atypical mitoses) occurs more commonly in older patients and correlates with their overall worse prognosis. Chemotherapy and radiation therapy, plus surgical resection, provide long-term survival rates of 90%.

Renal Cell Carcinoma Is the Most Common Primary Cancer of the Kidney

RCC is a malignant neoplasm of renal tubular or ductal epithelial cells. It accounts for 80% to 90% of primary renal cancers. More than 30,000 cases occur each year in the United States.

MOLECULAR PATHOGENESIS: Most RCCs are sporadic, but about 5% are inherited. Hereditary RCCs occur in the context of three distinct syndromes:

- **von Hippel–Lindau (VHL) syndrome,** an autosomal dominant cancer syndrome (see Chapter 5), that includes cerebellar hemangioblastomas, retinal angiomas, clear cell RCCs (40% of cases of VHL disease), pheochromocytomas, and cysts in various organs
- **Autosomal dominant RCC,** in which a clear cell tumor is the main manifestation; it occurs in 1/2 of at-risk patients with genetic abnormalities like those in VHL syndrome
- **Hereditary papillary RCC,** an autosomal dominant inherited cancer characterized by multiple bilateral papillary tumors
- **Birt–Hogg–Dube (BHD) syndrome,** a hereditary disease with risk for bilateral, multifocal chromophobe RCC

Hereditary RCCs tend to be multifocal and bilateral, and appear in younger patients than do sporadic RCCs. A family history of RCC increases the risk for RCC four- to fivefold.

Several translocations involving a breakpoint on chromosome 3 contribute to VHL and autosomal dominant

RCC syndromes. Patients with sporadic RCC may have deletions and LOH in the short arm of chromosome 3 (3p) in the tumor tissue. Finally, the *VHL* tumor suppressor gene is at 3p25. *In virtually all (98%) sporadic clear cell RCCs, one VHL allele is lost; VHL mutations occur in more than 50% of these tumors.* Thus, loss of *VHL* tumor-suppressor function plays a key role in clear cell RCC tumorigenesis.

Abnormal *VHL* gene function causes the transcriptional regulatory molecule, hypoxia-inducible factor-α (HIF-α), to accumulate. In turn, genes that make proteins that activate kinase-dependent signaling pathways are transcriptionally upregulated. Components of these pathways are targets for kinase inhibitors and mTOR (see Chapter 5) inhibitors, which have proven useful for treating RCC.

Unlike clear cell RCC, hereditary papillary RCC is not linked to *VHL*. Trisomies or tetrasomies of chromosomes 7, 16, and 17, and loss of the Y chromosome, occur in many cases. Mutations in c-*met* proto-oncogene (*MET*) at 7q31 are implicated in the development of hereditary papillary RCC.

Chromophobe RCCs derive from intercalated cells of renal collecting ducts, and collecting duct RCCs originate in the ducts of Bellini of the medullary pyramids. Patients with BDH syndrome have germline inactivating mutations in the *BHD* gene, which produces folliculin (FLCN). The function of this protein is not clear but it appears to act as a tumor suppressor. These patients are at risk for developing bilateral, multifocal chromophobe RCCs.

Tobacco, whether smoked or chewed, increases the risk of RCC: 1/3 of RCCs are linked to tobacco use. Inherited and acquired renal cystic diseases may lead to RCC, especially papillary RCC. The cancer has also been tied to analgesic nephropathy.

PATHOLOGY: The pathologic variants of RCC reflect differences in histogenesis and predict different outcomes. The most common histologic categories of RCC are shown in Table 22-16.

- **Clear cell RCC** is the most common type. It arises from proximal tubular epithelial cells. Its gross appearance is typically yellow-orange, solid or focally cystic; focal hemorrhage and necrosis are common (Fig. 22-92). The removal of abundant cytoplasmic lipids and glycogen during tissue preparation for light microscopy accounts for the tumor cells' clear cytoplasm (Fig. 22-93). The cells are often arranged in round or elongated collections

TABLE 22-16	
CATEGORIES OF RENAL CELL CARCINOMA	
Category	**Frequency (%)**
Clear cell type	70–80
Papillary type	10–15
Chromophobe type	5
Collecting duct type	1

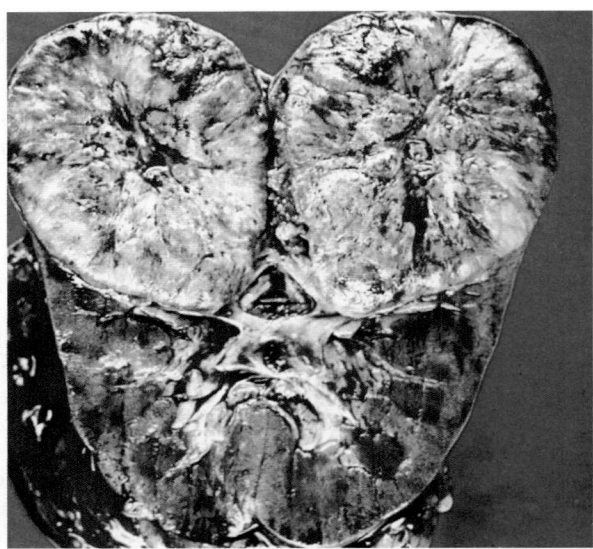

FIGURE 22-92. Clear cell renal cell carcinoma. This kidney contains a large irregular neoplasm with a variegated cut surface. Yellow areas correspond to lipid-containing cells.

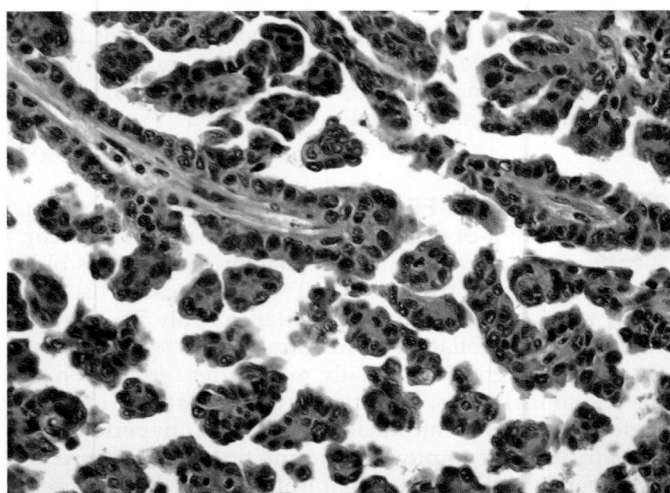

FIGURE 22-94. Papillary renal cell carcinoma. This tumor consists of papillary fronds covered by neoplastic cells.

demarcated by a network of delicate vessels. Little cellular or nuclear pleomorphism is present.

- **Papillary RCC** contains tumor cells on fibrovascular stalks. Type 1 papillary RCC has small basophilic cells, and type 2 has large acidophilic cells. The latter is more aggressive, with a worse prognosis. Cytoplasm may be eosinophilic or basophilic. These tumors arise from proximal tubular epithelial cells (Fig. 22-94).
- **Chromophobe RCC** has a mixture of acidophilic granular cells and pale transparent cells with prominent cell borders, which impart a plant cell–like appearance (Fig. 22-95). Many cytoplasmic vesicles are filled with a distinctive mucopolysaccharide that stains with the Hale colloidal iron technique. These vesicles displace other organelles to the periphery, causing central cytoplasmic pallor. Chromophobe RCCs appear to arise from intercalated cells of the renal collecting ducts.
- **Collecting duct RCC** is a rare variety that originates in medullary collecting ducts (ducts of Bellini) but may extend into the cortex. It contains tubular and papillary

structures lined by a single layer of cuboical cells with a hobnail appearance. Renal medullary carcinomas are variants of collecting duct carcinomas that develop almost exclusively in blacks who have sickle cell trait or disease.

- **Sarcomatoid changes** may occur in any RCC, correspond with a higher mutation burden, and carry a worse prognosis.

Histologic grading for RCC follows the World Health Organization/International Society of Urological Pathology (WHO/ISUP) grading classification system, which has the greatest outcome predictive value in clear cell and papillary RCC:

- **Grade I:** RCC cell nucleoli absent or inconspicuous and basophilic at 400× magnification
- **Grade II:** RCC cell nucleoli conspicuous and eosinophilic at 400× magnification and visible but not prominent at 100× magnification

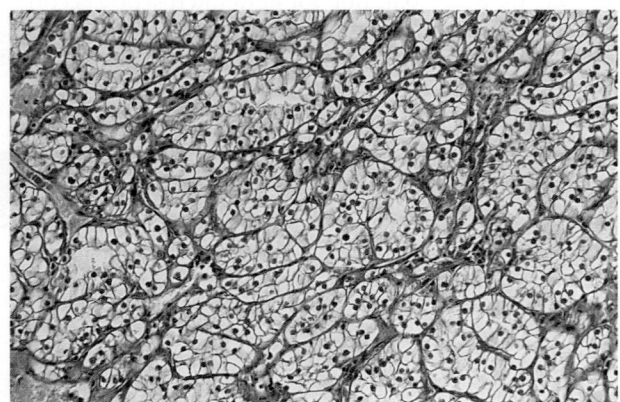

FIGURE 22-93. Clear cell renal cell carcinoma. This tumor consists of islands of neoplastic cells with abundant clear cytoplasm.

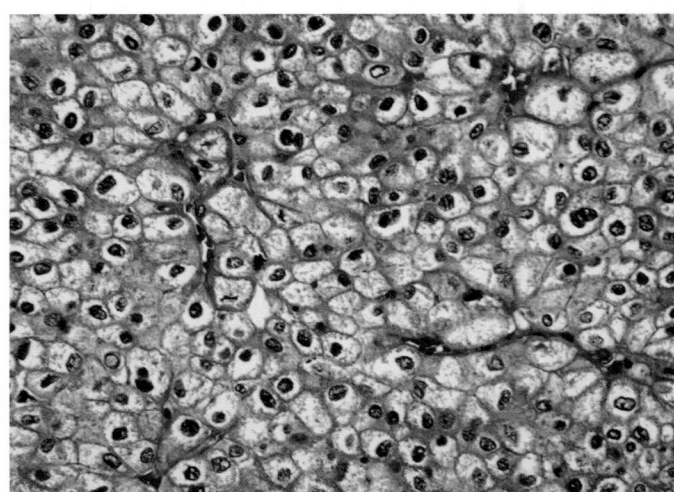

FIGURE 22-95. Chromophobe renal cell carcinoma. This tumor consists of pale acidophilic granular cells with prominent cell borders.

- **Grade III** RCC cell nucleoli conspicuous and eosinophilic at 100× magnification
- **Grade IV:** RCC with extreme nuclear pleomorphism, multinucleated giant cells and/or sarcomatoid and/or rhabdoid differentiation

CLINICAL FEATURES: The incidence of RCC peaks in the sixth decade, and it occurs twice as often in men as in women. *Hematuria is the most common presenting sign, but incidental discovery is common in imaging studies of the abdomen done for other reasons. The classic clinical triad of hematuria, flank pain, and a palpable abdominal mass occurs in fewer than 10% of patients.* RCC is known as a "great mimic," and it produces ectopic hormones that may cause fever and paraneoplastic syndromes. For example, secretion of a PTH-like substance leads to symptoms of hyperparathyroidism, production of erythropoietin causes erythrocytosis, and RCC secretion of renin results in hypertension. Patients with RCC often come to medical attention because of symptoms from a metastasis. A sudden convulsion or a cough in a previously healthy person leads to discovery of an unsuspected tumor in the brain or lung, which on further examination proves to be metastatic RCC.

Prognosis for RCC reflects tumor size, extent of invasion and metastasis, histologic type, and nuclear grade. Patients whose tumors show prominent sarcomatoid features rarely survive more than 1 year. By contrast, 1-year survival after nephrectomy for clear cell RCC is 50%. Papillary and chromophobe types have better prognoses than clear cell tumors, whereas collecting duct tumors have a worse prognosis. *Tumor stage is the single most important prognostic factor.* If RCC remains within the renal capsule, 5-year survival is 90%. This drops to 30% if there are distant metastases. The tumor spreads most frequently to the lungs and bones.

Renal medullary carcinomas are rapidly growing neoplasms that are almost always associated with sickle cell disease.

Transitional Cell Carcinoma

Between 5% and 10% of primary kidney cancers are transitional cell carcinomas of the pelvis or calyces (see Chapter 23). These are morphologically identical to the more common transitional cell carcinomas of the urinary bladder and are associated with them in 1/2 of cases. Fewer than 5% of transitional cell carcinomas occur in the collecting system proximal to the bladder.

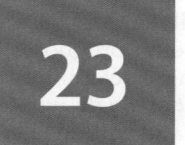

23 | The Lower Urinary Tract and Male Reproductive System

Kim HooKim, Peter A. McCue

Anatomy and Embryology

LOWER URINARY TRACT

The ureters, urinary bladder, and urethra—collectively known as the lower urinary tract—are the outflow portion of the urinary system (Fig. 23-1). In males, the lower urinary tract is closely related to the reproductive system. The embryologic development of the urinary tract and male reproductive system is shown in Figure 23-1.

The Urinary Bladder Is in the Retroperitoneal Space of the Lower Abdomen

The urinary bladder is an epithelial-lined muscular viscus that can store up to 500 mL of urine. The epithelial lining is composed of up to seven layers of stratified urothelial cells,

and the muscular wall consists of interlacing bundles of smooth muscle fibers. In males, the urinary bladder is anterior to the rectum and superior to the prostate (Fig. 23-2). In females, it is anterior to the lower uterine corpus and anterior vaginal fornix.

The bladder is subdivided anatomically into the apex (dome), midportion, and base, the latter comprising the trigone and bladder neck (Fig. 23-3). The apex is located behind the symphysis pubis and is linked in the midline to the umbilicus by the umbilical ligament, a fibrous remnant of the fetal **urachus which involutes shortly before or after birth**. Before involution, the urachus is a tubular structure, derived from the allantois, that connects the dome of the bladder to the umbilicus. The bladder neck in males rests on the upper surface of the prostate, where the smooth muscle fibers of the two organs intertwine. Inside the bladder, the **trigone** is the triangular area at the posterior aspect of the bladder base. It lacks mucosal folds and appears flattened. Superiorly, the

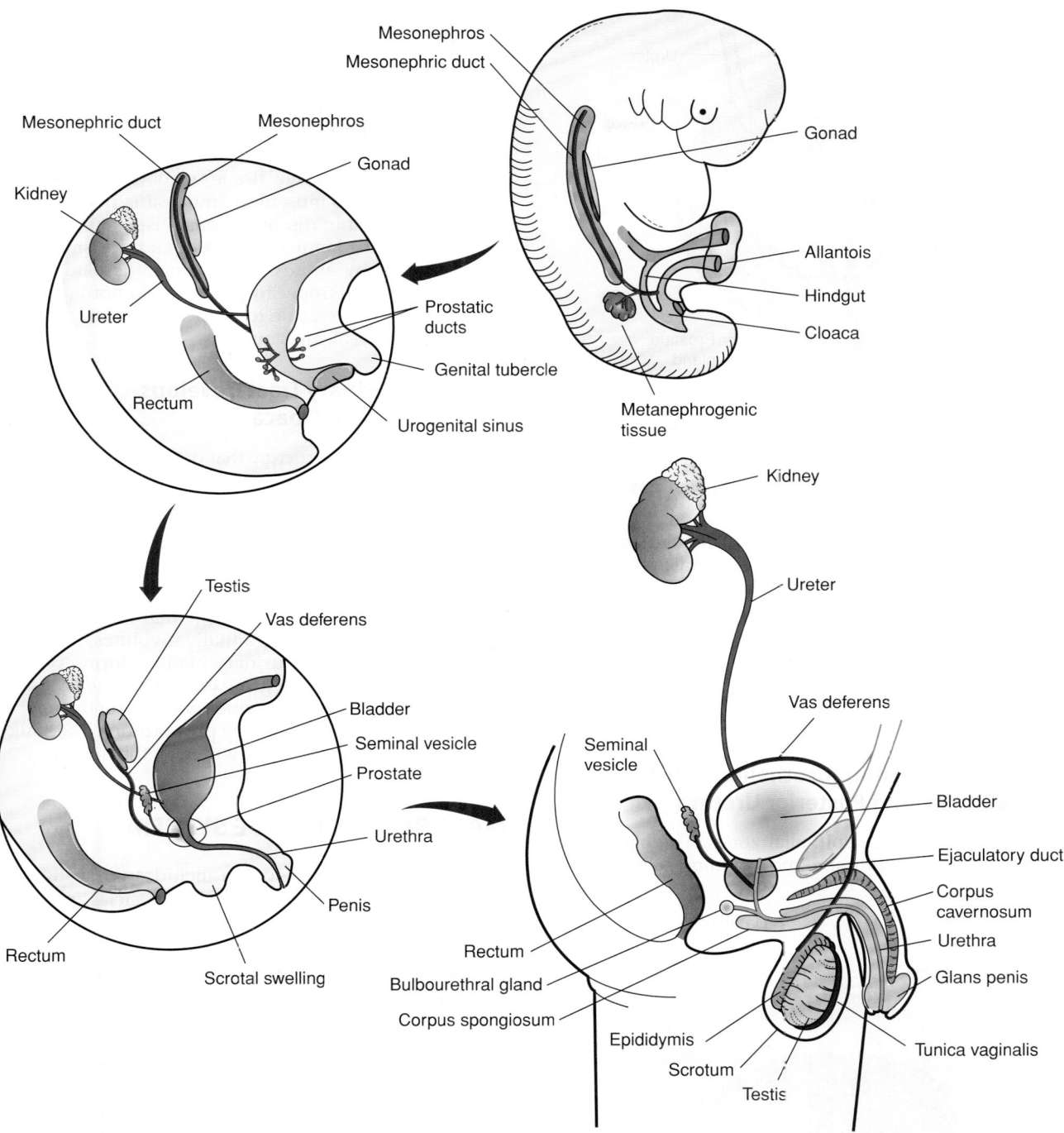

FIGURE 23-1. Embryologic development of the urinary tract and male reproductive system.

trigone is bound by a muscular ridge joining the laterally placed orifices of the ureters. The inferior tip of the trigone is formed by the funnel-shaped internal orifice of the urethra.

The Ureters Are in the Posterior Retroperitoneal Space, Lateral to the Vertebrae

The ureters are paired organs linking each renal pelvis to the bladder. The lowermost part of each ureter is obliquely embedded in the smooth muscular wall of the urinary bladder, which acts as sphincters known as the **ureterovesical**

valves. These valves let urine pass downward into the bladder but not in the opposite direction.

The Urethra Is the Terminal Outflow Conduit of the Urinary Tract

The male urethra averages 20 cm long and has three parts: (1) **prostatic urethra**, traversing the prostate; (2) **membranous urethra**, penetrating the pelvic floor; and (3) **spongy or penile urethra**, in the central portion of the penis. The prostatic urethra contains ostia of the ejaculatory and prostatic ducts. The posterior part of the penile urethra, also called the **bulbous**

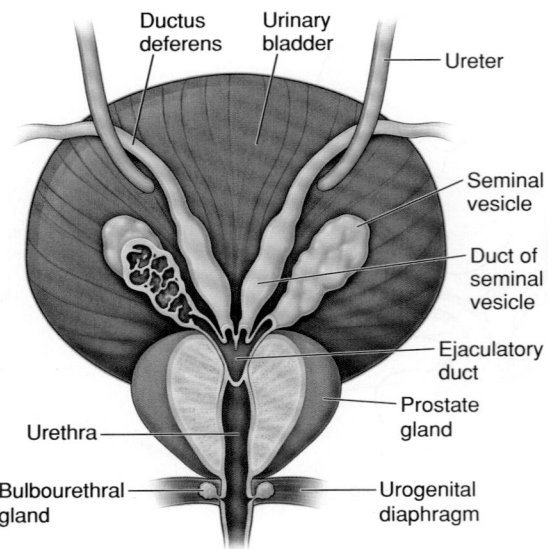

FIGURE 23-2. Gross anatomy of the male reproductive system.

urethra, receives secretions from the mucous bulbourethral (Cowper) glands. The anterior part of the penile urethra contains scattered mucus-secreting glands of Littré. The penile urethra terminates in the fossa navicularis, just proximal to the external orifice, or meatus, on the tip of the penis.

The female urethra is shorter, only 3 to 4 cm in length. It extends from its internal orifice at the urinary bladder to its external orifice in the vulva, immediately below the clitoris. The wall of the female urethra also contains mucous glands.

Transitional Epithelium (Urothelium) Lines the Ureters, Bladder, and Posterior Urethra

The urothelium has three epithelial zones. The **basal layer** lies on a basement membrane and contains cells that can

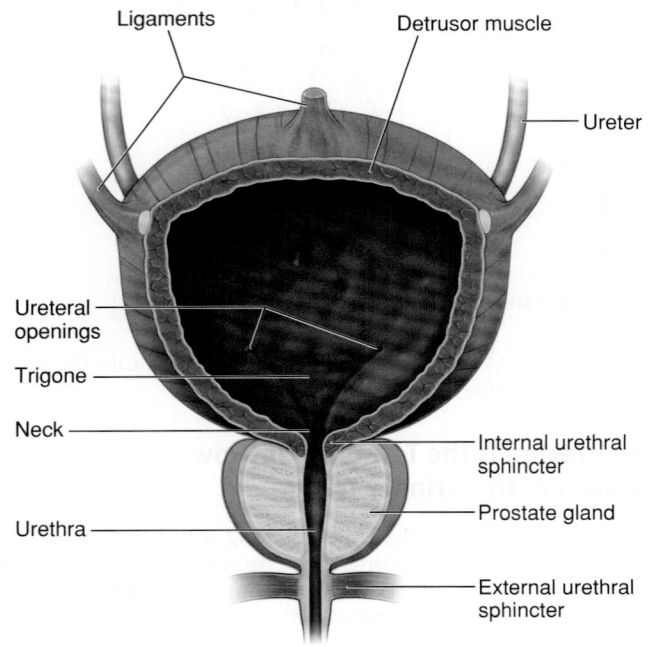

FIGURE 23-3. Gross anatomy of the bladder.

divide and replace damaged or sloughed superficial cells. Above the basal layer is the **intermediate zone**, composed of three to four layers of polygonal cells. Both basal and polygonal cells can flatten when the bladder dilates. The **superficial layer** consists of "umbrella cells," which are resistant to the urine that constantly bathes them.

Under the epithelium, the lamina propria contains mainly loose connective tissue, smooth muscle cells, and blood vessels. The muscularis mucosa is poorly developed and consists of thin discontinuous wisps of smooth muscle cells. Beyond the lamina propria lies a thick smooth muscle layer, covered by an adventitia. Since the bladder, ureters, and urethra are retroperitoneal, they do not have an external serosa. However, due to its location, part of the bladder dome has a serosal covering.

The Lower Urinary Tract Develops Mostly From the Cloaca

The **cloaca** is a fetal structure that becomes partitioned early in ontogenesis into an anterior part, the **urogenital sinus**, and a posterior part, which is the primordium of the rectum (Fig. 23-1). The urogenital sinus is the anlage of the urinary bladder, proximal urethra, and **urachus**, the latter being a temporary fetal structure that connects the dome of the bladder and umbilicus. Caudally, the urogenital sinus makes contact with an invagination of the urogenital membrane, to form the urethra. The urachus gradually involutes into the umbilical ligament. The fetal urinary bladder forms symmetrical lateral **ureteric buds** that grow cranially. When these epithelial buds reach the nephrogenic zone, they induce formation of the metanephros, the kidney primordium. The stalk of the ureteric bud elongates distally to form the ureter.

MALE REPRODUCTIVE SYSTEM

The male reproductive system includes the testis, epididymis, ductus (vas) deferens, seminal vesicles, prostate, and penis (Fig. 23-1).

Testes Are Linked to the Epididymis and Are Located in the Scrotum

Testes are paired oval organs measuring roughly $4 \times 3 \times 3$ cm. Each is invested with a **tunica vaginalis**, a layer of mesothelial cells that covers the outer fibrous capsule of the testis, which is called the **tunica albuginea**. This capsule has internal septal ramifications that divide the testis into about 250 **lobules** (Fig. 23-4A). Each lobule consists of coiled seminiferous tubules and loose interstitial tissue containing blood vessels and Leydig interstitial cells (Fig. 23-4B).

Testicular arteries originate from the abdominal aorta and nourish the testes. The right internal spermatic vein empties into the inferior vena cava, while the left drains into the left renal vein. This anatomic difference has several clinical implications discussed below.

Spermatogenesis Occurs in the Seminiferous Tubules

These tubules are the principal functional unit of the testes. They contain seminiferous epithelium and **Sertoli cells**, which

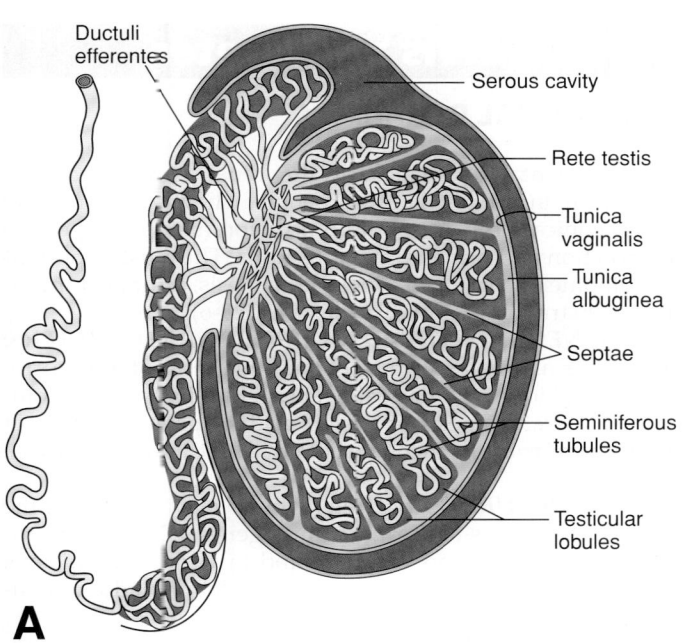

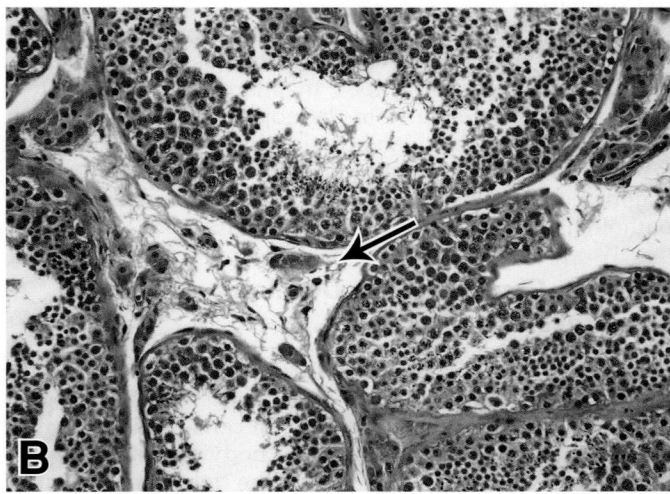

FIGURE 23-4. Cross section of normal testis showing epididymis, rete testis, and testis. A. Testis is encased by a fibrous capsule called the tunica albuginea which is surrounded by a mesothelial-lined cavity called the tunica vaginalis. The testis is divided by fibrous septae into lobules containing seminiferous tubules. **B.** Histologic section of normal testis showing seminiferous tubules which are the sites of spermatogenesis and Sertoli cells. The interstitial tissue contains aggregates of pink cells called Leydig cells (*arrow*) which produce testosterone.

support spermatogenesis. Sertoli cells also secrete **inhibin**, which communicates with the pituitary to regulate secretion of **gonadotropins** (i.e., follicle-stimulating hormone [FSH] and luteinizing hormone [LH]). The interstitial spaces of the testis contain **Leydig cells**, the primary source of testosterone.

In prepubertal testes, seminiferous tubules contain primitive **germ cells** (spermatogonia) and Sertoli cells. At puberty, LH stimulates testosterone production by Leydig cells to initiate spermatogenesis, and FSH acts on germ cells and Sertoli cells to drive spermatogenesis.

Hormonal stimuli increase numbers of germ cells, primarily **spermatogonia** which begin differentiating into **primary spermatocytes**. Meiotic division of the diploid primary spermatocytes produces **secondary spermatocytes**, which carry a haploid number (23) of chromosomes. Secondary spermatocytes mature to **spermatids**, and then to **spermatozoa**, which are discharged through the channels of rete testis into the epididymal ducts.

Each **epididymis** lies along the posterior-lateral aspect of the testis and extends into the ductus deferens. In the epididymis, spermatozoa are admixed with fluid secreted by epididymal lining cells and travel through the **vas deferens**, which empties its contents into the urethra. Finally, semen is ejaculated through the penile urethra as a mixture of spermatozoa in epididymal secretions and fluids made by **accessory glands**, namely, the seminal vesicles, prostate, Cowper bulbourethral glands, and urethral glands.

The Prostate Is an Accessory Gland Located in the Pelvis

It contacts the posterior and inferior external layers of the urinary bladder, close to the rectum. Posteriorly it is attached to **seminal vesicles**. Microscopically it is a tubuloalveolar

gland with a rich fibromuscular stroma. It develops under the influence of testosterone, which is essential for maintaining its production of seminal fluid.

Functionally, the prostate is organized into three distinct zones. The **transition zone** surrounds the prostatic urethra. The **central zone** sits slightly posterior and extends toward the seminal vesicles. The **peripheral zone** envelops the other zones and defines the boundaries of the gland (Fig. 23-5).

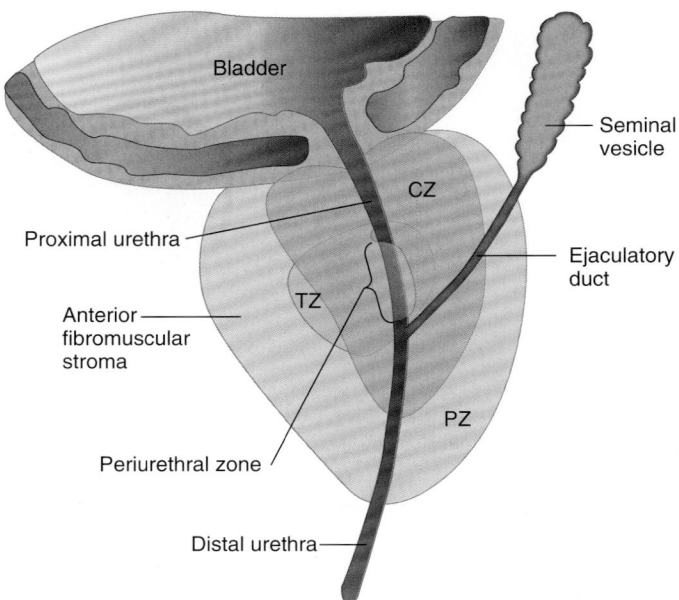

FIGURE 23-5. Normal prostate gland. Prostate gland contains four distinct regions. Central zone (*CZ*), peripheral zone (*PZ*), transitional zone (*TZ*), and nonglandular anterior fibromuscular stroma.

Precise anatomic boundaries of the zones may be difficult to discern by light microscopy, but biologic discrimination is important, as most cancers arise in the peripheral zone, while hyperplasia generally arises in the transition zone.

The prostate lacks a true **capsule**. In some areas, a concentric band of fibromuscular tissue blends into the adjacent glandular stroma. At the apex, the margin of the prostate is essentially inseparable from the adjacent soft tissue. Thus, what constitutes capsular invasion by tumor is somewhat arbitrary, and this carries important implications in cancer staging both for the surgeon who removes the organ and the pathologist assessing the extent of disease.

The Male Genital System Develops From Several Primordia

The testes develop from **genital ridges**, which arise on the posterior surface of the celomic cavity. These ridges are populated by migratory **primordial germ cells** (initially formed in the yolk sac) that enter the fetal body through the midline, and then migrate laterally into the right and left genital ridges. Complex interactions between germ cells and stromal cells in the genital ridges lead to formation of the fetal testes on the posterior wall of the mid abdomen. At the same time, the testes connect with the future epididymis and vas deferens, which develop from the **wolffian ducts**. At that point, the testes begin a gradual descent into the inguinal canal and to the scrotum.

The **scrotum** and **penis** develop simultaneously with the testes but from a different anlage that resides mostly in the genital tubercle and partly in the anterior urogenital sinus. These primordia of the external genital organs are initially identical in both sexes. In a male fetus, testosterone drives their development into penis, penile urethra, and scrotum; in a female fetus, they become clitoris, labia minora, and labia majora.

Renal Pelvis and Ureter

CONGENITAL DISORDERS

Developmental anomalies of the renal pelvis and ureters occur in 2% to 3% of all people. They do not usually cause clinical problems, but on occasion may predispose to obstruction and urinary tract infections. The most important developmental anomalies include agenesis, ectopia, duplications, obstructions, and dilations (Fig. 23-6).

AGENESIS OF THE RENAL PELVIS AND URETERS: This rare anomaly always entails agenesis of the corresponding kidney. Unilateral agenesis is usually asymptomatic. Bilateral agenesis of ureters and kidneys, a feature of **Potter syndrome**, is incompatible with extrauterine life (see Chapter 22).

ECTOPIC URETERS: Ureteric buds may develop at the wrong anatomic site during embryogenesis. The lower orifices of ectopic ureters can be found in various anomalous places, such as the midportion of the urinary bladder, seminal vesicles, urethra, or vas deferens.

DUPLICATIONS: Ureteral duplication is the most common congenital abnormality of the urinary system. Duplicate or multiple ureteric buds may originate on the side of the fetal bladder and may be unilateral or bilateral, complete, or partial. Usually there are two parallel ureters, each with its own renal pelvis and separate vesical orifice. **Bifid ureters** (subdivided by a septum), **bifurcate ureters**, and many variations thereof may be encountered, but most are of no clinical significance.

URETERAL OBSTRUCTION: Obstructions can be traced to congenital **atresia** or abnormal **ureteral valves**. However, congenital **obstruction of the ureteropelvic junction (UPJ)**, which is the most common form of hydronephrosis in infants and children, is thought to be related to abnormal layering of smooth muscle cells and/or fibrous tissue replacing the

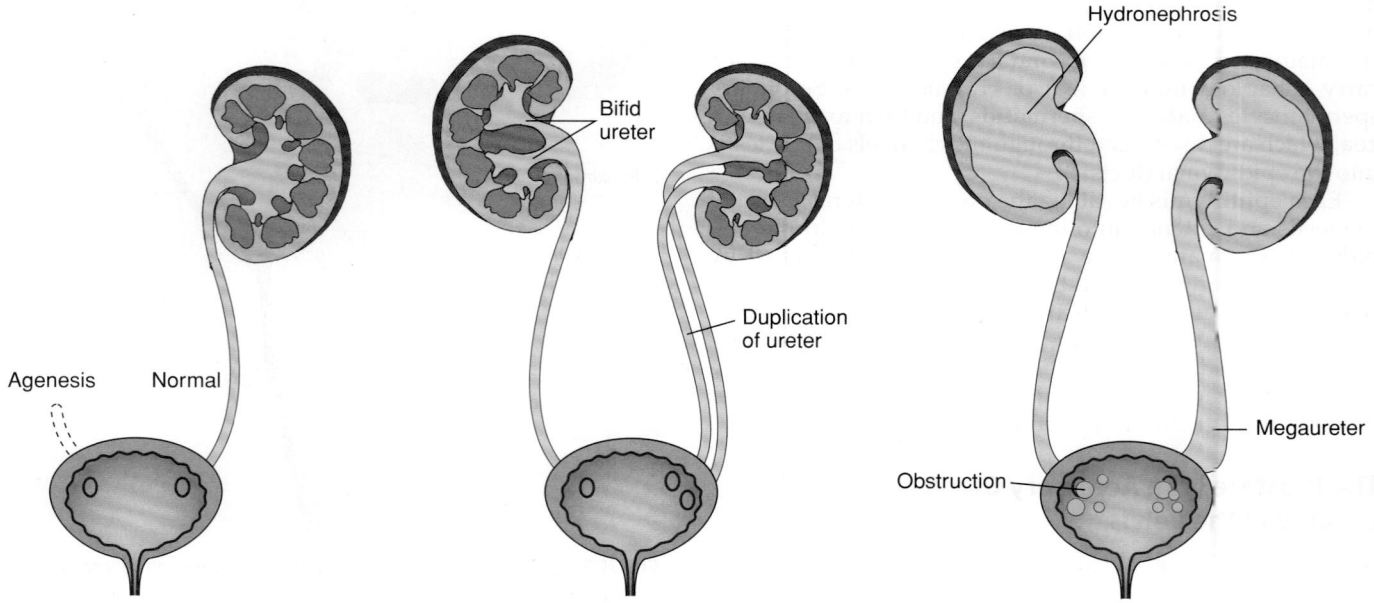

FIGURE 23-6. Anomalies of renal pelvis and ureters.

smooth muscle cells at the UPJ. Urinary obstruction in these children is usually unilateral but is bilateral in 20% of cases. Obstruction is more common in boys than girls and is usually diagnosed during the first 6 months of life. Congenital UPJ obstruction is often associated with other urinary tract anomalies, including, in some cases, agenesis of the contralateral kidney.

DILATIONS OF THE RENAL PELVIS OR URETERS: Localized dilations of the renal pelvis or ureters are called **diverticula**. Generalized dilation of the entire ureter, referred to as **congenital megaureter**, may be unilateral or bilateral. Affected ureters are tortuous and lack peristalsis. Resulting stagnation of urine **(hydroureter)** is typically associated with progressive hydronephrosis, ultimately leading to renal failure.

URETERITIS AND URETERAL OBSTRUCTION

Ureteritis, or inflammation of the ureters, is a complication of descending infections from the kidneys or ascending infections due to vesicoureteric reflux (VUR). Ureteritis is often associated with ureteral obstruction, which may be intrinsic or extrinsic (Fig. 23-7).

Intrinsic ureteral obstruction may be caused by calculi, intraluminal blood clots, fibroepithelial polyps, inflammatory strictures, amyloidosis, or tumors of the ureter.

Examples of extrinsic causes of ureteral obstruction include uterine enlargement during pregnancy, aberrant renal vessels to the lower pole of the kidney that cross the ureter, or endometriosis. Tumors that compress the ureters usually originate from the digestive and female genital tracts and may compress the ureters by direct extension or through metastases to retroperitoneal lymph nodes.

Ureteral obstruction can also result from diseases of the urinary bladder, prostate, and urethra (e.g., bladder cancer near a ureteral orifice or bladder neck, neurogenic bladder, and prostatic hyperplasia or cancer). Proximal causes of ureteral obstruction tend to be unilateral, while more distal ones, such as prostatic diseases, lead to bilateral hydronephrosis, with the possibility of renal failure in untreated cases.

Idiopathic retroperitoneal fibrosis (Ormond disease) is a rare cause of ureteral obstruction. It is characterized by dense fibrosis of retroperitoneal soft tissues and modest, nonspecific, chronic inflammation. On occasion, idiopathic retroperitoneal fibrosis is accompanied by inflammatory fibrosis in other areas, including Riedel struma (thyroid), primary sclerosing cholangitis (liver), and mediastinal fibrosis. Some of these multisystemic cases are associated with elevated serum immunoglobulin G4 (IgG4), and thus belong to the group of **IgG4-related diseases**. The fibrotic lesions are infiltrated with IgG4-positive plasma cells, which may play a pathogenetic role in fibrogenesis although the responsible mechanisms are undefined. The disease may respond to treatment with corticosteroids or immunosuppression. **Secondary retroperitoneal fibrosis** resembles the idiopathic form of the disease clinically and pathologically and may evolve as a complication of surgery or radiation therapy, or as an adverse reaction to certain drugs such as methysergide or β-adrenergic blockers.

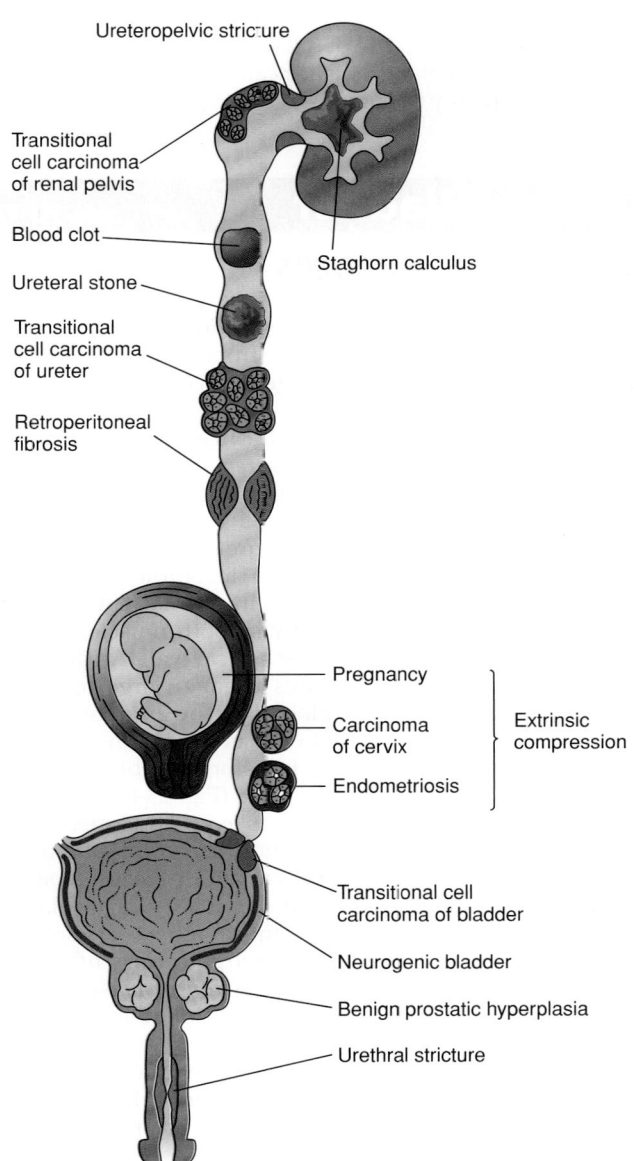

FIGURE 23-7. Common causes of ureteral obstruction.

TUMORS OF THE RENAL PELVIS AND URETER

Tumors of the renal pelvis and ureter resemble those of urinary bladder (see below) except that they are 1/10 as common. Most (>90%) are **urothelial (transitional) cell carcinomas**. Etiologies associated with such tumors of the renal pelvis and ureter are similar to those found in bladder cancer, suggesting a "field effect" in which the entire urothelial mucosa is a continuous "target organ." About 2% to 4% of tumors are bilateral, and almost half of treated patients develop subsequent urothelial bladder tumors.

CLINICAL FEATURES: Patients most often present in their sixth and seventh decades with hematuria (80%) and flank pain (25%). Treatment of urothelial cell carcinoma of the ureter or renal pelvis requires radical nephroureterectomy. The entire ureter must be removed because of the high frequency of concurrent and subsequent urothelial carcinomas. Prognosis is determined mainly by tumor stage at the time of diagnosis.

Urinary Bladder

CONGENITAL DISORDERS

Congenital developmental malformations of the urinary bladder include (1) bladder exstrophy, (2) diverticula, (3) urachal remnants, and (4) congenital vesicoureteral valve incompetence.

EXSTROPHY OF THE BLADDER: This malformation is characterized by absence of the anterior bladder wall and part of the anterior abdominal wall. It occurs in 1 in 50,000 births. In some boys it is associated with **epispadias** (i.e., incomplete formation of the penile urethra).

Bladder exstrophy results from incomplete resorption of the anterior cloacal membrane. In normal embryogenesis, this membrane is replaced by smooth muscle, but if it persists, it constitutes the anterior vesical wall. As the membrane is thin, it ultimately ruptures to leave a large defect that is accompanied by defective closure of the anterior abdominal muscular wall. These two defects expose the posterior bladder wall to the exterior and transform the bladder into a cup-like organ that cannot hold urine (Fig. 23-8). The posterior wall of the exstrophic bladder is exposed to mechanical injury and prone to frequent infection, causing squamous or glandular metaplasia. Exstrophy can be surgically repaired, but the metaplastic mucosa is at increased risk of bladder cancer, even 50 to 60 years after surgical repair of exstrophy.

DIVERTICULA: These sac-like outpouchings of bladder wall are related to incomplete formation of muscular layers. They can be solitary or multiple. Urine retained within such diverticula is commonly infected, which may lead to urinary stone formation. Congenital diverticula must be distinguished from **acquired vesical diverticula**, which typically occur in long-standing urinary tract obstruction due to prostatic hyperplasia in adults.

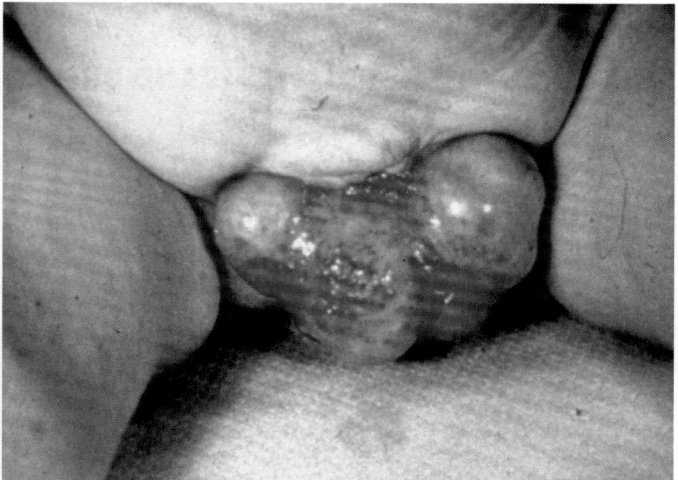

FIGURE 23-8. Exstrophy of the urinary bladder. (From Weiss MA, Mills SE. *Atlas of Genitourinary Tract Diseases*. New York: Gower Medical Publishers; 1988.)

URACHAL REMNANTS: The urachus is the fetal allantoic stalk connecting the bladder and umbilicus. If it persists and remains patent throughout, it forms a *vesical–umbilical fistula*. Incomplete regression of the urinary end, midportion, or umbilical end of the urachus leads to a **urachal diverticulum, umbilical–urachal sinus**, or **urachal cyst**, respectively. The columnar epithelium of urachal remnants may give rise to **adenocarcinomas**. Only 0.2% of bladder cancers—but one-third of bladder adenocarcinomas—arise in such remnants.

CONGENITAL VESICOURETERAL VALVE INCOMPETENCE: This anomaly results from an abnormal junction between the ureters and the urinary bladder. The ureters normally enter the bladder wall obliquely and have a long intravesical portion. The muscular layer of the bladder compresses the ureters and acts as a sphincter, to prevent backflow of urine into ureters. However, if ureters enter the bladder at right angles, they have a short intravesical segment that does not adequately prevent urine backflow during micturition. **VUR** is more common in young girls than boys and is often familial. In 75% of cases, VUR is asymptomatic, but it may lead to reflux pyelonephritis. Congenital VUR is distinguished from acquired VUR which can occur during pregnancy or with bladder hypertrophy.

CYSTITIS

Cystitis is inflammation of the bladder. It may be acute or chronic. It is the most common urinary tract infection. Cystitis often occurs in hospitalized patients, especially those who have had indwelling bladder catheters.

 ETIOLOGIC FACTORS: *Cystitis is usually secondary to infection of the lower urinary tract.* Factors related to bladder infection include a patient's age and gender, the presence of bladder calculi, bladder outlet obstruction, diabetes mellitus, immunodeficiency, prior instrumentation or catheterization, radiation therapy, and chemotherapy. *The risk of cystitis is greater in females, especially during pregnancy, because of their short urethra.* Bladder outlet obstruction due to prostatic hyperplasia predisposes men to cystitis. Instrumentation (cystoscopy) may introduce pathogens into the bladder, and cystitis is especially common in patients in whom indwelling catheters remain for prolonged periods.

Coliform bacteria are the most common cause of cystitis, mostly *Escherichia coli, Proteus vulgaris, Pseudomonas aeruginosa*, and *Enterobacter* spp. Tuberculosis of the bladder is rarely seen in the Western world today and almost always follows renal tuberculosis. Fungal cystitis may be seen in immunosuppressed patients. Gas-forming bacilli, usually in people with diabetes, may produce characteristic interstitial bubbles in the lamina propria of the urinary bladder (**emphysematous cystitis**). Schistosomiasis is a common cause of cystitis in North Africa and the Middle East, where *Schistosoma haematobium* is endemic.

Iatrogenic cystitis is common after radiation therapy and chemotherapy. **Radiation cystitis** usually develops 4 to 6 weeks following irradiation of pelvic tumors, and is most often seen in patients with uterine, rectal, or bladder cancer. Inflammation of the bladder is usually associated with epithelial cell atypia, which is usually transient and should not be mistaken for malignancy. Late consequences of radiation cystitis include extensive fibrosis, which may be transmural and incapacitating.

Drug-induced cystitis is most common after cyclophosphamide treatment, which typically produces hemorrhagic cystitis. Other cytotoxic drugs can also cause cystitis, but the injury is less prominent. These drugs also induce cytologic atypia, which is usually transient.

PATHOLOGY: Stromal edema, hemorrhage, and a neutrophilic infiltrate of variable intensity are typical of acute cystitis (Fig. 23-9). Focal petechial mucosal hemorrhages **(hemorrhagic cystitis)** are often seen in acute bacterial cystitis. Bleeding diatheses (e.g., leukemia or treatment with cytotoxic drugs) and disseminated intravascular coagulation often cause extensive hemorrhagic cystitis. *Acute cystitis that does not resolve is associated with chronic cystitis, including an infiltrate of mainly lymphocytes and plasma cells (Fig. 23-10), and fibrosis of the lamina propria.* Occasionally, an inflamed bladder mucosa may contain lymphocytic follicles **(follicular cystitis)** or dense infiltrates of eosinophils **(eosinophilic cystitis)**. **Granulomatous cystitis** is characteristic of tuberculosis, but may also be seen in patients with bladder cancer treated with intravesical instillation of attenuated *Mycobacterium tuberculosis,* bacillus Calmette–Guérin (BCG). Ova of *S. haematobium* can cause simultaneous granulomatous reactions and eosinophilic infiltrates. Specific forms of chronic cystitis include:

- **Ulcerative cystitis:** Chronic irritation caused, for example, by indwelling catheters or traumatic cystoscopy may lead to ulceration and focal mucosal hemorrhage. **Solitary mucosal ulcer** is also found in interstitial cystitis (see below).

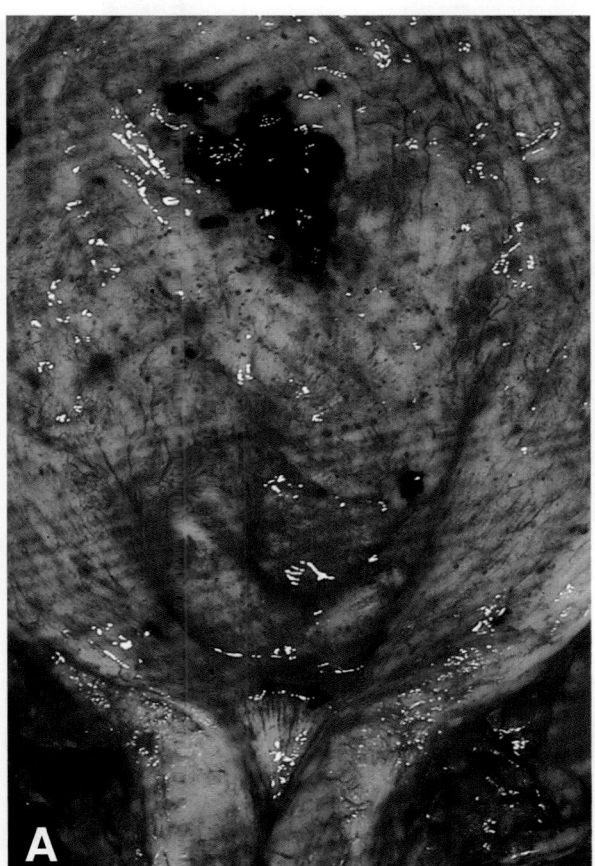

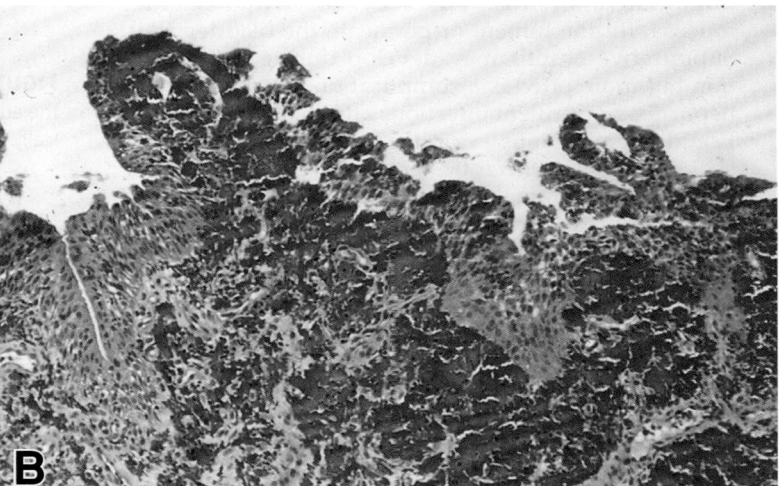

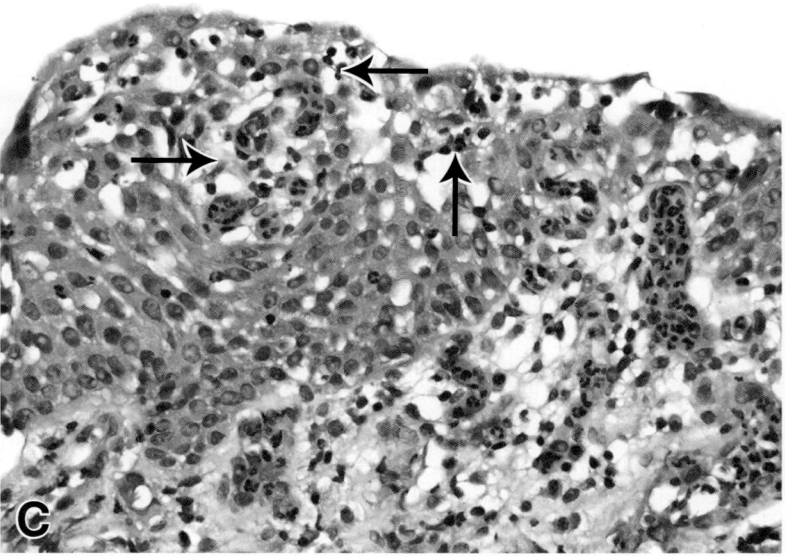

FIGURE 23-9. Acute cystitis. In this example, cystitis was caused by an indwelling catheter. **A.** Foci of hemorrhage are seen on the surface of the hyperemic bladder mucosa. **B.** Microscopic view of mucosal hemorrhage. **C.** Polymorphonuclear leukocytes (*arrows*) infiltrating the mucosa.

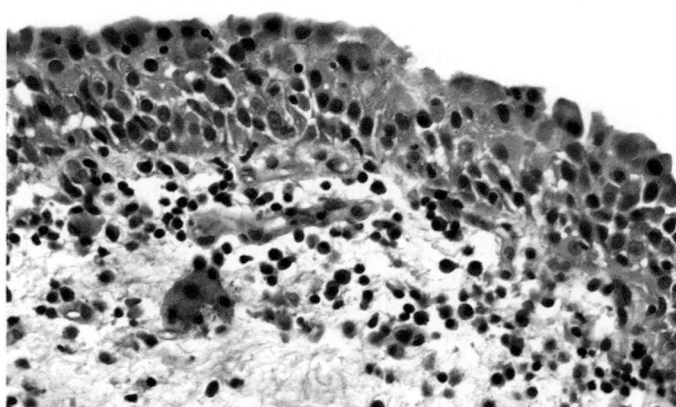

FIGURE 23-10. Chronic cystitis. A chronic inflammatory infiltrate of lymphocytes and plasma cells is present in the edematous lamina propria.

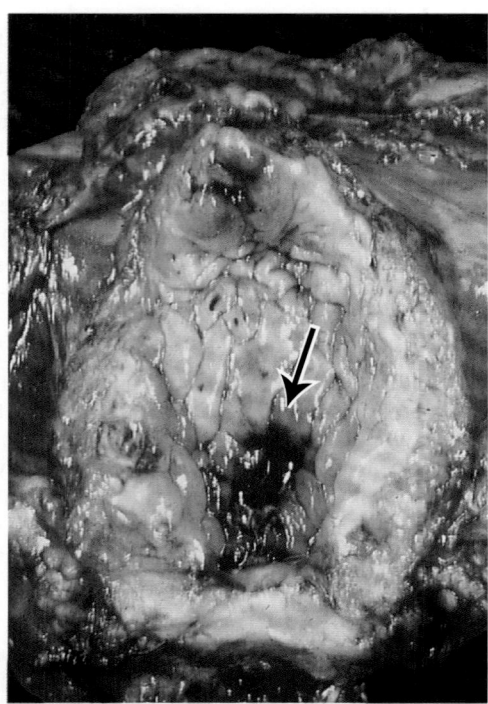

FIGURE 23-11. Interstitial cystitis. The hemorrhagic defect (*arrow*) in the edematous mucosa of the posterior wall of the bladder is known clinically as a Hunner ulcer.

- **Suppurative cystitis:** Pus may cover the bladder mucosa, fill the lumen, or permeate the bladder wall. Suppurative cystitis may develop during local infection but more often is a complication of sepsis, pyelonephritis, or purulent infections after bladder surgery.
- **Pseudomembranous cystitis:** Pseudomembranes—shaggy layers of necrotic, gray, or yellow cell detritus; fibrin; inflammatory cells; and blood—sometimes cover the bladder mucosa. The underlying mucosa is hemorrhagic and ulcerated. Pseudomembranous cystitis typically complicates infections that follow treatment with cytotoxic drugs, such as cyclophosphamide.
- **Calcific cystitis:** This form of chronic inflammation is typically found in schistosomiasis. Calcification of ova produces bladder wall encrustations resembling grains of sand. These gradually coalesce, to transform the entire urinary bladder into a calcified rigid vessel.

CLINICAL FEATURES: Virtually all patients with acute or chronic cystitis complain of excessive urinary frequency, painful urination **(dysuria)**, and lower abdominal or pelvic discomfort. The urine usually contains inflammatory cells, and the causative agent can be identified by urine culture. Most cases of acute cystitis respond well to treatment with antimicrobial agents. Recurrent and chronic cystitis may pose therapeutic problems.

CHRONIC INTERSTITIAL CYSTITIS: This persistent painful inflammation of the bladder affects over 100,000 middle-aged women in the United States. It has no known cause, and presents with suprapubic pain, the urge for frequent urination, hematuria, and dysuria. During cystoscopic dilation of the bladder, the mucosa typically develops hemorrhagic cracks and petechial hemorrhages. Urine cultures are almost always negative. In chronic stages of the disease, transmural inflammation of the bladder wall is occasionally associated with mucosal ulceration **(Hunner ulcer)** (Fig. 23-11). Chronic inflammation, including fibrosis and increased mast cells,

is common in the mucosa and muscularis. Hunner ulcers contain intense acute inflammation. The disease is typically persistent and refractory to therapy.

*MALAKOPLAKIA (from the Greek, **malakos**, "soft"; **plax**, "plaque"): This is an uncommon inflammatory disorder of unknown etiology.* Originally described in the bladder, malakoplakia may be seen in many other sites, within and outside the urinary tract. It occurs at all ages, with peak incidence in the fifth to seventh decades, and has a marked female preponderance.

Malakoplakia is often associated with urinary tract infection by *E. coli*, although a direct causal relationship is dubious. A clinical background of immunosuppression, chronic infections, or cancer is common.

PATHOLOGY: Malakoplakia is characterized by soft, yellow plaques on the mucosal surface of the bladder. There is a striking chronic inflammatory cell infiltrate mainly of large macrophages with abundant, eosinophilic cytoplasm containing periodic acid–Schiff (PAS)-positive granules (Fig. 23-12). Ultrastructurally, these granules are engorged lysosomes that contain fragments of bacteria, suggesting that malakoplakia may reflect an acquired defect in lysosomal degradation. Some of these macrophages have laminated, basophilic calcospherites, called **Michaelis–Gutmann bodies**, caused by calcium salt deposition in the enlarged lysosomes.

The clinical symptoms of malakoplakia of the bladder are indistinguishable from those of other forms of chronic cystitis. Treatment is ineffective.

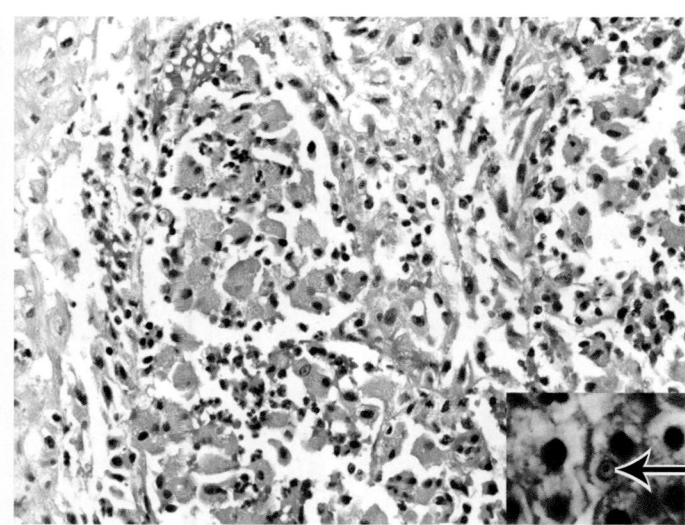

FIGURE 23-12. Malakoplakia. Inflammatory cells include mainly macrophages, with fewer lymphocytes. *Inset.* A Michaelis–Gutmann body (*arrow*) is seen at high magnification.

BENIGN PROLIFERATIVE AND METAPLASTIC UROTHELIAL LESIONS

Benign proliferative and metaplastic lesions of urothelium occur mostly in the urinary bladder but may be found anywhere in the urinary tract. Normal urothelium is composed of epithelial cells that vary from 3 to 7 cells in thickness with a distinct basal layer and a luminal layer of flattened umbrella cells (Fig. 23-13A). Nonneoplastic lesions may show hyperplasia (Fig. 23-13B) or combined hyperplasia and metaplasia, mostly in association with chronic inflammation due to urinary tract infections, calculi, neurogenic bladder, and (rarely) bladder exstrophy. They may also occur without a known pre-existing inflammatory condition. Such nonneoplastic lesions include the following types:

- **Brunn buds** are bulbous invaginations of the surface urothelium into the lamina propria (Fig. 23-13C). They are found in more than 85% of bladders and are considered normal variants of the urothelium. **Brunn nests** are similar to Brunn buds, but the urothelial cells are seen within the lamina propria, detached from the surface.
- **Cystic lesions of the urinary bladder (cystitis cystica)** appear as fluid-filled groups of cysts. Similar cysts can be seen in the urethra or ureter (**urethritis cystica, ureteritis cystica**) (Fig. 23-14). Cystitis cystica is found in 60% of otherwise normal bladders. Histologically, these lesions correspond to cystic Brunn nests, lined by normal urothelium. Transitional epithelium may undergo metaplasia into mucus-secreting epithelium, which is then referred to as **cystitis glandularis** (Fig. 23-13D).
- **Squamous metaplasia** (Fig. 23-13E) is a reaction to chronic injury and inflammation and is particularly associated with calculi. It is seen in up to half of normal women and 10% of men.
- **Nephrogenic metaplasia** is a lesion caused by transformation of transitional epithelium to resemble renal tubules (Fig. 23-13F). It is most common in the urinary bladder but is also seen in the urethra and ureter. Many small tubules clustered in the lamina propria create a

papillary exophytic nodule. The histogenesis is unclear, but some cases seem to result from implants of detached renal tubular cells carried downstream by urine. The lesion may produce tumor-like protrusions in the bladder, which may obstruct the ureters and require surgical treatment.

CLINICAL FEATURES: These proliferative and metaplastic urothelial lesions should not be confused with cancer. However, patients with such changes have higher risk of urothelial bladder carcinoma and, in the case of cystitis glandularis, of **adenocarcinoma** as well. Yet there is no evidence to suggest that these lesions themselves are preneoplastic.

TUMORS OF THE URINARY BLADDER

The most important facts about bladder cancer are:

- The urinary bladder is the most common site of urinary tract tumors.
- They mostly occur in older patients (median, 65 years) and are rare in patients under age 50.
- Tumors are much more common in men than in women.
- Most tumors (90%) are urothelial malignant neoplasms (formerly, "transitional cell" neoplasms). Squamous cell cancers, adenocarcinomas, neuroendocrine malignancies, and sarcomas are rare.
- Tumors are often multifocal and can occur in any part of the urinary tract lined by transitional epithelium, from the renal pelvis to the posterior urethra.
- Local treatment is often followed by tumor recurrence.
- Tumor invasion into the muscularis propria markedly decreases 5-year survival rate.

EPIDEMIOLOGY: Bladder cancer represents 7% of all new cancers in men and 2% in women. It accounts for 4% of all cancer-related deaths in men and 2% in women. Bladder cancer shows significant geographic and sex differences throughout the world. The highest frequencies are among urban whites in the United States and Western Europe. It is less common in Japan and among American blacks.

A high incidence of bladder cancer in Egypt, Sudan, and some other African countries is due to endemic schistosomiasis. Most schistosomiasis-related cases are squamous cell carcinomas.

Bladder cancer may occur at any age, but most patients (80%) are 50 to 80 years old. Men are affected three times as often as women. In men over 80 years of age, bladder cancer is the fourth leading cause of cancer-related deaths. There is no genetic predisposition to bladder cancer and no hereditary factors have been identified in the vast majority of cases.

The most important risk factors are:

- Cigarette smoking (fourfold increased risk)
- Industrial exposure to azo dyes
- Infection with *S. haematobium* (in endemic regions)
- Drugs, such as cyclophosphamide and analgesics
- Radiation therapy (following cervical, prostate, or rectal cancer)

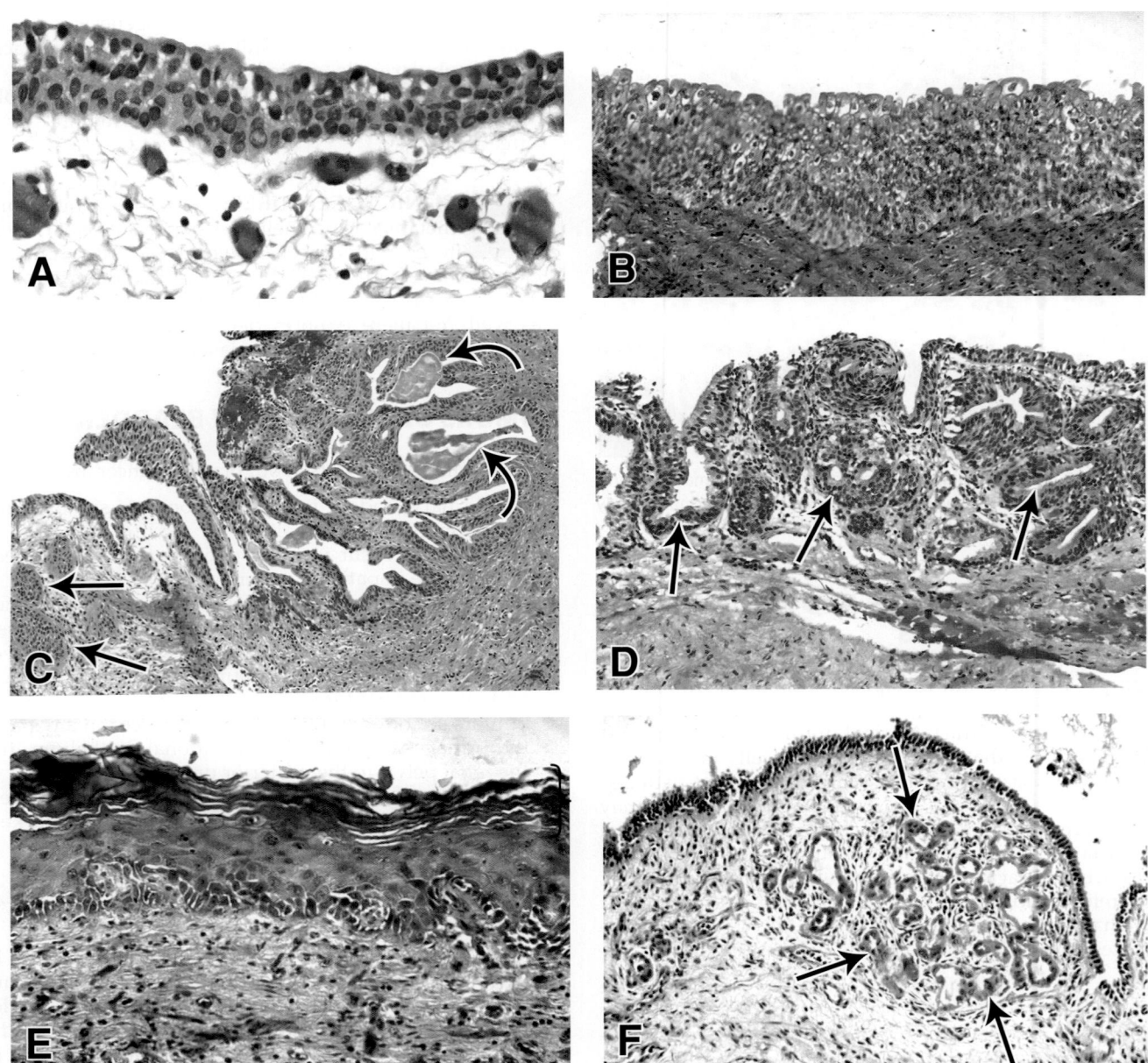

FIGURE 23-13. Proliferative and metaplastic changes of the urinary bladder. A. Normal bladder mucosa. B. Hyperplasia. Note the expansion of the normal 6–7 layers of urothelial cells. **C. Cystitis cystica.** Brunn nests (*straight arrows*) and cysts (*curved arrow*) protrude into the lamina propria. **D. Cystitis glandularis.** Metaplastic glandular mucosa is highlighted by the *arrows*. **E. Squamous metaplasia.** Note the keratinizing layer on the superficial epithelium (*bracket*). **F. Nephrogenic metaplasia** (*arrows*).

ETIOLOGIC FACTORS: Bladder cancer following occupational exposure to certain organic chemicals was described in 1895 among workers in the German aniline dye industry and was subsequently confirmed in similar workers in the United States. This was one of the first occupational cancers known. Increased risk of bladder cancer was later noted in the leather, rubber, paint, and organic chemical industries. Improved industrial hygiene has reduced this risk. *Today, polycyclic hydrocarbons from cigarette smoke are the most important risk factor for bladder carcinoma.*

A role for chemicals in bladder cancer has been strengthened by the demonstration that β-naphthylamine, to which the dye industry workers were exposed, produces bladder cancer in dogs. The metabolism of naphthylamines explains their organ specificity. Arylamines are conjugated to glucuronic acid in the liver, and the conjugates are excreted in the urine. In the bladder, β-glucuronidase in acidic urine hydrolyzes the glucuronic acid conjugate, producing reactive arylnitrenium ions that act as mutagens by binding guanines in DNA.

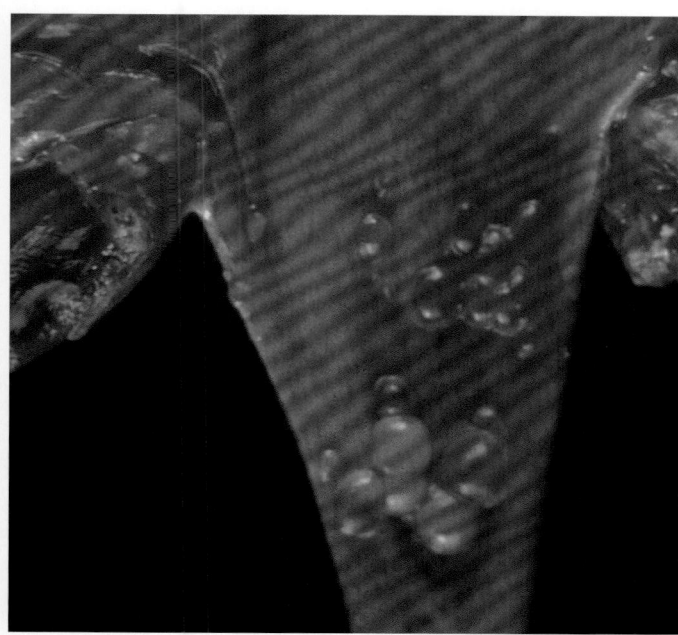

FIGURE 23-14. Ureteritis cystica. The mucosa of the proximal ureter exhibits multiple cystic structures. (From Weiss MA, Mills SE. *Atlas of Genitourinary Tract Diseases*. New York: Gower Medical Publishers; 1988.)

MOLECULAR PATHOGENESIS: The molecular pathology of bladder cancer is heterogeneous, and variants in several genes and genetic pathways have been implicated. Gene expression analysis of bladder cancer has shown that these genetic aberrations are important and provide the basis for classification of bladder tumors according to tumor biology, morphology, and clinical behavior. The molecular characteristics of flat and papillary tumors are distinct from each other, and low-grade nonmuscle invasive carcinomas differ from high-grade muscle invasive carcinomas. Therefore, bladder cancers are characterized as either flat lesions or elevated with papillary formations, as low or high grade, and as nonmuscle or muscle invasive tumors.

Specific cytogenetic abnormalities occur in 50% of bladder cancers. These often include early mutational events in urothelial neoplasia which involve chromosome 9, such as deletion of chromosome 9, or its short (p), or long arm (q) (thus, 9p- or 9q-), and deletions of 11p, 13p, 14q, or 17p, as well as aneuploidy of chromosomes 3, 7, and 17. Deletions within 9p, which contains the **tumor suppressor gene *p16***, are consistently found in low-grade papillary tumors and flat carcinomas in situ. Low-grade papillary urothelial carcinomas are also associated with mutations in genes involved in cell growth and proliferation, including the mitogen-activated protein kinase (MAPK) and phosphoinositide 3-kinase (PI3K) pathways. Flat carcinoma in situ and invasive tumors show additional distinct mutations in tumor suppressor genes that regulate the cell cycle, such as deletions in 17p, the site of the tumor suppressor gene *TP53*.

These genetic abnormalities suggest that cell cycle dysregulation due to mutated *p53* allows propagation of genetically abnormal urothelial cells. Unregulated proliferation reflects accumulated mutations in other cell cycle regulators, such as cyclin-dependent kinase inhibitors (e.g., p16/INK4a) or deletion of the tumor suppressor gene *RB1* (Fig. 23-15).

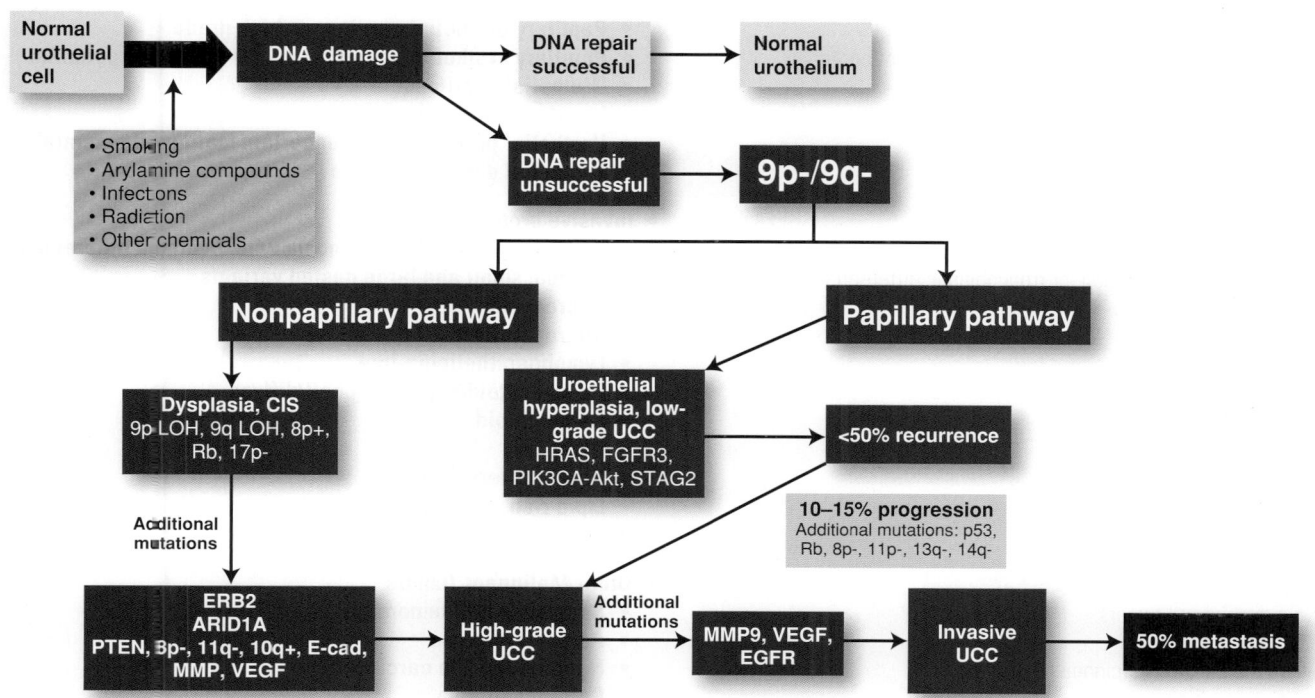

FIGURE 23-15. Molecular model of urothelial neoplasia. The transition from normal urothelium to carcinoma occurs gradually in several steps.

PATHOLOGY: Over 90% of primary bladder tumors are epithelial in origin. Most are urothelial carcinomas. However, neoplastic urothelial lesions arising from the bladder mucosa comprise a spectrum. One end includes benign papillomas and low-grade exophytic papillary carcinomas and the other end is invasive transitional cell carcinomas and highly malignant tumors (Fig. 23-16). Other tumors (Table 23-1) are considerably less common.

Urothelial Papilloma Is a Rare Benign Tumor

These papillomas are usually discovered incidentally in men aged 50 or older, during cystoscopy for an unrelated condition or for painless hematuria. They represent less than 1% of bladder tumors and have two forms: classical exophytic papilloma and inverted papilloma.

Exophytic papilloma features papillary fronds lined by transitional epithelium, virtually indistinguishable from normal urothelium. On cystoscopy, most patients show single lesions 2 to 5 cm in diameter, but some tumors may be multiple. Although considered benign, some recur or progress to carcinoma, mandating regular follow-up. Most "recurrences" are new tumors that develop elsewhere in the urinary bladder.

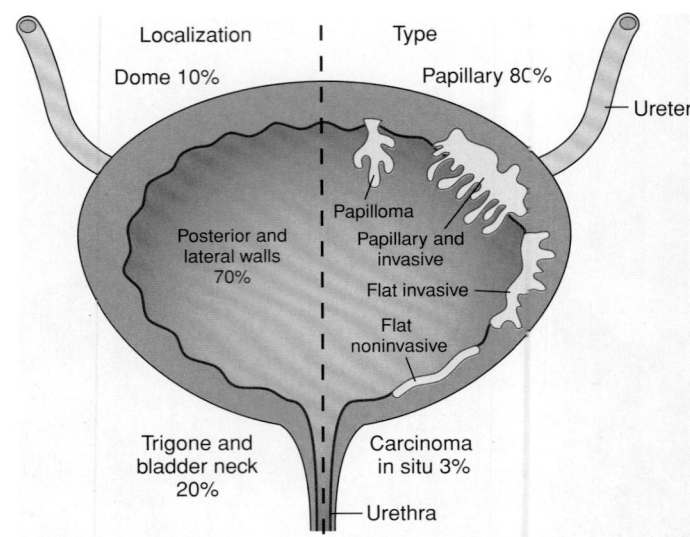

FIGURE 23-16. Urothelial neoplasms. Most tumors arise in the posterior and lateral walls; trigone and bladder neck are involved less often and the dome least. Malignant tumors may be papillary or flat. Both flat and papillary tumors may be invasive or noninvasive. Benign transitional cell papillomas are rare.

TABLE 23-1	
THIRD AND FOURTH EDITIONS OF WHO CLASSIFICATION OF TUMORS OF THE UROTHELIAL NEOPLASMS	
Third Edition	**Fourth Edition**

• Noninvasive urothelial lesions
  • Urothelial carcinoma in situ
  • Papillary urothelial carcinoma, low grade
  • Papillary urothelial carcinoma, high grade
  • Papillary urothelial neoplasm of low malignant potential
  • Urothelial papilloma
  • Inverted urothelial papilloma
	• **Noninvasive urothelial lesions**
	  • **Urothelial carcinoma in situ**
	  • **Papillary urothelial carcinoma, low grade**
	  • **Papillary urothelial carcinoma, high grade**
	  • **Papillary urothelial neoplasm of low malignant potential**
	  • **Urothelial papilloma**
	  • **Inverted urothelial papilloma**
	  • **Urothelial proliferation of uncertain malignant potential**
	  • **Urothelial dysplasia/atypia**

• Invasive urothelial tumors
  • Infiltrating urothelial carcinoma with squamous differentiation, or glandular differentiation, or trophoblastic differentiation
  • Nested
  • Microcystic
  • Micropapillary
  • Lymphoepithelioma-like
  • Lymphoma-like
  • Plasmacytoid
  • Sarcomatoid
  • Giant cell
  • Undifferentiated
	• **Invasive urothelial tumors**
	  • **Infiltrating urothelial carcinoma with divergent differentiation**
	  • **Nested, small and large nested variants**
	  • **Microcystic**
	  • **Micropapillary**
	  • **Lymphoepithelioma-like**
	  • **Plasmacytoid/signet ring cell/diffuse**
	  • **Sarcomatoid**
	  • **Giant cell**
	  • **Poorly differentiated**
	  • **Lipid rich**
	  • **Clear cell**

• Other Malignant Tumors
  • Squamous cell tumors
  • Adenocarcinoma
  • Neuroendocrine carcinoma
  • Carcinosarcoma
  • Sarcomas
	• **Other Malignant Tumors**
	  • **Squamous cell tumors**
	  • **Adenocarcinoma**
	  • **Neuroendocrine carcinoma**
	  • **Carcinosarcoma**
	  • **Sarcomas**

Inverted papillomas are rare and typically present as nodular mucosal lesions, usually in the trigone area. They have also been observed in the renal pelvis, ureter, and urethra. Inverted papillomas are covered by normal urothelium, from which cords of transitional epithelium descend into the lamina propria. These lesions are most common in men in their sixth and seventh decades. Hematuria of recent onset is the usual clinical presentation. Inverted papillomas are benign tumors and are usually cured by simple excision.

Urothelial Carcinomas Vary From Flat, Noninvasive Carcinomas In Situ to Noninvasive Papillary Carcinomas, and From Superficially Invasive to Deeply Invasive Carcinomas

PATHOLOGY: Papillary cancers arise most frequently in the lateral or posterior bladder walls. Grossly, tumors may be small, delicate, low-grade papillary lesions limited to the mucosal surface or larger, high-grade, solid masses that are invasive and ulcerated (Fig. 23-17).

They are graded as papillary urothelial neoplasms of low malignant potential (PUNLMP) and papillary urothelial carcinomas, low grade and high grade. The latter may be invasive.

- **Papillary urothelial neoplasms of low malignant potential:** These papillary tumors resemble urothelial papillomas but show increased cellularity. They are considered intermediate between benign papillomas and low-grade papillary urothelial carcinomas. These lesions are usually larger than papillomas but lack the architectural and cytologic atypia characteristic of low-grade carcinomas. PUNLMP may recur (<50%) or occasionally progress to higher-grade tumors (<5%).
- **Low-grade papillary urothelial carcinoma:** Low-grade tumors have fronds lined by neoplastic urothelial epithelium with minimal architectural and cytologic atypia (Fig. 23-18A). The cells are moderately hyperchromatic with little nuclear pleomorphism and low mitotic activity. Papillae are long and delicate. Fusion of papillae is focal and limited. Invasion of the lamina propria or the deep muscularis propria occurs in 10%. The recurrence rate is 50% and the risk of progression is 5% to 10%.

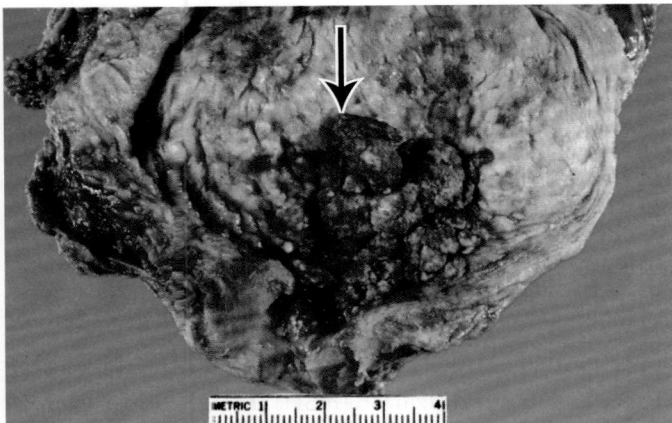

FIGURE 23-17. Urothelial carcinoma of the urinary bladder. A large exophytic tumor (*arrow*) is situated above the bladder neck.

- **High-grade papillary urothelial carcinoma:** These tumors show significant nuclear hyperchromasia and pleomorphism. The epithelium is disorganized (Fig. 23-18B) with mitoses in all layers. Approximately 80% of high-grade tumors invade the lamina propria and, less often, the muscularis propria or through the entire thickness of the bladder wall. Regional lymph nodes contain metastatic tumor in half of patients with these invasive tumors.
- **Urothelial carcinoma in situ is a flat, full-thickness intraepithelial lesion:** *This term is reserved for full-thickness lesions in which malignant changes are confined to nonpapillary bladder mucosa with no evidence of invasion.* The involved urothelium is of variable thickness, with cellular atypia from the basal layer to the surface (Fig. 23-18C). Atypia entails loss of nuclear polarity, nuclear irregularity, enlargement, hyperchromatism, and prominent nucleoli. *The basement membrane is intact and there is no invasion into underlying stroma.* One-third of carcinomas in situ of the bladder are associated with subsequent invasive carcinoma. In turn, most invasive transitional cell carcinomas arise from carcinoma in situ rather than from papillary transitional cell cancers. Confined to the mucosal surface, in situ lesions typically appear as multiple, red, velvety, flat patches that are often near exophytic papillary transitional cell carcinomas (see below). Concurrent in situ cancers elsewhere in the bladder or ureters, urethra, and prostatic ducts are common. Carcinoma in situ is often multifocal at the time of discovery, or similar lesions may develop shortly thereafter. Lesions involving the bladder neck or the urethra may extend into the periurethral prostatic ducts.
- **Invasive urothelial carcinoma:** These highly malignant tumors may evolve from papillary lesions or flat carcinomas in situ (Fig. 23-18D). In many cases, the nature of the initial lesion is unknown. Depth of invasion into the bladder wall, or beyond, determines the prognosis.

Bladder cancers are staged according to the tumor–node–metastasis (TNM) system (Table 23-2), with depth of invasion determining the T stage of the tumor (Fig. 23-19). In order of decreasing frequency, metastases involve regional and periaortic lymph nodes, liver, lung, and bone.

CLINICAL FEATURES: Urothelial carcinoma of the bladder typically manifests as sudden **hematuria** and, less often, **dysuria**. Cystoscopy reveals one or more tumors. At the time of presentation, 85% of tumors are confined to the urinary bladder; 15% show regional or distant metastases.

The probability of tumor extension and subsequent recurrence increases with:

- Increased tumor size
- High stage
- High grade
- Presence of multiple tumors
- Vascular or lymphatic invasion
- Urothelial dysplasia (including carcinoma in situ) at other sites in the bladder

The overall 10-year survival rate with noninvasive or superficially invasive low-grade urothelial tumors

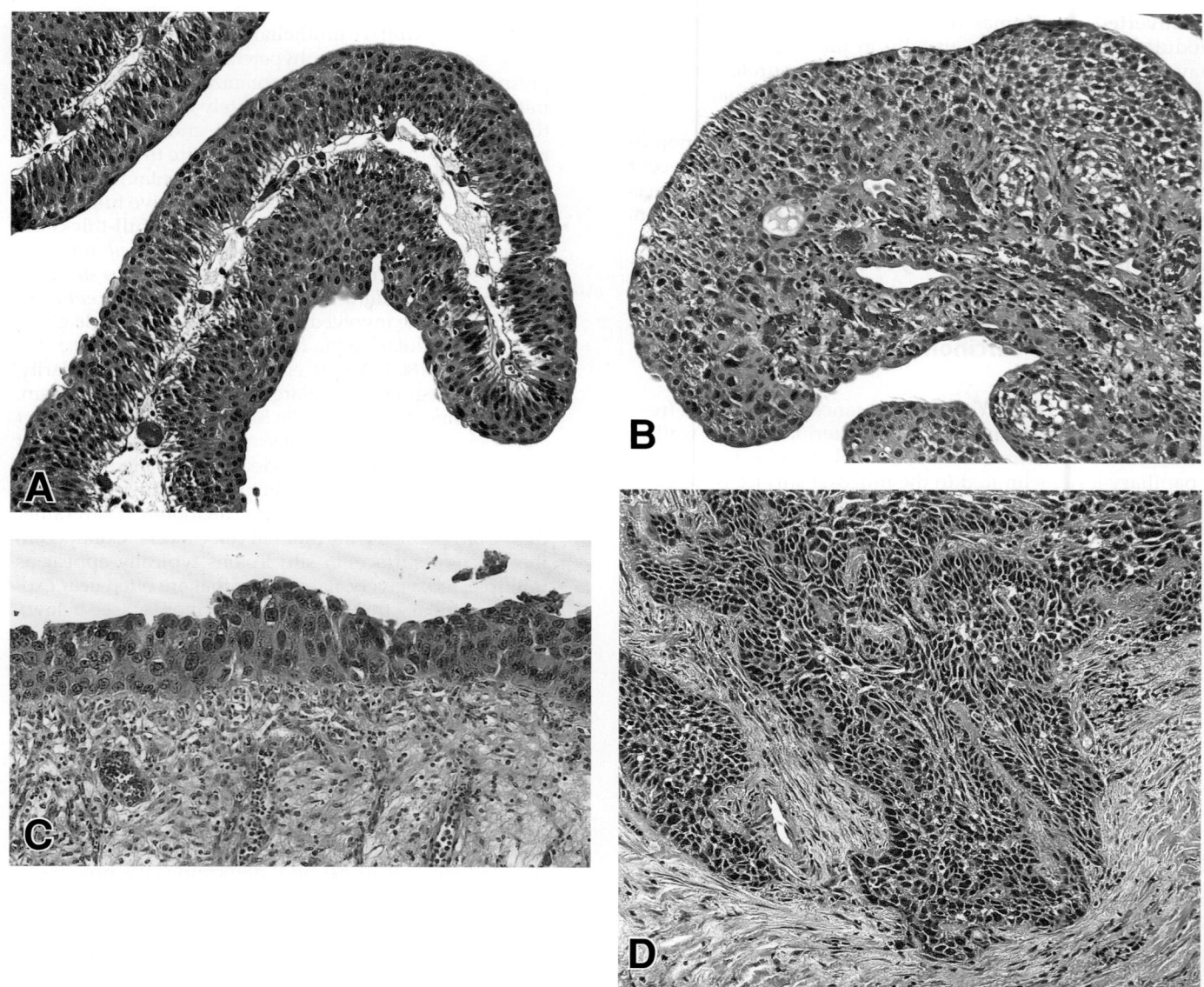

FIGURE 23-18. Urothelial tumors of the urinary bladder. A. Low-grade papillary urothelial carcinoma consists of exophytic papillae that have a central connective tissue core and are lined by slightly disorganized transitional epithelium. **B.** High-grade papillary urothelial carcinoma at higher magnification shows architectural disorder and pleomorphic hyperchromatic nuclei. **C.** Urothelial carcinoma in situ is a flat lesion with marked nuclear pleomorphism and loss of polarity from the basal layer to the surface. **D.** Invasive high-grade papillary urothelial carcinoma consists of irregular nests of hyperchromatic cells invading into the muscularis.

exceeds 95% irrespective of the number of recurrences. Only 10% of low-grade tumors progress to higher-grade tumors, and thus there is a worse prognosis.

Nonmuscle invasive tumors (papillary tumors limited to the epithelium surface with no invasion, Ta; carcinoma in situ, Tis; or invasion of mucosa or lamina propria, T1) are usually treated conservatively by fulguration via transurethral resection, intravesical immunotherapy with bacillus Calmette–Guérin (BCG) or other chemotherapy agents, along with close monitoring for disease recurrence and progression. Radical cystectomy is reserved for patients whose tumors show muscle invasion (T2), and occasionally for advanced-stage tumors. Invasive tumors or those refractory to conservative therapy are treated by cystectomy, possibly with adjuvant systemic chemotherapy. Tumors invading the bladder muscle are associated with 25% to 30% overall mortality. In bladder cancer patients, the most common causes of death are uremia (from urinary outflow tract obstruction), extension into adjacent organs, and effects of distant metastases.

Recurrent or progressive disease is detected by cystoscopy and biopsy, or by less invasive techniques such as urinalysis for tumor markers, urine cytology, and cytogenetic analysis of desquamated cells. The latter analyzes cells from the patient's urine for ploidy values of specific chromosomal regions (see above) by fluorescence in situ hybridization (FISH) (Fig. 23-20; see Chapter 6). Currently, aneuploidy for chromosomes 3, 7, and 17 and loss of 9p21 are detected as diagnostic markers.

TABLE 23-2

TNM STAGING OF UROTHELIAL CARCINOMA OF URINARY BLADDER

T—Primary Tumor

T0 No grossly visible tumor

Ta Noninvasive papillary carcinoma

Tis Carcinoma in situ

T1 Invasion of the lamina propria

T2 Invasion of the muscularis propria
    T2a Superficial invasion of the muscularis (inner half)
    T2b Invasion of deep muscle (outer half)

T3a Microscopic invasion of the perivesical tissue
T3b Macroscopic invasion of the perivesical tissue

T4a Extravesical spread into adjacent organs: prostate, seminal vesicles, uterus, vagina, rectum
T4b Extravesical spread into pelvic or abdominal wall

N—Regional Lymph Nodes

N0 No lymph node involvement

N1 Single lymph node metastasis

N2 Multiple regional lymph node metastasis

N3 Metastasis to common iliac lymph nodes

M—Distant Metastases

M0 No metastases

M1a Distant metastases to lymph nodes beyond the common iliac lymph nodes
M1b Nonnodal distant metastases

Nonurothelial Bladder Cancers Are Rare

Squamous cell bladder carcinomas develop in foci of squamous metaplasia, usually due to schistosomiasis. Bladder wall invasion is common at the time of initial presentation and prognosis is poor.

Adenocarcinomas account for 1% of malignant bladder tumors. They derive from urachal epithelial remnants, foci of cystitis glandularis, or intestinal metaplasia. Most bladder adenocarcinomas are deeply invasive when they initially present and are not curable.

Neuroendocrine carcinoma, resembling small cell lung carcinoma, occurs uncommonly in the urinary bladder. It is highly malignant and has a poor prognosis.

Sarcomas of the bladder are rare. They are highly malignant, form bulky masses and are often inoperable. **Leiomyosarcoma** is the most common form in adults.

Rhabdomyosarcoma, typically of the embryonal type, occurs mostly as **sarcoma botryoides** in children, as edematous, mucosal, polypoid masses resembling a cluster of grapes. Combined treatment with radiation therapy and chemotherapy has greatly increased survival rates.

Penis, Urethra, and Scrotum

CONGENITAL DISORDERS OF THE PENIS

Developmental anomalies of the penis include anomalies of the penile urethra and prepuce, as well as rare and infrequent conditions such as agenesis or hypoplasia.

HYPOSPADIAS: In this congenital anomaly, the urethra opens on the underside (ventral) of the penis; the meatus is thus proximal to its normal location on the tip of the penis. It results from incomplete closure of the urethral folds of the urogenital sinus.

Hypospadias occurs in 1 in 350 male babies. Most cases are sporadic but familial occurrence is known. It may be associated with other urogenital anomalies and complex, multisystemic, developmental syndromes. In 90% of cases, the meatus is located on the underside of the glans, or the corona (Fig. 23-21). Less often, it occurs mid shaft, in the scrotum or even in the perineum. Surgical repair is usually uncomplicated.

EPISPADIAS: In this rare congenital anomaly, the urethra opens on the upper side (dorsum) of the penis. In its most common form, the entire penile urethra is open along the whole shaft. Severe epispadias may be associated with bladder exstrophy (Fig. 23-8). In its mildest form, the defect is limited to the glandular urethra. Surgical treatment of epispadias is more complicated than that of hypospadias.

PHIMOSIS: The orifice of the prepuce may be too narrow to allow retraction over the glans penis. Phimosis may be congenital or acquired. The latter is usually a consequence of recurrent infections or trauma of the prepuce in uncircumcised men. Phimosis predisposes to penile infections. A narrow prepuce, if forcefully retracted, may strangulate the glans and impede the outflow of venous blood, a condition called **paraphimosis**. Circumcision is curative.

SCROTAL MASSES

Scrotal masses and conditions that lead to scrotal swelling or enlargement often reflect abnormalities of testicular, epididymal, and scrotal development. Clinical problems related to these conditions are most often seen in children but may be found in adults (Fig. 23-22).

HYDROCELE: This is a collection of serous fluid in the mesothelial lined scrotal sac between the two layers of the tunica vaginalis. Hydroceles may be congenital or acquired.

Congenital hydrocele reflects patency or incomplete obliteration of the processus vaginalis testis. This is the most common cause of scrotal swelling in infants and is often associated with inguinal hernia.

Acquired hydrocele in adults is due to some other disease affecting the scrotum, such as infection, tumor, or trauma. The diagnosis is made by ultrasound or by transluminating the fluid in the cavity. Hydrocele is a benign condition that disappears once the cause has been addressed. However, long-standing hydroceles may cause testicular atrophy or compress the epididymis, or the fluid may become infected and lead to **periorchitis**.

HEMATOCELE: Blood may accumulate between the layers of tunica vaginalis after trauma or hemorrhage into a hydrocele, or as a result of testicular tumors and infections.

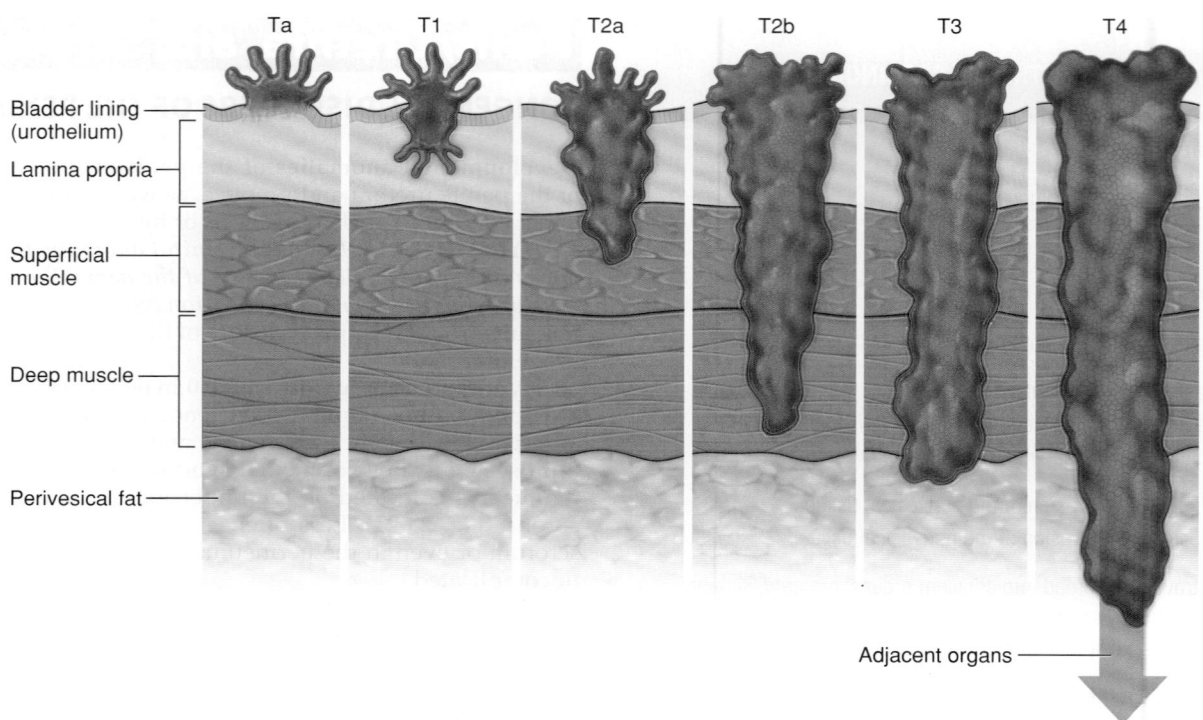

FIGURE 23-19. TNM staging of urothelial carcinoma. Carcinoma in situ (CIS) is flat, noninvasive high-grade urothelial carcinoma staged as Tis. Papillary, noninvasive high-grade urothelial carcinoma is staged as Ta. High-grade urothelial carcinoma with invasion into lamina propria is T1. High-grade urothelial carcinoma with invasion into muscularis propria is T2. Invasion into perivesical soft tissue is T3. High-grade urothelial carcinoma with invasion into perivesical adipose tissue is T4.

SPERMATOCELE: This is a cyst formed from protrusions of widened efferent ducts of the rete testis or epididymis. It manifests as a hilar paratesticular nodule or a fluctuating mass filled with milky fluid. The cyst is lined by cuboidal epithelium that contains spermatozoa in various stages of degeneration.

VARICOCELE: This dilation of testicular veins appears as a nodularity on the lateral side of the scrotum. Most are asymptomatic and are discovered during physical examination of infertile men. Massive varicocele is described as resembling a "bag of worms." Varicoceles are considered a common cause of infertility and oligospermia, although it is unclear why dilation of veins should have such effects. Testicular atrophy occurs only rarely and only in long-standing cases. Surgical ligation of the internal spermatic vein often improves reproductive function.

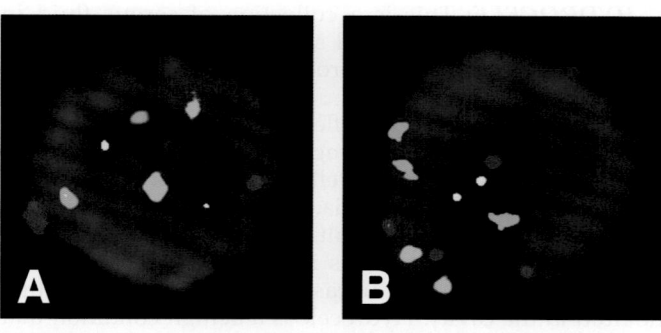

FIGURE 23-20. Fluorescence in situ hybridization of bladder cancer. A. Normal. In this single urothelial cell collected from the urine of a normal person, *red* fluorescence represents chromosome 3, *green* is chromosome 7, *aqua* is chromosome 17, and *gold* marks the 9p21 locus. All probe signals are present in two copies indicating euploidy. **B. Urothelial carcinoma of the bladder.** Multiple *green* and *red* probes indicate aneuploidy of chromosomes 3 and 7. Chromosome 17 and the 9p21 locus are euploid.

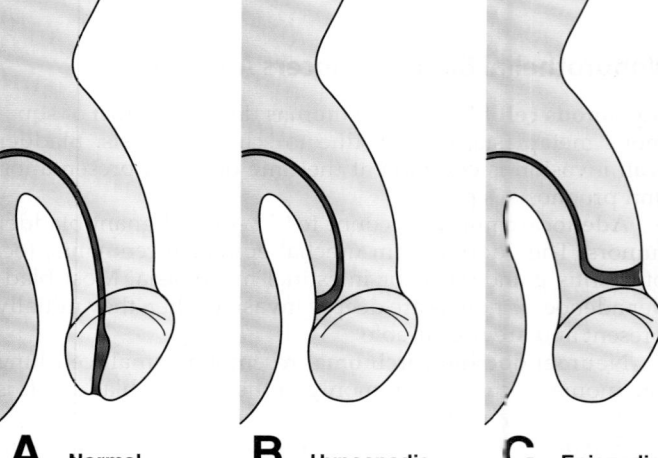

A. Normal   **B.** Hypospadia   **C.** Epispadia

FIGURE 23-21. Congenital anomalies of the penis. A. Normal penis has the urethral opening on the tip of the glans. **B.** Hypospadias is characterized by a urethral opening on the ventral side of the penis. **C.** Epispadias is characterized by a urethral opening on the dorsal side of the penis. (From Bulock BA, Henze RL. *Focus on Pathophysiology.* Philadelphia, PA: Lippincott Williams & Wilkins; 2000.)

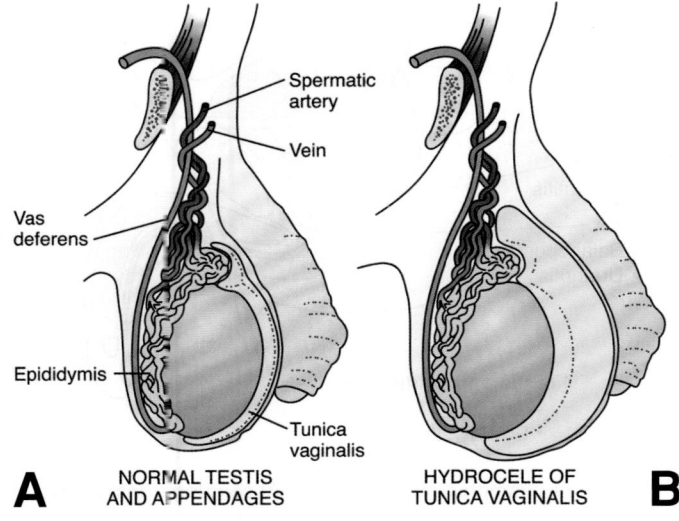

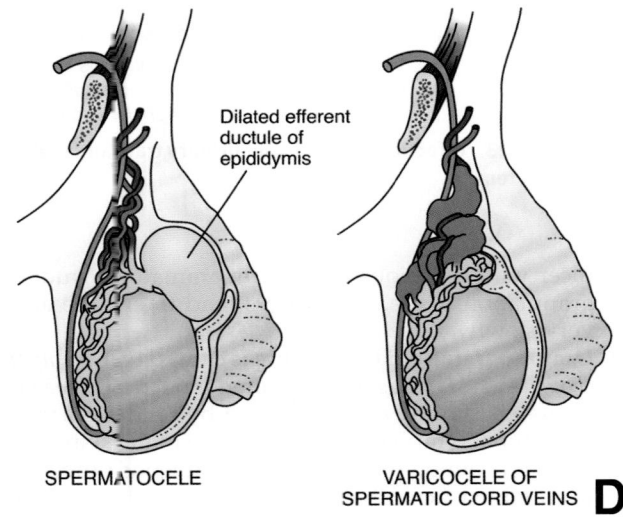

FIGURE 23-22. Scrotal masses. **A.** Normal testis. **B.** Hydrocele. **C.** Spermatocele. **D.** Varicocele of spermatic cord veins.

SCROTAL INGUINAL HERNIA: Intestinal protrusion into the scrotum through the inguinal canal is a scrotal hernia. The bowel may be repositioned, but if it remains untreated, such a hernia may cause adhesions or testicular atrophy. Hernias can only be repaired surgically.

CIRCULATORY DISTURBANCES

SCROTAL EDEMA: Lymph or serous fluid may accumulate in the scrotum from obstruction to lymphatic or venous drainage. **Lymphedema** from lymphatic obstruction can be caused by pelvic or abdominal tumors, surgical scars, or infections such as filariasis. **Transudation** of plasma into the scrotum is common in patients with heart failure, anasarca due to cirrhosis, or nephrotic syndrome. Fluid accumulates in the loose connective tissue and the cavity lined by the tunica vaginalis testis.

ERECTILE DYSFUNCTION: This condition, also known as impotence, is the *inability to achieve or maintain an erection sufficient for satisfactory sexual performance.* Its prevalence increases with age, from 20% at age 40 years to 50% by age 70.

Erection requires adequate filling of the penile corpora cavernosa and spongiosa with blood. Penile tumescence is the result of a complex interaction of mental, neural, hormonal, and vascular factors. Filling of these vascular spaces depends on nitric oxide (NO•)-mediated relaxation of vascular smooth muscle cells in the erectile cylinders. NO• release is related to cyclic guanosine monophosphate (cGMP), so drugs that inhibit the phosphodiesterase that degrades cGMP (e.g., sildenafil [Viagra], vardenafil hydrochloride [Levitra], or tadalafil [Cialis]) are used to treat erectile dysfunction. Disorders associated with erectile dysfunction are listed in Table 23-3.

PRIAPISM: Priapism is *continuous penile erection unrelated to sexual excitation.* It may be primary or secondary. Primary priapism is idiopathic and painful. Treatment is usually ineffective. Secondary priapism may occur in (1) pelvic diseases that impede outflow of blood from the penis (e.g., pelvic tumors or hematomas, thrombosis of pelvic veins, infections); (2) hematologic disorders (e.g., sickle cell anemia, polycythemia vera, leukemia); and (3) brain and spinal cord diseases (e.g., tumors, syphilis).

TABLE 23-3
DISORDERS ASSOCIATED WITH ERECTILE DYSFUNCTION
Neuropsychiatric
Psychiatric disorders (e.g., depression)
Spinal cord injury
Nerve injury during surgery (e.g., pelvic or perineal surgery)
Endocrine
Hypogonadism
Pituitary diseases (e.g., hyperprolactinemia)
Hypothyroidism, Cushing syndrome, Addison disease
Vascular
Diabetic microangiopathy
Hypertension
Atherosclerosis
Drugs
Antihypertensives
Psychotropic drugs
Estrogens, anticancer drugs, etc.
Idiopathic
"Performance anxiety"
Age-related "impotence"

INFLAMMATORY DISORDERS

The most important inflammatory diseases of the penis are (1) sexually transmitted diseases (STDs); (2) nonspecific infections; (3) diseases of unknown etiology, such as balanitis xerotica obliterans; (4) dermatoses; and (5) dermatitis of the penile shaft and scrotum (Table 23-4).

Sexually Transmitted Diseases Cause Discrete Penile Lesions

STDs (see Chapter 9) involving lower urinary tract infections (Fig. 23-23) include the following:

- **Genital herpes** is most often caused by herpes simplex virus (HSV)-2 or, less commonly, by HSV-1. It is the most common STD affecting the glans and manifests typically as grouped vesicles that ulcerate and transform into crusts.
- **Primary syphilis,** caused by a spirochete, *Treponema pallidum,* may manifest as a solitary, soft ulcer **(chancre)** accompanied by palpable inguinal lymphadenopathy.
- **Chancroid** is caused by *Haemophilus ducreyi* and presents as a papule that transforms into a pustule and finally ulcerates. Shallow ulcers on the glans or the skin of the shaft are often associated with painful suppurative inguinal lymphadenitis.
- **Granuloma inguinale** is a tropical disease caused by *Calymmatobacterium granulomatis.* It appears as a raised

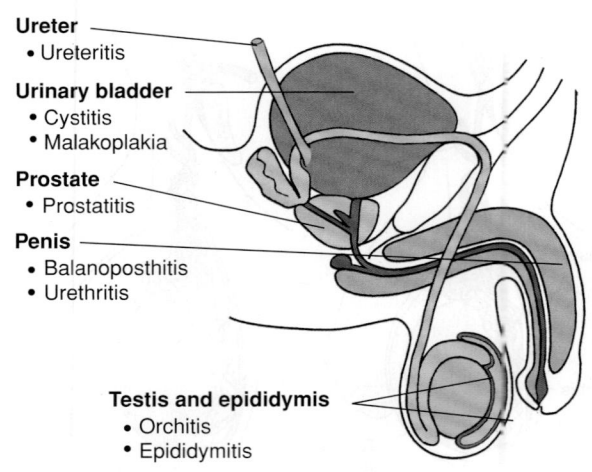

FIGURE 23-23. Infections of the lower urinary tract and male reproductive system.

ulcer with a copious chronic inflammatory exudate and granulation tissue. Such ulcers tend to enlarge and heal very slowly.
- **Lymphogranuloma venereum** is caused by *Chlamydia trachomatis.* It starts as a small, often innocuous, vesicle that ulcerates, typically accompanied by tender enlargement of inguinal lymph nodes that adhere to the skin and form sinuses draining pus and serosanguineous fluid.
- **Condyloma acuminatum** is caused by human papillomavirus (HPV) type 6 or, less often, 11. It appears as flat-topped warts on the shaft (Fig. 23-24), small polyps on the glans and urethral meatus, or larger cauliflower-like tumors that may be confused with verrucous carcinoma.

Balanitis Is Inflammation of the Glans Penis

In uncircumcised men, balanitis usually extends from the glans to the foreskin and is called **balanoposthitis**. Mostly it is caused by bacteria, but it may also be caused by fungi in diabetics or immunosuppressed people. Balanitis typically reflects poor hygiene. Significant complications of chronic balanoposthitis are meatal stricture, phimosis, and paraphimosis.

BALANITIS XEROTICA OBLITERANS: This idiopathic chronic inflammatory condition is equivalent to lichen sclerosus of the vulva (see Chapter 24) and is characterized by fibrosis and sclerosis of subepithelial connective tissue. The affected portion of the glans is white and indurated. Fibrosis may constrict the urethral meatus or cause phimosis.

CIRCINATE BALANITIS: In oculo-urethro-synovial syndrome (OUS) (see below), the glans may show circular, linear, or confluent plaque-like discolorations, occasionally associated with superficial ulcers.

TABLE 23-4
INFLAMMATORY LESIONS OF THE PENIS
Sexually Transmitted Diseases
Herpes genitalis
Syphilis
Chancroid
Granuloma inguinale
Lymphogranuloma venereum
Human papillomavirus infections
Nonspecific Infectious Balanoposthitis
Bacterial, fungal, viral
Diseases of Unknown Etiology
Balanitis xerotica obliterans
Circinate balanitis
Plasma cell balanitis (Zoon balanitis)
Peyronie disease
Dermatitis Involving the Shaft of the Penis and Scrotum
Infectious (bacterial, viral, fungal)
Noninfectious (e.g., lichen planus, bullous skin diseases)

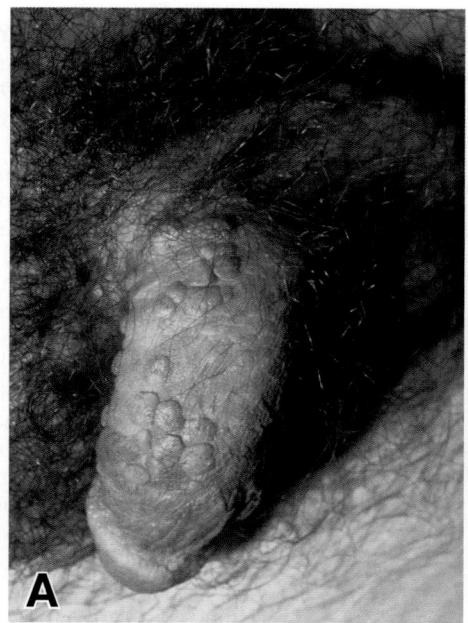
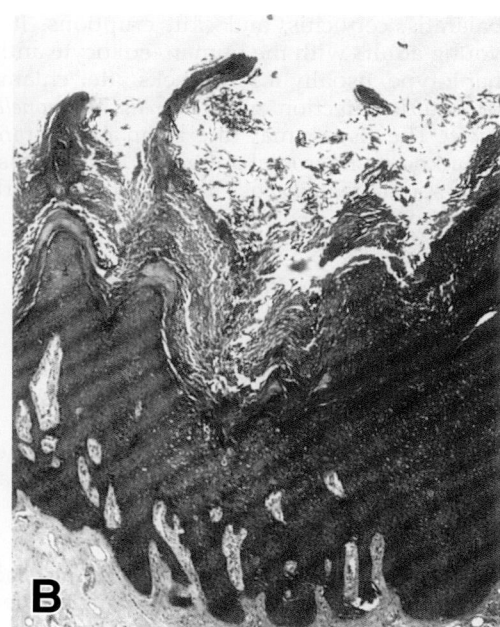

FIGURE 23-24. Condylomata acuminata of the penis. A. Raised, circumscribed lesions are seen on the shaft of the penis. **B.** Microscopic view of a lesion shows epidermal hyperkeratosis, parakeratosis, acanthosis, and papillomatosis.

PLASMA CELL BALANITIS: This chronic, innocuous disease of unknown origin (also called Zoon balanitis) causes macular discoloration or painless papules on the glans. Plasma cell and lymphocytic infiltrates are seen beneath a thickened overlying epithelium.

DERMATOSES: Many inflammatory skin diseases may involve the penis. Such conditions are discussed in Chapter 28.

Peyronie Disease Is an Idiopathic Fibrous Induration of the Penis

It is characterized by focal, asymmetric fibrosis of the penile shaft. During erections, the penis becomes curved and painful. Typically, it presents as an ill-defined induration of the penile shaft in a young or middle-aged man, with no change in the overlying skin. Microscopically, dense fibrosis is associated with sparse, nonspecific, chronic inflammatory infiltration. Collagen focally replaces muscle in the septum of the corpus cavernosum.

Peyronie disease affects 1% of men over age 40. In most instances, it is mild and does not interfere with sexual function. However, severe cases may be so incapacitating as to require surgery in which the outcome is not always satisfactory.

URETHRITIS AND RELATED CONDITIONS

Urethritis is acute or chronic inflammation of the urethra.

SEXUALLY TRANSMITTED URETHRITIS: Urethritis presenting as urethral discharge is the most common sign of STDs in men. Women rarely notice distinct urethral discharge and usually complain of vaginal discharge.

Gonococcal and **nongonococcal** urethritis have an acute onset, related to recent sexual intercourse. The discharge is typically purulent and greenish yellow. Symptoms include pain or tingling at the meatus of the urethra and pain on micturition (**dysuria**). Meatal redness and swelling are common in both sexes. Acute gonococcal and nongonococcal urethritis can both become chronic.

The diagnosis is made by identifying the causative agent. In gonococcal urethritis, the discharge contains *Neisseria gonorrhoeae,* which can be identified microscopically in smears of urethral exudates. Nongonococcal urethritis is mostly caused by *C. trachomatis* or *Ureaplasma urealyticum* but may be related to a variety of other pathogens.

NONSPECIFIC INFECTIOUS URETHRITIS: Uropathogens such as **E. coli** *and* **P. aeruginosa** *can cause urethritis.* Typically infection is associated with cystitis but may be caused by other diseases (e.g., prostatic hyperplasia or urinary stones). In men, infectious urethritis may be the only sign of prostatitis. In women, it may be a complication of vaginitis and vulvitis. In hospitalized patients, it commonly follows cystoscopy and other urologic procedures and is almost inevitable in patients with indwelling urethral catheters.

Nonspecific infectious urethritis manifests clinically with urgency and a burning sensation during urination. Usually there is no discharge, but men may express some milky fluid by "stripping" or "milking" the urethra.

URETHRAL CARUNCLES: Polypoid inflammatory lesions near the female urethral meatus cause pain and bleeding. They are idiopathic and occur only in women, mostly after menopause. Urethral mucosal prolapse and attendant chronic inflammation may be implicated.

Urethral caruncles present as 1- to 2-cm exophytic, often ulcerated, polypoid masses, at or near the urethral meatus. They show acutely and chronically inflamed granulation tissue and ulceration and hyperplasia of transitional cell or squamous epithelium. Complex patterns of papillomatosis and occasional dysplastic epithelium may suggest a superficial resemblance to carcinoma, but this inflammatory lesion does not lead to cancer. Treatment is surgical excision.

REACTIVE ARTHRITIS (PREVIOUSLY REITER SYNDROME): Reactive arthritis is a triad of urethritis, conjunctivitis, and arthritis of weight-bearing joints (e.g., knee, intervertebral joints). Other findings may include circinate balanitis, cervicitis, and skin eruptions. It tends to affect young adults with the human leukocyte antigen (HLA)-B27 haplotype, usually a few weeks after chlamydial urethritis or enteric infection with *Shigella, Salmonella,* or *Campylobacter*. The disease may thus be an aberrant immune reaction to unknown microbial antigen(s). Symptoms usually disappear spontaneously in 3 to 6 months, but arthritis recurs in half of patients.

TUMORS

Urethral Cancers May Arise From Squamous or Transitional Epithelia

These uncommon tumors usually occur in elderly women. Some penile cancers arise in the terminal part of the penile urethra.

 PATHOLOGY: Most urethral cancers are squamous carcinomas originating in the distal urethra. Urothelial carcinomas, like those in the bladder, arise in the proximal urethra.

 CLINICAL FEATURES: Urethral cancer develops most often in the sixth and seventh decades. Patients present with urethral bleeding and dysuria. Most tumors have spread to adjacent tissues or lymph nodes by the time of presentation. Radical surgery is the main therapy.

Cancer of the Penis Occurs Mostly in Uncircumcised Men

Cancer of the penis originates from the squamous mucosa of the glans and contiguous urethral meatus or the prepuce and skin covering the penile shaft.

 EPIDEMIOLOGY: In the United States, invasive squamous cell carcinoma of the penis is uncommon, accounting for less than 0.5% of all cancers in men. The average age of patients is 60 years. Penile cancer is much more common in less developed countries. In some parts of Africa and Asia and South America, it constitutes 10% of cancers in men. It is virtually unknown in men circumcised at birth.

 ETIOLOGIC FACTORS: No single agent has been identified as the cause of penile cancer. Current interest centers on the possible influence of smegma, the whitish material composed of accumulated keratin debris and secretion of the preputial (Tyson) glands that accumulates beneath the prepuce. Human papillomavirus (HPV) DNA has been found in 50% of all invasive carcinomas of the penis, suggesting that HPV types 16 and 18 play a role in some penile cancers. Cigarette smoking is also associated with a higher risk of penile cancer.

 PATHOLOGY: Penile carcinoma may be preinvasive (in situ) or invasive.

SQUAMOUS CELL CARCINOMA IN SITU: Carcinoma in situ of the penis is similar to that in other sites (see Chapter 28). Grossly, it may present as Bowen disease or erythroplasia of Queyrat. **Bowen disease** is a sharply demarcated, erythematous, or grayish white plaque on the shaft. **Erythroplasia of Queyrat** appears as solitary or multiple, shiny, soft, erythematous plaques on the glans and foreskin. Both of these resemble **squamous cell carcinoma in situ** elsewhere. They show cytologic atypia among keratinocytes of all layers of the epidermis, parakeratosis, or hyperkeratosis; papillomatosis with broad epidermal papillae; and thinning of the granular layer. By definition, there is no invasion of the underlying dermis. Progression to invasive squamous cell carcinoma is estimated to occur in less than 10% of cases.

Bowenoid papulosis of the penis is caused by HPV and affects young, sexually active men. In contrast to the solitary lesion of Bowen disease, bowenoid papulosis appears as multiple brownish or violaceous papules. Microscopically, it resembles other squamous carcinomas in situ, but there are some differences. Most carcinomas in situ slowly merge at the margins with normal epithelium, but bowenoid papulosis is sharply demarcated from normal epidermis, like HPV-induced warts. The altered epidermis shows some superficial stratification and maturation and may contain giant keratinocytes with multinucleated atypical nuclei. HPV type 16 can be demonstrated in 80% of patients, and type 18 is occasionally implicated. Virtually all these lesions regress spontaneously and do not progress to invasive carcinoma.

INVASIVE SQUAMOUS CELL CARCINOMA: This tumor presents as (1) an ulcer; (2) an incurated crater; (3) a friable hemorrhagic mass; or (4) an exophytic, fungating, papillary tumor. It usually involves the glans or prepuce and less commonly the penile shaft. Extensive destruction of penile tissue, including the urethral meatus, is seen when the tumor has been left untreated. Microscopically, these are typically well-differentiated, focally keratinizing, squamous cell carcinomas. Invasive tumors are usually associated with underlying dense, chronic inflammation. The adjacent epidermis often shows dysplastic changes. The tumor may invade deeply along the shaft and spread to inguinal lymph nodes, then to iliac nodes, and ultimately to distant organs.

VERRUCOUS CARCINOMA: This tumor is distinguished from other penile cancers because it is a cytologically benign but clinically malignant exophytic squamous cell carcinoma (Fig. 23-25). Grossly and cytologically, it resembles **condyloma acuminatum**, but unlike the latter, it shows local invasion. Verrucous carcinoma rarely metastasizes. Surgery is curative.

CLINICAL FEATURES: Most squamous cell cancers are confined to the penis at the time of presentation. Occult metastases to inguinal lymph nodes are not uncommon, but half of patients with enlarged regional lymph nodes do not have nodal metastases, but rather only reactive changes due to tumor-associated inflammation.

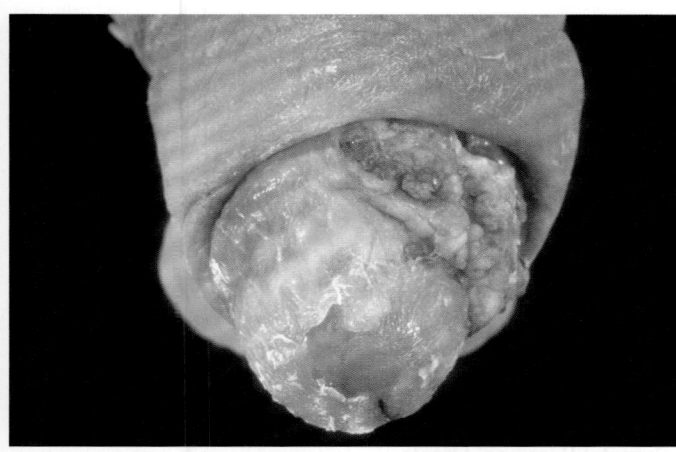

FIGURE 23-25. Carcinoma of the penis. This verrucous carcinoma on the glans appears as an exophytic mass.

Survival in patients with penile cancer is related to the clinical stage and, to a lesser degree, histologic grade of the tumor. Amputation of the penis is usually necessary. Patients with superficially invasive cancer have 90% 5-year survival; inguinal lymph node metastases reduce 5-year survival to 20% to 50%, depending on the extent of spread. HPV infection is seen in at least half of cases.

Cancer of the Scrotum Is Quite Uncommon

In 1775, Sir Percival Pott introduced the idea of chemical carcinogenesis by reporting scrotal cancer as an occupational disease of chimney sweeps (see Chapter 8). Many industrial chemicals were found to be causative. Improved industrial hygiene has made this a rare tumor.

Squamous carcinoma of the scrotum typically affects men mostly in their 50s and 60s. At presentation, many show invasion of the scrotal contents and metastases to regional nodes. Therapy is by surgical excision. As in penile cancer, HPV has been implicated in the pathogenesis of scrotal squamous carcinomas.

Testis, Epididymis, and Vas Deferens

CRYPTORCHIDISM

Cryptorchidism, clinically known as **undescended testis,** *is a congenital abnormality in which one or both testes are not in the scrotum.* It is the most common urologic condition requiring surgical treatment in infants. The testes are not in the scrotum or are easily retracted in 5% of term male infants and 30% of those born prematurely. In the large majority, the testes descend into the scrotum in the first year of life. Thus, the prevalence of cryptorchidism from the end of the first year of life into adulthood is about 1%. It is bilateral in 30% of affected men.

 ETIOLOGIC FACTORS: Testicular maldescent is usually an isolated idiopathic developmental disorder. It may rarely be associated with other congenital anomalies.

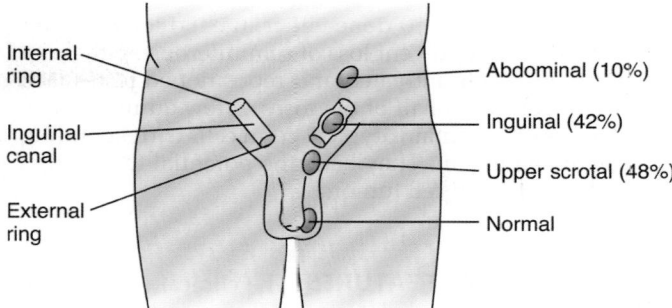

FIGURE 23-26. Cryptorchidism. In most instances, the testis has an upper scrotal location. It may also be retained in the inguinal canal and uncommonly in the abdominal cavity.

 PATHOLOGY: Testicular descent may become arrested at any point from the abdominal cavity to the upper scrotum (Fig. 23-26). Cryptorchid testes are classified by their location as **abdominal, inguinal, or upper scrotal.** Rarely, the testes are located in unusual locations, such as the perineum or calf.

Cryptorchid testes are smaller than normal even at an early age, and differences between the affected and unaffected testes increase with age. The affected testes are firm and show fibrosis.

The histology of cryptorchid testes varies with age. In infancy and early childhood, seminiferous tubules in affected testes are smaller, with fewer than normal germ cells. Postpubertal testes also show decreased germ cells, and spermatogenesis is limited to a minority of tubules. Hyaline thickening of tubular basement membranes and prominent stromal fibrosis are observed (Fig. 23-27). Eventually, tubules lose spermatogenic cells and become entirely hyalinized. **Orchiopexy** (surgical placement of a

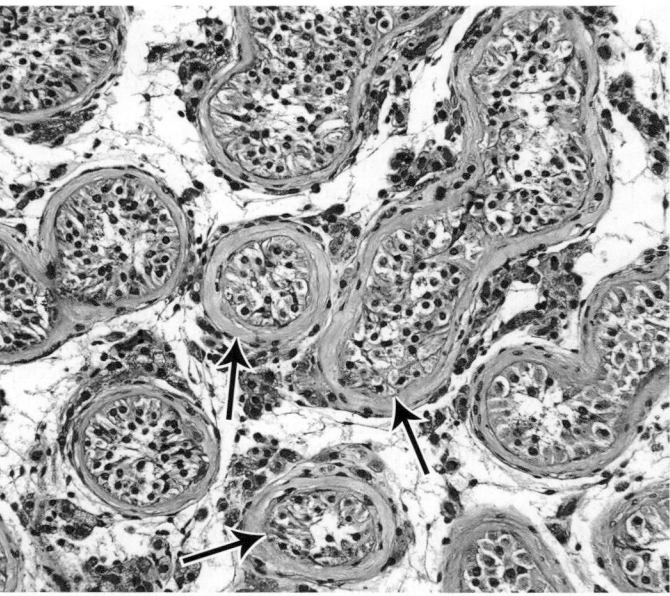

FIGURE 23-27. Cryptorchidism. Microscopic view of a testis removed from a postpubertal man with cryptorchidism shows markedly thickened hyalinized basement membranes (*arrows*) of seminiferous tubules, with no evidence of spermatogenesis.

testis into the scrotum) done either in childhood or after puberty does not prevent loss of seminiferous epithelium and tubules; both untreated and repositioned testes lack spermatogenesis in half of the cases. A few adult cryptorchid testes (2%) contain atypical germ cells corresponding to carcinoma in situ. They have the potential to progress to malignant germ cell tumors.

CLINICAL FEATURES: The clinical significance of undescended testes includes increased incidences of **infertility** and **germ cell neoplasia**. All men with bilateral cryptorchid testes have **azoospermia** and are infertile. Unilateral cryptorchidism is associated with **oligospermia**, defined as a sperm count below 20 million/mL, in 40% of cases. Although oligospermia reduces fertility, most men with one normal testis can father children. Orchiopexy done in childhood or after puberty has no effect on the sperm count. Most urologists recommend orchiopexy between 6 months and 1 year of age, but it is not clear that this improves the eventual sperm count.

Cryptorchidism is associated with a 20- to 40-fold increased risk for testicular cancer. Conversely, 10% of patients with germ cell neoplasia have cryptorchid testes. Intra-abdominal testes are at higher risk than those retained in the inguinal canal; in turn, inguinal testes are at higher risk than those high in the scrotum. A contralateral, normally descended testis is also at risk, about four times that in normal men. Unfortunately, orchiopexy does not reduce cancer risk.

ABNORMALITIES OF SEXUAL DIFFERENTIATION

Disorders of gonadogenesis and formation of external genital organs, as well as development of secondary sex characteristics, can pertain to:

- Genetic sex; the presence or absence of X and Y chromosomes
- Gonadal sex; the presence or absence of testes or ovaries
- Genital sex; the appearance of external genital organs
- Psychosocial sexual orientation

Various conditions are listed in Table 23-5. Some of these, such as Klinefelter and Turner syndromes, are discussed in Chapter 6.

HERMAPHRODITISM: This rare developmental disorder is characterized by ambiguous genitalia in someone who has both male and female gonads. Gonads may become ovotestes (combination of ovary and testis) or one gonad may be testis and the other ovary. Half of these patients have a female karyotype (46,XX). The others are genetic males (46,XY) or mosaics or have a missing sex chromosome (45,X).

FEMALE PSEUDOHERMAPHRODITISM: Virilization of external genitalia may occur in genetic females (46,XX) who have normal ovaries and internal female genital organs. The vulva may fuse into scrotal folds and clitoromegaly is common. This phenotype is most often seen in the adrenogenital syndrome caused by 21-hydroxylase deficiency (see Chapter 27). Lack of this enzyme leads to excess androgen

TABLE 23-5
DISORDERS OF SEXUAL DIFFERENTIATION
Sex Chromosomal Abnormalities
Klinefelter syndrome and its variants
Turner syndrome 46,XX males
Single-Gene Defects
Adrenogenital syndromes
Androgen insensitivity syndromes
Müllerian inhibitory substance deficiency
Prenatal Hormonal Effects
Exogenous hormones during pregnancy
Maternal hormone-producing tumors
Idiopathic Conditions
Hermaphroditism
Gonadal dysgenesis

production in the adrenal gland during fetal life, and the ambiguous genitalia are seen at birth. Excess androgens in a pregnant woman can have the same effects on the external genitalia of the female baby in utero.

A 46,XX karyotype is found in 1 of 25 patients with classical signs of Klinefelter syndrome. These 46,XX males carry the locus for the sex-determining region of chromosome Y (SRY) on one of their X chromosomes. It is not known how this translocation occurs.

MALE PSEUDOHERMAPHRODITISM: A spectrum of congenital disorders affects genetic males who have a normal 46,XY karyotype. The gonads are cryptorchid testes, but external genitalia appear feminine or ambiguously female with some virilization. Male pseudohermaphroditism occurs most often in **androgen insensitivity syndromes** due to defects in the androgen receptor (AR). This is also known as **testicular feminization syndrome**.

MALE INFERTILITY

Infertility is empirically defined as inability to conceive after 1 year of coital activity with the same sexual partner without contraception. Some 15% of couples are childless in the United States, but the true prevalence of infertility is difficult to assess because it is confounded by cultural and social issues. The male is infertile in 20% of couples, the female in 40%, and both partners in 20%. In the remaining 20% of infertile couples, no apparent cause can be identified. The causes of male infertility are listed in Table 23-6 and illustrated in Figure 23-28.

Supratesticular causes of infertility affect hormonal and metabolic aspects of spermatogenesis. The best examples are injuries in the hypothalamic–pituitary area. Infertility can result from transection of the pituitary stalk, destruction

TABLE 23-6
CAUSES OF MALE INFERTILITY

Supratesticular Causes

Disorders of the hypothalamic–pituitary–gonadal axis

Endocrine disease of the adrenal, thyroid; diabetes

Metabolic disorders

Major organ diseases (e.g., renal, hepatic, cardiopulmonary diseases)

Chronic infectious and debilitating diseases (e.g., tuberculosis, AIDS)

Drugs and substance abuse

Testicular Causes

Idiopathic: hypospermatogenesis or azoospermia

Developmental (cryptorchidism, gonadal dysgenesis)

Genetic disorders (e.g., Klinefelter syndrome)

Orchitis (immune and infectious)

Iatrogenic testicular injury (radiation, cytotoxic drugs)

Trauma of the testis and surgical injury

Environmental (possibly phytoestrogens)

Posttesticular Causes

Congenital anomalies of the excretory ducts

Inflammation and scarring of excretory ducts

Iatrogenic or posttraumatic lesions of excretory ducts

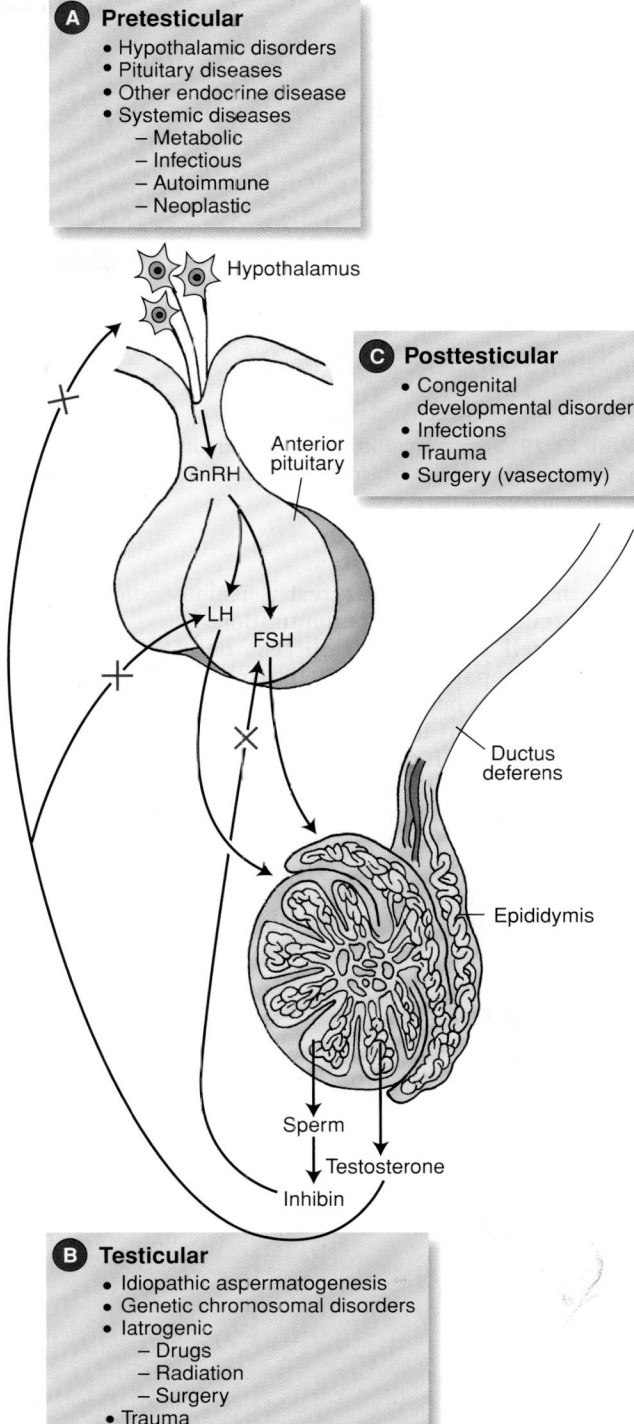

FIGURE 23-28. Causes of male infertility. A. Pretesticular infertility. *FSH* = follicle-stimulating hormone; *GnRH* = gonadotropin-releasing hormone; *LH* = luteinizing hormone. **B.** Testicular infertility. **C.** Posttesticular (obstructive) infertility.

of the hypothalamus by a brain tumor, or pressure on the pituitary by a craniopharyngioma. A pituitary tumor secreting prolactin (prolactinoma) may act as a mass lesion that destroys gonadotropin-secreting pituitary cells or compresses the pituitary stalk. It also secretes prolactin, which suppresses spermatogenesis.

Testicular infertility, the most common variety of male infertility, is related to pathologic changes in the testis. A male infertility (andrologic) workup includes urologic examination, sonography, semen analysis, hormonal studies, and in some cases testicular biopsy.

Posttesticular infertility entails blockage of excretory ducts through which sperm reach the urethra. Chronic infections of the epididymis or vas deferens, previous trauma, and congenital atresia are the causes.

 PATHOLOGY: Testicular biopsy may identify causes of infertility, such as the following:

- **Immaturity of seminiferous tubules** is seen in hypogonadotropic hypogonadism caused by pituitary or hypothalamic diseases (Fig. 23-29). Seminiferous tubules show no spermatogenesis and resemble those of prepubertal testes.

- **Decreased spermatogenesis (hypospermatogenesis)** occurs in several systemic and endocrine diseases, including malnutrition and AIDS. Hypospermatogenesis is also found in cryptorchid testes and after vasectomy.

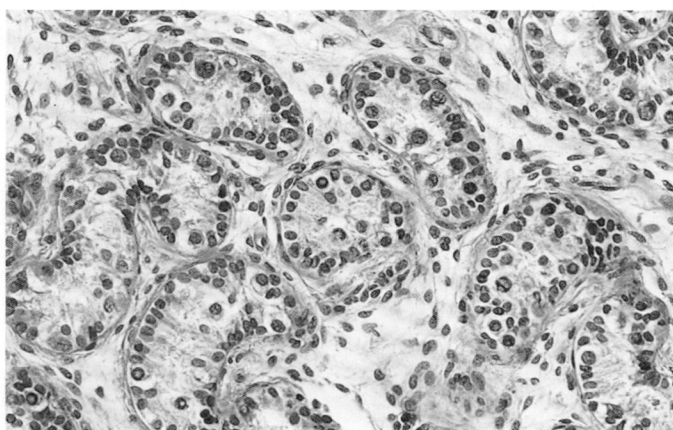

FIGURE 23-29. Hypogonadotropic hypogonadism. The testis of this 25-year-old man is composed of immature seminiferous tubules similar to those seen in prepubertal boys.

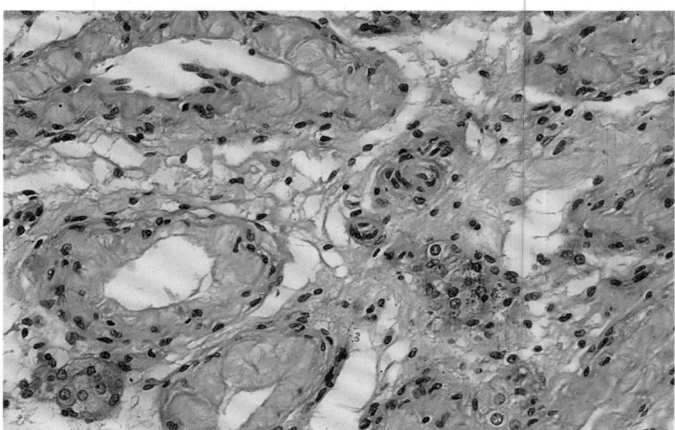

FIGURE 23-31. Postirradiation tubular atrophy of the testis. Seminiferous tubules are hyalinized, and there is no evidence of spermatogenesis.

- **Germ cell maturation arrest** is usually idiopathic. It can occur at any stage of maturation.
- **Germ cell aplasia** ("Sertoli cells only" syndrome) is mostly idiopathic (Fig. 23-30). An underlying genetic mutation has been identified in some patients involving deletions in the azoospermia factor region of the Y chromosome. It can also be seen in drug-induced and toxic injuries of the seminiferous epithelium.
- **Orchitis** is caused by viruses (e.g., mumps) or autoimmune diseases.
- **Peritubular and tubular fibroses** may be related to congenital disorders such as cryptorchidism or to previous infection, ischemia, or radiation (Fig. 23-31).

EPIDIDYMITIS

Epididymitis is acute or chronic inflammation of the epididymis, usually caused by bacteria.

Bacterial epididymitis in young men most often occurs in an acute form as a complication of gonorrhea or a sexually acquired *Chlamydia* infection. It is characterized by suppurative inflammation (Fig. 23-32). In older men, *E. coli* from associated urinary tract infections is a more common culprit. Patients present with intrascrotal pain and tenderness, with or without associated fever. Epididymitis of recent origin shows the hallmarks of acute inflammation. Persistent chronic epididymitis is associated with accumulation of plasma cells, macrophages, and lymphocytes and, ultimately, with fibrotic obstruction of infected ducts. Gonorrheal epididymitis is a common cause of acquired male infertility.

Tuberculous epididymitis is now uncommon and is usually associated with established pulmonary and renal tuberculosis. It manifests as palpable enlargement of the epididymis and beading of the vas deferens caused by confluent caseating granulomas.

Spermatic granulomas result from intense inflammatory responses to sperm outside of their usual channels. Traumatic rupture of epididymal ducts may play a role. Patients present with scrotal pain and swelling, frequently for weeks or months. The epididymis contains a mixed inflammatory cell infiltrate with many sperm fragments and macrophages phagocytosing sperm. Ultimately, inflammation results in interstitial fibrosis, ductal obstruction, and infertility.

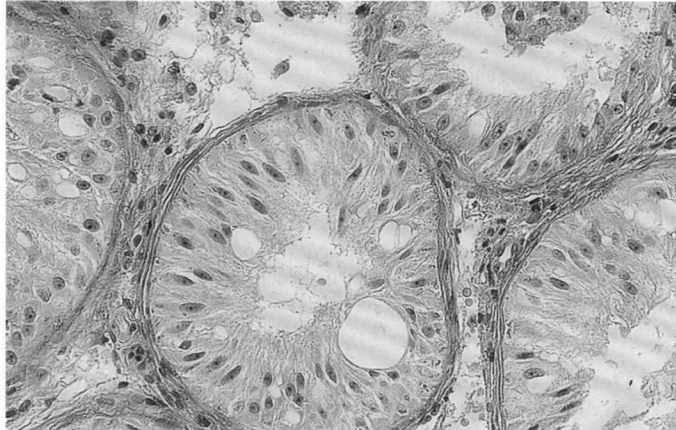

FIGURE 23-30. Germ cell aplasia–Sertoli cell-only syndrome. The seminiferous tubules are lined by Sertoli cells and do not contain germ cells.

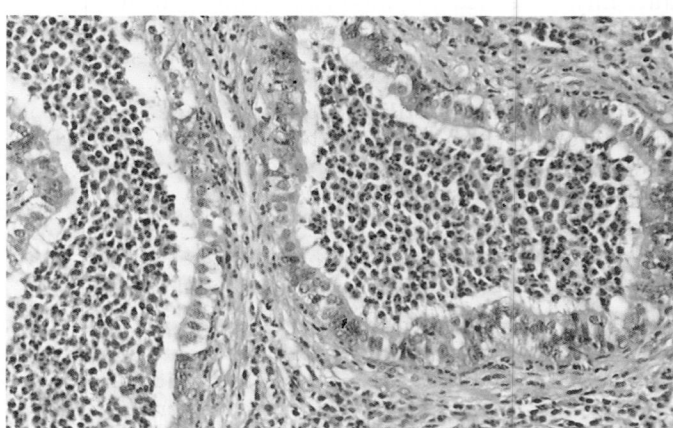

FIGURE 23-32. Bacterial epididymitis. The epididymal ducts contain numerous polymorphonuclear leukocytes.

ORCHITIS

Orchitis is acute or chronic inflammation of the testis. It may occur as part of epididymo-orchitis, usually caused by ascending infection, or as isolated testicular inflammation. The latter is usually due to hematogenous spread of pathogens, but may be of autoimmune origin.

- **Gram-negative bacterial orchitis** is the most common form of the disease. It is often secondary to urinary tract infection and is typically associated with epididymitis. Infection may also manifest as intratesticular abscess or peritesticular suppuration and fibrosis.
- **Syphilitic orchitis** has two forms: (1) interstitial perivascular inflammation, with plasma cells, lymphocytes, and macrophages; or (2) granulomatous inflammation (gummas).
- **Mumps orchitis** occurs in 20% of men who develop mumps but is now uncommon because of widespread immunization against mumps. Viral infection is characterized by testicular pain and gonadal swelling, most often unilateral. Interstitial inflammation leads to destruction and loss of seminiferous epithelium (Fig. 23-33).
- **Granulomatous orchitis** of unknown cause is an uncommon disorder of middle-aged men that presents acutely as painful testicular enlargement or insidiously as induration. It shows noncaseating granulomas but with neither organisms nor sperm remnants that might act as inciting agents. Variable numbers of seminiferous tubules become destroyed by the inflammatory process, which is considered to be a type IV (cell-mediated) hypersensitivity reaction.
- **Malakoplakia** of the testis has the same microscopic features and presumably the same histogenesis as malakoplakia elsewhere. It is typically related to *E. coli* infection.

TUMORS OF THE TESTIS

Tumors of the testis account for less than 1% of all cancers in men. More than 90% of these tumors are characterized by:

- Diagnosis between 25 and 45 years of age
- Neoplasms of germ cell origin
- Neoplasms of sex cord stromal origin

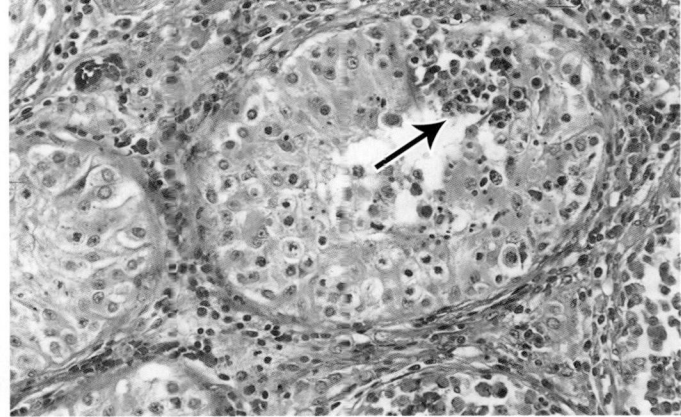

FIGURE 23-33. Viral orchitis. The interstitial spaces are infiltrated with mononuclear cells that spill focally into the lumen of seminiferous tubules (*arrow*). Note that the inflammation has interrupted normal spermatogenesis and seminiferous tubules do not contain sperm.

- Curable by a combination of surgery and chemotherapy
- Cytogenetic marker, namely, isochromosome p12
- Metastasis first to periaortic abdominal lymph nodes

The two major groups of invasive testicular germ cell tumors are seminoma and nonseminomatous tumors. The nonseminomatous tumors include embryonal carcinoma, yolk sac tumor, choriocarcinoma, and teratoma.

MOLECULAR PATHOGENESIS: The etiology of these tumors is not known. However, intrinsic and environmental factors may predispose to developing testicular germ cell tumors.

There is a geographic variation in the incidence of testicular cancer. The highest incidence occurs in Denmark, Sweden, and Norway, but it is low in Finland and southern European countries. Testicular tumors are five times more common among Americans of European descent than in those of African origin. Unlike prostatic adenocarcinoma, this incidence pattern does not change with migration. Familial testicular cancers have been documented but are rare.

The majority of postpubertal testicular germ cell tumors show full or partial gains in short arm of chromosome 12 (12p). Up to 80% of germ cell tumors show isochromosome 12p mutation i(12p), which consists of simultaneous loss of 12q and gain of 12p. Other known risk factors are disorders of gonadal development, such as **cryptorchidism, androgen insensitivity syndrome, intersex syndromes, gonadal dysgenesis, and previous history of germ cell tumor**. In these conditions, intrinsic and/or environmental factors are believed to delay or block maturation of primordial germ cells or gonocytes which causes infertility and promotes development of germ cell tumors. Primordial germ cells show similar gene expression profile to malignant germ cells and are morphologically similar to seminoma cells. Embryonic carcinoma cells also share significant similarities with human embryonic stem cells.

These suboptimally differentiated germ cells later develop into precursor lesions of testicular germ cell tumors and are called **germ cell neoplasia in situ (GCNIS)**, which consists of undifferentiated malignant germ cells confined to seminiferous tubules. GCNIS is seen in 2% to 4% of patients with cryptorchidism. Similar to invasive germ cell tumors, GCNIS is also associated with i(12p). GCNIS may also evolve into intermediate precursor lesions which are intratubular forms of seminoma or embryonal carcinoma before invasive disease is established. Seminoma and embryonal carcinoma contain primitive pluripotent stem cells that can differentiate into somatic tissue or extraembryonic tissue forming mixed germ cell tumors, teratomas, yolk sac tumors, or choriocarcinomas (Fig. 23-34).

GCNIS is not found in testes harboring spermatocytic tumors (spermatocytic seminoma), teratomas of prepubertal testes, or yolk sac tumors of infancy. Rather, it is thought that these neoplasms develop directly from altered germ cells without an in situ phase. It is possible that some migratory primordial germ cells may not find their way into the seminiferous tubules during fetal testicular organogenesis and become progenitors of yolk sac tumors and teratomas. Such "misplaced" cells may also give rise to midline extragonadal germ cell tumors in the retroperitoneum, sacral region, anterior mediastinum, and area of the pineal gland.

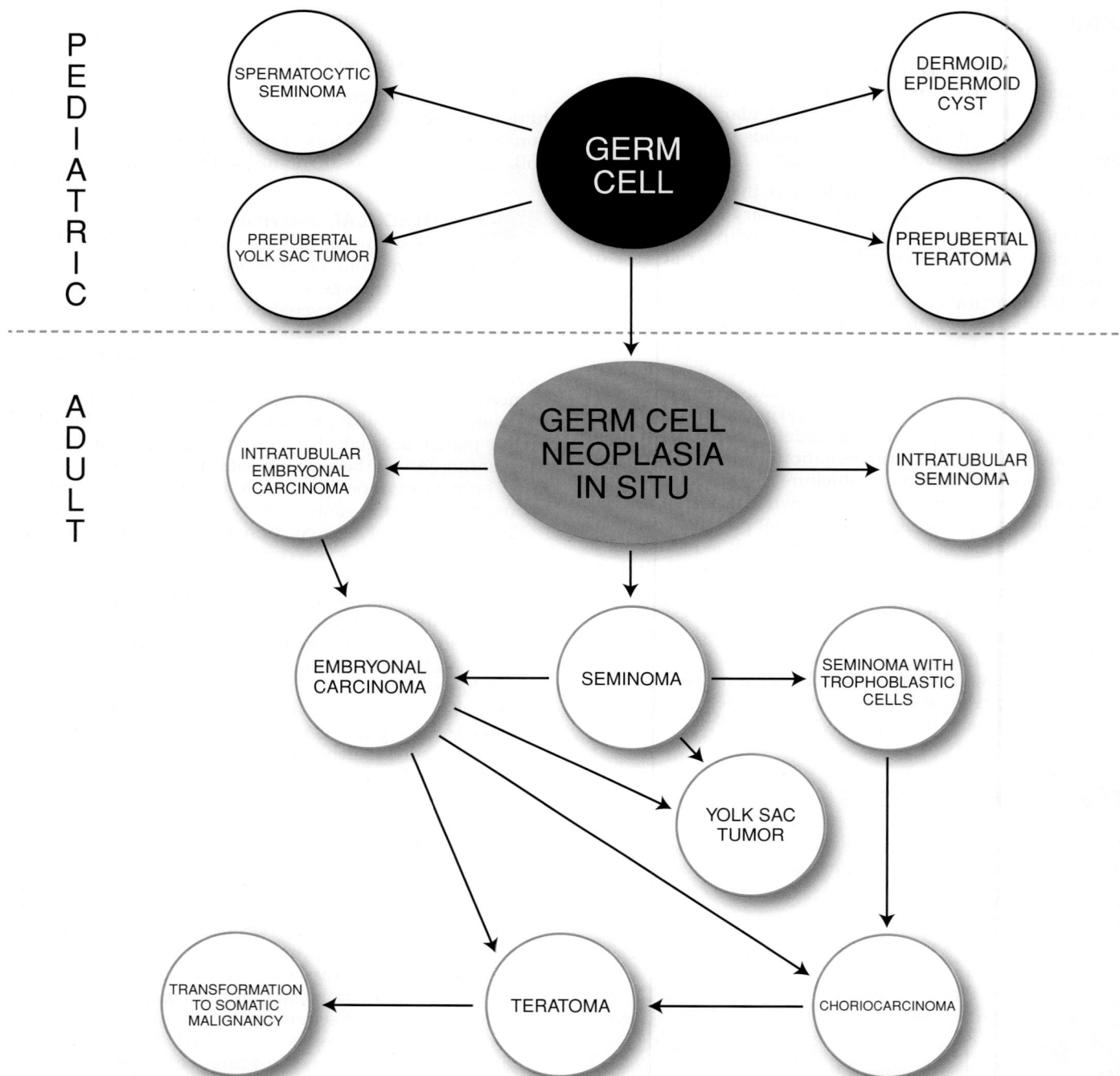

FIGURE 23-34. Testicular germ cell neoplasia pathways. Pediatric tumors and spermatocytic tumor are derived from germ cells and are not associated with germ cell neoplasia in situ. Germ cell tumors of adult testes can be classified as seminomas (40%) or nonseminomatous germ cell tumors (NSGCTs) (35%) and are preceded by a carcinoma in situ stage known as germ cell neoplasia in situ (GCNIS). Seminoma and embryonal carcinoma can give rise to a variety of other germ cell tumors. In 15% of cases, seminomatous elements are intermixed with NSGCT, forming mixed germ cell tumors of the testis, epididymis, and related structures. Tumors originating from sex cord stromal cells (Leydig and Sertoli cell tumors) account for 5% of testicular tumors. Epididymal tumors, tumors of the mesothelial lining of the tunica vaginalis (adenomatoid tumors) and metastases are rare.

TABLE 23-7
TESTICULAR TUMORS

Germ Cell Tumors—90%

Seminoma (40–50%)

Nonseminomatous germ cell tumors (NSGCTs)
Embryonal carcinoma (5%)
Choriocarcinoma (<1%)

Mixed germ cell tumors (30–50%)

Teratoma (1%)

Spermatocytic tumor (1%)

Yolk sac tumor of infancy (2%)

Sex Cord Cell Tumors—5%

Leydig cell tumors (60%)

Sertoli cell tumors (40%)

Metastases—2%

Other Rare Tumors—3%

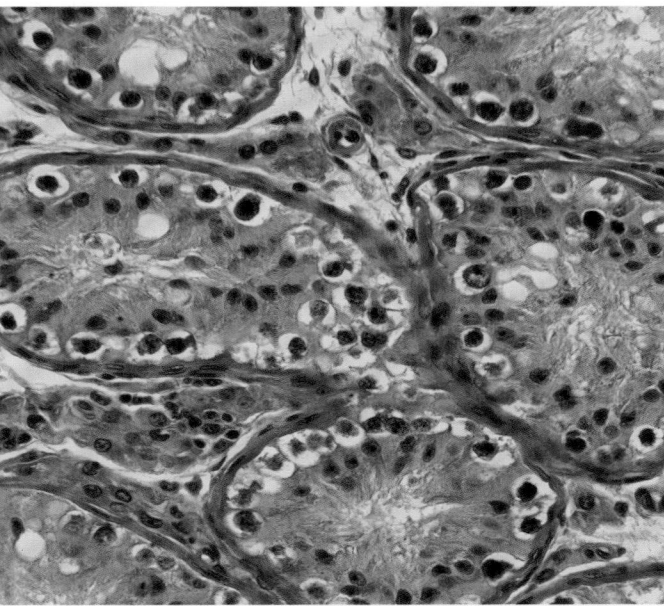

FIGURE 23-35. Germ cell neoplasia in situ (GCNIS). Seminiferous tubules show no evidence of spermatogenesis but instead contain large atypical cells indicating germ cell neoplasia in situ.

 PATHOLOGY: Testicular tumors are classified histogenetically on the basis of their cell of origin into several groups (Table 23-7).

Germ Cell Neoplasia In Situ Is Testicular Carcinoma In Situ

GCNIS represents a preinvasive form of germ cell tumors.

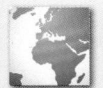 **EPIDEMIOLOGY:** GCNIS can be seen as (1) an isolated focal histologic change in 2% of cryptorchid testes or testicular biopsies performed for infertility, (2) widespread carcinoma in situ adjacent to almost all invasive germ cell tumors, and (3) lesions in 5% of contralateral testes in patients who undergo orchiectomy for a testicular germ cell tumor.

 PATHOLOGY: GCNIS occurs in a patchy distribution, usually affecting less than 10% to 30% of tubules. Seminiferous tubules harboring this lesion have thick basement membranes and contain no sperm. Normal germ cells are replaced by neoplastic ones that are broadly attached to the basal lamina (Fig. 23-35). Tumor cells of GCNIS resemble spermatogonia or fetal germ cells but are much larger and have central, polyploid nuclei with finely dispersed chromatin and prominent nucleoli. Their cytoplasm is abundant and its clear appearance reflects the presence of considerable glycogen. Nuclear DNA content is increased, consistent with the cells being triploid. Plasma membranes are distinct. Like fetal germ cells, these cells express placental-like alkaline phosphatase (PLAP) and CD117 on their surface and OCT3/4 in their nuclei. The transcription factor OCT3/4 is a reliable marker for nuclei of GCNIS cells.

 CLINICAL FEATURES: GCNIS is a precursor of invasive carcinoma, but the invasive tumor develops at an unpredictable pace. Half of men with GCNIS develop invasive cancer within 5 years and 70% in 7 years. In infertile men with a history of cryptorchid testes, GCNIS can persist unchanged for 5 to 10 years, after which the neoplastic cells acquire invasive properties, penetrate tubular basement membranes, and give rise to infiltrating malignant tumors. Diagnosis of GCNIS on testicular biopsy is an indication for prophylactic orchiectomy.

Seminomas Contain Monomorphous Cells That Resemble Spermatogonia

 EPIDEMIOLOGY: Seminomas are the most common testicular cancer, making up 40% of all germ cell tumors. Peak incidence is 30 to 40 years. They are not found before prepuberty, except in those who have dysgenetic gonads.

 PATHOLOGY: Seminomas are solid, firm, rubbery, bosselated masses that are usually sharply demarcated from normal tissue, which may become compressed, atrophic, and fibrotic. On cross section, the tumors look lobulated and homogeneous tan or grayish yellow (Fig. 23-36). Areas of necrosis or hemorrhage are infrequent but may be seen in larger tumors.

Seminomas resemble **ovarian dysgerminoma** (see Chapter 24) microscopically. They feature a single population of uniform polygonal cells with central vesicular nuclei. Their ample cytoplasm may be pale and eosinophilic or clear, since it has considerable glycogen and

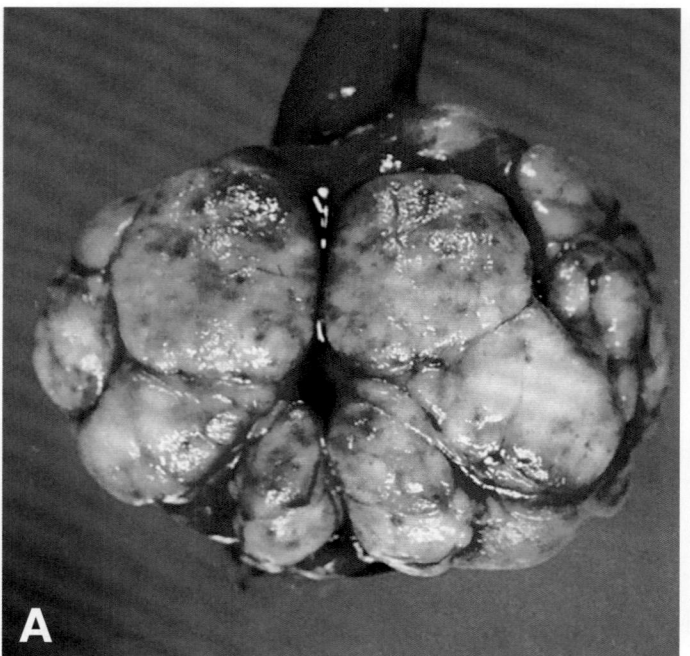

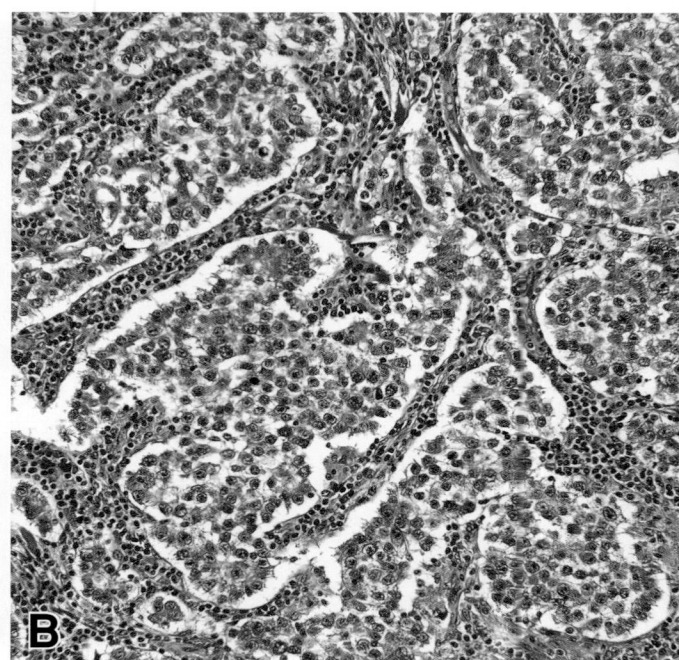

FIGURE 23-36. Seminoma. A. The cut surface of this nodular tumor is tan and bulging, reflecting the fact that the tumor is firm and rubbery. **B.** Groups of tumor cells are surrounded by fibrous septa infiltrated with lymphocytes. Tumor cells have vesicular nuclei, which are much larger than the small round nuclei of the lymphocytes.

some lipid. Cells grow in nests or sheets separated by fibrous septa infiltrated with lymphocytes, plasma cells, and macrophages. Septa may contain granulomas with giant cells. Tumor cells invade the testicular parenchyma and spread through seminiferous tubules into rete testis. The epididymis is involved later in the disease, usually before spread to abdominal lymph nodes.

Seminoma cells resemble immature spermatogonia. Like fetal spermatogonia and primordial germ cells in the fetus, they express PLAP on the plasma membrane. Seminoma cells also react with antibodies to c-Kit (CD117) and OCT3/4, which are reliable markers for this tumor.

Two subtypes of seminoma are defined pathologically: (1) **seminoma with syncytiotrophoblastic giant cells** and (2) **anaplastic seminoma**. The first subtype includes the 20% of tumors that contain syncytiotrophoblastic cells. These multinucleated giant cells are best demonstrated with antibodies to human chorionic gonadotropin (hCG). Although they secrete hCG, blood hCG levels are usually below detectable limits. Some 5% of seminomas show brisk mitotic activity and nuclear pleomorphism and are classified as **anaplastic seminoma**. Despite the distinct pathologic differences, however, there are no significant clinical differences between classical seminomas and these two microscopic tumor variants.

CLINICAL FEATURES: Seminomas are usually progressively growing scrotal masses. They are often diagnosed while still curable by orchiectomy, with or without abdominal lymph node dissection. They are highly radiosensitive, and radiotherapy is important in treating tumors not cured by surgery alone. In advanced stages of dissemination, chemotherapy can

be curative. *The cure rate for all histologic subtypes of seminoma is now better than 90%.*

Spermatocytic tumor, previously known as spermatocytic seminoma, is a rare tumor, which, despite its original name, is unrelated to classical seminoma. These are benign tumors of men over age 40. They are not associated with GCNIS and do not elicit lymphocytic reactions. Spermatocytic tumors contain three cell types described as large, small, and intermediate cells. These cells do not express typical seminoma markers. Orchiectomy is curative.

Nonseminomatous Germ Cell Tumors May Be Derived From GCNIS, Embryonal Cells, or Seminoma

Nonseminomatous germ cell tumors (NSGCTs) of the testis include several entities, two of which account for most of the cases: (1) pure embryonal carcinoma and (2) **mixed germ cell tumor** in which any combination of more than one germ cell tumor type is seen in a mass. Therefore, any combination of seminoma, teratoma, embryonal carcinoma, yolk sac tumor, and choriocarcinoma may be seen. In fact, up to one-third of testicular germ cell tumors have both seminoma and nonseminomatous elements. These tumors are treated clinically as nonseminomatous neoplasms even if they contain a component of seminoma. The other NSGCTs, **pure choriocarcinoma** and **pure yolk sac carcinoma of the adult testis**, are rare.

EPIDEMIOLOGY: NSGCTs constitute 55% of all testicular germ cell tumors. All other tumors of this group are extremely rare. Like seminomas, NSGCTs have a peak incidence in the third to fourth decades. At diagnosis, these patients are usually somewhat younger than those with seminomas.

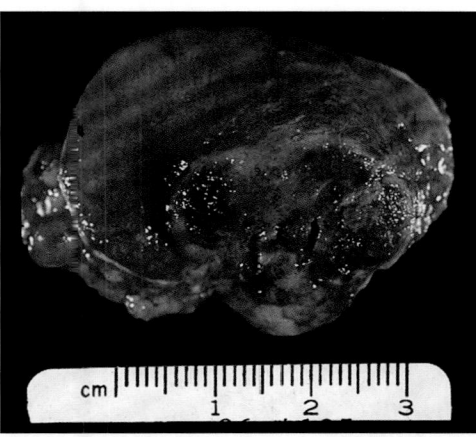

FIGURE 23-37. Nonseminomatous germ cell tumor (NSGCT) of the testis. The cut surface of this 1.5 cm testicular tumor shows considerable heterogeneity, varying in color from white to dark red.

PATHOLOGY: NSGCTs vary in size and shape. They may be solid or partially cystic. Solid areas vary from white to yellow to red, indicating that they are composed of viable tumor cells, foci of necrosis, and hemorrhage, respectively (Fig. 23-37).

The histology of NSGCTs is highly variable. Pure embryonal carcinomas contain exclusively undifferentiated embryonal carcinoma cells similar to those seen in preimplantation-stage embryos (Fig. 23-38). Because the tumor cells have little cytoplasm, their hyperchromatic, disproportionately large nuclei seem to overlap. Embryonal carcinoma cells may grow as broad solid sheets, cords, gland-like tubules and acini, and sometimes even line papillary structures. Mitoses and apoptotic cells are

common. Embryonal carcinomas invade the testis, epididymis, and blood vessels and metastasize to abdominal lymph nodes, lungs, and other organs. Embryonal carcinomas, like seminomas, react with antibodies to PLAP and OCT3/4. Unlike seminomas and other tumors, they express cytokeratins and CD30, but not c-KIT (CD117).

In other cases, embryonal carcinoma cells differentiate into the three embryonic germ layers (ectoderm, mesoderm, and endoderm) with formation of somatic tissue elements of adult (mature) or fetal (immature) development (Figs. 23-39 and 23-40). These tumors are called **teratomas**. Ectoderm differentiates into skin, central nervous system, retinal pigment cells, and other related tissues. Mesoderm gives rise to smooth and striated muscle, cartilage, and bone. Endoderm forms intestinal tissue, bronchial epithelium, salivary glands, and so forth. Teratomas may contain variable proportions of different tissues derived from these three germ cell layers (Figs. 23-39A and 23-40). Immature and mature elements are frequently encountered together. **Epidermoid cysts** and **dermoid cysts** are subtypes of teratomas in which only ectodermal elements are present with no evidence of other germ cell tumors, GCNIS, or immature somatic tissue. Epidermoid cysts are lined by keratinized squamous epithelium, and dermoid cysts are lined by keratinized squamous epithelium and contain pilosebaceous units. **Malignant teratomas** may develop if any of the somatic elements undergo malignant transformation, in which case they may give rise to squamous cell carcinomas, adenocarcinomas, or sarcomas.

Extraembryonic derivatives of embryonal carcinoma cells give rise to chorionic epithelium (cytotrophoblast and syncytiotrophoblast) and yolk sac–like epithelium. These complex tumors are composed of undifferentiated malignant embryonal cells and their somatic and extraembryonic derivatives are **teratocarcinomas** or **malignant teratomas**. Tumors that contain highly malignant cytotrophoblast and syncytiotrophoblast, have overgrown other elements, and are composed of a single tumor type are classified as **choriocarcinomas** (Fig. 23-39A,C). Likewise, clones of malignant yolk sac epithelium produce **yolk sac carcinoma** (Fig. 23-39B). Yolk sac tumors are composed of cells arranged into structures reminiscent of parts of fetal yolk sac. Diagnosis is based on recognizing multiple microscopic tumor patterns and glomeruloid **Schiller–Duval bodies** (Fig. 23-41). These neonatal tumors resemble those of the yolk sac elements in NSGCTs. Unlike seminomas, NSGCTs often contain yolk sac and syncytiotrophoblastic components.

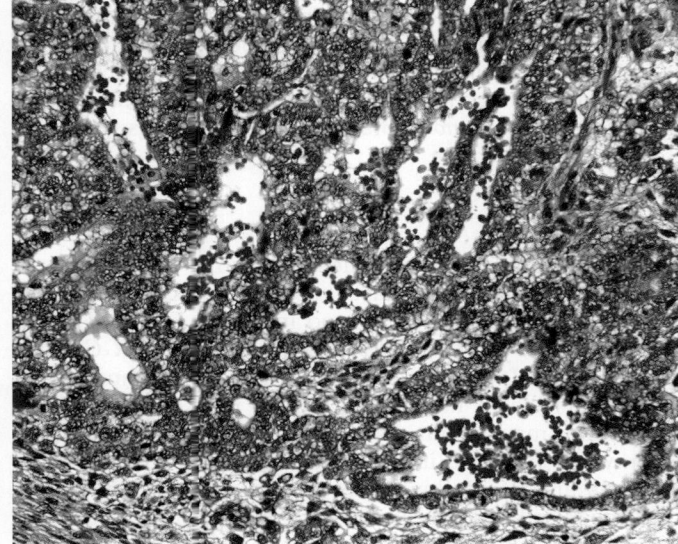

FIGURE 23-38. Embryonal carcinoma component of a nonseminomatous germ cell tumor (NSGCT). Because these undifferentiated cells have scant cytoplasm, their hyperchromatic nuclei impart a bluish color to stained sections. The nuclei appear crowded and seem to overlap each other. The cells form cords and sheets surrounding dilated vascular channels filled with red blood cells.

CLINICAL FEATURES: Most NSGCTs present as testicular masses. They tend to grow faster than seminomas and metastasize more readily and more widely. Hence, for some NSGCTs, metastases may be the first clinically apparent sign of the neoplasm.

Testicular Tumors Are Rare in Prepubertal Boys

TERATOMAS: In the first 4 years of life, most testicular neoplasms are yolk sac tumors, occurring mainly in boys under 2 years. Benign teratomas are the most common testicular tumor between ages 4 and 12 years. Pure teratomas

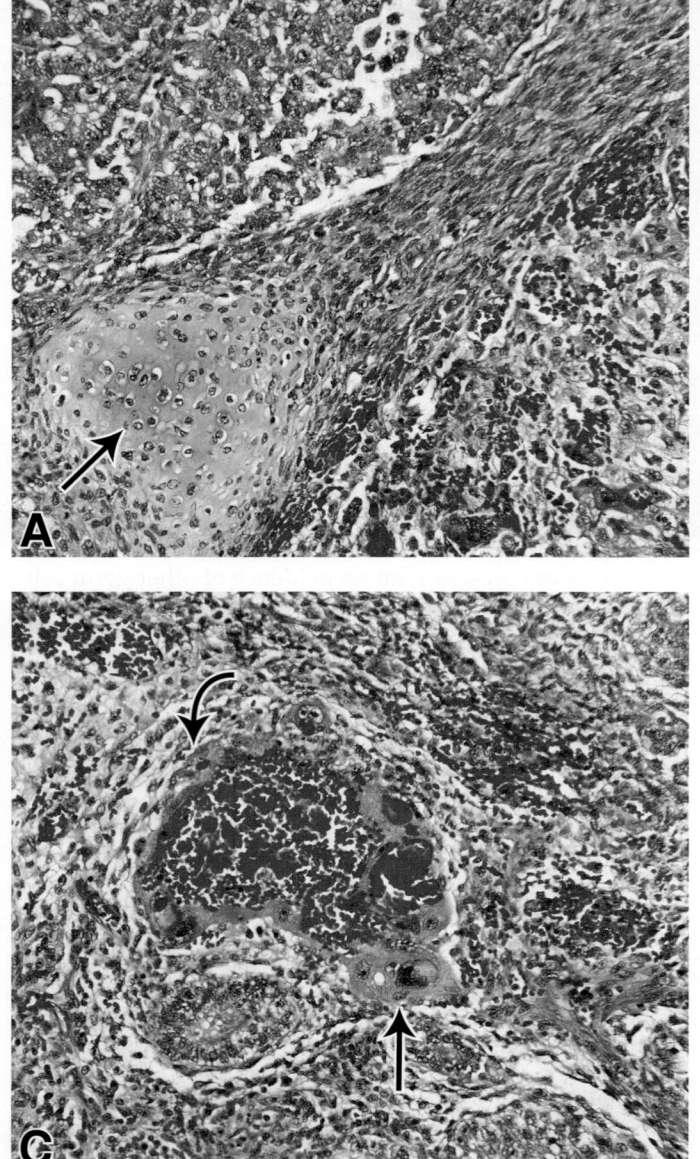

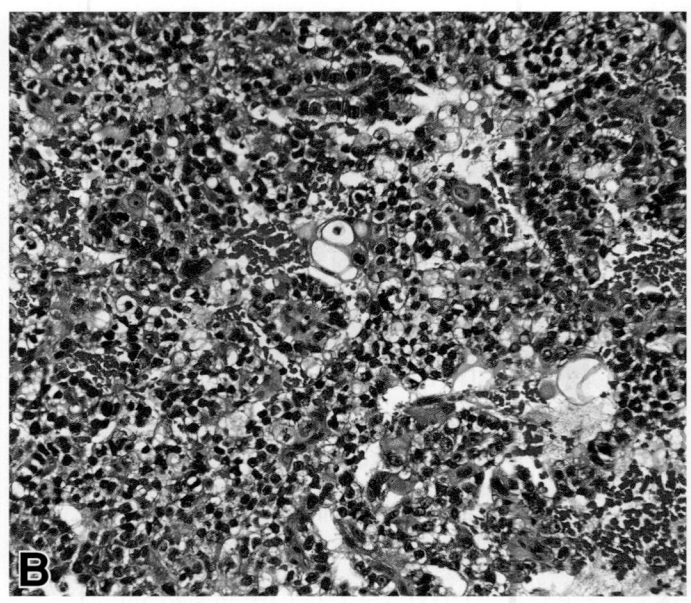

FIGURE 23-39. Nonseminomatous germ cell tumor (NSGCT).
A. Somatic tissue of this tumor includes well-differentiated cartilage (*arrow*) and nondescript connective tissue separating the embryonal carcinoma (**upper left corner**) from the hemorrhagic choriocarcinoma (**right lower corner**). **B.** Yolk sac component consists of interlacing cords of epithelial cells surrounded by loose stroma resembling the early yolk sac. **C.** Choriocarcinoma component of the NSGCT consists of multinucleated syncytiotrophoblastic giant cells (*straight arrow*) and mononuclear cytotrophoblastic cells (*curved arrow*). Invasive growth of trophoblasts is usually associated with hemorrhage.

comprise about one-third of testicular germ cell tumors in children, and, in this clinical setting, tend to have a benign clinical course. Orchiectomy and even testis-sparing surgery are curative.

By contrast, pure teratomas represent less than 5% of testicular germ cell tumors in postpubertal patients and may metastasize even in the absence of immature elements. That is, histologically benign teratomas of postpubertal young men may exhibit a malignant clinical course, even though they appear to contain only mature somatic tissues, without embryonal elements (Fig. 23-40). Therefore, unlike ovarian teratoma, there is no clinical significance in distinguishing mature versus immature testicular teratomas in postpubertal males.

YOLK SAC TUMORS: Yolk sac cells secrete α-fetoprotein (AFP), a fetal protein not normally found in the blood. Yolk sac tumors of infancy and early childhood are considered

malignant, but timely orchiectomy cures over 95% of patients. Syncytiotrophoblast cells release hCG, a hormone of pregnancy not typically found in males. *Elevated serum AFP or hCG is found in 70% of patients with NSGCTs and is thus a useful tumor marker.* Serum AFP, hCG, and lactate dehydrogenase (a nonspecific tumor marker that reflects total tumor mass) are measured in all patients before orchiectomy and included in clinical staging of the tumor. These antigens are also followed in postoperative patients who have been treated for NSGCT. Persistently elevated AFP and/or hCG indicates persistent tumor. If initially high levels of AFP and hCG normalize after treatment but later rise, metastatic spread is likely. AFP is a relatively insensitive marker of recurrence as elevated serum AFP is found only in 70% of patients with recurrent cancer.

Treatment of NSGCT includes orchiectomy to remove the primary tumor, followed by platinum-based chemotherapy

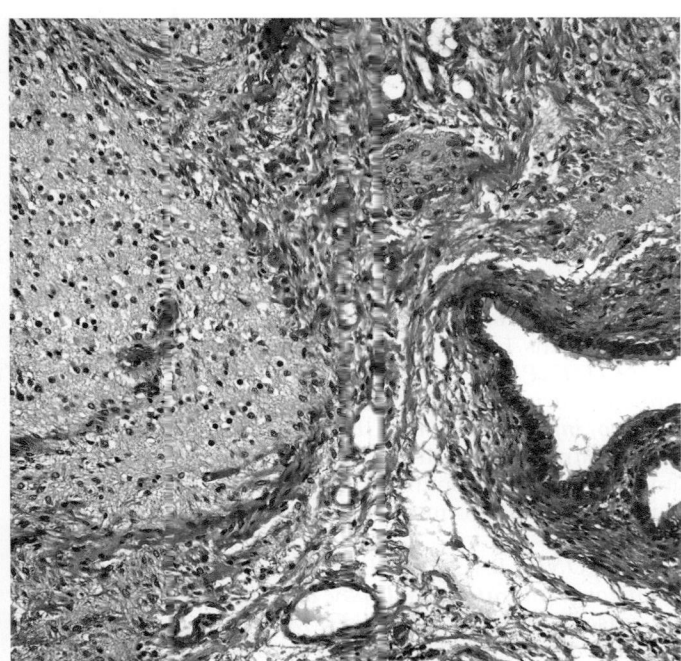

FIGURE 23-40. Teratoma. The tumor consists of neural tissue (**left**), connective tissue smooth muscle cells (**midportion**) and glands lined by columnar epithelium (**right side of the picture**).

and, if indicated, surgical dissection of abdominal lymph nodes. Chemotherapy usually eliminates metastatic embryonal carcinoma cells, but differentiated tissues originating from them are resistant, particularly teratoma which may progress (growing teratoma syndrome). Such tissues do not grow and are not likely to endanger the patient. Nevertheless, it is better to eliminate residual tumor rather than take a

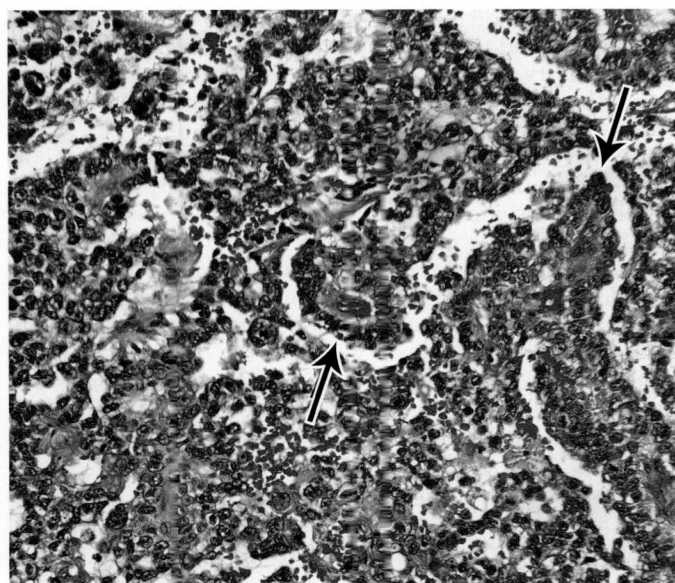

FIGURE 23-41. Yolk sac tumor. This childhood tumor is composed of interlacing strands of epithelial cells surrounded by loose connective stroma. Glomeruloid structures (Schiller–Duval bodies) are marked by *arrows*.

chance that a few malignant tumor cells might be lurking in lymph nodes. *Complete cures of NSGCTs are now achieved in over 90% of cases.*

Gonadal Stromal/Sex Cord Tumors Are Composed of Cells That Resemble Sertoli or Leydig Cells

Gonadal stromal/sex cord tumors make up 5% of testicular tumors.

LEYDIG CELL TUMORS: These rare neoplasms are composed of cells resembling interstitial (Leydig) cells of the testis. They can secrete androgens, estrogens, or both. Leydig cell tumors occur at any age, with distinct peaks in childhood and then in adults from the third to the sixth decade.

PATHOLOGY: Leydig cell tumors vary from 1 to 10 cm and are circumscribed; some appear encapsulated. The cut surface is yellow to brown, and larger tumors have fibrous trabeculae, giving them a lobular appearance. Microscopically, Leydig tumor cells are uniform, with round nuclei and well-developed eosinophilic or vacuolated cytoplasm (Fig. 23-42). **Reinke crystals**—rectangular, eosinophilic, cytoplasmic inclusions—are characteristic of normal Leydig cells and are seen in 30% of tumors. Most (90%) Leydig cell tumors are benign, but it is difficult to predict their biologic behavior on histologic grounds.

CLINICAL FEATURES: Androgenic effects of testicular Leydig cell tumors in prepubertal boys lead to precocious physical and sexual development. By contrast, feminization and gynecomastia are seen in some adults with this tumor. Either estrogen or testosterone levels may be elevated, but there is no characteristic pattern. All Leydig cell tumors in children and almost all tumors in adults are cured by orchiectomy.

SERTOLI CELL TUMORS: Some testicular sex cord stromal cell tumors contain neoplastic Sertoli cells. Most (90%) are benign, however, and produce few if any hormonal symptoms.

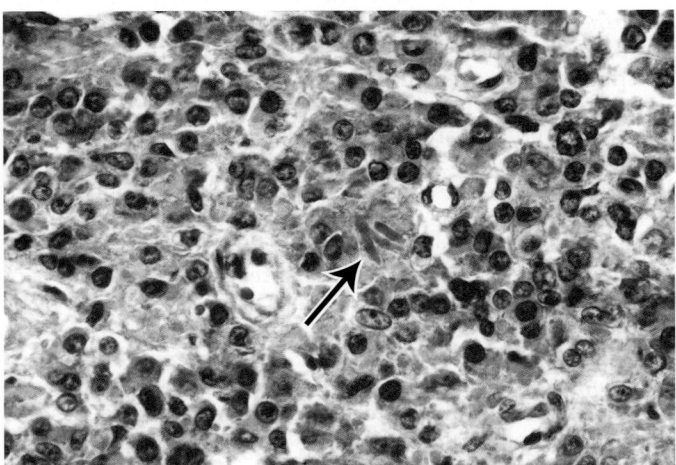

FIGURE 23-42. Leydig cell tumor. Tumor cells have uniform round nuclei and well-developed eosinophilic cytoplasm. Three cytoplasmic Reinke crystals are seen in the center of the field (*arrow*).

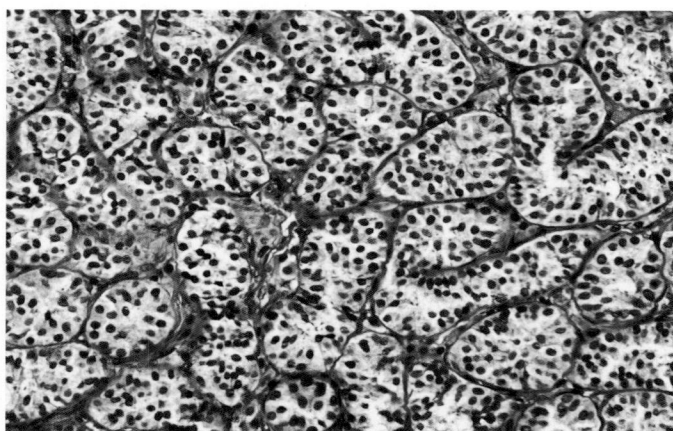

FIGURE 23-43. Sertoli cell tumor. Neoplastic cells are arranged in tubules surrounded by a basement membrane. These structures are reminiscent of seminiferous tubules devoid of germ cells.

PATHOLOGY: Sertoli cell tumors are small (1 to 3 cm), solid, yellow-gray, well-circumscribed nodules. They contain columnar tumor cells arranged into tubules or cords in a fibrous trabecular framework (Fig. 23-43). The rare malignant variant shows greater cellular pleomorphism, focal necrosis, and few cords and tubules. Most patients with Sertoli cell tumors are younger than age 40 and come to medical attention because of a scrotal mass. Endocrine effects are uncommon and, if present, are vague. Orchiectomy is curative.

All Other Germ Cell Tumors Are Rare

Tumors may originate from the epithelium of the epididymis, connective tissue stroma, mesothelium, and tunica vaginalis testis. All these tumors are rare. Metastatic tumors, including lymphomas, are also uncommon. Together, these tumors account for less than 5% of all scrotal masses.

ADENOMATOID TUMOR: Adenomatoid tumor (benign mesothelioma) is a benign tumor that originates from the mesothelium of the testicular tunica vaginalis. These neoplasms usually occur in the upper pole of the epididymis, with fewer involving the tunica vaginalis or spermatic cord. They are well-demarcated nodules found by palpating the testis or epididymis. Microscopically, they contain mesothelial cells in cords or small duct-like structures embedded in dense fibrous stroma. Malignant mesotheliomas of tunica vaginalis testis are very rare.

METASTASES: Most of these spread from primary cancers of the prostate, large intestine, or bladder (i.e., organs that are located in the pelvis and close to the testes).

MALIGNANT LYMPHOMA: This cancer is the most common neoplasm in the testes of men older than 60 years. It may be primary in the testis. More often, it reflects seeding of lymphoma from other sites or occurs in patients with leukemia. Diffuse large B-cell lymphoma is the most common form of lymphoma involving the testis. Most patients with lymphomatous involvement of the testis have a poor prognosis.

Prostate

The pathologic processes affecting the prostate can be simplified by considering just three processes: (1) inflammation, (2) hyperplasia, and (3) neoplasia.

PROSTATITIS

Prostatitis is inflammation of the prostate. There are acute and chronic forms. Prostatitis is usually caused by coliform uropathogens, but often no etiology is found.

ACUTE PROSTATITIS: Typically a complication of other urinary tract infections, acute prostatitis results from reflux of infected urine into the prostate. An acute inflammatory infiltrate is seen in prostatic acini and stroma. It causes intense discomfort on urination and is often associated with fever, chills, and perineal pain. Most patients respond well to antibiotics.

CHRONIC BACTERIAL PROSTATITIS: This infection is of longer duration and may or may not be preceded by an episode of acute prostatitis. Most patients complain of dysuria and burning at the urethral meatus. Suprapubic, perineal and low back pain, and nocturia may be also present. The urine usually contains bacteria. In addition to reflux of urine, prostatic calculi and local prostatic duct obstruction may contribute to development of chronic bacterial prostatitis. Infiltrates of lymphocytes, plasma cells, and macrophages are the rule. Prolonged antibiotic therapy is often, but not always, curative.

NONBACTERIAL PROSTATITIS: Sometimes, no causative organism is identified in chronic prostatitis. This is the most common form of prostatitis encountered in prostatic biopsies, prostatectomy specimens, or at autopsy. Nonbacterial prostatitis typically affects men older than 50 years but can be seen at any age. Some cases may be due to *C. trachomatis, Mycoplasma,* or *U. urealyticum*. However, in practice, nonbacterial prostatitis is a diagnosis of exclusion. The most common histology shows dilated glands filled with neutrophils and foamy macrophages surrounded by chronic inflammatory cells. The condition may be asymptomatic or it may cause symptoms like those of chronic bacterial prostatitis. Specific therapy is usually not available.

GRANULOMATOUS PROSTATITIS: In most cases, the cause of granulomatous prostatitis cannot be established. Rarely, this disease can be traced to specific causative agents, including *M. tuberculosis,* BCG, or fungi such as *Histoplasma capsulatum.* A granulomatous lesion resembling rheumatoid nodules has been related to previous transurethral resection of a portion of the prostate. The symptoms of chronic granulomatous prostatitis are vague and the diagnosis is made histologically. Caseating or noncaseating granulomas are associated with localized destruction of prostatic ducts and acini and, in later stages, with fibrosis.

CLINICAL FEATURES: As indicated above, symptoms of chronic prostatitis are highly variable and treatment may be ineffective. Most importantly, it may cause elevated serum prostate-specific antigen (PSA), a worrisome suggestion of prostatic malignancy (see below). Thus, the diagnosis is often made by biopsy done to exclude carcinoma

NODULAR HYPERPLASIA OF THE PROSTATE

Nodular prostatic hyperplasia, also called benign prostatic hyperplasia (BPH), is a common disorder characterized clinically by obstruction of urinary outflow and pathologically by proliferation of glands and stroma.

EPIDEMIOLOGY: BPH is most common in Western Europe and the United States and least common in Asia. Its prevalence in the United States is higher among blacks than among whites. Clinical prostatism (i.e., BPH severe enough to interfere with urination) peaks in the seventh decade. However, prevalence of BPH is far greater at autopsy than is suggested by clinically apparent prostatism. In fact, 75% of men over age 80 have some degree of prostatic hyperplasia. The disorder is rare in men younger than 40 years of age.

MOLECULAR PATHOGENESIS: The earliest pathogenic events in BPH remain unclear. Testosterone is necessary for prostatic development and to maintain secretory function. The active androgen form, dihydrotestosterone (DHT), is a product of the enzyme 5α-reductase. DHT binds nuclear receptors in glandular and stromal cells and promotes growth of prostatic stromal and glandular tissues. Therefore, drugs that block 5α-reductase (e.g., finasteride or dutasteride) can reduce the size of the prostate in men with BPH. Given the key role that androgens play in prostatic growth, it is not surprising that BPH is not observed before puberty or in castrated men. Prepubertal castration prevents development of age-related BPH and completely protects against prostate cancer. Interestingly, exogenous testosterone does not induce hyperplasia and does not even stimulate atrophic glands. With aging, circulating testosterone levels decline in men with and without BPH. As well, no change in serum DHT is seen in men with BPH, although the ratio of circulating testosterone to DHT may be low.

PATHOLOGY: Early nodular hyperplasia begins in the submucosa of the proximal urethra **(the transitional zone)**. Enlarging nodules compress the centrally located urethral lumen and the more peripherally located normal prostate (Fig. 23-44). In well-developed BPH, the normal part of the gland is actually limited to an attenuated rim of tissue beneath the capsule. Individual nodules are demarcated by enveloping fibrous pseudocapsules (Fig. 23-45). Larger nodules may show focal hemorrhage or infarction. Small stones may be seen as well.

In BPH, proliferation of epithelial cells of acini and ductules, smooth muscle cells, and stromal fibroblasts is all seen in variable proportions. Typical fibromyoadenomatous nodules contain variably sized hyperplastic prostatic acini randomly scattered throughout their stroma. The epithelial (adenomatous) component contains a double layer of cells, with tall columnar cells overlying a basal layer (Fig. 23-45C) and often showing papillary hyperplasia. Chronic inflammation and corpora amylacea

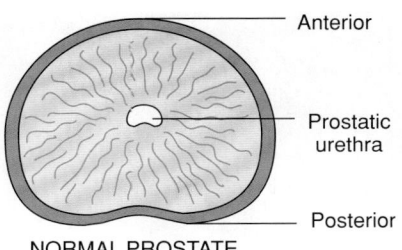

NORMAL PROSTATE

Anterior

Prostatic urethra

Posterior

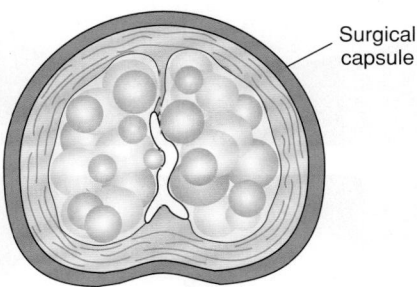

NODULAR PROSTATIC HYPERPLASIA

Surgical capsule

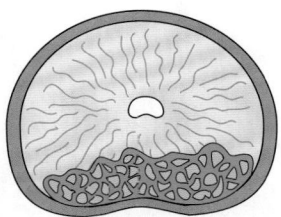

ADENOCARCINOMA OF PROSTATE

FIGURE 23-44. Normal prostate, nodular hyperplasia, and adenocarcinoma. Prostatic hyperplasia involves predominantly the periurethral part of the gland. Hyperplastic nodules compress and distort the urethra. Expansion of the central prostatic glands leads to compression of the peripheral parts and fibrosis, resulting in the formation of a so-called surgical capsule. Prostatic carcinoma usually arises from peripheral glands, and compression of the urethra is a late clinical event.

(eosinophilic laminated concretions) are frequently seen within acini. In the uninvolved peripheral region of the prostate, glands are often atrophic and compressed by the expanding nodules.

Nonspecific prostatitis is common in nodular hyperplasia. It typically consists of a dense intraglandular and periglandular infiltrate of lymphocytes, plasma cells, and macrophages, often with acute inflammatory cells and focal gland destruction. Focal infarcts of varying age are present in 20% of cases. Squamous metaplasia of ductal epithelium at the periphery of infarcts is typical.

CLINICAL FEATURES: Symptoms of nodular hyperplasia result from compression of the prostatic urethra and consequent bladder outlet obstruction (Fig. 23-46). A history of decreased vigor of the urinary stream and increasing urinary frequency is

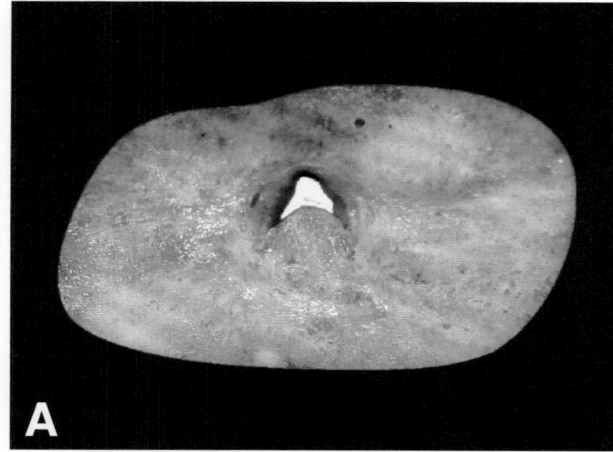

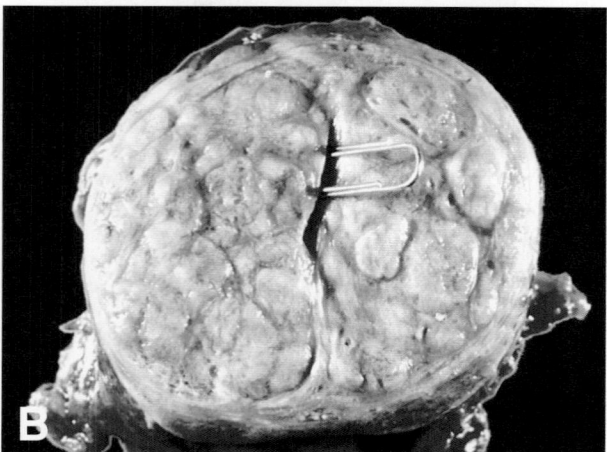

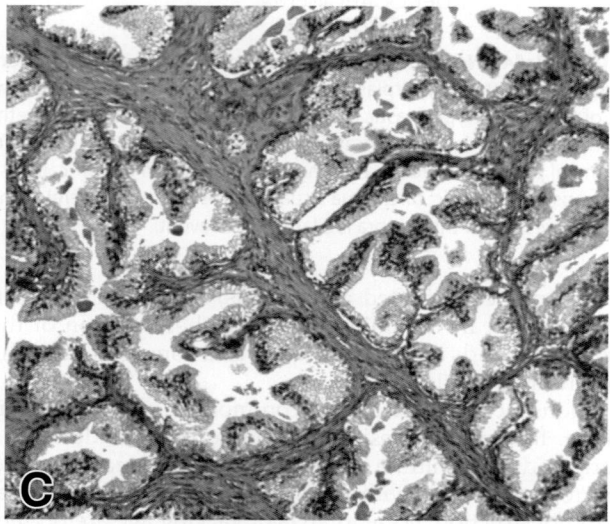

FIGURE 23-45. Nodular hyperplasia of the prostate. A. Normal prostate. **B.** The cut surface of a prostate enlarged by nodular hyperplasia shows numerous well-circumscribed nodules of prostatic tissue surrounded by pseudocapsules. The prostatic urethra (*paper clip*) has been compressed to a narrow slit. **C.** Hyperplastic prostate glands in nodular hyperplasia. The columnar epithelium lining the acini is composed of two cell layers: polarized clear cuboidal cells lining the acinar lumen and flattened basal cells interposed between the cuboidal acinar cells and the stroma. Hyperplastic cells line papillary projections protruding into the lumina of the acini.

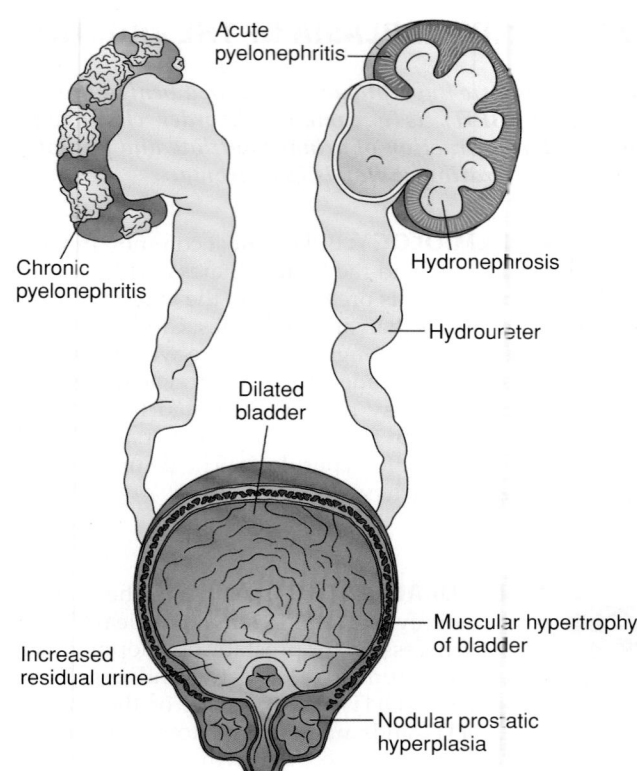

FIGURE 23-46. Complications of nodular prostatic hyperplasia.

typical. Rectal examination reveals a firm, enlarged, nodular prostate. If obstruction is severe and prolonged, back pressure can lead to hydroureter, hydronephrosis, and ultimately renal failure and death.

Treatment of BPH includes surgery or drugs that block 5α-reductase. In addition, some patients receive α$_1$-adrenergic blockers which relax smooth muscle in the prostate and bladder neck and thereby enhance urine flow. Transurethral resection, radiofrequency ablation, and cryotherapy are the interventional treatment choices. Other treatment options include surgically implanted luminal tie-backs and transurethral heating of the hyperplastic tissue.

IN SITU AND INVASIVE ADENOCARCINOMA OF THE PROSTATE

EPIDEMIOLOGY: Adenocarcinoma of the prostatic acini is the most common prostatic malignancy, and here, is simply referred to as prostatic adenocarcinoma. *In 1990, prostatic adenocarcinoma surpassed lung cancer to become the most frequently diagnosed cancer in American men.* An estimated 164,690 new cases are diagnosed yearly in the United States. About 29,430 American men die annually from it, a figure equivalent to that of colorectal carcinoma. Prostate cancer is largely a disease of elderly men: 75% of patients are 60 to 80 years of age. Autopsy studies confirm that the tumor is more common with advancing age. Prostate cancer is diagnosed at autopsy in 20% of men in their 40s, and in

70% of men over age 70. The cumulative lifetime probability of being diagnosed with latent or symptomatic prostatic carcinoma is one in six for American men. There is considerable variation in age-related death rates for adenocarcinoma of the prostate throughout the world, the highest being in the United States and Scandinavian countries where the incidence of prostate cancer is high, and the lowest in Mexico, Greece, and Japan where the incidence is less frequent. Most western European countries have intermediate rates. Also, American blacks, have the highest prostate carcinoma–related death rates in the world—twice as high as that of white Americans. Ethnic genetic factors likely may play a role in pathogenesis, but environmental factors and disparities in access to health care also impact risk. In the United States, descendants of Polish and Japanese immigrants have a higher incidence of prostatic carcinoma than men in their original countries. Similarly, mortality from prostatic carcinoma among black American men exceeds that of blacks in Africa.

In addition to geographic, racial, and age differences, hereditary factors and possibly diet (red meat, animal fat) affect prostate cancer risk. One-tenth of cases have familial tendencies, and the risk is significantly increased in men with first-degree relatives with prostate cancer. Dietary fat may increase the risk of prostate cancer, but mechanisms underlying possible environmental or dietary factors have not been defined.

The clinical course of prostate cancer is often capricious. Some tumors are amenable to therapy, while others are not. Many prostate cancers are so indolent (or latent) that they may never become clinically significant during the patient's lifetime. For this reason, the value of screening for prostate cancer using blood PSA levels remains controversial.

MOLECULAR PATHOGENESIS: The pathogenesis of prostate adenocarcinoma is complex and multiple factors, including hereditary, environmental, hormonal, and genetic, have been implicated. Androgenic control of normal prostatic growth and the responsiveness of prostate cancer to castration and exogenous estrogens indicate a role for male hormones. However, patients with prostate cancer do not typically have higher levels of circulating androgens. In fact, elevated urinary estrone-to-testosterone ratios have been reported. The gene encoding AR shows considerable variation in CAG repeats in exon 1. Men with fewer CAG repeats are at greater risk for developing prostate cancer although the underlying mechanism is not well understood. Some tumors show somatic mutations that place the transcription factor gene *ETV1* under the control of the androgen-regulated *TMPRSS2* promoter. Other cases show hypermethylation of the gene for the antioxidant enzyme glutathione S-transferase. Altered regulation of STAT transcription factors and dysregulation of the *PTEN* tumor suppressor have been documented. Mutations in *BRCA1* and *BRCA2*, known to increase risk of breast and ovarian cancer in women, have also been implicated in prostate cancer risk in men.

Intraductal dysplastic epithelial proliferation, termed **prostatic intraepithelial neoplasia (PIN),** is now considered

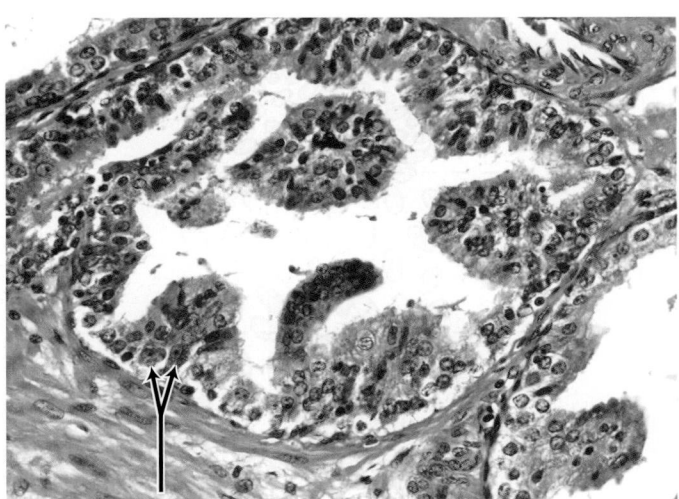

FIGURE 23-47. High-grade prostatic intraepithelial neoplasia (HGPIN). The large duct in the center is lined by atypical cells with enlarged nuclei and prominent nucleoli (*arrows*).

to be a precursor lesion of prostatic adenocarcinoma. *PIN describes prostatic ducts lined by cytologically atypical luminal cells and a concomitant decrease in basal cells.* Nuclei of high-grade PIN are enlarged and show nucleoli and marked crowding (Fig. 23-47). Substantial data indicate that PIN lesions are premalignant and progress to adenocarcinoma. High-grade PIN may precede invasive cancer within two decades.

Considerable morphologic evidence links PIN to invasive prostate cancer. Both lesions arise in a mainly peripheral distribution in the prostate. Cytologically, high-grade PIN closely resembles invasive cancer, and there is close topographic proximity of high-grade PIN to invasive cancer. Finally, PIN lesions are more frequent in prostates with cancer than in those without tumors. Both high-grade PIN and invasive cancers show aneuploidy and express similar biochemical markers such as TGFα and type IV collagenase, and genetic markers such as *bcl-2* and *c-erb-b2* oncogenes). Recognition of high-grade PIN on needle biopsy is important because many patients with high-grade PIN on initial biopsy have invasive carcinoma on follow-up biopsy.

PATHOLOGY: Adenocarcinomas account for the vast majority of all primary prostatic tumors. They are commonly multicentric in distribution and located in the peripheral zones in over 70% of cases. The cut surface of a carcinomatous prostate may show vague irregular, yellow-white lesions, but the majority of cases show no distinctive macroscopic findings and are therefore difficult to detect on gross examination.

HISTOLOGIC FEATURES OF INVASIVE CARCINOMA: Most prostatic adenocarcinomas are of acinar origin and feature small- to medium-sized glands that lack basal cells, are poorly circumscribed, and infiltrate the stroma. Normal prostatic glands contain basal cells, but malignant glands have no basal cells and no longer grow in a lobular pattern. Well-differentiated tumors

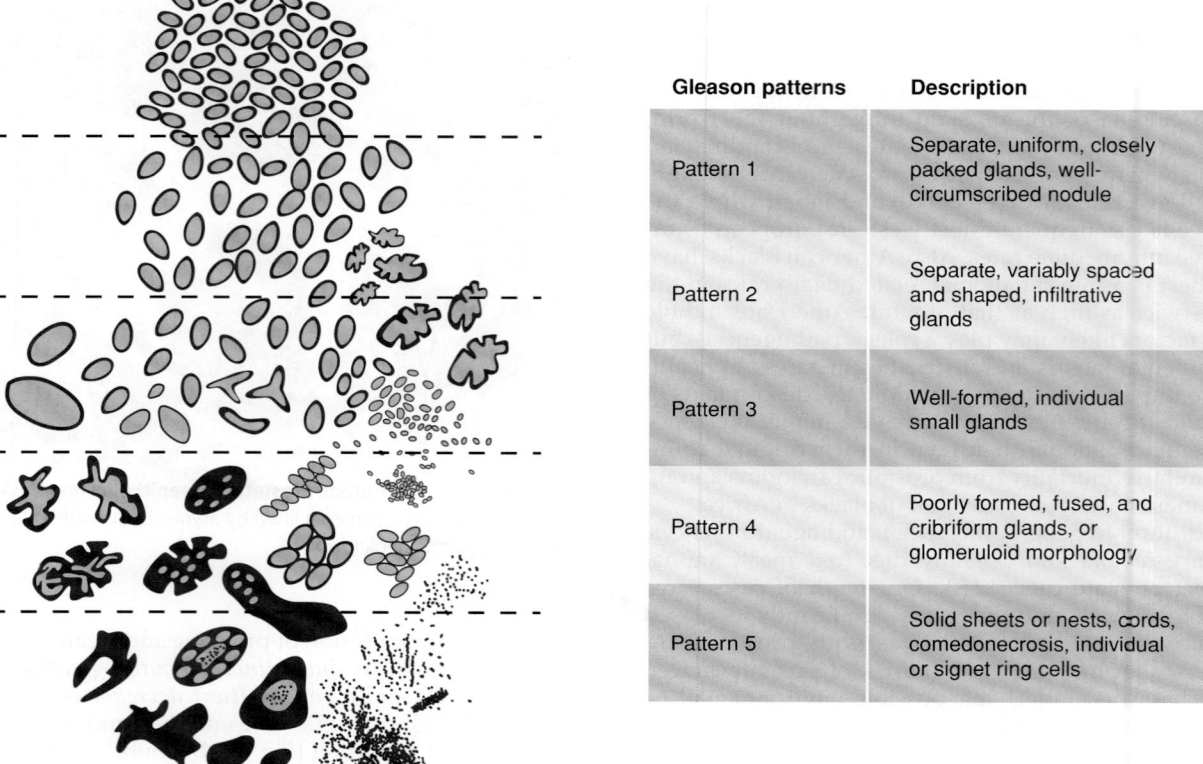

Gleason patterns	Description
Pattern 1	Separate, uniform, closely packed glands, well-circumscribed nodule
Pattern 2	Separate, variably spaced and shaped, infiltrative glands
Pattern 3	Well-formed, individual small glands
Pattern 4	Poorly formed, fused, and cribriform glands, or glomeruloid morphology
Pattern 5	Solid sheets or nests, cords, comedonecrosis, individual or signet ring cells

FIGURE 23-48. Updated Gleason grading system depicting patterns 1 to 5.

show uniform medium-sized or small glands lined by a single layer of neoplastic epithelial cells (Fig. 23-48). Immunohistochemistry using antibodies detecting **high–molecular-weight cytokeratin** and **p63** for basal cells will show no staining in malignant glands due to the absence of basal cells, and positive staining in benign glands (Fig. 23-49A). Also, unlike benign glands, premalignant HGPIN and prostatic adenocarcinoma express **alpha-methylacyl-coenzyme A racemase (AMACR)** as demonstrated by immunohistochemical staining (Fig. 23-49B). The presence or absence of basal cells and AMACR is particularly useful in diagnosing prostate cancer in challenging prostate biopsies.

Progressive loss of differentiation of prostatic adenocarcinomas is characterized by:

- Increasing variability of gland size and configuration.
- Papillary and cribriform patterns.
- Rudimentary (or no) gland formation, with only solid cords of infiltrating tumor cells. Uncommonly, a prostate cancer may be composed of small undifferentiated cells growing individually or in sheets, without evidence of any structural organization.

CYTOLOGIC FEATURES: The presence of pleomorphic and hyperchromatic nuclei is highly variable. One or two conspicuous nucleoli in a background of chromatin clumped near the nuclear membrane is the most frequent nuclear feature. The cytoplasm stains slightly eosinophilic or may be so vacuolated that it simulates clear cells of renal cell carcinoma. Cell borders are distinct in

better-differentiated tumors but are not well demarcated in poorly differentiated ones.

GRADING: Prostatic adenocarcinoma is most commonly classified according to its histologic grade using the **Gleason grading system** (Figs. 23-48 and 23-50), which is based on five histologic patterns of tumor gland formation and infiltration. The most well-differentiated tumors containing well-formed glands are assigned Gleason patterns 1 and 2. However, these are rare and difficult to differentiate from benign glands. The most commonly diagnosed Gleason pattern is 3, which consists of smaller, separate, infiltrating malignant glands (Fig. 23-50A). As tumors become less differentiated, higher Gleason patterns are assigned. Gleason pattern 4 consists of more complex and abnormal gland formations, such as fused glands, cribriform glands, and glomeruloid formations (Fig. 23-50B). Gleason pattern 5 is the highest grade and is assigned when gland formation is not seen and malignant cells grow in solid sheets. It is also assigned in adenocarcinomas with comedo necrosis, single cells, and cords (Fig. 23-50C).

Recognizing the high frequency of mixed tumor patterns, a **Gleason score** provides an overall assessment of tumor histologic grade and is calculated as the sum of the most prominent Gleason pattern and that of the second most prominent minority pattern. The Gleason score has been shown to be a powerful predictor of clinical behavior. The most well-differentiated tumors with the lowest Gleason scores (scores 2–6) are most likely to have prolonged recurrence-free progression. Less well-differentiated

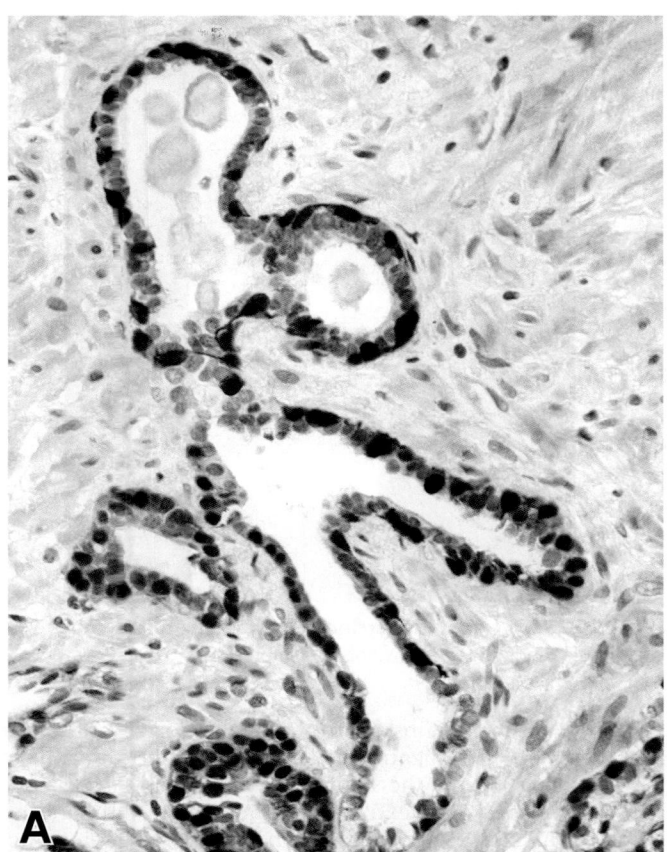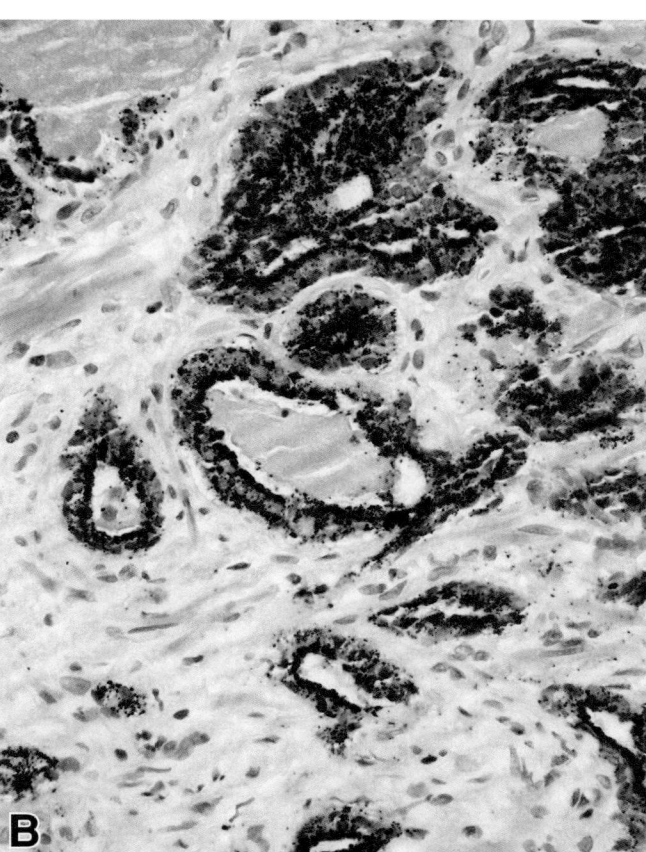

FIGURE 23-49. Immunohistochemical stains on benign glands and prostatic adenocarcinoma. A. Benign prostatic glands show positive staining with basal cell markers (*brown* chromogen) and are negative for AMACR (*red* chromogen). **B.** Small infiltrating glands of prostatic adenocarcinoma lack basal cell markers and are positive for AMACR (*red* chromogen).

prostatic adenocarcinoma with higher Gleason scores (7–10) are less likely to have prolonged recurrence-free progression. Risk stratification grade groups from 1 to 5 have been devised to reflect the increased risk associated with histologic grade. Gleason score 6 or less is assigned the lowest-risk grade group of 1; Gleason score 3 + 4 = 7 is grade group 2; Gleason score 4 + 3 = 7 is grade group 3; Gleason score 8 (4 + 4; 3 + 5; 5 + 3) is grade group 4; and Gleason score 9 or 10 (4 + 5; 5 + 4; 5 + 5) is grade group 5. Combined with tumor stage, Gleason grading has prognostic value: lower scores, risk grade groups, and lower stage all correlate with better prognoses.

INVASION AND METASTASIS: The high frequency of invasion of the prostatic capsule by adenocarcinoma reflects the tumor's subcapsular site of origin. Perineural tumor invasion within the prostate and in adjacent tissues is commonly seen. Since peripheral nerves are devoid of perineural lymphatic channels, this mode of invasion represents contiguous spread of the tumor along a tissue space that offers a plane of low resistance.

The seminal vesicles are almost always involved by direct extension of prostate cancer. Invasion of the urinary bladder tends to occur later in the clinical course. The earliest metastases appear in the obturator lymph nodes, and then in iliac and periaortic lymph nodes. Metastases to the lung reflect further lymphatic spread via the thoracic duct and dissemination from the prostatic venous plexus

to the inferior vena cava. Bony metastases, particularly to the vertebral column (Fig. 23-51), ribs, and pelvic bones, are painful and difficult to manage.

CLINICAL FEATURES: Current screening programs for prostate cancer use digital rectal examination in combination with serum PSA levels. PSA is a glycoprotein produced by the prostate. It is a serine protease involved in liquefying seminal ejaculate. It maintains a baseline serum level in men. Serum levels are increased by prostate inflammation, hypertrophy, and neoplasia. Patients with elevated serum PSA levels are typically evaluated further by needle biopsies. *Preoperative PSA levels correlate with cancer volume.* Since most prostate cancers are asymptomatic, PSA screening is the most common detection method. Uncommonly, patients with prostate cancer present with bladder outlet obstruction or symptoms referable to metastatic tumor.

At present, guidelines for prostate cancer screening are in flux. Widespread screening leads to more cancer diagnoses and treatment. With treatment come side effects and quality-of-life issues. Several large epidemiologic studies have reported conflicting results regarding the benefit of active prostate cancer therapy. The high frequency of side effects associated with aggressive screening

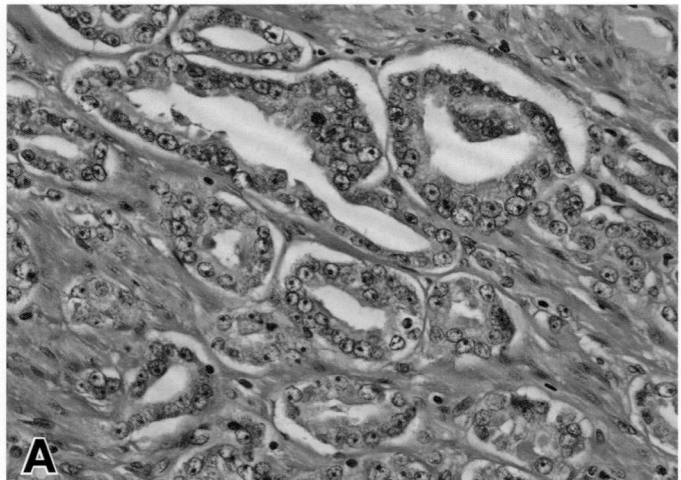

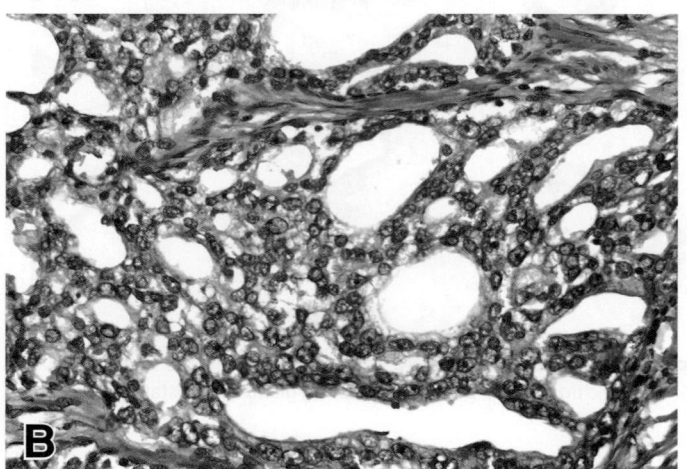

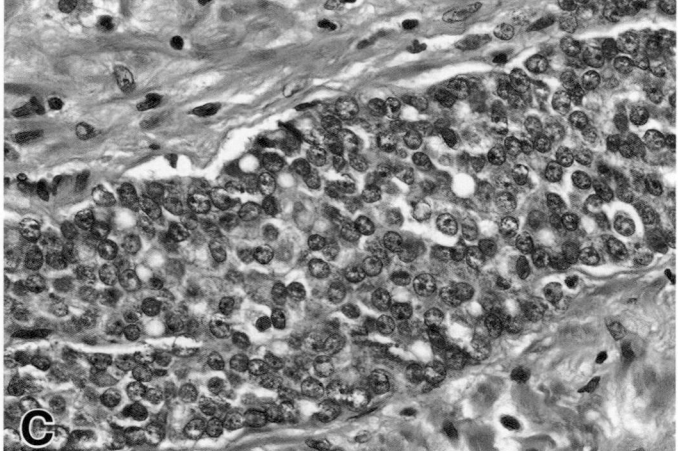

FIGURE 23-50. Gleason grading system. A. Gleason grade 3. **B.** Gleason grade 4. **C.** Gleason grade 5.

and treatment (e.g., incontinence, impotence) cannot be ignored. In 2018, the U.S. Preventive Service Task Force (USPSTF) updated their 2012 guidelines and concluded that there was insufficient evidence to recommend routine prostate cancer screening (and, by default, therapy).

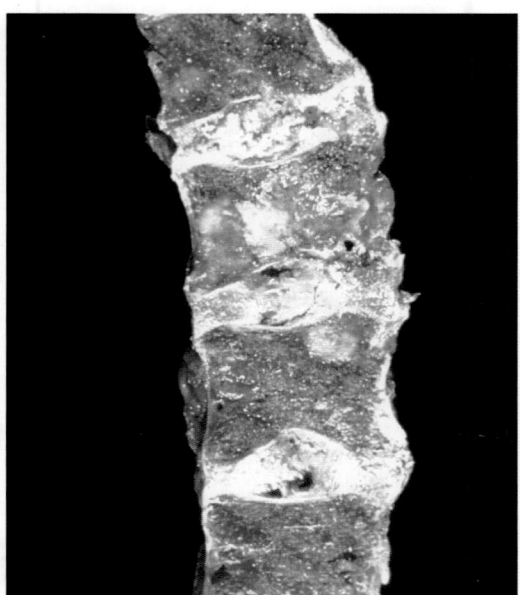

FIGURE 23-51. Prostatic carcinoma metastatic to the spine. Vertebral bodies contain several osteoblastic metastases.

This position remains controversial, however, and other professional organizations such as the American College of Physicians and the American Urological Association have adopted less extreme guidelines, recommending individualized patient evaluation and selective screening.

The principles of clinical staging (TNM) of prostate cancer are shown in Figure 23-52 and Table 23-8. At initial presentation, 10% of prostate cancers are clinical stage T1 (clinically unapparent localized tumor). Stage T2 applies

TABLE 23-8

TNM STAGING OF PROSTATIC CARCINOMA

T—Primary Tumor

T1 No clinically detectable tumor
    T1a Histologic tumor found in 5% or less of tissue examined
    T1b Histologic tumor found in more than 5% of tissue examined

T2 Tumor confined to the prostate

T3 Tumor extends through the capsule
    T3a Extracapsular extension only
    T3b Tumor extends into seminal vesicles

T4 Tumor invades adjacent structures other than seminal vesicles

N—Regional Lymph Nodes

N0 No regional lymph node involvement

N1 Regional lymph node metastases present

M—Distant Metastases

M0 No distant metastases

M1 Distant metastases present

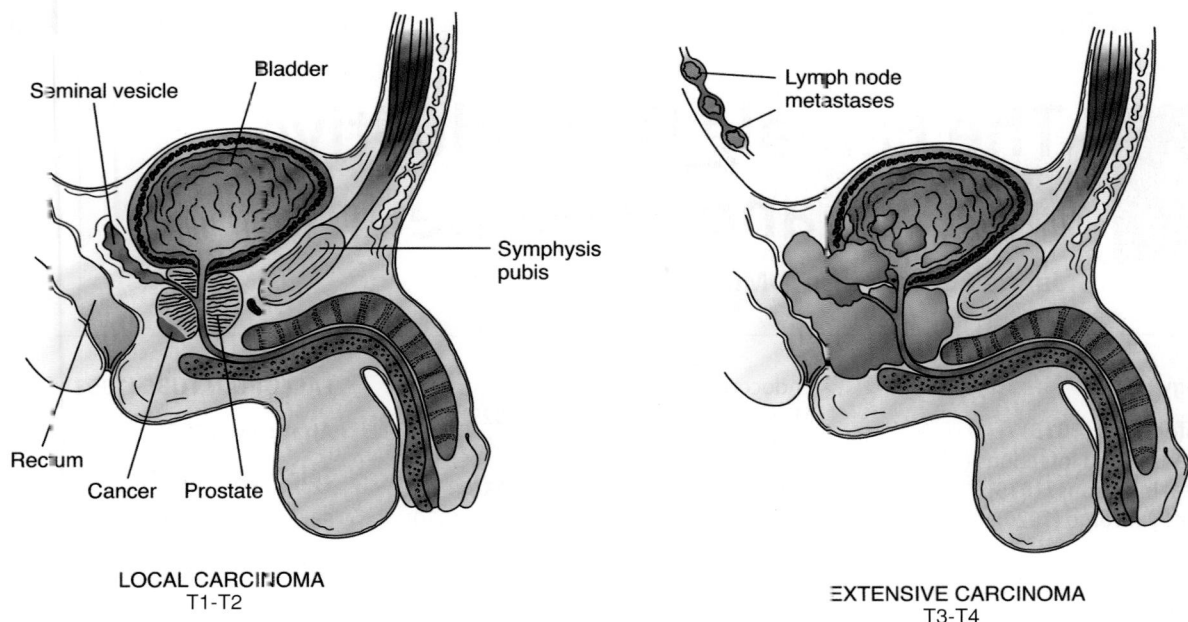

LOCAL CARCINOMA
T1-T2

EXTENSIVE CARCINOMA
T3-T4

FIGURE 23-52. Staging of prostatic carcinoma. The tumor–node–metastasis (TNM) system is widely used for staging of prostate carcinoma. Stage T1 and T2 tumors are localized to the prostate, whereas stage T3 and T4 tumors have spread outside the prostate.

to patients with clinically palpable localized prostatic tumors. However, 60% of patients initially staged as T2 show microscopic evidence of capsular penetration or seminal vesicle invasion and are therefore stage T3. Metastases are found in lymph nodes bones, lung, and liver, in order of decreasing frequency. Widespread tumor dissemination (carcinomatosis), with pneumonia or sepsis, is the most common cause of death.

Immunohistochemical demonstration of **PSA** in metastatic tumors is useful in identifying the prostate as the primary site of a tumor. PSA is also detectable in the serum of patients with prostate cancer. A rising serum PSA level is an indicator of recurrent disease after therapy. AMCAR is also a useful marker for identifying prostatic adenocarcinoma inside the gland as well as in metastatic sites. **Serum alkaline phosphatase** levels are elevated in patients with osteoblastic bony metastases, because this enzyme is released from osteoblasts forming new bone at a site of metastasis.

Therapy for prostate cancer is highly controversial, owing to recent studies indicating that many tumors may best be left alone. Considerable difficulty remains in identifying tumors likely to benefit from treatment. Treatment generally depends on tumor stage. Patients with stage T1 and T2 cancers are treated by radical prostatectomy, radiofrequency ablation, cryogenic procedures, or radiation therapy. Radiation therapy may be either external beam or intraglandular (brachytherapy). In stage T3 tumors, radiation therapy, combined with androgen deprivation therapy, is the treatment of choice, acknowledging that half of these patients have occult pelvic lymph node metastases (and possibly further systemic dissemination), which cannot be cured by surgical means alone. Patients with low-grade, low-volume tumors may opt to be managed by active surveillance only.

For patients with metastatic disease or whose tumors progress clinically, traditional chemotherapy combined with androgen deprivation is the main strategy. Bone metastases can be treated using local radiation, bisphosphonates, RANKL inhibition, and supplements of calcium and vitamin D.

The 5-year survival rates depend on stage and Gleason grade. Using staging data, survival is as follows: stages T1 and T2, 90%; stage T3, 40%; and stage T4, 10%.

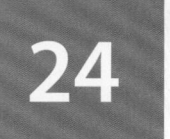

24 The Female Reproductive System and Peritoneum

Jaime Prat, George L. Mutter

EMBRYOLOGY

The gonadal anlage forms as a swelling of the embryonic urogenital ridge, initially in an indifferent state. The gonad is derived from mesoderm except for the germ cells, which are of extraembryonic (yolk sac) origin. Both sex chromosomes and autosomal chromosomes determine whether gonadal stromal cells will differentiate into testis or ovary. If the gonadal stroma is male, a gene on the Y chromosome (sex-determining region Y [SRY]) interacts with the primitive gonad to initiate development of a testis. An ovary develops if gonadal stroma is female and there is no stimulus to form a testis. Ovaries and testes become histologically distinct by about day 40.

Wolffian (mesonephric) ducts begin to develop at about day 25, regardless of the embryo's sex. If stimulated by testosterone (secreted by Leydig cells starting at about day 70), the ducts differentiate into vas deferens, epididymis, and seminal vesicle. If not stimulated by day 84, the ducts regress and remain as vestigial rests in the female. They may form cysts in the cervix or vagina **(mesonephric cyst)**.

Müllerian (paramesonephric) ducts, the anlage of the fallopian tubes, uterus and vaginal wall, appear at about day 37 as funnel-shaped openings of celomic epithelium. They develop into paired, undifferentiated tubes, using the wolffian ducts as "guide wires" to reach the area of the future hymen. If a wolffian duct is absent, as in renal agenesis, the vagina and cervix are almost always abnormal or absent. At day 54, müllerian ducts fuse into a straight uterovaginal canal.

A central tenet of genital tract development in both sexes is that müllerian ducts develop along female lines unless specifically impeded by embryonic testicular factors. In males, Sertoli cells in developing testes produce **antimüllerian hormone**, also called **müllerian-inhibiting substance**, which causes müllerian ducts to regress. This hormone, a glycoprotein in the TGFβ superfamily, is structurally related to inhibin and activin, which exert opposing actions on FSH synthesis and secretion, and also participate in regulating cell proliferation, differentiation, and apoptosis.

External genitalia assume masculine form if testosterone is converted locally to dihydrotestosterone. Otherwise (i.e., in a state of relative estrogen excess), female external genitalia persist. The genital tubercle develops into the clitoris, genital folds into the labia minora and genital swellings into the labia majora. The basic layout of the female genital tract is established by day 120.

GENITAL INFECTIONS

Most Genital Infections Are Sexually Transmitted

Infectious diseases of the female genital tract are common and are caused by many organisms (Table 24-1; also **see Chapter 9**). Most of the important infectious diseases of the female genital tract are sexually transmitted.

Bacterial Infections

Gonorrhea

Gonorrhea is caused by *Neisseria gonorrhoeae*, a fastidious, gram-negative diplococcus. A million cases of gonorrhea occur yearly in the United States. The infection is a frequent cause of acute salpingitis and pelvic inflammatory disease (PID) (Fig. 24-1).

  ETIOLOGIC FACTORS AND PATHOLOGY: The organisms ascend through the cervix and endometrial cavity, where they cause **acute endometritis**. They then attach to mucosal cells in the fallopian tube and elicit acute inflammation, which is confined to the mucosal surface **(acute salpingitis)**. Infection may then spread to the ovary, sometimes causing a **tuboovarian**

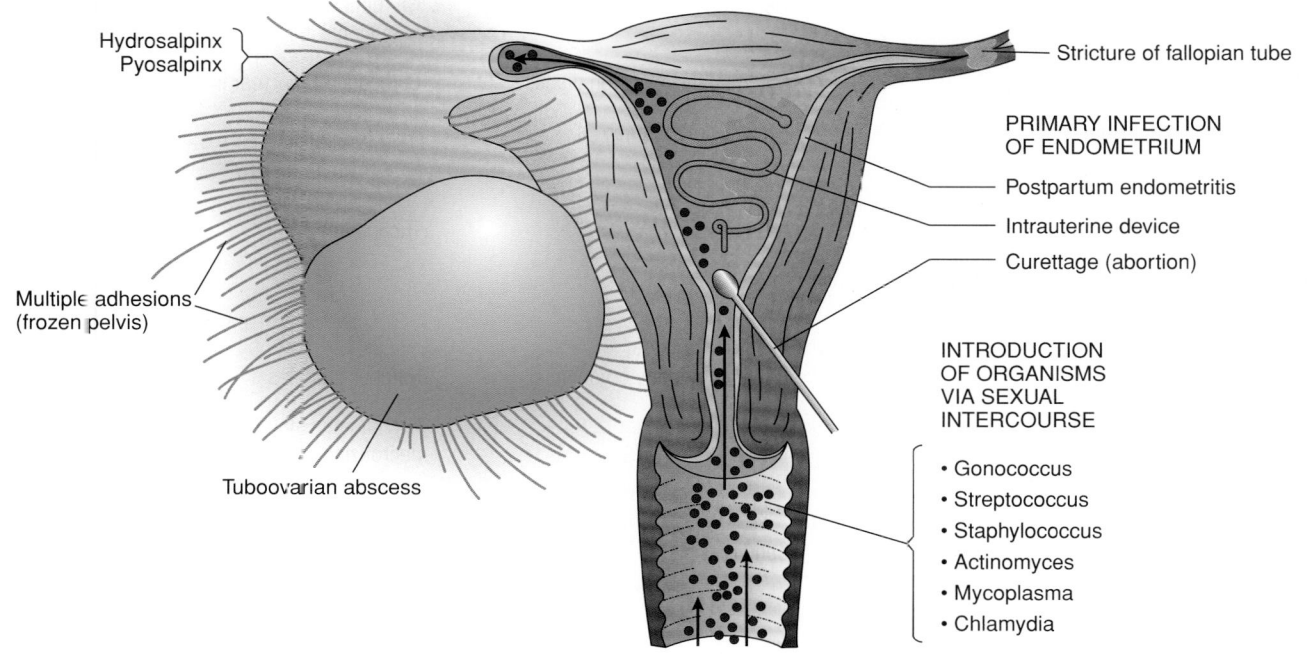

FIGURE 24-1. Pelvic inflammatory disease.

Hydrosalpinx
Pyosalpinx

Stricture of fallopian tube

PRIMARY INFECTION OF ENDOMETRIUM

Postpartum endometritis

Intrauterine device

Curettage (abortion)

Multiple adhesions (frozen pelvis)

Tuboovarian abscess

INTRODUCTION OF ORGANISMS VIA SEXUAL INTERCOURSE

• Gonococcus
• Streptococcus
• Staphylococcus
• Actinomyces
• Mycoplasma
• Chlamydia

TABLE 24-1

INFECTIOUS DISEASES OF THE FEMALE GENITAL TRACT

Organism	Disease	Diagnostic Feature
Sexually Transmitted Diseases		
Gram-negative rods and cocci		
Calymmatobacterium granulomatis	*Granuloma inguinale*	Donovan body
Gardnerella vaginalis	*Gardnerella infection*	Clue cell
Haemophilus ducreyi	Chancroid (soft chancre)	
Neisseria gonorrhoeae	Gonorrhea	Gram-negative diplococcus
Spirochetes		
Treponema pallidum	Syphilis	Spirochete
Mycoplasmas		
Mycoplasma hominis	Nonspecific vaginitis	
Ureaplasma urealyticum	Nonspecific vaginitis	
Rickettsiae		
Chlamydia trachomatis types D–K	Various forms of pelvic inflammatory disease (PID)	
Chlamydia trachomatis type L_{1-3}	Lymphogranuloma venereum	
Viruses		
Human papillomavirus (HPV)	Condyloma acuminatum/planum Neoplastic potential	Koilocyte
Types 6, 11, 40, 42, 43, 44, 57	Low risk for cancer	Low-grade squamous intraepithelial lesion (LSIL)
Types 16, 18, 31, 33, 35, 39, 45, 51, 52, 56, 58, 66	High risk for cancer	High-grade squamous intraepithelial lesion (HSIL)
Herpes simplex type 2	Herpes genitalis	Multinucleated giant cell with intranuclear homogenization and inclusion bodies
Cytomegalovirus (CMV)	Cytomegalic inclusion disease	Bulbous intranuclear inclusion body
Molluscum contagiosum	Molluscum infection	Molluscum body
Protozoa		
Trichomonas vaginalis	Trichomoniasis	Trichomonad
Selected Nonsexually Transmitted Diseases		
Actinomyces and related organisms		
Actinomyces israelii	PID (one of many organisms)	Sulphur granules
Mycobacterium tuberculosis	Tuberculosis	Granulomas (nonnecrotizing in endometrium, necrotizing elsewhere)
Fungi		
Candida albicans	Candidiasis	*Candida* sp.

abscess. Pelvic and abdominal cavities may be affected, leading to subdiaphragmatic and pelvic abscesses.

Systemic complications of gonorrhea include septicemia and septic arthritis. At all sites of infection, the organisms induce purulent inflammatory reactions that rarely resolve completely. Dense fibrous adhesions often remain, distorting and destroying the plicae of the fallopian tube and frequently leading to sterility.

Syphilis

Syphilis (**see Chapter 9**) is caused by *Treponema pallidum*, a thin, motile spirochete. Spread is via sexual contact with an infected person or transplacental spread (congenital syphilis). *T. pallidum* penetrates small cuts in the skin or normal mucosal surfaces. Untreated, syphilis persists, often waxing and waning, through three stages.

- In the **primary stage**, a **chancre** usually appears after about 3 weeks at the portal of bacterial entry. It is a painless, indurated papule, 1 to several cm in diameter, surrounded by an inflammatory cuff that breaks down to form an ulcer. The lesion may persist for 2 to 6 weeks. It then heals spontaneously.
- **Secondary syphilis** appears after a latent period of several weeks to months, and features low-grade fever, headache, malaise, lymphadenopathy, and highly infectious lesions called **condylomata lata** (syphilitic warts). These secondary lesions heal after 2 to 6 weeks and symptoms disappear spontaneously.
- The **tertiary stage** develops any time thereafter and may entail severe damage to the cardiovascular and nervous systems

 PATHOLOGY: The hallmark of syphilis in biopsy specimens is a dense inflammatory infiltrate with lymphocytes and plasma cells, particularly adjacent to blood vessels. Silver impregnation techniques (Warthin–Starry stain or its modifications), or organism-specific immunostain demonstrate the spirochetes. More advanced stages of disease show greater obliterative endarteritis and subsequent tissue destruction.

Granuloma Inguinale

This is caused by *Calymmatobacterium granulomatis*, a sexually transmitted, gram-negative, encapsulated rod. The disease occurs with equal frequency in women and men.

 PATHOLOGY: The primary lesion begins as a painless, ulcerated nodule involving genital, inguinal, or perianal skin. The organisms invade through skin abrasions and spread initially by direct extension, destroying skin, and underlying tissues. Extensive local spread and lymphatic permeation occur later. Vacuolated macrophages teem with characteristic intracellular bacteria (**Donovan bodies**). The organism, best seen with the Wright stain, resembles a closed safety pin. Hyperplasia of overlying squamous epithelium may be exuberant enough to be misinterpreted as a squamous cell carcinoma. Relapses following antibiotic therapy are common.

Chancroid

Also called **soft chancre**, chancroid is caused by *Haemophilus ducreyi*, a gram-negative bacillus. It is rare in the United States but common in underdeveloped countries.

 PATHOLOGY: Single or sometimes multiple small, vesiculopustular lesions appear on the cervix, vagina, vulva, or perianal region 3 to 5 days after sexual contact with an infected partner. At this stage histologic examination shows granulomatous inflammation. The lesion may rupture to form a painful, purulent ulcer that bleeds easily. Inguinal lymphadenopathy, fever, chills, and malaise may occur. A major complication is scarring during the healing phase, which may cause urethral stenosis.

Gardnerella

Sexual transmission of *Gardnerella vaginalis*, a gram-negative coccobacillus, causes many cases of "nonspecific vaginitis." Since the organism does not penetrate the mucosa, it causes no inflammation and biopsies appear normal. A wet mount specimen of a vaginal discharge or a Papanicolaou-stained smear (Pap smear) can identify the bacteria. **Clue cells**, squamous cells covered by coccobacilli, are pathognomonic.

Mycoplasma

Mycoplasmas (**see Chapter 9**) are minute pleomorphic organisms that resemble the so-called L bacterial forms (i.e., bacteria that lack cell walls) but they are distinct and do not originate from such L forms. They are common oropharyngeal and urogenital tract commensals and colonize the lower genital tract through sexual contact. *Ureaplasma urealyticum* can be isolated from the lower genital tract in 40% of healthy women. It may cause infertility and lead to adverse effects on pregnancy and perinatal infections. *Mycoplasma hominis* is found in the lower genital tract of 5% of healthy women and causes a small proportion of cases of symptomatic cervicitis and vaginitis. *M. hominis* is often isolated in association with *G. vaginalis* or *Trichomonas vaginalis* infection. Although the role of mycoplasma in genital tract infections is not completely understood, the organisms are encountered in PID, acute salpingitis, spontaneous abortion, and puerperal fever. Affected tissue is usually unremarkable histologically.

Chlamydia Infections

Chlamydia trachomatis is a common, venereally transmitted gram-negative obligate intracellular rickettsia. Fifteen serotypes are known. *C. trachomatis* causes several disorders in women, men, and infants. It has been found in the genital tracts of about 8% of asymptomatic women and 20% of women with symptoms of lower genital tract infection. Chlamydial disease is easily confused with gonorrhea, as the symptoms of both diseases are similar.

 PATHOLOGY: Serotypes D through K cause the more common genital infections. Cervical mucosa is severely inflamed, and endocervical and metaplastic squamous cells contain small inclusion bodies. Cytologically, perinuclear intracytoplasmic inclusions with distinct borders and intracytoplasmic **coccoid bodies** are seen. Complications include ascending infection of the endometrium, fallopian tube, and ovary, which may result in tubal occlusion and infertility. Chlamydia may also infect Bartholin glands and cause acute urethritis. Infants delivered vaginally to infected mothers may develop conjunctivitis, otitis media, and pneumonia.

Lymphogranuloma Venereum

This is a venereal infection of men and women, endemic in tropical countries. It is caused by the L form of *C. trachomatis*, serotypes L1 through L3.

 PATHOLOGY: After a few days to a month, a small painless vesicle forms at the site of inoculation. It heals rapidly and often is not even noticed. In the second stage, inguinal lymph nodes become enlarged and may rupture to form suppurative fistulas. Perirectal lymph nodes in women become matted and painful. In untreated patients, a third stage may appear after latency lasting several years. In this phase, scarring causes lymphatic obstruction, resulting in genital elephantiasis and rectal strictures. Infected tissues in the second and third stages show necrotizing granulomas and neutrophil infiltrates. Inclusion bodies within macrophages may also be seen.

Viral Infections

Human Papillomavirus

Human papillomavirus (HPV) is a DNA virus that infects genital skin and mucosal surfaces to produce wart-like lesions referred to as **condylomata acuminatum** or flat lesions known as **squamous intraepithelial lesions (SILs)**. Over 100 HPV serotypes are known, one-third of which cause genital tract lesions. The median time from infection to first detection of HPV is 3 months. In the United States, as many as two-thirds of women graduating college have genital HPV infections, which result from sexual contact with an infected person. Even in women who have had only one sex partner, the risk of cervical HPV by 3 years after first intercourse is 50%. HPV prevalence among women 14 to 59 years old exceeds 25%. About 20 million people are currently infected with HPV in this country; serotypes 6 and 11 account for over 80% of visible condylomata.

Several strains of HPV are the major etiologic factors for squamous cell cancer in the female lower genital tract, as well as anal and oropharyngeal cancers in both sexes. Types 16, 18, 31, and 45 are most often linked to high-grade squamous intraepithelial lesions (HSILs) and invasive cancer (see below). Vaccines to prevent infection with high-risk HPV serotypes 6, 11, 16, and 18 have been available since 2006 and now account for the lower infection rates in teenage girls.

Most cases of HPV are diagnosed by cervical Pap smear. Recent tests directly detect HPV DNA. Treatment is based on the histology of lesions (low vs. high grade), which predicts those at greatest risk for progression to carcinoma.

 PATHOLOGY: Lesions in the vulva, perianal region, perineum, vagina, and cervix caused by HPV infection are separated into low and high grades based on the appearance of the affected epithelium, which may be flat or exophytic. The warty form of low-grade squamous intraepithelial lesion (LSIL) is known as condylomata acuminatum. Acuminate warts are generally caused by low-cancer-risk viral subtypes and may present as papules, plaques, or nodules, which eventually become spiked or cauliflower-like excrescences (Fig. 24-2A). LSIL is characterized by koilocytes (from the Greek *koilos*, "hollow"), epithelial cells with a perinuclear halo and a wrinkled nucleus bearing HPV particles (Fig. 24-2B). Viral DNA typically remains episomal (i.e., not incorporated into epithelial cell chromosomal DNA). Extensive virus replication causes cytoplasmic injury, creating koilocytes (Fig. 24-2C). HSILs are discussed below.

Herpesvirus

Herpes simplex type 2 is a very large double-stranded DNA virus that commonly causes sexually transmitted genital infections. After an incubation period of 1 to 3 weeks, small vesicles develop on the vulva and erode into painful ulcers. Similar lesions occur in the vagina and cervix. Epithelial cells adjacent to intraepithelial vesicles show ballooning degeneration and many contain large nuclei with eosinophilic viral inclusions.

Herpesvirus infections follow relapsing, remitting courses. While latent, the virus resides in spinal (sacral) ganglia. If it becomes reactivated during pregnancy, passage through the birth canal may transmit the virus to the newborn infant, often with fatal consequences. Active vaginal herpetic lesions at the time of delivery are therefore an indication for cesarean section.

Cytomegalovirus

Cytomegalovirus (CMV) is a ubiquitous double-stranded DNA virus of the *Herpesvirus* family. More than 80% of people over the age of 35 have antibodies to CMV. Several lines of evidence suggest that many cases are sexually transmitted: (1) seroprevalence of CMV has risen in young adults, (2) the virus is recovered more often from cervical secretions and semen than from any other body sites, and (3) viral titers in semen are 100,000 times higher than in urine. Still, CMV only rarely causes genital infections in women. Infection in the endometrium may result in spontaneous abortion or infection of the newborn. Infected cells exhibit characteristic large, eosinophilic, intranuclear inclusions and, occasionally, cytoplasmic inclusions.

Molluscum Contagiosum

Molluscum contagiosum (**see Chapter 28**) is a highly contagious double-stranded DNA poxvirus. Infection leads to multiple smooth, gray-white nodules that are centrally umbilicated and exude a cheesy material. Lesions occur predominantly in the genital region but may be found elsewhere as well. Large, cytoplasmic viral inclusions (**molluscum bodies**) are seen in infected epithelial cells. Most lesions regress spontaneously, but untreated ones may persist for years.

Trichomoniasis

T. vaginalis is a large, pear-shaped, flagellated protozoan that often causes vaginitis. It is transmitted sexually, and 25% of infected women are asymptomatic carriers. Infection causes a heavy, yellow-gray, thick, foamy discharge with severe itching, dyspareunia (painful intercourse), and dysuria (painful urination). Motile trichomonads are identified on wet mount preparations and may also be seen in Pap smears.

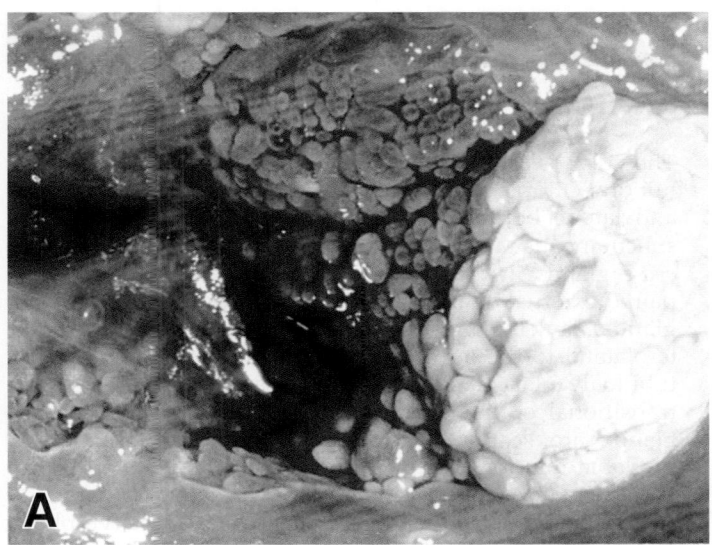

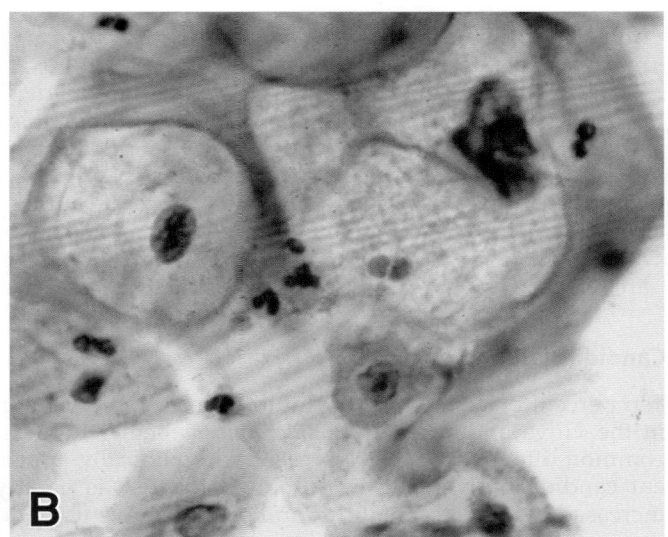

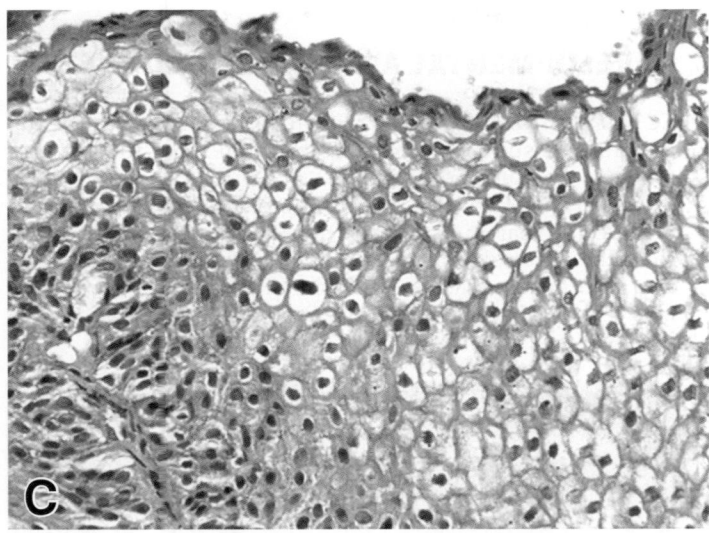

FIGURE 24-2. Human papillomavirus-induced condylomatous infections. A. Condyloma acuminatum on the cervix, visible with the naked eye as cauliflower-like excrescences. **B.** A cervical smear contains characteristic koilocytes, with a perinuclear halo and a wrinkled nucleus that contains viral particles. **C.** Biopsy of the condyloma shows koilocytes with perinuclear halos and significant nuclear pleomorphism and altered chromatin density.

Pelvic Inflammatory Disease

PID is infection of pelvic organs due to extension of one of several microorganisms above the uterine corpus (Fig. 24-1). Ascending infection results in bilateral acute salpingitis, pyosalpinx, and tuboovarian abscesses. **N. gonorrhoeae *and* Chlamydia *are the main organisms responsible for PID, but most infections are polymicrobial.*** PID is less common in monogamous women than in others. Occasionally, it occurs after postpartum endometritis or as a complication of endometrial curettage.

 CLINICAL FEATURES: Patients with PID typically present with lower abdominal pain. Physical examination reveals bilateral adnexal tenderness and marked discomfort when the cervix is manipulated (chandelier sign). Complications of PID include (1) rupture of a tuboovarian abscess, which may result in life-threatening peritonitis; (2) infertility from scarring of the healed tubal plicae; (3) increased rates of ectopic pregnancy; and (4) intestinal obstruction from fibrous bands and adhesions.

Some Genital Infections Are Not Transmitted Sexually

Tuberculosis

Mycobacterium tuberculosis may infect any part of the female genital tract. Genital tuberculosis occurs in 1% of infertile women in the United States and in over 10% of such women in less developed countries. Detecting acid-fast bacilli (AFB) confirms the diagnosis.

PATHOLOGY: *TUBERCULOUS SALPINGITIS:* Salpingitis is usually the initial lesion of tuberculous genital infection, due to hematogenous dissemination from the respiratory tract. Tuberculous salpingitis results in fibrinous adhesions and scarring of the fallopian tube. These complications lead to multiple functional abnormalities (e.g., infertility, ectopic gestation, pelvic pain). The tubes may become nodular. **Pyosalpinx** (fallopian tube distended with pus) and **hydrosalpinx**

(fluid-filled tube) are late sequelae, and the adjacent ovary may become infected.

TUBERCULOUS ENDOMETRITIS: Endometritis complicates half of the cases of tuberculous salpingitis. Although the endometrium may show well-formed granulomas with caseous necrosis and characteristic Langhans giant cells, menstrual shedding limits the time during which such mature granulomas may develop. Thus, noncaseating, poorly formed granulomas with rare giant cells are typical.

Candidiasis

Ten percent of women are asymptomatic carriers of fungi in the vulva and vagina, *Candida albicans* being the most common offender. Only 2% present with clinically apparent candidal vulvovaginitis, although the risk is greatly increased by diabetes mellitus, oral contraceptive use, and pregnancy. Infection causes vulvar itching and a white discharge. Clinical examination reveals firmly adherent, small white plaques on mucous membranes ("thrush"). Biopsy shows submucosal edema and chronic inflammation. Fungi do not penetrate the epithelium; rather, the white patches are foci of desquamated, necrotic epithelial cells containing cellular debris; bacterial flora; candidal spores; and pseudohyphae. Characteristic spores and pseudohyphae in a wet mount preparation or with a Pap stain are diagnostic. Untreated infections wax and wane and often disappear after delivery.

Actinomycosis

Genital tract actinomycosis is uncommon but is increasingly reported in association with use of intrauterine devices (IUDs). *Actinomyces israelii,* the causative organism, is a gram-positive rod found in 4% of normal genital tracts. It enters the uterine cavity via the tail of the IUD; ascends to the fallopian tube, ovary, and broad ligaments; and forms a tuboovarian abscess. Suppurating lesions display drainage tracts that contain dense microcolonies of organisms ("sulfur granules"). Actinomycosis results in extensive fibrosis and scarring of the female genital tract.

Toxic Shock Syndrome Is due to Vaginal Staphylococcal Infection

Toxic shock syndrome is an acute, sometimes fatal disorder characterized by fever, shock, and a desquamative erythematous rash. Vomiting, diarrhea, myalgias, neurologic signs, and thrombocytopenia are common clinical features. Certain strains of *Staphylococcus aureus* release an exotoxin called **toxic shock syndrome toxin-1**, which impairs the ability of mononuclear phagocytes to clear other potentially toxic substances, such as endotoxin. Pathologic alterations are characteristic of shock, and lesions of disseminated intravascular coagulation are usually prominent. Toxic shock syndrome was first recognized when long-acting tampons were introduced, allowing sufficient time for staphylococci to proliferate. Contraceptive "sponges" were also implicated. The incidence of toxic shock syndrome has decreased markedly since recognition of the role of tampons in promoting colonization of the vagina by *S. aureus.*

Vulva

ANATOMY

The vulva is composed of the mons pubis, labia majora and minora, clitoris, and vestibule. At puberty, the mons pubis and lateral borders of the labia majora acquire increased subcutaneous fat and grow coarse hair. Sebaceous and apocrine glands in these regions develop concomitantly. The paired external openings of the paraurethral glands **(Skene glands)** flank the urethral meatus. **Bartholin glands,** just posterolateral to the introitus, are branching, mucus-secreting, tubuloalveolar glands drained by a short duct lined by transitional epithelium. In addition, microscopic mucous glands are scattered throughout the area bounded by the labia minora. Inguinal and femoral lymph nodes provide primary lymph drainage routes, except for the clitoris (the homolog of the penis), which shares the lymphatic drainage of the urethra.

DEVELOPMENTAL ANOMALIES AND CYSTS

ECTOPIC BREAST TISSUE: Small, isolated nodules of ectopic breast tissue may extend in the "milk line" to the vulva and enlarge during pregnancy.

BARTHOLIN DUCT CYST: The paired Bartholin glands produce a clear mucoid secretion that continuously lubricates the vestibular surface. The ducts are prone to obstruction and consequent cyst formation (Fig. 24-3). Cyst infection may lead to **abscess formation**. Bartholin gland abscess was

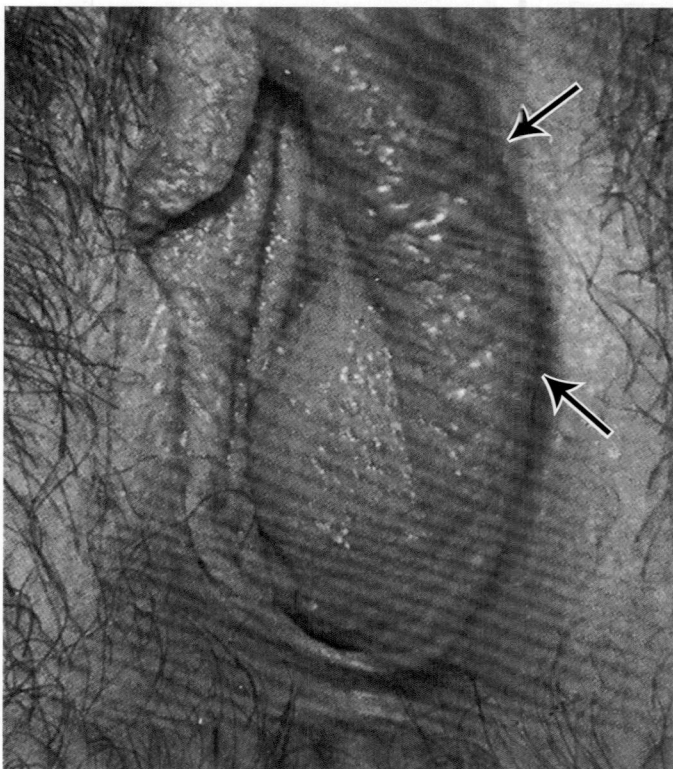

FIGURE 24-3. Bartholin gland cyst. The 4-cm lesion (*arrows*) is posterior to the vaginal introitus.

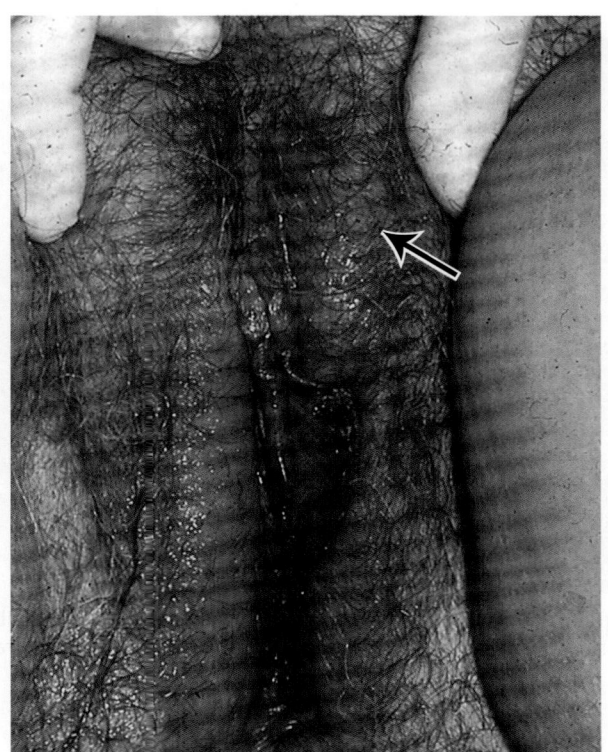

FIGURE 24-4. Vulvar acute dermatitis (eczema). Erythema, edema, and weeping vesicles (*arrow*) are present. (Reprinted with permission from Stanley J. Robboy, MD, and Gynecologic Pathology Associates, Durham and Chapel Hill, North Carolina.)

formerly associated with gonorrhea, but staphylococci, chlamydia, and anaerobes are now more frequently the cause. Treatment consists of incision, drainage, marsupialization, and appropriate antibiotics.

FOLLICULAR CYSTS: Follicular cysts recapitulate the most distal portion of the hair follicle. Also called **epithelial inclusion cysts** or **keratinous cysts**, follicular cysts frequently appear on the vulva, especially the labia majora. They contain a white cheesy material and typically are lined by stratified squamous epithelium.

MUCINOUS CYSTS: Vulvar mucinous glands occasionally become obstructed and develop cysts. Mucinous columnar cells line the cyst and may become infected.

DERMATOSES

Vulvar Acute Dermatitis Appears as Reddened Vesiculated Skin

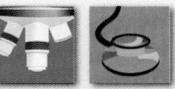 **PATHOLOGY:** As vesicles rupture (Fig. 24-4), the fluid forms a crust on the skin surface. The epidermis contains various inflammatory cells, and spongiotic areas form vesicles that rupture to produce the exudative lesions. The dermis shows a perivascular lymphocytic infiltrate and edema, with separation of collagen fibers. Dilated lymphatics and capillaries are typical.

The most common endogenous types of acute dermatitis are **atopic (hypersensitivity) dermatitis** and

seborrheic dermatitis, seen as a scaly macular eruption. Dermatitides with exogenous causes include irritant dermatitis (e.g., urine on the vulvar skin) and contact allergic dermatitis (type 4 delayed hypersensitivity reaction) and are manifest as either acute or chronic dermatitis.

Chronic Dermatitis, or Lichen Simplex Chronicus, Is the End Stage of Many Vulvar Inflammatory Diseases

Vulvar chronic dermatitis (Fig. 24-5) follows many diseases that are clinically pruritic and thus subject to repeated scratching in their active phase. These include lichen planus, psoriasis, and lichen sclerosus (**see Chapter 28**). The skin is thickened and white with exaggerated markings ("lichenification") as a result of marked hyperkeratosis. Scaling is generally present, and excoriations due to recent scratching are often seen.

LICHEN SCLEROSUS: This is an inflammatory disease associated with autoimmune disorders such as vitiligo, pernicious anemia, and thyroiditis. Autoimmune etiology of lichen sclerosus is further suggested by the presence of activated T cells in the dermis.

PATHOLOGY AND CLINICAL FEATURES: The condition is characterized by white plaques and atrophic skin with a parchment-like or crinkled appearance and, occasionally, marked contracture of vulvar tissues (Fig. 24-6A).

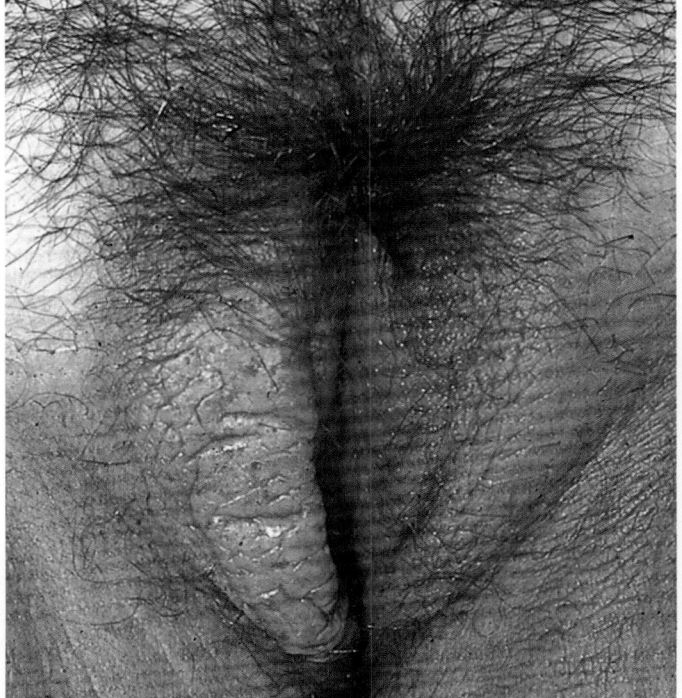

FIGURE 24-5. Lichen simplex chronicus of the right labium majus. There is thickening and accentuation of skin markings, with surface excoriation due to recent scratching. (Reprinted with permission from Stanley J. Robboy, MD, and Gynecologic Pathology Associates, Durham and Chapel Hill, North Carolina.)

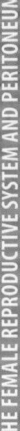

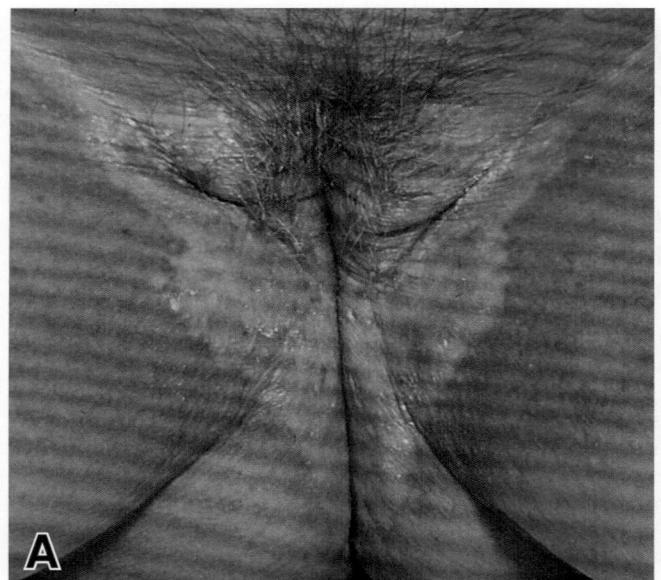
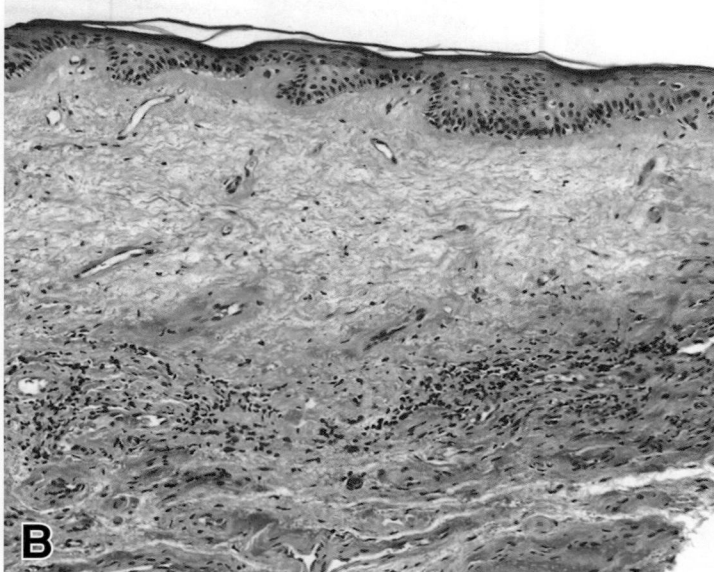

FIGURE 24-6. Lichen sclerosus of vulva. A. The sharply demarcated white lesion affects the vulva and perineum. **B.** The epidermis is thin and exhibits hyperkeratosis and a lack of the normal rete pattern. The dermis displays an acellular, homogeneous zone overlying a mild chronic inflammatory infiltrate.

Hyperkeratosis, loss of rete ridges, epithelial thinning with flattening of rete pegs, cytoplasmic vacuolation of the basal layer and a homogeneous, acellular collagenous zone in the upper dermis are seen (Fig. 24-6B). A band of lymphocytes with few plasma cells typically underlies this layer. The disease develops insidiously and is progressive, often causing itching and dyspareunia. Women with symptomatic lichen sclerosus have a 15% chance of developing squamous cell carcinoma.

BENIGN TUMORS

HIDRADENOMA: This benign apocrine sweat gland tumor appears chiefly in the labia majora as a well-circumscribed nodule, rarely larger than 1 cm. Microscopically, it is composed of papillary tubules and acini lined by two layers of cells: an inner layer of apocrine columnar cells and an outer one of myoepithelial cells.

SYRINGOMA: An adenoma of eccrine glands, syringoma manifests as a flesh-colored papule within the dermis of labia majora. This asymptomatic tumor is composed of a proliferation of small ducts embedded in a dense fibrous stroma (**see Chapter 28**). Duct walls have two layers of cells: an inner layer of serous cells and an outer one of myoepithelial cells. The lumen contains amorphous eosinophilic material.

CONNECTIVE TISSUE TUMORS: **Senile hemangiomas** (cherry hemangiomas) are small, purple skin papules, which may bleed following surface trauma. **Lobular capillary hemangioma** (formerly called pyogenic granuloma), previously thought to be a reaction to superficial wound infection, is a variant of hemangioma. Secondary infection occurs, as the surface of the lesion is fragile and easily disrupted. Soft tissue tumors found elsewhere in the body also occur in the vulva, including granular cell tumor, leiomyoma, fibroma, lipoma, and histiocytoma.

PIGMENTED VULVAR LESIONS: **Lentigo** occurs in about 10% of women and presents as small macules. **Nevi** and **seborrheic keratosis** also occur in this area (Chapter 28).

MALIGNANT TUMORS AND PREMALIGNANT CONDITIONS

Vulvar Intraepithelial Neoplasia Is a Precursor of Invasive Squamous Cell Carcinoma

Vulvar carcinoma, mostly squamous cell carcinoma, accounts for 3% of all female genital cancers and occurs mainly in women over age 60. These tumors are divided into keratinizing squamous cell carcinomas unrelated to HPV (>70% of cases) and warty basaloid carcinomas associated with high-risk HPV (<25% of cases). Classic vulvar intraepithelial neoplasia (VIN) lesions associated with HPV are also known as high-grade vulvar squamous intraepithelial lesions (vulvar HSILs), whereas intraepithelial precursor lesions unassociated with HPV are called "differentiated VIN."

  ETIOLOGIC FACTORS AND CLINICAL FEATURES: Keratinizing squamous carcinomas frequently develop in older women (mean age, 76 years), sometimes in the context of long-standing lichen sclerosus. The precursor lesion is called **differentiated vulvar intraepithelial neoplasia (dVIN)** (Fig. 24-7A), which carries a high risk of developing cancer. Carcinomas arise as nodules or masses in a background of **"leukoplakia"** (*white plaques*, a nonspecific, descriptive term). Cases of lichen sclerosus, differentiated VIN, and invasive squamous cell carcinoma with identical p53 gene (*TP53*) mutations have been reported; however, p53 gene mutation is an uncommon late event in vulvar carcinogenesis.

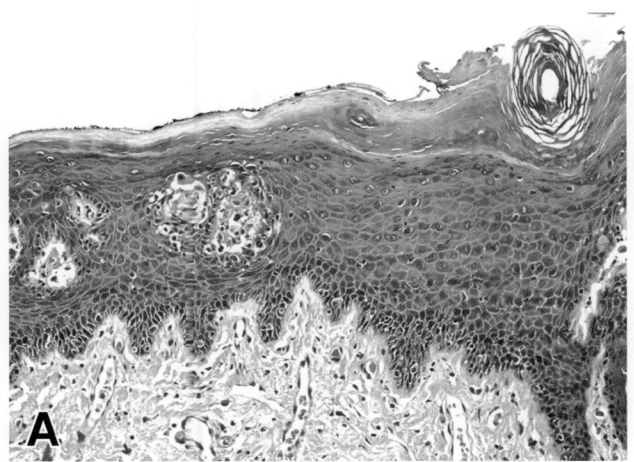
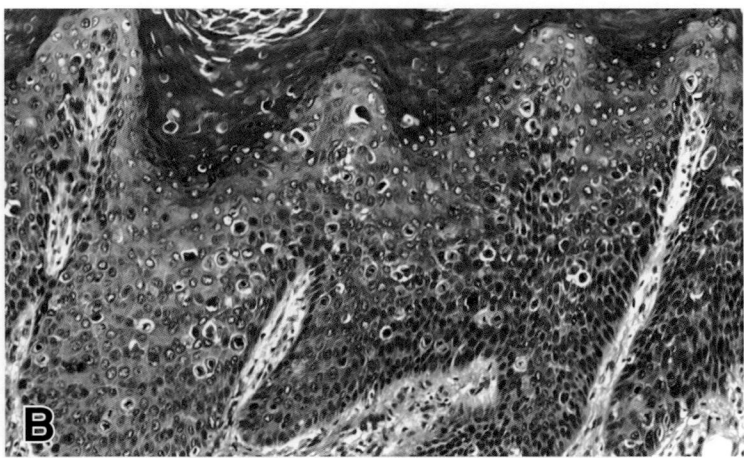

FIGURE 24-7. Vulvar intraepithelial neoplasia (VIN). A. Differentiated VIN is not associated with human papillomavirus (HPV) and demonstrates atypia accentuated in the basal and parabasal layers. There is striking epithelial maturation in the superficial layers. **B.** Classic VIN is caused by HPV and includes features of full-thickness atypia, numerous mitoses and often, as in this example, hyperkeratosis.

By contrast, the less common HPV-associated warty and basaloid carcinomas develop from a precursor lesion called **classic VIN** (Fig. 24-7B). Since 1980, the incidence of classic VIN has increased 5- to 10-fold in women under age 40, typically related to **HPV 16**. HPV-associated VIN lesions have a low risk of progression to invasive carcinomas (6%), except in older or immunosuppressed women. Lesions associated with oncogenic HPV types generally demonstrate activated p16. Women with VIN may have squamous neoplasms similar to VIN elsewhere in the lower genital tract.

PATHOLOGY: VIN reflects a spectrum of neoplastic changes from minimal to severe cellular atypia with differing pathogenesis as described above. These lesions may be single or multiple, and macular, papular or plaque-like. Histologic grades of VIN I, II, and III correspond to mild, moderate, and severe dysplasia, respectively. However, grade III, which includes squamous cell carcinoma in situ (CIS), is by far the most common. Differentiated VIN shows severe nuclear atypia of the basal layer with striking epithelial maturation in the superficial layers (Fig. 24-7A). Keratinocytes of the latter contain rounded nuclei with enlarged nucleoli and ample eosinophilic cytoplasm with prominent intercellular bridges. Rete pegs often contain keratin pearls.

Terminology for HPV-related lesions has recently been standardized throughout the anogenital tract along the lines of what has been applied to the cervix: LSIL and HSIL. This has not been adopted universally, however, and there is the additional complication that most vulvar squamous precancerous lesions are not HPV related (differentiated VIN). In the vulva, LSILs include acuminate warts and bland flat lesions that may only have rare diagnostic koilocytes. As in comparable lesions in the cervix (see below), criteria used in establishing the grade of classic VIN include (1) nuclear size and atypia, (2) number and severity of atypical mitoses, and (3) loss of cytoplasmic differentiation toward the epithelial surface. In the undifferentiated form seen in younger women, the entire epithelium consists of cells with highly atypical nuclei and negligible cytoplasm. Mitoses, often atypical, are common (Fig. 24-7B). **Bowen disease**, a term still used in the dermatologic literature, is a synonym for VIN III.

Keratinizing squamous cell carcinomas usually follow differentiated VIN. Two-thirds of larger tumors are exophytic (Fig. 24-8A); the remainder are ulcerative and endophytic. The tumor is composed of invasive nests of malignant squamous epithelium with central keratin pearls (Fig. 24-8B). The tumors grow slowly, extending to contiguous skin, vagina, and rectum. They metastasize initially to superficial inguinal lymph nodes and then to deep inguinal, femoral, and pelvic lymph nodes.

CLINICAL FEATURES: Most patients with VIN present with vulvar itching and burning with raised, well-defined skin lesions of variable sizes, which may be pink, red, brown, or white. Carcinomas, but not VIN, may develop ulceration, bleeding, and secondary infection. Spontaneous regression of VIN has been reported, most often in younger women.

Prognosis for patients with vulvar cancer is generally good, with 70% overall 5-year survival. Tumor grade, size, location and, most importantly, the number of lymph node metastases, predict survival. Two-thirds of women with inguinal node metastases survive 5 years, but only one-fourth of those with pelvic node metastases live that long. Better-differentiated tumors have a better mean survival, approaching 90% if nodes are negative.

Verrucous Carcinoma Is a Well-Differentiated Squamous Cancer

Vulvar verrucous carcinoma is a distinct variety of squamous cell carcinoma that grows as a large fungating mass resembling a giant condyloma acuminatum. HPV, usually type 6 or 11, is commonly involved. The tumor is very well

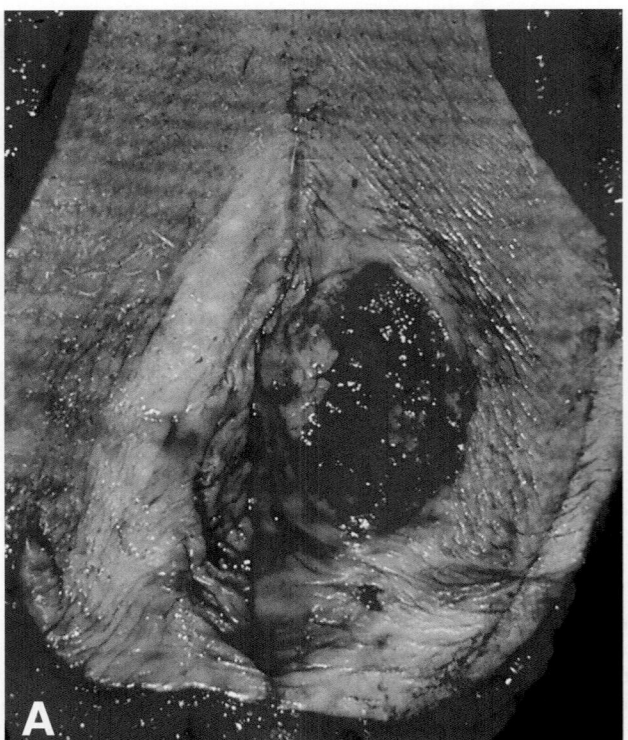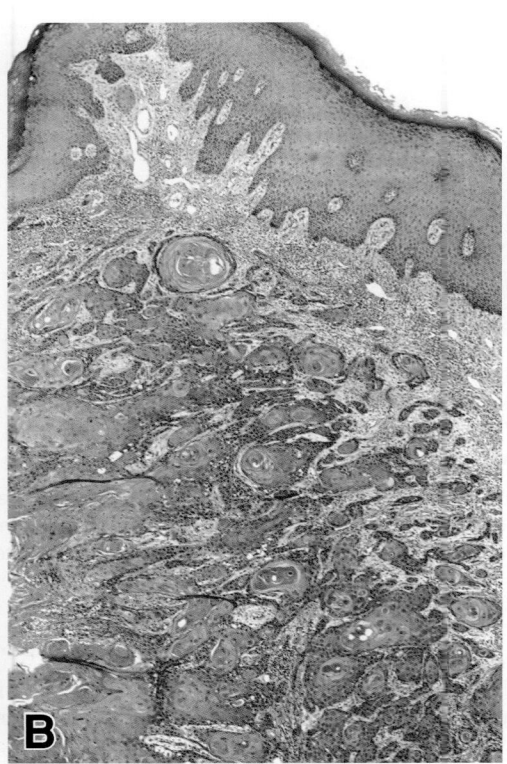

FIGURE 24-8. Squamous cell carcinoma of vulva. A. The tumor is situated in an extensive area of lichen sclerosus (*white*). **B.** Nests of neoplastic squamous cells, some with keratin pearls, are evident in this well-differentiated tumor.

differentiated, with large nests of squamous cells with abundant cytoplasm and small, bland nuclei. Squamous pearls are common and mitoses are rare. The tumor invades along broad fronts, and lymphocytes and plasma cells often heavily infiltrate the stromal interface. Verrucous carcinomas rarely metastasize. Wide local surgical excision is the treatment of choice, but other forms of therapy (cryosurgery and retinoids) have been successful.

Basal Cell Carcinoma

Basal cell carcinomas of the vulva are identical to those in the skin. They are not associated with HPV, rarely metastasize and are usually cured by surgical excision.

Malignant Melanoma

Although uncommon, malignant melanoma is the second most frequent cancer of the vulva (5%). It occurs in the sixth and seventh decades but is occasionally found in younger women. It has biologic and microscopic characteristics of melanomas occurring elsewhere in the body. It is highly aggressive, and the prognosis is poor.

Extramammary Paget Disease Resembles Similar Tumors of the Breast and Elsewhere

This disorder usually occurs on the labia majora in older women. Women with Paget disease of the vulva complain of pruritus or a burning sensation for many years.

 PATHOLOGY: The lesion is large, red, moist, and sharply demarcated. Diagnostic cells (Paget cells) may arise in the epidermis or epidermally derived adnexa. They have pale, vacuolated cytoplasm (Fig. 24-9) with abundant glycosaminoglycans; they stain with periodic acid–Schiff (PAS) and mucicarmine and express carcinoembryonic antigen (CEA). They appear as large single cells or, less often, as clusters of cells that lack intercellular bridges and are usually confined to the epidermis.

Intraepidermal Paget disease may be present for many years and is often far more extensive throughout the epidermis than preoperative biopsies indicate. Unlike Paget disease of the breast, which is almost always associated with underlying duct carcinoma, extramammary Paget disease is only rarely associated with carcinoma of the skin adnexa. Metastases occur rarely, so treatment requires only wide local excision or simple vulvectomy.

Vagina

ANATOMY

The vagina extends from the uterus to the vestibule of the vulva and is lined by hormone-responsive squamous epithelium. Estrogens stimulate, and progestogens inhibit, vaginal epithelial proliferation and maturation. Thus, in the secretory phase of the menstrual cycle or during pregnancy, when progesterone levels are high, intermediate cells, rather than

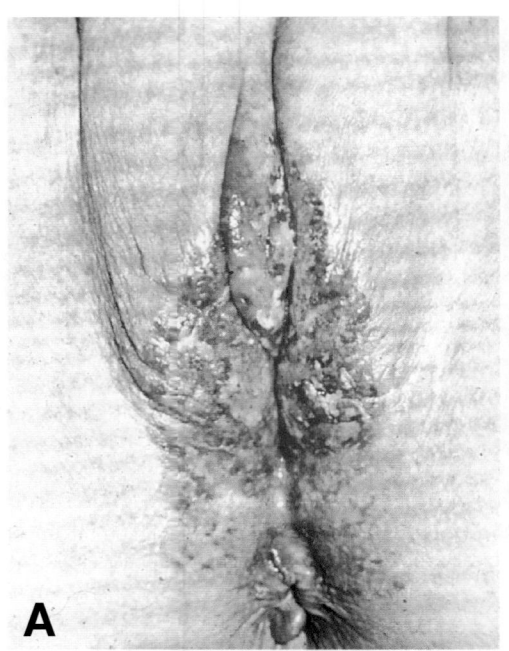
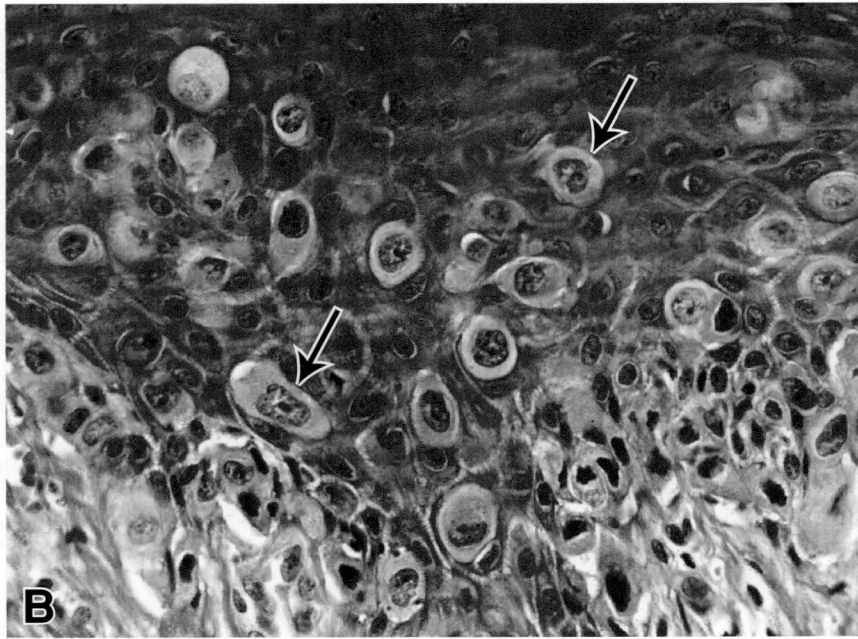

FIGURE 24-9. Paget disease of the vulva. A. The lesion is red, moist and sharply demarcated. **B.** Individual Paget cells (*arrows*), characterized by an abundant pale cytoplasm, infiltrate the epithelium and are interspersed among normal keratinocytes.

superficial ones, predominate in vaginal smears. Maturing epithelial cells accumulate glycogen, giving their cytoplasm a clear appearance.

Lymph drains through the lateral perivaginal plexus. Lymphatics from the vaginal vault and upper vagina join branches from the cervix, to drain into pelvic and then paraaortic nodes. The lower vagina also drains to inguinal and femoral nodes.

NONNEOPLASTIC CONDITIONS AND BENIGN TUMORS

Congenital Anomalies of the Vagina Are Rare

Congenital absence of the vagina is generally associated with anomalies of the uterus and urinary tract. If there is a functional uterus, absence of a vagina may lead to accumulation of menstrual blood in the uterus.

Septate vagina results from failure of embryonic müllerian ducts to fuse properly, and the resulting median wall is not resorbed.

Vaginal atresia and imperforate hymen prevent the vaginal embryonic lining from maturing from müllerian to squamous epithelium, which can cause vaginal adenosis.

Diminished Estrogen Stimulation Causes Atrophic Vaginitis

Atrophic vaginitis is thinning and atrophy of the vaginal epithelium. The thinned epithelium is a poor barrier to infections or abrasions. This occurs most commonly in postmenopausal women with low estrogen levels. Dyspareunia and vaginal spotting are common symptoms.

Vaginal Adenosis Occurred in Females Exposed to Diethylstilbestrol In Utero

In vaginal adenosis, the glandular epithelium that normally lines the embryonic vagina fails to be replaced during fetal life by squamous epithelium. In the 1970s, use of diethylstilbestrol (DES) to prevent miscarriages in women who were prone to repetitive abortions led to a substantial increase in this disorder in daughters of those women. Between the 10th and 18th weeks of gestation, upgrowth of squamous epithelium from the urogenital sinus replaces the glandular (müllerian) linings of the vagina and exocervix. DES exposure during this critical time arrests this process and some glandular tissue (i.e., adenosis) remains.

Adenosis manifests as red, granular patches on the vaginal mucosa. Microscopically, these are composed of mucinous columnar cells (resembling those lining the endocervix) and ciliated cells (like those lining the endometrium and fallopian tubes). Many of these lesions disappear as young women grow older. Rare cases of **clear cell adenocarcinoma** of the vagina (Fig. 24-10) have also occurred in the daughters of women treated with DES, typically arising in the upper third of the vagina. Clear cell adenocarcinomas are almost invariably curable when small and asymptomatic, but in more advanced stages, may spread by hematogenous or lymphatic routes.

Fibroepithelial Polyp

Vaginal polyps are uncommon benign growths with a connective tissue core and an outer lining of vaginal squamous epithelium. They are usually single, gray-white and smaller than 1 cm in diameter. Simple excision is usually curative. Torsion of benign fibroepithelial polyps may yield a loose edematous stroma resembling the myxomatous stroma of

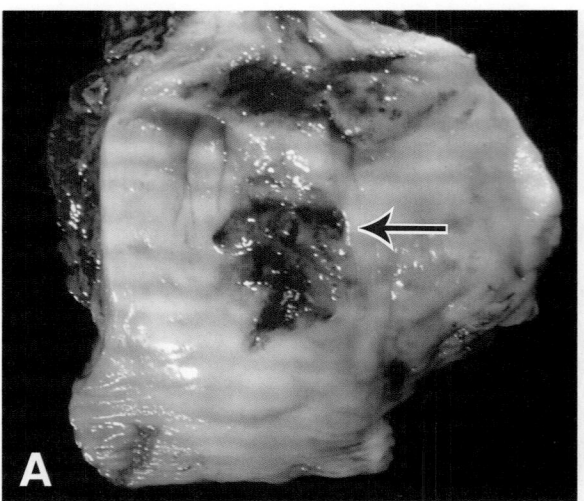
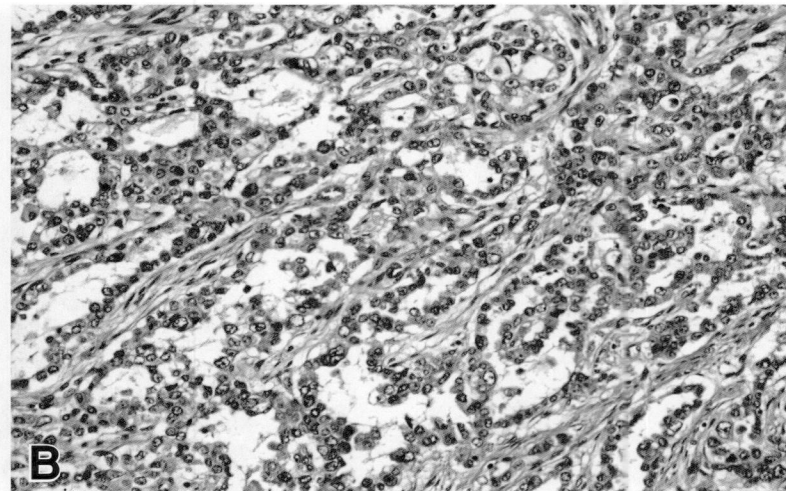

FIGURE 24-10. Clear cell adenocarcinoma of the vagina (in utero exposure to diethylstilbestrol [DES]). A. The tumor has arisen on the upper third of the anterior wall (*arrow*), corresponding to the most frequent site of adenosis. **B.** Microscopically, tubular glands are lined by hobnail cells.

angiomyxoma. Benign polyps demonstrate a vascular core rather than a distributed vascular network, and lack the infiltrating borders of angiomyxoma.

Benign Mesenchymal Tumors

Most benign vaginal tumors resemble those elsewhere in the female genital tract and include leiomyomas, rhabdomyomas, and neurofibromas. These are solid submucosal tumors usually less than 2 cm in diameter.

MALIGNANT TUMORS OF THE VAGINA

Primary malignant tumors of the vagina are uncommon, constituting about 2% of all genital tract tumors. **Most (80%) vaginal malignancies represent metastatic spread.** The most common symptoms are vaginal discharge and bleeding during coitus, but advanced tumors may cause pelvic or abdominal pain and edema of the legs. Tumors confined to the vagina are usually treated by radical hysterectomy and vaginectomy.

Over 90% of Primary Vaginal Cancers Are Squamous Carcinomas

It is generally a disease of older women, with peak incidence between the ages of 60 and 70. It is most common in the anterior wall of the upper third of the vagina, where it usually grows as an exophytic mass. High-grade **vaginal intraepithelial lesion** (vaginal HSIL), a term replacing both "vaginal dysplasia" and "carcinoma in situ," frequently precedes invasive carcinoma. Vaginal squamous cell carcinoma may develop some years after cervical or vulvar carcinoma, suggesting a carcinogenic field effect in the lower genital tract, related to HPV infection.

Since most preinvasive and early invasive cancers are clinically silent, routine use of vaginal cytology is the most effective method to detect squamous carcinoma of the vagina. Prognosis is related to the extent of tumor spread at the time of discovery. Five-year survival in patients with tumors confined to the vagina (stage I) is 80%, but it is only 20% for those with extensive spread (stages III/IV).

Rhabdomyosarcoma Is a Rare Vaginal Tumor in Children

This tumor typically consists of confluent polypoid masses resembling a bunch of grapes, and hence has been called sarcoma botryoides (from the Greek *botrys*, "grapes") (Fig. 24-11A). It occurs almost exclusively in girls under 4 years old. It arises in the lamina propria of the vagina and consists of primitive spindle rhabdomyoblasts (Fig. 24-11B), some of which show cross-striations. Myosin and actin myofibrils are often demonstrable. A dense zone of round rhabdomyoblasts (the cambium layer) is present beneath the vaginal epithelium (Fig. 24-11C). Deep to this layer, the stroma is myxomatous and shows fewer neoplastic rhabdomyoblasts. The tumor is usually detected because of spotting on the child's diaper. Tumors under 3 cm in greatest dimension tend to be localized and may be cured by wide excision and chemotherapy. Larger tumors often spread to adjacent structures, regional lymph nodes or distant sites. Even in advanced cases, half of patients survive following radical surgery and chemotherapy.

Cervix

ANATOMY

The cervix (from the Latin *collare*, "neck") is the inferior part of the uterus that connects the corpus to the vagina (Fig. 24-12). Its exposed portion (the **exocervix, ectocervix,** or **portio vaginalis**) protrudes into the upper vagina and is covered by glycogen-rich squamous epithelium. The **endocervix** is the canal that leads to the endometrial cavity. It is lined by longitudinal mucosal ridges made of fibrovascular cores covered by a single layer of mucinous columnar cells. Occasionally, the outlet of an endocervical gland becomes blocked and mucin is retained. This produces cystic dilations

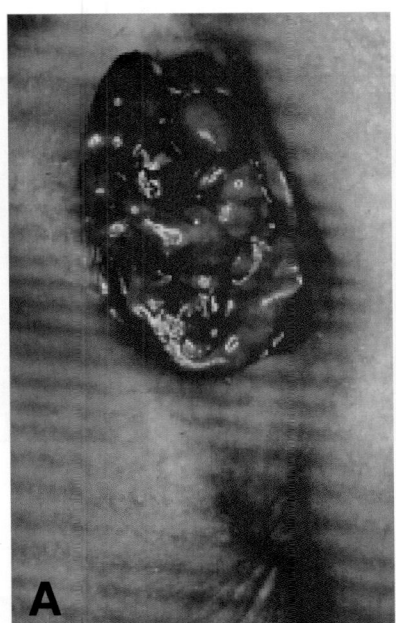

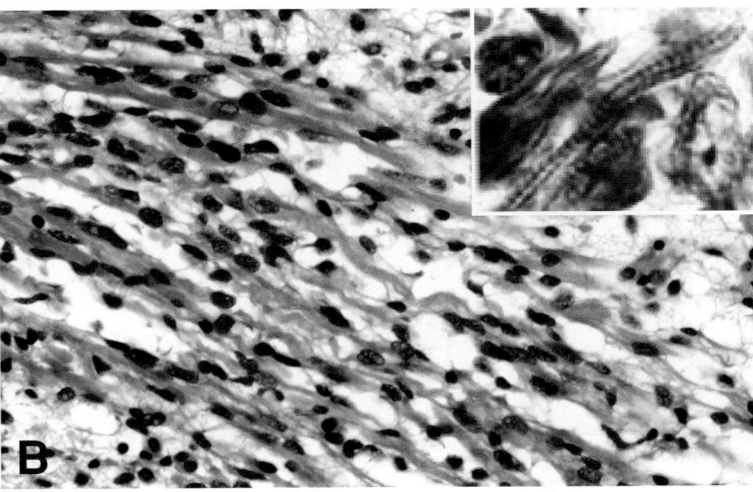

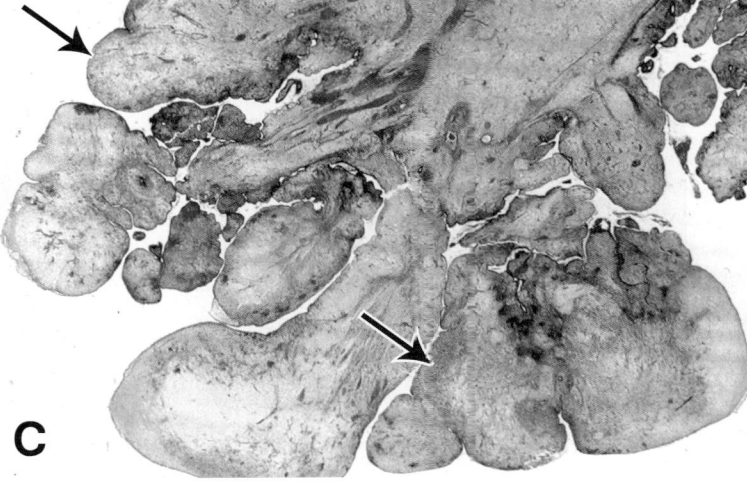

FIGURE 24-11. Embryona rhabdomyosarcoma (sarcoma botryoides) of vagina. A. The grape-ike tumor protrudes through the introitus. **B.** The tumor cells are composed of elongated, primitive rhabdomyoblasts, with cross-striations seen at high magnification in the *inset*. **C.** A section of the tumor shows a dense layer of neoplastic stroma termed the cambium layer (*arrows*) beneath the surface epithelium of the vagina. A loose neoplastic stroma is present beneath the cambium layer.

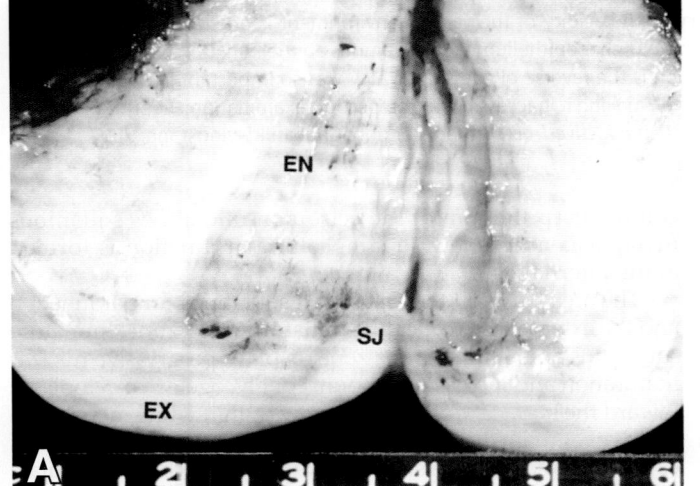

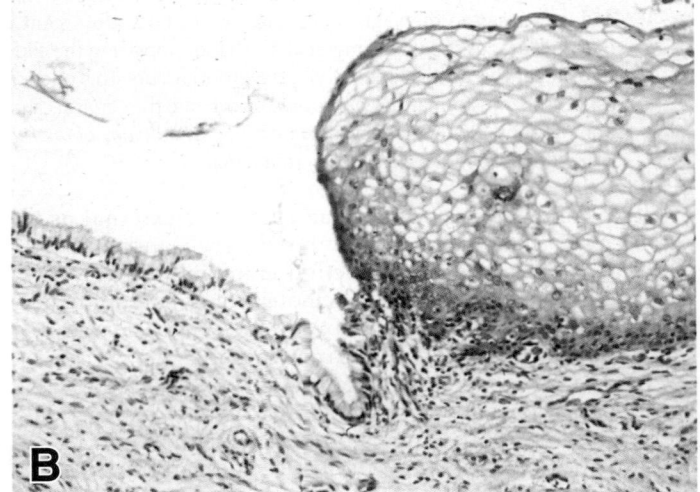

FIGURE 24-12. Anatomy of the cervix. A. The cervix has been opened to show the endocervix (*EN*), squamocolumnar junction (*SJ*), and exocervix (*EX*). The thick layer of squamous cells covering the exocervix accounts for its white color. **B.** A microscopic view of the squamocolumnar junction. The endocervix is lined by a single layer of columnar mucus-producing cells (seen on left side of image) that abruptly meets the exocervix lined by mature squamous cells (right side). *Note:* In specimens in which the squamocolumnar junction is on the ectocervix or in the endocervical canal, the region between it and the external os is called the *transformation zone* (see Fig. 24-13).

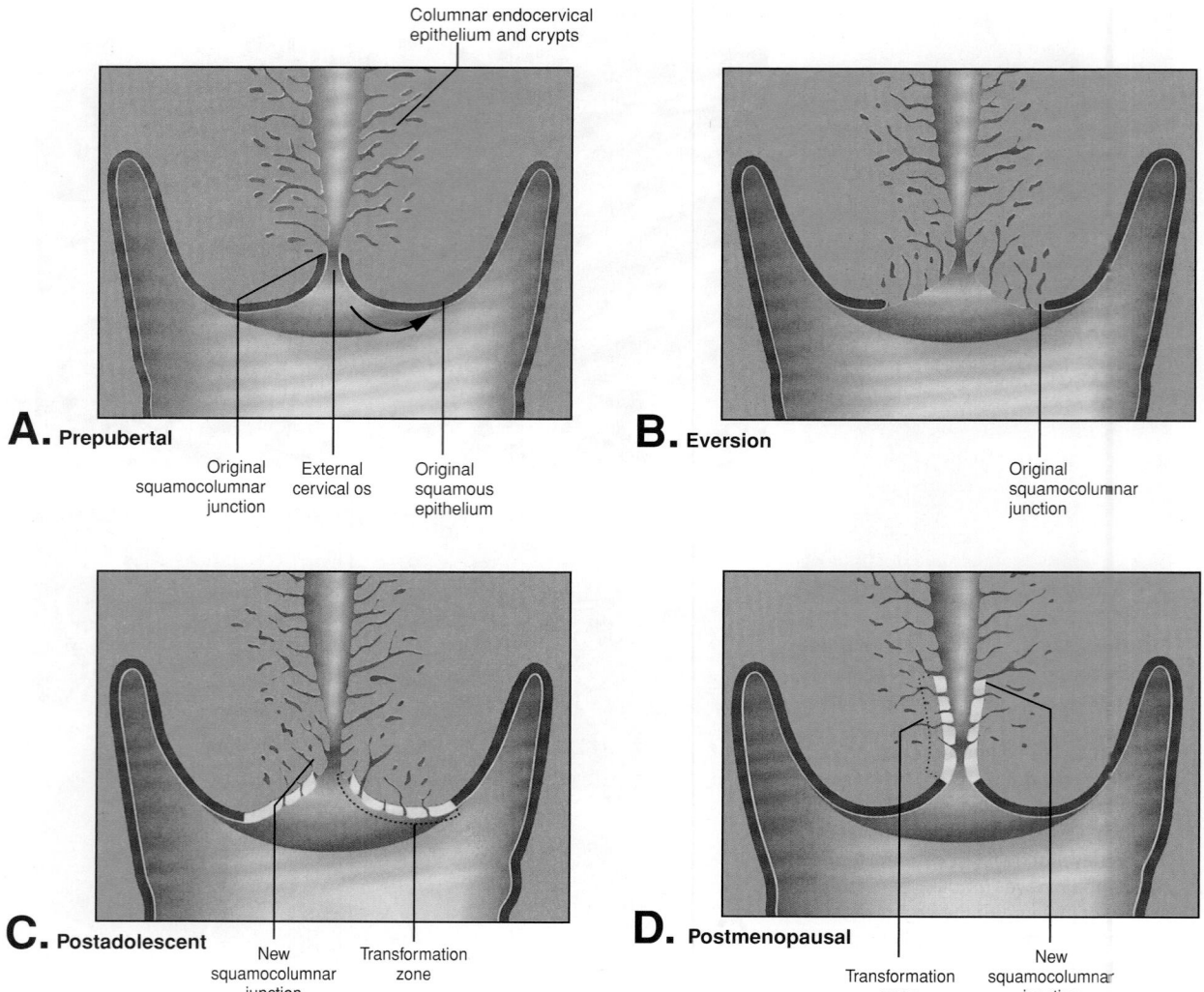

FIGURE 24-13. The transformation zone of the cervix. A. Prepubertal cervix. The squamocolumnar junction is situated at the external cervical os. The *arrow* shows the direction of the movement that takes place as a result of the increase in bulk of the cervix during adolescence. **B. The process of eversion.** On completion, endocervical columnar tissue lies on the vaginal surface of the cervix and is exposed to the vaginal environment. **C. Postadolescent cervix.** The acidity of the vaginal environment is one of the factors that encourages squamous metaplastic change, replacing the exposed columnar epithelium with squamous epithelium. **D. Postmenopausal cervix.** At this time, cervical inversion occurs. This phenomenon is the reverse of eversion, which was so important in adolescence. The transformation zone is now drawn into the cervical canal, often making it inaccessible to colposcopic examination. (Reprinted from Robboy SJ, Anderson MC, Russell P, eds. *Pathology of the Female Reproductive Tract.* 4th ed. London: Churchill-Livingstone; 2002. Copyright © 2002 Elsevier. With permission.)

of these glands, termed **nabothian cysts**. The **external os** is the *macroscopic* junction between the exocervix and endocervix. The **squamocolumnar junction** is the *microscopic* junction of the squamous and mucinous columnar epithelia. The area between the endocervix and endometrial cavity is called the **isthmus** or **lower uterine segment**.

The exocervix remodels continuously throughout life. During embryonic development, upward migration of squamous cells meets columnar epithelium of the endocervix to form the initial squamocolumnar junction (Fig. 24-13). In some young women, this "original" squamocolumnar junction is located at the internal os. In most, however, the columnar epithelium extends onto the exocervix, in which case, the areas of the exocervix lined by columnar epithelium are termed **endocervical ectropion** and appear by colposcopic examination as reddish discolorations. With age, the columnar epithelium of the ectropion undergoes squamous metaplasia and a new squamocolumnar junction is formed at the internal os.

The area between the distalmost squamocolumnar junction and the external os is called the **transformation zone**. Immature squamous epithelium of this zone displays progressive nuclear maturation and increasing amounts of glycogen-free cytoplasm toward the surface. Colposcopy shows a thin white membrane, which eventually becomes thicker and whiter as the squamous epithelium matures (Figs. 24-13 and 24-14). As cells accumulate glycogen, they become indistinguishable from normal squamous epithelium lining the exocervix. The transformation zone is the site of cervical squamous carcinoma (see below).

Examination of the transformation zone by iodine staining is the basis of the **Schiller iodine test**. Normal mature (glycogen-rich) squamous cells lining the exocervix stain

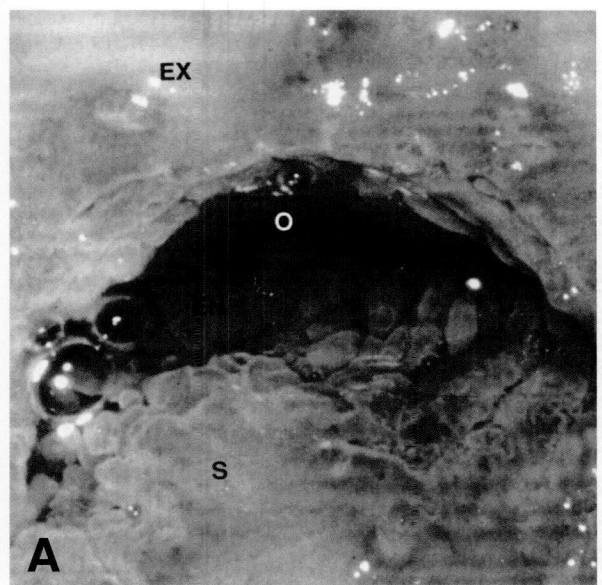

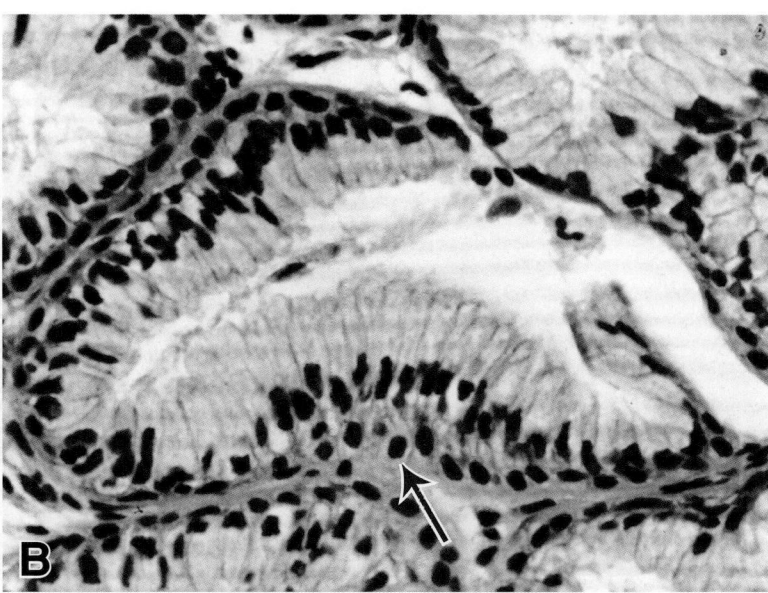

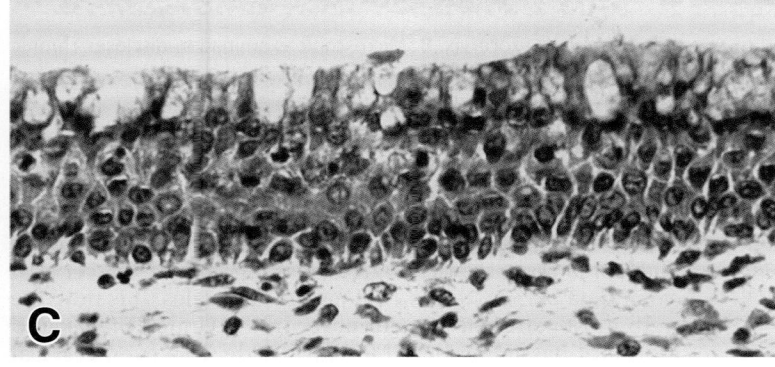

FIGURE 24-14. Squamous metaplasia in the transformation zone. A. In this colposcopic view of the cervix, a white area of metaplastic squamous epithelium (*S*) is situated between the exocervix (*EX*) and the mucinous endocervix (*EN*), which terminates at the internal os (*O*). **B.** In early stages of squamous metaplasia of the transformation zone, reserve cells, which normally constitute a single layer, begin to proliferate (*arrow*). **C.** At a later stage, proliferating reserve cells displace the glandular epithelium. As a final step, metaplastic cells mature into glycogen-rich squamous cells, resembling those in Figure 24-12B.

with iodine and the exocervix appears mahogany brown. If they are immature (glycogen poor), no iodine staining occurs and the exocervix is pale.

CERVICITIS

Inflammation of the cervix is common and is related to constant exposure to bacterial flora in the vagina. Acute and chronic cervicitis are caused by many organisms, particularly endogenous vaginal aerobes and anaerobes, *Streptococcus*, *Staphylococcus*, and *Enterococcus*. Other specific organisms include *C. trachomatis*, *N. gonorrhoeae*, and occasionally herpes simplex type 2. Some agents are sexually transmitted; others may be introduced by foreign bodies, such as residual fragments of tampons and pessaries.

> **PATHOLOGY:** In **acute cervicitis**, the cervix is grossly red, swollen, and edematous, with copious pus "dripping" from the external os. Microscopically, the tissues exhibit extensive polymorphonuclear leukocyte infiltration and stromal edema.
>
> **Chronic cervicitis** is more common. The cervical mucosa is hyperemic (Fig. 24-15) and may show true epithelial erosions. The stroma is infiltrated, principally by lymphocytes and plasma cells. Metaplastic squamous

epithelium of the transformation zone may extend into endocervical glands, forming clusters of squamous epithelium, which must be differentiated from carcinoma.

BENIGN TUMORS AND TUMOR-LIKE CONDITIONS OF THE CERVIX

Endocervical Polyps Are Usually Benign

Endocervical polyps are the most common cervical growths (Fig. 24-16). They appear as single smooth or lobulated masses, usually under 3 cm in greatest dimension. They typically manifest as vaginal bleeding or discharge. The lining epithelium is mucinous, with variable squamous metaplasia, but may feature erosions and granulation tissue if they cause symptoms. Simple excision or curettage is curative. Cancer rarely arises in an endocervical polyp (0.2% of cases).

Microglandular Hyperplasia Reflects Progestational Stimulation

Cervical microglandular hyperplasia is a benign condition showing closely packed vacuolated glands lacking intervening stroma and mixed with a neutrophilic infiltrate. The glands vary in size and are lined by a flattened-to-cuboidal

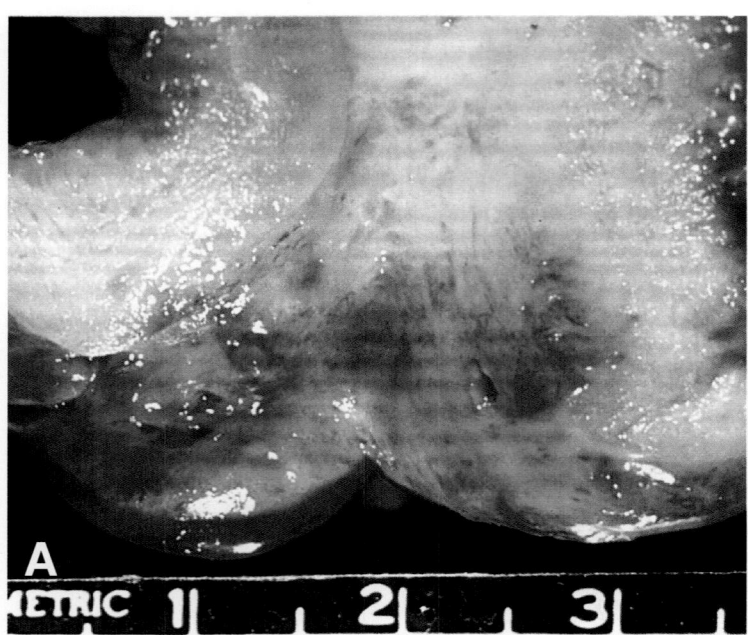

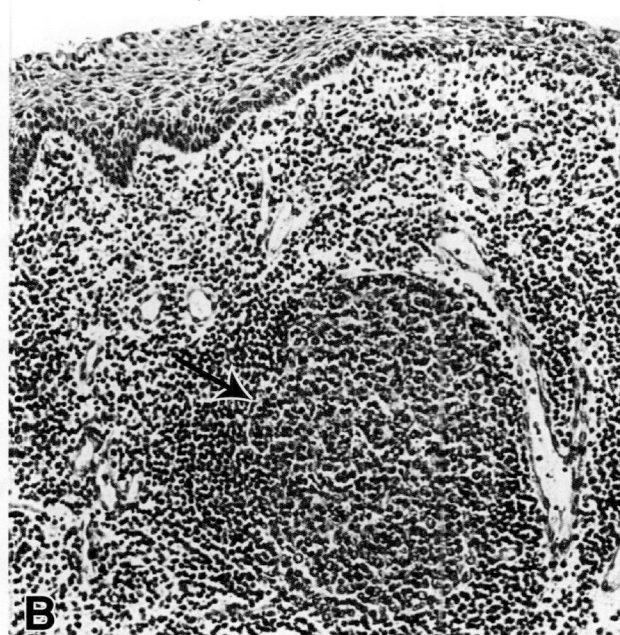

FIGURE 24-15. Chronic cervicitis. A. The cervix has been opened to reveal the reddened exocervix. **B.** Microscopic examination discloses chronic inflammation and the formation of a lymphoid follicle (*arrow*).

epithelium (Fig. 24-17). Nuclei are uniform, and mitoses are rare. Squamous metaplasia and reserve cell hyperplasia are common. It should not be confused with well-differentiated adenocarcinoma. Microglandular hyperplasia is usually asymptomatic and, because it is typically associated with progestin stimulation, it usually occurs during pregnancy, in the postpartum period and in women taking oral contraceptives.

Leiomyomas Can Cause Cervical Bleeding

Cervical leiomyomas can prolapse into the endocervical canal and cause uterine contractions and pain resembling the early phases of labor. The appearance is similar to that of uterine leiomyomas (see below).

SQUAMOUS CELL NEOPLASIA

Fifty years ago, cervical cancer was the leading cause of cancer death in American women. The introduction and widespread use of cytologic screening decreased cervical carcinoma by 50% to 85% in Western countries. It is now the sixth most common female cancer in the United States, and mortality has fallen by 70%. Worldwide, however, cervical cancer remains the second most common cancer in women.

Squamous Intraepithelial Lesions Are Precursors of Invasive Cancer

SILs of the cervix are the effects of human papilloma virus and are designated as low grade (LSILs) or high grade (HSILs) based on the corresponding infecting viral subtype

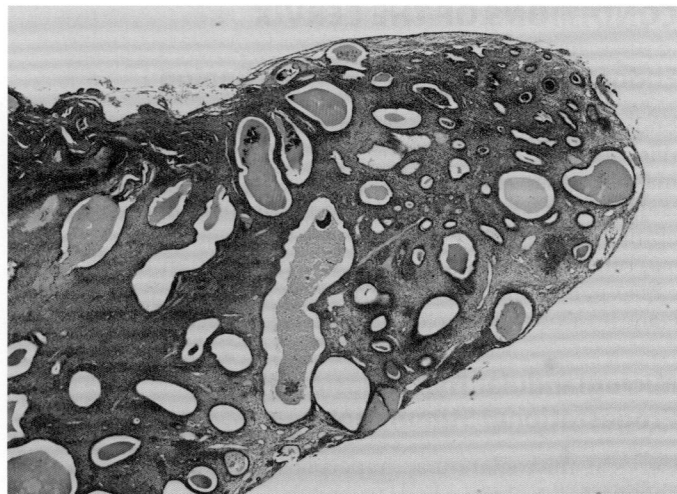

FIGURE 24-16. Endocervical polyp. An epithelial lining covers a fibrovascular core.

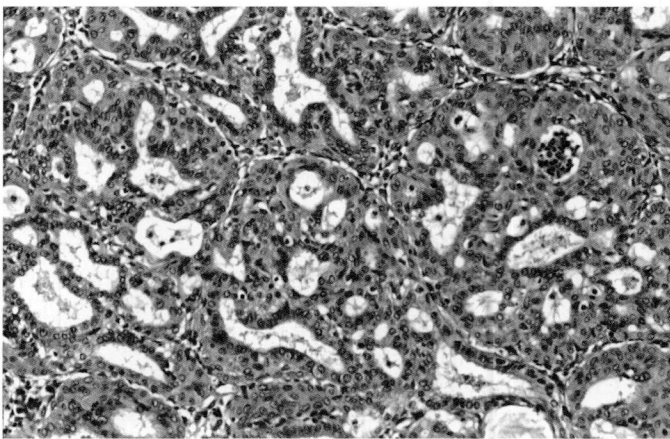

FIGURE 24-17. Microglandular hyperplasia. Small proliferated glands are admixed with a neutrophilic infiltrate.

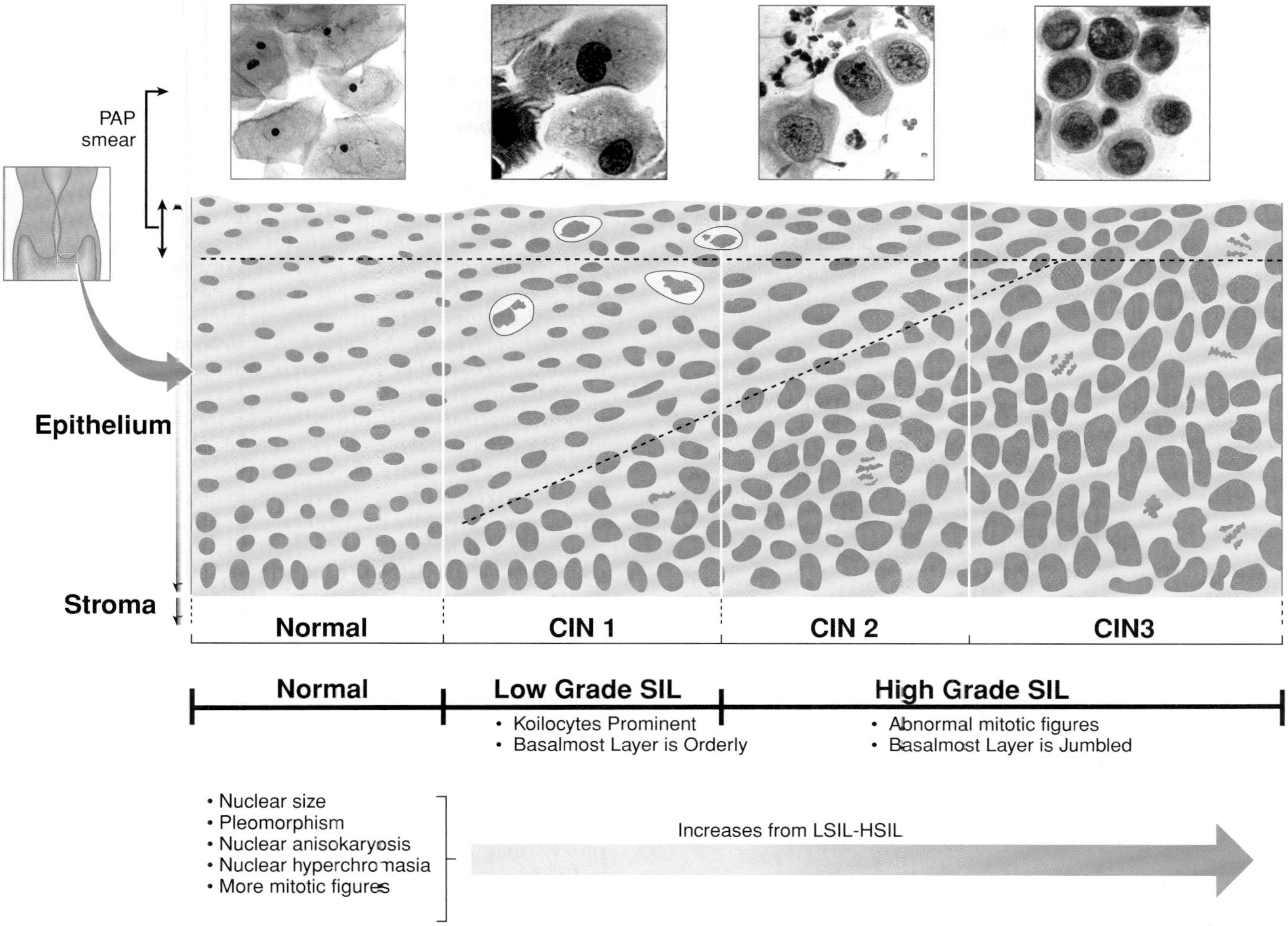

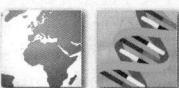

FIGURE 24-18. The Bethesda system for designation of premalignant cervical disease as squamous intraepithelial lesions (SILs). This system integrates multiple aspects across the normal–LSIL (low-grade squamous intraepithelial lesion) and LSIL–HSIL (high-grade squamous intraepithelial lesion) interfaces, which correspond to therapeutic thresholds. It lists qualitative and quantitative features that distinguish low-cancer-risk (LSIL) from high-cancer-risk (HSIL) lesions, which are generally caused by different subtypes of human papillomavirus. It also illustrates approximate counterparts for the legacy cervical intraepithelial neoplasia (CIN) system, which was based on a model of continuous progression rather than dichotomous viral subtypes. Finally, the scheme illustrates the corresponding cytologic smear resulting from exfoliation of the most superficial cells, indicating that even in the mildest disease state, abnormal cells reach the surface and are shed. (Reprinted from Robboy SJ, Anderson MC, Russell P, eds. *Pathology of the Female Reproductive Tract.* 4th ed. London: Churchill-Livingstone; 2002. Copyright © 2002 Elsevier. With permission.)

and risk of progression to invasive squamous cell carcinoma (Fig. 24-18). Squamous precancer terminology was standardized across all anogenital sites in 2012 by the Lower Anogenital Squamous Terminology (LAST) group under the sponsorship of the College of American Pathologists, although legacy terms of cervical intraepithelial neoplasia (CIN), dysplasia, and CIS are commonly used interchangeably.

*Cervical SIL carries a risk for **malignant transformation*** that varies between low- and high-grade subtypes (Figs. 24-18 and 24-19). The disease spectrum is primarily driven by the nature of the infecting virus, with each class demonstrating its own disease spectrum. The grades of SIL are:

- LSIL: CIN-1: mild dysplasia
- HSIL: CIN-2, moderate dysplasia; CIN-3, severe dysplasia, carcinoma in situ. LSIL (CIN-1, mild dysplasia) rarely progresses in severity and commonly disappears. HSIL describes more severe histologic lesions (CIN-2 and

CIN-3), which tend to progress and require treatment. Early phases of infection with all HPV types likely involve episomal viral propagation throughout a polyclonal epithelial field, with an LSIL cytology. Oncogenic types of HPV are prone to subsequent genomic integration of virus and promotion of monoclonal outgrowth of cells driven by transforming viral proteins (E6/E7) with progression to HSIL.

EPIDEMIOLOGY AND MOLECULAR PATHOGENESIS: Epidemiologic features of SIL and invasive cancer are similar. Cervical cancer usually manifests in women 40 to 60 years old (mean 54), but SIL generally occurs before age 40. *The critical factor is HPV infection, which correlates with multiple sexual partners and early age at*

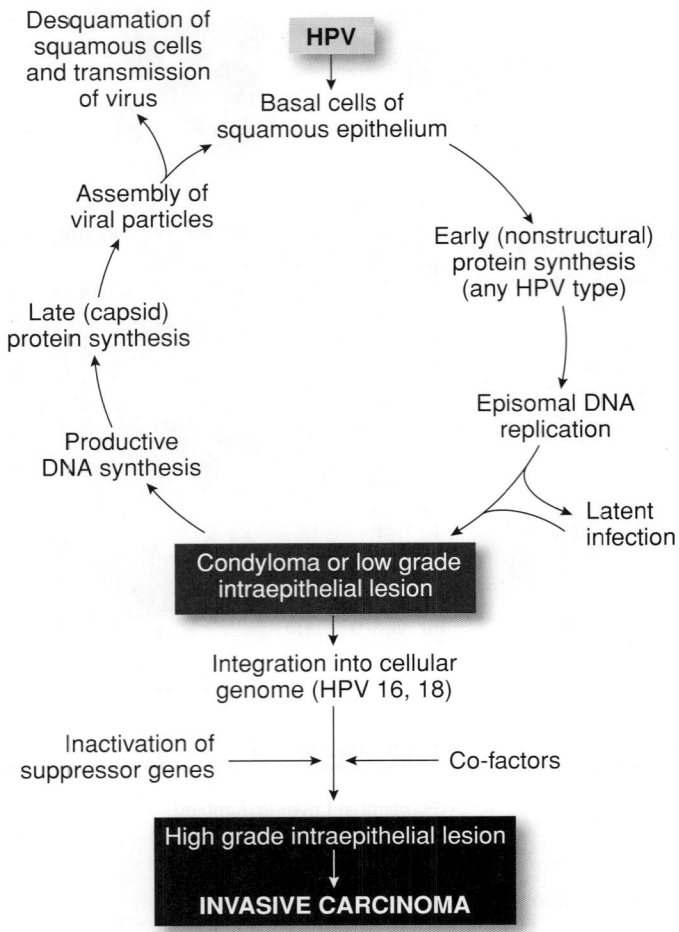

FIGURE 24-19. Role of human papillomavirus (HPV) in the pathogenesis of cervical neoplasia.

first coitus. Thus, SIL is essentially a **sexually transmitted disease**. Smoking increases the incidence of cancer of the cervix, but the mechanism is obscure.

HPV infection leads to SIL and cervical cancer (Fig. 24-19). In LSIL, HPV is episomal and replicates freely to cause cell death. Huge numbers of virus must accumulate in the cytoplasm before being visible as a koilocyte. In most cases of HSIL, viral DNA integrates into the cell genome. Proteins encoded by HPV-16 E6 and E7 genes bind and inactivate p53 and Rb proteins, respectively, and mitigate their tumor suppressor functions (**see Chapter 5**). Once HPV integrates into host DNA, copies of intact virus do not accumulate and koilocytes are absent in many cases of high-grade dysplasia and all invasive cancers.

Roughly 85% of LSIL lesions have low-risk HPV. Genital warts (condylomata acuminata) of the cervix often contain HPV-6 or -11, both considered low-risk HPV types. By contrast, cells in HSIL usually contain HPV types 16, 18, 31, 33, 35, 39, 45, 51, 52, 56, 58, 59, and 68. **HPV types 16 and 18** are found in 70% of invasive cancers; additional high-risk types account for another 25%.

Hormonally induced eversion of the cervix and an acidic vaginal environment encourage development of the transformation zone. Without HPV, benign squamous

metaplasia is the eventual outcome. But in the presence of HPV or other carcinogenic agents, transformation zone stem cells are diverted into SIL and may progress to invasive carcinoma, depending on the subtype and host factors.

PATHOLOGY: The HPV-susceptible cell type has been identified as a cytokeratin 7–expressing stem cell located in the region of the cervical transformation zone between the columnar endocervix and squamous exocervix. *It is the location of the transformation zone and its component cell types on the exposed portion of the cervix that determines the distribution of SIL, and hence cervical cancer.*

The normal process by which cervical squamous epithelium matures is disturbed across the full thickness of SIL, as evidenced by changes in cellularity, differentiation, polarity, nuclear features, and mitotic activity. While the height to which the basaloid cells extend upward in the epithelium generally differs between LSIL and HSIL, this is an oversimplification. For example, the most dramatic changes in **LSIL (CIN-1)** occur not in the base, but rather in koilocytes of the superficial epithelium, which show ballooned cytoplasm and irregular large nuclei caused by episomal virus propagation within differentiated squamous cells that are absent in the base. Features in the basal region related to genomic integration of virus in propagating basal cells are prominent in **HSIL (CIN-2/-3)**. These include disorganization of basal cell alignment along the basement membrane and nuclear changes that persist as cells are pushed upward in the epithelium. Abnormal mitotic figures, pathognomonic of chromosomal aneuploidy, may also be present in HSILs. Thus, grading of individual lesions as HSIL and LSIL requires consideration of all features described in Figure 24-18. The differing histologic changes of LSIL and HSIL are shown in Figure 24-20.

Since abnormal cells are present throughout the epithelium in women with SIL, they are shed into the Pap smear. Nuclear abnormalities and the degree of cytoplasmic differentiation in exfoliated abnormal cells are used to identify SIL and subclassify it as LSIL or HSIL. That this distinction can usually be made in shed cells indicates that morphologic differences between HSIL and LSIL are reflected in superficial as well as deep aspects of the epithelium. But while the Pap smear is an exquisitely sensitive screen for SIL lesions, it is only a screen. Definitive classification is best made in a histologic specimen where the architecture of the full epithelium can be assessed.

Altered vasculature and epithelial changes in cervical SIL can be seen on colposcopic examination. Mosaicism (irregular surface resembling inlaid woodwork) (Fig. 24-21) and vascular punctation are two patterns most often seen in HSIL. The oncogenic process occurs more often on the anterior than the posterior cervical lip and often involves the endocervical glands.

 CLINICAL FEATURES: The mean age at which women develop SIL has declined over the past few decades and is now 25 to 30 years. Seventy percent of cases of LSIL regress, 6% progress to HSIL, and less than 1% become invasive cancer. Progression of

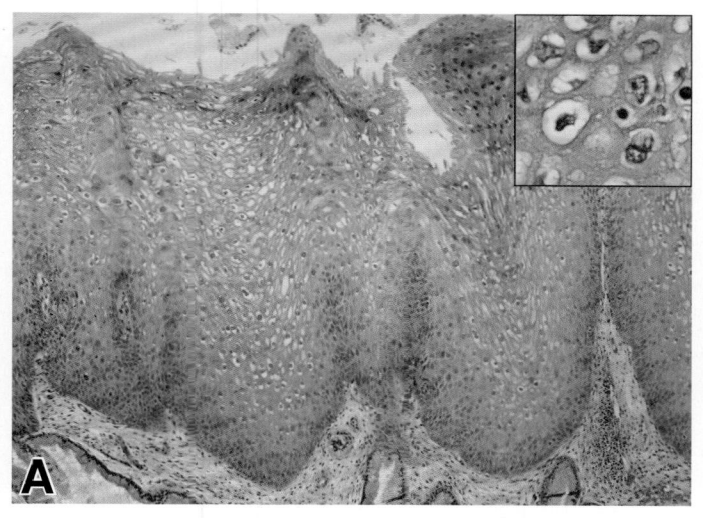

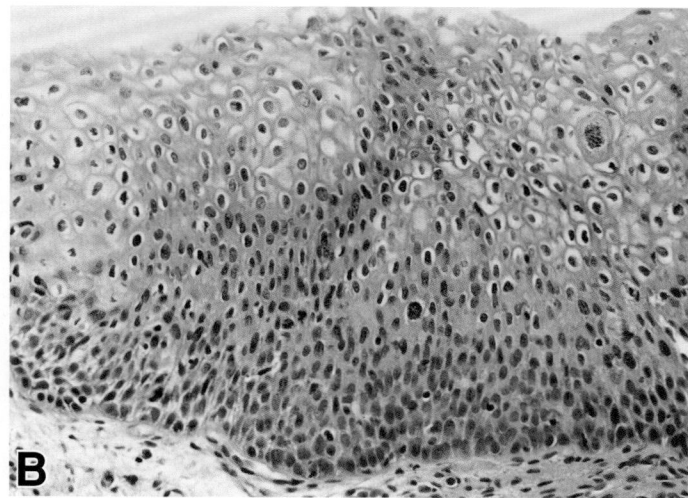

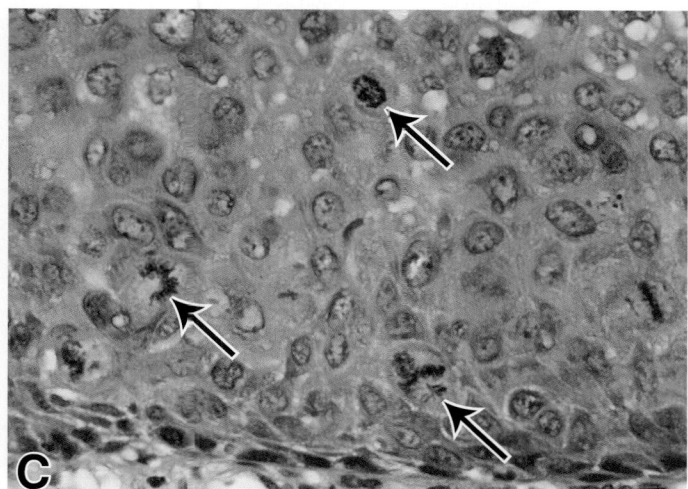

FIGURE 24-20. Cervical squamous intraepithelial lesions (SILs). A. Low-grade SIL (LSIL/CIN-1). The cervical epithelium shows pronounced vacuolated koilocytes (*inset*) in the upper epithelium and a thin basal zone that maintains polarity against the basement membrane. **B.** High-grade SIL (HSIL/CIN-2/-3). Basal cells with integrated HPV proliferate as neoplastic clones through the entire epithelium. Basal cells are disorganized and extend upward to a higher level without differentiation. Koilocytes may occur but are infrequent. **C.** Atypical mitoses (*arrows*) in this HSIL indicate an aneuploid genotype, seen with high-risk viruses. Horseshoe, multipolar, and unequal metaphases are seen.

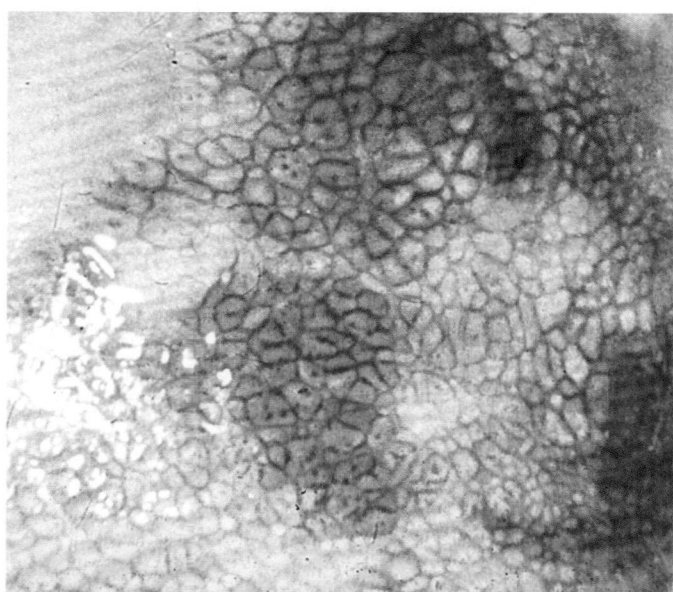

FIGURE 24-21. High-grade squamous intraepithelial lesion (HSIL) of the cervix. Examination with the colposcope discloses a mosaic pattern resembling inlaid woodwork.

HSIL to invasive squamous carcinoma occurs with greater frequency and over a shorter interval, but the exact figures vary with intervening management. *Ten to 20% of cases of HSIL progress to invasive carcinoma if untreated.*

Biopsy is indicated when SIL is discovered on Pap smear. Targeted biopsies may be visually directed by colposcopy, or the entire transformation zone can be removed by a wire "loop" electrosurgical excision procedure (LEEP). LEEP may fulfill both diagnostic and therapeutic functions. Diagnostic endocervical curettage also helps determine the extent of endocervical involvement. Women with LSIL are often followed conservatively (i.e., repeated Pap smears plus close follow-up), although some gynecologists advocate local ablative treatment. High-grade lesions are treated by ablation methods determined by their anatomic distribution. LEEP may be sufficient, if margins are negative. Cervical conization (removal of a cone of tissue around the external os), cryosurgery and (rarely) hysterectomy may also be done. Follow-up smears and clinical examinations should continue for life, as vaginal or vulvar squamous cancer may develop later.

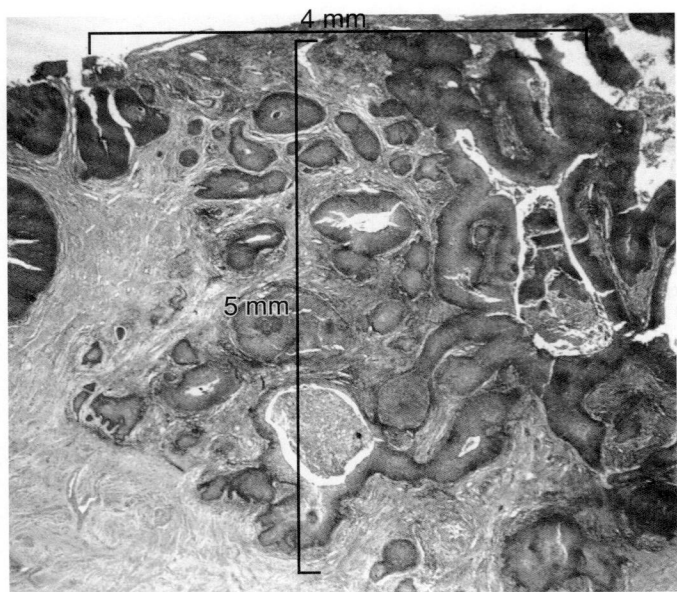

FIGURE 24-22. Invasive squamous cell carcinoma. The tumor invades 5 mm deep and 4 mm wide, exceeding the 3-mm depth limit placed on superficially invasive tumors.

Superficially Invasive Squamous Cell Carcinoma Is the Earliest Stage of Invasive Cervical Cancer

In this setting, stromal invasion usually arises from overlying HSIL. About 7% of specimens removed for CIS show focal superficially invasive cancer. Superficially invasive disease is based on depth of invasion, defined by the International Federation of Gynecology and Obstetrics (FIGO) as invasion less than 5 mm from the basement membrane point of origin (Table 24-2).

The earliest recognizable invasive changes are tiny irregular epithelial buds emanating from the base of HSILs (Fig. 24-22), previously described as being "microinvasive" (Fig. 24-23). The presence of these small (<1 mm) tongues of neoplastic

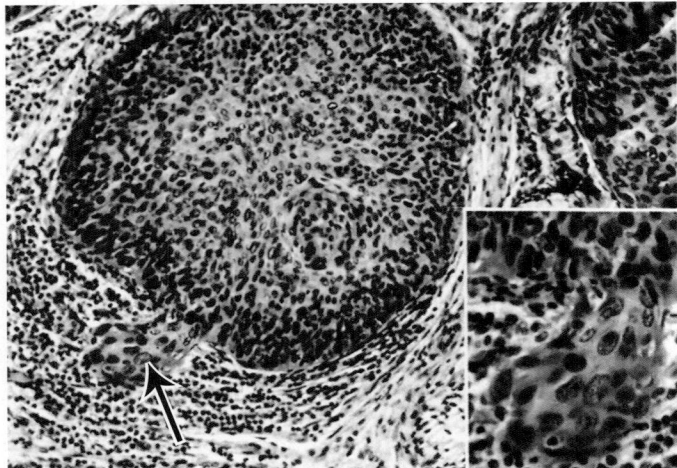

FIGURE 24-23. Early ("microinvasive") stromal invasion in a superficially invasive squamous cell carcinoma. Section of the cervix shows that high-grade squamous intraepithelial lesion (HSIL) in an endocervical gland has broken through the basement membrane (*arrow*) to invade the stroma. *Inset.* A higher-power view of the early invasive focus.

TABLE 24-2

FIGO (2018) STAGING OF CARCINOMA OF THE UTERINE CERVIX

Stage	Anatomic Distribution
Stage I	Carcinoma confined to the uterine cervix (extension to the uterine corpus is disregarded)
IA	Invasive carcinoma that can be diagnosed only microscopically, with deepest invasion <5 mm[a]
IA1	Measured stromal invasion of <3.0 mm
IA2	Measured stromal invasion of ≥3.0 mm and <5.0 mm
IB	Invasive carcinoma with deepest invasion ≥5.0 mm (greater than stage IA), lesions limited to the cervix uteri[b]
IB1	Invasive carcinoma ≥5.0 mm depth of invasion and <2.0 cm in greatest dimension
IB2	Invasive carcinoma ≥2.0 cm and <4.0 cm in greatest dimension
IB3	Invasive carcinoma ≥4.0 cm in greatest dimension
Stage II	Tumor invades beyond the uterus, but not to the pelvic wall or the lower third of the vagina
IIA	Without parametrial invasion
IIA1	Invasive carcinoma <4.0 cm in greatest dimension
IIA2	Invasive carcinoma ≥4.0 cm in greatest dimension
IIB	With parametrial invasion
Stage III	Tumor involves lower third of the vagina and/or extends to the pelvic wall and/or causes hydronephrosis or nonfunctioning kidney and/or involves pelvic and/or paraaortic lymph nodes[c]
IIIA	Tumor involves lower third of the vagina, with no extension to the pelvic wall
IIIB	Tumor extension to the pelvic wall and/or hydronephrosis or nonfunctioning kidney
IIIC	Involvement of pelvic and/or paraaortic lymph nodes, irrespective of tumor size and extent (with r and p notations)[c]
IIIC1	Pelvic lymph node metastasis only
IIIC2	Paraaortic lymph node metastasis
Stage IV	Tumor has extended beyond the true pelvis or has involved (biopsy proven) the mucosa of the bladder or rectum
IVA	Spread to adjacent organs
IVB	Spread to distant organs

[a]Imaging and pathology can be used, where available, to augment clinical findings with respect to tumor size and extent, in all stages.

[b]Involvement of vascular/lymphatic spaces does not change the staging.

[c]Adding notation of r (imaging) and p (pathology) to indicate findings used to allocate the case to stage IIIC.

FIGO = International Federation of Gynecology and Obstetrics.

epithelial cells does not affect the prognosis of HSILs; hence, both can be treated similarly with conservative surgery. The LAST consensus group further limits use of the term "superficially invasive squamous cell carcinoma" to tumors that are not grossly visible. Conization or simple hysterectomy generally cures superficially invasive squamous cell carcinomas.

If the maximum dimensions described above are exceeded, the lesion is no longer considered "superficially invasive," but rather "invasive" squamous cell carcinoma of the cervix (Fig. 24-22; see below). The International Federation of Gynecology and Obstetrics (FIGO) clinical staging criteria (Table 24-2) are widely used to guide management of gynecologic malignancies.

Invasive Squamous Cell Carcinoma Remains Common Worldwide

EPIDEMIOLOGY: Squamous cell carcinoma is by far the most common type of cervical cancer. In the United States (Table 24-3), roughly 13,000 new cases occur annually, which are less than either endometrial or ovarian cancer. However, in underdeveloped areas, where cytologic screening is less available, cervical squamous cancer is still a major cause of cancer death. *Widespread HPV vaccination has the potential to reduce cervical cancer incidence around the world by as much as 90%. Vaccination may also reduce screening intervals and subsequent medical care.* Vaccinated women have reduced rates of HPV-associated precancers.

PATHOLOGY: Early stages of cervical cancer are often poorly defined, granular, eroded lesions or nodular and exophytic masses (Fig. 24-24A). If the tumor resides mainly within the endocervical canal, it can be an endophytic mass that infiltrates stroma and causes diffuse enlargement and hardening of the cervix. Most tumors are nonkeratinizing, with solid nests of large malignant squamous cells and no more than individual

TABLE 24-3				
INCIDENCE OF GYNECOLOGIC CANCER IN THE UNITED STATES (2018, ESTIMATED)				
	New Cases		Death	
	Cases	%ᵃ	Cases	%ᵃ
Endometrium	63,230	3.6	11,350	1.9
Ovary	22,440	1.3	14,080	2.3
Cervix, invasive	13,240	0.8	4,170	0.7
Vulva, invasive	6,190	0.4	1,200	0.2
Vagina and other, invasive	5,170	<1	1,330	<1

ᵃ% = percentage of all cases of cancer in females.
American Cancer Society Statistics.

cell keratinization. Most remaining cancers show nests of keratinized cells in concentric whorls, the so-called keratin pearls (Fig. 24-24B). The least common, and most aggressive, tumor is small cell carcinoma. It consists of infiltrating masses of small, cohesive, nonkeratinized, malignant cells, and has the worst prognosis.

Cervical cancer spreads by direct extension or through lymphatic vessels (Fig. 24-25) and only rarely by the hematogenous route. Local extension into surrounding tissues (parametrium) (stage IIIB) may result in **ureteral compression** and cause clinical complications of hydroureter, hydronephrosis, and renal failure, the most common cause of death (50% of patients). Bladder and rectal involvement (stage IVA) may lead to fistula formation. Lymphatic spread leads to metastases in paracervical, hypogastric, and external iliac nodes. Overall, tumor growth and spread are relatively slow; the average age for patients with stage 0 tumor (HSIL) is 35 to 40 years; for stage IA, 43 years; and for stage IV, 57 years.

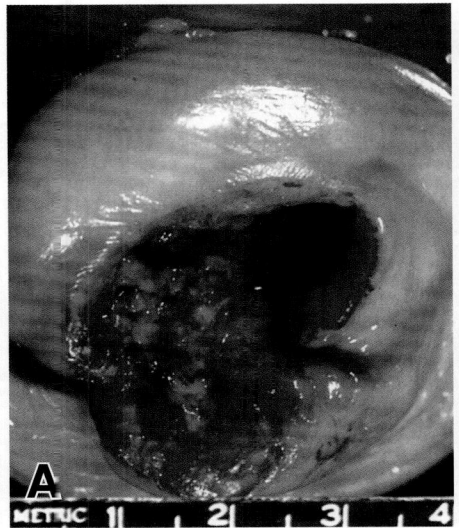
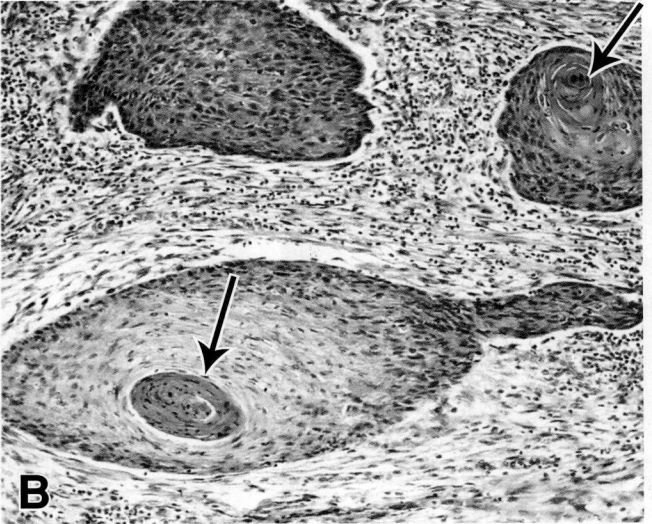

FIGURE 24-24. Squamous cell cancer. A. The cervix is distorted by the presence of an exophytic, ulcerated squamous cell carcinoma. **B.** The keratinizing pattern of the tumor is manifested as whorls of keratinized cells ("keratin pearls") (*arrows*).

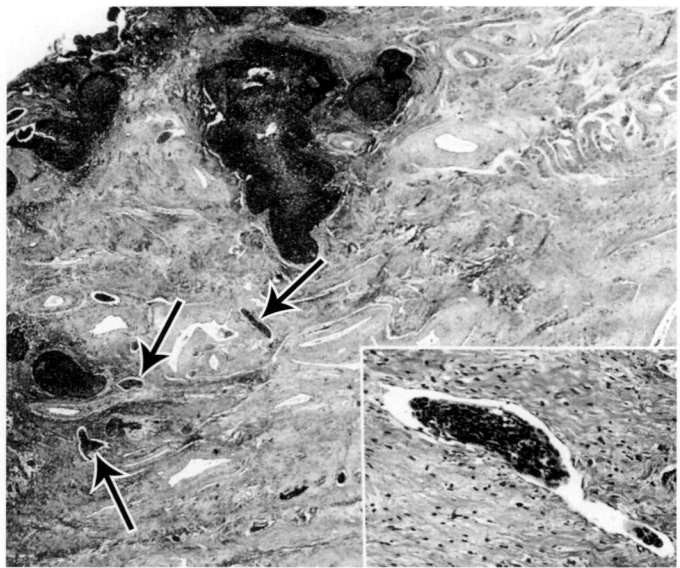

FIGURE 24-25. Squamous cell cancer of the cervix with lymphatic invasion. Low magnification shows a squamous cell carcinoma that has invaded the stroma and permeated lymphatics (*arrows*). *Inset.* A high-power view of lymphatic invasion.

CLINICAL FEATURES: In early stages of cervical cancer, patients complain most often of vaginal bleeding after intercourse or douching. With more advanced tumors, symptoms are referable to the route and degree of spread. The Pap smear remains the most reliable screening test for detecting cervical cancer.

The anatomic stage of cervical cancer is the best predictor of survival (Table 24-2): 5-year survival is 90% in stage I; 75% in II; 35% in III; and 10% in VI, for an overall 5-year survival rate of 60%. About 15% of patients develop recurrences on the vaginal wall, bladder, pelvis, or rectum within 2 years of therapy. Radical hysterectomy is favored for localized tumor, especially in younger women; radiation therapy or combinations of the two are used for more advanced tumors.

Endocervical Adenocarcinoma Accounts for 20% of Malignant Cervical Tumors

The incidence of cervical adenocarcinoma has increased recently, with a mean age of 56 years at presentation. Most tumors are of endocervical cell (mucinous) type, but the various subtypes have little bearing on overall survival. Adenocarcinoma shares epidemiologic factors with squamous carcinoma of the cervix and spreads similarly. They are often associated with adenocarcinoma in situ and contain HPV types 16 or 18.

PATHOLOGY: *ADENOCARCINOMA IN SITU:* Also called **cervical glandular intraepithelial neoplasia**, this lesion generally arises at the squamocolumnar junction and extends into the endocervical canal. The pattern of spread and involvement of endocervical glands resemble those of cervical SIL. Adenocarcinoma in situ is intraepithelial, maintaining normal endocervical gland architecture. The cells show slight enlargement, atypical hyperchromatic nuclei, increased nuclear-to-cytoplasmic ratio, apoptosis, and variable mitoses. Abrupt transitions help distinguish neoplastic from neighboring normal endocervical cells. Squamous HSIL occurs in 40% of cases of adenocarcinoma in situ.

INVASIVE ADENOCARCINOMA: This tumor typically presents as a fungating polypoid (Fig. 24-26A) or papillary mass. Exophytic tumors often have a papillary pattern (Fig. 24-26B), whereas endophytic ones display tubular or glandular patterns. Most endocervical adenocarcinomas (usual-type; 75%) are HPV-related, whereas the remaining tumors include the gastric-type and clear cell carcinomas which are unrelated to HPV infection and are more aggressive neoplasms.

Adenocarcinoma of the endocervix spreads by local invasion and lymphatic metastases, but overall survival is somewhat worse than for squamous carcinoma. Treatment is similar to that for squamous carcinoma.

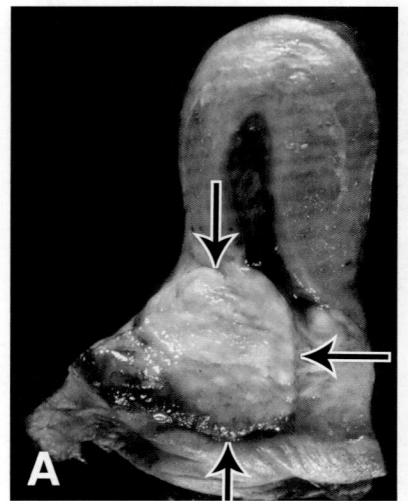
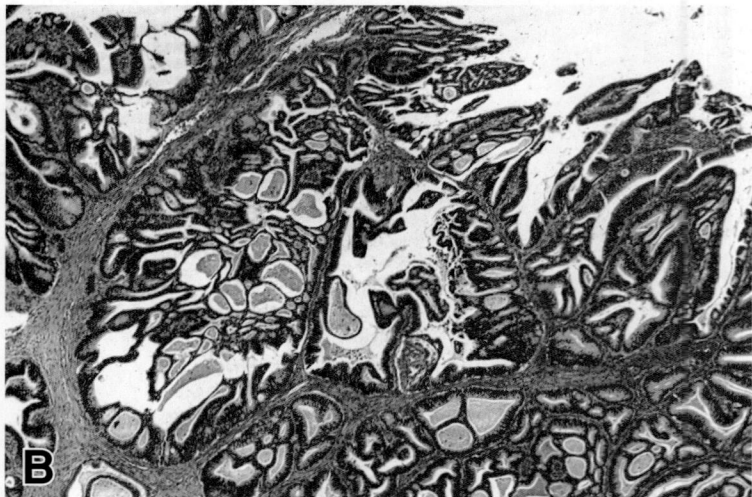

FIGURE 24-26. Endocervical adenocarcinoma. A. The endocervical tumor appears as a polypoid mass (*arrows*). **B.** Microscopic view of endocervical adenocarcinoma showing a papillary pattern of growth.

Uterus

ANATOMY

The uterine corpus (body) is smaller than the cervix at birth and during childhood but increases rapidly in size after puberty. The endometrium is composed of glands and stroma. It is thin at birth, when it consists of a continuous surface of cuboidal epithelium that dips to line a few sparse tubular glands. After puberty, it thickens. The superficial two-thirds, the "zona functionalis," responds to hormones and is shed with each menstrual phase. The deepest third, the basal layer is the germinative portion that regenerates a new functional zone with each cycle.

The endometrium is supplied by arcuate arteries that traverse the outer myometrium and give off two sets of vessels, one to the myometrium and the other, the radial arteries, to the endometrium. In turn, the radial arteries branch into two types of vessels. The basal arteries supply the basal endometrium and the spiral arteries nourish the superficial two-thirds.

THE MENSTRUAL CYCLE

Normal endometrium undergoes sequential changes that support growth of implanted fertilized ova (zygotes). If conception does not occur, the endometrium is shed, and then regenerated to support a fertilized ovum in the next cycle (Fig. 24-27).

MENSTRUAL PHASE: Without a blastocyst to secrete human chorionic gonadotropin (hCG), ovarian granulosa and thecal cells degenerate. Progesterone levels fall. The endometrium becomes desiccated, spiral arteries collapse, and stroma disintegrates. Menses start at day 28, last 3 to 7 days and result in loss of about 35 mL of blood. The denuded surface is regenerated by extension of the residual glandular epithelium.

PROLIFERATIVE PHASE: The endometrium responds to estrogenic stimulation during days 3 to 15 of the menstrual cycle. Tubular to coiled glands in the functional zone are evenly distributed and supported by a cellular, monomorphic stroma (Fig. 24-27A). Glands are narrow early in the proliferative phase but coil and increase slightly in caliber over time. Columnar cells lining tubules increase from one layer in thickness to a mitotically active pseudostratified epithelium. The glands secrete a watery alkaline fluid that facilitates passage of sperm through the endometrium into the fallopian tubes. The stroma is also mitotically active. Spiral arteries are narrow and inconspicuous.

SECRETORY PHASE: Ovulation occurs about 14 days after the last menstrual period. The graafian follicle that discharged its ovum becomes a corpus luteum. Granulosa cells of the corpus luteum secrete progesterone, which transforms the endometrium from a proliferative to a secretory state.

Day of Cycle		3–15	15–16	17	18	19–22	23	24–25	26–27	1–2
Post-ovulatory day			1–2	3	4	5–8	9	10–11	12–13	14+
Cycle phases		Proliferative	Interval	Early secretory		Mid-secretory			Late secretory	Menstrual
Key feature		Mitoses	Mitoses and subnuclear vacuoles	Maximum subnuclear vacuoles	Subnuclear vacuoles present	Stromal edema	Focal predecidua around spiral arteries	Patchy predecidua	Extensive predecidua	Stroma crumbling
Microscopic features of functional zone	Stroma	Loose stroma. Mitoses	Same as proliferative	Loose stroma. Scanty mitoses	Loose stroma	Stromal edema	Focal predecidua around spiral arteries. Edema prominent	Predecidua throughout stroma. Some edema	Extensive predecidua. Prominent granulated lymphocytes	Stroma crumbling. Hemorrhage
	Glands	Straight to tightly coiled tubules. Mitoses	Some subnuclear vacuoles, otherwise as proliferative	Extensive subnuclear vacuoles	Dilated glands. Some subnuclear vacuoles	Dilated glands with irregular outline. Luminal secretion		'Saw tooth' glands	Prominent 'saw tooth' glands	Disrupted glands. Secretory exhaustion. Regenerating epithelium
Appearances		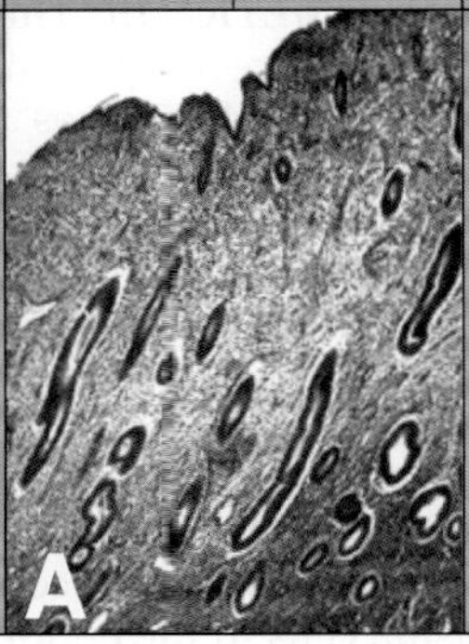				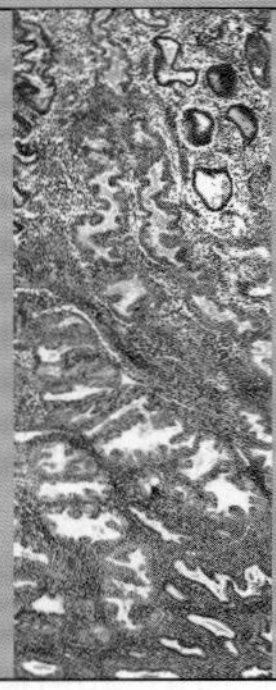			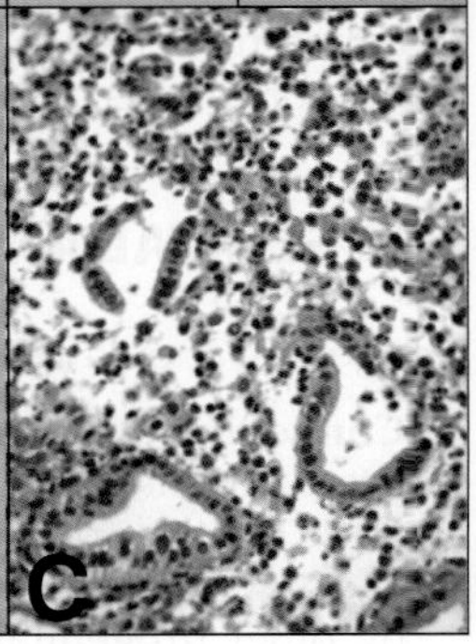	

FIGURE 24-27. Main histologic features of the endometrial phases of the normal menstrual cycle. A. Proliferative phase. Straight tubular glands are embedded in a cellular monomorphic stroma. **B.** Secretory phase, day 24. Dilated tortuous glands with serrated borders are situated in a predecidual stroma. **C.** Menstrual endometrium. Fragmented glands, dissolution of the stroma and numerous neutrophils are evident. (Reprinted from Robboy SJ, Anderson MC, Russell P, eds. *Pathology of the Female Reproductive Tract.* 4th ed. London: Churchill-Livingstone; 2002. Copyright © 2002 Elsevier. With permission.)

- **Days 17–19 (postovulatory days 3 to 5):** Endometrial glands enlarge, dilate, and become more coiled. The lining cells develop abundant and prominent, glycogen-rich, subnuclear vacuoles (day 17). Over the next several days, these cells produce copious secretions that support the zygote as it develops early chorionic villi capable of invading the endometrium.
- **Days 20–22 (postovulatory days 6 to 8):** The endometrium displays prominent stromal edema. Cells lining the glands have homogeneous cytoplasm with a few discrete vacuoles and the glands are dilated and more tortuous.
- **Day 23 (postovulatory day 9):** Stromal cells surrounding spiral arterioles enlarge and exhibit large, round, vesicular nuclei and abundant eosinophilic cytoplasm ("vascular cuffing"). With time, these cells become more extensively distributed until they fill the functionalis. They are precursors of the decidual cells of pregnancy and are referred to as "predecidua."
- **Day 27 (postovulatory day 13):** The entire stroma is now predecidualized and ready for menstruation. Tubular glands continue to dilate and develop serrated (sawtoothed) borders.

ATROPHIC ENDOMETRIUM: After menopause, the number of glands and quantity of stroma diminish. Remaining glands have a thin epithelium and the stroma contains abundant collagen. Glands of the atrophic endometrium are often quite dilated, and this condition is called **senile cystic atrophy of the endometrium.**

ENDOMETRIUM OF PREGNANCY

The corpus luteum of pregnancy requires continuous stimulation by hCG secreted by placental trophoblast of the developing embryo. Trophoblast begins to develop at about day 23. Under hCG stimulation, the corpus luteum increases its progesterone output, stimulating secretion of fluid by endometrial glands. In the hypersecretory endometrium of pregnancy, highly dilated glands are lined by cells with abundant glycogen. These features can persist for up to 8 weeks after delivery.

The hypersecretory response may be exaggerated with intrauterine pregnancy, ectopic pregnancy, or trophoblastic disease. Glandular cell nuclei may enlarge and appear bulbous and polyploid, owing to DNA replication without cell division. These nuclei protrude beyond the apparent cellular cytoplasmic limits into the gland lumen, an appearance referred to as the **Arias-Stella phenomenon** (Fig. 24-28). Enlarged nuclei are polyploid rather than aneuploid, a condition sometimes seen in adenocarcinoma.

CONGENITAL ANOMALIES OF THE UTERUS

Congenital anomalies of the uterus are rare.

- **Congenital absence of the uterus (agenesis)** reflects failure of müllerian ducts to develop. Since elongation of these ducts during embryonic life requires wolffian ducts as guides, uterine agenesis is almost always accompanied by other urogenital tract anomalies and agenesis of the vagina and fallopian tubes.
- **Uterus didelphys** is a double uterus, due to failure of the two müllerian ducts to fuse in early embryonic life. A double vagina commonly accompanies this anomaly.

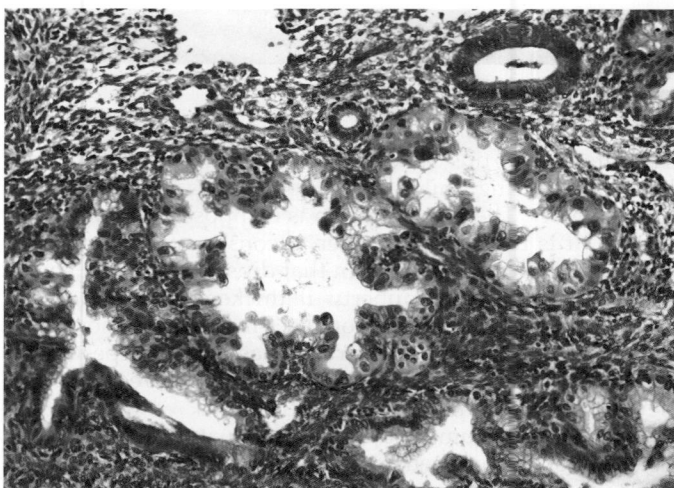

FIGURE 24-28. Arias-Stella reaction of pregnancy associated with human chorionic gonadotropin (hCG) stimulation. A section of endometrium shows enlarged, bulbous nuclei that protrude into the gland lumen.

- **Uterus duplex bicornis** is a uterus with a common fused wall between two distinct endometrial cavities. The common wall between the apposed müllerian ducts fails to degenerate to form a single uterine cavity.
- **Uterus septus** is a single uterus with a partial septum, due to incomplete resorption of the wall of the fused müllerian ducts. These patients have increased risk for habitual abortion.
- **Bicornuate uterus** refers to a uterus with two cornua (horns) and a common cervix. Didelphic and bicornuate uterine fusion defects increase the risk of premature birth only slightly.

ENDOMETRITIS

In endometritis, or an inflamed endometrium, there is an abnormal inflammatory infiltrate in the endometrium. It must be distinguished from the normal presence of neutrophils during menstruation and mild lymphocytic infiltrates at other times. In most cases of endometritis, findings are nonspecific and rarely point to a specific cause.

ACUTE ENDOMETRITIS: This condition is defined as the abnormal presence of polymorphonuclear leukocytes in the endometrium. Most cases result from an ascending infection from the cervix (e.g., after the usually impervious cervical barrier is compromised by abortion, delivery, or medical instrumentation). Curettage is diagnostic and often curative, because it removes necrotic tissue that has served as the nidus of the ongoing infection. Of little significance now, acute endometritis was dangerous before the availability of antibiotics.

CHRONIC ENDOMETRITIS: Although lymphocytes and lymphoid follicles occur occasionally in normal endometrium, plasma cells in the endometrium are diagnostic of chronic endometritis (Fig. 24-29). The disorder is associated with IUDs, PID, and retained products of conception after an abortion or delivery. Without a culture, the pathologic findings alone do not distinguish between infective and

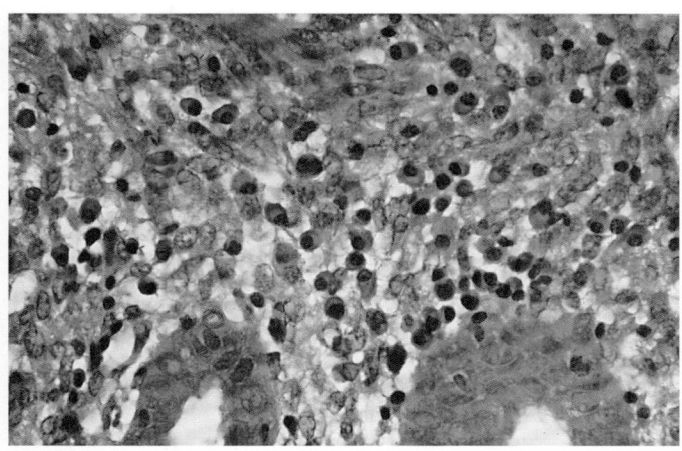

FIGURE 24-29. Chronic endometritis. The inflammatory infiltrate is composed largely of lymphocytes and plasma cells. (Reprinted with permission from Stanley J. Robboy, MD, and Gynecologic Pathology Associates, Durham and Chapel Hill, North Carolina.)

noninfective causes. Patients usually complain of bleeding and/or pelvic pain. The condition is generally self-limited.

PYOMETRA: Defined as pus in the endometrial cavity, pyometra is associated with gross anatomic defects such as fistulous tracts between bowel and uterine cavity, bulky or perforating malignancies or cervical stenosis. Long-standing pyometra may rarely be associated with development of endometrial squamous cell cancer.

TRAUMATIC LESIONS

INTRAUTERINE DEVICE: IUDs predispose to (1) increased menstrual flow, (2) uterine perforation, and (3) spontaneous abortion if conception occurs with the IUD in place. However, IUD use reduces endometrial cancer risk by half. Much

of the adverse publicity about IUDs was related to early devices. Only 1% of women who desire contraception now use an IUD.

INTRAUTERINE ADHESIONS (ASHERMAN SYNDROME): Intrauterine fibrous adhesions sometimes develop after curettage, particularly for postpartum complications or therapeutic abortion. These bands traverse, but do not necessarily obliterate, the endometrial cavity. Additional complications include amenorrhea or, in the event of a subsequent pregnancy, increased abortion rates, preterm labor, and placenta accreta.

ADENOMYOSIS

Adenomyosis is the presence of endometrial glands and stroma within the myometrium. Pain, dysmenorrhea, or menorrhagia correlates with adenomyosis if the glands are 1 mm or more beneath the endometrial myometrial junction, and symptoms become more severe as glands penetrate more deeply into the myometrium. Pain develops as foci of adenomyosis enlarge when blood is entrapped during menses. One-fifth of all surgically removed uteri show some adenomyosis.

PATHOLOGY: The uterus may be enlarged. The myometrium contains small, soft, tan areas, some of which are cystic (Fig. 24-30). Microscopic examination shows glands lined by proliferative to inactive endometrium and surrounded by endometrial stroma with varying degrees of fibrosis. Secretory changes are rare, except during pregnancy or in patients treated with progestins. The adjacent myometrium is often hypertrophic and nodular. The uterus may also become enlarged from cyclic bleeding into these foci. Extension of hyperplastic or neoplastic endometrium from the endometrial functionalis into adenomyotic foci may occur.

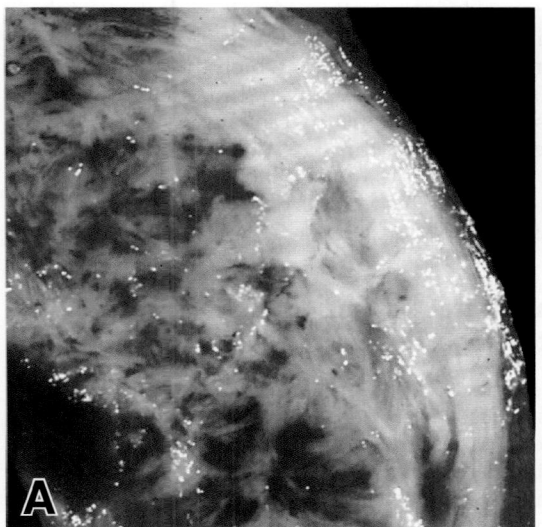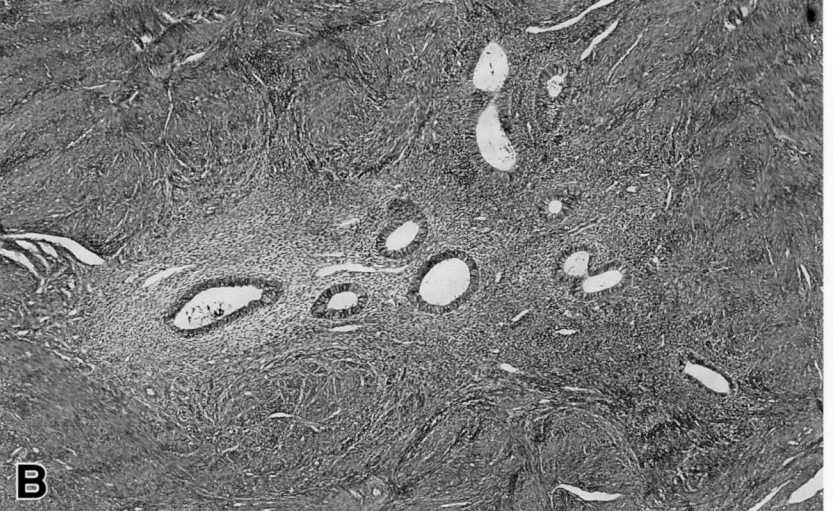

FIGURE 24-30. Adenomyosis. A. The cut surface of the uterus reveals small, red areas corresponding to endometrial glands in the myometrium. (Reprinted from Fobboy SJ, Anderson MC, Russell P, eds. *Pathology of the Female Reproductive Tract.* 4th ed. London: Churchill-Livingstone; 2002. Copyright © 2002 Elsevier. With permission.) **B.** A microscopic view shows endometrial glands and stroma within the myometrium.

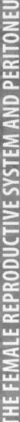

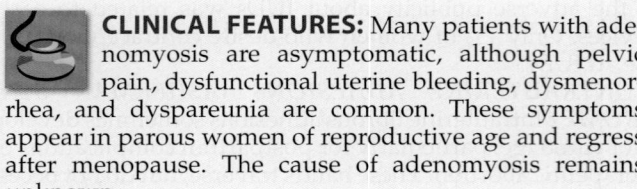 **CLINICAL FEATURES:** Many patients with adenomyosis are asymptomatic, although pelvic pain, dysfunctional uterine bleeding, dysmenorrhea, and dyspareunia are common. These symptoms appear in parous women of reproductive age and regress after menopause. The cause of adenomyosis remains unknown.

HORMONAL EFFECTS

Contraceptive Steroids Prevent Pregnancy and Many Gynecologic Cancers

Oral contraceptive agents induce endometrial changes depending on the types, potencies and dosages of estrogens and progestins in individual formulations. Combined preparations generally contain potent progestins and weak estrogens. Pseudodecidual change thus appears early and overshadows the weak glandular growth. After several cycles, endometrial glands atrophy. Newer contraceptive combinations contain lower doses of hormones and elicit less change. Women who use contraceptives containing progestational agents have significantly lower rates of endometrial and ovarian cancer, reflecting the growth-inhibiting properties of progesterone and fewer ovulations (see below).

Dysfunctional Uterine Bleeding Occurs During or Between Menstrual Periods

Dysfunctional bleeding is among the most common gynecologic disorders of women of reproductive age but it remains poorly understood. Its causes lie outside the uterus. Most cases are related to a disturbance in the hypothalamic–pituitary–ovarian axis (Table 24-4). Ovarian dysfunction also occurs, especially in the presence of anovulation.

Some causes of menstrual irregularity are intrinsic to the uterus and are not considered dysfunctional. These include (1) growths (e.g., carcinoma, endometrial intraepithelial neoplasia [EIN], submucosal leiomyomata, and polyps), (2) inflammation (e.g., endometritis), (3) pregnancy (e.g., complications of intrauterine or ectopic pregnancy), and (4) the effects of IUDs (Table 24-4).

Anovulatory Bleeding Is the Most Common Form of Dysfunctional Bleeding

Anovulatory bleeding is a complex syndrome of many causes that manifests as the absence of ovulation during the reproductive years. It occurs most often at either end of reproductive life (i.e., menarche and menopause).

  ETIOLOGIC FACTORS AND PATHOLOGY: In an anovulatory cycle, failure of ovulation leads to excessive and prolonged estrogen stimulation, without a postovulatory rise in progesterone. As a result, the endometrium remains in a proliferative state dominated by a disordered, cystic glandular appearance, and excessive bulk. Lacking progesterone, the spiral arteries of the endometrium do not develop normally. "Breakthrough bleeding"

TABLE 24-4	
CAUSES OF ABNORMAL UTERINE BLEEDING (INCLUDING UTERINE AND EXTRAUTERINE CAUSES)	
Newborn	Maternal Estrogen
Childhood	Iatrogenic (trauma, foreign body, infection of vagina)
	Vaginal neoplasms (sarcoma botryoides)
	Ovarian tumors (functional)
Adolescence	Hypothalamic immaturity
	Psychogenic and nutritional problems
	Inadequate luteal function
Reproductive age	Anovulatory
	Central: psychogenic, stress
	Systemic: nutritional and endocrine disease
	Gonadal: functional tumors
	End-organ: benign endometrial hyperplasia
	Pregnancy: ectopic, retained placenta, abortion, mole
	Ovulatory
	Organic: neoplasia, infections (PID), leiomyomas
	Polymenorrhea: short follicular or luteal phases
	Iatrogenic: anticoagulants, IUD
Menopause	Irregular shedding
Postmenopause	Carcinoma, EIN, benign hyperplasias, polyps, leiomyomata

EIN = endometrial intraepithelial neoplasia; IUD = intrauterine device; PID = pelvic inflammatory disease.

can occur from damage to these fragile spiral arterioles. Thrombosis causes local tissue breakdown resembling that of menstrual endometrium, which the patient experiences as symptomatic bleeding out of synchrony with other areas of the endometrium. Elevated estrogen levels usually decline, either through delayed ovulation or involution of the stimulatory follicle. If the decline is rapid, the endometrium undergoes a heavy synchronized menstrual flow.

Luteal Phase Defect Is Caused by Inadequate Progesterone

Luteal phase defect results in an abnormally short cycle in which menses occur 6 to 9 days after the surge of luteinizing hormone (LH) associated with ovulation. It occurs when a corpus luteum develops improperly or regresses prematurely. Luteal phase defects are responsible for 3% of cases of infertility and must be considered in assessing infertility or abnormal uterine bleeding. A biopsy showing an endometrium over 2 days delayed from the chronologic day of the menstrual cycle confirms the diagnosis.

ENDOMETRIAL TUMORS

Endometrial Polyps Are Benign Stromal Neoplasms

Polyps occur mostly in the perimenopausal period and not before menarche. They are monoclonal outgrowths of endometrial stromal cells altered by chromosomal translocation, with secondary induction of polyclonal glandular elements. Stroma and glands of endometrial polyps respond poorly to hormonal stimulation and do not slough upon menstruation.

PATHOLOGY: Most endometrial polyps arise in the fundus (Fig. 24-31) but can occur anywhere within the endometrium. They vary in size from several millimeters to growths filling the entire endometrial cavity. Most are solitary, but 20% are multiple. Polyp cores are composed of (1) endometrial glands, often cystically dilated and hyperplastic; (2) fibrous endometrial stroma; and (3) thick-walled, coiled, dilated blood vessels, derived from a straight artery that normally would have supplied the basal zone of the endometrium. Cores are covered by endometrial epithelium, usually out of cycle from adjacent normal endometrium.

CLINICAL FEATURES: Endometrial polyps typically present with intermenstrual bleeding, owing to surface ulceration or hemorrhagic infarction. Since bleeding in an older woman may indicate endometrial cancer, this sign must be evaluated thoroughly. Endometrial polyps are not ordinarily precancerous, but up to 0.5% harbor adenocarcinoma.

Endometrial Hyperplasia Is Two Diseases, One of Which Is Neoplastic

The 2014 WHO classification of endometrial hyperplasias divides lesions into etiologic subgroups based on cancer risk and treatment options. **Nonatypical endometrial hyperplasia** is a functionally normal endometrium that responds to excess estrogen; **endometrial intraepithelial neoplasia** (**EIN**, also called **atypical endometrial hyperplasia**) is composed of mutated precancerous cells that grow as a neoplastic clone.

- **Nonatypical hyperplasia:** Nonatypical endometrial hyperplasia includes a spectrum of changes, dependent upon the duration and dose of estrogen exposure. Glands are irregularly distributed and punctuated by cysts, creating a variably increased ratio of glands to stroma. Cytologic changes, when they occur, mostly involve metaplasia distributed in a scattered, nongeographic, or random fashion. Carcinoma develops in 1% to 3%.
- **EIN (atypical hyperplasia):** Endometrial intraepithelial neoplasia, or atypical endometrial hyperplasia, is a clonal outgrowth of genetically altered endometrial glands with an increased risk of future endometrioid endometrial carcinoma through malignant transformation. EIN is composed of crowded aggregates of cytologically altered tubular or slightly branching glands. Within the geographic confines of the lesion, the area of glands exceeds that of stroma, with altered cytology compared to residual background normal glands, which may be adjacent to and/or admixed with the lesion. Thirty-seven percent of patients with EIN will develop carcinoma, almost always of the endometrioid type.

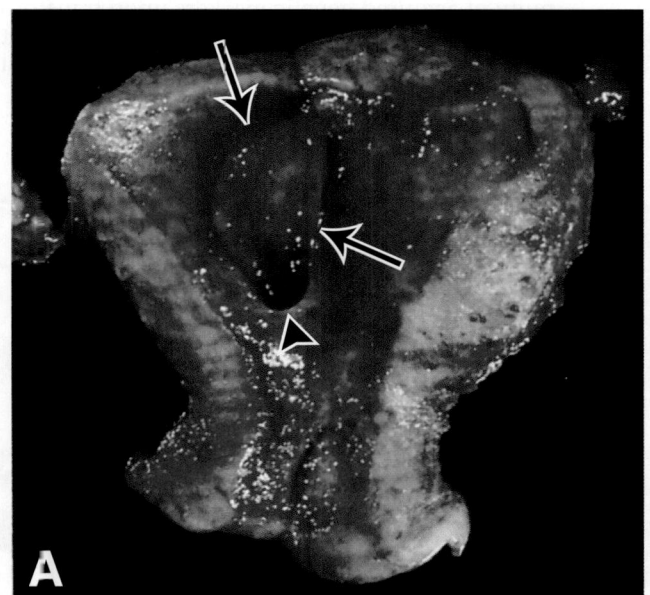
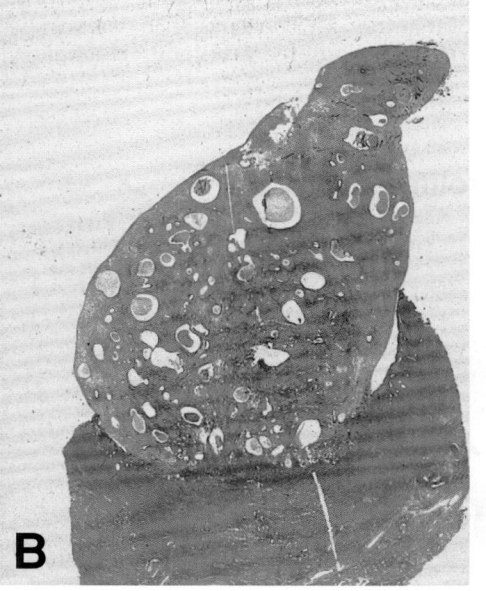

FIGURE 24-31. **Endometrial polyp. A.** A single polyp (*arrows*) extends into the endometrial cavity. The necrotic tip (*arrowhead*) is responsible for clinical bleeding. **B.** On microscopic section, a polyp exhibits slightly dilated endometrial glands embedded in a markedly fibrous stroma. (Reprinted with permission from Stanley J. Robboy, MD, and Gynecologic Pathology Associates, Durham and Chapel Hill, North Carolina.)

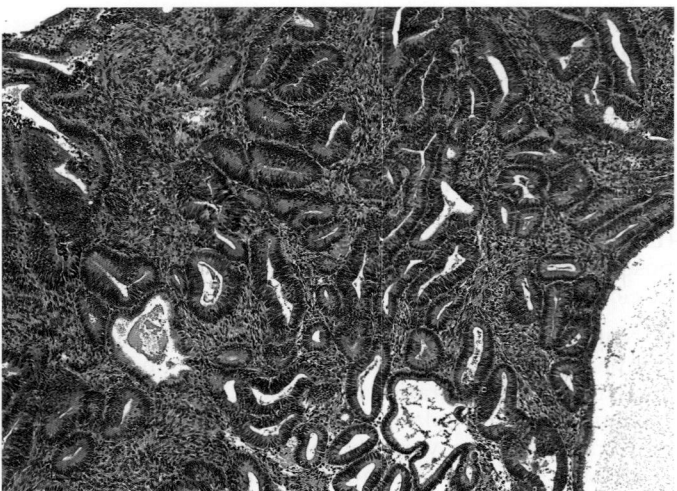

FIGURE 24-32. Nonatypical endometrial hyperplasia. Proliferative endometrial glands are irregularly distributed and randomly dilated. Gland density varies locally, but crowded and uncrowded areas have a consistent cytology throughout. This is a benign endometrium altered by unopposed estrogen.

Nonatypical Endometrial Hyperplasia Is Caused by Abnormal Estrogenic Stimulation

It is characterized by diffuse architectural and randomly distributed cytologic changes (Fig. 24-32). Estrogenic stimulation of the endometrium beyond the normal 2-week proliferative phase causes progressive changes associated with a 2- to 10-fold increased risk of endometrial cancer.

PATHOLOGY: Nonatypical endometrial hyperplasia affects the entire endometrium, in which remodeling of glands and stroma creates an irregular density of commingled cystic, slightly branching, and tubular glands. The earliest changes are isolated cystic expansion of scattered proliferative glands without a substantial change in gland density, often designated **disordered proliferative** endometrium. Morphologic transition to **nonatypical endometrial hyperplasia** is gradual and arbitrarily defined but can be said to occur when gland density becomes irregular throughout, with some regions having more glands than stroma.

As long as circulating estrogens persist, glands remain proliferative. Scattered glands may develop tubal differentiation with cilia formation. With increasing estrogen exposure, stroma breaks down and glands collapse, often associated with fibrin vascular thrombi. Architectural and metaplastic changes can persist after gradual weaning from a hyperestrogenic state. Sudden loss of estrogen leads to massive shedding with attendant heavy menses.

CLINICAL FEATURES: Nonatypical endometrial hyperplasia may result from anovulatory cycles, polycystic ovary syndrome, an estrogen-producing tumor, estrogen administration or obesity. Therapy directed at the primary cause may alleviate estrogenic stimulation. Large doses of progestins can produce temporary symptomatic relief or objective remission, depending on persistence of the underlying hormonal condition. Short-term risk of endometrial cancer is low, if extensive sampling of the endometrium shows no EIN/atypical hyperplasia. Long-term risks of refractory nonatypical endometrial hyperplasia are best assessed by repeat biopsy.

Endometrial Intraepithelial Neoplasia (Atypical Endometrial Hyperplasia) Is a Clonal Precancer

EIN is a monoclonal neoplastic growth of genetically altered cells with greatly increased risk of becoming endometrioid type of endometrial carcinoma (Fig. 24-33). It shows a continuity of acquired genetic markers upon transformation into a malignant phase. EIN and nonatypical endometrial hyperplasia coexist in many patients but have different histologic features.

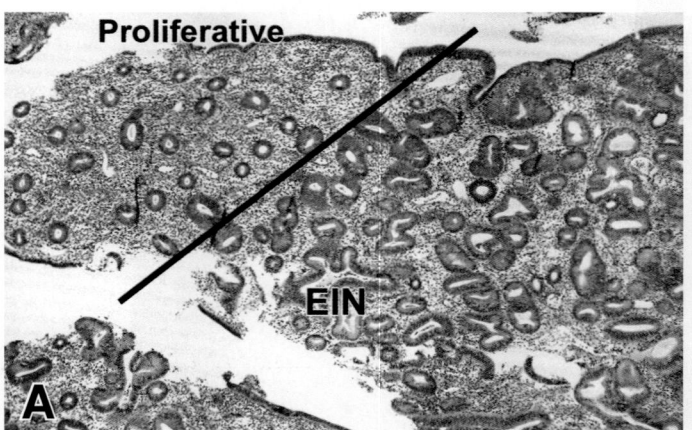

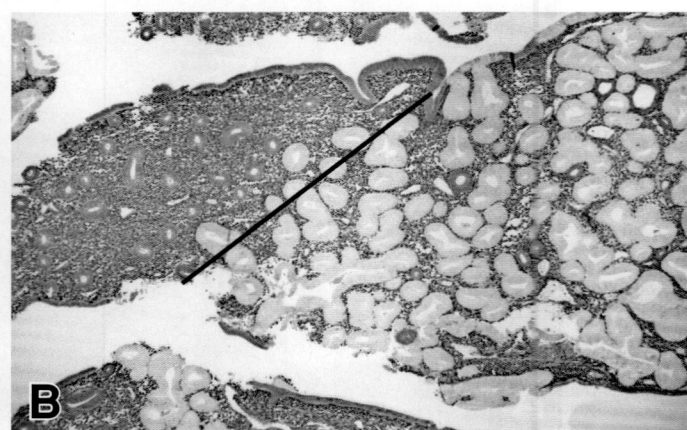

FIGURE 24-33. Endometrial intraepithelial neoplasia (EIN, atypical endometrial hyperplasia). A. Tight clusters of cytologically altered neoplastic endometrial glands with abundant cytoplasm and rounded nuclei (*right*) are offset from the background endometrium (*left*) in this geographic focus of EIN. Measurement across the perimeter of this aggregate of individual tubular glands exceeds 1 mm, and features of adenocarcinoma such as cribriform, maze-like, or solid architecture are lacking. **B.** Glands affected by EIN show loss of PTEN expression by immunohistochemistry (loss of brown staining).

PATHOLOGY: EIN lesions begin at a single point and then expand centripetally as proliferating neoplastic glands that displace and separate normal glands The densely crowded EIN glands differ cytologically from the background endometrium, have areas exceeding their stromal areas and measure more than 1 mm in dimension in a single fragment. Cytologic changes are evident in crowded glands by comparison with flanking normal glands and usually include alterations in nuclear size, shape, and texture. Malignant transformation is evident when glands develop solid, cribriform, or maze-like patterns characteristic of carcinoma.

CLINICAL FEATURES: Women newly diagnosed with EIN (atypical hyperplasia) have a 37% chance of having endometrial cancer diagnosed within 1 year. In most cases, cancer is probably present at the time of the initial biopsy, lending credence to the clinical adage "not cancer but better out."

The goals of management are to rule out concurrent and prevent future cancer. Hysterectomy, usually the therapy of choice, meets both goals if a woman does not want more children. Those who want more children or are poor operative risks may be treated with progestins.

There Are Two Main Types of Endometrial Carcinomas

EPIDEMIOLOGY: Endometrial carcinoma is the fourth most frequent cancer in American women and the most common gynecologic cancer (Table 24-5). It caused 10,920 deaths in the United States in 2017 (4% of all cancers in women). Incidence of this cancer was stable from 1950 to 1970, but by 1975 it had increased by 40%, possibly related to use of estrogens for easing symptoms of menopause. By 1985, rates had returned nearly to 1950 levels, a trend that correlated with use of lower doses of estrogen, incorporation of progestins (estrogen antagonists) into estrogen replacement regimens and increased surveillance of women treated with estrogens.

The incidence of endometrial cancer varies with age, from 12 cases per 100,000 women at age 40 to 34 cases per 100,000 women at age 60. Three-quarters of women with endometrial cancer are postmenopausal. The median age at diagnosis is 62.

Endometrial carcinoma is broadly grouped into two histologic types (Fig. 24-34 and Table 24-5). Type I tumors (about 80%), endometrioid carcinomas, often arise from EIN/atypical hyperplasia precursors and are associated with estrogenic stimulation. They occur mainly in pre- or perimenopausal women and are associated with obesity, hyperlipidemia, anovulation, infertility, and late menopause. Most endometrioid carcinomas are confined to the uterus and follow a favorable course. In contrast, type II tumors (about 10%) are nonendometrioid, largely serous carcinomas, arising occasionally in endometrial polyps. A preinvasive form of disease, serous endometrial intraepithelial carcinoma (serous EIC) can metastasize to the peritoneum by exfoliation and surface spread. Type II tumors are not associated with estrogen stimulation or hyperplasia, readily invade myometrium and vascular spaces and are highly lethal. The molecular alterations of endometrioid (type I) carcinomas are different from those of the nonendometrioid (type II) carcinomas.

These tumors overlap in clinical, pathologic, immunohistochemical, and molecular characteristics. Some nonendometrioid (type II) carcinomas may arise from pre-existing endometrioid carcinomas and share pathologic and molecular features of both types I and II endometrial carcinomas. The type II tumor category consists primarily of serous carcinomas but also includes rarer clear cell carcinoma and carcinosarcoma histotypes that have distinct molecular and clinical features.

Endometrial cancer is the most common extracolonic cancer in women with hereditary nonpolyposis colon cancer (Lynch) syndrome, a defect in DNA mismatch repair (**see Chapter 19**) also associated with breast and ovarian cancers.

MOLECULAR PATHOGENESIS: A dualistic model of endometrial carcinogenesis has been proposed in which normal endometrial cells transform into endometrioid carcinoma by accumulating mutations in oncogenes and tumor suppressor genes. The most commonly affected genes and mechanisms of genetic damage differ between endometrioid (type I) and nonendometrioid (type II) cancers.

Genetic alterations accumulate in the type I carcinoma pathway, during the transition from normal to EIN (atypical hyperplasia) to endometrioid carcinoma (Fig. 24-35). These may occur over a period of years and involve a combination of deletions, point mutations, and epigenetic modifications of cells that maintain normal or near-normal karyotypes. *PTEN*, which encodes a phosphatase that regulates the cell cycle, is the most frequently inactivated tumor suppressor gene

TABLE 24-5		
CLINICOPATHOLOGIC FEATURES OF ENDOMETRIAL CARCINOMA		
	Type I: Endometrioid Carcinoma	**Type II: Serous Carcinoma**
Age	Pre- and perimenopausal	Postmenopausal
Unopposed estrogen	Present	Absent
Hyperplasia precursor	Present	Absent
Grade	Low	High
Myometrial invasion	Superficial	Deep
Growth behavior	Stable	Progressive
Genetic alterations	Microsatellite instability, PTEN, PIK3CA, β-catenin	p53 mutations, loss of heterozygosity (LOH)

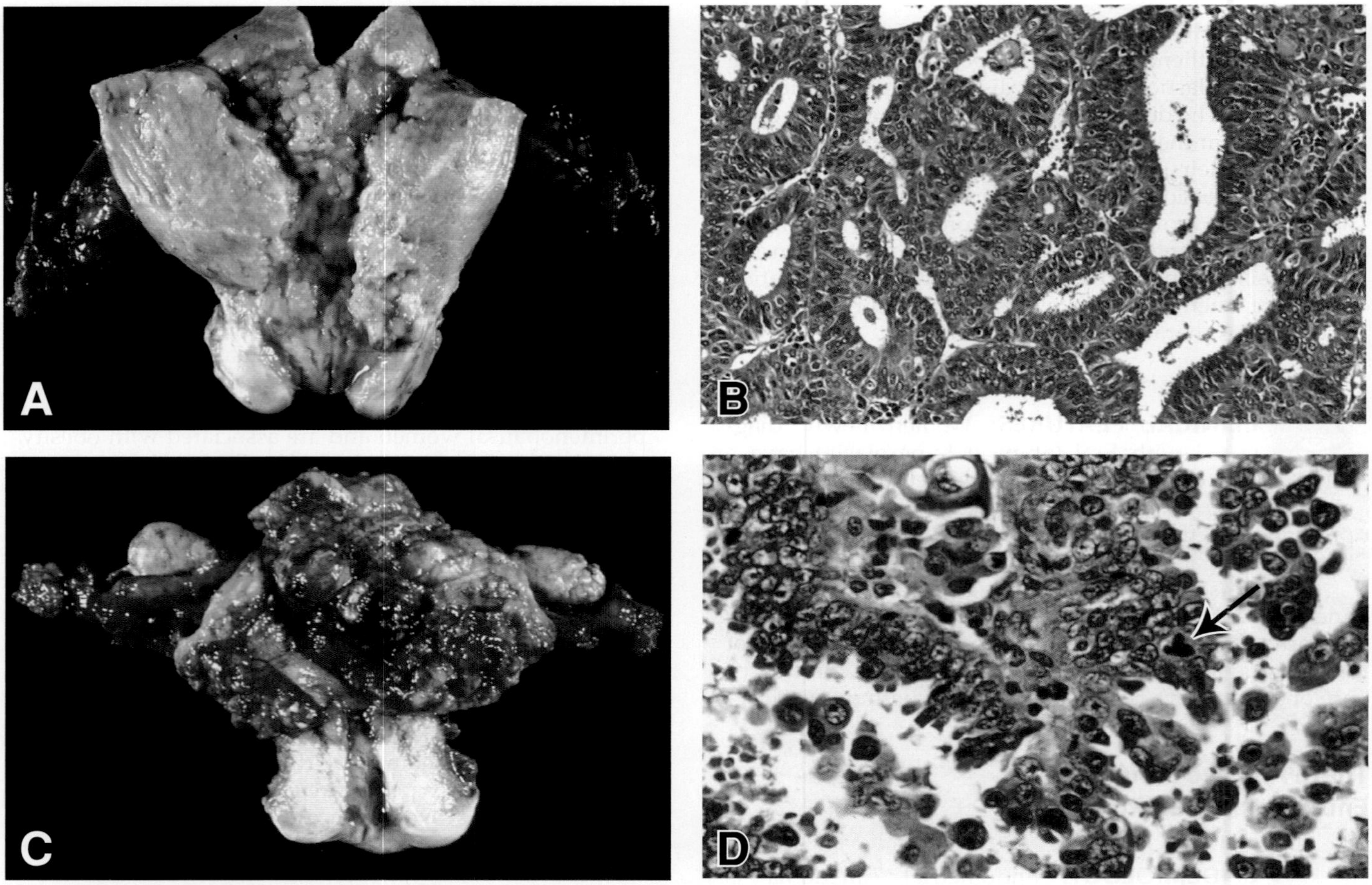

FIGURE 24-34. Adenocarcinoma of the endometrium. A, B. Endometrioid carcinoma. Polypoid tumor with only superficial myometrial invasion. In this well-differentiated (grade 1) adenocarcinoma, the neoplastic glands resemble normal endometrial glands. **C, D. Nonendometrioid carcinoma.** Large hemorrhagic and necrotic tumor with deep myometrial invasion. This serous carcinoma (severe cytologic atypia) exhibits stratification of anaplastic tumor cells and abnormal mitoses (*arrow*).

in endometrial tumorigenesis (2/3 of cases), resulting from deletion, mutation and/or promoter hypermethylation (Figs. 24-33 and 24-35). *PIK3CA*, which encodes the p110α subunit of phosphatidyl inositol 3-kinase

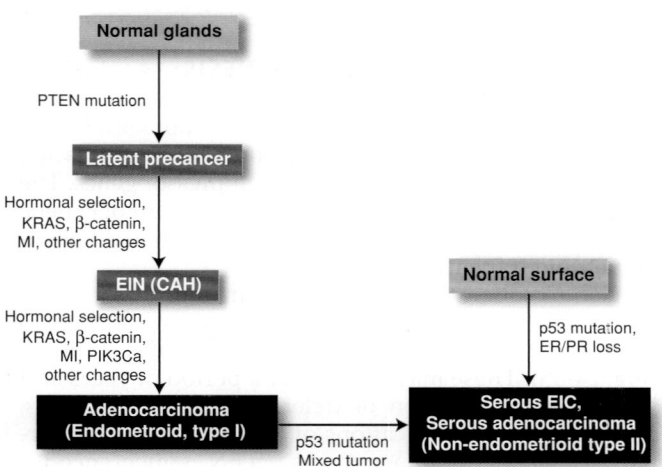

FIGURE 24-35. From endometrial hyperplasia to endometrioid carcinoma: molecular and genetic events. *MI* = microsatellite instability.

(PI3K), is the most commonly activated oncogene (by mutation, in up to 39% of cases) in endometrial carcinoma. *PTEN* inactivation frees the PI3K-Akt pathway, evading apoptosis and resulting in tumor growth advantage; *PIK3CA* mutations are rarely seen in such cases. Other frequently mutated genes include *KRAS* (10% to 30%) and β-catenin (*CTNNB1*) with nuclear protein accumulation (25% to 38%). *TP53* mutations are rare (5% to 10%). In a quarter of sporadic tumors, a specific type of genetic damage, microsatellite instability (MSI), results from promoter hypermethylation of *MLH1* (a gene involved in DNA repair) and leads to microsatellite instability and accelerated mutation in several critical target genes that regulate apoptosis, cell proliferation, and differentiation. The wide range of resultant mutations, in both microsatellite-stable and -unstable endometrioid tumors, creates genetically heterogeneous tumors.

Over 90% of type II nonendometrioid carcinomas have p53 mutations, and 80% lose estrogen and progesterone receptors. Mechanisms of DNA damage are different from endometrioid tumors. MSI is rare (<5%), and gross structural and numerical chromosomes abnormalities are more common. Nonendometrioid carcinomas may also develop from endometrioid tumors via p53 mutations and other means.

PATHOLOGY: Endometrial cancers usually show diffuse or exophytic growth (Fig. 24-34). Large tumors are typically hemorrhagic and necrotic.

ENDOMETRIOID CARCINOMA OF THE ENDOMETRIUM: This type of endometrial cancer, composed entirely of glandular cells, is the most common histologic variant (80% to 85%). The FIGO system categorizes this tumor into three grades depending on the ratio of glandular to solid elements, the latter signifying poorer differentiation (Fig. 24-36).

- **Grade 1:** Well differentiated; almost only neoplastic glands, with minimal (<5%) solid areas
- **Grade 2:** Moderately differentiated; 5% to 50% of malignant epithelium forms glands
- **Grade 3:** Poorly differentiated; large (>50%) areas of solid tumor

Nuclei of endometrial carcinoma cells range from bland to markedly pleomorphic, usually with prominent nucleoli. Mitoses are abundant and may be abnormal in less differentiated tumors. Tumor cells that grow in solid sheets are poorly differentiated. The FIGO system also defines stages of endometrial cancer (Table 24-6).

VARIANTS OF ENDOMETRIOID CARCINOMA: One-third of endometrial carcinomas contain squamous cells as well as glands. If the squamous element shows only minimal atypia, the tumor is a **well-differentiated**

TABLE 24-6	
FIGO (2009) STAGING OF CANCER OF THE ENDOMETRIUM	
Stage	**Anatomic Distribution**
Stage I	Tumor confined to the corpus uteri
IA	No myometrial invasion or invasion <50% of myometrium thickness
IB	Tumor invades ≥50% of myometrium thickness
Stage II	Tumor invades cervical stroma but does not extend beyond the uterus
Stage III	Local and/or regional spread of the tumor
IIIA	Tumor invades the serosa of the corpus uteri and/or adnexa
IIIB	Vaginal and/or parametrial involvement
IIIC	Metastases to pelvic and/or paraaortic lymph nodes
Stage IV	Tumor invades bladder and/or bowel mucosa, and/or distant metastases
IVA	Tumor invasion of bladder and/or bowel mucosa
IVB	Distant metastases, including intra-abdominal metastases and/or inguinal lymph nodes

FIGO = International Federation of Gynecology and Obstetrics.

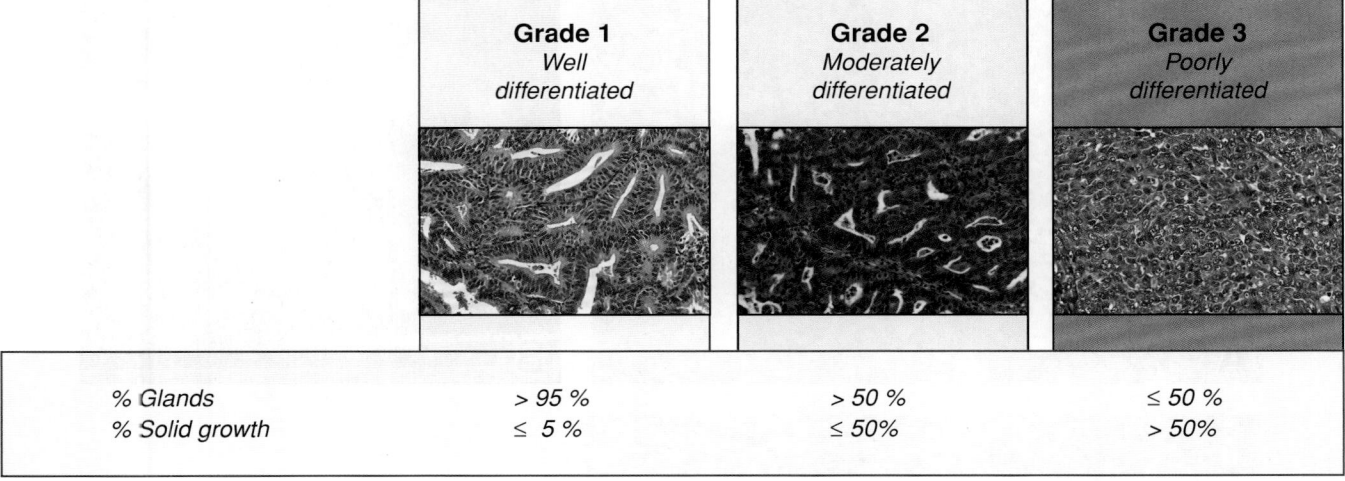

	Grade 1 *Well differentiated*	Grade 2 *Moderately differentiated*	Grade 3 *Poorly differentiated*
% Glands	> 95 %	> 50 %	≤ 50 %
% Solid growth	≤ 5 %	≤ 50%	> 50%

Significant
NUCLEAR ATYPIA
if present
increases the grade

Nuclear atypia
Round nuclei
Variation in shape and size
Variation in staining
Hyperchromasia
Coarsely clumped chromatin
Prominent nucleoli
Frequent mitoses
Abnormal mitoses

FIGURE 24-36. Grading of endometrial adenocarcinoma. The grade depends primarily on the architectural pattern, but significant nuclear atypia changes a grade 1 tumor to grade 2, and a grade 2 tumor to grade 3. Nuclear atypia is characterized by round nuclei; variation in shape, size, and staining; hyperchromasia; coarsely clumped chromating; prominent nucleoli; and frequent and abnormal mitoses. Significant nuclear atypia if present increases the tumor grade.

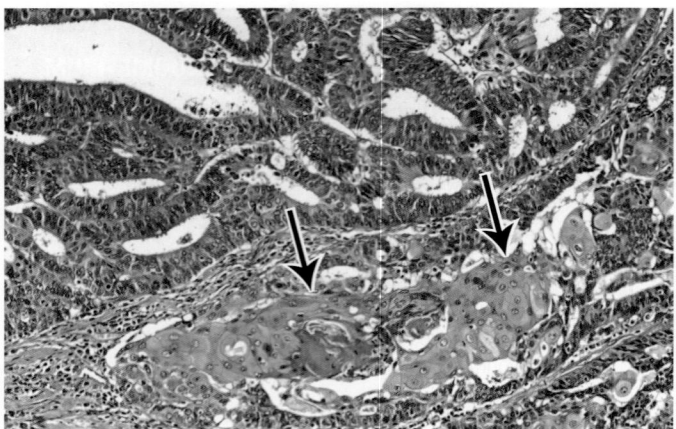

FIGURE 24-37. Squamous differentiation in endometrioid adenocarcinoma of the endometrium. Well-differentiated squamous cells (*arrows*) show minimal atypia. This pattern has been called adenoacanthoma when squamous cells form squamous morules and nests among glands.

carcinoma with squamous differentiation (previously, **adenoacanthoma**) (Fig. 24-37). If the squamous element appears malignant, the tumor is **poorly differentiated carcinoma with squamous differentiation** (also known

as **adenosquamous carcinoma**). These variants represent 22% and 7% of all endometrial cancers, respectively.

An extremely well-differentiated but otherwise typical endometrial carcinoma that exhibits large subnuclear vacuoles of glycogen is called **secretory type**. This variant occurs in premenopausal women, in some cases owing to progesterone stimulation, and has the most favorable prognosis.

NONENDOMETRIOID ENDOMETRIAL CARCINOMA: Nonendometrioid types of endometrial carcinoma are less common and not associated with estrogen exposure. They are aggressive as a group, and histologic grading is not clinically useful as all cases are considered high grade.

- **Serous carcinoma** histologically resembles, and behaves like, serous carcinoma of the ovary (Fig. 24-34D). It often shows transtubal spread to peritoneal surfaces. A noninvasive form is termed "serous endometrial intraepithelial carcinoma" (serous EIC).
- **Clear cell carcinoma** is a tumor of older women. It contains large cells with abundant cytoplasmic glycogen ("clear cells") or cells with bulbous nuclei that line glandular lumens ("hobnail cells") (Fig. 24-38A). Serous and clear cell carcinomas have poor prognoses.

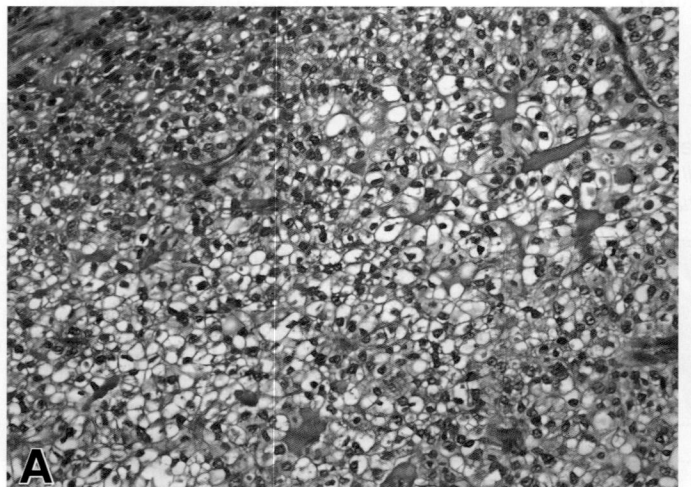

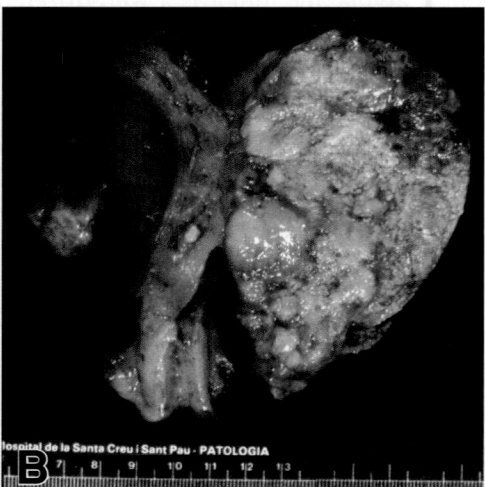

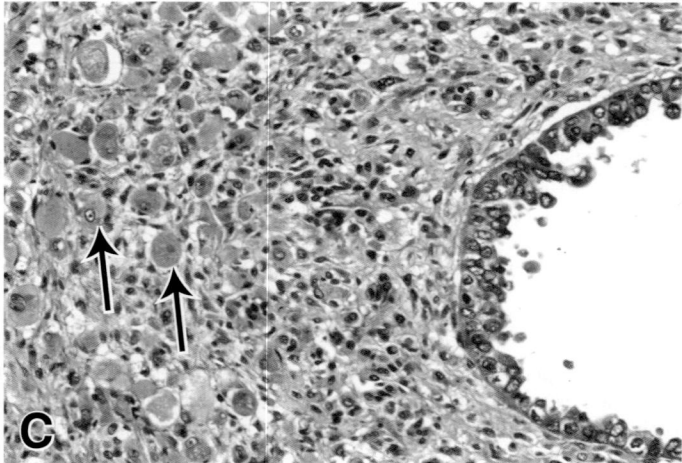

FIGURE 24-38. Nonendometrioid types of endometrial adenocarcinoma. A. Clear cell endometrial adenocarcinoma. The clear appearance of the cytoplasm is due to extraction of glycogen during specimen processing for microscopic examination. Tumor cells have round and eccentric nuclei. **B.** Carcinosarcoma (malignant mixed müllerian tumor). Solid, partially cystic and necrotic mass that expands the uterine cavity. **C.** Rhabdomyoblasts (heterologous elements, *arrows*) appear as pleomorphic, rounded cells with ample eosinophilic cytoplasm adjacent to malignant epithelium.

TABLE 24-7

GENOMIC-BASED CLASSIFICATION OF ENDOMETRIAL CARCINOMA BY THE CANCER GENOME ATLAS (TCGA) (2013)

Molecular Classification	Molecular Definition	Histopathology
Ultramutated/polymerase ε (POLE)	High mutation rate and hot-spot mutations in POLE	High-grade endometrioid carcinomas
Hypermutated/MSI	MSI, due to MLH1 promoter methylation	Endometrioid (Lynch syndrome–associated) carcinomas
Low-copy number abnormalities	MSS; frequent CTNNB1 mutations	Endometrioid carcinomas
High-copy number abnormalities	TP53 mutations	Serous, high-grade endometrioid, and mixed carcinomas

MSI = microsatellite instability; MSS = microsatellite stability.

- **Carcinosarcoma (malignant mixed mesodermal tumor):** In this highly malignant tumor (Fig. 24-38B), pleomorphic **epithelial** cells commingle with areas showing **mesenchymal** differentiation (Fig. 24-38C). These mixed neoplasms are derived from a common clone believed to be of epithelial origin. Overall 5-year survival is 25%.

Integrated Genomic Characterization of Endometrial Carcinoma: Two Histologic Subgroups Resolve Into Four Molecular Subgroups

By combining morphology and molecular genetics, The Cancer Genome Atlas (TCGA) Research Network report on endometrial carcinoma (Table 24-7) underlines the importance of histotype in determining clinical outcome. It classifies endometrial carcinoma into four types which carry different prognosis:

1. **Ultra-mutated endometrial carcinoma** with recurrent mutations in the exonuclease domain of **DNA polymerase epsilon (POLE)**, a gene involved in nuclear DNA replication and repair. These tumors have extremely high somatic mutation frequencies (>100 mutations per megabase [Mb]) in most cases. They are high-grade endometrioid endometrial carcinomas with prominent tumor-infiltrating lymphocytes (TILs).

2. **Hypermutated endometrial carcinoma, with microsatellite instability** (MSI) due to dysfunctional mismatch repair (MMRd) proteins: MLH1, PMS2, MSH2, and MSH6. The predominant underlying mechanism is epigenetic silencing of MLH1 by promoter hypermethylation. In rare cases, the MMRd is caused by somatic or germline mutations in mismatch repair (MMR) genes, the latter being diagnostic for Lynch syndrome, an autosomal-dominant cancer susceptibility disorder associated with a markedly increased risk of colorectal carcinoma and endometrial carcinoma. MMRd leads to high mutation frequencies, usually >10 mutations per Mb. Endometrial carcinomas with MSI or MMRd are mostly of endometrioid subtype. Like POLE-mutant endometrial carcinomas, these tumors typically show TILs.

3. The third molecular subgroup, designated as **low somatic copy number abnormalities (SCNAs)**, is genomically relatively stable, MMR-proficient, and has a moderate number of mutations, mostly within the PI3K/Akt and Wnt signaling pathways. This subgroup is almost exclusively composed of endometrioid carcinomas with estrogen (ER) and progesterone receptor (PR) positivity by immunohistochemistry.

4. The fourth subgroup has **high SCNA**, very similar to high-grade serous ovarian carcinomas, and frequent TP53 mutations (92%). The tumors are high-grade (grade 3) endometrial carcinomas, including most serous carcinomas, but interestingly endometrioid carcinomas (26%) were also classified in this group, justifying the term "serous-like cancers."

Ultramutated tumors have excellent prognosis even though most are grade 3 endometrioid carcinomas. The copy number-high group (serous-like), composed mostly of serous carcinomas and grade 3 endometrioid carcinomas, has the worst prognosis. TCGA revealed significant genotypic overlap between FIGO grade 3 endometrioid and serous carcinomas. In fact, 24% high-grade (G3) endometrioid carcinomas, classified by histopathology, exhibited TP53 mutations, and behaved as serous carcinomas (serous-like). These patients require adjuvant therapy in addition to surgical resection.

Most endometrial carcinomas arise in the uterine corpus, but a small proportion originate in the lower uterine segment (isthmus). These isthmus tumors often occur in women under the age of 50 and are often high grade and deeply invasive. They lack ER expression and are associated with Lynch syndrome in 29% of cases (versus 1% to 2% for carcinomas of the corpus).

CLINICAL FEATURES: Endometrial cancers usually occur in peri- or postmenopausal women. The chief complaint is commonly abnormal uterine bleeding, especially in the early stages of tumor growth confined to the endometrium. Unfortunately, cervicovaginal cytologic screening does not efficiently detect early endometrial cancer. Fractional curettage is needed to assess spread to the cervix, whereas peritoneal washing detects tubal reflux and abdominal contamination. Transvaginal ultrasound is valuable diagnostically in postmenopausal patients in whom an endometrium

TABLE 24-8

STAGE, GRADE AND SURVIVAL FOR ENDOMETRIAL CANCER

	5-Year Survival (%)		
Stage	G-1[a]	G-2	G-3
I	90	69	52
II	80	42	12
III, IV	25	33	17

[a]G = FIGO (International Federation of Gynecology and Obstetrics) grade.

greater than 5 mm thick is considered highly suspicious. Unlike cervical cancer, endometrial cancer may bypass pelvic lymph nodes and spread directly to paraaortic nodes. Patients with advanced cancers may also have pulmonary metastases (40% of cases with metastases).

Women with well-differentiated cancers confined to the endometrium are usually treated by simple hysterectomy. Postoperative radiation is considered if the tumor is poorly differentiated or nonendometrioid in type, the myometrium is deeply invaded, the cervix is involved or lymph nodes contain metastases.

Survival in endometrial carcinoma depends on tumor stage and histotype. For endometrioid tumors, additional prognostic factors include histologic grade and age. High

tumor levels of estrogen and progesterone receptors and low mitotic rates correlate with a better prognosis. Actuarial survival for all patients with endometrial cancer following treatment is 80% after 2 years, decreasing to 65% after 10 years. Tumors that have penetrated the myometrium or invaded lymphatics are more likely to have spread beyond the uterus. Endometrial cancers involving the cervix have a poorer prognosis. Spread outside the uterus carries the worst outlook (Table 24-8).

Fewer Than 2% of Uterine Cancers Are Endometrial Stromal Tumors

Some endometrial stromal tumors are pure sarcomas; in others, sarcomatous (stromal) and epithelial elements are intermingled. The nomenclature of these tumor types, the spectrum of their histologic components and the correlation of each tumor type with its potential for malignant behavior are presented in Table 24-9.

Endometrial Stromal Sarcoma

Pure stromal tumors are divided into two major categories, based on whether the tumor margin is expansile or infiltrating. Expansile lesions that do not invade are **benign stromal nodules**, which carry little clinical significance. Tumors with infiltrating margins are termed **stromal sarcomas** and are classified into low-grade (most common) and high-grade categories.

TABLE 24-9

NOMENCLATURE OF UTERINE TUMORS

Tumor	Epithelium	Stroma	Clinical Behavior
Epithelium and Stroma			
Endometrial polyp	Polyclonal benign	Neoplastic	Benign
Nonatypical endometrial hyperplasia	Polyclonal benign	Polyclonal benign	Benign
Endometrial intraepithelial neoplasia	Neoplastic	—	Premalignant
Endometrial adenocarcinoma	Neoplastic	—	Malignant
Endometrial stromal nodule	—	Neoplastic	Benign
Endometrial stromal sarcoma	—	Neoplastic	Low-grade malignant
Undifferentiated sarcoma	—	Neoplastic	Malignant
Adenosarcoma	Unknown	Neoplastic	Low-grade malignant
Carcinosarcoma	Neoplastic	Neoplastic, transformed epithelial cells	Malignant
Smooth Muscle			
Leiomyoma	—	Neoplastic	Benign
Cellular leiomyoma	—	Neoplastic	Benign
Intravenous leiomyomatosis	—	Neoplastic	Locally aggressive
Leiomyosarcoma	—	Neoplastic	Malignant

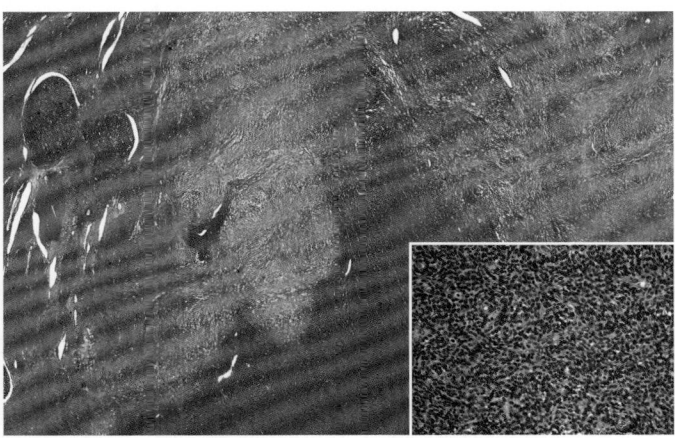

FIGURE 24-39   Endometrial stromal sarcoma, low grade. The myometrium is irregularly permeated by the tumor, which invades vascular spaces. *Inset.* A higher-power view shows typically small tumor cells with scant cytoplasm and uniform round to oval nuclei. There are numerous small arterioles.

PATHOLOGY: Low-grade endometrial stromal sarcomas may be polypoid and fill the endometrial cavity, or they may diffusely invade the myometrium. Large masses of spindle cells with scant cytoplasm dissect the myometrium and invade vascular channels (Fig. 24-39). Tumor cells resemble endometrial stromal cells in the proliferative phase and show little or no cytologic atypia and low mitotic activity. Expression of CD10 and estrogen and progesterone receptors (ER and PR) helps confirm the diagnosis. Most low-grade endometrial stromal sarcomas harbor t(7;17)(p21;q15), which results in a fusion between *JAZF1* and *SUZ12* (the former encodes a nuclear factor that represses transcription, and the latter participates in polycomb repressive complexes that mediate epigenetic regulation via histone methylation). By contrast, the high-grade endometrial stromal sarcomas, characterized by the recurrent aberration t(10;17)(q22;p13), exhibit an atypical round cell (predominant) and a low-grade spindle cell component. CD10, ER, and PR are negative, but cyclin D1 is strongly positive. Higher-grade sarcomas originating in the endometrium lose all antigenic and morphologic resemblance to endometrial stroma and are thus designated as **undifferentiated uterine sarcoma**.

CLINICAL FEATURES: Many years may elapse before low-grade endometrial stromal sarcomas recur clinically, and metastases may occur even if the original tumor was confined to the uterus at initial surgery. Recurrences usually involve the pelvis first, followed by lung metastases. Prolonged survival and even cure are feasible despite metastases. By contrast, high-grade endometrial stromal and undifferentiated uterine sarcomas recur early, generally with widespread metastases, even if there had been little myometrial invasion. Low-grade endometrial stromal sarcomas can be treated successfully with surgery and progestin therapy, with 90% survival 10 years after diagnosis.

Uterine Adenosarcoma

Uterine (müllerian) adenosarcoma is a distinctive low-grade tumor with benign glandular epithelium and malignant stroma (Fig. 24-40). It differs from carcinosarcoma, in which both epithelial and stromal elements are malignant (see above).

Adenosarcomas typically present as polypoid masses within the endometrial cavity. The glandular epithelium resembles proliferative phase endometrial glands, but occasionally squamous epithelium and mucinous-type epithelium are seen. The stroma is cellular and may exhibit mitotic activity. It is often densest about the glandular epithelium (periglandular cuffing) and resembles endometrial stromal cells in the proliferative phase of the cycle. One-fourth of patients with adenosarcomas eventually succumb to local recurrence or metastatic spread. In these patients, myometrial invasion and/or high-grade sarcomatous overgrowth usually occur.

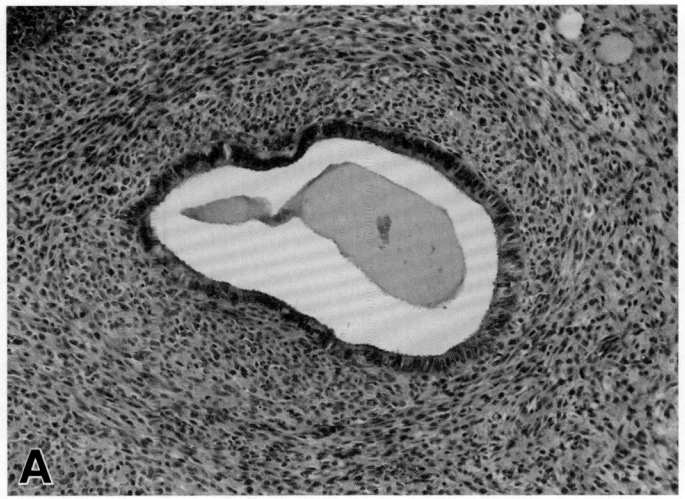
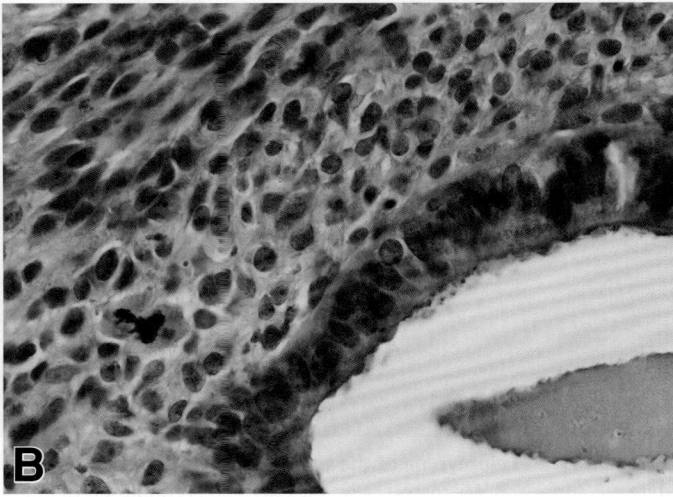

FIGURE 24-40.   Adenosarcoma. A. This tumor involves periglandular cuffing by atypical stromal cells. **B.** Tumor cells show increased mitotic activity.

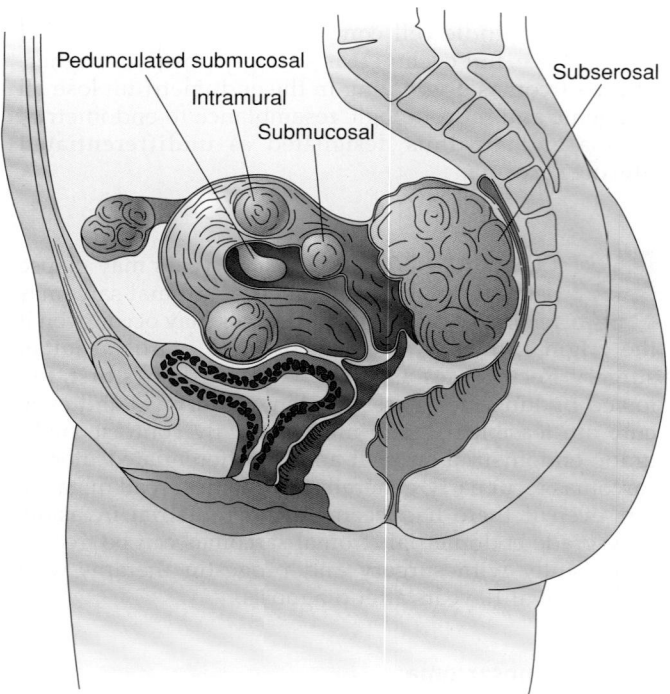

FIGURE 24-41. Leiomyomas of the uterus. Leiomyomas can be intramural, submucosal (which may appear as a pedunculated endometrial polyp) and subserosal (which can compress the bladder or the rectum).

Leiomyomas Are the Most Common Female Genital Tract Tumors

Leiomyomas, benign tumors of smooth muscle origin, are colloquially known as "myomas" or "fibroids." Including minute tumors, leiomyomas occur in 75% of women over age 30. They are rare before age 20, and most regress after menopause. Although often multiple, each tumor is monoclonal (**see Chapter 5**). Estrogen promotes their growth but does not initiate them.

PATHOLOGY: Grossly, leiomyomas are firm, pale gray, whorled, and without encapsulation (Figs. 24-41 and 24-42A). They vary from 1 mm to over 30 cm in diameter. Their cut surface bulges, and borders are smooth and distinct from neighboring myometrium. Most leiomyomas are intramural, but some are submucosal, subserosal, or pedunculated. Many, especially larger ones, show areas of degenerative hyalinization that are sharply demarcated from adjacent normal myometrium. Leiomyomas show little mitotic activity (<4 mitoses per 10 high-power fields [HPFs]), lack nuclear atypia and geographical necrosis and have little or no malignant potential. A **"mitotically active leiomyoma"** is one that shows brisk mitotic activity but is relatively small. It is sharply demarcated from adjacent normal myometrium and lacks both geographical necrosis and significant cellular atypia. It is usually benign.

Microscopically, leiomyomas exhibit interlacing fascicles of uniform spindle cells containing elongated nuclei with blunt ends (Fig. 24-42B). Cytoplasm is abundant, eosinophilic and fibrillar. The cells of leiomyomas and adjacent normal myometrium are cytologically identical, but leiomyomas are easily distinguished by their circumscription, nodularity, and denser cellularity.

CLINICAL FEATURES: Submucosal leiomyomas may cause bleeding owing to ulceration of thinned, overlying endometrium, or become pedunculated and protrude through the cervical os, eliciting cramping pains. Many intramural leiomyomas are symptomatic because of their sheer bulk, and large ones may interfere with bowel or bladder function or cause dystocia in labor. Pedunculated leiomyomas on the uterine serosa may interfere with the function of neighboring viscera. Leiomyomas may also infarct and become painful if they undergo torsion.

Leiomyomas usually grow slowly but occasionally enlarge rapidly during pregnancy. Large symptomatic

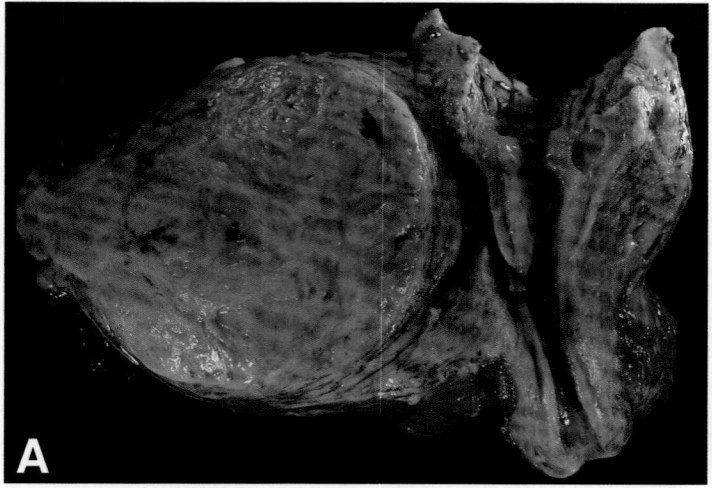
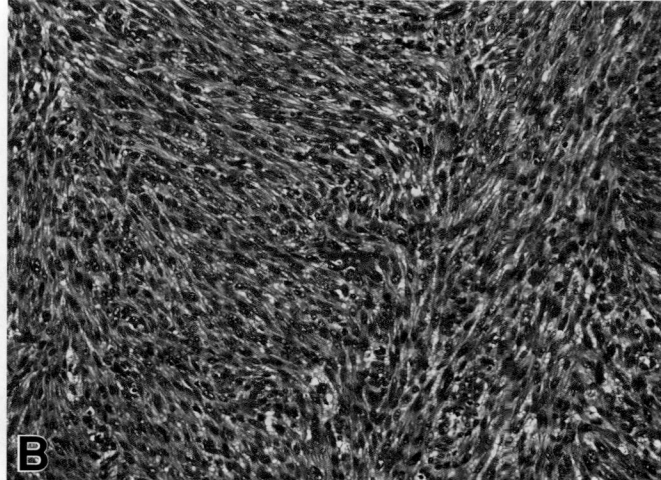

FIGURE 24-42. Leiomyoma of the uterus. A. This bisected uterus displays a prominent, sharply circumscribed tumor with a whorled homogeneous white cut surface. **B.** Microscopically, a leiomyoma is composed of intertwined bundles of smooth muscle cells, some of which are cut longitudinally (elongated nuclei) and others transversely (round to oval nuclei).

leiomyomas are removed by myomectomy or hysterectomy. Ablation by arterial thrombosis may also been used.

Intravenous Leiomyomatosis Does Not Metastasize

Intravenous leiomyomatosis is a rare condition in which benign smooth muscle grows within uterine and pelvic veins. It may develop after vascular invasion by a uterine leiomyoma or from growth of venous smooth muscle. At surgery, it appears as worm-like extensions near the external uterine surface or as projections into uterine veins in the broad ligament. Although they may grow extensively within blood vessels, these neoplasms do not metastasize. Rare fatalities have resulted from direct extension of leiomyomas from pelvic veins into the inferior vena cava and right atrium. Treatment consists of total abdominal hysterectomy.

Leiomyosarcomas Are Very Rare Compared to Leiomyomas

Leiomyosarcoma is a smooth muscle malignancy whose incidence is 1/1,000th of its benign counterpart. It accounts for 2% of uterine cancers. Its pathogenesis is uncertain, but at least some appear to arise within leiomyomas. Women with leiomyosarcomas are on average more than a decade older (age above 50) than those with leiomyomas, and the malignant tumors are larger (10 to 15 cm vs. 3 to 5 cm) (Fig. 24-43A).

PATHOLOGY: Leiomyosarcoma should be suspected when an apparent leiomyoma is soft, shows areas of necrosis on gross examination, has irregular borders (invasion of adjacent myometrium) or fails to protrude above the surface when cut. Evidence that a uterine smooth muscle tumor is a leiomyosarcoma includes (1) presence of geographical necrosis with a sharp transition from viable tumor (Fig. 24-43B); (2) 10 or more mitoses per 10 HPFs (Fig. 24-43C), if the tumor is more than 5 cm in diameter; (3) 5 or more mitoses per 10 HPFs, with geographical necrosis and diffuse cytoplasmic/nuclear atypia; and (4) myxoid and epithelioid smooth muscle tumors with 5 or more mitoses per 10 HPFs.

Size is important: tumors under 5 cm in diameter almost never recur. However, most leiomyosarcomas are large and advanced when detected and are usually fatal despite surgery, radiation therapy and/or chemotherapy. Nearly half of recurrences first present in the lung, and 5-year survival is about 20%.

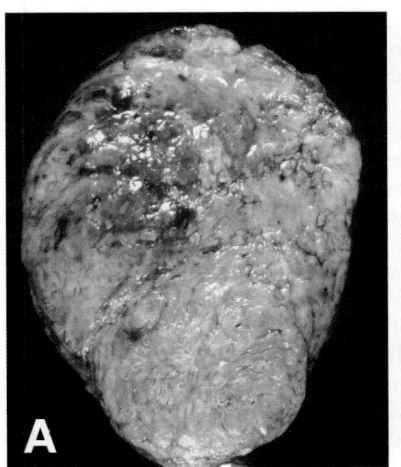
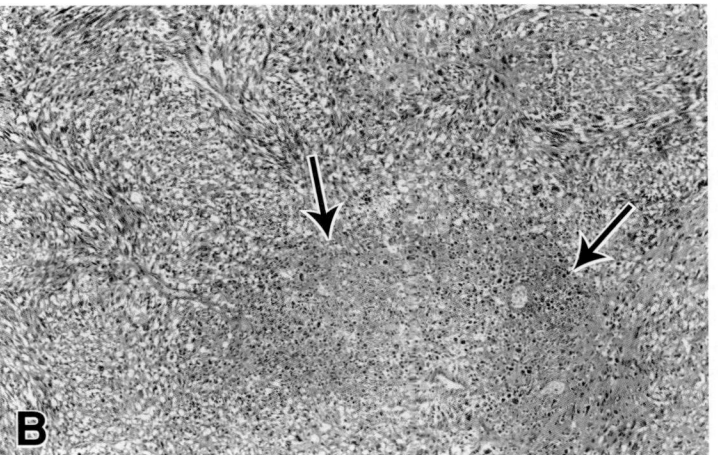
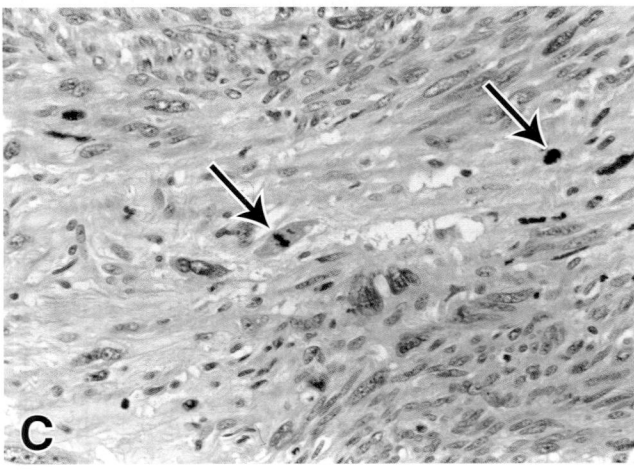

FIGURE 24-43. Leiomyosarcoma of the uterus. A. The myometrium of this uterus has been replaced by a large, soft leiomyosarcoma with extensive necrosis. **B.** A zone of coagulative tumor necrosis (*arrows*) appears demarcated from the viable tumor. **C.** The tumor shows considerable nuclear atypia and abundant mitotic activity (*arrows*).

Fallopian Tube

ANATOMY

The fallopian tubes extend from the uterine fundus to the ovaries. An interstitial portion, the **isthmus**, lies within the cornua of the uterus and connects the uterine cavity with the straight portion of the tube. As the tube extends to the ovary, it increases in diameter to form the **ampulla**, which merges with the **infundibulum**. The fimbriated end opens like the bell of a trumpet and has finger-like extensions that envelop the ovary. The lining cells are ciliated and play an important role in transport of ova.

SALPINGITIS

Salpingitis is inflammation of the fallopian tubes, typically due to infections ascending from the lower genital tract. The most common causative organisms are *N. gonorrhoeae, Escherichia coli, Chlamydia,* and *Mycoplasma,* and most infections are polymicrobial. Acute episodes of salpingitis (particularly if due to chlamydia) may be asymptomatic. A fallopian tube damaged by prior infection is very susceptible to reinfection. In most cases, chronic salpingitis develops only after repeated episodes of acute salpingitis.

 PATHOLOGY: In acute salpingitis, there is marked neutrophil infiltration, edema, and congestion of mucosal folds (plicae). In chronic salpingitis, the inflammatory infiltrate is mainly lymphocytes and plasma cells; edema and congestion are usually minimal. In late stages, the fallopian tube may seal and become distended with pus **(pyosalpinx)** or a transudate **(hydrosalpinx)**.

The fallopian tube allows infections from the lower genital tract to ascend and enter the peritoneal cavity, leading to peritonitis and PID. Fibrinous adhesions between the fallopian tube serosa and surrounding peritoneal surfaces organize into thin fibrous bands ("violin string" adhesions). The adjacent ovary may also be involved, sometimes as a **tuboovarian abscess**. Destruction of the fallopian tube epithelium or deposition of fibrin on its surface leads to fibrin bridges interconnecting the plicae. In severe chronic salpingitis, dense adhesions cause the end of the tube to become blunted and clubbed. A blocked lumen may lead to hydrosalpinx or pyosalpinx. The damage wrought by chronic salpingitis may also impair tubal motility and passage of sperm, resulting in **infertility**. Chronic salpingitis is a common cause of **ectopic pregnancy**, since adherent mucosal plicae create pockets in which ova become entrapped.

ECTOPIC PREGNANCY

Ectopic pregnancy is implantation of a fertilized ovum outside the endometrium. The frequency of ectopic pregnancy in the United States has increased threefold, to 1.5% of live births, during the past two decades, although mortality has sharply declined. **Over 95% of such pregnancies are in the fallopian tube, mostly in the distal and middle thirds.**

PATHOLOGY: Ectopic pregnancy results when passage of a conceptus along a fallopian tube is impeded, for example, by mucosal adhesions or abnormal tubal motility due to inflammatory disease or endometriosis. The trophoblast readily penetrates the tubal mucosa and musculature. Blood from the tubal implantation site enters the peritoneum, causing abdominal pain. Ectopic pregnancy is also associated with anomalous uterine bleeding after a period of amenorrhea and Arias-Stella cells in the endometrium. The thin tubal wall usually ruptures by the 12th week of gestation. *Tubal rupture is life-threatening as it can lead to rapid exsanguination.*

Rupture of the tube's interstitial portion produces greater intra-abdominal hemorrhage than rupture in other locations because vasculature there is richer and rupture occurs later in gestation. In the isthmus, the tube ruptures early (within the first 6 weeks), because its thick muscular wall does not allow much distention. Tubal pregnancies in the ampulla tend to be of longer duration, since the distensible tubal wall can accommodate a growing pregnancy for a longer time.

Ectopic pregnancy must be treated promptly with surgery or chemotherapy. Administration of methotrexate terminates ectopic pregnancy and is used when the conceptus is smaller than 4 cm.

FALLOPIAN TUBE TUMORS

Benign tumors arising within the fallopian tube are rare. The most common is the small, circumscribed **adenomatoid tumor**, which is of mesothelial origin. It arises in the mesosalpinx and is composed of benign mesothelial cells that line slit-like spaces.

Thorough evaluation of the fallopian tube in women at heightened hereditary risk for "ovarian" cancer (BRCA mutation) has shown that some resultant cancers arise in the tubal fimbria as **serous tubal intraepithelial carcinoma** (STIC) (Fig. 24-44A). Tubal fimbria have also been shown to be sites of early involvement of some sporadic (nonhereditary) serous carcinomas. STIC lesions are physically small, often grossly inapparent and composed of mitotically active regions of atypical epithelium expressing mutant *TP53* (Fig. 24-44B). An unknown proportion of **high-grade serous carcinomas** previously classified as ovarian or peritoneal primary tumors may in fact be tubal carcinomas metastatic to those sites. This revised biologic model of serous carcinogenesis has identified new targets for prevention in the fallopian tube. Clinical tumor staging at these sites has been revised to consider ovarian and tubal carcinomas in an integrated fashion (Table 24-10).

Fallopian tube involvement by metastases or implants from adjacent ovarian and uterine neoplasms also occurs. Most primary malignancies that involve the fallopian tubes secondarily are serous carcinomas, with peak incidence among 50- to 60-year-olds.

Ovary

ANATOMY AND EMBRYOLOGY

The ovaries are paired organs that flank the uterus. They are attached to the posterior surface of the broad ligament in a

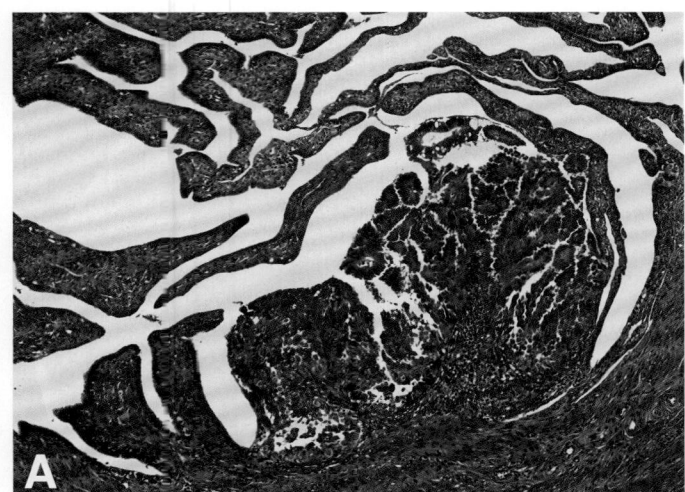

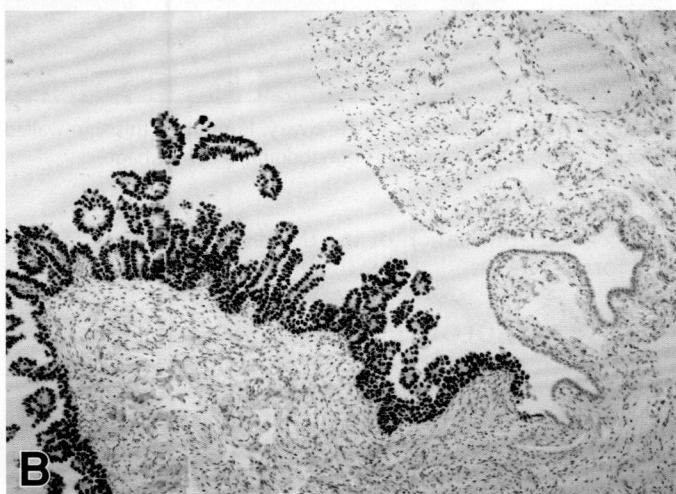

FIGURE 24-44. Serous tubal intraepithelial carcinoma (STIC) of the tubal fimbria. A. This noninvasive papillary tumor shows dark mitotically active atypical epithelial cells. **B.** Tumor cell nuclei exhibit strong p53 overexpression.

TABLE 24-10	
FIGO (2014) STAGING OF CANCER OF THE OVARY, FALLOPIAN TUBE AND PERITONEUM	
Stage	**Anatomic Distribution**
Stage I	Tumor confined to ovaries or fallopian tube(s)
IA	Tumor limited to one ovary (capsule intact) or fallopian tube Surface free of tumor and washings negative
IB	Tumor limited to both ovaries (capsules intact) or fallopian tubes Surface free of tumor and washings negative
IC	Tumor limited to one or both ovaries or fallopian tubes, with any of the following:
IC1	Surgical spill intraoperatively
IC2	Capsule ruptured before surgery or tumor on ovarian or fallopian tube surface
IC3	Malignant cells in the ascites or peritoneal washings
Stage II	Tumor involves one or both ovaries or fallopian tubes with pelvic extension (below pelvic brim) or primary peritoneal cancer
IIA	Extension and/or implants on the uterus and/or fallopian tubes and/or ovaries
IIB	Extension to other pelvic intraperitoneal tissues
Stage III	Cytologically or histologically confirmed spread to the peritoneum outside the pelvis and/or metastasis to the retroperitoneal lymph nodes
IIIA	Metastasis to the retroperitoneal lymph nodes with or without microscopic peritoneal involvement beyond the pelvis
IIIA1	Positive retroperitoneal lymph nodes only (cytologically or histologically proven)
IIIA1 (i)	Nodal metastasis ≤10 mm in greatest dimension
IIIA1 (ii)	Nodal metastasis >10 mm in greatest dimension
IIIA2	Microscopic extrapelvic (above the pelvic brim) peritoneal involvement with or without positive retroperitoneal lymph nodes
IIIB	Macroscopic peritoneal metastases beyond the pelvic brim ≤2 cm in greatest dimension with or without positive retroperitoneal nodes
IIIC	Macroscopic peritoneal metastases beyond the pelvic brim >2 cm in greatest dimension with or without positive retroperitoneal nodes
Stage IV	Distant metastasis excluding peritoneal metastases
IVA	Pleural effusion with positive cytology
IVB	Metastases to extra-abdominal organs (including inguinal lymph nodes and lymph nodes outside of abdominal cavity)

FIGO = International Federation of Gynecology and Obstetrics.

shallow peritoneal fossa between the external iliac vessels and the ureter. Each ovary has an epithelial surface, a mesenchymal stroma containing steroid-producing cells and germ cells, an outer cortex and an inner medulla.

Ovaries appear early in fetal life as swellings of the genital ridges. At the 19th gestational day, germ cells migrate from the primitive yolk sac to the gonads and multiply by mitotic division. By the 40th day, ovaries and testes are histologically distinct. Toward the third trimester of fetal life, germ cells stop multiplying and instead continue to proliferate by meiosis. Of 1 million primordial follicles present at birth, only 70% remain by puberty and fewer than 15% persist to age 25 years. Only some 450 ova are actually shed during a woman's average 35-year reproductive lifetime.

The ovarian cortex mesenchyme consists of spindle-shaped, fibroblast-like cells. These give rise to granulosa and theca cells, which form a functional unit about each ovum (theca interna and theca externa). The complex of a germ cell and supporting granulosa cells is known first as a **primordial follicle**. During the reproductive period, a dominant follicle develops every month into a **graafian follicle**, which then ruptures during ovulation. Ovulation itself is often associated with mild cramping pain, which, if severe, is called **mittelschmerz** (i.e., midcycle pain). It is frequently confused with appendicitis. After ovulation, the follicle granulosa cells luteinize, that is, they become hypertrophied and accumulate lipid. They then produce and secrete progesterone in addition to estrogens. The collapsed follicle turns bright yellow and becomes the **corpus luteum** (yellow body).

Cells of ovarian stromal origin include hilus cells and those resembling luteinized cells of the theca interna, both of which respond to pituitary hormones. These specialized cells make and secrete both androgens and estrogens, which stimulate proliferation in end-organs (e.g., uterus). They inhibit hypothalamic function by negative feedback loops.

CYSTIC LESIONS OF THE OVARIES

Cysts usually arise from invaginated surface epithelium (serous cysts) and are the most common cause of enlarged ovaries. Almost all of the rest derive from ovarian follicles.

Follicle Cysts Tend to Be Asymptomatic

Follicle cysts are thin-walled, fluid-filled structures lined internally by granulosa cells and externally by theca interna cells. They occur at any age up to menopause, are unilocular and may be single or multiple, unilateral, or bilateral. They arise from ovarian follicles and are probably related to abnormalities in pituitary gonadotropin release.

 PATHOLOGY: Follicle cysts rarely exceed 5 cm. In an unstimulated state, granulosa cells of the cyst have uniform, round nuclei and little cytoplasm. Thecal cells are small and spindle shaped. Occasionally, the layers may be luteinized, and the lumen wall contains fluid high in estrogen or progesterone. If the cyst persists, hormonal output can cause precocious puberty in a child and menstrual irregularities in an adult. The only significant complication is mild intraperitoneal bleeding (Fig. 24-45).

Corpus Luteum Cysts Can Bleed

A corpus luteum cyst results from delayed resolution of a corpus luteum's central cavity. Continued progesterone synthesis by the luteal cyst leads to menstrual irregularities. Rupture of a cyst can cause mild hemorrhage into the abdominal cavity. A corpus luteum cyst is typically unilocular, 3 to 5 cm in size with a yellow wall. Cyst contents vary from serosanguineous fluid to clotted blood. Microscopic examination shows numerous large, luteinized granulosa cells. The condition is self-limited.

Theca Lutein Cysts Relate to High Gonadotropin Levels

Theca lutein cysts, also called *hyperreactio luteinalis,* are often multiple and bilateral. They are associated with high levels of circulating gonadotropin (as in pregnancy, hydatidiform mole, choriocarcinoma, or exogenous gonadotropin therapy) or physical impediments (dense adhesions, cortical fibrosis) to ovulation. Excessive gonadotropin levels lead to

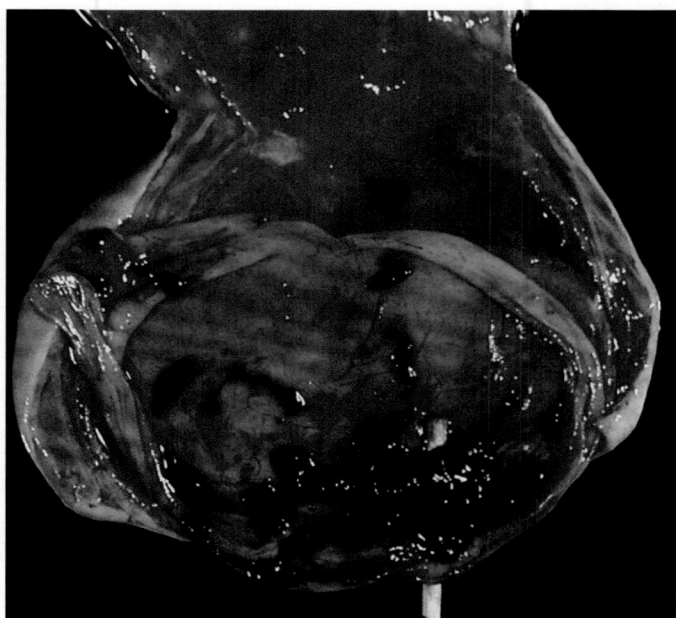

FIGURE 24-45. Follicle cyst of the ovary. Rupture of this thin-walled follicular cyst (dowel stick) led to intra-abdominal hemorrhage.

exaggerated stimulation of the theca interna and extensive cyst formation.

 PATHOLOGY: Multiple thin-walled cysts filled with clear fluid and lined by a markedly luteinized layer of theca interna replace both ovaries. Ovarian parenchyma shows edema and foci of luteinized stromal cells. Intra-abdominal hemorrhage due to torsion or rupture of the cyst may require surgical intervention.

POLYCYSTIC OVARY SYNDROME

Polycystic ovary syndrome, or **Stein–Leventhal syndrome**, reflects (1) excess secretion of androgenic hormones, (2) persistent anovulation, and (3) many small subcapsular ovarian cysts. It was first described as a syndrome of **secondary amenorrhea, hirsutism, and obesity**, but clinical presentations are now known to be far more variable and include amenorrheic women who appear otherwise normal and, even rarely, have ovaries lacking polycystic features. *This condition is a common cause of infertility: up to 7% of women experience polycystic ovary syndrome.*

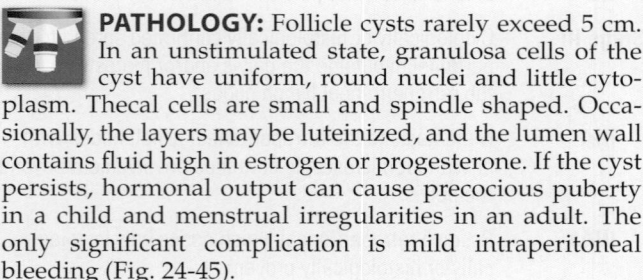 **PATHOPHYSIOLOGY:** Polycystic ovary syndrome is a state of functional ovarian hyperandrogenism with elevated levels of LH, although increased LH is probably a result, rather than a cause, of ovarian dysfunction (Fig. 24-46).

1. The central abnormality is thought to be increased ovarian production of androgens, although adrenal hypersecretion of androgens may also occur. The rate-limiting enzyme in androgen biosynthesis, cytochrome $P450_{c17\alpha}$ (17α-hydroxylase), expressed in both the ovary and the adrenal gland, is abnormally regulated.

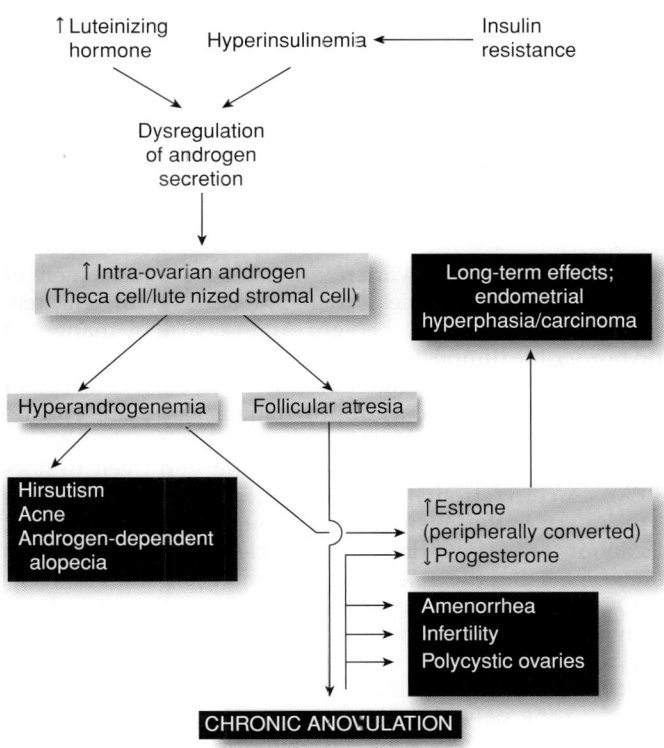

FIGURE 24-46. Pathogenesis of polycystic ovary syndrome.

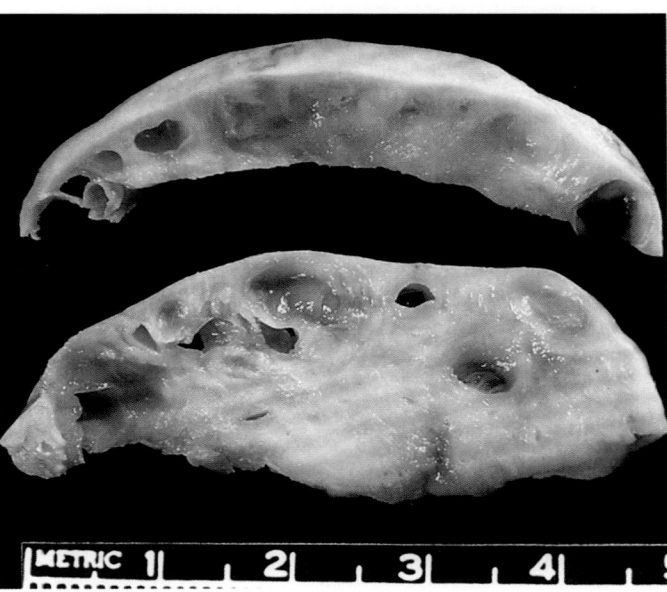

FIGURE 24-47. Polycystic disease of the ovary. Cut surfaces of this ovary show numerous cysts embedded in a sclerotic stroma.

2. Excess ovarian androgens act locally to cause (1) premature follicular atresia, (2) multiple follicular cysts, and (3) a persistent anovulatory state. Impaired follicular maturation results in decreased secretion of progesterone. Peripherally, hyperandrogenism leads to hirsutism, acne, and male-pattern (androgen-dependent) alopecia. Affected patients may have high serum levels of androgens, such as testosterone, androstenedione, and dehydroepiandrosterone sulfate. There are individual variations, however, and some patients have normal androgen levels.

3. Excess androgens are converted to estrogens in peripheral adipose tissue, an effect that is exaggerated by obesity. Acyclic estrogen production and progesterone deficiency increase pituitary secretion of LH.

4. Women with polycystic ovary syndrome exhibit marked peripheral insulin resistance, out of proportion to the degree of obesity. The mechanism appears to involve a post–insulin-receptor defect, possibly related to decreased expression of a glucose transporter. In any event, the resulting hyperinsulinemia seems to contribute to increased ovarian hypersecretion of androgens and direct stimulation of pituitary LH production.

PATHOLOGY: Both ovaries are enlarged. The surface is smooth, owing to lack of ovulation. On cut section, the cortex is thickened and contains numerous theca lutein–type cysts, typically 2 to 8 mm in diameter, arranged peripherally around a dense

core of stroma or scattered throughout an expanded stroma (Fig. 24-47). Microscopic features include (1) numerous follicles in early developmental stages; (2) follicular atresia; (3) increased stroma, occasionally with luteinized cells (hyperthecosis); and (4) features of anovulation (thick, smooth capsule and absence of corpora lutea and corpora albicantia). Many subcapsular cysts show thick zones of theca interna, in which some cells may be luteinized.

CLINICAL FEATURES: *Nearly three-quarters of women with anovulatory infertility have polycystic ovary syndrome.* Patients are typically in their 20s and tell of early obesity, menstrual problems and hirsutism. Half of women with polycystic ovary syndrome are amenorrheic and most others have irregular menses. Only 75% are actually infertile, however, indicating that some do occasionally ovulate. Unopposed acyclic estrogen activity increases incidence of endometrial hyperplasia and carcinoma.

Treatment of polycystic ovary syndrome targets two common problems in reproductive endocrinology—hirsutism and anovulation. Therapy is mostly hormonal and seeks to interrupt the constant excess of androgens. Wedge resection of the ovary provides temporary remission of the syndrome but is rarely used today.

STROMAL HYPERTHECOSIS

Stromal hyperthecosis is focal luteinization of ovarian stromal cells. These stromal cells are often functional and cause **virilization**. The condition is most common in postmenopausal women and, in a microscopic form, is found in one-third of postmenopausal ovaries.

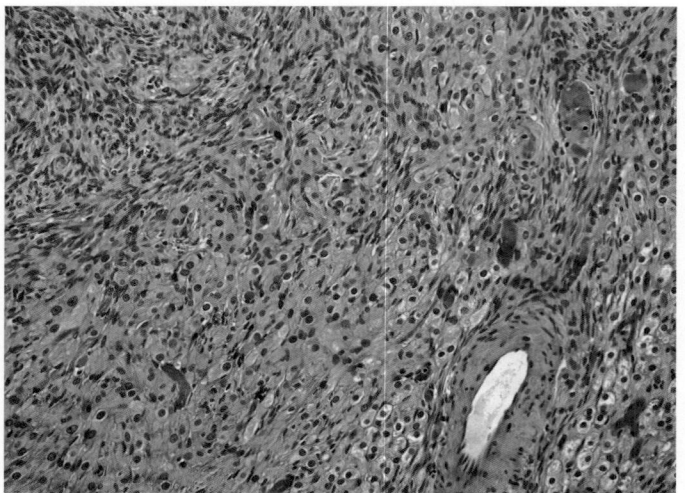

FIGURE 24-48. Hyperthecosis of the ovary. Numerous nests of luteinized (lipid-rich) stromal cells are present.

PATHOLOGY: If stromal hyperthecosis is detected clinically, usually owing to masculinizing signs, both ovaries may be enlarged, sometimes up to 8 cm in greatest dimension. The serosa is smooth, and the cut surface is homogeneous, firm, and brown to yellow. Single nests or nodules of luteinized stromal cells with deeply eosinophilic, often vacuolated

cytoplasm are seen in the cortex or medulla (Fig. 24-48). Luteinized cells have a large central nucleus and a prominent nucleolus, features shared with all hormonally active stromal cells in the ovary.

OVARIAN TUMORS

About two-thirds of ovarian tumors occur in women of reproductive age and less than 5% develop in children. Approximately 80% are benign. Almost 90% of malignant and borderline tumors are diagnosed after the age of 40 years.

Ovarian tumors are classified by the ovarian cell type of origin (Fig. 24-49). Most (approximately 60%) are **epithelial tumors** that arise directly or indirectly from müllerian epithelium. Other important groups are germ cell tumors (30%), sex cord/stromal tumors (8%), and tumors metastatic to the ovary. In the Western world, epithelial tumors account for about 90% of ovarian malignancies, high-grade serous carcinoma being the most common among these.

Ovarian cancer is the second most frequent gynecologic malignancy after endometrial cancer and carries a higher mortality rate than all other female genital cancers combined (Table 24-3). Over three-fourths of patients have tumor spread to the pelvis or abdomen at the time of diagnosis (Stage III), and an early and curable stage is rarely encountered. Approximately 22,000 new cases of ovarian cancer are diagnosed each year in the United States, and more than 14,000 women die from the disease (Table 24-3). Lifetime risk

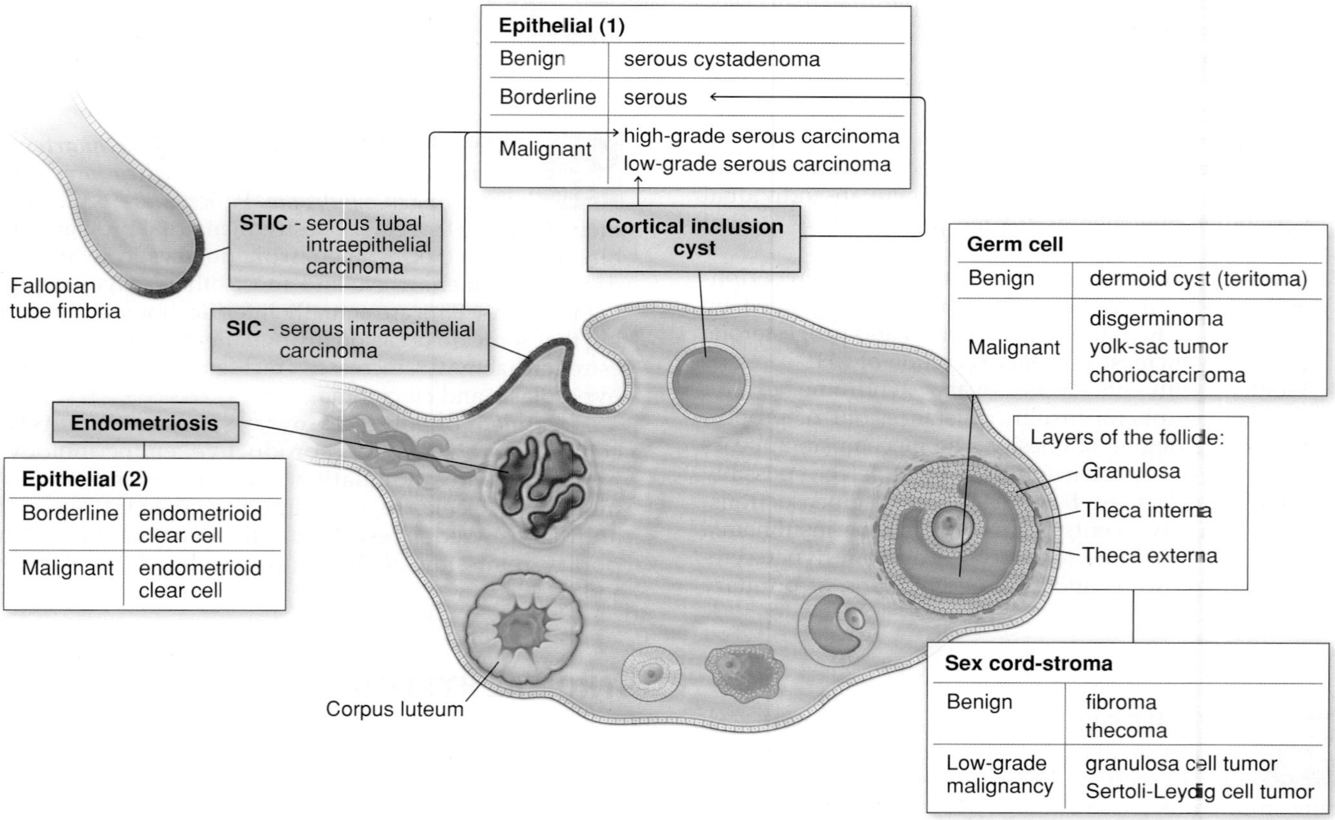

Epithelial (1)

Benign	serous cystadenoma
Borderline	serous
Malignant	high-grade serous carcinoma low-grade serous carcinoma

STIC - serous tubal intraepithelial carcinoma

SIC - serous intraepithelial carcinoma

Cortical inclusion cyst

Fallopian tube fimbria

Endometriosis

Epithelial (2)

Borderline	endometrioid clear cell
Malignant	endometrioid clear cell

Corpus luteum

Germ cell

Benign	dermoid cyst (teritoma)
Malignant	disgerminoma yolk-sac tumor choriocarciroma

Layers of the follicle:
- Granulosa
- Theca interna
- Theca externa

Sex cord-stroma

Benign	fibroma thecoma
Low-grade malignancy	granulosa cell tumor Sertoli-Leydig cell tumor

FIGURE 24-49. Classification of ovarian tumors based on cell of origin.

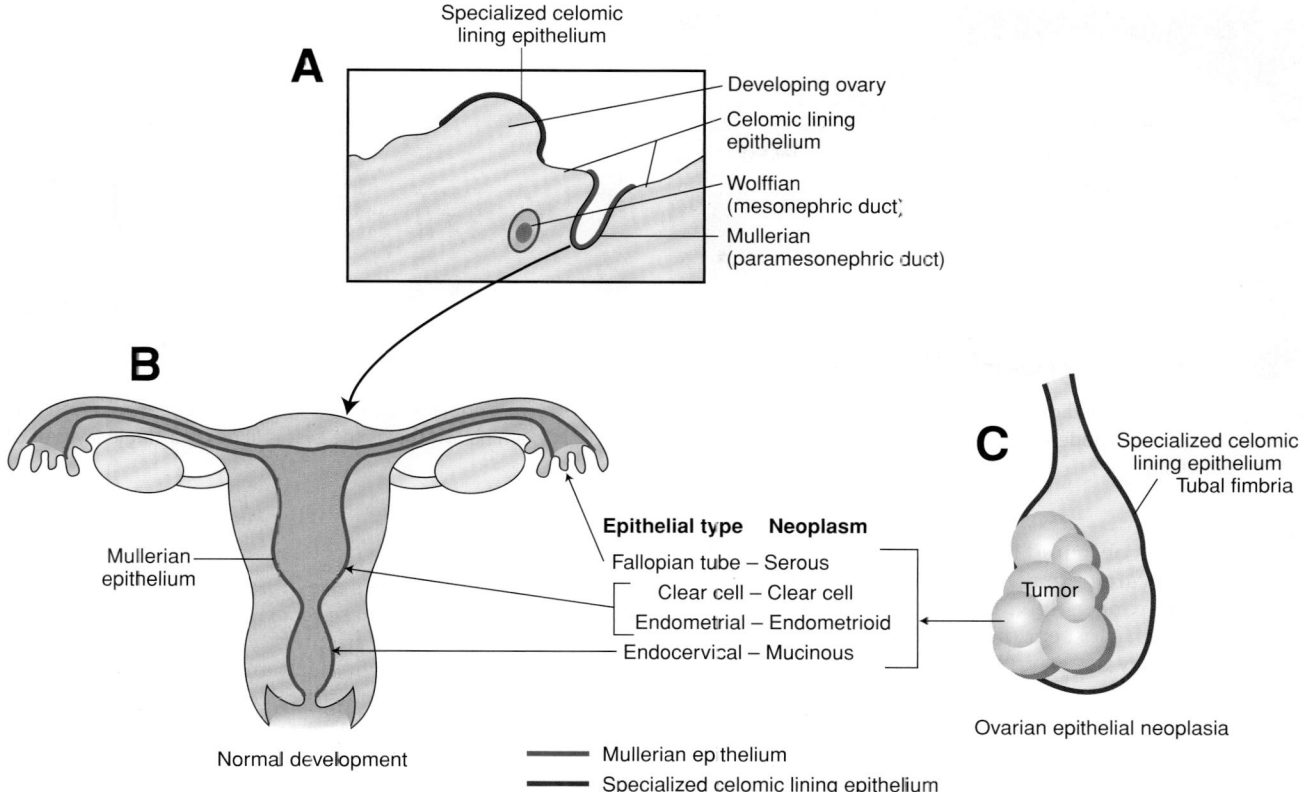

FIGURE 24-50. Histogenesis of ovarian epithelial/stromal tumors.

of developing ovarian cancer is 2%. These tumors predominate in women older than 60 years but may occur in younger women with a family history of the disease.

Epithelial Tumors Account for Over 90% of Ovarian Cancers

Tumors of epithelial origin are broadly classified, according to cell proliferation, degree of nuclear atypia and presence or absence of stromal invasion, as being: (1) **benign**, (2) of **borderline malignancy**, or (3) **malignant** (i.e., carcinomas) (Fig. 24-50).

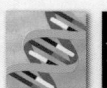 **MOLECULAR PATHOGENESIS AND ETIOLOGIC FACTORS:** Epithelial neoplasms are apparently related to repeated disruption and repair of the epithelial surface resulting from cyclic or "incessant" ovulation. Thus, tumors occur most commonly in nulliparous women and least often in women in whom ovulation has been suppressed (e.g., by pregnancy or oral contraceptives). Persistent, high concentrations of pituitary gonadotropins after menopause may stimulate proliferation of surface epithelial cells, thereby promoting accumulation of genetic changes and carcinogenesis. Irritants, such as talc or asbestos, transported up the reproductive tract to the ovaries have also been implicated.

Epithelial tumors, particularly serous carcinomas, are thought to arise from ovarian surface epithelium (mesothelium) or serosa. During embryonic life, the celomic cavity is lined by mesothelium, parts of which specialize to form the serosal epithelium covering the gonadal ridge. The same mesothelial lining gives rise to müllerian ducts, from which the fallopian tubes, uterus, and vagina arise (Fig. 24-49). Thus, as the ovary develops, the surface epithelium may extend into the ovarian stroma to form glands and cysts, and in some cases, these inclusion cysts become neoplastic and show a variety of müllerian-type differentiations (Fig. 24-50).

Approximately 10% of patients with high-grade serous carcinoma (HGSC) have a family history of ovarian cancer. If a first-degree relative had ovarian cancer, a woman's risk of developing ovarian cancer is increased 3.5-fold. Women with a history of ovarian carcinoma are also at greater risk for breast cancer and vice versa. Defects in repair genes implicated in hereditary breast cancers, BRCA1 and BRCA2, are incriminated in familial ovarian cancers as well. Ovarian carcinomas arising in patients with germline BRCA1 or BRCA2 mutations are almost invariably of high-grade serous type. Women with BRCA1 mutations tend to develop ovarian cancers at younger ages than those who develop sporadic ovarian tumors, but BRCA1-related tumors have a better prognosis.

The traditional view that HGSCs arise exclusively from ovarian surface epithelium or epithelial inclusion cysts has been challenged recently by the identification, in women with BRCA1 or BRCA2 germline mutations, of STIC (Fig. 24-44) in the distal fimbriated end of the fallopian tube as a malignant lesion related to advanced HGSC. Currently, the relative proportion of HGSC of ovarian and tubal derivation is unknown mainly because

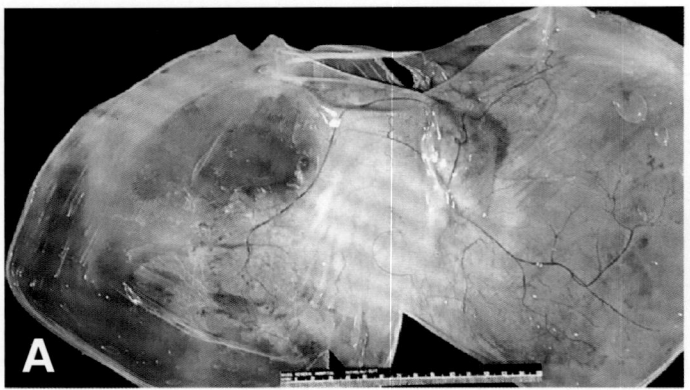
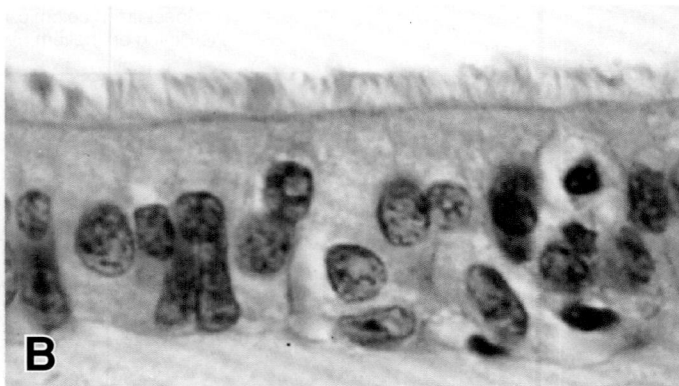

FIGURE 24-51. Serous cystadenoma of the ovary. A. Gross appearance of serous cystadenoma of the ovary. The fluid has been removed from this huge unilocular serous cystadenoma. The wall is thin and translucent. **B.** Microscopic examination shows the cyst is lined by a single layer of ciliated tubal-type epithelium.

the primary site is obscured in advanced stage cancers. As for endometrial carcinoma, women with hereditary non-polyposis colon cancer (HNPCC) are also at greater risk for ovarian cancer. Most endometrioid and clear cell carcinomas of the ovary are thought to originate from ovarian endometriosis.

 PATHOLOGY: In order of decreasing frequency, the **epithelial ovarian tumors** are:

- **Serous tumors** that resemble fallopian tube epithelium
- **Mucinous tumors** that mimic the mucosa of the endocervix or that of the gastric pylorus
- **Endometrioid tumors** that are similar to the glands of the endometrium
- **Clear cell tumors** with glycogen-rich cells like endometrial glands in pregnancy
- **Transitional cell tumors** that resemble the mucosa of the bladder
- **Mixed tumors**

Cystadenomas

Benign epithelial tumors are almost always serous or mucinous adenomas and generally arise in women 20 to 60 years old. These tumors are frequently large, often 15 to 30 cm in diameter. Some, particularly mucinous ones, reach massive proportions, exceeding 50 cm in diameter, and may mimic the appearance of a term pregnancy. Benign epithelial tumors are typically cystic, hence the term **cystadenoma**. Serous cystadenomas are more often bilateral (15%) than mucinous cystadenomas and tend to be unilocular (Fig. 24-51). By contrast, **mucinous tumors** usually contain hundreds of small cysts (locules) (Fig. 24-52). Unlike their malignant counterparts, benign ovarian epithelial tumors tend to have thin walls and lack solid areas. A single layer of tall columnar epithelial cells lines the cysts. Papillae, if present, have a fibrovascular core covered by a layer of tall columnar epithelium identical to the cyst lining.

Transitional Cell Tumor (Brenner Tumor)

The typical Brenner tumor is benign and occurs at all ages. Half of cases present in women over the age of 50. Size

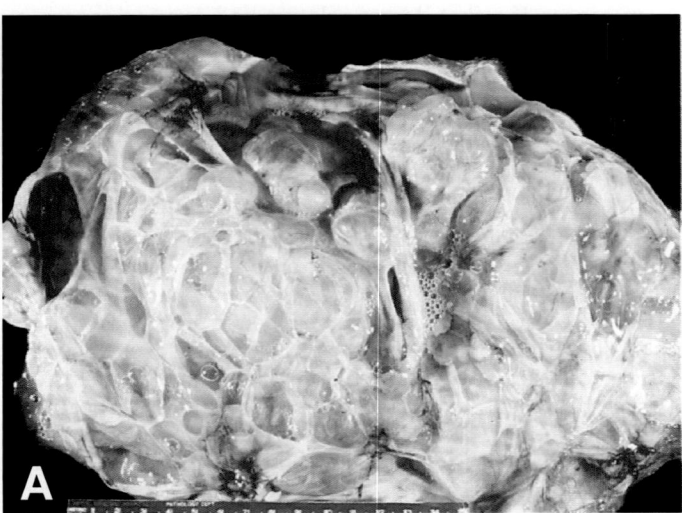
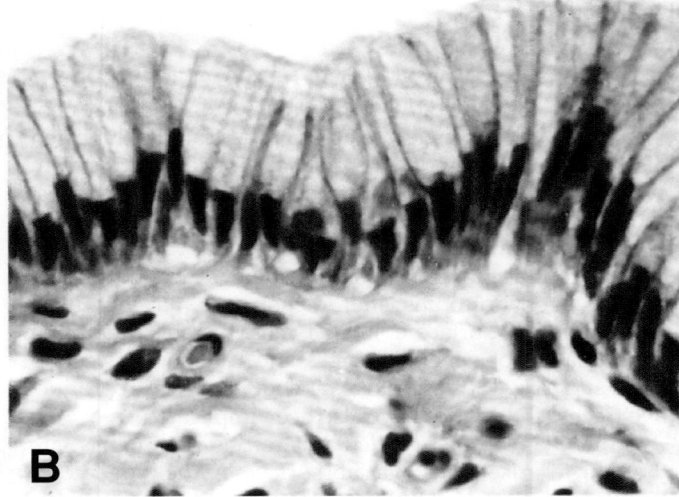

FIGURE 24-52. Mucinous cystadenoma of the ovary. A. The tumor is characterized by numerous cysts filled with thick, viscous fluid. **B.** A single layer of mucinous epithelial cells lines the cyst.

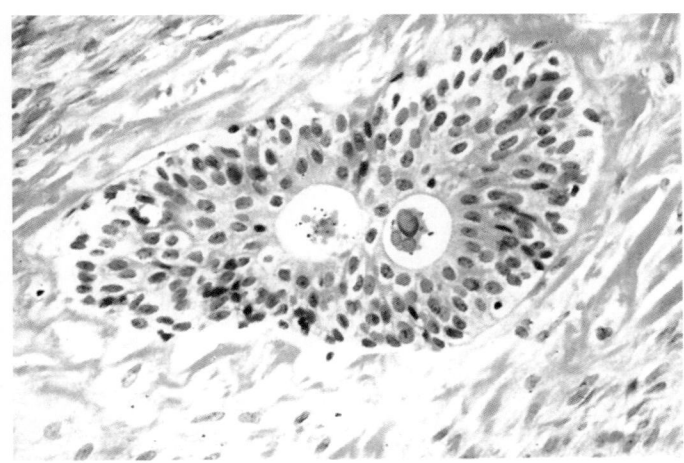

FIGURE 24-53. Brenner tumor. A nest of transitional-like cells is embedded in a dense, fibrous stroma.

varies from microscopic foci to masses 8 cm or more in diameter. Brenner tumors are adenofibromas, typically showing solid nests of transitional-like (urothelium-like) cells encased in a dense, fibrous stroma (Fig. 24-53). Epithelial nests are often cavitated and the most superficial epithelial cells may exhibit mucinous differentiation (Fig. 24-53).

Borderline Tumors

"Borderline tumors" are a well-defined group of ovarian tumors characterized by epithelial cell proliferation and nuclear atypia but without destructive stromal invasion. Despite histologic features suggesting aggressiveness, they share an excellent prognosis. Serous borderline tumors generally occur in women 20 to 50 years old (average, 46 years) but are also seen in older women.

Serous tumors of borderline malignancy are more commonly bilateral (34%) than mucinous ones (6%) or other types. The tumors vary in size, although mucinous ones

may be gigantic. In serous tumors of borderline malignancy, papillary projections, ranging from fine and exuberant to grape-like clusters arising from the cyst wall, are common (Fig. 24-54). These structures resemble the papillary fronds seen in benign cystadenomas, but they show epithelial stratification, moderate nuclear atypia and mitotic activity. The same criteria apply to borderline mucinous tumors, although papillary projections are less conspicuous. *By definition, the presence of more than focal microinvasion (i.e., discrete nests of epithelial cells <3 mm into the ovarian stroma) identifies a tumor as low-grade invasive serous carcinoma, rather than a borderline tumor.*

Despite the lack of ovarian stromal invasion, serous borderline tumors, particularly those with exophytic growth, implant on peritoneal surfaces in 30% of cases (Fig. 24-55). The vast majority (90%) of peritoneal implants are noninvasive and benign (Fig. 24-55A,B); however, approximately 10% progress to LGSC and invade underlying tissues (Fig. 24-55C). *Invasive peritoneal implants and LGSC are histologically identical and are distinguished only by the timing of the disease and the volume of the tumor. Whereas invasive peritoneal implants are early superficial lesions of microscopic or small macroscopic size (≤1 to 2 cm), LGSC frequently presents as bulky disease or peritoneal carcinomatosis.*

Surgical cure is almost always possible if the serous borderline tumor is confined to the ovaries. Even when it has spread to the pelvis or abdomen, 90% of patients are alive after 10 years. Lymph node involvement does not change the favorable prognosis. The risk of recurrence or development of a second serous borderline tumor is only 5% to 10%. Tumors rarely recur beyond 10 years. Late progression to low-grade serous carcinoma (LGSC) occurs in approximately 7% of cases. Almost all patients dying of recurrent tumor had invasive peritoneal implants, which is the key feature associated with a poor prognosis.

Malignant Epithelial Tumors

Carcinomas of the ovary are most common in women 40 to 60 years old and rare in women under the age of 35. *Based*

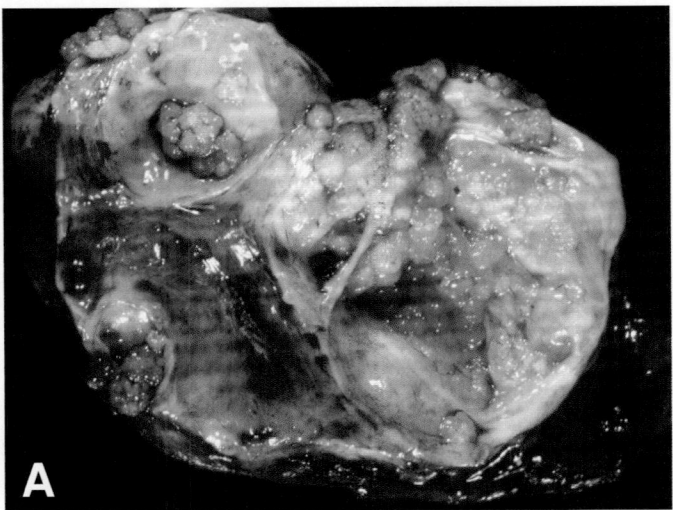

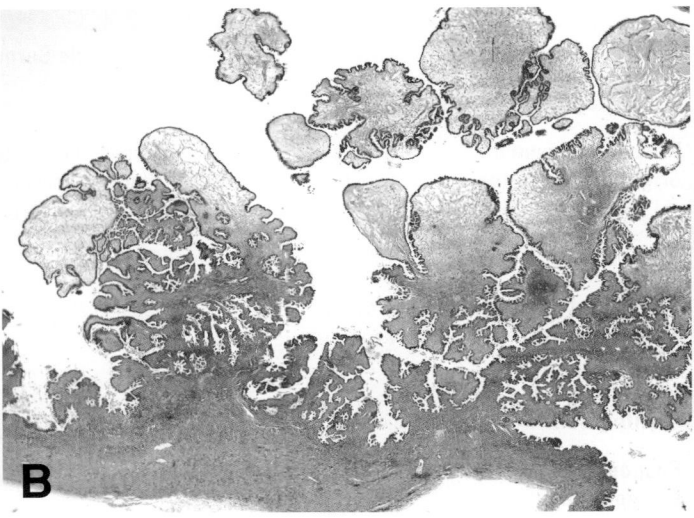

FIGURE 24-54. Serous cystic borderline tumor. A. The inner surface of the cysts is partly covered by closely packed papillae (endophytic growth). **B.** Microscopic view of the papillary tumor shows complex, hierarchical branching of papillae without stromal invasion. Some papillae have fibroedematous stalks.

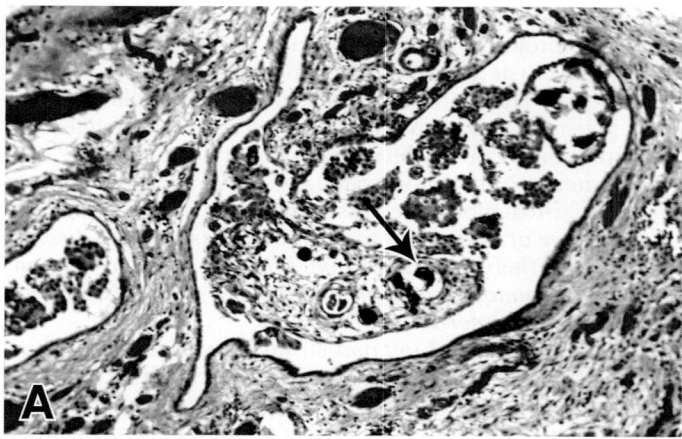

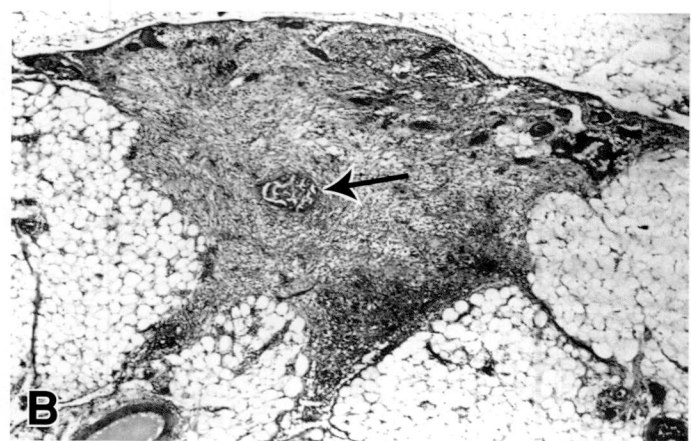

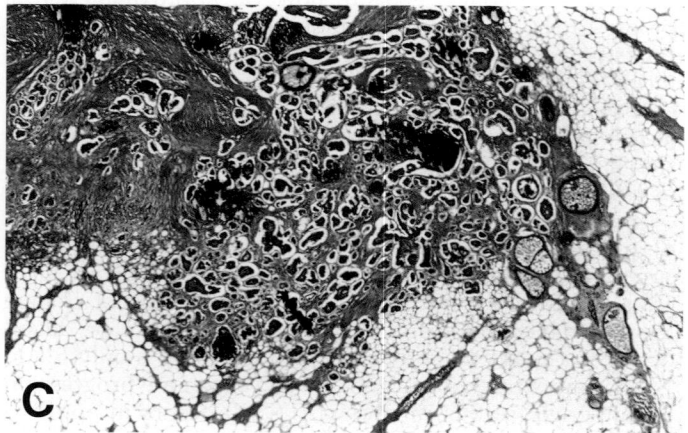

FIGURE 24-55. Peritoneal implants of serous borderline tumor. A. Noninvasive epithelial implant within a smoothly contoured invagination of the peritoneum. The epithelial proliferation contains psammoma bodies (*arrow*) and resembles the primary ovarian tumor. **B.** Noninvasive desmoplastic implant. The implant invaginates between adjacent lobules of omental fat. A few nests of tumor cells (*arrow*) are present within a loose fibroblastic stroma. **C.** Invasive omental implant. The tumor glands and papillae appear disorderly and resemble a low-grade serous carcinoma. They are distributed within a dense fibrous stroma.

on light microscopy and molecular genetics, ovarian carcinomas are classified into five main subtypes (Table 24-11), which, in descending order of frequency, are **high-grade serous carcinomas** (>70%), **endometrioid carcinomas** (10%), **clear cell carcinomas** (10%), **mucinous carcinomas** (3% to 4%) and **low-grade serous carcinomas** (<5%). These subtypes, which account for 98% of ovarian carcinomas, can be reproducibly diagnosed and categorized based on differences in epidemiologic and genetic risk factors, precursor lesions, patterns of spread, molecular events during

TABLE 24-11

MAIN SUBTYPES OF OVARIAN CARCINOMA

	Low-Grade Serous	High-Grade Serous	Clear Cell	Endometrioid	Mucinous
Usual stage at diagnosis	Early or advanced	Advanced	Early	Early	Early
Presumed tissue of origin/precursor lesion	Serous borderline tumor	Fallopian tube or tubal metaplasia in inclusions of ovarian surface epithelium	Endometriosis, adenofibroma	Endometriosis, adenofibroma	Adenoma–borderline–carcinoma sequence; teratoma
Genetic risk	?	*BRCA1/2*	?	HNPCC	?
Significant molecular abnormalities	*BRAF* or *KRAS*	*TP53* and *BRCA*	HNF-1β *ARID1A* *PIK3CA* *PTEN*	*PTEN* β-catenin *ARID1A KRAS* MI	*KRAS ERBB2*
Proliferation	Low	High	Low	Low	Intermediate
Response to primary chemotherapy	26–28%	80%	15%	?	15%
Prognosis	Favorable	Poor	Intermediate	Favorable	Favorable

HNF-1β = hepatocyte nuclear factor-1β; HNPCC = hereditary nonpolyposis colon cancer.

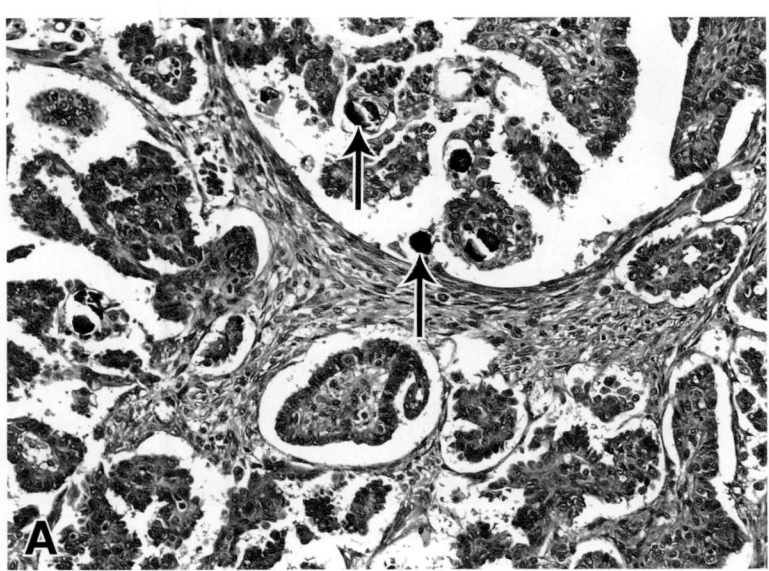
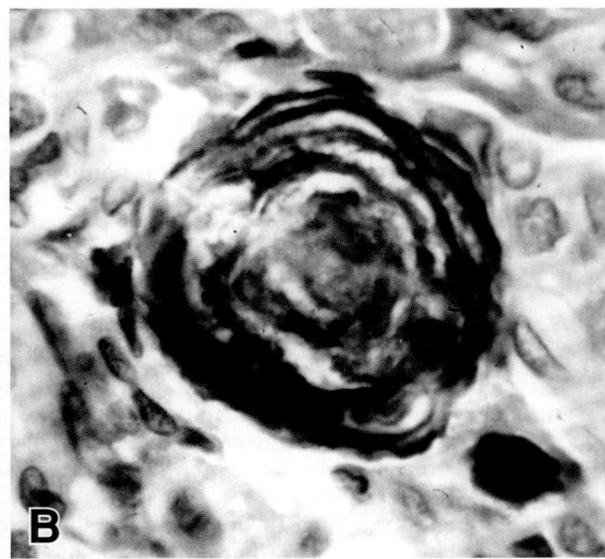

FIGURE 24-56. Low-grade serous carcinoma. A. Nests of tumor cells are distributed in a disorderly fashion and appear surrounded by clefts. In contrast to high-grade serous carcinoma, the nuclei are low grade. Psammoma bodies (*arrows*) are seen. **B.** A higher-power view shows the laminated structure of a psammoma body.

oncogenesis, responses to chemotherapy and outcomes. Advances in subtype-specific management of ovarian cancer make accurate subtype assignment increasingly important.

SEROUS CARCINOMAS:

MOLECULAR PATHOGENESIS: Low- and high-grade serous carcinomas are fundamentally different tumors. Whereas low-grade tumors are frequently associated with serous borderline tumors and have mutations in *KRAS* or *BRAF* oncogenes, most high-grade serous carcinomas lack identifiable precursor lesions and have a high frequency of mutations in *p53*, but not in *KRAS* or *BRAF*. Interestingly, carcinomas arising in patients with germline *BRCA1* or *BRCA2* mutations (hereditary ovarian cancers) are almost invariably the high-grade serous type and commonly have *p53* mutations. A significant number of *BRCA1*- or *BRCA2*-related tumors arise from epithelium of the fimbriated end of the fallopian tube (Fig. 24-44), suggesting that at least some sporadic high-grade ovarian and the so-called "primary" peritoneal serous carcinomas may actually develop from the distal fallopian tube and "spill over" onto adjacent tissues.

PATHOLOGY: Low-grade serous carcinomas are characterized by irregular invasion of the ovary by small, tight nests of tumor cells with variable desmoplasia (Fig. 24-56). Nuclear uniformity is the principal criterion for distinguishing low- and high-grade serous carcinomas. Psammoma bodies are often present. Low-grade serous carcinomas rarely progress to high-grade tumors.

High-grade serous carcinomas are mainly solid, multinodular masses, usually containing areas of necrosis and hemorrhage (Fig. 24-57A). The tumor often spreads

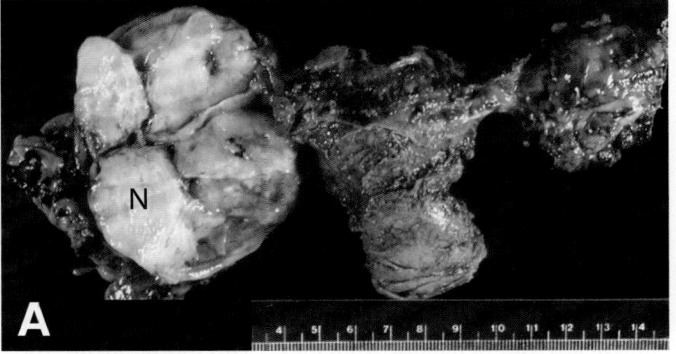
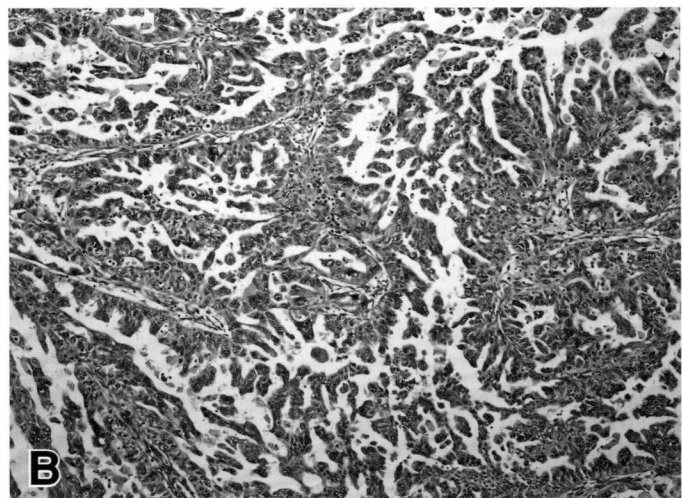

FIGURE 24-57. High-grade serous carcinoma. A. In addition to containing cysts (*left*), this ovary is enlarged by a solid tumor that exhibits extensive necrosis (*N*). **B.** Microscopic examination shows complex papillae, lined by markedly atypical nuclei.

beyond the ovary and seeds the peritoneum. Two-thirds of serous cancers with extraovarian spread are bilateral. High-grade serous cancers typically show obvious stromal invasion. Most tumors have a high nuclear grade with irregularly branching, highly cellular papillae with little or no stromal support and slit-like glandular lumens within more solid areas (Fig. 24-57B). The mitotic rate is very high.

MUCINOUS CARCINOMA:

MOLECULAR PATHOGENESIS: Mucinous ovarian tumors are often heterogeneous. Benign, borderline, noninvasive, and invasive carcinoma components may coexist within the same tumor. Such a morphologic continuum suggests progression from cystadenoma and borderline tumor to noninvasive, microinvasive, and invasive carcinomas.

KRAS mutations, which are an early event in mucinous tumorigenesis, occur in 43.6% of mucinous carcinomas and 78.8% of mucinous borderline tumors. Overexpression/amplification of *HER2* has been found in 18.8% of mucinous carcinomas and 6.2% of mucinous borderline tumors. Interestingly, *KRAS* mutations are near mutually exclusive of *HER2* amplification. Approximately 34% of mucinous carcinomas have neither *HER2* amplification nor *KRAS* mutation and these cases are associated with worse prognosis. *KRAS* mutations remain the most frequent alteration among mucinous carcinomas and mucinous borderline tumors.

PATHOLOGY: Mucinous carcinomas are usually large, unilateral, multilocular, or unilocular cystic masses containing mucinous fluid. They often include papillary and solid areas that may be soft and mucoid, or firm, hemorrhagic and necrotic. Since these tumors are bilateral in only 5% of cases, finding bilateral or unilateral mucinous tumors smaller than 10 cm raises suspicion of metastatic mucinous carcinoma from the gastrointestinal tract or elsewhere.

The category of mucinous borderline tumor with intraepithelial carcinoma is reserved for tumors that lack architectural features of invasive carcinoma but focally show unequivocal malignant cells lining glandular spaces. Mucinous borderline tumors with intraepithelial carcinoma have a very low likelihood of recurrence.

Mucinous adenocarcinomas may be further subdivided into (1) **expansile** or **confluent glandular pattern**, lacking destructive stromal invasion (Fig. 24-58) but showing back-to-back or complex malignant glands with minimal or no intervening stroma, and (2) **infiltrative**, with obvious glandular stromal invasion. The expansile pattern appears to have a more favorable prognosis than the infiltrative type. The combination of extensive, infiltrative stromal invasion; high nuclear grade; and tumor rupture is a strong predictor of recurrence for stage I mucinous adenocarcinomas.

Pseudomyxoma peritonei is a clinical condition of abundant gelatinous or mucinous ascites in the peritoneum, fibrous adhesions, and frequently mucinous tumors involving the ovaries. The appendix is involved by

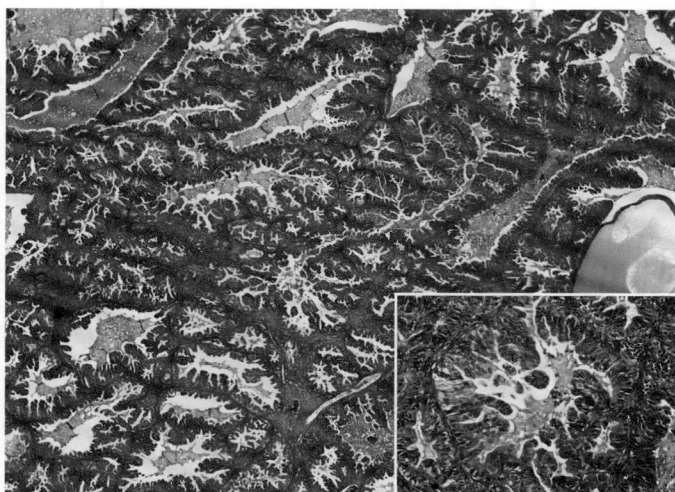

FIGURE 24-58. Mucinous carcinoma. The tumor shows expansile (confluent) invasion. *Inset.* Complex mucinous glands with cytologic atypia form a confluent or expansile pattern.

a similar mucinous tumor in 60% of the cases and appears normal in the remaining 40%. In most cases, the ovarian tumors are metastases from the appendiceal lesions. Concordant *KRAS* mutations have been found in both the appendiceal and ovarian tumors of individual patients.

ENDOMETRIOID CARCINOMA: Endometrioid carcinoma histologically resembles its endometrial counterpart (Fig. 24-59A), and may have areas of squamous differentiation. It is second only to serous adenocarcinoma in frequency, and accounts for 10% of all ovarian cancers. These tumors occur most commonly after menopause. Unlike serous and mucinous neoplasms, most endometrioid tumors are malignant. Up to one-half of these cancers are bilateral and, at diagnosis, most are confined either to the ovary or within the pelvis.

MOLECULAR PATHOGENESIS: Endometrioid carcinomas are thought to arise by malignant transformation of endometriosis, rather than from the ovarian surface epithelium (Fig. 24-59B). Mutations in the AT-rich interactive domain 1A gene (*ARID1A*) have been implicated not only in endometrioid and clear cell carcinomas but also in adjacent endometriosis. *ARID1A* behaves as a tumor suppressor. Loss of expression of the BAF250 protein, encoded by *ARID1A*, may increase risk of developing clear cell or endometrioid ovarian cancer. Other common genetic abnormalities in sporadic endometrioid carcinoma of the ovary are somatic mutations of β-catenin (*CTNNB1*) and *PTEN* genes and microsatellite instability. Endometrioid borderline tumors also have β-catenin mutations.

PATHOLOGY: Endometrioid carcinomas vary in size from 2 cm to more than 30 cm. Most are largely solid with areas of necrosis, although they may be cystic. Endometrioid tumors are graded like their endometrial counterparts. Between 15% and 20% of

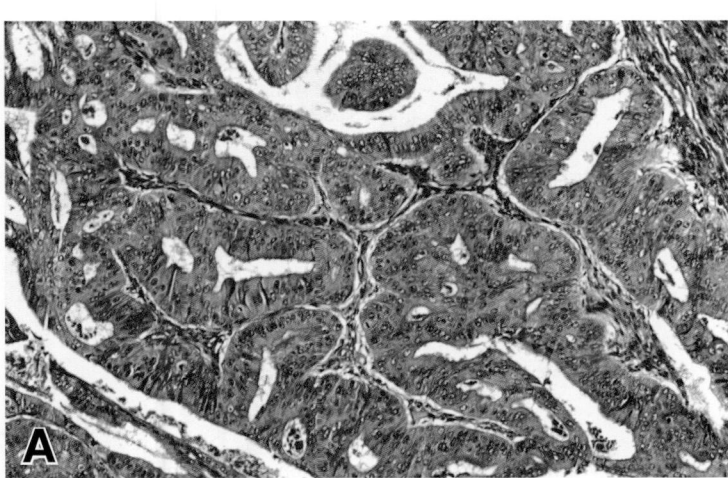
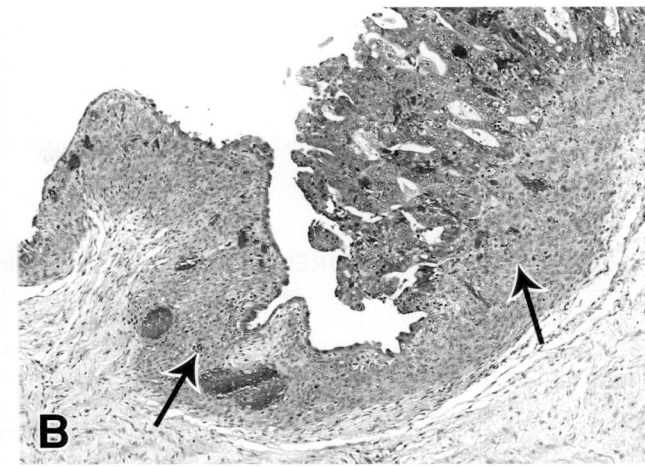

FIGURE 24-59. Endometrioid carcinoma. A. Crowded neoplastic glands are lined by stratified non–mucin-containing epithelium. Nuclear atypia is moderate to severe. **B.** Endometrioid carcinoma (*right*) arising in endometriosis. Note the stromal cells of endometriosis (*arrows*).

patients with endometrioid carcinoma of the ovary also harbor an endometrial cancer. If ovarian and endometrial cancers coexist, they generally arise independently, although one may be metastatic from the other. This distinction has important prognostic implications. An alternative explanation is that the ovarian endometrioid carcinomas may arise from ovarian endometriosis or from endometrial stem cells that reached the ovary through menstrual reflux. Molecular diagnostic methods including loss of heterozygosity (LOH), gene mutation and clonal X-inactivation analysis can help distinguish these possibilities. The 5-year survival exceeds 85% in synchronous tumors. As with all malignant epithelial tumors of the ovary, prognosis depends on the stage at which it presents.

CLEAR CELL CARCINOMA: This enigmatic ovarian cancer is closely related to endometrioid adenocarcinoma and often occurs in association with endometriosis (Fig. 24-60A). It constitutes 5% to 10% of all ovarian cancers usually occurring after menopause.

Roughly half of clear cell carcinomas (46% to 57%) carry *ARID1A* mutations and lack BAF250 protein. Other common genetic abnormalities are inactivating *PTEN* mutations and activating *PIK3CA* mutations. Hepatocyte nuclear factor-1β (HNF-1β) regulates several specific genes in clear cell carcinoma, including those that encode dipeptidyl peptidase IV (involved in glycogen synthesis), osteopontin (a progesterone-regulated endometrial secretory protein), angiotensin-converting enzyme 2 (involved in ferritin induction, iron deposition, antiapoptosis), annexin 4 (paclitaxel resistance), and UGT1A1 (a UDP glucuronosyltransferase involved in detoxification).

Although patients typically present with stage I or II disease, clear cell carcinomas have a poor prognosis compared with other low-stage ovarian carcinomas. Tumors range in size from 2 to 30 cm, and 40% are bilateral. Most are partially cystic and show necrosis and hemorrhage in the solid areas.

Clear cell carcinomas of the ovary resemble their counterparts in the vagina and have sheets or tubules of

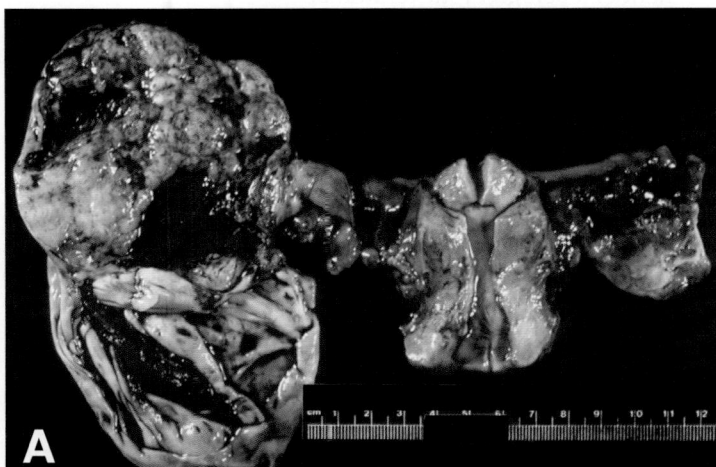
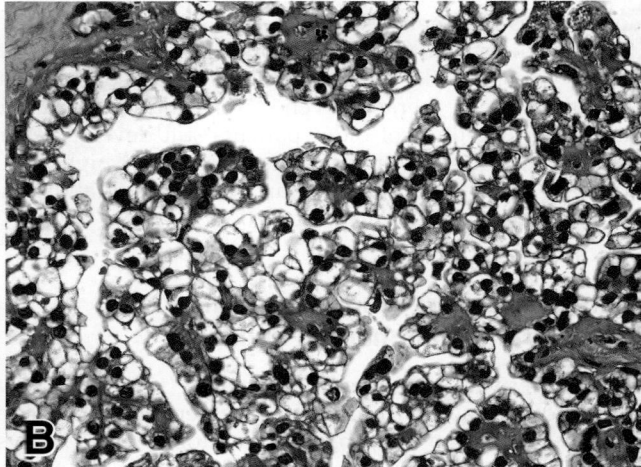

FIGURE 24-60. Clear cell carcinoma. A. Clear cell carcinoma arising as an ovarian mass in a large, hemorrhagic endometriotic cyst. **B.** The clear cells are polyhedral and have eccentric, hyperchromatic nuclei without prominent nucleoli.

malignant cells with clear cytoplasm (Fig. 24-60B). In the tubular form, malignant cells often display bulbous nuclei that protrude into the lumen of the tubule ("hobnail cell"), resembling an Arias-Stella reaction in gestational endometrium (Fig. 24-28). The clinical course parallels that of endometrioid carcinoma.

CLINICAL FEATURES: Most ovarian tumors do not secrete hormones. However, the cancer antigen, CA-125, is detectable in the serum in about half of epithelial tumors confined to the ovary and about 90% that have spread. The specificity of this test is highest when combined with transvaginal ultrasonography.

Ovarian masses rarely produce symptoms until they become large and distend the abdomen to cause pain, pelvic pressure, or compression of regional organs. By the time ovarian cancers are diagnosed, many have metastasized to (i.e., implanted on) the surfaces of the pelvis, abdominal organs, or bladder. Evaluation of a patient with an epithelial ovarian cancer requires knowledge of staging, grading, and routes of tumor spread. For example, ovarian tumors have a tendency to implant in the peritoneal cavity on the diaphragm, paracolic gutters, and omentum. Lymphatic spread preferentially involves paraaortic lymph nodes near the origin of the renal arteries and to a lesser extent external iliac (pelvic) or inguinal lymph nodes. In addition to local symptoms, metastatic cancers may cause ascites, weakness, weight loss, and cachexia.

Survival in patients with malignant ovarian tumors is generally poor. The most important prognostic index is the surgical stage of the tumor at the time of detection (Table 24-10). Overall, 5-year survival is only 35%, because more than half of tumors have spread to the abdominal cavity (stage III) or elsewhere by the time they are discovered. Prognostic indices for epithelial tumors also include grade, histologic type, and the size of the residual neoplasm.

Surgery to remove the primary tumor, establish the diagnosis and determine the extent of spread, is the mainstay of therapy. The peritoneal surfaces, omentum, liver, subdiaphragmatic recesses and all abdominal regions must be visualized, and as much metastatic tumor removed as possible. Adjuvant chemotherapy is used to treat distant occult sites of tumor spread.

At some time after the initial operation, another exploratory (second-look) laparotomy may be used to assess effectiveness of therapy. Even if no residual disease is apparent, one-third of older patients still develop recurrences. Risk factors for recurrence include (1) high stage, (2) high grade, and (3) more than 2 cm of residual disease remaining after the primary operation.

Germ Cell Tumors Tend to Be Benign in Adults and Malignant in Children

Tumors derived from germ cells make up 1/4 of ovarian tumors. In adult women, ovarian germ cell tumors are virtually all benign (mature cystic teratoma, dermoid cyst), but in children and young adults, they are largely cancerous. *In children, germ cell tumors are the most common ovarian cancer (60%); they are rare after menopause.*

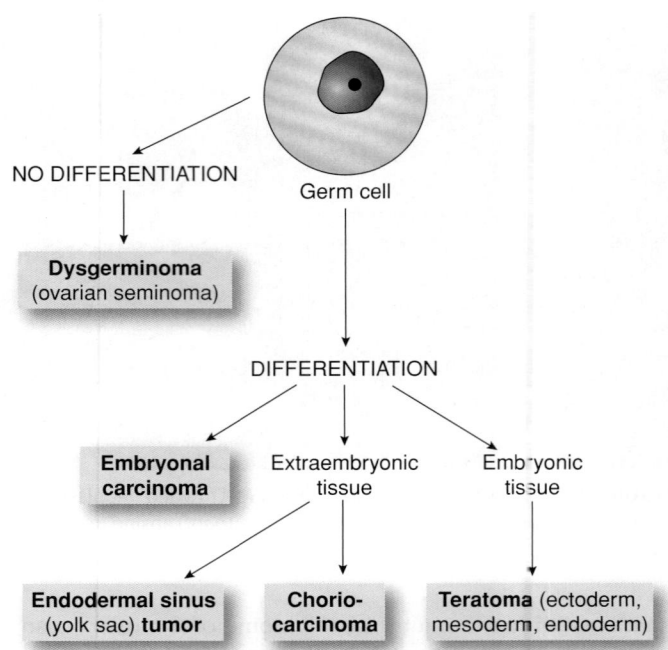

FIGURE 24-61. Classification of germ cell tumors of the ovary.

Neoplastic germ cells may differentiate along several lines (Fig. 24-61):

- **Dysgerminomas** are composed of neoplastic germ cells, similar to oogonia of fetal ovaries.
- **Teratomas** differentiate toward somatic (embryonic or adult) tissues.
- **Yolk sac tumors** form extraembryonic endodermal and mesenchymal tissue.
- **Choriocarcinomas** feature cells similar to those covering the placental villi.

Germ cell tumors in infants tend to be solid and immature (e.g., yolk sac tumor and immature teratoma). Tumors in young adults show greater differentiation, as in mature cystic teratoma. Malignant germ cell tumors in women older than 40 years usually result from transformation of a component of a benign cystic teratoma.

Malignant germ cell tumors are very aggressive. Solid ovarian germ cell tumors were once always fatal, but now over 80% of patients survive with chemotherapy.

Dysgerminoma

Dysgerminoma, the ovarian counterpart of testicular seminoma, is composed of primordial germ cells. It accounts for less than 2% of ovarian cancers in all women, but constitutes 10% in women younger than 20 years. Most patients are between 10 and 30. The tumors are bilateral in about 15% of cases.

PATHOLOGY: Dysgerminomas are often large and firm and have a bosselated external surface. The cut surface is soft and fleshy. They contain large nests of monotonously uniform tumor cells with clear glycogen-filled cytoplasm and irregularly flattened

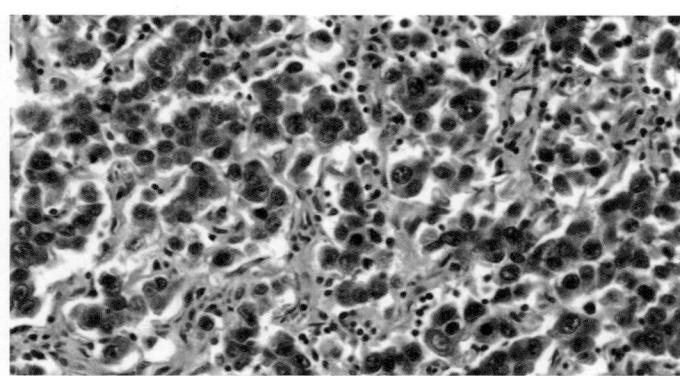

FIGURE 24-62. Dysgerminoma. Neoplastic germ cells are distributed in nests separated by delicate fibrous septa. The stroma contains lymphocytes.

central nuclei (Fig. 24-62). Fibrous septa containing lymphocytes traverse the tumor. Diffuse positive nuclear staining for the stem cell/primitive germ cell nuclear transcription factors OCT-4 and SALL4 is seen.

Dysgerminomas are treated surgically; 5-year survival for patients with stage I tumor approaches 100%. Because the tumor is highly radiosensitive and also responsive to chemotherapy, even higher-stage tumors have 5-year survival rates exceeding 80%.

Teratoma

Teratoma is a tumor of germ cell origin that differentiates toward somatic structures. Most contain tissues from at least two, and usually all three, embryonic layers.

MATURE TERATOMA (MATURE CYSTIC TERATOMA, DERMOID CYST): This benign neoplasm accounts for 1/4 of all ovarian tumors, with peak incidence in the third decade. Mature teratomas develop by **parthenogenesis**. Haploid (postmeiotic) germ cells endoreduplicate to give rise to diploid genetically female tumor cells (46,XX).

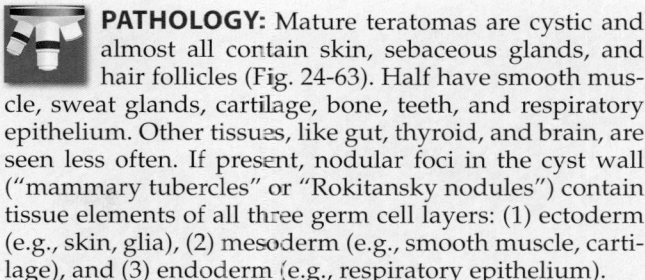

PATHOLOGY: Mature teratomas are cystic and almost all contain skin, sebaceous glands, and hair follicles (Fig. 24-63). Half have smooth muscle, sweat glands, cartilage, bone, teeth, and respiratory epithelium. Other tissues, like gut, thyroid, and brain, are seen less often. If present, nodular foci in the cyst wall ("mammary tubercles" or "Rokitansky nodules") contain tissue elements of all three germ cell layers: (1) ectoderm (e.g., skin, glia), (2) mesoderm (e.g., smooth muscle, cartilage), and (3) endoderm (e.g., respiratory epithelium).

Struma ovarii is a cystic lesion composed mainly of thyroid tissue. It occurs in 5% to 20% of mature cystic teratomas. Rarely hyperthyroidism can occur in struma ovarii.

Very few (1%) dermoid cysts become malignant. These cancers usually occur in older women and correspond to the tumors that arise in other differentiated tissues of the body. Three-fourths of cancers that arise in dermoid cysts are squamous cell carcinomas. The remainder are carcinoid tumors, basal cell carcinomas, thyroid cancers and others. Rarely, functional gut derivatives may cause carcinoid syndrome. The prognosis of patients with malignancies in mature cystic teratoma is related largely to the stage of the cancer.

IMMATURE TERATOMA: Immature teratomas of the ovary contain elements derived from the three germ layers. However, unlike mature cystic teratomas, immature teratomas contain embryonal tissues. These tumors account for 20% of malignant tumors at all sites in women under the age of 20 but become progressively less common in older women.

PATHOLOGY: Immature teratomas are predominantly solid and lobulated, with numerous small cysts. Solid areas may contain grossly recognizable immature bone and cartilage. Multiple tumor components are usually seen, including those differentiating toward nerve (neuroepithelial rosettes and immature glia) (Fig. 24-64), glands and other structures found in mature cystic teratomas. Grading is based on the amount of immature neural tissue present. Metastases of immature teratomas are

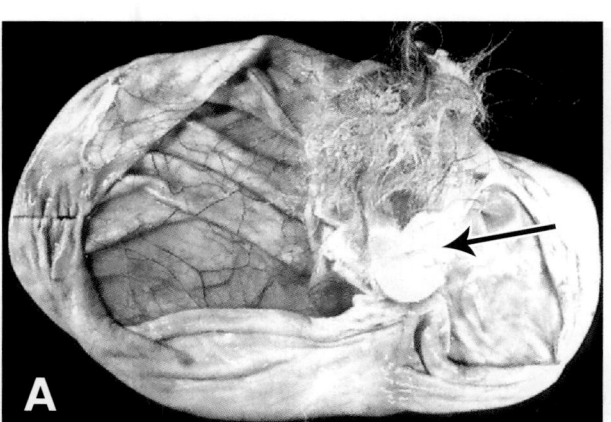
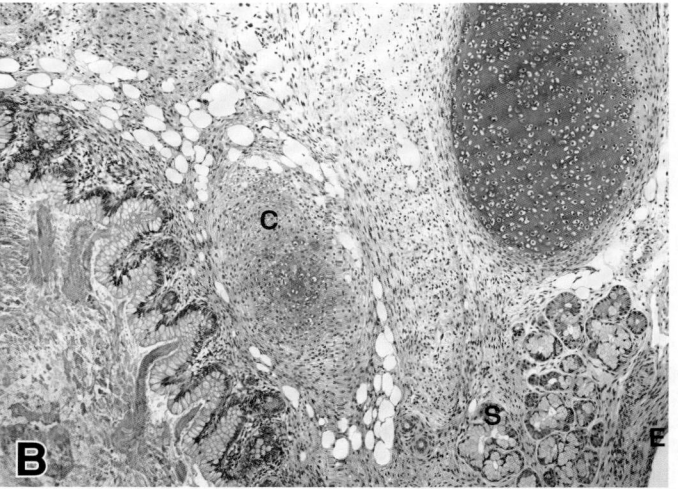

FIGURE 24-63. Mature teratoma of the ovary. A. A mature cystic teratoma has been opened to reveal a solid knob (*arrow*) from which hair projects. **B.** Microscopic view of a mature teratoma exhibiting gastrointestinal glands (*left side of image*), fetal-type cartilage (*C*), mixed seromucinous salivary glands (*S*), and tissue resembling skin with an epidermins (*E*) overlying dermal structures.

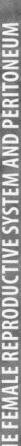

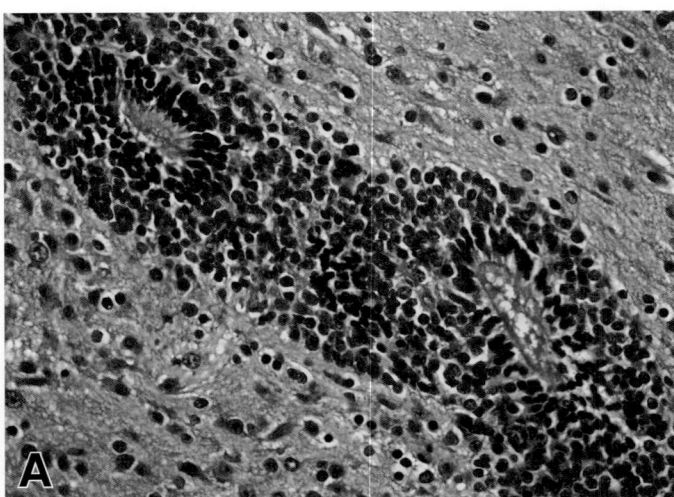
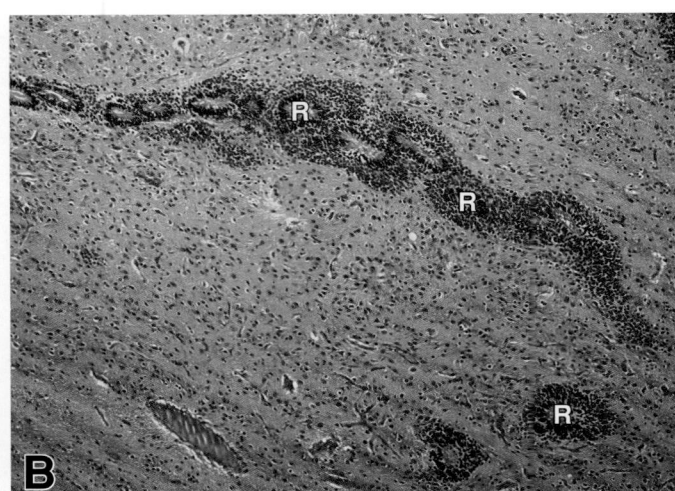

FIGURE 24-64. Immature teratoma of the ovary. A. Embryonal glia display densely packed, atypical nuclei. **B.** Immature neural tissue exhibits rosettes (*R*) with multilayered nuclei.

composed of embryonal, usually stromal, tissues. By contrast, rare metastases of mature cystic teratomas resemble epithelial adult-type malignancies.

Survival reflects tumor grade. Well-differentiated immature teratomas have a good prognosis, but high-grade tumors (mainly embryonal tissue) are often lethal.

Yolk Sac Tumor (Primitive Endodermal Tumor)

Yolk sac tumors are highly malignant tumors of women under the age of 30 that histologically resemble mesenchyme of the primitive yolk sac. They are the second most common malignant germ cell tumors and are almost always unilateral.

PATHOLOGY: Yolk sac tumors are large, with extensive necrosis and hemorrhage. Several patterns are seen. The most common is a reticular, honeycombed structure of communicating spaces lined by primitive epithelial cells with glycogen-rich, clear cytoplasm and large hyperchromatic nuclei (primitive

endoderm). Glomerular or **Schiller–Duval bodies** (Fig. 24-65A) are found sparingly in a few tumors but, when seen, are highly characteristic. They consist of papillae that protrude into a space lined by tumor cells, resembling the glomerular Bowman space. The papillae are covered by a mantle of embryonal cells and contain a fibrovascular core and a central blood vessel.

Yolk sac tumors should not be confused with embryonal cell carcinomas, which are common in the testis but rare in the ovary. The former secretes α-fetoprotein, which can be demonstrated histochemically (Fig. 24-65B). Detection of α-fetoprotein in the blood is useful for diagnosis and for monitoring the effectiveness of therapy. Yolk sac tumors also express glypican-3, SALL4, and villin. Although once uniformly fatal, 5-year survival with chemotherapy for stage I yolk sac tumors now exceeds 80%.

Choriocarcinoma

Choriocarcinoma of the ovary is a rare tumor that mimics the epithelial covering of placental villi, namely, cytotrophoblast

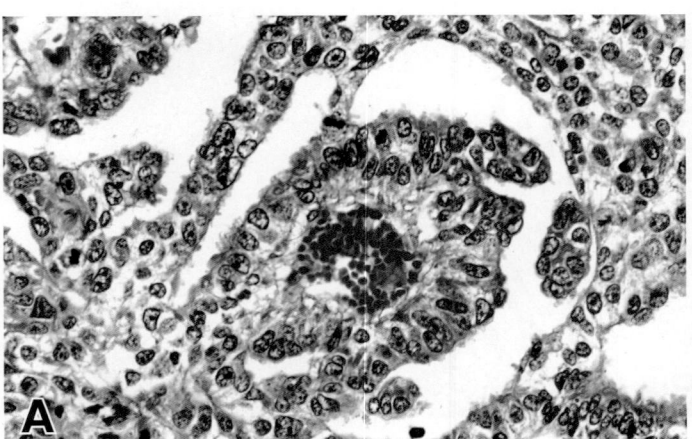
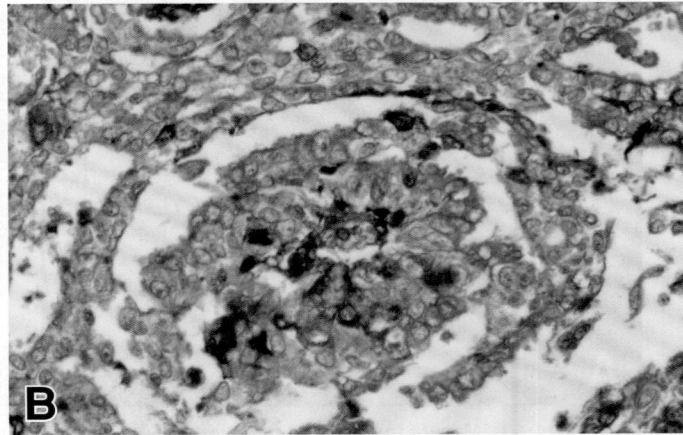

FIGURE 24-65. Yolk sac tumor of the ovary. A. Glomeruloid Schiller–Duval body that resembles the endodermal sinuses of the rodent placenta and consists of a papilla protruding into a space lined by tumor cells. **B.** Strong immunoreaction (brown signal) for α-fetoprotein.

and syncytiotrophoblast. If it arises before puberty or together with another germ cell tumor, it is most likely of germ cell origin. Young girls may show precocious sexual development, menstrual irregularities, or rapid breast enlargement. In women of reproductive age, however, it may also be a metastasis from an intrauterine gestational tumor.

PATHOLOGY: Choriocarcinoma is unilateral, solid, and widely hemorrhagic. Microscopically, it shows a mixture of malignant cytotrophoblast and syncytiotrophoblast (see placenta, choriocarcinoma, below). The syncytial cells secrete hCG, which accounts for the frequent finding of a positive pregnancy test result. Bilateral theca lutein cysts, a result of hCG stimulation, may also be found. Serial serum hCG determinations are useful both for diagnosis and follow-up. The tumor is highly aggressive but responds to chemotherapy.

Gonadoblastoma

Gonadoblastoma is a rare ovarian tumor that is distinctively associated with gonadal dysgenesis, especially in women who bear a Y chromosome. It occurs in phenotypic women under 30 years of age, although 20% are found in phenotypic men with cryptorchidism, hypospadias, and female internal sex organs. Most affected women are virilized and suffer from primary amenorrhea and developmental abnormalities of the genitalia. Cellular nests show a mixture of germ cells and sex cord derivatives that resemble immature Sertoli and granulosa cells, suggesting that the tumor is an in situ form of germinoma. In half of cases, it is overgrown by dysgerminoma. Gonadoblastomas do not metastasize, but their overgrowths do.

Sex Cord/Stromal Tumors Are Clinically Functional

Tumors of sex cord and stroma originate from either primitive sex cords (which originate from epithelium of the two gonadal ridges) or from mesenchymal stroma of developing gonads. They represent 10% of ovarian tumors, vary from benign to low-grade malignant and may differentiate toward female (granulosa and theca cells) or male (Sertoli and Leydig cells) structures.

Fibroma

Fibromas account for 75% of all stromal tumors and 7% of all ovarian tumors. They occur at all ages, peaking in the perimenopausal period, and are almost always benign.

PATHOLOGY: Tumors are solid, firm, and white (Fig. 24-66). The cells resemble the stroma of the normal ovarian cortex, being well-differentiated spindle cells, with variable amounts of collagen. Half of the larger tumors are associated with ascites and, rarely, with ascites and pleural effusions **(Meigs syndrome)**.

Thecoma

Thecomas are functional ovarian tumors of postmenopausal women and are almost always benign. They are closely related to fibromas, but additionally contain varying amounts of steroidogenic cells that in many cases produce estrogens or androgens.

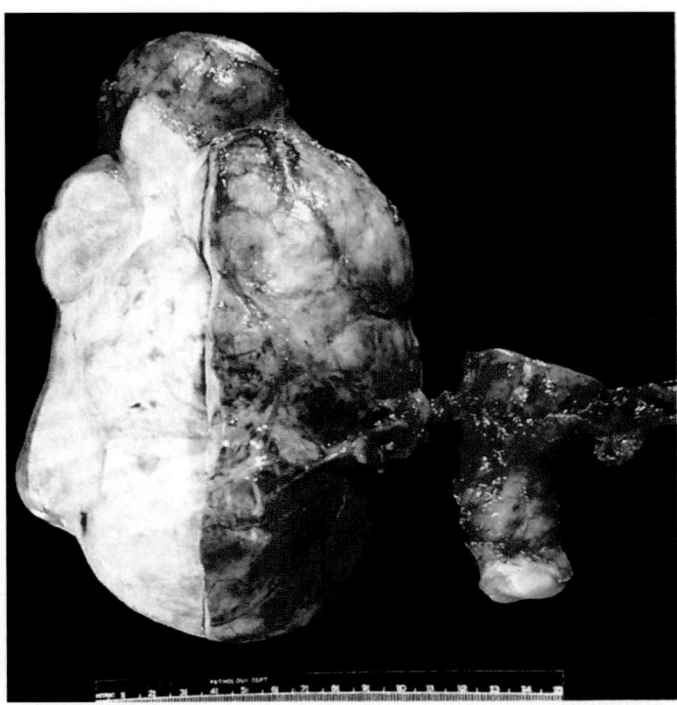

FIGURE 24-66. Fibroma of the ovary. This ovary is conspicuously enlarged by a firm, white, bosselated tumor.

PATHOLOGY: Thecomas are solid, and typically 5 to 10 cm in diameter. Cut section is yellow, owing to the many lipid-laden theca cells, which are large and oblong to round, with lipid-rich vacuolated cytoplasm (Fig. 24-67). Bands of hyalinized collagen separate nests of theca cells.

Because they produce estrogen, thecomas in premenopausal women may cause irregular menstrual cycles and breast enlargement. Endometrial hyperplasia and cancer are well-recognized complications.

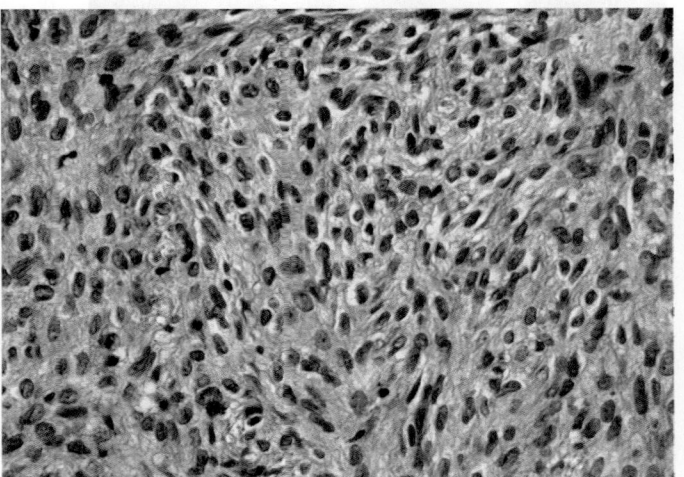

FIGURE 24-67. Thecoma of the ovary. Oblong cells are invested by collagen (reddish material) The cytoplasm contains lipid.

Granulosa Cell Tumor

Granulosa cell tumors are the prototypical functional neoplasms of the ovary associated with estrogen secretion. They should be considered malignant because of their potential for local spread and the rare occurrence of distant metastases.

ETIOLOGIC FACTORS: Most granulosa cell tumors occur after menopause (adult form) and are unusual before puberty. A juvenile form in children and young women has distinct clinical and pathologic features (hyperestrinism and precocious puberty). Development of granulosa cell tumors is linked to loss of oocytes. Oocytes appear to regulate granulosa cells, and tumorigenesis occurs when follicles become disorganized or atretic.

PATHOLOGY: Adult-type granulosa cell tumors, like most ovarian tumors, are large and focally cystic to solid. The cut surface shows yellow areas, owing to lipid-rich luteinized granulosa cells, white zones of stroma and focal hemorrhages (Fig. 24-68). Granulosa cell tumors show diverse growth patterns: (1) diffuse (sarcomatoid), (2) insular (islands of cells), or (3) trabecular (anastomotic bands of granulosa cells). Random nuclear arrangement about a central degenerative space (**Call–Exner bodies**) gives a characteristic follicular pattern (Fig. 24-68B). Tumor cells are typically spindle shaped and have a cleaved, elongated nucleus (coffee bean appearance). They secrete **inhibin**, a protein that suppresses pituitary release of follicle-stimulating hormone (FSH). These tumors can also express **calretinin**, a primarily neuronal protein, which suggests possible neural differentiation or derivation for these neoplasms. Somatic missense point mutations in the *FOXL2* gene (402 C to G) occur in more than 90% of adult granulosa cell tumors.

CLINICAL FEATURES: *Three-fourths of granulosa cell tumors secrete estrogens.* Thus, endometrial hyperplasia is a common presenting sign. EIN or endometrial adenocarcinoma may develop if a functioning granulosa cell tumor remains undetected. At diagnosis, 90% of granulosa cell tumors are within the ovary (stage I). Over 90% of these patients survive 10 years. Tumors that have extended into the pelvis and lower abdomen have a poorer prognosis. Late recurrence 5 to 10 years after surgical removal is not uncommon and is usually fatal.

Sertoli–Leydig Cell Tumors

Ovarian Sertoli–Leydig cell tumors (**arrhenoblastoma** or **androblastoma**) are rare androgen-secreting mesenchymal neoplasms of low malignant potential that resemble embryonic testis. Tumor cells typically secrete weak androgens (dehydroepiandrosterone), so tumors are usually quite large before patients complain of masculinization. Sertoli–Leydig cell tumors occur at all ages but are most common in young women of childbearing age.

PATHOLOGY: Sertoli–Leydig cell tumors are unilateral, usually 5 to 15 cm, and tend to be lobulated, solid and brown to yellow. They vary from well to poorly differentiated and some contain heterologous elements (e.g., mucinous glands and, rarely, even cartilage). Large Leydig cells have abundant eosinophilic cytoplasm and a central round to oval nucleus with a prominent nucleolus. Tumor cells are embedded in a sarcomatoid stroma (Fig. 24-69). The stroma in some areas often differentiates into immature solid tubules of embryonic Sertoli cells. Mutations in *DICER1*, a gene encoding an RNase III endoribonuclease involved in microRNA production, are found in 60% of Sertoli–Leydig cell tumors.

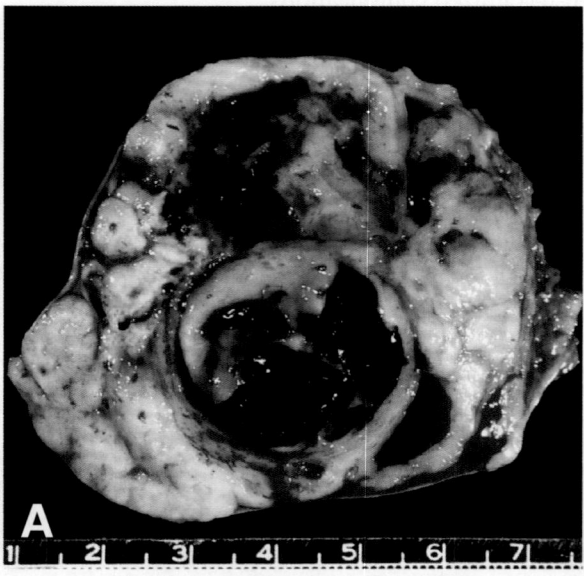

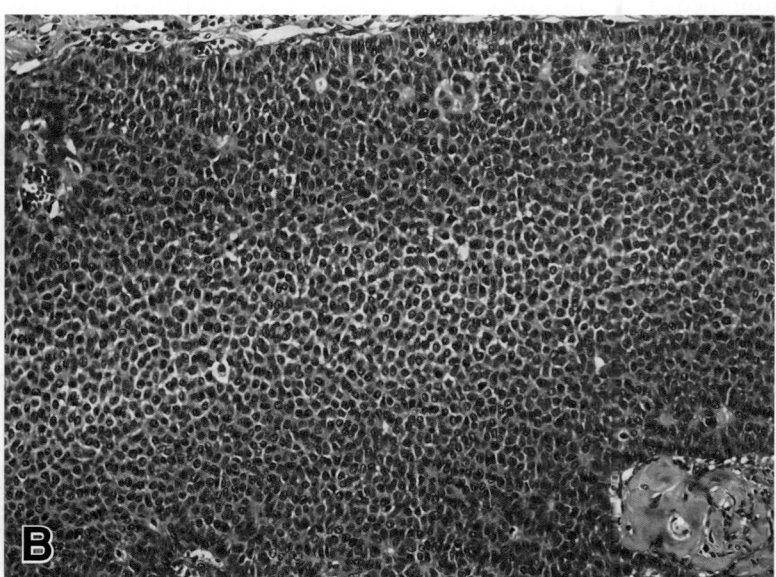

FIGURE 24-68. Granulosa cell tumor of the ovary. A. Cross-section of this enlarged ovary shows a variegated solid tumor with focal hemorrhages. Yellow areas represent collections of lipid-laden luteinized granulosa cells. **B.** Tumor cells have uniform, oval-to-round, cleaved (coffee bean nuclei) nuclei. The orientation of tumor cells about central spaces results in the characteristic follicular pattern (Call–Exner bodies) (*top and right lower corner*).

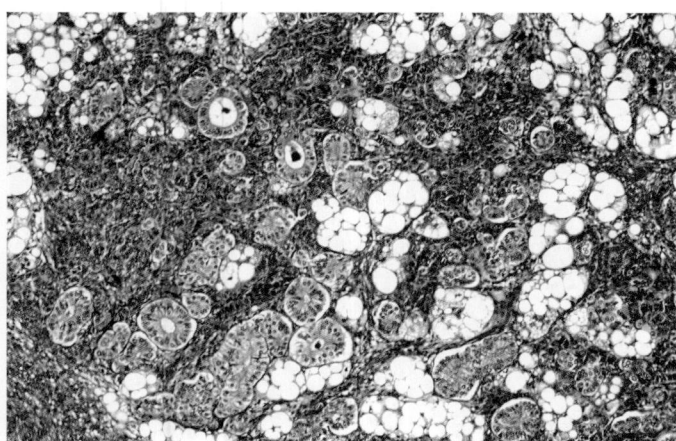

FIGURE 24-69. Sertoli–Leydig cell tumor, well differentiated. Hollow tubules are lined by mature Sertoli cells. The intervening stroma contains numerous Leydig cells with vacuolated cytoplasm.

> **CLINICAL FEATURES:** Nearly half of all patients with Sertoli–Leydig cell tumors exhibit signs of virilization: hirsutism, male escutcheon, enlarged clitoris, and deepened voice. Initial signs are often defeminization, manifested as breast atrophy, amenorrhea, and loss of hip fat. Once the tumor is removed, these signs disappear or lessen. Well-differentiated tumors are virtually always cured by surgical resection, but poorly differentiated ones may metastasize.

Steroid Cell Tumor

Steroid cell tumors of the ovary, also called **lipid cell** or **lipoid cell tumors**, are composed of cells that resemble lutein cells, Leydig cells, and adrenal cortical cells. Most steroid cell tumors are hormonally active, usually with androgenic manifestations. Some secrete testosterone; others synthesize weaker androgens. **Hilus cell tumor** is a specialized form of steroid cell tumor that is typically a benign neoplasm of Leydig cells. It arises in the hilus of the ovary, usually after menopause. Because it secretes testosterone, the most potent of the common androgens, masculinizing signs are frequent (75%), even with small tumors. Most hilus cell tumors contain "crystalloids of Reinke" (rodlike cytoplasmic structures).

Tumors Metastatic to the Ovary May Mimic a Primary Tumor

About 3% of cancers found in the ovaries arise elsewhere, mostly in the breast, large intestine, endometrium, and stomach, in descending order. These tumors vary from microscopic lesions to large masses. Those from the breast are usually tiny and are seen in 10% of ovaries removed prophylactically in cases of advanced breast cancer. Metastatic tumors large enough to cause symptoms originate most often in the colon (Fig. 24-70). Commonly, the tumor cells stimulate ovarian stroma to differentiate into hormonally active cells (luteinized stromal cells), leading to androgenic and sometimes estrogenic symptoms.

Krukenberg tumors are metastases to the ovary, composed of nests of mucin-filled "signet-ring" cells in a cellular stroma derived from the ovary (Fig. 24-71). The stomach is the primary site in 75% of cases and most of the rest are from the colon.

Bilateral ovarian involvement and multinodularity suggest a metastatic carcinoma, and both ovaries are grossly involved in 75% of cases. Even an ovary that appears uninvolved grossly may contain surface implants or minute foci of tumor within the parenchyma. Thus, when metastasis to one ovary is documented, the other should also be removed.

Peritoneum

The peritoneum is a nearly continuous membrane that lines the peritoneal cavity and separates viscera from the

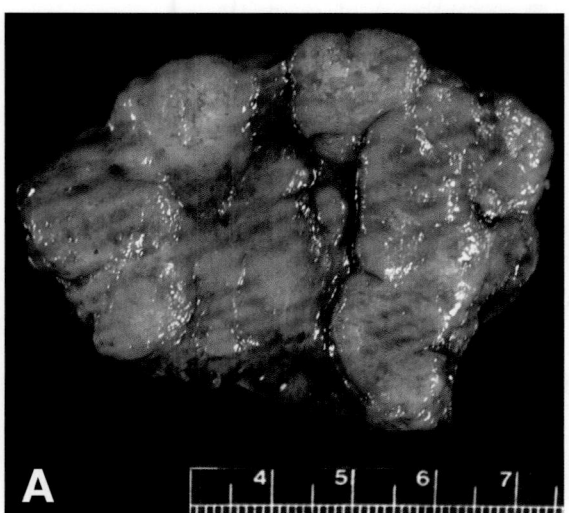

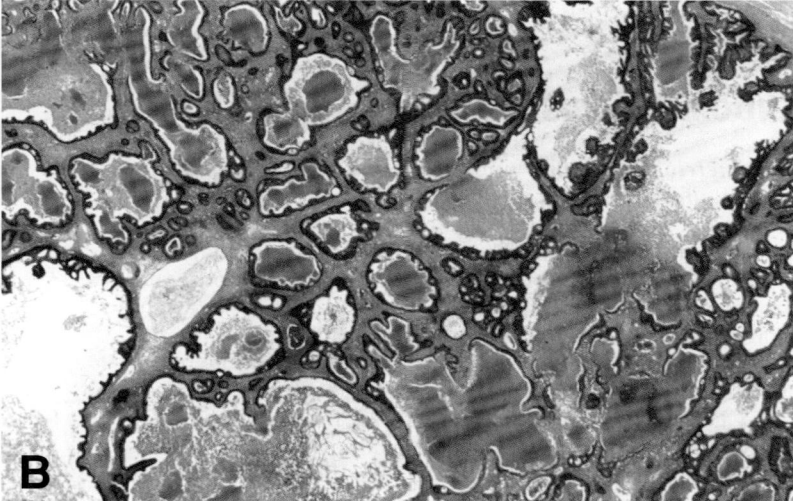

FIGURE 24-70. Metastatic adenocarcinoma from colon. A. The ovary is replaced by multinodular tumor which appears solid on cut surfaces. **B.** Microscopically, the tumor shows a garland-like glandular pattern with focal segmental necrosis and abundant necrotic debris.

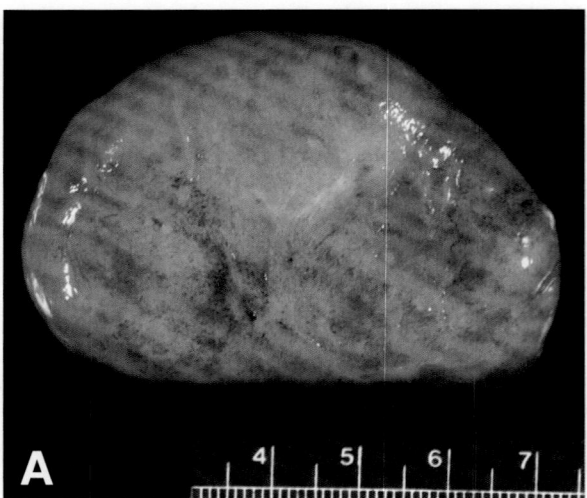
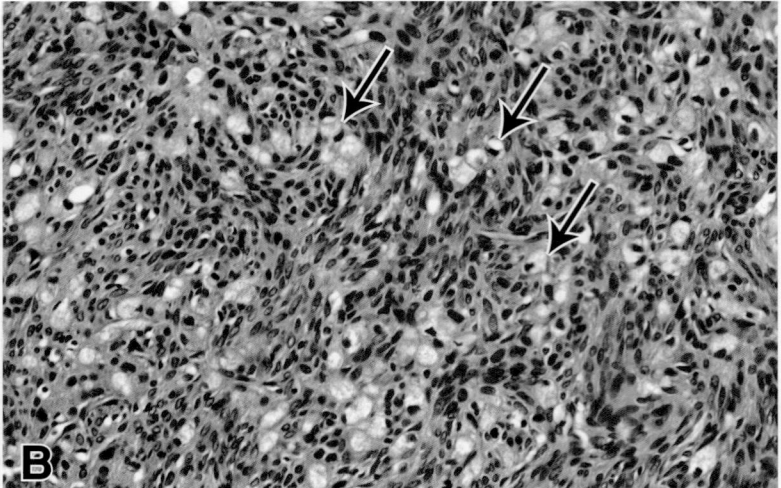

FIGURE 24-71. Krukenberg tumor. A. The ovary is enlarged and the cut surface appears solid, pale yellow and partially hemorrhagic. **B.** Microscopic examination reveals mucinous (signet-ring) cells (clear cells, *arrows*) infiltrating the ovarian stroma.

abdominal wall. In men, the peritoneum is a closed system. In women, it is an "open system" interrupted in the pelvis by the fallopian tubes, which provide a final conduit for transmission of pathogens and chemicals from the genital tract to the peritoneal cavity.

The cells that line the peritoneal cavity and those that form the serosa of the ovary are both of celomic epithelial origin. *Thus, it is unclear whether tumors and tumor-like lesions of peritoneum and ovary (i.e., müllerian epithelial lesions) are the same entity in both locations.*

Many inflammatory lesions involve the peritoneum. Granulomatous peritonitis develops as a response to foreign materials such as sutures, surgical glove powder, or radiologic contrast media. Exposure to intestinal contents after perforation (e.g., in Crohn disease or diverticulitis); rupture of a mature cystic teratoma (dermoid cyst) of the ovary; and, of course, tuberculosis can also cause peritoneal inflammation. Reactive mesothelial proliferation occurs with the slightest irritation. Peritonitis is discussed in Chapter 19.

ENDOMETRIOSIS

Endometriosis is the presence of benign endometrial glands and stroma outside the uterus. It afflicts 5% to 10% of women of reproductive age and regresses after natural or artificial menopause. The mean age range at diagnosis is in the late 20s to early 30s, although it may appear any time after menarche. Sites most frequently involved are the ovaries (>60%), other uterine adnexa (uterine ligaments, rectovaginal septum, pouch of Douglas) and the pelvic peritoneum covering the uterus, fallopian tubes, rectosigmoid colon, and bladder (Fig. 24-72). Endometriosis can be even more widespread and occasionally affects the cervix, vagina, perineum, bladder, and umbilicus. Even pelvic lymph nodes may contain foci of endometriosis. Rarely, distant areas such as lungs, pleura, small bowel, kidneys, and bones contain lesions.

 PATHOPHYSIOLOGY: The pathogenesis of endometriosis is uncertain. Several mechanisms, not necessarily mutually exclusive, have been proposed:

1. **Transplantation** of endometrial fragments to ectopic sites
2. **Metaplasia** of the multipotential celomic peritoneum
3. **Induction** of undifferentiated mesenchyme in ectopic sites to form lesions after exposure to substances released from shed endometrium

TRANSPLANTATION: The most widely accepted theory holds that menstrual endometrium refluxes through the fallopian tubes and implants at ectopic sites. It

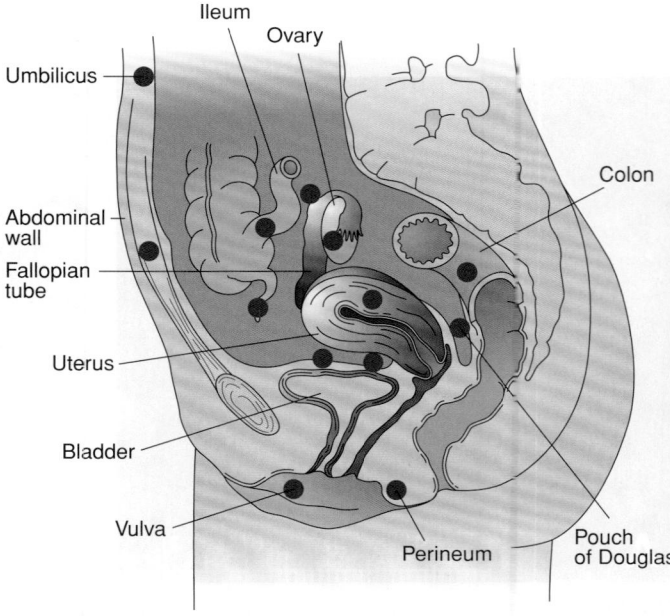

FIGURE 24-72. Sites of endometriosis.

is known that retrograde menstruation through the fallopian tubes occurs in 90% of women. A mechanism involving lymphatic and hematogenous dissemination would explain endometriosis in lymph nodes and at distant organ sites like the lungs and kidneys. The observation that pulmonary endometriosis occurs almost exclusively in women who have had uterine surgery supports this contention.

CELOMIC METAPLASIA: This theory proposes that endometriosis arises by endometrial metaplasia of peritoneal serosa or serosa-like structures. Thus, if appropriately stimulated, the pelvic peritoneum may differentiate into any type of müllerian epithelium.

INDUCTION THEORY: This concept suggests that one or more factors secreted by the endometrium promotes development of endometrial epithelium and stroma at ectopic sites.

PATHOLOGY: The earliest lesions of endometriosis may appear as yellow-red stains, reflecting breakdown of blood products. Red lesions, which also occur early in the disease, are actively growing foci of endometriosis (Fig. 24-73). Operative specimens usually contain black lesions showing some degree of resolution. These 1- to 5-mm foci on the ovary and peritoneal surfaces are called "mulberry" nodules. With repeated cycles of hemorrhage and subsequent fibrosis, affected surfaces may scar and become grossly brown ("powder burns"). Over time, fibrous adhesions may become more pronounced and lead to complications, such as intestinal obstruction. Repetitive hemorrhage in the ovaries may turn endometriotic foci into cysts up to 15 cm in diameter containing inspissated, chocolate-colored material ("chocolate cysts").

Endometriosis is characterized by ectopic normal endometrial glands and stroma (Fig. 24-73). Occasionally, healed foci may contain only fibrous tissue and hemosiderin-laden macrophages, which by themselves are not diagnostic. Immunohistochemical demonstration of CD10 can be diagnostic.

CLINICAL FEATURES: Symptoms of endometriosis depend on where implants are located. Dysmenorrhea, caused by implants on uterosacral ligaments, is common. Lesions swell just before or during menstruation, producing pelvic pain. Half of women with dysmenorrhea have endometriosis. Other symptoms include dyspareunia and cyclical abdominal pain.

Infertility is the primary complaint in a third of women with endometriosis (Fig. 24-74). The hormonal milieu in a woman who does not achieve pregnancy encourages development of endometriosis. In turn, once endometriosis develops, it contributes to the infertile state and a vicious circle is established. Conversely, pregnancy may alleviate the disease. Conservative surgery to restore pelvic anatomy helps many women with endometriosis to become pregnant.

Malignancy occurs in about 1% to 2% of cases of endometriosis (Fig. 24-60). Clear cell and endometrioid tumors are the most frequent forms. Adenosarcoma, although rare, is the most common sarcoma.

MESOTHELIAL TUMORS

Mesothelial tumors range from benign to multicentric aggressive malignancies.

Adenomatoid Tumors Are Benign Mesothelial Neoplasms, Mainly of Fallopian Tubes

They are encountered in the fallopian tubes and in subserosal tissue of the uterine corpus near the fallopian tubes. They are rare elsewhere in the peritoneum.

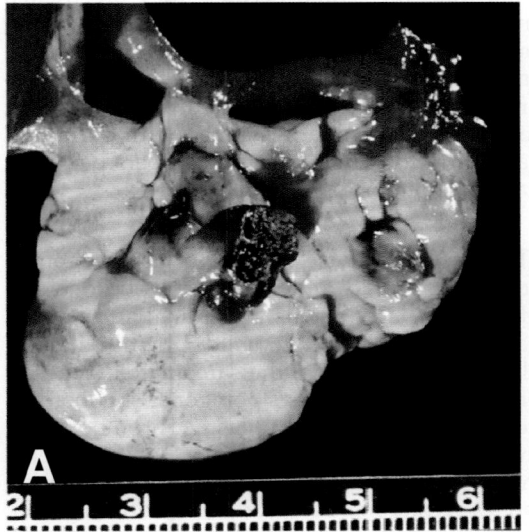 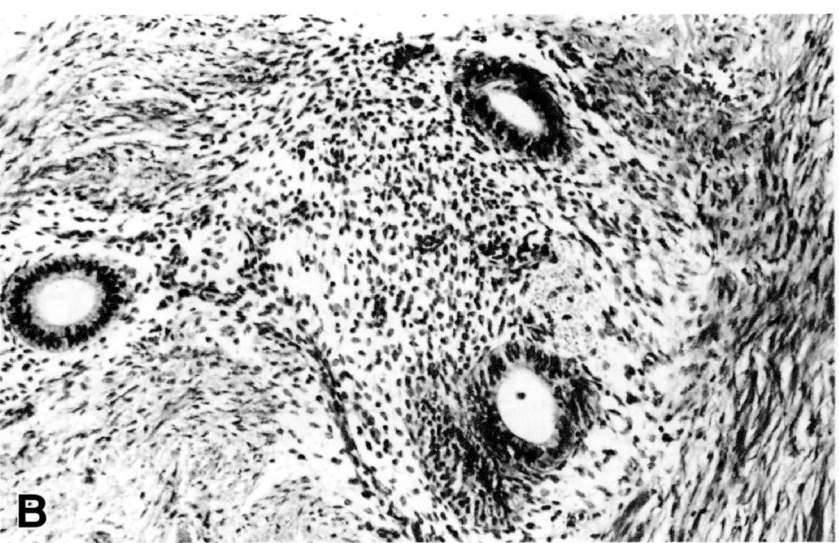

FIGURE 24-73. Endometriosis. A. Implants of endometriosis on the ovary appear as red-blue nodules. **B.** Microscopic view shows endometrial glands and stroma in the ovary.

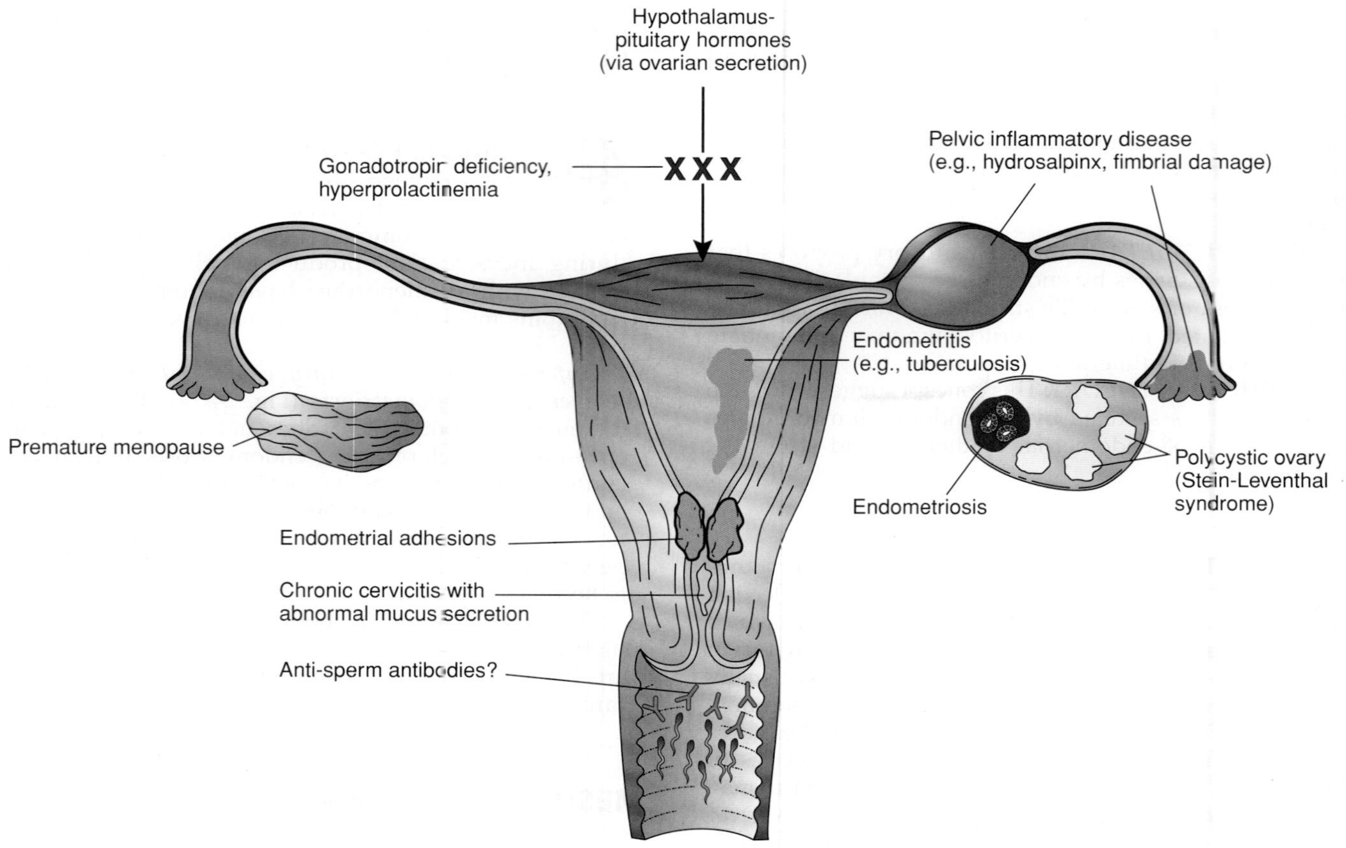

Hypothalamus-
pituitary hormones
(via ovarian secretion)

Gonadotropin deficiency,
hyperprolactinemia

XXX

Pelvic inflammatory disease
(e.g., hydrosalpinx, fimbrial damage)

Premature menopause

Endometritis
(e.g., tuberculosis)

Polycystic ovary
(Stein-Leventhal
syndrome)

Endometriosis

Endometrial adhesions

Chronic cervicitis with
abnormal mucus secretion

Anti-sperm antibodies?

FIGURE 24-74. Causes of acquired infertility.

Well-Differentiated Papillary Mesotheliomas Are Benign

Well-differentiated papillary mesotheliomas are rare in women of reproductive age. They are typically asymptomatic and usually found incidentally at operation. These tumors are solitary, small, broad-based, wart-like polypoid, or nodular excrescences with a single layer of small bland cuboidal cells covering thick papillae (Fig. 24-75). They often resemble serous epithelial tumors of the ovary, but the two are treated differently.

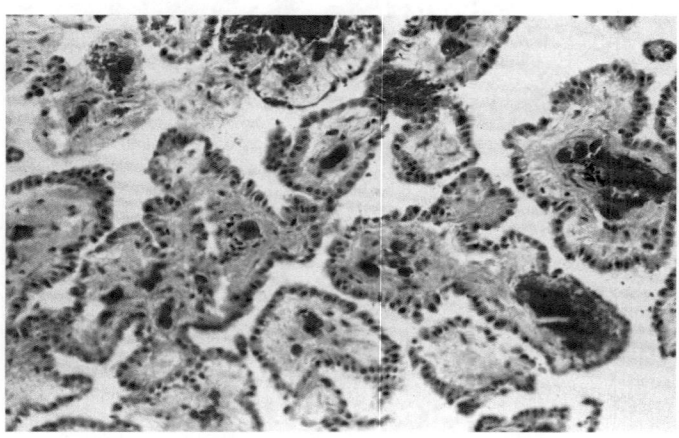

FIGURE 24-75. Well-differentiated peritoneal mesothelioma. Cuboidal epithelium lines papillae.

Diffuse Peritoneal Malignant Mesotheliomas Are Invariably Fatal

These tumors arise from peritoneal mesothelium. They are rare in women and constitute only a small proportion of all malignant mesotheliomas, most of which are pleural. They must be distinguished from serous adenocarcinomas, including those arising from the peritoneal surface itself and those metastatic from the ovary, because they are treated differently and have much different survival rates. Most patients are middle-aged or postmenopausal with nonspecific symptoms such as ascites, abdominal discomfort, digestive disturbances, and weight loss. Unlike pleural tumors, asbestos exposure is uncommon in women with peritoneal mesothelioma, but up to 2 million asbestos fibers per gram wet weight have been reported in some tumors.

 PATHOLOGY: Diffuse malignant mesothelioma extensively involves and thickens the peritoneum and serosa of the various abdominal and pelvic organs. It has a tubulopapillary to solid growth pattern. Unlike in pleural mesothelioma, the sarcomatoid type is rare. The epithelial variant displays polygonal or cuboidal neoplastic cells with abundant cytoplasm. Thrombomodulin, calretinin, cytokeratin 5/6, and HBME-1 are markers of malignant mesothelioma, whereas CA-125, CEA, and estrogen and progesterone receptors (ER and PR) are markers of ovarian epithelial tumors. No effective treatment is available.

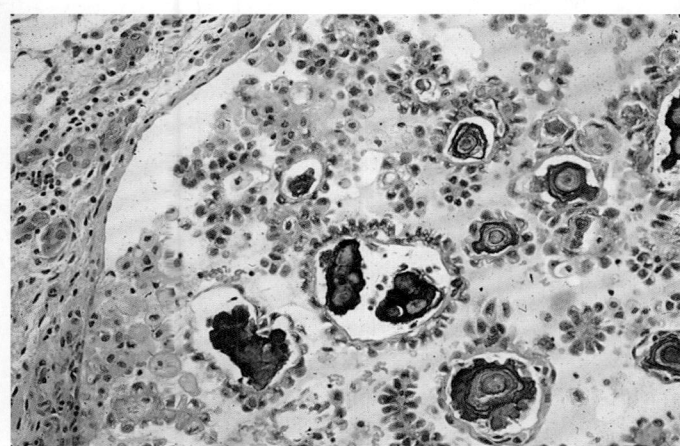

FIGURE 24-76. Noninvasive implants of borderline serous tumor on the peritoneum. The tumor exhibits epithelial tufts and psammoma bodies (compare to Fig. 24-56B). (Reprinted with permission from Stanley J. Robboy, MD, and Gynecologic Pathology Associates, Durham and Chapel Hill, North Carolina.)

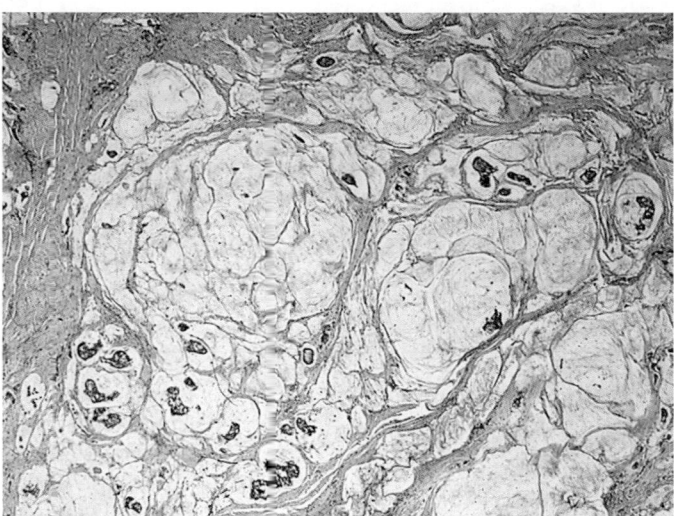

FIGURE 24-77. Pseudomyxoma peritonei. Multiple clusters of tumor cells are present in the mucinous material. (Reprinted with permission from Stanley J. Robboy, MD, and Gynecologic Pathology Associates, Durham and Chapel Hill, North Carolina.)

SEROUS TUMORS (PRIMARY AND METASTATIC)

Unlike the ovary, which features a wide range of tumors, serous tumors are virtually the only type found in the peritoneum. Mucinous tumors involving the peritoneum are metastases from primary cancers of the appendix or ovary.

Serous Borderline Tumors Resemble the Corresponding Ovarian Neoplasms

Most serous borderline tumors in the peritoneum are metastases from the ovary, but some may be primary in the peritoneum. In the latter case, serous peritoneal tumors without invasion are usually benign; those that are invasive carry a worse prognosis.

PATHOLOGY: Whether in the ovary or the peritoneum, borderline serous tumors are characterized by papillary processes, small clusters of cells, cell stratification, detached cellular clusters, nuclear atypia, and mitotic activity in the absence of invasion. Implants appear as fine granularities or small nodules with clusters of blunt papillae or glandular structures, often having complex cellular tufts (Fig. 24-76). Psammoma bodies are common and may fill the core of the papillae. Mild to severe cytologic atypia with some stratification is common but is substantially less frequent than that seen in adenocarcinoma.

Serous Carcinoma Occurs in Women With Normal Ovaries

The frequency of serous carcinomas arising de novo in the peritoneum is estimated as 10% of its counterpart in the ovary. The mean age of women with this tumor is 50 to 65 years. The diagnosis of a primary peritoneal tumor requires demonstration of normal ovaries. Abdominal pain and ascites are frequent presentations. Like ovarian cancer, serous carcinoma primarily in the peritoneum may have a familial basis and can metastasize to distant locations.

PSEUDOMYXOMA PERITONEI

Pseudomyxoma peritonei is the accumulation of jelly-like mucus in the pelvis or peritoneum. Previously interpreted as spread from mucinous ovarian tumors, pseudomyxoma peritonei is now understood to derive largely from mucus-producing adenocarcinomas of the appendix.

PATHOLOGY: This condition may be extensive and appear as semisolid gelatin covering all abdominal structures, or there may be little more than a slightly thickened gelatinous coat over a focal area of bowel or omentum. The appendix is commonly enlarged or adherent to an omentum covered with the gelatinous material. Within the gelatin are strips of well-differentiated, intestinal-type, mucinous epithelium (Fig. 24-77). If only isolated foci are present, the epithelium may be so well differentiated that it resembles a simple mucinous adenoma. Cribriform patterns or other histologic features of malignancy, such as signet-ring cells or glands, are seen on occasion and warrant a diagnosis of adenocarcinoma.

Low-grade tumors are usually treated for cure, which entails aggressive surgical debulking and intraperitoneal chemotherapy. The 5-year survival is under 50%.

25 The Breast

Anna Marie Mulligan, Frances P. O'Malley

DEVELOPMENT, ANATOMY AND PHYSIOLOGIC CHANGE

The human breast first appears during the 5th week of embryonic development, when ectodermal thickenings—the mammary ridges, or "milk lines"—extend from the axilla to the medial part of the thigh. Regression follows in all regions except in the 4th intercostal space, where the breast will later develop. By the 9th week of gestation, cords of epithelial cells grow from the epidermal layer into the underlying mesenchyme. From about the 20th to 32nd weeks of gestation, these solid cellular invaginations become canalized and, under the influence of maternal hormones, form a network of about 15 to 25 branching, primary, mammary ducts. Near the end of gestation, maternal and placental steroid hormones and prolactin may produce secretory activity, and stimulate breast development which may be transiently prominent in male and female newborns. After birth, the breast tissue returns to an inactive state. Further breast development accelerates at puberty, when ducts begin to elongate and branch (Fig. 25-1A). Estrogen and progesterone cause terminal end buds and connective tissue stroma to proliferate, differentiate, and remodel to form the terminal duct lobular unit (TDLU) of the adult breast (Fig. 25-1B).

The breasts are situated on the upper chest wall between the 2nd and the 6th ribs. They extend medially to the sternum and laterally to the anterior axillary line, although a tail of breast tissue may extend further into the axilla. Each breast is composed of skin, subcutaneous adipose tissue, and the functional component composed of ducts, lobules, and stroma. Collecting ducts, through which milk is secreted, open at the nipple. The nipple–areolar complex is centrally placed and contains abundant sensory nerves and sebaceous and apocrine glands. The nipple consists mainly of dense fibrous tissue mixed with smooth muscle. The latter gives the nipple its erectile capability and contributes to expression of milk. Pigmentation increases in the nipple and areola at puberty and increases further during pregnancy. Stratified squamous epithelium that lines the nipple skin extends superficially into the collecting ducts before it transitions abruptly to glandular epithelium. The latter contains an inner luminal secretory epithelial cell layer and an outer myoepithelial cell layer.

Just beneath the nipple, collecting ducts dilate to form lactiferous sinuses, which subdivide into 15 to 25 lobes with segmental and subsegmental ducts. These terminate in the TDLUs, where milk is made. The TDLU consists of (1) terminal ductules or acini, whose epithelium differentiates into secretory acini in pregnant or lactating glands; (2) the intralobular collecting duct; and (3) specialized intralobular stroma (Fig. 25-1B).

The TDLU is a dynamic structure that changes cyclically during the menstrual cycle. These periodic alterations include epithelial proliferation and apoptosis, and changes in the intralobular stroma. In the follicular phase of the menstrual cycle, terminal ducts are few and lined by a simple, two-cell layer of epithelium with surrounding myoepithelium. After ovulation, mitoses increase in the luminal epithelium, and the intralobular stroma becomes edematous. Myoepithelial cells become more prominent, owing to cytoplasmic accumulation of glycogen. These changes may cause progressive fullness and tenderness of the breast. TDLUs return to their follicular phase state during menses, when declining estrogen and progesterone levels cause apoptosis. During this time, lymphocytes infiltrate the intralobular stroma.

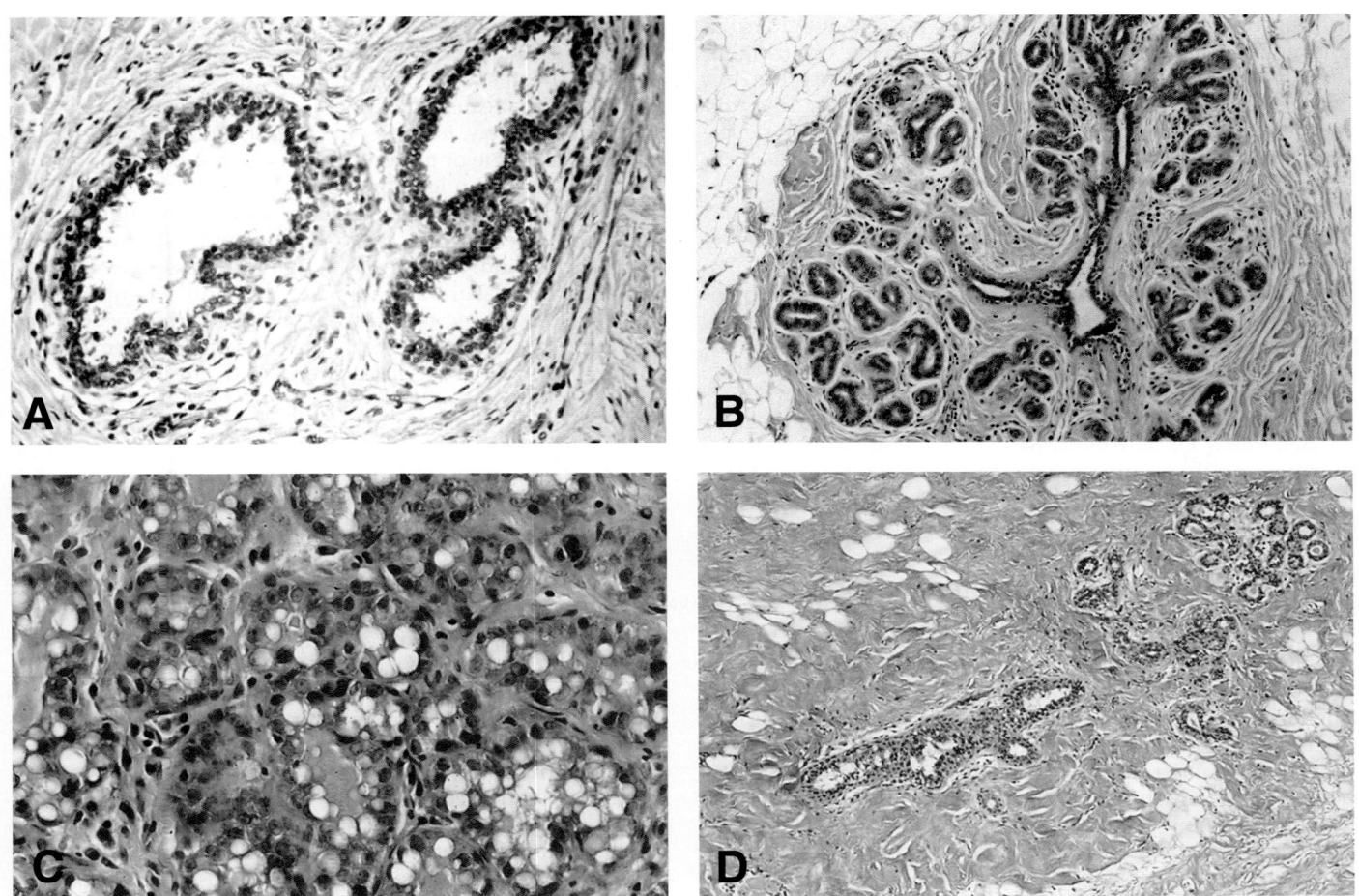

FIGURE 25-1. Normal breast architecture at various ages. A. Adolescent breast. Large and intermediate-size ducts are seen within a dense fibrous stroma. Lobular units are not yet present. **B.** Postpubertal breast. The terminal duct lobular unit (TDLU) consists of small ductules arrayed around an intralobular duct. The two-cell-layered epithelium shows no secretory or mitotic activity. The intralobular stroma is dense and confluent with the interlobular stroma. **C.** Lactating breast. The terminal duct lobular units are conspicuously enlarged, with inapparent interlobular and intralobular stroma. The individual terminal ducts, now termed acini, show prominent epithelial secretory activity (cytoplasmic vacuolization). The acinar lumens contain secretory material. **D.** Postmenopausal breast. The terminal duct lobular units are absent. The remaining intermediate ducts and larger ducts are commonly dilated.

Full functional breast development occurs only with the hormonal changes of pregnancy and lactation. During pregnancy, glandular tissue increases markedly in comparison to fibrous and fatty connective tissue. Early in pregnancy, TDLUs grow rapidly. Stromal vascularity and chronic inflammatory cells increase. In later pregnancy, lobular epithelial cells become vacuolated owing to increased secretion into distended lobular units. This effect is more pronounced with lactation (Fig. 25-1C). Once lactation ceases, the gland involutes dramatically, as pronounced cell death and tissue remodeling occur, and eventually the breast returns to its pre-pregnancy state.

After menopause, TDLUs atrophy, but large and intermediate-sized ducts persist (Fig. 25-1D). Fat predominates over fibrous tissue, but the latter typically cuffs the remaining ducts. Fat increases as a percentage of total breast mass as a woman ages.

Other than TDLUs, nonspecialized collagenous connective tissue and fat make up the bulk of the breast tissue. Intralobular stroma is more cellular than interlobular stroma. Mucopolysaccharides in extracellular matrix are also more abundant in intralobular stroma, which also includes a few lymphocytes, plasma cells, mast cells, and macrophages.

The breast is highly vascular and contains a complex lymphatic network, draining mainly into axillary lymph nodes, with a minority communicating with internal mammary nodes.

DEVELOPMENTAL ABNORMALITIES

Complete bilateral or unilateral absence of breast development is rare, but hypoplasia is more common. Minor asymmetry between breasts occurs frequently. Less often, breasts may differ markedly in size owing to hypoplasia of one breast or unusual enlargement of the other (juvenile hypertrophy). However, such enlargement is usually bilateral. Unless there is an underlying hormonal abnormality, juvenile breast hypertrophy regresses spontaneously. The most common anomaly of breast development is supernumerary nipples, or polythelia, with or without associated breast tissue (polymastia), which results from persistent epidermal thickenings (mammary ridges). These mostly occur along the milk line, which extends from the axilla to the groin, but other sites may rarely be involved. Congenitally inverted nipple results from failure of nipple eversion during development, usually unilaterally.

INFLAMMATORY DISEASES OF THE BREAST

Acute Mastitis Is a Complication of Breast Feeding

Acute mastitis typically occurs early in the postpartum period and is due to bacterial infection, usually with *Staphylococcus* or *Streptococcus*. Patients experience pain, swelling, or redness, often with fever and malaise. Cracks in the skin or lactational stasis predispose to infection. When minor, mastitis usually resolves with antibiotics and continued lactation. If it is severe or left untreated, abscesses or systemic infection may occur.

Squamous Metaplasia of Lactiferous Ducts Presents as a Painful Red Mass

It is unrelated to lactation, age, or history of pregnancy. It produces a painful subareolar mass and overlying erythema. The large majority of patients are cigarette smokers. Nipple ducts show keratinizing squamous metaplasia. A keratin plug can become trapped and lead to duct rupture. Keratinous debris spills into the stroma where it elicits a chronic foreign body inflammatory response, which may become secondarily infected. Recurrences are common and can lead to fistulas. Surgical excision is curative.

Granulomatous Mastitis Has Diverse Etiologies

Granulomatous inflammation (Fig. 25-2) of the breast can be infectious (mycobacteria, parasites, fungi) or noninfectious (foreign material, sarcoidosis, idiopathic granulomatous mastitis). Tuberculosis of the breast is rare in Western countries but is still seen in developing countries, where the infection is endemic. Patients typically present with a mass or sinus that may be mistaken clinically for invasive carcinoma. Other organisms that cause granulomas are discussed in Chapter 9. Sarcoidosis rarely involves the breast, but when it does, it presents as single or multiple breast masses.

Silicone gel can leak from breast implants and cause foreign body granulomatous inflammation, with a fibrous capsule. Severe cases may be associated with skin retraction, nipple inversion, and formation of hard masses, which may simulate or obscure a malignancy. Draining lymph nodes may enlarge, owing to spread of vacuolated histiocytes containing refractile particles. The use of saline, rather than silicone, in implants has greatly reduced implant-associated granulomatous mastitis.

Gross sectioning reveals a rim of firm tissue surrounding the ruptured implant. Fat necrosis and a foreign body giant cell reaction, with varying degrees of inflammation and fibrosis, are characteristic. The tissue may be gritty if calcification is present. During tissue processing for microscopic examination, the silicone is largely lost from the tissue, leaving behind clear spaces. However, these spaces, and nearby macrophages, may contain birefringent particles of silicone material. The fibrous capsule is formed by a band of frequently calcified, collagenous tissue. Some capsules around implants develop synovial metaplasia, with a lining that resembles synovium, with or without papillary hyperplasia (Fig. 25-3).

Idiopathic granulomatous mastitis is rare. It typically occurs in women 20 to 40 years old who have recently been pregnant. It is bilateral in up to 25% of patients. Granulomas in this setting are centered within lobules, often with superimposed acute inflammation and microabscesses (Fig. 25-4). These features of idiopathic granulomatous mastitis show overlap with cystic neutrophilic granulomatous mastitis (CNGM), which typically presents as a clinical or radiologic breast mass in young, parous women. The key distinguishing feature of CNGM is the presence of small cystic spaces within the granulomas surrounded by neutrophils, within which, gram-positive bacteria (usually *Corynebacteria*) may be found.

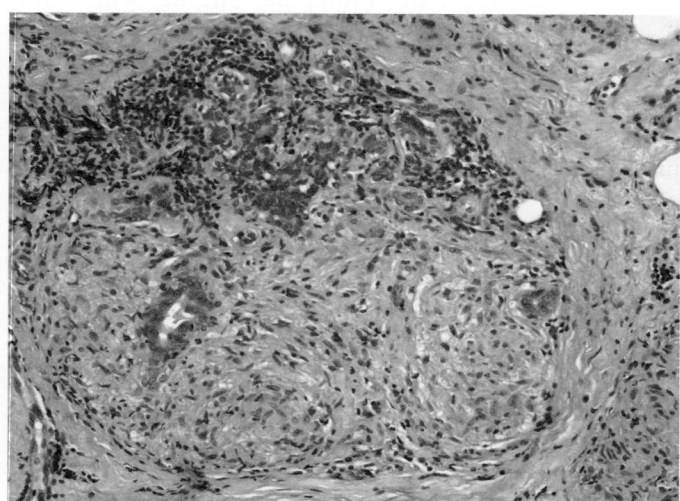

FIGURE 25-2. Breast lobule showing florid granulomatous inflammation characterized by collections of epithelioid histiocytes.

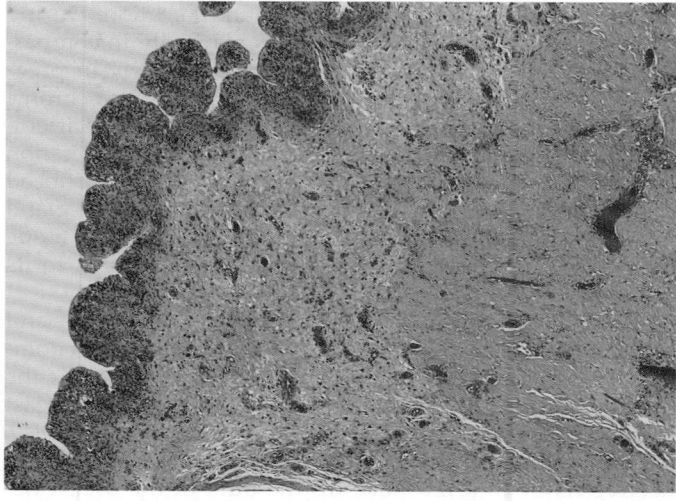

FIGURE 25-3. Capsule around breast implant showing synovial metaplasia with papillary hyperplasia and chronic inflammation.

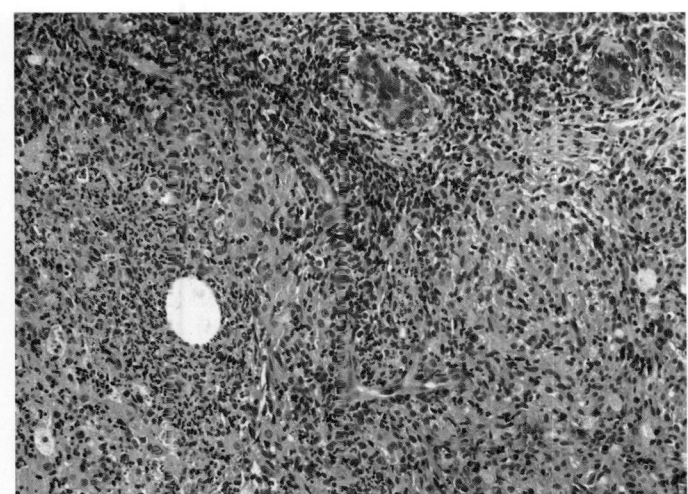

FIGURE 25-4. Cystic neutrophilic granulomatous mastitis. Histologic features of CNGM include granulomatous inflammation centered on a breast lobule with a prominent acute inflammatory cell infiltrate surrounding a clear space.

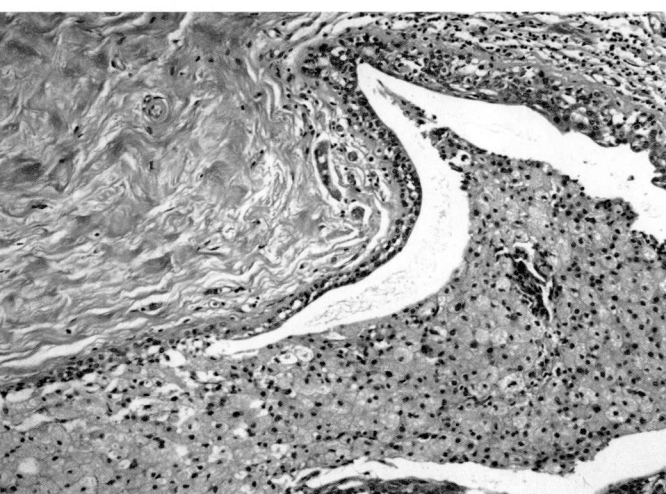

FIGURE 25-6. Duct ectasia. A dilated duct is filled with foamy histiocytes. The duct epithelium is infiltrated focally by histiocytes, and the periductal stroma shows chronic inflammation.

Lymphocytic Mastopathy Is an Autoimmune Reaction

Lymphocytic mastopathy, also called sclerosing lymphocytic lobulitis, is uncommon. It is often associated with other autoimmune diseases, in particular type 1 diabetes mellitus and Hashimoto thyroiditis. Clinically, most patients exhibit a hard mass, which may be tender and sometimes bilateral. Histologically, it shows circumscribed aggregates of small lymphocytes surrounding lobules, ducts, and vessels. Lobular atrophy, basement membrane thickening, and fibrosis are also evident (Fig. 25-5). Interlobular stroma shows dense fibrosis and epithelioid myofibroblasts.

IgG4-related sclerosing mastitis is part of the family of IgG4-related diseases. Unilateral or bilateral painless masses consisting of a dense nodular lymphoplasmacytic infiltrate with lymphoid follicles and IgG4-positive plasma cells are

typical. Affected individuals may have elevated serum levels of IgG4.

Duct Ectasia May Lead to Duct Rupture

Duct ectasia is characterized by dilation and periductal inflammation, with fibrosis of large and intermediate breast ducts, which contain inspissated material. Peri- or postmenopausal women are more likely to be symptomatic, experiencing serous or bloody nipple discharge, mass, or pain. As disease progresses, duct wall fibrosis may cause the nipple to retract. Episodes of acute inflammation may be complicated by abscess or sinus formation. Dilated ducts contain amorphous debris and foamy macrophages (Fig. 25-6). The lining epithelium and periductal stroma is infiltrated by inflammatory cells and foamy macrophages. Duct rupture incites a chronic inflammatory response, often with foreign body granulomas. Over time, fibrosis increases and may obliterate ducts.

Fat Necrosis May Mimic Cancer

Like carcinoma of the breast, fat necrosis often presents as a hard mass, frequently associated with skin tethering. Some patients may give a history of trauma. Necrotic fat cells, acute inflammation, cholesterol clefts, and hemorrhage are evident early in the course of fat necrosis. Foamy macrophages and multinucleated giant cells that engulf lipid droplets gradually accumulate (Fig. 25-7). With time, fibrosis and dystrophic calcification develop.

BENIGN EPITHELIAL LESIONS

Classification of benign epithelial lesions of the breast is based on their risk of subsequent cancer development. Lesions not associated with increased risk are nonproliferative breast changes (e.g., fibrocystic change). Proliferative conditions without atypia entail a 1.5- to 2-fold increased risk of developing carcinoma over 5 to 15 years and are classified

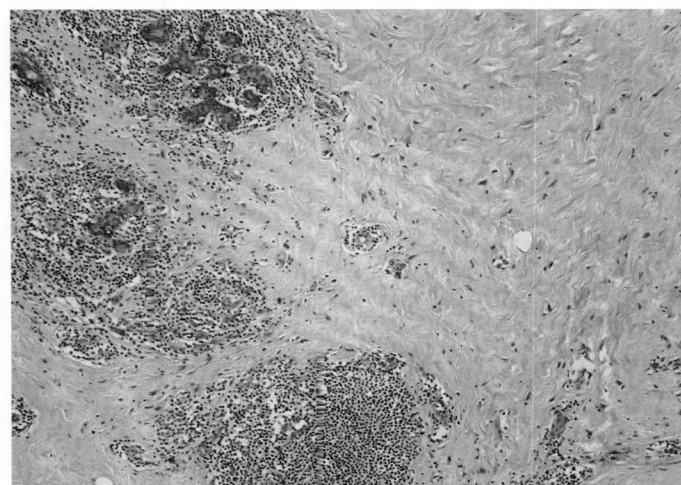

FIGURE 25-5. Lymphocytic mastopathy. Characteristic features include prominent periductal and perivascular lymphocytic infiltration in a dense fibrous stroma.

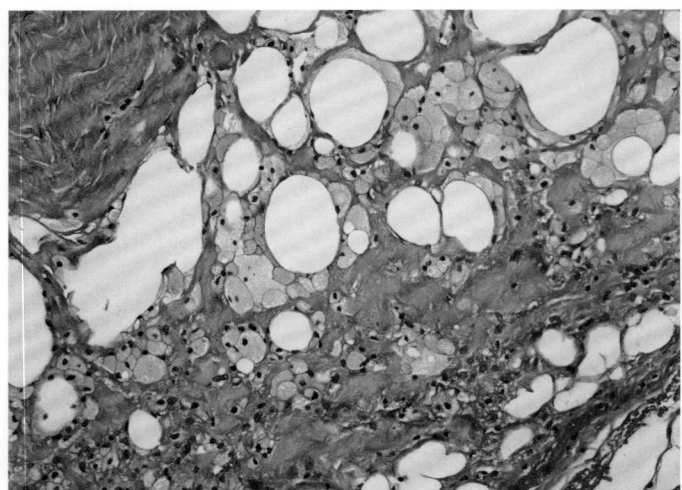

FIGURE 25-7. Fat necrosis. Necrotic fat cells with abundant foamy histiocytes.

simply as proliferative breast diseases. Proliferative lesions with atypia involve even greater relative risk (three- to five-fold). Patients with these lesions require close clinical monitoring. Those at high risk may consider medical treatment options (e.g., estrogen antagonists).

Fibrocystic Change Is an Exaggerated Physiologic Response

Fibrocystic change (FCC) is a nonproliferative change that includes gross and microscopic cysts, apocrine metaplasia, mild epithelial hyperplasia (≤4 cell layers above the basement membrane), and an increase in fibrous stroma. FCC affects over one-third of women 20 to 50 years old, and then declines after menopause. Most women with FCC are asymptomatic, but some present with nodularity and, occasionally, pain. FCC is typically multifocal and bilateral.

PATHOLOGY: The breast in FCC consists grossly of firm fibrofatty tissue containing multiple clear cysts or "blue dome" cysts that arise within TDLUs (Fig. 25-8A,B). The latter cysts contain a dark, thin fluid that imparts a blue color when unopened. Cysts vary from 1 mm to several centimeters in diameter. They may lack an epithelial lining or be lined by attenuated epithelium and myoepithelium (Fig. 25-8C). Their lining may include large apocrine-type cells with abundant, granular, eosinophilic cytoplasm and basally located nuclei (Fig. 25-8D). The surrounding stroma is often sclerotic. Cyst rupture may incite an inflammatory response. Mild "usual" ductal hyperplasia (see below) is frequently present (Fig. 25-8C).

Proliferative Breast Disease Variably Increases Risk of Cancer

Usual Epithelial Hyperplasia

Usual epithelial hyperplasia is associated with a 1.5- to 2-fold increase in the risk of breast cancer, which may subsequently arise in either breast. Usual epithelial hyperplasia occurs within the TDLU or, less commonly, extralobular ducts. Its hallmark is increased cellularity, relative to the basement membrane (Fig. 25-8E,F). Proliferation exceeds four cell layers, and often traverses duct lumens. Nuclei may exhibit a streaming pattern. Secondary spaces within the hyperplastic lesions are slit-like, irregular, and typically peripheral in location (Fig. 25-8F). Both luminal and basal epithelial cells proliferate, the latter expressing high–molecular-weight ("basal") cytokeratins. Usual epithelial hyperplasia does not show consistent genetic alterations, and the characteristic alterations seen in atypical ductal hyperplasia (ADH) and low-grade ductal carcinoma in situ (DCIS) are absent (see below).

Sclerosing Adenosis

Adenosis refers to a benign proliferative condition in which acini become enlarged and more numerous. In sclerosing adenosis (SA), the TDLU shows disordered epithelial, myoepithelial, and stromal components. Lesions vary from microscopic foci to palpable masses that may be mistaken clinically and radiologically for carcinoma. SA often calcifies, which may prompt a core biopsy when seen on mammography. However, it is not a precursor of invasive cancer, and is grouped with proliferative lesions without atypia for risk assessment purposes.

PATHOLOGY: SA lesions show disorderly proliferation of ducts, tubules, and intralobular stromal cells, resulting in distortion and expansion of lobules and obliteration of duct spaces (Fig. 25-9). The lobulocentric architecture of the TDLU is maintained. Some cases may be difficult to distinguish from invasive carcinoma, but immunohistochemistry can be used to demonstrate preservation of myoepithelial cells around distorted ducts.

Columnar Cell Lesions

Columnar cell lesions are often encountered in core biopsies targeting mammographic calcifications. They are further categorized as columnar cell change, columnar cell hyperplasia, and flat epithelial atypia (FEA; encompassing columnar cell change with atypia and columnar cell hyperplasia with atypia). They all have in common enlargement of TDLUs and dilatation of acini. The dilated acini often show irregular contours and may contain secretory material and calcifications. The TDLUs are lined by one or two layers of columnar cells with uniform, ovoid to elongated nuclei, oriented perpendicular to the basement membrane. Nucleoli are inconspicuous and mitoses rare. While the cytologic features of columnar cell hyperplasia are similar in the various categories, more than two cell layers may occur with crowding and overlapping of cells. In such cases, apical blebs on the luminal surface of the columnar epithelial cells may be prominent. FEA is diagnosed when low-grade cytologic atypia is present. Here, cells show uniform round nuclei and a slight increase in the nuclear-to-cytoplasmic ratio. Cell polarity is lost, and nucleoli are variably prominent. However, architectural complexities, including micropapillae, bridges, bars, or cribriform structures, are absent (Fig. 25-10).

FEA may coexist with ADH, DCIS, atypical lobular hyperplasia/lobular carcinoma in situ (ALH/LCIS), and

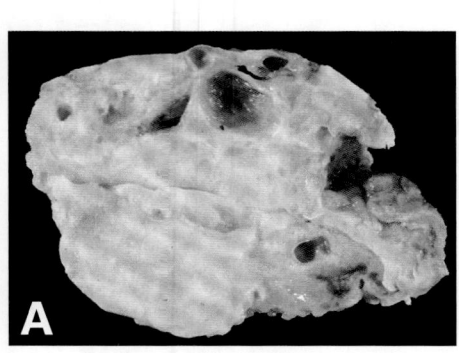

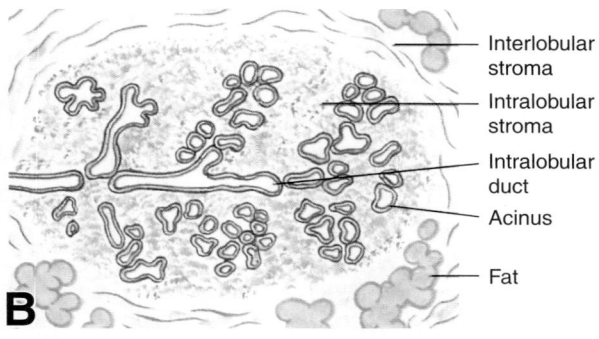

Interlobular stroma

Intralobular stroma

Intralobular duct

Acinus

Fat

Terminal duct lobular unit

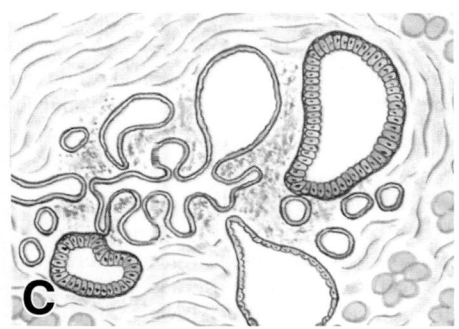

Nonproliferative fibrocystic change

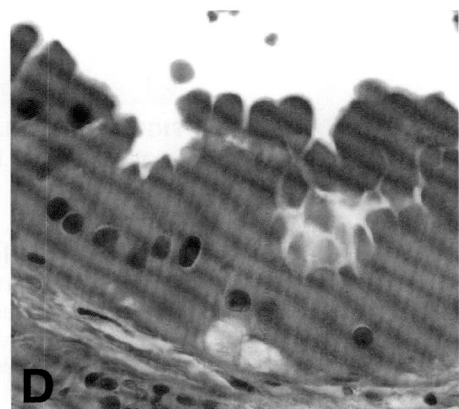

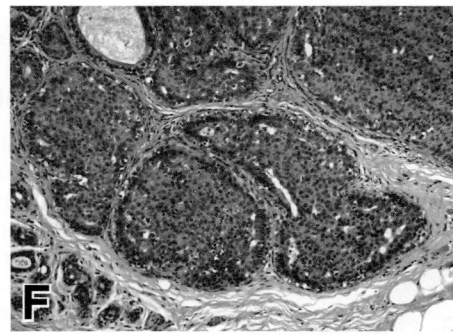

Proliferative breast disease

FIGURE 25-8. Fibrocystic change. A. Cysts of various sizes are dispersed in dense, fibrous connective tissue. Some cysts are large and contain old blood-tinged proteinaceous debris. **B.** Normal terminal duct lobular unit. **C.** Nonproliferative fibrocystic change combines cystic dilation of the terminal ducts with varying degrees of apocrine metaplasia of the epithelium and increased fibrous stroma. **D.** Apocrine metaplasia. Epithelial cells have apocrine features with eosinophilic cytoplasm. **E.** Proliferative breast disease. Terminal duct dilation and intraductal epithelial hyperplasia are present. **F.** Florid epithelial hyperplasia of usual type. The epithelium within the ducts proliferates and nearly fills the duct lumen, with residual "secondary" spaces remaining as peripheral slit-like spaces. Cytoplasmic borders are indistinct and nuclei appear round to oval and frequently overlap, resulting in a streaming pattern.

invasive carcinoma, especially tubular carcinoma. The cells of FEA are similar in morphology to those in coexisting in situ and invasive carcinomas. Loss of heterozygosity (LOH) occurs in most cases that coexist with DCIS or invasive carcinoma. The characteristic 16q loss seen in low-grade DCIS and invasive carcinoma is the most frequently detected recurrent change in FEA. Limited clinical outcome data in patients with FEA suggest that local recurrence and progression to invasive carcinoma are uncommon. Furthermore, FEA does not appear to be associated with an increased risk of breast cancer beyond that attributable to coexisting proliferative breast lesions.

Microglandular Adenosis

Microglandular adenosis (MGA) is an uncommon form of adenosis characterized by round tubular structures containing secretory material dispersed within fibrous stroma and

fat. The glands are lined by a single layer of epithelial cells and lack a myoepithelial cell layer, although the underlying basement membrane is preserved. While it is considered a benign lesion, atypical MGA can occur and in situ and invasive carcinoma can arise in this setting. As with the benign counterpart, the cancers that arise in MGA are negative for estrogen receptor (ER), progesterone receptor (PR), and human epidermal growth factor receptor 2 (HER2). They also exhibit *TP53* mutations and copy number alterations.

Radial Scar/Complex Sclerosing Lesion

Radial scar is a benign sclerosing lesion composed of a central fibroelastotic scar and peripheral radiating ducts and lobules. If the lesion is over 1 cm, it is called a complex sclerosing lesion. Larger lesions may be detected mammographically as stellate or spiculated structures with radiolucent central areas that may be difficult to distinguish from cancer.

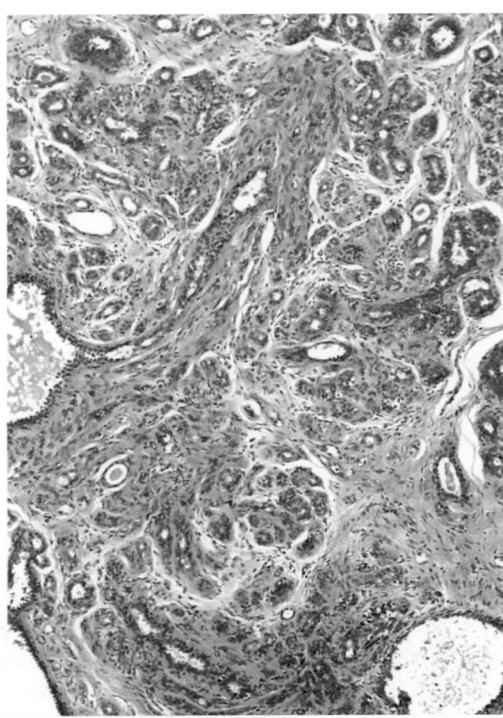

FIGURE 25-9. Sclerosing adenosis. This lesion is characterized by proliferation of small, abortive, duct-like structures, and expansion by myoepithelial cells which distort the lobule in which it arises. The lesion is well circumscribed, in contrast to a cancerous lesion.

PATHOLOGY: Radial scars are characterized by central fibroelastotic cores containing entrapped small, distorted ducts (Fig. 25-11). At the edges, radiating ducts and lobules show various benign alterations. Occasionally, atypical hyperplasia or carcinoma may be present within the lesion.

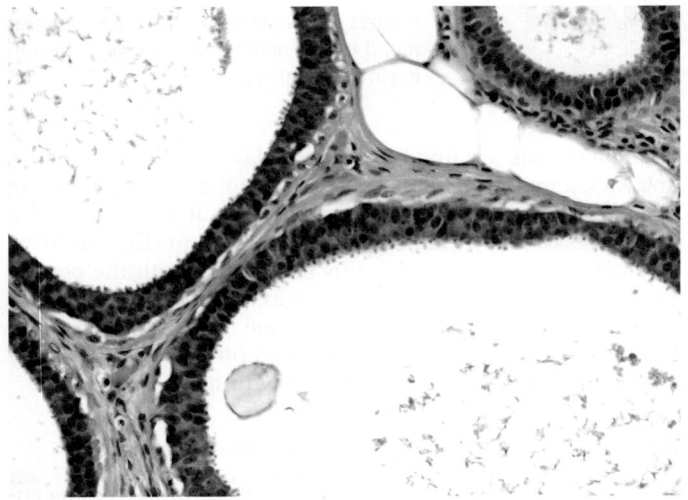

FIGURE 25-10. Flat epithelial atypia. The terminal duct lobular unit (TDLU) is enlarged as a result of dilatation of lobular acini. The acini are lined by one to two layers of epithelial cells showing low-grade cytologic atypia. Nuclei appear round with variably conspicuous nucleoli, and they exhibit loss of their basal location (loss of polarity). Architectural complexity is not a feature.

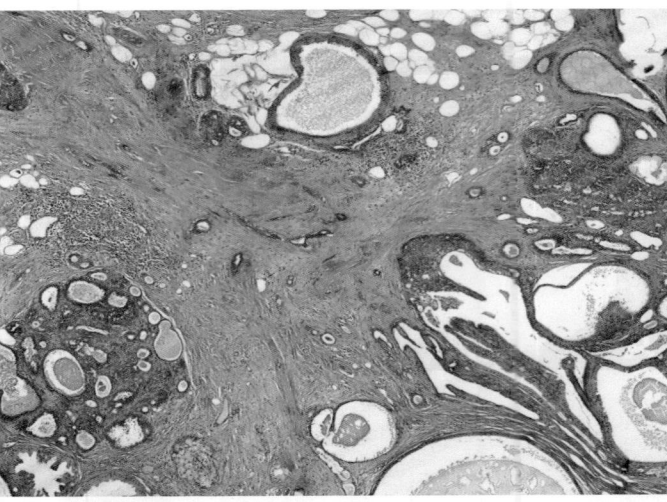

FIGURE 25-11. Radial scar. Angulated glands in a fibroelastotic center are surrounded by a radial distribution of benign ducts and apocrine cysts.

CLINICAL FEATURES: Radial scars carry a twofold increase in breast cancer risk, which is even greater in women with coexisting proliferative disease, with and without atypia. This increased risk pertains to both ipsilateral and contralateral breasts, indicating that radial scars are markers of generally increased susceptibility to breast cancer. Since cancer can occur in radial scars, surgical excision is usually recommended, although recent data suggest that small, incidental radial scars without atypia may be followed.

Intraductal Papilloma

Intraductal papillomas are benign lesions characterized by the presence of finger-like fibrovascular cores. They can be divided into central papillomas, which involve large lactiferous ducts and tend to be solitary, and peripheral papillomas, which originate in TDLUs and are usually multiple. Patients may present with a mass lesion or a bloody nipple discharge. On mammography, central papillomas appear as well-circumscribed masses. Peripheral papillomas may be seen as clustered calcifications or small nodular masses. Ultrasound often shows larger lesions as well-defined hypoechoic masses, with solid and cystic components, near dilated ducts.

PATHOLOGY: Papillomas vary from microscopic foci to masses several centimeters across (Fig. 25-12A). Larger lesions frequently have foci of hemorrhage or necrosis. Dilated duct spaces contain multiple branching papillae with fibrovascular cores. The ducts are lined by a layer of myoepithelium, on which one or more layers of epithelium reside (Fig. 25-12B). Florid epithelial hyperplasia of usual type or ADH may be present (Fig. 25-13). Papillomas often contain areas of apocrine change and, less often, squamous metaplasia. Sclerosis of papillae or duct walls is variable, but it can be marked, and entrap and distort benign epithelium at the periphery, thus mimicking an invasive process.

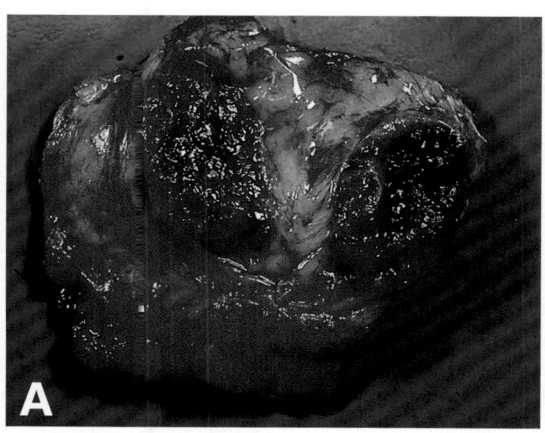
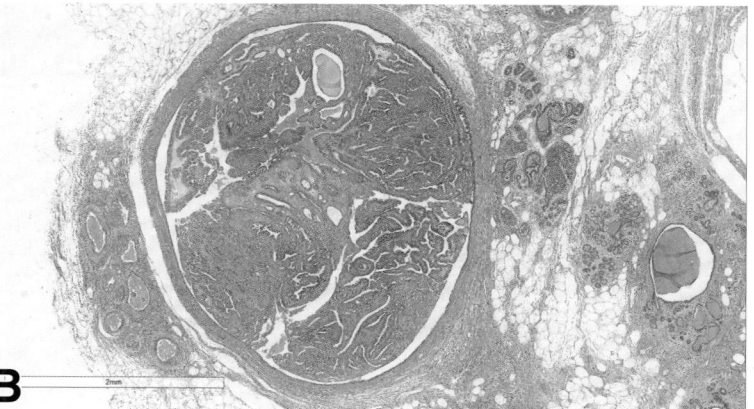

FIGURE 25-12. **Intraductal papilloma. A.** A large papillary mass is seen within dilated ducts. **B.** Dilated subareolar duct containing multiple branching papillae with fibrovascular cores.

CLINICAL FEATURES: Peripheral papillomas are more often associated with concurrent or subsequent breast cancer. The relative risk of a malignancy is twofold in patients with central papillomas and threefold if papillomas are peripheral. If atypia is present, relative risks increase to five- and sevenfold, respectively. Papillomas with atypia diagnosed on a core biopsy require excision, but management of papillomas without atypia is less clearly defined. Some centers opt for surveillance as an alternative to immediate excision.

Proliferative Lesions With Atypia

Atypical Ductal Hyperplasia

PATHOLOGY: ADH is an intraductal epithelial proliferation with a dual population of low-grade neoplastic epithelial cells and benign cells. The benign population may comprise normal lining cells or proliferating cells showing epithelial hyperplasia of usual type. The neoplastic population consists of monomorphic, evenly spaced small cells with well-defined cytoplasmic borders and uniform round, hyperchromatic nuclei. They form architecturally complex structures, such as micropapillae, rigid bridges, bars, solid sheets, or cribriform arrays (Fig. 25-14). If a duct is completely filled by neoplastic cells, and if two duct spaces are involved over a distance of at least 2 mm, the lesion is considered low-grade DCIS. However, if these criteria are not fulfilled, most pathologists would designate the lesion as ADH.

MOLECULAR PATHOGENESIS: One-third to one-half of ADH lesions show no apparent genetic changes. The others, however, exhibit several recurrent genetic alterations that overlap with those seen in low-grade DCIS. Common patterns of genetic alterations in proliferative breast lesions are summarized in Table 25-1.

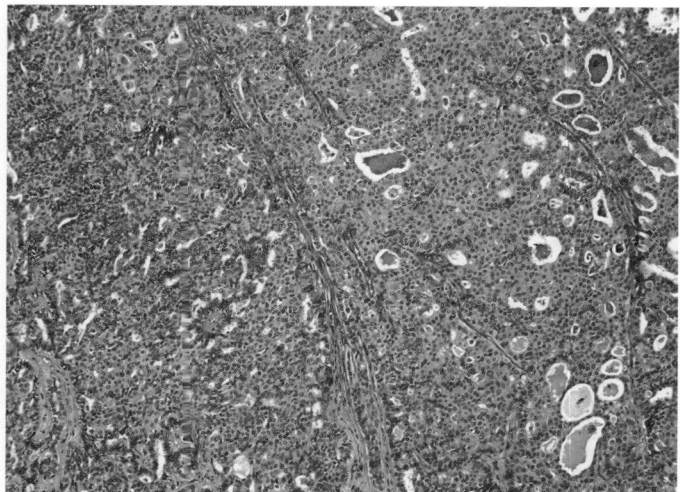

FIGURE 25-13. **Intraductal papilloma** with focus (*on right of image*) showing low-grade cytologic atypia and architectural atypia in keeping with atypical ductal hyperplasia occurring within a papilloma (atypical papilloma).

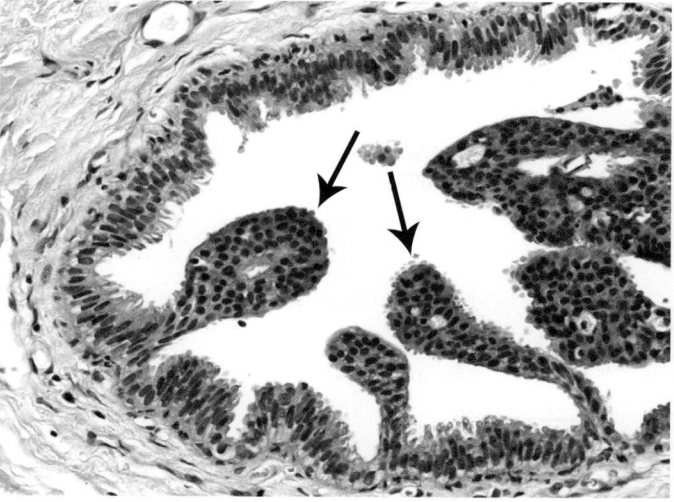

FIGURE 25-14. **Atypical ductal hyperplasia (ADH).** Micropapillae (*arrows*) project into the duct lumen and consist of cells with an increased nuclear-to-cytoplasmic ratio and nuclear hyperchromasia. Residual benign columnar cells are seen lining the duct.

TABLE 25-1

COMMON GENETIC ALTERATIONS ASSOCIATED WITH BREAST LESIONS

Lesion Type	Other	Alteration
ADH	Loss	16q, 17p
	Gain	1q
Phyllodes tumors	Gain	1q, 5p
	Loss	6q, 13q, 9p,10p
	Mutation	*MED12, TERT*
Familial adenomatous polyposis	Mutation	*APC*, β-catenin
	Loss	5q
Familial breast cancer, high penetrance		*BRCA1, BRCA2*
	Li–Fraumeni	*TP53*
	Cowden	*PTEN*
	Hereditary diffuse gastric cancer	*CDH1*
	Peutz–Jeghers	*STK11*
Familial breast cancer, moderate penetrance	Ataxia telangiectasia	*ATM*
		PALB2
		RAD51C/D
	Li–Fraumeni variant	*CHEK2*
Low-grade DCIS	Gain	1q
	Loss	16q
High-grade DCIS	Gain	17q, 8q, 5p
	Loss	11q, 14q, 8p, 13q
	Amplifications	17, 6, 8, 11
Encapsulated papillary carcinoma		LOH, 16q, 1q
Lobular neoplasia	Gain	1q, 6q
	Loss	16p, 16q (especially 16q22.1), 17p, 22q
Pleomorphic LCIS	Gains and losses	Same as lobular neoplasia
	Amplification	8q24, 17q12
	LOH	16q22.1, *TP53, HER2, BRCA1*
Invasive ductal NST, low grade	Loss	16q
	Gain	1q, 16p
Invasive ductal NST, high grade		Heterogeneous and aneuploid
Invasive lobular carcinoma	Loss	16q
	Gain	1q, 16p
Invasive lobular carcinoma, high grade		Same as invasive lobular carcinoma
	Amplification	8q24, 17q12, 20q13
Tubular carcinoma	Loss	16q (8p, 3p, 11q)
	Gain	1q, 16p
Medullary carcinoma	Mutations (acquired)	*TP53, BRCA1*
	Epigenetic inactivation	*BRCA1*
Micropapillary	Gain	8q, 17q, 20q
	Loss	6q, 13q
Metaplastic carcinoma	Mutations	*TP53*
Male breast cancer	Inherited mutations	*BRCA2*
	Acquired mutations	*TP53, PTEN, CHEK2*

ADH = atypical ductal hyperplasia; DCIS = ductal carcinoma in situ; LCIS = lobular carcinoma in situ; LOH = loss of heterozygosity; NST = no specific type.

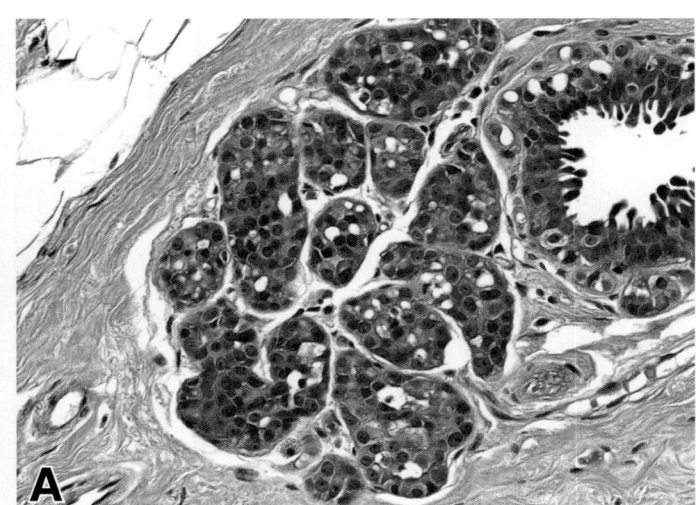
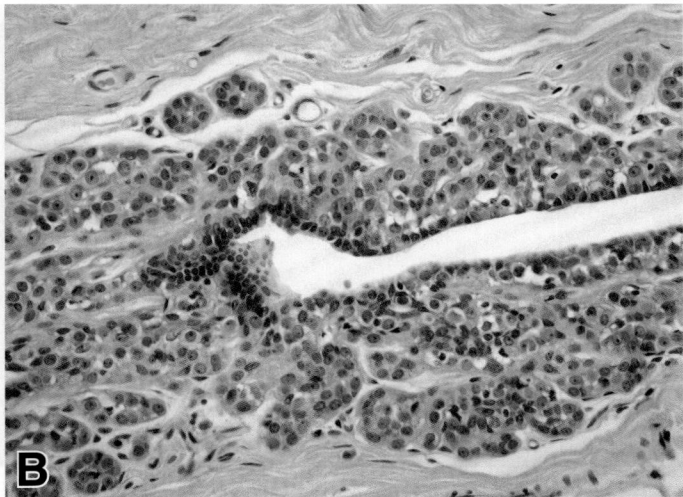

FIGURE 25-15. A. Atypical lobular hyperplasia (ALH). There is minimal distension of the lobular acini by a uniform population of cells with intracytoplasmic lumens and round nuclei containing small nucleoli. **B.** Pagetoid spread of lobular neoplastic cells into the terminal duct. Here the atypical cells lie beneath an attenuated surface layer of luminal epithelial cells.

The relative risk of subsequent breast cancer in patients with ADH is increased three- to fivefold over that in age-matched controls. Cancers occur in both ipsilateral and contralateral breasts, although they may arise more frequently in the ipsilateral breast. Patients with ADH are followed with active surveillance. Hormonal therapy may reduce the risk of developing breast cancer. Identification of ADH on a core biopsy generally requires surgical excision of the radiologic abnormality in view of the risk of upgrade to DCIS or invasive carcinoma.

Atypical Lobular Hyperplasia

ALH is usually an incidental finding in a biopsy or excision performed for other reasons such as reduction mammoplasty. In ALH, cells are indistinguishable from those seen in LCIS (see below), but the degree of involvement of the TDLU is less in ALH than in LCIS; fewer acini are involved and less than 50% within the lobule are distended (Fig. 25-15A). As in LCIS, cells of ALH can spread in a pagetoid (i.e., "upward") fashion to involve ducts (Fig. 25-15B). ALH morphology and associated risk of subsequent breast cancer are discussed below.

FIBROEPITHELIAL LESIONS

These arise from intralobular stroma and contain both stromal and epithelial elements.

Fibroadenoma

Fibroadenomas are common, mobile, painless, breast lumps that most often affect 20- to 35-year-old women. Clinically silent lesions are particularly common and are usually identified by mammography. They are typically well-defined solitary masses, which may be calcified. However, they can be multiple and bilateral, most often in Afro-Caribbean women.

PATHOLOGY: Fibroadenomas are round to ovoid in shape and rubbery in consistency (Fig. 25-16A). They are sharply demarcated from surrounding breast tissue. Most are less than 3 cm, but rarely, can be up to 20 cm in young women or adolescents. Fibroadenomas have both stromal and epithelial components (Fig. 25-16B). The stroma typically contains spindle cells of variable, but usually low, cellularity. In younger women, the stroma is often myxoid. With age, stroma may become denser and calcify. The epithelial component arises from normal TDLU constituents, and epithelial and myoepithelial layers are preserved. The epithelial component usually consists of hyperplasia, especially in young women. Rarely, ADH, lobular neoplasia, or DCIS can occur within fibroadenomas. The relationship of the stroma to the epithelium is typically uniform throughout. Two growth patterns are recognized. In the intracanalicular pattern, stromal growth compresses ducts into curvilinear slits. The pericanalicular pattern is characterized by ducts that maintain a tubular configuration, surrounded by stromal proliferation. These growth patterns carry no prognostic significance. Complex fibroadenomas show benign changes, including epithelial calcifications, sclerosing adenosis (Fig. 25-17), papillary apocrine change or cysts greater than 3 mm.

Variants of fibroadenomas include tubular adenomas, in which small tubular structures are surrounded by a loosely cellular vascularized stroma (Fig. 25-18), and juvenile fibroadenomas, which are most common in adolescents. The latter grow rapidly and may reach 20 cm, causing clinical concern. Juvenile fibroadenomas resemble fibroadenomas histologically, but with more cellular stroma and more prominent epithelial hyperplasia. Lactating adenoma, also called nodular lactational hyperplasia, occurs in pregnancy and the postpartum period. In most instances, it represents coalescence of enlarged lobular units with lactational changes.

Fibroadenomas are surgically excised if they are of clinical or radiologic concern. They can recur. However,

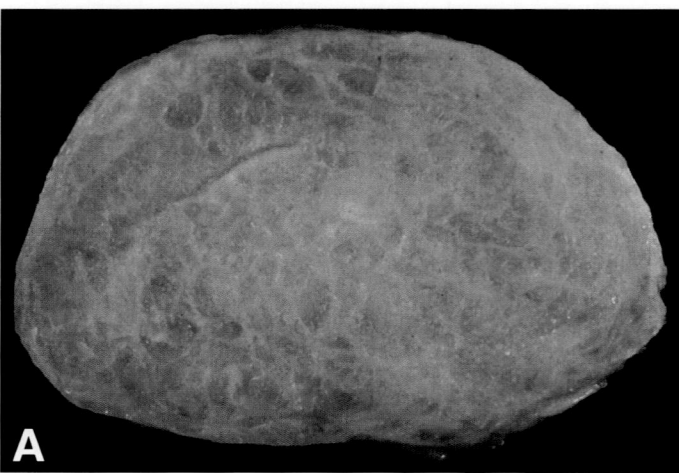
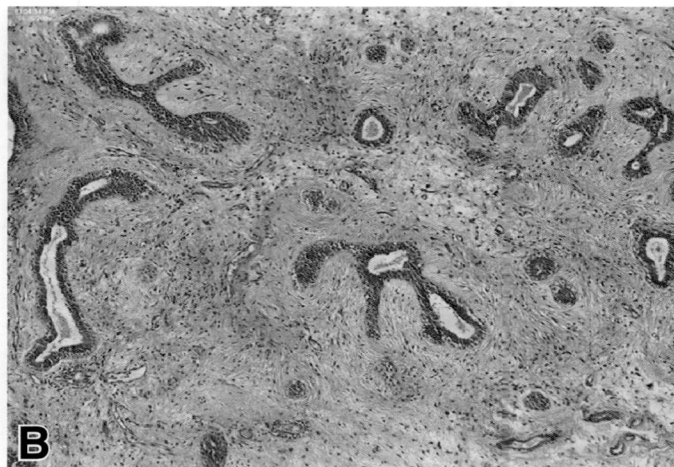

FIGURE 25-16. Fibroadenoma. A. This well-circumscribed tumor was easily enucleated from the surrounding tissue during surgery. The cut surface is characteristically glistening tannish-white with a septate appearance. **B.** Microscopic examination shows elongated epithelial duct structures within a loose, myxoid stroma.

risk of subsequent breast cancer is not increased in the vast majority of cases.

Phyllodes Tumor

These usually benign tumors are rare, making up less than 1% of breast tumors. They have epithelial and stromal components, the latter being neoplastic. The name is derived from the Greek word *phyllos*, meaning "leaf," because they show a leaf-like growth pattern. They can occur at any age but are most common in the 6th decade. Phyllodes tumors present as rapidly growing breast masses. On mammography, they are well circumscribed or lobulated. Ultrasound may show internal hyperechoic areas in a hypoechoic mass.

PATHOLOGY: Phyllodes tumors vary in size from a few to 20 cm in diameter. Most phyllodes tumors are benign and are sharply circumscribed. Their cut surfaces are firm, glistening, and grayish white.

Clefts may be prominent. On microscopy, fronds of mild or moderately hypercellular stroma with mild cytologic atypia and few mitosis form leaf-like structures, which project into cystic spaces (Fig. 25-19). These spaces are lined by a dual layer of benign epithelium and myoepithelium. The stroma ranges from benign and hypercellular to frankly sarcomatous. Malignant lesions often show infiltrative margins. Phyllodes tumors are considered malignant when the following five features are all present: (1) marked stromal cytologic atypia, (2) stromal hypercellularity, (3) abundant mitoses (>10 per 10 HPFs), (4) stromal overgrowth, and (5) infiltrative margins. If malignant heterologous elements, such as bone, cartilage, or fat, are present, the lesion is considered malignant, regardless of the presence of the other histological features. Tumors that contain some, but not all, of the five histological features listed above are called borderline.

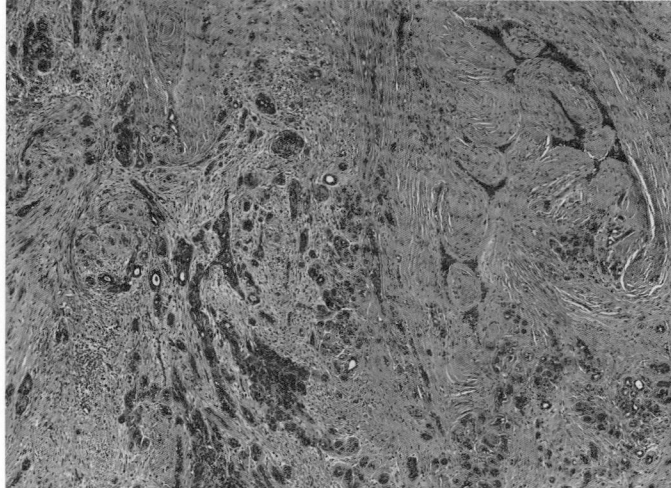

FIGURE 25-17. Fibroadenoma involved by sclerosing adenosis.

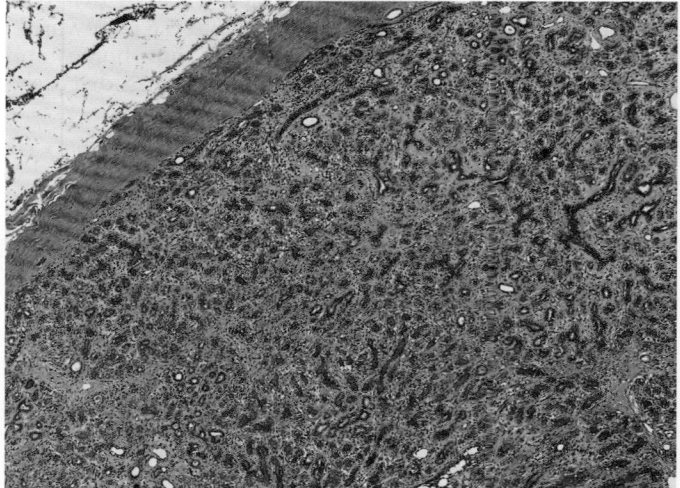

FIGURE 25-18. Tubular adenoma. This well-circumscribed fibroepithelial lesion contains closely packed round tubules with little intervening stroma.

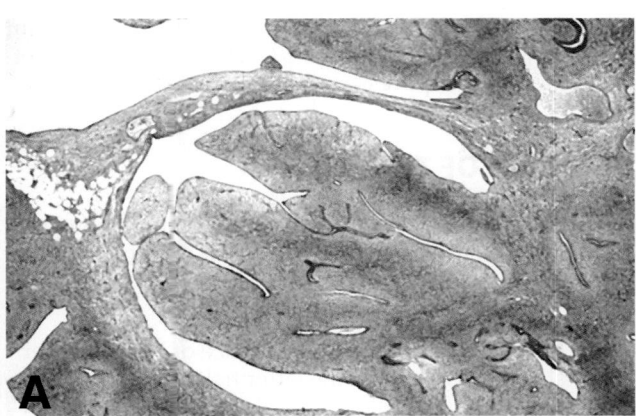
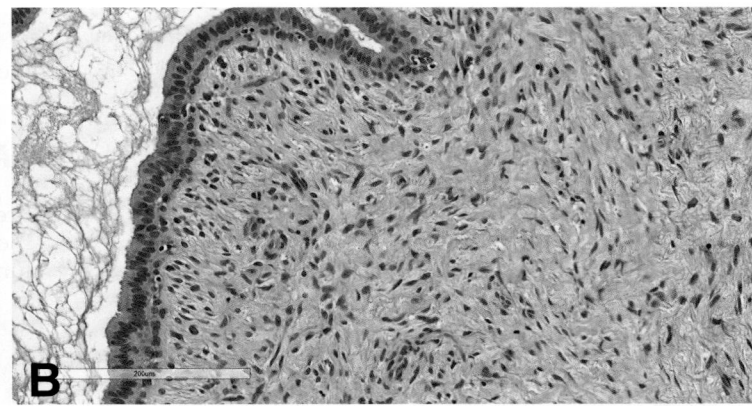

FIGURE 25-19. Phyllodes tumor. A. A polypoid tumor with a leaf-like pattern expands a duct. **B.** The stromal component adjacent to ductal epithelium is similar to that seen in a fibroadenoma, but is more cellular. The residual ductal structure is benign.

MOLECULAR PATHOGENESIS: Epithelial–stromal interactions in phyllodes tumors appear to influence stromal growth. Upregulation of transcriptionally active β-catenin and downstream effectors such as cyclin D1 via Wnt pathway signaling occurs in these tumors along with recurrent gains in 1q and 5p and losses in 6q, 13q, 9p, and 10p with pattern of alterations being shown to be grade specific in some studies. Mutations in mediator complex subunit 12 (*MED12*), which regulates activities of one or more cyclin-dependent kinases, have been identified in both fibroadenomas and phyllodes tumors, suggesting its role as an early event in fibroadenoma and phyllodes tumor pathogenesis. *TERT* promoter mutations, frequently associated with *MED12* variants, are identified with increasing malignancy in fibroepithelial lesions suggestive of a mechanistic role in progression. Such variants in *TERT* promoters inappropriately activate the core catalytic component of telomerase.

The main risk of benign phyllodes tumors is local recurrence, which happens 10% to 17% of the time. Local recurrence is more common with malignant lesions (23% to 30%). Metastases are rare overall (≤2%) and mostly limited to malignant phyllodes tumors. Only stromal components are seen in metastases. Axillary lymph node metastases are very rare.

STROMAL LESIONS

Stromal lesions arise from nonspecialized interlobular stroma. Mesenchymal lesions that occur outside the breast, such as lipomas or vascular tumors, can also occur here as well. Stromal lesions specific to the breast, such as pseudoangiomatous stromal hyperplasia (PASH) and myofibroblastoma, are also found.

Pseudoangiomatous Stromal Hyperplasia Mimics a Vascular Lesion

PASH is a benign process that is usually found incidentally in biopsies done for other reasons. It occasionally presents clinically as a firm painless mass. It may be seen in fibroepithelial lesions and commonly occurs in gynecomastia. Most female patients are premenopausal, suggesting that hormonal factors may play a role in PASH development and growth.

PATHOLOGY: PASH lesions are circumscribed, with homogeneous tan cut surfaces. They vary from 1 to 7 cm. Interanastomosing spaces, which rarely contain red blood cells, are seen in dense collagenous stroma (Fig. 25-20). Myofibroblasts close to these spaces mimic endothelial cells. True vascular channels may occur in the stroma.

Fibromatosis Consists of Fibroblasts and Myofibroblasts

Fibromatosis can be locally aggressive but does not metastasize. The lesion usually presents as a unilateral, painless, firm to hard mass. Most patients are in their 40s, but any age group can be affected. Mammography shows a stellate mass, mimicking carcinoma.

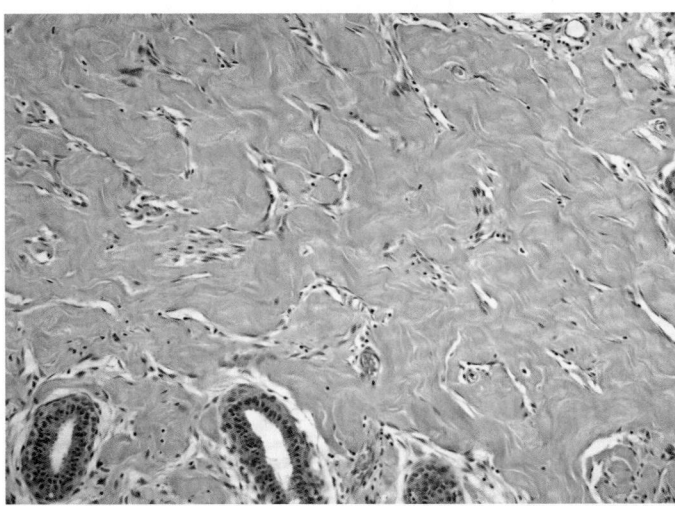

FIGURE 25-20. Pseudoangiomatous stromal hyperplasia. Slit-like spaces occur within a collagenized stroma. Myofibroblasts, distributed singly at the margins of the spaces, resemble endothelial cells. True capillaries are also evident.

MOLECULAR PATHOGENESIS: Fibromatosis is usually sporadic but may be seen in association with familial adenomatous polyposis (FAP) and Gardner syndrome. FAP is caused by mutations in the adenomatous polyposis coli (*APC*) gene, which negatively regulates nuclear translocation of β-catenin. Sporadic and FAP-associated lesions show genetic alterations in APC or β-catenin, affecting the Wnt/β-catenin pathway, with β-catenin mutation or mutation or allelic loss of 5q, the location of the APC gene (Table 25-1).

PATHOLOGY: Grossly, fibromatosis is poorly defined and firm, with infiltrative margins. It varies in size from less than 1 cm to greater than 10 cm. Histologically, it is characterized by broad sweeping fascicles and interlacing bundles of bland-appearing spindle or oval cells (Fig. 25-21). Collagen may be prominent. Adjacent normal breast tissue is infiltrated by proliferating spindle cells, and collections of lymphocytes are commonly seen at the periphery. Cellular atypia is absent and mitotic figures are rare (<3 per 10 HPFs). Immunohistochemical demonstration of abnormal nuclear localization of β-catenin may aid in diagnosis, but is neither highly sensitive nor specific.

Fibromatosis recurs locally in 20% to 30% of patients. While wide local excision was previously recommended, close surveillance is now practiced in many centers.

Myofibroblastoma

Myofibroblastoma is an uncommon benign tumor of the breast that affects men and women equally. It is most common in postmenopausal women and elderly men. It presents as a slow-growing well-circumscribed mobile mass that may be mistaken for fibroadenomas clinically and radiologically. On histology, they are well-circumscribed, non-encapsulated lesions consisting of short fascicles of bland spindle cells admixed with bands of brightly eosinophilic collagen. Mature fat and mast cells are variably present.

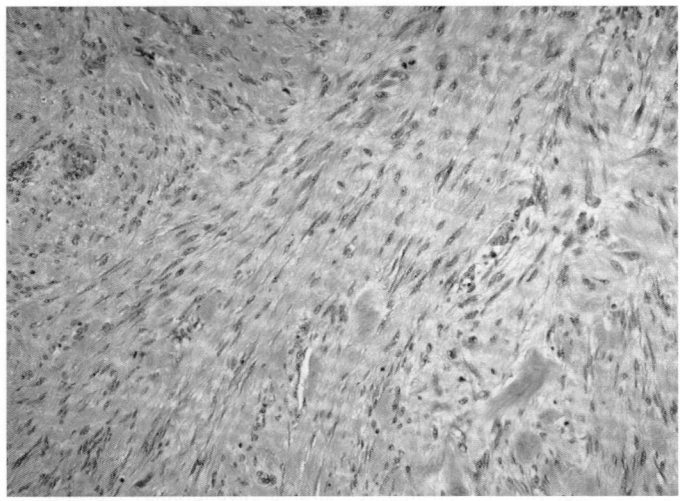

FIGURE 25-21. Fibromatosis. Interlacing bundles of spindle cells, without nuclear atypia, are admixed with focal bands of collagen.

Mitotic activity is inconspicuous. Deletion or rearrangement of 13q14 with subsequent loss of *Rb1*, which encodes the retinoblastoma tumor suppressor, characterizes these lesions.

CARCINOMA OF THE BREAST

Breast cancer is the most common malignancy of women in the United States; its mortality, in women, is second only to lung cancer.

EPIDEMIOLOGY: The incidence of breast cancer slowly increased in the latter half of the 20th century but has leveled off or declined in developed countries. Women in the United States have a one in eight risk of developing breast cancer; however, as this represents lifetime risk, it overestimates actual risk for an individual woman. Overall, one in five women with breast cancer will die of their disease; however, racial/ethnic disparities exist with black women having the highest mortality rate (31%). Age-specific incidence rates increase dramatically after 40 years of age. In industrialized countries with high rates of breast cancer, incidence continues to increase with age, finally plateauing at 75 to 80 years. In some populations, including Hispanic and black women, that plateau is reached at a younger age. Breast cancer is uncommon before the age of 35 in all populations. The incidence of ER-negative cancers increases rapidly until age 50, after which it flattens or decreases. By contrast, ER-positive breast cancer continues to rise after that age. Thus, peak ages of onset for ER-negative and ER-positive breast cancers are 50 and 70, respectively.

Breast cancer occurs four to five times more commonly in Western industrialized countries than in the developing world. Risk in daughters and granddaughters of women who migrated from countries of low incidence to Western countries increases in successive generations.

Widespread use of screening mammography in the 1980s led to a sharp increase in the diagnosis of noninvasive breast lesions (i.e., DCIS). The frequency of small invasive cancers has also increased. However, although widespread screening mammography greatly increased detection of early breast cancers, it has not appreciably decreased the incidence of late-stage breast cancers. Overall mortality has declined from 30% to 20%, and stage-specific mortality has also improved. More effective targeted therapies have contributed greatly to the decline in breast cancer mortality.

ETIOLOGIC FACTORS: Multiple risk factors for breast cancer have been identified, some of which cannot be modified and others can be mitigated (Table 25-2). Women can be stratified by level of breast cancer risk. Those who carry a germline *BRCA* mutation (see below) or who have a history of chest radiation are considered high risk; women who have had multiple family members with breast cancer or who have multiple risk factors are at moderate risk.

Nonmodifiable risk factors include age, race (greatest in non-Hispanic white population), family history, genetic factors (germline mutations in *BRCA1* or *BRCA2*),

TABLE 25-2

RISK FACTORS FOR BREAST CANCER DEVELOPMENT

Not Modifiable	Modifiable
Age	Body mass index
BRCA germline mutations	Diet
Family history	Alcohol
Chest radiation	Exogenous estrogen
Race/ethnicity	Exercise
Height	Smoking
Age at menarche	Reproductive history
Age at menopause	Age at first full-term delivery
Breast density	Lactation
Atypia on prior breast biopsy	

breast density, and early age at menarche. Modifiable risk factors are late age at first live birth, diet, high body mass index, alcohol consumption, and use of exogenous hormones.

SPORADIC BREAST CANCER: Only about 25% of sporadic breast cancers have identifiable risk factors. Factors affecting the hormonal milieu modify breast cancer risk.

- The majority of breast cancers are stimulated by estrogen. Cumulative lifetime exposure to estrogen determines the level of this risk. Thus, early menarche (younger than 11 years), late menopause, and older age at first-term pregnancy increase risk. Pregnancy before age 20 is protective; nulliparity and deferring childbearing until after 35 years of age are associated with two- to three-fold increased relative risk. Longer intervals of lactation reduce risk of breast cancer. Oophorectomy before age of 35, but not afterward, dramatically lowers risk of breast cancer. Antiestrogens, including tamoxifen and aromatase inhibitors, decrease the development of ER-positive breast cancer. Oral contraceptives do not increase breast cancer risk, although hormone replacement therapy (HRT) increases risk slightly, by 1.2 to 1.7 times.
- Radiation increases risk of breast cancer, as documented in survivors of the atomic bomb blasts in World War II, and in women who received irradiation for Hodgkin lymphoma. Irradiation earlier in life (i.e., in childhood or adolescence) poses the greatest risk; exposure after the age of 40 years has not been shown to increase incidence.
- Although the influence of dietary fat on breast cancer risk has been studied extensively, data suggesting that total fat increases risk after menopause are limited. If such an association exists, the risk is likely to be small. The effect is postulated to occur through modifying levels of circulating estrogens. Prospective studies of dietary carbohydrate consumption have not shown consistent associations with breast cancer risk.

- Alcohol consumption consistently predicts higher breast cancer rates although the increase is relatively modest. Results from the Nurses' Health Study showed that low levels of alcohol consumption (3 to 6 drinks per week) are associated with a minute increase in breast cancer risk (relative risk 1.15). The most relevant measure was cumulative average alcohol consumption over long periods of time, and both drinking earlier and later in adult life were independently associated with breast cancer risk. An association with binge drinking was also found.
- Postmenopausal women who are overweight or obese are at greater risk for breast cancer. Central adiposity has been positively correlated with risk. Interestingly, obesity appears to have an opposite effect on breast cancer risk among premenopausal women. Weight loss after menopause that is maintained is associated with reduced risk of breast cancer, particularly ER-positive tumors.
- Active smoking, particularly if begun at an early age and continued for a prolonged interval, increases risk of developing breast cancer by approximately 20%. This risk is strongly associated with a polymorphism in *NAT2*, the gene that encodes N-acetyltransferase 2, which results in reduced metabolism (slow acetylation) of carcinogens in cigarette smoke. Risk of breast cancer associated with passive smoking is less well established, but some studies suggest that younger, mainly premenopausal, nonsmoking women with significant exposure for extended times may have increased risk.
- Mammographic breast density reflects the relative amounts of stroma and epithelium versus fat in breast tissue. Patients with denser breasts (≥75% density) have a four- to fivefold greater risk of breast cancer. Density is influenced by age, parity, body mass index, and menopausal status, although genetic factors likely also play a role.
- Higher levels of physical activity are associated with a reduction in breast cancer risk, with most studies showing evidence of a dose-response relationship. The benefit of activity is independent of race or ethnicity. The mechanism is not well understood.
- Prior breast biopsies showing atypical hyperplasia or nonatypical proliferative breast disease increase relative risk by 4 to 5 times and 1.5 to 2 times, respectively (see above). Women with a previous breast cancer have a 10-fold increased risk of developing a second primary tumor in the ipsilateral or contralateral breast. Hormonal treatment with antiestrogens decreases this risk.

 MOLECULAR PATHOGENESIS: FAMILIAL BREAST CANCER: The strongest association with increased risk for breast cancer is a family history of breast cancer at a young age in first-degree relatives. The risk is greater if the relative was affected at a young age or had bilateral breast cancer. Familial disease accounts for 10% of breast cancers. Pathogenic variants in two high-risk breast cancer susceptibility genes, *BRCA1* and *BRCA2*, account for 20% to 50% of familial tumors.

Some inherited breast cancer susceptibility is part of more generalized familial cancer susceptibility syndromes (Table 25-1). Common inherited polymorphisms have been identified through genome-wide association studies, but the 20 most common low-risk alleles identified thus far account for less than 5% of familial risk.

BRCA1 and *BRCA2* are tumor suppressor genes that display an autosomal dominant pattern of inheritance with variable penetrance. *BRCA1*, on chromosome 17q21, is involved in DNA repair, transcriptional regulation, chromatin remodeling, and protein ubiquitination. Pathogenic germline mutations in *BRCA1* confer a lifetime breast cancer risk of between 37% and 85% by age 70 years, with over half of the cancers occurring before age 50. In women older than 70 years, pathogenic *BRCA1* germline mutations account for less than 2% of cancers; however, 30% of cancers in women under 45 years of age occur in mutation carriers. Carriers are also at significantly increased risk of other cancers, most notably ovarian cancer, with a lifetime risk of 15% to 40%. The incidence of cancers of the cervix, endometrium, fallopian tube, and stomach is elevated, and prostate cancer is more common in male carriers. About 0.1% of the population has a pathogenic *BRCA1* germline mutation, but rates are higher in Ashkenazi Jews and French Canadians. Breast cancers that develop in patients with germline mutations are typically high-grade, invasive ductal carcinomas, of no special type (NST); however, they show many of the features present in medullary-like cancers, with pushing margins, prominent inflammatory responses, absent tubule formation, high mitotic counts, and significant nuclear pleomorphism (Fig. 25-22). In *BRCA1* carriers, the majority of cancers are negative for ER, PR, and HER2, and p53 mutations are more common. Young age at onset is typical.

Pathogenic germline mutations in *BRCA2*, located on chromosome 13q12, are associated with a 30% to 40% lifetime risk of developing breast cancer and an increased risk of ovarian cancer. Moreover, the incidence of uveal tract and skin melanomas and cancers of the pancreas and biliary tract is also increased. Male carriers of *BRCA2* mutations are also at risk for breast and prostatic cancers. Women mostly develop high-grade invasive ductal tumors of NST, which as defined below show no specific or "special" histologic features. *BRCA2*-related cancers are more commonly positive for ER and PR than are *BRCA1* cancers. HER2 gene amplification is rare. Like *BRCA1*, *BRCA2* encodes a protein involved in DNA repair. It may also fulfill other functions that are important in suppressing carcinogenesis.

Breast cancer is not a single disease. For example, molecular phenotyping suggests that ER-positive and ER-negative breast cancers are distinct entities. Furthermore, breast cancer evolution is thought to follow two different grade-based pathways, referred to as low-grade and high-grade neoplasia pathways. Low-grade tumors express hormone receptors and lack HER2 overexpression. Their karyotypes are diploid or near diploid and they exhibit recurrent copy number changes including 16q deletion and 1q and 16p gains. High-grade tumors, by contrast, are a more heterogeneous group. They frequently lack hormone receptor expression, show HER2 overexpression or are negative for ER, PR, and HER2 (i.e., they are triple negative or TN). They often demonstrate aneuploidy and complex karyotypes. Only a relatively few gene mutations are actually present in a high percentage of tumors (see Chapter 5). These include *PTEN*, *PIK3CA*, and *TP53*. Genetic comparisons of matched primary and metastatic tumors show that tumors are largely mosaics of subclones of cancer cells, and metastases may derive from genetically distinct subpopulations in the primary tumor (see Chapter 5).

Ductal Carcinoma In Situ Is a Nonobligate Precursor of Invasive Cancer

Carcinoma of the breast may occur in situ (confined by the gland's basement membrane) or be invasive, in which the malignant cells have breached the basement membrane and infiltrated into the adjacent breast stroma. Further subclassification is based on morphology, immunohistochemistry, and molecular profiling. Of women with biopsy-proven DCIS who receive no further therapy, 20% to 30% subsequently develop invasive cancer.

Ductal Carcinoma in Situ

DCIS identifies a heterogeneous group of lesions that vary in their architectural and cytologic features, as well as in their natural history. These abnormalities are considered nonobligate precursors of invasive carcinoma, and the chance of progressing to invasion varies with the histologic subtype, grade, and extent. The incidence of DCIS has soared with the advent of widespread screening mammography in the mid-1980s. It represented about 5% of breast cancers beforehand, but now accounts for 25% of breast cancers in screened populations. However, increased detection of DCIS has not been associated with decreased incidence of advanced breast cancers, and precursor–product relationship between lesions categorized as DCIS and invasive breast cancer remains unclear.

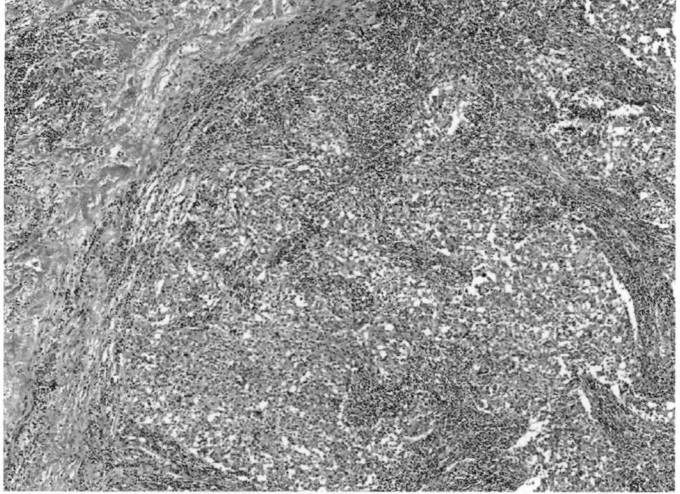

FIGURE 25-22. ***BRCA1*-associated breast cancer.** High-grade invasive ductal carcinoma, no special type, characterized by pushing margins and a prominent lymphocytic infiltrate.

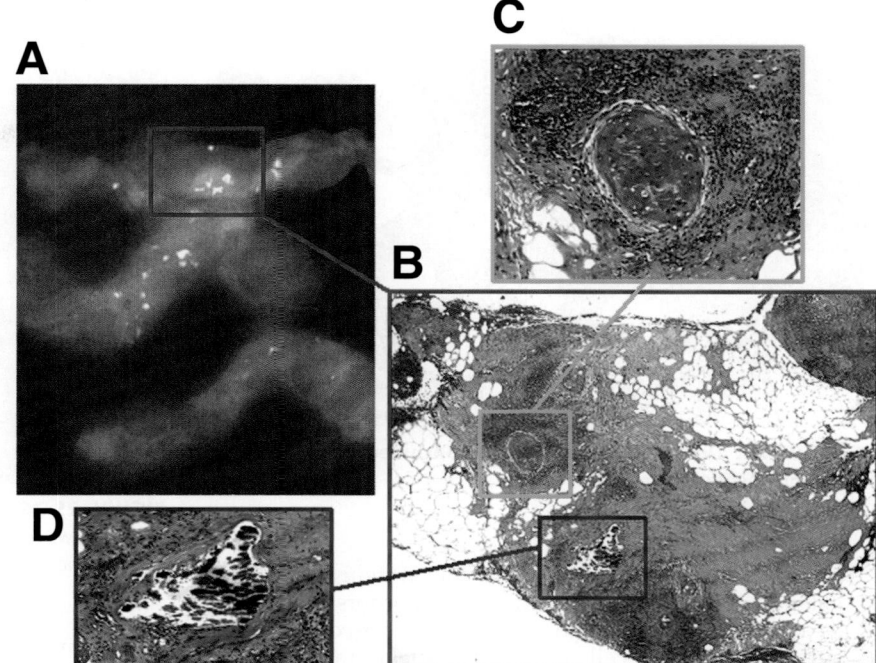

FIGURE 25-23. Ductal carcinoma in situ. A. Radiograph of a core biopsy specimen shows linear and punctate calcifications that are highly suspicious for cancer. **B.** Low-power photomicrograph showing high-grade in situ ductal carcinoma. **C.** High-power image of a duct expanded by in situ ductal carcinoma. **D.** High-power photomicrograph of tissue calcification.

MOLECULAR PATHOGENESIS: In some cases, DCIS appears to be a precursor of invasive breast carcinoma. In such cases, DCIS is often seen together with invasive carcinomas. The noninvasive tumors and their invasive counterparts often show similar cytologic appearance and nuclear grade. They also share distinct molecular and cytogenetic alterations. Nevertheless, mechanisms responsible for potential progression of DCIS to invasive carcinoma are poorly understood. Furthermore, molecular analyses have identified differences in the numbers and types of chromosomal changes in low- and high-grade DCIS (Table 25-1). More numerous alterations are seen in the latter but they do not necessarily overlap with those seen in low-grade lesions. Intermediate-grade DCIS shares alterations of both groups. Invasive carcinomas occurring in association with DCIS share grade and molecular alterations. Low-grade and high-grade DCIS are therefore fundamentally distinct entities, and one does not appear to evolve into the other. The same appears to be true for low- and high-grade invasive cancer. Multiple pathways of carcinogenesis and progression are likely.

PATHOLOGY: DCIS predominantly involves ducts but can extend into lobules. It is characterized by proliferation of malignant epithelial cells showing a range of histologic features (Fig. 25-23). Growth pattern types include cribriform, micropapillary, papillary, solid, and comedo, and multiple architectural patterns can coexist in one lesion. More important prognostically is the nuclear grade which is categorized as low, intermediate, and high. Heterogeneity in grade is not uncommon, however.

- High-grade DCIS is composed of large, pleomorphic cells with marked variation in size and shape. They have abundant cytoplasm and irregular nuclei with prominent nucleoli and coarse chromatin. They proliferate rapidly. Intraductal necrosis is common (Fig. 25-24) and appears grossly as distended ducts containing white necrotic material resembling comedos—hence the term comedo necrosis. The cellular necrotic debris often undergoes dystrophic calcification, which may be seen on mammography as linear, branching calcifications. The cells remain in duct spaces, but periductal chronic inflammation and new vessel formation may

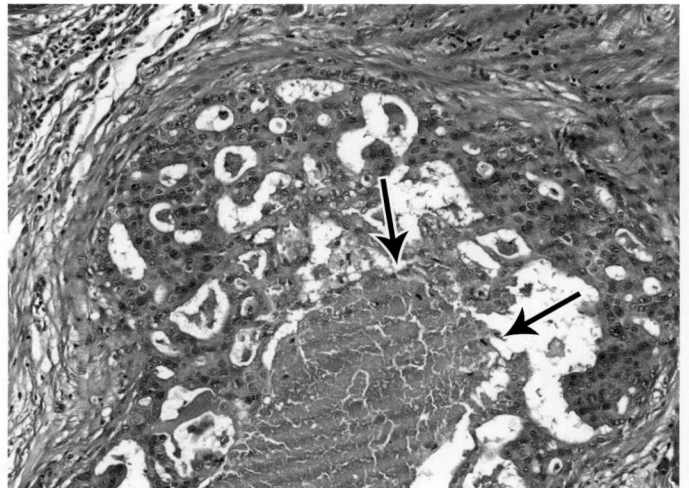

FIGURE 25-24. Ductal carcinoma in situ (DCIS) with comedo necrosis. Intraductal carcinoma with a cribriform architecture and central comedo necrosis (*arrows*).

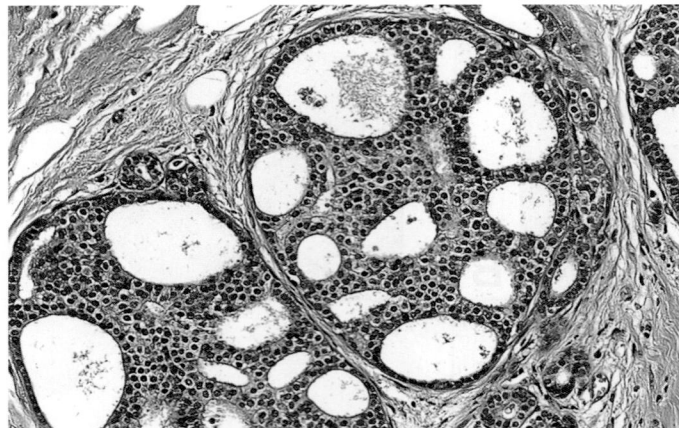

FIGURE 25-25. Ductal carcinoma in situ noncomedo type. A cribriform arrangement of tumor cells is evident.

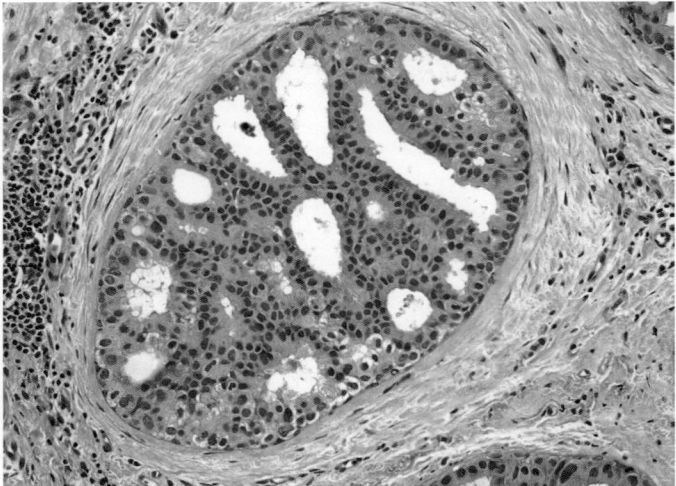

FIGURE 25-26. Intermediate-grade ductal carcinoma in situ. This grade shows moderate nuclear pleomorphism and some polarization of cells around secondary spaces.

occur. DCIS spreads through the duct system and often extends beyond clinically detected borders, making clear margins difficult to obtain in breast-conserving surgery. Malignant cells with high nuclear grade can be seen in any of the above growth patterns.

- Low-grade DCIS: At the other end of the histologic spectrum, cells in low-grade DCIS are uniform, small, and evenly spaced, with round, regular hyperchromatic nuclei (Fig. 25-25). Mitoses are infrequent. Micropapillary or cribriform growth patterns predominate, and solid growth patterns are less common. Although necrosis is uncommon, foci of punctate or comedo necrosis can be seen.
- Intermediate-grade DCIS: This grade falls between high- and low-grade DCIS. Cells show moderate pleomorphism but maintain some degree of polarization (Fig. 25-26). Solid or cribriform growth is typical.
- Microinvasive carcinoma: This pattern is defined as one or more foci of invasive carcinoma, none of which exceeds 1 mm in diameter (Fig. 25-27). This lesion typically occurs in the setting of high-grade DCIS.

Immunohistochemistry may occasionally be of help in the diagnosis of DCIS. For example, the vast majority of DCIS lacks high–molecular-weight cytokeratins, although some high-grade DCIS may express "basal," high–molecular-weight cytokeratins. Stains for myoepithelial cell markers (smooth muscle myosin heavy chain, calponin, p63, etc.) will confirm that the lesion is in situ and helps in cases with foci suspicious for microinvasion.

Low- and intermediate-grade DCIS typically show strong diffuse staining for ER. High-grade lesions show less frequent ER staining but often (up to 60% of cases) overexpress HER2. This is greater than the frequency seen in invasive carcinoma.

CLINICAL FEATURES: DCIS is most often visualized on mammography as calcifications. A small proportion of women present symptomatically

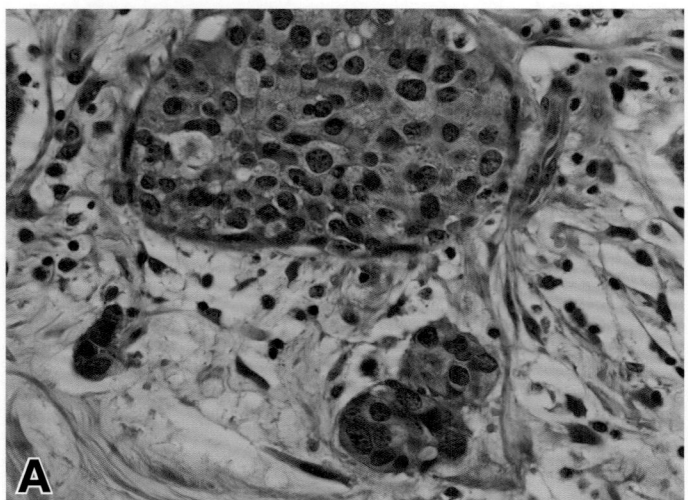

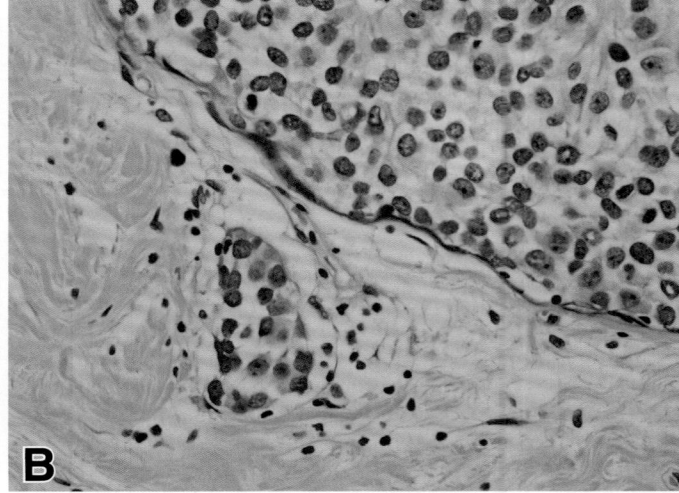

FIGURE 25-27. Ductal carcinoma in situ. A. An adjacent focus of microinvasive carcinoma. **B.** Immunohistochemical staining for smooth muscle myosin heavy chain (*brown signal*) confirms the absence of a myoepithelial cell layer around the microinvasive stromal cluster.

with a mass lesion, a nipple discharge, or Paget disease of the nipple (see below).

DCIS is treated by surgical excision. Mastectomy is typically reserved for women with extensive disease. Breast-conserving surgery is possible in many cases, and adjuvant radiation reduces the risk of recurrence. In some patients with low-risk DCIS, excision alone may be adequate. Ongoing clinical trials are evaluating active surveillance rather than excision in selected women with low-risk DCIS.

When DCIS recurs, it generally does so at the site of the previous surgery. It recurs as invasive carcinomas 50% of the time. Lymph node metastases occur in less than 1% of patients with DCIS. Such cases raise the possibility that foci of invasion were missed when the primary lesions were examined. Antihormone therapy reduces the risk of recurrence or progression for hormone receptor–positive DCIS. In all, the critical prognostic factors for patients with DCIS include lesion size, nuclear grade, the presence of comedo necrosis, and margin status. Cancer-specific mortality is extremely low, with 1.0% to 2.6% dying from invasive cancer 8 to 10 years after diagnosis of DCIS.

Encapsulated Papillary Carcinoma Is an Indolent Tumor

Encapsulated papillary carcinoma covers lesions previously called intracystic or encysted papillary carcinoma. Immunohistochemical studies demonstrate an absence of myoepithelial cells at their periphery, however, and whether these tumors are truly in situ or invasive is unclear. Limited data show that they exhibit LOH at 16q and 1q. These tumors are not aggressive, and metastases are rare. While still controversial, the current approach is to stage them as Tis (carcinoma in situ) disease. If there is any indication of conventional invasive carcinoma, the tumor stage is based on the extent of the invasive component.

Grossly, they are well-circumscribed, partially cystic, frequently hemorrhagic, solid masses. Microscopically, the lesion consists of fibrovascular cores that are lined by one or more layers of malignant epithelial cells, with no intervening myoepithelial cell layer (Fig. 25-28). The cells are usually low to intermediate grade. At its edge, the tumor has a smooth pushing border and is surrounded by a capsule. If frank

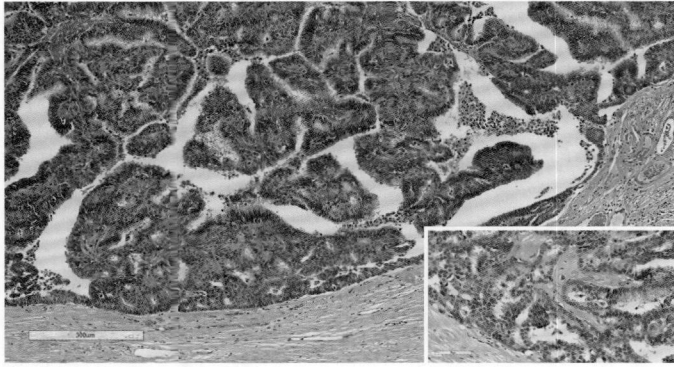

FIGURE 25-28. Encapsulated papillary carcinoma. Fibrovascular cores lined by malignant epithelial cells, without an intervening myoepithelial cell layer. *Inset:* The edge of the tumor has a pushing front, without evidence of stromal invasion.

stromal invasion occurs, the lesion is categorized as typical invasive carcinoma of NST.

Paget Disease of the Nipple Reflects Extension of DCIS or Invasive Cancer

In Paget disease of the nipple, malignant glandular cells penetrate the epidermis of the nipple and areola. It is invariably associated with underlying DCIS, with or without invasive ductal carcinoma. This disease is rare, occurring in 1% to 4% of breast cancers.

Paget disease presents as erythema or an eczematous change to the nipple and areola (Fig. 25-29A), sometimes with nipple retraction. Half of patients have palpable masses.

Malignant glandular epithelial cells are present in the epidermis, singly or in small groups (Fig. 25-29B). They are large cells, with abundant cytoplasm containing mucin globules, and pleomorphic nuclei with prominent nucleoli. They express epithelial membrane antigen (EMA) and low–molecular-weight cytokeratins. They almost always overexpress HER2. ER and PR are positive in 40% and 30% of cases, respectively. Genetically, Paget cells resemble the underlying tumor cells in the vast majority of cases. Prognosis is a function of the stage of the underlying breast cancer rather than the presence of Paget cells.

Lobular Neoplasia Encompasses LCIS and ALH

In their classic forms, LCIS and ALH (see above) reflect the same atypical proliferations of loosely cohesive epithelial cells, but they differ in the relative risk of developing breast cancer. Rare cases demonstrate variant features such as comedo necrosis or pleomorphic cells.

EPIDEMIOLOGY: Since classic LCIS is generally asymptomatic, its true incidence is unknown. Estimated incidence is 1% to 4%. It is bilateral in up to 30% of patients and multicentric in 85%. ALH and LCIS are often considered to be risk factors because the cancers that develop are typically not at the same site as these lesions and may be in the contralateral breast. Relative risk of subsequent cancer is 3- to 5.5-fold for ALH and 7- to 10-fold for LCIS. For LCIS, this means an absolute risk of 1% to 2% per year and a lifetime risk of 30% to 40%. Some evidence supports a precursor role for these lesions, albeit not an obligate one: a disproportionately high number of tumors that develop are invasive lobular carcinoma, and two-thirds occur in the ipsilateral breast. Furthermore, coexistent LCIS and invasive lobular carcinomas often show the same genetic changes, suggesting that at least some LCIS lesions give rise to invasive carcinoma.

MOLECULAR PATHOGENESIS: LCIS and ALH exhibit genetic and karyotypic abnormalities (Table 25-1). These include recurrent 16q22.1 loss in LCIS, ALH, and invasive lobular carcinoma, for which the target gene is *CDH1*. This gene encodes E-cadherin, a protein that plays an essential role in cell adhesion and in cell cycle regulation through the Wnt/β-catenin pathway. *CDH1* may be inactivated via various mechanisms including

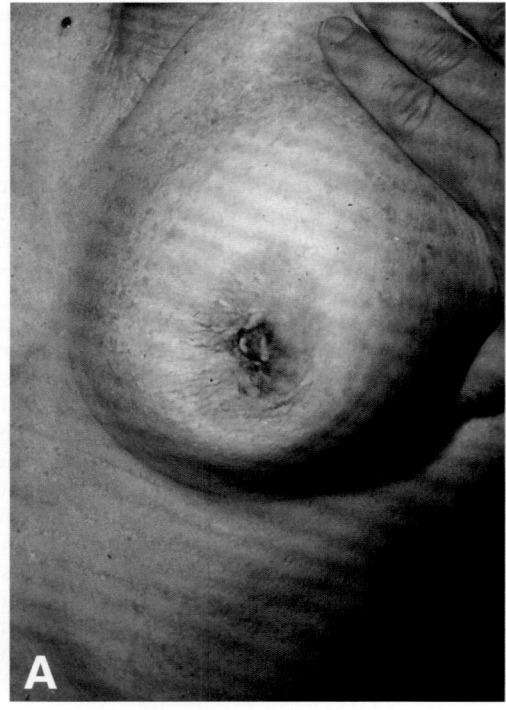

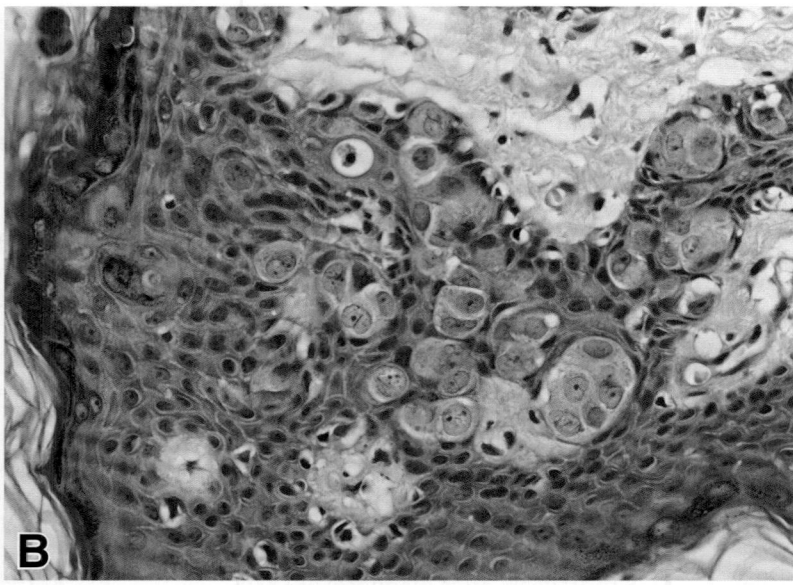

FIGURE 25-29. Paget disease of the nipple. A. The nipple is involved with an erythematous, scaly, and weeping "eczema." **B.** The epidermis contains clusters of ductal-type carcinoma cells that are considerably larger and have more abundant pale cytoplasm than surrounding keratinocytes.

physical loss of chromosomal regions, missense mutations, or gene promoter methylation. Patients with germline mutations in *CDH1* are at a high risk of developing lobular breast carcinoma and gastric signet ring cell carcinoma. Pleomorphic LCIS shares recurrent genomic alterations with classic LCIS, including LOH at 16q22.1 (Table 25-1), but also harbors greater genomic instability with some cases demonstrating LOH at *p53*, *HER2*, and *BRCA1* loci. LCIS and ILC can show similar somatic mutations, with *PIK3CA* and *CDH1* being the most frequently mutated genes.

LCIS is not detected mammographically but associated calcifications may be present in residual nonneoplastic luminal epithelial cells. In rare variants, such as pleomorphic LCIS and classic LCIS with comedo necrosis, dystrophic calcifications associated with central necrosis are detectable on mammography.

PATHOLOGY: The cells of classic LCIS are monotonous and small, with regular round nuclei and minute nucleoli, although larger cells with conspicuous nucleoli occasionally dominate (Fig. 25-30). Cytoplasmic mucin vacuoles may be surrounded by a distinct halo. Unlike DCIS, the cells of LCIS do not form complex patterns but rather grow in clusters that pack and distend lobular acini. This growth pattern is loosely cohesive or dyshesive. Gaps between individual cells reflect loss of cell–cell adhesion (see above). Pagetoid spread of lobular neoplastic cells is common in LCIS, with cells tracking beneath native luminal epithelial cells of the duct.

ALH and LCIS are distinguished by the degree of filling and distention of acini. In LCIS, at least 50% of acini in a lobular unit are completely involved and distended by the atypical cell population, in contrast to less than 50% in ALH. A variant form of LCIS may be associated

with central, comedo necrosis. Constituent cells retain the cytologic features of classic rather than pleomorphic LCIS (Fig. 25-31).

Pleomorphic LCIS shows a much greater degree of nuclear atypia than is seen in classic LCIS. Nuclei vary in size and shape, and nucleoli and mitotic figures are often prominent (Fig. 25-32). Central comedo necrosis, often with microcalcifications, is typical.

Distinguishing LCIS from low-grade solid DCIS may be difficult. Negative immunostaining for E-cadherin in LCIS and ALH may help (Fig. 25-33), as DCIS cells retain cell membrane staining for E-cadherin.

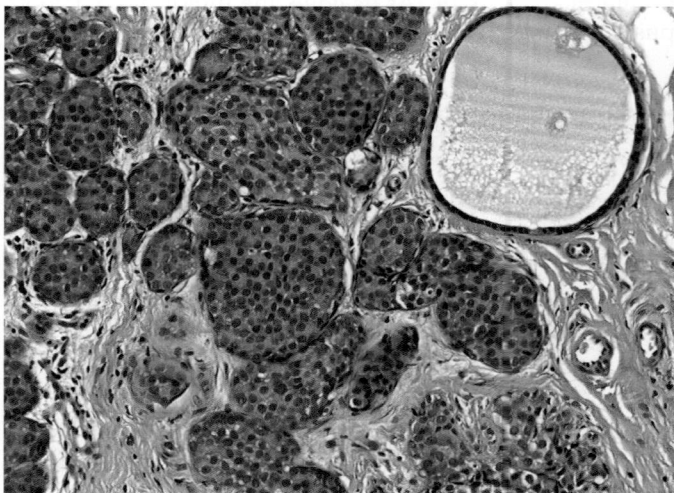

FIGURE 25-30. Lobular carcinoma in situ. The lumens of terminal duct lobular units are distended by tumor cells, which exhibit round nuclei and small nucleoli. Cytoplasmic mucin vacuoles are present.

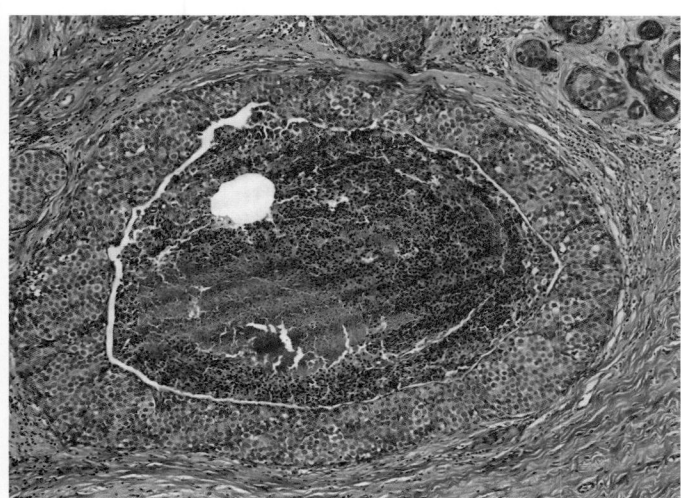

FIGURE 25-31. Lobular carcinoma in situ. This example shows classic nuclear features but also exhibits central expansile comedo necrosis.

CLINICAL FEATURES: Management of patients with LCIS is controversial. Those with classic LCIS are usually managed by active surveillance with or without chemoprevention. However, little is known about the natural history of variants of LCIS. Limited data suggest that these variants are more commonly associated with invasive carcinoma. Thus, treatment of lesions with more aggressive morphologic features should perhaps be more akin to that for DCIS, but this remains an unresolved issue.

Invasive Breast Carcinoma Is Derived From the TDLU

Breast cancer can occur anywhere in the breast but the most frequent site is the upper outer quadrant. Patients present most commonly with an ill-defined breast mass, which may

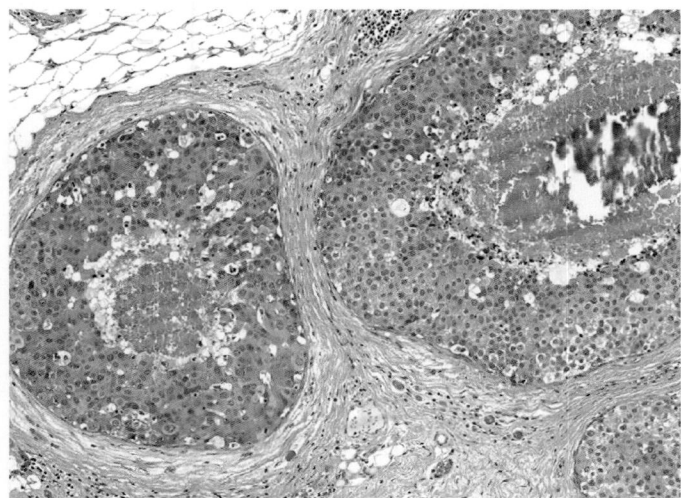

FIGURE 25-32. Pleomorphic lobular carcinoma in situ (PLCIS). A dyscohesive population of markedly atypical epithelial cells with central comedo necrosis fill and distend the ducts. Dissociation of the neoplastic cells creates spaces that may be misinterpreted as secondary spaces. E-cadherin expression is absent.

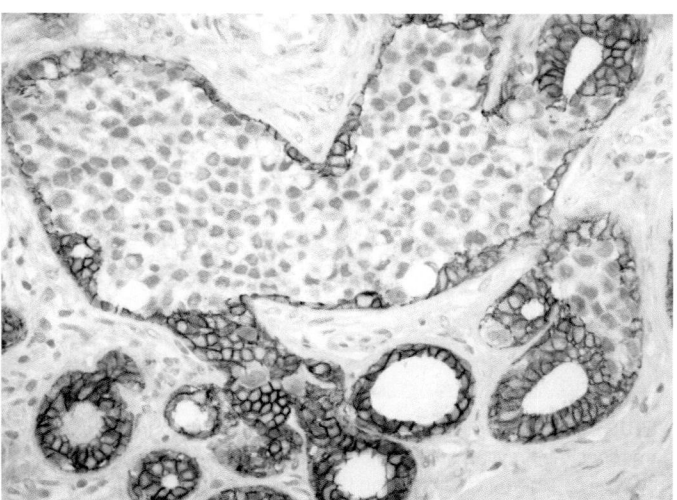

FIGURE 25-33. E-cadherin in lobular carcinoma in situ (LCIS). Membranous E-cadherin expression is seen in residual luminal epithelial cells, but the lobular neoplastic cells show loss of staining.

be adherent to the skin or underlying muscle. Nonpalpable asymptomatic tumors are usually detected by mammography. These mostly appear radiologically as spiculated masses or architectural distortion, with or without associated microcalcifications.

Most invasive breast cancers are classified as carcinomas of NST. The remainder are special types of carcinomas or have mixed morphologic features.

Invasive Ductal Carcinoma, No Special Type

The proportion of invasive breast cancers in this category varies from 47% to 70%, with women younger than 35 years having this tumor type more than older patients. This is a heterogeneous group of tumors that do not show characteristics of a specific or "special" histologic type. The term "invasive carcinoma of no special type (ductal NST)" is preferred by the World Health Organization (WHO) Working Group.

Ductal NSTs present as irregular, dense masses on mammography or ultrasound (Fig. 25-34A). Grossly, they are usually moderately or poorly defined, are nodular or stellate, and have firm to hard cut surfaces (Fig. 25-34B). Tumor cells form trabeculae, sheets, nests, and glands (Fig. 25-34C). Nuclear pleomorphism and mitotic counts vary. Surrounding stroma varies from desmoplastic to collagenous. Higher-grade lesions may show tumor necrosis. If a special-type component comprises over 50% of the tumor, the tumor is considered mixed (i.e., ductal with special-type features). DCIS is present in up to 80% of cases and is typically of the same nuclear grade as the invasive component.

Most ductal NSTs (70% to 80%) are ER-positive, and 15% are HER2-positive. Specific genetic lesions or alterations are associated in some cases with a particular histologic type or grade. Low-grade invasive NSTs are usually diploid or near diploid, with trends in chromosomal variations (Table 25-1), while high-grade tumors tend to be less easily categorized. Since deletions of 16q are found in only about one-third of low-grade NSTs, progression from low- to high-grade cancer is probably relatively uncommon.

Overall, 35% to 50% of patients with ductal NSTs survive 10 years, varying according to tumor and lymph node stage,

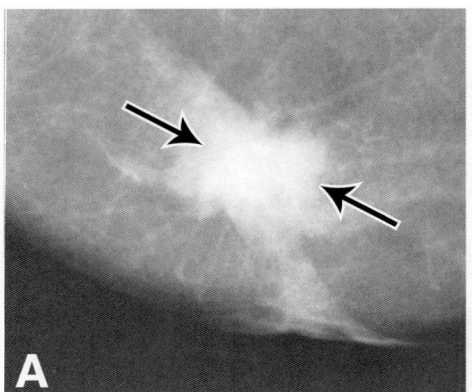
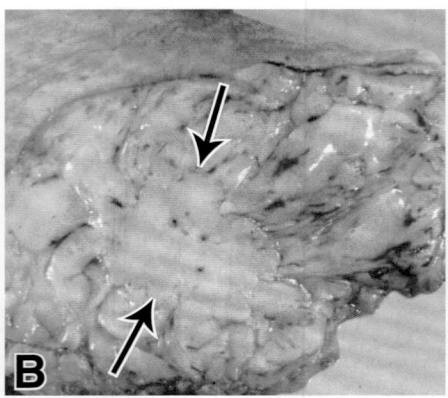
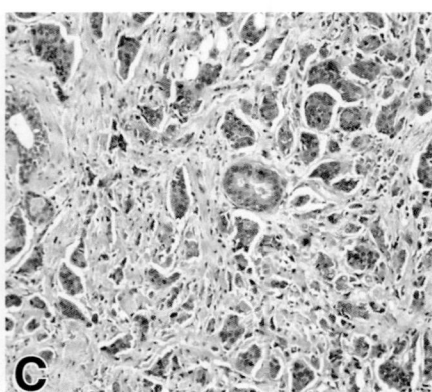

FIGURE 25-34. Carcinoma of the breast. A. Mammography shows a dense, irregularly shaped mass (*arrows*) in this otherwise fatty breast. **B.** Mastectomy specimen reveals an irregular, firm white mass (*arrows*) surrounded by fatty tissue. **C.** Microscopically, the tumor consists of irregular cords and nests of ductal carcinoma cells invading the stroma.

tumor grade, and the presence or absence of lymphovascular invasion.

Invasive Lobular Carcinoma

Invasive lobular carcinoma is the second most common form of invasive breast cancer, accounting for 5% to 15% of all invasive carcinomas. Some studies report that multicentricity and bilaterality are more common, while others suggest the risk to be similar to that seen with NST cancers (i.e., 5% to 10%). Because stromal desmoplasia and fibrosis may be minimal, clinical and mammographic detection can be challenging. Some cases present with a poorly defined thickening of the breast.

Invasive lobular cancers characteristically show dyscohesive malignant epithelial cells that infiltrate the stroma diffusely (Fig. 25-35). They often form single files and may show a periductal "targetoid" arrangement. They do not form ducts, but rather solid sheets, trabeculae, or nests. Neoplastic cells typically contain intracytoplasmic lumens and eccentric nuclei and resemble the cells of LCIS.

Invasive lobular carcinomas are more often ER-positive than are ductal NSTs, although high-grade lobular cancers

may lack ER and overexpress HER2. E-Cadherin expression is usually low or absent, reflecting biallelic loss of the tumor suppressor gene that encodes this protein. Patterns of genetic changes in invasive lobular carcinoma differ from those in ductal carcinomas (Table 25-1).

These carcinomas show a particular pattern of metastases with a tendency to spread to the peritoneum, retroperitoneum, ovary and uterus, leptomeninges, and gastrointestinal tract (Fig. 25-36). Matched for grade and stage, their prognosis is similar to that of ductal NST cancers.

Tubular Carcinoma

Tubular carcinomas represent only 1% to 2% of invasive breast cancers, although their detection by mammography is disproportionately greater. Tubular carcinomas form well-defined stellate masses whose cellular composition consists almost entirely of open and angulated tubules, lined by a single layer of mildly atypical epithelial cells (Fig. 25-37A). Over 95% of tubular carcinomas are ER-positive and HER2-negative. Tubular carcinomas share some patterns of karyotypic changes with other tumor types (Table 25-1). Lymph node metastases are rare, and the prognosis is excellent.

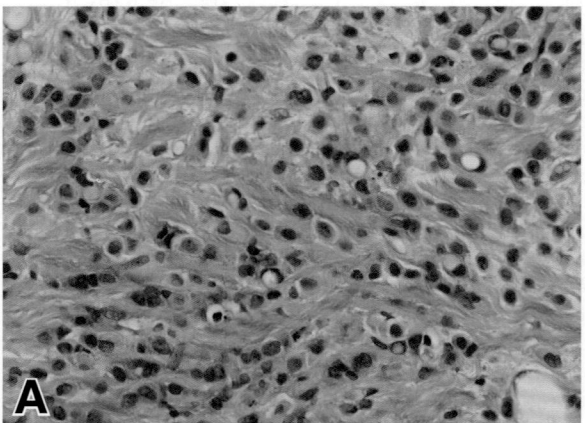
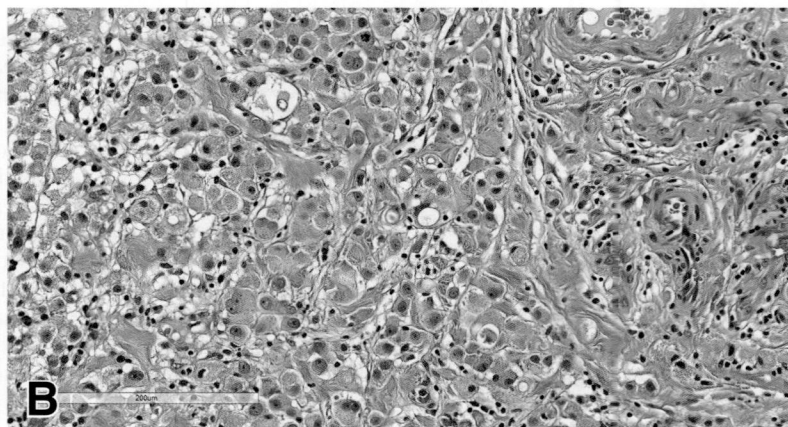

FIGURE 25-35. Lobular carcinoma. A. Invasive lobular carcinoma. In contrast to invasive ductal carcinoma, the cells of lobular carcinoma tend to form single strands that invade between collagen fibers in a diffuse pattern. The tumor cells are similar in appearance to those seen in lobular carcinoma in situ. **B.** Invasive lobular carcinoma, high histologic grade. The tumor consists of large dyscohesive cells with abundant cytoplasm, marked nuclear pleomorphism, and frequent mitoses.

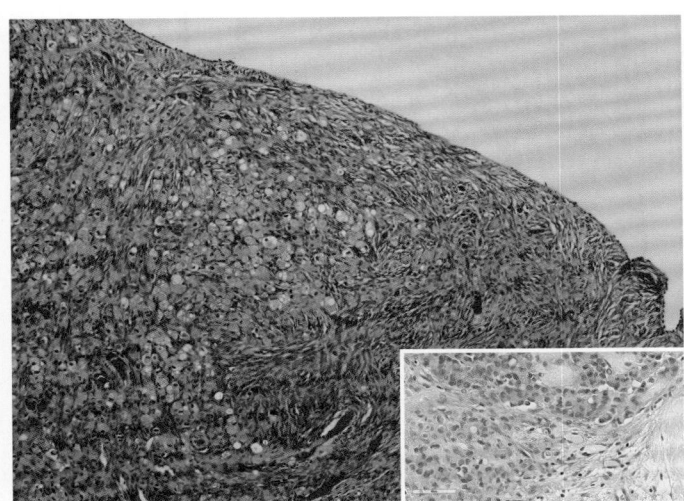

FIGURE 25-36. Metastatic lobular carcinoma. This ovary contains metastatic dyscohesive lobular carcinoma cells with eccentric nuclei and intracytoplasmic lumens. *Inset:* These features are seen at higher magnification.

Mucinous Carcinoma

Patients with mucinous carcinoma are typically older than those with other tumor types. These tumors make up 1% to 6% of breast cancers, depending on criteria used for diagnosis. Grossly, they are well circumscribed, with a gelatinous texture. Low-grade malignant epithelial cells form acini, nests, or trabeculae, which appear to float in pools of extracellular mucin (Fig. 25-37B). The malignant epithelial cells do not invade stroma directly. Pure mucinous carcinomas show little genomic instability or recurrent amplifications. They are uniformly of low histologic grade. Most are ER-positive and HER2-negative. Patients with pure mucinous carcinoma have an excellent prognosis.

Carcinomas With Medullary Features

Classic medullary carcinomas are exceptionally rare, although other types of carcinoma may show medullary features. Almost one-half of patients are younger than 50. Medullary tumors are well circumscribed and soft and include all of the following: (1) grade 2 to 3 nuclei; (2) circumscribed, pushing margins; (3) syncytial growth pattern in greater than 75% of the tumor; (4) a moderate or marked lymphoplasmacytic infiltrate; and (5) no tubule formation (Fig. 25-37C). DCIS is an uncommon concomitant. Medullary cancers are typically ER-, PR-, and HER2-negative ("triple negative"). P53 overexpression is part of a characteristic pattern of genetic changes (Table 25-1). Tumors arising in patients with pathogenic *BRCA1* germline mutations often show medullary features, but only 13% of tumors with medullary features are associated with such mutations.

The prognosis for pure medullary carcinoma is better than for high-grade ductal NST tumors, and lymph node metastases occur less frequently. Most women who die from their disease do so within 5 years of diagnosis.

Micropapillary Carcinoma

Pure micropapillary carcinomas occur rarely, but micropapillary areas are more often admixed with ductal NST carcinoma. As micropapillary tumors invade lymphatic vessels and metastasize to lymph nodes readily, recognizing even a minor component of micropapillary carcinoma is important. The high frequency of lymph node metastases notwithstanding, it is unknown if micropapillary tumors have an inherently poorer prognosis. In these tumors, malignant epithelial nests or acini are surrounded by a clear space (Fig. 25-37D). The vast majority of micropapillary carcinomas are ER- and PR-positive. Up to one-third shows HER2 positivity. Common genetic changes seen in these tumors are shown in Table 25-1.

Metaplastic Carcinoma

Metaplastic carcinomas are heterogeneous tumors with malignant spindle cells, squamous cell carcinoma, or heterologous elements, such as bone or cartilage (Fig. 25-37E). Adenocarcinoma may be absent, but cytokeratin immunoreactivity is at least focally positive. These tumors typically cluster with the basal molecular subgroup on gene expression profiling (see below).

Metaplastic tumors are usually ER- and HER2-negative and show complex patterns of chromosomal gains and losses (Table 25-1). Subtypes of metaplastic carcinomas are associated with better or worse prognosis when compared with ductal NSTs. Low-grade, fibromatosis-like, metaplastic carcinoma and low-grade adenosquamous metaplastic carcinoma are associated with a favorable outcome. Other metaplastic subtypes respond poorly to adjuvant chemotherapy and fare worse than other forms of triple-negative breast cancer.

PROGNOSTIC FACTORS

Breast Cancer Staging

Breast cancer spreads by direct extension (e.g., to chest wall); via lymphatics to axillary, internal mammary, and infra- and supraclavicular lymph nodes; and hematogenously to distant sites. Breast cancer survival is strongly influenced by tumor stage, expressed as the TNM classification (tumor [T], regional lymph nodes [N], and distant metastasis [M]; Table 25-3). This TNM staging system of the American Joint Commission of Cancer (AJCC) was recently updated (8th edition, 2017). While the updated staging system is still based on the anatomic factors of TNM, increasing evidence on the impact of tumor grade, proliferation rate, ER/PR/HER2 status, and gene expression prognostic panels on prognosis warrants their inclusion in the staging system as well. For example, patients with ER-/PR-/HER-negative (triple negative) carcinomas have survival rates comparable to patients whose tumors are one stage higher, but express either HER2, ER, or PR. Similarly, patients with stage-II T2, lymph node–negative tumors with a low Oncotype DX recurrence score (and thus biologically low-risk), are downgraded to stage I.

Tumor Size

Prognosis varies with tumor size (T in the TNM protocol) such that patients with larger tumors show poorer survival. In assessing tumor size, only the invasive part is considered. Some locally advanced tumors are staged T4, based on skin or chest wall invasion, regardless of tumor size.

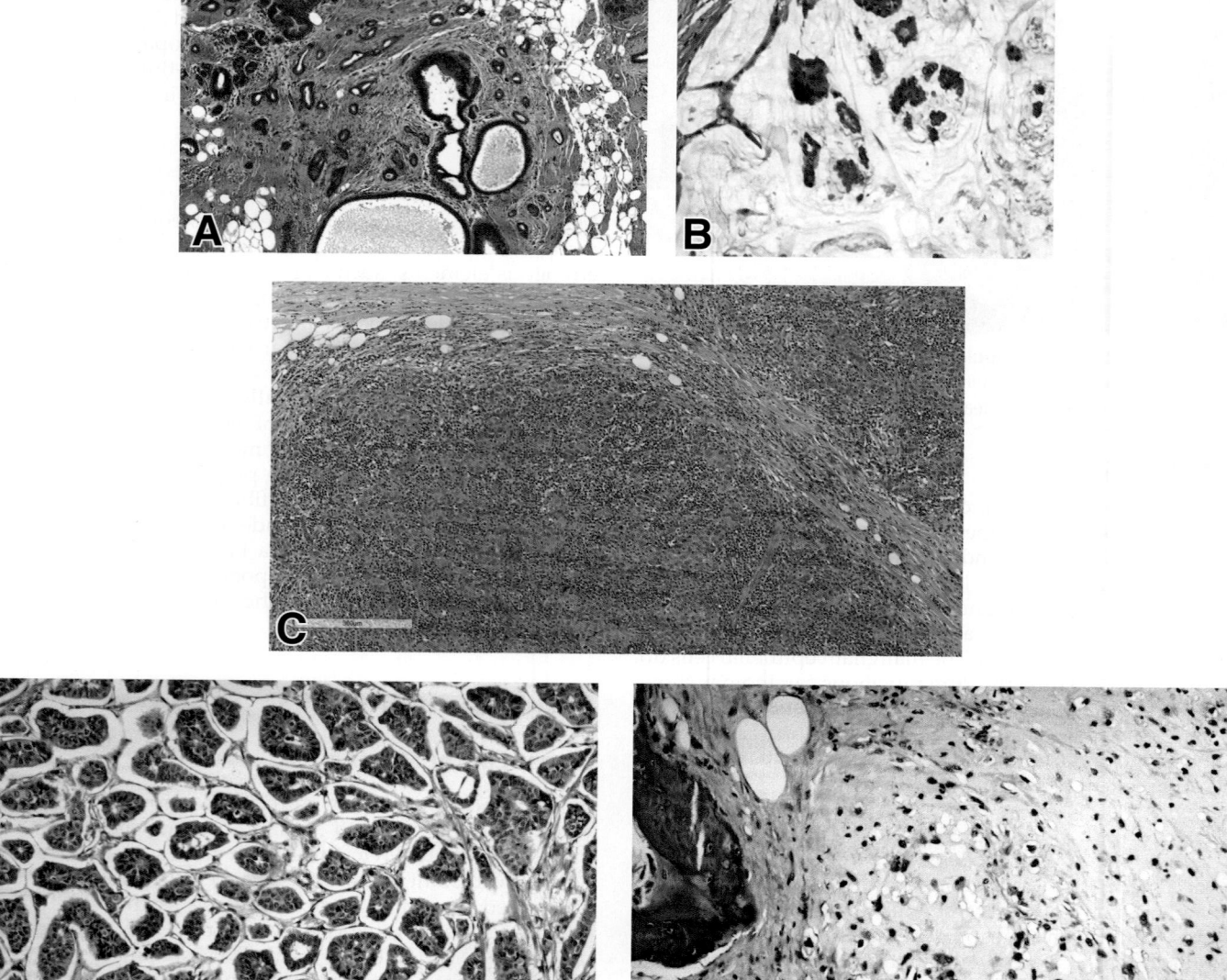

FIGURE 25-37. Patterns of breast carcinoma. A. Tubular carcinoma. Open and angulated malignant glands are dispersed between normal lobules and extend into the adjacent fat. A single layer of epithelium lines the tubules, and myoepithelial cells are absent. **B.** Mucinous carcinoma. Clusters of malignant cells float in large pools of extracellular mucin. **C.** Medullary carcinoma. The malignant cells are pleomorphic and grow in solid sheets, forming a blunt margin. There is no gland formation. Numerous mitoses are present. The tumor is surrounded by a dense lymphocytic infiltrate. **D.** Micropapillary carcinoma. A sponge-like pattern of empty spaces contains glands and small clusters of malignant epithelium. **E.** Metaplastic carcinoma. Cartilaginous and osseous matrix occur as heterologous elements in a metaplastic carcinoma. Present elsewhere in this tumor were foci of poorly differentiated adenocarcinoma.

TABLE 25-3
PATHOLOGIC TUMOR STAGING (8TH EDITION AJCC TNM CLASSIFICATION)

TX	Primary tumor cannot be assessed
T0	No evidence of primary tumor
Tis (DCIS)	Ductal carcinoma in situ
Tis (Paget)	Paget disease of the nipple NOT associated with DCIS or invasive carcinoma
T1mic	Microinvasion (≤1 mm)
T1a	Invasive tumor >1 mm but ≤5 mm (round any measurement from >1.0–1.9 mm to 2 mm)
T1b	Invasive tumor >5 mm but ≤1 cm
T1c	Invasive tumor >1 cm but ≤2 cm
T2	Invasive tumor >2 cm but ≤5 cm
T3	Invasive tumor >5 cm
T4	Edema or tumor ulcerating through skin or satellite skin nodules (invasion of the dermis alone does not qualify as T4); and/or chest wall invasion[a] or inflammatory breast carcinoma.

[a]Does not include invasion of the pectoralis muscle.
Data from Amin MB, Edge S, Greene F, et al., eds. *AJCC Cancer Staging Manual*. 8th ed. New York: Springer; 2017.

"Inflammatory breast cancer" has a particularly poor prognosis. This tumor features edema, erythema, induration, warmth, and tenderness of overlying skin, resulting in an orange peel–like ("peau d'orange") appearance. Arm edema and pain may also occur, probably because of lymphatic obstruction by tumor. These findings reflect tumor invasion of dermal lymphatic vessels.

Lymph Node Status

The presence or absence of axillary lymph node metastases is a key prognostic indicator for patients with breast cancer and requires pathologic evaluation of surgically resected lymph nodes. Axillary dissection can lead to significant postoperative morbidity (e.g., lymphedema and nerve damage). Sentinel lymph node (SLN) biopsy reduces this risk. This procedure involves injection of a dye and radioactive isotope to intraoperatively map lymphatic drainage and identify the "sentinel" lymph node, the node most likely to contain breast cancer metastases. If this node is negative, axillary dissection can safely be avoided. Immunohistochemical staining can help identify cytokeratin-positive epithelial cells in lymph nodes that may not be seen otherwise. Such detailed SLN evaluation has improved detection of micrometastases (>0.02 cm, <0.2 cm, or >200 cells) and isolated tumor cells (ITCs). However, the actual impact on prognosis of micrometastases and/or ITCs is small compared with node-negative women. Thus, the general consensus is of little value in performing additional levels or immunohistochemical studies on SLNs.

Distant Metastases

Distant metastases portend a poor prognosis. The site of distant metastases is bone in 25% of cases and, of women who die from their disease, 70% eventually develop bone involvement. The underlying mechanisms are incompletely understood but include complex interactions between circulating tumor cells and bone marrow stromal cells promoting epithelial-to-mesenchymal transition and expression of parathyroid hormone by the cancer cells. Less frequent sites of metastases include lung, liver, central nervous system (CNS), skin, and adrenal glands.

Tumor Grade

Histopathologic grading of breast tumors is a critical component of prognostication. The Nottingham grading system, also called the modified Bloom and Richardson method, is most widely used. It combines scores for tubule formation, nuclear pleomorphism, and mitotic count into a final grade of 1, 2, or 3 corresponding to low-, intermediate-, and high-grade carcinomas, respectively (Fig. 25-38). Patients with grade 1 tumors have significantly better survival than those with grade 2 or grade 3 tumors.

Other Prognostic Features

- Lymphovascular invasion (LVI): Finding tumor cells within lymphovascular spaces correlates well with lymph node metastases (Fig. 25-39) and is a poor prognostic sign. If both LVI and nodal metastases are present, prognosis is worse than either alone. Furthermore, LVI is present in 15% of patients without axillary nodal metastases and is a more important prognostic factor in this group.
- Proliferative index and ploidy: Tumors with high proliferative indices have worse prognoses. Proliferation in breast cancers is measured by (1) mitotic index, assessed histologically; (2) the proportion of cells in S phase of the cell cycle determined by flow cytometry; (3) immunohistochemical detection of proteins such as Ki67 expressed by actively proliferating cells (Fig. 25-40); and (4) thymidine labeling index. Aneuploidy, detected by cell cycle analysis in two-thirds of breast cancers, confers a poorer prognosis. Notably, much of the prognostic impact of multigene predictor signatures (discussed below) comes from proliferation genes.
- Response to neoadjuvant therapy: Response to therapy in patients who receive systemic treatment before surgery (neoadjuvant therapy) is a strong prognostic factor. Patients who show a complete pathologic response (i.e., who lack pathologic evidence of residual breast or nodal disease) have excellent long-term survival. Poorly differentiated tumors with high proliferation indices are more likely to respond to neoadjuvant treatment than low-grade cancers. A pathologically complete response occurs in 10% to 30% of patients, little or no response in 10% to 15% of patients, and partial response in the remainder.
- Estrogen and progesterone receptor expression: Steroid receptor proteins are expressed by normal breast epithelium and in 70% to 80% of breast cancers (ER > PR). ER and PR status is determined by immunohistochemistry, which uses antibodies to detect these nuclear receptors (Fig. 25-41). Hormone receptor positivity is defined as ≥1% staining tumor cells. ER and PR bind their respective

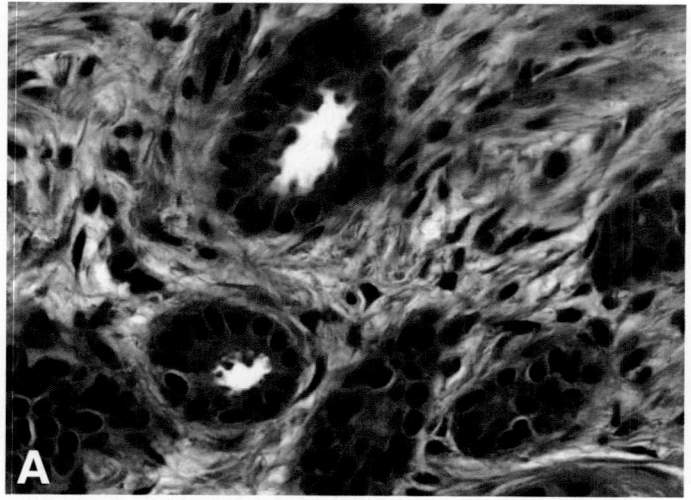

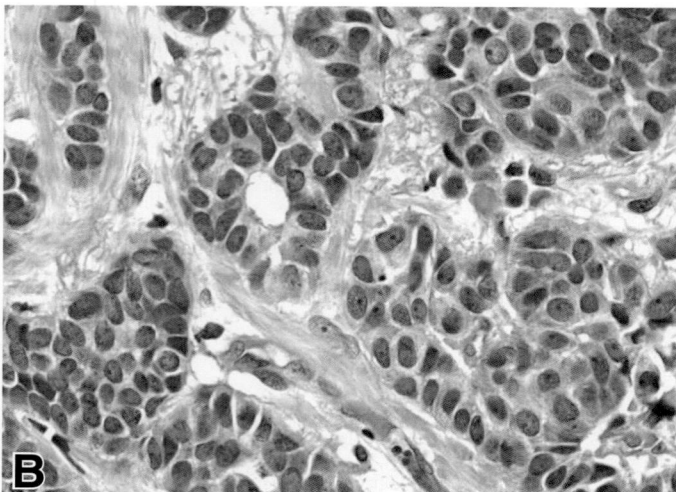

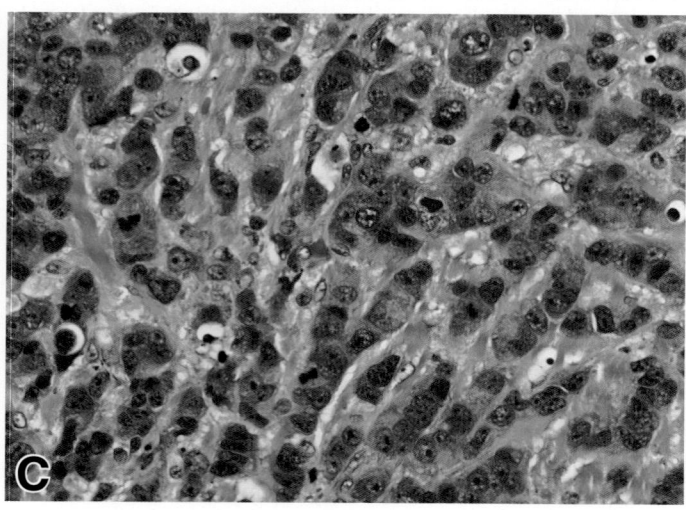

FIGURE 25-38. Tumor histologic grade. A. Low-grade invasive carcinoma is characterized by good tubule formation, mild nuclear pleomorphism, and inconspicuous mitoses. **B.** Moderately differentiated carcinoma shows less tubule formation, moderate nuclear pleomorphism, and variably prominent mitoses. **C.** Poorly differentiated carcinoma has absent tubule formation, marked nuclear pleomorphism, and frequent mitotic figures.

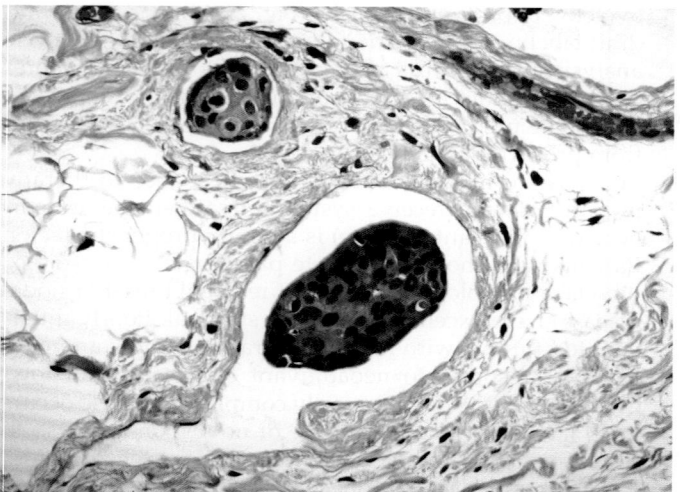

FIGURE 25-39. Lymphovascular invasion. Lymphatic channels lined by endothelial cells contain tumor emboli.

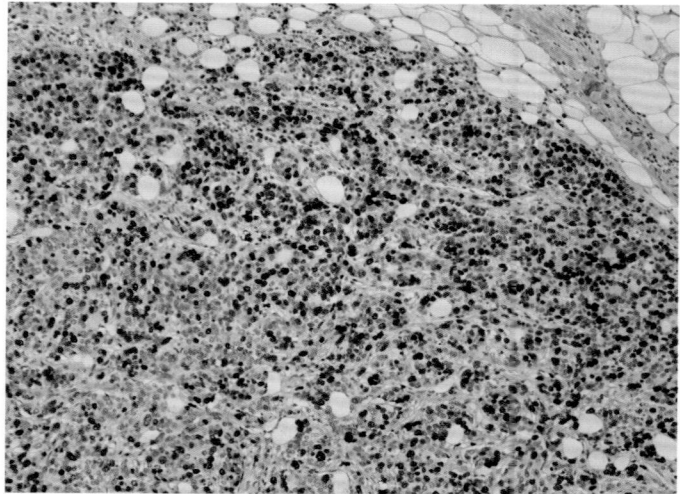

FIGURE 25-40. Ki-67 staining as a marker of proliferation in invasive carcinoma. This example shows a high percentage of cell nuclei staining.

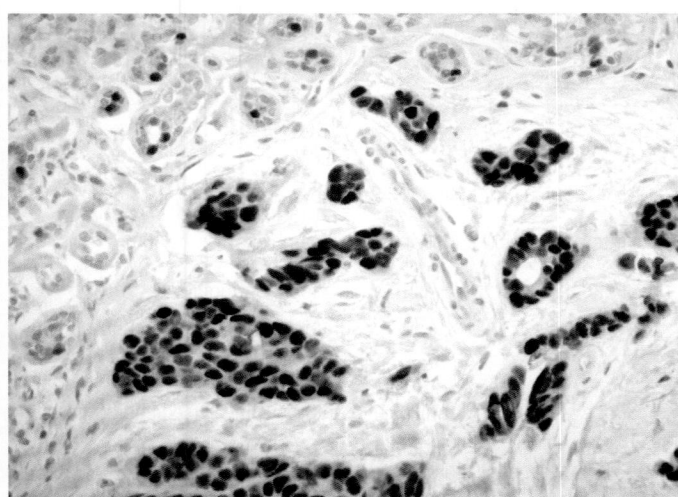

FIGURE 25-41. Estrogen receptor (ER). Strong nuclear immunohistochemical staining for estrogen receptor is seen in this moderately differentiated invasive ductal carcinoma. Positive staining is also seen in normal breast lobules in the upper left-hand corner.

ligands (estrogen and progesterone) and stimulate cell growth. The greatest value of assessing hormone receptor status in breast cancer is its predictive ability. Patients with ER-/PR-negative tumors are unlikely to respond to hormonal therapies with antiestrogens while ER-/PR-positive tumors show a greater probability of response.

- HER2 expression: Overexpression or gene amplification (see Chapter 5) of HER2 occurs in approximately 15% of newly diagnosed breast cancers, and is an adverse prognostic factor irrespective of lymph node status. Overexpression of cell membrane HER2 can be detected by immunohistochemistry and gene amplification is determined by in situ hybridization. HER2-positive patients can be treated with monoclonal antibodies or tyrosine kinase inhibitors that target HER2. However, as with hormone receptor status, many patients who express HER2 show de novo or eventual resistance to such drugs (Fig. 25-42).
- Tumor-infiltrating lymphocytes (TILs): Evidence of the prognostic value of TILs in predicting the response to

neoadjuvant chemotherapy is increasing, particularly in triple-negative and HER2+ breast cancer. Higher levels of TILs are associated with improved prognosis in these subtypes, in both the early and advanced stages, and a higher probability of achieving pathologic complete response (pCR) in the neoadjuvant setting. Analysis of TILs in residual disease after neoadjuvant therapy also has prognostic value, and TILs may play a role in predicting response to immune checkpoint blockade.

Molecular Subtypes

Microarray gene expression profiling and other techniques have identified a set of genes, an "intrinsic gene list," within which several molecular subgroups (Table 25-4) appear to predict clinical outcome and response to therapy.

- Luminal A: The luminal groups (A and B) are characterized by gene expression patterns similar to normal breast luminal epithelial cells, including low–molecular-weight cytokeratins 8/18, and ER and ER-associated genes. Luminal A tumors are typically low grade and have an excellent prognosis.
- Luminal B: These tumors also express ER and ER-associated genes, but are usually higher grade than luminal A tumors. They exhibit higher proliferative indices and have a poorer prognosis. Although they respond better to chemotherapy than luminal A tumors, both luminal subtypes generally respond poorly to chemotherapy.
- HER2: Tumors that overexpress HER2 protein, express genes in the HER2 pathway and are usually ER-negative. These tumors behave aggressively, but targeting with anti-HER2 therapies, has significantly increased patient longevity.
- Basal-like cancers: These highly aggressive tumors constitute 10% to 20% of invasive breast carcinomas. They are mainly ER-/PR- and HER2-negative. Their name derives from their consistent expression of genes characteristic of the basal or myoepithelial cells of the breast, including high–molecular-weight cytokeratins 5/6, 14, and 17; caveolins 1 and 2; nestin; p63; and EGFR. These tumors are distinctive, with high nuclear grade, many mitoses, pushing margins, central areas of necrosis or fibrosis, and

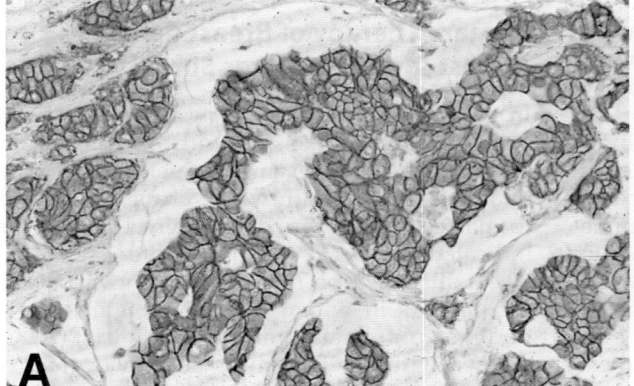
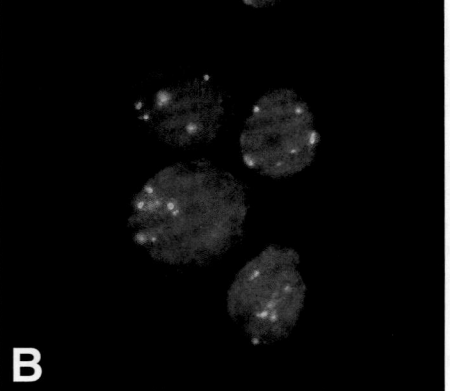

FIGURE 25-42. HER2/neu abnormalities in a breast cancer. A. Immunohistochemical staining shows overexpression of the *HER2* (erbB-2) protein in an invasive ductal carcinoma. **B.** Fluorescence in situ hybridization (FISH) identifies the number of gene copies for *HER2* (erbB-2) (red probe) in cancer cells. Normal cells have two copies. The presence of more than two copies indicates *HER2* gene amplification. The green probe identifies the centromeric region of chromosome 17.

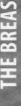

TABLE 25-4

MOLECULAR SUBTYPES OF BREAST CANCER

Molecular Subgroup	ER	PR	HER2	Proliferation Index	Other	Prognosis	Treatment
Luminal A	+	+	−	Low	CK8/18	Excellent	Endocrine therapy
Luminal B	+	+	−/+	Moderate	CK8/18	Intermediate	Endocrine and chemotherapy
HER2+	−	−	+	High	AR	Poor	Anti-HER2 monoclonal antibodies Anti-HER2 small-molecule kinase inhibitors Anthracyclines
Basal	−	−	−	Very high	CK5/6, CK14, vimentin, EGFR, c-kit	Poor	Platinum- and anthracycline-based chemotherapy PARP inhibitors Anti-PD-L1 monoclonal antibodies

+ positive; − negative; −/+ sometimes positive; AR = androgen receptor; ER = estrogen receptor; PARP = poly(adenosine diphosphate-ribose) polymerase; PR = progesterone receptor.

a lymphocytic infiltrate. Cancers with medullary features and metaplastic carcinomas are typically basal-like. Most cancers arising in patients with germline *BRCA1* mutations are basal-like. However, some tumors classified as basal are associated with a favorable outcome (e.g., secretory carcinoma and adenoid cystic carcinoma).

- Additional subtypes of ER-negative breast cancers have emerged: molecular apocrine, claudin-low, and interferon-rich. Molecular apocrine tumors are androgen receptor–positive and frequently HER2-positive. They demonstrate prominent apocrine features, with abundant eosinophilic cytoplasm and prominent nucleoli. Claudin-low tumors express high levels of genes involved in epithelial-to-mesenchymal transition, including vimentin, Snail, and TWIST, and downregulation of genes involved in cell adhesion (E-cadherin, claudins 3, 4, and 7). These tumors also display stem cell–like features. Tumors of the interferon-rich subtype express high levels of interferon-regulated genes, including STAT1. The clinical importance of these additional subgroups has yet to be elucidated.

Gene Expression Profiling Prognostic Assays

Multigene prognostic assays are now widely used as both prognostic tools and in predicting response to various therapies in patients with ER-positive breast cancer. Importantly, in guiding treatment decisions and evaluating prognosis, these tools complement, but do not replace, histopathology and clinical analyses.

One example is Oncotype DX (Genomic Health, Inc.), an RT-PCR assay that measures mRNA levels of 21 genes in formalin-fixed, paraffin-embedded tumor tissue. It compares 16 cancer-related genes and five reference genes to determine a "recurrence score" that predicts low, high, or intermediate risk of developing distant recurrence at 10 years after 5 years of antiestrogen therapy. It was initially used to assess prognosis in ER-positive, node-negative women treated with tamoxifen (an ER receptor antagonist), but it also predicts therapeutic responses in women treated with aromatase-inhibitors (which block conversion of testosterone to estradiol) and those with nodal metastases. Its main clinical use is in predicting the likelihood of benefit from adjuvant chemotherapy in select women.

MammaPrint (Agendia) is a 70-gene microarray-based prognostic signature that can be used on unfixed frozen tissue or formalin-fixed, paraffin-embedded tumor samples. It predicts prognosis in invasive breast cancer based on expression levels of 70 cancer-related genes and 1,800 reference genes. Results are reported as low or high risk for distant metastases at 10 years without adjuvant treatment. It thus identifies patients in whom withholding chemotherapy may be warranted.

The Prosigna assay (NanoString) is a clinical application of the intrinsic subtype analysis involving luminal A and B tumors, HER2-positive tumors, and basal-like tumors. It calculates a continuous risk of recurrence score based on expression of 50 cancer genes and eight housekeeping genes. It uses RNA extracted from formalin-fixed, paraffin-embedded tumor tissue.

High-throughput next-generation sequencing permits sequencing of large numbers of potential cancer genes to identify predictive or prognostic (actionable) variants. Its current use is largely in patients with advanced disease to identify mutations that may be targeted with novel therapies and/or for entry into clinical trials.

PROGNOSTIC FACTORS

Primary Therapy of Breast Cancer Almost Always Involves Surgery

In general, patients with early stage breast cancer undergo primary surgical excision with or without adjuvant radiation. Breast conserving surgery (i.e., lumpectomy or quadrantectomy) with whole breast radiation is equivalent to mastectomy in terms of survival in this population. As indicated above, SLN sampling often replaces more extensive axillary lymph node chain removal, which is reserved for patients in whom the SLN contains tumor. Based on findings from a randomized clinical trial (ACOSOG Z0011), women with T1/T2 tumors and fewer than three positive SLNs who undergo lumpectomy and will receive whole breast radiation, can also forego additional axillary lymph node surgery. Systemic therapies including hormonal, chemotherapy and targeted molecular modalities are essential in managing patients with breast cancer. Patients with the worst prognoses usually gain the greatest benefit from such systemic therapies. Targeted therapies rely on the presence of particular targets in the tumor (e.g., ER, PR, and HER2).

Preoperative chemotherapy (neoadjuvant therapy) does not by itself enhance survival. However, it can render inoperable tumors resectable and downstage tumors in patients with large tumors making breast-conserving surgery feasible.

Emerging Therapeutic Targets

Therapies may target the intrinsic properties of the tumor cells or the tumor microenvironment in which complex interactions between the malignant epithelial component and the nonmalignant stromal and inflammatory components determine important biologic processes. Tumor cell therapeutic candidates include those that target the PI3K/AKT/mTOR pathway, which regulates cell proliferation, differentiation, and death, in addition to being implicated in endocrine resistance. *PIK3CA* is one of the most frequently mutated genes in all subtypes of cancer. Everolimus, a rapamycin analog that inhibits mTOR kinase activity, is the first FDA-approved agent targeting this pathway. Small molecule inhibitors targeting different components of this pathway are being investigated in clinical trials.

PARP1 plays a key role in DNA single-strand break repair via base excision repair (BER) and has been implicated in other pathways such as nucleotide excision repair (NER) and mismatch repair (MMR). Inhibiting PARP1 is most potent in BRCA-associated cancers. Olaparib is an FDA-approved PARP inhibitor for germline *BRCA1*-associated metastatic breast cancer. Second-generation PARP inhibitors are being evaluated in clinical trials.

Androgen receptor (AR) is a nuclear receptor which is commonly seen in women with breast cancer. While AR is commonly expressed in ER-positive disease, a subclass of "triple negative" breast cancer has been identified as the luminal androgen receptor (LAR) subtype. Trials using AR antagonists are ongoing with most focusing on AR-positive metastatic triple-negative tumors.

Stromal cells in the tumor microenvironment play important roles in tumor progression and metastasis. Thus, drugs that target tumor–stromal interactions and/or enhance the host immune response are in development. Targets include tumor-infiltrating immune cells, vascular endothelial cells, and cancer-associated fibroblasts (CAFs). Emerging immunotherapies include vaccines to stimulate an immune response against tumor-associated antigens and immune checkpoint blockade, such as those modulating activities of cytotoxic T lymphocyte–associated antigen 4 (CTLA-4) and programmed cell death protein 1 (PD-1). Monoclonal antibodies targeting PD-1 or PD-L1 have demonstrated promising results in metastatic triple-negative tumors.

THE MALE BREAST

Gynecomastia Is Enlargement of the Male Breast

Male breast tissue has receptors for androgens, estrogens, and progesterone. Estrogen stimulates duct development and progesterone stimulates lobular development in the presence of luteinizing hormone, follicle-stimulating hormone, and growth hormone. Androgens antagonize the effects of estrogen. Testosterone can be converted to estradiol by the enzyme aromatase, which is abundant in adipose tissue.

Physiologic gynecomastia occurs in most neonates, stimulated by circulating maternal and placental estrogen and progesterone. Transient gynecomastia also affects over half of boys during puberty, because estrogen production peaks earlier than that of testosterone. With increasing age, free testosterone decreases, and adipose tissue expands, increasing the prevalence of breast enlargement.

Gynecomastia is benign enlargement of the male breast, with proliferation of ductal and stromal elements. It is due to relatively decreased androgens and/or increased estrogen effect. Breast enlargement caused by accumulation of adipose tissue is called pseudogynecomastia. Nonphysiologic gynecomastia results from drugs or disorders associated with low testosterone levels, high conversion of testosterone to estrogens, elevated estrogen levels, and increased estrogen effect due to increased sex hormone–binding globulin levels that lower free testosterone. It may occur in patients with hyperthyroidism, cirrhosis, renal failure, chronic lung disease, and certain hormone-producing tumors, including Leydig and Sertoli cell tumors, testicular germ cell tumors, and cancers of the liver and lung. Drugs implicated in gynecomastia include digitalis, cimetidine, spironolactone, marijuana, and tricyclic antidepressants. Klinefelter syndrome is the most common chromosomal disorder associated with gynecomastia.

Gynecomastia presents as a rubbery discrete mass or ill-defined area of induration. Histologically, it may display a florid or fibrous phase (Fig. 25-43). The florid phase typically occurs early, within 6 months of onset, and is characterized by epithelial hyperplasia with flat or micropapillary architecture. Periductal stroma is hypercellular and edematous, with increased vascularity and chronic inflammation.

The fibrous phase is seen after 1 year or more. It lacks epithelial proliferation, and the stroma is more collagenous. Mixtures of both phases may be seen. PASH may be seen in either phase.

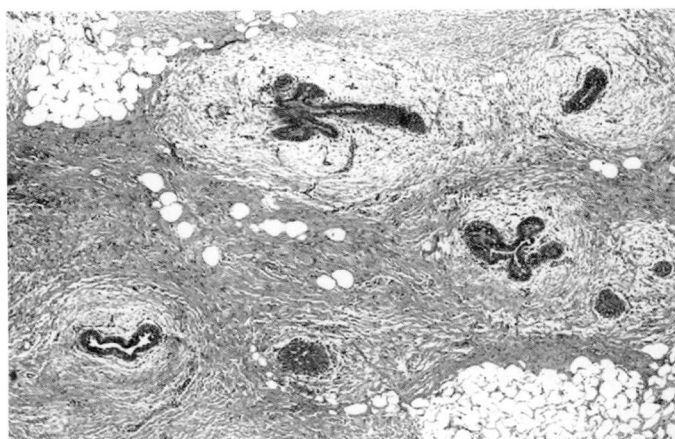

FIGURE 25-43. Gynecomastia. There is proliferation of branching, intermediate-sized ducts. The ductal epithelium is hyperplastic, and mitoses are seen. A concomitant increase in the surrounding fibrous tissue produces a palpable mass.

Male Breast Cancers Often Reflect Hyperestrogen States

EPIDEMIOLOGY: These tumors make up 1% of breast cancers in the United States, whereas in sub-Saharan Africa, they make up 7% to 14% of breast cancers. The difference may be attributable to endemic diseases causing liver damage and secondary hyperestrogenism. In the United States, rates are highest in black men, intermediate in non-Hispanic white men and Asian-Pacific Islanders, and lowest in Hispanic men. The mean age at presentation is 65.

The risk of breast cancer is greater in high-estrogen states. Men with Klinefelter syndrome have a 58-fold higher risk than normal men and an absolute risk of up to 3%. Male–female transsexuals following castration and high-dose estrogen and men treated with estrogen for prostate cancer also are at greater risk. Ionizing radiation has been implicated as a causal factor. For example, breast cancer occurred in Japanese men after nuclear fallout and in patients treated with therapeutic chest irradiation at a young age. Men with pathogenic germline mutations in *BRCA2* show a 7% cumulative risk of developing breast cancer by age 80 years. The risk of developing breast cancer for male *BRCA1* carriers is much less.

PATHOLOGY: Most breast cancers in males are invasive carcinoma, NST; however, papillary carcinoma is disproportionately represented in men. Invasive lobular carcinoma is rare. Ninety percent of cancers are ER- and PR-positive. Androgen receptor positivity is frequently seen.

CLINICAL FEATURES: Most patients present with a painless lump. Nipple involvement, including retraction, discharge or ulceration, is an early event. Paget disease is a presenting feature in 1% of affected men.

Management of breast cancer in men is based largely on results of clinical studies done in women: simple mastectomy and SLN biopsy or axillary dissection. Postoperative radiation may be given for large tumors or those with close margins. Hormonal therapy with tamoxifen is frequently administered. There is limited experience in treating male breast cancer with aromatase inhibitors. Adjuvant chemotherapy with or without trastuzumab, which targets HER2, may be indicated, depending on the aggressiveness of the disease and HER2 status.

26 | Hematopathology

Parul Bhargava, David Hudnall, Olga Weinberg, Alina Dulau Florea

Bone Marrow

NORMAL MYELOPOIESIS: EMBRYOLOGY

Hematopoietic stem and progenitor cells (HSPCs) give rise to all blood and immune cells throughout our entire life. Normal individuals maintain approximately 11,000 hematopoietic stem cells (HSCs), of which approximately 30% actively contribute to hematopoiesis. The rest remain as a pool of immature, slowly cycling HSCs. Steady-state hematopoiesis arises primarily from long-lived multipotent progenitors and short-term HSCs. During embryonic development, hematopoiesis occurs sequentially in several anatomic sites. It begins in the yolk sac, and subsequently arises in the aorta–gonad–mesonephros region, the placenta, and in the vitelline and umbilical arteries. Around the 11th week of embryogenesis HSCs accumulate in the fetal liver. HSCs and erythroid precursors make up most of the hematopoietic tissue during the early stages of blood cell formation in the fetal liver. Production of megakaryocytes and mature neutrophils soon follows. A switch from the production of red blood cell (RBC) embryonic hemoglobins to fetal hemoglobins also occurs during the hepatic phase of erythropoiesis. HSCs migrate from the liver to the bone marrow around the 17th week of embryogenesis, and soon before birth, the bone marrow becomes the main hematopoietic organ; this persists throughout adult life. From birth to puberty, all skeletal bone marrow is densely packed with hematopoietic tissue (**red marrow**), which produces all blood cell types. Red marrow subsequently becomes largely confined to the proximal epiphyseal regions of the humerus and femur and the flat bones that form the skull, scapula, clavicles, sternum, ribs, vertebrae, and pelvis. In adults, adipose tissue (inactive "yellow marrow") occupies most available space in the medullary cavities of the skeleton. The bone marrow in the axial skeleton continues to be active until old age, when resorption of cancellous bone enlarges marrow cavities and leads to further fatty replacement. Remarkably, in healthy individuals, normal peripheral blood counts are maintained even as the amount of red marrow declines.

Most HSCs remain in an immature and quiescent/slow-cycling state, and a small pool of HSCs will self-renew a few times during the lifetime. Local expansion of hematopoietic progenitors in red (cellular) marrow and reactivation of peripheral yellow marrow allow the hematopoietic system to meet physiologic demands for increased blood cell formation. If the hematopoietic system cannot respond to stress/demand, there is probably an abnormality of one or more hematopoietic lineages. Reactivation of hepatic and splenic hematopoiesis rarely occurs in adult life. Significant extramedullary hematopoiesis (EMH) in adulthood usually suggests a clonal (malignant) disorder, rather than a reactive process.

HEMATOPOIETIC DEVELOPMENT

Hematopoietic Cells Derive From Multipotent Stem Cells

Bone marrow is composed of a complex network of solid cords separated by sinusoids (Fig. 26-1). The cords contain stromal and hematopoietic cells, knitted together by extracellular matrix. A semipermeable barrier between sinusoids and cords consists of an endothelial cell layer, a thin basement membrane, and an outer layer of interrupted reticular adventitial cells. The latter branch extensively throughout the cords and help anchor stromal and hematopoietic cells. Bone marrow stromal cells include macrophages, endothelial cells, and fibroblasts.

Islands of erythroblasts, usually arranged in concentric rings around a macrophage that stores excess iron, are present within the cords. The erythroid islands lie close to sinusoid walls, as do megakaryocytes. Granulocyte precursors reside deeper in the cords, adjacent to bony trabeculae.

STEM CELLS: Pluripotent HSCs have two properties, self-renewal and differentiation, and it is this multipotency property that allows them to differentiate and proliferate into more committed progenitors and precursors (Fig. 26-2). Within the bone marrow, HSCs represent only a small proportion of total hematopoietic cell mass, the remaining cells being progenitors and more mature hematopoietic cells.

HSCs are small, mononuclear and difficult to identify by microscopy. Local factors regulate the fate of HSCs toward quiescence ("dormant" HSCs), self-renewal or differentiation ("active" HSCs) into progenitor cells of specific lineages as needed. When marrow elements are injected into irradiated mice, stem cells form visible colonies in the spleen (**"colony-forming unit, spleen" [CFU-S]**). In bone marrow cultures, stem cells form colonies containing **multipotential cells** called granulocyte, erythroid, macrophage and megakaryocyte elements (**CFU-GEMM**) and lymphoid precursor cells (**CFU-L**).

HSCs are also the cells responsible for long-term engraftment and reconstitution potential after bone marrow transplantation.

PROGENITOR CELLS: Like stem cells, progenitor cells are small to medium-sized mononuclear cells that resemble mature lymphocytes. In culture, they give rise to colonies of differentiated progeny. Progenitor cells committed to RBC production form luxuriant burst-shaped colonies (**"burst-forming unit, erythroid" [BFU-E]**). Each subsequent generation of BFU-E makes smaller colonies, until a final progenitor cell, the "colony-forming unit, erythroid" (**CFU-E**), produces only a small clone of mature erythroblasts.

Granulocytic and **monocytic** cell lines derive from a single progenitor cell. This cell, named "colony-forming unit, granulocyte-monocyte" (**CFU-GM**), makes a colony with both granulocytic and monocytic cells. As the cell matures, its progeny are increasingly committed to polymorphonuclear leukocyte (**CFU-G**) or monocyte/macrophage (**CFU-M**) lineages. **Eosinophils** and **basophils** also have specific progenitor cells (**CFU-Eo** and **CFU-Ba**, respectively). "Megakaryocytic progenitor cells" (**CFU-Meg**) produce colonies in vitro consisting of four to eight megakaryocytes.

REGULATION OF HEMATOPOIESIS: Bone marrow hematopoiesis responds to fluctuating needs for blood cells and maintains the size of the circulating blood cell mass. **Transcription factors** and **hematopoietic cytokines** mediate this responsiveness by regulating the rate of cellular proliferation, primarily in the progenitor cell compartment (Fig. 26-2).

- **Scl, Runx1, CBFβ, Lmo2,** and **GATA2** are transcription factors essential for HSC fate regulation.
- **Stem cell factor** (SCF, or c-KIT ligand) and **Flt3 ligand** (Flt3L) support survival and proliferation of pluripotent stem cells, CFU-GEMM, and various progenitor cells.
- **Interleukin (IL)-3** and **granulocyte-macrophage colony-stimulating factor (GM-CSF)** are important for proliferation of CFU-GEMM and multiple CFUs.
- **Granulocyte colony-stimulating factor (G-CSF)** and **macrophage colony-stimulating factor (M-CSF)** promote granulocyte and monocyte maturation from CFU-G and CFU-M, respectively.
- **Erythropoietin (EPO),** released by renal interstitial peritubular cells in response to hypoxia, activates erythroid progenitor cells.
- **Thrombopoietin (TPO)** primarily facilitates production and maturation of megakaryocytes, but also stimulates other lineages.
- *Deficiencies in one or more blood cell populations (e.g., postchemotherapy pancytopenia, especially neutropenia; stem cell mobilization prior to bone marrow transplantation; renal failure; see below) are treated with various growth factors, mainly GM-CSF, G-CSF, EPO, and TPO.*

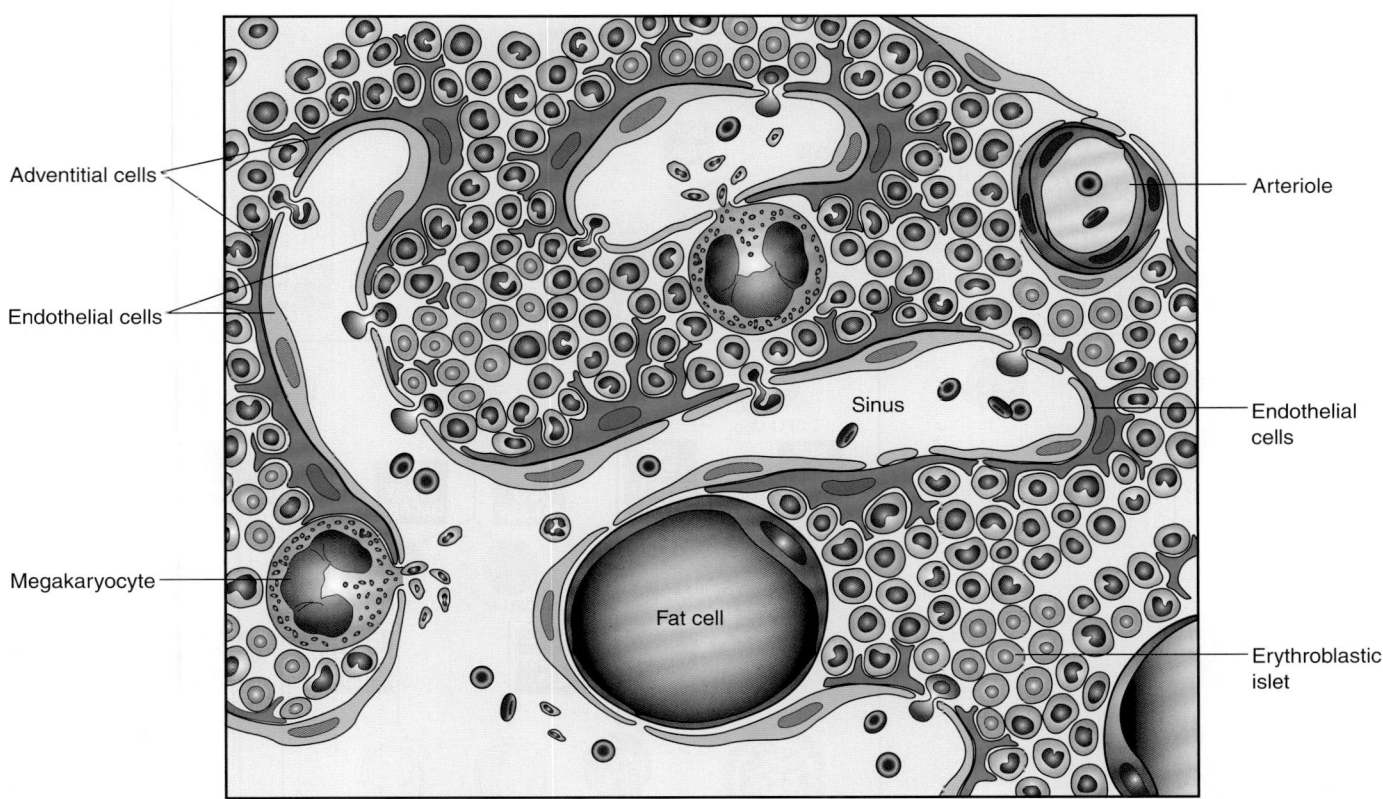

FIGURE 26-1. Structure of normal bone marrow. The sinusoids represent the major point of egress of hematopoietic cells from the bone marrow. Note that the bone marrow does not have lymphatic channels.

- *PRECURSOR CELLS:* Progenitor cells mature into precursor cells, or **blasts**. *Starting at the precursor stage, and continuing beyond, cells are morphologically recognizable in terms of their lineage.* Maturation of precursor cells to mature cells entails progressive nuclear changes and cytoplasmic maturation to reflect cellular functions (e.g., oxygen carriage in RBCs, cytotoxic enzymes in neutrophils). In parallel, lineage-related cell surface proteins/antigens appear. The latter help to identify both cell types and stages of maturation.

- **Erythroid precursor cells:** The **proerythroblast** is the first stage in RBC maturation. Like other committed blast cells, proerythroblasts are relatively few in number, compared to more mature red cell forms. Proerythroblasts have large round nuclei, fine open chromatin with visible nucleoli, and intensely basophilic (blue) cytoplasm. Maturation in the erythroid series is marked by a progressive decrease in cell size with each division, decreased nuclear size, increased nuclear chromatin density, and progressive hemoglobinization of the cytoplasm. With hemoglobin accumulation, the cytoplasm color gradually changes from blue to pink. All erythrocytes express glycophorin, which helps define the erythroid lineage. **Orthochromatic erythroblasts** extrude their nuclei to create **reticulocytes,** whose cytosol has mitochondria and hemoglobin-producing polyribosomes. Reticulocytes represent the final stage of erythroid cell maturation in the bone marrow. After leaving the bone marrow, reticulocytes lose the capacity for aerobic metabolism and hemoglobin synthesis, and become mature erythrocytes within 1 to 2 days. Of note, bone marrow is the only site of adult erythropoiesis, but under erythroid stress conditions, the spleen may be used to expand the erythropoietic capacity. Normal blood contains approximately 5×10^6 erythrocytes per microliter (μL), and these cells live an average of 120 days. As the main oxygen transporters, mature erythrocytes have a biconcave shape that creates a large surface area for gas exchange. Their small size allows them to enter capillaries in tissues.

- **Granulocytic precursors: Myeloblasts** have round to oval nuclei with delicate chromatin, multiple visible nucleoli and a blue-gray cytoplasm. **Promyelocytes,** the next stage, have similar nuclei, but their cytoplasm contains primary (azurophilic) granules. Maturation from **promyelocytes** to mature **neutrophils** involves (1) progressive nuclear chromatin condensation, (2) increasing nuclear lobulation, and (3) the appearance of secondary (specific) granules. **Basophils** and **eosinophils** derive from specific progenitor and precursor cells and are distinguished by their secondary granules, which are dark blue in basophils and salmon-red in eosinophils. Granulocyte precursors express CD13 and CD33 and progressively lose CD34 as they mature.

- **Monocytic precursors:** Monoblasts are mononuclear cells that are morphologically indistinguishable from granulocytic blasts. Gradual differentiation of monocytes from monoblasts involves a condensation process that changes nuclei from round/oval to C-shaped with folds, and leads

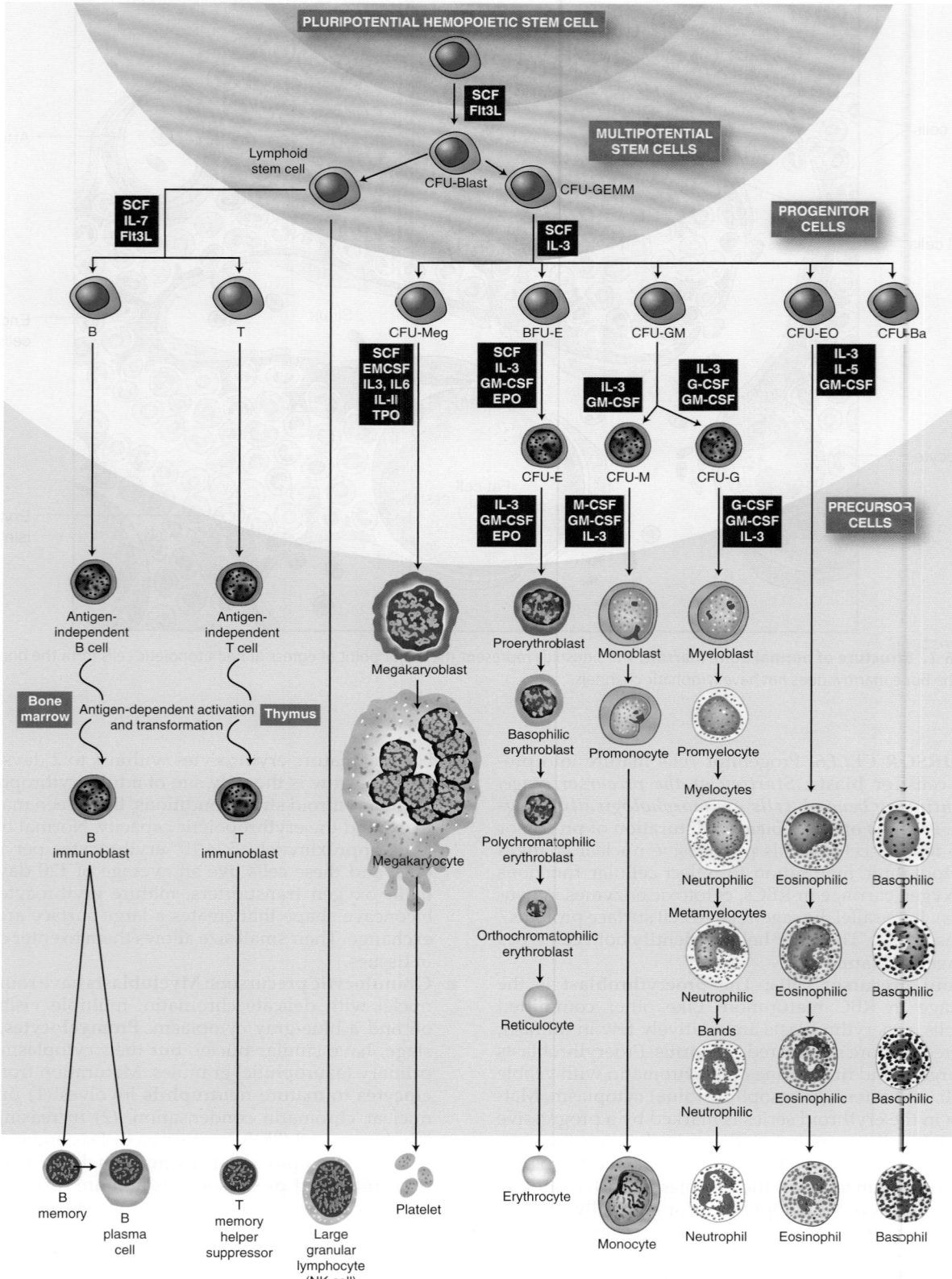

FIGURE 26-2. Cellular differentiation and maturation of the lymphoid and myeloid components of the hematopoietic system. Only the precursor cells (blasts and maturing cells) are identifiable by light microscopic evaluation of the bone marrow. *BFU* = burst-forming unit; *CFU* = colony-forming unit (*Ba* = basophils; *E* = erythroid; *Eo* = eosinophils; *G* = polymorphonuclear leukocytes; *GM* = granulocyte-monocyte; *M* = monocyte/macrophages; *Meg* = megakaryocytic); *EPO* = erythropoietin; *GM-CSF* = granulocyte-macrophage colony-stimulating factor; *IL* = interleukin; *NK* = natural killer; *SCF* = stem cell factor; *TPO* = thrombopoietin.

to the disappearance of nucleoli. The cytoplasm becomes gray, with rare pink or purple granules. **Once monocytes leave the blood, they migrate to tissues.** Although a small subset picks up antigens and transports them to regional lymph nodes without becoming macrophages, **most monocytes differentiate into macrophages that are characteristic for the tissue in which they reside. Examples of such tissue-specific macrophages include alveolar macrophages in the lung, Kuppfer cells in the liver, osteoclasts in bone, and microglia in the brain.** They may function as **phagocytic cells** (fixed or wandering) or in immunoregulation (e.g., dendritic reticulum cells, Langerhans cells).

■ **Megakaryocytic precursors:** Marrow megakaryoblasts, the earliest megakaryocytic lineage-committed cells, differentiate into megakaryocytes, which undergo endomitotic divisions (incomplete mitoses with failure of both nuclear and cytoplasmic division) and increase their ploidy. Mature megakaryocytes are large cells with multilobulated, polyploid nuclei. After reaching a certain ploidy, the cytoplasm becomes stippled and azurophilic, eventually to be released into the sinusoids as long, platelet-containing ribbons. Some intact megakaryocytes are also released, and platelet production occurs after they localize in the pulmonary microcirculation.

RELEASE FROM THE MARROW: After they mature, hematopoietic cells leave the bone marrow through sinusoids and enter the blood (Figs. 26-1 and 26-2). *Hematopoietic homeostasis is highly regulated by cell–cell interactions in the bone marrow and/or by stimulatory and inhibitory cytokines.* The cellular release mechanism in the bone marrow responds to the needs of the peripheral circulation and can quickly provide a boost of mature cells in an emergency (e.g., RBCs and/or reticulocytes during acute hemorrhage or neutrophils in acute infection).

Biopsy and Aspirate Smear Allow Complementary Analyses of Bone Marrow

The posterior iliac crest (or, rarely, the sternum) is the most common site of bone marrow biopsy for analysis in adults. In infants, the anterior tibia may also be used. Bone marrow core biopsy sections allow evaluation of the amount of hematopoietic elements and marrow architecture (Fig. 26-3A), while the several bone marrow cell lineages are identified and evaluated in stained smears made from aspirated liquid bone marrow (Fig. 26-3B). The ratio of hematopoietic cells to fat is estimated as the **bone marrow cellularity,** which varies with age. In a normal middle-aged adult, about half of bone marrow core biopsy volume is adipocytes; the other half is actively dividing and differentiating hematopoietic cells. Marrow cellularity is higher in children and lower in the elderly.

Bone marrow cellularity mostly consists of maturing granulocyte precursors, erythroid precursors, and megakaryocytes, called **trilineage hematopoiesis.** The ratio of myeloid to erythroid cells (i.e., the **M:E ratio**) is normally 2:1 to 3:1 (Table 26-1). There are usually 2 to 5 megakaryocytes per high-power field. Monocytic cells, lymphocytes, and plasma cells are normally present in low numbers. Normal bone marrow has less than 3% plasma cells, up to 20% lymphocytes and only rare mast cells and macrophages. Blasts are usually

TABLE 26-1
NORMAL ADULT BONE MARROW (AGE 18–70 YEARS)
Fat-to-cell ratio: 50:50 ± 15%
Myeloid-to-erythroid ratio: 2:1 to 4:1

Cell distribution (% surface area)
    Fat cells: 35–65% (roughly % fat = age in years)
    Erythroid series: 10–20%
    Granulocytic (myeloic) series: 40–65%

Megakaryocytes: 1–4/high-power field
Plasma cells: <3% of nucleated cells
Lymphocytes: <20% of nucleated cells
No fibrosis

less than 3% of marrow cells in normal adults, and comprise a mixture of early but committed, erythroid, granulocytic ("myeloblasts"), and B-lymphoid precursors.

Changes in the normal number and distribution of mature cells toward immature cells are referred to as **left shifts**. These can occur in both reactive and neoplastic processes. *The number of blasts in the bone marrow helps to distinguish these two broad categories, as reactive states do not significantly increase the number of blasts in the marrow.* In addition to evaluating cellularity and the proportions of the various cell types, bone marrow examination includes assessment of normal progressive maturation of hematopoietic precursors. *Dyssynchronization or aberration in the highly regulated process of nuclear and cytoplasmic maturation is evidence of bone marrow disease.*

Bone marrow iron stores are assessed by staining a smear with Prussian blue. In normal individuals, iron storage occurs in sideroblastic iron granules in the cytoplasm of macrophages and nucleated RBC precursors. Finally, marrow infiltration by abnormal cells, such as metastatic tumor cells, malignant hematopoietic cells or infectious granulomas, can be identified on microscopic examination.

Abnormal Non-Neoplastic Myelopoiesis

DISORDERS OF NEUTROPHILS

Quantitative Abnormalities of Neutrophils Reflect the Absolute Neutrophil Count (ANC)

Neutropenia is defined as a circulating absolute neutrophil count (ANC) below 1,500/μL. The automated ANC is obtained multiplying the white blood cell count by the percentage of polymorphonuclear cells and band forms on the differential count.

Clinical manifestations of neutropenia depend on its severity. ANCs of 1,000 to 1,500/μL are considered mild;

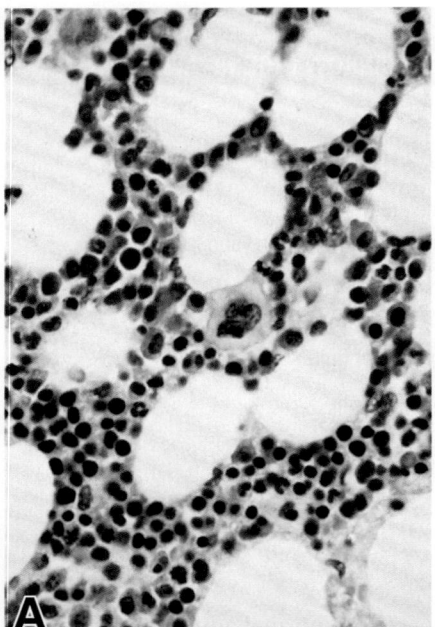
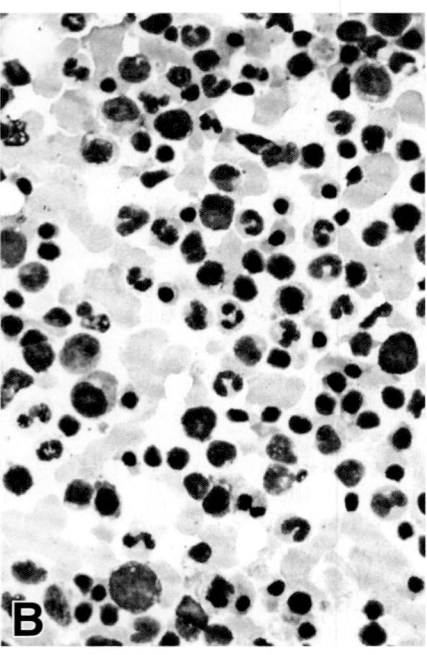

FIGURE 26-3. Normal bone marrow. A. Tissue section showing the normal relationship of cellular hematopoietic elements to fat cells, a normal myeloid-to-erythroid ratio (2:1) and a megakaryocyte in the center of the field hematoxylin and eosin stain). **B.** Bone marrow aspirate smear from the same patient demonstrating normal hematopoietic elements in varying stages of differentiation (Wright–Giemsa stain).

ANCs of 500 to 1,000/µL are moderate, and ANCs less than 500/µL indicate severe neutropenia. In mild neutropenia, the number of neutrophils is adequate to defend against microorganisms. With moderate neutropenia, patients become vulnerable to microbial infections. In severe neutropenia, the risk of serious infection is high. **Agranulocytosis** is the term used to indicate severe neutropenia, although granulocytes comprise neutrophils, eosinophils, and basophils.

Neutropenia is usually due to either decreased production or increased destruction of neutrophils (Table 26-2). Most cases are asymptomatic and unexplained, and are referred to as **chronic benign neutropenia**. A rare condition called myelokathexis, is characterized by adequate production of bone marrow granulocytes but failure of release into the blood, resulting in accumulation of neutrophils within the marrow.

DECREASED NEUTROPHIL PRODUCTION: Radiation or chemotherapeutic drugs suppress normal hematopoiesis and thus interfere with generation of neutrophils and their bone marrow precursors. Certain drugs, such as phenothiazines, phenylbutazone, antithyroid drugs, and indomethacin, can cause **idiosyncratic** marrow suppression. Viral infection and alcohol intake may also suppress myelopoiesis.

MOLECULAR PATHOGENESIS: Decreased granulocyte production can also result from constitutional genetic alterations in several rare hereditary disorders, including **Kostmann syndrome** and **infantile genetic agranulocytosis**. The genetic causes of several of these diseases are known. Mutations in *ELANE*, the gene encoding neutrophil elastase, cause the most common form of congenital agranulocytosis. Mutations in *HAX*, a gene regulating apoptosis, are responsible for Kostmann syndrome. Ineffective myelopoiesis occurs in the neutropenia of megaloblastic anemias and myelodysplastic syndromes (MDSs). In **cyclic neutropenia**, episodes recur regularly about every 21 days.

INCREASED NEUTROPHIL DESTRUCTION: Accelerated elimination of granulocytes is caused by:

- Increased consumption of neutrophils in infections
- Chronic splenomegaly with increased sequestration (hypersplenism)
- Increased destruction by antibodies directed against neutrophils (immune causes)

TABLE 26-2
PRINCIPAL CAUSES OF NEUTROPENIA

Decreased Production
Irradiation
Drug induced (long and short term)
Viral infections
Congenital
Cyclic

Ineffective Production
Megaloblastic anemia
Myelodysplastic syndromes

Increased Destruction
Isoimmune neonatal
Autoimmune
  Idiopathic
  Drug induced
  Felty syndrome
  Systemic lupus erythematosus
  Dialysis (induced by complement activation)
  Splenic sequestration
  Increased margination

Bacterial infections usually produce leukocytosis. However, some infections including typhoid fever, brucellosis, tularemia, and tuberculosis, are associated with neutropenia.

Viral infections can lead to neutropenia. These include infections caused by respiratory syncytial virus (RSV), measles, rubella, influenza A and B, parvovirus, infectious mononucleosis (caused by Epstein–Barr virus [EBV]), cytomegalovirus, and hepatitis A.

Rickettsial infections and some **parasitic infections** such as kala-azar caused by Leishmania donovani, cause neutropenia, either isolated or as part of pancytopenia.

Hemophagocytic syndrome: Neutropenia (but usually, pancytopenia) can occur when macrophages become activated in response to infections (commonly EBV). This is accompanied by splenomegaly and cytopenia(s). Another term describing this process is hemophagocytic lymphohistiocytosis (HLH).

Many **drugs** can cause immune-mediated neutrophil destruction, especially sulfonamides, phenylbutazone and indomethacin. The toxic effects result from attachment of circulating antigen–antibody complexes to granulocyte surfaces, with subsequent complement-mediated injury.

Neutropenia is common in HIV infection, either from autoimmune destruction or as a side effect of antiretroviral drugs administration (e.g., zidovudine). Lymphopenia is more common, however, due primarily to decreased CD4 T-cells.

Neutrophilia is defined as an ANC above 7,000/μL. It can be primary (occurring in myeloproliferative disorders) or secondary (Table 26-3), and reflects (1) **increased mobilization** of neutrophils from bone marrow storage, (2) **demargination** of peripheral blood neutrophils (release of neutrophils from the vascular endothelium to which they reversibly adhere), or (3) **increased bone marrow production**. Increased mobilization of neutrophils from the marrow or peripheral marginal pools occurs in settings of acute trauma or infections.

Acute bacterial infections usually cause leukocytosis with neutrophilia and an increased number of band forms (a left shift). Additionally, the neutrophils can contain toxic granulations (prominent dark blue granulation of the cytoplasm), Döhle bodies (large pale blue cytoplasmic inclusions), and cytoplasmic vacuoles.

LEUKEMOID REACTION: In response to infections and occasionally during severe hemorrhage or acute hemolysis, white blood counts (mostly neutrophils and bands) may be so high (up to 50,000/μL) as to be mistaken for leukemia, especially chronic myeloid leukemia (CML). Such non-neoplastic increases in leukocyte counts are called **leukemoid reactions,** which can be recognized by several features: presence of toxic granulations and/or Döhle bodies in neutrophils, a high LAP (leukocyte alkaline phosphatase) score, resolution of leukocytosis in response to therapy, and absence of cytogenetic abnormalities such as translocation t(9;22) and Philadelphia chromosome (see below).

Inflammation. Both acute and chronic inflammatory disorders can cause neutrophilia. Examples include

TABLE 26-3
PRINCIPAL CAUSES OF NEUTROPHILIA

Infections
  Primarily bacterial

Immunologic/Inflammatory
  Rheumatoid arthritis
  Rheumatic fever
  Vasculitis

Neoplasia

Hemorrhage

Drugs
  Glucocorticoids
  Colony-stimulating factors (CSFs)
  Lithium

Hereditary
  CD18 deficiency

Metabolic
  Acidosis
  Uremia
  Gout
  Thyroid storm

Tissue Necrosis
  Infarction
  Trauma
  Burns

Kawasaki disease, rheumatoid arthritis, Crohn disease, ulcerative colitis, and Sweet syndrome.

Medications can cause neutrophilia. Administration of G-CSF (filgrastim) is common in clinical practice to increase ANC and reduce the incidence of infections. Glucocorticoids and the immunostimulant drug plerixafor promote release of granulocytes from the bone marrow. Catecholamines cause demargination of neutrophils within blood vessels, and are associated with mild neutrophilia.

Genetic or inherited disorders causing neutrophilia are suspected when other family members present similar hematologic and/or somatic abnormalities. Hereditary chronic neutrophilia is associated with a mutation in *CSFR*, resulting in constitutive activation of G-CSFR, the G-CSF receptor.

Qualitative Disorders of Neutrophils Are Associated With Impaired Function

If granulocyte functionality (their killing ability or chemotactic cell movement) is impaired, resistance to infection may decrease despite a normal granulocyte count. Such rare hereditary disorders of granulocyte killing ability include chronic granulomatous disease, myeloperoxidase deficiency, and Chédiak–Higashi syndrome (see Chapter 2). Intrinsic disorders of chemotaxis include hyperimmunoglobulin E syndrome, leukocyte adhesion defects, and Shwachman–Diamond syndrome.

Disorders of Other White Blood Cell Series

Eosinophils, components of the granulocytic lineage, develop and differentiate in the bone marrow under the influence of eosinophil growth factors (IL-5 and IL-3). After being released into the blood, they are recruited to tissues including the gastrointestinal tract, respiratory tract, and skin. This process is mediated by eotaxins (a family of chemokines). The exact functions of eosinophils in health are not well understood. Their normal level in blood is 0 to 500 cells/μL. They respond to chemotactic substances made by mast cells or are induced by persistent antigen–antibody complexes. The main causes of eosinophilia are listed in Table 26-4.

Eosinophilia, an increase in eosinophils in the peripheral blood or tissues, arises by two mechanisms: clonal expansion driven by a genetic defect in a hematopoietic stem or progenitor cell, or polyclonal expansion due to overproduction of IL-5 in multiple conditions.

Clonal hypereosinophilia in which eosinophilia is part of a myeloid/lymphoid neoplasm due to cytogenetic or molecular genetic abnormalities (such as acute eosinophilic leukemia with inversion 16, myeloid neoplasms with mutations in *PDGFRA, PDGFRB,* or *FGFR1*), is discussed in a later section. Eosinophilia can also be associated with CML and systemic mastocytosis.

Polyclonal hypereosinophilia may accompany neoplastic diseases including Hodgkin or non-Hodgkin lymphomas, in which eosinophilia results from dysregulation of cytokine production by lymphocytes, or solid tumors. Other common causes of peripheral eosinophilia are parasitic or other infections, drug reactions, adrenal insufficiency, and connective tissue/rheumatologic diseases.

Hypereosinophilic syndrome is defined as an absolute eosinophil count of ≥1,500/μL accompanied by organ dysfunction attributable to eosinophilia. Accumulation of eosinophils in tissues often leads to necrosis or fibrosis, particularly in the myocardium, where it produces endomyocardial disease (see Chapter 17). Neurologic dysfunction may also develop. Eosinophil-mediated tissue injury is due to release of toxic eosinophil granule products, particularly major basic protein and cationic protein, release of cytokines, or production of lipid mediators (see Chapter 2).

In **idiopathic hypereosinophilic syndrome,** circulating eosinophils exceed 1,500/μL for more than 5 months without evident underlying disease. Eosinophil counts in this condition may reach 50,000 to 100,000/μL. If untreated, the prognosis is grave; only 10% of untreated patients survive 3 years. With aggressive corticosteroid therapy, 70% live more than 5 years, even with cardiac involvement.

Basophilia Occurs in Allergic Reactions and Myeloproliferative Diseases

Basophils are the least abundant of all leukocytes. They differentiate in the bone marrow, circulate briefly in the blood and then localize into tissues. Their relationship to mast cells is controversial. Basophil granules contain several preformed inflammatory mediators, including histamine and chondroitin sulfate. When stimulated, basophils also synthesize leukotrienes and other mediators. Basophilia occurs most often in immediate-type hypersensitivity reactions and in chronic myeloproliferative neoplasms (MPNs). The major causes of basophilia are listed in Table 26-5.

Monocytosis Occurs in Both Malignant and Inflammatory Conditions

Monocytosis is defined by a circulating monocyte count that exceeds 800/μL. The main causes include hematologic

TABLE 26-4
PRINCIPAL CAUSES OF EOSINOPHILIA
Allergic Disorders
Skin Diseases
Parasitic (Helminth) Infestations
Malignant Neoplasms Hematopoietic Solid tumors
Collagen Vascular Disorders
Miscellaneous Hypereosinophilic syndromes Eosinophilia–myalgia syndrome Interleukin-2 therapy

TABLE 26-5
PRINCIPAL CAUSES OF BASOPHILIA
Allergic (Drug, Food)
Inflammation Juvenile rheumatoid arthritis Ulcerative colitis
Infection Viral (chickenpox, influenza) Tuberculosis
Neoplasia Myeloproliferative syndromes Basophilic leukemia Carcinoma
Endocrine Diabetes mellitus Myxedema Estrogen administration

malignancies, infections, immunologic and inflammatory conditions, and solid cancers. Malignant monocytes and monoblasts will be discussed in the section on myeloid malignancies. Differentiation of macrophages from monocytes is accentuated in response to infection or cancer. Tissue macrophages can differentiate into either proinflammatory, microbicidal (M1), or anti-inflammatory (M2) subtypes. Macrophages are part of the innate immune system, and play important roles in digesting microbes and presenting microbial antigens to lymphocytes to initiate an adaptive immune response to the microbial agent. Macrophages also secrete numerous proteins that mediate host defense and inflammation.

Proliferative Disorders of Mast Cells Release Inflammatory Mediators

Mast cells are the initial tissue-based effector cells of the immediate allergic reaction. They also play a role in innate and acquired immunity, in wound healing and in tumor angiogenesis. They arise from a pluripotent hematopoietic cell in the bone marrow, where they differentiate under the influence of Kit and its ligand SCF. They then migrate to tissue sites and mature. They localize in proximity to the epithelial surface of the skin and respiratory tract, in the gastrointestinal and genitourinary tracts, and in perivascular sites (see Chapter 2). Their role in allergic reactions is facilitated by high-affinity receptors for IgE. They can also be activated by non-IgE factors and nonimmunologic factors. Activation of mast cells leads to release of their granules, which contain biologically active mediators such as histamine, heparin, leukotrienes, and cytokines. Symptoms of mast cell proliferative diseases are related to release of these substances and include flushing, pruritus, and hives. Secretion of heparin also causes bleeding from the nasopharynx or GI tract.

Reactive mast cell hyperplasia is a non-neoplastic process that occurs in immediate- and delayed-type hypersensitivity reactions and in lymph nodes that drain malignant tumors. It is also observed in Waldenström macroglobulinemia, in the bone marrow of women with postmenopausal osteoporosis, in MDSs, and after chemotherapy for leukemia.

Disorders of Hematopoietic Stem Cells

BONE MARROW FAILURE

Disorders of HSC/Bone Marrow Failure May Manifest in Multiple Hematopoietic Series

Aplastic Anemia

Aplastic anemia is a disorder of pluripotent hematopoietic stem cells that leads to bone marrow failure and peripheral cytopenias. All main blood cell lineages (red cells, neutrophils, and platelets) are decreased, a condition known as **pancytopenia**.

  PATHOPHYSIOLOGY AND ETIOLOGIC FACTORS: Aplastic anemia (AA) is a rare condition that results from inherited or acquired injury of HSCs. It is acquired in the majority of cases. Most acquired cases are idiopathic, with no clear identifiable etiology, although in 10% to 20% of cases, a recent marrow insult such as viral infection (e.g., hepatitis viruses), drugs, chemicals, or ionizing radiation, can be documented (Table 26-6). The pathogenic mechanism is often immune-mediated destruction of hematopoietic progenitors by hyperactive T-cells that suppress hematopoiesis. Cytokines secreted by these T-cells contribute to marrow suppression.

PATHOLOGY: The bone marrow in AA is hypocellular or acellular, and all three cell lines (myeloid, erythroid precursors, and megakaryocytes) are decreased, with a relative increase in lymphocytes and plasma cells. As marrow cellularity declines, there is a corresponding increase in fat (Fig. 26-4). These changes are reflected in low numbers of circulating cells resulting in anemia, neutropenia, and thrombocytopenia. Even in the face of elevated erythropoietin (EPO) levels, reticulocytosis is absent, which underscores the underlying stem cell defect.

CLINICAL FEATURES: Patients with aplastic anemia show signs and symptoms due to pancytopenia (i.e., weakness, fatigue, infection, and bleeding). Untreated, the prognosis is grim, with a 3- to

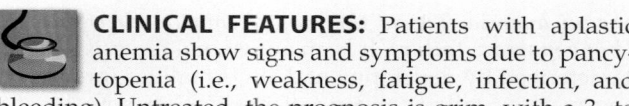

TABLE 26-6
ETIOLOGY OF APLASTIC ANEMIA

Idiopathic (two-thirds of cases)
Ionizing radiation

Drugs
    Chemotherapeutic agents
    Chloramphenicol
    Anticonvulsants
    Nonsteroidal anti-inflammatory agents
    Gold

Chemicals
    Benzene

Viruses
    Hepatitis C virus (HCV)
    Epstein–Barr virus (EBV)
    HIV
    Parvovirus B19

Hereditary
    Fanconi anemia

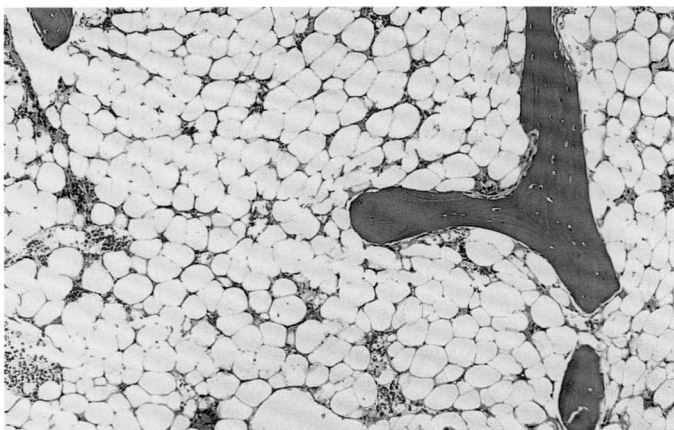

FIGURE 26-4. Aplastic anemia. The bone marrow consists largely of fat cells and lacks normal hematopoietic activity.

6-month median survival. Immunosuppressive therapy with antithymocyte globulin and cyclosporine, in combination with agents that stimulate hematopoiesis (eltrombopag), leads to transient remissions. Stem cell transplantation is curative.

Fanconi Anemia

Fanconi anemia (FA) is the most frequent inherited cause of bone marrow failure. It is an autosomal recessive disease characterized by developmental abnormalities, progressive bone marrow failure and predisposition to both hematologic and solid malignancies. Fifteen FA disease alleles have been identified. They are labeled *FANC* (for Fanconi complementation group), followed by A, B, and so forth. *FANCD1* is also known as *BRCA2* (see Chapters 5 and 25). FA genes encode proteins involved in DNA replication and repair. They form a complex with other downstream FA proteins such as ATM, ATR, NBS, and BRCA1 (see Chapter 5) in response to DNA damage and mediate repair of altered DNA by homologous recombination. Mutations in these genes produce chromosome fragility with defective DNA repair.

Because FA genes are also necessary for normal development of several organs, affected patients usually present at a young age with diverse abnormalities including malformations of their thumbs and radii, abnormal skin pigmentation (hypopigmentation or café au lait spots), and cardiac, renal, and other malformations. Decreased fertility and bone marrow failure are also common features, but may not be apparent at birth. Presentation in adult life has been demonstrated recently by identifying germline mutations in *FANC* genes in patients presenting with bone marrow failure syndrome, but without a suggestive family history or syndromic stigmata. The reported incidence of FA is less than 1 per 100,000 live births, although the condition is probably underdiagnosed.

Bone marrow failure associated with FA affects all hematopoietic series, but in contrast to idiopathic AA, Fanconi patients do not respond to immunosuppressive treatments. Some patients respond to androgen therapy, but HSC transplantation is the treatment of choice. Unfortunately, the sen-

sitivity of FA patients to DNA damaging agents complicates pretransplant conditioning. More recent therapeutic options include gene therapy, or genome editing using genetic recombination or engineered nucleases.

FA patients who survive hematopoietic failure have a high risk of developing hematopoietic malignancies (MDSs and acute myelogenous leukemia, as described below) or solid tumors in their second or third decade of life.

Dyskeratosis Congenita

Dyskeratosis congenita (DC) usually presents during childhood, but this varies and it may present in older patients. When diagnosed at an early age, patients often exhibit thrombocytopenia or aplastic anemia, and characteristically short telomeres. Some but not all display a diagnostic triad of dysplastic nails, lacy reticular skin pigmentation, and oral leukoplakia. Older DC patients may be diagnosed because of pulmonary fibrosis or hepatopulmonary syndrome. DC patients have an increased risk of malignancies including MDSs, acute myeloid leukemia (AML), or squamous cell carcinomas of the head and neck or anogenital region. HSC transplantation is the best therapeutic choice for patients who develop bone marrow failure, MDS or AML, with careful choice of the pretransplant regimens due to potential pulmonary toxicity from irradiation and chemotherapy. Unfortunately, the risk of solid tumors is increased following stem cell transplantation.

Some HSC Disorders Affect One Series Preferentially

Pure Red Cell Aplasia

Pure red cell aplasia (PRCA) is selective marrow suppression of committed erythroid precursors. White blood cells and platelets are unaffected.

 PATHOPHYSIOLOGY: PRCA most often results from immune suppression of red cell production, the etiology of which is usually unknown. On occasion, it is due to viral infection (usually parvovirus B19) or thymic lesions (e.g., thymoma, thymic hyperplasia). The P antigens on red cell membranes are receptors for parvovirus, which explains the restricted infection of erythroid precursors.

Diamond–Blackfan anemia is usually diagnosed early in life (within the first 2 years or even in utero) with symptoms of anemia. Physical anomalies such as cleft lip or palate, micrognathia, limb abnormalities, and short stature, may be present but are often subtle. It is caused by de novo or inherited (germline) mutations in genes that encode ribosomal proteins. At least eight different genes for both large and small ribosomal subunit proteins have been implicated. Approximately 25% of cases are due to mutations in *RPS19*, which encodes a small subunit protein. Anemia is the result of diminished responsiveness by defective erythroid precursors to erythropoietin and decreased erythroid burst- and colony-forming capacities.

PATHOLOGY: Bone marrow cellularity is normal in PRCA, but erythroid precursors are absent or markedly decreased, and arrested in maturation at the pronormoblast stage. In cases caused by parvovirus B19, proerythroblasts exhibit intranuclear viral inclusions and the infection can be detected by PCR. Myeloid and megakaryocytic precursors are adequate in number and show normal maturation.

Anemia in PRCA is moderate to severe, often with macrocytic indices. Despite increased EPO, there is no accompanying reticulocytosis.

CLINICAL FEATURES: Acquired PRCA manifests as an acute self-limited illness or a chronic relapsing process. **Acute self-limited PRCA** is often due to parvovirus B19. This condition may not be clinically apparent unless the patient suffers from an underlying chronic hemolytic anemia (e.g., hereditary spherocytosis [HS], sickle cell anemia). Such cases may be complicated by an aplastic "crisis" (i.e., sudden worsening of anemia). Immunocompromised patients cannot clear parvovirus infection and anemia may be prolonged. **Chronic relapsing PRCA** may be idiopathic or associated with an underlying thymic lesion. In such cases, thymectomy may correct the anemia.

Diamond–Blackfan anemia is usually treated with corticosteroids or transfusions, with attendant risks associated with iron overload and chronic use of steroids. Interestingly, about 20% of patients may have spontaneous remission.

Paroxysmal Nocturnal Hemoglobinuria

Paroxysmal nocturnal hemoglobinuria (PNH) is an acquired clonal, nonmalignant stem cell disorder characterized by episodic intravascular hemolytic anemia and thromboses.

MOLECULAR PATHOGENESIS: The underlying defect in PNH involves somatic mutations in *PIG-A*, on the X chromosome (Xp22.1) (see Table 26-14 later in the chapter). This gene encodes a protein called phosphatidylinositol glycan class A, which is crucial in the synthesis of the glycosylphosphatidylinositol (GPI) anchor, which normally attaches many proteins (e.g., CD14, CD16, CD55, CD59) to the membranes of blood cells. As a consequence of the genetic defect, GPI is not synthesized and all blood cells derived from affected HSC clones lack the surface proteins mentioned above. Some of these proteins, such as **decay acceleration factor** (CD55) and **membrane inhibitor of reactive lysis** (CD59), are important complement regulators, and red cells lacking these proteins are susceptible to lysis by complement. Leukocytes and platelets derived from the abnormal stem cells also lose GPI-linked membrane proteins. PNH platelets fix complement and become activated, potentially leading to thrombosis.

PNH may arise as a primary disorder or in association with aplastic anemia (AA/PNH). Although the *PIG-A* mutation itself is benign, patients with PNH, especially if associated with AA, may progress to **myelodysplasia** or overt **acute leukemia** (see below). The mechanism of malignant transformation usually involves acquisition of additional somatic mutation(s), either in the PNH cells that already harbor *PIG-A* mutations, or in cells unaffected by PNH.

PATHOLOGY: During hemolytic episodes, patients develop varyingly severe normocytic or macrocytic anemia. Reticulocyte counts, which reflect the adequacy of bone marrow response to hemolysis, are often inadequate. Thus, erythropoiesis in the marrow does not adequately compensate for the red cell lysis by complement, and this explains why PNH is included as a subtype of bone marrow failure. Because the hemolysis is intravascular, hemoglobinuria is present, and iron deficiency may develop over time from recurrent iron loss in the urine. *PNH is diagnosed by flow cytometric demonstration that blood cells lack GPI-anchored proteins (CD16, CD14, CD55, CD59).*

CLINICAL FEATURES: Patients may have intermittent intravascular hemolysis. Venous and arterial thrombosis, notably Budd–Chiari syndrome (hepatic vein thrombosis; see Chapter 20), are increased in PNH because of complement-mediated platelet activation. Treatment involves agents that block complement activation, such as eculizumab. Despite its high efficacy, however, the high cost and short acting effect of this biologic limit wide utilization. Bone marrow transplantation is curative.

Red Blood Cells

NORMAL STRUCTURE AND FUNCTION

RBCs, or erythrocytes, transport oxygen to tissues. Mature RBCs are anucleate cells measuring 7- to 8-μm diameter, similar in size to small lymphocyte nuclei (Fig. 26-5). They are round, biconcave disks with reddish, eosinophilic cytoplasm, and centers paler than their outer rims. The pale center comprises roughly one-third of the total diameter of the cell. Their main cytoplasmic component is hemoglobin, which imparts the red color. Erythrocytes are released from the marrow as reticulocytes, which are larger than mature RBCs and have a bluish-gray cytoplasmic hue, called **polychromatophilia**. This bluish hue is due to the presence of RNA and cytoplasmic organelles including ribosomes, mitochondria, and Golgi complex. Once released into the blood, reticulocytes lose cytoplasmic RNA within 24 hours and become mature RBCs.

As in all cells, the RBC membrane is a phospholipid bilayer. It is attached to an underlying cytoskeletal network comprised of horizontally arranged interconnected spectrin protein dimers, and stabilizing proteins, including ankyrin,

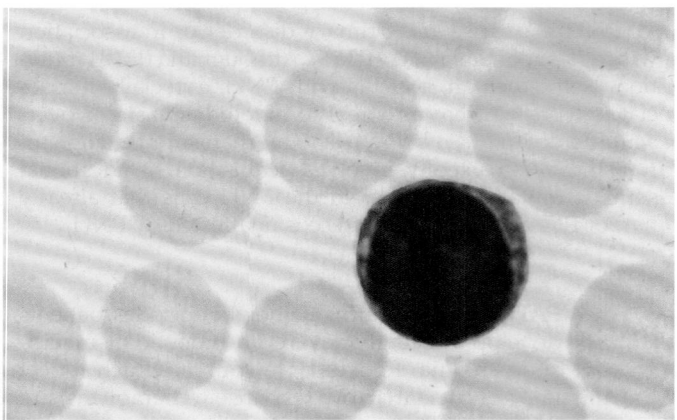

FIGURE 26-5. Normal red blood cells are approximately the same size as the nucleus of a small lymphocyte (≈7 to 8 μm).

actin, and band 4.1 (Fig. 26-6). These cytoskeletal proteins allow RBCs to deform as they traverse narrow capillaries. *Changes in this membrane–cytoskeletal unit may lead to characteristic abnormalities in RBC shape, increased cell rigidity, and premature destruction of circulating RBCs.* Transmembrane receptors, channels and anchors for other membrane components also insert into the lipid bilayer. *Different RBC membrane proteins and their modifications with carbohydrate groups produce the various red cell antigen groups.*

Hemoglobin accounts for the oxygen-carrying capacity of RBCs. Each hemoglobin molecule has four heme groups and four globin chains and, when fully saturated, transports four molecules of oxygen. The heme part of the molecule consists of a porphyrin ring (protoporphyrin IX), with one ferrous ion (Fe^{2+}). The globin portion consists of pairs of two different protein chains, usually two alpha (α)-globin chains and two

non-alpha globin chains. Two α-globin chains pair with two beta (β)-globin chains in hemoglobin A, the most abundant normal hemoglobin in adults. Hemoglobin A_2, present in minor amounts in healthy adults, is comprised of two α- and two delta (δ)-globin chains. Hemoglobin F, present in minor amounts in healthy adults but in major amounts at birth, is made of two α- and two gamma (γ)-globin chains. Synthesis and assembly of each hemoglobin molecule requires multiple biochemical steps involving distinct enzymes.

Each heme group interacts with a hydrophobic pocket in one globin chain, resulting in a globular tertiary structure for the complete molecule. Deoxygenated hemoglobin has low oxygen-binding affinity and requires increased oxygen tension for heme–oxygen binding to occur. After this initial interaction, hemoglobin molecules undergo a conformational change that facilitates subsequent oxygen binding to the remaining heme groups. This progressive increase in oxygen-binding affinity is reflected in the sigmoid shape of the oxygen dissociation curve (Fig. 26-7). Acidosis shifts the curve to the right, which increases tissue oxygen delivery. Increased 2,3-diphosphoglycerate (2,3-DPG) (a product of an alternate pathway of glycolysis) has a similar effect. Alkalosis shifts the curve to the left, increasing the affinity for oxygen binding.

The average life span of blood erythrocytes is 120 days. Changes in membrane proteins and phospholipid accumulation in aged red cells serve as signals for their removal by mononuclear phagocytes.

The erythroid component of the blood is best analyzed by a complete blood count (CBC) plus microscopic examination of a blood smear (Table 26-7). The CBC includes measurements of **hemoglobin** (Hgb), **RBC count**, and **hematocrit** (Hct). Additional parameters include RBC indices such as **mean corpuscular volume** (MCV = Hct/RBC), **mean corpuscular hemoglobin** (MCH = Hgb/RBC) and **mean corpuscular hemoglobin concentration** (MCHC = Hgb/Hct). Variability in RBC size, or red cell distribution width (RDW),

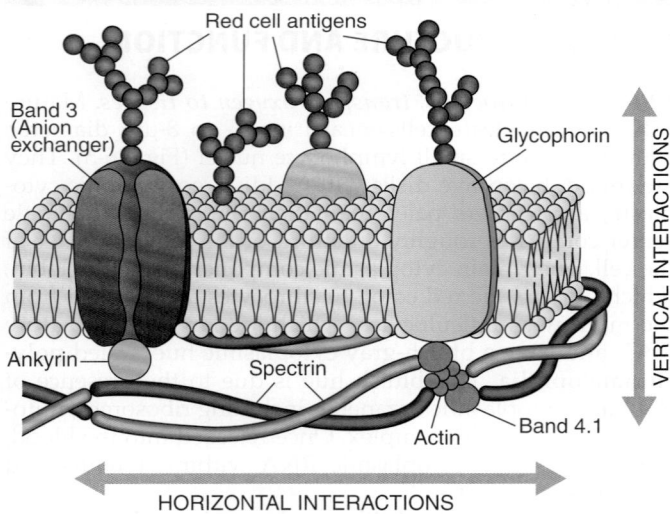

FIGURE 26-6. Structure of the erythrocyte plasma membrane. The membrane is stabilized by a number of interactions. The two vertical interactions are spectrin-ankyrin–band 3 and spectrin-protein 4.1–glycophorin. The two horizontal connections are spectrin heterodimers and spectrin-actin–protein 4.1.

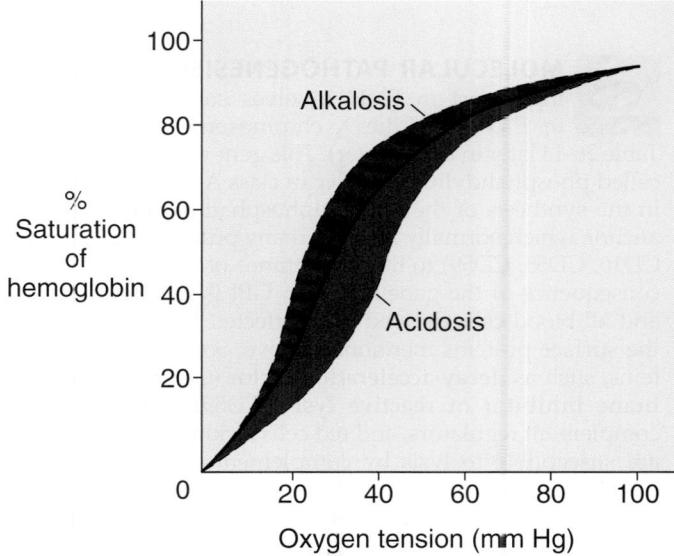

FIGURE 26-7. Oxygen dissociation curve of hemoglobin. With decreasing pH (acidosis), the oxygen affinity declines (shifts right); with increasing pH (alkalosis), the affinity increases (shifts left).

TABLE 26-7
COMPLETE BLOOD COUNT (CBC): NORMAL ADULT VALUES

Erythrocytes

Hemoglobin	Male, 14–18 g/dL Female, 12–16 g/dL
Hematocrit	Male, 40–54% Female, 35–47%
Red blood cell (RBC) count	Male, $4.5–6 \times 10^6/\mu L$ Female, $4–5.5 \times 10^6/\mu L$
Reticulocytes	0.5–2.5%

Indices

Mean corpuscular volume	82–100 μm^3
Mean corpuscular hemoglobin	27–34 pg
Mean corpuscular hemoglobin concentration	32–36%

	Absolute Count/μL	Differential Count (%)
Leukocytes		
White blood cells (WBCs)	4,000–11,000	
Neutrophil granulocytes	1,800–7,000	50–60
Neutrophil bands	0–700	2–4
Lymphocytes	1,500–4,000	30–40
Monocytes	0–800	1–9
Basophils	0–200	0–1
Eosinophils	0–450	0–3

Platelets

Quantitative normal value: 150,000–400,000/μL

Qualitative estimation on smear: Number of platelets/oil immersion field × 10,000 = estimated platelet count

Normal ratio of RBC to platelets = 15:1 to 20:1

is also derived. Reticulocytes can be accurately quantified using supravital dyes that stain their cytoplasmic ribosome aggregates. Automated analyzers can also measure the immature reticulocyte fraction (percentage of reticulocytes that are the most immature) and/or hemoglobin content of reticulocytes (CHr).

ANEMIA

Anemia is reduced circulating erythrocyte mass; it is diagnosed by a low hemoglobin concentration, Hct or RBC count. Anemia leads to decreased oxygen transport by the blood and, if severe, tissue hypoxia.

 CLINICAL FEATURES: In the face of anemia, compensatory mechanisms act to enhance oxygen delivery to tissues. These include:

- Increased cardiac output
- Increased respiratory rate
- Shunting of blood flow to increase perfusion of vital organs
- Decreased hemoglobin–oxygen affinity
- Increased marrow erythrocyte production in response to EPO stimulation

Clinical signs and symptoms (tachycardia, shortness of breath, systolic murmurs) may reflect these compensatory processes. If anemia is severe (i.e., hemoglobin <7 g/dL), tissue hypoxia is insufficiently compensated and additional clinical findings may include easy fatigability, faintness, angina, and dyspnea on exertion.

Anemias Are Classified by Morphology or Pathophysiology

Morphologic classification of anemia is based on RBC appearance, as determined by automated blood counters and microscopy. RBC size (generally measured by analyzers) is reflected in the MCV, which divides anemias into three groups: (1) **microcytic** (decreased MCV), (2) **normocytic,** and (3) **macrocytic** (increased MCV) (Table 26-8). Abnormally shaped RBCs **(poikilocytes)** are seen on blood smears in many anemias, and poikilocyte characteristics can aid in diagnosis (Fig. 26-8).

Pathophysiologic classification of anemia includes five main groups (Table 26-9):

1. **Acute Blood loss**
2. **Decreased production** of red cells by the bone marrow, either by **progenitor cell defects or lack of available nutrients**

TABLE 26-8
MORPHOLOGIC CLASSIFICATION OF ANEMIA

Macrocytic

Nutritional deficiency	Hypothyroidism
Alcohol use	Reticulocytosis
Liver disease	Primary bone marrow disease

Microcytic

Iron deficiency

Thalassemias

Sideroblastic

Normocytic

Anemia of chronic disease/inflammation

Anemia of renal disease

Acute blood loss

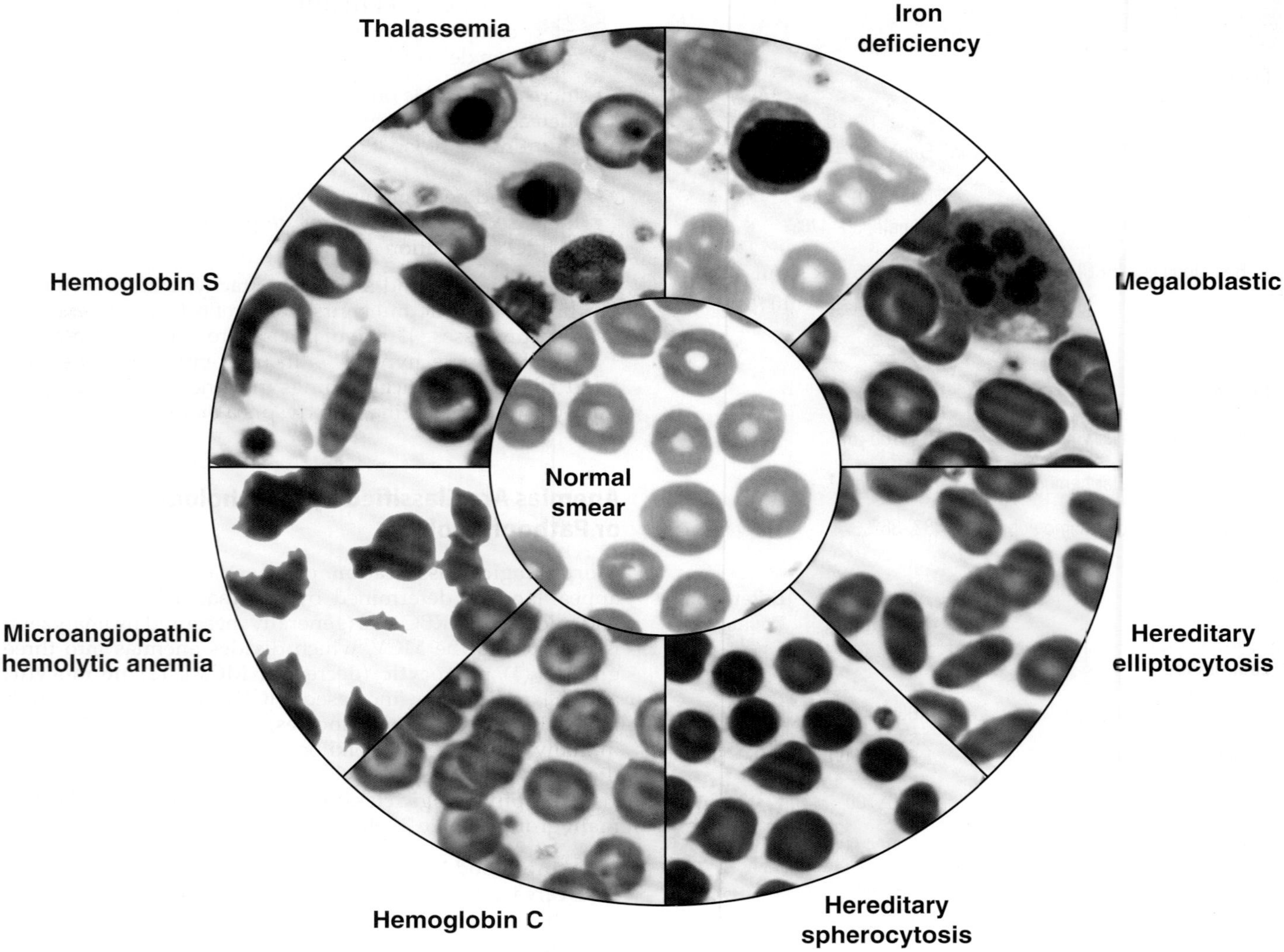

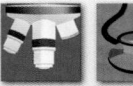

FIGURE 26-8. Abnormal red blood cell morphologies associated with various types of anemia. The morphology of normal erythrocytes is shown in the center. **Clockwise from 12:00: A. Iron deficiency (disturbance in hemoglobin synthesis; lack of iron):** Hypochromic, microcytic erythrocytes. A small lymphocyte is present for comparison. **B. Megaloblastic anemia (disturbance in DNA synthesis, most often caused by deficiency of vitamin B$_{12}$ or folic acid):** Oval macrocytes, some irregularly shaped cells and hypersegmented neutrophils. **C. Hereditary elliptocytosis (membrane defect):** Elliptocytes. **D. Hereditary spherocytosis (membrane defect):** Spherocytes lacking central pallor. **E. Hemoglobin C disease (abnormal globin chain):** Target cells. **F. Microangiopathic hemolysis (mechanical damage to erythrocytes;** disseminated intravascular coagulation [DIC], thrombocytic thrombocytopenic purpura [TTP], heart valve prosthesis sequela): Schistocytes/fragments. **G. Sickle cell (hemoglobin S) disease (abnormal globin chain):** Sickle cells. **H. Thalassemia (disturbance in hemoglobin synthesis):** Hypochromic, microcytic erythrocytes; poikilocytosis; basophilic stippling; target cells, nucleated red blood cells (RBCs).

3. **Ineffective hematopoiesis** with reduced release of erythrocytes from marrow
4. **Increased RBC destruction** outside the marrow, either from **intracorpuscular** or **extracorpuscular** causes
5. **Sequestration**

Circulating reticulocytes are elevated (**reticulocytosis**) as a response to hypoxia in anemias from non–marrow-based causes, such as blood loss or increased RBC destruction. Reticulocytosis does not occur in other causes of anemia. Expanded plasma volume results in decreased measured hemoglobin concentration, RBC counts, and Hct, but this form of "dilutional anemia" is not true anemia as red cell mass is preserved or even increased in some situations (such as in late pregnancy).

Acute Blood Loss

 PATHOLOGY AND CLINICAL FEATURES: Initial signs of acute blood loss reflect volume depletion and decreased tissue perfusion. Since whole blood is lost, the severity of the anemia may not be appreciated at first. Within 24 to 48 hours after significant hemorrhage, however, fluid is

TABLE 26-9
PATHOPHYSIOLOGIC CLASSIFICATION OF ANEMIA

Acute Blood Loss

Decreased Production

Stem Cell and Progenitor Cell Defects

Iron deficiency	Leukemia
Anemia of chronic disease	Myelodysplastic syndromes
Aplastic anemia	Marrow infiltration
Pure red cell aplasia	Lead poisoning
Paroxysmal nocturnal hemoglobinuria	Anemia of renal disease

Ineffective Hematopoiesis

Megaloblastic anemia	Thalassemia
Myelodysplastic syndromes	

Increased Destruction

Intracorpuscular

Membrane defect	Hemoglobinopathies
Enzyme defect	

Extracorpuscular

Immunologic

Autoimmune	Alloimmune

Nonimmunologic

Mechanical	Infectious
Hypersplenism	Chemical
Thermal	

Sequestration

mobilized from extravascular locations into the intravascular space to restore overall blood volume. This is when the extent of the anemia becomes apparent, since red cell replacement is not as rapid. *Acute anemia reflects blood loss from the intravascular compartment.*

Acute blood loss leads to normocytic, normochromic anemia. If the underlying bleeding is stopped, EPO-driven bone marrow erythroid hyperplasia will gradually correct the anemia. The blood smear shows no specific abnormalities, but polychromasia reflecting reticulocytosis occurs during the recovery phase.

Decreased RBC Production

Decreased RBC production may be due to:

- **Lack of nutrients** (e.g., iron deficiency, vitamin B_{12}, or folate deficiency)

- **Bone marrow pathologies** including primary marrow defects such as aplastic anemia, or marrow infiltration by metastatic disease (inherited and acquired diseases of HSCs or of their committed derivatives are discussed above).
- **Marrow suppression** from medications, irradiation, etc.
- **Lack of marrow stimulatory hormones** (e.g., low erythropoietin from chronic kidney disease, hypothyroidism, or low androgens)
- **Anemia of inflammation,** which leads to low bioavailability of iron for erythropoiesis, mildly decreased erythropoietin and mildly decreased RBC lifespan

Iron-Deficiency Anemia
Iron deficiency interferes with normal heme (hemoglobin) synthesis and leads to impaired erythropoiesis and anemia. Iron deficiency is the most common cause of anemia worldwide.

 ETIOLOGIC FACTORS: The normal daily Western adult diet contains about 20 mg of iron. Approximately 1- to 2-mg iron is absorbed by the duodenum and proximal jejunum (see Chapter 20) to compensate for physiologic losses via sloughing of iron containing skin or mucosal cells. Anemia (especially with ineffective erythropoiesis) triggers increased intestinal absorption. About 85% of absorbed iron is transported by a carrier protein, transferrin, to be incorporated into developing red cells via transferrin receptors on their surface. As senescent red cells are removed from circulation, hemoglobin is broken down into its components, and iron is recycled. Excess iron is stored as **hemosiderin** and **ferritin**. Hemosiderin consists of large aggregates of iron with a disorganized structure; ferritin is complexed with protein (apoferritin) and appears highly organized.

Many underlying conditions cause iron deficiency. In infants and children, dietary iron may be insufficient for growth and development. Iron requirements also increase during **pregnancy** and **lactation**. In adults, iron deficiency typically results from **chronic blood loss** or, less often, **intravascular hemolysis.** Two milliliters of whole blood contain 1 mg of iron, which is lost with bleeding. In women of reproductive age, **gynecologic blood loss** (menstruation, parturition, vaginal bleeding) is most common. In postmenopausal women and men, unexplained iron deficiency should prompt a search for gastrointestinal **tumors** or **vascular lesions,** as this is the most common site of chronic blood loss.

 PATHOLOGY: Iron deficiency causes a **microcytic, hypochromic** anemia (Fig. 26-9). Variations in RBC size (**anisocytosis**) and shape (**poikilocytosis**) are reflected in increased RDW. **Ovalocytes** may be found; some of these are very thin and are called **pencil cells.** Iron deficiency causes an RBC production defect, so marrow erythroid hyperplasia occurs but blood reticulocytosis does not. Prussian blue staining of marrow aspirates shows absence of storage iron and erythroid iron.

Serum iron and ferritin levels are low in iron deficiency, while total iron-binding capacity (TIBC) is increased (because of increased serum transferrin levels). As a result, transferrin saturation is conspicuously lower (often <5%).

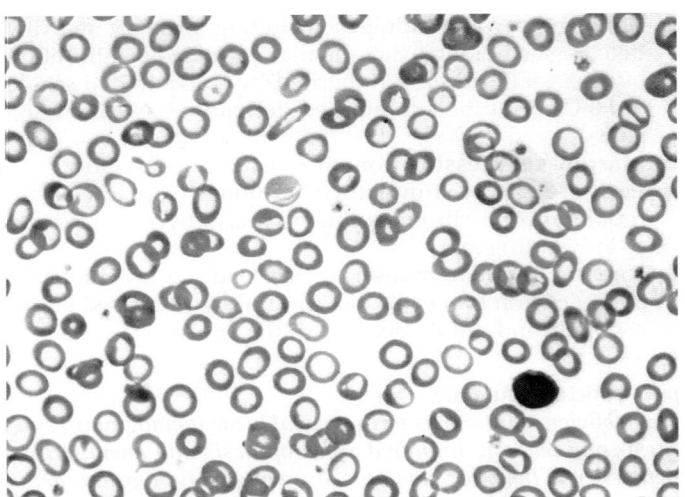

FIGURE 26-9. Microcytic hypochromic anemia caused by iron deficiency. Red blood cells (RBCs) are significantly smaller than the nucleus of a small lymphocyte, and they have increased central pallor (normal central pallor is about one-third of the RBC diameter).

CLINICAL FEATURES: Symptoms of iron deficiency are those of anemia in general. With advanced disease, a smooth and glistening tongue (**atrophic glossitis**) and inflammation at the corners of the mouth (**angular stomatitis**) may occur, as may a spoon-shaped deformity of the fingernails (**koilonychia**). Treatment requires identification and cessation of the source of chronic blood loss, and oral or parenteral iron supplementation.

Anemia of Inflammation

Anemia of inflammation (also known as anemia of chronic disease) occurs in acute and chronic inflammatory states, including critical illness, chronic infections, malignancies, autoimmune diseases, renal disease, obesity, and aging.

PATHOPHYSIOLOGY: Inflammatory cytokines (e.g., IL-6, IL-1β) increase hepatic production of hepcidin, a 25-amino acid peptide that serves as a key regulator of iron homeostasis. Hepcidin blocks release of iron from macrophages to developing erythroid precursors and reduces intestinal absorption of iron, leading to a functional iron deficiency, even though iron stores may be normal or even increased. Other factors that may contribute to anemia of inflammation are shorter RBC life span, blunted renal EPO response to tissue hypoxia and poor bone marrow response to erythropoietin. *Thus, both iron sequestration and impaired erythropoiesis lead to anemia of inflammation.*

PATHOLOGY: Anemia of chronic disease is typically mild to moderate; red cells are often normocytic and normochromic, but can be microcytic. Prussian blue staining of marrow aspirates shows normal or increased iron in macrophages, but reduced erythroid iron. Serum iron levels tend to be low. However, unlike iron-deficiency anemia, TIBC also tends to be decreased (as is serum albumin). Reticulocyte counts are not appropriately increased for the degree of anemia. Successful treatment of the underlying disease restores normal hemoglobin levels.

Anemia of Renal Disease

PATHOPHYSIOLOGY: Some patients with chronic renal diseases develop anemia due to **decreased renal production of EPO**. The severity of anemia is proportional to the extent of renal insufficiency. Administration of recombinant EPO is the treatment of choice. A "uremic toxin," that suppresses erythroid precursors, and a minor hemolytic component, may contribute to the anemia of chronic renal disease.

PATHOLOGY: Anemia of chronic renal disease is normocytic and normochromic Erythrocytes may develop scalloped cell membranes (**Burr cells**). If renal insufficiency is due to malignant hypertension, red cells may be fragmented and form schistocytes.

Anemia Associated With Marrow Infiltration (Myelophthisic Anemia)

Myelophthisic anemia is a hypoproliferative anemia associated with marrow infiltration.

ETIOLOGIC FACTORS: Any infiltrative process (e.g., myelofibrosis, hematologic malignancies, metastatic carcinoma, or granulomatous disease) may replace normal hematopoietic elements and cause anemia (and often leukopenia and thrombocytopenia). In an attempt to maintain blood cell production, EMH may develop, mostly in the spleen and liver.

PATHOLOGY: Bone marrow infiltration causes moderate to severe normocytic anemia, with anisopoikilocytosis and teardrop cells. Circulating immature granulocytes and nucleated erythrocytes (**leukoerythroblastosis**) are common.

Anemia of Lead Poisoning

Lead poisoning results in anemia by interfering with several enzymes involved in heme synthesis (see Chapter 8).

In Ineffective Red Cell Production, There Are Fewer Circulating Erythrocytes

Various anemias result from abnormal erythrocyte production caused by ineffective hematopoiesis. In such cases, the bone marrow erythrocyte precursor pool is expanded. Thus, sufficient erythroid precursors are formed in the bone marrow, but erythrocytes do not enter the circulation.

Megaloblastic Anemias

Megaloblastic anemias are caused by impaired DNA synthesis, usually because of vitamin B$_{12}$ or folic acid deficiency.

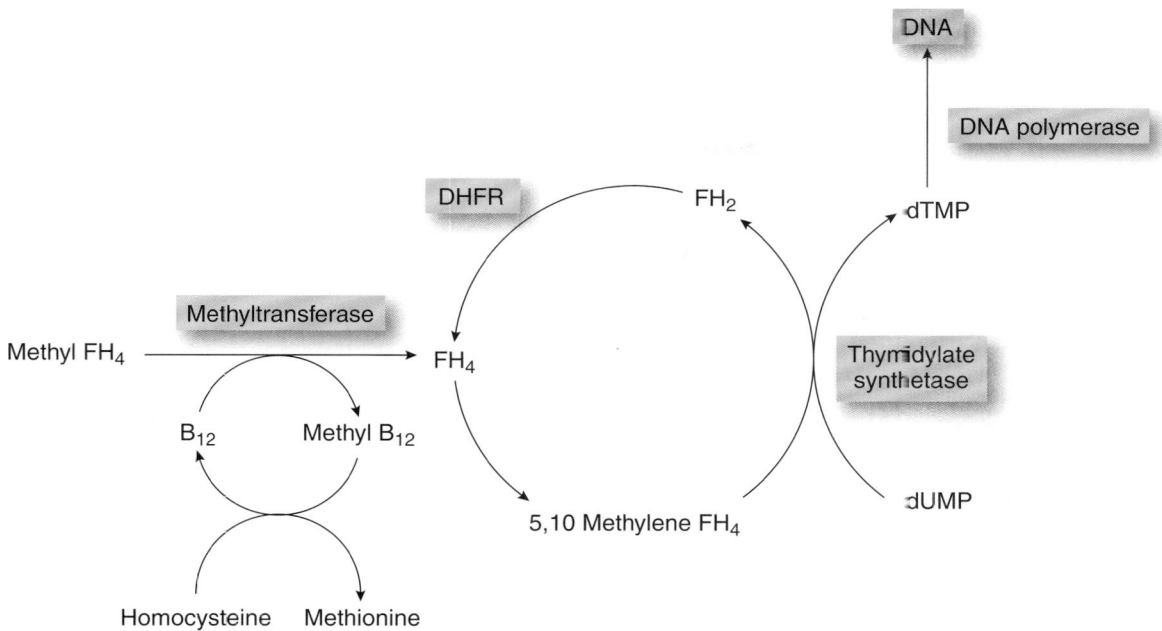

FIGURE 26-10. Relationship of folic acid to vitamin B$_{12}$. A 1-carbon transfer mediated by folic acid methylates dUMP to dTMP, which is then used for the synthesis of DNA. To enter this cycle, folate (methyl FH$_4$) is demethylated to FH$_4$, vitamin B$_{12}$ acting as the cofactor. Thus, both vitamin B$_{12}$ and folic acid deficiencies lead to impaired DNA synthesis and megaloblastic anemia. *DHFR* = dihydrofolate reductase: *dTMP* = deoxythymidine monophosphate; *dUMP* = deoxyuridine monophosphate; *FH$_2$* = dihydrofolate; *FH$_4$* = tetrahydrofolate.

 PATHOPHYSIOLOGY AND ETIOLOGIC FACTORS: Megaloblastic anemias are a group of diseases characterized by hallmark megaloblasts, which are abnormally large erythroid precursors. Impaired DNA synthesis leads to abnormal nuclear maturation. This, in turn, leads to ineffective erythrocyte maturation and anemia. All proliferating cell types, including myeloid precursors and cervical and gastrointestinal mucosal cells, are affected.

Megaloblastic anemia is most commonly due to vitamin B$_{12}$ or folate deficiency. Some chemotherapeutic agents (methotrexate, hydroxyurea) or antiretroviral drugs (5-azacytidine) may also be responsible. Inherited defects in purine or pyrimidine metabolism may rarely be involved.

Folate and vitamin B$_{12}$ are critical for normal DNA synthesis. The enzyme thymidylate synthetase converts uridylate to thymidylate using tetrahydrofolate as a cofactor. Tetrahydrofolate is converted from methyl tetrahydrofolate by methyltransferase, with vitamin B$_{12}$ as a cofactor. Vitamin B$_{12}$ is also required for the conversion of homocysteine to methionine (Fig. 26-10).

With impaired DNA synthesis, nuclear development is delayed, but the cytoplasm matures normally with progressive hemoglobinization. This leads to **nuclear-to-cytoplasmic asynchrony** and formation of large nucleated erythrocyte precursors (**megaloblasts**). Since these megaloblasts do not mature enough to be released into the blood, they undergo intramedullary destruction. Released erythrocytes are macrocytic.

Vitamin B$_{12}$ (cyanocobalamin) cannot be synthesized from precursors by humans and must come from diet.

It occurs in a variety of animal food sources and is also produced by intestinal microorganisms. Proper vitamin B$_{12}$ absorption requires intrinsic factor, which is produced in the stomach (see Chapter 19) and protects vitamin B$_{12}$ from degradation by intestinal enzymes (Fig. 26-11). The intrinsic factor–vitamin B$_{12}$ complex is absorbed in the distal ileum via specific receptors. In the blood, the vitamin is transported by proteins called **transcobalamins**, of which transcobalamin II is the most important. The daily usage of vitamin B$_{12}$ is 1 μg. Therefore, normal body stores of 1,000 to 5,000 μg provide several years of reserve.

Inadequate dietary intake of vitamin B$_{12}$ is rare and usually occurs only in strict vegetarians (vegans). *Most often, lack of intrinsic factor impairs its absorption.* Surgery that involves resection of the gastric fundus removes the source of intrinsic factor.

Pernicious anemia, an autoimmune disorder in which patients develop antibodies against parietal cells and intrinsic factor (see Chapter 19), leads to intrinsic factor deficiency. Antiparietal cell antibodies also cause atrophic gastritis with achlorhydria. Primary intestinal disorders (inflammatory bowel disease) or previous intestinal surgery (ileal bypass) can impair vitamin B$_{12}$ absorption. Microbiologic competition (e.g., from bacterial overgrowth of a blind loop or infestation by the fish tapeworm, *Diphyllobothrium latum*) can also lead to vitamin B$_{12}$ deficiency.

Folic acid is present in leafy vegetables, meat, and eggs. Dietary folic acid exists in a polyglutamate form but is deconjugated to monoglutamates in the intestines and absorbed primarily in the jejunum. Folate is then reduced and methylated to 5-methyl tetrahydrofolate, which is transported in the blood by folate-binding protein. The

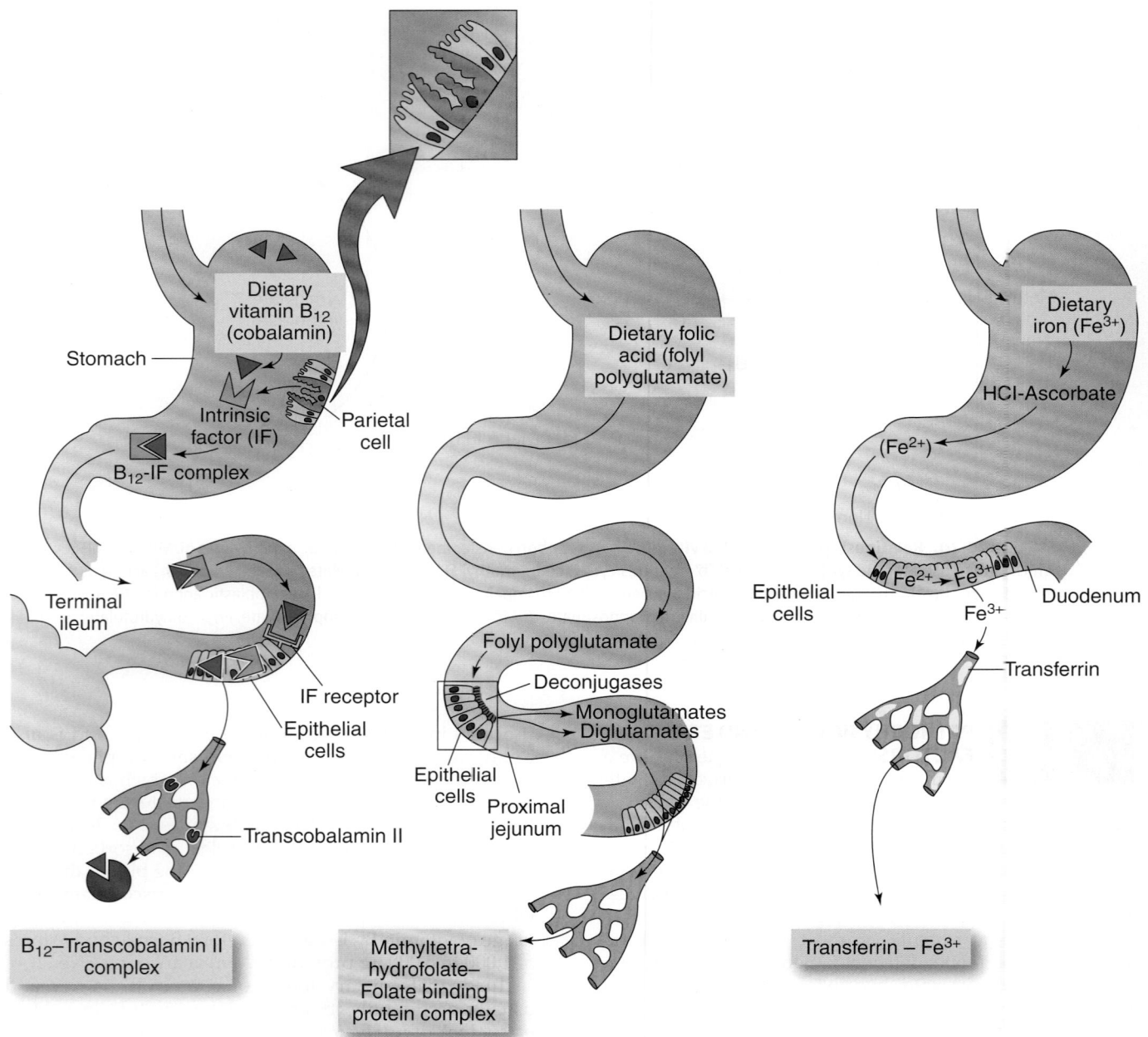

FIGURE 26-11. Absorption of vitamin B$_{12}$, folic acid, and iron. Absorption of vitamin B$_{12}$ requires initial complexing with intrinsic factor (IF), which is produced by the parietal cells of the gastric mucosa. Absorption then occurs in the terminal ileum, where there are receptors for the IF–B$_{12}$ complex. Dietary folic acid is conjugated by conjugase enzymes to polyglutamate. Absorption occurs in the jejunum following deconjugation in the intestinal lumen. Reduction and methylation result in the generation of methyl tetrahydrofolate, which is then transported by folate-binding protein. Dietary ferric iron (Fe^{3+}) is reduced to ferrous iron (Fe^{2+}) in the stomach and absorbed principally in the duodenum. Iron is transported by transferrin in the circulation.

daily requirement for folate is about 50 µg. Body stores of folate average 2,000 to 5,000 µg, providing a few months' reserve before signs of deficiency develop.

The most common cause of folic acid deficiency is inadequate dietary intake. This occurs mostly in patients with poor diets (alcoholics, recluses). Demand for folic acid is increased in pregnancy, lactation, periods of rapid growth, and chronic hemolytic disease. During such times, folate deficiency may occur unless folate supplementation is provided. Primary intestinal diseases (inflammatory bowel disease, sprue) may interfere with folic acid absorption. Various medications can also impair folic acid absorption (phenytoin) or metabolism (methotrexate).

PATHOLOGY: The hematologic manifestations of folic acid and vitamin B$_{12}$ deficiencies are identical. Hematopoiesis in the bone marrow tends to be increased, but the marrow releases insufficient mature, functional cells because of increased intramedullary cell

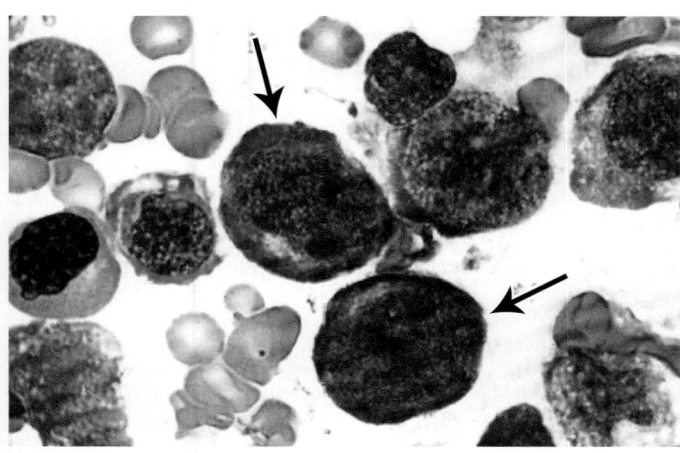

FIGURE 26-12. Megaloblastic anemia. A bone marrow aspirate from a patient with vitamin B₁₂ deficiency (pernicious anemia) shows prominent megaloblastic erythroid precursors (*arrows*).

death. This is called **ineffective hematopoiesis**. RBC precursors show megaloblastic maturation, in which cells enlarge (Fig. 26-12). The cytoplasm matures with progressive hemoglobinization but nuclear maturation lags and nuclei remain large, with more open, granular chromatin. The myeloid series shows similar dyssynchrony, with giant bands and metamyelocytes, and hypersegmented nuclei in mature granulocytes. Megakaryocytes may also be large.

The magnitude of anemia varies but may be severe. Erythrocytes are macrocytic and may be oval (oval macrocytes). Anisopoikilocytosis is usually prominent, sometimes with teardrop cells. Circulating neutrophils often show nuclear hypersegmentation (>5 lobes) (Fig. 26-13). Reticulocytes are not increased, but platelet counts may be decreased.

Because of massive intramedullary destruction of red cell precursors, serum levels of lactate dehydrogenase (LDH), especially isoenzyme 1, and bilirubin are elevated.

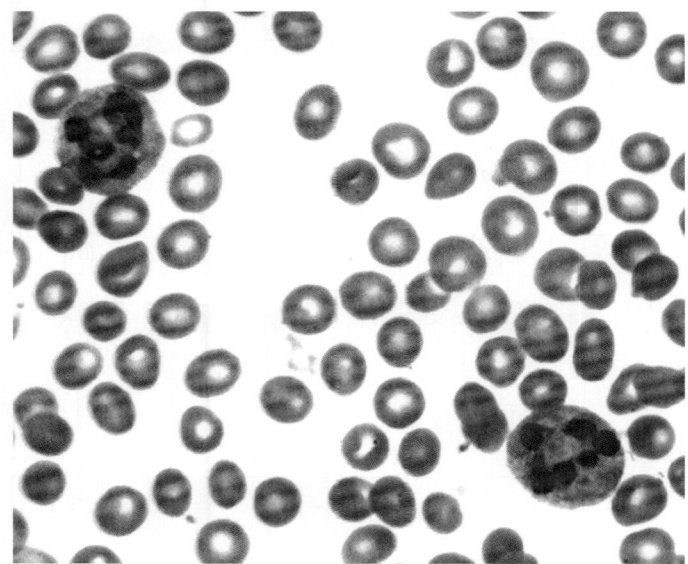

FIGURE 26-13. Hypersegmented granulocytes in a patient with vitamin B₁₂ deficiency.

Folate and vitamin B₁₂ deficiencies are usually distinguished by measuring serum levels of these vitamins. Red cell folate levels are not affected by recent dietary intake and provide information regarding folate levels in the preceding 3 to 4 months. However, low RBC folate can also be seen in vitamin B₁₂ deficiency.

Serum B₁₂ assays may yield false-positive and false-negative results and are particularly problematic in patients with intrinsic factor antibodies. Serum **homocysteine** and **methyl malonic acid (MMA)** are elevated in a majority of patients with untreated clinical vitamin B₁₂ deficiency and are therefore useful in diagnosis, particularly in patients with borderline B₁₂ levels. MMA is more sensitive and specific. Circulating **antibodies against gastric parietal cells or intrinsic factor** are present in cases of pernicious anemia. The former antibody is more often detected, but the latter is more specific for pernicious anemia. The Schilling test was used historically to determine the cause of B₁₂ deficiency. It involved measuring radiolabeled vitamin B₁₂ absorption, with or without intrinsic factor, along with urinary B₁₂ (this test is no longer employed). Chronic atrophic gastritis can be diagnosed by endoscopic biopsy, elevated fasting serum gastrin level or a low level of serum pepsinogen I.

CLINICAL FEATURES: The clinical presentation of megaloblastic anemia is similar, whether due to B₁₂ or folate deficiency. The latter tends to develop more rapidly (months) than the former (years). The most important difference clinically is that B₁₂ deficiency is complicated by neurologic symptoms, owing to posterior and lateral column demyelination in the spinal cord. This may cause sensory and motor deficiencies (see Chapters 8 and 32). Unless treated quickly, these neurologic symptoms may become irreversible. Folate deficiency involves no such complications.

Thalassemias

Thalassemias are congenital anemias caused by deficient globin chain synthesis. Depending on the affected globin chain, α-thalassemia (defective α-chain production), β-thalassemia (defective β-chain production), δβ-thalassemia (defective δ- and β-chain production) or γδβ-thalassemia (defective γ-, δ-, and β-chain production) result.

The basic defect is generally a "quantitative abnormality" with reduced or absent production of the respective globin chains (i.e., reduced levels of β-globin in β-thalassemia or α-globin in α-thalassemia). A minority of thalassemia cases have "qualitative abnormalities" with structural hemoglobin variants yielding unstable globins with effective decreases in quantity. Since α- and β-chains normally pair to form hemoglobin tetramers, the lack of one type of chain leads to unpaired normal globin chains in thalassemic erythrocytes. In β-thalassemia, excess normal α-chains form an unstable structure that precipitates at the cell membrane. This makes the RBCs very fragile, and they are destroyed within the bone marrow. In α-thalassemia, excess β-chains (appearing in extrauterine life) form tetramers called HbH (β4). In intrauterine life, excess γ-chains form tetramers called HbBarts (γ4). Both of these abnormal hemoglobins are unstable and there is excessive RBC destruction.

TABLE 26-10

MAJOR FORMS OF HEMOGLOBIN AND THEIR CHAIN COMPOSITION

Type of Hemoglobin	Contribution of Globin Chains						Explanation
	ζ	ε	α	β	γ	δ	
Very early fetal life (4–8 weeks of gestation)							
Gower 1	2	2					Two ζ (zeta) chains are the α-like chains which combine with two ε (epsilon) chains; replaced by fetal hemoglobin after 8 weeks of gestation
Gower 2		2	2				Replaced by fetal hemoglobin after 8 weeks of gestation
Portland	2				2		Hemoglobin present very early in fetal life. May persist in very severe α-thalassemia.
Fetus and early infancy							
F			2		2		Normal hemoglobin for most of intrauterine life. Production usually ends by early infancy; hemoglobin F is largely undetectable after 6 months of age. Persists in β-thalassemia.
Late infancy to adults							
A			2	2			Principal normal hemoglobin (>95% of total) in postnatal life.
A_2			2			2	Usually <3% of total hemoglobin, but may be slightly increased in β-thalassemia.
Abnormal hemoglobins							
H				4			Mainly seen in α-thalassemia, where deficiency of α-chains leads to hemoglobins composed of β-chain tetramers. Responsible for formation of Heinz bodies.
Bart's					4		Seen in babies with α-thalassemia. Heinz bodies seen.

EPIDEMIOLOGY: Thalassemia is most common in the Mediterranean area, especially in Italy and Greece. However, it has a wide distribution, particularly in areas where malaria has been endemic (Middle East, India, Southeast Asia, China). Heterozygosity for thalassemia may help protect against malaria and increase the reproductive potential of heterozygotes, which may explain how these disease alleles persist. In many geographic areas where thalassemia is common, other structural hemoglobin defects (e.g., hemoglobin S [HgbS]) are also frequent. This can lead to double heterozygosity (e.g., sickle thalassemia), which demonstrates features of both disorders.

There are four α-genes, two on each chromosome 16. Non–α-genes are on chromosome 11, two γ–, one δ–, and one β-gene per chromosome. Embryonic globin genes zeta (ζ) (α equivalent) and epsilon (ε) (non–α equivalent) are on chromosomes 16 and 11, respectively. The most important types of hemoglobin and the globin chains that contribute to each are presented in Table 26-10.

MOLECULAR PATHOGENESIS: Normal hemoglobin contains four globin chains: two α- and two non–α-chains. There are three normal hemoglobin variants, based on the nature of the non–α-chains (Fig. 26-14). *Adult hemoglobin is 95% to 98% HgbA ($\alpha_2\beta_2$), plus small amounts of HgbF ($\alpha_2\gamma_2$) and A_2 ($\alpha_2\delta_2$).*

Thalassemias are generally classified by the affected globin chain. The two most clinically significant forms involve deficits of α- and β-chains. Thalassemias involving γ- and δ-globin chain synthesis occur but are not common.

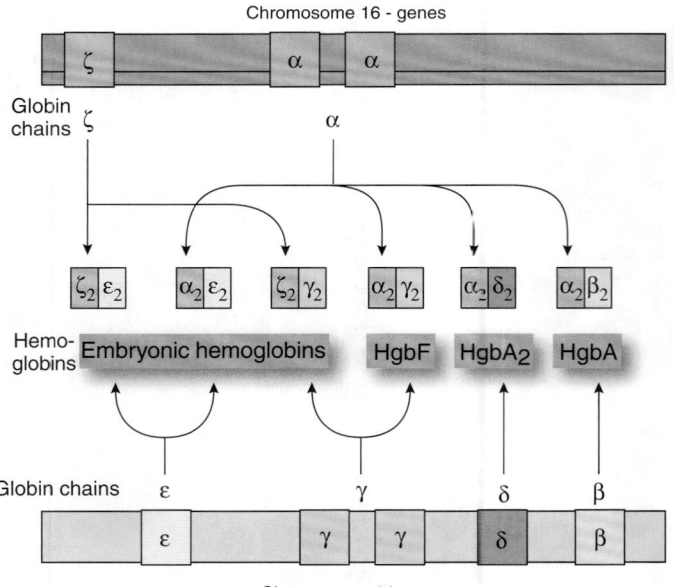

FIGURE 26-14. Hemoglobin assembly scheme using globin chains coded on chromosomes 11 and 16.

β-Thalassemia

MOLECULAR PATHOGENESIS: β-Thalassemias are a heterogeneous group of disorders that are mostly caused by point mutations in *HBB*, the β-globin gene. Mutations may reside in the promoter region, at a splice site or in other coding regions, or may lead to creation of an inappropriate stop codon. The result is that transcription of the gene is entirely (β⁰) or partly (β⁺) suppressed. Occasionally, a mutation may also affect the adjacent δ-globin gene, *HBD*, leading to a βδ-thalassemia, or the γ- and δ-genes, leading to γδβ-thalassemia.

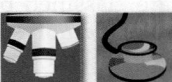

PATHOLOGY AND CLINICAL FEATURES: Homozygous β-thalassemia (Cooley anemia) is characterized by moderate to severe, microcytic and hypochromic anemia (Figs. 26-15 and 26-16). There is a marked excess of α-chains, which form unstable tetramers (α_4) that precipitate in the cytoplasm of developing erythroid precursors. In the β⁰ type, most hemoglobin is fetal hemoglobin ($\alpha_2\gamma_2$), although increased (5% to 8%) HgbA₂ ($\alpha_2\beta_2$) is also present. In the β⁺ type, some HgbA may be present (depending on the nature of the underlying defect) and HgbA₂ is mildly increased. A modest increase in HgbA₂ is characteristic of all forms of β-thalassemia, as δ-globin genes are upregulated.

Blood smears show microcytosis, hypochromia and striking anisopoikilocytosis (uneven size and shape) with target cells, basophilic stippling and circulating normoblasts (especially after splenectomy). The increased oxygen-binding affinity of HgbF plus the underlying anemia, impairs oxygen delivery and elicits increased EPO. The latter causes marked bone marrow erythroid hyperplasia. The marrow space is expanded, which can cause facial and cranial bone deformities. EMH contributes to hepatosplenomegaly and may cause soft tissue masses.

Excess erythropoiesis stimulates iron absorption. This, together with repeated transfusions, causes iron overload. Excess iron deposition in tissues leads to morbidity and mortality in thalassemic patients and often requires aggressive chelation therapy.

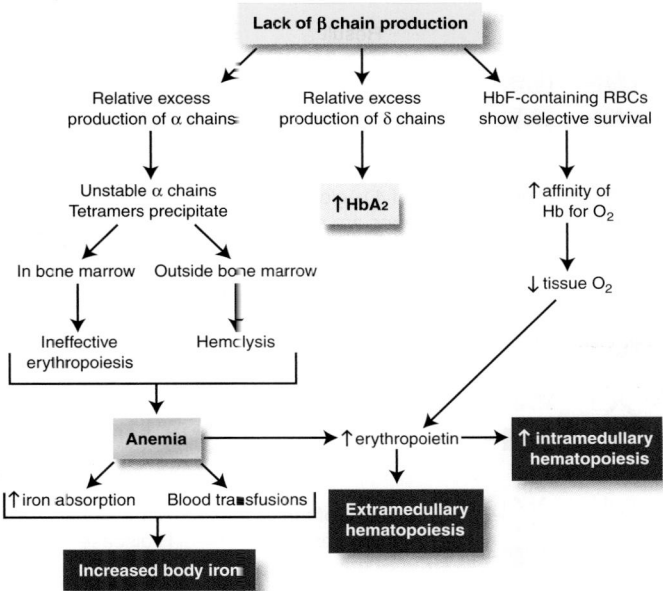

FIGURE 26-16. Pathogenesis of disease manifestations in β-thalassemia.

Heterozygous β-thalassemia (heterozygous carrier of β-thalassemia) is associated with microcytosis and hypochromia. The degree of microcytosis is disproportionate to the severity of the anemia, which is generally mild or absent. Erythrocytosis (increased RBC count) with minimal anisocytosis (normal RDW) is common. Target cells, basophilic stippling, increased reticulocytes and a mild increase in HgbA₂ (3.5% to 6%) are present. Most patients are asymptomatic. Iron absorption is increased.

α-Thalassemia

MOLECULAR PATHOGENESIS: α-Thalassemias are most often due to gene deletions. More syndromes are clinically observed because of the potential number (up to four) of α-globin genes that may be affected. The genetics of the several α-thalassemias are illustrated in Figure 26-17. α-Thalassemia is associated with excess β- or γ-chains, which can form tetrameric HgbH (β_4) and Hgb Bart (γ_4). Hemoglobins H and Bart are both unstable and precipitate in the cytoplasm, forming Heinz bodies, but to a lesser degree than α_4 tetramers. Further, they have high oxygen affinities and cause decreased tissue oxygen delivery. The relative amount of these tetrameric hemoglobins depends on the number of α-genes involved and the patient's age. Because of the underlying impairment in hemoglobin synthesis, circulating red cells usually are microcytic and hypochromic.

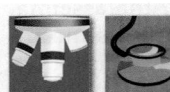

PATHOLOGY AND CLINICAL FEATURES:

- **Silent carrier α-thalassemia** (one gene affected) is difficult to diagnose, because the only hematologic abnormality is small amounts of Hgb Bart (γ4), detectable

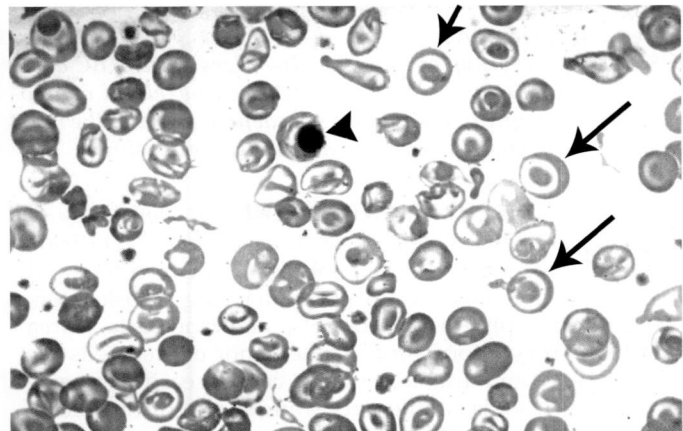

FIGURE 26-15. Thalassemia. The peripheral blood erythrocytes are hypochromic and microcytic and show anisopoikilocytosis with frequent target cells (*arrows*) and circulating nucleated red blood cells (*arrowhead*).

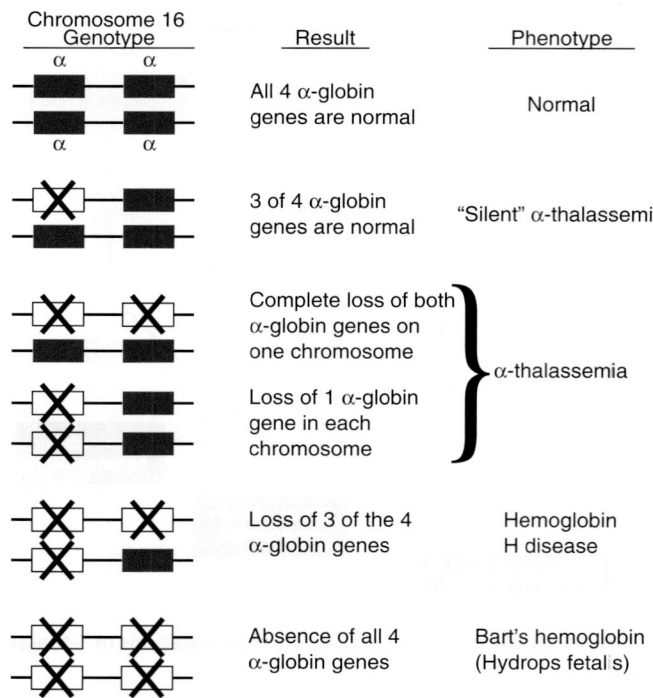

Chromosome 16 Genotype	Result	Phenotype
α α	All 4 α-globin genes are normal	Normal
	3 of 4 α-globin genes are normal	"Silent" α-thalassemia
	Complete loss of both α-globin genes on one chromosome	α-thalassemia
	Loss of 1 α-globin gene in each chromosome	
	Loss of 3 of the 4 α-globin genes	Hemoglobin H disease
	Absence of all 4 α-globin genes	Bart's hemoglobin (Hydrops fetalis)

FIGURE 26-17. Genetics of α-globin deficiencies and their manifestations.

only in infancy. There is no anemia and patients are asymptomatic.

- **α-Thalassemia trait** (two genes affected) is associated with a mild microcytic anemia. Like heterozygous β-thalassemia, the degree of microcytosis is disproportionately low compared to the degree of anemia. HgbA$_2$ is not increased, allowing distinction between α- and β-thalassemia traits. Up to 5% Hgb Bart can be seen during infancy.

    Two different genotypes are possible in heterozygous α-thalassemia. A single gene may be deleted from each chromosome 16 (i.e., in *trans*) or, alternatively, both genes may be deleted from the same chromosome 16 (i.e., in *cis*). The former is more common in people of Mediterranean and African descent, while the latter occurs more often in Southeast Asia. Clinically, both genotypes present similarly, but homozygous α-thalassemia (see below) can only develop if both genes are deleted from the same chromosome.

- **Hemoglobin H disease** (three genes affected) is associated with moderate microcytic anemia. Increased Hgb Bart (up to 25% in infancy) and variable levels of HgbH (β$_4$) are seen. Both HgbH and Hgb Bart give characteristic patterns on hemoglobin electrophoresis, since they migrate faster than HgbA. Precipitated HgbH (Heinz bodies) appears on supravital staining of blood smears.

- **Homozygous** (all four genes affected) **α-thalassemia,** also called α hydrops fetalis or Bart fetalis, is incompatible with life. After the first trimester, when production of embryonal hemoglobin declines, HgbF (α$_2$γ$_2$) production cannot take place due to lack of α-globin chains. Affected fetuses develop severe anemia, marked anisopoikilocytosis and large amounts of Hgb Bart (γ$_4$).

Severe impairment in tissue oxygen delivery is associated with heart failure and generalized edema. Massive hepatosplenomegaly is due to EMH. A woman carrying a fetus with Hgb Bart has increased risk for obstetric complications, including eclampsia and postpartum bleeding. Affected fetuses die in utero, generally by late second trimester, or shortly after birth.

Hemolytic Anemias Result From Increased Red Cell Destruction

Hemolysis (i.e., premature elimination of circulating RBCs) causes **hemolytic anemia**. These anemias are classified by the site of red cell destruction. In **extravascular hemolysis,** the monocyte/macrophage system in the spleen and, to a lesser extent, the liver, is involved. In **intravascular hemolysis,** RBCs are destroyed while circulating.

Hemolytic anemias are characterized by a compensatory increase in red cell production and release. In the blood, this manifests as red cell polychromasia because of increased reticulocytes. Other laboratory findings commonly associated with hemolysis include increased LDH (particularly isoenzyme 1) and unconjugated (indirect) bilirubin, decreased haptoglobin, free (extracellular) hemoglobin in the blood and urine, increased urobilinogen and urine hemosiderin.

Hemolytic anemias may be caused by factors "extrinsic" to the RBC (e.g., immune, mechanical, thermal, osmotic causes) or factors "intrinsic" to the RBCs (e.g., defects in the RBC membrane, hemoglobinopathies, or enzymopathies).

Erythrocyte Membrane Defects

Normal erythrocyte membranes are remarkably deformable, which allows red cells to pass unimpaired through the microcirculation and splenic vasculature. The red cell membrane consists of a phospholipid bilayer linked to an underlying cytoskeleton, composed primarily of a dimer of α- and β-spectrin subunits and other erythrocyte specific cytoskeletal components (Fig. 26-6). Ankyrin (band 2.1) anchors spectrin to transmembrane proteins (band 3, anion exchanger proteins), while spectrin is bound to actin and glycophorin by protein 4.1. *Alterations in any part of the red cell membrane can impair RBC plasticity, impacting the "vertical linkages" and rendering erythrocytes susceptible to hemolysis.*

Hereditary Spherocytosis
HS is a diverse group of inherited disorders of the RBC cytoskeleton, in which spectrin or another cytoskeletal component (ankyrin, protein 4.2, band 3) is deficient. HS is the most common congenital hemolytic anemia in Caucasians.

 MOLECULAR PATHOGENESIS: Deficiency of any cytoskeletal protein leads to a **"vertical"** defect in red cell membranes, in which the lipid bilayer is uncoupled from the underlying cytoskeleton. The result is progressive loss of membrane surface area and **spherocyte** formation. These abnormal red cells are more rigid and fragile, and so cannot easily traverse splenic sinusoids. While circulating through the spleen, spherocytes lose additional surface membrane, become trapped and ultimately succumb to extravascular hemolysis. About 75% of HS cases are inherited as autosomal

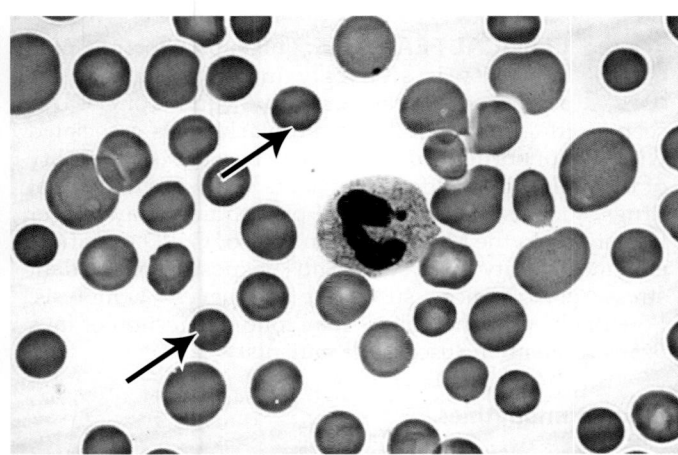

FIGURE 26-18. Hereditary spherocytosis. The peripheral blood smear shows frequent spherocytes with decreased diameter, intense staining, and lack of central pallor (*arrows*).

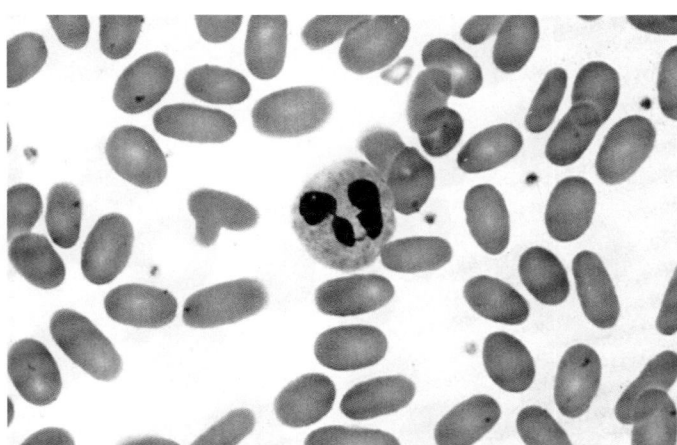

FIGURE 26-19. Hereditary elliptocytosis. A peripheral blood smear reveals that virtually all of the erythrocytes are elliptical with parallel sides.

dominant traits involving variants in at least five genes. About half of cases are related to dominant mutations in *ANK1*, which encodes the ankyrin that links spectrin to specific transmembrane proteins. Rare recessive cases of HS involve defects in the spectrin α-subunit.

PATHOLOGY: Most patients with HS have a moderate normocytic anemia. Conspicuous spherocytes that appear hyperchromic (no central pallor) are typical, along with polychromasia and reticulocytosis (Fig. 26-18). The bone marrow shows erythroid hyperplasia. Although typical spherocytes have low MCV because of membrane loss and cell dehydration, these patients may have normal MCV due to the presence of increased reticulocytes (which are larger than average RBCs).

Spherocytes show greater **osmotic fragility** than normal erythrocytes. Laboratory findings are typical of hemolysis: decreased haptoglobin, increased indirect bilirubin, increased LDH.

CLINICAL FEATURES: Most patients have splenomegaly caused by chronic extravascular hemolysis. They may appear jaundiced, and up to 50% develop cholelithiasis, with pigmented (bilirubin) gallstones. Despite chronic hemolysis, transfusion is not usually needed. An exception is a sudden decline in hemoglobin and reticulocytes, which herald **aplastic crisis** (usually caused by infection by parvovirus B19). Anemia may also become more severe in the so-called **hemolytic crisis,** when hemolysis accelerates transiently. Patients with HS can be managed effectively by splenectomy, although spherocytes still persist in the circulation. Splenectomy, however, renders patients more susceptible to certain infections, particularly with *Streptococcus* spp.

Hereditary Elliptocytosis
Hereditary elliptocytosis (HE) is a diverse group of inherited disorders affecting the erythrocyte cytoskeleton.

MOLECULAR PATHOGENESIS: HE is characterized by elliptical or oval RBCs. The most commonly described HE variants include defects in self-assembly of spectrin, spectrin–ankyrin binding, protein 4.1, and glycophorin C. RBCs have an area of central pallor, since there is no loss of the lipid bilayer (as seen in HS). Most forms of HE are autosomal dominant. Most cases are due to mutations in genes encoding α-spectrin (*SPTA1*), β-spectrin (*SPTB*), or protein 4.1 (*EPB41*).

PATHOLOGY AND CLINICAL FEATURES: HE is more common in malaria endemic regions of West Africa. Patients with HE usually have only mild normocytic anemia. Many are asymptomatic. Blood smears show many elliptocytes with only minimal reticulocytosis (Fig. 26-19). Generally, HE has less hemolysis and subsequent anemia than are seen with HS. Occasional patients with more severe hemolysis may require splenectomy.

Acanthocytosis
Acanthocytosis results from a defect within the red cell membrane lipid bilayer and features irregularly spaced spiny projections of the surface, which may be associated with hemolysis.

PATHOPHYSIOLOGY: The most common cause is chronic liver disease, in which increased free cholesterol accumulates in cell membranes. Acanthocytes also occur in abetalipoproteinemia, an autosomal recessive disorder with lipid membrane abnormalities (see Chapter 19).

PATHOLOGY AND CLINICAL FEATURES: Abnormalities in their lipid membranes cause erythrocytes to deform and develop irregular spiny surface projections and centrally dense cytoplasm (no central pallor) (Fig. 26-20). These **acanthocytes** (spur cells) should be distinguished from burr

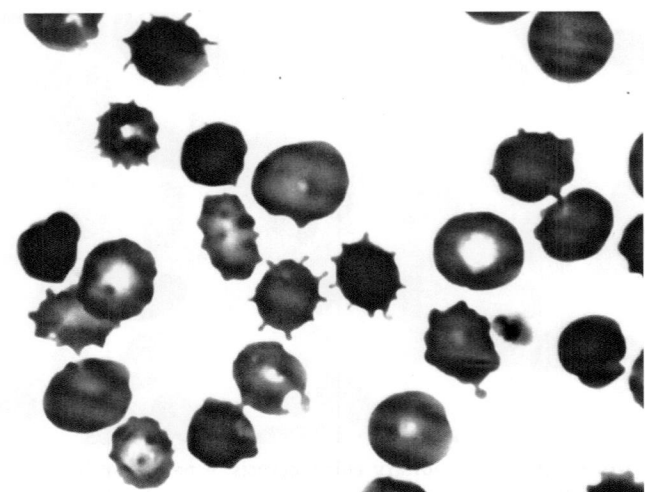

FIGURE 26-20. Acanthocytes. The red cells lack central pallor and display irregular spikes on the surface.

cells (crenated cells, **echinocytes**), which show more uniform membrane scalloping and maintain their central pallor. Hemolysis and anemia are mild in acanthocytosis.

Enzyme Defects

Erythrocytes generate ATP mainly by glycolysis. Inherited defects of enzymes in the glycolytic pathway can predispose circulating red cells to hemolysis. The most common enzyme defect involves glucose-6-phosphate dehydrogenase (G6PD), which catalyzes conversion of glucose-6-phosphate to 6-phosphogluconate. Deficiencies of other glycolytic enzymes are rare and have autosomal recessive inheritance. Among these, pyruvate kinase deficiency is the most common. Clinically, these defects cause variable degrees of anemia and are classified as **hereditary nonspherocytic anemias**.

G6PD deficiency is an X-linked disease in which RBCs are abnormally sensitive to oxidative stress, which triggers hemolytic anemia. G6PD deficiency is most common in areas where malaria is historically endemic, notably Africa and the Mediterranean. The various *G6PD* mutations appear to protect somewhat against malaria.

PATHOPHYSIOLOGY: Since G6PD helps to recycle reduced glutathione, red cells deficient in this enzyme are susceptible to oxidative stress (e.g., as caused by infections, drugs, or fava bean ingestion [favism]). Hemoglobin oxidation generates methemoglobin, in which Fe^{2+} ions are converted to ferric (Fe^{3+}) ions. Methemoglobin cannot transport oxygen, is unstable and precipitates in the cytoplasm as Heinz bodies. These precipitates increase cell rigidity and lead to hemolysis.

PATHOLOGY: In quiescent periods, erythrocytes in G6PD deficiency appear normal. But, in a hemolytic episode precipitated by oxidative stress, Heinz bodies appear with supravital staining. Passage through the spleen may remove part of RBC membranes, to form the so-called **bite cells**.

CLINICAL FEATURES: Full expression of G6PD deficiency is seen only in males; females are asymptomatic carriers. The A variant of G6PD is seen in 10% to 15% of American blacks. It is associated with 10% of normal enzyme activity because of instability of the molecule. In affected patients, exposure to oxidant drugs, such as the antimalarial primaquine, may trigger hemolysis. In the Mediterranean type of G6PD mutation, enzyme activity is absent. Thus, exposure to oxidant stress sets off more sustained and severe hemolysis. Potentially lethal hemolysis may follow ingestion of fava beans **(favism)** in susceptible patients.

Hemoglobinopathies

Most clinically relevant hemoglobinopathies are caused by point mutations in the β-globin chain gene.

Sickle Cell Disease

In sickle cell disease, an abnormal hemoglobin, HgbS, causes RBCs to sickle upon deoxygenation.

EPIDEMIOLOGY: HgbS is most common in people of African ancestry, although the gene is also present in Mediterranean, Middle Eastern and Indian people. In some regions of Africa, up to 40% of the population is heterozygous for HgbS. Ten percent of African-Americans are heterozygous and 1 in 650 is homozygous. Heterozygosity for HgbS may partially protect against falciparum malaria. Infected erythrocytes selectively sickle and are removed from the circulation by splenic and hepatic macrophages, effectively destroying the parasite.

MOLECULAR PATHOGENESIS: A point mutation in *HBB*, the gene for the β-globin chain, substitutes valine for glutamic acid at the 6th amino acid. This single change makes an unstable molecule that polymerizes upon deoxygenation. Polymerization of HgbS transforms the cytoplasm into a rigid filamentous gel and produces less deformable sickle-shaped erythrocytes.

The rigidity of sickled erythrocytes obstructs the microcirculation, leading to tissue hypoxia and ischemic injury in many organs. The inflexibility of sickled cells also renders them susceptible to destruction (hemolysis) during passage through the spleen. Thus, the two primary manifestations of sickle cell disease are recurrent ischemic events and chronic extravascular hemolytic anemia.

At first, reoxygenation reverses sickling, but after several cycles of sickling and unsickling, the process becomes irreversible. Sickled erythrocytes also have changes in their membrane phospholipids, and so adhere more strongly to endothelial cells. This further impairs capillary blood flow.

People homozygous for HgbS show the full clinical picture of sickle cell disease. A sickling disorder also occurs in patients who are doubly heterozygous (i.e., are compound heterozygotes) for two β-chain mutations (e.g., HgbSC disease, sickle/β-thalassemia). Heterozygotes for HgbS (sickle trait), however, do not develop red cell sickling, because their HgbA prevents HgbS polymerization. HgbF

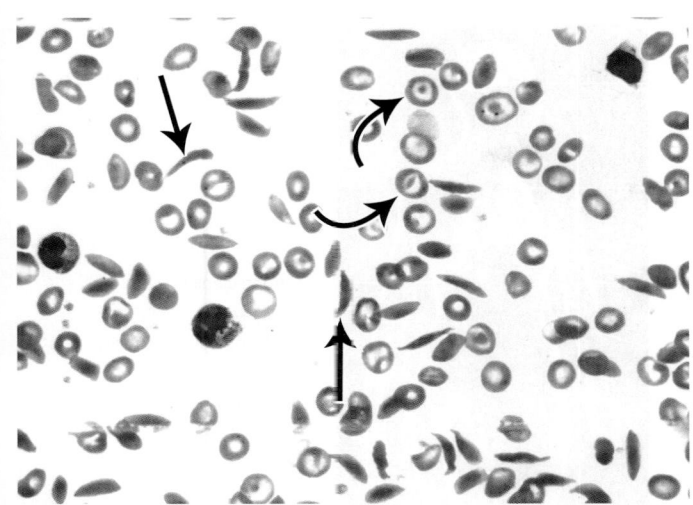

FIGURE 26-21. Sickle cell anemia. Sickled cells (*straight arrows*) and target cells (*curved arrows*) are evident in the blood smear.

also interferes with HgbS polymerization, and patients who are homozygous for HgbS and have increased HgbF have a milder form of disease.

PATHOLOGY: Homozygous patients (HgbSS) have severe normocytic or macrocytic anemia. The macrocytosis reflects increased numbers of reticulocytes, owing to chronic hemolysis. Blood smears show marked anisopoikilocytosis and polychromasia. There are classic sickle cells and target cells, as well as other abnormally shaped erythrocytes (Fig. 26-21). Howell–Jolly bodies, which represent nuclear remnants, are evident in most patients beyond childhood and reflect hyposplenism because of ischemic infarction of splenic tissue.

Electrophoretic analysis shows that HgbS accounts for 80% to 95% of total hemoglobin; HgbA is absent. HgbF and HgbA$_2$ make up the remaining hemoglobin.

CLINICAL FEATURES: Infants with SS hemoglobin are asymptomatic for the first 8 to 10 weeks of life, because they have high levels of HgbF. Clinical symptoms first appear in children as synthesis of γ-globin chains declines. This decline is somewhat delayed in homozygous S patients. Although patients suffer from lifelong hemolysis, adaptation occurs over time and most may not require regular transfusions. Instead, the clinical picture is dominated by sequelae of repeated **vaso-occlusive disease**. In an attempt to minimize these complications by decreasing the amount of HgbS in circulation, chronic exchange transfusions may be necessary. Sickle cell anemia is a systemic disorder and eventually impairs the functions of most organ systems and tissues (Fig. 26-22).

Patients with sickle cell disease develop episodic painful crises, which vary in number. Capillary occlusion leads to ischemia and hypoxic cell injury, which cause severe pain, especially in the chest, abdomen, and bones. Painful crises can be triggered by various stimuli (e.g., underlying infection, acidosis, or dehydration).

APLASTIC CRISIS: In aplastic crisis, the bone marrow fails to compensate for the high level of red cell loss. Hemoglobin levels drop rapidly, with no reticulocyte response. Parvovirus B19 is the most frequent cause of an aplastic crisis, although other viral and bacterial infections may also cause transient bone marrow suppression.

SEQUESTRATION CRISIS: In this situation, sudden pooling of erythrocytes, especially in the spleen, decreases circulating blood volume and lowers hemoglobin levels. The etiology is unclear, but it occurs most often in young children who still have functioning spleens. This complication is followed by hypovolemic shock and is the most common cause of death early in life. Organs affected by sickle cell disease include:

- **Heart:** Chronic demand for increased cardiac output may lead to cardiomegaly and heart failure. In addition, obstruction of coronary microcirculation may cause myocardial ischemia. Myocyte function may also be impaired by excess iron deposition, owing to chronic hemolysis and repeated transfusions.
- **Lungs:** Up to 1/3 of patients with sickle cell anemia may rapidly lose respiratory function, with pulmonary infiltrates on chest radiography. This **acute chest syndrome** may be fatal. Pulmonary infarction can occur, and sickle cell patients are more susceptible to a variety of pulmonary infections.
- **Spleen:** Splenomegaly often occurs in childhood, but repeated splenic infarction leads to functional autosplenectomy. In most adults, only a small fibrous remnant of the spleen remains. The asplenic state increases susceptible to infections with encapsulated bacteria, especially *Pneumococcus*.
- **Brain:** Patients with sickle cell anemia develop neurologic complications related to vascular obstruction, including transient ischemic attacks, strokes, and cerebral hemorrhages. Occlusion of retinal microvasculature may lead to retinal hemorrhage and detachment, proliferative retinopathy and blindness.
- **Kidney/GU tract:** The hypoxic, acidotic, and hypertonic environment in the renal medulla often leads to sickling there. This impairs the ability to concentrate the urine and causes renal infarcts and papillary necrosis. Men may develop priapism, which, if not treated promptly, may lead to permanent erectile dysfunction.
- **Liver:** As in any form of chronic hemolytic anemia, patients with sickle cell anemia have increased levels of unconjugated (indirect) bilirubin, which can predispose to formation of pigmented bilirubin gallstones. Cholelithiasis may lead to cholecystitis and require cholecystectomy. Hepatomegaly and increased hepatic iron deposition are also seen.
- **Extremities:** Cutaneous ulcers over the lower extremities, especially near the ankles, are common and reflect obstruction of dermal capillaries. Children may develop "hand–foot syndrome," with self-limited swelling of the hands and feet because of underlying bone infarcts. Avascular necrosis of the femoral head requires corrective hip surgery. Sickle cell disease is also associated with increased incidence of osteomyelitis, particularly with *Salmonella typhimurium*, possibly because of the underlying impairment in splenic function.

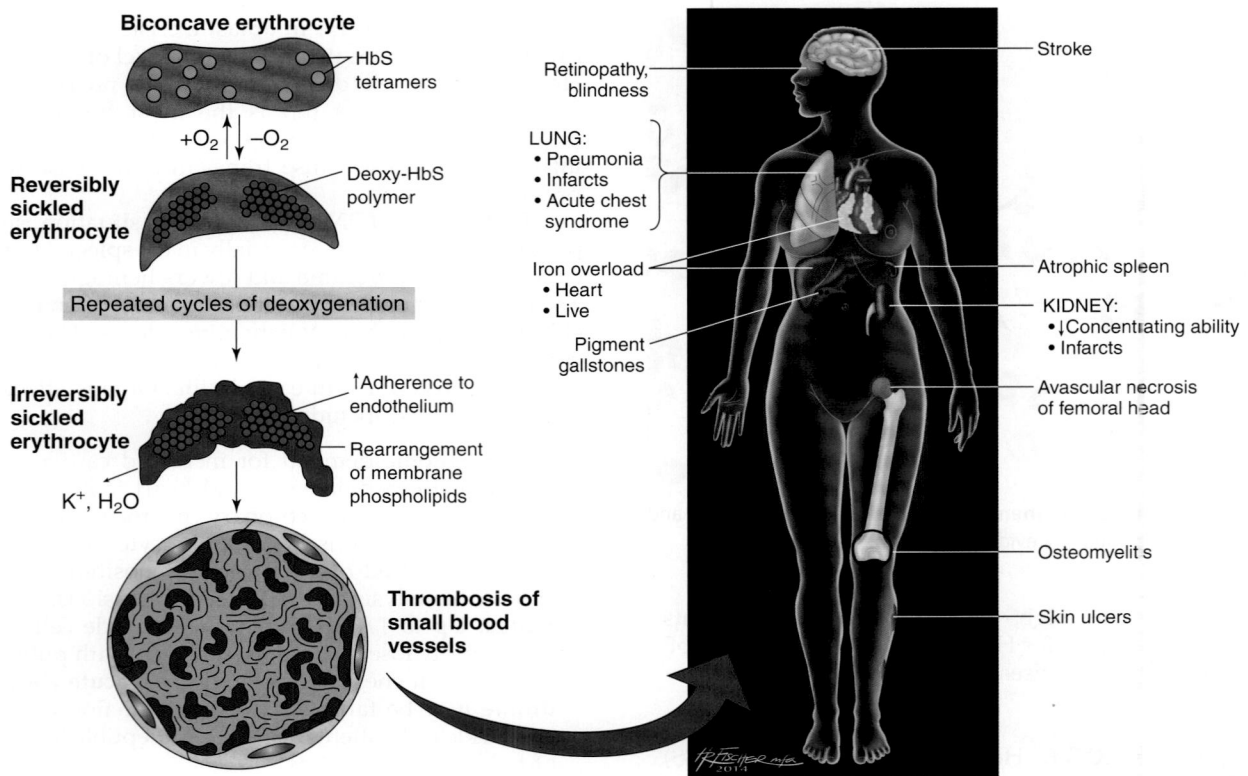

FIGURE 26-22. Pathogenesis of the vascular complications of sickle cell anemia. Substitution of valine for glutamic acid leads to an alteration in the surface charge of the hemoglobin molecule. Upon deoxygenation ($-O_2$), sickle hemoglobin (HbS) tetramers aggregate to form poorly soluble polymers. The erythrocytes change shape from a biconcave disk to a sickle form with the polymerization of HbS. This process is initially reversible upon reoxygenation ($+O_2$), but with repeated cycles of deoxygenation and reoxygenation, the erythrocytes become irreversibly sickled. Irreversibly sickled cells display a rearrangement of phospholipids between the outer and inner monolayers of the cell membrane, in particular an increase in aminophospholipids in the outer leaflet. Potassium (K^+) and water (H_2O) are lost from the cells. The erythrocytes are no longer deformable and are more adherent to endothelial cells, properties that predispose to thrombosis in small blood vessels. The resulting vascular occlusions lead to widespread ischemic complications.

Sickle Cell Trait

Heterozygosity for the Hgb-S mutation is called sickle cell trait.

 PATHOPHYSIOLOGY: Patients who are heterozygous for HgbS normally have about 40% HgbS and rest is HgbA. The HgbA in their red cells prevents HgbS polymerization, so their erythrocytes do not normally sickle. However, under extreme conditions (e.g., high altitudes, deep-sea diving), their RBCs may sickle. Heterozygotes are clinically asymptomatic, do not develop hemolytic anemia and live normal life spans.

Double Heterozygosity for HgbS and Other Hemoglobinopathies

Some patients with a sickling disorder are actually heterozygous for both HgbS and other abnormal hemoglobins (e.g., HgbC or HgbD), or for thalassemia.

 PATHOPHYSIOLOGY: The presence of an additional abnormal hemoglobin or thalassemic allele does not prevent HgbS polymerization, and the clinical expression and severity of disease may be affected.

People who are doubly heterozygous may have less frequent crises, higher baseline hemoglobin values, microcytic red cell indices, or persistent splenomegaly into adult life.

 CLINICAL FEATURES: Double heterozygosity for HgbS and HgbC causes a milder sickle phenotype than does homozygosity for HgbS. These patients have episodic skeletal or abdominal pain. However, they develop a retinopathy that is relatively common and severe. They are also prone to undergo necrosis of their femoral heads. These features probably reflect the high blood viscosity conferred by HgbSC.

Blood smears from hemoglobin SC patients reveal mild reticulocytosis, target cells, and relatively few sickled erythrocytes. However, RBCs with hemoglobin crystals caused by hemoglobin C are seen.

Double heterozygosity for HgbS and β-thalassemia is either Hgb Sβ⁰ thalassemia, in which β-globin is absent, or Hgb Sβ⁺ thalassemia, in which β-globin is present but reduced. Hgb Sβ⁰ thalassemia is clinically similar to sickle cell disease in severity. Sβ⁺ thalassemia is milder than HgbSC disease.

Hemoglobin C Disease

HgbC disease results from homozygous inheritance of a structurally abnormal hemoglobin, which increases erythrocyte rigidity and causes mild chronic hemolysis.

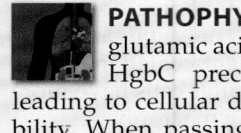 **PATHOPHYSIOLOGY:** In HgbC, lysine replaces glutamic acid at the sixth amino acid of β-globin. HgbC precipitates in erythrocyte cytoplasm, leading to cellular dehydration and decreased deformability. When passing through the spleen, the abnormal red cells are removed from the circulation, causing mild anemia and splenomegaly. HgbC has reduced oxygen affinity, so tissue oxygen delivery is increased. This mitigates the severity of disease. HgbC is mostly found in the same populations as HgbS, although it occurs less commonly.

 PATHOLOGY: Homozygosity for HgbC disease (CC) causes a mild normocytic anemia. Hemoglobin may be unevenly distributed within red cells, and dense, rhomboidal crystals (precipitated HgbC) occur in some erythrocytes. Hemoglobin electrophoresis reveals no HgbA and greater than 90% HgbC.

Two to 3% of African-Americans are heterozygous for HgbC and are asymptomatic (HgbC trait). In such people, about 40% of hemoglobin is HgbC. Red cell morphology is normal, except for some target cells.

Hemoglobin E Disease

HgbE disease is a result of homozygosity for a structurally abnormal hemoglobin, leading to a thalassemia-like defect associated with mild chronic hemolysis.

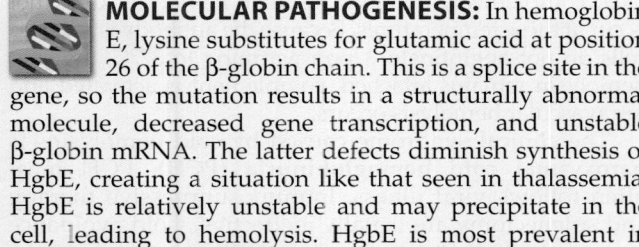 **MOLECULAR PATHOGENESIS:** In hemoglobin E, lysine substitutes for glutamic acid at position 26 of the β-globin chain. This is a splice site in the gene, so the mutation results in a structurally abnormal molecule, decreased gene transcription, and unstable β-globin mRNA. The latter defects diminish synthesis of HgbE, creating a situation like that seen in thalassemia. HgbE is relatively unstable and may precipitate in the cell, leading to hemolysis. HgbE is most prevalent in Southeast Asia and globally is second in incidence only to HgbS. HgbE may help protect against malaria.

PATHOLOGY: Patients homozygous for HgbE (EE) have a mild microcytic anemia. MCV is decreased, and there is often erythrocytosis because of the thalassemia-like component. Their RBCs are microcytic and hypochromic and include target cells. More than 90% of hemoglobin is HgbE.

Other Hemoglobinopathies

Several hundred additional known hemoglobin variants result from mutations in α- or β-globin genes. These mutations may lead to structural abnormalities and/or functional derangements in the hemoglobin molecule.

 PATHOPHYSIOLOGY: Some mutations alter hemoglobin tertiary structure, destabilizing it and causing it to precipitate in the cytoplasm. These **unstable hemoglobins** are often named after the place where they were first discovered (e.g., hemoglobin Köln). Unstable hemoglobins precipitate and form Heinz bodies within erythrocytes that can be visualized with supravital staining. Heinz bodies bind to cell membranes, increasing their rigidity and leading to mild chronic hemolysis. Patients may suffer jaundice and splenomegaly.

Other hemoglobin mutations cause **abnormal oxygen affinity. Increased oxygen affinity** decreases tissue oxygen delivery. Resulting hypoxia elicits increased EPO production and bone marrow erythroid hyperplasia. This, in turn, causes erythrocytosis. Patients are mostly asymptomatic, but some may have symptoms related to hyperviscosity. Abnormal hemoglobins with **decreased oxygen affinity** readily release oxygen in tissues. EPO levels are low, and most patients have mild anemia. Because of increased deoxyhemoglobin, patients may appear cyanotic.

Immune and Autoimmune Hemolytic Anemias

In immune hemolytic anemias, red cell destruction (hemolysis) is caused by antibodies against erythrocyte surface antigens. The red cells themselves are intrinsically normal but are targets for immune-mediated attack. Immune hemolytic anemia can involve auto- or allo-antibodies, and the site of hemolysis may be **extravascular** or **intravascular**. A common cause of anemia in the elderly is autoimmune hemolytic anemia (AIHA), which may be associated with chronic lymphocytic leukemia/small lymphocytic lymphoma.

In AIHA, there are autoantibodies against red cells. Autoantibodies can be classified as either **warm** or **cold antibodies**.

Warm Antibody Autoimmune Hemolytic Anemia

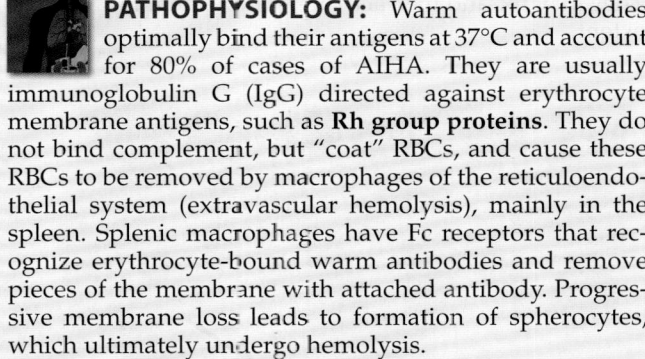 **PATHOPHYSIOLOGY:** Warm autoantibodies optimally bind their antigens at 37°C and account for 80% of cases of AIHA. They are usually immunoglobulin G (IgG) directed against erythrocyte membrane antigens, such as **Rh group proteins**. They do not bind complement, but "coat" RBCs, and cause these RBCs to be removed by macrophages of the reticuloendothelial system (extravascular hemolysis), mainly in the spleen. Splenic macrophages have Fc receptors that recognize erythrocyte-bound warm antibodies and remove pieces of the membrane with attached antibody. Progressive membrane loss leads to formation of spherocytes, which ultimately undergo hemolysis.

Warm antibody AIHA affects women more than men. Half of cases are idiopathic. In the remaining cases, the antibody reflects an underlying condition (e.g., infection, collagen vascular disease, lymphoproliferative disorders, and drug reactions).

Drug-induced warm antibodies arise by several mechanisms (see Chapter 4). In the **hapten** mechanism, a drug such as penicillin attaches to RBC surfaces. With this modification, the red cell–drug complex elicits antibodies, some of which react with the erythrocyte itself. In the **immune complex** mechanism, a drug (like quinidine) reacts with specific circulating antibody to form immune complexes, which then bind to red cell membranes. In the **autoantibody** mechanism, a drug (e.g., α-methyldopa) elicits antibodies that cross-react with red cell membrane components. In hapten and immune-complex models, the drug is required for hemolysis, while in the autoantibody model, hemolysis occurs in the absence of the initiating drug.

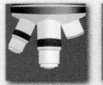 **PATHOLOGY AND CLINICAL FEATURES:** Warm antibody AIHA is associated with normocytic or occasionally macrocytic anemia, with spherocytes and polychromasia. Extravascular hemolysis leads to increased serum bilirubin, mostly unconjugated bilirubin; hemoglobinemia (free hemoglobin in the blood) and hemoglobinuria (hemoglobin in the urine) are uncommon. The direct antiglobulin (Coombs) test is usually positive and helps distinguish immune from nonimmune spherocytosis. In the direct Coombs test, a patient's red cells are incubated with anti-human immunoglobulin. Agglutination indicates antibody is present on the cell surface. Warm antibody AIHA is treated with immunosuppression. Refractory cases may require splenectomy or transfusions.

Cold Antibody Autoimmune Hemolytic Anemia

Cold antibodies have maximal reactivity at 4°C. Some 20% of cases of AIHA are caused by cold IgM or IgG antibodies, which occur as cold agglutinins or hemolysins.

 PATHOPHYSIOLOGY: Cold agglutinins may be idiopathic or may be due to an underlying condition, usually infections (EBV, *Mycoplasma*) or lymphoproliferative disorders. Cold agglutinins are mostly IgMs directed against I/i antigens on red cells. At cooler temperatures in the peripheral circulation, these antibodies may bind and agglutinate red cells (Fig. 26-23). They may fix, and then activate, complement to a variable extent.

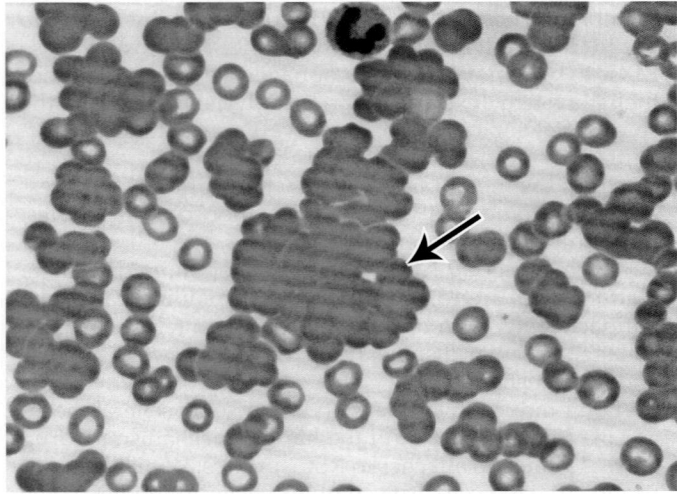

FIGURE 26-23. Red blood cell clumping (agglutination) caused by cold agglutinins (*arrow*). Note that this is not the same phenomenon as rouleaux formation.

The entire complement cascade may be activated (through the membrane attack complex). This process leads to intravascular hemolysis, resulting in hemoglobinemia, hemoglobinuria, and decreased haptoglobin levels (free hemoglobin released into the circulation binds haptoglobin, which causes a decline in haptoglobin).

Alternatively, complement may only be activated through C3. In that case, complement-coated red cells are removed in the liver, because Kupffer cells have more complement receptors than do splenic macrophages.

  PATHOLOGY AND CLINICAL FEATURES: Cold agglutinins are often activated when blood cools to room temperature, and erythrocytes agglutinate in blood smears (Fig. 26-22). Agglutination leads to falsely low RBC counts and Hct, and falsely elevated MCV and MCHC values determined by laboratory analyzers. Warming a blood sample to 37°C before analysis corrects the spurious results. The direct Coombs test is positive but usually only for the presence of complement on red cells. Significant hemolysis is uncommon with cold agglutinins and patients are more likely to develop peripheral vascular symptoms (e.g., Raynaud phenomenon; see Chapter 11), owing to red cell agglutination with cold exposure.

Cold Hemolysin Disease (Paroxysmal Cold Hemoglobinuria)

 PATHOPHYSIOLOGY: Cold hemolysins (Donath–Landsteiner antibodies) are usually biphasic IgGs directed against P antigens on red cells. Cold hemolysins have biphasic activity and rarely cause AIHA. The antibody binds to erythrocytes at low temperatures and fixes complement, but intravascular hemolysis does not occur at these temperatures. Because the antibody is IgG, red cells do not agglutinate. Upon warming to 37°C, the cold hemolysin remains attached, complement is activated and intravascular hemolysis occurs.

The clinical syndrome caused by cold hemolysins is **paroxysmal cold hemoglobinuria (PCH)**. PCH most often follows viral illness. Immunosuppressive therapy and splenectomy are usually ineffective. Cold avoidance and supportive therapy such as RBC transfusions are required.

 PATHOLOGY: Patients with PCH may develop severe anemia, decreased haptoglobin levels and hemoglobinuria due to intravascular hemolysis. The direct Coombs test is positive for complement but may be negative for IgG, since cold hemolysins may readily dissociate from red cells in vitro.

Hemolytic Transfusion Reactions

An **immediate hemolytic transfusion** reaction occurs when a patient with preformed alloantibodies receives grossly incompatible blood, usually because of a clerical error. Massive hemolysis of the transfused blood may cause severe complications, including hypotension, renal failure and death. Hemolytic transfusion reaction and hemolytic disease in the newborn (see below, Chapter 6) are examples of **alloimmune hemolytic anemia,** in which alloantibodies cause destruction of red cells.

Delayed hemolytic transfusion reactions usually involve antibodies to minor red cell antigens. After a first exposure to such antigens, antibody levels rise, but then may fall and become undetectable by routine pretransfusion screening. Subsequent reexposure to the offending antigen elicits an anamnestic antibody response and hemolysis occurs several days later. Delayed hemolytic transfusion reactions are usually less severe than immediate reactions and may be clinically undetectable. In both types of hemolytic transfusion reactions, the direct antiglobulin test is positive.

Hemolytic Disease of the Newborn

Hemolytic disease of the newborn (HDN) reflects incompatibility of blood types between a mother and her developing fetus; the mother lacks an antigen present on fetal RBCs. Maternal IgG alloantibodies can cross the placenta and cause hemolysis of fetal erythrocytes. Erythroblastosis is visible in peripheral blood smears (Fig. 26-24). Erythroblasts (immature RBCs) are released from the fetal bone marrow in an effort to compensate for the RBC loss. HDN antibodies are mostly directed against ABO or Rh antigens.

With ABO-type HDN, the mother is type O and the fetus is usually type A. Naturally occurring maternal anti-A antibodies cause hemolysis in the fetus. No prior exposure through pregnancy or transfusion is required for hemolysis to develop. The anemia associated with ABO incompatibility is usually mild. Affected babies develop hyperbilirubinemia, spherocytosis, and a positive direct antiglobulin test.

With Rh-type HDN, the mother is Rh negative and the fetus is Rh positive. The D antigen is most frequently involved, although minor Rh antigens can also cause disease. Prior maternal exposure occurs via previous pregnancy or transfusion. Disease severity varies, but hemolysis in Rh incompatibility is generally more significant than in ABO-type HDN. Severely affected fetuses may develop **hydrops fetalis,** with heart failure, generalized edema, ascites, and intrauterine death (see Chapter 6). Fortunately, most cases of D-related HDN can be prevented by passive immunization

of Rh-negative mothers during pregnancy with injections of Rh immune globulin. Laboratory findings are similar to those described above for ABO HDN.

Nonimmune Hemolytic Anemias

In nonimmune hemolytic anemias, factors other than antibodies to red cell antigens destroy RBCs (e.g., red cell fragmentation syndromes and "march" hemoglobinuria).

Mechanical Red Cell Fragmentation Syndromes (Microangiopathic Hemolytic Anemias)
In red cell fragmentation syndromes, intrinsically normal erythrocytes are damaged mechanically as they circulate in the blood (intravascular hemolysis).

 ETIOLOGIC FACTORS: In **thrombotic microangiopathic** hemolytic anemia, red cells are fragmented mechanically either by contact with an abnormal surface (e.g., prosthetic heart valve, synthetic vascular graft) or by altered small blood vessel endothelial surfaces associated with microthrombosis, fibrin deposition, and platelet aggregation. As RBCs travel through such damaged vessels, these fibrin meshworks cause them to fragment (Fig. 26-8). Classic examples of microangiopathic hemolysis include **disseminated intravascular coagulation** (DIC), **thrombotic thrombocytopenic purpura** (TTP), and **hemolytic–uremic syndrome** (HUS). Altered blood flow dynamics, as occurs in malignant hypertension or vasculitis, may also lead to mechanical fragmentation of erythrocytes.

Long-distance running or walking ("march hemoglobinuria") or prolonged vigorous exercise can cause repetitive trauma to red cells and lead to hemolysis.

 PATHOLOGY: Laboratory findings in microangiopathic hemolytic anemia include a mild to moderate microcytic or normochromic anemia with appropriate reticulocyte response. Blood smears show fragmented erythrocytes (schistocytes) and polychromasia (Fig. 26-25). Abnormalities in coagulation and thrombocytopenia characterize DIC, while thrombocytopenia alone is seen in cases of TTP (see below).

Hypersplenism
Mild hemolytic anemia may develop in patients with hypersplenism and congestive splenomegaly. Splenomegaly causes pooling of blood and delayed transit of blood cells through the splenic circulation. Prolonged exposure of red cells to splenic macrophages may lead to their premature destruction.

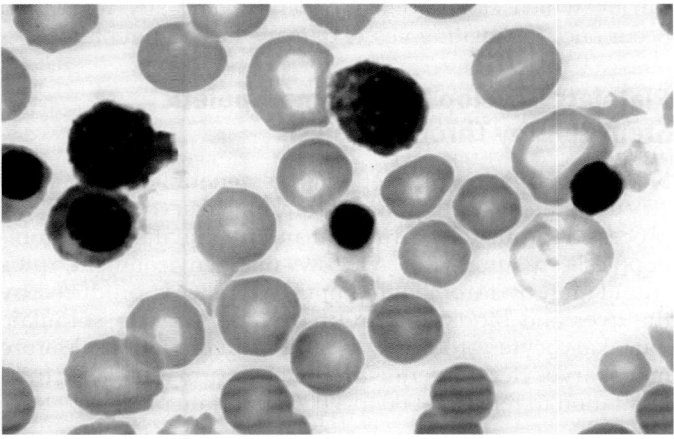

FIGURE 26-24. Hemolytic disease of the newborn (HDN). The presence of nucleated red blood cells in the peripheral blood beyond the first few days of life is abnormal. They are often present in various types of hemolytic disorders, but are particularly numerous in HDN.

 PATHOLOGY AND CLINICAL FEATURES: The anemia of hypersplenism shows no specific morphologic features. Leukopenia and thrombocytopenia are common and are caused by sequestration rather than destruction of these elements in the enlarged spleen. Bone marrow shows compensatory hyperplasia of all cell lines.

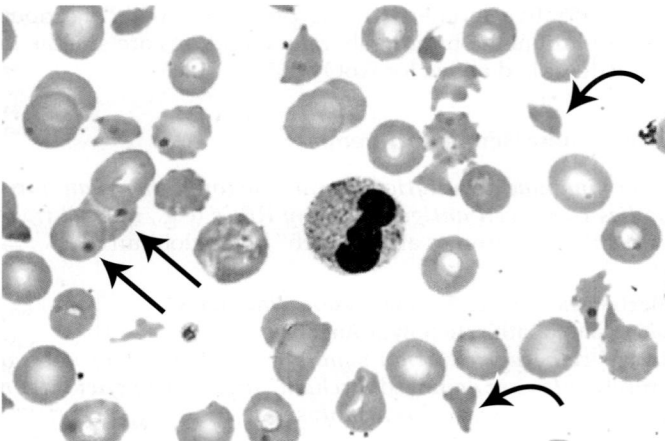

FIGURE 26-25. Microangiopathic hemolytic anemia (MAHA). Irregular, fragmented erythrocytes (schistocytes, *curved arrows*) are seen in the blood smear of a patient with disseminated intravascular coagulation. Howell–Jolly bodies are also present (*straight arrows*).

Other Hemolytic Anemias

Thermal burns lead to intravascular RBC hemolysis. Normal red cell membranes are disrupted and fragmented at temperatures over 49°C. Blood smears show schistocytes, microspherocytes, and polychromasia. Direct Coombs tests are negative. **Fresh water drowning** can cause intravascular osmotic lysis of red cells.

Infection can cause both pancytopenia and isolated anemia. Several **infectious microorganisms** specifically parasitize erythrocytes and can cause hemolysis. All species of *Plasmodium* have an intraerythrocytic life cycle, which ultimately causes RBC lysis (see Chapter 9). Infected red cells are also removed from circulation by splenic macrophages. *Babesiosis,* found in more temperate climates (northeastern United States), is also associated with hemolysis once the intraerythrocytic life cycle is completed. In both cases, blood smears reveal parasites within red cells.

POLYCYTHEMIAS

Polycythemia (erythrocytosis) is an increase in RBC mass.

 ETIOLOGIC FACTORS: Polycythemia is defined arbitrarily as an elevated Hct of greater than 49% in men and greater than 48% in women, or increased hemoglobin exceeding 16.5 g/dL in men and 16.0 g/dL in women. Blood viscosity increases exponentially at Hcts over 50%, and cardiac function and peripheral blood flow may be impaired. If the Hct exceeds 60%, blood flow may be so compromised as to cause tissue hypoxia.

Polycythemia can be further divided into relative and absolute categories on the basis of overall red cell mass.

- **Relative polycythemia** occurs in dehydration. Plasma volume is decreased, but red cell mass is normal. This is sometimes called Gaisböck syndrome, or spurious polycythemia. It is not a true increase in red cell mass, but rather a reflection of altered total blood volume.
- **Absolute polycythemia** is a true increase in red cell mass. It can be primary or secondary.

- **Primary polycythemia,** or **polycythemia vera (PV),** is autonomous, EPO-independent proliferation of erythroid cells caused by an acquired, clonal, HSC disorder. PV is an MPN (see below).
- **Secondary polycythemia** arises from EPO stimulation of erythropoiesis, usually to compensate for general tissue hypoxia. Tissue hypoxia may arise from chronic lung disease, cigarette smoking, residence at high altitudes, a right-to-left cardiac shunt or an abnormal hemoglobin with high oxygen affinity.

Secondary polycythemia can also occur under certain circumstances unrelated to tissue hypoxia. For example, some tumors secrete ectopic EPO as a paraneoplastic syndrome (see below), particularly renal cell carcinoma, hepatocellular carcinoma, cerebellar hemangioblastoma, and uterine leiomyoma. Some non-neoplastic conditions of the kidney may cause secondary polycythemia. Renal cysts or hydronephrosis may exert direct pressure on the kidney, leading to localized hypoxia and increasing EPO production. Some athletes use EPO to enhance their maximal exercise capacity.

Platelets and Hemostasis

NORMAL HEMOSTASIS

Normal hemostasis requires that platelets, endothelial cells, coagulation factors, endogenous anticoagulants, and thrombolytics maintain a resting nonthrombotic state but they must respond instantly to vascular damage and form a clot. After blood vessel injury, the primary phase of hemostasis occurs within seconds and involves vasoconstriction to divert blood away from the damage. A large circulating protein called von Willebrand factor (vWF) adheres to exposed subendothelial collagen, and platelets then adhere to both collagen-bound vWF and collagen to form a platelet monolayer. Activated platelets recruit and activate additional platelets to form a **platelet aggregate**. Secondary hemostasis occurs in minutes and involves activation of the coagulation cascade to form fibrin which stabilizes platelet aggregates. The tertiary phase of hemostasis occurs over hours or days during which clot stabilization and eventually resorption occur once the inciting vessel damage has been repaired.

Platelets Develop From Hematopoietic Stem Cells by Thrombopoiesis

Normal circulating platelet count is generally 150 to 400 × 10^3/μL. Platelets are derived from megakaryocytes via the process of proplatelet formation and fragmentation. Thrombopoiesis requires the marrow microenvironment, plus stimulation by thrombopoietin (TPO). TPO is produced by the liver and binds the TPO receptor, c-Mpl, to stimulate megakaryocyte proliferation and differentiation. Mature megakaryocytes undergo proplatelet formation and fragmentation to release 1,000 to 4,000 anucleate platelets.

Morphology and Function

Platelets are small discoid cells, 2 to 3 μm in diameter (Fig. 26-26), with a life span of about 7 to 10 days. On Wright-stained

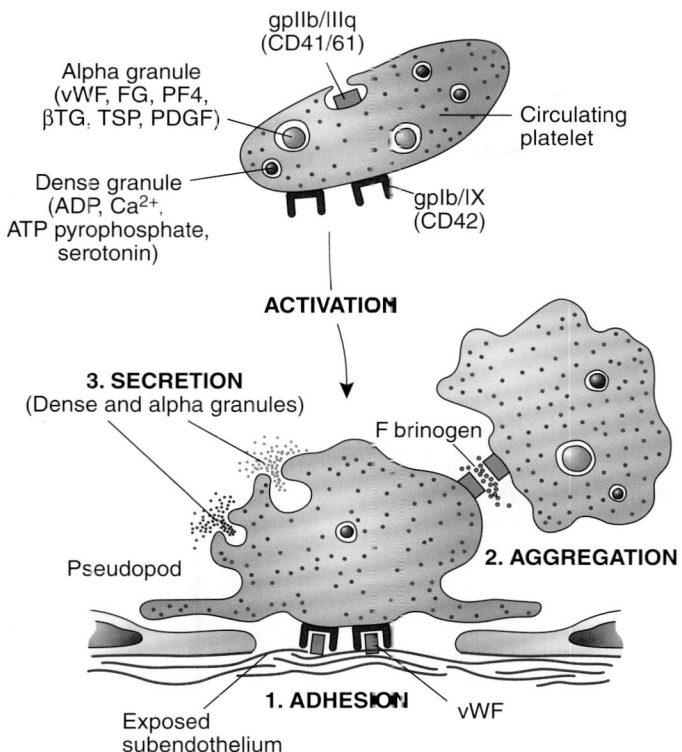

FIGURE 26-26. Platelet activation involves three overlapping mechanisms. 1. Adhesion to the exposed subendothelium is mediated by the binding of von Willebrand factor (vWF) to glycoprotein (Gp) Ib/IX (CD42) and is the initiation signal for activation. **2.** Exposure of Gp IIb/IIIa (CD41/61) to the fibrinogen (FG) receptor on the platelet surface allows for platelet aggregation. **3.** At the same time, platelets secrete their granule contents, which facilitates further activation. α-Granules contain vWF, fibrinogen, platelet factor 4 (PF4), thromboglobulin (TG), thrombospondin (TSP), and platelet-derived growth factor (PDGF).

smears they appear pale blue with faint pink granules. They are anucleate but contain cytoplasmic organelles including mitochondria, glycogen particles, and granules. They contain two types of granules: dense granules and α-granules.

1. **Dense granules** are submicroscopic and contain adenosine diphosphate (ADP), a potent aggregating molecule; adenosine triphosphate (ATP); calcium; histamine; serotonin; and epinephrine.
2. **α-Granules** are visible by light microscopy. They are numerous (40 to 60/platelet) and membrane-bound. They express the adhesive proteins P-selectin on their membranes and contain fibrinogen, vWF, fibronectin and thrombospondin, as well as the chemokines platelet factor 4, neutrophil-activating peptide 2, platelet-derived growth factor (PDGF), and transforming growth factor-α (TGF-α).

Platelet Activation

When vascular endothelium is disrupted, platelets respond by creating a platelet plug to minimize bleeding. After contact with the extracellular matrix, particularly type I collagen, as well as vWF, platelets undergo a sequence of steps involved in platelet activation (Fig. 26-26):

1. **Platelets adhere** to subendothelial matrix proteins via binding of specific platelet surface glycoproteins (Gp).

Major adhesive ligands include collagen (via the Gp Ia/IIa [$\alpha_2\beta_1$ integrin] and Gp VI receptors) and vWF (via Gp Ib/IX).
2. **Platelet shape changes** after initial adhesion, from discoid to spherical to stellate.
3. **Secretion of platelet granule contents from both the dense granules and α-granules** results in the release of ADP, epinephrine, calcium, vWF, and PDGF.
4. **Thromboxane A$_2$** is generated by cyclooxygenase 1.
5. **Membrane changes** expose P-selectin and procoagulant anionic phospholipids such as phosphatidylserine.
6. **Aggregation of platelets** occurs by fibrinogen receptor Gp IIb/IIIa cross-linking.

Each of these functional steps has specific consequences. Initial adhesion signals platelet activation. Secreted granule contents and thromboxane A$_2$ provide positive feedback to activate additional platelets via their surface receptors. The stellate shape projects the procoagulant membrane surface and activated Gp IIb/IIIa/fibrinogen to the site of interaction with coagulation factors and other platelets, respectively. *Thus, the surface of activated platelets is an optimal environment for propagating assembly of the coagulation–factor complex, including the prothrombinase complex. The resulting thrombin has many consequences, particularly further platelet activation.* Finally, P-selectin participates in binding leukocytes and localizing them to participate in healing, together with substances secreted by platelets such as PDGF. *As a result of these concerted steps, activated platelets form a strong primary plug and then an aggregate within a platelet–fibrin meshwork, which stops bleeding and begins healing.*

Activation of the Coagulation Cascade Completes Blood Clot Formation

Platelets and leukocytes circulate in an inactive state. Similarly, coagulation factors are present as inactive zymogen forms. Activation of platelets and coagulation factors is concerted and highly constrained in space and time, to prevent clots from spreading through the circulation. Localization of coagulation–factor complexes to activated surfaces of blood cells, especially platelets, accelerates activation of coagulation factors at the site of injury and avoids the many anticoagulant factors in plasma.

Activation of the coagulation cascade by damaged tissue exposes tissue factor and culminates in conversion of prothrombin (factor II) to thrombin (factor IIa), and generation of fibrin from fibrinogen (Fig. 26-27). Thrombin has additional roles. It activates both platelets and factors that sustain coagulation (see Chapter 16).

Generally, each active enzyme in the cascade is assisted by a cofactor and localized to a phospholipid surface (PL). The coagulation pathways are presented in detail in Chapter 16. There are three essential procoagulant complexes and one anticoagulant complex (Figs. 26-27 and 26-28).

PROCOAGULANT PATHWAYS: Two complexes activate factor X. These are the so-called "Xase complexes":

1. The complex of **tissue factor (TF) and factor VIIa** initiates coagulation. Its activation is controlled by exposure to subendothelial cells or activated monocytes and endothelial cells. Microparticles derived from activated leukocytes and endothelial cells contribute to a pool of circulating TFs that participates in hemostasis and thrombosis. TF/VIIa/PL initiates factor X activation but

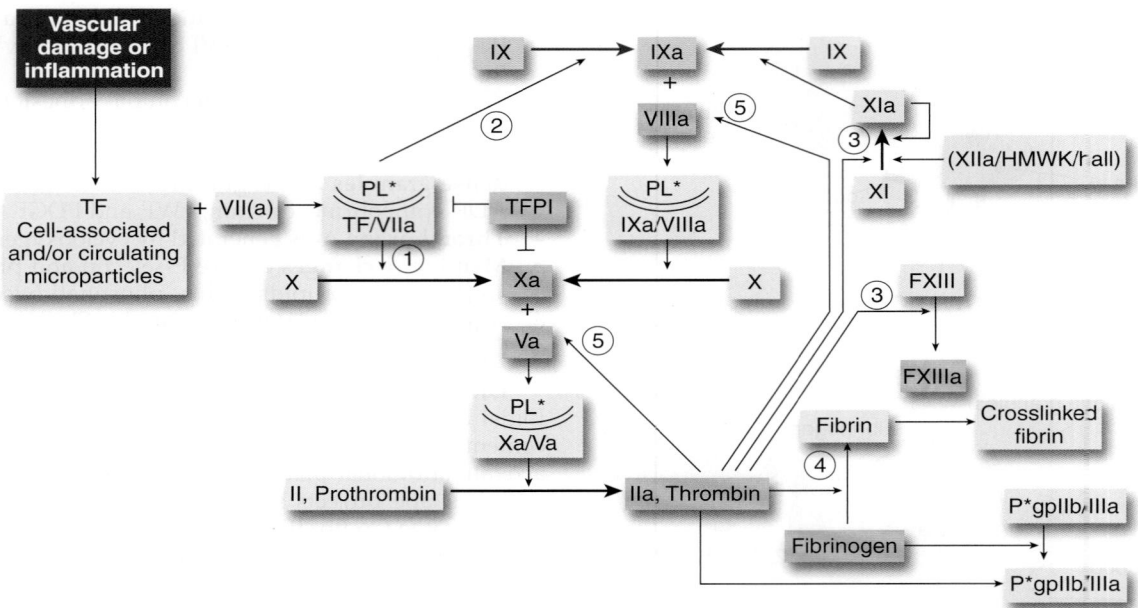

FIGURE 26-27. Hemostasis and thrombosis. Following injury to a vessel, rupture of an atherosclerotic plaque or the presence of major inflammation, coagulation is initiated when tissue factor (TF) binds to circulating factor VII, a small proportion of which is activated (VIIa). TF is located on cells (subendothelial or activated endothelial cells or leukocytes) or circulating microparticles. The TF/VIIa complex is activated by localizing to an activated phospholipid surface (PL*) such as that provided by activated platelets. TF/VIIa activates factor X to form Xa (*1*) and IX to form IXa (*2*). However, TF pathway inhibitor (TFPI) inhibits both (*1*) and (*2*). Sustained amplification is achieved through the actions of factors XI, IX, and VIII. Factor XI is activated through the small amount of initial thrombin formed and, to a limited extent, by autoactivation or factor XIIa. Cofactors V and VIII, when activated by thrombin, form complexes with X (Xa/Va) and IX (IXa/VIIIa), respectively, on activated PL surfaces. Note the central and multiple roles for thrombin (*4*), which converts fibrinogen to fibrin, activates cofactors V and VIII (*5*), activates factors XI and XIII (*3*), and activates platelets. Fibrinogen binds to the Gp IIb/IIIa integrin receptor on activated platelets (P*). Note the extensive control in time and space of these concerted surface reactions. The combined result is the platelet–fibrin thrombus.

is then rapidly shut off by **TF pathway inhibitor (TFPI)** (Fig. 26-28). The TF/VIIa/PL complex also cleaves and thus activates a small amount of factor IX.

2. The **IXa/VIIIa/PL** complex also initiates factor X activation, with ongoing activation of factor IX by XIa.

The third procoagulant pathway involves factor Xa, together with its cofactor Va (**Xa/Va complex**, also known as the **prothrombinase complex**), which cleaves factor II (prothrombin) to IIa (thrombin). Note that thrombin activates the Xase complexes by activating factors XI, VIII, and V. *In summary, the three procoagulant complexes are the prothrombinase complex, Xa/Va/PL, and the two Xase complexes, TF/VIIa/PL and IXa/VIIIa/PL.*

ANTICOAGULANT PATHWAYS: The two main natural anticoagulant systems are the protein C/S system and antithrombin.

An anticoagulant complex (α-thrombin–thrombomodulin) activates protein C (Fig. 26-28). The **protein C$_{ase}$ complex** contains thrombin and thrombomodulin within endothelial cell plasma membranes. Endothelial protein C receptor also participates in forming this cell surface complex. Activated protein C, with its cofactor protein S, inactivates the key cofactors VIIIa and Va, thus limiting further generation of Xa and IIa (see Chapter 16).

Antithrombin inhibits thrombin activity. Antithrombin also cleaves activated factors IXa, Xa, XIa, and XIIa. In vivo this effect is accentuated by heparan sulfate proteoglycans and, most dramatically, by therapeutic administration of heparin.

Thrombolysis Is Mediated by Plasminogen Activation

Once a thrombus is firmly established, its further growth is curtailed by removal of platelet-activating factors and coagulation proteins. Endothelial cells near the thrombus produce plasminogen activators. The two major plasminogen activators, **tissue plasminogen activator** (t-PA) and **urokinase-type plasminogen activator** (u-PA), convert circulating plasminogen to plasmin and initiate thrombolysis (i.e., **fibrinolysis**). Together, the protease plasmin and the activity of macrophages dissolve the thrombus. Plasmin targets specific sites in the fibrin meshwork for degradation, helping to localize its activity to sites where it is needed (see Chapter 16).

The factors that limit clot formation are themselves kept in check by several naturally occurring inhibitors. Plasminogen activator inhibitor-I (PAI-I), antiplasmin and thrombin-activatable fibrinolysis inhibitor (TAFI) all block plasminogen cleavage to plasmin and thus limit plasmin action temporally and spatially.

Thrombolysis coincides with the initiation of wound repair (see Chapter 7). The latter involves influx and proliferation of fibroblasts and endothelial cells, secretion

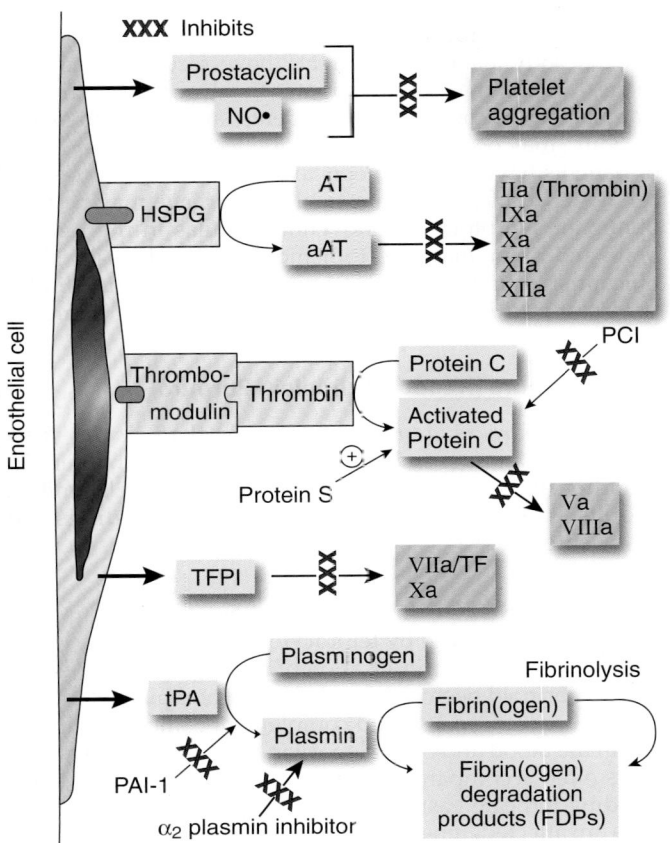

FIGURE 26-28. The role of endothelium in anticoagulation, platelet inhibition, and thrombolysis. The endothelial cell plays a central role in the inhibition of various components of the clotting mechanism. Heparan sulfate proteoglycan potentiates the activation of antithrombin (AT) 15-fold. Thrombomodulin stimulates the activation of protein C by thrombin 30-fold. *HSPG* = heparan sulfate proteoglycan; *NO•* = nitric oxide; *PAI-I* = plasminogen activator inhibitor-I; *PCI* = protein C inhibitor; *tPA* = tissue plasminogen activator.

of new extracellular matrix components, and restoration of blood vessel patency. Angiogenesis (i.e., new blood vessels budding from existing ones) occurs in the setting of tissue ischemia or damage. Indeed, many products of coagulation and fibrinolysis are potent angiogenic agents.

Blood Vessels and Endothelial Cells Interact With Platelets

The above discussion highlights the many roles of endothelial cells in regulating platelets and coagulation (Fig. 26-28). Endothelial cells rest on a basement membrane containing collagens, elastin, laminin, fibronectin, vWF, and other structural and adhesive proteins. Subendothelial cells are a potent source of TF. When exposed, the intimal basement membrane matrix is intensely thrombogenic. Its adhesive proteins bind corresponding platelet membrane glycoprotein receptors, which then adhere to the exposed matrix. TF binds circulating activated factor VIIa to activate factors X and IX (Fig. 26-27).

The normal endothelium provides a smooth, nonthrombogenic surface. It synthesizes anticoagulant molecules and prevents unstimulated platelets from adhering to, or penetrating, the endothelial barrier. Endothelial cells also

synthesize prostacyclin (also known as prostaglandin I2), a potent vasodilator that also inhibits platelet activation. Nitric oxide (NO) exerts similar effects. These actions prevent clots from forming unless endothelial injury exposes subendothelial tissue (see Chapters 2 and 16).

HEMOSTATIC DISORDERS

Defects in hemostasis occur when the balance of procoagulant and anticoagulant activities tilts toward one or the other. Such defects are either **hemostatic** disorders or **thrombotic** disorders. If hemostasis fails to restore an injured vessel's integrity, the result is **bleeding**. Inability to maintain the fluidity of blood causes **thrombosis**.

Clinical manifestations of hemorrhage associated with disorders of each component of the hemostatic system tend to be distinctive (Table 26-11). Defects in *primary hemostasis* (e.g., from defects in blood vessels, vWF, platelets) tend to cause spontaneous bleeding, producing both petechiae and

TABLE 26-11		
PRINCIPAL CAUSES OF BLEEDING		
Vascular Disorders		
Senile purpura		
Purpura simplex		
Glucocorticoid excess		
Dysproteinemias		
Allergic (Henoch–Schönlein) purpura		
Hereditary hemorrhagic telangiectasia		
Platelet Abnormalities		
Thrombocytopenia (see Table 26-7)		
Qualitative disorders		
Inherited		**Acquired**
Glycoprotein IIb/IIIa deficiency (Glanzmann thrombasthenia)		Uremia
Glycoprotein Ib/IX/V deficiency (Bernard–Soulier syndrome)		Drugs
Storage pool diseases (α and δ)		Cardiopulmonary bypass
Abnormal arachidonic acid metabolism		Myeloproliferative disorders
Liver disease		
Coagulation Factor Deficiencies		
Inherited factor deficiencies (XI, IX, VIII, X, VII, V, II, I)		
von Willebrand disease		
Acquired factor inhibitors		
Vitamin K deficiency/antagonism		
Liver disease		
Disseminated intravascular coagulation		
Decreased Clot Stability/Increased Fibrinolysis		
Factor XIII deficiency		
Plasminogen activator inhibitor (PAI-1) deficiency		

purpuric hemorrhages in the skin and mucous membranes. Deficiencies of coagulation factors, or defects of *secondary hemostasis*, lead to hemorrhage into muscles, viscera and joint spaces, often associated with trauma. *Tertiary hemostasis* defects often accelerate clot breakdown, leading to delayed bleeding post trauma or surgery. Examples of tertiary hemostasis defects are factor XIII deficiency leading to insufficient cross linking of clot and thus producing an unstable clot, or hyperactive plasmin due to deficiency of its inhibitors (e.g., PAI-1 deficiency or alpha-2-antiplasmin deficiency).

Hemostatic Disorders of Blood Vessels Reflect Vascular or Extravascular Dysfunction

Dysfunction of the extravascular or vascular tissues may cause hemorrhages ranging from cosmetic blemishes to life-threatening blood loss.

Extravascular Dysfunction

SENILE PURPURA: The most common disorder in extravascular dysfunction, senile purpura, is age-related atrophy of supporting connective tissues. Senile purpura is associated with superficial, sharply demarcated, persistent purpuric spots (purple or red bruises in light skin) on the forearms and other sun-exposed areas.
PURPURA SIMPLEX: A similar type of purpura occurs principally in women during menses. Purpura simplex occurs in the deep dermis and resolves quickly.
SCURVY: Vitamin C deficiency (scurvy) impairs collagen synthesis and leads to purpura (see Chapter 8). Perifollicular hemorrhages are characteristic.

Vascular Dysfunction

Deposition of immunoglobulin fragments in vessel walls occurs in **amyloidosis** (see Chapter 15), **cryoglobulinemia** and other **paraproteinemias** and can weaken vessel walls and cause purpura. Certain **arteritides** also injure vessel walls and may lead to hemorrhage (see Chapter 16).

Hereditary Hemorrhagic Telangiectasia (Rendu–Osler–Weber Syndrome)

Hereditary hemorrhagic telangiectasia (HHT) is an autosomal dominant disorder of blood vessel walls (venules and capillaries) in which arteriovenous malformations (AVMs) and telangiectases (dilated, tortuous small blood vessels) form in solid organs, mucous membranes, and dermis. The incidence is 1 to 2 individuals per 10,000.

MOLECULAR PATHOGENESIS: The underlying defect is dilation and thinning of vessel walls due to inadequate elastic tissue and smooth muscle. The disorder is caused by mutations in TGF-β family members, including *ENG*, which encodes endoglin and *ALK1*, which makes activin receptor–like kinase 1.

CLINICAL FEATURES: At first, telangiectasias appear as punctate reddish spots on the lips and nose, up to 0.5 cm in diameter. They can remain as

such or progress to AVMs or aneurysmal dilations throughout the body. Patients with HHT have recurrent hemorrhages. These may occur spontaneously or after trivial trauma. As a consequence, patients are often anemic. Bleeding may occur at the site of any lesion, but over 80% of patients have recurrent epistaxis, beginning at an early age. Later in life, gastrointestinal hemorrhage may be the dominant symptom. Arteriovenous fistulas in the lungs, brain and retina may lead to hemorrhage or clinically significant shunting of blood. Recurrent bleeding may limit physical activities, but death from exsanguination is rare.

Allergic Purpura (Henoch–Schönlein Purpura)

Allergic purpura is a vascular disease that results from immunologic damage to blood vessel walls (see Chapter 22). In children, it often follows viral infections and is self-limited. In adults, it often reflects exposure to a variety of drugs and may be chronic.

PATHOLOGY: Henoch–Schönlein purpura is characterized by **leukocytoclastic vasculitis,** with perivascular infiltration of neutrophils and eosinophils, fibrinoid necrosis of vessel walls, and platelet plugs in vascular lumens. IgA and complement complexes circulate in the blood and often deposit in vessel walls. Purpuric spots often accompany raised urticarial lesions. Colic and bleeding indicate gastrointestinal involvement. If the kidneys are affected, renal failure may ensue.

Platelet Disorders May Result From Insufficient Production, Excessive Destruction, or Impaired Platelet Function

Clinical manifestations of platelet disorders include easy bruising; mucocutaneous bleeding, including gingival bleeding, epistaxis and menorrhagia; or life-threatening bleeds into the gastrointestinal (GI) tract, genitourinary tract and brain. Petechiae are characteristic of platelet disorders but may also accompany vascular diseases. They are non-blanching, red lesions less than 2 mm in diameter. They usually occur in the legs and dependent parts of the body, on the buccal mucosal and soft palate and at pressure points (waistband, wristwatch band).

Thrombocytopenia

Thrombocytopenia, defined as a platelet count under 150,000/μL, results from either decreased production or increased destruction. Manifestations of thrombocytopenia include spontaneous bleeding, with normal prothrombin time (PT) and normal activated partial thromboplastin time (APTT). Lower platelet counts are associated with greater risk of bleeding. Patients with less than 10,000 platelets/μL are at greatest risk of spontaneous hemorrhage (Table 26-12).

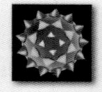

ETIOLOGIC FACTORS AND MOLECULAR PATHOGENESIS: Decreased platelet production can result from multiple congenital or acquired defects in megakaryocytopoiesis,

TABLE 26-12

PRINCIPAL CAUSES OF THROMBOCYTOPENIA

Decreased Production

Aplastic anemia

Bone marrow infiltration (neoplastic, fibrosis)

Bone marrow suppression by drugs or radiation

Ineffective Production

Megaloblastic anemia

Myelodysplasias

Increased Destruction

Immunologic (idiopathic, HIV, drugs, alloimmune, post-transfusion purpura, neonatal)

Nonimmunologic (DIC, TTP, HUS, vascular malformations, drugs)

Increased Sequestration

Splenomegaly

Dilutional

Blood and plasma transfusions

DIC = disseminated intravascular coagulation; HUS = hemolytic–uremic syndrome; TTP = thrombocytic thrombocytopenic purpura.

including diseases that affect the marrow generally, abnormalities that selectively impair platelet production and defects that lead to ineffective megakaryocytopoiesis. Marrow infiltration by malignant cells or bone marrow failure (e.g., in patients with aplastic anemia or who received radiotherapy or chemotherapy) may cause pancytopenia, including thrombocytopenia. Certain viral infections, such as cytomegalovirus (CMV) and HIV, and certain drugs impair platelet production (HIV may also increase platelet destruction; see below). Megaloblastic anemia and myelodysplasia may cause thrombocytopenia due to ineffective megakaryopoiesis.

May–Hegglin anomaly is a congenital form of thrombocytopenia that entails decreased platelet production. It is the most common of a family of inherited thrombocytopenias called myosin heavy chain 9 (MYH9)-related platelet disorders. They result from mutations in *MYH9*, which encodes a contractile cytoskeletal protein, nonmuscle myosin heavy chain IIA (NMMHC-IIA). There are three other overlapping disorders: Epstein syndrome, Fechtner syndrome, and Sebastian platelet syndrome. These all lead to abnormal megakaryocyte maturation and abnormally large platelets (macrothrombocytopenia). Neutrophils are also slightly abnormal and show blue cytoplasmic inclusions (**Döhle-like bodies;** true Döhle bodies occur in acute infections).

Increased platelet destruction can result from immune-mediated damage with consequent removal of circulating platelets, as in idiopathic thrombocytopenic purpura (ITP) and drug-induced thrombocytopenia. Excessive platelet destruction can also occur by nonimmunologic conditions such as intravascular platelet aggregation (e.g., in TTP).

Abnormal platelet distribution, or pooling, is seen in disorders of the spleen and hypothermia.

Idiopathic (Autoimmune) Thrombocytopenic Purpura

In ITP, antibodies against platelet or megakaryocytic antigens cause thrombocytopenia. It is, thus, more fittingly called **immune thrombocytopenic purpura**. ITP occurs in two forms: an acute, self-limited, hemorrhagic syndrome in children and a chronic bleeding disorder in adolescents and adults. The autoantibodies often recognize the platelet membrane glycoproteins, Gp IIb/IIIa or Ib/IX, which are involved in platelet adhesion and clot formation.

 PATHOPHYSIOLOGY: Like AIHA, ITP reflects antibody-mediated destruction of platelets or their precursors. In most cases, these are IgGs, but IgM antiplatelet antibodies also occur.

Acute ITP typically appears in children of either sex after a viral illness and is likely caused by virus-induced changes in platelet antigens that elicit autoantibodies. Complement bound at the surface lyses platelets in the blood or mediates their phagocytosis and destruction by splenic and hepatic macrophages.

Chronic ITP occurs mainly in adults (male-to-female ratio = 1:2.6) and may be associated with autoimmune (e.g., systemic lupus erythematosus [SLE]) or malignant lymphoproliferative (e.g., chronic lymphocytic leukemia; see below) diseases. It is also common in people infected with HIV. The magnitude of thrombocytopenia in ITP reflects the balance between (1) levels of antiplatelet antibodies; (2) the extent to which platelet production in the marrow is impaired, as some antibodies may bind to megakaryocytes; and (3) expression of Fc and complement receptors at macrophage cell surfaces. This expression is upregulated in infection and pregnancy but is restored by certain drugs, including corticosteroids, danazol and intravenous γ-globulin, all of which are used to treat ITP.

 PATHOLOGY: In acute ITP, the platelet count is typically less than 20,000/μL. In chronic adult ITP, platelet counts vary from a few thousand to 100,000/μL. Peripheral blood smears show many large platelets, owing to accelerated release of young platelets by bone marrow actively engaged in platelet production. Bone marrow thus shows compensatory increases in megakaryocytes (Fig. 26-29). Platelets carry detectable IgG in more than 80% of patients with chronic ITP; in half of these, platelet-associated C3 is also detectable.

CLINICAL FEATURES: Children with **acute ITP** experience sudden onset of petechiae and purpura but are otherwise asymptomatic. Spontaneous recovery occurs within 6 months in over 80% of cases. The major threat (<1% of cases) is intracranial hemorrhage. Treatment is rarely necessary, but with serious disease, corticosteroids and intravenous immunoglobulin (IVIG) may be needed. Glucocorticoids decrease antiplatelet antibody production and downregulate macrophage Fc receptors. IVIG inhibits clearance of IgG-coated platelets from the circulation via multiple mechanisms.

Chronic ITP in adults manifests as bleeding episodes, such as epistaxis, menorrhagia or ecchymoses, and

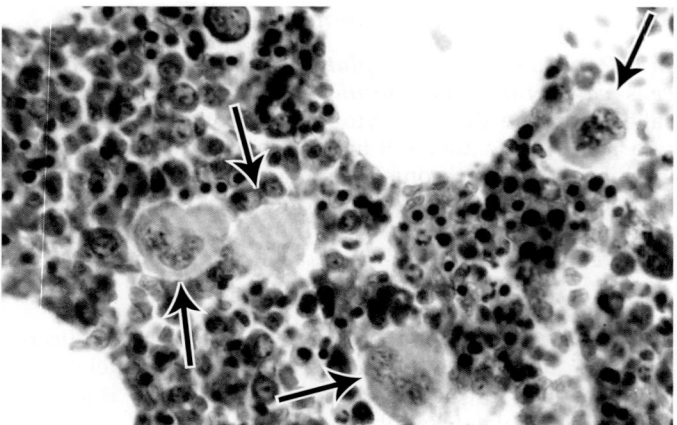

FIGURE 26-29. Idiopathic thrombocytopenic purpura. A section of the bone marrow reveals increased megakaryocytes (*arrows*).

excessive bleeding after trauma and minor procedures (e.g., tooth extraction). Life-threatening hemorrhages are uncommon. Occasionally, asymptomatic people are discovered to have thrombocytopenia on a routine blood cell count. Most adults with chronic ITP improve with corticosteroids and IVIG. Danazol (a synthetic anabolic steroid) acts like glucocorticoids. In 70% of patients who do not respond adequately to drug therapy within 2 to 3 months, splenectomy produces complete or partial remission. Other second-line therapies used in ITP include thrombopoietic agents that activate the TPO receptor, such as rituximab, or other immunosuppressive therapies.

Drug-Induced Autoimmune Thrombocytopenia

Many drugs cause immune-mediated platelet destruction: quinine, quinidine, heparin, sulfonamides, gold salts, antibiotics, sedatives, tranquilizers, and anticonvulsants. The drugs often complex with a platelet-related protein to make a neoepitope that elicits antibody production. Chemotherapeutic agents, ethanol and thiazides cause thrombocytopenia by directly suppressing platelet production.

Heparin-induced thrombocytopenia (HIT) is a distinct type of drug-induced thrombocytopenia. It has two types. About 25% of patients experience mild, transient thrombocytopenia 2 to 5 days after heparin treatment starts. This mild form of HIT is self-limited, entails aggregation of platelets by nonimmune mechanisms and follows a relatively benign course.

Type II HIT is immunologically mediated. It is caused by acquired IgG antibodies against platelet factor 4–heparin complexes. It occurs in 1% to 3% of patients treated with unfractionated heparin. After 4 to 10 days of therapy, these patients develop severe consumptive thrombocytopenia, but also platelet activation and, thus, a hypercoagulable state. Because this form of HIT entails hypercoagulability, platelet aggregation predisposes to arterial and venous thromboembolic events that may be lethal.

In both cases, heparin seemingly paradoxically activates platelet aggregation. In type I HIT, it is the heparin itself that induces platelets to aggregate. In type II HIT, heparin acts as a hapten, binding platelet membranes and eliciting antibodies. These antibodies, in turn, trigger platelet aggregation. Thus, the principal complication of HIT is thrombosis.

Pregnancy-Associated Thrombocytopenia

Minimal thrombocytopenia occurs often during the third trimester of pregnancy, owing to dilution of platelets. Since platelet counts are usually above 100,000/μL, no special management is needed. Conversely, preeclampsia/eclampsia syndromes can result in maternal thrombocytopenia. A condition related to preeclampsia is called **HELLP** (hemolysis, elevated liver enzyme tests and low platelets; see Chapter 14). The latter two syndromes can be life-threatening.

Neonatal Thrombocytopenia

Neonatal thrombocytopenias are either **inherited** or **acquired**.

Inherited causes associated with increased platelet destruction include **Wiskott–Aldrich syndrome** (WAS), an X-linked recessive disorder caused by variants in *WASP*, the gene that makes the Wiskott–Aldrich syndrome protein. Affected boys have small platelets, eczema, and immunodeficiency. A variant of WAS is **X-linked thrombocytopenia,** with mutations in the same gene, but which only involves thrombocytopenia. Other inherited defects associated with poor platelet production include amegakaryocytic thrombocytopenia, thrombocytopenia-absent radius syndrome, and Fanconi anemia. Thrombocytopenia can also be seen in infants with trisomy 13, 18, or 21.

Fanconi anemia (see above) is an inherited, autosomal recessive, bone marrow failure disorder that often includes thrombocytopenia and RBC macrocytosis. The family of Fanconi genes mediates DNA double-strand break repair and genetic stability. There is a high incidence of malignancies as well as congenital anomalies, such as skin hypopigmentation and hyperpigmentation, short stature, microcephaly, microphthalmia, and radial/thumb abnormalities (see Chapters 5 and 6).

Neonatal alloimmune thrombocytopenia (NAIT) is caused by increased destruction of platelets, because of alloimmunization to the human platelet antigen HPA-1a and other platelet-specific antigens that occurs during pregnancy. In NAIT, antibodies made by an HPA-1a–negative mother recognize a paternal HPA-1a antigen on the fetus's platelets. The fetus or neonate, but not the mother, develops thrombocytopenia. NAIT predisposes to fetal and neonatal intracranial hemorrhage.

Nonimmune causes of thrombocytopenia in the neonate are like those in adults, but in the context of additional considerations affecting neonates such as birth asphyxia, hypoxic injury, sepsis/DIC, necrotizing enterocolitis, hemangiomas, and thrombosis.

Posttransfusion Purpura

This complication of blood transfusion typically develops in women who are HPA-1-negative, and who were sensitized to HPA-1 as a result of previous pregnancies. It may also occur in men who have had previous blood transfusions. Thus, HPA-1–negative people may develop antibodies to HPA-1–positive platelets, either after pregnancy or transfusion with HPA-1–positive platelets. Any HPA-1–positive platelets infused thereafter become destroyed by those antibodies. Curiously, the patient's own HPA-1–negative platelets are also destroyed. They may acquire the antigen passively or immune complexes may localize to host platelet membranes. In any event, a self-limited thrombocytopenia occurs about a week after the transfusion.

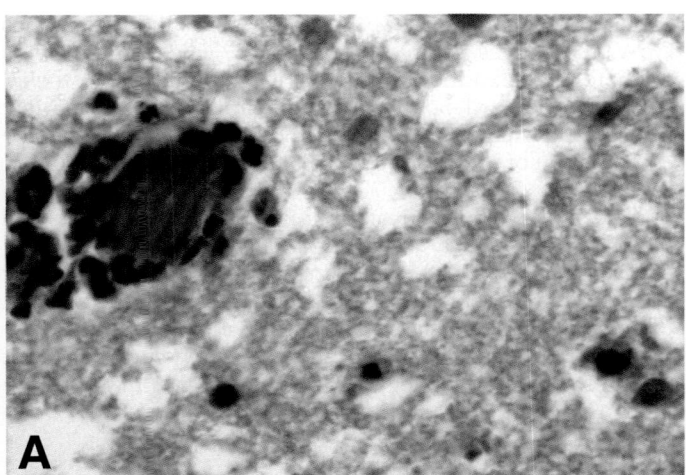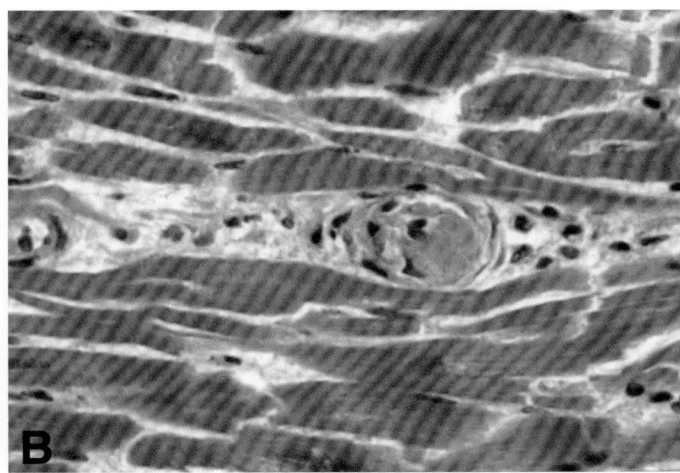

FIGURE 26-30 **Thrombotic thrombocytopenic purpura.** Microthrombi are present in the brain (**A**) and heart (**B**) of a patient who died of thrombotic thrombocytopenic purpura.

Thrombotic Thrombocytopenic Purpura

Thrombotic microangiopathies (TMAs) are a heterogeneous group of syndromes characterized by microthrombi in small blood vessels and capillaries leading to thrombocytopenia and microangiopathic hemolytic anemia. Patients often have neurologic symptoms, fever, and renal impairment. TMAs include TTP and HUS. Their pathology reflects widespread platelet aggregation and deposition of hyaline thrombi in the microcirculation.

MOLECULAR PATHOGENESIS: In TTP, ultralarge molecular weight vWF multimers released from injured endothelial cells are inadequately cleaved, leading to intravascular platelet aggregates. vWF monomers are normally assembled into multimeric molecules of varying size (up to millions of daltons) within endothelial cells and released locally in response to endothelial stimulation. The metalloprotease ADAMTS13 normally cleaves large vWF multimers. *In TTP, ADAMTS13 is deficient, causing ultra-large vWF multimers to accumulate. These multimers bind platelets, which form thrombi in the microvasculature, depleting platelets and causing thrombocytopenia.* ADAMTS13 is genetically absent or defective in familial TTP because of mutations of the *ADAMTS13* gene. The protein is inactivated by autoantibodies in idiopathic TTP. Prophylactic plasma infusion, which replaces the missing ADAMTS13 protein, is most effective in familial forms of TTP, and plasma exchange is preferred in acquired types.

Although most cases arise in otherwise normal people, TTP may also complicate systemic diseases such as autoimmune collagen vascular disorders (e.g., SLE, rheumatoid arthritis, Sjögren syndrome), drug-induced hypersensitivity reactions and malignant hypertension. It can also be triggered by infections, cancer chemotherapy, bone marrow transplantation, and pregnancy in HELLP syndrome (see Chapter 12).

PATHOLOGY: In TTP, periodic acid–Schiff (PAS)-positive hyaline microthrombi deposit in arterioles and capillaries throughout the body,

mainly in the heart, brain, and kidneys (Fig. 26-30). These microthrombi contain platelet aggregates, fibrin, and a few erythrocytes and leukocytes. Unlike immune-mediated vasculitis, there is no inflammation in TTP. Fragmented erythrocytes (schistocytes) always appear in peripheral blood smears (Fig. 26-31) and are caused by shearing of RBCs in vessels narrowed by thrombi. RBC polychromasia is also a feature and reflects an increase in reticulocytes in response to anemia. Hemolysis increases serum LDH and unconjugated bilirubin levels.

CLINICAL FEATURES: TTP may occur at any age but is most common in women in the fourth and fifth decades. It may be chronic and recurrent for years or, more frequently, occur as an acute, fulminant disease that can be fatal. Most patients present with neurologic symptoms, including seizures, focal

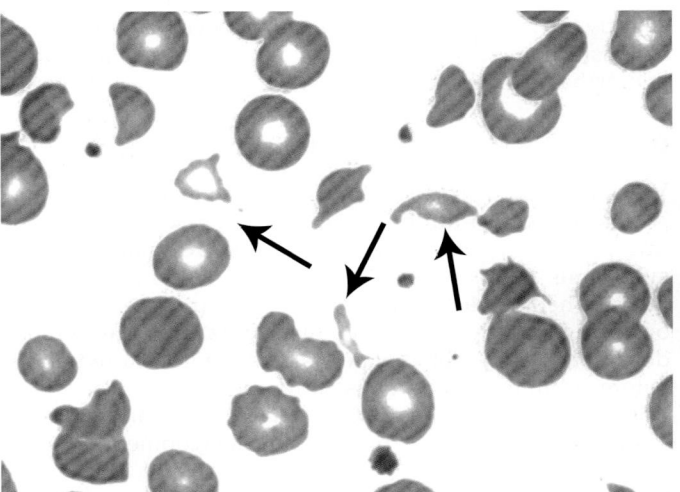

FIGURE 26-31. Microangiopathic hemolytic anemia. Numerous schistocytes (*arrows*) are present in a patient with thrombotic thrombocytopenic purpura. Schistocytes are fragmented RBCs with two or more points and reduced central pallor. Also note thrombocytopenia.

weakness, aphasia, and alterations in consciousness. Widespread purpura is often present and vaginal bleeding may occur in women. Hemolytic anemia is a constant feature; hemoglobin levels are often below 6 g/dL. Jaundice caused by hemolysis may be severe. Renal dysfunction includes proteinuria, hematuria, and mild renal insufficiency.

More than half of patients with TTP have platelet counts below 20,000/μL. Despite the presence of aggregated platelets, the coagulation cascade is not activated. Thus, the PT (monitors the extrinsic coagulation pathway), the APTT (monitors the intrinsic coagulation pathway), and fibrinogen all remain normal. These parameters distinguish this syndrome from DIC (see below). With plasma infusion and plasmapheresis, about 89% of patients survive this once almost uniformly fatal disease.

Hemolytic–Uremic Syndrome

HUS is a thrombotic microangiopathy that resembles TTP, but its pathogenesis is entirely different. HUS is characterized by thrombocytopenia, microangiopathic hemolysis, and acute renal failure.

Classic HUS occurs in children, usually after an acute infectious hemorrhagic gastroenteritis caused by *Escherichia coli* strain O157:H7 or *Shigella dysenteriae* (see Chapter 22). Production of a Shiga-like toxin damages vascular endothelium and activates platelets. Fibrinogen then binds activated platelet Gp IIb/IIIa complex, and platelets aggregate. In HUS, aggregated platelet thrombi accumulate primarily in the renal microvasculature. Kidney failure, rather than neurologic abnormalities, is the main clinical feature.

Splenic Sequestration of Platelets

Many patients with splenomegaly, irrespective of the cause, show **hypersplenism**. This syndrome includes sequestration of platelets in the spleen. One-third of platelets are normally stored temporarily in the spleen, but in massive splenomegaly, up to 90% of the total platelet pool may be sequestered in that organ. Interestingly, platelet life span is normal, or only slightly reduced. Thrombocytopenia associated with hypersplenism is rarely severe and by itself does not produce a hemorrhagic diathesis.

Other Causes of Thrombocytopenia

Vascular malformations, including hemangiomas and AVMs, can cause thrombocytopenia. Platelet consumption due to hemangiomas has been called **Kasabach–Merritt syndrome**. Platelet loss also occurs in patients who have massive hemorrhage, such as in bleeding from a peptic ulcer or during surgery with heavy blood loss. Transfused blood does not contain viable platelets because it is stored at 4°C before administration. Thus, thrombocytopenia occurs in transfused patients because of platelet loss and dilution. Platelet transfusion may prevent this development.

Hereditary Disorders of Platelets

Bernard–Soulier Syndrome (Giant Platelet Syndrome)

This is an autosomal recessive disorder in which platelets have a quantitative or qualitative defect in the membrane glycoprotein complex (Gp Ib/IX [CD42] and sometimes Gp V) that serves as a receptor for vWF. This complex helps mediate platelet adhesion to vWF in injured subendothelial tissues. In Bernard–Soulier syndrome, platelets vary widely in size and shape, and the diagnosis is suggested by the combination of *thrombocytopenia and giant platelets* on a blood smear.

The syndrome manifests in infancy or childhood with a bleeding pattern characteristic of *abnormal platelet function*: ecchymoses, epistaxis, and gingival bleeding. At a later age, traumatic hemorrhage, gastrointestinal bleeding, and menorrhagia occur. Many patients have only a mild bleeding disorder, but others suffer more severe hemorrhage that requires frequent platelet transfusions and that may even be fatal.

Glanzmann Thrombasthenia

This is an autosomal recessive defect in platelet aggregation caused by a quantitative or qualitative abnormality in the glycoprotein complex IIb/IIIa (CD41/61). In normal platelets, this complex is activated during platelet adhesion. It acts as a receptor for fibrinogen and vWF, to mediate platelet aggregation and generate a solid plug. The IIb/IIIa complex is also linked to the platelet cytoskeleton and transmits the force of contraction to adherent fibrin, which promotes clot retraction. In Glanzmann thrombasthenia, impaired aggregation and clot retraction hampers hemostasis and causes bleeding, despite a normal platelet count.

The disease becomes clinically apparent shortly after birth when an infant exhibits mucocutaneous or gingival hemorrhage, epistaxis or bleeding after circumcision. Later, patients may suffer unexpected hemorrhage after trauma or surgery. Disease severity varies, and only a few patients experience life-threatening hemorrhage. Platelet transfusions correct the condition temporarily.

Alpha Storage Pool Disease (Gray Platelet Syndrome)

Alpha storage pool disease is a rare inherited disease in which platelets lack morphologically recognizable α-granules. The defect is in granule membranes, which are abnormal. Thrombocytopenia is common; platelets are large, pale/gray and agranular appearing under light microscopy. The bleeding diathesis tends to be mild.

Delta Storage Pool Disease

This heterogeneous illness is caused by absence of platelet dense granules (also known as delta granules), or abnormal secretion of their contents. It is sometimes associated with other multisystem hereditary disorders, including Chédiak–Higashi syndrome or Hermansky–Pudlak syndrome (both of which include oculocutaneous albinism). Bleeding manifestations are mild to moderate. Since delta granules are not normally visible under light microscopy, electron microscopy is required to establish the diagnosis.

Acquired Qualitative Platelet Disorders

Several acquired disorders may impair platelet function:

- **Drugs:** Various drugs can impair platelet activity. Aspirin irreversibly acetylates cyclooxygenase (COX), primarily COX-1, and thus blocks production of platelet thromboxane A_2, which is important for platelet aggregation. Platelets cannot synthesize cyclooxygenase, so the aspirin effect lasts for the life span of platelets (7 to 10 days). Non-steroidal analgesics, such as indomethacin or ibuprofen, impair platelet function, but as their inhibition of cyclooxygenase is reversible, their effect on platelets is short lived. Antibiotics, particularly β-lactams (penicillin and cephalosporins), can cause platelet dysfunction. Ticlopidine markedly impedes platelet function and is used to treat thromboembolic disease. However, it may cause TTP.

- **Renal failure:** Qualitative platelet defects leading to prolonged bleeding times and a tendency toward hemorrhage may complicate kidney disease. These platelet abnormalities are heterogeneous and are aggravated by uremic anemia. Reestablishing a normal Hct using EPO may return bleeding time to normal without correcting the azotemia.
- **Cardiopulmonary bypass:** Use of extracorporeal circuit during bypass surgery may impair platelet function by activating and fragmenting platelets.
- **Hematologic malignancies:** Platelet dysfunction in chronic MPNs and MDSs reflects intrinsic platelet defects. In dysproteinemias, platelets are coated with plasma paraprotein, impairing function.

Thrombocytosis

Reactive Thrombocytosis
Increases in platelet counts occur in association with (1) iron-deficiency anemia, especially in children; (2) splenectomy; (3) cancer; and (4) chronic inflammatory disorders. Reactive thrombocytosis is rarely symptomatic, but it may trigger thrombotic episodes, especially in patients bedridden after splenectomy.

Clonal Thrombocytosis
MPNs (see below) such as polycythemia vera and essential thrombocythemia (ET) entail malignant proliferations of megakaryocytes. Resulting increases in circulating platelets may lead to episodic thrombosis or bleeding.

Coagulopathies Are Caused by Deficient or Abnormal Coagulation Factors

Quantitative and qualitative disorders of all of the coagulation factors are known, and may be **inherited** or **acquired**. Most result from deficiency of the protein factor, leading to inadequate hemostasis and concomitant bleeding. Occasionally the protein factor is present but dysfunctional. The more commonly encountered hereditary deficiencies include those of vWF, factor VIII (hemophilia A), and factor IX (hemophilia B).

Hemophilia is an X-linked recessive disorder of blood clotting that results in joint and muscle bleeding. Classic hemophilia is actually two distinct diseases resulting from mutations in *F8* and *F9*, the genes for **factor VIII (hemophilia A)** and **factor IX (hemophilia B)**, respectively.

Hemophilia is one of the oldest genetic diseases recorded, having been described in the Talmud almost 2000 years ago. Male infants of Jewish families with a history of fatal bleeding after circumcision were excused from this ritual. Transmission of a bleeding tendency to boys from unaffected mothers has been known for 200 years. Dissemination of hemophilia throughout Europe's royal families by Queen Victoria's daughters highlighted this disease.

Hemophilia A (Factor VIII Deficiency)

 MOLECULAR PATHOGENESIS: *Hemophilia A is the most common X-linked inherited bleeding disorder (1 per 5,000 to 10,000 males).* The gene for factor VIII was cloned in 1984. Causative mutations in the very large *F8* gene at the tip of the long arm of the X chromosome (Xq28) include deletions, inversions, point mutations, and insertions. Each family with a history of hemophilia actually harbors a different mutation (private mutant allele). In half of cases, hemophilia A can be traced through many generations, but the other half represent de novo mutations arising within two generations of the index case. In most cases of de novo mutations, an origin in the mother, maternal grandfather, or maternal grandmother can be identified.

CLINICAL FEATURES: Patients with hemophilia A have mild, moderate, or severe bleeding tendencies. In most, the severity of the illness parallels factor VIII activity in the blood. Half of patients have virtually no factor VIII activity and often suffer spontaneous bleeding. A third of patients, with 1% to 5% of normal factor VIII activity, will only occasionally bleed spontaneously, but do so often after minor trauma. One-fifth have factor VIII activity levels from 5% to 40% of normal and bleed only after significant trauma or surgery.

The most frequent complication of hemophilia A is a degenerative joint disease caused by repeated bleeding into many joints. Although uncommon, bleeding into the brain was formerly the most common cause of death. Hematuria, intestinal obstruction and respiratory obstruction may all occur with bleeding into the respective organs.

Management consists of factor VIII replacement, either prophylactically to prevent bleeding or therapeutically in response to bleeding episodes. The aim is to correct factor VIII levels to control bleeding and prevent long-term sequelae. Unfortunately, in the 1980s, many of these patients developed AIDS and viral hepatitis from contamination of pooled factor VIII preparations (from plasma-derived concentrates). Screening blood donors for HIV, heat-treating purified factor VIII to inactivate HIV and, now, the use of human recombinant factor VIII, have eliminated these complications. Screening to detect female carriers and prenatal diagnosis using DNA markers are highly accurate.

Hemophilia B

 MOLECULAR PATHOGENESIS: *Hemophilia B is an X-linked inherited disorder of factor IX deficiency.* It is 1/4 as common as hemophilia A, at 1 in 20,000 male births, and accounts for 15% of cases of hemophilia. Factor IX is a vitamin K–dependent protein made in the liver. Many different mutations in the responsible gene, *F9*, from single base substitutions to gross deletions, may cause hemophilia B.

 CLINICAL FEATURES: Bleeding manifestations in hemophilia B are like those of hemophilia A. Treatment relies on infusion of purified or recombinant factor IX concentrates.

von Willebrand Disease

von Willebrand disease (vWD) is a heterogeneous complex of hereditary bleeding disorders related to deficiency or abnormality of vWF. Over 20 distinct subtypes are known. A simplified classification (see below) recognizes three major categories. Variable expression of vWF (especially type I) confounds estimates of prevalence, but some experts consider vWD to be the most common inherited coagulopathy (1% to 2% of the population).

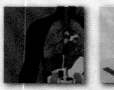 **PATHOPHYSIOLOGY AND MOLECULAR PATHOGENESIS:** vWF is an adhesive molecule made by endothelial cells and megakaryocytes as a 250-kd monomer. It polymerizes to form multimers with molecular weights in the millions. vWF is stored in cytoplasmic Weibel–Palade bodies in endothelial cells, from which it is released into subendothelial tissues and plasma. After endothelial insult, vWF binds subendothelial collagen. It then binds platelet glycoprotein receptors (Gp Ib/IX or CD42), triggering platelet adhesion and sealing the injury (Fig. 26-32). Both vWF and fibrinogen bind Gp IIb/IIIa (CD41/61) to promote platelet aggregation. Separately, in plasma, vWF serves to carry factor VIII, protecting it from clearance. Thus, factor VIII levels drop in vWF deficiency.

vWD is an autosomal disease, affecting men and women. The *vWF* gene on chromosome 12 is large and complex (180 kb with 52 exons). Three major types of the disease are recognized, each of which is heterogeneous:

- **Type I vWD:** These variants constitute 75% of cases of vWD and are inherited as autosomal dominant traits with variable penetrance. Type I vWD is a **quantitative deficiency in vWF. The number of vWF multimers is reduced (i.e., vWF antigen levels are decreased) with a parallel reduction in vWF activity (generally 5% to 30% of normal).** All multimers are reduced in amount, but their relative proportions remain unchanged.
- **Type II vWD: Qualitative defects in vWF** characterize type II variants, which account for 20% of vWD. In type II disease, interactions of vWF with the blood vessel wall, platelets or factor VIII are defective. While the number of vWF molecules (i.e., vWF antigen levels) may be normal or mildly reduced, vWF activity is disproportionately reduced because of the functional defect. In type IIa, higher–molecular-weight multimers are absent from platelets and plasma. In type IIb, an abnormal vWF has increased affinity for platelets, leading to aberrant binding of the highest–molecular-weight (HMW) multimers to platelets. Clearance of such HMW vWF-platelet complexes causes selective loss of HMW multimers and thrombocytopenia. In type IIM, all multimers are present but their function is defective. Type IIN involves a mutation in the factor VIII–binding site leading to extremely low factor VIII levels and a hemophilia like clinical picture.

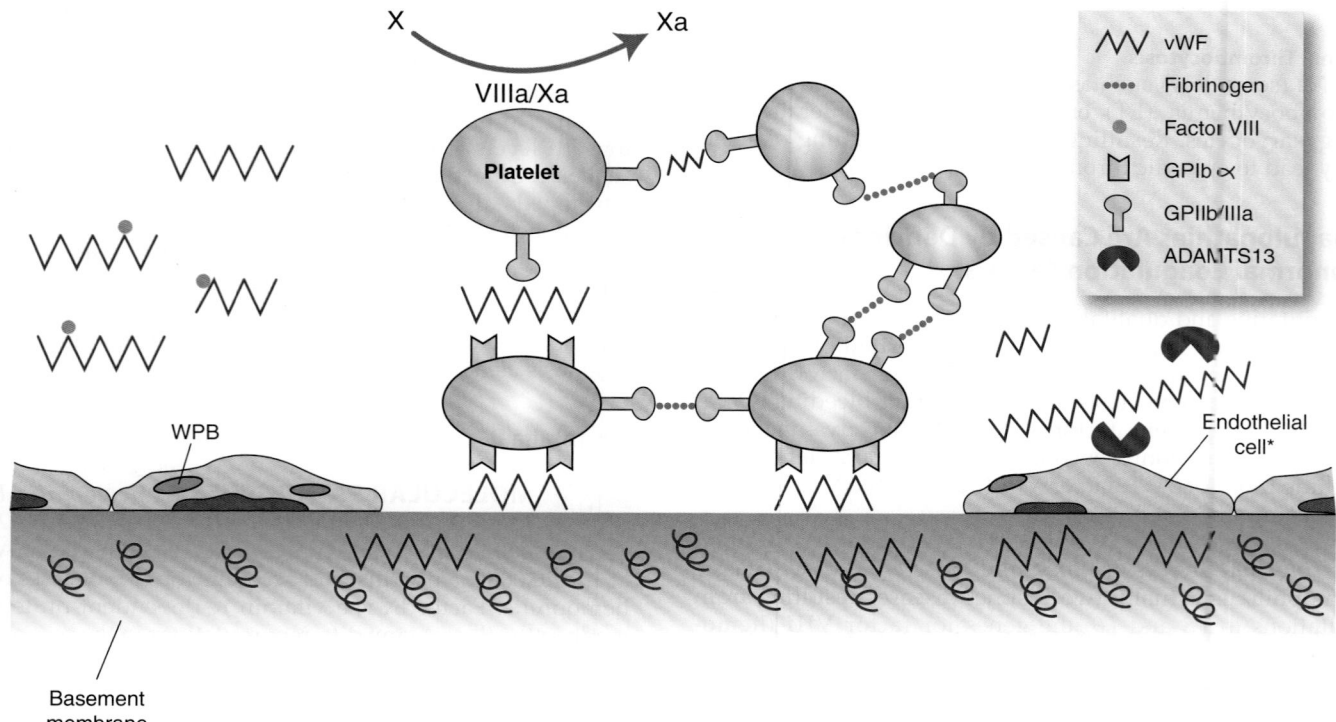

FIGURE 26-32. von Willebrand factor (vWF). vWF is stored in Weibel–Palade bodies (WPBs) of endothelial cells and is secreted from activated endothelial cells (*) into the subendothelial space. vWF is also secreted from platelet α-granules. After endothelial injury, vWF binds to subendothelial collagen and then platelet adhere to vWF via glycoprotein (Gp) receptors Gp Ibα/IX. Released vWF stabilizes platelet adhesion to the damaged vessel wall and promotes platelet–fibrin interactions. vWF also binds Gp IIB/IIA on the activated platelet surface to promote platelet aggregation. ADAMTS13 is the protease that cleaves ultra-large multimers of vWF. In plasma, vWF also protects factor VIII.

- **Type III vWD:** This least common form of the disease is **a severe quantitative deficiency** of vWD. It is inherited as an autosomal recessive trait, but some patients are compound heterozygotes with different mutations in the two vWF alleles. vWF activity is extremely low (<5%) and plasma factor VIII levels are less than 10% of normal

 CLINICAL FEATURES: Except for type III, most cases of vWD entail only a mild bleeding diathesis.

By contrast to hemophilia-related bleeding, patients with vWD show immediate mucocutaneous bleeding, easy bruising, epistaxis, GI bleeding, and (in women) menorrhagia. The presenting symptom is often excessive hemorrhage after trauma or surgery. Patients with type III vWD can have life-threatening hemorrhage from the gut; hemarthroses like those that occur in hemophilia are not unusual.

All forms of vWD respond well to supplementation with vWF concentrates or cryoprecipitate. The vasopressin analog desmopressin (DDAVP) is the treatment of choice in types I and IIa, because it increases release of preformed vWF from endothelial storage pools. DDAVP intranasal sprays are now available.

Other Coagulation Factor Deficiencies

Deficiencies of all coagulation factor proteins, including factors VII, X, V, XI and II (prothrombin) and fibrinogen, have been reported in humans. As expected, the severity of bleeding usually correlates with the level of functional protein activity. Prolonged PT (extrinsic coagulation pathway) or APTT (intrinsic coagulation pathway) in patients who bleed excessively helps identify a problem with coagulation factors. Factor-specific assays confirm the diagnosis. The thrombin time helps to screen for deficiency or dysfunction of fibrinogen. Deficiency of fibrinogen causes bleeding. By contrast, dysfibrinogenemia may cause bleeding but more often leads to thrombosis.

Deficiency of factors XII and contact factors (high–molecular-weight kininogen and prekallikrein) do not cause bleeding manifestations. However, since these are needed ex vivo in the APTT reaction, they do cause marked prolongations of APTT.

Liver Disease

Many coagulation factors are produced by the liver (e.g., II, V, VII, IX, X). In addition, the liver plays a key role in vitamin K absorption. Severe liver disease may thus impair secretion of coagulation factors, as a manifestation of the general protein synthetic defect. In this case, levels of all liver-synthesized coagulation factors are low, affecting the intrinsic and extrinsic pathways. PT and APTT are both prolonged, but because vitamin K–dependent factors are disproportionately affected in liver disease, the PT is much more affected than the APTT. This is unlike the situation in DIC (see below).

Vitamin K Deficiency

Liver-derived coagulation factors depend on vitamin K as an essential cofactor in γ-carboxylation of glutamic acid to form γ-carboxyglutamate (Gla) residues. The secreted proteins are functional only if Gla residues are present. By contrast, factor V is made in the liver but does not require vitamin K. Thus, in vitamin K deficiency (see Chapter 8), activities of factors II, VII, IX, and X are low but factor V activity is normal. Severe liver disease will, however, decrease activities of all of these factors because of a general impairment of hepatic protein synthesis.

 CLINICAL FEATURES: Levels of vitamin K are physiologically low in neonates, and it is standard practice to administer vitamin K to newborns to prevent hemorrhagic disease. In adults, vitamin K deficiency may reflect poor dietary intake. Since colonic bacteria produce the form of vitamin K that is best absorbed, prolonged antibiotic intake or large colonic resections may also lead to vitamin K deficiency.

Inhibitors of Coagulation Factors

Acquired inhibitors of coagulation factors, **circulating anticoagulants,** are usually IgG autoantibodies. Most are directed against factor VIII and vWF, but rarely antibodies to any of the other coagulation factors can be present. In hereditary coagulation disorders, especially hemophilia, circulating anticoagulants are alloantibodies due to exposure to exogenous factors used therapeutically. Autoantibodies to clotting factors may also develop in some patients with autoimmune disorders (e.g., SLE, rheumatoid arthritis; see Chapter 11), or those with lymphoproliferative disorders, presumably owing to abnormal immune regulation. Finally, acquired anticoagulants often appear in apparently normal people.

 CLINICAL FEATURES: Acquired anticoagulants may cause life-threatening hemorrhage. These autoantibodies are difficult to eliminate, but 1/3 of patients remit spontaneously. Treatment is two pronged, including control of bleeding (administration of factor concentrates, activated prothrombin complex, activated factor VII a) and elimination of the inhibitor using immunosuppression (e.g., corticosteroids, cyclophosphamide, rituximab).

Disseminated Intravascular Coagulation

DIC is widespread intravascular activation of coagulation, generating thrombin and microvascular fibrin thrombi and triggering fibrinolysis. Platelets and clotting factors are consumed, so patients also tend to hemorrhage. DIC is serious and often fatal. It may complicate massive trauma, burns, sepsis from diverse organisms (see Chapter 12) and obstetric emergencies. It is also associated with metastatic cancer, hematopoietic malignancies, cardiovascular and liver disease, and many other conditions.

 PATHOPHYSIOLOGY: DIC begins with activation of clotting cascades within the vascular compartment by tissue injury and/or endothelial damage. *Subsequent generation of substantial amounts of thrombin (Fig. 26-33), combined with the failure of natural inhibitory mechanisms to neutralize thrombin, trigger DIC.* With consequent uncontrolled intravascular

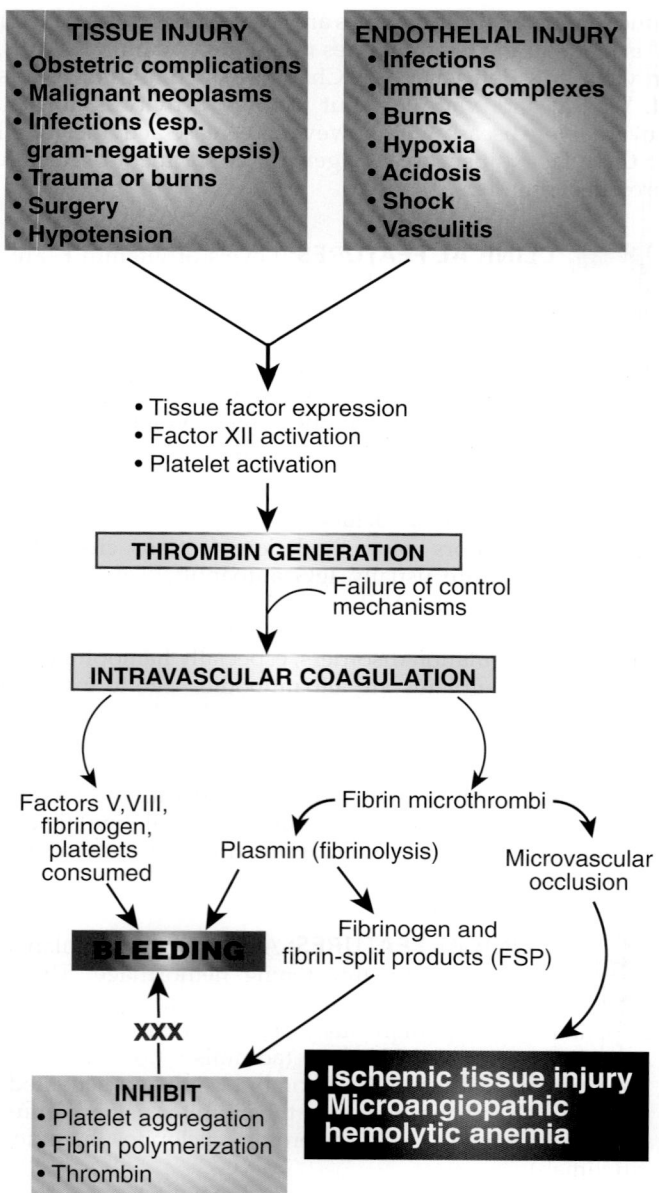

FIGURE 26-33. The pathophysiology of disseminated intravascular coagulation (DIC). The DIC syndrome is precipitated by tissue injury, endothelial cell injury or a combination of the two. These injuries trigger increased expression of tissue factor on cell surfaces and activation of clotting factors (including XII and V) and platelets. With the failure of normal control mechanisms, generation of thrombin leads to intravascular coagulation.

coagulation, the delicate balance between coagulation and fibrinolysis goes awry. This leads to consumption of clotting factors, platelets and fibrinogen, and a resultant hemorrhagic diathesis.

Procoagulant TF is released into the circulation after many kinds of injury, including direct trauma, brain injury, and obstetric accidents (e.g., premature separation of the placenta) (see Chapter 14). **Bacterial endotoxin** stimulates macrophages to release TF (see Chapter 12) and certain **tumor cells** cause DIC by releasing TF. With activation of the clotting cascade, intravascular fibrin

microthrombi deposit in the smallest blood vessels. Stimulation of the fibrinolytic system by fibrin generates fibrin split (degradation) products, which possess anticoagulant properties and further contribute to the bleeding diathesis.

Endothelial injury often plays an important role in the development of DIC. The anticoagulant properties of the endothelium (Fig. 26-28) are impaired by diverse injuries, including (1) TNF in gram-negative sepsis; (2) other inflammatory mediators, such as activated complement, IL-1, or neutrophil proteases; (3) viral or rickettsial infections; and (4) trauma (e.g., burns).

PATHOLOGY: Arterioles, capillaries, and venules throughout the body are occluded by **microthrombi** made of fibrin and platelets (Fig. 26-34). However, because fibrinolysis is activated, these thrombi may no longer be detectable at the time of autopsy. Microvascular obstruction is associated with widespread **ischemic changes,** particularly in the brain, kidneys, skin, lungs, and GI tract. These organs are also sites of bleeding, which, in the case of the brain and gut, may be fatal.

Erythrocytes become fragmented (**schistocytes**) in passing through webs of intravascular fibrin, resulting in **microangiopathic hemolytic anemia**. Consumption of activated platelets leads to **thrombocytopenia**, while **depletion of clotting factors** prolongs PT and APTT, and decreases plasma fibrinogen. Plasma fibrin split products also prolong the thrombin time. Fibrinopeptide A- and D-dimers are elevated (as markers of coagulation and fibrinolytic activation, respectively).

CLINICAL FEATURES: DIC symptoms reflect both microvascular thrombosis and a bleeding tendency. Ischemic injury in the brain leads to seizures and coma. Depending on the severity of DIC, renal symptoms range from mild azotemia to fulminant acute renal failure. Acute respiratory distress syndrome

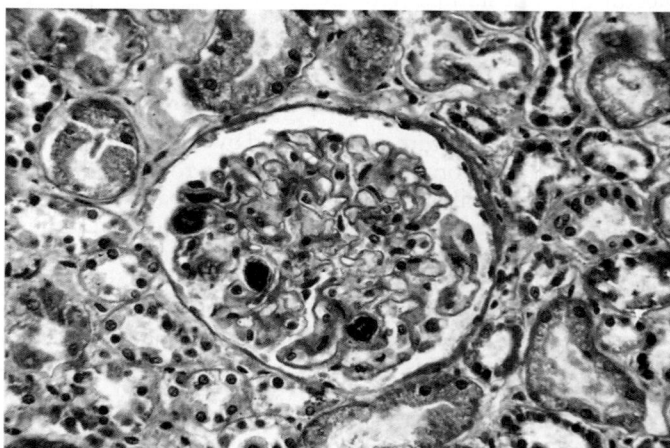

FIGURE 26-34. Disseminated intravascular coagulation. A section of a glomerulus stained with phosphotungstic acid hematoxylin (PTAH), which colors fibrin deep purple, demonstrates several microthrombi.

(see Chapter 18) may supervene, and acute mucosal ulcers in the gut may bleed. The bleeding diathesis is evidenced by cerebral hemorrhage, ecchymoses, and hematuria. Patients with DIC are treated with heparin anticoagulation to interrupt the cycle of intravascular coagulation, and replenishment of platelets and clotting factors to control the bleeding.

Hypercoagulability Causes Widespread Thrombosis

Hypercoagulability is increased tendency to form clots, compared to normal. A possible hypercoagulable state should be explored when unexplained thrombotic episodes arise in any of the following contexts:

- Recurrence
- Development at a young age
- Family history of thrombotic episodes
- Thrombosis in unusual anatomic locations
- Difficulty in controlling with anticoagulants

Hypercoagulable states are either inherited or acquired (Table 26-13).

Inherited Hypercoagulability

This reflects alterations in the natural anticoagulant pathways. A hereditary tendency to clot excessively, regardless of its origin, is referred to as **thrombophilia**.

- **Activated protein C (APC) resistance—factor V Leiden:** A point mutation in *F5*, the factor *V* gene, known as factor V Leiden renders it resistant to inhibition by APC.

TABLE 26-13
PRINCIPAL CAUSES OF HYPERCOAGULABILITY

Inherited
Activated protein C resistance (factor √ Leiden)
Antithrombin deficiency
Protein C deficiency
Protein S deficiency
Dysfibrinogenemias
Prothrombin mutation
High factor VIII

Acquired
Antiphospholipid antibody syndrome
Malignancy
Nephrotic syndrome
Smoking
Factor concentrates
Heparin-induced thrombocytopenia with thrombosis (HITT)
Oral contraceptives
Hyperlipidemia
Thrombotic thrombocytopenic purpura
Pregnancy
Stasis

Resistance to APC action is the most common genetic hypercoagulability disorder. It accounts for up to 65% of patients with venous thrombosis. The factor V Leiden mutation occurs worldwide, but more so in whites (up to 5% of the general population) and much less so in Africans (near 0%). Compared with normal people, heterozygotes for factor V Leiden have seven times the risk for deep venous thrombosis. In homozygotes, the increased risk is 80-fold.

- **Antithrombin (AT) deficiency:** This autosomal dominant disorder, which has incomplete penetrance, occurs in 0.2% to 0.4% of the general population and can result in either a quantitative or a qualitative effect on AT. The risk of a thrombotic event (usually venous) is increased by 20% to 80% in different families.
- **Protein C and protein S deficiencies:** Homozygous protein C deficiency causes life-threatening neonatal thrombosis with **purpura fulminans**. Up to 0.5% of the general population has heterozygous protein C deficiency, but many affected individuals are symptom free. Clinically, deficiencies of proteins C and S resemble AT deficiency.
- **Other causes of hypercoagulability:** A variant (G20210A) in the 3′-untranslated region of *F2*, the prothrombin gene, is associated with thrombosis. The mechanism is unclear, but it causes excessively high prothrombin levels. Unusually high levels of fibrinogen and factors VII and VIII are also associated with thrombosis, as are some dysfibrinogenemias.

Acquired Hypercoagulability

Venous stasis contributes to hypercoagulability associated with prolonged immobilization and congestive heart failure. Increased platelet activation probably accounts for excessive clotting in patients with myeloproliferative disorders, heparin-associated thrombocytopenia and TTP.

Antiphospholipid Antibody Syndrome

This autoimmune disorder is characterized by **clinical events involving thrombosis** (arterial, venous or placental, the latter manifesting as fetal loss and other pregnancy complications) and **laboratory demonstration of antibodies** against several negatively charged protein/phospholipid complexes.

In this syndrome, antibodies (mainly IgG or IgM) react with proteins bound to anionic phospholipids, such as phosphatidylserine (PS) or cardiolipin. These membrane lipids are only exposed when cells such as platelets are activated. Many plasma proteins (e.g., β2-glycoprotein 1) and Gla domain–containing procoagulant proteins (e.g., prothrombin) bind to PS and related anionic phospholipids.

Laboratory diagnosis entails detection of (1) lupus-type anticoagulant activity, (2) anticardiolipin antibodies, and (3) antibodies to plasma protein β_2-glycoprotein 1 (GP1). Anticardiolipin antibodies bind β_2-GP1 in the presence of cardiolipin.

Lupus anticoagulants are antibodies that bind to phospholipid-bound proteins, and prolong phospholipid-dependent clotting assays such as the APTT. The term "lupus anticoagulant" is a misnomer; these antibodies are not restricted to patients with SLE (see Chapter 11) and can occur in patients with other autoimmune conditions, or in otherwise asymptomatic people. Although they prolong APTT in vitro, and thus appear to be an "anticoagulant," they are in fact procoagulant in patients.

Antiphospholipid antibody syndrome is the leading acquired hematologic cause of thrombosis. Resulting thromboses may occur via several mechanisms, including platelet activation, endothelial cell activation, and altered coagulation factor assembly on membranes. Thrombosis in the uteroplacental vasculature is the likely mechanism in recurrent fetal loss.

Neoplastic Disorders of Myelopoiesis

Malignant leukocytes originate from either myeloid or lymphoid cells.

NON-ACUTE MYELOID PROLIFERATIONS

Malignant proliferations of myeloid cells are derived from bone marrow cells and manifest as **AMLs, MDSs,** or **MPNs**. **Malignant lymphocytes** may arise anywhere there are lymphoid cells. World Health Organization (WHO) classifications are based on morphology, immunophenotype, cytogenetics, and molecular abnormalities. In 2008 and 2016, the WHO made significant changes to the classification of hematopoietic malignancies.

Myeloproliferative Neoplasms Are Clonal Stem Cell Disorders

MPNs are clonal HSC disorders with unregulated, increased proliferation of one or more myeloid lineages (granulocytes, erythrocytes, megakaryocytes, or mast cells). The WHO recognizes four well-established (1-4), and four additional (5-8), entities: (1) **chronic myelogenous leukemia, BCR-ABL1 positive; (2) polycythemia vera; (3) primary myelofibrosis (PMF); (4) ET; (5) chronic neutrophilic leukemia; (6) chronic eosinophilic leukemia; (7) mastocytosis; and (8) unclassifiable MPN** (Table 26-14).

MPNs typically affect adults 40 to 80 years old. They are relatively uncommon, with a yearly incidence of 6 to 10 cases per 100,000, which increases with age. Radiation and benzene exposure are implicated in a subset of cases, but the cause is usually unknown. There is also evidence of inherited predisposition to develop MPNs. Characteristic pathologic features depend on the stage but generally include bone marrow hypercellularity with effective hematopoietic maturation and increased numbers of red cells, granulocytes, and/or platelets. Bone marrow fibrosis of different degrees and splenomegaly often accompany MPNs. Specific oncogene mutations and/or translocations are diagnostic of certain MPNs (see below).

Chronic Myelogenous Leukemia

CML is derived from an abnormal pluripotent bone marrow stem cell and results in prominent neutrophilic leukocytosis over the full range of myeloid maturation. A **Philadelphia chromosome,** or molecular or cytogenetic demonstration of the **BCR/ABL fusion gene,** is required to establish the diagnosis. CML is the most common MPN and accounts for 15% to 20% of all cases of leukemia.

 MOLECULAR PATHOGENESIS: The cause of CML is usually unknown. Radiation exposure and myelotoxic agents, such as benzene, have been implicated in a small number of cases. Conventional cytogenetic and/or fluorescence in situ hybridization (FISH) techniques identify a reciprocal balanced translocation in 95% of cases. This translocation involves exchange of genetic material between chromosomes 9 and 22, resulting in a Philadelphia chromosome [t(9;22)(q34;q11)] (Table 26-15; Fig. 26-35A). This chromosome itself is a derivative (shortened) chromosome 22 [der(22q)]. The *BCR* (breakpoint cluster region) gene on chromosome 22 is fused to the *ABL* gene on chromosome 9 to form a *BCR/ABL* fusion gene. A small number of cases have cryptic translocations involving 9q34 and 22q11 that cannot be identified by conventional cytogenetics. In these cases, *BCR/ABL* fusion is detected by FISH (Fig. 26-35B) or by molecular techniques, such as reverse transcriptase polymerase chain reaction (RT-PCR).

In the vast majority of cases, the abnormal BCR/ABL fusion gene encodes a 210-kd fusion protein (p210), which is a constitutively active tyrosine kinase that is central to the pathogenesis of the neoplasm. This activated tyrosine kinase autophosphorylates and then activates downstream signaling pathways that trigger cell proliferation, differentiation, survival, and adhesion. Much less commonly, the *BCR/ABL* fusion gene results from a breakage in the minor breakpoint cluster regions yielding alternative fusion proteins such as p190 and p230 (often associated with prominent neutrophilic maturation and/or thrombocytosis). While small amounts of p190 (often associated with monocytosis) fusion product occur in CML, this form of BCR/ABL is more often seen in **Philadelphia chromosome-positive acute lymphoblastic leukemia occurring outside the setting of CML.** RT-PCR can identify the specific BCR/ABL product fusion present in the leukemic cells and quantify the fusion product. The latter parameter is useful for monitoring patient responses to therapy. Identification of additional chromosomal abnormalities (e.g., a second Philadelphia chromosome, trisomy 8, etc.), usually heralds progression to more aggressive phases of the disease.

 PATHOLOGY: CML may present in **chronic, accelerated,** or **blast phases**.

- **CML, chronic phase (CP):** Patients present with leukocytosis and the bone marrow shows predominance of myeloid cells in all stages of maturation with increased numbers of myelocytes. By definition, blasts make up less than 10% of circulating or bone marrow leukocytes. Basophilia and eosinophilia are common. Platelets are normal or increased, and may exceed $10^6/\mu L$. Bone marrow biopsies show hypercellularity, usually with total effacement of the marrow space by mostly myeloid cells and their precursors (Fig. 26-36). Megakaryocytes are often small with nuclear hypolobation; these are referred to as "dwarf" megakaryocytes. Reticulin fibers are normal or moderately increased.
- **CML, accelerated phase (AP):** AP represents disease progression from CML-CP. CML-AP is defined by one or more of the following criteria: (1) persistent or

TABLE 26-14

MYELOPROLIFERATIVE NEOPLASMS[a]

	Chronic Myelogenous Leukemia, BCR-ABL1 Positive	Polycythemia Vera	Primary Myelofibrosis	Essential Thrombocythemia
Clinical Features				
Peak age range (years)	25–60	40–60	50–70	50–70
Splenomegaly	90%	75%	100%	30% (slight)
Hepatomegaly	50%	40%	80%	40% (slight)
Acute leukemic conversion	80%	5–10%	5–10%	2–5%
Median survival (years)	3–4	13	5	>10
Bone Marrow				
Histopathology	Panhyperplasia (predominantly granulocytic)	Panhyperplasia (predominantly erythroid)	Panhyperplasia with fibrosis	Large megakaryocytes in clusters
M:E ratio	10:1 to 50:1	≤2:1	2:1 to 5:1	2:1 to 5:1
Fibrosis	<10%	15–20%	90–100%	<5%
Laboratory Findings				
Hemoglobin	Mild anemia	>20 g/dL	Mild anemia	Mild anemia
RBC morphology	Slight aniso- and poikilocytosis	Slight aniso- and poikilocytosis	Immature erythrocytes and marked aniso- and poikilocytosis	Hypochromic microcytes
Granulocytes	Moderate to markedly increased with spectrum of maturation	Normal to mildly increased; may show a few immature forms	Normal to moderately increased; some immature WBCs	Normal to slightly increased
Platelets	Normal to moderately increased	Normal to moderately increased	Increased to decreased	Markedly increased with abnormal forms
Genetics	Philadelphia chromosome: *BCR/ABL* gene rearrangement	JAK2 activating mutation	JAK2 activating mutation	JAK2 activating mutation

M:E ratio = ratio of myeloid to erythroid, RBC = red blood cell; WBC = white blood cell.

[a]Other myeloproliferative neoplasms include chronic neutrophilic leukemia, chronic eosinophilic leukemia, mastocytosis and myeloproliferative neoplasm, unclassifiable.

increasing WBC count unresponsive to therapy, (2) persistent or increasing splenomegaly unresponsive to therapy, (3) persistent thrombocytopenia or thrombocytosis unresponsive to therapy, (4) additional chromosomal abnormalities, (5) 20% or more blood basophils, and/or (6) 10% to 19% blasts in the blood or bone marrow. Response to therapy parameters are also now included as provisional criteria.

- **CML, blast phase (BP):** This phase represents the evolution to acute leukemia and features (1) 20% or more blasts in the blood or bone marrow, (2) extramedullary proliferation of blasts (skin, lymph nodes, spleen, bone, brain), and (3) clusters of blasts in the bone marrow. Blast phase heralds a poor prognosis. In 70% of blast crises, the leukemic blasts show myeloid morphology and immunophenotype; in 30%, they are lymphoblasts, usually of B-cell precursor lymphoblast immunophenotype (expressing CD10, CD19, CD34, and terminal deoxynucleotidyl transferase [TdT]). Transformation to accelerated phase or blast crisis usually entails additional cytogenetic alterations (Table 26-14).

CLINICAL FEATURES: Peak incidence is in the fifth and sixth decades, with a slight male predominance. Patients with CML report fatigue, anorexia, weight loss, and vague abdominal discomfort caused by hepatosplenomegaly. Acute left upper quadrant pain is often a symptom of splenic infarction. Blood findings include mild to moderate anemia, leukocytosis, and absolute basophilia Peripheral granulocytes are markedly increased with a full maturation range with peaks in myelocytes and segmented neutrophils. Clinical deterioration often heralds blast phase.

TABLE 26-15

COMMON GENETIC ABNORMALITIES ASSOCIATED WITH MYELOID PROLIFERATIONS

Disease	Associated Genetic/Chromosomal Abnormality	Importance
Paroxysmal nocturnal hemoglobinuria (PNH)	PIG-A mutations	Characteristic of PNH
Chronic myeloid leukemia (CML)	t(9;22)(q34;q11) (Philadelphia chromosome)	Largely defines CML
	Trisomy 8; trisomy 19; isochromosome 17q; second Philadelphia chromosome	Occur in some cases in blast phase of CML
Polycythemia vera	Trisomy 8 or 9; del 20q; del 13q; del 9p	Associated in some cases
	JAK2 V617F	Seen in 95% of polycythemia vera cases
Primary myelofibrosis (PMF)	del(13)(q12–22)	Associated in some cases
	der(6)t(1;6)(q21–23;p21.3)	Strongly associated in some cases
	JAK2 V617F	Seen in 50% of PMF
Essential thrombocythemia (ET)	del 20q; trisomy 8	Diagnostically helpful if present
	JAK2 V617F	Seen in 40% of ET cases
	MPL mutations	Seen in rare cases of ET
Myelodysplastic syndromes	5q–	Suggests favorable prognosis
	7q–	Suggests unfavorable prognosis
Acute myelogenous leukemia (AML)	t(8;21)(q22;q22); inv(16)(p13;q22); t(16;16)(p13.1;q22); t(9;11)(p22;q23); t(6;9)(p3;q34); inv(3)(q21;q26.2)	Seen in some cases of AML with recurring chromosomal abnormalities
Acute promyelocytic leukemia (APL)	t(15;17)(q22;q12)	Defines APL
Acute monocytic leukemia (AMoL)	del(11q); t(9;11); t(11;19)	Seen in some cases of AMoL
Acute myelomonocytic leukemia (AMML)	inv(16)(p13;q22); del(16q)	Seen in some cases of AMML
Acute megakaryoblastic leukemia	t(1:22)(p13;q13)	Seen in some cases, particularly in children
Myeloid sarcoma	Translocations involving (11q23), NPM mutations	Seen in some cases, not unique to myeloid sarcomas

CML is a model of targeted drug therapy in human malignancies. The drug imatinib, a tyrosine kinase inhibitor (TKI), blocks the ATP-binding site on BCR/ABL tyrosine kinase, and thereby inactivates it. Survival of 70% to 90% is typical in patients treated with imatinib. However, increasingly, subclones with point mutations within the ATP-binding pocket emerge and demonstrate resistance to imatinib. Second-generation TKIs and allogeneic bone marrow transplantation have greatly improved the outcome in CML patients. In the current era of TKI therapy, the most important prognostic indicator is response to treatment as monitored by hematologic, cytogenetic, and molecular assays.

Polycythemia Vera

PV is a chronic MPN arising from a clonal HSC and characterized by autonomous production of RBCs independent of the mechanisms that normally regulate erythropoiesis. It is a clonal proliferation not only of erythroid elements but also of megakaryocytes and granulocytes in the bone marrow. As secondary polycythemia and other MPNs resemble PV both clinically and pathologically, the WHO established diagnostic criteria for polycythemia. A diagnosis of PV requires that either all three major criteria or the first two major criteria and the minor criterion be present. Major criteria include (1) increased RBC mass or Hgb greater than 16.5 g/dL in men or greater than 16.0 g/dL in women; (2) bone marrow biopsy showing age-adjusted hypercellularity with trilineage increase (panmyelosis); and (3) the gain-of-function V617F variant in *JAK2,* which encodes Janus kinase 2, or a similar mutation in exon 12 of *JAK2.* The minor criterion is a subnormal serum EPO level.

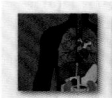 **PATHOPHYSIOLOGY AND MOLECULAR PATHOGENESIS:** PV derives from malignant transformation of a single stem cell with primary commitment to the erythroid lineage. Proliferation of the neoplastic clone occurs mainly

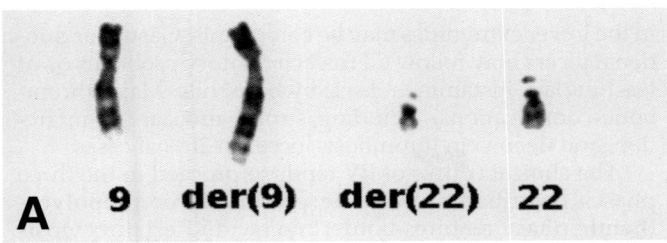

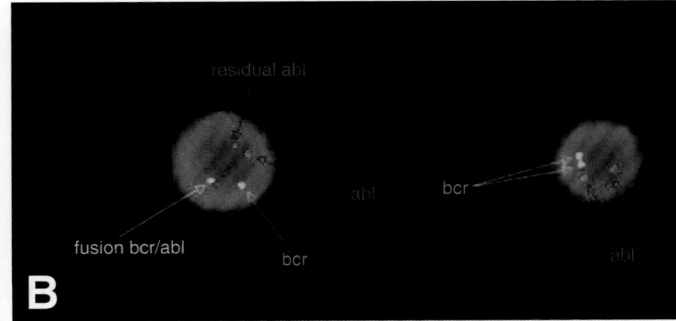

FIGURE 26-35. Chronic myelogenous leukemia. A. The Philadelphia chromosome der(22) is shown. **B.** Fluorescence in situ hybridization (FISH) in a patient with t(9;22) (Philadelphia chromosome)-positive chronic myeloid leukemia. *Right image.* A normal cell contains two separate bcr (chromosome 22) and abl (chromosome 9) genes. *Left image.* A leukemic cell with a fusion bcr/abl signal; residual abl signal; and two normal abl and bcr signals derived from normal chromosomes 9 and 22, respectively.

in the bone marrow but may involve extramedullary sites in the spleen, lymph nodes, and liver (**myeloid metaplasia**). The abnormal myeloproliferation of PV is sustained by a constitutively active JAK/STAT signal transduction pathway. In some cases, PV may be driven by loss of negative regulation of JAK activation caused by mutations in *LNK*, which encodes an adaptor protein that negatively regulates JAK/STAT signaling, or mutations in the *SOCS* (suppressor of cytokine signaling) family of tumor suppressor genes. The current view suggests that several other cooperating genetic hits might be required. Among

others, mutations involving *EZH2*, which makes a histone methyltransferase involved in epigenetic regulation, or *TET2*, which functions as a transcriptional regulator, have also been described in PV.

EPO is the primary regulator of erythropoiesis and its synthesis by the kidney is triggered by tissue hypoxia. The neoplastic erythroid progenitor cells of PV are sensitive to EPO, like their normal counterparts. When exposed to EPO in culture, they form luxuriant clusters of erythroid cells (BFU-E). However, at the more mature colony-forming stage (CFU-E), cultured PV neoplastic cells form erythroid colonies even without EPO stimulation. These autonomous erythroid colonies, "endogenous CFU-E," characterize PV throughout the disease and stand in contrast to normal erythroid progenitors, in which CFU-Es require added EPO ("exogenous CFU-E").

Autonomous (EPO-independent) proliferation of PV cells gives them a proliferative advantage. Their increased RBC mass suppresses EPO secretion and thus the proliferation of normal RBC progenitors. Serum EPO levels in PV are normal or low, while in secondary (functional) erythrocytosis EPO is increased.

Over 95% of patients with PV have the V617F somatic mutation in exon 14 of *JAK2* and most of the others (4% of PV) have different mutations in exon 122. These gain-of-function mutations occur in HSCs and cause constitutive activation of JAK/STAT signaling and hypersensitivity to growth factors and cytokines, including EPO. The JAK2 family of transcription factors plays a critical role in cytokine signaling in normal hematopoietic cells mainly by triggering signal transducers and activators of transcription (STAT) proteins. In vitro studies indicate that the activating *JAK2* mutation confers proliferative and survival advantages to hematopoietic precursors. The JAK2 V617F mutation is not specific for PV; it also occurs in other MPNs. Patients with the *JAK2* mutation have a longer duration of disease and higher risk for bleeding complications and fibrosis.

Abnormal cytogenetic karyotypes occur in 20% of patients with PV, the most common of which are presented in Table 26-14. Philadelphia chromosome and

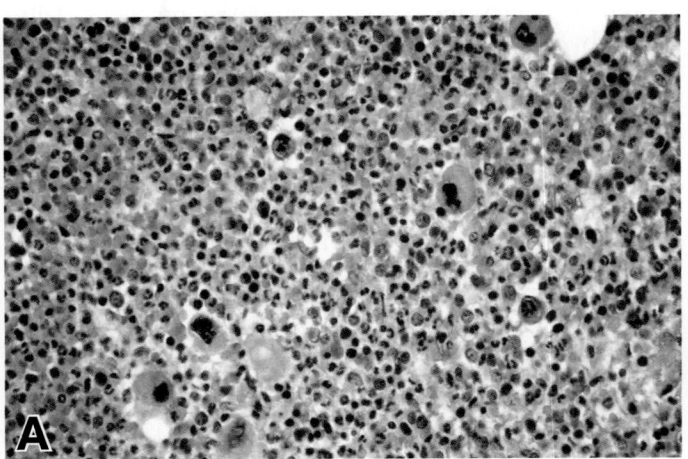

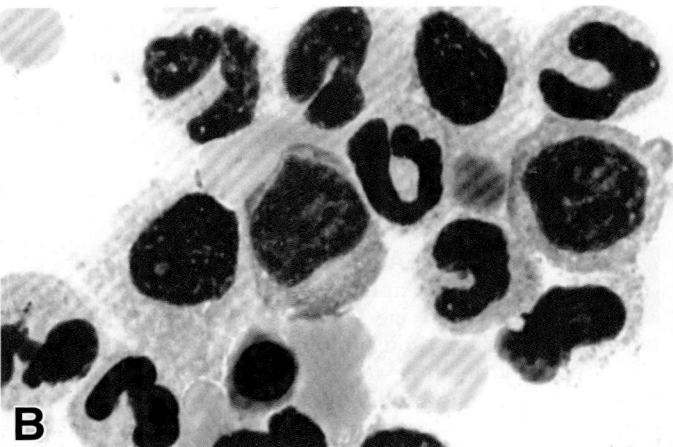

FIGURE 26-36. Chronic myelogenous leukemia. A. The bone marrow is markedly hypercellular because of an increase in myeloid precursors, mature neutrophils, and megakaryocytes. **B.** A smear of the bone marrow aspirate from the same patient reveals numerous granulocytes at various stages of development with prominence of myelocytes.

BCR/ABL fusion protein do not occur in PV but rare cases of *JAK2*-mutant PV may acquire a *BCR-ABL* rearrangement, the significance of which is uncertain.

PATHOLOGY: Bone marrow in PV is hypercellular and shows an increased number of erythroid, myeloid, and megakaryocytic lineages (Table 26-15). Panmyelosis is characteristic but morphologic findings and clinical course vary, depending on the stage of disease. As explained below, PV occurs in three stages: the **prepolycythemic stage**, the **overt polycythemic stage,** and the **postpolycythemic (post-PV MF) myelofibrosis stage**. In pre- and polycythemic stages, erythroid precursors predominate, and the myeloid-to-erythroid ratio is decreased. Both erythroid and myeloid series both show normal maturation. Megakaryocytes are typically increased in number, are of variable size, and tend to cluster in the biopsy. In over 95% of cases, marrow-stainable iron is decreased or absent. A mild to moderate increase in reticulin is common in the early stages. In the later stage of postpolycythemic myelofibrosis, also called the "spent phase," erythropoiesis decreases and the marrow becomes replaced by reticulin and collagen fibrosis.

The spleen is typically enlarged, with prominent accumulation of erythrocytes in the red pulp cords and sinuses. In the polycythemic phase, there is minimal EMH. However, EMH, with blood cell precursors outside the marrow, increases in the postpolycythemic myelofibrotic phase. Although the main site of EMH is the spleen, the liver and lymph nodes may contain foci of erythroid precursors, immature granulocytes and megakaryocytes, especially in patients with advanced PV.

Blood hemoglobin concentrations may exceed 20 g/dL, and the Hct can surpass 60% (Table 26-14). Initially, there is mild to moderate leukocytosis (10,000 to 25,000/μL) in most cases, and mild to moderate thrombocytosis (400,000 to 800,000/μL) in half of cases, often with abnormal platelet morphology. Anemia occurs in the later, spent phase of PV. Hyperuricemia and secondary gout may also arise, due to rapid cell turnover.

Peripheral blood smears in the polycythemic phase show crowding of usual normochromic, normocytic RBCs. Hypochromia and microcytosis also develop in a setting of concurrent iron deficiency, which is common in PV, since stored iron is diverted to erythropoiesis or is lost to phlebotomy or bleeding from the GI tract. In the later stages of PV, anemia develops and the peripheral blood shows a leukoerythroblastic picture with poikilocytosis with teardrop-shaped RBCs.

CLINICAL FEATURES: The annual incidence of PV in North America is 8 to 10 cases per million with a mean age at diagnosis of 60 years. Onset tends to be insidious, and symptoms are generally nonspecific, typically relating to increased erythrocyte mass. Plethora and splenomegaly are early findings. Headache, dizziness and visual problems reflect hypertension and/or vascular disturbances in the brain and retina. Angina pectoris, from slowing of coronary blood flow, and intermittent claudication caused by sluggish peripheral blood flow

in the lower extremities may be complaints. Gastric or duodenal ulcers may follow GI tract circulatory problems or, at least in part, histamine release by basophils. Major thrombotic complications, including stroke, myocardial infarction, and deep vein thrombosis, occur in 20% of cases.

The clinical course of PV tends to proceed in the three phases described above. The prodromal or **prepolycythemic phase** features borderline or mild erythrocytosis with mild erythroid hyperplasia, but not to an extent that is diagnostic of PV. The diagnosis can be based on a low EPO level, *JAK2* or similar mutation or endogenous erythroid colony formation. However, at this stage, the bone marrow findings may be nonspecific. Later, when red cell mass is definitively increased, the disease has entered the **polycythemic stage**. This ongoing progression includes a low incidence of evolution to the **postpolycythemic (spent) phase** in which excessive erythroid proliferation ceases, and anemia occurs. Another 10% of cases progress to myelofibrosis with EMH, as in other MPNs **(postpolycythemic myelofibrosis)**. **Acute myelogenous leukemia (AML)** or **myelodysplasia** occurs in up to 15% of cases of PV and may, in part, be caused by treatment with ^{32}P or alkylating agents. Disease progression is often associated with karyotypic evolution and acquisition of complex chromosomal abnormalities.

Median survival of patients with PV is 13 years. Specific causes of death related to the disease itself include thrombosis, hemorrhage, AML, and consequences of the spent phase. Repeated phlebotomy or chemotherapy to reduce erythrocyte mass is effective management in most cases. JAK2 inhibitors have shown encouraging results.

Primary Myelofibrosis

PMF is a clonal MPN characterized by proliferation of abnormal megakaryocytes and granulocytes with bone marrow fibrosis.

MOLECULAR PATHOGENESIS: As in other MPNs, exposures to benzene or radiation have been implicated in some cases of PMF. The neoplastic megakaryocytes in PMF produce PDGF and TGFβ, both of which are powerful fibroblast mitogens. Ultimately, although fibroblasts are not part of the clonal stem cell disorder, their stimulation by those cytokines causes the entire marrow space to be replaced by connective tissue. In the fibrotic phase, clonal stem cells enter the circulation to cause EMH at multiple sites, especially the spleen. Approximately 50% to 60% of PMF cases carry the *JAK2* V617F mutation, about 30% have a mutation in *CALR*, the gene for calcium regulatory protein calreticulin, and 8% have a mutation in *MPL*, which encodes the thrombopoietin receptor protein. About 12% of cases are triple negative for these mutations. Some chromosomal abnormalities suggest, but are not diagnostic of, PMF (Table 26-14).

PATHOLOGY: PMF evolves through two stages, an early **prefibrotic stage**, and a **fibrotic stage**. Most patients are diagnosed at the latter stage, but 30% to 40% are first detected in a prefibrotic stage, which

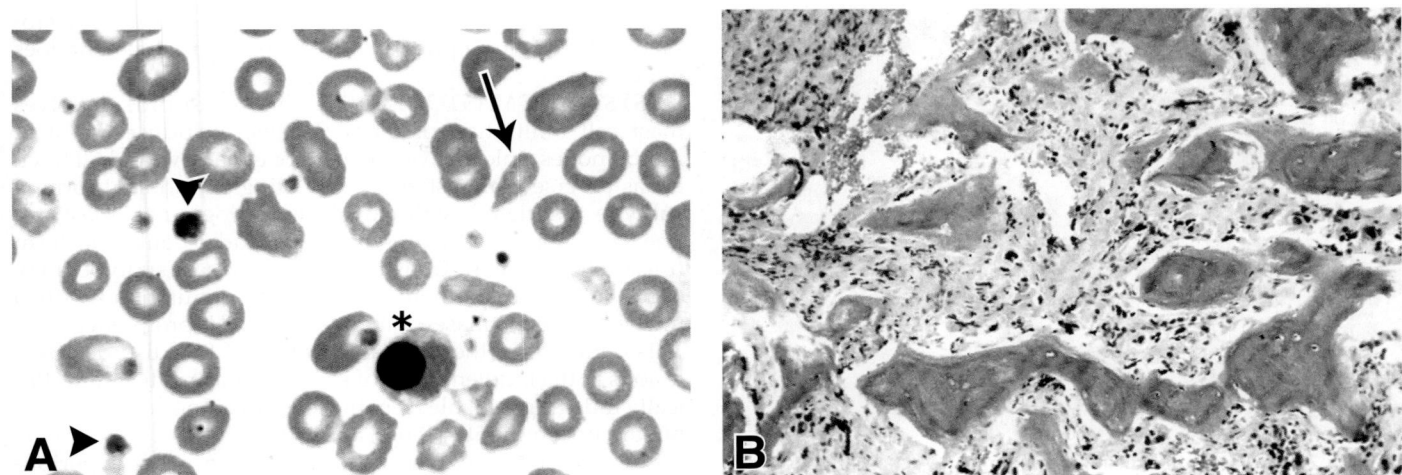

FIGURE 26-37. Chronic idiopathic myelofibrosis. A. Peripheral smear shows anisocytosis (red blood cells of different size), poikilocytosis with teardrop forms (*arrow*), and nucleated erythrocytes. Large to giant platelets are also present. **B.** A section of bone marrow shows collagenous fibrosis, osteosclerosis, and numerous abnormal megakaryocytes.

usually presents with unexplained thrombocytosis. The hypercellular bone marrow shows prominent neutrophilic and megakaryocytic proliferation, but only minimal fibrosis. Megakaryocytes are densely clustered and atypically lobated with a high nuclear-to-cytoplasmic ratio and occasionally "cloud-like" nuclei. In the **fibrotic stage,** the blood shows leukopenia or marked leukocytosis, with myeloid precursors and nucleated RBCs (leukoerythroblastosis). Red cells exhibit poikilocytosis and teardrop forms (Fig. 26-37A). Bone marrow cellularity gradually decreases, and foci of hematopoiesis containing mostly atypical megakaryocytes alternate with hypo- or acellular regions. Conspicuous reticulin or collagen fibrosis in the marrow defines this stage (Fig. 26-37B). EMH leads to splenomegaly, hepatomegaly and lymphadenopathy, and may be seen in other organs.

The WHO requires three major criteria and at least one minor criterion for the diagnosis of PMF. Major criteria include (1) megakaryocyte proliferation and atypia with or without fibrosis; (2) absence of features of other well-defined MPNs and (3) a clonal genetic marker, such as *JAK2, CALR,* or *MLP* mutations. Minor criteria include anemia, leukocytosis, leukoerythroblastosis, elevated serum lactate dehydrogenase, and splenomegaly.

 CLINICAL FEATURES: The annual incidence of idiopathic myelofibrosis is 0.5 to 1.5 per 100,000. Its peak incidence is in the seventh decade. Up to 30% of patients with idiopathic myelofibrosis are asymptomatic at diagnosis, with the disease being detected by splenomegaly on physical examination or by the presence of teardrop red cells or thrombocytosis on a blood smear. Early clinical symptoms are nonspecific and include fatigue, low-grade fever, night sweats and weight loss. Platelet function may be impaired and associated with either increased platelet aggregation and thrombosis or decreased platelet aggregation with a bleeding diathesis. Transformation to AML occurs in 5% to 30% of cases (Table 26-14).

Essential Thrombocythemia

ET is an MPN in which megakaryocytes proliferate without restraint. It is characterized by sustained thrombocytosis (>450,000/μL) in peripheral blood, and recurrent episodes of thrombosis and hemorrhage are common. The disease affects middle-aged people of both genders (Table 26-14).

 MOLECULAR PATHOGENESIS: ET is a clonal disorder believed to derive from neoplastic transformation of a single HSC with principal, but not exclusive, commitment to megakaryocytic lineage. The disease features a marked proliferation of megakaryocytes, with a 15-fold or greater increase in platelet production leading to marked thrombocytosis (sometimes >10^6/μL). About 50% to 60% have the *JAK2* V617F mutation, 30% have a mutation in *CALR*, and 3% have a variant in *MPL*; 12% are "triple negative." Chromosomal abnormalities, including del(20q) and trisomy 8, are identified in approximately 5% to 10% of cases.

PATHOLOGY: In diagnosing ET, other chronic MPNs and reactive thrombocytosis must be excluded. Abnormalities of platelet function are common in primary thrombocythemia. Recurrent episodes of thrombosis in arteries or veins are attributed to severe thrombocytosis, and hemorrhage reflects defective platelet function. Thromboses in the spleen, with subsequent infarction, may cause splenic atrophy. Iron-deficiency anemia follows hemorrhage from GI or urogenital tracts. The bone marrow in most cases is normocellular or moderately hypercellular, with fewer fat cells (Fig. 26-38). Increased numbers of large, hyperlobulated, "stag-horn–shaped" megakaryocytes with abundant mature cytoplasm form cohesive clusters or sheets in the marrow. Marrow reticulin is normal or slightly increased. Post-ET myelofibrosis is rare. Iron stores are normal or low.

The spleen is mildly enlarged in 50% of cases of ET. EMH is common, but extensive myeloid metaplasia

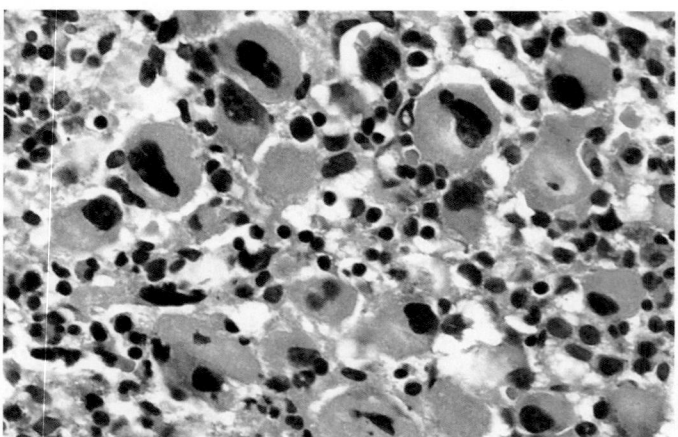

FIGURE 26-38. Essential thrombocythemia. A section of bone marrow exhibits a marked increase in the number of megakaryocytes, which display atypical features and hyperlobated forms.

occurs only once myelofibrosis develops. The peripheral blood shows thrombocytosis.

CLINICAL FEATURES: The clinical course of ET is indolent, with median survival exceeding 10 to 15 years. Microvascular occlusion can lead to transient ischemic attacks. Thrombosis of large arteries and veins is common in untreated cases, especially in the legs, heart, intestine, and kidneys. Hemorrhage, usually from mucosal surfaces, is less common and mild, rather than life threatening. AML supervenes in up to 5% of cases. The disease is treated with platelet pheresis and myelosuppressive chemotherapy.

Mastocytosis

Mastocytosis is a clonal hematopoietic disorder in which neoplastic mast cells accumulate in certain tissues, mainly skin and bone marrow. It is characterized by an abnormal mast cell infiltrate, which often contains multifocal compact clusters or cohesive aggregates. The disorder is heterogeneous with manifestations ranging from skin lesions that can spontaneously regress to highly aggressive disease associated with multiorgan failure and poor survival. Subtypes of mastocytosis are characterized by distinct tissue involvement and clinical manifestations.

CUTANEOUS MASTOCYTOSIS: Cutaneous mastocytosis is most common in children and can be manifest at birth. It presents with either single or multiple lesions. In the former case, there is a tan-brown, cutaneous nodule in newborns; in the latter, groups of skin nodules or disseminated brown-red macular or papular lesions occur in young children. The most common type of cutaneous mastocytosis is **urticaria pigmentosa**, which occurs as multiple, symmetrically distributed, tan-brown cutaneous macules or papules in infants and young children. The skin of the trunk is mostly affected, but any skin site may be involved. Skin biopsy shows aggregates of spindle-shaped mast cells filling the papillary dermis and extending into the reticular dermis. A perivascular and periadnexal distribution of mast cells is often seen. Spontaneous resolution of cutaneous mastocytosis usually occurs at puberty and systemic involvement does not ensue.

SYSTEMIC MASTOCYTOSIS: This rare disorder involves mast cell infiltration of many organs, including the skin, lymph nodes, spleen, liver, bones, bone marrow, and GI tract. It has diverse manifestations, including an indolent form, a subtype associated with clonal hematologic non–mast cell lineage disease, an aggressive form and a leukemic form (mast cell leukemia). Transitions between these subtypes may occur. In most cases there is an activating mutation (D816V) in the tyrosine kinase domain of the *KIT* proto-oncogene. This underscores the neoplastic nature of this disorder. Skin lesions in the indolent form of systemic mastocytosis are clinically indistinguishable from those in cutaneous mastocytosis but are uncommonly seen in adults.

In mast cell leukemia, the bone marrow and peripheral blood show a significant increase in atypical mast cells (≥20% in the marrow) and depletion of fat and normal hematopoietic elements in the marrow. The circulating cells often exhibit cytologic atypia, including a round rather than a spindle shape, hypogranulation and/or nuclear irregularity, or less differentiated forms with blast-like morphology.

PATHOLOGY: Although lymph nodes are rarely involved in systemic mastocytosis, they may show perifollicular and perivascular infiltration by mast cells (Fig. 26-39). Compact aggregates of mast cells within paracortical areas can also be seen. The spleen shows nodular aggregates of mast cells with accompanying dense fibrosis in both red and white pulp. In the liver, portal triads are involved first. The distribution of involvement in the bone marrow may be peritrabecular, perivascular or diffuse, and there is often accompanying fibrosis and eosinophilia.

CLINICAL FEATURES: Systemic mastocytosis occurs at any age, but adults in the sixth and seventh decades are most commonly affected. Symptoms reflect the overproduction of mediators normally

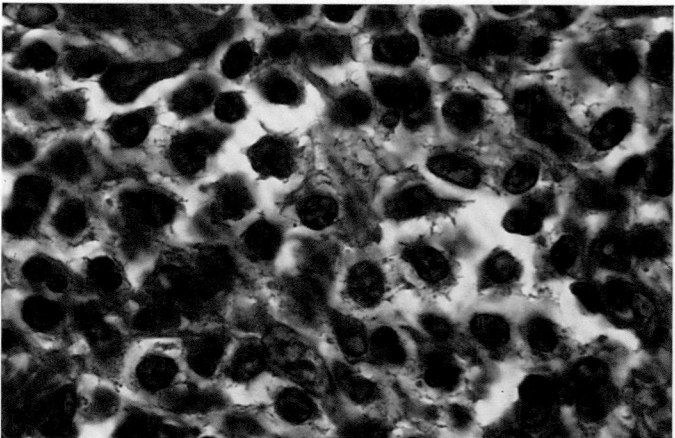

FIGURE 26-39. Mastocytosis. A section of lymph node shows effacement of the normal architecture by sheets of masT-cells. The centrally situated nuclei are round to elongated, and occasionally indented. The cytoplasm is pale pink and finely granular.

made by mast cells and basophils, including histamine, prostaglandin D_2, and thromboxane B_2. Most people experience gastrointestinal pain and diarrhea. Serum tryptase levels are usually elevated. Anaphylactic episodes, with pruritus, flushing, hypotension, and asthmatic symptoms, are common. Extensive mast cell infiltration of the bone marrow leads to secondary anemia, neutropenia, and thrombocytopenia. Physical findings at initial diagnosis may include splenomegaly, lymphadenopathy, and hepatomegaly. Prognosis is variable, depending on subtype. The indolent form has a chronic course, and half of patients survive 5 years or more. Symptomatic relief is obtained, at least partially, with H_1- and H_2-receptor antagonists to counteract effects of histamine. However, there is no effective therapy for the underlying disease process.

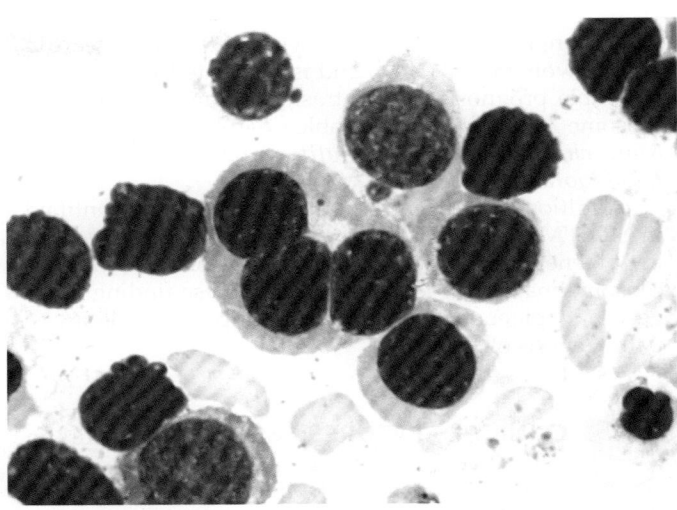

FIGURE 26-40. Myelodysplastic syndrome. Dysplastic, multinucleated, megaloblastoid erythroid precursors are shown.

Myelodysplastic Syndromes Are Clonal Disorders of Ineffective Hematopoiesis

MDSs are a group of clonal HSC diseases characterized by peripheral blood cytopenia, dysplasia in one or more lineages, and a generally hypercellular marrow with ineffective hematopoiesis. Recurrent genetic abnormalities and increased risk of transformation to AML are characteristic features. The apparent discrepancy between the paucity of peripheral blood elements and the hypercellularity in the bone marrow occurs because ineffective hematopoiesis leads to increased apoptosis in the marrow.

Subtypes of MDSs are defined by the involved cell lineage(s) and the percentage of blasts in the blood or bone marrow. *All subtypes show refractory anemia and/or other cytopenias. The recommended threshold for cytopenias is established by the original International Prognostic Scoring System (IPSS) for risk stratification. Erythrocytosis, leukocytosis, and thrombocytosis typically do not occur in MDS, unlike the MPNs (see above).* Thrombocytosis is recognized in MDS associated with cytogenetic abnormalities including isolated del(5q), in(3)(q21.3q26.2), or t(3;3)(q21.3;q26.2). In addition to showing features of dysplasia, an increased number of blasts may be present in MDS. However, the percentage of blasts is always less than 20% in the blood or bone marrow, beyond which the requisite threshold recommended for the diagnosis of AML is fulfilled. Progression of MDS to AML (i.e., progression from ineffective hematopoiesis to a proliferative state) occurs in 30% to 40% of cases and is usually associated with underlying genetic instability and increased numbers of blasts. This progression coincides with acquisition of additional genetic abnormalities. Some low-grade MDSs subsets have more stable clinical courses and do not progress, or only rarely progress to AML.

ETIOLOGIC FACTORS: MDSs may be either primary (de novo) or secondary (therapy related). Patients with secondary MDSs have typically received radiation or chemotherapy (particularly alkylating agents or topoisomerase II inhibitors). Other risk factors include benzene exposure, cigarette smoking, and congenital disorders such as Fanconi anemia or Kostmann syndrome.

PATHOLOGY: *The morphologic hallmark of MDS is dysplasia in one or more lineages.* Subclassification of MDS is based on the number of cytopenias at presentation, the number of dysplastic lineages, and the presence of ringed sideroblasts and the percentage of blasts in bone marrow and blood. Dysplasia is most often seen in erythroid precursors, which show megaloblastoid changes, multinucleation, nuclear budding, bridging between nuclei and karyorrhexis (Fig. 26-40). Erythroid precursors with iron-laden mitochondria around the nuclei **(ringed sideroblasts)** occur in several subtypes of MDSs (Fig. 26-41A) and are associated with mutations in *SF3B1*, which encodes a protein involved in mRNA splicing. Dysgranulopoietic features include nuclear hyposegmentation (pseudo-Pelger–Huët cells) and cytoplasmic hypogranulation. Dysplastic megakaryocytes may be small and hypolobated or show nuclear separation (Fig. 26-41B). Careful elucidation of the blast percentage is important in assigning an MDS subcategory and predicting the clinical course of the disease. Only one cytogenetic abnormality, del(5q), is used to define a specific subtype of MDS.

Cytogenetic and molecular studies are essential to diagnosing, treating, and assessing prognosis of MDS. Conventional cytogenetic tests identify clonal abnormalities in half of cases. The combination of isolated deletion of the long arm of chromosome 5 (5q–), macrocytic anemia, megaloblastoid erythropoiesis with or without ringed sideroblasts and normal or increased platelets

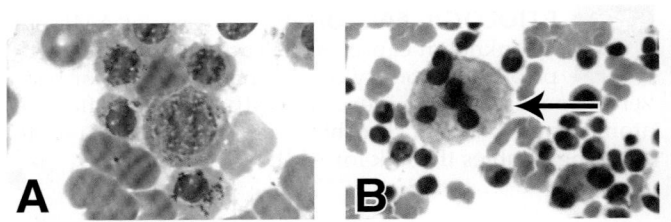

FIGURE 26-41. Myelodysplastic syndrome. A. Smear of a bone marrow aspirate stained with Prussian blue shows an erythroid precursor cell containing iron-laden mitochondria that encircle the nuclei (ringed sideroblast). **B.** Dysplastic megakaryocyte with nuclear separation (*arrow*).

with monolobated megakaryocytes is typically seen in elderly women with MDS and is associated with a more favorable prognosis. By contrast, abnormalities of chromosome 7 confer an unfavorable prognosis (Table 26-14). *More chromosomal abnormalities are associated with less favorable outcomes.*

Additional recurrent mutations have been identified in MDS. Most involve genes encoding proteins involved in epigenetic regulation or components of the RNA spliceosome machinery (see Chapter 5). These findings suggest that epigenetic factors play an important role in the pathogenesis of MDS.

CLINICAL FEATURES: MDS usually occurs in older patients, with a median age of 70. The WHO classification of MDS subtypes is beyond the scope of this discussion. *However, in general, MDS presents with symptoms related to peripheral blood cytopenias: weakness in anemia, recurrent infections in neutropenia and bleeding in thrombocytopenia. Up to 40% of MDS patients progress to AML.* Progression to AML and overall prognosis depend on the morphologic subtype of MDS. Increased numbers of blasts, complex cytogenetic abnormalities, and specific mutations including those involving *TP53* all confer a worse prognosis.

ACUTE MYELOID LEUKEMIA

Acute Myeloid Leukemia Is a Clonal Proliferation of Myeloblasts

A diagnosis of AML requires at least 20% myeloblasts in the blood or bone marrow. However, this diagnostic requirement is relaxed in AML types associated with specific cytogenetic abnormalities (Table 26-14). AML with t(15;17)(q22;q12) is called acute promyelocytic leukemia (APL). Such types are defined as AML regardless of blast cell count. If fewer than 20% blasts are present in AMLs without specific recurrent cytogenetic abnormalities, the disease is more appropriately classified as MDS or MPN. There are six distinct types of AML (Table 26-16):

1. **AML with recurrent genetic abnormalities**
2. **AML with myelodysplasia-related changes**
3. **Therapy-related myeloid neoplasms**
4. **AML, not otherwise specified**
5. **Myeloid sarcoma**
6. **Myeloid proliferations related to Down syndrome**

ETIOLOGIC FACTORS: Most cases of AML are of unknown cause. Some cases are attributed to prior radiation, cytotoxic chemotherapy, or benzene exposure. The incidence of AML increased after the atomic bomb blasts in Hiroshima and Nagasaki. Cigarette smoking doubles the risk for AML (see Chapter 8).

PATHOLOGY: Myeloblasts are present in the bone marrow and, usually, in the peripheral blood. Myeloblasts are medium to large in size

---

TABLE 26-16

WHO CLASSIFICATION OF ACUTE MYELOID LEUKEMIA (AML)

Acute Myeloid Leukemia with Recurrent Genetic Abnormalities

AML with t(8;21)(q22;q22); RUNX1-RUNX1T1

AML with abnormal bone marrow eosinophils inv(16)(p13q22) or t(16;16)(p13;q22); CBFβ/MYH11

Acute promyelocytic leukemia [AML with t(15;17)(q22;q12)(PML/RARα)] and variants **(M3)**

AML with (9;11)(p22;q23); MLLT3-MLL

AML with t(6;9)(p23;q34); DEK-NUP214

AML with inv(3)(q21q24.2) or t(3;3)(q21;126.2); RPN1-EVI1

AML (megakaryoblastic) with t(1;22)(p13;q13); RBM15-MKL1

AML with gene mutations (NPM1, CEBPA, FLT3, etc.)

Acute Myeloid Leukemia with Myelodysplasia-Related Changes

Following a myelodysplastic syndrome or myelodysplastic syndrome/myeloproliferative disorder

Without antecedent myelodysplastic syndrome

Therapy-Related Myeloid Neoplasms

Alkylating agent related

Topoisomerase type II inhibitor related (some may be lymphoid)

Other types

Acute Myeloid Leukemia Not Otherwise Categorized

AML minimally differentiated **(M0)**

AML without maturation **(M1)**

AML with maturation **(M2)**

Acute myelomonocytic leukemia (M4)

Acute monoblastic and monocytic leukemia **(M5)**

Acute erythroid leukemia **(M6)**

Acute megakaryoblastic leukemia **(M7)**

Acute basophilic leukemia

Acute panmyelosis with myelofibrosis

Myeloid Sarcoma

Myeloid Proliferations Related to Down Syndrome

PML = promyelocytic leukemia; RAR = retinoic acid receptor; WHO = World Health Organization.

---

with round or slightly irregular nuclei and immature nuclear chromatin. Typically, myeloblasts displace normal hematopoietic cells in the bone marrow (Fig. 26-42). In a subset of AML cases, blasts show slender, eosinophilic cytoplasmic inclusions, called *Auer rods,* which are coalesced primary granules (Fig. 26-43). Auer rods are specific for the myeloid lineage and their presence thus precludes a diagnosis of lymphoblastic leukemia.

Immunophenotyping by flow cytometry, chromosomal analysis (cytogenetic studies), and molecular studies are essential for accurate WHO classification of AML. Myeloid antigens frequently expressed include CD13, CD15, CD33, and CD117 (*c-kit*), in addition to the progenitor cell marker CD34. AML with megakaryoblastic differentiation may express the platelet/megakaryocyte

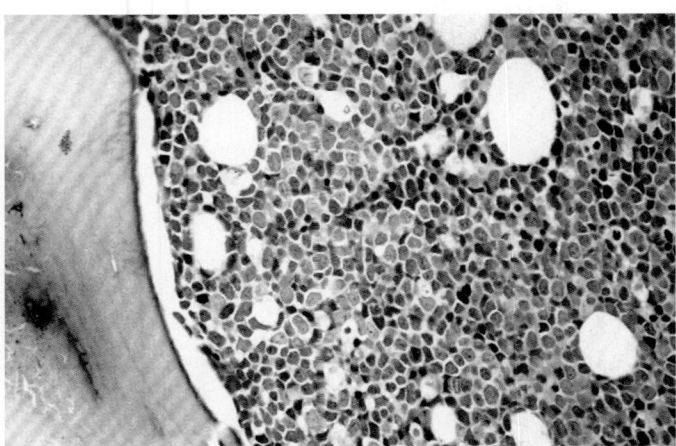

FIGURE 26-42. Acute myelogenous leukemia. A hypercellular bone marrow showing effacement of the normal architecture by sheets of myeloblasts.

markers CD41 and CD61 (platelet Gp IIb/IIIa complex). Monocytic markers include CD64, CD11b, and CD14. Cytochemical staining for myeloperoxidase, Sudan black (lipids), and nonspecific esterase (NSE), remain helpful in classifying AML cases.

CLINICAL FEATURES: Most cases of AML occur in adults, with a median age of 67 at onset. AML involves progressive accumulation in the marrow of immature myeloid blasts cells that cannot differentiate and mature further. Although leukemic myeloblasts divide more slowly than do normal hematopoietic precursor cells, they also undergo spontaneous cell death less often than normal cells. Thus, an expanded pool of abnormal leukemic blasts eventually overwhelms the marrow and suppresses normal hematopoiesis. As a result, the major clinical presenting problems in AML are leukopenia, thrombocytopenia, and anemia. Infections, especially with opportunistic organisms (e.g., fungi), are common, as are

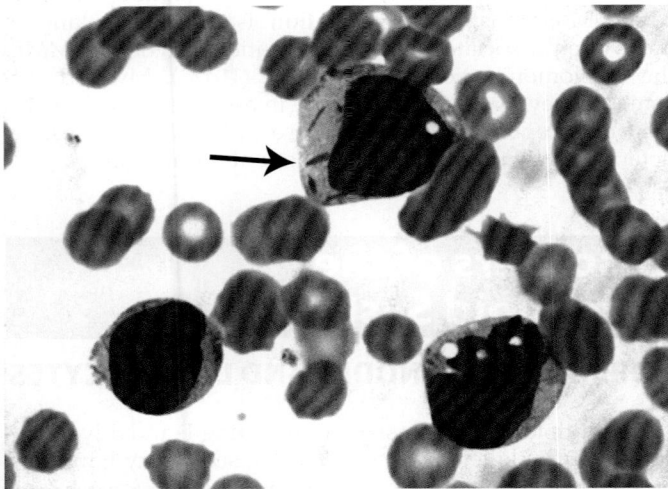

FIGURE 26-43. Acute promyelocytic leukemia. Blasts show prominent auer rods (*arrow*).

cutaneous bleeding (petechiae and ecchymoses) and serosal hemorrhages in the abdominal viscera. Untreated AML has a dismal prognosis. Chemotherapy leads to remission in over half of patients, but relapses are common and overall 5-year survival in AML patients is under 40%. Bone marrow transplantation is a common mode of treatment for high-risk forms of AML and for AML in relapse.

Selected Acute Myeloid Leukemia Subtypes

AML WITH RECURRENT GENETIC ABNORMALITIES: Multiple cytogenetic abnormalities are associated with this category of AML (Table 26-14). These include AML with mutated *NPM1* or biallelic *CEBPA* mutations. AML with *RUNX1* mutations is considered as a provisional category.

AML with t(15;17)(q22;q12) is defined as **APL.** It mainly affects middle-aged patients and accounts for 5% to 10% of AMLs. *It involves a translocation of the* **promyelocytic leukemia 1 (PML1) gene at 15q22 and the retinoic acid receptor-α (RARA) gene at 17q12.**

APL is a paradigm for a molecular disease in which the underlying genetic defect determines the type of treatment. The t(15;17)(q22;q12) translocation results in production of a *PML/RARA* fusion gene, that makes a functional retinoic acid receptor. Targeting this receptor with all-*trans*-retinoic acid (ATRA) causes tumor cells to mature. The bone marrow is packed with tumor cells with promyelocytic morphologic features. Auer rods are abundant and abnormal promyelocytes are strongly positive for myeloperoxidase or Sudan black. *Patients with APL frequently present with DIC.* Senescent leukemic cells degranulate and activate the coagulation cascade. By inducing maturation of tumor cells, treatment with ATRA prevents degranulation and DIC. The prognosis for APL is more favorable than for all other types of AMLs.

THERAPY-RELATED MYELOID NEOPLASMS: Cytotoxic radiation or chemotherapy for a prior malignancy can induce mutational changes that lead to secondary hematopoietic neoplasms one to several years after treatment. This category includes AMLs, MDSs, and MPNs related to prior mutagenic therapies grouped as one entity. Alkylating agents and radiation most often give rise to myelodysplasia and subsequent AML after 5 to 10 years. In contrast, topoisomerase II inhibitors (epipodophyllotoxins) lead to overt AML with latencies of 1 to 5 years. Most therapy-related myeloid neoplasms have cytogenetic abnormalities and poor prognoses.

ACUTE MYELOID LEUKEMIA, WITH MYELODYSPLASIA RELATED CHANGES: AML with myelodysplasia-related changes (AML MRC) has morphologic features of dysplasia with *at least* 20% blasts in peripheral blood or bone marrow. This type of AML occurs in patients with a prior history of MDS or a mixed MDS/MPN, with MDS-related cytogenetic abnormalities or with findings of multilineage dysplasia in >50% of cells in at least two lineages. AML MRC often presents with severe pancytopenia.

ACUTE MYELOID LEUKEMIA, NOT OTHERWISE SPECIFIED: These leukemias do not fulfill diagnostic criteria for the defined subtypes of AML and are grouped together based on the older French–American–British (FAB) classification. The WHO classification incorporates the FAB scheme (Fig. 26-44):

■ **AML with minimal differentiation:** The leukemic cells are immature myeloblasts with no defining morphologic

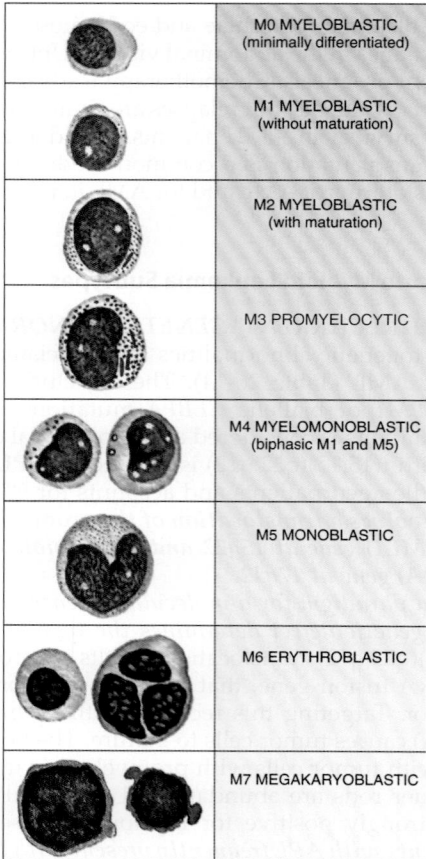

	M0 MYELOBLASTIC (minimally differentiated)
	M1 MYELOBLASTIC (without maturation)
	M2 MYELOBLASTIC (with maturation)
	M3 PROMYELOCYTIC
	M4 MYELOMONOBLASTIC (biphasic M1 and M5)
	M5 MONOBLASTIC
	M6 ERYTHROBLASTIC
	M7 MEGAKARYOBLASTIC

FIGURE 26-44. Morphology of acute myeloid leukemia (AML) in the traditional French–American–British (FAB) classification, now within the framework of the World Health Organization (WHO) classification "AML-not otherwise specified."

or cytochemical criteria of the myeloid lineage. Immunophenotyping by flow cytometry establishes the myeloid nature of blasts with expression of CD34, CD38, CD13, or CD117, and 60% express CD33 but lack evidence of myeloid and monocytic maturation such as CD11b, CD15, CD14, and CD65. The prognosis is unfavorable.

- **AML without maturation:** Blasts usually express myeloperoxidase but less than 10% of the myeloid cells are promyelocytes or more mature myeloid cells. This disease occurs most often in middle-aged people.
- **AML with maturation:** In addition to blasts, more than 10% maturing myeloid cells (promyelocytes and later) are present.
- **Acute myelomonocytic leukemia (AMML):** This tumor is composed of a mixture of neutrophils and their precursors, plus monocytes and their precursors. The latter make up 26% to 80% of tumor cells. AMML accounts for 5% to 10% of AMLs.
- **Acute monoblastic/monocytic leukemia (AMoL):** At least 80% of myeloid leukemic cells have monocytic differentiation, including monoblasts, abnormal promonocytes, and monocytes. AMoL constitutes 5% to 8% of AMLs and is seen in younger patients.
- **Acute erythroid leukemia:** Acute erythroid leukemias feature prominent erythroid proliferation and are characterized by neoplastic immature cells committed to

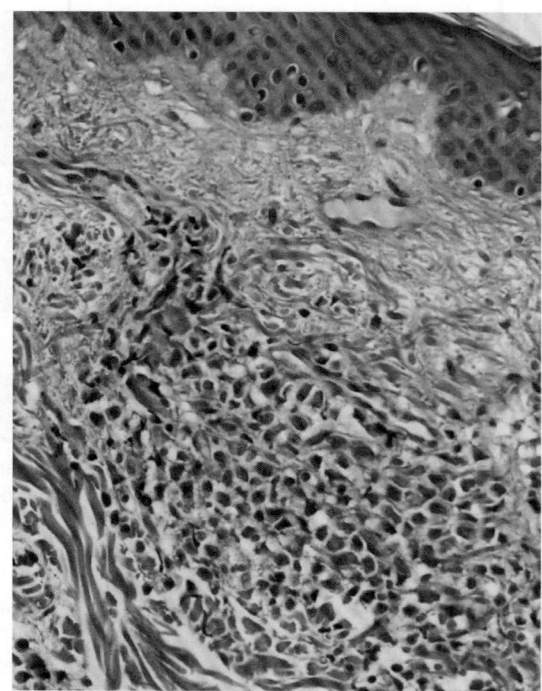

FIGURE 26-45. Myeloid sarcoma. The skin from a patient with acute monoblastic leukemia (leukemia cutis) shows neoplastic myeloid cells.

erythroid lineage making up more than 80% of nucleated bone marrow cells.
- **Acute megakaryoblastic leukemia (AMegL):** At least 50% of the blasts have a megakaryocytic immunophenotype as shown by expression of CD61 and CD42b.
- **Acute basophilic leukemia:** AML with primary differentiation to basophils.
- **Acute panmyelosis with myelofibrosis:** Acute panmyeloid proliferation is characterized by increased blasts to at least 20% of cells in bone marrow or peripheral blood.

MYELOID SARCOMA: Myeloid sarcoma is an extramedullary solid tumor of myeloblasts or monoblasts (Fig. 26-45). This entity is sometimes called a **chloroma** (because of its greenish color), **granulocytic sarcoma,** or **monoblastic sarcoma. Monoblastic differentiation** is uncommon and is most often associated with translocations involving *MML,* the myelomonocytic leukemia gene (11q23). Myeloid sarcoma may evolve de novo or arise in association with AML, or it may represent the blast phase in MPNs. Prognosis is determined by the underlying genetic abnormality.

Disorders of the Lymphoid System

NORMAL LYMPH NODES AND LYMPHOCYTES

The lymphoid system consists of circulating T- and B-lymphocytes, natural killer (NK) cells and the secondary lymphoid organs, which mainly include lymph nodes, spleen, and thymus. In addition to the tonsils in the oro- and nasopharynx (Waldeyer ring), there are mucosa-associated lymphoid tissue (MALT) aggregates in extranodal sites, such as the gut, lungs and skin, for example, Peyer patches of the terminal ileum.

Lymphocytes arrive in tonsils and Peyer patches by migrating through the tall endothelial cells of vessels, which are comparable to the postcapillary venules in lymph nodes. *MALT plays an important role in immune defenses in areas vulnerable to potential invaders.* IgA secretion is a key facet of this protection.

All three major types of lymphocytes (T-cells, B-cells, and NK-cells) develop from lymphoid stem cells in the bone marrow (see Fig. 26-2). T-cells mature and differentiate in the thymus. B-cells undergo activation, transformation, and selection in the lymph nodes and spleen. NK-cells forego thymic or lymph node education phases, but are released into the peripheral circulation, as large granular lymphocytes. All lymphocyte development entails a tightly controlled sequence of gene expression and silencing that leads to sequential gain and loss of nuclear material and changes cytoplasmic and/or surface antigen expression. *Patterns of antigenic expression identify lineage and maturational stages of normal and neoplastic lymphoid cells* (see below, Chapter 4).

LYMPH NODES: Lymph nodes are nodular structures composed of lymphoid tissue, located along lymphatic vessels throughout the body. They filter circulating lymph and participate in immune reactions. Normal lymph nodes are oval to bean-shaped, and normally under 1 cm. Larger nodes are considered clinically enlarged and may be abnormal microscopically. Lymph nodes are organized in regional collections—chains or groups (e.g., cervical lymph node chain). Sometimes many nodes within a chain or group may be enlarged (e.g., during infection), and/or matted together, for example, in cancer.

Individual lymph nodes are surrounded by a thin fibrous capsule with internally radiating trabeculae, which provides structural support (Fig. 26-46). Subjacent to the fibrous capsule the subcapsular sinus receives lymph fluid (potentially containing antigens) from **afferent lymphatic vessels** that penetrate the node at several points along the outer capsule. The **subcapsular sinus** is continuous with the penetrating fibrous trabeculae, forming trabecular sinuses, which ultimately connect to the efferent lymphatic vessels. Nodal sinuses are lined by macrophages, which are involved in antigen presentation (see Chapter 4). The arrangement of the sinuses maximizes contact between foreign antigens and macrophages and immunoreactive lymphocytes.

Lymph nodes have an **outer cortex** and an **inner medulla** (Fig. 26-46). The cortex contains mostly B-cells arranged in nodular lymphoid follicles. The paracortex is a T-cell predominant area between B-cell follicles and extending deeply into the cortex. Other cells in the paracortex are rare transformed immunoblasts (T or B), interdigitating dendritic cells (IDCs), plasmacytoid dendritic cells, and postcapillary venules. IDCs process and present antigens to T-lymphocytes.

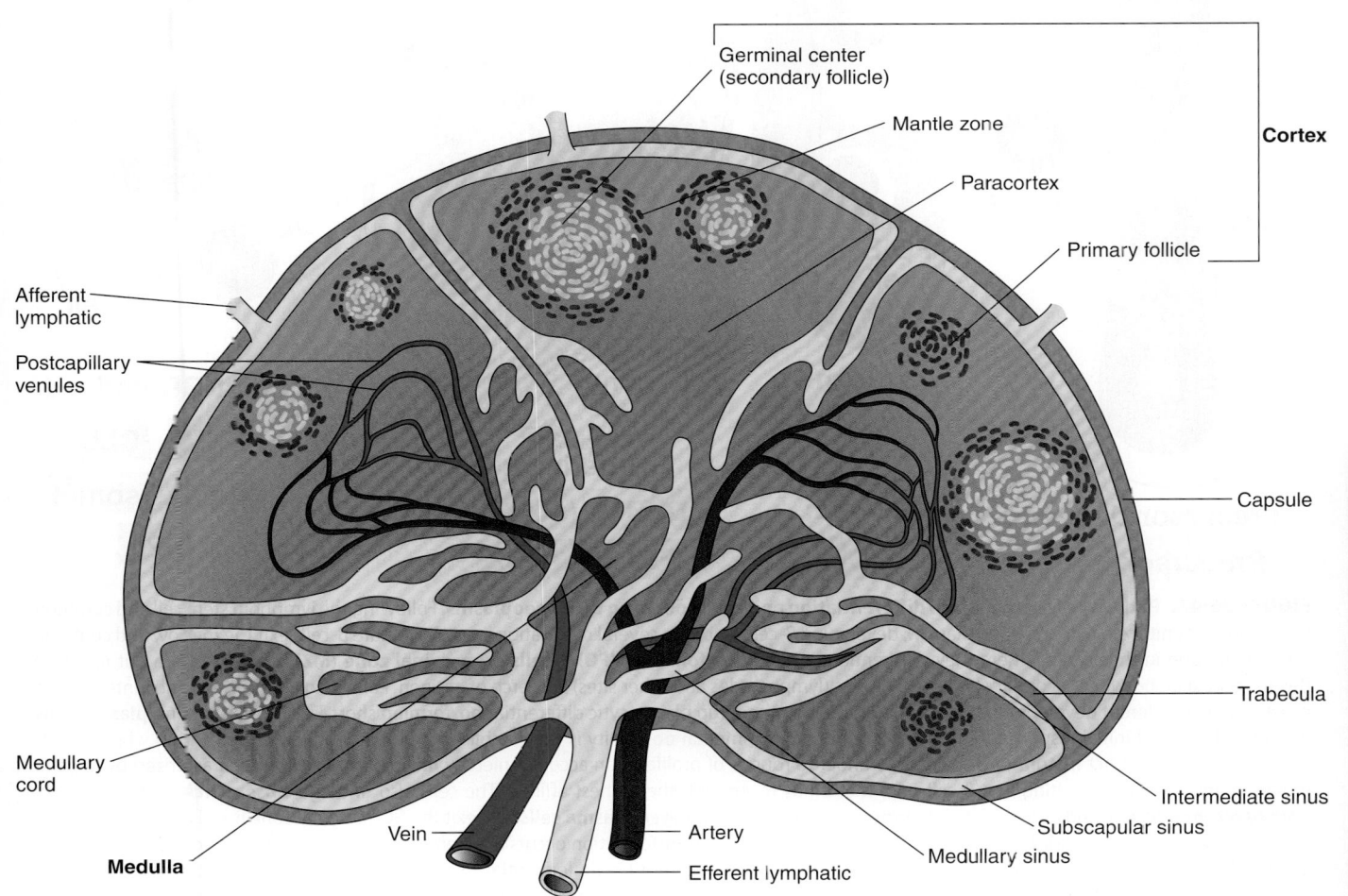

FIGURE 26-46. Structure of normal lymph node.

Lymphocytes from the circulation enter the lymph node cortex by migrating through the tall endothelial cells of the postcapillary venules in the **paracortex**. T-cells tend to remain in the paracortex, while B-lymphocytes home to **follicle germinal centers**.

The B-cell–rich cortex contains two types of follicles: (1) immunologically inactive **primary follicles**, containing antigen-naïve cells; and (2) immunologically active **secondary follicles**, which respond to antigenic stimulation. Primary follicles are aggregates of small lymphocytes without well-defined germinal centers or mantle zones. Secondary follicles contain germinal centers in which large noncleaved lymphocytes **(centroblasts)** mingle with smaller lymphocytes with cleaved nuclei **(centrocytes)**. Normal germinal centers also contain scattered macrophages with phagocytized nuclear and cytoplasmic debris ("tingible body" macrophages) and **follicular dendritic cells (FDCs)** that are stellate cells with long cytoplasmic processes. FDCs present antigens to follicular lymphocytes. Macrophages, and to a lesser extent dendritic cells, provide growth factors for activated B-cells.

The medulla is the most central region of the lymph node, adjacent to the hilum. It mostly contains small B- and T-lymphocytes, and mature plasma cells, all arranged into cords surrounding medullary sinuses. These sinuses contain histiocytes.

B-LYMPHOCYTE DEVELOPMENT: B-lymphocytes are a central component of the adaptive humoral immune system, and protect against numerous pathogens, by producing antigen-specific immunoglobulins. The "B" represents the Bursa of Fabricius, the main site of B-cell development in birds. Mammalian **B-cell progenitors** arise in the bone marrow (Fig. 26-47) (called hematogones) from hematopoietic precursors cells. Their numbers vary with age: they are more numerous in children than in adults. Their phenotype resembles the cells of **precursor B-cell acute lymphoblastic leukemia (B-ALL):**

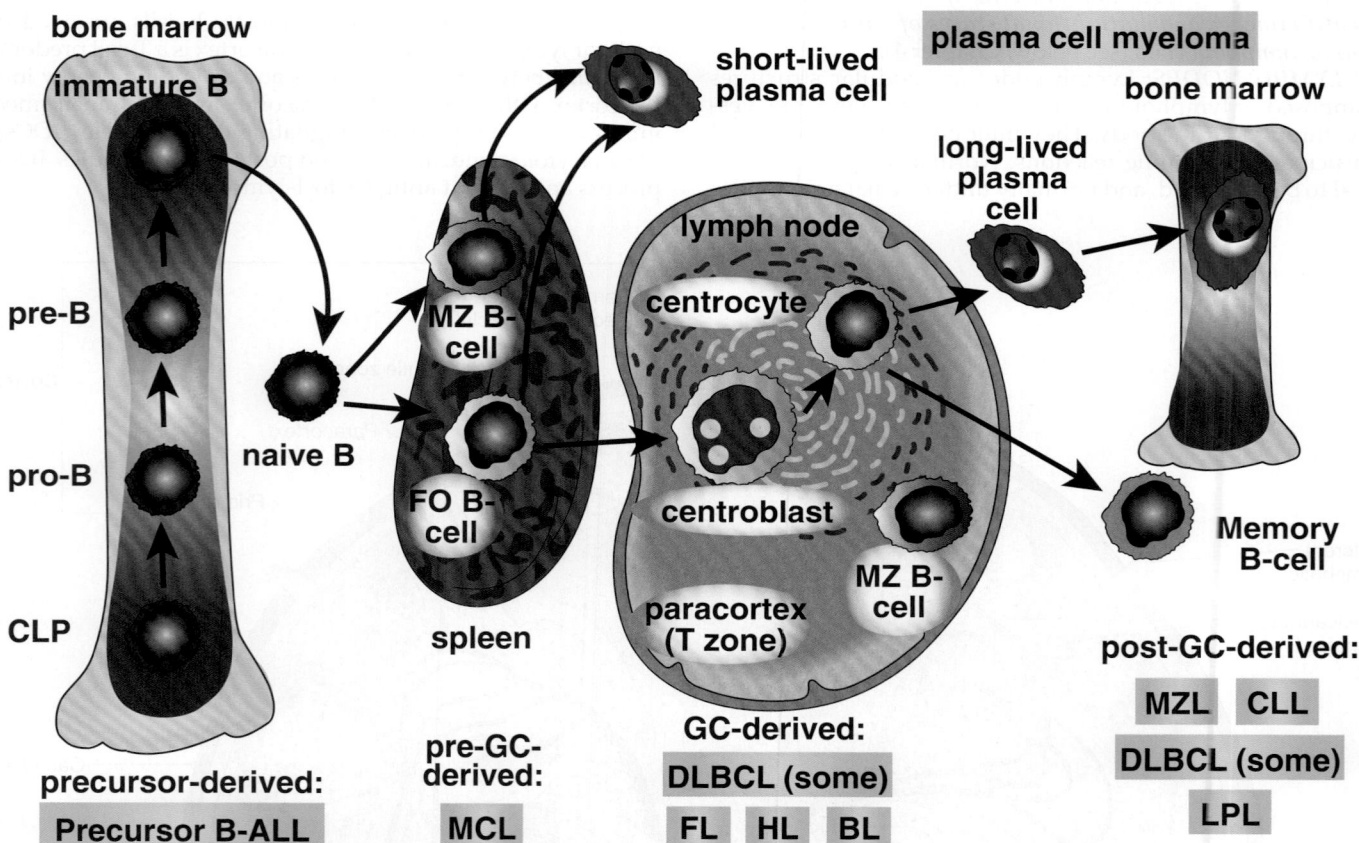

FIGURE 26-47. Pathway of normal B-cell differentiation and corresponding B-cell neoplasms. Following the lymphoid stem cell and common lymphoid progenitor stage in the bone marrow, developing B-cells undergo several maturation steps. Immature B-cells exit the marrow and continue their maturation in the spleen, where they differentiate into mature **follicular (FO) B-cells** or **marginal zone (MZ) B-cells**. Mature but naïve FO B-cells recirculate between secondary lymphoid organs (lymph nodes and other sites) in search of antigen. Following antigen (Ag) encounter, B-cells can experience different developmental possibilities: they can undergo plasmacytic differentiation, forming short-lived, IgM-secreting **plasma cells** that provide a rapid initial response to antigen. Another developmental possibility is the establishment of a germinal center, within which B-cells engage in several distinct maturations steps: they undergo rounds of proliferation accompanied by **affinity maturation,** characterized by Ig gene mutation and selection resulting in a B-cell pool that binds to Ag with the highest affinity. The cells also undergo **class switch (Ig heavy chain switch) recombination,** and differentiate into **memory B-cells** and long-lived **plasma cells** that exit the GC. Marginal zone B-cells home to mucosa-associated lymphoid tissue (MALT) sites and bone marrow. Neoplastic transformation occurs at all phases of B-cell differentiation. *Precursor B-ALL* = acute B-lymphoblastic leukemia/lymphoma; *B-CLL* = B-cell chronic lymphocytic leukemia; *Ig* = immunoglobulin; *CLP* = common lymphoid progenitor; *DLBCL* = Diffuse large B-cell lymphoma; *MCL* = mantle cell lymphoma; *MZL* = marginal zone lymphoma; *LPL* = lymphoplasmacytic lymphoma.

both hematogones and B-ALL cells express the early B-cell surface antigens **CD10** (common acute leukemia/lymphoma antigen [CALLA]) and **CD19**, and the nuclear enzyme **TdT**. Early B-cell precursors lack CD20, which gradually acquired at later stages and is expressed in all mature B-cells. It is important to differentiate normal B-cell precursors from B-ALL: the former differentiate and mature progressively, while B-ALL cells (lymphoblasts) are usually arrested in maturation at a certain stage (see below). B-cell progenitor initial development within the bone marrow reflects functional rearrangement of immunoglobulin (Ig) gene segments, which generates a B-cell repertoire expressing antibodies capable of recognizing millions of different antigens. There are three recognized developmental bone marrow stages (see Chapter 4): **pro–B-cells** with germline (unrecombined) DNA and no surface Ig; **pre–B-cells** that rearrange their μ-**heavy chain** gene segment, and after a few divisions, rearrange the gene segments encoding κ– and λ–**light (L) chains**. Light chains combine with the μ-chain to form an IgM molecule, which is expressed on the surface of **immature B-cells**. In precursor B-cells, IgM is expressed in the cytoplasm. **Mature (but naïve) B-cells** express surface Ig light (L) and heavy (H) chains in addition to pan B-cell antigens CD19, CD20, and CD22.

Reactive increases in B-cell precursors (hematogones) occurs during viral infections and in bone marrow recovery after chemotherapy or stem cell transplantation.

Regulation of early B-cell development depends on the activity of several factors including recombination-activating gene (RAG-1 and RAG-2), Bruton tyrosine kinase (BTK), and B-cell linker protein (BLNK).

B-cells must find a balance between specific responses against a vast number of pathogens and avoiding potentially harmful autoreactivity. This balance is achieved by clonal anergy and deleting the pre–B-cell receptor (pre-BCR).

Mature but naïve, bone marrow–derived B-cells exit the marrow and migrate to the spleen as transitional B-cells, where further development occurs by differentiating into either follicular or marginal zone B-cells. Follicular B-cells home to B-cell follicles within lymph node, where they encounter antigens, become activated and develop inside **germinal centers (GCs)**. GCs are where B-cells are activated (with the help of T-lymphocytes) and expand clonally. Several important events take place in GCs: somatic hypermutation, affinity maturation, and class switch. **Somatic hypermutation** entails point mutations in the variable genes of heavy chains (VH) and light (VL) chains, thereby increasing B-cell receptor affinity for antigens. During **affinity maturation,** B-cells with increased affinity for antigen are preferentially activated and survive. **Class-switching** consists of changing the isotype from IgM to IgG, IgA, or IgE. **Class-switched memory B-cells** and **plasma cells** develop in GCs; memory B-cells leave lymph nodes, while plasma cells migrate to the B-cell–dependent lymph node medullary cords. Independently of T-cells, marginal zone B-cells in the spleen, upon contact with antigen, develop into short-lived plasma cells.

Plasma cells have eccentric nuclei with clumped chromatin, marginated at the nuclear membrane, traditionally described as "clock-face chromatin." They have abundant blue-purple cytoplasm, with a pale paranuclear zone where the Golgi complex resides. Normal plasma cells no longer express CD20 or surface Ig.

Regulatory elements for B-cell development after the BM stage include adhesion molecules and chemokine receptors.

These regulate B-cell homing to follicles, GC formation, and exit of B-cells from tissues back into the bloodstream. **Activation-induced cytidine deaminase (AID)** is critical for somatic hypermutation.

T-LYMPHOCYTES: T-cells are derived from HSCs in the bone marrow. T-cell progenitors migrate from there to the thymus. The developing progenitors within the thymus—thymocytes—are exposed to a number of thymic hormones that induce sequential expression of pan T-cell surface antigens such as CD2, CD3, CD5, and CD7, and CD4 or CD8 (Fig. 26-48). *T-cell receptor gene rearrangement generates a diverse population of T-cells, each of which recognizes a single antigen.* T-cells that interact with antigen/MHC with high affinity survive, while T-cells that cannot bind a foreign antigen (have weak affinity), as well as T-cells that recognize self-antigens, are eliminated via apoptosis (see Chapter 4). Once mature and educated, T-cells exit the thymus and circulate in the blood, lymph nodes, and spleen as **postthymic T-cells**.

When exposed to foreign (non-self) receptor-specific antigen in the context of MHC class II molecules, CD4+ T-cells become activated via release of mitogenic growth factors, for example, IL-1, IL-2. The antigens presented to T-helper cells are peptide fragments derived from partial digestion of foreign proteins by macrophages and/or other antigen-presenting cells. Most CD4+ T-cells function as helper cells: they interact with B-lymphocytes that express the same antigenic specificity and induce the latter to proliferate and differentiate into plasma cells, which produce antigen-specific antibody.

CD8+ cells are activated when their receptors recognize peptide antigens presented in association with MHC class I. Most CD8+ T-cells then become suppressor/cytotoxic cells. CD8+ cells limit expansion of activated B-cells and stop their immune response in a negative feedback response loop.

NATURAL KILLER AND CYTOTOXIC LYMPHOCYTES: A small subset of lymphocytes lack the usual T- or B-cell antigens. These are **NK-cells**. NK-cells are cytotoxic effectors that do not require antigen recognition to initiate their killing function. They are large lymphocytes with granular cytoplasm (i.e., **large granular lymphocytes**) (Fig. 26-49). They differ from mature T-cells in that they lack surface CD3 and possess other surface antigens, like CD16 and CD56.

Lymphocytes have diverse morphologies in stained peripheral blood and bone marrow smears, as well as in tissue sections. Like other blast cells, immature lymphoid cells have high nuclear-to-cytoplasmic ratios, fine chromatin, and visible nucleoli. During maturation and differentiation, lymphoid cells can range from large to small, but they generally show more clumped nuclear chromatin and variable amounts of cytoplasm (with or without granules) compared to their immature (blast-like) precursors. While a variety of cell sizes (including many large transformed or activated cells) occur normally in secondary lymphoid organs, lymphocytes that circulate in the blood and those in the bone marrow are mainly small and heterogeneous (Fig. 26-49).

In peripheral blood smears, transformed cytotoxic T-cells are **variant lymphocytes** (sometimes called "atypical lymphocytes"). Variant lymphocytes tend to have abundant blue-gray cytoplasm and multiple nucleoli in Wright–Giemsa-stained smears. The same cells in tissue sections stained with hematoxylin and eosin (H&E) have round-to-oval nuclei, one to several eosinophilic nucleoli apposed to their nuclear membranes and abundant clear to purple cytoplasm. *T- and B-cells appear identical in routinely stained smears or tissue sections. Precise identification and characterization*

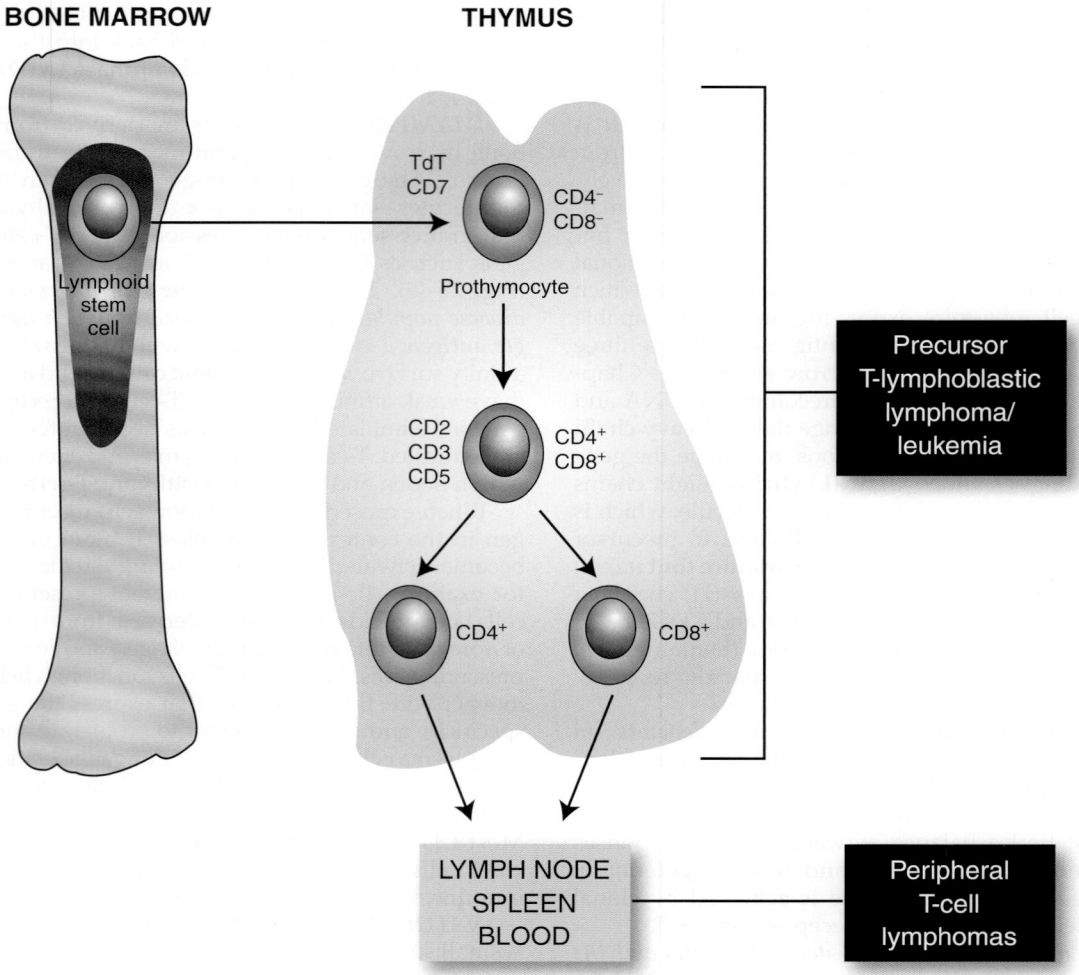

FIGURE 26-48. Pathways of normal T-cell development and corresponding T-cell neoplasms. *CD* = cluster designation; *TdT* = terminal deoxynucleotidyl transferase.

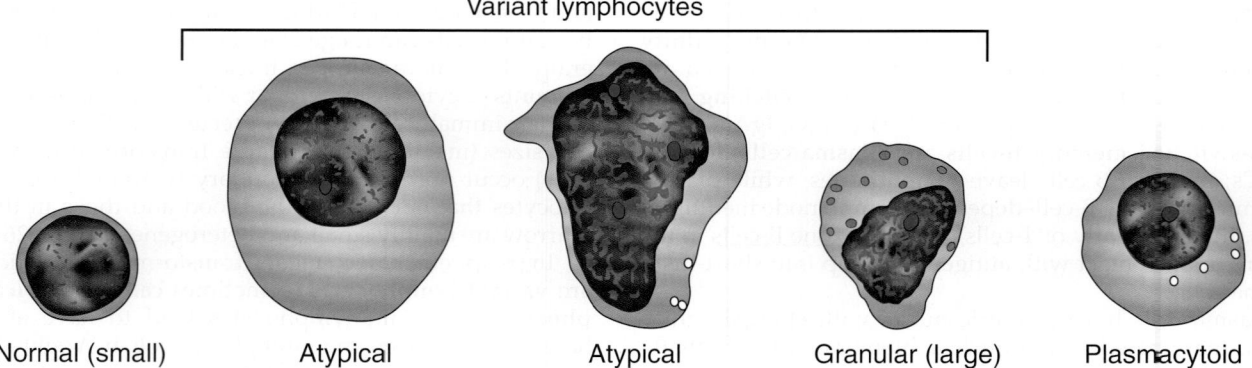

FIGURE 26-49. Lymphocyte morphology. The term "variant lymphocytes" covers atypical lymphocytes and large granular lymphocytes. Atypical lymphocytes are large and exhibit deep blue to pale gray cytoplasm; they are seen in benign reactive processes. Large granular lymphocytes are medium to large lymphoid cells with some pink cytoplasmic granules. They are suppressor T-lymphocytes, some with natural killer (NK) function, and may be increased in benign or malignant disorders. Plasmacytoid lymphocytes have abundant blue cytoplasm and are seen in some reactive disorders.

of lymphoid cells requires flow cytometric or immunohistochemical analysis. In the blood, 60% to 80% of circulating lymphocytes are T-cells, 10% to 15% are B-cells, and the rest are NK-cells.

BENIGN DISORDERS OF THE LYMPHOID SYSTEM

In Benign Lymphocytosis, Absolute Numbers of Circulating Lymphocytes Are Transiently Increased

The upper limits of normal are 4,000/μL in adults, 7,000/μL in children, and 9,000/μL in infants. Lymphocytosis may reflect increased production, redistribution (from bone marrow or secondary lymphoid organs) or decreased cell death. Increased production of benign lymphocytes occurs most commonly in response to infections or inflammation. Benign reactive lymphocytes are morphologically heterogeneous, and include "atypical" lymphocytes (Figs. 26-49 and 26-50). Infectious mononucleosis due to EBV infection is the most common cause of reactive lymphocytosis, but other viral infections can produce similar syndromes (e.g., CMV). Other less common causes of reactive lymphocytosis include pertussis, chronic bacterial infections such as tuberculosis and brucellosis, stress and cigarette smoking. Persistent absolute lymphocytosis of greater than 4,000/μL, particularly in adults, raises suspicion for a lymphoproliferative disorder and deserves further evaluation. Malignant lymphocytes are usually uniform in size and shape because of their clonal nature.

Bone Marrow Plasmacytosis May Signify a Plasma Cell Disorder

- **Plasma cells in peripheral blood:** Plasma cells are terminally differentiated B lineage cells, and circulate in the blood infrequently. When seen, they are usually part of the spectrum of lymphoid cells in infectious mononucleosis-

like syndromes caused by viruses other than EBV. Circulating plasma cells in adults, raise suspicion for plasma cell neoplasms, such as plasma cell myeloma (PCM) or plasma cell leukemia (see below).

- **Reactive bone marrow plasmacytosis:** Plasma cells normally account for less than 3% of bone marrow cells. Plasmacytosis may be polyclonal or monoclonal, which distinction can be made by flow cytometry: in benign conditions plasma cells make Ig with different light chains restriction and preserve normal surface antigens. In children and young adults, plasmacytoses are mostly reactive, due to chronic infections or systemic inflammatory disorders, particularly autoimmune diseases. Plasmacytosis may also accompany a metastatic neoplasm in the bone marrow. *Bone marrow plasmacytosis exceeding 10% typically reflects plasma cell neoplasia.* In both reactive and neoplastic plasma cell proliferations, immunoglobulin may accumulate in the cytoplasm to form prominent eosinophilic globules, called **Russell bodies**. Similarly, benign and neoplastic plasma cells may contain nuclear pseudoinclusions (**Dutcher bodies**), which represent immunoglobulin invaginated into the nucleus and seen in cross-section.

Lymphocytopenia Usually Reflects Decreased T-Helper Lymphocytes

Peripheral blood lymphocytopenia is defined as a blood lymphocyte count less than 1,500/μL in adults or less than 3,000/μL in children. Since T-helper (CD4$^+$) cells are the most abundant lymphocytes in the blood, lymphocytopenia generally means decreased CD4$^+$ T-cells. Evaluation of lymphocytopenia includes clinical history, physical examination, assessment of lymphocyte subpopulations and immunoglobulin levels. There are several mechanisms of lymphocytopenia:

- **Decreased lymphocyte production:** Several congenital and acquired immunodeficiency syndromes entail reduced lymphocyte generation.
- **Increased lymphocyte destruction:** Certain therapies—for example, irradiation, chemotherapy, antithymocyte globulin, and corticosteroids—destroy lymphocytes. Some infections, particularly HIV and bacterial or fungal sepsis, are also common causes. In sepsis, in addition to apoptosis, lymphocytes decrease in blood because they migrate and redistribute toward affected tissues.
- **Loss of lymphocytes:** Disorders associated with damage to intestinal lymphatics can lead to loss of lymph fluid and lymphocytes into the gut lumen. Such diseases include protein-losing enteropathies, Whipple disease, and conditions of increased central venous pressure (e.g., right-sided heart failure, chronic constrictive pericarditis). Immunologic damage to lymphocytes may occur in collagen vascular diseases, like SLE.

Acute suppurative lymphadenitis occurs in lymph nodes that drain sites of acute bacterial infections. Such nodes enlarge rapidly because of edema and hyperemia, and are usually tender because their capsules become distended. They are basically abscesses, with neutrophils, fibrin, bland macrophages, and necrotic tissue. Less acute and more localized suppurative lymphadenitis may accompany fungal infections.

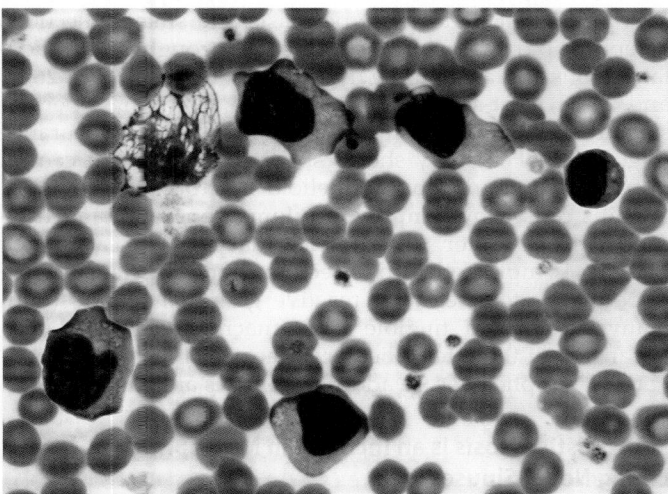

FIGURE 26-50. Infectious mononucleosis. An absolute lymphocytosis caused by a heterogeneous population of small and larger lymphoid cells, including atypical lymphocytes, is characteristic of this Epstein–Barr virus–driven disorder.

Reactive Lymphoid Hyperplasia Is Benign and Reversible Lymph Node Enlargement due to Antigenic Stimulation

Common causes of enlarged lymph nodes include: infections, autoimmune disorders, certain medications, Castleman disease (see below), histiocytosis, Kikuchi lymphadenitis, and sarcoidosis. Lymph node hyperplasia may involve certain or all components. Thus, four patterns are recognized: follicular pattern (mainly B-cells), diffuse paracortical (T zone) hyperplasia, sinus histiocytosis, or mixed pattern (Fig. 26-51). Fine-needle aspiration, core biopsy, or best, excisional biopsy, aid in diagnosis, but the patient's age and clinical history are crucial in evaluating any lymphadenopathy.

The histology and magnitude of lymph node enlargement in reactive hyperplasia reflect the age of the patient (children tend to show greater immunoreactivity than adults), the immunologic competence of the host and the inciting stimulus.

The location of the nodes involved in reactive lymphadenopathy often provides a clue to its cause. For example, posterior auricular lymph nodes are commonly enlarged in rubella infection; occipital lymph nodes in scalp infections; posterior cervical lymph nodes in toxoplasmosis; axillary lymph nodes in infections of the arms or chest wall; and inguinal lymph nodes in venereal infections and infections of the legs. Generalized lymphadenopathy may occur in systemic infections, hyperthyroidism, drug hypersensitivity reactions, and autoimmune diseases.

Reactive Follicular Hyperplasia

Hyperplasia of secondary follicles (enlarged follicles with prominent germinal centers) indicates B-cell immunoreactivity. In **nonspecific reactive follicular hyperplasia,** prominent hyperplastic follicles expand the lymph node cortex. Nodal architecture is distorted but not entirely effaced (Figs. 26-51 and 26-52). Follicles are round or irregularly shaped and may coalesce. Activated B-cells in these follicles range from small cells with irregular, cleaved nuclei to large cells: centroblasts and immunoblasts. Mitotic figures are frequent and reflect rapid proliferation of activated B-lymphocytes. Scattered benign macrophages—tangible body macrophages, with abundant pale cytoplasm containing pyknotic nuclear and cytoplasmic debris—are also characteristic of benign follicular hyperplasia. A well-defined mantle of normal small B-cells surrounds follicles, sharply separating them from interfollicular regions.

The trigger for nonspecific reactive follicular hyperplasia is often unknown. It could be a virus, drug, or inflammatory process. The clinical course involves complete resolution of lymphadenopathy after the inciting stimulus disappears.

Reactive lymphadenopathy (either localized or generalized) characterized by follicular hyperplasia and interfollicular plasmacytosis is common in rheumatoid arthritis. It also occurs early in HIV infection. Lymph nodes in patients with HIV/AIDS show a high incidence of lymphomas (e.g., diffuse B-cell lymphoma, Burkitt lymphoma (BL), classical Hodgkin lymphoma; see below), Kaposi sarcoma or opportunistic infection (e.g., with atypical mycobacteria or CMV).

Paracortical Hyperplasia

Paracortical (interfollicular) hyperplasia of the deep cortex or paracortex, is characteristic of T-lymphocyte immunoreactivity.

Nonspecific reactive diffuse (interfollicular) paracortical hyperplasia (Fig. 26-51) is most commonly caused by viral infections or immunologic reactions. Although the precise cause is often unknown, the condition usually resolves promptly. Common viral triggers include varicella-herpes zoster infection, measles, and herpes simplex virus.

Lymphadenopathy in **SLE** is characterized by interfollicular hyperplasia with prominent immunoblasts and plasma cells, and variably pronounced necrosis or hemorrhage. Arteriolitis with fibrinoid necrosis of vessel walls is common. "Hematoxylin bodies," which are extracellular 5 to 12 micron clumps of amorphous, necrotic material, are common. Unlike acute suppurative lymphadenitis, SLE-related lymphadenitis lacks neutrophils. The clinical picture is informative, with cytopenias, splenomegaly, and autoantibodies commonly present.

Dermatopathic Lymphadenopathy Occurs in Chronic Dermatoses

Dermatopathic lymphadenopathy is a paracortical T-cell proliferation caused by certain chronic skin diseases. Lipid, melanin, and hemosiderin drain from affected skin to regional lymph nodes. The draining lymph nodes show an immune reaction to antigenic material arriving there from the skin, and mainly accumulating in paracortical macrophages. A heterogeneous cell population expands the paracortex, including Langerhans cells, IDCs, and histiocytes. The histiocytes contain lipid or pigments such as melanin. Medullary sinuses are distended and filled with histiocytes, plasma cells, and eosinophils.

Mixed Patterns of Reactive Lymph Node Hyperplasia

Some infectious diseases are associated with mixed patterns of lymphoid hyperplasia, in which several different features are prominent. For example, in **toxoplasmosis,** one sees prominent follicular hyperplasia and small collections of epithelioid macrophages scattered through interfollicular regions and around the hyperplastic follicles (Figs. 26-51 and 26-53). **Cat-scratch disease** elicits follicular hyperplasia and suppurative granulomas with a stellate appearance (Fig. 26-54). Histology shows small abscesses with central necrosis surrounded by epithelioid macrophages. Lymphadenitis caused by **lymphogranuloma venereum** and **tularemia** (see Chapter 9) resembles that seen in cat-scratch disease. Lymph nodes in **infectious mononucleosis** have hyperplastic follicles with reactive germinal centers (with many B-cells and tingible body macrophages), and also expansion of the interfollicular paracortex by sheets of activated T-lymphocytes. In addition, sinuses are often dilated.

Sinus Histiocytosis Is an Increase in Macrophages Lining Nodal Sinuses

In sinus histiocytosis, tissue macrophages in nodal subcapsular and trabecular sinuses are more prominent (Figs. 26-51 and 26-55). Sinus histiocytes derive from blood monocytes. Sinus histiocytosis is common in lymph nodes draining

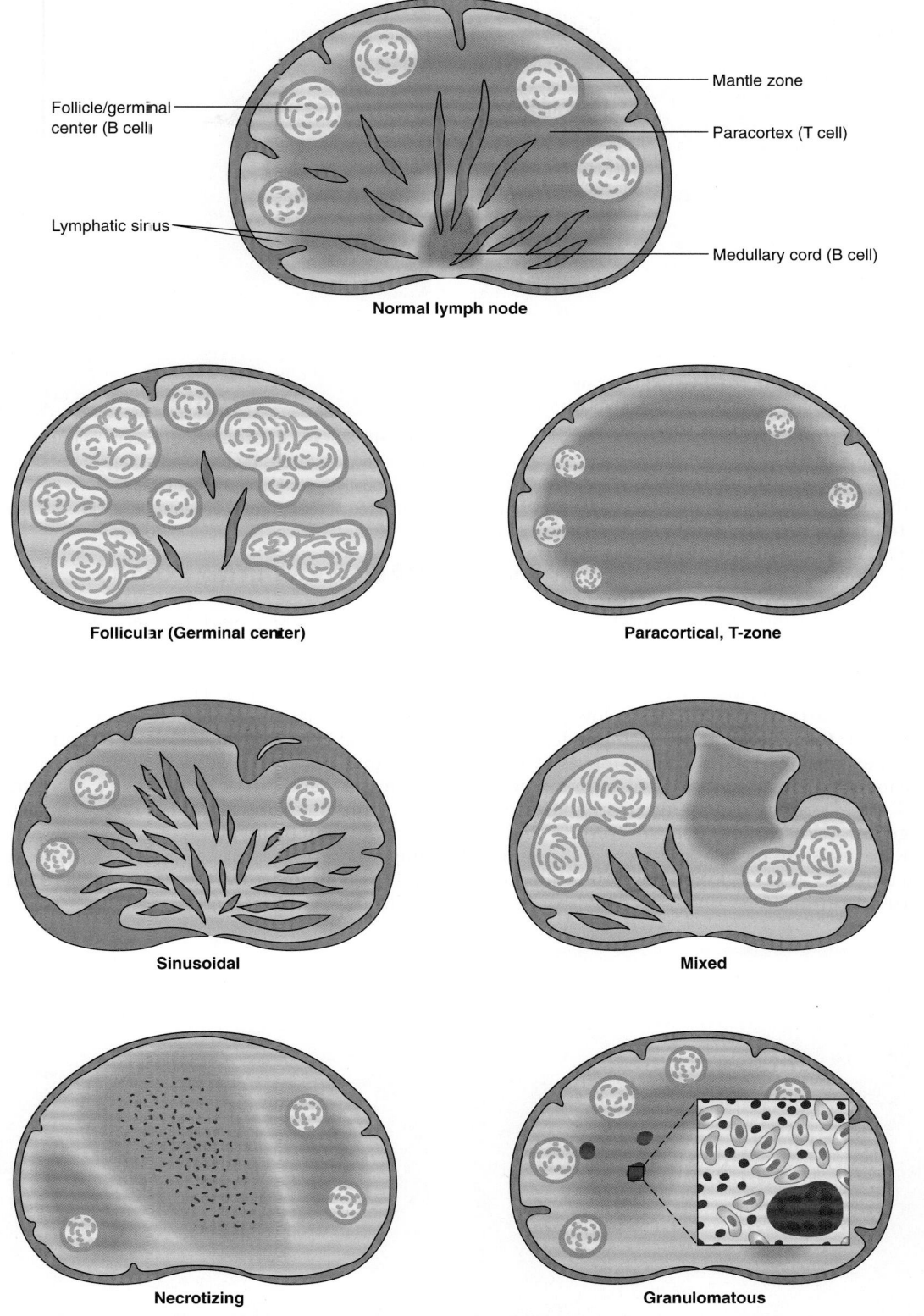

FIGURE 26-51 Patterns of reactive lymphadenopathy. The major patterns of reactive hyperplasia are contrasted with the architecture of a normal lymph node. Follicular hyperplasia, with an increased number of enlarged and irregularly shaped follicles, is characteristic of B-cell immunoreactivity. Interfollicular hyperplasia with expansion of the paracortex is typical of T-cell immunoreactivity. The sinusoidal pattern is typified by expansion of sinuses by bland macrophages. This pattern is seen in reactive proliferations of the mononuclear–phagocyte system. A mixed pattern of follicular, interfollicular, and sinusoidal hyperplasia is common in a variety of complex immune reactions. In necrotizing lymphadenitis, variable zones of necrosis are found within the lymph nodes, with or without the presence of neutrophils. Cohesive clusters of macrophages and occasional multinucleated gianT-cells are characteristic of the granulomatous inflammation pattern.

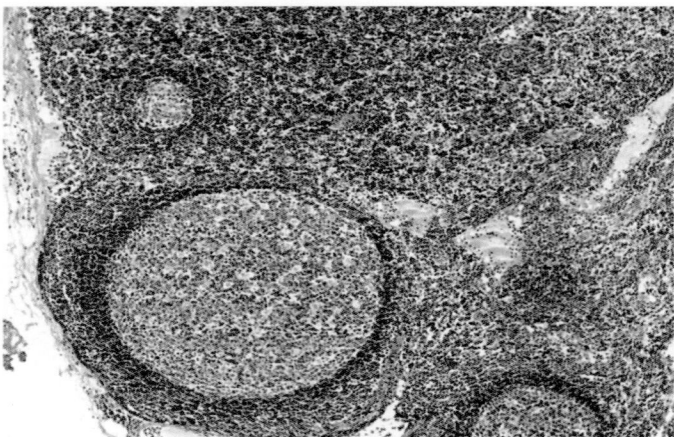

FIGURE 26-52. Lymph node with reactive follicular hyperplasia. A section of a hyperplastic lymph node shows prominent follicles (germinal centers) containing numerous macrophages with pale cytoplasm.

carcinomas and, less often, inflammatory and infectious foci. The nature of the phagocytic debris in the cytoplasm of such macrophages helps identify the origin of the process. For example, anthracotic pigment accumulates in macrophages in mediastinal lymph nodes showing sinus histocytosis. Macrophages containing erythrocytes and hemosiderin pigment characterize AIHAs and sites draining hemorrhages.

Sinus histiocytosis may or may not cause lymph node enlargement. Common sinus histiocytosis should not be confused with **sinus histiocytosis with massive lymphadenopathy (Rosai–Dorfman disease**, see below), in which prominent bilateral (usually cervical) lymphadenopathy reflects a marked expansion of lymph node sinuses by histocytes that have ingested intact lymphocytes (emperipolesis). Most cases of Rosai–Dorfman disease occur in adolescents, sometimes together with a short febrile episode and/or night sweats. Rare cases are more aggressive, with immune dysfunction manifested as auto-antibodies, joint inflammation, or glomerulonephritis.

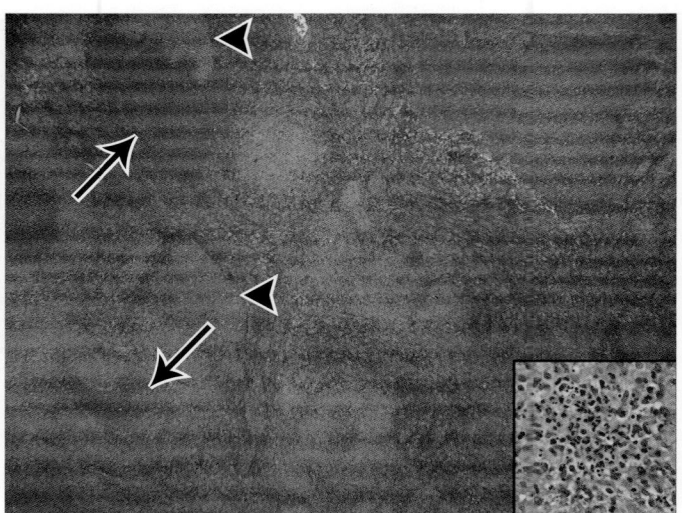

FIGURE 26-54. Cat-scratch disease. Follicular hyperplasia (*arrowheads*) is punctuated by irregularly shaped granulomas (*arrows*), which occasionally impinge on the germinal centers. *Inset*. The granulomas are composed of central cores of neutrophils with surrounding macrophages.

MALIGNANT LYMPHOMAS

Lymphomas are clonal lymphocytic malignancies. B-cell, T-cell, and NK-cell lymphomas may be **immature** (derived from precursor cells; lymphoblasts) or **mature** (derived from mature effector cells). The latter are more common. While all lymphomas are malignant, they show a wide spectrum of clinical behavior: some follow an indolent clinical course (and may not even require treatment), while others are very aggressive (and can cause death in a short time, if untreated).

Lymphomas mostly affect lymph nodes, but any tissue or organ may be involved (e.g., GI tract, thyroid, liver, skin, lungs, brain). If lymphoma cells are present in the blood and/or bone marrow, the tumor is "leukemic" or "peripheralized."

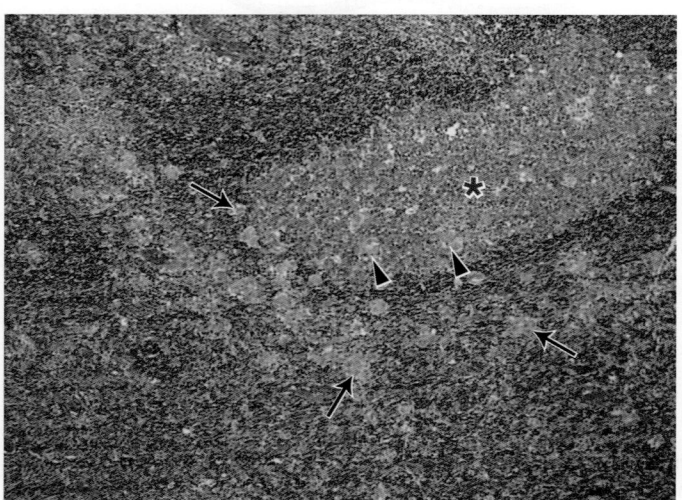

FIGURE 26-53. Toxoplasmosis. The pattern of toxoplasmosis in lymph nodes characteristically features follicular hyperplasia (*), with clusters of pink epithelioid macrophages that are scattered, seemingly splattered randomly amid germinal centers (*arrowheads*) and areas in the mantle and marginal zones, as well as throughout the node (*arrows*).

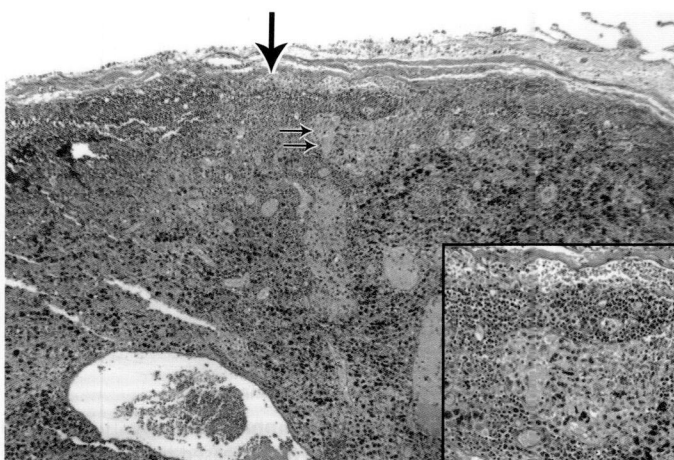

FIGURE 26-55. Sinus histiocytosis. In this hilar lymph node, macrophages are prominent in the subcapsular sinus (*single arrow*) and also in draining sinuses (*double arrows*). *Inset*. A higher-power view demonstrates the large, pink macrophages both at the bottom of the subcapsular sinus and in the draining sinus.

Beyond the broad categories of B-cell, T-cell, and NK-cell types, lymphomas are further classified by their postulated cells of origin, normal cellular counterpart, immunophenotype, molecular/genetic alterations, clinical features, and morphology. Hodgkin lymphoma (HL) is classified separately from non-Hodgkin lymphoma (NHL). The WHO classification of lymphoid tumors takes all of these parameters into account and is currently used by pathologists and clinicians alike. The major recognized types of B-, T-, and NK-cell lymphomas are shown in Table 26-17. Selected examples are discussed below.

Precursor B-Cell Lymphoblastic Leukemia/Lymphoma (B-LBLL) Is a Malignant Neoplasm of Precursor B-Lymphoblasts

The malignanT-cells in B-LBLL are precursor B-cells (**lymphoblasts**). B-lymphoblastic tumors that present with bone marrow and blood involvement are **B-lymphoblastic leukemias (or B-ALL)**. B-lymphoblastic tumors that present with extramedullary disease (e.g., lymph nodes, thymus, skin) are **B-lymphoblastic lymphomas**. Normal B-lymphoblasts, or **hematogones** (see above), resemble neoplastic

---

TABLE 26-17

2016 WHO CLASSIFICATION OF MATURE LYMPHOID, HISTIOCYTIC, AND DENDRITIC NEOPLASMS

Mature B-Cell Neoplasms

Chronic lymphocytic leukemia/small lymphocytic lymphoma
Monoclonal B-cell lymphocytosis
B-cell prolymphocytic leukemia
Splenic marginal zone lymphoma
Hairy cell leukemia
Splenic B-cell lymphoma/leukemia, unclassifiable
   Splenic diffuse red pulp small B-cell lymphoma
   Hairy cell leukemia-variant
Lymphoplasmacytic lymphoma
   Waldenström macroglobulinemia
Monoclonal gammopathy of undetermined significance (MGUS), IgM
μ heavy-chain disease
γ heavy-chain disease
α heavy-chain disease
Monoclonal gammopathy of undetermined significance (MGUS), IgG/A
Plasma cell myeloma
Solitary plasmacytoma of bone
Extraosseous plasmacytoma
Monoclonal immunoglobulin deposition diseases
Extranodal marginal zone lymphoma of mucosa-associated lymphoid tissue (MALT lymphoma)
Nodal marginal zone lymphoma
   Pediatric nodal marginal zone lymphoma
Follicular lymphoma
   In situ follicular neoplasia
   Duodenal-type follicular lymphoma
Pediatric-type follicular lymphoma
Large B-cell lymphoma with IRF4 rearrangement
Primary cutaneous follicle center lymphoma
Mantle cell lymphoma
   In situ mantle cell neoplasia
Diffuse large B-cell lymphoma (DLBCL), NOS
   Germinal center B-cell type
   Activated B-cell type
T-cell/histiocyte-rich large B-cell lymphoma
Primary DLBCL of the central nervous system (CNS)

Primary cutaneous DLBCL, leg type
EBV+ DLBCL, NOS
EBV+ *mucocutaneous ulcer*
DLBCL associated with chronic inflammation
Lymphomatoid granulomatosis
Primary mediastinal (thymic) large B-cell lymphoma
Intravascular large B-cell lymphoma
ALK+ large B-cell lymphoma
Plasmablastic lymphoma
Primary effusion lymphoma
HHV8+ *DLBCL, NOS*
Burkitt lymphoma
Burkitt-like lymphoma with 11q aberration
High-grade B-cell lymphoma, with MYC and BCL2 and/or BCL6 rearrangements
High-grade B-cell lymphoma, NOS
B-cell lymphoma, unclassifiable, with features intermediate between DLBCL and classical Hodgkin lymphoma

Mature T and NK Neoplasms

T-cell prolymphocytic leukemia
T-cell large granular lymphocytic leukemia
Chronic lymphoproliferative disorder of NK-cells
Aggressive NK-cell leukemia
Systemic EBV+ T-cell lymphoma of childhood
Hydroa vacciniforme–like lymphoproliferative disorder
Adult T-cell leukemia/lymphoma
Extranodal NK-/T-cell lymphoma, nasal type
Enteropathy-associated T-cell lymphoma
Monomorphic epitheliotropic intestinal T-cell lymphoma
Indolent T-cell lymphoproliferative disorder of the GI tract
Hepatosplenic T-cell lymphoma
Subcutaneous panniculitis-like T-cell lymphoma
Mycosis fungoides
Sézary syndrome
Primary cutaneous CD30+ T-cell lymphoproliferative disorders
   Lymphomatoid papulosis
   Primary cutaneous anaplastic large cell lymphoma

(*continued*)

TABLE 26-17

2016 WHO CLASSIFICATION OF MATURE LYMPHOID, HISTIOCYTIC, AND DENDRITIC NEOPLASMS (CONTINUED)

Primary cutaneous γδ T-cell lymphoma	**Posttransplant Lymphoproliferative Disorders (PTLD)**
Primary cutaneous CD8⁺ aggressive epidermotropic cytotoxic T-cell lymphoma	Plasmacytic hyperplasia PTLD
Primary cutaneous acral CD8⁺ T-cell lymphoma	Infectious mononucleosis PTLD
Primary cutaneous CD4⁺ small/medium T-cell lymphoproliferative disorder	Florid follicular hyperplasia PTLD
Peripheral T-cell lymphoma, NOS	Polymorphic PTLD
Angioimmunoblastic T-cell lymphoma	Monomorphic PTLD (B- and T-/NK-cell types)
Follicular T-cell lymphoma	Classical Hodgkin lymphoma PTLD
Nodal peripheral T-cell lymphoma with TFH phenotype	**Histiocytic and Dendritic Cell Neoplasms**
Anaplastic large-cell lymphoma, ALK⁺	Histiocytic sarcoma
Anaplastic large-cell lymphoma, ALK	Langerhans cell histiocytosis
Breast implant–associated anaplastic large-cell lymphoma	Langerhans cell sarcoma
	Indeterminate dendritic cell tumor
Hodgkin Lymphoma	Interdigitating dendritic cell sarcoma
Nodular lymphocyte predominant Hodgkin lymphoma	Follicular dendritic cell sarcoma
Classical Hodgkin lymphoma	Fibroblastic reticular cell tumor
Nodular sclerosis classical Hodgkin lymphoma	Disseminated juvenile xanthogranuloma
Lymphocyte-rich classical Hodgkin lymphoma	Erdheim–Chester disease
Mixed cellularity classical Hodgkin lymphoma	
Lymphocyte-depleted classical Hodgkin lymphoma	

Reprinted with permission from Swerdlow SH, Campo E, Pileri SA, et al. The 2016 revision of the World Health Organization classification of lymphoid neoplasms. *Blood.* 2016;127(20):2375--2390

B-lymphoblasts, in morphology and immunophenotype. Hematogones, like neoplastic B-lymphoblasts, produce nuclear TdT (see above) and express early B-cell surface antigens CD10 and CD19. Unlike leukemic B-cells, hematogones are polyclonal. B-cell clonality can be assessed by PCR amplification of the immunoglobin heavy chain (IgH) variable region gene locus using primers upstream and downstream of the rearranged VDJ locus. Amplified DNA from hematogones is composed of multiple VDJ fragments that vary in length (polyclonal); amplified DNA from B-lymphoblastic tumors is composed of a single rearranged VDJ fragment that derives from a single B-cell clone (monoclonal).

 EPIDEMIOLOGY: *B-ALL is the most common childhood leukemia.* Although it can present at any age, 75% of cases occur in children under age 6. Several environmental and genetic factors have been implicated as risk factors, including Down syndrome, Bloom syndrome, ataxia-telangiectasia, neurofibromatosis type I, in utero exposure to ionizing radiation and organic solvents such as benzene. Most cases present as leukemia rather than lymphoma, unlike its T-cell counterpart.

MOLECULAR PATHOGENESIS: Chromosomal abnormalities are present in most cases of precursor B-cell ALL, including both numerical and structural abnormalities (Table 26-18). Translocations are common, including t(9;22), *BCR/ABL* fusion. Unlike the 210-kDa fusion protein in adult B-LBL and CML, the fusion

protein (p190) is smaller in childhood B-ALL. Other chromosomal changes may impact prognosis (Table 26-18).

 PATHOLOGY: Lymphoblasts are small to medium-sized cells with high nucleus-to-cytoplasm (N:C) ratio, fine chromatin, inconspicuous nucleoli, and agranular cytoplasm (Fig. 26-56). They typically comprise at least 20% of bone marrow cellularity, with variable numbers of blasts in blood. Immunophenotypic patterns are variable and reflect the different stages of early B-cell maturation (Fig. 26-47), including the earliest antigens that indicate B-cell differentiation—CD10, CD19, and TdT—and no surface Ig.

 CLINICAL FEATURES: The leukemic cells of B-ALL proliferate in the bone marrow, where they displace normal marrow elements and cause anemia, thrombocytopenia, and neutropenia (pancytopenia). Organomegaly and central nervous system (CNS) involvement are common. The rapid growth within the marrow induces bone pain and arthralgias, which may be the earliest presenting symptoms in children.

The prognosis of childhood B-ALL is generally excellent. Complete remission rates exceed 90%. Among other variables, age younger than 1 year or older than 12 years, older adult onset and/or the presence of certain cytogenetic abnormalities [e.g., t(9;22), t(1;19), t(4;11), hypodiploidy] are poor prognostic indicators. Translocations

TABLE 26-18

COMMON GENETIC ABNORMALITIES ASSOCIATED WITH PROLIFERATIONS OF LYMPHOID CELLS

Disease	Associated Genetic/Chromosomal Abnormality	Importance
B-lymphoblastic leukemia/lymphoma	t(9;22) translocations involving *MLL* at 11q23	Children often make p190 bcr/abl, while adults make p210 bcr/abl from t(9;22)
	Hyperdiploidy	Better prognosis
	Hypodiploidy	Worse prognosis
T-lymphoblastic leukemia/lymphoma	TCR genes translocate to sites involving *MYC, TAL1, RBTN1, RBTN2, HOX11*	Disturbed transcriptional regulation results
B-cell chronic lymphocytic leukemia/small lymphocytic lymphomas	del 13q12–14; frequent IgVH gene rearrangements	
	del 11q; trisomy 12; del 17p	17p locus encodes p53; these changes imply worse prognosis
Follicular lymphoma	t(14;18)(q32 q21)	Characteristic, leads to overexpression of Bcl-2
	Inactivation of p53; activation of *MYC*	Transformation to more aggressive phenotype
Mantle cell lymphoma	t(11;14)(q13 q32)	Primary genetic event, upregulates cyclin D1
	Mutation at 11q22–23	Inactivates *ATM*
Marginal zone lymphoma	t(11;18); t(1;14)	No longer responds to antibiotic treatment alone
	Mutations of IgV region genes; trisomy 3	
Lymphoplasmacytic Lymphoma	MYD88 L265P mutation	
	BRAF V600E mutation	
Hairy cell leukemia	BRAF V600E or MAP2K1 mutation	
Langerhans cell histiocytosis		
Diffuse large B-cell lymphoma	Rearrangements involving 3q27	3q27 carries *BCL6* locus
	t(14;18) rearrangements involving *MYC*	Tend to portend worse prognosis
Burkitt lymphoma	Rearrangements involving *MYC*: t(8;14) or t(2;8) or t(8;22)	Characteristic rearrangement
Plasma cell myeloma	Clonal rearrangements involving Ig H and L genes	
	Abnormalities of chromosome number	Poor prognosis
	IgH translocations with *cyclin D1, C-MAF, FGFR3, cyclin D3, MAFB*; monosomy or partial deletion of chromosome 13	
	t(4;14); t(14;16); t(14;20); del 17p	Poorer prognosis
Anaplastic large cell lymphoma	t(2;5) (involving anaplastic lymphoma kinase and *NPM* genes)	Tends to occur in younger patients, upregulates *ALK*, better prognosis

H = heavy; Ig = immunoglobulin; L = light; TCR = T-cell receptor.

involving the *MLL* gene at 11q23 are associated with a poor prognosis regardless of age.

Precursor T-Cell Acute Lymphoblastic Leukemia/Lymphoma Is a Neoplasm of T Lymphoblasts

Whether it presents as T-cell acute lymphoblastic leukemia (**T-ALL**) or T-cell lymphoblastic lymphoma (**T-LBL**), the malignant T-cells are immature T-cells. As with precursor B-ALL, the decision to call the tumor leukemia or lymphoma is often arbitrary.

 EPIDEMIOLOGY: T-ALL occurs at any age. It accounts for 15% of childhood ALL and affects adolescents more often than younger children. T-ALL is more common in males than females. In adults, 25% of acute lymphoblastic leukemias are T-ALL. Compared

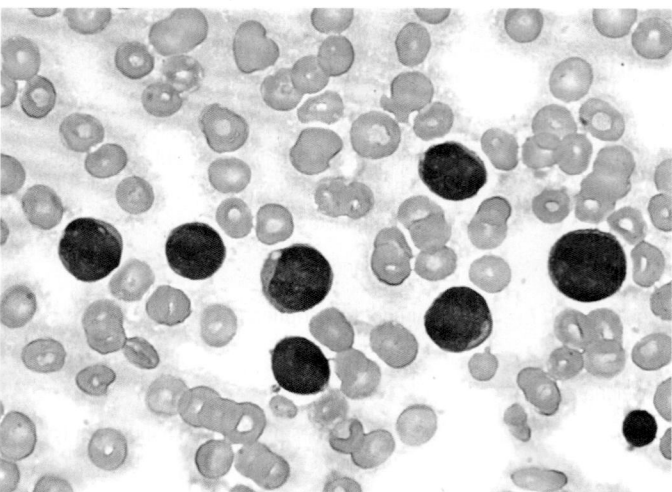

FIGURE 26-56. Acute lymphoblastic leukemia. The lymphoblasts in peripheral blood have irregular and indented nuclei with fine nuclear chromatin, visible nucleoli and variable amounts of agranular cytoplasm.

to its B-cell counterpart, precursor T-cell ALL is more likely to present as a lymphoma.

MOLECULAR PATHOGENESIS: The genes encoding the four T-cell receptor chains (α-, β-, γ-, δ-chains) often participate in chromosomal translocations with genes encoding transcription factors (Table 26-18). Juxtaposition of T-cell receptor loci to transcription factor genes often leads to transcriptional dysregulation.

PATHOLOGY: T-lymphoblasts resemble B-lymphoblasts morphologically; proper identification requires immunophenotype analysis (Fig. 26-56). T-ALL immunophenotype reflects normal T-cell differentiation and maturation in the bone marrow and thymus (Fig. 26-48). The earliest expressed T-cell antigen is CD7, followed by CD2 and CD5. During early thymic differentiation, T-cells express CD1a and cytoplasmic CD3 (cCD3; CD3ε). Early cortical thymocytes express both CD4 and CD8, while medullary thymocytes express either CD4 or CD8. Like precursor B-cell AL, lymphoblasts in most cases of T-cell ALL express TdT.

CLINICAL FEATURES: Peripheral lymphocyte (lymphoblast) counts are usually high, and a mediastinal mass or other tissue mass may be present. Lymphadenopathy and organomegaly are common, as are pleural effusions. **Mediastinal adenopathy** occurs often in adolescent males. Mediastinal involvement may sometimes present with respiratory distress due to compression of the central airways or superior vena cava syndrome due to compression of the vena cava.

Mature B-Cell Lymphomas Are the Most Common Lymphomas in the Western World

Mature B-cell malignancies are clonal proliferations of differentiated B-cells. As B-cells progress through the steps of differentiation and maturation from naive B-lymphocytes to memory B-cells and plasma cells, lymphomas may arise at any point along the way (Fig. 26-47).

EPIDEMIOLOGY: Mature B-cell lymphomas represent over 90% of lymphoid neoplasms worldwide. Frequencies of specific types of B-cell lymphoma vary in different parts of the world. For example, BL is endemic in malarial–endemic regions of equatorial Africa and New Guinea, but accounts for only 1% to 2% of lymphomas in industrialized nations. Similarly, follicular lymphoma (FL) occurs more frequently in the United States and Western Europe than South America, eastern Europe, and Asia. *Worldwide, the most common lymphomas are diffuse large cell lymphoma (37%), FL (29%), exclusive of Hodgkin lymphoma, and PCM (Table 26-19).*

Most mature B-cell lymphomas occur in older adults. A variant of diffuse large B-cell lymphoma (DLBCL), mediastinal large B-cell lymphoma, is an exception, with a median age of 35. Mature B-cell lymphomas other than BL and DLBCL are uncommon in children.

Risk factors for B-cell lymphoma include immunodeficiency (e.g., HIV infection, iatrogenic immunosuppression, congenital immunodeficiency), autoimmune disease, infectious agents (e.g., EBV, HHV-8, hepatitis C

TABLE 26-19	
FREQUENCY OF B- AND T-/NK-CELL LYMPHOMAS	
Diagnosis	**% of Total Cases**
Diffuse large B-cell lymphoma	30.6
Follicular lymphoma	22.1
MALT lymphoma	7.6
Mature T-cell lymphomas (except ALCL)	7.6
Chronic lymphocytic leukemia/small lymphocytic lymphoma	6.7
Mantle cell lymphoma	6.0
Mediastinal large B-cell lymphoma	2.4
Anaplastic large cell lymphoma	2.4
Burkitt lymphoma	2.5
Nodal marginal zone lymphoma	1.8
Precursor T-cell lymphoblastic lymphoma	1.7
Lymphoplasmacytic lymphoma	1.2
Other types	7.4

ALCL = anaplastic large cell lymphoma; MALT = mucosa-associated lymphoid tissue; NK = natural killer.

virus, *Helicobacter pylori*, *Chlamydia*), environmental exposures (e.g., herbicides, pesticides), and genetic polymorphisms of immunoregulatory genes.

PATHOPHYSIOLOGY: Most peripheral B-cell lymphomas occur without apparent cause; however, immunologic impairment and certain infectious agents are often associated (Table 26-20). Immunodeficiency caused by HIV infection and therapeutic immunosuppression in allograft recipients favor development of high-grade EBV-positive large B-cell lymphoma or BL. Low-grade B-cell lymphomas tend to develop in patients with **autoimmune disease.** For example, patients with Sjögren disease or Hashimoto thyroiditis (see Chapters 11, 27, and 29) may develop extranodal marginal zone B-cell lymphoma (MALT lymphoma). **EBV** is linked to endemic BL, HIV-associated lymphomas, and immunosuppression-related lymphomas. Human herpesvirus 8 (HHV-8) and hepatitis C virus also predispose to B-lymphomas—primary effusion lymphoma and lymphoplasmacytic lymphoma (LPL) associated with type 2 cryoglobulinemia, respectively. MALT lymphomas are often associated with gastric *H. pylori* infections (see Chapter 19) and often regress after antibiotic treatment.

Lymphomas are classified according to their respective normal lymphocyte counterparts (Fig. 26-47). After precursor stage, B-cells undergo immunoglobulin *VDJ* gene rearrangements and mature to surface IgM- and IgD-positive naive B-cells that often express CD5. These mature but naïve B-cells may give rise to some cases of **CLL/SLL** and to **mantle cell lymphoma (MCL)**, with overexpression of the cell cycle activator cyclin D1 (due to cyclin D1 translocation). **FLs** derive from germinal center B-cells (centroblasts and/or centrocytes) that over-express the apoptosis inhibitor Bcl-2 (due to Bcl-2 translocation), giving them a survival advantage. **BL** and **DLBCL of GC type** also derive from germinal center B-cells.

Late-stage memory B-cells reside in marginal zones of lymphoid follicles. **Marginal zone lymphomas** include **splenic marginal zone lymphoma, nodal marginal zone lymphoma,** and **MALT lymphoma**. MALT lymphomas arise in extranodal sites such as the stomach, skin, lung, conjunctiva, and salivary glands. Memory B-cells can also give rise to a subset of cases of chronic lymphocytic leukemia/small lymphocytic lymphoma **(CLL/SLL)**. Plasma cells are terminally differentiated germinal center B-cells. They are produce and release copious amounts of antibody protein (immunoglobulin). Plasma cells, unlike B-cells, lack detectable cell surface immunoglobulin (sIg), expressing instead cytoplasmic Ig (cIg). Plasma cells populate lymph nodes, spleen, GI tract, and bone marrow, where they may give rise to plasma cell tumors including **monoclonal gammopathy of undetermined significance (MGUS), multiple myeloma,** and **plasmacytoma.**

CLINICAL FEATURES: Clinical behavior of B-cell lymphoma is largely based on extent of disease (stage), organ involvement, pathology (morphology and immunophenotype), and genetic abnormalities. *B-cell lymphomas composed of small mature lymphocytes usually follow an indolent clinical course, but B-cell lymphomas composed of large cells are usually aggressive.* Thus, indolent B-cell lymphomas include CLL/SLL, FL, extranodal MALT lymphoma, and LPL. Examples of aggressive B-cell lymphomas include DLBCL, BL, and MCL. Conversely, although indolent lymphomas progress slowly, they are usually incurable using standard therapy, unlike aggressive lymphomas, which progress rapidly, but are often curable with conventional therapies.

Our subsequent discussion of B-cell lymphomas follows B-cell development paradigms outlined in Figure 26-47.

B-Cell Chronic Lymphocytic Leukemia (CLL)/Small Lymphocytic Lymphoma (SLL)

B-cell CLL/SLL is a low-grade, often asymptomatic, lymphoid malignancy, mostly of elderly adults. The tumor cells are clonal CD5+CD23+ B-cells, comprising a monomorphic population of small mature lymphocytes with few admixed large cells—called prolymphocytes (in the blood) or paraimmunoblasts (in tissue). CLL/SLL may involve blood, bone marrow, lymph nodes, and/or extranodal sites. Disease limited to blood and marrow (leukemia) is **CLL**. If lymph nodes and/or solid tumor masses predominate, the term **SLL** is preferred. B-CLL/SLL generally follows an indolent clinical course.

TABLE 26-20

DISORDERS WITH INCREASED RISK OF SECONDARY MALIGNANT LYMPHOMA

Sjögren syndrome

Hashimoto thyroiditis

Renal and cardiac transplant recipients

AIDS

EBV infection

HHV-8 infection

Helicobacter pylori–positive gastritis

Hepatitis C

Congenital immune deficiency syndromes
    Chediak–Higashi
    Wiskott–Aldrich
    Ataxia-telangiectasia
    IgA deficiency
    Severe combined immune deficiency

α Heavy-chain disease

Celiac disease

Hodgkin lymphoma (posttreatment)

EBV = Epstein–Barr virus; HHV = human herpesvirus; Ig = immunoglobulin.

EPIDEMIOLOGY: *B-cell CLL is the most common form of leukemia in adults in the Western world. Average age at diagnosis is 65 with a male predominance.*

MOLECULAR PATHOGENESIS: The vast majority of B-cell CLL/SLL have cytogenetic abnormalities. The most common are shown in Table 26-18. B-CLL can be classified as mutated or unmutated. Unmutated cases have no somatic mutations in IgH variable-region genes (*IgVH*), a germline genotype consistent with naive B-cells. Mutated cases have somatic IgVH mutations (*IgVH* gene rearrangement), which genotype is consistent with post-germinal center B-cells. Unmutated cases tend to behave more aggressively than mutated cases.

PATHOLOGY: Lymph nodes involved by B-cell CLL/SLL are effaced by a proliferation of mostly small lymphocytes in a vaguely nodular pattern (Fig. 26-57A). The blood shows absolute lymphocytosis, mostly small mature lymphocytes, disrupted smudge cells, an artifact of smear preparation (Fig. 26-57B) and a variable number (usually <10%) of large prolymphocytes with prominent nucleoli.

To establish a diagnosis of B-CLL in the absence of tissue-based disease, circulating monoclonal B-cells must exceed 5,000/μL. Circulating clonal B-cell counts under 5,000/μL represent a **monoclonal B-cell lymphocytosis**.

The vaguely nodular pattern of CLL/SLL is due to lighter-staining zones called proliferation centers, which contain large cells called para-immunoblasts (Fig. 26-57C). Large confluent sheets of para-immunoblasts or other large lymphoid cells may be worrisome for transformation to high-grade DLBCL (see below). CLL/SLL infiltrates the spleen and portal areas of the liver. Bone marrow involvement ranges from complete marrow space effacement to patchy interstitial or nodular infiltrates.

The immunophenotype of CLL/SLL is distinctive. *The neoplastic cells express pan B-cell antigens (CD19, weak CD20) as well as CD5, CD23, and weak surface immunoglobulin light chain.* CLL/SLL is negative for cyclin D1 (positive in MCL) and CD10 (positive in FL). CD38 and ZAP-70 expression are surrogate markers for unmutated CLL/SLL.

CLINICAL FEATURES: Most patients with CLL/SLL are asymptomatic, and many cases are diagnosed incidentally. Often the first hint of the disease is absolute lymphocytosis (≥5,000 clonal B-cells/μL). Erythrocyte and platelet counts are initially normal, but as the disease advances, anemia, thrombocytopenia, and/or neutropenia can develop. Up to 20% of cases develop immune-mediated hemolytic anemia. A small monoclonal paraprotein may be present, mostly of IgM heavy-chain type in contrast to IgG paraprotein in multiple myeloma.

Immune deficiency (hypogammaglobulinemia, impaired delayed-type hypersensitivity) is common, leading to increased risk of infection. The disease course and prognosis are variable. Certain genetic abnormalities may suggest a favorable, or unfavorable, prognosis (Table 26-18).

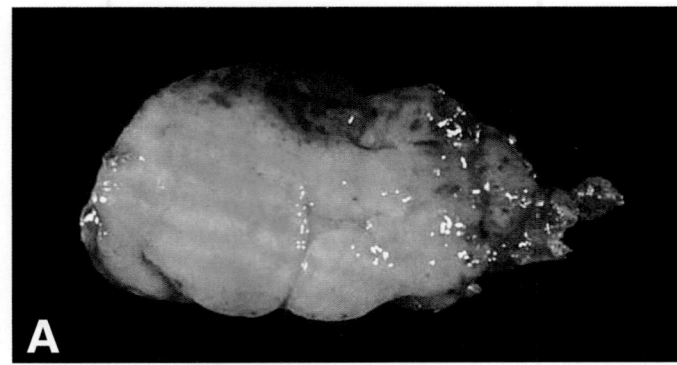

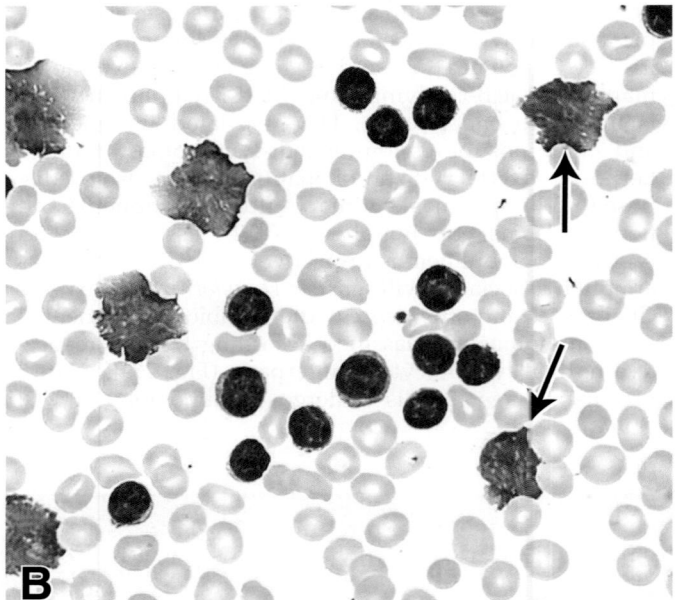

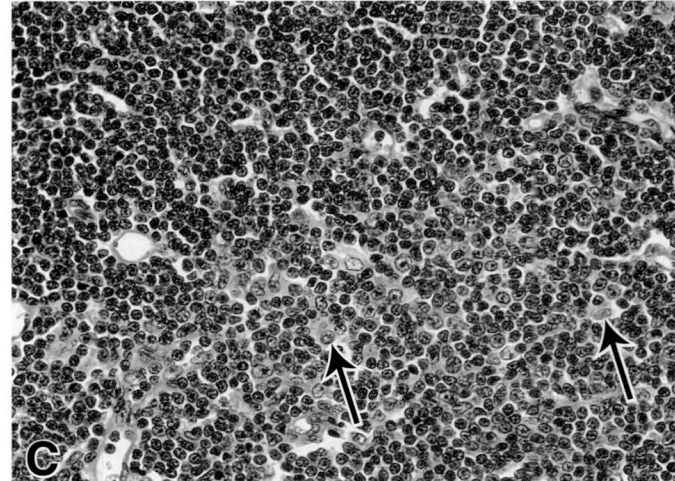

FIGURE 26-57. B-Cell small lymphocytic lymphoma/chronic lymphocytic leukemia. A. Gross image of a bisected, enlarged lymph node shows the characteristic uniform, glistening, fish-flesh appearance seen in tissues involved by lymphoma. **B.** A smear of peripheral blood exhibits numerous small to medium-sized lymphocytes with clumped nuclear chromatin. Scattered smudge cells (osmotically fragile cells) are present (*arrows*). **C.** On microscopic examination, the nodal architecture is replaced by a diffuse proliferation of small lymphocytes admixed with a low number of larger cells known as paraimmunoblasts (*arrows*) found in scattered proliferation centers.

Transformation to prolymphocytic leukemia or DLBCL is associated with rapid disease progression. Prolymphocytic leukemia is heralded by worsening cytopenias, increasing splenomegaly and progressive increases in circulating prolymphocytes or para-immunoblasts in lymph nodes or other tissues. Transformation to DLBCL (**Richter syndrome**) is marked by a rapidly enlarging mass and worsening systemic symptoms. Most patients who develop prolymphocytic or Richter transformation survive less than 1 year.

Follicular Lymphoma

FL is a mature B-cell lymphoma of germinal center B-cells. FL must have at least a partially follicular (nodular) architecture to meet diagnostic criteria. The neoplastic cells are heterogeneous: a mix of small centrocytes and large centroblasts. Tumor behavior varies from indolent to aggressive, largely reflecting histologic grade, which in turn reflects the number of centroblasts in neoplastic follicles (increased large cells suggest aggressive disease).

EPIDEMIOLOGY: FL is the second most common lymphoma worldwide, but in the United States it is the most common non-Hodgkin lymphoma, constituting 20% of adult lymphomas. It is mainly a disease of adults with peak incidence in the sixth decade. It is rare in people under age 20, and affects women more than men.

MOLECULAR PATHOGENESIS: The t(14:18) is the characteristic genomic abnormality in FL. It is found in up to 90% of grade 1 and 2 tumors (the so-called low-grade FLs; Table 26-18). Placed under the control of the highly active IgH promotor on chromosome 14, increased transcription of the Bcl-2 gene on chromosome 18 leads to overexpression of the Bcl-2 antiapoptotic protein. *Bcl-2 inhibits apoptosis and provides a survival advantage to the lymphoma cells.* In addition to the *Bcl-2/IgH* rearrangement, several other genetic alterations may occur in FL, some of them being associated with progression/transformation from low-grade indolent forms to more aggressive grade 3 FL or DLBCL (Table 26-18)

PATHOLOGY: Lymph nodes (or other tissues) involved by FL have a distinctly nodular (follicular) pattern or a combination of nodular and diffuse architectural patterns (Fig. 26-58). Neoplastic follicles are present in high density, often in a back-to-back arrangement with little intervening paracortex. The neoplastic follicle centers contain both small and large cells with irregular nuclear contours (centrocytes/cleaved cells) and scattered centroblasts, which have round nuclear contours and multiple nucleoli at the nuclear membrane.

There are three histologic grades of FL, distinguished by the number of centroblasts per high-power field, and which help predict prognosis (Fig. 26-59). Diffuse areas

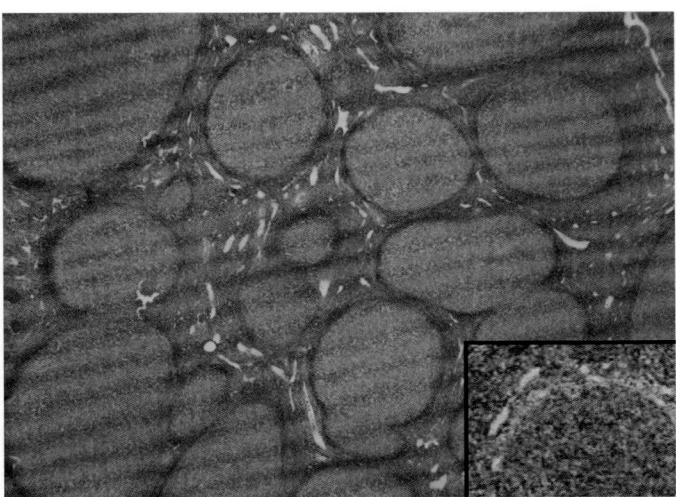

FIGURE 26-58. Follicular lymphoma. The normal lymph node architecture is replaced by malignant lymphoid follicles in a back-to-back pattern. *Inset.* Malignant lymphoid follicle germinal centers can be distinguished from normal/reactive germinal centers using immunohistochemistry for Bcl-2.

occur in FL but generally do not affect prognosis unless they are composed of large B-cells, in which case a diagnosis of concurrent DLBCL is made. The bone marrow is involved in 40% to 60% of cases, in a characteristic paratrabecular pattern in most positive bone marrow core biopsies. FL cells circulate in the blood in 10% of cases; they show prominent nuclear irregularity and deep nuclear clefts.

FLs express pan B-cell antigens including CD19, CD20, CD22, CD79a, PAX-5, and cell surface Ig, which in most cases contain only one type of light chain (κ or λ). In addition, FLs also express germinal center cell markers CD10 and Bcl-6, as would be expected since they originate from follicle centers. Unlike MCL and B-cell CLL/SLL, FLs do not express CD5. FL cells express Bcl-2 protein in over 90% of cases (Fig. 26-58, *inset*). The latter finding may help to distinguish FL from follicular hyperplasia, since the latter is negative for Bcl-2.

CLINICAL FEATURES: Most patients with FL present with generalized adenopathy. Over 80% have stage III or IV disease at diagnosis. Extranodal presentations are relatively uncommon, compared to other B-cell lymphomas. The lymphadenopathy is painless and may have followed a waxing and waning course before the patient seeks medical attention. Some patients will report having fevers, fatigue, and night sweats (B symptoms).

Most cases of FL follow an indolent clinical course. Therefore, and because the disease is usually incurable, treatment is not always needed at diagnosis. Overall median survival is 7 to 9 years, which does not improve dramatically with high-dose chemotherapy. As discussed above, the clinical course is linked to histologic grade, and progression/transformation to more aggressive disease may occur in 50% of cases.

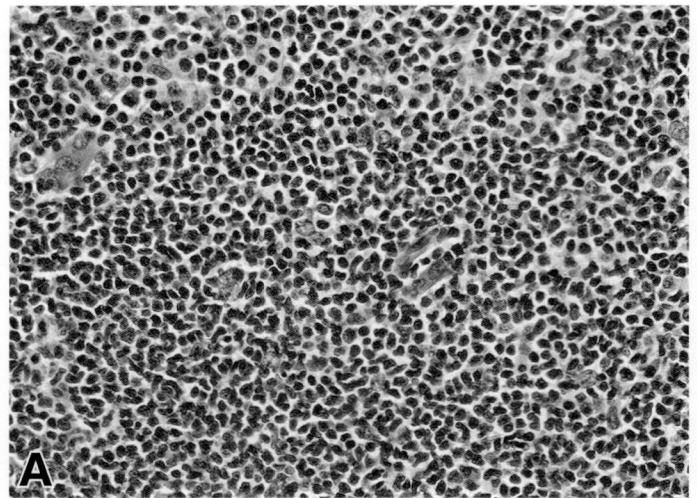

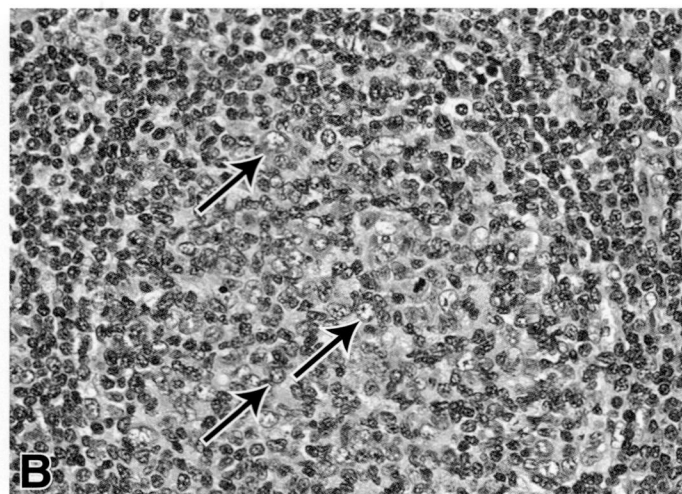

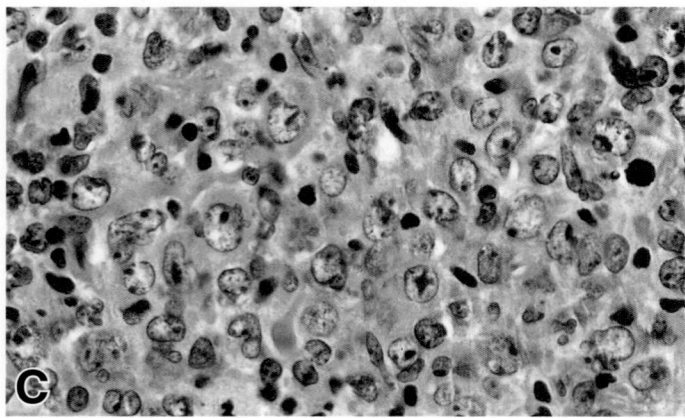

FIGURE 26-59. Follicular lymphoma grading. A. Follicular lymphoma, grade 1. The neoplastic follicles are composed of predominantly small cleaved cells (centrocytes) and only a few scattered centroblasts are present. **B. Follicular lymphoma, grade 2.** The neoplastic follicle shows a mixture of small and large cleaved cells and centroblasts characterized by multiple nucleoli (*arrows*). **C. Follicular lymphoma, grade 3.** The neoplastic follicle shows a predominance of centroblasts with only rare admixed centrocytes. The persistence of a follicular pattern helps distinguish this entity from diffuse large B-cell lymphoma.

Mantle Cell Lymphoma

MCL is composed of monotonous small to medium-sized lymphocytes with irregular nuclear contours.

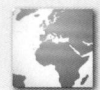

EPIDEMIOLOGY: MCL accounts for under 10% of B-cell lymphomas. This is a disease of adults, with a median age of 60, and affects men twice as often as women. MCL does not occur in children.

MOLECULAR PATHOGENESIS: The reciprocal chromosomal translocation t(11;14) is considered the primary genetic event in nearly all cases of MCL (Table 26-18). It causes overexpression of cyclin D1. Cyclin D1 drives cell cycle progression at the G_1-to-S-phase transition, by binding to Cdk4/6. This event leads to phosphorylation of retinoblastoma (Rb) and subsequent activation of transcription factors promoting cell cycle progression from the G_1 to S phase (see Chapter 5). Several other oncogenic changes may occur in MCL (see Table 26-18).

PATHOLOGY: Lymph nodes involved by MCL show a diffuse to vaguely nodular lymphoid infiltrate of small to medium-sized B-cells with irregular nuclear contours. In some cases, MCL lymphocytes are round and resemble the cells of B-cell CLL/SLL, which is often in the differential diagnosis, especially since they also both aberrantly coexpress CD5. One of the characteristic features in typical cases of MCL is the striking monotony of the lymphoma cells in size and shape (Fig. 26-60A). Unlike many other small B-cell lymphomas, large transformed cells and/or centroblasts are absent or rare. Scattered epithelioid histiocytes and hyalinized small blood vessels completes the picture of typical cases.

There are three major variants: one with a more nodular-appearing pattern with a mantle zone–like infiltrate surrounding germinal centers (**mantle zone pattern**), one with immature lymphoblast-like features (**blastoid variant**) and another with irregular pleomorphic tumor cells (**pleomorphic variant**). The mantle zone pattern behave less aggressively than the typical type, while the blastoid variant is more aggressive. MCL is mainly a node-based disease, but may involve several tissues and organs, particularly the spleen, bone marrow, and gut. Multifocal mucosal small intestinal and colonic involvement may produce is called **lymphomatous polyposis**.

MCLs express B-cell markers CD19 and CD20 with surface light-chain restriction. The lymphoma cells also express CD5, but not CD10 or CD23. *MCL cells are usually positive for cyclin D1* (Fig. 26-60B). Cyclin D1-negative

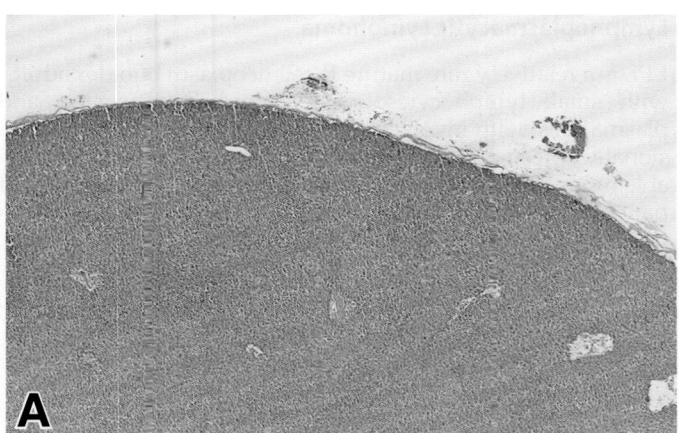

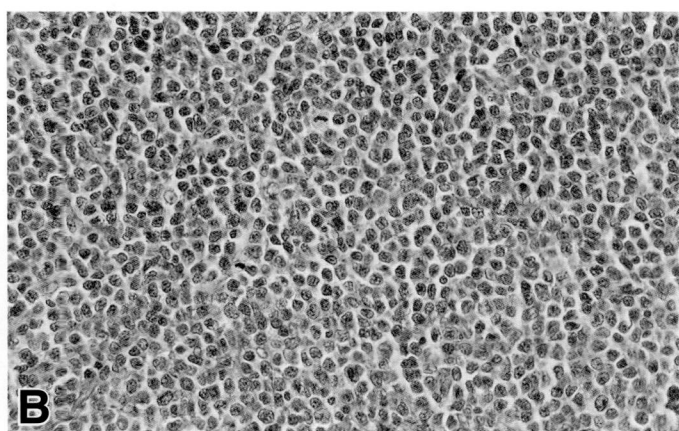

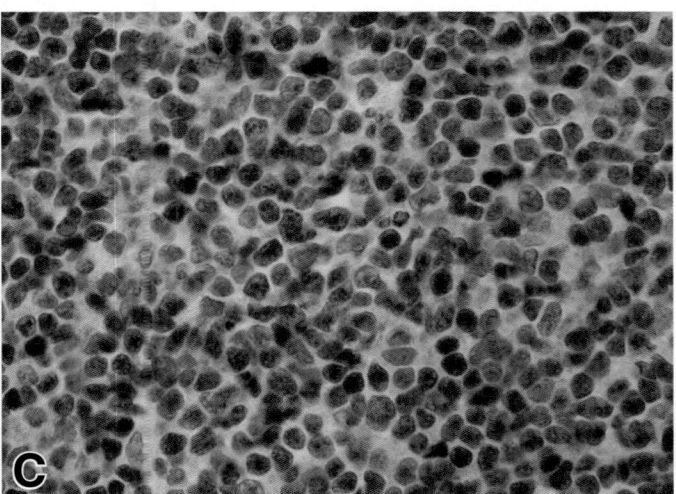

FIGURE 26-60. Mantle cell lymphoma (MCL). A. Lymph node architecture is completely effaced by a small lymphocytic infiltrate. **B.** At closer examination, the population of lymphocytes consists of monotonous, small cells with irregular nuclei. Unlike small lymphocytic lymphomas, MCL has very few admixed larger cells. **C.** A nuclear stain for Bcl-1 (cyclin D1) is positive. This finding correlates with the presence of t(11;14), the typical translocation in MCL.

cases usually express SOX-11. Its immunophenotype and morphologic features distinguish MCL from other small B-cell lymphomas with a more indolent course.

 CLINICAL FEATURES: Most patients with MCL present with high-stage disease (III or IV). About 1/3 have peripheral blood involvement at diagnosis. Despite its small cell morphology, MCL is clinically aggressive and considered incurable by standard chemotherapy.

Marginal Zone Lymphomas

Marginal zone lymphomas are a heterogeneous group of mature B-cell tumors that arise in lymph nodes, spleen, and extranodal tissues. The lymphoma cells are thought to arise from the GC marginal zone, which contains post-GC memory B-cells. Regardless of the primary site of involvement, marginal zone lymphomas all share similar morphology and immunophenotype. Prototypical marginal zone lymphomas are extranodal marginal zone B-cell lymphomas arising in MALT, the so-called **MALT lymphomas**.

These are generally indolent B-cell lymphomas with a heterogeneous population of small B-cells including centrocyte-like cells (marginal zone cells), monocytoid lymphocytes, small lymphocytes, and scattered larger lymphoid cells resembling centroblasts and immunoblasts. These tumors often occur at extranodal sites, like the GI tract, salivary glands, ocular adnexa, lungs, and skin. Plasma cell differentiation may be variably present.

EPIDEMIOLOGY: MALT lymphomas account for 5% to 10% of B-cell lymphomas and are the most common type of gastric lymphoma. Most occur in adults with a median age of 60; they are rare in children and young adults. There is a slight female predominance in part because they may occur at sites of autoimmune disease (e.g., parotid gland in Sjögren syndrome, thyroid in Hashimoto thyroiditis). Immunoproliferative small intestinal disease (IPSID), also called α-chain disease or **Mediterranean lymphoma,** a subtype of MALT lymphoma, produces α-heavy chains (absent light chains).

PATHOPHYSIOLOGY AND MOLECULAR PATHOGENESIS: MALT lymphomas are monoclonal B-cell tumors that arise in the setting of chronic inflammation, most often due to autoimmunity or infection. What initially begins as a benign polyclonal B-cell reaction over time accumulates transforming mutations and chromosome defects. *The* *prototypical infection-driven MALT is gastric lymphoma associated with H. pylori gastritis* (see Chapter 19). Gastric MALT lymphomas at their earliest phases of development may regress with antibiotic therapy to eradicate *H. pylori*. MALT lymphomas that have progressed to acquire other chromosomal translocations (Table 26-18) no longer respond to antibiotic therapy alone. Dissemination to distant sites and/or transformation to DLBCL occur as additional genetic lesions accrue.

PATHOLOGY: In early-stage MALT lymphoma increased marginal zone lymphocytes surround and infiltrate the germinal centers of reactive B-cell follicles. The malignant B-cells are heterogeneous and include varying proportions of small lymphocytes, medium-sized monocytoid lymphocytes with abundant cytoplasm, plasmacytoid lymphocytes, and admixed clonal plasma cells. The tumor cells also invade glandular epithelia, causing **lymphoepithelial lesions** (Fig. 26-61). Indolent MALT lymphomas may occasionally transform into large cell B-cell lymphomas.

MALT lymphomas have no specific immunophenotype. Most tumor cells express IgM and show light-chain restriction. They express B-cell–associated antigens and are negative for CD5, CD10, CD23, and cyclin D1, which distinguish them from CLL/SLL, MCL, FL, and MCL.

Common cytogenetic abnormalities (see Table 26-18), along with clonal *IgH* gene rearrangements, may help to establish the diagnosis if gastric infiltrates are subtle.

CLINICAL FEATURES: MALT lymphoma may involve the stomach, respiratory tract, salivary glands, ocular adnexa, skin, thyroid, and breast. The tumors usually remain localized for prolonged periods and follow an indolent clinical course. Transformation to DLBCL is associated with more aggressive disease.

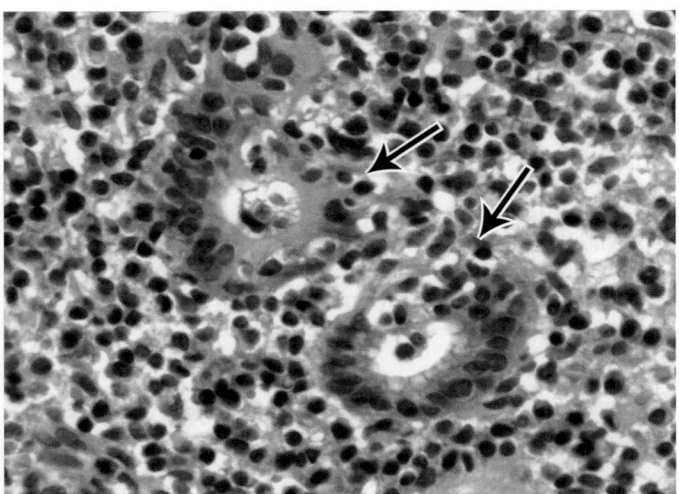

FIGURE 26-61. Mucosa-associated lymphoid tissue (MALT) lymphoma. A stomach biopsy showing the characteristic lymphoepithelial lesions seen in MALT lymphomas (*arrows*). The infiltrating lymphocytes are B-cells.

Lymphoplasmacytic Lymphoma

LPL is a relatively rare mature B-cell neoplasm of older adults, with small lymphocytes, plasmacytoid lymphocytes, and plasma cells, with involvement of the bone marrow, and occasionally spleen and lymph nodes. Most LPLs produce a sizeable monoclonal serum paraprotein (usually IgM). A subset of patients with LPL develop clinical **Waldenström macroglobulinemia** (see below), associated with **hyperviscosity syndrome**.

PATHOLOGY: LPL in the bone marrow is a variably dense heterogeneous lymphoid infiltrate of small lymphocytes, plasmacytoid lymphocytes, and mature plasma cells, often with admixed mast cells. Lymphoplasmacytic cells with nuclear pseudo-inclusions of immunoglobulin (Dutcher bodies) are common in tissue sections. Absolute lymphocytosis is rare. Affected lymph nodes show an interfollicular pattern of involvement, and nodal architecture is generally preserved.

LPLs express pan B-cell antigens, while negative for CD5, CD10, CD23, and cyclin D1. The plasma cell component expresses the plasma cell marker, CD138. Plasma cell clonality is demonstrable in tissue sections using immunostains for κ- and λ-light chains.

 MOLECULAR PATHOGENESIS: Nearly all LPL cases carry a *MYD88* L265P mutation. The mutation also occurs in IgM MGUS and some cases of DLBCL.

CLINICAL FEATURES: Fatigue, weakness, and weight loss are the most common presenting complaints of people with LPL. These nonspecific findings are usually related to anemia caused by marrow infiltration or immune-mediated hemolysis. About half of patients have lymphadenopathy and/or organomegaly at diagnosis. Most patients have a serum IgM paraprotein, but some may have IgG or IgA paraproteins. Increased blood viscosity due to macroglobulinemia occurs in 30% of patients, and may cause visual impairment, neurologic problems, bleeding, and cryoglobulinemia (Waldenstrom macroglobulinemia). LPL is an indolent disease that is slowly progressive. In a small number of patients, it may transform into DLBCL.

Hairy Cell Leukemia (HCL)

HCL is a clonal B-cell neoplasm of small to medium-sized lymphocytes (with abundant pale cytoplasm and hair-like cell cytoplasmic protrusions) involving bone marrow, spleen, and peripheral blood (Fig. 26-62A). The neoplastic cells arise from a post-germinal center B-cell (late activated memory B-cell). HCL is uncommon, and affects mainly middle-aged to elderly men. Marked splenomegaly and pancytopenia are common.

PATHOLOGY: Involved bone marrow contains a subtle interstitial infiltrate with fine reticulin fibrosis. The marrow architecture is largely undisturbed. The tumor cells have small bean-shaped nuclei and abundant clear cytoplasm which gives them a "fried egg"

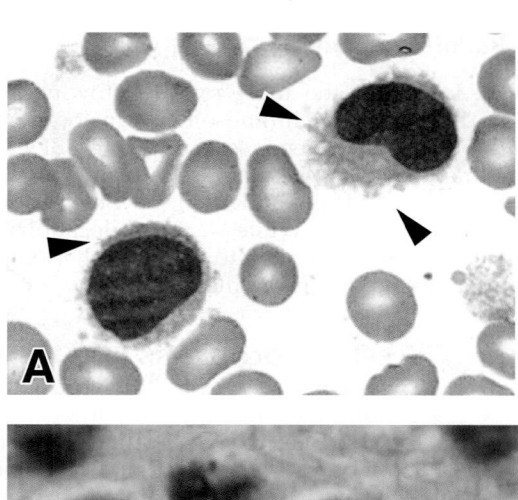

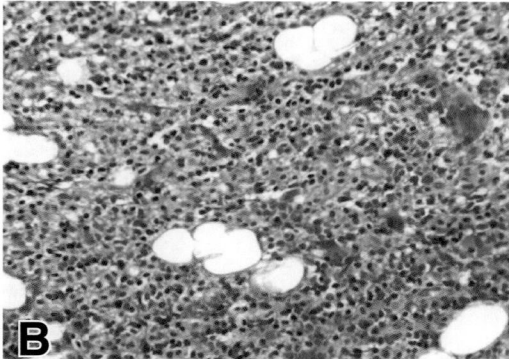

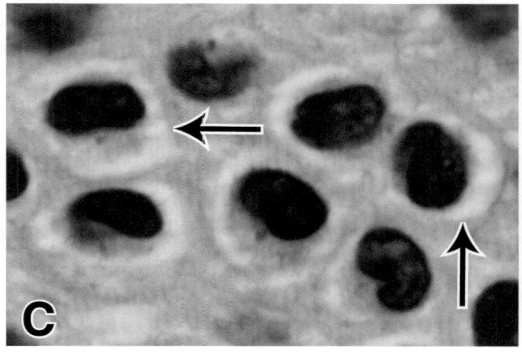

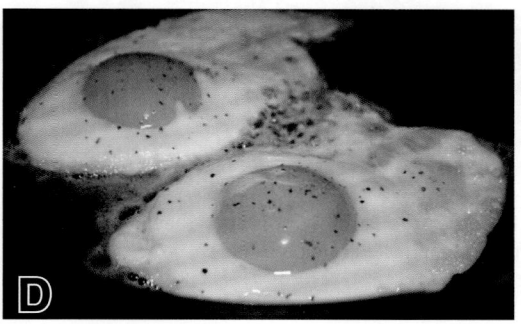

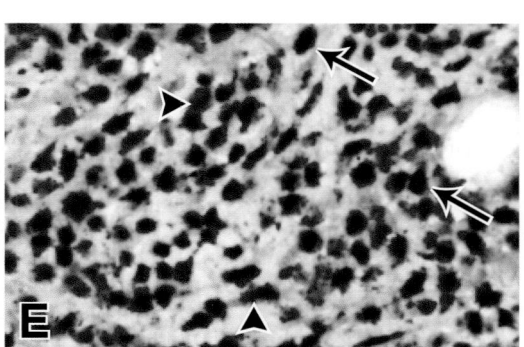

FIGURE 26-62. Hairy cell leukemia. A. Peripheral smear highlighting "hairy" projections (*arrowheads*) of the leukemic cells. **B.** Bone marrow biopsy, showing infiltration by small to medium-sized lymphocytes with oval to reniform nuclei and pale cytoplasm. **C.** Higher-power photomicrograph of hairy cell lymphocytes infiltrating the bone marrow. Typical "fried egg" cells, with round-oval to kidney-shaped nuclei, are shown (*arrows*). **D.** Fried eggs, for comparison. **E.** Bone marrow biopsy doubly stained for tartarate-resistant acid phosphatase (TRAP), red cytoplasmic staining (*arrowheads*), and brown nuclear staining (*arrows*) for PAX5 B-cell activation-related transcription factor.

appearance in tissue sections (Fig. 26-62B,C). In blood smears, hairy cells display delicate (hairy) cytoplasmic extensions. HCL generally spares lymph nodes but involves liver and spleen prominently. The leukemic cells express pan B-cell antigens as well as CD25, CD103, and TRAP (tartrate-resistant acid phosphatase). Some cases may show variable expression of CD5, CD10, and cyclin D1.

 MOLECULAR FEATURES: Virtually all HCL cases carry an activating BRAF V600E mutation. The mutant BRAF protein is hyperactive, leading to uncontrolled cell proliferation.

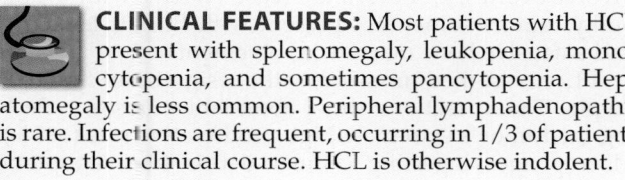 **CLINICAL FEATURES:** Most patients with HCL present with splenomegaly, leukopenia, mono-cytopenia, and sometimes pancytopenia. Hepatomegaly is less common. Peripheral lymphadenopathy is rare. Infections are frequent, occurring in 1/3 of patients during their clinical course. HCL is otherwise indolent.

Diffuse Large B-Cell Lymphomas (DLBCLs)

DLBCLs are a heterogeneous group of aggressive B-cell tumors. Their heterogeneity is evident at the morphologic, immunophenotypic, genetic, and clinical levels. While some cases of DLBCL arise de novo, others represent transformation or progression from more indolent types of lymphoma.

 EPIDEMIOLOGY: DLBCLs are the most common type of B-cell lymphoma worldwide. They occur at all ages, but are most prevalent between the ages of 60 and 70.

 PATHOPHYSIOLOGY AND MOLECULAR PATHOGENESIS: The cause of DLBCL is unknown, but immunodeficiency, chronic inflammation, and viral infection (EBV, HHV-8) play a role in some cases. EBV-positive cases are most common in immunosuppressed patients and in

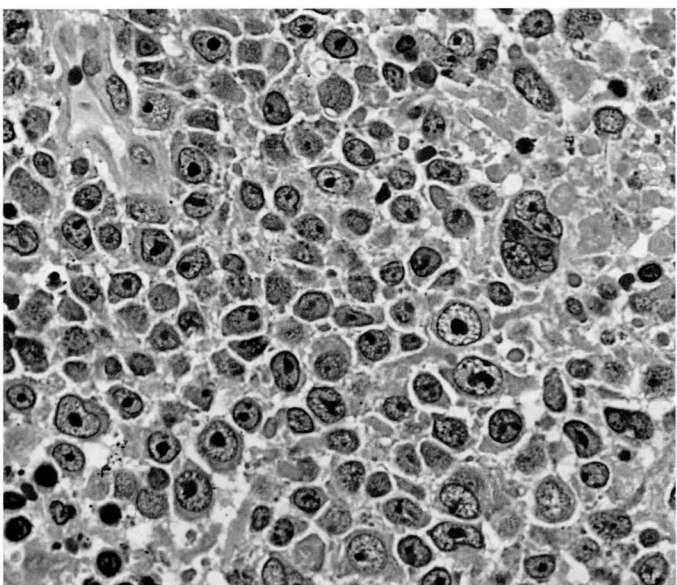

FIGURE 26-63. Diffuse large B-cell lymphoma. Sheets of large lymphoma cells with prominent nucleoli are present.

those over 50. Several chromosomal rearrangements are seen in DLBCL (Table 26-18), some of which involve genes that dysregulate cell growth and impair apoptosis.

PATHOLOGY: In DLBCL, there is a diffuse infiltrate of large neoplastic B-cells (Fig. 26-63). DLBCL may be morphologically classified as centroblastic (most common), immunoblastic, or anaplastic (pleomorphic). *While DLBCL most often involves lymph nodes, extranodal sites, especially the GI tract, may be involved.*

In nearly all cases the large tumor cells express pan B-cell antigens, such as CD19, CD20, CD79a, and PAX-5. However, accumulated genetic defects may cause aberrant loss of expression of common markers. DLBCL can be subclassified into germinal center (GC) type and activated B cell (ABC) type, distinguished by their expression patterns of three markers (CD10, BCL-6, and MUM1). All cases are negative for TdT and cyclin D1, distinguishes DLBCL from B-cell lymphoblastic lymphoma (TdT positive) and MCL (cyclin D1 positive).

CLINICAL FEATURES: Patients with DLBCL present most often with a rapidly growing tumor in nodal and/or extranodal sites. Bone marrow involvement is usually a late event. Symptoms reflect the site(s) of involvement. For example, a large mass in the colon can cause obstruction or bowel perforation, while a rapidly growing mediastinal mass can impinge on the superior vena cava to cause SVC syndrome. Systemic manifestations such as fever, fatigue, and night sweats ("B symptoms") occur often in patients with DLBCL.

Because these tumors are highly proliferative, they are sensitive to chemotherapeutic agents that target rapidly dividing cells. Most patients achieve complete remissions.

Burkitt Lymphoma

BL is one of the most rapidly growing malignancies. It is defined by a chromosomal translocation that activates the c-*MYC* oncogene (see Chapter 5). BLs often present at extranodal sites, contain a monomorphic population of medium-sized cells and often show blood and/or bone marrow involvement. While MYC translocation is highly characteristic, it is not limited to BL, and other diagnostic features are required to confirm the diagnosis.

EPIDEMIOLOGY: BL occurs in three distinct variants, each with different clinical presentations, morphology, and pathogenesis. In equatorial Africa and Papua, New Guinea, **endemic BL** is the most common childhood malignancy. Its peak incidence is in 4- to 7-year-olds, and commonly involves the jaw, facial bones, and abdominal viscera. **Sporadic BL** occurs worldwide, mainly affecting children and young adults. In the Western world, Sporadic BL is uncommon but accounts for nearly half of childhood lymphomas. The median age of adult patients is 30. Unlike endemic BL, sporadic BL often presents as an abdominal mass involving the ileocecum. **Immunodeficiency-associated BL** mainly occurs in HIV infection and may be the initial manifestation of AIDS.

MOLECULAR PATHOGENESIS: All cases are associated with translocations that upregulate c-*MYC* expression. The gene on chromosome 8 is upregulated by a translocation that places it under the control of IgH [t(8;14)] or IgL [t(2;8 for κ) or t(8;22 for λ)] promoters (Table 26-18). In endemic cases, the breakpoint on chromosome 14 occurs in the heavy-chain–joining region, as seen in early B-cells. In sporadic BL, the translocation occurs in the Ig switch region, which is more characteristic of mature B-cells. Excessive c-*MYC* expression is driven by the highly active Ig heavy-chain or light chain promoters, causing uncontrolled tumor cell growth (see Chapter 5).

EBV is present in virtually all cases of endemic BL but in less than 30% of sporadic and immunodeficiency-related cases. Many endemic BL patients experience prodromal polyclonal B-cell activation caused by opportunistic bacterial, viral or parasitic infections (e.g., malaria).

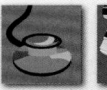 **CLINICAL FEATURES AND PATHOLOGY:** BL typically produces extranodal tumors rather than lymphadenopathy. All variants carry a high risk for CNS involvement. The classic presentation for endemic BL is a destructive tumor in the jaws or other facial bones (Fig. 26-64A). Sporadic BL typically presents with abdominal masses. All types may involve ovaries, kidneys, and breast. Patients with sizable bulky tumors sometimes present with Burkitt leukemia and extensive bone marrow involvement.

BL cells are medium sized, without significant cytologic atypia. Tissue sections show abundant mitoses, reflecting the tumor's extremely high proliferative rate (>95%). Macrophages ingesting cellular debris from apoptotic

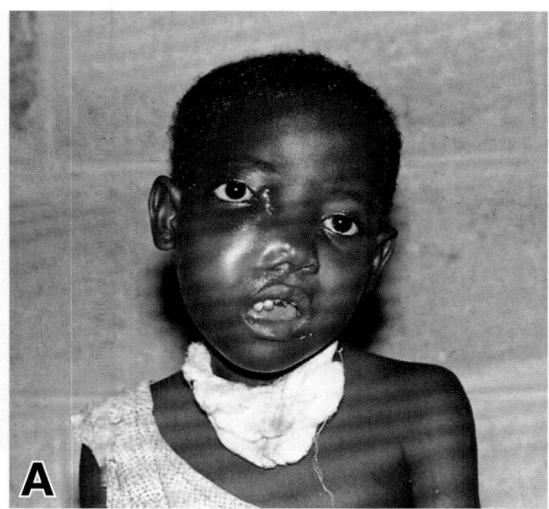

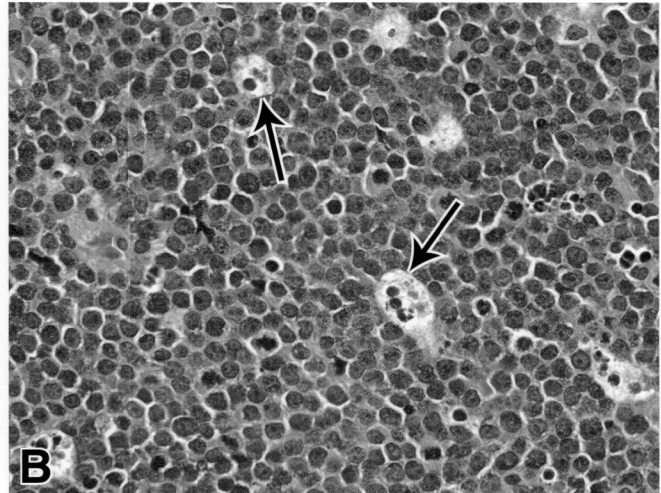

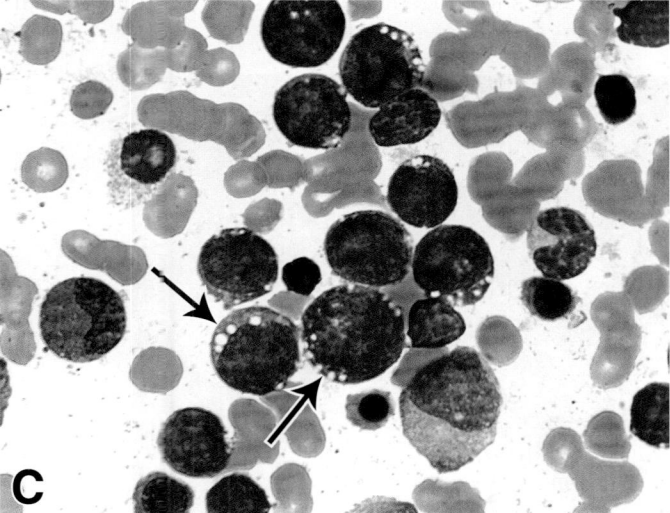

FIGURE 26-64. Burkitt lymphoma. A. A tumor of the jaw distorts the child's face. **B.** Lymph node is effaced by neoplastic lymphocytes with several starry-sky macrophages (*arrows*). **C.** Bone marrow aspirate smear showing typical cytologic features of Burkitt lymphoma. Note the deeply basophilic cytoplasm and lipid vacuoles (*arrows*).

tumor cells are scattered throughout the tumor, imparting a "starry sky" microscopic appearance (Fig. 26-64B). Aspirate smears stained with Wright–Giemsa show lipid vacuoles in the deeply basophilic tumor cell cytoplasm (Fig. 26-64C).

BL cells express surface IgM, Ig light chain, and common B-cell antigens (CD19, CD20, CD22). They also express CD10 and BCL-6, which suggest that they originate from germinal centers. They do not express TdT, helping to distinguish these tumors from precursor B-cell acute lymphoblastic leukemia/lymphoma (see above).

All variants of BL are highly aggressive, and most patients have bulky extranodal tumors and disseminated disease at presentation. BL responds well to intensive chemotherapy, reflecting its high proliferative rate. Up to 90% of people with early stage disease and 60% to 80% of those with high-stage disease may be cured. Children and young adults with BL tend to fare better than older adults. Massive treatment-related tumor cell lysis may trigger a potentially lethal complication—tumor lysis syndrome (hyperuricemia, hyperuricosuria, hyperkalemia, and hyperphosphatemia leading to renal failure).

Plasma Cell Neoplasia

Plasma cell neoplasms result from clonal expansion of plasma cells. Thus, these terminally differentiated B-lymphocytes usually produce a monoclonal paraprotein (**monoclonal gammopathy**). The major plasma cell neoplasms include MGUS, PCM (multiple myeloma), plasmacytoma, and immunoglobulin deposition disease (amyloidosis and light-chain disease). Plasma cell neoplasms almost exclusively affect adults.

ETIOLOGY:
- **Genetic predisposition.** Increased incidence of multiple myeloma in first-degree relatives of patients with plasma cell neoplasia and higher frequency of multiple myeloma in people of African origin.
- **Ionizing radiation.** Long-term survivors of the bombing of Hiroshima and Nagasaki had a fivefold greater incidence of multiple myeloma.
- **Chronic antigenic stimulation.** Some cases of multiple myeloma follow chronic infections and chronic inflammatory disorders (e.g., osteomyelitis, rheumatoid arthritis). Such ongoing reactive polyclonal B-cell proliferation may render the cells susceptible to later mutagenic events, that may establish a single malignant clone.

Monoclonal Gammopathy of Undetermined Significance (MGUS)

MGUS occurs in older adults. Criteria for MGUS diagnosis include:

- monoclonal paraproteinemia of less than 3.0 g/dL;
- less than 10% clonal plasma cells in the marrow;
- lack of end-organ damage (CRAB: hypercalcemia, renal insufficiency, anemia, bone lesions); and
- exclusion of other B-cell neoplasms or diseases that may generate monoclonal paraproteins (CLL/SLL, LPL).

IgM MGUS is most often associated with a clone of immunoglobulin-secreting B-cells and can progress to a small B-cell lymphoma with plasma cell differentiation such as LPL. Non-IgM MGUS is most often associated with clonal plasma cells and may progress to a bona fide malignant plasma cell neoplasm. MGUS progresses to overt PCM in about 1% of patients per year.

Plasma Cell Myeloma (PCM)

PCM is a malignancy of plasma cells, almost always with a serum and/or urine paraprotein. PCM is primarily bone marrow based, and varies from asymptomatic and indolent to highly aggressive with leukemic involvement. Combined radiographic, clinical and laboratory findings establish the diagnosis.

EPIDEMIOLOGY: PCM accounts for 10% of hematologic malignancies. Men are more affected than women, and the disease occurs proportionately in African-Americans twice as commonly as in whites. Over 90% of cases affect people over 50. It does not affect children and is extremely rare in adults under age 30. There is a familial predisposition: people with a first-degree relative with PCM are at fourfold greater risk.

PATHOLOGY: PCM produces multifocal destructive bone lesions (lytic or "punched out" radiographically) throughout the skeleton, most often affecting the vertebral column, ribs, skull, pelvis, femurs, clavicles, and scapulae. Plasma cells focally fill the medullary cavity, erode cancellous bone and eventually destroy the bony cortex, causing pathologic fractures. The affected bone contains gelatinous red-brown soft tissue masses that are sharply demarcated from the surrounding normal tissue (Fig. 26-65).

Pathologic examination of the bone marrow is essential in diagnosing PCM. The plasma cells (often >30%

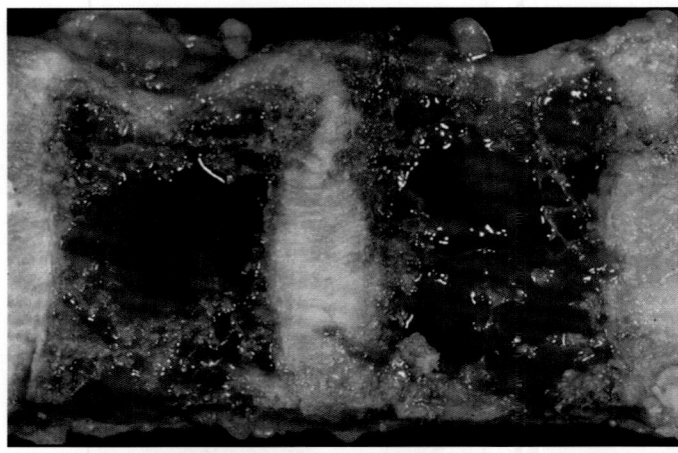

FIGURE 26-65. Plasma cell myeloma. Multiple lytic bone lesions are present in the vertebra. Bones such as this are prone to pathologic fracture.

of marrow cellularity) form interstitial clusters, nodules and/or confluent sheets of plasma cells in bone marrow core biopsies. In contrast, clonal plasma cells in MGUS comprise <10% of marrow cellularity.

Immunostaining for the plasma cell marker CD138 may help to enumerate marrow plasma cells. Marrow involvement may be spotty, with heavily involved areas interspersed with normal marrow. Thus, marrow aspirate smears may show variable plasmacytosis. Neoplastic plasma cells may resemble normal plasma cells (Fig. 26-66A), or they may show immature, plasmablastic, or pleomorphic features (Fig. 26-66B). Cytoplasmic and nuclear inclusions of accumulated immunoglobulin are occasionally present.

Erythrocyte rouleaux (Fig. 26-67) in peripheral blood smears reflect the type and quantity of circulating paraprotein. High levels of paraprotein cause RBCs on blood smears to stick together like a stack of coins. Small

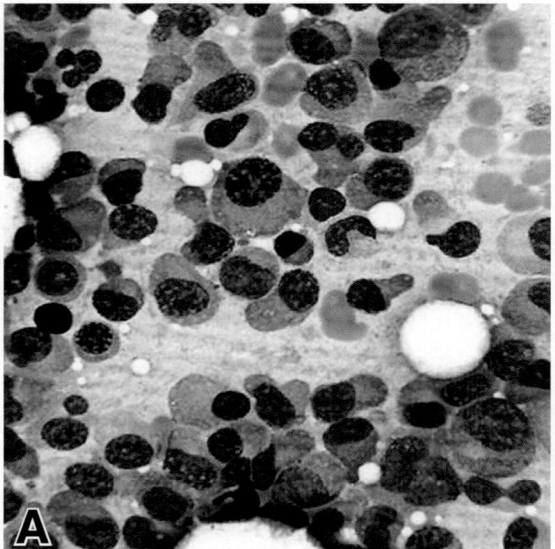
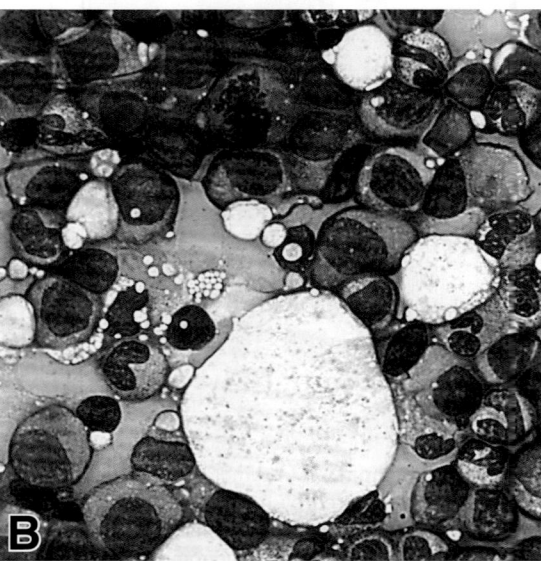

FIGURE 26-66. Plasma cell myeloma (PCM). Neoplastic plasma cells can show variable cytologic features ranging from normal-appearing cells (**A**) to cells resembling blasts (**B**). Total number, clonality, and clinicopathologic findings help distinguish PCM from other plasma cell proliferations.

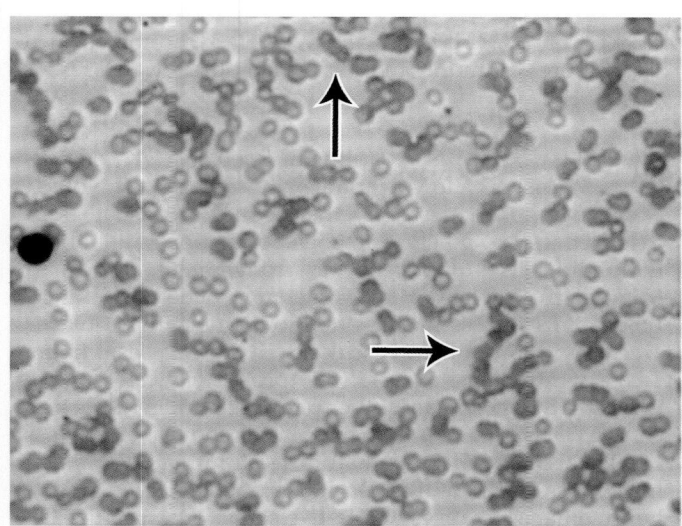

FIGURE 26-67. Plasma cell myeloma, rouleaux in peripheral blood. In plasma cell myeloma, the peripheral blood commonly shows red blood cells seemingly stacked on each other, like coins in a roll. These are rouleaux (*arrows*).

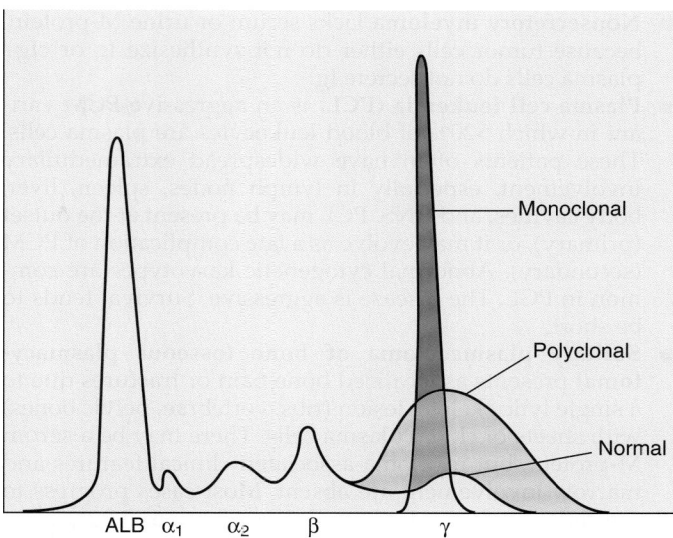

FIGURE 26-68. Abnormal serum protein electrophoretic patterns contrasted with a normal pattern. Polyclonal hypergammaglobulinemia, characteristic of benign reactive processes, shows a broad-based increase in immunoglobulins as a result of immunoglobulin secretion by myriad reactive plasma cells. Monoclonal gammopathy of unknown significance (MGUS) or plasma cell neoplasia shows a narrow peak, or spike, as a result of the homogeneity of the immunoglobulin molecules secreted by a single clone of aberrant plasma cells. *ALB* = albumin.

numbers of plasma cells may circulate in the blood in a minority of PCM cases. Plasma cell leukemia is diagnosed if marked peripheral blood plasmacytosis occurs.

Plasma cells in PCM, like normal plasma cells, express the B-cell marker CD79a, plasma cell markers CD38, and CD138 and monotypic *cytoplasmic* immunoglobulin. Unlike normal plasma cells, myeloma cells may aberrantly express the NK-cell marker CD56 and the immature myeloid cell marker CD117, and lack the B-cell marker CD19. In most cases, the heavy chain in the monoclonal paraprotein is IgG or IgA. IgD or IgE paraproteins are rare. The neoplastic plasma cells usually produce complete antibody molecules (called **M-proteins**, with intact H and L chains). Rarely, they only secrete light chains (**light-chain disease**), or no paraprotein at all (**non-secretory myeloma**).

Serum (or urine) paraprotein can be identified by serum (or urine) protein electrophoresis followed by immunofixation (Fig. 26-68). After electrophoresis, clonal immunoglobulin protein is identified in the gel as a single narrow peak (spike) of protein (M-spike). Immunofixation identifies the Ig components by heavy chain type and as monoclonal κ- or λ-light chains. Most cases are IgG, followed by IgA, light chain only, IgD and IgE.

MOLECULAR PATHOGENESIS: PCMs show clonal rearrangement of Ig L- and H-chain genes, and may have both numerical and structural chromosomal abnormalities. The IgH gene is often involved in translocations that activate oncogenes (Table 26-18). Half of cases show partial or complete loss of chromosome 13.

CLINICAL FEATURES: As stated above, diagnosing PCM usually entails a constellation of clinical and pathologic findings. The most important disorder to consider in the differential diagnosis of PCM is MGUS.

Symptomatic myeloma is characterized by hypercalcemia, renal failure, anemia, bone lesions (usually lytic), amyloidosis and immune deficiency–related infections, hyperviscosity syndrome, treatment-related myeloid neoplasia, and/or coagulation defects. PCM commonly presents with pathologic bone fractures, in part because malignant plasma cells secrete osteoclast-activating factor. Calcium released from resorbed bone may precipitate in the kidneys and impair renal function (nephrocalcinosis). Monoclonal light-chain proteinuria can damage renal tubular epithelium, leading to kidney failure. M-proteins can suppress normal antibody responses and predispose to infectious complications. Patients may be anemic because of both marrow replacement and EPO deficiency due to kidney disease. Serum and/or urine have detectable M-proteins in 97% of patients, the isotype of which predicts disease progression.

- **IgG myeloma.** Infectious complications are common.
- **IgA myeloma.** Serum hyperviscosity due to dimeric IgA.
- **IgD myeloma.** Aggressive disease in middle-aged men.
- **IgE myeloma.** Aggressive disease in young adult men.
- **Light-chain disease.** Aggressive disease with light chain proteinuria and renal disease.

Total disease burden (reflected in serum β_2-microglobulin and albumin levels) and genetic abnormalities (Table 26-18) most accurately predict outcome.

Clinical Variants of Plasma Cell Myeloma

- **Asymptomatic myeloma** meets diagnostic criteria (clonal plasma cell percentage in marrow, paraprotein levels), but patients lack detectable end-organ damage (hypercalcemia, renal disease, anemia, bone lesions).

- **Nonsecretory myeloma** lacks serum or urine M-protein, because tumor cells either do not synthesize Ig or cIg+ plasma cells do not secrete Ig.
- **Plasma cell leukemia (PCL)** is an aggressive PCM variant in which >20% of blood leukocytes are plasma cells. These patients often have widespread extramedullary involvement, especially in lymph nodes, spleen, liver, body cavities, and CNS. PCL may be present at the outset (primary), or it may evolve as a late complication of PCM (secondary). Abnormal cytogenetic karyotypes are common in PCL. The disease is aggressive. Survival tends to be short.
- **Solitary plasmacytoma of bone (osseous plasmacytoma)** presents as localized bone pain or fractures due to a single lytic skeletal lesion (ribs, vertebrae, pelvic bones) with sheets of clonal plasma cells. There may be a serum M-protein, but myeloma-associated clinical features and marrow involvement are absent. Most cases progress to multiple myeloma. **Extramedullary (extraosseous) plasmacytomas** are localized plasma cell tumors outside of bone and marrow. Most arise in the upper respiratory tract, including nasal sinuses, nasopharynx, and tonsils. Other sites include lungs, breast, and lymph nodes. Given their anatomic distribution, they must be distinguished from B-cell lymphomas with plasma cell differentiation such as MALT lymphomas. Most do not progress to PCM.
- **Primary amyloidosis (AL amyloid, see Chapter 15)** is a disease of older adults (median age, 65), caused by tissue deposition of insoluble aggregates of λ-light chains, leading to end-organ damage. Light-chain amyloid is produced by neoplastic plasma cells in myeloma or B-cell lymphomas with plasmacytic differentiation. Of patients with amyloidosis, 20% have PCM, but most only meet criteria for MGUS. Clinical presentations reflect organ sites where amyloid deposits and causes organomegaly or organ dysfunction (e.g., congestive heart failure, nephrotic syndrome, malabsorption). Purpura, bone pain, peripheral neuropathy, and carpal tunnel syndrome may be early signs of disease. Over 90% of cases have M-proteins, and most have λ-light chains. Tissues infiltrated by amyloid look dense and lardaceous. Patients with primary amyloidosis have median survivals of 2 years. Those with PCM and amyloidosis fare worse than those with either alone. Amyloid-related cardiac disease is the most common cause of death.

Peripheral T-Cell, NKT-Cell, and NK-Cell Lymphomas Originate From Postthymic T-Cells, NKT-Cells and NK-Cells

This heterogeneous group of peripheral T-cell lymphomas (PTCLs) arises in lymph nodes, spleen, gut, and skin (Fig. 26-48), and are relatively rare, compared to B-cell lymphomas. They generally have a poorer prognosis.

EPIDEMIOLOGY: Mature T-cell tumors represent 12% of non-Hodgkin lymphomas worldwide. They are more common in Asia than in the Western world. Risk factors include human T-cell leukemia virus type 1 (HTLV-1) and EBV (see Chapter 5). HTLV-1 is endemic in southwestern Japan (8% to 10%) with a lifetime risk for adult T-cell leukemia/lymphoma

(ATLL) of 5%. EBV-associated T-cell lymphomas also occur more commonly in Asians than other ethnicities.

PATHOLOGY: Peripheral T-cell and NK-cell neoplasms show variable morphology. Involved lymph nodes and other tissues are usually diffusely effaced by a heterogeneous population of abnormal lymphoid cells. Tumor cells vary from small to large, and from relatively bland to overtly anaplastic in appearance. Eosinophils and histiocytes often comingle with neoplastic T-cells, with prominent vascularity in many cases. Mature T-cell lymphomas express the prototypic cell surface marker CD3 (sCD3) and other pan T-cell antigens such as CD2, CD5, and CD7. Often, tumor cells show aberrant loss of CD2, CD5, or CD7. As mature T-cell tumors, PTCLs do not express TdT, unlike T-cell lymphoblastic leukemia/lymphoma. Most cases of PTCL express CD4 and αβ TCR heterodimers. γδ T-cell lymphomas are far less common, and express both CD3 and the NK-cell marker CD56, but are negative for CD4 and CD8. γδ T-cells normally are <5% of T-cells, and congregate at epithelial surfaces and in splenic red pulp. Some mature T-cell lymphomas express a **cytotoxic T-cell** phenotype, expressing cytolytic granule-associated proteins perforin, granzyme B and T-cell intracellular antigen (TIA-1). **NK-cells** lack surface CD3, but express intracellular CD3 ε-subunit plus other T-cell–associated markers (CD2, CD7, CD8, CD16, CD56).

CLINICAL FEATURES: Peripheral T-cell and NK-cell tumors are grouped into leukemic, nodal, extranodal, and cutaneous forms. *T-cell/NK-cell neoplasms are usually widely disseminated at presentation (high stage) and so generally more aggressive than B-cell neoplasms.* Systemic manifestations like fever, pruritus, eosinophilia, fever, and weight loss are common. T- and NK-cell lymphomas are treated with multiagent chemotherapy like other aggressive lymphomas; however, most respond poorly. Overall 5-year survival is 20% to 30%.

Adult T-Cell Leukemia/Lymphoma (ATLL)

ATLL is caused by a human retrovirus, **HTLV-1**. The normal counterparts of ATLL cells are mature activated CD4+ T-cells.

EPIDEMIOLOGY: In addition to southwestern Japan, ATLL is endemic in the Caribbean basin and parts of Central Africa. Worldwide, it accounts for 10% of mature T-cell neoplasms. Most cases are endemic, but sporadic cases also occur. The disease has a long latency period. Exposure to HTLV-1 occurs early in life in endemic regions, but the disease does not manifest until adulthood, with a mean age of 58. The virus may be transmitted in breast milk, blood, and blood products.

PATHOLOGY: ATLL is usually widespread at presentation, often involving lymph nodes, spleen, bone marrow, peripheral blood, and

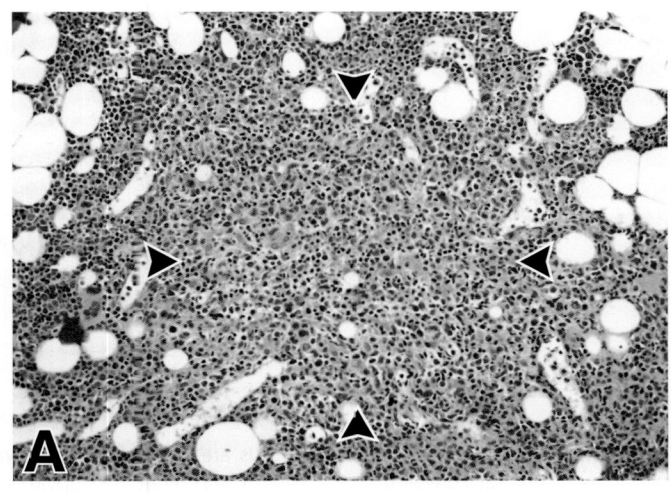

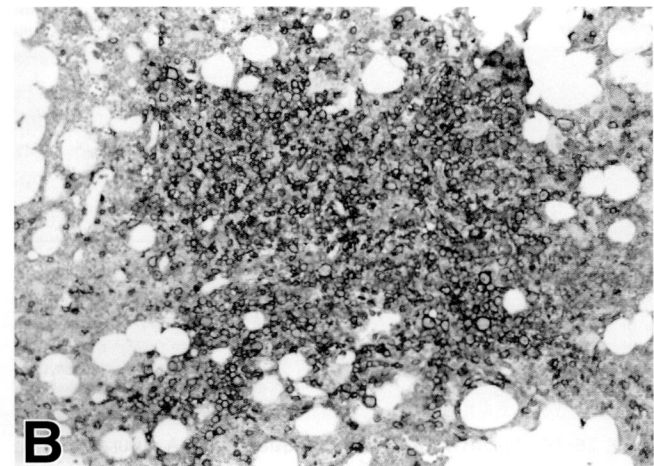

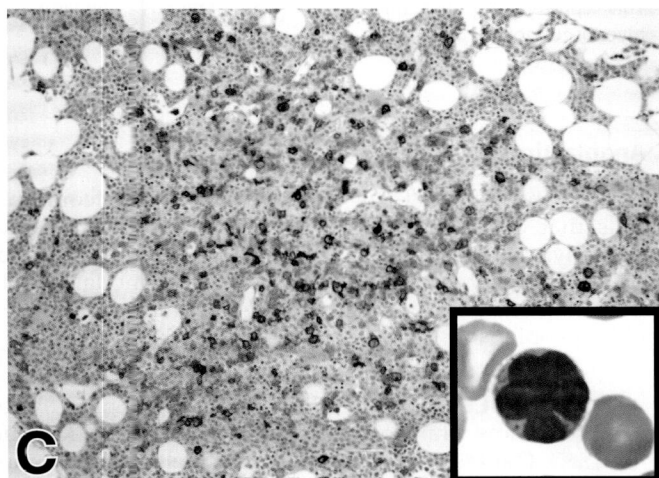

FIGURE 26-69. Adult T-cell leukemia/lymphoma (ATLL). This disease is characterized by proliferation of malignant T-lymphocytes. **A.** Routine H&E-stained bone marrow shows an abnormal aggregate of cells (outlined by *arrowheads*) somewhat larger than the surrounding hematopoietic elements in the marrow. **B.** The same aggregate is positive for CD4. **C.** Many cells in the aggregate are also positive for CD25. *Inset.* Peripheral blood smear showing malignant T-cell with extremely irregular, flower-like nuclear contour.

skin. Skin involvement is the most common extralymphatic site of disease. The neoplastic lymphoid cells vary widely in appearance (Fig. 26-69). They commonly have prominent nuclear convolutions (called flower cells), express T-cell–associated antigens CD2, CD3, CD4, and CD5, but usually not CD7. Nearly all cases strongly express CD25. *Tumor cells carry clonal T-cell receptor gene rearrangements and clonally integrated HTLV-1.* A viral protein, p40 (Tax), directs transcriptional activation of several genes in infected lymphocytes. HTLV-1 infection is not sufficient for tumor development. Other genetic lesions are required to progress from infection to malignancy.

CLINICAL FEATURES: ATLL is a systemic disease with multiorgan manifestations and peripheral leukocytosis. Acute, smoldering, and chronic variants occur. Hypercalcemia, with or without lytic bone lesions, is typical. Acute ATLL has a poor prognosis: most patients survive under 1 year, despite aggressive chemotherapy. Death frequently occurs from infectious complications, like those in AIDS patients. Chronic and smoldering forms have a somewhat better prognosis.

Mycosis Fungoides (MF) and Sézary Syndrome

MF is the most common primary cutaneous T-cell lymphoma (CTCL). Malignant CD4+ T-cells with marked nuclear folding infiltrate the epidermis. Sézary syndrome, a variant of MF, features a triad of erythroderma, generalized lymphadenopathy and lymphoma cells circulating in blood (Sézary cells).

EPIDEMIOLOGY: Mycosis fungoides occurs mainly in adults and the elderly. It affects men twice as often as women.

CLINICAL FEATURES: MF is an indolent lymphoma that progresses slowly over many years from skin patches to skin plaques to mass lesions.

- The **premycotic or eczematous stage** lasts years and is difficult to distinguish from many benign chronic dermatoses. Skin biopsies may not be diagnostic, but instead may show nonspecific perivascular and periadnexal lymphocytic infiltration with eosinophils and plasma cells.
- The **plaque stage** follows, with well-demarcated, raised cutaneous plaques. It is usually possible to diagnose MF at this stage (see below).

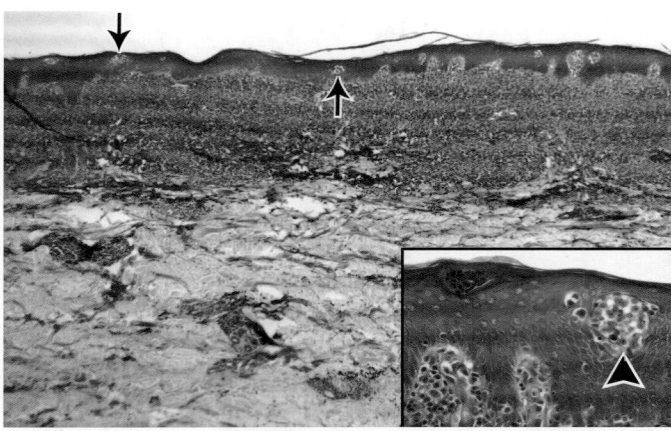

FIGURE 26-70. Mycosis fungoides, plaque phase. A diffuse infiltrate of neoplastic lymphocytes is present in the upper dermis and may occasionally invade the epidermis, as small Pautrier microabscesses (*arrows*). The lower dermis is often spared. A higher magnification of a Pautrier microabscess is shown in the *inset* (*arrowhead*).

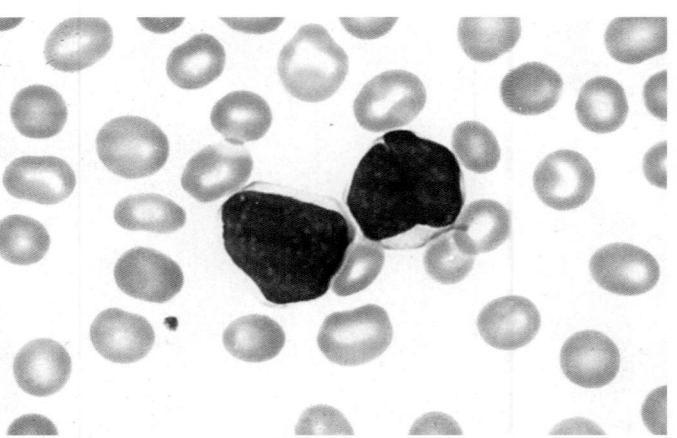

FIGURE 26-71. Sézary cells. Typical cells are medium to large with prominent nuclear convolutions resulting in a cerebriform appearance. This represents the leukemic phase of the cutaneous T-cell lymphoma, mycosis fungoides.

- In the **tumor stage,** there are raised cutaneous tumors, mostly on the face and in body folds. These frequently ulcerate and may become secondarily infected. The name, **mycosis fungoides,** reflects the raised, fungating, mushroom-like appearance. Extracutaneous involvement is common, particularly of lymph nodes, spleen, liver, bone marrow, and lungs.

    Extracutaneous involvement augurs a poor prognosis. The 5-year survival in Sézary syndrome is 10% to 20%.

PATHOLOGY: The histologic features of MF vary with the stage of the disease (see Chapter 28). A superficial band-like (lichenoid) infiltrate with early intra-epithelial involvement characterizes the initial patch stage. In the plaque stage, there is pronounced infiltration of the epidermis (epidermotropism), with lymphocytes arrayed densely in the upper dermis (Fig. 26-70). The tumor cells have very irregular nuclear contours, reminiscent of the cerebral cortical surface (cerebriform nuclei). These distinctive cells with hyperchromatic cerebriform nuclei are **mycosis cells. Pautrier microabscesses** in the epidermis are highly characteristic but are not common.

Diffuse dermal infiltrates of small, medium, and/or large lymphoma cells and loss of epidermotropism characterize the tumor stage. Identification of MF cells in extracutaneous sites like lymph nodes may be difficult, and T-cell receptor gene rearrangement studies are important adjuncts to histologic evaluation.

The characteristic cerebriform nuclei of Sézary cells facilitate their identification in peripheral blood smears (Fig. 26-71).

MF cells have a T-helper cell immunophenotype, and generally express CD2, CD3, CD5, CD4, and TCR-αβ. Like other mature T-cell lymphomas, the pan T-cell antigen, CD7, is absent. Clonal T-cell receptor gene rearrangements help to distinguish subtle cases of MF from benign inflammatory dermatoses.

Anaplastic Large Cell Lymphoma (ALCL)

ALCLs are mature T-cell tumors with large pleomorphic cells that express the CD30 lymphoid activation marker. These lymphomas often involve both nodal and extranodal sites (especially skin). This disease has a bimodal age distribution: one peak occurs in young people and a second in older people.

MOLECULAR PATHOGENESIS: Some cases show translocations involving the *ALK* gene (Table 26-18) and have a relatively good prognosis. ALK-negative ALCLs tend to be more aggressive. Their prognosis is like that of unspecified types of PTCL.

PATHOLOGY: The histology of ALCL is variable, but all cases have cells with irregularly shaped nuclei (often horseshoe or kidney shaped) and abundant cytoplasm called **hallmark cells** (Fig. 26-72). ALCL tumors express CD30, ALK (subset), and cytotoxic proteins (TIA-1, granzyme B), but usually lack CD3. Nearly all cases show clonal T-cell receptor rearrangements.

CLINICAL FEATURES: Most patients present with advanced disease (stage III or IV). Lymphadenopathy, extranodal and bone marrow involvement are common. Patients often present with fever. ALK-positive ALCL is more aggressive than ALK-negative ALCL.

Angioimmunoblastic T-Cell Lymphoma (AITL)

AITL is a peripheral (mature) T-cell lymphoma. Patients present with generalized lymphadenopathy and systemic autoimmune symptoms. Neoplastic T-cell infiltrates expand the paracortical regions of lymph nodes and are associated with eosinophilia and proliferation of high endothelial

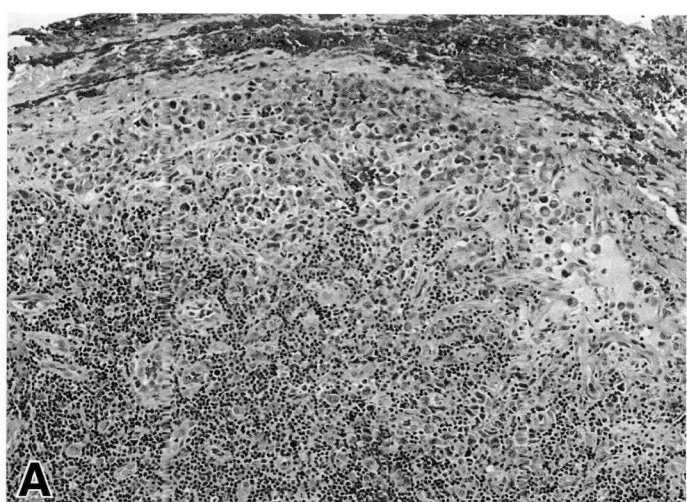
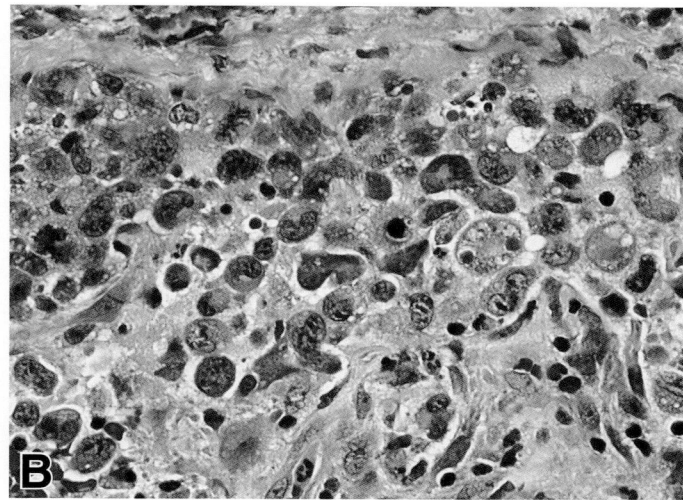

FIGURE 26-72. Anaplastic large cell lymphoma (ALCL). A: Partially effaced lymph node with accumulation of malignanT-cells in the subcapsular sinus. This common ALCL pattern may be confused with metastatic carcinoma. **B:** The intrasinusoidal lymphoma cells are large and pleomorphic. Cells with kidney-shaped nuclei and an eosinophilic zone near the nucleus are known as hallmark cells and are seen in all variants of ALCL.

venules. Benign EBV-infected B-cells are present in nearly all cases.

CLINICAL FEATURES: AITL occurs in adults. Most patients have extensive disease at the outset, including generalized lymphadenopathy, hepatosplenomegaly, pruritic rash, bone marrow involvement, hypergammaglobulinemia, and body cavity effusions. Laboratory findings include cold agglutinins, hemolytic anemia, circulating immune complexes, and rheumatoid factor. This is an aggressive lymphoma; median patient survival is under 3 years. Patients often die from infections. Some develop large B-cell lymphomas.

PATHOLOGY: Lymph nodes involved by AITL show partial or complete architectural effacement by a heterogeneous population of atypical small to medium-sized cells, in a setting of prominent, arborizing high endothelial venules. Some cases contain lymphoma cells with abundant clear cytoplasm and minimal atypia, and others contain a population of atypical large lymphoid cells (Fig. 26-73). Tumor cells express CD4 and most pan–T-cell antigens (but sometimes not CD5 or CD7), with a follicular T-helper cell phenotype (CD10, Bcl-6, CXCL13, PD-1). Clonal TCR rearrangement occurs in most AITL, and a minority also show clonal Ig gene rearrangement (reflecting a clonal expansion of EBV-positive B-cells).

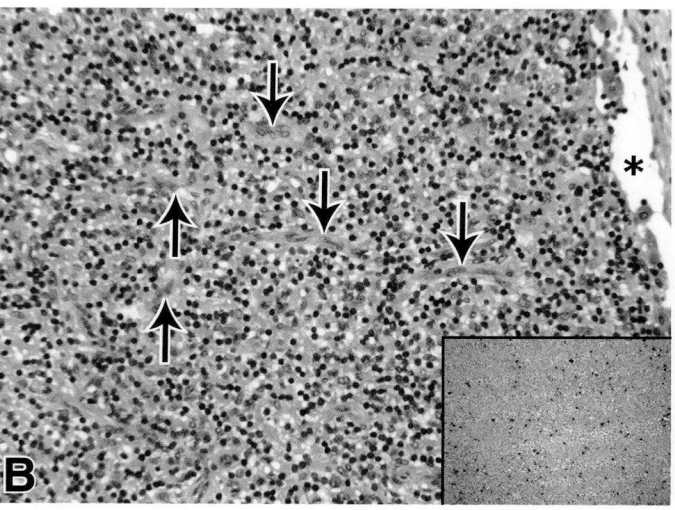

FIGURE 26-73. Angioimmunoblastic T-cell lymphoma. A. Complete effacement of lymph node architecture by an infiltrate that includes a mixture of neoplastic T-cells, prominent blood vessels, and Epstein–Barr virus (EBV)–positive B-lymphocytes. The lymph node capsule is at the top. **B.** Higher magnification showing the blood vessels (representative vessels are highlighted by *arrows*) and their prominent endothelial cells. The subcapsular sinus is identified (*). *Inset.* In situ hybridization for EBV transcript, demonstrating the scattered EBV-positive B-lymphocytes scattered throughout the neoplastic T-cell proliferation.

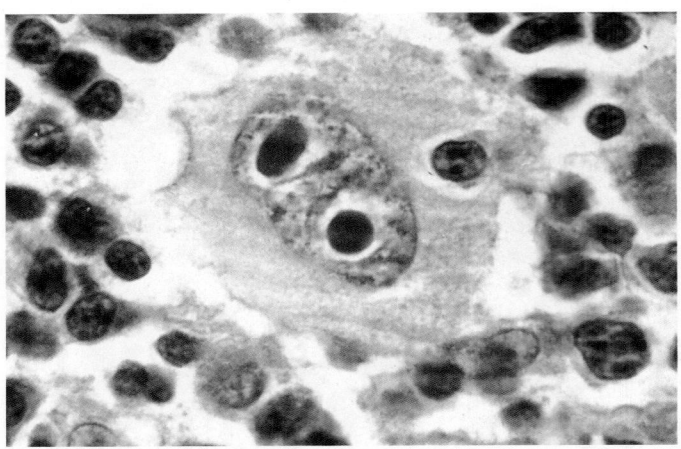

FIGURE 26-74. Classic Reed–Sternberg cell. Mirror-image nuclei contain large eosinophilic nucleoli.

Classical Hodgkin Lymphomas (HL) Are Composed of a Prominent Inflammatory Background and Scattered Malignant Hodgkin Reed–Sternberg Cells

Classic Hodgkin Reed–Sternberg (HRS) cells are large binucleated cells with prominent nucleoli (Fig. 26-74); there are two types of HL: **classical Hodgkin lymphoma** and **nodular lymphocyte-predominant Hodgkin lymphoma**. Unlike non-Hodgkin lymphomas, classical HL usually arise in a single lymph node region and spread in a contiguous fashion, mostly in adolescents and young adults. They contain relatively few neoplastic cells, amid a prominent mixed inflammatory infiltrate of small T-lymphocytes, histiocytes, and eosinophils. *In virtually all cases, the neoplastic cells in HL are derived from germinal center B-cells and express CD30 and CD15 markers (Fig. 26-75).*

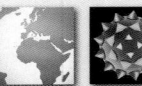

EPIDEMIOLOGY AND ETIOLOGIC FACTORS: *HL is the most common malignancy in the United States between the ages of 10 and 30.* Geographic variation in HL incidence, plus some clinical and pathologic features resembling an infectious process, suggest a viral etiology. Reports of several self-limited "mini-epidemics" of HL in children suggest horizontal transmission (i.e., by interpersonal contact) of an infectious agent. A possible link between HL and EBV infection has been suggested. Young adults with a recent history of EBV-associated infectious mononucleosis have a threefold higher risk of developing HL. The EBV genome is frequently identified in Reed–Sternberg cells.

Genetic factors may contribute. Certain HLA subtypes, particularly HLA-B18, are more common in patients with HL. Moreover, siblings of HL patients have a 7-fold greater risk of HL, which rises to 100-fold for monozygotic twins.

Immune status also seems to be a factor, at least in some cases. HL occurs more often in people with altered immunity or autoimmune diseases, such as rheumatoid arthritis. Also, HL accounts for 7% of malignancies in immunodeficient ataxia-telangiectasia patients.

EBV may be detected in HRS cells by immunohistochemistry for LMP1 protein (Fig. 26-75) or by in situ hybridization for EBER RNA (not shown). EBV-positive RS cells are seen in 70% to 80% of mixed-cellularity HL, but in under 40% of nodular sclerosis HL.

Classical Hodgkin Lymphoma

This lymphoma is a B-cell neoplasm composed (in most cases) of mononuclear Hodgkin cells and multinucleate Reed–Sternberg cells (Fig. 26-74) in a reactive inflammatory background of small lymphocytes (mostly T-cells), plasma cells, histiocytes, and eosinophils. Fibrosis is variably prominent,

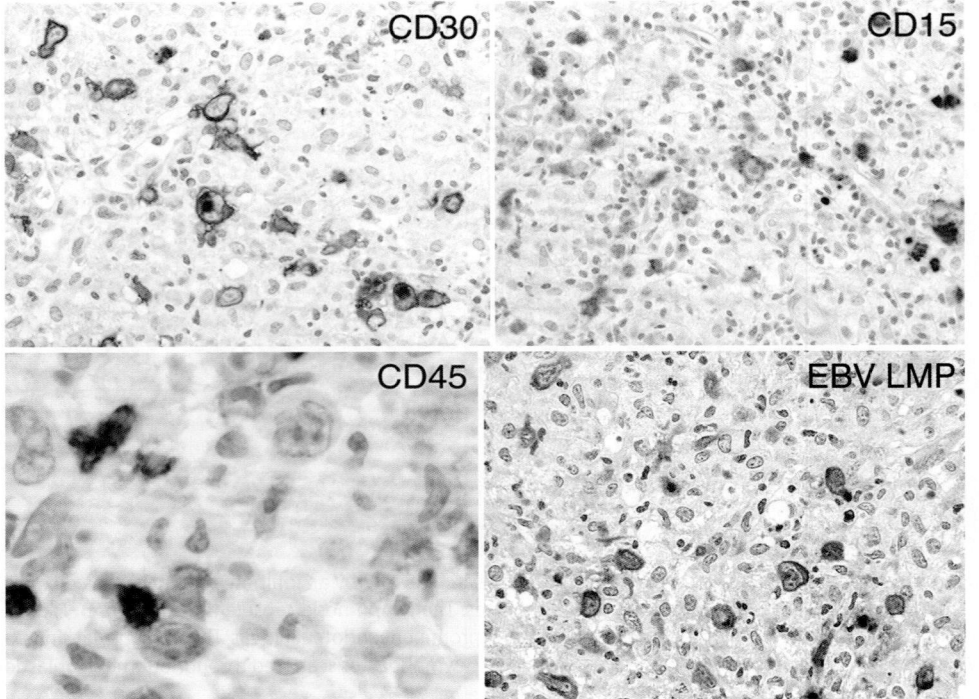

FIGURE 26-75. Reed–Sternberg and Hodgkin cells. The Hodgkin/Reed–Sternberg (HRS) cells are uniformly positive for CD30, CD15, and Epstein–Barr virus latent membrane protein antigen (EBV LMP) (immunohistochemistry; red chromogen). Common leukocyte antigen CD45 is not expressed on HRS cells.

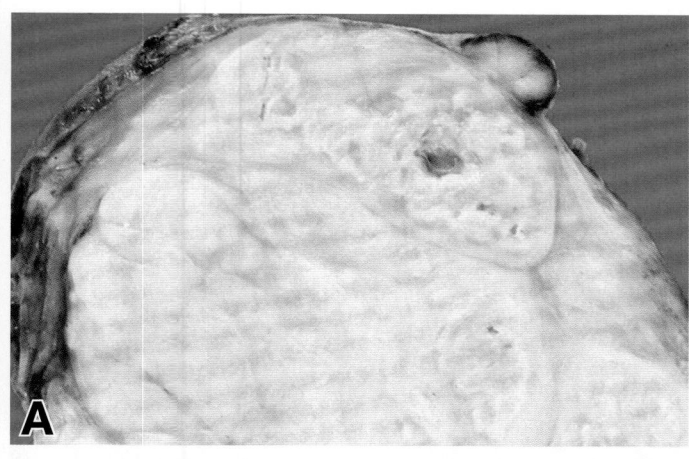

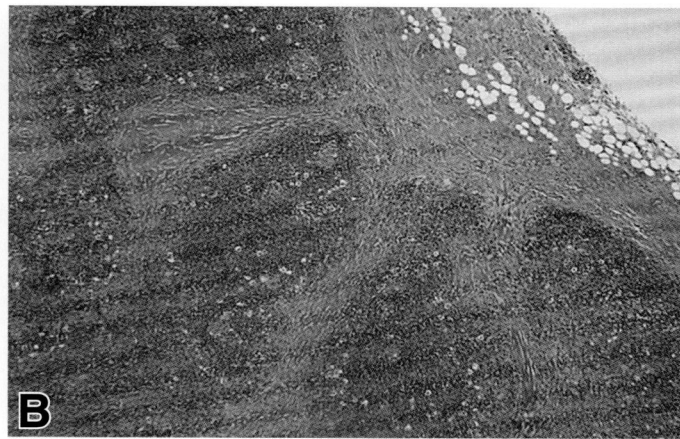

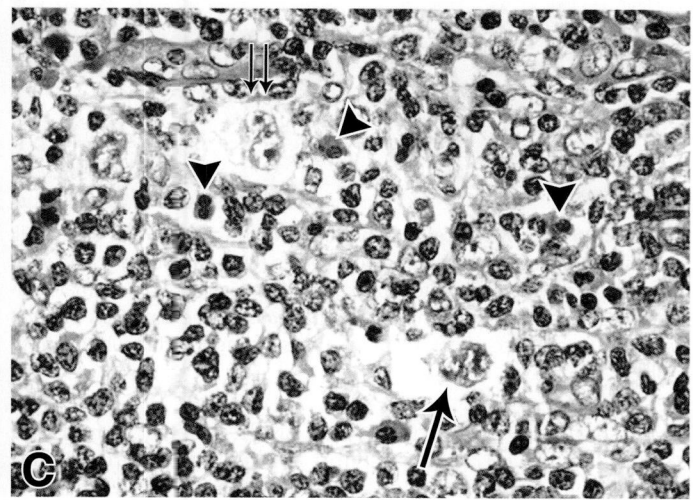

FIGURE 26-76. Nodular sclerosis Hodgkin lymphoma (NSHL). A. Gross photograph showing an enlarged lymph node with a thickened capsule and broad bands of fibrosis dividing the parenchyma into distinct nodules. Several foci of necrosis are evident (red-brown discolorations). **B.** A low-power photomicrograph demonstrates broad bands of fibrosis. There is a dense inflammatory background. Reed–Sternberg cells are rare. **C.** A photomicrograph of NSHL shows a mixed inflammatory background with eosinophils (*arrowheads*), Reed–Sternberg cells (*double arrow*) and lacunar cells (*arrow*).

with or without broad bands of collagen (Fig. 26-76). HRS cells are usually scattered, and sometimes form syncytial aggregates. Classical HL encompasses four histologic subtypes, largely reflecting the associated inflammatory background and the appearance of HRS cells. These subtypes are *nodular sclerosis, mixed cellularity, lymphocyte-rich,* and *lymphocyte-depleted* (in order of prevalence). HRS cells in all subtypes share a unique immunophenotype not seen in non-Hodgkin lymphomas.

EPIDEMIOLOGY: Classical Hodgkin lymphomas represent 95% of HLs. The disease has a bimodal age distribution: one peak is at 15 to 35 years and another in older adults. People with recent histories of infectious mononucleosis are at increased risk of classical HL.

PATHOLOGY: Lymph nodes involved by classical HL show architectural effacement by a mixed inflammatory cell infiltrate with variable fibrosis (sclerosis) (Fig. 26-76). HRS cells are large, with at least two nuclear lobes or nuclei and abundant light blue cytoplasm (Fig. 26-74). Their nuclei have irregular contours and prominent eosinophilic nucleoli with perinucleolar

haloes, resembling "owl's eyes." HRS cells may undergo apoptosis, resulting in mummified-appearing cells with condensed cytoplasm and pyknotic nuclei. Despite their unique appearance, when few in number, HRS cells may be difficult to identify in standard H&E-stained tissue sections. Immunostains for CD15, CD30, CD45, and PAX-5 help to identify them and distinguish them from imposters seen in many other conditions.

HRS cells almost always express CD30 lymphoid activation marker (Fig. 26-75), and the CD15 macrophage/monocyte marker in most cases. Unlike non-Hodgkin lymphoma cells, HRS cells do not usually express the pan-leukocyte marker CD45, B-cell antigens CD20 and CD79a, T-cell antigens (CD2, CD3), or histiocyte antigens (CD68, CD163).

The unique HRS immunophenotype, not shared with any normal cell counterpart, delayed identification of the cell lineage of HRS cells for many years. Only after development molecular diagnostic techniques in the late 1990s did their origin from clonal germinal center cells become clear. *HRS cells in almost all HL cases show clonal Ig gene rearrangement.*

Cytokines from HRS cells induce the characteristic inflammatory background. IL-5 and eotaxin attract eosinophils, IL-6 recruits plasma cells and TGFβ induces fibrosis.

TABLE 26-21

ANN ARBOR STAGING SYSTEM FOR HODGKIN DISEASE

Stage I A or B[a]	I	Involvement of a single lymph node region
		or
	I_E	A single extralymphatic organ or site
Stage II A or B	II	Involvement of two or more lymph node regions on the same side of the diaphragm
		or
	II_E	With localized contiguous involvement of an extralymphatic organ site
Stage III A or B	III	Involvement of lymph node regions on both sides of the diaphragm
		or
	III_E	With localized contiguous involvement of an extralymphatic organ or site
		or
	III_S	With involvement of spleen
		or
	III_ES	Both extralymphatic organ or site and spleen involvement
Stage IV A or B	IV	Diffuse or disseminated involvement of one or more extralymphatic organs with or without associated lymph node involvement

[a]A = asymptomatic; B = presence of constitutional symptoms (fever, night sweats, and weight loss exceeding 10% of baseline body weight in preceding 6 months).

Nodular Sclerosis Hodgkin Lymphoma (NSHL)

In **NSHL,** lymph node capsules show fibrous thickening, and collagen bands extend from the capsule into the nodal cortex, to form nodules (Fig. 26-76A). **Lacunar HRS cells**, due to a retraction artifact in formalin-fixed tissues, are characteristic of NSHL (Fig. 26-76C). The nodules surrounded by fibrosis contain mixed inflammatory cells, described above, with variable numbers of classical HRS and lacunar cells. NSHL represents 70% of classical HL cases, occurring most often between ages 15 and 30. Most patients present with mediastinal involvement, and 40% have B symptoms (Table 26-21). Bone marrow involvement and EBV positivity are uncommon, relative to other HL types.

Mixed Cellularity Hodgkin Lymphoma (MCHL)

In **MCHL**, relatively abundant HRS cells sit amid a mixed inflammatory background of eosinophils, neutrophils, macrophages, and plasma cells (Fig. 26-77). Nodular fibrosis, as in NSHL, is lacking. *MCHL is the most frequent HL subtype in HIV-1–infected patients, and shows the highest association with EBV.* MCHL is most common in the fourth and fifth decades. Mediastinal involvement is uncommon.

Lymphocyte-Rich Hodgkin Lymphoma

In **lymphocyte-rich Hodgkin lymphoma (LRHL)**, scattered classical HRS cells are surrounded by a nodular (rarely diffuse) lymphoid infiltrate of small B-cells. The reactive inflammatory background typical of NSHL and MCHL is absent. Only 5% of classical HL are LRHL, which tends to occur in

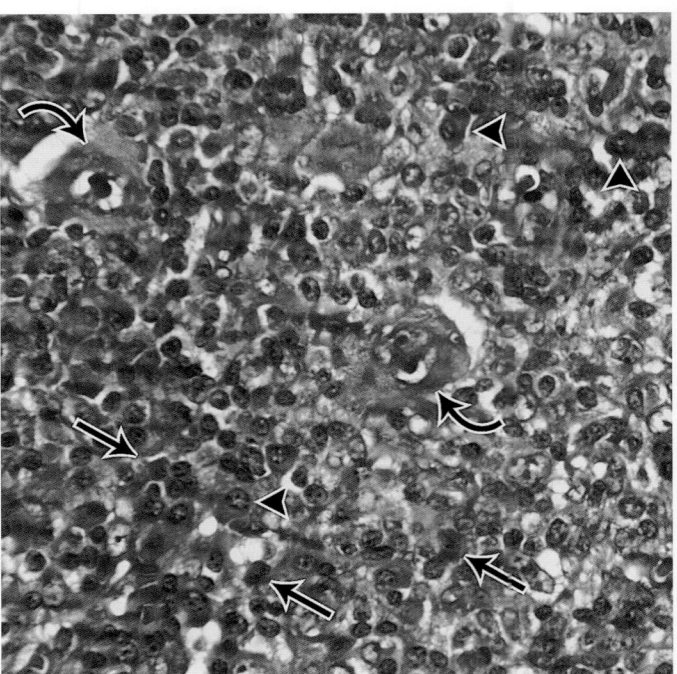

FIGURE 26-77. Mixed cellularity Hodgkin lymphoma. This type of HL shows frequent mononuclear and binucleated Reed–Sternberg cells (*curved arrows*) in a mixed inflammatory background that includes many small lymphocytes (T-cells), plus plasma cells (*arrowheads*), and eosinophils (*straight arrows*). The absence of fibrotic bands helps distinguish this subtype from NSHL.

older people. Overall survival for LRHL is better than for all other classical HL subtypes, and is like survival in nodular lymphocyte-predominant HL (see below).

Lymphocyte-Depleted Hodgkin Lymphoma (LDHL)

This is the least common classical HL subtype. In LDHL, HRS cells predominate. Against a background of diffuse fibrosis and numerous histiocytes, lymphocytes are largely absent (Fig. 26-78). Typical patients are 30- to 40-year-old

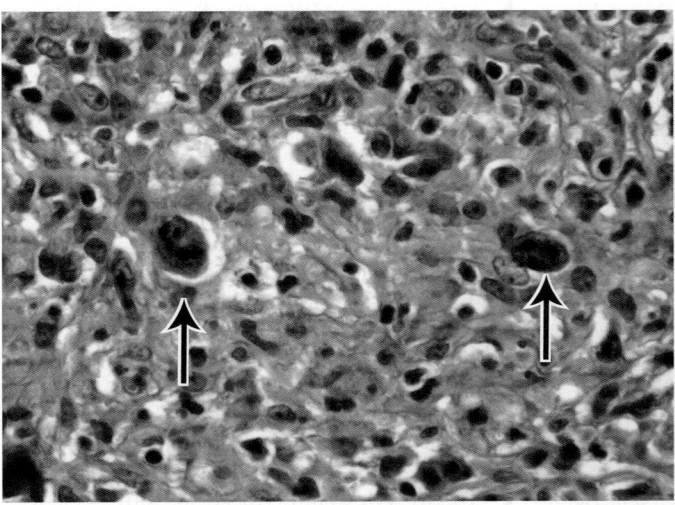

FIGURE 26-78. Lymphocyte-depleted Hodgkin lymphoma. Two Hodgkin/Reed–Sternberg cells are seen (*arrows*). The number of reactive lymphocytes in the fibrotic background is markedly reduced. The differential diagnosis in cases like this includes large cell lymphoma.

men. This subtype, like MCHL, is often associated with HIV infection. Unlike other forms of HL, LDHL not infrequently involves retroperitoneal lymph nodes, and infiltrates abdominal organs and bone marrow. Patients with associated HIV infection fare poorly. In some cases, distinction from non-Hodgkin lymphoma may be difficult.

CLINICAL FEATURES: HL usually presents as nontender peripheral adenopathy in a single lymph node or group of nodes. Cervical and mediastinal nodes are involved in most cases. The anterior mediastinum is frequently involved, especially in NSHL. Axillary, inguinal, and retroperitoneal lymph nodes are less often affected. Peripheral node groups, for example, antecubital, popliteal, and mesenteric lymph nodes, are usually spared. Initially, HL spreads between contiguous lymph node groups via efferent lymphatics. With progression, spread becomes less predictable because of vascular invasion and hematogenous dissemination (Fig. 26-79).

About 40% of patients show constitutional ("B") symptoms: low-grade fever, night sweats, and weight loss. Pruritus may occur as disease progresses. Patients with HL often have deficient T-lymphocyte function. Subtle defects of delayed-type hypersensitivity (such as skin test anergy), which can be detected in most patients even at presentation, often get worse as disease progresses. Absolute lymphocytopenia (<1,500 cells/μL) is present in half of cases, mostly in advanced HL. Humoral immunity usually remains intact until late in the disease.

HL prognosis depends mainly on patient age and anatomic extent (stage) of the disease. Good prognostic factors include (1) young age, (2) low clinical stage, and (3) lack of B symptoms. The comprehensive Ann Arbor Staging System (Table 26-21) includes clinical, radiographic, and pathologic criteria (including bone marrow biopsy) to assign stage.

Complications of HL include compromise of vital organs by enlarging tumor, plus secondary infections due to primary defective delayed-type hypersensitivity and immunosuppressive effects of therapy. Second malignancies (aggressive non-Hodgkin lymphoma, AML) may arise after therapy.

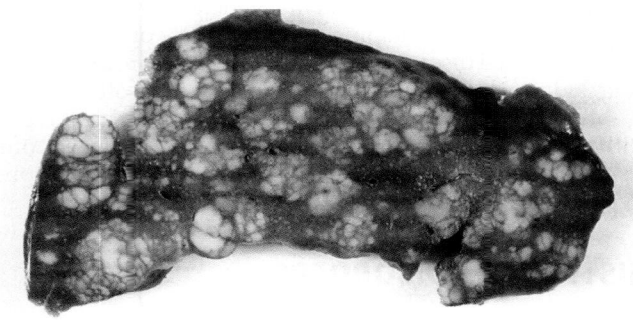

FIGURE 26-79. Hodgkin lymphoma involving the spleen. Multiple masses replace the normal splenic parenchyma. Laparotomy and splenectomy are no longer routinely performed for diagnostic and staging purposes.

Nodular Lymphocyte–Predominant Hodgkin Lymphoma (NLPHL)

This type of Hodgkin lymphoma is distinct from classical HLs. Although classified as a Hodgkin lymphoma, many of its clinical and pathologic features resemble indolent B-cell non-Hodgkin lymphomas. NLPHL tumor cells are large B-cells called **LP cells**, or "popcorn cells," because of their popcorn kernel appearance. As in most classical HLs, neoplastic LP cells of NLPHL are not abundant in tissue sections.

LP cells like HRS cells derive from germinal center B-cells. Unlike classical HRS cells, LP cells express B-cell lineage antigens (CD20, CD79a, surface Ig), almost always show clonal Ig rearrangement, but are negative for CD15 and CD30.

NLPHL is uncommon, accounting for only 5% of HL cases. It mainly affects men 30 to 50 years old, but may also occur in younger people, including children. It is typically localized at the time of diagnosis (i.e., stage I), commonly affecting cervical, axillary, or inguinal lymph nodes. Mediastinal, splenic, visceral, and bone marrow involvement are rare. NLPHL often skips node groups when it spreads. Only 20% of cases present with B symptoms. These tumors follow an indolent clinical course. Ten-year survival for patients with low-stage disease (stage I or II) is more than 80%. Complications include recurrent disease (common) and progression to DLBCL (uncommon).

Lymphoproliferative Disorders Are Associated With Immune Deficiencies

Several types of non-Hodgkin and Hodgkin lymphomas occur in patients with immune dysfunction, but there is a specific group of lymphoproliferative diseases that develop in patients with primary immune defects, HIV infection, organ transplants, and iatrogenic immunosuppression.

Post-Transplant Lymphoproliferative Disorders (PTLD)

Post-transplant lymphoproliferative disorders are secondary to immunosuppressive drug therapy in organ transplant recipients. PTLD infiltrates range from plasmacytic lesions resembling infectious mononucleosis to overt large B-cell lymphomas. T-cell and HL-like PTLDs are rare. *Most of these disorders are associated with EBV infection, and the key risk factor is EBV seronegativity prior to transplantation.*

EPIDEMIOLOGY: Several factors increase the risk of developing PTLD, reflecting patient characteristics, allograft types, EBV seropositivity, and immunosuppressive regimens, which may vary from institution to institution. Patients with renal allografts have the lowest risk of PTLD, while those with heart/lung or intestinal allografts have the highest risk. Patients with stem cell or bone marrow allografts have a low risk of PTLD. The risk in these individuals reflects the degree of HLA matching: unrelated or HLA-mismatched transplants are more likely to develop PTLD. PTLD occurs more often in children, probably because children are more often EBV seronegative at the time of transplant.

MOLECULAR PATHOGENESIS: Most cases are caused by EBV, with an average latency period of <1 year. However, EBV-negative cases may occur 5 or more years after transplantation. In solid organ recipients, PTLD develops from EBV+ recipient lymphocytes, while in marrow or stem cell allograft recipients, PTLD develops from EBV+ donor lymphocytes.

PATHOLOGY: The histology of PTLD is diverse and includes:

- **Early lesions:** These show plasmacytic hyperplasia or infectious mononucleosis–like changes. They tend to occur in younger—particularly EBV-negative—patients. Early lesions involve lymph nodes or tonsils and adenoids. These lesions are usually polyclonal and regress spontaneously or with reduction in immunosuppression; however, some infectious mononucleosis–like lesions may occasionally be fatal.
- **Polymorphic PTLD:** These lesions contain heterogeneous cellular populations, including immunoblasts, plasma cells, and small to medium-sized lymphocytes (Fig. 26-80). The atypical lymphoplasmacytic/immunoblastic proliferation tends to efface lymph node architecture and/or form destructive extranodal masses. This type of PTLD is most common in children, following primary EBV infection. Variable numbers of cases regress with reduction in immunosuppression, while others progress and require cytotoxic chemotherapy. The atypical cells in polymorphic PTLD show clonally rearranged Ig genes, although detectable clones are less prominent, compared to levels in monomorphic PTLD (see below).
- **Monomorphic PTLD:** These are proliferations of large B-lymphocytes or plasma cells that qualify as DLBCL, BL, or PCM/plasmacytoma. Virtually all show clonal Ig gene rearrangements; most have clonal EBV genomes.

Cytogenetic abnormalities are common. The majority require treatment for lymphoma; this type of PTLD does not typically respond to reduction in immunosuppression, unlike PTLD types discussed above.

- **Classical Hodgkin lymphoma–type PTLD:** This rare type of PTLD occurs more often in renal transplant patients, is almost always EBV positive and resembles classical HL (see above).

CLINICAL FEATURES: Patients with PTLD present with lethargy, malaise, weight loss and fever, often with lymphadenopathy and allograft dysfunction. Enlarged tonsils may cause airway obstruction in some patients, mostly children. In addition to lymph nodes and tonsils, PTLDs often involve extranodal sites, particularly the gut, lungs, and liver. The allograft itself may be affected, which may cause diagnostic confusion with allograft rejection. The prognosis of PTLD depends largely on the type of lesion. Early lesions tend to regress as immunosuppression is reduced, without graft loss. Reducing immunosuppression may be useful treating other forms that more closely resemble lymphomas, but many require additional cytotoxic therapy. EBV viral load monitoring of seronegative patients is common practice in many transplant centers and has decreased the incidence of disseminated PTLD.

Iatrogenic Immunodeficiency-Associated Lymphoproliferative Disorders

These disorders occur mostly in patients receiving immunosuppressive drugs for autoimmune diseases or other conditions (excluding transplantation). Lymphoid proliferations in these patients resemble those in patients with PTLD, and vary from polymorphic disorders to DLBCLs, PTCLs, or classical HL. Methotrexate, which has long been used to treat rheumatoid arthritis (RA), was the first immunosuppressive agent linked to a lymphoproliferative disorder. Newer agents used to treat RA, such as the TNFα antagonists, also increase the risk of lymphoma, compared to healthy age-matched people. Like most PTLDs, the iatrogenic lymphoproliferative disorders are often associated with EBV, but EBV is not the only important risk factor. Chronic antigenic stimulation, thus with lymphoproliferation, and patients' genetic backgrounds, also affect lymphoma development. Almost 50% of cases present with extranodal disease, often in the GI tract, skin, liver, spleen, lung, kidney, thyroid gland, bone marrow, and soft tissues.

Many of these tumors resemble DLBL or classical HL. As with PTLD, iatrogenic lymphoproliferative disorders often respond, at least partially, to withdrawing immunosuppressive medications, especially in EBV-positive cases.

HISTIOCYTIC DISORDERS

Histiocytic Proliferations May Be Benign or Neoplastic

Benign histiocytic disorders include Rosai–Dorfman disease (sinus histiocytosis with massive lymphadenopathy), lipid storage disorders such as Niemann–Pick disease and Gaucher disease (see Chapter 6) and hemophagocytic syndromes.

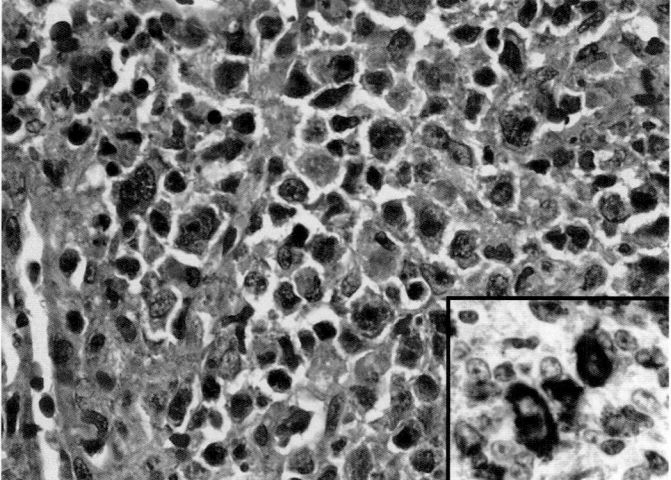

FIGURE 26-80. Posttransplant lymphoproliferative disorder (PTLD). Polymorphic-type PTLD is characterized by a heterogeneous population of atypical lymphocytes with clonal immunoglobulin gene rearrangements. *Inset.* Atypical lymphocytes are positive for Epstein–Barr virus latent membrane protein (EBV LMP) by immunohistochemistry.

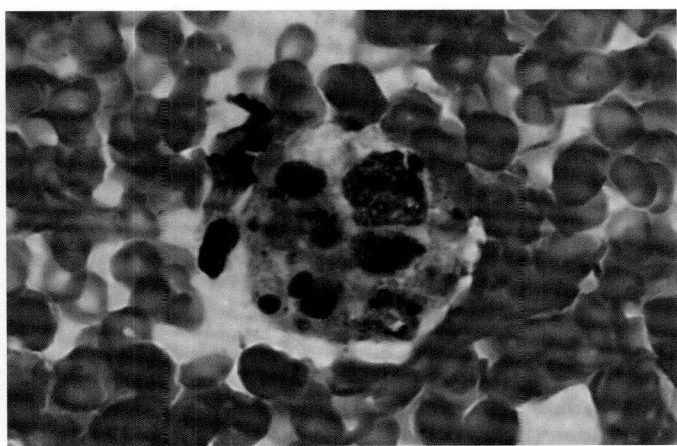

FIGURE 26-81. Hemophagocytic syndrome. This disorder is characterized morphologically by phagocytosis of hematopoietic cells by tissue macrophages. Shown here is a macrophage engulfing bone marrow cells.

Hemophagocytic Disorders

All hemophagocytic disorders are due to immune dysregulation with overproduction of proinflammatory cytokines and unregulated T-cell activation and proliferation of hemophagocytic histiocytes. Proinflammatory cytokines (see Chapter 4) include TNFα, IL-6 and, IFNγ.

Hemophagocytic syndromes may be inherited (primary) or acquired (secondary).

Primary hemophagocytic syndrome (HLH) is due to several mutations, including in *PFR1* (perforin) gene mutation, and typically presents in young childhood.

Diagnosis is based upon combined clinical and pathologic criteria: high fever, splenomegaly, anemia, thrombocytopenia, hypertriglyceridemia and hypofibrinogenemia, plus abundant histiocytes with ingested leukocytes and red cells in the bone marrow, spleen or lymph nodes (Fig. 26-81). Hemophagocytosis of bone marrow cells often leads to pancytopenia. Acquired hemophagocytic syndromes may also occur with severe infections (viral, bacterial, fungal), autoimmune disease and malignancy.

Histiocytic Neoplasms Are Rare Tumors Derived From Neoplastic Histiocytes or Dendritic Cells

This group of neoplasms includes Langerhans cell histiocytosis (LCH), FDC sarcoma, and IDC sarcoma.

Langerhans Cell Histiocytosis (LCH) Is a Neoplastic Proliferation of Langerhans Cells

Clinical presentations range from asymptomatic involvement at a single site (bone or lymph nodes), to aggressive systemic multiorgan disease. Langerhans cells are bone marrow–derived antigen presenting cells that populate the epidermis and squamous mucosa. Their role is to carry foreign antigens from skin and mucosal sites to lymph node paracortical T-cells. Langerhans cells that remain in the lymph node paracortex mature into IDCs.

LCH occurs most often in infants, children, and young adults. The extent of disease and rate of progression correlate inversely with age at presentation. The most common and least aggressive form of LCH (**eosinophilic granuloma**) is a localized, usually self-limited, disorder that usually involves a single bone or, less often, lymph nodes, skin, and lung. This form of LCH affects older children and young adults.

Sometimes, the tumor is a multifocal, but indolent disorder confined to one tissue, usually bone or soft tissue. Seen in young children, this form of LCH was once called **Hand–Schüller–Christian disease**.

The rarest form of LCH, seen in infants and young children, is an acute condition with disseminated disease. Skin lesions, hepatosplenomegaly, lymphadenopathy, bone lesions, and pancytopenia are typical. It was once called **Letterer–Siwe** disease.

 PATHOLOGY: LCH tumors are composed of Langerhans cells, admixed with reactive eosinophils, histiocytes, and small T-lymphocytes (Fig. 26-82). Langerhans cells are medium to large cells with distinctive grooved nuclei. Electron microscopy shows Birbeck granules—distinctive rod-shaped or tubular cytoplasmic bodies called. The Langerhans cells express S-100 protein and CD1a.

 MOLECULAR PATHOGENESIS: Most cases of LCH carry mutually exclusive mutations of either BRAF or MAP2K1.

CLINICAL FEATURES: Clinical manifestations of LCH reflect the sites involved. Skin involvement, mainly in Letterer–Siwe disease, resembles seborrheic or eczematoid dermatitis, and affects the scalp, face, and trunk most prominently. Painless localized or generalized lymphadenopathy and hepatosplenomegaly are common. Bone pain is caused by lytic bone lesions (see Chapter 30). Proptosis (protrusion of the eyeball) may reflect infiltration of the orbit. If the hypothalamic–pituitary axis is affected, diabetes insipidus may develop. Prognosis in LCH depends on age at presentation, extent of disease and rate of progression. LCH is usually self-limited in older people (eosinophilic granuloma), but children under 2 years (Letterer–Siwe disease) tend to do poorly.

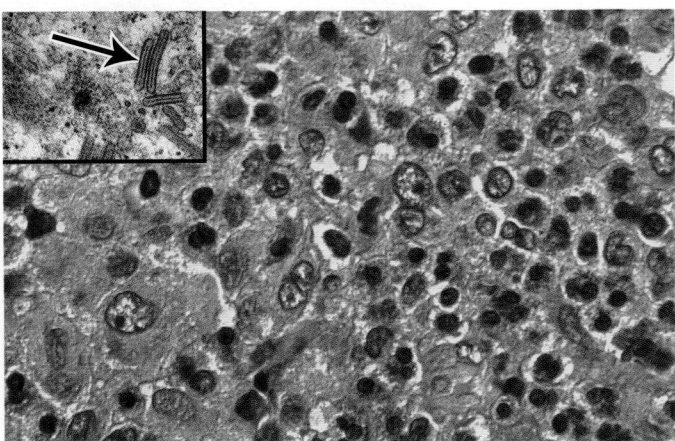

FIGURE 26-82. Eosinophilic granuloma. A section of an affected rib shows proliferated Langerhans cells and numerous eosinophils. *Inset.* Electron micrograph showing a Birbeck granule (*arrow*) in Langerhans histiocytosis.

HEMATOPATHOLOGY

Spleen

ANATOMY AND FUNCTION

The spleen is a lymphoid organ that plays a major role in clearing pathogens from the blood, removing abnormal or senescenT-cells, immune complexes, and opsonized bacteria. It is also a major site for B-lymphocyte development. A normal spleen weighs 100 to 170 g. It is not palpable on physical examination. The spleen's supporting structure includes a fibrous capsule, radiating fibrous trabeculae and a delicate stromal framework of reticulum fibers (Fig. 26-83). The splenic artery enters at the hilum and branches into trabecular arteries, following the course of the fibrous trabeculae. The spleen is divided into red and white pulp, which is useful, because most diseases affect either one or the other.

THE WHITE PULP: The white pulp is the spleen's lymphoid tissue, with masses of T- and B-lymphocytes, ensheathing a central artery. T-cells are mainly in the periarteriolar lymphoid sheath, while the B-cell domain has follicles and a perifollicular marginal zone. Follicular arteries arise from the central artery and enter B-cell follicles and end in marginal sinuses where the white and red pulp meet. Circulating lymphocytes exit the vascular system from the marginal sinus and travel to their respective B- and T-cell domains. Lymphocytes leave the white pulp and enter the red pulp via the same marginal sinuses.

Effector B- and T-cells of the white pulp carry out immunologic functions as in lymph nodes. The white pulp is (1) the source of protection from blood-borne infection; (2) a major site for synthesis of opsonizing IgM antibody; and (3) a place for lymphocyte and plasma cell production.

THE RED PULP: The red pulp contains a network of stromal cords and vascular sinuses. Blood from the penicilliary arteries empties directly into the sinuses (closed circulation), then drains into trabecular veins, and ultimately into the splenic vein. A small fraction (5% to 10%) is diverted into splenic cords (open circulation) and slowly percolates through a meshwork studded with phagocytic macrophages. Blood then reenters the sinusoids through narrow slits of longitudinally oriented, slender endothelial cells and radially oriented ring fibers.

The red pulp is mainly a filter that screens and eliminates defective or foreign cells. There, mononuclear phagocytes scrutinize erythrocytes, which must be deformable enough to traverse the narrow interstices between the lining endothelial cells. The RBCs must also be able to withstand hypoxia, hypoglycemia, and acidosis that characterize the stromal cord microenvironment. Splenic macrophages identify and eliminate senescent and damaged erythrocytes. The spleen normally removes half of aged erythrocytes; the liver, bone

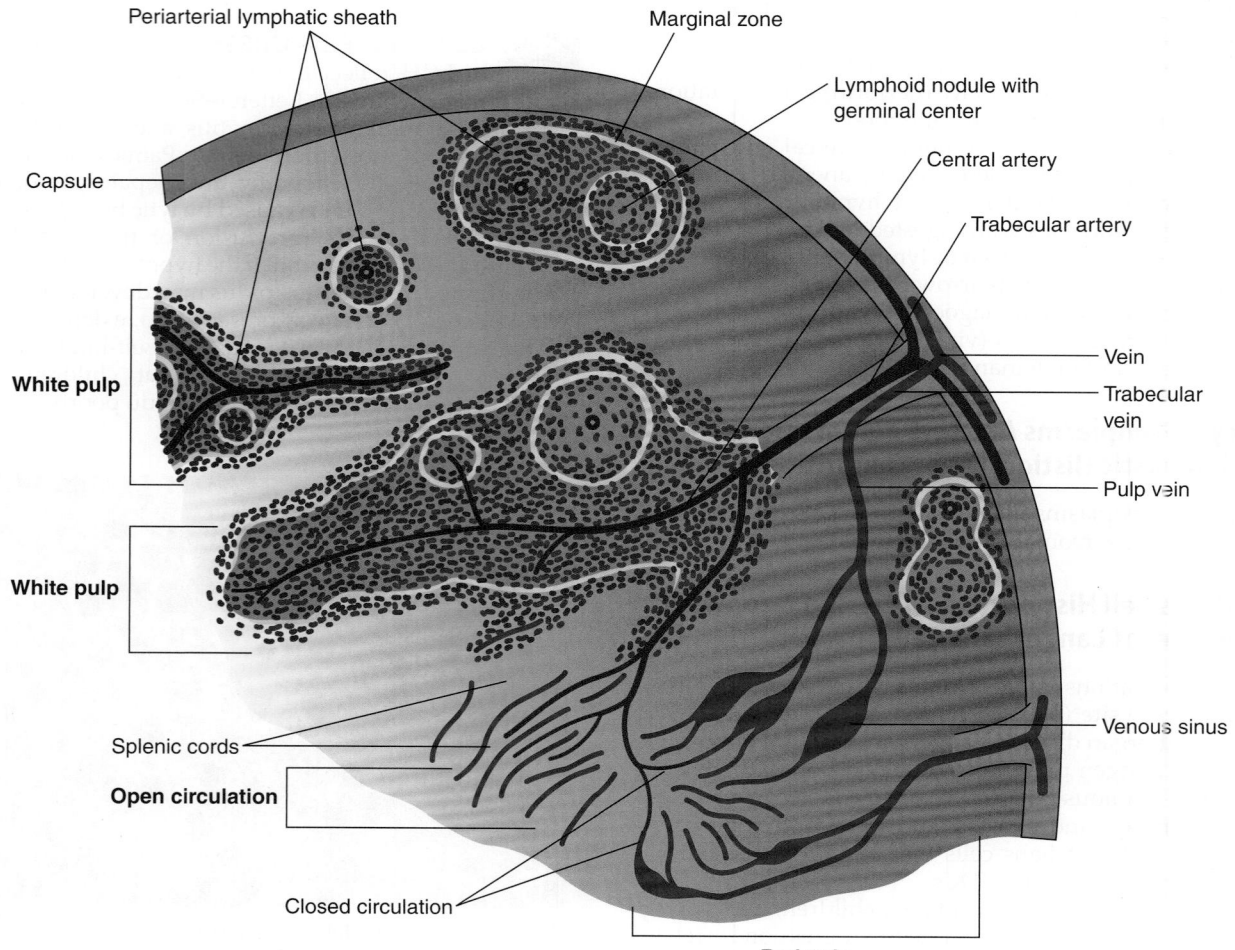

FIGURE 26-83. Structure of the normal spleen.

marrow, and other organs eliminate the rest. After phagocytosing and breaking down erythrocytes, macrophages first store the resulting iron as hemosiderin. This pigment then binds to transferrin, leaves the macrophages and travels to the bone marrow to be reused in erythropoiesis.

Splenic macrophages also identify abnormal erythrocyte inclusions, like Howell–Jolly bodies (remnants of nuclear DNA), Heinz bodies (denatured hemoglobin) and siderotic granules (iron), and remove them without destroying the erythrocytes.

Some membrane lipids of maturing erythrocytes are removed in the red pulp. Without this function, such as after splenectomy, RBC membrane may accumulate, relative to the amount of hemoglobin. This causes central hemoglobin pools, imparting a "target cell" appearance.

Most normal erythrocytes survive, as do granulocytes and platelets. They ultimately enter trabecular veins and leave the hilum via the splenic vein. One-third of blood platelets and a small fraction of granulocytes normally reside, undamaged, in the spleen. The spleen does not significantly sequester erythrocytes, so that splenectomy leads to thrombocytosis and granulocytosis, not erythrocytosis.

DISORDERS OF THE SPLEEN

Hypersplenism is a functional disorder, which presents (see hemolytic anemias, above) with anemia, leukopenia, thrombocytopenia, and compensatory bone marrow hyperplasia. In **hyposplenism,** normal splenic functions are impaired by diseases such as immune disorders, or malignancies. The spleen's normal filtering function is impaired or absent, increasing risk of severe bacteremia and causes mild leukocytosis and thrombocytosis. Circulating erythrocytes contain nuclear remnants and Howell–Jolly bodies.

Asplenia is complete loss of splenic function. It may be anatomical or functional. Congenital absence of a spleen occurs once in 40,000 births, and often accompanies other congenital anomalies. Anatomical asplenia may be due to surgical splenectomy, for example, for trauma or to treat hemolytic anemias or immune thrombocytopenia (ITP). Functional asplenia occurs most frequently in sickle cell disease, due to multiple infarctions causing splenic atrophy and hyposplenism. Episodic infarction is often painful because of secondary fibrinous perisplenitis. Without a spleen to sequester erythrocytes and remove redundant materials from them, excess membrane and intracellular debris persist. Many red cells assume target shapes and carry nuclear remnants (see above).

Accessory spleens are common congenital anomalies due to incomplete fusion of the spleen during embryogenesis. They are usually solitary, near the splenic hilum, the tail of the pancreas or the gastrosplenic ligament. After splenectomy, accessory spleens may enlarge, but they rarely become large enough to replace a lost spleen functionally. Other congenital anomalies include polysplenia with multiple small splenic masses, fusion, hamartomas, and cysts.

Splenomegaly

The spleen is a key member of both lymphopoietic and mononuclear phagocyte systems. Thus, splenomegaly is common in many unrelated benign and malignant diseases (Table 26-22).

TABLE 26-22
PRINCIPAL CAUSES OF SPLENOMEGALY

Infections
  Acute
  Subacute
  Chronic

Immunologic Inflammatory Disorders
  Felty syndrome
  Lupus erythematosus
  Sarcoidosis
  Amyloidosis
  Thyroiditis

Hemolytic Anemias

Immune Thrombocytopenia

Splenic Vein Hypertension
  Cirrhosis
  Splenic or portal vein thrombosis or stenosis
  Right-sided cardiac failure

Primary or Metastatic Neoplasm
  Leukemia
  Lymphoma
  Hodgkin disease
  Myeloproliferative syndromes
  Sarcoma
  Carcinoma

Storage Diseases
  Gaucher
  Niemann–Pick
  Mucopolysaccharidoses

Reactive Splenomegaly

Acute splenitis occurs in many blood-borne infections: the spleen becomes congested, with red and white pulp infiltrated by neutrophils and plasma cells. In most cases the spleen is moderately enlarged (400 g).

In acute and chronic parasitemias, splenic red pulp may be engorged with parasites and their breakdown products. The spleen may be massively enlarged in chronic malaria (up to 10 kg), with fibrous thickening of the capsule and trabeculae, with slate gray to black coloration of the pulp from phagocytosed malarial pigment (hematin).

In infectious mononucleosis, half of patients have splenomegaly. Reactive lymphocytes infiltrate the capsular and trabecular systems and blood vessels, weaken the spleen's supporting structure and predispose it to traumatic rupture. A polymorphic population of T and B immunoblasts, which may include large multinucleated forms, permeates the red pulp cords and sinuses. Such splenomegaly may rarely cause potentially fatal splenic rupture.

In chronic inflammatory disorders, white pulp hyperplasia causes splenomegaly. Germinal centers are prominent, as in rheumatoid arthritis. The red pulp has a parallel increase in mononuclear phagocytes, immunoblasts, plasma cells, and eosinophils. Fibrinoid necrosis of the capsule and concentric, or "onion skin," thickening of penicilliary arteries and central white pulp arterioles of the white pulp may occur in SLE.

Congestive Splenomegaly

Chronic passive congestion of the spleen causes splenomegaly and hypersplenism. This occurs most often in patients with portal hypertension due to cirrhosis, thrombosis of the hepatic portal or splenic veins, or right-sided heart failure. Splenic congestion also complicates hereditary hemolytic anemias and hemoglobinopathies. In many of these diseases, erythrocyte shape is rigid, so RBCs are trapped as they attempt to pass through splenic cords.

The Spleen in Sickle Cell Anemia

The spleen is modestly enlarged (300 to 700 g), with a thickened, fibrotic capsule. Focal accentuation of the capsular fibrosis leads to a "sugar-coated" appearance. The cut surface is firm, and the color varies from pink to deep red, depending on the extent of fibrosis. Venous sinuses are distended with red cells and surrounded by hemosiderin-laden macrophages. Later, because of hypoxia and infarcts, splenic parenchyma becomes atrophic and fibrotic. Foci of old hemorrhage persist as **Gamna–Gandy bodies**, fibrotic nodules with iron and calcium salts encrusted on collagen and elastin fibers.

Infiltrative Splenomegaly

Increased cellularity or deposits of extracellular material, as in amyloidosis, may cause splenomegaly. Splenic macrophages accumulate in chronic infections, hemolytic anemias and a variety of storage diseases (see Chapter 6). Diverse neoplastic and reactive bone marrow diseases may lead to EMH and corresponding increases in spleen size. Malignant cells may infiltrate the spleen in hematologic proliferations, like leukemias and lymphomas, and in virus-associated hemophagocytic syndrome.

Splenomegaly Caused by Cysts and Tumors

Splenic cysts are rare. They are lined by epithelial cells, in contrast to pseudocysts, which are more common and have fibrous walls. Hydatid, or echinococcal, cysts are the most common cysts worldwide, in areas endemic for *Echinococcus granulosus* (see Chapter 9). They are quite rare in the United States.

Primary splenic neoplasms are also rare. Vascular tumors are the most common nonhematopoietic neoplasms of the spleen, including such benign tumors as **hemangiomas** and **lymphangiomas**. Hemangiomas, from minute to very large, are usually cavernous (see Chapter 16), with large endothelium-lined spaces. Other benign tumors include littoral cell angiomas and hemangioendotheliomas.

The most common primary malignant tumors of the spleen are angiosarcomas. Splenic angiosarcomas are rare, highly malignant neoplasms of vascular endothelial cells that tend to metastasize to the liver via the portal drainage. Other malignancies, such as malignant non-Hodgkin lymphomas or HL, usually affect the spleen as part of generalized disease. Two exceptions are worth mentioning: **Splenic marginal zone lymphoma**, a B-cell neoplasm, and **hepatosplenic T-cell lymphoma**, an aggressive lymphoma of

cytotoxic T-cells of γ/δ T-cell receptor type. These two lymphomas, originate in the spleen, and lymphadenopathy and extranodal sites are usually absent.

Despite its large blood supply and filtering function, the spleen is only rarely involved by metastatic solid tumors, and then only in the setting of wildly metastatic cancers.

Thymus

The thymus elaborates many factors (thymic hormones) that play key roles in maturation of the immune system and development of immune tolerance. On this basis, we discuss certain entities associated with thymus abnormalities in this chapter.

ANATOMY AND FUNCTION

The thymus derives embryologically from the third pair of pharyngeal pouches, with inconstant contributions from the fourth pair. The organ is irregularly pyramidal, with its base inferiorly and its two lobes fused in the midline. Its fibrous capsule extends into the parenchyma, forming septa that delimit lobules. It is largest, relative to body size and weight, at birth, when it averages ≈15 g. It grows until puberty, when it may weigh 30 to 40 g.

Thymic lobules have outer cortices densely with packed lymphocytes (**thymocytes**) and inner medullas, with many more epithelial cells and fewer thymocytes. Thymocytes mingle with a few epithelial and mesenchymal cells. **Hassall corpuscles** are medullary structures that are focally keratinized, concentric aggregates of epithelial cells

The thymus is the key site for T-lymphocyte differentiation (see Chapter 4). It also has a small population of neuroendocrine cells, which may explain how neuroendocrine tumors arise there. There is also a complement of myoid cells of uncertain function, which resemble striated muscle cells but are felt to be epithelial cells.

The thymus starts to involute at puberty. Initially, cortical thymocytes are decreased relative to epithelial cells. Eventually, the thymus is little more than islands of epithelial cells with few lymphocytes, and with aggregates of Hassall corpuscles separated by adipose tissue. As a result of involution, numbers of naïve T-cells leaving the thymus decrease significantly and are much lower after age 45 to 50.

In older adults, diminished T-cell function has significant consequences. Dramatically decreased T-cell receptor diversity reduces the repertoire needed to protect from new viral infections. Decreased numbers of CD4 T-cells impair antibody responses, because CD4 (helper) T-cells are important in stimulating B-cells. Also, decreased T regulatory cells (Tregs) leads to increased autoimmunity, since Tregs help to keep the immune system "in check" by limiting autoimmune responses.

AGENESIS AND DYSPLASIA

Abnormal thymus structure may vary from complete absence (agenesis) or severe hypoplasia to a small thymus, but with normal architecture. Some small glands may show thymic dysplasia: they lack thymocytes, have few if any Hassall corpuscles and contain only epithelial components. Various

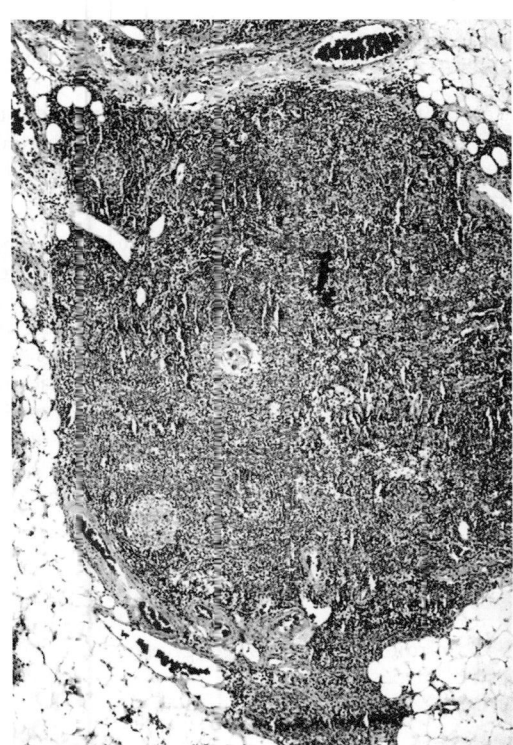

FIGURE 26-84. Thymic hyperplasia. This thymus removed from a patient with myasthenia gravis shows lymphoid follicles with germinal centers.

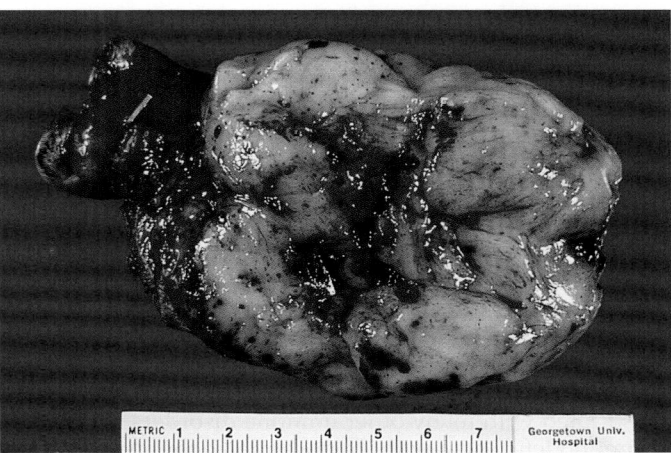

FIGURE 26-85. Thymoma. The tumor in cross-section is whitish and has a bulging surface with areas of hemorrhage. Note the attached portion of normal thymus.

developmental anomalies are associated with immune deficiencies (see Chapter 4) and hematologic disorders.

THYMIC HYPERPLASIA

The presence of lymphoid follicles in the thymus defines thymic hyperplasia (Fig. 26-84). The total gland weight is usually normal, but it may be slightly increased. The follicles contain germinal centers, largely with B-lymphocytes producing IgM and IgD. These follicles tend to occupy and distort medullary zones.

Thymic hyperplasia occurs in 2/3 of patients with myasthenia gravis (see Chapter 31). Interestingly, thymic epithelial and myoid cells contain nicotinic acetylcholine receptor protein, which may stimulate development of antibodies against that receptor. Thymic follicular hyperplasia also occurs in other autoimmune diseases, for example, Graves disease, Addison disease, SLE, scleroderma, and rheumatoid arthritis.

THYMOMA

Thymomas are neoplasms of thymic epithelial cells. Most thymomas occur in adult life and most (80%) are benign. There are no known risk factors, but there is strong association with myasthenia gravis and other paraneoplastic syndromes.

PATHOLOGY: Most thymomas arise in the anterior mediastinum, but rarely occur in the neck, middle and posterior mediastinum, and pulmonary hilus. Benign thymomas are irregularly shaped

masses of a few centimeters to 15 cm or more. They are encapsulated, firm and gray to yellow tumors that are divided into lobules by fibrous septa (Fig. 26-85). Large thymomas may have foci of hemorrhage, necrosis, and cystic degeneration.

Thymomas contain a mixture of neoplastic epithelial cells and nontumorous T-lymphocytes (Fig. 26-86). Proportions of these elements vary from case to case, and even among different lobules. Epithelial cells are plump or spindle shaped, with vesicular nuclei. If epithelial cells predominate, they may show organoid arrangement, including perivascular spaces with lymphocytes and macrophages, tumor cell rosettes and whorls suggesting abortive Hassall corpuscles. Because normal thymus contains immature T-cells, differentiating a thymoma—with tumor epithelial cells admixed with immature benign T-cells—from ATLL, a malignant tumor of immature T-cells without an epithelial component—may be challenging.

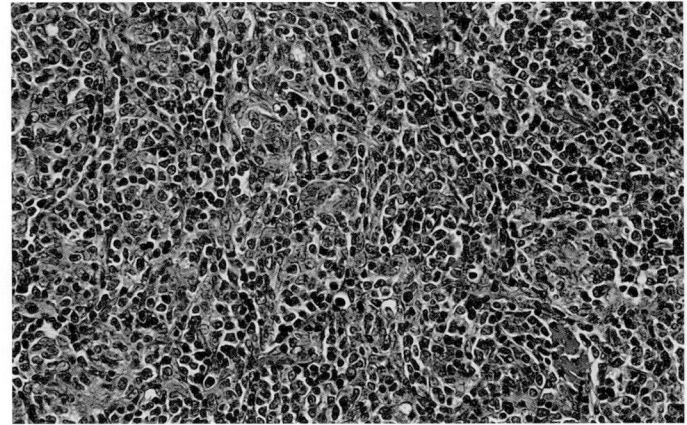

FIGURE 26-86. Microscopic features of thymomas. The tumor consists of a mixture of neoplastic epithelial cells and nontumorous lymphocytes.

MYASTHENIA GRAVIS: Myasthenia gravis (MG) is an autoimmune condition in which antibodies against neuromuscular junction acetylcholine receptors of voluntary muscle interfere with neurotransmission. It presents as weakness, fatigue, diplopia, ptosis, and dysphagia. Fifteen percent of MG patients have thymomas. Conversely, up to 1/2 of patients with thymomas develop myasthenia gravis.

Thymomas associated with myasthenic symptoms, show plump—rather than spindly—epithelial cells. Thymic hyperplasia is almost always present in the nontumorous thymic tissue, and lymphoid follicles may even be present in the thymoma itself.

OTHER ASSOCIATED DISEASES: Thymomas are associated with many other immune disorders including immunodeficiency with hypogammaglobulinemia and pure white cell aplasia, or PRCA. Unlike patients with MG, in such patients the epithelial component of the thymoma is spindle shaped. Other thymoma-associated signs and symptoms are skin eruptions, chronic diarrhea, and elevated liver enzymes.

The prognosis for benign thymomas is generally good. The presence or absence of myasthenic symptoms has little prognostic value.

Thymic Carcinomas Invade Locally and May Metastasize

Thymic carcinomas are overtly malignant epithelial tumors with cytologic atypia, invasive margins, and distorted lobular architecture.

PATHOLOGY: Pathology of thymic carcinomas is very variable, although all have a characteristic dense fibrocollagenous stroma without organotypical features in the carcinoma component Necrosis is common. Thymic carcinomas are: squamous cell carcinomas, undifferentiated carcinomas, lymphoepithelioma-like carcinomas (identical to those in the oropharynx; see Chapter 29), spindle cell (sarcomatoid) carcinoma and other rare patterns.

CLINICAL FEATURES: Thymic carcinomas are treated by surgical excision and radiation. Chemotherapy is added in cases with distant metastases. For thymic carcinomas, prognosis correlates with the extent of disease.

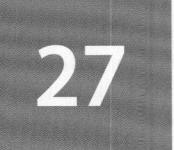

27 The Endocrine System

Krzysztof Glomski, Vania Nosé

Endocrine Signaling Integrates the Body's Functions

The main function of the endocrine system is communication of physiologic messages. Although the nervous and endocrine systems use some common soluble mediators and sometimes overlap functionally, the endocrine system is unique in its ability to communicate at a distance using soluble mediators, called hormones.

The term **hormone** (from the Greek, *horman,* "set in motion") applies to chemicals secreted by "ductless" (i.e., endocrine or neuroendocrine) cells within an endocrine organ *directly into the circulation* to deliver hormones to target tissues, which, in turn, enact physiologic responses through the binding of *hormone receptors*. To qualify as a hormone, a chemical messenger must bind a receptor, whether on a cell's surface (such as thyroid-stimulating hormone receptor [TSHR]) or inside of it (as in steroid hormone receptors). Anatomically, hormones may act over short distances on specific targets (e.g., hypothalamic hormones travel in the hypothalamic–pituitary portal system to affect the adjacent pituitary gland), or travel great distances and generate global effects (e.g., catecholamines generated by the adrenal medulla leading to a "fight or flight" response).

Hormones may act either on the final effector target or on glands that, in turn, produce their own hormones. For instance, TSH released by the pituitary gland promotes thyroid hormone secretion by the thyroid gland. Thyroid hormone affects metabolism in many types of cells in the body and also provides *feedback inhibition* to the pituitary gland to decrease TSH production.

As illustrated in the above example, hormones may lead to stimulation/production/activation of an effector pathway or inhibition/downregulation of that pathway. The exquisite balance of stimulatory and inhibitory feedback is constantly at work across all endocrine pathways to maintain homeostasis.

Clinically, endocrine disorders are divided into those caused by excess hormone production/signaling and those resulting from failure of a hormone pathway to function (lack of hormone, its target receptor, or intracellular components required for downstream effects). Mechanisms of endocrine disorders are diverse and include (but are not limited to): developmental anomalies or genetic mutations, infections, vascular pathologies, neoplasms, autoimmune diseases, toxins, and medical interventions (surgery and/or medications). As individual endocrine organs and diseases are reviewed, understanding normal signaling and feedback components allows intuitive deduction of the effects and manifestations of endocrine pathologies.

Pituitary Gland

THE PITUITARY GLAND PLAYS A MAJOR ROLE IN ENDOCRINE SIGNALING

The pituitary gland (also called *hypophysis*) is a small ($1.3 \times 0.9 \times 0.5$ cm) gland that weighs approximately 0.5 g. It is located in the anteroinferior, midline surface of the brain near the optic nerve and cavernous sinuses. It resides deep in the skull within a bony cavity called the sella turcica. Because of its location near the optic chiasm and cranial nerves III, IV, V, and VI, pituitary enlargement may alter vision or cause nerve palsies through compression.

Anatomically, the pituitary is composed of two lobes: an anterior and a posterior. The anterior lobe, or **adenohypophysis**, arises from the ectoderm, comprises about 80% of the gland volume, and is populated by various hormone-producing epithelial cells within a rich vascular network. The anterior lobe develops from the **Rathke pouch**, an evagination from the developing oral cavity (the craniopharyngeal duct). Along its migration tract, the craniopharyngeal duct may leave squamous epithelial rests that can give rise to tumors known as **craniopharyngiomas**.

The anterior pituitary gland relies on a portal venous system through which it is connected to the hypothalamus. The hypothalamus controls release of hormones by the anterior pituitary gland by releasing its own hormones from hypothalamic neurons into the hypothalamic–pituitary portal circulation, which then stimulate (or inhibit) anterior pituitary epithelial cells. Venous drainage from the pituitary flows through the cavernous sinus to bilateral inferior petrosal sinuses, which then joins the general circulation at the internal jugular veins, leading to dissemination of pituitary hormones throughout the body.

The posterior lobe, or **neurohypophysis**, originates from the neuroectoderm as a prolongation of the hypothalamus. The posterior lobe begins as a downward projection of the brain and remains connected to the hypothalamus via the hypophyseal stalk by way of axons and unmyelinated nerve fibers (hypothalamohypophysial tract) (Fig. 27-1). These nerves regulate secretion of **arginine vasopressin (antidiuretic hormone [ADH])** and **oxytocin**, which are made in

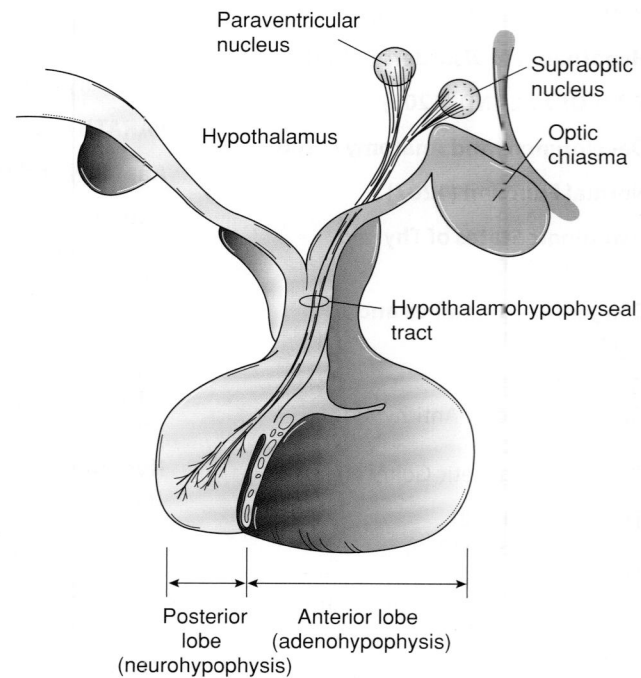

FIGURE 27-1. Anatomy of the pituitary gland. The anterior pituitary gland is immediately inferior to the optic chiasm. The hypothalamohypophyseal tract connects the hypothalamus to the posterior pituitary gland.

the hypothalamus, stored in the posterior pituitary lobe, and released into the systemic circulation upon stimulation. ADH promotes water resorption from distal renal tubules; oxytocin stimulates contraction of the pregnant uterus at term and also of cells around lactiferous ducts in the breasts.

The anterior pituitary produces six major hormone products (**adrenocorticotropic hormone, follicle-stimulating hormone (FSH), luteinizing hormone (LH), prolactin, growth hormone (GH), and TSH**) from various anterior pituitary cell types under the control of hypothalamic signals. These anterior pituitary hormones have downstream effects on numerous target organs, as summarized in Figure 27-2.

Traditionally, the cell types of the anterior pituitary were subclassified by their staining patterns in routine histologic sections (basophilic, acidophilic, or chromophobe). Immunohistochemistry is now used to subcategorize these cells by staining of hormones and/or transcription factors.

The cell types of the anterior pituitary include:

- **Corticotrophs:** These basophilic cells secrete **proopiomelanocortin (POMC)** under the control of corticotropin-releasing hormone (CRH) from the hypothalamus. POMC is then cleaved into derivatives including **adrenocorticotropic hormone (ACTH, corticotropin)**, which controls adrenal secretion of **corticosteroids**,

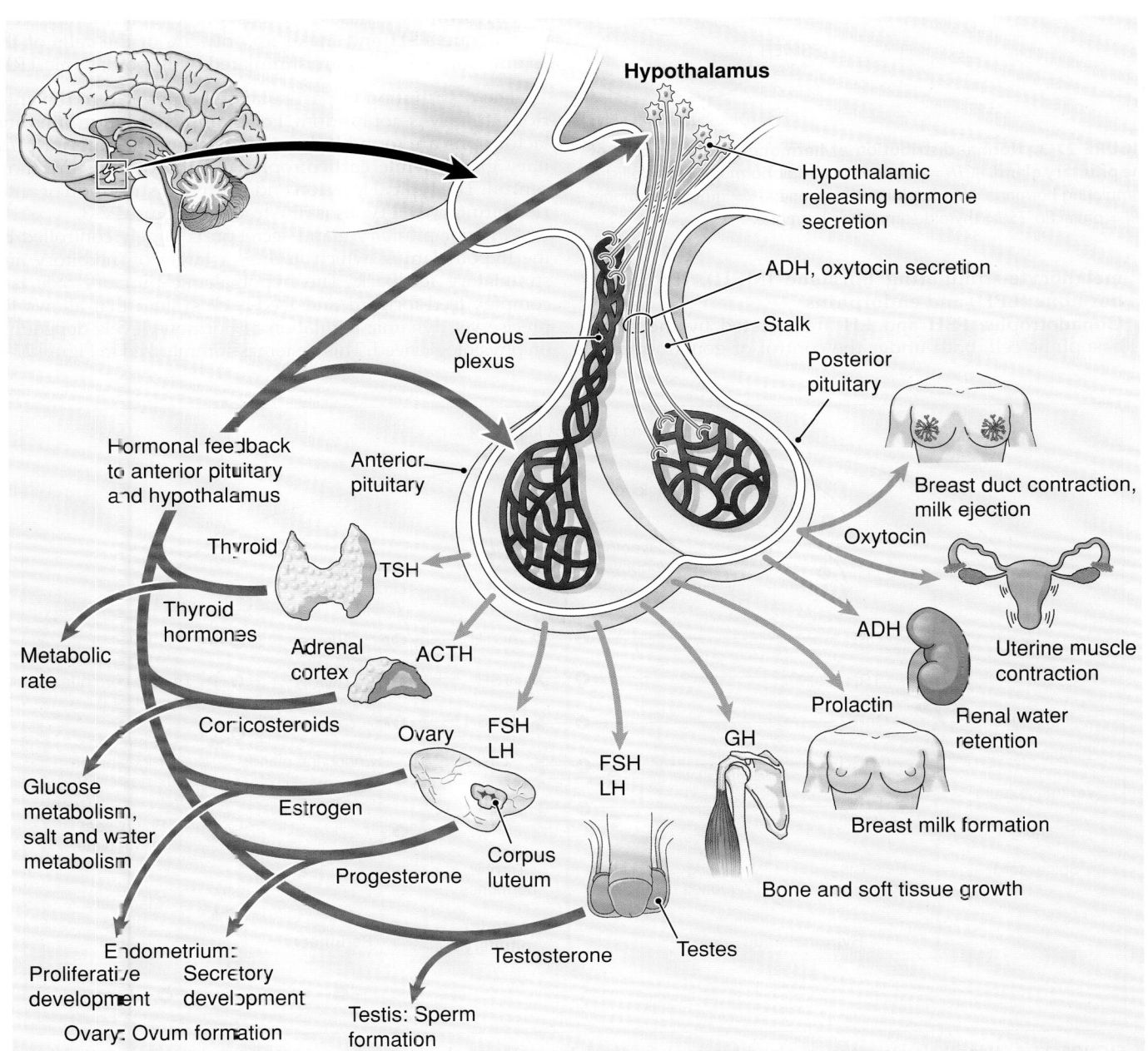

FIGURE 27-2. The hypothalamic–pituitary axis showing target-organ stimulation by pituitary hormones. *ADH* = antidiuretic hormone; *ACTH* = adrenocorticotropic hormone; *FSH* = follicle-stimulating hormone; *LH* = luteinizing hormone; *GH* = growth hormone; *TSH* = thyroid-stimulating hormone. (Reprinted with permission from McConnell TH. *The Nature of Disease Pathology for the Health Professions.* 2nd ed. Philadelphia, PA: Wolters Kluwer; 2014.)

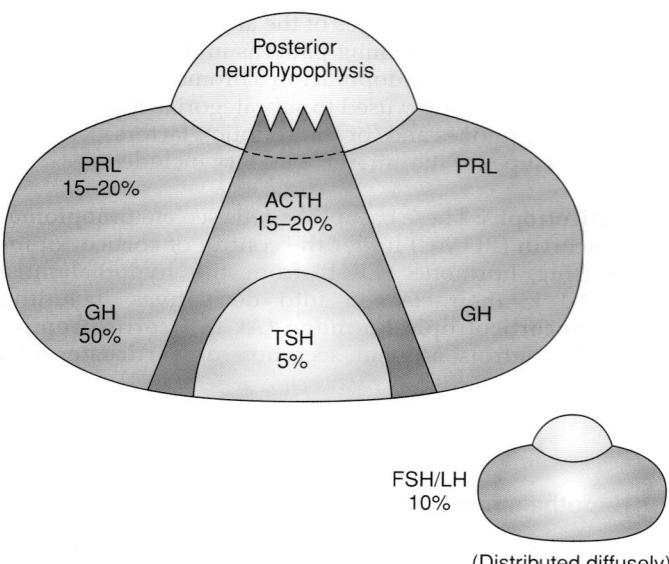

FIGURE 27-3. Normal distribution of hormone-producing cells of the pituitary gland. *ACTH* = adrenocorticotropic hormone; *FSH* = follicle-stimulating hormone; *LH* = luteinizing hormone; *GH* = growth hormone; *PRL* = prolactin; *TSH* = thyroid-stimulating hormone.

melanocyte-stimulating hormone (MSH), lipotropic hormone (LPH) and **endorphins**.

■ **Gonadotrophs: FSH** and **LH** are secreted by the same basophilic cell, both under the control of gonadotropin-

releasing hormone (GnRH) from the hypothalamus. FSH and LH are critical for gonadal development and function in both sexes.

■ **Lactotrophs:** These acidophilic cells secrete **prolactin**, which is essential for lactation and other metabolic activities. Its production is regulated by hypothalamic release of numerous factors including thyrotropin-releasing hormone (TRH) (stimulatory) and dopamine (inhibitory).

■ **Somatotrophs:** These acidophilic cells produce and secrete **GH** and constitute half of the hormone-producing cells of the adenohypophysis. GH has global effects on musculoskeletal growth. Hypothalamic GH-releasing hormone (GHRH) regulates GH secretion.

■ **Mammosomatotrophs:** Cells that secrete both prolactin and GH.

■ **Thyrotrophs:** These pale basophilic/amphophilic cells generate **TSH** and make up only 5% of the cells of the anterior lobe. They are stimulated by hypothalamic TRH.

The distribution of particular cell types within the anterior pituitary is not random. For example, somatotrophs and lactotrophs are found in lateral aspects of the anterior pituitary gland, while corticotrophs and thyrotrophs are more central. The typical location and relative distribution of anterior pituitary cell types is illustrated in Figure 27-3.

Anterior pituitary gland secretion is largely controlled by the hypothalamus, which itself is a target of inhibitory and stimulatory feedback. The hypothalamic–pituitary axis is a complex feed-forward and feed-back system that allows for precise yet dynamic regulation of hormone levels depending on physiologic need. This system is summarized in Figure 27-4.

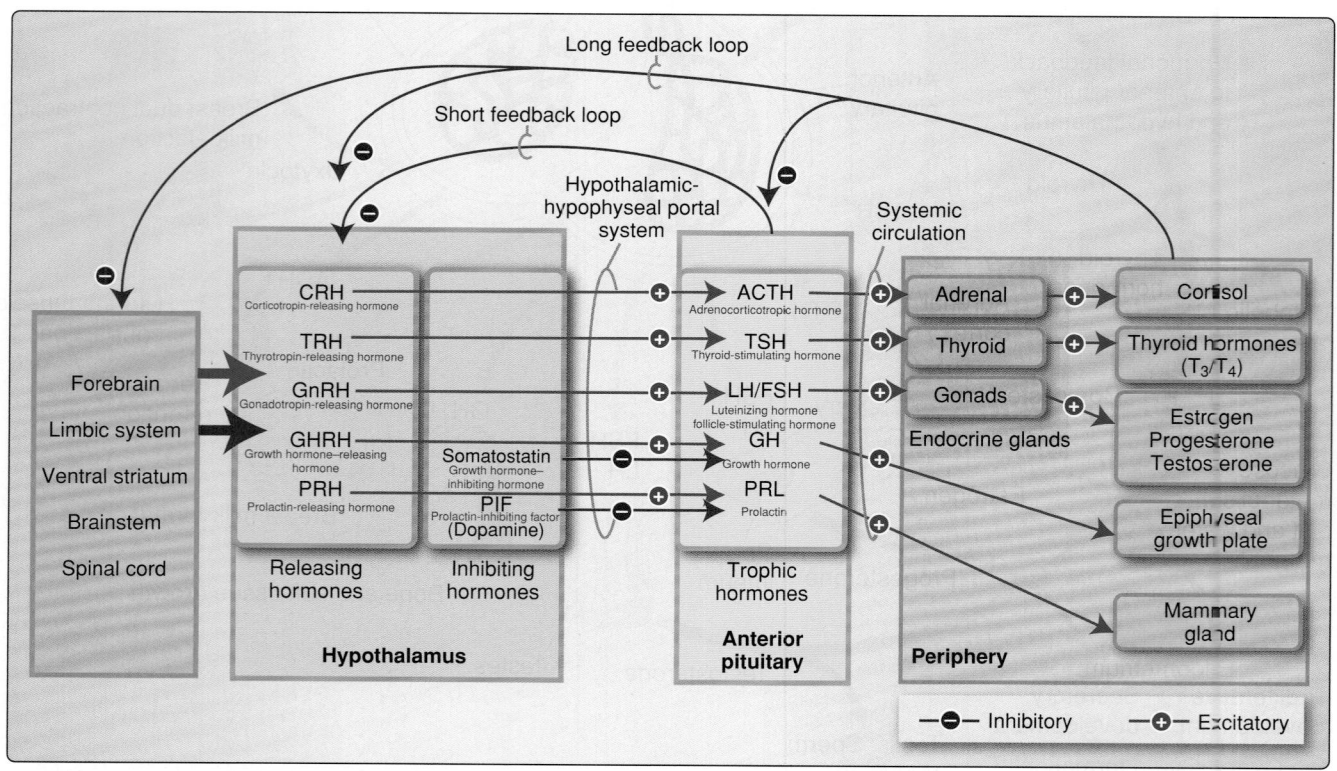

FIGURE 27-4. Hypothalamic–pituitary gland hormone feedback loops. Hypothalamic stimulating hormones induce pituitary hormone production. These hormones stimulate target organs and simultaneously inhibit the hypothalamus (short feedback loop). The products of target organs in the periphery provide negative feedback to both the pituitary gland and hypothalamus (long feedback loop). (Reprinted with permission from Krebs C, Weinberg J, Akesson E. *Lippincott's Illustrated Reviews: Neuroscience.* 1st ed. Philadelphia, PA: Lippincott Williams & Wilkins; 2012.)

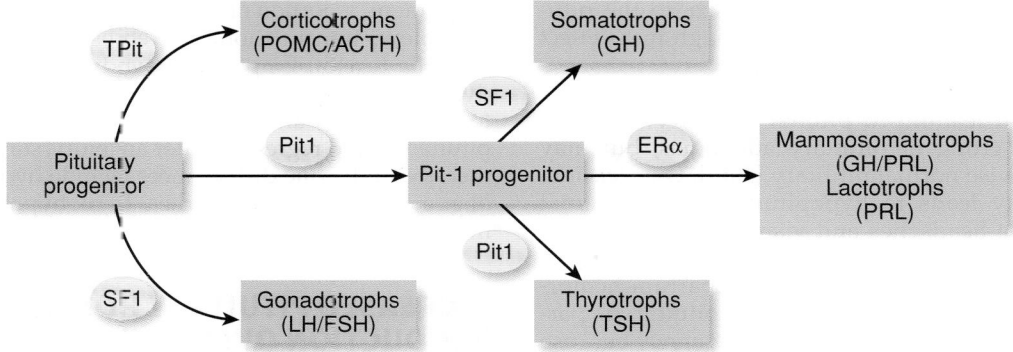

FIGURE 27-5. Transcription factors involved in pituitary epithelial-cell development and differentiation. *ACTH* = adrenocorticotropic hormone; *POMC* = proopiomelanocortin; *FSH* = follicle-stimulating hormone; *LH* = luteinizing hormone; *GH* = growth hormone; *PRL* = prolactin; *TSH* = thyroid-stimulating hormone.

All anterior pituitary cells derive from a common stem cell. Differentiation of these stem cells into specific cell types is controlled by several transcription factors, including Pit-1, Tpit, and SF-1. Pit-1 is a master transcription factor regulating expression of GH in somatotrophs, TSH in thyrotrophs (in conjunction with TEF and GATA2), and prolactin in mammotrophs (in conjunction with ERα). Tpit is critical for POMC production in corticotrophs, while SF-1 is important for LH and FSH production in gonadotrophs (Fig. 27-5).

INSUFFICIENT PITUITARY HORMONE PRODUCTION INTERRUPTS ENDOCRINE FUNCTION

Hypopituitarism is a rare disorder in which the pituitary secretes insufficient amounts of one or more hormones. It has many causes and various clinical presentations. Most often, only one or a few pituitary hormones are deficient. Occasionally **panhypopituitarism** occurs, in which the gland fails totally. The effects of hypopituitarism vary with the extent of the loss, specific hormones involved and age of the patient. In general, symptoms relate to deficient function of the thyroid and adrenal glands and the reproductive system. In children, growth retardation and delayed puberty are also seen. Deficiencies of pituitary hormones are treated with supplementation.

Anomalous Pituitary Development May Lead to Hypothyroidism

Several mutations targeting transcription factors during embryogenesis may lead to combined pituitary hormone deficiencies. Loss-of-function mutations in several genes have been identified, including *PROP1* (causing deficiency in LH, FSH, GH, PRL, and TSH), *PIT1* (deficiency in GH, prolactin, and TSH), and *HESX1* (midline forebrain abnormalities, optic nerve hypoplasia, and deficiencies in GH, TSH, and ACTH).

Congenital GH deficiency constitutes a unique group of disorders. It may occur in isolation, as in **isolated growth hormone deficiency** (IGHD), or together with other pituitary hormone deficiencies (as above). There are four types of familial and sporadic IGHD, differentiated by severity, inheritance pattern and causative gene. Inheritance can be autosomal recessive (AR), autosomal dominant (AD) or X-linked recessive. Inherited IGHD is linked to mutations, including

deletions, amino acid substitutions and splice site variants in genes for human GH or growth hormone–releasing hormone (GHRH) receptor signaling. Replacement with recombinant GH is the treatment of choice for children with this disorder.

Hypopituitarism Has Many Causes

Pituitary hypofunction is often due to extrinsic factors impeding or impinging on the gland, and include neoplastic, vascular, infectious, inflammatory, or traumatic causes.

Over half of hypopituitarism in adults is caused by pituitary tumors, usually adenomas, which may be nonfunctional (nonhormone secreting) and result in adjacent gland compression with subsequent hypofunction. Occasionally, cystic lesions, including **Rathke cleft cysts**, may manifest as hypopituitarism through similar compressive mechanisms (Fig. 27-6). Due to the rich vascular supply of the pituitary

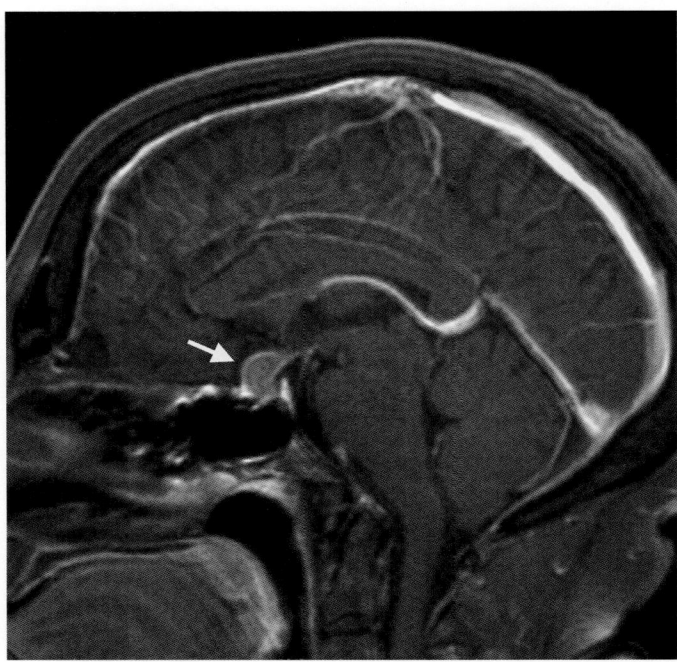

FIGURE 27-6. Rathke cleft cyst. A magnetic resonance image of a cystic lesion in the region of the pituitary gland (*arrow*) represents a Rathke cleft cyst that caused compressive hypopituitarism.

gland, advanced carcinomas may metastasize to the pituitary gland and cause hypopituitarism through mass effect or infarction.

Pituitary apoplexy describes either hemorrhage or vascular occlusion leading to pituitary failure. Typically, it occurs in the setting of pituitary adenomas, but may occur in an otherwise normal pituitary gland. On occasion, pituitary apoplexy leads to hypopituitarism. The initial symptoms include headaches and visual problems. **Sheehan syndrome** describes ischemic necrosis of the pituitary gland secondary to hypotension from postpartum hemorrhage or, rarely, after normal delivery. The pituitary is particularly vulnerable to ischemia during pregnancy because of its marked enlargement, and even small changes in blood pressure to the gland may result in irreversible ischemic necrosis and hypopituitarism. Agalactia, amenorrhea, hypothyroidism, and adrenocortical insufficiency may develop. Sheehan syndrome is rare in developed countries.

Bacteria, fungi, mycobacteria, and viruses may damage the pituitary either by primary infection or as part of a disseminated infection (as in fungemia, bacterial sepsis, or active tuberculosis). Other etiologies include vasculitides such as granulomatosis with polyangiitis, autoimmune conditions (e.g., sarcoidosis, Crohn disease), deposition diseases (e.g., Wilson disease, amyloidosis, hemochromatosis), Langerhans cell histiocytosis, or primary lymphocytic hypophysitis.

Therapy-related (iatrogenic) hypophysitis may be caused by radiation, medications, surgeries, or intravascular interventions. These therapeutic interventions may damage the pituitary gland directly, or affect its blood supply, leading to neuroendocrine abnormalities, including hypopituitarism. Similarly, high-energy traumatic injuries may result in hypopituitarism and other endocrinopathies secondary to vascular or gland trauma.

Empty sella syndrome is primarily a radiologic term for an enlarged sella containing a thin, flattened pituitary at the base (Fig. 27-7). It is due to a congenitally defective or absent sellar

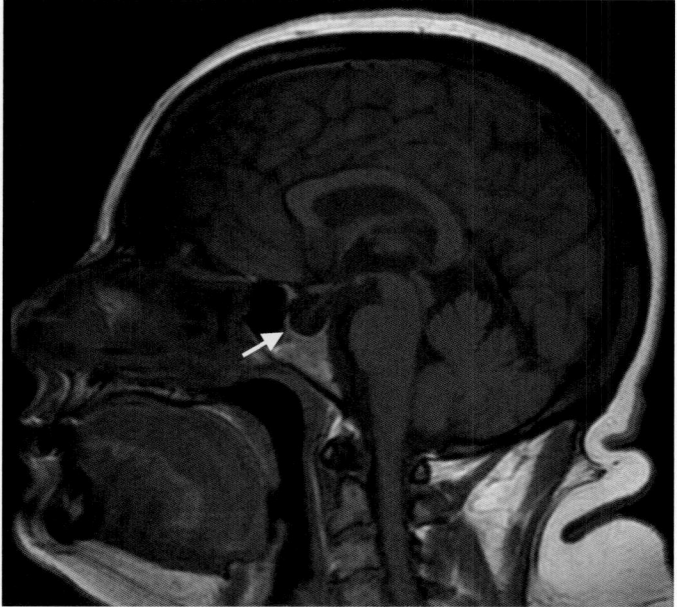

FIGURE 27-7. Empty sella syndrome. A sagittal magnetic resonance image demonstrating the absence of pituitary gland in the empty bony sella turcica (*arrow*).

diaphragm, a portion of the dura mater with a circular orifice that allows transmission of cerebrospinal fluid pressure into the sella turcica. Empty sella syndrome can cause pituitary dysfunction and endocrine abnormalities. It has been linked to both pituitary and nonpituitary causes and can result from pituitary gland regression after an injury, surgery, or radiation therapy. Endocrine disturbances include hyperprolactinemia, oligomenorrhea or amenorrhea, frank hypopituitarism, acromegaly, diabetes insipidus, and Cushing syndrome.

INCREASED PITUITARY HORMONE PRODUCTION OVERSTIMULATES THE ENDOCRINE SYSTEM

Excess production of one or more pituitary hormones is known as hyperpituitarism and may be due to pituitary hyperplasia or pituitary neoplasia (most commonly adenoma). Pituitary hyperplasia is defined as expansion of an adenohypophyseal cell population due to an extrapituitary stimulus, which is reversible if the stimulus is removed. Pituitary hyperplasia occurs in the context of normal pituitary architecture (the fibrovascular support structure of the pituitary is maintained) and may be physiologic (e.g., pregnancy) or pathologic (e.g., CRH-producing tumor). By contrast, pituitary adenomas are neoplasms of adenohypophyseal cells that arise within the pituitary gland, grow independent of external stimuli, and alter or destroy the underlying architecture of the gland and possibly surrounding structures.

Pituitary Hyperplasia

Lactotroph hyperplasia is most commonly physiologic, as in the pregnancy/postpartum period, when lactotrophs expand in size and number to meet lactational demand. In addition, antidopaminergic agents, such as those used in certain psychiatric medications, disinhibit the usual inhibitory stimulus dopamine imparts on lactotrophs, and may lead to lactotroph hyperplasia.

Corticotroph hyperplasia is most commonly due to CRH-producing tumors, either in the hypothalamus, or, more commonly, from neuroendocrine tumors of other sites. Corticotroph hyperplasia may result in excess ACTH production and hypercortisolism (Cushing syndrome, see below). Similarly, somatotroph hyperplasia is most commonly secondary to neuroendocrine tumors that produce GHRH, which results in excess GH production and may lead to acromegaly or gigantism (see below).

Thyrotroph and/or gonadotroph hyperplasia usually arises from a lack of feedback inhibition by thyroid hormone and/or sex hormones, respectively, on the hypothalamus. Normally, secretion of TRH by the hypothalamus is inhibited by the thyroid hormone. Thus, absence of the thyroid hormone (e.g., in hypothyroidism or postthyroidectomy) results in high TRH production by the hypothalamus and thyrotroph hyperplasia. An analogous mechanism occurs in gonadotroph hyperplasia, with GnRH secretion by the hypothalamus as the stimulus in the setting of gonadal hypofunction or absence.

Pituitary Adenomas Are Benign Pituitary Tumors That May Produce Hormone

Pituitary adenomas are benign neoplasms of the anterior lobe of the pituitary gland. They often secrete one or more

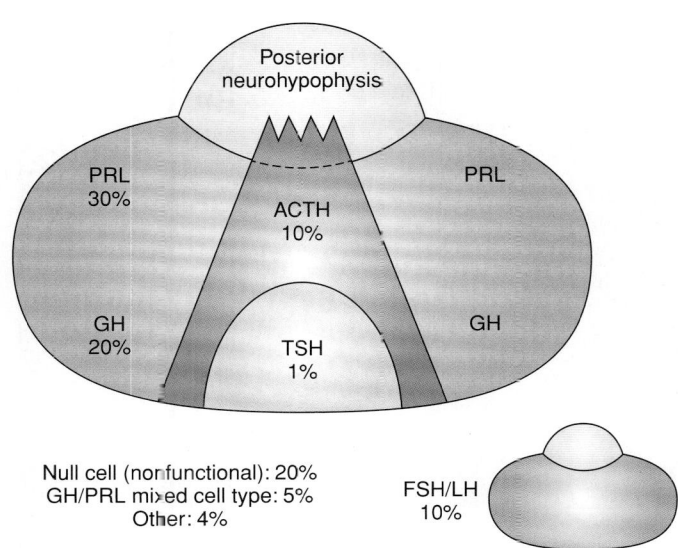

Null cell (nonfunctional): 20%
GH/PRL mixed cell type: 5%
Other: 4%

FIGURE 27-8. Relative incidence and distribution of pituitary adenomas in the pituitary gland. *ACTH* = adrenocorticotropic hormone; *FSH* = follicle-stimulating hormone; *LH* = luteinizing hormone; *GH* = growth hormone; *PRL* = prolactin; *TSH* = thyroid-stimulating hormone.

pituitary hormones which may be manifest clinically as end-organ/target organ hyperfunction. Pituitary adenomas occur in both sexes and are more common in adults. **Lactotroph adenomas** are the most common hormone-secreting tumors of adults and children while **gonadotroph adenomas** are more frequent in the elderly. Small, **nonfunctioning pituitary adenomas** are found incidentally at autopsy in up to 25% of adults without a clinical history of endocrinopathy or pituitary compressive symptoms. The relative incidence of pituitary adenoma subtypes is summarized in Figure 27-8.

 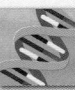 **ETIOLOGY AND MOLECULAR PATHOGENESIS:** The pathogenesis of pituitary adenomas is multifaceted, and involves hormonal, environmental, and genetic factors.

Sporadic pituitary adenomas (95% of cases) have been linked to gain-of-function mutations in *GNAS* which encodes the alpha subunit of the stimulatory G protein (G$_s$), and thus produce high levels of cAMP thought to stimulate cell proliferation. Other tumors show dysregulation of the fibroblast growth factor (FGF) and epidermal growth factor receptor (EGFR) pathways, as well as mutations in *RB1*, *CYCLIN-D1* and *p16*.

A minority of pituitary adenomas occur in familial syndromes (~5%), including multiple endocrine neoplasia type 1 (**MEN-1**), multiple endocrine neoplasia type 4 (**MEN-4**), **Carney complex, hereditary paraganglioma-pheochromocytoma**, and **familial isolated pituitary (somatotroph) adenoma syndrome** (see Table 27-1).

PATHOLOGY: In general, pituitary adenomas grow in broad sheets and disrupt lobulation of the anterior pituitary gland (Fig. 27-9A,B). In smear preparations, pituitary adenomas disperse into monolayers of homogenous cells, typically with "salt and pepper" chromatin (numerous fine and course puncta of chromatin distributed evenly in the nucleus) (Fig. 27-9C). Previously, pituitary adenomas were classified by their hematoxylin and eosin staining properties (acidophil, basophil, or chromophobe), but are now identified by immunohistochemical staining of transcription factors and hormone products (Figs. 27-5 and 27-9D). Adenomas may be classified as "atypical" if they show a proliferation index above 3% by Ki-67 staining, and/or diffuse p53 expression. Atypical adenomas are more likely to be locally invasive and/or recur.

TABLE 27-1
ENDOCRINE SYNDROMES WITH PITUITARY GLAND ADENOMA

Syndrome	Gene	Inheritance	Pituitary Adenoma Types	Other Manifestations
Multiple neuroendocrine neoplasia type 1	*MEN1*	Autosomal dominant	Lactotroph most common, nonfunctional, somatotroph, and corticotroph	Pancreatic and duodenal neuroendocrine tumors, parathyroid adenomas
Multiple neuroendocrine neoplasia type 4	*CDKN1B*	Autosomal dominant	Somatotroph most common	Pancreatic and duodenal neuroendocrine tumors, parathyroid adenomas
Carney complex	*PRKAR1A*	Autosomal dominant	Lactotroph and somatotroph most common	Skin pigmentation, soft tissue and atrial myxomas, pigmented nodular adrenocortical disease, large cell calcifying testicular Sertoli cell tumors, pigmented melanotic schwannomas, thyroid adenomas and carcinomas
Hereditary paraganglioma-pheochromocytoma syndrome	*SDHB, SDHC, SDHD*	Autosomal dominant	Somatotroph most common	Sympathetic paraganglioma (both adrenal and extra-adrenal). Some forms associated with gastrointestinal stromal tumor (Carney–Stratakis syndrome) and SDH-deficient renal cell carcinoma
Familial isolated pituitary adenoma syndrome	*AIP*	Autosomal dominant	Somatotroph and non-functioning	None

THE ENDOCRINE SYSTEM

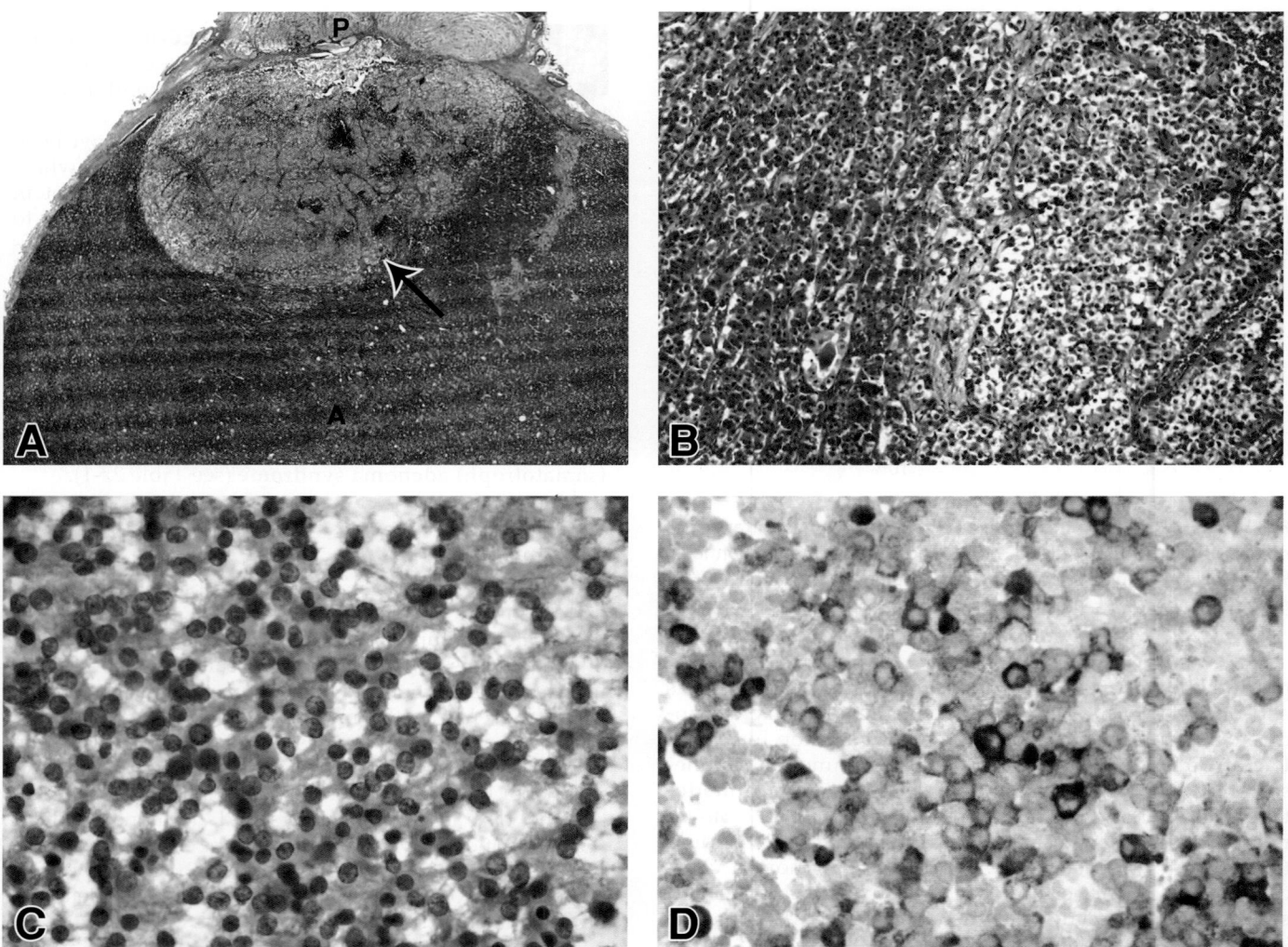

FIGURE 27-9. Pituitary adenomas. A: Pituitary adenoma arising from the central-posterior pituitary gland (*arrow*), with surrounding anterior pituitary (*A*) and posterior pituitary (*P*). **B:** Higher-power image showing expanded growth of monotonous cells (*right side* of image) adjacent to normal anterior pituitary (*left side* of image). **C:** Monotonous adenoma cells have "salt-and-pepper" type nuclear chromatin. **D:** Immunohistochemistry for ACTH reveals positivity in this corticotroph adenoma.

Pituitary adenomas range in size from small lesions that do not enlarge to expansive tumors that erode the sella turcica and impinge on adjacent cranial structures. In general, adenomas less than 1 cm are called microadenomas while larger tumors are macroadenomas. Microadenomas are typically asymptomatic unless they secrete hormones, while macroadenomas tend to cause local compression due to their size and systemic manifestations owing to overproduction of hormones.

CLINICAL FEATURES: In general, symptoms reflect the hormone produced. Pituitary macroadenomas may compress the optic chiasm, causing severe headaches, bitemporal hemianopsia and loss of central vision. Oculomotor palsies occur when a tumor invades the cavernous sinuses. Large adenomas may invade the hypothalamus, interfere with normal hypothalamic input to the pituitary and lead to loss of temperature regulation, hyperphagia and hormonal syndromes.

Lactotroph Adenomas Secrete Prolactin

Lactotroph adenomas are the most common pituitary adenomas, accounting for approximately 30% of all adenomas. They are most often symptomatic in young women who may experience amenorrhea, galactorrhea, and infertility due to disruption of normal LH surges necessary for ovulation. Men often present at an older age and tend to suffer from decreased libido and impotence. Functional lactotroph microadenomas are often treated with dopamine agonists (bromocriptine), which reduces PRL secretion and may shrink the adenoma significantly. Adenomas that do not respond to medical therapy or are large enough to cause compressive symptoms may require surgery. Prognosis is typically favorable, though less so for men than women.

PATHOLOGY: Lactotroph adenomas tend to be chromophobic and contain spheroid nuclei with prominent nucleoli. They are sparsely granulated and may show diffuse or papillary growth patterns.

They may contain endocrine amyloid (see Chapter 15) or psammoma bodies (calcospherites). Lactotroph adenomas stain for PRL in a dot-like "Golgi pattern" by immunohistochemistry and are also positive for nuclear Pit-1 and estrogen receptor. They have not been linked to characteristic mutations although abnormal expression of genes regulating the cell cycle (e.g., *RB, CDKN2A*) and FGF pathways has been reported.

Somatotroph Adenomas Overproduce GH

Somatotroph adenomas secrete GH. Excess GH secretion stimulates production of insulin-like growth factor 1 (IGF-1) in the liver, which promotes growth of muscle, bones, skin, lungs, and abdominal organs. A somatotroph adenoma arising in a child or adolescent before epiphyses close causes **gigantism**, a condition of extremely tall stature. Somatotroph adenomas arising in adults after long bone epiphyses have fused results in **acromegaly**, characterized by gradual development of coarse facial features with overgrowth of the mandible (prognathism) and maxilla, increased space between upper incisor teeth, a thickened nose, and large hands and feet (Fig. 27-10).

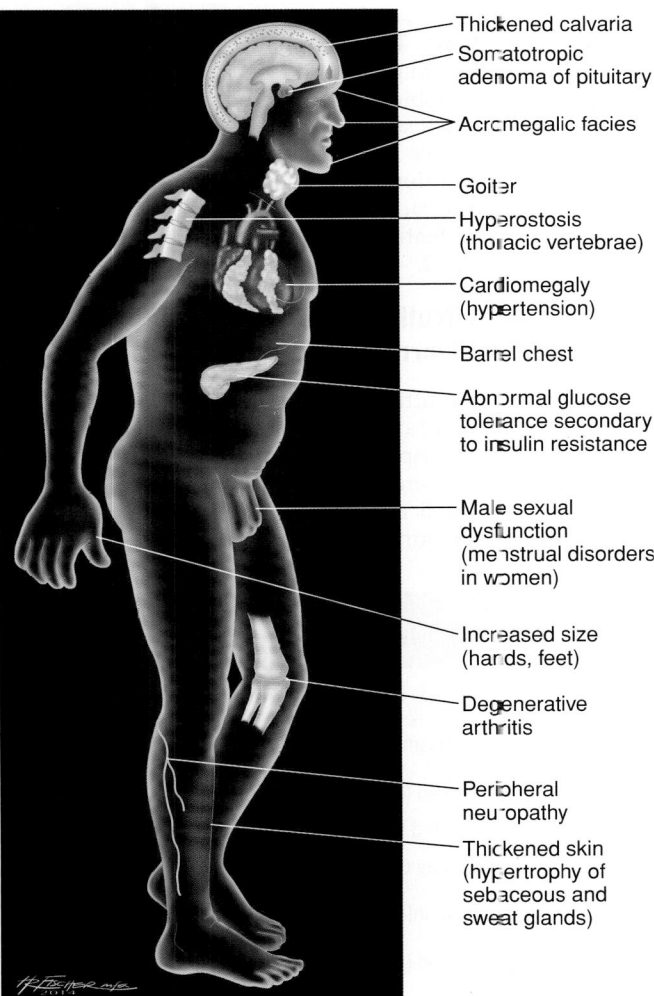

- Thickened calvaria
- Somatotropic adenoma of pituitary
- Acromegalic facies
- Goiter
- Hyperostosis (thoracic vertebrae)
- Cardiomegaly (hypertension)
- Barrel chest
- Abnormal glucose tolerance secondary to insulin resistance
- Male sexual dysfunction (menstrual disorders in women)
- Increased size (hands, feet)
- Degenerative arthritis
- Peripheral neuropathy
- Thickened skin (hypertrophy of sebaceous and sweat glands)

FIGURE 27-10. Clinical manifestations of acromegaly (growth hormone excess).

 PATHOLOGY: Of patients with acromegaly, 75% have a somatotroph macroadenoma, typically located laterally in the gland. Multiple histologic variants of somatotroph adenomas (densely granulated, sparsely granulated, mammosomatotroph, mixed somatotroph–lactotroph) have a different propensity for aggressive behavior and different responses to therapy.

Densely granulated somatotroph adenomas are more commonly associated with acromegaly and are composed of acidophilic cells with granular cytoplasm and a diffuse growth pattern. They show strong, diffuse immunohistochemical reactivity for GH and Pit-1, low proliferative indices, and tend to be less aggressive than sparsely granulated somatotropin adenomas. **Sparsely granulated somatotroph adenomas** have highly pleomorphic, chromophobe cells with prominent spheroid cytoplasmic inclusions called "fibrous bodies." They stain strongly for Pit-1 and faintly for GH. This variant tends to grow rapidly and is more likely to invade adjacent bone.

In **mixed somatotroph–lactotroph adenomas** (rare), two distinct cell types elaborate GH and PRL, respectively. **Mammosomatotroph adenomas** are monomorphous with a single cell type expressing both GH and PRL, with expression of both Pit-1 and estrogen receptor.

 CLINICAL FEATURES: Acromegaly is uncommon, with an annual incidence of three cases per million. It is usually sporadic, but may arise in MEN1 or Carney complex (see above). Acromegaly has serious complications; cardiovascular, cerebrovascular, and respiratory deaths are increased. Most acromegalics have neurologic and musculoskeletal symptoms, including headaches, paresthesias, arthralgias, and muscle weakness. One-third has hypertension, and half of normotensive acromegalics have increased left ventricular mass and are at risk for heart failure. Visceral hypertrophy is common. Diabetes and hypercalciuria with renal stones occur in up to 20%.

Definitive therapy for somatotroph adenomas is surgical resection via transsphenoidal hypophysectomy. Preoperative medical therapy with somatostatin analogs (to inhibit GH release from somatotrophs) and GH receptor antagonists (to block the effects of GH in target tissues) is designed to shrink adenomas prior to resection. Signs and symptoms resolve slowly after successful surgery, with good long-term prognosis in most cases.

Corticotroph Adenomas Produce ACTH

Corticotroph adenomas produce ACTH, which induces adrenal cortisol hypersecretion and **Cushing disease** (see below). Corticotroph adenomas account for approximately 10% of all pituitary adenomas and are usually located centrally in the gland.

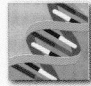 **MOLECULAR PATHOGENESIS:** The molecular pathogenesis of ACTH-producing adenomas is still emerging, though mutations in the EGFR pathway component *USP8*, which increases EGFR signaling, is believed to be a major driver.

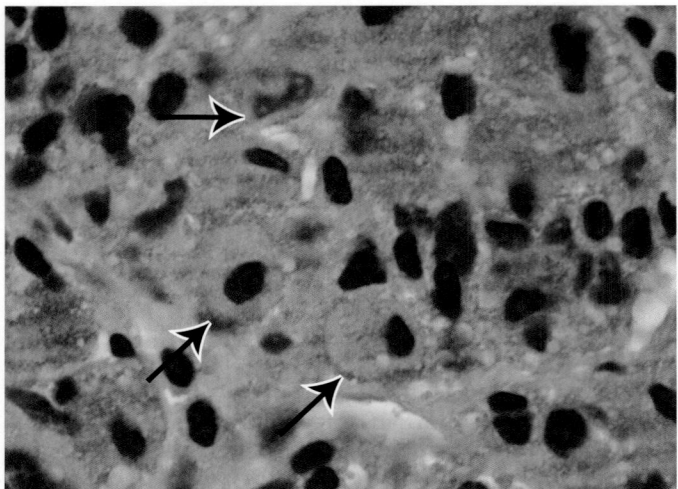

FIGURE 27-11. Micrograph of a corticotroph adenoma with Crooke hyaline change (*arrows*).

Pathologically, tumors are typically microadenomas composed of nests of basophilic and periodic acid–Schiff (PAS) positive cells. Immunohistochemistry shows ACTH (cytoplasmic), low–molecular-weight keratin (cytoplasmic), NeuroD1, and Tpit (nuclear) staining. There are numerous subtypes of corticotroph adenomas. **Densely granulated corticotroph adenomas**, the most common subtype, are basophilic and characteristically show strong staining for ACTH and PAS. **Sparsely granulated corticotroph adenomas** are chromophobic and more aggressive than densely granulated counterparts and may show pleomorphic features with apoptosis. They typically will show weaker ACTH staining and strong Tpit staining by immunohistochemistry.

By electron microscopy, basophilic adenomas contain many secretory granules and perinuclear bundles of fine, keratin-positive intermediate filaments (type I filaments). These filaments may be abundant enough to be visible by light microscopy as **Crooke hyalinization** (Fig. 27-11), which reflects suppression of ACTH secretion by high levels of circulating cortisol. **Crooke adenomas** are ACTH-producing tumors with massive cell hyaline deposition between cells, and ACTH and keratin staining typically peripheral to the cell membrane.

Surgical excision is definitive therapy, though relapse may occur, necessitating re-excision or radiation therapy.

Gonadotroph Adenomas May Produce FSH and/or LH

Most of these tumors are hormonally inactive (nonsecretory) macroadenomas and are detected either incidentally or because of local compressive effects due to suprasellar extension. They comprise approximately 10% of all pituitary adenomas and may occur anywhere in the gland. Clinical presentations include headache, visual disturbance, and hypopituitarism.

Gonadotroph adenomas are usually chromophobic and PAS-negative. They grow in a diffuse pattern with low proliferation index. Tumor cells are positive for FSH and/or LH immunostaining in the cytoplasm, and SF-1 in the nucleus. Definitive therapy is surgical.

Thyrotroph Adenomas Secrete TSH

These are the rarest of pituitary adenomas, accounting for <1% of all adenomas. They come to medical attention by producing symptoms associated with hyperthyroidism with goiter or a pituitary mass lesion. Circulating TSH *and* thyroid hormone levels are usually elevated (whereas hyperthyroidism due to primary thyroid disease causes low TSH through feedback inhibition). Thyrotroph adenomas are predominantly macroadenomas and can be invasive and fibrotic. They are chromophobic, with polyhedral or columnar cells that may form calcifications. They stain for α- and β-TSH, Pit-1, and tend to have high proliferative indices.

Surgical intervention is the therapy of choice. Infiltrative tumors may require radiation therapy.

The pathologic features of pituitary adenomas are summarized in Table 27-2.

Nonfunctional (Null-Cell) Adenomas Do Not Secrete Hormone

Approximately one-fifth of pituitary tumors does not secrete excess hormones and do not have specific lineage specificity defined by transcription factor staining. They are slowly growing macroadenomas that typically occur in older people and come to medical attention because of mass effect on the pituitary or surrounding structures.

TABLE 27-2

HISTOLOGIC AND MOLECULAR FEATURES OF PITUITARY ADENOMAS

Adenoma Type	Location	Hormone	Transcription Factors	Histologic Appearance
Lactotroph	Lateral-posterior	Prolactin	Pit1, ER	Chromophobic, psammoma bodies and amyloid may be present
Corticotroph	Central, posterior	ACTH	Tpit	Densely granulated (basophilic, indolent)
				Sparsely granulated (chromophobic, infiltrative)
				Crooks hyaline may be present
Gonadotroph	Diffuse	LH/FSH	SF1	Chromophobic, indolent
Somatotroph	Lateral-anterior	GH	Pit1, SF1	Densely granulated (indolent) and sparsely granulated (infiltrative) types
Thyrotroph	Central-anterior	TSH	Pit1	Chromophobic, high

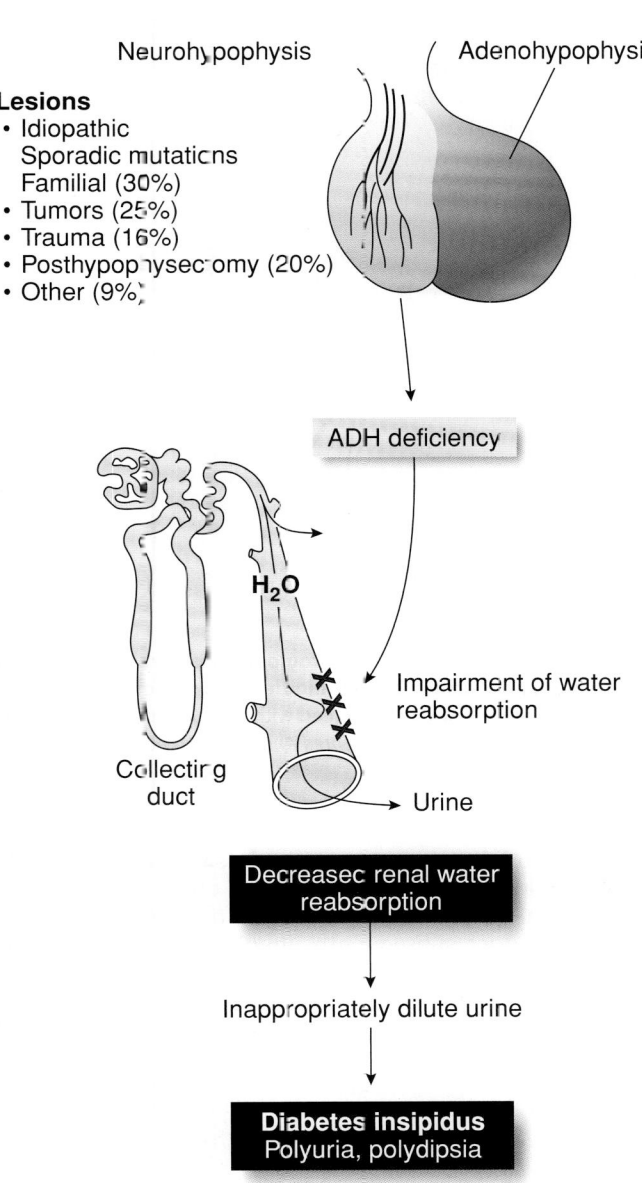

Lesions
- Idiopathic
  Sporadic mutations
  Familial (30%)
- Tumors (25%)
- Trauma (16%)
- Posthypophysectomy (20%)
- Other (9%)

FIGURE 27-12. Mechanism of central diabetes insipidus.

Null cell adenomas are usually chromophobic and arise in the adenohypophysis. They are PAS-negative and grow in a pseudopapillary pattern. While tumor cells are negative for anterior pituitary hormones and transcription factors, they do express chromogranin A and synaptophysin.

Oncocytomas are variants of nonfunctional null cell adenoma. They are composed of enlarged, eosinophilic cells, often with granular cytoplasm (called "oncocytes"). They are typically large at presentation and may extend outside the sella. Visual impairment and symptoms of hypopituitarism are common. Neoplastic cells of oncocytomas are packed with mitochondria, producing a granular appearance, but are otherwise similar to other null cell adenomas.

Pituitary Carcinoma Is Extremely Rare

It is not possible to distinguish pituitary adenomas and carcinomas on morphologic grounds, as they may appear identical. Pituitary carcinomas declare their malignant nature by spreading to cerebrospinal and/or extracranial sites (bone, lung, liver). Most pituitary carcinomas are functional (i.e., they secrete hormones) and produce endocrinopathies as seen in adenomas. Imaging studies may show tumor extension beyond the sella turcica into surrounding brain or skull base. Pituitary carcinoma carries a poor prognosis.

POSTERIOR PITUITARY DYSFUNCTION INCLUDES DIABETES INSIPIDUS

Central diabetes insipidus (C-DI) (Fig. 27-12) is the only significant disease associated with the posterior pituitary. Affected patients cannot concentrate their urine due to lack of ADH production by the posterior pituitary gland. ADH typically acts at the distal nephron to reabsorb water from urine. Patients with C-DI have chronic water diuresis (polyuria), hypernatremia, thirst, and polydipsia. ADH is secreted by the posterior pituitary under the influence of the hypothalamus. One-third of C-DI cases are of unknown etiology or are caused by sporadic or familial mutations in *AVP*, the vasopressin–neurophysin II gene.

One-fourth of C-DI cases are associated with brain tumors, especially **craniopharyngiomas** (Fig. 27-13; see Chapter 32). These tumors arise above the sella turcica from remnants of

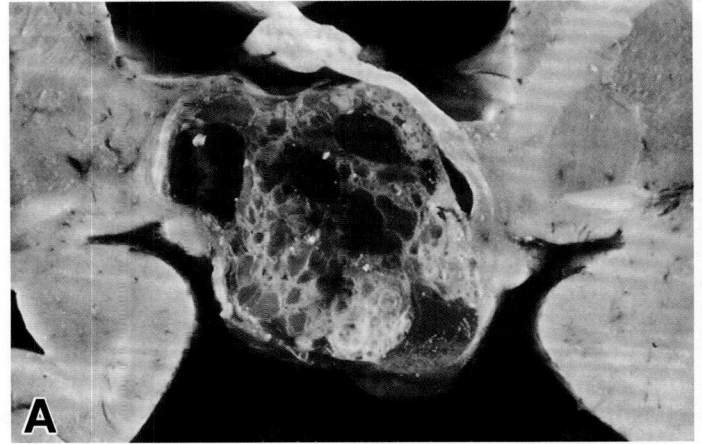

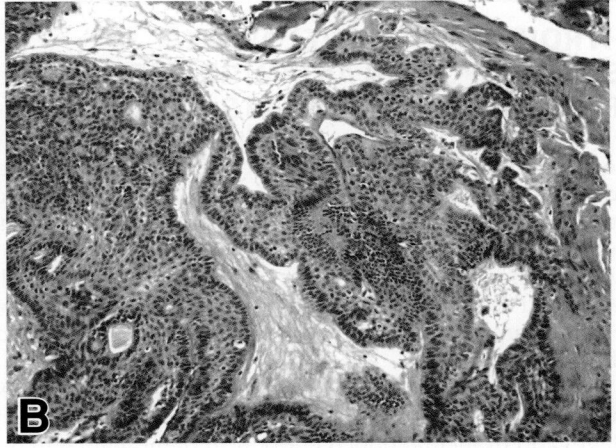

FIGURE 27-13. Craniopharyngioma. A: Gross cross-section of a craniopharyngioma showing complex material within a cystic lesion. **B:** Microscopic image of a craniopharyngioma showing islands of epithelial cells with interspersed loose keratinaceous debris.

the Rathke pouch and invade and compress adjacent tissues. Trauma and hypophysectomy for anterior pituitary tumors account for most remaining cases of diabetes insipidus. Less often, localized hemorrhage or infarction, Langerhans cell histiocytosis (see Chapter 26) or granulomatous infiltrates (as seen in sarcoidosis or tuberculosis) involve the posterior pituitary stalk or body, leading to C-DI. Polyuria may be controlled by intranasal vasopressin. A syndrome of inappropriate ADH secretion (SIADH) may be caused by paraneoplastic secretion of ADH by neuroendocrine tumors of various organs (see below).

Deletion mutations in AVPR2, the gene for the vasopressin V2 receptor, and *AQP2*, which encodes the vasopressin-sensitive aquaporin-2 water channel, may cause **nephrogenic diabetes insipidus (N-DI)**, which is characterized by normal ADH production by the posterior pituitary gland without proper response by the kidney. Other causes of N-DI include interstitial nephritis, hypercalcemia, hypokalemia, and numerous drugs (lithium, amphotericin, colchicine).

HYPOTHALAMIC DISORDERS ARE A RARE CAUSE OF PITUITARY DYSFUNCTION

The hypothalamus may be injured by primary and metastatic tumors, viral infections, and granulomatous inflammations, as well as by degenerative and hereditary disorders. Hypothalamic dysfunction may also occur without an identifiable anatomic abnormality. Clinical manifestations of hypothalamic dysfunction include hypogonadism, precocious puberty, amenorrhea, and eating disorders (obesity or anorexia) due to altered communication between the hypothalamus and pituitary gland.

A rare disorder of GnRH deficiency (Kallmann syndrome) is characterized by a deficiency in GnRH-producing neurons in the hypothalamus due to a defect in proper migration during development. This defect results in anosmia and abnormalities of sexual development (hypogonadism, amenorrhea) due to impaired LH and FSH secretion by the anterior pituitary gland.

Thyroid Gland

THYROID GLAND DEVELOPMENT RELIES ON FUSION AND MIGRATION OF MULTIPLE COMPONENTS

The thyroid is one of the largest endocrine organs in the body. In adults, it is bilobed and located in the lower neck, with the right and left lobes situated lateral to the trachea (and inferior to the thyroid cartilage) with a thin isthmus of thyroid tissue connecting the two lobes anteriorly. In adults, the thyroid weighs approximately 15 to 25 g and each lobe measures approximately 2 to 2.5 cm in width and 4 to 5 cm in length.

The thyroid gland becomes identifiable by the third week (day 24) of development. It derives from the foregut (medial anlage) and branchial pouch endoderm (lateral anlage) near the base of the tongue (foramen cecum). After forming, the medial and lateral anlage fuse and the developing thyroid

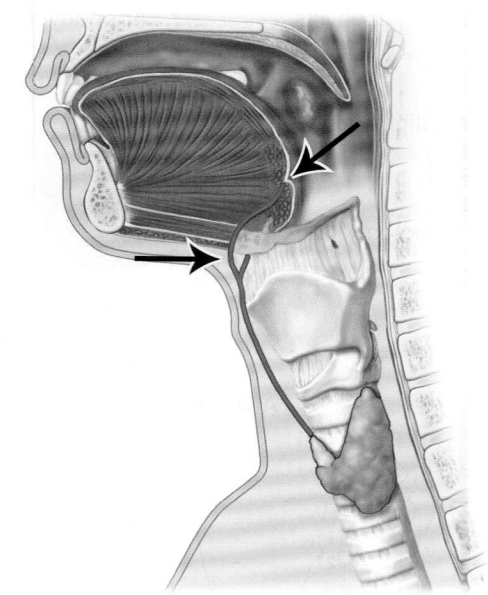

FIGURE 27-14. Course of the thyroglossal duct from the root of the tongue (*upper arrow*) to the middle neck. The duct passes over the hyoid bone (*lower arrow*). (Modified with permission from Moore KL, Dalley AF, Agur AMR. *Clinically Oriented Anatomy*. 8th ed Baltimore, MD: Wolters Kluwer; 2018: Fig B9.6A.)

descends caudally along the thyroglossal duct (Fig. 27-14) toward the lower neck; it arrives at its final position in the lower/lateral neck by the seventh week of development. The thyroglossal duct subsequently involutes, fragments, and becomes obliterated in adults. However, a small remnant persists in most adults as the pyramidal lobe of the thyroid, a superior extension of thyroid tissue contiguous with the isthmus (Fig. 27-15). Thyroid gland follicles form at approximately 12 weeks of development, and thyroid hormone is produced by the fetus.

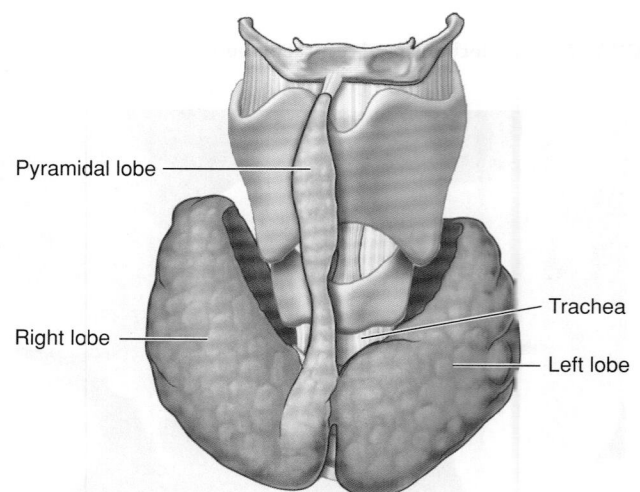

FIGURE 27-15. Anatomy of the thyroid gland. The gland is bi-lobed and commonly has a pyramidal lobe. (Modified with permission from Moore KL, Dalley AF, Agur AMR. *Clinically Oriented Anatomy*. 8th ed. Baltimore, MD: Wolters Kluwer; 2018: Fig B9.8B.)

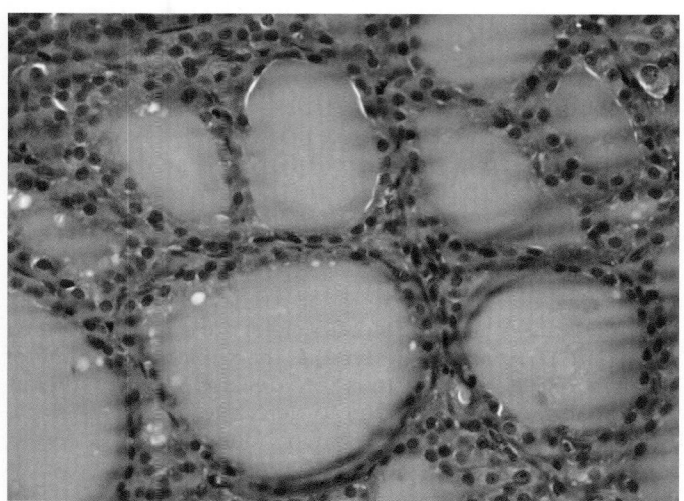

FIGURE 27-16. Normal thyroid follicles.

Grossly, the cut surface of the thyroid is glistening, light brown, and lobulated. In its early development, the gland contains cords of cells that become the follicles or acini that are the functional units of the thyroid gland. Follicles average 200 μm in diameter. They consist of a single layer of cuboidal cells surrounded by a delicate basement membrane and covering a roughly spherical mass of homogenous, proteinaceous colloid material, representing secreted/stored thyroglobulin from which active thyroid hormones are released (Fig. 27-16). A thyroid lobule is composed of 20 to 40 follicles supplied by a lobular artery and sustained by a diffuse mesh of fibrous stroma, lymphatics, and connective tissue.

Staining for thyroglobulin is a sensitive and specific immunohistochemical method to identify follicular cells. Other markers used to identify follicular epithelium include thyroid transcription factor-1 (TTF1, also called NKX2.1) and Pax-8 (paired box gene 8).

In addition to follicular epithelial cells, the thyroid contains parafollicular or C-cells interspersed among thyroid follicles mainly in lateral aspects of the upper portion of both thyroid lobes. Derived from the neural-crest, C-cells are closely associated with the branchial pouch endoderm (lateral anlage) during development. The region of fusion of the lateral and medial anlage corresponds to the distribution of C-cells. In children, discrete nests of C-cells can be readily identified, whereas in adults, they are typically more dispersed.

C-cells produce calcitonin, a calcium-lowering hormone. They also secrete smaller amounts of other peptides such as serotonin and somatostatin. C-cells are difficult to identify using routine stains but are readily seen by immunostaining for calcitonin or neuroendocrine markers such as chromogranin and synaptophysin-A.

THYROID HORMONE IS A GLOBAL REGULATOR OF METABOLISM

The main function of **follicular cells** in the thyroid gland is to make the thyroid hormones **triiodothyronine** (T_3) and tetraiodothyronine (**thyroxine**, T_4). T_4 is principally a prohormone while the major effector of thyroid function is T_3. These molecules are formed by iodination of tyrosine residues in thyroglobulin by follicular cells. Iodinated thyroglobulin is then secreted into the follicle lumen. Alone among endocrine glands, the thyroid can store a large amount of preformed hormone.

Upon stimulation by TSH, follicular cells reabsorb thyroglobulin and liberate T_4 and T_3 into the blood. Most secreted hormone is T_4, which is deiodinated in peripheral tissues to its more active form, T_3. Thyroid hormones in the blood are both free and bound to thyronine-binding globulin (TBG). Peripheral cells take up only free hormone, which binds to nuclear receptors and orchestrates changes in gene expression.

Thyroid hormone affects almost all organs. It stimulates basal metabolic rate and metabolism of carbohydrates, lipids, and proteins. It increases body heat and hepatic glucose production by increasing gluconeogenesis and glycogenolysis. It promotes synthesis of structural proteins, enzymes, and other hormones. Glucose use, fatty acid synthesis in the liver, and adipose tissue lipolysis all increase. Thyroid hormone upregulates both anabolic and catabolic activities.

Thyroid function is governed mainly by pituitary TSH. In turn, thyroid hormone suppresses TSH and TRH secretion via an inhibitory feedback loop. Normal thyroid hormone production requires an adequate dietary supply of iodine.

PATHOLOGIC STATES OF THYROID FUNCTION INCLUDE HYPOTHYROIDISM AND HYPERTHYROIDISM

Hypothyroidism is the clinical state of thyroid hormone deficiency. It is characterized by weight gain, *myxedema* (prominent edema of the face, hands, feet, and tongue), mental and physical slowness, constipation, bradycardia, sex hormone dysfunction, and fatigue (Fig. 27-17). If hypothyroidism occurs perinatally, it may cause severe developmental and intellectual disability. Conceptually, any process

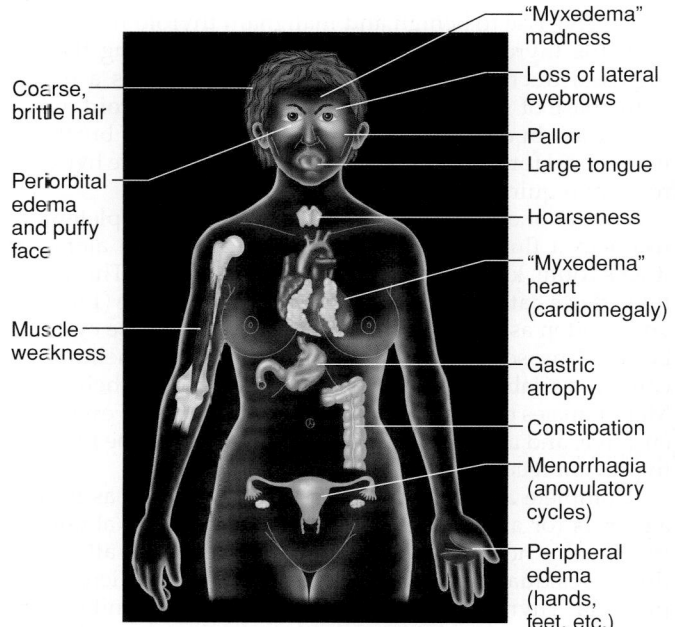

FIGURE 27-17. Clinical manifestations of severe hypothyroidism.

that affects thyroid hormone synthesis (genetic deficiencies, congenital absence of the thyroid, infections, autoimmune/immune insults, medications, surgical removal) or its regulation (pituitary failure) may result in hypothyroidism. Hypothyroidism is detected by T_3 and T_4 measurement in the blood. TSH will often be elevated (unless the pituitary is incapable). Therapy is designed to target the underlying cause, which if irreversible, requires exogenous thyroid hormone replacement.

Hyperthyroidism is the state of excess thyroid hormone release by the thyroid gland. It may result in weight loss, tachycardia, tremor, insomnia, muscle weakness, hyperreflexia, and exophthalmos. Hyperthyroidism may be caused by autoimmune conditions (most commonly Graves disease), autonomously functioning toxic (multinodular) goiter, exogenous hormone administration, or, rarely, by TSH overproduction by the pituitary. T_3 and T_4 levels are high and TSH is low (unless the process is TSH-driven). Hyperthyroidism is managed both medically and surgically, with the goal of removing the source of thyroid hormone.

CONGENITAL ANOMALIES LEAD TO STRUCTURAL AND FUNCTIONAL ABNORMALITIES OF THE THYROID

Heterotopic/ectopic thyroid refers to thyroid tissue that resides outside the typical location of the thyroid gland. Such ectopic sites may involve lymph nodes, soft tissues of the upper neck, base of tongue (see below), mediastinum, and even pericardium. Ectopic thyroid tissue is functionally and histologically normal and can produce thyroid hormone. Small nodules of ectopic tissue are typically without consequence and are usually discovered incidentally (if ever), though pathologic lesions, including malignant tumors, may develop in ectopic thyroid.

Occasionally, mature cystic teratomas of the ovary may show thyroid differentiation (termed struma ovarii) and rarely give rise to benign and malignant thyroid neoplasms.

If the thyroid fails to initiate its descent along the thyroglossal duct during embryogenesis, it remains a nodule at the base of the tongue, known as **lingual thyroid**, which may result in difficulty speaking, swallowing, or breathing. Its removal for symptomatic relief lead to complete hypothyroidism requiring hormone supplementation.

Failure of a thyroglossal duct to involute completely can result in a fluid-filled cystic remnant anywhere along the duct's route, known as a **thyroglossal duct cyst**. This condition affects patients in all age groups, varies in size (1 to 4 cm) and is often associated with the hyoid bone. These cysts can be lined by squamous or respiratory-type epithelium and contain variable amounts of thyroid tissue in their walls. Malignancies can develop in these cysts. Surgical excision is curative, and a portion of the hyoid bone should be removed to prevent recurrence.

Complete absence of thyroid tissue is known as **thyroid agenesis** (or athyrosis). This is a rare congenital abnormality, usually not discovered until several weeks after birth due to residual maternal thyroid hormone supplied via the placenta. Thyroid agenesis leads to severe congenital hypothyroidism as the child is unable to generate endogenous thyroid hormone.

Endemic congenital hypothyroidism is due to inadequate maternal dietary iodine required for proper thyroid hormone production. In this circumstance, the mother is typically severely deficient in iodine and has endemic goiter (see below). The child, while possessing a thyroid gland, is unable to synthesize thyroid hormone without proper iodine stores.

Symptoms of congenital hypothyroidism start in the early weeks of extrauterine life. Infants are apathetic and sluggish. Their abdomens are large and often show umbilical hernias. Body temperatures are often below 35°C (95°F), and the skin is pale and cold. Refractory anemia and dilated hearts are common. By 6 months, the clinical syndrome of congenital hypothyroidism is well developed. Mental retardation, stunted growth (due to defective osseous maturation) and characteristic facies are evident. Serum T_4 and T_3 are low and TSH levels are high (unless hypothyroidism is due to defective TSH secretion by the pituitary).

Prompt thyroid hormone replacement therapy is required to prevent mental retardation and stunted growth. Although treatment may prevent dwarfism, its effects on mental development are more variable. Children in whom hypothyroidism is detected early with neonatal screening respond well to thyroid hormone treatment and are normal mentally while delayed treatment leads to severe neurocognitive disability.

GOITER REFERS TO CLINICAL THYROID GLAND ENLARGEMENT OF ANY ETIOLOGY

Goiters (from the Latin, *guttur*, "throat") may be nodular, multinodular, or involve the gland diffusely. Depending on the etiology, pathophysiology, and stage of a particular disease, a goiter may result in hyperthyroidism, hypothyroidism, or be euthyroid (normal levels of thyroid hormone). Goiters may be categorized by etiology (idiopathic, inflammatory, autoimmune, infiltrative/deposition diseases, neoplasms) and/or thyroid functional status (hypothyroid, euthyroid, or hyperthyroid). A "toxic" goiter generates excessive thyroid hormone, while a "nontoxic" goiter does not.

Sporadic (nontoxic) goiter, also called simple, colloid, or multinodular goiter or nodular hyperplasia, is a benign enlargement of the thyroid gland that is often idiopathic, though genetic factors have been implicated. Sporadic goiter may occur as a uniform enlargement of the gland, typically seen in young women (8:1 F:M ratio) or as a multinodular growth (known as multinodular nontoxic goiter) typically seen in older adults (>50 years). Multinodular nontoxic goiter typically develops over time.

Endemic goiter is a benign, typically diffuse thyroid enlargement that may exist in communities where natural water and soil iodination is poor, typically affecting a large proportion of the population (over 10%). Deficient dietary iodine is believed to be the etiologic factor and is most common in mountainous regions of Southeast Asia, Central America, and Africa.

 CLINICAL FEATURES: Patients with simple or endemic (nontoxic) goiters come to medical attention because of a neck mass (Fig. 27-18A), which may cause dysphagia (esophagus), inspiratory stridor

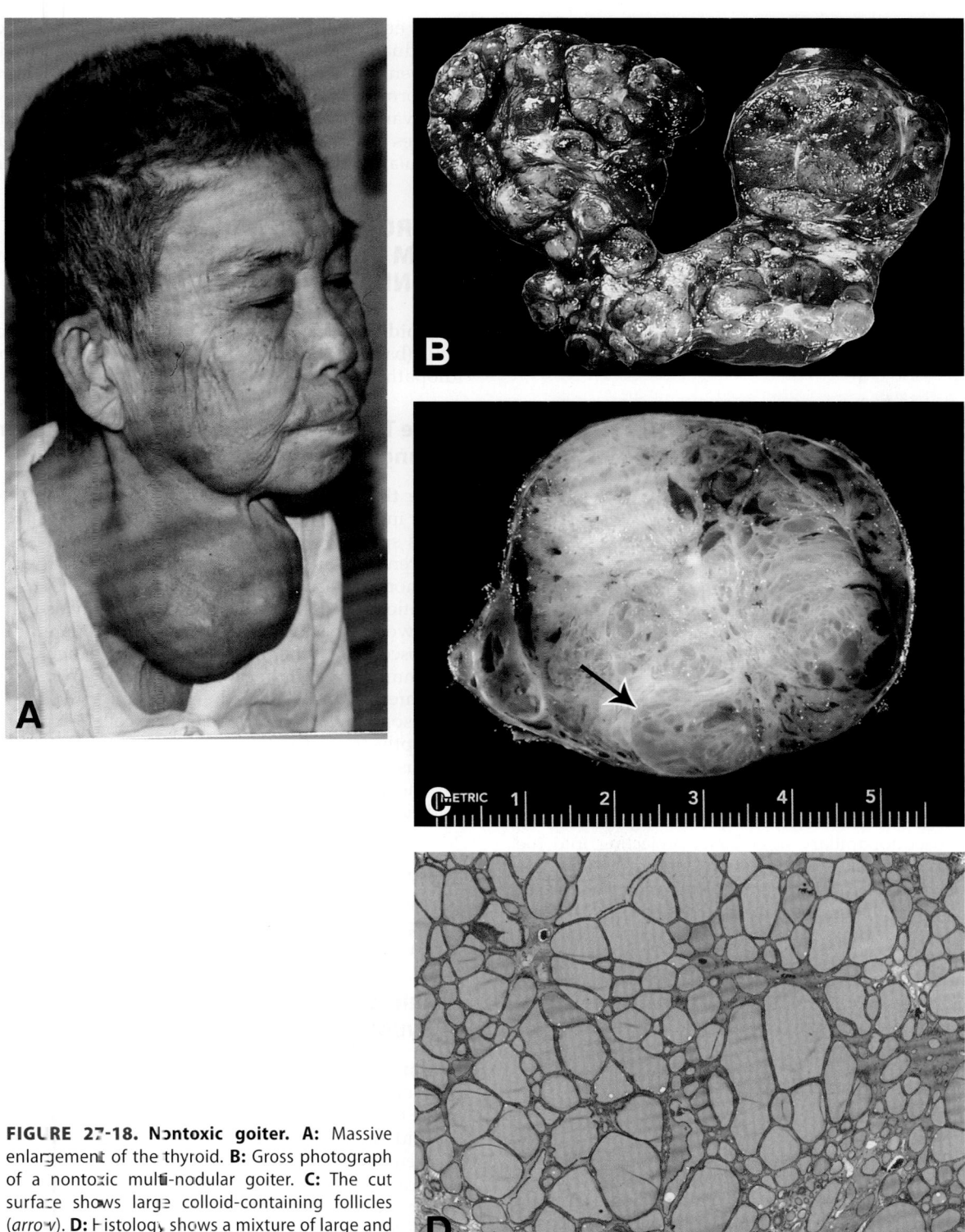

FIGURE 27-18. Nontoxic goiter. A: Massive enlargement of the thyroid. **B:** Gross photograph of a nontoxic multi-nodular goiter. **C:** The cut surface shows large colloid-containing follicles (*arrow*). **D:** Histology shows a mixture of large and small follicles.

(trachea), venous congestion of the head and face (neck veins), or hoarseness (recurrent laryngeal nerve). Hemorrhage into a nodule or cyst may cause local pain. Patients are usually euthyroid, with blood T$_4$, and T$_3$ in the low-normal range, while TSH may be normal or slightly elevated. If left untreated, patients may eventually develop hyperthyroidism due to autonomous production of thyroid hormone within a nodular goiter, in which case the term **toxic multinodular goiter** (see below) is applied.

PATHOPHYSIOLOGY: The pathophysiology of sporadic and endemic goiters is similar. Deficiencies in iodine or thyroid hormone production, whether dietary, genetic, chemical (or idiopathic), result in compensatory TSH production by the pituitary gland, which stimulates thyroid follicles. The resulting enlargement of thyroid follicles produces diffuse enlargement of the gland. Follicles may develop differential sensitivities to TSH stimulation resulting in asymmetric hyperplasia, with large and small follicles interspersed within the gland and some areas enlarging more than others. Eventually, a follicle may become *autonomous* (i.e., grow without TSH stimulus), leading to the development of toxic multinodular goiter. Unlike sporadic goiter, endemic goiter rarely becomes toxic.

MOLECULAR PATHOGENESIS: Mutations in *TG*, the thyroglobulin gene, occur in some families who have simple goiter. Linkage analysis has also identified variants in *MNG-1*(multinodular goiter-1) in chromosome 14q and at another locus (Xp22) as possible genetic causes of multinodular goiter. Mutations in the TSH receptor gene (*TSHR*) have also been implicated.

Histopathology: Nontoxic goiters range in size from roughly double the mass of a normal gland (40 g) to thyroids weighing hundreds of grams (Fig. 27-18A,B). In early disease, the thyroid typically enlarges symmetrically. Follicles are small, with tall columnar cells and little colloid. As the disease progresses, asymmetric multinodular growth dominates. Grossly, the cut surface is glistening, yellow-red, and shows many irregular, soft nodules filled with yellow-green colloid, with varying amounts of intervening fibrous tissue. Microscopically, follicles vary in size and shape. They contain abundant colloid and are lined by attenuated flat-to-cuboidal cells (Fig. 27-18C) that occasionally form pseudopapillary aggregates projecting into the follicle space. Hemosiderin deposition, hemorrhage, chronic inflammation, and cholesterol granulomas may all be seen.

Therapy: Nontoxic goiters are usually treated with exogenous thyroid hormone to reduce TSH levels and thereby shrink the goiter. However, hormone replacement may be ineffective if nodules transition toward autonomous (toxic) growth. Surgery may be required if a goiter becomes clinically symptomatic (dysphagia, obstruction/compression).

Goitrogens Are Agents That Induce Thyroid Enlargement

Several drugs and naturally occurring chemicals are *goitrogenic* in that they suppress thyroid hormone synthesis, resulting in TSH elevation and thyroid enlargement. Common goitrogenic drugs include **lithium**, phenylbutazone, and *p*-aminosalicylic acid. Certain cruciferous vegetables (turnips, rutabaga, cassava) also contain goitrogens and can potentiate an iodine-deficient diet to produce goitrous hypothyroidism.

Dyshormonogenetic Goiter Results From Congenital Deficiencies in Thyroid Hormone Synthesis

Dyshormonogenetic goiter is most commonly due to defects in iodination of thyroid hormone (often due to mutations in genes encoding thyroid peroxidase [TPO], ductal oxidase-2, and dual oxidase maturation factor 2). Thyroid enlargement ensues secondary to chronic TSH stimulation. Grossly, dyshormonogenetic thyroid glands are large, tan, and firm, with variably sized nodules. Microscopically, nodules vary in sizes and contain hypercellular aggregates and cords of follicular epithelial cells with *minimal-to-no colloid*.

THYROIDITIS IS A DESCRIPTIVE TERM INDICATING THYROID GLAND INFLAMMATION

Thyroiditis may be due to a number of causes, including infectious (bacterial, fungal, viral), autoimmune, drug-induced, or idiopathic.

Acute Thyroiditis Is Caused by Bacterial, Viral, or Fungal Infection of Thyroid Tissue

Acute thyroiditis typically arises from an antecedent systemic infection that reaches the thyroid through hematogenous spread (sepsis). It occurs in patients of all ages, but children, the elderly, or immunocompromised are most commonly affected.

Patients present with fever, chills, malaise, and a painful, swollen neck mass that may be unilateral or diffuse. Microscopically, the gland shows diffuse acute and chronic inflammation with focal microabscess formation. Rarely, the infection may spread into the trachea, mediastinum, and esophagus. The prognosis is excellent if the infection is promptly treated with antibiotics. Patients with acute thyroiditis are typically euthyroid.

The most common causative organisms in acute thyroiditis are *Streptococcus, Staphylococcus,* and *Pneumococcus* species. Other causes include disseminated fungal infection (second most common), tuberculous, and cytomegalovirus (CMV) infections, particularly in patients with immune suppression (as in HIV infection, bone marrow ablation prior to transplantation, or chronic immune suppression after solid organ transplantation).

Hashimoto Thyroiditis Is the Most Common Cause of Hypothyroidism in the United States

Hashimoto thyroiditis (HT) is an autoimmune condition characterized by humoral- and cellular-mediated autoimmune destruction of thyroid parenchyma resulting in hypothyroidism and goiter. It is typically seen in middle-aged women and is the most common cause of goiter in children. Clinically, the patient may present with a firm, nodular goiter, serum "antithyroid" antibodies (most commonly anti-TPO, and/or antithyroglobulin) and elevated TSH. Occasionally, active thyroid destruction may produce transient hyperthyroidism.

HT is associated with other autoimmune conditions (MEN2, Sjögren syndrome, diabetes mellitus, pernicious anemia, Addison disease, and myasthenia gravis) and often occurs in patients with HLA-DR3 and HLA-DR5 alleles. Certain genetic conditions, including Down syndrome, Turner syndrome, and familial Alzheimer disease are also associated with HT. Family members of patients with HT may have detectable antithyroid antibodies.

MOLECULAR PATHOGENESIS: Both cellular and humoral immunity are involved. The autoimmune process in HT arises from activation of CD4 (helper) T-lymphocytes sensitized to thyroid antigens. These CD4⁺ cells stimulate proliferation of autoreactive cytotoxic (CD8⁺) T-cells, which attack follicular epithelial cells and induce apoptosis. The activated lymphocytes also secrete interferon-γ, causing thyroid cells to express MHC class II molecules and thereby further expanding the autoreactive T-cell population. These mechanisms explain the striking accumulation of lymphocytes often seen in the glands of patients with autoimmune thyroiditis.

Activated CD4 cells also recruit autoreactive B-cells to produce antibodies against thyroid antigens. These include antibodies against TPO (95%), thyroglobulin (60%), TSH receptor (inhibitory), and thyroid microsomal antigen. Cytotoxic antibodies that fix complement have been described in some patients, and antibody-dependent cell-mediated cytotoxicity may contribute to thyroid injury.

PATHOLOGY: The gland in patients with HT is diffusely, symmetrically enlarged, and firm, weighing 60 to 200 g. The cut surface is pale-tan, and often fleshy with vague nodularity. Microscopically, the thyroid shows a prominent lymphoplasmacytic infiltrate with germinal centers and destruction/atrophy of follicles with oxyphilic (Hürthle cell) or squamous metaplasia (Fig. 27-19). Occasionally, nuclear atypia or nuclear clearing mimicking cancer may be seen. Prominent fibrosis (fibrous variant HT) like that seen in IgG₄-related thyroiditis (see below) may occur but it is limited to the thyroid and not associated with obliterative phlebitis within the gland. HT is confirmed by the presence of anti-TPO antibodies and antimicrosomal, antithyroglobulin, and cell membrane antibodies. The thyroid eventually undergoes atrophy in some patients, who are left with a small, fibrotic gland infiltrated by lymphocytes.

Therapy: Thyroid hormone is given to treat hypothyroidism and decrease the size of the gland. Surgery is reserved for patients who do not respond to suppressive hormone therapy or have local thyroid enlargement resulting in pressure symptoms.

Subacute Thyroiditis (de Quervain or Granulomatous Thyroiditis) Is a Painful Thyroiditis

Subacute thyroiditis, also known as de Quervain or granulomatous thyroiditis, is an uncommon self-limited disorder characterized by granulomatous inflammation within the thyroid parenchyma. It typically occurs after upper respiratory viral infections (influenza, adenovirus, echovirus, or coxsackievirus) suggesting, at least in part, a viral etiology. Symptoms of subacute thyroiditis include neck/thyroid/jaw pain, fever, myalgia, and exquisite thyroid tenderness. The disease progresses through three phases: hyperthyroid, hypothyroid, and recovery. The hyperthyroid phase is associated with inflammation-mediated damage and release of stored thyroid hormone. The hypothyroid phase results from extensive thyroid parenchymal damage. Most patients recover thyroid function completely within months without specific therapy.

PATHOLOGY: The thyroid is often asymmetrically enlarged to 40 to 60 g with firm and pale cut surfaces. Acute inflammation, often with microabscesses, is followed by a patchy infiltrate of lymphocytes, plasma cells, and macrophages throughout the gland. Destruction of follicles releases colloid, which elicits a conspicuous granulomatous reaction (Fig. 27-20). Abundant foreign body–type multinucleated giant cells, often containing colloid, are present. Fibrosis may follow resolution of the inflammatory reaction, but over time, normal thyroid architecture is usually restored.

Riedel Thyroiditis Is Associated With Extensive Thyroid Gland Fibrosis

The "thyroiditis" in Riedel thyroiditis (RT) is believed to be part of an IgG₄-related systemic disease that causes extensive

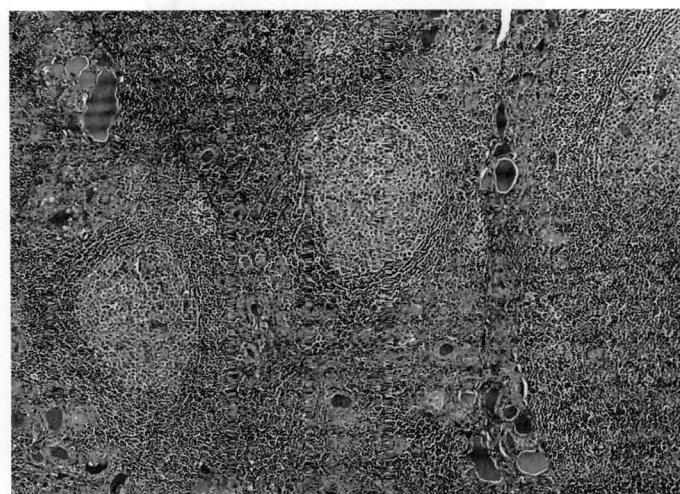

FIGURE 27-19. Hashimoto thyroiditis. A microscopic section reveals a conspicuous chronic inflammatory infiltrate and many atrophic thyroid follicles. Inflammatory cells form prominent lymphoid follicles with germinal centers.

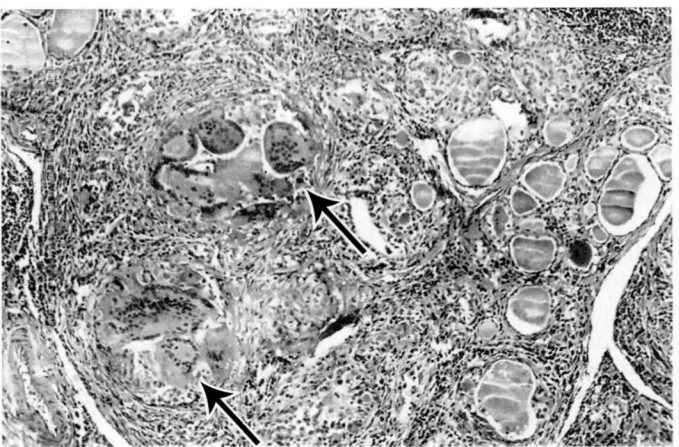

FIGURE 27-20. Subacute thyroiditis. Release of colloid into the interstitial tissue has elicited a prominent granulomatous reaction, with numerous foreign body giant cells (*arrows*).

fibrosis in affected organs and typically involves both the thyroid gland as well as extrathyroidal tissues of the neck, including salivary glands, retroperitoneum, mediastinum, and orbit. Patients typically present with a large, hard mass in the neck that may enlarge rapidly and cause local compressive symptoms of dysphagia, hoarseness, or stridor. The pathogenesis is poorly understood but is believed to be inflammatory and may respond to immunosuppressive therapy. Most typically, surgical resection for localized symptoms is performed.

PATHOLOGY: The thyroid is asymmetrically enlarged, pale, and hard with a *"woody"* texture. Surgical resection may be difficult due to dense fibrosis that typically extends to extrathyroidal tissues (fat, muscle, nerves parathyroid glands). Histologically, RT typically shows diffuse thyroidal and extrathyroidal fibrosis, variable plasmacytic infiltrate rich in IgG$_4$-positive plasma cells, and obliterative phlebitis. Interestingly, the fibrous variant of HT also contains an increased number of IgG$_4$-positive plasma cells, but unlike RT, is limited to the thyroid and not associated with systemic fibrosis.

Silent Thyroiditis Is a Painless Enlargement of the Thyroid With Lymphocytic Inflammation

Silent thyroiditis, also called **painless/atypical subacute thyroiditis** or **lymphocytic thyroiditis**, is a self-limited hyperthyroid state characterized by multifocal destruction of follicles with lymphocytic infiltration. Thus, while it resembles subacute thyroiditis clinically by progressing through hyperthyroid, hypothyroid, and recovery states (though without pain), it is closer to HT pathologically. Silent thyroiditis differs from the latter by the lack of antithyroid antibodies or other evidence of autoimmune thyroiditis. As in subacute thyroiditis, the hyperthyroid state reflects release of preformed thyroid hormone from the injured gland. Silent thyroiditis mainly affects women, often in the postpartum period, causing hyperthyroidism that usually persists for 2 to 4 months. Most cases resolve completely.

HYPERTHYROIDISM IS DUE TO OVERPRODUCTION OF THYROID HORMONE

Graves Disease Is the Most Common Cause of Hyperthyroidism in the United States

CLINICAL FEATURES: Also known as diffuse toxic goiter, **Graves disease** (GD) is one of the most common autoimmune diseases, affecting 0.5% to 1% of the population under 40. There is a significant female predilection (7 to 10:1 F:M ratio) and it typically develops in the fourth decade of life. A family history of autoimmune thyroid disease, smoking, emotional stress, postpartum status, and a personal history of other autoimmune conditions are all strongly associated with GD.

Clinically, GD is characterized by goiter, resting tremor, tachycardia, proximal myopathy, hyperreflexia, weight loss, dermopathy (warm, moist skin) and/or pretibial myxedema (uncommon) (Fig. 27-21). Up to half of patients exhibit ophthalmopathy including exophthalmos

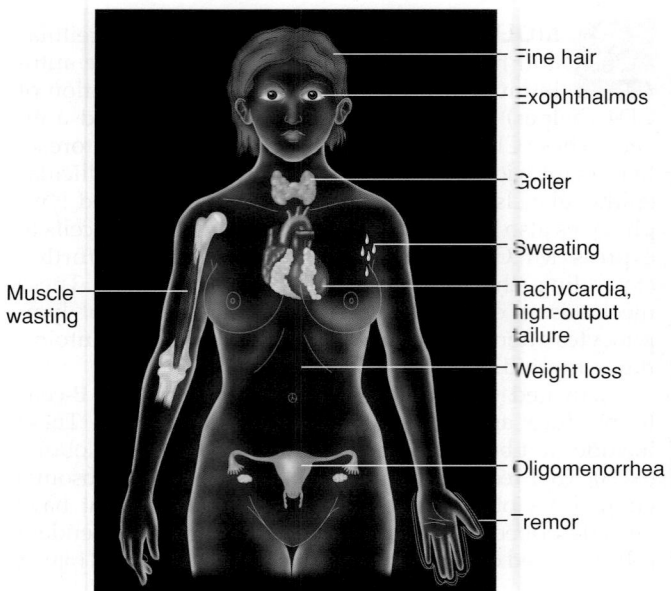

FIGURE 27-21. Clinical manifestations of Graves disease.

(Fig. 27-22), eyelid swelling, and lid lag. Additional symptoms may include nervousness, weight loss, heat intolerance, palpitations, and hyperhidrosis. Occasionally, skeletal myopathy or heart failure may develop due to increased cardiac output triggered by thyroid hormone.

On physical examination, patients have a symmetrically enlarged, nontender thyroid gland that may exhibit a vascular bruit or palpable thrill. Laboratory studies show elevated T3 and T4 levels, markedly decreased TSH levels and, in most cases, serum (activating) autoantibodies against the TSHR. The clinical course is characterized by exacerbations and remissions. Untreated, hyperthyroidism may eventually lead to progressive thyroid failure and hypothyroidism.

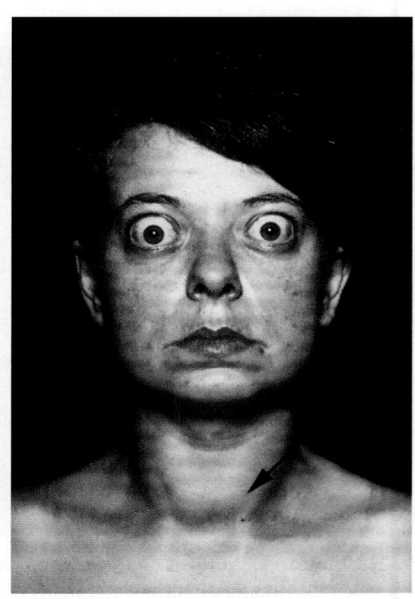

FIGURE 27-22. Exophthalmos associated with Graves disease. (Sandoz Pharmaceutical Corporation.)

PATHOPHYSIOLOGY: The main drivers in GD are activating autoantibodies against the TSHR, which stimulate thyroid follicular cells to proliferate and produce thyroid hormone in the absence of TSH (which is extremely low in GD due to negative feedback on the hypothalamic–pituitary axis). Chronic activation of TSHR causes diffuse, symmetrical thyroid enlargement and increases vascularity within the gland (resulting in bruit or palpable thrill). The targets of thyroid hormone are global, leading to increased metabolism, increased sensitivity to catecholamines, and growth. The cause of exophthalmos is less well understood, but is thought to be due to proliferation of fibroblasts within orbital fat and accumulation of fluid and glycosaminoglycans within the orbital soft tissues. Fluid retention by glycosaminoglycans has also been implicated in the development of pretibial myxedema.

Elaboration of thyroid-stimulating antibodies requires thyroid-specific helper (CD4+) T-cells that recognize multiple TSH receptor epitopes and stimulate autoreactive B-cells. These then produce thyroid-stimulating immunoglobulins. Patients with GD have decreased levels of suppressor CD8+ cells, which may play a role in the lack of immune tolerance.

Graves autoantibodies are heterogeneous. Some stimulate thyroid hormone secretion while others seem to be cytotoxic and may cause thyroid failure that often follows long-standing GD. These include antibodies against thyroglobulin, TPO, and the sodium–iodide symporter, all of which may also play roles in the pathogenesis of HT. Thus, both GD and HT are driven by autoimmune mechanisms but with opposing manifestations (Fig. 27-23).

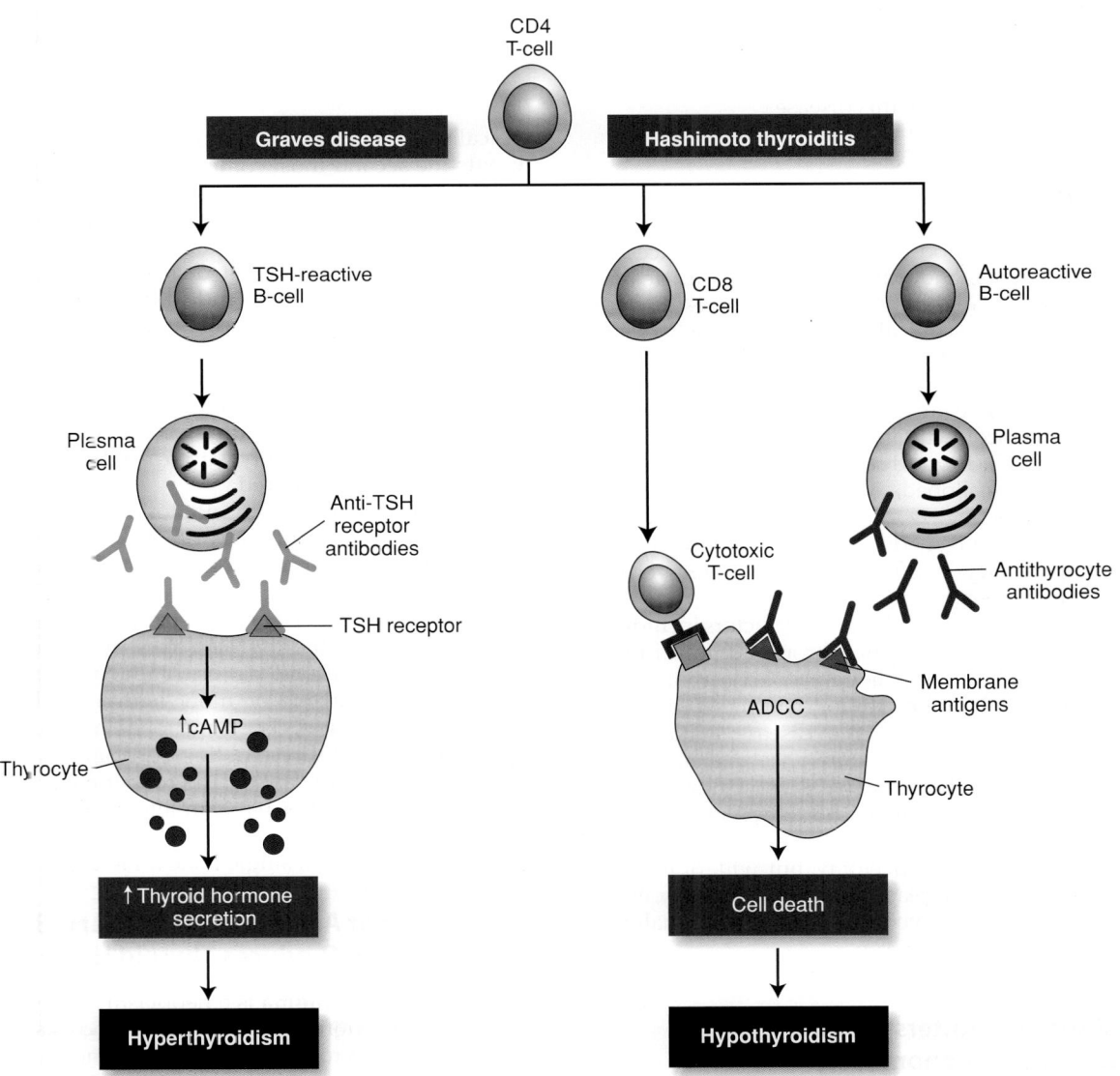

FIGURE 27-23. Immune mechanisms of Graves disease and Hashimoto thyroiditis. CD4+ T-cells stimulate antibody production by autoreactive B-cells. Anti–thyroid-stimulating hormone (TSH) receptor antibodies stimulate thyroid hormone synthesis in Graves disease. Antibodies induce thyrocyte cell death in Hashimoto thyroiditis by complement-dependent cytotoxicity and antibody-dependent cell-mediated cytotoxicity (ADCC). Thyrocyte death also results from attack by CD8+ (cytotoxic) T-cells. *cAMP* = cyclic adenosine 3′,5′-monophosphate.

MOLECULAR PATHOGENESIS: The strongest risk factor for GD is a positive family history. However, no single genetic abnormality has been found to be necessary or sufficient. The concordance rate in monozygotic twins is only 30% to 50%, while in dizygotic twins it is 5%. Thus, environmental factors likely play important pathogenic roles.

A number of genetic associations have been described in GD. HLA-B8, HLA-DR3, and HLA-DQA1 alleles have a stronger association with the development of GD in Caucasians, while Chinese patients are more likely to be positive for HLA-Bw46, and Japanese patients for HLA-Bw35. Other genetic factors have been linked to GD, but their exact role in pathogenesis remains poorly understood. They include polymorphisms or mutations in genes that make cytotoxic T-lymphocyte antigen-4 (*CTLA-4*), protein tyrosine protein tyrosine phosphatase nonreceptor type 22 (*PTPN22*), CD25, CD40, and thyrotropin receptor. Patients with GD and their relatives have a much higher incidence of other autoimmune diseases (e.g., pernicious anemia and HT). Asymptomatic, first-degree relatives of these patients may also show increased ^{131}I uptake, further emphasizing the genetic underpinnings of this disease.

PATHOLOGY: The thyroid is symmetrically enlarged and usually weighs 35 to 100 g, with firm, vaguely nodular dark red cut surfaces in undertreated patients, and paler cut surfaces in treated patients. Diffuse follicular hyperplasia and increased vascularity are seen microscopically. Thyroid epithelial cells are tall and columnar, and are arrayed on papillae that project into the lumens of the follicles but lack fibrovascular cores. These papillae are more prominent in untreated cases and may be incorrectly interpreted as papillary thyroid carcinoma (PTC). Thyroid colloid tends to be depleted and appears pale, scalloped, or "moth-eaten" where it abuts epithelial cells (Fig. 27-24), although may be abundant in patients following medical therapy prior to surgery. Focal lymphoplasmacytic infiltrate with scattered germinal centers may be seen.

Therapy: Treatment depends on many factors including response to medical management. Chronic administration of antithyroid medications (methimazole, carbimazole, and propylthiouracil) inhibit thyroid hormone production and thereby lead to regression of disease. Radioactive iodine therapy is an alternative to medical management. It ablates highly metabolically active thyroid tissue, leading to remission, although it may lead to hypothyroidism. Lastly, patients with severe symptoms resistant to medical therapy may undergo thyroidectomy, but will, of course, require thyroid hormone replacement. Unfortunately, even if hyperthyroidism is relieved surgically, exophthalmos often persists or may even worsen.

Toxic Multinodular Goiters Produce Thyroid Hormone Autonomously

Many patients with long-standing nontoxic multinodular goiter may eventually develop toxic (thyroid hormone–producing) multinodular goiter after many years. Toxic multinodular goiter is more common in women (8:1) and

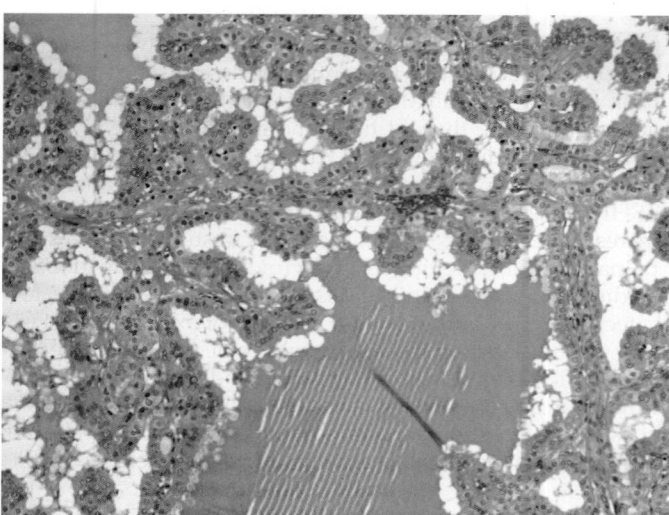

FIGURE 27-24. Graves disease. Follicles are lined by hyperplastic, tall columnar cells with papillary-like growth. Colloid is pink and scalloped at the periphery adjacent to follicular cells.

typically develops in patients over 50 years of age. It represents the second most common cause of hyperthyroidism in adults behind Graves disease.

Patients with toxic multinodular goiter often have less severe symptoms of hyperthyroidism than those with Graves disease, and do not develop exophthalmos. Since patients with toxic goiter tend to be older, cardiac complications, including atrial fibrillation and heart failure, may dominate the clinical presentation. Serum T_4 and T_3 levels are only minimally elevated, and radiolabeled iodine uptake may be normal or only slightly increased. Radiolabeled iodine after a course of antithyroid therapy is the most common therapy. Occasionally, surgical resection for localized symptoms may be required.

Mechanisms by which nontoxic multinodular goiter assumes functional autonomy are not fully understood but two pathologic patterns are often seen. In some patients, the thyroid shows groups of small hyperplastic follicles mixed with other nodules of varying size that appear to be inactive, even though the thyroid takes up radioactive iodine diffusely. In the second pattern, radiolabeled iodine accumulates focally in one or more nodules, which suppress the rest of the gland. The functional nodules show large hyperplastic follicles resembling adenomas that are clearly distinct from inactive areas. The functional nodules are not neoplastic (they do not have an alteration causing autonomous growth), but the clinical picture is similar to that of a normal thyroid with a single toxic follicular adenoma (FA).

Toxic Follicular Adenoma Is a Solitary, Benign Neoplasm That Produces Thyroid Hormone

Toxic follicular adenoma is a neoplasm that typically arises in an otherwise normal thyroid gland and is an uncommon cause of hyperthyroidism (see below). Such tumors display autonomous function independent of TSH and are not suppressed by exogenous thyroid hormone.

Toxic thyroid adenoma is most common in the fourth and fifth decades, and tends to present when the nodule is sizable (above 3 cm). Spontaneous necrosis and hemorrhage within an adenoma may relieve the hyperthyroidism. A toxic adenoma eventually suppresses the rest of the thyroid, which then atrophies. [131]I scintigraphy shows a solitary focus of iodine uptake ("hot nodule") in a background of minimal uptake. Many, but not all, toxic adenomas carry a variety of somatic activating mutations of the TSH receptor.

Since the normal thyroid tissue is suppressed, toxic adenomas are treated effectively with radiolabeled iodine. Large nodules may be excised surgically, especially in young patients, to minimize risk of thyroid cancer that may occur many years after radiolabeled iodine administration.

THYROID NEOPLASMS ARE CATEGORIZED AS FOLLICULAR, PAPILLARY, OR MEDULLARY

Follicular Adenomas Are Benign, Encapsulated, Noninvasive Neoplasms

FA are the most common thyroid tumors and are derived from follicular epithelial cells. They typically present sporadically in euthyroid patients as solitary "cold" nodules (i.e., that do not take up radioiodine, unless they are toxic FAs, see above) and come to clinical attention once they grow to palpable size, although they may also be detected incidentally by imaging. Small FAs are clinically silent and may never be detected, making the true incidence of FA difficult to assess. Autopsy studies suggest an incidence of up to 5% in the general population. There is a female predominance, and they are usually detected in the fifth or sixth decade.

Radiation exposure and/or iodine deficiency may be associated with development of FA many years (or decades) later. Patients with PTEN-hamartoma tumor syndrome (Cowden syndrome) have a high propensity of developing *multiple* FAs at a young age due to deficiency of *PTEN* tumor-suppressor activity.

MOLECULAR PATHOGENESIS: Mutations in *RAS* oncogenes are common in FA (seen in ~30%), most often involving codon 61 of *HRAS*, and least frequently involving *KRAS*. Somatic mutations of *PTEN* are seen in approximately 5% of all FAs. Other

mutations may involve *Pax8/PPARG* or trisomy of chromosome 7.

Grossly, FAs are solitary nodules completely enclosed by a fibrous capsule (Fig. 27-25A). The cut surface of an FA is soft, grey-white or red, and usually paler than the surrounding gland. Hemorrhage, fibrosis, and cystic changes are common. Microscopically, FAs have a fibrous capsule encasing epithelial cells of various histologic patterns, most commonly microfollicular (Fig. 27-25B). The tumor cells are typically monotonous and cuboidal, and have round basophilic nuclei. Importantly, there is *no invasion* into vessels or into the fibrous capsule (these are characteristic features of follicular carcinoma and must be excluded through thorough examination of the capsule). There are several distinctive histologic variants of FA, including lipoadenomas (containing mature adipose tissue), FAs with bizarre nuclei (seen in patients treated with radioactive iodine), signet-ring cell FA (cells with eccentric nuclei and large prominent intracytoplasmic vacuoles), clear-cell FA (cells with clear cell changes), and spindle-cell FA. These subtypes may be confused with malignant tumors. Surgical excision (thyroid lobectomy) is definitive therapy, with no risk of recurrence.

Noninvasive Follicular Thyroid Neoplasm With Papillary-Like Nuclear Features (NIFTP) Are Indolent Tumors With Variant Nuclear Features

NIFTP is an encapsulated or well-circumscribed noninvasive neoplasm with a purely follicular growth pattern and nuclear features of PTC (enlarged, crowded, elongated with nuclear membrane irregularities, nuclear pseudoinclusions, and clear marginated chromatin) (Fig. 27-26). Thorough examination of the neoplastic capsule is required to exclude vascular and capsular invasion, which would indicate carcinoma (i.e., an invasive encapsulated follicular variant of PTC [FVPTC]). NIFTPs have a high prevalence of *RAS* oncogene mutations and behave extremely indolently, similarly to FAs. Surgical excision of NIFTP (thyroid lobectomy) is essentially curative with an extremely low probability of recurrence.

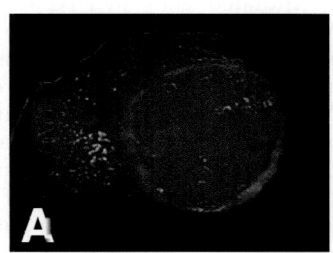

FIGURE 27-25. Follicular adenoma. A: Gross photograph of a follicular adenoma shows a well-circumscribed tan-red lesion within the beefy-red normal thyroid gland. **B:** Microscopically, follicular adenomas show microfollicles (*left side of image*) bound by a distinct capsule.

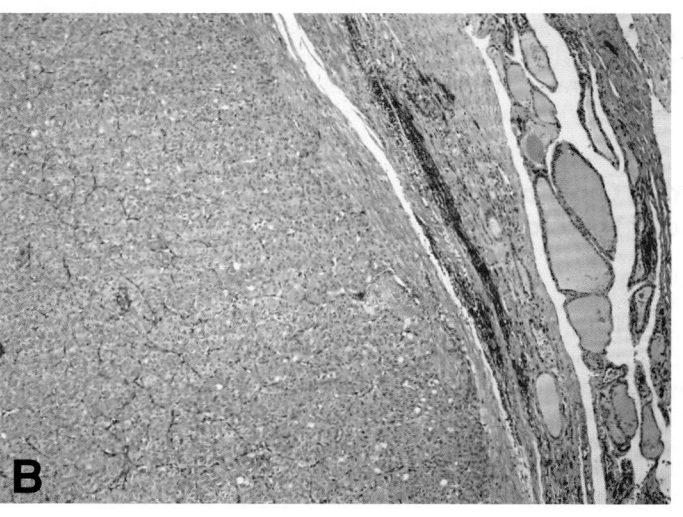

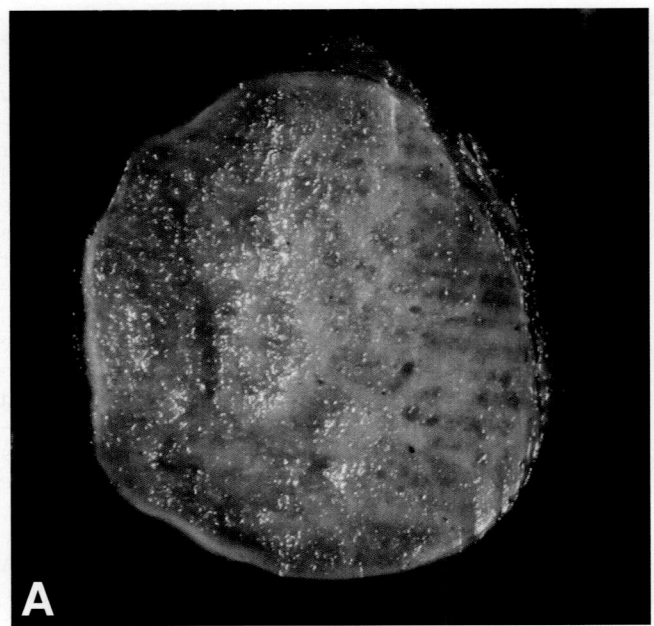

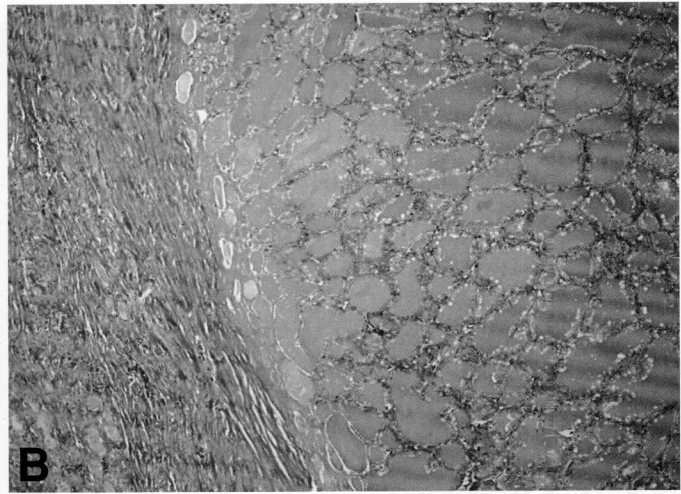

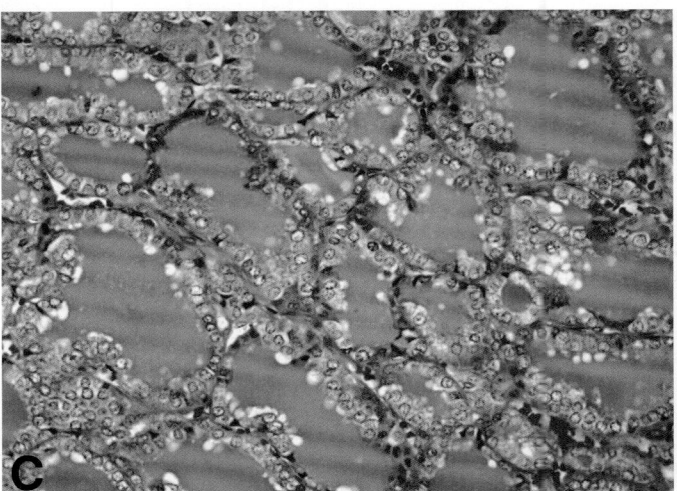

FIGURE 27-26. Noninvasive follicular neoplasm with papillary-like features (NIFTP). A: Grossly, NIFTP is homogenous, well circumscribed, and bound by a capsule. **B:** Microscopically, NIFTP shows follicles bound by a capsule akin to follicular adenoma. **C:** The nuclear features of NIFTP are "papillary-like" with crowded nuclei, cleared chromatin, and nuclear grooves.

THYROID CARCINOMAS ARE UNCOMMON TUMORS WITH INCREASING INCIDENCE

The incidence of thyroid malignancy has nearly tripled since the late 1980s to 13.5 cases per 100,000 people. Despite the increased incidence, survival is high. Nearly 98% of patients are alive at 5-year follow-up, although high-risk subtypes carry worse prognoses. No single etiologic factor is responsible for thyroid carcinoma, but genetic factors, environmental exposures (radiation, nitrates, smoking, iodine), and comorbidities (diabetes, obesity) are all believed to play a role.

Papillary Thyroid Carcinoma Is the Most Common Type of Thyroid Carcinoma

PTC is a malignant tumor of follicular epithelial cells that show distinctive changes associated with a variety of architectural subtypes. PTC accounts for approximately 85% of sporadic thyroid carcinomas in the United States. It occurs most often between the ages of 20 and 50, with a female-to-male ratio of 3:1. However, it may arise at any age and is the most common thyroid malignancy in children and young adolescents. Both excess iodine administration and exposure to ionizing radiation have been associated with development

of PTC. In general, the younger the age of radiation exposure, the higher the probability of developing PTC will be. Family members of patients with PTC also carry an increased risk of developing the disease.

MOLECULAR PATHOGENESIS: The most commonly mutated gene in PTC is *BRAF*, seen in approximately 70% of cases. Some PTC subtypes, including the classical and tall cell variants have a much higher proportion of *BRAF* mutations than other subtypes such as the FVPTC. The most common mutation in *BRAF* is a valine-to-glutamic acid substitution at position 600 (***BRAF V600E***), although other mutations near codon 600 may also occur. As part of the Raf family of kinases, *BRAF* plays an important role in MAP kinase pathways, which regulate cell growth and division. Codon 600 resides in a protein region that normally "locks" *BRAF* in an inactive state until it becomes phosphorylated by upstream kinases. Mutations at or near codon 600 can destabilize this critical region resulting in constitutive *BRAF* activation and dysregulated cell growth and division.

Chromosomal rearrangements resulting in activating **fusion** events involving the oncogenic ***RET*** gene (known as **RET/PCT rearrangement**) are also observed in PCT

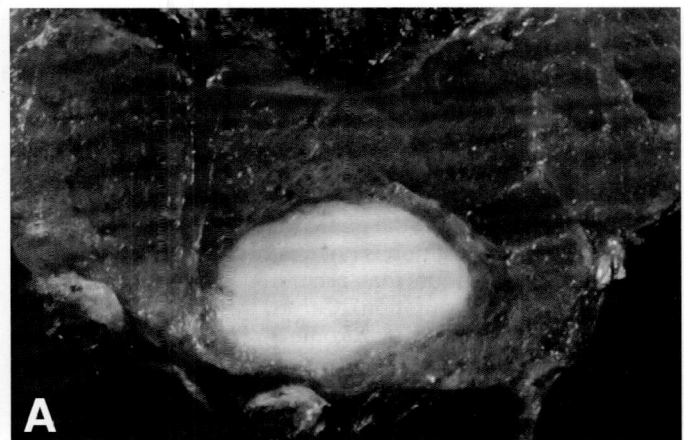

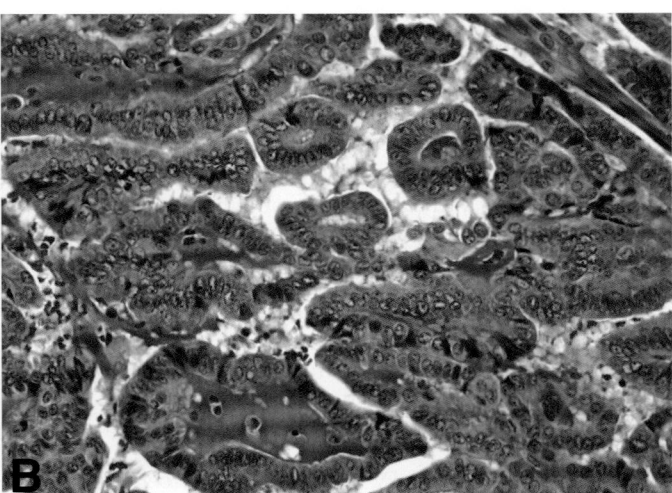

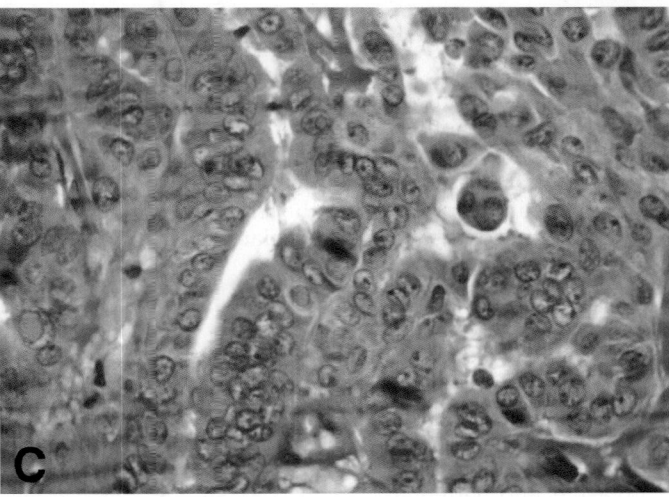

FIGURE 27-27. Papillary carcinoma of the thyroid. A: The cut surface of a surgically resected thyroid displays a well-circumscribed pale tan mass. **B:** Branching papillae are lined by neoplastic columnar epithelium with crowded, overlapping nuclei. **C:** Nuclear clearing, longitudinal grooves, and nuclear inclusions are evident on high magnification.

(5% to 30%) and are typically exclusive of *BRAF* mutations. *RET* encodes a receptor tyrosine kinase; fusions result in constitutive tyrosine kinase activity, which drives cell growth.

Mutations in the *RAS* oncogene also occur, but are more common in the FVPTC.

PATHOLOGY: PTCs vary from microscopic lesions detected incidentally at autopsy to tumors larger than a normal gland. Papillary cancers may occur in either lobe or the isthmus and are associated with lymph node metastases on presentation in up to 25% of patients. Macroscopically, they are firm, solid, white-yellowish masses with irregular and infiltrative borders and occasionally a gritty texture caused by focal calcifications (Fig. 27-27A).

PTC typically invades lymphatics and spreads to regional cervical lymph nodes. Lymph node metastases vary from tiny foci in otherwise normal lymph nodes to large masses that dwarf the primary lesion. Hematogenous metastases are rare in PTC, but are more common in other thyroid cancers, including follicular thyroid carcinoma (FTC).

Various PCT subtypes have been described, with **conventional (classical) PCT** being the most common. Major variants include **follicular variant, diffuse sclerosing variant, tall cell variant, columnar variant, cribriformmorular variant**, and **hobnail variant**. PTC with a size less than 1 cm is termed a "**papillary microcarcinoma**" and is typically indolent, particularly if not associated with lymph node metastases.

Conventional (classical) PCT is defined microscopically by papillary architecture and distinctive nuclear features. Papillae are structures that contain a *fibrovascular core* and are lined by a neoplastic epithelial cell population (Fig. 27-27B). While they are required for a diagnosis of classical PCT, a variety of morphologies including nests, cords, and follicles may also be seen. Occasionally papillae may undergo degenerative calcification to form psammoma bodies, concentrically laminated calcific particles commonly seen in classical PTC. Prominent fibrotic reaction often accompanies PCT, particularly if it is invasive.

Nuclear atypia is an extremely important diagnostic feature in PCT. It includes enlarged, overlapping nuclei, marginated chromatin giving the nucleus a clear (**ground-glass** or **Orphan Annie**) appearance, and irregularities in the nuclear membrane including pseudoinclusions (round deformations of the nuclear membrane by cytoplasm) and longitudinal nuclear grooves ("coffee bean" nuclei) (Fig. 27-27C).

FVPTC has exclusively follicular architecture (no papillae) with nuclear features of PTC. It may be infiltrative or have a capsule that has been invaded by tumor. These tumors are morphologically identical to NIFTP (see above) and differ only in their invasive behavior. FV-PCT behaves similarly to PCT in that they often have lymph node metastases and carry a favorable prognosis.

Diffuse sclerosing variant develops in young patients and involves a majority of the thyroid with diffuse thyroid enlargement on clinical examination which may mimic thyroiditis. Dense sclerosis, numerous psammoma bodies with widely infiltrative disease and nests of squamous metaplasia are characteristic. This subtype is associated with more lymph node metastases and extrathyroidal extension, with a lower 10-year survival (93%) than classical PTC.

Tall cell variant of PCT contains large cells that are three times as tall as they are wide, have abundant oncocytic (pink) cytoplasm, and are typically arranged in a single layer on a long fibrovascular core. This subtype is more common in older patients. It is associated with extrathyroidal extension, distant metastases, and overall lower survival.

Columnar cell variant contains pseudostratified epithelial cells with dark, elongated, overlapping nuclei that contrast with those of other PCT variants (clear with irregular membranes). Morphologically, these tumors can mimic adenomas of the GI tract. When localized, they carry a good prognosis, but this worsens with disease spread.

Cribriform-morular variant of PCT is associated with familial adenomatous polyposis (FAP). It shows diverse architectural patterns (cribriform, papillary, solid, follicular) with very little colloid, and round nests of cells with squamous morphology (squamous morules) interspersed throughout the tumor. FAP patients can develop multiple tumors, but sporadic cases do occur and are usually solitary.

Hobnail variant of PCT shows papillary and micropapillary (small papillae without fibrovascular cores) structures lined by large cells with eosinophilic cytoplasm, large nuclei, and prominent nucleoli. The cells show decreased intercellular cohesion, causing an irregular "humped" contour produced by individual cells protruding away from the surface of the papillae. This variant is more likely to recur and show disseminated disease. It carries a worse prognosis.

Surgery is the primary form of therapy. Complete removal of the primary tumor and any associated involved lymph nodes carries a good prognosis. Radioactive iodine may be given following thyroid resection to ablate microscopic residual disease. Long-term follow-up is necessary, as recurrence may develop years or decades later.

Follicular Thyroid Carcinoma Is the Second Most Common Thyroid Carcinoma

FTC is a follicular-patterned malignant neoplasm without cytologic or architectural feature of PTC that demonstrates invasive growth. It accounts for 5% to 10% of thyroid carcinomas. Most patients are older than 40 and female (3:1) and it is rare in children. A painless neck mass is the most common presentation, although local compressive symptoms may develop. FTC is usually confined to the thyroid, but hematogenous spread to distant sites (lung, bone, brain) may occur and rarely be the presenting sign.

ETIOLOGIC FACTORS: Incidence of follicular carcinoma is higher in iodine-deficient areas. Irradiation to the gland may precede FTC in some cases, but the association is not as strong as for PTC. Genetically, follicular tumors may occur in patients with Cowden syndrome (*PTEN* mutation), Carney syndrome (*PRKAR1A* mutation), and Werner syndrome (*WRN* mutation).

MOLECULAR PATHOGENESIS: Point mutations in oncogenes of the *RAS* family (*NRAS, KRAS, HRAS*) occur in 30% to 50% of FTC. *HRAS* codon 61 is the most frequently affected hotspot. *PAX8/ PPARγ* (paired box 8/peroxisome proliferator–activated receptor γ) rearrangement with a t(2;3)(q13;p25) translocation affects another 20% to 30% of patients. *PIK3CA* mutations are found in an additional 10%, and PTEN mutations are also found in approximately 10% of tumors. Mutations in the promoter of the telomerase gene *TERT* is found in 20% of cases and is associated with more aggressive behavior.

PATHOLOGY: Follicular cancers vary in size. They are yellow-tan with thick white fibrous capsules, and may also show areas of hemorrhage and necrosis, and foci of cystic degeneration. They are subdivided into minimally invasive, encapsulated angioinvasive, and widely invasive FTCs.

Minimally invasive and **encapsulated angioinvasive FTCs** are well-defined, encapsulated tumors with thick fibrous capsules. Most show close resemblance to FAs, although they tend to contain more microfollicular or trabecular patterns and mitoses may be common. More importantly, however, unlike FAs, FTC show invasion. In minimally invasive FTC, tumor extends through the fibrous capsule in a "mushroom"-like pattern into the surrounding tissue (Fig. 27-28). In encapsulated angioinvasive tumors, tumor cells invade vessels. They often have a covering of endothelial cells associated with fibrin thrombus or red blood cells. FTC with only transcapsular invasion have an excellent prognosis, while vascular invasion increases the risk of distant metastases many years or decades later, often to bone and visceral organs. The more vascular invasion identified, the worse the prognosis.

Widely invasive FTC shows frank infiltrative invasion of surrounding thyroid and/or extrathyroidal tissue. They may show extensive vascular invasion of both veins and arteries. These tumors are typically large and do not pose the sort of diagnostic challenge seen in minimally invasive FCT. They carry a worse prognosis than encapsulated angioinvasive FCT. Therapy involves surgical excision. Postoperative radio-iodine may be particularly efficacious due to high uptake of iodine by follicular lesions.

Oncocytic (Hürthle cell) tumors are follicular neoplasms containing cells with distinctive morphology.

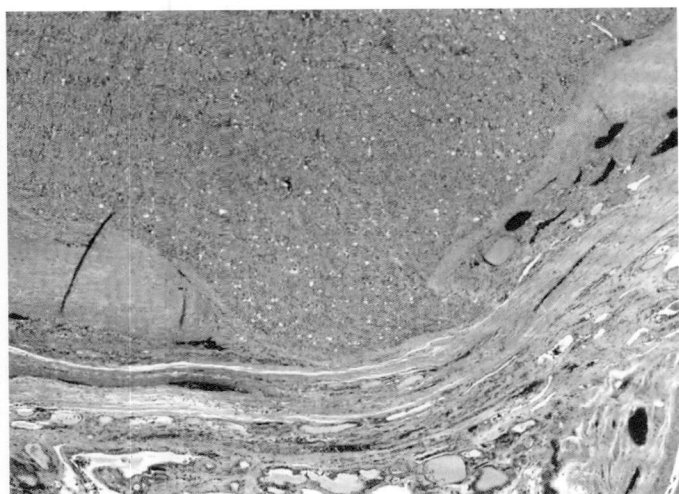

FIGURE 27-28. Follicular carcinoma of the thyroid shows proliferation in microfollicles in dense nests with rupture and invasion through the surrounding fibrous capsule.

Hürthle cells are large with highly abundant eosinophilic and granular cytoplasm, round-to-oval nuclei with prominent nucleoli. These tumors are usually encapsulated, unless extensively invasive. As for FAs and carcinomas, the malignant potential of Hürthle cell tumors is dictated by the degree of capsular or vascular invasion. Tumors without invasion are Hürthle cell adenomas. Those that invade through the fibrous capsule are minimally invasive, and widely invasive tumors show frank intrathyroidal or extrathyroidal extension. Hürthle cell carcinomas may metastasize to regional lymph nodes and distant sites through hematogenous spread. They tend to have a higher frequency of capsule and vascular invasion than FAs of similar size and carry a worse prognosis.

Anaplastic (Undifferentiated) Thyroid Carcinoma Is an Aggressive Tumor With Poor Prognosis

Anaplastic thyroid cancer (ATC) is composed of undifferentiated follicular thyroid cells without discernible thyroid differentiation by histomorphology. They often lack immunohistochemical markers of thyroid origin. They are thought to arise from undifferentiated thyroid follicular precursor cells by "dedifferentiation" of a PTC or FTC into a more primitive state.

Patients are often elderly and present with a large, rapidly growing infiltrative neck mass with localized compressive symptoms, often with metastases to distant sites. Macroscopically, these tumors are usually tan, firm, fleshy, and widely infiltrative. Microscopically, anaplastic thyroid carcinomas are highly atypical with large, pleomorphic cells reminiscent of high-grade sarcomas (Fig. 27-29). Occasionally giant cell or squamous differentiation is seen. Necrosis, high mitotic rate, and vascular invasion are all common.

Anaplastic thyroid carcinomas often carry *p53* mutations (up to 70%), as well as *BRAF* (~20%), *RAS* (~20%), *PIK3CA* (~10%), and *PTEN* (10%) mutations, as seen in other thyroid malignancies. Immunohistochemical markers of thyroid differentiation (thyroglobulin, TTF-1) are typically negative in ATC, though Pax-8 may be positive. The prognosis, despite therapy, is extremely poor with <10% survival at 5 years.

Poorly Differentiated (Insular) Thyroid Carcinoma Has Intermediate Prognosis

Poorly differentiated thyroid carcinoma (PDTC) is a follicular neoplasm with minimal follicular differentiation, and morphologic and prognostic parameters between well-differentiated (FTC, PTC) and anaplastic thyroid carcinomas. These tumors often occur in adults and typically present with a large, solitary thyroid mass that shows extrathyroidal extension and vascular invasion, but to a lesser extent than seen in anaplastic carcinoma.

Microscopically, PDTC is defined by the Turin criteria, which require the growth of tumor cells in cords, sheets, or nests without nuclear features of PCT. Three or more mitotic

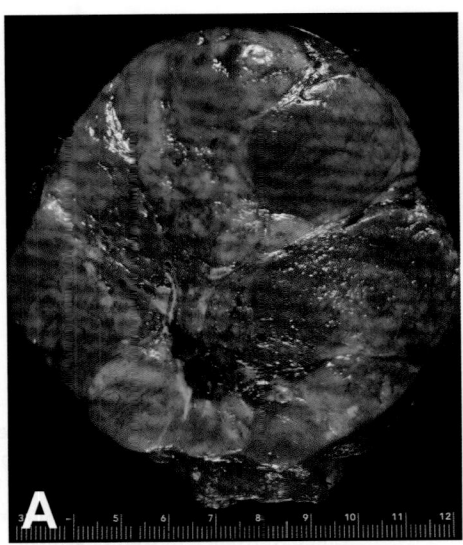

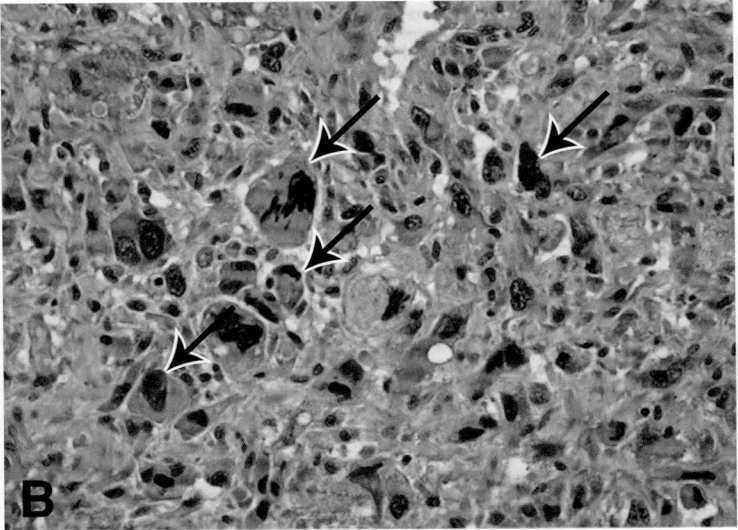

FIGURE 27-29. Anaplastic carcinoma of the thyroid. A: The tumor in transverse section partially surrounds the trachea and extends into the adjacent soft tissue. **B:** The tumor is composed of bizarre spindle and giant cells with polyploid nuclei and prominent mitotic activity (*arrows*).

TABLE 27-3			
NEUROENDOCRINE SYNDROMES WITH MEDULLARY THYROID CARCINOMA			
Syndrome	Gene	Inheritance	Manifestations
Multiple neuroendocrine neoplasia type 2a	*RET* (C634R) most common	Autosomal dominant	Medullary thyroid carcinoma Pheochromocytoma Parathyroid hyperplasia
Multiple neuroendocrine neoplasia type 2b	*RET* (M918T) most common	Autosomal dominant	Medullary thyroid carcinoma Pheochromocytoma Marfanoid habitus Mucosal neuromas, intestinal ganglioneuromas
Familial medullary thyroid carcinoma	*RET* (E768D and V804L) *NTRK1*	Autosomal dominant	Medullary thyroid carcinoma

figures per high-powered field, necrosis, or nuclear irregularity are required to fulfill diagnostic criteria. Nuclei are typically small and monotonous. PDTCs are important to recognize as they may progress to anaplastic thyroid carcinomas.

PDTCs harbor mutations in *p53* (up to 35%), *RAS* (up to 50%), *BRAF*, *PIK3CA*, and *PTEN*. Immunohistochemically, these tumors typically stain for TTF-1 and Pax-8, but not thyroglobulin. Patient with PDTC have a 60% to 70% 5-year survival. Older patient age, larger tumors, advanced local disease, and metastases are all poor prognostic factors.

Medullary Thyroid Carcinomas Are Tumors of Neoplastic C-Cells

Medullary thyroid carcinomas (MTC) represent fewer than 3% of all thyroid cancers and occur in both sporadic and familial forms. They most frequently produce calcitonin, which may result in hypocalcemia. They may also express other hormones such as serotonin, ACTH, CRH, and somatostatin.

MTC is sporadic in ~70% of cases and occurs in the fifth or sixth decades of life with a slight female predominance. Inherited MTC (30% of all cases) occurs in younger patients in the context of the AD MEN2 syndromes (MEN2a, MEN2b, and familial MTC [FMTC], see below), which are caused by gain-of-function mutations in the proto-oncogene *RET*.

Patient most often presents with a painless nodule that is "cold" on scintigraphy, often with regional lymph node metastases. High levels of calcitonin are often seen with concomitant hypocalcemia. Diarrhea and flushing may occur in serotonin-secreting tumors, and Cushing syndrome may occur secondary to ACTH or CRH secretion.

MTC Genetic Predisposition Syndromes: Heritable MTC is seen in multiple endocrine neoplasia 2 (MEN2) syndrome, which is subdivided into **MEN2A**, **MEN2B**, and FMTC based on clinical features (Table 27-3). Importantly, the location and nature of a given *RET* mutation manifests in various ways (Fig. 27-30).

Sporadic MTC is commonly associated with somatic point mutations in the *RET* gene (M918T is seen in up to 60%

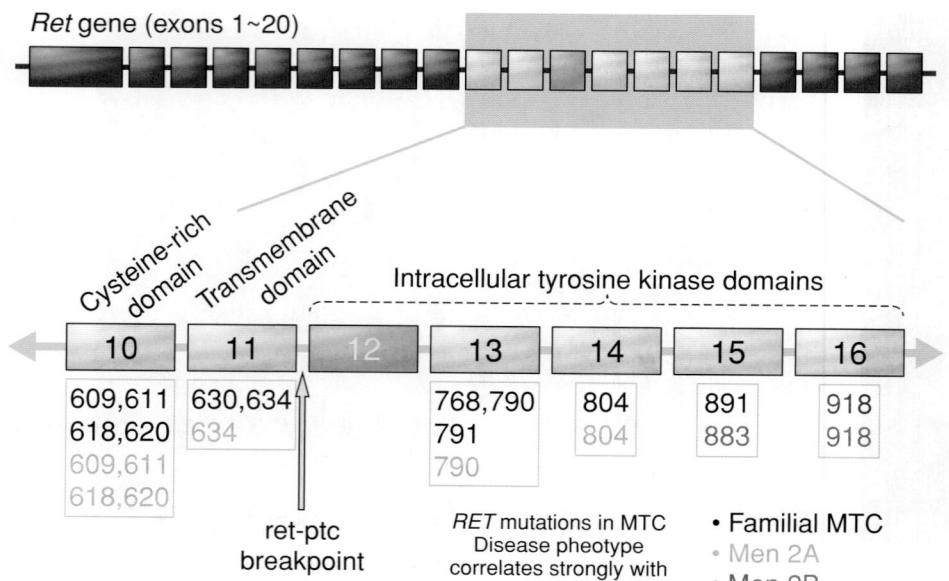

FIGURE 27-30. Schematic representation of the *RET* oncogene. The most commonly associated mutations occur in Exons 10 to 16. Substitution at various codon positions is associated with different syndrome manifestations, including MEN2A, MEN2B, and familial MTC. Several sporadic mutations in the *RET* gene are also detected in nonsyndrome-related MTCs.

of cases) and mutations in *RAS* (in up to 15%). *RET* fusions may also be present.

PATHOLOGY: MTC tends to occur in the mid-to-upper region of the thyroid, where C-cells arise. In the setting of MEN2, tumors are often multicentric and bilateral. MTCs are typically not encapsulated, but they often appear well-circumscribed, and have firm, grey-white cut surfaces. They may be grossly infiltrative (Fig. 27-31). Microscopically, they may show highly variable morphologies that can mimic other tumors. MTC can grow in solid, lobular, or corded patterns and may contain polygonal, spindled, or round cells (or any mixture therein) with finely granular cytoplasm (Fig. 27-31B). Dense fibrosis and stromal amyloid deposition composed of full-length calcitonin (procalcitonin) are seen in >90% of MTCs (Fig. 27-31C). Focal calcification may be extensive enough to be detected radiologically. Local invasion into adjacent tissues and lymph node metastases are common.

Seen by electron microscopy, neoplastic C-cells have dense-core secretory granules that are positive for several endocrine markers, including calcitonin, synaptophysin, chromogranin, and neuron-specific enolase. Nearly all of these tumors express carcinoembryonic antigen (CEA), which may be used to monitor for recurrence.

C-cell hyperplasia is the precursor lesion of FMTCs. It consists of clusters of C-cells with clear cytoplasm located near follicular cells. Mutations may be present in these early lesions. Thus, patients with MEN types 2A and 2B (see section on adrenal medulla) who are at risk for MTC are monitored by periodic measurements of serum calcitonin, CEA and sometimes chromogranin. If these are elevated, the patient may receive a total thyroidectomy.

MTC is treated with total thyroidectomy and lymph node dissection due to the high incidence of lymph node metastases. Hematogenous spread may also occur, most often to the lungs, bone, and liver. Five-year survival for patient with MTC is approximately 75%.

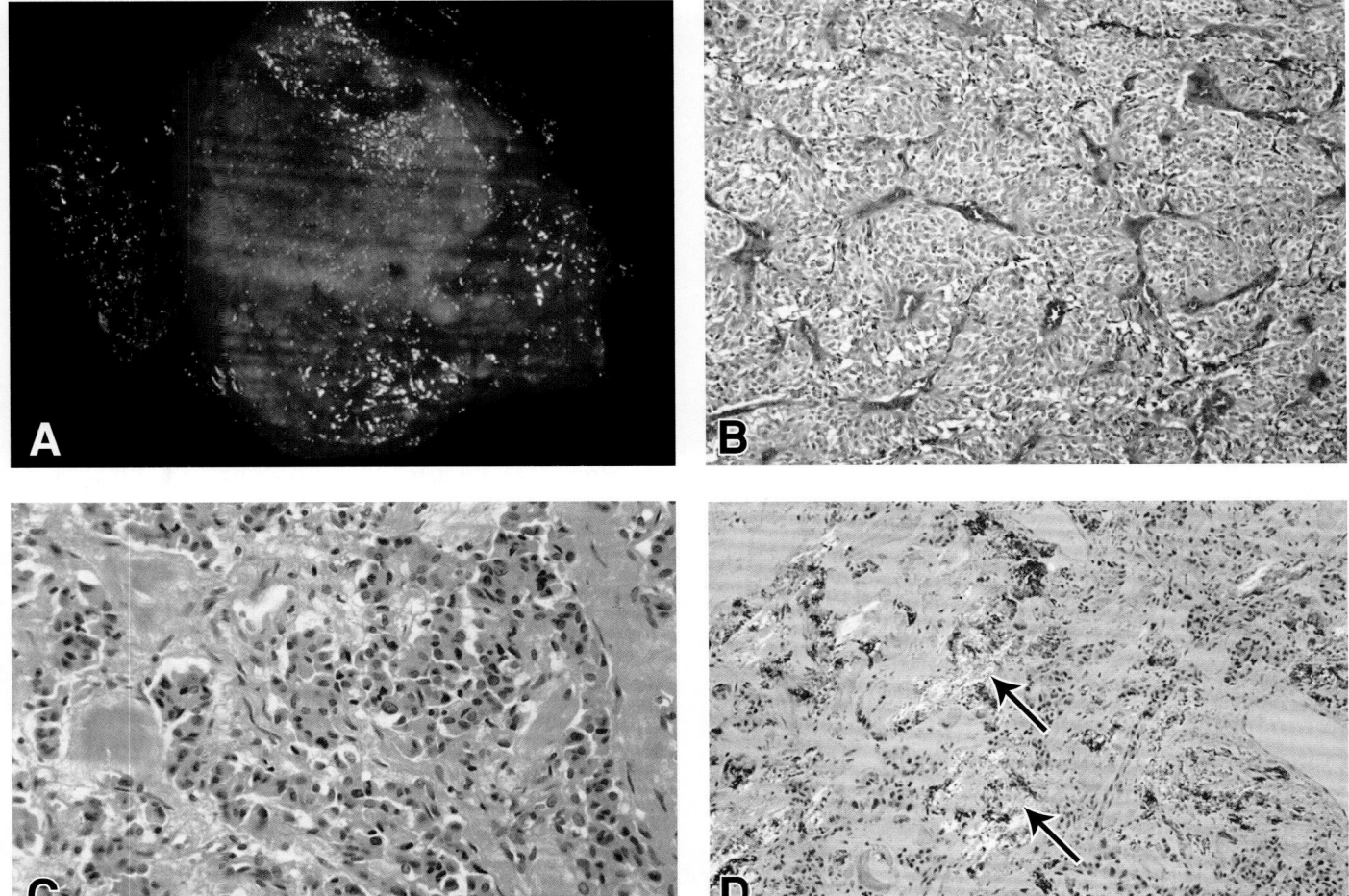

FIGURE 27-31. Medullary thyroid carcinoma. A: Grossly, medullary thyroid carcinoma is often a tan-yellow, irregular mass adjacent to normal red-brown thyroid tissue. **B:** Microscopically, the morphology of medullary thyroid carcinoma varies, and may include elongated, spindled cells (as in this figure) or flat, rounded (epithelioid) cells. **C, D:** Amyloid, as seen as amorphous reddish deposits in panel **C**, is detectable as birefringent material by Congo-Red staining (*arrows* in **D**).

THE ENDOCRINE SYSTEM

Parathyroid Glands

PARATHYROID GLANDS WORK IN CONCERT WITH THE KIDNEY TO REGULATE CALCIUM

The parathyroid glands are derived from the third and fourth branchial pouches. Most people have 4 glands (2 superior and 2 inferior), but numbers vary from 1 to 12. They are normally located on the posterior surface of the thyroid gland, but may occur within the thyroid or in ectopic locations such as mediastinum, pericardium, or near the recurrent laryngeal nerve.

A parathyroid gland is typically $5 \times 2 \times 2$ mm and weighs 20 to 50 mg. Approximately 75% of the cells are chief and oxyphil cells and the remaining cells are mature adipocytes. The amount of fat varies throughout life; before puberty, parathyroid glands are highly cellular with minimal fat, but in older adults fat may predominate.

Chief cells secrete parathyroid hormone (PTH) and parathyroid hormone–related protein (PTHrP). Chief cells are polyhedral with pale, eosinophilic-to-amphophilic cytoplasm that contains glycogen and fat droplets. Electron microscopy reveals membrane-bound cytoplasmic secretory granules. These cells stain positively for cytokeratin, chromogranin A, synaptophysin, and PTH. They are negative for TTF-1 and thyroglobulin.

Chief cells are highly sensitive to serum calcium concentrations. They respond to low blood levels of ionized calcium by releasing PTH which acts on renal tubular cells to increase calcium reabsorption. PTH also stimulates expression of *CYP27B1* which produces 1-α-hydroxylase in proximal convoluted tubules. This enzyme converts 25-hydroxyvitamin D (calcifediol) to biologically active 1,25-dihydroxyvitamin D_3 (calcitriol), leading to increased intestinal absorption of calcium and release of calcium in bone into the blood. PTH secretion is inhibited by high levels of calcium or calcitriol in the serum or very low magnesium levels.

Clear cells are chief cells whose cytoplasm is packed with glycogen. **Oncocytes** appear after puberty, are larger than chief cells and have deeply eosinophilic cytoplasm, owing to many mitochondria. They have no secretory granules and do not secrete PTH.

As seen in other endocrine organs, parathyroid glands can exhibit pathologic overactivity (hyperparathyroidism) or underactivity (hypoparathyroidism).

HYPERPARATHYROIDISM IS DEFINED BY EXCESS PTH PRODUCTION

Primary Hyperparathyroidism Refers to Autonomous PTH Production by the Parathyroid Glands Irrespective of Calcium Levels

This condition is uncommon, with an apparent incidence of 1 in 1,000. It occurs most commonly in women in the fifth decade. Primary hyperparathyroidism may be due to **parathyroid adenoma** (80% to 90% of cases), **hyperplasia** of all parathyroid glands (10% to 15%) or (rarely) **parathyroid carcinoma** (~1%). Primary hyperparathyroidism may be sporadic or a component of familial syndromes.

Clinical features are highly variable. Some patients exhibit asymptomatic hypercalcemia (detected on routine

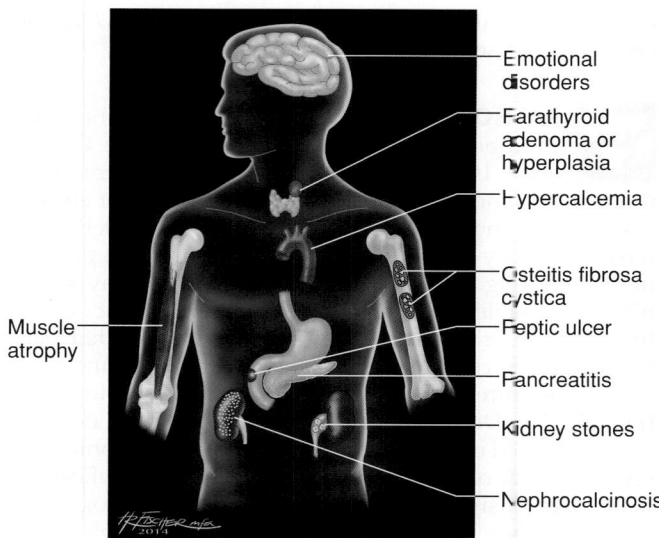

FIGURE 27-32. Clinical features of hyperparathyroidism.

blood analysis), while others show florid systemic, renal, and skeletal diseases (Fig. 27-32). Hypercalcemia and hypophosphatemia are typical. High PTH levels increase serum calcium by promoting reabsorption of calcium in the kidney and increasing calcitriol (vitamin D_3) levels, which induces release of calcium from bones and increases intestinal calcium absorption. Common symptoms include nausea, vomiting, fatigue, weight loss, anorexia, polyuria, and polydipsia. A neck mass may be palpable in some patients.

Skeletal, renal, nervous, and gastrointestinal systems are all affected by hyperparathyroidism. The characteristic bone lesions of hyperparathyroidism, osteitis fibrosa cystica (see Chapter 30), occur in a minority of patients who have an accelerated and serious form of the disease. These patients present with bone pain, bone cysts, pathologic fractures, and localized bone swellings (brown tumors). Renal colic due to kidney stones brings 10% of patients with primary hyperparathyroidism to medical attention. Nephrocalcinosis, observed radiologically as diffuse renal calcification, may also occur (see Chapter 22). Polyuria is caused by hypercalciuria and leads to polydipsia. Psychiatric changes including depression, emotional lability, poor mentation, and memory defects are common. Reflexes may be hyperactive and peripheral neuropathy with type 2 skeletal muscle fiber atrophy leads to weakness. Peptic ulcer disease is increased in patients with hyperparathyroidism, possibly because hypercalcemia increases serum gastrin, thus stimulating gastric acid secretion. Hypercalcemia may also cause constipation and chronic pancreatitis. The clinical manifestations of hyperparathyroidism may thus be summarized as "painful bones, renal stones, psychiatric moans, and abdominal groans."

Parathyroid Adenoma Is the Most Common Cause of Primary Hyperparathyroidism

Parathyroid adenoma is a benign proliferation of chief cells or oncocytes (or a mixture of both) which occurs much more commonly in women than men (3:1 ratio).

TABLE 27-4
SYNDROMES OF PARATHYROID NEOPLASIA AND HYPERPLASIA

Syndrome	Gene	Inheritance	Manifestations
Multiple neuroendocrine neoplasia type 1	MEN1	Autosomal dominant	Parathyroid adenomas Pituitary adenomas (Lactotroph most common) Pancreatic and duodenal neuroendocrine tumors
Multiple neuroendocrine neoplasia type 4	CDKN1B	Autosomal dominant	Parathyroid adenomas Pituitary adenomas (Somatotroph most common) Pancreatic and duodenal neuroendocrine tumors
Hyperparathyroidism-jaw tumor syndrome	CDC73 (HRPT/Parafibromin)	Autosomal dominant	Parathyroid adenoma Parathyroid carcinoma Ossifying fibromas of mandible/maxilla
Multiple neuroendocrine neoplasia type 2a	RET (C634R) most common	Autosomal dominant	Parathyroid hyperplasia Medullary thyroid carcinoma Pheochromocytoma
Familial isolated hyperparathyroidism	CASR CDC73 MEN1	Autosomal dominant	Parathyroid hyperplasia Parathyroid carcinoma

MOLECULAR PATHOGENESIS: Parathyroid adenomas are clonal proliferations that arise sporadically (80%) or in the context of familial syndromes (~20% of adenomas). Sporadic parathyroid adenomas are associated with mutations in the gene encoding the cell-cycle regulatory protein cyclin D1 (*CCND1*) in up to 40% of cases. Somatic inactivation of the tumor suppressor *MEN1* is seen in up to 35%.

Familial endocrine syndromes associated with parathyroid adenomas include MEN1, MEN4, and hyperparathyroidism-jaw tumor (HPT-JT) syndromes (summarized in Table 27-4).

PATHOLOGY: Macroscopically, parathyroid adenomas are circumscribed, red-brown, solitary masses that are typically ovoid and may be surrounded by a thin fibrous capsule. They may show hemorrhage and cystic change. They are usually between 0.6 to 3 cm in greatest dimension, weighing between 0.1 and 1 g, but may be much larger. Larger tumors are associated with more severe symptoms (Fig. 27-33A).

Microscopically, adenomas are composed of sheets of neoplastic chief cells within a rich capillary network. Chief cells are usually polyhedral with round nuclei and "salt-and-pepper" chromatin typical of endocrine cells. Occasionally cells within an adenoma may be spindled. A rim of normal parathyroid tissue is usually evident outside the capsule and distinguishes adenomas from parathyroid hyperplasia (Fig. 27-33B). Intracellular lipid droplets in parathyroid adenoma cells are considerably decreased compared to normal chief cells.

Histologic variants of parathyroid adenomas include *oncocytic adenomas*, which contain large cells with abundant eosinophilic cytoplasm and small round nuclei and *parathyroid lipoadenomas*, which contain fat, fibrosis, and inflammatory cells in addition to neoplastic chief cells.

Parathyroid adenomas are treated by surgical removal which provides immediate relief of the symptoms of hyperparathyroidism (PTH levels drop within minutes). Nonadenomatous parathyroid glands tend to be atrophic but regain normal structure and function once the offending gland(s) has been removed. Most parathyroid adenomas only involve one gland, but may rarely involve two. Adenomas can also occur within the thyroid gland or in ectopic parathyroid tissue. Once removed completely, parathyroid adenomas do not recur.

Primary Parathyroid Hyperplasia Is Characterized by Increased Cellularity and Size of All Parathyroid Glands

Primary parathyroid hyperplasia results in autonomous secretion of PTH leading to symptoms of hyperparathyroidism. It is responsible for 15% of cases of hyperparathyroidism and is two to three times more common in women.

Primary hyperparathyroidism is usually sporadic and its etiology is not fully understood. Approximately 20% of cases occur in familial syndromes associated with other endocrine tumors, including MEN2A and familial isolated hyperparathyroidism (FIPTH) (Table 27-4). FIPTH is associated with mutations in *CASR* (encoding a calcium-sensing receptor), which causes parathyroid hyperplasia and autonomous PTH production by interfering with the ability of chief cells to sense serum calcium levels.

One-third of sporadic primary parathyroid hyperplasia cases are associated with widespread proliferation of clones of chief cells, suggesting diffuse neoplastic proliferation. In such instances, chief cell hyperplasia and multiple small

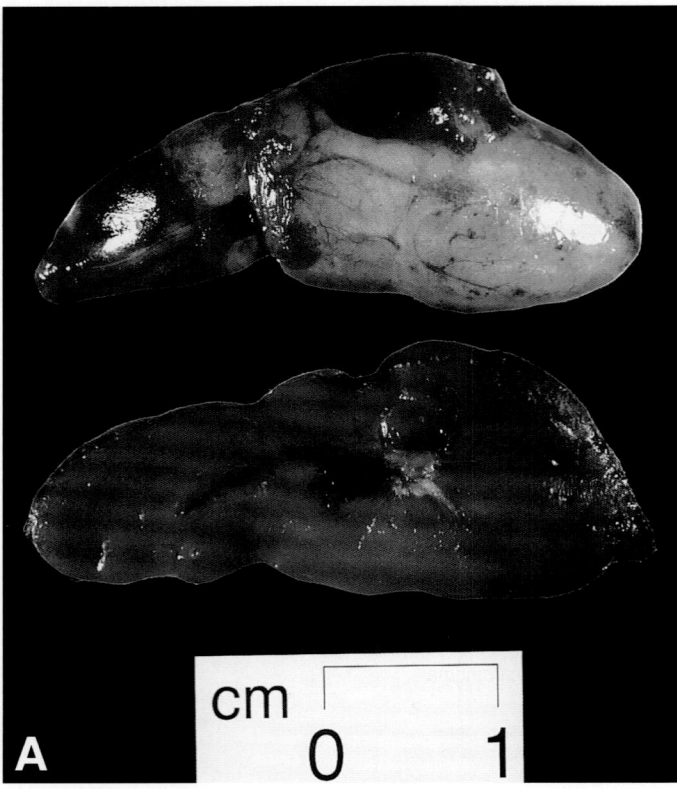

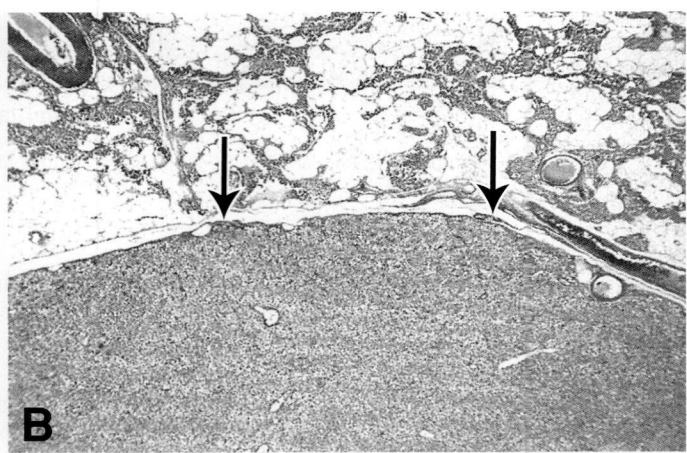

FIGURE 27-33. Parathyroid adenoma. A: External (*top*) and cross-section (*bottom*) views show a tan fleshy tumor. **B:** The tumor consists of sheets of neoplastic chief cells (seen at the bottom of this image) separated from normal parenchyma by a thin capsule (*arrows*).

adenomas occur in the same gland. Factors associated with sporadic primary hyperparathyroidism include exposure to ionizing radiation and lithium ingestion.

PATHOLOGY: All four parathyroid glands are enlarged, with combined weights from less than 1 to 10 g. In half of patients, one gland may be noticeably larger than the others, which may complicate the distinction from adenoma. Normal glandular adipose tissue is replaced by hyperplastic chief cells arranged in sheets, or in trabecular or follicular patterns (Fig. 27-34). Scattered oxyphil cells are common, and small foci of adipose tissue may remain. Intracellular lipid droplets are often decreased, but not to the same extent as that seen in adenomas. As opposed to adenomas, there is no "rim" of normocellular parathyroid gland, and surgical removal of one gland does not normalize PTH levels.

Treatment of primary hyperparathyroidism is surgical, often necessitating removal of all parathyroid glands. A small portion of one hyperplastic gland may be left behind in an attempt to restore normal PTH levels and normalize calcium homeostasis.

Parathyroid Carcinoma Is a Rare Malignant Neoplasm

Parathyroid carcinomas are derived from parathyroid cells, with an average age at diagnosis of 58 years and without sex predilection. Most cases occur in patients with PTH-JT and FIHP syndromes, but sporadic cases do occur.

Clinically, parathyroid carcinomas are functioning tumors producing high PTH levels and symptoms of hyperparathyroidism. Hypercalcemia in these patients is often severe, with serum calcium in excess of 14 mg/dL. Patients may show symptoms of profound bone mineral loss, renal failure with stones, weakness, psychiatric symptoms, and weight loss.

MOLECULAR PATHOGENESIS: The most common alteration in parathyroid carcinomas is an inactivating mutation in the tumor suppressor *CDC73* gene (also known as *HRPT2*), both in sporadic cases and syndrome cohorts (PTH-JT and FIHP) (Table 27-4). Ten-to-fifteen percent of patients with PTH-JT syndrome will develop parathyroid carcinoma in their lifetime.

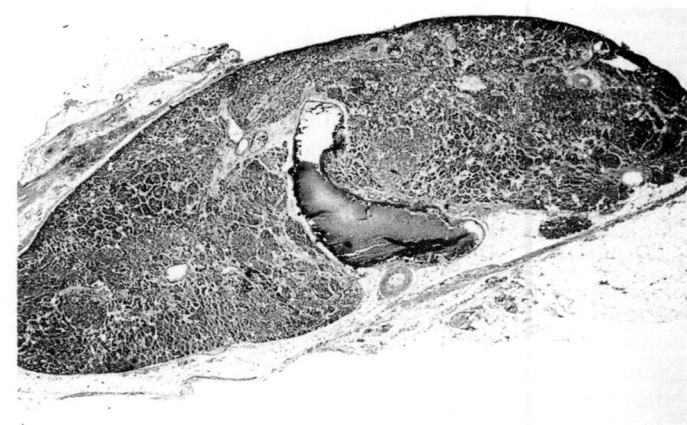

FIGURE 27-34. Primary parathyroid hyperplasia. The normal adipose tissue of the gland has been replaced by sheets and trabeculae of hyperplastic chief cells.

PATHOLOGY: Macroscopically, parathyroid carcinomas are poorly circumscribed, firmly adherent masses in the lateral neck. They tend to be larger than parathyroid adenomas, often showing multilobulated growth and characteristically infiltrate adjacent thyroid or soft tissues of the neck or metastasize to other organs, most commonly lung, liver, and cervical lymph nodes.

Microscopically, these tumors are composed of pleomorphic chief cells arranged in sheets or trabeculae. It may be difficult to distinguish parathyroid adenoma from carcinoma purely by cytomorphology. Often, carcinomas will show increased mitotic figures and contain dense fibrous bands running throughout the tumor. Cystic changes in parathyroid carcinoma is associated with HPT-JT. Necrosis and the presence of large nucleoli are features associated with aggressive behavior. Definitive diagnosis may require correlation with aggressive local invasive behavior or metastases.

Treatment of parathyroid carcinoma involves surgery but local recurrence is common. About one-third of patients develop metastases to the regional lymph nodes, lungs, liver, and bone. The risk of recurrence rises with the size of the primary tumor. When fatal, death is more often due to hyperparathyroidism than carcinomatosis. Ten-year survival is 50% to 70%.

Secondary Hyperparathyroidism Is most Commonly due to Renal Failure

Secondary parathyroid hyperplasia is a reactive hyperplasia that results from persistent stimulation of PTH production due to hypocalcemia. The most common cause is chronic renal failure, which decreases calcitriol activation by proximal tubular epithelial cell and reduces renal tubular reabsorption of calcium. Other associated factors include vitamin D deficiency, intestinal malabsorption, Fanconi syndrome, and renal tubular acidosis (Fig. 27-35), all of which may result in chronic hypocalcemia and, thereby, stimulate the parathyroid glands.

Secondary hyperplasia of all parathyroid glands leads to excess levels of PTH, which produces the main clinical manifestations of skeletal pain and deformities, osteomalacia, and osteitis fibrosis cystica. These osseous manifestations of hyperparathyroidism are called **renal osteodystrophy** (see Chapter 30).

Pain, swelling, and joint stiffness may be due to calcium deposits around joints. The gross and microscopic appearance of parathyroid glands in secondary hyperplasia resembles those of primary hyperparathyroidism. Relief of the underlying stimulus of excess PTH production, usually achieved by treating renal disease or correcting vitamin D deficiency, is the primary mode of therapy. If the underlying pathology cannot be managed medically, then surgical removal is performed.

Tertiary Hyperparathyroidism Arises From Prolonged Secondary Hyperparathyroidism

Tertiary hyperthyroidism is a condition of autonomous parathyroid secretion of PTH following long-standing secondary hyperparathyroidism, usually in patients with chronic renal failure. In such cases, parathyroid hyperplasia may not regress after renal transplantation, and parathyroidectomy may be required to control calcium levels. Pathologically, tertiary hyperparathyroidism is similar in appearance to primary hyperparathyroidism.

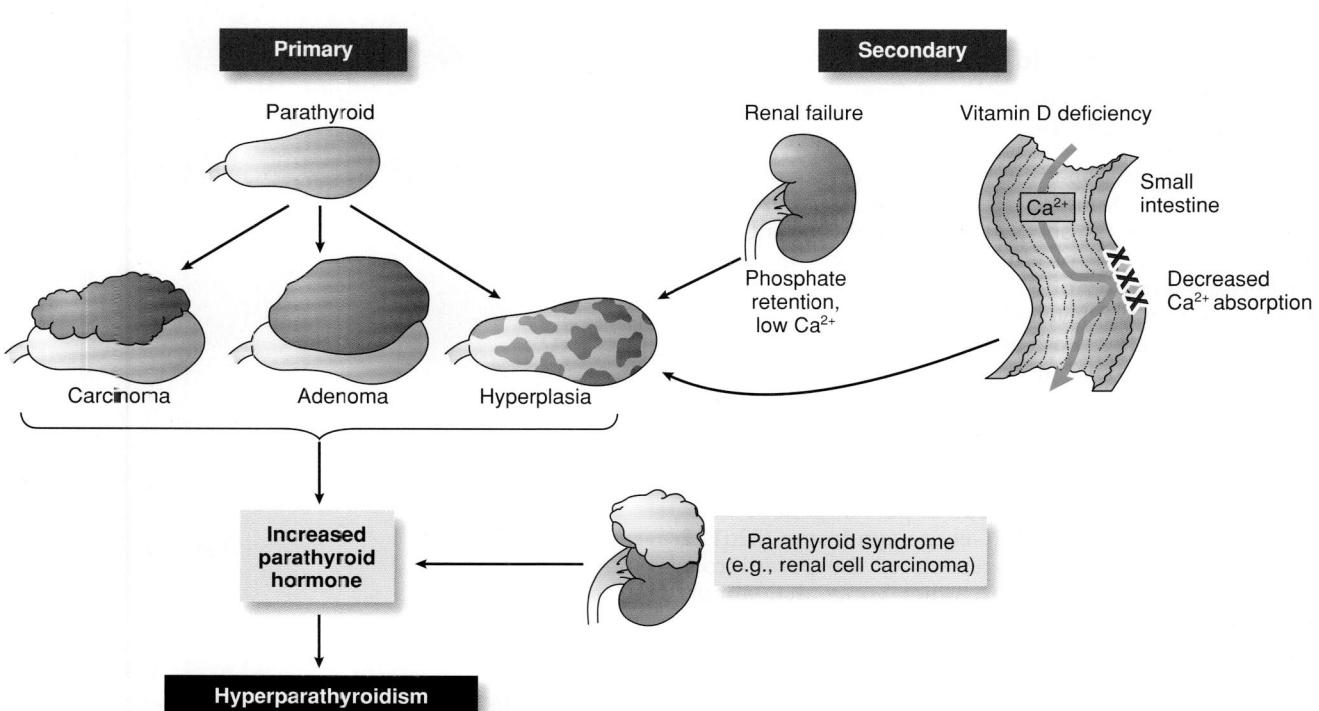

FIGURE 27-35. Pathogenic pathways leading to clinical primary and secondary hyperparathyroidism.

Paraneoplastic Hyperparathyroidism Is Driven by PTHrP

Occasionally, solid neoplasms including squamous cell carcinoma, breast carcinoma, renal cell carcinoma, and prostatic carcinoma may liberate PTHrP, which acts on osteoclasts in the bone to resorb calcium and increase serum calcium levels. This causes a paraneoplastic syndrome seen clinically as hyperparathyroidism, but unlike PTH elevation in hyperparathyroidism, excess PTHrP does not typically increase calcitriol levels.

HYPOPARATHYROIDISM IS CHARACTERIZED BY HYPOCALCEMIA AND HYPERPHOSPHATEMIA

Hypoparathyroidism results from decreased secretion of PTH or end-organ insensitivity to it (pseudohypoparathyroidism), whether congenital or acquired.

Traumatic/Iatrogenic Hypoparathyroidism Is the Most Common Cause of Hypoparathyroidism

Surgical excision of the parathyroid glands in patients with trauma, thyroid disease, or hyperparathyroidism is the most common etiology of hypoparathyroidism in the United States. Symptoms of hypocalcemia that arise in hypoparathyroidism include increased neuromuscular excitability associated with tingling in the hands and feet, severe muscle cramps, tetany, laryngeal stridor, and convulsions. Neuropsychiatric manifestations include depression, paranoia, and psychoses. High cerebrospinal fluid pressure and papilledema may mimic a brain tumor. Patients with all forms of hypoparathyroidism are treated with vitamin D and calcium supplementation.

Genetic Hypoparathyroidism Includes Familial Isolated Hypoparathyroidism and DiGeorge Syndrome

Familial isolated hypoparathyroidism is a group of rare diseases with AD, X-linked recessive, or AR patterns of inheritance that result in abnormalities of parathyroid gland development or PTH production. Mutations in *GCM2*, which encodes a transcription factor that plays a fundamental role in parathyroid development, have been identified in some affected families. Loss-of-function mutations in *PTH*, the PTH gene itself, may cause defective production or result in a nonfunctional hormone. Gain-of-function mutations in *CASR*, which encodes a calcium-sensing receptor, may reduce PTH secretion despite low levels of calcium, due to aberrant calcium sensing.

Hypoparathyroidism can occur as part of genetic deletion syndromes such as the **DiGeorge syndrome** (22q11.2 deletion), in which there is agenesis of the parathyroid glands and thymus along with other congenital abnormalities including cardiac defects. Mutations in *AIRE*, which encodes a protein that drives negative selection of self-recognizing T-cells, have been linked to autoimmune polyglandular failure syndrome type 1, which includes hypoparathyroidism, adrenal insufficiency, and mucocutaneous candidiasis.

Pseudohypoparathyroidism Is a Phenotype of Albright Hereditary Osteodystrophy

Pseudohypoparathyroidism describes a group of hereditary conditions characterized by hypocalcemia, hyperphosphatemia, and *increased* serum concentration of PTH. It arises due to tissue insensitivity to PTH and is most commonly caused by loss-of-function mutations in *GNAS1*, resulting in low activity of G_s, the stimulatory G protein that couples hormone receptors to adenylyl cyclase. As a result, cAMP production in response to PTH in renal tubular epithelium is impaired, causing inadequate calcium resorption. Patients with pseudohypoparathyroidism (PHP) are also often resistant to other cAMP-coupled hormones, including TSH, glucagon, FSH and LH. These patients have a characteristic phenotype (**Albright hereditary osteodystrophy**) including short stature, obesity, mental retardation, subcutaneous calcification, and congenital anomalies of bone, particularly abnormally short metacarpals and metatarsals (Fig. 27-36).

Pseudopseudohypoparathyroidism reads like a typographical error, but it refers to rare cases in which the phenotype of Albright hereditary osteodystrophy is associated with normal PTH, vitamin D, and calcium levels. This condition is caused by paternal imprinting of a mutated *GNAS1* gene. When passed to his children, there is differential utilization of paternal and maternal *GNAS1* alleles. In the kidney, the normal maternal copy is utilized, allowing for proper PTH signaling and calcium homeostasis, while the defective copy is utilized in remaining tissues, generating the Albright hereditary osteodystrophy phenotype.

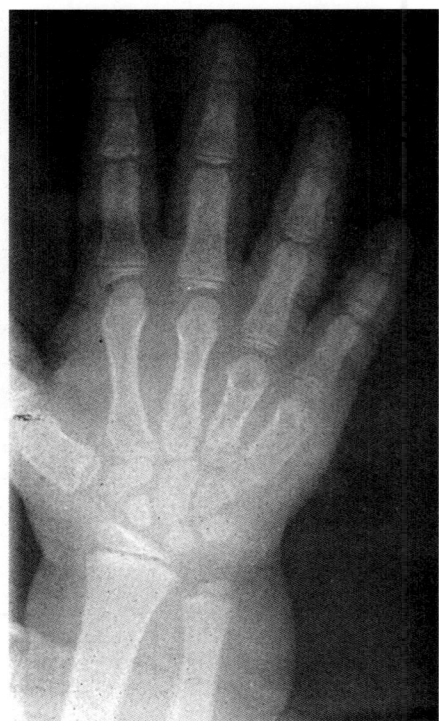

FIGURE 27-36. Pseudohypoparathyroidism. A radiograph of the hand reveals the characteristic shortness of the fourth and fifth metacarpal bones.

Adrenal Cortex

THE ADRENAL GLAND PRODUCES MINERALOCORTICOIDS, GLUCOCORTICOIDS, AND SEX HORMONES

Each adrenal (or suprarenal) gland contains two independent endocrine organs: the outer adrenal cortex and the inner adrenal medulla. They are distinct anatomically, functionally, and embryologically. The cortex arises from celomic mesodermal cells near the urogenital ridge, while the adrenal medulla arises from neural crest cells.

During early fetal development an (inner) fetal zone and outer definitive zone form. At this time, the fetal zone comprises most of the gland mass and generates large amounts of dehydroepiandrosterone, an estrogen precursor utilized by the placenta. Over time, the fetal zone is invaded by neural crest progenitors that will become the adrenal medulla. A second wave of mesodermal cells that will give rise to the glomerular and fascicular zones envelops the developing cortex. At birth, the fetal zone regresses and is replaced by neuroendocrine cells of the medulla. The three layers of the adrenal cortex (glomerular, fascicular, reticular) mature and thicken over the first years of life. Mature development of the adrenal cortex relies on trophic actions of ACTH. The fully developed adrenal cortex secretes steroid hormones such as aldosterone, cortisol, and testosterone important in homeostasis and sexual development.

Adult adrenal glands are pyramidal organs located above each kidney. They are covered by perirenal fascia and reside in the retroperitoneum. At birth, adrenal glands weigh as much at 6 to 7 g, but over the course of months reduce to ~4 to 5 g due to regression of the fetal zone. In adults, adrenal glands weigh 4 to 6 g.

Grossly, the adrenal cortex has a yellow color because of steroid and lipid deposits while the medulla is red-purple due to the rich blood supply enveloping nests of neuroendocrine cells. The cortex contains three layers or zones:

- The **zona glomerulosa** is the outermost layer. It produces aldosterone in response to angiotensin generated by the kidney. It is also stimulated by low serum potassium levels. Aldosterone production is inhibited by atrial natriuretic peptide and somatostatin. The zona glomerulosa makes up 5% to 15% of the cortex. It is composed of indistinct spherical nests of cells with dark-staining nuclei and moderate numbers of cytoplasmic fat droplets.
- The **zona fasciculata** makes up 75% of the cortex. It produces glucocorticoids, such as cortisol under the control of ACTH from the pituitary gland. It is not distinctly separated from the zona glomerulosa. It consists of radial cords of larger cells with small nuclei and abundant foamy cytoplasm containing stored lipids.
- The **zona reticularis**, the innermost layer of cortex adjacent to the medulla, secretes androgens critical for sexual development. It consists of irregular anastomosing cords of compact cells with bland nuclei and lipid-poor, slightly granular eosinophilic cytoplasm.

Production of adrenal cortical hormones is complex and hierarchical. It involves multiple biochemical synthetic pathways in which the steroid hormone precursor cholesterol is transformed into physiologically active hormones

(Fig. 27-37). Excessive action or deficiency of each of these pathways underlies the pathophysiology of adrenal cortical diseases.

The **medulla** is in the center of the gland, surrounded by cortex. Microscopically, the cells of the adrenal medulla are monomorphic, with round nuclei with "salt-and-pepper" chromatin. They are arranged in ball-like clusters (termed "zellballen"), with a rich vasculature and supporting cells surrounding each cluster. Adrenal medullary cells secrete epinephrine and norepinephrine.

DEVELOPMENTAL ANOMALIES AND DISEASES

Heterotopic adrenal tissue is adrenal tissue outside the adrenal glands, typically occurring along the migration path of gonadal tissue, which, like the adrenals, also arises from the urogenital ridge. Common locations of ectopic adrenal tissue include the retroperitoneum, the broad ligament near the ovary, bladder, epididymis, kidneys, and the liver. Heterotopic adrenal tissue usually contains only cortical tissue which may give rise to benign or malignant tumors.

Adrenal gland fusion, whereby both glands are joined at the midline near the aorta, occurs rarely, typically in conjunction with renal abnormalities. Occasionally, **adrenal gland adhesion** may result in firm attachment of the gland to adjacent liver and kidney, potentially complicating surgical procedures.

X-linked adrenal hypoplasia is a rare condition caused by inactivating mutations in *NROB1*, which encodes DAX1, a nuclear receptor protein essential for development of the adrenal glands and the pituitary gland. This rare condition may accompany renal agenesis. It causes decreased sex hormone production leading to hypogonadotropic hypogonadism in adolescents.

DISORDERS OF ADRENAL CORTICAL HORMONE EXCESS MAY BE DUE TO HYPERPLASIA OR NEOPLASIA

Most adrenal masses are nonfunctional and are detected incidentally during imaging studies for other purposes or at autopsy. Excess mineralocorticoid (aldosterone) production is mainly due to cortical hyperplasia or adenoma. The most common cause of elevated glucocorticoid (cortisol) levels is iatrogenic administration of steroids for therapeutic (anti-inflammatory) indications, but other causes include ACTH-producing pituitary adenomas, ectopic ACTH-producing tumors, and adrenal cortical neoplasms. Excess sex-hormone production is most often seen in hyperplasia (most typically congenital adrenal hyperplasia [CAH]) or in cortical neoplasms, including adrenal cortical carcinoma (ACC).

Hyperaldosteronism

Primary Hyperaldosteronism Is the Autonomous Secretion of Aldosterone by the Adrenal Gland

Primary aldosteronism, or **Conn syndrome**, is caused by cortical hyperplasia (65%) or adrenal cortical adenomas (33%).

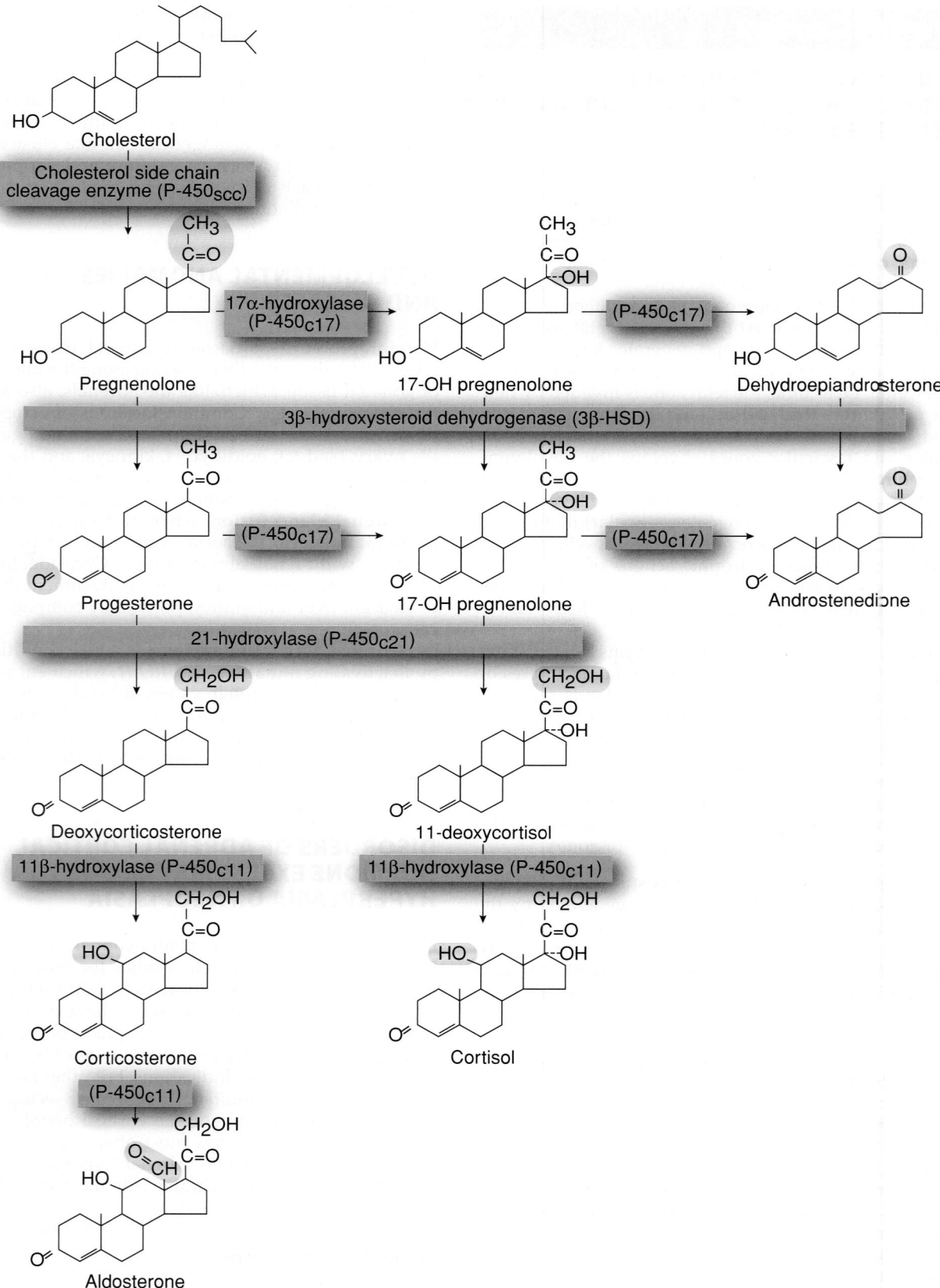

FIGURE 27-37. Biosynthetic pathways in the synthesis of adrenal corticosteroids.

In both cases, aldosterone secretion is autonomous and causes hypertension due to sodium retention. It may also cause hypokalemia due to potassium wasting in the distal nephron with associated metabolic alkalosis.

Hyperaldosteronism is typically diagnosed by comparing plasma renin and aldosterone levels. The aldosterone to renin ratio (PAC/PRC) is abnormally high in primary hyperaldosteronism, indicating autonomous aldosterone production. Patients often present in early to mid-adulthood with unexplained hypertension. Adrenal hyperplasia is typically bilateral, but may rarely be unilateral. High-resolution imaging studies may show enlarged, thickened, or nodular adrenal glands. The molecular pathogenesis of hyperplasia with hyperaldosteronism is not well understood. Most cases are sporadic. Patients with hyperplasia are treated with aldosterone antagonists such as eplerenone and spironolactone.

Familial hyperaldosteronism (FH) syndromes account for a small proportion (<5%) of cases of primary hyperaldosteronism. These are subdivided into three categories. **Type 1 FH**, also known as glucocorticoid suppressible FH, is an AD syndrome caused by fusion of two closely located genes on chromosome 8: *CYP11B1* which encodes aldosterone synthase, and *CYP11B2*, the 11β-hydroxylase gene which is regulated by ACTH. The result is abnormal production of aldosterone stimulated by ACTH. Interestingly, administration of glucocorticoids, which decreases plasma ACTH, reduces the activity of the fusion gene and thereby suppresses aldosterone production. **Type 2 FH** is not well understood. It is apparently transmitted in an AD pattern. **Type 3 FH** is associated with germline mutations in *KCNJ5* which makes GIRK4 potassium channels. The mutant channels have impaired ion selectivity. They allow abnormal sodium entry into zona glomerulosa cells which stimulates production of aldosterone independent of angiotensin signaling.

Aldosterone-producing cortical adenomas are common tumors of the adrenal gland, seen in up to 10% of the adult population, but the great majority do not produce hormone. Occasionally, they may generate aldosterone autonomously, leading to signs and symptoms of hyperaldosteronism. Such adenomas are more common in women than men (3:1) and usually occur between the ages of 30 and 50 years.

MOLECULAR PATHOGENESIS: About 40% of aldosterone-producing adenomas are caused by somatic mutations in *KCNJ5*, the same gene in which germline mutations cause type 3 FH. Gain-of-function mutations in genes for other membrane ion channels (*ATP1A1, ATF2B3, CACNA1D*) have also been implicated in aldosterone-producing adenomas.

PATHOLOGY: Cortical adenomas that produce aldosterone are often solitary masses, usually less than 5 cm, and contiguous with normal-appearing adrenal cortex (nonatrophic). They typically have a yellow or orange color (Fig. 27-38). Microscopically, they are composed of large cells with abundant intracytoplasmic lipid, and small, round nuclei with occasional pleomorphism. They typically grow in cords and nests enveloped in a network of reticulin fibers (Fig. 27-39).

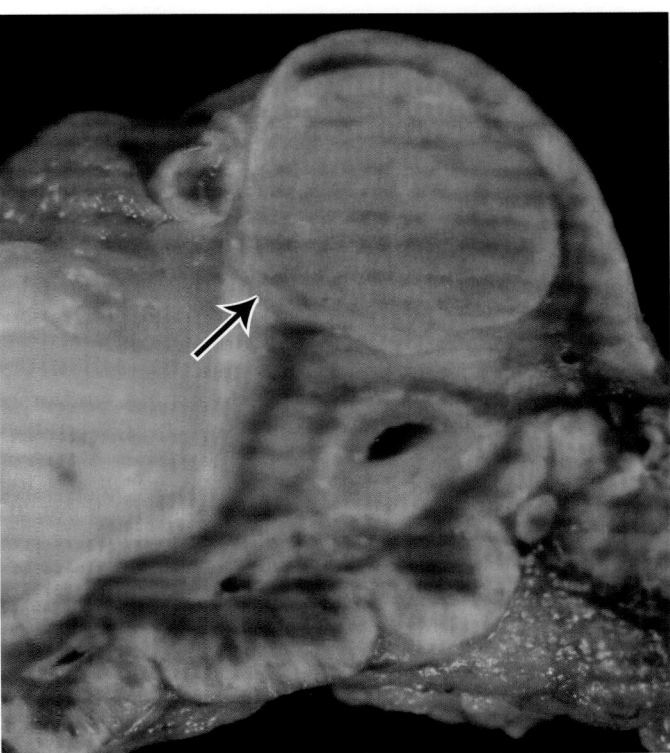

FIGURE 27-38. Adrenal cortical adenoma. Grossly, an adrenocortical adenoma is a well-circumscribed nodule (*arrow*) with the same yellow-tan color as the surrounding adrenal cortex.

Surgical excision of aldosterone-producing adenomas is definitive therapy, with very low probability of recurrence.

Hyperaldosteronism may be *secondary* to a **juxtaglomerular cell tumor**, an extremely rare tumor derived from the juxtaglomerular apparatus in the kidney that secretes renin. The increased renin induces the production of aldosterone by the adrenal gland and leads to symptoms of hyperaldosteronism. These tumors occur in children and young adults, more commonly in females.

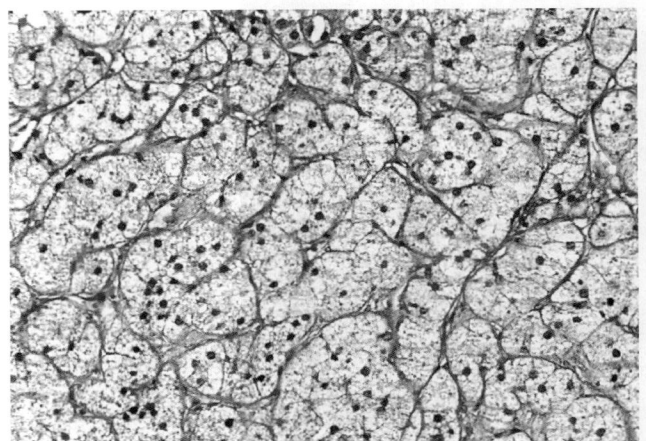

FIGURE 27-39. Adrenal cortical adenoma. A micrograph of an adrenal cortical adenoma reveals nests of clear, lipid-laden cells with small, monotonous nuclei.

Biochemical testing shows elevated renin and aldosterone levels. Surgical resection is curative.

Hypercortisolism Is Also Known as Cushing Syndrome

Excess cortisol causes characteristic clinical signs and symptoms (Fig. 27-40). These include central truncal obesity with purple striae over the abdomen, facial, and upper back fat pad expansion ("moon facies" and "buffalo hump"), thin atrophic skin with propensity to bruise, osteoporosis with propensity for fractures, hyperglycemia, mild virilization, and muscle weakness. Psychiatric disturbances include mental slowness, irritability, and depression. Collectively, these signs and symptoms are referred to as Cushing syndrome. Their extent and severity are proportional to the duration and degree of cortisol excess.

The most common cause of Cushing syndrome in the United States is glucocorticoid administration for the treatment of inflammatory and autoimmune conditions. In this circumstance, known as exogenous Cushing syndrome, ACTH is low and the adrenal cortex may be atrophic.

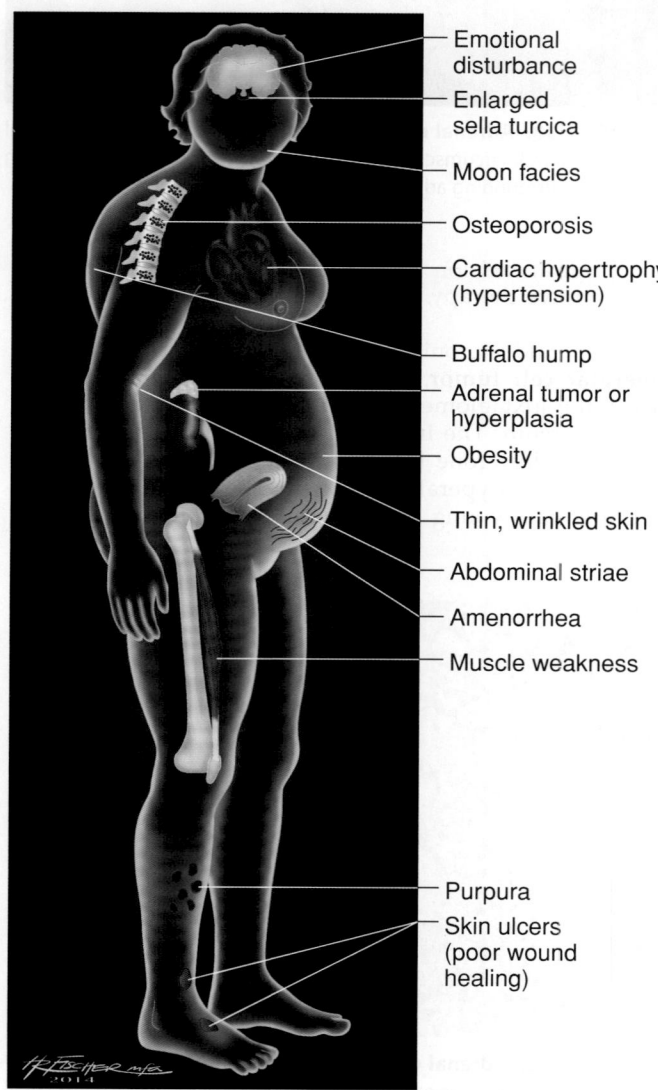

- Emotional disturbance
- Enlarged sella turcica
- Moon facies
- Osteoporosis
- Cardiac hypertrophy (hypertension)
- Buffalo hump
- Adrenal tumor or hyperplasia
- Obesity
- Thin, wrinkled skin
- Abdominal striae
- Amenorrhea
- Muscle weakness
- Purpura
- Skin ulcers (poor wound healing)

FIGURE 27-40. Clinical manifestations of Cushing syndrome.

Endogenous Cushing syndrome refers to intrinsic pathologies leading to excess cortisol production. It is a rare disease, with an incidence of six to seven cases per million person-years. Approximately 80% of cases are caused by excess ACTH production, which stimulates the adrenal gland to produce and secrete cortisol (**ACTH-dependent** Cushing syndrome). Of these, most are related to corticotrope pituitary adenomas (Fig. 27-41). Ectopic ACTH secretion from a neuroendocrine tumor (often small cell lung carcinoma) accounts for the remaining cases. Rarely, a CRH-producing tumor, either in the hypothalamus or elsewhere, may cause ACTH-dependent Cushing syndrome. Adrenal glands in patients with ACTH-dependent Cushing syndrome may be symmetrically enlarged due to persistent stimulation.

ACTH-independent Cushing syndrome, accounting for ~20% of cases of endogenous Cushing syndrome cases, is usually due to autonomous cortisol producing adrenal tumors, either adrenal cortical adenomas or ACCs (Fig. 27-41). Rarely, diffuse hyperplasia of adrenal glands may be the source of excess cortisol in ACTH-independent Cushing syndrome.

Laboratory testing in Cushing syndrome includes measurement of urine-free cortisol over 24 hours, overnight serum cortisol levels (which are normally low), or dexamethasone-suppression testing.

Cushing Disease Is Defined as Cushing Syndrome Caused by an ACTH-Producing Pituitary Adenoma

Cushing disease accounts for approximately 10% of all pituitary adenomas. There is a female predominance with peak incidence in the fourth to sixth decades. Corticotroph adenomas are the most common pituitary adenomas in children, and cause most cases of Cushing syndrome in this age group with male predominance.

The molecular pathogenesis, pathology, and treatment of corticotroph adenomas are described above. As part of the laboratory diagnosis of Cushing syndrome, a high-dose dexamethasone suppression test will often show suppression of cortisol production if the source of ACTH is the pituitary gland, while cortisol will remain elevated in the case of an ectopic ACTH-producing tumor (see below)

Ectopic ACTH May Be Produced by Many Tumor Types

Ectopic ACTH production in tumors other than pituitary adenomas accounts for approximately 10% of endogenous Cushing syndrome cases. Most tumors generating ectopic ACTH are intrathoracic. Pulmonary neuroendocrine tumors (small cell carcinoma, bronchial neuroendocrine tumors) account for approximately half of cases, and thymic neuroendocrine tumors for approximately 10%. About 20% are caused by pancreatic neuroendocrine tumors. Theoretically, any tissue with neuroendocrine cells has the potential to become neoplastic and act as a source of ectopic ACTH.

Surgical excision of ACTH-producing tumors is usually curative, but relapse may occur if the resection is incomplete. Localizing the source of ectopic ACTH can sometimes be difficult.

Cortisol-Secreting Adrenal Cortical Tumors May Cause ACTH-Independent Cushing Syndrome

Cortisol-secreting adenomas and ACCs are both causes of autonomous cortisol production. In these circumstances,

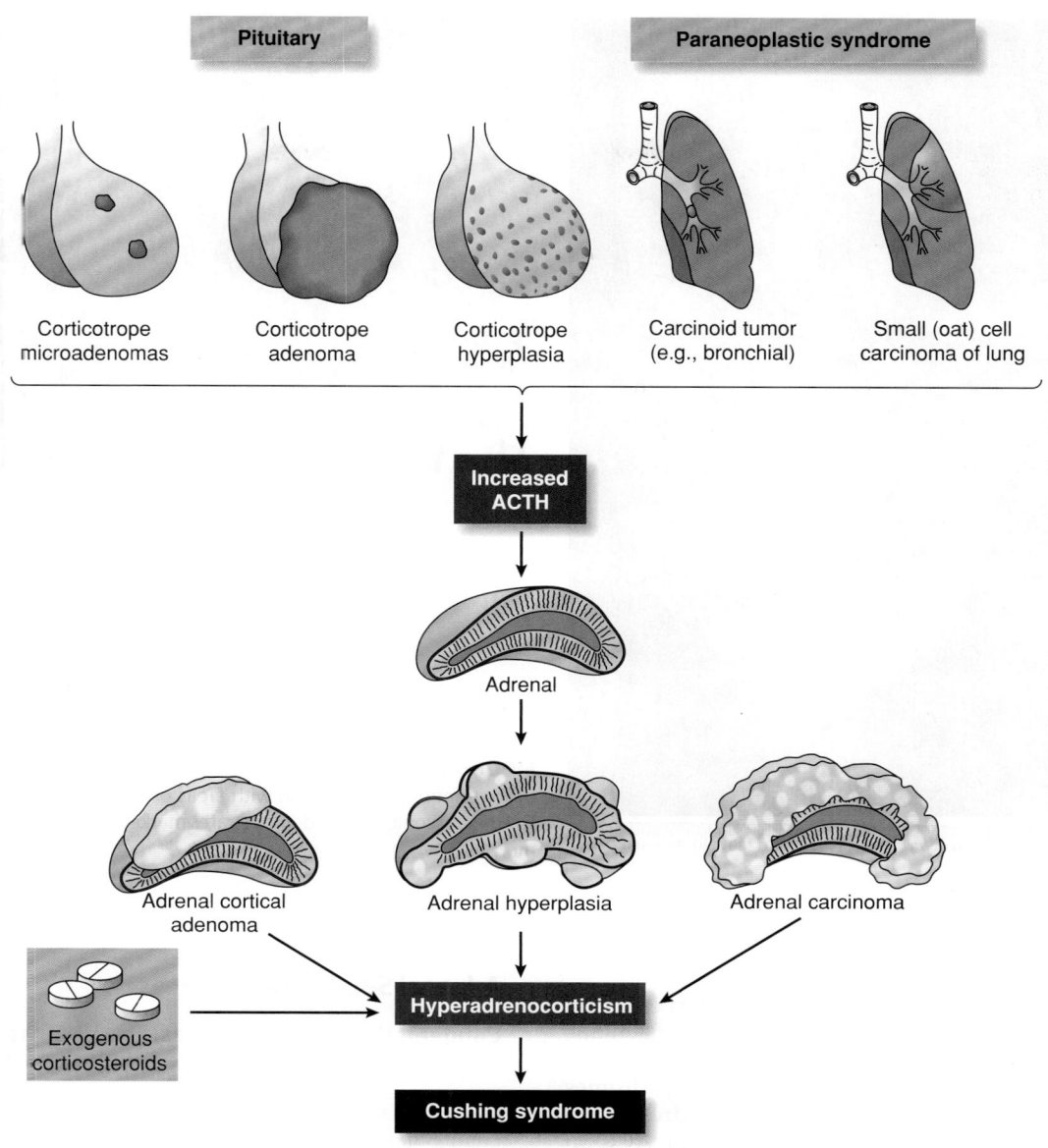

FIGURE 27-41. Pathogenic pathways in Cushing syndrome. The ACTH-dependent pathway is called Cushing disease. *ACTH* = adrenocorticotropic hormone (corticotropin).

ACTH is low while urine free and plasma cortisol levels are elevated. Dexamethasone does not suppress cortisol-producing adenomas and carcinomas.

About half of cortisol-producing adrenal cortical adenomas are linked to mutations in *PRKACA* which encodes a catalytic subunit of protein kinase A. Grossly, these tumors are tan-brown in color, usually less than 5 cm in diameter and contiguous with the adjacent adrenal cortex, which is often atrophic due to low serum levels of ACTH. Microscopically, they are composed of pale, lipid-rich cells with uniform nuclei and "salt-and-pepper" chromatin, arranged in nests, cords, and sheets without features suggestive of ACC (see below).

ACC is a rare malignant neoplasm of adrenal cortical cells in adults with a female predilection. Most patients (40% to 60%) present with symptoms attributable to hormone excess, most commonly cortisol and/or sex hormones. The remaining cases have symptoms related to the presence of a large mass (30%) or are discovered incidentally by imaging studies (15% to 20%).

ACCs tend to be large, commonly over 10 cm, and often displace and/or invade adjacent organs (pancreas, liver, kidney). Grossly, they appear as variegated, nodular masses with focal necrosis and hemorrhage (Fig. 27-42). They are often surrounded by a thick fibrous capsule. Microscopically, they are composed of sheets or nests of highly atypical cells that invade the fibrous capsule, vascular structures, and nearby organs. The mitotic rate is above 5 per 50 high-powered microscopic fields, and those with more than 20 per 50 high-power fields show more aggressive behavior. Immuno-histochemically, ACCs are positive for inhibin, SF1, Melan-A, synaptophysin-A, and calretinin. Chromogranin, keratins, and EMA are often negative. Distinguishing ACCs from adrenal cortical adenomas is critical, as the prognosis for ACC is poor, with a 5-year survival of approximately 40%.

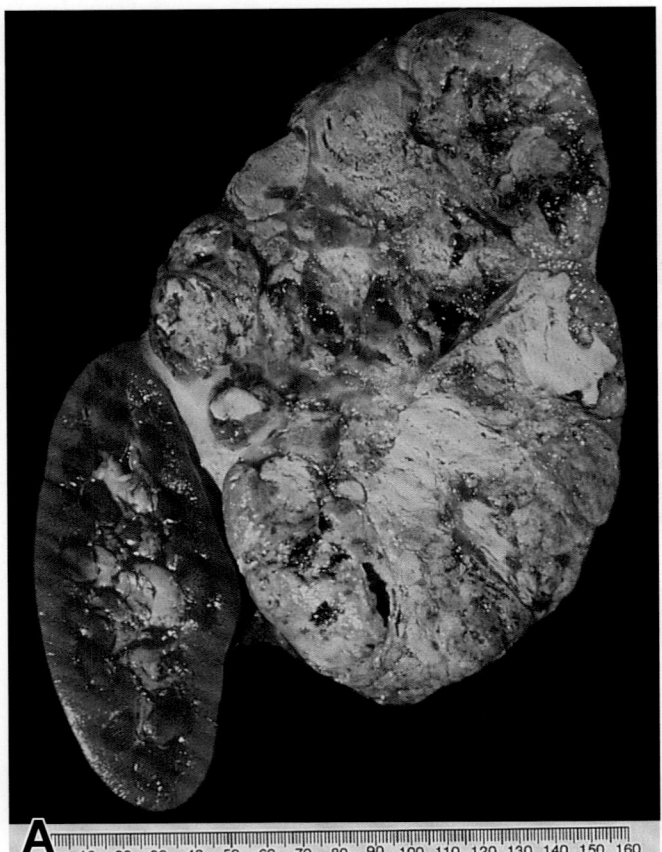

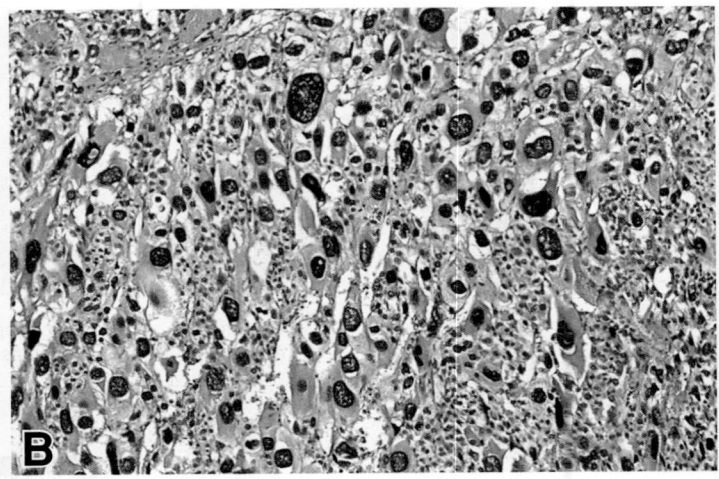

FIGURE 27-42. Adrenal cortical carcinoma. A: The cut surface of this bulky tumor is yellow to tan with areas of necrosis and cystic degeneration. **B:** A microscopic section demonstrates marked anisocytosis and nuclear pleomorphism.

MOLECULAR PATHOGENESIS: Most cases are sporadic. They show a high incidence of somatic mutations in *p53*, overexpression of IGF-2, and WNT signaling pathway defects. Familial syndromes associated with ACC include Li–Fraumeni syndrome (*p53* deficiency), which accounts for a majority of ACC in children (80%), Lynch syndrome (mismatch-repair defects), MEN1, and Carney syndrome (*PRKAR1A* activating mutation).

Bilateral Adrenal Cortical Micronodular Hyperplasia Is a Manifestation of Carney Syndrome

Carney syndrome or **primary pigmented nodular adrenocortical disease** is a rare cause of ACTH-independent Cushing syndrome. It is usually seen in children or young adults, who present at age 10 to 20 with skin and/or atrial myxomas, facial and labial lentigines, large-cell calcifying Sertoli cell tumors, pituitary somatotroph adenomas, and multiple thyroid nodules. The adrenals contain small, brown, or black nodules, up to 0.5 cm, with large eosinophilic cells filled with lipofuscin granules (primary pigmented nodular adrenocortical disease). Carney complex/syndrome is due to activating mutations in the tumor suppressor gene, *PRKAR1A*, which encodes a regulatory subunit of protein kinase A, leading to autonomous production of cortisol.

Adrenal Sex-Hormone Excess

Congenital Adrenal Hyperplasia Is the Most Common Cause of Sex-Hormone Excess in Children

CAH is a state of differential adrenocortical hormone deficiency *and* hormone excess caused by genetic abnormalities in normal steroid biosynthesis pathways. The incidence of CAH varies from 1 in 10,000 among whites to 1 in 500 in Alaskan Eskimos.

The great majority of cases (90% to 95%) are linked to mutations in *CYP21A2* resulting in **deficiency in 21-hydroxylase**. This enzyme normally converts 17-hydroxyprogesterone to 11-deoxycortisol, a precursor of cortisol. It also catalyzes conversion of progesterone to 11-deoxycorticosterone, a precursor of aldosterone. Thus, deficient 21-hydroxylase activity leads to accumulation of both 17-hydroxyprogesterone and progesterone, which are shunted into an androgen synthesis pathway making androstenedione and testosterone. The resulting deficiencies in cortisol and aldosterone cause symptoms of adrenal insufficiency (Addison disease, see below) and compensatory adrenal hyperplasia due to persistent stimulation by ACTH.

In addition to causing reduced cortisol and aldosterone levels, complete loss of 21-hydroxylase activity leads to excessive production of androgens. The resulting phenotype, known as **salt-wasting CAH**, is characterized by ambiguous genitalia (clitoromegaly, labial fusion) in female neonates (Fig. 27-43A) as well as life-threatening hyponatremia,

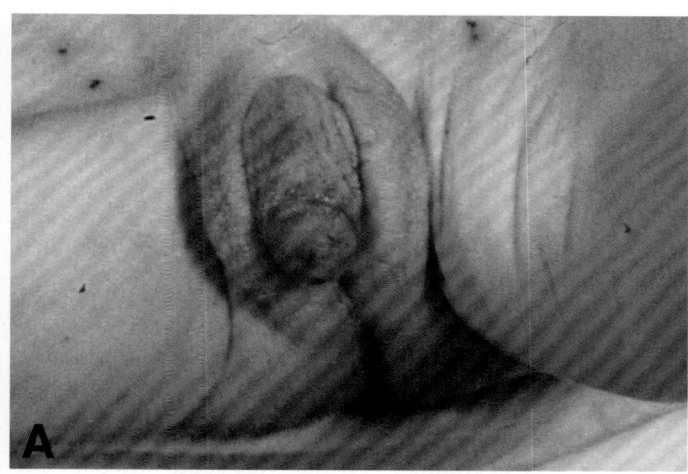

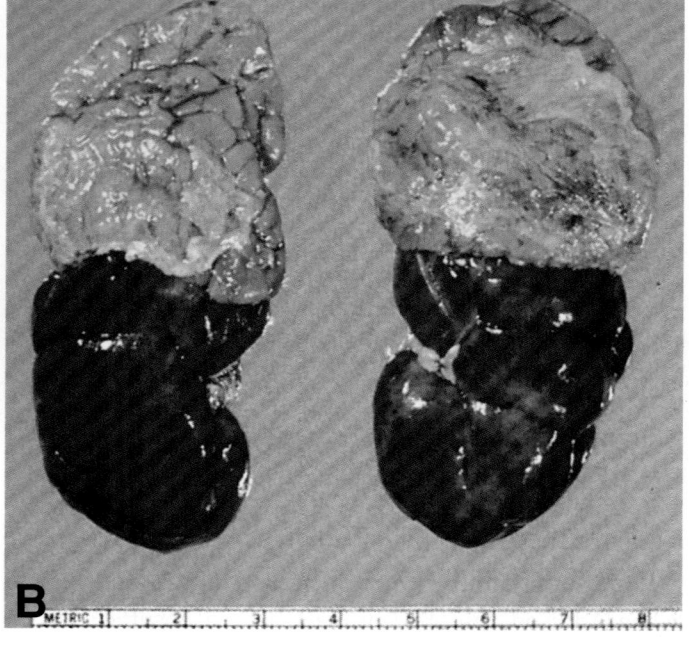

FIGURE 27-43. Congenital adrenal hyperplasia. A: A female infant is markedly virilized with hypertrophy of the clitoris and partial fusion of labioscrotal folds. **B:** A 7-week-old male died of severe salt-wasting congenital adrenal hyperplasia. At autopsy, both adrenal glands were markedly enlarged.

hyperkalemia, and hypoglycemia (Addisonian crisis, see below), which may be rapidly fatal if not treated. Newborn males with salt-wasting CAH show normal genital anatomy, but suffer from severe electrolyte abnormalities.

Less than complete 21-hydroxylase deficiency, with residual activity ~2% of normal, produces a less severe phenotype known as **simple virilizing CAH**, in which female neonates may show ambiguous genitalia, but no electrolyte abnormalities. Female external genitalia are not necessarily abnormal at birth, but infant girls may develop a syndrome of androgen excess, with clitoral enlargement and pubic hair. Infant boys may exhibit sexual precocity. Eventually, the high levels of adrenal androgens lead to premature closure of epiphyses and short stature. Adult women with CAH tend to be infertile because elevated levels of androgens and progestogens interfere with the hypothalamic–pituitary–gonadal axis, disturb the menstrual cycle, and inhibit ovulation. Men with CAH may be fertile, but some have azoospermia.

In **nonclassic CAH**, patients do not present with virilization at birth nor do they show signs of cortisol or aldosterone deficiency. Instead, they present in adolescence or adulthood with virilization during puberty. Females may display hirsutism, menstrual irregularity, and polycystic ovarian syndrome. Men with nonclassic CAH may be clinically normal but may have abnormalities in spermatogenesis. Many cases in men may be undiagnosed.

PATHOLOGY: The adrenal glands are enlarged, weighing as much as 30 g (Fig. 27-43B). Grossly, they are soft, tan to brown in color, and either diffusely enlarged or nodular. The cortex shows widening between the medulla and zona glomerulosa. The hyperplastic zone is filled with compact, granular eosinophilic cells. In most cases, the zona glomerulosa is also hyperplastic, but not to the same extent as seen in the other

zones, especially the zona fasciculata secondary to ACTH stimulation. Ectopic adrenal tissues or nodules, if present, may be also hyperplastic, and if stimulation persists, adenomas can develop.

Therapy for classic CAH includes supplementation with glucocorticoids and mineralocorticoids to suppress ACTH and normalize steroid hormone function. Reconstructive surgery for virilized females may be performed. Treatment for nonclassic CAH includes glucocorticoids to reduce hyperplasia and mitigate overproduction of androgens or mineralocorticoids.

A small number of CAH cases (5%) are caused by AR **11β-hydroxylase deficiency**. This is an unusual condition in the general population, but is the most common cause of CAH among Jews of Iranian or Moroccan ancestry in Israel. 11β-hydroxylase catalyzes the terminal hydroxylation of cortisol in its biosynthesis pathway. Deficient activity results in accumulation of 11-deoxycortisol and 17-hydroxyprogesterone, the latter of which has virilizing effects similar to those seen in 21-hydroxylase deficiency. Elevated levels of 11-deoxycortisol, a weak mineralocorticoid, may cause sodium retention and hypertension which, if present, help distinguish 11β-hydroxylase from 21-hydroxylase deficiency. However, these patients may also experience symptoms of cortisol deficiency (Addison disease, below).

Rare forms of CAH are caused by genetic deficiencies in enzymes in adrenocorticosteroid biosynthesis pathways (17-α hydroxylase, 3β hydroxysteroid dehydrogenase, P450 oxidoreductase, and aldosterone synthase among others). These lead to diverse phenotypes of electrolyte abnormalities and anomalies of the sex organs depending on the particular branch of the steroid biosynthesis pathway that is affected. Treatment involves lifelong glucocorticoid replacement to prevent adrenal insufficiency.

Sex-Hormone Secreting Adrenal Neoplasms Include Adrenal Cortical Adenomas and Carcinomas

Adrenal neoplasms only rarely produce sex hormones. The type of sex hormone produced determines the clinical picture. Androgen-producing tumors may result in virilizing symptoms in females; estrogen-producing tumors may result in gynecomastia and infertility in men. Rarely, tumors may produce both estrogens and androgens.

In general, sex-hormone producing adrenal tumors are more likely to be ACCs than adenomas. ACCs typically present later in life unless there is a genetic predisposition. They carry a poor prognosis (see above).

ADRENAL CORTICAL HORMONE INSUFFICIENCY

Addison Disease Is Also Known as Primary Adrenal Insufficiency

When Addison described primary adrenal insufficiency in 1855, the most common cause of the syndrome was tuberculosis involving the adrenal glands. Worldwide, tuberculosis remains a common cause of chronic adrenal insufficiency, but in Western societies, autoimmunity is responsible for up to 90% of cases some of which may be related to polyglandular autoimmune syndromes (see below).

Other causes of adrenal destruction include metastatic carcinoma, amyloidosis, hemorrhage, sarcoidosis, and infections (bacterial, fungal, mycobacterial). In idiopathic Addison disease, the biochemical defect of adrenoleukodystrophy (see Chapter 32) is common. Rarely, adrenal insufficiency is due to congenital adrenal hypoplasia (see above) or familial glucocorticoid deficiency (defective ACTH receptor).

Addison disease is categorized as primary, secondary, tertiary, or iatrogenic. The primary disease relates to insufficient adrenal gland function, as seen in autoimmune, infectious, genetic, ischemic, or traumatic etiologies. The secondary disease is due to insufficient ACTH production by the pituitary gland. The tertiary disease is caused by hypothalamic dysfunction with decreased CRH production, and iatrogenic disease is due to abrupt withdrawal of chronic corticosteroid therapy.

Addison disease may develop acutely (known as adrenal crisis or Addisonian crisis) or more gradually and persistently (chronic adrenal insufficiency), depending on the nature and severity of the etiology. Infections and vascular events, for example, can cause acute adrenal crisis.

Acute Adrenal Insufficiency Is a Sudden Failure of Adrenal Function

Signs and symptoms of adrenal crisis include profound hypotension and shock, nausea/vomiting, weakness, abdominal pain, mental confusion, lethargy, and ultimately, coma and death within a short window of time.

Adrenal crisis occurs in three settings:

- Abrupt withdrawal of corticosteroid therapy in patients with adrenal atrophy due to long-term steroid administration. Chronic administration of corticosteroids results in shrinkage and atrophy of the adrenal glands. Once atrophic, they are incapable of producing the appropriate levels of steroid hormones when faced with abrupt withdrawal of exogenous corticosteroids. This represents the most common cause of acute adrenal insufficiency.
- Stress caused by infection or surgery may precipitate sudden, devastating worsening of chronic adrenal insufficiency, particularly if adrenal vascular supply is compromised or the adrenal cortex has been injured by trauma.
- **Waterhouse–Friderichsen syndrome** is an acute, bilateral, hemorrhagic infarction of the adrenal cortex. It most often occurs as a complication of meningococcal or Pseudomonas septicemia (see Chapter 7). Adrenal hemorrhage in these circumstances is thought to be a local manifestation of a generalized Shwartzman reaction with disseminated intravascular coagulation. Acute adrenal insufficiency due to adrenal hemorrhage is also seen in newborns subjected to birth trauma. Patients with acute adrenal hemorrhage may present with shock, abdominal/flank pain, fever, disorientation, and abdominal tenderness with rigidity.

Adrenal crisis is almost always fatal unless diagnosed quickly, and treated promptly and aggressively with corticosteroids and supportive measures.

Chronic Adrenal Insufficiency Includes Primary Autoimmune and Secondary Causes

Chronic adrenal insufficiency develops more slowly than adrenal crisis. Patients may present with weight loss, profound fatigue, abdominal pain with nausea, hypoglycemia, and musculoskeletal pain. In chronic *primary* adrenal failure, ACTH and pro-opiomelanocortin levels are elevated due to lack of steroid hormone feedback on the hypothalamus and pituitary gland. Thus, patients with primary, but not secondary or tertiary, adrenal insufficiency may have skin hyperpigmentation. Patients with primary adrenal insufficiency also develop postural hypotension, hyponatremia, hyperkalemia, and salt craving due to mineralocorticoid deficiency. Secondary and tertiary adrenal insufficiency patients do not show these signs, as their mineralocorticoid production is preserved. Normal life expectancy can be achieved with glucocorticoid and mineralocorticoid replacement therapy.

Primary Autoimmune Addison Disease Is Driven by Autoantibodies Against Adrenal Antigens

The most common cause of primary adrenal insufficiency in the United States and other western countries is autoimmune Addison disease, accounting for up to 90% of cases. Primary autoimmune Addison disease is rare (~14 cases per 100,000). It is caused by anti-adrenal autoantibodies (most commonly against 21-hydroxylase), which promote immune-mediated adrenal destruction. The disease usually develops in middle-aged females and is associated with other autoimmune conditions, such as autoimmune thyroid disease, type-1 diabetes mellitus, and hypoparathyroidism in ~50% of cases. A genetic predisposition to primary autoimmune Addison disease is seen in patients with polyglandular autoimmune syndrome, predominantly type II (see below).

Primary autoimmune Addison disease develops insidiously, typically affecting mineralocorticoid (zona glomerulosa) production before cortisol (zona fasciculata) production. Lymphocytic infiltrates with evidence of tissue damage accumulate in the respective zones prior to the onset of symptoms. As cortical tissue damage progresses, a compensatory rise in renin and ACTH levels may occur, followed by clinical features of adrenal insufficiency and abnormal skin and mucous membrane pigmentation. Over 90% of the adrenal gland must be destroyed before chronic adrenal insufficiency becomes symptomatic. The diagnosis of primary autoimmune Addison disease is made by documenting abnormal cortisol levels in the blood levels after ACTH stimulation, and identifying antiadrenal autoantibodies.

Autoimmune Addison disease causes the adrenal glands to become pale, irregular, and shrunken, weighing 2 to 3 g or less. The medulla is intact but surrounded by fibrous tissue containing only small islands of atrophic cortical cells. Depending on the stage of the disease, variably intense lymphoid infiltrates, mainly T-cells, may be seen.

The main therapy for primary autoimmune Addison disease is glucocorticoid and mineralocorticoid replacement. Patients have an excellent prognosis and normal life expectancy.

Polyendocrine Autoimmune Syndrome Also Causes Adrenal Insufficiency

Half of patients with autoimmune adrenal insufficiency suffer from other autoimmune endocrine diseases. These are grouped into two polyendocrine syndromes.

Type I polyendocrine autoimmune syndrome or **candidiasis–hypoparathyroidism–Addison disease syndrome** is a rare AR condition with a slight female predominance. It is seen in older children and adolescents. In addition to adrenal insufficiency, most (60%) patients have hypoparathyroidism and chronic mucocutaneous candidiasis. Insulin-dependent diabetes (type 1) is common. Premature ovarian failure, hypothyroidism, infertility, malabsorption syndromes, pernicious anemia, chronic hepatitis, alopecia totalis, and vitiligo are also frequent.

Type I polyendocrine disease is prevalent among Finns and Iranian Jews. The affected gene is *AIRE* (autoimmune regulator; see Chapter 11) on chromosome 21q22. This gene is expressed in thymus, lymph nodes, and fetal liver. It encodes a protein involved in negative selection of self-recognizing T-cells and, thus, plays an important role in immune system maturation and immune tolerance. Like the common form of autoimmune Addison disease, sera from patients with type I polyendocrine disease recognize steroidogenic autoantigens and other targets.

Type II polyendocrine autoimmune syndrome (Schmidt syndrome) is more common than type I and always includes adrenal insufficiency. Women are affected twice as often as men. The disorder usually presents in young adults, ages 20 to 40. Half of cases are familial, but several modes of inheritance are known. HT and occasionally Graves disease occur in over two-thirds of cases. Insulin-dependent diabetes mellitus and premature ovarian failure are common.

Secondary Adrenal Insufficiency Is due to Pituitary Failure

Secondary failure of the pituitary gland may be due to pituitary tumors, craniopharyngioma, empty sella syndrome, and pituitary infarction. Trauma, surgery, and radiation therapy may also cause loss of pituitary function. Isolated ACTH deficiency is often associated with autoimmune endocrinopathies.

Tertiary Adrenal Insufficiency

Any disorder that interferes with secretion of corticotropin (ACTH)-releasing hormone (CRH) by the hypothalamus (e.g., tumors, sarcoidosis) can lead to inadequate ACTH secretion, and thus adrenal insufficiency. The fact that patients can secrete glucocorticoids in response to ACTH distinguishes this from primary adrenal insufficiency. Pigment and electrolyte abnormalities are typically absent in secondary adrenal insufficiency because these processes are not regulated by ACTH.

MISCELLANEOUS ADRENAL CORTICAL TUMORS

Nonfunctional adrenal cortical adenomas are found in as many as 10% of adult autopsies and are of no clinical significance. Progression to ACC is extraordinarily rare. Nonfunctional adenomas are macroscopically and microscopically identical to their functional counterparts, and are often removed following incidental detection by imaging studies for other indications.

Adrenal myelolipomas are mixtures of mature adipose tissue and functional hematopoietic marrow. They are benign neoplasms that may come to clinical attention by causing symptoms due to mass effect.

Adrenal cysts are rare. Most are actually pseudocysts derived from degeneration in benign adrenal tumors or resolution of hemorrhage. In some cases, they represent remnants of an underlying vascular lesion.

Metastatic cancers to the adrenal glands usually originate in the lungs or breasts, or may be malignant melanomas. The adrenal gland is the fourth most common site of metastatic disease after the lung, bone, and liver. The glands may be unilaterally or bilaterally enlarged, and weigh up to 20 to 45 g. They are largely replaced by cancer, often with associated necrosis and hemorrhage (Fig. 27-44). Sufficient functional adrenal cortex usually remains so that Addison disease does not develop, at least not in view of the limited survival of many of these patients.

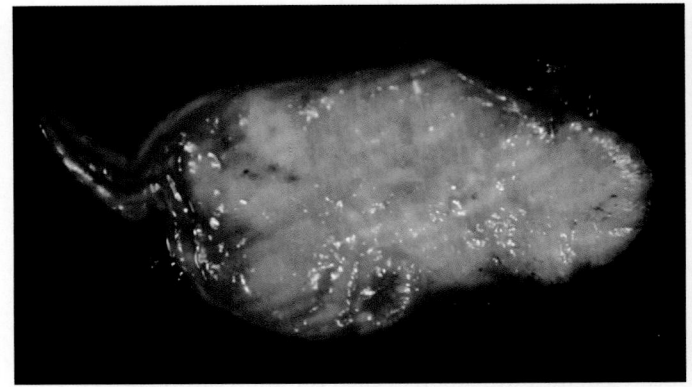

FIGURE 27-44. Metastatic carcinoma to the adrenal gland. A yellow-tan, infiltrating lesion is commonly seen in metastatic carcinoma to the adrenal gland.

Adrenal Medulla and Paraganglia

PARAGANGLIA MAY BE SYMPATHETIC OR PARASYMPATHETIC AND ARE CLOSELY INTEGRATED WITH THE NERVOUS SYSTEM

The adrenal glands and paraganglia are neuroendocrine organs that share a neural crest origin. Broadly speaking, paraganglia may be divided into sympathetic (chromaffin cell) paraganglia or parasympathetic (glomus cell) paraganglia. Strictly speaking, the adrenal medulla is a sympathetic paraganglion surrounded by adrenal cortex. Extra-adrenal sympathetic paraganglia are distributed laterally (and occasionally anteriorly) to the spinal column in close association with sympathetic ganglia. Parasympathetic paraganglia in the head and neck are associated with major nerves (vagus and hypoglossal nerves) and comprise anatomically distinct paraganglia, including the carotid, aortic, and jugulotympanic bodies.

Sympathetic paraganglia (including the adrenal medulla) are composed of **chromaffin** cells, which secrete catecholamines (primarily epinephrine and norepinephrine) in times of physical, physiologic, or emotional stress. The adrenal medulla accounts for 10% of the adrenal gland volume. It is the largest aggregate of chromaffin cells in adults and the most common site of tumors of sympathetic paraganglia (pheochromocytomas). Extra-adrenal sympathetic paraganglia become atrophic in adulthood and are difficult to locate, although they may still give rise to tumors of sympathetic paraganglioma origin (extra-adrenal pheochromocytomas). In fetal life, a sympathetic extra-adrenal paraganglion known as the **organ of Zuckerkandl** (located near the origin of the inferior mesenteric artery) is considerably larger than in adults and serves as a major source of catecholamines in fetal life.

Microscopically, sympathetic paraganglia are composed of chromaffin cells arranged in small ball-like nests (zellballen). Chromaffin cells are polyhedral in shape with pale amphiphilic cytoplasm and small, round, vesicular nuclei. Enveloping each nest of chromaffin cells is a fibrovascular network (sustentacular network) that provides a rich vascular supply and support structure. Chromaffin cells are filled with numerous electron-dense (100 to 300 nm) catecholamine-containing granules, resembling those at sympathetic nerve endings. Epinephrine accounts for 85% of the content of these granules, with the remainder being norepinephrine and noncatecholamine hormones. Stored catecholamines are secreted upon sympathetic stimulation as a response to stress (exercise, cold, fasting, trauma) or emotional excitation accompanying fear and anger.

The adrenal medulla is supplied by arterial and portal venous circulations that originate in the zona reticularis of the cortex. Most of the blood supply to the hormonally active cells of the medulla comes from the portal venous system. Paraganglia are innervated by cholinergic preganglionic sympathetic neurons, which synapse directly onto sympathetic paraganglia to stimulate release of catecholamines.

Parasympathetic paraganglia in the head and neck are named by their anatomic location or association. For example, the carotid bodies are major parasympathetic paraganglia located at the bifurcation of each common carotid artery. They play an important role in sensing low oxygen tension and/or high carbon dioxide in the blood and relay signals to increase heart rate and ventilation. In general, neither parasympathetic paraganglia nor tumors that arise from them are hormonally active. Histologically, parasympathetic paraganglia are composed of nests of chief cells with pale cytoplasm and small vesicular nuclei. They are supported by a sustentacular network, analogous to the pattern in sympathetic paraganglia.

PHEOCHROMOCYTOMA IS A TUMOR OF CHROMAFFIN CELLS

If the cell of origin is an intra-adrenal chromaffin cell, the tumor is known as a *pheochromocytoma*; if the cell of origin comes from an extra-adrenal sympathetic paraganglion, the tumor is known as a sympathetic (extra-adrenal) paraganglioma or *extra-adrenal pheochromocytoma*.

Pheochromocytomas are rare tumors, with roughly equal sex distribution. They occur most commonly in the fourth and fifth decades, although they arise at younger ages as a component of various hereditary syndromes (see below). Pheochromocytomas generate catecholamines (most importantly epinephrine) which cause severe hypertension, either episodically or continuously. Typically, episodic catecholamine release leads to paroxysms or crises, lasting up to several hours, with severe throbbing headache, sweating, palpitations, tachycardia, abdominal pain, and vomiting. Blood pressure may be elevated to an extreme degree. Paroxysms can be triggered by activities that place pressure on the tumor, such as exercise, lifting, bending, or vigorous abdominal palpation. Anxiety reactions can develop during a paroxysm but are not an initiating factor. Orthostatic hypotension may occur due to decreased plasma volume and poor postural tone. Increased basal metabolism, sweating, heat intolerance, and weight loss may mimic hyperthyroidism. Angina and myocardial infarction due to excessive stimulation of β-adrenergic pathways can occur in the absence of coronary artery disease. The cardiac complications also include contraction band necrosis and features reminiscent of Takotsubo cardiomyopathy (see Chapter 17) caused by elevated catecholamine levels (**catecholamine cardiomyopathy**) and calcium overload in cardiac myocytes.

Pheochromocytomas are mostly sporadic, but up to 30% develop in patients with hereditary syndromes. Thorough workup of patients with these tumors may, therefore, include genetic testing and family member screening for the most common syndromes associated with familial pheochromocytoma. These include von Hippel–Lindau syndrome (*VHL* gene), MEN types 2A or 2B (*RET* gene), familial paraganglioma–pheochromocytoma (mutations in *SDHB, SDHC* and *SDHD* genes, which encode succinate dehydrogenase subunits mutations), and neurofibromatosis type 1 (*NF1* gene mutation) (Table 27-5).

PATHOLOGY: In sporadic pheochromocytomas, 80% of tumors are unilateral, 10% are bilateral, and 10% occur in extra-adrenal locations as sympathetic paragangliomas; 10% are malignant and 10% occur in children. Tumors occurring in the context of MEN syndromes are usually bilateral. They may become large masses of more than 2 kg, but most are 5 to 6 cm in diameter and weigh 80 to 100 g.

Grossly, pheochromocytomas tend to be encapsulated, spongy, and reddish, with prominent central scars and foci of hemorrhage and cystic degeneration (Fig. 27-45A). Their histology is highly variable. Typically, they are composed

TABLE 27-5

MOST COMMON SYNDROMES WITH PARAGANGLIOMA/PHEOCHROMOCYTOMA

Syndrome	Gene	Inheritance	Manifestations
Von Hippel–Lindau	*VHL*	Autosomal dominant	Pheochromocytoma Paraganglioma Hemangioblastoma Clear cell renal cell carcinoma Pancreatic neuroendocrine tumors
Multiple neuroendocrine neoplasia type 2a	*RET* (C634R) most common	Autosomal dominant	Pheochromocytoma Paraganglioma Medullary thyroid carcinoma Parathyroid hyperplasia
Multiple neuroendocrine neoplasia type 2b	*RET* (M918T) most common	Autosomal dominant	Pheochromocytoma Paraganglioma Medullary thyroid carcinoma Marfanoid habitus, mucosal neuromas Intestinal ganglioneuromas
Multiple neuroendocrine neoplasia type 4	*CDKN1B*	Autosomal dominant	Pituitary adenomas (somatotroph most common) Pancreatic and duodenal neuroendocrine tumors Parathyroid adenomas
Neurofibromatosis type 1	*NF1*	Autosomal dominant	Pheochromocytoma Neurofibromas, café-au-lait spots Pancreatic neuroendocrine tumor (somatostatinoma) Gastrointestinal stromal tumors (GIST)
Paraganglioma-pheochromocytoma syndrome	*SDHB, SDHC, SDHD*	Autosomal dominant	Sympathetic paraganglioma (both adrenal and extra-adrenal)
Carney triad	*SDHC*	Sporadic	Paraganglioma Gastrointestinal stromal tumors Pulmonary chondroma

of circumscribed nests (**zellballen**) of polyhedral to fusiform neoplastic cells containing granular, amphophilic or basophilic cytoplasm, and vesicular nuclei (Fig. 27-45B). Eosinophilic cytoplasmic globules are common. Cellular pleomorphism may be prominent, including multinucleated tumor giant cells. These tumors are highly vascular, with many capillaries running in a supportive sustentacular network. Electron microscopy shows membrane-bound, dense core granules containing stored catecholamines. Immunostains show strong and diffuse positivity for chromogranin-A in neoplastic chromaffin cells and strong positivity for S100 in sustentacular cells (Fig. 27-45C).

Of adrenal pheochromocytomas, 5% to 10% are malignant, and most commonly associated with *SDHB* mutations. Malignancy in pheochromocytomas is defined by its metastatic behavior and not by its histology. Both benign and malignant pheochromocytomas may show mitoses, cellular pleomorphism, capsular or vascular invasion, and necrosis. Malignant tumors spread most often to regional lymph nodes, bone, lung, and liver. Five-year survival for metastatic tumors is approximately 50%.

The diagnosis of pheochromocytoma includes biochemical and radiologic assessment. Increased levels of urinary catecholamine metabolites, particularly vanillylmandelic acid (VMA), metanephrine, and unconjugated catecholamines, help confirm the presence of a pheochromocytoma. Imaging studies including those with iodine–metaiodobenzylguanidine, an analog of guanethidine that identifies several neuroendocrine tumors, may be useful in locating tumors once they are identified biochemically. Complete surgical removal is curative and β-adrenergic blocking agents are often used to control hypertensive crises.

Sympathetic (extra-adrenal) paragangliomas may arise in paraganglia in any location outside of the adrenal gland, most commonly (85% of cases) below the diaphragm near the adrenal gland or organ of Zuckerkandl. Their incidence is approximately one-tenth of that of pheochromocytomas. They are most common in

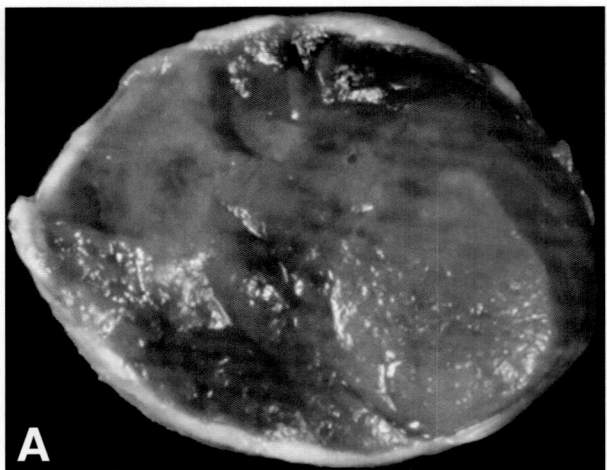

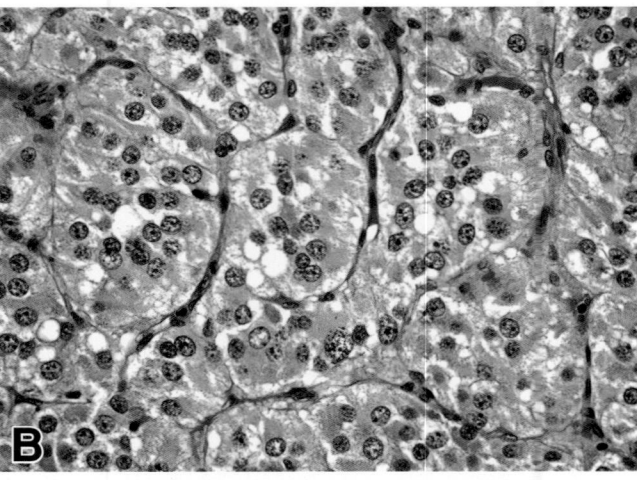

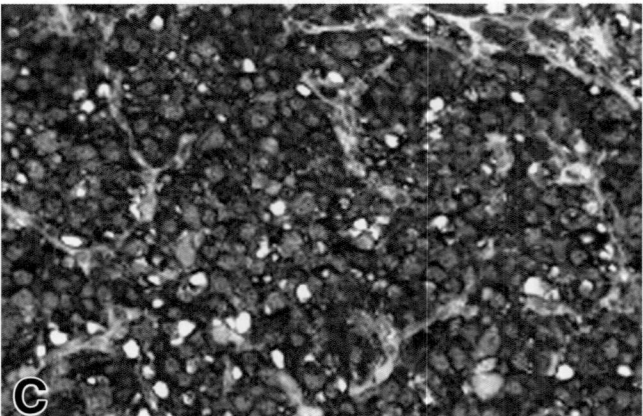

FIGURE 27-45. Pheochromocytoma. A: The cut surface of an adrenal tumor from a patient with episodic hypertension is reddish brown with a prominent area of fibrosis. Foci of hemorrhage and cystic degeneration are evident. **B:** A photomicrograph of the tumor shows polyhedral tumor cells with ample finely granular cytoplasm. Note the enlarged hyperchromatic nuclei. **C:** Many of the tumor cells show positive immunohistochemical staining for chromogranin A, a marker of neuroendocrine differentiation.

middle-aged adults. Like pheochromocytomas, a significant proportion arise in familial syndromes (see above). Clinically, they may produce catecholamines and cause symptoms identical to intra-adrenal pheochromocytoma. Histologic, immunohistochemical, and diagnostic features are also identical to those described for pheochromocytoma. Complete resection is curative.

HEAD AND NECK PARAGANGLIOMA ARE PARASYMPATHETIC

Head and neck (parasympathetic) paragangliomas (HNPGLs) most commonly arise from the carotid body or the jugulotympanic body. These tumors tend to occur in adult women, particularly in regions in which there is low partial oxygen pressure (e.g., high altitude). Most are nonfunctional, but may rarely (<5%) generate catecholamines. HNPGLs have a strong hereditary component. A great majority (80%) are linked to mutations in *SDHD*, which may be germline in familial cases and associated with familial paraganglioma–pheochromocytoma syndrome (Table 27-5).

Grossly, HNPGLs are well circumscribed and rubbery in texture. They may occasionally infiltrate surrounding tissues. Histologically, a zellballen pattern of growth of chief cells is seen, with an accompanying sustentacular cell network. Immunohistochemically, neuroendocrine markers (synaptophysin, chromogranin A, CD56) are positive in

chief cells and S100 highlights the sustentacular network. HNPGLs are treated surgically. Tumors that harbor *SDHB* disease alleles are more likely to metastasize than those with other *SDH* mutations.

NEUROBLASTOMA ARE EMBRYONAL MALIGNANT TUMORS OF NEURAL CREST ORIGIN

They originate in the adrenal medulla, paravertebral sympathetic ganglia, and sympathetic paraganglia. They are composed of neoplastic neuroblasts, which are derived from primitive sympathogonia at an intermediate stage in the development of sympathetic ganglion neurons. Neuroblastomas are the most common solid extracranial neoplasms of early childhood; 90% of cases are diagnosed before age 5 and overall incidence peaks in the first 3 years (1 in 7,000 live births).

Clinical presentations are highly variable, reflecting the many sites where the primary tumors may develop and metastasize. They arise most commonly in the adrenal glands (40%) and abdominal/thoracic ganglia (40%). Neck and pelvic tumors are less common. The first sign is often an enlarging abdomen in a young child. Examination discloses a firm, irregular, nontender mass. Metastases involve liver, bone, and other organs. Spinal cord compression may lead to gait disturbance and sphincter dysfunction. Tumors may cause a number of paraneoplastic syndromes including watery diarrhea, hypokalemia, and achlorhydria (collectively known as WDHA syndrome) caused by vasoactive intestinal peptide (VIP) secretion and/or hypertension from catecholamine secretion. Urinary catecholamines and their metabolites are almost invariably elevated, particularly **norepinephrine, VMA, homovanillic acid (HVA)**, and **dopamine**. Some patients show paraneoplastic opsoclonus–myoclonus syndrome, which usually indicates an excellent prognosis, although some may develop permanent neurologic deficits. Prognosis is determined by numerous histologic categories, epidemiologic factors, and genetic lesions.

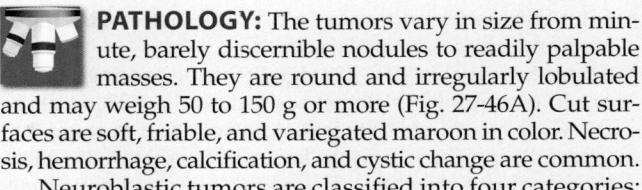

MOLECULAR PATHOGENESIS: Neuroblastomas are congenital in some cases and account for half of cancers diagnosed in the first month of life. A majority of neuroblastomas are sporadic. Embryogenesis of the adrenal medulla and presumably of other parts of the sympathetic nervous system continues during the first year of life. Persistence and transformation of these embryonal structures may be related to the pathogenesis of these tumors.

Rare familial cases have been associated with linkage to chromosome 16p12, mutations in *PHOX2A* (a cell-cycle regulator) or *ALK*. Those genetically predisposed to this disease usually have multifocal tumors at an early age and follow AD inheritance.

Neuroblastomas may show marked variation in chromosomal content; hyperploid tumors tend to have better outcomes. Loss of heterozygosity of chromosome 1 (1p35-36) is seen in about 30% of cases, and trisomy of chromosome 17q is seen in 60% of cases.

Amplifications in the *MYCN* gene, seen in approximately a quarter of cases, are associated with aggressive tumor behavior. Mutations in *ATRX*, which encodes an ATP-dependent helicase that remodels chromatin, are seen in approximately half of neuroblastomas in patients 1 year or older, and are also associated with a poor prognosis.

PATHOLOGY: The tumors vary in size from minute, barely discernible nodules to readily palpable masses. They are round and irregularly lobulated and may weigh 50 to 150 g or more (Fig. 27-46A). Cut surfaces are soft, friable, and variegated maroon in color. Necrosis, hemorrhage, calcification, and cystic change are common.

Neuroblastic tumors are classified into four categories:

- **Neuroblastoma** (Schwannian stroma-poor)
- **Ganglioneuroblastoma, intermixed** (Schwannian stroma-rich)
- **Ganglioneuroma** (Schwannian stroma-dominant)
- **Ganglioneuroblastoma, nodular** (composite, Schwannian stroma-rich/stroma dominant and Schwannian stroma poor).

Neuroblastomas contain dense sheets of small, round to fusiform cells with scant cytoplasm, and hyperchromatic nuclei, resembling lymphocytes. There is little or no Schwannian proliferation, and mitoses are frequent. Characteristic Homer–Wright rosettes are defined by a rim of dark tumor cells in a circumferential arrangement around a central pale fibrillar core (Fig. 27-46B). By electron microscopy, malignant neuroblasts show peripheral dendritic processes with longitudinally oriented microtubules and neurosecretory granules and filaments.

Neuroblastomas readily infiltrate surrounding structures and metastasize to regional lymph nodes, liver, lungs, bones, and other sites. The tumors may differentiate into ganglioneuromas (see below).

Several factors are useful in predicting the outcome of neuroblastomas:

- **Age:** Age at diagnosis is one of the most important predictors of survival. Children under 1 year have better outcomes than older patients with the same stage of disease. Spontaneous tumor regression occurs commonly at this age.

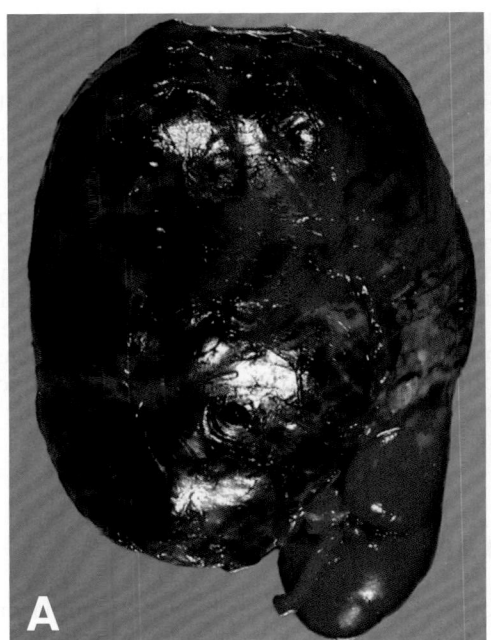

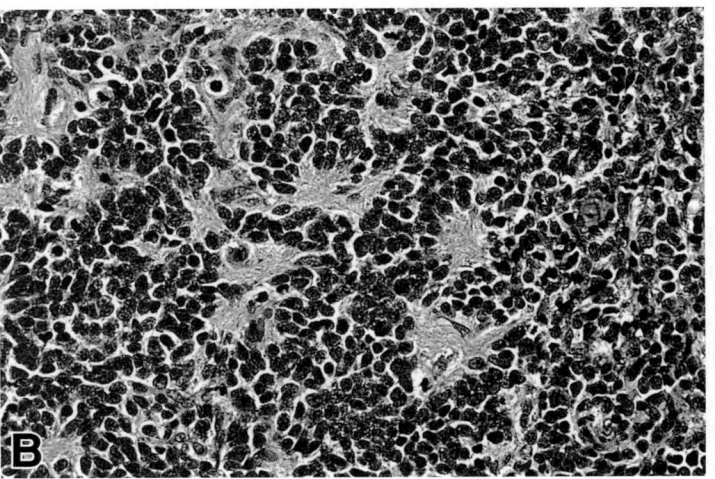

FIGURE 27-46. Neuroblastoma. A: A large, lobulated, hemorrhagic and cystic tumor, adherent to the upper pole of the kidney was removed from a child who presented with an abdominal mass. **B:** A photomicrograph illustrates the characteristic rosettes formed by small, regular, dark tumor cells arranged around a central, pale fibrillar core.

- **Site:** Extra-adrenal tumors tend to be better differentiated and, thus, less aggressive.
- **Stage:** Survival is 90% in stage I (tumor confined to the organ of origin) but decreases to less than 3% in stage IV (widespread metastases). An exception is stage IVS (special), in which tumors lack the characteristic chromosomal abnormalities. Even with liver and bone marrow metastases, patients with stage IVS may undergo spontaneous remissions and have 60% to 90% survival.
- **Tumor histology:** Low-grade (better-differentiated) tumors do better than high-grade (undifferentiated) tumors. If the **VMA/HVA ratio** is less than 1, the tumor is deficient in dopamine β-hydroxylase and likely to be more aggressive.
- **DNA ploidy:** A DNA index near the diploid/tetraploid range is unfavorable, but hyperdiploid or near-triploid neuroblastomas have a good prognosis. DNA ploidy has less prognostic significance in patients older than 2 years.
- **Genomic alterations:** *MYCN* amplification occurs in 20% to 25% of cases and suggests poor outcome. Tumors with *MYCN* amplification often have chromosome 1p deletions (especially del 1p36.3). Allelic gain of 17q implies aggressiveness.

Neuroblastomas can express several tyrosine kinase neurotrophin receptors: TrkA, TrkB, and TrkC. High levels of TrkA correlate with younger age, lower stage, absence of *MYCN* amplification and favorable prognosis. Conversely, TrkB expression correlates with an invasive phenotype, high-risk disease, and chemoresistance. TrkC occurs in lower-stage tumors. High-level expression of *EFNB2* and *EFNB3* (which encode ephrins, proteins that regulate growth of migrating axons, *EPHB6* (encodes an ephrin receptor), and *CD44* makes a cell adhesion protein), correlates with good clinical outcome.

Prognosis also correlates with cytogenetic findings:

- Lack of significant chromosome changes portends excellent survival.
- Tumors with any chromosome copy number changes tend to relapse.
- Tumors with segmental alterations, *MYCN* amplification, 1p and 11q deletions and 1q gain have overall poor survival.

Localized neuroblastomas are treated by surgical resection alone. Patients with disseminated tumors may receive chemotherapy and sometimes radiation therapy.

Ganglioneuromas Are Benign Tumors of Neural Crest Origin

They occur in older children and young adults and arise in sympathetic ganglia, typically in the posterior mediastinum. Up to 30% develop in the adrenal medulla. In keeping with their degree of differentiation, ganglioneuromas do not manifest chromosomal abnormalities characteristic of neuroblastomas (see above).

PATHOLOGY: Ganglioneuromas are well encapsulated, with myxoid, glistening cut surfaces. They show well-differentiated, mature ganglion cells associated with spindle cells in a loose, abundant

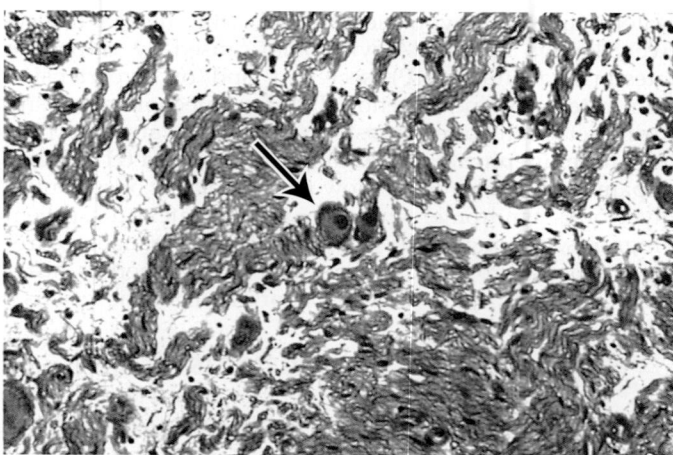

FIGURE 27-47. Ganglioneuroma. A photomicrograph shows mature ganglion cells (*arrow*) interspersed among wavy spindle cells embedded in a myxoid matrix.

fibrillar stroma (Fig. 27-47). The fibrils are neurites extending from tumor cell bodies. Cytoplasmic processes of ganglion cells contain neurosecretory granules and may form synaptic junctions. Typical neuroendocrine substances, such as neuron-specific enolase and certain peptide hormones, are abundant. Neuroblastomas may differentiate into ganglioneuromas.

Pineal Gland

ANATOMY AND FUNCTION

The pineal gland is a 5- to 7-mm cone-shaped organ located below the posterior edge of the corpus callosum, suspended from the roof of the third ventricle over the superior colliculi. It has a lobulated architecture, compartmentalized by fibrovascular septa, and contains cords and clusters of large epithelial-like cells called **pinealocytes**. These have modified photosensory and neuroendocrine functions. Astrocytes make up 10% of pineal gland cellularity.

The pineal gland produces several neurotransmitters, of which **melatonin** is among the most abundant. Melatonin levels are distinctly higher at night than during waking hours, and it is thought to act as a sleep inducer.

Serotonin and several other substances are also produced by the pineal. The most significant of these is arginine vasotocin, a hormone that has important antigonadotropic activity.

Beginning at about the time of puberty, calcifications (corpora arenacea or "brain sand") develop in the pineal gland, and may be visualized in autopsy specimens or by radiographic techniques. These mineralized concretions accumulate with age and are accompanied by cystic degeneration and gliosis.

NEOPLASMS OF THE PINEAL GLAND ARE RARE

Tumors of the pineal gland include: (1) neoplasms originating from the pineal parenchyma, presumably from pinealocytes; (2) tumors residing in the pineal gland region (**astrocytomas**) but derived from cells other than pinealocytes; and, rarely, (3) metastases from other sites.

PATHOLOGY:
- **Germ cell tumors:** These are the most common pineal neoplasms. They apparently derive from misplaced germ cells within the pineal parenchyma. Of these, 60% are seminomas. Germ cell tumors often show immunopositivity for OCT3/4 and SALL4; within the germ cell tumor category, seminomas are CD117- and PLAP-positive.
- **Pineocytomas:** These benign tumors are solid, well-circumscribed masses that replace the pineal body. Small tumor cells with round nuclei and eosinophilic cytoplasm grow in nests and rosettes separated by thin strands of connective tissue (Fig. 27-48). They resemble paragangliomas, but lack neurosecretory granules.
- **Pineoblastomas:** These highly malignant tumors are extremely rare and occur in young adults. Grossly, they are soft masses with hemorrhagic areas and necrosis. They infiltrate surrounding structures. Microscopically, they are composed of clusters of densely packed small oval cells in occasional rosettes with dark nuclei and scant cytoplasm, resembling medulloblastomas or neuroblastomas. Mitoses are abundant. Metastasis to the central nervous system and spine are common.

CLINICAL FEATURES: Regardless of histologic type, pineal gland tumors present with signs and symptoms owing to their impact on surrounding structures, including headaches and visual and behavioral disturbances. In children, these tumors may precipitate

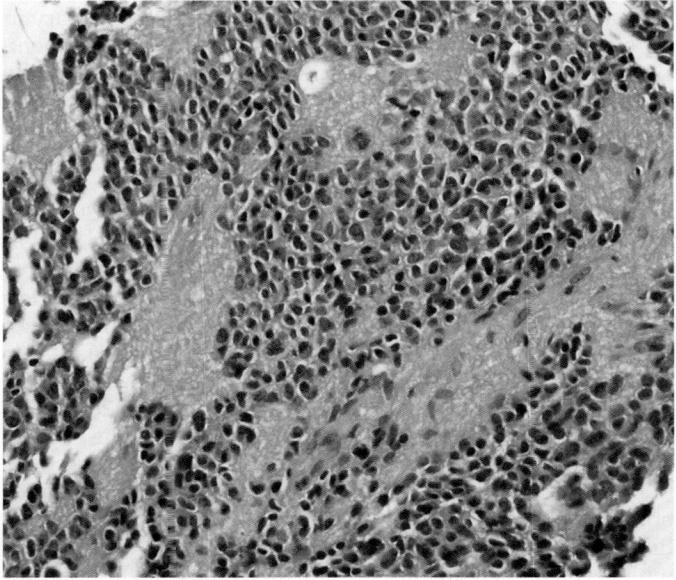

FIGURE 27-48. Pineocytoma. A photomicrograph shows nests of tumor cells with round nuclei and eosinophilic cytoplasm separated by connective tissue.

precocious puberty, especially in boys. The prognosis of pineoblastoma is poor. However, even benign pineal tumors and nonneoplastic pineal cysts carry guarded prognoses and pose a great threat due to their deep location within the brain.

Paraneoplastic Syndromes With Endocrine Function

Malignant tumors may produce diverse peptide hormones whose secretion is not under normal regulatory control. Most of these hormones are normally present in the brain, gastrointestinal tract, or endocrine organs. Their inappropriate secretion can cause a variety of effects, largely detailed above.

Ectopic secretion of ACTH by a tumor leads to features of Cushing syndrome, including hypokalemia, hyperglycemia, hypertension, and muscle weakness. ACTH production is most commonly seen with cancers of the lung, particularly small cell carcinoma. It also complicates carcinoid tumors and other neuroendocrine tumors, such as pheochromocytomas, neuroblastomas, and MTCs.

Inappropriate diuresis due to production of arginine vasopressin (ADH) by a tumor may cause sodium and water retention to such an extent that it is manifested as water intoxication, resulting in altered mental status, seizures, coma, and sometimes death. The tumor that most often produces this syndrome is small cell lung carcinoma. It is also reported with carcinomas of the prostate, gastrointestinal tract, and pancreas, and with thymomas, lymphomas, and Hodgkin disease.

Hypercalcemia afflicts 10% of cancer patients and is usually caused by metastatic tumor invasion of bone. However, in about one-tenth of cases, it occurs in the absence of bony metastases. The most common cause of paraneoplastic hypercalcemia is secretion of a parathormone-like peptide by an epithelial tumor, usually squamous-cell lung carcinoma or breast adenocarcinoma. In multiple myeloma and lymphomas, hypercalcemia is attributed to secretion of osteoclast-activating factor.

Cancer-induced hypocalcemia is actually more common than hypercalcemia, and complicates osteoblastic metastases from cancers of the lung, breast, and prostate. The cause of hypocalcemia is less well understood. Low calcium levels have been reported in association with calcitonin-secreting medullary carcinomas of the thyroid.

Gonadotropins may be secreted by germ cell tumors, gestational trophoblastic tumors (choriocarcinoma, hydatidiform mole), and pituitary tumors. Less commonly, gonadotropin secretion is observed with hepatoblastomas in children, and cancers of the lung, colon, breast, and pancreas in adults. High gonadotropin levels lead to precocious puberty in children, gynecomastia in men and oligomenorrhea in premenopausal women.

The best-understood cause of hypoglycemia associated with tumors is excessive insulin production by pancreatic islet cell tumors (see Chapter 21). Other tumors, especially large mesotheliomas, pleomorphic sarcomas, and primary hepatocellular carcinomas, are associated with hypoglycemia.

28 The Skin

Ronnie M. Abraham, Emily Y. Chu, David E. Elder

INTRODUCTION

The skin is an optimal organ for studying fundamental principles of pathology because lesions on its surface are readily apparent and easily biopsied. Most classes of disease manifest in the skin. Some diseases, such as the blistering diseases, are largely confined to the skin.

ANATOMY AND PHYSIOLOGY OF THE SKIN

The skin is a protective barrier *par excellence*. Microorganisms find it nearly impossible to penetrate intact epidermis from the outside, and water loss is limited from the inside. It plays a vital role in regulating temperature and protecting against ultraviolet (UV) light. Diverse sensory receptors communicate details of the immediate environment. The skin plays a prominent role in immune regulation through its associated lymphoid tissues, which include lymphocytes and antigen-presenting cells that travel between the skin and regional lymph nodes via the lymphatics and bloodstream. Keratinocytes, Langerhans cells, mast cells, lymphocytes, and macrophages all participate in immune responses. Epidermal keratinocytes produce many cytokines, notably interleukin 1α (IL-1α) and IL-1β, eicosanoids, and melanocortin. The ability of keratinocytes to participate in immunity, inflammation, and pigment production by melanocytes is necessary in an organ relentlessly exposed to the external environment. Langerhans cells, the dendritic antigen-presenting cells of the skin, are bone marrow–derived, epidermal immigrant cells. They are central to development and regulation of immune responses including contact hypersensitivity, allograft rejection, and graft-versus-host disease.

KERATINOCYTES: The epidermis is a multilayered sheet of keratin-producing cells. It forms undulating folds at the interface with the dermis, called dermal papillae. A progressive change in morphology occurs from the replicating columnar cells of the basal layer **(stratum basalis)** through the spinous layer **(stratum spinosum)** and the granular layer **(stratum granulosum)** to the nonviable flattened cells of the cornified layer **(stratum corneum)** (Figs. 28-1 and 28-2). The basal cells exhibit most of the mitotic activity of the epidermis. As keratinocytes approach the surface, they lose their nuclei and form flattened plates of dead cells on the outer boundary of the skin (the cornified or keratin layer). Keratinocytes synthesize sulfur-poor, filamentous **tonofibrils**, which are related to the keratin molecules of the stratum corneum. More than 30 different keratins are responsible for forming diverse structures such as the stratum corneum, hair, and nails. Bundles of tonofibrils converge on, and

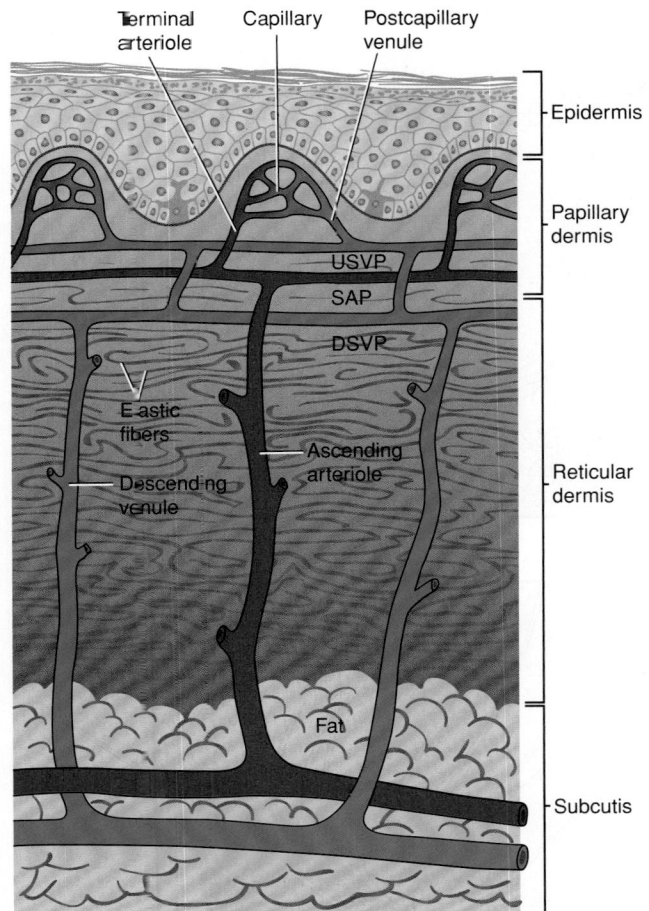

FIGURE 28-1. The dermis and its vasculature. The dermis is divided into two distinct anatomic regions. The papillary dermis with its vascular plexus and the epidermis usually react together in diseases that are primarily limited to the skin. The reticular dermis and the subcutis are altered in association with systemic diseases that manifest in the skin. *USVP* = upper superficial venular plexus; *SAP* = superficial arterial plexus; *DSVP* = deep superficial venular plexus.

terminate at, the plasma membrane in attachment plates called **desmosomes** (Fig. 28-3).

Keratinocytes produce two other specialized structures: "**keratohyalin granules**" and "**Odland bodies**," also known as keratinosomes or membrane-coating granules. Keratohyalin granules are the defining feature of the granular layer and are composed of a histidine-rich, electron-dense, basophilic protein—profilaggrin—which is associated with intermediate filaments (Fig. 28-3). Odland bodies and their discharged lamellated products are related to epidermal barrier function in the outer granular layer.

The epidermis harbors cells of neuroectodermal and mesenchymal origin or differentiation that have their own highly distinctive organelles. Their numbers vary among the several different levels of the epidermis. Two of these cell types, **melanocytes** and **Langerhans cells**, are dendritic immigrants. The third, the **Merkel cell**, may be epidermal-derived and is associated with a terminal neuronal axon (Fig. 28-2).

MELANOCYTES: Melanocytes are dendritic cells of neural crest origin that largely determine skin color. They lie in the basal layer of the epidermis, separated from the dermis by the epidermal basement membrane zone. A single melanocyte may supply dendrites to over 30 keratinocytes (Fig. 28-4).

The **melanosome** is a cytoplasmic membrane–bound complex in which melanin is synthesized. When melanin synthesis is active, melanosomes contain filaments in parallel arrays along the long axis of the organelle (Fig. 28-4). As melanosomes mature, their orderly internal structure becomes obliterated, and they are converted into electron-opaque granules. These are transferred to keratinocytes, where they form a supranuclear cap, protecting the nuclear material from ultraviolet light.

Skin color is largely based on the number, size, and packaging of melanosomes in keratinocytes.

LANGERHANS CELLS: These cells arrive in embryonic skin in the last month of the first trimester, following the melanocytes by a month. These HLA-DR-positive cells allow skin to recognize and process antigens, and so are a part of the immune system. They are uncommon in the dermis but

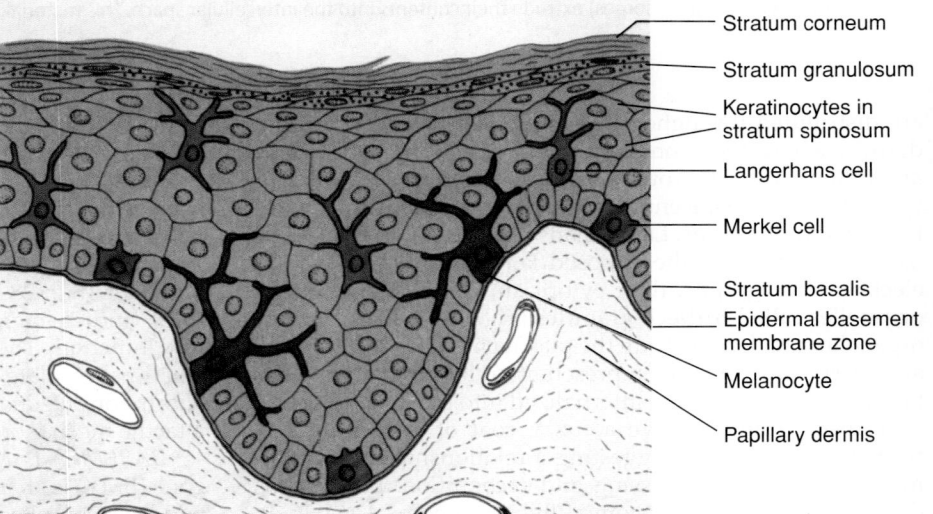

FIGURE 28-2. Normal epidermis and epidermal immigrant cells. Keratinocytes form the multilayered epidermis, protecting against water loss and bacterial invasion. Melanocytes provide pigment as well as protection against ultraviolet radiation. Langerhans cells are among the cells responsible for the skin's function as an immunologic organ. Merkel cells may represent one of the enablers of tactile function of the skin.

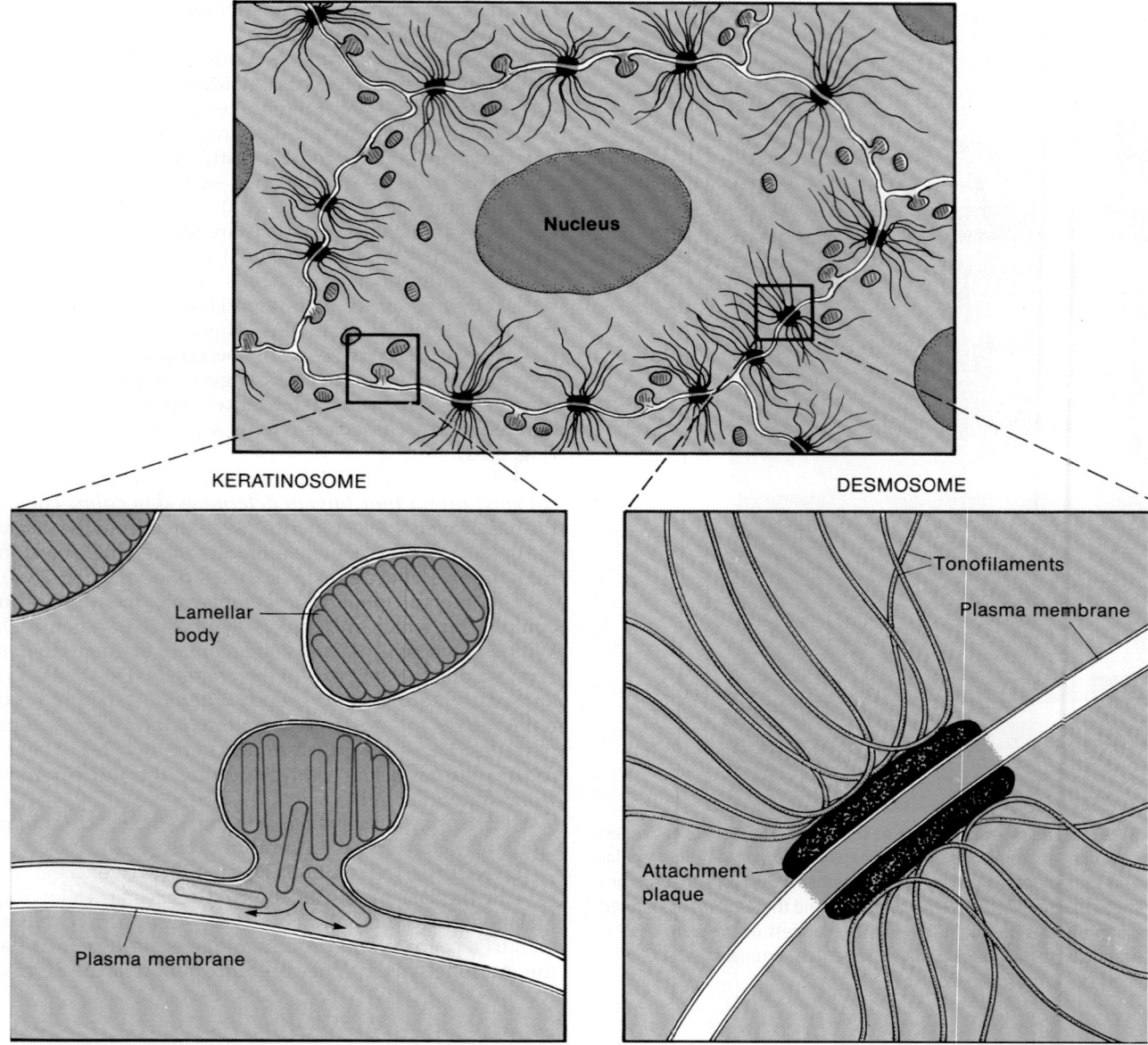

FIGURE 28-3. The keratinocyte, keratinosome, and desmosome. Keratinocyte cytoplasm is dominated by delicate keratin fibrils, the tonofilaments. These are part of the cytoskeleton of the cell and loop within the attachment plaque of the desmosome. Lamellar bodies of keratinocytes (keratinosomes) extrude their contents into the intercellular space. This material may play a role in cellular cohesion.

are distributed throughout the nucleated layers of the epidermis, where they constitute about 4% of the cells. They are difficult to see by routine light microscopy because their cytoplasm is translucent and they are composed of a perikaryon and dendrites. Langerhans cells do not have specialized attachments to the apposed keratinocytes. As seen in electron micrographs, their cytoplasm contains specialized organelles called **Birbeck granules** (Fig. 28-5). These unique organelles are derived from the plasma membrane and probably participate in antigen presentation by Langerhans cells (antigenic material being internalized into Birbeck granules).

Birbeck granules have a fuzzy coat of clathrin, a feature of "coated pits," suggesting a relationship to receptor-mediated antigen processing and recognition. Langerhans cells express major histocompatibility complex I (MHC-I),

MHC-II and receptors for Fc IgG and Fc IgE. They express CD1a, Langerin, and, less specifically, S-100 protein.

MERKEL CELLS: Merkel cells occur in special regions such as the lips, oral cavity, external root sheaths of hair follicles and palmar skin of the digits. They have a distinctive organelle, a membrane-bound, dense-core granule, 100 nm or wider (Fig. 28-6). Immunohistochemical and ultrastructural studies suggest that Merkel cells fulfill a neurosecretory function. The basal aspect of the cell is apposed to a small nerve plate that connects to a myelinated axon by a short, nonmyelinated axon. This complex structure may be a tactile mechanoreceptor.

BASEMENT MEMBRANE: The basement membrane zone (BMZ) is an interface between the dermis and epidermis and is as complex in function as it is in structure (Fig. 28-7).

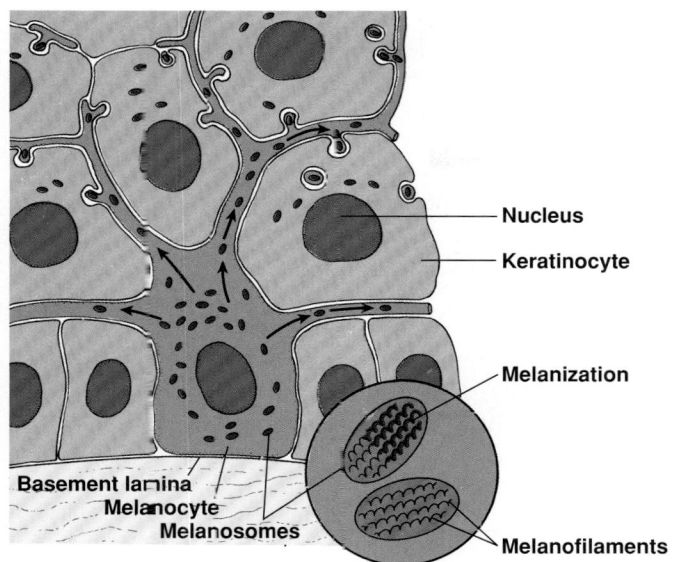

FIGURE 28-4. A single melanocyte supplies over 30 keratinocytes with melanin granules by way of complex dendritic cytoplasmic extensions. Melanin granules are transferred to keratinocytes and come to lie in a supranuclear cap, a site indicating their protective function. Pigment granules are actually formed in the melanocytes within distinctive organelles—the melanosomes. Pigment is synthesized on small filaments (melanofilaments) within these organelles (*inset*).

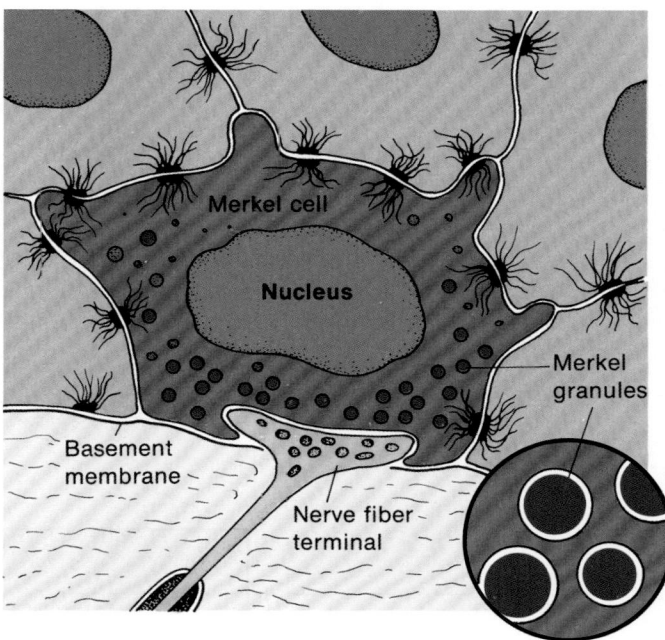

FIGURE 28-6. The Merkel cell, which differs from other immigrant cells, forms desmosomes with keratinocytes and is attached to a small nerve plate (nerve fiber terminal). Membrane-delimited, dense core granules (Merkel granules) are distinctive neurosecretory structures in these cells (*inset*).

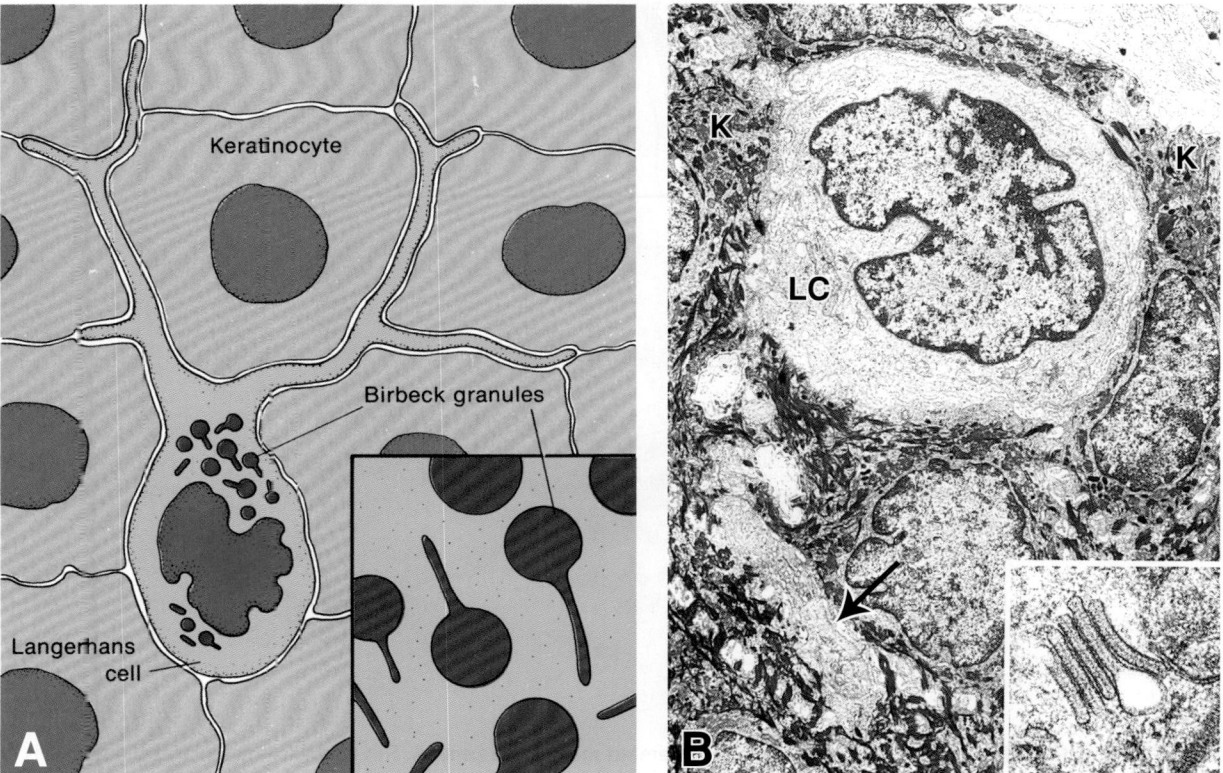

FIGURE 28-5. Dendritic Langerhans cells recognize and process antigens. A. Unique racket-shaped organelles, called *Birbeck granules,* may be important in antigen presentation. **B.** An electron micrograph of a Langerhans cell shows these racket-shaped organelles (*inset*). The Langerhans cell body (LC) is pale compared to the surrounding keratinocytes (K), whose cytoplasm contains electron-dense packets of tonofilaments.

THE SKIN

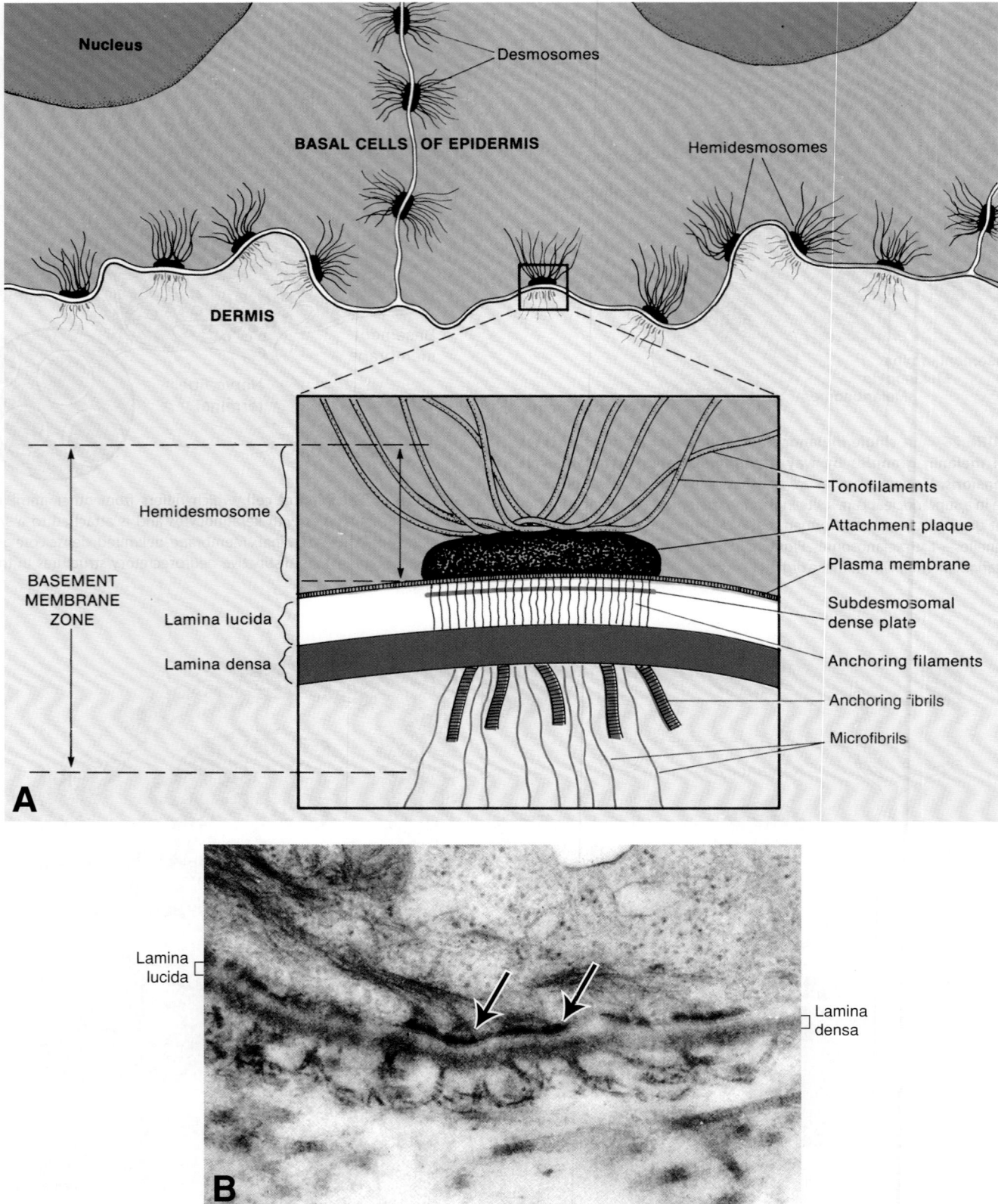

FIGURE 28-7. The dermal–epidermal interface and the basement membrane zone. A. This epithelial–mesenchymal interface is the site of the basement membrane zone, a complex structure synthesized mostly by the basal cells of the epidermis. Each of its components is a site of change in specific disease, from tonofilaments and attachment plaques of basal cells to anchoring fibrils and microfibrils. **B.** An electron micrograph shows the hemidesmosomal attachment plaques with their inserting tonofilaments (*arrow*). The subdesmosomal dense plates, the lamina lucida, the lamina densa, and the subjacent anchoring fibrils are well demonstrated.

It mediates dermal–epidermal adherence and probably acts as a selective macromolecular filter as well. It is also a site of immunoglobulin and complement deposition in certain cutaneous diseases. Most structures of the BMZ are elaborated by epidermal cells. The basal lamina is the primary organizational feature of the BMZ and is responsible for epithelial cell polarity as well as some keratin gene expression. Ultrastructurally, the basal lamina includes:

- **Deep aspects of basal keratinocytes** including plasma membrane and tonofilaments, which attach to the deep face of the hemidesmosome
- **Hemidesmosome**, with its subdesmosomal dense plate
- **Anchoring filaments**, comprised of laminin 5 and 8 which extend from subdesmosomal dense plates across the lamina lucida and insert into the lamina densa
- **Lamina lucida**, an electron-lucent layer containing adhesion proteins
- **Lamina densa**, composed principally of type IV collagen
- **Anchoring fibrils**, which are arrays of type VII collagen extending from the inner face of the lamina densa for a short distance into the papillary dermis
- **Microfibrils**, which feature delicate, long, elastic fibrils that blend with the underlying elastic fibrillary system of the skin

Various antigenic components have been identified in the BMZ, some of which play roles in cutaneous disease, particularly blistering disorders. **Laminin** is a glycoprotein in the lamina lucida and lamina densa of all BMZs. It helps to organize BMZ macromolecules and promotes cell attachment to extracellular matrix. Laminin binds **type IV collagen**.

Bullous pemphigoid (BP) antigens were identified with antibodies from patients with the blistering disorder BP, described later. The antigens BPAG1 and BPAG2 **(type XVII collagen)** are normal constituents of the dermal–epidermal junction but are absent in BMZs around adnexal structures and blood vessels. These BP antigens localize in hemidesmosomes and cytoplasm of basal keratinocytes. **Type IV collagen**, in the lamina densa of all BMZs, is the most superficial component of the complex collagen fiber network of the dermis. It is important in dermal–epidermal attachment. **Type VII collagen** is present on the deep aspect of the basal lamina in anchoring fibrils. Anchoring fibril antigens (AF-1 and AF-2) reside within anchoring fibrils and possibly within the lower lamina densa.

The **dermis** is a complex organization of connective tissue deep to the BMZ, containing mostly collagen, which is embedded in a ground substance rich in hyaluronic acid. The dermis has two zones:

PAPILLARY DERMIS: The papillary dermis is a narrow zone just below the BMZ of the epidermis. It has a pale pink eosinophilic appearance and has little organization when viewed with the light microscope (Figs. 28-1 and 28-2). Delicate collagen fibrils are the most apparent structures. This delicate connective tissue extends into the dermal papillae, and also forms a sheath about blood vessels, nerves, and adnexal structures. This entire network of collagen is known as the **adventitial dermis**.

The papillary dermis is generally altered in epidermal diseases and disorders affecting the superficial vascular bed. The epidermis, papillary dermis, and superficial vascular bed react jointly and influence each other in complex ways. Some primary skin diseases, such as bullous disorders, psoriasis and lichen planus (LP), involve mainly or exclusively these superficial structures.

RETICULAR DERMIS: The reticular dermis is deep to the papillary dermis and contains most of the dermal collagen, which is predominantly **type I collagen** and is organized into coarse bundles and associated with elastic fibers (Fig. 28-1). The reticular dermis and **subcutis** (also recognized as a cutaneous structure) are less common sites of pathologic change. If they are diseased, it is often as a manifestation of systemic disorders such as scleroderma (progressive systemic sclerosis) and erythema nodosum.

CUTANEOUS VASCULATURE: Circulating blood in the skin serves a number of functions. The skin, via its vascular network, is important in temperature regulation. In addition, many aspects of cutaneous inflammation involve the superficial cutaneous vasculature.

Ascending arterioles arise from arteries in the subcutis and directly cross much of the reticular dermis (Fig. 28-1). In the outer part of the reticular dermis, in conjunction with other similar ascending arterioles, a superficial arteriolar plexus is formed. Each terminal arteriole extends from this plexus into a dermal papilla, where an arterial capillary is formed. The arterial capillary makes a U-turn and on its descent becomes a venous capillary and then a postcapillary venule. These venules join to form a complex venular plexus in the reticular dermis, just under the papillary dermis. The venular end of this vascular structure is important in cutaneous inflammatory responses.

Cutaneous lymphatic vessels form a random network, starting as lymphatic capillaries near the epidermis. A superficial lymphatic plexus then sends forth lymphatic channels that drain to regional lymph nodes. Lymphatic channels are involved in drainage of tissue fluids but also in metastasis of cutaneous cancers, especially malignant melanoma. Cutaneous lymphatics have, at best, an incomplete basal lamina.

Mast cells, derived from bone marrow, are normally present around dermal venules. They release vasoactive and chemotactic substances that participate in many inflammatory reactions. They also proliferate in a spectrum of diseases, called **urticaria pigmentosa** (Fig. 28-8).

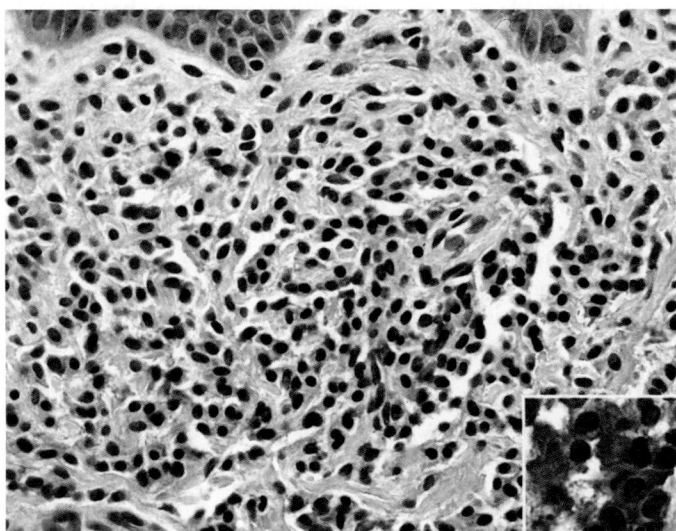

FIGURE 28-8. Urticaria pigmentosa. Mast cells fill and expand the papillary dermis. The cytoplasm of mast cells contains granules rich in chloroacetate esterase, producing a red hue in this Leder stain (*inset*), a useful distinguishing feature.

A few lymphocytes and histiocytes are normally present in the skin, as are dermal dendritic cells and stromal cells such as fibroblasts, smooth muscle cells, pericytes, and endothelial cells. Dermal dendritic cells may be antigen-presenting cells, and some express the clotting factor XIIIa.

HAIR FOLLICLES: Hair follicles originate in the primitive epidermis. They grow downward through the dermis and upward through the epidermis. Growing hairs of the scalp and beard have bulbs of epithelial and mesenchymal tissue firmly embedded in the subcutis. A vertical cross-section of a bulb reveals a cap of actively dividing, keratin-synthesizing cells that become arrayed in layers that join at the top of the bulb to form the cylindrical hair shaft. The differentiating hairs form the roof of the epithelial bulb and interact with an island of melanocytes that contribute melanin to the passing keratinocytes, resulting in hair coloration. The colored keratinocytes lose their nuclei as they form the final product, the cylindrical hair shaft. Curly hair is formed from angulated bulbs; straight hair develops from round bulbs.

THE HAIR CYCLE: Hair grows in a cyclical fashion. At any given time, 90% of hairs are normally in the actively growing, or **anagen**, phase. These are interspersed with hairs that show no evidence of active growth, called **telogen** hairs. Hairs in the process of ceasing growth, **catagen** hairs, still have hair shafts. Catagen or "club" hairs end in the lower reticular dermis as slightly widened club-like structures, each surrounded by a rim of nucleated keratinocytes. Hair bulbs are no longer evident, and the lamina densa around the catagen hair is strikingly thickened.

As the **telogen** phase (resting follicle) is reached, the end of the hair retreats to the level of the arrector pili muscle. The hair shaft may be missing: it is no longer tethered at the base and leaves only a remnant of the original follicle. However, a delicate vascularized mesenchymal tract, the telogen tract, extends from the attenuated tip. At the top of this tract, an early anagen hair forms again from follicular stem cells. With growth, it follows the delicate pathway through the reticular dermis into the panniculus, there forming a mature anagen follicle and a new hair.

ALOPECIA: Alopecia, commonly known as baldness, is loss of hair. **Androgenetic alopecia**, or **common** or **"pattern" alopecia**, affects both men and women and results from a complex and poorly understood interaction of heritable and hormonal factors involving androgens. Loss of scalp hair leads to replacement of large terminal hair follicles by tiny "vellus" hair follicles, the source of the delicate "fuzz" on the cheeks of women and the upper cheeks of men.

Growing hair is a site of active mitosis. Many systemic diseases inhibit hair mitosis and give rise to alopecia. If the condition passes, mitotic activity is renewed and hair regrows. In patients treated with potent antimitotic drugs (e.g., chemotherapy), hair follicles stop growing, hair is lost and a telogen follicle follows. When therapy stops, hair cycling resumes. Almost any kind of follicular inflammation can trigger the telogen phase. The synchronous onset of telogen in multiple follicles may result in rapid hair loss, called "telogen effluvium." In "**scarring alopecia**," fibrosis distorts the telogen tract (the regrowth pathway), and permanent loss of that follicle's function is the result.

Alopecia areata is a circumscribed area of hair loss, usually on the scalp, although other body areas may be involved. Brisk lymphocytic infiltrates around the hair bulb result in formation of telogen hairs and hair loss. This histologic pattern and the association of this phenomenon with the inheritance of HLA class II alleles (especially HLA-DQ3) have been interpreted as evidence for an autoimmune etiology. Generally, scarring does not occur and hair may regrow normally after varying time periods. **Alopecia totalis** is an autoimmune disease that causes loss of all body hair. Aside from cosmetic concerns, it is harmless.

VELLUS HAIRS: These fine hairs may play a role in touch perception in many mammals, but in humans they have no function. Vellus hairs are diminutive anagen hairs, with a small active bulb high in the reticular dermis, together with small sebaceous glands.

SEBACEOUS FOLLICLES: These structures develop with puberty and are the sites of **acne**. Sebaceous follicles have a minute vellus hair at the base. The central face has large sebaceous glands that dwarf the vellus hairs and fill the follicular canal with sebum.

DISEASES OF THE EPIDERMIS

Ichthyoses Feature Epidermal Thickening and Scales

Ichthyosiform dermatoses, many of which are heritable, are diverse diseases showing striking thickening of the stratum corneum. The term **ichthyosis** reflects the similarity of the diseased skin to coarse, fish-like scales (Fig. 28-9). Several rare ichthyoses are associated with other abnormalities, such as abnormal lipid metabolism, neurologic or bone diseases and cancer. For example, some inborn errors of lipid metabolism alter keratinocyte adhesion and impair the barrier function of the skin. Such actions may promote epidermal hyperplasia.

MOLECULAR PATHOGENESIS: Three general defects are involved in excessive epidermal cornification of ichthyoses:

- **Increased cohesiveness** of the cells of the stratum corneum, possibly reflecting altered lipid metabolism
- **Abnormal keratinization,** manifested as impaired tonofilament formation and keratohyalin synthesis, and excessive cornification
- **Increased basal cell proliferation,** associated with a decrease in transit time of keratinocytes across the epidermis

PATHOLOGY: In ichthyoses, the stratum corneum is typically disproportionately thick compared to the nucleated epidermal layers.

Ichthyosis Vulgaris

Ichthyosis vulgaris is an autosomal dominant keratinization disorder characterized by hyperkeratosis and reduced or absent epidermal keratohyalin granules (Fig. 28-10). Scaly skin results from increased cohesiveness of the stratum corneum. The attenuated stratum granulosum is a single layer with small, defective keratohyalin granules *Decreased or absent synthesis of* **profilaggrin,** *a keratin filament "glue," is responsible for these defects.*

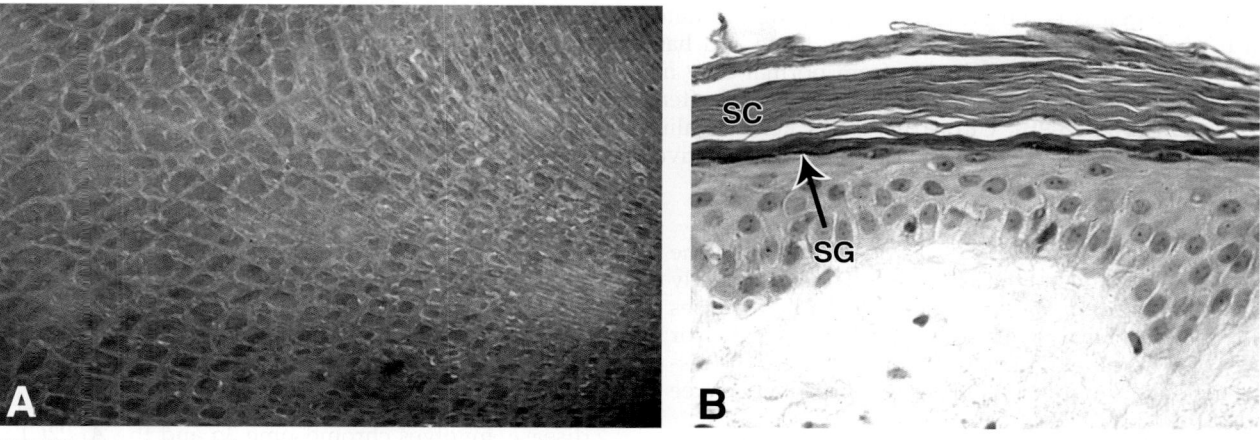

FIGURE 28-9. Ichthyosis vulgaris. A. Noninflammatory fish-like scales are evident on the thigh of a patient with a strong family history of ichthyosis vulgaris. (From Elder DE, Elenitsas R, Johnson BL, et al. *Synopsis and Atlas of Lever's Histopathology of the Skin*. Philadelphia, PA: Lippincott Williams & Wilkins; 1999.) **B.** There is disproportionate thickening of the stratum corneum (*SC*) relative to the normal thickness of the nucleated epidermal layer. The stratum granulosum (*SG*) is thin and focally absent.

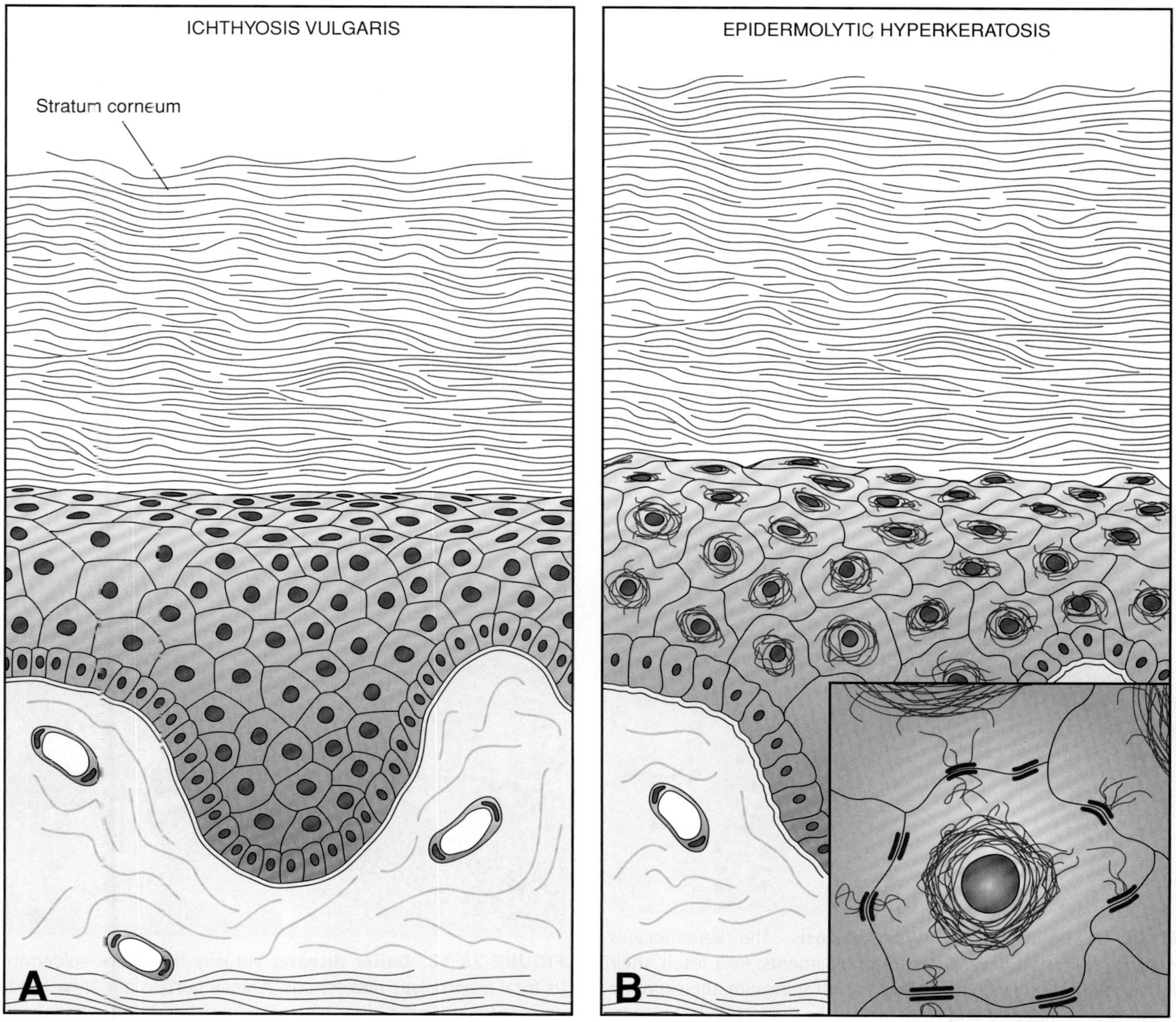

ICHTHYOSIS VULGARIS

Stratum corneum

EPIDERMOLYTIC HYPERKERATOSIS

FIGURE 28-10. A. Ichthyosis vulgaris. B. Epidermolytic hyperkeratosis. Both diseases are characterized by thickening of the stratum corneum relative to the nucleated layers. Epidermolytic hyperkeratosis is characterized by abnormal keratin synthesis, manifested by whorled keratin filaments about the nucleus (*inset*).

Ichthyosis vulgaris is the prototype of disproportionate corneal thickening. The stratum corneum is loose and has a basket-weave appearance, differing from normal only in amount. The granular layer is greatly diminished and often appears absent (Fig. 28-9B). Ultrastructurally, keratohyalin granules appear small and sponge-like, indicating defective synthesis.

CLINICAL FEATURES: Ichthyosis vulgaris is the most common of the ichthyoses. It begins in early childhood, often in people with family histories of this condition. Small white scales occur on the extensor surfaces of extremities and on the trunk and face. The disease is lifelong, but most patients can be maintained free of scales with topical treatment.

States similar to ichthyosis vulgaris may accompany other diseases or may follow certain drugs. Ichthyosis may occur with lymphomas, especially Hodgkin disease, other cancers, systemic granulomatous disorders, and connective tissue disease. Drugs may produce ichthyosis by interfering with similar pathways of lipid metabolism.

X-Linked Ichthyosis

This is a recessive heritable epidermal disorder characterized by delayed dissolution of desmosomal discs in the stratum corneum, owing to deficiency of steroid sulfatase. Steroid sulfatase normally degrades the Odland body product, cholesterol sulfate, which provides cellular adhesion in the lower stratum corneum. Failure of this action leads to persistent cohesion of the stratum corneum with preservation of the granular layer.

Other examples of ichthyotic disorders, each caused by one of several possible single gene defects affecting keratins in the suprabasal epidermis, and lamellar body function, respectively, include *lamellar ichthyosis* and *epidermolytic hyperkeratosis* (which can also be seen as an incidental focal finding in otherwise normal skin (Fig. 28-11).

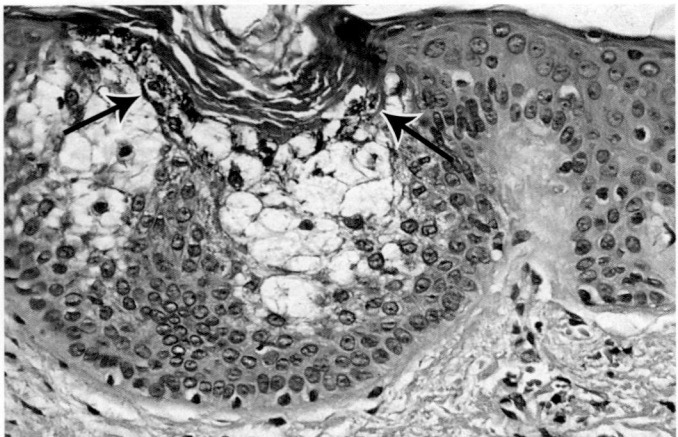

FIGURE 28-11. Epidermolytic hyperkeratosis. The keratinocytes of the stratum spinosum have clumped tonofilaments. As a result, their cytoplasm is relatively clear. In the outer stratum spinosum, the clumped fibrils are further compacted and whorl about the nuclei (*arrows*), resulting in dark cytoplasm condensed about the nuclei. These cells separate from each other to produce epidermolysis. A normal portion of epidermis is seen on the *right*.

Darier Disease Is an Autosomal Dominant Disorder of Keratinization

Also called **keratosis follicularis**, this disease is characterized by multifocal keratoses.

 MOLECULAR PATHOGENESIS: Darier disease is a familial dermatosis linked to a defect in the intercellular matrix. The *ATP2A2* gene on chromosome 12q23-24 encodes a calcium pump of the endoplasmic reticulum, and its mutation may exert a direct effect on calcium-dependent desmosome assembly. These patients may have neuropsychiatric problems, also probably related to *ATP2A2* mutations.

A similar autosomal dominant disorder, Hailey–Hailey disease, involves chromosome 3q and the *ATP2C1* gene, which is also believed to govern keratinocyte desmosomal interactions.

 PATHOLOGY: The warty papule of Darier disease has a suprabasal cleft. Above and to the side of the cleft, dyskeratotic keratinocytes with eosinophilic cytoplasm contain keratin fibrils that whorl about the nucleus, forming characteristic "corps ronds" (round bodies) and "grains" (Fig. 28-12). The roof of the cleft is formed by a column of compact keratotic material. Similar lesions may occur as an isolated scaly nodule called a "warty dyskeratoma." Lesions in Hailey–Hailey disease resemble those of Darier disease, albeit with more acantholysis, or keratinocyte dyshesion. This results in a characteristic "dilapidated brick wall" appearance (Fig. 28-13).

CLINICAL FEATURES: Darier disease first appears late in childhood or in adolescence as skin-colored papules that later become crusted. Affected areas have many warty elevations, 2 to 4 mm in diameter, largely on the chest, nasolabial folds, back, scalp, forehead, ears, and groin.

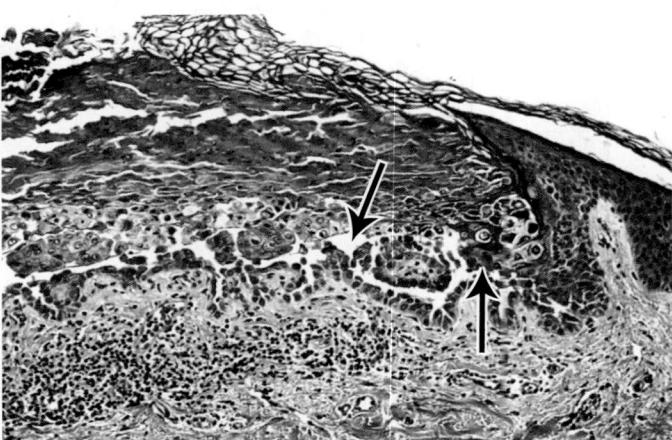

FIGURE 28-12. Darier disease. Virtually the entire epidermis exhibits focal acantholytic dyskeratosis. A small portion of normal epidermis is present (*right*). In the lesion, there is a suprabasal cleft (*arrows*) with a few dyshesive (acantholytic) keratinocytes surmounted by hyperkeratosis and parakeratosis. The cleft is not a vesicle because true vesicles contain inflammatory cells and tissue fluid. Dyskeratosis is present above the cleft.

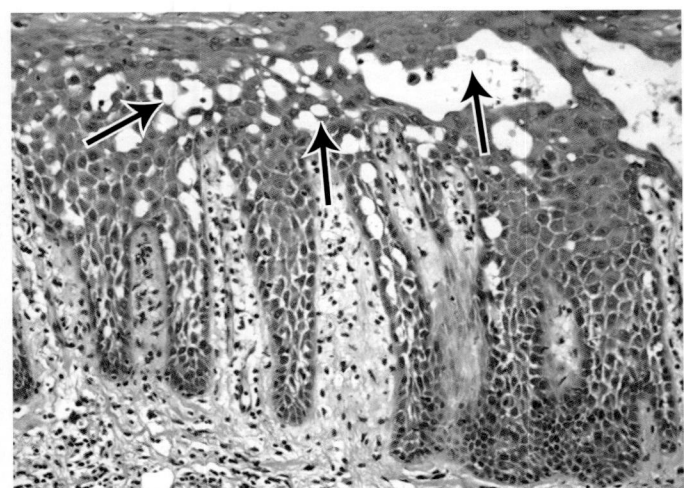

FIGURE 28-13. Hailey–Hailey disease. Hailey–Hailey disease shows acantholysis of the epidermis (*arrows*) with dyskeratosis of keratinocytes, yielding a characteristic "dilapidated brick wall" appearance on histology.

Psoriasis Is a Proliferative Skin Disease With Persistent Epidermal Hyperplasia

Psoriasis is a chronic, frequently familial disorder that features large, erythematous, scaly plaques, commonly on extensor cutaneous surfaces. It affects 1% to 2% of the population worldwide. Psoriasis may arise at any age but shows a peak in late adolescence. Interestingly, the condition is not seen among Native Americans and is infrequent among Asians.

MOLECULAR PATHOGENESIS: The pathogenesis of psoriasis is multifactorial, with genetic, immunologic and environmental factors contributing to the development of psoriatic lesions.

GENETIC FACTORS: Psoriasis unquestionably has a genetic component, although only 1/3 of patients with psoriasis have a family history of the disease. The more severe the illness, the greater is the likelihood of a familial background. The incidence is increased among relatives of patients with psoriasis, and there is 65% concordance in monozygotic twins. The incidence is also increased in individuals with certain HLA haplotypes. A 300-kb segment in the MHC-I region of chromosome 6p21, referred to as the major psoriasis susceptibility locus or PSORS1, is felt to be a major genetic determinant of risk.

IMMUNOLOGIC FACTORS: T lymphocytes are crucial in the pathogenesis of psoriatic lesions. T$_H$1 and T$_H$17 cells, subtypes of CD4$^+$ T cells, appear to drive the inflammatory response and subsequent dermatosis. These subsets of T cells, in addition to effector CD8$^+$ T cells and antigen-presenting dendritic cells, secrete proinflammatory cytokines and growth factors. For these reasons, therapeutics targeting cytokines, such as TNFα inhibitors, or those targeting IL-6, IL-17, and IL-23 are currently being used.

ENVIRONMENTAL FACTORS: Clinical lesions may occur anywhere on the skin. Stimuli such as physical injury ("Köbner phenomenon"), infection, certain drugs, and photosensitivity may produce psoriatic lesions in apparently normal skin.

PATHOLOGY: The most distinctive pathology is seen at the edges of chronic psoriatic plaques. The epidermis is thickened, with **hyperkeratosis** and **parakeratosis** (persistence of nuclei in cells of the stratum corneum, which occurs with increased epidermal turnover). Parakeratosis may be circumscribed and focal, or it may be diffuse, in which case the granular layer is diminished or absent. The nucleated layers of the epidermis are thickened severalfold in the rete pegs and are frequently thinner over dermal papillae (Fig. 28-14). In turn, the papillae are elongated and appear as sections of cones, with their apices toward the dermis. In chronic lesions, dermal papillae may appear as bulbous "clubs" with short handles (Figs. 28-14 and 28-15). The rete ridges of the epidermis have a profile reciprocal to that of the dermal papillae, resulting in interlocked dermal and epidermal "clubs," with alternately reversed polarity. Capillaries of dermal papillae are dilated and tortuous (Fig. 28-15). In very early lesions, changes may be limited to capillary dilation, with a few neutrophils "squirting" from the capillaries into the epidermis. Epidermal hyperplasia and hyperkeratosis occur mainly in chronic lesions.

Neutrophils may become localized in the epidermal spinous layer or in small microabscesses (of Munro) in the stratum corneum and may be associated with limited areas of parakeratosis (Fig. 28-16). The dermis below the papillae contains variable mononuclear inflammation, mostly lymphocytes, around the superficial vascular plexus. The inflammatory process does not extend into the subjacent reticular dermis.

Virtually all diseases characterized by thickening of the nucleated epidermal layers also exhibit hyperkeratosis. For example, chronic scratching or rubbing of normal skin causes a thickened epidermis, hyperkeratosis, and dermal fibrosis, a "psoriasiform" condition known as **lichen simplex chronicus**. Psoriasiform histology is common in cutaneous pathology. Seborrheic dermatitis, lichen simplex chronicus, subacute and chronic spongiotic dermatitis (eczema), and cutaneous T-cell lymphoma (mycosis fungoides) all may exhibit such change. However, these usually do not mimic psoriasis precisely.

CLINICAL FEATURES: The initial presentation of psoriasis is variable and disease activity is intermittent. Familial psoriasis tends to be more severe than sporadic types, but disease severity varies from annoying scaly lesions over the elbows to a serious debilitating disorder involving most of the skin and often associated with arthritis. A single lesion of psoriasis may be a small focus of scaly erythema or an enormous confluent plaque covering much of the trunk (Fig. 28-14A). A typical plaque is 4 to 5 cm, sharply demarcated at its margin and covered by a surface of silvery scales. If the scales are detached, pinpoint foci of bleeding from the dilated capillaries in the dermal papillae dot the underlying glossy erythematous surface ("Auspitz sign").

Seronegative arthritis develops in 7% of patients with psoriasis. The tendency to arthropathy is linked to several HLA haplotypes, particularly HLA-B27. Psoriatic arthritis closely resembles its rheumatoid counterpart, but it is usually milder and causes little disability.

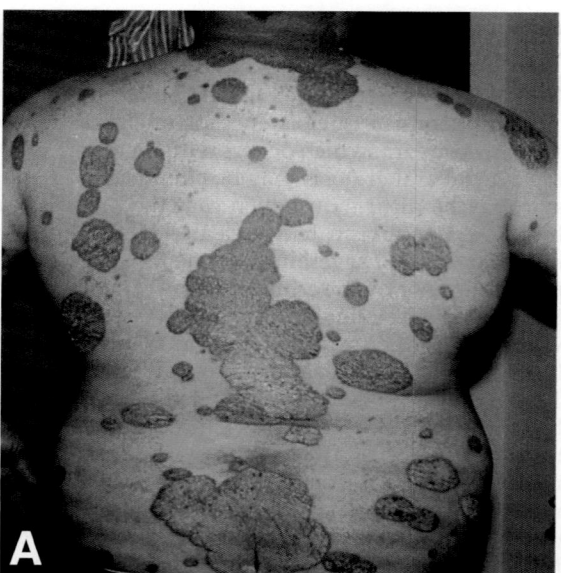

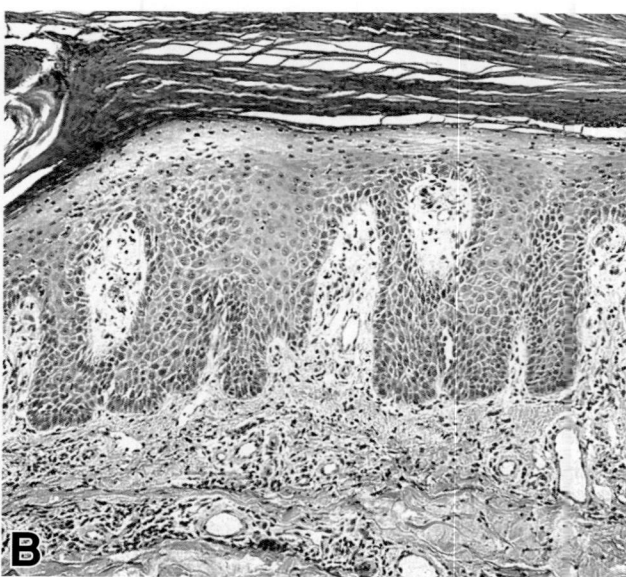

FIGURE 28-14. Psoriasis. This disorder is the prototype of psoriasiform epidermal hyperplasia. **A.** A patient with psoriasis shows large, confluent, sharply demarcated, erythematous plaques on the trunk. **B.** Microscopic examination of a lesion demonstrates that the rete ridges are uniformly elongated, as are the dermal papillae, giving an interlocking pattern of alternately reversed "clubs." The dermal papillae are edematous and reside beneath a thinned epidermis (suprapapillary thinning). There is striking parakeratosis (persistent nuclei in cells of the stratum corneum), which is the scale observed clinically.

In some variations of the disease, neutrophilic pustules (of Kogoj) dominate **(pustular psoriasis)**. Severe intractable psoriasis has been observed in some patients with AIDS.

Pemphigus Vulgaris Is a Blistering Disease due to Antibodies to Keratinocytes

Dyshesive disorders are cutaneous diseases in which blisters form because of diminished cohesiveness between epidermal keratinocytes. Pemphigus vulgaris (PV) (Greek, *pemphix,*

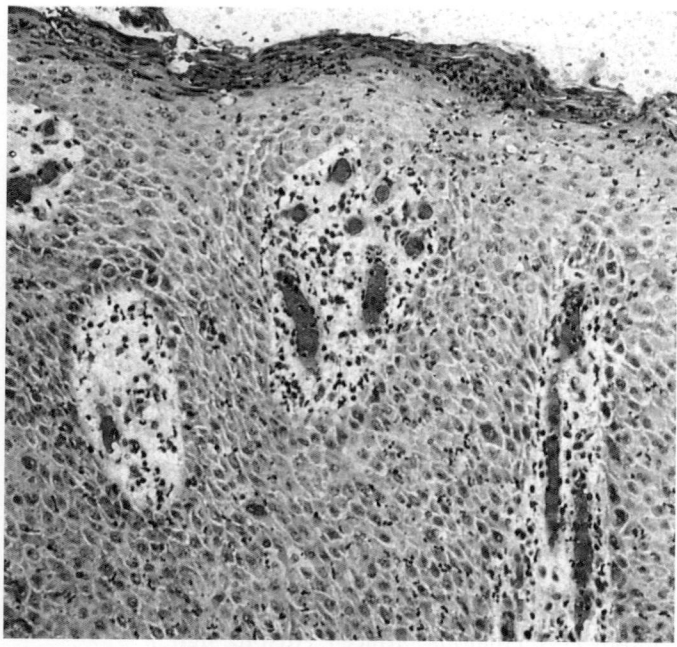

FIGURE 28-15. Psoriasis. The clubbed papillae contain tortuous dilated venules. The prominent venules are part of the venulization of capillaries, which may be of importance in the pathogenesis of psoriasis. The papilla to the *right* contains a single cross-section of its superficial capillary venule loop, which is normal. The papilla in the *center* shows numerous cross-sections of its venule, indicating striking tortuosity.

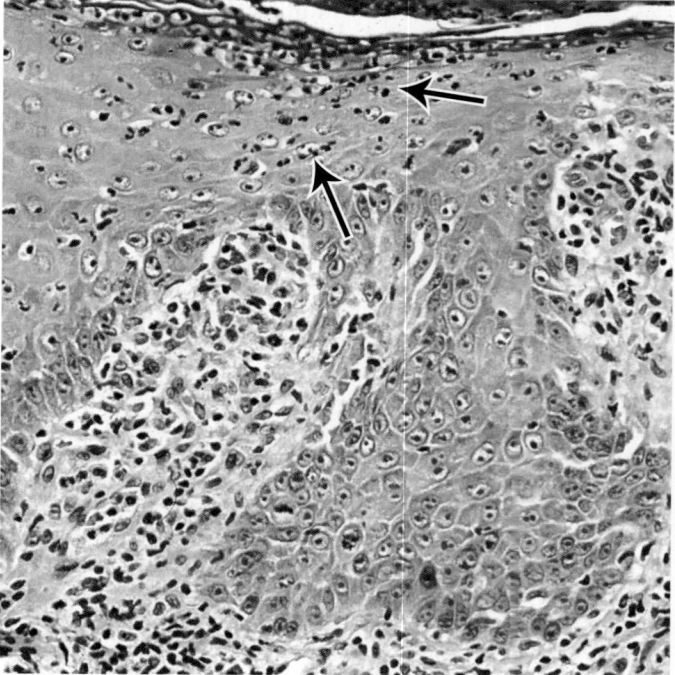

FIGURE 28-16. Psoriasis. Neutrophils migrate into the epidermis, emerging from venulized capillaries at the tips of the dermal papillae. They migrate to the upper stratum spinosum and stratum corneum (*arrows*). In some forms of psoriasis, pustules are common clinical lesions.

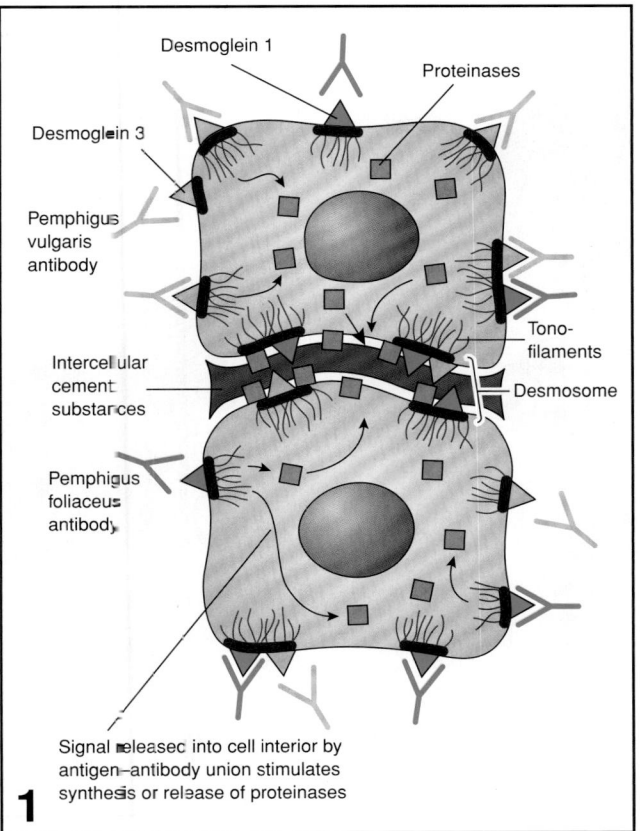

FIGURE 28-17. Mechanism of suprabasal dyshesion in pemphigus vulgaris. 1. Circulating autoantibodies bind to antigen at desmosomes on the outer leaflet of the plasma membranes of keratinocytes, especially in basal regions. **2.** Antigen–antibody union results in release of a proteinase (plasmin). **3.** The proteinase disrupts cell–cell adhesion at desmosomes (intercellular cement substances), initiating dyshesion. (*continued*)

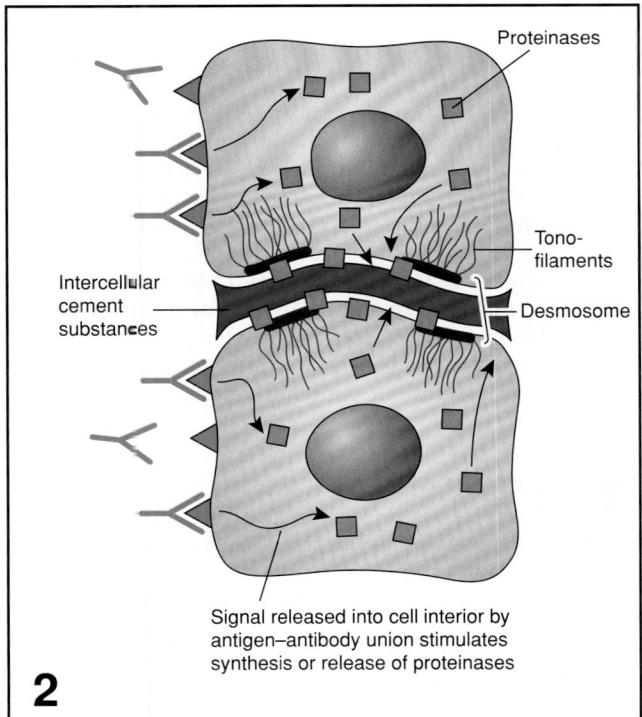

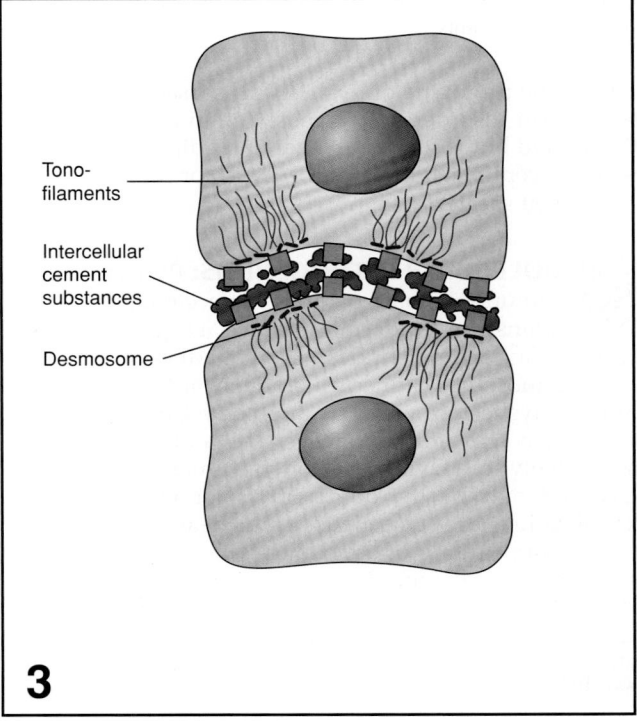

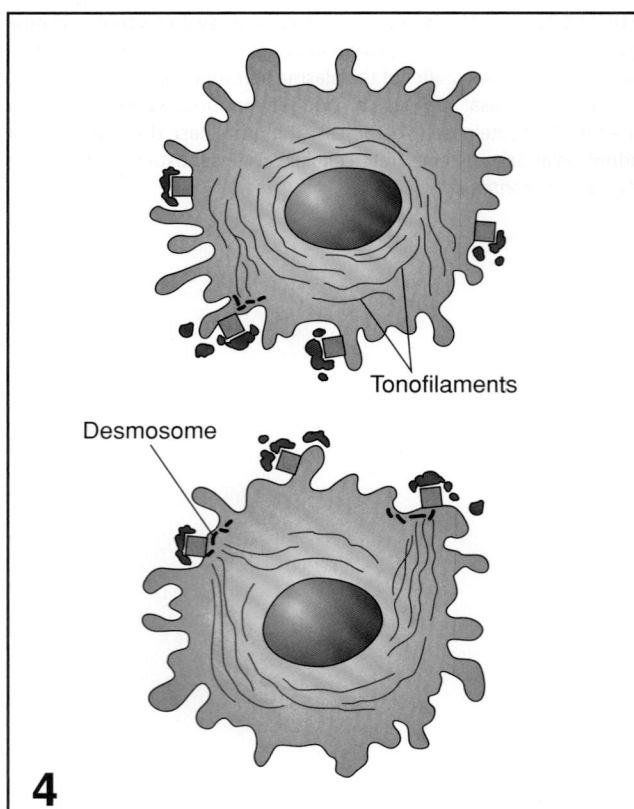

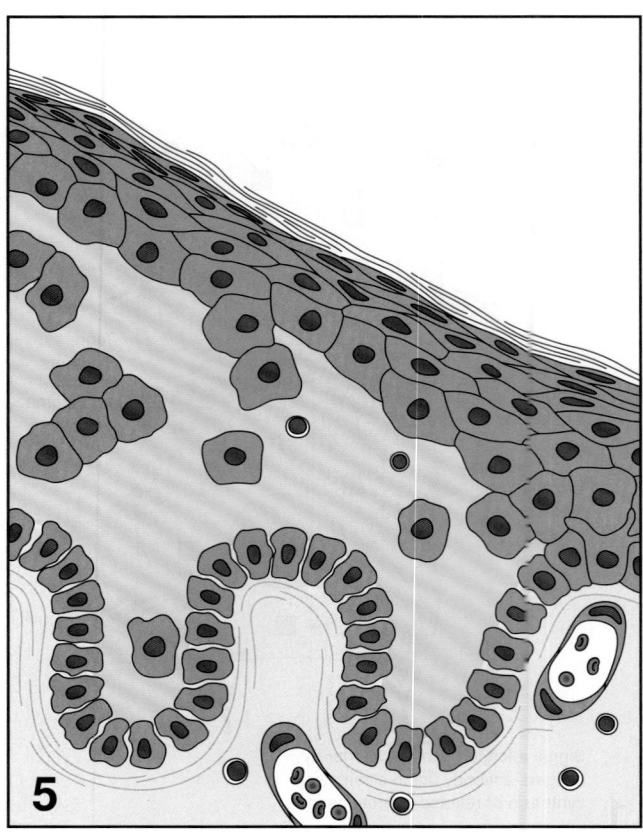

FIGURE 28-17. (*Continued*) **4.** Desmosomes deteriorate, tonofilaments clump about keratinocyte nuclei, the cells round up and separation is complete. **5.** A vesicle, usually suprabasal, forms. Alternatively, acantholysis may occur by direct interference with desmosomal and adherence junction attachments.

"bubble"), the prototype of dyshesive diseases, is a chronic, blistering skin disorder that is most common in people 40 to 60 years old but is seen at all ages, including children. All races are susceptible, but people of Jewish or Mediterranean heritage are at greatest risk.

MOLECULAR PATHOGENESIS: PV is an autoimmune disease; patients have circulating IgG against an epidermal surface antigen, **desmoglein-3**, a Ca²⁺-dependent desmosomal adhesion protein (i.e., a desmosomal cadherin). Antigen–antibody union results in dyshesion, which is augmented by release of plasminogen activator and, hence, activation of plasmin. This proteolytic enzyme acts on the intercellular substance and may be the dominant factor in dyshesion. Internalization of pemphigus antigen–antibody complexes, disappearance of attachment plaques and retraction of perinuclear tonofilaments may all act in concert with proteinases to cause dyshesion and vesiculation (Fig. 28-17). Blisters in PV are intraepidermal. In other blistering disorders that affect the basement membrane zone, discussed below, subepidermal blisters are formed.

PATHOLOGY: The outer epidermal layers separate from the basal layer. This suprabasal dyshesion results in a blister with an intact basal layer as a floor and the remaining epidermis as a roof (Fig. 28-18).

Desmoglein-3 is concentrated in the lower epidermis, explaining the location of the blister. The blister contains moderate numbers of lymphocytes, macrophages, eosinophils, and neutrophils. Distinctive, rounded keratinocytes, or **acantholytic cells**, are shed into the vesicle during dyshesion. Basal cells remain adherent to the basal lamina and form a layer of "tombstone cells." Dyshesion may extend along dermal adnexa and is not always strictly suprabasal. The subjacent dermis shows a moderate infiltrate of lymphocytes, macrophages, eosinophils and neutrophils, predominantly around the capillary venular bed.

CLINICAL FEATURES: The characteristic lesion of PV is a large, easily ruptured blister that leaves extensive denuded or crusted areas. They are most common on the scalp and mucous membranes and in periumbilical and intertriginous areas. Without corticosteroid treatment, PV is progressive and usually fatal. Much of the skin surface may become denuded. Immunosuppression is also useful for maintenance therapy. With appropriate treatment, the 10-year mortality rate for PV is less than 10%.

Other diseases caused by dyshesion that have pathogenetic mechanisms like PV include **pemphigus foliaceus, pemphigus erythematosus**, and **drug-induced pemphigus** (often associated with penicillamine or captopril). In pemphigus foliaceus, antibodies against **desmoglein-1**,

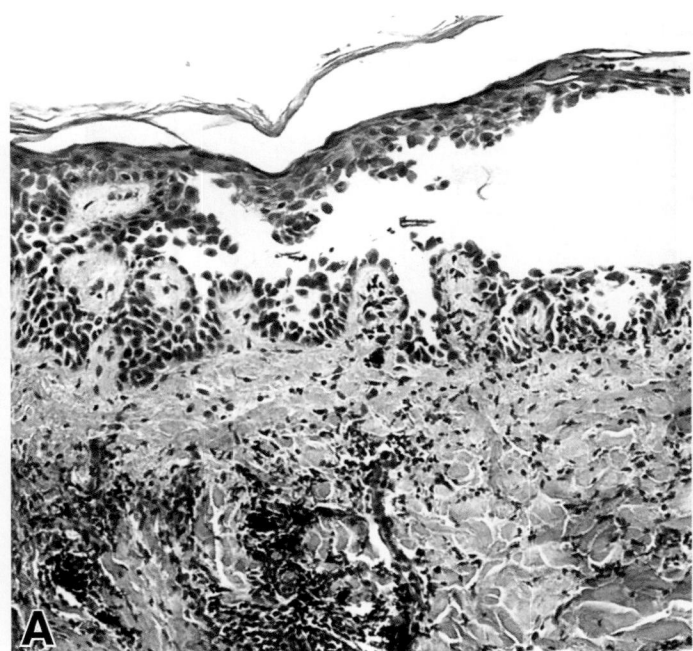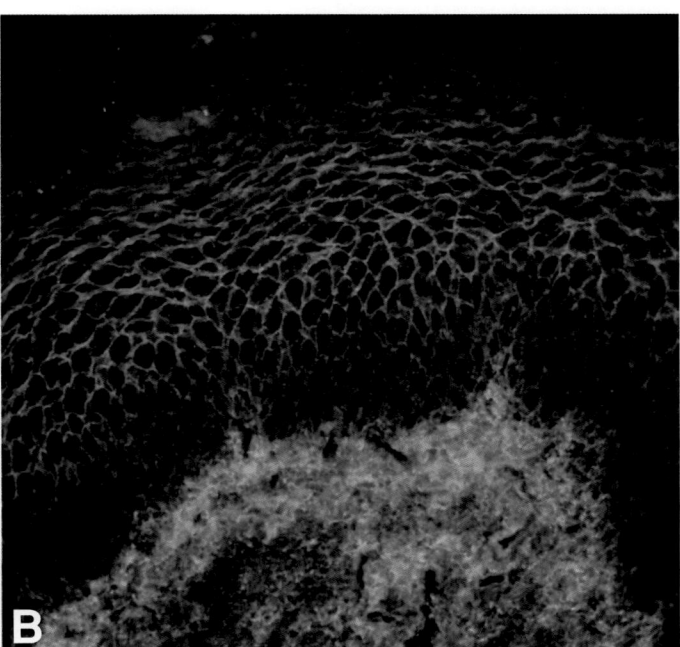

FIGURE 28-18. Pemphigus vulgaris. A. Suprabasal dyshesion leads to an intraepidermal blister containing acantholytic keratinocytes. Basal keratinocytes are slightly separated from each other and totally separated from the stratum spinosum. The basal keratinocytes are firmly attached to the epidermal basement membrane zone. **B.** Direct immunofluorescence examination of perilesional skin reveals deposition of antibodies, usually of the immunoglobulin G (IgG) type, in the intercellular substance of the epidermis, yielding a lace-like pattern outlining the keratinocytes.

a related desmosomal cadherin, cause dyshesion in the outer spinous and granular epidermal layers (vs. suprabasal dyshesion in PV) (Fig. 28-19). In pemphigus foliaceus and pemphigus erythematosus, dyshesion occurs in the spinous layer. **Paraneoplastic pemphigus** may occur with some cancers, usually lymphoproliferative tumors, and shows variable patterns of dyshesion and antigenic targets.

Pemphigus may accompany other autoimmune diseases, such as myasthenia gravis and lupus erythematosus, and may also be seen with benign thymomas. Other diseases may mimic the histology of PV, namely, familial benign chronic pemphigus (Hailey–Hailey disease) and transient acantholytic dermatosis (Grover disease). However, antibodies do not react with epidermal antigens in these entities.

DISEASES OF THE BASEMENT MEMBRANE ZONE (DERMAL–EPIDERMAL INTERFACE)

In Epidermolysis Bullosa Blisters Form in the Basement Membrane Zone

Epidermolysis bullosa (EB) is a heterogeneous group of disorders loosely bound by their hereditary nature and by a tendency to form blisters at sites of minor trauma. The clinical spectrum ranges from a minor annoyance to a widespread, life-threatening blistering disease. *These blisters are almost always present at birth or shortly thereafter.* Classification of these disorders is based on a combination of clinical features and site of blister formation in the BMZ. Different mechanisms of blister formation underlie each of the four major categories of EB (Fig. 28-20).

Epidermolytic Epidermolysis Bullosa

Also known as **EB simplex**, this is a group of autosomal dominant and autosomal recessive skin diseases in which blisters form because of disruption of basal keratinocytes. Blisters develop after minor trauma, such as merely rubbing the skin, but heal without scarring (thus the term "simplex"). Epidermolytic EB is cosmetically disturbing and sometimes debilitating but is not life-threatening.

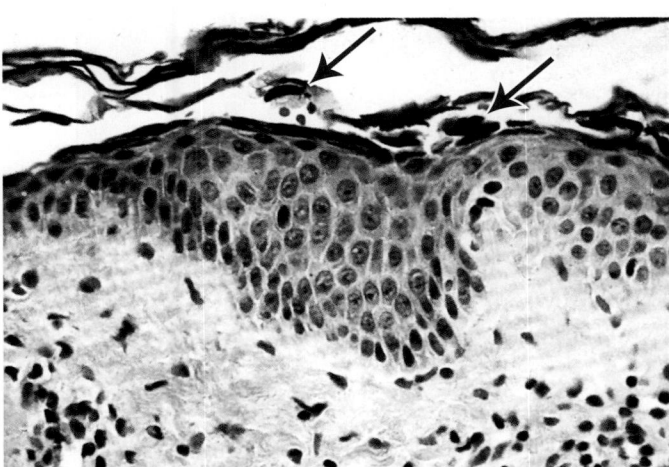

FIGURE 28-19. Pemphigus foliaceus. Dyshesion develops in the outer stratum spinosum and stratum granulosum. (Compare with that of pemphigus vulgaris, Fig. 24-18.) Dyshesive and dyskeratotic keratinocytes of the stratum granulosum (*arrows*) are important hallmarks.

EPIDERMOLYTIC EB

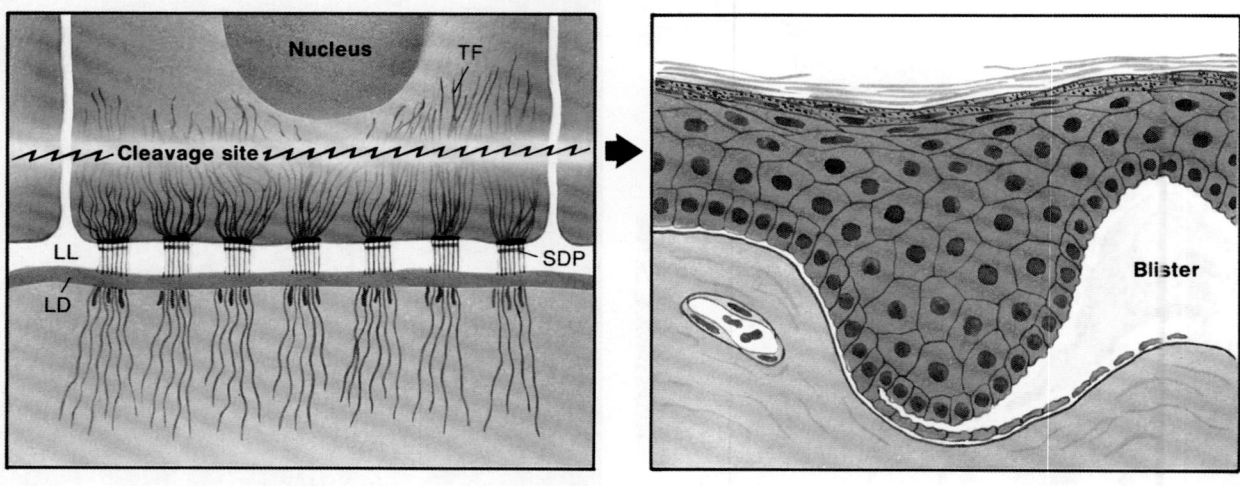

JUNCTIONAL EB

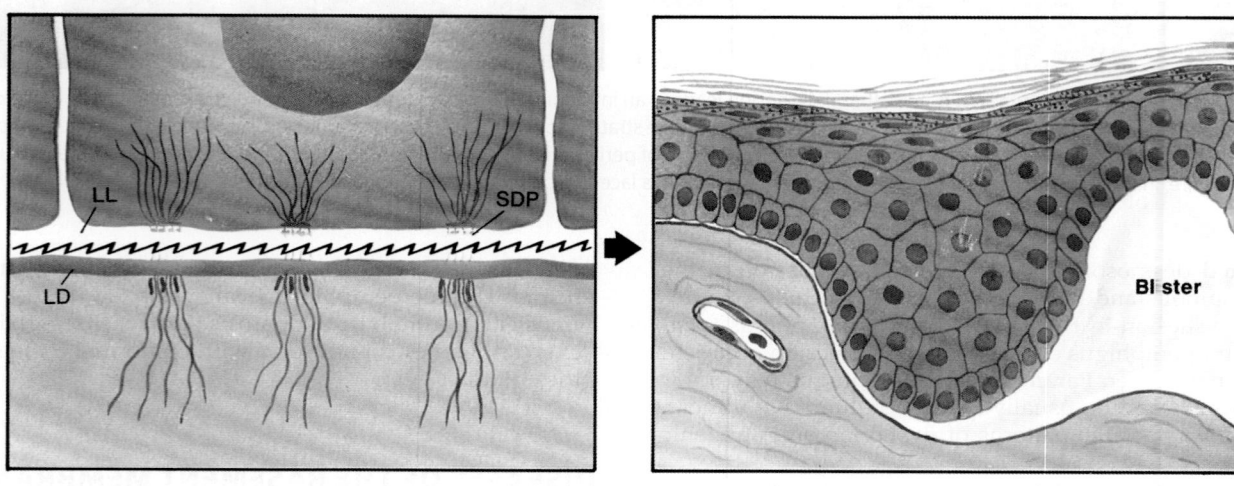

DERMOLYTIC EB

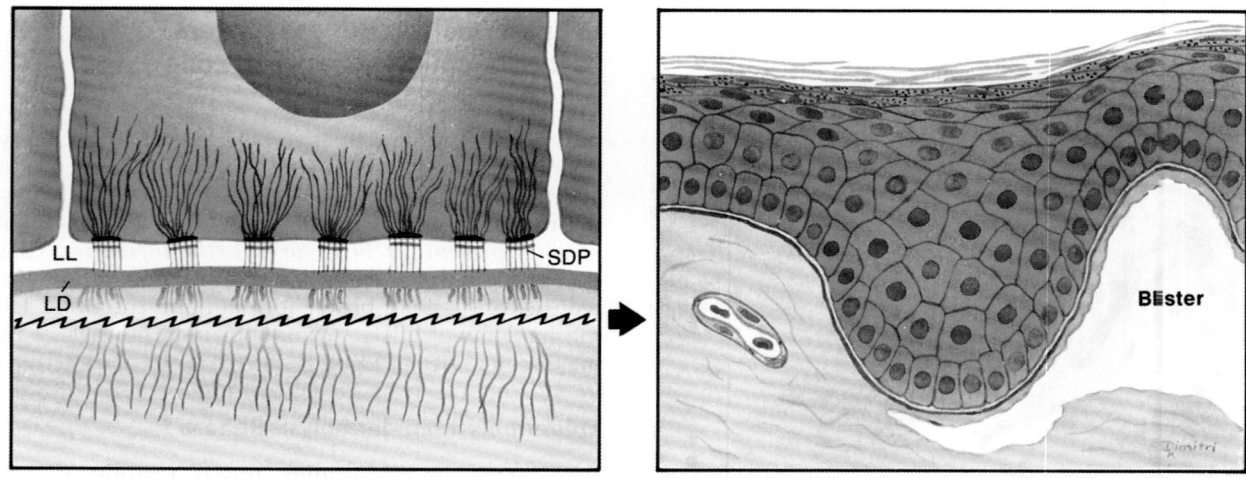

FIGURE 28-20. Epidermolysis bullosa (EB). Three distinct mechanisms of blister formation are shown. Electron microscopic images showing cleavage sites are diagrammed on the *left;* light microscopic images are diagrammed on the *right.* **Epidermolytic EB** is caused by disintegration of the lowermost regions of the epidermal basal cells. The bottom portions of basal cells cleave, and the remainder of the epidermis lifts away. Small fragments of basal cells remain attached to the basement membrane zone. **Junctional EB** is characterized by cleavage in the lamina lucida. **Dermolytic EB** is associated with rudimentary and fragmented anchoring fibrils within the dermis. The entire basement membrane zone and epidermis split away from the dermis in relationship to these flawed anchoring fibrils. *LL* = lamina lucida; *LD* = lamina densa; *SDP* = subdesmosomal dense plate.

MOLECULAR PATHOGENESIS: Epidermolytic EB has been attributed to mutations in *KRT5* and *KRT14*, usually inherited in an autosome dominant fashion. These genes encode keratins 5 and 14, respectively, which assemble into intermediate filaments that normally provide mechanical stability to the epidermis. The mutant proteins do not assemble properly and instead aggregate around keratinocyte nuclei. This produces subnuclear cytoplasmic vacuoles which gradually enlarge and coalesce. The plasma membrane ruptures when the large vacuole reaches it, after which the cell is lysed. Cytolysis of basal keratinocytes causes the blisters in the epidermolytic variety of EB.

 PATHOLOGY: An intraepidermal vesicle results from lysis of several basal keratinocytes. The roof of the vesicle is an almost intact epidermis with a fragmented basal layer. The vesicle floor has bits of basal cell cytoplasm attached to the lamina densa, which appears as a well-preserved pink line at the base of the vesicle. Inflammatory cells are sparse.

Junctional Epidermolysis Bullosa

This type of EB is a group of autosomal recessive skin diseases in which blisters form within the lamina lucida. Clinical expression ranges from a benign disease with no effect on life span to a severe condition that may be fatal within the first 2 years of life. There may be associated abnormalities of the nails and teeth.

 MOLECULAR PATHOGENESIS: A severe form of the disease is caused by mutations in *LAMA3*, *LAMB3*, and *LAMC2* all of which encode subunits of laminin 332, a protein that links the epidermis to the basement membrane. Mutations in any of these genes produce an abnormal protein that greatly increases the fragility of the epidermis. A more benign form of the disease is caused by mutations in *COL17A1*, the gene for type XVII collagen. Both types heal without scarring but may cause residual atrophy of the skin.

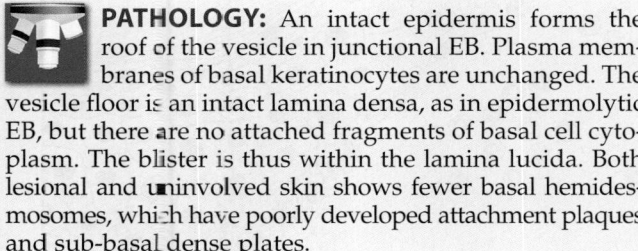 **PATHOLOGY:** An intact epidermis forms the roof of the vesicle in junctional EB. Plasma membranes of basal keratinocytes are unchanged. The vesicle floor is an intact lamina densa, as in epidermolytic EB, but there are no attached fragments of basal cell cytoplasm. The blister is thus within the lamina lucida. Both lesional and uninvolved skin shows fewer basal hemidesmosomes, which have poorly developed attachment plaques and sub-basal dense plates.

Dermolytic Epidermolysis Bullosa

Also known as **dystrophic EB**, dermolytic EB is a group of autosomal dominant and autosomal recessive diseases in which blisters occur immediately deep to the lamina densa. The recessive variant is more severe. In both types, healed blisters show atrophic ("dystrophic") scarring. Nails and teeth may be involved.

 MOLECULAR PATHOGENESIS: Dermolytic EB is attributed to a defect in anchoring fibrils. These fibrils are abnormally arranged and reduced in number in apparently normal skin of affected newborns. The basic defect is a mutation in *COL7A1*, the gene for collagen type VII (3p21). Collagen type VII is the main component of anchoring fibrils which make up a net in the upper dermis, through which collagen types I and III fibers course. This structure anchors the epidermis to the underlying dermis. Its disruption results in subepidermal bullae arising in the sublamina densa zone.

 PATHOLOGY: The vesicle roof is normal epidermis with an attached, intact lamina lucida and lamina densa. The base of the vesicle is the outer part of the papillary dermis. Ultrastructurally, there are fewer anchoring fibrils in the dominant type and virtually none in the recessive form. A corresponding decrease in anchoring fibril proteins AF-1 and AF-2 occurs in the two variants.

Kindler Syndrome

This type of EB shows autosomal recessive transmission and blisters with mixed cleavage planes. Distinctive clinical findings that differentiate it from other inherited EB types include poikiloderma (mottled pigmentation of the skin) and photosensitivity.

 MOLECULAR PATHOGENESIS: This entity results from a mutation in *FERMT1* (20p12), which encodes kindlin-1, a protein involved in adhesion between basal keratinocytes.

Bullous Pemphigoid (BP) Is a Subepidermal Blistering Disease Caused by Autoantibodies Against Basement Membrane Proteins

BP is a common, autoimmune, blistering disease, which has clinical similarities to PV (hence the term "pemphigoid"), but which lacks acantholysis (loss of intercellular junctions). The disease is most common in the later decades of life and affects all races and both genders.

 MOLECULAR PATHOGENESIS: Like PV, BP is an autoimmune disease, but here complement-fixing IgG antibodies are against BPAG1 and BPAG2 basement membrane proteins. BPAG1, also known as dystonin (encoded by the *DST* gene), is a 230-kd protein in the intracellular portion of the basal cell hemidesmosome. BPAG2 is another name for collagen type XVII (made by *COL17A1*). It is a 180-kd protein that traverses the plasma membrane and extends into the upper lamina lucida. The antigen–antibody complex may injure the basal cell plasma membrane via the C5b–C9 membrane attack complex (see Chapter 4). This damage may in turn interfere with elaboration of adhesion factors by basal keratinocytes. More importantly, anaphylatoxins C3a and C5a are released in complement activation. They trigger mast cell degranulation and release of factors chemotactic for eosinophils, neutrophils, and lymphocytes. Levels of IL-5 and eotaxin, which play significant roles in recruitment and function of eosinophils, are elevated in the blister fluid of patients with BP. Eosinophil granules contain tissue-damaging substances, including eosinophil peroxidase and major basic protein. These molecules, together with neutrophil and mast cell proteases, cause dermal–epidermal separation within the lamina lucida (Fig. 28-21).

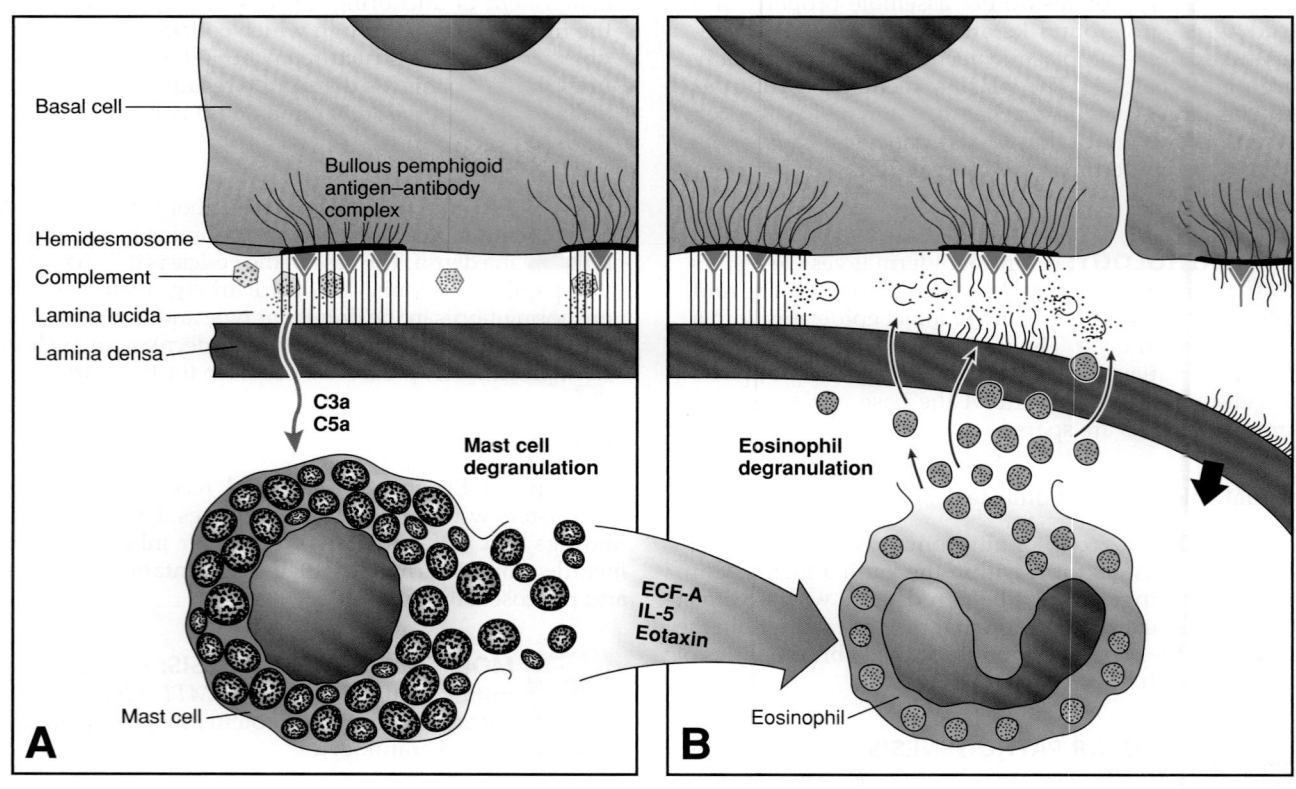

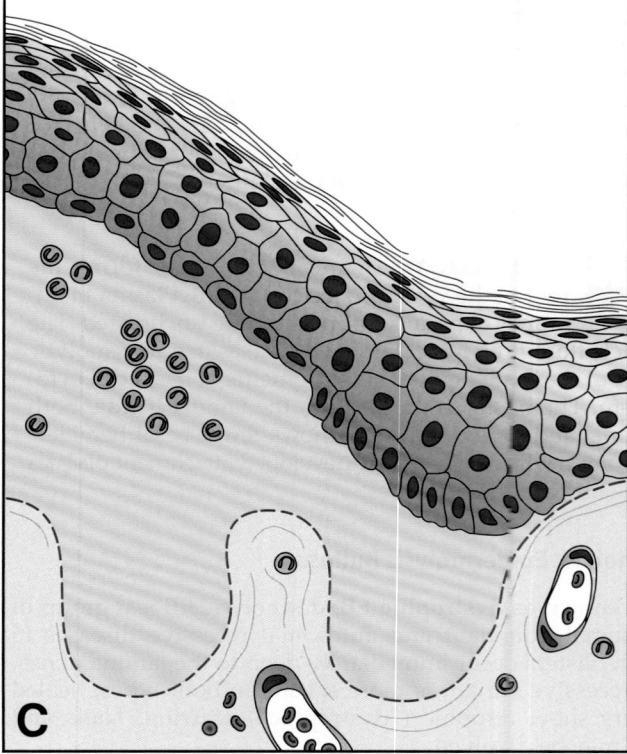

FIGURE 28-21. Mechanisms of blister formation in bullous pemphigoid (BP). Circulating antibodies to an apparently normal glycoprotein—BP antigen—in the lamina lucida mediate pathogenic events in bullous pemphigoid. **A.** Antigen–antibody union activates complement, and the anaphylatoxins C3a and C5a are produced. These cause mast cells to degranulate, resulting in the release of eosinophilic chemotactic factors. **B, C.** Tissue-damaging substances of eosinophilic granules lead to vesicle formation at the lamina lucida, with some breakdown of the lamina densa. *ECF-A* = eosinophil chemotactic factor-A.

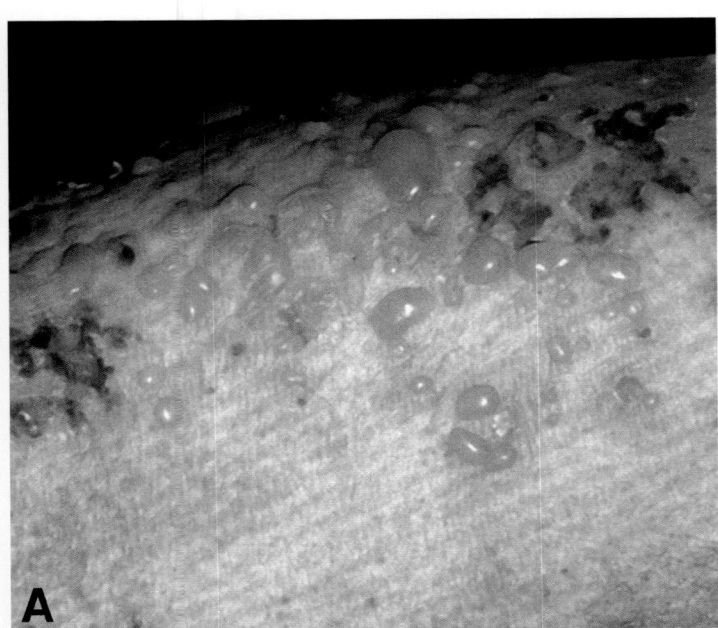
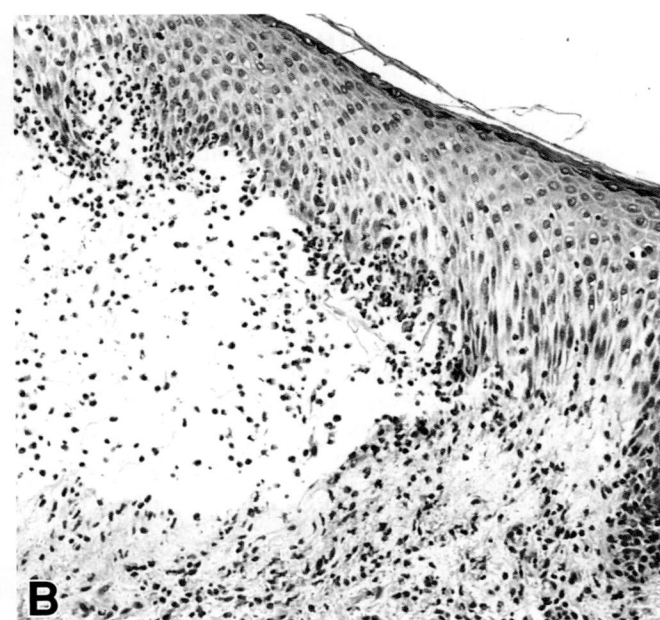

FIGURE 28-22. Bullous pemphigoid. A. The skin shows multiple tense bullae on an erythematous base and erosions, distributed primarily on the medial thighs and trunk. (From Elder DE, Elenitsas R, Johnson BL, et al. *Synopsis and Atlas of Lever's Histopathology of the Skin*. Philadelphia: Lippincott Williams & Wilkins, 1999.) **B.** A subepidermal blister has an edematous papillary dermis as its base. The roof of the blister consists of the intact, entire epidermis, including the stratum basalis. Inflammatory cells (including many eosinophils), fibrin and fluid fill the blister.

PATHOLOGY: The blisters of BP are subepidermal; the roof is intact epidermis and the base is the lamina densa of the BMZ (Fig. 28-22). The blisters contain many eosinophils, plus fibrin, lymphocytes, and neutrophils. In BP, apparently normal skin shows migration of mast cells from venules toward the epidermis. With the onset of erythema, eosinophils appear in the upper dermis and may be arrayed along the epidermal BMZ. Ultrastructurally, dermal–epidermal separation begins with disruption of anchoring filaments of the lamina lucida. Immunofluorescence shows linear deposition of C3 and IgG at the epidermal BMZ (Fig. 28-23), and serum antibodies against BPAG1 and BPAG2 can be demonstrated by ELISA assays.

CLINICAL FEATURES: The blisters of BP are large and tense and may appear on normal-appearing skin or on an erythematous base (Fig. 28-22). The medial thighs and flexor aspects of the forearms are commonly affected, but the groin, axillae, and other cutaneous sites may also develop blisters. The disease is self-limited but chronic, and the patient's general health is usually unaffected. Systemic glucocorticoid treatment greatly shortens the course of the disease.

Dermatitis Herpetiformis Reflects Gluten Sensitivity and Immune Complex Deposition

Dermatitis herpetiformis (DH) is an intensely pruritic eruption of urticaria-like plaques and small subepidermal vesicles over the extensor surfaces of the body.

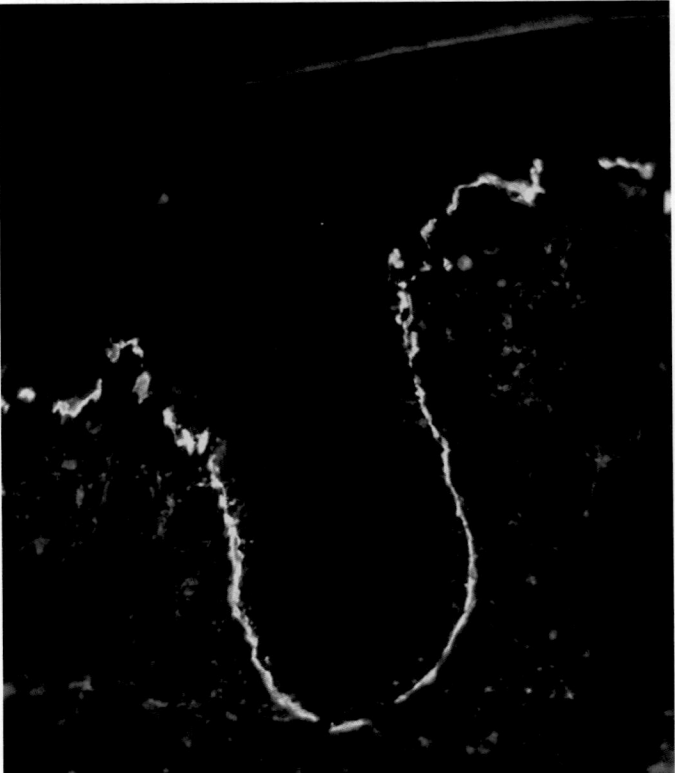

FIGURE 28-23. Bullous pemphigoid. Direct immunofluorescence analysis shows linear deposition of immunoglobulin G (IgG) (and C3) along the dermal–epidermal junction. Ultrastructural examination reveals that these antibodies and complement are present in the lamina lucida.

MOLECULAR PATHOGENESIS: It accompanies gluten sensitivity in patients with HLA-B8, HLA-DR3, and HLA-DQw2 haplotypes. Although gluten-sensitive enteropathy may be subclinical in patients with DH, most will exhibit features of celiac disease on small intestinal biopsy (see Chapter 19). DH cutaneous lesions show granular deposits of IgA, mainly at the tips of dermal papillae (Fig. 28-24). These IgA immune complexes are more prominent in perilesional skin than in normal-appearing skin. Gluten-free diets control the disease; reintroduction of gluten provokes new lesions.

Genetically predisposed patients may develop IgA antibodies to components of gluten in the intestines. Resulting IgA complexes then gain access to the circulation and deposit in dermal papillae (Fig. 28-24). Patients with DH have increased levels of IgA autoantibodies to tissue transglutaminase, suggesting that a dermal autoantigen is related to tissue transglutaminase. Antibodies to smooth muscle endomysium are also increased in many patients with DH. Neutrophils attracted to the site release lysosomal enzymes that degrade laminin and type IV collagen, cleaving the epidermis from the dermis and eventually causing blisters (Fig. 28-24).

CLINICAL FEATURES: The lesions of DH are especially prominent over the elbows, knees, and buttocks (Fig. 28-25A). These intensely pruritic vesicles may become grouped similarly to those of herpes simplex infections (hence, "herpetiformis") and are almost invariably rubbed until broken. Thus, patients may present with only crusted lesions and no intact vesicles. DH is of varying severity and characterized by remissions, but it is disturbingly chronic. Healing lesions often leave scars. Besides a gluten-free diet, dapsone or sulfapyridine may control the signs and symptoms of DH by an unknown mechanism. An increased risk of lymphoproliferative disorders and systemic lupus erythematosus has been reported.

PATHOLOGY: A delicate perivenular lymphocytic infiltrate appears first, together with a row of neutrophils just deep to the lamina densa in the dermal papillae. During the next 12 hours, neutrophils aggregate in clusters of 10 to 25 at the tips of the dermal papillae to create a diagnostic histologic appearance.

There are two related mechanisms of dermal–epidermal separation. One is associated with the sheetlike spread of a layer or two of neutrophils at the dermal–epidermal interface. In this case, the entire epidermis detaches from the papillary dermis (Fig. 28-25B). The vesicle roof contains the epidermis; the floor is composed of the lamina densa and the papillary dermis. Unlike in BP, eosinophils are uncommon early in the course of DH. In the second route of vesicle formation, many neutrophils accumulate rapidly in the tips of the dermal papillae. Release of their lysosomal enzymes into the superficial portion of the dermal papillae uncouples the epidermis from the dermis at the tips of dermal papillae, disrupts the BMZ in the lamina lucida and superficial part of the papillae, and causes the epidermis to tear across the adjacent rete ridges. Roofs of resulting vesicles have alternating tears across their epidermal covering, and their floors have residual epidermal pegs alternating with the basal half of dermal papillae. In both cases, granular IgA is deposited at the dermoepidermal junction (Fig. 28-25C).

Erythema Multiforme Is Often a Reaction to a Drug or Infection

Erythema multiforme (EM) is an acute, self-limited disorder that varies from a few annular or ring-like and targetoid erythematous macules and blisters (EM minor) to a life-threatening, widespread ulceration of the skin and mucous membranes (EM major; Stevens–Johnson syndrome, SJS also known as toxic epidermal necrolysis or TEN). *It is usually a reaction to a drug or an infectious agent, in particular, herpes simplex virus infection.*

ETIOLOGIC FACTORS: Numerous agents may provoke EM, including herpesvirus, *Mycoplasma* and sulfonamides, but precipitating factors are identified in only half of cases. In postherpetic EM, viral antigens, IgM and C3 deposit perivascularly, and at the epidermal BMZ. The combination of infiltrating lymphocytes and antigen–antibody complexes within the lesions suggests that humoral and cellular hypersensitivity are both involved.

PATHOLOGY: The dermis in EM shows a sparse lymphocyte infiltrate about the superficial vascular bed and at the dermal–epidermal interface. The characteristic morphologic feature in the epidermis is apoptotic ("dyskeratotic") keratinocytes, with pyknotic nuclei and eosinophilic cytoplasm. Apoptosis may be extensive and associated with a subepidermal vesicle, whose roof is an almost completely necrotic epidermis. Because of the acute onset of the disease, in most cases there is little or no change in the stratum corneum. There is a superficial dermal perivascular lymphocytic infiltrate, without eosinophils. The histology of SJS and TEN is identical to that of EM except for their extent; especially in a small biopsy, the diagnosis requires clinicopathologic correlation.

CLINICAL FEATURES: The characteristic "target" or "iris" lesions of EM have a central, dark red zone, occasionally with a blister, surrounded by a paler area (Fig. 28-26). In turn, the latter is encompassed by a peripheral red rim. Urticarial plaques are common. The presence of vesicles and bullae usually predicts a more severe course. EM is a common condition, with a peak incidence in the second and third decades of life. It is occasionally encountered in association with other presumably immunologic cutaneous disorders, including erythema nodosum, toxic epidermal necrolysis, and necrotizing vasculitis. **SJS** and **TEN** refer to unusually severe forms of EM that involve mucosal surfaces and internal organs and are frequently fatal, without effective treatment.

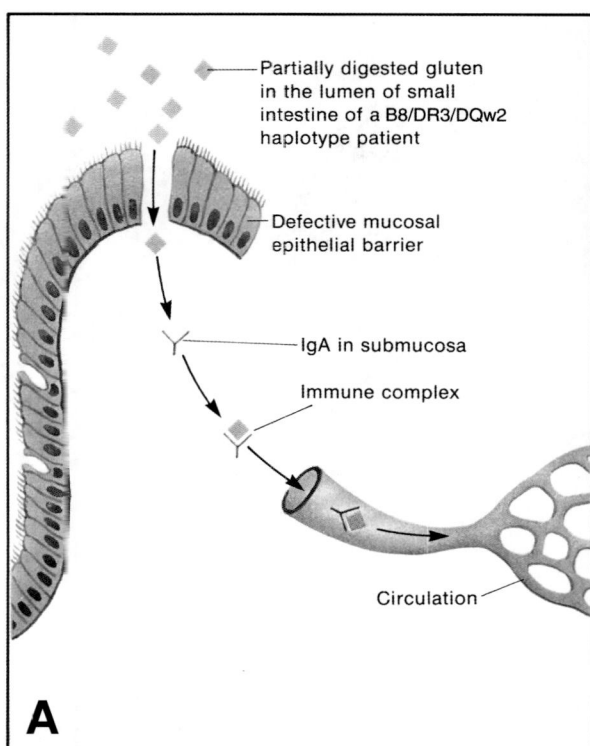

1. Formation of immune complexes in submucosa of small intestine. Passage of immune complexes into **the circulation.**

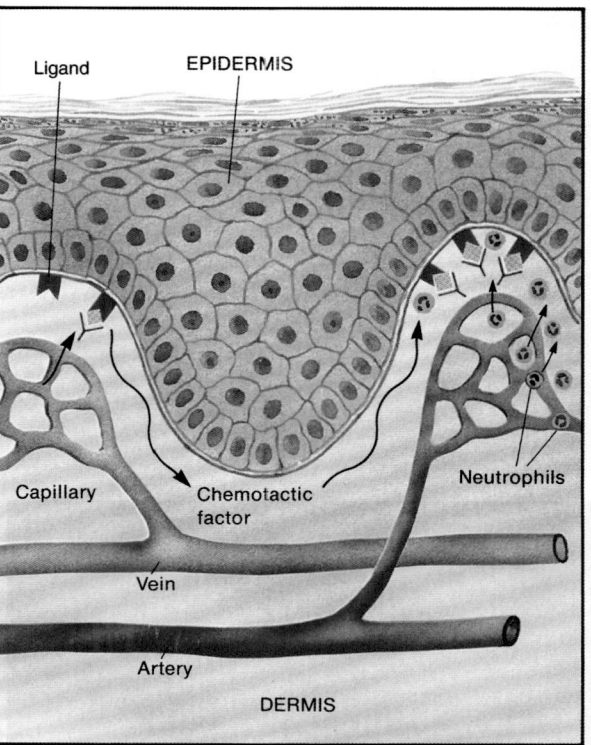

2. Ligand–immune complex union releases neutrophil chemotactic factor. Neutrophils migrate to the tips of the papillae.

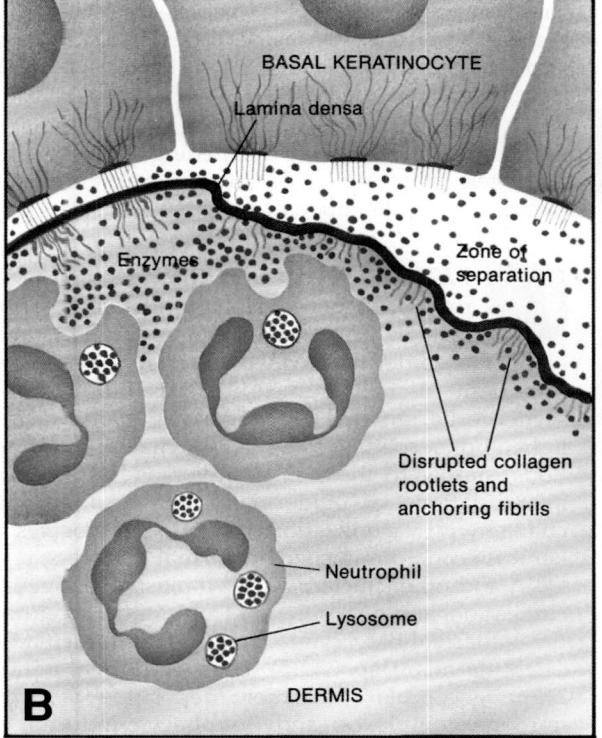

3. Dissolution of basal rootlets and anchoring fibrils by enzymes released by neutrophils. Early dermo-epidermal separation.

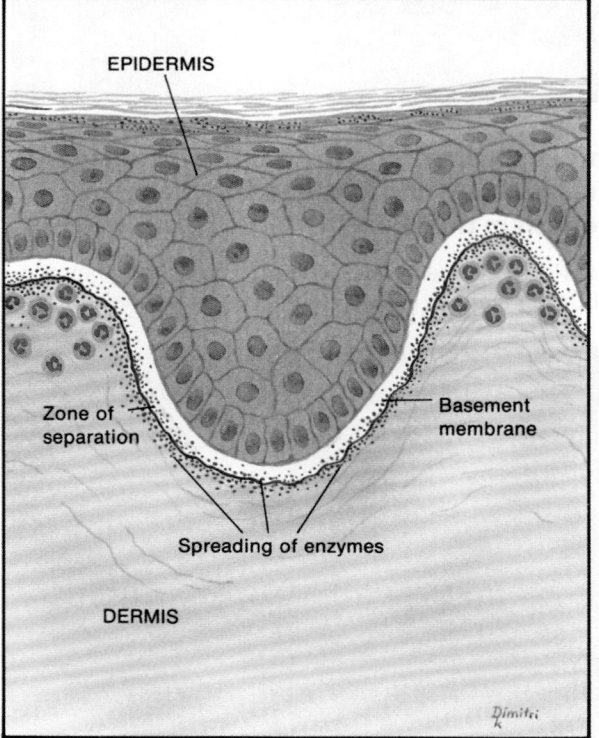

4. Concentration of neutrophils at the tips of the papillae. Spreading of enzymes along basement membrane. Lifting away of lamina densa.

FIGURE 28-24. Pathogenesis of cutaneous lesions in dermatitis herpetiformis. A. The disease is initiated in the small intestine and is expressed in the skin likely because of the presence of a ligand immediately deep to the lamina densa. Engagement of this ligand in the skin by immunoglobulin A originating in the submucosa of the gut produces chemotactic factors that attract neutrophils. *IgA* = immunoglobulin A. **B.** Enzymes released by neutrophils destroy anchoring fibrils and promote dermoepidermal separation.

THE SKIN

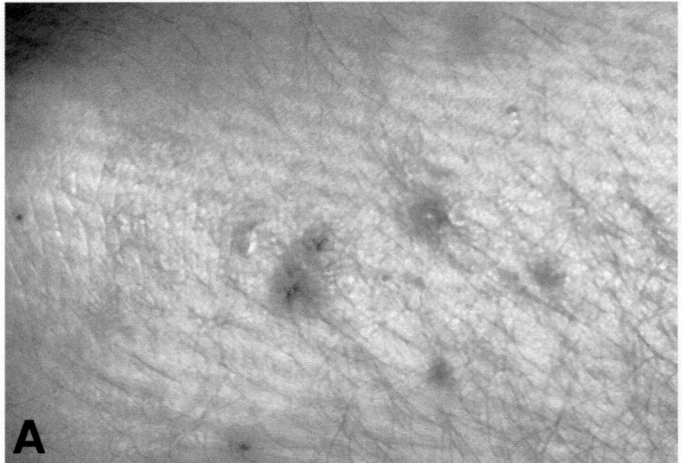

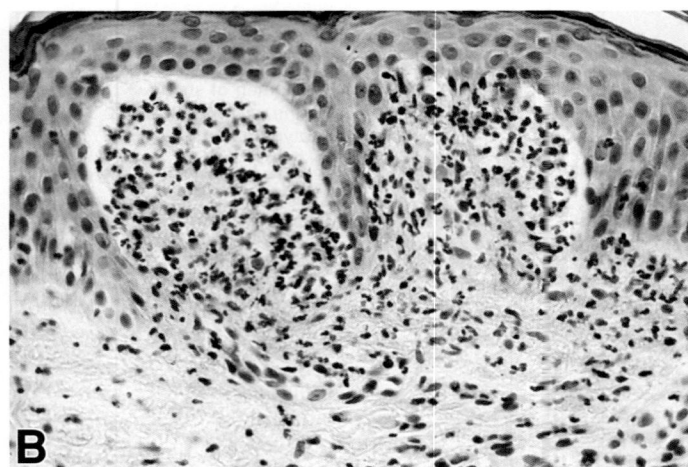

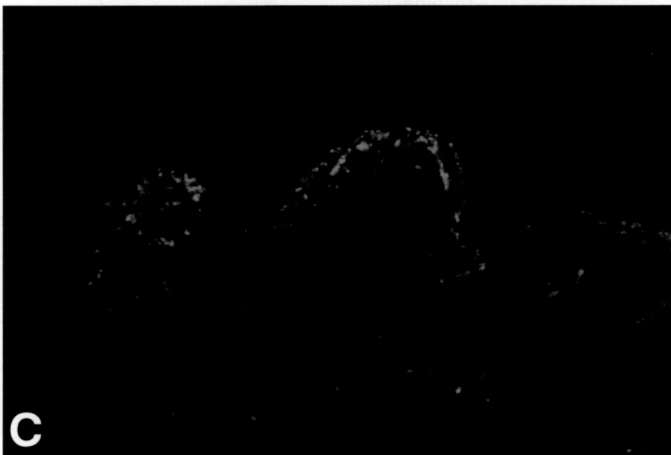

FIGURE 28-25. Dermatitis herpetiformis. A. Pruritic, symmetric, grouped vesicles on an erythematous base are seen on the elbows and knees. (From Elder DE, Elenitsas R, Johnson BL, et al. *Synopsis and Atlas of Lever's Histopathology of the Skin.* Philadelphia, PA: Lippincott Williams & Wilkins; 1999.) **B.** Dermal papillary abscesses of neutrophils with vesicle formation at the dermal–epidermal junction are characteristic. **C.** Direct immunofluorescence reveals deposition of immunoglobulin A (IgA) in dermal papillae in association with (but not necessarily directly upon) anchoring fibrils and elastic tissue fibers. This is the site of neutrophil infiltration and subepidermal vesicle formation.

Systemic Lupus Erythematosus Is Characterized by Autoantibodies and Immune Complexes That Deposit in the Skin

Cutaneous involvement in systemic lupus erythematosus (SLE; see Chapter 11) may be severe and cosmetically

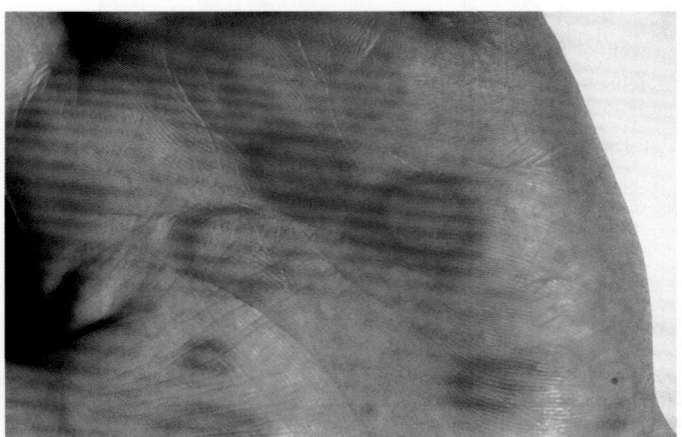

FIGURE 28-26. Erythema multiforme. Steroid-responsive "target" papules, characterized by central bullae with surrounding erythema, appeared in this patient after antibiotic therapy. (From Elder DE, Elenitsas R, Johnson BL, et al. *Synopsis and Atlas of Lever's Histopathology of the Skin.* Philadelphia, PA: Lippincott Williams & Wilkins; 1999.)

devastating but it is not life threatening. However, the nature and pattern of immune reactants in the skin are an excellent indicator of the likelihood of systemic disease.

PATHOPHYSIOLOGY: Immune complexes are present in both lesional and normal-appearing skin in SLE. Deposition of immune reactants along the epidermal BMZ of normal-appearing skin is important in making the diagnosis. Epidermal injury seems to be initiated by exogenous agents such as UV light and perpetuated by cell-mediated immune reactions, similar to those in graft-versus-host disease. The manifestations of epidermal injury include **interface change** with vacuolization of basal keratinocytes, hyperkeratosis, and diminished epidermal thickness, release of DNA and other nuclear and cytoplasmic antigens to the circulation, and deposition of DNA and other antigens in the epidermal BMZ (lamina densa and immediately subjacent dermis) (Fig. 28-27). Thus, epidermal injury, local immune complex formation, deposition of circulating immune complexes, and lymphocyte-induced cellular injury all seem to act in concert.

The various forms of cutaneous lupus are classified according to their chronicity, but considerable overlap in features is possible. There is an inverse relationship between the prominence of skin lesions and the extent of systemic disease.

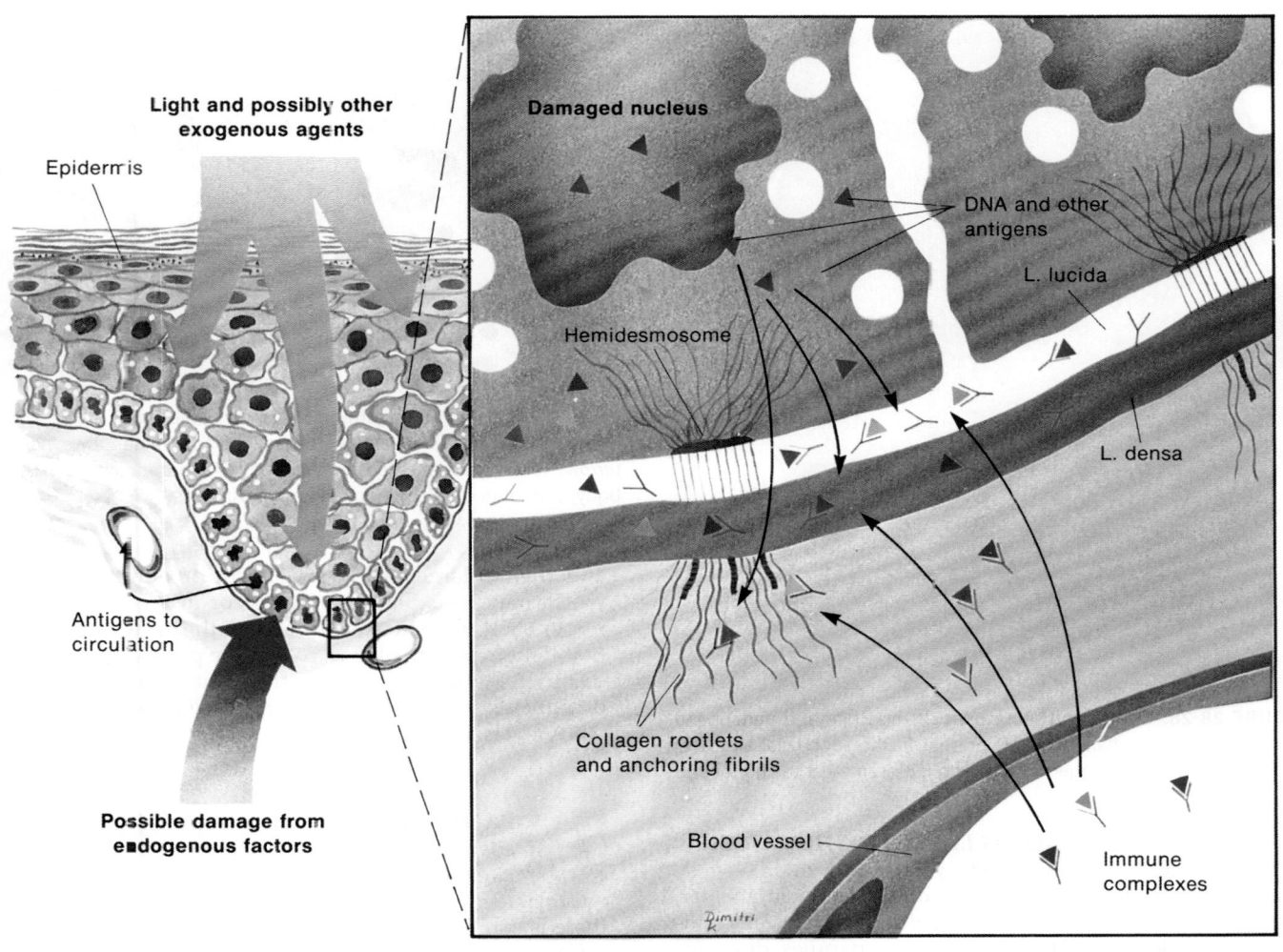

FIGURE 28-27. Lupus erythematosus. A cell-mediated immune reaction leads to epidermal cellular damage when initiated by light or other exogenous agents as well as endogenous ones. Such injury releases a large number of antigens, some of which may return to the skin in the form of immune complexes. Immune complexes are also formed in the skin by a reaction of local DNA with antibody that may also be deposited beneath the epidermal basement membrane zone. *L* = lamina.

CHRONIC CUTANEOUS (DISCOID) LUPUS ERYTHEMATOSUS: This form of lupus is usually limited to the skin. It generally affects skin above the neck, on the face (especially the malar area), scalp, and ears. Lesions begin as slightly elevated violaceous papules with a rough scale of keratin. They enlarge to assume a disc shape, with a hyperkeratotic margin and a depigmented center. The cutaneous lesions may culminate in disfiguring scars. Elevated circulating antinuclear antibody (ANA) levels are seen in less than 10% of patients.

PATHOLOGY: In discoid lupus, nucleated epidermal layers are modestly thickened or somewhat thin. Hyperkeratosis, without prominent parakeratosis, and plugging of hair follicles are prominent. The rete–papillae pattern of the dermal–epidermal interface is partially effaced. There is interface change with vacuolar change of basal keratinocytes, and eosinophilic apoptotic bodies are noted. The lamina densa is greatly thickened and reduplicated. On periodic acid–Schiff (PAS)

staining, multiple layers of lamina densa extend into the subjacent dermis. The excessive quantity of lamina densa, a product of basal keratinocytes, reflects a response of basal cells to damage. These changes all suggest that injury to basal keratinocytes is an essential pathogenic characteristic of skin disease associated with lupus (Figs. 28-28 to 28-30).

Basal keratinocytes and BMZ contain a diffuse lymphocytic infiltrate that penetrates the basal layer focally, resulting in the vacuolar interface changes. Deeper in the dermis, dense patches of helper and cytotoxic/suppressor T lymphocytes, often with plasma cells, are commonly found especially around skin appendages (Fig. 28-28). Immune complexes occur mainly deep to the lamina densa but also as granular deposits on the lamina densa and within the lamina lucida. This pattern contrasts with that of BP in which there are only two potential antigens, both in the lamina lucida and characterized by a linear rather than granular staining pattern.

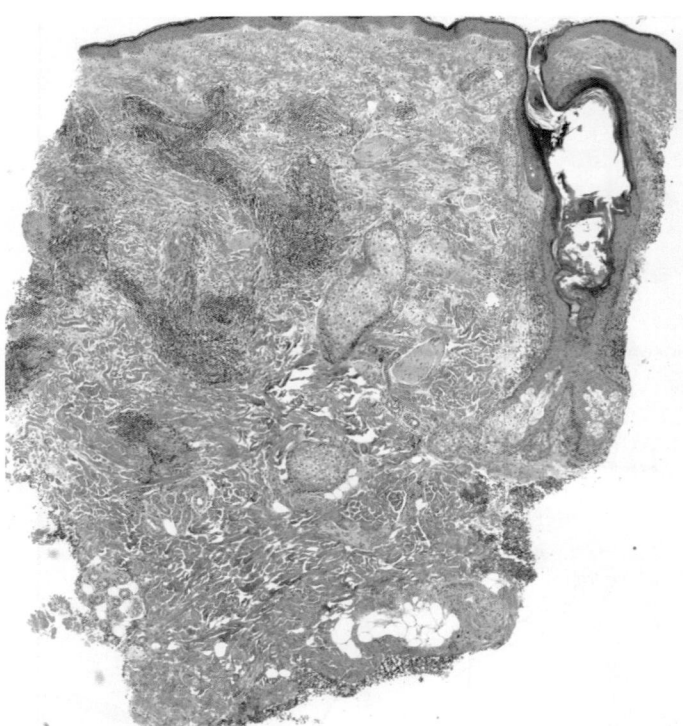

FIGURE 28-28. Lupus erythematosus. Perivascular and periappendageal lymphocytic inflammation is present in the superficial and deep dermis. A hair follicle plugged with keratin is present near the right edge.

SUBACUTE CUTANEOUS LUPUS ERYTHEMATOSUS: This disorder primarily afflicts young and middle-aged white women. Unlike discoid lupus, subacute cutaneous lupus may also involve the musculoskeletal system and kidneys. Initially, scaly erythematous papules develop

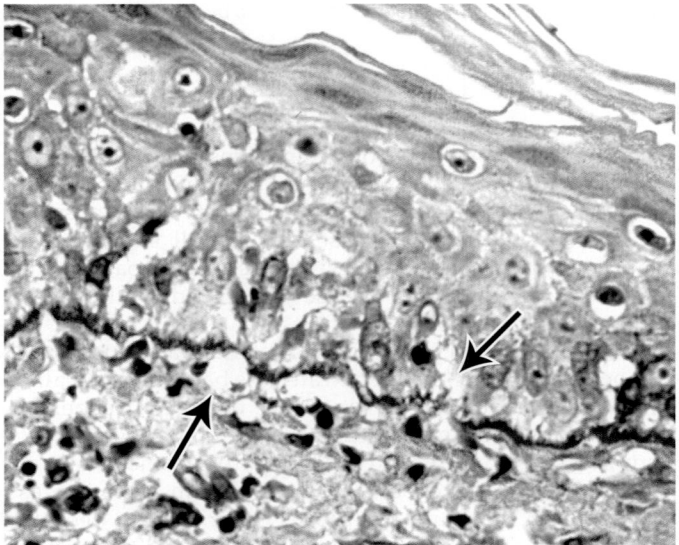

FIGURE 28-29. Lupus erythematosus. Basal cell necrosis with resultant basal keratinocytic migration and synthesis of new basement membrane zone leads to thickening of the epidermal basement membrane zone (BMZ), as evidenced by the red material in this periodic acid–Schiff (PAS) stain. Notice the vacuoles (*arrows*) on either side of the BMZ, an indicator of cellular injury.

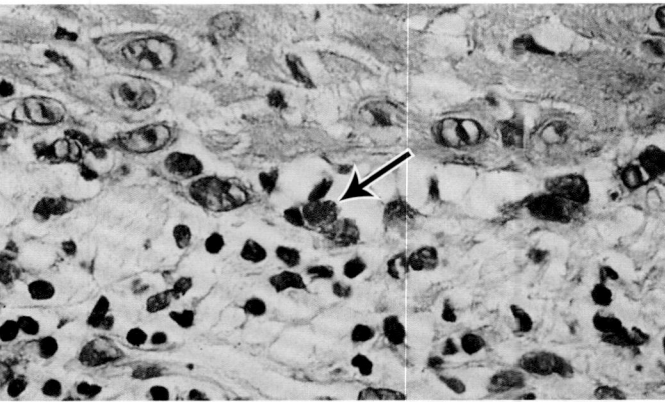

FIGURE 28-30. Lupus erythematosus. An active lesion shows striking interface changes with basal vacuolization, and keratinocyte necrosis (*arrow*) forming a dense eosinophilic body (apoptotic/fibrillary/colloid body) surrounded by lymphocytes (satellitosis).

and then enlarge into psoriasiform or annular lesions, which may fuse. Skin changes occur in the upper chest, upper back and extensor surfaces of the arms, suggesting that light exposure plays a role in the pathogenesis of the disorder. Significant scarring does not occur. About 70% of patients have circulating anti-Ro (SS-A) antibodies. ANA levels are elevated in 70%.

PATHOLOGY: Subacute cutaneous lupus features edema of the papillary dermis, thickening of the lamina densa and prominent interface change with vacuolar degeneration of basilar keratinocytes. Although there is some lymphocytic infiltration of the BMZ, deeper infiltrates of lymphocytes are not observed.

ACUTE SYSTEMIC LUPUS ERYTHEMATOSUS: Over 80% of patients with SLE have acute skin disease during their illness, in association with disease of the kidneys and joints. The rash is often the first manifestation of the disease and may precede the onset of systemic symptoms by a few months. The typical "butterfly" rash of SLE is a delicate erythema of the malar area of the face, which may pass in a few hours or a few days. Many patients have a maculopapular eruption of the chest and extremities, often following sun exposure. Both rashes heal without scarring. Lesions indistinguishable from discoid lupus may occur. ANA levels are elevated in more than 90% of patients.

PATHOLOGY: The earliest malar blush of acute cutaneous lupus may show only edema of the papillary dermis. More often, changes resemble those of subacute lupus. The histopathologic picture of lupus can be indistinguishable from **dermatomyositis**, another connective tissue disease with prominent interface changes. In **bullous SLE**, blisters may occur subepidermally and beneath the lamina densa. An autoantibody against type VII collagen, a component of anchoring fibrils in this location, is deposited and is associated with an infiltrate of neutrophils at the junction.

Lichen Planus Is a Cell-Mediated Immune Reaction at the Dermal–Epidermal Junction

"Lichenoid" tissue reactions are so named because the clinical lesions resemble certain lichens that form scaly growths on rocks or tree trunks. Lichenoid infiltrates are characterized by a band-like aggregation of lymphocytes that obscures the dermal–epidermal junction. Epidermal turnover is decreased, leading to hyperkeratosis without parakeratosis. LP is the prototypic disorder of this group, which includes entities such as lichen nitidus and lichenoid drug eruptions.

 ETIOLOGIC FACTORS: The etiology of LP is unknown. It is occasionally familial and may also accompany autoimmune disorders, such as SLE and myasthenia gravis. LP is more common in patients with ulcerative colitis and may coexist with hepatitis C infection. Some drugs, such as gold compounds, chlorothiazide, and chloroquine, may induce lichenoid reactions, in which case eosinophils may be present. External agents such as photographic chemicals may also evoke a lichenoid response. LP-like lesions often occur in later stages of chronic graft-versus-host disease. Thus, it seems that immunologic mechanisms play a role in the pathogenesis of LP (Fig. 28-31). The presence of apoptotic bodies and reduced epidermal cell turnover suggest that the lesions of LP result from basal layer cell destruction, creating reduced and subsequent reactive epidermal proliferation. Evidence suggests that LP is a delayed type of hypersensitivity reaction (see Chapter 4), initiated and amplified by cytokines such as IFNγ and IL-6, produced both by infiltrating lymphocytes and by stimulated keratinocytes.

PATHOLOGY: The epidermis in LP features compact hyperkeratosis with little or no parakeratosis, the lack of which correlates with reduced epidermal turnover associated with damage to basal keratinocytes. The stratum granulosum is thickened, frequently in a distinctive, focal, wedge-shaped pattern, with the base of the wedge abutting the stratum corneum. The stratum spinosum is variably thickened.

The distinctive pathology of LP is at the dermal–epidermal interface. The basal row of cuboidal cells is replaced by flattened or polygonal keratinocytes. The undulating interface between the dermal papillae and the rounded profiles of the rete ridges is obscured by a dense infiltrate of helper/inducer lymphocytes and macrophages, many of the latter containing melanin pigment **(melanophages)** (Fig. 28-32). Plasma cells are absent; their presence in association with basal keratinocyte atypia would suggest a lichenoid actinic keratosis, a form of epidermal dysplasia. Sharply pointed ("saw-toothed") rete ridges of keratinocytes project into the inflammatory infiltrate.

Commonly admixed with the infiltrate (in the epidermis or dermis) are globular, fibrillary, eosinophilic bodies, 15 to 20 μm in diameter (Fig. 28-32C), which represent apoptotic keratinocytes. These structures are variably called *apoptotic, colloid, Civatte* or *fibrillary bodies,* or *dyskeratotic cells.* The fibrils within the apoptotic bodies are keratin filaments. Epidermal Langerhans cells are increased early in LP.

 CLINICAL FEATURES: LP is a chronic eruption with violaceous, flat-topped papules, usually on the flexor surfaces of the wrists (Fig. 28-32A). White patches or streaks may also be present on oral mucous membranes (Wickham striae). The pruritic lesions usually resolve in less than a year but may occasionally persist longer.

INFLAMMATORY DISEASES OF THE SUPERFICIAL AND DEEP VASCULAR BED

Urticaria and Angioedema Are IgE-Dependent Hypersensitivity Reactions

These reactions are initiated by degranulation of mast cells sensitized to a specific antigen. **Urticaria** ("hives") are raised, pale, well-demarcated pruritic papules and plaques that appear and disappear within a few hours. The lesions represent edema of the superficial dermis. **Angioedema** is caused by edema in the deeper dermis or subcutis, resulting in an egg-like swelling. Both entities have a rapid onset and range in severity from simply annoying lesions to life-threatening anaphylactic reactions. The mainstays of treatment are avoiding the offending agent and prompt administration of antihistamines.

Dermatographism is a linear hive with a rich pink flare produced by briskly stroking the skin. It occurs in 4% of the population. It represents an exaggerated IgE-dependent response. One may write on the skin of such individuals and create a hive in the form of a legible word.

 ETIOLOGIC FACTORS: Most cases of urticaria are IgE dependent and reflect exaggerated venule permeability due to mast cell degranulation. An almost endless list of materials may react with IgE antibodies on the surface of mast cells. Urticaria may occur in both atopic (i.e., allergic) and nonatopic people. Atopic patients experience intensely pruritic skin eruptions, and have a family history of similar eruptions and a personal or family history of allergies. They commonly have elevated circulating IgE.

When mast cells degranulate and release their vasoactive mediators, cutaneous venules respond initially by becoming more permeable. This leads to rapidly forming edema. If the reaction persists, inflammatory cells are attracted to the area, causing an urticarial plaque (lasting more than a day).

Hereditary angioedema is a serious autosomal dominant disorder caused by loss-of-function mutations in *SERPING1,* which encodes a C1-esterase inhibitor. Reduced activity of this protein results in elevated levels of bradykinin which increases vascular permeability and induces inflammation. Some cases are caused by gain-of-function mutations in *F12,* which encodes coagulation factor VII. Increased factor VII activity also generates high levels of bradykinin.

PATHOLOGY: In urticaria, collagen fibers and fibrils are splayed apart by excess fluid. Lymphatic vessels are dilated; venules show margination of neutrophils and eosinophils. Vessels are cuffed by a few lymphocytes. In persistent urticaria, lymphocytes and eosinophils are increased, but neutrophils are sparse.

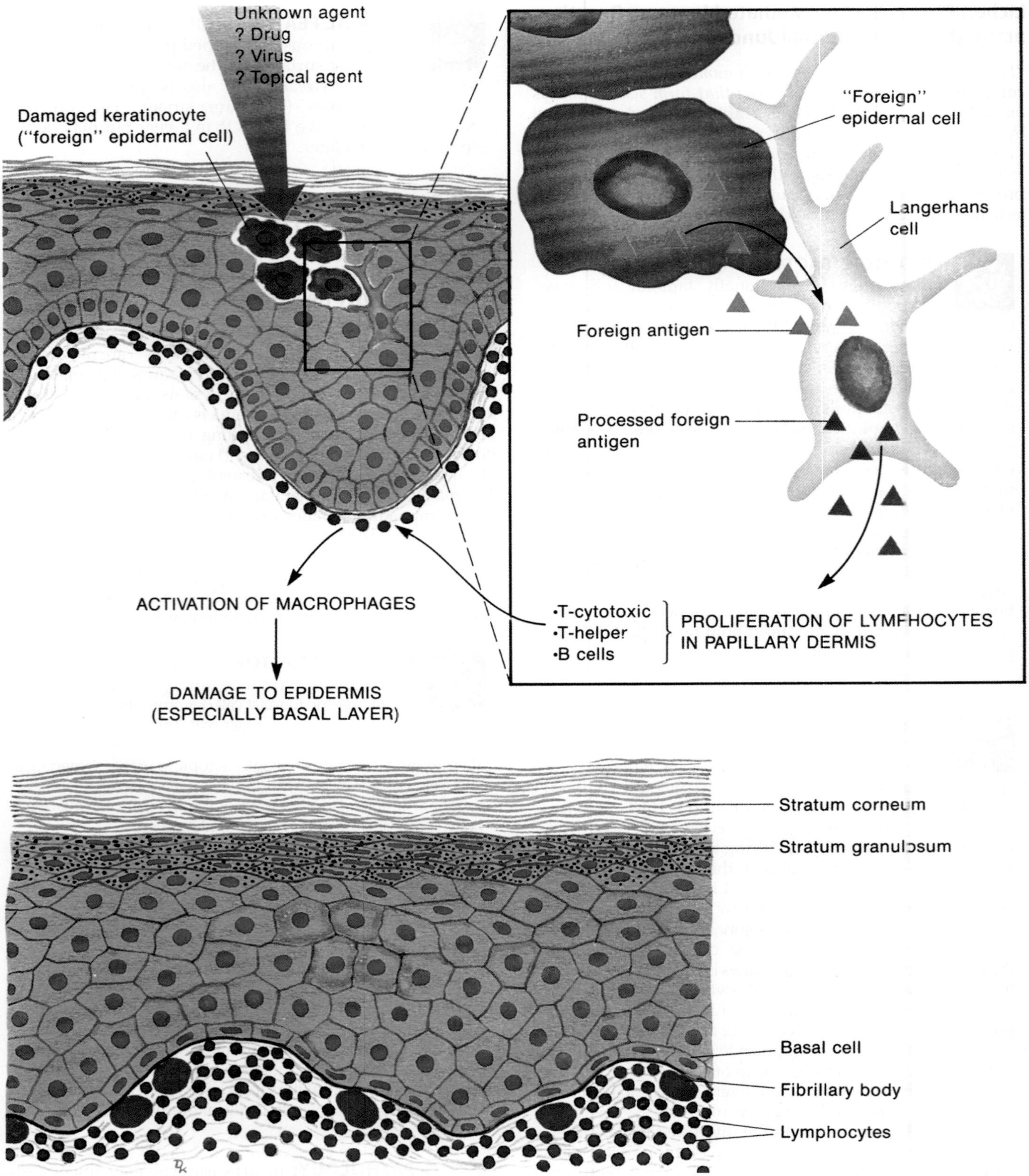

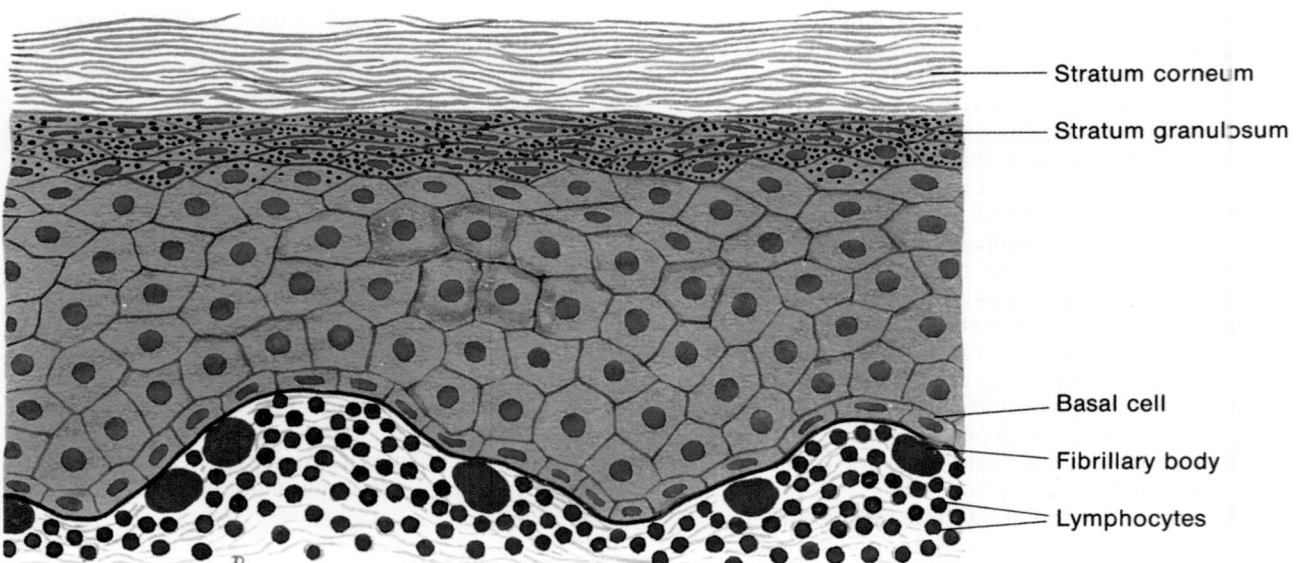

Unknown agent
? Drug
? Virus
? Topical agent

Damaged keratinocyte
("foreign" epidermal cell)

"Foreign" epidermal cell

Langerhans cell

Foreign antigen

Processed foreign antigen

ACTIVATION OF MACROPHAGES

• T-cytotoxic
• T-helper
• B cells

PROLIFERATION OF LYMPHOCYTES IN PAPILLARY DERMIS

DAMAGE TO EPIDERMIS
(ESPECIALLY BASAL LAYER)

Stratum corneum

Stratum granulosum

Basal cell

Fibrillary body

Lymphocytes

FIGURE 28-31. Pathogenic mechanisms in lichen planus. The disease is apparently initiated by epidermal injury, which causes some epidermal cells to be recognized as "foreign." Processing of antigens in the damaged epidermis by Langerhans cells induces lymphocytic proliferation and macrophage activation. Macrophages, along with T lymphocytes, kill epidermal basal cells, resulting in a reactive epidermal proliferation and formation of fibrillary (apoptotic/dyskeratotic/Civatte) bodies.

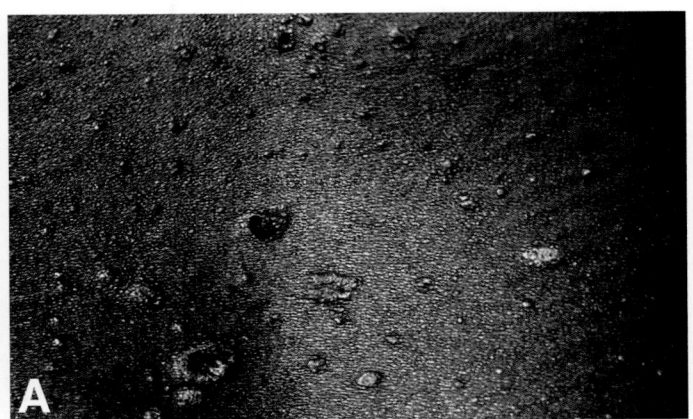

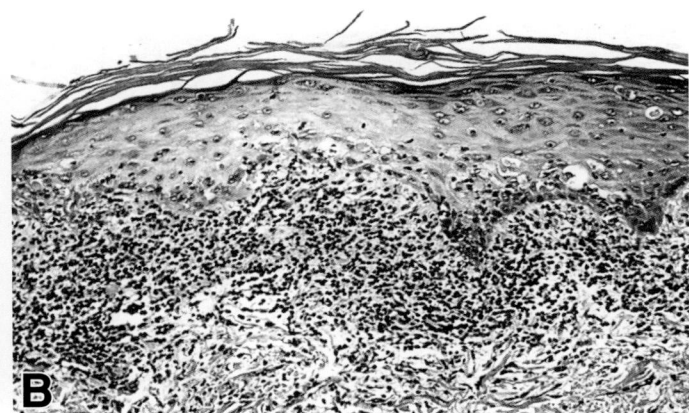

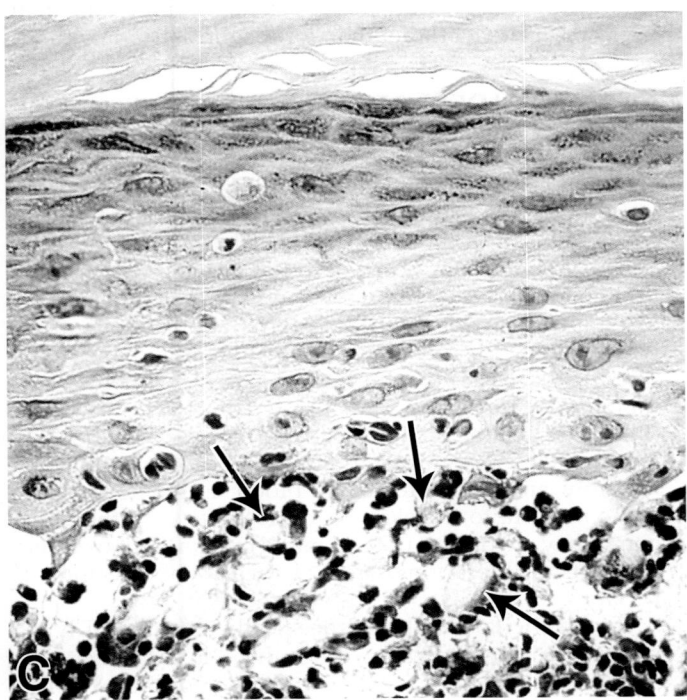

FIGURE 28-32. Lichen planus. A. The skin displays multiple flat-topped violaceous polygonal papules. (From Elder DE, Elenitsas R, Johnson BL, et al. *Synopsis and Atlas of Lever's Histopathology of the Skin*. Philadelphia, PA: Lippincott Williams & Wilkins; 1999.) **B.** A cell-rich, band-like, lymphocytic infiltrate disrupts the stratum basalis. Unlike lupus erythematosus, there is usually epidermal hyperplasia, hyperkeratosis, and wedge-like hypergranulosis. **C.** Hypergranulosis (increased thickness of the stratum granulosum) and loss of rete ridges are conspicuous features. A striking infiltrate of lymphocytes, many of which surround apoptotic keratinocytes (*arrows*) occurs at the dermal–epidermal junction, which is the site of pathologic injury.

Cutaneous Leukocytoclastic Vasculitis Is an Immune Reaction With Neutrophil Inflammation of Vessel Walls

Cutaneous leukocytoclastic vasculitis (LCV) presents as **"palpable purpura"** and has also been called **allergic cutaneous vasculitis, cutaneous necrotizing vasculitis**, and **hypersensitivity angiitis**.

ETIOLOGIC FACTORS: In LCV, circulating immune complexes deposit in vessel walls at sites of injuries, at branch points where turbulence is increased or where venous circulation is slowed, as in the lower extremities. Elaborated C5a complement component attracts neutrophils, which degranulate and release lysosomal enzymes, causing endothelial damage and fibrin deposition (Fig. 28-33).

LCV may be primary, without a known precipitating event in about half of the cases, or associated with a specific infectious agent (e.g., hepatitis B or C viruses). Or, it may be a secondary process in a variety of chronic diseases, such as rheumatoid arthritis, SLE, and ulcerative colitis. LCV may also be associated with (1) underlying malignancies such as lymphoma, (2) a drug or some other allergy, or (3) a postinfectious process such as Henoch–Schönlein purpura.

PATHOLOGY: Lesions of LCV show vessel walls obliterated by a neutrophilic infiltrate. Endothelial cells are difficult to visualize and vessel damage is manifested by fibrin deposition and erythrocyte extravasation (Fig. 28-34). Many neutrophils are also damaged, resulting in dust-like nuclear remnants, a process known as "leukocytoclasia." Collagen fibers between affected vessels are separated by neutrophils, eosinophils, and leukocytoclastic cellular remnants, as well as the extravasated erythrocytes that account for the characteristic palpable purpura, and by edema fluid, which results in dilatation of lymphatics.

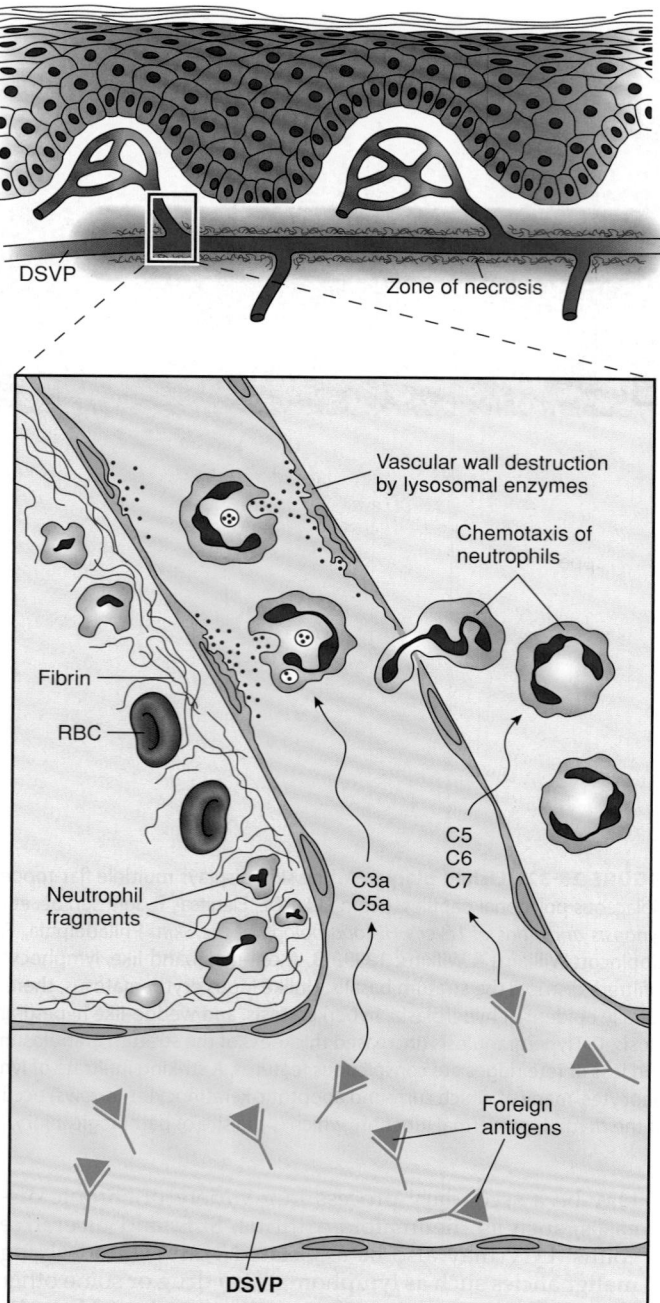

FIGURE 28-33. Pathogenesis of cutaneous necrotizing vasculitis. The site of vascular injury is indicated in the *upper diagram*. Circulating immune complexes activate complement, which results in neutrophilic chemotaxis (*C5a*) and neutrophilic destruction. Vascular damage leads to extravasation of erythrocytes, fibrin deposition, and accumulation of neutrophilic fragments (leukocytoclasia). *DSVP* = deep superficial venular plexus; *RBC* = red blood cell.

CLINICAL FEATURES: LCV is distinguished by 2- to 4-mm red, palpable lesions that do not blanch under pressure ("palpable purpura") (Fig. 28-34). Multiple lesions characteristically appear in crops on the legs or at sites of pressure. Lesions may be confined to the skin in an otherwise healthy person or may involve small blood vessels in the joints, gastrointestinal

tract, or kidneys. Individual lesions persist for up to a month, then resolve, leaving hyperpigmentation or atrophic scars. Despite removal of the offending agent, episodes of CNV may recur.

Allergic Contact Dermatitis Is Cell-Mediated Hypersensitivity to Exogenous Sensitizing Agents

Members of the *Rhus* genus of plants are common sensitizing agents, so that 90% of the population of the United States is sensitive to the common offenders: *Rhus radicans* (poison ivy), *Rhus diversiloba* (poison oak), and *Rhus vernix* (poison sumac). These plant dermatitides are so well known that the resultant disease is commonly labeled according to the offending plant. Patients state, "I have poison ivy" and go to physicians for relief rather than for diagnosis.

 ETIOLOGIC FACTORS: The offending plant contains low–molecular-weight haptens (see Chapter 4), in particular, oleoresins. They are active in sensitization only when they combine with a carrier protein. This likely happens at the Langerhans cell membrane in the **sensitization phase**, a process that has been studied as a prototype of antigenic sensitization in delayed-type hypersensitivity (DTH). Formation of a **hapten–carrier complex** requires about 1 hour, after which it is processed as an antigen by Langerhans cells. These cells carry the antigen through lymphatics to regional lymph nodes and present it to CD4$^+$ T cells (Fig. 28-35). After 5 to 7 days, some of these sensitized T lymphocytes recognize the antigen, become activated, multiply and circulate in the blood as memory cells. Some migrate to the skin, ready to react with the antigen if they encounter it. IL-1, made by Langerhans cells, supports proliferation of CD4$^+$ T$_H$1 cells, the effectors of DTH.

In the **elicitation phase**, specifically sensitized T lymphocytes in the circulation enter the skin. At the site of antigen challenge, Langerhans cells, endothelial cells, perivascular dendritic cells, and monocytes process the antigen and present it to the specifically sensitized T cells, which then migrate into the epidermis. Cytokine production promotes accumulation of more T cells and macrophages, which are responsible for epidermal cell injury.

PATHOLOGY: Allergic contact dermatitis is a type of **spongiotic dermatitis**. In the 24 hours after re-exposure to the offending plant (elicitation phase), lymphocytes and macrophages congregate about superficial venules and extend into the epidermis, a process called **exocytosis**. Epidermal keratinocytes are partially separated by edema fluid, creating a sponge-like appearance (**spongiosis**) (Fig. 28-36). The stratum corneum contains coagulated eosinophilic fluid and plasma proteins. Later, many mononuclear inflammatory cells and eosinophils accumulate. Vesicles containing lymphocytes and macrophages are present, and abundant eosinophilic coagulated fluid accrues in the stratum corneum.

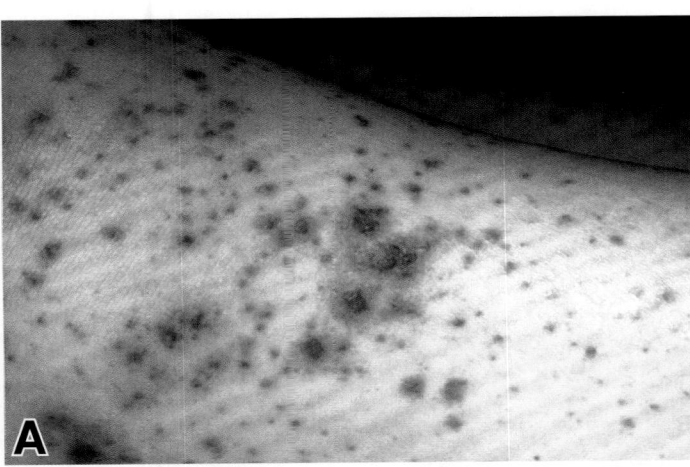
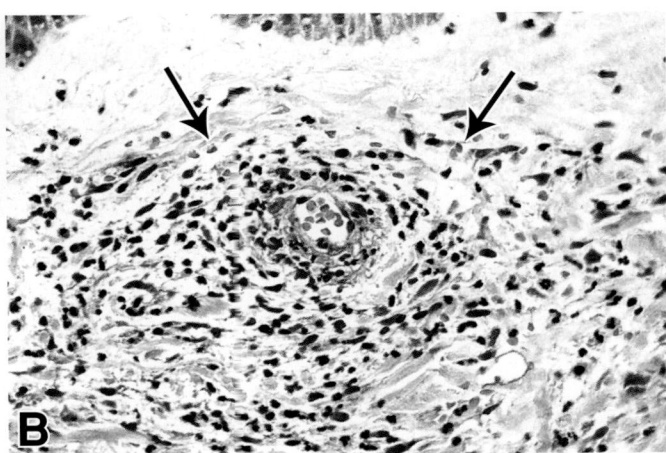

FIGURE 28-34. Cutaneous necrotizing vasculitis. A. Palpable purpuric tender papules on the legs of a 25-year-old woman. The condition resolved after therapy for streptococcal pharyngitis. (From Elder DE, Elenitsas R, Johnson BL, et al. *Synopsis and Atlas of Lever's Histopathology of the Skin*. Philadelphia, PA: Lippincott Williams & Wilkins; 1999.) **B.** A dermal vessel is surrounded by pink fibrin and neutrophils, many of which have disintegrated (leukocytoclasis). Extravasated red blood cells (*arrows*) and inflammation give the classic clinical appearance of "palpable purpura."

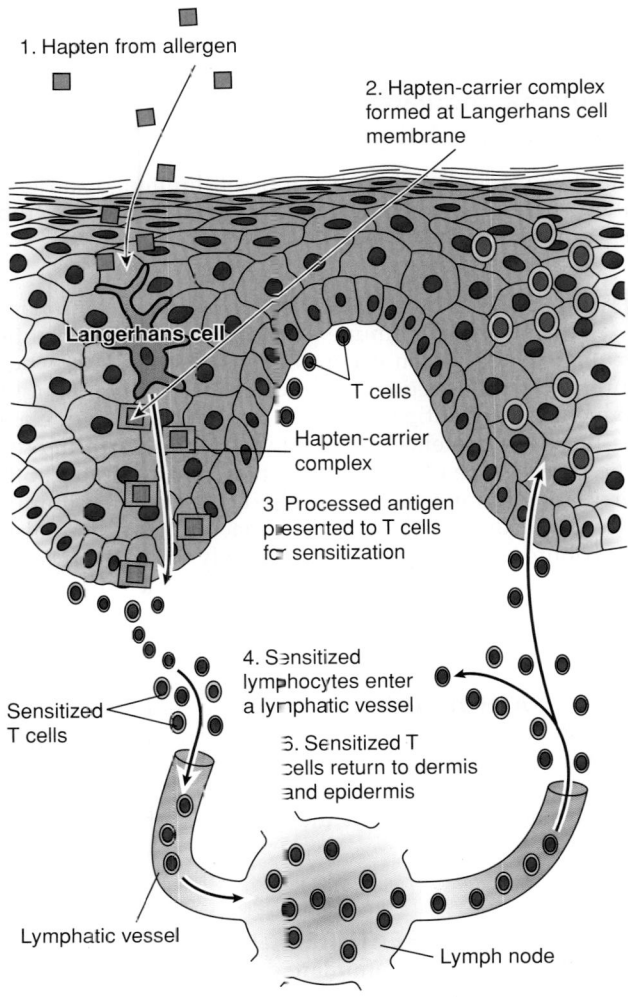

FIGURE 28-35. Pathogenic mechanisms in allergic contact dermatitis.

1. Hapten from allergen

2. Hapten-carrier complex formed at Langerhans cell membrane

Langerhans cell

T cells

Hapten-carrier complex

3. Processed antigen presented to T cells for sensitization

Sensitized T cells

4. Sensitized lymphocytes enter a lymphatic vessel

5. Sensitized T cells return to dermis and epidermis

Lymphatic vessel

Lymph node

5. Sensitized lymphocytes transported to regional lymph nodes, where T cell hyperplasia is induced

CLINICAL FEATURES: At first contact with poison ivy, for example, there is no immediate reaction. Five to 7 days after an exposure, the site of contact becomes intensely pruritic. Then, erythema and small vesicles rapidly develop (Fig. 28-36). Over the next few days, the area enlarges, becomes fiery red, develops vesicles, and exudes a large amount of clear proteinaceous fluid. The entire process lasts about 3 weeks. Exudation gradually subsides and the area is covered by an irregular crust that eventually falls off. Pruritus diminishes and healing occurs without scarring.

When a sensitized patient again comes into contact with poison ivy, the process is faster. Lesions appear within 1 to 2 days, spread rapidly and produce the same clinical appearance. However, the reaction is usually more intense. Lesions again clear in about 3 weeks. Allergic contact dermatitis responds to topical or systemic corticosteroids.

Granulomatous Dermatitis Is a Response to Indigestible Antigens

Granulomas, generally defined as localized collections of epithelioid macrophages (see Chapter 1), form in response to insoluble or slowly released antigens that produce either a focal nonallergic response or an allergic response in sensitized people. Implicated antigens include substances implanted accidentally into the skin (which produce **foreign-body granulomas**) or endogenous antigens such as keratin. Other common causes include mycobacteria and other infections. Often, for example, in **sarcoidosis** and **granuloma annulare**, an inciting antigen may not be known. Phagocytosis of the foreign particulate matter, or processing of protein antigens, is central to activation of tissue macrophages, as they become the characteristic granulomatous epithelioid cells.

Sarcoidosis Is a Systemic Disease That May Lead to Skin Lesions

Sarcoidosis is a granulomatous disorder of unknown etiology that mainly affects the lungs but may also involve the

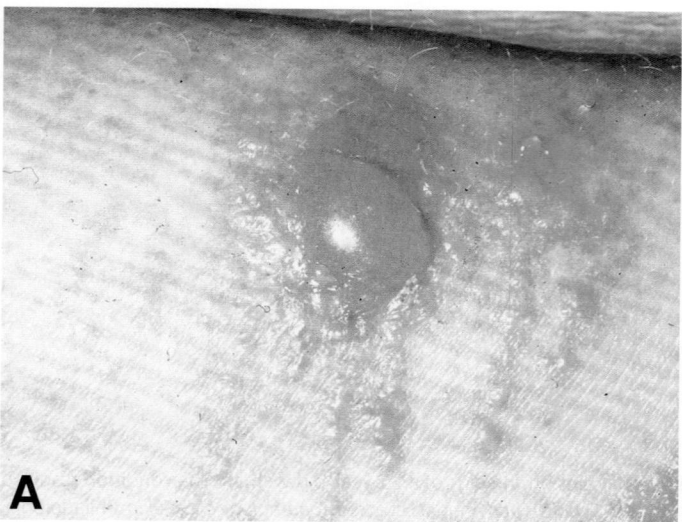
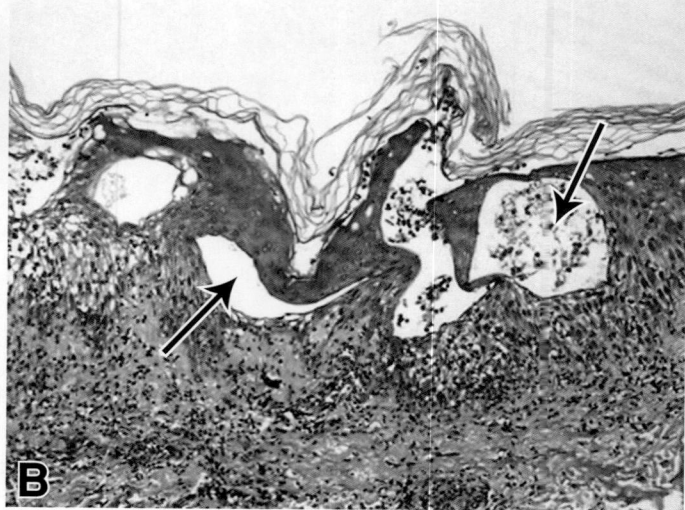

FIGURE 28-36. Allergic contact dermatitis. A. Vesicles and bullae developed on the volar forearm after application of perfume. [From Elder DE, Elenitsas R, Johnson BL, et al. *Synopsis and Atlas of Lever's Histopathology of the Skin*. Philadelphia, PA: Lippincott Williams & Wilkins; 1999.) **B.** Epidermal spongiosis and spongiotic vesicles (*arrows*) are seen in this biopsy of "poison ivy." Infiltrating lymphocytes and eosinophils are present in the dermis and extend into the epidermis ("exocytosis"), where they elicit the cell-mediated delayed hypersensitivity reaction.

skin, lymph nodes, spleen, heart, eyes, and other organs. Sarcoidal granulomas are the classic epithelioid cell type, without necrosis (Fig. 28-37). Cutaneous manifestations of sarcoidosis are asymptomatic papules, plaques and nodules in the dermis and subcutis. Some dermal plaques may be annular, and those that involve the subcutis appear as irregular nodules. In severe cases, cutaneous lesions may be so prominent that they simulate a diffusely infiltrative neoplasm.

FIGURE 28-37. Sarcoidosis. Numerous large granulomas fill the reticular dermis. Around some of the granulomas are small cuffs of lymphocytes (*arrows*). The granulomas are composed of epithelioid macrophages, some of which are multinucleated (*inset*).

Granuloma Annulare Is a Reaction to an Unknown Antigen

Granuloma annulare is a benign, self-limited disorder of unknown etiology, characterized by palisading "necrobiotic" granulomas in the skin.

ETIOLOGIC FACTORS: Granuloma annulare may be an immune reaction to an unknown antigen(s). It can occur after insect bites, sun exposure, and viral infections. Offending antigens are thought to include viral antigens, altered dermal collagen or elastic fibers, or proteins in the saliva of biting arthropods. The precise type of immune reaction is unclear, but both circulating immune complexes and cell-mediated immunity may participate. Activated macrophages may also contribute to the process by releasing lysosomal enzymes and cytokines, which in turn cause the characteristic focal collagen degeneration ("necrobiosis").

PATHOLOGY: Well-developed lesions contain a central area of acellular degenerated collagen and mucin in the superficial to mid reticular dermis (Fig. 28-38B). This central area is surrounded by palisaded macrophages, with the long axis of their nuclei radiating outward.

CLINICAL FEATURES: The most common type of granuloma annulare occurs on the dorsum of the hands and feet, primarily in children and young adults (Fig. 28-38A). The disease features asymptomatic, skin-colored or erythematous annular plaques. About 15% of patients have disseminated granuloma annulare, with 10 or more lesions involving the trunk and

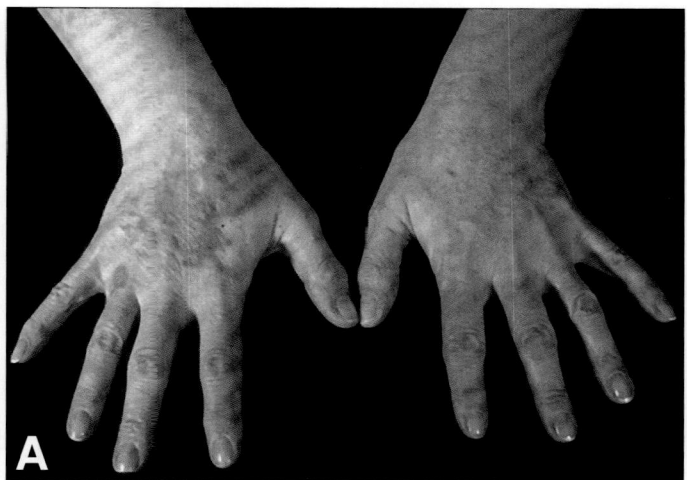 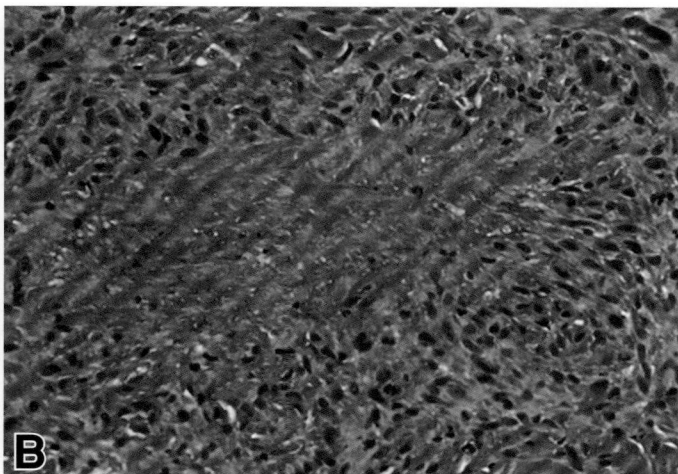

FIGURE 28-38. Granuloma annulare. A. The skin exhibits a typical annular plaque on the dorsal right hand. (From Elder DE, Elenitsas R, Johnson BL, et al. *Synopsis and Atlas of Lever's Histopathology of the Skin*. Philadelphia, PA: Lippincott Williams & Wilkins; 1999.) **B.** A central acellular area of degenerated collagen is surrounded by palisaded macrophages with the long axes of their nuclei radiating outward.

neck. **Granuloma annulare rarely requires treatment and usually has no medical consequences.**

SCLERODERMA: A DISORDER OF THE DERMAL CONNECTIVE TISSUE

Scleroderma (Greek, *skleros,* "hard") also displays variable structural and functional involvement of internal organs, including the kidneys, lungs, heart, esophagus, and small intestine. **Morphea** is similar to scleroderma but involves only patchy, circumscribed areas of the skin. The pathogenesis and systemic manifestations of scleroderma are discussed elsewhere (see Chapters 4 and 12).

PATHOLOGY: The initial cutaneous lesions of scleroderma arise in the lower reticular dermis, but eventually the entire reticular dermis and even the papillary dermis are involved. Space among collagen bundles in the reticular dermis is diminished and they tend to become enlarged and parallel to each other, causing the reticular dermis to appear hypocellular. A patchy lymphocytic infiltrate containing a few plasma cells is common and may also be present in the underlying subcutaneous tissue. Sweat ducts become entrapped in the thickened fibrous tissue, and the fat that usually surrounds them is lost. Hair follicles are completely obliterated (Fig. 28-39). In late stages of the disease, large areas of subcutaneous fat are replaced by newly formed collagen.

CLINICAL FEATURES: Scleroderma has a peak incidence in people 30 to 50 years old. Women are afflicted four times as often as men. Patients with early scleroderma usually present with Raynaud phenomenon or nonpitting edema of the hands or fingers. Affected areas become hard and tense. Thickened

skin on the face causes it to become mask-like and expressionless, and the skin around the mouth exhibits radial furrows. In late stages of the disease, the skin over large parts of the body is thickened, densely fibrotic and fixed to the underlying tissue. Prognosis is related to the extent of disease in visceral organs, particularly the lungs and kidneys.

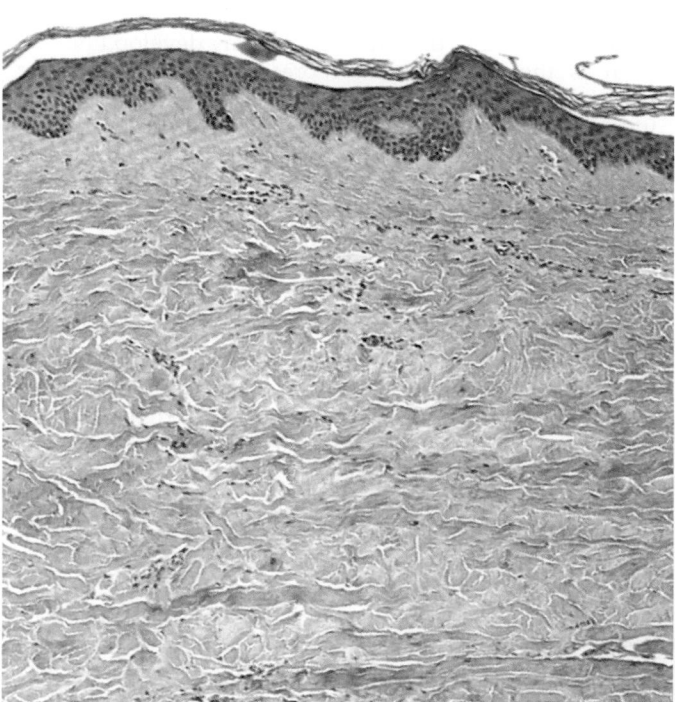

FIGURE 28-39. Scleroderma. The dermis is characterized by large, reticular collagen bundles oriented parallel to the epidermis. The large size of these collagen bundles and loss of basket-weave pattern are abnormal. No appendages (e.g., hair follicles and sebaceous glands) are apparent because such structures have been destroyed.

INFLAMMATORY DISORDERS OF THE PANNICULUS

Panniculitis denotes a diverse group of diseases characterized by inflammation, mainly in the subcutis (panniculus). Disorders gathered under the umbrella of panniculitis are classified according to the location of the inflammation. **Septal panniculitis** is inflammation in connective tissue septa, while **lobular panniculitis** entails involvement of fat lobules. These two patterns may be mixed and occur with or without accompanying vasculitis.

Erythema Nodosum Is Related to Toxic and Infectious Agents

Erythema nodosum (EN) is a cutaneous disorder that manifests as nonsuppurative, self-limited, tender nodules over extensor surfaces of the legs. It has a peak incidence in the third decade of life and is three times more common in women than in men.

 ETIOLOGIC FACTORS: EN is triggered by a variety of agents, such as drugs and microorganisms, and it accompanies a number of benign and malignant systemic diseases. Common infections complicated by EN include streptococcal diseases (especially in children), tuberculosis and *Yersinia* infection. In endemic areas, deep fungal infections (blastomycosis, histoplasmosis, coccidioidomycosis) are common causes. EN also frequently occurs after acute respiratory tract infections of unknown etiology, but which are likely viral. Agents most commonly implicated in drug-induced EN are sulfonamides and oral contraceptives. Finally, people with Crohn disease and ulcerative colitis may develop EN.

It is thought that EN represents an immunologic response to foreign antigens, although the evidence is indirect. Early acute inflammation suggests that it may be a response to complement activation, with resulting neutrophil chemotaxis. Subsequent chronic inflammation, foreign-body giant cells, and fibrosis are due to adipose tissue necrosis at the interface of septa and lobules.

PATHOLOGY: Early EN lesions occur in fibrous septa of the subcutaneous tissue, where neutrophilic inflammation is associated with extravasation of erythrocytes. In chronic lesions, the septa are widened, with focal collections of giant cell macrophages around small areas of altered collagen and an ill-defined lymphocytic infiltrate (Fig. 28-40). Giant cells and inflammatory cells extend into the lobule from the interface between the septum and the fat lobule.

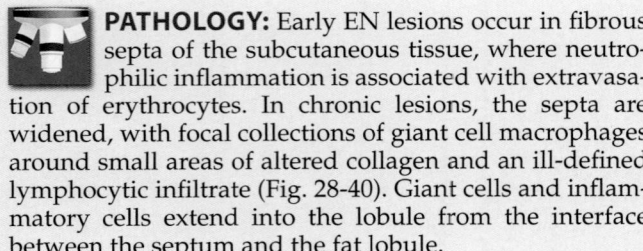 **CLINICAL FEATURES:** EN typically manifests acutely on the anterior aspects of the legs as dome-shaped, exquisitely tender, erythematous nodules. These eventually become firm and less tender and disappear in 3 to 6 weeks. As some nodules heal, others may arise, but all lesions resolve without residual scarring within 6 weeks.

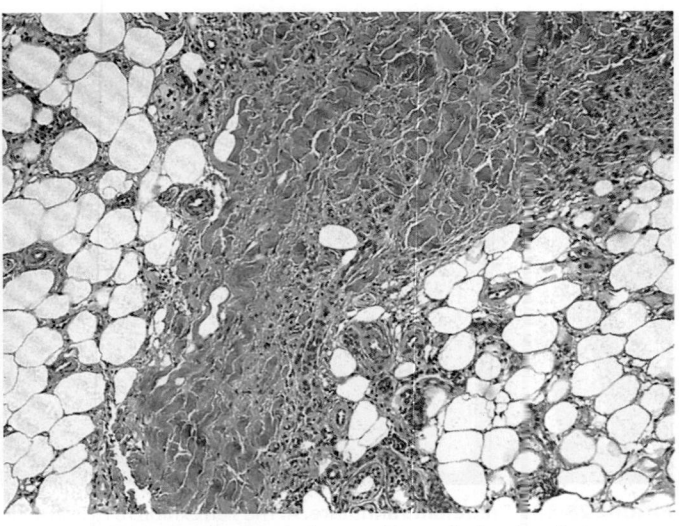

FIGURE 28-40. Erythema nodosum. The reticular dermis is present in the *upper right*. Within the panniculus is a widened septum (*extending through the middle of the field*). Lymphocytes and macrophages are present at its interface with the adipose tissue lobules. Vessels palisading along the interface of the septum are infiltrated by lymphocytes.

Erythema Induratum Is Often Associated With *Mycobacterium tuberculosis*

Erythema induratum (EI) refers to chronic, recurrent subcutaneous nodules or plaques on the legs, predominantly in women. EI was traditionally considered a "tuberculid" (i.e., a hypersensitivity reaction to mycobacteria or associated antigens, but at a distant site). Although lesional tissue does not contain intact mycobacteria, specific *Mycobacterium tuberculosis* DNA is present in greater than 75% of skin biopsies with EI.

PATHOLOGY: In contrast to EN, which is a septal panniculitis, EI is a lobular panniculitis initially, which arises secondary to a vasculitis that produces ischemic necrosis of the fat lobule (Fig. 28-41). The panniculus exhibits a dense, chronic inflammation within lobules, which can form prominent tuberculoid granulomas or areas of coagulative necrosis. Septa around the lobules are relatively spared. Vascular changes may be extensive and include (1) prominent infiltration of small and medium-sized arteries and veins by a dense lymphoid or granulomatous infiltrate; (2) endothelial swelling, which may progress to thrombosis; and (3) fibrous thickening of the intima. Thus, another name for this condition is "nodular vasculitis." Extensive ischemic necrosis provokes subsequent ulceration of the overlying epidermis. Eventually, lesions heal by fibrosis.

CLINICAL FEATURES: Patients with EI present with recurrent, tender, erythematous, subcutaneous nodules on the legs, particularly the calves (as opposed to the shins, which are the usual location of EN). Lesions tend to ulcerate and heal producing an atrophic scar. The course may last many years. Systemic steroids are usually necessary to control the disease.

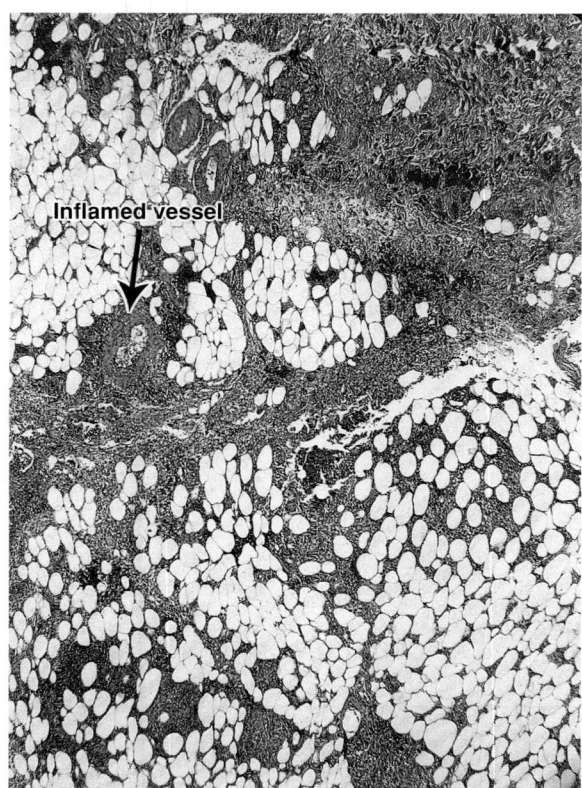

FIGURE 28-41. Erythema induratum/nodular vasculitis. There is predominantly lobular panniculitis with inflammation spilling into a septum, and with an inflamed vessel in the upper panniculus. (Reprinted with permission from Elder DE, Elenitsas R, Rubin AI, Ioffreda M, Miller J, Fred Miller III O. *Atlas and Synopsis of Lever's Histopathology of the Skin.* 3rd ed. Philadelphia, PA: Lippincott Williams & Wilkins; 2012.)

Acne Vulgaris Is a Disorder of the Pilosebaceous Unit

Acne vulgaris is a self-limited, inflammatory disorder of sebaceous follicles that typically afflicts adolescents, results in intermittent formation of discrete papular or pustular lesions and may lead to scarring. It is cosmetically disfiguring and often psychologically debilitating. Acne is so common that many regard it as a "rite of passage" through adolescence. In some cases, acne extends to the third decade.

 ETIOLOGIC FACTORS AND PATHOLOGY: The development of acne is related to (1) excessive hormonally induced production of sebum, (2) abnormal cornification of portions of the follicular epithelium, (3) a response to the anaerobic diphtheroid *Propionibacterium acnes*, and (4) follicle rupture and subsequent inflammation. The sebaceous follicle contains a vellus hair and prominent sebaceous glands. Changes in hormonal status at puberty generate sebum production in the follicle and altered cornification in the neck of the sebaceous follicle (infundibulum). These effects lead to dilation of the follicular canal. Another round of excessive sebum production is associated with desquamation of squamous cells and accretion of keratinous debris, providing a rich environment for *P. acnes* proliferation.

These combined changes produce a distended, plugged follicle called a **comedone**. Neutrophils may be attracted to the area by chemotactic factors released by *P. acnes* and release hydrolytic enzymes to form a follicular abscess **(pustule)**. They also attack the follicle wall, thus permitting escape of sebum, keratin and bacteria into perifollicular tissue, where they stimulate further acute inflammation and a perifollicular abscess (Fig. 28-42). The development of allergy to *P. acnes* intensifies the inflammatory response. Fully evolved lesions show intense neutrophilic inflammation surrounding a ruptured sebaceous follicle. Abundant macrophages, lymphocytes, and foreign-body giant cells may also accumulate in response to sebaceous follicle rupture.

 CLINICAL FEATURES: Acne vulgaris features a variety of skin lesions in different stages of development, including comedones, papules, pustules, nodules, cysts, and pitted scars. Comedones, the primary noninflammatory lesions of acne, are either open **(blackheads)** or closed **(whiteheads)**. More advanced inflammatory lesions vary from small, erythematous papules to large, tender, purulent nodules, and cysts.

INFECTIONS AND INFESTATIONS

The skin is under constant assault from countless marauders and is an effective but imperfect barrier against them; bacteria, fungi, viruses, parasites, and insects sometimes penetrate this first line of defense.

Impetigo Is a Cutaneous Infection by Staphylococci or Streptococci

Superficial bacterial infections of the skin, known as **impetigo**, occur mostly in children, who are often infected through minor breaks in the skin. Adults tend to contract impetigo after an underlying disease process compromises the barrier function of the skin. Honey-colored crusted erosions or ulcers, often with central healing, occur most commonly on exposed areas such as the face, hands, and extremities (Fig. 28-43). A combination of topical and systemic antimicrobial agents against staphylococci or streptococci is the mainstay of therapy.

PATHOLOGY: In impetigo, neutrophils accumulate beneath the stratum corneum. Bacteria may be visualized with special stains. Vesicles or bullae form and eventually rupture, allowing a thin, seropurulent discharge to appear on the skin surface. This discharge dries and forms the characteristic layers of exudate containing neutrophils and cell debris. Reactive epidermal changes (spongiosis, elongation of rete ridges) and superficial dermal inflammation are usually present.

Ecthyma is more typically caused by *Pseudomonas aeruginosa* (ecthyma gangrenosum) and several other organisms. It occurs when the organisms enter the superficial aspects of the skin from the bloodstream to form a localized necrotizing ulcerated lesion. Neutrophils are

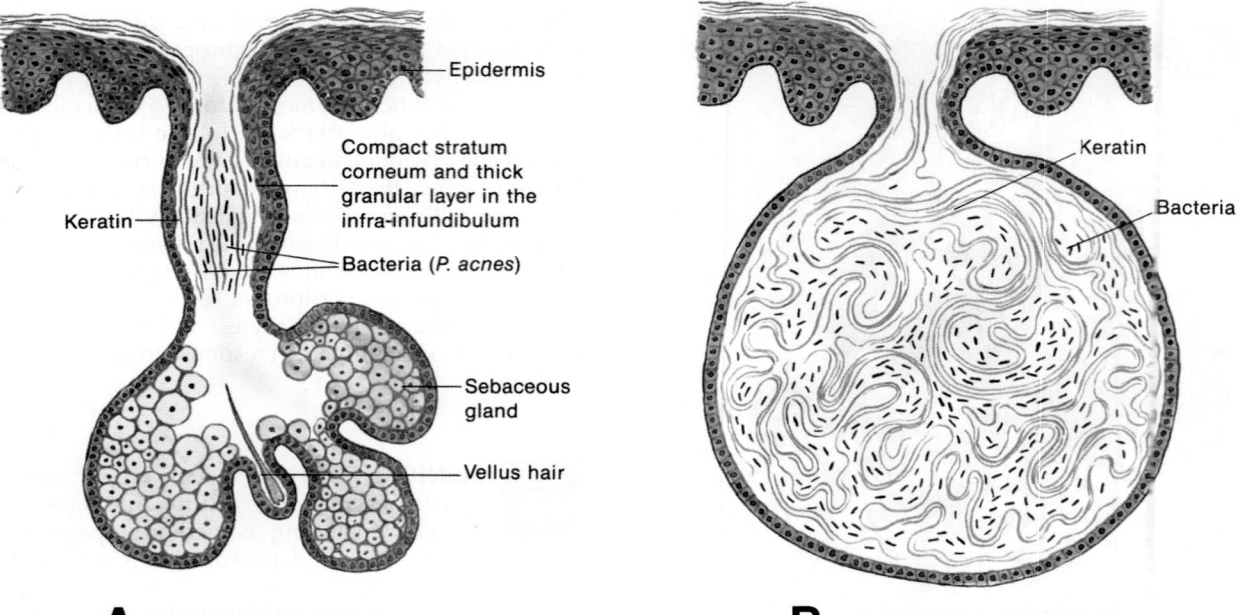

A. MICROCOMEDOME

B. CLOSED COMEDONE

C. OPEN COMEDONE

D. INVASION OF FOLLICLE BY NEUTROPHILS

FIGURE 28-42. Pathogenesis of acne vulgaris. Acne is a disease of the follicular canal of a sebaceous follicle. Initial formation of a comedone (clogged sebaceous follicle) occurs with a compact stratum corneum and a thickened granular layer in the infra-infundibulum. Microcomedones develop first **(A)** eventually leading to formation of closed **(B)** and open **(C)** comedones. Excessive sebum is secreted, and proliferation of the bacterium *Propionibacterium acnes* produces chemotactic factors, leading to neutrophil migration into the intact comedone **(D)**.

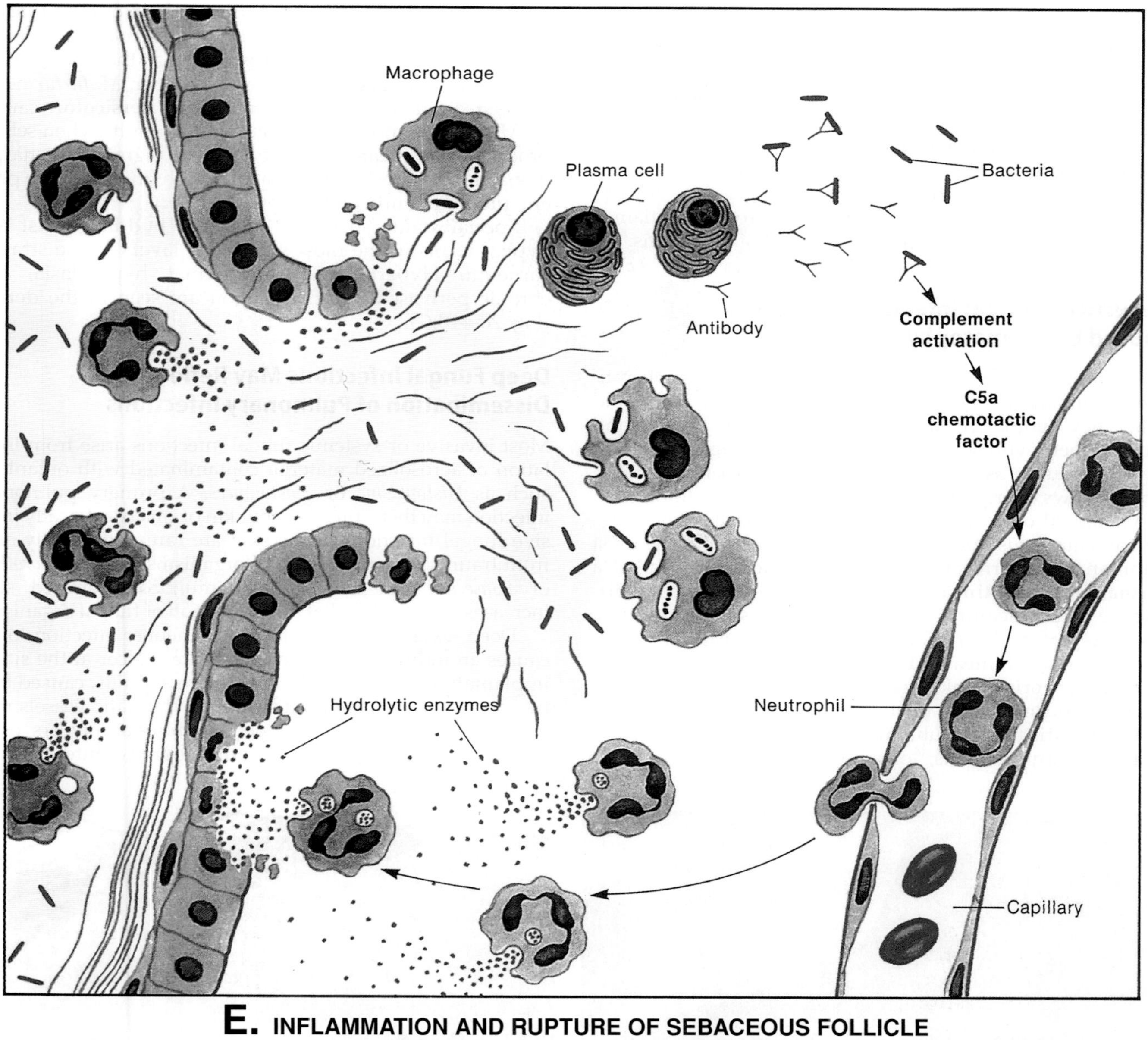

E. INFLAMMATION AND RUPTURE OF SEBACEOUS FOLLICLE

FIGURE 28-42. (*Continued*) Neutrophilic enzymes are released, and the comedone ruptures, inducing a cycle of chemotaxis and intense neutrophilic inflammation (**E**).

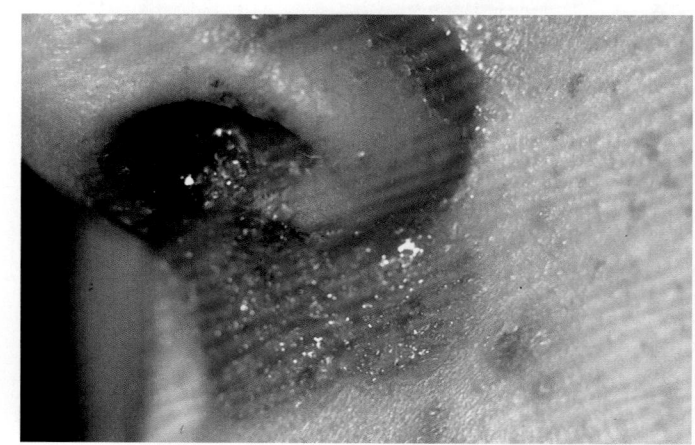

FIGURE 28-43. Impetigo contagiosa. Honey-colored crusts secondary to rupture of vesicopustules are seen in the nasal area of a child, a site frequently colonized by *Staphylococcus aureus*. (From Elder DE, Elenitsas R, Johnson BL, et al. *Synopsis and Atlas of Lever's Histopathology of the Skin.* Philadelphia, PA: Lippincott Williams & Wilkins; 1999.)

present in the floor of the ulcer and in the dermis, and bacteria are often seen migrating through vessel walls.

Spreading infections of the skin caused by invasive organisms such as streptococci, staphylococci, and others are termed **erysipelas** (more superficial) and **cellulitis** (deeper). **Necrotizing fasciitis** is a life-threatening condition caused by organisms that invade into deep tissue compartments, often from an origin in the skin. All of these conditions are characterized by neutrophilic inflammation with exudation, and the presence of organisms.

Superficial Fungal Infections May Be Caused by Dermatophytes

Dermatophytes are fungi that can infect nonviable keratinized epithelium, including stratum corneum, nails, and hair. They synthesize keratinases that digest keratin and provide them with sustenance. Superficial fungal infections are often caused by a change in the skin microenvironment, which allows overgrowth of transient or resident flora.

Of the 10 or so dermatophyte species that often cause human cutaneous infection, *Trichophyton rubrum* is the most common. A superficial dermatophyte infection is called a **dermatophytosis, tinea**, or **ringworm**. The tineas have distinctive clinical features depending on the site of infection. They are categorized as follows: (1) **tinea capitis** (scalp; "ringworm"), (2) **tinea barbae** (beard), (3) **tinea faciei** (face), (4) **tinea corporis** (trunk, legs, arms or neck), (5) **tinea manus** (hands), (6) **tinea pedis** (feet; "athlete's foot"; Fig. 28-44A), (7) **tinea cruris** (groin, pubic area and thigh; "jock itch"), and (8) **tinea unguium** (nails; "onychomycosis").

Other causes of superficial fungal infections are *Candida* sp. and *Malassezia furfur*. *Candida* sp. require a warm, moist environment in which to flourish, such as that found when a baby's bottom is encased in a wet diaper. *M. furfur* needs a moist, lipid-rich environment. **Tinea versicolor**, caused by *M. furfur*, is more common in young adults when sebum production is greatest. Variably sized, pigmented, sharply demarcated, round or oval macules with fine scales are present, predominantly on the upper trunk.

Special stains such as PAS show budding yeast and hyphal forms in the most superficial layers of the stratum corneum. Hyperkeratosis, epidermal hyperplasia, and chronic perivascular inflammation are seen in the dermis (Fig. 28-44B,C).

Deep Fungal Infections May Reflect Dissemination of Pulmonary Infections

Most invasive or systemic fungal infections arise from inhalation of aerosolized material contaminated with organisms such as *Histoplasma* or *Blastomyces*. A primary pulmonary infection may then spread to the skin or mucosa. Locally invasive fungal infections of the skin are rare and usually arise from traumatic implantation of organisms such as *Sporothrix* or *Fonsecaea*. An underlying immunocompromised state increases the likelihood of dissemination of fungal organisms.

Deep extension of a local cutaneous infection often causes an indurated (i.e., "chancre-like") ulcer at the site of implantation, as prototypically seen in syphilis, caused by a treponeme (*T. pallidum*). Intervening lymphatic vessels may become indurated and thickened. Nodules and ulcers, especially if bilateral, suggest an internal source of infection.

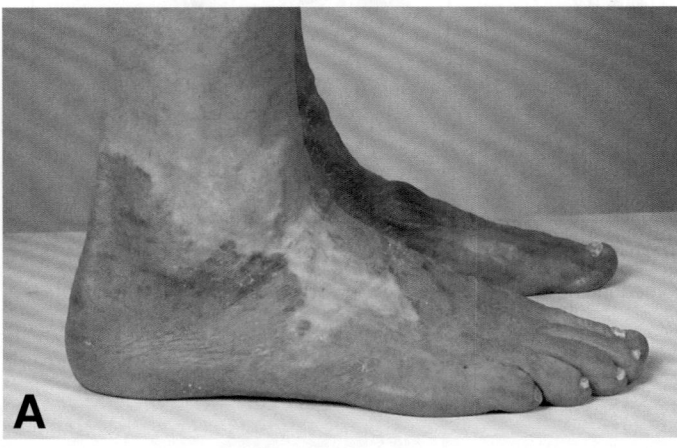

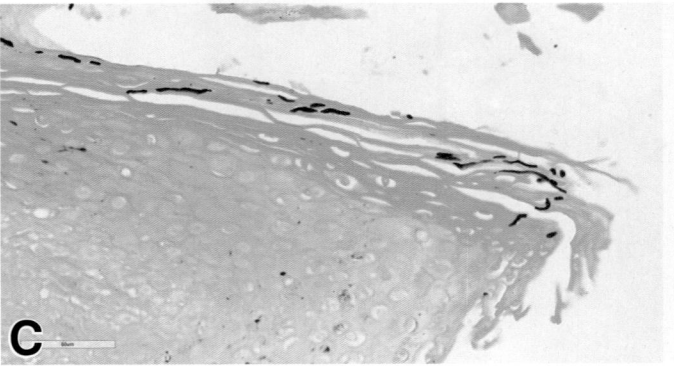

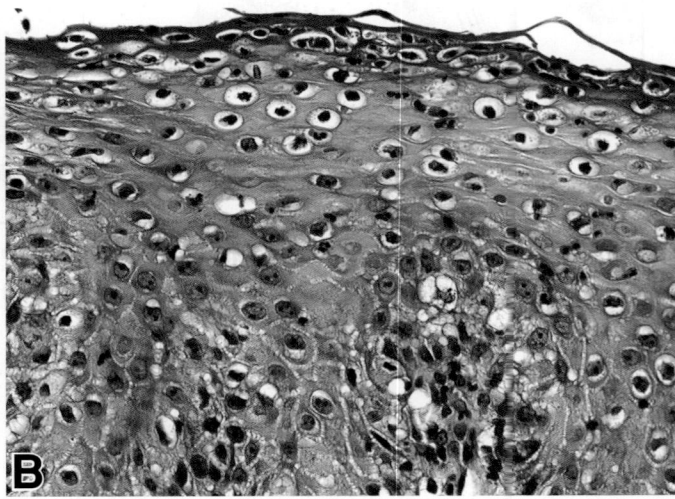

FIGURE 28-44. Dermatophytosis. A. Tinea pedis. A leading edge of scale and erythema in a moccasin distribution characterizes this infection, most commonly caused by *Trichophyton rubrum*. (From Elder DE, Elenitsas R, Johnson BL, et al. *Synopsis and Atlas of Lever's Histopathology of the Skin*. Philadelphia, PA: Lippincott Williams & Wilkins; 1999.) **B.** A few neutrophils in the upper epidermis or especially in the stratum corneum can be a subtle sign of the presence of dermatophytes. **C.** Fungal hyphae (*black structures*) in the stratum corneum.

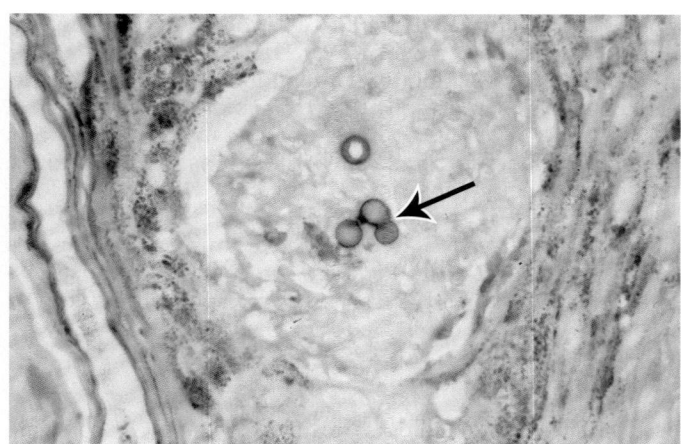

FIGURE 28-45. Blastomycosis. A Gomori methenamine silver stain highlights the organisms, which are thick-walled spores 8 to 15 microns in diameter. One of the organisms demonstrates broad-based budding (*arrow*). (From Elder DE, Elenitsas R, Johnson BL, et al. *Synopsis and Atlas of Lever's Histopathology of the Skin.* Philadelphia, PA: Lippincott Williams & Wilkins; 1999.)

The presence of certain morphologic features or staining patterns may provide clues about the identity of the organism. For example, the yeast form of *Blastomyces dermatitidis* has notably refractile walls and a broad-based budding pattern, whereas the yeast form of *Histoplasma capsulatum* is much smaller, is often found within macrophages and shows a narrow-based budding pattern. Staining a smear with India ink, or a tissue biopsy with mucicarmine, may show the thick capsule characteristic of the yeast *Cryptococcus neoformans.* Marked epidermal hyperplasia, intraepidermal microabscesses, and suppurative-granulomatous inflammation in the dermis are often associated with these deep-seated fungal infections (Fig. 28-45).

Viral Skin Infections Cause Diverse Clinical Manifestations

Some viruses (see Chapter 9), such as the poxvirus **molluscum contagiosum** or **human papillomaviruses** (HPVs),

cause transient benign epithelial proliferations that resolve spontaneously. Others (e.g., measles or *parvovirus* [**erythema infectiosum**]) produce febrile illnesses with self-limited cutaneous eruptions **(exanthems)**. Primary infection by most **human herpesviruses** is often asymptomatic but results in a state of latent infection. Upon reactivation, these viruses cause a painful, vesicular eruption.

Molluscum contagiosum is a common infection among children and sexually active adults. It is self-limited and easily spread by direct contact. Firm, dome-shaped, smooth-surfaced papules with a characteristic central umbilication are usually found on the face, trunk, and anogenital area. Epidermal cells contain large intracytoplasmic inclusion bodies ("molluscum bodies") within cup-shaped areas that also exhibit verrucous (papillomatous) epidermal hyperplasia. Numerous viral particles are present within these inclusion bodies (Fig. 28-46).

Arthropod Infestations Produce Pruritic Skin Lesions

Mites and lice, other insects and spiders cause local lesions that may be very pruritic.

- *Scabies* is a severely pruritic, eczematous dermatitis caused by the mite *Sarcoptes scabei.* The female mite burrows beneath the stratum corneum on the fingers, wrists, trunk, and genital skin (Fig. 28-47). Intense lymphocytic and eosinophilic dermatitis is induced as a hypersensitivity reaction to the mite and its eggs and feces.
- *Pediculosis,* another pruritic dermatosis, may be caused by a variety of human lice. Eggs ("nits") of the lice may be found attached to hair shafts.
- **Biting or stinging insects** and other arthropods produce lesions that vary from small, pruritic papules to large, weeping nodules. The "arthropod assault reaction" varies with the responsible arthropod species and the host immune response. For example, tick bites tend to be large, with a striking lymphocytic and eosinophilic infiltrate. Lymphoid follicles may also form. Flea bites are usually urticarial, with a scant neutrophilic infiltrate. Venoms injected by arthropods such as the brown recluse spider may give rise to severe local tissue necrosis.

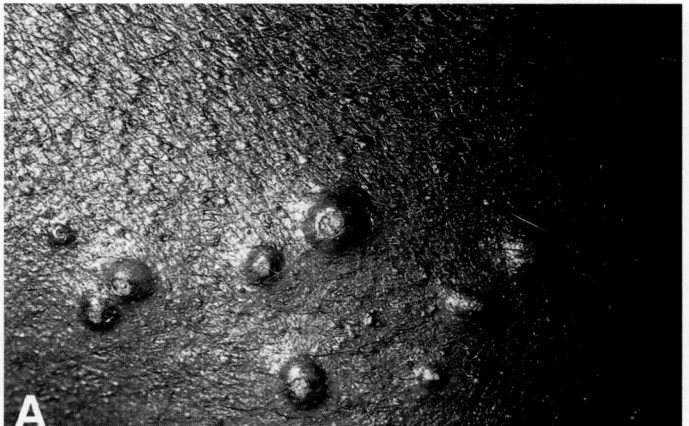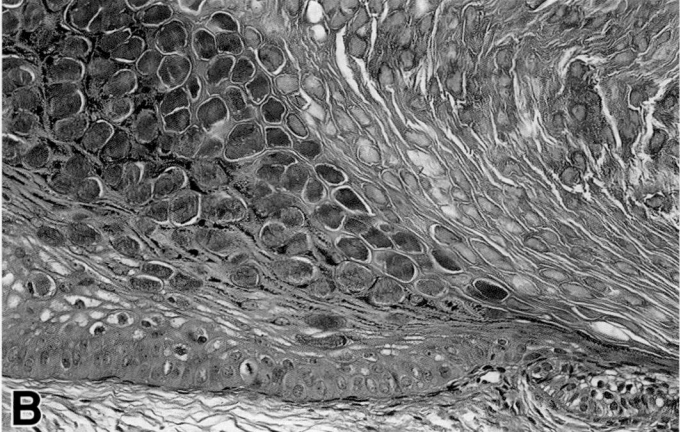

FIGURE 28-46. Molluscum contagiosum. A. Multiple umbilicated papules in an HIV-positive patient. **B.** Keratinocytes infected with this poxvirus show large eosinophilic cytoplasmic inclusions called "molluscum bodies." (From Elder DE, Elenitsas R, Johnson BL, et al. *Synopsis and Atlas of Lever's Histopathology of the Skin.* Philadelphia, PA: Lippincott Williams & Wilkins; 1999.)

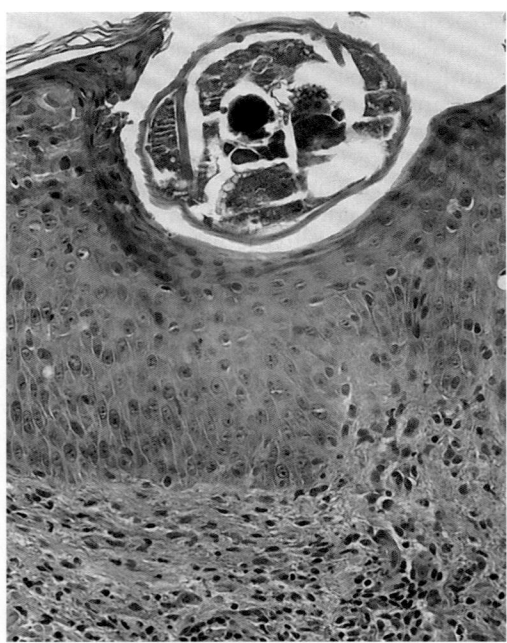

FIGURE 28-47. Scabetic nodule. A scabies mite is present in the stratum corneum. (From Elder DE, Elenitsas R, Johnson BL, et al. *Synopsis and Atlas of Lever's Histopathology of the Skin.* Philadelphia, PA: Lippincott Williams & Wilkins; 1999.)

PRIMARY NEOPLASMS OF THE SKIN

Prognosis in Malignant Melanoma Reflects the Depth of Invasion (Thickness)

Malignant melanoma is a neoplasm of melanocytes. The term "melanoma" in current practice is synonymous with "malignant melanoma." Malignant melanoma, although not one of the most common cancers overall, is a leading cause of cancer mortality in young adults. It is rare in adolescence and exceedingly rare in childhood. The incidence of melanoma is increasing rapidly. It is estimated that over 1% of those born today will develop melanoma.

Melanomas may progress through two major stages. In the "radial growth phase" (RGP), the lesion spreads (as viewed clinically) along the radii of an imperfect circle in the skin but remains superficial and thin, as measured by micrometer in the method described by Breslow. In the "vertical growth phase" (VGP), there is a focal area in which the lesion expands in a more or less spherical manner to form a tumor mass, with increasing Breslow thickness.

Melanomas like other neoplasms are dependent on a genetic "driver" such as an activated oncogene. Most of the oncogenes involved in melanoma in one way or another activate mitogen-activated protein kinase (MAP kinase) pathways, which are constitutively activated in most melanomas. The histopathologic subtypes of melanoma, discussed below, are related to the particular oncogenes involved in their pathogenesis. These oncogenes are also activated in melanocytic nevi, benign tumors of melanocytes that may be simulants, risk markers, and potential precursors for melanomas. Loss of one or more tumor suppressors, most commonly p16, occurs as melanomas develop, leading to unrestrained proliferation, which further increases the

potential for genomic instability and thereby promotes progression "from bad to worse."

Excision for histologic examination is the gold standard for diagnosis of melanoma, and complete excision with a "safety margin" is the mainstay of therapy. The prognosis of most melanomas is excellent if lesions are recognized and excised before entering a vertical growth phase. However, risk of dying from metastatic disease is increased if the tumor exceeds a critical depth in the dermis, and it increases further with increasing thickness, presumably because distant spread has already occurred before the primary tumor is excised.

Radial Growth Phase Melanoma

The clinical and histologic features of the RGP correlate with the epidemiology and the genomic landscape of the various forms of melanoma, characterized as "Pathways to Melanoma" in the 2018 WHO Classification of Melanomas of the Skin (Table 28-1). The term "pathway" is a reflection of epidemiologic events, sequential genomic events, and morphologic tumor progression stages that give rise to melanoma. These stages include a potential precursor nevus, a potential intermediate lesion such as a dysplastic nevus, the in situ or superficially invasive radial growth phase, the vertical growth phase, and metastases. Not all melanomas pass through all of these stages, but this progression has been shown to correlate with increasing numbers of critical genomic events.

The classification incorporates consideration of the role of sun exposure. Morphologically, the extent of "cumulative sun damage (CSD)," as measured by the degree of solar elastosis seen in a skin biopsy, separates the most common melanomas in Western populations into two categories, low and high CSD melanomas. The other pathways to melanoma seem not to depend on chronic solar damage and the incidence of these lesions is lower overall but is relatively consistent across populations. Table 28-1 summarizes the classification of melanoma.

TABLE 28-1
CLASSIFICATION OF MELANOMA

Melanomas arising in sun-exposed skin

Low-CSD melanoma, melanoma in skin with a low degree of cumulative sun damage

    Pathway I: Low-CSD melanoma/superficial spreading melanoma/SSM

High-CSD melanoma, melanoma in skin with a high degree of cumulative sun damage

    Pathway II: High-CSD melanoma/Lentigo maligna melanoma/LMM

    Pathway III: Desmoplastic melanoma

Melanomas arising at sun-shielded sites or without known etiologic associations with UV radiation exposure

    Pathway IV: Malignant Spitz tumor (Spitz melanoma)

    Pathway V: Acral melanoma

    Pathway VI: Mucosal melanoma

    Pathway VII: Melanoma arising in congenital nevus

    Pathway VIII: Melanoma arising in blue nevus

    Pathway IX: Uveal melanoma

MOLECULAR PATHOGENESIS: Several genetic mutations are implicated in the pathogenesis of melanoma, involving many different molecular pathways; however involvement of the MAP kinase pathway is a common feature. As is also true of benign nevi (see sections following), activating *BRAF* mutations are seen in 40% to 50% of melanomas, and *NRAS* mutations (mutually exclusive) are seen in 10% to 20%. These genes encode kinases that both utilize the MAPK pathway, which regulates cell proliferation. Upstream from both NRAS and BRAF is the receptor tyrosine kinase c-Kit, in which mutations account for only 1% of melanomas overall. However, it is a more common mutation in acral and mucosal subtypes, and also in lentigo maligna melanoma. Downstream from NRAS is the phosphatidylinositol-3-kinase (PI3K)/AKT pathway, which regulates cell survival and is suppressed by PTEN (see Chapter 5). In this context, *PTEN* mutations occur in 60% of cases. Mutations in the tumor suppressor *CDKN2A* are common in sporadic and familial melanomas. *CDKN2A* encodes two tumor suppressors, including p16^{INK4A}, which inhibits CDK4 and CDK6, and p14 which has a role in the

p53 pathway. The function of p16 may be impaired by additional mechanisms such as genomic deletion or less often epigenetic changes involving methylation, as alternatives to actual mutations of its gene. As the same activating mutations occur in both benign nevi and melanomas, malignant transformation likely entails a combination of these mutations, followed by inactivation of senescence/suppressor genes (like p16), and other alterations, including mutations of the *PTEN* pathway, P53 and *TERT* (telomerase) which occur in most melanomas in early and later stages of evolution.

Increased understanding of melanoma molecular mechanisms has spurred developments of **targeted therapies** aimed at inhibiting specific aberrant pathways, including tyrosine kinase inhibitors of the *BRAF, MEK,* and *KIT* oncogenes, with many more in clinical development (Fig. 28-48).

A lymphocytic response is seen in most melanomas, at least in part as a reaction to mutated genes, and this serves as a diagnostic clue compared to nevi. Spontaneous partial regression of the RGP is common in melanomas, while regression of the VGP or metastatic melanoma occurs more rarely. However, the recent introduction of **immune checkpoint therapy** may result in a "complete pathologic response" in which a deposit of metastatic melanoma is replaced by an infiltrate of lymphocytes, melanophages, and other cells (the lesion may seem to persist clinically because of the presence of these cells). In checkpoint therapy, monoclonal antibodies are used to block receptors that block the immune response, like CTLA-4 and PD-1. These markers can be demonstrated on tumor cells and host responding cells by immunohistochemistry.

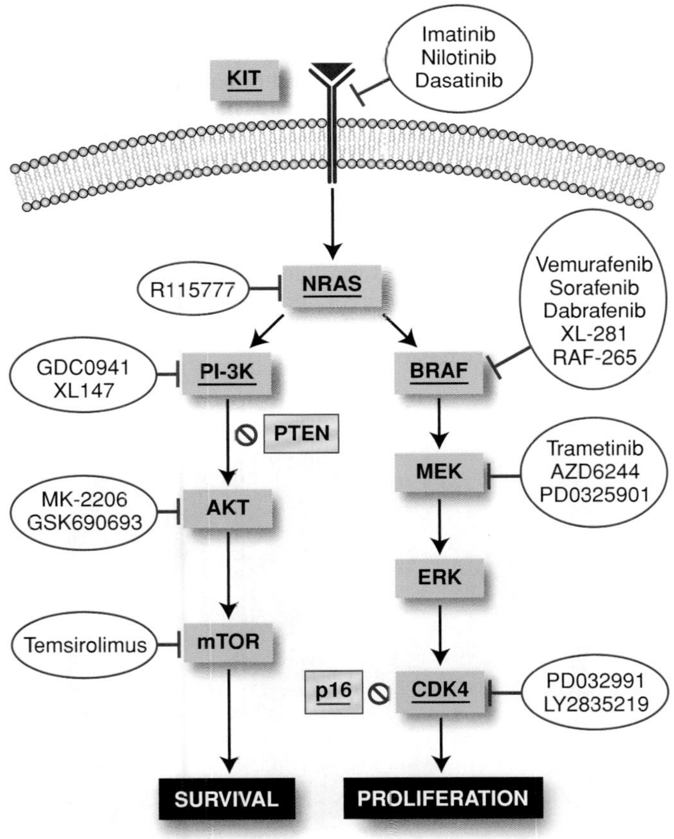

Superficial Spreading Melanoma

The most common type of melanoma is **superficial spreading melanoma (SSM)**, which can present in the radial growth phase with or without VGP (Fig. 28-49). Most of the morphologic features used to classify melanomas are attributes of the radial growth phase.

FIGURE 28-48. Simplified melanoma molecular pathway schema. Melanoma pathogenesis involves derangements in mitogen-activated protein kinase (MAPK) and phosphatidylinositol-3-kinase (PI3K)/AKT pathways, which regulate predominantly cell proliferation and cell survival, respectively. Red ovals contain examples of targeted therapeutic agents currently in use or in clinical trials. Underlined pathway proteins are products of genes with proven mutations in melanoma.

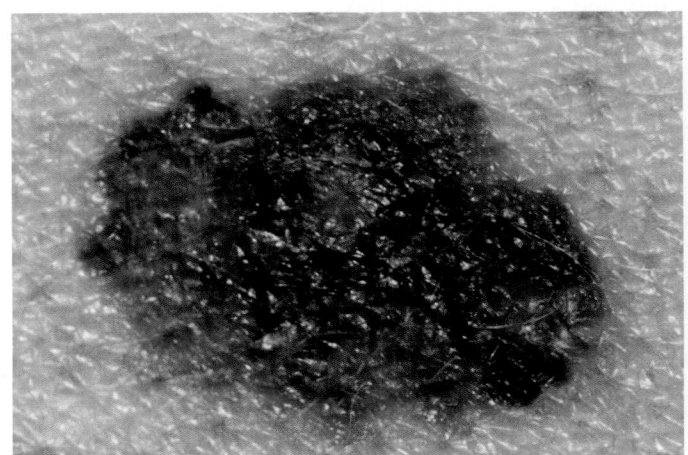

FIGURE 28-49. Clinical appearance of the radial growth phase in malignant melanoma of the superficial spreading type. The larger diameter is 1.8 cm.

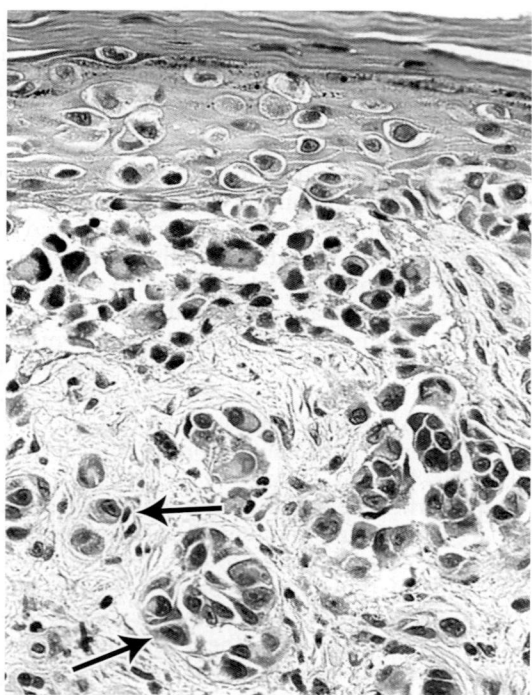

FIGURE 28-50. Malignant melanoma, superficial spreading type, radial growth phase. Melanocytes grow singly within the epidermis at all levels and as large, irregularly sized nests at the dermal–epidermal junction. Tumor cells are present in the papillary dermis (*arrows*), but no individual nest shows preferential growth over the others, or over the larger nest in the overlying epidermis.

PATHOLOGY: In the RGP of an SSM, large, often pigmented epithelioid melanocytes are dispersed in nests and as individual cells through the entire thickness of the epidermis ("pagetoid scatter") and not just along the basal layer, as occurs in nevi and in lentiginous forms of melanoma described below. These melanocytes may be limited to the epidermis **(melanoma in situ)** or they may invade into the papillary dermis. In the RGP, no nest has growth preference (larger size) over the other nests (Fig. 28-50). The cells tend to grow evenly in all directions: upward in the epidermis, peripherally in the epidermis, and into the dermis **(invasion)**. Mitoses are not seen in dermal melanocytes, except by definition when the VGP is present, but may be present in the epidermal component. Histologically, the "radial" component appears as a horizontal proliferation along the epidermis and superficial dermis, while the VGP, if present, is seen as an expansile nodule (Figs. 28-51 and 28-52), with increasing Breslow thickness. A brisk lymphocytic infiltrate often accompanies melanocytes in the radial growth phase. Pure RGP lesions rarely if ever metastasize.

CLINICAL FEATURES: The incidence of SSM is correlated with a history of intermittent sun exposure and sunburn. Childhood sun exposure is the most important, even though the melanomas occur in adulthood. Melanomas in the radial growth phase have slightly elevated and palpable borders. The neoplasm is usually variably and haphazardly pigmented. Some parts

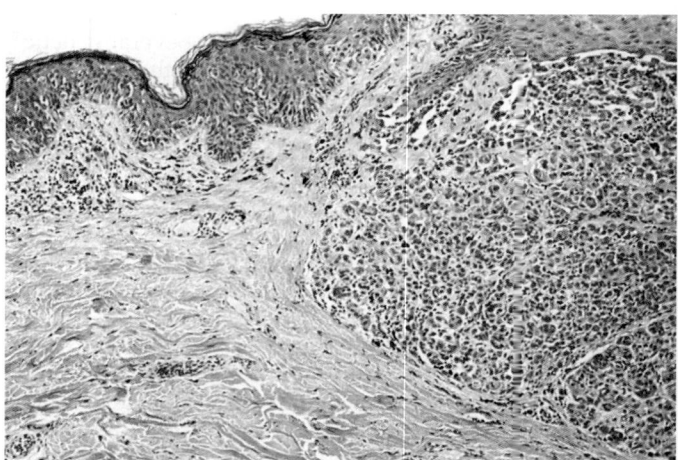

FIGURE 28-51. Malignant melanoma, superficial spreading type, vertical growth phase. Vertical growth is manifested by the distinct spheroid tumor nodule to the *right*. This focus of melanocytes clearly has a growth advantage (larger size of the aggregate) over nests in the adjacent radial growth phase (*left*).

are black or dark brown, while other areas may be lighter brown, possibly mixed with pink or light blue tints (Figs. 28-49 and 28-52). Patients often report that a change occurred in a nevus that is eventually documented to be a melanoma. Such alterations can include itching, increase in size, or darkening. Bleeding and oozing tend to appear later. With or without such observations on the part of the patient, any lesion that prompts clinical suspicion of melanoma warrants an excisional biopsy. The "ABCDE rule" is a convenient mnemonic to help recognize changes in nevi that require medical attention: **a**symmetry of shape, **b**order irregularity, **c**olor variation, and a **d**iameter more than 6 mm. "E" can stand for "**e**levation" or more importantly "**e**volution." However, not all early melanomas exhibit these attributes, and any changing lesion should be evaluated for excisional biopsy.

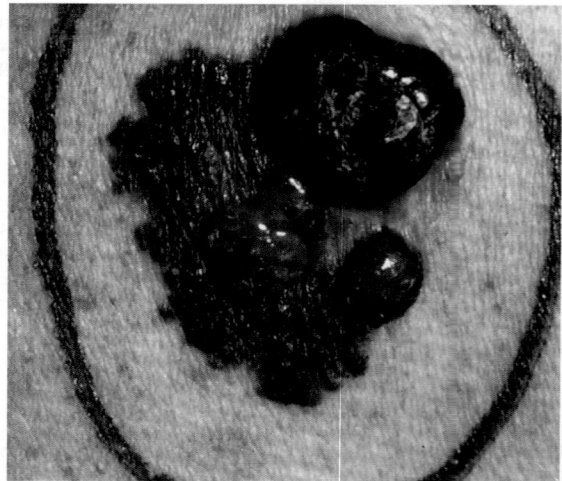

FIGURE 28-52. Malignant melanoma. The superficial spreading type is represented by the relatively flat, dark, brown–black portion of the tumor (seen on the *left* side). Three areas in this lesion are characteristic of the vertical growth phase. All are nodular in configuration; two have a pink coloration, and the largest is a rich, ebony black.

Lentigo Maligna Melanoma

Lentigo maligna melanoma (LMM), also known as **Hutchinson melanotic freckle**, typically presents as a large, pigmented macule on sun-damaged skin. It occurs almost exclusively in fair-skinned, usually elderly whites, often with a history of working outdoors. Because it occurs on exposed body surfaces and is associated with severe CSD, it is probably related to chronic ultraviolet light exposure. Lentigo maligna melanoma, like acral and mucosal melanomas (see below), is less likely than superficial spreading melanoma to be associated with mutations of *BRAF*, while *NRAS* mutations are more common. Some have activating mutations of the receptor tyrosine kinase gene *KIT* and thus may be responsive, at least for a time, to c-Kit inhibitors.

PATHOLOGY: In the radial growth phase, lentigo maligna melanoma (LMM) is a flat, irregular, poorly circumscribed brown to black patch that may cover a large part of the face or dorsal hands (Figs. 28-53 and 28-54). The cells of the radial growth phase are predominantly in the basal layer, often forming contiguous rows of atypical single melanocytes, characterized as a "lentiginous" pattern because of resemblance to the pattern of proliferation in a lentigo. This pattern of proliferation has been related to the expression of certain genes (e.g., NRAS, KIT), in benign as well as malignant lesions. Occasionally there are small nests that hang down into the papillary dermis (Fig. 28-55). Although cells of the radial growth phase of LMM vary in size, they tend to be smaller and less pigmented than those of SSM and are usually associated with effacement of rete ridges and thinning of the epidermis. The subjacent dermis often shows a sparse lymphocytic infiltrate, and severe solar degeneration of the connective tissue (elastosis, CSD) (Fig. 28-55).

The clinical appearance of LMM in the vertical growth phase is shown in Figure 28-54. Histologically, cells in the VGP tend to be spindle shaped. They occasionally provoke a connective tissue response to form a firm plaque

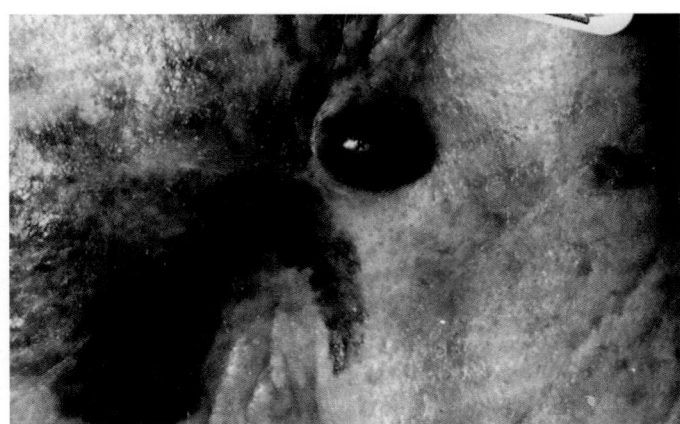

FIGURE 28-54. Lentigo maligna. The clinical appearance of the radial and vertical growth phase in malignant melanoma of the lentigo maligna type is shown. The lesion is very broad.

(desmoplastic melanoma), which may mimic a scar or a neuroma and be difficult to diagnose histologically. Desmoplastic melanomas have a very high mutation burden (related to chronic UV exposure), which may result in the presence of characteristic nodules of lymphocytes within them, and potential responsiveness to immune therapy. Cells of the VGP, in any melanoma but especially in LMM and other lentiginous melanomas may also grow along small nerves ("neurotropism").

Acral Melanoma

Acral lentiginous melanomas occur with about equal frequency in all races. It is thus the most common form of melanoma in dark-skinned people. As the name implies, it is generally limited to palms, soles, and subungual regions. Increased copy numbers and often mutations in *CCND1*, the gene for the cell cycle marker cyclin D, are common findings in these lesions. Pagetoid and *BRAF*-mutated melanomas may also occur in acral skin.

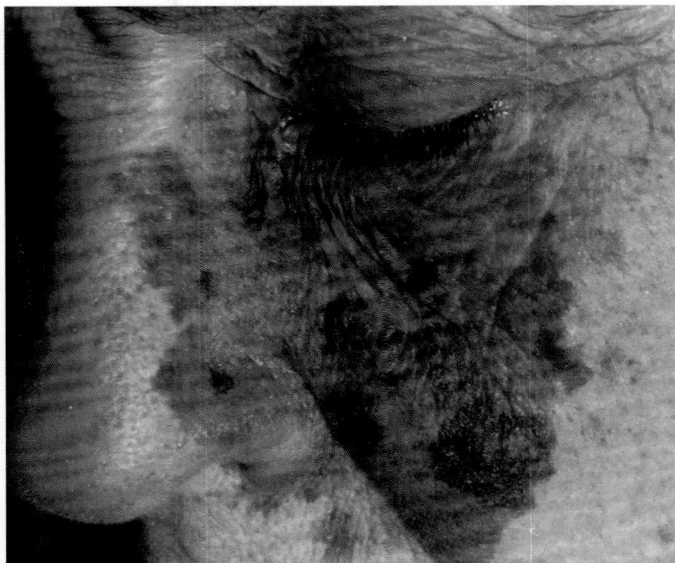

FIGURE 28-53. Malignant melanoma of the lentigo maligna type, radial growth phase.

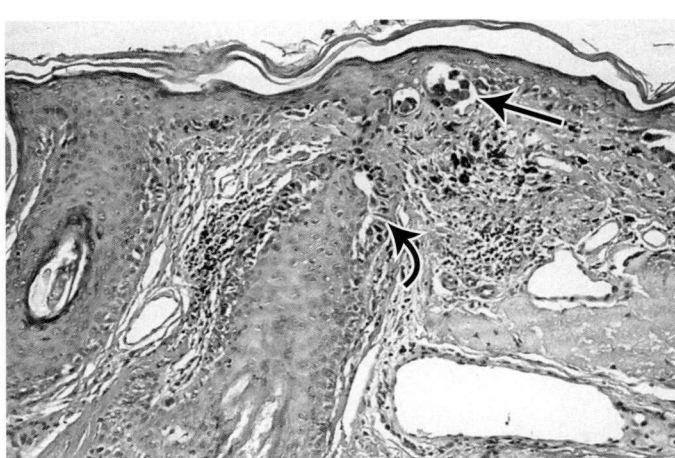

FIGURE 28-55. Lentigo maligna. Atypical melanocytes grow mostly at the dermal–epidermal interface (*straight arrow*), with extension down the external root sheath of follicles (*curved arrow*). Upward growth of melanocytes is much less prominent than in SSM. The gray material in the mid-dermis to the right of the image is "severe" solar elastosis.

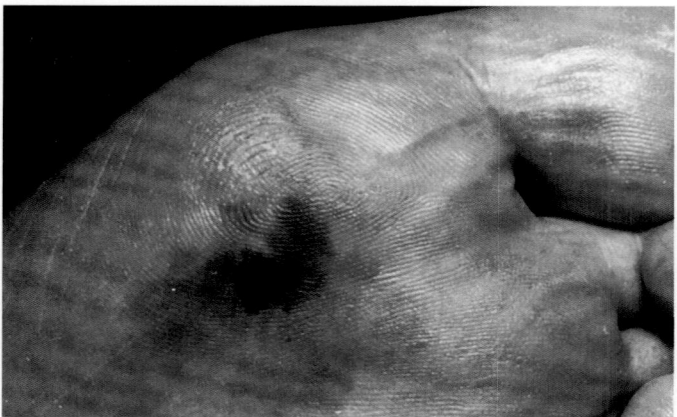

FIGURE 28-56. Malignant melanoma, acral lentiginous type (radial growth phase). The clinical appearance of a large asymmetric, variably pigmented lesion of the sole of the foot is illustrated.

PATHOLOGY: In the radial growth phase, acral lentiginous melanoma forms an irregular, poorly circumscribed brown to black patch that covers a part of the palm or sole (Fig. 28-56) or arises under a nail, usually on a thumb or great toe ("subungual melanoma"). Tumor cells are confined mostly to the basal layer of the epidermis and tend to maintain long dendrites (Figs. 28-57 and 28-58). A lichenoid lymphocytic infiltrate is often seen.

The vertical growth phase (Figs. 28-59 and 28-60) is like that of lentigo maligna melanoma, in that it commonly consists of spindle cells and occasionally includes desmoplasia and neurotropism.

Vertical Growth Phase (VGP) Melanoma

After a variable time (usually 1 to 2 years), the character of growth may begin to change in an RGP melanoma of any pathway. Melanocytes exhibit mitotic activity in both the epidermal and dermal components and grow as expanding spheroid nodules in the dermis (Fig. 28-51). The net direction of growth tends to be perpendicular to that of the radial

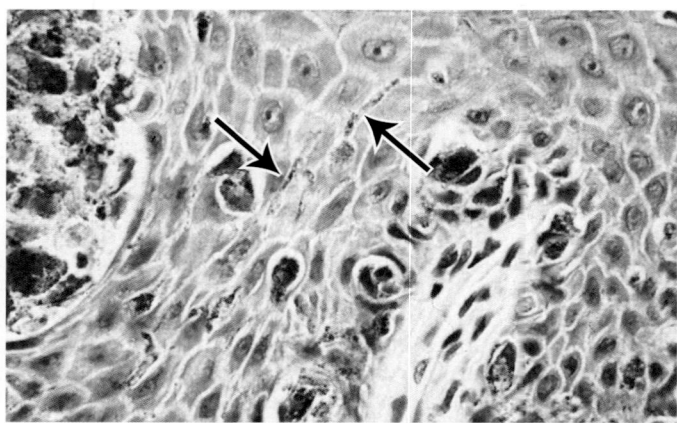

FIGURE 28-58. Malignant melanoma, acral lentiginous type, in situ in this image. Large melanocytes with prominent dendrites (*arrows*) are present in the basilar region of the epidermis. Tumor cells contain numerous melanosomes, causing perinuclear and dendritic cytoplasm to appear brown.

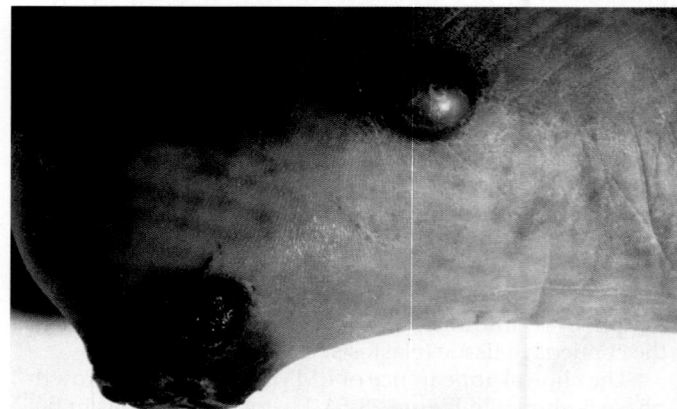

FIGURE 28-59. Malignant melanoma, acral lentiginous type. The lesion on the heel is the primary tumor. The flat portion represents the radial growth phase, while the elevated portion indicates the vertical growth phase. The dark nodule on the instep is a metastasis.

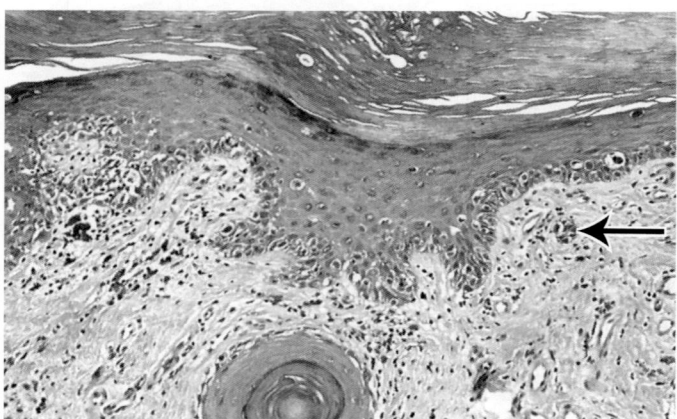

FIGURE 28-57. Malignant melanoma, acral lentiginous type, predominantly intraepidermal radial growth. Atypical melanocytes are present along the dermal–epidermal junction. A small dermal nest of atypical melanocytes is present (*arrow*).

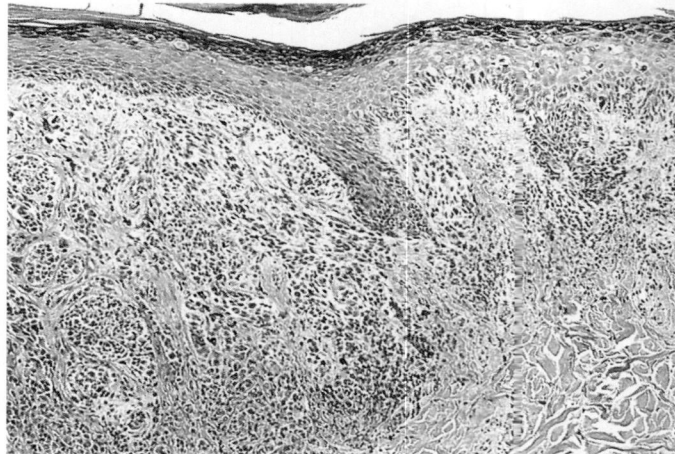

FIGURE 28-60. Malignant melanoma, acral lentiginous type, vertical growth phase. Confluent growth of atypical dermal melanocytes filling and expanding the papillary dermis and infiltrating the reticular dermis is seen on the *left*; on the *right* is the (horizontal) radial growth phase.

growth phase as viewed clinically, hence the designation **vertical** (Figs. 28-51 to 28-53).

> **PATHOLOGY:** The VGP is characterized by a cellular aggregate in the dermis that is larger than the clusters of melanocytes that form the epidermal and dermal (invasive) components of the RGP (Fig. 28-51). Invasion can occur in both the radial growth phase and vertical growth phase, but the dominant direction of tumor growth shifts from the epidermis to the dermis in the vertical growth phase. This property of expansile growth in the dermis is called *tumorigenicity*. Mitotic figures are common in the VGP and, along with tumorigenicity, form one of its two defining attributes. Markers of cell cycle progression, such as Ki-67, and phosphohistone mitosis markers increase in cells of the vertical growth phase. Melanocytes tend to look different from those of the RGP. For example, they may contain little or no pigment, while cells in the RGP are melanotic. Host response (i.e., lymphocytic inflammation) may be absent or reduced at the base of the VGP, compared to the RGP.
>
> Not all tumors in the VGP possess the propensity to metastasize. In fact, VGP melanomas less than 1 mm thick that lack mitoses rarely metastasize. The risk of metastasis can be predicted, albeit imperfectly, through the use of prognostic and staging models. The American Joint Commission on Cancer (AJCC) staging model depends on Breslow thickness and the presence or absence of ulceration to categorize melanomas into stages and substages at differing risk of causing melanoma-related death, for which different treatment strategies can be offered.

Nodular Melanoma (NM)

Occasionally, a melanoma "bypasses" the stepwise tumor progression described above and manifests all of its malignant characteristics in the initial lesion. NM is an uncommon form of the tumor (10%), which appears as a circumscribed, elevated, spheroidal nodule (Fig. 28-61). It does not develop through a perceptible radial growth phase but is in the vertical growth phase when initially observed (Fig. 28-62). These lesions lack most of the ABCD criteria. They may be advanced in thickness, and thus at high risk of metastasis at the time of diagnosis, despite being often small in diameter,

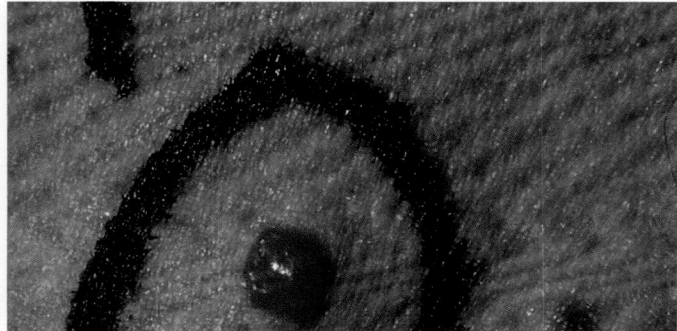

FIGURE 28-61. Malignant melanoma of the nodular type. The primary focus of growth of this 0.5-cm lesion is in the dermis, elevating the epidermis to form a symmetrical, well circumscribed pink nodule.

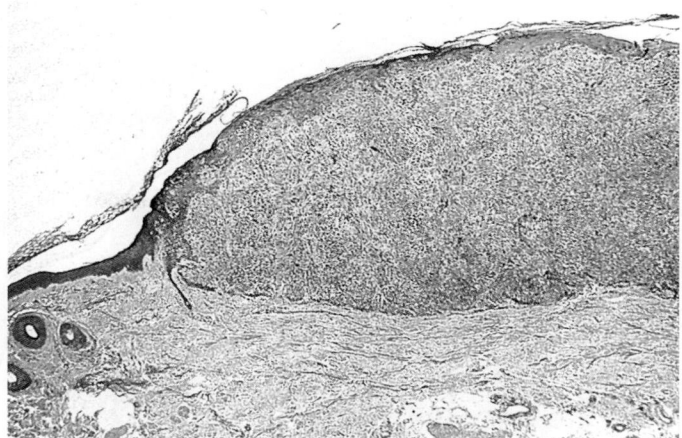

FIGURE 28-62. Malignant melanoma, nodular type. Intraepidermal growth is essentially absent. There is no radial growth lateral to the nodule. The tumor expands the papillary dermis and distorts the reticular dermal junction; it is therefore level III.

symmetric, and homogeneous in color. They are therefore difficult to detect in a curable stage.

Metastatic Melanoma

Metastatic melanoma arises from melanocytes of the vertical growth phase in any of the various forms of melanoma. Initial metastases usually involve regional skin and/or lymph nodes, although hematogenous spread to organs is also possible. When the latter occurs, metastases are unusually widespread in comparison with other neoplasms; virtually any organ may be involved. Metastatic melanomas may remain dormant and clinically undetectable for long periods after the apparently successful excision of a primary melanoma, only to reappear years later (see Chapter 5).

Staging and Prognosis of Melanoma

Prognosis for a patient with a melanoma can be related to many factors; only the first two listed below are used in standard staging of a primary melanoma:

TUMOR THICKNESS: Tumor thickness, originally described by Breslow, is the strongest prognostic variable for melanomas that are apparently confined to their primary sites (stages 1 and 2 in the staging system of the AJCC). The "Breslow thickness" of a melanoma is measured from the most superficial aspect of the stratum granulosum to the point of maximal thickness (Fig. 28-63). Outcome can be predicted with some accuracy by dividing tumors based on thickness. Cutoffs occur at 1-mm intervals, although the 0.76-mm cutoff (now rounded to 0.8 mm) originally proposed by Breslow is used as a stage modifier for optimal separation of the lowest-risk melanomas (Stage 1a).

Prognosis up to 10 years after removal of the primary lesion may be estimated from Table 28-2.

ULCERATION: Ulceration in a primary melanoma is associated with decreased survival. In one study, survival rates were 66% and 92% for patients with and without ulceration, respectively. Ulceration is a stage modifier in the AJCC system; its presence raises a lesion to the next stage in each thickness group.

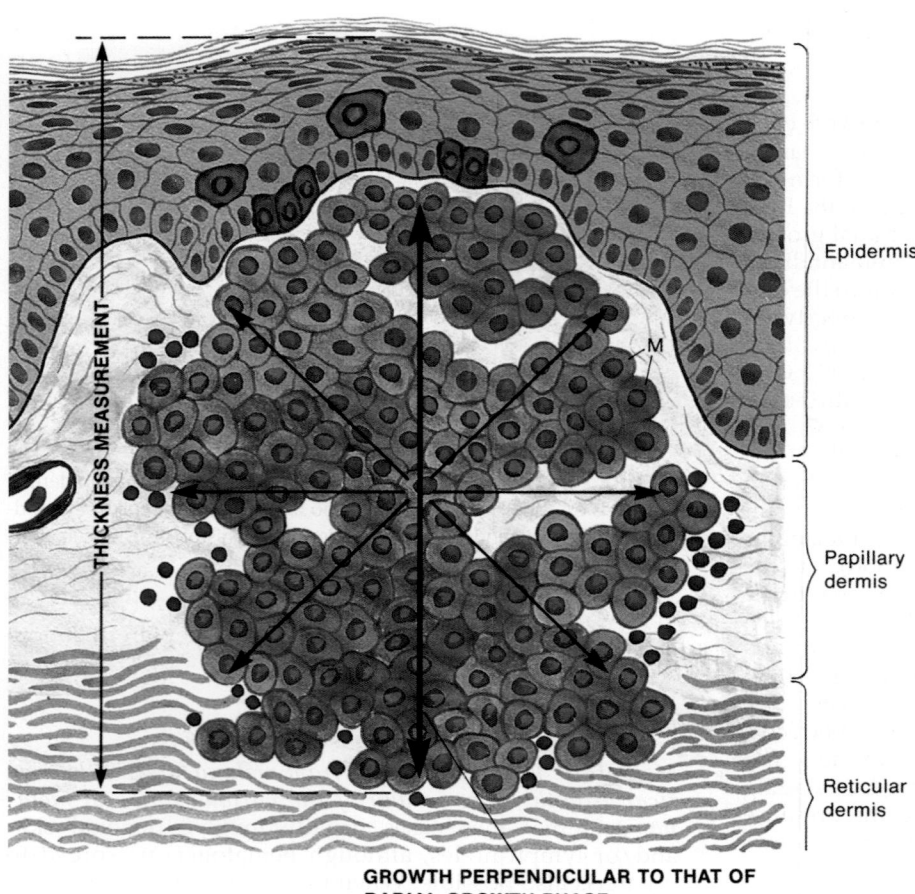

GROWTH PERPENDICULAR TO THAT OF RADIAL GROWTH PHASE

FIGURE 28-63. Malignant melanoma. The evolution of the vertical growth phase in malignant melanoma of the superficial spreading type is shown schematically, with an indication of how thickness is measured. In this illustration, the vertical growth phase has extended into the reticular dermis. Small nodules of tumor cells that clearly have a growth preference over other tumor cells are a manifestation of the vertical growth phase. Thickness is measured from the most superficial aspect of the granular layer across the tumor at its thickest point to its deepest point of invasion.

DERMAL MITOTIC RATE: Survival becomes progressively worse as the mitotic rate increases. The 5-year survival is 99% for node-negative patients whose tumors have no mitoses, and 84% if the mitotic rate is $\geq 11/\text{mm}^2$. However,

this and the other attributes listed below are not included in the current AJCC staging system, which is the standard of care.

LYMPHOCYTIC INFILTRATE: Interaction of lymphocytes with tumor cells in the vertical growth phase (tumor-infiltrating lymphocytes [TILs]) is an important prognostic indicator. Lymphocytes are said to be "infiltrative" when they actually penetrate and disrupt the tumor, sometimes forming rosettes around tumor cells (Figs. 28-64 and 28-65). The more prevalent the TILs, the better is the prognosis.

REGRESSION: In many primary melanomas there is evidence of spontaneous regression in the RGP component, indicated clinically by a color change to blue-white or white. Such regression entails a widened papillary dermis, containing melanophages and a lymphocytic infiltrate, with no melanoma cells in the epidermis overlying these dermal changes. The prognostic significance of RGP regression is unclear, as a progressing VGP may co-exist. Regression is uncommon in the VGP, and in metastases, except after effective immune therapy, and is probably an effect of TILs within the tumor, as discussed above.

LOCATION: Melanomas on the extremities have a better prognosis than those on the head, neck, or trunk (axial). However, melanomas on the sole of the foot or the subungual region have a prognosis similar to, or worse than, axial lesions.

SEX: Women generally have better prognoses than men. For example, women with axial melanomas 0.8 to 1.7 mm

TABLE 28-2

TUMOR STAGE AS PREDICTOR OF OUTCOME 10 YEARS AFTER DEFINITIVE THERAPY OF PRIMARY MELANOMA, IN PATIENTS WITH NEGATIVE SENTINEL NODES[a]

Stage	Thickness (mm)	Ulceration	10-yr Survival (%)
T1a	≤1.0	No	98
T1b	<0.8	Yes	96
T2a	>1.0–2.0	No	92
T2b	>1.0–2.0	Yes	86
T3a	>2.0–4.0	No	88
T3b	>2.0–4.0	Yes	81
T4a	>4.0	No	83
T4b	>4.0	Yes	75

[a]Patients with T1N0 melanomas are included whether or not they had sentinel node biopsy.

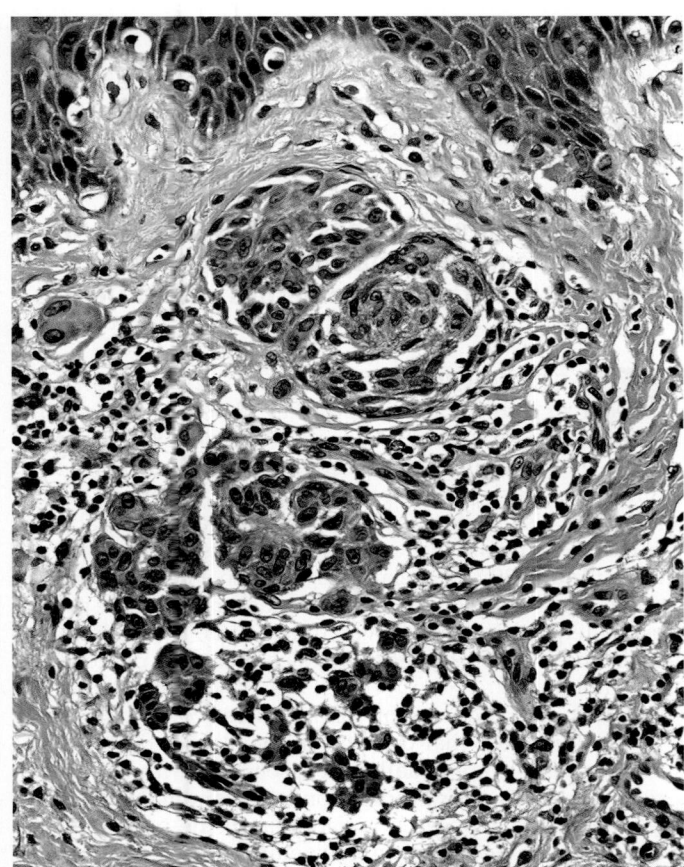

FIGURE 28-64. Malignant melanoma, early vertical growth phase. The host response consists of lymphocytes infiltrating amid the melanocytes ("tumor-infiltrating lymphocytes").

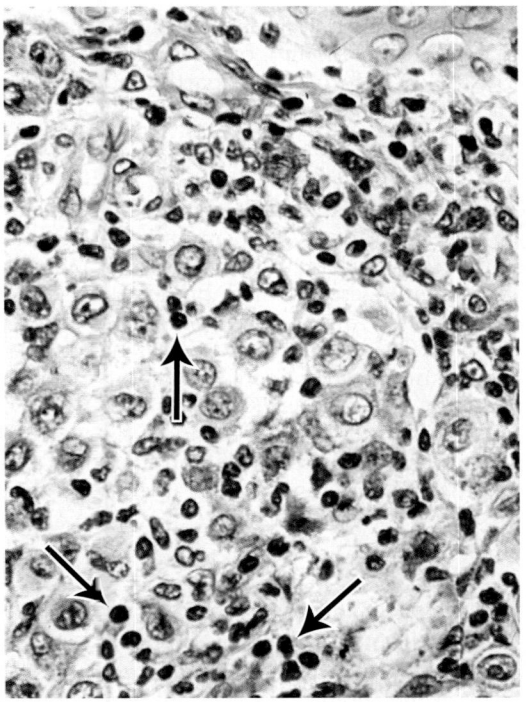

FIGURE 28-65. Malignant melanoma, vertical growth phase. Numerous tumor-infiltrating lymphocytes (*arrows*) are arranged among individual tumor cells.

thick have nearly 90% 10-year survival after excision of the lesion, while the comparable figure for men is 60%.

LEVELS OF INVASION: The Clark level system describes the degree of tumor penetration within the anatomic layers of the skin. The Clark levels (I to V) are not as accurate as tumor thickness in predicting risk of metastasis and are not included in the AJCC system. However, levels have prognostic significance in some subsets of cases.

LYMPHATIC INVASION: Although intuitively important, this property has not been included in prognostic models because it is rarely seen in routine sections. However, lymphatic invasion may be more common than previously thought when enhanced detection techniques are used, and it may be prognostically significant.

STAGE: The stage of the disease is the most important single factor influencing a patient's survival.

The tumor–node–metastasis (TNM) system of tumor staging incorporates features of the primary tumor, regional lymph nodes, and soft tissues and distant metastases. The **T** (primary tumor) attributes of tumor thickness, presence or absence of ulceration, and mitogenicity are classified histologically after excision of the melanoma. Numbers of lymph nodes with metastatic tumor and characterization of this tumor by size are the basis of the **N** (node) classification. Metastasis to regional lymph nodes is now determined routinely by sentinel lymph node staging, which involves biopsy of a single node that lies first in the regional node drainage pattern. Lymph node involvement implies a 26% decrease in 10-year survival, compared with patients with clinically localized tumors. The number of involved lymph nodes is also highly predictive of prognosis. Patients with 1 positive node have a 10-year survival of 75%, compared with 68% with 2 or 3 positive nodes, and 47% with 4 or more nodes involved. **Micrometastases** are nodal metastases diagnosed after sentinel or elective lymphadenectomy; **macrometastases** are clinically detectable nodal metastases. The term "submicroscopic" metastasis has been proposed for sentinel node involvement below certain thresholds of size and penetration into the node. The **M** (metastasis) properties incorporate results of evaluation for distant metastases at various anatomic sites. **TNM classification** is based primarily on thickness and modified by ulceration, and the presence and distribution of metastases. For localized primary melanomas and for regional and systemic metastatic disease, it helps define the pathologic stage of disease, which in turn reflects the probability of survival.

Current guidelines regarding surgical excision of confirmed melanomas recommend that a 5-mm margin of uninvolved tissue be obtained with in situ melanoma, a 1-cm margin with a tumor thickness of 1 mm or less and a 2-cm margin with a tumor thickness greater than 1 mm. However, margins are typically adjusted so as to spare important structures, such as the eyes. Sentinel lymph node sampling is generally considered with tumors of thickness greater than 1 mm or with other risk factors, including ulceration or increased dermal mitotic activity, especially in tumors 0.8 mm or thicker. If metastatic disease ensues, targeted therapeutics, such as *BRAF* inhibitors, can be employed. Immunomodulatory drugs are also used, such as antibodies to CTLA-4 (cytotoxic T-lymphocyte antigen 4) and PD-1 (programmed cell death 1), to boost immune responses against malignancy.

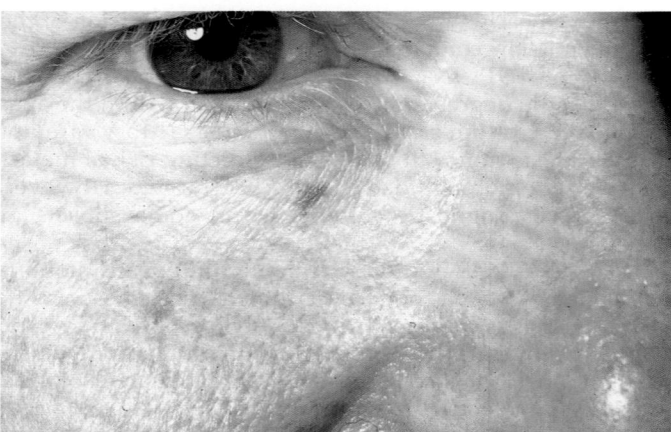

FIGURE 28-66. Freckle. A fair-complexioned man has a prominent brown macule that darkens in sunlight. (From Elder DE, Elenitsas R, Johnson BL, et al. *Synopsis and Atlas of Lever's Histopathology of the Skin*. Philadelphia, PA: Lippincott Williams & Wilkins; 1999.)

Benign Tumors of Melanocytes and Pigmented Lesions May Mimic Melanoma and Be Markers of Risk for Melanoma

Freckle and Lentigo

Freckles, or **ephelides**, are small, brown macules that occur on sun-exposed skin, especially in people with fair skin (Fig. 28-66). They usually appear at about age 5. The pigmentation of a freckle deepens with exposure to sunlight and fades when light exposure ceases. A **lentigo** is a discrete, brown macule that appears at any age and on any part of the body (though a **solar lentigo** appears at an older age after long-term sun exposure) (Fig. 28-67). Histologically, ephelides show hyperpigmentation of basal keratinocytes without concomitant increases in the number of melanocytes. Lentigines, on the other hand, display elongated rete ridges, increased melanin pigment in both basal keratinocytes and melanocytes, and increased numbers of melanocytes. Larger

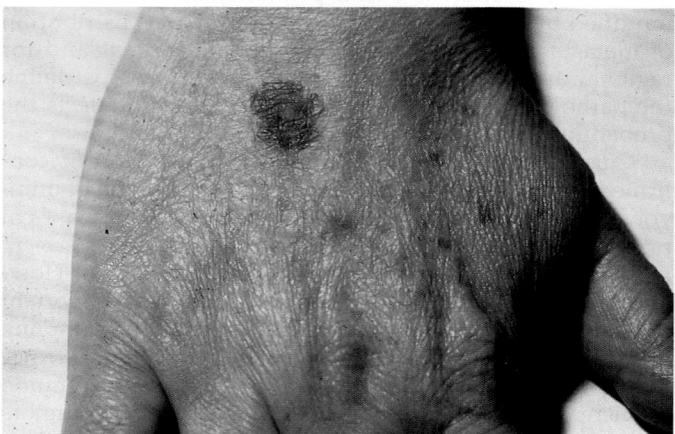

FIGURE 28-67. Lentigo. A 1-cm irregular patch of slightly variegated hyperpigmentation is present on a background of chronic solar damage (seen as wrinkling of the skin). (From Elder DE, Elenitsas R, Johnson BL, et al. *Synopsis and Atlas of Lever's Histopathology of the Skin*. Philadelphia, PA: Lippincott Williams & Wilkins; 1999.)

lesions may need to be biopsied to rule out lentigo maligna melanoma.

Lentigines, often called freckles by the public and by clinicians, are strong risk factors for melanoma, acting synergistically with nevi, dysplastic nevi and other risk factors, and are also potential "lookalikes" or simulants.

Common Acquired Melanocytic Nevi (Moles) Are Localized Benign Neoplastic Proliferations of Melanocytes Within the Epidermis and/or Dermis

 ETIOLOGIC FACTORS: Most people, regardless of skin color, develop 10 to 50 nevi on their skin. The total number depends on light exposure and innate susceptibility. Except for occasional cosmetic significance, nevi are important mainly as markers of increased risk of developing melanoma, as potential precursors of melanoma and as simulants of melanoma. Even though 30% of melanomas arise in a nevus, nevi are much more common than melanomas, and most are stable or undergo senescence over time. Thus, indiscriminate excision of nevi is not effective as a means of preventing melanoma.

Black skin can develop nevi, but less commonly than white skin. Nevi that develop in the skin of darkly pigmented people are usually not associated with increased risk of melanoma or progression to melanoma. However, the risk of developing a melanoma on the palms of the hands, the soles of the feet, the genital skin, or in mucous membranes is the same in all races and is generally low and not related to nevi. Like melanomas, nevi do not ordinarily develop in areas protected from light by at least two layers of clothing, such as the buttocks. There is an unequivocal causal relationship between exposure to ultraviolet light and risk of developing melanocytic nevi (and malignant melanoma), but the relationship is complex. The ability to form nevi is partly under genetic control, but this is poorly understood.

MOLECULAR PATHOGENESIS: A majority of nevi have an activating mutation of the oncogene *BRAF*, which can lead to growth stimulation through the mitogen-activated protein kinase (MAPK) pathway. However, after an initial period of growth, nevi become stable lesions that may regress or senesce. Such senescence is mediated by increased activity of p16, which is encoded by the gene *CDKN2A* on chromosome 9p21 and is an inhibitor of cyclin-dependent kinase 4 (CDK4). The p16 protein suppresses cell proliferation and promotes end-stage differentiation of the nevus cells (see Chapter 5).

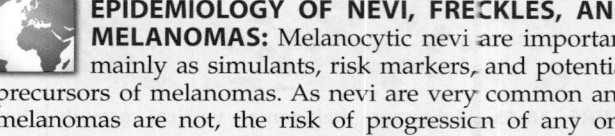 **EPIDEMIOLOGY OF NEVI, FRECKLES, AND MELANOMAS:** Melanocytic nevi are important mainly as simulants, risk markers, and potential precursors of melanomas. As nevi are very common and melanomas are not, the risk of progression of any one nevus to melanoma is small. As potentially close simulants,

nevi must be distinguished from melanoma clinically and histologically, as discussed below.

Nevi are important as risk markers for development of melanomas. Someone with 100 or more nevi that are 2 to 5 mm in diameter has a threefold greater risk of developing melanoma than a person with fewer than 25 similar nevi. Patients with clinically atypical-appearing nevi or histologically proven dysplastic nevi are at even greater risk for melanoma. Having only 10 or more such clinically atypical or dysplastic nevi may be associated with a 12-fold increased risk for melanoma. Other important risk factors include a family history of melanoma, a history of sun exposure and sunburns, and the presence of numerous solar lentigines or "freckles" which are caused by sun exposure in susceptible individuals. Such susceptibility is associated with polymorphisms in *MC1R*, the gene that encodes the melanocortin-1 receptor, and with subsequent variation in the ratio of pheomelanin to eumelanin. These pigments are associated with red and brown hair, respectively, and also with susceptibility to burning and tanning. At least two separate (but overlapping) profiles distinguish individuals at risk for melanoma. One group prototypically has skin that may burn but does tan and has an increased number of nevi. The other group consists of red-haired, blue-eyed people with milk-white skin, who are exquisitely sensitive to light and do not tan well. However, they form freckles and do not develop a significant number of nevi.

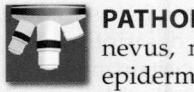 **CLINICAL FEATURES:** Melanocytic nevi begin to appear between the first and second years of life and continue to emerge for the first two decades of life. A nevus first appears as a small tan dot no bigger than 1 to 2 mm. During the next 3 to 4 years, the dot enlarges to become a uniform tan to brown circular or oval area. The peripheral outline usually remains regular. When it reaches 4 to 5 mm in diameter, it is flat or slightly elevated, stops enlarging peripherally and is sharply demarcated from surrounding normal skin. Over the next 10 years, the lesion elevates and its color pales to the point of becoming a tan tag-like protrusion. For the next decade or two, it gradually flattens and the skin may approximate a normal appearance. In most people, the number of nevi gradually decreases over time. Notably, many melanoma patients tend to retain increased numbers of nevi, including atypical ones, in later decades of life.

PATHOLOGY: At the inception of a melanocytic nevus, melanocytes are increased in the basal epidermis, with subsequent hyperpigmentation. They eventually form nests, frequently at tips of rete ridges, and then migrate into the dermis where they form small clusters. As the lesion becomes elevated, the dermal nevus cells begin to differentiate in a manner reminiscent of Schwann cells (melanocytes like Schwann cells are derived from embryonic neural crest and they express some of the same transcription factors), an evolution that gradually encompasses the entire dermal component, leaving a core of delicate neuromesenchyme. The nevus may eventually flatten and possibly even disappear. The

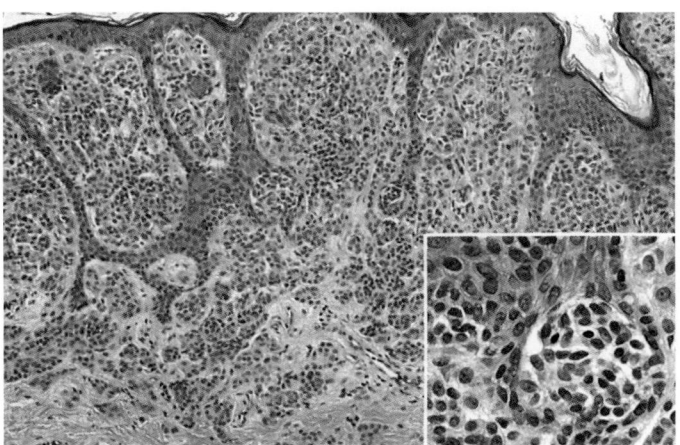

FIGURE 28-68. Compound melanocytic nevus. Melanocytes are present as nests within the epidermis and dermis. An intraepidermal nest of melanocytes is surrounded by keratinocytes (*inset*).

histologic classification of melanocytic nevi reflects their evolution:

- **Junctional nevus:** Melanocytes form nests at the tips of epidermal rete ridges. They are then by definition known as "nevus cells," and they also tend to lose their dendritic morphology and retain pigment in their cytoplasm.
- **Compound nevus:** Nests of melanocytes are seen in the epidermis and some of the cells have migrated into the dermis (Fig. 28-68).
- **Dermal nevus:** Intraepidermal melanocytic growth has ceased and melanocytes are present only in the dermis (Fig. 28-69). Pigment tends to be lost at this stage, but the presence of a residual nested architecture is an important clue to the diagnosis of a nevus versus another tumor.

Dysplastic (Atypical) Nevi Are Risk Markers for Melanoma

An increased number of total nevi is a significant risk factor for melanoma, as is the presence of large nevi. Some acquired nevi do not follow the pattern of growth, differentiation, and disappearance described above but instead

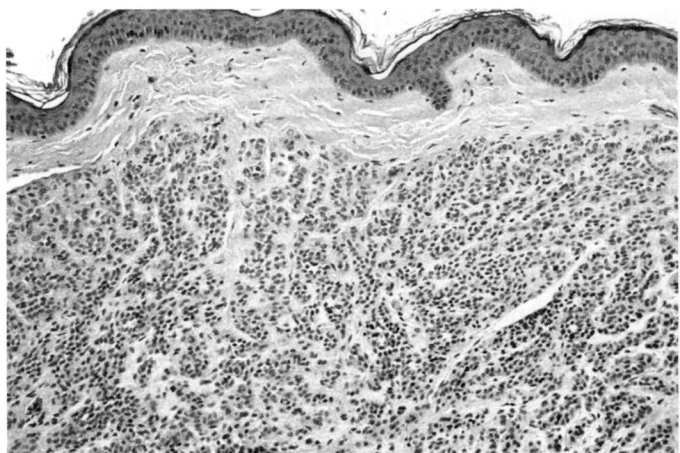

FIGURE 28-69. Dermal melanocytic nevus. Melanocytes are entirely confined to the dermis.

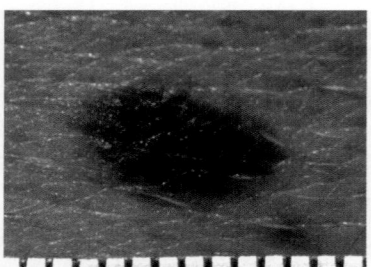

FIGURE 28-70. Clinically dysplastic nevus. This lesion fulfills criteria for a dysplastic nevus: size >5 mm; a macular component with an indefinite border; and variegated pigmentation. (Reprinted with permission from Elder DE, Elenitsas R, Rubin AI, Ioffreda M, Miller J, Fred Miller III O. *Atlas and Synopsis of Lever's Histopathology of the Skin*. 3rd ed. Philadelphia, PA: Lippincott Williams & Wilkins; 2012.)

exhibit atypical features. These are called "dysplastic nevi." They are examples of "intermediate lesions" that have acquired one or more genomic abnormalities in addition to the initiating oncogene mutation. Dysplastic nevi are especially strong risk factors for melanoma. They are also potential precursors, but the risk of progression for any one dysplastic nevus is very low. They tend not to undergo senescence (or do so less frequently) and are often larger than 5 mm. They may contain foci of aberrant melanocytic growth and become larger and somewhat irregular peripherally (although less so than melanomas) (Fig. 28-70). The peripheral area is flat (macular) and extends symmetrically from the parent nevus. Some clinically dysplastic nevi are entirely macular.

Dysplastic nevi were first described in melanoma kindreds, families with a greatly increased incidence of melanoma. In these families and in the general population, patients with dysplastic nevi are at increased risk of developing melanoma. Not all patients with dysplastic nevi develop melanomas, and not all melanomas occur in patients with dysplastic nevi. The magnitude of this risk varies with the number of dysplastic nevi and is especially high in patients with a prior melanoma or family history of melanoma. The genetics of dysplastic nevi are not completely understood, but contributions from multiple genomic abnormalities have been implicated.

Melanocytic Dysplasia Features Architectural Disorder and Cytologic Atypia

Dysplastic nevi are characterized by junctional proliferation of nevoid to epithelioid melanocytes arranged singly and in nests, with nests predominating. These lesions occur mainly near the dermal–epidermal junction and at the tips and sides of elongated rete ridges. A band of eosinophilic connective tissue ("concentric eosinophilic fibroplasia") is seen around the rete ridges. Horizontal nests of lesional cells extend from some rete to adjacent rete ("bridging"). As these architectural features become more prominent, melanocytes with large atypical nuclei resembling those of malignant cells may also appear in areas of architectural disorder, but remain a minority population and constitute "random cytologic atypia." The combination of architectural disorder and cytologic atypia defines a dysplastic nevus (Fig. 28-71). Areas of dysplasia may also be associated with a subjacent lymphocytic infiltrate. More than 1/3 of malignant melanomas have precursor nevi, most of which have melanocytic dysplasia.

However, most dysplastic nevi are stable and never progress to melanoma. In other words, dysplastic nevi are much more common in the population than melanomas. Between 7% and 20% of the population has at least one dysplastic nevus, depending on the diagnostic criteria applied. Controversy about the significance of dysplastic nevi largely reflects diagnostic variation. Moderate and severe histologic dysplasia, but not mild dysplasia, are associated with increased risk of developing melanoma. Mild histologic dysplasia is therefore considered, as in other sites in the body, to be a common lesion of little or no prognostic or diagnostic significance. In the 2018 WHO Classification of Skin Tumours, the category of mild dysplasia is no longer used, and moderate and severe dysplasia are categorized as low-grade and high-grade dysplasia, respectively.

Congenital Melanocytic Nevus

About 1% of white children are born with some form of pigmented skin lesion, sometimes as inconspicuous as a small patch of pale tan hyperpigmentation. Much more rarely, the trunk or an extremity is covered by a large pigmented patch or plaque that is cosmetically deforming ("giant hairy" or "garment" nevus). Such areas display a striking increase in intraepidermal and dermal melanocytes, which may extend deep into the subcutaneous tissue. True congenital nevi are usually associated with activating mutations of *NRAS*. Malignant melanomas may develop in these large congenital melanocytic nevi, although not in the majority of cases. These melanomas may occur in childhood. Attempts are sometimes made to remove these large lesions, but their size may make surgical removal problematic.

Spitz Nevi and Tumors

Spitz nevi (also known as spindle and epithelioid cell nevi) occur in children or adolescents and, less often, in adults. They are elevated, spheroid, pink, smooth nodules, usually on the head or neck. Spitz tumors grow rapidly, reaching 3 to 5 mm in 6 months or less. They are composed of large spindle or epithelioid melanocytes in the epidermis and dermis (Fig. 28-72). The cells, although to some extent stereotypic, are so atypical that an incorrect diagnosis of melanoma may be made, even though melanoma is rare in childhood. Most Spitz tumors are benign and are called Spitz nevi. Some, especially in adults, have atypical features, and are called atypical Spitz tumors (AST). Those that metastasize, although usually not beyond regional nodes, and the very small number that progress and cause death, are termed "Spitz melanomas." Therefore, the prognosis is to some extent uncertain, especially in adults. Sometimes in these lesions, as in other rare categories of melanocytic tumors, a descriptive diagnosis, such as "melanocytic tumor of uncertain malignant potential" (MELTUMP), is all that can be rendered. Genomic assessment of copy number variation in tumor cell nuclei can be of assistance in decision making regarding therapy. Most Spitz tumors have fusion gene rearrangements forming constitutively activated chimeric oncogenes, rather than the point mutations of oncogenes that are the rule in melanomas. Common fusion partners include genes often seen in aggressive malignancies such as leukemia or lung cancer, including, for example *ALK*, *NTRK1*, *ROS*, and also occasionally *BRAF*; these abnormalities do not correlate with aggressive behavior in Spitz nevi.

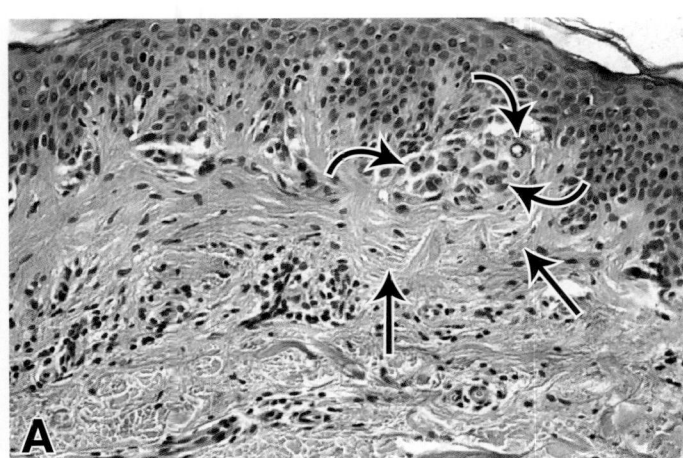

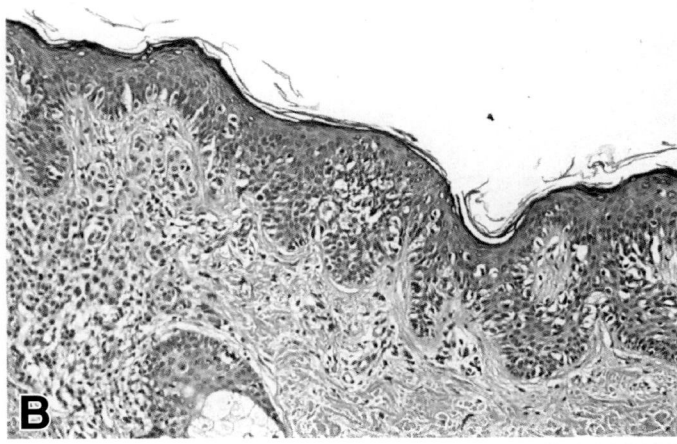

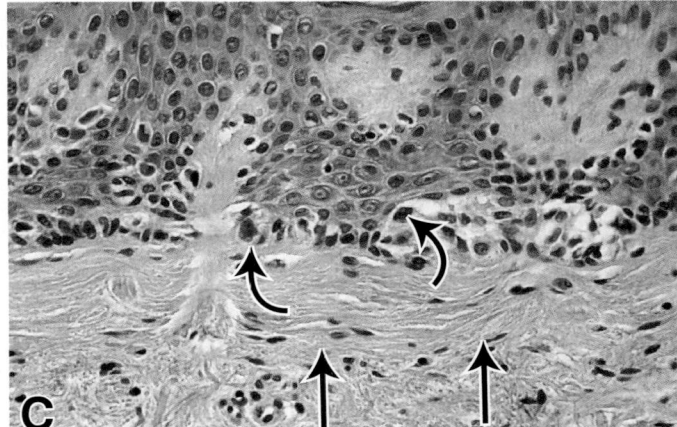

FIGURE 28-71. Dysplastic nevus. A. Features include bridging of rete ridges by nests of melanocytes, melanocytes with cytologic atypia (*curved arrows*), lamellar fibroplasia (*straight arrows*), and a scant perivascular lymphocytic infiltrate **B.** On the *left* is a zone containing typical dermal nevus cells of a compound melanocytic nevus. The epidermis on the *right* contains a proliferation of atypical melanocytes with lamellar fibroplasia. This photomicrograph is taken at the junction of the papular and macular components of this dysplastic nevus. Dysplasia usually develops in the macular portion, which takes up most of the field. **C.** Irregular melanocytic nests resting above lamellar fibroplasia (*straight arrows*) exhibit large epithelioid melanocytes with atypia (*curved arrows*).

Blue Nevus

Blue nevi appear in childhood or late adolescence as dark blue, gray or black, firm, well-demarcated papules or nodules on the dorsal hands or feet or on the buttocks, scalp, or face. They are benign neoplasms characterized by an activating mutation of a specific gene, usually *GNAQ* or *GNA11* (which encode α-subunits of the regulatory G proteins, G_q or G_{11}, respectively), differing from other nevi, and resembling the genomic landscape of ocular melanoma. Their clinical appearance may prompt an excisional biopsy to rule out nodular

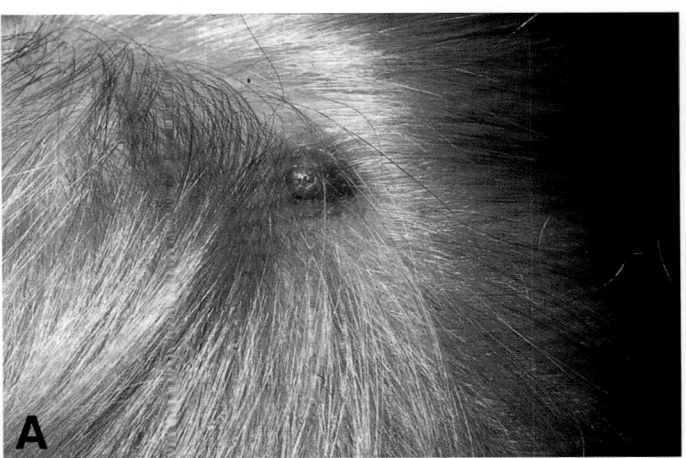

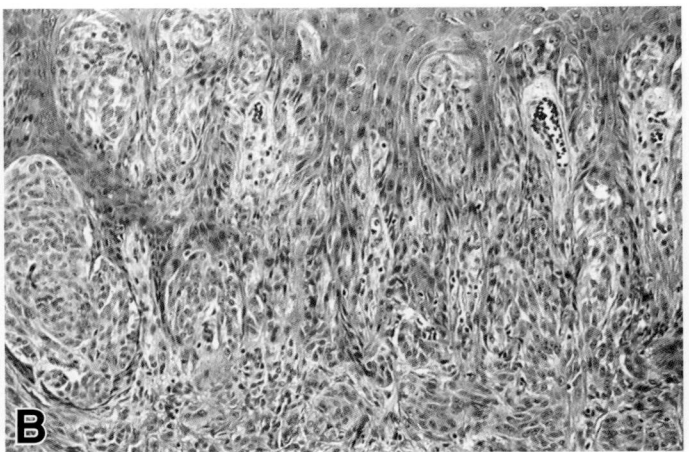

FIGURE 28-72. Spindle and epithelioid cell (Spitz) nevus. A. A symmetric pink nodule appeared suddenly on the scalp of a child and then remained stable for several weeks before it was excised. (From Elder DE, Elenitsas R, Johnson BL, et al. *Synopsis and Atlas of Lever's Histopathology of the Skin.* Philadelphia, PA: Lippincott Williams & Wilkins; 1999.) **B.** Spitz tumors are composed of large melanocytes with prominent nuclei. The melanocytes are present in large nests within a hyperplastic epidermis. Even though the cells are large and, at first glance, suggest melanoma, they are much more uniform than the cells of most malignant melanomas.

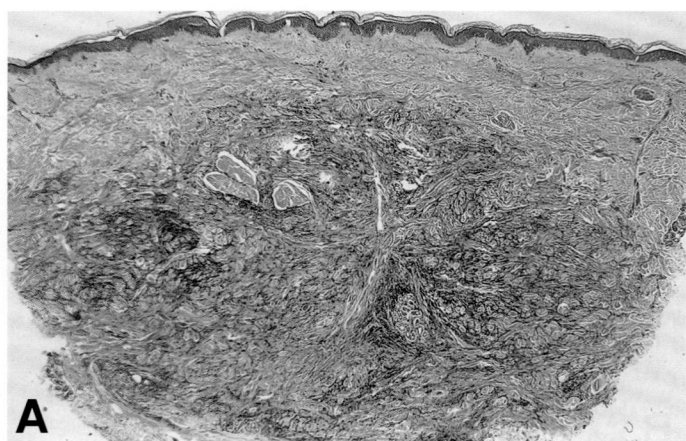

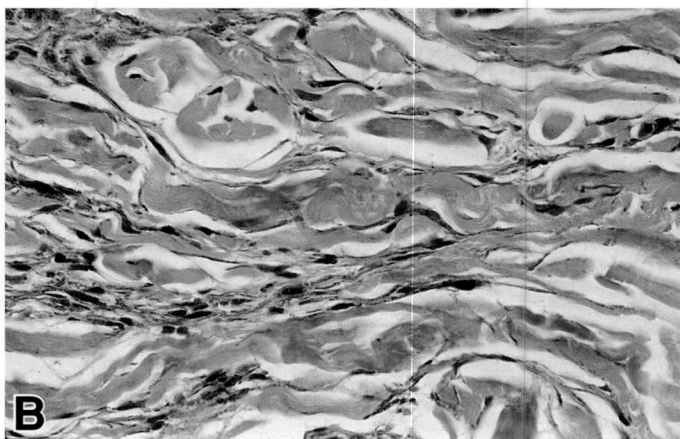

FIGURE 28-73. Blue nevus. A. Within the dermis there is a poorly defined but symmetric spindle cell proliferation that appears dark brown. **B.** The lesion is composed of elongated cells with heavily pigmented dendrites and small bland nuclei. (From Elder DE, Elenitsas R, Johnson BL, et al. *Synopsis and Atlas of Lever's Histopathology of the Skin*. Philadelphia, PA: Lippincott Williams & Wilkins; 1999.)

melanoma. Melanin-containing melanocytes with long, thin dendrites are present in the superficial to mid-dermis, where they are often admixed with numerous melanin-containing macrophages (Fig. 28-73). There are also rare examples of "cellular blue nevi" and "malignant blue nevi."

Verrucae Are Warts Caused by Human Papillomavirus (HPV)

Verrucae are cutaneous tumors. They are elevated, circumscribed, symmetric, epidermal proliferations that often appear papillary. *They are caused by HPV.*

PATHOLOGY:

- **Verruca vulgaris,** or the **common wart,** is an elevated papule with a verrucous (papillomatous) surface. A papilla, the defining feature of a papilloma, is a finger of connective tissue usually containing a vessel, covered by a glove of epithelium. Such lesions

may be single or multiple and occur most on the dorsal surfaces of the hands or on the face. Verruca vulgaris displays hyperkeratosis and papillary epidermal hyperplasia with columns of parakeratosis above the papillae (Fig. 28-74). **Koilocytes** (i.e., enlarged keratinocytes with pyknotic nuclei surrounded by a halo-like cleared areas, constituting a viral cytopathic effect) are seen within the upper epidermis. Viral inclusions are difficult to identify (Fig. 28-75). HPV, especially serotypes 2 and 4, can be identified in verruca vulgaris. There is no malignant potential.

- **Plantar warts** are benign, frequently painful, hyperkeratotic nodules on the soles of the feet. Occasionally, similar lesions appear on the palms of the hands **(palmar warts)**. Plantar warts are endophytic or exophytic, papillary, squamous epithelial proliferations. The cells contain abundant cytoplasmic inclusions that resemble the darker-staining keratohyalin granules. The nuclei of keratinocytes near the base of these warts also contain pink nuclear inclusions. HPV type 1 is the etiologic agent.

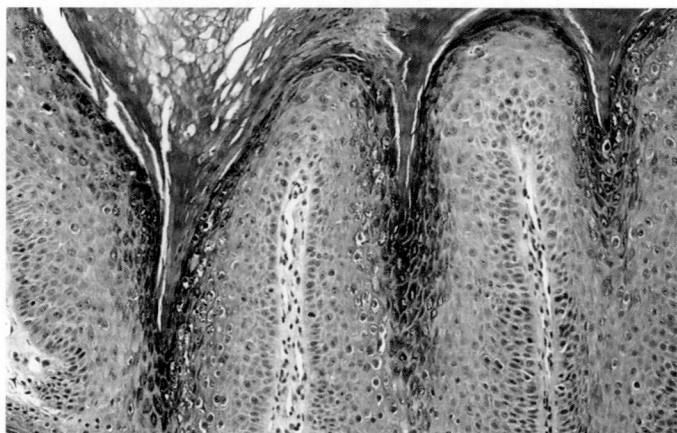

FIGURE 28-74. Verruca vulgaris. This is the prototype of papillary epidermal hyperplasia. It is composed of squamous epithelial-lined fronds with fibrovascular cores. Blood vessels within the cores extend close to the surface of verrucae, making them susceptible to traumatic hemorrhage and the resultant black "seeds" that patients observe.

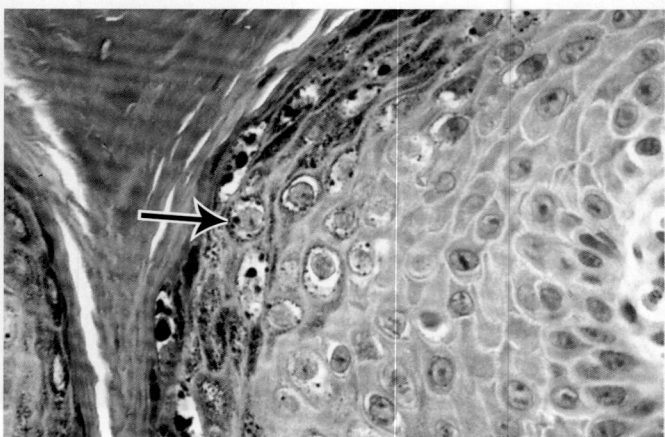

FIGURE 28-75. Verruca vulgaris. Characteristic cytopathic changes occur in the outer portion of the stratum spinosum and stratum granulosum, in which there is perinuclear vacuolization and prominent keratohyalin granules, with homogeneous blue inclusions (*arrow*).

- **Verruca plana,** or "flat warts," are small flat papules that typically appear on the face. They display slight elongation of rete ridges (acanthosis), striking hypergranulosis and superficial koilocyte formation. HPV types 3 and 10 often elicit these lesions. They do not progress to cancer.
- **Condyloma acuminatum** is a venereally transmitted wart usually caused by HPV serotypes 6 and 11 and occurring primarily around the genitalia. These are papillary squamous proliferations. Koilocytosis and an almost continuous cap of parakeratosis are usually present. Squamous carcinomas may develop, especially when HPV types 16 and 18 are involved.
- **Bowenoid papulosis,** also caused by HPV types 16 and 18, is characterized by multiple hyperpigmented papules on the genitalia. Lesions may be histologically identical to squamous cell carcinoma (SCC) in situ in that they display disordered epithelial maturation and scattered keratinocyte atypia. The lesions also exhibit parakeratosis and irregular acanthosis. Although Bowenoid papulosis often regresses, it may progress to dysplasia or malignancy.
- **Epidermodysplasia verruciformis** is a rare autosomal recessive disease characterized by impaired cell-mediated immunity and consequent enhanced susceptibility to HPV infection. It has been linked to mutations in *EVER1* or *EVER2*, genes that encode transmembrane channel proteins involved in zinc metabolism and homeostasis. Warts similar to those of verruca plana, with confluence into patches, are widespread. It first appears in childhood, and squamous cell carcinoma develops in 30% to 60% of patients. HPV types 5, 8, 9, and 47 are most common.

A Keratosis Is a Benign Horny Growth Composed of Keratinocytes

Seborrheic Keratosis

Seborrheic keratoses are scaly, frequently pigmented, elevated papules or plaques with scales that are easily rubbed off. They are common later in life but their etiology is unknown. Seborrheic keratoses tend to be familial. Clinically and microscopically, they appear "pasted on" and contain broad anastomosing cords of mature stratified squamous epithelium, forming papillae and associated with small cysts of keratin (horn cysts) (Fig. 28-76). Seborrheic keratoses are innocuous but are a cosmetic nuisance to some. The sudden appearance of many seborrheic keratoses may be associated with internal malignancies ("sign of Leser-Trélat"), especially gastric adenocarcinoma.

Actinic Keratosis

Actinic keratoses ("from the sun's rays") are keratinocytic neoplasms that develop in sun-damaged skin as circumscribed keratotic patches or plaques, commonly on the backs of the hands or the face. The stratum corneum no longer has a loose basketweave structure, and is replaced by a dense parakeratotic scale. Basal keratinocytes are atypical (Fig. 28-77). Actinic keratoses may evolve into squamous carcinomas in situ and finally into invasive cancers, but most are stable and many regress.

Keratoacanthoma

Keratoacanthomas are rapidly growing keratotic papules on sun-exposed skin that develop over 3 to 6 weeks into crater-like nodules. They reach a maximum size of 2 to

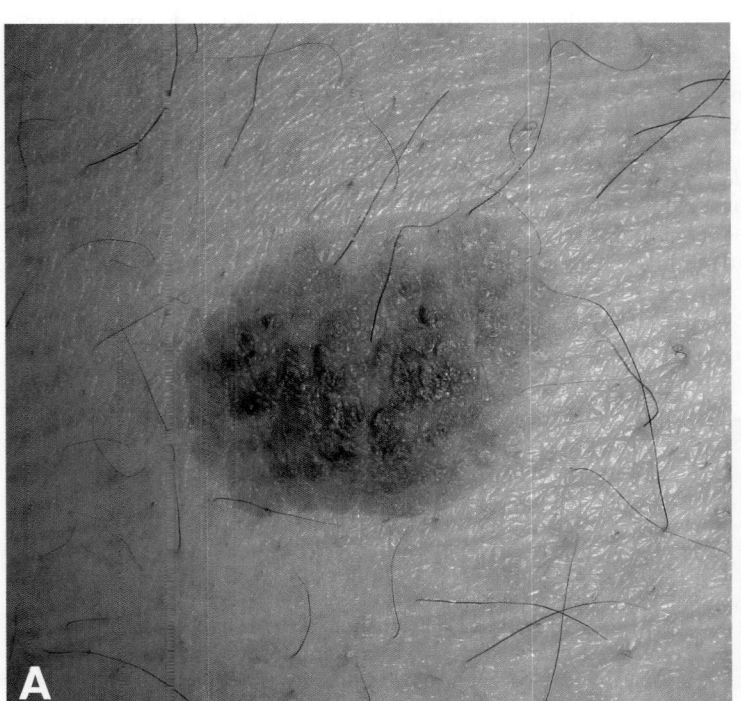
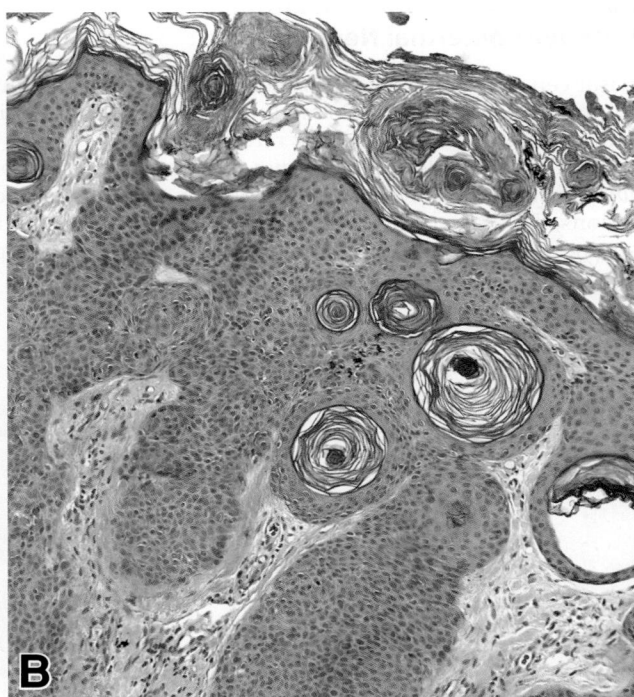

FIGURE 28-76. Seborrheic keratosis. A. Sharply defined, "stuck-on" brown lesions are a common presentation. **B.** Broad anastomosing cords of mature stratified squamous epithelium are associated with small keratin cysts.

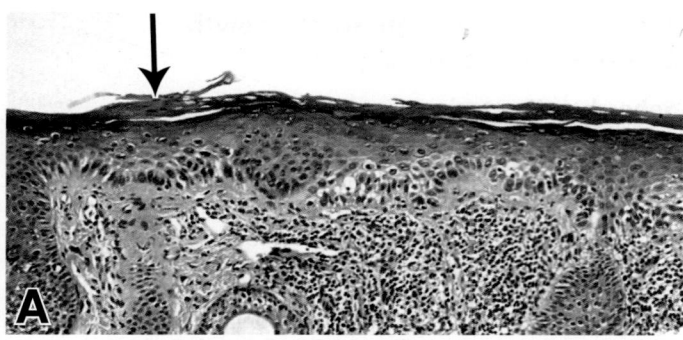

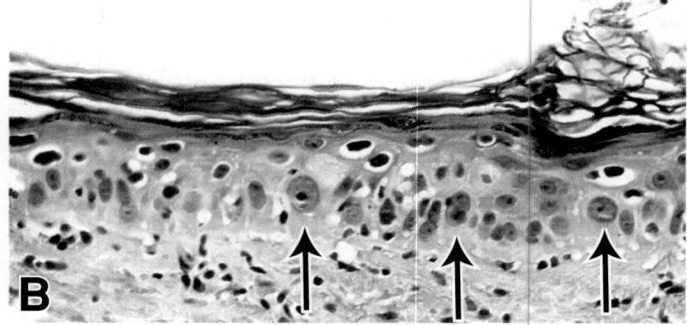

FIGURE 28-77. Actinic keratosis. A. A low-power view reveals cytologic atypia within the stratum basalis and lower stratum spinosum with loss of polarity. A lichenoid, band-like, lymphocytic infiltrate is frequently present. Parakeratosis is present here only in a small focus (*arrow*). **B.** High-power examination reveals striking cytologic atypia of basal keratinocytes (*arrows*), the hallmark of actinic keratoses.

3 cm. Spontaneous regression usually follows within 6 to 12 months, leaving an atrophic scar. Some lesions may cause considerable damage before they regress, and some fail to regress. Keratoacanthomas are now considered to be (usually) self-resolving variants of squamous cell carcinoma.

PATHOLOGY: Histologically, keratoacanthomas are endophytic proliferations of keratinocytes. The lesion is cup shaped, with a central, keratin-filled umbilication and overhanging ("buttressing") epidermal edges (Fig. 28-78). Keratinocytes at the base are large and have abundant homogeneous, eosinophilic ("glassy") cytoplasm. At the lower aspect of the lesion, irregular tongues of squamous epithelium infiltrate the collagen of the reticular dermis. Microabscesses of neutrophils and entrapped dermal elastic fibers are often present within the lesion.

Basal Cell Carcinoma Is a Locally Invasive Epidermal Neoplasm

Basal cell carcinoma (BCC) is the most common malignant tumor in people with pale skin. It may be locally aggressive, but metastases are exceedingly rare.

BCC usually develops on sun-damaged skin of people with fair skin and freckles. However, unlike squamous lesions, BCC also arises on areas not exposed to intense sunlight. It is unusual to find BCC on the fingers and dorsal

surfaces of the hands. The tumor is thought to derive from pluripotential cells in the basal layer of the epidermis, more specifically, in the bulge region of the hair follicle.

In several heritable syndromes, BCC originates on skin that has had little light exposure. In **nevoid BCC syndrome**, multiple tumors occur in the context of a complex multisystem disease. The syndrome also includes pits (dyskeratoses) on the palms and soles, mandibular cysts, hypertelorism and a predisposition to other neoplasms, including medulloblastoma. The BCCs of this syndrome appear at a young age and may number in the hundreds.

MOLECULAR PATHOGENESIS: Germline mutations in the *PTCH* tumor suppressor gene on chromosome 9q22 cause nevoid BCC syndrome. This gene encodes patched-1, a protein that interacts with sonic hedgehog to regulate cell growth, differentiation, and patterning. Somatic mutations in *PTCH* have been implicated in up to 90% of sporadic BCCs and may be targeted in therapy of advanced lesions.

PATHOLOGY: BCCs contain nests of deeply basophilic epithelial cells with narrow rims of cytoplasm that are attached to the epidermis and protrude into the subjacent papillary dermis (Fig. 28-79).

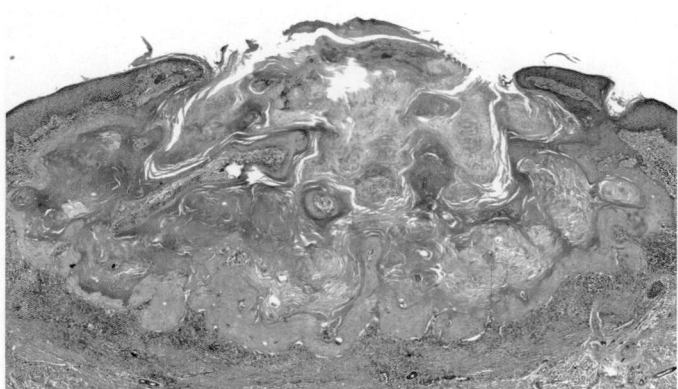

FIGURE 28-78. Keratoacanthoma. A keratin-filled crater (*center*) is lined by glassy proliferating keratinocytes.

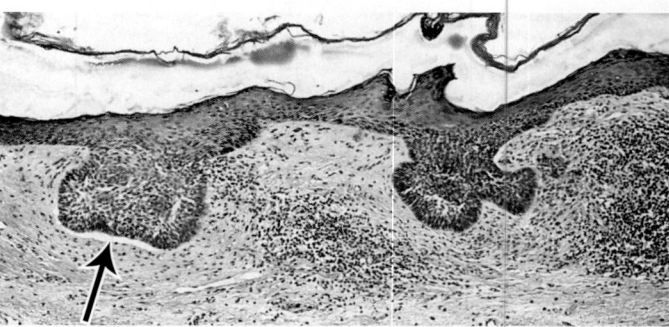

FIGURE 28-79. Basal cell carcinoma, superficial type. Buds of atypical basaloid keratinocytes extend from the overlying epidermis into the papillary dermis. Peripheral keratinocytes mimic the stratum basalis by palisading. Separation artifact (*arrow*) is present because of poorly formed basement membrane components and a hyaluronic acid-rich stroma that contains collagenase.

The lesions are commonly ulcerated. At least in early lesions, there is typically a specialized loose mucinous stroma containing fibroblasts and lymphocytes. Clefting artifact between the epithelial cells of the tumor and the stroma may sometimes help to distinguish BCC from other adnexal neoplasms with basaloid cell proliferation. The central part of each nest contains closely packed keratinocytes that are slightly smaller than normal epidermal basal keratinocytes and have occasional apoptoses and mitoses. The periphery of each nest has an organized layer of polarized, columnar keratinocytes, with the long axis of each cell perpendicular to the surrounding stroma ("peripheral palisading"). **Superficial, multicentric BCC** is composed of apparently isolated, but actually interconnected, nests that usually remain confined to the papillary dermis and manifest clinically as a spreading plaque (Fig. 28-79). **Nodulocystic BCC** is also attached to the epidermis and exhibits the same cytologic and architectural features as the superficial type of BCC but grows more deeply into the dermis. Usually, tumor cells of the dermal islands are associated with a mucinous ground substance and are surrounded by an array of fibroblasts and lymphocytes. It is important to distinguish BCCs with pushing borders from those with an infiltrative pattern, because **infiltrating BCC** tumors may be more likely to recur locally and progress. Infiltrating BCCs with particularly dense sclerotic stroma are called **morpheaform BCCs** because of a clinical resemblance to scar-like lesions of localized scleroderma (also known as "morphea").

CLINICAL FEATURES: Common forms of BCC are categorized as follows:

- **Pearly papule** is the prototypic nodulocystic type of lesion, so named because it resembles a 2- to 3-mm pearl. It is covered by tightly stretched epidermis and is laced with small, delicate, branching vessels (telangiectasia) (Fig. 28-80A).
- **Rodent ulcer** is a small crater in the center of the pearl (Fig. 28-80A).

- **Superficial BCC** appears as a scaly, red, sharply demarcated plaque.
- **Morpheaform BCC** is a pale, firm, scar-like tumor that is ill defined on and especially beneath the skin surface, making it particularly difficult to eradicate (Fig. 28-80B).
- **Pigmented BCC** may grossly resemble malignant melanoma. The pigment comes from reactive melanocytes that populate the tumor.

Treatment of BCC usually involves various excision or eradication procedures.

Cells of Squamous Cell Carcinomas May Resemble Differentiated Keratinocytes

SCCs are second only to BCCs in skin cancer incidence. SCCs are most common on sun-damaged skin of fair individuals with light hair and freckles, and often originate in actinic keratoses. They are exceedingly rare on normal black skin.

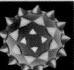

ETIOLOGIC FACTORS: SCCs have multiple causes, UV light being the most common, but also including ionizing radiation, chemical carcinogens, and HPV. SCCs arising in sun-damaged skin rarely metastasize (<2%). They may also arise in chronic scarring processes, such as osteomyelitis sinus tracts, burn scars ("Marjolin ulcers") and areas of radiation dermatitis. In these settings, they metastasize more often. Over 90% of SCCs, and many actinic keratoses, have mutated *TP53* genes.

PATHOLOGY: Tumor cells in SCC mimic epidermal stratum spinosum in varying degrees and extend into the subjacent dermis, forming a crusted tumor (Fig. 28-81A). The edges of many tumors have changes typical of actinic keratosis, namely, a variably thickened epidermis with parakeratosis and significant atypia of basal keratinocytes, or there may be fully evolved squamous cell carcinoma in situ (Fig. 28-81B).

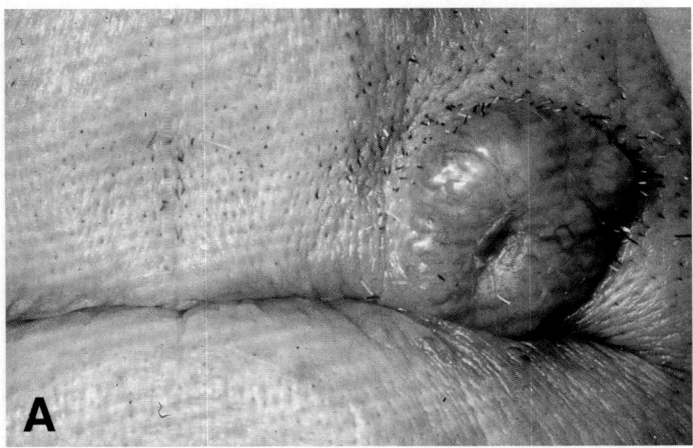

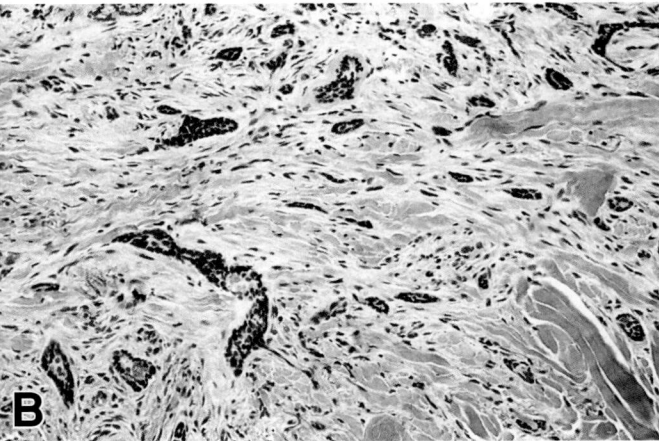

FIGURE 28-80. Basal cell carcinoma (BCC). A. Pearly papule: the tumor exhibits typical rolled pearly borders with telangiectases and central ulceration. (From Elder DE, Elenitsas R, Johnson BL, et al. *Synopsis and Atlas of Lever's Histopathology of the Skin.* Philadelphia, PA: Lippincott Williams & Wilkins; 1999.) **B.** Microscopic examination of morpheaform BCC shows a sclerosing and infiltrative lesion. Irregularly branching strands of tumor cells permeate the dermis, with induction of a cellular, fibroblastic, hyaluronic acid–rich stroma.

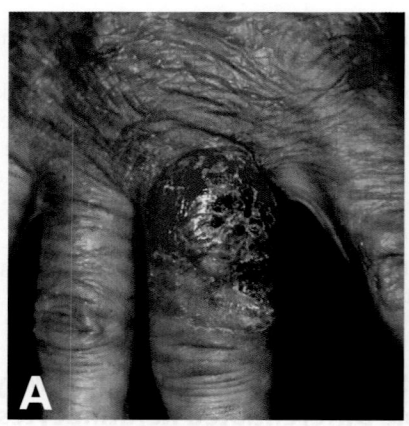
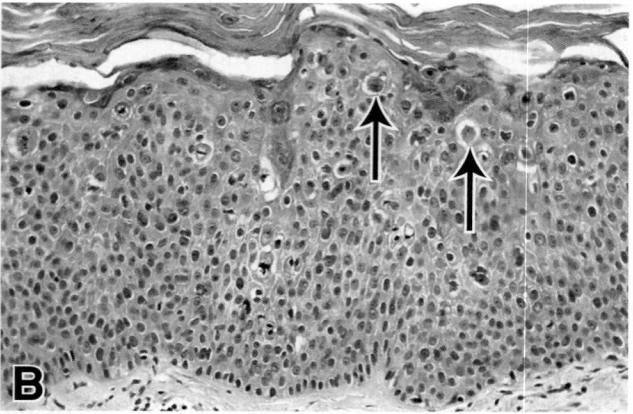

FIGURE 28-81. Squamous cell carcinoma. A. An ulcerated, encrusted and infiltrating lesion is seen on the sun-exposed dorsal aspect of a finger. **B.** A microscopic view of the periphery of the lesion shows squamous cell carcinoma in situ. The entire epidermis is replaced by atypical keratinocytes. Mitoses are apparent, as is apoptosis (*arrows*).

CLINICAL FEATURES: SCCs characteristically arise in chronically sun-exposed areas such as the backs of the hands, face, lips, and ears (Fig. 28-81A). Early lesions are small, scaly or ulcerated, erythematous papules, which may be pruritic. They are usually treated by excision, or sometimes by electrosurgery, topical chemotherapy, or radiation therapy.

Merkel Cell Carcinomas Are Aggressive Tumors of Neuroendocrine Cells That Have Epithelial Differentiation

These are typically solitary, dome-shaped, red to violaceous nodules or indurated plaques on the skin of the head and neck in elderly white patients. Merkel cell carcinomas (MCCs) are aggressive tumors that are lethal in 25% to 70% of patients within 5 years.

PATHOLOGY: Most MCCs have large nests of undifferentiated cells that resemble small cell carcinoma of the lung (Fig. 28-82). Peripherally, the tumors may show a trabecular pattern. Nuclear chromatin is dense and evenly distributed; cytoplasm is scant and mitotic figures and nuclear fragments are common. Cytokeratin 20 is distributed in a "perinuclear dot" cytoplasmic pattern. Tumor cells also express neuroendocrine markers such as chromogranin and synaptophysin.

MOLECULAR PATHOGENESIS: The genome of Merkel cell polyoma virus (MCV) is present in 75% of MCCs and may play a role in tumorigenesis (see Chapter 5). Tumorigenicity is associated with a truncating mutation of the MCV *Tag* gene which encodes a viral T antigen recognized by the immune system in MCV infection. The mutation promote tumorigenesis and impairs T cell responses to MCV.

Adnexal Tumors Differentiate Toward Skin Appendages

Adnexal tumors appear as elevated small skin nodules that may occur in people with family histories of similar tumors. They often appear at puberty. Although most are benign, malignant behavior is sometimes observed.

Sebaceous Neoplasms

Sebaceous neoplasms, including sebaceous adenomas, sebaceous epitheliomas (sebaceomas), and sebaceous carcinomas, are all tumors of sebaceous gland derivation, with varying degrees of differentiation. Clinically, sebaceous adenomas and epitheliomas are small, slow-growing papules or nodules commonly on the head and neck. Sebaceous carcinomas, however, often present larger than 1 cm and have a predilection for periocular sites. Sebaceous adenomas comprise a well-circumscribed proliferation of sebaceous

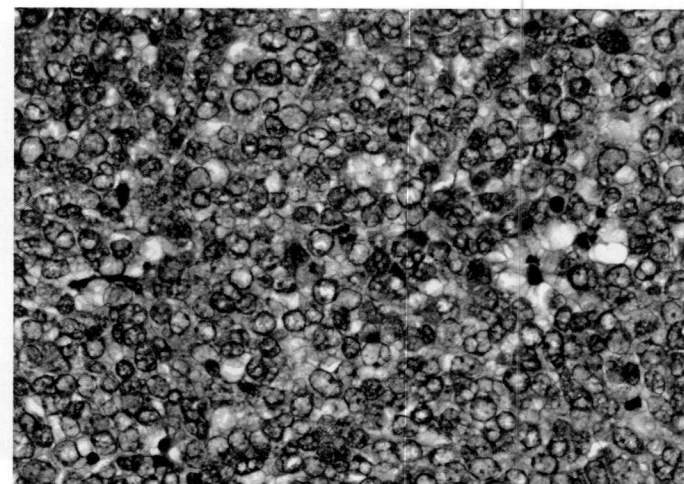

FIGURE 28-82. Merkel cell carcinoma. The tumor is composed of solid nests of undifferentiated cells that resemble small cell carcinoma of the lung.

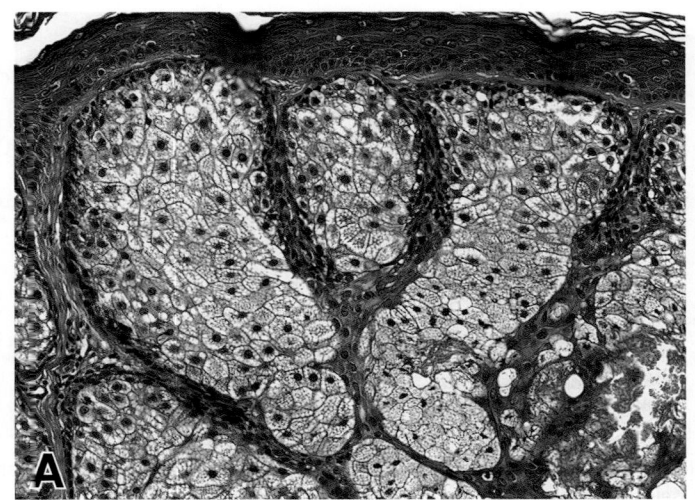
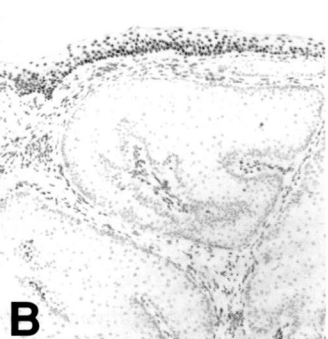

FIGURE 28-83. Sebaceous Adenoma. A. Microscopic view of a sebaceous adenoma showing large sebaceous lobules composed primarily of clear sebocytes lined by basaloid germinative cells. **B.** Immunohistochemical staining for mismatch repair protein MSH6 shows loss of nuclear staining in the neoplastic sebaceous cells with intact staining in the benign surface epithelium and in intermixed dermal fibroblasts. These findings indicate this patient may have Muir–Torre syndrome.

lobules, primarily composed of mature sebocytes with some germinative basaloid cells. Sebaceous epitheliomas have a preponderance of germinative cells (Fig. 28-83). Sebaceous carcinomas exhibit histologic features of malignancy, such as severe cytologic atypia, high mitotic activity, and infiltrative growth.

 MOLECULAR PATHOGENESIS: Patients with Muir–Torre syndrome, a variant of hereditary nonpolyposis colorectal carcinoma (HNPCC), may present with sebaceous neoplasms. HNPCC (or Lynch syndrome) is associated with inherited germline defects in mismatch repair genes such *MLH1*, *MSH2*, and *MSH6*. These mutations promote microsatellite instability and increase the rate of mutations in cancer cells. See Chapters 5 and 19 for more about HNPCC.

Cylindroma

Cylindromas are benign adnexal neoplasms with features of sweat gland differentiation. They may be solitary or multiple elevated nodules around the scalp. Occasionally, they become large and cluster about the head ("turban tumors"). Cylindromas have sharply circumscribed nests of deeply basophilic cells surrounded by a hyalinized, thickened BMZ (Fig. 28-84). Brocke–Spiegler syndrome is a rare autosomal dominant genetic condition that results in a range of skin appendage tumors including hair follicle and sweat gland tumors, as well as tumors in other sites including salivary glands. The syndrome includes the limited variants, familial cylindromatosis, and multiple familial trichoepitheliomas (MFT1). This has been linked to germline mutations in the tumor suppressor CYLD, which encodes a protein that regulates NFκB signaling in apoptosis.

Syringoma

Syringomas typically occur about the eyelid and upper cheek as small, elevated, flesh-colored papules. Small ducts resembling intraepidermal portions of eccrine sweat ducts are seen (Fig. 28-85).

Poroma

Poroma is a solitary usually endophytic neoplasm comprised of basaloid to squamoid cells with narrow ductal lumina and occasional cystic spaces. The pattern has been interpreted as eccrine sweat gland differentiation. These tumors are firm, flat, or raised lesions, usually less than 2 cm in diameter, that develop on the sole or sides of the foot or on the hands or fingers. Poromas extend from the lower portion of the epidermis into the dermis as broad, anastomosing bands of uniform, cuboidal cells. Occasional malignant lesions with similar differentiation are called **porocarcinomas**.

Trichoepithelioma

Trichoepithelioma is a neoplasm that differentiates toward hair structures. It is usually a solitary lesion, but in "multiple trichoepithelioma syndrome," it occurs as an autosomal dominant trait. This syndrome has been linked to mutations

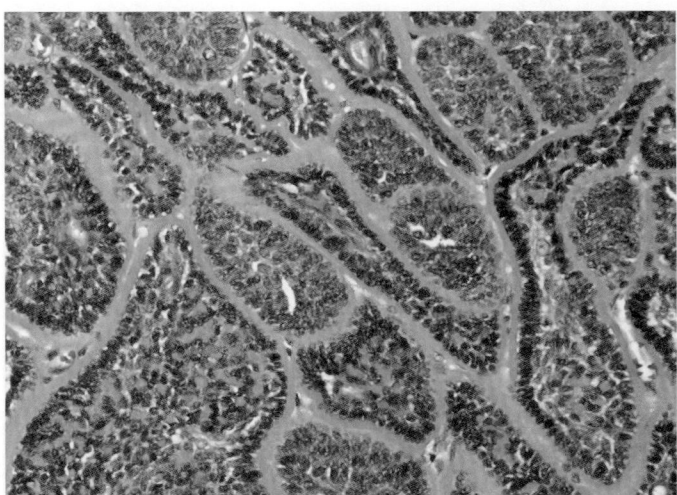

FIGURE 28-84. Cylindroma. Sharply circumscribed islands of basophilic epithelial cells reside in a jigsaw puzzle–like array. Dense eosinophilic hyaline sheaths surround each island.

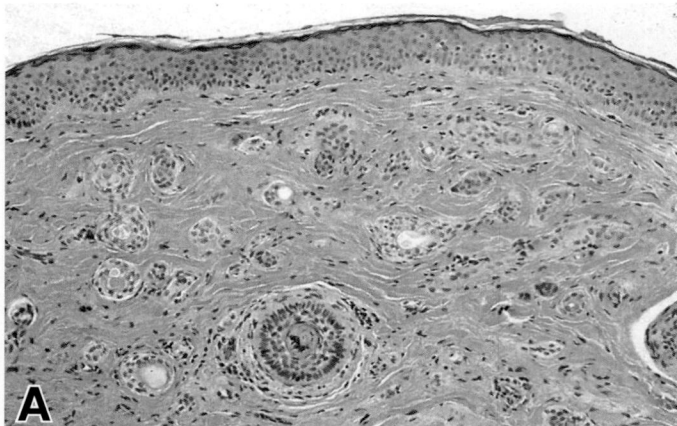
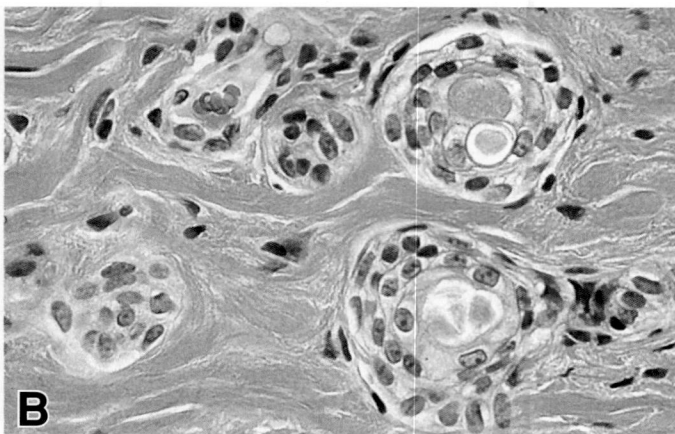

FIGURE 28-85. Syringoma. A. Within the upper dermis is an epithelial proliferation forming ducts, tubules, and solid islands amid a dense fibrous stroma. **B.** The ductal differentiation closely mimics that of the straight dermal eccrine duct, with a central lumen and cuticle (amorphous eosinophilic material) formation.

in *CYLD,* the gene also implicated in familial cylindromatosis (described above), and some authorities regard the two clinical syndromes as different forms of the same disease. Lesions begin to appear at puberty, on the face, scalp, neck, and upper trunk. Trichoepitheliomas resemble BCCs but lack atypia and contain many "horn cysts" (keratinized centers surrounded by basophilic epithelial cells).

Fibrohistiocytic Tumors of the Skin Have a Varied Spectrum of Differentiation

Dermatofibroma

Dermatofibroma is a common, benign tumor of fibroblast-like cells and macrophages. The former are the neoplastic cells. These tumors occur on the extremities as dome-shaped, firm

nodules with ill-defined borders and pink to dark brown pigmentation. They rarely exceed 5 mm. The papillary and reticular dermis are replaced by fibrous tissue that forms ill-defined small cartwheels, with small central vascular spaces (Fig. 28-86). The tumors are not well demarcated and blend into the surrounding dermis. The overlying epidermis is hyperplastic and often hyperpigmented.

Dermatofibrosarcoma Protuberans

Dermatofibrosarcoma protuberans (DFSP), a tumor with intermediate malignant potential, is a slowly growing nodule or indurated plaque that appears mostly on the trunk of young adults. Local recurrence after attempted complete excision is common, but metastases are rare. The most common histologic pattern is a poorly circumscribed, monotonous

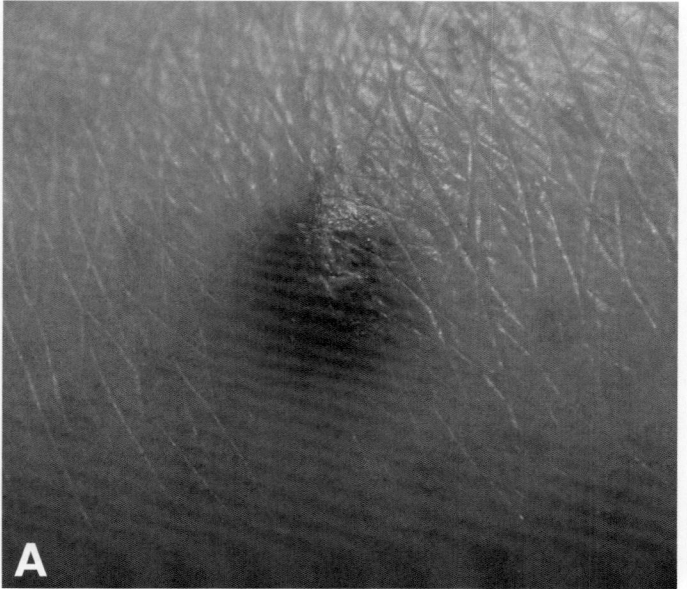
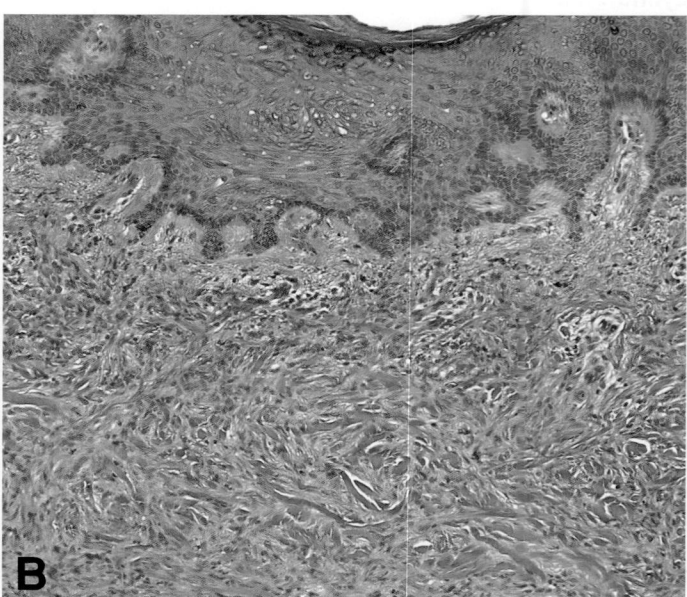

FIGURE 28-86. Dermatofibroma. A. A brown dome-shaped nodule on the lower leg is a common clinical presentation. **B.** Fibrous tissue replaces the dermis and forms poorly defined cartwheels, with overlying epidermal hyperplasia and basaloid proliferation, resembling basal cell carcinoma.

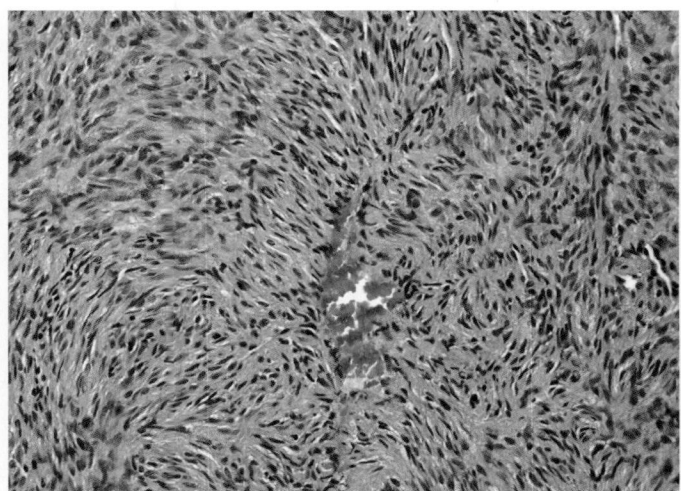

FIGURE 28-87. Dermatofibrosarcoma protuberans. Tumor cells form small cartwheels with central vascular spaces.

population of spindle cells arranged in a dense "storiform" (pinwheel-like) array (Fig. 28-87). The tumor extends into the subcutis along fat septa and interstices, creating an infiltrative, honeycomb-like pattern. Tumor cells display CD34, a marker of endothelial cells, and some neural tumor cells, as well as dermal fibroblast-like dendritic cells, the probable cell of origin. Positivity for CD34 may help distinguish this tumor from a dermatofibroma, which does not express this antigen.

MOLECULAR PATHOGENESIS: More than 90% of DFSPs have a chromosomal translocation t(17;22), which fuses the collagen gene (*COL1A1*) with the *PDGF-B* gene. This balanced translocation creates a fusion gene product that causes transcriptional upregulation of the *PDGF-B* gene and increased neoplastic growth.

Mycosis Fungoides Is a Variant of Cutaneous T-Cell Lymphoma

The etiology of mycosis fungoides (MF) is unknown, but this malignancy of helper T cells (CD4⁺) may be a pathologic response initiated by chronic exposure to an antigen.

PATHOLOGY: In the early stages of the disease, delicate, erythematous plaques appear, often by the buttocks. These plaques show psoriasiform changes in the epidermis. The early inflammatory cell infiltrates in the dermis are polymorphic and are often not diagnostic of MF.

Skin involvement becomes progressively more prominent and infiltrative (Fig. 28-88). The most important histologic feature of MF is the presence of atypical lymphocytes in the epidermis ("epidermotropism"). In later stages, the dermal infiltrate becomes dense to the point of forming tumor nodules. Increasing numbers of atypical lymphocytes that display hyperchromatic, convoluted ("cerebriform") nuclei are seen in the papillary dermis

and epidermis. Circumscribed nests of these atypical lymphocytes ("Pautrier microabscesses") eventually involve the epidermis. T-cell receptor gene rearrangement studies define a clonal cell population.

Sézary syndrome is a systemic dissemination of cutaneous T-cell lymphoma. The characteristic feature is the presence of cerebriform lymphocytes in the peripheral blood.

CLINICAL FEATURES: MF affects older people, has a slight male predominance, and preferentially affects blacks over whites. It is classically divided into three stages: patch, plaque, and tumor. In the patch stage, which may persist for months, eruptions consist of scaly, erythematous macules that may be slightly indurated. They usually involve the lower abdomen, buttocks, and upper thighs as well as women's breasts, and can mimic other dermatitides such as psoriasis or eczema (Fig. 28-87A). Plaque-stage lesions are more infiltrated and circumscribed. As these coalesce, involvement becomes more widespread. Large, variably shaped tumor nodules can form on existing indurated plaques or on apparently normal skin. Large cell transformation, spread to lymph nodes, or visceral involvement portend reduced survival. Therapy includes UV light, topical nitrogen mustard and electron beam therapy.

HIV Infection Is Associated With Various Skin Diseases

Kaposi Sarcoma

This malignant tumor of endothelial cells of blood vessels was once seen only in older people of Mediterranean descent or in Africans. With the advent of HIV infection, Kaposi sarcoma (KS) is most often seen in patients with AIDS. *Human herpesvirus 8 (HHV8) is the etiologic agent of KS.*

PATHOLOGY: All cases of Kaposi sarcoma, whether associated with HIV or not, evolve through three stages: patch, plaque, and nodule. In the patch stage, a subtle proliferation of irregular vascular channels, lined by a single layer of mildly atypical endothelial cells, radiates from pre-existing blood vessels and extends almost imperceptibly into the surrounding reticular dermis. Extravasated red blood cells, hemosiderin deposition, and a sparse inflammatory infiltrate of lymphocytes and plasma cells are common.

In the plaque stage (Fig. 28-89), the entire reticular dermis is involved, with frequent extension into the subcutis and formation of bundles of spindle cells. In the nodule stage (Fig. 28-90), well-circumscribed dermal nodules are composed of anastomosing fascicles of spindle cells surrounding numerous slit-like spaces. HHV8 nuclear expression can be readily demonstrated with an immunohistochemical stain.

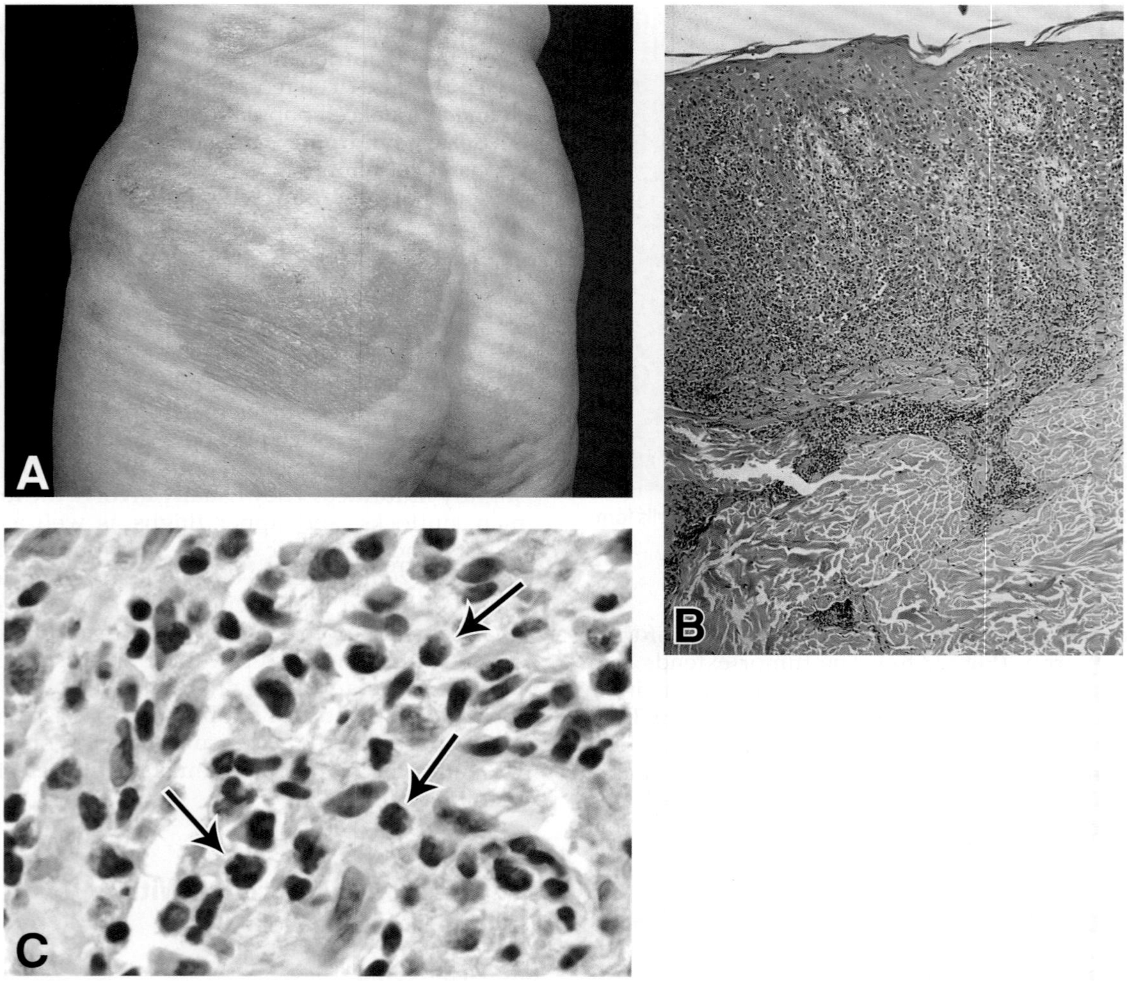

FIGURE 28-88. Mycosis fungoides. A. A 66-year-old woman presented with a 30-year history of erythematous scaly patches and plaques with telangiectases, atrophy, and pigmentation. (From Elder DE, Elenitsas R, Johnson BL, et al. *Synopsis and Atlas of Lever's Histopathology of the Skin*. Philadelphia: Lippincott Williams & Wilkins; 1999.) **B.** An atypical infiltrate of lymphocytes expands the papillary dermis and extends into the epidermis ("epidermotropism"). **C.** Some lymphocytes display hyperchromatic and convoluted ("cerebriform") nuclei (*arrows*).

Bacillary Angiomatosis

Bacillary angiomatosis is a pseudoneoplastic proliferation of capillaries that arises in response to infection with *Bartonella* species. Patients with late-stage AIDS are at risk for infection with these organisms. The proliferative lesions are red to brown papules, often in large numbers, and may be confused with Kaposi sarcoma. Silver impregnation stains highlight dense masses of bacilli within the basophilic deposits. Lesions clear with antibiotic treatment.

Eosinophilic Folliculitis

Eosinophilic folliculitis (EF) is a chronic pruritic eruption of papules, centered on hair follicles. Patients infected with HIV are a distinct population that displays EF, although variants of EF not related to HIV infection occur in other populations. Lesions occur most often on the trunk and proximal extremities. An infiltrate of lymphocytes, macrophages, and many eosinophils is present in intrafollicular and perifollicular areas and around dermal blood vessels.

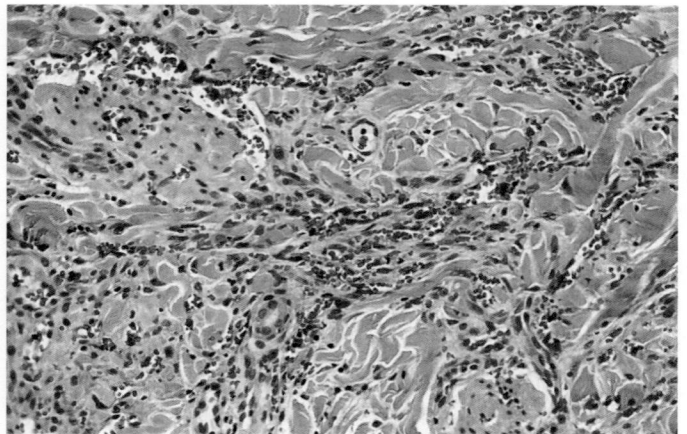

FIGURE 28-89. Kaposi sarcoma, plaque stage. A proliferation of endothelial cells extends along dermal vascular arcades and amid reticular dermal collagen. They form delicate vascular channels filled with red blood cells. Some endothelial cell collections are not canalized (have not formed lumens).

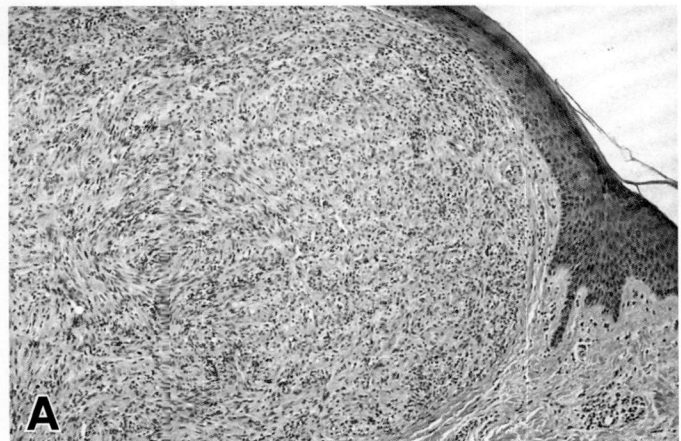

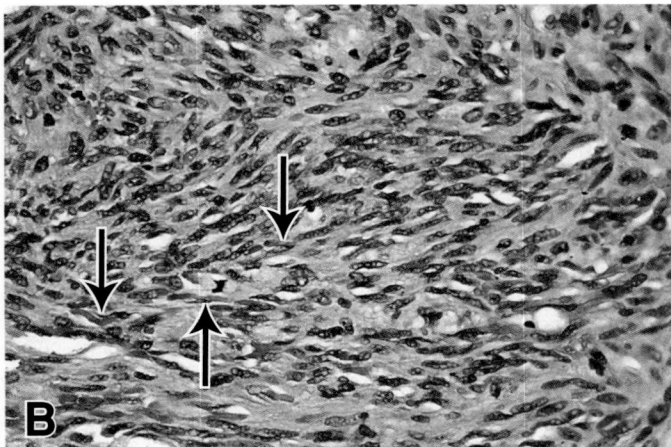

FIGURE 28-90. Kaposi sarcoma, nodule stage. A. A large nodule is composed of proliferating endothelial cells forming fascicles and vascular spaces. **B.** A higher-power view shows cytologic atypia of the spindle cells. Red blood cells appear agglutinated (*arrows*). The endothelial cells, in which the agglutinated red blood cells are present, form slit-like spaces.

PARANEOPLASTIC SYNDROMES INVOLVING THE SKIN

Diverse dermatologic manifestations may complicate internal malignancies, often preceding detection of the tumor itself. Certain pigmented lesions and keratoses are well-recognized paraneoplastic effects.

- **Acanthosis nigricans** is marked by hyperkeratosis and pigmentation of the axilla, neck, flexures, and anogenital region. *It is of particular interest because some patients with acanthosis nigricans have cancer.* The onset of acanthosis nigricans may precede, accompany, or follow detection of the cancer. More than 90% of cases occur in association with gastrointestinal carcinomas, and more than half accompany cancers of the stomach. Other cases may be associated with obesity, diabetes, and other conditions, or present as an isolated phenomenon.
- **Dermatomyositis or polymyositis** has a five- to sevenfold greater incidence in cancer patients than in the general population. The association is most conspicuous in affected men older than 50 years, among whom more than 70% have cancer. In most cases, the muscle disorder and cancer present within a year of each other. In men, lung and gastrointestinal cancers are most often associated with dermatomyositis, whereas in women, the most common association is with breast cancer.
- **Sweet syndrome** is a combination of elevated neutrophil count, acute fever and painful red plaques in the anus, neck and face, histologically characterized by a neutrophilic infiltrate. About 1/5 of cases occur with malignancies, particularly those of the hematopoietic system (see Chapter 26).

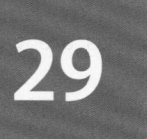

29 The Head and Neck

Joaquín J. García, Diane L. Carlson

Oral Cavity

The oral cavity extends from the lips to the pharynx (Fig. 29-1). Its boundaries are:

- The vermilion border of the lips (anterior)
- A line from the junction of the hard and soft palate to the circumvallate papillae of the tongue (posterior)
- The hard palate until its junction with the soft palate (superior)
- The anterior two-thirds of the tongue to the line of the circumvallate papillae (inferior)
- The buccal mucosa of the cheeks (lateral)

The oral mucosa is composed of keratinized epithelia of the attached gingiva, hard palate mucosa, and specialized keratinized gustatory mucosa of the dorsum of the tongue. It also includes nonkeratinized mucosal surfaces of the inner lip and inner cheek, the nonattached, movable gingiva that continues into the maxillary and mandibular sulci, ventral tongue, floor of the mouth, soft palate, and tonsillar pillars. The epithelium is three to four times the thickness of epidermis. Under the epithelium is a lamina propria of fibrous tissue and blood vessels, beneath which is the densely fibrous periosteum of the hard palate or the alveolus of the maxilla and mandible. The term **submucosa** is sometimes loosely applied to the deep connective tissue just above the

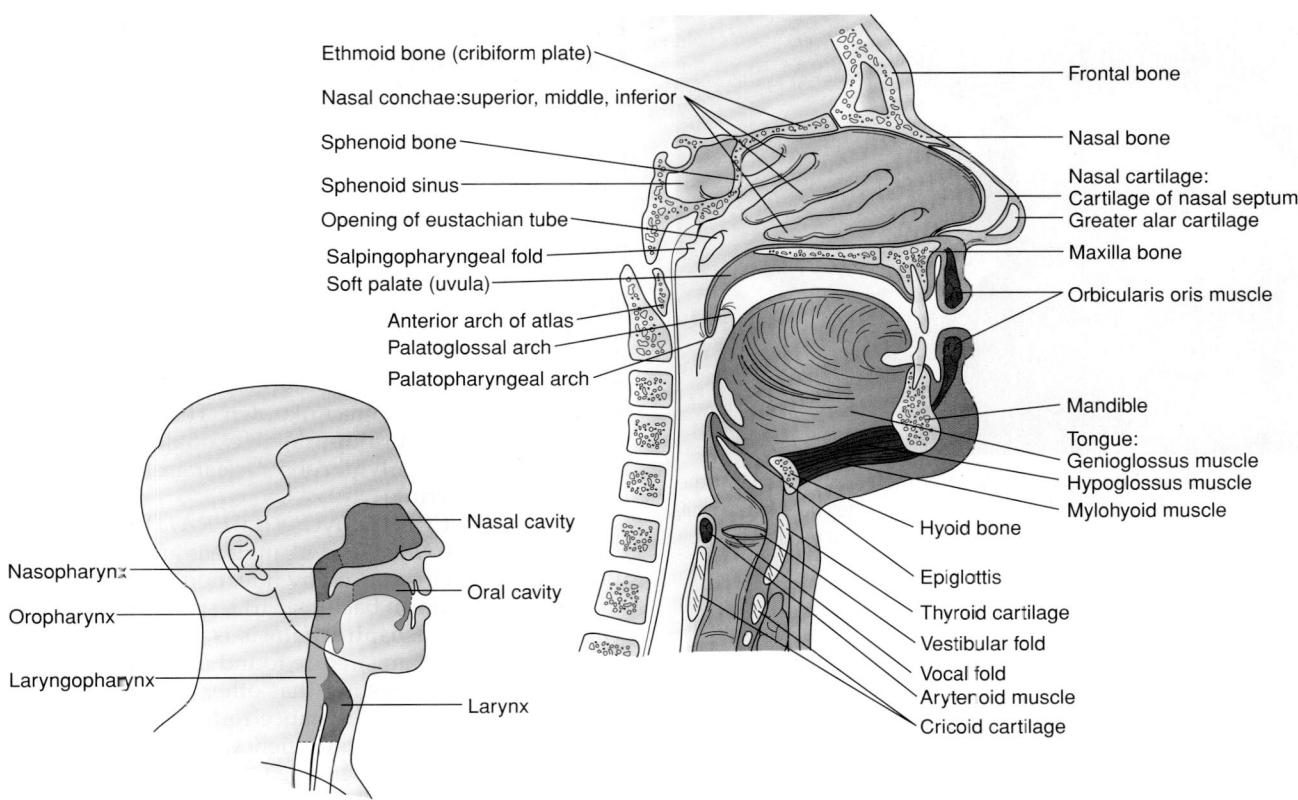

FIGURE 29-1. Structure of the oral cavity, oropharynx, and larynx. Schematic diagram of the oral cavity, palate, oropharynx, and larynx.

muscle layer, in which the minor salivary glands are often embedded.

Minor salivary glands, both mucous and serous, are scattered throughout the oral cavity as unencapsulated small lobules within the mucosa and submucosa. Mucous glands occur in the lamina propria, particularly in the posterior hard palatal mucosa. Minor salivary glands of pure mucous type exist in the anterior ventral portion of the tongue (called Blandin, or Nunn, glands). Serous salivary glands lie near circumvallate papillae on the posterior and lateral tongue (von Ebner glands). Mixed mucoserous and mainly mucous glands predominate in the rest of the oral cavity. Minor salivary glands also occur in the retromolar mandibular ridge, but not the anterior hard palate or gingiva.

The anterior two-thirds of the dorsum of the tongue is covered by keratinized stratified squamous epithelium that is specialized to form **filiform papillae** (pointed projections of keratin). Between these are **fungiform papillae,** mushroom-shaped mucosal elevations containing taste buds. **Circumvallate papillae** separate the anterior two-thirds of the tongue from the posterior one-third and contain taste buds at their base. The final group is the **foliate papillae,** in the posterior lateral tongue in a series of ridges. Each taste bud is a barrel-shaped collection of modified epithelial cells that extend vertically from the basal lamina to the epithelial surface, opening via a taste pore.

DEVELOPMENTAL ANOMALIES

FACIAL CLEFTS: If facial structures fail to fuse in the 7th week of embryonic life, facial clefts form. The most common of these is cleft upper lip **(harelip).** It may be unilateral or bilateral and is often associated with cleft palate (see Chapter 6).

Crouzon syndrome (craniofacial dysostosis) and **Apert syndrome** (acrocephalosyndactyly) are autosomal dominant disorders associated with craniosynostosis (premature fusion of the cranial sutures). This can lead to **brachycephaly** (flat head), **scaphocephaly** or **dolichocephaly** (the head is disproportionately long and narrow or "boat" shaped) or **trigonocephaly** (triangular shaped). Severe craniosynostosis may result in **Kleeblattschädel deformity** ("cloverleaf" skull). *Both syndromes reflect mutations in fibroblast growth factor receptor 2 (FGFR2), on the long arm of chromosome 10.*

MOLECULAR PATHOGENESIS: The FGFR2 gene encodes a G-protein–coupled receptor that, upon binding its ligands, signals to induce bone maturation. In **Apert syndrome,** a mutant FGFR2 protein is produced, which promotes premature bone fusion in the calvarial (skull) bones.

HAMARTOMAS AND CHORISTOMAS: These lesions are common in the oral cavity. Fordyce granules are aggregates of sebaceous glands in the oral cavity **(choristoma).** They occur on the buccal mucosa, lingual surface and lip in 70% to 95% of adults; rarely, they coalesce to form mass lesions.

Abnormal descent of the thyroid during development may create submucosal foci of **ectopic thyroid** between the tongue and suprasternal notch. The base of the tongue between the foramen cecum and epiglottis is the most common site for ectopic thyroid **(lingual thyroid).**

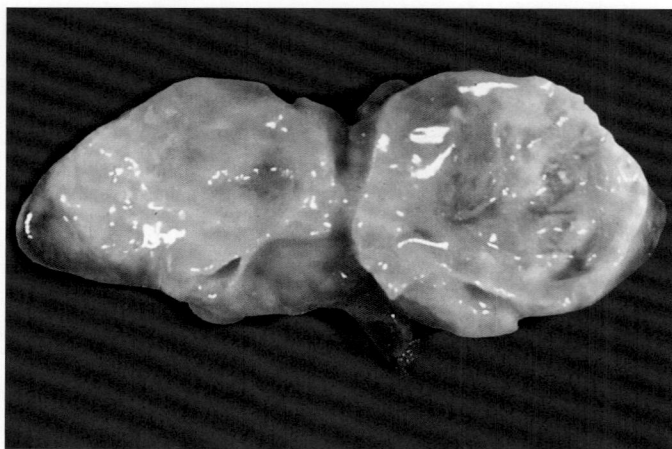

FIGURE 29-2. Branchial cleft cyst. Most of these cysts arise from the second branchial cleft and occur laterally in the neck. They have a thin wall, contain turbid fluid and are lined by stratified squamous or respiratory-type epithelium.

Over 75% of patients with lingual thyroid lack a cervical thyroid ("total migration failure"). Thus, surgically removing a lingual thyroid may lead to hypothyroidism and stunted physical growth and mental development (**cretinism**; see Chapter 6). In fact, 70% of patients with symptomatic lingual thyroid are hypothyroid and 10% suffer from cretinism. Malignancies in ectopic thyroid glands are rare but are generally papillary carcinomas. An abnormally descended thyroid may also affect parathyroid gland development and localization.

Thyroglossal duct cysts result from persistence and cystic dilatation of the thyroglossal duct midline in the neck. This anomaly usually occurs above the thyroid isthmus but below the hyoid bone. Patients, usually under age 40, present clinically with a palpable 4- to 5-cm midline nodule, which moves up and down upon swallowing. Surgery is the treatment of choice. Malignancies, predominantly papillary thyroid carcinomas, arise in up to 1% of thyroglossal duct cysts.

BRANCHIAL CLEFT CYST: Branchial cleft cysts originate from branchial arch remnants. They occur in the lateral anterior neck or parotid gland, mostly in young adults, and contain thin, watery fluid and mucoid or gelatinous material (Fig. 29-2). These cysts are usually lined by squamous epithelium, with occasional foci of ciliated respiratory or pseudostratified columnar epithelium.

INFECTIONS OF THE ORAL CAVITY

Bacteria and spirochetes are present normally in the oral cavity and are generally harmless. If the mucosa is injured or immunity is impaired, otherwise normal oral flora may become pathogenic (see Chapter 9 for further discussion).

These terms are used to describe localized inflammation of the oral cavity:

- **Cheilitis** (lips)
- **Gingivitis** (gum)
- **Glossitis** (tongue)
- **Stomatitis** (oral mucosa)

Bacterial and Fungal Infections of the Oral Cavity May Involve Both Commensal and Invasive Species

SCARLET FEVER: Scarlet fever is mainly a childhood disease caused by β-hemolytic streptococci (*Streptococcus pyogenes*). Damage to vascular endothelium by the erythrogenic toxin results in a rash on the skin and oral mucosa. The tongue acquires a white coating, through which hyperemic fungiform papillae project as small red knobs ("strawberry tongue"). Untreated scarlet fever can lead to glomerulonephritis and heart disease (**acute rheumatic fever**; see Chapters 11 and 17).

APHTHOUS STOMATITIS (CANKER SORES): Aphthous stomatitis is a common disease characterized by small, painful, recurrent, solitary, or multiple ulcers of oral mucosa. Its cause remains unknown. The lesion is a shallow ulcer covered by a fibrinopurulent exudate, with underlying mononuclear and polymorphonuclear inflammation. They heal without scarring.

ACUTE NECROTIZING ULCERATIVE GINGIVITIS (VINCENT ANGINA): Vincent angina is an acute necrotizing ulcerative gingivitis caused by infection with two symbiotic organisms, a fusiform bacillus and a spirochete (*Borrelia vincentii*). The term **fusospirochetosis** is used to designate this infection. These organisms are found in the mouths of many healthy people, suggesting that other factors are involved, particularly decreased resistance to infection due to inadequate nutrition, immunodeficiency, or poor oral hygiene. Vincent angina is characterized by punched-out erosions of the interdental papillae. The process tends to spread and eventually involves all gingival margins, which become covered by a necrotic pseudomembrane.

LUDWIG ANGINA: Ludwig angina is a rapidly spreading cellulitis originating in the submaxillary or sublingual space but extending to involve both. Several aerobic and anaerobic oral bacteria have been implicated. Ludwig angina is a potentially life-threatening inflammatory process. It is uncommon in developed countries except in patients with chronic illnesses associated with immunosuppression.

Ludwig angina is most often related to dental extraction or trauma to the floor of the mouth. After extraction of a tooth, hairline fractures may occur in the lingual cortex of the mandible, providing microorganisms ready access to the submaxillary space. Infection may dissect into the parapharyngeal space along fascial planes and from there into the carotid sheath. This may lead to a mycotic internal carotid artery aneurysm, erosion of which may cause massive hemorrhage. The inflammation may also dissect into the superior mediastinum to involve the pleural space and pericardium.

DIPHTHERIA: Infection with *Corynebacterium diphtheriae* is characterized by a patchy pseudomembrane, which often begins on the tonsils and pharynx but may also involve the soft palate, gingiva, or buccal mucosa (see Chapter 9).

TUBERCULOSIS: Primary tuberculosis of the oral mucosa is rare. Most lesions spread from the lung, with bacilli carried in sputum and entering small breaks in the mucosa. There, they produce irregular, painful ulcers, mostly on the tongue. Caseating granulomatous inflammation is typical.

SYPHILIS: Primary syphilitic chancres may form on the lips, tongue, or oropharyngeal mucosa after contact with an infectious lesion (see Chapter 9). Regional lymphadenitis follows and heals by itself in a few weeks. A diffuse mucocutaneous eruption of the secondary stage follows. Syphilitic lesions in the oral mucosa are multiple gray-white patches overlying ulcerated surfaces. They may remit and also recur spontaneously. **Gummas** on the palate and tongue may appear years after initial infection as firm nodular masses that ulcerate and may cause palatal perforation.

ACTINOMYCOSIS: Actinomycetes are common denizens of the oral cavity in healthy people. Invasive actinomycosis is most often caused by *Actinomyces bovis*, but *Actinomyces israelii* is sometimes seen. The organisms produce chronic granulomatous inflammation and abscesses that drain by fistula formation, with suppurative infection containing characteristic yellow "sulfur granules." In cervicofacial actinomycosis, soft tissue infection may extend to adjacent bones, most often to the mandible.

CANDIDIASIS: Also called **thrush** or **moniliasis**, oral candidiasis is caused by *Candida albicans* (see Chapter 9), which commonly resides on mucosal surfaces of the oral cavity, gastrointestinal tract, and vagina. To cause disease, the fungus must penetrate tissues, albeit superficially. Oral candidiasis may be seen in patients with diabetes and those with compromised immune systems. The incidence in patients with AIDS is 40% to 90%. Lesions are white, slightly elevated, soft patches that consist mainly of fungal hyphae.

Oral Viral Diseases Are Mostly Recurrent Herpesvirus Infections

HERPES SIMPLEX VIRUS TYPE 1: Herpes labialis (cold sores, fever blisters) and herpetic stomatitis are caused by herpes simplex virus (HSV) type 1 and are among the most common viral infections of the lips and oral mucosa in children and young adults. Transmission is via aerosol, and the virus can be recovered from saliva of infected people. Disease starts with painful inflammation of affected mucosa, followed shortly by formation of vesicles. These result from "ballooning degeneration" of epithelial cells, some of which show intranuclear inclusions (Fig. 29-3). The vesicles rupture to form shallow, painful, 1- to 10-mm ulcers, which heal spontaneously without scarring.

Once HSV enters the body, it remains dormant in the trigeminal ganglion until it becomes reactivated by stresses such as trauma, allergy, menstruation, pregnancy, exposure to ultraviolet light or other viral infections. Recurrent

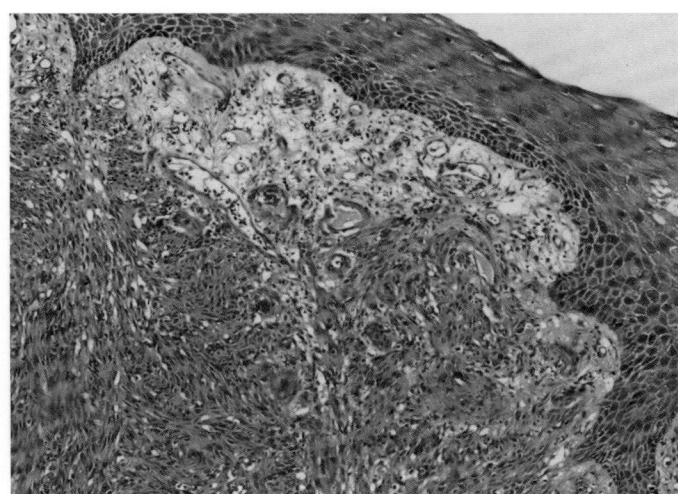

FIGURE 29-4. Kaposi sarcoma. This palate biopsy demonstrates an intact overlying squamous mucosa. Within the underlying lamina propria, there is a malignant spindle cell proliferation forming slit-like spaces filled with extravasated red blood cells.

oral cavity vesicles almost invariably develop on a mucosa that is tightly bound to periosteum, for example, the hard palate.

HUMAN PAPILLOMAVIRUS (HPV)–RELATED DISEASES: The HPV family of viruses (see Chapter 9) causes epithelial proliferations including papillomas (e.g., sinonasal, Schneiderian papillomas, and other papillomas of upper aerodigestive tract sites). "High-risk" HPV, mainly types 16 and 18, as well as 31, 33, and 35, is strongly associated with oropharyngeal squamous cell carcinoma (SCC, see below).

EPSTEIN BARR VIRUS–RELATED DISEASES: Epstein–Barr virus (EBV) is a member of the Herpesvirus family that causes oral hairy leukoplakia, various lymphoid diseases (see Chapter 20) and epithelial cancers in the nose and pharynx (see below).

HUMAN HERPES VIRUS 8 (HHV8): HHV8 is associated with **Kaposi sarcoma** (KS). This tumor occurs most often in the skin (see Chapter 24) but can also involve, among other places, the tongue and oral cavity. These tumors resemble their cutaneous counterparts (Fig. 29-4). Immunosuppressed patients (e.g., transplant recipients or patients infected with HIV-1) are at very high risk for this disease. It is also seen in elderly men of Mediterranean/East European descent and in non–HIV-infected middle-aged adults and children in equatorial Africa.

 MOLECULAR PATHOGENESIS: Details of herpesvirus molecular pathogenesis are presented in Chapter 9.

Bullous Lesions of the Oral Cavity Resemble Those in the Skin

PEMPHIGUS VULGARIS: Autoantibodies against desmogleins (desmosomal adhesion molecules) disrupt intercellular bridges between squamous cells in the skin and oral mucosa, causing the blisters, or *bullae*, of **pemphigus vulgaris**. The oral cavity is often the site of initial presentation, with cutaneous bullae developing later. These blisters are

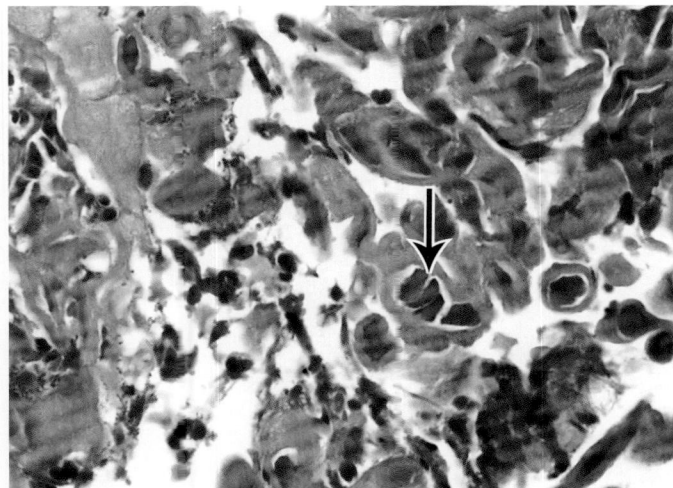

FIGURE 29-3. Herpes simplex virus type 1. A biopsy from a nonhealing ulcer on the tongue demonstrates intranuclear viral inclusions (*arrow*) within squamous cells infected by the virus.

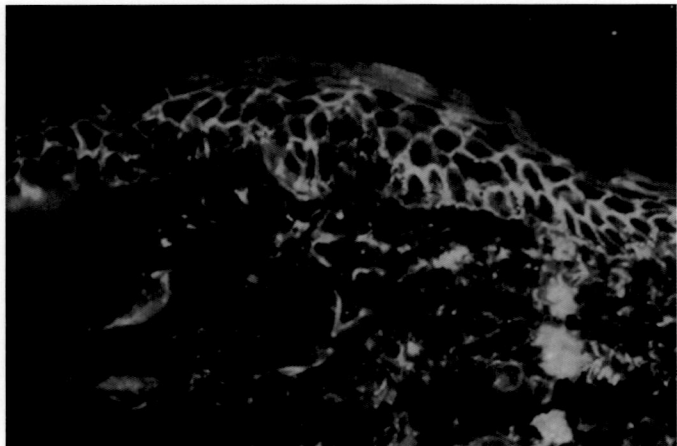

FIGURE 29-5. Pemphigus vulgaris. Direct immunofluorescence of auto-IgG antibodies demonstrates a lace-like pattern of reactivity. Antidesmoglein autoantibodies produced induce acantholysis, leading to vesicle formation in the oral cavity and the skin.

very fragile and rupture so easily that one sees scabs more often than intact bullae. The disease occurs primarily in adults between 30 and 60 years old and is the most common type of pemphigus (*vulgaris* comes from the Latin meaning "common" or "derived from the common people"). It can be life-threatening. The diagnosis is made by observing an immunofluorescence pattern of a lace-like outline of the epidermal cells (Fig. 29-5). Treatment includes steroids or other immunosuppressive agents.

BULLOUS PEMPHIGOID: Clinically, this disease resembles pemphigus, but in bullous pemphigoid, autoantibodies are directed against the epidermal basement membrane. Immunofluorescence reveals a line along the base of the epidermis. Resulting bullae are subepidermal, and thus less fragile than in pemphigus vulgaris. This is a disease of older patients and does not usually manifest in the mouth; the bullae are less likely to get infected as they do not rupture as easily. Rarely, pemphigus may be caused by medications.

BENIGN TUMORS

Benign tumors found elsewhere in the body (e.g., nevi, fibromas, hemangiomas, lymphangiomas, and squamous papillomas) may also occur in the oral cavity. Trauma may lead to ulceration of the lesions, causing bleeding or infection.

PAPILLOMA: Squamous papillomas are benign, exophytic epithelial tumors composed of branching fronds of squamous epithelium and fibrovascular cores (Fig. 29-6A). They are the most common benign oral cavity neoplasms and have been associated with HPV types 6 and 11, which are low-risk serotypes not associated with malignancy (Fig. 29-6B). They occur mainly in the third to fifth decades. The tongue, palate, buccal mucosa, tonsil, and uvula are most often involved.

BENIGN MINOR SALIVARY GLAND TUMORS: **Pleomorphic adenoma** (benign mixed tumor) is the most common oral salivary gland tumor (see below). Monomorphic adenomas such as myoepithelioma or oncocytoma are less common.

LOBULAR CAPILLARY HEMANGIOMA (PYOGENIC GRANULOMA): Lobular capillary hemangiomas are benign polypoid capillary hemangiomas that occur mainly on the skin, mucous membranes and, most often, gingiva. The term "pyogenic granuloma" is a misnomer: it is neither infectious nor granulomatous. In the mouth, they are elevated, soft, red or purple lesions, ranging in size from a few millimeters to a centimeter, with smooth, lobulated, ulcerated surfaces. They are composed of lobules or clusters of submucosal vessels, with central capillaries and smaller ramifying tributaries. In time, they may become less vascular and resemble fibromas.

An identical lesion in the gingiva **("pregnancy tumor")** may occur in pregnant women near the end of the third trimester. It may or may not regress after delivery.

PRENEOPLASTIC OR PRECURSOR EPITHELIAL LESIONS

Premalignant lesions of the upper aerodigestive tract include leukoplakia, erythroplakia, or speckled leukoplakia, terms

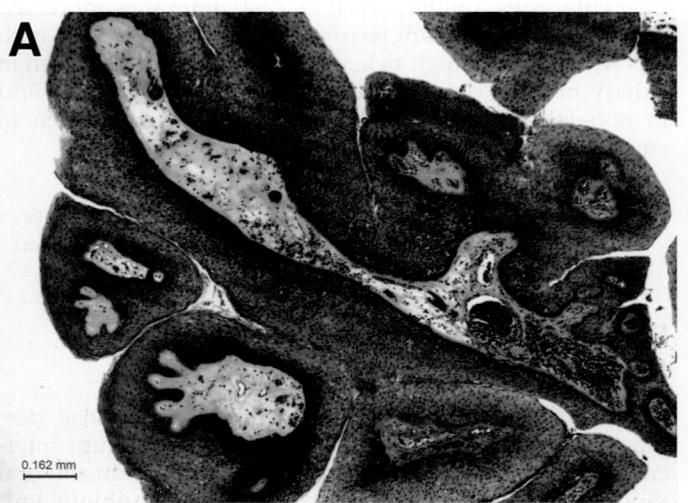

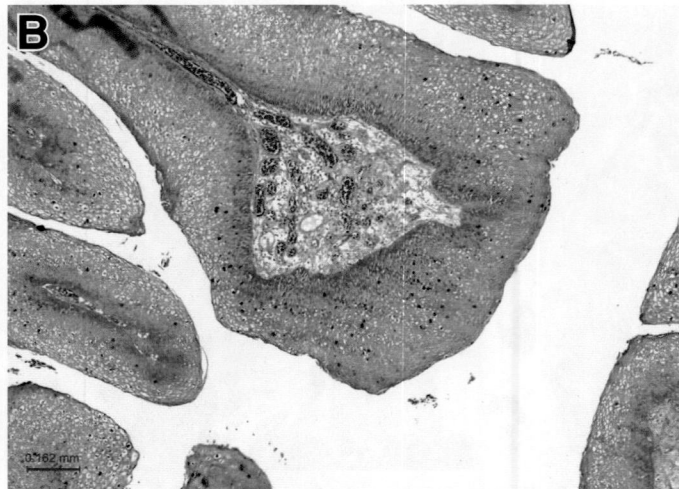

FIGURE 29-6. A. Squamous papilloma. This exophytic frond-like papillary tumor arose from the patient's uvula. **B.** In situ hybridization for low-risk human papillomavirus (LR-HPV) demonstrates nuclear localization.

describing white, red or mixed white/red epithelial lesions, respectively. *Leukoplakia* (*from the Greek, leukos, "white," and plax, "plaque"*) *is an asymptomatic white lesion on the surface of a mucous membrane*. It affects both sexes equally, mostly after the third decade. Some may become SCCs. Diverse diseases appear clinically as leukoplakia, including various keratoses and squamous carcinoma in situ. *Thus, leukoplakia is a descriptive clinical term, not a pathologic diagnosis*. Other diseases may also cause white plaques on the oral mucosa (e.g., candidiasis, lichen planus, psoriasis, syphilis). The causes of leukoplakia include tobacco use, alcoholism, and local irritation. The same factors are important in the pathogenesis of oral carcinoma.

Erythroplakia is the red equivalent of leukoplakia but occurs less often. Red areas associated with leukoplakic lesions are **speckled leukoplakia (speckled mucosa; erythroleukoplakia)**. Erythroplakia may represent moderate to severe epithelial dysplasia or carcinoma. However, not all red erythroplakic lesions indicate dysplasia/carcinoma, as many may be inflammatory.

PATHOLOGY: Leukoplakia (Fig. 29-7) occurs mostly on the buccal mucosa, tongue, and floor of the mouth. Plaques may be solitary or multiple, small lesions to large patches. Erythroplakia is often associated with ominous histopathologic features, including severe dysplasia, carcinoma in situ, or invasive SCC. In contrast, leukoplakic lesions may show a spectrum of histopathologies, from increased surface keratinization without dysplasia to invasive keratinizing squamous carcinoma. Leukoplakias, unlike erythroplakic lesions, tend to have well-demarcated margins. The risk of malignancy with leukoplakia is 10% to 12%. The chance of speckled leukoplakia becoming cancer is intermediate between "pure" leukoplakic and "pure" erythroplakic lesions, but speckled leukoplakia should be considered a variant of erythroplakia.

Oral hairy leukoplakia has shaggy parakeratosis and edema, with or without associated inflammation. It occurs mainly in people who are HIV-1 positive, usually with candidiasis. EBV-infected squamous cells are seen just beneath the keratin layer and have dense central eosinophilic inclusions and vacuolated cytoplasm. Oral hairy leukoplakia and candidiasis together suggest low CD4$^+$ lymphocyte counts and high viral load.

SQUAMOUS CELL CARCINOMA

SCCs are the most common malignant tumors of the oral mucosa and may occur at any site. Over 40,000 cases occur yearly in the United States, most often involving the tongue, then, in descending order: the floor of the mouth, alveolar mucosa, palate, and buccal mucosa. The male-to-female ratio is 2:1 for the gums, but 10:1 for the lips. The geographic distribution of oral cancer varies widely: it is the most common cancer of men in India, where it is associated with chewing of betel leaves (quid), also known as *pan*, or *Areca* nuts, also called Betal nuts.

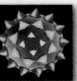 **MOLECULAR PATHOGENESIS AND ETIOLOGIC FACTORS:** Use of tobacco, alcoholism, iron deficiency (Plummer–Vinson syndrome), Fanconi anemia, physical and chemical irritants, chewing betel leaves and nuts, ultraviolet light on the lips and poor oral hygiene (dental caries, gingivitis, and ill-fitting dentures), all predispose to oral SCC. Not surprisingly, several of these factors are also connected with leukoplakia. Multiple separate SCCs may arise simultaneously (synchronous) or occur at intervals (metachronous) in the oral mucosa ("field cancerization"). Worldwide, 35% to 50% of head and neck SCCs are associated with high-risk HPV, particularly HPV-16.

Midline carcinomas of the upper aerodigestive tract linked to rearrangement of the *nuclear protein of the testis (NUT)* gene (NUT midline carcinoma) were first described in children, but are now being identified increasingly in adults. These tumors have a balanced translocation (t15;19), creating a BRD4-NUT oncogene. They tend to occur in midline structures of the upper aerodigestive tract (e.g., sinonasal tract) and non–head and neck sites (e.g., mediastinum) but may be away from the midline (e.g., parotid gland). NUT midline carcinomas are mainly undifferentiated or poorly differentiated SCCs.

PATHOLOGY: *Invasive oral cavity SCC resembles the same tumor in other sites. It is generally preceded by carcinoma in situ*. It ranges from well to poorly differentiated, plus undifferentiated and sarcomatoid variants. Well-differentiated, or grade I, tumors are frequently keratinizing (Fig. 29-8). At the opposite end of the spectrum, tumors may be so poorly differentiated that their origin is difficult to determine.

Oral SCC mainly metastasizes to submandibular, superficial, and deep cervical lymph nodes. At autopsy

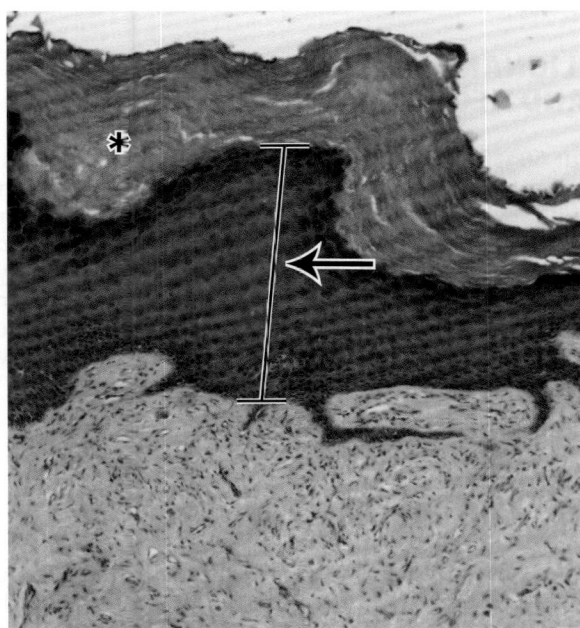

FIGURE 29-7. Leukoplakia. This lesion (*region within bracket*) was seen as a white patch on the buccal mucosa of a heavy smoker. Histologically, epithelial hyperplasia (*arrow*) and hyperkeratosis (*) are evident.

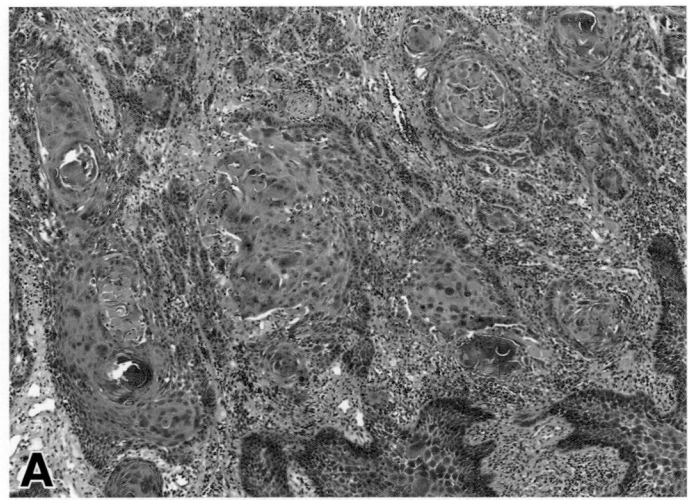

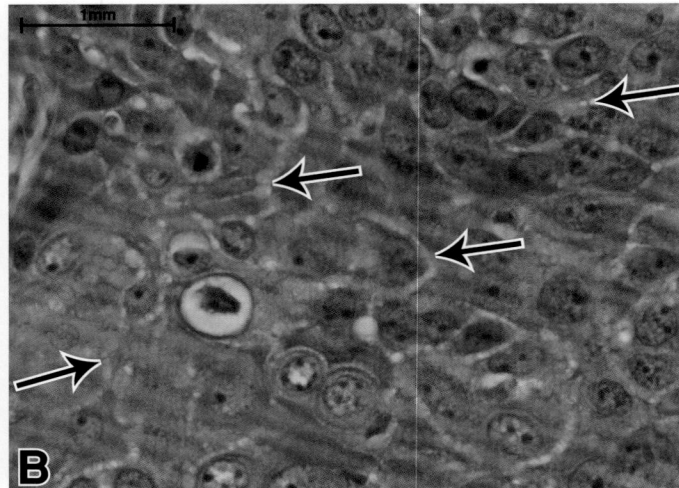

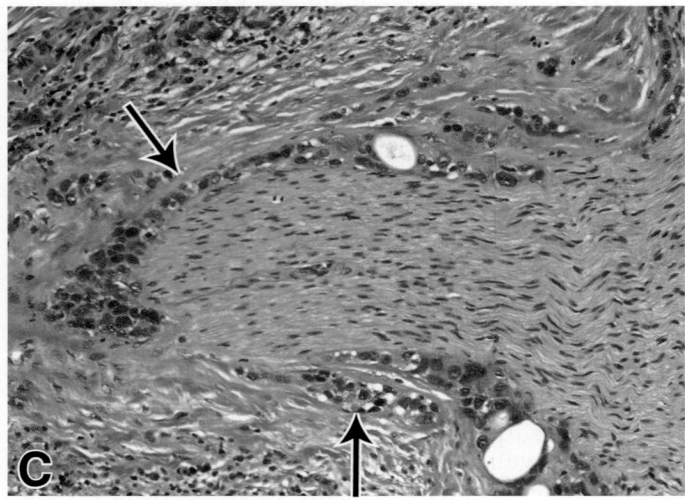

FIGURE 29-8. Invasive squamous cell carcinoma. A. This infiltrative neoplasm is composed of cohesive nests of tumor. **B.** A less differentiated tumor displays cells with pleomorphic nuclei, prominent nucleoli, brightly eosinophilic cytoplasm indicating keratinization and intercellular bridges (*arrows*) connecting adjacent cells. **C.** Perineural invasion by squamous cell carcinoma. Tumor (*arrows*) surrounds a nerve bundle.

18% of patients also have axillary metastases. More than half who die of head and neck SCC have distant, blood-borne metastases, most often in lungs, liver, and bones.

Local recurrence is predicted by a tumor's pattern of infiltration: single-cell invasion is less favorable than a broad, "pushing" border. Other prognostic factors include depth of tumor invasion, perineural invasion, and lymphovascular tumor emboli. Negative resection margins are important in local and regional control of the tumor.

Verrucous carcinomas (VCs) are highly differentiated variants of SCC that generally occur in the sixth and seventh decades; they are locally destructive but do not usually metastasize. They may arise anywhere in this region but are most common on the buccal mucosa, gingiva, and larynx. These tumors are usually white, warty to fungating, or exophytic and generally have broad bases (Fig. 29-9A). They are composed of benign-appearing squamous epithelium (without dysplasia or atypia), with marked surface keratinization and a pushing border of bulbous rete pegs (Fig. 29-9B). These tumors carry a good prognosis if completely removed.

MALIGNANT MINOR SALIVARY GLAND NEOPLASMS

About 50% of intraoral minor salivary gland tumors are malignant. These include mucoepidermoid carcinomas, adenoid cystic carcinomas (ACCs) and polymorphous adenocarcinomas (see below). Some common malignancies of major salivary glands occur less frequently in minor salivary glands (e.g., acinic cell adenocarcinoma). Polymorphous adenocarcinoma and clear cell carcinoma are more common in the palate than in major salivary glands.

BENIGN DISEASES OF THE LIPS

The lips are affected by many degenerative, inflammatory, and proliferative processes. Some, particularly those expressed in the skin and mucous membranes, are systemic; others reflect localized disease. A **mucocele** is a mucus-filled cystic lesion of the minor salivary glands that is often caused by trauma (Fig. 29-10).

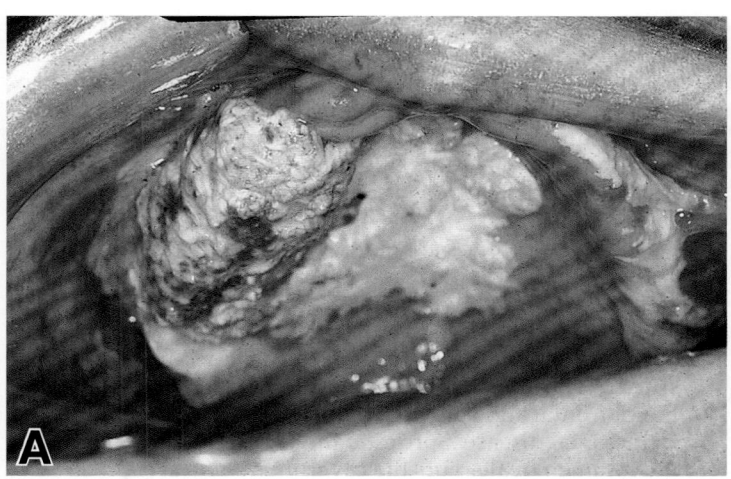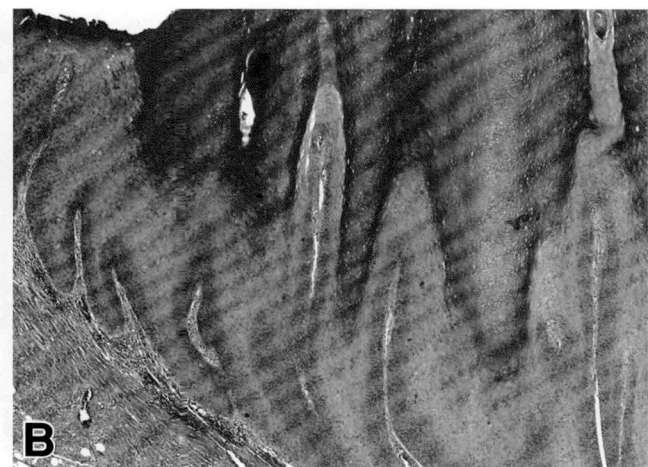

FIGURE 29-9.   Verrucous carcinoma. A. The tumor is white with an exophytic appearance involving the alveolar ridge, between the teeth and the hard palate. Note the confluent flat white (leukoplakic) appearance of the palate. **B.** Microscopically, there is prominent surface keratinization ("church-spire" keratosis) composed of bland-appearing uniform squamous cells without dysplasia, and broad or bulbous rete pegs with a pushing margin into the submucosa.

BENIGN DISEASES OF THE TONGUE

MACROGLOSSIA: All parts of the tongue may be involved in localized or systemic diseases, some of which can cause tongue enlargement. When present at birth, macroglossia is usually due to diffuse lymphangioma (Fig. 29-11) or hemangioma, although it may rarely be caused by congenital neurofibromatosis or true muscle hypertrophy. An enlarged tongue that protrudes from the mouth occurs in congenital hypothyroidism, Hurler syndrome, glycogen storage disease type II (Pompe disease), Beckwith–Wiedemann syndrome, and Down syndrome. Acquired macroglossia may be due to amyloidosis, acromegaly, or infiltration or lymphatic obstruction by tumors.

GLOSSITIS: Inflammation of the tongue can be caused by infectious or chemical agents, physical effects or systemic diseases. It may also occur in vitamin deficiencies involving, for example, vitamin B_{12}, riboflavin, niacin (B_3), and pyridoxine (B_6).

ODONTOGENIC CYSTS AND TUMORS

Odontogenic lesions are related to tooth development. Odontogenic cysts, arising from the odontogenic epithelium, may be inflammatory or developmental. Most common are

FIGURE 29-10.   Mucocele of lower lip. This cystic lesion is associated with the minor salivary glands (*upper part of image*) and was probably caused by trauma that allowed escape of mucus. The cyst has a fibrous wall and is lined by granulation tissue (*arrow*). The lumen is filled with mucus that contains numerous macrophages (*lower part of image*).

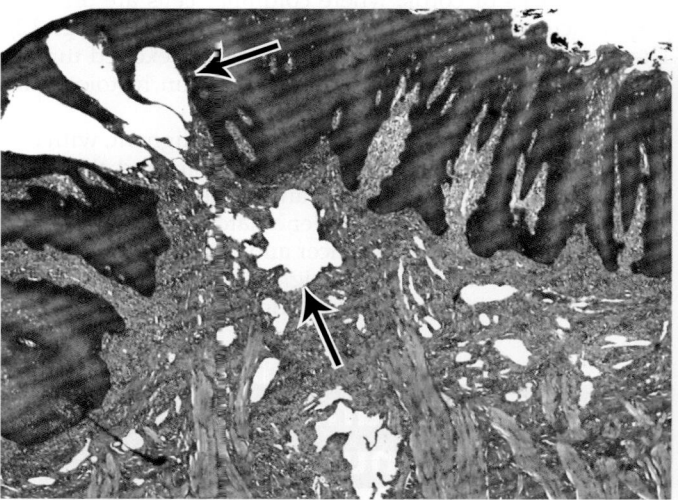

FIGURE 29-11.   Lymphangioma of the tongue. Submucosal dilated lymphatics (*arrows*) splay skeletal muscle fibers.

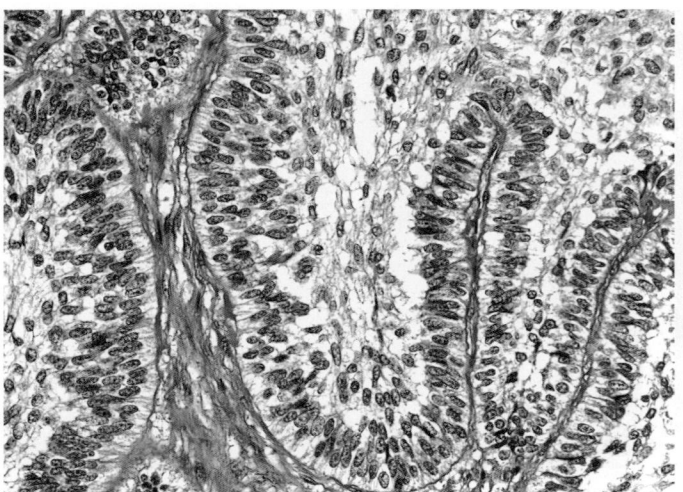

FIGURE 29-12. Ameloblastoma. A common histologic pattern is characterized by islands of odontogenic epithelium with a central stellate reticulum-like area, surrounded by basal cells with a "picket fence" appearance, due to subnuclear vacuoles.

radicular (apical, periodontal) cysts, involving tooth apices, usually after infection of the dental pulp.

Dentigerous cysts are associated with the crowns of impacted, embedded, or un-erupted teeth, most often involving mandibular and maxillary third molars. They form after the crown has completely developed; fluid accumulates between the crown and overlying enamel epithelium. Dentigerous cysts may be complicated by ameloblastoma or SCC.

Ameloblastomas are tumors of odontogenic epithelia and are the most common clinically significant odontogenic tumors. They are slow growing and locally invasive, generally following a benign clinical course, even as they can be locally destructive. Most arise in the mandibular ramus or molar area, maxilla or floor of the nasal cavity. The tumors grow slowly as central lesions of bone, showing a characteristic "soap bubble" radiographic appearance. Ameloblastomas resemble the enamel organ in its various stages of differentiation, and a single tumor may show several histologic patterns. Thus, tumor cells resemble ameloblasts at the edges of epithelial nests or cords, where columnar cells are oriented perpendicularly to the basement membrane (Fig. 29-12). The prognosis is favorable, but incompletely excised tumors recur. Some may metastasize and yet remain histologically benign (metastasizing ameloblastoma).

Ameloblastic carcinomas are frankly malignant, with cellular atypia, necrosis, nuclear pleomorphism, and abundant mitoses. Nuclei may show aberrant β-catenin expression. A missense mutation in *APC* (adenomatous polyposis coli), which plays a role in colon cancer and normally participates in the canonical Wnt-β-catenin signaling pathway, may also contribute to the pathogenesis of odontogenic tumors.

Nasal Cavity and Paranasal Sinuses

ANATOMY: The **nostril apertures** (anterior nares) lead into the **nasal vestibule,** a space lined by skin that contains hairs and sebaceous glands. Beyond the nares, the median septum divides the nasal cavity into two symmetric chambers, the **nasal fossae.** Each nasal fossa has an **olfactory region,** consisting of the superior nasal concha and the opposed part of the septum, and a **respiratory region,** which form the rest of the cavity. Laterally, the inferior, middle and superior nasal conchae **(turbinates)** overhang the corresponding nasal passages or meatus.

Paranasal sinuses are paired air spaces that communicate with the nasal cavity. The respiratory portion of the nasal cavity is covered by ciliated, columnar epithelium with interspersed goblet cells.

These anatomic interrelations determine routes of disease spread (Fig. 29-13). Infections can spread to maxillary, ethmoid, frontal and sphenoid sinuses, causing intraorbital and intracranial disease. Spread to the vein of Vesalius, medial to the foramen ovale, puts the cavernous sinus at risk.

NONNEOPLASTIC DISEASES OF THE NOSE AND NASAL VESTIBULE

Virtually all diseases of the skin can occur on the external nose, including lesions due to solar damage (e.g., actinic keratosis, basal cell carcinoma, SCC, and malignant melanoma). The many sebaceous glands of the nose are commonly affected in acne vulgaris.

Rosacea is a chronic skin disorder of the cheeks, nose, chin, and central forehead, characterized by telangiectasias (abnormally widened venules), flushing, erythema, papules, pustules, rhinophyma (a protuberant bulbous mass on the nose) and ocular manifestations. Bacteria (e.g., *Bacillus oleronius* and *Staphylococcus epidermidis*), as well as Demodex mites, have all been implicated. Inflammation is central to this disease, although the initiating factors and etiology of rosacea remain unknown. Antibiotics, such as tetracycline and metronidazole, are common therapies.

Rhinophyma is caused by marked hyperplasia of sebaceous glands and chronic inflammation of the skin in acne rosacea.

Nosebleed (epistaxis) is most often due to trauma but has many causes, including hypertension, diverse hematologic abnormalities, inflammatory conditions, and nasal mucosal tumors. Epistaxis often originates in a triangular area of the anterior nasal septum called "Little area," where the epidermis is thin and the anterior ethmoid, greater palatine, sphenopalatine, and superior labial arteries anastomose to form the **Kiesselbach plexus.** Many dilated blood vessels, or telangiectasias, are often apparent. Ulcers and perforations, which may be caused by various diseases or by trauma to the septum, occur here (Table 29-1).

NONNEOPLASTIC DISEASES OF THE NASAL CAVITY AND SINUSES

Rhinitis Is Usually Viral or Allergic

Rhinitis is inflammation of the mucous membranes of the nasal cavity and sinuses. Its causes range from the common cold to unusual infections such as diphtheria, anthrax, or glanders (see Chapter 9).

VIRAL RHINITIS: The most common cause of acute rhinitis is viral infection, typically the common cold **(acute**

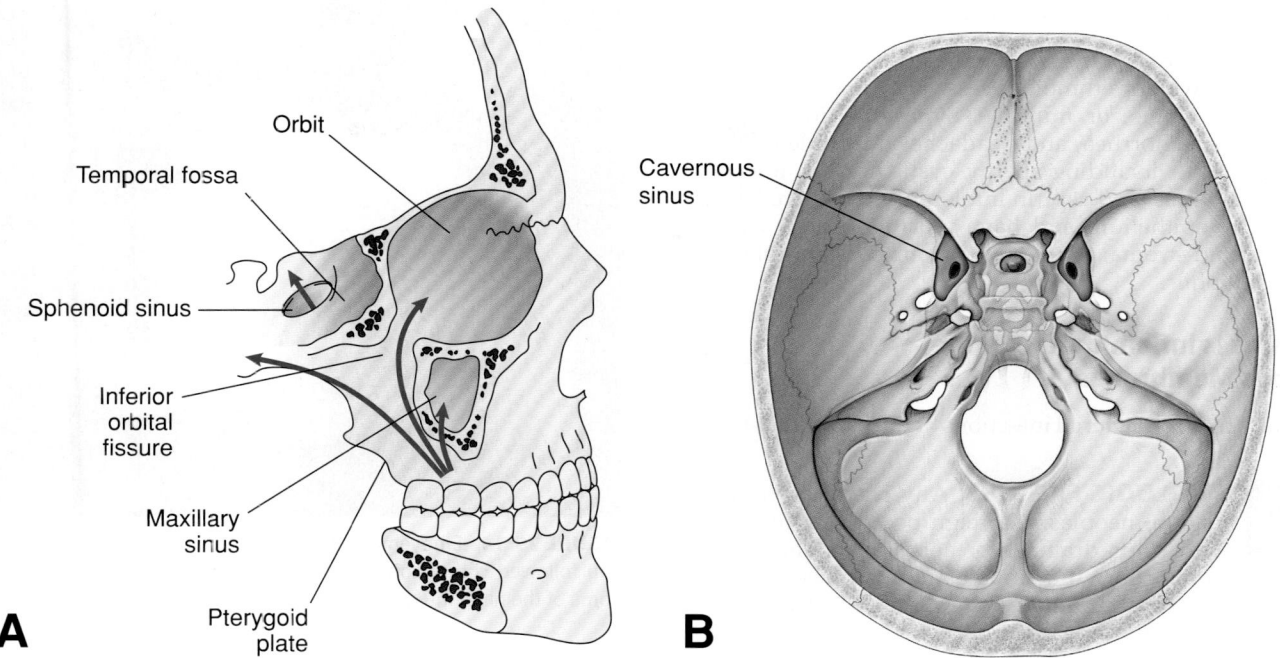

FIGURE 29-13. Osseous pathways of infection from the jaws to the intracranial cavity. *Arrows* indicate the direction of spread from the teeth to the maxillary sinus and through the inferior orbital fissure to the orbit. A deeper route is along the lateral pterygoid plate up to the base of the skull, where, medial to the foramen ovale, a small aperture admits the vein of Vesalius. Through this small vein, the pterygoid plexus communicates with the cavernous sinus.

coryza). Virus replication in epithelial cells causes degenerating cells to be shed. The mucosa becomes edematous and engorged, infiltrated by neutrophils and mononuclear cells. Clinically, mucosal swelling is felt as nasal stuffiness. Abundant mucus secretion and increased vascular permeability lead to **rhinorrhea** (free discharge of a thin watery mucus or "runny nose").

Secondary infection caused by normal nasal and pharyngeal flora may follow viral rhinitis by a few days. The abundant serous discharge then becomes mucopurulent, after which the surface epithelium is shed. Once inflammation subsides, the epithelium regenerates rapidly.

ALLERGIC RHINITIS (HAY FEVER): Allergens are ubiquitous in our environment, and sensitivity to any one of them can cause allergic rhinitis. Allergic rhinitis may be acute and seasonal, or chronic and perennial.

TABLE 29-1
CAUSES OF NASAL SEPTUM PERFORATION
Trauma
Specific infections (tuberculosis, syphilis, leprosy)
Wegener granulomatosis
Lupus erythematosus
Chronic exposure to dust (containing arsenic, chromium, copper, etc.)
Cocaine abuse
Malignant tumors

 MOLECULAR PATHOGENESIS: Plasma cells of the nasal mucosa produce immunoglobulin E (IgE), which is bound by specific receptors on mast cells in the nasal mucosa. When air-borne allergens (e.g., pollens, molds, animal dander) deposit there, they activate IgE molecules bound to mast cells or free in nasal secretions specifically directed against those allergens. Thus triggered, mast cells release cytoplasmic granules containing diverse chemical mediators and enzymes. Some preformed mediators act rapidly (e.g., histamine); others (such as heparin or trypsin) elute slowly from the granule matrix; still others (e.g., leukotrienes) are newly synthesized. Thus, an immediate, rapid response is followed by a prolonged inflammatory reaction as the various mediators exert their effects, causing the signs and symptoms of allergic rhinitis. Many of these responses are due to histamine, acting through its H_1 receptor.

PATHOLOGY: Vasodilators increase vascular permeability which leads to edema of the nasal mucosa, especially of the inferior turbinates. Many eosinophils may be seen in the nasal mucosa or secretions. The late phase of mast cell–mediated reactions is associated with persistent mucosal edema and manifests clinically as nasal obstruction.

CHRONIC RHINITIS: Repeated bouts of acute rhinitis may lead to chronic rhinitis. In this condition, the nasal mucosa is thickened by persistent hyperemia, mucous gland hyperplasia, and infiltration with lymphocytes and plasma cells.

Inflammatory Polyps Are Nonneoplastic Swellings

These polyps arise in the nose and sinuses, mostly from the lateral nasal wall or ethmoid recess. They may be unilateral or bilateral, single, or multiple. Symptoms include nasal obstruction, rhinorrhea, and headaches. Multiple etiologies are responsible, including allergy, cystic fibrosis, infections, diabetes mellitus, and aspirin intolerance. They are lined by respiratory epithelium and have mucous glands within a loose mucoid stroma, containing plasma cells, lymphocytes, and eosinophils.

Sinusitis Is Inflammation of the Mucous Membranes

It usually reflects bacterial infections of the paranasal sinuses.

 ETIOLOGIC FACTORS: Any condition (inflammation, neoplasm, foreign body) that interferes with sinus drainage or aeration renders it susceptible to infection. If a sinus ostium is blocked, secretions or exudate accumulate behind the obstruction.

Acute sinusitis is a disorder of less than 3 weeks' duration, caused largely by extension of infection from the nasal mucosa. *Haemophilus influenzae* and *Branhamella catarrhalis* are the most common organisms. Maxillary sinusitis may also be caused by odontogenic infections: bacteria from the roots of the first and second molars penetrate the thin bony plate that separates them from the floor of the maxillary sinus. Incomplete resolution of infection or recurrent acute sinusitis may lead to chronic sinusitis, in which the purulent exudate almost always contains anaerobic bacteria.

 PATHOLOGY: Complications of acute or chronic sinusitis may include:

- **Mucocele:** This is an accumulation of mucous secretions in a nasal sinus. If infected, a mucocele may cause a sinus to fill with mucopurulent exudate, called a **pyocele.** Purulent exudation in a sinus is **empyema** (Fig. 29-14). Mucoceles occur most often in the anterior compartments ("cells") of frontal and ethmoid sinuses. They develop slowly and the pressure of their expansion causes bone resorption. Mucoceles of anterior ethmoid or frontal sinuses may be large enough to displace the contents of the orbit and occasionally, erode into the central nervous system.
- **Osteomyelitis:** Suppurative infection of nasal sinus walls may spread through Volkmann canals to the periosteum, producing periostitis and subperiosteal abscess. If these occur on the orbital side of the bone, an orbital cellulitis or abscess forms. Overlying skin is often markedly edematous, and subcutaneous cellulitis or a subcutaneous abscess also may develop. Osteomyelitis also may spread rapidly between the outer and inner tables of the skull.
- **Septic thrombophlebitis:** Sinus infections that penetrate the bone may spread to frontal and diploe venous systems. Resulting septic thrombophlebitis may involve the cavernous venous sinus through the superior

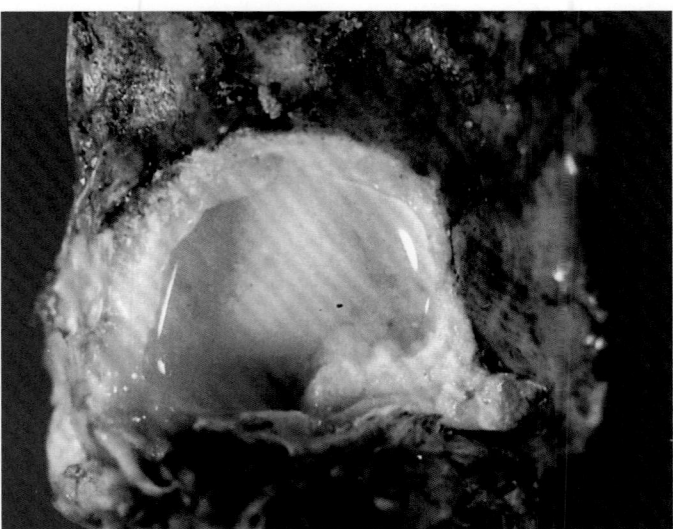

FIGURE 29-14. Empyema of the maxillary sinus (sagittal section). Infection followed chronic obstruction of the orifice caused by adenocarcinoma of the nasal mucosa.

ophthalmic veins and is a potentially life-threatening condition.
- **Intracranial infections:** Sinusitis may also spread infection to the cranial cavity. Lesions include epidural, subdural and cerebral abscesses and purulent leptomeningitis. Spread may be via lymphatics and veins and need not involve extensive destruction of bone.

Syphilis May Destroy the Nasal Bridge

Primary chancres in the nose are rare, but mucosal lesions of secondary syphilis are common in the nose and nasopharynx. In tertiary syphilis, inflammation may involve large portions of the nasal mucosa, underlying cartilage and bone. Perichondrial or periosteal gummas may destroy nasal cartilage and bone, causing the nasal bridge to collapse and producing "saddle nose." Destruction of nasal bony walls may also lead to perforation of the nasal septum, hard palate, wall of the orbit, or maxillary sinus.

Leprosy Is Spread Through Nasal Secretions

Mycobacterium leprae multiplies best at lower temperatures and so prefers cooler body sites, like the nares and anterior nasal mucosa. Nasal involvement is often the first manifestation of leprosy. Tuberculoid and intermediate forms of leprosy account for most cases (see Chapter 9). The skin around the nares and anterior nasal mucosa shows nodules, ulceration, or perforations. Nasal involvement is important as leprosy is spread via nasal secretions teeming with bacilli.

Rhinoscleroma (Scleroma) Is a Chronic Bacterial Infection

Rhinoscleroma is a chronic inflammatory process caused by a gram-negative diplobacillus, *Klebsiella rhinoscleromatis*. It begins in the nose and usually remains localized but may extend slowly into the nasopharynx, larynx, and trachea.

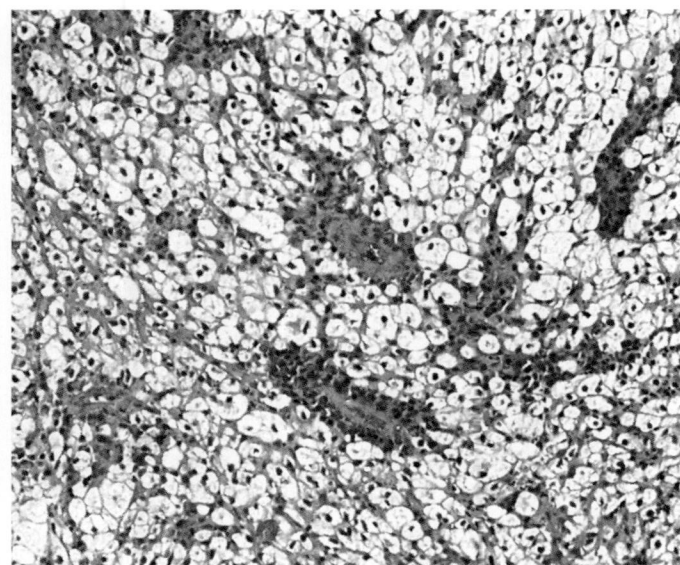

FIGURE 29-15. Rhinoscleroma. Granulation tissue contains numerous foamy macrophages (Mikulicz cells).

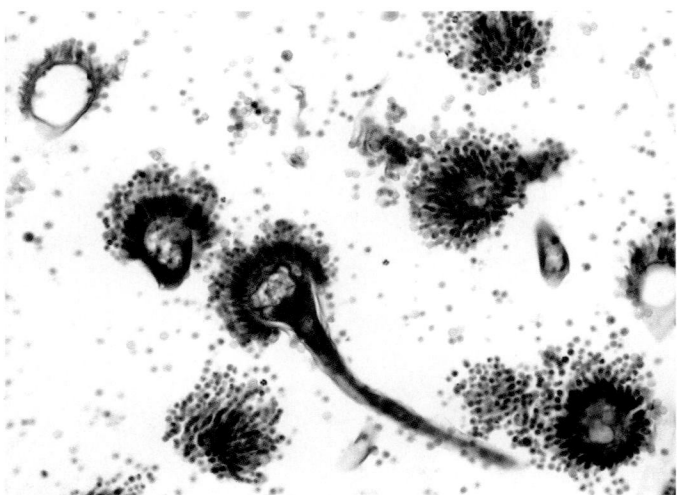

FIGURE 29-16. Aspergillus. This microscopic view of a green, nasal mass in a patient with lymphoma demonstrates abundant fruiting bodies.

It rarely involves other sites, such as the paranasal sinuses, orbital tissues, skin, lips, oral mucosa, cervical lymph nodes, and gastrointestinal tract. Scleroma is endemic in parts of the Mediterranean basin, Asia, Africa, and Latin America. Indigenous cases also occur in the United States. It affects both sexes at any age, and often reflects poor personal hygiene.

PATHOLOGY: Infected tissues are firm, thickened, irregularly nodular, and often ulcerated. The granulation tissue is very rich in plasma cells, lymphocytes, and foamy macrophages (Fig. 29-15). Characteristic large macrophages or Mikulicz cells, contain masses of phagocytosed bacilli. The disease is treatable with antibiotics.

Most Fungal Infections of the Nose and Sinuses Are Opportunistic

Pathogenic fungi may involve the nose and paranasal sinuses as part of cutaneous or mucocutaneous infection, particularly in a setting of immunodeficiency (see Chapter 9). **Candidiasis** is the most common fungus infection of the nasal mucosa. It usually accompanies oral and pharyngeal candidiasis **(thrush)**. **Aspergillosis** is uncommon, and when it occurs it generally involves a paranasal sinus. Fungi may disseminate to venous sinuses, meninges, and the brain. Aspergillosis of the sinonasal tract may be noninvasive or invasive, including angioinvasive. Noninvasive aspergillus sinusitis includes **allergic fungal sinusitis** (AFS) and **sinus mycetoma** (the so-called fungus ball).

Allergic Fungal Sinusitis

Allergic fungal sinusitis (AFS) reflects hypersensitivity to fungal antigens, such as allergic bronchopulmonary aspergillosis (see Chapter 12). AFS occurs at all ages but is most common in children or young adults, especially those who are atopic or immunologically "hypercompetent." Any sinus may be affected, but maxillary and ethmoid sinuses are most often involved.

Fungus balls, or **aspergillomas**, occur in immunologically normal patients, usually with chronic sinusitis and poor drainage. In this setting, fungi proliferate to form a dense mass of hyphae that causes nasal obstruction. Bone destruction and ocular symptoms may occur.

Invasive Fungal Sinusitis

Invasive fungal sinusitis usually affects immunocompromised patients (Fig. 29-16). In the rare **rhinocerebral aspergillosis**, the organisms penetrate venous sinuses and spread to the meninges and brain. Few patients survive.

Mucormycosis is a potentially life-threatening infection, particularly in diabetic and immunosuppressed patients. It typically involves the nasopharynx but can invade the skin, bone, orbit, and brain.

Nasal **rhinosporidiosis** is caused by the fungus *Rhinosporidium seeberi*. The disease is endemic in Sri Lanka and parts of India, and Central and South America. Affected nasal mucosa contains vascular polyploid masses that show marked chronic inflammation and characteristic spherical 50- to 350-μm-diameter sporangia (Fig. 29-17).

Leishmaniasis (Also Known as Kala-Azar)

Mucocutaneous leishmaniasis, due to Leishmania braziliensis, commonly affects the nose (see Chapter 9). The nasal disease, known as **espundia**, occurs in Central and South America. Initial skin sores heal within a few months, to be followed in some patients by mucocutaneous lesions of the nose or upper lip months or years later. Infection most likely spreads by nasal contact with contaminated fingers. Early in infection, the mucosa has polypoid inflammatory lesions, and superficial ulcers with macrophages contain parasites. Later, tuberculoid granulomatous responses develop, with few recognizable parasites. Bacterial infection may supervene and lead to soft tissue destruction and collapse of the anterior cartilaginous nasal septum.

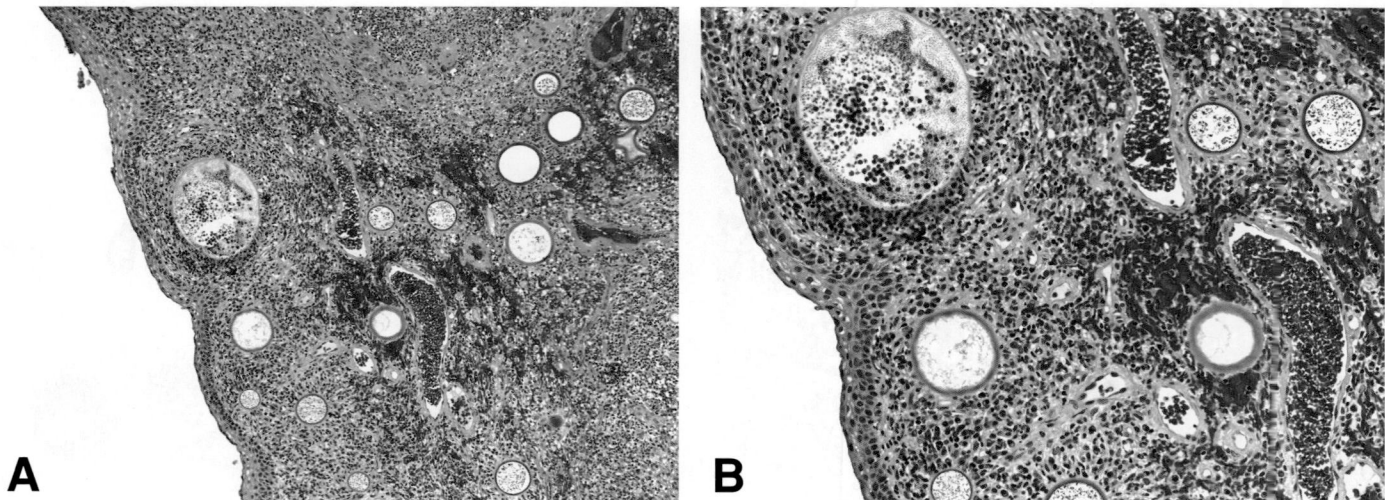

FIGURE 29-17. Rhinosporidiosis. A. Squamous metaplasia of the intact mucosal surface on the *left* can be seen overlying "punched out" appearing spaces. **B.** Higher magnification further illustrates thick-walled sporangia filled with endospores, which are approximately 6 to 10 microns in greatest diameter.

Granulomatosis With Polyangiitis Is a Systemic Disease That Affects the Nose and Lower Airways

PATHOLOGY: This condition, previously called Wegener granulomatosis, may affect many organs (see Chapters 10, 12, and 17). The sinonasal tract may be the only involved site, or it may be part of systemic disease. Septal perforation and mucosal ulceration may be followed by slowly progressive destruction of the nose and paranasal sinuses, leading to a saddle nose deformity. Constitutional symptoms, such as fever, malaise, and weight loss, may accompany resulting "runny nose," sinusitis and nosebleeds. Nasal lesions show ischemic-type necrosis, vasculitis, mixed chronic inflammation, scattered multinucleated giant cells, and microabscesses. Well-formed granulomas are not seen. Elevated serum antineutrophil cytoplasmic antibodies (ANCAs; see Chapter 4) and proteinase 3 (PR3) are associated with active disease.

Benign Tumors of the Nasal Cavity and Paranasal Sinuses

SQUAMOUS PAPILLOMA: This is the most common benign tumor of the nasal cavity. It resembles a wart (verruca vulgaris) and almost always occurs in the nasal vestibule.

SCHNEIDERIAN PAPILLOMAS: These benign neoplasms arise from the sinonasal (Schneiderian) mucosa and are composed of a squamous or columnar epithelial proliferation with associated mucous cells. Three morphologically distinct lesions are collectively called Schneiderian papillomas: **inverted, oncocytic** (cylindrical or columnar cell) and **fungiform** (exophytic, septal) papillomas. Schneiderian papillomas represent less than 5% of sinonasal tract tumors (Fig. 29-18).

INVERTED PAPILLOMA: This tumor involves the lateral nasal wall and may spread to the paranasal sinuses. Inverted papillomas occur mainly in middle-aged people. As

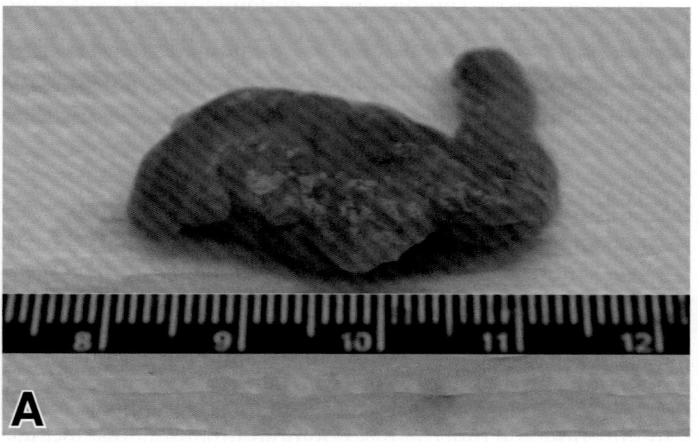

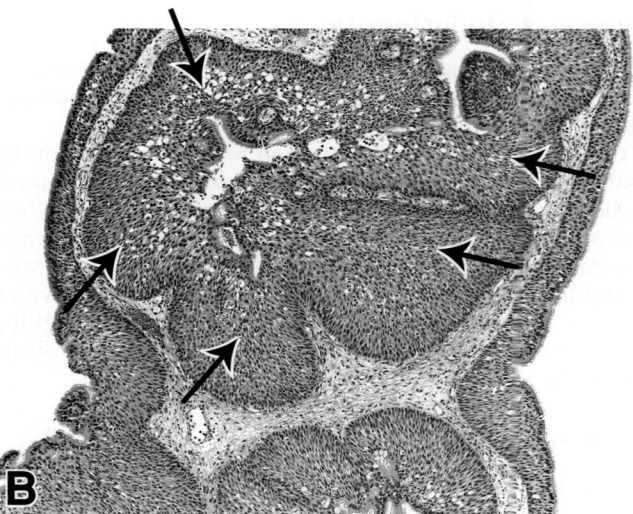

FIGURE 29-18. Sinonasal inverted papilloma. A. Gross photograph of sinonasal inverted papilloma. **B.** Epithelial nests are growing downward (inverted) into the submucosa in the direction of the *arrows*. They are composed of a uniform cellular epithelial proliferation, with scattered inflammatory cells and microcysts.

the name implies, they show inversion of surface epithelium into underlying stroma (Fig. 29-18B). HPV types 6 and 11 and, rarely, types 16, 18, 33, 40, or 57 are detected but are of uncertain significance. Although benign, these tumors may erode bone by pressure. Surgical resection must extend beyond the boundaries of grossly visible lesions, or they may recur. In 5% of cases, inverted papillomas give rise to SCC.

MALIGNANCIES OF THE NASAL CAVITY AND PARANASAL SINUSES

SCC Is Often Associated With Occupational Risk Factors

Over half of nasal cavity and paranasal sinus cancers arise in the maxillary sinus antrum, one-third in the nasal cavity, 10% in the ethmoid sinus and 1% in sphenoid and frontal sinuses.

Most are keratinizing or nonkeratinizing SCCs (Table 29-2). Some 15% are adenocarcinomas, or undifferentiated carcinomas. Maxillary sinus tumors can lead to obvious facial deformity by invasion of adjacent tissues. Involvement of the facial nerve can cause drooping of the mouth on one side due to facial nerve paralysis.

 ETIOLOGY: Several industrial chemicals may cause cancers of the nose and sinuses, including nickel, chromium, and aromatic hydrocarbons. Occupational settings associated with increased risk for cancer of the nose and sinuses (but for which a specific chemical agent has not been identified) are woodworking in the furniture industry, use of cutting oils, and leather textile industries.

Nickel workers are prone to SCCs, mostly arising in the middle turbinate, with latencies from 2 to over 30 years. Most other occupational exposures lead mainly to adenocarcinomas and occur predominantly in the maxillary and ethmoid sinuses. Because of these occupational risk factors, cancers of the nose and sinuses occur far more often in men and after age 50. These tumors grow relentlessly and invade adjacent structures but typically do not metastasize. Survival is usually only a few years.

TABLE 29-2
VARIANTS OF SQUAMOUS CELL CARCINOMA
Acantholytic squamous cell carcinoma
Adenosquamous carcinoma
Basaloid squamous cell carcinoma
Carcinoma cuniculatum
Papillary squamous cell carcinoma
Spindle cell squamous carcinoma
Verrucous carcinoma
Lymphoepithelial carcinoma (non-nasopharyngeal)

Olfactory Neuroblastoma Is of Neural Crest Origin

This tumor, also called esthesioneuroblastoma, is uncommon. It has a slight male predominance. Although it may occur at almost any age, a bimodal distribution in the second and sixth decades is most common.

PATHOLOGY: This cancer arises from the olfactory mucosa covering the superior third of the nasal septum, cribriform plate (Fig. 29-19A), and superior turbinate. Its growth pattern is usually polypoid and highly vascular, and it shows diverse histologies, depending on the amount of intercellular neurofibrillary material. Tumor cells are slightly larger than lymphocytes,

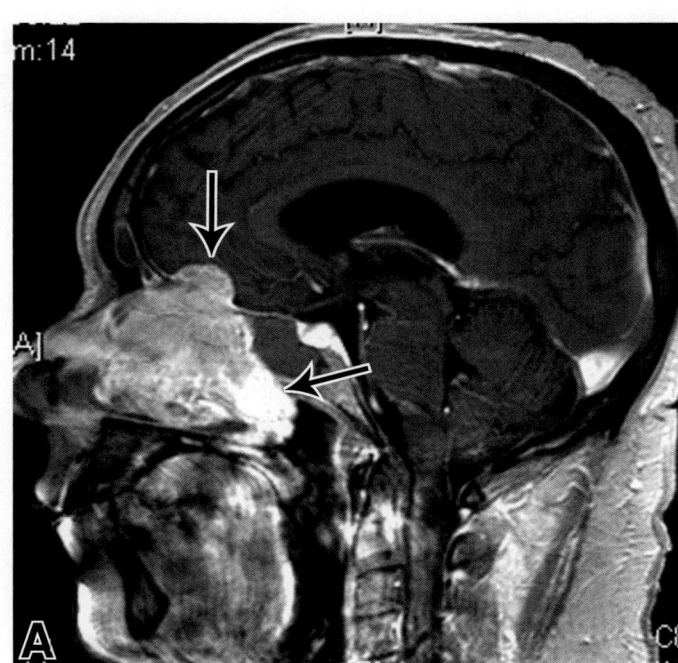

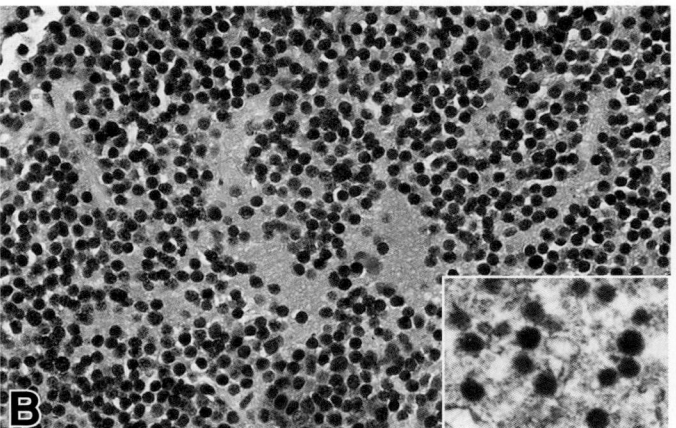

FIGURE 29-19. Olfactory neuroblastoma. A. Sagittal T1 postcontrast magnetic resonance image (MRI) showing a hyperintense mass (*arrows*) arising from the cribriform plate and filling the nasal cavity. **B.** The tumor is composed of small round cells with hyperchromatic nuclei and a background eosinophilic stroma representing neurofibrillary matrix. *Inset.* An electron micrograph shows intracytoplasmic, secretory-type, membrane-bound granules with dense cores.

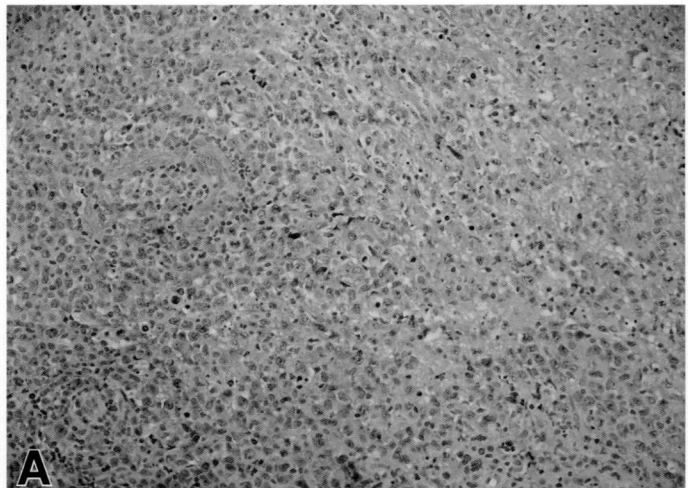 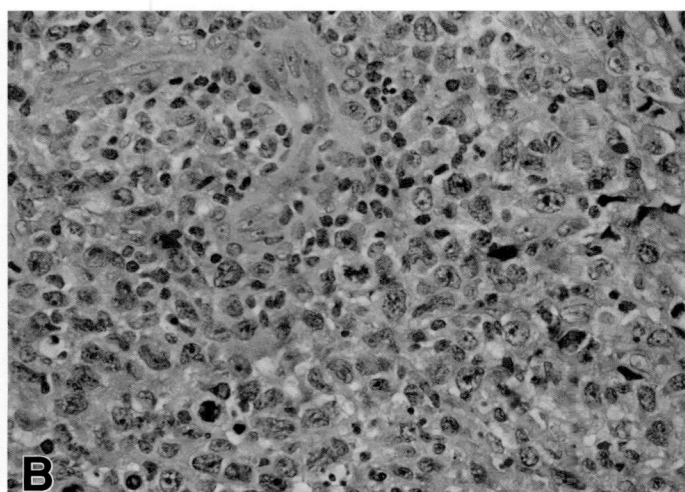

FIGURE 29-20. NK/T-cell Angiocentric lymphoma. A. Low-power magnification demonstrates an atypical lymphocytic infiltrate with vascular invasion and areas of necrosis. **B.** Higher magnification demonstrates abnormal mitoses and marked nuclear pleomorphism. (Photographs courtesy of Dr. Kyle Bradley, Emory University Hospital, Atlanta, GA.)

with round nuclei and inconspicuous cytoplasm (Fig. 29-19B). They may form pseudorosettes (Homer Wright rosettes) or true neural rosettes (Flexner–Wintersteiner rosettes). In 2017, the World Health Organization adopted a four-tiered grading system, based on lobular architecture, mitosis, necrosis, nuclear pleomorphism, fibrillary matrix, and rosettes. Olfactory neuroblastomas express synaptophysin and neuron-specific enolase (NSE) but not cytokeratin and epithelial membrane antigen (EMA). S-100 protein often surrounds nests or lobules (**sustentacular cells**), mostly in lower-grade tumors. The cells of olfactory neuroblastomas have intracytoplasmic neurosecretory granules like those of neuroblastomas at other sites.

CLINICAL FEATURES: Olfactory neuroblastomas invade and destroy bony structures slowly. They spread readily via lymphatics to regional and distant lymph nodes. Hematogenous spread occurs less often. Prognosis usually corresponds to tumor grade. Complete removal is critical, and craniofacial resection with chemotherapy and/or radiation therapy provides 85% 5-year survival.

Nasal-Type Angiocentric Natural Killer/T-Cell Lymphoma Is Highly Lethal

These tumors, once called **lethal midline granulomas**, midline malignant reticulosis and polymorphic reticulosis, are now recognized as malignant lymphomas.

PATHOLOGY: The characteristic lymphoid infiltrate is necrotizing and polymorphic. Similar infiltrates may occur in the upper airways, lungs, and alimentary tract, but any organ can be involved. Tumor cells surround small- to medium-sized blood vessels (angiocentric); infiltrate through their walls (angioinvasion), often occluding vessel lumens like a thrombus; and cause

necrosis in adjacent tissues (ischemic type) (Fig. 29-20). *EBV infection is associated with this type of lymphoma.*

CLINICAL FEATURES: Nasal-type natural killer (NK)/T-cell lymphoma usually begins insidiously as nonspecific rhinitis or sinusitis. Gradually, the nasal mucosa becomes focally swollen, indurated, and eventually ulcerated. Ulcers are covered by a black crust, under which cartilage and bone are eroded, producing defects of the nasal septum, hard palate, and nasopharynx, with serious functional consequences. The skin of the midface is often involved. Half of patients have localized disease, but wide dissemination is common. Death is usually due to secondary bacterial infection, aspiration pneumonia or hemorrhage from eroded large blood vessels. These lymphomas are, at least initially, radiosensitive, and remission with cytotoxic agents has also been reported.

Nasopharynx and Oropharynx

ANATOMY: The nasopharynx is continuous anteriorly with the nasal cavities; its roof is formed by the body of the sphenoid bone and its posterior wall by the cervical vertebrae. Eustachian tube openings are on the lateral walls of the nasopharynx. In newborns, the nasopharynx is covered by pseudostratified ciliated columnar epithelium. With advancing age, this is replaced by a stratified squamous epithelium over large areas (80%). The mucosa contains many mucous glands and abundant lymphoid tissue.

Waldeyer ring is a circular band of lymphoid tissue at the opening of the oropharynx into the respiratory and digestive tracts. Lymphoid tissue on the superior posterior wall forms the nasopharyngeal tonsils, which, when hyperplastic, are called **adenoids**. The palatine tonsils are lateral, where the pharynx connects with the oral cavity. They are covered by stratified squamous epithelium, often referred to as *lympho-epithelium*, which lines infoldings (**tonsillar crypts**) into the lymphoid tissue. Crypts normally contain desquamated epithelium, lymphocytes, some neutrophils and saprophytic organisms, such as bacteria, *Candida* and actinomycetes. Pathogens (e.g., *Corynebacterium diphtheriae*, meningococcus) may also be seen in the pharynx of healthy people.

Waldeyer ring is well developed in children and its follicles have germinal centers. In fact, the tonsils represent the largest collections of B lymphocytes in a normal child. Pharyngeal lymphoid tissue diminishes considerably by adulthood. It gradually involutes with age but does not totally disappear.

PHARYNGEAL LYMPHOID HYPOPLASIA AND HYPERPLASIA

Bruton sex-linked agammaglobulinemia (see Chapter 4) affects only males, who have minimal or no lymphoid tissue in their tonsils, pharynx, and intestines (Peyer patches and appendix). They have a normally developed thymus.

Atrophy of pharyngeal lymphoid tissue is common in chronically immunosuppressed patients. Local radiation therapy also causes marked loss of lymphoid tissue in the Waldeyer ring.

Hyperplasia of nasopharyngeal lymphoid tissue follows infections or chronic irritation due to dust, smoke, and fumes. Tonsils may enlarge in some primary immunodeficiencies (dysgammaglobulinemia type I or nodular lymphoid hyperplasia), presumably reflecting an adaptive response by the immune system.

INFECTIONS

Pharyngitis and tonsillitis are among the most common diseases of the head and neck. Nasopharyngeal inflammation occurs mainly in children but is also common in adolescents and young adults. Viral or bacterial infections may be limited to the palatine tonsils but may also involve nasopharyngeal tonsils or adjacent pharyngeal mucosa, often as part of a general upper respiratory tract infection. Viruses are the usual culprits: influenza, parainfluenza, adenovirus, respiratory syncytial virus, and rhinovirus, spread by droplet or by direct contact.

S. pyogenes is the most important cause of pharyngitis and tonsillitis because it may cause serious suppurative and nonsuppurative sequelae. **Diphtheria** still produces pharyngitis in some countries. These infections are characterized by an exudate or, in the case of diphtheria, a pseudomembrane on the tonsils and pharynx.

Acute tonsillitis is usually due to *S. pyogenes* (group A β-hemolytic streptococci). In **follicular tonsillitis**, pinpoint exudates may be extruded from the crypts.

In **pseudomembranous tonsillitis**, a necrotic mucosa is covered by a coat of exudate, as in diphtheria or **Vincent angina**. The latter is caused by fusiform bacilli and spirochetes that are part of the normal oral flora. They become pathogenic when local or systemic resistance is low (e.g., after mucosal injury or in malnutrition).

Recurrent or chronic tonsillitis is not as common as once believed, and enlarged tonsils in children do not necessarily signify chronic tonsillitis. However, repeated infections can cause tonsils and adenoids to enlarge and obstruct air passages. Repeated streptococcal tonsillitis may lead to rheumatic fever or glomerulonephritis in children, who may benefit from tonsillectomy.

Peritonsillar abscesses (also referred to as quinsy) are collections of pus behind the posterior capsule of the tonsil, usually due to α- and β-hemolytic streptococci. About one-third of patients have histories of tonsillitis. Untreated, such abscesses may be life-threatening since (1) aided by gravity, they may dissect inferiorly to the pyriform sinus to obstruct, or rupture into, the airway; (2) they may extend laterally into the parapharyngeal space (parapharyngeal abscess) and weaken the carotid artery wall; or (3) they may penetrate along the carotid sheath inferiorly into the mediastinum or, superiorly, to the base of the skull or cranial cavity, with disastrous consequences.

Infectious mononucleosis (mostly due to EBV) often presents with exudative tonsillitis, pharyngitis, and posterior cervical lymphadenopathy. **Adenoids** represent chronic inflammatory hyperplasia of pharyngeal lymphoid tissue. This condition is often accompanied by chronic tonsillitis or rhinitis, almost always in children. Enlarged adenoids may partly or completely obstruct the eustachian tube, leading to otitis media.

NEOPLASMS

Nasopharyngeal Angiofibroma Is a Tumor of Adolescent Boys

These tumors, once called "juvenile nasopharyngeal angiofibromas," are uncommon, highly vascular neoplasms of the nasopharynx. They are histologically benign but locally aggressive. These tumors most often arise in adolescent males but are not restricted to this age group.

 PATHOLOGY: Angiofibromas are multinodular, lobulated, or smooth pink-white masses, which may show surface ulceration and obvious blood vessels (Fig. 29-21A). They typically arise in the submucosa of the **posterolateral nasal wall** and tend to expand into adjacent structures, causing local mass effects. They may grow into fissures and foramina of the skull or destroy bone and spread into adjacent structures, such as the nasal cavity, paranasal sinuses, orbit, middle cranial fossa, or pterygomaxillary fossa.

Angiofibromas have vascular and stromal components (Fig. 29-21B). Blood vessels vary in size and shape; the smooth muscle in their walls is not layered, but rather arranged irregularly. Stromal fibroblasts express aberrant nuclear β-catenin (Fig. 29-21C).

CLINICAL FEATURES: Many angiofibromas regress spontaneously after puberty. They respond to estrogen therapy, and so may be hormonally regulated and androgen dependent. Vessel wall defects impair vasoconstriction, leading to brisk bleeding after trauma. Biopsies may thus be dangerous and are contraindicated. Radiation therapy is also effective. Preoperative

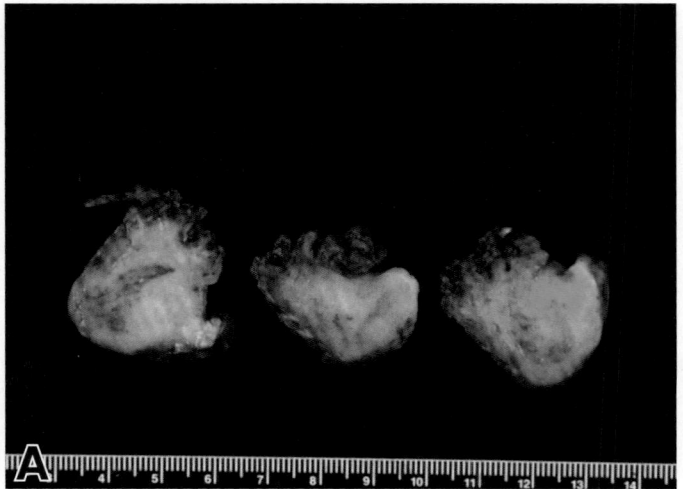

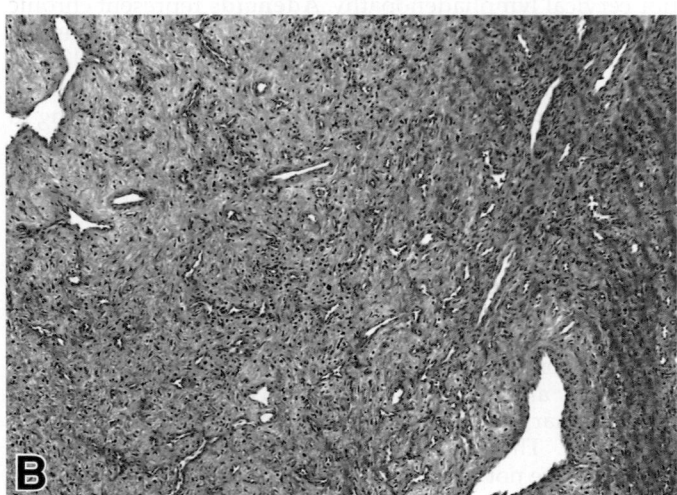

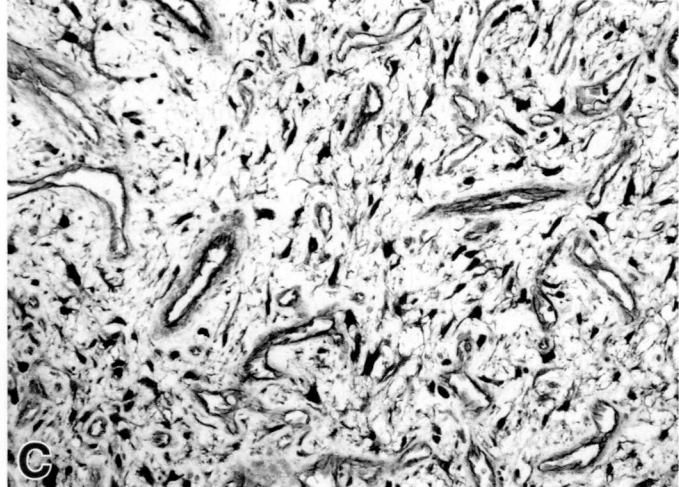

FIGURE 29-21. Nasopharyngeal angiofibroma. A. The cut surface of the tumor appears dense and spongy. **B.** Microscopically, it is composed of slit-like vascular structures in a collagenous stroma. **C.** Immunohisto-chemistry for β-catenin demonstrates aberrant nuclear labeling.

embolization may be used to reduce vascularity prior to surgery. These tumors have a familial tendency; they occur 25 times more often in patients with familial adenomatous polyposis (FAP) syndrome.

Oropharyngeal SCCs Are Usually Associated With HPV

In the United States, 80% of oropharyngeal SCCs are associated with high-risk HPV serotypes. These cancers, called HPV-associated head and neck squamous cell carcinomas (HPV-HNSCCs), arise mainly from palatine and lingual tonsils and are nonkeratinizing tumors of the basaloid cell type (Fig. 29-22A). Such tumors may be small and difficult to detect and often present as metastatic cancer in a cervical lymph node.

Compared to non–HPV-HNSCCs, HPV-HNSCCs tend to occur in younger people without the risk factors for HNSCC as often seen in older patients (i.e., smoking, alcohol). HPV-HNSCCs also are radiosensitive and have better overall better prognosis than non–HPV-associated HNSCCs (Fig. 29-22B,C).

The pathogenic roles played by cancer-associated HPV serotypes and their associated proteins are described elsewhere (see Chapters 5 and 18).

Nasopharyngeal Carcinoma Is Related to Epstein–Barr Virus

Nasopharyngeal carcinoma (NPC) is divided into keratinizing and nonkeratinizing types. The latter are associated with EBV infection and may be differentiated or undifferentiated.

EPIDEMIOLOGY: *Undifferentiated nonkeratinizing carcinomas are particularly common in southeast Asia and parts of Africa.* By far the most common cancer of the nasopharynx, NPC is the most common of all cancers in China. In Hong Kong, it represents 18% of all malignancies, compared with 0.25% worldwide. Chinese born in the United States have a 20-fold greater mortality from this tumor than do other ethnicities.

MOLECULAR PATHOGENESIS: Environmental risk factors for NPC have remained elusive. The A2/sin human leukocyte antigen (HLA) profile is more common in Chinese patients, suggesting a genetic susceptibility. Frequent deletions in several chromosomes, in particular 3p, 9p, and 14q, occur in NPCs.

About 85% of patients with NPC have antibodies to EBV. The virus genomes are detected in 75% to 100% of nonkeratinizing and undifferentiated types of NPC. EBV is more variable in keratinizing NPCs (see Chapters 5 and 9 for more detail).

PATHOLOGY: Differentiated nonkeratinizing NPCs have a stratified appearance and distinct cell margins. By contrast, in undifferentiated tumors, clusters of poorly delimited or syncytial cells have large oval nuclei and scant eosinophilic cytoplasm (Fig. 29-23A). Lymphoid infiltrates may be prominent in

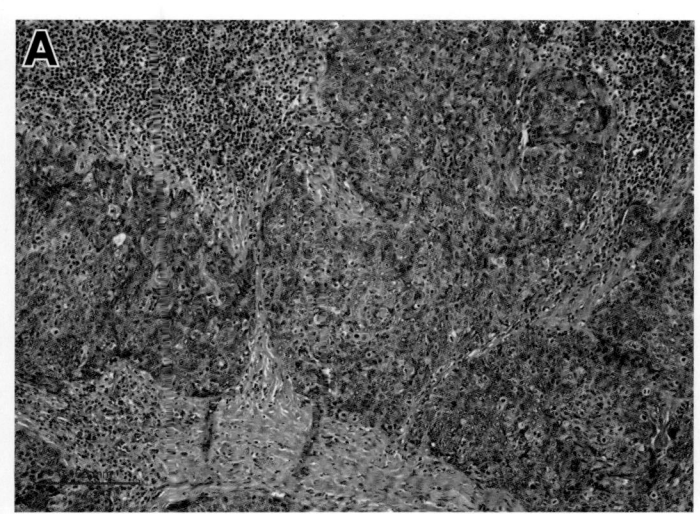

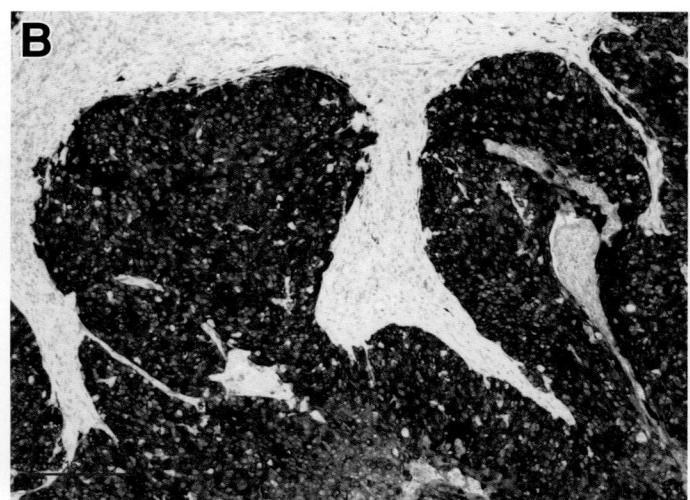

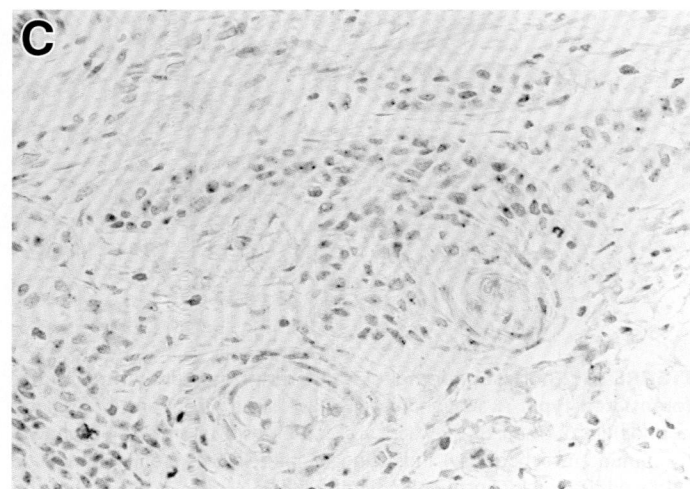

FIGURE 29-22. Human papillomavirus (HPV)–associated squamous cell carcinoma of the tonsil. A. Nests of invasive carcinoma are positive for p16 immunohistochemistry (**B**). **C.** In situ hybridization for high-risk HPV RNA (including types 16 and 18) demonstrates nuclear and cytoplasmic localization (*brown dots*).

undifferentiated tumors, accounting for the obsolete (and misleading) term "lymphoepithelioma." Both subtypes express cytokeratin (Fig. 29-23B), but not hematologic or lymphoid markers. In situ hybridization studies usually identify EBV DNA (Fig. 29-23C).

CLINICAL FEATURES: Owing to their location, most NPCs are asymptomatic for a long time and in half of patients first present as palpable cervical lymph node metastases. Even then, many patients have no complaints referable to the nasopharynx. Tumors invade adjacent structures, such as the parapharyngeal space, orbit, and cranial cavity, causing neurologic symptoms and hearing disturbances. Invasion of the base of the skull leads to cranial nerve involvement. Tumors in the fossa of Rosenmüller and the lateral wall of the nasopharynx cause symptoms referable to the middle ear. Eustachian tube obstruction is common. The abundant local lymphatic network gives rise to frequent and early metastases to cervical lymph nodes.

Undifferentiated NPC is radiosensitive, and most patients with tumors restricted to the nasopharynx survive 5 years or more. Cranial nerve involvement or metastases to cervical lymph nodes or beyond portend poor survival.

Lymphomas of the Waldeyer Ring Are Mostly Diffuse B-Cell Tumors

Lymphomas account for 5% of head and neck cancers. The Waldeyer ring is by far the most common site of origin of lymphoma in this region: the palatine tonsils first, then the nasopharynx and base of the tongue. These lymphomas are histologically diffuse (90%), and over half are large cell lymphomas. In the United States and Asia, the vast majority are of B-cell origin.

Most Extramedullary Plasmacytomas Occur in the Head and Neck

These tumors occur in the nasopharynx, nasal cavity, and paranasal sinuses and behave like other extramedullary plasmacytomas. Head and neck plasmacytomas may remain localized or evolve into systemic plasma cell myelomas (see Chapter 20).

Chordomas Are Derived From Remnants of Embryonic Notochord

Chordomas are uncommon cancers in people under age 40. In the cranial region, they originate from the area of the sphenooccipital synchondrosis or **clivus**, and in one-third

THE HEAD AND NECK

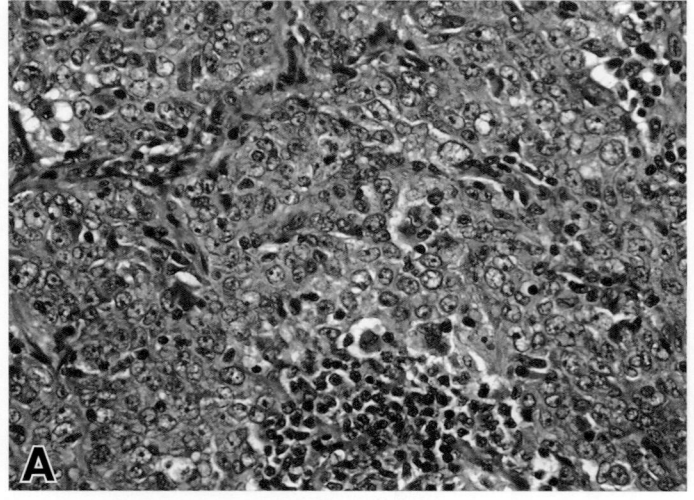

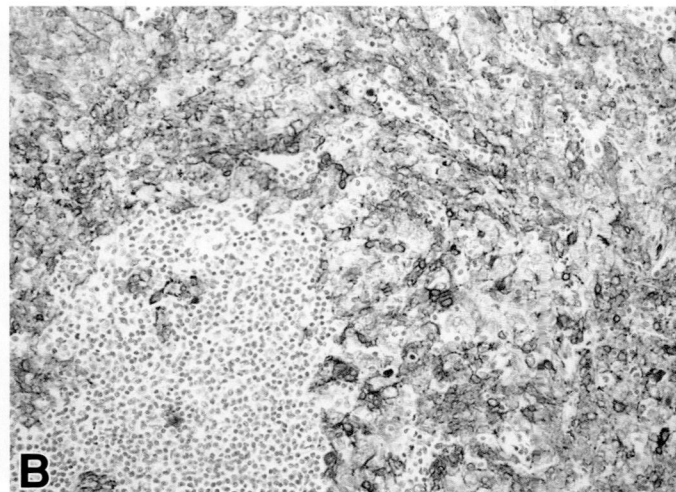

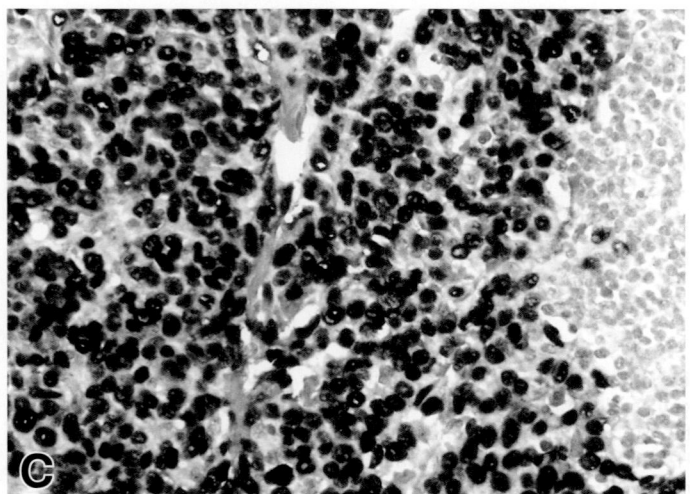

FIGURE 29-23. Nasopharyngeal nonkeratinizing carcinoma, undifferentiated type. A. Malignant cells have large nuclei and prominent eosinophilic nucleoli. **B.** They are cytokeratin positive (brown stain shown by immunohistochemistry), indicating an epithelial cell proliferation. **C.** In situ hybridization for Epstein–Barr virus (EBER-ISH).

of cases, extend into the nasopharynx. They are composed of large vacuolated **(physaliferous)** cells, surrounded by abundant intercellular matrix (Fig. 29-24). Chordomas grow slowly, but they infiltrate bone and are difficult to excise

completely by surgery. Patients with cranial region chordomas rarely survive more than 5 years.

Other Malignancies of the Nasopharynx Are Rare

They may derive from various components of mucosa or adjacent supportive soft tissues and skeleton. **Embryonal rhabdomyosarcomas** (Fig. 29-25) are highly malignant tumors of pharyngeal tissues of young children. They invade contiguous structures and metastasize via the bloodstream and lymphatics. Nasopharyngeal **Kaposi sarcomas** may occur in patients with AIDS, in association with HHV8.

Larynx and Hypopharynx

INFECTIONS

EPIGLOTTITIS: Inflammation of the epiglottis is most commonly caused by *H. influenzae* type B. It occurs in infants and young children and may be a life-threatening emergency. Swelling of an acutely inflamed epiglottis may obstruct airflow. Inspiratory stridor (loud wheezing on inspiration) and

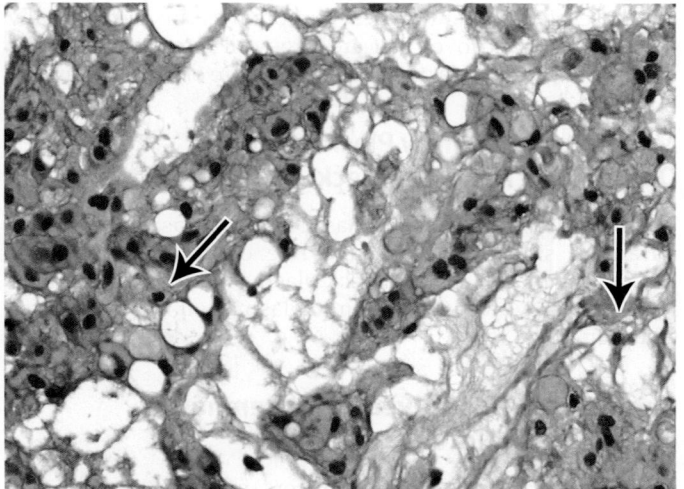

FIGURE 29-24. Chordoma. Large vacuolated (physaliferous) tumor cells (*arrows*) are evident.

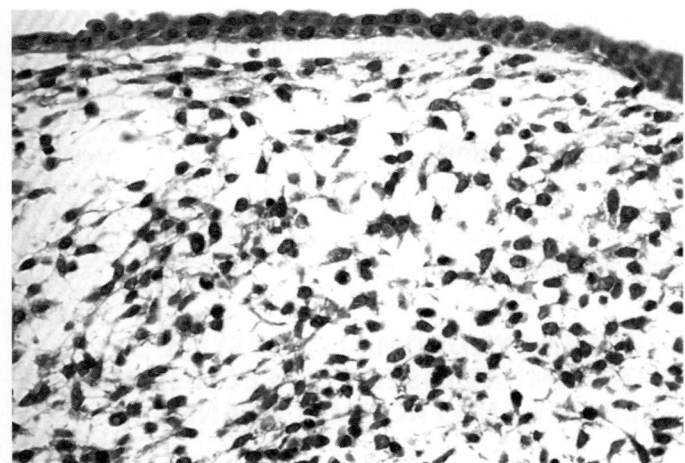

FIGURE 29-25. Embryonal rhabdomyosarcoma from a 3-year-old girl. This highly malignant tumor arose in the parapharyngeal space and invaded the adjacent structures. The oval or tadpole-shaped tumor cells under the epithelium have hyperchromatic, eccentric nuclei and immunohistochemical and ultrastructural features of rhabdomyoblasts.

the onset of cyanosis may indicate airway obstruction so severe as to require tracheostomy.

CROUP: Croup is a laryngotracheobronchitis of young children who have symptoms of inspiratory stridor, cough, and hoarseness, due to varying degrees of laryngeal obstruction. It is a complication of an upper respiratory infection, with marked laryngeal edema and a "barking cough." This was once a deadly complication of diphtheria. However, antibiotics and immunizations have helped prevent or treat it, and today, it is most commonly caused by the parainfluenza viruses.

VOCAL CORD NODULE AND POLYP

Also called *singer's nodules*, these are stromal reactions related to inflammation and/or trauma. They may be seen in all age groups but occur most commonly between the third and sixth decades (Fig. 29-26). Symptoms caused by vocal cord polyps and nodules are similar: hoarseness or voice changes ("cracking" of the voice). Lesions arise after voice abuse, infection (laryngitis), excessive alcohol consumption, smoking, or endocrine dysfunction (e.g., hypothyroidism). Edematous fibromyxoid stroma is seen in early stages, while hyalinized, densely fibrotic stroma occurs later.

NEOPLASMS OF THE LARYNX

SQUAMOUS PAPILLOMA AND PAPILLOMATOSIS: These are solitary or multiple papillary growths of mature squamous cells that line the surfaces of fibrovascular cores. They may be multiple in children or adolescents (**juvenile laryngeal papillomatosis**) and may extend into the trachea and bronchi. HPV, especially serotypes 6 and 11, are the main causes. The condition may cause life-threatening respiratory obstruction and, rarely, evolve into overt SCC, particularly in smokers or after radiation therapy. Surgical excision may not be curative, as the viral infection is often widespread, and these tumors tend to recur over many years. Solitary laryngeal squamous papilloma occurs in adults, mostly men, and is usually cured surgically.

SQUAMOUS CELL CARCINOMA: Almost all laryngeal cancers are SCCs, predominantly in men, most of whom smoke cigarettes. HPV is found in a quarter of cases.

- **Glottic carcinoma** is limited to one or both true vocal cords and accounts for two-thirds of laryngeal SCCs. It metastasizes late to lymph nodes and has a good prognosis.
- **Supraglottic carcinomas** arise in the ventricle, false cords or epiglottis and, by definition, do not involve the true cords. Up to one-third of laryngeal cancers arise in this location. Nodal metastases are more common than in glottic tumors.
- **Transglottic carcinoma** by definition involves true and false cords (Fig. 29-27). It spreads to lymph nodes and often requires total laryngectomy.
- **Infraglottic carcinomas** are uncommon. Found below the true cords or involving the true cords with infraglottic extension and frequent extension into the trachea, they commonly spread to lymph nodes. Total laryngectomy is usually required.

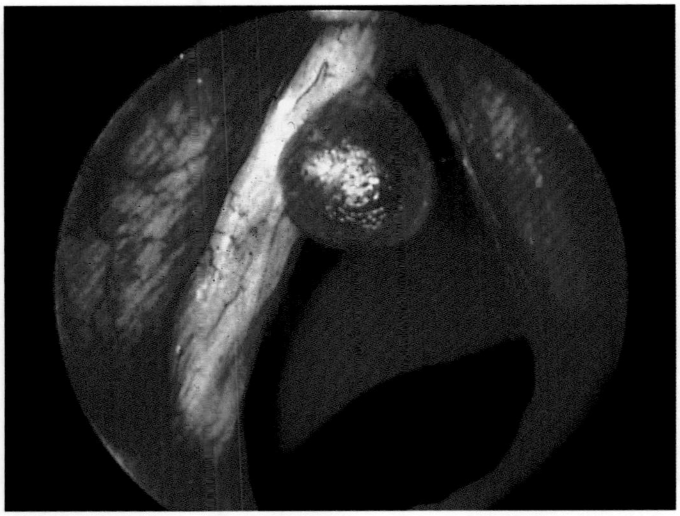

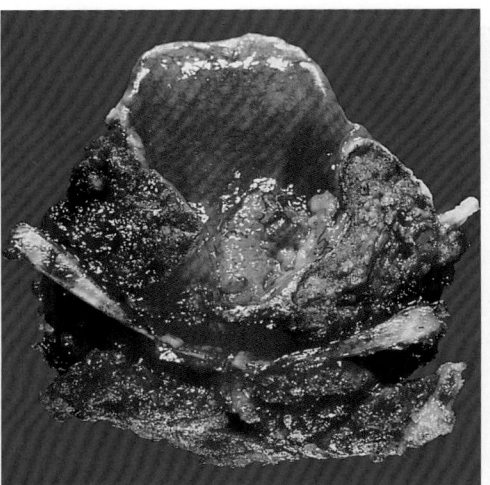

FIGURE 29-27. Supraglottic laryngectomy specimen for squamous cell carcinoma. The carcinoma appears as an irregular raised granular-appearing area in the right supraglottic larynx.

FIGURE 29-26. Vocal cord polyp. A solitary polypoid lesion with a glistening appearance is seen arising from the true vocal cord.

CHONDROSARCOMA: Chondrosarcomas account for 75% of nonepithelial laryngeal malignancies. In the larynx, they grow as exophytic, polypoid masses and can cause airway obstruction. Most patients are men in their 70s. It also occurs in the nasopharynx, mandible, maxilla, and nasal and paranasal sinuses. Patients present with hoarseness, airway obstruction, and dyspnea.

Salivary Glands

The salivary glands develop from buds of oral ectoderm to form tubuloalveolar structures that secrete saliva. Major salivary glands are paired organs. Parotid glands secrete serous saliva, and submandibular and sublingual glands make mixed serous and mucous saliva. Minor salivary glands are widespread beneath the mucosa of the lips, cheeks, palate, and tongue. Lymph nodes are normally embedded in the parotid gland and may be involved in inflammatory, reactive, proliferative, or malignant processes.

XEROSTOMIA: Xerostomia or chronic mouth dryness due to lack of saliva has many causes. Diseases of the major salivary glands that lead to xerostomia include mumps, Sjögren syndrome, sarcoidosis, radiation-induced atrophy (Fig. 29-28), and drug sensitivity (e.g., antihistamines, tricyclic antidepressants, phenothiazines).

SIALORRHEA: Increased salivary flow is associated with many conditions, including acute inflammation of the oral cavity (e.g., as in aphthous stomatitis), Parkinson disease, rabies, Down syndrome, nausea, and pregnancy.

ENLARGEMENT: Unilateral enlargement of major salivary glands is usually caused by cysts, inflammation, or neoplasms. Bilateral enlargement may be due to inflammation (mumps, Sjögren syndrome; see below), granulomatous disease (sarcoidosis), or diffuse neoplastic involvement (leukemia or lymphoma).

SIALOLITHIASIS: Calcific stones in salivary gland ducts mostly occur in the submandibular gland. They obstruct ducts, leading to inflammation distally.

PAROTITIS: Bacteria (usually Staphylococcus aureus) may ascend from the oral cavity when salivary flow is reduced and cause acute suppurative parotitis. This occurs most often in debilitated or postoperative patients. Salivary duct stricture or obstruction by stones may cause acute or chronic parotitis. Stagnant secretions serve as a medium for retrograde bacterial invasion.

Epidemic parotitis (mumps) is an acute viral disease of the parotid glands that spreads via infected saliva. Submandibular and sublingual glands may be affected. Involved glands show dense lymphocytic and macrophage infiltrates, epithelial degeneration, and necrosis.

SJÖGREN SYNDROME IS A SYSTEMIC AUTOIMMUNE DISEASE AFFECTING THE SALIVARY AND LACRIMAL GLANDS

The disease may be limited to these sites, or may be associated with a systemic autoimmune disease (see Chapter 11). In the salivary glands, it leads to xerostomia. Involvement of the lacrimal glands causes dry eyes (**keratoconjunctivitis sicca**). The pathogenesis and clinical features of Sjögren syndrome are discussed in Chapters 4 and 11.

 PATHOLOGY: In Sjögren syndrome, parotid glands, and sometimes submandibular glands, are enlarged unilaterally or bilaterally, but their lobulation is preserved. Initial periductal chronic inflammation gradually extends into the acini, until the glands are completely replaced by a sea of polyclonal lymphocytes, immunoblasts, germinal centers, and plasma cells. Proliferating myoepithelial cells surround remnants of damaged ducts and form the so-called epimyoepithelial islands (**lymphoepithelial sialadenitis**; Fig. 29-29). Similar changes occur in the lacrimal glands and minor salivary glands. Focal lymphocytic sialadenitis may also occur in minor salivary glands. Late in the course of the disease, affected glands become atrophic, with fibrosis and fatty infiltration of the parenchyma. Lymphocytes in Sjögren syndrome may show restricted immunoglobulin types and remain localized, without invasion.

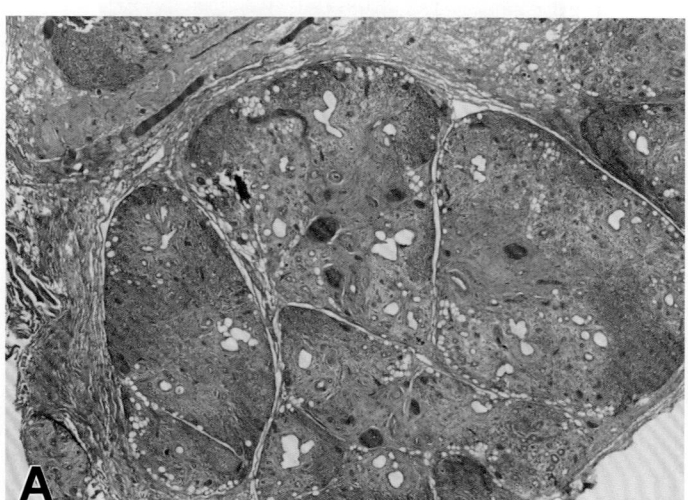

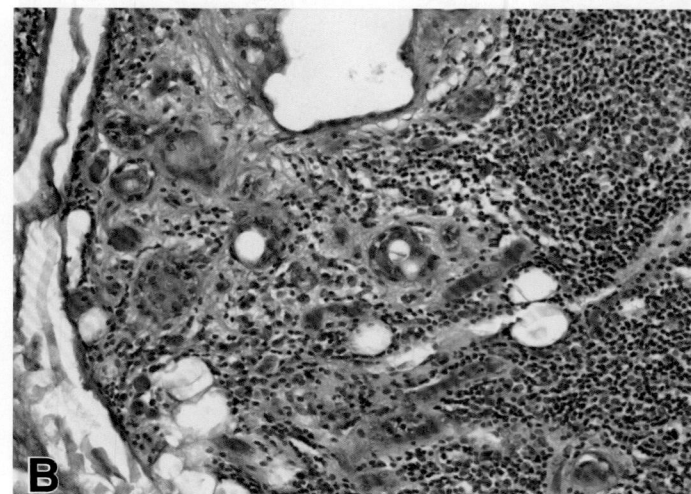

FIGURE 29-28. Chronic sialadenitis. Severe chronic inflammation, stromal fibrosis, and marked atrophy of the submandibular gland are present after irradiation of an adjacent oral cancer. The atrophic acini have been replaced by fat. (Magnification **A.** 50× and **B.** 200×).

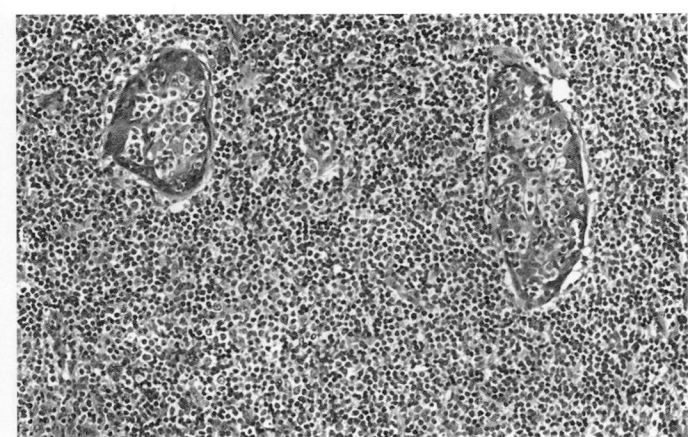

FIGURE 29-29. Sjögren syndrome. There is infiltration of the involved salivary gland by a mixed chronic inflammatory cell infiltrate. Extension of the infiltrate into epithelial (ductal) structures results in metaplasia and characteristic epimyoepithelial islands.

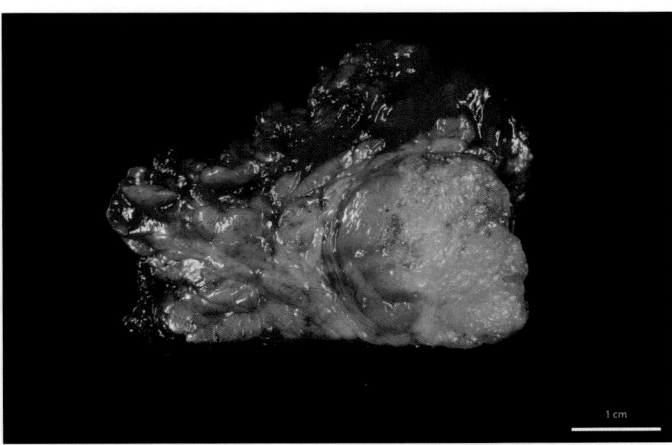

FIGURE 29-30. Pleomorphic adenoma of the parotid. The bisected surgical specimen demonstrates a white, glistening, homogenous, well-circumscribed tumor.

BENIGN SALIVARY GLAND NEOPLASMS

Pleomorphic Adenoma Is the Most Common Salivary Gland Tumor

These neoplasms, also called **mixed tumors**, are benign proliferations with admixed epithelial and stromal elements. Two-thirds of major salivary gland tumors, and about half of those in the minor glands, are pleomorphic adenomas. They occur nine times more often in the parotid than in the submandibular gland and usually arise in the superficial lobe of the former. Middle-aged people and women are most affected.

MOLECULAR PATHOGENESIS: Loss of heterozygosity of chromosome 8q17p and rearrangements in 3p21 and 12q13-15 have been found in pleomorphic adenomas. In most of these tumors, *PLAG1* (pleomorphic adenoma gene 1), which encodes a zinc finger protein, is activated by reciprocal chromosomal translocations involving 8q12. Carcinomas that develop from pleomorphic adenomas may have 8q12 rearrangements, alterations in 12q13-15 and mutations in *HMGIC* and *MDM2* genes. *HMGIC* encodes a non-histone protein component of chromatin, and *MDM2* encodes a nuclear-localized E3 ubiquitin ligase that targets tumor suppressors such as p53 for proteasomal degradation.

 PATHOLOGY: Pleomorphic adenomas are slowly growing, painless, movable, firm masses with smooth surfaces (Fig. 29-30). Those arising deep in the parotid may grow between the ramus of the mandible, the styloid process and the stylomandibular ligament into the parapharyngeal space and appear as swellings of the lateral pharyngeal or tonsillar regions. These tumors show epithelial tissue mingled with myxoid, mucoid, or chondroid areas (Fig. 29-31A), hence the older term **benign mixed tumor**. However, the neoplastic component is considered to be of epithelial origin.

The epithelial component consists of myoepithelial and ductal cells. Cells that line the ducts form tubules or small cystic structures and contain clear fluid or eosinophilic, periodic acid–Schiff (PAS)-positive material. Around ductal epithelial cells are smaller myoepithelial cells, which are the main cellular component. These cells form well-defined sheaths, cords or nests and are often separated by a ground substance that resembles cartilaginous, myxoid, or mucoid material.

CLINICAL FEATURES: Pleomorphic adenomas have fibrous capsules which form by condensation of surrounding fibrous tissue as the tumors grow. The tumors expand and often protrude focally into adjacent tissues, becoming nodular and occasionally forming "podocytes" (Fig. 29-31B). These tumor projections can be retained if a tumor is not fully excised with its capsule intact along with an adequate margin of gland parenchyma. Tumor implanted during surgery or tumor nodules left behind continue to grow and recur in scars from previous operations. Recurrences usually represent local regrowth, rather than malignancy. Definitive surgery may require sacrificing the facial nerve.

Rarely, carcinomas may arise in pleomorphic adenomas (**carcinoma ex pleomorphic adenoma**). In such cases, a tumor that was present for many years begins to grow rapidly or becomes painful. These carcinomas are most frequently high-grade malignancies. Virtually any type of salivary gland malignancy may occur in this setting, including mucoepidermoid or ACCs. If the malignancy is contained within the tumor capsule and does not invade adjacent normal salivary gland tissue, it is considered **in situ or noninvasive carcinoma ex pleomorphic adenoma**. If it invades beyond the tumor capsule but not more than 1.5 mm, it is called **minimally invasive carcinoma ex pleomorphic adenoma**. These entities have an excellent prognosis. By contrast, tumors invading beyond 1.5 mm (i.e., ***widely invasive***) act aggressively, recur often, metastasize and have a poor prognosis.

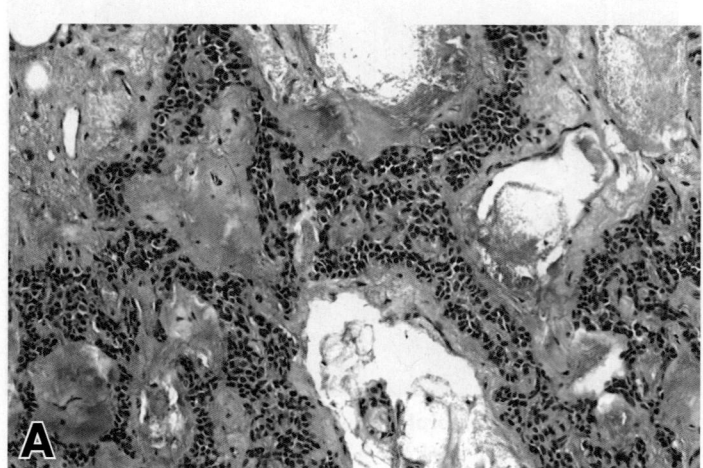
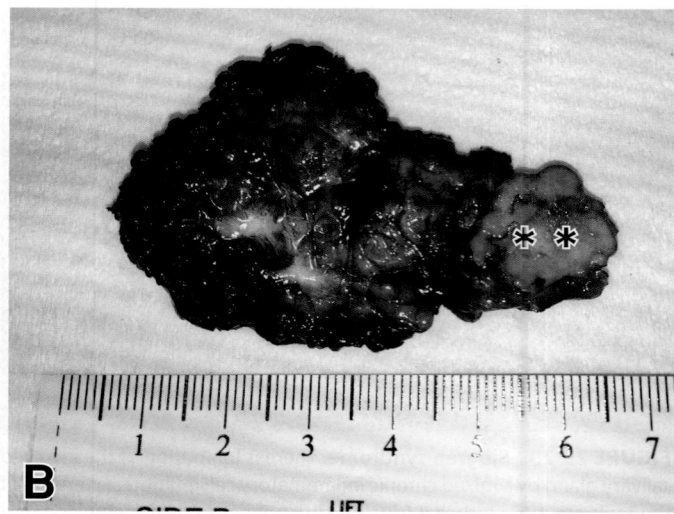

FIGURE 29-31. Pleomorphic adenoma of the parotid gland. A. Cellular components of pleomorphic adenomas include an admixture of glands and myoepithelial cells within a chondromyxoid stroma. **B.** The tumor (**) contains characteristic myxoid and chondroid portions. The tumor is partly encapsulated, but a nodule protruding into the parotid gland lacks a capsule. If such nodules are not included in the resection, the tumor will recur.

Monomorphic Adenomas Represent 5% to 10% of Benign Salivary Gland Tumors

In monomorphic adenomas, the epithelium is arranged in a regular, usually glandular, pattern without a mesenchymal component. Monomorphic adenomas include (1) Warthin tumors, (2) basal cell adenomas, (3) oxyphilic adenomas or oncocytomas, (4) canalicular adenomas, (5) myoepitheliomas, and (6) clear cell adenomas.

Warthin Tumor (Papillary Cystadenoma Lymphomatosum)

Warthin tumors, the most common type of monomorphic adenoma, are benign parotid gland neoplasms composed of cystic glandular spaces within dense lymphoid tissue. Clearly benign, they may be bilateral (15% of cases) or multifocal within one gland. They are the only salivary gland tumors that are more common in men than in women. They generally occur after age 30, and most arise after age 50.

PATHOLOGY: Warthin tumors have glandular spaces that tend to become cystic, with papillary projections. The cysts are lined by eosinophilic epithelial cells (oncocytes), surrounded by dense lymphoid tissue with germinal centers (Fig. 29-32).

The histogenesis of this tumor is uncertain. Lymph nodes are normally found in the parotid gland and its immediate vicinity and usually contain a few ducts or small islands of salivary gland tissue. Warthin tumors may arise from proliferation of these salivary gland inclusions.

Oncocytoma (Oxyphil Adenoma)

Oncocytes are benign epithelial cells swollen with mitochondria, which impart a granular light microscopic appearance to the cytoplasm. They are normally scattered or in small clusters among epithelial cells of various organs (e.g., thyroid, parathyroid). Oncocytes first appear in early adulthood and increase in number with age. Rare adenomas are composed of nests or cords of oncocytes occur in parotid glands in the elderly.

MALIGNANT SALIVARY GLAND TUMORS

Salivary gland tumors account for 5% of all head and neck cancers. Most (75%) arise in the parotid glands, 10% in the submandibular glands and 15% in the minor salivary glands of the upper aerodigestive tract. Malignancies of the sublingual glands are rare.

Mucoepidermoid Carcinomas Show Mixed Cell Populations

Mucoepidermoid carcinomas (MECs) are derived from ductal epithelium, which has a great potential for metaplasia (Fig. 29-33). They account for 5% to 10% of major salivary gland tumors and 10% of tumors in minor salivary glands. Over half of MECs in the major glands arise in the parotid. In the minor salivary glands, they develop mostly in the palate. Most MECs arise in adult women but may occur in adolescents.

MOLECULAR PATHOGENESIS: Over 60% of MECs are characterized by a t(11;19)(q21-22;p13) translocation (Fig. 29-34). This recombination generates a fusion gene (*MECT1–MAML2* fusion) in which the cAMP responsive domain of the transcriptional coactivator MECT1 is fused to the transactivation domain of the Notch coactivator MAML2. This presumably dysregulates Notch signaling in the tumors.

PATHOLOGY: Mucoepidermoid carcinomas grow slowly and present as firm, painless masses. Low-grade tumors contain irregular solid, duct-like and cystic spaces that include squamous cells, mucus-secreting cells and intermediate cells (Fig. 29-33). Intermediate-grade tumors tend to grow in more solid patterns, with more epidermoid and intermediate cells and fewer mucus-secreting cells. High-grade MECs are very pleomorphic with minimal differentiation, and only rare scattered glandular cells.

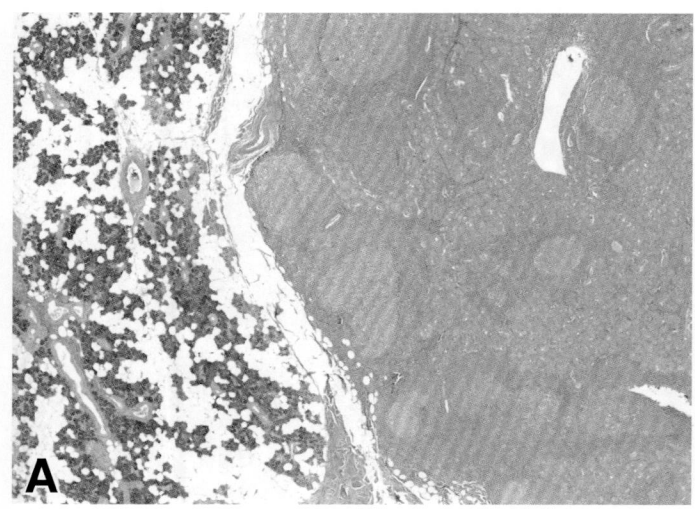

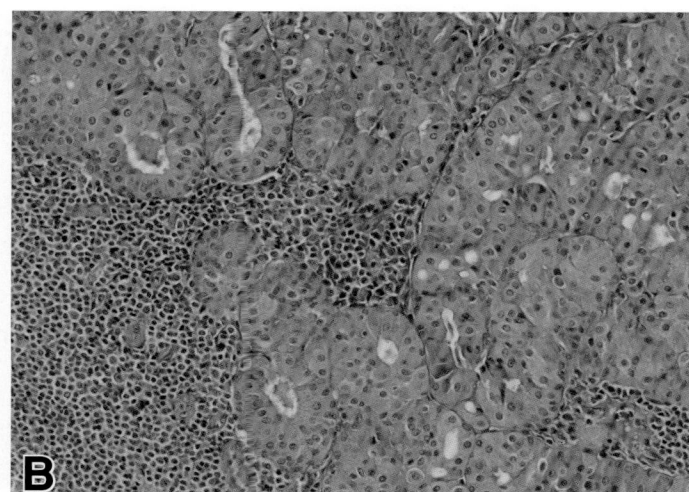

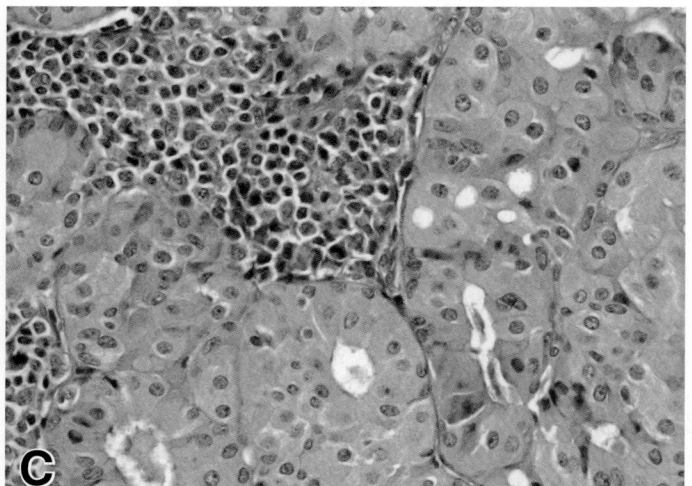

FIGURE 29-32. Warthin tumor. A. Low power (50×) demonstrates normal parotid gland tissue on the *left* side of the image. **B.** Follicular lymphoid tissue is present. **C.** Higher magnification (400×) shows cystic spaces and duct-like structures lined by oncocytes.

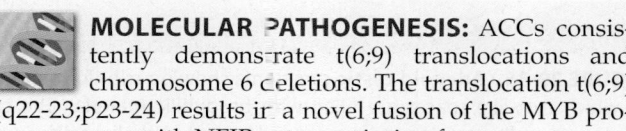 **CLINICAL FEATURES:** Even low-grade mucoepidermoid carcinomas may metastasize, but over 90% of patients survive 5 years, regardless of the primary site. Survival with high-grade tumors is much worse (20% to 40%). Treatment is dictated by grade; low-grade tumors are treated surgically, but high-grade tumors require both surgery and radiation therapy.

Adenoid Cystic Carcinomas Invade Locally and Often Recur After Resection

ACCs tend to grow slowly. One-third arise in the major salivary glands and two-thirds in the minor ones. They represent 5% of major salivary gland tumors and 20% of those of the minor salivary glands. ACCs may occur not only in the oral cavity but also in the lacrimal glands, nasopharynx, nasal cavity, paranasal sinuses, and lower respiratory tract. They are most common in people 40 to 60 years old.

MOLECULAR PATHOGENESIS: ACCs consistently demonstrate t(6;9) translocations and chromosome 6 deletions. The translocation t(6;9) (q22-23;p23-24) results in a novel fusion of the MYB proto-oncogene with NFIB, a transcription factor.

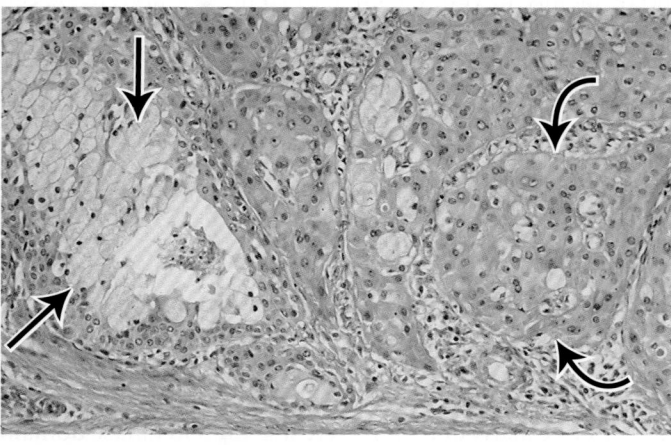

FIGURE 29-33. Mucoepidermoid carcinoma is characterized by an admixture of mucocytes (*straight arrows*), epidermoid cells (*curved arrows*), and intermediate cells. The mucocytes are clustered and have clear cytoplasm with eccentrically situated nuclei. Epidermoid cells are squamous-like cells but lack keratinization and intercellular bridges. Intermediate cells (best seen at lower left) are smaller than epidermoid cells.

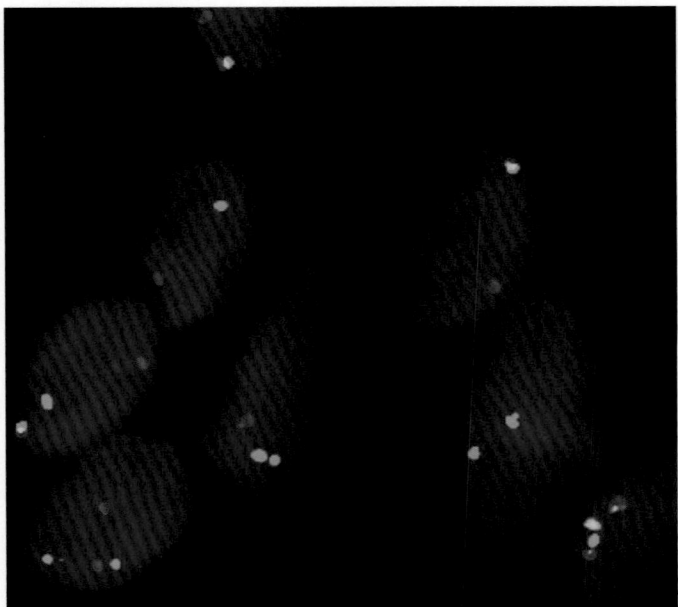

FIGURE 29-34. Mucoepidermoid carcinoma fluorescence in situ hybridization (FISH) MAML2-positive case. The green and red break-apart probes are both designed for the *MAML2* gene of chromosome 11. Yellow signals indicate an intact *MAML2* gene, whereas the solitary green and red probes are consistent with gene disruption or translocation.

PATHOLOGY: ACCs show variable histology. The tumor cells are small, have scant cytoplasm and grow in solid sheets or as small groups, strands, or columns. Within these structures, tumor cells interconnect to enclose cystic spaces, resulting in solid, tubular, or cribriform (sieve-like) patterns (Fig. 29-35). Grading ACCs depends on the proportions of tubular and cribriform patterns, with over 30% solid growth defining "high grade." Such high-grade tumors have a 5-year survival rate of about 15%. Tumor cells

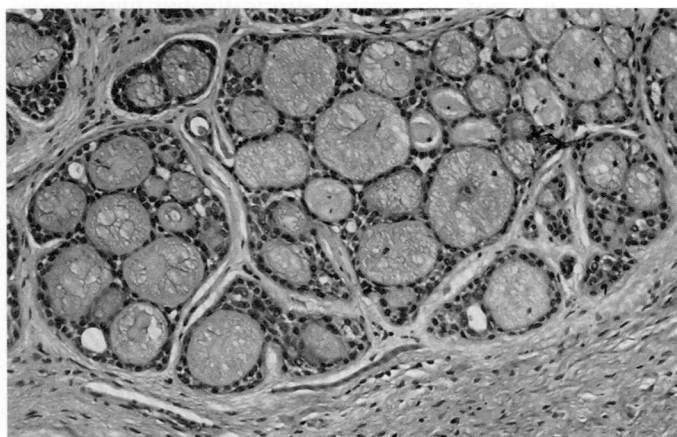

FIGURE 29-35. Adenoid cystic carcinoma showing cribriform growth in which cyst-like spaces are filled with basophilic material. The cyst spaces are really pseudocysts surrounded by myoepithelial cells.

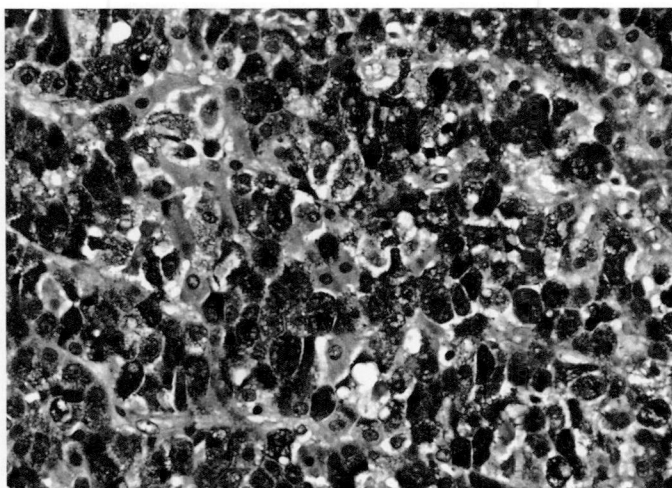

FIGURE 29-36. Acinic cell carcinoma. This tumor demonstrates a solid growth pattern and is composed of basophilic cells with abundant cytoplasm filled with zymogen granules.

produce a homogeneous basement membrane material that gives them the characteristic "cylindromatous" appearance.

ACCs probably arise from cells that differentiate toward intercalated ducts and myoepithelium. *They tend to infiltrate perineural spaces and thus are often painful.* Most do not metastasize for years, but they are often diagnosed late, are difficult to eradicate completely and have a poor long-term prognosis.

Acinic Cell Adenocarcinomas Arise From Secretory Cells

These uncommon parotid tumors (10% of salivary gland tumors) arise occasionally in other salivary glands. They occur mainly in young men ages 20 to 30 years. Acinic cell carcinomas are encapsulated, round masses, usually under 3 cm, and may be cystic. They are composed of uniform cells with small central nuclei and abundant basophilic cytoplasm, similar in appearance to the secretory (acinic) cells of normal salivary glands (Fig. 29-36). They may spread to regional lymph nodes. Most (90%) patients survive 5 years with surgery, but one-third experience local recurrences. Only half survive for 20 years.

Secretory Carcinomas Resemble ACCs

These tumors comprise a distinct histologic entity. They have an associated unique translocation t(12;15)(p13;q25) that leads to the *ETV6–NTRK3* fusion oncogene. This results in constitutive activation of the tyrosine protein kinase domain of NTRK3 which leads to increased cyclin D1 activity and cell cycle progression, and also activation of MAPK mitogenic pathways and PI3K pathways that promote AKT-dependent cell survival. Secretory carcinomas mainly arise in the parotid gland.

The Ear

EXTERNAL EAR

ANATOMY: The outer portion of the external ear includes the auricle or pinna, leading into the external auditory canal. The external auditory canal or meatus extends from the concha medially to the tympanic membrane (eardrum). Its lateral wall is cartilage and connective tissue, and its medial wall is bone. The eardrum sits obliquely at the end of the external auditory canal, separating the external ear and the middle ear.

The auricle is composed of keratinizing, stratified squamous epithelium with associated adnexa (hair follicles, sebaceous glands, eccrine sweat glands). The outer third of the external auditory canal also has ceruminal glands, modified apocrine glands that produce cerumen (ear wax). They are composed of clusters of cuboidal cells with eosinophilic cytoplasm, often containing granular, golden yellow pigment and secretory droplets at their luminal border. Peripheral to the secretory cells are flattened myoepithelial cells. Ceruminal gland ducts end in hair follicles or on the skin. The inner portion of the external auditory canal has no adnexa. The eardrum is airtight. Its outer surface is made of squamous epithelium, continuous with the skin of the external ear canal. Its inner surface is lined by cuboidal epithelium. Between these two is a middle layer of dense fibrous tissue.

KELOIDS: Keloids often form on the ear lobes after piercing for earrings or other trauma (see Chapter 3). They are far more common in blacks and Asians than in whites. Keloids can attain considerable size and tend to recur. They are composed of thick, hyalinized bundles of collagen in the deep dermis (see Chapter 3).

CAULIFLOWER EARS: These deformities, especially common in wrestlers and boxers, result from repeated mechanical trauma to the external ear. Blows to the ears cause subperichondrial hematomas, which organize and deform the ears.

RELAPSING POLYCHONDRITIS: This rare, chronic disorder of unknown origin is characterized by intermittent inflammation that destroys hyaline, elastic or fibrocartilage of the ears, nose, larynx, tracheobronchial tree, ribs, and joints.

The etiology of relapsing polychondritis is obscure; immune mechanisms are suspected. During acute attacks, patients may have serum antibodies to cartilage, type II collagen, and chondroitin sulfate. Immune complexes can be detected in involved cartilage. Relapsing polychondritis may occur alone or with other connective tissue diseases. Noncartilaginous tissues, such as the sclera and cardiac valves, may also be affected. Aortic involvement can lead to fatal rupture.

PATHOLOGY: The perichondrium is infiltrated by lymphocytes, plasma cells, and neutrophils, which also extend into the adjacent cartilage (Fig. 29-37). Chondrocytes die and the cartilaginous matrix degenerates and fragments. Ultimately, the cartilage is replaced by granulation tissue and fibrosis.

"MALIGNANT" OTITIS EXTERNA: This infection of the external auditory canal is caused by *Pseudomonas aeruginosa*. Infection may spread through the skin and cartilage to cause mastoiditis or osteomyelitis of the skull, venous sinus thrombosis, meningitis, and death. Malignant otitis externa occurs mainly in elderly diabetics but is also seen in patients with blood dyscrasias (e.g., leukemia, granulocytopenia).

AURAL POLYPS: These benign inflammatory lesions arise in the external ear canal or extrude into the canal from the middle ear. Aural polyps are ulcerated, and are composed of inflamed granulation tissue, which bleeds readily. Those arising in the middle ear result from chronic otitis media.

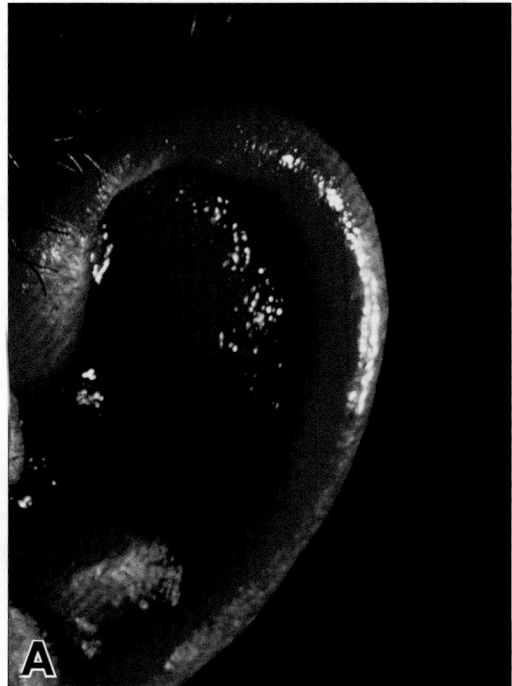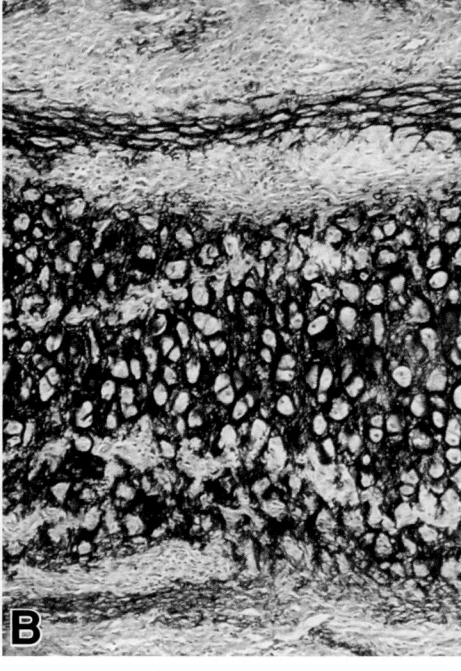

FIGURE 29-37. Relapsing polychondritis. A. The ear is beefy red. **B.** The perichondrium and elastic cartilage are infiltrated and partially destroyed by inflammatory cells and replaced by fibrosis.

NEOPLASMS: Benign and malignant tumors of the external ear include the gamut of skin-related neoplasms: squamous papillomas, seborrheic keratosis, basal cell carcinoma, SCC, and benign and malignant adnexal tumors.

Ceruminal gland tumors are unique to this area. Benign tumors include ceruminal gland adenomas and salivary gland–type tumors (e.g., pleomorphic and monomorphic adenomas). Malignant tumors include adenocarcinoma and malignant salivary gland–type tumors (e.g., adenoid cystic and mucoepidermoid carcinomas).

MIDDLE EAR

ANATOMY: The middle ear, or tympanic cavity, is an oblong space in the temporal bone lined by a mucous membrane. Together with the mastoid air sinuses, it forms a closed mucosal compartment, also called the **middle ear cleft**. Most of its lateral wall is the tympanic membrane. Anteriorly, the eustachian tube connects the middle ear to the nasopharynx. This air passage allows air pressure on both sides of the tympanic membrane to equalize. The three auditory ossicles—the malleus, incus, and stapes—are a chain that connects the tympanic membrane with the oval window located at the medial wall of the tympanic cavity. They conduct sound across the middle ear. Free motion of the ossicles, mainly the stapes in the oval window, is more important for hearing than is an intact tympanic membrane. The middle ear opens posteriorly into the mastoid antrum, a honeycomb of small, aerated, bony compartments (air cells) lined by a thin mucous membrane continuous with that of the middle ear.

Otitis Media Often Follows Obstruction of the Eustachian Tube

Otitis media is inflammation of the middle ear. It usually results from upper respiratory tract infections that spread from the nasopharynx. Obstruction of the eustachian tube is important in production of middle ear effusions. When the pharyngeal end of the eustachian tube is swollen, air cannot enter the tube. Air in the middle ear is absorbed through the mucosa, and negative pressure causes transudation of plasma and occasional bleeding. Antibiotics usually cure or suppress the condition.

ETIOLOGY: Acute otitis media may be due to viral or bacterial infection or sterile obstruction of the eustachian tube. Viral otitis media may resolve without suppuration, or can lead to secondary invasion by pus-forming bacteria. Microorganisms ascend from the nasopharynx, through the eustachian tube, to the middle ear. Otitis media almost invariably penetrates the mastoid antrum into the mastoid cells.

ACUTE SEROUS OTITIS MEDIA: Obstruction of the eustachian tube may result from sudden changes in atmospheric pressure (e.g., while flying in an aircraft or deep-sea diving). This effect is particularly severe if there is an upper respiratory tract infection, acute allergic reaction, or viral or bacterial infection at the eustachian tube orifice. Inflammation may also occur without bacterial invasion of the middle ear. Over half of children in the United States have at least one bout of serous otitis media

before their third birthday. Repeated otitis media in early childhood often leads to residual (usually sterile) fluid in the middle ear, which contributes to unsuspected hearing loss.

CHRONIC SEROUS OTITIS MEDIA: The same conditions that cause acute obstruction of the eustachian tube also cause recurrent or chronic middle ear serous effusions. Carcinoma of the nasopharynx may cause chronic serous otitis media in adults and should be suspected if a unilateral middle ear effusion occurs in an adult.

ACUTE SUPPURATIVE OTITIS MEDIA: One of the most common infections of childhood, acute suppurative otitis media, is caused by pyogenic bacteria that invade the middle ear, usually via the eustachian tube. The most common culprit in all age groups (30% to 40%) is *Streptococcus pneumoniae* (pneumococcus). *H. influenzae* causes about 20% of cases, but less often with increasing age. Accumulating purulent exudate in the middle ear may rupture the eardrum, causing a purulent discharge. In most cases, infection is self-limited and may resolve without therapy.

ACUTE MASTOIDITIS: Infection of the mastoid bone was once a common complication of acute otitis media, before the advent of antibiotics. It is still seen, rarely, if otitis media is not treated adequately. Mastoid air cells become filled with pus, and their thin osseous intercellular walls are destroyed. Serious complications may ensue if infection spreads to contiguous structures (Fig. 29-38).

CHRONIC SUPPURATIVE OTITIS MEDIA AND MASTOIDITIS: Neglected or recurrent middle ear and mastoid infections may lead to chronic inflammation of the mucosa or destruction of the periosteum of the ossicles. Chronic otitis media occurs much more commonly in people who had ear disease in early childhood, which may have arrested normal development of the air cells in the mastoid.

PATHOLOGY: In chronic serous otitis media, mucus-producing (goblet) cell metaplasia may be seen in the mucosal lining of the middle ear. Hemorrhage (e.g., in the mastoid cells) may accompany

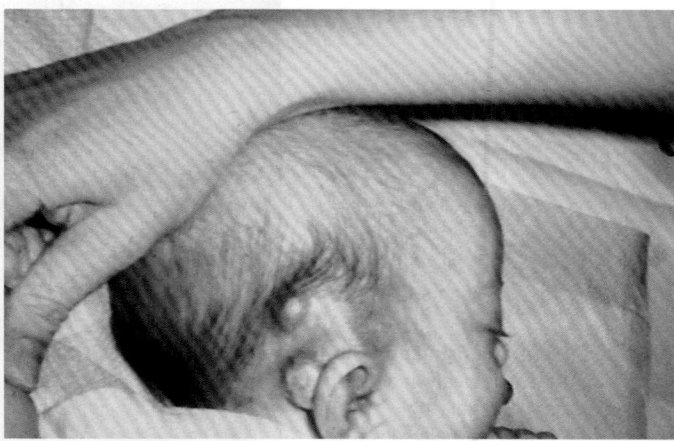

FIGURE 29-38. Acute mastoiditis. An unusual complication of otitis media, acute mastoiditis, appears as large bulging lesions above the child's ear.

acute obstruction. Extravasation of blood and degradation of erythrocytes liberate cholesterol. Cholesterol crystals stimulate a foreign-body response and production of granulation tissue, called a **cholesterol granuloma**. If large, these granulomas may destroy tissue in the mastoid or antrum. If allowed to persist for months, the granulation tissue may become fibrotic, which may eventually lead to complete obliteration of the middle ear and mastoid by fibrous tissue. Inflammation tends to be insidious, persistent, and destructive. In chronic otitis media, by definition, the eardrum is always perforated. Painless discharge **(otorrhea)** and variable hearing loss are constant symptoms. Exuberant granulation tissue may form polyps, which can extend through the perforated eardrum into the external ear canal.

A **cholesteatoma** is a mass of accumulated keratin and squamous mucosa due to growth of squamous epithelium from the external ear canal through a perforated eardrum into the middle ear. There, it continues to produce keratin. Cholesteatomas are identical to epidermal inclusion cysts. They are surrounded by granulation tissue and fibrosis. The keratin mass often becomes infected and protects bacteria from antibiotics. The main dangers of cholesteatoma arise from bony erosion, which may destroy important contiguous structures (e.g., auditory ossicles, facial nerve, labyrinth).

COMPLICATIONS OF ACUTE AND CHRONIC OTITIS MEDIA: Antibiotic therapy has made complications of otitis media uncommon. However, suppurative middle ear infections may still cause serious complications:

- Destruction of the facial nerve
- Deep cervical or subperiosteal abscess, if cortical bone of the mastoid process is eroded
- Petrositis, when infection spreads to the petrous temporal bone through the chain of air cells
- Suppurative labyrinthitis, due to infection of the internal ear
- Epidural, subdural or cerebral abscess, when infection extends through the inner table of the mastoid bone
- Meningitis, when infection reaches the meninges
- Sigmoid sinus thrombophlebitis, if infection traverses the dura to the posterior cranial fossa

Jugulotympanic Paragangliomas Arise From Middle Ear Paraganglia

Jugulotympanic paragangliomas are the most common benign tumors of the middle ear. They grow slowly but, over years, may destroy the middle ear and extend into the internal ear and cranial cavity. Metastases are rare.

Middle ear paragangliomas resemble those arising elsewhere, with characteristic lobules of cells in richly vascular connective tissue (Fig. 29-39). Paraganglial cells are of neural crest origin and contain varying amounts of catecholamines, mostly epinephrine and norepinephrine.

INTERNAL EAR

ANATOMY: The petrous portion of the temporal bone contains the labyrinth, which shelters the end organs for hearing **(cochlea)** and equilibrium **(vestibular labyrinth)**. The complex cavities of the osseous labyrinth contain the

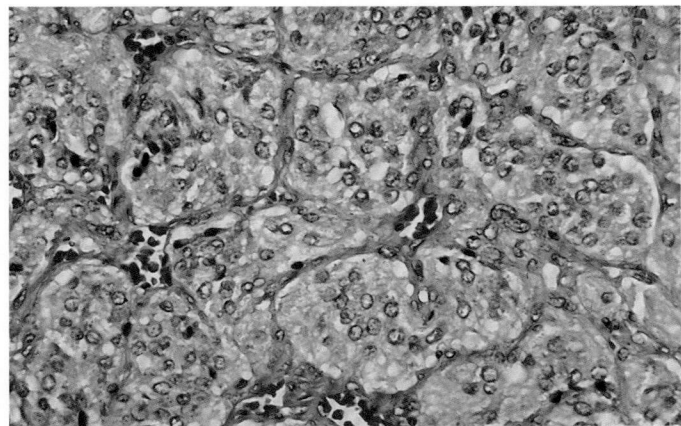

FIGURE 29-39. Jugulotympanic paraganglioma. Tumor cell nests are composed of cells with ill-defined cell borders and prominent eosinophilic cytoplasm (chief cells).

membranous labyrinth, a series of communicating membranous sacs and ducts. The osseous labyrinth connects to the subarachnoid space via the cochlear aqueduct. It is filled with perilymph, a clear fluid that mingles with cerebrospinal fluid. The membranous labyrinth contains a different fluid, the endolymph, which circulates in a closed system. Because there are no barriers between the cochlear and vestibular labyrinths, injury or disease of the inner ear frequently affects both hearing and equilibrium.

The **cochlea** is coiled upon itself like a snail shell and makes 2-1/2 turns. It has three compartments: two that contain perilymph and a third (the cochlear duct) with endolymph. The cochlear duct encompasses the end organ of hearing, **the organ of Corti,** which rests on the basement membrane and is arranged as a spiral, with three rows of outer hair cells and a row of inner hair cells. When hairs of these neuroepithelial cells are bent or distorted by vibration, the mechanical force is converted into electrochemical impulses and interpreted in the temporal cortex as sound. The vestibular part of the membranous labyrinth consists of the utricle, saccule, and semicircular canals, each with specialized neuroepithelium that determines equilibrium.

Otosclerosis Is Formation of New Spongy Bone About the Stapes

Otosclerosis causes progressive deafness. *It is an autosomal dominant hereditary defect and is the most common cause of conductive hearing loss in young and middle-aged adults in the United States.* This disorder affects 10% of white and 1% of black adult Americans, although 90% of cases are asymptomatic. The female-to-male ratio is 2:1, and both ears are usually affected.

PATHOLOGY: Although any part of the petrous bone may be affected, otosclerotic bone tends to form at particular points. The most frequent (85%) site is immediately anterior to the oval window. The focus of sclerotic bone extends posteriorly and may infiltrate and replace the stapes, progressively immobilizing

THE HEAD AND NECK

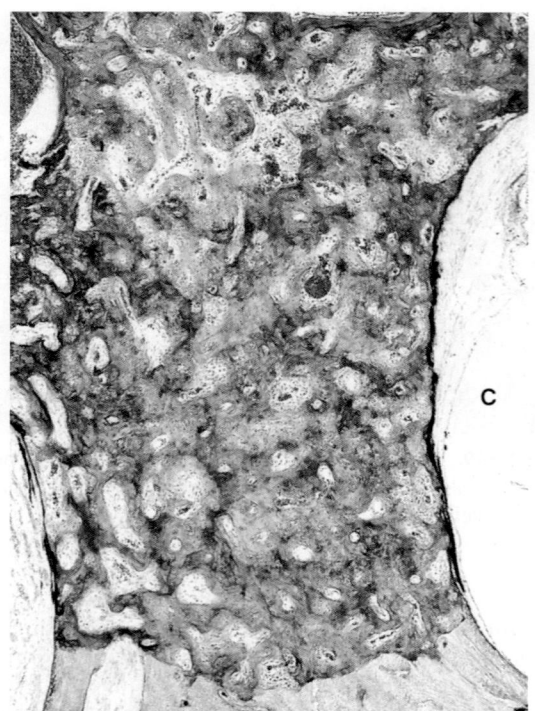

FIGURE 29-40. Otosclerosis. In the lateral wall of the cochlea, the basophilic and more vascular bone is well demarcated. C = organ of Corti.

the footplate of the stapes. The developing bony ankylosis is manifested functionally as slowly progressive conductive hearing loss.

Otosclerosis begins with resorption of bone and formation of highly cellular fibrous tissue, with wide vascular spaces and osteoclasts. The resorbed bone is later replaced by immature bone, which, with repeated remodeling, becomes mature (Fig. 29-40). Otosclerosis is treated by surgical mobilization of the auditory ossicles.

Ménière Disease Is a Triad of Vertigo, Sensorineural Hearing Loss and Tinnitus

Several etiologies have been suggested, but the cause of **Ménière disease** is uncertain. About 45,500 new cases are diagnosed in the United States annually. Viral etiologies, vascular causes and, possibly, autoimmune mechanisms have all been suggested. Tinnitus is usually unilateral and is most frequent between 40 and 60 years of age. A familial association suggests an underlying genetic predisposition.

PATHOLOGY: The earliest change is dilatation of the cochlear duct and saccule. As the disease **(hydrops)** progresses, the entire endolymphatic system dilates and the membranous wall may tear (Fig. 29-41). Ruptures can be followed by collapse of the membranous labyrinth, but atrophy of sensory and neural structures is rare. Symptoms occur when endolymphatic hydrops causes rupture, and endolymph escapes into the perilymph.

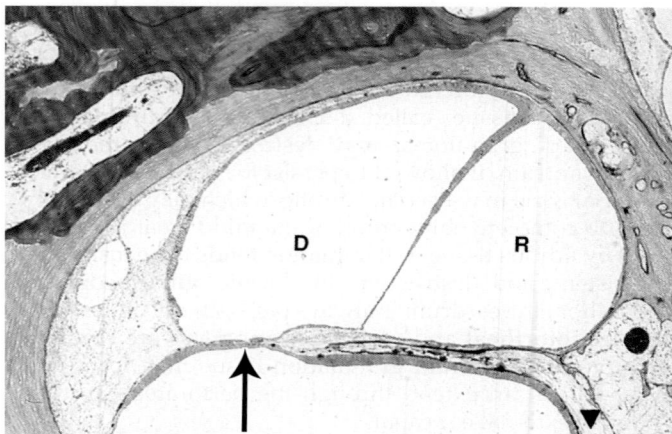

FIGURE 29-41. Ménière disease. The cochlear duct (*D*) is markedly distended, and the Reissner membrane (*R*) is pushed back by endolymphatic hydrops. Neither the organ of Corti (*arrow*) nor the spiral ganglion (*arrowhead*) is in its usual location.

CLINICAL FEATURES: Attacks of vertigo, often with incapacitating nausea and vomiting, last less than 24 hours. Repeat episodes may be separated by weeks or months. In time, remissions become longer. Hearing loss is recovered between attacks but later may become permanent. Ménière disease may improve with a low-salt diet and diuretics.

Labyrinthine Toxicity Is a Cause of Drug-Induced Deafness

Aminoglycoside antibiotics are the most common ototoxic drugs, producing irreversible damage to vestibular or cochlear sensory cells. Other antibiotics, diuretics, antimalarials, and salicylates may also lead to transient or permanent sensorineural hearing loss. Among antineoplastic drugs, cisplatin causes temporary or permanent hearing loss.

The labyrinth of the developing embryo is very sensitive to some drugs. Maternal use of antimalarials and other drugs may cause congenital deafness.

Viral Labyrinthitis Can Result in Congenital Deafness

Viral infections may cause inner ear disorders, particularly deafness. This is mostly due to viral invasion of the labyrinth. CMV and rubella are the best-known prenatal viral infections that cause congenital deafness via maternal-to-fetal transmission.

Mumps is the most common postnatal viral cause of deafness. It can cause rapid hearing loss, which is unilateral in 80% of cases. By contrast, prenatal infection of the labyrinth with rubella is usually bilateral, with permanent loss of cochlear and vestibular function. Other viruses are suspected to cause labyrinthitis, including influenza and parainfluenza viruses, EBV, herpesviruses, and adenoviruses. Such cases show severe damage to the organ of Corti, with almost total loss of inner and outer hair cells.

Acoustic Trauma

Noise-induced hearing loss is a significant problem in industrialized countries. Occupational or recreational exposure to loud noises may impair hearing temporarily or permanently, for example, people exposed to jet engines or loud music. The external hair cells of the organ of Corti are damaged earliest. Loss of sensory hairs is followed by deformation, swelling, and disintegration of the hair cells.

Schwannoma Is the Most Common Tumor of the Inner Ear

SCHWANNOMA: Nearly all schwannomas in the internal auditory canal arise from the vestibular nerves. Vestibular schwannomas, which account for about 10% of all intracranial tumors, are slow growing and encapsulated. Larger tumors protrude from the internal auditory meatus into the cerebellopontine angle and may deform the brainstem and adjacent cerebellum. Schwannomas cause slowly progressive vestibular and auditory symptoms. In neurofibromatosis type 2 (see Chapter 28), bilateral vestibular schwannomas identical to other vestibular schwannomas occur frequently.

MENINGIOMA: Meningiomas of the cerebellopontine angle originate from the meningothelial cells in the arachnoid villi. The favored sites for these tumors are the sphenoid ridge and petrous pyramid. Meningiomas may extend into the adjacent temporal bone or dural sinuses (see Chapter 28).

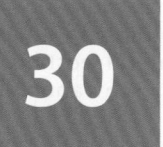

30 Bones, Joints, and Soft Tissue

Roberto A. Garcia, Michael J. Klein, Elizabeth G. Demicco, Alan L. Schiller

Bones

The functions of bone are mechanical, mineral storage, and hematopoietic. Mechanical functions include protection for the brain, spinal cord, and chest organs; rigid internal support for limbs; and deployment as lever arms for skeletal muscles. Bone is the principal reservoir for calcium and it stores other ions such as phosphate, sodium, and magnesium. Bones also serve as hosts for hematopoietic bone marrow.

The mechanical properties of bone are related to its construction and internal architecture. Although extremely light, it has high-tensile strength. This combination of strength and light weight results from its hollow tubular shape, layering of bone tissue, and internal buttressing of the matrix.

The term **bone** can refer to both an organ and a tissue. The "organ" is composed of bone tissue, cartilage, fat, marrow elements, vessels, nerves, and fibrous tissue. Bone "tissue" is described in microscopic terms and is defined by the relation of its collagen and mineral structure to the bone cells.

ANATOMY

Macroscopically, two types of bone are recognized:

- **Cortical bone** is dense, compact bone, whose outer shell defines the shape of the bone. It composes 80% of the skeleton. Because of its density, its functions are mainly biomechanical.
- **Coarse cancellous bone** (also called **spongy, trabecular,** or **medullary bone**) is found at the ends of long bones within the medullary canal. Cancellous bone has a high surface-to-volume ratio and contains many more bone cells per unit volume than cortical bone. **Changes in the rate of bone turnover are manifested principally in cancellous bone.**

All bones contain both cancellous and cortical elements (Fig. 30-1), but their proportions differ. The body or shaft of a long tubular bone, such as the femur, is composed of cortical bone and its marrow is mainly fat. Toward the ends of the femur, the cortex becomes thin, and coarse cancellous bone becomes the predominant structure. By contrast, the skull is formed by outer and inner tables of compact bone, with only a small amount of cancellous bone, called the **diploë**, within the marrow space.

The anatomy of bone is defined in relation to the growth plate (**physis**), a transverse structure which is present in the growing child (Fig. 30-2A–C). The terms **epiphysis, metaphysis**, and **diaphysis** are defined in relation to the growth plate.

- The **epiphysis** is the area of the bone that extends from the subarticular bone plate to the base of the growth plate.
- The **metaphysis** contains coarse cancellous bone. It extends from the side of the growth plate away from the joint to form the area where the bone develops a fluted or funnel shape.
- The **diaphysis** corresponds to the body or shaft of the bone. The metaphysis blends into the diaphysis in the area where coarse cancellous bone dissipates. This area of bone is particularly important in hematogenous infections, tumors, and skeletal malformations.

Two additional terms are essential to an understanding of bone organization:

- **Endochondral ossification** is the process by which bone tissue replaces cartilage.
- **Intramembranous ossification** refers to the mechanism by which bone tissue supplants membranous or fibrous tissue laid down by the periosteum.

All bones are formed by at least some intramembranous ossification, which accounts for the formation of compact bone. Some bones (e.g., the calvaria of the skull) are forged purely by intramembranous ossification. Longitudinal growth of long bones is accounted for by endochondral ossification.

The Bone Marrow Resides in the Marrow Space or Medullary Canal

The marrow space is enclosed by cortical bone. It is supported by a delicate connective tissue framework that enmeshes marrow cells and blood vessels. Three types of marrow are evident to the naked eye:

- **Red marrow** corresponds to hematopoietic tissue and is found in virtually all bones at birth. At adolescence, it becomes confined to the axial skeleton (the skull, ribs, and vertebrae). Its presence in appendicular bones (the portion of the skeleton that supports the limbs including the pelvis and pectoral girdle) may also be pathologic, depending on the patient's age and the site of the marrow. For example, red marrow in the femoral diaphysis of a 55-year-old man is abnormal and may reflect underlying disease, such as leukemia.
- **Yellow marrow** is fat tissue and is found in the limb bones. It is abnormal at any age in a hematopoietic site, such as a vertebral body.
- **Gray or white marrow** is deficient in hematopoietic elements and is often fibrotic. *It is always a pathologic tissue in a nongrowing adult bone or in areas distant from the growth plate in a child.*

Blood Supply Enters Bone Through Specialized Canals

The long tubular bones are provided with blood from two sources and contain canals to supply the tissues.

- **Nutrient arteries** enter bone through a nutrient foramen and supply the marrow space and the internal one-third to one-half of the cortex.
- **Perforating arteries** are small straight vessels that extend inward from periosteal arteries on the external surface of the periosteum (the fibrous capsule of the bone). Perforating arteries anastomose in the cortex with branches from nutrient arteries coming from the marrow space.
- **Haversian canals** are spaces in cortical bone that course parallel to the long axis of the bone for a short distance and then branch and communicate with other similar canals. Each canal contains one or two blood vessels, and some nerve fibers (Fig. 30-2D).
- **Volkmann canals** (Fig. 30-2E) are spaces within the cortex that run transversely to the long axis of the cortex to connect adjacent Haversian canals. Volkmann canals also contain blood vessels.

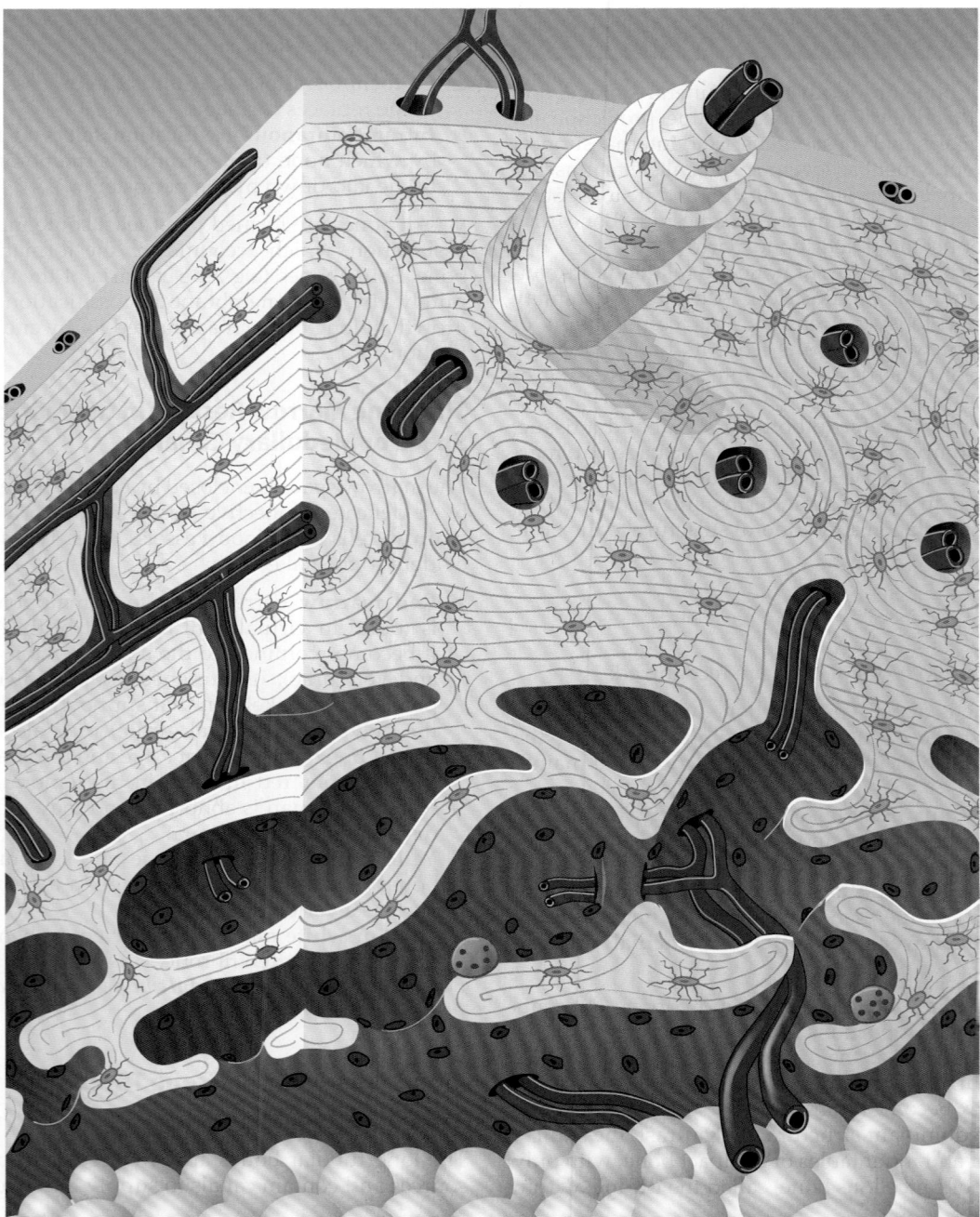

FIGURE 30-1. Anatomy of bone. A schematic representation of cortical and trabecular bone. The longitudinal section (*left*) shows the vasculature entering the periosteum via the periosteal perforating arteries and coursing through the bone perpendicular to the long axis in Volkmann canals. The vessels that proceed longitudinally, or parallel to the long axis, are located in Haversian canals. Each artery is accompanied by a vein. Within the cortex, osteocytes reside in lacunae, and their cell processes extend into the canaliculi. The cross-sectional view (*right*) illustrates the various types of lamellar bone in the cortex. Circumferential lamellar bone is located adjacent to the periosteum and borders the marrow space. Concentric lamellar bone surrounds the central Haversian canals to form an **osteon**. Each layer of the concentric lamellar bone displays a change in the pitch of the collagen fibers, such that each layer has a different arrangement of collagen. The interstitial lamellar bone occupies the space between osteons. The marrow space is filled with fat, and its trabecular bone is contiguous with the cortex. Multinucleated osteoclasts are present, and palisaded osteoblasts surround the bone surfaces. The perforating arteries from the periosteum and the nutrient artery from the marrow space communicate within the cortex via Haversian and Volkmann canals.

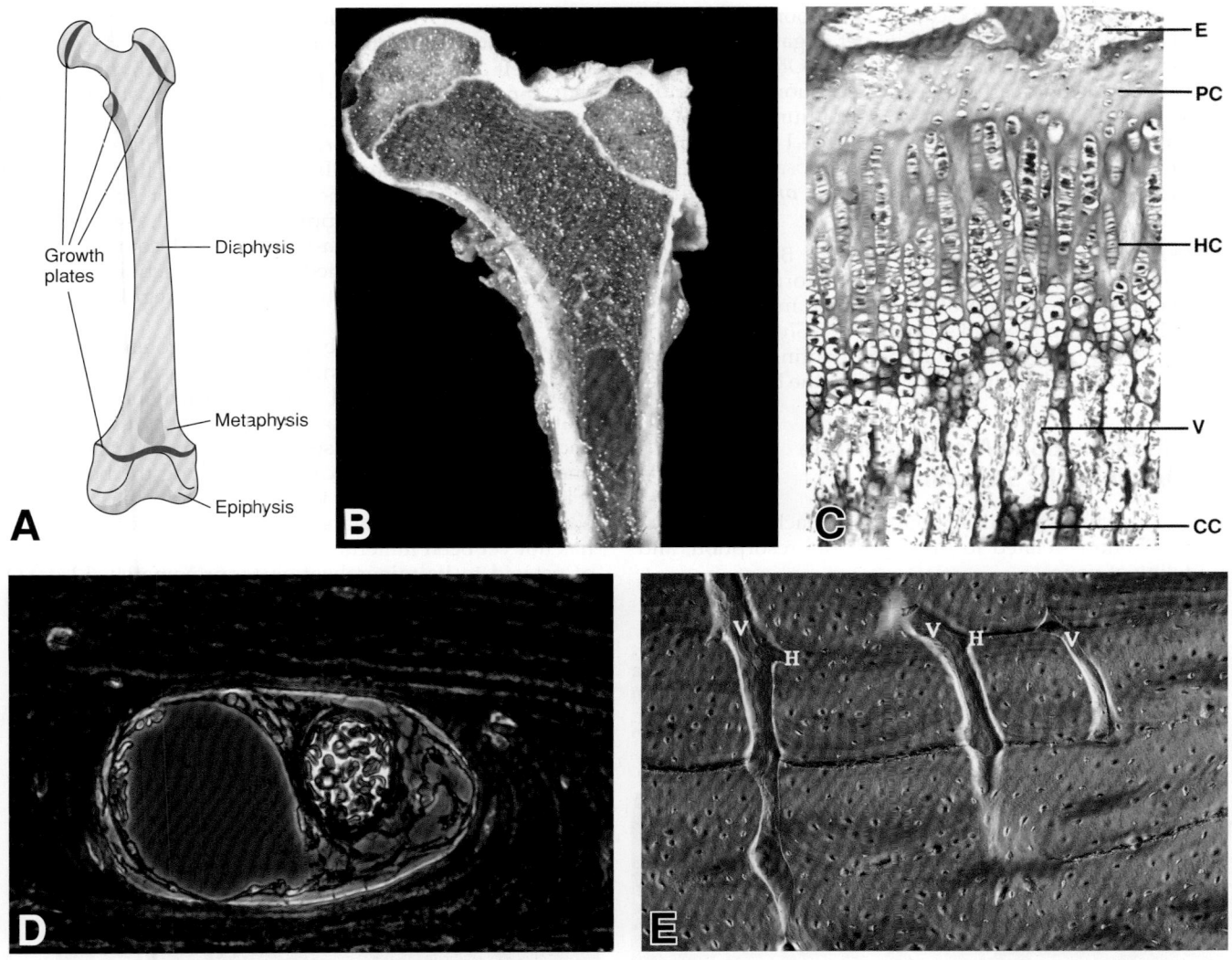

FIGURE 30-2. Anatomy of a long bone. A. Diagram of the femur illustrates the various compartments. **B. Coronal section of the proximal femur** illustrates the various anatomic parts of a long bone. The epiphysis of the femoral head and the apophysis of the greater trochanter are separated from the metaphysis by their respective growth plates. The cortex and the medullary cavity are well visualized. The medullary cavity contains cancellous bone until the metaphysis narrows into the diaphysis (shaft) of the bone, which is almost completely devoid of bone and filled with marrow. **C. A section of the epiphysis** with a zone of proliferating cartilage cells. Beneath this zone, the hypertrophic cartilage cells are arrayed in columns. At the *bottom,* the calcifying matrix is invaded by blood vessels. *CC* = calcified cartilage; *E* = epiphysis; *HC* = hypertrophic cartilage; *PC* = proliferative cartilage; *V* = vascular invasion. **D. Haversian canal** containing a venule (thin-walled wider vessel on *left*) and an arteriole (thicker-walled narrow vessel on the *right*). **E. Volkmann canals.** Three Volkmann canals are seen running parallel to each other (*V*) and perpendicular to the cortex. The openings of two Haversian canals (*H*) are visible.

Each artery has its paired vein and, sometimes, associated free nerve endings. Venous drainage proceeds from the cortex outward to periosteal veins, or inward into the marrow space and out via nutrient veins (which are paired with nutrient arteries).

Periosteum Covers All Bones and Can Form Bone

The periosteum is the fibrous tissue that envelops the outer surface of the bone and demarcates it from the surrounding soft tissue. It is connected to the bone by collagenous fibers called **Sharpey fibers.** The internal layer of the periosteum, the **cambium layer,** is applied to the surface of the bone and consists of loosely arranged collagenous bundles, with spindle-shaped connective tissue cells and a network of thin elastic fibers. The

outer **fibrous layer** is contiguous with adjacent soft-tissue planes and fascia. It is composed of dense connective tissue containing blood vessels. The cambium layer is responsible for the process of intramembranous ossification and formation of the cortex. If the periosteum is injured (e.g., infection, trauma or tumor), it can respond by producing a significant amount of reactive bone that can be seen radiographically.

Bone Matrix Is Organic and Heavily Mineralized

Bone tissue is composed of cells (10% by weight), a mineralized phase (hydroxyapatite [HA] crystals, representing 60% of the total tissue) and an organic matrix (30%). *Thus, except for its cells, bone is a composite structure composed of an organic and an inorganic matrix.*

The **mineralized matrix** consists of poorly crystalline HA, $Ca_{10}(PO_4)_6(OH)_2$. Because of its net negative charge, it can neutralize substantial amounts of acid. Other important ions in bone include carbonate, citrate, fluoride, chloride, sodium, magnesium, potassium, and strontium.

The **organic matrix** consists of 88% type I collagen, 10% other proteins and 1% to 2% lipids and glycosaminoglycans. *Thus, type I collagen basically defines the organic matrix.* Other proteins include:

- **Osteocalcin** is produced by osteoblasts. Blood levels of this protein are a useful marker of bone formation.
- **Osteopontin** and **sialoprotein** are bone matrix proteins containing the amino acid sequence *Arg-Gly-Asp*, which is recognized by **integrins**. Thus, osteopontin and bone sialoprotein probably help anchor cells to the bone matrix.

The Cells of the Bone Are Responsible for Maintaining Its Structure

There are four types of cells in bone tissue, each of which has specific functions related to the formation, resorption, and remodeling of bone:

OSTEOPROGENITOR CELL: The osteoprogenitor cell differentiates ultimately into osteoblasts and osteocytes. It is itself derived from a primitive mesenchymal stem cell that can develop into adipocytes, myoblasts, fibroblasts, or osteoblasts. Osteoprogenitor cells are found in marrow, periosteum and all supporting structures within the marrow cavity. They are not readily recognized by light microscopy as they are small, nonspecific, stellate, or spindle-shaped cells. In response to an appropriate signal, osteoprogenitor cells give rise to osteoblasts. Osteoblast commitment and differentiation are controlled by complex activities involving signal transduction and transcriptional regulation of gene expression

OSTEOBLAST: Osteoblasts are the protein-synthesizing cells that produce and mineralize bone tissue. As mentioned above, they are derived from mesenchymal progenitors that also give rise to chondrocytes, myocytes, adipocytes, and fibroblasts. Osteoblasts are large mononuclear, polygonal cells that are arrayed in a line along the bone surface (Fig. 30-3A). Underlying the layer of osteoblasts is a thin, eosinophilic zone of organic bone matrix, called **osteoid**, that has not yet been mineralized. The time from the deposition of osteoid to its mineralization (approximately 12 days) is

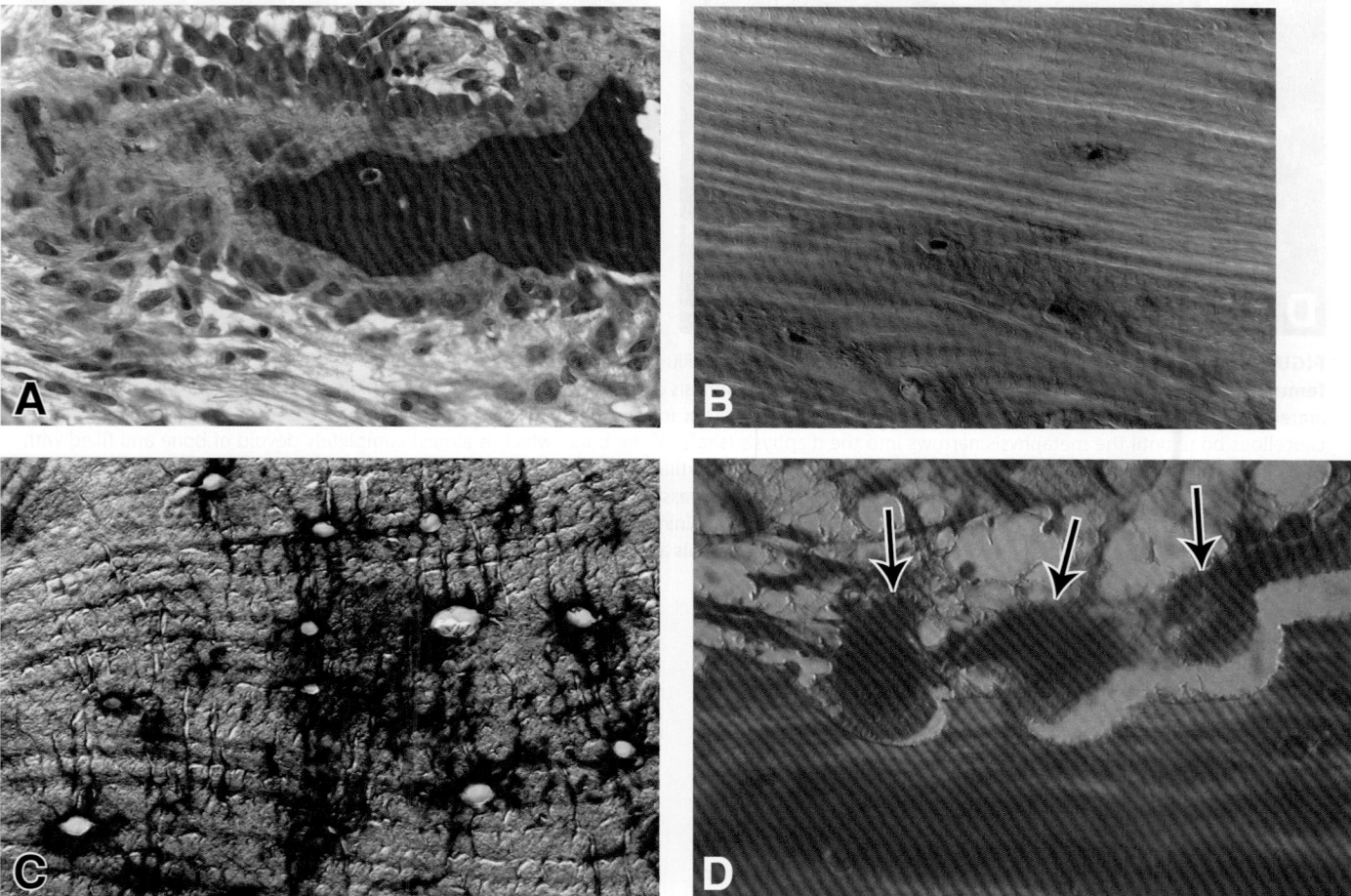

FIGURE 30-3. The cells of bones. A. A **developing bone spicule** demonstrates a prominent layer of plump osteoblasts lining the pink osteoid seam. The dark purple structure within the osteoid seam is mineralized bone. **B. Osteocytes.** Osteocytes represent trapped osteoblasts surrounded by bone matrix. The space surrounding the cell is called a **lacuna. C.** Extensive **intercommunication of osteocyte processes** via their canalicular network in cortical bone is visible in this section. **D. Osteoclasts.** These multinucleated giant cells (*arrows*) are found on bone surfaces within small scalloped reabsorption pits, called **Howship lacunae.**

known as the **mineralization lag time**. The protein synthetic capacity of an osteoblast is reflected in its abundant endoplasmic reticulum, prominent Golgi apparatus, and mitochondria with calcium-containing granules. Cytoplasmic processes that extend into the osteoid contact cells embedded in the matrix called **osteocytes**. Osteoblasts contain alkaline phosphatase, manufacture osteocalcin and express parathyroid hormone (PTH) receptors. Collagenase secreted by osteoblasts may also facilitate osteoclastic activity. They also produce a number of growth factors and cytokines, including transforming growth factor-β (TGF-β), insulin-like growth factor-I (IGF-I), IGF-2, platelet-derived growth factor (PDGF), interleukin-1 (IL-1), fibroblast growth factor (FGF), and tumor necrosis factor-α (TNF-α), which regulate bone growth and differentiation. Osteoblasts also express surface receptors for various hormones (e.g., PTH, vitamin D, estrogen, glucocorticoids, etc.), as well as for cytokines and growth factors. When an osteoblast is inactive, it flattens on the surface of bone tissue. *The osteoblast ultimately controls the activation, maturation, and differentiation of the osteoclast through a paracrine cell signaling mechanism (see Osteoclast below).*

OSTEOCYTE: The osteocyte is an osteoblast that has become surrounded by bone matrix and is isolated in a lacuna (Fig. 30-3B). Osteocytes deposit small quantities of bone around lacunae, but with time, they lose the capacity for protein synthesis. They have small hyperchromatic nuclei and numerous processes that extend through bony canals called **canaliculi**, which communicate via gap junctions with cell processes from other osteocytes (Fig. 30-3C). *The osteocytes may be the bone cells that recognize and respond to mechanical forces and are important regulators of bone remodeling.*

OSTEOCLAST: Osteoclasts are the exclusive bone-resorptive cells. They arise from hematopoietic progenitor cells and are members of the monocyte/macrophage family. Three major factors are required for osteoclastogenesis: (1) TNF-related receptor RANK (receptor activator for nuclear factor-κB [NFκB]); (2) RANK ligand (RANKL); and (3) macrophage colony-stimulating factor (M-CSF). RANK is expressed by osteoclast precursors. RANKL and M-CSF are produced by osteoblasts and stromal cells. Binding of RANKL to RANK activates NFκB signaling, which stimulates osteoclastogenesis. M-CSF is required for survival of cells of macrophage/osteoclast lineage. **Osteoprotegerin**, another protein produced by osteoblasts and also a member of the TNF family, blocks interactions between RANK and RANKL and thus inhibits osteoclastogenesis.

Osteoclasts are multinucleated cells that contain many lysosomes and are rich in hydrolytic enzymes. They are found in small depressions on bone surfaces called **Howship lacunae** (Fig. 30-3D). As seen by electron microscopy, an osteoclast forms a polarized-ruffled plasmalemmal membrane (Fig. 30-4) when it comes in contact with and is actively degrading bone. Osteoclastic resorption is a multistep process that first involves attachment of the cell to bone by integrins. A tight gasket-like seal isolates an extracellular compartment that forms between bone and the osteoclast-ruffled membrane. A proton pump then acidifies this compartment to a pH of 4.5, in effect creating a giant extracellular lysosome. This proton-rich milieu mobilizes bone mineral, and thereby exposes the organic bone matrix to degradation by lysosomal enzymes. Degraded fragments of

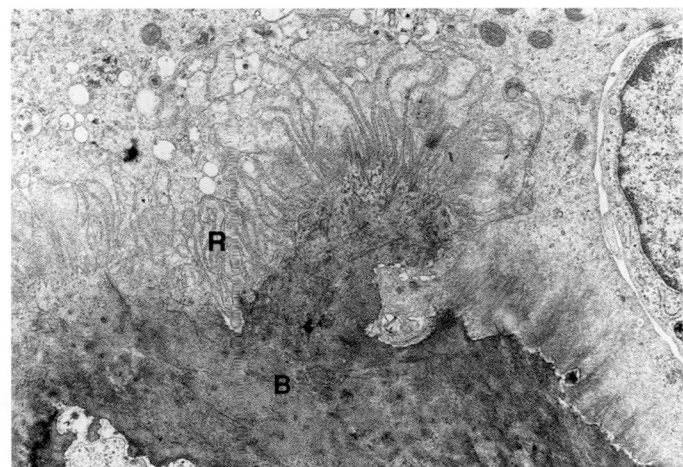

FIGURE 30-4. Osteoclast. This electron micrograph shows the ruffled membrane (*R*) of an osteoclast, which consists of a complex infolding of the plasma membrane juxtaposed to bone (*B*).

bone are transported to the opposite side of the osteoclasts and then released to the extracellular space.

Although the machinery of an osteoclast is superbly suited for bone resorption, it functions only if the matrix is mineralized. *In fact, any bone that is lined by osteoid or unmineralized cartilage is protected from osteoclastic activity.* In rickets, for example (see below), the growth plate does not calcify normally; it thus grows without osteoclastic resorption and becomes very thick.

Constant bone remodeling is a normal part of skeletal maintenance (Fig. 30-5). It is initiated by activation of the cytokine receptor RANK on osteoclasts. PTH and soluble factors released during bone resorption aid in recruitment and activation of osteoblasts at sites of new bone formation. Osteoclasts

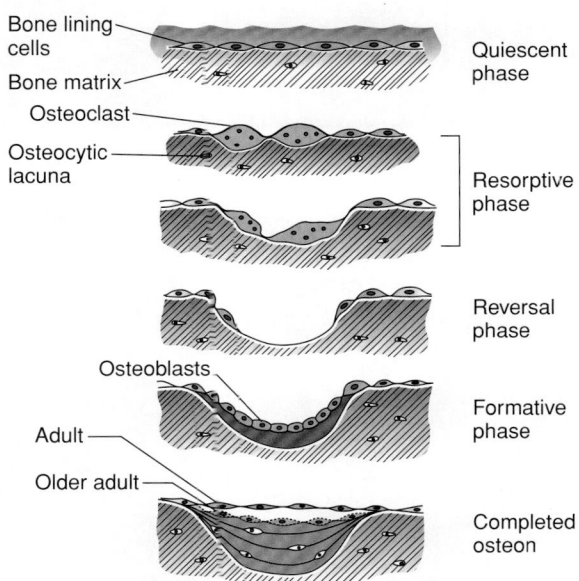

FIGURE 30-5. Bone-remodeling sequence. Bone remodeling is initiated by osteoclasts on a bone surface previously lined by fusiform cells. After creating a resorption bay, osteoclasts are replaced by osteoblasts, which deposit new bone. Bone loss that attends aging (senile osteoporosis) is due to incomplete filling of resorption bays.

express receptors for **calcitonin**, which inhibits osteoclast activity. *Thus, bone remodeling involves replacing old bone with newly formed bone via the functional coupling of osteoclasts and osteoblasts, called the bone-remodeling unit.* Bone remodeling enables bone to adapt to mechanical stress, maintain its strength, and regulate calcium homeostasis.

Microscopic Organization of Bone Tissue: Lamellar Bone and Woven Bone

Both may be mineralized or unmineralized. Unmineralized bone is called **osteoid**.

Lamellar Bone

Lamellar bone is made slowly and is highly organized. As the stronger bone tissue, it forms the adult skeleton. *Anything other than lamellar bone in the adult skeleton is abnormal.* Lamellar bone is defined by: (1) a parallel arrangement of type I collagen fibers; (2) few osteocytes in the matrix; and (3) uniform osteocytes in small lacunae parallel to the long axis of the collagen fibers. There are four types of lamellar bone (Fig. 30-6):

- **Circumferential bone** forms the outer periosteal and inner endosteal lamellar envelopes of the cortex.
- **Concentric lamellar bone** is arranged around the Haversian canals. In two dimensions, concentric lamellar bone and its Haversian artery and vein constitute the **osteon** (Fig. 30-1). In three dimensions, osteons make up the **Haversian system**. These cylinders of bone arranged around Haversian canals run parallel to the long axis of the cortex and are the strongest bone made. Osteons form only if there is appropriate stress.
- **Interstitial lamellar bone** represents remnants of either circumferential or concentric lamellar bone that have been remodeled and are wedged between osteons.
- **Trabecular lamellar bone** forms the coarse cancellous bone of the medullary cavity. It exhibits plates of lamellar bone perforated by marrow spaces.

Woven Bone

Woven bone is identified by: (1) an irregular arrangement of type I collagen fibers—hence the term *woven*; (2) numerous osteocytes in the matrix; and (3) variation in osteocyte size and shape (Fig. 30-7A,B).

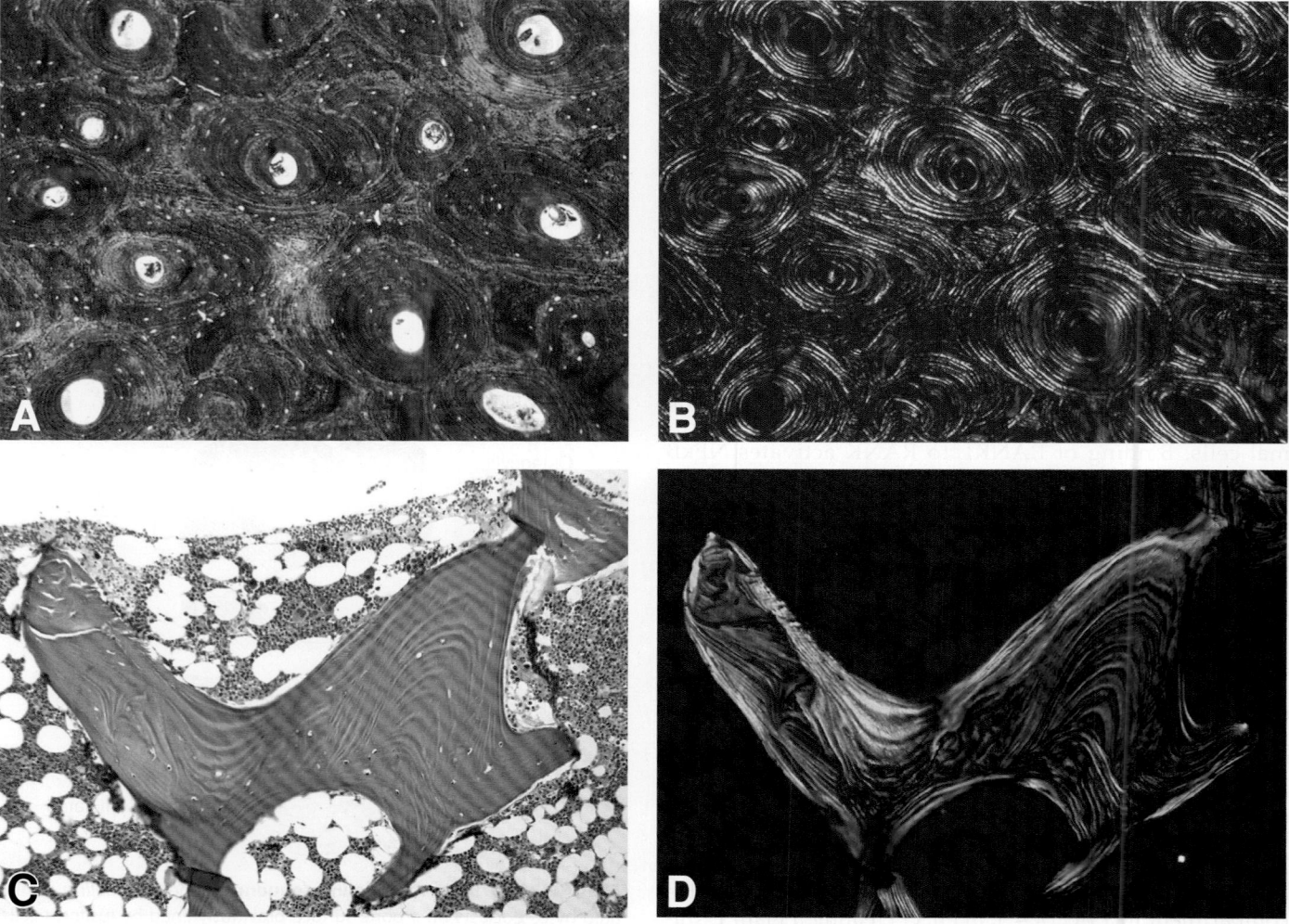

FIGURE 30-6. Cortical lamellar bone. A. Lamellae of the compacta (cortex) are arranged concentrically about Haversian canals. **B.** The same field viewed in polarized light shows alternating light and dark layers of collagen fibers. **C. Lamellae of the spongiosa** in a single mature trabecula are shown in a bright field view. **D.** Polarized light demonstrates lamellae arranged in light and dark layers in long plates rather than in a concentric arrangement.

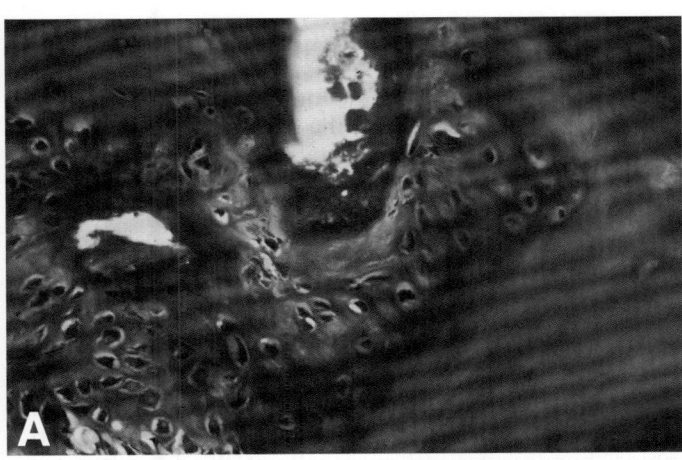 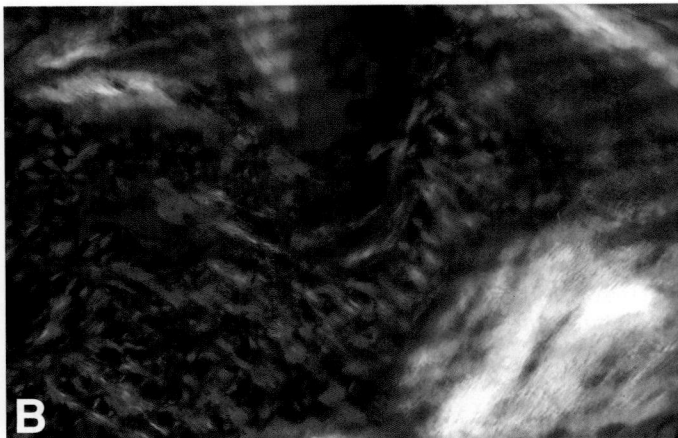

FIGURE 30-7. Woven bone. A. Woven bone in early fracture repair contains many osteocytes that vary in size but are mainly large with prominent lacunae (compare with area of lamellar bone at *lower right*). **B.** The same section viewed in polarized light shows collagen fibers resembling the loose fiber pattern of coarsely woven burlap.

Woven bone is deposited more rapidly than lamellar bone. It is haphazardly arranged and of low tensile strength, serving as a temporary scaffolding for support. It is not surprising that woven bone is found in the developing fetus, in areas surrounding tumors and infections, and as part of a healing fracture. *Its presence in the adult skeleton is always abnormal and indicates that reactive tissue has been produced in response to some stress in the bone.*

Cartilage, Unlike Bone, Contains No Blood Vessels, Nerves, or Lymphatics

Cartilage may be focally calcified to provide some internal strength in the appropriate areas.

Cartilage Matrix

Like bone, cartilage may be viewed as an organic and inorganic composite material. The inorganic phase is composed of calcium HA crystals, similar to those found in bone matrix, but only present in a few foci of the cartilage. The organic matrix consists mainly of two types of macromolecules, type II collagen and proteoglycans, which constitute roughly 20% of its weight. The proteoglycans are hyperhydrated such that water comprises the remaining 80% of the total weight of the matrix. This water content is extremely important in the function of articular cartilage as it enhances resilience and lubrication of the joint. Proteoglycans are complex macromolecules composed of a central linear protein core, to which long side arms of polysaccharides, called **glycosaminoglycans**, are attached. The linear protein cores are attached to macromolecules of hyaluronic acid via link proteins. These macromolecules are polyanionic because of the regular presence of carboxyl groups and sulfates, and their strong negative charge accounts for their ability to bind large amounts of water (hydrophilia). Cartilage glycosaminoglycans comprise three long-chain, unbranched, repeating, polydimeric saccharides: chondroitin-4-sulfate, chondroitin-6-sulfate, and keratan sulfate. The chondroitin sulfates are the most abundant, accounting for 55% to 90% of the cartilage matrix, depending on the age of the tissue.

Types of Cartilage

There are three types of cartilage:

- **Hyaline cartilage:** This is the prototypic cartilage, constituting the articular cartilage of joints; cartilaginous anlage of developing bones; growth plates; costochondral cartilages; cartilages of the trachea, bronchi, and larynx; and nasal cartilages.
- **Fibrocartilage:** This tissue is essentially dense connective tissue whose cells resemble chondrocytes. It contains less glycosaminoglycan than hyaline cartilage, and includes type I collagen which provides tensile and structural strength. It is found in the annulus fibrosus of the intervertebral disc, tendinous and ligamentous insertions, menisci, symphysis pubis, and insertions of joint capsules.
- **Elastic cartilage** is found in the epiglottis, in the arytenoid cartilages of the larynx and in the external ear. It resembles hyaline cartilage but its chondrocytes are enveloped in elastic fibers which help to impart its shape memory.

Chondrocytes

Chondrocytes are derived from primitive mesenchymal cells that are similar to the precursors of bone cells. The chondroblast gives rise to the chondrocyte. Activation of SOX9 transcription factor is essential for chondrocyte formation, and SOX9 is expressed in cartilaginous neoplasms. As in bone, the cell that resorbs calcified cartilage is the osteoclast.

BONE FORMATION AND GROWTH

Bone tissue grows only by appositional growth, defined as deposition of new matrix on a pre-existing surface by adjacent surface osteoblasts. By contrast, virtually all other tissues, especially cartilage, increase by interstitial cell proliferation within the matrix as well as by appositional growth.

Bone development in the fetus follows a stereotypical sequence. Most of the skeleton (except the calvaria and clavicles) forms from cartilage anlagen present during fetal development. This cartilage is eventually resorbed and replaced by bone during **endochondral ossification**. Development of bone can be illustrated by using a limb as an example.

The Process of Primary Ossification Follows a Defined Temporal Sequence

1. **Cartilage anlage:** By 5 weeks of gestation, a thin layer of mesenchymal cells forms between the ectoderm and endoderm of the limb bud and condenses into a core of hyaline cartilage. This cartilaginous anlage is the precursor of the future long bone of that limb. The fibrous capsule of the cartilage anlage is called a **perichondrium**. The width of the cartilaginous anlage is increased by appositional growth of chondroblasts, which deposit cartilage matrix on the internal surface of the perichondrium. At the same time, the anlage increases in length by both appositional and interstitial growth of the chondrocytes. At this stage, the long "bone" is actually composed of cartilage.
2. **The primary center of ossification:** The vascular bed increases, and the perichondrium deposits woven bone on the surface of the cartilage core at the midportion of the future bone. This circumferential sleeve of woven bone is the primary center of ossification, because it is the first bone tissue to be formed. The perichondrium then becomes **periosteum** (Fig. 30-8A).
3. **Cylinderization:** Within the cartilaginous anlage, chondrocytes form proliferating columns, which eventually undergo focal calcification. Calcification is the signal for osteoclastic resorption and invasion of vessels into the cartilaginous mass. Thus, the earliest endochondral ossification occurs after the cartilage is hollowed out from the center of the anlage. This "cavitation" of the cartilaginous core forms the future marrow space. The progressive hollowing of the diaphysis is called **cylinderization**.
4. **Primary spongiosum:** The swollen, hypertrophied chondrocytes within the central cartilage begin to die. Capillary invasion increases. The surfaces of the calcified cartilage cores become enveloped by woven bone laid down by osteoblasts, which arrive from the pluripotential mesenchymal tissue that enters with the capillaries. This cartilaginous core, surrounded by woven bone, is

called **primary spongiosum**, or **primary trabecula.** It is the first bone formed after the replacement of cartilage.

Cavitation continues along the future diaphysis toward each end of the bone. Meanwhile, the bone enlarges in width by appositional bone growth from the ever-increasing periosteal sleeve, which makes additional woven bone for the future cortex.

In Secondary Ossification, Cartilage Is Stimulated and Transformed Into Bone

Programmed events similar to those in the primary spongiosum take place in the cartilaginous ends of the future bone. Resting (reserve) cartilage is stimulated to become columns of proliferating cartilage, which then progress to hypertrophied chondrocytes and, eventually, calcified cartilage.

1. **The secondary center of ossification** (Fig. 30-8B): Also called the **epiphyseal center of ossification**, this structure is formed at the ends of the bone when cartilage is resorbed.
2. **Formation of the growth plate:** As the bony ends expand during endochondral ossification, a zone of cartilage remains between the ossifying end of the bone and the diaphysis. This cartilage is destined to become the **growth plate** (Fig. 30-9A), a layer of modified cartilage between the diaphysis and epiphysis. Its structure is essentially unchanged from early fetal life to skeletal maturity. *The growth plate controls the longitudinal growth of bones and ultimately determines adult height.*
3. **Structure of the growth plate:** Chondrocytes of the growth plate are arranged in vertical rows, which, in three dimensions, are really helices. Viewed longitudinally, the growth plate, proceeding from epiphysis to metaphysis, is divided into zones (Figs. 30-2C and 30-9).
   - The **reserve (resting) zone** is supplied by epiphyseal arteries and has small chondrocytes and very little matrix. An additional peripheral zone, known as the **zone of Ranvier,** lies directly under the perichondrium.
   - The **proliferative zone** is the next deeper zone, in which active proliferation of chondrocytes occurs both longitudinally and transversely (although the main

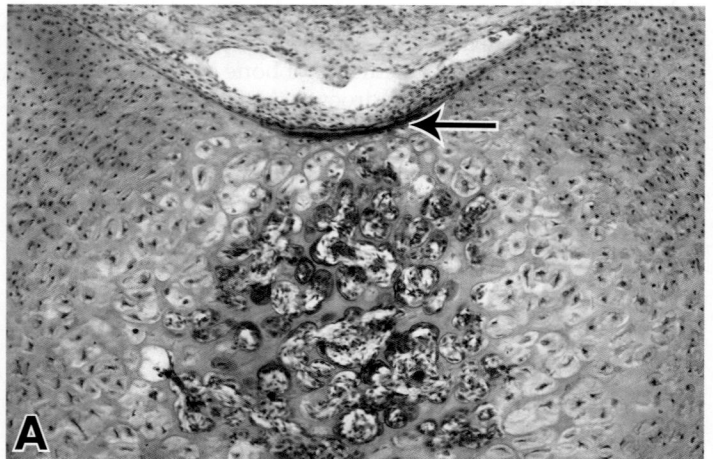
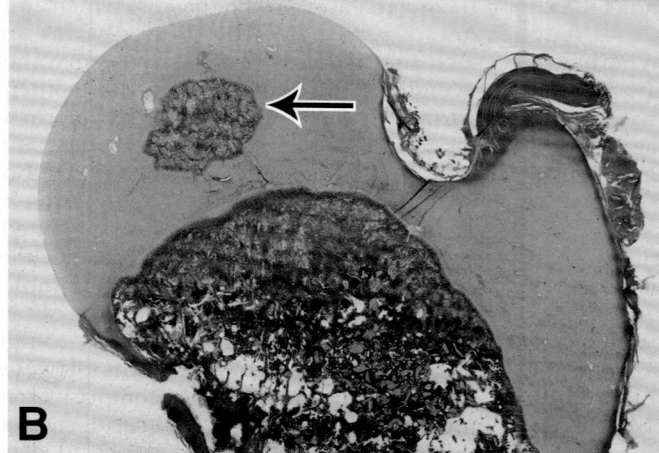

FIGURE 30-8. Primary ossification. A. This section of a short tubular bone demonstrates the first true bone tissue (*arrow*) deposited on the outside of the midshaft of the cartilage model along with early hollowing of the center of the cartilage model to form mixed spicules of cartilage and bone (primary spongiosa). **B.** The **secondary ossification center** (*arrow*) is demonstrated in this femoral head.

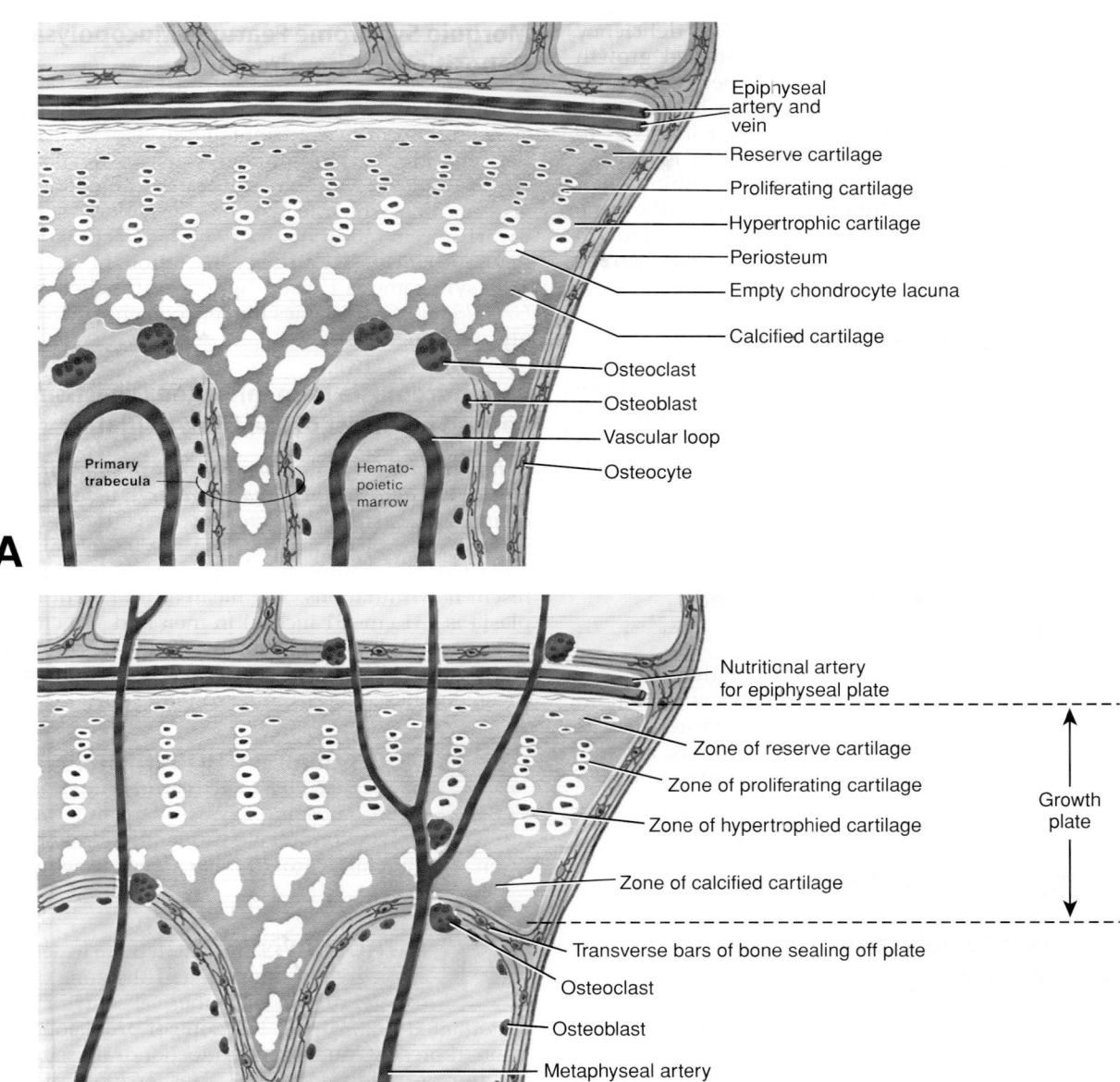

FIGURE 30-9. Anatomy of the epiphyseal growth plate. A. Normal growing epiphyseal plate. The epiphysis is separated from the epiphyseal plate by transverse plates of bone that seal the plate so that it grows only toward the metaphysis. The various zones of cartilage are illustrated. As calcified cartilage migrates toward the metaphysis, chondrocytes die, and lacunae become empty. At the interface of the epiphyseal plate and the metaphysis, osteoclasts bore into the calcified cartilage, accompanied by a capillary loop from the metaphyseal vessels. Osteoblasts follow the osteoclasts and lay down woven bone on the cartilage core, thereby forming the primary spongiosum or primary trabeculae. **B. Normal closure.** The epiphyseal cartilage has ceased to grow, and metaphyseal vessels penetrate the cartilage plate. Transverse bars of bone separate the plate from the metaphysis.

growth thrust is longitudinal). In a very active growth plate, proliferative zones account for over half the thickness of the growth plate.

■ The **hypertrophic zone** is next and demonstrates a substantial increase in chondrocyte size. The intercellular matrix is prominent, and a dense zone, the **territorial matrix,** surrounds chondrocytes.

■ The **zone of calcification** is the cartilaginous zone closest to the metaphysis, where the matrix becomes mineralized.

■ The **zone of ossification** is the area where a coating of bone is laid down on the surface of the calcified cartilage. Capillaries grow into the calcified cartilage and provide access to osteoclasts, which resorb much of the calcified matrix. Residual vertical walls of calcified cartilage act as scaffolding for the deposition of bone.

Molecular mechanisms governing endochondral growth are beginning to be understood. PTH-related protein (PTHrP) is secreted from perichondrial cells and chondrocytes and maintains chondrocyte proliferation. PTHrP deficiency leads to severe growth retardation and distorted growth plates. The developmental regulator Indian hedgehog (Ihh) is also involved in growth plate maturation by acting in conjunction with PTHrP. A third major factor involved in growth plate regulation is FGF. Activation of FGF receptor-3 (FGFR3) in proliferating chondrocytes leads to inhibition of growth plate proliferation. Mutations in *FGFR3* (the gene that encodes FGFR3 protein) are associated with growth arrest (e.g., achondroplasia or other forms of dwarfism) or growth acceleration.

Tapering of the Epiphysis to Diaphysis

This begins at the ring of Delacroix, a periosteal cuff of bone surrounding the epiphyseal cartilage. A wave of periosteal osteoclasts resorbs the cortex, and at the same time, endosteal osteoblastic bone is deposited to keep pace with, and offset, some of the osteoclastic resorption. The net result is that the wide end of the bone tapers into the hollow cylindrical diaphysis, resembling a funnel.

The Growth Plate Is Normally Obliterated at a Specific Age for Each Bone

Closure of the growth plate (Fig. 30-9B) is induced by sex hormones and occurs earlier in females. Renewal of chondrocytes slows and ultimately ceases. The entire plate is eventually replaced by bone. In some individuals, a transverse bony plate representing the site of closure can be seen by radiography.

DISORDERS OF THE GROWTH PLATE

Cretinism Leads to Defective Cartilage Maturation

Cretinism results from **maternal iodine deficiency** (see Chapter 27) and has profound effects on the skeleton. Thyroid hormone plays a role in chondrocytes, osteoblasts, and osteoclasts by regulating their production of cytokines and other factors involved in bone development and growth. Linear growth is severely impaired, resulting in dwarfism, with limbs disproportionately short in relation to the trunk. Delayed closure of the fontanelles of the skull causes an unusually large head. There is delay in closure of the epiphyses, as well as radiologic stippling of these zones. Shedding of deciduous teeth and eruption of permanent teeth are retarded.

 PATHOLOGY: In cretinism, chondrocytes do not follow the orderly endochondral sequence. Instead, maturation of the hypertrophied zone is retarded, and the zone of proliferative cartilage is narrow. Endochondral ossification, therefore, does not proceed appropriately, and transverse bars of bone in the metaphysis seal off the growth plate. Although growth plates may remain open, failure of endochondral ossification produces severe dwarfism. The misshapen epiphyses seen by radiography reflect incomplete penetration of the secondary centers of ossification of the epiphysis.

Morquio Syndrome Features Mucopolysaccharide Deposition in Chondrocytes

Many of the mucopolysaccharidoses (see Chapter 6) involve skeletal deformities, attributable to deposition of mucopolysaccharides (glycosaminoglycans) in developing bones. An example is Morquio syndrome (mucopolysaccharidosis type IV), which leads to a particularly severe form of dwarfism, in addition to dental defects, corneal opacities, and increased urinary excretion of keratan sulfate. This syndrome is caused by loss-of-function mutations in *GALNS* and *GLB1*, genes that encode enzymes that degrade glycoaminoglycans.

Achondroplasia Is an Inherited Dwarfism Caused by Arrest of the Growth Plate

Achondroplasia refers to a syndrome of short-limbed dwarfism and macrocephaly and represents a failure of normal epiphyseal cartilage formation. It is the most common genetic form of dwarfism (1 in 15,000 live births) and is inherited as an autosomal dominant trait. Most cases represent new mutations. The mean adult height in achondroplasia is 131 cm (51 inches) in men and 125 cm (49 inches) in women. Achondroplastic dwarfs have normal mentation and average life spans. However, some patients develop severe kyphoscoliosis and its complications.

 MOLECULAR PATHOGENESIS: Achondroplasia is caused by an **activating** mutation in *FGFR3* on chromosome 4(p16.3). The mutation constitutively inhibits chondrocyte differentiation and proliferation, which retards growth plate development.

PATHOLOGY: The growth plate in achondroplasia is greatly thinned, and the zone of proliferative cartilage is either absent or markedly attenuated (Fig. 30-10). The zone of provisional calcification, if present, undergoes endochondral ossification, but at a greatly reduced rate. A transverse bar of bone often seals off the growth plate, thus preventing further bone formation and causing dwarfism. Interestingly, the secondary centers of ossification and the articular cartilages are normal. Because intramembranous ossification is undisturbed, the periosteum functions normally and the bones become very short and thick. For the same reasons, the heads of affected patients appear unusually large, compared with the bones formed from the cartilage of the face. The spine is of normal length, but limbs are abnormally short.

Scurvy Results From Dietary Deficiency of Vitamin C

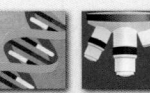 **MOLECULAR PATHOGENESIS AND PATHOLOGY:** Hydroxyproline and hydroxylysine are important in stabilizing the helical structure of collagen and in cross-linking tropocollagen fibers into the proper molecular structure of collagen. Vitamin C is a cofactor in hydroxylation of

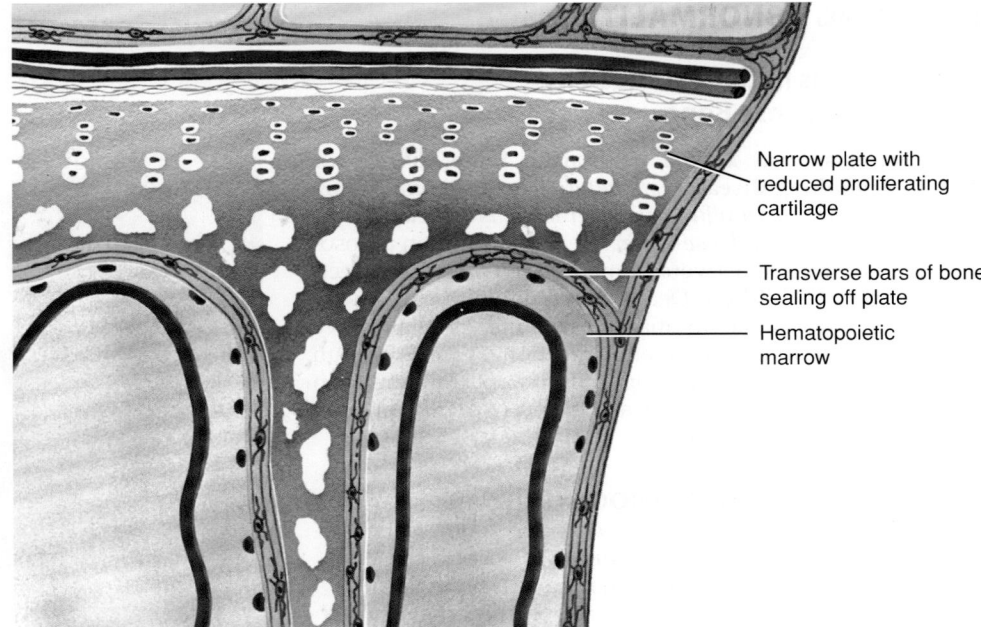

Narrow plate with reduced proliferating cartilage

Transverse bars of bone sealing off plate

Hematopoietic marrow

FIGURE 30-10. The epiphyseal growth plate of an achondroplastic dwarf. In achondroplasia, the epiphyseal plate is reduced in thickness, and zones of proliferating cartilage are attenuated (compare to Fig. 30-9). Osteoclastic activity is inconspicuous, and the interface between the plate and the metaphysis is often sealed by transverse bars of bone that prevent further endochondral ossification. As a result, the bones are shortened.

proline and lysine. The skeletal changes of vitamin C deficiency (scurvy) reflect the lack of osteoblastic function. New bone is not formed because osteoblasts cannot produce and normally cross-link collagen. Chondrocytes at the growth plate continue to grow and the zone of calcified cartilage may actually become more prominent, because it is more heavily calcified. Osteoclasts resorb this zone, but the primary spongiosum does not form properly, and there is irregular vascular perforation of the cartilage plate.

 CLINICAL FEATURES: Today, scurvy is a rare disease (see Chapter 8). Wound healing and bone growth are impaired in patients with scurvy. Capillary basement membranes are also damaged and widespread capillary bleeding is common. Subperiosteal hemorrhage may occur, leading to joint and muscle pain.

Asymmetric Cartilage Growth Causes Spinal Disorders and Tumors

Asymmetric cartilage growth, such as occurs in patients with knock-knees and bowed legs, develops when one part of the growth plate, either medial or lateral, grows faster than the other. Most cases are hereditary, but mechanical forces such as trauma near the growth plate may stimulate one side to grow faster or in an asymmetric fashion. Aside from the cosmetic appearance, these conditions may require correction to prevent future incongruity, eventual loss of articular cartilage, and joint destruction.

Scoliosis and Kyphosis

Scoliosis *is an abnormal lateral curvature of the spine, usually affecting adolescent girls.* **Kyphosis** *refers to an abnormal anteroposterior curvature.* When both conditions are present, the term **kyphoscoliosis** is used.

ETIOLOGIC FACTORS: A vertebral body grows in length (height) from the endplates of the vertebrae, which correspond to the growth plates of long tubular bones. As in tubular bones, vertebral bodies increase in width by appositional bone growth from the periosteum. In scoliosis, for unknown reasons, one portion of the endplate grows faster than the other, producing lateral curvature of the spine.

CLINICAL FEATURES: Treatment involves application of appropriate stress on the vertebral body through use of braces or internal fixation to straighten the spine. If kyphoscoliosis is severe, the patient may eventually develop chronic pulmonary disease because of thoracic deformity and impaired breathing mechanics, cor pulmonale, and joint problems, particularly involving the hip.

Hemihypertrophy

Hemihypertrophy describes several conditions in which one limb's growth plate is stimulated to undergo rapid and prolonged endochondral ossification. That limb becomes much longer than the contralateral one. Infection in the metaphyseal area may stimulate the growth plate to grow rapidly. An arteriovenous malformation may also cause one growth plate to grow faster than its counterpart, as may fractures and tumors near the growth plate. In some cases, hemihypertrophy is part of an inherited syndrome, most commonly attributed to loss-of-function mutations in *CDKN1C*, a tumor suppressor that regulates cell growth. Children with isolated hemihypertrophy are at increased risk for neoplasms.

MODELING ABNORMALITIES

Osteopetrosis Is Characterized by Abnormally Dense Bone

Osteopetrosis, *also known as* **marble bone disease** *or* **Albers-Schönberg disease,** *is a heterogeneous group of rare inherited disorders in which skeletal mass is increased as a result of abnormally dense bone.* The most common autosomal recessive form is a severe, sometimes fatal disease affecting infants and children. Death of infants with this severe variant is attributable to marked anemia, cranial nerve entrapment, hydrocephalus, and infection. A more benign form, transmitted as an autosomal dominant trait and seen in adulthood or adolescence, is associated with mild anemia or no symptoms at all.

 MOLECULAR PATHOGENESIS: *The sclerotic skeleton of osteopetrosis is the result of failed osteoclastic bone resorption.* The disease is caused by mutations in genes that govern osteoclast formation or function. The most common mutations cause defects in bone acidification, which is necessary for osteoclastic bone resorption. These include mutations in *TCIRG1* (which makes an osteoclast proton pump; autosomal dominant); *CLCN7* (osteoclast chloride channel; autosomal recessive); and the **carbonic anhydrase II** gene (*CA-11*, autosomal recessive). Other mutations that cause osteopetrosis involve genes for transcription factors or cytokines necessary for osteoclast differentiation.

PATHOLOGY: Because osteoclast function is arrested, osteopetrosis is characterized by: (1) retention of the primary spongiosum with its cartilage cores; (2) deficient normal tapering of the metaphysis; and (3) a thickened cortex. The result is short, block-like, radiodense bones, and hence the term **marble bone disease** (Fig. 30-11A). These bones are extremely radiopaque and weigh two to three times more than normal bone. However, they are structurally weak because of internal disorganization and failure to remodel along lines of stress. The overmineralized cartilage is also brittle, so that bones in osteopetrosis fracture easily. Grossly, these bones are widened in the metaphysis and diaphysis, causing a characteristic "Erlenmeyer flask" deformity (Fig. 30-11A,B). Histologically, the bone tissue is extremely irregular, and almost all areas contain cartilage cores (Fig. 30-11C). Marrow spaces are obliterated. Depending on the mutation, osteoclasts may be absent, present in normal numbers, or even abundant. In osteopetrosis with normal or increased numbers of osteoclasts, the molecular defect lies in a gene involved in the osteoclast function, rather than in their formation.

CLINICAL FEATURES: Suppression of hematopoiesis in osteopetrosis is due to obliteration of the marrow cavity by bone and calcified cartilage. Marrow suppression in patients with the malignant form of osteopetrosis may lead to severe anemia or pancytopenia. To compensate for loss of marrow hematopoiesis, extramedullary hematopoiesis occurs in the liver,

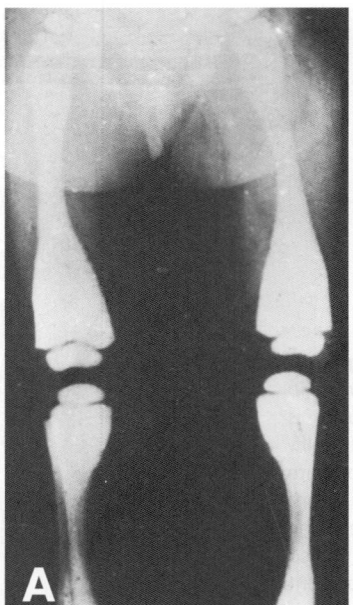
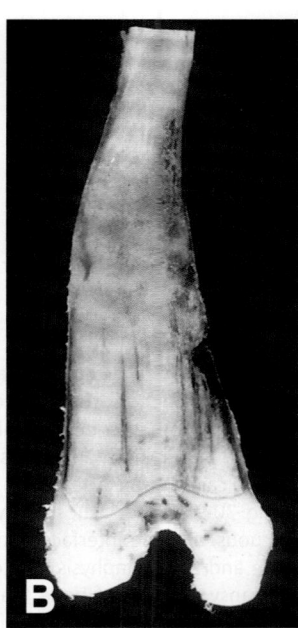
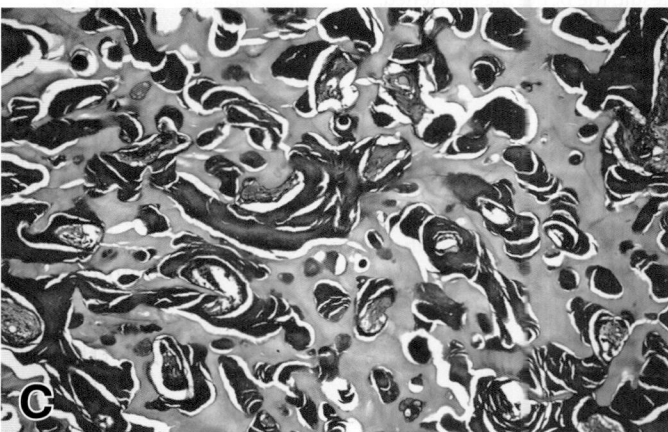

FIGURE 30-11. Osteopetrosis. A. This radiograph of a child shows markedly misshapen and dense bones of the lower extremities, characteristic of "marble bone disease." **B.** A gross specimen of the femur shows obliteration of the marrow space by dense bone. **C.** A photomicrograph of bone in a child with autosomal recessive osteopetrosis demonstrates disorganization of bony trabeculae by retention of primary spongiosa (mixed spicules) and further obliteration of the marrow space by secondary spongiosa. The result is complete disorganization of trabeculae and absence of marrow.

spleen, and lymph nodes, which become enlarged. Narrowing of neural foramina causes cranial nerve encroachment which leads to blindness and deafness. Osteopetrosis has been treated by bone marrow transplantation, which may give rise to new clones of functional osteoclast precursors.

Progressive Diaphyseal Dysplasia Features Thickened Long Bones

Progressive diaphyseal dysplasia (Camurati–Engelmann disease) is an autosomal dominant disorder of children in which cylinderization does not proceed appropriately, resulting in symmetric thickening and increased diameter of the diaphyses of long bones. These changes are due to increased bone formation driven by activating mutations in *TGFB1*, which produce a constitutively active form of TGF-β. The disease particularly affects the femur, tibia, fibula, radius, and ulna. Patients have pain over the affected areas, fatigue, muscle wasting, atrophy, and gait abnormalities.

DELAYED MATURATION OF BONE

Osteogenesis Imperfecta Is Characterized by Abnormal Type I Collagen

Osteogenesis imperfecta (OI) refers to a heterogeneous group of inherited disorders of connective tissue, characterized by low bone mass and consequently increased bone fragility. Most types are caused by mutations in the gene for type I collagen, affecting the skeleton, joints, ears, ligaments, teeth, sclerae, and skin (see Chapter 6). There are at least eight types of OI, most with different genetic structural mutations and different clinical severity.

 MOLECULAR PATHOGENESIS: Most cases of OI result from mutations in *COL1A1* and *COL1A2*, which encode the α_1- and α_2-chains of type I procollagen, the major structural protein of bone. These genes are on chromosome 17 (17q21.3–q22) and chromosome 7 (7q21.3–q22), respectively. A point mutation that affects a glycine residue in either *COL1A1* or *COL1A2* is the most common abnormality found in OI. Mutations in *COL1A1* affect three-fourths of the type I collagen molecules, with half of the molecules containing one abnormal pro–α_1-chain and one-quarter containing two abnormal pro–α_1-chains. By contrast, mutations in *COL1A2* affect only half of the synthesized collagen molecules. The resulting phenotypes range from mild to lethal depending on which gene is affected, the location in the collagen triple helix at which the substitution occurs, and which amino acid is substituted for glycine.

Osteogenesis Imperfecta Type I

OI type I is the mildest phenotype. It is inherited as an autosomal dominant trait, characterized by multiple fractures after birth, blue sclera, and hearing abnormalities. In some patients, abnormalities of the teeth are also conspicuous (dentinogenesis imperfecta).

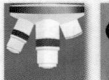 **PATHOLOGY AND CLINICAL FEATURES:** Fractures usually first occur after the infant begins to sit and walk. Hundreds of fractures may occur each year following minor movement or trauma. Radiologic examination shows extremely thin, delicate, and abnormally curved bones (Fig. 30-12A). The mutant collagen has reduced tensile strength and bone mineralization is defective. The combination of these abnormalities accounts for the brittleness of OI bone. In OI, insufficient bone is formed, leading to decreased cortical thickness and reduced trabecular bone. When a fracture occurs, the fracture callus may be extensive enough to resemble a tumor (Fig. 30-12B). As the child grows, fractures tend to decrease in severity and frequency, and stature is generally unaffected.

The sclerae are very thin, with a blue color attributable to the underlying choroid. Progressive hearing loss, culminating in total deafness in adulthood, results from fusion of the auditory ossicles. Joint laxity associated eventually leads to kyphoscoliosis and flat feet. Because of hypoplasia of the dentine and pulp, the teeth are misshapen and bluish yellow.

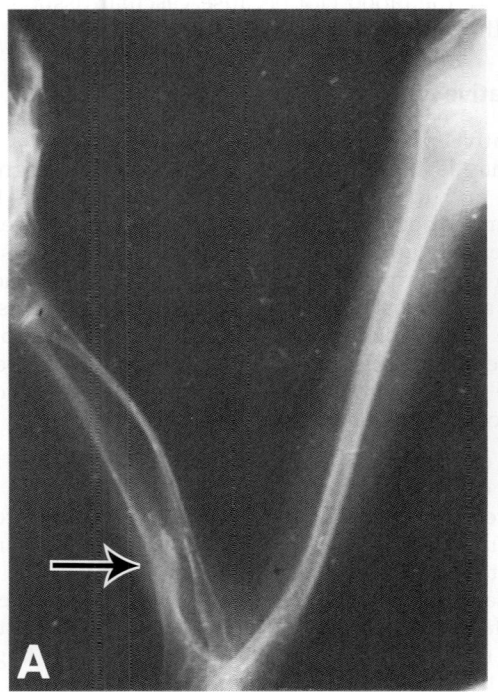
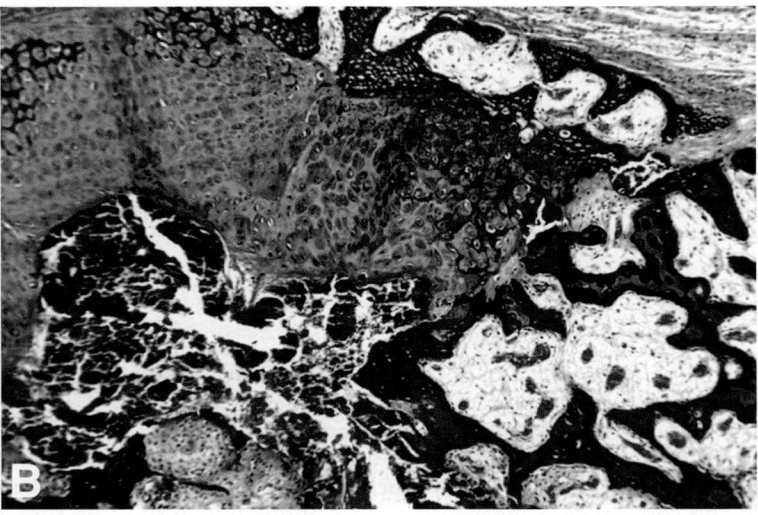

FIGURE 30-12. Osteogenesis imperfecta. A. This radiograph illustrates the markedly thin and attenuated humerus and bones of the forearm. A fracture callus (*arrow*) is seen in the proximal ulna. **B.** A photomicrograph of the fracture callus shows prominent cartilage (*upper left*). The cortex is thin and composed of hypercellular woven bone.

Osteogenesis Imperfecta Type II

OI type II is a lethal, autosomal dominant, perinatal disease. Affected infants are stillborn or die within a few days after birth, in a sense being crushed to death. They are markedly short in stature, with severe limb deformities. Nearly all bones sustain fractures during delivery or during uterine contractions in labor. As in OI type I, sclerae are blue.

Osteogenesis Imperfecta Type III

OI type III is the progressive, most severely deforming type of disease and is characterized by many bone fractures, growth retardation, and severe skeletal deformities. Inheritance is usually autosomal dominant, although rare autosomal recessive forms have been reported. Fractures are present at birth, but bones are less fragile than in the type II form. These patients eventually develop severe shortening of their stature because of progressive bone fractures and severe kyphoscoliosis. Sclerae may be blue at birth, but become white shortly thereafter. Dental abnormalities are common.

Osteogenesis Imperfecta Type IV

OI type IV is similar to type I except that sclerae are normal. Clinical presentation is heterogeneous, and there may or may not be dental disease. In this disorder, abnormal cross-linkages of collagen result in thin, delicate, and weak collagen fibrils. This defective collagen does not allow the bone cortex to mature, so that at birth the cortex of the bone resembles that of a fetus, and is composed of woven bone and small areas of lamellar bone. The cortex eventually matures, but this may not occur until adolescence or even later. In any event, the frequency of fractures tends to decrease over a prolonged interval. Treatment involves orthopedic devices, including rods inserted into the medullary cavities, to prevent the dwarfing effect of multiple fractures.

Additional types of OI (types V, VI, VII, and VIII) have been identified from within the heterogeneous type IV group, based on distinct clinical, genetic, and bone histologic features.

There is no mechanism-based treatment for OI. Osteoprogenitor cells for bone marrow transplantation, growth factors, bisphosphonates, and gene therapy to improve collagen synthesis are undergoing clinical trials in efforts to modify the course and severity of the disease. Because of the exuberant fracture callus formation, some cases of OI have been misdiagnosed as malignant bone tumors.

FRACTURE

The most common bone lesion is a fracture, which is defined as a discontinuity of the bone. A force perpendicular to the long axis of the bone results in a **transverse fracture.** A force along the long axis of the bone yields a **compression fracture.** Torsional force results in **spiral fractures,** and combined tension and compression shear forces cause angulation and displacement of the fractured ends.

A force powerful enough to fracture a bone also injures adjacent soft tissues. In this situation, there is often: (1) extensive muscle necrosis; (2) hemorrhage because of shearing of capillary beds and larger vessels of soft tissues; (3) tearing of tendinous insertions and ligamentous attachments; and (4) even nerve damage, caused by stretching or direct tearing of nerves.

Fracture Healing Is Divided Into Inflammatory, Reparative, and Remodeling Phases

The duration of each phase (Fig. 30-13) depends on the patient's age, the site of fracture, the patient's overall health and nutritional status, and the extent of soft-tissue injury. Local factors, such as vascular supply and mechanical forces at the site, also play a role in healing. *In repairing a bone fracture, formation of anything other than bone tissue at the fracture site represents incomplete healing.*

The Inflammatory Phase

Rupture of blood vessels in the periosteum and adjacent muscle and soft tissue leads to extensive hemorrhage in the first 1 to 2 days after a fracture. Disruption of large vessels in the bone and interruption of cortical vessels (i.e., Volkmann and Haversian canals) can also cause extensive bone necrosis at the fracture site. *Dead bone is characterized by the absence of osteocytes and empty osteocyte lacunae.*

By 2 to 5 days after fracture, the hemorrhage forms a large clot, which must be absorbed so that the fracture can heal. Neovascularization begins at periphery of this blood clot, and by the end of the first week, most of the clot is becoming organized by invasion of blood vessels and early fibrosis.

The earliest bone, which is invariably woven bone, is formed after 7 days. *This corresponds to the "scar" of bone.* Since bone formation requires a good blood supply, woven bone spicules begin to appear at the periphery of the clot. Pluripotent mesenchymal cells derived from adjacent soft tissue and within the bone marrow give rise to the osteoblasts that synthesize woven bone. In most fractures, cartilage also is formed and is eventually resorbed by endochondral ossification. Granulation tissue containing bone or cartilage is called a **callus.** Woven bone also forms inside the marrow cavity at the edge of the blood clot because vascular tissue is also present in that location.

The Reparative Phase

The reparative phase follows the first week after a fracture and may last for months, depending on the degree of movement and the fixation of the fracture. By this time, acute inflammation has subsided. Pluripotent progenitor cells differentiate into fibroblasts and osteoblasts. As is proceeds from the periphery toward the center of the fracture site, repair accomplishes two objectives: (1) it organizes and resorbs the blood clot and, more importantly; (2) it supplies blood vessels to the developing callus, which will eventually bridge the fracture site. The reparative phase involves orchestration of the following processes:

1. Armies of osteoclasts within the Haversian canals form **cutting cones** that bore into the cortex toward the fracture site. New vessels accompany the cutting cones, supplying nutrients to these cells and providing more pluripotent cells for cell renewal.
2. At the same time, the external callus, which is formed on the surface of the bone and arises from the periosteum and the soft-tissue mesenchymal cells, continues to grow toward the fracture site.

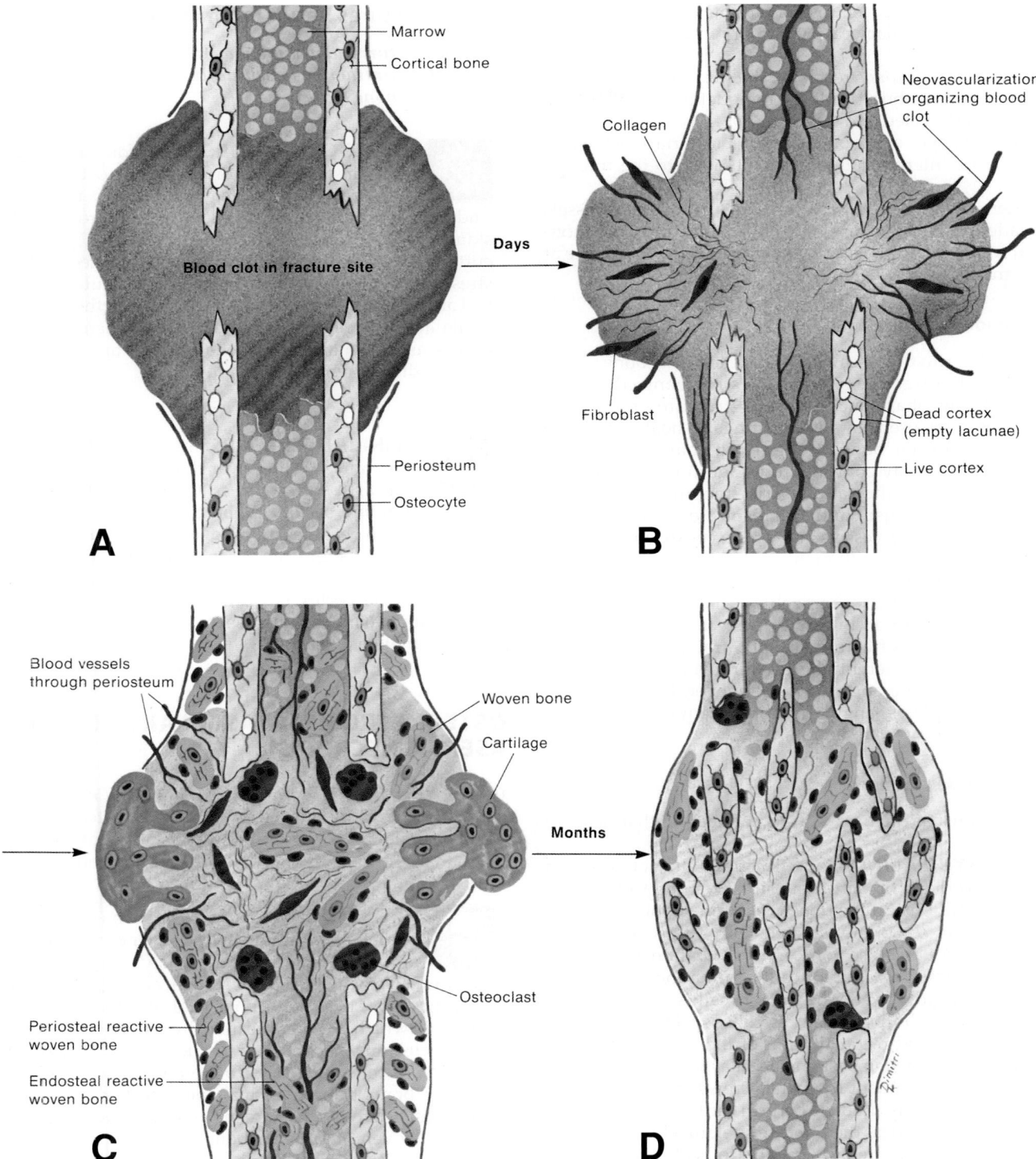

FIGURE 30-13. Healing of a fracture. A. Soon after a fracture is sustained, an extensive blood clot forms in the subperiosteum and soft tissue, as well as in the marrow cavity. The bone at the fracture site is jagged. **B.** The **inflammatory phase** of fracture healing is characterized by neovascularization and early organization of the blood clot. Because osteocytes in the fracture site are dead, their lacunae are empty. Osteocytes of the cortex are necrotic well beyond the fracture site, owing to the traumatic interruption of perforating arteries from the periosteum. **C.** The **reparative phase** of fracture healing is characterized by formation of a callus of cartilage and woven bone near the fracture site. The jagged edges of the original cortex have been remodeled and eroded by osteoclasts. The marrow space has been revascularized and contains reactive woven bone, as does the periosteal area. **D.** During the **remodeling phase**, the cortex becomes revitalized by reactive bone that may be lamellar or woven. The new bone is organized along stress lines as determined by mechanical forces. Extensive osteoclastic and osteoblastic cellular activity is maintained.

3. Simultaneously, an endosteal or internal callus forms within the medullary cavity and grows outward toward the fracture site.
4. Cortical cutting cones reach the fracture site and the ends of the fractured bone undergo remodeling by osteoclasts to become beveled and smooth.
5. Similar changes occur on the endosteal surface of the cortex, as the internal callus works its way to the fracture site.
6. If there are large areas of cartilage, new blood vessels invade the calcified cartilage, after which the endochondral sequence duplicates the normal formation of bone at the growth plate.

The Remodeling Phase

Once the ingrowth of callus has sealed the bone ends, the bone at the fracture site becomes reorganized during the remodeling phase such that the structure of the original cortex is restored. In some settings, a healed fracture may regain normal bone strength but may not become fully healed and may continue to undergo remodeling for years. For instance, the callus of rib fractures may persist throughout life because continual respiratory movement of the ribs shears blood vessels and preserves extensive cartilage callus. In a child with open growth plates, the normal modeling of growing bone overtakes the callus, such that a fracture may not be recognizable in later life. Similarly, normal modeling in a child may correct abnormal angulation of a bone at a fracture site. If a fracture occurs near the growth plate, differential growth rates within the plate may also correct the angulation. However, in adults with closed growth plates, angulation often requires correction with external or internal devices.

Special Considerations

There are unusual nuances to fracture healing that deserve mention.

PRIMARY HEALING: Some fractures do not result in bone displacement or soft-tissue injury. For example, an orthopedic drill hole in the bone cortex or a controlled fracture, such as an osteotomy created with a fine saw during surgery, does not displace bone. In this situation, there is little if any soft-tissue reaction or callus formation because the bone remains rigidly fixed. The fracture callus grows directly into the fracture site by a process called **primary healing**. This results in rapid reconstitution of the cortex, including restoration of Haversian systems. Similarly, if a fracture site is held in rigid alignment by metal screws and plates, little external callus forms. Rather, cortical cutting cones play a prominent role and heal the fracture site quickly.

NONUNION: Failure of a fracture to heal is called **nonunion**. Causes of nonunion include interposition of soft tissues at the fracture site, excessive motion, infection, poor blood supply, and other factors mentioned above. Continued movement at the unhealed fracture site may also lead to **pseudoarthrosis**, a condition in which tissue similar to that in a joint is formed. In this situation, pluripotent progenitor cells give rise to cells that are histologically indistinguishable from synovial cells, secrete synovial fluid and form a joint-like structure. In such cases, the fracture never heals and the abnormal tissue must be removed surgically for the fracture to heal properly.

Stress Fractures Result From Microfractures

In these fractures, also known as **fatigue** *or* **march fractures***, repeated microfractures eventually result in a true fracture through the bone cortex.*

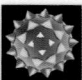 **ETIOLOGIC FACTORS:** Stress fractures occur in bones in which the cortex has few osteons. If the ill-prepared cortex (e.g., in the 5th metatarsal) undergoes repeated mechanical stress (e.g., from jogging, skiing or ballet dancing), the bone responds by producing cutting cones in an attempt to implant osteons. If the stress continues and microfractures accumulate, periosteal and endosteal calluses develop to strengthen the bone while active remodeling takes place. An actual fracture occurs as the final event if the stresses are continually applied during remodeling.

 CLINICAL FEATURES: Stress fractures produce pain and swelling over the affected bone. *At the site of a future stress fracture, a callus forms before a fracture occurs.* When the actual fracture takes place, the pain becomes more severe. In the early stages of this condition, before the actual fracture, the radiologic appearance may resemble that of a tumor. A biopsy will show that the cortex is riddled with cutting cones for remodeling, which is also seen in reactive bone at the edge of an invasive tumor.

OSTEONECROSIS (AVASCULAR NECROSIS, ASEPTIC NECROSIS)

Osteonecrosis refers to the death of bone and marrow in the absence of infection (Fig. 30-14). Causes of osteonecrosis are listed in Table 30-1. Necrotic bone heals differently in the cortex than in the underlying coarse cancellous bone.

 PATHOLOGY: Osteonecrosis is characterized by death of bone and marrow. The necrotic bone has empty lacunae lacking osteocyte nuclei, and the marrow displays dystrophic calcification (Fig. 30-14B). Necrotic coarse cancellous bone heals by **creeping substitution**, in which the necrotic marrow is replaced by invading or creeping neovascular tissue, which provides the pluripotent cells needed for bone remodeling. Although necrotic bony trabeculae may be resorbed directly by osteoclastic activity, they are more commonly surrounded by new woven or lamellar bone generated by the osteoblastic activity of granulation tissue. Eventually, the sandwich of necrotic bone surrounded by viable bone is remodeled by osteoclastic activity, and new bone is laid down through intramembranous bone formation.

Necrotic cortical bone is healed by a cutting cone. The cutting cone, as discussed above, forms by way of pre-existing vascular channels in the cortex. Chemical signals from the necrotic bone reach this vascular channel and stimulate neovascularization by surrounding pluripotent mesenchymal tissue. Osteoclasts make their way into the necrotic compact cortical bone, with osteoblasts trailing behind. As a

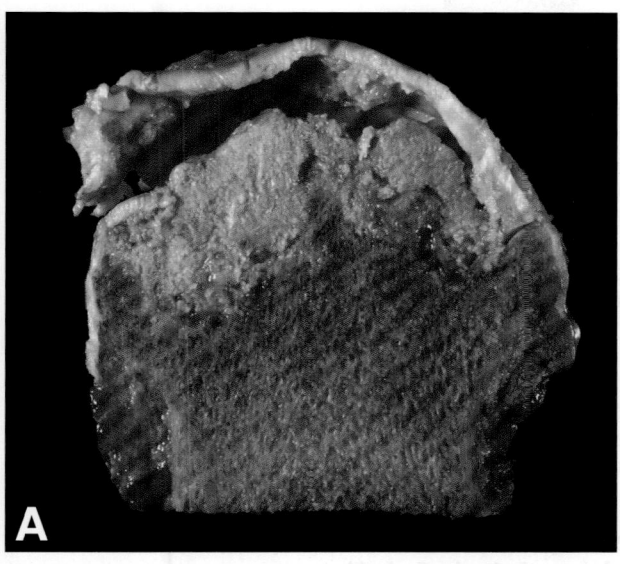
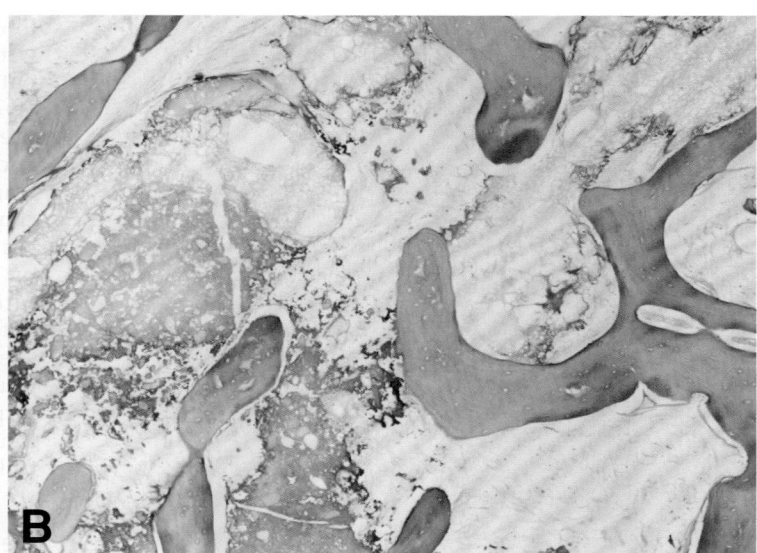

FIGURE 30-14. Osteonecrosis of the head of the femur. A. Coronal section shows a circumscribed area of subchondral infarction with partial detachment of the overlying articular cartilage and subarticular bone. **B.** Microscopically, the necrotic bone is characterized by empty lacunae and necrotic marrow with dystrophic calcification (*purple areas*).

result, tunnels bore their way into the necrotic cortex, leading to new bone formation. This is a slow process, and the bone is often laid down *de novo* as lamellar bone.

Legg–Calvé–Perthes disease is osteonecrosis in the femoral head in children; **idiopathic osteonecrosis** occurs

in a similar location in adults. In both conditions, collapse of the femoral head may create joint incongruity and, eventually, severe osteoarthritis. Collapse of the subchondral bone results from several mechanisms:

- Necrotic bone may sustain stress fractures and compaction over a long period.
- The portion peripheral to the necrotic bone may undergo neovascularization. Radiologic examination shows a lucent area surrounding the necrotic zone.
- The rigid articular cartilage and subchondral bone may actually crack as the subchondral necrotic zone collapses, producing a fracture.

A radiograph in avascular necrosis often shows the necrotic zone to be radiodense because of: (1) relative osteoporosis in the surrounding viable bone compared with the unchanged necrotic bone; (2) addition of new bone through creeping substitution; (3) formation of calcium soaps (insoluble Ca^{2+} salts of fatty acids), which arise as a result of the necrosis of marrow fat; and (4) actual compaction of the pre-existing dead bone.

REACTIVE BONE FORMATION

Reactive bone is intramembranous bone formed in response to stress on bone or soft tissue. Conditions such as tumors, infections, trauma, or generalized or focal disease can stimulate bone formation.

 PATHOLOGY: The periosteum may respond with a so-called **sunburst** pattern (Fig. 30-15), as seen with certain tumors, or progressive layering of the periosteum, which yields an **onionskin pattern** of the cortex. The endosteal or the marrow surface may produce new bone, so that by radiolography, the cortex appears to be thickened, and the coarse cancellous bone is denser.

TABLE 30-1
CAUSES OF OSTEONECROSIS

Trauma, including fracture and surgery

Emboli, producing focal bone infarction

Systemic diseases, such as polycythemia, lupus erythematosus, Gaucher disease, sickle cell disease and gout

Radiation, either internal or external

Corticosteroid administration

Specific focal bone necrosis at various sites—as in the head of the femur (Legg–Calvé–Perthes disease) or in the navicular bone (Köhler disease)

Organ transplantation, particularly renal, in patients with persistent hyperparathyroidism

Osteochondritis dissecans, a condition of unknown etiology in which a fragment of articular cartilage and subchondral bone breaks off into a joint. This is thought to occur when a focal area of bone undergoes necrosis and eventually detaches

Autografts and allografts

Thrombosis of local vessels caused by pressure from adjacent tumors or other space-occupying lesions

Idiopathic factors, as in the high incidence of osteonecrosis of the head and the femur in alcoholics. Necrotic bone heals differently in the cortex and in the underlying coarse cancellous bone

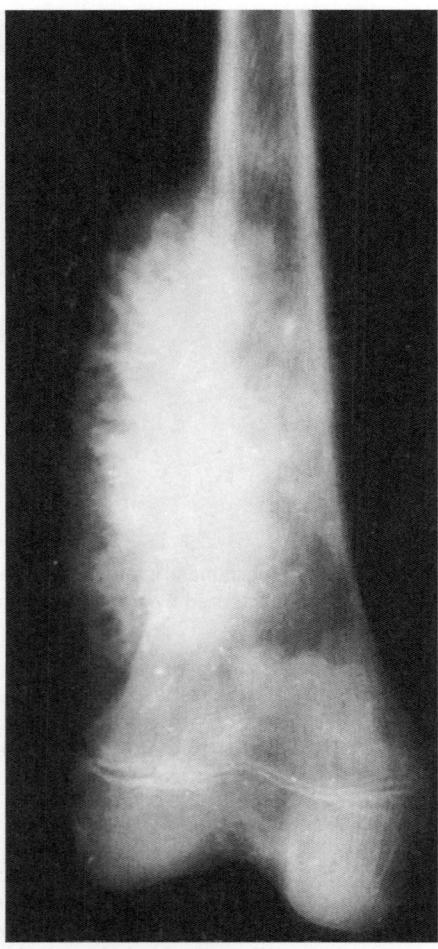

FIGURE 30-15. Reactive bone formation. This radiograph of a resected femur bearing an osteosarcoma shows a sunburst pattern of hyperdense new bone in the distal diaphysis and metaphysis. This radiodensity is due to woven bone produced by the sarcoma and the periosteal reaction of the host bone. The epiphyseal plate is seen as a transverse lucent line separating the metaphysis from the epiphysis. Radiating radiodense bone extends beyond the periosteum into the adjacent soft tissues, obscuring the underlying bone architecture.

Reactive bone may be either woven or lamellar, depending on the rates of deposition of the reactive bone. For example, if the bone has time to respond to persistent stress, as in chronic osteomyelitis, reactive bone may be laid down *de novo* as lamellar bone from the periosteum. Similarly, a benign tumor may cause a lamellar bone reaction. By contrast, a rapidly enlarging tumor is more likely to promote woven bone. In any case, the reactive bone is invariably of the intramembranous type, because it is derived from the periosteum or the endosteal tissue of the marrow.

Heterotopic Ossification Is Bone Formation Outside the Skeletal System

Heterotopic ossification (HO) is formation of reactive bone (woven or lamellar) in extraskeletal sites such as the skin, subcutaneous tissue, skeletal muscle, and fibroconnective tissue around joints. HO is not associated with any metabolic disease, as reflected by the fact that patients have normal serum calcium and phosphorous levels. HO occurs in five major clinical settings: genetic predisposition, posttraumatic, neurogenic, postsurgical, and as distinctive reactive lesions such as **myositis ossificans**. A genetic disorder known as **fibrodysplasia ossificans progressiva** is characterized by massive deposits of bone around multiple joints and in ligaments. It is caused by dominant mutations in *ACVR1*, which lead to constitutive activation of type I receptors for bone morphogenetic protein (BMP). HO may also form in hematomas or skeletal muscle after trauma. Neurogenic HO occurs in muscle and periarticular fibrous tissue at multiple sites in patients with head trauma, spinal cord injury, or prolonged coma. HO can also form in periarticular soft tissue following joint surgery.

Heterotopic Calcification Is Deposition of Calcium Salts in Soft Tissues

HO and heterotopic calcification have a distinctive radiographic appearance. Bone formation is characterized by a spicular or trabeculated pattern, whereas heterotopic calcification has an irregular, splotchy, amorphous appearance. Heterotopic calcification tends to occur in necrotic soft tissue or in cartilage and on radiography is usually denser than bone. Heterotopic calcification appears in two forms:

- **Metastatic calcification** occurs when there is an increase in the calcium–phosphorus product. Thus, hypercalcemic states or hyperphosphatemic conditions predispose normal soft tissues to calcification.
- **Dystrophic calcification** is seen in abnormal or damaged soft tissues (e.g., tumors), degenerative diseases such as arteriosclerosis and areas subjected to trauma. Loss of neurologic function, as seen in quadriplegia and hemiplegia, also predisposes affected areas to soft-tissue calcification.

Myositis Ossificans Is Formation of Reactive Bone in Muscle After Injury

Myositis ossificans is a distinctive form of HO that affects young people and, although entirely benign, it often mimics a malignant neoplasm. It is a self-limited process and carries an excellent prognosis. Spontaneous regression has been observed. No treatment is required once the diagnosis is established.

 ETIOLOGIC FACTORS: The lesion typically results from blunt trauma to the muscle and soft tissues, usually of the lower limb. However, some cases occur spontaneously. Peripheral neovascularization and fibrosis at the site of tissue damage, in combination with local hemorrhage, promote to bone spicule formation. These changes are similar to those that develop within the initial hematoma in a healing fracture. Because myositis ossificans often occurs near a bone such as the femur or tibia, it may be misdiagnosed on radiography as a malignant bone-forming tumor.

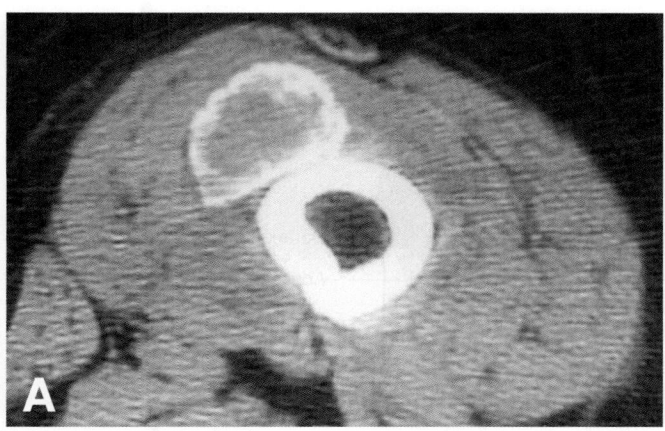
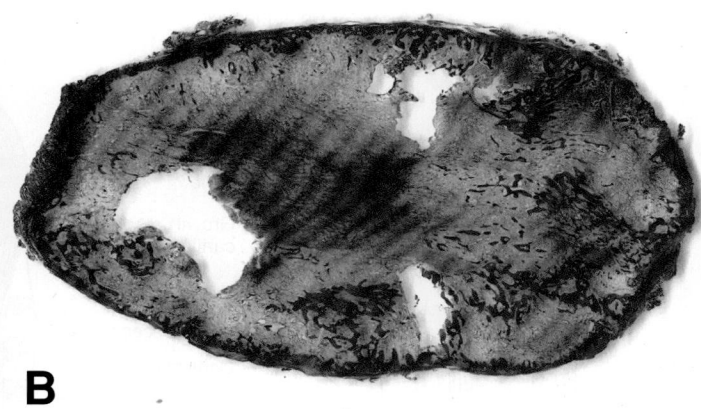

FIGURE 30-16. Myositis ossificans circumscripta. A. Computed tomography scan of the thigh shows an axial view of an ovoid, intramuscular mass adjacent to the femoral cortex with a radiolucent center and ossification that becomes denser at the periphery. **B.** Viewed at low magnification, the mass contains woven bone at the periphery and fibrous tissue (*pale material*) in the center.

PATHOLOGY: Histologically, woven bone is formed within granulation tissue and reactive fibrous tissue (Fig. 30-16B). The core of an early lesion of myositis ossificans is characterized by proliferating fibroblasts and more peripheral osteoblastic cells that begin to form woven bone. The fibroblasts are often cytologically atypical and show abundant mitoses, features reminiscent of a malignant tumor. *The key feature that distinguishes myositis ossificans from a neoplasm is that the bone matures peripherally, while in the center of the lesion it remains immature or not ossified at all.* The phenomenon of peripheral maturity with central immaturity, the **zonation effect**, clearly indicates a reactive process. In well-developed lesions, this phenomenon may be readily apparent by radiography (Fig. 30-16A). A neoplasm has the opposite zonation effect; the most mature tissue of the tumor is located centrally.

The growth pattern of myositis ossificans reflects the ingrowth of neovascular tissue from the periphery into the center of the damaged area. In the late stages, the lesion may contain cartilage and even lamellar bone. Thus, in a well-developed lesion, it may mimic a sesamoid bone in the soft tissue.

INFECTIONS

Osteomyelitis Is Inflammation of Bone Secondary to Bacterial Infection

Any infectious agent may be responsible, but the most common pathogens are *Staphylococcus* sp. (60% to 80%). Other organisms, such as *Kingella kingae, Escherichia coli, Neisseria gonorrhoeae, Haemophilus influenzae* and *Salmonella* sp., are also seen. Organisms gain entry via the bloodstream or by direct introduction into the bone.

Direct Penetration

Infection by direct penetration or extension of bacteria is now the most common cause of osteomyelitis in the United States. Bacteria can be introduced directly into bone by penetrating wounds, open fractures, or surgery. Staphylococci and streptococci are still commonly incriminated, but anaerobic organisms are involved in 25% of postoperative infections. Rarely, a gram-negative organism may seed a hip after urologic or gastrointestinal surgery or instrumentation.

Hematogenous Osteomyelitis

Infectious organisms may reach the bone via the bloodstream from a source elsewhere in the body. The primary focus itself (e.g., a skin pustule or infected teeth and gums) may pose little threat.

The most common sites affected by hematogenous osteomyelitis are the metaphyses of the long bones, such as in the knee, ankle, and hip. The infection principally affects boys aged 5 to 15 years, but is occasionally seen in older age groups as well. Drug addicts may develop hematogenous osteomyelitis from infected needles.

 ETIOLOGIC FACTORS AND PATHOLOGY: Hematogenous osteomyelitis primarily affects the metaphyseal area because of the unique vascular supply in this region (Fig. 30-17). Normally, arterioles enter the calcified portion of the growth plate, form a loop, and then drain into the medullary cavity without establishing a capillary bed. This loop system causes slowing and sludging of blood flow, which allows bacteria enough time to penetrate blood vessel walls and establish infective foci within the marrow. Proliferation of virulent organisms increases pressure on adjacent thin-walled vessels which lie in the closed space of the marrow cavity. This further compromises vascular supply in this region and promotes bone necrosis. Necrotic areas coalesce into an avascular zone, which further facilitates bacterial proliferation.

If infection is not contained, pus and bacteria extend into the endosteal vascular channels that supply the cortex and spread throughout the Volkmann and Haversian canals of the cortex. Eventually, pus forms beneath the periosteum, shearing off the perforating arteries of the periosteum and further devitalizing the cortex. Pus flows between the periosteum and the cortex, isolating more bone from its blood supply, and may even invade the joint. Eventually, it

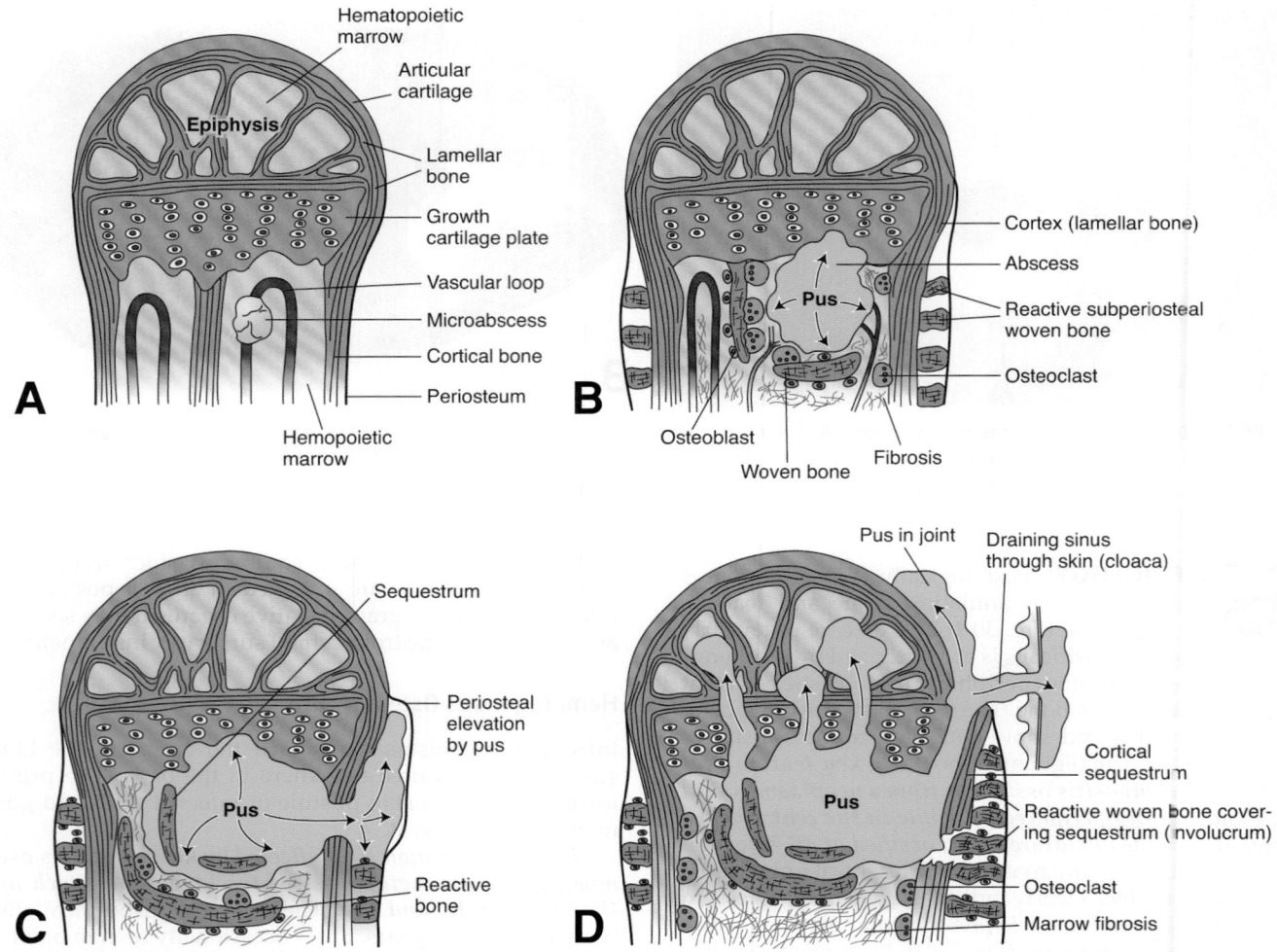

FIGURE 30-17. Pathogenesis of hematogenous osteomyelitis. A. The epiphysis, metaphysis and growth plate are normal. A small, septic microabscess is forming at the capillary loop. **B.** Expansion of the septic focus stimulates resorption of adjacent bony trabeculae. **Woven bone** begins to surround this focus. The abscess expands into the cartilage and stimulates reactive bone formation by the periosteum. **C.** The **abscess,** which continues to expand through the cortex into the subperiosteal tissue, shears off perforating arteries that supply the cortex, causing necrosis of the cortex. **D.** Extension of this process into the joint space, the epiphysis and the skin produces a **draining sinus.** The necrotic bone is called a **sequestrum.** The viable bone surrounding a sequestrum is termed the **involucrum.**

penetrates the periosteum and forms a draining sinus that discharges through the skin (Figs. 30-17D and 30-18). Epidermis can grow into the sinus tract that connects the skin to the discharging hole in the bone (cloaca). When the sinus tract becomes epithelialized, it invariably remains open, continually draining pus, necrotic bone, and bacteria.

Periosteal new bone formation and reactive bone formation in the marrow tend to wall off the infection. At the same time, osteoclastic activity resorbs bone. If the infection is virulent, this attempt to contain it is overwhelmed and it races through the bone, with virtually no bone formation but extensive bone necrosis. More commonly, pluripotent cells differentiate into osteoblasts in an attempt to wall off the infection. Several lesions may develop:

- **Cloaca** is the hole that arises in the bone during formation of a draining sinus.
- **Sequestrum** is a fragment of necrotic bone that is embedded in the pus.

- **Brodie abscess** consists of reactive bone derived from the periosteum and the endosteum, which surrounds and contains the infection.
- **Involucrum** refers to a lesion in which periosteal new bone formation forms a sheath around the necrotic sequestrum. An involucrum that involves an entire bone may exist for years before a patient seeks medical attention.

In very young children (1 year old or younger) afflicted with osteomyelitis, the adjacent joint is often involved (septic arthritis). This occurs because the periosteum is loosely attached to the cortex, and metaphyseal vessels penetrate the open growth plate to join epiphyseal vessels, which allows infectious organisms to reach the subchondral bone. From the age of 1 year to puberty, subperiosteal abscesses are common. Spread of infection to adjacent joints and subchondral bone regions also occur in adults.

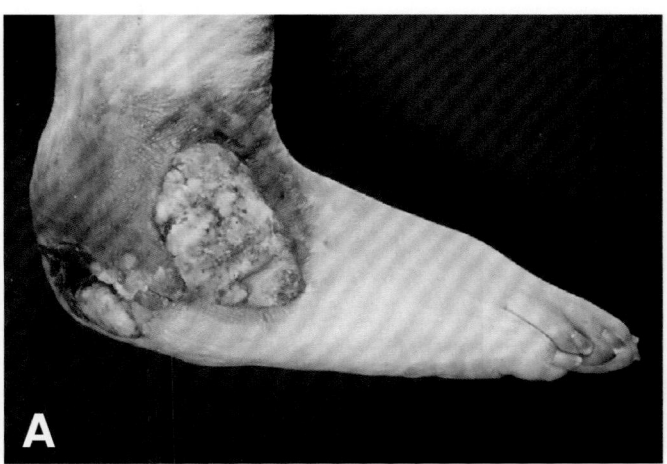
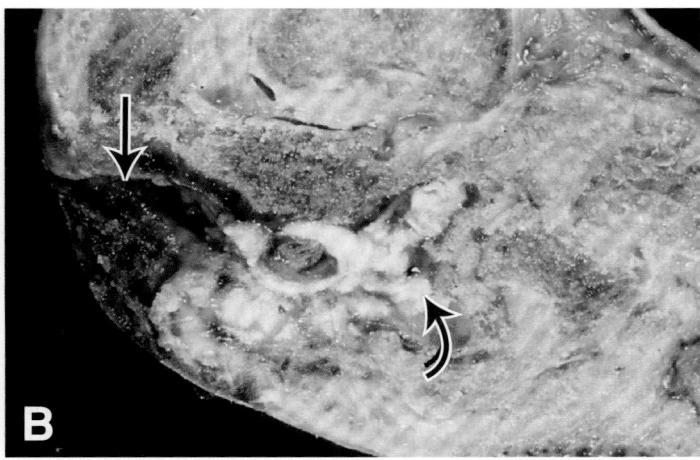

FIGURE 30-18. Chronic osteomyelitis. A. In this patient with chronic osteomyelitis, the skin overlying an infected bone is ulcerated and a draining sinus (*dark area*) is evident over the heel. **B.** Sagittal section of the amputated foot shows a draining sinus (*straight arrow*) connecting the infected bone with the surface of the ulcerated skin. The white tissue (*curved arrow*) is invasive squamous cell carcinoma, which arose in the skin. (From Bullough PG. *Atlas of Orthopaedic Pathology*. 2nd ed. New York: Gower Medical Publishing, 1992 Copyright Lippincott Williams & Wilkins.)

Vertebral Osteomyelitis

In adults, osteomyelitis frequently involves vertebral bodies (Fig. 30-19). The intervertebral disc is not an effective barrier to bacterial osteomyelitis, particularly those involving staphylococcal infection. Infections directly traverse the disc and travel from one vertebra to the next. The intervertebral disc itself may be the primary source of infection, so-called discitis. The disc expands with pus and is eventually destroyed as the pus bores into adjacent vertebral bodies.

Half or more of cases of vertebral osteomyelitis are caused by *Staphylococcus aureus*. Twenty percent involve *E. coli* and other enteric organisms, often originating from the urinary tract. *Salmonella* sp. are also seen in the vertebral bodies, as are *Brucella* sp and *Pseudomonas* in intravenous drug abusers. Predisposing factors include intravenous drug abuse, upper urinary tract infections, urologic procedures, and hematogenous spread of organisms from other sites. Back pain, with point tenderness over the area of infection, is associated with low-grade fever and serum markers of inflammation. Occasionally, a paravertebral abscess draining the bone may "point" and emerge in the groin or elsewhere. Vertebral osteomyelitis may lead to: (1) vertebral collapse and paravertebral abscesses; (2) spinal epidural abscesses, with cord compression from the abscess or from displaced fragments of the infected bone; and (3) compression fractures of the vertebral body, leading to neurologic deficits.

Complications

The complications of osteomyelitis include:

- **Septicemia:** Dissemination of organisms through the bloodstream may occur as a result of bone infection. It is unusual for osteomyelitis to result from septicemia.
- **Acute bacterial arthritis:** Joint infection secondary to osteomyelitis can occur at all ages. Direct digestion of cartilage by inflammatory cells destroys the articular cartilage and produces osteoarthritis. Rapid intervention to prevent this complication is mandatory.

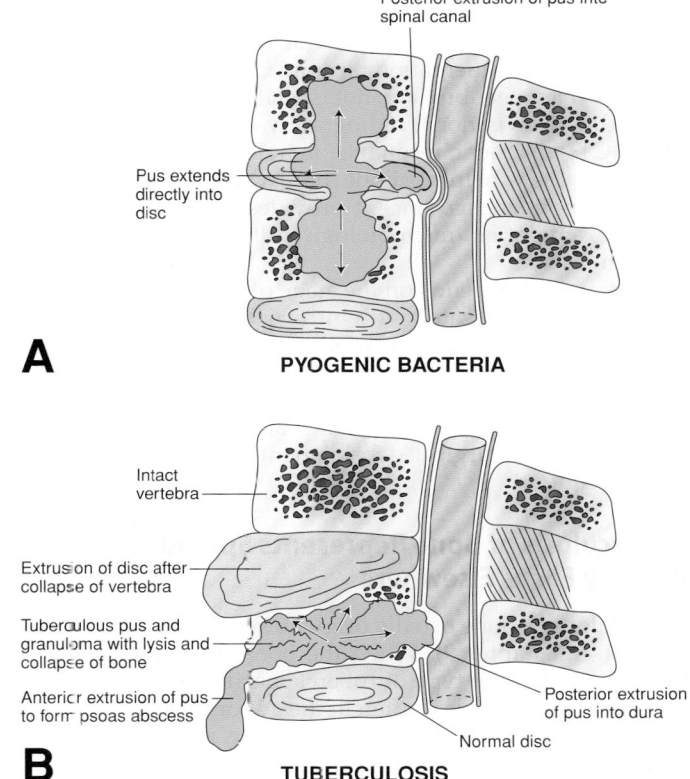

FIGURE 30-19. Osteomyelitis of the vertebral body. A. Bacterial osteomyelitis expands from one vertebral body to the next by direct invasion of the intervertebral disc. It may also push posteriorly into the spinal canal. The sequence of events in the marrow cavity is similar to that in a long bone. **B.** In **tuberculous osteomyelitis,** bone is destroyed by resorption of bony trabeculae, which results in mechanical collapse of the vertebrae and extrusion of the intervertebral disc. Tuberculous organisms cannot penetrate the intervertebral disc directly, but they extend from one vertebra to the next once mechanical forces have destroyed and extruded the intervertebral disc.

- **Pathologic fractures:** Osteomyelitis may lead to fractures, which heal poorly and may require surgical drainage.
- **Chronic osteomyelitis:** Chronic osteomyelitis (Fig. 30-18) may follow acute osteomyelitis. It is difficult to treat, especially if it involves the entire bone, because necrotic bone or sequestra function as foreign bodies in avascular areas, and antibiotics do not reach the bacteria. Chronic osteomyelitis is, therefore, treated symptomatically with surgery or antibiotics for the duration of the patient's life.
- **Squamous cell carcinoma:** This cancer can develop in the bone or the sinus tract of long-standing chronic osteomyelitis, often years after the initial infection. It derives from cells of the skin lining the sinus tract that undergo malignant transformation (Fig. 30-18B).
- **Amyloidosis:** This used to be a common consequence of chronic osteomyelitis but is now rare in industrialized countries.

CLINICAL FEATURES: Hematogenous osteomyelitis in children occurs as a sudden illness, with fever and systemic toxicity, or as a subacute illness in which local manifestations predominate. Swelling, erythema, and tenderness over the involved bone are characteristic. The leukocyte count is often conspicuously increased, but may be normal in so many cases that absence of leukocytosis does not rule out the disease. Erythrocyte sedimentation rate and C-reactive protein are usually elevated but are not specific. Imaging studies including conventional radiography, computed tomography (CT), magnetic resonance imaging (MRI), and bone scan are very helpful. Bone biopsy is necessary for a definitive diagnosis, since it provides material for histologic examination, microbiologic cultures, and antibiotic sensitivity.

Treatment depends on the stage of the infection. Early osteomyelitis is treated with intravenous antibiotics for 6 or more weeks. Surgery is used to drain and decompress the infection within the bone or to drain abscesses that do not respond to antibiotic therapy. In long-standing, chronic osteomyelitis, antibiotics alone are not curative and extensive surgical debridement of necrotic bone is often required.

Tuberculosis of Bone Represents Spread From a Primary Focus Elsewhere

Tuberculosis of bone usually originates in the lungs or lymph nodes (see Chapter 9). When the bone infection is caused by the rarer bovine type of tubercle bacillus (*Mycobacterium bovis*), the initial focus is often in the gut or tonsils. Mycobacteria spread to the bone hematogenously, and only rarely is there direct spread from the lungs or lymph nodes.

Tuberculous Spondylitis (Pott Disease)

Tuberculous spondylitis (i.e., infection of the spine) is a feared complication of childhood tuberculosis. The disease affects vertebral bodies, sparing the lamina, spinous processes, and adjacent vertebrae (Figs. 30-19B and 30-20). Thoracic vertebrae are usually affected, especially the 11th thoracic vertebra. Lumbar and cervical vertebrae are less frequently involved. With current antibiotic treatment, Pott disease is now rare.

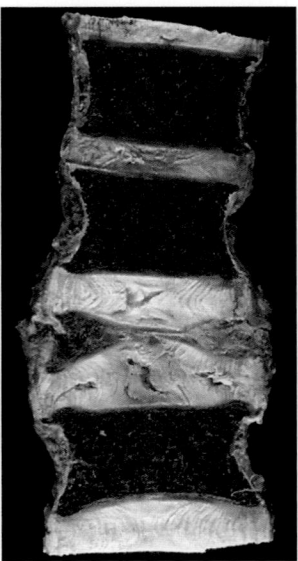

FIGURE 30-20. Tuberculous spondylitis (Pott disease). A vertebral body is almost completely replaced by tuberculous tissue. Note preservation of the intervertebral discs.

PATHOLOGY: The pathology of tuberculous spondylitis is similar to tuberculosis at other sites. Granulomas with caseous necrosis first appear in the bone marrow, which leads to slow resorption of bony trabeculae and occasionally to formation cystic spaces in the bone. Since there is little or no reactive bone formation, affected vertebrae tend to collapse, leading to kyphosis and scoliosis. Intervertebral discs are crushed and destroyed by the compression fracture, rather than by invasion of organisms. The typical "hunchback" of bygone days was often the victim of Pott disease.

If the infection ruptures into the soft tissue anteriorly, pus and necrotic debris drain along the spinal ligaments and form a **cold abscess** (i.e., an abscess lacking acute inflammation). A **psoas abscess** (Fig. 30-19B), which forms near the lower lumbar vertebrae and dissects along the pelvis to emerge through the skin of the inguinal region as a draining sinus, may be the first manifestation of tuberculous spondylitis. Paraplegia can occur as a result of vascular insufficiency of the spinal nerves, rather than from direct pressure.

Tuberculous Arthritis

Hematogenous spread of tuberculosis may bring organisms to the joint capsule, synovium, or intracapsular portion of the bone. Granulomas form in synovial tissue, which then becomes edematous and papillary and may fill the entire joint space. Massive destruction of articular cartilage results from undermining granulation tissue in the bone. The destroyed joint is replaced by bone, an effect that produces an immovable joint **(bony ankylosis)**.

Tuberculous Osteomyelitis of the Long Bones

Infection of long bones is the least common bone manifestation of tuberculosis. This infection occurs near the joint, where it also produces arthritis. For unknown reasons, the greater trochanter of the femur is a common site for this disease.

Syphilis of Bone Is Rare Today

Syphilis causes a slowly progressive, chronic, inflammatory disease of bone, characterized by granulomas, necrosis, and marked reactive bone formation. It may be acquired through sexual contact or transmitted transplacentally from mother to fetus (see Chapter 9). The bone changes in syphilis depend on the patient's age, endosteal and periosteal changes and the presence or absence of gummas.

Congenital Syphilis

PATHOLOGY: Bone involvement in congenital syphilis may appear as early as the fifth month of gestation and is fully developed at birth. Spirochetes are ubiquitous in the epiphysis and periosteum, where they produce osteochondritis (epiphysitis) and periostitis, respectively (Fig. 30-21). In severe disease, an epiphysis may become dislocated, leaving the child with a functionless limb **(pseudoparalysis of Parrot)**.

The knee is most often affected by congenital syphilis. The growth plate is irregularly widened and displays a yellow discoloration. After the zone of calcified cartilage is destroyed, a sea of lymphocytes, plasma cells, and spirochetes fills the marrow spaces. Because the periosteum is stimulated to produce reactive new bone, the thickness of the cortex may actually be doubled. The inflammatory infiltrate permeates the cortex through the Volkmann and Haversian canals and settles in the elevated periosteum. Ultimately, as the affected bones grow, they become short and deformed.

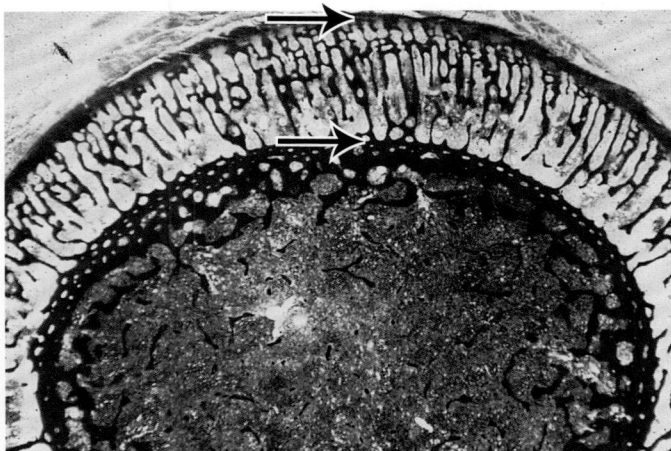

FIGURE 30-21. Congenital syphilis of bone. A cross-section of a tubular bone infected by syphilis shows marked periosteal new bone formation (*area between arrows*). The medullary cavity is filled with a lymphoplasmacytic infiltrate that replaces the normal marrow fat. The cortex is irregularly destroyed by osteoclastic resorption, a process that stimulates periosteal new bone formation.

Acquired Syphilis

Acquired syphilis in adults produces lesions of the bone early in the tertiary stage, 2 to 5 years after inoculation of the organisms. Periostitis is the predominant feature because the growth plates have already closed. The bones most commonly affected are the tibia, nose, palate, and skull. Tibial lesions are marked by periostitis, with deposition of new bone on the medial and anterior aspects of the shaft, which leads to the **saber shin** deformity. The skull thickness also increases because of periosteal stimulation.

Gumma formation is seen most often in tertiary syphilis. Bone adjacent to gummas is slowly replaced by fibrous marrow. Ultimately, perforations occur through the cortex. Markedly thickened, irregular periosteal surfaces perforated by pits and serpiginous ulcerations are characteristic of syphilis. Lysis and collapse of nasal and palatal bones produce the classic **saddle nose**—perforation, destruction, and collapse of the nasal septum (see Chapter 29).

Metabolic Bone Diseases

Metabolic bone diseases are defined as disorders of metabolism that result in secondary structural effects on the skeleton, including diminished bone mass due to decreased synthesis or increased resorption, reduced bone mineralization, or both. Because metabolic bone diseases are systemic, a biopsy of any bone should reveal the abnormality, even though severity may differ in various parts of the skeleton (Fig. 30-22).

OSTEOPOROSIS

Osteoporosis is a metabolic bone disease in which normally mineralized bone is decreased in mass to the point that it no longer provides adequate mechanical support. Although osteoporosis has a number of causes, it is always characterized by loss of skeletal mass. The remaining bone has a normal ratio of mineralized to nonmineralized (i.e., osteoid) matrix. Bone loss and eventually fractures are the hallmarks of osteoporosis, regardless of the underlying cause (Fig. 30-23). Factors promoting bone loss are diverse and include menopause, smoking, vitamin D deficiency, low body mass index, hypogonadism, sedentary lifestyle, and glucocorticoid therapy.

EPIDEMIOLOGY: Osteoporosis and its complications have become major public health problems as life expectancy has increased. Bone mass normally peaks between the ages of 25 and 35 and begins to decline in the fifth or sixth decade. Bone loss with age occurs in all races, but because blacks have higher peak bone mass, they are less prone to osteoporosis than are Asians and whites. Bone loss during normal aging in women has been divided into two phases: menopausal and aging. The latter affects men as well as women. At a certain point, loss of bone becomes sufficient to justify the label **osteoporosis** and renders weight-bearing bones susceptible to fractures, which occur mostly commonly in the neck and intertrochanteric region of the femur

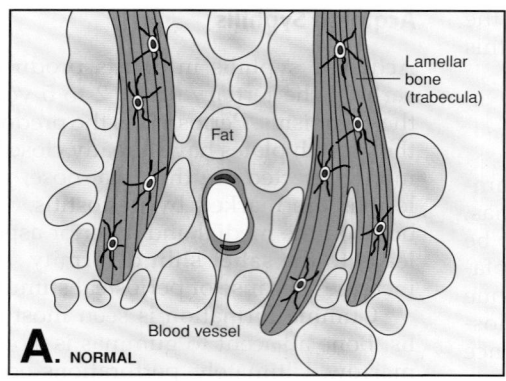

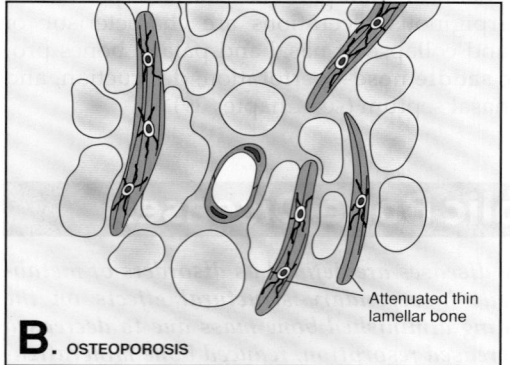

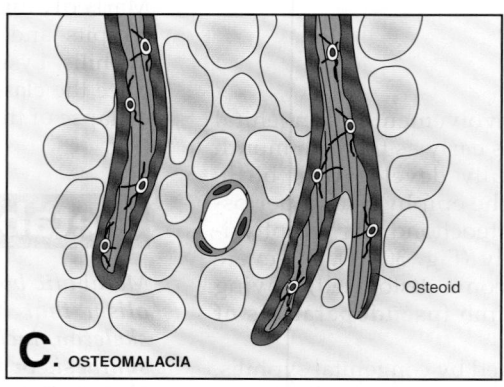

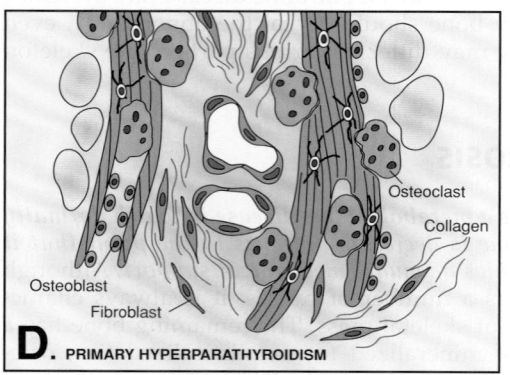

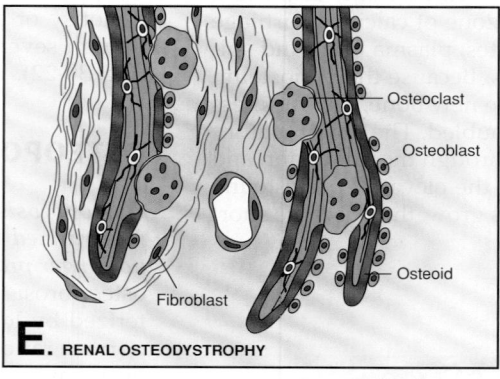

FIGURE 30-22. Metabolic bone diseases. A. Normal trabecular bone and fatty marrow. Trabecular bone is lamellar and contains evenly distributed osteocytes. **B. Osteoporosis.** Lamellar bone trabeculae are discontinuous and thin. **C. Osteomalacia.** Lamellar bone trabeculae contain abnormal amounts of nonmineralized bone (osteoid). The osteoid seams are thickened and cover an abnormally large area of the trabecular bone surface. **D. Primary hyperparathyroidism.** Lamellar bone trabeculae are actively resorbed by numerous osteoclasts that bore into each trabecula. The presence of osteoclasts dissecting into trabeculae, a process termed **dissecting osteitis,** is diagnostic of hyperparathyroidism. Osteoblastic activity is also pronounced. The marrow is replaced by fibrous tissue adjacent to the trabeculae. **E. Renal osteodystrophy.** The morphologic appearance is similar to that of primary hyperparathyroidism, except that prominent osteoid covers the trabeculae. Osteoclasts do not resorb unmineralized bone, and wherever an osteoid seam is lacking, osteoclasts bore into the trabeculae. Osteoblastic activity is also prominent.

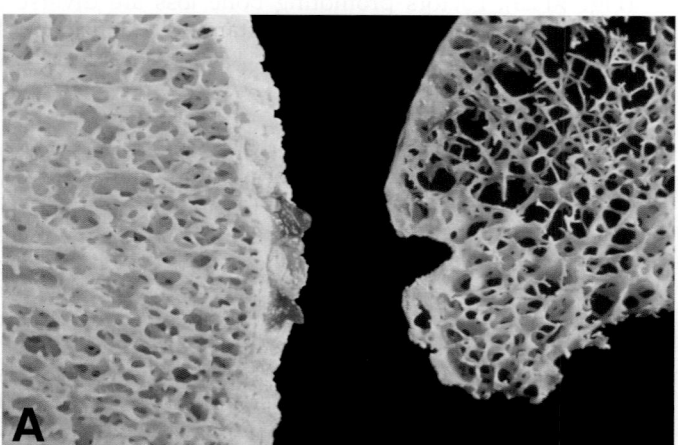

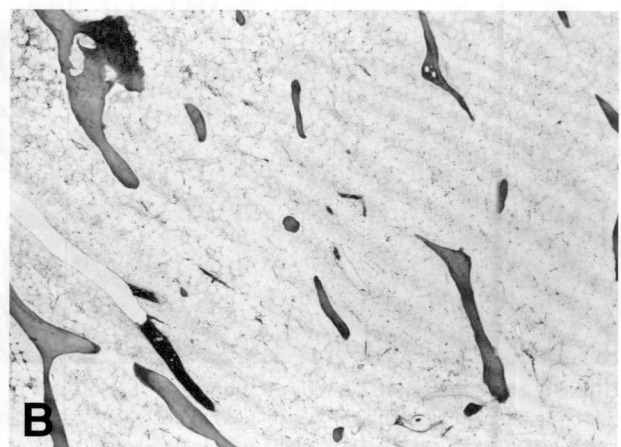

FIGURE 30-23. Osteoporosis. A. Femoral head of an 82-year-old woman with osteoporosis who sustained a femoral neck fracture (*right*) compared with a normal femoral head cut to the same thickness (*left*). **B.** Microscopically, bone trabeculae are reduced in size and thickness, and show loss of connectivity.

(hip fracture), vertebral bodies **(compression fracture)**, and distal radius **(Colles fracture)**. By age 80, 15% of whites in the United States have had a hip fracture, and this increases to 25% by age 90. Women have twice the risk of hip fracture as men, although among blacks and some Asian populations, the incidence is equal between sexes. Compared with other osteoporotic fractures, hip fractures incur the greatest morbidity, mortality (up to 20% within a year), and direct medical costs. The female predominance of 8:1 is particularly striking for vertebral fractures. A subset of women in the early postmenopausal years is at particular risk of vertebral fractures, which are rare in middle-aged men. The propensity of men to sustain hip fractures as opposed to vertebral fractures is related to factors other than reduced bone mass, such as loss of proprioception.

  ETIOLOGIC FACTORS AND MOLECULAR PATHOGENESIS: *Regardless of the cause of osteoporosis, it always reflects enhanced bone resorption relative to formation.* Thus, this family of diseases should be viewed in the context of the remodeling cycle. Bone resorption and bone formation exist simultaneously. Osteoblasts and osteoclasts belong to a unique temporary structure, known as the **basic multicellular unit** (BMU or **bone-remodeling unit**), which is responsible for bone remodeling throughout life. Individuals younger than 35 or 40 years completely replace bone resorbed during the remodeling cycle. With increasing age, however, less bone is replaced in resorption bays than is removed, leading to a small deficit at each remodeling site. Given the thousands of remodeling sites in the skeleton, net bone loss, even in a short time, can be substantial.

Osteoporosis is classified as either primary or secondary. **Primary osteoporosis**, by far the more common variety, is of uncertain origin and occurs principally in postmenopausal women (type 1) and elderly people of both sexes (type 2). **Secondary osteoporosis** is a disorder associated with a defined cause, including a variety of endocrine and genetic abnormalities.

Type 1 primary osteoporosis is due to an absolute increase in osteoclast activity. Since osteoclasts initiate bone remodeling, the number of remodeling sites increases in this state of enhanced osteoclast formation, a phenomenon known as **increased activation frequency**.

The increase in osteoclasts in the early postmenopausal skeleton is a result of estrogen withdrawal, but the effects are not targeted directly to the osteoclast. Instead, the mechanism involves reduced secretion of estrogen sensitive cytokines that recruit osteoclasts from the bone marrow, including IL-1, IL-6, TNF-α, and M-CSF.

Type 2 primary osteoporosis, also called **senile osteoporosis**, has a more complex pathogenesis than type 1. Type 2 osteoporosis generally appears after age 70 and reflects decreased osteoblast function. Thus, even if osteoclast activity is not increased, the number of osteoblasts and amount of bone produced per cell are insufficient to replace bone removed in the resorptive phase of the remodeling cycle.

Primary Osteoporosis Is Caused by a Number of Factors

Primary osteoporosis has been linked to multiple factors that influence peak bone mass and the rate of bone loss:

- **Genetic factors:** Interactions between environmental and genetic factors play a role in determining peak bone mass and risk of osteoporosis. The onset of clinically significant osteoporosis is related, in largest part, to the maximal amount of bone that develops in a given person, referred to as the **peak bone mass**. In general, peak bone mass is greater in men than in women and in blacks than in whites or Asians. There is a higher concordance of peak bone mass in monozygotic than in dizygotic twins. Women of reproductive age whose mothers have postmenopausal osteoporosis exhibit a lower **bone mineral density** (BMD) than do women in the general population. BMD is the most commonly used index for defining and studying osteoporosis. Genetic factors are thought to play an important role in regulating BMD. In fact, genetic variations explain as much as 70% of the variance in BMD. Sequence variants in genes for the vitamin D receptor (*VDR*), type I collagen (*COL1A1*), estrogen receptor-α (*ESR1*), IL-6 and low-density lipoprotein receptor–related protein-5 (*LRP5*) are all associated with differences in BMD. Furthermore, the vitamin D receptor and IL-6 interact with environmental and hormonal factors (e.g., calcium intake, estrogen) to modulate BMD.
- **Calcium intake:** Average calcium intake in postmenopausal women in the United States is below the recommended value of 800 mg/day. However, whether this apparent shortfall contributes to development of osteoporosis remains controversial. Nevertheless, it has been recommended that both premenopausal and postmenopausal women increase the intake of calcium and vitamin D.
- **Calcium absorption and vitamin D:** Intestinal absorption of calcium decreases with age. Because calcium absorption is largely under the control of vitamin D, attention has been directed to the role of this steroid hormone in osteoporosis. Patients with osteoporosis have reduced circulating levels of 1,25-dihydroxyvitamin D [1,25(OH)$_2$D], the active form of vitamin D that promotes calcium absorption in the intestine. This has been attributed to age-related decreases in 1α-hydroxylase activity in the kidney, the enzyme that catalyzes formation of 1,25(OH)$_2$D. Lower 1α-hydroxylase activity has, in turn, been attributed to diminished stimulation of the enzyme by PTH, as well as an age-related decrease in responses of renal tubules to PTH. Interestingly, estrogen replacement in postmenopausal women with osteoporosis increases both circulating 1,25(OH)$_2$D and calcium absorption. It has been suggested that decreased 1α-hydroxylase activity in the kidney may stimulate PTH secretion, and so contribute to bone resorption.
- **Exercise:** Physical activity is necessary to maintain bone mass, and athletes often have increased bone mass. By contrast, immobilization of a bone (e.g., prolonged bed rest, application of a cast) elicits accelerated bone loss. The weightlessness of space flight results in severe bone loss (33% of trabecular bone mass in 25 weeks). Yet vigorous exercise in this setting does not seem to increase bone mass substantially or prevent osteoporosis.

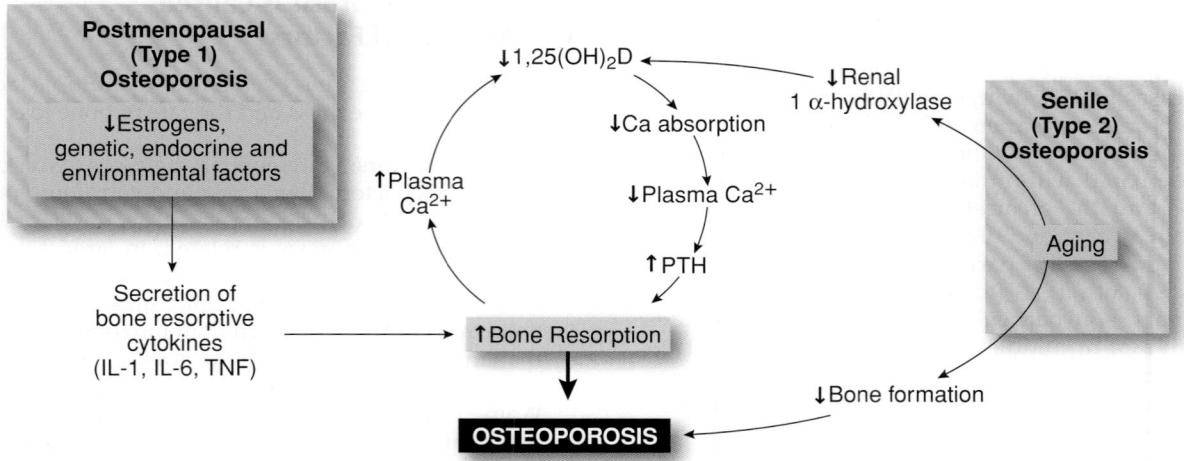

FIGURE 30-24. Pathogenesis of primary osteoporosis. *Ca²⁺* = calcium; *IL* = interleukin; *PTH* = parathyroid hormone; *TNF* = tumor necrosis factor.

- **Environmental factors:** Cigarette smoking in women has been correlated with an increased incidence of osteoporosis. Decreased levels of active estrogens caused by smoking may be responsible for this effect.

In summary, the two major determinants of primary osteoporosis are estrogen deficiency in postmenopausal women and the aging process in both sexes. Potential mechanisms for these effects are summarized in Figure 30-24.

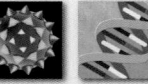 **PATHOLOGY:** *The ratio of osteoid to mineralized bone is normal in individuals with osteoporosis.* Because of the abundance of cancellous bone in the spine, osteoporotic changes are generally most conspicuous there. In vertebral body fractures caused by osteoporosis, the vertebra is deformed, with anterior wedging and collapse. Even if the vertebral body is not fractured, there is a general outline of both endplates, with a virtual absence of cancellous bone.

Osteoporosis is characterized histologically by decreased thickness of the cortex and a reduction in the number and size of trabeculae of the coarse cancellous bone (Fig. 30-23). Although senile osteoporosis tends to feature reduced trabecular thickness, postmenopausal osteoporosis exhibits disrupted connections between trabeculae. The loss of trabecular connectivity, which is attended by diminished biomechanical strength and ultimately provokes fracture, is due to perforation of trabeculae by resorbing osteoclasts in remodeling sites. In histologic sections, the loss of connectivity results in the appearance of "isolated" islands of bone (Figs. 30-22B and 30-23B).

CLINICAL FEATURES: Postmenopausal osteoporosis is usually recognizable within 10 years after onset of the menopause; senile osteoporosis generally becomes symptomatic after age 70 years. Until recently, most patients were unaware of their disease until they had a fracture of a vertebra, hip or other bone. However, use of sensitive screening techniques to measure bone mineral density permits early diagnosis. Vertebral body compression fractures often occur after trivial trauma or may even follow lifting a heavy object. With each compression fracture, the patient becomes shorter and develops kyphosis **(dowager hump)**. Serum calcium and phosphorus levels remain normal.

Estrogen therapy is an effective yet controversial means of preventing postmenopausal osteoporosis. Because hormone treatment carries with it increased risks of breast and endometrial cancers, other bone-specific antiosteoporotic drugs have been developed. **Bisphosphonates** are currently the most popular therapeutic agents used. All successful antiosteoporotic agents developed thus far block or slow the rate of bone resorption but do not stimulate bone formation. Thus, these drugs may prevent disease progression but cannot cure a patient who already has osteoporosis. Dietary calcium and vitamin D supplementation in elderly patients reduces the risk of osteoporotic fractures by half.

Secondary Osteoporosis Reflects Extraosseous Metabolic Disorders

ETIOLOGIC FACTORS AND MOLECULAR PATHOGENESIS: Causes of secondary osteoporosis include adverse effects of drug therapy, endocrine abnormalities, eating disorders, immobilization, marrow-related conditions, diseases of the gastrointestinal or biliary tracts, renal insufficiency, and cancer.

- **Endocrine conditions:** The most common form of secondary osteoporosis is iatrogenic and results from corticosteroid administration. Bone loss may also result from an excess of endogenous glucocorticoids, as in Cushing disease (see Chapter 27). Corticosteroids inhibit osteoblastic activity, thus reducing bone formation. They also impair vitamin D–dependent intestinal calcium absorption, an effect that leads to increased secretion of PTH and enhanced bone resorption.

Estrogen is a key hormone for maintaining bone mass, and its deficiency is the major cause of age-related bone loss in both sexes; estrogen deficiency or a low level of bioavailable estrogen decreases bone mass in elderly males. Estrogen stimulates production of various cytokines known to act via estrogen receptors on both osteoblasts and osteoclasts. These include IL-1, IL-6, TNF-α, RANKL, granulocyte-macrophage colony-stimulating factor (GM-CSF), M-CSF, and prostaglandin E_2 (PGE$_2$).

- **Hyperparathyroidism** stimulates osteoclast recruitment and increases osteoclastic activity, resulting in secondary osteoporosis (see below). In both sexes, hyperparathyroidism secondary to calcium malabsorption increases remodeling, worsens cortical bone thinning and porosity, and predisposes to hip fractures.
- **Hyperthyroidism** increases osteoclastic activity and causes accelerated turnover of bone. Although thyrotoxicosis is associated with some secondary osteoporosis, bone loss is limited.
- **Hypogonadism** in both men and women is accompanied by osteoporosis. In women with primary gonadal failure (Turner syndrome) or with secondary amenorrhea as a result of pituitary disease, estrogen deficiency is likely the cause. Hypogonadal men (e.g., Klinefelter syndrome, hemochromatosis) are at risk of osteoporosis because of deficiency of anabolic androgens. Similarly, hypogonadism contributes to bone loss in 25% of elderly males. Decreased bone density also occurs in men treated with androgen deprivation therapy for prostate cancer.
- **Hematologic malignancies:** Various hematologic cancers are accompanied by significant bone loss. This is especially prominent in multiple myeloma in which malignant plasma cells secrete osteoclast-activating factors. Nonhematologic malignancies are also associated with secondary osteoporosis. Even in the absence of skeletal metastases, some neoplasms (e.g., squamous cell carcinoma of lung) are associated with severe hypercalcemia due to bone resorption. Osteoclastic activity is enhanced in these patients, owing to secretion of PTH-related protein by the tumor (paraneoplastic syndrome).
- **Malabsorption:** Gastrointestinal and hepatic diseases that cause malabsorption often contribute to osteoporosis, probably because of impaired absorption of calcium, phosphate and vitamin D.
- **Alcoholism:** Chronic alcohol abuse also has been linked to development of osteoporosis. Alcohol is a direct inhibitor of osteoblasts and may also inhibit calcium absorption.

OSTEOMALACIA AND RICKETS

Osteomalacia (soft bones) *is a disorder of adults characterized by inadequate mineralization of newly formed bone matrix.* **Rickets** *refers to a similar disorder in children, in whom the growth plates (physes) are open.* Thus, children with rickets manifest defective mineralization not only of bone (osteomalacia) but also of the cartilaginous matrix of the growth plate. Diverse conditions associated with osteomalacia and rickets include abnormalities in vitamin D metabolism, phosphate deficiency states and defects in the mineralization process itself.

Vitamin D Metabolism Influences Bone Mineralization

MOLECULAR PATHOGENESIS: Vitamin D is ingested in food or synthesized in the skin from 7-dehydrocholesterol under the influence of ultraviolet light (Fig. 30-25). The vitamin is first hydroxylated in the liver to form its major circulating metabolite, 25-hydroxyvitamin D, and then hydroxylated again in proximal renal tubules to produce the active hormone 1,25(OH)$_2$D. Exposure to sunlight provides sufficient vitamin D for bone growth and mineralization, even if there is an inadequate dietary source.

Receptors for 1,25(OH)$_2$D are present not only in classic targets, such as intestine, bone, and kidney, but in many other cell types as well. Vitamin D is a general inducer of differentiation, for example, influencing maturation of hematopoietic and dermal cells, and also affecting many cancers. In the intestine, 1,25(OH)$_2$D stimulates calcium and phosphate absorption. It is also essential for osteoclast maturation. Regardless of mechanism, 1,25(OH)$_2$D, in concert with PTH, maintains blood calcium and phosphate at levels that are required for proper mineralization of bone. *The key determinant of 1,25(OH)$_2$D production is blood calcium concentration.* Decreases in blood calcium

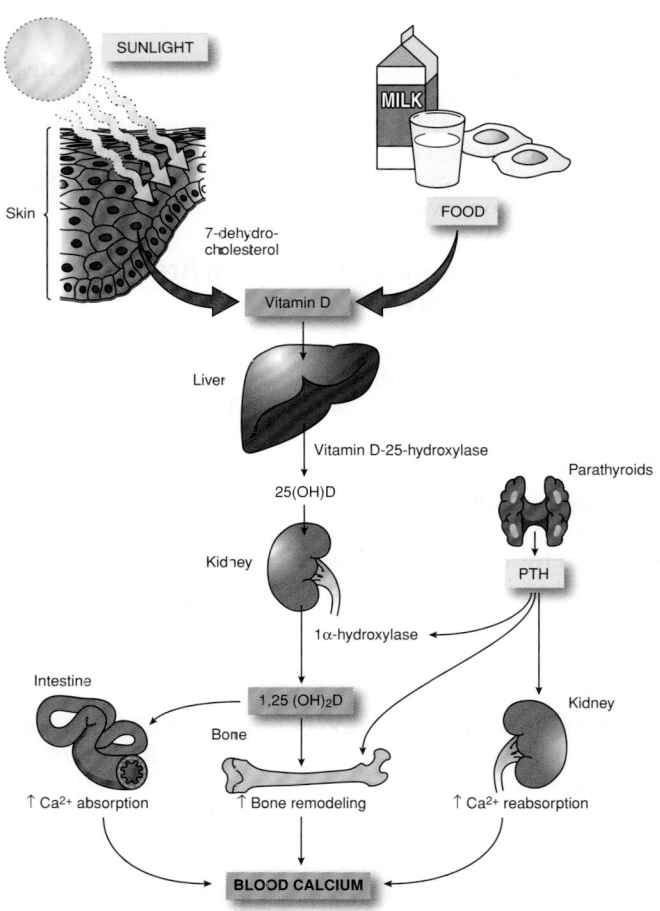

FIGURE 30-25. Metabolism of vitamin D and regulation of blood calcium.

stimulate release of PTH, which augments renal synthesis of 1,25(OH)₂D.

Hypovitaminosis D can result from: (1) inadequate exposure to sunlight; (2) deficient dietary intake; or (3) defective intestinal absorption. There are also hereditary and acquired disorders of vitamin D metabolism.

Dietary Deficiency of Vitamin D and Inadequate Exposure to Sunlight Cause Rickets

Rickets plagued some 85% of children in the industrial cities of Europe from the 17th century through the 19th century. These children had insufficient sun exposure and their dietary intake of vitamin D was inadequate. Use of vitamin D–rich cod liver oil and later fortification of milk and other foods with vitamin D effectively ended widespread rickets in Western countries. However, nutritional vitamin D deficiency remains a problem elsewhere in the world, in the neglected elderly and in food faddists.

Intestinal Malabsorption Decreases the Availability of Vitamin D

In industrialized countries, diseases associated with intestinal malabsorption are a greater cause of osteomalacia than poor nutrition. *Intrinsic diseases of the small intestine, cholestatic disorders of the liver, biliary obstruction, and chronic pancreatic insufficiency are the most frequent causes of osteomalacia in the United States.*

Malabsorption of vitamin D and calcium complicates a number of small-intestinal diseases, including celiac disease, Crohn disease, scleroderma, and the postsurgical blind-loop syndrome. In obstructive jaundice, the lack of bile salts in the intestine impairs absorption of lipids and lipid-soluble substances, among which is fat-soluble vitamin D.

Disorders of Vitamin D Metabolism Are Inherited or Acquired

Vitamin D metabolism can be disturbed either by defective 1α-hydroxylation of vitamin D in the kidney or by insensitivity of the target organ to 1,25(OH)₂D. Two autosomal recessive diseases associated with rickets are together known as **vitamin D–dependent rickets**.

- **Vitamin D–dependent rickets type I** results from an inherited deficiency of renal 1α-hydroxylase activity caused by autosomal recessive mutations in *CYP2R1*. The clinical and biochemical changes of rickets appear during the first year of life, and these children exhibit hypocalcemia, hypophosphatemia, and high levels of serum PTH and alkaline phosphatase. The disease can be controlled by the administration of 1,25(OH)₂D.
- **Vitamin D–dependent rickets type II** involves inherited recessive mutations in *VDR*, the gene for the vitamin D receptor, so that end organs are insensitive to 1,25(OH)₂D. The disease usually manifests early in life but may appear at any time up to adolescence. Serum concentrations of 1,25(OH)₂D are very high. Patients do not respond to 1,25(OH)₂D but are helped by repeated intravenous administration of calcium.
- **Acquired alterations in vitamin D metabolism** include defective renal 1α-hydroxylation and end-organ insensitivity. Some of the causes of impaired α-hydroxylation are

hypoparathyroidism, tumor-induced osteomalacia, chronic renal diseases, and osteomalacia of old age. Osteomalacia occasionally complicates the treatment of epilepsy with anticonvulsant drugs, particularly phenobarbital and phenytoin. It is believed that these drugs block the action of 1,25(OH)₂D on target organs.

Renal Disorders of Phosphate Metabolism Interfere With Vitamin D Metabolism

Both rickets and osteomalacia may result from impaired reabsorption of phosphate by proximal renal tubules, with resulting hypophosphatemia.

 MOLECULAR PATHOGENESIS: *X-LINKED HYPOPHOSPHATEMIA:* This condition, also known as **vitamin D–resistant rickets** or **phosphate diabetes**, is the most common type of hereditary rickets. It is caused by dominant mutations in the *PHEX* (phosphate-regulating) gene on the X chromosome (Xp22). *PHEX* encodes a protease that inactivates fibroblast growth factor-23 (FGF23). Its loss of function increases levels of FGF23 which promotes renal phosphate wasting by impairing transport of phosphate across the luminal membrane of proximal renal tubular cells. Although renal phosphate wasting is central to the disease, osteoblast function is also impaired. In boys, florid rickets appears during childhood, but girls often suffer only hypophosphatemia. Treatment consists of lifelong administration of phosphate and 1,25(OH)₂D. Microscopically, the bones of patients with X-linked hypophosphatemia show severe osteomalacia and wide osteoid seams. They also exhibit characteristic hypomineralized areas surrounding osteocytes, known as **halos**. The presence of these structures indicates that osteocytes are responsible for the terminal mineralization of bone.

FANCONI SYNDROMES: These inborn errors of metabolism are characterized by renal wastage of phosphate, glucose, bicarbonate. and amino acids. They are all characterized by renal tubular acidosis and lead to rickets and osteomalacia. Fanconi syndromes include Wilson disease, tyrosinemia, galactosemia, glycogen storage disease, and cystinosis. Renal tubular damage that leads to phosphate wastage may also be acquired, as in lead or mercury intoxication, amyloidosis, and Bence–Jones proteinuria.

TUMOR-ASSOCIATED OSTEOMALACIA: This disorder is a phosphate-wasting paraneoplastic syndrome that is associated with predominantly benign and occasionally malignant tumors of soft tissue and bone. Tumor-derived phosphaturic factors, known as **phosphatonins**, cause renal tubular phosphate wasting and prevent tubular conversion of 25-hydroxyvitamin D into 1,25(OH)₂D. Typical laboratory features are hypophosphatemia, hyperphosphaturia, low serum concentrations of 1,25-(OH)₂D, and elevated serum alkaline phosphatase. Phosphatonins thus appear to have the same effect as germline mutations in *PHEX* seen in X-linked hypophosphatemia. Phosphate wastage causes secondary osteomalacia but removal of the primary tumor is often curative. FGF23 has been implicated as a phosphatonin.

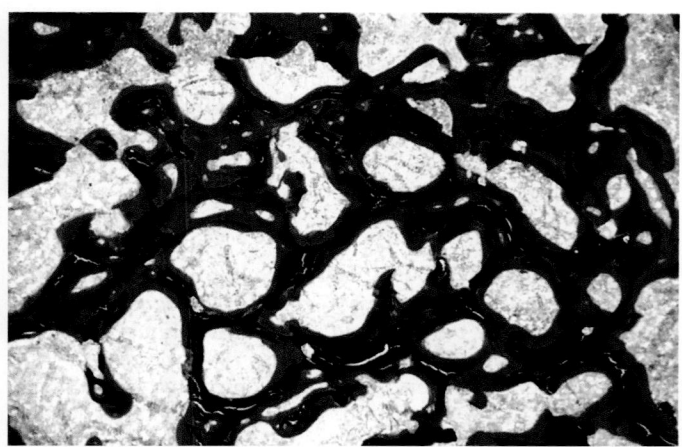

FIGURE 30-26. Osteomalacia. The surfaces of bony trabeculae (*black*) in this section prepared with the von Kossa stain are covered by an abnormally thick layer of osteoid (*red*).

PATHOLOGY: *OSTEOMALACIA:* Osteomalacia, like osteoporosis, causes an osteopenic radiographic pattern. The only findings may be vertebral compression fractures and decreased bone thickness, as in osteoporosis. However, some specific findings may be seen in osteomalacia, including the pseudofractures of **Milkman–Looser syndrome.** These are radiolucent transverse defects that are most common on the medial side of the neck of the femur, ischial and pubic rami, ribs, and scapula.

Microscopically, defective mineralization in osteomalacia results in **exaggeration of osteoid seams**, both in thickness and in the proportion of trabecular surface covered (Figs. 30-22C and 30-26). Osteoid seams reflect a time lag between the deposition of collagen and the appearance of the calcium salt. Although adults add 1 μm of new matrix to the surfaces of bone every day, it takes approximately 10 days for this new matrix to become mineralized. The normal thickness of osteoid seams, therefore, does not exceed 12 μm. Areas of pseudofracture display abundant osteoid and may function as stress points for true fractures. These areas do not evoke formation of callus and do not extend through the entire diameter of the bone.

RICKETS: Rickets is a disease of children and thus causes extensive changes at the physeal plate (Fig. 30-27), which does not become adequately mineralized. The calcified cartilage and zones of hypertrophy and proliferative cartilage continue to grow because osteoclastic activity does not resorb the poorly mineralized growth plate cartilage. As a consequence, the growth plate is conspicuously thickened, irregular, and lobulated. Endochondral ossification proceeds very slowly and preferentially at peripheral portions of the metaphysis. The result is a flared, cup-shaped epiphysis. The largest part of the

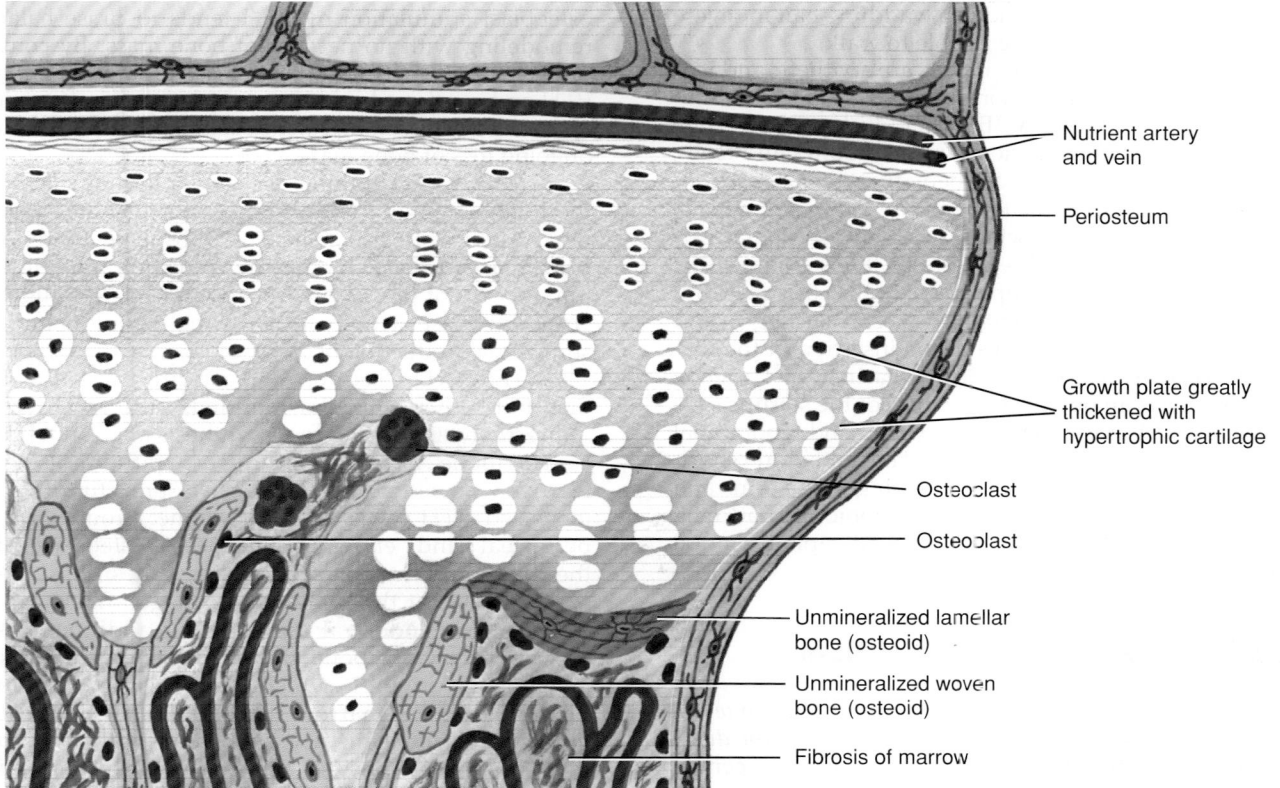

Nutrient artery and vein

Periosteum

Growth plate greatly thickened with hypertrophic cartilage

Osteoclast

Osteoblast

Unmineralized lamellar bone (osteoid)

Unmineralized woven bone (osteoid)

Fibrosis of marrow

FIGURE 30-27. The growth plate in rickets. The growth plate is thickened and disorganized, with a large zone of hypertrophic cartilage cells. Irregular perforation of the cartilage plate by osteoclasts occurs because there is little calcified cartilage. Woven bone on the surface of some primary trabeculae is unmineralized and therefore easily fractured. Such microfractures often lead to hemorrhage at the interface between the plate and the metaphysis.

primary spongiosum is composed of lamellar or woven bone that, importantly, remains unmineralized.

Microscopically, the growth plate exhibits striking changes. The resting zone is normal, but the zones of proliferating cartilage are greatly distorted. The ordered progression of helix-forming chondrocytes is lost and is replaced by a disorderly profusion of cells separated by small amounts of matrix. Resulting lobulated masses of proliferating and hypertrophied cartilage are associated with increasing width of the growth plate, which may be 5 to 15 times the normal width. The zone of provisional calcification is poorly defined, and only a minimal amount of primary spongiosum is formed. Masses of proliferating cartilage extend into the metaphyseal region, without any apparent vascular invasion and with little osteoclastic activity.

CLINICAL FEATURES: *OSTEOMALACIA:* The clinical diagnosis of osteomalacia is often difficult. Patients have nonspecific complaints, such as muscle weakness or diffuse aches and pains. In mild forms of the disease, only slowly progressive changes in bone are seen, and many patients remain totally asymptomatic for years. In advanced cases, poorly localized bone pain and tenderness are common, especially in the spine, pelvis, and proximal parts of the extremities. In such cases, the diagnosis may be made only after occurrence of an acute fracture, the most common sites being the femoral neck, pubic ramus, spine, or ribs. Muscular weakness and hypotonia lead to a waddling gait in severe cases, and some patients are unable to walk.

RICKETS: Children with rickets are apathetic and irritable and have short attention spans. They are content to be sedentary, assuming a "Buddha-like" posture. They are short, with characteristic changes of bones and teeth. Flattening of the skull, prominent frontal bones (**frontal bossing**) and conspicuous suture lines are typical. Delayed dentition is associated with severe dental caries and enamel defects. The chest has the classic **rachitic rosary** (a grossly beaded appearance of the costochondral junctions due to enlargement of the costal cartilages) and indentations of the lower ribs at the insertion of the diaphragm (**Harrison groove**). **Pectus carinatum** ("pigeon breast") reflects an outward curvature of the sternum.

The overall musculature is weak, and abdominal weakness generates a "potbelly." The limbs are shortened and deformed, with severe bowing of the arms and forearms and frequent fractures. The femoral head may dislocate from the growth plate (slipped capital femoral epiphysis).

PRIMARY HYPERPARATHYROIDISM

Primary hyperparathyroidism is a metabolic bone disease characterized by generalized bone resorption due to inappropriate secretion of PTH. Early in the 20th century, bone disease in primary hyperparathyroidism was often advanced and crippling because the connection between parathyroid glands, bone, and calcium was not known. With routine screening of patients for abnormalities of serum calcium, severe primary hyperparathyroidism is now rarely

encountered and presentations with clinically significant bone disease are unusual.

Histologic changes of primary hyperparathyroidism include paratrabecular marrow fibrosis, which accompanies the markedly accelerated bone remodeling and may also be seen in Paget disease, in hyperthyroidism and even in some patients with postmenopausal osteoporosis.

 ETIOLOGIC FACTORS: *Some 90% of cases of primary hyperparathyroidism are caused by one or more parathyroid adenomas. Hyperplasia of all four glands accounts for only 10%.* Because PTH increases renal conservation of calcium and stimulates osteoclastic bone resorption, high serum calcium levels are characteristic; and because calcium and phosphate levels are inversely related, phosphate levels are often low. A familial type of primary hyperparathyroidism is associated with mutations in the calcium-sensing receptor (*CASR*) gene, located on chromosome 3 (3q13.3).

The effects of PTH are mediated by its effects on bone, kidney, and (indirectly) intestine.

BONE: PTH mobilizes calcium from bone (the major reservoir of calcium in the body) by stimulating osteoclastic activity and recruiting new osteoclasts from preosteoclastic mesenchymal cells. The mechanism involves PTH-stimulated secretion of RANKL by osteoblasts, which binds to RANK receptors in osteoclasts and osteoclast precursors, and thereby leads to bone resorption. Under physiologic circumstances, PTH secretion is shut down by increases in ionic calcium. At the same time, osteoblast stimulation by PTH tends to cause balanced remodeling with no net loss of bone mass. By contrast, under pathologic conditions, release of large amounts of PTH and continued RANKL secretion prevent osteoclast apoptosis, and prolong osteoclast life and activation, with ongoing loss of bone mass.

KIDNEY: PTH stimulates reabsorption of calcium by the thick ascending and granular portions of the distal renal tubules. It also enhances phosphate excretion in proximal and distal tubules by directly inhibiting sodium-dependent phosphate transport. PTH also augments 1α-hydroxylase activity in proximal tubules and thus stimulates production of 1,25(OH)$_2$D.

INTESTINE: PTH does not act directly on the intestine, but rather enhances intestinal calcium absorption indirectly by increasing renal synthesis of 1,25(OH)$_2$D.

The bone histology of hyperparathyroidism varies over time. Initially, osteoclasts are stimulated by increased PTH levels to resorb bone. From both subperiosteal and endosteal surfaces, osteoclasts bore their way into the cortex as cutting cones (Figs. 30-22D and 30-28A). At the same time, collagen fibers are laid down in the endosteal marrow and additional osteoclasts penetrate the bone. By contrast to myelofibrosis of hematologic origin, in which fibrous tissue is randomly distributed in the marrow space, the collagen of osteitis fibrosa (i.e., bone disease associated with hyperparathyroidism) is deposited adjacent to trabeculae, which suggests that the stromal cells depositing matrix material are osteoblast precursors. Later, the trabecular bone is resorbed and marrow is replaced by loose fibrosis, hemosiderin-laden macrophages, areas of hemorrhage

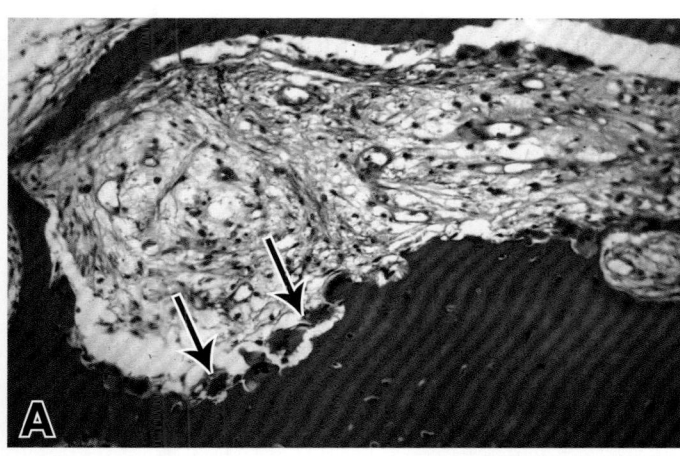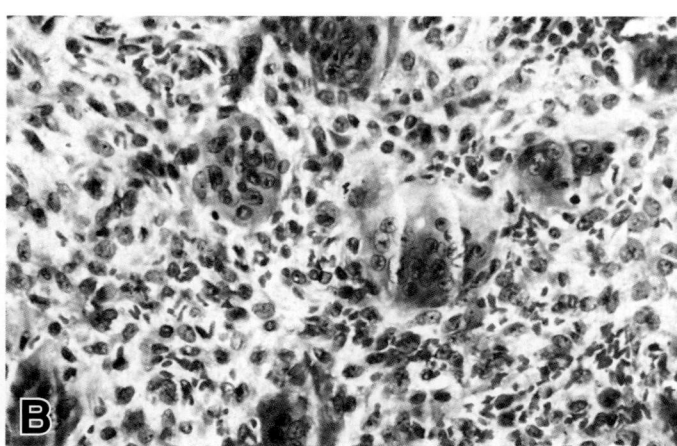

FIGURE 30-28. Primary hyperparathyroidism. A. Section through compact bone shows tunneling resorption of a Haversian canal. Numerous osteoclasts (*arrows*) and stromal fibrosis are evident. **B.** A section of a "brown tumor" reveals numerous giant cells in a cellular fibrous stroma. Scattered erythrocytes are present throughout the tissue.

from microfractures and reactive woven bone. As primary hyperparathyroidism progresses and hemorrhage continues, cystic degeneration ultimately occurs, evoking the final stage of the disease. Areas of fibrosis containing reactive woven bone and hemosiderin-laden macrophages often display many osteoclastic giant cells. Because of its brown macroscopic appearance, this lesion has been dubbed **brown tumor** (Fig. 30-28B). This is not a true neoplasm, but rather an attempted repair reaction at the end stage of hyperparathyroidism. A single lesion taken in isolation may be histologically mistaken for a primary giant cell tumor of bone.

Skeletal radiographs of most patients with primary hyperparathyroidism are normal, but some exhibit mottled bone cortices with an irregular frayed surface in the outer table of the skull, tufts of the terminal digits, and shafts of the metacarpals (Fig. 30-29). A distinctive radiographic peculiarity, referred to as **subperiosteal bone resorption**, is evident in the subperiosteal outer surface

of the cortex and reflects dissecting bone resorption. Resorption around tooth sockets causes the lamina dura of the teeth to disappear, a well-known finding on imaging studies.

 CLINICAL FEATURES: Symptoms of primary hyperparathyroidism are related to abnormal calcium homeostasis and have been summarized as "stones, bones, moans, and groans." The "stones" refer to kidney stones and the "bones" to the skeletal changes. The "moans" describe psychiatric depression and other abnormalities associated with hypercalcemia. The "groans" characterize the gastrointestinal irregularities associated with a high serum calcium level.

Primary hyperparathyroidism is treated by surgical removal of the parathyroid adenomas. If diffuse parathyroid hyperplasia is the cause, three and a half glands are usually removed. The remaining fragment suffices to protect against hypocalcemia. After surgery, the histologic appearance of the affected skeleton gradually normalizes.

RENAL OSTEODYSTROPHY

Renal osteodystrophy is a complex metabolic bone disease that occurs in the context of chronic renal failure. Severe renal osteodystrophy is most common in patients maintained on long-term dialysis, because they live long enough to develop conspicuous bone disease.

 ETIOLOGIC FACTORS AND MOLECULAR PATHOGENESIS: The pathogenesis of renal osteodystrophy is similar to that of osteomalacia, with secondary hyperparathyroidism exerting its influence by way of osteoclastic bone resorption (Fig. 30-22E). The development of renal osteodystrophy is summarized as follows:

1. In chronic renal disease, reduced glomerular filtration rate leads to retention of phosphate, and produces

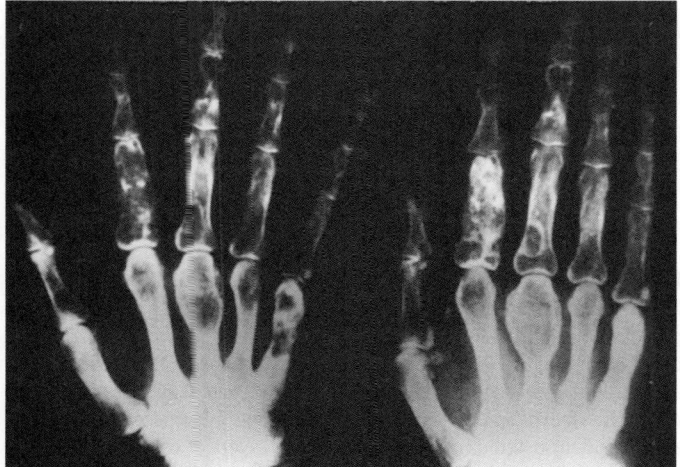

FIGURE 30-29. Primary hyperparathyroidism. A radiograph of the hands reveals bulbous swellings ("brown tumors") and numerous cavities, both representing bone resorption.

hyperphosphatemia. High serum phosphate levels drive down serum calcium levels.

2. Renal tubular injury reduces 1α-hydroxylase activity, resulting in 1,25(OH)$_2$D deficiency.

3. Intestinal calcium absorption is, in turn, decreased, worsening **hypocalcemia**.

4. Hypocalcemia stimulates **PTH production**. In fact, most patients with end-stage renal disease have substantial hyperparathyroidism. However, PTH does not effectively promote intestinal calcium absorption or renal tubular resorption of calcium because the diseased kidneys cannot make adequate 1,25(OH)$_2$D.

5. Disturbances in the vitamin D pathway may cause osteomalacia. This can lead to accumulation of new bone collagen (osteoid) and a substantial increase in unmineralized bone mass with reduction in only those areas that were mineralized prior to the development of osteomalacia. The sclerotic process may be particularly prominent in vertebrae where the radiographic appearance of alternating bands of radiopaque and normally dense bone has been named "rugger jersey" spine.

The **adynamic variant of renal osteodystrophy (ARO)** is characterized by arrested bone remodeling. More than 40% of adults who are treated with hemodialysis and more than 50% of those who are treated with peritoneal dialysis have bone biopsy evidence of ARO. Adynamic bone is characterized microscopically by an overall reduction in cellular activity in bone, with fewer or absent osteoblasts and osteoclasts. These changes are often due to overzealous control of secondary hyperparathyroidism with oral phosphate binders which impairs PTH-dependent osteoblast activity, or because of direct inhibitory effects of systemic factors on osteoblast function. Older, fatigued bone accumulates because it is being not remodeled. The result is structural compromise of the skeleton and increased tendency to fractures.

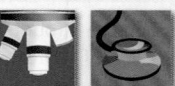 **PATHOLOGY AND CLINICAL FEATURES:** Renal osteodystrophy in the setting of chronic renal failure is characterized by varying degrees of hyperparathyroid bone disease, osteomalacia, osteosclerosis, and adynamic bone disease (Fig. 30-30). Combinations of osteitis fibrosa and osteomalacia are particularly common. Hyperphosphatemic patients with terminal chronic renal disease may display metastatic calcification at various sites, especially in areas that develop pH gradients with local alkalinity.

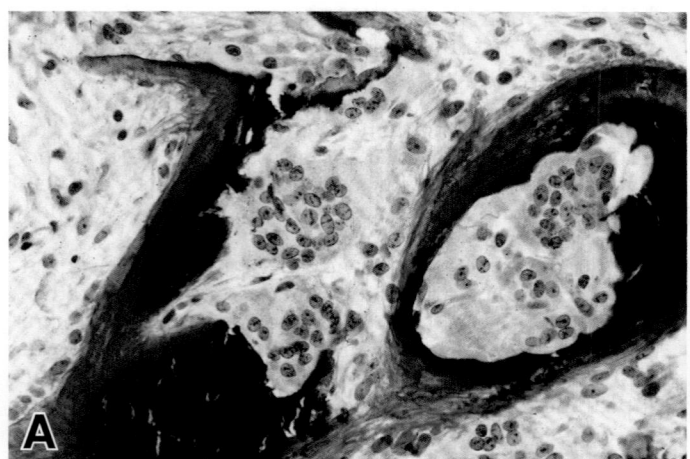

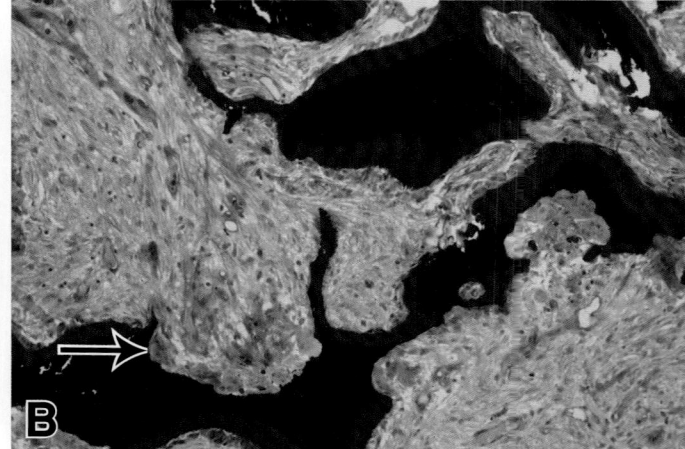

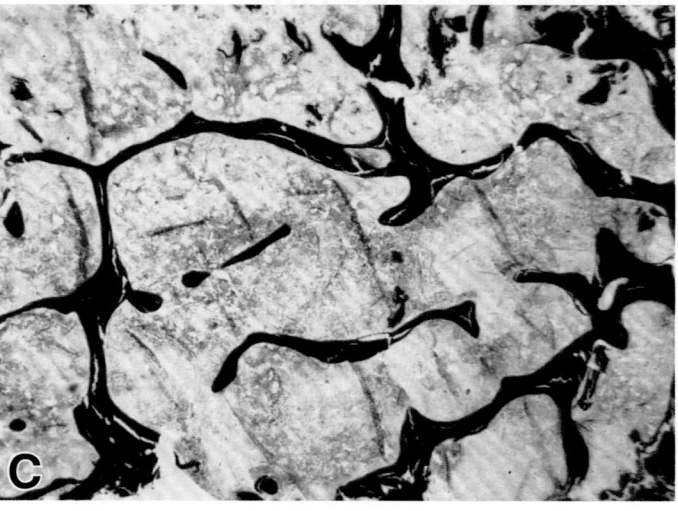

FIGURE 30-30. Renal osteodystrophy. A. Osteitis fibrosa. Several large multinucleated osteoclasts are resorbing bone spicules, and the paraosseous tissue is fibrotic. Note that osteoclastic resorption takes place only on mineralized (*blue*) portions of the trabeculae. In this undecalcified section, unmineralized bone (osteoid) appears *red.* **B. Osteomalacia.** A von Kossa stain of an undecalcified section shows mineralized bone (*black*) and abundant osteoid (*magenta*). Thickened layers of osteoid line a large proportion of the bone surfaces. Surfaces not covered by osteoid demonstrate scalloped Howship lacunae and contain abundant osteoclasts (*arrow*). **C. Adynamic bone disease** in which remodeling is attenuated, shows a paucity of osteoblasts, osteoclasts, and osteoid (von Kossa stain).

Management of renal osteodystrophy involves not only treatment of the underlying cause(s) of renal failure but also control of phosphate levels by appropriate drug therapy and infusions. Occasionally, parathyroidectomy is required to control the hyperparathyroidism, and administration of vitamin D may also be necessary.

PAGET DISEASE OF BONE

Paget disease is a chronic condition characterized by disordered bone remodeling, in which excessive bone resorption initially results in lytic lesions, followed by disorganized and excessive bone formation.

EPIDEMIOLOGY: Paget disease generally affects men and women older than 50 years. In predisposed populations, 3% of the elderly are affected by the disease. It has an unusual worldwide distribution, afflicting populations of the British Isles and following their migrations throughout the world. People of English descent living in the United States, Australia, New Zealand, and Canada have a high incidence of the disease. Northern Europeans have more Paget disease than southern Europeans. The disorder is almost nonexistent in Asia and in the indigenous populations of Africa and South America. For unknown reasons, the incidence of Paget disease appears to have decreased worldwide over the last several decades.

James Paget coined the term **osteitis deformans** for this disease over a century ago, but until recently its etiology has been obscure. Paget disease resembles a metabolic bone disease histologically and there is an increase in bone turnover in affected patients. However, its clinical tendency to involve a portion of one bone or only a few bones does not fulfill the definition of a metabolic disorder.

MOLECULAR PATHOGENESIS: The epidemiology of Paget disease is highly suggestive of genetic underpinnings, and a hereditary predisposition has been supported by reports of nearly 100 families in whom Paget disease is transmitted as an autosomal dominant trait with incomplete age-dependent penetrance. There is evolving evidence that Paget disease and some related diseases are caused by mutations in genes encoding proteins in the RANK signaling pathway. Specifically, mutations in *SQSTM1* have been found in familial and sporadic forms of Paget disease. This gene encodes a protein, p62, that acts as a scaffold in the RANK signaling pathway. How mutated p62 leads to accelerated osteoclast activity is unclear, but inactivating mutations in *SQSTM1* disrupt RANKL-induced osteoclastogenesis, suggesting a significant role for this protein in osteoclast function.

Additional evidence suggests that Paget disease may be related to viral infection. Inclusions consistent with viral structures are seen in the nuclei of osteoclasts and osteoclast precursors in virtually all patients. They consist of microfilaments in a paracrystalline array and are reminiscent of inclusions in the brains

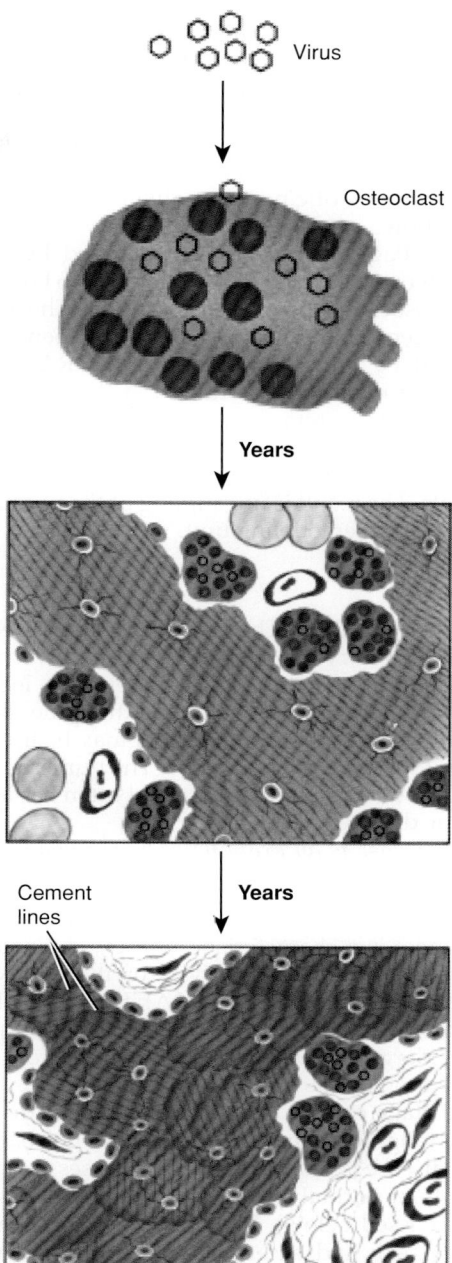

FIGURE 30-31. Hypothetical viral etiology of Paget disease of bone. Viral infection of osteoclastic progenitors or osteoclasts in a genetically predisposed individual stimulates osteoclastic activity, thereby leading to excessive resorption of bone. Over a period of years, the bone develops a characteristic mosaic pattern, produced by chaotically juxtaposed units of lamellar bone that form irregular cement lines. The adjacent marrow is often fibrotic, and a mixture of osteoclasts and osteoblasts is seen on the surface of the bone.

of patients with subacute sclerosing encephalitis (see Chapter 32). This similarity suggests that a slow virus may be involved (Fig. 30-31). Support for this hypothesis has come from the finding that the marrow of Paget disease patients contains paramyxovirus nucleocapsid transcripts. Infection of osteoclast precursor cells with paramyxovirus can increase expression of RANK and thereby increase osteoclastic activity. In addition, paramyxoviruses stimulate osteoblasts to produce IL-6, which contributes to osteoclastogenesis. Although a viral etiology seems plausible, actual live viruses have not been isolated from pagetic bone, and it is difficult to explain monostotic bone involvement by a systemic viral infection.

Overall, Paget disease is characterized by localized increases in osteoclast formation that lead to bone resorption and associated osteoblastic activity. The increased osteoclastogenic nature of the bone microenvironment is mediated by enhanced IL-6 and the RANK signaling. These pathways are perturbed in Paget disease as a result of genetic factors such as *SQSTM1* mutations and possibly a slow virus infection that may act as a catalyst driving the pagetic phenotype in genetically predisposed individuals. The result is uncoupling of the normal osteoclast/osteoblast remodeling unit.

PATHOLOGY: The lesions of Paget disease may be solitary (monostotic) or involve multiple bones (polyostotic). They tend to localize in bones of the axial skeleton, including the spine, skull, and pelvis. The proximal femur and tibia may be involved in the polyostotic form of the disease. The humerus is rarely involved in solitary Paget disease, but often has lesions in polyostotic disease.

Paget disease is an example of bone remodeling gone awry. It develops in three phases:

1. **"Hot"** or **osteoclastic resorptive stage:** Radiographically, there is a characteristic, sharply defined, flame-shaped or wedge-shaped lysis of the cortex, which may mimic a tumor (Fig. 30-32A). Histologically, there is widespread **osteolysis** with marked resorption by bizarre, large osteoclasts, along with marrow fibrosis, and dilation of marrow sinusoids.
2. **Mixed stage of osteoblastic and osteoclastic activity:** By imaging, the bones are larger than normal. In fact, Paget disease is one of only two diseases that produce **larger than normal bones** (the other is fibrous dysplasia, discussed below). The cortex in the mixed phase is thickened, and accentuation of the coarse cancellous bone makes the bone look heavy and enlarged (Fig. 30-32B,C). Involvement of vertebral bodies evokes a "picture frame" appearance (Fig. 30-32D), as cortices and endplates become greatly exaggerated compared to the coarse cancellous bone of the vertebral body. Although the bone is abnormal, the distorted, coarse cancellous bone and cortex still tend to align along stress lines. The pelvis is often thickened in the area of the acetabulum. Histologically, there is evidence of both increased osteoclastic and osteoblastic activity (Figs. 30-31 and 30-33B).
3. **"Cold"** or **burnt-out stage:** This phase is characterized histologically by little cellular activity and radiographically by thickened and disordered bones.

The disease need not progress through all three stages, and in polyostotic disease, various foci may appear in different stages.

The osteoclast is the pathologic cell of Paget disease, and its appearance is characteristic. Normal osteoclasts contain fewer than a dozen nuclei, but those of Paget disease are huge and may have more than 100 (Fig. 30-33B). As noted previously, nuclei may contain intranuclear inclusions that contain virus-like particles (Fig. 30-33B,C).

Because active Paget disease is a disorder of accelerated remodeling, its histologic features resemble those of hyperparathyroidism. Numerous large osteoclasts, active osteoblasts, and peritrabecular marrow fibrosis are seen (Fig. 30-33B). Rapid remodeling disrupts trabecular architecture, and trabeculae become distorted and irregular, with a high surface-to-volume ratio. Bone collagen is often arranged in a woven rather than lamellar pattern.

With time, the lesions of Paget disease burn out and become inactive. The diagnostic hallmark of this stage is an abnormal arrangement of lamellar bone, in which islands of irregular bone formation resembling pieces of a jigsaw puzzle are separated by prominent irregular **cement lines** (Fig. 30-33A), resulting in a **mosaic pattern** of the bone. Osteons in the cortex of an affected bone tend to become destroyed, and concentric lamellae are incomplete. Although these histologic changes in lamellar bone are diagnostic, it is common to see woven bone as part of the pathologic process. In this situation, the woven bone is a reactive phenomenon, as in a microcallus, and represents a temporary bridge between islands of the mosaic bone of Paget disease.

CLINICAL FEATURES: The most common focal symptom of Paget disease is pain in the affected bone, although its cause is not clear. It may be related to microfractures, stimulation of free nerve endings by dilated blood vessels adjacent to the bones, or weight bearing in weaker bones. The diagnosis is primarily made by imaging studies and bone biopsy is seldom necessary.

SKULL: Involvement of the skull is particularly common. It exhibits localized lysis, called **osteoporosis circumscripta**, generally in the frontal and parietal bones. Alternatively, there may be thickening of the outer and inner tables, which is most pronounced in the frontal and occipital bones. Hearing loss follows involvement of the middle ear ossicles and bony impingement on the 8th cranial nerve at the foramen. **Platybasia** (flattening of the base of the skull) may impinge on the foramen magnum, compressing the medulla and upper spinal cord.

The jaws may become grossly misshapen and teeth may fall out. Often, facial bones increase in size, especially the maxillary bones, producing the so-called **leontiasis ossea** (lion-like face).

PAGETIC STEAL: Occasionally, patients feel light-headed, due to so-called pagetic steal. In this situation, blood from the internal carotid system is shunted to the bones rather than being directed to the brain.

FRACTURES AND ARTHRITIS: Fractures are common in Paget disease, the bones snapping transversely like a piece of chalk. Incomplete fractures without displacement are called **infractions**. Involvement of the pelvis engenders hip problems. Bone deformity, joint incongruity and loss of subchondral bone compliance causes secondary osteoarthritis.

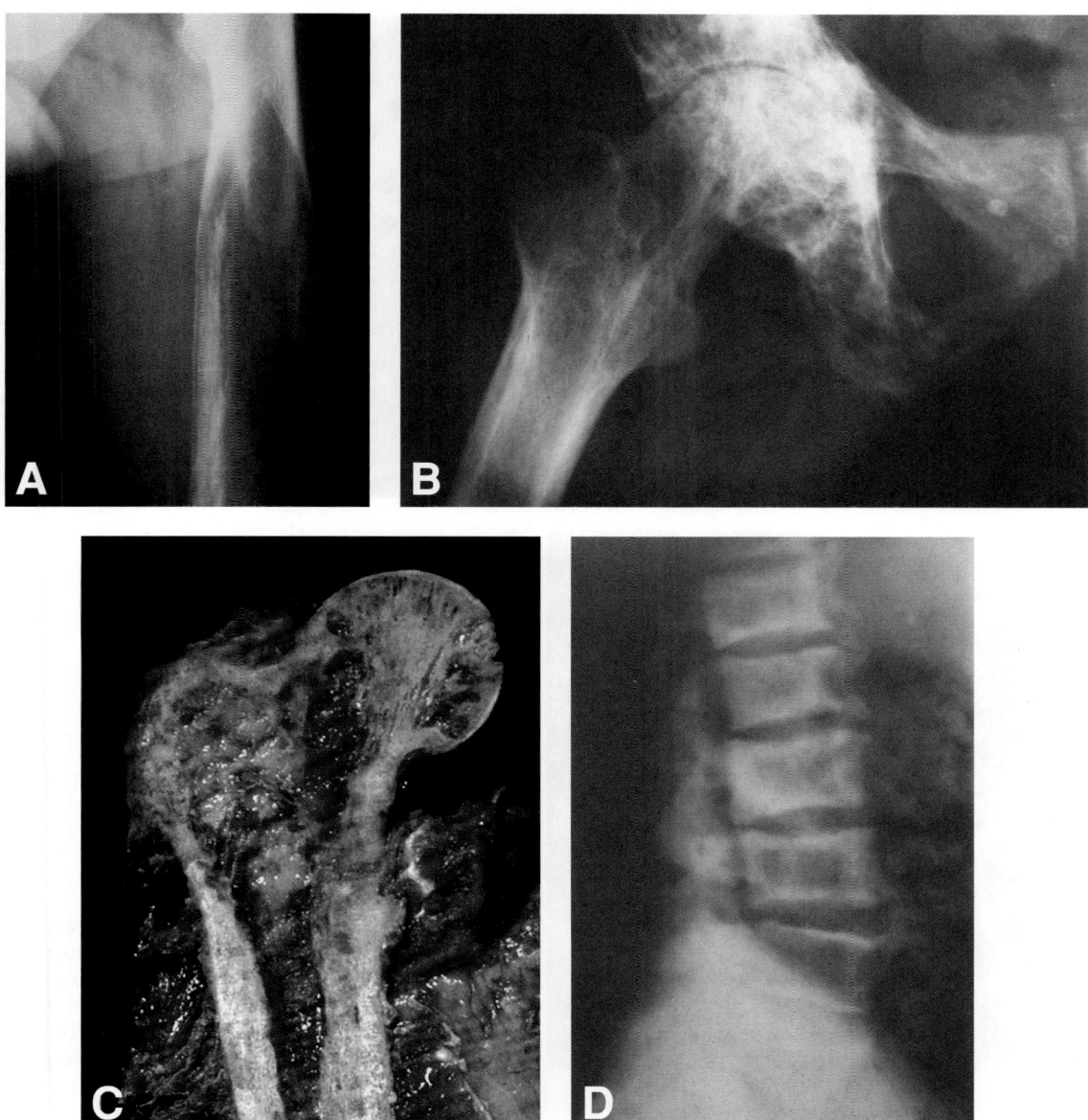

FIGURE 30-32. Paget disease. A. A radiograph of early Paget disease shows cortical dissolution, increased diameter of the diaphysis and an advancing wedge-shaped area of cortical resorption ("flame sign"). Proximal to the edge of this wedge, the femur appears entirely normal. **B.** Later, Paget disease of the proximal femur and pelvis shows cortical disorganization and irregular coarse trabeculations. **C.** Gross specimen of proximal femur showing cortical thickening and coarse trabeculations of the femoral head and neck. **D.** Paget disease of the spine shows shortening and widening of lumbar vertebral bodies. Their cortices and endplates are thickened and have a "picture frame" appearance.

HIGH-OUTPUT CARDIAC FAILURE: With extensive Paget disease, blood flow to the bones and subcutaneous tissue increases remarkably, requiring increased cardiac output. In the presence of underlying myocardial disease, it may be severe enough to result in heart failure.

SARCOMATOUS CHANGE: Neoplastic transformation may occur in Paget disease, usually in the femur, humerus, or pelvis. This complication occurs in less than 1% of all cases and usually arises in patients with severe polyostotic disease. Nevertheless, the incidence of bone sarcoma is 1,000 times higher than that in the general population. Interestingly, the skull and vertebrae, the bones most commonly involved by Paget disease, rarely undergo sarcomatous change. The tumors are usually osteosarcoma but may be fibrosarcoma or chondrosarcoma. They all carry a poor prognosis.

Serum calcium and phosphorus levels in Paget disease are normal, even though bone turnover increases by more than 20-fold. Hypercalcemia is rare, but does occur if a patient is immobilized. The collagen structure of bone in Paget disease is entirely normal, but because of the accelerated bone turnover, levels of collagen breakdown

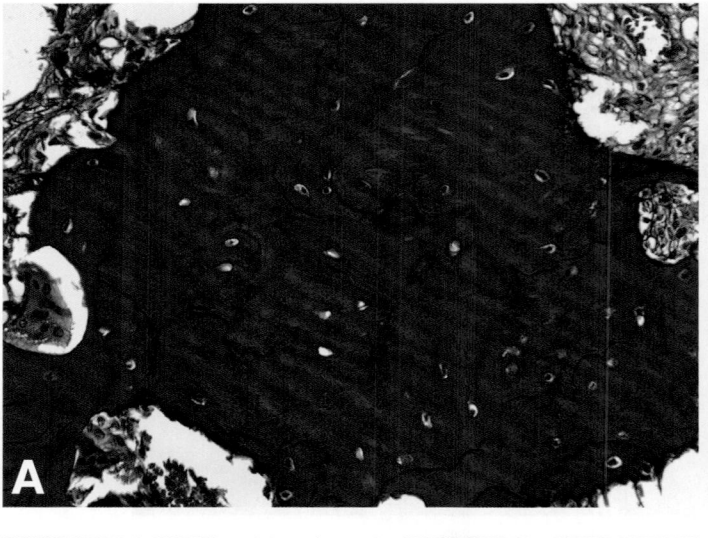

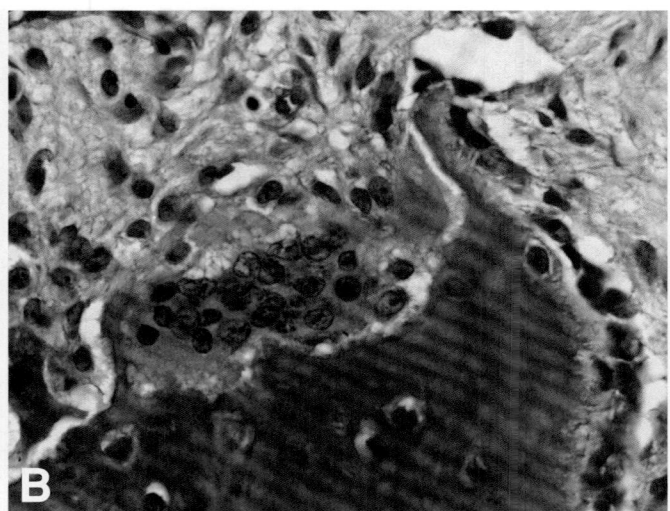

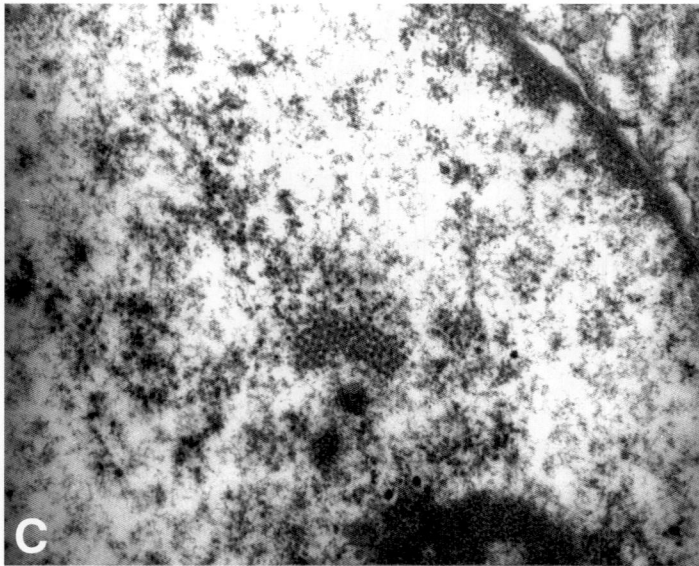

FIGURE 30-33. Paget disease. A. A section of bone shows prominent and irregular basophilic cement lines and numerous lining osteoclasts and osteoblasts. **B.** An osteoclast in pagetic bone contains many more nuclei than a usual osteoclast. A few of the nuclei contain intranuclear inclusion-like particles. **C.** Electron microscopy of osteoclast nuclei reveals particles that resemble paramyxovirus in shape and orientation.

products (hydroxyproline and hydroxylysine) increase in the serum and urine. Hydroxyproline excretion may reach 1,000 mg/day (normal, <40 mg). Serum alkaline phosphatase activity is the most useful laboratory test in monitoring disease activity. Alkaline phosphatase activity is disproportionately high with skull involvement but tends to be lower when only the pelvis is affected. A sudden increase in serum alkaline phosphatase level may reflect sarcomatous change within a lesion.

Fortunately, most patients with Paget disease are asymptomatic and require no treatment. Fractures, osteoarthritis, and other orthopedic complications are treated symptomatically. Drugs that mitigate abnormal osteoclast hyperfunction, including calcitonin and bisphosphonates, are useful.

GIANT CELL TUMOR IN PAGET DISEASE: Giant cell tumors may arise in Paget disease. They are not true neoplasms but rather arise as a result of a reactive phenomenon similar to the "brown tumor" of hyperparathyroidism. Giant cell tumors reflect an overshoot

of osteoclastic activity with an associated fibroblastic response.

GAUCHER DISEASE

This autosomal recessive hereditary storage disease is discussed in Chapter 6. It is caused by mutations in *GBA* which encodes an enzyme, β-glucocerebrosidase, that breaks down glucocerebrosides into glucose and ceramide. Loss of function in *GBA* leads to accumulation of glucocerebrosides in multiple sites including the marrow cavities which produce skeletal manifestations. These include:

- **Failure of remodeling:** This is the most common and least problematic skeletal abnormality. Flaring from epiphysis to diaphysis is abnormal, giving rise to an Erlenmeyer flask shape of the distal femur and proximal tibia.
- **Bone crisis:** This rare but very painful event results from acute infarction of a large segment of one or more bones, often after an acute viral illness. There is insufficient bone

blood flow owing to marrow infiltration by Gaucher cells. These cells, of monocyte-macrophage origin, accumulate large amounts of intracellular glucocerebrosides. Bone crisis lasts about 2 weeks and then gradually improves.

- **Localized and diffuse bone loss:** Radiolucent lesions with overlying cortical thinning are usually asymptomatic unless a fracture occurs at the site. These lesions are packed with Gaucher cells.
- **Osteosclerotic lesions:** These reflect increased bone formation, usually in the medullary cavity of the long bones and pelvis. Reactive new bone formation following osteonecrosis may be involved.
- **Corticomedullary osteonecrosis:** This disabling complication of Gaucher disease is most common in patients between 8 and 35 years old. It mostly involves the femoral head or proximal humerus. Extensive marrow infiltration by Gaucher cells restricts blood flow to the bone.
- **Pathologic fractures:** Vertebrae, long bones, and even the pelvis may show spontaneous fractures, owing to bone necrosis or osteopenia.
- **Osteomyelitis and septic arthritis:** Commonly caused by coliform or anaerobic organisms, spread via bloodstream to the bones and joints of Gaucher patients is common, especially after surgery.

LANGERHANS CELL HISTIOCYTOSIS

Langerhans cell histiocytosis (LCH) is a generic term (previously referred to as **histiocytosis X**) for three entities characterized by proliferation of Langerhans cells in various tissues: (1) **eosinophilic granuloma**, a localized form; (2) **Hand–Schüller–Christian disease**, a disseminated variant; and (3) **Letterer–Siwe disease**, a fulminant and often fatal generalized disease (see Chapter 26).

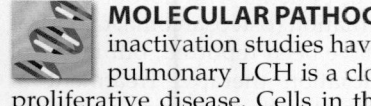 **MOLECULAR PATHOGENESIS:** X-chromosome inactivation studies have demonstrated that nonpulmonary LCH is a clonal and likely neoplastic proliferative disease. Cells in the lesion are diploid and show no consistent cytogenetic abnormalities. *BRAF V600E* somatic mutations are found in about 60% of LCH cases.

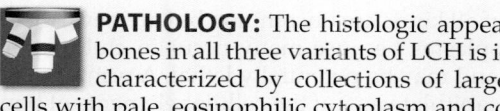 **PATHOLOGY:** The histologic appearance of the bones in all three variants of LCH is identical. It is characterized by collections of large, histiocytic cells with pale, eosinophilic cytoplasm and convoluted or grooved nuclei (see Fig. 18-68B). By immunohistochemistry, the histiocytic cells stain with CD1a, Langerin, and S-100 protein. On electron microscopy these cells have the typical racquet-shaped, tubular structures, "Birbeck granules," which occur in normal Langerhans cells of the skin. There are many eosinophils throughout these lesions, occasionally forming collections called "eosinophilic abscesses." Multinucleated osteoclast-like giant cells are often observed, as are chronic inflammatory cells and neutrophils. The lesions of LCH may occur anywhere in the body, including bones, skin, brain, lungs, lymph nodes, liver, and spleen. Radiographic findings in the bones in all three diseases are identical. Lesions may occur in the

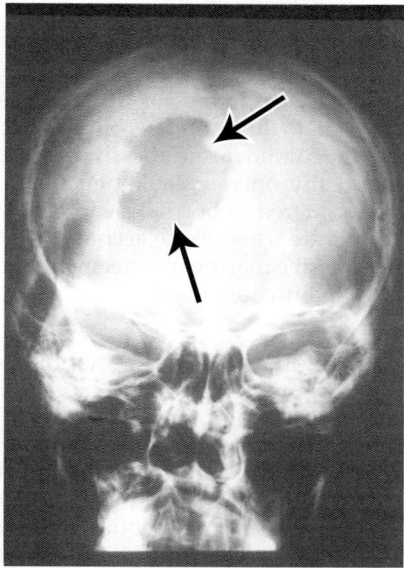

FIGURE 30-34. Eosinophilic granuloma. This radiograph of the skull shows a large, lytic lesion (*arrows*).

metaphysis or diaphysis of long bones, or in a flat bone, especially in the skull (Fig. 30-34). They are punched-out lytic defects, with virtually no reactive bone. Such lesions may precipitate fractures and periosteal callus formation.

Eosinophilic Granuloma Is a Self-Limited Disease

Eosinophilic granuloma, in either its solitary or multiple varieties, accounts for 70% of all cases of LCH. It is usually seen in the first two decades of life but occasionally occurs in older individuals. Typically, one or two lytic areas occur in bones of the axial or appendicular skeleton (Fig. 30-34) or the vertebrae. These lesions may cause mild pain or may be incidental findings on routine chest radiographs. Foci of disease in the lower thoracic or upper lumbar vertebrae may lead to collapse and pathologic fractures. Eventual recovery is the rule.

Hand–Schüller–Christian Disease Is a Multiorgan Disease of Childhood

Hand–Schüller–Christian disease occurs in children 2 to 5 years old and represents some 20% of all cases of LCH. The lesions are more widespread than in eosinophilic granuloma. Radiolucent bony lesions characterize the disorder, occurring most frequently in the calvaria, ribs, pelvis, and scapulae. Infiltration of the retro-orbital space causes exophthalmos; infiltration of the hypothalamic stalk brings about diabetes insipidus. One-fifth of patients have lymphadenopathy and lung infiltrates. Crusty, red, weepy skin lesions occur at the hairline and on the extensor surfaces of the extremities, the abdomen, and occasionally the soles of the feet. Deafness results from involvement of the external auditory canal and mastoid air cells. One-third of affected patients have disease in the liver and spleen, and 40% have bone lesions, half of which involve the skull. Thus, the classic triad of Hand–Schüller–Christian disease, namely: **(1) radiolucent lesions of the skull; (2) diabetes insipidus; and (3) exophthalmos**, occurs in only one-third of patients.

Letterer–Siwe Disease Is an Aggressive, Potentially Fatal Disease of Infants

Letterer–Siwe disease accounts for 10% of cases of LCH. Affected children fail to thrive and become cachectic. Multiple organ involvement culminates in massive hepatosplenomegaly, lymphadenopathy, anemia, leukopenia, and thrombocytopenia. Widely scattered, seborrheic skin lesions, which are often hemorrhagic, are usual. Bone lesions are not prominent initially, but progressive marrow replacement and pulmonary infiltration occasionally cause death.

CLINICAL FEATURES: Eosinophilic granuloma is a self-limited disease, and most lesions disappear if left alone. A bone lesion may have to be curetted and packed with bone chips. Sometimes biopsy itself can stimulate repair of the lytic lesion. A collapsed vertebra may actually reconstitute itself over time. Hand–Schüller–Christian disease may require radiation therapy for some bone and retro-orbital lesions. Diabetes insipidus seems to be irreversible, even after irradiation of the pituitary region. Corticosteroids, cyclophosphamide, and tumoricidal agents may also be used to treat Hand–Schüller–Christian disease. Aggressive chemotherapy for Letterer–Siwe disease seems to improve the prognosis.

FIBROUS DYSPLASIA

Fibrous dysplasia was historically viewed as a developmental abnormality characterized by a disorganized mixture of fibrous and osseous elements in the medullary region of affected bones. It is now known to be secondary to specific gene mutations. It occurs in children and young adults and may affect one (monostotic) or multiple bones (polyostotic) or other systems (McCune–Albright syndrome).

MOLECULAR PATHOGENESIS: Activating mutations in *GNAS1*, the gene encoding the α subunit of the stimulatory G protein (G$_s$), have been described in bone cells from patients with fibrous dysplasia and McCune–Albright syndrome. The result is constitutive activation of adenylyl cyclase and increased levels of the second messenger cyclic adenosine 3′,5′-monophosphate (cAMP). This enhances signaling via multiple downstream targets including c-*fos* and c-*jun* proto-oncogenes, IL-6, and IL-11.

CLINICAL FEATURES: *MONOSTOTIC FIBROUS DYSPLASIA:* This is the most common form of the disease, and is most often seen in the second and third decades, with no sex predilection. It typically involves the proximal femur, tibia, ribs, and facial bones, although any bone may be affected. It may be asymptomatic or lead to a pathologic fracture.

POLYOSTOTIC FIBROUS DYSPLASIA: One-fourth of patients with fibrous dysplasia exhibit disease in multiple bones, including the facial bones. Symptoms usually arise in childhood, and almost all patients have pathologic fractures, limb deformities, or limb-length discrepancies. Polyostotic fibrous dysplasia is more common in females.

Sometimes the disease becomes quiescent at puberty, and pregnancy tends to stimulate the growth of lesions.

MCCUNE-ALBRIGHT SYNDROME: This condition is characterized by polyostotic fibrous dysplasia and endocrine dysfunction, including acromegaly, Cushing syndrome, hyperthyroidism, and vitamin D–resistant rickets. The most common endocrine abnormality is precocious puberty in girls (boys rarely have McCune–Albright syndrome). As a result, premature closure of the growth plates leads to abnormally short stature. The most common extraskeletal manifestations of McCune–Albright syndrome are characteristic skin lesions composed of pigmented macules ("café-au-lait" spots) with irregular ("coast of Maine") borders that do not cross the midline of the body and are usually located over the buttocks, back, and sacrum. These often overlie the skeletal lesions. Polyostotic fibrous dysplasia may also be associated with soft-tissue myxomas (**Mazabraud syndrome**).

The radiographic features of fibrous dysplasia are distinctive. Bone lesions have a lucent ground-glass appearance with well-marginated borders and a thin cortex. Affected bones may be ballooned, deformed, or enlarged, and involvement may be focal or encompass the entire bone (Fig. 30-35A).

PATHOLOGY: All forms of fibrous dysplasia have an identical histologic pattern (Fig. 30-35B,C). This includes benign fibroblastic tissue arranged in a loose, whorled pattern in which irregularly arranged, purposeless spicules of woven bone that lack osteoblastic rimming are embedded. In 10% of cases, irregular islands of hyaline cartilage are also present. Occasionally, cystic degeneration occurs, with hemosiderin-laden macrophages, hemorrhage, and osteoclasts congregated about the cyst. Rare cases (<1% of patients with fibrous dysplasia) of malignant transformation (osteosarcoma, chondrosarcoma, fibrosarcoma) have been reported, but many of these involved prior radiation therapy. Treatment of fibrous dysplasia consists of curettage, repair of fractures and prevention of deformities.

BENIGN TUMORS OF BONE

Bone tumors of all kinds are uncommon but are nevertheless important neoplasms because many occur in children and young adults and may be potentially lethal. A primary bone tumor may recapitulate any of the cellular elements of bone. Most neoplasms of bone occur near the metaphyseal area, and more than 80% of primary tumors are found in the distal femur or proximal tibia (Fig. 30-36). In a growing child, these areas show conspicuous growth activity.

Nonossifying Fibroma Is a Solitary Lesion of Childhood

Nonossifying fibroma, also called **fibrous cortical defect** or **metaphyseal fibrous defect**, is a benign tumor that occurs in the metaphysis of a long bone, most commonly the tibia or femur. It is very common and may occur in as many as 25% of all children between the ages of 4 and 10 years, after which it characteristically regresses. Nonossifying fibroma

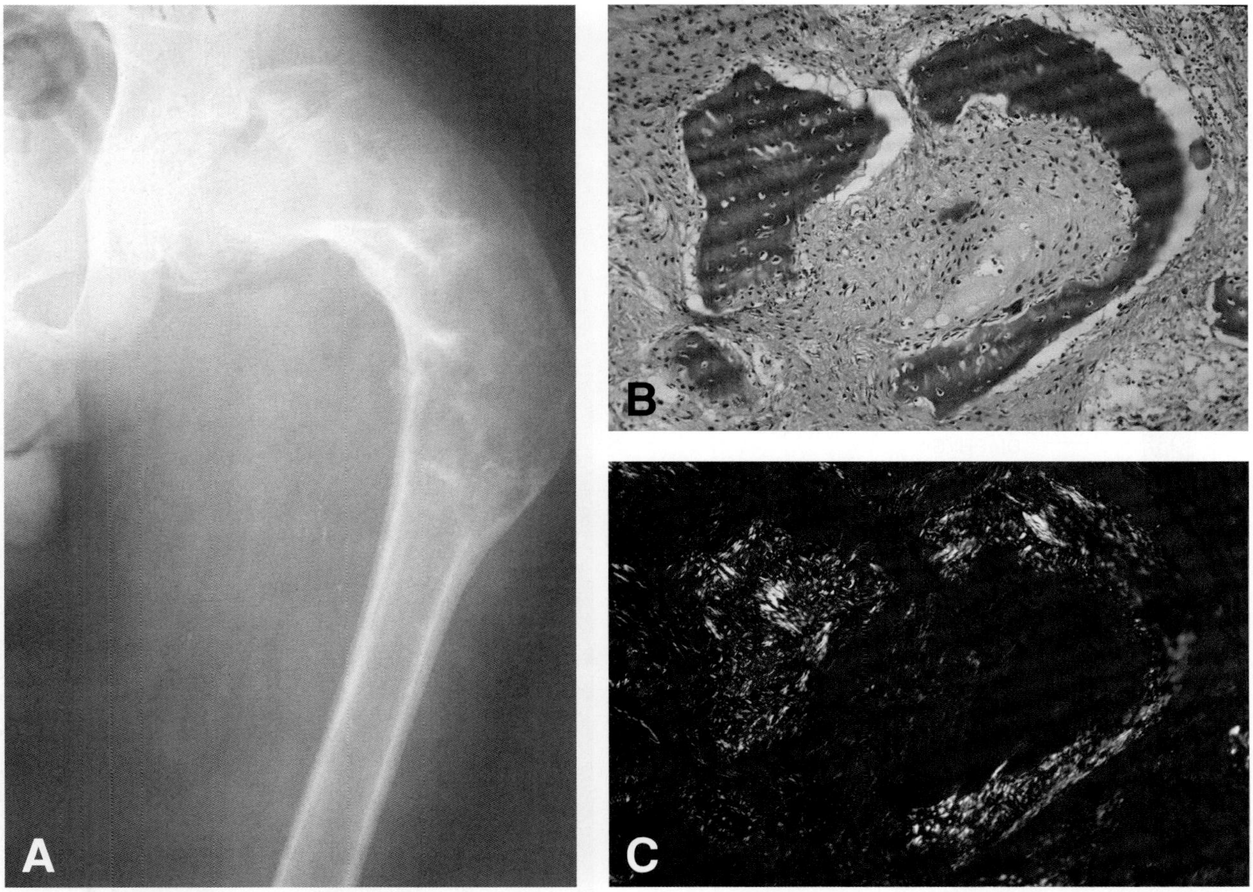

FIGURE 30-35. Fibrous dysplasia. A. A radiograph of the proximal femur shows the "shepherd's crook" deformity caused by fractures sustained over the years. Irregular, marginated, ground-glass lucencies are surrounded by reactive bone. The appearance of the shaft has been likened to a soap bubble. **B.** Histologically, fibrous dysplasia consists of moderately cellular fibrous tissue in which irregular, curved spicules of woven bone develop without discernible appositional osteoblast activity. **C.** The same section viewed in polarized light demonstrates not only that the spicules are woven but also that their fiber pattern extends imperceptibly into the fiber pattern of the surrounding stroma.

is considered to be a developmental lesion and not a neoplasm. Most cases are asymptomatic, although pain or fracture through the thin cortex overlying the lesion occasionally calls attention to the condition. Multiple nonossifying fibromas may be seen with neurofibromatosis type 1 and in the **Jaffe–Campanacci syndrome (associated with café au lait spots)**. Radiographically, nonossifying fibromas show a cortical, eccentric position, and well-demarcated, central lucent zones surrounded by scalloped, sclerotic margins (Fig. 30-37A).

PATHOLOGY: On gross examination, the lesion is granular and dark red to brown. Microscopically, it is composed of bland spindle cells arranged in an interlacing, whorled pattern, with scattered multinucleated giant cells and foamy macrophages (Fig. 30-37B).

CLINICAL FEATURES: Spontaneous regression is common. Radiographic follow-up is sufficient management in most cases. The rare, symptomatic or expanded lesions that are prone to fracture are treated with curettage and bone grafting.

Simple Bone Cyst Occurs in Children and Adolescents

Simple, unicameral, or solitary bone cysts are benign, fluid-filled, unilocular lesions. There is a male predilection (3:1), and 80% occur in the first two decades of life. More than two-thirds of all solitary bone cysts are located in the proximal humerus, proximal femur, or proximal tibia, usually in the metaphysis adjacent to the growth plate.

ETIOLOGIC FACTORS: Solitary bone cysts are not neoplasms but rather disturbances of bone growth with superimposed trauma. Secondary organization of a hematoma or some abnormality of the metaphyseal vessels causes accumulation of fluid. The "tumor" then grows by expansion of the fluid cavity. The resulting pressure causes bone resorption, mediated by neighboring osteoclasts. The process is slow, so that as the endosteal surface of the cortex is resorbed, a thin periosteal shell of new bone is laid down. This sequence results in a thin, well-marginated, radiolucent bone lesion (Fig. 30-38), which is never greater in diameter

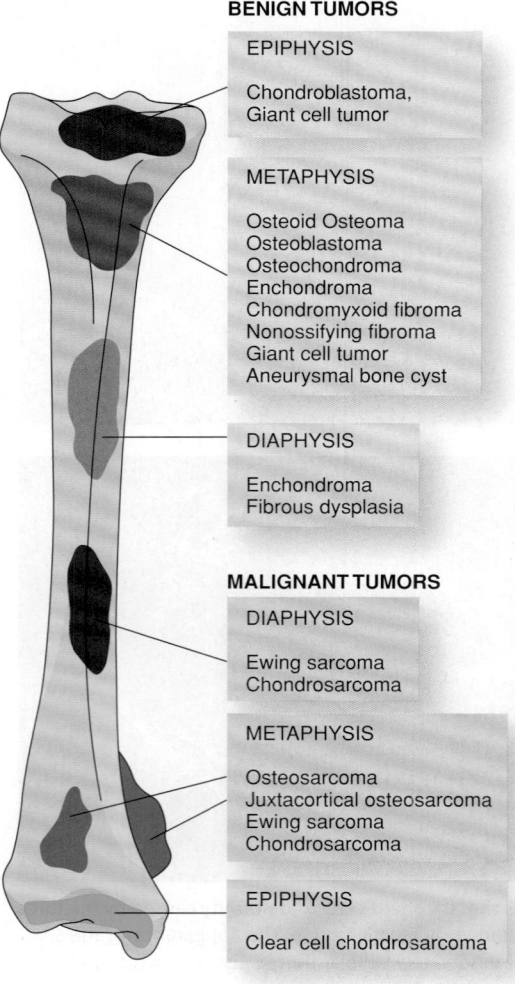

BENIGN TUMORS

EPIPHYSIS

Chondroblastoma,
Giant cell tumor

METAPHYSIS

Osteoid Osteoma
Osteoblastoma
Osteochondroma
Enchondroma
Chondromyxoid fibroma
Nonossifying fibroma
Giant cell tumor
Aneurysmal bone cyst

DIAPHYSIS

Enchondroma
Fibrous dysplasia

MALIGNANT TUMORS

DIAPHYSIS

Ewing sarcoma
Chondrosarcoma

METAPHYSIS

Osteosarcoma
Juxtacortical osteosarcoma
Ewing sarcoma
Chondrosarcoma

EPIPHYSIS

Clear cell chondrosarcoma

FIGURE 30-36. Location of primary bone tumors in long tubular bones.

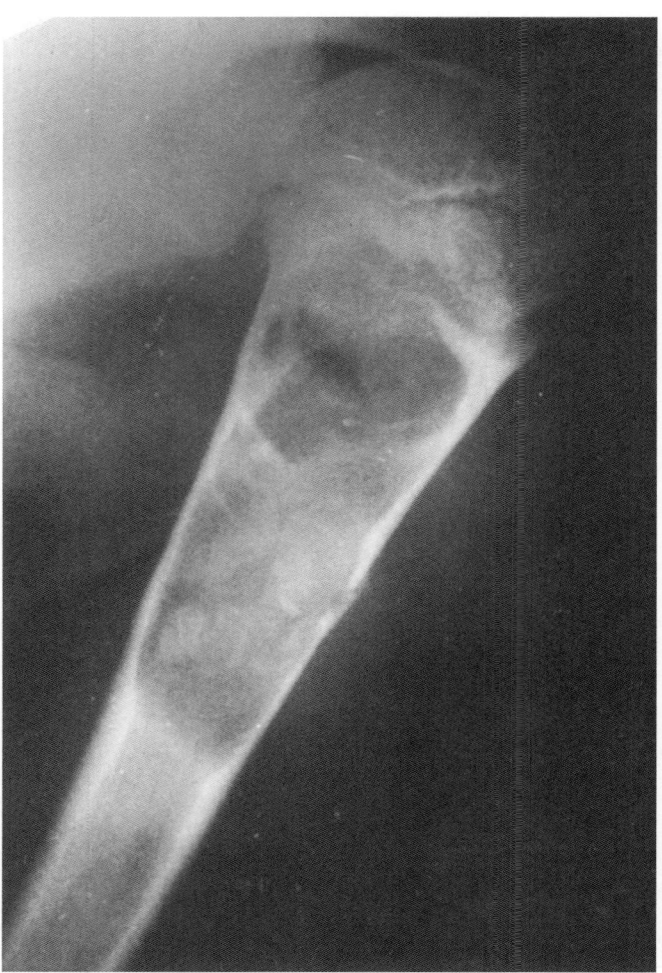

FIGURE 30-38. Solitary bone cyst. A radiograph of the proximal humerus of a child (note the epiphyseal plate) shows a large, well-demarcated, lytic epiphyseal and diaphyseal lesion. The cortex is thinned, but there is no cortical distortion or malformation of the shape of the bone.

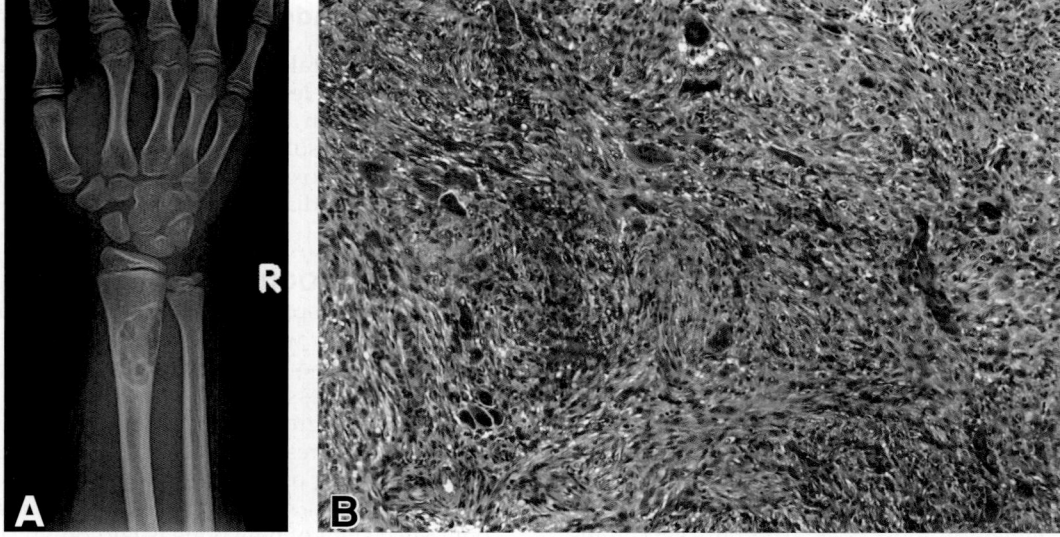

FIGURE 30-37. Nonossifying fibroma. A. A radiograph of the distal radius of a child shows an eccentric, metaphyseal lytic lesion with scalloped and sclerotic margins. **B.** Microscopically, the lesion is composed of bland spindle cells arranged in interlacing fascicles, with scattered, multinucleated, osteoclast-type giant cells.

than the growth plate and is particularly susceptible to pathologic fracture.

PATHOLOGY: Solitary bone cyst is not a true cyst because it lacks a distinct cell lining. Rather, it is lined by fibrous tissue, a few osteoclastic giant cells, hemosiderin-laden macrophages, chronic inflammatory cells and reactive bone. Osteoclasts are present in the advancing front of the cyst and allow expansion of the lesion. The cyst wall may contain characteristic masses of amorphous, calcified, fibrinous material resembling cementum.

CLINICAL FEATURES: Most simple bone cysts are entirely asymptomatic until a pathologic fracture calls attention to them. Once the diagnosis is confirmed by imaging studies and by finding clear fluid by needle aspiration, intralesional corticosteroids may be given. Currently, curettage and bone grafting are the preferred treatment.

Aneurysmal Bone Cyst May Be Primary or Secondary

Aneurysmal bone cysts (ABCs) are uncommon, benign, expansive, and often destructive lesions arising within a bone or on its surface. They usually occur in children and young adults, with a peak incidence in the second decade. Although the lesion has been observed at every skeletal site, it is most frequent in the metaphysis of long bones and in the vertebral column. Solid and extraskeletal variants have been described. Radiographically, ABC presents as a lytic, expansile mass with well-defined margins. Magnetic resonance imaging shows a multiloculated lesion with internal septation and fluid-fluid levels which develop as blood cells separate from plasma (Fig. 30-39A).

MOLECULAR PATHOGENESIS: The pathogenesis of ABC is controversial. Some cases represent cystic and hemorrhagic transformation of an underlying lesion, most commonly chondroblastoma, osteoblastoma, fibrous dysplasia, giant cell tumor, and osteosarcoma ("secondary ABC"). Other cases have no

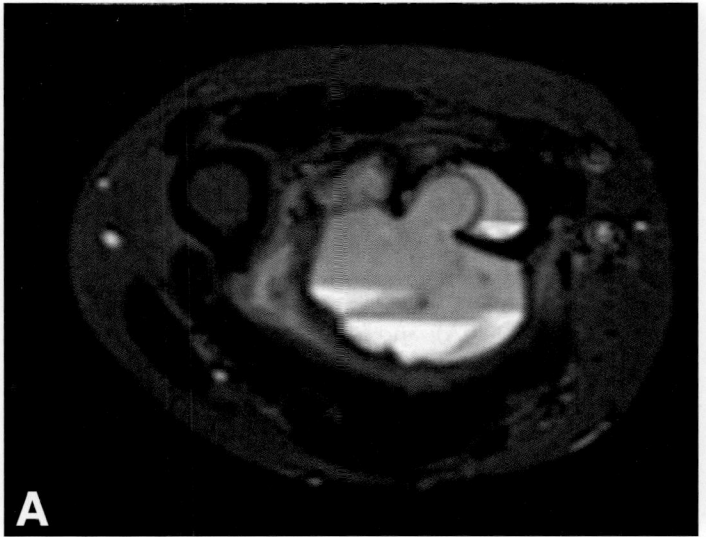
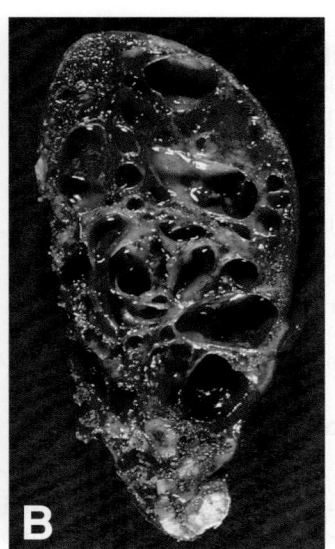

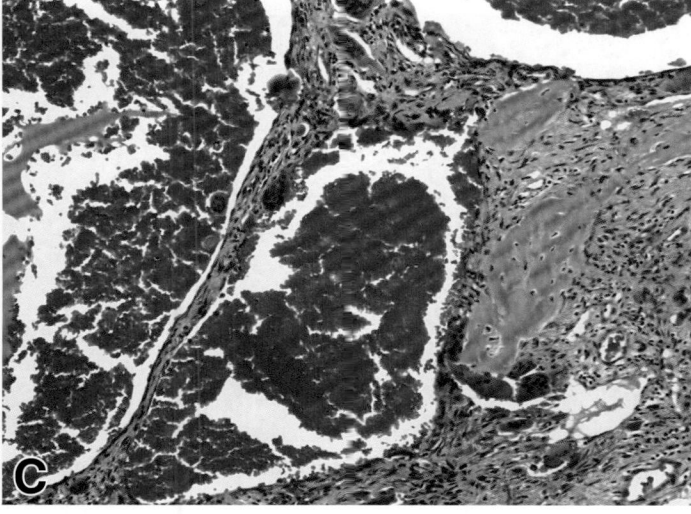

FIGURE 30-39. Aneurysmal bone cyst. A. A magnetic resonance image shows fluid–fluid levels that develop when blood cells separate from plasma. **B.** In cross-section, the lesion consists of a spongy mass containing multiple blood-filled cysts. Some septa between the cysts contain bony tissue. **C.** Microscopically, the blood-filled spaces are separated by cellular fibrous septa with scattered osteoclast-type giant cells and reactive bone. (39B from Bullough PG. *Atlas of Orthopaedic Pathology.* 2nd ed. New York: Gower Medical Publishing, 1992. Copyright Lippincott Williams & Wilkins.)

detectable associated lesion ("primary ABC"). Primary ABC is now considered a true neoplasm, since it is frequently associated with a recurring chromosomal translocation t(16;17)(q22;p13). This anomaly fuses the promoter region of the osteoblast cadherin 11 gene (*CDH11*) on chromosome 16q22 to the coding sequence of the ubiquitin protease gene (*USP6*) on chromosome 17p13. Other fusion genes have been described (involving *TRAP150*, *ZNF9*, *OMD* and *COL1A1*). *USP6* is thought to play a role in regulating actin remodeling. However, the mechanism of neoplastic transformation mediated by upregulation of *USP6* has not been elucidated. *USP6* gene rearrangements are not found in secondary ABC.

PATHOLOGY: The periosteum around an aneurysmal bone cyst is ballooned but intact. The cut surface of the multiloculated cyst resembles a sponge permeated with blood and blood clots (Fig. 30-39B). Microscopically, it is composed of blood-filled cystic spaces separated by fibrous septa. The walls and septa are composed of moderately cellular fibrous tissue with bland spindle cells, multinucleated osteoclast-like giant cells and reactive bone (Fig. 30-39C).

CLINICAL FEATURES: Some aneurysmal bone cysts tend to grow slowly, but most expand rapidly, and may attain a large size. They usually manifest with pain and swelling, sometimes in relation to trauma, and often develop in a short period of time. A bone cyst may "blow out," that is, rupture and produce local hemorrhage. Treatment is usually excision and curettage with bone grafting. Recurrence rate is variable (20% to 70%). Incising the cyst at surgery decreases its internal pressure which may cause brisk bleeding that is difficult to control. In sites such as the vertebral column or the pelvis, selective arterial embolization has been successful.

Osteoma Is a Benign Tumor Composed of Compact Cortical Bone

Osteomas are benign, slow-growing tumors composed of dense compact bone. These lesions can be divided into four major clinicopathologic subtypes: (1) calvarial and mandibular osteomas; (2) osteomas of the sinonasal and orbital bones; (3) bone islands occurring in medullary bone; and (4) surface osteomas of long bones. Some osteomas are likely hamartomas that arise during development. However, sinonasal osteomas may be benign osteoblastic neoplasms. Interestingly, multiple osteomas are associated with familial adenomatous polyposis in Gardner syndrome (see Chapter 19) and may, therefore, be driven by altered Wnt/β-catenin signaling. Osteomas and bone islands are usually asymptomatic and seldom require surgical treatment.

Osteoid Osteoma Is a Benign, Painful Lesion

Osteoid osteomas are composed of immature osseous tissue (the nidus) surrounded by a halo of dense reactive bone. The typical patient is between 5 and 25 years old. Males are affected more often than females (3:1). The lesion frequently arises in the diaphyseal cortex of the tubular bones of the leg but may occur elsewhere. Osteoid osteomas have limited growth potential and do not metastasize. Radiographically, they are small, well-demarcated sclerotic lesions with a radiolucent halo surrounded by dense sclerosis and periosteal reaction.

MOLECULAR PATHOGENESIS: Chromosomal analysis of a few osteoid osteomas has disclosed structural abnormalities of chromosome 22q13 and loss of part of 17q, which suggests that the lesions are neoplasms.

PATHOLOGY: Osteoid osteomas are spherical, hyperemic tumors, about 1 cm in diameter, that are considerably softer than the surrounding bone (Fig. 30-40A) and easily enucleated at surgery. Microscopically, the center of the tumor (nidus) is composed of thin, irregular trabeculae of woven bone within a cellular and vascular fibrous stroma containing many osteoblasts and osteoclasts (Fig. 30-40B). The trabeculae are more mature in the center, which is often partially calcified. Reactive sclerotic bone surrounds the nidus.

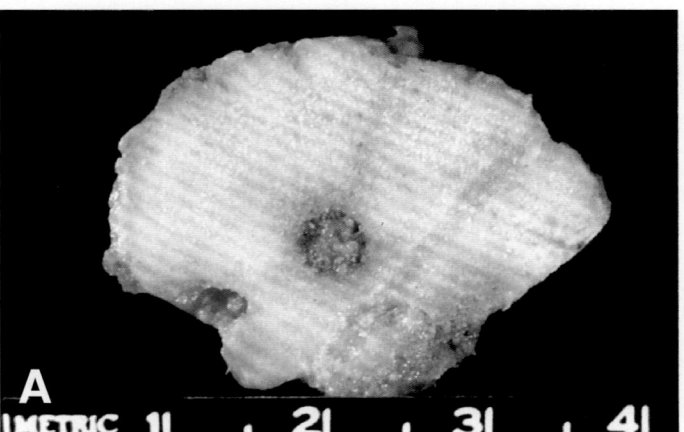
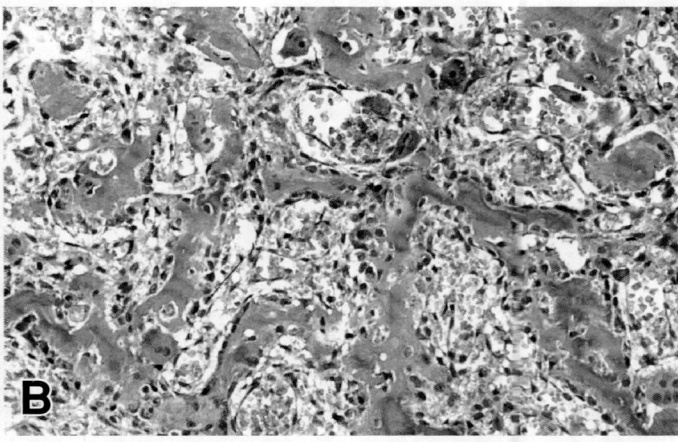

FIGURE 30-40. Osteoid osteoma. A. A gross specimen of an osteoid osteoma shows the central nidus embedded in dense bone. **B.** A photomicrograph of the nidus reveals irregular trabeculae of woven bone surrounded by osteoblasts, osteoclasts and fibrovascular marrow.

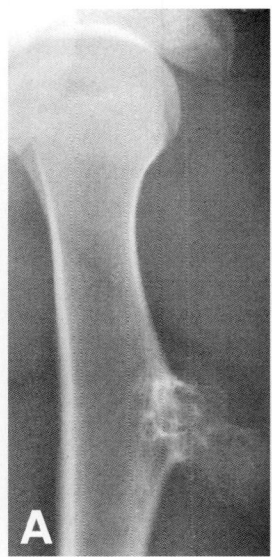
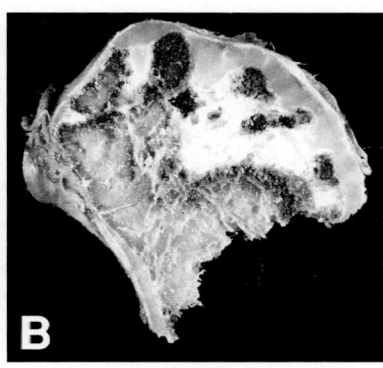
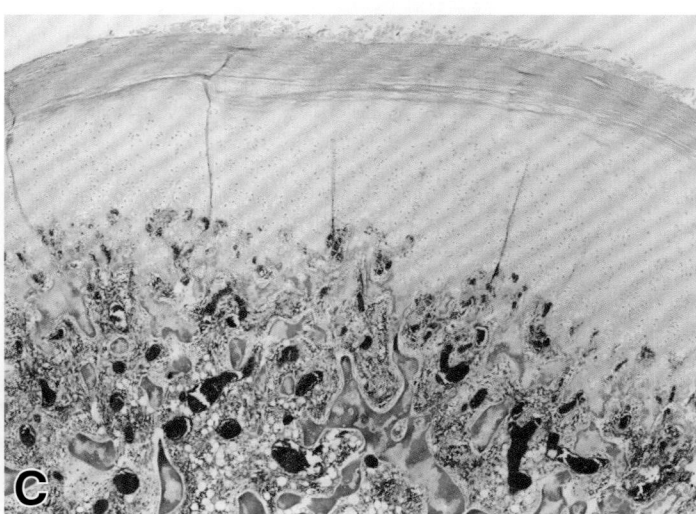

FIGURE 30-41. Osteochondroma. A. A radiograph of an osteochondroma of the humerus shows a lesion directly contiguous with the marrow space. **B.** Cross-section of an osteochondroma shows a cap of calcified cartilage overlying poorly organized cancellous bone. **C.** Microscopically, the cartilaginous cap is covered by a fibrous membrane (perichondrium). It also shows endochondral ossification.

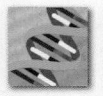 **CLINICAL FEATURES:** Pain is typically nocturnal and out of proportion to the size of the lesion. Interestingly, the pain is often exacerbated by drinking alcohol and promptly relieved by aspirin or other anti-inflammatory drugs, possibly because of the high prostaglandin content and abundant nerve fibers within the tumor. Complete surgical excision or radiofrequency ablation are effective treatment modalities. Recurrence is exceedingly rare.

Osteoblastoma Is Larger Than Osteoid Osteoma but Less Painful

Osteoblastoma is an uncommon, benign neoplasm that is histologically similar to osteoid osteoma but larger (usually >2 cm) and with a tendency to progressive growth. It is not accompanied by the characteristic nocturnal pain of osteoid osteoma, although dull pain sometimes occurs. It stimulates less bone reaction and appears mostly as a purely radiolucent lesion, with only a thin shell of surrounding bone. Osteoblastoma occurs between the ages of 10 and 35 years, is more common in males, and mainly affects the spine and long bones. The histologic features of osteoblastoma are similar to those of osteoid osteoma. Secondary ABCs may be seen. Curettage may be adequate treatment for small osteoblastomas, but larger lesions require wide resection. Recurrences are uncommon and prognosis is excellent.

 MOLECULAR PATHOGENESIS: Several chromosomal and molecular abnormalities have been described in osteoblastoma, but no consistent abnormality has emerged. Aneuploid to hyperdiploid karyotypes have been demonstrated.

Osteochondroma

Osteochondroma is a benign tumor consisting of a bony projection with a cartilaginous cap arising on the surface of the bone. It occurs in the metaphysis of bones formed by endochondral ossification (especially the long bones of the extremities) and was viewed for many years as a developmental defect of the growth plate. Most are solitary but 15% are multiple and hereditary. Recently described gene mutations in solitary and multiple osteochondromas favor a neoplastic nature. Solitary osteochondroma is one of the most common benign bone tumors and is more frequent in young males. Most osteochondromas are asymptomatic, but some may require surgical excision if cosmetically displeasing or if they compress an artery or nerve. Recurrence is very rare. Osteochondromas stop growing when the growth plates close at the end of puberty. They tend to grow away from the nearest joint. In radiographs, the cortex and medullary cavity of an osteochondroma is in continuity with the parent bone (Fig. 30-41A).

 MOLECULAR PATHOGENESIS: Cytogenetic aberrations in sporadic and hereditary osteochondromas occur on chromosomes 8q24.1, 11p11–12, and 19p, where the tumor suppressor genes *EXT1*, *EXT2*, and *EXT3* are located, respectively. The *EXT* genes may control chondrocyte proliferation and differentiation by regulating the Indian hedgehog–PTH-related protein (Ihh–PTHrP) pathway, which is vital for proper development of endochondral bones. *EXT* mutations increase chondrocyte proliferation in the cartilage cap and disrupt the differentiation process, which may alter the direction of chondrocyte growth and promote development of osteochondromas.

PATHOLOGY: On gross examination, osteochondromas have a cartilage cap with underlying cortical and cancellous bone (Fig. 30-41B). The marrow cavity of the lesion is in continuity with that of the bone in which it arose. The bony mass is surrounded by a surface fibrous membrane, which is perichondrium

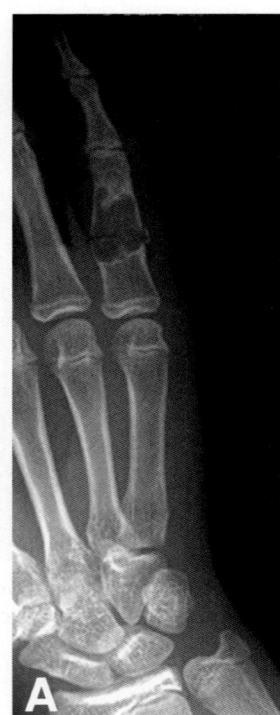

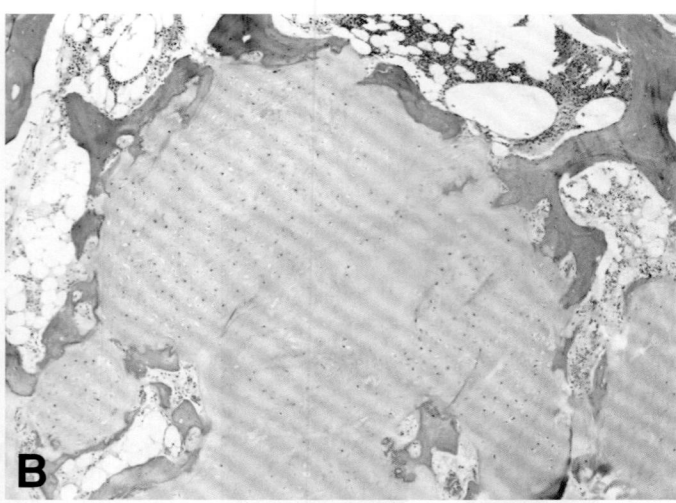

FIGURE 30-42. Enchondroma. A. A radiograph of an enchondroma shows a well-demarcated, lytic lesion in the diaphysis of a proximal phalanx with internal calcification and associated pathologic fracture. **B.** Histologically, the tumor is composed of lobules of hypocellular hyaline cartilage without atypia.

overlying the cartilage and periosteum overlying the bone. Histologically, the cap is composed of benign hyaline cartilage with active endochondral ossification, which is morphologically similar to that seen in the epiphyseal growth plate (Fig. 30-41C). The bony stalk is composed of cortical lamellar bone, and the medullary cavity contains lamellar bone trabeculae with fatty and/or hematopoietic marrow.

HEREDITARY MULTIPLE OSTEOCHONDROMA-TOSIS: This inherited autosomal dominant disorder is characterized by multiple osteochondromas and associated skeletal deformities. Hereditary multiple osteochondromatosis (HMO) is one of the most common inherited musculoskeletal disorders and is caused by loss of *EXT1* or *EXT2* gene function (see Molecular Pathogenesis above). Although not as common as solitary osteochondroma, the heritable variety is not exceedingly rare, with an incidence of about 1 in 50,000. It occurs predominantly in males, but because of its variable penetrance, a seemingly unaffected female from an afflicted family may transmit the disorder to her offspring.

PATHOLOGY: Individual lesions in HMO are identical to a solitary osteochondroma. In severe cases, dwarfism may result because of lateral displacement of longitudinal growth plates by osteochondromas. Metacarpals may be shortened, and fixed pronation or supination may develop if the lesions occur in the forearm and interfere with wrist function. Further difficulties may be caused by unequal leg length and disturbed joint function because of encroaching osteochondromas. Secondary peripheral chondrosarcoma is a rare complication.

Solitary Chondroma Is a Benign Tumor of Mature Hyaline Cartilage

These benign cartilage tumors are called **enchondromas** when intramedullary and **periosteal chondromas** when they arise on the bone surface. They may occur at any age and many cases are asymptomatic and discovered incidentally. Most occur in the metacarpals and phalanges of the hands, and the remainder can arise in almost any other tubular bone. The tumor is usually small and grows slowly. Radiographically, it appears as an well-delimited, intramedullary, radiolucent area, sometimes containing stippled or ring-like calcifications (Fig. 30-42A).

PATHOLOGY: On gross examination, solitary enchondromas have the semitranslucent appearance of hyaline cartilage, often with a few calcified areas. Microscopically, the cartilaginous tissue is well differentiated with sparse uniform chondrocytes, extensive cartilaginous matrix, and a lobular configuration with lamellar bone at the periphery of the lobules (Fig. 30-42B). Asymptomatic enchondromas are best left untreated and followed radiographically. When pain or pathologic fracture occurs, curettage and bone grafting are the treatment of choice. Recurrences are uncommon.

Enchondromatosis Is Marked by Multiple Cartilaginous Tumors

Enchondromatosis *or* **Ollier disease** *is characterized by development of multiple cartilaginous masses that lead to bony deformities.* The condition is not hereditary and usually manifests in early childhood. It commonly affects the long and short bones of the appendicular skeleton with the development of multiple intramedullary enchondromas (Fig. 30-43).

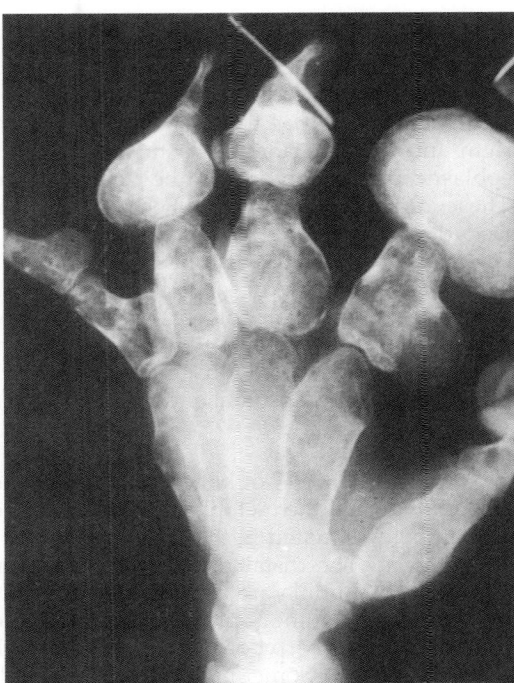

FIGURE 30-43. Multiple enchondromatosis (Ollier disease). A radiograph of the hand shows bulbous swellings formed by nodular masses composed of hyaline cartilage, which may be admixed with more primitive myxoid cartilage.

These tumors tend to be metaphyseal and result in deformity, limb asymmetry, and occasional pathologic fractures.

There is a strong tendency for malignant transformation, mostly into chondrosarcoma. Therefore, a patient with enchondromatosis who has increasing pain and/or an actively growing lesion should be evaluated to rule out an underlying sarcoma.

Solitary enchondroma and enchondromas of Ollier disease are histologically similar but the latter tend to be more cellular and atypical.

Maffucci syndrome is characterized by multiple enchondromas and cavernous or spindle-cell hemangiomas of soft tissue. It usually manifests in early childhood and may produce significant skeletal deformities. Chondrosarcomas develop in up to half of all patients with Maffucci syndrome. The incidence of extraskeletal malignant tumors of various types (i.e., carcinomas, gliomas, etc.) is also greatly increased in patients with Maffucci syndrome.

 MOLECULAR PATHOGENESIS: Approximately 50% of solitary enchondromas and 90% of enchondromas of Ollier disease and Maffucci syndrome have mutations in *IDH1* and *IDH2*, genes that encode isozymes of isocitrate dehydrogenase. *IDH1* mutations are the most common and are also frequently found in gliomas of the central nervous system and acute myeloid leukemia. The mutations lead to gain of function and increased production of the oncometabolite D-2-hydroxyglutarate as well as DNA hypermethylation and downregulation of several genes in enchondromas. In addition, less than 5% of patients with enchondromatosis have mutations in *PTHR1*, the gene encoding a receptor for PTH and PTHrP. These mutations result in substitutions in the receptor's extracellular domain that increase cAMP signaling. Mutant receptors may delay chondrocyte differentiation by activating Hedgehog signaling, and thereby promote formation of the multiple cartilaginous masses characteristic of the disease.

Chondroblastoma Is a Benign Tumor of the Epiphyses of Long Bones

Chondroblastomas are uncommon, chondrogenic tumors with predilection for the epiphyses of the proximal femur, tibia, and humerus. They are more common in males than in females (2:1), and 90% of cases occur in young patients between the ages of 5 and 25. They grow slowly; imaging studies show an eccentric, radiolucent lesion with sharply defined borders (Fig. 30-44A).

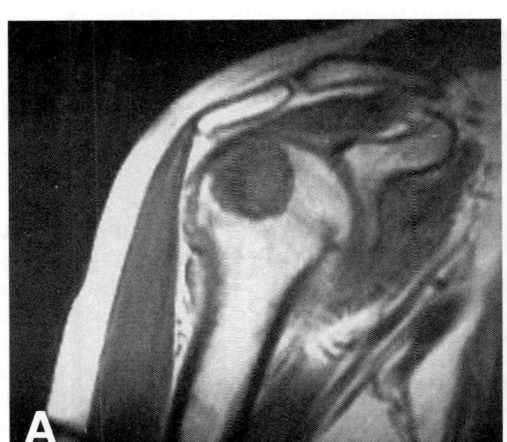
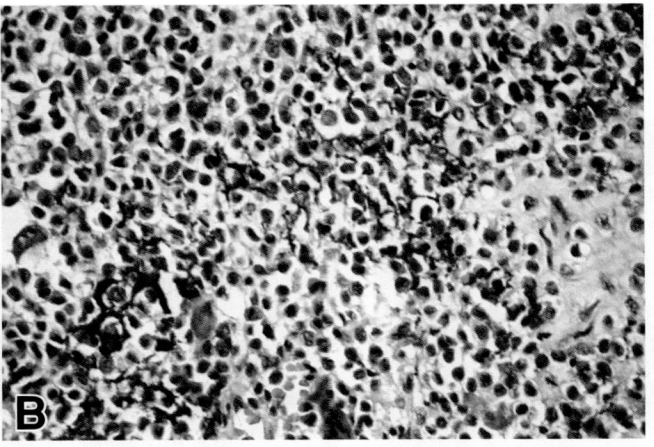

FIGURE 30-44. Chondroblastoma. A. A magnetic resonance image of the shoulder of a child shows a prominent lytic lesion of the head of the humerus that involves the epiphysis and extends across the epiphyseal plate. **B.** Histologically, chondroblastomas are characterized by plump, round cells (chondroblasts) surrounded by mineralized primitive chondroid matrix.

MOLECULAR PATHOGENESIS: Specific somatic driver mutations in *H3F3B* have been detected in 95% of chondroblastomas. *H3F3B* encodes H3.3, a member of the histone 3 family, which plays important roles in chromatin structure and epigenetic regulation. Affected individuals express an aberrant form of H3.3, but how this may promote tumor pathogenesis is unclear. Structural abnormalities involving chromosomes 5 and 8 have also been described.

PATHOLOGY: On gross examination, the tumor is soft and compact with scattered gray or hemorrhagic areas. Microscopically, it is composed of primitive chondroblasts arranged as sheets of round to polyhedral cells with well-defined cytoplasmic borders and large, ovoid nuclei, often with prominent nuclear grooves (Fig. 30-44B). Osteoclast-like giant cells are frequently present. The usually scanty cartilage matrix is variably calcified and appears primitive. This accounts for the mottled pattern often seen in CT scans. Well-developed hyaline cartilage as seen in enchondroma is not found in chondroblastoma. The tumor causes bone destruction by stimulating osteoclastic resorption and may perforate the cortex but tends to remain confined by the periosteum.

CLINICAL FEATURES: Because of its para-articular location, chondroblastoma tends to cause joint pain with mild swelling and functional limitation of joint movement. If neglected, it may (rarely) attain a large size, destroy the epiphyseal area and invade the joint. Curettage is the treatment of choice. Local recurrence occurs in over 10% of the cases.

Giant Cell Tumors of Bone Rarely Metastasize

Giant cell tumor (GCT) of bone is a benign, locally aggressive neoplasm characterized by the presence of osteoclast-like multinucleated giant cells, randomly and uniformly distributed in a background of proliferating mononuclear cells. It usually occurs in the third and fourth decades, has a slight predilection for women, and seems to be more common in Asia than in Western countries. Paget disease may produce a giant cell reactive lesion that closely resembles a true GCT.

MOLECULAR PATHOGENESIS: GCT is composed of numerous large reactive osteoclast-like giant cells and two lineages of mononuclear cells. One population is believed to be of macrophage-monocyte origin and is likely nonneoplastic. The other has a preosteoblastic phenotype and is the neoplastic cell of GCT. These tumor cells produce RANKL and induce osteoclast formation (hence the large number of giant cells). Driver mutations of the histone-related gene *H3F3A* have been detected in 92% of giant cell tumors of bone. The exact pathophysiologic role of these mutations is unknown. The majority of giant cell tumors show random or clonal chromosomal aberrations, most commonly telomeric associations (chromosomal end-to-end fusion).

In most cases (90%), GCT of bone originates at the junction of the epiphysis and the metaphysis of a long bone, with more than half being situated in the knee area (distal femur and proximal tibia). The distal radius, proximal humerus, sacrum, and proximal fibula are also occasionally involved. Radiographically, these tumors present as eccentric, expansile, lucent lesions with sharp borders that extend to the end of the bone (Fig. 30-45A). Sometimes, they have a multiloculated or "soap bubble" appearance, produced by endosteal resorption of the bone.

PATHOLOGY: On gross examination, GCT is clearly circumscribed and its cut surface is soft and light brown, without bone or calcification. The presence of numerous hemorrhagic areas creates the appearance of a sponge full of blood. Cystic cavities and necrotic areas are seen in some cases. GCT is often limited by the periosteum, although aggressive forms penetrate the cortex and the periosteum, even reaching the joint capsule and the synovial membrane. Microscopically, GCT exhibits two types of cells (Fig. 30-45B). The mononuclear ("stromal") cells are plump and oval, with large nuclei and scanty cytoplasm. Large osteoclast-like multinucleated giant cells, some with more than 100 nuclei, are scattered evenly throughout the richly vascularized stroma. Diffuse interstitial hemorrhage is common. Secondary aneurysmal bone cyst may also be seen. On low-power microscopic examination, the tumor often appears as a syncytium of

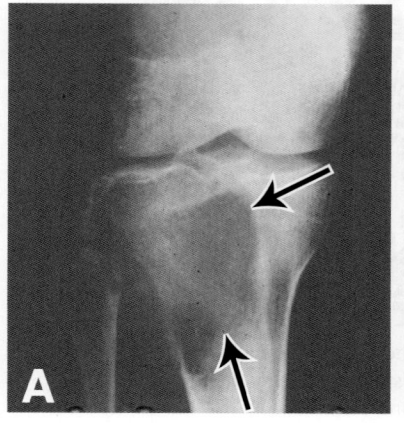

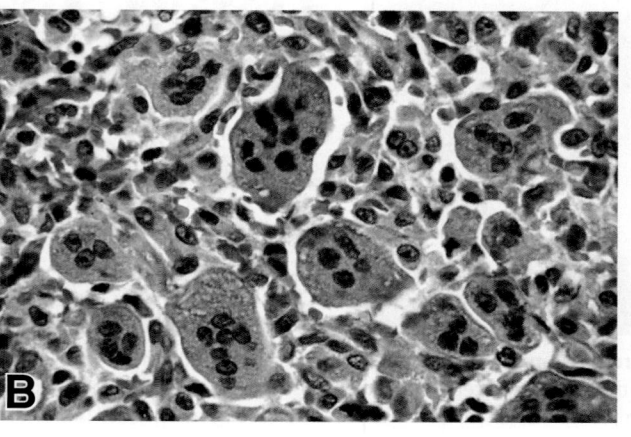

FIGURE 30-45. Giant cell tumor of bone. A. This radiograph of the proximal tibia shows an eccentric lytic lesion with virtually no new bone formation (*arrows*). The tumor extends to the subchondral bone plate and breaks through the cortex into the soft tissue. **B.** A photomicrograph shows osteoclast-type giant cells and plump, oval, mononuclear cells. The nuclei of both types of cells appear identical.

nuclei with poor demarcation of cytoplasmic borders and random distribution of the giant cells. It is evident that the mononuclear cells are the neoplastic and proliferative components of GCT (mitotic activity is common in the mononuclear cells but is not observed in the giant cells).

CLINICAL FEATURES: The vast majority of GCTs are considered benign, but aggressive tumors have the potential to recur locally (30% to 40%) after simple curettage. They rarely metastasize to distant sites (1% to 2%), but when this occurs, the lungs are usually involved. Virtually all metastases arise after initial surgical intervention and they show benign histology resembling the primary tumor. Pulmonary metastases usually do not cause patient death and they can be surgically removed. Taken together, these observations suggest that local recurrence reflects incomplete tumor resection rather than biologic aggressiveness, and distant metastases result from dislodgment of tumor fragments during surgery with venous transport to the lungs.

True malignancy in GCT is observed in only 1% of cases, either as a sarcomatous lesion arising in a typical GCT or a pure sarcoma after a GCT has been curetted. Recurrence as pure sarcoma may occur spontaneously or after local radiation therapy.

GCTs present with pain, usually in the joint adjacent to the tumor. Microfractures and pathologic fractures are frequent, owing to thinning of the cortex. The tumor is treated with thorough curettage and bone grafting, although more aggressive management, including en bloc resection or even amputation, may be necessary.

MALIGNANT TUMORS OF BONE

Osteosarcoma Is the Most Common Primary Malignant Bone Tumor

Osteosarcoma, or **osteogenic sarcoma,** *is a highly malignant bone tumor characterized by formation of bone matrix by tumor cells.* It represents one-fifth of all bone cancers and is most frequent in adolescents between 10 and 20 years old, affecting males more often than females (2:1).

MOLECULAR PATHOGENESIS: Conventional osteosarcomas have complex karyotypes, with multiple nonspecific numerical and structural chromosomal aberrations. Osteosarcomas are associated with mutations in tumor suppressor genes; almost two-thirds show mutations in *Rb,* the retinoblastoma gene (see Chapter 5) and many have mutations in the *p53* gene. Many other chromosomal and molecular abnormalities pertaining to apoptosis, replicative potential, insensitivity to growth inhibitory signals, and cell cycle regulation contribute in some part to the development of the tumor. For example, amplification of *MDM2, CDK4,* and *PRIM1,* as well as overexpression of *MET* and *FOS,* have been detected in a significant proportion of cases.

ETIOLOGIC FACTORS: The etiology of osteosarcoma is unknown. It occurs with increased incidence in association with several genetic syndromes including Li-Fraumeni, hereditary retinoblastoma and Rothmund-Thomson among others. The tumors are more common in tall people and interestingly, they occur more frequently in tall breeds of dogs. They frequently arise in areas of active growth like the distal femur and proximal tibia. In older people, they usually occur in the context of Paget disease or following radiation exposure (secondary osteosarcoma). For example, radium watch dial painters, who pointed their brushes by licking them, developed osteosarcomas many years later, owing to radium deposition in their bones. Today, secondary osteosarcoma often develops in adults and children previously subjected to external therapeutic radiation for some other malignancy. Several pre-existing benign bone lesions are associated with an increased risk of developing osteosarcoma, including fibrous dysplasia, osteomyelitis, and bone infarcts. Although trauma may call attention to an existing osteosarcoma, there is no evidence that it ever causes the tumor.

PATHOLOGY: Osteosarcomas often arise near the knee, in the distal femur (Fig. 30-46A), proximal tibia, or fibula, although any metaphyseal area of a long bone may be affected. The proximal humerus is the second most common site; 75% of tumors arise adjacent to the knee or shoulder. Only rarely do they arise in extraskeletal sites.

Radiographic evidence of bone destruction and bone formation by osteosarcoma is characteristic, the latter representing neoplastic bone. Often, the periosteum produces an incomplete rim of reactive bone adjacent to the site where it is lifted from the cortical surface by the tumor. The radiographic appearance of a shell of bone intersecting the cortex at one end and open at the other end is referred to as **Codman triangle**. A "sunburst" periosteal reaction is often superimposed (Fig. 30-15).

The gross appearance of osteosarcoma is highly variable, depending on the proportions of bone, cartilage, fibrous stroma, and blood vessels. The cut surface may show any combination of hemorrhagic, cystic, fibrous, cartilaginous, and bony areas. The tumor often spreads within the marrow cavity, breaks through the cortex invading into adjacent soft tissues, elevates or perforates the periosteum, may extend into the epiphysis, and sometimes even reach the joint space (Fig. 30-46A).

Histologic examination reveals a hypercellular tumor composed of malignant polygonal to spindled cells with osteoblastic differentiation, producing very irregular woven bone (Fig. 30-46B). The tumor cells have large hyperchromatic and pleomorphic nuclei with a high nucleus to cytoplasmic ratio. Numerous mitoses, including atypical mitoses are commonly seen. The tumor cells stain prominently for alkaline phosphatase, osteocalcin, and osteonectin. The tumorous bone is laid down haphazardly and is not aligned along stress lines. Often, foci of malignant cartilage or pleomorphic giant

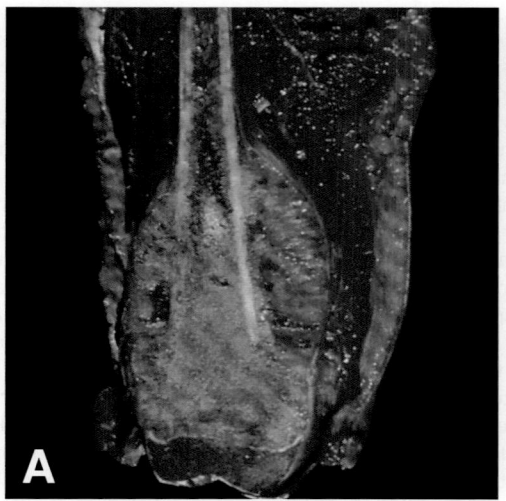
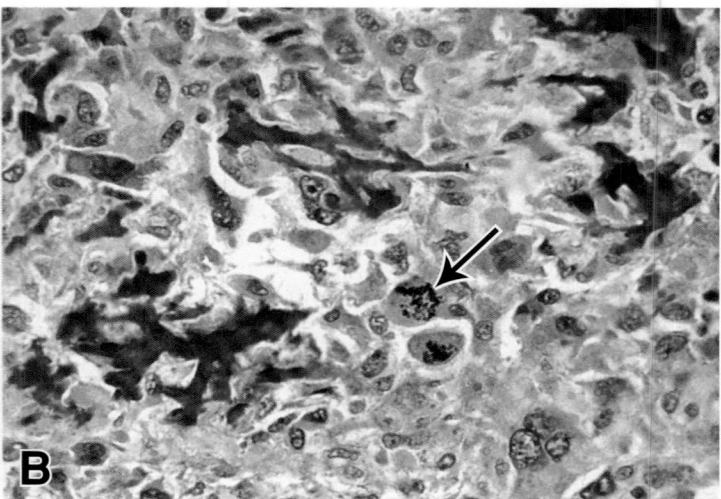

FIGURE 30-46. Osteosarcoma. A. The distal femur contains a dense osteoblastic malignant tumor that extends through the cortex into the soft tissue and the epiphysis. **B.** A photomicrograph reveals pleomorphic malignant cells, tumor giant cells, and bizarre mitoses (*arrow*). The tumor cells produce woven bone that is focally calcified.

cells are intermixed. In areas of osteolysis, nonneoplastic osteoclasts are found at the advancing front of the tumor.

Osteosarcoma spreads through the bloodstream to the lungs. In fact, nearly all patients (98%) who die of this disease have lung metastases. Less commonly, the tumor metastasizes to other bones (35%), the pleura (33%), and the heart (20%).

CLINICAL FEATURES: Osteosarcoma presents with mild or intermittent pain around the involved area and a palpable mass. As pain intensifies, the area becomes swollen and tender. The adjacent joint becomes functionally limited. Pathologic fractures may occur. Serum alkaline phosphatase is increased in half of patients and may decrease after amputation, only to increase again with recurrence or metastasis. Metastatic disease heralds rapid clinical deterioration and death.

Historically, osteosarcoma was treated exclusively by amputation or disarticulation of the involved limb, but the prognosis for 5-year survival did not exceed 20%. Today, standard therapy with preoperative chemotherapy and limb-sparing surgery gives 5-year disease-free rates from 60% to 80%. Resection of isolated pulmonary metastases may prolong survival.

Parosteal osteosarcoma or juxtacortical osteosarcoma is a rare variant of osteosarcoma that occurs on the surface of the bone, especially the lower posterior metaphysis of the femur (70% of cases). Unlike classic osteosarcoma, most patients are older than 25 years, and the tumor is more common in women. Parosteal osteosarcoma usually does not invade the bone and grows external to the shaft. Codman triangles are not evident radiologically, because the periosteum is not elevated. Most parosteal osteosarcomas are low-grade, well-differentiated bone forming tumors that do not require adjuvant chemotherapy. Surgical excision is the treatment of choice. The prognosis is good, with a 5-year survival of better than 80%.

MOLECULAR PATHOGENESIS: Cytogenetic analysis of parosteal osteosarcomas typically reveals supernumerary ring chromosomes containing amplified material from chromosomal region 12q13-15 and consequently, amplification of *CDK4* and *MDM2*, genes involved in cell cycle progression. These gene amplifications can be detected by immunohistochemistry and fluorescence *in situ* hybridization. The same finding is seen in low-grade (well-differentiated) intramedullary osteosarcoma.

Other rare variants of osteosarcoma include telangiectatic and small-cell osteosarcoma, which are high-grade tumors, and periosteal osteosarcoma which is intermediate grade.

Chondrosarcoma Is a Cartilaginous Malignancy Whose Grade Determines Prognosis

Chondrosarcoma is a malignant tumor of cartilage that may arise from a pre-existing cartilage rest or a pre-existing lesion like an enchondroma. Some patients have a history of multiple enchondromas, solitary osteochondroma, or hereditary multiple osteochondromas. Most have no known pre-existing lesion. *Chondrosarcoma is the second most common primary malignant bone tumor and is slightly more common in males.* It is most frequently seen in the fifth to seventh decades and most patients are older than 50.

MOLECULAR PATHOGENESIS: Numerous nonrandom structural and numerical chromosomal abnormalities have been discovered in chondrosarcoma. Recently, mutations in the isocitrate dehydrogenase genes *IDH1* and *IDH2* have been described in central chondrosarcomas but not in peripheral chondrosarcoma. The exact role of these mutations in tumorigenesis is unknown. Different molecular mechanisms appear to be involved in central chondrosarcomas and secondary peripheral chondrosarcomas (tumors arising in the cartilaginous cap of an osteochondroma; see below). The latter may develop by upregulation of PTHrP and Bcl-2 expression in an osteochondroma, along with mutations in other genes such as *p53* and nonspecific chromosomal abnormalities. By contrast, central chondrosarcoma is related, at least in part, to abnormalities of chromosome 9p12-22, which may involve the *CDKN2A* tumor suppressor gene. The transcription factor gene *SOX9*, which plays a critical role in normal chondrocyte development, is expressed in chondrosarcomas.

PATHOLOGY: Chondrosarcoma occurs in three anatomic variants:

CENTRAL CHONDROSARCOMA: This form arises in the medullary cavity of pelvic bones, ribs, and long bones, although any site may be affected. Radiographically, these tumors show poorly defined borders, a thickened shaft, and perforation of the cortex. Stippled or ring-like radiopacities representing calcifications or endochondral ossification in the tumor are usually seen (Fig. 30-47A). Although central chondrosarcoma may penetrate the cortex, extension beyond the periosteum is uncommon. Grossly, the neoplastic cartilaginous tissue is compressed inside the bone and exhibits areas of necrosis, cystic change, and hemorrhage (Fig. 30-47B). The cortex of the bone and intertrabecular spaces of the marrow are infiltrated by the tumor.

Central chondrosarcomas present with deep pain, which becomes more intense with time. They are only rarely palpable, but in untreated cases, large masses may eventually form.

PERIPHERAL CHONDROSARCOMA: This form is less common than the central variety of chondrosarcoma. It arises outside the bone, almost always in the cartilaginous cap of an osteochondroma. It occurs after the age of 20 years and almost never before puberty. The most frequent location of peripheral chondrosarcoma is the pelvis, followed by the femur, vertebrae, sacrum, humerus, and other long bones. Only rarely does it arise distal to the knee or elbow. Radiographically, it usually shows the same characteristic radiopacities seen in central chondrosarcoma. Macroscopically, peripheral chondrosarcomas tend to be large bosselated masses that surround the base of an osteochondroma and may invade and destroy the bone.

Peripheral chondrosarcomas are usually seen as a slowly growing mass. Expansion of the mass causes pain and local symptoms. In the pelvis, the lumbosacral plexus may be compressed, and tumors in the vertebrae may cause paraplegia.

JUXTACORTICAL CHONDROSARCOMA: This is the least common variety of chondrosarcoma and is similar

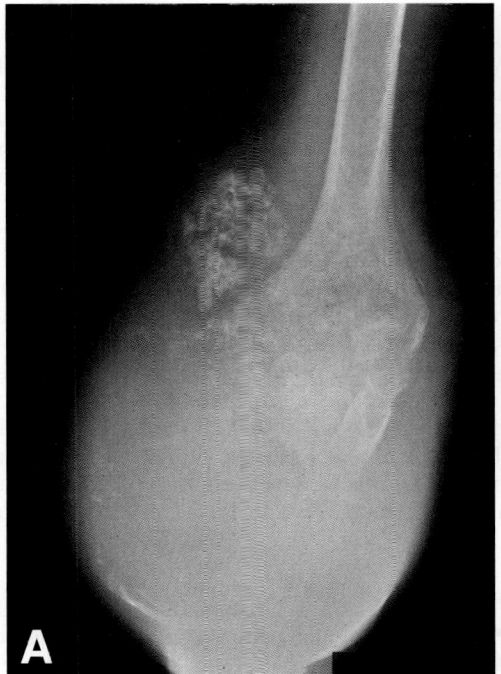

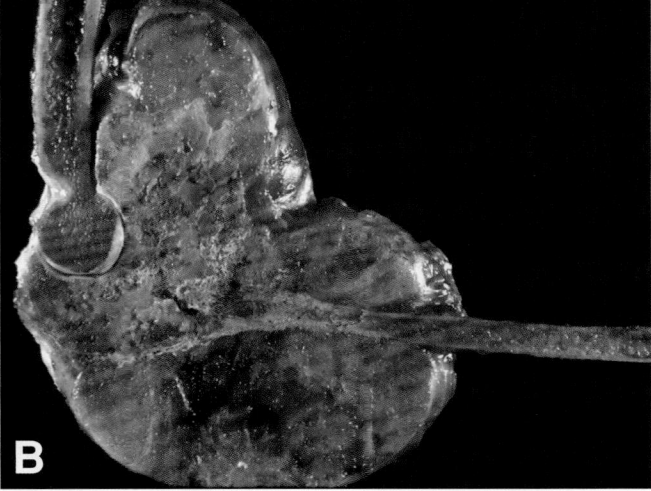

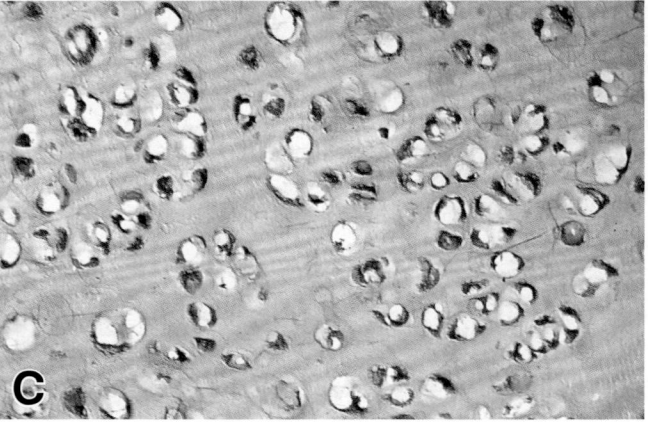

FIGURE 30-47. Chondrosarcoma. A. Radiograph demonstrates a large, destructive mass replacing the proximal ulna. The soft-tissue component of the mass contains aggregates of ring-shaped and popcorn-like calcifications. **B.** Resected gross specimen demonstrates lobulated hyaline cartilage with calcifications, ossification, and focal liquefaction. **C.** A photomicrograph of a chondrosarcoma shows malignant chondrocytes with pronounced atypia.

to central chondrosarcoma in its predilection for middle-aged men. It tends to be situated in the metaphysis of long bones, lying on the outer surface of the cortex. Thus, it is probably periosteal or parosteal in origin. Radiographically, it may be entirely translucent or focally calcified. Symptoms of juxtacortical chondrosarcoma are dominated by swelling, with little accompanying pain.

Histologically, chondrosarcomas are composed of chondrocytes with enlarged nuclei and sometimes multiple nuclei in various stages of maturity (Fig. 30-47C). Giant chondrocytes and mitotic activity are infrequent; their presence increases the histologic grade. Occasionally, a well-differentiated chondrosarcoma is difficult to distinguish from a benign enchondroma on cytologic grounds alone. Zones of calcification are often conspicuous and are seen radiographically as splotches or bulky masses. Chondrosarcomas expand by stimulating osteoclastic resorption of bone and often break through the cortex. Most are slowly growing and localized, but hematogenous metastases to the lungs are common in poorly differentiated variants.

The histologic grade and morphologic features of chondrosarcomas correlate with their degree of karyotypic complexity. Trisomy 7 and rearrangement of the short arm of chromosome 17 are associated with high-grade chondrosarcomas. Alterations in 12q13 are found in tumors that exhibit myxoid features.

OTHER VARIANTS OF CHONDROSARCOMA: The forms of chondrosarcoma described above are all characterized by a hyaline cartilage matrix. Uncommon histopathologic variants of chondrosarcoma include **clear-cell chondrosarcomas**, which occur almost exclusively in the proximal epiphysis of the femur or humerus and are composed of chondrocytes with abundant clear cytoplasm, areas of woven trabecular bone formation and focal regions with a hyaline cartilage matrix. The prognosis for this tumor following complete excision is close to that of a conventional low-grade chondrosarcoma. **Dedifferentiated chondrosarcomas** are defined as high-grade nonchondrogenic pleomorphic sarcomas (e.g., osteosarcomas or fibrosarcomas) that arise in association with a low-grade conventional chondrosarcomas or enchondromas. These tumors usually arise in flat bones of the pelvis or long bones of the extremities and have a dismal prognosis, with less than 10% of patients surviving 5 years. Another variant, **mesenchymal chondrosarcoma**, is histologically characterized by two distinct components. The first is a high-grade malignant, small, round, blue-cell tumor that resembles Ewing sarcoma. Sheets of tumor cells are interrupted by the second component, discrete islands of low- to intermediate-grade malignant hyaline cartilage histologically similar to conventional chondrosarcoma. The bones of the jaw and the chest wall are the most commonly affected sites. About one-third of the cases are extraskeletal. The prognosis for these tumors is poor. Mesenchymal chondrosarcomas express a specific fusion gene, *HEY1-NCOA2*, which may alter nuclear signaling and Notch pathways.

CLINICAL FEATURES: Patients generally present with pain at the affected site. Chondrosarcoma is one of the few tumors in which microscopic grading carries significant prognostic value.

The 5-year survival rate for low-grade conventional chondrosarcomas is 80%, for moderate-grade tumors 50% and for high-grade tumors only 20%. Wide excision is the usual treatment, since response to radiation and chemotherapy is poor.

Ewing Sarcoma Is a Primitive Neuroectodermal Tumor of Childhood

Ewing sarcoma (EWS) is an uncommon malignant bone tumor composed of small, uniform, round cells. It represents only 5% of all bone tumors and occurs in children and adolescents, with two-thirds of cases in patients younger than 20 years. Males are affected more often than females (2:1). EWS is very rare in blacks. About 10% to 20% of EWSs are extraskeletal.

MOLECULAR PATHOGENESIS: EWS is thought to arise from primitive marrow elements or immature mesenchymal cells. Most (90%) of these tumors have a reciprocal translocation between chromosomes 11 and 22 [t(11;22)(q24;q12)], resulting in the fusion of the amino terminus of *EWS1* to the carboxy terminus of *FLI-1*. The resulting fusion protein, EWS/FLI-1, is an aberrant transcription factor whose target genes are not yet fully identified. A less common translocation, t(21;22)(q22;q12), generates *EWS/ERG* gene fusion. Other chromosomal rearrangements seen in EWS are listed in Table 30-2.

EWS is primarily a tumor of the long bones in childhood, especially the humerus, tibia, and femur, where it occurs as a midshaft or metaphyseal lesion. It tends to parallel the distribution of red marrow, so when it arises in the third decade or later, it affects the pelvis and spine. However, no bone is immune from involvement.

The radiographic findings are variable and depend on the interaction of the tumor with the host bone. There is often a destructive process causing the border between normal bone and the lesion to become indistinct. Periosteal reaction and a soft-tissue mass are also commonly seen (Fig. 30-48A). The onion-skin pattern of periosteal bone sometimes seen radiographically represents circumferential discontinuous layers of periosteal new bone associated with a lytic lesion in the medulla and endosteal surface of the cortex. Some patients present with fever and weakness as well as bone pain, so it is not surprising that EWS may be mistaken for osteomyelitis.

PATHOLOGY: Grossly, EWS is typically soft and grayish white, often studded by hemorrhagic foci and necrotic areas. It may infiltrate medullary spaces without destroying bony trabeculae. It may also diffusely infiltrate cortical bone or form nodules in which the bone is completely resorbed. In many cases, the tumor mass penetrates the periosteum and extends into adjacent soft tissues.

Microscopically, EWS cells appear as sheets of closely packed, small, round cells with little cytoplasm. They are up to twice the size of lymphocytes (Fig. 30-48B). Fibrous strands separate the sheets of cells into irregular nests.

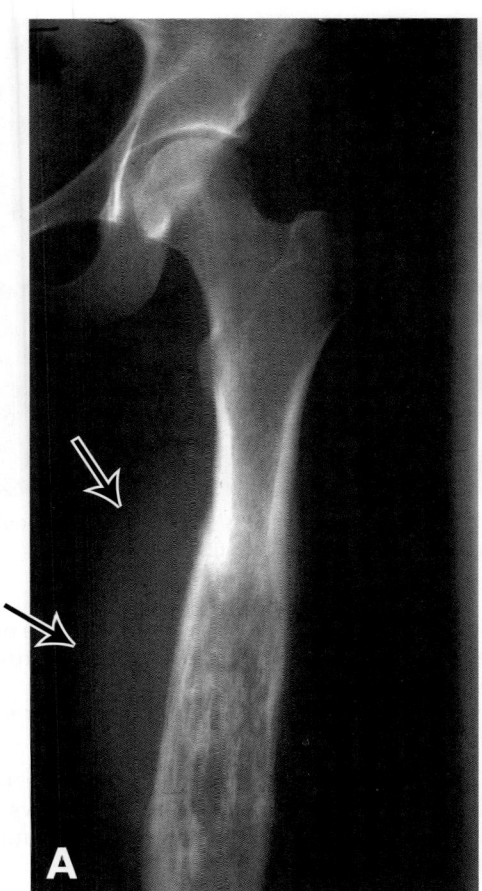

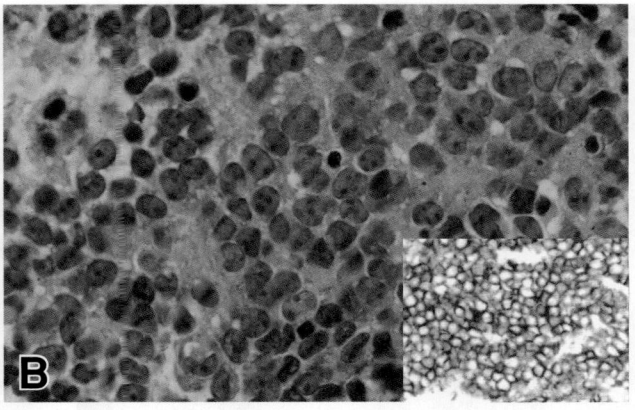

FIGURE 30-48. Ewing sarcoma. A. A radiograph demonstrates expansile cortical destruction with poor circumscription and a delicate interrupted periosteal reaction (*arrows*). **B.** Histology shows fairly uniform small cells with round, dark blue nuclei and poorly defined cytoplasm. Immunohistochemical stain for CD99 shows a membranous (i.e., cell surface) pattern (*inset*).

There is little or no interstitial stroma, and mitoses are infrequent. In some areas, the neoplastic cells tend to form rosettes. An important diagnostic feature is the presence of substantial amounts of glycogen in the cytoplasm of the tumor cells, which is well visualized with the periodic acid–Schiff (PAS) stain. EWS cells also express characteristic antigens that can be detected by immunohistochemistry (Fig. 30-48B, *inset*), some of which are fusion gene products (e.g., CD99 and FLI-1).

EWS metastasizes to many organs, including the lungs and brain. Other bones, especially the skull, are common sites of metastases (50% to 75% of cases).

CLINICAL FEATURES: EWS initially presents with mild pain, which becomes more intense and is followed by swelling of the affected area. Nonspecific symptoms, including fever and leukocytosis, commonly follow. In some cases, a soft-tissue mass is detected.

EWS prognosis used to be dismal, but current chemotherapy and radiation protocols and limb-sparing surgery in patients without metastases have increased 5-year disease-free survival rates to 60% to 75%.

Plasma Cell Myeloma Produces Lytic Lesions in Bone

Malignant plasma cell tumors may be either localized (plasmacytoma) or diffuse (multiple myeloma, see Chapter 26).

Multiple myeloma occurs mostly in older people (average age, 55) and affects men twice as often as women. Because myeloma cells secrete cytokines that recruit osteoclasts, the lesions are unique in that they are almost exclusively radiolucent. The bones most frequently involved are the skull (Fig. 30-49A), spine, ribs, pelvis, and femur. Pathologic fractures are common. Microscopic examination reveals sheets of plasma cells with varying degrees of maturity (Fig. 30-49B). Amyloid deposits, derived from monoclonal antibodies produced by tumor cells, are seen in 10% of patients in both skeletal and extraskeletal sites.

With newer therapies, median survival of patients with multiple myeloma now is about 5 years. Death is usually due to infection or renal failure. Solitary plasmacytoma has a better prognosis, with 60% 5-year survival.

Metastatic Tumors Are the Most Common Malignant Tumors in Bone

In adults, most metastatic lesions to bone are carcinomas, particularly of the prostate, breast, lung, thyroid, and kidney. In children, the most common bone metastases are from rhabdomyosarcoma, neuroblastoma, Wilms tumor, and clear-cell sarcoma of the kidney. It is estimated that skeletal metastases occur in at least 85% of cancer cases that have run their full clinical course. The vertebral column is the most common location in adults (Fig. 30-50A), and the appendicular skeleton is the most common site in children. Tumor cells usually gain access to bones via the bloodstream; in spinal metastases, they are often transported by vertebral veins.

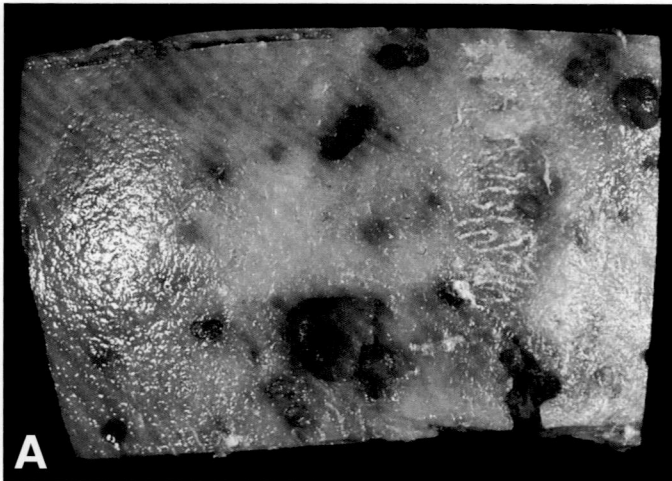
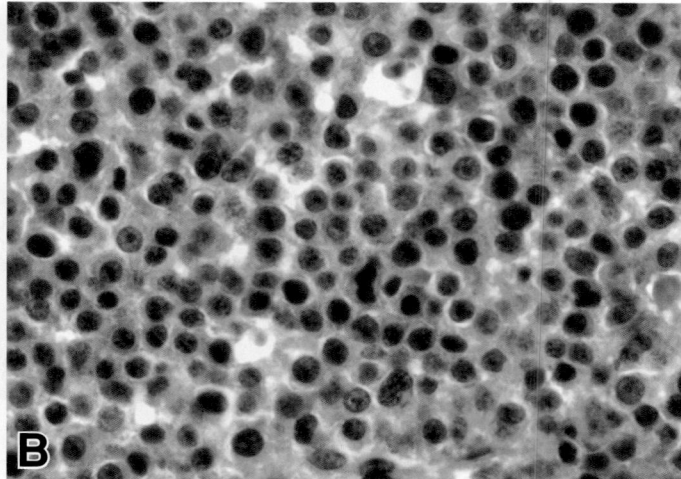

FIGURE 30-49. Multiple myeloma. A. A portion of the skull from a patient with multiple myeloma reveals numerous punched-out, lytic lesions. **B.** Microscopically, the lesions are composed of sheets of plasma cells with atypia, binucleation, and discernible nucleoli.

Some tumors (e.g., thyroid, gastrointestinal tract, kidney, and neuroblastoma) produce mostly lytic lesions by stimulating osteoclasts (Fig. 30-50B). A few neoplasms (e.g., prostate, breast, lung, stomach) stimulate osteoblastic components to make bone, thus creating dense foci seen on imaging studies (blastic or sclerotic lesions). However, most metastatic tumors in the bones show a mixture of both lytic and blastic elements.

Joints

A joint (or articulation) is a union between two or more bones, whose construction varies with the function of that joint. There are two types of joints: (1) a **synovial** or **diarthrodial** joint, which is a movable joint, such as the knee or elbow, that is lined by a synovial membrane; and (2) a **synarthrosis**, which is a joint that has little movement.

Synarthroses are further divided into four subclassifications:

- A **symphysis** is an articulation joined by fibrocartilaginous tissue and firm ligaments that allows little movement. Examples are the symphysis pubis and the ends of vertebral joints.
- A **synchondrosis** is found at the ends of bones and has articular cartilage but is not associated with synovium or a significant joint cavity (e.g., the sternal manubrial joint).
- A **syndesmosis** connects bones by fibrous tissue without any cartilaginous elements. The distal tibiofibular articulation and the cranial sutures are syndesmoses.

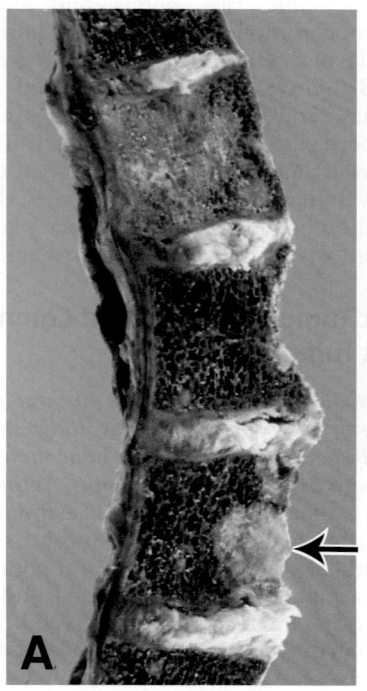
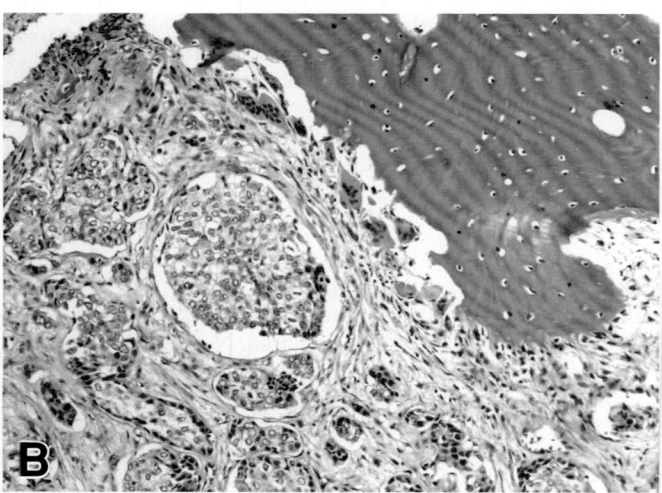

FIGURE 30-50. Metastatic carcinoma to bone. A. A section through the vertebral column reveals conspicuous tan nodules of metastatic tumor (*arrow*). **B.** Tumor-induced osteolysis. Breast cancer metastatic to bone recruits numerous osteoclasts, which resorb bone and cause osteolytic lesions.

■ A **synostosis** is a pathologic bony bridge between bones as, for example, in ankylosis of the spine.

Diseases of diarthrodial joints are among the oldest pathologic conditions known, having been found in the fossil bones of dinosaurs. One-third of the population of the United States older than 50 years develops some form of clinically significant joint disease.

CLASSIFICATION OF SYNOVIAL JOINTS

The synovial, or diarthrodial, joints are classified according to the type of movement they permit.

■ A **uniaxial joint** allows movement around only one axis. Examples include a hinge joint such as the elbow and a pivot (rotational) joint such as the radioulnar joint.
■ A **biaxial joint** allows movement around two axes, as the condyloid joint of the wrist axis is oriented in the long diameter and the other along the short diameter of the articular surfaces. This allows four-way movement: flexion, extension, abduction, and adduction. In a saddle joint, such as the carpometacarpal joint of the thumb, joint surfaces allow movement as in a condyloid joint.
■ **Polyaxial joints** permit movement in virtually any axis. In a ball-and-socket joint, such as is found in the shoulder and hip, all movements, including rotation, are possible.
■ A **plane joint,** represented by the patella, allows articular surfaces to glide over one another.

UNIT LOAD: **The concept of unit load is the most important principle in understanding joint function.** The unit load is the compressive force experienced by the joint, expressed as kilograms per cubic centimeter of articular cartilage. It is fairly constant over the hip, knee and ankle (20 to 26 kg/cm^3 along the articular surfaces). Because the articular cartilage is injured if a load exceeds these values, several mechanisms protect a joint from exceeding the unit load.

Adjacent muscles are the major shock-absorbing structures that protect the joint. Deformation, even to the extent of microscopic fractures of the coarse cancellous bone, also helps protect the joint. Joint deformation allows the contact area to increase with increasing load. Diarthrodial joints may have intra-articular structures, such as ligaments and menisci. Menisci hold distributed force along the articular surface and allow two planes of motion, such as flexion and rotation. However, 90% or more of energy absorption across the knee joint is by active muscle contraction, and only 10% or less is by secondary mechanisms, such as by the coarse cancellous bone of the knee joint. A properly functioning joint also requires support from ligaments and tendons, periarticular connective tissues such as the joint capsule and nerves that provide proprioception. Thus, to protect the articular cartilage from forces that exceed the critical unit load, virtually any structure is sacrificed, even to the point of a bone fracture.

Once an insult occurs to one component of the joint, the resulting dysfunction can lead to degeneration of other components of the joint. For example, knee ligament injuries sustained by athletes, such as a torn anterior cruciate ligament, can result in joint instability. Over time, this situation contributes to degeneration of articular cartilage, owing to changes in movement and load on the joint (secondary osteoarthritis).

ARTHRITIS: Arthritis refers to joint inflammation, usually accompanied by pain, swelling and sometimes changes in joint structure. Arthritis is divided into two major forms: (1) **inflammatory arthritis** usually involves the synovium and is mediated by inflammatory cells (e.g., rheumatoid arthritis [RA]); and (2) **noninflammatory arthritis**, as featured in primary osteoarthritis, which may involve cytokines in its pathogenesis (see below).

STRUCTURES OF THE SYNOVIAL JOINT

Movement plays a major role in joint formation. Lack of movement retards joint development and may cause **arthrogryposis**, a rare but crippling disease characterized by joint fusion.

Synovium

Synovial joints are partially lined on their internal aspects by the synovium. Synovial linings are not true membranes since they lack basement membranes to separate synovial lining cells from subsynovial tissue. The synovium is composed of one to three layers of lining cells and includes two cell types distinguishable by electron microscopy. **Type A cells** are macrophages with lysosomal enzymes and dense bodies. **Type B cells** secrete hyaluronic acid. Synovial cell membranes are disposed in villi and microvilli, an arrangement that creates an enormous surface area. It is estimated that the knee alone has 100 m^2 of synovial lining.

The synovium controls: (1) diffusion in and out of the joint; (2) ingestion of debris; (3) secretion of hyaluronate, immunoglobulins and lysosomal enzymes; and (4) lubrication of the joints through secretion of hyaluronate and glycoproteins. Synovial fluid is clear, sticky, and viscous. It is present only in small amounts, not exceeding 1 to 4 mL, and is the main source of nourishment for chondrocytes of the articular cartilage, which lacks a blood supply. It is an ultrafiltrate that acts as a molecular sieve. It does not contain tissue thromboplastin and so cannot clot. Hyaluronate is a long-chain polymer of dissacharide units of Na-glucuronate-N-acetylglucosamine. Its polyanionic form has a high affinity for water and it produces a viscoelastic solution that serves as a lubricant.

Articular Cartilage

The hyaline cartilage that covers the articular ends of bones does not participate in endochondral ossification and is well suited for its dual role of absorbing shocks and lubricating the surfaces of movable joints. On gross examination, the articular cartilage is glistening, smooth, white and semirigid, and is generally not thicker than 6 mm.

Joint Histology

The articular surface appears smooth to the eye, but scanning electron microscopy reveals gentle waves and pits that correspond to the underlying lacunae of the surface chondrocytes. There are four zones in articular cartilage (Fig. 30-51).

■ **Tangential** or **gliding zone:** This is the region closest to the articular surface, where chondrocytes are elongated, flattened, and oriented parallel to the long axis of the surface. Within this zone, a condensation of type II collagen fibers forms the so-called skin of the articular cartilage.

BONES, JOINTS, AND SOFT TISSUE

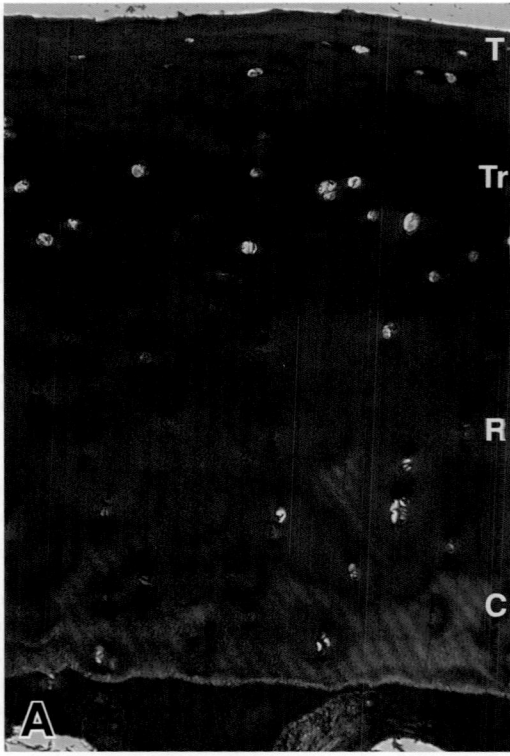

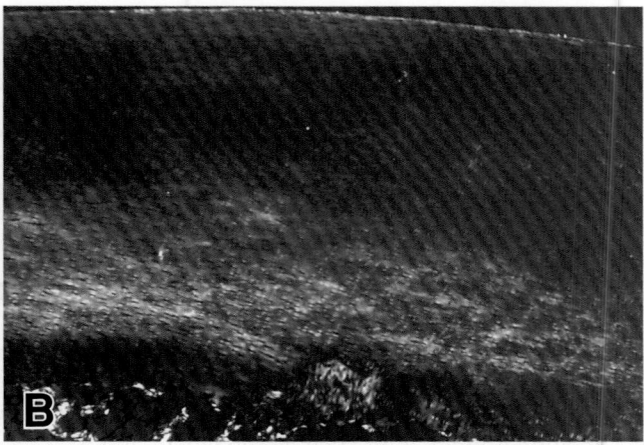

FIGURE 30-51. Articular hyaline cartilage. A. Hyaline cartilage that covers articular ends of bones consists of a tangential zone (*T*), transitional zone (*Tr*), radial zone (*R*), and calcified zone (*C*). Chondrocyte lacunae change shape in conformation with the direction of collagen arcades within the cartilage. **B.** Viewed with polarized light, tangential and radial zones of articular cartilage have the highest concentration of collagen fibers and appear bright yellow.

- **Transitional zone:** Chondrocytes in this slightly deeper zone are larger, ovoid, and more randomly distributed than those in the tangential zone. The standard hyaline cartilage matrix is present, and by electron microscopy, collagen fibers are arranged transverse to the articular surface.
- **Radial zone:** The next deeper zone is the radial zone, where small chondrocytes are arranged in short columns like those seen in the epiphyseal plate. In this area, collagen fibers are large and oriented perpendicular to the long axis of the articular surface.
- **Calcified zone:** Small chondrocytes and a heavily calcified matrix characterize the deepest region.

The calcified zone is separated from the radial zone by a transverse, undulating, heavily calcified "blue line" (evident on hematoxylin–eosin staining), called the **tidemark**. The tidemark is the interface between mineralized and unmineralized cartilage. Above the tidemark on the joint side, all of the cartilage is nourished by diffusion from the synovial fluid. Deep to the tidemark, the calcified cartilage is supplied by epiphyseal blood vessels.

The tidemark is the area where cartilage cells are renewed by cell division. This causes true articular chondrocytes to migrate upward toward the joint surface. Cell division below the tidemark occurs in the calcified cartilage, if there is appropriate stimulation. For example, in acromegaly, when the epiphyseal plates have already closed, the bones may grow in minute increments, because growth hormone stimulates the calcified cartilage remnant of the epiphyseal cartilage anlage. Because the joints in acromegaly do not keep pace, joint incongruity leads to severe osteoarthritis. Deep to the calcified cartilage, the transverse bony plate, called the **subchondral bone plate**, supports the articular cartilage. It is directly contiguous with the coarse cancellous bone of the epiphysis.

OSTEOARTHRITIS

Osteoarthritis (OA), also known as degenerative joint disease (DJD), is a slowly progressive destruction of articular cartilage that affects weight-bearing joints and fingers of older individuals or the joints of younger people subjected to trauma. OA is the single most common form of joint disease and the major form of noninflammatory arthritis. It encompasses a group of conditions that have in common the mechanical destruction of a joint.

In **primary OA**, destruction of joints results from intrinsic defects in the articular cartilage. The prevalence and severity of primary OA increase with age. About 4% of people aged 18 to 24 are affected, versus 85% of those 75 to 79 years. Before age 45, the disease mainly affects men. After age 55, OA is more common in women. Many cases of primary OA exhibit a familial clustering, suggesting genetic determinants of disease.

In primary OA, progressive degradation of articular cartilage leads to joint narrowing, subchondral bone thickening, and eventually a nonfunctioning painful joint. Although OA is not primarily an inflammatory process, a mild inflammatory reaction may occur within the synovium.

Secondary OA has a known underlying cause, including congenital or acquired incongruity of joints, trauma, crystal deposits, infection, metabolic diseases, endocrinopathies, chronic inflammatory diseases, osteonecrosis and hemarthrosis.

Chondromalacia is a term applied to a subcategory of OA that affects the patellar surface of the femoral condyles of young people and produces pain and stiffness of the knee.

ETIOLOGIC FACTORS: *INCREASED UNIT LOAD:* Abnormal force on the cartilage has many causes but it is often attributable to incongruities of the joint. Thus, in congenital hip dysplasia, a fairly common abnormality, the socket of the acetabulum is shallow, covering only 35% of the femoral head (normal, 50%). Less surface area is covered by articular cartilage, which thus bears an increased load. When the critical unit load is exceeded, chondrocyte death leads to degradation of articular cartilage.

RESILIENCE OF THE ARTICULAR CARTILAGE: Because articular cartilage binds extensive amounts of water, it normally has a swelling pressure of at least 3 atmospheres. Disruption in water bonding leads to decreased resilience.

STIFFNESS OF SUBCHONDRAL COARSE CANCELLOUS BONE: The structure of bone adjacent to a joint is important in maintaining articular cartilage. Mechanical forces are not transferred to articular cartilage by normal stress, but rather are dissipated by microfractures of coarse cancellous bone. Thus, damage to this structure can increase unit load on the cartilage because of increased stiffness of subchondral bone (e.g., in Paget disease).

 MOLECULAR PATHOGENESIS: *BIOCHEMICAL ABNORMALITIES:* The biochemical changes of OA mainly involve proteoglycans. Proteoglycan content and aggregation decrease, and glycosaminoglycan chain length is reduced. Collagen fibers are thicker than normal and the water content of osteoarthritic cartilage increases. Reduced proteoglycan content allows more water to be bound to collagen. Thus, osteoarthritic cartilage, or any cartilage that is fibrillated, swells more than normal cartilage.

Although matrix synthesis by chondrocytes increases early in OA, protein synthesis eventually declines, suggesting that the cells reach a point at which they fail to respond to reparative stimuli. Similarly, chondrocytes replicate early OA but this diminishes with advanced disease. Acid cathepsins, which attack the protein cores of matrix macromolecules, increase in osteoarthritic cartilage. Collagenase is absent in normal cartilage but is expressed in osteoarthritic cartilage.

Chondrocyte apoptosis, decreased type II collagen synthesis and breakdown of extracellular matrix also occur in association with local increases in IL-1β and TNF-α. In turn, these cytokines induce expression of matrix metalloproteinases (MMPs), nitric oxide, and PGE$_2$. Mechanical stress appears to be the triggering factor for these signaling cascades.

Studies of identical twins have demonstrated genetic contributions to the prevalence of OA. Genetic analysis of patients with a type of familial, early-onset OA revealed a variety of variants in the gene for type II collagen (*COL2A1*), the major collagen species of articular cartilage.

 PATHOLOGY: Joints commonly affected by OA are the proximal and distal interphalangeal joints, and the joints of the arms, knees, hips, and cervical and lumbar spine. Radiologically, OA is characterized

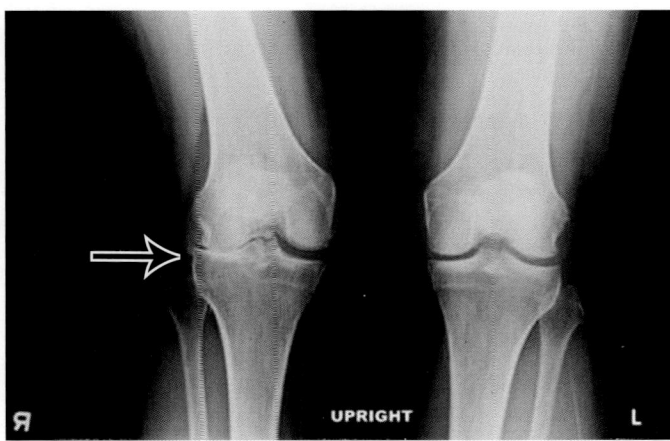

FIGURE 30-52. A radiograph of a patient with osteoarthritis of the right knee shows marked narrowing of the joint space, increased density of subchondral bone, and osteophyte formation laterally (*arrow*).

by: (1) narrowing of the joint space, reflecting loss of articular cartilage; (2) increased thickness of the subchondral bone; (3) subchondral bone cysts; and (4) large peripheral growths of bone and cartilage, called **osteophytes** (Fig. 30-52). Histologic changes follow a well-described sequence.

1. The earliest histologic evidence of OC is loss of proteoglycans from the surface of the articular cartilage, seen as decreased metachromatic staining. At the same time, empty lacunae in articular cartilage indicate that chondrocytes have died (Fig. 30-53A). Viable chondrocytes enlarge, aggregate into groups or clones (Fig. 30-53C) and become surrounded by basophilic staining matrix called the **territorial matrix**.

2. OA may arrest at this stage for many years before progressing to the next stage, which is characterized by fibrillation (i.e., development of surface cracks parallel to the long axis of the articular surface). These fibrillations may persist for many years before further progression occurs (Fig. 30-53B).

3. As fibrillations propagate, synovial fluid begins to flow into the defects. The cracks are progressively oriented more vertically, parallel to the long axis of the collagen fibrils. Synovial fluid penetrates deeper into the articular cartilage along these cracks. Eventually, fragments of articular cartilage break off and lodge in the synovium, inducing inflammation and a foreign body giant cell reaction. The result is a hyperemic and hypertrophied synovium.

4. As the crack extends down toward the tidemark and eventually crosses it, neovascularization from the epiphysis and subchondral bone extends into the area of the crack, inducing subchondral osteoclastic bone resorption (Fig. 30-53C). Adjacent osteoblastic activity also occurs and results in a thickening of the subchondral bone plate in the area of the crack. As neovascularization extends into the area of the crack, mesenchymal cells invade and fibrocartilage forms as a poor substitute for the articular hyaline cartilage (Figs. 30-53D and 30-54A). These fibrocartilaginous plugs may persist where formed, or be swept into the joint. The subchondral bone becomes exposed and burnished as it grinds

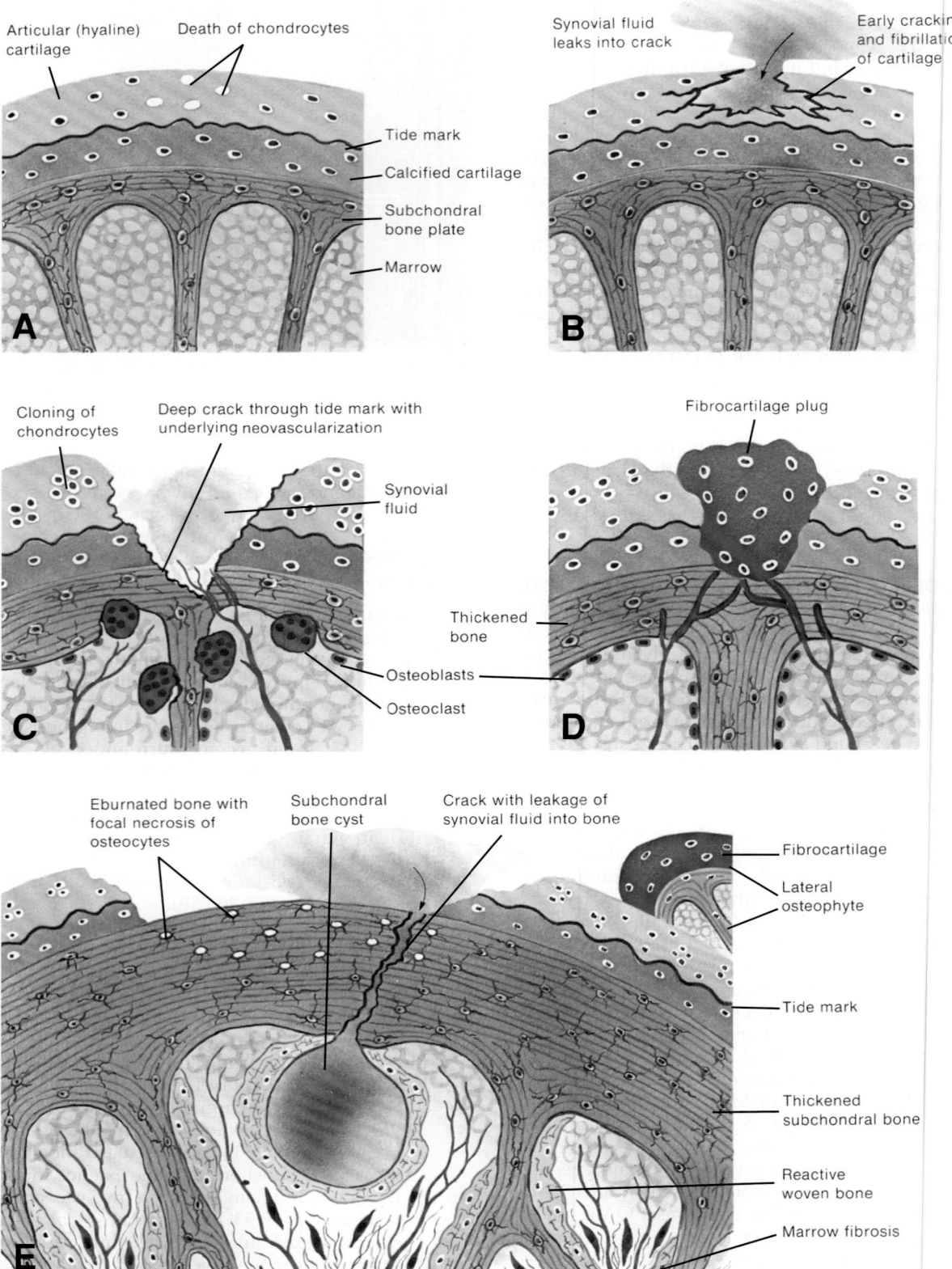

FIGURE 30-53. Histogenesis of osteoarthritis. A, B. The death of chondrocytes leads to a crack in the articular cartilage followed by an influx of synovial fluid and further loss and degeneration of cartilage. **C.** As a result of this process, cartilage is gradually worn away. Below the tidemark, new vessels grow in from the epiphysis, and fibrocartilage (**D**) is deposited. **E.** The fibrocartilage plug is not mechanically sufficient, however, and may be worn away, thus exposing the subchondral bone plate, which becomes thickened and eburnated (i.e., ivory like). If a crack forms in this region, synovial fluid leaks into the marrow space and produces a subchondral bone cyst. Focal regrowth of the articular surface leads to formation of osteophytes.

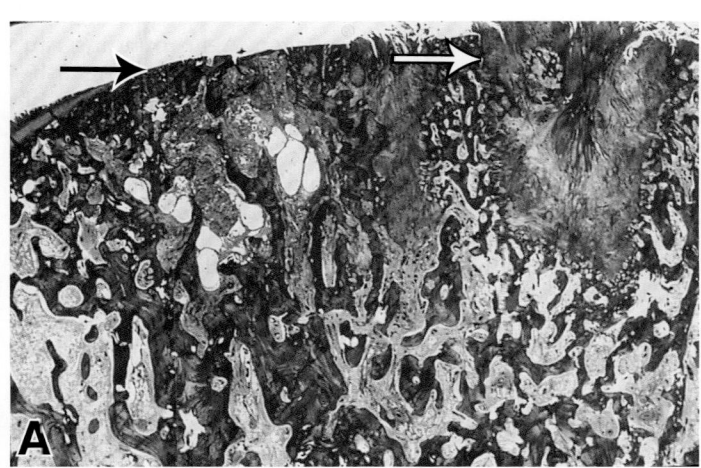 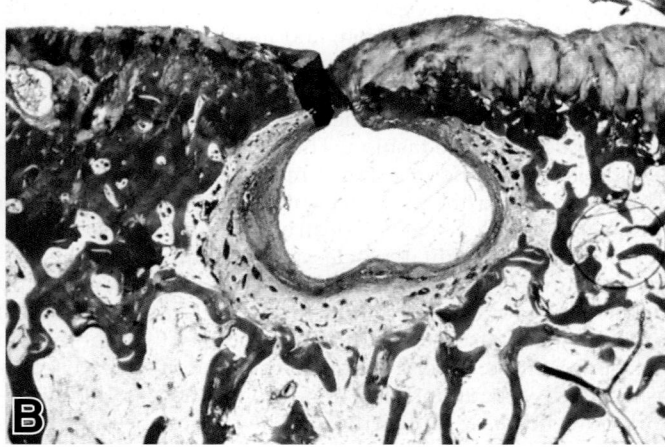

FIGURE 30-54. Osteoarthritis. A. A femoral head with osteoarthritis shows a fibrocartilaginous plug (*white arrow*) extending from the marrow onto the joint surface. Eburnated bone is present over the remaining surface (*black arrow*). **B.** A section through the articular surface of an osteoarthritic joint demonstrates focal absence of the articular cartilage, thickening of subchondral bone (*left*) and a subchondral bone cyst. (54B from Bullough PG. *Atlas of Orthopaedic Pathology.* 2nd ed. New York: Gower Medical Publishing, 1992. Copyright Lippincott Williams & Wilkins.)

against the opposite joint surface, which undergoes the same process. These thick, shiny, smooth areas of subchondral bone are referred to as **eburnated** (ivory-like) bone.

5. In some areas, the eburnated bone cracks, allowing synovial fluid to extend from the joint surface into the subchondral bone marrow, where it eventually produces a **subchondral bone cyst** (Figs. 30-53E and 30-54B). These cysts increase in size as synovial fluid is forced into the space but cannot exit. Eventually, osteoclasts resorb bone and osteoblasts attempt to wall off the area. The result is a subchondral bone cyst filled with synovial fluid, with a well-marginated wall of reactive bone.

6. An osteophyte develops, usually in the lateral portions of the joint, when the mesenchymal cells of the synovium differentiate into osteoblasts and chondroblasts to form a mass of cartilage and bone. Osteophytes are pearly grayish bone nodules on the periphery of the joint surface. Also known as bony spurs, osteophytes can occur at lateral edges of intervertebral discs, extending from the adjacent vertebral bodies. They produce the "lipping" pattern seen on radiologic studies as OA of the spine. In the fingers, osteophytes at the distal interphalangeal joints are called **Heberden nodes**.

CLINICAL FEATURES: Signs and symptoms of OA depend on the location of the involved joints and the severity and duration of the joint deterioration. Physical findings vary. The involved joints may be enlarged, tender, and boggy and may produce crepitus. The clinical hallmark of OA is deep, achy joint pain that follows activity and is relieved by rest. Pain is usually a sign of significant joint destruction. It arises in periarticular structures, as articular cartilage lacks nerve supply. Discomfort also is caused by short periods of stiffness, which frequently occurs in the morning or after periods of minimal activity. Restricted joint motion indicates severe disease. It may result from joint or muscle contractures, intra-articular loose bodies, large osteophytes, and loss of congruity of the joint surfaces.

At present, OA cannot be prevented or arrested. Therapy is directed at specific orthopedic conditions and includes exercise, weight loss, and other supportive measures. In disabling osteoarthritis, joint replacement may be necessary. Such procedures are increasing greatly in economically advanced societies as the population ages.

NEUROPATHIC JOINT DISEASE (CHARCOT JOINT)

Neuropathic joint disease is a form of noninflammatory arthritis characterized by progressive joint destruction due to a primary neurologic disorder, such as peripheral neuropathy or central motor abnormality. In the mid-19th century, Jean-Martin Charcot described destruction of knee joints in patients with syphilitic tabes dorsalis (Charcot joint). *Today, the most common form of neuropathic joint disease is destruction of foot joints in people with diabetic peripheral neuropathy.* Destruction of shoulder or other upper extremity joints can occur in patients with syringomyelia, an abnormality affecting the cervical spinal cord.

Neuropathic joint disease can be viewed as a rapid and severe form of secondary OA in which a joint essentially fragments. Microscopically, there is marked destruction of articular cartilage and subchondral bone, inciting subchondral sclerosis, cyst formation, and large amounts of cartilage and bone detritus within hyperplastic synovium. Although the pathogenesis remains uncertain, it is most likely that loss of innervation to the joint structures brings on a lack of proprioception and pain, and this leads to abnormal joint mechanics and ultimately joint destruction.

RHEUMATOID ARTHRITIS

RA is a systemic, chronic inflammatory disease in which chronic polyarthritis involves diarthrodial joints, symmetrically and bilaterally (see Chapter 11). The proximal interphalangeal and metacarpophalangeal joints, elbows, knees, ankles, and spine are most commonly affected. RA may occur at any age but usually begins in the third or fourth decade, and prevalence increases until age 70. It afflicts 1% to 2% of the adult population, and its incidence is greater in premenopausal women than in men (3:1). After menopause, the frequency for men and women is about the same. Commonly, joints of the extremities are simultaneously affected, often in a symmetric fashion. The course of the disease varies and is often punctuated by remissions and exacerbations. The broad spectrum of clinical manifestations ranges from barely discernible to severe, destructive, mutilating disease.

It is now thought that classic RA comprises a heterogeneous group of disorders. Patients who are persistently seronegative for rheumatoid factor (RF; IgM autoantibodies) probably have disease of a different etiology than those who are seropositive. There are also rheumatoid-like diseases associated with underlying conditions, such as inflammatory bowel disease and cirrhosis. The pathogenesis of RA is presented in Chapter 11.

PATHOLOGY: The early synovial changes of RA are edema and accumulation of plasma cells, lymphocytes, and macrophages (Fig. 30-55B). Vascularity increases, with exudation of fibrin into the joint space, which may result in small fibrin nodules that float in the joint (**rice bodies**).

PANNUS FORMATION: Synovial lining cells, normally only one to three layers thick, undergo hyperplasia and form layers 8 to 10 cells deep. Multinucleated giant cells are often found among the synovial cells. The synovial lining is thus thrown into numerous villi and frond-like folds that fill the peripheral recesses of the joint (Figs. 30-55C and 30-56A,B). This inflammatory synovium, which now contains mast cells, creeps over the surface of the articular cartilage and adjacent structures and is termed **pannus** (cloak). Pannus covers the articular cartilage and isolates it from the synovial fluid (Fig. 30-55D). Lymphocytes aggregate and eventually develop follicular centers (Figs. 30-55C and 30-56B). The pannus erodes the articular cartilage and adjacent bone, probably through the action of collagenase produced by the pannus. In addition, PGE_2 and IL-1 produced in the rheumatoid synovium may mediate bone erosion by stimulating osteoclasts.

The characteristic bone loss of RA is juxta-articular; that is, immediately adjacent to both sides of the joint. The pannus penetrates the subchondral bone where it may involve tendons and ligaments, and thereby lead to deformities and instabilities. Eventually, the joint is destroyed and undergoes fibrous fusion, or **ankylosis** (Figs. 30-55E and 30-57). Long-standing cases feature bony bridging of the joint (**bony ankylosis**). The pannus may destroy cartilage by depriving it of nourishment. It may also stimulate T lymphocytes to secrete a factor that promotes release of lysosomal enzymes which further contributes to secondary OA.

Changes in synovial fluid include a massive increase in volume, increased turbidity, and decreased viscosity. The protein content and the number of inflammatory cells in the fluid increase, correlating with the activity of the rheumatoid process. In some cases, the leukocyte count exceeds 50,000/μL, with 95% polymorphonuclear leukocytes.

RHEUMATOID NODULES: RA is a systemic disease that involves tissues other than joints and tendons. A characteristic lesion, the "rheumatoid nodule," is found in extra-articular locations. It has a central core of fibrinoid necrosis, which is a mixture of fibrin and other

proteins, such as degraded collagen. A surrounding rim of macrophages is arranged in a radial or palisading fashion (Fig. 30-58). Beyond the macrophages is a circle of lymphocytes, plasma cells, and other mononuclear cells. The overall appearance resembles a peculiar granuloma surrounding a core of fibrinoid necrosis. Rheumatoid nodules are usually found in areas of pressure (e.g., the skin of elbows and legs). They are movable, firm, rubbery, and occasionally tender. A large nodule may ulcerate. They often recur after surgical removal.

Rheumatoid nodules may also be seen in lupus erythematous and rheumatic fever. They are sometimes found in visceral organs, such as the heart and/or pericardium, lungs, intestinal tract, and even the dura. Nodules in the bundle of His may cause cardiac arrhythmias; in the lungs, they produce fibrosis and even respiratory failure (see Chapter 18). RA also may be accompanied by **acute necrotizing vasculitis**, which can affect any organ.

CLINICAL FEATURES: The clinical diagnosis of RA is imprecise. It is based on a number of clinical, radiographic, and laboratory criteria, such as the number and types of joints involved, the presence of rheumatoid nodules and RF, and radiographic features characteristic of the disease.

The onset of RA may be acute, slowly progressing, or insidious. Most patients experience slowly developing fatigue, weight loss, weakness, and vague musculoskeletal discomfort, which eventually localizes to the involved joints. Diseased joints tend to be warm, swollen, and painful. The pain is heightened by motion and is most severe after periods of disuse. Unabated disease causes progressive destruction of the joint surfaces and periarticular structures. Eventually, severe flexion and extension deformities develop, leading to joint subluxation and, ultimately, joint ankylosis.

The natural history of RA is variable. In most patients, disease activity waxes and wanes. One-fourth of patients seem to recover completely. Another quarter have only slight functional impairment for many years. However, half develop serious progressive and disabling joint disease, with increased mortality from infection, gastrointestinal hemorrhage and perforation, vasculitis, heart and lung involvement, amyloidosis, and subluxation of the cervical spine. In fact, survival of patients with active RA is comparable to that in Hodgkin disease and diabetes.

Three types of drugs are used to suppress synovial inflammation and induce remission:

- **Nonsteroidal anti-inflammatory drugs (NSAIDs).**
- **Corticosteroids**, which have both anti-inflammatory and immunoregulatory activity.
- **Disease-modifying antirheumatic drugs (DMARDs)**, which have been shown to alter the course of the disease and improve outcome. These include methotrexate, leflunomide, cyclosporin, cyclophosphamide, azathioprine, sulfasalazine, gold salts, penicillamine, antimalarial drugs (hydroxychloroquine), TNF inhibitors, T-cell costimulatory blockers, B-cell–depleting agents, and IL-1 receptor antagonists. Used early in the course of the disease, they prevent progression, induce remission, and prevent joint deformities and functional disabilities.

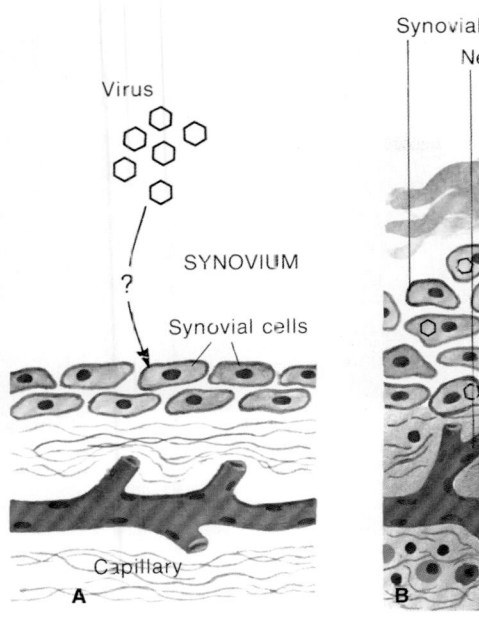

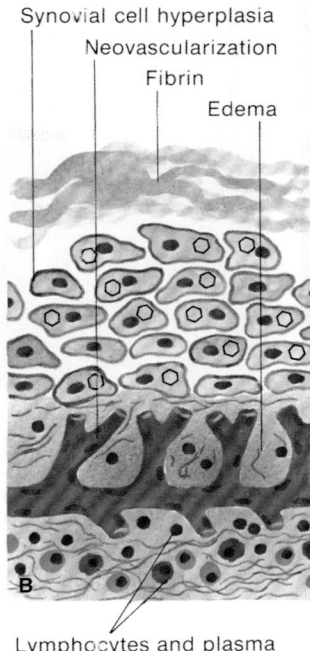

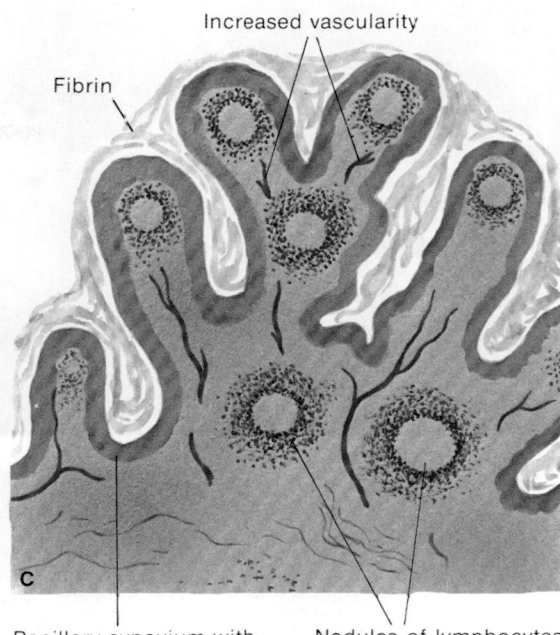

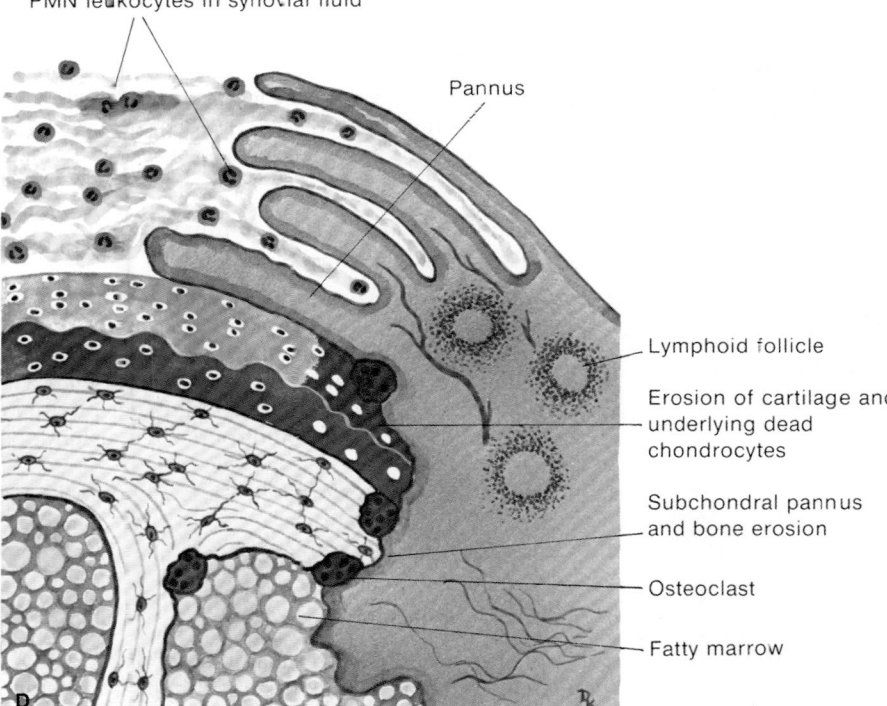

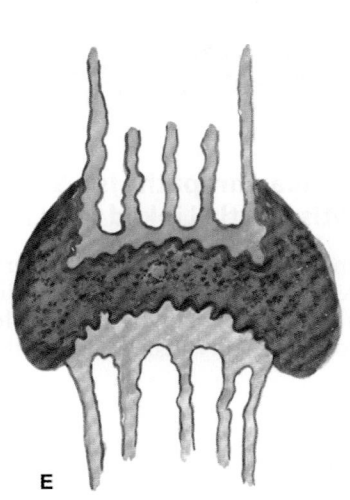

FIGURE 30-55. Histogenesis of rheumatoid arthritis. A. A virus or an unknown stress may stimulate synovial cells to proliferate. **B.** Influx of lymphocytes, plasma cells, and mast cells, together with neovascularization and edema, leads to hypertrophy and hyperplasia of the synovium. **C.** Lymphoid nodules are prominent. **D.** Proliferating synovium extends into the joint space, burrows into the bone beneath the articular cartilage and covers the cartilage as a pannus. Articular cartilage is eventually destroyed by direct resorption or deprivation of its nutrient synovial fluid. Synovial tissue continues to proliferate in the subchondral region, and within the joint. **E.** Eventually, the joint is destroyed and becomes fused, a condition termed **ankylosis.**

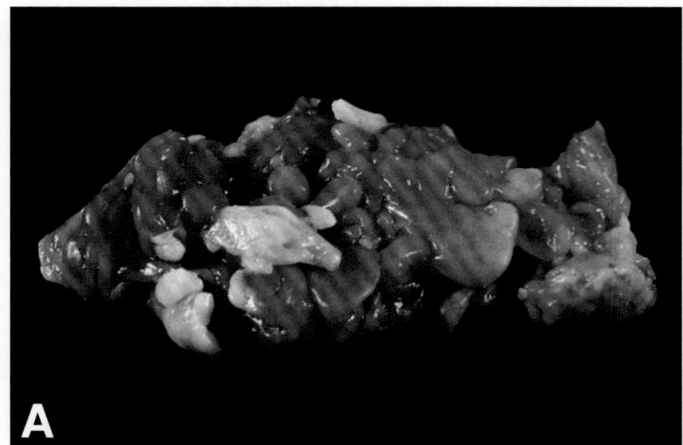

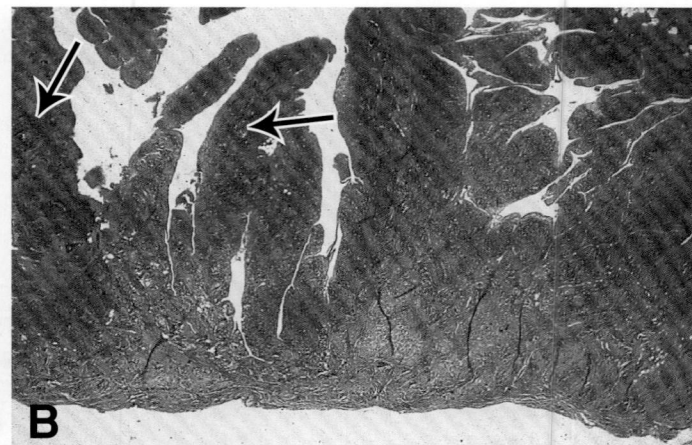

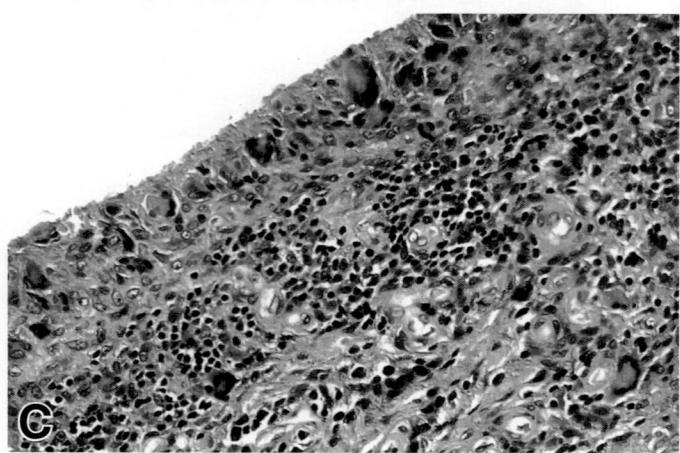

FIGURE 30-56. Rheumatoid arthritis. A. Hyperplastic synovium from a patient with rheumatoid arthritis shows numerous finger-like projections, with focal pale areas of fibrin deposition. The brownish color of the synovium is attributable to hemosiderin accumulation from previous hemorrhage. **B.** A microscopic view reveals prominent lymphoid follicles (Allison–Ghormley bodies; *arrows*), synovial hyperplasia and hypertrophy, villous folds, and thickening of the synovial membrane by fibrosis and inflammation. **C.** A higher-power view of the inflamed synovium demonstrates hyperplasia and hypertrophy of the lining cells. Numerous giant cells are on and below the surface. The stroma is chronically inflamed.

Spondyloarthropathy Is a Seronegative Arthritis Mostly Linked to HLA-B27

A number of clinical entities formerly classified as variants of RA are now recognized to be distinct disorders. These forms of arthritis, known as **spondyloarthropathies**, include ankylosing spondylitis, reactive arthritis, psoriatic arthritis, and arthritis associated with inflammatory bowel disease. They share several features:

- Seronegativity for RF and other serologic markers of RA
- Association with class I histocompatibility antigens, particularly human leukocyte antigen (HLA)-B27
- Sacroiliac and vertebral involvement
- Asymmetric involvement of only a few peripheral joints
- A tendency to inflammation of periarticular tendons and fascia
- Inflammation of other organs, especially associated with uveitis, carditis, and aortitis
- Preferential onset in young men

Ankylosing Spondylitis

Ankylosing spondylitis is an inflammatory arthropathy of the vertebral column and sacroiliac joints. It may be accompanied by asymmetric, peripheral arthritis (30% of patients), and systemic manifestations. It is most common in young men, with peak incidence at about age 20. Over 90% of patients have HLA-B27 (present in 4% to 8% of the normal population), although the disorder affects only 1% of people with this haplotype.

PATHOLOGY: Ankylosing spondylitis begins at the sacroiliac joints bilaterally, and then ascends the spinal column by involving the small joints of the posterior elements of the spine. The result is destruction

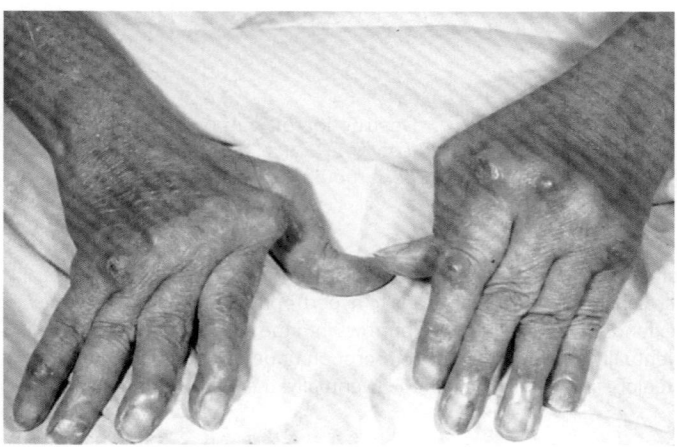

FIGURE 30-57. Rheumatoid arthritis. The hands of a patient with advanced arthritis show swelling of the metacarpophalangeal joints and the classic ulnar deviation of the fingers.

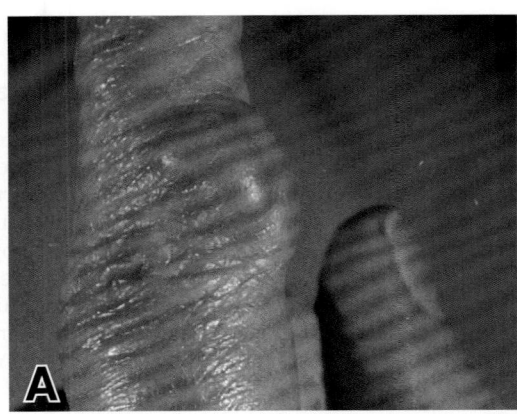
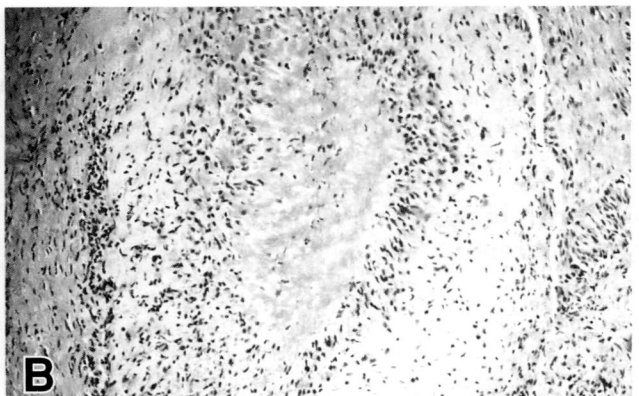

FIGURE 30-58. Rheumatoid nodule. A. A subcutaneous mass on a digit in a patient with rheumatoid arthritis. **B.** Microscopic view of a rheumatoid nodule shows a central area of necrosis surrounded by palisaded macrophages and chronic inflammatory infiltrate.

of these joints, after which the spine becomes fused posteriorly. The unburdened vertebral bodies become square and osteoporotic, because the main force of gravity is borne by the fused posterior elements. In such cases, intervertebral discs undergo ossification and may disappear. Eventually, bony fusion of the vertebral bodies ensues (Fig. 30-59).

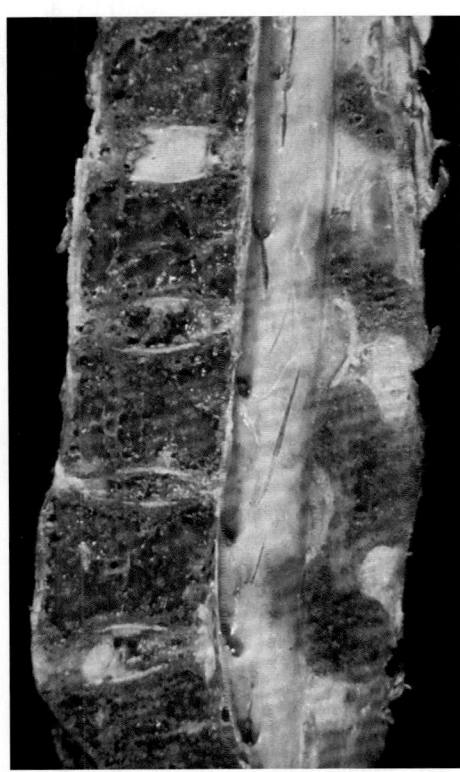

FIGURE 30-59. Ankylosing spondylitis. The vertebrae have been cut longitudinally. The vertebral bodies are square and have lost most of their trabecular bone, owing to osteonecrosis from disuse. Bone bridges fuse one vertebral body to the next across the intervertebral discs. Portions of the intervertebral discs are replaced by bone marrow. Bony bridges also fuse the posterior elements (**ankylosis**). (From Bullough PG. *Atlas of Orthopaedic Pathology*. 2nd ed. New York: Gower Medical Publishing, 1992. Copyright Lippincott Williams & Wilkins.)

A few patients with ankylosing spondylitis rapidly develop crippling spinal disease, but most are able to maintain functionality and live a normal life span. However, up to 5% develop AA amyloidosis and uremia and a few manifest severe cardiac involvement.

Reactive Arthritis

Reactive arthritis (previously, Reiter syndrome) is a triad of: (1) seronegative polyarthritis; (2) conjunctivitis/uveitis; and (3) nonspecific urethritis. It occurs almost exclusively in men and usually follows venereal exposure or an episode of bacillary dysentery. As in ankylosing spondylitis, this syndrome is associated with HLA-B27 in 90% of patients. In fact, after an attack of dysentery, 20% of HLA-B27–positive men develop reactive arthritis.

The pathologic features of this syndrome are comparable to those of RA. More than half of patients develop mucocutaneous lesions similar to those of pustular psoriasis (**keratoderma blenorrhagica**) over the palms, soles, and trunk. In most patients, the disease remits within a year, but 20% develop progressive arthritis, including ankylosing spondylitis.

Psoriatic Arthritis

About 7% of patients with psoriasis develop an inflammatory seronegative arthritis. It arises more commonly in patients with severe disease. HLA-B27 has been linked to psoriatic spondylitis and inflammation of distal interphalangeal joints, and HLA-DR4 has been associated with a rheumatoid pattern of involvement. Joint disease is usually mild and slowly progressive, although a mutilating form is occasionally encountered.

Enteropathic Arthritis

Ulcerative colitis and Crohn disease are accompanied by seronegative peripheral arthritis in 20% of cases and spondylitis in 10%. This form of arthritis also is seen in patients with Whipple disease and after certain bacterial infections of the gut. No particular tissue type is associated with peripheral arthritis, but most patients with ankylosing spondylitis are HLA-B27 positive. It has been proposed that HLA-B27 and proteins from enteric bacteria are structurally related in a manner that affects antigen presentation to the T-cell receptor. Resection of the affected bowel in ulcerative colitis relieves the arthritis, but in Crohn disease, this complication often does not resolve.

Juvenile Arthritis Includes any Inflammatory Arthritis in Children

Several different chronic arthritic conditions in children are included in this designation, also called **Still disease**. In addition to RA, many children with juvenile arthritis eventually develop ankylosing spondylitis, psoriatic arthritis, and other connective tissue diseases.

- **Seropositive arthritis:** Fewer than 10% of children with arthritis are positive for RF and have a polyarticular presentation. Females predominate (80%) among children with seropositive Still disease, and in most cases (75%), antinuclear antibodies are present. HLA-D4 is often present, and more than half of these children eventually develop severe arthritis.
- **Polyarticular disease without systemic symptoms:** One-fourth of juvenile arthritis patients (90% female) have disease of several joints, but are seronegative and do not manifest systemic symptoms. Fewer than 15% of these patients eventually develop severe arthritis.
- **Polyarticular disease with systemic symptoms:** Twenty percent of children with polyarticular arthritis have prominent systemic symptoms, including high fever, rash, hepatosplenomegaly, lymphadenopathy, pleuritis, pericarditis, anemia, and leukocytosis. Most (60%) are males who are negative for RF, and one-fourth suffer with severe arthritis.
- **Pauciarticular arthritis:** Children with involvement of only a few large joints, such as the knee, ankle, elbow, or hip girdle, account for half of all cases of juvenile arthritis. They fall into two general groups. The larger group (80%) mainly comprises females who are negative for RF but exhibit antinuclear antibodies and are positive for HLA-DR5, HLA-DRw6, or HLA-DRw8. Of these patients, one-third have ocular disease, characterized by chronic iridocyclitis (inflammation of the iris and ciliary body). Only a small minority of these children have residual polyarthritis or ocular damage. The smaller group of children with a pauciarticular presentation is composed almost exclusively of males who are negative for both RF and antinuclear bodies and are positive for HLA-B27 (75%). A few have acute iridocyclitis, which typically resolves spontaneously. Some of these patients subsequently develop ankylosing spondylitis.

LYME DISEASE

Lyme disease usually involves the knee or other large joints and is caused by the spirochete Borrelia burgdorferi transmitted by the Ixodes tick (see Chapter 9). Patients generally present with joint effusion and other manifestations of Lyme disease. Although there may be a transient arthritis with acute infection, some patients can develop chronic Lyme arthritis, which is microscopically identical to RA.

GOUT

Primary Gout Is a Disorder of Uric Acid Metabolism

Gout is a heterogeneous group of diseases characterized by increased serum uric acid and urate crystal deposition in joints and kidneys. All such patients have hyperuricemia, but fewer than 15% of people with hyperuricemia have gout. It is characterized by acute and chronic arthritis. Gout is classified as primary or secondary, depending on the etiology of hyperuricemia. In **primary gout**, hyperuricemia occurs without any other disease; **secondary gout** occurs in association with another illness that results in hyperuricemia.

MOLECULAR PATHOGENESIS: Uric acid is a product of purine catabolism. It can accumulate as a result of a high-purine diet or increased *de novo* synthesis. There is a tight balance between uric acid production and tissue deposition of urates. Uric acid is eliminated only in the urine. Thus, the blood uric acid level (normal, <7.0 mg/dL in men, <6.0 mg/dL in women) reflects the difference between the amount of purines ingested and synthesized and renal excretion. Gout can result from: (1) overproduction of purines; (2) increased catabolism of nucleic acids due to greater cell turnover; (3) decreased salvage of free purine bases; or (4) decreased urinary uric acid excretion (Fig. 30-60). High dietary intake of purine-rich foods (e.g., meat) by an otherwise normal person does not lead to hyperuricemia and gout.

Most cases (85%) of idiopathic gout result from an as-yet-unexplained impairment of renal uric acid excretion. In the remainder, primary overproduction of uric acid is the cause, but the underlying abnormality is identified only in a minority of cases.

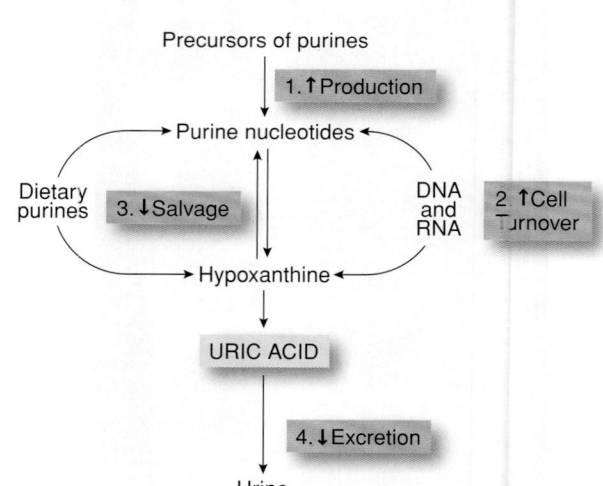

FIGURE 30-60. Pathogenesis of hyperuricemia and gout. Purine nucleotides are synthesized *de novo* from nonpurine precursors or derived from preformed purines in the diet. Purine nucleotides are catabolized to hypoxanthine or incorporated into nucleic acids. The degradation of nucleic acids and dietary purines also produces hypoxanthine. Hypoxanthine is converted to uric acid, which in turn is excreted in the urine. Hyperuricemia and gout result from: (*1*) increased *de novo* purine synthesis; (*2*) increased cell turnover; (*3*) decreased salvage of dietary purines and hypoxanthine; and (*4*) decreased uric acid excretion by the kidneys.

A *familial tendency* to gout has been recognized since the time of Galen. Hyperuricemia is common among relatives of patients with gout. Primary hyperuricemia in some people is apparently inherited as an autosomal dominant trait with variable expression, in some as an X-linked abnormality and in others as a result of polygenic determinants. Precocious gout exhibits a strong familial tendency. The consensus today is that multiple genes control the level of serum uric acid.

Gout Can Be due to Inborn Errors of Metabolism

The rate-limiting step in purine synthesis is condensation of glutamine with phosphoribosyl pyrophosphate (PP-ribose-P) to form phosphoribosylamine. Increased intracellular PP-ribose-P accelerates purine biosynthesis. PP-ribose-P, through the activity of hypoxanthine phosphoribosyl transferase (HPRT), also condenses with, and so salvages, purine bases (hypoxanthine and guanine) derived from catabolism of nucleic acids. Although the specific cause of an abnormally high rate of urate production is not known in most cases of primary gout, two inborn errors of metabolism are known to lead to elevated PP-ribose-P.

Lesch–Nyhan syndrome is an inherited, X-linked (Xq26-q27) deficiency of HPRT, a defect that leads to accumulation of PP-ribose-P, and in turn to enhanced purine synthesis. Children with this syndrome are clinically normal at birth but exhibit developmental delays and neurologic dysfunction within the first year. Most are mentally retarded and exhibit self-mutilation. They are hyperuricemic and eventually develop gouty arthritis. Obstructive (urate related) nephropathy and hematologic abnormalities also occur.

Secondary Gout Often Results From DNA Turnover

A number of conditions result in hyperuricemia and secondary gout. As in primary gout, secondary hyperuricemia may reflect overproduction or decreased urinary excretion of uric acid. Increased production is most often associated with increased nucleic acid turnover, as seen in leukemias and lymphomas and after chemotherapy. Accelerated turnover of adenosine triphosphate (ATP), which occurs in glycogen storage diseases and tissue hypoxia, may also lead to overproduction of uric acid. Ethanol intake evokes secondary hyperuricemia, in part owing to accelerated ATP catabolism and (to a lesser degree) decreased renal excretion of uric acid. Reduced urate excretion may also result from primary renal disease. Dehydration and diuretics increase tubular reabsorption of uric acid and induce hyperuricemia. In fact, various drugs are implicated in 20% of patients with hyperuricemia.

Saturnine gout was described in 18th-century England, where this disease was prevalent among the upper classes with lead plumbing in their houses (Saturn is the symbol for lead). It is now recognized that these patients were afflicted with lead nephropathy. The Romans had a similar problem, because they drank from vessels containing lead.

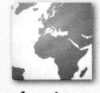 **EPIDEMIOLOGY:** Primary gout usually afflicts adult men; only 5% of cases occur in women. It is rare in children before puberty and in women during the reproductive years. Peak incidence is in the fifth decade. This sex distribution can be traced to the fact that at all ages, mean serum urate concentrations in women are lower than in men, although they increase after menopause. Many patients have a family history of gout, but environmental factors are also important. Positive correlations exist between the prevalence of hyperuricemia in a population and mean weight, protein intake, alcohol consumption, social class, and intelligence. Thus, gout is a disease that exemplifies the interplay between genetic predisposition and environmental influences.

 PATHOLOGY: When sodium urate crystals precipitate from supersaturated body fluids, they adsorb fibronectin, complement, and a number of other proteins on their surfaces. Neutrophils that have ingested urate crystals release activated oxygen species and lysosomal enzymes, which mediate tissue injury and promote an inflammatory response.

The presence of long, needle-shaped crystals that are negatively birefringent under polarized light is diagnostic of gout (Fig. 30-61). Monosodium urate monohydrate crystals may be found intracellularly in leukocytes of the synovial fluid. A **tophus** is an extracellular soft-tissue deposit of urate crystals surrounded by foreign body giant cells and an associated inflammatory cell response. These granuloma-like areas are found in cartilage, in any of the soft tissues around joints and even in the subchondral bone marrow adjacent to joints.

Macroscopically, any chalky white deposit on intraarticular surfaces, including articular cartilage, suggests gout (Fig. 30-61B). Radiologically, gouty arthritis exhibits characteristic, punched-out, juxta-articular, lytic ("rat bite") lesions with only minimal reactive new bone (Fig. 30-62). In contrast to RA, there is no juxta-articular osteopenia in gout.

Renal urate deposits occur between the tubules, especially at the apices of the medulla. These areas are grossly visible as small, shiny, golden-yellow, linear streaks in the medulla.

CLINICAL FEATURES: The clinical course of gout is divided into four stages: (1) asymptomatic hyperuricemia; (2) acute gouty arthritis; (3) intercritical gout; and (4) chronic tophaceous gout. Renal stones may occur in any stage except the first. In most cases, symptomatic gout appears before renal stones, which usually require 20 to 30 years of sustained hyperuricemia.

- **Asymptomatic hyperuricemia** often precedes clinically evident gout by many years.
- **Acute gouty arthritis** was well characterized by Thomas Sydenham, who described his own disease in the 1600s. It is a painful condition that usually involves one joint, without constitutional symptoms. Later in the course of the disease, polyarticular involvement with fever is common. At least half of patients present with a painful and red 1st metatarsophalangeal joint (great toe), designated **"podagra."** Eventually, 90% of all patients have such an attack. Commonly, a gouty attack begins at night and is exquisitely painful, simulating an acute

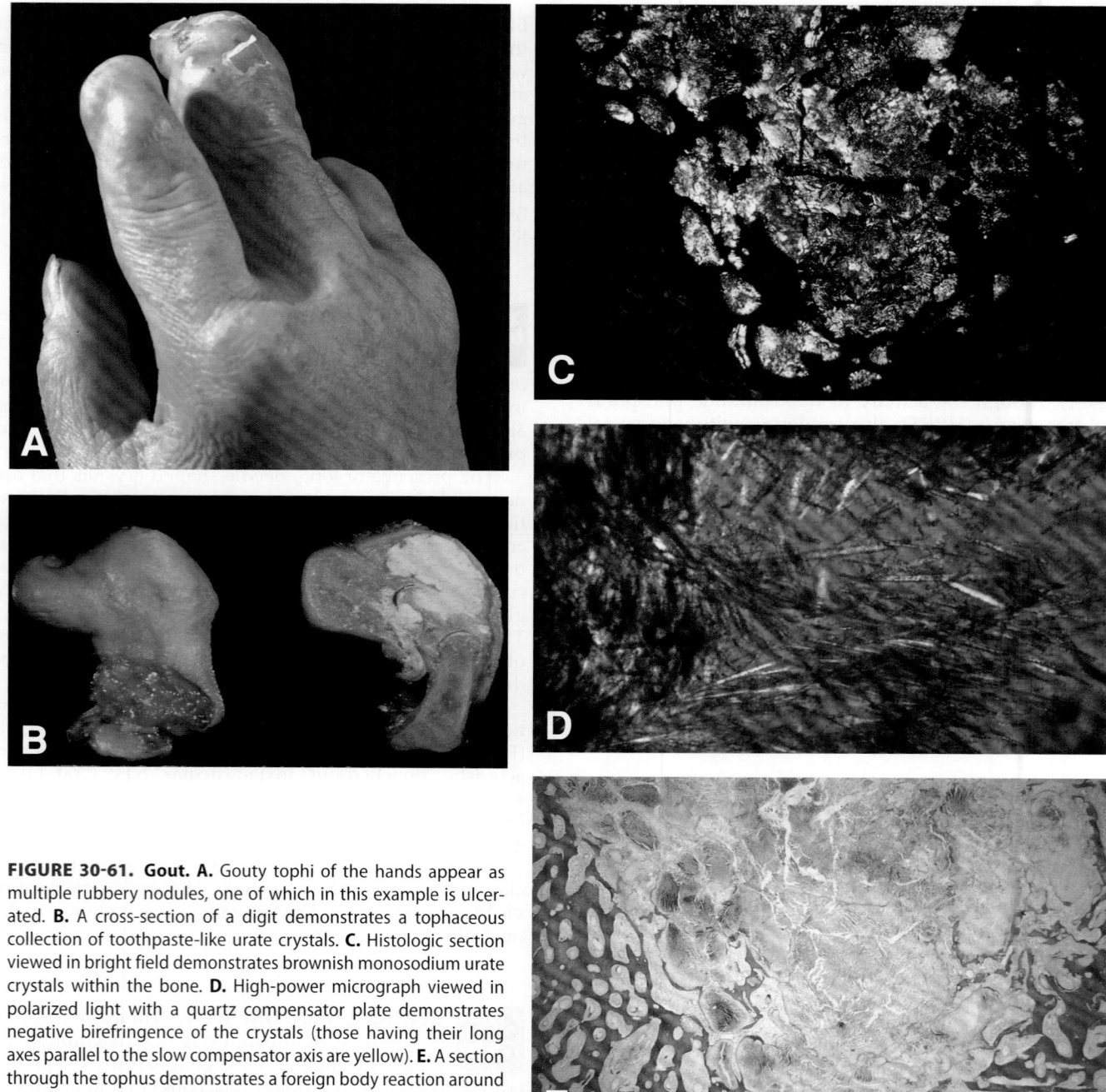

FIGURE 30-61. Gout. A. Gouty tophi of the hands appear as multiple rubbery nodules, one of which in this example is ulcerated. **B.** A cross-section of a digit demonstrates a tophaceous collection of toothpaste-like urate crystals. **C.** Histologic section viewed in bright field demonstrates brownish monosodium urate crystals within the bone. **D.** High-power micrograph viewed in polarized light with a quartz compensator plate demonstrates negative birefringence of the crystals (those having their long axes parallel to the slow compensator axis are yellow). **E.** A section through the tophus demonstrates a foreign body reaction around a pink, amorphous lesion from which urate crystals have been dissolved during usual aqueous tissue processing for microscopy.

bacterial infection of the affected joint. A large meal or drinking alcoholic beverages may trigger an attack, but other specific events such as trauma, certain drugs, and surgery may also be responsible. Even when untreated, acute attacks of gout are self-limited.

- The **intercritical period** is the asymptomatic interval between the initial acute attack and subsequent episodes. These periods may last up to 10 years, but later attacks tend to be increasingly severe, prolonged, and polyarticular.

- **Tophaceous gout** eventually appears in the untreated patient in the form of tophi in the cartilage, synovial membranes, tendons, and soft tissues.

Renal failure is responsible for 10% of deaths in patients with gout. One-third of patients have mild albuminuria, reduced glomerular filtration and decreased renal concentrating ability. However, the contribution of urate nephropathy to chronic renal dysfunction is unclear, and hypertension, pre-existing kidney disease, and intake of

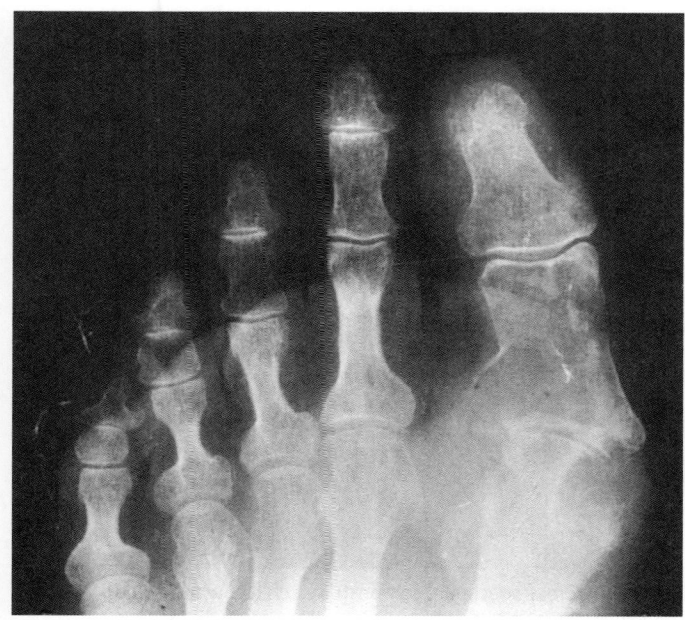

FIGURE 30-62. Gout. A radiograph of the 1st metatarsophalangeal joint shows a lytic lesion that has destroyed the joint space. There is an adjacent soft-tissue tophus and edema.

analgesic drugs may be more important. In patients with severe gout caused by inherited enzyme deficiencies and in those with a precocious presentation, urate nephropathy is a prominent feature. **Urate stones** constitute 10% of all renal calculi in the United States and up to 40% in Israel and Australia. The prevalence of urate stones correlates with the serum concentration of uric acid and affects 25% of gout patients. Patients also have an increased frequency of calcium-containing stones, in which uric acid may serve as a nidus for calcium stone formation.

Treatment of gout is designed to: (1) decrease the severity of acute attacks; (2) reduce serum urate; (3) prevent future attacks; (4) promote dissolution of urate deposits; and (5) alkalinize the urine to prevent stone formation. Nonsteroidal anti-inflammatory drugs are used to interrupt the inflammatory process, and prevent or mitigate acute attacks. Colchicine has been used for hundreds of years as a prophylactic agent to prevent recurrent episodes. Uricosuric drugs that interfere with urate reabsorption by the renal tubules are often useful.

Allopurinol is a competitive inhibitor of xanthine oxidase, the enzyme that converts xanthine and hypoxanthine to uric acid. It produces a prompt decrease in uricosemia and uricosuria and is used in people with renal insufficiency and those who are resistant to other uricosuric drugs. It is also used in patients undergoing chemotherapy for hematopoietic proliferative disorders, which increases the rate of urate production.

CALCIUM PYROPHOSPHATE DIHYDRATE DEPOSITION DISEASE (CHONDROCALCINOSIS AND PSEUDOGOUT)

Calcium pyrophosphate dihydrate (CPPD) deposition disease involves accumulation of this compound in synovial membranes, joint cartilage (chondrocalcinosis), ligaments

and tendons. It can be idiopathic, associated with trauma, linked to a number of metabolic disorders or, in rare cases, hereditary. When symptomatic, it is called pseudogout.

CPPD deposition disease is principally a condition of old age; half of those over age 85 are afflicted. Most cases in the elderly are asymptomatic. Because fully two-thirds of these patients manifest pre-existing joint damage, it is thought that trauma and the aging process in cartilage promote nucleation of CPFD crystals. In asymptomatic cases, punctate or linear calcifications may occur in any fibrocartilage or hyaline cartilage surface. For example, radiography of the knee may disclose linear streaks that outline the menisci.

MOLECULAR PATHOGENESIS: The major predisposing abnormality in patients with CPPD deposition disease is excessive inorganic pyrophosphate in synovial fluid. This material derives from hydrolysis of nucleoside triphosphates in joint chondrocytes. Increased pyrophosphate in synovial fluid can result from either increased production or decreased catabolism.

CPPD deposition is commonly found in the knees after trauma and after surgical removal of the menisci. Nucleotides released by injured articular cartilage may act as substrates for nucleotide triphosphate pyrophosphohydrolase (NTP), thus increasing production of pyrophosphate. A number of other disorders lead to deposition of CPPD crystals, including hyperparathyroidism, hypothyroidism, hemochromatosis, Wilson disease, and ochronosis. Iron and copper inhibit pyrophosphatase, thus accounting for decreased degradation of pyrophosphate.

Loss-of-function mutations in *ANKH* cause familial autosomal dominant CPPD chondrocalcinosis. This gene encodes a membrane pyrophosphate transporter that inhibits mineralization in several tissues including joints, articular cartilage, and tendons. Mutated ANKH elevates intracellular pyrophosphate and reduces extracellular pyrophosphate.

Hypophosphatasia is a heritable condition arising from deficient alkaline phosphatase (the enzyme that hydrolyzes pyrophosphate) activity in serum and tissue. As a result, pyrophosphate is not adequately metabolized and accumulates in synovial fluid.

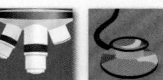

PATHOLOGY AND CLINICAL FEATURES: A minority of patients symptomatic with CPPD deposition disease are classified according to the nature of joint involvement.

- **Pseudogout** refers to self-limited attacks of acute arthritis lasting from 1 day to 4 weeks and involving one or two joints. Some 25% of patients with CPPD deposition disease experience acute onset of gout-like symptoms such as inflammation and swelling of the knees, ankles, wrists, elbows, hips, or shoulders. Metatarsophalangeal joints, frequently affected in gout, are usually spared. Synovial fluid exhibits abundant leukocytes containing CPPD crystals.
- **Pseudorheumatoid arthritis** is a variant of CPPD deposition disease in which multiple joints are chronically involved. Symptoms are mild and resemble those of RA.

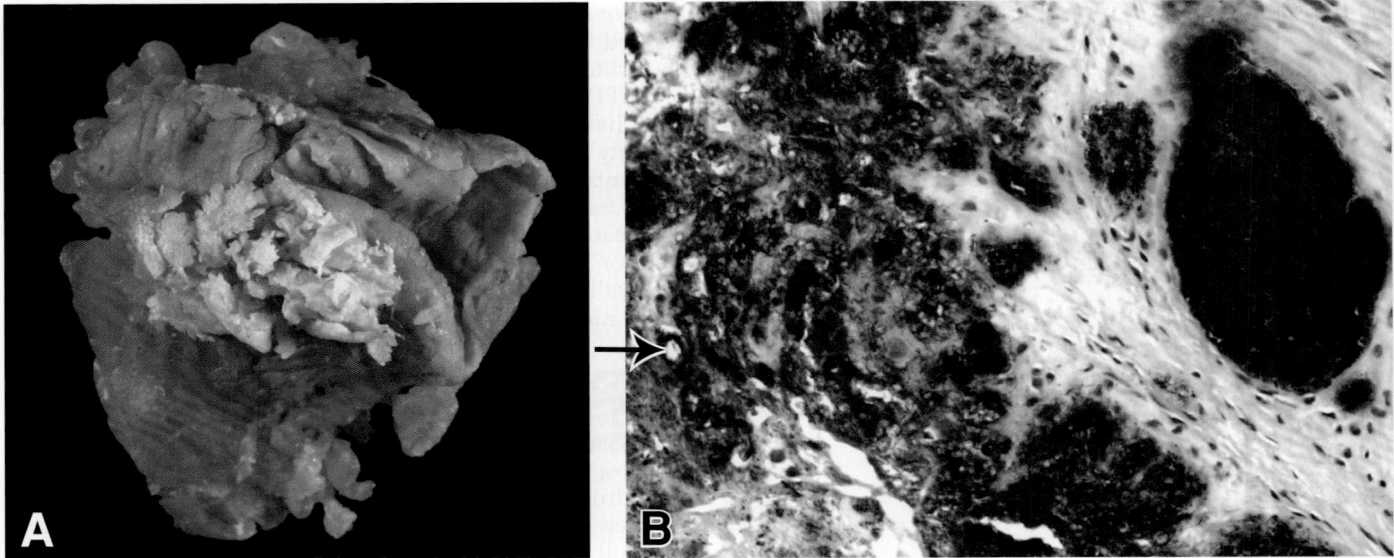

FIGURE 30-63. Calcium pyrophosphate dihydrate (CPPD) deposition disease. A. Gross specimen demonstrates chalky-white calcific material. **B.** Microscopically, the deposits are deep purple with discernible rhomboid-shaped crystals (*arrow*).

- **Pseudo-osteoarthritis** has symptoms similar to those of osteoarthritis.
- **Pseudoneurotrophic disease** is characterized by joint destruction severe enough to resemble a neurotrophic joint.

On gross examination, CPPD deposits appear as chalky white areas on cartilaginous surfaces (Fig. 30-63A). Unlike needle-shaped urate crystals, they are stubby, short, and rhomboid ("coffin shaped") and display weak positive birefringence under polarized light. In contrast to urate crystals, CPPD crystals are less soluble in water and are easily found in tissue sections within purple calcific deposits (Fig. 30-63B). Only a few mononuclear cells and macrophages surround foci of crystal deposition.

Treatment of CPPD is largely symptomatic pain control. Nonsteroidal anti-inflammatory drugs and steroids are commonly used.

CALCIUM HYDROXYAPATITE DEPOSITION DISEASE

Calcium HA deposition disease is an acute or chronic arthritis characterized by HA crystals within inflammatory cells in joint tissue and synovial fluid. Calcium HA, the major mineral of bone and teeth, is also deposited in dystrophic and metastatic calcification. HA crystals are frequently encountered in the synovial fluid of joints involved by osteoarthritis, but severe HA deposition appears to be a distinct entity. Joints most frequently involved are the knee, shoulder, hip, and fingers. Attacks may last several days.

HEMOPHILIA, HEMOCHROMATOSIS, AND OCHRONOSIS

Hemophilia, hemochromatosis, and ochronosis (see Chapter 6) all produce joint disease associated with degradation of the matrix and destruction of the articular cartilage.

- **Hemophilia** gives rise to severe forms of arthritis because of extensive bleeding into joints (hemarthrosis), particularly the knees, elbows, ankles, shoulders, and hips. This damages the articular cartilage matrix and promotes synovial proliferation that resembles RA.
- **Hemochromatosis** is complicated by arthritis in half of affected patients. The hands, hips, and knees may be involved in recurrent attacks.
- **Ochronosis** is a rare, autosomal recessive disease caused by a defect in homogentisic acid oxidase. Deposition of homogentisic acid produces polymers in the cartilage of the joints, including the intervertebral discs, eventually causing them to become brittle and degenerate. Homogentisic acid is excreted in the urine, causing it to become black upon standing or with alkalinity. This phenomenon is called **alkaptonuria**.

TUMORS AND TUMOR-LIKE LESIONS OF JOINTS

True neoplasms of the joints are rare. The most common malignant lesions of the synovium are metastatic carcinomas, particularly adenocarcinoma of the colon, breast, and lung. Lymphoproliferative diseases (e.g., leukemia) may also involve the synovium, mimicking other conditions, such as RA. It is unusual for primary malignant bone tumors to extend into the joint, although they may invade the joint capsule from the soft tissues.

A Ganglion Is a Small Fluid-Filled Cyst

A ganglion is a thin-walled, simple cyst containing clear mucinous fluid. Ganglion cysts occur most commonly on the extensor surfaces of the hands and feet, especially the wrist. They are more common in women between the ages of 25 and 45 years. They arise either from the synovium or from areas of myxoid change in the connective tissue, possibly after trauma. The cyst wall is composed of fibrous tissue, and there is no cell lining. They may be painful and can be readily removed surgically.

A **Baker cyst** is a herniation of the synovium of the knee joint into the popliteal space. It is most often seen in association with various forms of arthritis, in which intra-articular pressure is increased. The cyst contains synovial fluid and microscopically demonstrates a synovial cell lining.

Synovial Chondromatosis Features Cartilage Nodules in a Joint

Synovial chondromatosis is a benign, self-limited disease in which hyaline cartilage nodules form in the synovium, become detached and float free in the synovial fluid. Chronic irritation produced by these "loose" bodies stimulates the synovium to secrete large amounts of synovial fluid and also causes bleeding in the synovial membrane. Synovial chondromatosis involves the large diarthrodial joints of young and middle-aged men, affecting the knee in most cases, but also the hip, elbow, shoulder, ankle, and temporomandibular joints. Patients complain of pain, stiffness, and locking of the joint, with associated bloody effusions.

Unlike cartilage that detaches from articular surfaces in osteoarthritis, fragments of hyaline cartilage in synovial chondromatosis are formed *de novo* in the synovium (Fig. 30-64). They do not have a tidemark and thus differ morphologically from true articular cartilage. Occasionally, cartilage nodules being formed in the synovium undergo endochondral ossification, in which case the disease is called **synovial osteochondromatosis**. If these nodules detach, the bony portions undergo necrosis, but the cartilage fragments remain viable and enlarge because they are nourished by synovial fluid. The condition is treated by evacuating the joint and performing a synovectomy. Recurrence is seen in 15% to 20% of the cases, but malignant transformation is very rare.

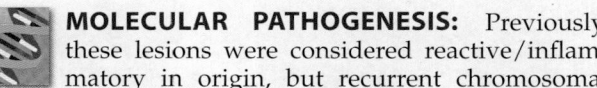 **MOLECULAR PATHOGENESIS:** Dysregulation of Sonic Hedgehog signaling, known to occur in various benign cartilaginous tumors, has been implicated in development of synovial chondromatosis in animal models. Thus, this condition may be a benign neoplasm. Clonal karyotypic abnormalities have been detected in a few cases of synovial chondromatosis, with diploid or near-diploid complements, chromosome 6 anomalies, rearrangements of 1p22 and 1p13, and extra copies of chromosome 5.

Tenosynovial Giant Cell Tumor Is a Benign Neoplasm of Synovial Lining

This is the most common neoplasm of the synovium and tendon sheath. It has both localized and diffuse forms and the lesions may be intra- or extra-articular.

- **Localized tenosynovial GCT or GCT of the tendon sheath** involves the hands and feet. In fact, it is the most common soft-tissue tumor of the hand. It occurs mostly in young and middle-aged women (30 to 50 years) and involves flexor surfaces of the middle or index fingers. These tumors are usually well circumscribed and grow slowly.
- **Diffuse tenosynovial GCT or pigmented villonodular synovitis (PVNS)** is characterized by an ill-defined, exuberant proliferation of synovial lining cells arising from periarticular soft tissues, with extension into the subsynovial tissue. It involves a single joint, usually in young adults, and is seen equally in men and women. The most common site is the knee (80%), but it also occurs in the hip, ankle, calcaneocuboid joint, elbow, and less frequently tendon sheaths of the fingers and toes.

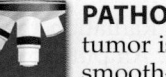 **MOLECULAR PATHOGENESIS:** Previously, these lesions were considered reactive/inflammatory in origin, but recurrent chromosomal aberrations have been described in both forms, supporting a neoplastic nature. Translocations involving the short arm of chromosome 1 have been detected, most commonly t(1;2)(p11;q35-36) or (p13;q37), leading to fusion of *CSF-1*, which encodes colony-stimulating factor-1, and *COL6a3* which makes a component of type IV collagen involved in extracellular matrix and basement membrane formation. Trisomies for chromosomes 5 and 7 have been found only in the diffuse form. The association of these anomalies with tumor pathogenesis is unclear.

PATHOLOGY: Localized tenosynovial giant cell tumor is typically a small (<4 cm), multinodular, smooth-contoured, partially encapsulated, exophytic mass attached to a tendon sheath. Tumors in the diffuse form are usually larger than 5 cm and poorly circumscribed. They invade joints and erode bone (Fig. 30-65A). They may insinuate through joint capsules into soft tissue and encompass nerves and arteries, sometimes necessitating radical surgical excision. The synovium develops enlarged folds and nodular excrescences, which are brown in color owing to their iron pigment content (Fig. 30-65B). Microscopically, both types of tumors have similar histology. They are composed of bland mononuclear cells resembling macrophages, admixed with scattered multinucleated giant cells, fibroblasts, and foam cells. Hemosiderin-laden macrophages reflect previous hemorrhage (Fig. 30-65C,D). The diffuse form extensively infiltrates surrounding tissues and frequently displays a villous configuration.

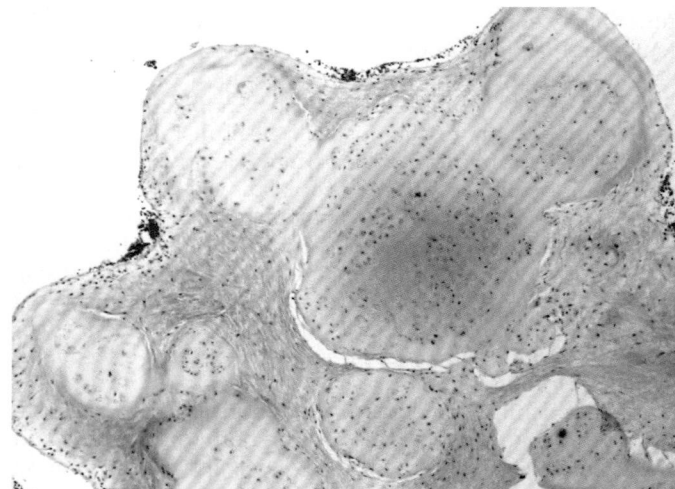

FIGURE 30-64. Synovial chondromatosis. Nodules of benign hyaline cartilage form in the synovium.

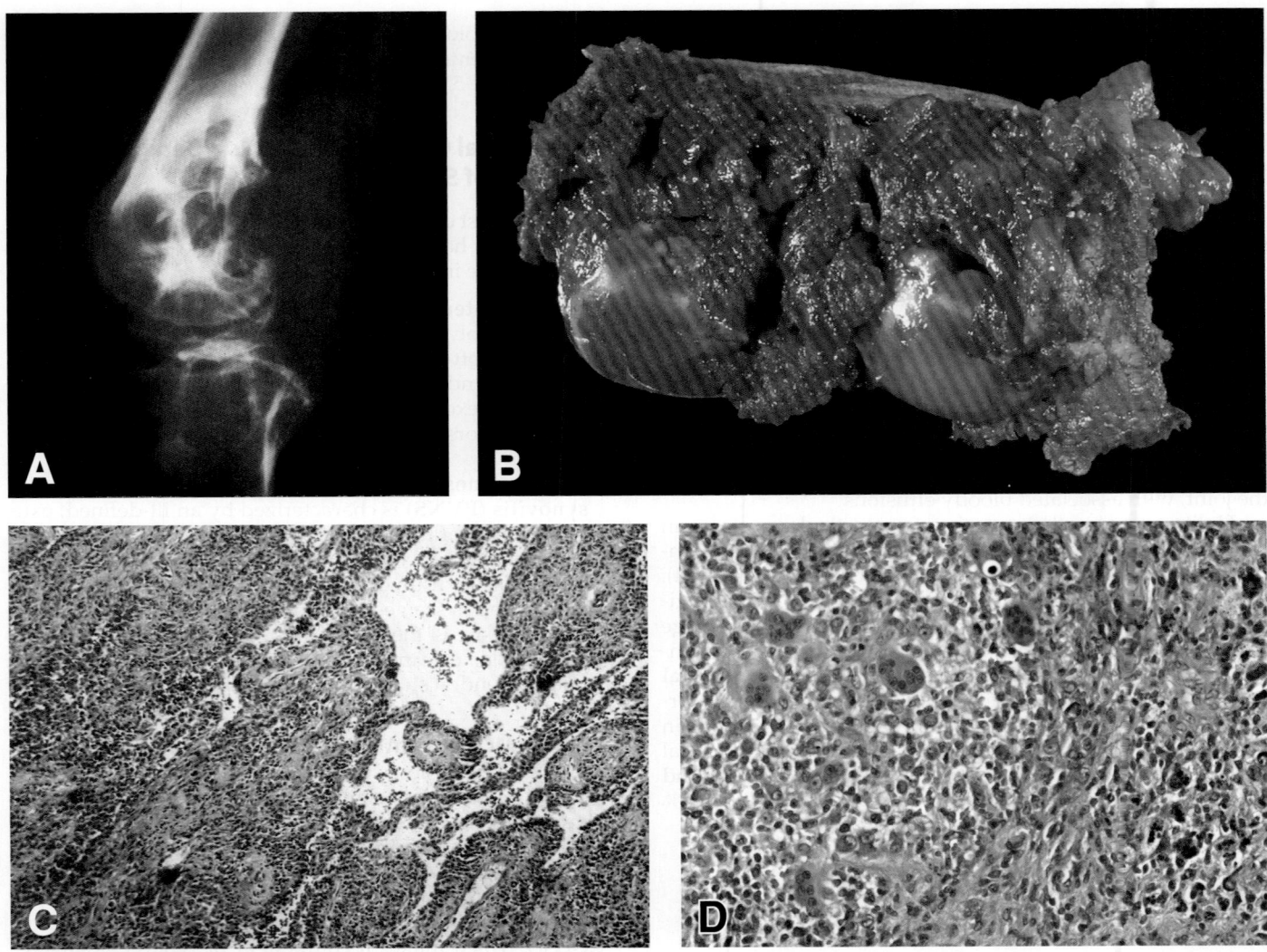

FIGURE 30-65. Pigmented villonodular synovitis. A. Radiograph of the knee demonstrates confluent erosions of the distal femur and proximal tibia and a soft-tissue mass within the joint. **B.** Gross specimen shows massive destruction of the femoral condyles. Note brown color and nodular thickenings. **C.** Low-power microscopy demonstrates thickened villous synovium. **D.** At higher power, the cellular infiltrate mainly consists of mononuclear histiocytic synoviocytes, many of which contain brown hemosiderin pigment, and multinucleated giant cells.

Treatment involves surgical excision. Radiation therapy has been used in unresectable cases. Amputation is occasionally necessary for local control. Tumors recur in 10% to 20% of cases of localized tenosynovial giant cell tumor, in contrast to 40% to 50% in the diffuse form. Metastases do not occur. A malignant counterpart has been described, but it is very rare.

Soft-Tissue Tumors

Soft-tissue tumors are mesenchymal neoplasms that can arise anywhere in the body but are most commonly found within skeletal muscle, fat, fibrous tissue, or blood vessels. Tumors of peripheral nerves (see Chapter 31) and other tumors of neuroectodermal differentiation may be included in the category of soft-tissue tumors. Soft-tissue tumors are thought to arise from pluripotent mesenchymal stem cells residing in soft tissues and bone marrow. While some tumors may show evidence of differentiation toward a particular cell type (fibroblastic, adipocytic, vascular, myoid, etc.), many tumors have no defined line of differentiation. However, many exhibit characteristic and unique genomic abnormalities that are diagnostically useful (Table 30-2).

Soft-tissue tumors may be benign, locally aggressive or malignant. Benign soft-tissue neoplasms are 100 times more common than malignant ones (sarcomas), which account for <1% of all malignancies in the United States. Locally aggressive tumors invade and may recur locally (e.g., fibromatosis). Malignant soft-tissue tumors (sarcomas) can metastasize via the bloodstream, usually to the lungs or bone. ***Patients generally die of metastatic disease rather than local invasion at the primary tumor site.***

Distinguishing sarcomas from benign mimics is key to prognostication; outcome depends on both tumor grade and stage. Several grading schemes have been published, among which the Fédération National des Centres de Lutte Contre le Cancer (FNCLCC) system is widely accepted. FNCLCC grading is based on cellular phenotype (histologic tumor

TABLE 30-2

SELECTED CHROMOSOMAL ABNORMALITIES IN SOFT-TISSUE TUMORS

Tumor Type	Chromosomal Abnormality	Gene(s)
Fibroblastic Tumors		
Nodular fasciitis	t(17;22)(p13;q13)	*MYH9-USP6*
Congenital/infantile fibrosarcoma	t(12;15)(p13;q25)	*ETV6-NTRK3*
Dermatofibrosarcoma protuberans	t(17;22)(q21;q13)	*COLIA1-PDGFB*
Low-grade fibromyxoid sarcoma	t(7;16)(q33;p11)	*FUS-CREB3L2*
	t(11;16)(p11;p11)	*FUS-CREB3L1*
Sclerosing epithelioid fibrosarcoma	t(7;16)(p22;q24)	*FUS-CREB3L2*
Inflammatory myofibroblastic tumor	t(1;2)(q22;p23)	*TPM3-ALK*
	t(2;19)(p23;p13)	*TPM4-ALK*
	t(2;17)(p23;q23)	*CLTC-ALK*
	t(2;2)(p23;q13)	*RANBP2-ALK*
	t(2;11)(p23;p15)	*CARS-ALK*
	inv(2)(p23;q35)	*ATIC-ALK*
Lipogenic Tumors		
Well-differentiated liposarcoma/atypical lipomatous tumor/dedifferentiated liposarcoma	12q14-15 (ring chromosomes, giant marker chromosomes)	Amplification of *MDM2, CDK4, HMGA2, GLI, SAS*
Myxoid-/round-cell liposarcoma	t(12;16)(q13;p11)	*FUS-DDIT3*
	t(12;22)(q13;q12)	*EWSR1-DDIT3*
Myogenic Tumors		
Alveolar rhabdomyosarcoma	t(2;13)(q35;q14)	*PAX3-FKHR*
	t(1;13)(p36;q14)	*PAX7-FKHR*
	t(X;2)(q13;q35)	*PAX3-AFX*
Spindle-cell/sclerosing rhabdomyosarcoma	t(6;8)(p12, q11.2)	*SRF-NCOA2*
	t(8;11)(q11.2;p15.3)	*TEAD1-NCOA2*
		MYOD1 mutation
Neuroectodermal Tumors		
Clear-cell sarcoma	t(12;22)(q13;q12)	*EWSR1-ATF1*
	t(2;22)(q33;q12)	*EWSR1-CREB1*
Ewing sarcoma; primitive neuroectodermal tumor (PNET)	t(11;22)(q24;q12)	*EWSR1-FLI1*
	t(21;22)(q22;q12)	*EWSR1-ERG*
	t(7;22)(p22;q12)	*EWSR1-ETV1*
	t(2;22)(q33;q12)	*EWSR1-FEV*
	t(16;21)(p11;q22)	*FUS-ERG*
	t(2;16)(q35;p11)	*FUS-FEV*
Synovial sarcoma	t(X;18)(p11;q11)	*SS18-SSX1, SSX2, SSX4*

type and degree of differentiation), mitotic activity, and presence of tumor necrosis as indicators of aggressive behavior. Grade is then combined with site-specific tumor size criteria and metastatic status to determine overall staging and predict risk.

As detailed below, genetic determinants have been identified in some soft-tissue tumors including neurofibromatosis type 1, tuberous sclerosis, Osler–Weber–Rendu disease, Li-Fraumeni syndrome, and Gardner syndrome. Radiation injury also contributes to the development of sarcomas, in particular angiosarcoma, osteosarcoma, or undifferentiated sarcoma, years after exposure. There is no evidence to support the association of trauma with the development of soft-tissue tumors, and injury merely draws attention to a pre-existing tumor.

A few important general principles relate to soft-tissue tumors:

- Superficial tumors tend to be benign.
- Deep lesions are often malignant.
- Large tumors are more often malignant than small ones.
- Rapidly growing tumors are more likely to be malignant than tumors that develop slowly.
- Calcification may exist in both benign and malignant tumors.
- Benign tumors are relatively avascular, while most malignant ones are hypervascular.
- Some soft-tissue tumors are classified on the basis of genetic or molecular findings.

TUMORS AND TUMOR-LIKE CONDITIONS OF FIBROUS ORIGIN

Nodular Fasciitis Is a Benign Lesion That May Mimic a Sarcoma

Nodular fasciitis is a rapidly growing but self-limited tumor that commonly affects superficial tissues of the forearm, trunk, and back and is characterized by rearrangement of the USP6 gene. Most cases occur in young adults who come to medical attention because of the rapid growth of the lesion. Histologically, nodular fasciitis may be mistaken for a sarcoma, as it is hypercellular and has abundant mitoses and numerous immature, spindle-shaped fibroblasts, and myofibroblasts in a myxoid stroma (Fig. 30-66). Long thought to be a posttraumatic reactive condition, nodular fasciitis is now known to be a neoplasm driven by overexpression of USP6, an oncogenic protein with possible roles in inflammation and proliferation. USP6 overexpression in nodular fasciitis most commonly results from chromosomal rearrangement fusing the *MYH9* promoter to *USP6,* although alternative gene fusions have been reported. Despite the underlying genetic alterations, nodular fasciitis is self-limited and is cured by surgical excision.

Fibromatosis Is a Locally Aggressive Proliferation of Fibroblasts

Fibromatosis is a locally invasive, slowly growing mass that may occur virtually anywhere in the body. Although histologically similar, superficial and deep "aggressive" variants of fibromatosis differ genetically. Fibromatosis does not metastasize, but surgical resection of deep tumors is often followed by local recurrence. Diabetics, alcoholics, and

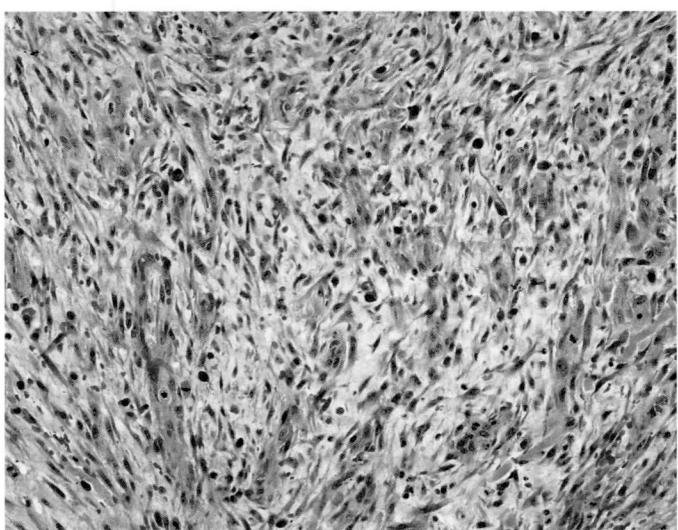

FIGURE 30-66. Nodular fasciitis. Elongated spindle and stellate cells are arranged haphazardly in a loose myxoid stroma, giving the lesion a "tissue culture–like" appearance. Extravasated erythrocytes and scattered lymphocytes are a common finding. Mitotic figures may be prominent.

epileptics have an increased incidence of fibromatosis, as do patients with familial adenomatous polyposis.

 MOLECULAR PATHOGENESIS: Fibromatosis results from signaling alterations in the Wnt pathway. Mutations involving *APC* or *CTNNB1* occur in deep aggressive fibromatosis (desmoid tumor) but not in superficial variants. Inactivating mutations in *APC* are found mostly in cases of fibromatosis associated with familial adenomatous polyposis. The APC protein binds β-catenin and enhances its proteasomal degradation. Loss of APC thus indirectly stabilizes β-catenin and promotes its translocation to cell nuclei where it interacts with TCF/LEF transcription factors to alter gene expression. Normally, β-catenin plays a key role in the canonical Wnt signaling pathway, which modulates developmental genes. Abnormal activation of this pathway can also promote fibromatosis. Most sporadic cases of desmoid tumor have activating (gain-of-function) mutations in *CTNNB1,* the gene encoding β-catenin, which render it resistant to inhibitory effects of APC. Thus, mutations in both the *APC* and *CTNNB1* genes result in persistent stabilization of β-catenin.

PATHOLOGY: Grossly, the lesions of fibromatosis tend to be large, firm and whitish, with poorly demarcated borders and a whorled appearance on cut surfaces. Microscopic examination reveals sheets and interdigitating fascicles of benign-appearing spindle cells (fibroblasts) with little mitotic activity (Fig. 30-67). Because microscopic tongues of tumor interdigitate with normal structures, surgical "shelling out" of these lesion is followed by recurrences in half of cases.

Specific forms of fibromatosis are identified by their characteristic locations:

- **Palmar fibromatosis** (Dupuytren contracture) is the most common form of fibromatosis. It affects 1% to 2%

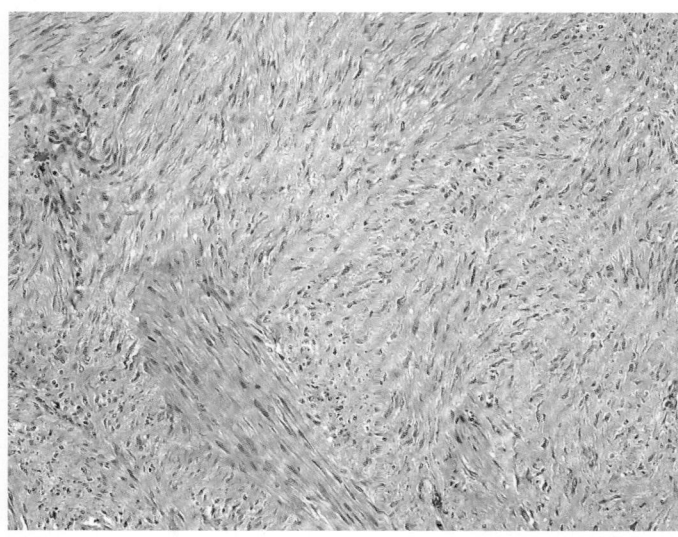

FIGURE 30-67. Fibromatosis. The lesion is composed of fascicles of bland spindle cells arrayed in long sweeping fascicles in a collagenous stroma.

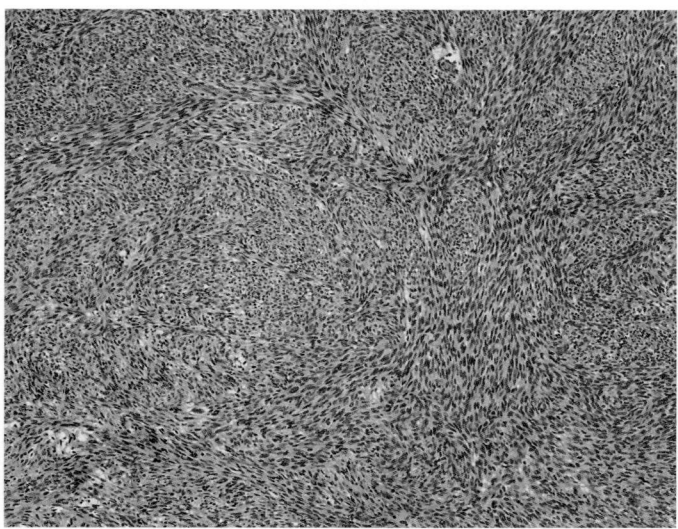

FIGURE 30-68. Fibrosarcoma. Irregularly arranged malignant fibroblasts are characterized by dark, irregular, and elongated nuclei of varying sizes.

of the general population but as many as 20% of people older than 65. In half of cases, the lesion is bilateral, and in 10% of cases, it is associated with fibromatosis in other locations. Fibrous nodules and cord-like bands in the palmar fascia eventually lead to flexion contractures of the fingers, particularly the fourth and fifth digits.

- **Plantar fibromatosis** is similar to palmar fibromatosis, except it is less frequent and involves the plantar aponeurosis.

- **Penile fibromatosis** (Peyronie disease) is the least common of the localized fibromatoses. It is characterized by induration of, or a mass in, the penile shaft, causing it to curve toward the affected side **(penile strabismus)**. It can lead to urethral obstruction and pain on erection.

- Deep aggressive fibromatosis (desmoid tumor) frequently involves fascia and muscular aponeuroses of the extremities or abdominal wall musculature. It may also arise in the mesentery. Lesions are highly infiltrative and difficult to resect completely, accounting for high recurrence rates. Mesenteric fibromatosis is more commonly associated with APC mutations, whereas abdominal fibromatosis shows a predilection for women.

Fibrosarcoma Is a Malignant Tumor Demonstrating Fibroblastic Differentiation

Many subtypes of sarcoma show evidence of fibroblastic differentiation. Pure adult fibrosarcoma is a diagnosis of exclusion, in part because it has no characteristic cytogenetic abnormalities. It accounts for less than 3% of adult sarcomas. Congenital (infantile) fibrosarcoma is characterized by a chromosomal translocation, t(12;15)(p13;q26), that fuses *ETV6* and *NTRK3* genes. *NTRK3* encodes a cell surface receptor for neurotropin-3, which regulates growth and development in the central nervous system but also fulfills other roles. *ETV6* makes a transcription factor involved in early hematopoiesis and angiogenesis. Fusion of these genes results in a chimeric oncoprotein with abnormal tyrosine kinase activity that apparently promotes congenital fibrosarcoma, although the

mechanism is not well understood. Fibrosarcomas arise from deep connective tissue, such as fascia, scar tissue, periosteum, and tendons. Macroscopically, they are sharply demarcated tumors and often exhibit necrosis and hemorrhage. Microscopic examination shows malignant-appearing fibroblasts (Fig. 30-68), typically forming densely interlacing bundles and fascicles in a "herringbone" pattern. The prognosis for high-grade adult fibrosarcomas is guarded; survival at 5 years is only 40% and at 10 years is 30%. Infantile fibrosarcomas rarely metastasize, and have a mortality rate of less than 5%.

Other variants of fibroblastic sarcomas include low-grade fibromyxoid sarcoma, myofibroblastic sarcoma, and myxofibrosarcoma, among others, each with its own distinct pathologic features and clinical course.

Undifferentiated Sarcoma Is a Diagnosis of Exclusion

Undifferentiated sarcomas include undifferentiated pleomorphic sarcoma (UPS), undifferentiated spindle-cell sarcoma (USS), undifferentiated epithelioid sarcoma (UES), and a phenotypically heterogeneous group of sarcomas characterized by complex chromosomal copy number alterations and rearrangements reflecting a high degree of genomic instability. Several oncogenes also play a role in the pathogenesis of UPS, including sarcoma amplified sequence ([SAS]; encodes a cell surface protein in the tetraspanin family that controls growth), *TP53*, *RB1*, and *CDKN2A*, among others. Historically, UPSs were known as malignant fibrous histiocytomas (MFH), and were considered to be a distinct diagnostic entity. However, it is now known that UPS comprises pleomorphic variants of liposarcoma, leiomyosarcoma, or rhabdomyosarcoma, and high-grade myxofibrosarcoma. A small proportion of cases remains unclassifiable and may truly represent the most primitive undifferentiated form of sarcoma. Efforts to classify such tumors are important, however, as pleomorphic rhabdomyosarcoma or leiomyosarcoma may have a slightly worse prognosis. Collectively, UPS is the most common sarcoma in patients over the age

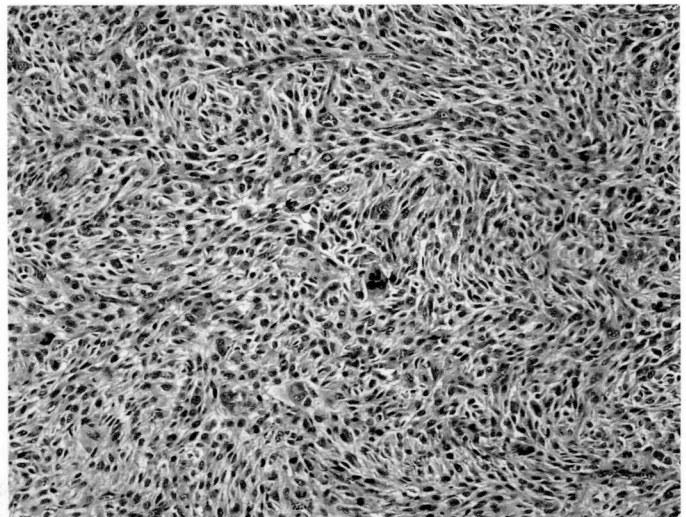

FIGURE 30-69. Undifferentiated pleomorphic sarcoma. An anaplastic tumor exhibits spindle cells, plump polygonal cells, bizarre tumor giant cells, and scattered chronic inflammatory cells. A similar appearance can be seen in pleomorphic sarcomas with other lines of differentiation (e.g., pleomorphic liposarcoma).

of 40, but cases have been documented at all ages. In half of the cases, tumors arise in the deep fascia or within skeletal muscle of the lower limbs.

 PATHOLOGY: Adult UPSs are usually unencapsulated, gray-white, or tan tumors that may contain areas of hemorrhage and necrosis. Microscopically, they may exhibit highly variable morphologic features, with areas of spindle-shaped cells arrayed in an irregularly whorled (storiform) pattern adjacent to fields with bizarre pleomorphic cells (Fig. 30-69). The spindle cells tend to be better differentiated and often show focal fibroblastic features. Mitoses are abundant. Nonneoplastic tumor-infiltrating inflammatory cells are often seen, including xanthomatous, dendritic, or histiocytic cells and a chronic inflammatory reaction. Some tumors contain numerous tumor giant cells, which exhibit intense cytoplasmic eosinophilia. The amount of collagen deposition varies and sometimes dominates the microscopic pattern. Necrosis is often present and may be extensive. A few tumors have a conspicuous myxoid stroma, indicating their likely progression from myxofibrosarcoma. Immunohistochemical and ultrastructural studies are generally used to identify a specific line of differentiation (smooth muscle, skeletal muscle, adipose tissue, etc.). If no such differentiation can be demonstrated, then the tumor is considered to be an **undifferentiated pleomorphic sarcoma**.

Prognosis in adult UPS depends on the degree of cytologic atypia, extent of mitotic activity, and degree of necrosis. Local recurrence after surgery occurs in almost half of these patients, and a comparable proportion later develops metastatic disease, mainly involving the lungs. Overall 5-year survival range is about 50%.

Radiation-induced sarcomas are a form of adult UPS that arise in bone or soft tissue, usually 10 to 20 years after radiotherapy for a malignancy in that field. A typical scenario is development of UPS or osteosarcoma of a rib or vertebral body (uncommon sites for *de novo* osteosarcomas) after radiation to the thorax as treatment for mediastinal lymphoma or breast cancer. The incidence of postradiation sarcoma is low (<1% of irradiated patients).

TUMORS OF ADIPOSE TISSUE

Lipomas Are the Most Common Soft-Tissue Mass and Closely Resemble Normal Fat

Composed of mature adipocytes, these benign, circumscribed tumors can originate at any site in the body that contains adipose tissue. Most occur in subcutaneous tissues of the upper half of the body, especially the trunk and neck. They are seen mainly in adults, and patients with multiple tumors often have relatives with a similar history.

 MOLECULAR PATHOGENESIS: Numerous cytogenetic abnormalities have been documented in lipomas. In general, the tumors can be subclassified into three major groups: (1) aberrations involving 12q13–15; (2) abnormalities involving 6p21–23; and (3) loss of portions of 13q. Some tumors have the translocation t(3;12)(q27–28;q13–15), which results in the generation of a fusion gene involving *HMGIC* (which encodes a member of the high-mobility group of proteins) and *LPP* (which makes a zinc finger LIM protein). The resultant fusion protein acts as a transcriptional activator. Some lipomas have no cytogenetic abnormalities and may represent localized adipocyte hyperplasia.

 PATHOLOGY: On gross examination, lipomas are encapsulated, soft, yellow lesions. They vary in size and may become quite large. Deeper tumors are often poorly circumscribed. Histologically, a lipoma is often indistinguishable from normal adipose tissue (Fig. 30-70). Adequate treatment is simple local excision.

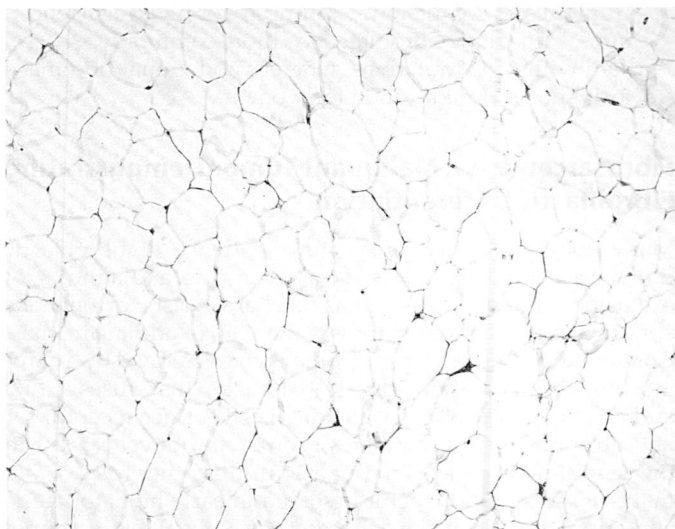

FIGURE 30-70. Lipoma. The tumor is composed of mature adipocytes with small eccentric nuclei.

An **angiolipoma** is a small, well-circumscribed, sub-cutaneous lipoma with extensive vascular proliferation. They usually occur in the upper extremities and trunk of young adults, and are often multiple and painful.

Liposarcomas Are the Second Most Common Sarcoma in Adults

Liposarcomas account for 25% of all malignant soft-tissue tumors. They arise after age 50 years, most commonly in the deep thigh and retroperitoneum. They tend to grow slowly but may become extremely large. Subtypes of liposarcoma include myxoid-/round-cell liposarcoma, well-differentiated liposarcoma, and pleomorphic liposarcoma.

 MOLECULAR PATHOGENESIS: Myxoid-/round-cell liposarcomas exhibit a translocation between chromosomes 12 and 16, [t(12;16)(q13;p11)], fusing *TLS/FUS* on chromosome 16 with *DDIT3* on chromosome 12. The *TLS/FUS* gene product is a novel RNA-binding protein, with substantial homology to the EWS protein of Ewing sarcoma, while the DDIT3 protein is a transcriptional repressor. Atypical lipomatous tumors and well-differentiated liposarcomas are defined by a giant marker chromosome, or a supernumerary ring chromosome with amplification of the 12q14–15 region, which includes the *MDM2* and *CDK4* genes, among others. MDM2 is involved in regulating growth and cell survival, in part by inhibiting p53 (see Chapter 5), while CDK4 is a regulatory factor promoting cell cycle progression. Pleomorphic liposarcomas have complex genomic rearrangements.

 PATHOLOGY: Gross appearances of liposarcoma subtypes vary depending on the proportions of adipose, mucinous, and fibrous tissue. Well-differentiated tumors may resemble normal fat or show fibrotic or gelatinous cut surfaces. Dedifferentiated or pleomorphic liposarcomas can appear grossly as soft, gelatinous masses, with necrosis, hemorrhage, and cysts. Microscopically, all types of liposarcomas may show *lipoblasts*, early adipocytes with univacuolated or multivacuolated cytoplasmic fat vesicles indenting the nucleus. While frequently seen in liposarcoma, lipoblasts may also be present in reactive or regenerative conditions and are neither necessary nor sufficient for the diagnosis of liposarcoma.

WELL-DIFFERENTIATED/DEDIFFERENTIATED LIPOSARCOMA: Well-differentiated liposarcomas are typically 5 to 10 cm in diameter, although retroperitoneal tumors may reach gigantic proportions (up to 40 cm in diameter and weighing in excess of 20 kg). Well-differentiated liposarcomas are often composed of large amounts of mature fat, and therefore can be confused with lipomas if sampled inadequately. Sclerosis, prominent lymphoid aggregates, or inflammatory infiltrates may also be seen. The defining feature of a well-differentiated liposarcoma is the presence of atypical neoplastic stromal cells with large, irregular nuclei, and hyperchromatic chromatin (Fig. 30-71). Dedifferentiated liposarcomas arise in pre-existing well-differentiated tumors and are usually composed of a monotonous population of mitotically active spindle cells, although some tumors may resemble UPS or myxofibrosarcoma.

MYXOID/ROUND CELL LIPOSARCOMA: These tumors arise most frequently in the proximal extremities. They are exceedingly rare in the retroperitoneum. Microscopically, they contain univacuolated "signet ring" lipoblasts and variable amounts of primitive ovoid to round cells embedded in a vascularized myxoid stroma. Round-cell liposarcomas represent a poorly differentiated form of myxoid liposarcoma and contain a high proportion of primitive round cells in a scant myxoid stroma.

PLEOMORPHIC LIPOSARCOMA: Pleomorphic liposarcomas have a UPS-like histologic appearance with numerous large, bizarre tumor cells, and foci of pleomorphic lipoblasts.

Well-differentiated liposarcoma is known as atypical lipomatous tumor in the extremities, where complete resection results in low recurrence rates. Retroperitoneal tumors cannot be completely resected and frequently recur. Well-differentiated liposarcomas almost never metastasize. Myxoid liposarcomas and differentiated liposarcomas have an intermediate risk of local recurrence and metastasis, whereas round cell and pleomorphic liposarcomas have a high frequency of local recurrence and metastasis. Pleomorphic liposarcoma has the worst outcome, with less than 20% 5-year survival, compared to better than 70% for well-differentiated or pure myxoid variants.

RHABDOMYOSARCOMA

Rhabdomyosarcoma is a malignant tumor that displays striated muscle differentiation. It is uncommon in mature adults but is the most frequent soft-tissue sarcoma of children and young adults.

 PATHOLOGY: Most cases can be classified in one of five subtypes. In addition to their characteristic light microscopic features, all subtypes of rhabdomyosarcomas show immunohistochemical evidence of skeletal muscle differentiation. Tumors may express nonspecific myoid markers, such as actin and desmin, but most demonstrate at least focal expression of skeletal muscle—specific markers, such as the transcription factors myogenin and MyoD1.

EMBRYONAL RHABDOMYOSARCOMA: This form is most common in children between 3 and 12 years old and frequently involves the head and neck, genitourinary tract, and retroperitoneum. Its appearance varies from that of a highly differentiated tumor containing rhabdomyoblasts, with large eosinophilic cytoplasm and cross-striations (Fig. 30-72A), to that of a poorly differentiated small-cell neoplasm.

BOTRYOID EMBRYONAL RHABDOMYOSARCOMA: This tumor, also known as **sarcoma botryoides** (from Greek, shaped like a bunch of grapes), is distinguished by its formation of polypoid, grape-like tumor masses. Microscopically, malignant cells are scattered in an

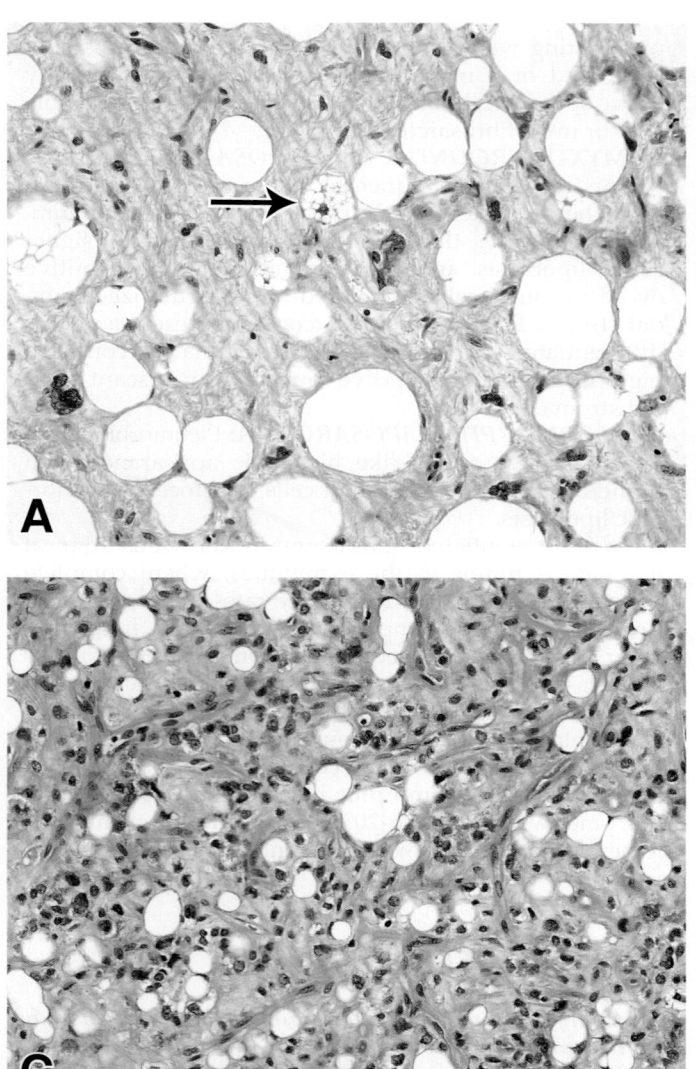

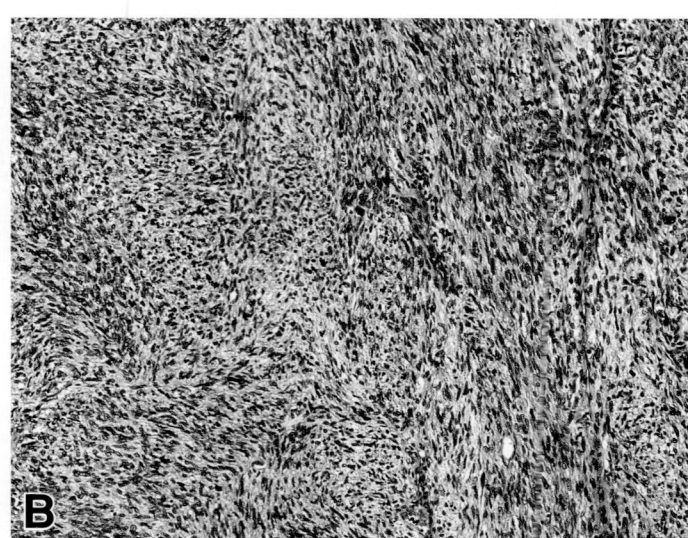

FIGURE 30-71. Liposarcoma. A. Well-differentiated liposarcoma. Atypical stromal cells with enlarged hyperchromatic nuclei reside within collagenous stroma surrounding mature adipocytes. Lipoblasts, containing multiple cytoplasmic lipid vacuoles that indent the nucleus (*arrow*), are present in this example but are not required for diagnosis. **B.** Dedifferentiated liposarcoma. The tumor is composed of a hypercellular proliferation of nondescript spindle cells, without evidence of lipogenic differentiation. **C.** Myxoid liposarcoma. The tumor is composed of a mixture of small round adipocyte precursors, univacuolated lipoblasts, and mature adipocytes arrayed in a myxoid stroma with a prominent plexiform vascular network.

abundant myxoid stroma. Botryoid foci may occur in any type of embryonal rhabdomyosarcoma, but are most common in tumors forming in hollow visceral organs, including the vagina (see Chapter 24) and urinary bladder.

ALVEOLAR RHABDOMYOSARCOMA: This subtype is less frequent than the embryonal type. It principally affects young people between ages 10 and 25, and is only rarely seen in elderly patients. It occurs most commonly in the upper and lower extremities, but may have a similar distribution as the embryonal type. Typically, it contains club-shaped tumor cells arranged in clumps outlined by fibrous septa. The loose arrangement of cells in the center of the clusters generates an "alveolar" pattern (Fig. 30-72B). Tumor cells exhibit intense eosinophilia, and occasional multinucleated giant cells are identified. Malignant rhabdomyoblasts, recognizable by their cross-striations, occur less commonly in the alveolar subtype than in embryonal rhabdomyosarcoma, being present in only 25% of cases.

MOLECULAR PATHOGENESIS: Most alveolar rhabdomyosarcomas express *PAX3-FOXO1* or *PAX7-FOXO1* gene fusions, resulting from t(2;13)(q35;q14) or t(1;13)(p36;q14) translocations, respectively. Either arrangement leads to abnormal expression of transcription factors. In patients with localized tumors, the type of fusion does not correlate with the clinical outcome. However, in metastatic disease, *PAX3-FOXO1*–positive tumors have a worse prognosis than do tumors positive for *PAX7-FOXO1*.

SPINDLE-CELL/SCLEROSING RHABDOMYOSARCOMA: Once thought to represent a variant of embryonal rhabdomyosarcoma, spindle-cell rhabdomyosarcoma is distinct subtype characterized by fascicles of monotonous spindle cells within a dense collagen stroma. A subset of spindle-cell rhabdomyosarcoma arising in infants is characterized by *NCOA2* gene rearrangements, while those affecting children and adults are typified by *MYOD1* mutations. Both promote abnormal expression of transcription factors.

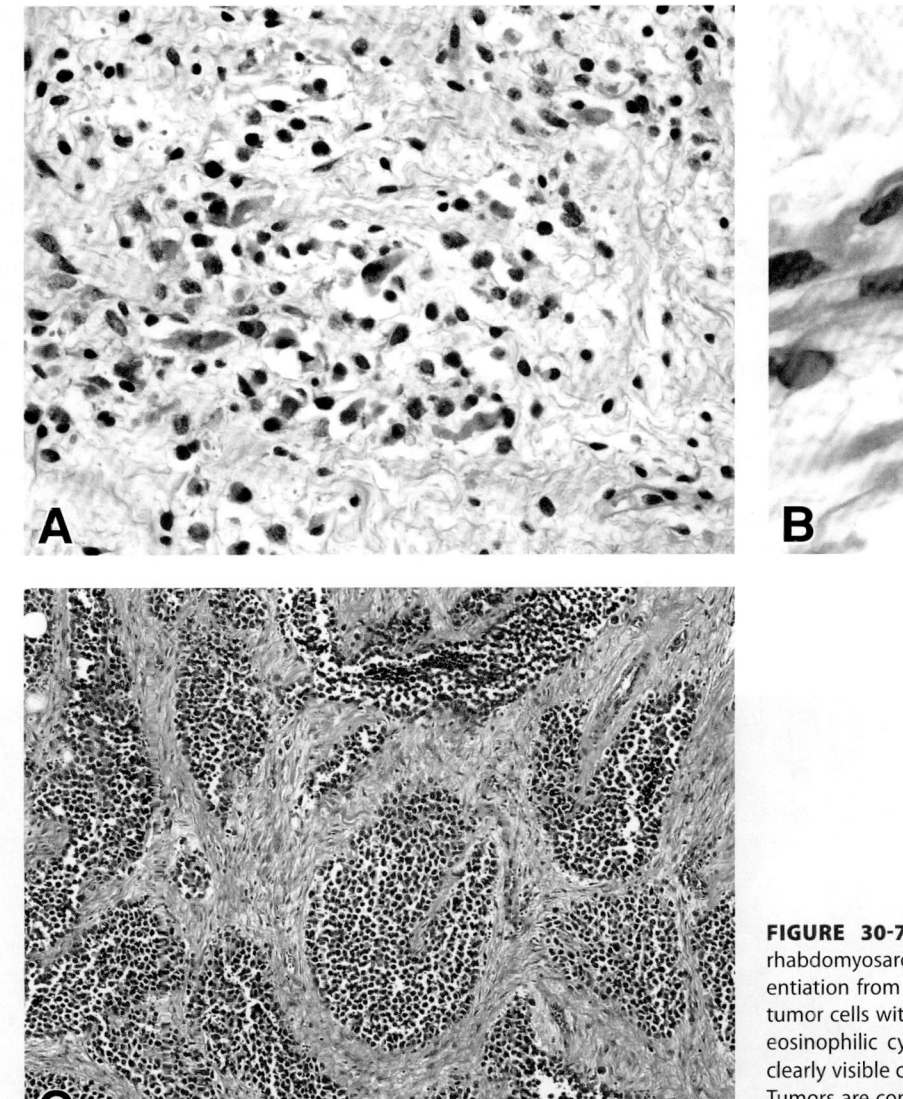

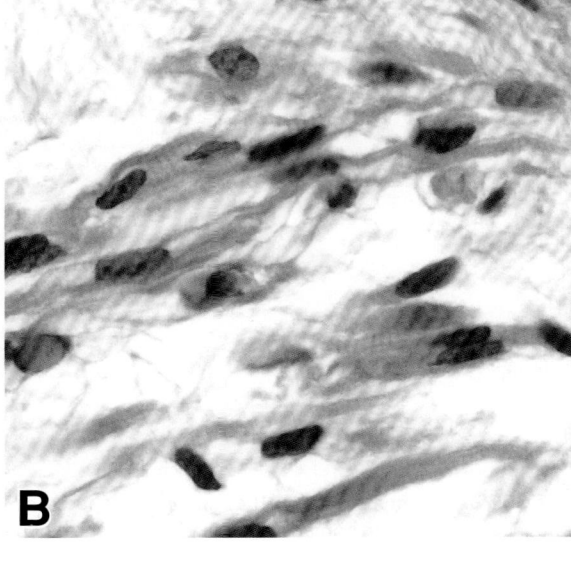

FIGURE 30-72. Rhabdomyosarcoma. A, B. Embryonal rhabdomyosarcoma. Tumors may show a spectrum of differentiation from (**A**) primitive small round cells and polyhedral tumor cells with enlarged, hyperchromatic nuclei, and deeply eosinophilic cytoplasm to (**B**) differentiated strap cells with clearly visible cross-striations. **C.** Alveolar rhabdomyosarcoma. Tumors are composed of primitive small round cells arranged in discohesive nests within a fibrous stroma.

PLEOMORPHIC RHABDOMYOSARCOMA: This least common form of rhabdomyosarcoma arises in skeletal muscles of older individuals, often in the thigh. It differs from other types of rhabdomyosarcoma by the degree of pleomorphism in its irregularly arranged cells and, thus, can be categorized as a type of adult undifferentiated pleomorphic sarcoma. Large, granular, eosinophilic rhabdomyoblasts, together with multinucleated giant cells, are commonly seen. Cross-striations are virtually nonexistent.

The dismal prognosis previously associated with most rhabdomyosarcomas has improved in the past two decades. Combinations of more effective types of surgery, radiation and chemotherapy now cure more than 80% of patients with localized or regional disease. Factors associated with worse prognosis include age older than 10, tumor size greater than 5 cm, alveolar and pleomorphic histologic subtypes and advanced stage of disease.

SMOOTH MUSCLE TUMORS

These tumors are characterized histologically by fascicles of spindled cells with brightly eosinophilic cytoplasm, cylindrical nuclei and immunohistochemical expression of smooth muscle actin, muscle-specific actin and desmin.

LEIOMYOMA: This benign soft-tissue tumor usually arises in sites associated with normal smooth muscle, including erector pili muscles in the dermis, blood vessel walls in subcutaneous or deep somatic tissues and the muscular wall of the esophagus or uterus. Leiomyomas appear as firm, gray-white, well-circumscribed nodules. Dermal or subcutaneous tumors may be painful. Microscopically, they are composed of intersecting fascicles of uniform spindled cells with cigar-shaped nuclei and very low mitotic activity. Simple excision is curative.

LEIOMYOSARCOMA: This malignant soft-tissue neoplasm typically arises within blood vessel walls in the soft tissue of the extremities or retroperitoneum of adults, or in the uterus. Macroscopically, leiomyosarcomas tend to be well circumscribed but are larger and softer than leiomyomas and

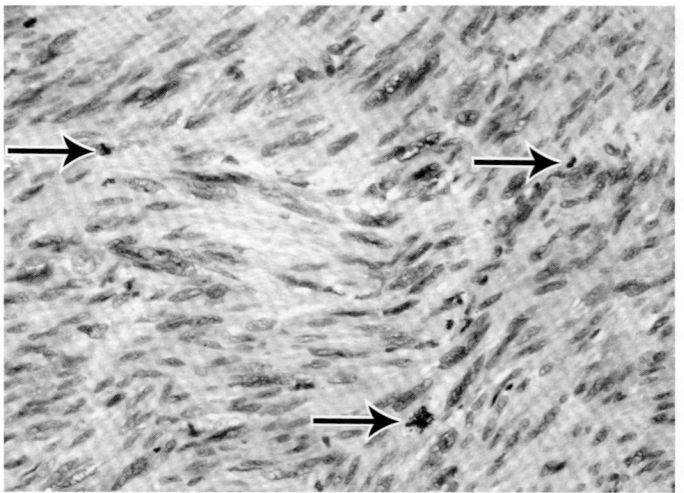

FIGURE 30-73. Leiomyosarcoma. The tumor is composed of spindle cells with elongated hyperchromatic nuclei, a variable degree of pleomorphism and frequent mitoses (*arrows*).

often exhibit necrosis, hemorrhage and cystic degeneration. Histologically, tumor cells are arranged in broad, intersecting fascicles. Well-differentiated tumor cells have elongated nuclei and eosinophilic cytoplasm; poorly differentiated ones show marked increased cellularity and severe cytologic atypia (Fig. 30-73). Most deep leiomyosarcomas eventually metastasize, although dissemination may occur as late as 15 or more years after resection of the primary tumor. Leiomyosarcomas have complex chromosomal rearrangements and numerous somatic mutations, but no characteristic alterations have been defined. Retroperitoneal and uterine tumors have a poor prognosis.

VASCULAR TUMORS

Benign vascular tumors (hemangiomas) are among the most common soft-tissue tumors and are the most frequent neoplasms of infancy and childhood. By contrast, angiosarcomas account for less than 1% of all sarcomas and are more common in older adults. Vascular tumors are discussed in detail in Chapter 16.

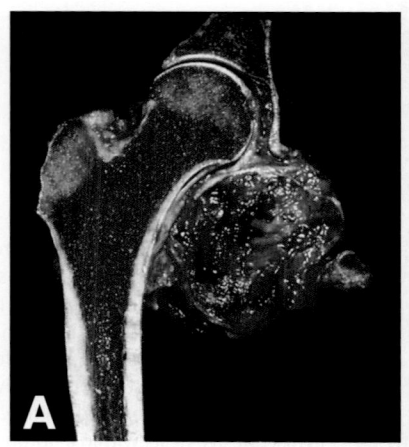

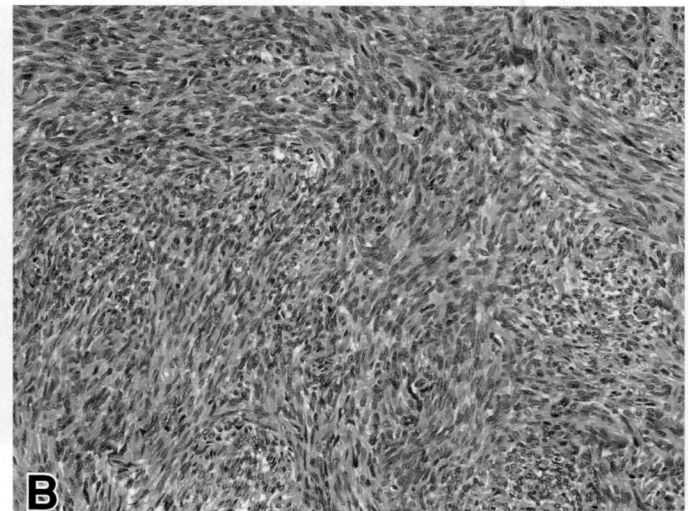

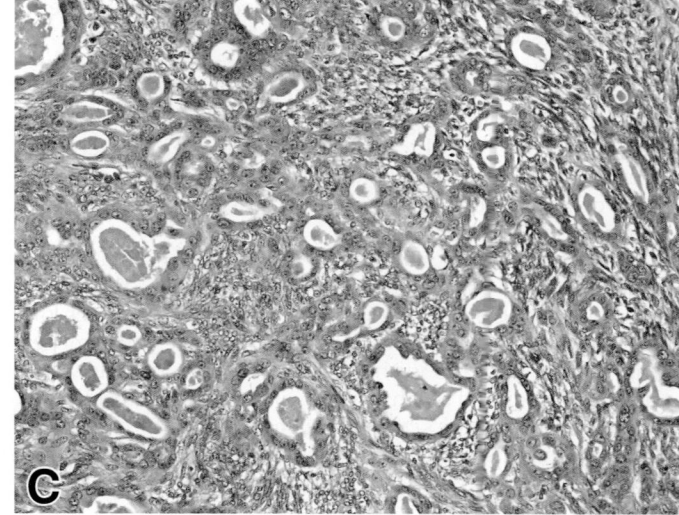

FIGURE 30-74. Synovial sarcoma. A. Section of the upper femur and acetabulum reveals a tumor adjacent to the hip joint and the neck of the femur. **B, C.** Synovial sarcomas may be monophasic (**B**), composed of swirling fascicles of plump spindle cells with monomorphic, hyperchromatic nuclei, or biphasic (**C**), displaying both spindle-cell mesenchymal differentiation and epithelial differentiation in the form of irregular glands containing eosinophilic proteinaceous material. (74A from Bullough PG. *Atlas of Orthopaedic Pathology*. 2nd ed. New York: Gower Medical Publishing, 1992. Copyright Lippincott Williams & Wilkins.)

SYNOVIAL SARCOMA

Synovial sarcomas are highly malignant soft-tissue tumors associated with a specific translocation between chromosomes X and 18. They may arise anywhere in the body but are commonly located in deep soft tissues near joints, tendon sheaths or joint capsules. They occur principally in young adults and usually present as a painful mass in the extremity.

Despite the name, synovial sarcomas neither arise from synovial tissues nor show synoviocyte differentiation. Expression of TLE1, a transcription factor associated with cell fate determination, is characteristic and may account for the dual epithelial and mesenchymal differentiation often seen in synovial sarcoma.

MOLECULAR PATHOGENESIS: Synovial sarcomas display a specific, balanced chromosomal translocation involving chromosomes X and 18 (t[x;18][p11.2;q11.2]). This translocation results in fusion of the *SS18/SYT* (synteny) gene on chromosome 18 to the *SSX* gene (a transcriptional repressor) on the X chromosome, leading to production of a hybrid protein, SS18-SSX1, SS18-SSX2 or, rarely, SS18-SSX4. These fusion proteins exert effects through complex mechanisms involving abnormal transcriptional regulation and chromatin remodeling. The SS18-SSX2 protein is associated with a better prognosis if the disease is localized.

PATHOLOGY: On gross examination, synovial sarcomas are usually circumscribed, round, or multilobular masses attached to tendons, tendon sheaths, or the exterior walls of joint capsules (Fig. 30-74A). They tend to be surrounded by a glistening pseudocapsule and in many instances are cystic. Areas of hemorrhage, necrosis, and calcification may be seen. They range from small nodules to masses of 15 cm or more in diameter, the average being 3 to 5 cm.

Microscopically, synovial sarcomas classically have a **biphasic pattern** (Fig. 30-74B). Fluid-filled glandular spaces lined by epithelial tumor cells are embedded in a sarcomatous background, comprised of plump spindle cells in swirling fascicles with a "school of fish" appearance. These elements vary in proportion, distribution, and cellular differentiation, with the spindle cells usually considerably more numerous than the glandular elements. If the epithelial component is lacking, the tumor is referred to as **monophasic synovial sarcoma**. Calcifications and thick collagenous bands may be conspicuous within the tumor. Poorly differentiated morphology imparts a poorer prognosis. Synovial sarcomas usually express cytokeratin or epithelial membrane antigens, further evidence of epithelial differentiation.

The recurrence rate is high, and metastases occur in over 60% of cases. The 5-year survival rate is 50%, and those who die usually have extensive lung metastases.

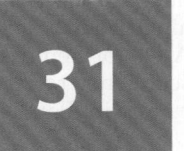

31 Skeletal Muscle and Peripheral Nervous System

Lawrence C. Kenyon, Thomas W. Bouldin

Skeletal Muscle

EMBRYOLOGY AND ANATOMY

The myoblast is a primitive cell that fuses with other myoblasts to form a cylindrical multinucleated myotube. The periphery of the myotube rapidly accumulates myofibrils, containing myosin and actin, which become arrayed in the cross-banded pattern characteristic of striated muscle (Fig. 31-1). The myofiber has a distinctive ultrastructural architecture (Fig. 31-2).

The myotube matures completely when it is innervated by the terminal axon of a lower motor neuron. Before innervation, the sarcolemma of the myotube contains diffusely distributed nicotinic receptors for acetylcholine (ACh) on its surface membrane. Upon innervation, these receptors become highly concentrated at the motor endplate. An individual muscle fiber is innervated by only a single nerve ending, but each motor neuron innervates many muscle fibers. After innervation, the

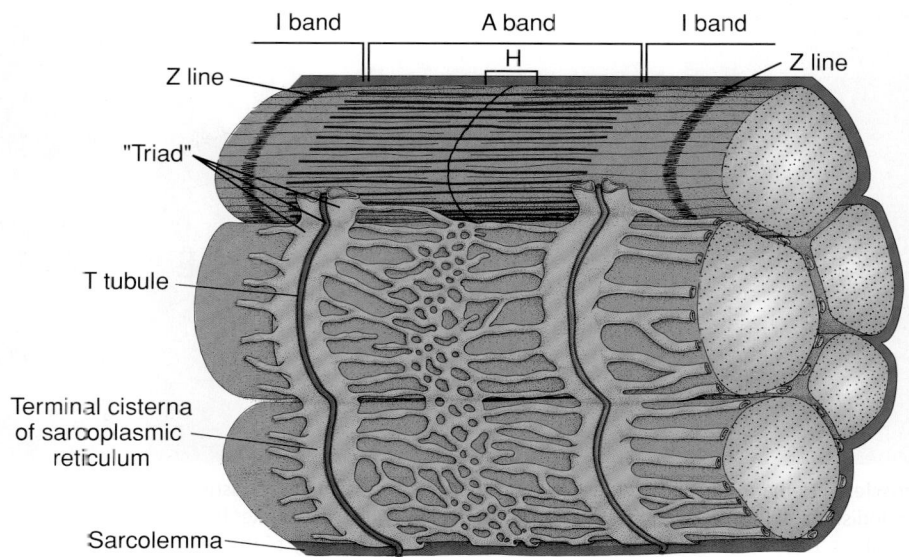

FIGURE 31-1. Normal striated muscle. Cross-striations of striated muscle are created by the arrangement of the myofilaments of the myofibril (compare to Fig. 31-2). The dark A band results from the thick myosin filaments and the thinner, partially overlapping actin filaments. In the middle portion of the myosin filaments where the actin does not overlap, there is a lighter band called the H zone or H band. In the middle of the H band, the center of each myosin filament thickens, forming intermolecular bridging with the adjacent myosin filament and giving rise to the M line (see Fig. 31-2). The finer actin filaments are anchored on the dark Z disk of the lighter I band. With contraction, the myosin filaments pull the actin filaments, causing the H zone to disappear, the I band to shrink, and the A band to remain the same. Mitochondria (not shown in this figure) are scattered throughout the sarcoplasm among the myofibrils. The endoplasmic reticulum (sarcoplasmic reticulum) forms an extensive, complex tubular network with periodic dilations (cisternae) around each myofibril. The cisternae are closely apposed to transverse (T) tubules, which are invaginations of the cell membrane (sarcolemma) that form a transverse network, resembling chicken wire, around each myofibril, thereby providing extensive communication between the internal and external environments. A triad consists of a T tubule and an adjacent terminal cisternae of the sarcoplasmic reticulum. (From Ross MH, Pawlina W. *Histology: A Text and Atlas.* 5th ed. Philadelphia, PA: Lippincott Williams & Wilkins; 2006.)

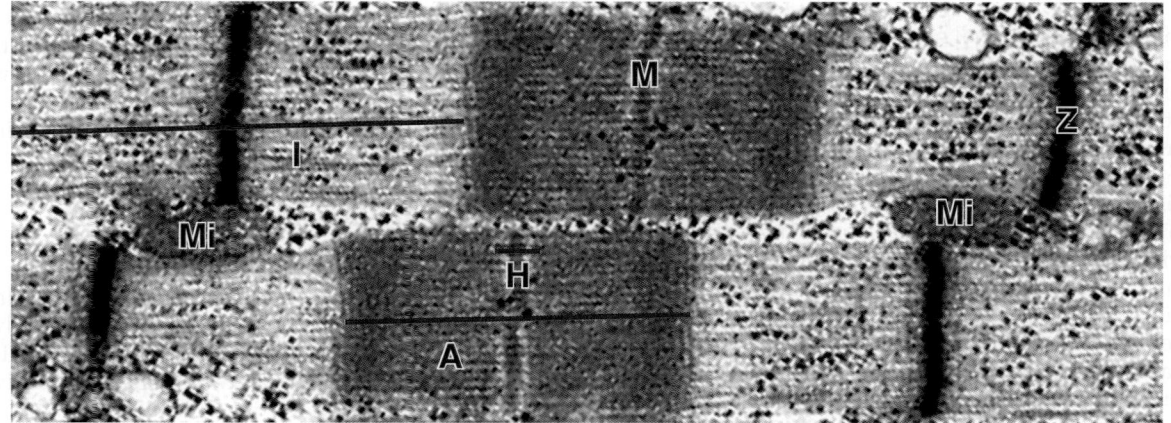

FIGURE 31-2. Normal muscle. This electron micrograph of quadriceps muscle demonstrates the ultrastructure of the sarcomere. The thin dark band, the Z disk (*Z*), bisects the broad, pale I band (*I*), a zone composed of the thin actin filaments. The broad, dark band, made up of the thick myosin filaments and overlapping actin filaments, is the A band (*A*). The middle of the A band consists of the pale H zone (*H*), which in turn is bisected by a slightly darker M line (*M*), representing a zone of intermolecular bridging of myosin. Mitochondria (*Mi*) tend to be located between myofibrils at the level of the I bands.

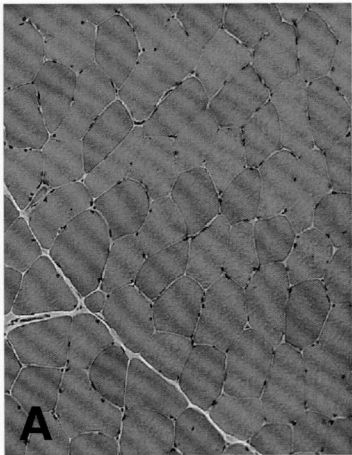
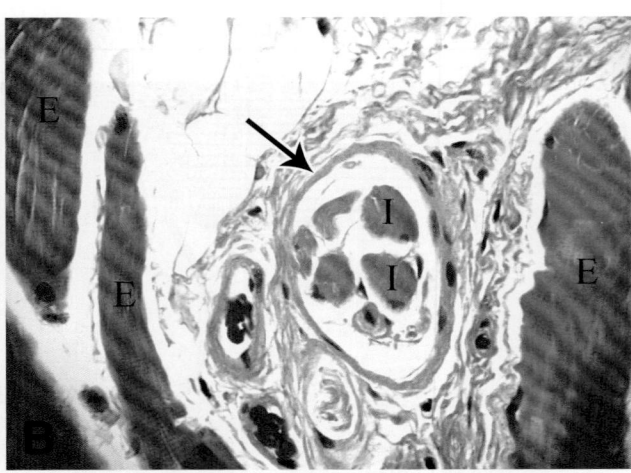
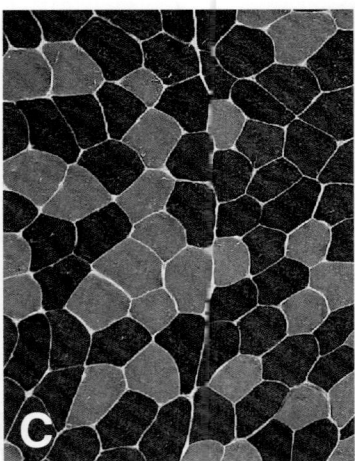

FIGURE 31-3. Normal muscle. A. Hematoxylin and eosin stain. In this transverse section of the vastus lateralis muscle, polygonal myofibers are separated from each other by an indistinct, thin layer of connective tissue, the endomysium. The thicker band of connective tissue, the perimysium, demarcates bundles or fascicles of fibers. All of the nuclei in this field are located at the periphery of the cells. Satellite cell nuclei are contained within the basement membrane of the muscle cell and cannot be distinguished from those of the myofibers by light microscopy. **B. Muscle spindle organ (stretch receptor).** The *arrow* marks the capsule of the muscle spindle organ. *I* = intrafusal fibers; *E* = extrafusal fibers. **C. Myofibrillar (myosin) ATPase.** Type I fibers are pale at high (alkaline) pH; type II fibers are dark. Note the intermixture of fiber types.

myofiber nuclei move from the center to arrange themselves in a regular pattern beneath the sarcolemma (Fig. 31-3A). Mature skeletal muscle cells are syncytia (multiple nuclei within a single cytoplasm) and can be several centimeters in length.

Muscle fibers responsible for movement are **extrafusal fibers**, while those in stretch receptors (muscle spindle organs, Fig. 31-3B) are **intrafusal fibers**. *In most primary myopathies, the damage affects extrafusal fibers but not intrafusal fibers.* Thus, muscle spindle organs, which are usually inconspicuous in routine histologic preparations, become relatively more prominent as extrafusal fibers disappear.

Myofiber Structure

The myofiber consists of distinct functional units (Figs. 31-1 and 31-2):

- **Sarcomere:** The functional myofibril unit, extending from one Z band to the next.
- **Z disk:** A distinct electron-dense disk that anchors the thin actin filaments.
- **I (Isotropic) band:** Zone where actin filaments extend from the Z band into the A band.
- **A (Anisotropic) band:** Structure composed of the thick myosin filaments. Actin filaments overlap myosin filaments to a variable extent, depending on the degree of muscle contraction. The thin filaments form a hexagonal array around each thick filament (best seen in cross-section).
- **H zone:** Pale region in the midportion of the A band where actin filaments end.
- **M line:** Zone of intermolecular bridging and thickening of myosin filaments at the midline of the A band, which forms a thin, slightly darker electron-dense band.

During contraction, actin filaments slide past myosin filaments. The sliding actin filaments advance farther into the A band, decreasing sarcomere length. As a result, the I band and H zone shorten, while the A band remains nearly constant. Many filamentous proteins make up the sarcomeres, and multiple proteins anchor sarcomeres to the sarcolemma.

These proteins may be mutated or abnormally regulated in muscular dystrophies (see below).

The **sarcoplasmic reticulum** surrounds each myofibril and forms an elaborate membranous network with irregular dilations (cisternae) juxtaposed to a transverse tubular network derived from the sarcolemma (Fig. 31-1). The **transverse tubular system** (T-tubule system) is arranged across the fiber like chicken wire, each ring wrapping around an individual myofibril. This arrangement allows an electrical stimulus (action potential) to proceed along the muscle fiber surface membrane and become diffusely and rapidly internalized via the T-tubular system. The electrical signal is translated into a chemical signal between the T-tubule and the cisternae of the sarcoplasmic reticulum. This process releases calcium from the sarcoplasmic reticulum into the vicinity of myofibrils, triggering muscle contraction.

The lower motor neurons and the fibers they innervate are the **motor units**, which vary in size. In limb muscles, one motor unit can include several hundred myofibers. By contrast, each motor unit of extraocular muscles may have only 20 myofibers. Eye muscles are also exceptional in that one fiber may have more than one motor endplate.

Myofibers Are Classified as Slow Twitch or Fast Twitch

After innervation, a characteristic metabolic profile develops for different muscle fibers. Muscle fiber types are broadly classified by the rate of contraction and fatiguability, as type I or type II, or slow-twitch fibers and fast-twitch fibers, respectively. These can be further subdivided into slow twitch, fatigue resistant (type I); fast twitch, fatigue resistant (type IIA), and fast twitch, fatigue sensitive (type IIB). There are also type IIC fibers, which are an immature fiber type. In lower mammals, some muscles are deep red (type I), while others are pale (type II).

TYPE I FIBERS (RED, SLOW TWITCH). When a nerve stimulates a dark (red) muscle, the resulting contraction is slower and more prolonged than when a nerve excites a pale (white) muscle. For this reason, red muscles have been classified as "slow twitch." Type I fibers tend to have more mitochondria and more myoglobin, the red, oxygen-storing pigment. Krebs cycle enzymes and electron-transport–chain carrier proteins are all more abundant in slow-twitch muscle than in fast-twitch muscle. The alkaline histochemical reaction for myosin adenosine triphosphatase (ATPase) gives a crisp distinction between the two fiber types. Type I fibers stain poorly at high (alkaline) pH, but type II fibers stain darkly (Fig. 31-3C).

Functionally, type I muscles have a greater capacity for long, sustained contractions and resist fatigue. A training program that increases endurance produces little change in the *size* of type I fibers, but conditioning of these fibers causes mitochondrial proliferation and increased capacity for generating energy.

TYPE II FIBERS (WHITE, FAST TWITCH): Stimulating type II fibers elicits faster, shorter, and stronger contractions than with type I fibers. Glycogen and phosphorylase and other enzymes that produce energy by anaerobic glycolysis are present in higher concentrations in white muscle. Type II muscle fibers are used for rapid, brief contractions. They hypertrophy during strength training and in response to androgenic steroids, and undergo selective atrophy after disuse.

A good way to remember the distinction between fiber types is to consider a chicken. The breast muscles are pale (white) compared to those of the back or legs. The breast muscles are fast twitch since they flap the wings during flight (granted, domesticated chickens have been bred to be too heavy to fly), while the darker muscles of the legs and back correspond to slow-twitch fibers since their function includes sustained contraction against gravity: standing and maintaining posture.

The lower motor neuron influences fiber type. During embryonic development, early muscle cells begin to express type-specific contractile proteins before muscle is innervated. Thus, the phenotype of a myofiber seems to be an autonomous characteristic of the cell, rather than one induced by the nerve supply. However, the kind of innervation can alter the types of myofibers. For example, after denervation injury, reinnervation of a slow-twitch muscle (type I) by a nerve from a fast-twitch muscle (type II) causes the newly innervated type I fibers to resemble type II fibers. It is thought that the pattern or rate of discharge of lower motor neurons plays an important role in this process. Because lower motor neurons can determine fiber type, it follows that all muscle fibers in a given motor unit are of the same type. A cross-section of muscle stained with alkaline ATPase reaction (see above) shows a random mixture of fiber types (Fig. 31-3C), because motor units interdigitate extensively with each other.

In humans, no muscles are composed exclusively of one fiber type. However, proportions of fiber types vary from muscle to muscle. For example, the soleus muscle contains mainly (≥80%) type I fibers. The pattern of fiber types in a given muscle is apparently genetically determined and varies between people. Some evidence indicates that changing the use of a muscle through lengthy, intensive training may alter the pattern of muscle fiber types.

MUSCLE BIOPSY: Since normal muscle patterns are more constant within a specific muscle, the same muscles are biopsied from case to case. Samples from the quadriceps femoris or biceps brachii are suitable for biopsy diagnosis in most primary muscle diseases (myopathies). Biopsies of the sural nerve and gastrocnemius muscle are often done if a peripheral neuropathy is suspected. However, as some neuromuscular conditions are more focal, locations for muscle biopsies vary.

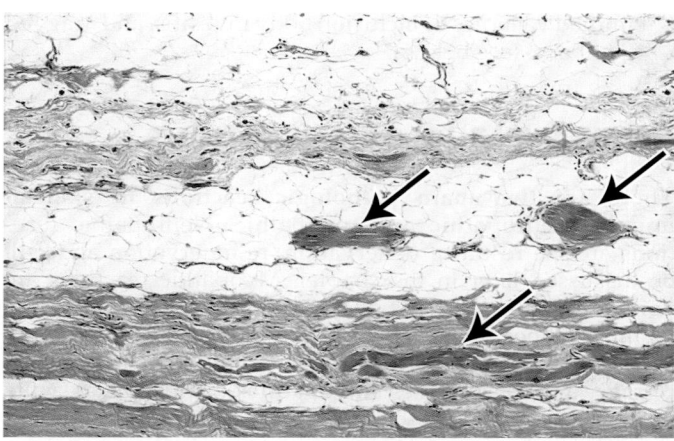

FIGURE 31-4. End-stage neuromuscular disease. In this section of the deltoid muscle stained by hematoxylin and eosin, skeletal muscle has been largely replaced by fibrofatty connective tissue. The few surviving muscle fibers (*arrows*) have a deeper eosinophilia than does the abundant collagenous component.

Biopsy sampling of a moderately affected muscle is most informative. Muscles that are uninvolved may show few or no pathologic changes, while very weak muscles may show end-stage changes and be replaced largely by fat and fibrous connective tissue (Fig. 31-4).

Evaluation of a muscle biopsy typically involves analysis of formalin-fixed, unfixed frozen, and glutaraldehyde-fixed tissue (the latter for potential electron microscopy). Several frozen section histochemical stains are used, many of which measure enzymatic activity using colorimetric assays. Unlike immunohistochemical stains that tell whether a protein is present or not, histochemical stains allow visualization of an enzyme's function. Some of the usual histochemical reactions used to evaluate skeletal muscle are:

- **Nonspecific esterase:** Important for identifying denervation atrophy and the presence of neuromuscular junctions.
- **NADH-tetrazolium reductase (NADH-TR):** Type I fibers appear dark owing to abundant mitochondria. This stain is useful in identifying central cores and signs of denervation.
- **Succinate dehydrogenase (SDH):** Sensitive histochemical index of mitochondrial proliferation.
- **Cytochrome C oxidase:** Fibers containing abnormal mitochondria lacking the final enzyme of the electron transport chain will fail to stain.
- **Alkaline phosphatase:** Regenerating fibers are selectively stained.
- **Acid phosphatase stain:** Identifies lysosomal activity within muscle fibers and macrophages.
- **Myosin ATPase:** Depending on the pH, helps to differentiate fiber types.

Some of the usual non-histochemical stains typically used in the analysis of muscle biopsies include:

- **Periodic acid–Schiff (PAS):** Helpful in identifying glycogen and diagnosing glycogen storage diseases (see below).
- **Oil red orcein (oil red O):** Marks neutral lipid and is particularly useful in assessing lipid storage myopathies such as carnitine deficiency (see below).
- **Modified Gomori trichrome stain:** Versatile stain in evaluating myopathies. It helps in assessing nemaline bodies,

rimmed vacuoles of inclusion body myositis, and "ragged red fibers" (see below).

GENERAL PATHOLOGIC REACTIONS

There are two main pathologic reactions in skeletal muscle—neuropathic and myopathic. Neuropathic reactions are the result of denervation/re-innervation and will be discussed later in the chapter. Myopathic reactions are nonneuropathic reactions related more directly to the skeletal muscle fibers themselves.

Necrosis is a common response of myofibers to injury in primary muscle diseases (**myopathies**). Widespread acute necrosis of skeletal muscle fibers (*rhabdomyolysis*) releases cytosolic proteins, including myoglobin, into the circulation, which may lead to myoglobinuria and cause acute renal failure. In many human myopathies, segmental necrosis occurs along the length of a fiber, with intact muscle flanking the site of damage (Fig. 31-5). The injury quickly elicits two responses: influx of blood-borne macrophages into the necrotic areas and activation of satellite cells, a population of dormant myoblasts nearby each fiber. As monocytes gradually phagocytose and remove necrotic debris, satellite cells proliferate and become active myoblasts. Within 2 days, they begin to fuse to each other and to the ends of the intact fiber remnants to form a joining multinucleated segment. This regenerating fiber is narrower than the parent fiber and has basophilic cytoplasm (owing to increased ribosomes) and large, vesicular nuclei with prominent nucleoli arranged in long chains (see below).

Regeneration can restore normal structure and function of muscle fibers within a few weeks after a single episode of injury. With subacute or chronic disorders, fiber necrosis proceeds concurrently with fiber regeneration, gradually leading to atrophy of muscle fibers and fibrosis.

MUSCULAR DYSTROPHY

In the middle of the 19th century, physicians discovered that progressive weakness of voluntary muscles could be caused by either a disorder of the nervous system or primary muscle degeneration. The latter was called **muscular dystrophy**. It was found to be frequently hereditary (or at least familial) and relentlessly progressive. Muscles from these patients showed fiber necrosis, with regeneration, progressive fibrosis, and infiltration by fatty tissue (Fig. 31-4). Little or no inflammation was seen. Subsequently, many variants of this type of muscle disease were found, and several hereditary, progressive, noninflammatory degenerative conditions of muscle have been classified.

Duchenne and Becker Muscular Dystrophies Are Severe, Progressive, X-Linked Diseases

Duchenne muscular dystrophy is characterized by progressive degeneration of muscles, particularly in the pelvic and shoulder girdles. It is the most common noninflammatory myopathy in children. A milder form of the disease is known as **Becker muscular dystrophy** (see Chapter 6 for the genetics of both diseases). Serum creatine kinase is usually greatly increased in both conditions.

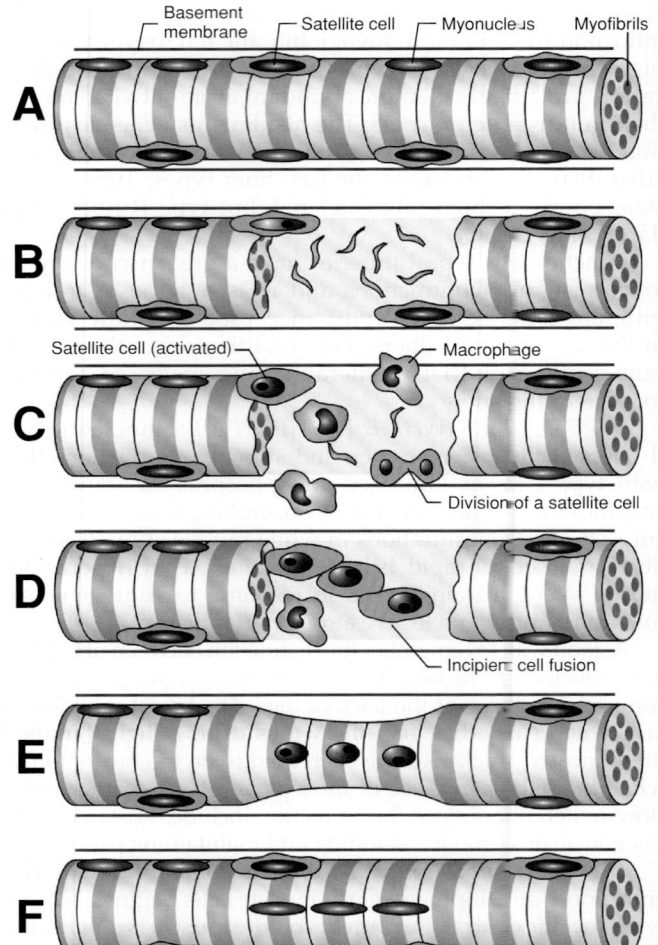

FIGURE 31-5. Segmental necrosis and regeneration of a muscle fiber. A. A normal muscle fiber contains myofibrils and subsarcolemmal nuclei and is covered by a basement membrane. Scattered satellite cells are situated on the surface of the sarcolemma, within the basement membrane. These cells are dormant myoblasts, capable of proliferating and fusing to form differentiated fibers. They constitute 3% to 5% of the nuclei, as observed in a cross-section of skeletal muscle. **B.** In many muscle diseases (e.g., Duchenne muscular dystrophy or polymyositis), injury to the muscle fiber causes segmental necrosis with disintegration of the sarcoplasm, leaving a preserved basement membrane and nerve supply (not shown). **C.** The damaged segment attracts circulating macrophages that penetrate the basement membrane and begin to digest and engulf the sarcoplasmic contents (myophagocytosis). Regenerative processes begin with the activation and proliferation of satellite cells, forming myoblasts within the basement membrane. Macrophages gradually leave the site of injury with their load of debris. **D.** At a later stage, myoblasts become aligned in close proximity to one another in the center of the fiber and begin to fuse. **E.** Regeneration of the fiber segment is prominent, as indicated by large, pale, vesicular, centrally located nuclei. **F.** The fiber is nearly normal except for a few persistent central nuclei. Eventually, the normal state (**A**) is restored.

> **MOLECULAR PATHOGENESIS:** Duchenne and Becker muscular dystrophies are caused by several loss-of-function mutations in *DMD*, a large gene on the short arm of the X chromosome (Xp21). This

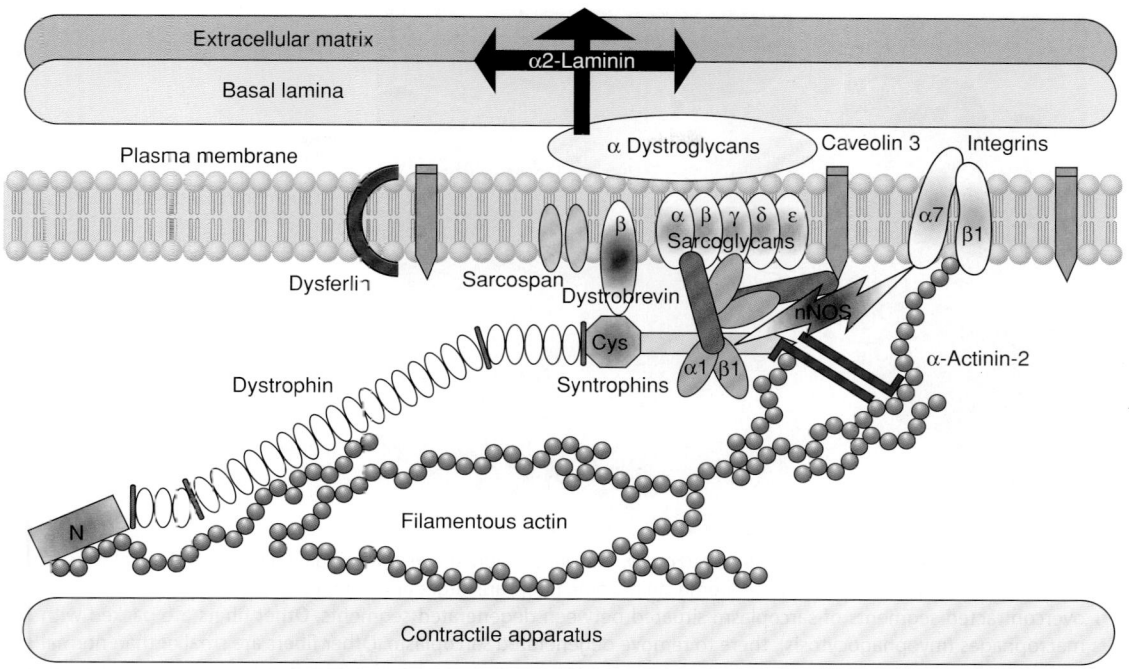

FIGURE 31-6. Proteins linking dystrophin to the plasma membrane and the contractile apparatus. Mutations in genes for several of these linking proteins are associated with known myopathies (Table 31-1). (Redrawn with permission from Rahman P. Structural and molecular basis of skeletal muscle diseases. *J Clin Neuromuscul Dis.* 2002;4[2]:104.)

gene encodes **dystrophin**, a 427-kd protein at the inner sarcolemmal surface. Dystrophin links the subsarcolemmal cytoskeleton to the exterior of the cell via a transmembrane complex of proteins and glycoproteins that binds to laminin (Fig. 31-6). If dystrophin is absent or greatly decreased, often owing to deletions of the gene (Fig. 31-7), the normal interaction between the sarcolemma and extracellular matrix is lost. This may cause the observed increase in osmotic fragility of dystrophic muscle, excessive influx of Ca^{2+}, and release of soluble muscle enzymes such as creatine kinase into the serum. Breakdown of the sarcolemma precedes muscle cell necrosis, and the basal lamina seems to separate from the sarcolemma early in the course of Duchenne muscular dystrophy.

Dystrophin genes may show point mutations, deletions, or duplications, leading to altered, usually truncated, proteins. Some mutated proteins may retain sufficient function to localize correctly to the muscle fiber surface but may distribute abnormally at the cell surface (Fig. 31-7). Such partly active proteins tend to produce less severe disease. Some patients have mutations affecting transmembrane proteins or glycoproteins that normally link the cytoskeleton and extracellular matrix (Fig. 31-6). In such affected fibers, dystrophin may be decreased or abnormally localized because its binding partners are abnormal, thus complicating diagnosis (see below).

Because Duchenne muscular dystrophy is inherited as an X-linked recessive disease, the abnormal gene is passed from heterozygous carrier mothers. About 30% of cases are due to spontaneous somatic mutation. Until recently, female carriers were best detected by repeatedly measuring serum creatine kinase, which is moderately increased in 75% of heterozygotes. Expression of the carrier state

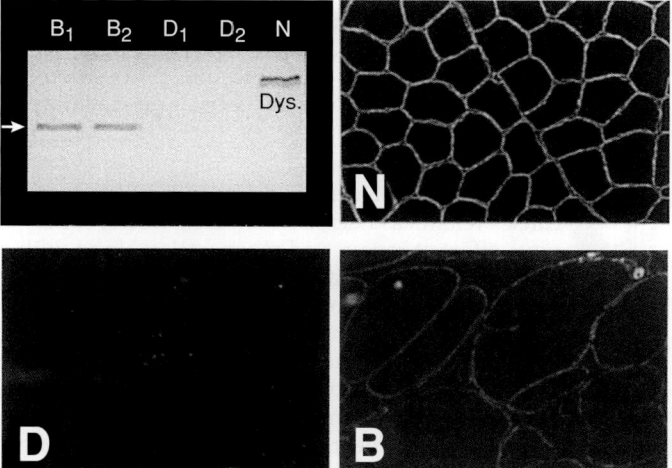

FIGURE 31-7. Dystrophin analysis in Duchenne and Becker muscular dystrophies. Immunofluorescence staining for dystrophin is shown in sections of skeletal muscle from a normal subject (*N*), a patient with Duchenne muscular dystrophy (*D*) and one with Becker muscular dystrophy (*B*). Dystrophin is normally concentrated at the surface membrane of every muscle fiber, but in Duchenne muscular dystrophy, the protein is absent or is only barely detected in a small proportion of muscle fibers. Becker muscular dystrophy exhibits hypertrophic muscle fibers with reduced expression of dystrophin. The immunoblot (*upper left*) of normal muscle shows a band near the top of the gel corresponding to the 427-kd protein dystrophin. Dystrophin is undetectable in Duchenne muscular dystrophy (two patients, D_1, D_2). In Becker muscular dystrophy, a weaker band has migrated farther down the gel relative to the normal protein, and it corresponds to a smaller, truncated protein (two patients, B_1, B_2). The combined analysis (immunolocalization and immunoblot) of the dystrophin protein is diagnostic of this group of dystrophies (*dystrophinopathies*).

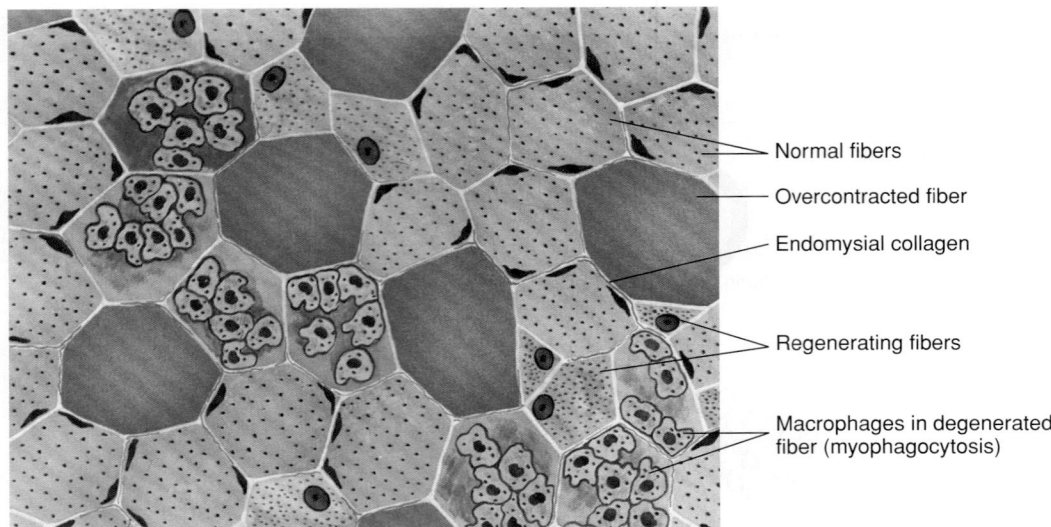

- Normal fibers
- Overcontracted fiber
- Endomysial collagen
- Regenerating fibers
- Macrophages in degenerated fiber (myophagocytosis)

FIGURE 31-8. Duchenne muscular dystrophy. This illustration shows pathologic changes in skeletal muscle stained with the modified Gomori trichrome stain. Some fibers are larger and darker than normal. These represent overcontracted segments of sarcoplasm situated between degenerated segments. Other fibers are packed with macrophages (myophagocytosis), there to remove degenerated sarcoplasm. Other fibers are smaller than normal and have granular sarcoplasm. These fibers have enlarged, vesicular nuclei with prominent nucleoli and represent regenerating fibers. Developing endomysial fibrosis is represented by the deposition of collagen around individual muscle fibers. The changes are those of a chronic, active noninflammatory myopathy.

is very variable, probably because of fluctuations in the random inactivation of the X chromosome. Dystrophin immunolocalization on muscle biopsy also identifies some carriers who show a characteristic mosaic pattern of deficient and normal myofibers. Molecular probes detect more than two-thirds of people who carry large deletions.

PATHOLOGY: Duchenne muscular dystrophy causes relentless necrosis of muscle fibers, continuous effort at repair, and regeneration along with progressive fibrosis. Degeneration eventually outstrips the regenerative capacity of the muscle. The number of muscle fibers then progressively decreases, to be replaced by fibro-fatty connective tissue. In the end stage, skeletal muscle fibers disappear almost completely (Fig. 31-4), but muscle spindle fibers (intrafusal fibers) are relatively spared.

Early in the disease, necrotic fibers and regenerating fibers tend to occur in small groups, together with scattered, large, hyalinized dark fibers. The latter are overly contracted and are thought to precede fiber necrosis (Figs. 31-8 and 31-9). Breakdown of the sarcolemma is one of the earliest ultrastructural changes. Macrophages invade necrotic fibers and reflect a scavenging function rather than an inflammatory process.

CLINICAL FEATURES: Analysis of genomic DNA establishes the diagnosis of Duchenne dystrophy. In usual clinical practice, this method only detects large deletions of the gene. About 30% of patients have small rearrangements or point mutations and are evaluated by muscle biopsy, which shows little or no detectable dystrophin by immunoblot or immunohis-

tochemistry. If there is an affected family member, prenatal diagnosis using chorionic villi may be useful.

Boys with Duchenne muscular dystrophy have markedly increased serum creatine kinase levels from birth and morphologically abnormal muscle even in utero. Clinical weakness is not detectable during the first year but is usually evident by 3 or 4 years of age, mainly around pelvic and shoulder girdles (proximal muscle weakness). The disease progresses relentlessly. "Pseudohypertrophy"

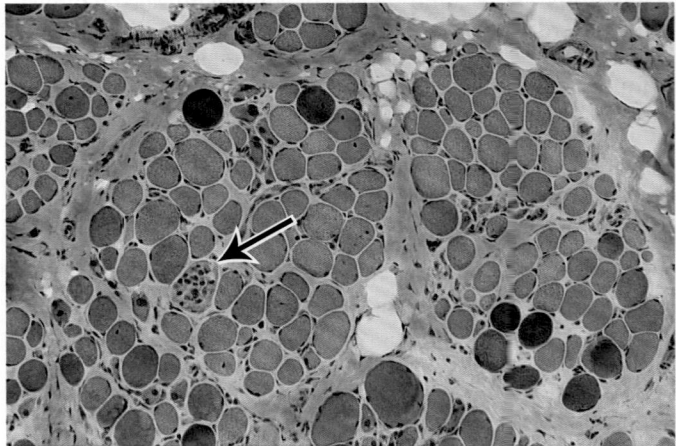

FIGURE 31-9. Duchenne muscular dystrophy. A section of vastus lateralis muscle, stained with modified Gomori trichrome, shows necrotic muscle fibers, some of which have been invaded by macrophages (*arrow*). Dark-staining, enlarged fibers represent overly contracted fibers. This is triggered by calcium influx across the defective sarcolemma which overwhelms mechanisms that maintain a normal low resting Ca^{2+} concentration. Amorphous material between the fascicles of muscle represents fibrosis. There is conspicuous perimysial and endomysial fibrosis.

(enlargement of a muscle when muscle fibers are replaced by fibroadipose tissue) of calf muscles eventually develops. Patients are usually wheelchair bound by age 10 and bedridden by 15. Death is usually from complications of respiratory insufficiency caused by muscular weakness or cardiac arrhythmia due to myocardial involvement. Other extraskeletal manifestations include gastrointestinal dysfunction (from degeneration of smooth muscle) and intellectual impairment. Many boys with Duchenne dystrophy show variably severe mental retardation, apparently due to lack of dystrophin in the central nervous system (CNS).

While the clinical presentation of patients with Becker muscular dystrophy is typically milder and of later onset, affected individuals often have exercise intolerance with muscle cramping, occasional rhabdomyolysis, and myoglobinuria. In Becker muscular dystrophy, dystrophin is present as a truncated protein unlike Duchenne muscular dystrophy, in which dystrophin is absent (Fig. 31-7).

Limb-Girdle Muscular Dystrophies Are Caused by Mutations in Diverse Proteins

Limb-girdle muscular dystrophies (LGMDs) are a group of disorders with several defective proteins and modes of inheritance (Table 31-1). Defects in many proteins have been implicated, but these patients show similar clinical features that include pelvic and shoulder girdle weakness. Onset may be in childhood or adulthood, with variable muscle weakness. Patients may have difficulty walking, running, or rising from a sitting position. Cardiac involvement is common. The histology resembles all muscular dystrophies, but some variants show unusual features including inflammation (LGMD2B, Miyoshi myopathy) and rimmed vacuoles (LGMD1A) like those seen in inclusion body myositis (see below). As a result, proper diagnosis requires detailed clinical histories and physical examination, plus immunohistochemical, immunoblotting, and genetic tests. LGMD (2C through 2F) are also known as the sarcoglycanopathies (Fig. 31-6).

Congenital Muscular Dystrophies Present in the Perinatal Period

These diseases are characterized by hypotonia, weakness, and contractures (Table 31-2). Depending on the variant, patients may also present with a leukoencephalopathy (white matter brain disease), brain malformations, and eye involvement.

Pathologically, these diseases resemble other muscular dystrophies, with variable fibrosis and fatty infiltration of muscle. Many of these disorders reflect mutations in extracellular matrix proteins (e.g., collagens, laminin, integrins) or abnormal glycosylation of α-dystroglycan (α-dystroglycanopathies) and sarcoplasmic reticulum (rigid spine muscular dystrophy). Some affected proteins also cause certain LGMDs, albeit with different **mutations**.

Nucleotide Repeat Syndromes May Cause Muscular Dystrophies

Several human genetic diseases are caused by abnormal numbers of intragenic oligonucleotide repeats. Myotonic dystrophy and oculopharyngeal muscular dystrophy are trinucleotide repeat syndromes with very different muscle pathologies.

TABLE 31-1		
LIMB-GIRDLE MUSCULAR DYSTROPHIES		
Limb-Girdle Muscular Dystrophies[a]	**Defective Protein**	**Subcellular Location**
LGMD1A	Myotilin	Sarcomere
LGMD1B	Lamin A/C	Nuclear envelope
LGMD1C	Caveolin 3	Sarcolemma
LGMD1D	Desmin	Cytoskeleton, periphery of Z-disk
LGMD1E	DNAJB6	Z-disk
LGMD1F	Transportin 3	Nuclear membrane
LGMD1G	HNRPDL	Ribonucleoprotein
LGMD2A	Calpain 3	Sarcoplasm
LGMD2B/Miyoshi	Dysferlin	Sarcolemma
LGMD2C	γ-Sarcoglycan	Sarcolemma
LGMD2D	α-Sarcoglycan	Sarcolemma
LGMD2E	β-Sarcoglycan	Sarcolemma
LGMD2F	δ-Sarcoglycan	Sarcolemma
LGMD2G	Telethonin	Sarcomere
LGMD2H	TRIM32	Sarcoplasm
LGMD2I	Fukutin-related protein	Golgi
LGMD2J	Titin	Sarcomere
LGMD2K	POMT1	Endoplasmic reticulum
LGMD2L	Anoctamin 5	Probably sarco-lemmal
LGMD2M	Fukutin	Golgi

[a]LGMD1s show autosomal dominant inheritance, while LMGD2s show autosomal recessive inheritance. This is a partial list as new LGMDs are being identified. For a more comprehensive list, see www.musclegenetable.fr

Adapted from Diseases of muscle. In Love S, Ironside J, Budka H, Perry A, eds. *Greenfield's Neuropathology.* 9th ed. Boca Raton, FL: CRC Press; 2015.

Both, however, exhibit "anticipation" (i.e., increasingly earlier ages at onset and more severe symptoms in successive generations, as numbers of repeats increase; see Chapter 6).

Myotonic Dystrophy Is the Most Common Adult Muscular Dystrophy

Myotonic dystrophy is an autosomal dominant disease characterized by slowed muscle relaxation (myotonia), progressive muscle weakness and wasting. Its prevalence is about 14 per 100,000, although minimally affected individuals are difficult to diagnose, so this estimate may be low. Age at onset and severity of symptoms vary greatly.

TABLE 31-2

CONGENITAL MYOPATHIES CAUSED BY ABNORMALITIES IN THE SARCOLEMMA OR EXTRACELLULAR MATRIX

Congenital Muscular Dystrophy (CMD)	Protein	Location and/or Function of Protein
Merosin-deficient CMD	Laminin α2	Extracellular matrix
Ullrich syndrome	Collagen VI	Extracellular matrix
Integrin α7 deficiency	Integrin α7	Plasma membrane
Fukuyama CMD	Fukutin	Possible substrate for glycosyltransferase
Muscle–eye–brain	POMGnT1 (*O*-mannose β-1,2-*N*-acetylglucosaminyl-transferase	Glycosyltransferase
Walker–Warburg syndrome	POMT1 (protein-*O*-mannosyl-transferase) Fukutin-related protein	Glycosyltransferase Possible putative glycosyl/phosphoryl ligand transferase
Rigid spine syndrome	Selenoprotein N1	Glycoprotein of the endoplasmic reticulum

Adapted from Diseases of muscle. In Love S, Louis DN, Ellison DW, eds. *Greenfield's Neuropathology*, 8th ed. New York: Oxford University Press; 2008.

MOLECULAR PATHOGENESIS: The two forms of myotonic dystrophy (DM1, DM2) both follow autosomal dominant inheritance and reflect mutations in different genes. DM1 is due to expansion of a CTG repeat near the 3′ end of the DM protein kinase (*DMPK*) gene, which encodes a serine–threonine kinase. Normally, there are fewer than 30 copies of this repeat, but in minimally affected myotonic dystrophy patients, there may be 50 or more copies. The greater the number of repeats (sometimes as many as 4000), the more severe the disorder. The mechanism of injury brought about by expansion of CTG repeats in myotonic dystrophy, as in other trinucleotide repeat disorders, may be related to interference of the abnormal RNA (containing repeats) and RNA-binding proteins. DM2 is caused by expansion of the tetranucleotide repeat CCTG in the first intron of the *ZNF9* gene. DM1 may be either adult onset or congenital whereas DM2 is not congenital.

PATHOLOGY: Pathology in adult myotonic dystrophy is highly variable, even in muscles from the same patient. Most patients show type I fiber atrophy and type II fiber hypertrophy. In contrast, most muscle disorders show relative type II fiber atrophy. Internally situated nuclei are a constant feature. The myosin ATPase and NADH-TR stains show many ring fibers, with circumferential concentration of heavily stained sarcoplasm. In these fibers, outer sarcomeres are circumferential, instead of their usual longitudinal arrangement along the fiber axis (Fig. 31-10). Necrosis and regeneration, although occasionally present, are not prominent (as they are in Duchenne muscular dystrophy). Ring fibers are more common in DM1 than in DM2. DM2 also affects type II fibers more than type I fibers.

Muscles in congenital myotonic dystrophy show myofiber atrophy, frequent central nuclei, and failure of fiber differentiation. These features closely resemble those of the X-linked recessive type of myotubular myopathy (see below).

CLINICAL FEATURES: People with DM1 experience slowly progressive muscle weakness and stiffness, principally in the distal limbs (proximal weakness is more common in DM2). Facial and neck weakness as well as ptosis are typical of DM1, but less common in DM2. Extraskeletal features sometimes present in myotonic dystrophy include frontal balding, gonadal atrophy, cataracts, personality degeneration, and endocrine abnormalities. Cardiac arrhythmias and, less often, cardiomyopathy may occur. A few patients exhibit involvement of smooth muscle, with disorders of the gastrointestinal tract, gallbladder, and uterus.

Diagnosis is based on clinical features, family history, and characteristic electromyography, which exhibits

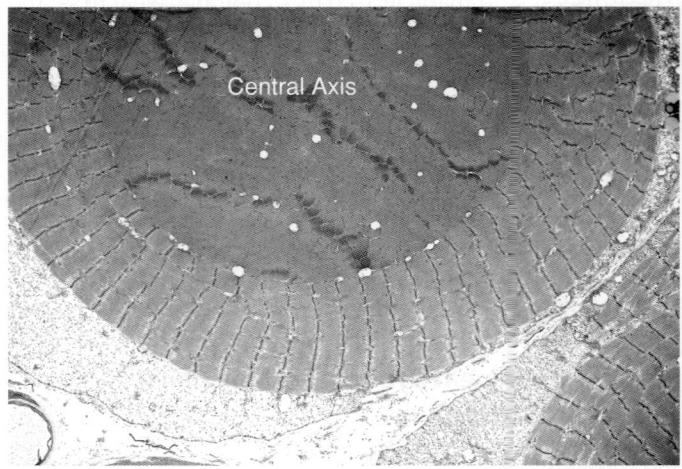

FIGURE 31-10. Ring fiber. This low-power electron micrograph (magnification ×1900) shows outer sarcomeres oriented perpendicular to the long axis of the myofiber.

myotonic discharges. Identifying an expanded CTG repeat (DM1) or CCTG (DM2) is predictive in utero and can be diagnostic in patients.

Congenital myotonic dystrophy is seen only in children of women with DM1 who themselves show symptoms of myotonic dystrophy. Affected infants have severe muscle weakness at birth. Myotonia is inconspicuous or absent but appears in later childhood. Many of these patients suffer mental retardation. Congenital DM2 has not been identified.

Oculopharyngeal Muscular Dystrophy Usually Presents in Adults

Oculopharyngeal muscular dystrophy (OPMD) is typically diagnosed in middle age (over 45 years) and mostly shows autosomal dominant inheritance. However, an autosomal recessive form does exist. Patients develop slowly progressive eyelid ptosis and dysphagia, and weakness of other muscle groups including the face and limbs. The autosomal dominant form is prevalent among French Canadians in Quebec and Bukhara Jews (formerly from central Asia), now living in Israel. Both autosomal dominant and recessive forms are due to abnormally increased numbers of GCG repeats in the poly(A) binding protein nuclear 1 gene (*PABPN1*), but differ in where these increased repeats are within the gene. Biopsies show intranuclear inclusions, rimmed vacuoles, and filamentous inclusions similar to those in inclusion body myositis (see below). Unlike the latter, the intranuclear inclusions contain 8.5-nm filaments.

Facioscapulohumeral Muscular Dystrophy Usually Presents in Childhood

Facioscapulohumeral muscular dystrophy (FSHD) is a relatively common muscular dystrophy inherited as an autosomal dominant disease that begins in childhood or young adulthood. Patients suffer from facial and shoulder girdle weakness. Scapular winging is prominent. Other muscles may also be affected. Life expectancy is usually normal. Extraskeletal involvement includes bundle branch block, hearing loss, and retinal vasculopathy. FSHD is caused by deletion of part of a repetitive DNA fragment in the subtelomeric region of chromosome 4q: affected patients have fewer repeats than normal. Chronic inflammation is prominent, resembling an inflammatory myopathy such as polymyositis (see below), but does not correlate with the disease course. A detailed clinical history is essential to making the proper diagnosis; otherwise, a patient with muscle weakness and a lymphocytic inflammatory infiltrate could easily be misdiagnosed as suffering from polymyositis.

CONGENITAL MYOPATHIES

A newborn occasionally shows generalized hypotonia, decreased deep tendon reflexes, and muscle bulk. Many of these children have a difficult perinatal period because of pulmonary complications of weak respiration. Many of the muscle diseases already described are "congenital" in the sense that they are due to germline mutations present at birth. However, such disorders are not clinically evident

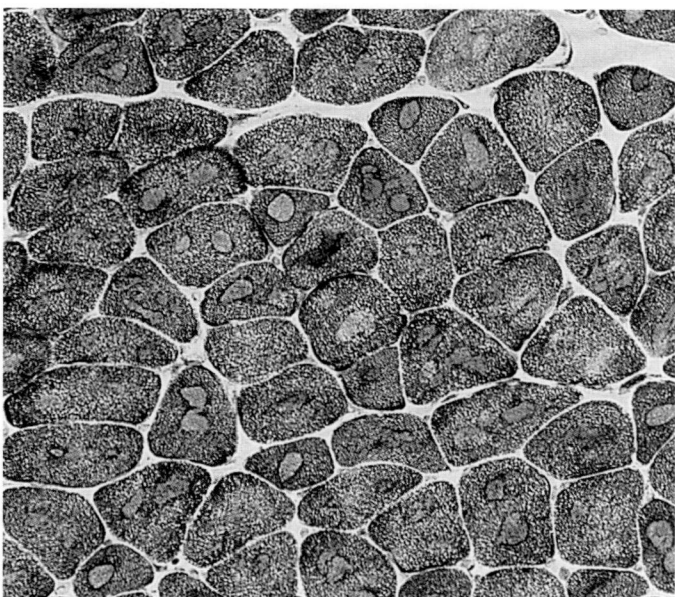

FIGURE 31-11. Central core disease. This section of vastus lateralis muscle stained for NADH-tetrazolium reductase shows a distinct circular zone of pallor in the center of most muscle fibers. A thin zone of excessive staining surrounds the core lesion. All of the myofibers in this case are type I, as demonstrated by the mycfibrillar ATPase stain (not shown). Note the close resemblance of the core lesions to the target formations found in the muscle fibers of neurogenic disorders (compare with Fig. 31-25).

until much later. In contrast, congenital myopathies, as described here, are evident at birth. Some have progressive "malignant" hypotonia, which results in death within the first year of life, for example, **infantile acid maltase deficiency (Pompe disease)**.

In other hypotonic patients, hypotonia may persist with little or no progression. These people become ambulatory and live a normal life span, although sometimes with secondary skeletal complications of hypotonia such as severe scoliosis. Muscle from these patients rarely reveals distinctive structurally abnormal myofibers. Three of the most common forms of congenital myopathies are **central core disease** (Fig. 31-11), **nemaline (rod) myopathy** (Fig. 31-12), and **central nuclear myopathy** (Fig. 31-13). All show congenital hypotonia, decreased deep tendon reflexes, decreased muscle bulk, and delayed motor milestones. In all three conditions, abnormal muscle morphology is usually limited to type I fibers with type I fiber predominance in some disorders and type I hypotrophy in others. Often, type I fibers are unusually predominant, or possibly, type II fibers fail to develop. There is no active myofiber necrosis or fibrosis, and patients have normal serum creatine kinase.

Central Core Disease Is an Autosomal Dominant Condition With Congenital Hypotonia and Proximal Muscle Weakness

 MOLECULAR PATHOGENESIS: Afflicted patients have decreased deep tendon reflexes and delayed motor development. The disease has been traced to mutations in *RYR1* on the long arm of chromosome 19

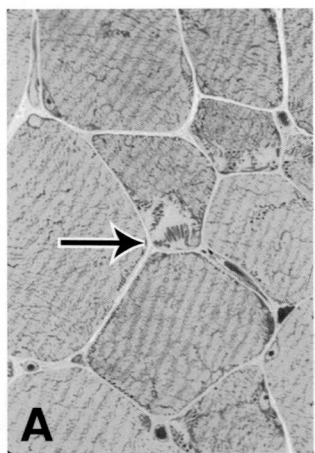

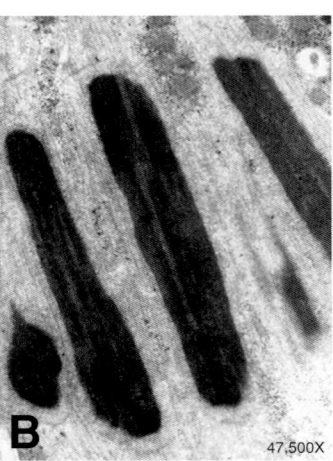

FIGURE 31-12. Rod (nemaline) myopathy. A. Muscle fibers contain dark rod-shaped aggregates (toluidine blue, 1000×). **B.** An electron micrograph shows that the rod-like structures are derived from the Z disk (47,500×).

(19q13.1) that codes for the ryanodine receptor, the calcium release channel of the sarcoplasmic reticulum. Occasional cases are sporadic or show autosomal recessive inheritance. Typical patients become ambulatory, but muscle strength remains less than normal.

PATHOLOGY: There is a striking predominance of type I fibers, often showing a central zone of degeneration with loss of NADH-TR reaction staining (Fig. 31-11) extending the entire length of the fiber. By electron microscopy, mitochondria and other membranous organelles are lost in the central cores with or without myofibril disorganization. Membranous organelles tend to condense around the margin of the central core. The periphery of the fiber is unremarkable.

Central core anomalies may resemble the target fibers seen in active denervating conditions (see below), although target fibers typically have dark rims around the areas of pallor and there is no evidence of denervation in central core disease.

Mutations in *RYR1* also cause **malignant hyperthermia**, a potentially fatal disorder that is triggered by succinylcholine and some anesthetic agents, particularly halothane. It is characterized by hyperpyrexia and rhabdomyolysis (see Chapter 8). Central core disease and malignant hyperthermia may coexist in some patients. Therefore, patients with central core disease may be at risk for malignant hyperthermia. However, patients with malignant hyperthermia often have no abnormal histologic changes. Malignant hyperthermia is suspected by family history and confirmed by an in vitro caffeine–halothane contracture test.

Rod Myopathy Sarcoplasmic Inclusions Derive From Z Bands

Rod myopathy includes a group of diseases in which rod-like inclusions accumulate within skeletal muscle sarcoplasm. The tangled, thread-like appearance of the inclusions led to the original name, "nemaline" (having the form of threads) myopathy. In reality, they are clusters of rod-shaped structures.

MOLECULAR PATHOGENESIS: Autosomal dominant and recessive inheritance patterns have been described. Genes responsible for rod myopathy include *NEB* (nebulin) (most common), *ACTA1* (skeletal muscle α-actin), *TPM1* and *TPM2* (α- and β-tropomyosin), and *TNNT1* (slow troponin T). Mutations in the ryanodine receptor gene may also lead to nemaline rod formation.

PATHOLOGY: There is variable predominance of type I fibers containing rod-shaped structures in their sarcoplasm. Aggregates of these inclusions often occur in subsarcolemmal regions near nuclei. They

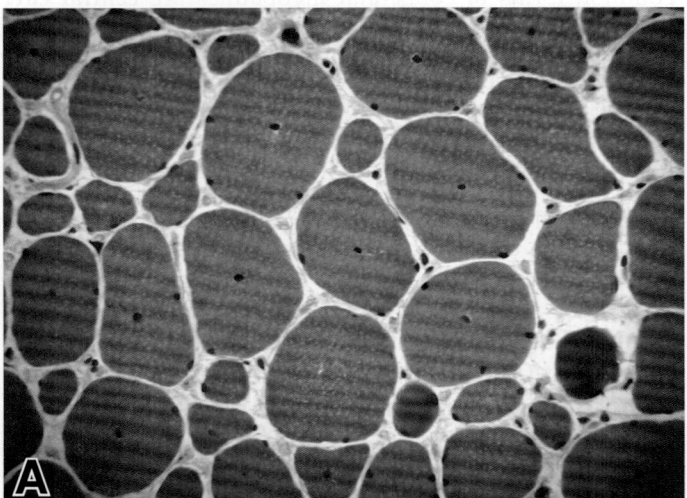

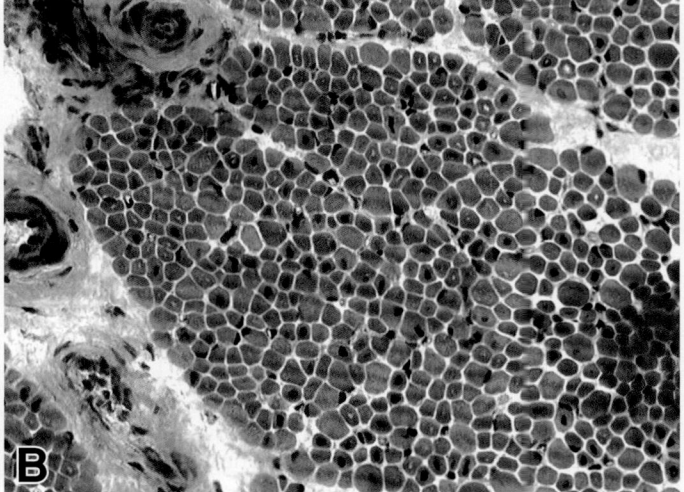

FIGURE 31-13. Central nuclear myopathy. A. Many muscle fibers in this section stained with hematoxylin and eosin contain a single central nucleus and many of the affected muscle fibers are abnormally small. **B.** This biopsy from a male newborn with severe hypotonia shows myotubular myopathy. Nuclei are absent in several fibers, which show a pale hollow where they had previously been.

are brilliant, red to dark red, when using modified Gomori trichrome stain, or blue on toluidine blue stain (Fig. 31-12A), but are often not visible with hematoxylin and eosin. The inclusions are rod shaped and arise from the Z band, which they resemble ultrastructurally (Fig. 31-12B).

Rods are described in several neuromuscular diseases, including denervation atrophy, muscular dystrophy, and inflammatory myopathies. Experimental tenotomy (cutting a tendon) induces formation of rods in the muscle when the nerve supply remains intact. In rod myopathy, however, inclusions are the main pathologic feature. Other abnormalities (inflammation, denervation) are absent.

 CLINICAL FEATURES: In the classic congenital form of rod myopathy, patients show congenital hypotonia, delayed motor milestones of variable clinical severity, and secondary skeletal changes such as kyphoscoliosis. Some exhibit severe involvement of muscles of the face, pharynx, and neck. Later-onset (childhood and adult) forms tend to be associated with some muscle degeneration, increased serum creatine kinase levels, and a slowly or nonprogressive course.

Central Nuclear Myopathy and Myotubular Myopathy Resemble the Myotubular Stage of Embryogenesis

  MOLECULAR PATHOGENESIS AND CLINICAL FEATURES: Central nuclear myopathy is a group of clinically and genetically heterogeneous inherited conditions in which skeletal muscle cells have centrally located nuclei. Autosomal recessive and autosomal dominant varieties are known. The latter tend to manifest in adolescence and show modestly increased serum creatine kinase. They progress slowly and, like rod myopathy, resemble the LGMDs (see above). Some patients exhibit striking involvement of facial and extraocular musculature. Bilateral ptosis is almost always present. The gene responsible, *DNM2* (dynamin 2), is involved in endocytosis and membrane trafficking as well as centrosome and actin assembly.

Myotubular myopathy is an X-linked disorder caused by *MTM1* (myotubularin) gene mutations. Myotubularin is a phosphatase expressed in most tissues and involved in phosphatidylinositol signaling. Clinically, myotubular myopathy is characterized by marked neonatal hypotonia and respiratory failure at birth. Pathologically, like central nuclear myopathy, there are centrally placed nuclei within both fiber types. The fibers in the central nuclear myopathies, including myotubular myopathies, resemble the myotubular stage in skeletal muscle embryogenesis.

 PATHOLOGY: Later-onset forms of central nuclear myopathy are characterized morphologically by muscle fibers that are normal size or larger, have numerous myofibrils, and display single central nuclei that appear mature (Fig. 31-13A). Biopsies of X-linked myotubular myopathies (Fig. 31-13B), typically from neonates, demonstrate small fibers with central nuclei.

IDIOPATHIC INFLAMMATORY MYOPATHIES

Inflammatory myopathies are a heterogeneous group of acquired disorders, all of which feature symmetric proximal muscle weakness, increased serum levels of muscle-derived enzymes, and nonsuppurative inflammation of skeletal muscle.

These are uncommon diseases, the annual incidence being 1 in 100,000. *Dermatomyositis afflicts children and adults, but polymyositis almost always begins after 20 years of age.* Both disorders occur more often in females than males. In contrast, inclusion body myositis is usually a disease of men over age 50.

These myopathies are thought to have an autoimmune origin (see Chapter 11) because (1) they often occur in association with other autoimmune and connective tissue diseases, (2) the pathology suggests autoimmune cellular injury, (3) serum autoantibodies can be detected, and (4) polymyositis and dermatomyositis (but not inclusion body myositis) respond to immunosuppressive therapy. No specific target autoantigens in muscle or blood vessels have been identified, but antinuclear and anticytoplasmic antibodies against several different antigens exist in all. By contrast, the recently described immune-mediated necrotizing myopathy (IMNM) generally shows little or no lymphocytic inflammatory reaction and is associated, in some cases, with specific autoantibodies.

The inflammatory myopathies are characterized by (1) the presence of inflammatory cells (although few if any lymphocytes in IMNM), (2) necrosis and phagocytosis of muscle fibers, (3) a mixture of degenerating, regenerating, and atrophic fibers and, in late stages, (4) fibrosis.

 CLINICAL FEATURES: All inflammatory myopathies manifest as insidious, often symmetric muscle weakness, gradually increasing over weeks to months. Patients have problems with simple activities that require use of proximal muscles, including lifting objects, climbing steps, or combing hair. Dysphagia and difficulty in holding up the head reflect involvement of pharyngeal and neck-flexor muscles. Some patients with inclusion body myositis have distal muscle weakness of the limbs that equals or exceeds that of proximal muscles. Myocardial involvement may occur. In advanced cases, respiratory muscles may be affected. Interstitial lung disease may also compromise respiratory function in 10% of polymyositis and dermatomyositis patients. Weakness progresses over weeks or months and leads to severe muscular wasting. Unlike cells in normal muscle, muscle cells in inflammatory myopathies express major histocompatibility complex (MHC) I antigens, which can promote an autoimmune reaction. There is an increased association of malignancy in adults with dermatomyositis. By contrast, the risk of malignancy in polymyositis and inclusion body myositis is considerably less, though nonzero.

Muscle Damage in Polymyositis Is Mediated by Cytotoxic T Cells

 MOLECULAR PATHOGENESIS: In polymyositis, there is no detectable microangiopathy as is seen in dermatomyositis (see below). In these

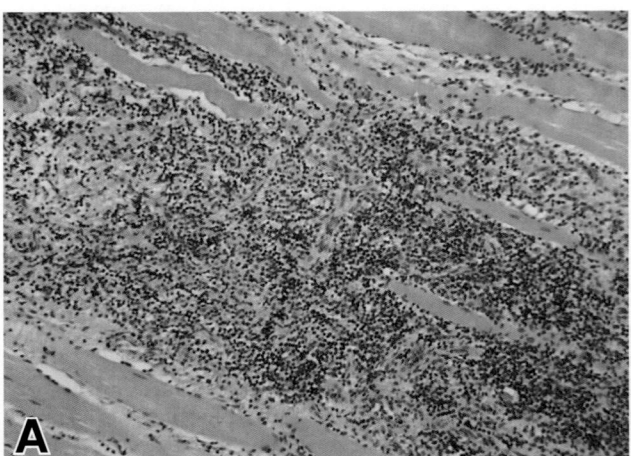
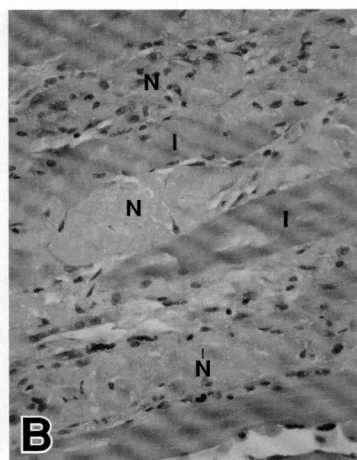
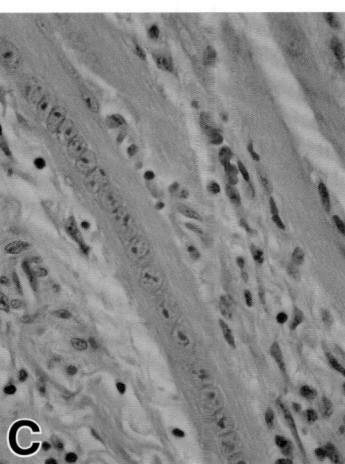

FIGURE 31-14. Polymyositis. A. A section of affected muscle stained with hematoxylin and eosin shows an inflammatory myopathy. Mononuclear inflammatory cells infiltrate chiefly the endomysium. The field includes single-fiber necrosis. **B.** A region of healing in an inflammatory myopathy demonstrates intact fibers (*I*) and necrotic fibers (*N*). The uppermost necrotic fiber is heavily infiltrated with macrophages. **C.** A regenerating fiber displays a linear array of enlarged centrally placed nuclei. Such enlarged nuclei are also represented diagrammatically in Figure 31-5E.

disorders, healthy muscle fibers are initially surrounded by CD8+ T lymphocytes (Fig. 31-14) and macrophages, after which the fibers degenerate.

The pathogenetic role of autoantibodies against nuclear antigens and cytoplasmic ribonucleoproteins in muscle injury is unknown. Polymyositis often has detectable anti-Jo-1, an antibody against histidyl-transfer RNA (tRNA) synthetase, with concomitant interstitial lung disease, Raynaud phenomenon, and nonerosive arthritis.

Viral infections may precede polymyositis, but virus cultures of muscle are negative. An inflammatory myopathy may also occur in many cases of HIV-1 infection, but the role of the virus is unclear.

PATHOLOGY: Inflammatory cells infiltrate connective tissue mostly within fascicles (i.e., endomysial inflammation) and invade apparently healthy muscle (Fig. 31-14). Angiopathy is absent. Isolated degenerating or regenerating fibers are scattered throughout fascicles. Perifascicular atrophy does not occur in polymyositis (see below).

Inclusion Body Myositis Is Characterized by Filamentous Inclusions and Amyloid Deposits

Inclusion body myositis typically occurs in older patients (>50 years) and is the most common inflammatory myopathy of the elderly. It resembles polymyositis pathologically, showing single-fiber necrosis and regeneration, with predominantly endomysial cytotoxic T cells. Basophilic granular material is seen at the edge of vacuoles (rimmed vacuoles) within muscle fibers (Fig. 31-15A,B). Such rimmed vacuoles are seen only on cryostat sections (i.e., sections of frozen, unfixed tissue). They are not present in formalin-fixed tissue. Curiously, muscle fibers in these patients contain intracellular amyloid that is immunoreactive for several amyloidogenic proteins typically associated with neurodegenerative diseases. These include the β-amyloid protein, the same type of amyloid seen in senile plaques in

Alzheimer disease. Other proteins associated with Alzheimer disease are also present including phosphorylated tau, and presenilins (see Chapter 32). Parkin, which accumulates in hereditary Parkinson disease, α-synuclein (idiopathic Parkinson disease and Lewy body disease), ubiquitin, TDP-43 (associated with frontotemporal degeneration and amyotrophic lateral sclerosis [ALS]), and the prion precursor protein have also been localized to the inclusions. Interestingly, these patients have no increased risk of neurodegeneration than age-matched controls.

The pathogenic role of these inclusions is unclear as similar neurodegenerative disease–associated protein accumulation has been observed in other rare myopathies (X-linked Emery–Dreifuss muscular dystrophy, oculopharyngeal muscular dystrophy [see above] and myofibrillar myopathies) as well as in chronic denervation. Unique features of inclusion body myositis include Congo red–positive inclusions (Congo red stains most amyloids), the characteristic cytoplasmic (or rarely nuclear) filaments in muscle fibers, and an inflammatory infiltrate, though the latter may be slight. By electron microscopy, the granules of rimmed vacuoles contain membranous whorls and adjacent distinctive filaments (Fig. 31-15C). An autosomal recessive hereditary form of the disease shows similar features but may present in late adolescence or adulthood. Despite the presence of inflammation, immunosuppressive therapy does not mitigate the disease, but intravenous immunoglobulin (IVIG) may be therapeutically useful.

Dermatomyositis Is an Immune-Mediated Microangiopathy

Dermatomyositis differs from other myopathies in having a characteristic rash on the upper eyelids, face, trunk, and sometimes elsewhere. It may occur alone or together with scleroderma, mixed connective tissue disease, or other autoimmune conditions.

PATHOPHYSIOLOGY: Dermatomyositis is characterized by (1) deposition of immune complexes of IgG, IgM, and complement components,

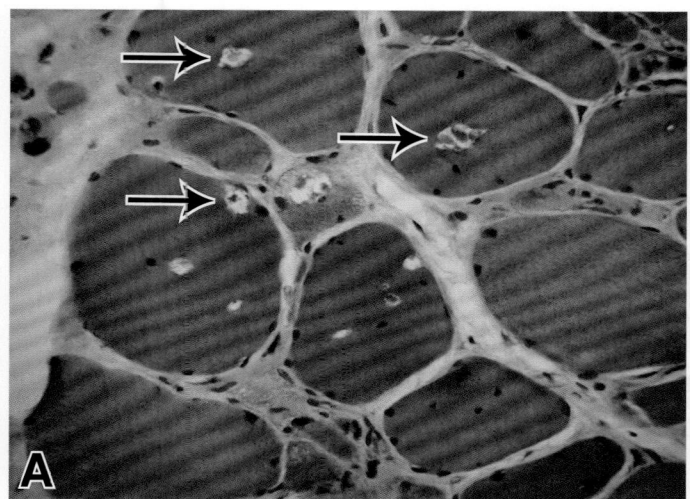
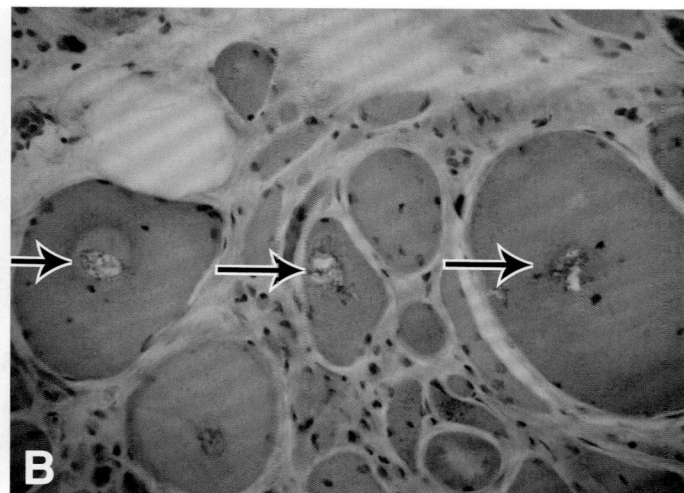

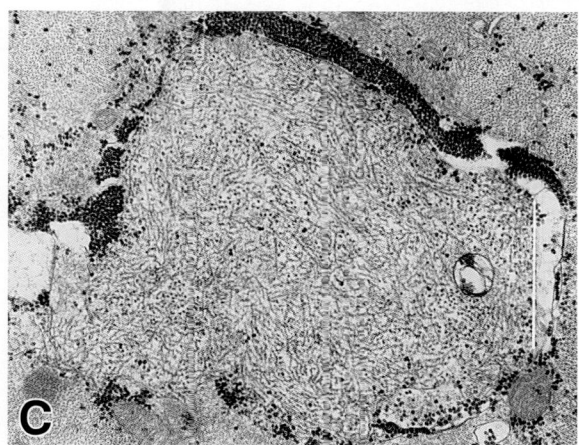

FIGURE 31-15. Inclusion body myositis (IBM). A. IBM as seen in this hematoxylin- and eosin-stained frozen section resembles polymyositis, but the muscle fibers also exhibit rimmed vacuoles (*arrows*) corresponding to enlarged lysosomes. **B.** The modified Gomori trichrome stain shows granular basophilic rimming of vacuoles. **C.** Electron microscopy shows the characteristic filaments of the amyloid inclusions.

including membrane attack complex C5b-9 in the walls of capillaries and other blood vessels; (2) microangiopathy with loss of capillaries; (3) signs of injury and atrophy of myofibers; (4) perivascular infiltrates of B cells and CD4+ helper T cells; and (5) perifascicular atrophy (Fig. 31-16). These features suggest that muscle injury in dermatomyositis is mainly mediated by complement-fixing cytotoxic antibodies against skeletal muscle microvasculature. Complement deposition in capillary walls preceding inflammation or damage to muscle fibers is the most specific finding. This microangiopathy is thought to lead to ischemic injury of individual muscle fibers and eventually to fiber atrophy. True infarcts may result from involvement of larger intramuscular arteries. The rash clinically distinguishes dermatomyositis from the other inflammatory myopathies due to the same microangiopathy.

PATHOLOGY: B and T lymphocytes infiltrate around blood vessels and in perimysial connective tissue with a high CD4+ (helper):CD8+ (cytotoxic/suppressor) T-cell ratio. Immune complexes including IgG, IgM, and complement C5-9 membrane attack complex in the walls of blood vessels (Fig. 31-16, inset) are associated with the microangiopathy. Perifascicular atrophy (one or more layers of atrophic fibers at the periphery

of fascicles) is pathognomonic (Fig. 31-16) even if inflammation is lacking. The perifascicular atrophy is due to relative hypoperfusion of perifascicular zones.

Immune-Mediated Necrotizing Myopathy Is Also Known as Necrotizing Autoimmune Myositis

IMNM is a recently described group of myopathies characterized by myonecrosis, myophagocytosis (numerous macrophages consuming myofiber debris), regenerating fibers, and a few scattered endomysial and perimysial macrophages. Lymphocytic infiltration is minimal to absent. As in other forms of inflammatory myopathies, MHC-1 is upregulated. Clinically, patients present with subacute symmetrical proximal limb weakness (similar to polymyositis), moderate-to-severe weakness of acute or subacute onset, and an elevated creatine kinase in the thousands.

PATHOPHYSIOLOGY: IMNM is associated with anti-SRP (signal recognition particle) and anti HMGCR (β-hydroxy-β-methylglutaryl-COA reductase) antibodies. Anti-SRP patients have an overall poor response to therapy with approximately half recovering. Cardiac involvement has been described. Some patients treated chronically with statin drugs (HMG CoA

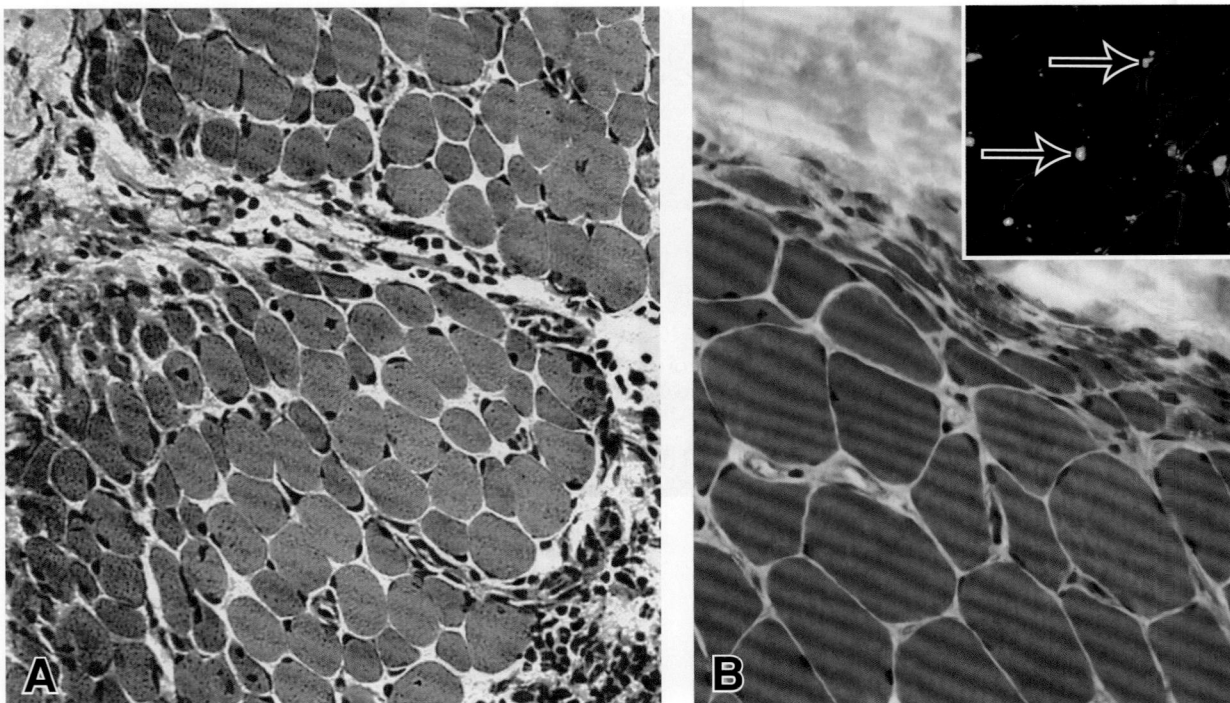

FIGURE 31-16. Dermatomyositis. A. Inflammatory cells infiltrate predominantly the perimysium rather than the endomysium. Peripheral regions of muscle fascicles show most of the muscle fiber atrophy and damage resulting in a pattern of injury characteristic of dermatomyositis termed *perifascicular atrophy*. **B.** High-magnification image of perifascicular atrophy shows flattening and shrinkage of fibers at the periphery of the fascicle. Immunofluorescence (*inset*) reveals that the walls of many capillaries display C5b-9 (membrane attack complex), reflecting the altered microvasculature typical of dermatomyositis.

reductase inhibitors) develop markedly elevated CKs, profound weakness, and anti-HMGCR antibodies despite discontinuation of the drugs. However, a large percentage of IMNM patients with anti-HMGCR antibodies have never been exposed to statins. IMNM patients with anti-HMGCR are at increased risk of malignancy. Some cases of IMNM are associated with viral infections including HIV and hepatitis C virus.

 PATHOLOGY: Muscle biopsies typically show scattered necrotic or degenerating fibers with endomysial macrophages and a lack of a lymphocytic inflammatory infiltrate. Often the clinical suspicion includes rhabdomyolysis. The mechanism of cell injury involves antibody-dependent complement-mediated lysis. Immunohistochemistry demonstrates deposits of MHC-1 and C5-9 complex on the sarcolemma in sharp contrast to the capillary C5-9 deposits seen in dermatomyositis. Macrophages are not the cause of injury; they merely remove the damaged myofibers. The histologic findings are not specific. Confirmation requires demonstration of anti-SRP or anti-HMGCR antibodies. INMN is responsive to immunosuppression.

Vasculitis in Skeletal Muscle May Be Part of Systemic Vasculitides

Vasculitis can be present in skeletal muscle in systemic inflammatory diseases of blood vessels including polyarteritis nodosa (PAN), granulomatosis with polyangiitis, collagen vascular diseases, and immune-mediated hypersensitivity states. In such instances, skeletal muscle may show neurogenic changes (see below) secondary to nerve damage.

MYASTHENIA GRAVIS

Myasthenia gravis is an acquired autoimmune disease in which antibodies to the ACh receptor at the neuromuscular junction cause abnormal muscular fatigability. It occurs in all races and is twice as common in women as in men. The disease typically begins in young adults, but first presentations may vary from childhood to old age.

PATHOPHYSIOLOGY: In myasthenia gravis, antibodies bind the ACh receptor of the motor endplate. Complement activation leads to shedding of the ACh receptor–rich terminal portions of the folds of the neuromuscular junction. The offending bivalent IgG antibodies also cross-link receptor proteins that remain in the postsynaptic membrane resulting in accelerated ACh receptor endocytosis such that the muscle cannot replace them. The combination of reduced postsynaptic membrane area, decreased numbers of ACh receptors per unit area, and widened synaptic space impairs signal transmission leading to muscle weakness and abnormal fatigability. However, the antireceptor antibodies do not directly block ACh binding its receptor.

Most patients with myasthenia gravis have anti–ACh receptor antibodies and thymic hyperplasia. About 15% have an associated thymoma. Surgical removal of the hyperplastic thymic tissue or the thymoma often causes the myasthenia gravis to remit. ACh receptors are present on the surface of some thymic cells in thymoma and thymic hyperplasia. Thus, thymic T cells may trigger production of antireceptor antibodies.

PATHOLOGY: Light microscopy may reveal atrophy of type II muscle fibers and focal collections of lymphocytes within fascicles. However, electron microscopy shows that most muscle endplates are abnormal, even in muscles that are not weakened. Sarcolemmal secondary folds are simplified with apparent breakdown, loss of the crests of the folds, and widening of the clefts.

CLINICAL FEATURES: The clinical severity of the condition is quite variable and symptoms tend to wax and wane as in other autoimmune diseases. Weakness of extraocular muscles is typically severe and causes ptosis and diplopia. Sometimes, myasthenia gravis may be limited to those muscles. More commonly, it progresses to other muscles (e.g., those associated with swallowing, the trunk and extremities). Patients with myasthenia gravis often have other autoimmune diseases.

The overall mortality from myasthenia gravis is about 10%, often because muscle weakness leads to respiratory insufficiency. In addition to thymectomy, treatment includes immunosuppression and anticholinesterase drugs that retard breakdown of ACh in the synaptic cleft. Plasmapheresis reduces anti–ACh receptor antibody titers, but any resultant clinical improvements are short-lived.

INHERITED METABOLIC DISEASES

Skeletal muscle is affected dramatically by many endocrine and metabolic diseases such as Cushing syndrome, Addison disease, hypothyroidism, hyperthyroidism (see Chapter 27), and conditions associated with hepatic or renal failure. Only primary hereditary abnormalities in metabolism of skeletal muscle resulting in abnormal muscular function are discussed here.

Glycogen Storage Diseases Are Genetic Disorders With Variable Effects on Muscle

Glycogen storage diseases (glycogenoses) are inherited autosomal recessive metabolic disorders characterized by defects in the ability to degrade glycogen (see Chapter 6). There are many glycogenoses, and only some affect skeletal muscle. Only the most important glycogenoses affecting skeletal muscle will be described.

Type II Glycogenosis (Acid Maltase [α-1,4-Glucosidase] Deficiency, Pompe Disease)

MOLECULAR PATHOGENESIS: Acid maltase is a ubiquitously expressed lysosomal enzyme that participates in glycogen degradation. Various mutations affect muscle acid maltase activity and lead to distinctly different clinical syndromes. When the enzyme is deficient, glycogen is not broken down, and it accumulates within lysosomes and remains membrane bound (Fig. 31-17).

PATHOLOGY: In all forms of glycogenosis due to acid maltase deficiency, the morphologic changes are distinctive and almost pathognomonic (Fig. 31-17). In the severe form, Pompe disease, muscle shows massive accumulation of membrane-bound glycogen. Myofilaments and other sarcoplasmic organelles disappear. There is very little regeneration and apparently inactive satellite cells are seen at the surfaces of muscle fibers that have been almost completely destroyed by the disease.

Late infantile, juvenile, and adult-onset forms of type II glycogenosis are milder with changes ranging from overt vacuolar myopathy to subtle accumulation of

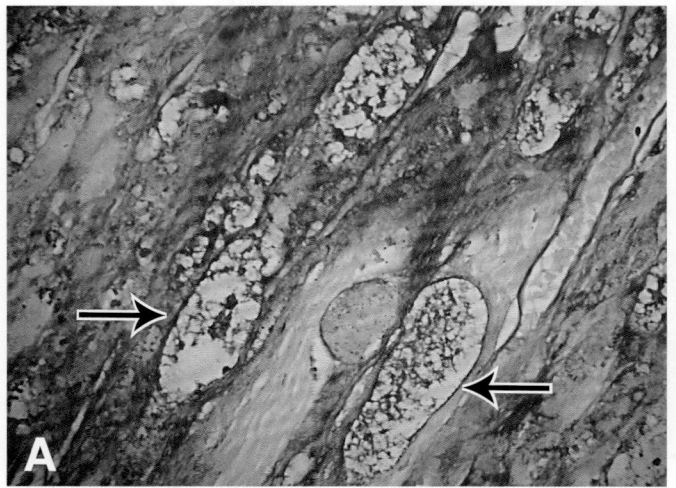
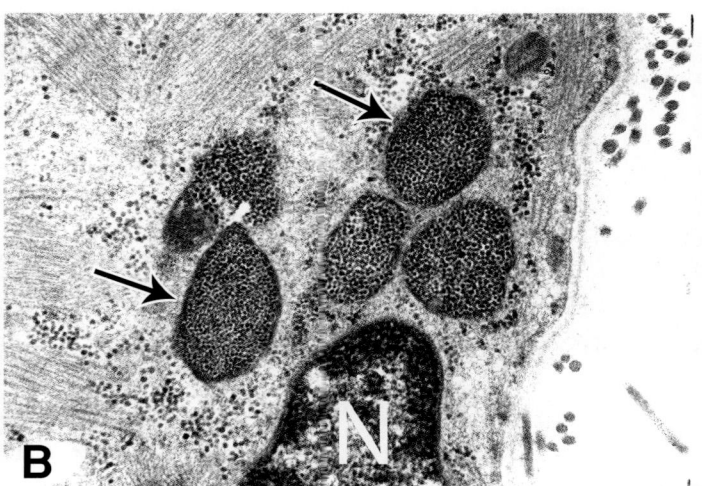

FIGURE 31-17. Acid maltase deficiency—adult onset. A. Periodic acid–Schiff (PAS) stain demonstrates large vacuoles filled with PAS-positive glycogen granules (*arrows*). **B.** Electron microscopy shows membrane-bound glycogen granules (*arrows*) adjacent to the cell nucleus (*N*).

membrane-bound glycogen particles detectable only by electron microscopy. Vacuoles seen by light microscopy are empty or contain glycogen.

 CLINICAL FEATURES: Pompe disease occurs in neonates or young infants and is the most extreme form of acid maltase deficiency. Patients have severe hypotonia and areflexia. Some have enlarged tongues and cardiomegaly and die of cardiac failure, usually within their first 2 years. Many tissues are affected, but skeletal and cardiac muscle, the CNS, and the liver are most involved. The serum creatine kinase level is slightly to moderately increased. Later-onset forms of the disease entail milder, but relentlessly progressive myopathy. Glycogen accumulates in other organs, but clinical expression of the disorder is usually limited to muscle.

Type III Glycogenosis (Debranching Enzyme Deficiency, Cori Disease, Limit Dextrinosis, Amylo-1,6-Glucosidase Deficiency)

 MOLECULAR PATHOGENESIS: Type III glycogenosis is a rare, autosomal recessive disease of children or adults. Because the debranching enzyme is absent, phosphorylase can hydrolyze 1,4-glycosidic linkages of the terminal glucose chains of glycogen, but not beyond branch points. Hepatomegaly and growth retardation are the rule. Muscle symptoms vary, and the most severe and consistent involvement is related to liver dysfunction in children.

Type V Glycogenosis (McArdle Disease, Myophosphorylase Deficiency)

MOLECULAR PATHOGENESIS: Type V glycogenosis is a more common metabolic myopathy that is usually not progressive or severely

debilitating. The deficient enzyme, myophosphorylase, is specific for skeletal muscle. Without this enzyme, skeletal muscle glycogen cannot be cleaved at 1,4-glycosidic chains to produce glucose for energy production during physical exertion. Thus, muscles cramp with exercise. Patients also cannot produce lactate during ischemic exercise which is the basis for a metabolic test for the condition.

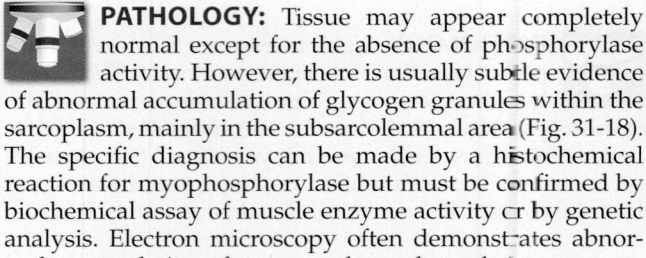 **PATHOLOGY:** Tissue may appear completely normal except for the absence of phosphorylase activity. However, there is usually subtle evidence of abnormal accumulation of glycogen granules within the sarcoplasm, mainly in the subsarcolemmal area (Fig. 31-18). The specific diagnosis can be made by a histochemical reaction for myophosphorylase but must be confirmed by biochemical assay of muscle enzyme activity or by genetic analysis. Electron microscopy often demonstrates abnormal accumulation of non–membrane-bound glycogen.

CLINICAL FEATURES: Myophosphorylase deficiency need not seriously interfere with patients' lives. However, prolonged, vigorous exercise can lead to widespread myofiber necrosis and release of soluble muscle proteins like creatine kinase and myoglobin into the blood. This can cause myoglobinuria and renal failure. Muscle biopsy should be performed several weeks after an episode of symptoms to allow regeneration of the muscle.

Type VII Glycogenosis (Phosphofructokinase Deficiency, Tarui Disease)

 MOLECULAR PATHOGENESIS: Phosphofructokinase (PFK) deficiency is less common than McArdle disease but causes the same syndrome. PFK converts fructose-6-phosphate to fructose-1,6-diphosphate and is a key enzyme in glycolysis. In muscle,

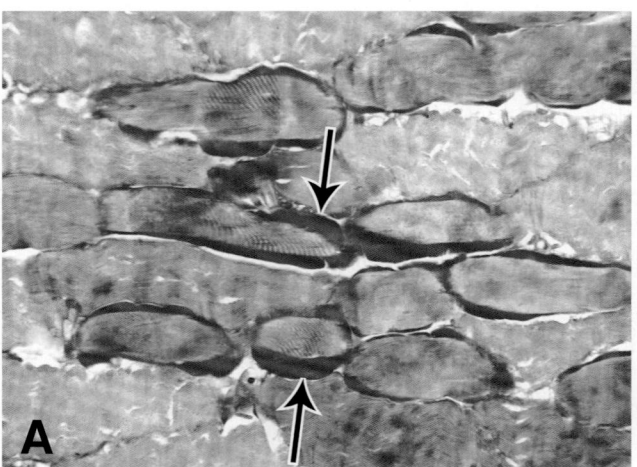

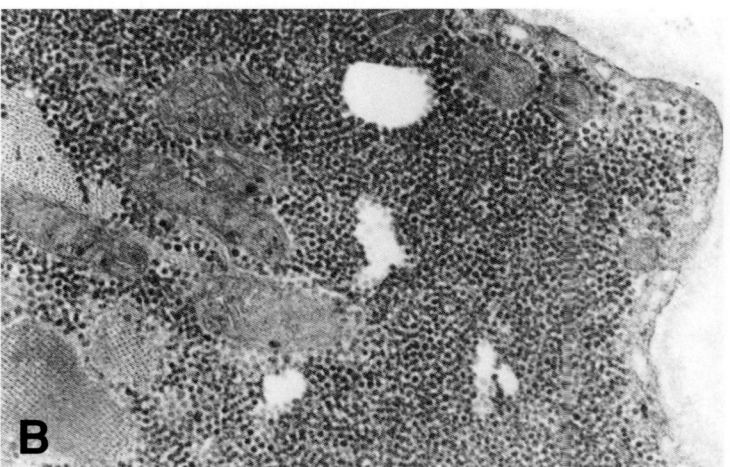

FIGURE 31-18. McArdle disease (myophosphorylase deficiency). A. Periodic acid–Schiff staining shows prominent glycogen accumulation in a subsarcolemmal distribution (*arrows*). **B.** Electron microcopy demonstrates a mass of glycogen particles just beneath the sarcolemma which, in contrast to the lysosomal glycogen storage of acid maltase deficiency shown in Figure 31-17B, is not surrounded by a membrane.

this enzyme has four identical subunits (M_4), while in erythrocytes, it has two different (M and L) subunits, each encoded separately. Genetic lack of the muscle subunit thus leads to complete absence of muscle PFK activity but reduces erythrocyte PFK by 50%. In red blood cells, the remaining active enzyme is composed of four normal L subunits.

Patients with type VII glycogenosis often have slight anemia or low-grade hemolysis, but muscle histology resembles that in McArdle disease except that phosphorylase activity is present. By contrast, histochemistry shows little or no PFK activity. The diagnosis is substantiated by biochemical assay of enzyme activity in muscle.

Lipid Myopathies Are Caused by Defective Fat Metabolism

A muscle biopsy from a patient with exercise intolerance or muscle weakness may sometimes show excess neutral lipids. This occurs in several metabolic disorders of lipid metabolism, more than a dozen of which are known. In brief, lipid myopathies may involve deficiencies in (1) fatty acid transport into mitochondria (carnitine deficiency syndromes, carnitine palmitoyl transferase deficiency), (2) various enzymes that mediate β-oxidation of fatty acids, (3) respiratory chain enzymes, and (4) triglyceride utilization.

Carnitine Deficiency

Carnitine is synthesized in the liver and occurs in large quantities in skeletal muscle. It is required for long-chain fatty acid transport into mitochondria. Muscle carnitine deficiency is an autosomal recessive condition associated with progressive proximal muscle weakness and atrophy often with signs of denervation and peripheral neuropathy. Without carnitine, lipid droplets accumulate massively in the sarcoplasm outside mitochondria and are readily seen in muscle biopsies (Fig. 31-19). Sometimes oral carnitine therapy alleviates symptoms. Carnitine deficiency in skeletal

muscle also occurs as part of a systemic disorder that can affect the CNS, heart, and liver. Structural abnormalities of mitochondria may be present.

Carnitine Palmitoyltransferase Deficiency

Patients with carnitine palmitoyltransferase deficiency cannot metabolize long-chain fatty acids owing to an inability to transport these lipids into mitochondria where they undergo β-oxidation. After heavy exercise, these patients have muscular pain that may progress to myoglobinuria. Prolonged fasting, which shifts energy production in muscle entirely to fatty acids, can produce the same symptoms. After such an episode, fibers regenerate and restore muscle structure. Biopsies are microscopically normal; the diagnosis requires biochemical assay of carnitine palmitoyltransferase activity.

In Mitochondrial Diseases, Nuclear or Mitochondrial DNA May Be Mutated

Inherited defects of mitochondrial metabolism are uncommon but conceptually important disorders. Historically, diseases of muscle were recognized first and designated mitochondrial myopathies, but others affect both CNS and muscle and are known as **mitochondrial encephalomyopathies**. The nervous system, skeletal muscle, heart, kidney, and other organs can be affected in different combinations as part of a multisystem disease.

Inherited diseases of mitochondria are divided into defects of **nuclear DNA** (nDNA) or **mitochondrial DNA** (mtDNA). Point mutations, deletions, and duplications of mtDNA have been linked to several mitochondrial encephalomyopathies.

MOLECULAR PATHOGENESIS: The genes for most mitochondrial proteins are in nDNA, but mtDNA encodes 13 of the 80 polypeptides in respiratory chain complexes. Defects in these proteins lead to mitochondrial encephalomyopathies.

Unlike Mendelian inheritance of nDNA genes, mtDNA diseases are inherited maternally since mtDNA is derived only from the oocyte. The zygote and its daughter cells have many mitochondria each of which contains maternally derived mtDNA. Mutations in this DNA are passed on randomly to later generations of cells. During fetal or later growth, some cells may thus contain only mutant genomes (mutant homoplasmy), others will have only normal genomes (wild-type homoplasmy), and still others receive mixed populations of mutant and normal mtDNA (heteroplasmy). Clinical expression of a disease due to a mutation in mtDNA depends on the proportion of the total content of mitochondrial genomes that is mutant. *The fraction of mutant mtDNA must exceed a critical value for a mitochondrial disease to be symptomatic.* This threshold varies in different organs and is related to cellular energy requirements.

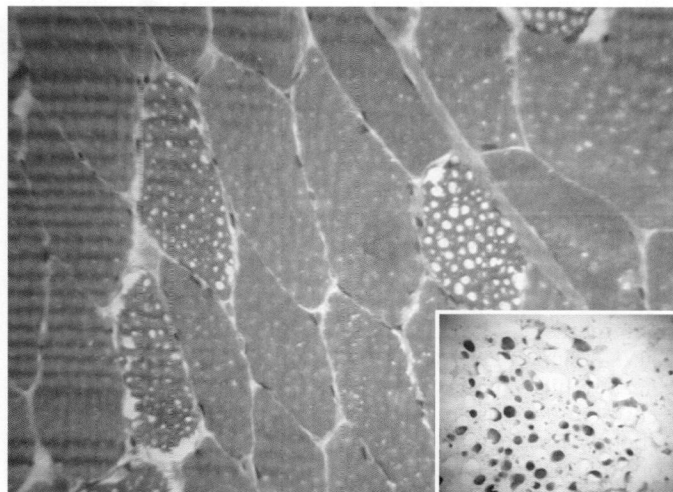

FIGURE 31-19. Lipid storage myopathy. Numerous cytoplasmic vacuoles are seen in muscle fibers in this frozen section stained with hematoxylin and eosin. Oil red-orcein stain (*inset*) demonstrates that the cytoplasmic vacuoles contain neutral lipid (seen as red stained material).

PATHOLOGY: In skeletal muscle, defects of mtDNA lead to accumulation of mitochondria, excessive numbers of which may appear as aggregates of reddish granular material in a subsarcolemmal

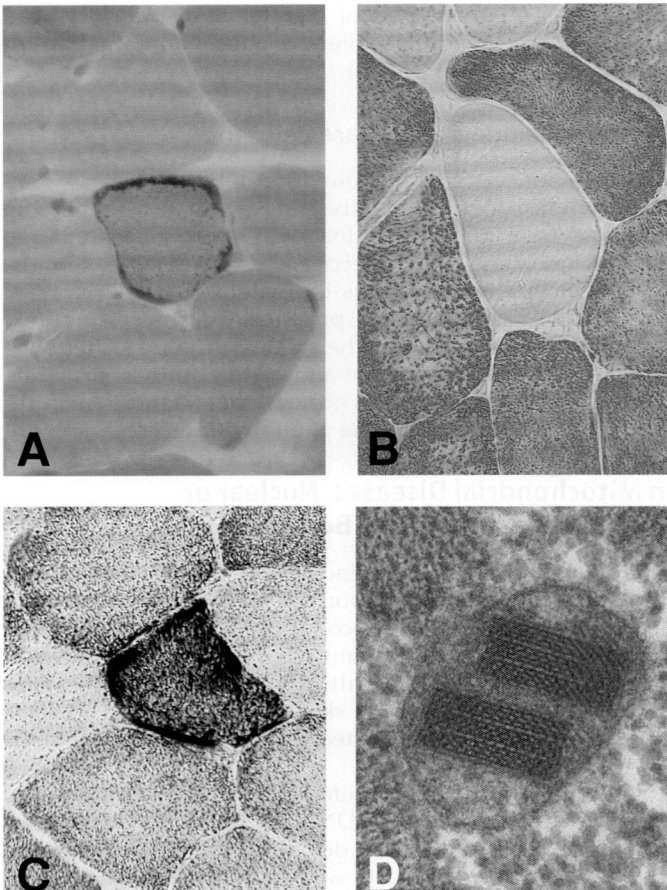

FIGURE 31-20. Mitochondrial myopathy caused by deletions of mitochondrial DNA (mtDNA). A. A ragged red fiber seen with the modified Gomori trichrome stain shows prominent proliferation of reddish, granular mitochondria, located chiefly in a subsarcolemmal region. **B.** A ragged red fiber displays lack of **histochemical staining for cytochrome oxidase** (central pale fiber). Three subunits of this electron-transport carrier are encoded by mtDNA, and the mutations have interfered with function in this fiber. **C.** Histochemical staining for **succinate dehydrogenase** activity shows that the ragged red fiber overexpresses this enzyme which is encoded only by nuclear DNA (nDNA). **D.** Electron microscopy reveals paracrystalline inclusions in mitochondria.

location (underneath the myocyte plasma membrane) with modified Gomori trichrome stain (Fig. 31-20A). These are called **ragged red fibers** because these deposits have an irregular contour at the fiber periphery. Three subunits of complex IV (cytochrome oxidase) are encoded by mtDNA and are required for the assembled electron transport chain to be functional. Pathogenic mutations of mtDNA may impair complex IV activity, such that ragged red fibers are often deficient in cytochrome oxidase activity (Fig. 31-20B). By contrast, ragged red fibers stain intensely for succinate dehydrogenase (SDH, complex II); this complex is encoded exclusively by nDNA (Fig. 31-20C). The increased SDH staining reflects mitochondrial proliferation. Such defects cause myofiber atrophy and accumulation of sarcoplasmic lipid and glycogen owing to impaired mitochondrial energy utilization. Ultrastructurally, mitochondria may display striking paracrystalline

inclusions (Fig. 31-20D), ring-shaped mitochondria, spiral cristae, and electron-dense deposits.

Increased ragged red fibers and cytochrome oxidase–negative fibers may also occur in elderly patients with unexplained muscle weakness ("mitochondrial cytopathy of old age"), presumably because of age related accumulation of mitochondrial mutations. Ragged red fibers, cytochrome oxidase–negative fibers, and intramitochondrial paracrystalline inclusions all suggest a mitochondrial disorder but are not specific as similar changes occur in some muscular dystrophies, in inclusion body myositis, and with certain drugs. Conversely, the absence of such changes does not exclude a mitochondrial disorder.

CLINICAL FEATURES: Clinical presentations of encephalomyopathies vary, but diseases may begin in children or adults. Some patients start with muscle weakness and then develop brain disorders. Others present with CNS disease with or without overt muscle weakness even though muscle biopsy shows mitochondrial pathology. Other organs such as the heart (arrhythmias) are often affected as part of a multisystem disorder. The number of known mitochondrial disorders is increasing rapidly. The discussion below of major mitochondrial myopathies is a small sample.

Four well-known mitochondrial syndromes include (1) **Kearns–Sayre syndrome** (KSS) (progressive ophthalmoplegia, retinitis pigmentosum, cardiac arrhythmias, diabetes mellitus, cerebellar ataxia, and multifocal neurodegeneration), (2) **chronic progressive external ophthalmoplegia**, (3) mitochondrial myopathy, encephalopathy, lactic acidosis and stroke-like episodes (**MELAS**), and (4) myoclonic epilepsy and ragged red fibers (**MERRF**). Most patients with KSS have large deletions of mtDNA that are usually nonfamilial. A related but clinically more benign condition, chronic progressive external ophthalmoplegia (CPEO) also has mitochondrial DNA deletions. Patients present with bilateral ptosis and weakness of eye muscles as in KSS. Clinically, the presence of cardiac arrhythmias in a CPEO patient predicts progression to KSS. The mitochondrial DNA deletions probably arise during oogenesis. All such affected people are heteroplasmic (i.e., they have a mixture of mutant and normal mitochondria) and the phenotype depends on the distribution and relative numbers of mutant mitochondria at birth. Despite the presence of these congenital mutations, symptoms typically appear in early adulthood (20 to 40 years). More severe forms (KSS) typically present in the second decade. Both KSS and CPEO patients have multiple mtDNA deletions that are secondary to mutations in a number of nuclear-encoded genes including *POLG* (DNA polymerase-γ, which replicates mitochondrial DNA), *TWNK* which encodes mitochondrial DNA helicase, and *ANT* which makes adenine nucleotide translocator-1. Thus, mutations in these nuclear-encoded genes subsequently produce mitochondrial DNA deletions. External ophthalmoplegia may also be present in other syndromes including MELAS and MERRF. MELAS and MERRF usually involve point mutations in mitochondrial genes for tRNAs, mostly—but not exclusively—leucine tRNA (MELAS) and lysine tRNA (MERRF). Mitochondrial genetic disorders like MELAS and MERRF are inherited from maternal mtDNA. Other syndromes affecting mitochondrial proteins encoded by nuclear genes show autosomal (such as CPEO) or X-linked patterns of inheritance.

Myoadenylate Deaminase Deficiency Causes Mild Weakness

 MOLECULAR PATHOGENESIS: There are large amounts of adenosine monophosphate deaminase (AMP-DA) in skeletal muscle, particularly in type II fibers. AMP-DA is important in regulating purine nucleotide cycles and maintaining the adenosine triphosphate–to–adenosine diphosphate (ATP:ADP) ratio during exercise. A subset of patients with mild proximal muscle weakness and exercise intolerance lack AMP-DA activity completely. It is a common, autosomal recessive condition, seen in 1% to 2% of all muscle biopsies. AMP-DA deficiency may thus not actually be a separate disease, but one that is unmasked by other neuromuscular diseases.

Familial Periodic Paralysis Reflects Impaired Electrolyte Flux

Familial periodic paralysis encompasses several autosomal dominant disorders in which episodic muscular weakness or even complete paralysis is followed by rapid recovery. These reflect abnormalities in sodium and potassium fluxes into and out of muscle cells. During an attack, muscle fibers cannot propagate action potentials, although calcium entry into the muscle fiber causes contraction. Muscle biopsies during an attack show no detectable abnormalities of recent onset. Later, permanent mild myopathic changes and sarcoplasmic vacuoles appear. These vacuoles are dilated or remodeled sarcoplasmic reticulum and transverse tubules. In some cases, a distinct subpopulation of fibers (type IIB) contains numerous tubular aggregates derived from the tubular network of the sarcoplasmic reticulum.

 MOLECULAR PATHOGENESIS: These dyskalemic episodic weakness syndromes include hypokalemic and hyperkalemic periodic paralysis. The former type is linked to mutations in several genes including a calcium channel (*CACNA1S*), a sodium channel (*SCN4A*), and a potassium channel (*KCNE3*). In the hyperkalemic form, the same sodium channel gene (*SCN4A*) is mutated, but the hyperkalemic form reflects a gain-of-function *SCN4A* mutation, while the hypokalemic form is due to a loss-of-function mutation in the same sodium channel gene. A previously described normokalemic periodic paralysis syndrome is now considered a variant of hyperkalemic periodic paralysis and demonstrates mutations in *SCN4A*.

RHABDOMYOLYSIS

Rhabdomyolysis is dissolution of skeletal muscle fibers and release of myoglobin into the blood. This may cause myoglobinuria and acute renal failure. The disorder may be acute, subacute, or chronic. During acute rhabdomyolysis, muscles are swollen, tender, and profoundly weak.

Episodes of rhabdomyolysis may be precipitated by diverse stimuli. They may complicate or follow bouts of influenza. Some patients develop rhabdomyolysis with apparently mild exercise and probably have some form of metabolic myopathy. A spectrum of muscle dysfunction, from pain (myalgia) to rhabdomyolysis, is also well known during treatment with statin cholesterol-lowering agents. Biopsies after recovery may show morphologically normal muscle. Rhabdomyolysis also may complicate heat stroke or malignant hyperthermia. Alcoholism is occasionally associated with either acute or chronic rhabdomyolysis.

Pathologically, rhabdomyolysis is an active, noninflammatory myopathy, with scattered muscle fiber necrosis and varying degrees of degeneration and regeneration. Macrophages, but no other inflammatory cells, are present in and around muscle fibers.

Type II Fiber Atrophy

Selective angular atrophy of type II fibers may resemble denervation atrophy in sections stained with hematoxylin and eosin. However, myosin ATPase stains show that all angular atrophic fibers are type II (Fig. 31-21) and these fibers are not heavily stained by nonspecific esterase or NADH-TR reactions. Type II fiber atrophy may be seen with chronic corticosteroid therapy, chronic disuse, or in the elderly. It may also be seen in cachexia, carcinoid myopathy, alcohol abuse, polymyalgia rheumatica, and myasthenia gravis.

STEROID MYOPATHY: Corticosteroid therapy can cause muscle weakness with type II fiber atrophy. This may be confusing clinically as patients with polymyositis often receive large doses of corticosteroids. If such a patient's weakness worsens, the physician must decide if this represents relapse of polymyositis, requiring more corticosteroids, or steroid myopathy, in which case the steroid dosage must be reduced.

Patients with corticosteroid toxicity do not have increased serum creatine kinase levels and biopsies show selective

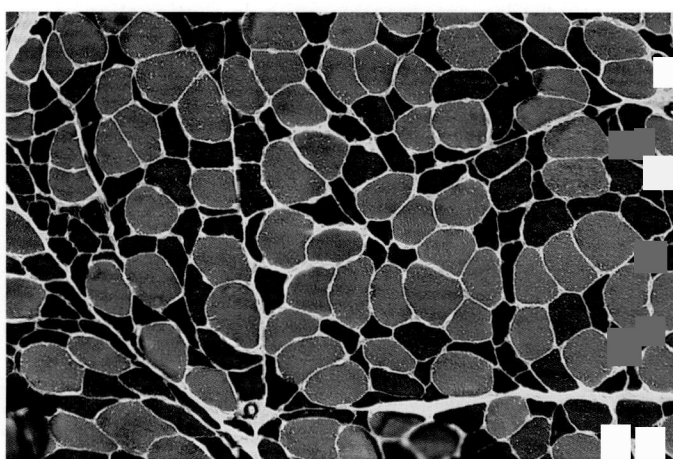

FIGURE 31-21. Type II fiber atrophy. This biopsy of the vastus lateralis muscle is from a 48-year-old man with proximal muscle weakness because of endogenous corticosteroid toxicity (Cushing syndrome). Virtually, all of the angular atrophic fibers are type II. This form of atrophy closely mimics denervation atrophy when visualized with the hematoxylin and eosin stain.

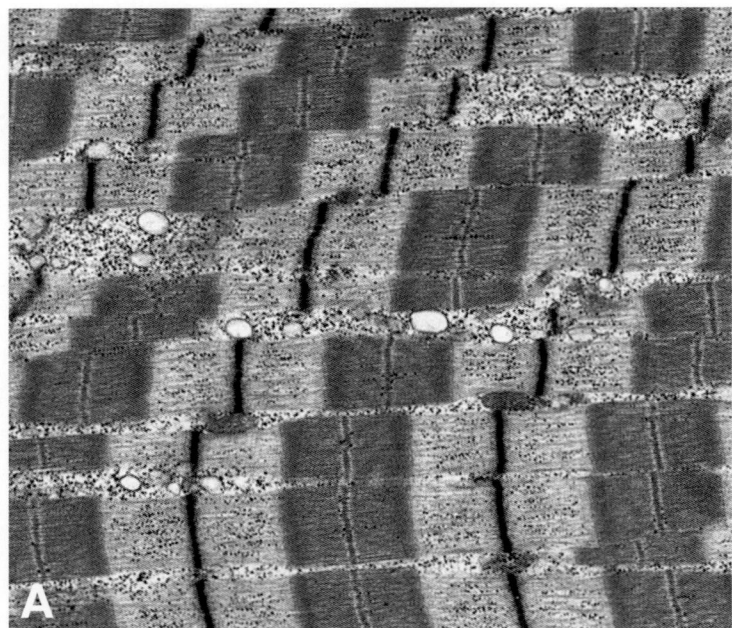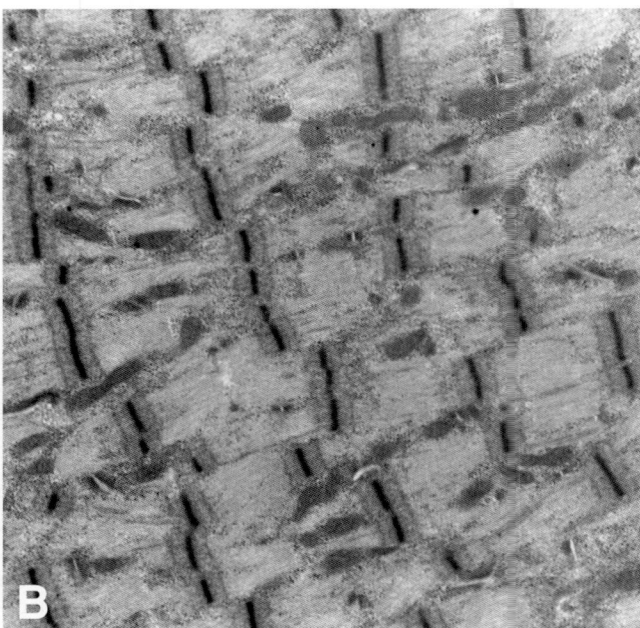

FIGURE 31-22. Critical Illness Myopathy. A. Electron microscopy of normal muscle shows sarcomeres composed of both thick (myosin) and thin (α-actin) filaments. **B.** Critical illness myopathy shows almost complete loss of thick myosin filaments, while α-actin (thin) filaments are intact. Note preservation of the Z disks.

atrophy of type II fibers, without muscle fiber degeneration or inflammation. By contrast, biopsies in recurrent polymyositis show fiber degeneration and inflammation associated with increased serum creatine kinase.

Critical Illness Myopathy

If patients being treated with high-dose steroids and neuromuscular blocking agents experience severe weakness despite removal of paralyzing agents, they may have **critical illness myopathy,** also known as **myosin heavy-chain depletion syndrome.** These patients show loss of thick myosin filaments from muscle fibers (Fig. 31-22). The underlying mechanism of the myosin depletion is unclear, although myosin thick filaments reappear with discontinuation of corticosteroids and muscle strength returns.

DENERVATION

The major differential diagnostic consideration in any patient with muscle weakness is whether the cause is myopathic or neurogenic. Myopathic conditions are those intrinsic to muscle and have been discussed above. Neurogenic causes of muscle weakness are due to denervation. The pathology of denervation reflects lesions of lower motor neurons and/or axons. Muscle biopsy detects lower motor neuron lesions, but patterns of denervation do not identify the cause of the lesion. The morphology may indicate whether denervation is recent or chronic but does not distinguish between, for example, ALS, a disorder of motor neurons, and neuropathy due to diabetes mellitus. Lesions of upper motor neurons, as in multiple sclerosis or stroke, lead to paralysis and atrophy but leave lower motor neurons intact. Pathologic changes thus reflect nonspecific diffuse atrophy rather than denervation atrophy.

When a skeletal muscle fiber becomes separated from contact with its lower motor neuron, it invariably atrophies, owing to progressive loss of myofibrils. On cross-section, atrophic fibers are characteristically angular, as though compressed by surrounding normal muscle fibers (Fig. 31-23). If a fiber is not reinnervated, atrophy progresses to complete loss of myofibrils, with nuclei condensing into aggregates. In the end stage, muscle fibers disappear and are replaced chiefly by fibroadipose tissue.

Early after denervation, fibers become irregularly scattered, angular, and atrophic. As the disease progresses, these fibers are first seen in small clusters of several fibers, and then in progressively larger groups (Fig. 31-23B). They stain excessively darkly for nonspecific esterase (Fig. 31-24) and NADH-TR, in contrast to atrophy caused by disuse or wasting. Groups of denervated fibers include both type I and type II fibers: **denervating conditions are not selective for only one type of motor neuron.**

"Target fibers" (Fig. 31-25) are seen transiently in 20% of cases of denervation. This change occurs during or shortly after denervation or reinnervation and indicates that the process is active. The lesion consists of central pallor of the muscle fiber surrounded by a condensed zone which, in turn, is surrounded by a normal zone of sarcoplasm. Target fibers are difficult to see with hematoxylin and eosin stain, but the NADH-TR stain shows greatly reduced staining in the central zone, reflecting reduced or absent mitochondria.

Denervation is always followed by an effort to reinnervate. If denervation proceeds slowly, reinnervation may keep pace. New sprouting nerve endings make synaptic contact with the muscle fiber at the site of the previous motor endplate. As in the myotubular phase of embryogenesis, nicotinic Ach receptors (extrajunctional receptors) cover muscle fibers soon after denervation. This denervated state induces sprouting of new nerve endings from adjacent surviving nerves. With reinnervation, extrajunctional receptors again

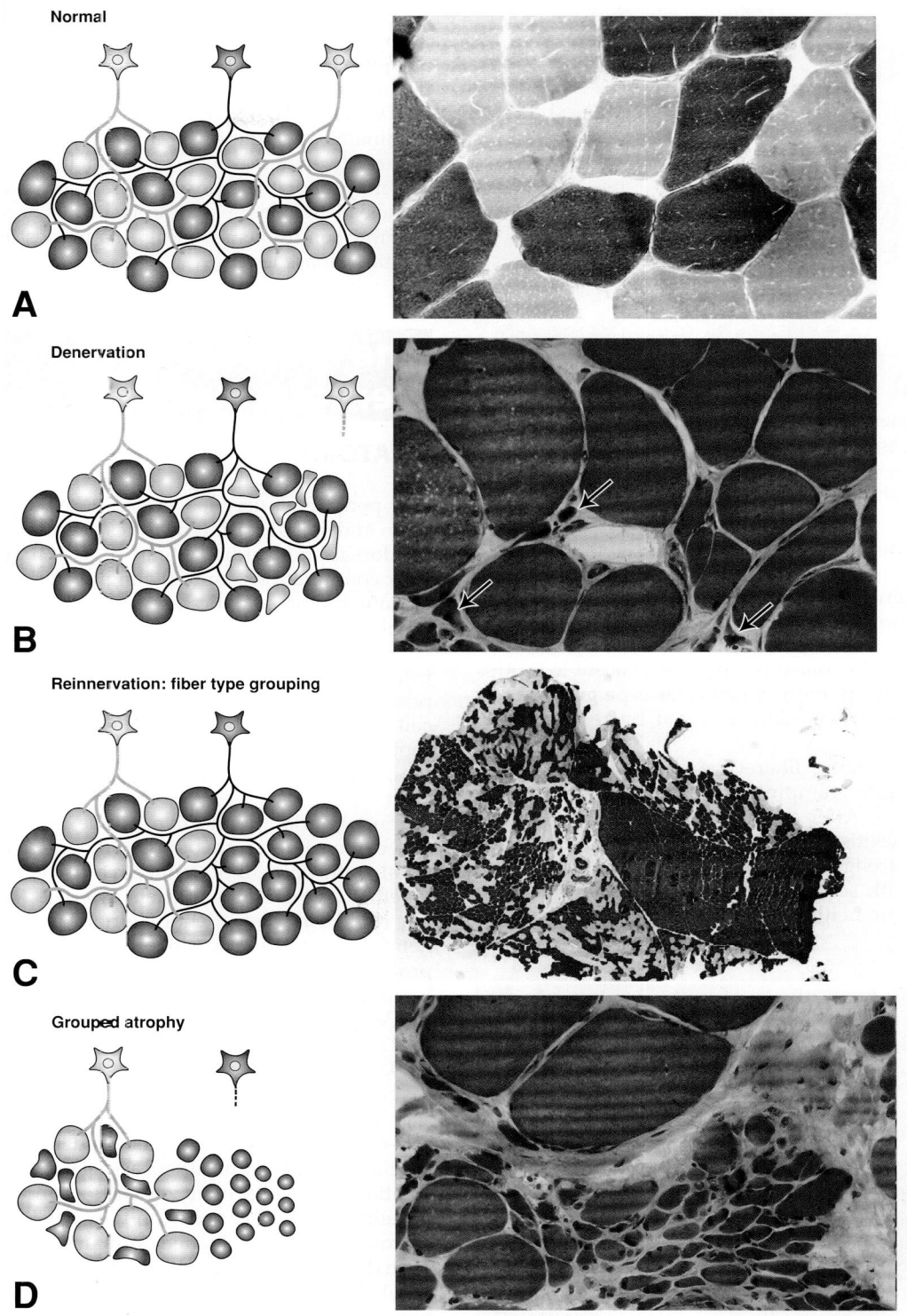

FIGURE 31-23. Denervation/reinnervation. A. ATPase staining shows that normal muscle contains intermixed type I (*pale*) and type II (*dark*) muscle fibers. In the drawing, two neurons (*pale*) innervate type I muscle fibers, and two neurons (*dark*) supply type II fibers. **B.** With early (mild) denervation, portions of the axonal tree degenerate resulting in angular atrophy of scattered type I and II muscle fibers depicted in the drawing and seen by hematoxylin and eosin staining (*arrows*). In this example, only type I fibers show angular atrophy because the injured neuron supplied only this fiber type. **C.** As neurons degenerate, surviving neurons sprout more nerve endings which reinnervate some denervated fibers. These fibers become either type I or type II, determined by the type of neuron that reinnervated them. The result is fewer, but larger, motor units and the appearance of clusters of fibers of one type adjacent to clusters of the other type, a pattern called "type grouping." The low power ATPase stained section shows such type grouping. If stained with hematoxylin and eosin, this field would appear normal except for the presence of a few atrophic fibers. **D.** With more advanced (severe, chronic) denervation, entire lower motor neurons or numerous axonal processes are lost, producing small groups of angular atrophic fibers (grouped atrophy) as illustrated in the photomicrograph.

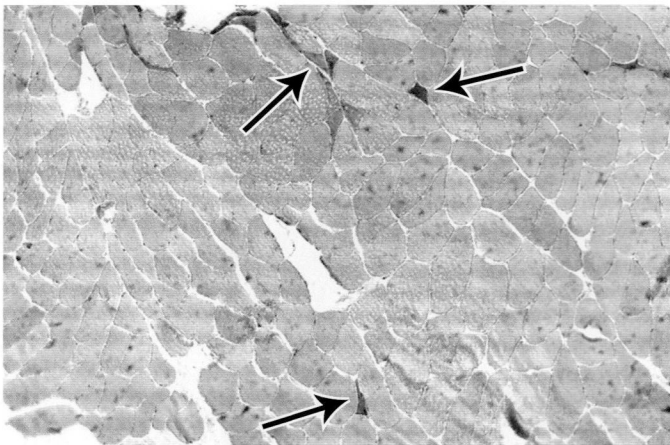

FIGURE 31-24. Denervation. This frozen section of the biceps muscle subjected to the nonspecific esterase reaction shows excessively dark staining in a few irregularly scattered, angular, atrophic fibers (*arrows*). This pattern is highly characteristic of atrophy due to denervation.

disappear from the sarcolemma, except at the point of synaptic contact.

In a chronic denervating condition, reinnervation of each surviving motor unit gradually enlarges. As a specific type of lower motor neuron takes over innervation of a given field of fibers, fiber groups of one type are seen adjacent to groups of another type. This pattern, called **fiber-type grouping**, is pathognomonic of denervation followed by reinnervation (Fig. 31-23C).

Patients with striking fiber–type grouping often have symptoms of muscle cramping in addition to progressive muscular weakness. After a single episode of denervation, such as in poliomyelitis, reinnervation often leads to remarkable recovery of strength. Years later, one sees conspicuoustype grouping, with scattered pyknotic nuclear clumps. In such cases, there are neither angular atrophic fibers nor target fibers.

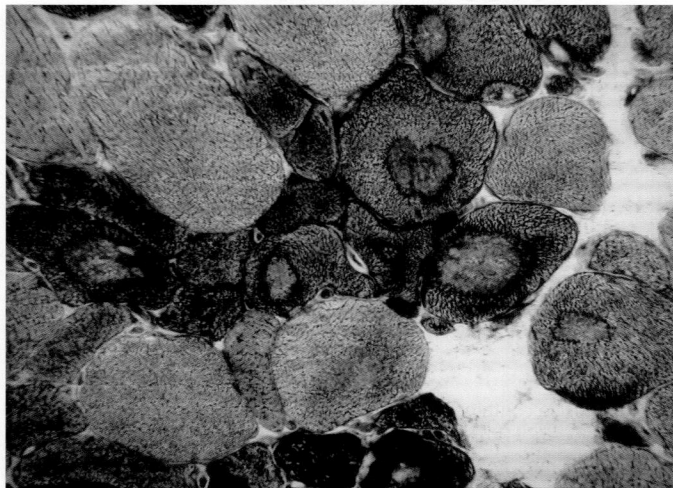

FIGURE 31-25. Target fiber. A cross-section of muscle treated with the NADH-tetrazolium reductase (NADH-TR) stain demonstrates "target fibers," a characteristic feature of some types of denervation. Because the enzyme reaction creates a colored product that selectively fixes to membranous organelles, the centers of the target areas appear devoid of mitochondria and sarcoplasmic reticulum. The myofibrils may or may not be intact.

If denervation continues after development of fiber-type grouping, large motor units become atrophic. Such **grouped atrophy** (Fig. 31-23D) is characteristic of chronic denervating disorders such as ALS.

Occasionally, one fiber type (either type I or type II) predominates over the other in **type predominance**. There is frequently evidence of denervation. In such cases, reinnervation may favor one type of lower motor neuron over another. Muscle fibers may uncommonly be lost or regenerate in neuropathic conditions resulting in a modest increase in serum creatine kinase levels.

The Peripheral Nervous System

ANATOMY

The peripheral nervous system (PNS) is external to the brain and spinal cord. It includes (1) cranial nerves III to XII, (2) dorsal and ventral spinal roots, (3) spinal nerves and their continuations, and (4) ganglia. Peripheral nerves carry somatic motor, somatic sensory, visceral sensory and autonomic axons.

Somatic motor and preganglionic autonomic axons arise from neuronal cell bodies within the CNS. Sensory and postganglionic autonomic axons originate from neuronal cell bodies within ganglia located on cranial nerves, dorsal roots, and autonomic nerves. PNS neurons, satellite cells of the ganglia, and all Schwann cells are derived from neural crest.

Endoneurial connective tissue surrounds individual nerve fibers, which are bundled into fascicles by a **perineurial sheath**. Epineurial connective tissue binds the fascicles together and contains nutrient arteries. A blood–nerve barrier (BNB), located in endoneurial capillaries and the perineurial sheath, and analogous to the blood–brain barrier, protects peripheral nerves, but not ganglia. There are no lymphatic vessels in nerve fascicles.

Peripheral nerve axons may be myelinated or unmyelinated (Fig. 31-26). Myelinated axons are 1 to 20 μm in diameter. Unmyelinated axons, at 0.4 to 2.4 μm, are much smaller. Myelin, made from Schwann cell plasmalemma, is necessary for optimal nerve conduction. The lipids in Schwann cell–derived PNS myelin and oligodendrocyte-derived CNS myelin are similar, but their associated proteins differ substantially. Myelin protein zero (MPZ) and peripheral myelin protein 22 (PMP22) occur only in the PNS. Schwann cells surround both myelinated and unmyelinated fibers. The axon determines whether the Schwann cell produces myelin. Myelin sheath thickness, internodal length (i.e., distance between two nodes of Ranvier), and conduction velocity are all proportional to axonal diameter.

REACTIONS TO INJURY

Peripheral nerve fibers show only a limited number of reactions to injury (Fig. 31-27). The major types of nerve fiber damage are axonal degeneration and segmental demyelination. PNS fibers differ from those in the CNS by being able to regenerate and remyelinate to recover function.

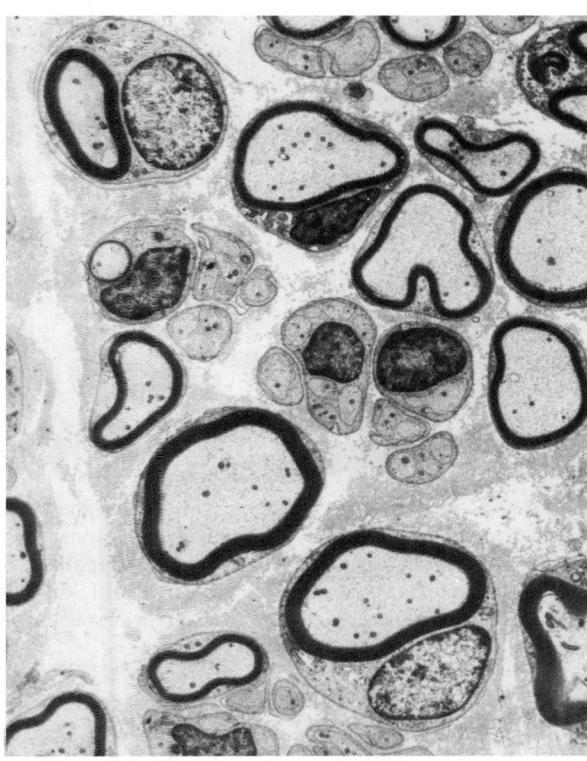

FIGURE 31-26. Structure of peripheral nerve. Electron microscopy of a peripheral nerve shows myelinated fibers (encircled by dark-staining myelin) interspersed with groups of unmyelinated fibers. Unlike myelinated axons, multiple unmyelinated axons may share a single Schwann cell.

Axonal Degeneration Reflects Injury to Axons or Neuronal Cell Bodies

Degeneration (necrosis) of the axon occurs in many neuropathies and may be limited to distal axons or involve both axons and neuronal cell bodies (Fig. 31-27). Immediately after an axon degenerates, the myelin sheath breaks down and Schwann cells proliferate. The latter initiate myelin degradation, which is completed by macrophages that

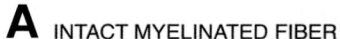

FIGURE 31-27. Basic responses of peripheral nerve fibers to injury. A. Intact myelinated fiber. The axon is insulated by the Schwann cell–derived myelin sheaths. **B. Distal axonal degeneration.** The distal axon has degenerated, and myelin sheaths associated with the distal axon have secondarily degenerated. The striated muscle shows denervation atrophy. **C. Degeneration of cell body and axon.** Degeneration involves the neuronal cell body and its entire axon. The myelin sheaths associated with the axon have also degenerated. **D. Segmental demyelination.** The myelin sheath associated with one Schwann cell has degenerated, leaving a segment of axon uncovered by myelin. The underlying axon remains intact and the skeletal muscle remains innervated. **E. Remyelination.** Proliferating Schwann cells cover the demyelinated segment of the axon and elaborate new myelin sheaths. The remyelinating Schwann cells have short internodal lengths. **F. Regenerating axon.** Regenerating axons sprout from the distal end of the disrupted axon. Ideally, regenerating axons reinnervate the distal nerve stump, where they will be ensheathed and myelinated by Schwann cells of the distal stump. **G. Regenerated nerve fiber.** The regenerated portion of the axon is myelinated by Schwann cells with short internodal lengths. The striated muscle is reinnervated.

infiltrate the nerve within 3 days after axonal degeneration. If injury is restricted to the distal axon, regenerating axons may sprout within 1 week from the intact, proximal axonal stump. There are several types of axonal degeneration.

DISTAL AXONAL DEGENERATION: In many neuropathies, axonal degeneration is initially limited to the distal ends of larger, longer fibers (**dying-back neuropathy** or

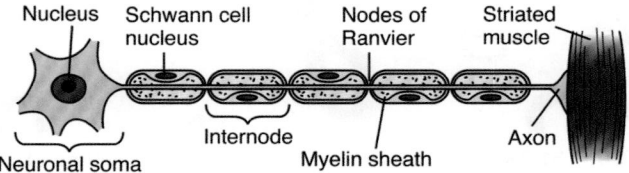

A INTACT MYELINATED FIBER

Nucleus · Schwann cell nucleus · Nodes of Ranvier · Striated muscle · Neuronal soma · Internode · Myelin sheath · Axon

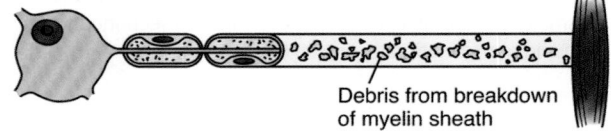

B DISTAL AXONAL DEGENERATION

Debris from breakdown of myelin sheath

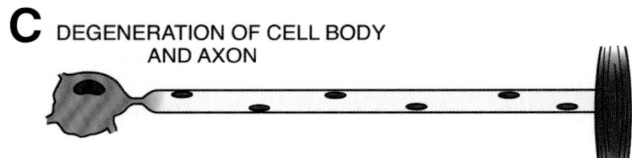

C DEGENERATION OF CELL BODY AND AXON

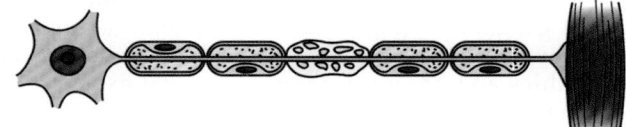

D SEGMENTAL DEMYELINATION

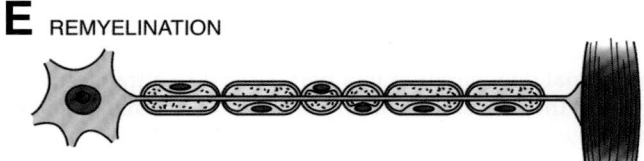

E REMYELINATION

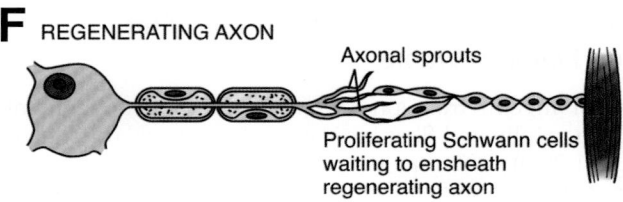

F REGENERATING AXON

Axonal sprouts

Proliferating Schwann cells waiting to ensheath regenerating axon

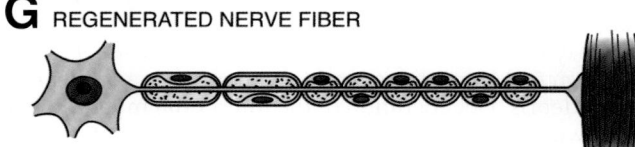

G REGENERATED NERVE FIBER

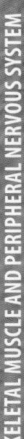

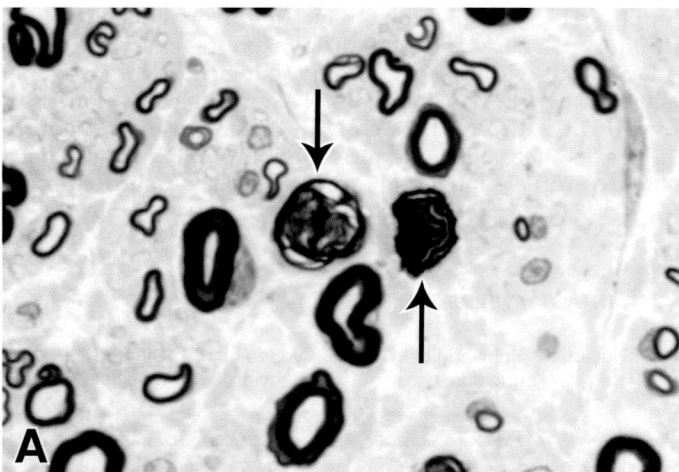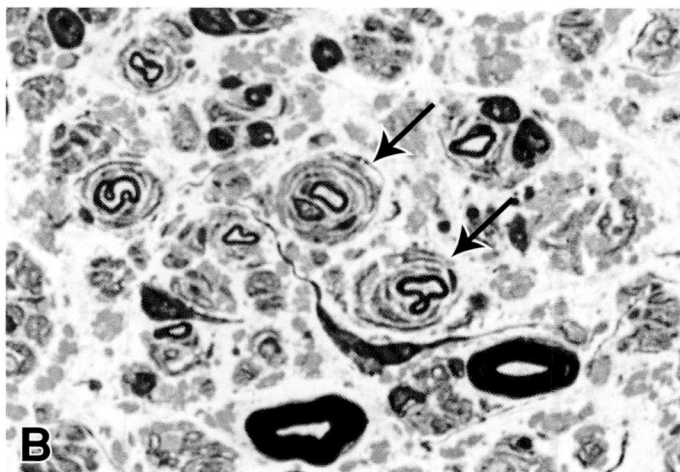

FIGURE 31-28. **A. Axonal degeneration in an axonal neuropathy.** A cross-section of sural nerve shows two degenerating myelinated fibers (*arrows*) in the center of the field. The axons are gone and their myelin sheaths have been reduced to rounded masses of myelin debris. In most axonal neuropathies, this type of axonal degeneration is limited to the distal axon. **B. Onion bulbs in chronic inflammatory demyelinating polyneuropathy.** Several remyelinating axons with thin myelin sheaths (*arrows*) are in the center of the field. They are surrounded by multiple concentric layers of Schwann cell cytoplasm, which resemble the concentric rings of a sectioned onion. Onion bulb formation is common in neuropathies with recurrent episodes of demyelination and remyelination.

distal axonopathy) (Figs. 31-27B and 31-28A). Peripheral neuropathies characterized by distal axonal degeneration typically present clinically as distal ("length-dependent" or "glove-and-stocking") neuropathies. In this setting, neuron cell bodies and proximal axons remain intact. Axons may thus regenerate and nerve function may return if the cause of the distal axonal degeneration is removed. This must occur before the dying-back degeneration reaches the proximal axon and causes the neuronal cell body to die.

NEURONOPATHY: Axonal degeneration may result from death of a neuronal cell body, as in autoimmune dorsal root ganglionitis (Fig. 31-27C). Peripheral neuropathies caused by selective damage to neuronal cell bodies are **neuronopathies** and are much rarer than distal axonopathies. Neuronopathies present clinically as proximal *and* distal (i.e., non–length-dependent) neuropathies. Death of the neuronal cell body precludes axonal regeneration, making recovery impossible.

WALLERIAN DEGENERATION: This term describes the axonal degeneration in a nerve distal to a transection or crush of the nerve. If the injury is not too proximal, the nerve may regenerate.

In Segmental Demyelination, the Myelin Sheath Breaks Down but the Underlying Axon Remains Viable

Loss of myelin from one or more internodes (segments) along a myelinated fiber indicates Schwann cell dysfunction (Fig. 31-27D). This may be due either to direct injury to the Schwann cell or myelin sheath (**primary demyelination**), or to underlying axonal abnormalities (**secondary demyelination**).

Loss of the myelin sheath does not cause the underlying axon to degenerate. Macrophages infiltrate the nerve and clear the myelin debris. Degeneration of the internodal myelin sheath is followed sequentially by Schwann cell proliferation, then remyelination of the demyelinated segments and finally

functional recovery. Remyelinated internodes have shortened internodal lengths (Fig. 31-27E). Repeated episodes of segmental demyelination and remyelination, as occur in chronic demyelinating neuropathies, cause proliferating Schwann cells that encircle the axons to form concentric rings (**onion bulbs**) (Fig. 31-28B) and produce clinically evident nerve enlargement (**hypertrophic neuropathy**).

PERIPHERAL NEUROPATHIES

A peripheral neuropathy is a process that affects the function of one or more peripheral nerves. It may be restricted to the PNS, involve both the PNS and CNS, or affect multiple organ systems. Peripheral neuropathies occur in all age groups and may be hereditary or acquired.

There are many causes of peripheral neuropathy (Table 31-3). ***Diabetes mellitus is the most common cause of generalized peripheral neuropathy in the United States.*** Other common causes include hereditary disorders, autoimmune diseases, alcoholism and nutritional deficiencies, chronic renal failure, neurotoxic drugs, monoclonal gammopathies, HIV infection, cancer, and trauma

PATHOLOGY: Pathologic findings in most neuropathies are limited to axonal degeneration, segmental demyelination, or both. If axonal degeneration predominates, the neuropathy is an **axonal neuropathy**; if segmental demyelination predominates, it is a **demyelinating neuropathy**. *Most (80% to 90%) neuropathies are axonal and of the dying-back type (distal axonal neuropathy).* Electrophysiologic studies often help to distinguish axonal and demyelinating neuropathies. Nerve conduction velocity is typically near normal in axonal neuropathies but is impaired in demyelinating neuropathies. The distinction between axonal and demyelinating neuropathies is useful clinically. Axonal neuropathies have

TABLE 31-3

ETIOLOGIC CLASSIFICATION OF NEUROPATHIES

Immune-mediated neuropathies

Acute inflammatory demyelinating polyradiculoneuropathy (Guillain–Barré syndrome)

  Acute motor (and sensory) axonal neuropathy (axonal form of Guillain–Barré syndrome)

  Fisher syndrome

  Chronic inflammatory demyelinating polyradiculoneuropathy (CIDP)

  Multifocal motor neuropathy

  Dorsal root ganglionitis (sensory neuronopathy)

  Immunoglobulin M (IgM) paraproteinemia-associated demyelinating neuropathy

  Vasculitic neuropathy (systemic vasculitis, connective tissue disease, cryoglobulinemia)

Metabolic neuropathies

  Diabetic polyneuropathy and mononeuropathies

  Uremic neuropathy

  Critical illness polyneuropathy

  Hypothyroid neuropathy

  Acromegalic neuropathy

Nutritional neuropathies

Neuropathy associated with deficiency of vitamin B_1, B_6, B_{12}, or E

Copper deficiency myeloneuropathy

Alcoholic neuropathy

Toxic and drug-induced neuropathies (see Table 31-4)

Amyloid neuropathy (AL amyloidosis and familial amyloid polyneuropathy)

Hereditary neuropathies (see Tables 31-5 and 31-6)

Neuropathies associated with infections

  Leprosy

  HIV

  Cytomegalovirus

  Hepatitis B and C (vasculitic neuropathy or CIDP)

  Herpes zoster

  Lyme disease

  Diphtheria (toxic neuropathy)

Paraneoplastic neuropathy

Sarcoid neuropathy

Radiation neuropathy

Traumatic neuropathy

Chronic idiopathic axonal polyneuropathy

many causes, but demyelinating neuropathies have a limited number of etiologies that are most likely to be hereditary or immunologically mediated.

The histopathology of many neuropathies does not indicate the underlying cause, so that clinical correlation is usually needed to establish causation. Less often, a specific etiology may be identified pathologically. These include necrotizing arteritis (vasculitic neuropathy), granulomatous inflammation (leprosy, sarcoid), amyloid deposition (amyloid neuropathy), abnormalities of the myelin sheath (IgM paraproteinemic neuropathy, hereditary neuropathy with liability to pressure palsies), or abnormal accumulations within Schwann cells (leukodystrophy), or axons (giant axonal neuropathy).

 CLINICAL FEATURES: Major clinical manifestations of peripheral neuropathy are muscle weakness and atrophy, sensory loss, paresthesia, pain, and autonomic dysfunction. Motor, sensory, and autonomic functions may be affected equally or selectively. Predominant involvement of large-diameter sensory fibers affects position and vibration sense, while injury to small-diameter fibers hinders pain and temperature sensation. A neuropathy may be acute (days to weeks), subacute (weeks to months), or chronic (months to years). It may affect one nerve (**mononeuropathy**) or several (**mononeuropathy multiplex**), dorsal root ganglia (**sensory neuronopathy**) or nerve roots (**radiculopathy**), and may involve multiple peripheral nerves (**polyneuropathy**), or nerve roots and peripheral nerves (**polyradiculoneuropathy**).

Peripheral Neuropathy Occurs in Nearly Half of Adults With Types 1 and 2 Diabetes Mellitus

Diabetic neuropathy may manifest as a distal sensorimotor polyneuropathy, autonomic neuropathy, mononeuropathy, or mononeuropathy multiplex. The mononeuropathies may involve cranial nerves (cranial neuropathy), nerve roots, or proximal peripheral nerves. *Distal, predominantly sensory, polyneuropathy is the most common form of diabetic neuropathy.*

 ETIOLOGIC FACTORS: How nerve fiber injury occurs in diabetes remains poorly understood (see Chapter 13). It has long been held that the distal symmetric polyneuropathy is due to the metabolic abnormalities of diabetes, while the mononeuropathies are caused by nerve ischemia from diabetic microvascular disease. However, local nerve ischemia also probably contributes to the symmetric polyneuropathy.

 PATHOLOGY: The distal symmetric polyneuropathy of diabetes is characterized by a mixture of axonal degeneration and segmental demyelination, with the former predominating. Axonal loss involves fibers of all sizes but may preferentially affect large myelinated fibers (**large-fiber neuropathy**) or small myelinated fibers and unmyelinated fibers (**small-fiber neuropathy**).

Uremic Neuropathy Often Complicates Chronic Renal Failure

Uremic neuropathy is a distal sensorimotor axonal polyneuropathy seen in half of patients with chronic renal failure. It shows both distal axonal degeneration and segmental demyelination, with the former predominating and mainly affecting large-diameter fibers. The pathogenesis of the axonal degeneration is not known, but uremic neuropathy often stabilizes or improves with long-term dialysis and resolves after renal transplantation.

Critical Illness Polyneuropathy Develops in Many Severely Ill Patients

It is associated with sepsis and multiorgan failure. The acute, predominantly motor, axonal neuropathy may first become apparent when a patient in the intensive care unit cannot be weaned from ventilatory support. A **critical illness myopathy** may also occur in these patients. The pathogenesis is obscure.

Neuropathy Is a Frequent Complication of Alcoholism

Alcoholic neuropathy is a distal sensorimotor axonal polyneuropathy, attributable to nutritional deficiencies and/or a direct toxic effect of ethanol on the PNS. Peripheral nerves show loss of nerve fibers due to axonal degeneration of the dying-back type.

Nutritional Neuropathy Is an Axonal Polyneuropathy With Multiple Causes

Nutritional neuropathy is associated with deficiencies in vitamins (B_1, B_6, B_{12}, or E) or copper. Copper deficiency may be a result of malnutrition, total parenteral nutrition, excessive ingestion of zinc, or bariatric surgery. Isoniazid therapy for tuberculosis interferes with pyridoxine (vitamin B_6) metabolism and may cause vitamin B_6 deficiency neuropathy. It is unclear if the chronic axonal neuropathy sometimes seen in celiac disease is due to malnutrition or reflects the underlying autoimmune process.

Acute Inflammatory Demyelinating Polyradiculoneuropathy May Be Immune Mediated

Guillain–Barré syndrome (GBS) is an acquired, acute immune-mediated demyelinating polyradiculoneuropathy (AIDP) that often follows bacterial, viral, or mycoplasmal infections. It may also follow immunization or surgery. Usually, there is an antecedent gastrointestinal or upper respiratory infection. Commonly associated infectious agents include *Campylobacter jejuni*, cytomegalovirus, Epstein–Barr virus, Zika virus, and *Mycoplasma pneumoniae*. GBS presents as an acute symmetric neuromuscular flaccid paralysis that often begins distally and ascends proximally. Sensory and autonomic disturbances may also occur, and 5% of cases present with the clinical triad of ophthalmoplegia, ataxia, and areflexia (**Fisher syndrome**). Muscular paralysis may cause respiratory dysfunction, and autonomic involvement may lead to cardiac arrhythmias and wide fluctuations in blood pressure. The neuropathy begins to resolve 2 to 4 weeks after onset, and most patients recover. Characteristically, the cerebrospinal fluid (CSF) contains increased protein but few white blood cells (albuminocytologic dissociation). The increased protein level is attributable to inflammation of spinal roots.

There are two pathologic variants of GBS. The demyelinating variant is an **acute inflammatory demyelinating polyradiculoneuropathy**. Immune-mediated demyelination may affect all levels of the PNS, including spinal roots, ganglia, craniospinal nerves, and autonomic nerves. The distribution of lesions varies. Involved regions show endoneurial infiltrates of lymphocytes and macrophages, segmental demyelination, and relative axonal sparing. Macrophages are frequently seen adjacent to degenerating myelin sheaths and can strip off and phagocytose superficial myelin lamellae. Such macrophage-mediated demyelination is rare in other neuropathies. The axonal variant of GBS is an **acute motor axonal neuropathy** or **acute motor and sensory axonal neuropathy**. Immune-mediated injury causes axonal degeneration accompanied by minimal endoneurial inflammatory infiltrates. The axonal variant is much less common than the demyelinating variant in North America and Europe but is more common in Asia. Axonal GBS often follows *C. jejuni* infection and shows serum antiganglioside antibodies (anti-GM_1, anti-GD1a). It is thought that molecular mimicry between an antigenic component of the infectious agent and a component of peripheral nerve fibers elicits a cross-reactive immune response that leads to axonal injury. Antiganglioside antibodies (anti-GQ1b, anti-GT1a) are also very common in Fisher syndrome. The role of antiganglioside antibodies in the demyelinating variant of GBS is less clear.

Chronic inflammatory demyelinating polyradiculoneuropathy (CIDP) is similar to AIDP but has a protracted course, with multiple relapses or slow continuous progression, and usually lacks evidence of antecedent infection. The neuropathy may occur sporadically (idiopathic CIDP) or be associated with paraproteinemia, HIV infection, chronic active hepatitis, connective tissue disease, inflammatory bowel disease, or Hodgkin lymphoma. The demyelinating neuropathy is symmetric, sensorimotor, and proximal and distal. Rarely, it may present as a mononeuropathy multiplex (**multifocal acquired demyelinating sensory and motor neuropathy**). Nerves and nerve roots in CIDP may show many onion bulbs owing to recurrent episodes of demyelination, Schwann cell proliferation, and remyelination (Fig. 31-28B). The pathogenesis of this immune-mediated neuropathy is obscure.

Multifocal motor neuropathy is a rare, slowly progressive, demyelinating mononeuropathy multiplex that may be mistaken clinically for motor neuron disease. There is often an associated increased titer of anti-GM_1 antibodies. This demyelinating neuropathy is immune mediated but is considered distinct from CIDP.

Dorsal Root Ganglionitis Is an Immune-Mediated Neuronopathy

This inflammatory ganglionopathy typically manifests as a subacute or chronic, non–length-dependent sensory polyneuropathy with sensory ataxia. It may occur sporadically (**idiopathic sensory neuronopathy**), in association with Sjögren syndrome or as a paraneoplastic neuropathy. Dorsal

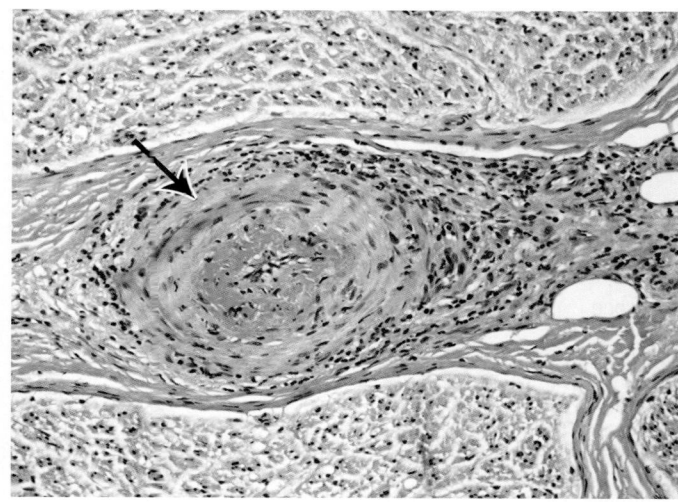

FIGURE 31-29. Vasculitic neuropathy. In this cross-section of a sural nerve from a patient with polyarteritis nodosa and mononeuropathy multiplex, an inflamed epineurial artery (*arrow*) shows fibrinoid necrosis of its wall. The resultant nerve ischemia causes axonal degeneration.

root ganglia show infiltration by lymphocytes and loss of sensory neurons. The pathogenesis of immune-mediated sensory neuronopathy is poorly understood.

Vasculitis Is a Principal Cause of Mononeuropathy Multiplex

Epineurial arteries of nerves may show necrotizing arteritis as a manifestation of systemic vasculitis. These include PAN, granulomatosis with polyangiitis (formerly called Churg–Strauss syndrome), eosinophilic granulomatosis with polyangiitis (formerly called Wegener granulomatosis), and microscopic polyangiitis. It also includes vasculitides associated with connective tissue diseases (rheumatoid arthritis, systemic lupus erythematosus, Sjögren syndrome), cryoglobulinemia, HIV infection, or cancer. In one-third of cases of vasculitic neuropathy, necrotizing arteritis is limited to the PNS (**nonsystemic vasculitic neuropathy**). The ischemic neuropathy is characterized pathologically by axonal degeneration (Fig. 31-29).

Monoclonal Gammopathies May Cause Several Types of Neuropathy

Monoclonal gammopathies, whether of undetermined significance (MGUS; see Chapter 26) or due to plasma cell myeloma, may cause amyloid neuropathy, cryoglobulinemia-associated vasculitic neuropathy, or a chronic demyelinating polyneuropathy. Chronic demyelinating polyneuropathy often occurs with an IgM MGUS or Waldenström macroglobulinemia, in which the IgM paraprotein binds myelin-associated glycoprotein (MAG). Anti-MAG antibodies may thus promote demyelination. Anti-MAG neuropathy is characterized by extensive segmental demyelination, a variable number of onion bulbs, axonal loss, and a distinctive widening of the myelin lamellae (Fig. 31-30).

Paraproteinemic neuropathy rarely presents as POEMS syndrome (polyneuropathy, organomegaly, endocrinopathy, monoclonal gammopathy and skin changes). Such patients

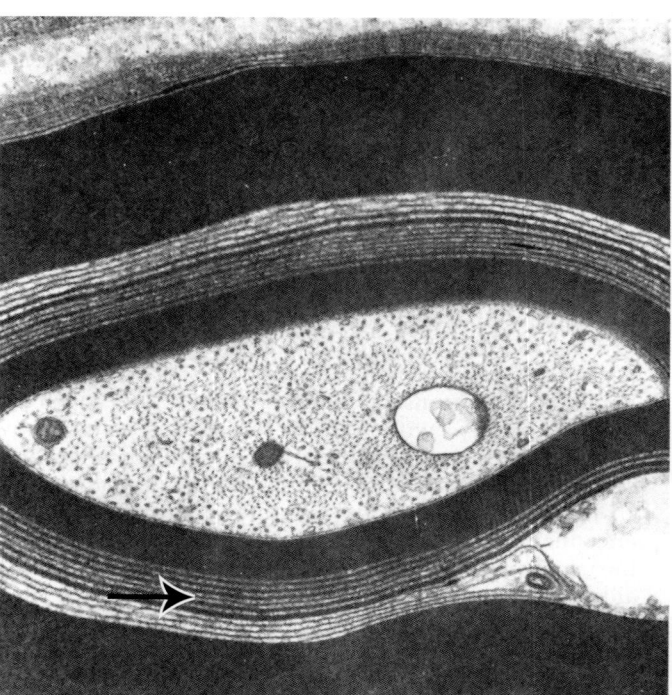

FIGURE 31-30. Anti–myelin-associated glycoprotein (MAG) IgM paraproteinemic demyelinating neuropathy. Electron microscopy shows multiple, abnormally widely spaced, myelin lamellae (*arrow*) in a myelinated fiber from a patient with an IgM monoclonal gammopathy of unknown significance and a chronic demyelinating neuropathy. Widely spaced myelin is a characteristic ultrastructural feature of anti-MAG paraproteinemic neuropathy.

show elevated serum levels of vascular endothelial growth factor (VEGF) and usually osteosclerotic myeloma.

Neuropathy Complicates Light-Chain and Familial Amyloidoses

In addition to its effects on sensory and motor nerves, amyloid infiltration of the PNS often leads to prominent autonomic dysfunction. The disorder may be hereditary but more often complicates light-chain amyloidosis (AL) in primary systemic amyloidosis or multiple myeloma. Familial amyloidosis is usually caused by a point mutation in the transthyretin gene, *TTR* (see Chapter 15), although mutations of the apolipoprotein A1 (*APOA1*) or gelsolin (*GSN*) genes are responsible in some cases.

Amyloid accumulates in endoneurial and epineurial extracellular spaces and vascular walls in peripheral nerves, dorsal root ganglia, and autonomic ganglia. Loss of myelinated and unmyelinated fibers ensues. Nerve-fiber damage may reflect direct mechanical injury of nerve fibers and ganglion cells by amyloid deposits, nerve ischemia caused by amyloid infiltration of vasa nervorum, or both.

Systemic amyloidosis may also cause **carpal tunnel syndrome** (CTS), a chronic entrapment neuropathy of the median nerve at the wrist. Nerve entrapment results from amyloid infiltration of the flexor retinaculum. CTS also occurs in many other settings, including occupational injuries, hypothyroidism, acromegaly, chronic renal failure (dialysis-related β_2-microglobulin amyloidosis), pregnancy, and rheumatoid arthritis. CTS is the most common cause of mononeuropathy.

Paraneoplastic Neuropathies Often Precede Discovery of a Cancer

Paraneoplastic nervous system diseases include polyneuropathy, chronic encephalomyelitis, necrotizing myelopathy, cerebellar degeneration, and the Eaton–Lambert syndrome. Several clinicopathologic types of paraneoplastic neuropathy have been defined.

- **Paraneoplastic sensorimotor polyneuropathy:** This distal polyneuropathy is the most common paraneoplastic neuropathy. It is characterized by axonal degeneration and demyelination, mainly the former. The cause of the nerve-fiber degeneration is unknown.
- **Paraneoplastic sensory neuronopathy:** This subacute polyneuropathy with sensory ataxia is caused by immune-mediated dorsal root ganglionitis. It often precedes discovery of cancer. Similar chronic inflammatory changes may also occur in the CNS (**paraneoplastic encephalomyelitis**). Small cell carcinoma of the lung is the usual culprit. The sensory neuronopathy and encephalitis are thought to be mediated mainly by anti-Hu antibodies (antineuronal autoantibodies).
- **Inflammatory demyelinating polyradiculoneuropathy:** Immune-mediated acute or chronic inflammatory demyelinating polyradiculoneuropathy may be associated with cancer.
- **Paraneoplastic vasculitic neuropathy:** Vasculitic neuropathy may rarely complicate cancer.

Not all cancer-associated neuropathies arise as remote effects of a distant neoplasm. Tumors may cause neuropathy by direct compression or infiltration of nerves or nerve roots. Cancer therapies may induce a toxic or radiation neuropathy.

Toxic Neuropathy Is Often Iatrogenic

A variety of environmental agents and industrial compounds cause peripheral neuropathy (Table 31-4), but most cases of toxic neuropathy result from drugs. Almost all toxic neuropathies are characterized by axonal degeneration, usually of the dying-back type. Notable exceptions are platinum compounds and pyridoxine, which produce a sensory neuronopathy, and diphtheria toxin, which leads to a demyelinating neuropathy. People with hereditary neuropathy (see below) may be especially vulnerable to drug-induced peripheral neuropathy.

The Most Common Chronic Neuropathies in Children Are Hereditary

Many inherited diseases include peripheral neuropathies (Tables 31-5 and 31-6), either as the sole manifestation of the hereditary disease or as part of a multisystem disease. Hereditary neuropathies may present as a motor and sensory neuropathy (HMSN), sensory and autonomic neuropathy (HSAN), or motor neuropathy (HMN).

Charcot–Marie–Tooth Disease

 MOLECULAR PATHOGENESIS: Charcot–Marie–Tooth disease (CMT) is a genetically and pathologically heterogeneous group of slowly progressive

TABLE 31-4	
AGENTS ASSOCIATED WITH TOXIC NEUROPATHY	
Drugs	**Environmental and Industrial Agents**
Amiodarone	Acrylamide
Bortezomib	Allyl chloride
Colchicine	Arsenic
Dapsone	Buckthorn toxin
Disulfiram	Carbon disulfide
Gold salts	Chlordecone
Isoniazid	Dimethylaminopropionitrile
Metronidazole	Diphtheria toxin
Misonidazole	Ethylene oxide
Nitrofurantoin	n-Hexane (glue sniffing)
Nucleoside analogs (antiretrovirals)	Methyl n-butyl ketone
Paclitaxel (taxanes)	Lead
Phenytoin	Mercury
Platinum compounds	Methyl bromide
Podophyllin	Organophosphates
Pyridoxine (vitamin B_6)	Polychlorinated biphenyls
Suramin	Thallium
Thalidomide	Trichloroethylene
Vincristine	Vacor

distal sensorimotor polyneuropathies that manifest in childhood or early adult life. It is the most common inherited neuropathy and among the most common inherited neurologic disorders, with a prevalence of 1 in 2,500. Classification of CMT is based on inheritance and pathology (**axonal** or **demyelinating**). **CMT1**, the most common form, is a chronic demyelinating polyneuropathy with autosomal dominant inheritance. The less common **CMT2** is also autosomal dominant but is a chronic axonal polyneuropathy. X-linked (**CMTX**) and autosomal recessive (**CMT4**) types also occur. CMT may be further subclassified by the specific genetic mutation. Thus, CMT1A is an autosomal dominant demyelinating neuropathy caused by duplication of the peripheral myelin protein 22 gene (*PMP22*) on chromosome 17, and CMT1B is an autosomal dominant demyelinating neuropathy caused by a heterozygous mutation in the myelin protein zero gene (*MPZ*). Mutations in over 40 different genes are associated with a CMT phenotype, but mutations in four genes (*PMP22*, *MPZ*, *GJB1*, and *MFN2*) are responsible for about half of all CMT cases. Approximately 75% of patients with CMT1 have mutations in *PMP22* (usually

TABLE 31-5

INHERITED DISEASES ASSOCIATED WITH NEUROPATHY

Ataxia-telangiectasia

Abetalipoproteinemia

Acute intermittent porphyria, hereditary coproporphyria, and variegate porphyria

Cerebrotendinous xanthomatosis

Fabry disease (α-galactosidase A deficiency)

Familial amyloid polyneuropathy (transthyretin, apolipoprotein A1, and gelsolin amyloidosis)

Friedreich ataxia

Giant axonal neuropathy

Hereditary motor and sensory neuropathies (Charcot–Marie–Tooth disease)

Hereditary motor neuropathies

Hereditary neuropathy with liability to pressure palsies

Hereditary sensory and autonomic neuropathies

Infantile neuroaxonal dystrophy

Leukodystrophies (metachromatic, globoid cell, and adrenoleukodystrophy)

Refsum disease (phytanic acid storage disease)

Tangier disease

a duplication) and roughly 10% have mutations in *MPZ*. Mutations in *MFN2* are the most common cause of CMT2. This gene encodes mitofuscin-2, a GTPase in the outer mitochondrial membrane. Nearly 90% of patients with CMTX have mutations in *GJB1*. This gene encodes the gap junction protein, connexin32, which is expressed in noncompact myelin at incisures and paranodes and forms gap junctions that facilitate molecular transport between layers of the Schwann cell myelin sheath. Classification is complex because mutations in diverse genes may produce the same phenotype, and different mutations in the same gene may lead to different phenotypes (Table 31-6).

Dejerine–Sottas syndrome (DSS, CMT3) resembles CMT1 but is much more severe, with onset in early infancy. Peripheral nerves show a severe demyelinating neuropathy with onion bulbs and axonal loss. Several genes are associated with this phenotype (Table 31-6).

Hereditary neuropathy with liability to pressure palsies (HNPP) typically manifests as recurrent mononeuropathies. Nerves show demyelination, distinctive sausage-shaped myelin sheath thickenings (tomacula) and axonal loss. Heterozygous deletion of *PMP22* on chromosome 17 causes HNPP, whereas duplication of *PMP22* causes CMT1A.

Peripheral Neuropathies Commonly Complicate HIV-1 Infection

HIV-1-associated peripheral neuropathies may manifest clinically as a distal symmetric polyneuropathy, autonomic neuropathy, lumbosacral polyradiculopathy, mononeuropathy, or mononeuropathy multiplex.

- **Distal symmetric polyneuropathy** (DSP) is the most common type of HIV-associated neuropathy and the most common neurologic complication of AIDS. It usually occurs in late stages of the disease. The mechanism responsible for the distal axonal degeneration is obscure, and there is no effective therapy.
- **Inflammatory demyelinating immune-mediated polyradiculoneuropathy** in HIV-infected people may be acute (AIDP) or chronic (CIDP). It typically occurs after HIV infection, before the onset of AIDS. It often responds to plasmapheresis, intravenous γ-globulin, or corticosteroids.
- **Cytomegalovirus infection** of the PNS is responsible for some of the mononeuropathies and lumbosacral polyradiculopathies associated with AIDS.
- **Vasculitic neuropathy** may cause a mononeuropathy or mononeuropathy multiplex in some patients with AIDS.

TABLE 31-6

CHARCOT–MARIE–TOOTH DISEASE (CMT) AND RELATED HEREDITARY MOTOR AND SENSORY NEUROPATHIES

Disease	Inheritance	Gene	Pathology
CMT1	Autosomal dominant	Peripheral myelin protein 22 (*PMP22*), myelin protein zero (*MPZ*) and others	Demyelinating neuropathy with onion bulbs; axonal loss also present
CMT2	Autosomal dominant	Mitofusin 2 (*MFN2*) and others	Axonal neuropathy
CMTX	X linked	Gap junction protein β1 (*GJB1*) (connexin 32) and others	Axonal loss, demyelination, and regenerating axons
Dejerine–Sottas syndrome (congenital hypomyelinating neuropathy)	Autosomal dominant or recessive	*PMP22, MPZ*, and others	Demyelinating neuropathy with onion bulbs; axonal loss also present
Hereditary neuropathy with liability to pressure palsies (HNPP)	Autosomal dominant	*PMP22*	Demyelinating neuropathy with tomacula; axonal loss also present

- **Toxic neuropathies** occur in response to several drugs used to treat AIDS (Table 31-4). Such antiretroviral-induced axonal neuropathies resemble HIV-associated DSP clinically.
- **Diffuse infiltrative lymphocytosis syndrome** may be complicated by an acute or subacute axonal polyneuropathy. Peripheral nerve shows perivascular CD8+ lymphocytic infiltrates.

Chronic Idiopathic Axonal Polyneuropathy Occurs in Older Patients

No cause can be identified for peripheral neuropathy, even with careful investigation, in a quarter of neuropathy patients, usually over age 50. Many of these patients have a slowly progressive, distal, sensory or sensorimotor, axonal polyneuropathy called chronic idiopathic axonal polyneuropathy (CIAP).

NERVE TRAUMA

Traumatic Neuromas Are Masses of Regenerating Axons and Scar Tissue

Traumatic neuromas form at the proximal stump of a nerve that has been physically disrupted. Within a week after transection of a peripheral nerve, regenerating axonal sprouts arise from the distal ends of the intact axons in the proximal nerve stump. If the severed ends of the proximal and distal nerve stumps are closely approximated, regenerating axonal sprouts may find and reinnervate the distal stump. Regenerating axons advance in the distal stump at a rate of about 1 mm/day. However, if the cut nerve ends are not closely apposed, or if there is an impediment (e.g., scar tissue) between the two stumps, regenerating sprouts may not reinnervate the distal stump. In that case, the regenerating axons grow haphazardly into the scar tissue at the end of the proximal stump to form a painful swelling: a **traumatic** or **amputation neuroma.**

Morton Neuroma Is a Painful Lesion in the Foot

Morton neuroma (plantar interdigital neuroma) is a sausage-shaped swelling of the plantar interdigital nerve between the second and third or third and fourth metatarsal bones. It is probably caused by repeated nerve compression, leading to endoneurial, epineurial, and perineurial fibrosis and loss of nerve fibers. The fibrotic mass does not contain regenerating axons, so it is not a true neuroma. Morton neuroma is particularly common in women who wear high heels or ill-fitting shoes.

TUMORS

Primary PNS tumors are of neuronal or nerve sheath origin. The former (e.g., neuroblastoma and ganglioneuroma) usually arise from the adrenal medulla or sympathetic ganglia. The common nerve sheath tumors are schwannoma and neurofibroma.

Schwannomas Are Benign Neoplasms of Schwann Cells

They are typically slowly growing, encapsulated tumors that originate in cranial nerves, spinal roots, or peripheral nerves (Fig. 31-31A). Schwannomas usually occur in adults and rarely become malignant.

VESTIBULAR SCHWANNOMA (ACOUSTIC SCHWANNOMA): Intracranial schwannomas account for 8% of all primary intracranial tumors and 85% of all **cerebellopontine angle tumors**. Most arise from the vestibular branch of the eighth cranial nerve within the internal auditory canal or at the meatus. They cause unilateral, sensorineural hearing loss; tinnitus; and vestibular dysfunction. The slowly growing tumor enlarges the meatus, extends medially into the subarachnoid space of the cerebellopontine angle, and compresses the fifth and seventh cranial nerves, brainstem, and cerebellum. The posterior fossa mass may also lead to increased intracranial pressure, hydrocephalus, and tonsillar herniation. Most vestibular schwannomas are unilateral and are not associated with neurofibromatosis (see Chapter 6). About 5% are bilateral and are a defining feature of NF2. Biallelic inactivating mutations in *NF2*, a tumor suppressor gene on chromosome 22, have been found in both NF2-related and sporadic vestibular schwannomas.

SPINAL AND PERIPHERAL SCHWANNOMAS: Spinal schwannomas are intradural, extramedullary tumors that arise most often from the dorsal (sensory) spinal roots. They produce radicular (root) pain and spinal cord compression. More peripherally located schwannomas usually arise on nerves of the head, neck, and extremities.

PATHOLOGY: Schwannomas tend to be oval and well demarcated and vary from a few millimeters to several centimeters. The nerve of origin, if large enough, may be identifiable. The cut surface is firm and tan-to-gray, often with focal hemorrhage, necrosis, xanthomatous change, and cystic degeneration. Proliferating Schwann cells form two distinctive histologic patterns (Fig. 31-31B).

- **Antoni A pattern** is characterized by interwoven fascicles of spindle cells with elongated nuclei, eosinophilic cytoplasm, and indistinct cytoplasmic borders. Nuclei may palisade (line up in a picket fence–like pattern) in areas to form structures known as **Verocay bodies**.
- **Antoni B pattern** has spindle or oval cells with indistinct cytoplasm in a loose, vacuolated matrix.

Degenerative changes in schwannomas are common and include collections of foam cells (macrophages with foamy cytoplasm), recent or old hemorrhage, focal fibrosis, and hyalinized blood vessels. Scattered atypical nuclei are frequently encountered in schwannomas, but mitotic figures are uncommon.

Neurofibromas May Be Sporadic or Part of Neurofibromatosis Type 1

Neurofibromas are benign, slowly growing tumors of peripheral nerve, composed of Schwann cells, perineurial-like cells, and fibroblasts. *Schwann cells are the neoplastic cells in these tumors.* Neurofibromas must be distinguished from schwannomas because the former are associated with NF1

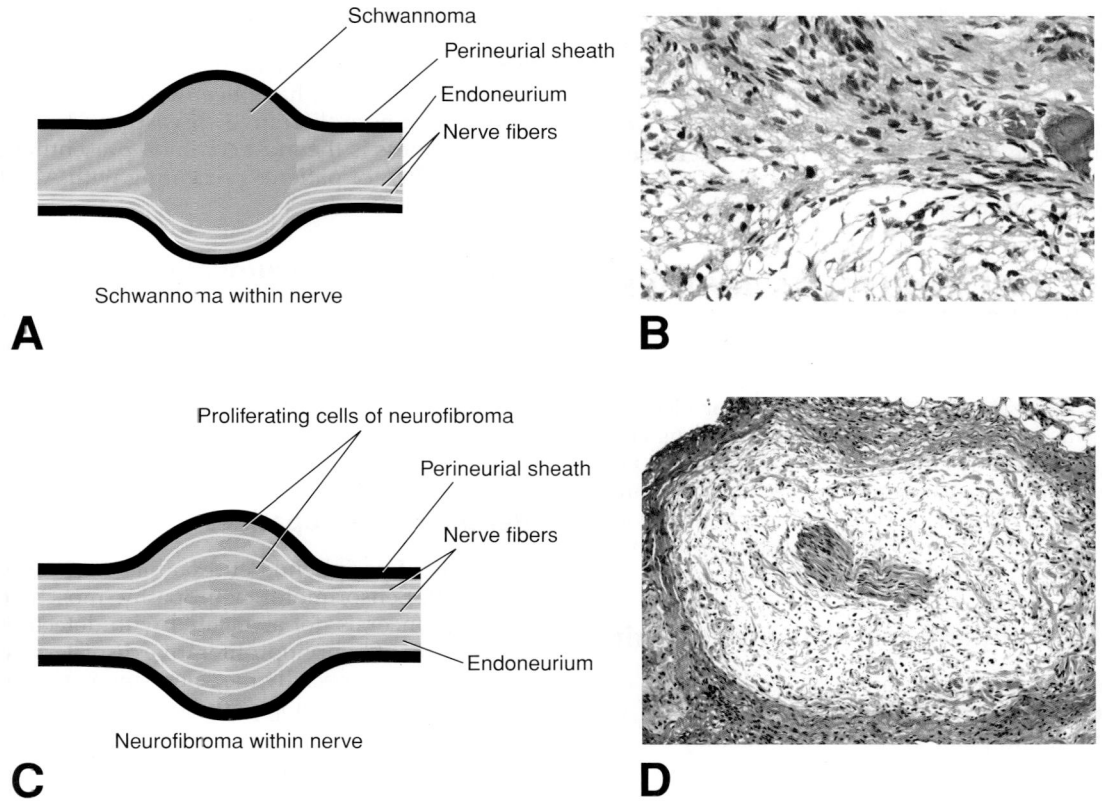

FIGURE 31-31. Schwannoma and neurofibroma growth patterns within peripheral nerves. A. Cellular proliferation in a schwannoma is well circumscribed and pushes surviving nerve fibers to the periphery of the tumor. **B.** A photomicrograph of a schwannoma shows the characteristically abrupt transition between the compact Antoni type A histologic pattern (*top*) and the spongy Antoni type B histologic pattern (*bottom*). **C.** Cellular proliferation in a neurofibroma is interspersed among surviving nerve fibers. **D.** A photomicrograph of neurofibroma shows proliferating spindle-shaped Schwann cells forming small strands that course haphazardly through a myxoid matrix. A small cluster of surviving nerve fibers is seen in the center of the neurofibroma.

and may become malignant peripheral nerve sheath tumors (MPNSTs).

Neurofibromas may be solitary or multiple and may arise on any nerve. They occur in children and adults. They mostly involve skin, subcutis, major nerve plexuses, large deep nerve trunks, retroperitoneum, and gastrointestinal tract. Most **solitary cutaneous neurofibromas** are not part of NF1 and do not degenerate into sarcomas. The presence of multiple neurofibromas or a single large plexiform neurofibroma strongly suggests NF1 and should prompt a search for other stigmata of the disease.

PATHOLOGY: Neurofibromas arising in large nerves are poorly circumscribed and fusiform (spindle shaped). A diffuse, intrafascicular growth of tumor within multiple nerve fascicles may so enlarge the fascicles that the nerve looks like a multistranded rope (**plexiform neurofibroma**). Neurofibromas may involve long stretches of a nerve, making complete surgical excision impossible. When they arise from small nerves, the nerve of origin may not be apparent. Cutaneous neurofibromas originate from dermal nerves and are seen as soft nodular or pedunculated skin tumors. These tumors are soft and light gray. Greatly enlarged, individual nerve

fascicles of the plexiform neurofibroma may be prominent. Tumors arising in large nerves are characterized by endoneurial proliferation of spindle cells with elongated nuclei, eosinophilic cytoplasm, and indistinct cell borders (Fig. 31-31D). The proliferating spindle cells include Schwann cells, fibroblasts, and perineurial-like cells. Mast cells are also increased. An extracellular myxoid matrix, wavy bands of collagen, and residual nerve fibers are interspersed among the spindle cells. The pattern of nerve fibers coursing through a neurofibroma contrasts with the pattern in schwannomas, in which nerve fibers are pushed peripherally into the tumor capsule (compare Fig. 31-31A,C). The neurofibromatous proliferation often extends beyond the nerve fascicle into adjacent tissue.

Some 5% of NF1-associated plexiform neurofibromas become MPNSTs. Increased cellularity, nuclear atypia, and mitotic figures herald malignant transformation.

Malignant Peripheral Nerve Sheath Tumor

MPNST is an aggressive, poorly differentiated spindle cell sarcoma of peripheral nerve of uncertain histogenesis. It may arise de novo or from malignant transformation of a neurofibroma. It may also arise at sites of previous irradiation. It is most common in adults and typically occurs in larger nerves of the trunk or proximal limbs. About half arise in patients with neurofibromatosis.

MPNSTs are unencapsulated, fusiform enlargements of a nerve. The tumors resemble fibrosarcomas, with closely packed spindle cells, nuclear atypia, mitotic figures and, often, foci of necrosis. MPNSTs are prone to local recurrence and blood-borne metastasis.

PARANEOPLASTIC SYNDROMES INVOLVING MUSCLE AND PERIPHERAL NERVES

Neurologic disorders are common in cancer patients, usually resulting from metastases or from endocrine or electrolyte disturbances. Vascular, hemorrhagic, and infectious conditions affecting the nervous system are also common. However, additional neurologic complications of malignancies are known and may appear before the underlying tumor is detected. Many of these are mediated by autoimmune mechanisms.

Sensory Neuropathy and Encephalomyeloneuritis

Patients afflicted with this paraneoplastic syndrome complain of numbness and paresthesias and, conversely, variably acute aching and pain. These symptoms may be focal, but often affect all extremities over time, and are often complicated by disorders of gait, confusion, and weakness. This syndrome may occur in patients with small cell lung cancer (see Chapter 18) and is caused by circulating antibodies against Hu, an RNA-binding protein. High titers of anti-Hu antibodies are almost exclusively detected in people with SCLC. Lymphocytic infiltration of dorsal root ganglia is seen. Symptoms tend to be treatable when the primary tumor is treated.

Paraneoplastic Autonomic Neuropathies

These are rare, but affect a quarter of patients with anti-Hu antibodies, and may be the initial presentation of the tumor. Systems affected, sometimes severely, include the vasculature, bowel, and bladder. Antibodies against the nicotinic ACh receptor are sometimes responsible.

Opsoclonus-Myoclonus

Nonvoluntary spasms of ocular and other muscles characterize this syndrome. Among children, about half of cases are associated with neuroblastoma. About 10% of adults with opsoclonus-myoclonus will have a malignancy, most often Hodgkin lymphoma.

Diseases of Upper and Lower Motor Neurons

These syndromes may be paraneoplastic in origin. Diverse tumor associations have been reported, the most frequent being lymphoproliferative diseases and anti-Hu antibodies. Weakness is the most common presenting symptom. As many as 10% of patients presenting with ALS have internal malignancies.

Subacute Motor Neuropathy

This is a disorder of the spinal cord characterized by slowly developing lower motor neuron weakness without sensory changes. It is so strongly associated with cancer that an intensive search for an occult neoplasm, often a lymphoma, should be made in patients who present with these symptoms.

Peripheral Neuropathies

An array of peripheral neuropathies may be paraneoplastic in origin. Sensorimotor neuropathy, most likely attendant to lung cancer, is not associated with detectable antibodies. Some types of lymphoproliferative disorders associated with paraproteins, especially the sclerosing variant of plasma cell myeloma, may develop peripheral neuropathies.

Neuromuscular Junction Disorders

The most common association is with thymomas. About 15% of patients with myasthenia gravis have thymomas, and about half of patients with thymomas suffer from myasthenia gravis. Autoantibodies against the nicotinic ACh receptor are the principal cause of this syndrome.

Eaton–Lambert Syndrome

This syndrome is a paraneoplastic disorder that manifests as muscle weakness, wasting, and fatigability of proximal limbs and trunk. Also called **myasthenic–myopathic syndrome**, it is usually associated with small cell lung carcinoma, but may also occur with other malignancies, and rarely in the absence of underlying cancer. Neurophysiologic evidence suggests a defect in Ach release at nerve terminals. IgG from patients can transfer the disease to mice. The pathogenic IgG autoantibodies target voltage-sensitive calcium channels expressed in motor nerve terminals and in the cells of the lung cancer. These calcium channels are necessary for ACh release and are greatly reduced in presynaptic membranes in these patients, thus reducing neuromuscular transmission. Lambert–Eaton syndrome responds to corticosteroid treatment.

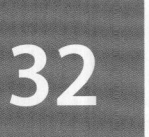

32 The Central Nervous System

Leomar Y. Ballester, Gregory N. Fuller, J. Clay Goodman

The Central Nervous System

The nervous system is the most complex organ system in the body. It is responsible for sensory processing and synthesis and motor control, and it is the organ of thought, emotion, and personality—in short, the basis of humanity itself. Disorders of the central nervous system (CNS) strike at the core of our being as sentient organisms, and so inspire fear and dread. Diseases of the nervous system are common throughout the human life span and contribute substantially to mortality and morbidity: stroke, Alzheimer disease, intellectual disability, traumatic brain and spinal cord injury, meningitis, and neoplasms.

TOPOGRAPHY: The functions of the nervous system have precise topographic localization, so that focal disease processes produce myriad signs and symptoms that permit a skilled clinician to locate the affected site. Selective vulnerability of different nervous system cells and CNS regions to specific disease processes is among the most profound unresolved enigmas of neurologic illnesses. For example, Huntington disease primarily causes degeneration of neurons in the caudate nuclei; Parkinson disease targets the nigrostriatal system; amyotrophic lateral sclerosis (ALS) selectively singles out upper and lower motor neurons of the cerebrum, brainstem, and spinal cord. Some infectious diseases prefer certain targets: poliomyelitis involves anterior horn cells of the spinal cord and motor nuclei of the brainstem, while herpes simplex virus preferentially affects the temporal lobes. Vascular and demyelinating diseases also have regional preferences within the CNS, as do some brain tumors. The basis of topographic vulnerability and protection for most such diseases is obscure.

AGE: The nervous system is affected by disorders throughout the life span, but individual diseases commonly affect selected age groups. Thus, inborn errors of metabolism and several posterior fossa tumors occur mainly in childhood. Reckless exuberance leads to a spike in traumatic brain and spinal cord injury in teens and young adults that subsides with maturity, only to return with the infirmities of age. Multiple sclerosis (MS) shows a strong preference for young adults, rarely beginning before puberty or after age 40. Neuropsychiatric disorders such as schizophrenia often appear in late adolescence and young adulthood when the brain undergoes striking neurodevelopmental changes. Huntington disease typically strikes youthful and middle-aged adults, while Parkinson and Alzheimer disease and stroke occur late in life.

CELLS OF THE NERVOUS SYSTEM

The diversity and complexity of the CNS is reflected at all levels in its organization, from the morphologic and functional subspecialization of the many unique cellular constituents to the regional localization of sensory, motor, and cognitive functions.

GRAY MATTER AND THE NEUROPIL: Gray matter includes all regions of the CNS rich in neurons: cerebral and cerebellar cortices, basal ganglia, and central gray matter of the spinal cord. Gray matter consists of cell bodies (perikarya) of neurons and supporting glial cell nuclei, plus the intervening delicate interwoven meshwork of neuronal and glial cell processes, the **neuropil** (Fig. 32-1). Circumscribed collections of neuronal cell bodies that share a common functional task are referred to as "nuclei."

WHITE MATTER: White matter consists of compact bundles **(tracts, fascicles)** of myelinated axons with many oligodendrocytes and interspersed astrocytes (Fig. 32-2).

NEURONS: The morphology of neuronal subtypes in the gray matter varies due to functional subspecialization, ranging from large motor and primary sensory neurons to tiny "granular cell" neurons (Fig. 32-3A). For example, pigmented neurons, which occur only in specific brainstem nuclei, are distinguished by brown cytoplasmic neuromelanin pigment, a byproduct of catecholaminergic neurotransmitter synthesis

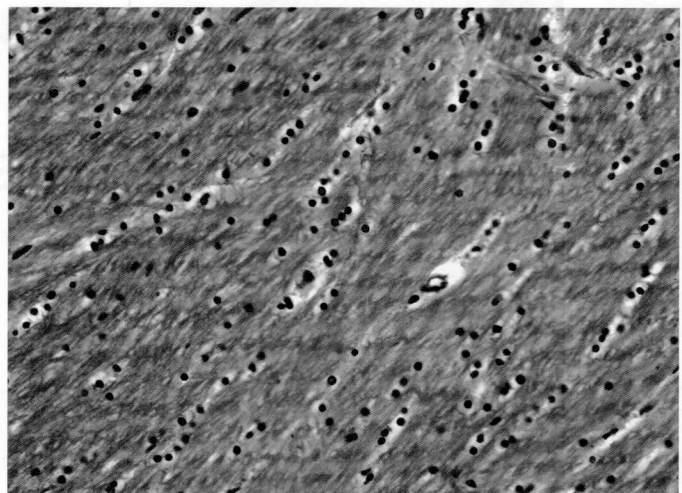

FIGURE 32-2. White matter. By contrast to gray matter, white matter is composed almost entirely of myelinated axons and the cells that produce and maintain their myelin sheaths, the oligodendroglia whose small round nuclei are seen between the fiber bundles.

(Fig. 32-3B). These clusters of pigmented catecholaminergic neurons are so dense as to be visible to the naked eye in the midbrain (substantia nigra) and pons (locus ceruleus).

ASTROCYTES: Astrocytes outnumber neurons at least 10:1 and play a critical supportive role in regulating the CNS microenvironment. They are also one of two primary CNS cell types that respond to many CNS insults (the other being microglia). Astrocytes respond to acute injury by upregulating synthesis of glial fibrillary acidic protein (GFAP) and assembling it into intracytoplasmic intermediate filaments, resulting in prominent cell bodies and cytoplasmic processes (Fig. 32-4A). With advancing age, astrocyte peripheral processes may accumulate spherical inclusion bodies called corpora amylacea which are composed of glucose polymers. They are especially numerous in subpial, subependymal and perivascular sites and in olfactory tracts (Fig. 32-4B). Cytoplasmic strap-like densities, Rosenthal fibers (Fig. 32-4C), appear in long-standing astrogliosis as densely compacted glial intermediate filaments with entrapped cytosol proteins.

OLIGODENDROGLIA: Oligodendroglia produce and maintain CNS axon myelin sheaths, and so are CNS counterparts of Schwann cells in the peripheral nervous system. Oligodendroglia cell bodies are dominated by uniform round nuclei that, in formalin-fixed paraffin-embedded tissue sections, are characteristically surrounded by only a small clear rim of vacuolated cytoplasm ("perinuclear halo") (Fig. 32-5).

MICROGLIA: Microglia are bone marrow–derived mononuclear phagocytes of the CNS. In health, they are inconspicuously distributed throughout the brain and spinal cord. But they respond quickly to CNS insults such as ischemia, trauma, or viral infection by developing thin, elongated nuclei, migrating through the CNS and localizing at sites of injury (Fig. 32-6).

EPENDYMA: The ependymal lining of the ventricular system forms a barrier between cerebrospinal fluid (CSF) and brain parenchyma and regulates fluid transfer between these two compartments. The normal ependyma is lined by ciliated cuboidal-to-columnar simple epithelium (Fig. 32-7).

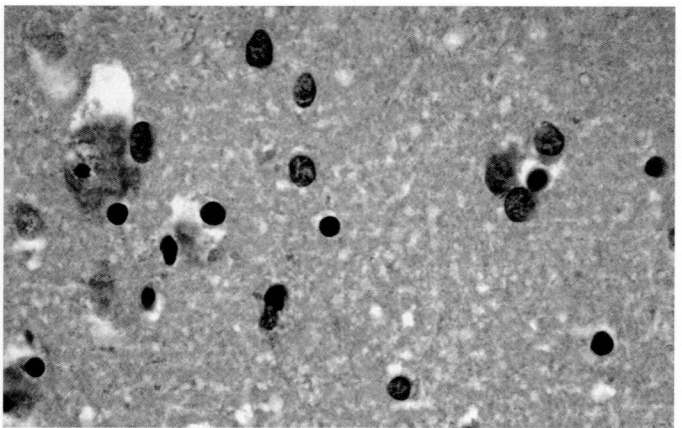

FIGURE 32-1. Gray matter and the neuropil. Gray matter by definition contains neuronal cell bodies. In addition, the nuclei of supporting glial cells, astrocytes, and satellite oligodendroglia, are present. The remaining finely fibrillar background meshwork is called the neuropil and consists of intimately intermingled axons, dendrites, and astrocytic cytoplasmic processes.

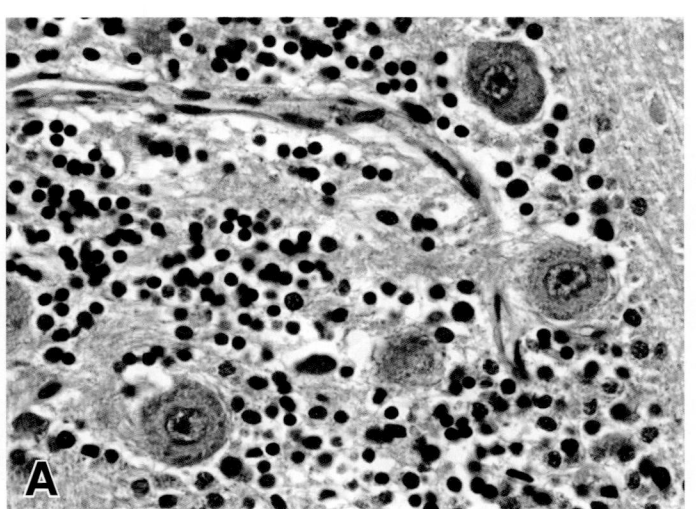
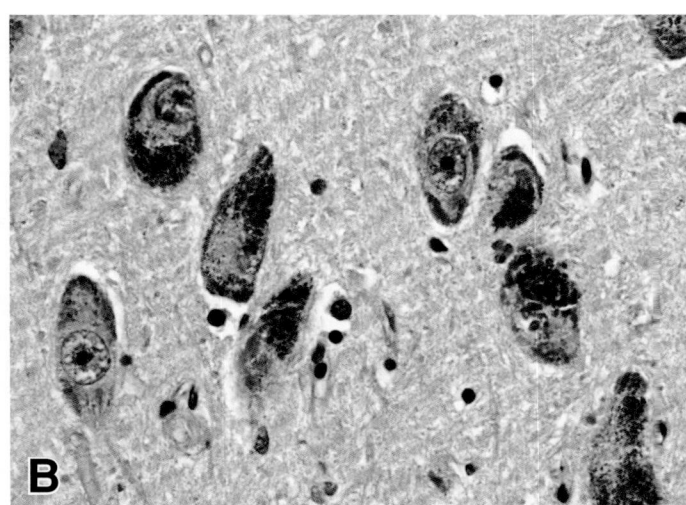

FIGURE 32-3. Neurons. A. The different neuronal populations of the central nervous system (CNS) subserve different functions, and this diversity is reflected in their morphology. Illustrative of the extremes are the large cell bodies of Purkinje cell neurons juxtaposed next to the diminutive granular cell neurons of the cerebellar cortex; the entire granular neuron cell body is not much bigger than the nucleolus of a Purkinje cell neuron! **B.** Pigmented catecholaminergic neurons with their prominent neuromelanin content serve are another striking example of diversity in form and function among CNS neuronal populations.

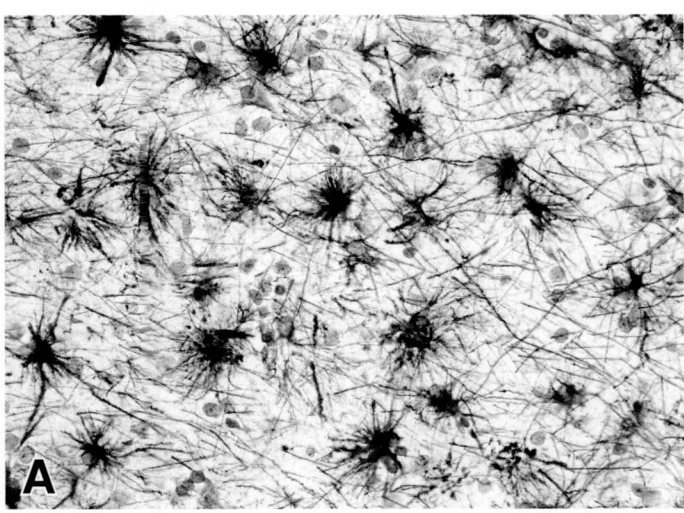
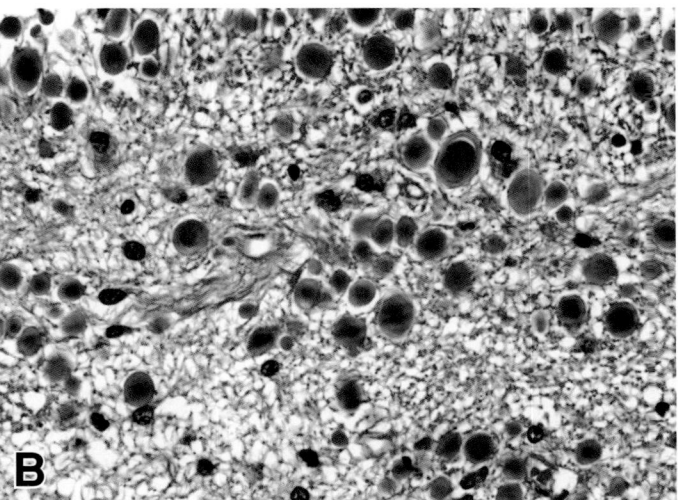

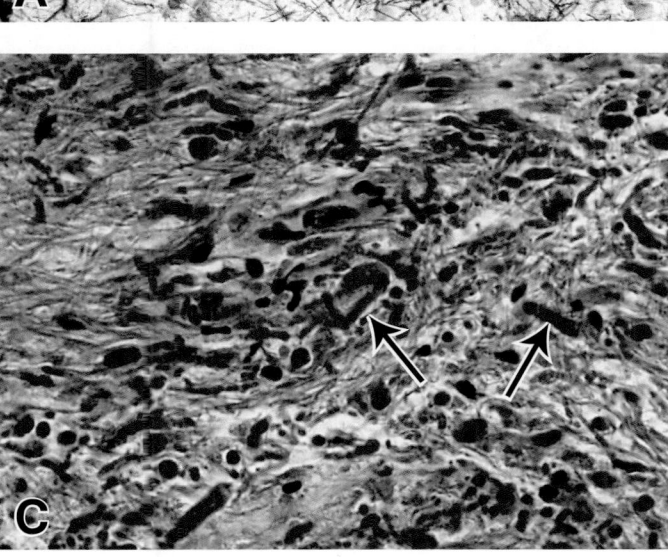

FIGURE 32-4. Astrocytes. A. Astrocytes have been called "the fibroblast of the central nervous system," referring to their role as the ubiquitous supporting cell of the brain and spinal cord that reacts to any pathologic insult. As seen in this immunostain directed against glial fibrillary acidic protein, astrocytes occupy adjacent domains and send cytoplasmic processes radiating out in all directions to fill their individual fiefdoms. **B.** With advancing age, astrocytes are prone to develop glucose polymer inclusion bodies, called corpora amylacea, in the distal distribution of their cell processes, particularly around blood vessels and subjacent to the pia and ependyma. **C.** Rosenthal fibers are another astrocytic inclusion body formed as a response to long-standing astrogliosis; they are composed of densely compacted glial intermediate filaments together with entrapped cytosolic proteins (*arrows*).

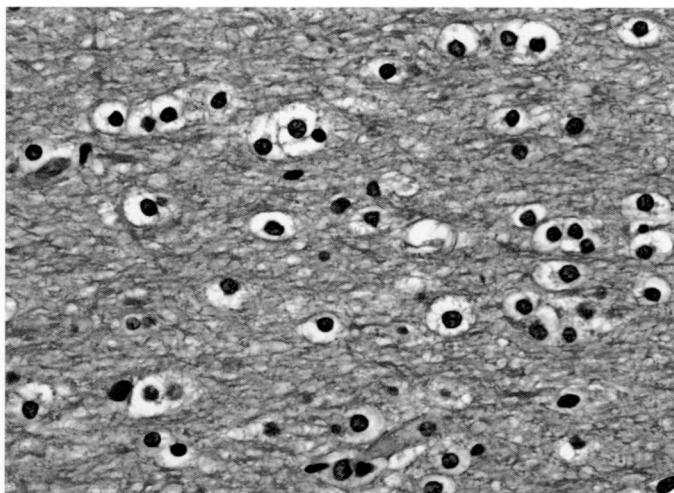

FIGURE 32-5. Oligodendroglia. Oligodendroglia are the myelin-forming glia of the central nervous system (CNS; including the optic "nerves," which are actually CNS tracts). On routine histologic imaging, oligodendroglia are easily recognized by their monotonous small dark round nuclei surrounded by a halo of vacuolated cytoplasm ("fried egg" appearance). This characteristic appearance is recapitulated in neoplastic oligodendrogliomas.

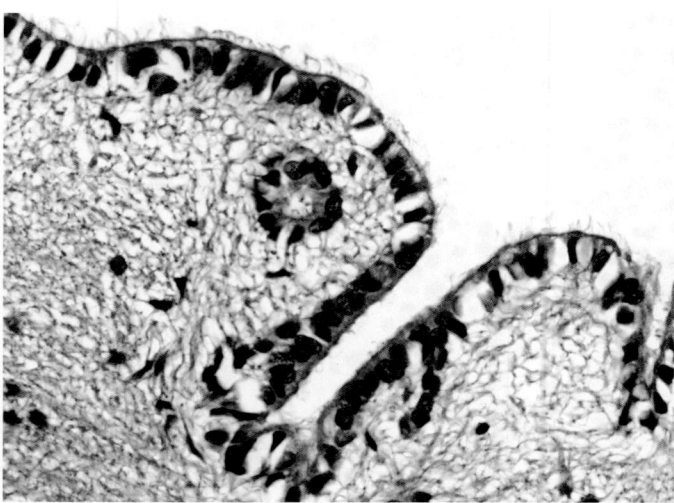

FIGURE 32-7. Ependyma. Ependymal cells form a ciliated cuboidal-to-columnar epithelium that lines the cerebral ventricles and spinal cord central canal. Ependymal cell clusters and true rosettes, as seen here, are commonly scattered beneath the ependymal lining.

SPECIALIZED REGIONS OF THE CENTRAL NERVOUS SYSTEM

CHOROID PLEXUS: The choroid plexus produces CSF. It resides in the cerebral ventricles, including the temporal horns bilaterally, interventricular foramen of Monro, the roof of the third ventricle and the roof and lateral recesses of the fourth ventricle. The choroid plexus is composed of cuboidal epithelium (derived from embryologic ependyma) that covers a fibrovascular core (Fig. 32-8A). The highly vascular

core is critical to CSF formation. It develops from leptomeninges (pia and arachnoid) and contains scattered nests of arachnoid (meningothelial) cells (Fig. 32-8B). Thus, the occasional "intraventricular" meningioma is actually a choroid plexus meningioma.

MENINGES: Three layers of meninges cover and protect the CNS. The **dura** is the tough outer fibrous membrane. It is composed primarily of collagen. Its outer surface is the inner periosteum of the cranial bones and its inner surface attaches weakly to the subjacent arachnoid via cell junctions. The two dural layers separate in several sites to form dural venous sinuses, the largest of which is the superior sagittal sinus. The underlying arachnoid is bound to the overlying dura by a loosely cohesive layer of cells, the **dural border cell (DBC) layer**. This layer is

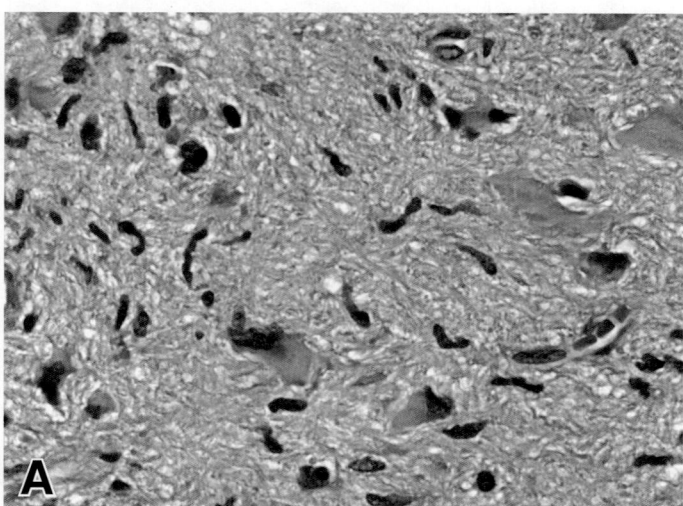

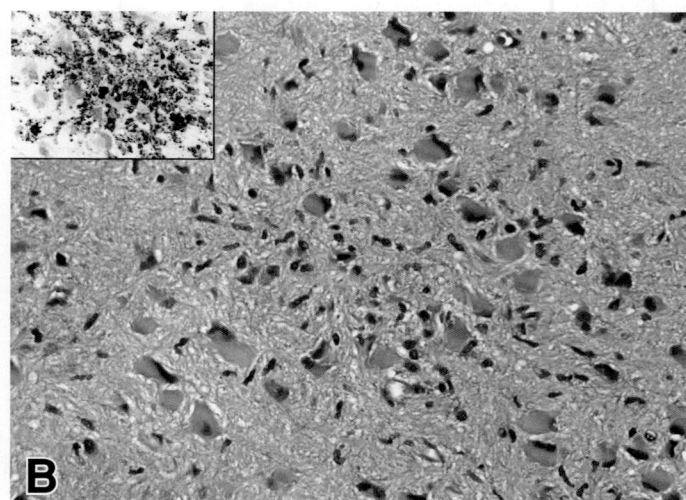

FIGURE 32-6. Microglia. A. Microglia are the resident representatives of the monocyte–macrophage system in the brain and spinal cord. While inconspicuous in normal healthy brain ("resting microglial"), they become prominent when responding to central nervous system (CNS) injury and are easily recognized by their elongated nuclei ("rod cells"), which reflect their infiltrative phenotype. **B.** Actively migrating through CNS parenchyma, they commonly cluster around foci of disease; such collections are known as "microglial nodules." Microglia demonstrate strong immunohistochemical reactivity for the macrophage marker CD68 (*inset*).

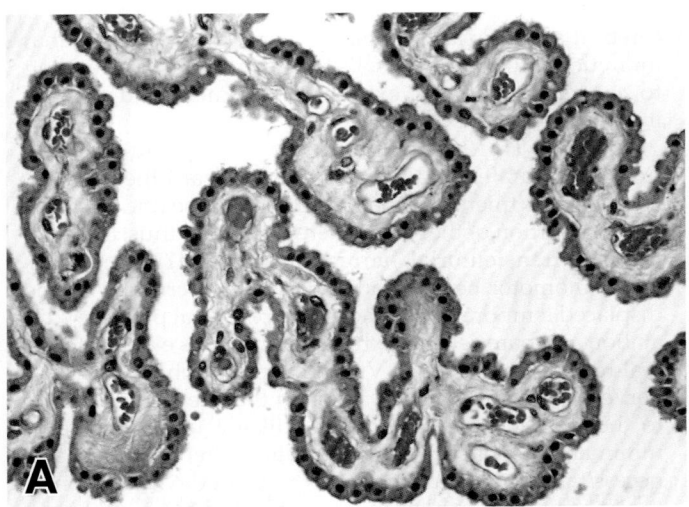
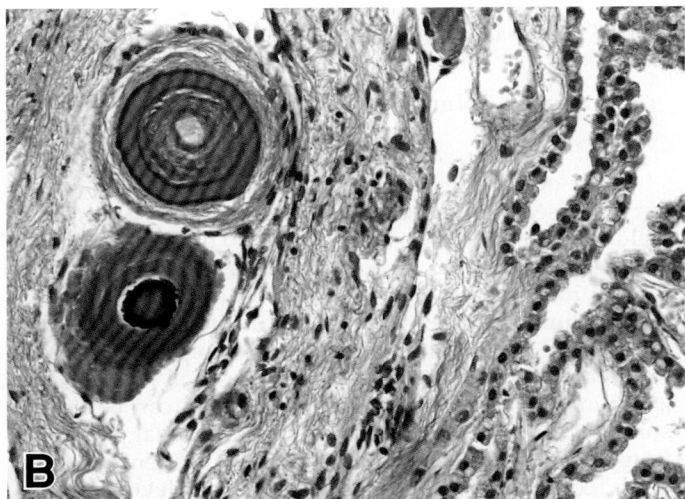

FIGURE 32-8. Choroid plexus. A. Choroid plexus is the central nervous system (CNS) organ responsible for producing cerebrospinal fluid. It consists of innumerable papillae with highly vascular cores covered by cuboidal epithelium derived embryologically from the ependyma. **B.** The cores also contain arachnoid (meningothelial) cell nests (by virtue of their embryologic derivation from the pia-arachnoid) that tend to mineralize with age, forming psammoma bodies (seen on the *left* side of the image).

the path of least resistance for pathologic fluids, which easily dissect the weak intercellular junctions to form the so-called subdural hematomas, hygromas, and empyemas. By contrast, the meningeal layer just beneath the DBC layer, the **arachnoid barrier cell (ABC) layer**, forms a cohesive outer limiting membrane of the subarachnoid space via abundant intercellular junctions (desmosomes) that weld together elongated, interlacing arachnoid (meningothelial) cell processes. Whorls of arachnoid cells are commonly seen in thicker areas of the arachnoid (Fig. 32-9); this feature is often recapitulated in arachnoid tumors (meningiomas).

PINEAL GLAND: The pineal gland (see Chapter 27) contains pineal parenchymal cells (pineocytes), plus supporting glial cells (pineal astrocytes), arranged in cell clusters separated by collagenous septa (Fig. 32-10). Inconspicuous autonomic peripheral nerve fibers coming from cell bodies in the superior cervical ganglia provide sympathetic (noradrenergic) innervation.

INCREASED INTRACRANIAL PRESSURE AND HERNIATION

ETIOLOGIC FACTORS: The most important pathophysiologic aspect of the brain is that it *lives in a closed box*! The brain, CSF, and blood going to and from the brain occupy the intracranial space which in adults is a rigidly fixed cavity. Any disease that occupies space does so at the expense of brain, CSF, or

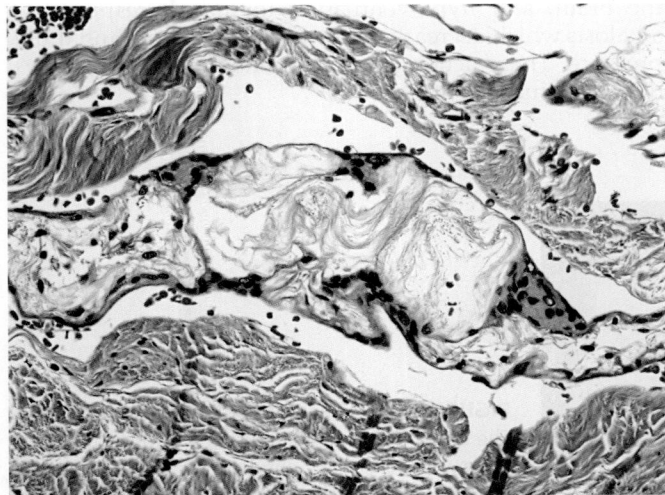

FIGURE 32-9. Arachnoid villi. The arachnoid membrane forms the outer boundary of the subarachnoid space and also protrudes into the dural venous sinuses, as seen here, to form arachnoid villi whose function is to return cerebrospinal fluid (CSF) into the venous circulatory system. The villi are covered by a layer of meningothelial cells, called arachnoid cap cells, that varies in thickness from a single cell to multilayered whorls.

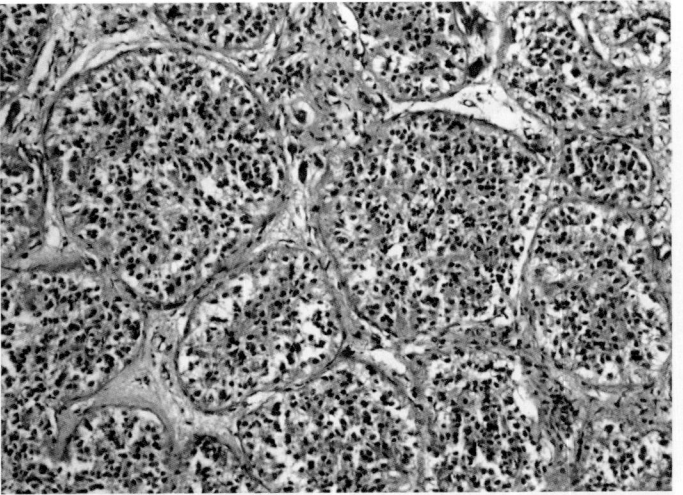

FIGURE 32-10. Pineal gland. The pineal is composed of pineal parenchymal cells (pineocytes) organized into lobules by fibrovascular septa.

blood. This is the anatomical basis of the Monro-Kellie hypothesis that states:

$$\text{Intracranial volume} = \text{Volume}_{CNS} + \text{Volume}_{CSF} + \text{Volume}_{blood} + \text{Volume}_{lesion}$$

Space-occupying lesions occur in every major category of disease except degenerative disorders. Examples include brain tumors, abscesses, swollen brain contusions following trauma and stroke with brain swelling.

The immediate and inevitable result of trying to fit more volume into the fixed space of the intracranial vault is increased intracranial pressure (ICP). Normal mean ICP for a patient in the lateral decubitus position is less than 200 mm H_2O or 15 mm Hg. This pressure can be measured by lumbar puncture or by an intracranial pressure transducer. As ICP increases, patients experience headaches, confusion and drowsiness and may develop papilledema. To compensate, CSF volume is reduced and, as a result, the ventricles become compressed to small slits and sulci are effaced.

If a lesion takes up more space than a reduction in CSF volume can accommodate, blood flow then decreases. Reduced cerebral blood flow may have an immediate adverse impact as the brain is critically dependent upon uninterrupted supply of oxygen and nutrients. If the lesion expands further, the only structure remaining to "give" is the brain itself. The intracranial compartment is subdivided by the dura—the tentorium cerebelli divides the vault into supra- and infratentorial compartments; and the falx divides the supratentorial compartment into right and left compartments. Depending on the location of the space-occupying lesion, the brain may be forced out of one compartment into another. Such shifts are called brain herniations.

CLINICAL FEATURES: *CINGULATE HERNIATION:* If a hemisphere is forced under the falx, the cingulate lobe is the first part of that hemisphere to be displaced. These situations are **subfalcine,** or **cingulate, herniations**. Clinical sequelae of such herniations include confusion and drowsiness. The anterior cerebral artery is also displaced beneath the falx, so that infarction within this vessel's territory may occur, leading to contralateral lower extremity weakness and urinary incontinence.

UNCAL HERNIATION: If one hemisphere is forced from the supratentorial compartment toward the infratentorial compartment, the medial temporal lobe (the uncus) is the first portion of the hemisphere displaced; thus, this is an **uncal,** or **transtentorial, herniation** (Fig. 32-11). The ipsilateral oculomotor nerve (cranial nerve III) is crushed by the displaced temporal lobe, leading to ipsilateral pupillary dilatation and paresis of all extraocular muscles except the lateral rectus (cranial nerve VI) and superior oblique (cranial nerve IV). The unopposed action of the lateral rectus leads to the eye "looking" laterally. A dilated unresponsive or minimally responsive pupil indicates extreme danger and necessitates immediate measures to arrest the herniation.

As medial displacement continues, the midbrain shifts away from the displaced hemisphere, and the contralateral cerebral pedicle is driven into the unyielding tentorium. This crushing injury of the cerebral pedicle **(Kernohan notch)** causes hemiparesis on the same side of the body as the offending mass. Because a hemispheric mass normally causes hemiparesis on the opposite side of the body, ipsilateral hemiparesis, can be clinically confusing, and is thus called a "false localizing" sign.

Downward and medial displacement of a hemisphere through the tentorial opening may also lead to compression of one or both posterior cerebral arteries as they travel from the infratentorial compartment to the now crowded supratentorial compartment. This can impair blood flow to the occipital lobes, resulting in infarction with attendant visual field disturbances bearing no obvious relationship to the inciting mass. This occipital lobe infarction and its attendant signs are also "false localizing."

Uncal herniation syndrome is ominous but is reversible with removal of the offending mass. Temporary measures to reduce intracranial pressure include administration of intravenous mannitol to osmotically shrink the brain, and hyperventilation to induce respiratory alkalosis which decreases cerebral blood volume and thus pressure. These actions may gain enough time to allow definitive surgical treatment.

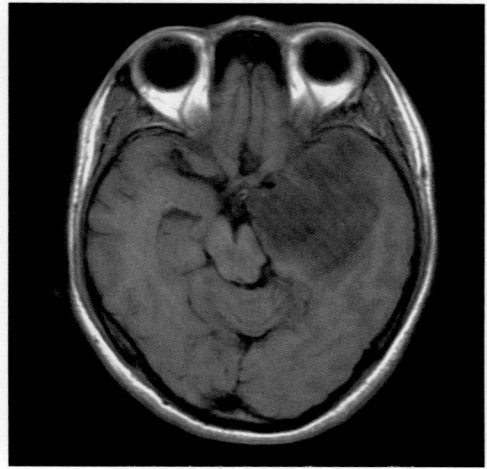
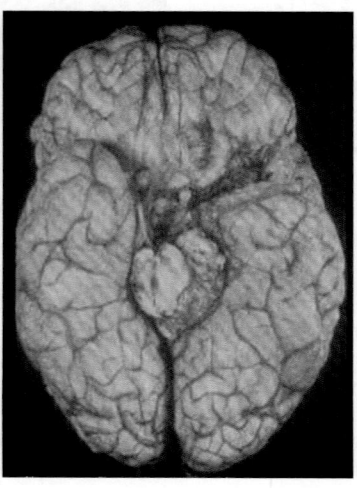

FIGURE 32-11. Uncal (transtentorial) herniation. The uncus of the parahippocampal gyrus is herniated downward to displace the midbrain, resulting in distortion of the midbrain with increased anterior-to-posterior and diminished left-to-right dimensions. The oculomotor nerve on the left is spared but on the right is compromised, leading to an ipsilateral third nerve palsy. The MRI (*left*) shows midbrain distortion due to herniation of a low signal intensity mass in the right temporal lobe.

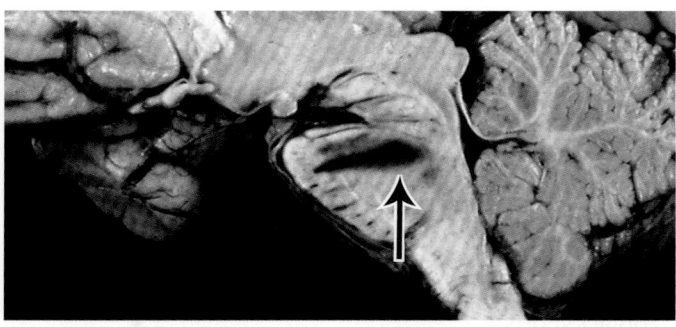

FIGURE 32-12. Duret hemorrhages (*arrow*) in a case of transtentorial herniation tend to be midline and occupy the brainstem from the upper midbrain to midpons. (Courtesy of Dr. F. Stephen Vogel, Duke University.)

CENTRAL HERNIATION: If both hemispheres herniate transtentorially, **central herniation syndrome** results. Both pupils dilate; flaccidity and coma ensue. The downward displacement of the brainstem may wrench vessels from their parenchymal beds within the midbrain and pons and cause multiple linear hemorrhages known as **Duret hemorrhages** or secondary hemorrhages of herniation (Fig. 32-12).

CEREBELLAR TONSILLAR HERNIATION: If the infratentorial compartment becomes crowded either from migrating supratentorial contents or from a mass arising in the infratentorial compartment, the brainstem and cerebellum may be forced through the foramen magnum. The compressed cerebellar tonsils and medulla may compress vital medullary centers and cause death. This bleak situation is **tonsillar herniation**.

FUNGUS CEREBRI: This refers to protrusion of the brain and dura through a traumatic or surgical defect in the skull.

Cerebral Edema May Be Cytotoxic, Vasogenic, or Interstitial

Cerebral edema results from an absolute increase in brain water volume resulting from a variety of neuropathologic processes. Cerebral edema can set up a self-perpetuating cycle in which edema increases intravascular pressure, which in turn begets more edema.

 ETIOLOGIC FACTORS: The amount of water in brain tissue is tightly controlled by the rates of CSF production, CSF outflow from the cranial vault and water flux across the blood–brain barrier (BBB). The BBB separates the brain from the blood so that only lipid-soluble molecules, or molecules that can access specialized transport systems, enter the brain. The structural basis of the BBB is endothelial cell tight junctions lining cerebral vessels. Water can enter the brain uncontrollably if the barrier is disrupted or if osmotic forces across it are sufficient to drive water into cerebral tissues. Three major forms of cerebral edema can occur:

- **Cytotoxic edema:** Water flows across an intact BBB by osmotic forces arising because injured cells in the brain can no longer maintain osmotic homeostasis or because of systemic water overload. In either case, water is driven down its concentration gradient into cerebral tissues until osmotic equilibrium is reestablished.
- **Vasogenic edema:** The BBB loosens, permitting uncontrolled entry of water into the tissues. *This is the most common cause of edema* and occurs with neoplasms, abscesses, meningitis, hemorrhage, contusions, and lead poisoning. A combination of cytotoxic and vasogenic edema is common in infarcts. The above processes may disrupt endothelial barrier activity, or vessels formed in neoplasms may be defective from their inception. Vasogenic edema often responds dramatically to administration of corticosteroids, which restore barrier integrity even in tumors.
- **Interstitial edema:** While cytotoxic and vasogenic edema involve water fluxes across the endothelium, interstitial edema involves overproduction of CSF or its failure to leave the cranial cavity, such that fluid seeps across the ependymal lining of the ventricles and accumulates in the white matter.

Hydrocephalus Can Be Noncommunicating or Communicating

Hydrocephalus is accumulation of CSF within the ventricles, causing them to dilate (Fig. 32-13). When ventricular distension is sufficiently advanced, fluid will leak trans-ependymally into the white matter, causing interstitial edema. CSF accumulation can arise from (1) *overproduction of CSF, which is very rare,* occurring only in the context of tumors of the choroid plexus; and (2) *failure of CSF to leave the cranial vault, which is more common.* If the blockage occurs within the ventricular system itself, ventricles proximal to the block dilate, while those downstream from the block are spared. This is **obstructive,** or **noncommunicating, hydrocephalus.** The most frequent site of block is at the ventricular system's narrowest strait—the aqueduct of Sylvius connecting the third and fourth ventricles.

A block may occur after the CSF leaves the ventricular system and travels over the cerebral convexities to the arachnoid granulations that usher the fluid into the venous sinuses. Then, all the ventricles dilate. This is **communicating**

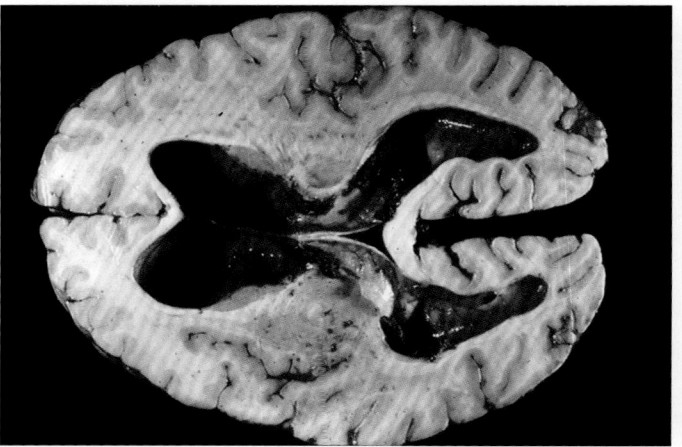

FIGURE 32-13. Hydrocephalus. Axial section of the brain from a patient who died of a brain tumor that obstructed the aqueduct of Sylvius shows marked dilation of the lateral ventricles.

hydrocephalus, meaning that ventricles are unobstructed in fluid flow. Communicating hydrocephalus may complicate subarachnoid hemorrhage (SAH) or inflammation, resulting in arachnoid scarring, or may result from thrombosis of the dural venous sinuses themselves.

 CLINICAL FEATURES: The clinical features of hydrocephalus depend on the patient's age. In infants and children, before cranial sutures have fused, the head enlarges sometimes to grotesque proportions as the ventricles dilate. As hydrocephalus is common in infants and treatable by shunting, measurement of the head circumference is a fundamental part of the pediatric physical examination.

After sutures fuse, hydrocephalus cannot enlarge the head, but rather increases intracranial pressure. This causes headache, confusion, drowsiness, papilledema, and vomiting. Ventricles enlarge at the expense of brain volume so that in advanced cases only a mantle of several millimeters' thickness remains. Remarkably, such individuals may retain substantial cognitive abilities, although spasticity may cloak the expression of this intelligence.

In older people, hydrocephalus may develop insidiously. Slow ventricular enlargement may appear clinically as progressive dementia, gait impairment and urinary incontinence as the long white matter fibers connecting portions of cortex to one another and lower motility centers are stretched apart by relentless expansion of the ventricles. This condition is usually accompanied by normal baseline intracranial pressure and so is called **normal-pressure hydrocephalus,** which may respond to shunting. If long-term CSF pressure is monitored, periodic waves of elevated intracranial pressure are seen.

All of the above forms of hydrocephalus result from disturbance of CSF dynamics and should be distinguished from **hydrocephalus ex vacuo,** which is compensatory ventricular enlargement due to loss of CNS tissue from other diseases. This occurs most often in diffuse cortical atrophy, but focal destruction such as occurs at the site of an old infarct may lead to focal compensatory ventricular enlargement.

TRAUMA

 EPIDEMIOLOGY: Physical injury to the brain, spinal cord, and peripheral nervous system is a major cause of loss of life and productivity. Populations at highest risk for such injuries include children, men in late adolescence, and early adulthood and the elderly. Such injuries are a signature of modern warfare. They are also the leading cause of death in childhood and young adulthood and a major concern for participants in contact sports.

 ETIOLOGIC FACTORS: The brain and spinal cord are encased protective bony cases that dissipate forces delivered to these delicate structures. Injury to the nervous system results from the transfer of kinetic energy to the neural tissues—the degree of injury correlates with the quantity of energy delivered and the time over which it was delivered. This energy transfer may directly disrupt tissues in penetrating injuries, or it may be translated into movement and compression of neural structures within the skull or spinal canal in a closed injury. Extreme injury of the brain and cord is possible with minimal disruption of overlying tissues. Conversely, superficial tissues can sustain dramatic injury while the nervous system underneath remains unscathed.

Epidural Hematomas Can Be Rapidly Fatal

Epidural hematomas usually result from blows to the head with skull fracture. Unless treated promptly, they can be fatal. The intracranial dura is securely bound to the inner aspect of the calvaria and so is analogous to the cranial periosteum. The middle meningeal arteries reside in grooves in the inner table of the bone between the dura and the calvaria, and their branches splay across the temporal–parietal area. The temporal bone, being one of the thinnest bones of the skull, is particularly vulnerable to fracture which may in turn lacerate branches of the middle meningeal artery, causing life-threatening epidural hemorrhage (Fig. 32-14).

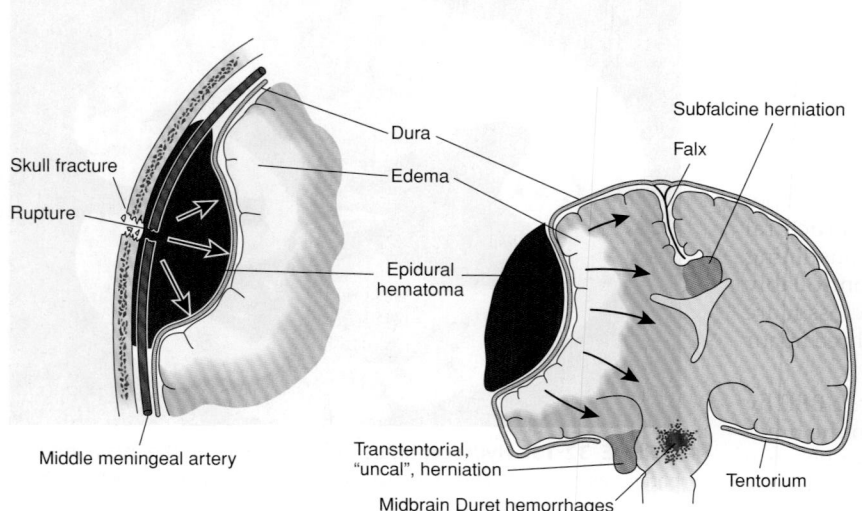

FIGURE 32-14. Development of an epidural hematoma. Laceration of a branch of the middle meningeal artery by the sharp bony edges of a skull fracture initiates bleeding under arterial pressure that dissects the dura from the calvaria and produces an expanding hematoma. After an asymptomatic period that may last several hours, subfalcine and transtentorial herniation occur, and if the hematoma is not evacuated, lethal herniation will occur.

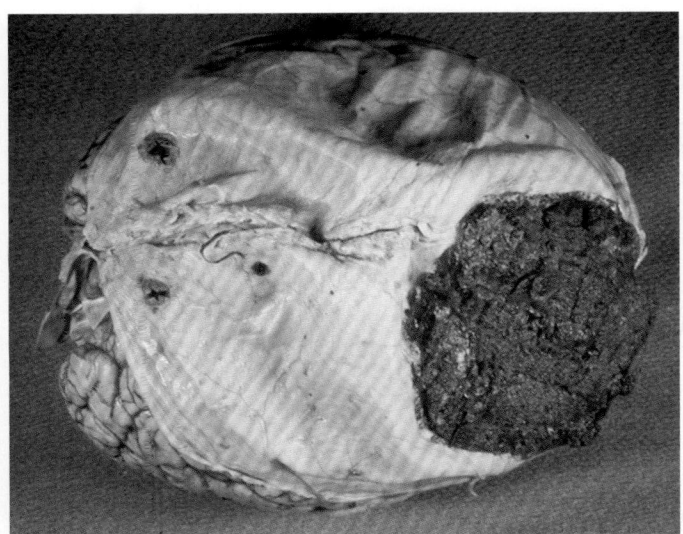

FIGURE 32-15. Epidural hematoma. A discoid mass of fresh hemorrhage overlies the dura covering frontal–parietal cortex but does not transgress the coronal sutures.

PATHOLOGY: Laceration of the middle meningeal artery allows blood under arterial pressure to escape into the epidural space that separates the dura from the calvaria. The dura is tightly bound to the calvarium at the coronal sutures. Thus, epidural bleeding does not extend beyond the suture lines. This leads to a lens-shaped accumulation of fresh blood that respects the coronal suture lines (Fig. 32-15).

CLINICAL FEATURES: Up to 1/3 of patients do not lose consciousness at the time of the precipitating injury and may have a "lucid interval" of unimpaired consciousness for several hours while epidural blood accumulates under arterial pressure. When the hematoma reaches 30 to 50 mL, symptoms of a space-occupying lesion appear. Epidural hematomas are invariably progressive and, when not recognized and evacuated, may be fatal within hours.

Subdural Hematomas Develop More Slowly Than Epidural Hematomas

Subdural hematomas are a significant cause of death associated with head injuries from falls, assaults, vehicular accidents, and sporting accidents. The hematomas expand more slowly than epidural hematomas, so their clinical tempo is slower, but once critical increased intracranial pressure is attained, clinical deterioration and death can occur with horrific rapidity.

PATHOLOGY: The cerebral hemispheres float in the CSF, tethered loosely by blood vessels and cranial nerves. Blood drains from cerebral hemispheres through veins that cross the subarachnoid space and arachnoid to breach the dura and enter the dural sinus.

There is no true subdural space per se, but the inner layer of meningothelial cells of the dura has fewer tight junctions than those in the outer layers of the dura. Shearing forces can separate these cells, allowing blood to seep between them. Since bleeding in this situation is under low venous pressure, it is slow to develop and may stop spontaneously from a local tamponade effect. The bleeding occurs within the dura itself and readily extends beyond the coronal sutures, causing a hematoma that can span the entire anterior to posterior dimensions of the calvarium (Fig. 32-16). Granulation tissue forms in reaction to the blood, and the delicate capillaries of this tissue may themselves leak. This leads to gradual accumulation of an ever enlarging subacute, and ultimately chronic, subdural hematoma.

The blood and granulation tissue become surrounded by a sheet of fibrous connective tissue—the "membranes" of a chronic subdural hematoma. Fibroblasts first create a membrane on the calvarial side of the hematoma, the **outer membrane**. Then they invade the subjacent hematoma to form a fibrous membrane subjacent to the blood clot. This **inner membrane** is visible in about 2 weeks (Fig. 32-17). A subdural hematoma may evolve in three ways. It may (1) be reabsorbed and leave only a trace of telltale hemosiderin; (2) remain static, and perhaps calcify; or (3) enlarge because of recurrent microhemorrhages in the granulation tissue.

Expansion of the hematoma, and onset of symptoms, commonly results from rebleeding, usually within 6 months. Granulation tissue is fragile and vulnerable to minor trauma, even that caused by shaking the head. Thus, subdural hematomas can re-bleed and create a new hematoma subjacent to the outer membrane. Episodes of sporadic re-bleeding expand these lesions periodically and at unpredictable intervals. Since the bleeding occurs in the inner dural border cell zone rather than an imaginary subdural space, no blood is seen in the CSF. In addition to granulation tissue and blood, other cellular constituents in the hematoma include plasma cells, lymphocytes, and extramedullary hematopoiesis. These may contribute to the cellular dynamics of the subdural hematoma by releasing cytokines and causing cerebral edema in the underlying brain.

CLINICAL FEATURES: Symptoms and signs of subdural hematomas are diverse. Stretching of meninges leads to headaches; pressure on the motor cortex produces contralateral weakness; and focal cortical irritation can initiate seizures. Subdural hematomas are bilateral in 15% to 20% of cases, and these may impair cognitive function and lead to a mistaken diagnosis of dementia. Ultimately expansion of a subdural hematoma can cause lethal transtentorial herniation (Fig. 32-16A).

Parenchymal Injuries Produce Variable Symptomatology

Traumatic brain and spinal cord injuries range in severity from temporary loss of function with little or no discernible structural damage in concussion, to intermediate damage with hemorrhage and necrosis of the tissue in contusions, to profound disruption of structure and function in lacerations.

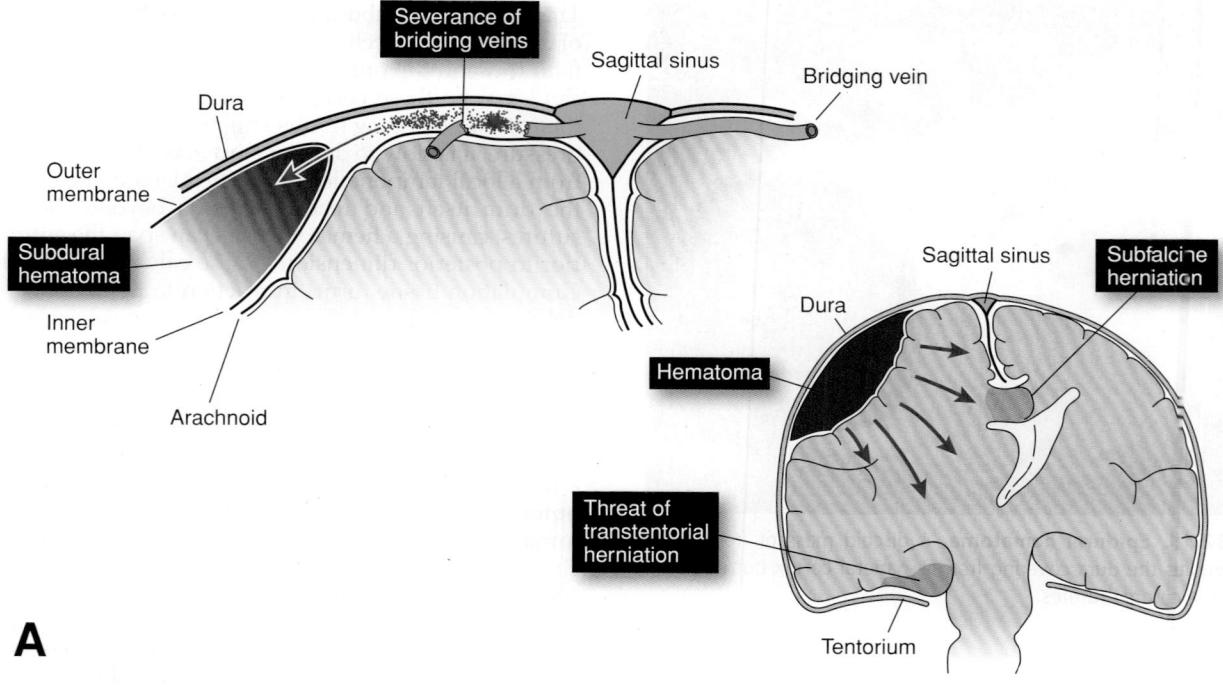

A

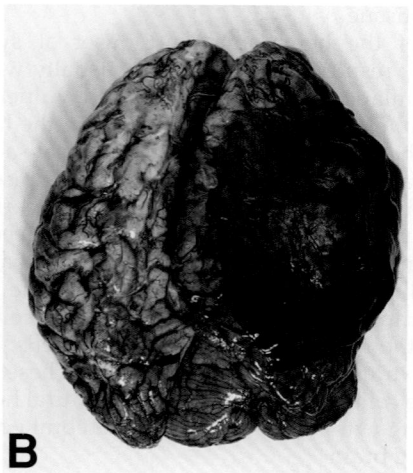

B

FIGURE 32-16. Development of a subdural hematoma. A. With head trauma, the dura moves with the skull, and the arachnoid moves with the cerebrum. As a result, bridging veins are sheared as they cross between the dura and the arachnoid. Venous bleeding creates a hematoma in the weak inner meningothelial cell layer. Subsequent transtentorial herniation is life threatening. **B.** The right hemisphere exhibits a large collection of blood in the "subdural space," owing to rupture of the bridging veins. In fact, the hemorrhage is intradural within the inner meningothelial cell layer where fewer tight junctions bind the cells together.

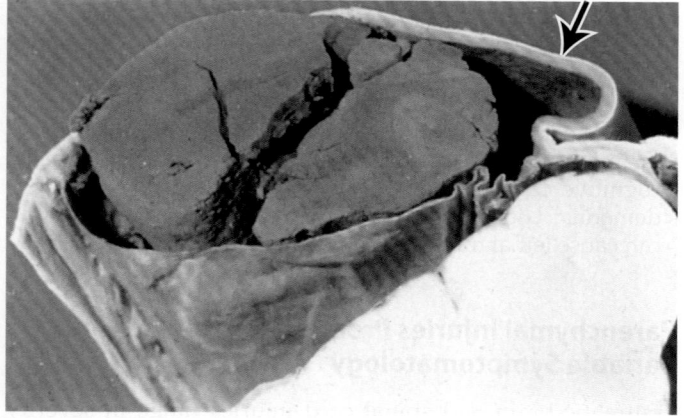

FIGURE 32-17. Chronic subdural hematoma with well-developed surrounding membranes. The thicker membrane (*arrow*) is the exterior membrane and the thinner membrane is adjacent to the brain (*lower right*). (Courtesy of Dr. F. Stephen Vogel, Duke University.)

Concussion

Concussion is transient loss of consciousness due to biomechanical forces acting on the CNS. A blow that causes an epidural hematoma does not necessarily produce a concussion. Consciousness depends on a functional brainstem reticular formation interacting with the cerebral hemispheres and is lost if either the reticular formation or both hemispheres are damaged. A classic example of concussion occurs in boxing, from a blow that deflects the head upward and posteriorly, often with a rotatory component. These motions impart quick rotational acceleration to the brainstem and cause dysfunction of reticular formation neurons. By contrast, a blow to the temporal–parietal area may cause a skull fracture and lethal epidural hematoma but may not cause loss of consciousness because lateral movement of the cerebral hemispheres does not occur.

Classically, concussion is not associated with gross neuropathology, and since the condition is not lethal, microscopic examination is not possible. Recent advances in diffusion tensor imaging (DTI) suggest that axonal injury functionally

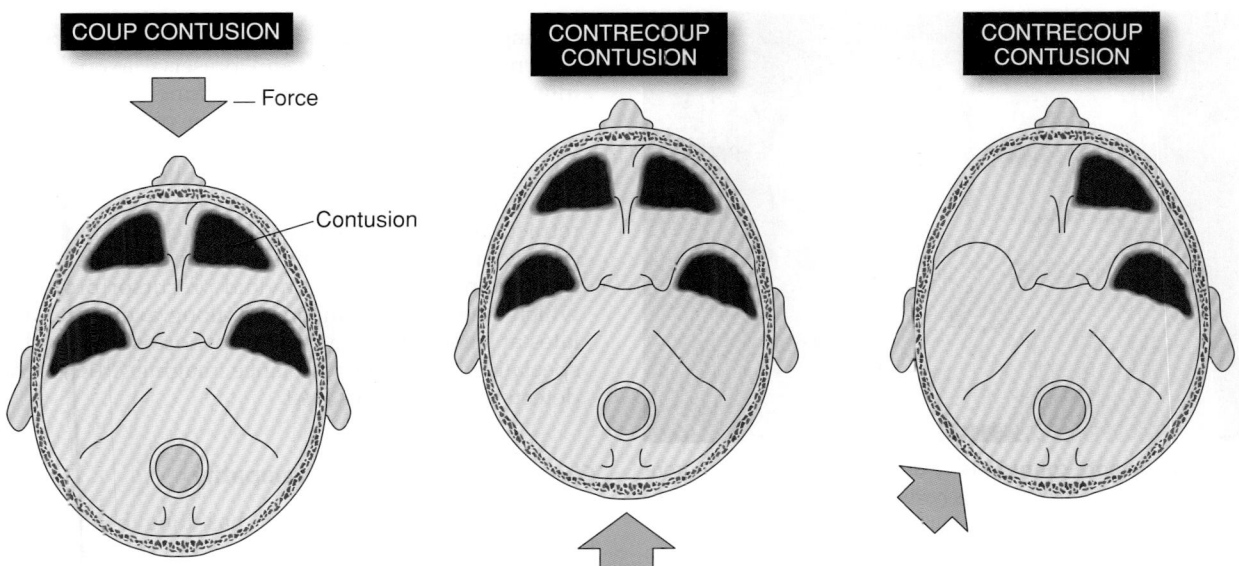

FIGURE 32-18. Biomechanics of cerebral contusion. The cerebral hemispheres float in the cerebrospinal fluid. Rapid deceleration or acceleration of the skull causes the cortex to impact forcefully into the anterior and middle fossae. The position of a contusion is determined by the direction of the force and the intracranial anatomy.

disconnects the reticular activating system from the cerebral hemispheres. Axonal injury and disconnection may also account for cognitive and memory difficulties, vertigo and the feelings that "things are just not quite right" that bedevil people who have sustained "mild" traumatic brain injury.

Cerebral Contusion

 ETIOLOGIC FACTORS: A cerebral contusion is a brain bruise—an area of tissue disruption and blood seepage—that usually occurs when the brain strikes the irregular bony contours of the skull because of abrupt acceleration or deceleration. If a moving object strikes the head, acceleration will be imparted to the skull and its delicate cargo, the brain. In contrast, a fall results in an abrupt deceleration. When a contusion

occurs at a point of impact, the lesion is a **coup** injury (French, *coup* = "blow") (Fig. 32-18). If the side of the brain opposite the impact site strikes the skull, resulting contusions are contralateral to the point of initial contact **(contrecoup)**. Coup injuries are maximal when the head is stationary and struck by an object, while contrecoup contusions are more severe when the head is in motion and abruptly stops. If an individual is struck by an assailant with a baseball bat, a large coup contusion will be present. In contrast, if a person falls off of a ladder, a large contrecoup contusion results.

PATHOLOGY: If the force of impact is mild, cerebral contusion is limited to the cortex and the crowns of gyri (Fig. 32-19A). Greater force destroys

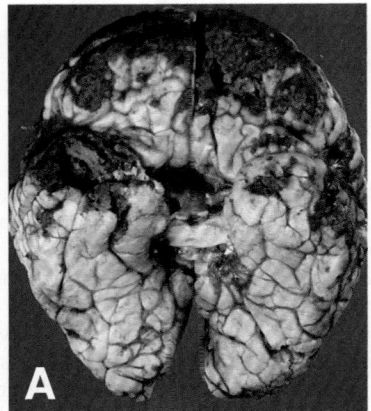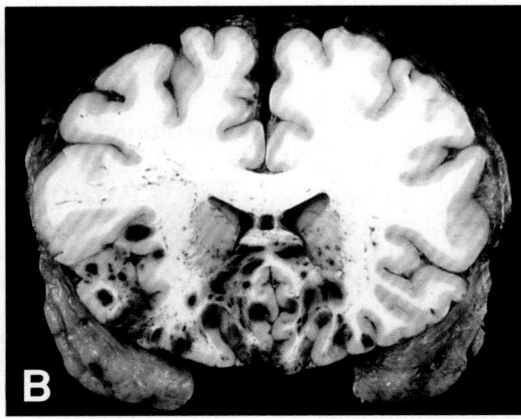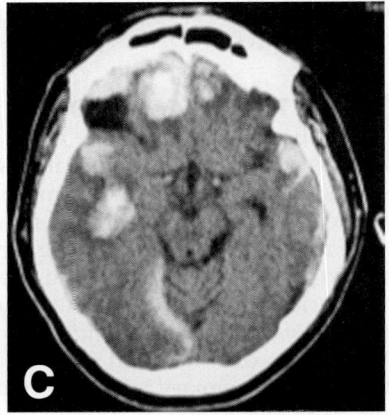

FIGURE 32-19. Acute contusions of the brain. A. After an automobile accident, the brain exhibits necrosis and hemorrhage involving the frontal and temporal lobes. (Courtesy of Dr. F. Stephen Vogel, Duke University.) **B.** In addition, there are some underlying white matter hemorrhages. (Courtesy of Dr. F. Stephen Vogel, Duke University.) **C.** Axial noncontrast computed tomography imaging shows acute contusions in the basal frontal and temporal tips regions. Hemorrhage is seen as the white signal in the frontal and temporal regions.

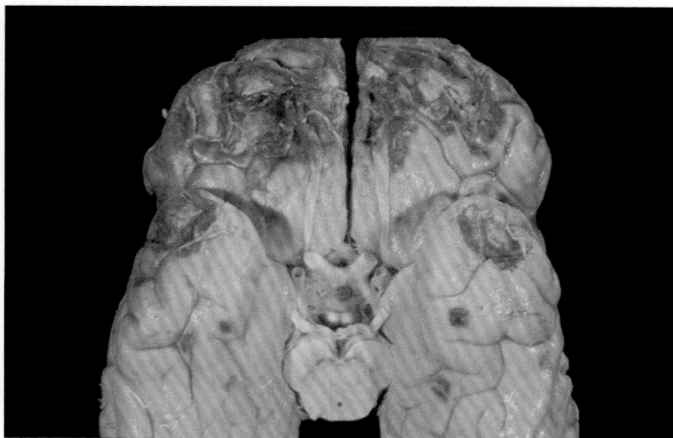

FIGURE 32-20. Remote contusions of the brain. Bilateral large frontal and smaller temporal tip contusions have been cleared out by macrophages, leaving residual hemosiderin-stained divots. Note involvement of the olfactory bulbs—anosmia (loss of sense of smell) is the most common cranial neuropathy following traumatic brain injury.

larger expanses of cortex, creating cavitary lesions that may extend into the white matter or lacerate the cortex, causing intraparenchymal hemorrhage (Fig. 32-19B). Together, edema and hemorrhage in a contusion may cause the contusion to expand over several days, which can become life threatening because of increased intracranial pressure.

Contusions leave permanent marks on the brain. Bruised, necrotic tissue is phagocytosed by macrophages. Astrocytosis then leads to local scar formation, which persists as telltale evidence of a prior contusion. Usually some residual hemosiderin imparts an orange brown hue to the old contusion (Fig. 32-20).

Diffuse Axonal Injury

Diffuse axonal injury (DAI) is a common result of traumatic brain injury and may lead to severe neurologic deficits and coma in patients without gross hematomas, contusions, or lacerations. Advances in imaging techniques allow better detection and quantification of these injuries, which are major contributors to morbidity and mortality. There is also increased interest in DAI as part of blast injuries.

 ETIOLOGIC FACTORS: The parasagittal cerebral hemispheres are anchored to arachnoid villi **(pacchionian granulations)**, while the lateral aspects of the cerebrum move more freely. This anatomic feature, together with the differential density of gray and white matter, allows for shearing forces between different brain regions, leading to axonal shearing injuries. Shearing injuries can distort or disrupt axons, causing immediate loss of function. Experimental studies indicate that DAI evolves over hours to days, so axons may be injured at the time of primary injury, with impaired axonal transport and cytoskeletal disruption leading to accumulation of axoplasm at sites of injury. Then, physical separation leads axons to form axonal retraction spheroids. Since DAI evolves over time, rather than being a catastrophic event

leading to immediately severed axons, it may be possible to arrest its progression and preserve axonal structural integrity. If an injury is severe, the functional loss of axonal activity may immediately render the patient comatose, but imaging may show only small hemorrhages and focal edema, particularly in the corpus callosum and midbrain. However, more widely distributed axonal swelling and retraction spheroids may be seen in cerebral white matter, corpus callosum, and brainstem. These can be highlighted by immunostaining for amyloid precursor protein (APP), which is normally transported along axons and accumulates at sites of injury where transport is impaired. DTI, a specialized magnetic resonance imaging (MRI) technique, detects and quantifies DAI.

Chronic Traumatic Encephalopathy

Acute traumatic brain injury has long been the primary focus of neurotrauma research, but long-term effects are now receiving overdue attention as large numbers of military service members return from Iraq and Afghanistan. In addition, the possible long-term neurodegenerative effects of repetitive head injury in sports—specifically chronic traumatic encephalopathy—has raised major concern in professional and amateur athletics. In 1928, it was recognized that boxers with repetitive head injury developed dementia and their brains showed neuronal loss and neurofibrillary tangles (NFTs).

This disorder, initially named "dementia pugilistica" but now called chronic traumatic encephalopathy (CTE), occurs in non-boxers experiencing varying degrees of repetitive head injury. Younger people (ages 20 to 40) tend to have a rapidly progressive course primarily involving behavioral and mood changes, while older people (ages 50 to 70) have slower disease progression involving primarily cognitive difficulties. There is a spectrum of abnormalities in individuals with CTE.

 PATHOLOGY: The most distinctive finding is deposition of tau, a microtubule-associated protein, in neurons and astrocytes at the depths of sulci and around blood vessels. Abnormal tau accumulation occurs in many neurodegenerative diseases, including Alzheimer disease, frontotemporal lobar degeneration (FTLD) and progressive supranuclear palsy (PSP), among others, but it is the distribution of NFTs in CTE that is unique. CTE may provide a mechanistic bridge between acute injury and progressive neurodegenerative disease.

Penetrating Traumatic Brain Injury

 PATHOPHYSIOLOGY: Penetrating objects like bullets and knives enter the cranium and traverse the brain with variable velocities. If there is no direct damage to vital brain centers, hemorrhage is the immediate threat to life (Fig. 32-21).

The damage done by a projectile depends on how much kinetic energy is involved ($E = mv^2$, where m = mass and v = velocity). Thus, projectile velocity is the key determinant of injury. The kinetic energy of a high-velocity bullet directly disrupts tissues by its own mass as well as by a centrifugal blast zone whose diameter is determined by the projectile's original kinetic energy. Thus, a high-velocity

A. HIGH-VELOCITY BULLET WOUND

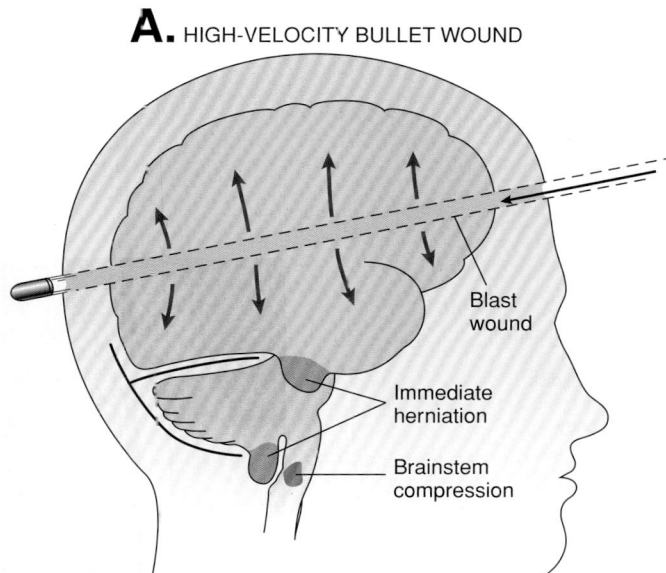

Blast wound

Immediate herniation

Brainstem compression

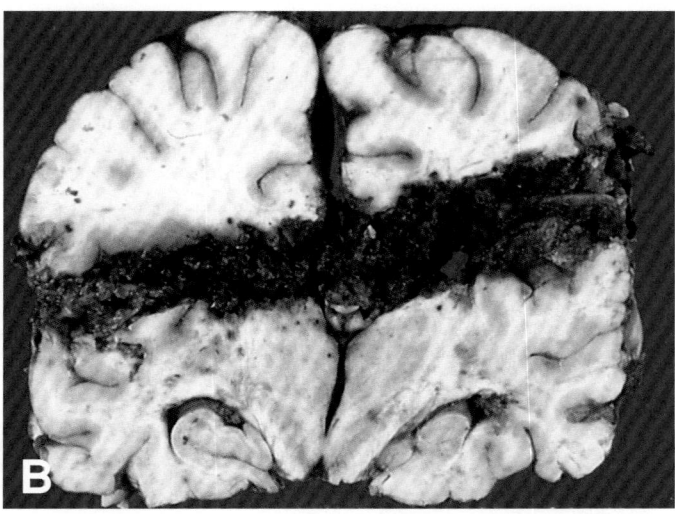

FIGURE 32-21. Consequences of high- and low-velocity bullet wounds. A. The "blast effect" of a high-velocity projectile causes an immediate increase in supratentorial pressure and results in death because of impaction of the cerebellum and medulla into the foramen magnum. A low-velocity projectile increases the pressure at a more gradual rate through hemorrhage and edema. **B.** Bullet track in a through-and-through penetrating injury. A penetrating, through-and-through high-velocity bullet track is seen traversing the brain. The trajectory is difficult to discern based on examination of the soft tissue of the brain but can be revealed by skull beveling. (Courtesy of Dr. F. Stephen Vogel, Duke University.)

bullet can cause an explosive increase in intracranial pressure, which forcefully herniates the cerebellar tonsils into the foramen magnum, causing immediate death.

Spinal Cord Injury

 ETIOLOGIC FACTORS: Traumatic lesions of the spinal cord may result from direct injury by penetrating wounds (e.g., stab wounds, bullets) or indirect injury from vertebral fractures or displacement. The spinal cord may be contused not only at the site of injury but also above and below the point of trauma. Compromised arterial supply to the cord, with resulting infarction, may complicate traumatic injury.

Vertebral bodies are separated by intervertebral discs and are stabilized in normal alignment by two longitudinal ligaments and the posterior bony processes. The anterior spinal ligaments adhere to the ventral surface of the vertebral bodies, while the posterior spinal ligament is affixed to the dorsal vertebral column. After extreme flexion or extension, the angulation of the bony vertebral column brings the spinal cord forcefully into contact with bone or interferes with regional circulation.

The consequences of a spinal cord injury depend on the severity of the trauma. **Spinal cord concussion** is the mildest injury, with transient, reversible functional disturbance. **Contusion of the spinal cord** results from more severe trauma, varying from minor transient bruises to hemorrhagic spinal cord necrosis (Fig. 32-22). Spinal cord necrosis and edema due to severe contusion are referred to as **myelomalacia**. A hematoma within the cord is a **hematomyelia. Lacerations and transections of the spinal cord** are usually caused by penetrating wounds

or severely displaced spinal fractures. They are irreversible and lead to complete loss of function below the spinal level of the injury. Whether paralysis affects only the legs **(paraplegia)** or all four extremities **(quadriplegia)** depends on the spinal level and extent of the injury. If even as little as 10% to 15% of the cross-sectional diameter of the spinal cord is spared, functional recovery is much better than with complete transection.

Neurotrauma is a process, not an event. The initial transfer of kinetic injury sets into motion a cascade of secondary injury mechanisms. Mitigation of secondary injury and facilitation of recovery continue to be major thrusts in neurotrauma.

CEREBROVASCULAR DISORDERS

Stroke is the third leading cause of death in the United States, after myocardial infarction and cancer. As elsewhere, vascular disease in the brain can result from vessel blockage, causing ischemia, or vascular leakage that results in hemorrhage. Vascular disorders of the nervous system lead to (1) globally or focally inadequate blood flow (ischemia), which, if sufficiently protracted, produces infarction; or (2) rupture of vascular structures that causes either intraparenchymal or subarachnoid hemorrhage.

Global Hypoperfusion Results in Hypoxic-Ischemic Encephalopathy

 ETIOLOGIC FACTORS: The brain receives about 20% of basal cardiac output. Aerobic glycolysis is virtually the sole source of energy of the mature

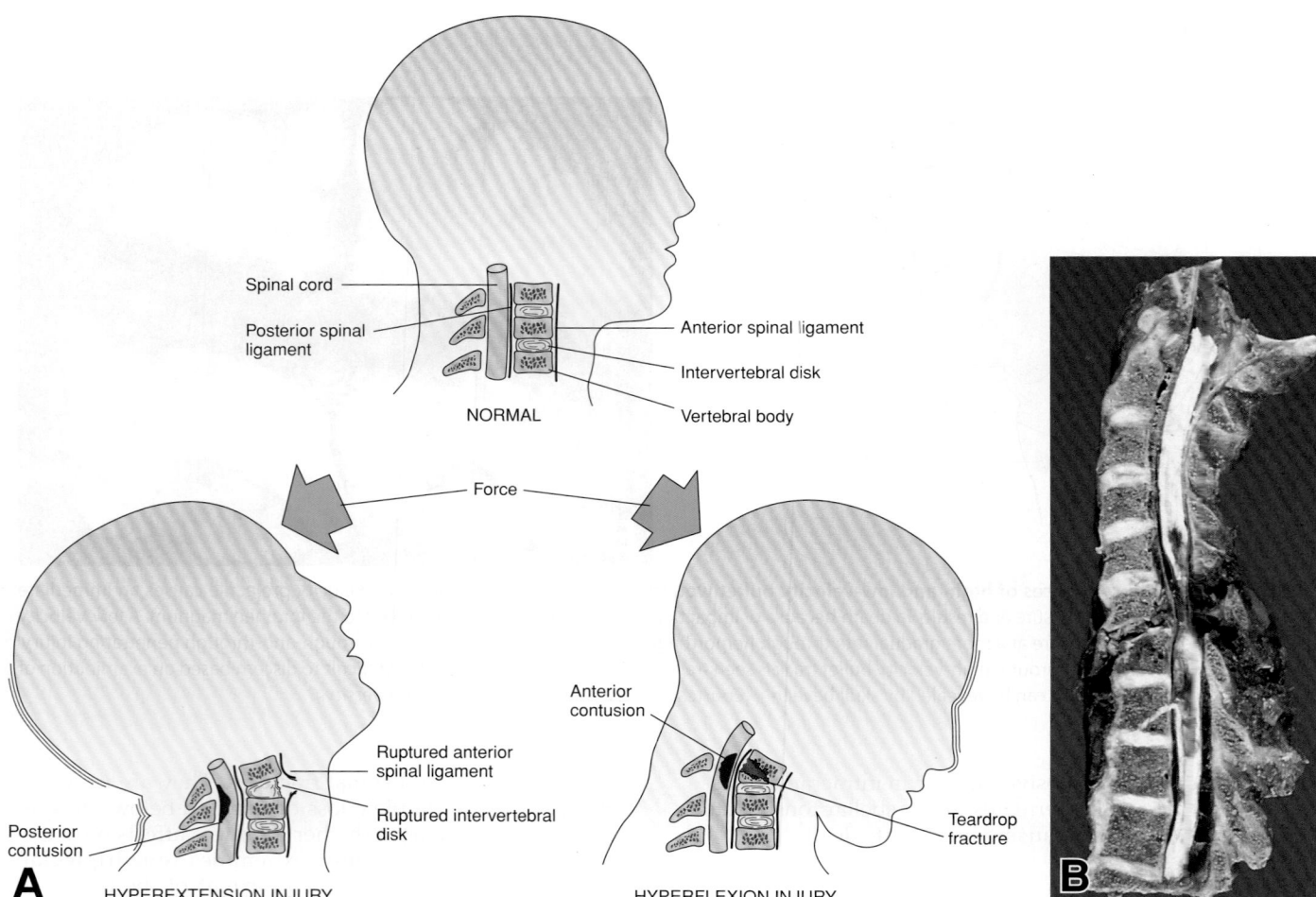

FIGURE 32-22. Spinal injury. A. Different angles of force can be applied to the highly vulnerable cervical spine. Posterior (hyperextension) and anterior (hyperflexion) injuries are the most common. Hyperextension injury causes rupture of the anterior spinal ligament and excessive posterior angulation. Hyperflexion injury causes compression associated with a "teardrop" fracture of a vertebral body and produces excessive forward angulation of the cord. **B.** Fracture dislocation of the spinal column may result in spinal cord contusion, laceration, necrosis, or frank transection. Preservation of a relatively small cross-sectional area of the spinal cord can have major beneficial effects on recovery. (Courtesy of Dr. F. Stephen Vogel, Duke University.)

brain. CNS glycogen reserves are meager and oxygen reserves are nil; hence, uninterrupted supply of oxygenated blood carrying sufficient glucose is essential for brain integrity. The brain's blood supply comes via paired internal carotid and vertebral arteries. The carotids, the "anterior circulation," supply most superficial and deep cerebral hemisphere structures; the vertebral arteries make up the "posterior circulation," feeding the brainstem, cerebellum, and territory of the posterior cerebral arteries. The posterior and anterior circuits connect via the circle of Willis. This anastomotic network at the base of the brain is quite variable, but in some fortunate individuals, the blood supply of the brain is sufficiently redundant that complete blockage of two carotids and one vertebral can be asymptomatic. Despite these elaborate hemodynamic precautions, many people experience global or focal ischemia leading to cerebral infarction.

*Global ischemia, which is usually due to cardiopulmonary arrest or extreme hypotension in severe shock, leads to widespread tissue injury, resulting in ischemic enceph-**alopathy.*** If perfusion failure is brief (minutes), neurologic functions may quickly be restored with only transient postischemic confusion. Some patients may come back more slowly and suffer subtle higher intellectual function impairments, which may preclude complete resumption of societal activities. More severe injury can lead to dementia and spasticity. If the ischemic period is protracted, the patient may not regain consciousness and show decorticate posturing and seizures and be in a coma indefinitely.

Although the entire brain is inadequately perfused, there is surprising focality to the pathologic alterations. Specific neuronal populations most vulnerable to ischemic injury include the large neurons in the Sommer sector of the hippocampus, Purkinje cells of the cerebellum and neurons of layers 3 and 5 of the cerebral cortex (Fig. 32-23).

The basis for this selective vulnerability is not clear. It may be related to local metabolic requirements, hemodynamic factors, and local neurotransmitters. When ischemia leads to brain energy depletion, membranes depolarize, permitting uncontrolled release of the amino

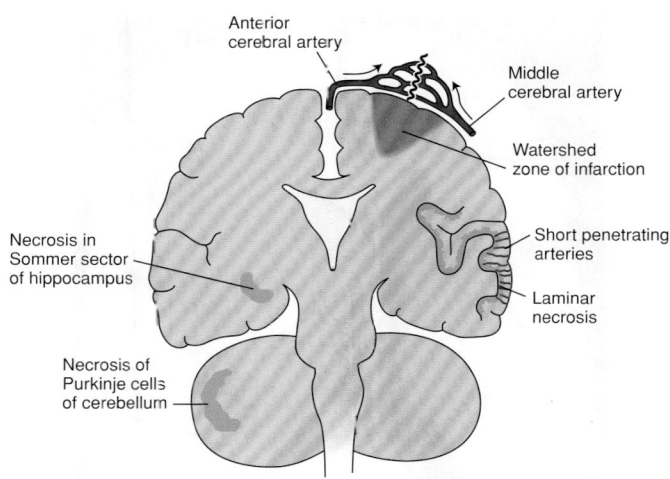

FIGURE 32-23. **Mechanisms of injury in global ischemia.** A global insult induces lesions that reflect the vascular architecture (watershed infarcts, laminar necrosis) and the selective vulnerability of individual neuronal systems (pyramidal cells of the Sommer sector, Purkinje cells, laminar necrosis). Both rheologic (blood flow) and neurochemical (excitotoxicity) factors play a role in laminar necrosis.

acid neurotransmitters glutamate and aspartate. These bind ligand-gated cation channels on postsynaptic cells, opening the floodgates for calcium and sodium entry, which depolarizes the cell membrane.

Calcium may activate intracellular proteases and quench mitochondrial energy production, propagating the energy failure and magnifying cellular injury. Injury done by abnormally released neurotransmitters, called **excitotoxicity,** may play a role in neurodegenerative disorders, epilepsy and stroke. In excitotoxicity, the areas of brain injury depend on the local use of potentially toxic neurotransmitters. For example, its high levels of amino acid neurotransmitters make the midcortex more vulnerable to ischemic injury, resulting in a midcortical band of necrosis with relatively preserved cortex in deep and superficial layers on either side of this band. As infarcted tissue is infiltrated by macrophages, it becomes apparent grossly as **laminar necrosis** (Fig. 32-24).

Hemodynamic factors cause **watershed** or **border zone infarcts,** which occur at junctions of major arterial supply zones (Fig. 32-25). These zones are at the precarious distal regions of arterial supply. If perfusion pressure drops, these are the first areas affected. The classic border zone lies between the distal territories of the anterior and middle cerebral arteries (Fig. 32-25). With global ischemia, these areas in both hemispheres may become infarcted, leading to symmetric wedge-shaped parasagittal high-convexity infarcts.

Regional Ischemia Causes Localized Cerebral Infarction

Occlusive cerebrovascular disease remains a major cause of morbidity and death because atherosclerosis is ubiquitous and progressive. *Atherosclerosis predisposes to vascular thrombosis and embolism, both of which result in localized ischemia and subsequent cerebral infarction.*

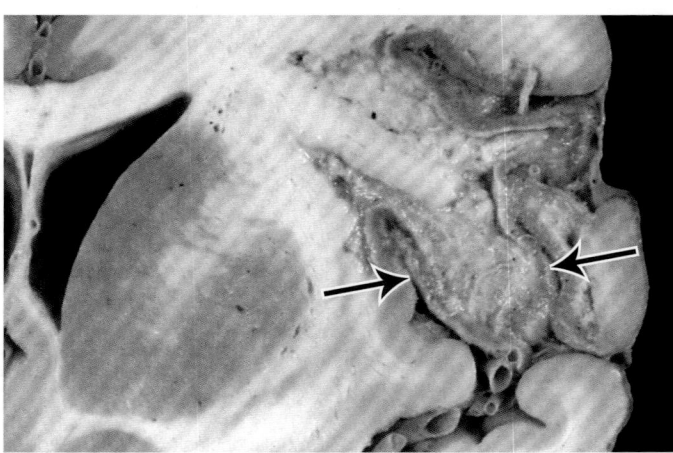

FIGURE 32-24. **Laminar necrosis.** A patient who suffered prolonged anoxia caused by a cardiac arrhythmia developed selective necrosis of middle layers in the cerebral cortex (*arrows*). (Courtesy of Dr. F. Stephen Vogel, Duke University.)

 ETIOLOGIC FACTORS: Cerebral infarcts are usually designated **hemorrhagic** or **bland.** *In general, infarcts caused by emboli are hemorrhagic, while those due to local thrombosis are ischemic (i.e., bland).* Emboli occlude vascular flow abruptly, after which the distal segments of affected blood vessels lose integrity and leak blood into the region during reperfusion (Fig. 32-26A). Atherothrombotic material complicating plaques in the common and internal carotid arteries may embolize. But the heart is also a rich source of emboli. These may derive from infected or defective valves, mural thrombi on inflamed, hypokinetic endocardial walls after myocardial infarction or atrial thrombi in atrial fibrillation, especially if there is associated mitral insufficiency. Fat emboli and deep vein thrombi from the systemic

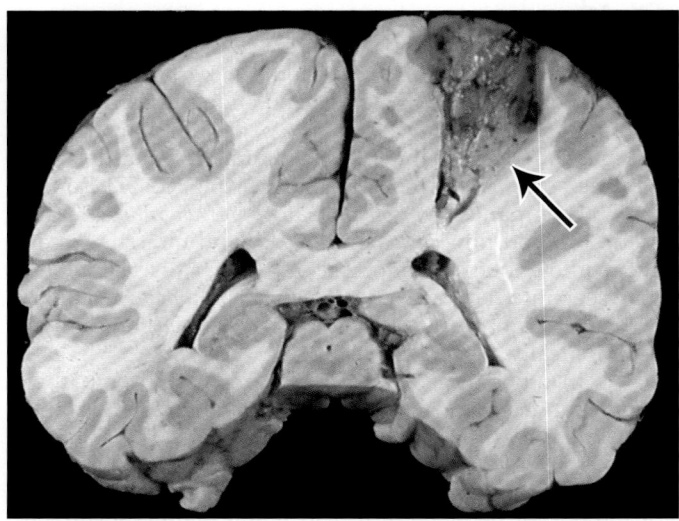

FIGURE 32-25. **Watershed infarct.** In global hypoperfusion, the most vulnerable perfusion zones are at the distal overlapping portions of the major cerebral vessels. Here an acute infarct is seen at the watershed of the anterior and middle cerebral arteries (*arrow*). (Courtesy of Dr. F. Stephen Vogel, Duke University.)

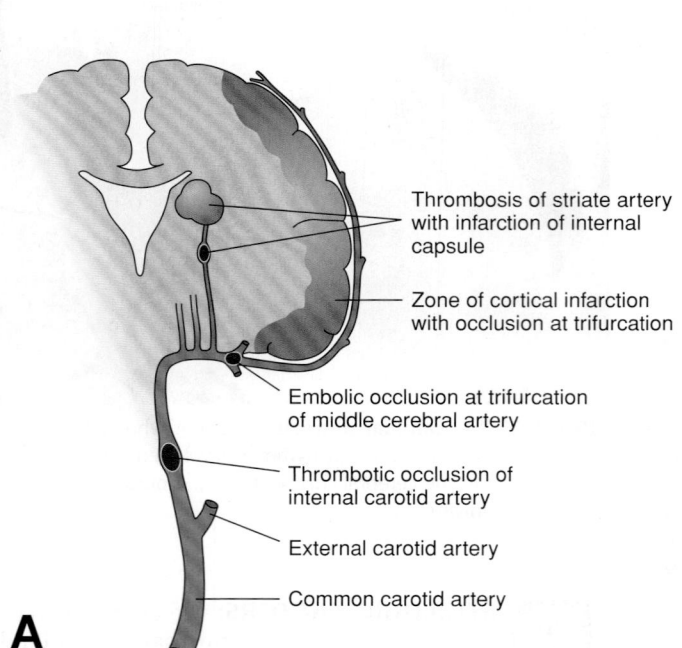

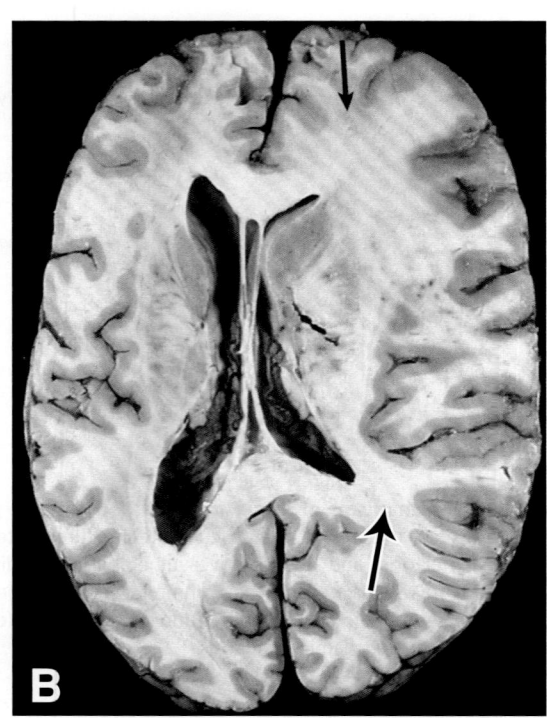

FIGURE 32-26. **A.** Distribution of cerebral infarcts. The normal distribution of the cerebral vasculature defines the pattern and size of infarcts and, consequently, their symptoms. Occlusion at the trifurcation causes cortical infarcts with motor and sensory loss and often aphasia. Occlusion of a striate branch damages the internal capsule and causes a motor deficit. **B.** Acute middle cerebral artery distribution infarct. An axial section of the brain of a patient who suffered thrombosis of the middle cerebral artery reveals a large infarct of the right hemisphere (*between arrows*) with swelling and focal dusky discoloration. (Courtesy of Dr. F. Stephen Vogel, Duke University.)

venous circulation may embolize paradoxically through a patent foramen ovale. Emboli of amniotic fluid or tumors (e.g., from atrial myxomas) also occur but are rare.

PATHOLOGY: Most infarcts caused by thrombosis are anemic or bland and are difficult to identify grossly for several hours, after which softening, and discoloration become increasingly prominent (Fig. 32-26B). Swelling and liquefaction follow within 3 to 5 days, which puts the patient in danger from the mass effect of the infarct. The infarct then matures into a cystic space over weeks to months (Fig. 32-27), sometimes accompanied by compensatory ventricular enlargement. If blood flow is restored to a bland infarct, as may occur in embolic or compressive vascular disease, blood may seep into the softened tissues. This may cause a hemorrhagic infarct, which is readily discernible grossly and radiologically (Fig. 32-28).

As in other tissues, an orderly procession of pathologic changes allows estimation of an infarct's age. If a patient survives for minutes to several hours, no changes are seen. If the patient survives for 6 to 24 hours, the infarct is slightly discolored and softened with blurring of the border between gray and white matter. Shrunken eosinophilic neurons ("red neurons") with nuclear pyknosis are present in the infarct (Fig. 32-29). These changes become more pronounced as the infarct ages. By 24 to 72 hours, neutrophils infiltrate the tissue and blood vessels

are prominent. The tissue is soft and edematous and may be sufficiently swollen to cause lethal mass effect.

By 3 to 4 days, macrophages replace neutrophils and clear debris in the infarct at a rate of about 1 mL per month. The infarct is now frankly mushy. In the second week, proliferating astrocytes join the macrophages. Over weeks to months, these astrocytes form a dense fibrillary glial meshwork around the dead tissue. The macrophages dispose of debris in the infarct over weeks to months. Simultaneously, the infarct evolves into a glial lined cyst, crossed at points by delicate glial sheets and small vessels and invested with residual lipid and hemosiderin-laden macrophages.

CLINICAL FEATURES: The diversity of neurologic deficits caused by strokes reflects the functional eloquence of the brain. For example, the lengthy and slender striate arteries, which take origin from the proximal middle cerebral artery, are commonly occluded by atherosclerosis and thrombosis. Resultant infarcts often impact the internal capsule to produce hemiplegia (Fig. 32-26A). Similarly, the middle cerebral artery trifurcation is a favored site for lodgment of emboli and thrombosis due to atherosclerosis. Middle cerebral artery occlusion at this site deprives much of the lateral hemispheric cortex of blood, producing motor and sensory deficits. If the dominant hemisphere is involved, aphasia may develop.

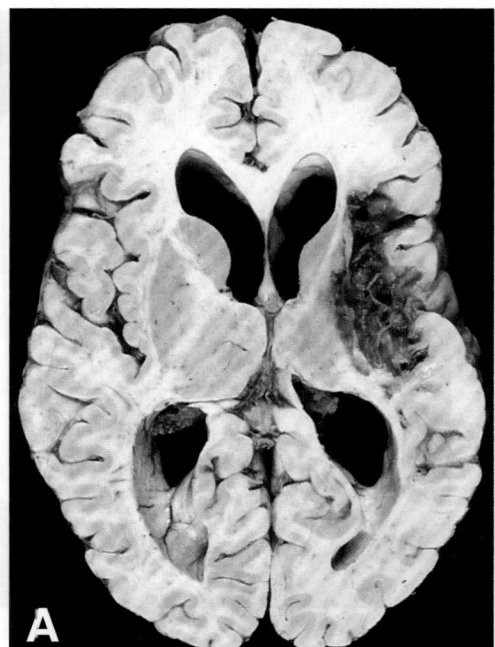 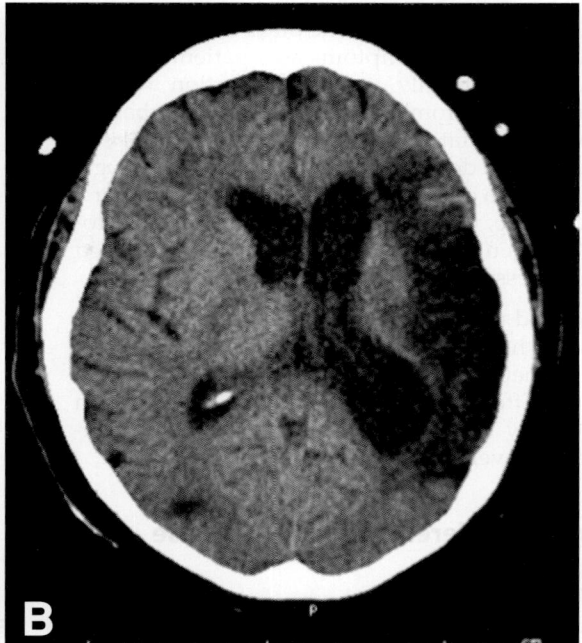

FIGURE 32-27. A. Remote middle cerebral artery distribution infarct. An axial section of the brain shows a remote middle cerebral artery distribution cystic infarct. The brain in Figure 32-26B would transform to this state as a result of clearing out of the large infarct by macrophages. (Courtesy of Dr. F. Stephen Vogel, Duke University.) **B.** Axial noncontrast computed tomography shows a remote middle cerebral artery distribution infarct resulting from a cardiogenic embolus that occluded the artery at the trifurcation. Note the low signal in the middle cerebral artery territory and the compensatory enlargement of the ventricles.

Localized ischemia may be associated with three distinct clinical syndromes:

- **Transient ischemic attack (TIA)** is focal cerebral dysfunction, lasting under 24 hours, and often only a few minutes. Although complete neurologic recovery follows, TIA heralds increased risk of cerebral infarction. TIAs, like angina, are warnings that all is not well with the cerebral blood supply. Their occurrence often triggers diagnostic and therapeutic activity. A patient with TIAs is at risk for later cerebral infarction; about 1/3 of

patients with TIAs will have a stroke within 5 years. The period of highest risk is the first 30 days after TIAs begin; in 1/3 of patients, the TIAs simply continue; and about 1/3 of patients will have no more TIAs, nor will they suffer a stroke. *TIAs often are harbingers of a stroke, but many people (50% to 85%) who develop cerebral infarcts never have a preceding TIA.* If a TIA lasts more than a few minutes, some tissue damage occurs as evidenced by MRI abnormalities on diffusion water inversion (DWI) sequences.

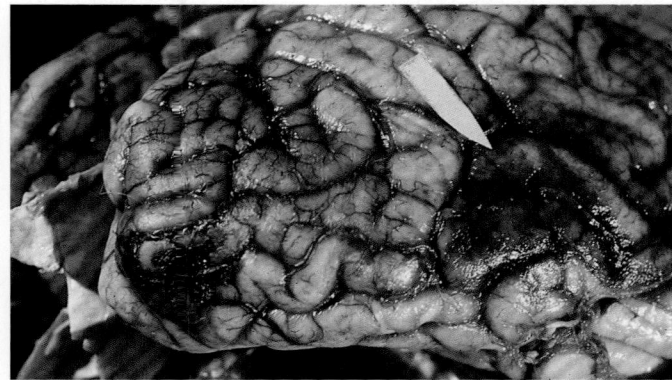 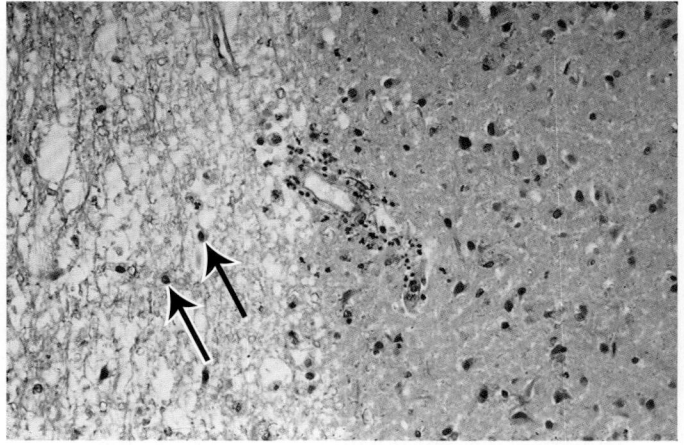

FIGURE 32-28. Hemorrhagic embolic infarct. Emboli from a carotid endarterectomy resulted in hemorrhagic infarcts in the territory of the middle cerebral artery (*arrow*). Such hemorrhagic infarcts may expand because of seepage of blood or frank hemorrhage and become life threatening.

FIGURE 32-29. Acute cerebral infarct histopathology. An 18-hour-old cerebral infarct (*left*) shows edema, eosinophilic neurons and perivascular polymorphonuclear leukocytes. Pyknotic nuclei of dying neurons are apparent (*arrows*).

- **Stroke in evolution** describes the often-stuttering progression of neurologic symptoms as a patient is being observed. This clinically unstable situation reflects propagation of a thrombus in the carotid or basilar arteries and necessitates urgent treatment.
- **Completed stroke** describes a stable or fixed neurologic deficit caused by a cerebral infarct. Two to 3 days after a completed stroke, there can be sufficient cerebral cytotoxic and vasogenic edema in the infarct that increased intracranial pressure and herniation become issues.

Our improved understanding of the basic pathophysiology of stroke has resulted in major advances in diagnosis and therapeutic intervention operating in a critical time window. Efforts directed at restoring circulation pharmacologically and through endovascular intervention have been proven to be effective.

Regional Occlusive Cerebrovascular Disease

 PATHOLOGY: The various occlusive cerebrovascular diseases that lead to cerebral infarcts may be classified by the caliber and nature of the vessel involved.

LARGE EXTRACRANIAL AND INTRACRANIAL ARTERIES: These arteries are often sites of atherosclerosis. Most notably, atherosclerotic plaques occur frequently in the common carotid artery at its bifurcation into external and internal branches. Occlusion or stenosis of an internal carotid artery affects the ipsilateral hemisphere, but this can be offset by variable collateral circulation through the anterior and posterior communicating arteries. Usually, carotid artery occlusion produces infarcts limited to all or part of the distribution of the middle cerebral artery. The consequences of large vessel disease depend on the configuration of the circle of Willis. Thus, a large anterior communicating artery can furnish collateral circulation to a frontal lobe whose blood supply is compromised by internal carotid artery occlusion. The middle cerebral artery is most often occluded by thrombosis complicating atherosclerosis in the circle of Willis. As a major stepdown in vascular caliber occurs at the trifurcation of the middle cerebral artery, this is the main site occluded by emboli.

While atherosclerosis is the primary substrate of ischemic stroke, both arterial dissection and vasculitis may also lead to stroke.

PARENCHYMAL ARTERIES AND ARTERIOLES: These vessels are less often severely atherosclerotic, but they are damaged by hypertension and can be narrowed by atherosclerosis. This causes small infarcts in the territories of the deep penetrating vessels. These **lacunar infarcts** are usually less than 15 mm. Depending on the functions of the small region supplied, symptoms can range from none to profound. They include, for example, contralateral hemiparesis from an infarct in the internal capsule or pure hemisensory loss caused by a thalamic lacunar infarct. When multiple, these minute infarcts can lead to impaired cognition, called **multiple infarct dementia**.

Hypertensive encephalopathy describes the acute neurologic complications of malignant hypertension. As in other affected organs, malignant hypertension can cause fibrinoid necrosis of small arteries and arterioles

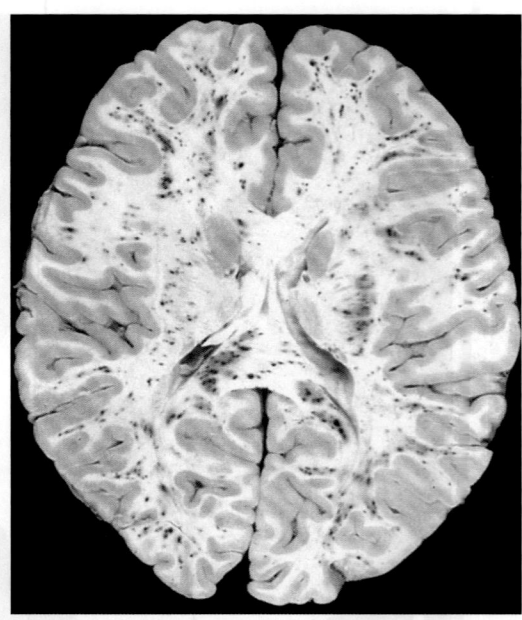

FIGURE 32-30. Fat emboli. An axial section of the brain in a trauma patient with multiple bone fractures leading to cerebral fat emboli shows numerous small petechiae throughout the white matter where fat emboli lodged in the microcirculation. (Courtesy of Dr. F. Stephen Vogel, Duke University.)

in the brain, as well as minute hemorrhages **(petechiae)**. Cerebral edema may complicate the vascular pathology. Hypertensive encephalopathy usually presents as headache and vomiting that progress to coma and death. With modern antihypertensive therapy, malignant hypertension is uncommon.

MICROCIRCULATION: Small emboli, composed, for example, of fat or air, may occlude capillaries **Fat emboli,** usually from fractured bones, travel through cerebral vessels until the size of the emboli exceeds that of the blood vessel, at which point they lodge and block blood flow. The distal capillary endothelium becomes hypoxic and permeable, and petechiae develop, mostly in the white matter (Fig. 32-30). **Air emboli** liberate many bubbles that further fragment as they encounter vascular bifurcations, until they impede vascular flow in small blood vessels. In this situation, petechiae are less restricted to white matter than those caused by fat emboli.

VENOUS CIRCULATION: The cerebral veins empty into large venous sinuses, the largest of which is the sagittal sinus, which accommodates venous drainage from the superior aspects of the cerebral hemispheres. Venous sinus thrombosis in the brain is a potentially lethal complication of diverse conditions including systemic dehydration, phlebitis caused by adjacent infections like mastoiditis, obstruction by a neoplasm such as a meningioma or sickle cell disease. Since venous obstruction causes stagnation upstream, abrupt sagittal sinus thrombosis leads to bilateral frontal lobe region hemorrhagic infarction (Fig. 32-31). More protracted occlusion of the sinus (e.g., due to invasion by a meningioma) allows recruitment of collateral circulation through the inferior sagittal sinus, which lies at the lower edge of the falx and empties into the straight sinus.

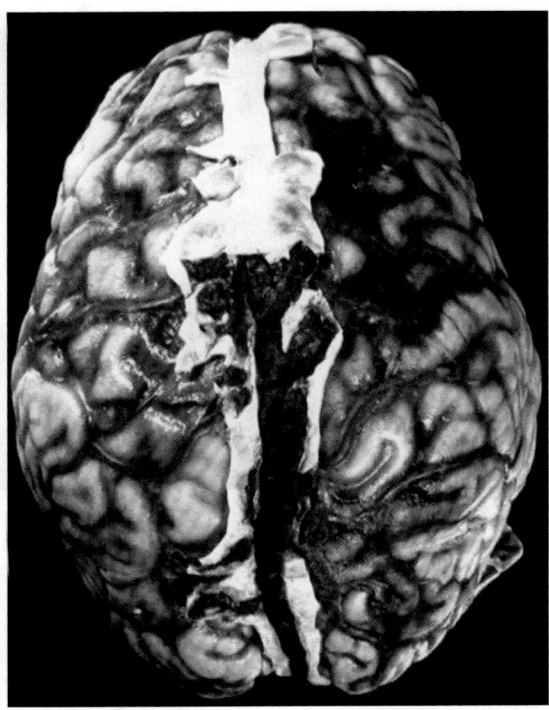

FIGURE 32-31. Superior sagittal sinus thrombosis. A thrombus, filling the superior sagittal sinus, impeded venous drainage of the cerebral hemispheres and caused bilateral hemorrhagic infarcts of the cerebral hemispheres. Venous thrombosis is seen in hypercoagulable states associated with dehydration, pregnancy, hereditary defects of thrombolysis, sickle cell disease or extension of an infection or neoplasm into the sinus. (Courtesy of Dr. F. Stephen Vogel, Duke University.)

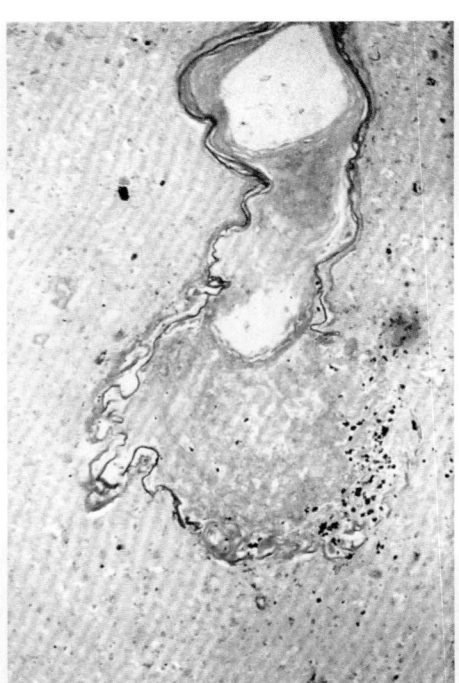

FIGURE 32-32. Charcot–Bouchard aneurysm. The combination of small penetrating cerebral vessels and high perfusion pressure leads to microaneurysms that may rupture and cause intracerebral hemorrhage. Effective treatment of hypertension reduces formation of microaneurysms and the risk of intracerebral hemorrhage. (Courtesy of Dr. F. Stephen Vogel, Duke University.)

Intracranial Hemorrhage Can Be Intraparenchymal or in the Subarachnoid Space

 ETIOLOGIC FACTORS: Intraparenchymal hemorrhage is called intracerebral hemorrhage and usually results from rupture of small fragile vessels or vascular malformations. SAH is mostly caused by rupture of aneurysms or vascular malformations.

Intracerebral Hemorrhage

PATHOLOGY: Cerebral hemorrhages that occur without trauma are usually caused by vascular malformations or are due to long-standing hypertension. **Hypertensive intracerebral hemorrhage (ICH)** occurs at preferential sites, which in order of frequency are (1) basal ganglia–thalamus (65%), (2) pons (15%), and (3) cerebellum (8%). Hypertensive ICH can also occur in the white matter of cerebral hemispheres, where it is called **lobar ICH**. Lobar ICH should suggest possible amyloid angiopathy, vascular malformation, coagulopathy or bleeding into a tumor, as well as simple hypertensive hemorrhage.

Hypertension compromises the integrity of cerebral arterioles by causing lipid and hyaline material to deposit in their walls: **lipohyalinosis**. Weakening of the wall leads to formation of **Charcot–Bouchard aneurysms,** which occur mainly along the trunk of an arteriole rather than at sites of bifurcation (Fig. 32-32).

CLINICAL FEATURES: The onset of symptoms of a hypertensive cerebral hemorrhage is abrupt. A patient may clutch his head complaining of severe headache and lapse into coma. Basal ganglion hypertensive ICHs may cause contralateral hemiparesis. If a hematoma expands progressively, as is common in the first day, death may occur when it reaches a critical volume of about 30 mL. An enlarging hematoma may cause death by transtentorial herniation. Rupture into a lateral ventricle may lead to massive intraventricular hemorrhage (Fig. 32-33).

INTRAVENTRICULAR HEMORRHAGE: Extension of the ICH into a ventricle rapidly distends the entire ventricular system with blood, including the fourth ventricle (Fig. 32-34). The blood may emerge from the foramina of Magendie and Luschka. Death may result from distension of the fourth ventricle and compression of vital centers in the medulla. Ventricular drainage allows reduction of intracranial pressure and removal of intraventricular blood.

PONTINE HEMORRHAGE: In this catastrophic event, loss of consciousness reflects damage to the reticular formation, an injury that overshadows all other specific cranial nerve deficits. The hemorrhage generally starts in the midpons (Fig. 32-35). It encroaches upon vital medullary centers with minimal enlargement, commonly causing death or severe disability.

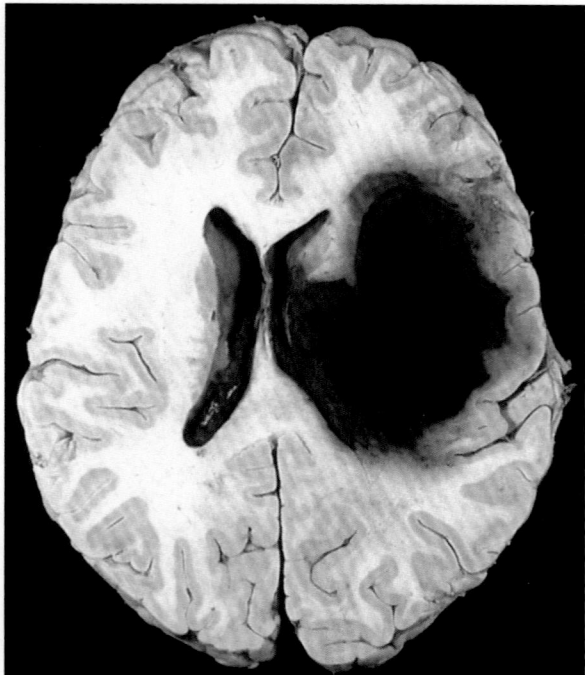

FIGURE 32-33. Intracerebral hemorrhage in the basal ganglia. A hypertensive patient bled into the basal ganglia, resulting in acute severe headache, contralateral hemiparesis, and rapid decline in level of consciousness. The deep cerebral nuclei (basal ganglia) and thalamus are the most common locations of intracerebral hemorrhages. (Courtesy of Dr. F. Stephen Vogel, Duke University.)

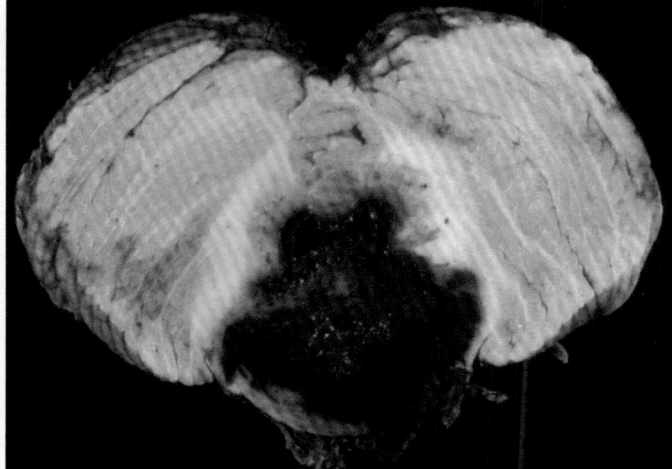

FIGURE 32-35. Pontine hemorrhage. Rupture of microaneurysms in the pons leads to rapid decline in level of consciousness because of disruption of the reticular activating system. This is often associated with multiple cranial neuropathies, dysconjugate gaze pupillary abnormalities, paralysis and dysregulation of respiration and cardiovascular function. The pons is the second most common site of intracranial hemorrhage, and bleeding there is often lethal. (Courtesy of Dr. F. Stephen Vogel, Duke University.)

CEREBELLAR HEMORRHAGE: Bleeding into the cerebellum leads to abrupt ataxia with a severe occipital headache and vomiting (Fig. 32-36). The expanding hematoma threatens life acutely by compressing the medulla or via cerebellar herniation through the foramen magnum. Surgical evacuation of the hematoma is life saving and

may leave few serious neurologic deficits, while surgical intervention for intracerebral hematomas in other locations has little or no demonstrated benefit.

Causes of spontaneous cerebral hemorrhages other than hypertension include leakage from an arteriovenous malformation, erosion of a blood vessel by a primary or secondary neoplasm, endothelial injury such as occurs in rickettsial infections, a bleeding diathesis or embolic infarction with consequent hemorrhage into the area of necrosis (hemorrhagic conversion).

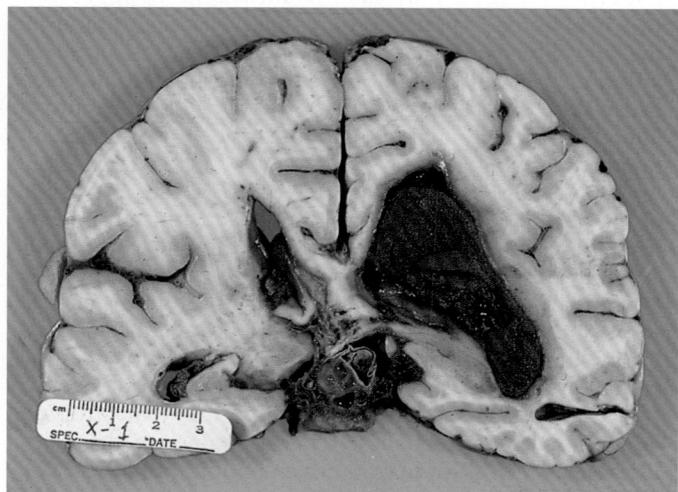

FIGURE 32-34. Intraventricular hemorrhage. A sagittal section of the brain shows ventricular chambers filled with blood that extended from a more anterior basal ganglionic intracerebral hemorrhage. The patient died rapidly from compression of the brainstem by blood in the fourth ventricle.

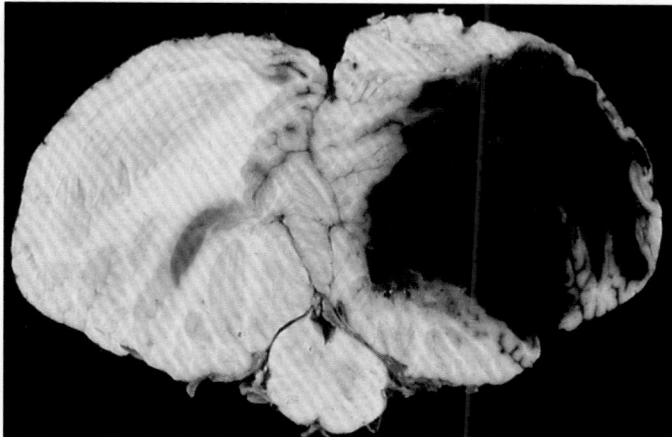

FIGURE 32-36. Cerebellar hemorrhage. Intracerebral hemorrhage in the cerebellum leads to acute-onset occipital headache, nausea, vomiting, vertigo, and ataxia. If the hematoma expands rapidly, fatal compression of the medulla may ensue. Surgical evacuation of the cerebellar intracranial hemorrhage can be lifesaving and is a neurosurgical emergency. (Courtesy of Dr. F. Stephen Vogel, Duke University.)

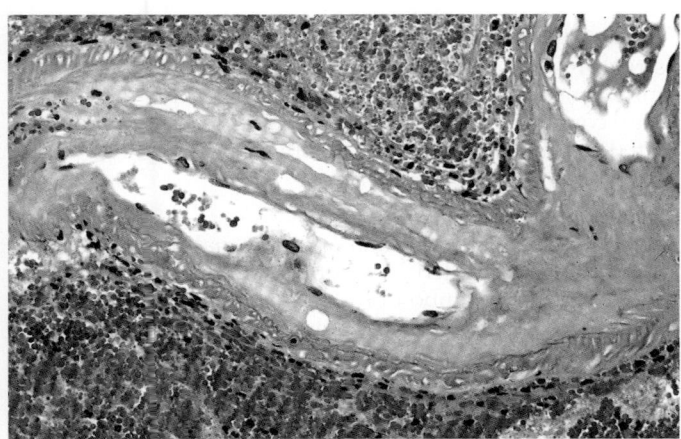

FIGURE 32-37 Amyloid angiopathy. While hypertension is the most common cause of intracerebral hemorrhage in the classic locations—basal ganglia and thalamus, pons, and cerebellum—hemorrhage in the white matter of the cerebral hemispheres has a broader range of possible etiologies. These hemorrhages, called lobar hemorrhages, may be caused by amyloid angiopathy in which β-amyloid protein is deposited in the walls of vessels. This leads to accumulation of amorphous glassy eosinophilic material shown here and weakens the vessel walls. This is the same protein involved in plaque formation in Alzheimer disease; amyloid angiopathy, and Alzheimer disease frequently coexist.

AMYLOID ANGIOPATHY: This vascular change results from deposition of β-amyloid protein in vascular walls, rendering them weak and friable (Fig. 32-37). Small intraparenchymal vessels in the lobar white matter are most affected, and their rupture may lead to lobar ICH. Amyloid angiopathy becomes more common with advancing age. It is an important cause of ICH in the elderly. It may coexist with Alzheimer disease, in which β-amyloid protein processing is abnormal (see below).

Subarachnoid Hemorrhage

Abnormal intravascular pressure and/or defects in arterial walls lead to formation of cerebral aneurysms that may rupture, leading to SAH. Ruptured aneurysms cause about 85% of SAH, while vascular malformations account for 15%.

Saccular (Berry) Aneurysms

Saccular aneurysms are balloon-like outpouchings of cerebral arteries that may rupture to cause catastrophic SAH. They tend to occur at branch points of the cerebral vasculature in or near the circle of Willis (Fig. 32-38).

 PATHOLOGY: When a developing blood vessel bifurcates into two branches, the muscularis layer may not adequately span the branch point. This leaves an area of congenital muscularis thinning, covered only by endothelium, the internal elastic membrane and a thin adventitia. Over time, pressure from the pulsatile blood flow from the parent vessel enlarges the defect. The internal elastic membrane may degenerate or fragment, after which a saccular aneurysm evolves that is precariously covered only by a layer of adventitia. Active vascular wall remodeling may contribute to the aneurysm's evolution.

More than 90% of saccular aneurysms occur at proximal branch points in the anterior circulation fed by the carotid system; however, some may arise on branches

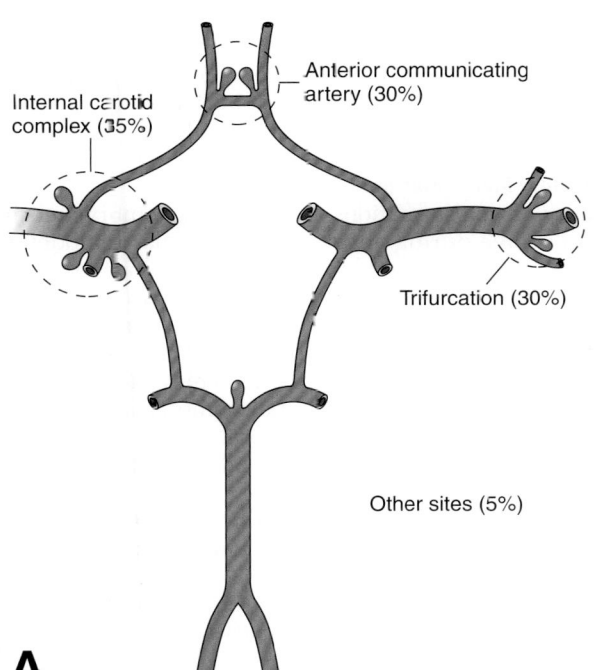

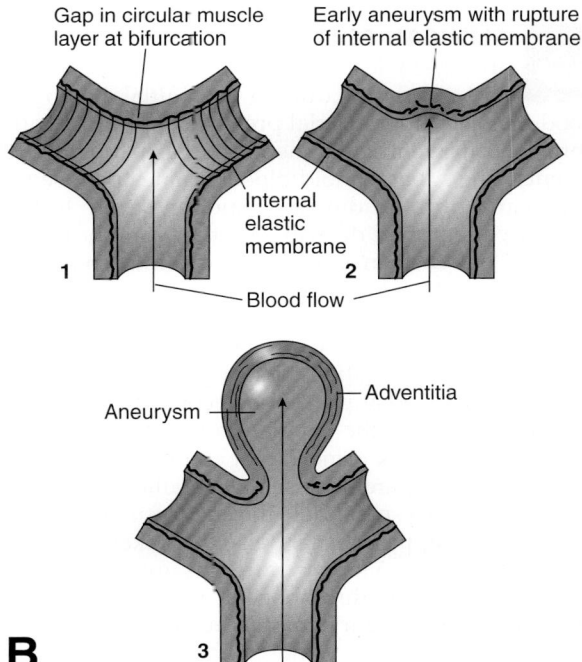

FIGURE 32-38. Pathophysiology of saccular aneurysm. A. The incidence of saccular aneurysms (berry aneurysms), which preferentially involve the proximal carotid tributaries, is shown. **B.** Lesions evolve as blood under pressure acts on an early embryonic defect of the vascular wall occurring at bifurcations.

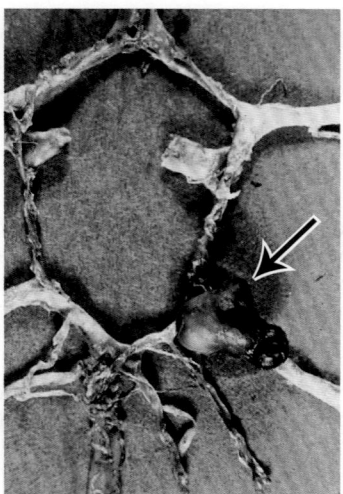

FIGURE 32-39. Berry aneurysm. A saccular aneurysm (*arrow*) arises from the posterior cerebral artery. The dark color is caused by subarachnoid blood that accumulated when the aneurysm ruptured.

of the posterior circulation, particularly on the posterior communicating and posterior cerebral arteries (Fig. 32-39). They are equally distributed at the junctions of the (1) anterior cerebral and anterior communicating arteries, (2) internal carotid–posterior communicating–anterior cerebral–anterior choroidal arteries and (3) trifurcation of the middle cerebral artery. Multiple aneurysms are present in 15% to 20% of cases. The incidence of cerebral aneurysms is increased in polycystic kidney disease, coarctation of the aorta, and Ehlers–Danlos syndrome, which may involve genetic defects in extracellular matrix proteins and/or signaling molecules.

CLINICAL FEATURES: Rupture of a saccular aneurysm leads to life-threatening SAH, with 35% mortality due to the initial hemorrhage. Blood may jet under arterial pressure to produce intracerebral or intraventricular hemorrhage in up to 1/3 of patients. The subarachnoid blood irritates pain-sensitive vessels and dura, leading to a sudden severe headache that the patient may describe as "the worst headache in my life," before then lapsing rapidly into coma. Those who survive 3 to 4 days may develop vasospasm, leading to fluctuating levels of consciousness and focal neurologic deficits. Survivors of the initial episode often rebleed within 21 days, and half of those who rebleed will perish. Therapy is directed at preventing rebleeding by isolating the aneurysm from the circulation by surgical occlusion of the vascular stalk or neck that connects the sac of the aneurysm to the parent vessel. A metallic clip across the neck of the aneurysm renders the aneurysm bloodless. An endovascular approach can also be taken: a catheter inserted through the femoral artery is guided to the cerebral circulation. Thin thrombogenic metallic coils are then threaded into the aneurysm sac, causing the blood in the aneurysm to clot. Aneurysmal coiling is less invasive than clipping and appears to be equally effective and durable.

At times, instead of rupturing, a saccular aneurysm can enlarge to form a mass that may compress cranial nerves and produce palsies or impinge on parenchymal structures and induce neurologic symptoms. Classically, for example, a posterior communicating artery aneurysm may compress the third cranial nerve, leading to an isolated oculomotor nerve palsy with dilated pupil.

Mycotic (Infectious) Aneurysms

Bacterial or fungal infections of an arterial wall may cause a focal dilatation called a mycotic aneurysm. These usually result from septic emboli originating in an infected cardiac valve. The embolus usually flows through the carotid circulation and lodges in the vasa vasorum of a distal branch of the middle cerebral artery, where microbes proliferate, induce inflammation, and destroy the affected arterial wall. This forms an aneurysm. Mycotic aneurysms occur in the distal cerebral circulation, unlike saccular aneurysms, which occur proximally. Rupture of the aneurysm can cause intracerebral or subarachnoid hemorrhage. Alternatively, microorganisms may be released and produce a cerebral abscess or meningitis.

Atherosclerotic Aneurysms

Aneurysms caused by atherosclerosis occur mainly in major cerebral arteries (vertebral, basilar, internal carotid) that are favored sites of atherosclerosis. Inflammation and accumulation of necrotic cores in atherosclerotic plaques damage the media and the internal elastic membrane and weaken the arterial wall to cause aneurysmal dilation. As they enlarge, atherosclerotic aneurysms take on a fusiform shape and elongate. An enlarging atherosclerotic aneurysm may compress cranial nerves or parenchyma, leading to focal neurologic deficits. Thus, atherosclerotic aneurysms of the basilar artery may encroach upon the cerebellopontine angle, compressing the eighth cranial nerve, and causing deafness and vertigo. Basilar aneurysms may compress cranial nerve V, leading to trigeminal neuralgia, or cranial nerve VII, leading to hemifacial spasm. Atherosclerotic aneurysms rarely rupture and cause SAH, but intraplaque hemorrhage may lead to vascular occlusion or a complicated plaque may lead to arterial thrombosis and ischemic stroke.

Vascular Malformations

Vascular malformations arise during embryogenesis but also evolve during angiogenesis, vascular remodeling, and recruitment of vessels from normal parenchyma. They are named according to the nature of the vascular channels in the malformation and the neuroglial parenchyma within the malformation which may be normal, gliotic, or absent altogether. Vascular malformations may bleed to cause subarachnoid or intraparenchymal hemorrhage or both. They may also irritate normal cerebral cortex, resulting in seizures, or divert blood flow from adjacent structures and produce focal neurologic deficits.

ARTERIOVENOUS MALFORMATION: An arteriovenous malformation (AVM) is a tangle of arteries and veins of varying calibers and wall thicknesses interspersed with abnormal gliotic parenchyma (Fig. 32-40). The abnormal vessels arise during embryogenesis from focal communications between cerebral arteries and veins without intervening capillaries. The resulting congeries of abnormal vessels are typically located in the cerebral cortex and the contiguous underlying white matter. AVMs enlarge with time and recruit vessels from adjacent tissue.

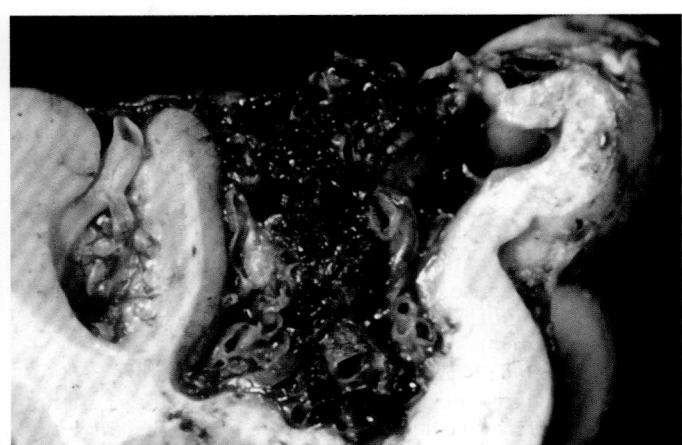

FIGURE 32-40. Arteriovenous malformation (AVM). A disorganized collection of arteries and veins is seen within the substance of the brain extending to the surface. AVMs may result in subarachnoid hemorrhage if they bleed on the surface or intraparenchymal hemorrhage if deeper vascular channels rupture. The hemorrhage is usually not as catastrophic as that seen in aneurysm subarachnoid hemorrhage or hypertensive intracerebral hemorrhage.

CLINICAL FEATURES: These include seizure disorders from irritation of neural tissue; focal neurologic deficits caused by vascular steal; and intracranial hemorrhages, usually subarachnoid or intracerebral, which commonly arise in the second or third decade. The hemorrhage is not often catastrophic but may be recurrent.

CAVERNOUS ANGIOMA: Cavernous angiomas are wide, irregular, thin-walled vascular channels with no intervening neural parenchyma. They are less common than AVMs. Although most are asymptomatic, they may cause intracranial bleeding, seizures, or focal neurologic disturbances. Cavernous angiomas may be multiple in 15% to 20% of cases. Many patients have autosomal dominant cerebral cavernous malformations (CCMs), the most common form of which, CCM1, results from loss-of-function mutations in the *KRIT* gene (also known as *CCM1*). The KRIT protein plays a role in regulating the actin cytoskeleton and maintaining cell–cell junctions. Mutations result in weakening of vascular cell junctions and leakage from blood vessels.

TELANGIECTASIA: These are focal aggregates of uniformly dilated, thin-walled, small capillary-sized vessels with normal intervening neural parenchyma. They only rarely initiate seizures or rupture. They are usually discovered incidentally during imaging for other conditions or at autopsy.

VENOUS ANGIOMA: This malformation consists of one or a few enlarged veins residing in normal parenchyma. They are distributed randomly in the spinal cord or brain and are generally asymptomatic.

Vascular malformations and their catastrophic consequences take a terrible toll. However, significant advances in understanding molecular genetic mechanisms of vascular remodeling in aneurysm formation and growth, vascular malformations and small vessels exposed to chronic hypertension have moved management of cerebrovascular disorders from pessimistic nihilism toward a scientifically driven, clinically optimistic outlook.

CNS INFECTIONS

Many infections of the CNS are devastating or lethal if untreated. Their clinical course can be swift and ferocious or indolent and progressive, and they may mimic many other disorders. Clinical vigilance, thorough diagnostic evaluation, and emphatic therapeutic response are all essential for effective management. The clinical context of nervous system infections is crucial. Patients' age, socioeconomic situation, risky behaviors, immune status, and travel history are critical in assessing infections of the CNS. Diverse factors such as AIDS, chemotherapy, economics, environmental change, bioterrorism, global travel, and immigration continue to change the face of infectious diseases.

Evaluation of CNS infections must include the location and extent of the infection, the nature of the host response, and the inciting organism.

Empyema in the epidural or subdural space is usually related to trauma or spread of a contiguous infection—usually bacterial—originating in the sinuses or ear.

In leptomeningitis (**meningitis**), the inflammatory response and most of the inciting organisms are within the subarachnoid space, floating in the CSF. The vigor of the inflammatory response may lead to parenchymal involvement (**cerebritis**) including cerebral edema and vasculitis with thrombosis, hemorrhage, or infarction. Long-term complications include effusions, obstruction of CSF flow with hydrocephalus and cranial neuropathies, particularly deafness from VIII nerve involvement.

Cerebritis is a purulent parenchymal infection that is usually bacterial or fungal. The involved brain tissue is soft and soupy and the borders of the infection cannot be easily discerned. If the process can be contained, the area of cerebritis is walled off to form a brain abscess. Abscesses have many neutrophils within a necrotic core, surrounded by granulation tissue, a dense fibrovascular capsule, and a gliotic rind.

Encephalitis, like cerebritis, is a parenchymal infection, but the term is usually reserved for viral infections with necrosis, perivascular lymphocytic cuffing, and microglial nodules. Intranuclear or cytoplasmic viral inclusions may be seen, as may gliosis, demyelination, and status spongiosus.

Different classes of infectious organisms produce distinctive host inflammatory responses. While not absolute, the inflammatory reaction provides clues about the inciting organism. Bacteria tend to induce vigorous polymorphonuclear (purulent) responses, while fungi and mycobacteria may elicit more indolent granulomatous reactions. In viral infections, lymphocytic responses predominate, while protozoa tend to incite lymphoplasmacytic infiltrates. Metazoan parasites generate eosinophilic and lymphocytic inflammation. Prions cause no inflammation but stimulate vigorous gliosis.

Bacterial Infections Produce Inflammation in the Subarachnoid Space

This response, called **leptomeningitis,** occurs between the pia and arachnoid layers of the meninges. CSF filling this compartment is an excellent culture medium for most bacteria. The inflammatory response to infections in the CSF varies with the virulence of the organism and the tempo of the infection. Changes occur in CSF cellular constituents and glucose and protein concentrations. Organisms are sometimes seen microscopically in the CSF and can be identified and characterized by culture, antigenicity, and in some cases polymerase chain reaction (PCR).

 CLINICAL FEATURES: Symptoms of meningitis include headache, vomiting, fever, altered mental status, and seizures. Classic signs of meningeal inflammation include neck rigidity, knee pain with hip flexion (Kernig sign), and knee/hip flexion when the neck is flexed (Brudzinski sign). At the extremes of age— newborn and senescence—clinical manifestations vary more widely. A newborn may have autonomic instability and fragmentary seizures, while the elderly may exhibit altered mental status without fever or headache.

Bacterial Meningitis

ETIOLOGIC FACTORS: Since most bacteria initiate purulent responses, the presence of neutrophils in the CSF is strong evidence of meningitis. CSF glucose is often decreased and protein elevated. Causes of bacterial meningitis depend on the age of the patient. *Escherichia coli* and β-hemolytic *Streptococcus* sp. predominate in neonates. In unvaccinated young children, *Haemophilus influenza* dominates, but vaccination programs against *H. influenzae* group B have changed the epidemiology, so that *Streptococcus pneumoniae* and *Neisseria meningitidis* have become more prevalent. *N. meningitidis* is most common in adolescents and young adults. *S. pneumoniae* is most common thereafter. Routes of entry to the intracranial vault are shown in Figure 32-41A.

ESCHERICHIA COLI: In newborns, whose resistance to gram-negative bacteria has not yet fully developed,

E. coli is a major cause of meningitis. Transplacental transfer of maternal immunoglobulin (Ig) G protects newborns from many bacteria, but *E. coli* and similar gram-negative organisms require IgM for neutralization, and IgM does not cross the placenta. Thus, in infants, gram-negative organisms quickly produce purulent meningitis with a high mortality.

HAEMOPHILUS INFLUENZAE: Environmental exposure to gram-negative *H. influenzae* is somewhat delayed. Thus, the incidence of meningitis peaks from 3 months to 3 years. *H. influenza* meningitis has decreased in recent years (see above).

STREPTOCOCCUS PNEUMONIAE: Later in life, *Pneumococcus* is the main cause of meningitis. Patients with a history of basilar skull fracture with CSF leak have a high incidence of pneumococcal meningitis, which often recurs after treatment. Alcoholics and patients who have undergone splenectomy are highly susceptible.

NEISSERIA MENINGITIDIS: Meningococci reside in the nasopharynx, and airborne transmission in crowded places (e.g., schools or barracks) causes "epidemic meningitis." Initially, bacteremia causes fever, malaise, and petechial rash, but intravascular coagulopathy may cause lethal adrenal hemorrhage **(Waterhouse–Friderichsen syndrome)**. Untreated meningococcal bacteremia can trigger acute fulminant meningitis. A polyvalent vaccine is recommended for all young people and is extremely effective. However, some strains of *N. meningitidis* are not covered by the vaccine, and vaccines are not widely available in many parts of the world. In 1996, sub-Saharan Africa experienced the largest epidemic of meningococcal meningitis in history, with over 250,000 cases and 25,000 deaths.

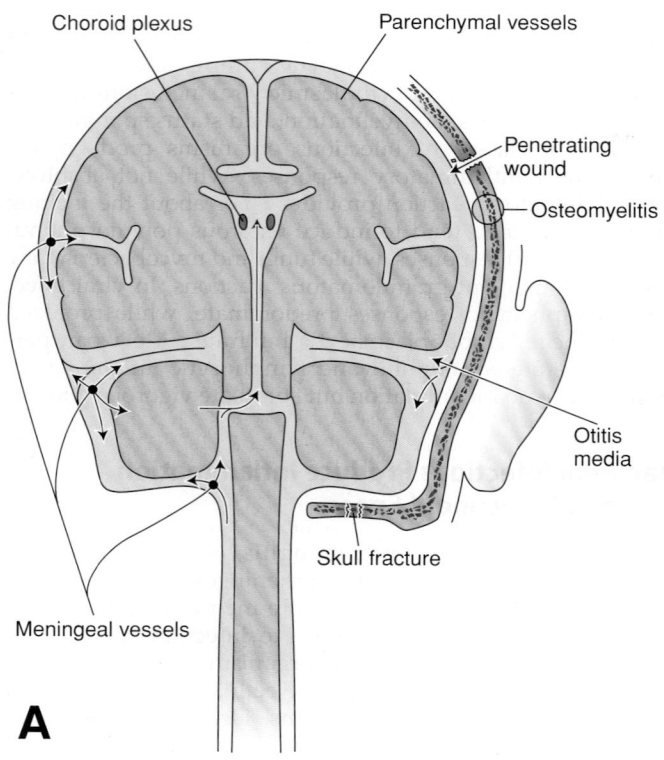

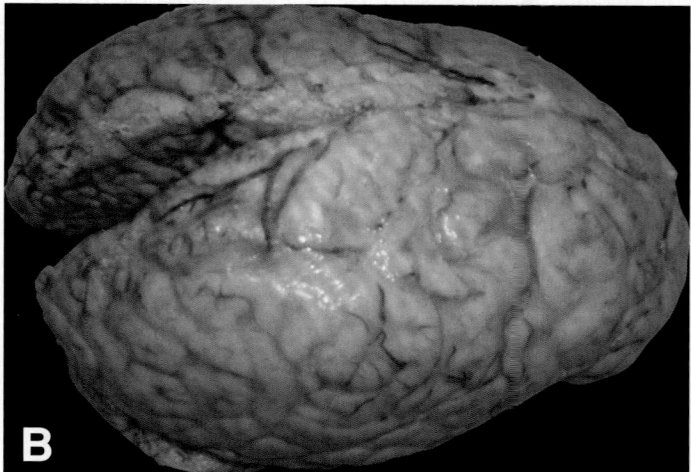

FIGURE 32-41. Purulent meningitis. A. Routes of entry of infectious organisms into the cranial cavity. **B.** A creamy exudate opacifies the leptomeninges in bacterial meningitis. The superficial veins are engorged and may develop thrombosis, and the arteries on the surface of the brain may also develop thrombosis, leading to infarcts.

LISTERIA MONOCYTOGENES: Listerial meningitis is increasing in all ages and may account for up to 10% of bacterial meningitis. Its course is less fulminant than other bacterial meningitides and CSF cellular responses may be lymphocyte predominant.

BACILLUS ANTHRACIS: Anthrax produces a fulminant hemorrhagic meningitis in up to 50% of cases. During the anthrax bioterrorism attacks in the United States in 2001, the index case was diagnosed as a result of the presence of large gram-positive rods in the CSF. Anthrax is a weaponizable biologic warfare agent.

 PATHOLOGY: In bacterial meningitis, an exudate of leukocytes and fibrin opacifies the arachnoid. This exudate varies from mild and equivocal to the naked eye to being prominent enough to obscure blood vessels. Purulent exudates are most conspicuous over the cerebral hemispheres (Fig. 32-41B) but may extend to the base of the brain and from intracranial to intraspinal and subarachnoid spaces. However, cerebral abscesses rarely occur as a complication of meningitis. The pia forms sleeves around blood vessels that penetrate the brain **(Virchow–Robin spaces)** in continuity with the subarachnoid space. The subarachnoid space including the Virchow–Robin domain is usually packed with neutrophils and organisms (Fig. 32-42). A vigorous host response is essential to clear the infection, but significant vascular and neuropil damage results from cytotoxic substances such as free radicals and cytokines released by inflammatory cells. Those cells may compete with the brain for glucose and low CSF glucose in bacterial meningitis mostly reflects glucose consumption by inflammatory cells. Corticosteroids may be given with antibiotics to mitigate host response–induced damage.

Cerebral Abscess

PATHOLOGY: A localized intraparenchymal abscess begins when bacteria or fungi lodge in the neuropil and incite an acute inflammatory and edematous reaction called **cerebritis**. The tissue becomes soft and soupy, and within days, liquefactive necrosis produces an expanding mass that may threaten life by herniation or rupture into a ventricle (Fig. 32-43). Vigorous reactive astrogliosis is triggered, and fibroblasts make a rare appearance in the brain by invading from cerebral microvasculature to encapsulate the nascent abscess.

As the abscess matures over days to weeks, three layers surround a central core of purulent debris: (1) an inner layer of vigorous granulation tissue where host and microbes engage in open warfare; (2) a second layer composed of a dense meshwork of fibroblasts and collagen that forms a tough rind around the core and granulation tissue; and (3) an outer zone of intense astrogliosis, microglial activation, and edema (Fig. 32-44). The granulation tissue layer lacks a BBB and thus leaks contrast material in radiographic imaging studies, causing a smooth ring of enhancement.

If an abscess is not drained or treated with antibiotics, increasing pressure within it may extrude microbes into adjacent parenchyma to spawn "daughter" abscesses. Or, the abscess may rupture catastrophically into the ventricles. Bacteria that cause brain abscesses are often anaerobic or microaerophilic, and thus may be difficult to culture. They often spread to the brain via the bloodstream from infections in the heart or lungs; as showers of organisms repeatedly enter the circulation, abscesses are multiple in 15% to 20% of cases. Brain invasion may also arise by contiguous spread from infected frontal or mastoid sinuses or neurosurgical wound infections.

Neurosyphilis

Syphilis is caused by a spirochete, *Treponema pallidum*. By aligning its transmission with host carnal impulses, *T. pallidum* has assured its status as a centuries-old scourge of mankind. The organism enters the bloodstream from the primary lesion, the chancre (see Chapter 9). Secondary syphilis is heralded by a maculopapular rash on the skin and mucous membranes. A few lymphocytes and plasma cells and increased protein in the CSF reflect entry of blood-borne spirochetes into the meninges, leading to transient and often asymptomatic meningitis. The organisms usually do not survive for long and the CSF reverts to normal. However, sometimes errant spirochetes initiate a meningeal fibroblastic response, accompanied by obliterative endarteritis that induces multiple small cerebral cortex or brainstem infarcts. The classical eponymic brainstem strokes described in the 18th and 19th centuries were largely due to an obliterative syphilitic endarteritis. Plasma cells, the inflammatory hallmark of syphilis,

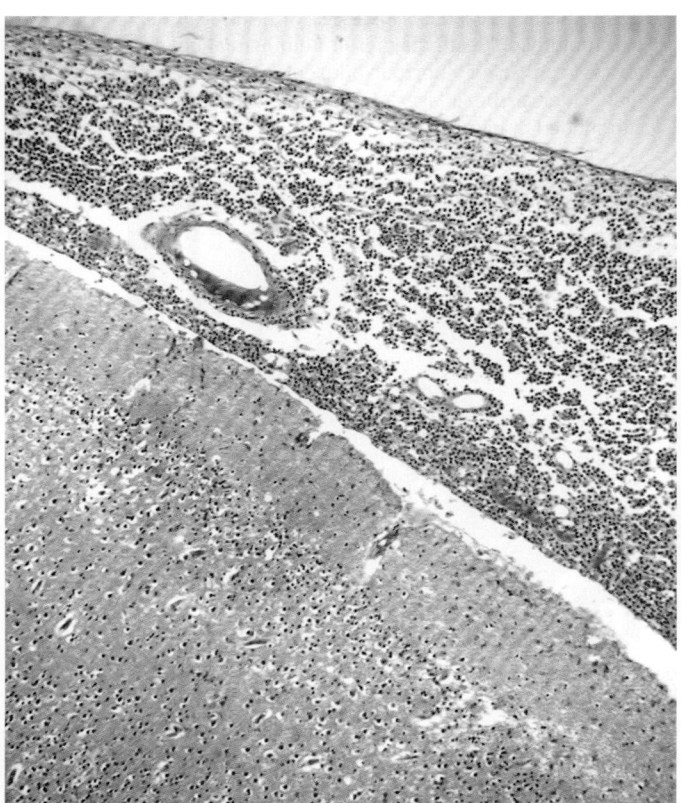

FIGURE 32-42. Bacterial meningitis. A microscopic section shows marked accumulation of neutrophils in the subarachnoid space.

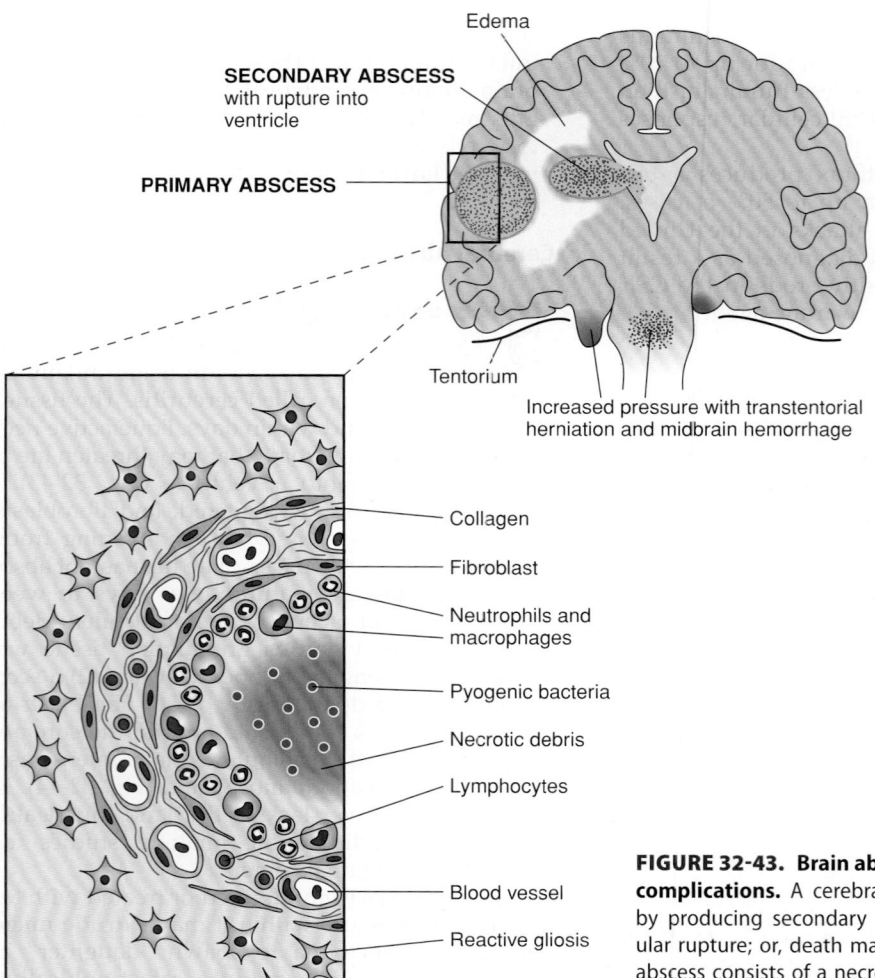

FIGURE 32-43. Brain abscess development and its complications. A cerebral abscess may cause death by producing secondary abscesses with intraventricular rupture; or, death may result from herniation. An abscess consists of a necrotic purulent core, a layer of granulation tissue, a layer of fibrosis, and finally, it is surrounded by gliosis.

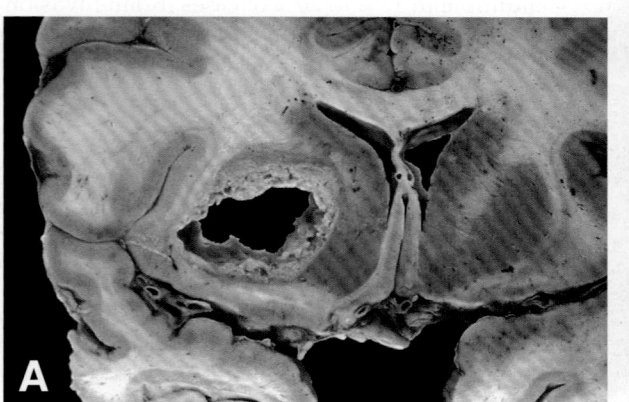

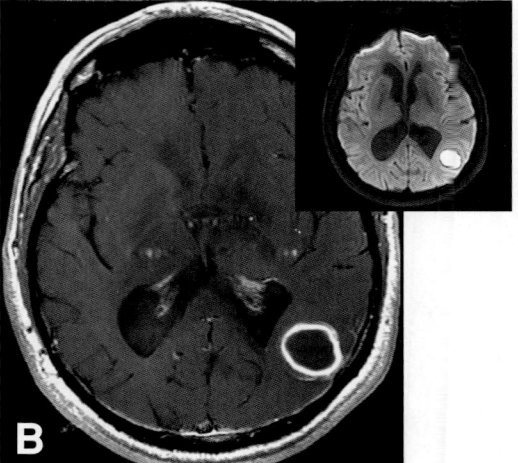

FIGURE 32-44. Cerebral abscess. A. An abscess in the left basal ganglia developed in a young man with bacterial endocarditis. **B.** Axial T1-weighted contrast-enhanced MR image of a similar patient shows a ring of enhancement of uniform thickness surrounding a central hypointense core. The smooth, uniform ring is highly suggestive of a pyogenic brain abscess. *Inset.* Additional evidence in support of this diagnosis is provided by diffusion-weighted MR imaging (DWI), which shows strong hyperintensity (bright signal) in the central core area. This is caused by restricted water molecule diffusion in this location due to water sequestration by neutrophils in the abscess core. By contrast, necrosis associated with metastases and malignant primary brain tumors does not show this degree of restricted diffusion, and the central necrotic zone thus remains dark on the DWI sequence. Other entities that show strongly restricted diffusion are cerebral infarcts, epidermoid cysts, and densely cellular tumors such as CNS lymphoma.

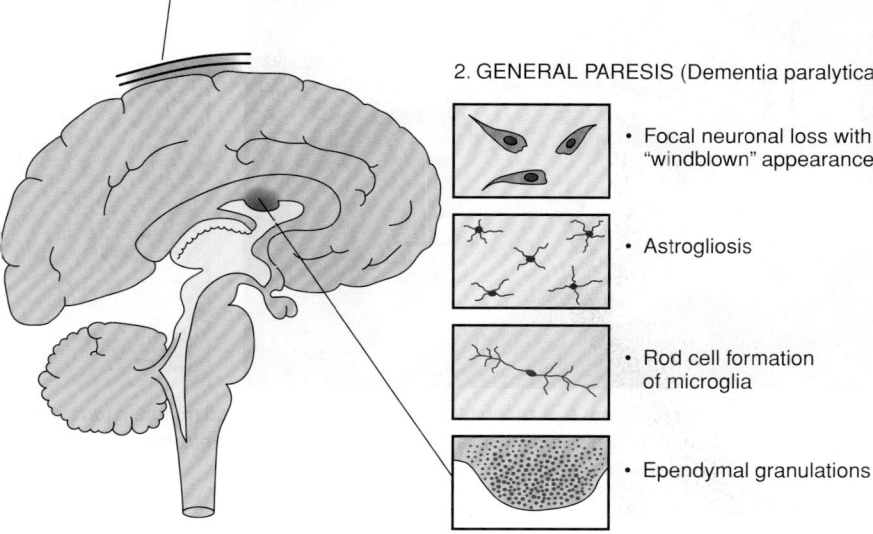

1. MENINGOVASCULAR SYPHILIS
* Thickened meninges
* Obliterative endarteritis with plasma cells

2. GENERAL PARESIS (Dementia paralytica)

* Focal neuronal loss with "windblown" appearance

* Astrogliosis

* Rod cell formation of microglia

* Ependymal granulations

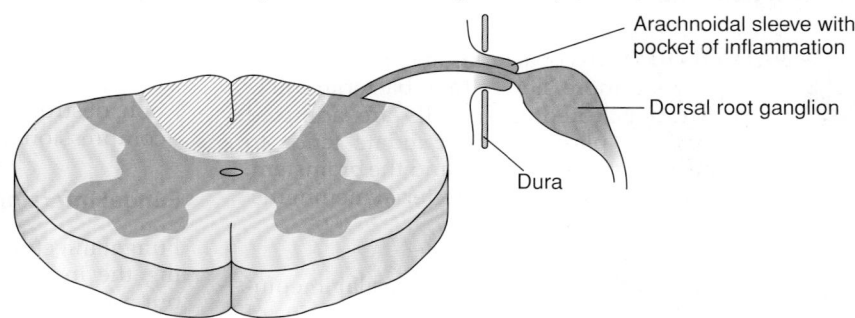

3. TABES DORSALIS (Posterior column degeneration)

Arachnoidal sleeve with pocket of inflammation

Dorsal root ganglion

Dura

FIGURE 32-45. Involvement of the central nervous system in syphilis. Hallmarks of neurosyphilis are (1) meningovascular inflammation leading to pachymeningitis and strokes caused by obliterative endarteritis; (2) intraparenchymal involvement leading to dementia; and (3) tabes dorsalis caused by inflammation of posterior roots and meninges.

surround arterioles of the cerebral cortex in meningovascular syphilis (Fig. 32-45).

Tabes Dorsalis

Tabes dorsalis is impairment of dorsal (posterior) spinal column function manifested by loss of joint position sense and fine touch (Fig. 32-46). Dorsal nerve roots proximal to dorsal root ganglia are met by a conical sleeve of arachnoid filled with CSF, which can be the site of syphilitic inflammation. Fibrous tissue triggered by the inflammation constricts nerve roots, causing axonal (wallerian) degeneration. Unlike spinothalamic afferents, axons that course cephalad in the posterior columns do not synapse with intramedullary neurons. Thus, wallerian degeneration initiated in the dorsal spinal nerves extends the length of the posterior fasciculi. The result is loss of position sense in the legs, and affected individuals come to rely on visual cues for the position of their feet and legs in space. In darkness or with eyes closed, patients become unsteady and may even fall. Inability to remain standing with eyes closed is called a positive Romberg sign and reflects severe posterior column dysfunction.

Luetic Dementia

T. pallidum may remain latent in the brain for decades. The spirochetes replicate sluggishly and escape eradication, resulting in dementia and psychosis years after the initial

infection. Morphologic features include focal loss of cortical neurons, disfigurement of residual nerve cells ("wind-blown appearance"), marked gliosis, and conversion of microglia into elongated forms encrusted with iron ("rod cells") associated with nodular ependymitis.

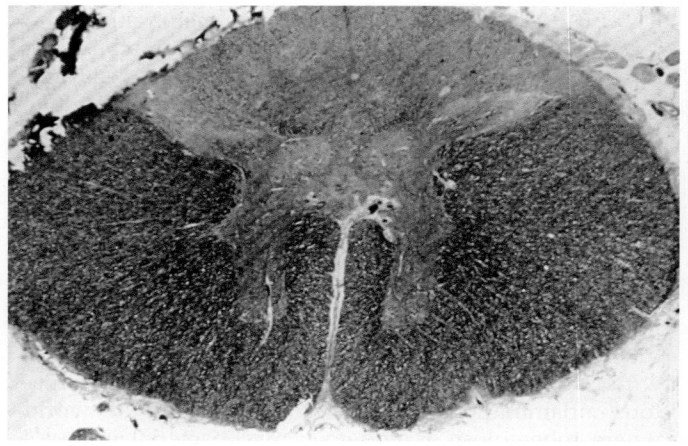

FIGURE 32-46. Tabes dorsalis. The spinal cord of a patient with tertiary syphilis displays posterior column degeneration (pale zones in this sliver impregnation stain). Because this leads to loss of proprioception, the patient is unable to walk without visual cues.

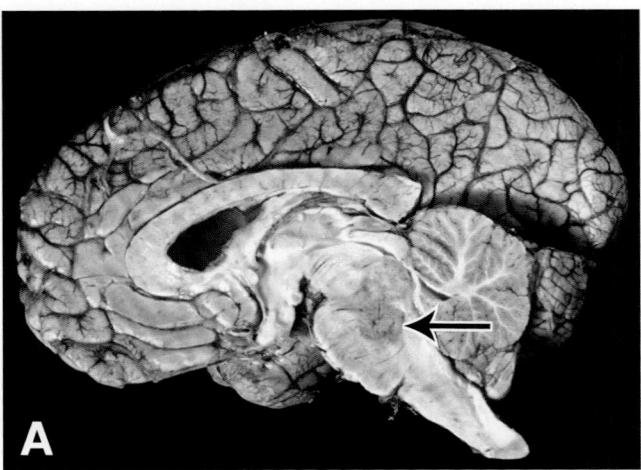
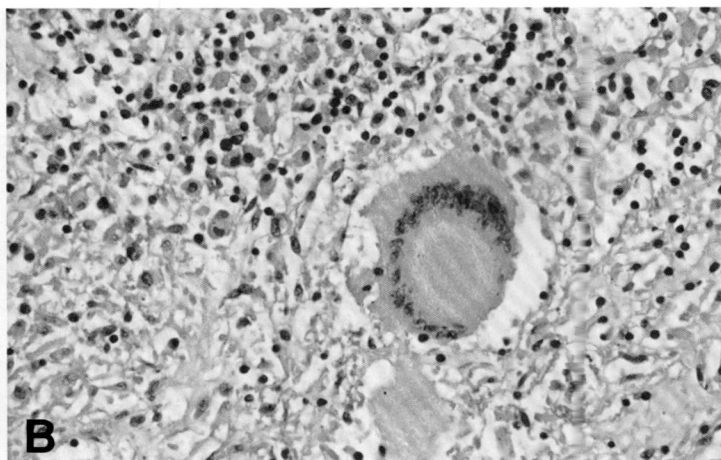

FIGURE 32-47. Tuberculoma. A. A tuberculoma is seen in the pons and midbrain (*arrow*). **B.** Microscopic examination shows caseous necrosis, macrophages, and Langhans giant cells. Rupture of a tuberculoma into the cerebrospinal fluid causes tuberculous meningitis to ensue.

Mycobacterial and Fungal Infections Elicit Granulomatous Responses

PATHOLOGY: Mycobacterial and fungal infections progress more slowly than bacterial infections. Multinucleated giant cells are admixed with lymphocytes and plasma cells. Exudate tends to accumulate at the base of the brain, around the brainstem, rather than over the convexities as in bacterial meningitis.

CLINICAL FEATURES: Chronic basilar meningitis may block CSF flow through the foramina of Magendie and Luschka, leading to hydrocephalus, headache, nausea, and vomiting. Cranial nerve palsies can occur as these nerves traverse the exudate where they emerge from the brainstem.

Tuberculous Meningitis and Tuberculomas

PATHOLOGY: Tuberculous meningitis is a chronic infection inciting a granulomatous host response with multinucleated giant cells and lymphocytes surrounding areas of caseous necrosis. Like neurosyphilis, mycobacterial meningitis may lead to meningeal fibrosis, communicating hydrocephalus and arteritis that may cause infarcts. As tuberculous meningitis preferentially affects the base of the brain, these infarcts are usually in the distribution of the penetrating striate and brainstem arteries. Untreated tuberculous meningitis is usually fatal in 4 to 6 weeks but may progress more rapidly in immunocompromised patients. Parenchymal tuberculosis produces **tuberculomas,** individual masses with central caseous necrosis surrounded by granulomatous inflammation (Fig. 32-47). In parts of the world where tuberculosis is endemic, mycobacterial granulomas are the most common brain masses (Fig. 32-48). In childhood, these granulomas congregate in the posterior fossa, which is also the most common site of childhood brain tumors. Confluent tuberculomas occur in miliary

tuberculosis. Tuberculous meningitis usually reflects hematogenous dissemination from an initial pulmonary focus, as intraparenchymal granulomas rupture into the CSF to produce meningitis. **Pott disease** is tuberculosis of the spine, in which epidural granulomatous inflammation destroys the bony spine, and leads to spinal cord compression (Fig. 32-49).

Fungal Infections

Fungal infections of the CNS are often opportunistic, reflecting the indolent saprophytic lifestyle of these organisms, but a few fungi are sufficiently virulent to cause disease in immunocompetent people. Fungi invading tissue may be round to oval, often budding, yeast forms, or branching hyphae. In some cases, yeast and hyphae both appear in infected tissues, facilitating tentative identification of fungi

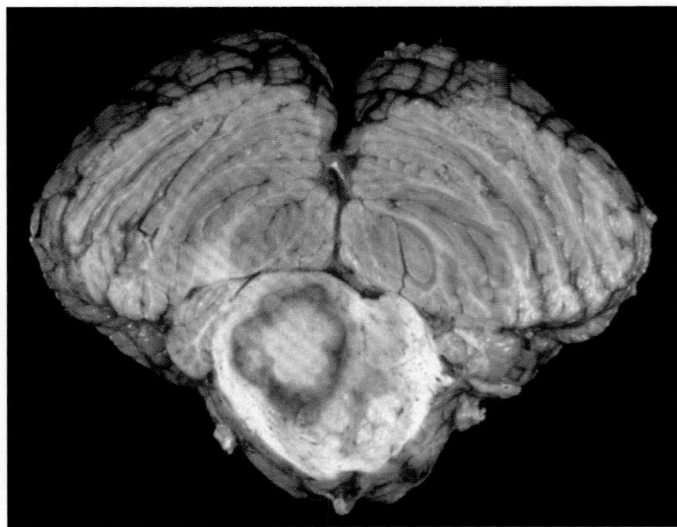

FIGURE 32-48. Tuberculoma. A focus of caseous necrosis is present in the pons and midbrain. In parts of the world where tuberculosis is endemic, tuberculomas are among the most common brain masses seen. (Courtesy of Dr. F. Stephen Vogel, Duke University.)

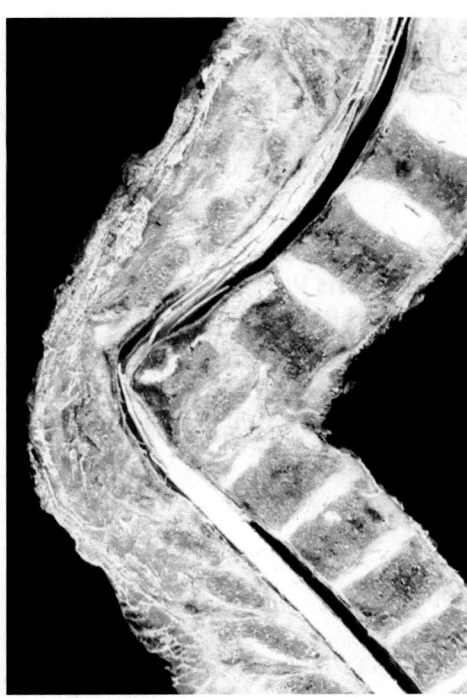

FIGURE 32-49. Pott disease. Tuberculosis involving the spinal column leads to slow vertebral collapse and acute angulation of the spine ("gibbus" deformity). Spinal cord compression may result, with myelopathic findings. (Courtesy of Dr. F. Stephen Vogel, Duke University.)

in tissue sections. However, ultimate speciation requires antigenic, PCR, or culture confirmation.

Cryptococcus

EPIDEMIOLOGY: Cryptococci are the most common fungal causes of meningitis. *Cryptococcus* often acts opportunistically in immunocompromised patients, but it can also establish meningitis in an immunologically competent host. Birds are the major reservoir of *Cryptococcus neoformans*. Inhalation of particles of fungus-laden bird excreta initiates a lung infection that may remain confined to the lungs or disseminate to involve other organs including the brain.

PATHOLOGY: *C. neoformans* typically elicits granulomatous responses, with infectious foci appearing as discrete white meningeal nodules, about 1 mm in diameter. Organisms may remain confined to the subarachnoid space, but infection sometimes spreads to the brain parenchyma. They may be abundant, particularly in the Virchow–Robin spaces. An occasional multinucleated giant cell, sometimes with phagocytosed organisms, accompanies scant epithelioid cells and a few lymphocytes. The organisms are encapsulated, budding yeast forms that are large by fungal standards (5 to 15 µm) and have an external gelatinous capsule that looks like a clear halo. The gelatinous capsule lends a clear, glistening appearance to microabscesses causing them to resemble soap bubbles (Fig. 32-50). Organisms can be highlighted by mixing contaminated CSF with India ink (Fig. 32-51).

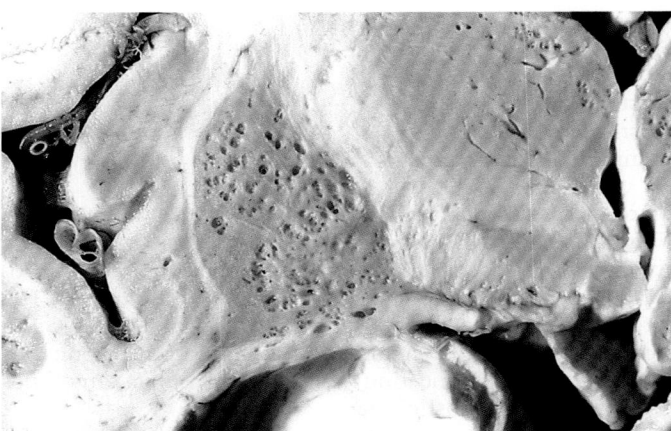

FIGURE 32-50. Cryptococcal "soap bubble" abscesses. The encapsulated organisms occur in great abundance in the Virchow–Robin space and in microabscesses within the parenchyma. The microbial capsule imparts a glistening clear appearance to these collections which has been likened to soap bubbles. (Courtesy of Dr. F. Stephen Vogel, Duke University.)

The capsules shield the organisms from host immune responses and account for the typically feeble inflammatory reaction. They also shed specific antigens that can be detected in the CSF by the latex cryptococcal antigen test.

Coccidioidomycosis

Coccidioides immitis is endemic in arid regions of the Southwest US and San Joaquin Valley in California. Initial pulmonary infection is usually asymptomatic and rarely spreads. It causes suppurative and granulomatous inflammation that sometimes includes an arteritis that may be complicated by infarction. The organism appears in tissue sections as an eye-catching refractile endosporulating spherule.

Histoplasmosis

Histoplasma capsulatum is endemic in the Mississippi basin and usually causes asymptomatic pulmonary infections. Rare CNS dissemination of this tiny, intracytoplasmic yeast form residing in macrophages may occur. A chronic

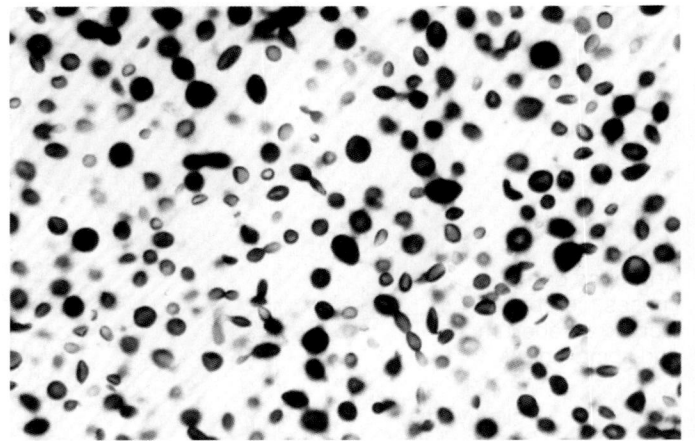

FIGURE 32-51. Cryptococcal meningitis. The cryptococcal organisms vary in size (5 to 15 microns in diameter), placing them among the largest of the yeast-form fungi (Gomori methenamine silver stain). They reproduce by budding. (Courtesy of Dr. F. Stephen Vogel, Duke University.)

meningitis ensues in which the surface of the brain may be studded by small granulomas.

Blastomycosis
Blastomyces dermatitidis is an uncommon cause of mycotic meningitis. The organisms are broad-based budding yeasts.

Mucormycosis (Zygomycosis)
Fungi of the order *Mucorales* are angioinvasive nonseptate hyphal forms that mostly cause disease in immunocompromised people or those with poorly controlled diabetes. The large vessels at the skull base, orbit, and neck are subject to invasion with occlusion and distal infarction. Blackening of the nasal mucosa indicating mucosal infarction is sometimes seen and is a diagnostic clue.

Aspergillosis
Aspergillus is an angiocentric septate hyphal fungus (usually, *Aspergillus fumigatus*) that mainly causes disease in immunocompromised hosts. Vascular involvement produces multiple gray necrotic abscesses within the parenchyma. The lung is the primary site of infection, but the brain is the second most commonly involved organ.

Candidiasis
Candida albicans is a ubiquitous opportunistic fungus that shows both yeast and pseudohyphae morphology in infected tissues. *Candida* produces many microabscesses, most often in immunocompromised patients. Systemic involvement is the rule, and in large hospital-based autopsy series, this is the most common systemic fungal infection.

Exserohilum rostratum: Infection From Contaminated Corticosteroid Injections
In 2012 and 2013, a serious epidemic of localized spinal and skull base fungal infections was traced to inadequate quality control in manufacturing of corticosteroids used for local articular, paraspinal, and epidural spinal injections for pain.

Exserohilum rostratum, a pigmented environmental fungus that rarely infects humans, was the culprit in most cases. It produced soft tissue and bone destruction with potential involvement of vertebral and basilar arteries. Approximately 700 patients were affected, with almost 60 deaths. This serious epidemic drew attention to inadequate quality control and nationwide dissemination of contaminated injectable compounds.

CNS Viral Infections Vary in Severity, Time Course, and Resolution

Manifestations of viral infections of the CNS are remarkably diverse, ranging from non–life-threatening viral meningitis to ominous viral encephalitis affecting the parenchyma. These diseases may unfold over a period of hours or span decades. In addition to producing infections, viruses have been implicated in some autoimmune and neurodegenerative diseases.

Viral Meningitis

Unlike bacterial meningitis, viral meningitis is usually benign and resolves without sequelae. The most common causative agents are enteroviruses (e.g., coxsackievirus B, echovirus), but mumps, lymphocytic choriomeningitis, Epstein–Barr and herpes simplex viruses cause many sporadic cases. Viral meningitis is mainly a disease of children and young adults. It begins as a sudden febrile illness with a severe headache. The CSF contains excess lymphocytes and a slight increase in protein but, unlike bacterial meningitis, no decrease in CSF glucose.

Viral Encephalitis

Manifestations of viral infections of CNS parenchyma are clinically and pathologically heterogeneous (Fig. 32-52). For example, poliomyelitis affects spinal and brainstem motor

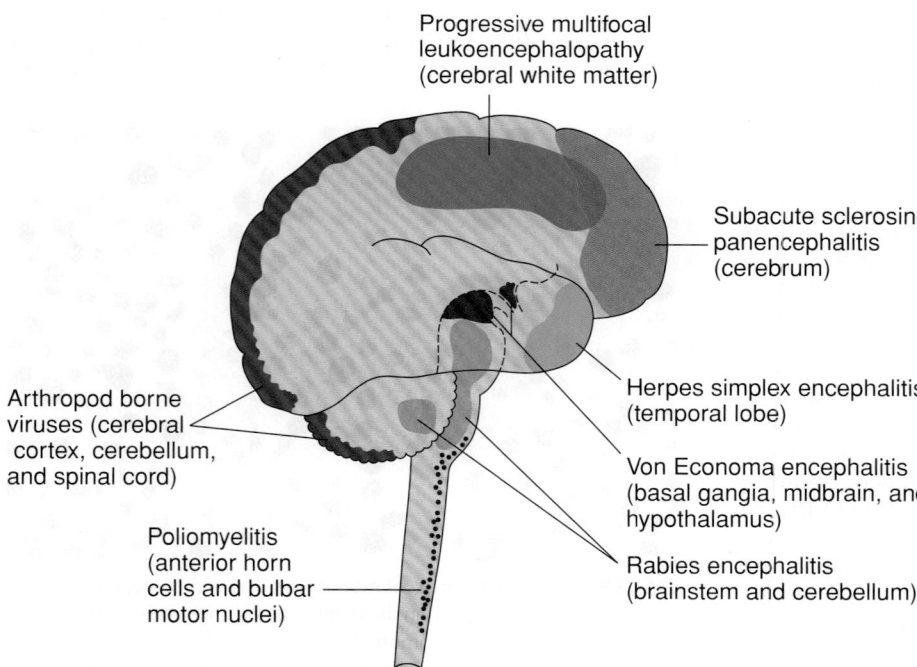

Progressive multifocal leukoencephalopathy (cerebral white matter)

Subacute sclerosing panencephalitis (cerebrum)

Arthropod borne viruses (cerebral cortex, cerebellum, and spinal cord)

Herpes simplex encephalitis (temporal lobe)

Von Economa encephalitis (basal gangia, midbrain, and hypothalamus)

Poliomyelitis (anterior horn cells and bulbar motor nuclei)

Rabies encephalitis (brainstem and cerebellum)

FIGURE 32-52. Distribution of lesions in viral encephalitis.

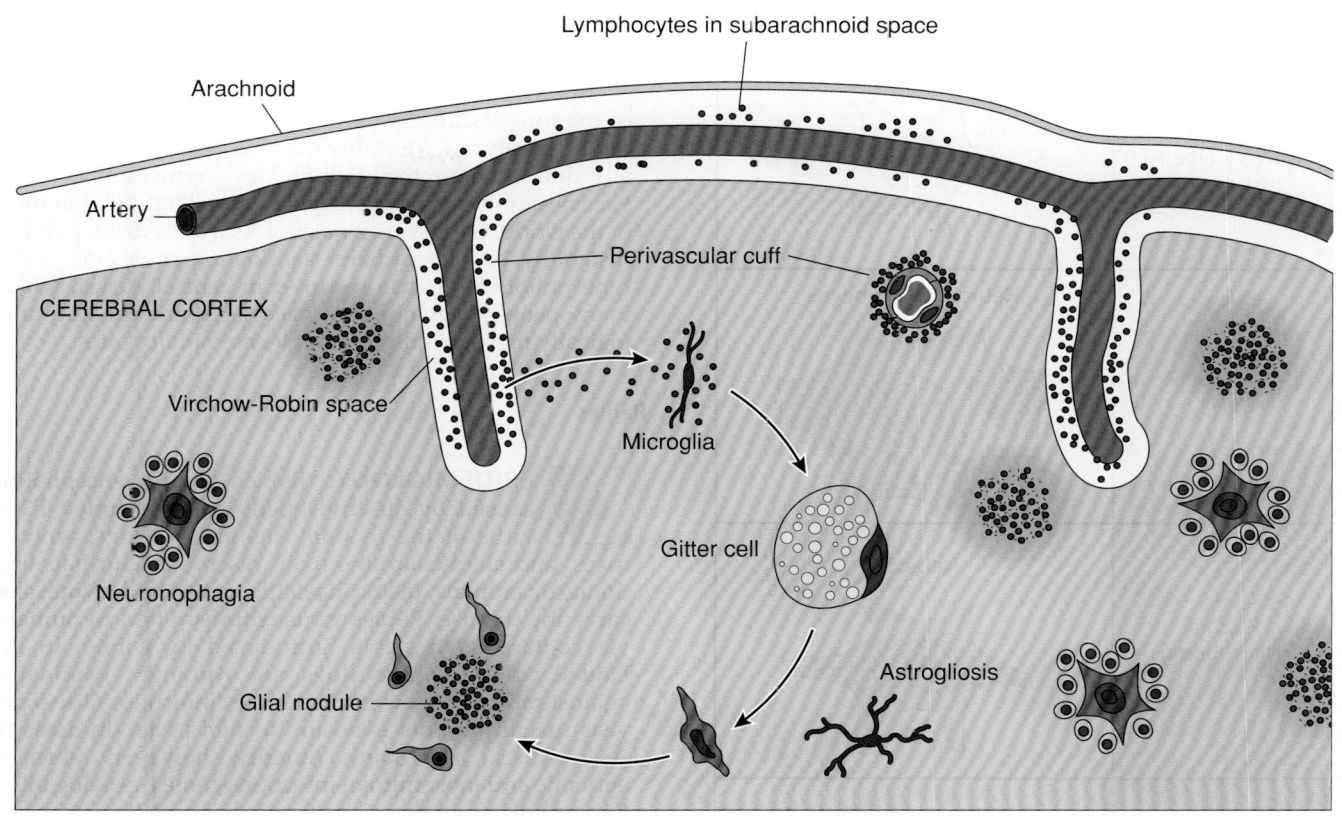

FIGURE 32-53. The lesions of viral encephalitis.

neurons, while herpes simplex targets the temporal lobes. Subacute sclerosing panencephalitis (SSPE) involves the gray matter, while progressive multifocal leukoencephalopathy (PML) is a white matter disorder. Mechanisms of viral tropism reflect specific binding interactions of viruses to plasma membrane receptors on specific CNS cells, their ability to remain latent, and their selective replication in specific intracellular microenvironments. Viruses may exploit axonal transport to travel to sites distant from their point of entry, as exemplified by rabies and herpes viruses.

PATHOLOGY: Most CNS viral infections elicit perivascular lymphocytes, macrophage and microglial activation (with formation of Gitter cells, microglial phagocytes laden with myelin debris) and gliosis (Fig. 32-53). Such changes are not specific for viral infections, but the presence of viral inclusions strongly suggests a viral infection (Fig. 32-54). Inclusion bodies do not occur with all viral infections. In situ hybridization, PCR, and immunochemistry are most often used to establish a diagnosis.

CLINICAL FEATURES: Most viral encephalitides begin abruptly. Specific neurologic deficits (e.g., paralysis of poliomyelitis, difficulty in swallowing in rabies) reflect the localization of the infection. Most encephalitides run a rapid course, but the tempo can vary. For example, the clinical course of SSPE may last years. Herpes simplex and varicella-zoster

viruses (VZVs) may be latent in sensory ganglia for years, only to be reactivated decades after initial infection.

Poliomyelitis

The term **poliomyelitis** describes any inflammation of the gray matter of the spinal cord. In common usage it implies an infection by poliovirus, which is one of the enteroviruses. These are small, nonenveloped, single-stranded RNA viruses.

Historical evidence suggests that poliomyelitis has occurred in epidemics since antiquity. Affected people shed large amounts of virus in their stools, and spread is by the fecal–oral route. The virus is acid-resistant and thus survives in the stomach. It initiates infection in the small intestine and gains access to the CNS via the blood stream.

PATHOLOGY: Virus enters motor neurons after binding CD155, a cell surface glycoprotein that functions as an adhesion molecule in cell–cell junctions in intestinal epithelial cells and is also expressed in motor neurons and dorsal root ganglia cells. Infected neurons may undergo chromatolysis, after which they are phagocytosed by macrophages (neuronophagia). Initial inflammatory responses briefly include neutrophils. Lymphocytes follow and surround blood vessels in the spinal cord and brainstem. The motor cortex usually shows no inflammation but may contain microglial nodules, which are focal collections of microglia and lymphocytes. Host immune responses to the virus, although limited, may

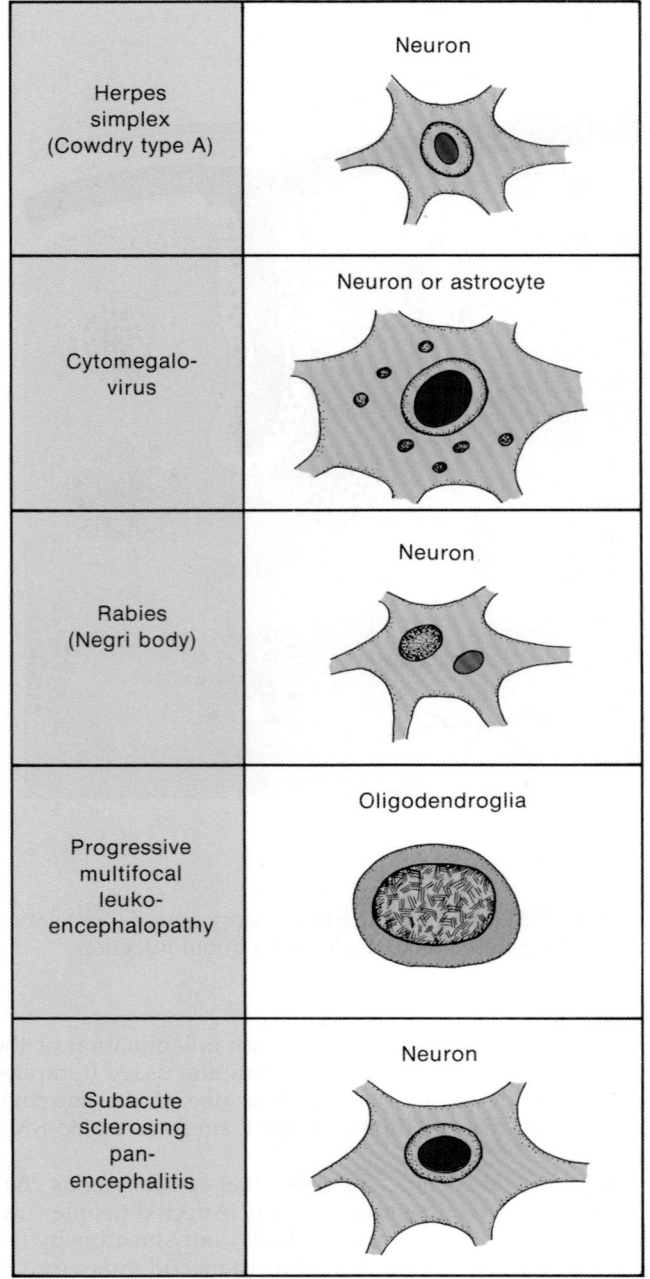

Herpes simplex (Cowdry type A)	Neuron
Cytomegalo-virus	Neuron or astrocyte
Rabies (Negri body)	Neuron
Progressive multifocal leuko-encephalopathy	Oligodendroglia
Subacute sclerosing pan-encephalitis	Neuron

FIGURE 32-54. Inclusion bodies in viral encephalitides.

halt progression of clinical disease. Sections of spinal cord in cases of healed poliomyelitis show loss of neurons, with secondary degeneration of corresponding ventral roots and peripheral nerves.

CLINICAL FEATURES: Nonspecific symptoms such as fever, malaise, and headache are followed in several days by signs of meningitis, and then by paralysis. In severe cases, the muscles of the neck, trunk, and all four limbs may be rendered powerless. Paralysis of the respiratory muscles may be life threatening.

Patients with milder disease may show asymmetric and patchy paralysis, most often in the legs.

Improvement begins in about a week, and only some of the muscles affected at the outset may remain permanently paralyzed. Mortality is 5% to 25%, with death usually due to respiratory failure. Development of effective vaccines in the 1950s has largely eliminated polio in most of the world. However, in parts of Asia and Africa, political instability has jeopardized vaccination programs. Wild-type poliomyelitis has recurred in central Africa, where many people have not been vaccinated and are immunologically naïve, resulting in high-case fatality rates.

Rabies

EPIDEMIOLOGY: Rabies is an encephalitis caused by an enveloped, single-stranded RNA virus of the rhabdovirus group. Dogs, wolves, foxes, and skunks are the main reservoirs, but bats and domestic animals, including cattle, goats, and swine, also carry the disease. Rabies virus is transmitted to humans via contaminated saliva, introduced by a bite. In the United States, where dogs are routinely vaccinated against rabies, the few human rabies infections (1 to 5 per year) usually follow exposure to rabid bats. In areas of Asia, Africa, and South America, however, rabies is endemic and most human infections come from dog bites. Rabies kills more than 50,000 people annually. Iatrogenic transmission has occurred, via corneal, solid organ and tendon transplants, and incubation periods may be extremely short or, mysteriously, as long as 18 months. Rabies is rare in industrialized countries, so the diagnosis may not be considered in potential organ donors. However, as the consequences of iatrogenic transmission of this uniformly fatal infection are so horrific, extreme caution is warranted in harvesting tissues from donors who die of strange or atypical neurologic disorders.

PATHOLOGY: The virus enters end terminals of motor neurons innervating skeletal muscle fibers and travels along axons to the neuronal cell bodies. It can spread from there throughout the spinal cord and brain and also into the salivary glands from which it can be transmitted to other hosts. Latent intervals vary in proportion to the distance of axonal transport, from 10 days to as long as 3 months.

Perivascular lymphocytes, scattered neurons with chromatolysis and neuronophagia and microglial nodules are seen. Inflammation is mainly in the brainstem and affects the cerebellum and hypothalamus. Eosinophilic cytoplasmic viral inclusion bodies in the hippocampus, brainstem, and cerebellar Purkinje cells **(Negri bodies)** confirm the diagnosis (Fig. 32-55).

CLINICAL FEATURES: Destruction of brainstem neurons by rabies virus initiates painful spasms of the throat, difficulty swallowing and a tendency to aspirate fluids that prompted the original name, "hydrophobia." Clinical symptoms also reflect a

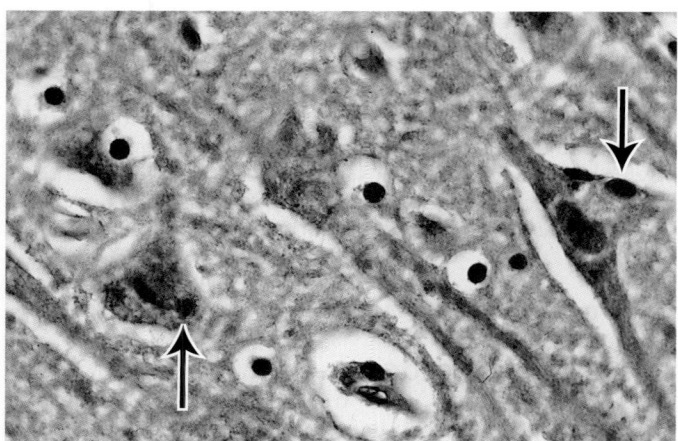

FIGURE 32-55. Negri bodies. Rabies encephalitis is characterized by round, eosinophilic cytoplasmic inclusions that resemble erythrocytes (*arrows*).

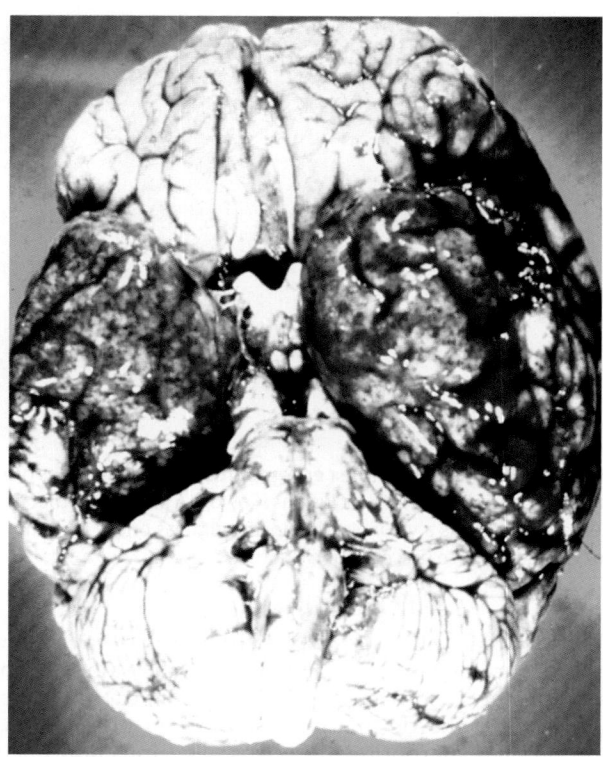

FIGURE 32-56. Herpes simplex encephalitis. The temporal lobes are grossly swollen, hemorrhagic, and necrotic. Selective involvement of the temporal lobes often leads to memory disturbances and complex partial seizures. (Courtesy of Dr. F. Stephen Vogel, Duke University.)

general encephalopathy, with irritability, agitation, seizures, and delirium. In up to 15% of cases, rabies may present in the paralytic form resembling Guillain–Barré syndrome rather than the encephalopathic form. The CSF displays a typical viral response, including (1) a modest increase in lymphocytes, (2) a moderate increase in protein, and (3) unaltered glucose and CSF pressure. Once symptoms develop, the illness progresses relentlessly to death within 1 to several weeks. Urgent rabies vaccination and hyperimmune globulin are administered for postexposure prophylaxis.

Herpes Viruses

Herpes viruses include herpes simplex (types 1 and 2), VZV, cytomegalovirus (CMV), Epstein–Barr virus (EBV), and simian B virus.

HERPES SIMPLEX TYPE 1: Herpes simplex virus type 1 (HSV-1) is largely responsible for "cold sores." The region of the vesicular lesion on the lip is innervated by sensory axons from the trigeminal ganglion. HSV-1 may reside latently in the trigeminal ganglion, where it proliferates during periods of stress and is transmitted centrifugally through the nerve trunk to the lip. Reactivation and spread of HSV-1 to the CNS results in herpes encephalitis, which is the most common sporadic (i.e., nonepidemic) viral encephalitis.

PATHOLOGY: Herpes encephalitis is a fulminant infection that localizes mainly in one or both temporal lobes. The temporal lobes become swollen, hemorrhagic, and necrotic (Fig. 32-56). Inflammation is mainly lymphocytic, with perivascular cuffing (Fig. 32-57). Small arteries and arterioles become hemorrhagic and edematous. Intranuclear eosinophilic inclusions, usually surrounded by a halo (Cowdry A), are seen in neurons and glial cells (Fig. 32-58). Viral protein detection by immunohistochemistry is diagnostically reliable. The diagnosis is often made by PCR of CSF and viral culture.

HERPES SIMPLEX TYPE 2: In women, herpes simplex virus type 2 (HSV-2) initiates a vesicular lesion on the vulva **(genital herpes),** coupled with a latent infection

in pelvic ganglia. Newborns acquire HSV-2 from active lesions (primary or recurrent) as they pass through the birth canal. Fulminant encephalitis with extensive liquefactive necrosis in the cerebrum and cerebellum may follow.

VARICELLA-ZOSTER: Varicella-zoster virus (VZV) causes childhood exanthem "chicken pox" whereupon VZV may become latent in dorsal root ganglia. In later

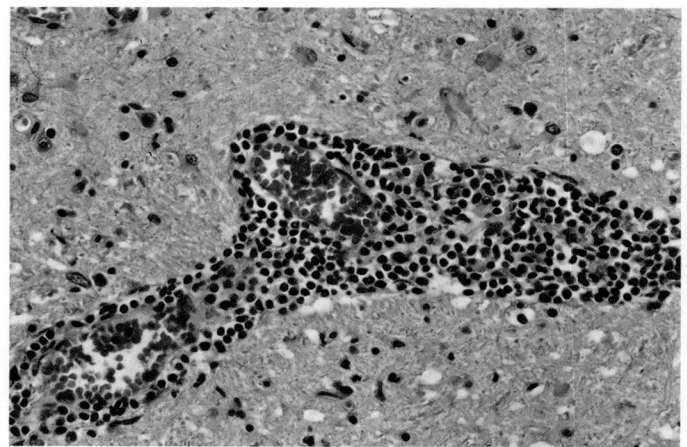

FIGURE 32-57. Herpes simplex encephalitis. Microscopically, the specimen exhibits pronounced perivascular lymphocytic inflammation. This finding reflects active inflammation but is not specific for any one viral etiology.

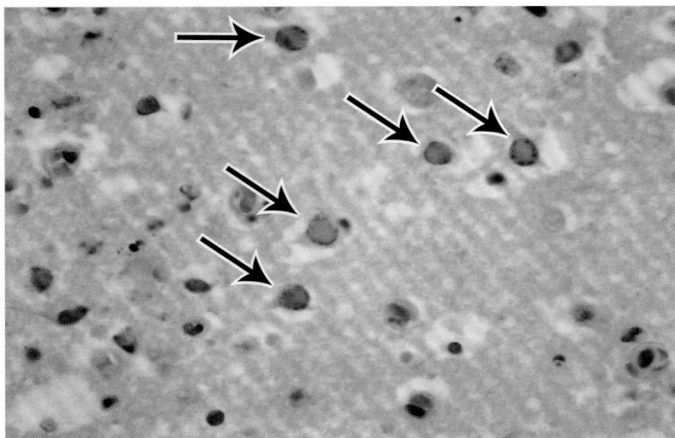

FIGURE 32-58. Herpes simplex encephalitis. Infected neurons display intranuclear, eosinophilic viral inclusions (Cowdry A inclusions) that fill the nuclei (*arrows*). This is a valuable diagnostic guide as only a limited number of viruses produce Cowdry A inclusions.

life, particularly after age 60, the virus may reactivate and be transported down sensory axons to the skin, causing an exquisitely painful cutaneous vesicular eruption called "shingles" in the dermatome distribution of the dorsal root ganglion harboring the virus. The infection elicits only mild inflammation and rarely spreads to the CNS. Intranuclear Cowdry A inclusions like those of HSV are present.

Rarely, VZV may cause a fatal encephalitis, and the virus has been implicated in isolated giant cell arteritis of the CNS leading to stroke. "Shingles" reflects reemergence of latent infection by the VZV and may be the initial manifestation of immune dysfunction. The pain and vesicular eruption can be severe and disabling, but a VZV vaccine is now available and is recommended for individuals over 60 years of age.

CYTOMEGALOVIRUS: CMV crosses the placenta to induce encephalitis in utero. Lesions in the embryonic

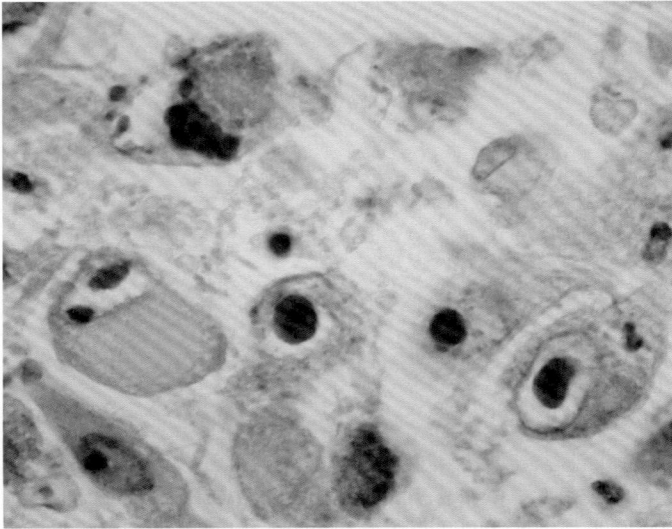

FIGURE 32-59. Cytomegalovirus ependymitis. Grotesquely enlarged infected ependymal cells display large intranuclear inclusions.

CNS are characterized by periventricular necrosis and calcification. Because of the proximity of these lesions to the third ventricle and the aqueduct, they may cause obstructive hydrocephalus. In adults, CMV encephalitis occurs in immunocompromised hosts. Eosinophilic nuclear and cytoplasmic viral inclusions are seen in astrocytes and neurons, most conspicuously in enlarged nuclei, where they are sharply defined and surrounded by a halo Fig. 32-59).

Arthropod-Borne Viral Encephalitis

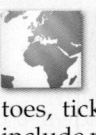 **EPIDEMIOLOGY:** Arthropod-borne viruses, or **arboviruses,** are transmitted between vertebrates by blood-sucking vectors (e.g., mosquitoes, ticks). Togaviridae, Bunyaviridae, and Flaviviridae include most of the arboviruses that cause human encephalitis. Arbovirus infections are zoonoses of animals; humans are infected when bitten by virus-harboring arthropods. Humans are not generally reservoirs, nor do they continue viral propagation. The various encephalitides caused by arboviruses are named principally for the location where they were first noted (Table 32-1), for example, Eastern, Western, and Venezuelan equine encephalitis; St. Louis encephalitis; Japanese B encephalitis; California encephalitis; and West Nile encephalitis. The latter has numerically eclipsed all other arbovirus encephalitides in the United States since it first appeared in 1999. West Nile encephalitis epidemics continue to occur, underscoring the importance of mosquito control. Most cases of West Nile infection are asymptomatic, so most infections are unrecognized. As infection can be transmitted by blood transfusion, it is now necessary to

TABLE 32-1
INSECT-BORNE VIRAL ENCEPHALITIS

Virus	Insect Vector	Distribution
St. Louis encephalitis	Mosquito	North and South America
Western equine encephalitis	Mosquito	North and South America
Venezuelan equine encephalitis	Mosquito	North and South America
Eastern equine encephalitis	Mosquito	North America
California encephalitis	Mosquito	North America
Murray Valley encephalitis	Mosquito	Australia, New Papua
Japanese B encephalitis	Mosquito	Eastern and southeastern Asia
Tick-borne encephalitis	Tick	Eastern Europe, Scandinavia
West Nile encephalitis	Mosquito	Global
Zika encephalitis	Mosquito	Caribbean, North and South America

screen blood for West Nile virus. Immunocompromised patients may have a fulminant course with the arboviral infections. Zika virus encephalitis emerged in the Caribbean, South America, and Central America in 2015. It produces devastating nervous system malformations in utero independent of the trimester when the mother is infected. The malformations including severe microcephaly and deep brain calcifications due to cytotoxic destruction in the germinal matrix. In addition to vector borne spread, Zika can be spread sexually and with blood transfusion. Intense efforts are now underway to develop an effective vaccine.

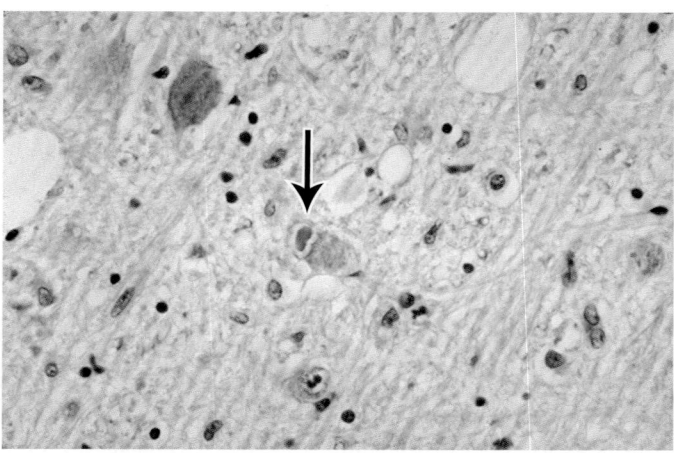

FIGURE 32-60. Subacute sclerosing panencephalitis. The brain shows loss of myelin and reactive gliosis. An intranuclear inclusion is present (*arrow*).

 PATHOLOGY: Lesions in the several arbovirus encephalitides resemble each other and vary from mild meningitis with scattered lymphocytes to severe inflammation of gray matter, thrombosis of small blood vessels, and prominent necrosis. No inclusions are seen in infected neurons. Neuronophagia is evident in necrotic foci, and if the patient survives, demyelination and gliosis may develop. West Nile encephalitis has a tropism for the spinal cord and may produce a syndrome clinically indistinguishable from classical poliomyelitis.

 CLINICAL FEATURES: Arthropod-borne encephalitides share many features, but each has a different course. For example, Eastern equine encephalitis is often a fulminant potentially lethal disease, but Venezuelan equine encephalitis tends to pursue a more benign course. Mild cases of arbovirus encephalitis may entail only a mild flu-like syndrome and not be diagnosed as encephalitis. In more severe cases, onset is abrupt, often with high fever, headache, vomiting and meningeal signs, followed by lethargy and coma. Death is more likely at the extremes of age, and those who survive may be left with cognitive impairment and recurrent seizures.

Subacute Sclerosing Panencephalitis

PATHOLOGY: SSPE is a consequence of infection with the measles virus, and most patients have a history of measles. It develops 6 to 8 years after the initial infection and is caused by a measles virus with defective expression of viral M (Matrix) protein. Nuclear inclusions occur in neurons and oligodendroglia, and marked gliosis affects gray and white matter, accompanied by patchy loss of myelin and ubiquitous perivascular lymphocytes and macrophages (Fig. 32-60). The intranuclear inclusions are basophilic, rimmed by a prominent halo. Affected neurons may have NFTs.

CLINICAL FEATURES: SSPE is a chronic, lethal, viral infection of the brain caused by measles virus. First recognized in 1933 as "subacute inclusion-body encephalitis," SSPE has an insidious onset, mainly in childhood, with cognitive and behavioral decline over months to years, ultimately leading to death.

The CSF typically has increased antibody to measles virus. The course is protracted, and inflammation occurs mainly in cerebral gray matter. In adults, SSPE may follow a more rapid course. SSPE is re-emerging as an infectious threat due to poorly informed failure of some to vaccinate their children.

Progressive Multifocal Leukoencephalopathy

PML is an increasingly common infectious demyelinating disease caused by a ubiquitous polyoma virus that infects oligodendrocytes and leads to cytolysis and patchy multifocal demyelination. Astrocytes are also infected, but instead of dying, they show extreme pleomorphism.

ETIOLOGIC FACTORS: JC virus is a polyoma virus, closely related to simian virus 40 (SV40). The "JC" derives from the initials of the first patient in whom the disease was described. Over 50% of people harbor JC virus, which resides in a latent state in the bone marrow after asymptomatic acquisition earlier in life. If the host becomes immunosuppressed, viremia ensues with specific neurovirulent viral strains.

CLINICAL FEATURES: PML occurs mostly in immunocompromised patients and manifests as dementia, weakness, visual loss, and ataxia, usually leading to death within 6 months. It is a terminal complication in immunosuppressed patients, such as those treated for cancer or lupus erythematosus, organ transplant recipients and especially people with AIDS. It may be a complication of drugs that inhibit T-cell adherence to endothelial cells as a treatment of immunologic disorders. One such drug, natalizumab, was temporarily withdrawn from the market after the appearance of PML in patients treated for MS or Crohn disease. It has been reintroduced to clinical use with stringent guidelines.

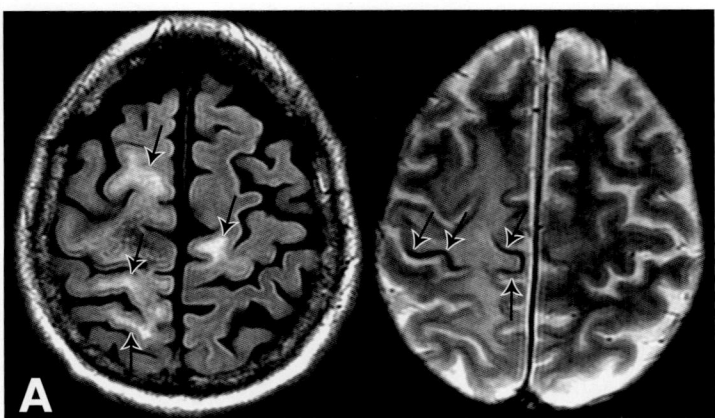
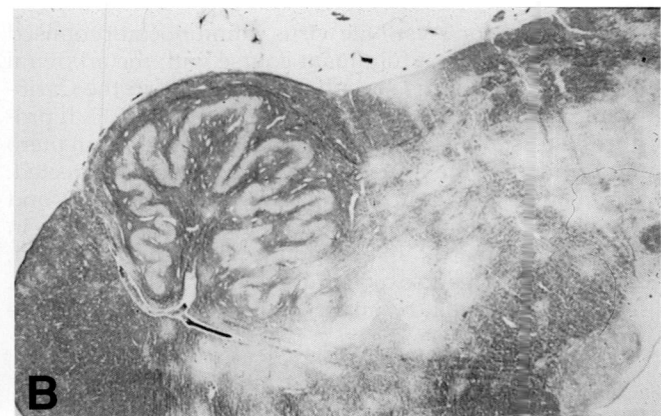

FIGURE 32-61. Progressive multifocal leukoencephalopathy. A. A T2-FLAIR (fluid attenuation inversion recovery) magnetic resonance imaging sequence shows patchy white matter hyperintensity (left panel, *arrows*), and a T2-GRE (gradient echo) sequence shows characteristic (although not pathognomonic) band-like gyriform hypointensity in the subcortical U-fiber region of the white matter (right panel, *arrows*). **B.** Luxol fast blue stain of the medulla reveals severe patchy loss of myelin.

PATHOLOGY: Typical lesions of PML appear as discrete widely scattered foci of demyelination near the gray–white junction in the cerebral hemispheres and brainstem (Fig. 32-61). They are several millimeters in diameter and spherical, with a central area largely devoid of myelin. Axons are retained, a few oligodendrocytes are seen and the lesion is infiltrated by macrophages. At the edges of the demyelinated areas, oligodendrocytes are seen with enlarged nuclei occupied by homogeneously dense, hyperchromatic, "ground-glass" intranuclear inclusions lacking a halo. Electron microscopy reveals crystalline intranuclear arrays of spherical 35- to 40-nm virions (Fig. 32-62). Infected astrocytes are highly pleomorphic, often with multiple irregular dark nuclei (Fig. 32-63) that may be confused as showing malignancy.

HIV

CNS disease is common in AIDS. Some patients have opportunistic CNS infections, such as toxoplasmosis, cytomegalovirus, herpes simplex or PML, or have EBV-driven primary CNS lymphoma (PCNSL). Cryptococcal meningitis is the most common fungal meningitis in AIDS patients, toxoplasmosis is the most common intracranial mass and PCNSL is the most common neoplasm. These are sentinels of AIDS; that is, any of these occurring in any patient should trigger diagnostic consideration of underlying AIDS. Many other opportunistic nervous system infections can occur in AIDS, and it is important to remember that the clinical presentation may be more fulminant or atypical than in immunocompetent individuals.

HIV Encephalopathy

Many AIDS patients have diffuse encephalopathy directly attributable to active CNS infection by HIV-1 retrovirus itself. This is variously called HIV encephalopathy (HIVE) or HIV-associated neurologic disease (HAND). Dementia was once the most common clinical manifestation of HIVE. It varies from mild to severe cognitive impairment with striking slowness of thought (bradyphrenia), often with marked bradykinesis mimicking Parkinson disease. CNS

FIGURE 32-62. Progressive multifocal leukoencephalopathy. An immunohistochemical stain for JC virus (*brown signal*) demonstrates numerous infected oligodendroglia in the white matter. Electron microscopy shows intranuclear paracrystalline arrays of viral particles (*insets*).

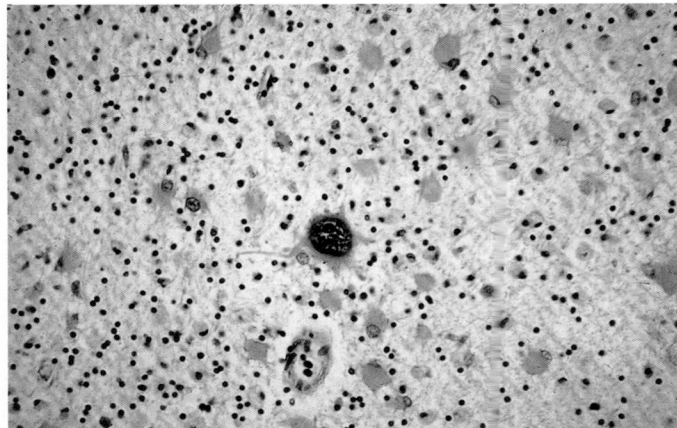

FIGURE 32-63. Progressive multifocal leukoencephalopathy (PML). This bizarre astrocyte (*center*) may suggest neoplasia but the presence of macrophages and ground-glass inclusions directs diagnostic consideration away from neoplasia and toward PML.

macrophages and microglial cells are productively infected by HIV-1. Infection of neurons and astrocytes is probably not clinically significant, but these cells are injured indirectly by neurotoxic viral proteins produced by infected cells or various cytokines, which cause oxidant-mediated cell injury.

The advent of highly active antiretroviral therapy (HAART) has dramatically extended the life span and quality of life of AIDS patients, including reducing opportunistic infections and primary CNS lymphoma. HAART drugs largely do not cross the BBB, and since the virus enters the CNS via infected blood monocytes soon after it enters the body, HAART has not altered the incidence of HAND. Rather, although frank dementia has become less common, a combination of sensory, motor, and other defects causing minor cognitive motor disease (MCMD) affects as many as 30% of HIV-1–positive patients. As these people age, this prevalence increases each year by an additional approximately 5% of the HIV-1–positive population. Initiation of HAART may also be complicated by immune reconstitution inflammatory syndrome (IRIS). In this syndrome, as the immune system recovers it mounts an overwhelming inflammatory response to an existing opportunistic infection. IRIS may lead to potentially lethal cerebral edema and exacerbation of focal symptoms and contribute to fulminant HIV encephalopathy.

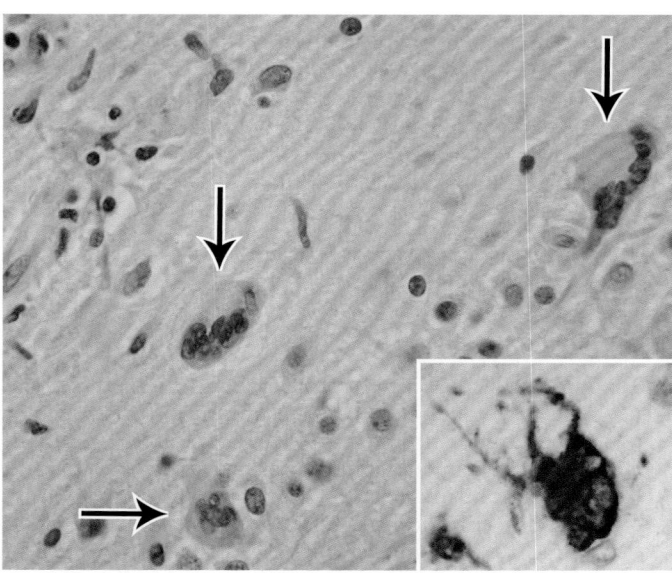

FIGURE 32-64. HIV encephalitis or encephalopathy (HIVE). Multinucleated giant cells (*arrows*) often in a perivascular location are characteristic of HIV encephalitis. *Inset.* Immunohistochemical stain for HIV anti-p24.

PATHOLOGY: HAND is characterized by mild cerebral atrophy, dilation of the lateral ventricles and slight prominence of gyri and sulci. Histologic changes are usually seen in subcortical gray and white matter. Multinucleated giant cells of monocyte/ macrophage lineage are associated with microglial nodules (Fig. 32-64). Myelin pallor, reflecting diffuse demyelination, intense astrogliosis, and loss of neurons are also common (Fig. 32-65).

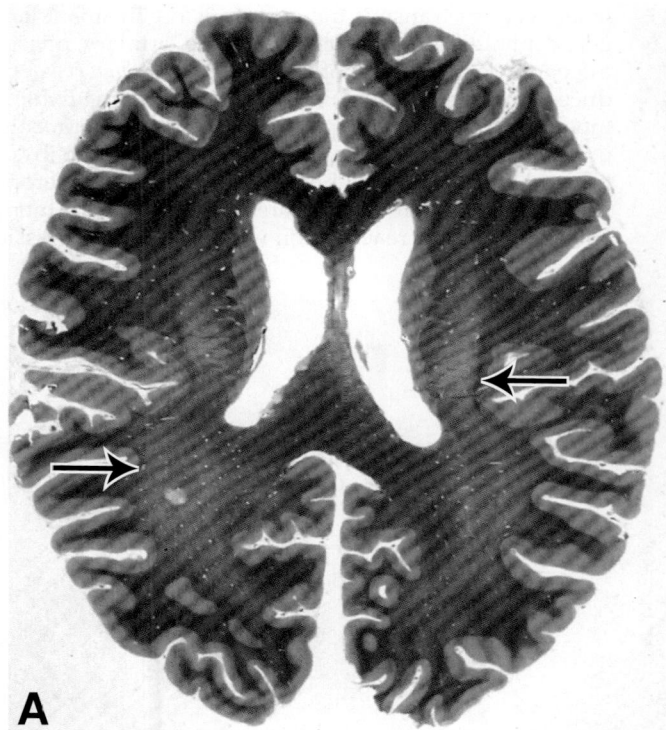

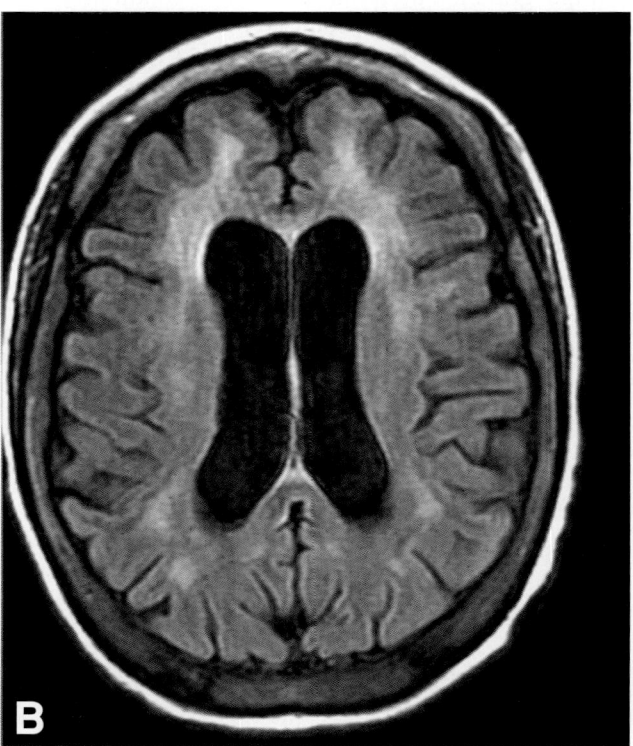

FIGURE 32-65. HIV encephalitis or encephalopathy (HIVE). A. An axial whole brain section in HIVE shows symmetric myelin pallor (*arrows*) caused by HIV-1. Demyelination caused by progressive multifocal leukoencephalopathy (PML) is less symmetric and has a patchy distribution. (Courtesy of Dr. F. Stephen Vogel, Duke University.) **B.** Axial magnetic resonance image shows bilateral white matter signal abnormalities in HIVE. The primary differential diagnosis is HIVE versus PML.

Vacuolar myelopathy is another disorder attributed to HIV infection, although it is less frequent than encephalopathy. It is characterized by marked vacuolation of the posterior and lateral columns, principally in the thoracic spinal cord. Ataxia and spastic paraparesis dominate the clinical presentation.

Protozoan and Metazoan Parasites Can Infect the CNS

Protozoan Infections

- **Toxoplasma** is a ubiquitous protozoan to which most of us have developed protective immunity. Immunocompromised patients lose the ability to contain these organisms. In toxoplasmosis, small comma-like tachyzoites and large polyorganismal cysts (bradyzoites) are seen in association with chronic inflammation, tissue necrosis, and vasculitis. Toxoplasmosis is the most common cause of multiple intracranial masses in AIDS patients (Fig. 32-66).
- *Naegleria* **spp.,** especially *Naegleria fowleri,* cause primary amebic meningoencephalitis, a fulminant and rapidly fatal disease with diffuse brain swelling. The amebae infect the nasal cavities of people who swim in warm stagnant freshwater ponds or who irrigate their sinus passages with inadequately decontaminated water. They enter the brain by migrating up the olfactory bulb, through the cribriform plate. *Naegleria* trophozoites resemble macrophages (Fig. 32-67).
- *Acanthamoeba* produces granulomatous amoebic encephalitis, a subacute, usually fatal illness characterized by multiple granulomatous abscesses. This condition is usually seen in immunocompromised hosts.
- *Entamoeba histolytica* leads to amebic brain abscess by spread from a gastrointestinal or hepatic locus. Amebae in tissue sections can be difficult to distinguish from foamy macrophages.
- **CNS malaria** is most commonly caused by *Plasmodium falciparum.* During attacks of cerebral malaria, the CSF shows elevated protein levels and pressure but pleocytosis is uncommon. In fatal cases, the brain is diffusely

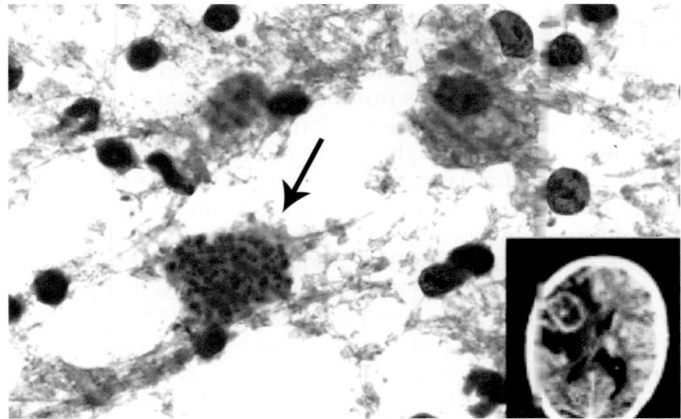

FIGURE 32-66. Toxoplasmosis in an HIV patient. Imaging studies in a previously asymptomatic patient showed an irregularly enhancing mass with surrounding edema (*inset*) that was initially thought to be a high-grade neoplasm. However, microscopic analysis showed *Toxoplasma gondii* bradyzoites (*arrow*) in a necrotic inflammatory background. Toxoplasmosis is the most common mass lesion in patients with AIDS and is an indicator disease of HIV infection.

swollen but may be otherwise unremarkable. However, it can show microinfarcts with gliosis (Dürck granulomata) in white matter or many small hemorrhages. Infarcts and microhemorrhages may arise from obstruction of blood flow in small vessels by parasitemia. Severity of cerebral malaria is also related to release of tumor necrosis factor-α by host cells.

- **Trypanosomal** infections include African sleeping sickness and American trypanosomiasis **(Chagas disease)**. Insect vectors transmit the infectious organisms. Meningoencephalitis may occur during the primary phase of infection. Reactivation of latent *Trypanosoma cruzi* produces multiple necrotic CNS lesions resembling toxoplasmosis. This occurs in people with AIDS and other forms of immunosuppression. Chagas disease is endemic in Central and South America, but 300,000 to 1,000,000 seropositive immigrants from those areas live in North America, and are at risk for reactivation with immunosuppression.

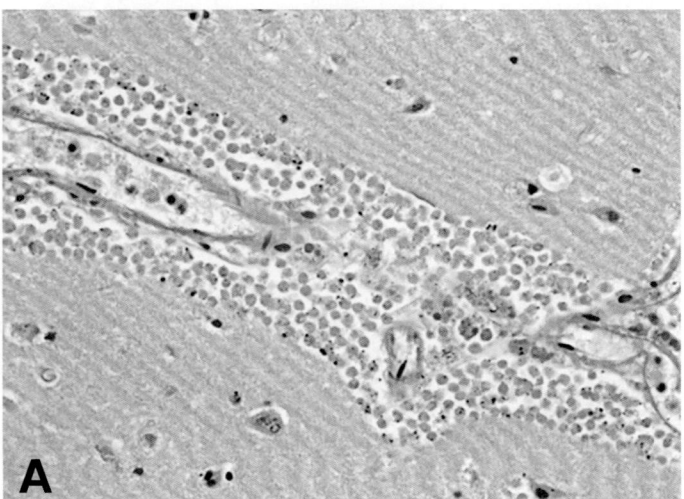

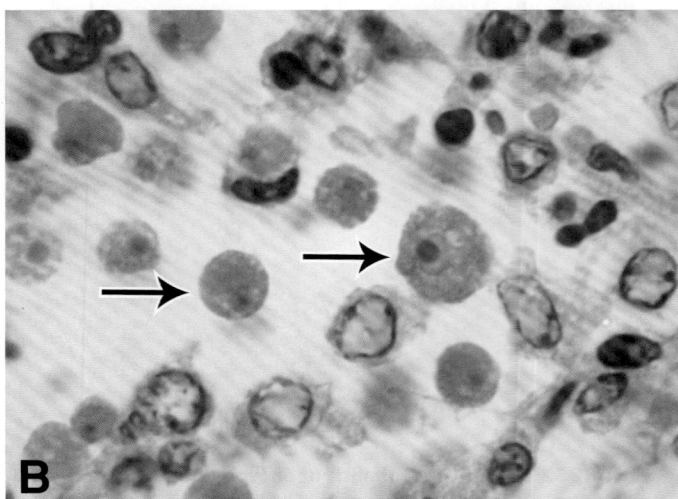

FIGURE 32-67. *Naegleria* **meningoencephalitis. A.** Abundant perivascular amebae are seen. **B.** Amebic organisms (*arrows*) resemble macrophages but have much more prominent nucleoli.

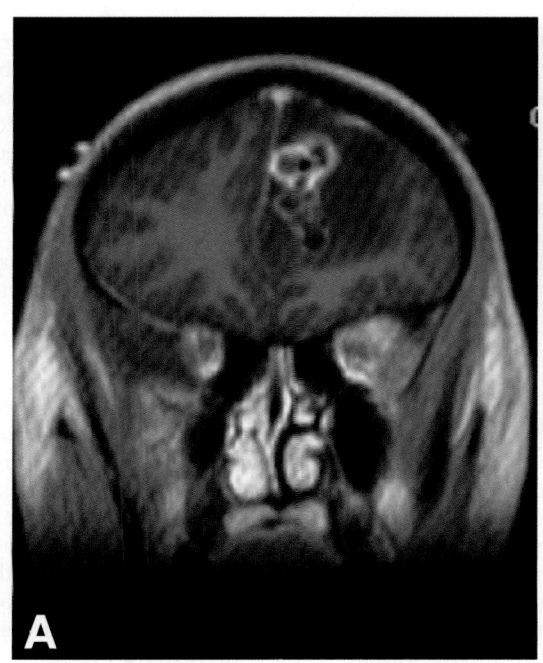

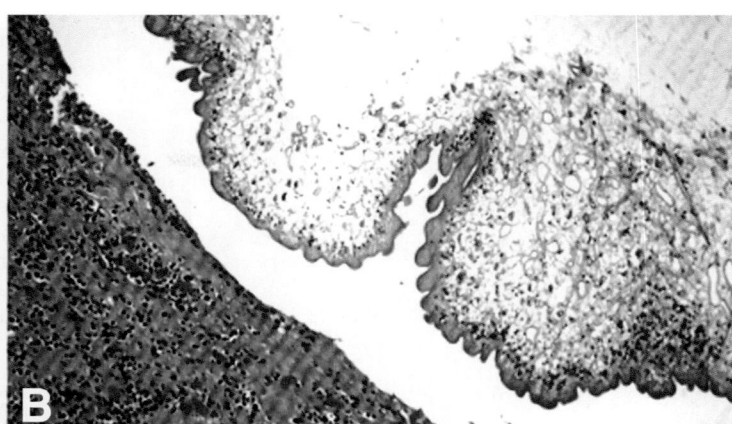

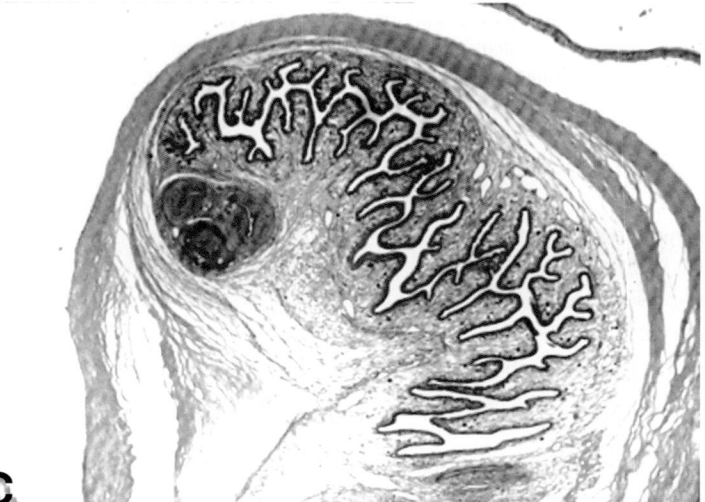

FIGURE 32-68. Neurocysticercosis. A. As seen radiographically, brain involvement by *Taenia solium* may result in solitary or multiple contrast-enhancing masses with surrounding edema. **B.** As seen microscopically, the cyst has a corrugated cuticular surface that interfaces with the adjacent brain, which has become inflamed as the parasites die and are detected by the host immune response. At this point, lesions may be symptomatic. **C.** At low magnification, a worm scolex can be seen in the gastrointestinal tract.

Since Chagas disease can be transmitted via blood transfusion, blood is now screened for this infection.

Metazoan Infections of the Nervous System

■ **Cysticercosis** is caused by infection with *Taenia solium*, the pig tapeworm. It can produce multiple parasitic cysts up to 1 cm in diameter involving the parenchyma, ventricles, or basal cisterns. Intraparenchymal disease usually becomes symptomatic when organisms die and are recognized immunologically by the host (Fig. 32-68). A peculiar form of this infection is extraparenchymal (racemose) neurocysticercosis, in which grape-like clusters and sheets of worm tissues are produced in the CSF without developed fully formed worms. Racemose cysticercosis is essentially invertebrate tissue culture in the CSF and it is resistant to therapy that is otherwise effective against intact parasites. Treatment of neurocysticercosis may lead to massive cerebral edema caused by host immune responses to the suddenly necrotic metazoan tissue. From a global health perspective, neurocysticercosis is one of the most common causes of epilepsy and intracranial mass lesions.
■ **Echinococcosis** results from *Taenia echinococcus* or *Echinococcus granulosus,* the dog tapeworm. It produces cerebral cysts that are usually solitary and may be huge, in contrast to the smaller multiple cysts of cysticercosis. The brain lesion is frequently accompanied by hepatic cysts.

■ **Trichinosis** is caused by *Trichinella spiralis* infection of skeletal and cardiac muscle, producing an acute eosinophilic myositis during the invasive phase. Larvae may then die and calcify, producing fibrosis and low-grade inflammation. The infection rarely encroaches on the CNS where it can produce lymphocytic-eosinophilic meningitis.

Prion Diseases (Spongiform Encephalopathies) Are Transmissible Neurodegenerative Diseases Caused by Modified Protein Particles

Prion diseases are characterized clinically by rapidly progressive ataxia and dementia and pathologically by accumulations of fibrillar or insoluble prion proteins, neuronal degeneration and vacuolization called **spongiform encephalopathy** (Fig. 32-69). The spongiform encephalopathies are biologically remarkable because the causative infectious agents, called **prions**, are proteinaceous particles and lack nucleic acids.

EPIDEMIOLOGY: The classic spongiform encephalopathies in humans include kuru, Creutzfeldt–Jakob disease (CJD), Gerstmann–Sträussler–Scheinker syndrome (GSS), and fatal familial insomnia (Table 32-2). Similar diseases occur in animals,

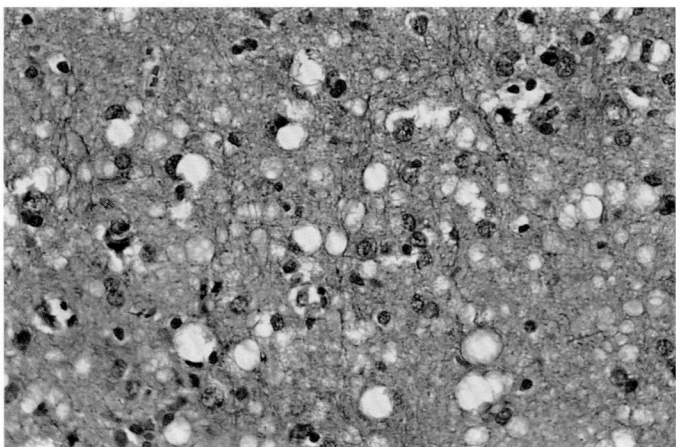

FIGURE 32-69. Creutzfeldt–Jakob disease. Spongiform degeneration of the gray matter is characterized by individual and clustered vacuoles, with no evidence of inflammation. (Courtesy of Dr. F. Stephen Vogel, Duke University.)

TABLE 32-2
PRION DISEASES

I. Human

A. Creutzfeldt–Jakob disease (CJD)

   1. Sporadic (85% of all CJD cases; incidence 1 per million worldwide)

   2. Inherited mutation of the prion gene, autosomal dominant transmission (15% of all CJD cases)

   3. Iatrogenic

      a. Hormone injection: human growth hormone, human pituitary gonadotropin

      b. Tissue grafts: dura mater, cornea, pericardium

      c. Medical devices: depth electrodes, surgical instruments (none definitely proven)

   4. New variant CJD (vCJD)

B. Gerstmann–Sträussler–Scheinker disease (GSS; inherited prion gene mutation, autosomal dominant transmission)

C. Fatal familial insomnia (FFI; inherited prion gene mutation, autosomal dominant transmission)

D. Kuru (confined to the Fore people of Papua New Guinea, formerly transmitted by cannibalistic funeral ritual)

II. Animal

A. Scrapie (sheep and goats)

B. Bovine spongiform encephalopathy (BSE; "mad cow disease")

C. Transmissible mink encephalopathy

D. Feline spongiform encephalopathy

E. Captive exotic ungulate spongiform encephalopathy (nyala, gemsbok, eland, Arabian oryx, greater kudu)

F. Chronic wasting disease of deer and elk

G. Experimental transmission to many species, including primates and transgenic mice

including scrapie in sheep and goats, bovine spongiform encephalopathy (BSE; mad cow disease), transmissible mink encephalopathy, and chronic wasting disease in mule deer and elk. BSE is of particular interest because it resulted from inadvertent introduction of prion-contaminated feed to cattle, thus establishing that prions can be transmitted by the oral route. BSE is also more easily transmitted and does not show the species selectivity of other prions. It decimated the cattle industry in the United Kingdom and spread to other regions of the world and to other species including zoo animals, pets, and humans.

MOLECULAR PATHOGENESIS: The signal molecular event in prion disorders is conversion of a native α-helix–rich protein into a pathogenic β-sheet–rich isoform that tends to polymerize with subsequent fibril formation (Figs. 32-70 and 32-71). Uniquely, conversion of the native protein to the pathogenic form is autocatalyzed by the pathogenic form itself. Thus, the pathogenic protein begets more pathogenic protein from the limitless supply of native protein! The native protein is produced by a human prion gene (*PRNP*) on the short arm of chromosome 20, which contains a single exon encoding 254 amino acid residues. The normal prion gene product, prion protein (PrP), is a constitutively expressed cell surface glycoprotein that attaches to the neuronal plasmalemma via a glycolipid anchor. PrP is made widely throughout the body, but the highest levels of PrP messenger RNA are in CNS neurons. Its function is unknown and prion-null mice have no apparent phenotype. Normal cellular prion protein, cellular PrP or PrP^C, and pathogenic (infectious) prion protein, known as scrapie PrP or PrP^{SC}, have the same primary amino acid sequence but different secondary structures and patterns of glycosylation. Specifically, PrP^C is rich in α-helix configuration, but the β-pleated sheet configuration predominates in PrP^{SC}. The pathogenic conformation is extremely stable so that PrP^{SC} strongly resists conventional microbial decontamination methods. It is also highly resistant to proteases. If PrP^{SC} enters the brain either through infectious transmission or by spontaneous misfolding of native protein, it will convert other PrP^C proteins into pathogenic PrP^{SC}, leading to autocatalytic, exponentially expanding accretion of abnormal PrP^{SC} (Fig. 32-70). Masses of PrP^{SC}

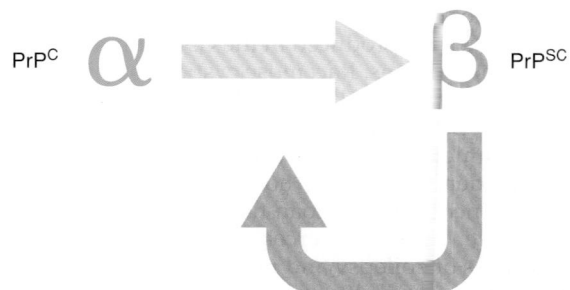

FIGURE 32-70. Creutzfeldt–Jakob disease. The unique mode of "reproduction" by prions is autocatalytic conversion of native α-helix–rich cellular prion protein into a β-sheet–rich pathogenic form that has a strong tendency toward aggregation.

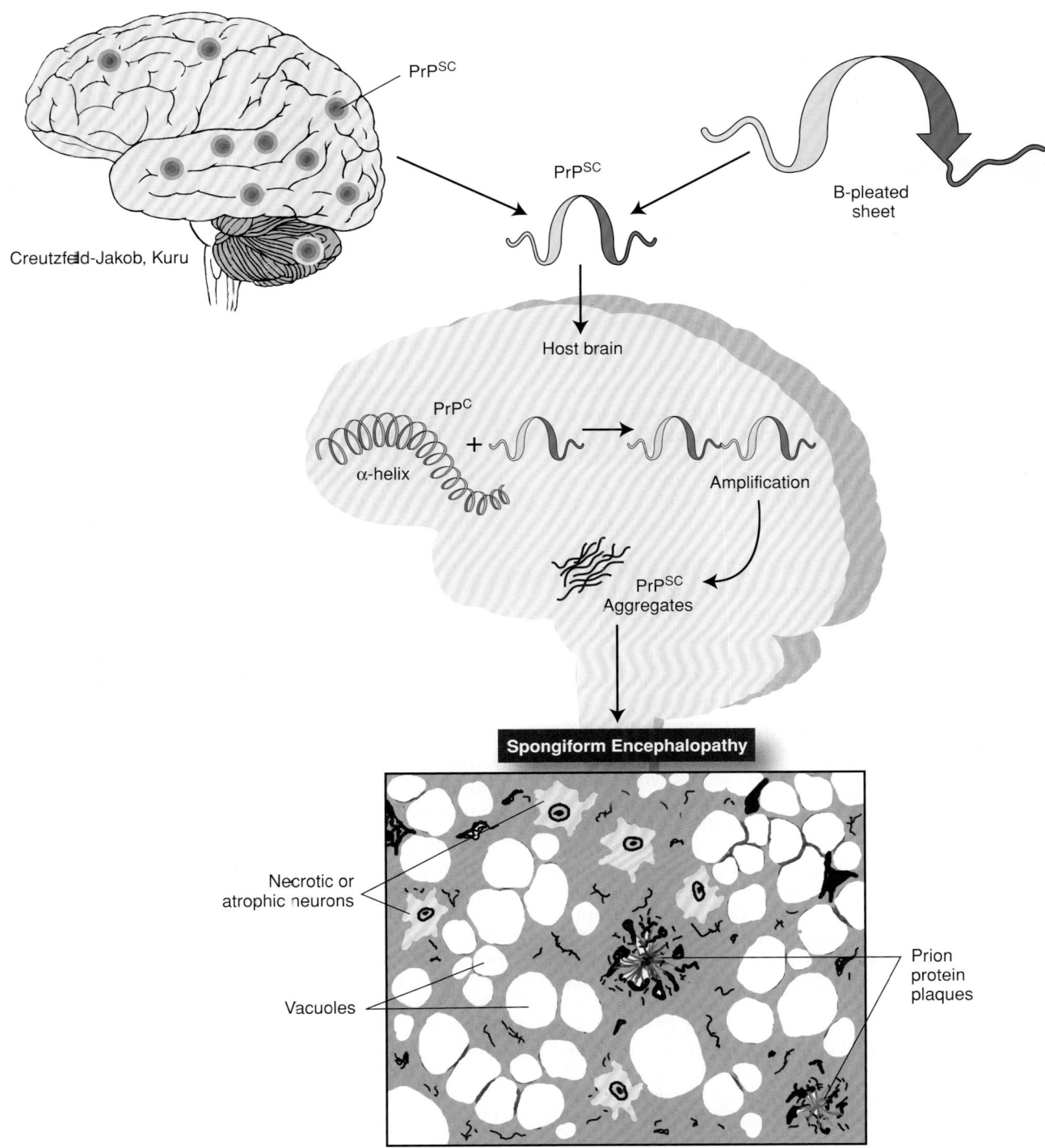

FIGURE 32-71. Molecular pathogenesis of prion disorders.

compromise cell function and cause neurodegeneration by mechanisms that remain to be elucidated but may be similar to those of other neurodegenerative diseases characterized by fibrillogenesis (Fig. 32-71).

All spongiform encephalopathies are transmissible, and inadvertent human transmission of CJD may follow administration of contaminated human pituitary growth hormone, corneal transplantation from a diseased donor,

poorly sterilized neurosurgical instruments, and surgical implantation of contaminated dura (Table 32-2).

PATHOLOGY: Prion diseases entail neuron degeneration, gliosis, spongiform degeneration, and accumulations of insoluble prions forming extracellular plaques. Many small, clear, often confluent microcysts occur in the neuropil (Figs. 32-69 and 32-71). Lesions develop mostly in cortical gray matter but also involve deeper nuclei of the basal ganglia, thalamus, hypothalamus, and cerebellum.

CLINICAL FEATURES: The several human prion diseases are distinct.

KURU: In 1956, a medical officer in New Guinea provided an account of kuru, a progressive, fatal neurologic disorder, in members of the isolated Fore tribe. The disease takes its name from the word "trembling" in their language. Transmission of kuru was linked to ritualistic funereal cannibalism in which women and children ate brains of deceased relatives.

Kuru was the first human prion disease shown to be transmissible. It attained epidemic proportions in the Fore people but was eliminated when cannibalism ceased. The initial and most prominent clinical feature of kuru is ataxia of the limbs and trunk, due to severe cerebellar involvement. In 70% of cases, insoluble, fibrillar prion proteins accumulate extracellularly in plaques. Spongiform change is present in both the cerebral hemispheres and cerebellum.

CREUTZFELDT–JAKOB DISEASE: CJD is the most common form of spongiform encephalopathy. Symptoms begin insidiously, but patients usually exhibit severe dementia leading to death within 6 months to 3 years. Cerebellar involvement produces ataxia, which helps to distinguish CJD from Alzheimer disease. Myoclonus often occurs for some weeks to months during the afflicted person's decline. Classification of CJD is based on etiology: sporadic, familial, iatrogenic, and new variant:

- **Sporadic CJD:** The sporadic form occurs worldwide, with an incidence of 1 per million, and accounts for 75% of CJD cases. The mode of acquisition is unknown; patients do not have the mutations associated with inherited forms of CJD or other prion diseases, and there is no history of iatrogenic exposure. A polymorphism in *PRNP* codon 129 confers differential susceptibility to CJD: homozygosity for either methionine (M) or valine (V) at this codon leads to disproportionate susceptibility to prion disorders, while heterozygotes (M/V) are resistant. Codon frequencies in the white population are 51% M/V, 37% M/M, and 12% V/V.
- **Inherited CJD: Familial CJD** accounts for 15% of prion diseases, with an incidence of 1 in 10 million. Several different *PRNP* mutations have been documented in various kindreds. In such cases, PrP^C has a greater tendency to misfold into the pathogenic isoform. Mutant forms of *PRNP* cause familial CJD, fatal familial insomnia, and Gerstmann–Sträussler–Scheinker disease.
- **Iatrogenic CJD:** As listed in Table 32-2, several iatrogenic causes of CJD are known, but most causes for iatrogenic CJD now have been eliminated. This has been achieved, for example, by replacing cadaveric human pituitary-derived preparations with recombinant human growth hormone for therapy. When brain biopsies or autopsies are done in prion disease cases, special protocols are used to limit exposure of staff and patients to prions. Disposable instruments are used if possible, and surfaces and instruments are treated with

concentrated NaOH. Conventional autoclaving and most standard disinfectants do not eradicate this hardy infectious agent.

- **New variant CJD (vCJD or nvCJD):** This form was identified by a surveillance program in the United Kingdom after the BSE epidemic (see above) between 1980 and 1996. A group of patients was identified that differed from other patients with sporadic CJD in several key characteristics, most importantly, age. The mean age at onset of symptoms for sporadic CJD is 65, but for vCJD it is 26. Also, vCJD patients had a longer duration of illness (median, 12 months vs. 4 months) and an atypical clinical presentation, including various behavioral changes or sensory disturbances (dysesthesias) and none of the usual electroencephalographic (EEG) findings of sporadic CJD. At autopsy, vCJD is characterized by prominent spongiform change in the basal ganglia and thalamus, and extensive PrP plaques in the cerebrum and cerebellum. The plaques are distinctive in that they resemble those of kuru. Finally, brains from vCJD patients contain much more PrP than brains of sporadic CJD patients. Physicochemical analysis showed that vCJD PrP^{SC} differed from CJD PrP^{SC}, but was similar to prions in BSE that were transmitted to mice and primates. Thus, BSE is considered to be the source of nvCJD. Current evidence suggests that vCJD cases have peaked and are declining. Essentially all vCJD cases occurred in codon 129 homozygotes (who are more susceptible), and a recent case in a heterozygote raises the unsettling specter of a longer incubation type of vCJD in this population. In addition, retrospective examination of surgical specimens of tonsils and appendices in the United Kingdom using PrP^{SC} has shown a significant number of asymptomatic individuals with pathogenic PrP that may become the nidus of a new epidemic of vCJD.

With globalization and diversification of economies, cultures, and populations, a global perspective is essential in considering infectious diseases. New disorders can emerge and disseminate rapidly. Many of these infections have an impact on the nervous system, as we have seen with HIV and H1N1 influenza. Ease of movement leads to infections previously thought of as exotic or tropic occurring unexpectedly in industrialized countries. Larger populations rendered immunocompromised due to HIV, cancer or immunosuppressive therapies provide fertile grounds for clinically atypical neurologic infectious disease. Finally, there is the ever present danger of manmade biologic agents being deployed.

DEMYELINATING DISEASES

Demyelinating diseases disrupt the myelin economy. This may involve flawed manufacture **(dysmyelination),** destruction of myelin **(demyelination),** or disruption of myelin metabolism **(leukodystrophies).** Central myelin is made by oligodendrocytes, while peripheral myelin is made by Schwann cells (see Chapter 31). These two types of myelin differ biochemically. Operationally, the border between the CNS and the peripheral nervous system can be considered as the point of transition between myelin made by oligodendrocytes and that made by Schwann cells. This transition usually occurs about 2 to 3 mm after a cranial nerve or spinal root exits the brainstem or spinal cord. Myelin disorders affect central or peripheral myelin, or both.

Multiple Sclerosis Is the Most Common Demyelinating Disease

EPIDEMIOLOGY: MS is a chronic demyelinating disease. With a prevalence of 1 per 1,000, it is the most common chronic CNS disease of young adults in the United States. It is characterized by exacerbations and remissions over many years. It becomes symptomatic at a mean age of 30, and women are afflicted almost twice as often as men.

MOLECULAR PATHOGENESIS: The etiology of MS remains incompletely understood, but genetic predisposition and immune dysfunction are probably involved. MS is mainly a disease of temperate climates. People who emigrate before age 15 from areas with a low prevalence to more temperate endemic areas assume the increased risk associated with their destinations, suggesting that environmental factors are important.

The disease tends to aggregate in families, with increased risk in second- and third-degree relatives of MS patients and 25% concordance for MS in monozygotic twins. Susceptibility is also linked to certain major histocompatibility complex (MHC) alleles (e.g., human leukocyte antigen [HLA]-DR2), implying that immune mechanisms are involved in the pathogenesis.

The microscopic appearance of MS lesions also suggests immune involvement. For example, chronic lesions show perivascular lymphocytes, macrophages and many CD4+ as well as CD8+ T cells (see Chapters 4 and 11). Moreover, CD4+ T cells in the CSF of MS patients tend to be oligoclonal. Although no target antigen has been identified, the data suggest an immune response to a specific CNS protein. Further support for immune mechanisms comes from an experimental antigen-specific, T-cell–

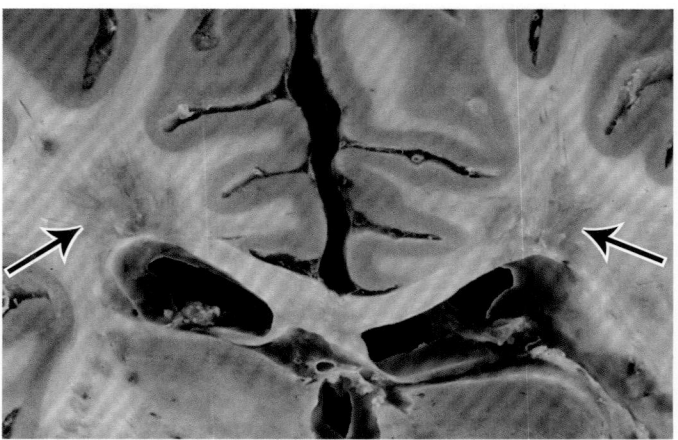

FIGURE 32-73. Multiple sclerosis. This fresh coronal section shows darker hues of the somewhat irregular periventricular plaques (*arrows*) reflecting loss of myelin, which normally imparts a glistening white appearance to white matter.

mediated, autoimmune disease, **experimental allergic encephalitis (EAE)**. Injecting myelin basic protein into animals, including nonhuman primates, elicits a demyelinating disorder similar to MS. However, unlike MS, EAE is a monophasic illness.

Although an assortment of viruses have been implicated in the etiology of MS, to date there is no compelling evidence for the involvement of any infectious agent.

PATHOLOGY: The demyelinated plaque is the pathologic hallmark of MS (Figs. 32-72 and 32-73). Plaques, rarely more than 2 cm across, accumulate in great numbers in the brain and spinal cord (Fig. 32-74). They are discrete, with smoothly rounded contours. They usually arise in white matter, although they may breach the gray matter. They preferentially affect the optic nerves, chiasm, paraventricular white matter, and spinal cord, but any part of the CNS may be involved.

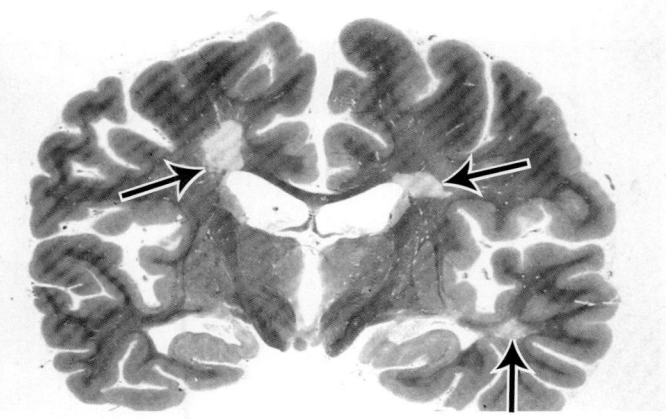

FIGURE 32-72. Multiple sclerosis. This myelin-stained coronal section of the brain of a patient with long-standing multiple sclerosis shows many discrete areas of myelin loss—plaques (*arrows*)—with characteristic periventricular demyelination especially prominent at the superior angles of the lateral ventricles. (Courtesy of Dr. F. Stephen Vogel, Duke University.)

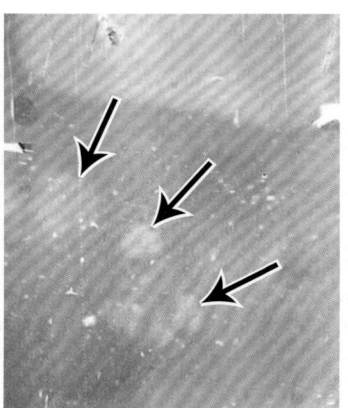

FIGURE 32-74. Multiple sclerosis. Subcortical white matter of a patient with multiple sclerosis shows multiple small irregular, partially confluent areas of demyelination (*arrows*). Normal intact myelin is blue in this Luxol fast blue–stained section.

Evolving plaques are marked by selective loss of myelin in regions of relative axonal preservation, lymphocytes clustering about small veins and arteries, influx of macrophages, and considerable edema.

Neuronal bodies within plaques are remarkably spared, but axons may degenerate. Numbers of oligodendrocytes are moderately decreased. As plaques age, they become more discrete and less edematous. This sequence emphasizes the focal nature of the injury and its selectivity and severity, as demyelination is total within a plaque. Axons within plaques usually lose their myelin abruptly. Old MS plaques are dense and gliotic.

CLINICAL FEATURES: MS usually begins in the third or fourth decade, after which patients experience abrupt episodes of disease progression, separated by periods of relative stability. The essential clinical criterion for MS is dissemination of lesions in space and time; that is, multiple separate areas of the CNS must be affected at differing times. Our understanding of disease activity in MS has been revolutionized by use of serial MRI studies, which show ongoing disease activity despite apparent clinical quiescence. New plaques emerge and regress, only occasionally causing clinical manifestations. Contemporary diagnostic criteria for MS strongly incorporate periodic imaging to visualize plaques scattered in space and time. Such imaging studies have taught us that MS is an ongoing active process even between clinical exacerbations. The therapeutic priority is now suppression of ongoing disease activity using a variety of immune system modulators and evidence of MRI efficacy as an endpoint in drug trials and clinical management. Neuropathologic studies have confirmed increased inflammatory activity in brains of MS patients between exacerbations.

Many patients with MS pursue relapsing remitting clinical courses, but some suffer a relentless course without remissions. Each exacerbation reflects the formation of additional demyelinated MS plaques. MS typically begins with symptoms relating to lesions in the optic nerves, brainstem, or spinal cord. Blurred vision or loss of vision in one eye as a result of optic neuritis is often the presenting complaint. When the initial lesion is in the brainstem, double vision and vertigo occur. In particular, internuclear ophthalmoplegia, caused by disruption of the medial longitudinal fasciculus, strongly suggests demyelinating disease when it occurs in a young person. Acute demyelination within the spinal cord is called **transverse myelitis** and produces weakness of one or both legs and sensory symptoms in the form of numbness in the lower extremities. Many of the initial symptoms are partially reversible within a few months.

Despite the fact that most patients have a chronic relapsing and remitting course, neurologic deficits accumulate gradually and relentlessly. Even in relatively quiescent plaques, axonal attrition can lead to irreversible lesions. In established cases, the degree of functional impairment is highly variable, ranging from minor disability to severe incapacity, with widespread paralysis, dysarthria, ataxia, severe visual defects, incontinence, and dementia. Patients with severe disability usually die of respiratory paralysis or urinary tract infections. Most patients survive 20 to 30 years after the onset of symptoms.

Neuromyelitis Optica Is a Demyelinating Disease due to Auto-Antibodies to Water Channels

Neuromyelitis optica (NMO) is a demyelinating disorder with a striking predilection for the optic nerves and spinal cord. Once regarded as a variant of MS, NMO is now recognized as resulting from autoantibodies against a water channel protein, aquaporin 4, which is expressed by astrocytes. Thus, NMO is pathophysiologically distinct from MS and it responds poorly to conventional MS therapy. New treatments based on disrupting autoantibody binding are being evaluated.

Postinfectious and Postvaccinal Encephalomyelitis Are Immune Responses to Microbial Antigens

Rarely, some viral infections (e.g., measles, varicella, rubella) may be followed by an encephalomyelitis that emerges 3 to 21 days after infection. The disease entails focal perivascular demyelination and conspicuous mononuclear cell infiltrates around small to medium-sized venules in brain and spinal cord white matter. It is thought to be immune mediated, but its precise pathogenesis remains unclear. Onset of postinfectious encephalomyelitis is heralded by headache, vomiting, fever, and meningismus that may be followed by paraplegia, incontinence, and stupor. Up to 15% to 20% of patients die. A similar syndrome, **postvaccinal encephalomyelitis**, may follow immunization against infectious agents (e.g., smallpox, rabies) (Fig. 32-75). Use of more highly purified vaccines, free of cross-reacting antigenic contaminants, has dramatically reduced the frequency of this complication.

Chronic Lymphocytic Inflammation With Pontine Perivascular Enhancement Responsive to Steroids (CLIPPERS) Affects the Brainstem

CLIPPERS is a rare, newly described disorder involving brainstem and cerebellar T-cell–predominant inflammation and demyelination. Imaging studies show symmetric curvilinear gadolinium enhancement scattered throughout the pons and extending variably into the medulla, cerebellum, midbrain, and occasionally spinal cord. Radiographic and clinical improvement occur with high-dose corticosteroid

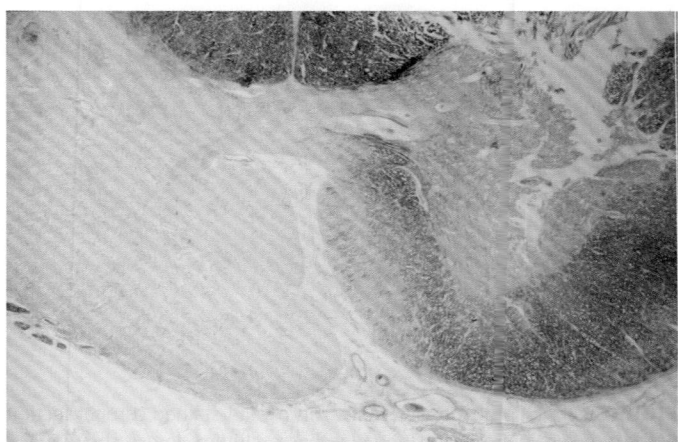

FIGURE 32-75. Post-vaccinal encephalomyelitis involving the spinal cord shows marked myelin loss in the lateral and anterior regions of the spinal cord on the left side.

therapy, but patients routinely worsen after steroids are tapered and often require chronic administration of steroids and/or other immunosuppressive therapy.

Leukodystrophies Are Inherited Defects of Myelin Biochemistry

These disorders often impact both central and peripheral myelin and usually manifest in infancy or childhood, although milder adult phenotypes may occur. Disruption of central myelin leads to blindness, spasticity, and loss of developmental milestones, while loss of peripheral myelin leads to weakness and loss of reflexes.

Metachromatic Leukodystrophy

Metachromatic leukodystrophy (MLD), the most common leukodystrophy, is an autosomal recessive disorder characterized by accumulation of a cerebroside (galactosyl sulfatide) in the white matter of the brain and peripheral nerves. MLD predominates in infancy, but rare juvenile or adult cases are described. It is lethal within several years. A clinical trial using gene-corrected bone marrow transplantation has shown promise in slowing MLD progression.

 PATHOPHYSIOLOGY: MLD is caused by deficiency in arylsulfatase A activity resulting in most cases from loss-of-function mutations in *ARSA*. Arylsulfatase A is a lysosomal enzyme involved in the degradation of myelin sulfatides. Accordingly, there is progressive accumulation of sulfatides within the lysosomes of myelin-forming Schwann cells and oligodendrocytes.

 PATHOLOGY: In MLD, accumulated sulfatides form spherical cytoplasmic granules, 15 to 20 µm in diameter, which stain metachromatically with cresyl violet and toluidine blue. Normal tissue staining is orthochromatic; that is, cresyl violet or toluidine blue stains tissue violet or blue. In metachromasia, polyanions (such as sulfatides) shift the dye color making tissue stained with cresyl violet or toluidine blue look rusty brown to red. The brain shows diffuse myelin loss, accumulation of metachromatic material in white matter and astrogliosis. Demyelination of peripheral nerves is less severe.

Krabbe Disease

Krabbe disease is a rapidly progressive, fatal, autosomal recessive neurologic disorder caused by mutations in the *GALC* gene leading to a deficiency in galactosylceramidase. This enzyme metabolizes galactolipids including galactosylceramide, which is an important component of myelin.

 PATHOLOGY: The brain is small, with widespread loss of myelin and preservation of the cerebral cortex. Astrogliosis is severe. Multinucleated "globoid cells" develop in the white matter and cluster around blood vessels, leading to the alternative

name, **globoid cell leukodystrophy**. The globoid cells are multinucleated macrophages full of undigested galactosylceramide. These cells are up to 50 µm in diameter, and contain up to 20 peripheral nuclei. In end-stage disease, numbers of globoid cells decline, and in areas of severe myelin loss, only scattered globoid cells remain. Marbled areas of partial and total demyelination are present. By electron microscopy, the globoid cells contain crystalloid-like inclusions with straight or tubular profiles.

 CLINICAL FEATURES: Krabbe disease appears in infancy and progresses to death within 1 to 2 years. Severe motor, sensory, and cognitive defects reflect diffuse involvement of the nervous system.

Adrenoleukodystrophy

 MOLECULAR PATHOGENESIS: Adrenoleukodystrophy (ALD) is an X-linked (Xq28) inherited disorder in which dysfunction of the adrenal cortex and nervous system demyelination are associated with high levels of saturated very-long-chain fatty acids (VLCFAs) in tissue and body fluids. The genetic defect involves mutations in *ABCD1*. This gene encodes the ALD protein, ALDP, which participates in transport of VLCFAs into peroxisomes. The resultant impairment in VLCFAs leads to abnormal accumulation of cholesterol esters and VLCFA toxicity.

 PATHOLOGY: The brain shows confluent, bilaterally symmetric demyelination. The most severe lesions occur in the subcortical white matter of the parieto-occipital region. They extend rostrally (while sparing cortex) and cause severe loss of myelinated axons and oligodendrocytes. Gliosis and perivascular infiltrates of mononuclear cells (mostly lymphocytes) are prominent in affected areas. Scattered macrophages contain periodic acid–Schiff (PAS)-positive and sudanophilic material composed of accumulated abnormal lipids. Peripheral nerves are affected, but to a lesser degree than the brain. High concentrations of VLCFAs are toxic to the adrenal cortex and the adrenal glands become atrophic. Electron microscopy of cortical cells shows pathognomonic cytoplasmic, membrane-bound, curvilinear inclusions, or clefts (lamellae) containing VLCFAs. Similar inclusions occur in Schwann cells and CNS macrophages.

 CLINICAL FEATURES: ALD occurs in children ages 3 to 10 years old, in whom neurologic symptoms precede signs of adrenal insufficiency. The disease progresses rapidly for 2 to 4 years, and the patient is quickly reduced to a vegetative state, which may persist for several years before death. Manipulation of dietary lipid composition and quantity using a 4:1 mixture of glycerol trioleate and glycerol trierucate ("Lorenzo's oil") reduces serum VLCFAs and slows progression of the disease in some cases. If the patient survives through childhood, the diet can be liberalized.

TOXIC AND METABOLIC DISORDERS

Given the enormous appetite of the brain for oxygen, glucose, amino acids, and other metabolic morsels, it is not surprising that it is liable to malfunction as a result of lack or misutilization of essential substances, intoxication, and hereditary metabolic diseases. These disorders are particularly important since correction of underlying metabolic derangements restores function. In most cases, dysfunction may be functionally profound but have no morphologic correlate; however, in some cases, pathologic changes occur.

Metabolic Storage Diseases Reflect Lack of Key Enzymes

Neuronal storage diseases are inherited enzyme defects in which normal metabolic products accumulate in lysosomes. Unlike leukodystrophies, which involve inherited enzyme defects in myelin metabolism (and produce blindness and spasticity), these diseases affect neurons and cause seizures and cognitive decline.

Tay–Sachs Disease

Tay–Sachs disease is a lethal, autosomal recessive disorder caused by mutations in the *HEXA* gene leading to deficiency of the lysosomal enzyme hexosaminidase A. This enzyme breaks down GM2 ganglioside, which accumulates in neurons to toxic levels. The disease is fatal in infancy and early childhood. Retinal involvement increases macular transparency and causes a **cherry-red spot** in the macula.

The brain is the major site of ganglioside storage, and it progressively enlarges in infancy. Lipid droplets in the cytoplasm distend CNS and peripheral neurons (Fig. 32-76A). Electron microscopy demonstrates the lipid within lysosomes as whorled "myelin figures" (Fig. 32-76B). The neural tissues develop diffuse astrogliosis. An affected infant appears normal at birth but by age 6 months shows delayed motor development. Thereafter, progressive deterioration leads to flaccid weakness, blindness, and severe intellectual impairment. Death usually supervenes before the end of the second year.

Hurler Syndrome

Hurler syndrome is an autosomal recessive disturbance in glycosaminoglycan metabolism caused by mutations in *IDUA* gene. The result is intraneuronal accumulation of mucopolysaccharides. Clinical variants of this syndrome are distinguished by variable involvement of visceral organs and the nervous system. The disease is typically expressed in infancy or early childhood as reduced stature, corneal opacities, skeletal deformities, and hepatosplenomegaly. Intraneuronal storage distends the cytoplasmic compartment and is accompanied by astrogliosis and progressive mental deterioration.

Gaucher Disease

Gaucher disease is an autosomal recessive genetic deficiency in which mutations in the *GBA* gene lead to deficiency of glucocerebrosidase and accumulation of glucocerebroside, principally in macrophages. The CNS is most severely involved in infantile (type II) Gaucher disease. Although intraneuronal accumulation of glucocerebroside is not conspicuous, neuronal loss is severe and is accompanied by diffuse astrogliosis. These infants fail to thrive and die at an early age.

Niemann–Pick Disease

Niemann–Pick disease is an autosomal recessive disorder in which inborn errors in the *SMPD1* gene result in deficiency of sphingomyelinase and intraneuronal storage of sphingomyelin. Symptoms occur early, with failure of the infant to develop and thrive. Mononuclear phagocytes throughout the body are the principle sites of storage, but symptoms related to the nervous system may predominate during infancy. The brain becomes atrophic, with marked astrogliosis. Retinal degeneration may produce a cherry-red spot, like that in Tay–Sachs disease.

Alexander Disease

Alexander disease is an astrocytic storage disease. It is an uncommon neurologic disorder of infants, children and

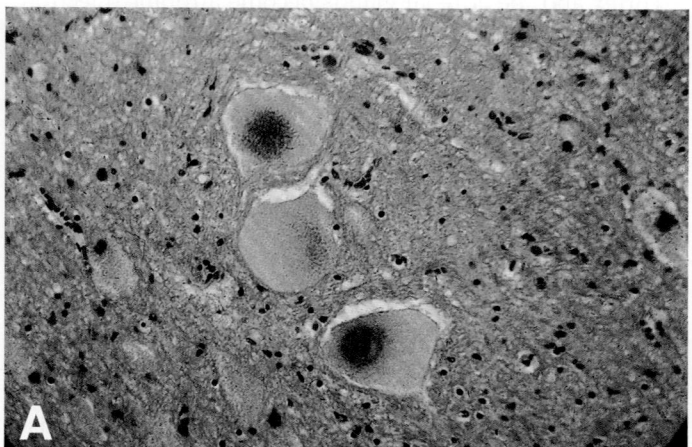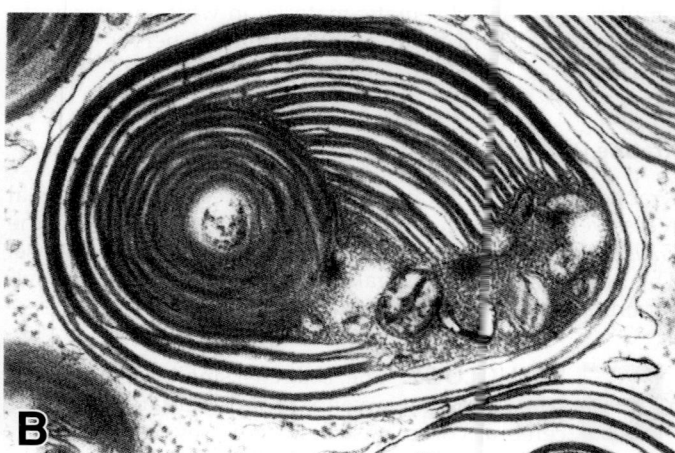

FIGURE 32-76. Tay–Sachs Disease. A. Neuron cytoplasm is distended by accumulation of eosinophilic storage material. **B.** Electron microscopy shows whorled "myelin bodies" composed of accumulated gangliosides within the cytoplasm.

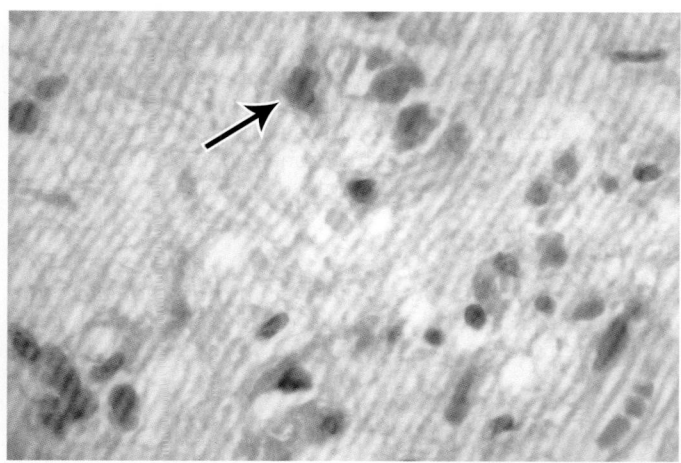

FIGURE 32-77. Alexander disease. This disease results from mutation in the gene for glial fibrillary acidic protein (*GFAP*). It is characterized by accumulation of aggregated GFAP into eosinophilic bodies called Rosenthal fibers (*arrow*). Rosenthal fibers are seen in Alexander disease, in pilocytic astrocytoma and as a reaction adjacent to chronic compressive lesions (also see Fig. 32-4C).

rarely adults, and is characterized by a loss of myelin in the brain. It is caused by mutations in the *GFAP* gene leading to striking eosinophilic collections of GFAP in astrocytic processes (Rosenthal fibers; Fig. 32-77), particularly in a perivascular and subpial distribution. Clinically, children exhibit psychomotor disability, progressive dementia and paralysis and eventually die. It is not yet clear how this process impairs myelin formation and induces degeneration of oligodendrocytes and myelin.

Phenylketonuria Is a Deficiency in Phenylalanine Hydroxylase

Phenylketonuria (PKU) is an autosomal recessive disease (see Chapter 6) caused by mutations in *PAH*. This gene makes phenylalanine hydroxylase which converts phenylalanine to tyrosine. As a result, phenylalanine accumulates in blood and tissues. Symptoms appear in the early months of life, with intellectual disability, seizures, and impaired physical development. Treatment involves restricting dietary phenylalanine. Untreated patients rarely obtain an IQ above 50, but those on the diet do well. Since the morbidity of PKU is preventable by a simple dietary intervention, all newborns are now screened for it. Although it shows no consistent morphologic alterations, the brain may be underweight and deficient in myelination.

Wilson Disease Is an Autosomal Recessive Disorder of Copper Metabolism

Wilson disease, or **"hepatolenticular degeneration,"** affects the brain and the liver. It is caused by mutations in the *ATP7B* gene which encodes a protein called copper-transporting ATPase2 (see Chapter 20). This protein plays a role in transport of copper from the liver to other parts of the body and in eliminating excess copper. Defective excretion of copper in the bile in Wilson disease leads to its deposition in the brain.

 CLINICAL FEATURES: Symptoms of cerebral involvement appear as a movement disorder with a tendency to choreoathetosis, usually in the second decade, but the disease may not become apparent until as late as the eighth decade. The movement disorder may be associated with psychosis. Before, during or after the appearance of neurologic symptoms, an insidiously developing cirrhosis may result in hepatic failure. Copper deposition in the limbus of the cornea produces a visible golden-brown band, the **Kayser–Fleischer ring**, seen on slit lamp examination.

Lenticular nuclei of the brain show a light golden discoloration, and 25% of cases have small cysts or clefts in the putamen or in deep layers of the neocortex. Mild neuron loss and gliosis are characteristic.

Some patients are "presymptomatic," and never develop high enough levels of copper to accumulate in the brain or eyes or developing cirrhosis. Diagnosis is critical as Wilson disease is treatable with chelating agents that promote renal excretion of copper. Failure to treat can lead to irreversible hepatic and CNS damage. Anyone presenting with a hyperkinetic movement disorder, particularly with onset in early adult life, in association with psychiatric or hepatic manifestations must be evaluated for Wilson disease.

Brain Dysfunction in Systemic Metabolic Disease Is Metabolic Encephalopathy

It may be caused by metabolic derangements produced by one or more cardiopulmonary, renal, hepatic, or endocrine diseases. Clinically, patients show declining level of consciousness, starting with inattentiveness that may include rowdiness, progressing to lethargy and finally lack of arousal, regardless of level of stimulation. The change in consciousness may be accompanied by tremor, asterixis, and changing multifocal neurologic signs. Computed tomography (CT) and MRI scans show no structural abnormality, and EEG shows progressive slowing of rhythmic cortical activity, sometimes accompanied by periodic high-amplitude discharges known as triphasic waves (which are seen most often in hepatic encephalopathy but are not specific for this condition). Biochemically, metabolic encephalopathy is characterized by lower cerebral glucose and oxygen utilization regardless of the underlying disorder. There are no specific morphologic features in metabolic encephalopathy, but presence of altered astroglia (**Alzheimer type II astrocytes**) suggests, but is not diagnostic of, hepatic encephalopathy.

Hepatic Encephalopathy

Hepatic encephalopathy is a common clinical manifestation of liver failure, with delirium, seizures, and coma. Symptoms generally greatly exceed their morphologic correlates in the brain, which are restricted to the appearance of Alzheimer type II astrocytes with enlarged nuclei and marginated chromatin, especially in the thalamus. These cells, which are also seen in Wilson disease, reflect metabolic abnormalities. They are not specifically associated with Alzheimer disease.

Osmotic Demyelination Syndrome (Central Pontine Myelinolysis)

This is a rare demyelinating disorder of the pons, where discrete areas of selective demyelination occur (Fig. 32-78). Lesions often are too small to manifest clinically and are evident only at autopsy. However, a few patients may develop quadriparesis, pseudobulbar palsy, or locked-in syndrome. Central pontine myelinolysis (CPM) arises from overly rapid correction of hyponatremia in alcoholics, malnourished people or patients with marked electrolyte instability, including liver transplant recipients and those with renal failure. Demyelination is not confined to the pons, and other extrapontine white matter areas may be involved. Thus, CPM is now considered part of a broader disorder called osmotic demyelination syndrome. A classical corpus callosal demyelination process, called Marchiafava–Bignami syndrome, is another example of an osmotic demyelination syndrome, and internal capsule, corona radiata and cerebellar white matter tracts may be involved as well.

Vitamin Deficiencies

Vitamin deficiencies and their systemic consequences are discussed in Chapter 8. Here, we consider effects on the nervous system.

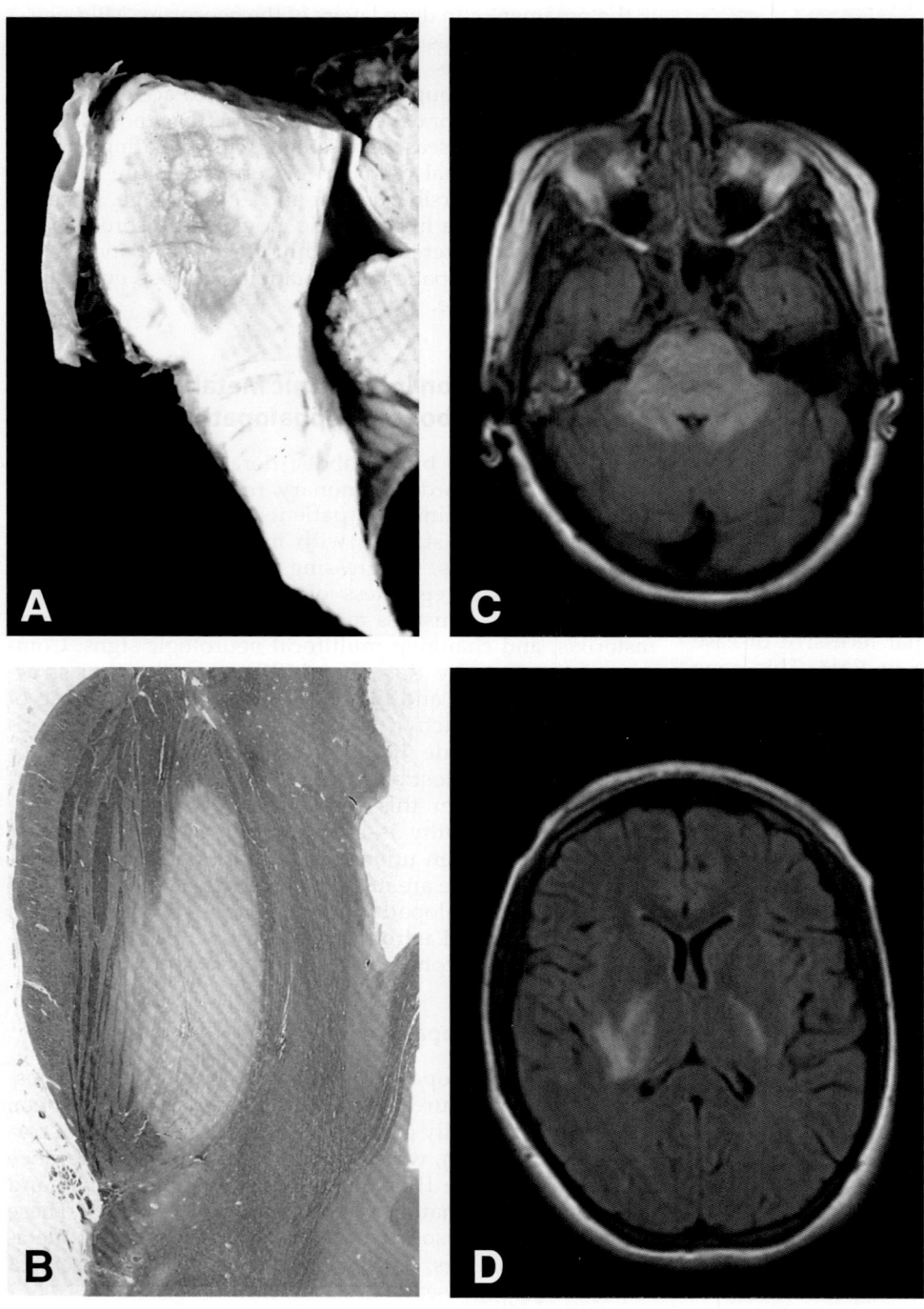

FIGURE 32-78. Osmotic demyelination syndrome with central pontine myelinolysis. A. This sagittal section of the brainstem shows a soft, discolored, midpontine lesion. (Courtesy of Dr. F. Stephen Vogel, Duke University.) **B.** A myelin-stained section reveals a sharply demarcated area of myelin loss appearing as a pink ovoid zone. (Courtesy of Dr. F. Stephen Vogel, Duke University.) **C, D.** Axial magnetic resonance images at the level of the pons and basal ganglia, respectively, show signal abnormalities in areas of demyelination.

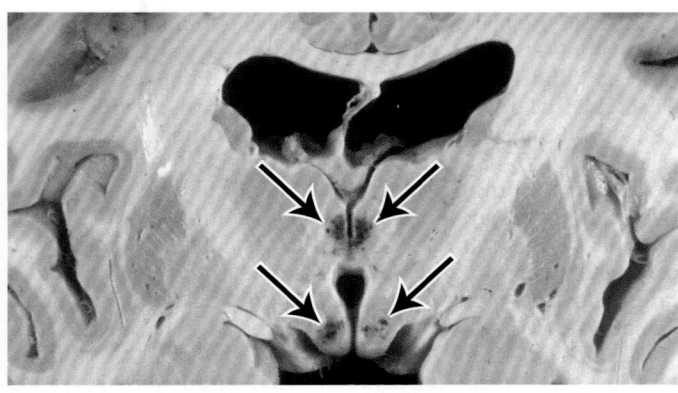

FIGURE 32-79. Wernicke encephalopathy. This coronal section shows hemorrhagic petechiae in the mamillary bodies and periventricular anterior thalamus (*arrows*). (Courtesy of Dr. F. Stephen Vogel, Duke University.)

Wernicke Syndrome

Wernicke syndrome results from thiamine (vitamin B_1) deficiency. It is characterized clinically by rapid onset of altered consciousness with dramatically impaired short-term memory, ophthalmoplegia, and nystagmus. Lesions are seen in the hypothalamus and mamillary bodies, the periaqueductal regions of the midbrain and the pontine tegmentum (Fig. 32-79). The syndrome is usually related to dietary insufficiency in chronic alcoholics but can occur in patients following bariatric surgery and in patients with severe morning sickness (hyperemesis gravidarum) in pregnancy. It may progress rapidly to death, but is reversed by administration of thiamine. In fatal cases, petechiae form around capillaries in the mamillary bodies, hypothalamus, periaqueductal region, and floor of the fourth ventricle (Fig. 32-80). Over time, hemosiderin deposition identifies regions where petechial hemorrhages had occurred. Neurons and myelin are generally spared, but mamillary body atrophy and capillary proliferation may be prominent.

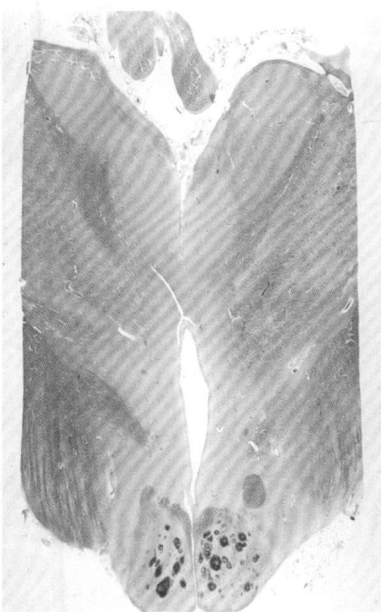

FIGURE 32-80. Wernicke encephalopathy with petechial hemorrhage in mammillary bodies. (Courtesy of Dr. F. Stephen Vogel, Duke University.)

Wernicke–Korsakoff syndrome is a state of disordered recent memory often compensated for by confabulation. It resembles Wernicke syndrome pathologically but may include degeneration of neurons in the medial–dorsal thalamic nucleus.

Many chronic alcoholics have cerebral atrophy of uncertain cause and for which the relative contributions of alcohol toxicity, malnutrition, and other factors are not defined. Similar uncertainties prevail with regard to atrophy of the Purkinje and granular cells of the cerebellum. These changes are common in chronic alcoholism and are the cause of truncal ataxia, which persists during periods of sobriety.

Subacute Combined Degeneration

Subacute combined degeneration of the spinal cord results from vitamin B_{12} deficiency (pernicious anemia) and leads to lesions in the posterolateral portions of the spinal cord. Initially, symmetric myelin and axonal loss occur in the thoracic spinal cord. Astrogliosis is mild in acute lesions, but with time, gliosis and atrophy develop, especially in posterolateral areas of the cord.

A burning sensation in the soles of the feet and other paresthesias herald the onset of this rapidly progressive and poorly reversible neurologic disorder. Weakness emerges in all four limbs, followed by defective postural sensibility, incoordination, and ataxia. Subacute combined degeneration may complicate a rare case of extensive gastric resection and other malabsorption syndromes. As vitamin B_{12} is not found in plants, some extreme vegetarians who eschew all animal products, including milk and eggs, develop subacute combined degeneration after many years on a restricted diet.

Iatrogenic, occupational or recreational exposure to the anesthetic gas nitrous oxide (N_2O) may lead to a condition that is clinically and morphologically indistinguishable from subacute combined degeneration. N_2O interferes with vitamin B_{12}–dependent enzymes. Hypocupric (low serum copper) myelopathy after bariatric surgery or zinc overdosage can produce a similar picture.

Intoxication

Neurotoxicology is a major aspect of contemporary neuropathology. The breadth of this topic far exceeds the scope of this chapter, so we concentrate on the more common and better-understood toxic injuries to the brain.

ETHANOL: Acute and chronic alcohol intake has widespread harmful effects and more widespread societal repercussions owing to its behavioral consequences. Acute alcohol intoxication signs and symptoms correspond to dose-related blood level, such that 0.05 to 0.1 mg/dL is associated with disinhibition and motor impairment; 0.1 to 0.3 mg/dL with frank inebriation and ataxia; and 0.3 to 0.35 mg/dL with extreme intoxication and sleepiness, nausea, and vomiting. Over 0.35 mg/dL is potentially lethal owing to respiratory depression and inability to protect the airway from aspiration. Lethal intoxication may tragically occur during competitive drinking among college students.

Chronic ethanol use is associated with neurologic complications caused by nutritional deficiencies, including Wernicke–Korsakoff syndrome and possibly peripheral neuropathy; liver failure with hepatic encephalopathy and non-Wilsonian hepatocerebral degeneration; and metabolic derangements including CPM from rapid correction of hyponatremia (Fig. 32-81). Alcoholics may also develop central necrosis of the corpus callosum or Marchiafava–Bignami

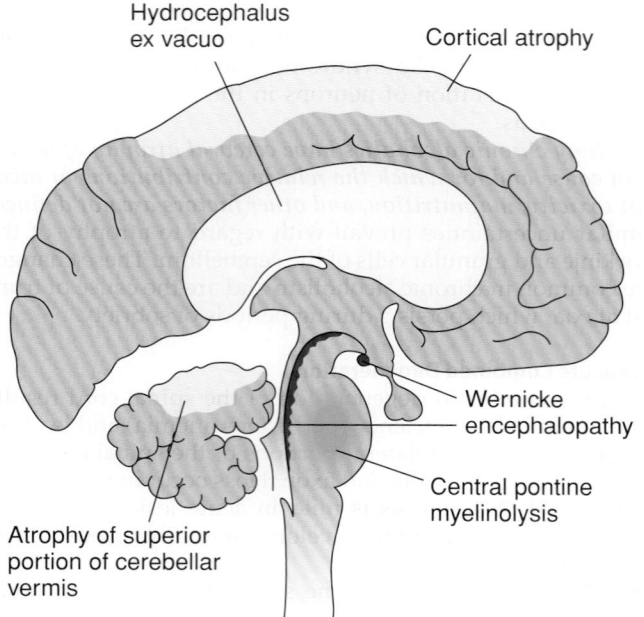

FIGURE 32-81. Lesions of the brain associated with chronic ethanol abuse.

disease (see above). This disease is part of the osmotic demyelination syndrome caused by overly rapid correction of hyponatremia. Less well understood is anterior superior vermal cerebellar degeneration, which occurs mainly in alcoholic men, presents with truncal ataxia and is grossly evident as atrophy of the vermis (Fig. 32-82).

METHANOL: In their quest for ethanol, alcoholics may from time to time drink methanol, which becomes oxidized to formaldehyde and formic acid. Patients dying of methanol intoxication have severe cerebral edema with hemorrhagic necrosis of the lateral putamen. Retinal edema and ganglion cell degeneration account for the blindness that afflicts these patients. Blindness may result from ingestion of as little as 4 mL. A lethal dose is in the range of 8 to 10 mL of pure methanol, although usually 70 to 100 mL is consumed in fatal cases.

ETHYLENE GLYCOL: Like methanol, ethylene glycol (found in automotive antifreeze) is sometimes consumed by alcoholics as an alternative to ethanol or by children or animals because of its sweet taste. Oxalate is its metabolic product. Severe organic acidosis may lead to coma and renal failure, and survivors may have residual neurologic deficits. Tissue oxalate crystal deposition can be seen.

CARBON MONOXIDE (CO): This colorless, odorless, tasteless gas is formed by incomplete combustion. CO binds hemoglobin far more avidly than oxygen. It thus displaces oxygen from hemoglobin, to form carboxyhemoglobin (COHb), which in turn reduces the oxygen-carrying capacity of blood. COHb is red and imparts a "cherry-red" hue to victims of CO poisoning. Severe intoxication causes virtually pathognomonic bilateral liquefactive necrosis of the globus pallidus. Other areas of CNS ischemic injury may be seen. The mechanism of the selective globus pallidus injury is unclear, but the recent discovery that CO may act as a neurotransmitter suggests that areas rich in heme-iron (such as the basal ganglia) may use CO under physiologic conditions for cell-to-cell signaling. As in amino acid excitotoxicity (see above), an excess neurotransmitter such as CO might injure areas in which it normally plays a physiologic role.

METAL INTOXICATION OR DEFICIENCY: Many metals employed in industry and medicine can cause neurologic disease. In addition, the biocidal properties of some of these substances, such as arsenic and thallium, have made them favorite tools of murderers, suicidal individuals, and pesticide users.

■ **Lead:** Acute lead poisoning produces an edema-based encephalopathy, especially in childhood. An amorphous

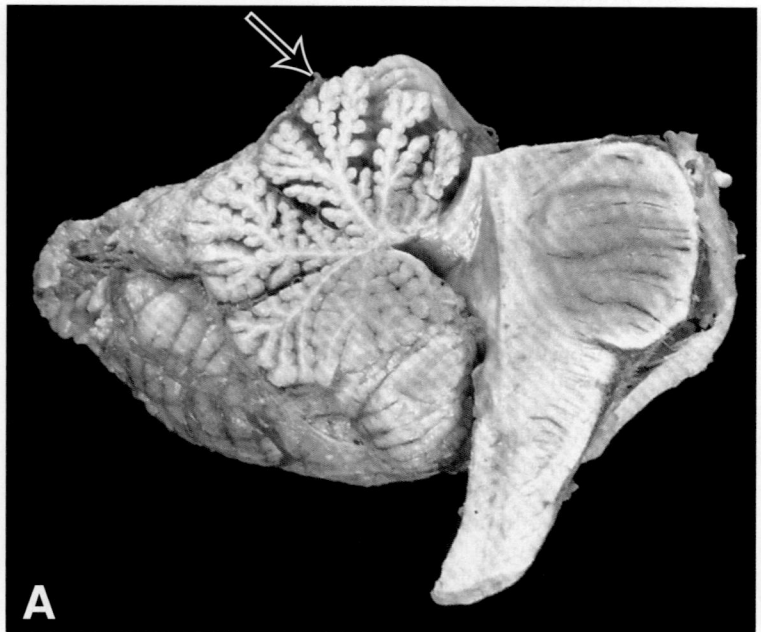

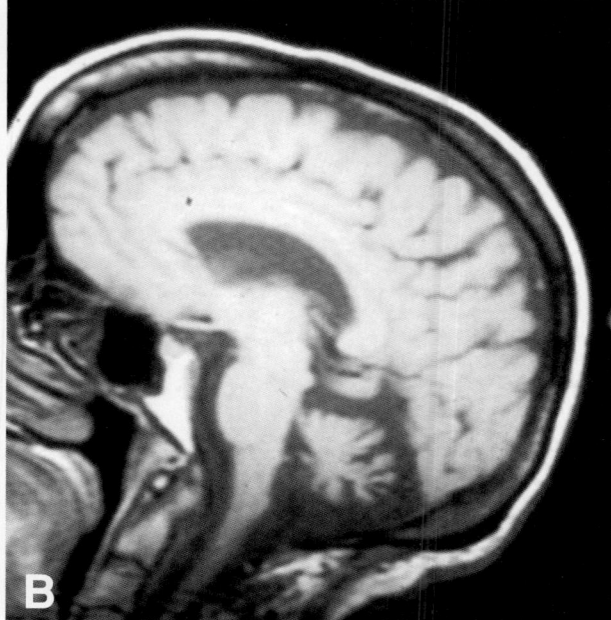

FIGURE 32-82. Chronic alcoholism. A. Superior and anterior portions of the cerebellar vermis are atrophic (*arrow*), leading to clinical signs of truncal ataxia. (Courtesy of Dr. F. Stephen Vogel, Duke University.) **B.** Coronal noncontrast computed tomography imaging shows profound vermal atrophy in an alcoholic individual.

exudate around microvessels may be seen, as may some vascular proliferation. Excess exposure in children may come from ingesting lead-based paint, fishing sinkers, and other lead weights. In adults, lead poisoning more commonly presents as a neuropathy rather than as an encephalopathy.

- **Mercury:** Chronic inorganic mercury intoxication may present with dementia, delirium, tremor, irritability, and insomnia. Now rare, mercury poisoning in the 19th-century decimated workers in cinnabar (mercury ore) mines, hat manufacturing ("mad as a hatter"), mirror silvering plants and manufacturing of scientific instruments. Cerebellar atrophy with loss of Purkinje cells was seen in these settings.
- **Organomercurial poisoning** is now more prevalent. In the 1950s and 1960s, for example, industrial mercuric chloride from the manufacture of vinyl chloride was dumped into Minamata Bay in Japan. The marine food chain concentrated the metal, and fishermen and local inhabitants then ate contaminated seafood. Many people were injured or died. These patients developed ataxia and blindness. Cerebellar and cerebrocortical atrophy occurred, with some cortical damage elsewhere. Congenital methylmercury neurotoxicity from in utero exposure results in severe intellectual disability, athetosis, ataxia, and spastic quadriparesis. Severe atrophy of the cerebrum with milder cerebellar atrophy is evident, with loss of the cortical lamellar organization perhaps indicating a defect in neuronal migration and organization in development.
- **Arsenic:** Arsenical intoxication manifests with gastrointestinal complaints including nausea, vomiting, and diarrhea. Cutaneous features including hyperkeratosis and increased pigmentation of the soles and palms and Mees lines on the nails. There is also a severe axonal neuropathy. In the brain, swelling and petechiae may be present. Long-term exposure has other risks (see Chapter 8).
- **Thallium:** Like arsenic, gastrointestinal disturbances are evident, with major cutaneous manifestations of late alopecia and Mees lines occasionally, and severe axonal neuropathy.
- **Manganese:** Basal ganglionic damage producing parkinsonism is seen in manganese miners. This may be associated with a psychosis known as "manganese madness."

Metal deficiencies can also injure the nervous system. For example, copper deficiency may follow bariatric surgery due to insufficient absorption or competitive malabsorption if the patient consumes excessive zinc or bismuth. This can cause hypocupric myelopathy with dorsal column and lateral column loss.

NEURODEGENERATIVE DISORDERS

Neurodegenerative disorders involve death of functionally related neurons; hence, these disorders can be classified by the primary functional system involved. **Cortical** degeneration leads to dementia, **basal ganglia** degeneration to movement disorders, **spinocerebellar** degeneration to ataxia and **motor neuron** degeneration to upper and lower motor neuron weakness. *Neuropathologically, there is loss of neurons in these systems. Characteristic neuronal inclusions and extracellular protein accumulations occur in these disorders associated with variable glial and microglial activation.*

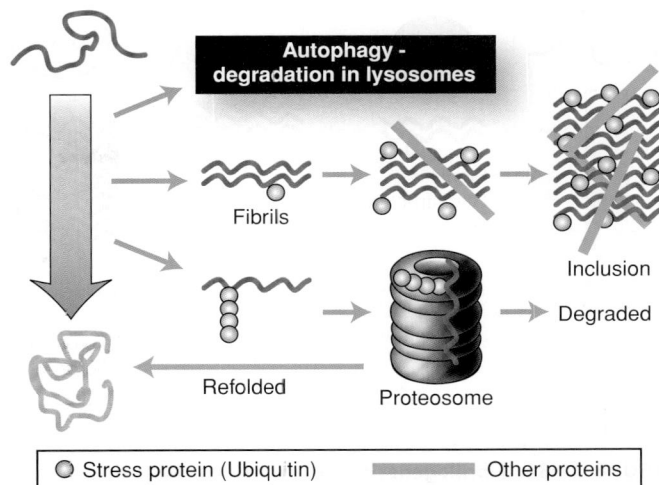

FIGURE 32-83. Possible fates of misfolded proteins. Many of the neurodegenerative diseases appear to be related, at least in part, to disorders of proteostasis, which involves cellular pathways that regulate protein synthesis, folding, trafficking, aggregation, disaggregation, and degradation.

 PATHOPHYSIOLOGY: Neurodegenerative disorders are classified according to which neuronal systems are most involved and the biochemistry of the proteins that accumulate in those neurons.

Intracellular, and particularly intracytoplasmic, inclusions have a history that is inextricably bound to neurodegenerative disorders, as these engaging features of diseased cells were among the first recognized histologic abnormalities of the nervous system. We now understand them to be markers of cellular stress: cytoplasmic landfills of abnormal cellular proteins and heat shock proteins. Abnormal protein homeostasis is probably central to the development of these disorders (Fig. 32-83; see Chapter 1).

When a neuron is stressed, its intermediate filament network collapses into perinuclear bundles or clumps. This may reflect increased protein phosphorylation or proteolysis stimulated by calcium influx into the stressed cell. If the stress is sub-lethal, the cell deploys an adaptive **heat shock response**. It produces stress-related proteins including crystallins and a family of heat shock proteins that help restore functional activity of partially denatured proteins or, if the insult is too severe to allow restoration, promote polyubiquitination of the damaged proteins for subsequent degradation. However, the highly stable β-pleated sheet conformation of the damaged proteins tends to support aggregation and prevent their effective removal by proteasomal or other means. If the proteins conjugated to the stress proteins are not successfully degraded, the conjugated complexes aggregate as intracellular inclusions.

The inclusions in neurodegenerative disorders *reflect damaged native cellular proteins and their stress response conjugates.* Cells activate stress responses whenever they are damaged; thus, stress response inclusions do not identify the inciting insult, but rather indicate that cells are trying to protect themselves. Neuropathologic inclusions are made from relatively few permutations of cytoskeletal and stress proteins—fewer, in fact, than the number of apparently discrete types of inclusions described. Ubiquitin is present in many intracellular inclusions. While not

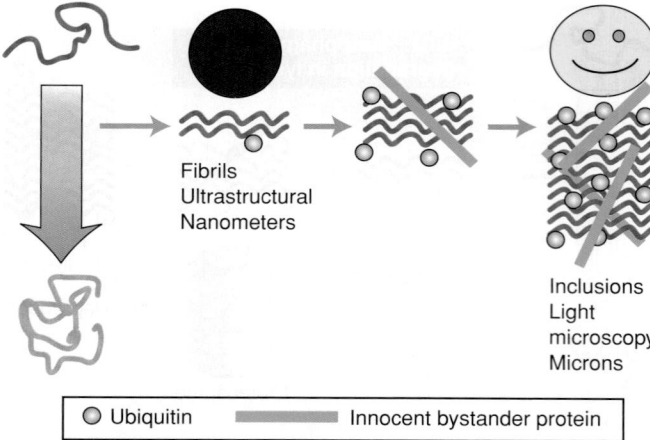

Ubiquitin ⬤   ▬▬▬ Innocent bystander protein

FIGURE 32-84. Fibrillogenesis and inclusions. Misfolded proteins with a tendency toward polymerization may form highly cytoxic fibrils visible only by electron microscopy. The cellular stress response may facilitate hyperaggregation to create inclusions that are visible by light microscopy. Such inclusions may be considered "toxic landfills" and because they sequester toxic fibrils may be protective.

"diagnostic" of any particular disease, ubiquitin immunostaining is the most sensitive technique for detecting such aggregated proteins. Combined with the morphology, cellular distribution and clinical context, it may be helpful diagnostically. Available antibodies allow identification of ubiquitinated proteins: tau, neurofilament, α-synuclein, and others. In summary, inclusions give limited data about the precise stress damaging the cell. Their biochemical compositions often overlap and final diagnostic categorization depends on clinical data, immunohistochemical characterization of inclusions and analysis of the cell populations affected.

Neuronal protein aggregates may cause disease (Fig. 32-84; Table 32-3) by several routes. Sequestration of specific proteins or other macromolecules makes them unavailable for their normal functions. As aggregates enlarge, they may physically obstruct axons, dendrites or interfere with movement of material within the cytoplasm. They may also act as ubiquitin sinks, depleting cell ubiquitin needed to target misfolded proteins for degradation. Thus, cellular protein recycling and homeostasis are impaired. As these proteins aggregate, they initially form fibrils that may be extremely cytotoxic. Thus, it appears that cellular stresses from a variety of causes may disrupt proteostasis and generate toxic fibrils that themselves can perpetuate and amplify the cellular stress.

Neurodegenerative disorders often begin focally and then spread in reasonably predictable ways throughout the CNS. This stereotypical pattern of dissemination likely involves actions of abnormally folded pathogenic proteins to recruit and transform native protein. This phenomenon is reminiscent of the molecular pathogenesis of prion diseases and is called "prion-like" protein misfolding or "templating."

At their core, the neurodegenerative diseases are largely disorders of proteostasis, involving impaired cellular pathways that control protein synthesis, folding, trafficking, aggregation, disaggregation, and degradation. Because of this unifying theme, fundamental pathogenetic insights derived from one neurodegenerative disease may be generalizable to others.

There Are Three Major Cerebral Cortical Neurodegenerative Diseases

Their clinical and pathologic features are distinctive, as different polymerized proteins accumulate (Fig. 32-85). These cortical degenerations ultimately lead to dementia.

TABLE 32-3

REPRESENTATIVE NEURODEGENERATIVE DISEASES WITH FIBRILLOGENESIS

Disease	Lesion	Components	Location
Alzheimer disease	Senile plaques	β-Amyloid	Extracellular
	Neurofibrillary tangles	Tau	Intracytoplasmic
Amyotrophic lateral sclerosis	Spheroids	Neurofilament	Intracytoplasmic
		Superoxide dismutase (SOD-1)	
		TDP43	
		FUS	
Dementia with Lewy bodies	Lewy bodies	α-Synuclein	Intracytoplasmic
Frontotemporal dementias	Neurofibrillary tangles	Tau	Intracytoplasmic
		TDP43, progranulin and other proteins	
Multiple system atrophy	Glial inclusions	α-Synuclein	Intracytoplasmic
Parkinson disease	Lewy bodies	α-Synuclein	Intracytoplasmic
Prion diseases	Prion deposits	Prions	Extracellular
Trinucleotide repeat diseases	Inclusions	Polyglutamine tracts	Intranuclear and cytoplasmic

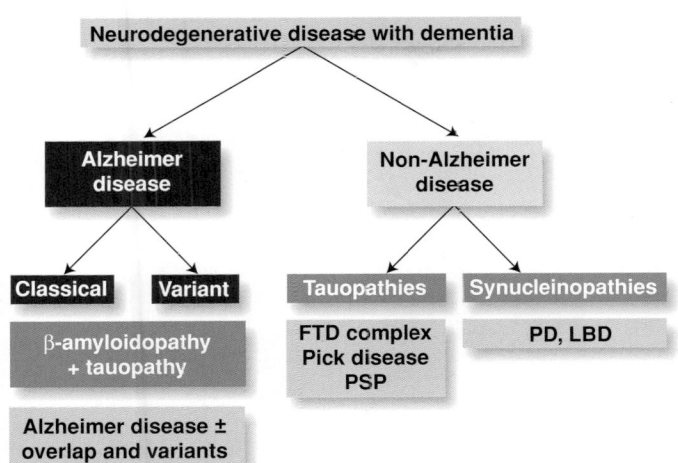

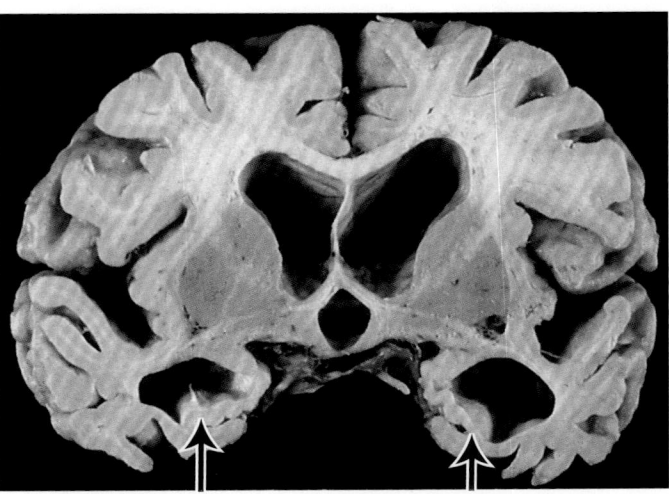

FIGURE 32-85. Protein fibrillogenesis. The dementias and other neurodegenerative diseases can now be classified on the basis of the proteins that undergo fibrillogenesis. Alzheimer disease (AD) is a combination of a β-amyloidopathy and a tauopathy. Most of the frontotemporal lobar degenerations (FTLDs) such as Pick disease and progressive supranuclear palsy (PSP) are pure tauopathies. Lewy body dementia (LBD) and Parkinson disease (PD) complex are α-synucleinopathies.

FIGURE 32-87. Cerebral atrophy with hydrocephalus ex vacuo in Alzheimer disease. Note also the severe atrophy of the hippocampus (*arrows*) which is associated with early memory disturbances in this disease. (Courtesy of Dr. F. Stephen Vogel, Duke University.)

- **Alzheimer disease (AD)** accounts for the majority of neurodegenerative dementia. It is characterized by abnormal accumulation of two proteins: β-amyloid and tau.
- **Pick disease,** which is the prototypical frontotemporal lobar dementia, is characterized by accumulation of abnormal tau without β-amyloid.
- **Lewy body dementia** features accumulation of α-synuclein.

Alzheimer Disease

EPIDEMIOLOGY: AD is an insidious progressive neurologic disorder characterized clinically by loss of memory, cognitive impairment and, eventually, dementia. Although Alzheimer's original patients were younger than 65 and suffered "presenile

dementia," the term is now used for dementia at any age with characteristic pathologic changes. *It is the most common dementia in the elderly, accounting for over half of cases.* The prevalence of the condition is closely related to age. In patients younger than 65, Alzheimer disease affects at most 1% to 2%, but it occurs in 40% or more of patients older than 85. Women are affected twice as often as men. Most cases are sporadic, but familial variants occur and can provide clues to pathogenic mechanisms.

PATHOLOGY: AD brains show cortical atrophy with hydrocephalus ex vacuo (Figs. 32-86 and 32-87). Gyri are narrowed, sulci widened, and cortical atrophy is especially apparent in the parahippocampal regions. However, as the disease progresses, atrophy of temporal, frontal, and parietal cortex becomes more severe.

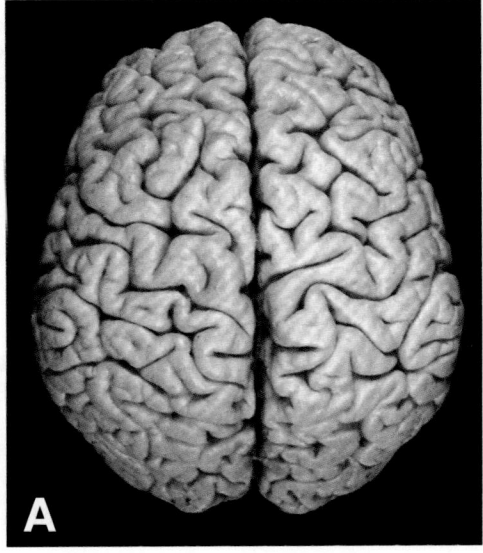 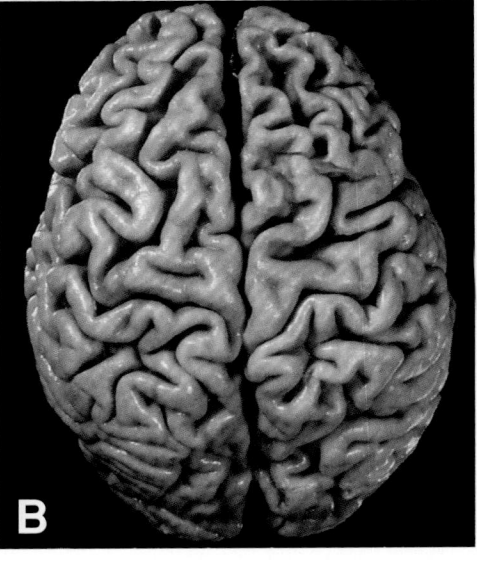

FIGURE 32-86. Cortical atrophy. A. Gyral structure in a normal adult brain. **B.** By contrast, the brain from a patient with Alzheimer disease shows cortical atrophy with thinning of the gyri and prominent sulci. (Photos courtesy of Dr. F. Stephen Vogel, Duke University.)

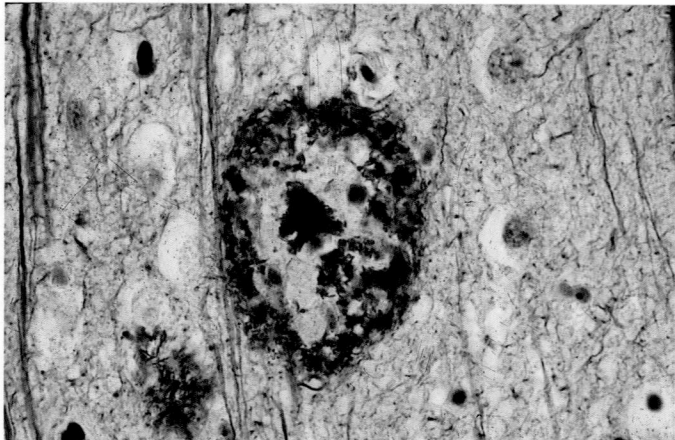

FIGURE 32-88. Neuritic plaques are extracellular accumulations of polymerized β-amyloid centrally with a rim of dystrophic neuritic processes. The number of plaques in the cerebral cortex does not correlate well with the severity of dementia in Alzheimer disease.

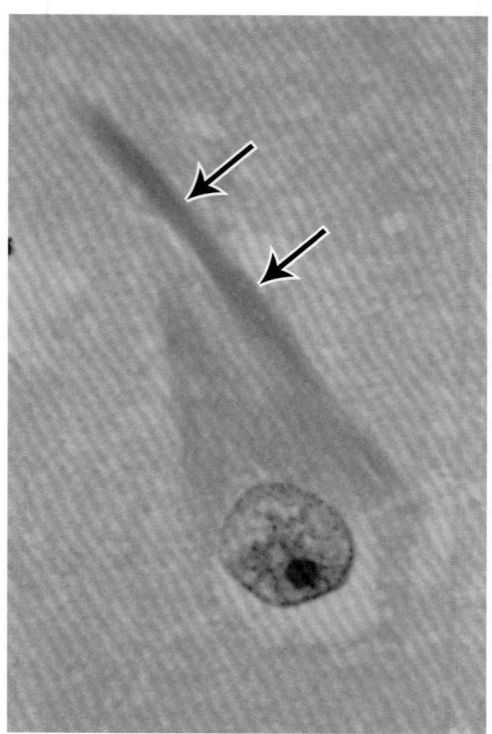

FIGURE 32-89. Neurofibrillary tangles are intracytoplasmic accumulations of polymerized hyperphosphorylated tau protein in neurons (*arrows*). The sites and extent of distribution of neurofibrillary tangles correlate with clinical symptoms.

Senile plaques and NFTs dominate the histology. Small numbers of plaques and tangles are common in elderly patients with mild forgetfulness and mild cognitive impairment (MCI), which in half of cases is a prodrome of AD.

NEURITIC PLAQUES: The most conspicuous histologic lesions, senile or neuritic plaques, are *extracellular* spherical deposits of β-amyloid several hundred microns in diameter. In end-stage disease, senile plaques occupy large volumes of affected cerebral gray matter (Fig. 32-88). They bind planar amyloid binding dyes such as Congo red and thioflavin S, and silver containing dyes (argentophilic), and are immunoreactive for β-amyloid protein (Aβ) at the core and periphery. They are surrounded by reactive astrocytes and microglia and display swollen distorted neuronal processes (dystrophic neurites). Identification of plaques is necessary to diagnose AD; their number and distribution do not correlate well with clinical disease severity.

NEUROFIBRILLARY TANGLES: NFTs are *intracytoplasmic* collections of polymerized tau filaments (Fig. 32-89). NFTs contain irregular bundles of fibrils that are positive by Congo red and thioflavin S and immunoreactive for tau. The tangles are paired, 10-nm-thick, helical filaments with abundant insoluble tau proteins. Their distribution correlates with the clinical severity of AD. Tangles in the entorhinal cortex and parahippocampal gyrus can be seen in asymptomatic people decades before the usual age of onset of AD and may represent the earliest expression of disease. As more temporal neocortex comes to possess tangles, MCI may develop. By the time large swaths of neocortex, deep nuclei and brainstem have become involved, full-blown AD is present. Based on this concept of gradual accretion of NFTs, efforts are increasingly directed at early diagnosis during the asymptomatic phase and development of drugs that can arrest progression.

NFTs are not unique to AD. They occur in other neurodegenerative diseases including dementia pugilistica (punch drunk syndrome in boxers), postencephalitic parkinsonism, Guam ALS/parkinsonism dementia complex,

Pick disease, corticobasal degeneration, sporadic frontotemporal dementias (FTDs), and hereditary frontotemporal lobe dementia with parkinsonism associated with mutations on chromosome 17 (FTDP-17). Collectively, these hereditary and sporadic neurodegenerative diseases showing abnormal tau aggregation are called **tauopathies.** They may share common mechanisms of brain degeneration. *Alzheimer disease is both a tauopathy and a β-amyloidopathy, leading to intracellular tangles and extracellular plaques, respectively, seen in this disorder.*

Minor histologic changes—granulovacuolar degeneration and Hirano bodies—occur in AD and normal aging. They can be visually arresting but lack diagnostic significance. **Granulovacuolar degeneration** is largely restricted to the cytoplasm of hippocampal pyramidal cells, where it is seen as circular clear zones containing basophilic and argentophilic granules (Fig. 32-90A). **Hirano bodies,** like granulovacuolar degeneration, occur almost exclusively in hippocampal pyramidal neurons, especially in their processes (Fig. 32-90B). Hirano bodies are 10- to 15-micron-thick eosinophilic rods composed of polymerized actin.

 PATHOPHYSIOLOGY AND MOLECULAR PATHOGENESIS: The cause of AD is not known, but the origins of associated amyloid and NFTs are increasingly understood.

- **β-Amyloid protein (Aβ):** Increasing evidence points to the importance of deposition of Aβ protein in **neuritic**

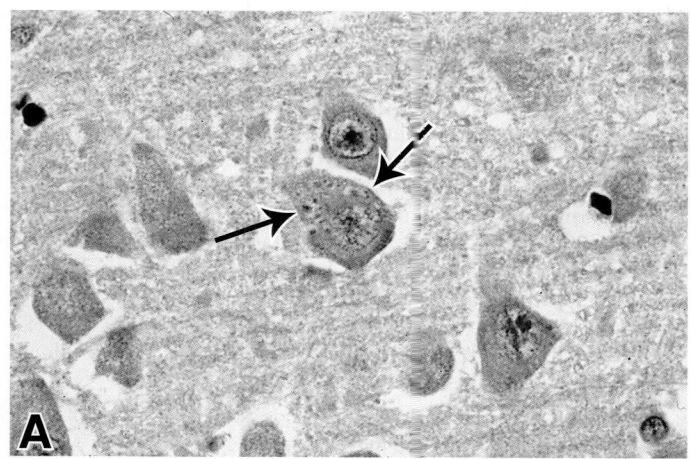
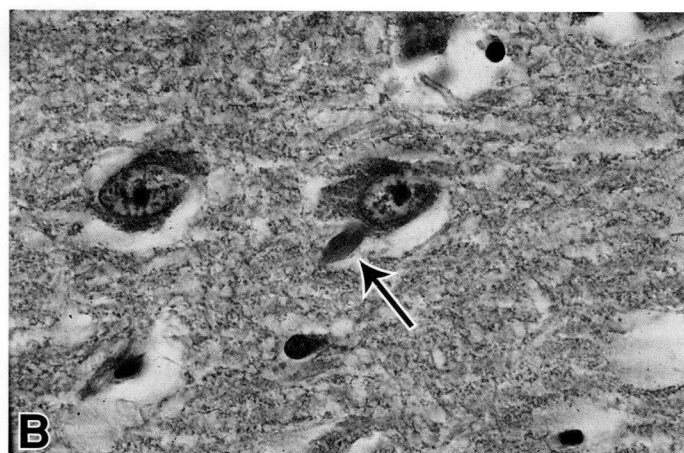

FIGURE 32-90. A. Granulovacuolar degeneration (*arrows*) is seen in hippocampal pyramidal neurons in both normal aging and Alzheimer disease. **B.** Hirano bodies are eosinophilic cytoplasmic accumulations of actin (*arrow*) seen in the cytoplasm of hippocampal pyramidal neurons in normal aging and Alzheimer disease.

plaques of Alzheimer disease. The core of these plaques contains a distinct form of Aβ peptide, which is mainly 42 amino acids long. Aβ is derived by proteolysis from a much larger (695 amino acids membrane-spanning **amyloid precursor protein** (APP). Full-length APP has an extracellular region, a transmembrane sequence and a cytoplasmic domain. The region comprising Aβ anchors the amino-terminal portion of APP to the membrane. The physiologic functions of APP and Aβ remain obscure.

Normal degradation of APP involves proteolytic cleavage in the middle of the Aβ domain, which produces a nonamyloidogenic fragment from the middle of the Aβ domain to the amino end of APP. Proteolysis at either end of the Aβ domain then releases intact and highly amyloidogenic Aβ which accumulates in senile plaques as amyloid fibrils.

Aβ deposition may be necessary for Alzheimer disease to develop because:

1. Patients with **Down syndrome** (trisomy 21) develop clinical and pathologic features of Alzheimer disease, including deposition of Aβ in neuritic plaques, generally by age 40. The gene for APP is on chromosome 21, and the additional dose of the gene product in trisomy 21 may predispose to precocious accumulation of Aβ.
2. Some patients with familial Alzheimer disease carry mutant *APP* genes or mutant presenilin genes. These mutations lead to increased production of Aβ, the amyloidogenic part of APP.
3. Transgenic mice expressing mutant human *APP* genes develop senile plaques in the brain highly reminiscent of those in Alzheimer disease. However, these mice lack other critical features of Alzheimer disease, such as NFTs, and evidence of neurodegeneration indicated by significant loss of neurons.

Neurons and glial cells are sites of APP synthesis in the brain, but Aβ also accumulates in cerebral blood vessel walls.

- **Neurofibrillary tangles:** NFTs are paired helical filaments that contain tau abnormally phosphorylated at aberrant sites. The resultant protein does not associate with microtubules but instead aggregates to form paired helical filaments. Release of tau from microtubules may deprive cells of its microtubule-stabilizing effects, thus impairing axonal transport and compromising neuron function. Alternatively, formation of fibrils of hyperphosphorylated tau aggregates may itself be cytotoxic.

Several genetic risk factors have been identified for AD. Mutations in the *APP* gene have been linked to early-onset familial variants of Alzheimer disease. Additional genetic associations (Table 32-4) involve variants in the apolipoprotein E gene (*APOE*) and genes for presenilin 1 (*PS1*) and 2 (*PS2*).

TABLE 32-4

GENETIC FACTORS IN ALZHEIMER DISEASE

Gene	Chromosome	Disease Association
Amyloid precursor protein (*APP*)	21	Mutations in *APP* are associated with early-onset familial Alzheimer disease
Presenilin 1 (*PS1*)	14	Mutations in *PS1* are associated with early-onset familial Alzheimer disease
Presenilin 2 (*PS2*)	1	Mutations in *PS2* are associated with Volga German familial Alzheimer disease
Apolipoprotein E (*APOE*)	19	Presence of the ε4 allele is associated with increased risk and younger age of onset of both inherited and sporadic forms of late-onset Alzheimer disease

APOLIPOPROTEIN E: Apolipoprotein E (apoE) has long been known for its role in cholesterol metabolism. In 1993, it was reported that specific apoE isoforms confer differential susceptibility to sporadic and late-onset familial subtypes of AD. The human apoE gene, *APOE*, is on chromosome 19 (19q13.2). Three common alleles—ε2, ε3, and ε4—occur in North American genotypes. Inheritance of the ε4 allele, particularly the homozygous ε4/ε4 genotype, confers increased risk of late-onset familial and sporadic AD. This genotype occurs in 2% of the population. Conversely, the ε2 allele may confer protection. The age at which symptoms appear in late-onset AD also correlates with the ε4 allele, with ε4/ε4 homozygotes showing the earliest onset (younger than 70) and patients with the ε2 allele having the latest onset (older than 90). The ε4 allele also correlates with increased numbers of senile plaques in patients with Alzheimer disease, but the *APOE* genotype is not an absolute determinant of the disease and does not predict who will develop it. How these different apoE alleles influence the risk of Alzheimer disease remains poorly understood.

PRESENILIN: Presenilins are protein subunits in the γ-secretase complex which is involved in proteolytic processing of AAP. Two presenilin genes with significant homology are associated with different kindreds of familial AD. Mutations in the *PS1* gene, on chromosome 14, are linked to the most common form of autosomal dominant early-onset Alzheimer disease. The *PS2* gene on chromosome 1 is associated with Alzheimer disease in Volga German pedigrees (Table 32-4). Presenilin mutations occur in half of cases of inherited AD, compared with only a few percent for mutant *APP* genes. There is some evidence that mutant PS1 and PS2 proteins alter processing of β-APP to favor increased production and deposition of Aβ. Cell processing of APP releases Aβ fragments of varying lengths, but the Aβ42 variant seems to be especially amyloidogenic. It is the Aβ molecule whose production is enhanced by mutant *PS1.*

Proposed mechanisms leading to development of AD are shown in Figure 32-91.

It is now recognized that AD evolves over a period of years, if not decades. In 2011, a National Institute on Aging/ Alzheimer Association (NIA/AA) consensus statement proposed that AD occurs in three stages:

1. **Presymptomatic:** At this early stage, patient have no cognitive impairment, but growing evidence indicates that extracellular β-amyloid is accumulating and tangles are beginning to form, especially in the hippocampus and adjacent temporal cortex.
2. **Mild cognitive impairment (MCI):** Patients experience mild deterioration of memory and cognitive function that may be worrisome but does not interfere with daily living. A significant number of patients with MCI go on to develop frank AD, but many do not. People with low levels of CSF β-amyloid 1–42 or high levels of amyloid load detected by positron emission tomography (PET) scanning appear more likely to progress to AD.
3. **Alzheimer disease:** These patients are frankly demented on clinical examination and neuropsychological evaluation. Activities of daily living are impaired.

In parallel with the development of these clinical consensus guidelines, new neuropathologic criteria for diagnosing

AD at autopsy have been developed. NFTs, neuritic plaques and β-amyloid distribution are assessed in standardized sections. β-Amyloid distribution is assessed by immunohistochemistry and described as absent (A0), neocortical and allocortical only (A1), diencephalon and striatum (A2), and brainstem and cerebellum (A3). The distribution of NFTs is categorized as absent (B0), trans-entorhinal (B1), limbic system and hippocampus (B2), and neocortical and brainstem (B3). Numbers of neuritic plaques are absent (C0), sparse (C1), moderate (C2), or frequent (C3). These changes are then combined as Ax, Bx, and Cx, with higher values in each dimension corresponding to a higher probability of AD. Comorbidities such as vascular disease, hippocampal sclerosis, and Lewy bodies are also described.

> **CLINICAL FEATURES:** Patients with AD come to medical attention because of gradual loss of memory and cognitive function, difficulty with language and changes in behavior. Those with MCI are increasingly being recognized, since they move on to full-blown dementia at a rate of about 15% per year. AD progresses inexorably, so that previously intelligent and productive people become demented, mute, incontinent, and bedridden. Bronchopneumonia, urinary tract infections, and pressure decubiti are common medical complications that lead to death.

Frontotemporal Lobar Degeneration: Pick Disease Complex

> **CLINICAL FEATURES:** The FTLDs are mainly tauopathies in which the frontal and temporal lobes bear the early brunt of the disease. The prototype eponymic disorder of the FTLDs is **Pick disease,** which manifests clinically as loss of frontal executive function causing disinhibition, loss of judgment about social propriety and inability to plan or foresee the consequences of one's actions. Most cases are sporadic, although Pick disease kindreds have been described. Sporadic Pick disease becomes symptomatic in midadult life and progresses relentlessly to death within 3 to 10 years. A respected pillar of the community may be reduced to a vulgar, disheveled derelict as this tragedy unfolds. Unlike AD, which generally begins with memory difficulties, FTLD starts with disruptive, inappropriate behavior. These dementias converge clinically at the end.

> **PATHOLOGY:** Cortical atrophy is mostly in the frontotemporal regions in Pick disease (Fig. 32-92). It may attain extreme proportions, so that affected gyri are reduced to thin slivers **(knife-edge atrophy).** The involved cortex is severely depleted of neurons and shows intense astrogliosis. Residual neurons contain intensely argentophilic and tau-immunoreactive-positive cytoplasmic inclusions called **Pick bodies** (Fig. 32-93). These are composed of densely aggregated straight tau filaments.

Pick disease is the prototypical FTLD, but others have begun to reveal their molecular secrets. In any cohort of patients with clinical FTLD, many have Pick disease, but a significant number do not. Often, their neurons

FIGURE 32-91. Mechanisms of amyloidosis and brain degeneration in Alzheimer disease. A. This schematic illustrates a hypothetical mechanism for the formation of senile plaques (SPs) from soluble Aβ peptides synthesized inside cells and secreted into the extracellular space. Amyloidogenic Aβ may encounter fibril-inducing cofactors and form A (aggregated) fibrils that are deposited in SPs (*far right*). SPs become surrounded by reactive astrocytes and microglial cells, which secrete cytokines that may further contribute to the toxicity of the SPs. These steps are potentially reversible. Thus, increasing Aβ clearance or reducing its production, as well as modulating the inflammatory response, may be effective therapeutic interventions for Alzheimer disease, in combination with therapies that target brain degeneration caused by neurofibrillary tangles (NFTs). **B.** This schematic illustrates a hypothetical mechanism promoting the conversion of normal tau protein overlying adjacent microtubules into paired helical filaments (PHFs). PHFs are generated in neuronal cell bodies and their processes. Overactive kinase(s) or hypoactive phosphatase(s) may contribute to this effect. Abnormally phosphorylated tau forms PHFs in neuronal processes (neuropil threads) and neuronal cell bodies (NFTs). Tau in PHFs loses the ability to bind microtubules, thus causing their depolymerization, disruption of axonal transport, and degeneration of neurons. Accumulation of PHFs in neurons could exacerbate this process by physically blocking transport in neurons. The death of affected neurons releases tau and increases the levels of tau in the cerebrospinal fluid (CSF) as seen in patients with Alzheimer disease. NFT formation may be reversible, and drugs that block NFT formation, reverse it or stabilize microtubules may be effective therapeutic interventions for Alzheimer disease. **C.** The National Institute on Aging/Alzheimer Association (NIA/AA) 2011 formulation on Alzheimer disease formally recognizes the temporal evolution of the disease from a long presymptomatic phase in which amyloid-β is accumulated and the pathophysiologic cascade is initiated. The pathogenic mechanisms interact to move the disease to mild cognitive impairment (MCI) and finally to frank dementia. Interventions attempted during the symptomatic phase may be too late to fundamentally change the trajectory of the disease. Increased attention is now being directed at the presymptomatic phase of the illness. Such a primary prevention approach is not unlike the highly successful presymptomatic intervention in myocardial infarction and stroke through exercise and pharmacologic control of hypertension and hyperlipidemia.

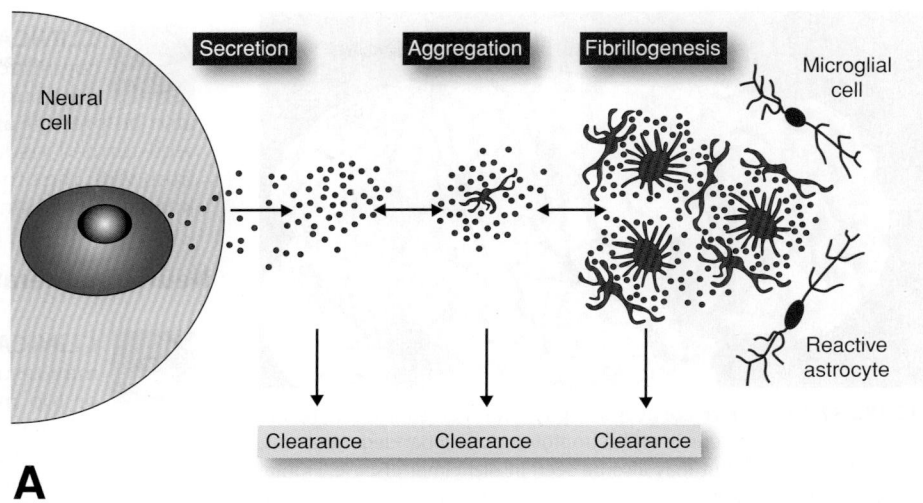

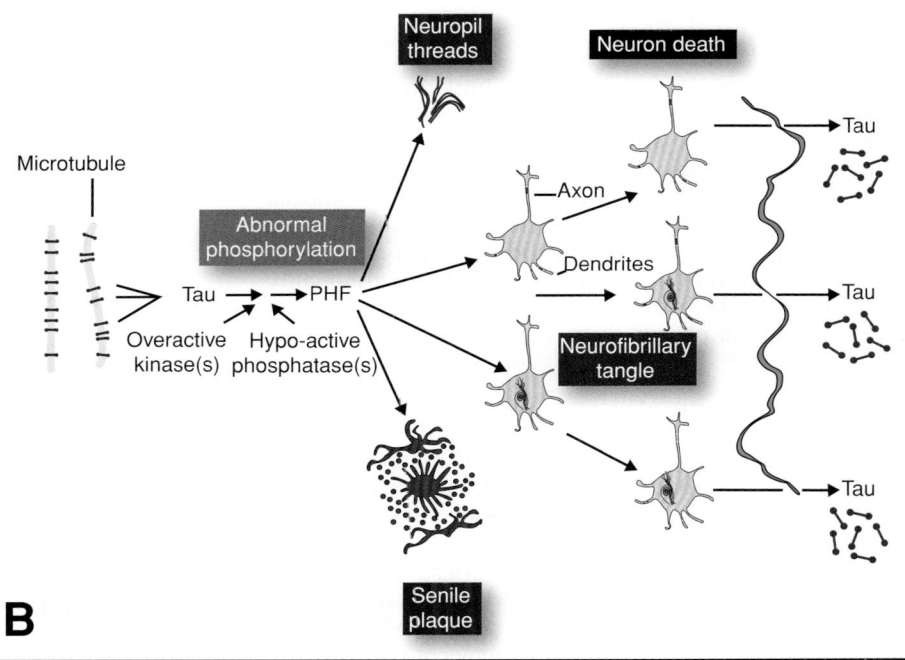

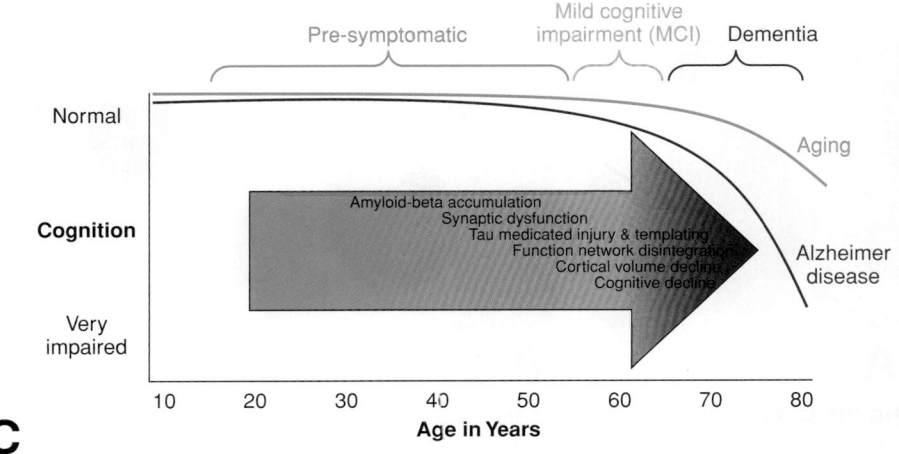

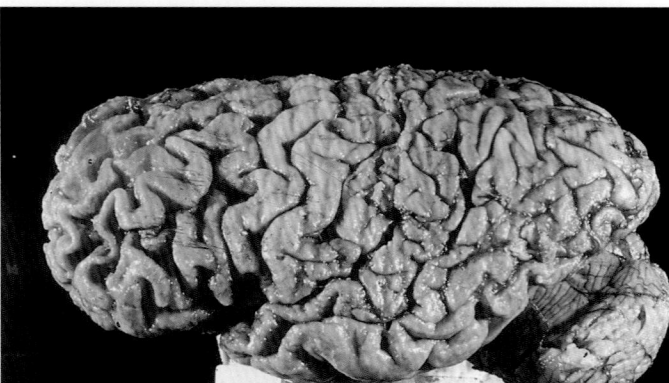

FIGURE 32-92. Severe cortical atrophy with marked frontotemporal involvement is characteristic of the frontotemporal lobar degenerations, such as Pick disease, but may also be seen in Alzheimer disease. Frontal atrophy correlates with loss of executive function, impaired judgment, and disinhibition.

are immunoreactive for ubiquitin, implying an as yet unidentified protein triggering an unfulfilled degradative response. These are classified at FTLD-U, the U for ubiquitin immunoreactivity. Several of these proteins have recently been identified. For example, abnormal accumulation of TDP43, a nuclear protein involved in various steps of protein production, occurs in both FTLD and motor neuron disease. This molecular commonality coincides with the increasingly recognized coexistence of FTLD and motor neuron disease.

Lewy Body Dementia

Lewy body dementia (LBD), also known as Lewy body disease or diffuse Lewy body disease, is characterized by intracytoplasmic α-synuclein inclusions in a relatively small number of cortical neurons, mostly in the cingulate cortex. These inclusions, referred to as Lewy bodies, are spherical, eosinophilic cytoplasmic inclusions. Also implicated in Parkinson disease, α-synuclein is a pre-synaptic neural protein whose normal function is not known. AD pathology may coexist with Lewy body inclusions at the end stage of the disease.

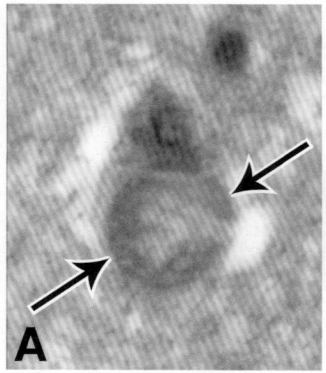 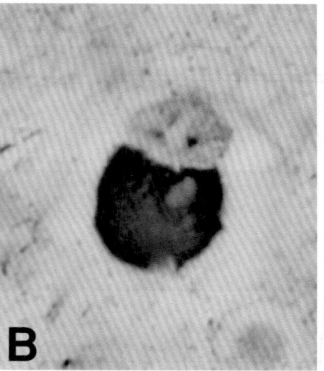

FIGURE 32-93. Pick bodies. A. In hematoxylin and eosin–stained sections, Pick bodies are basophilic, spherical, intracytoplasmic, intraneuronal aggregates of tau protein (*arrows*). **B.** They tend to be round rather than angular like the neurofibrillary tangles (NFTs) in Alzheimer disease, but like NFTs, they are argentophilic (silver impregnation).

 CLINICAL FEATURES: LBD is distinctive in that cognitive function fluctuates greatly from day to day. Subtle extrapyramidal manifestations may also be present and patients may experience fascinating well-formed visual hallucinations. LBD exists on a continuum with the other α-synucleinopathies that include Parkinson disease and multiple system atrophy (MSA).

Neurodegeneration of the Basal Ganglia

 CLINICAL FEATURES: Movement disorders may result in too little **(bradykinetic)** movement or too much involuntary **(hyperkinetic)** movement. **Parkinson disease** is the prototypical bradykinetic movement disorder, characterized by difficulty initiating and sustaining voluntary movement associated with resting tremor and postural instability. This clinical triad is referred to as **"parkinsonism,"** and while the most common cause is Parkinson disease, other disorders such as PSP, MSA, and even neuro-AIDS may produce parkinsonism.

The prototypical hyperkinetic movement disorder is **Huntington disease**, with progressive development of involuntary rapid twitching movements (chorea) and writhing dance-like movements (athetosis) that may conflate as choreoathetosis.

Parkinson Disease

First described in 1817, Parkinson disease (PD) is characterized clinically by tremors at rest, cogwheel rigidity, expressionless countenance, postural instability and, less often, cognitive impairment. Pathologically, neurons are lost, largely in the substantia nigra, and Lewy bodies, composed of filamentous aggregates of α-synuclein, accumulate. Dopaminergic neurons that project from the substantia nigra to the striatum are diminished.

 EPIDEMIOLOGY: PD typically appears in the sixth to eighth decades. It is common: 1% to 2% of the population in North America eventually become afflicted. Its prevalence has remained unchanged for at least the past 40 years. No racial differences are apparent, but men are affected more than women.

 PATHOPHYSIOLOGY: Most cases are sporadic, but missense mutations in *SCNA*, the α-synuclein gene cause rare autosomal dominant, early-onset, familial PD. Identification of wild-type α-synuclein as the major polymerized protein in Lewy bodies led to the idea of fibrillogenesis as a major contributor to the pathogenesis of neurodegenerative diseases. Accumulating evidence suggests that oxidative stress due to auto-oxidation of catecholamines during melanin formation injures neurons in the substantia nigra by promoting misfolding of α-synuclein and formation of filamentous inclusions.

In addition to occurring in PD, accumulation of filamentous α-synuclein inclusions is seen in other diseases, including MSA, dementia with Lewy bodies, progressive

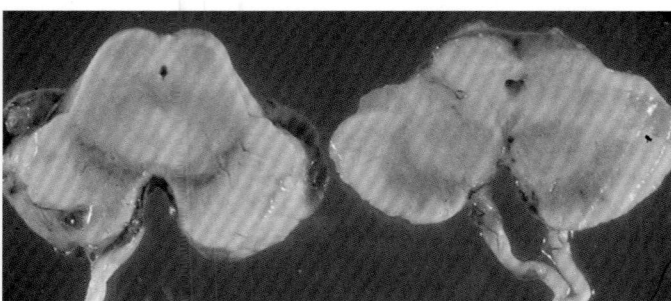

FIGURE 32-94. Parkinson disease. The normal substantia nigra (left) is heavily pigmented, while the substantia nigra in a patient with Parkinson disease (right) has lost pigmented neurons and the nucleus now blends inconspicuously into the adjacent midbrain. The locus ceruleus in the pons is also depigmented (not shown). (Courtesy of Dr. F. Stephen Vogel, Duke University.)

autonomic failure and rapid eye movement (REM) sleep behavior disorder. These disorders are now called **α-synucleinopathies** and, like the tauopathies, are considered brain-specific amyloidoses.

 PATHOLOGY: Brains of PD patients show loss of pigmentation in the substantia nigra and locus ceruleus (Fig. 32-94). Other brain regions are less affected. Pigmented neurons are scarce, and small extracellular deposits of melanin accrue from dying neurons. Some residual neurons are atrophic, and a few contain Lewy bodies (Fig. 32-95).

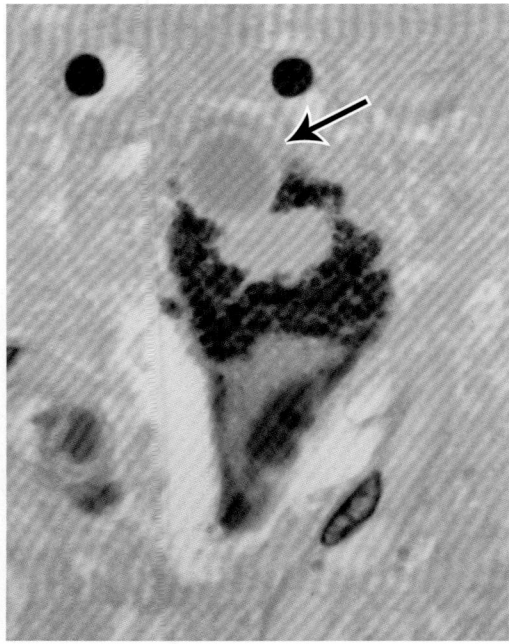

FIGURE 32-95. Lewy body in Parkinson disease. Residual neurons in the substantia nigra show intracytoplasmic, intraneuronal, spherical eosinophilic inclusions composed of polymerized α-synuclein called Lewy bodies (*arrow*). These inclusions often have a thin clear halo.

Other Disorders Causing Parkinsonism

PD is not the sole cause of parkinsonism. Other disorders share a common theme of loss of pigmented dopaminergic neurons in the substantia nigra. Normal aging is associated with some neuron loss in the substantia nigra and reduced dopamine levels, but these features are exaggerated in PD and these other causes of parkinsonism.

- **MPTP-induced parkinsonism** was discovered the late 1970s when there was an epidemic of parkinsonism among intravenous drug abusers that was ultimately linked to a toxic byproduct produced during illicit synthesis of a meperidine. That contaminant, 1-methyl-4-phenyl-1,2,3,6-tetrahydropyridine (MPTP), is metabolized by monoamine oxidase in the brain into a highly reactive free radical.
- **Post infectious parkinsonism** developed after viral encephalitis (von Economo encephalitis) associated with the influenza pandemic after World War I. It has not since recurred to a major degree. It was characterized by loss of substantia nigra neurons but Lewy bodies were not present. How this disorder develops is unknown, but it raises concerns that a similar combination of influenza antigens could lead to a recurrence of this epidemic. The 2009 H1N1 influenza virus, for example, was similar antigenically to that seen in the earlier pandemic. However, no apparent uptick in post infectious parkinsonism has been reported in association with the 2009 flu virus.
- **Striatonigral degeneration** is a rare disorder that closely mimics PD. At autopsy, the striatum (caudate and putamen) is visibly atrophied, with severe loss of neurons in this region. Changes in the substantia nigra and locus ceruleus are less severe. This condition may coexist with Shy–Drager disease (dysautonomia) and olivopontocerebellar atrophy (OPCA) as part of a unified disorder of **multiple system atrophy (MSA),** in which filamentous α-synuclein inclusions, known as **glial cytoplasmic inclusions,** accumulate primarily in oligodendroglia. They also occur to a lesser extent in neurons, where they resemble the Lewy bodies of PD and LBD.
- **Progressive supranuclear palsy (PSP)** is an uncommon disorder characterized by parkinsonism, severe postural instability with falls and progressive paralysis of vertical eye movements. Pathologic changes in the brain are more widespread than in PD, but the hallmark is atrophy of the midbrain tegmentum, leading to an exaggerated contribution of the cerebral peduncles to the profile of the midbrain in axial sections—a profile that is referred to by some as "Mickey Mouse" midbrain. Since the midbrain, as well as the substantia nigra, is the locus of integration of vertical eye movement, the combination of parkinsonism and vertical gaze dysfunction makes anatomic sense. PSP is a **tauopathy:** the sole inclusions are tau-rich NFTs. PSP spreads throughout the nervous system, and cognitive impairment complicates the disease course.

Huntington Disease

 EPIDEMIOLOGY: First described in 1872, Huntington disease (HD) is an autosomal dominant genetic disorder characterized by involuntary movements, deterioration of cognitive function, and often severe emotional disturbances. It mainly affects whites of northwestern European ancestry, with an incidence of 1 in 20,000. Genealogic studies indicate that all cases derive from an original founder in northern Europe; the disease is very rare in Asia and Africa.

 CLINICAL FEATURES: Symptoms of HD usually begin by age 40, but 5% of patients with the disorder develop neurologic signs before age 20, and a similar proportion first present after age 60. Cognitive and emotional disturbances precede the onset of abnormal movements by several years in over half of patients. Once it develops, choreoathetosis may be incapacitating. Cortical involvement leads to a severe loss of cognitive function and intellectual deterioration, often accompanied by paranoia and delusions. The interval from the onset of symptoms to death averages 15 years.

MOLECULAR PATHOGENESIS: The *HD* gene, on chromosome 4 (4p16.3), encodes the protein **huntingtin**. The aberration at this locus is expansion of a trinucleotide (CAG) repeat (see Chapter 6). The repeat is within a coding region of the gene and yields an altered protein, with a polyglutamine tract near the N-terminus. In agreement with the dominant mode of inheritance, the triplet expansion causes a toxic gain of function.

Huntingtin is widely expressed in tissues throughout the body and in all regions of the CNS by neurons and glia, but its normal function remains unknown. As with other CAG repeat expansion diseases (see Chapter 6), the longer the CAG repeat, the more severe the disease phenotype and the earlier the age of clinical onset. In HD, CAG length is more unstable and tends to be longer when inherited from the father than in maternal transmission. As a result, transmission of the *HD* mutation from the father results in clinical disease some 3 years earlier than when it is passed on from the mother. Of children with juvenile-onset HD, the ratio of those who inherit the expanded CAG allele from their father to those who inherit it from their mother is 10:1.

 PATHOLOGY: The frontal cortex is symmetrically and moderately atrophic, while the lateral ventricles are disproportionately large, owing to loss of the normal convex curvature of the caudate nuclei (Fig. 32-96). There is symmetric atrophy of the caudate nuclei, with lesser involvement of the putamen. Neuron populations of the caudate and putamen, especially the small neurons, are severely depleted, with accompanying astrogliosis. The cerebral cortical neurons are also lost, but less severely. Huntingtin aggregates in neurons, mainly in nuclei, but also in neuronal processes, potentially impairing axodendritic transport. The neurotransmitter γ-aminobutyric acid (GABA) and glutamic acid decarboxylase involved in its production are markedly decreased.

Nucleotide Repeat Expansion Disorders

HD is one of an ever-increasing group of neurologic diseases that are nucleotide repeat expansion syndromes (see Chapter 6). They are not rare. They include the most common cause of intellectual disability in boys (fragile X syndrome), the most common adult-onset muscular dystrophy (myotonic dystrophy) and the most common hereditary spinocerebellar ataxia (Friedreich ataxia).

MOLECULAR PATHOGENESIS: Trinucleotide repeats are a normal feature of many genes, and expansion of the number of triplet repeats confers pathogenicity. Some triplet repeat diseases show only a small expansion compared with their normal counterparts (e.g., Huntington disease), but in others, the expansion is quite large (e.g., fragile X syndrome and Friedreich ataxia). This class of diseases includes all forms of inheritance: X-linked, autosomal dominant, and autosomal recessive. In most of the autosomal dominant CAG expansion disorders, abnormal expansion in the coding region of a gene leads to production of an abnormal protein. In other disorders, the expansion is in a noncoding part of the gene where it may interfere with transcription or mRNA processing. This constitutes a loss-of-function mutation because it decreases protein levels (as appears to be the case with GAA expansion in Friedreich ataxia).

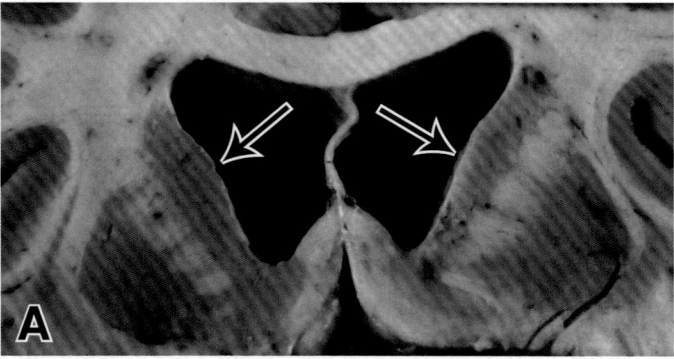
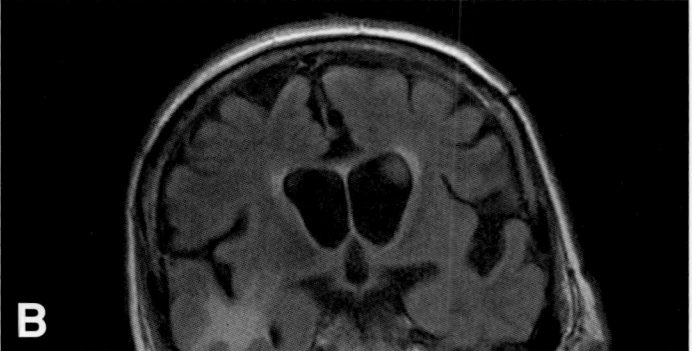

FIGURE 32-96. Huntington disease. A. The caudate nuclei (*arrows*) are atrophic bilaterally, leading to enlarged lateral ventricles. Some cortical atrophy is also seen, but it is usually not as severe as that seen in the primary cortical dementias such as Alzheimer and Pick diseases. **B.** Axial magnetic resonance imaging shows enlarged lateral ventricles accompanied by modest cortical atrophy. The square-shaped lateral ventricles of Huntington disease are sometimes called "box-car ventricles."

In myotonic dystrophy, a noncoding region expansion produces a transcript that interferes with proper mRNA splicing for multiple gene products, accounting for the multiorgan multiprotein manifestations of this condition.

Spinocerebellar Neurodegeneration

The spinocerebellar ataxias are a heterogeneous group of genetic disorders that impact cerebellar inflow and outflow pathways, or the cerebellar parenchyma itself. The cerebellum plays a key role helping the cerebral motor cortex and basal ganglia in motor functions, and ensuring smooth performance of repetitive motor tasks such as playing the piano, riding a bicycle or speaking. Once the cerebellum is exposed to motor tasks, it serves as a repository of motor programs (i.e., a "motor memory").

Cerebellar dysfunction leads to ataxia, the inability to execute motor tasks smoothly, particularly those requiring rapid alternating movement or precise motor control. Ataxia may result from defects in the major cerebellar input pathways including the middle cerebellar peduncle, which conveys motor execution commands from the cerebral motor and premotor cortex, and the inferior cerebellar peduncle, which receives proprioceptive data from the spinal cord via the spinocerebellar tracts. If the cerebellar parenchyma itself degenerates, ataxia will reflect a distribution congruent with the functional portion of the cerebellum involved—vermal degeneration leads to truncal ataxia, while cerebellar hemispheric degeneration leads to appendicular ataxia. Finally, the cerebral outflow—the dentatorubrothalamic pathway—may degenerate, leading to a peculiarly high-amplitude ataxia called "wing-beating ataxia."

Friedreich Ataxia

EPIDEMIOLOGY: Friedreich ataxia is the most common inherited ataxia. Its prevalence in European populations is 1 in 50,000. Inheritance is autosomal recessive, but many cases arise sporadically without prior family history.

CLINICAL FEATURES: Symptoms usually begin before age 25, followed by an unremittingly progressive course of about 30 years to death. Friedreich ataxia is a cerebellar inflow disorder with ataxia of both the upper and lower limbs, dysarthria, lower limb areflexia, extensor plantar reflexes, and sensory loss reflecting concurrent degeneration of spinal long tracts. Additional features include deformities of the skeletal system (e.g., scoliosis, pes cavus), hypertrophic cardiomyopathy (which commonly causes death) and diabetes mellitus.

MOLECULAR PATHOGENESIS: The genetic defect in Friedreich ataxia is autosomal recessive loss-of-function mutations in *FXN* which encodes **frataxin,** a mitochondrial protein involved in iron transport into mitochondria. In most cases the mutation is an unstable expansion of a trinucleotide (GAA) repeat in the first intron of this gene (9q13.3–21.1). The recessive

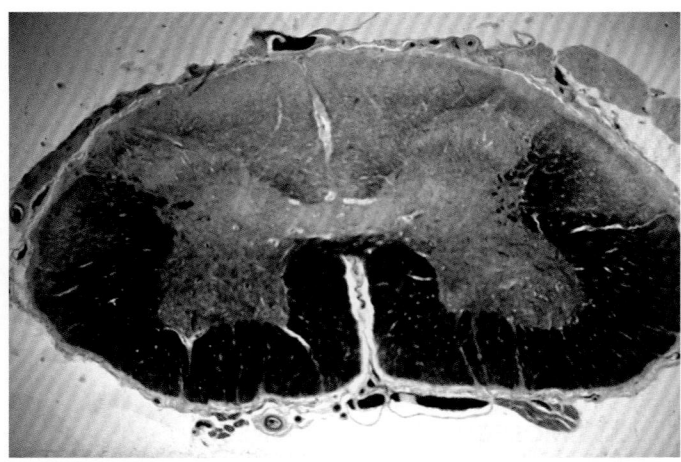

FIGURE 32-97. Friedreich ataxia. This is the most common hereditary ataxia. Myelin-stained sections of the spinal cord show secondary degeneration of the dorsal columns, lateral corticospinal tracts, and spinocerebellar tracts. This is predominantly an inflow ataxia and the cerebellum is usually not atrophic.

pattern of inheritance means that both frataxin alleles must bear the trinucleotide repeat expansion. Or, one may have the repeat expansion while the other allele may be compromised by a different mutation. The expansion mutation may impede transcription or mRNA processing. In unaffected people, levels of frataxin protein are highest in the heart and spinal cord. Loss of frataxin is thus probably responsible for both the neurologic and cardiac manifestations of Friedreich ataxia. Longer repeat expansion correlates with earlier age of disease onset, faster rate of progression, and greater frequency of hypertrophic cardiomyopathy.

PATHOLOGY: The most prominent postmortem findings in Friedreich ataxia are in the spinal cord, which shows degeneration of the posterior columns, corticospinal pathways, and spinocerebellar tracts (Fig. 32-97). Posterior column degeneration accounts for the sensory loss experienced by these patients and results from loss of the parent neuronal cell bodies in the dorsal root ganglia. In advanced cases, this is apparent grossly as shrinkage of dorsal spinal roots and posterior funiculi. Similarly, spinocerebellar tract atrophy, with attendant ataxia, follows neuronal degeneration in the dorsal nucleus of Clarke. Corticospinal tracts show the most pronounced degeneration more distally in the cord leading to weakness and release of the plantar extensor reflex.

Amyotrophic Lateral Sclerosis Is the Most Common Motor Neuron Disease

Amyotrophic Lateral Sclerosis

ALS is a degenerative disease of upper and lower motor neurons of the brain and spinal cord. It leads to progressive weakness and wasting of extremities and tongue, sometimes confusing combination of hyperreflexia and hyporeflexia and eventual impairment of respiratory muscles.

EPIDEMIOLOGY: ALS is a worldwide disease with an incidence of 1 in 100,000. It peaks in the fifth decade, and is rare in people before age 35. There is a 1.5- to 2-fold excess in men. Restricted geographic areas with a particularly high incidence exist in Guam and parts of Japan and Papua New Guinea, but these cases differ from ALS in the rest of the world. Cases in the Chamorro people indigenous to Guam are characterized by abundant accumulations of tau-rich NFTs and are now classified as **tauopathies**. Moreover, ALS in Guam is part of a spectrum of disorders that includes dementia and parkinsonism.

MOLECULAR PATHOGENESIS: Familial ALS cases account for 5% to 10% of ALS. An intronic GGGGCC repeat expansion in *C9orf72* is the most common cause of familial ALS and FTD. The C9ORF72 protein is highly expressed at presynaptic terminals. It plays complex roles in RNA transcription and translation and RNA transport. It also interacts with endosomes and is required for normal vesicle trafficking and lysosomal biogenesis. GGGGCC repeat expansion reduces *C9ORF72* expression, triggering neurodegeneration through two mechanisms: accumulation of glutamate receptors, leading to excitotoxicity, and impaired clearance of neurotoxic dipeptide repeat proteins derived from the repeat expansion. Familial ALS has also been associated with missense mutations in *SOD1*, the gene that encodes the cytosolic form of the antioxidant enzyme superoxide dismutase (Cu/Zn SOD, or SOD1; see Chapter 1). Since SOD1 is a key free radical detoxifying enzyme, *SOD1* mutations might lead to increased free radical damage. The extent to which enzyme activity is lost is limited, however, but mutant SOD1 protein is more prone to aggregation than wild-type SOD1, so this type of familial ALS appears to be a **protein conformational disorder**.

PATHOLOGY: ALS affects lower motor neurons, including anterior horn cells of the spinal cord and the motor nuclei of the brainstem, especially the hypoglossal nuclei; and the upper motor neurons of the cerebral cortex. Loss of upper motor neurons leads to degeneration of their axons, with secondary demyelination visualized in myelin-stained axial sections of the spinal cord as loss of the lateral and anterior corticospinal pathways (Fig. 32-98).

The main histologic change in ALS is loss of large motor neurons, with mild gliosis (Fig. 32-99). This is most apparent in the anterior horns of the lumbar and cervical enlargements of the spinal cord, and the hypoglossal nuclei. Giant pyramidal Betz cells in the cerebral motor cortex are also lost. Anterior nerve roots bearing the few remaining axons of the dying lower motor neurons become atrophic, and affected muscles become pale and shrunken, reflecting severe neurogenic atrophy.

CLINICAL FEATURES: ALS often begins asymmetrically as weakness and wasting of muscles of one hand. Irregular rapid involuntary contractions

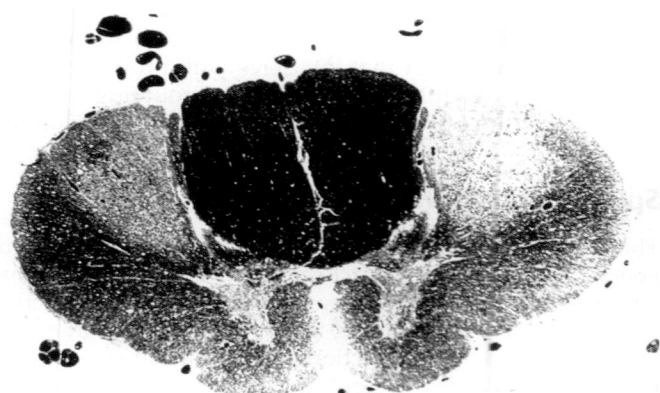

FIGURE 32-98. Amyotrophic lateral sclerosis (ALS) involves loss of upper motor neurons. This myelin-stained section of the spinal cord shows degeneration (pale staining) of the lateral corticospinal tracts reflecting degeneration of the axons of the upper motor neurons originating in the motor strip of the cerebral cortex. Note preservation of the dorsal columns, spinothalamic tracts, and spinocerebellar pathways.

of small muscle groups (fasciculations) are characteristic and are felt to arise from hyperirritability of terminal arborizations of dying lower motor neurons. The disease is inexorably progressive, with increasing weakness of the limbs leading to total disability. Speech may become unintelligible, and respiratory weakness supervenes. Despite the dramatic wasting of the body, intellectual capacity is preserved to the end, although some patients with ALS also suffer dementia of the frontotemporal lobar type. The clinical course does not usually exceed a decade.

Spinal Muscular Atrophy

Spinal muscular atrophy is the second most common lethal autosomal recessive condition in white populations. It usually presents in infancy with extreme muscle weakness and atrophy due to severe loss of anterior horn cells. It results from mutations in *SMN1* which encodes for survival motor neuron (SMN), a protein that inhibits neuronal apoptosis.

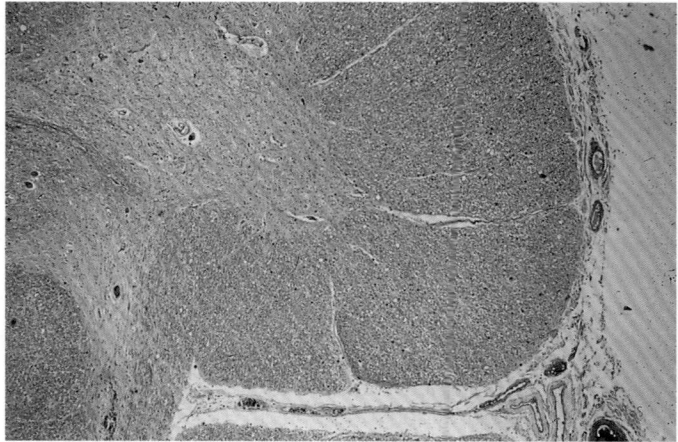

FIGURE 32-99. Amyotrophic lateral sclerosis (ALS) also involves loss of lower motor neurons in the spinal cord. The anterior horns of the spinal cord normally contain numerous large lower motor neurons. Loss of anterior horn cells occurs in ALS, accompanied by gliosis.

Loss-of-function of both copies of SMN1 causes neurons to have an increased susceptibility to programmed cell death. Classically, patients die from respiratory failure or aspiration pneumonia usually within a few months of diagnosis. Accurate diagnosis has become critical for genetic risk management and therapy considering major recent advances in anti-sense oligonucleotide therapy in this disorder. All individuals possess SMN2, a second gene in the SMN family, which codes for limited quantities of SMN but the majority of the protein is unstable due to alternative slicing.

Anti-oligonucleotide therapy with nusinersen prevents the alternative slicing and boosts production of SMN. Clinical progression is arrested or even reversed. Extremely high cost and the necessity of intrathecal administration of nusinersen are problematical, but this drug is a superb example of modern therapeutics driven by detailed molecular genetic information.

Figure 32-100 summarizes various neurodegenerative, infectious, and vitamin deficiency disorders that impact the spinal long tracts.

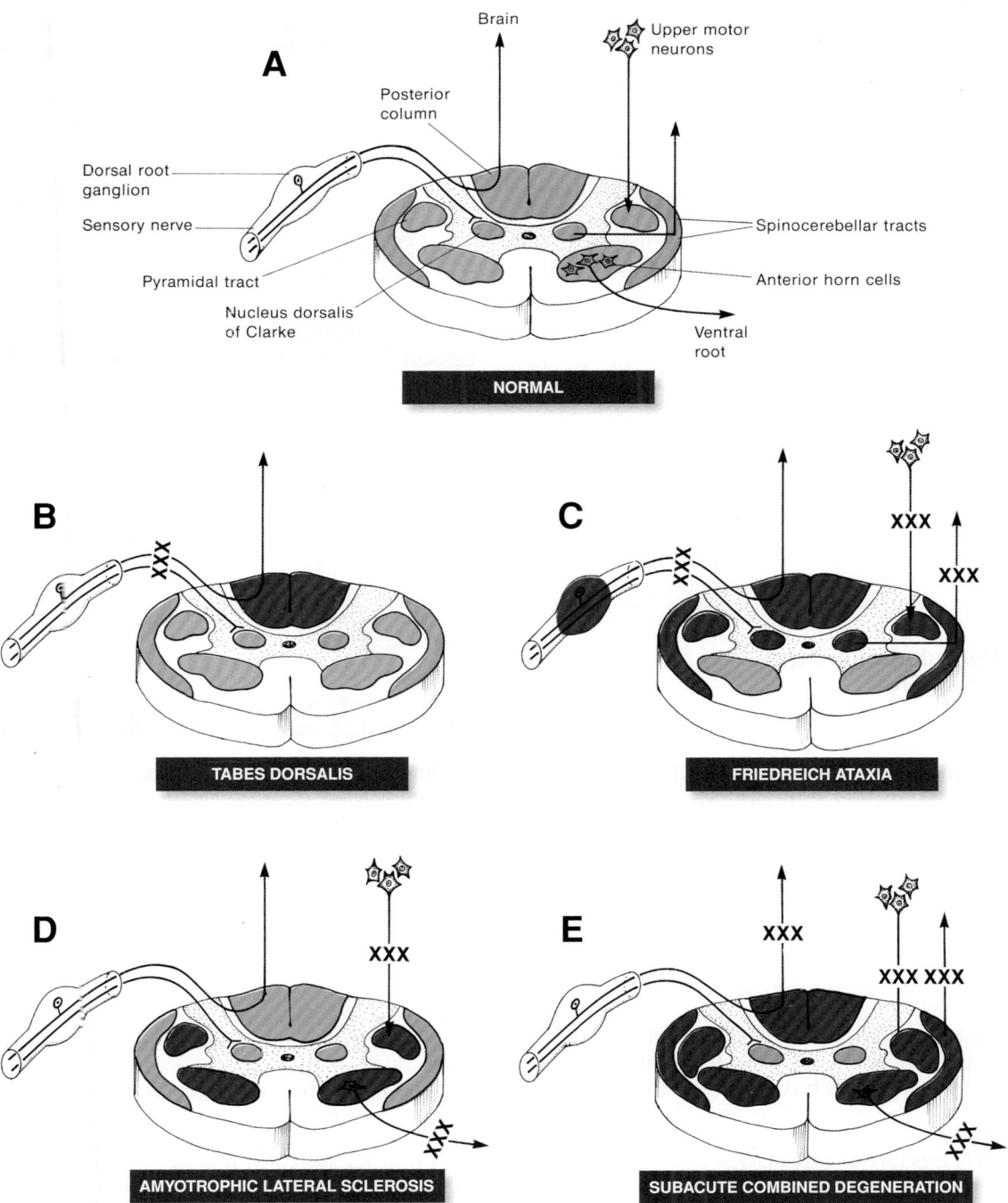

FIGURE 32-100. Tract degeneration in diseases of the spinal cord. Ascending sensory (*blue*) and descending motor (*green*) pathways travel through the spinal cord (**A**). These tracts may be differentially affected (*red*) depending on the nature of the underlying disease. Patterns of tract degeneration are shown for the four diseases we have considered, tabes dorsalis (**B**), Friedreich ataxia (**C**), amyotrophic lateral sclerosis (**D**) and subacute combined degeneration (**E**).

DEVELOPMENTAL MALFORMATIONS

CNS development unfolds according to a precise schedule, with each morphologic event serving as the foundation for those that follow. Thus, congenital anomalies reflect interruptions in the completion of developmental processes. *Congenital malformations are defined more by the timing than the specific nature of an insult.*

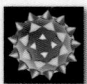 **ETIOLOGIC FACTORS:** CNS development occurs in three critical stages: (1) neurulation, (2) segmentation and cleavage, and (3) proliferation and migration. Neurulation consists of formation and closure of the neural tube and is complete by 4 weeks of gestation, often before a woman is aware that she is pregnant. This step establishes the cranial–caudal, dorsal–ventral and left–right axes of the embryo. From weeks 4 to 8, the neural tube segments into neighborhoods that will ultimately become the spinal cord, medulla, pons and cerebellum, midbrain, diencephalon, and telencephalon. The diencephalon and telencephalon then split into the paired basal ganglia, thalami, and cerebral hemispheres. By the end of 8 weeks of gestation, basic CNS architecture has been established. During the rest of gestation and beyond into postnatal life, cell proliferation creates the *trillions* of neuroglia that ultimately populate the mature CNS. These cells are mostly born in the periventricular germinal matrix and must successfully migrate to their ultimate destinations. In humans, defects of proliferation and migration mainly impact the formation of cerebral cortex and cause intellectual disability and seizures. Once neurons and glia reach their destinations, they must establish the proper wiring of the brain using mechanisms of axonal pathfinding and oligodendroglial myelination.

Defects of Neurulation Are the Neural Tube Defects

Anencephaly

Anencephaly is the congenital absence of all or part of the brain as a result of unsuccessful closure of the cephalad (anterior neuropore) portion of the neural tube.

 EPIDEMIOLOGY: Anencephaly is the second most common CNS malformation after spina bifida (0.5–2.0 per 1,000 births, with females predominating) and is the most common lethal CNS malformation. Anencephalic fetuses are stillborn or die in the first few days of life.

Anencephaly is a multifactorial birth defect exhibiting geographic variation in incidence. In the United States, it occurs in 0.3 per 1,000 live births and stillbirths. In Ireland, the frequency is 20-fold greater (5–6 per 1,000). Incidence declines to 2–3 per 1,000 among Irish immigrants to North America. It is rare among blacks.

ETIOLOGIC FACTORS: Anencephaly is a dysraphic defect of neural tube closure (Fig. 32-101). Its concurrence with other neural tube defects

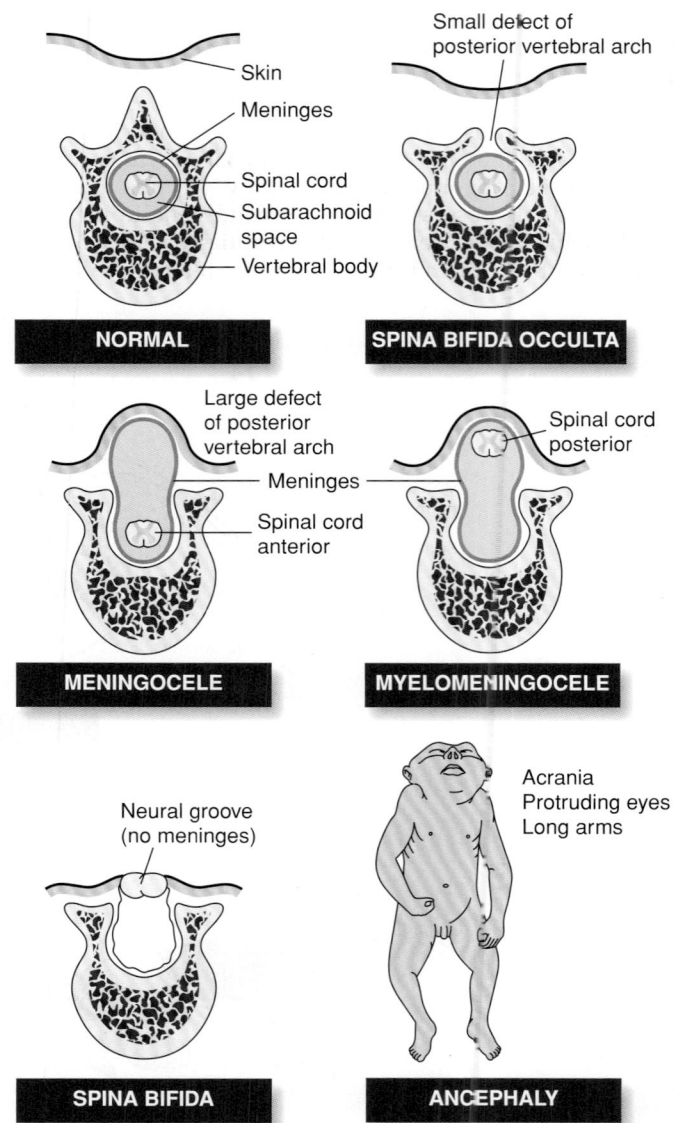

FIGURE 32-101. Defects of the neural tube. The first critical step in neural development is neurulation—formation and closure of the neural tube. Incomplete fusion of the neural tube and overlying bone, soft tissues or skin leads to several defects, varying from mild anomalies (e.g., spina bifida occulta) to severe anomalies (e.g., anencephaly).

(NTDs), such as spina bifida, suggests shared pathogenic mechanisms. During development, the neural plate invaginates and is transformed into the neural tube by fusion of the posterior surfaces. Mesenchymal tissue overlying the primitive neural tube then forms the skull and vertebral arches posterior to the spinal cord, while ectoderm forms the overlying skin. If the neural tube does not close, neither can the overlying bony structures of the cranium. The calvarium, skin, and subcutaneous tissues will thus be absent in this region. The exposed brain is incompletely formed or even entirely absent. Most often, the base of the skull has only bits of neural and ependymal tissue and residues of meninges.

Genetic factors contribute to the pathogenesis of anencephaly. The anomaly is twice as common in female as in male fetuses, and it occurs with higher frequency in certain families. The risk of a second anencephalic fetus is 2% to 5%. After bearing two anencephalic fetuses, the risk reaches 25% for each subsequent pregnancy.

Folic acid supplied in the periconceptional period lowers the incidence of NTDs. In 1998, the U.S. Food and Drug Administration began requiring supplemental folate to be added to enriched flour, bread, cereals, and some other products. This was associated with a significant decrease in the incidence of NTDs of all types (see Chapters 6 and 14).

PATHOLOGY: The cranial vault is absent. The cerebral hemispheres are replaced by a highly vascularized, disorganized neuroglial tissue, referred to as the **cerebrovasculosa** (Fig. 32-102), on the flattened base of the skull. Two well-formed eyes with well-differentiated retinas mark the anterior margin of disturbed organogenesis. Short segments of optic nerves extend posteriorly. The posterior aspect of the malformation forms a variable transitional zone with a recognizable midbrain, but the brainstem and cerebellum are usually rudimentary. The upper spinal cord is hypoplastic, and a dysraphic bony posterior spinal column defect **(rachischisis)** may affect the cervical area. Vertebral and basilar arteries usually are identifiable amid the meningeal vessels.

The cerebrovasculosa typically contains islands of immature neural tissue. It also encloses cavities partly lined by ependyma, with or without choroid plexus. However, the mass mainly consists of abnormal vascular channels that vary considerably in size.

Two-thirds of anencephalic fetuses die in utero; those that are alive at birth rarely survive more than a week. Screening of pregnant women for serum α-fetoprotein and ultrasonography detect virtually all anencephalic fetuses.

Spina Bifida

Spina bifida includes a group of NTDs that are due to failure of neural tube closure in the more caudal regions. These anomalies usually arise in the lumbar region and range in severity from asymptomatic to disabling. They are generally not lethal. They result from a developmental error occurring between the 25th and 30th days of gestation, reflecting the

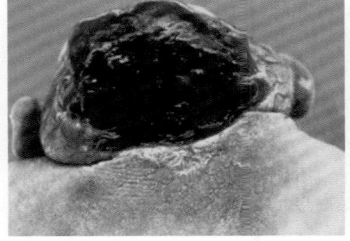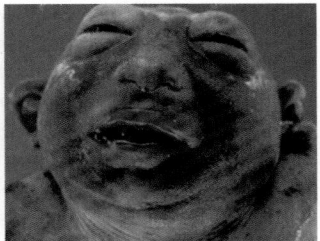

FIGURE 32-102. Anencephaly is the most severe defect of neurulation. The cerebral vault is absent (*right panel*), and the absence of a calvarium exposes a mass of vascularized tissue (cerebrovasculosa, *left panel*), in which there are rudimentary neuroectodermal structures. The lesion is bounded anteriorly by normally formed eyes and posteriorly by the brainstem.

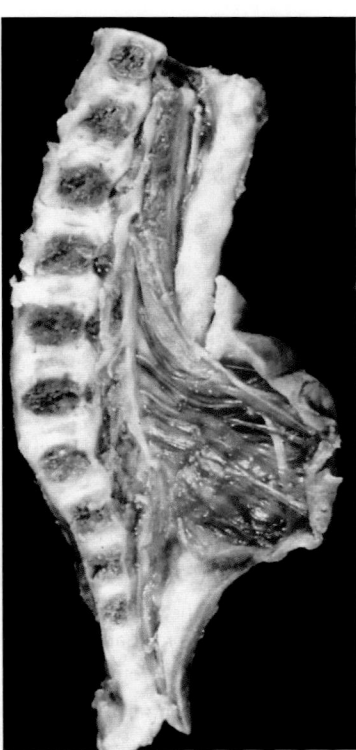

FIGURE 32-103. Meningomyelocele. This dysraphic defect, caused by lack of fusion of the spinal canal usually in the lumbar region, produces disorganized spinal cord tissue with entrapment of nerve roots in a cerebrospinal fluid–filled sac. (Courtesy of Dr. F. Stephen Vogel, Duke University.)

timing of neural tube closure. They are subclassified by the severity of the defect:

- **Spina bifida occulta:** This defect is restricted to the vertebral arches and is usually asymptomatic. It frequently manifests externally only by a dimple or small tuft of hair on the lower back.
- **Meningocele:** This condition entails a greater bone and soft tissue defect that permits the meninges to protrude as a fluid-filled sac visible on the external surface of the back, in the midline. The sides of the sac are usually covered by a thin layer of skin. Its apex may be ulcerated, allowing microorganisms to access the CSF.
- **Meningomyelocele:** This is an even more extensive defect that exposes the spinal canal and causes nerve roots (particularly those of the cauda equina) and spinal cord to be entrapped in an externalized protruding CSF-filled sac (Fig. 32-103). Usually, the spinal cord is a flattened, ribbon-like structure. Severe neurologic consequences include lower extremity motor and sensory defects and compromise of neurogenic bowel and bladder control.
- **Rachischisis:** In this extreme defect, the spinal column is a gaping canal, often without a recognizable spinal cord (Fig. 32-104). Rachischisis is usually lethal and seen in abortuses.

Spina bifida can be induced in rats and chicks at the 8th to 9th gestational day by chemicals such as trypan blue or by hypervitaminosis A. It presumably reflects failure of the neural tube to close, but this concept is not established. As mentioned above, maternal folate deficiency is implicated in NTDs. Some drugs, notably retinoids used to treat acne and valproic acid

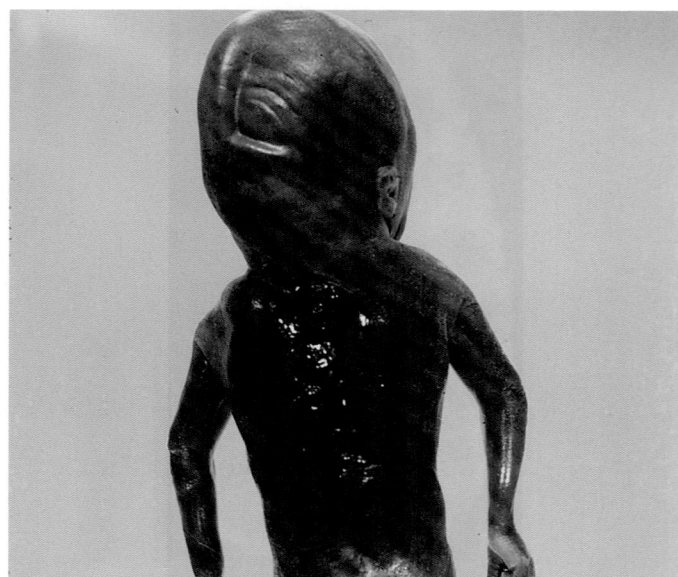

FIGURE 32-104. Rachischisis. The vertebral column shows a bony, cutaneous defect with segmental thoracic absence of the spinal cord and overlying vertebral arches and soft tissues.

used to manage seizures, must be avoided by women of child-bearing age because of their association with NTDs.

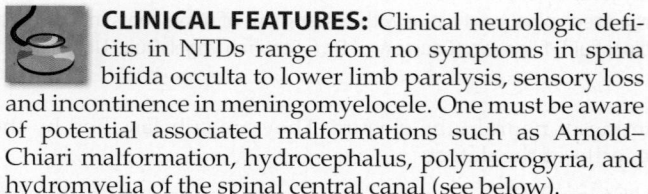**CLINICAL FEATURES:** Clinical neurologic deficits in NTDs range from no symptoms in spina bifida occulta to lower limb paralysis, sensory loss and incontinence in meningomyelocele. One must be aware of potential associated malformations such as Arnold–Chiari malformation, hydrocephalus, polymicrogyria, and hydromyelia of the spinal central canal (see below).

Malformations of the Spinal Cord

Some other spinal cord malformations are less apparent at birth than NTDs. These include rare total **(dimyelia)** to partial duplication of the spinal cord into two separate structures **(diastematomyelia)**. **Hydromyelia** is dilation of the central spinal cord canal.

Syringomyelia is a congenital malformation involving a tubular cavitation (syrinx) that extends for variable distances within the spinal cord and may or may not communicate with the central canal. It can first arise as a congenital malformation but progress slowly and present clinically in adults. Some cases of syringomyelia are not congenital in origin but are caused by trauma, ischemia, or tumors. The syrinx is filled with a clear fluid similar to CSF. **Syringobulbia** is a variant of syringomyelia in which the syrinx is located in the medulla.

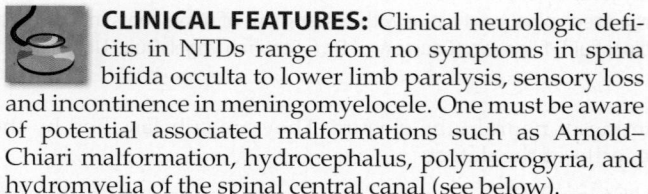**CLINICAL FEATURES:** Symptoms of syringomyelia occur at the spinal level of the syrinx where it disrupts the segmentally crossing secondary axons of the spinothalamic pathway. This leads to loss of pain and thermal sensation bilaterally at the spinal level of the syrinx with relative sparing of fine touch and proprioception as well as motor pathways.

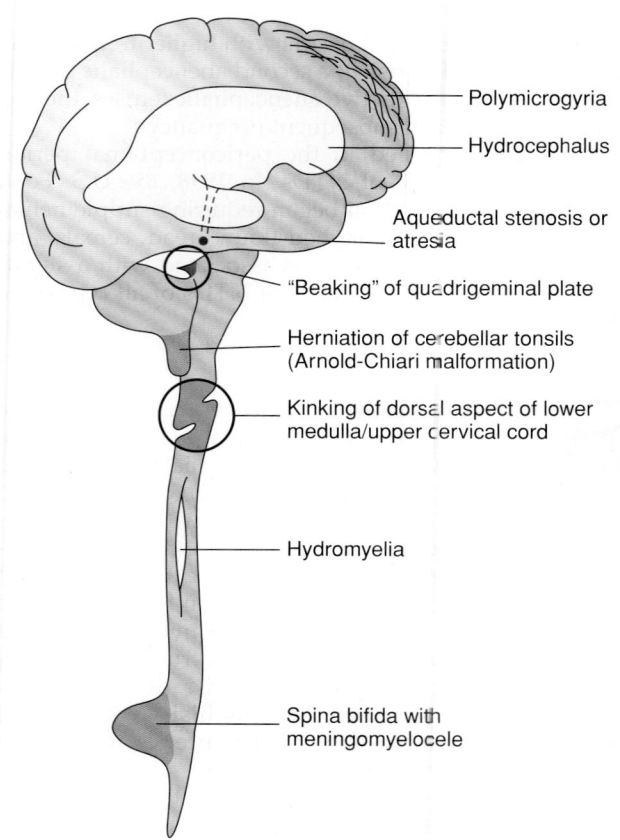

- Polymicrogyria
- Hydrocephalus
- Aqueductal stenosis or atresia
- "Beaking" of quadrigeminal plate
- Herniation of cerebellar tonsils (Arnold–Chiari malformation)
- Kinking of dorsal aspect of lower medulla/upper cervical cord
- Hydromyelia
- Spina bifida with meningomyelocele

FIGURE 32-105. Arnold–Chiari malformation and associated lesions.

Arnold–Chiari Malformation

Arnold–Chiari malformation is a complex condition in which the brainstem and cerebellum are compacted into a shallow, bowl-shaped posterior fossa with a low-positioned tentorium. It is often associated with syringomyelia or a lumbosacral meningomyelocele. Symptoms depend on the severity of the defect (Fig. 32-105). *Since this malformation involves segmentation of the medulla and cerebellum as well as neural tube closure, it represents a defect of both neurulation and segmentation.*

PATHOPHYSIOLOGY: The pathogenesis of Arnold–Chiari malformation is obscure. It has spawned much speculation, but no single hypothesis accounts for all features of the condition. One theory posits that a meningomyelocele anchors the lower end of the spinal cord, causing downward growth of the vertebral column, and creating traction on the medulla. However, this does not explain other facets of the malformation such as curvature of the medulla and beaking of the quadrigeminal plate (Fig. 32-105). Other proposals include increased intracranial pressure plus hydrocephalus or limited size of the posterior fossa.

PATHOLOGY: In Arnold–Chiari malformation, the caudal aspect of the cerebellar vermis is herniated through an enlarged foramen magnum and protrudes onto the dorsal cervical cord, often reaching

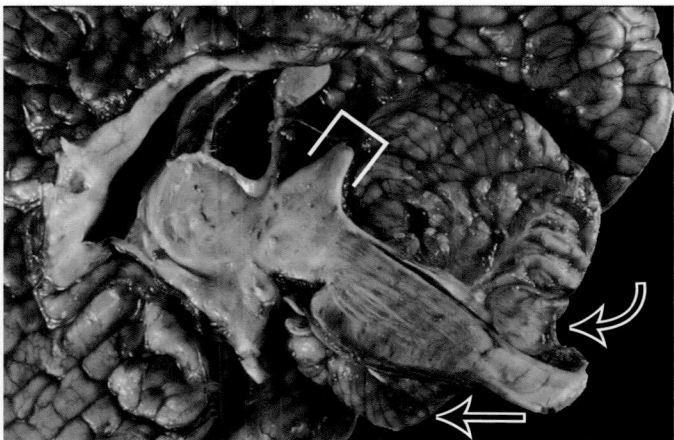

FIGURE 32-106. **Arnold–Chiari malformation.** The cerebellar vermis is herniated below the level of the foramen magnum (*arrow*). Downward displacement of the dorsal portion of the cord causes the obex of the fourth ventricle to occupy a position below the foramen magnum (*curved arrow*). The midbrain shows extreme "beaking" of the tectum and the four colliculi of the quadrigeminal plate are replaced by a single pyramidal-shaped structure (*bracket*).

C3–C5 (Fig. 32-105). The herniated tissue is held in position by thickened meninges and shows pressure atrophy exemplified by depletion of Purkinje and granular cells. The brainstem also is displaced caudally. Typically, this is more exaggerated dorsally than ventrally, and landmarks such as the obex of the fourth ventricle are more caudal than ventral structures such as the inferior olive. From a lateral perspective, the lower medulla is angulated in its midsegment, creating a dorsal protrusion. The foramina of Magendie and Luschka are compressed by the bony ridge of the foramen magnum, causing hydrocephalus. The cerebellum is flattened to a discoid contour, and the quadrigeminal plate is often deformed by a "beak-shaped" dorsal protrusion of the inferior colliculi.

Defects of Segmentation and Cleavage Cause Loss of Key Structures

Holoprosencephaly

This represents a series of defects in which the interhemispheric fissure is absent or only partly formed owing to a failure of the telencephalon to divide into the two hemispheres. Holoprosencephaly is a continuum: complete cleavage failure gives rise to **alobar holoprosencephaly**; partial failure leads to **lobar holoprosencephaly** and the subtlest form is failure of olfactory nerves to form, causing **arrhinencephaly**. Alobar holoprosencephaly produces a bulbous horseshoe-shaped cortical dome of fused frontal poles with gyri oriented in an irregular horizontal pattern (Fig. 32-107). A common ventricular chamber is created by lateral displacement of the posterior portions of the telencephalon. Bilobed caudate nuclei and thalami are prominent. In lobar holoprosencephaly, there is partial cleavage in the posterior portion of the telencephalon, but with a single gaping ventricular chamber. Holoprosencephaly is rarely compatible with life beyond a few weeks or months. Those who survive suffer severe intellectual disability and seizures.

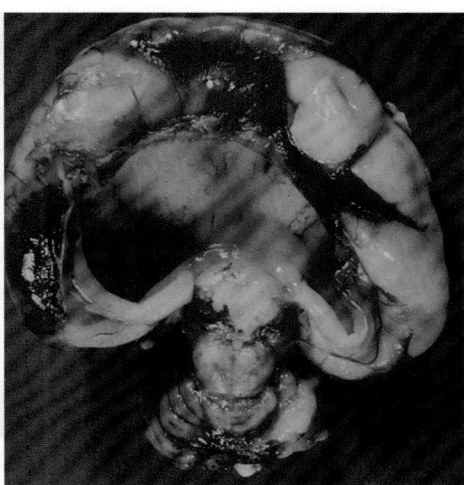

FIGURE 32-107. **Holoprosencephaly.** The brain exhibits a lack of separation of the hemispheres which creates a single large ventricle as seen here viewed from an anterior perspective. Because no interhemispheric fissure is present, this constitutes alobar holoprosencephaly.

 MOLECULAR PATHOGENESIS: About 25% to 50% of patients with holoprosencephaly have numerical or structural chromosomal abnormalities. Monogenic holoprosencephaly is sometimes associated with mutations in *SHH*, the gene encoding the morphogen sonic hedgehog which plays an important role in patterning in embryonic development.

Arrhinencephaly

The absence of the olfactory tracts and bulbs (rhinencephalon) is the least severe of the holoprosencephaly defects (Fig. 32-108).

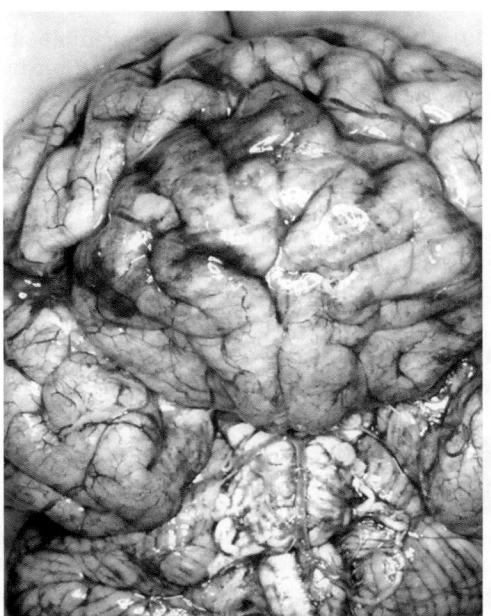

FIGURE 32-108. **Arrhinencephaly,** the least severe form of holoprosencephaly, consists grossly of absence of the olfactory bulbs and nerves (hence its name "a," *without,* and "rhinencephaly," *nose brain*). Subtle microscopic abnormalities also occur, and most of these individuals have some degree of intellectual disability. (Courtesy of Dr. F. Stephen Vogel, Duke University.)

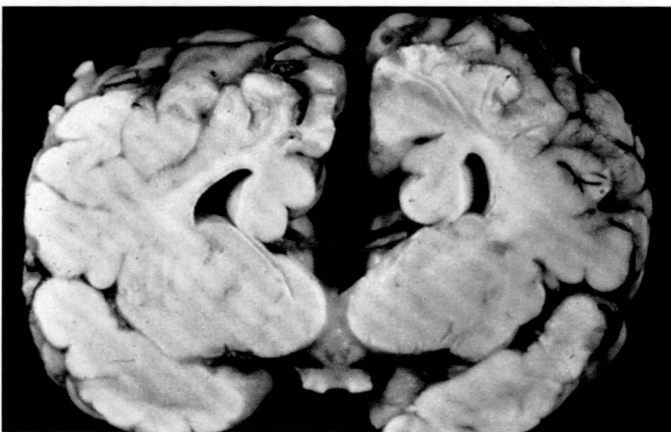

FIGURE 32-109. Congenital absence of the corpus callosum. A coronal section at the level of the thalamus reveals absence of the corpus callosum and "bat-wing" shape of the lateral ventricles. (Courtesy of Dr. F. Stephen Vogel, Duke University.)

It is clinically manifested by lack of a sense of smell **(anosmia)** and may be associated with intellectual disability.

Agenesis of the Corpus Callosum

This anomaly is a regular feature of holoprosencephaly but can also be a solitary lesion. Lack of a corpus callosum does not entail significant loss of interhemispheric functional coordination, but it is associated with seizures. The corpus callosum physically tethers and functionally interconnects the hemispheres, so its absence permits the lateral ventricles to drift outward and upward. This produces a diagnostic radiographic finding of "bat-wing" ventricles (Fig. 32-109).

Congenital Atresia of the Aqueduct of Sylvius

This is the most common cause of congenital obstructive hydrocephalus, occurring in 1 in 1,000 live births. It may result from deranged mesencephalic (midbrain) development. The brain is enlarged owing to grotesque ventricular dilatation, with thinning of the cerebral cortex and stretching of white matter tracts. The midbrain may show multiple atretic channels or an aqueduct narrowed by gliosis, which may arise due to developmental failure during segmentation or later in gestation as a result of transplacental transmission of infections that induce ependymitis.

Cortical Malformations Arise From Defects of Neuroglial Proliferation and Migration

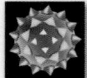 **ETIOLOGIC FACTORS:** Neuroglial proliferation and migration begin in the first trimester of embryonic development and continue throughout prenatal life. Primitive neurons and glia move centrifugally from the periventricular germinal matrix to populate the cortex. The number and positions of neurons in the cortex determine the cortical infolding that creates sulci and gyri.

Disorders of cortical development reflect the nature and severity of disruption of gyral patterning. A cortical defect may be global or focal, and there is a spatial destiny of neuroglial cells in a given region of germinal matrix such that portions of the germinal matrix induce formation of specific overlying portions of the cerebral cortex. If a focal region of germinal matrix is destroyed or damaged, the cortical destination of cells spawned in that region will reflect this damage. **Schizencephaly** is an example of such a failure of focal cortical development due to damage to the germinal matrix. Here, a patch of cortex is "missing" but cortex built from otherwise undamaged germinal matrix will be structurally normal. More global, often genetically determined defects of neuroglial proliferation and migration result in a more widespread and severe cortical defect, called lissencephaly, meaning "smooth brain."

- **Lissencephaly** is the most severe congenital disorder of cortical development. The cortical surface of the cerebral hemispheres is smooth or has imperfectly formed gyri. Some 60% of patients with lissencephaly show deletions in the *LIS1* gene on chromosome 17p13.3. This gene encodes a protein involved in cytoskeletal dynamics and loss-of-function mutations affect cell proliferation and motility which are of obvious importance in neuroglial proliferation and migration. The white matter in lissencephaly contains clusters of neurons that failed to reach the cortex.
- **Heterotopias** are focal disturbances in neuronal migration that lead to formations of nodules of ectopic neurons and glia, usually in white matter. They are often associated clinically with intellectual disability and seizures. They have been linked to maternal alcoholism.
- **Polymicrogyria** describes the presence of excessive small gyri (Fig. 32-110). The brain surface appears to be textured with many small bumps.
- **Pachygyria** is a condition in which gyri are reduced in number and unusually broad (Fig. 32-111).

Late-Term and Perinatal Insults May Lead to Severe Brain Damage

Sometimes the CNS develops successfully, only to suffer catastrophic damage late in pregnancy or in the perinatal

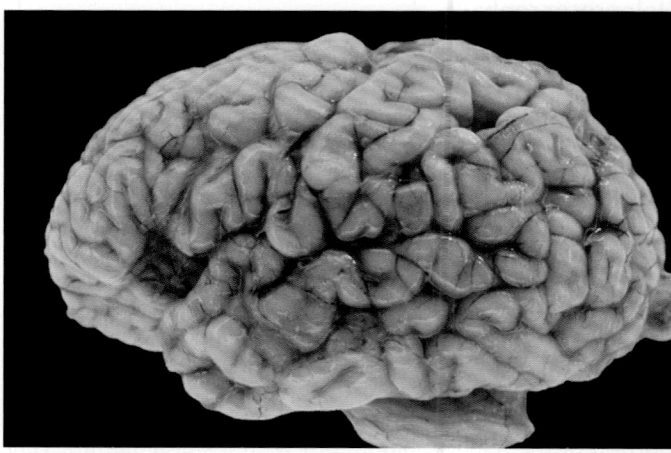

FIGURE 32-110. Polymicrogyria. The surface of the brain exhibits an excessive number of small, irregularly sized, randomly distributed gyral folds.

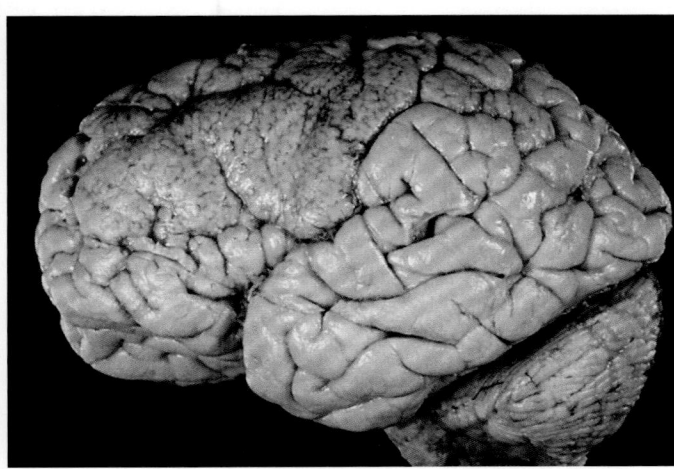

FIGURE 32-111. Pachygyria. Broad textured gyri are seen in the superior frontal region, indicating a defect in cortical formation. (Courtesy of Dr. F. Stephen Vogel, Duke University.)

period. If the brain is deprived of blood or oxygen, the cerebral hemispheres may liquefy, leaving a fluid-filled cranial cavity, a state called **hydranencephaly**. Head circumference reflects the largest size the brain attained before the insult occurred. The head can be transilluminated as no tissue remains to block the passage of light through the cranial vault. Cranial sutures may override as the nascent brain degenerates.

Less severe, but still devastating, is hypoxia/ischemia which can lead to late-term and perinatal cerebral infarcts. Developing brains are unique bioenergetically. In adults, the gray matter receives three times the blood and consumes three times the oxygen as the white matter. By contrast, the periventricular germinal matrix and streams of migrating neuroglia equalize bioenergetic demand in developing brains, so that deep structures and cerebral cortex have similarly huge energy and substrate requirements. The deep periventricular white matter is a watershed perfusion zone and is at highest risk for infarction. Thus, intrauterine or perinatal hypoxia ischemia may cause chalky white, sometimes calcific **periventricular leukomalacia**. Infarcted areas may undergo resorption, leading to **multicystic leukoencephalopathy**, with numerous interconnected cystic cavities deep in the white matter near the ventricles.

The germinal matrix is active during later phases of gestation but gradually involutes as term approaches. If a baby is born prematurely, its metabolically active germinal matrix is perfused by delicate capillaries floating in a frenzied sea of stem cells and newly spawned neuroglia. Such an infant is ill equipped for cerebrovascular regulation. These delicate vessels may be exposed to dramatic swings in perfusion pressure, leading to **germinal matrix hemorrhage**. Hemorrhage may remain confined to a small region of the germinal matrix or spread catastrophically as intraventricular hemorrhage. Germinal matrix hemorrhage is a major challenge in clinical management of premature newborns.

Congenital Defects May Be Associated With Chromosomal Abnormalities

Derangements of the larger autosomes, 1 through 12, are incompatible with sustained intrauterine life: affected fetuses are spontaneously aborted. Structural and functional abnormalities may be attributed to gross chromosomal derangements of the smaller autosomes (e.g., trisomies of chromosomes 13–15 and 21 [Down syndrome]). Trisomies 13 or 15 occur in 1 in 5,000 births, with a modest female predominance. The resultant congenital deformities involve the brain, heart, facial features, and extremities. Brain malformations include holoprosencephaly, arrhinencephaly, microphthalmia, and cyclopia.

CENTRAL NERVOUS SYSTEM NEOPLASIA

Primary CNS cancers represent 1.5% of all primary malignant tumors. Metastatic tumors to the CNS occur far more commonly than primary tumors and they present major challenges in clinical management. The broad spectrum of cellular constituents of the CNS—all of the diverse cell types that are represented in the CNS—is mirrored by the wide range of tumor types that arise within the brain and spinal cord and their overlying meninges. More than 130 different types of CNS neoplasms are recognized and formally codified by the World Health Organization (WHO), but most are very rare. By far the most common are meningiomas and gliomas, each of which accounts for 1/3 of CNS tumors (Table 32-5). While most brain tumors arise in adults, some are more common in childhood, the most prominent being medulloblastoma, pilocytic astrocytoma (PA), and diffuse pontine astrocytoma. Together, primary brain tumors are second only to leukemias as the most common childhood malignancy and they are the most common solid tumors in children.

Diagnosing a brain tumor entails preoperative consideration of a differential diagnosis of likely possibilities based on clinical and imaging findings (Table 32-6), followed by a definitive tissue-based diagnosis by biopsy or resection. Clinical management requires analysis of the key characteristics of different brain and spinal cord tumors and other kinds of diseases, plus the patient's age, the location of

TABLE 32-5
MAJOR TYPES OF PRIMARY CENTRAL NERVOUS SYSTEM (CNS) TUMORS
Meningioma
Gliomas (including diffuse and circumscribed astrocytomas, oligodendrogliomas, ependymomas, choroid plexus tumors, several rare glioma subtypes)
Medulloblastoma and other embryonal tumors
Craniopharyngiomas
Germ cell tumors
Hemangioblastomas
Neuronal and mixed glioneuronal tumors
Pineal tumors
Primary CNS lymphomas

TABLE 32-6

ESSENTIAL CLINICAL INFORMATION IN CENTRAL NERVOUS SYSTEM TUMORS

Patient age and gender
Anatomic location and compartment of the lesion
Neuroimaging (computed tomography, magnetic resonance imaging) features
Nature and time course of presenting signs and symptoms
Relevant clinical history

TABLE 32-7

MAJOR NEUROIMAGING (COMPUTED TOMOGRAPHY, MAGNETIC RESONANCE IMAGING) FEATURES

Anatomic location and compartment of the lesion(s)
Nature of the interface between the lesion and the surrounding parenchyma (e.g., sharply circumscribed vs. diffuse)
Presence or absence of enhancement following contrast agent administration
If contrast enhancing, the pattern of enhancement (e.g., solid uniform enhancement, ring enhancement around a central area of necrosis, C-shaped open ring enhancement, enhancing nodule within the wall of a cyst)

the lesion, specific neuroimaging features, the nature and time course of preceding clinical signs and symptoms and major elements of the clinical history, such as the presence of a systemic primary tumor or a tumor predisposition syndrome.

PATIENT AGE: Different types of brain tumors tend to arise at particular ages. The two most common brain tumors of childhood are medulloblastoma and PA. Rare tumors that also tend to occur in children include diffuse pontine glioma, atypical teratoid/rhabdoid tumor, and choroid plexus carcinoma. Metastatic carcinomas from the lung, breast, and colon mainly affect older adults. Other brain tumors, such as ganglioglioma and central neurocytoma, have a peak incidence in young adulthood. Some tumors may be most common in adults but spare no age group. For example, glioblastomas, the most common and most malignant of gliomas, can occur at any time of life.

PATIENT GENDER: Most primary brain tumors are more common in males. Two notable exceptions are pituitary adenomas and meningiomas, which are more common in young adult and middle-aged to older adult women, respectively. Primary tumors from other sites that metastasize to the brain follow the gender patterns of incidence of those tumor types (e.g., breast, prostate).

ANATOMIC LOCATION AND COMPARTMENT OF THE LESION: Anatomic localization of brain lesions includes two components: the region of the CNS involved, such as the cerebrum, cerebellum or spinal cord, and the compartment(s). Examples of the latter include intraparenchymal (e.g., within the brain substance), intraventricular or intradural–extra-axial (within the spinal subarachnoid space). Such information is of critical importance in formulating a differential diagnosis. For example, intradural, extra-axial spinal cord masses are likely meningiomas or peripheral nerve sheath tumors; masses within a cerebral lateral ventricle are more likely to be choroid plexus papillomas, ependymomas, or other tumors that frequent those haunts.

NEUROIMAGING FEATURES: Preoperative imaging of a CNS lesion provides critical data that bear directly on the differential diagnosis (Table 32-7; Fig. 32-112). The most obvious are the number and distribution of lesions, as noted above. The nature of the interface between the lesion and the surrounding brain is also important. For example, the borders of highly infiltrative tumors, such as fibrillary astrocytomas, oligodendrogliomas (ODGs), and lymphomas, are subtle and diffuse. By contrast, interfaces with the surrounding brain are more sharply circumscribed for metastases or minimally infiltrative primary tumors, such as PA or ganglioglioma.

Vascularity, assessed by administration of radiographic contrast agents, is also helpful, since some tumor types, such as glioblastoma, meningioma, medulloblastoma, and metastatic carcinomas, are more vascular, while others, such as low-grade diffuse fibrillary astrocytoma, are usually not so highly vascularized. Meningiomas and primary CNS lymphoma tend to show relatively solid, even enhancement, whereas ring enhancement around a central area of necrosis is more typical of glioblastomas. Nontumor diseases, many of which mimic tumor radiographically, also often have characteristic enhancement patterns. For example, demyelinating pseudotumors frequently present as mass lesions with "open ring" or "C-shaped" enhancement, while cerebral abscesses typically show a smooth-walled enhancing ring (Fig. 32-112).

NATURE AND TIME COURSE OF CLINICAL SIGNS AND SYMPTOMS: In general, a prolonged history of signs or symptoms, such as several years of poorly controlled seizures, favors more indolent or low-grade disease, while a relatively brief history, such as a 2-week history of headache, nausea and emesis with localizing signs, favors a higher-grade and more aggressively expanding lesion.

RELEVANT CLINICAL HISTORY: Information regarding previous non-CNS tumors, previous radiation to the CNS, systemic diseases, or tumor predisposition syndromes is also useful (Table 32-8).

GRADING OF CENTRAL NERVOUS SYSTEM TUMORS: Tumors in the brain and spinal cord are commonly graded according to criteria established in the *WHO Classification of Tumours of the Central Nervous System.* According to WHO criteria, tumor grades range from I to IV, with I being the lowest grade and IV the most malignant. The subjective and ill-defined term "benign" should be used with extreme caution, if at all, with respect to CNS tumors, including WHO grade I tumors. Anatomic location, growth pattern, and other factors can result in a clinical course for a grade I CNS tumor that entails considerable morbidity and even mortality. For example, most meningiomas are grade I, but those that grow en plaque (flat and plaque-like) along the skull base can surround cranial nerves and blood vessels as they enter and exit the cranial cavity. These can be very difficult to treat surgically and often do not respond favorably to radiation or chemotherapy. Similarly, the vast majority of low-grade diffuse

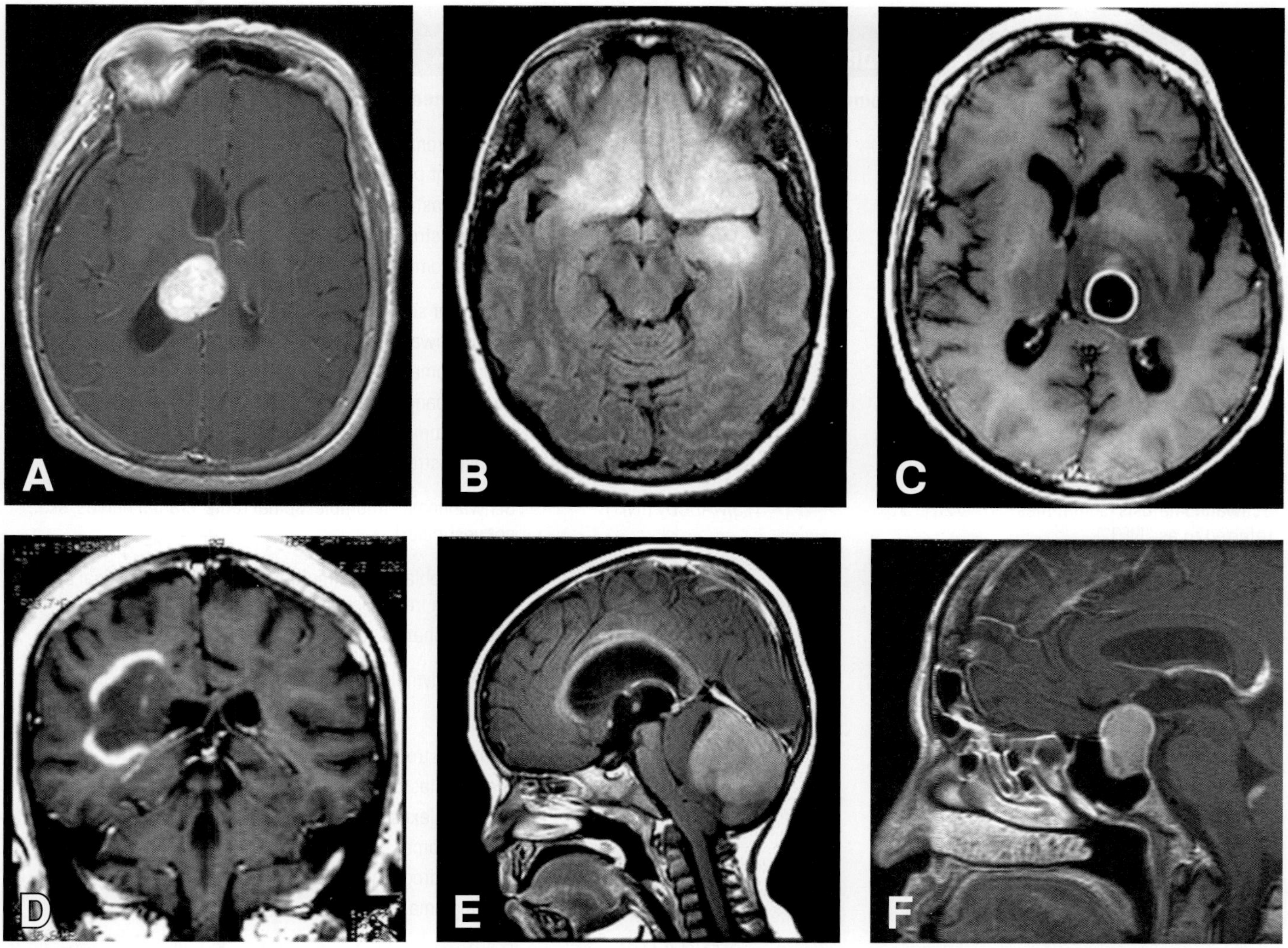

FIGURE 32-112. Neuroimaging—the modern pathologist's gross pathology. Contemporary neuroimaging provides the first look at the "gross pathology" of a central nervous system lesion and constitutes a rich source of information that enables the pathologist to formulate a refined differential diagnosis prior to surgical biopsy and tissue examination. Shown here are representative examples of magnetic resonance images that illustrate the highly informative features of six different brain lesions. **A.** A contrast-enhancing, circumscribed mass located within the lateral ventricle (choroid plexus meningioma). **B.** Diffuse hyperintensity involving both frontal lobes and the left temporal lobe (infiltrating glioma). **C.** Smooth-walled ring-enhancing mass in the left thalamus (pyogenic abscess). **D.** C-shaped open ring-enhancing lesion in the white matter of the right parietal lobe (demyelinating pseudotumor). **E.** Hyperintense midline mass of the cerebellar vermis and fourth ventricle (medulloblastoma). **F.** Contrast-enhancing midline mass of the sellar and suprasellar region (pituitary adenoma).

gliomas (WHO grade II) are ultimately fatal, even though this is the lowest grade for this subtype of glioma.

Meningiomas Are the Most Common Central Nervous System Tumors

Meningiomas are derived from the middle layer of arachnoid (meningothelial) cells that form the outer boundary of the subarachnoid space. Anatomic locations in which meningiomas occur thus parallel the distribution of the arachnoid membrane, and these tumors can arise at any CNS site where arachnoid cells are present—including the dural venous sinuses (such as the superior sagittal sinus), cerebral convexity, skull base, around the optic nerve and spinal cord, and even within the choroid plexus in the cerebral ventricles as mentioned earlier.

 MOLECULAR PATHOGENESIS: Meningiomas typically arise in one of three settings:

- **Sporadic:** *The vast majority of meningiomas arise sporadically.* Many show loss, partial deletion or other types of mutations in NF2 (22q12). Disturbances of this tumor suppressor gene may thus be involved not only in neurofibromatosis type 2 (NF2)–associated tumors but also in the origin of sporadic meningiomas (and schwannomas). Meningiomas without alterations in NF2 frequently have alterations in TRAF7 (involved in TNF signaling), KLF4 (encodes a transcription factor that regulates proliferation and migration), AKT1 (encodes a kinase that regulates proliferation and cell survival) and SMO (encodes smoothened, a G-protein–coupled

TABLE 32-8

MAJOR NERVOUS SYSTEM TUMOR PREDISPOSITION SYNDROMES

Syndrome	Chromosome Locus	Gene (Protein)	Associated Nervous System Tumors
Neurofibromatosis type 1 (NF1)	17q11.2	*NF1* (neurofibromin)	Neurofibromas (dermal and plexiform) Malignant peripheral nerve sheath tumor (MPNST) Pilocytic astrocytoma ("optic glioma") Diffuse astrocytoma Glioblastoma
Neurofibromatosis type 2 (NF2)	22q12	*NF2* (merlin/schwanomin)	Vestibular schwannomas (bilateral) Other schwannomas Meningiomas (multiple) Meningioangiomatosis Ependymoma of spinal cord Diffuse astrocytoma
Schwannomatosis (sometimes referred to as "NF3")	22q11.23	*SMARCB1* (INI1)	Schwannomas (multiple, spinal roots, cranial nerves, skin, not vestibular)
von Hippel–Lindau (vHL)	3p25–26	*VHL* (pVHL)	Hemangioblastomas (multiple) of cerebellum, spinal cord, brainstem, retina, spinal peripheral nerve roots Endolymphatic sac tumor
Tuberous sclerosis complex	9q34 16p13.3	*TSC1* (hamartin) *TSC2* (tuberin)	Subependymal giant cell astrocytoma
Li–Fraumeni syndrome	17p13	*TP53* (TP53 protein)	Diffuse astrocytomas, including glioblastoma Medulloblastoma Choroid plexus papilloma or carcinoma Ependymoma Oligodendroglioma Meningioma
Cowden disease	10q23	*PTEN/MMAC1* (PTEN protein)	Dysplastic gangliocytoma of the cerebellum (Lhermitte–Duclos disease)
Turcot type 1 syndrome (mismatch repair [MMR]/hereditary nonpolyposis colon cancer [HNPCC]–associated Turcot)	3p21.3 2p16 5q11–q13 2q32 7p22	*MLH1* *MSH2* and *MSH6 MSH3* *PMS1* *PMS2* *APC* (APC protein)	Glioblastoma
Turcot type 2 syndrome (familial adenomatous polyposis [FAP]–associated Turcot)	5q21		Medulloblastoma
Nevoid basal cell carcinoma (Gorlin) syndrome	9q22.3	*PTCH* (Ptch protein)	Medulloblastoma
Rhabdoid tumor predisposition syndrome	22q11.23	*SMARCB1* (INI1)	Atypical teratoid/rhabdoid tumor

receptor in the sonic hedgehog pathway). Tumors arising in the posterior skull base often have *NF2* alterations whereas those arising in the medial anterior skull base often display alterations in *AKT1* and *SMO*. *TERT* promoter mutations have been linked to more aggressive behavior in meningiomas. Although correlations between specific histologic subtypes (described below) and genetic alterations are limited, secretory meningiomas frequently carry mutations in both *TRAF7* and *KLF4*.

- **Iatrogenic:** Induction of meningiomas as a complication of radiation therapy generally involves a latent period of a decade or more and is directly related to radiation dosage. Until the early 1960s, low-dose scalp irradiation was used to treat tinea capitis. The average interval between treatment and detection of a meningioma for such patients was 35 years. With the higher radiation doses used for head and neck cancers, the interval may be as short as 5 years.
- **Tumor predisposition syndromes:** Meningiomas can occur in conjunction with genetic tumor predisposition syndromes, the most important being NF2. Rare multiple meningioma syndromes (meningiomatosis syndromes) have also been documented, some associated with mutations in *NF2*, *SMARCB1* or *SMARCE1* (both of which encode proteins involved in chromatin remodeling) or *SUFU* (which makes a negative regulator of hedgehog signaling).

PATHOLOGY: On MRI and gross examination, most meningiomas appear as well-circumscribed dura-based masses of variable size that compress, but do not invade, the underlying brain (Fig. 32-113A,B). The cut surface is fleshy and tan. The classic histologic hallmark of meningiomas is a whorled pattern, often in association with psammoma bodies (laminated, spherical calcospherites) (Fig. 32-113C,D). However, these tumors can show diverse morphologic patterns, and 13 subtypes are recognized by the WHO (Table 32-9). Most of these are WHO grade I, but two variants, clear cell and chordoid, behave more aggressively (WHO grade II), and two other variants, papillary and rhabdoid, are frankly anaplastic (WHO grade III). Meningiomas typically express epithelial membrane antigen (EMA) focally (Fig. 32-113C). They have many intercellular junctions, owing to their origin from the cohesive arachnoid barrier cell layer (Fig. 32-113E).

Mitotic activity, expressed as the number of mitoses in 10 high-power fields (typically at 400× magnification) is used as a way to assess the aggressiveness of meningiomas and as a criterion for determining WHO grade. For example, meningiomas with 4 or more mitoses per 10 high-power fields are assigned WHO grade II, whereas those with 20 or more mitoses per 10 high-power fields are assigned WHO grade III. Immunohistochemical staining for Ki67 antigen can also be used to evaluate tumor proliferation, but this is not a recognized part of the grading criteria established by the WHO.

CLINICAL FEATURES: The indolent growth of most meningiomas allows them to enlarge slowly for years before becoming symptomatic. During that time, they displace but usually do not infiltrate the brain (Fig. 32-114). Patients often develop seizures, particularly with tumors arising at parasagittal sites over the convexity of the hemispheres. In other locations, meningiomas compress a variety of structures and cause corresponding functional deficits. Thus, tumors in the olfactory groove produce anosmia; those in the suprasellar region cause visual deficits by compressing the optic chiasm; those in the cerebellopontine angle cause cranial nerve dysfunction; and those along the spinal cord compromise spinal nerve root and spinal cord function. Invasion of cranial bone, often accompanied by hyperostosis seen on CT scans, is relatively common, and growth through the calvarium may create a tumor mass beneath the scalp. As mentioned previously, meningiomas rarely invade the underlying brain but when this occurs, such aggressive behavior warrants upgrading to WHO grade II (atypical). Tumors that are not completely excised surgically tend to recur, and some may undergo anaplastic progression over time. Anaplastic (malignant) meningiomas (WHO grade III) may also rarely arise de novo.

TABLE 32-9

MENINGIOMA SUBTYPES

World Health Organization (WHO) Grade I: Benign Meningioma

Meningothelial

Fibrous

Transitional

Psammomatous

Angiomatous

Microcystic

Secretory

Lymphoplasmacyte rich

Metaplastic

WHO Grade II: Atypical Meningioma

Chordoid

Clear cell

WHO Grade III: Anaplastic (Malignant) Meningioma

Rhabdoid

Papillary

Astrocytomas Are the Most Common Malignant Primary Brain Tumors

They are categorized into two major types based on how diffusely they infiltrate the brain parenchyma. *Diffuse astrocytomas* infiltrate the brain widely. These include low-grade fibrillary astrocytoma, anaplastic astrocytoma and the most malignant astrocytic tumor, glioblastoma. Members of the other major category typically do not infiltrate the CNS but instead grow slowly as compact masses that cause symptoms by compressing adjacent structures. These include PAs, pleomorphic xanthoastrocytomas (PXAs), and subependymal giant cell astrocytomas (SEGAs).

Diffuse Astrocytoma

The defining biologic characteristic of diffuse astrocytomas, as the name implies, is the ability of individual tumor cells to infiltrate widely through brain and spinal cord parenchyma (Fig. 32-115). This property reaches its extreme in **gliomatosis**

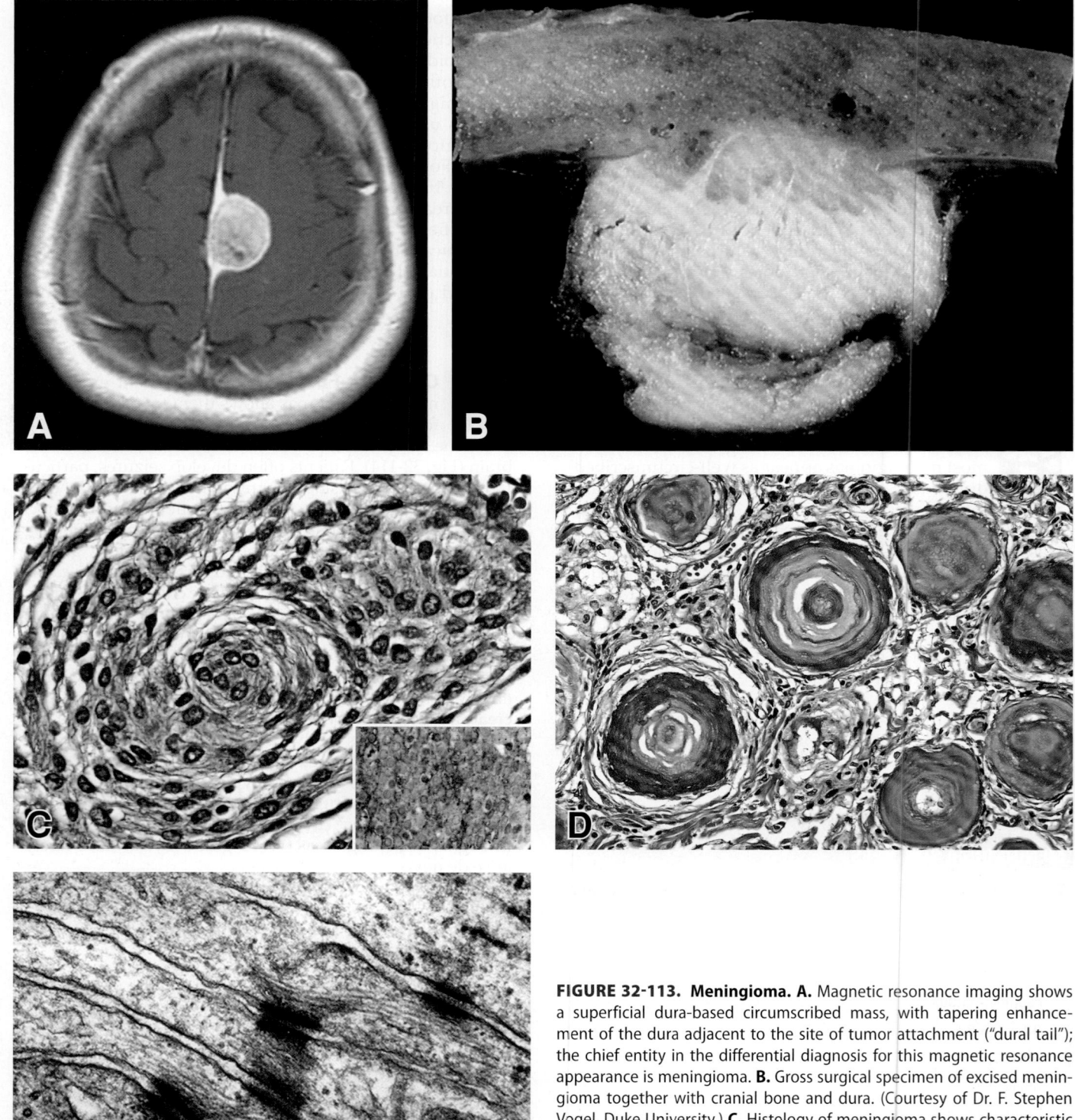

FIGURE 32-113. Meningioma. A. Magnetic resonance imaging shows a superficial dura-based circumscribed mass, with tapering enhancement of the dura adjacent to the site of tumor attachment ("dural tail"); the chief entity in the differential diagnosis for this magnetic resonance appearance is meningioma. **B.** Gross surgical specimen of excised meningioma together with cranial bone and dura. (Courtesy of Dr. F. Stephen Vogel, Duke University.) **C.** Histology of meningioma shows characteristic whorled, bland, plump spindle cells. Meningiomas are immunopositive for epithelial membrane antigen, which is a useful diagnostic adjunct in difficult cases (*inset*). **D.** Prominent psammoma body formation is typical of the "psammomatous" subtype of meningioma. **E.** The ultrastructural hallmark of meningiomas is numerous intercellular junctions (desmosomes), which tightly bind adjacent meningioma cell processes together.

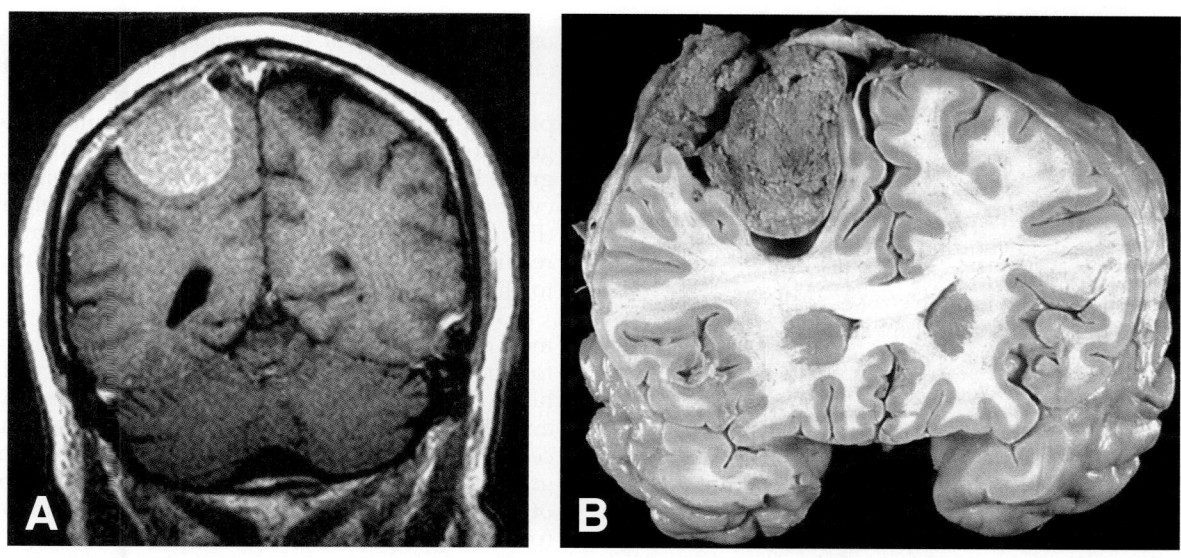

FIGURE 32-114. Meningioma. Meningiomas compress, but do not usually invade, the underlying brain. **A.** Magnetic resonance image. **B.** Gross specimen. (Courtesy of Dr. F. Stephen Vogel, Duke University.)

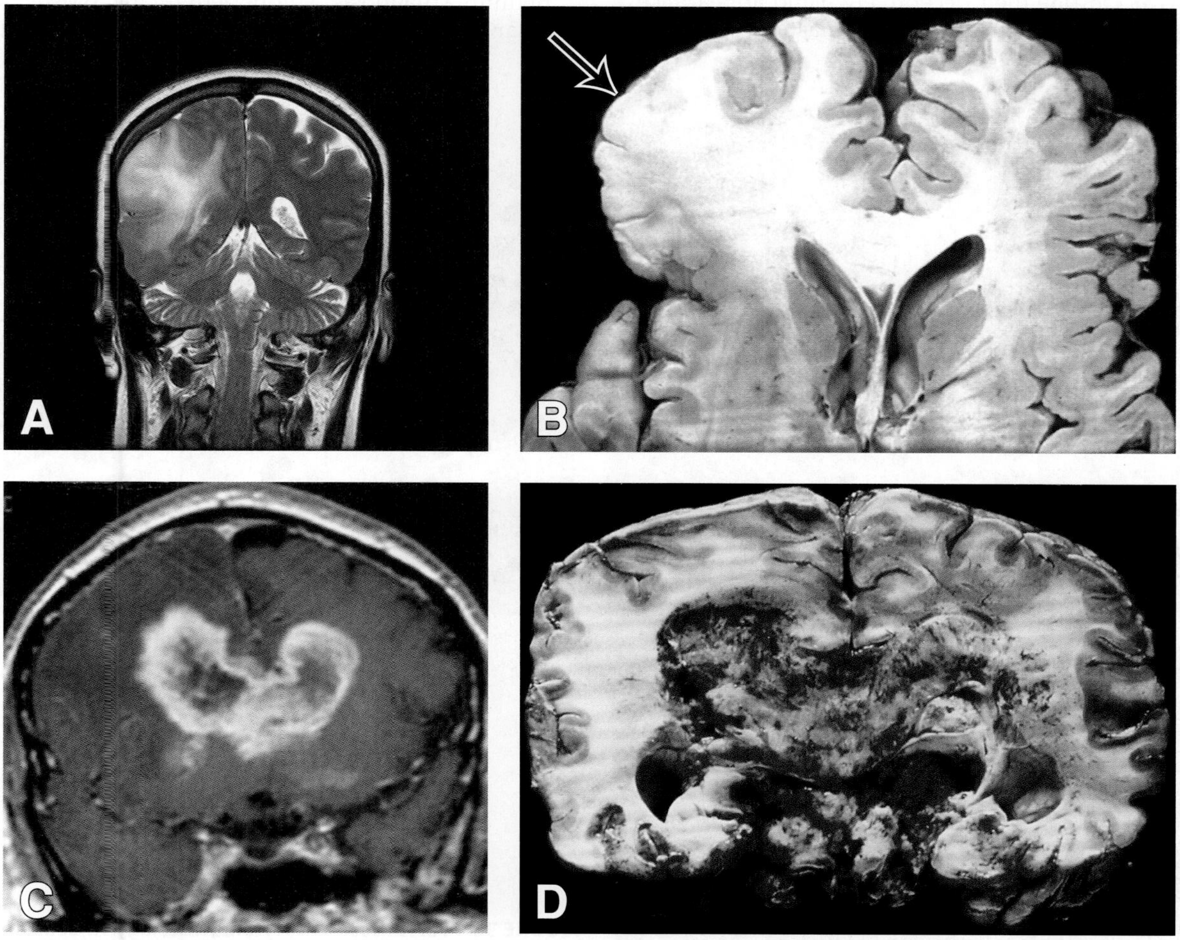

FIGURE 32-115. Gliomas. A. As seen by magnetic resonance imaging, **infiltrating astrocytomas** exhibit a diffuse, fuzzy interface with the adjacent brain tissue that is being invaded. **B.** This gross specimen shows "blurring" of the normally sharp interface between the gray matter and white matter, a manifestation of diffuse infiltration as astrocytoma cells overrun the cortex (*arrow*). (Courtesy of Dr. F. Stephen Vogel, Duke University.) **C.** In contrast to low-grade diffuse astrocytomas, **glioblastomas** show prominent irregular ring contrast enhancement and often infiltrate across the corpus callosum to involve the contralateral hemisphere ("butterfly" glioblastoma), as seen in this preoperative magnetic resonance image. **D.** Gross autopsy specimen of a lesion corresponding to image in panel C. (Courtesy of Dr. F. Stephen Vogel, Duke University.)

cerebri, in which infiltrating glioma cells (usually astrocytes but occasionally oligodendroglia) involve at least three cerebral lobes, and often more, with infiltration into both hemispheres, the brainstem, the cerebellum, and even the spinal cord. Diffuse tumor infiltration of brain and spinal cord explains why effective therapy for these tumors is lacking.

Glioblastomas typically present as large, ring-enhancing masses with an irregular central areas of necrosis and prominent edema of surrounding white matter. The infiltrating component of glioblastomas often crosses to the contralateral hemisphere via the corpus callosum; such cases are referred to as "butterfly" glioblastomas based on their appearance on coronal MRI (Fig. 32-115).

PATHOLOGY: Low-grade fibrillary astrocytomas (WHO grade II) are composed of well-differentiated astrocytic tumor cells with little nuclear atypia or cell proliferation. Gemistocytic astrocytoma is a distinctive subtype of low-grade astrocytoma in which the main population of cells has prominent globular cytoplasm filled with glial intermediate filaments (Fig. 32-116). Despite their deceptively bland appearance, diffuse astrocytomas often undergo anaplastic progression, usually over several years, into high-grade astrocytoma (anaplastic astrocytoma, WHO grade III) and, ultimately, into glioblastoma (WHO grade IV). This tendency for anaplastic progression is even more pronounced with the gemistocytic variant. **Anaplastic astrocytoma (WHO grade III)** is more cellular than low-grade fibrillary astrocytoma, and individual tumor cells are more pleomorphic (Fig. 32-116). Mitotic rates are greater and mitoses are readily seen. Anaplastic astrocytomas typically progress to glioblastomas within a few years.

Glioblastoma (GBM; WHO grade IV) is the single most common primary malignant brain tumor. It accounts for about 20% of all CNS tumors. GBMs are cytologically highly pleomorphic, and tumor cells vary greatly in size and shape, with large bizarre nuclei and multinucleated cells. They may arise by anaplastic progression from lower-grade diffuse astrocytomas (secondary glioblastoma; 5% of GBMs) or, much more commonly, as de novo tumors (primary glioblastoma; 95% of GBMs). Although usually solitary, they may rarely present as two separate epicenters of enhancement within the brain. Such cases may mimic metastases radiographically, but biopsy provides the definitive diagnosis. Mitotic activity in GBMs is high; vascular proliferation and foci of tumor necrosis surrounded

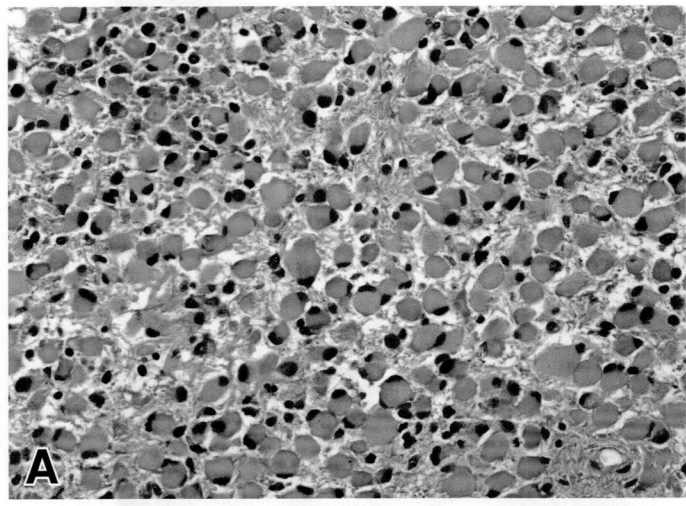

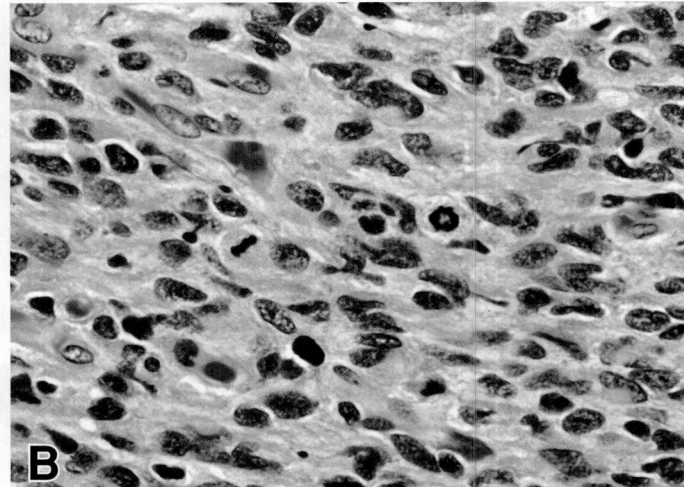

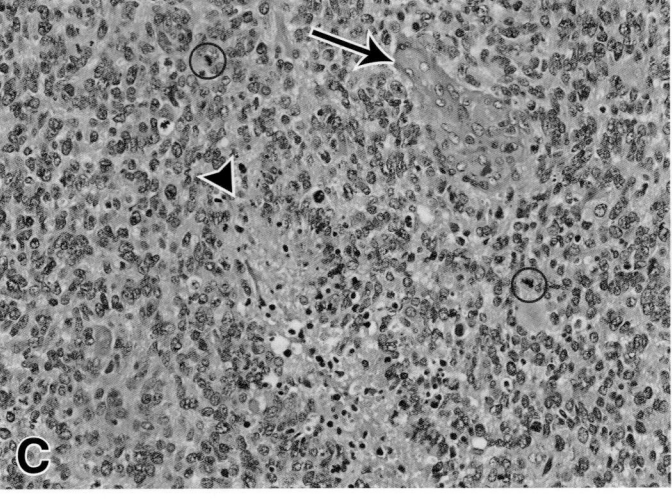

FIGURE 32-116. Diffuse astrocytoma histology. A. Gemistocytic astrocytomas are low-grade (World Health Organization [WHO] grade II) diffuse astrocytomas characterized by prominent globular cytoplasm. **B. Anaplastic astrocytomas (WHO grade III),** by contrast, are more cellular and more pleomorphic, in addition to having a higher proliferation rate. **C. Glioblastomas (WHO grade IV)** display mitotic activity (*red circles*), foci of tumor necrosis surrounded by hypercellular cuffs of tumor cells ("pseudopalisading necrosis") (*arrowhead*), and vascular proliferation (*arrow*).

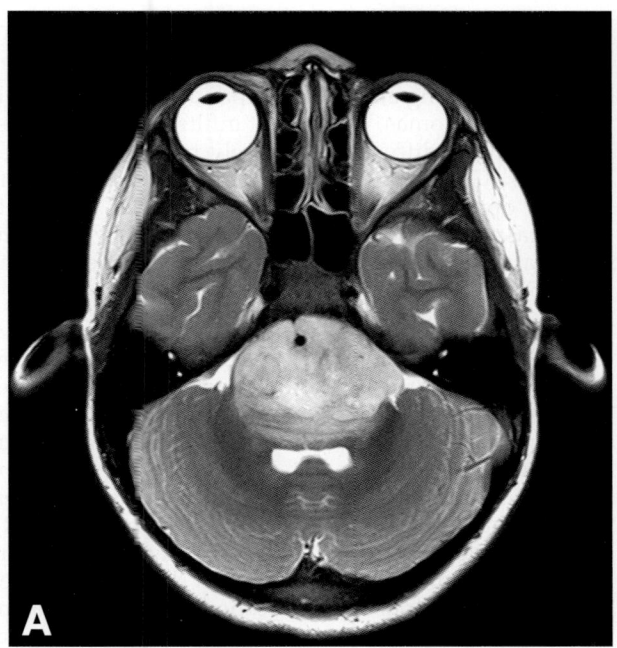
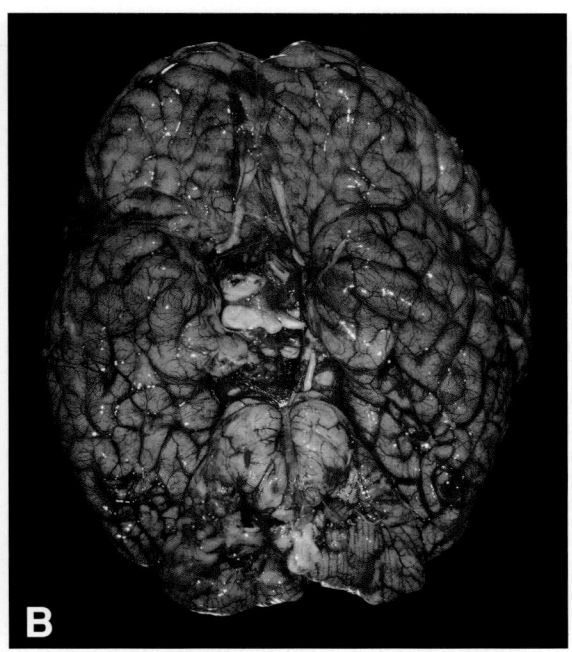

FIGURE 32-117. Diffuse pontine astrocytoma ("diffuse intrinsic pontine glioma"). Diffuse pontine astrocytomas of childhood infiltrate and expand the brainstem pons, often to the point of encircling the basilar artery. The majority of these tumors have mutations in the histone 3.3 gene *H3F3A* (specifically, H3.3 p.K27M). **A.** Magnetic resonance imaging. **B.** Autopsy gross specimen.

by a densely cellular cuff of tumor cells ("pseudopalisading necrosis") are characteristic (Fig. 32-116C).

Diffuse pontine astrocytoma (diffuse intrinsic pontine glioma or DIPG) is a lethal, diffusely infiltrating astrocytoma that arises in, and expands, the pons of the brainstem of young children (Fig. 32-117). The combination of MR imaging and clinical features is so distinctive that treatment is usually initiated without biopsy confirmation of the diagnosis. These tumors are assigned WHO grade IV because despite aggressive treatment, all cases ultimately exhibit growth, infiltration, and fatal compromise of vital brainstem structures. Molecular studies have demonstrated that the majority of these tumors harbor mutations in *H3F3A or HIST1H3B*, the genes that encode histone proteins H3.3 or H3.1. The most common mutation converts lysine 27 to methionine (K27M). Loss of methylation at lysine 27 alters chromatin structure and causes global changes in gene expression. As a result of the increased understanding of the molecular alterations in these tumors (Table 32-10), the 2016 WHO codified a new entity called Diffuse Midline Glioma, H3 K27-Mutant, which includes the majority of, though not all, DIPGs. Mutations in *TP53, PPM1D* (which encodes a protein phosphatase) and *ACVR1* (which makes a protein in the bone morphogenic protein [BMP] pathway) have also been implicated DIPGs.

MOLECULAR PATHOGENESIS: *The vast majority of GBMs are sporadic,* but a few arise in the setting of a genetic tumor predisposition syndrome (Table 32-8). Sporadic GBMs may arise de novo or via anaplastic progression from lower-grade astrocytoma (see above). Molecular characterization reveals differences

TABLE 32-10
MAJOR MOLECULAR ALTERATIONS IN PRIMARY BRAIN TUMORS

Tumor	Molecular Alterations
Pilocytic astrocytoma	*KIAA1549-BRAF* fusion, BRAF p.V600E
Ganglioglioma	*BRAF* (BRAF p.V600E), *KRAS*, FGFR1/FGFR2
Pleomorphic xanthoastrocytoma	BRAF p.V600E
Low grade diffuse astrocytoma	*IDH1/IDH2, ATRX, TP53*
Ependymoma	*C11orf95-RELA* fusion (supratentorial location)
Oligodendroglioma	*IDH1/IDH2, TERT* promoter, 1p deletion, 19q deletion
Glioblastoma (adults)	*EGFR, PTEN, CDKN2A, TERT* promoter, *NF1*
Glioblastoma (pediatric)	*H3F3A* (H3.3 p.K27M—midline location) (H3.3 p.G34R/V—hemispheric location)
Medulloblastoma	*CTNNB1, PTCH, TP53*
Embryonal tumors	C19MC amplification
Craniopharyngioma	Adamantinomatous type—*CTNNB1* Papillary type—BRAF p.V600E
Primary CNS lymphoma	*MYD88*

in the mutational landscape seen in these two major classes. Primary GBMs often show amplification of the epidermal growth factor receptor (*EGFR*) gene, and mutation of *PTEN* and telomerase reverse transcriptase (*TERT*) genes, whereas secondary GBM has a higher incidence of *TP53* mutations. Mutations in the isocitrate-dehydrogenase genes 1 or 2 (*IDH1*, *IDH2*), and especially in *IDH1*, are now recognized as common signatures of low-grade (grade II) and anaplastic (grade III) diffuse gliomas, and of the majority of secondary GBMs that arise from these lower-grade tumors (see Chapter 5). *IDH1/IDH2* mutations in astrocytomas or secondary glioblastomas frequently coexist with mutations in *TP53* and *ATRX* (which encodes a helicase involved in chromatin remodeling). Primary GBMs generally do not show *IDH* mutations. Other mutations in specific molecular subsets of GBM include deletion or mutation of the *NF1* gene and amplification of the *ERBB2* gene.

Similarly, molecular insight into the basis for resistance to treatment is also beginning to be understood. GBMs can be stratified into two groups based on whether the promoter for the DNA repair gene *MGMT* is methylated, and hence inactivated, or unmethylated, and so capable of repairing damage caused by alkylating agents used in chemotherapy. Patients with *MGMT* promoter methylation (inactivation) respond significantly better to treatment. The 2016 WHO classification of astrocytomas and glioblastomas was specifically modified to incorporate *IDH1/IDH2* mutation into the definitions and names, due the strong prognostic significance of these genetic alterations. Diffuse Astrocytoma, IDH-mutant (or IDH-wildtype), Anaplastic Astrocytoma, IDH-mutant (or IDH-wildtype) and Glioblastoma, IDH-mutant (or IDH-wildtype) are now formal diagnostic terms for these tumors. Patients who have an astrocytoma or glioblastoma with an IDH mutation have a better prognosis than patients whose gliomas are IDH-wildtype. Gliomas with both IDH mutation and 1p/19q whole arm codeletion have the most favorable prognosis and response to therapy of all diffuse gliomas; this molecular signature is the defining feature of oligodendroglioma and is considered a favorable predictive molecular marker.

Pilocytic Astrocytoma (WHO Grade I)

PAs are circumscribed gliomas that typically arise in children and young adults and expand very slowly. Unlike diffuse astrocytomas, PAs do not infiltrate brain or spinal cord parenchyma diffusely and rarely progress to higher-grade tumors. Common locations include the cerebellum, brainstem, optic nerves, and third ventricular region. PAs are contrast enhancing. They may show a cystic component and are well circumscribed on preoperative imaging studies (Fig. 32-118).

 PATHOLOGY: PAs consist of compact areas of tumor cells with elongated bipolar cytoplasmic processes (pilocytes) separated by prominent microcysts. The compact areas frequently have prominent **Rosenthal fibers** (see Fig. 32-4C), a histologic hallmark of PA. Vascular proliferation is typical and correlates with the contrast enhancement seen on preoperative MR imaging studies. Mitotic activity, vascular proliferation, and foci of necrosis in pilocytic areas do not carry the same negative prognostic significance as in diffuse astrocytomas. In favorable anatomic locations, such as the cerebellum, surgical resection may be curative. **Pilomyxoid astrocytoma** is a recognized variant of PA, primarily arising in the hypothalamic region, that may exhibit a more aggressive clinical behavior. Previously, pilomyxoid astrocytoma was assigned WHO grade II, but the current recommendation is to withhold grading this entity until more definitive evidence determines if they are truly more aggressive than conventional PAs.

MOLECULAR PATHOGENESIS: PAs in the cerebellum are frequently associated with *KIAA1549-BRAF* fusion (~75% of cases). This gene fusion results in increased activity of BRAF kinase and increased cell proliferation. Other alterations of the mitogen-activating protein kinase (MAPK) pathway can also be detected in PAs, including BRAF p.V600E mutation, *KRAS* mutations, and *NF1* mutations.

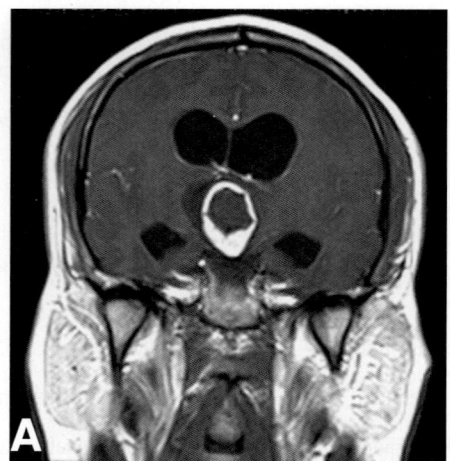
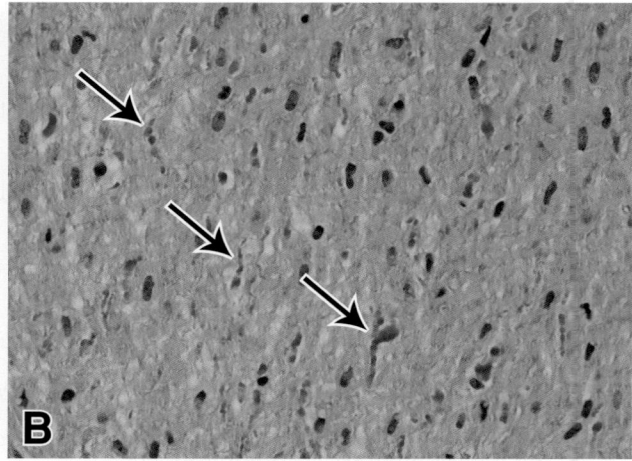

FIGURE 32-118. Pilocytic astrocytoma (World Health Organization grade I). A. Pilocytic astrocytomas are very low-grade circumscribed contrast-enhancing gliomas. **B.** Histologically, neoplastic pilocytes ("hair cells") exhibit greatly elongated bipolar cytoplasmic processes that are prone to Rosenthal fiber formation (*arrows*).

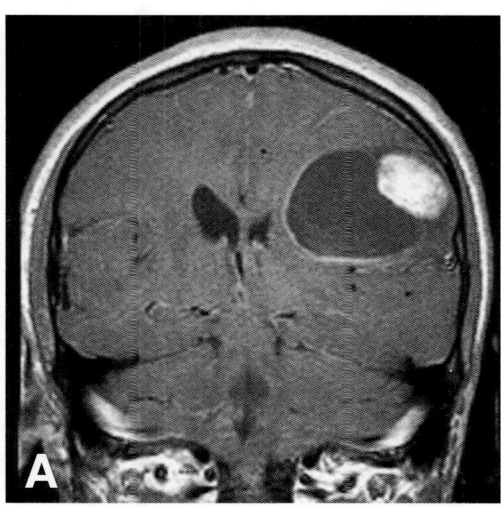
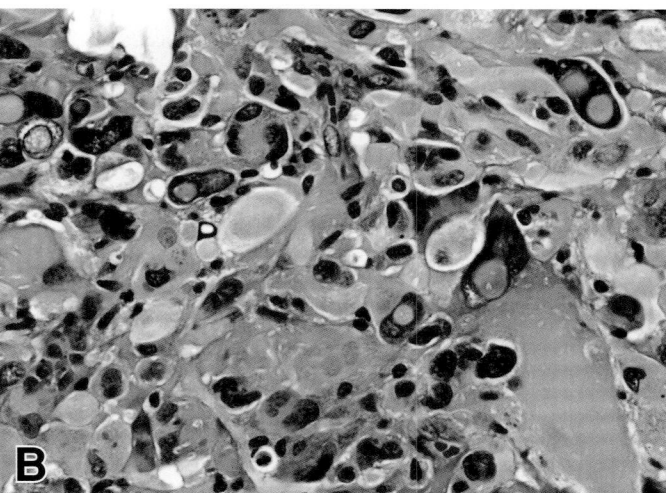

FIGURE 32-119. Pleomorphic xanthoastrocytoma (PXA). A. PXAs are low-grade (World Health Organization grade II) circumscribed astrocytomas. On imaging studies, they typically display a "cyst with enhancing mural nodule" pattern, similar to other low-grade tumors such as pilocytic astrocytomas and gangliogliomas. **B.** Microscopically, PXAs superficially resemble giant cell glioblastomas, with strikingly bizarre giant cells, but pursue a much more indolent clinical course. A subset of these tumors harbor the *BRAF* p.V600E mutation.

Pleomorphic Xanthoastrocytoma (WHO Grade II)

PXA is another circumscribed astrocytoma variant seen in children and young adults (Fig. 32-119A). There is usually a several-year history of poorly controlled seizure activity; the temporal lobe is the most common location. In favorable anatomic locations, PXAs, like PAs, are amenable to surgical resection, but incompletely resected tumors frequently recur. About 15% of these undergo anaplastic progression to high-grade diffuse astrocytoma. Approximately 66% or more of PXAs harbor a *BRAF* V600E mutation. Loss of expression of the tumor suppressor p16, in combination with *BRAF* p.V600E, can also be seen in the majority of PXAs.

 PATHOLOGY: PXA mimics giant cell glioblastoma in having strikingly pleomorphic tumor cells (Fig. 32-119B). Unlike GBM, however, mitotic

activity is very low, and vascular proliferation and necrosis are usually absent. The characteristic eosinophilic granular bodies, which are also seen in other low-grade circumscribed tumors such as PA and ganglioglioma, are a strong signature of PXA.

Subependymal Giant Cell Astrocytoma (WHO Grade I)

SEGA is a very indolent low-grade glioma that arises from the wall of the lateral ventricle. It grows slowly within the ventricular cavity and causes obstructive hydrocephalus with attendant signs and symptoms of increased intracranial pressure once it encroaches on the interventricular foramen of Monro (Fig. 32-120A). SEGAs are densely compact mixtures of very plump epithelioid cells, often intermixed with elongated spindle cells (Fig. 32-120B).

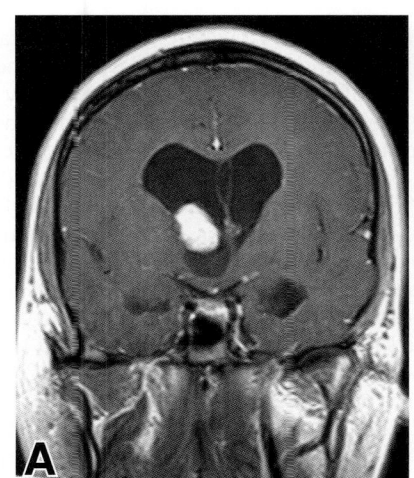
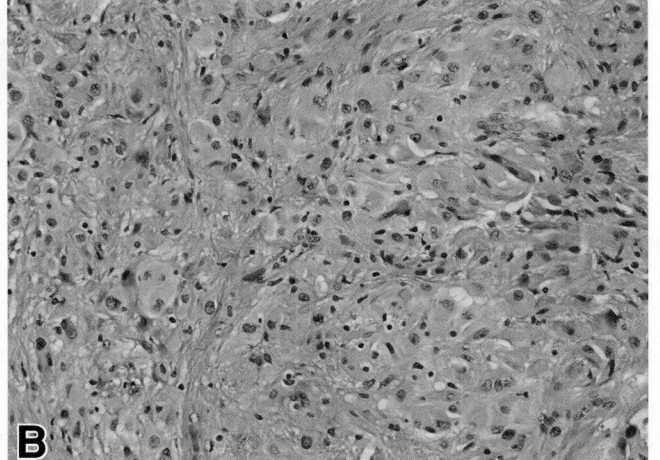

FIGURE 32-120. Subependymal giant cell astrocytoma (SEGA). A. This World Health Organization grade I astrocytoma arises within the lateral ventricle, often obstructing the interventricular foramen of Monro, and resulting in obstructive hydrocephalus. **B.** Microscopically, SEGAs have globular eosinophilic cytoplasm and nuclei often display single prominent nucleoli, thus mimicking gemistocytic astrocytoma or ganglion cell tumor. However, the anatomic location within the cerebral ventricle should preclude misdiagnosis.

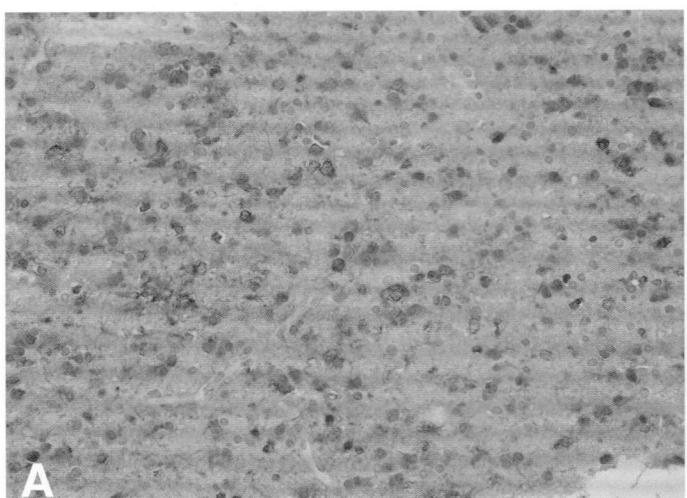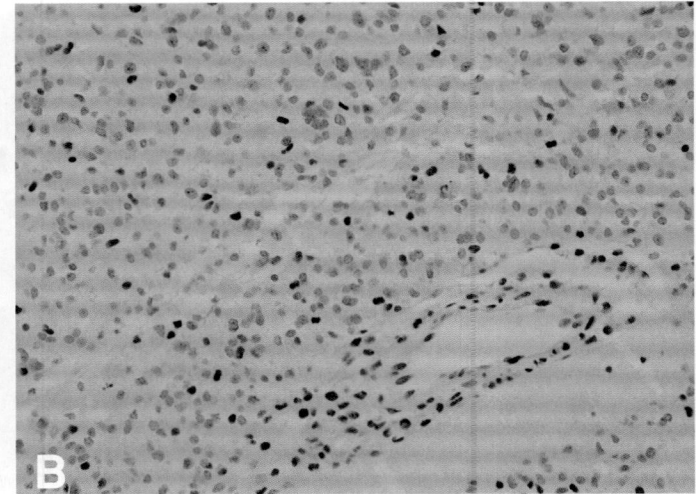

FIGURE 32-121. Molecular alterations in infiltrating astrocytomas. Lower-grade (WHO grade II and III) astrocytomas typically present in younger adult patients and have mutations in *IDH1* or *IDH2, ATRX* and *TP53*. The most common *IDH* mutation is the *IDH1* p.R132H which occurs in ~90% of IDH-mutant gliomas. **A.** IDH-mutant astrocytoma shows immunoreactivity for an antibody that specifically recognizes the *IDH1* p.R132H mutant protein but not the wildtype protein. Only infiltrating tumor cells show positive staining. Endothelial cells in blood vessels have a wildtype *IDH1* gene, and are negative. **B.** Immunoreactivity for the ATRX antibody is lost in tumor cells, but preserved in normal tissue constituents such as endothelial cells.

Based on histology alone, SEGAs could be mistaken for gemistocytic astrocytomas or gangliogliomas, but their intraventricular location, readily identified by preoperative imaging, in a young patient helps guide diagnosis. SEGAs are associated with **tuberous sclerosis** and may be the presenting feature in a child with otherwise inconspicuous stigmata of that disease. In keeping with its WHO grade I assignment and favorable location within the lateral ventricle, surgical resection of SEGA is curative. Tuberous sclerosis entails loss of *TSC1* or *TSC2* inhibition of mammalian target of rapamycin (mTOR) signaling. Thus, pharmacologic inhibitors of the mTOR pathway can shrink SEGAs and provide a medical approach in the management of these patients.

Oligodendrogliomas (WHO Grade II) Are Often More Indolent Than Diffuse Astrocytomas

Like diffuse astrocytomas, ODGs are highly infiltrative. However, their response to treatment and overall survival are much more favorable than for diffuse astrocytomas of similar grade. ODGs must, therefore, be distinguished from their diffuse astrocytic cousins.

MOLECULAR PATHOGENESIS: A translocation between chromosomes 1 and 19 is a defining molecular signature of ODGs, in combination with mutations in *IDH1* or *IDH2*. This translocation causes complete loss of the short arm of chromosome 1 (1p) and the long arm of chromosome 19 (19q). *Combined whole arm deletion of 1p and 19q, in combination with IDH1 or IDH2 mutation, is a favorable genetic signature in diffuse gliomas and correlates closely with classic ODG morphologic features. TERT* promoter mutations are also frequently seen in ODGs. While ODGs are characterized by a combination of *IDH1/IDH2* mutations, *TERT* promoter mutations, and 1p/19q codeletion, low-grade

astrocytomas, in contrast, are characterized by the presence of genetic variants in the triad of *IDH1/IDH2, TP53*, and *ATRX* (Fig 32-121). Identification of these distinct molecular signatures facilitates the diagnosis of these classes of infiltrating gliomas, which not infrequently can be difficult to distinguish histologically because of overlapping morphologic features. The 2016 WHO classification modified the names of ODGs to incorporate the defining molecular alterations (Table 32-11). The new diagnostic terms for these tumors are Oligodendroglioma, IDH-mutant and 1p/19q codeleted, WHO grade II or III; or Oligodendroglioma, NOS ("*not otherwise specified*"), WHO grade II or III, if the tumor has classical histologic features of ODG but the molecular signature has not been determined.

PATHOLOGY: Most ODGs arise in adults in the fourth and fifth decades, largely in the white matter of cerebral hemispheres. They commonly infiltrate into overlying cerebral cortex. They show a monotonous population of cells with regular round nuclei surrounded by a small rim of clear cytoplasm ("perinuclear halo" or "fried egg" appearance) like normal oligodendroglia (Fig. 32-122A). This halo is a diagnostically useful artifact created by processing tissue samples with formalin fixation and paraffin embedding. Other characteristic features of ODGs include a network of delicate, branching blood vessels ("chicken wire" pattern) and scattered microcalcifications. In areas of cortical infiltration, ODG cells tend to cluster around neuron cell bodies (perineuronal satellitosis) and blood vessels (perivascular satellitosis). They also form an infiltrating layer just beneath the pia (subpial growth). These features, described by Scherer in 1938, are still called "secondary structures of Scherer." Mitotic activity is inconspicuous in low-grade (WHO grade II) ODG, but these tumors recur and ultimately undergo anaplastic progression.

TABLE 32-11
MOLECULAR ALTERATIONS INCORPORATED IN THE DIAGNOSIS OF CNS TUMORS
Diffuse astrocytoma, IDH-mutant
Diffuse astrocytoma, IDH-wildtype
Diffuse astrocytoma, NOS
Anaplastic astrocytoma, IDH-mutant
Anaplastic astrocytoma, IDH-wildtype
Anaplastic astrocytoma, IDH-NOS
Glioblastoma, IDH-mutant
Glioblastoma, IDH-wildtype
Glioblastoma, NOS
Oligodendroglioma, IDH-mutant and 1p/19q-codeleted
Oligodendroglioma, NOS
Anaplastic Oligodendroglioma, IDH-mutant and 1p/19q-codeleted
Anaplastic Oligodendroglioma, NOS
Diffuse midline glioma, H3 K27M-mutant
Ependymoma, *RELA* fusion-positive
Medulloblastoma, WNT-activated
Medulloblastoma, SHH-activated and *TP53*-mutant
Medulloblastoma, SHH-activated and *TP53*-wildtype
Medulloblastoma, non-WNT/non-SHH
Embryonal tumor with multilayered rosettes, C19MC-altered
Embryonal tumor with multilayered rosettes, NOS

The NOS or not otherwise specified designation indicates that the tumor shows histologic features indicative of a particular tumor type, but has not been tested for the critical genetic alteration(s).

Anaplastic Oligodendroglioma (WHO Grade III)

Anaplastic oligodendrogliomas differ from WHO grade II ODGs by showing increased mitotic activity and microvascular proliferation. These features may sometimes be accompanied by foci of tumor necrosis (Fig. 32-122B).

Ependymomas (WHO Grade II) Derive From Ependymal Lining Cells

These are typically slow-growing tumors of children and young adults that originate in the cerebral ventricles or central canal of the spinal cord. In children, the posterior fossa fourth ventricle is the preferred location, while in adults most are in the supratentorial compartment and may arise in either the ventricle or in the cerebral hemisphere white matter. Ependymomas of the fourth ventricle tend to fill

the ventricle and grow into the lateral recesses, occasionally even flowing through the lateral foramina of Luschka into the subarachnoid space (Fig. 32-123A,B). In the spinal cord, ependymomas are the most common intra-axial tumors, followed by diffuse astrocytomas.

 PATHOLOGY: Ependymomas grow as relatively circumscribed masses, and so are amenable to surgical resection. Their histologic hallmark is perivascular pseudorosettes, cuffs of radiating tumor cell cytoplasmic processes around vessels (Fig. 32-123C). True ependymal rosettes, in which tumor cells surround a central lumen, can also be seen but are rarer. Ependymomas express epithelial membrane antigen (EMA; Fig. 32-123C, *inset*) and GFAP (Fig. 32-123D, *inset*). GFAP reactivity is often strongest in perivascular pseudorosettes, and—unlike the membranous pattern of EMA expression in meningiomas—ependymoma EMA positivity is characteristically in a cytoplasmic dot-like and ring-like distribution. This pattern correlates with the presence of intercellular lumens filled with microvilli and cilia and sealed by intercellular junctional complexes at the ultrastructural level. **Anaplastic ependymoma (WHO grade III)** shows increased mitotic activity and microvascular proliferation, although the prognostic significance of these features in ependymomas has been questioned and is uncertain.

 MOLECULAR PATHOGENESIS: Ependymomas can be classified according to the anatomic site in which they arise (supratentorial, infratentorial, and spinal cord). Approximately 70% of supratentorial ependymomas have a characteristic *C11orf95-RELA* fusion that drives NFkB signaling. The presence of this fusion is a marker of poor prognosis in supratentorial ependymomas. As a result, the 2016 WHO classification formally codified Ependymoma, RELA Fusion Positive, as a distinct entity.

Myxopapillary Ependymoma (WHO Grade I)

Myxopapillary ependymomas (MPEs) are unique low-grade variants of ependymoma that arise almost exclusively in the spinal cords of adults from ependymal remnants in the conus medullaris or filum terminale (Fig. 32-124A). These tumors enlarge slowly as discrete, well-circumscribed, elongated masses in the lumbar CSF cistern. They are covered by an outer layer of investing leptomeninges. Nests and ribbons of epithelioid and spindled ependymal tumor cells are interspersed between myxoid microcysts, and perivascular cuffs of myxoid material are also prominent (Fig. 32-124B). The immunophenotype is similar to other ependymomas: they express both glial (S-100, GFAP) and epithelial (EMA) markers. Because they are well circumscribed and arise in a favorable anatomic location in the lumbar cistern, complete surgical resection is the treatment of choice. Microscopic breach of the pial "capsule" may occur in some tumors before (or during) surgery, allowing locally disseminated tumor to grow around nerve roots in the cauda equina. These cases are difficult to treat with conventional irradiation or chemotherapy, as their slow growth rate makes them relatively resistant to cell cycle inhibitors.

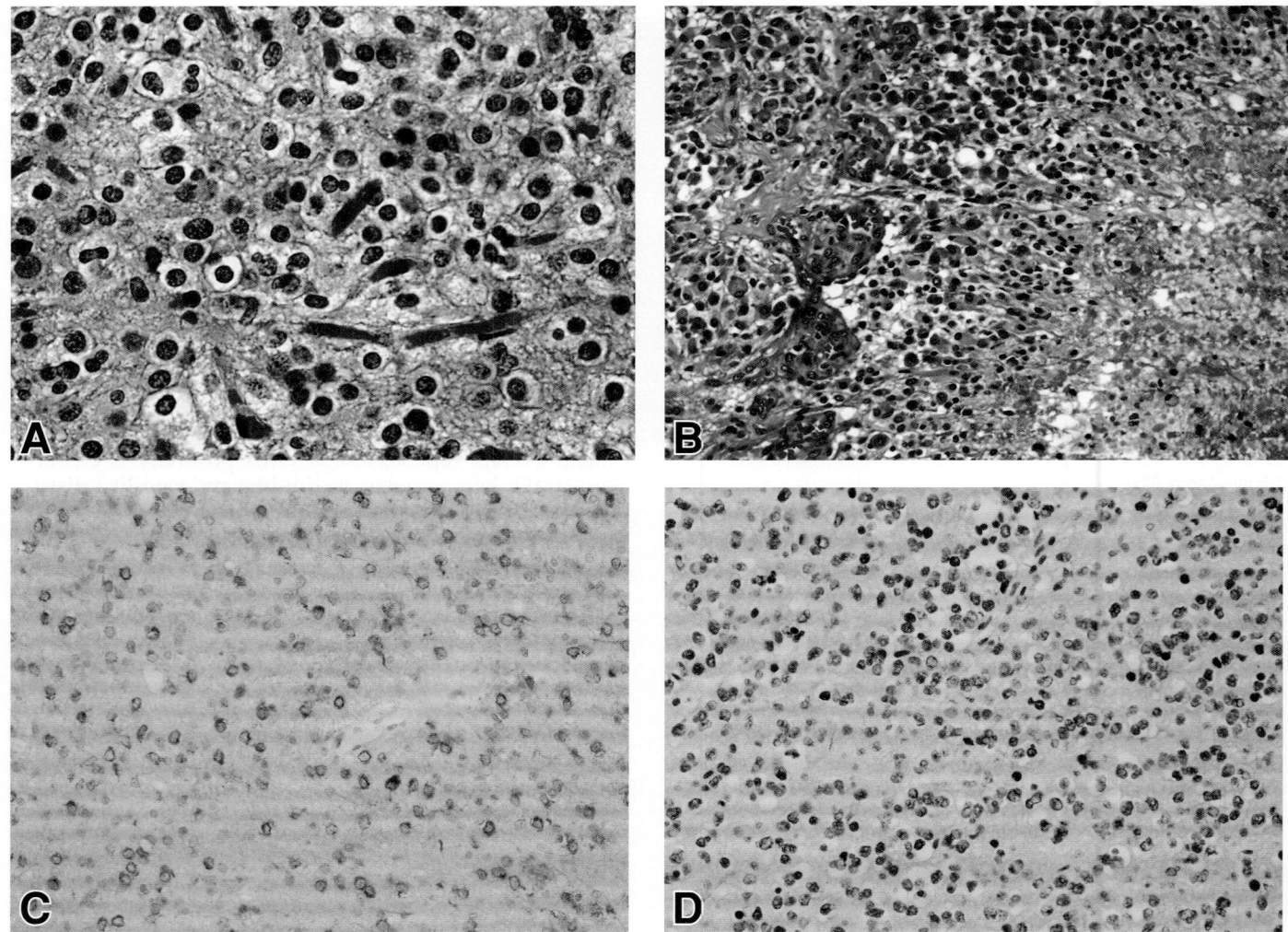

FIGURE 32-122. Oligodendroglioma. A. The cells of **low-grade oligodendrogliomas** (World Health Organization grade II) closely resemble normal oligodendrocytes, with regular round nuclei surrounded by perinuclear halos. **B. Anaplastic oligodendrogliomas** (AO) display increased cellularity and brisk mitotic activity, with some tumors also developing foci of necrosis (*seen on the right side of this image*) with tumor cell pseudopalisading. **C, D.** Molecular alterations in oligodendrogliomas include *IDH1/IDH2* mutations and 1p/19q codeletion. The *IDH1* p.R132H mutation is detected by immunohistochemistry (C). ATRX expression is retained in oligodendrogliomas (D). Taken together, these feature help distinguish oligodendroligomas from astrocytomas, which lose ATRX expression.

Subependymoma (WHO Grade I)

Subependymomas are indolent intraventricular gliomas of adults (rare cases may arise in the spinal cord). They are often small and asymptomatic and may be identified incidentally on imaging studies or at autopsy. Occasionally, however, they enlarge to block the interventricular foramen of Monro or fourth ventricle outlet foramina, causing obstructive hydrocephalus (Fig. 32-125A). Subependymomas show scattered clusters of small uniform glial cell nuclei separated by large zones of fibrillary matrix formed by tumor cell cytoplasmic processes (Fig. 32-125B). Surgical resection is curative.

Choroid Plexus Tumors Originate From Choroid Plexus Epithelium

Unlike other common childhood brain tumors, which favor the posterior fossa (cerebellum, fourth ventricle, and brainstem),

choroid plexus papillomas (CPPs; WHO grade I) in children arise most commonly in the lateral ventricles (Fig. 32-126A). In adults, the fourth ventricle is preferred. CPPs are benign and, given their location within ventricles, are potentially curable by surgery. However, CSF dissemination can occur, significantly worsening the prognosis in such cases.

PATHOLOGY: CPPs closely recapitulate the papillary architecture of the normal choroid plexus (Fig. 32-126B), but the tumor cells tend to be more crowded and commonly assume a columnar rather than cuboidal architecture (Fig. 32-126C). Their immunophenotype includes reactivity for glial markers (S-100, GFAP) and transthyretin (prealbumin). Two higher-grade choroid plexus tumors are **atypical CPP (WHO grade II)** (Fig. 32-126D), which has increased mitotic activity (2 mitoses or more per 10 high-power

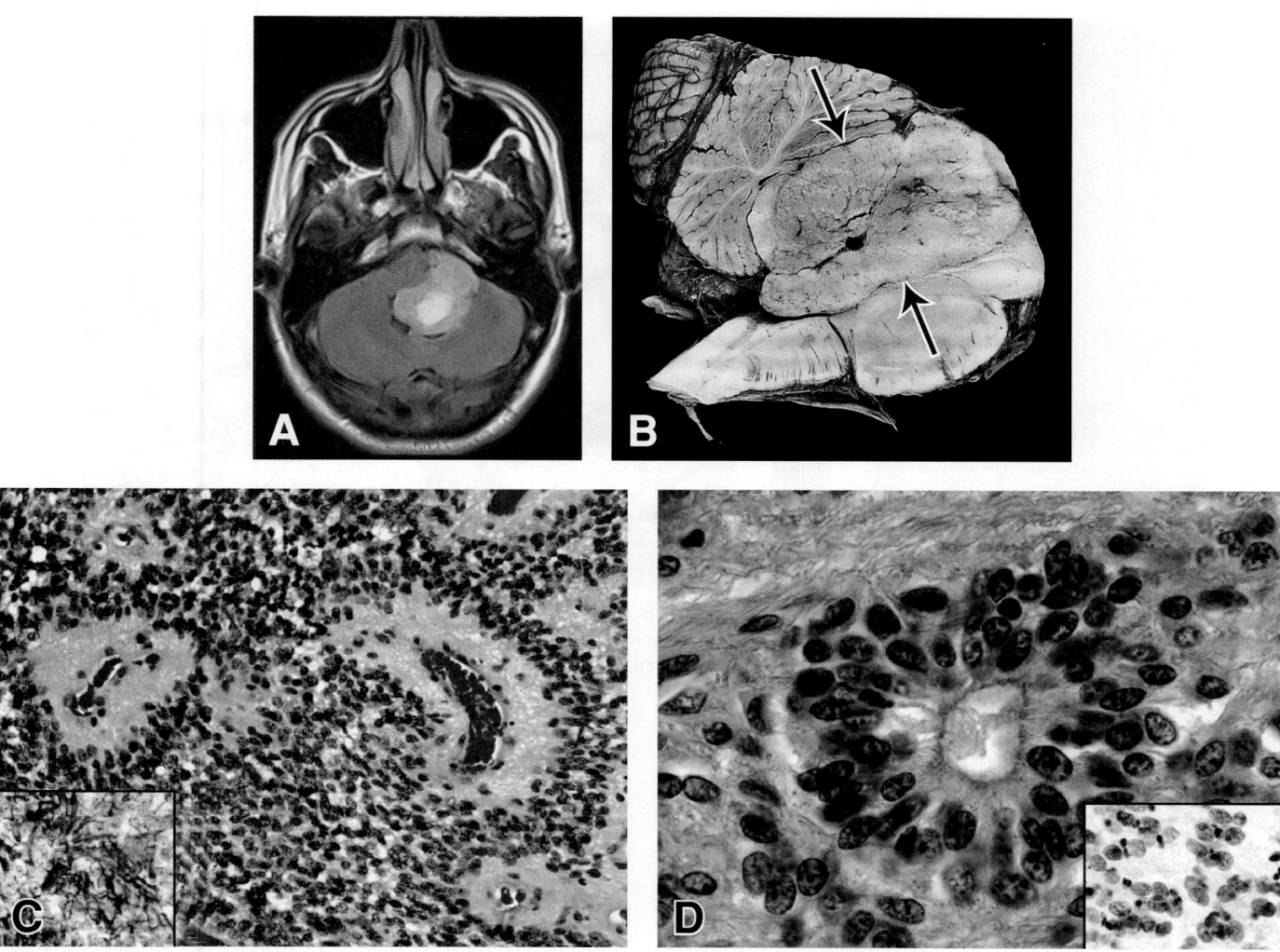

FIGURE 32-123. Ependymoma. A. Ependymomas can arise in the ventricles, the cerebral hemisphere or the spinal cord. Those located within the posterior fossa tend to grow through the ventricular outlet foramina (median foramen of Magendie and lateral foramina of Luschka) into the subarachnoid space, as seen in this magnetic resonance image. **B.** Autopsy gross specimen shows the tumor (*between the arrows*). (Courtesy of Dr. F. Stephen Vogel, Duke University.) **C.** Microscopically, the hallmark of ependymomas is the perivascular pseudorosette. The immunophenotype of ependymoma includes dot-like and ring-like positivity for epithelial membrane antigen (*inset*). **D.** This well-formed true ependymal rosette shows immunoreactivity for the glial marker glial fibrillary acidic protein (*inset*).

fields) compared to grade I tumors, and **choroid plexus carcinoma (WHO grade III),** which shows increased mitotic activity, loss of papillary architecture with a solid growth pattern, and often marked nuclear atypia and cellular pleomorphism (Fig. 32-126E). The latter tumors can invade adjacent brain parenchyma and also disseminate via the CSF. Choroid plexus carcinomas, in particular those occurring at an early age, may be associated with Li–Fraumeni syndrome (germline *TP53* mutation).

The choroid plexus may also host several other types of neoplastic and nonneoplastic mass lesions, including "intraventricular" meningiomas, metastatic carcinomas (especially renal cell carcinoma) and **xanthogranulomas** (reactive mass lesions probably related to microhemorrhage, and containing prominent cholesterol clefts and multinucleated giant cells).

Medulloblastoma and Other Embryonal Tumors (WHO Grade IV) Are Largely Tumors of Children

Of the several different types of embryonal tumors, or primitive neuroectodermal tumors (PNETs) recognized in the WHO classification, medulloblastoma (MB) is by far the most common. By definition, MBs arise in the cerebellum. Their peak incidence is at 7 years, but they also occur in 20- to 45-year-old adults. Childhood MBs commonly arise in the midline vermis, often expanding to fill the fourth ventricle (Fig. 32-127A). The adult versions prefer the cerebellar hemispheres. There are, however, many exceptions in both children and adults. About 1/3 of patients have leptomeningeal spread, a negative prognostic factor, at the time of presentation. Partial surgical resection, large cell or anaplastic morphology and amplification of the *MYCN* oncogene all portend poor prognosis.

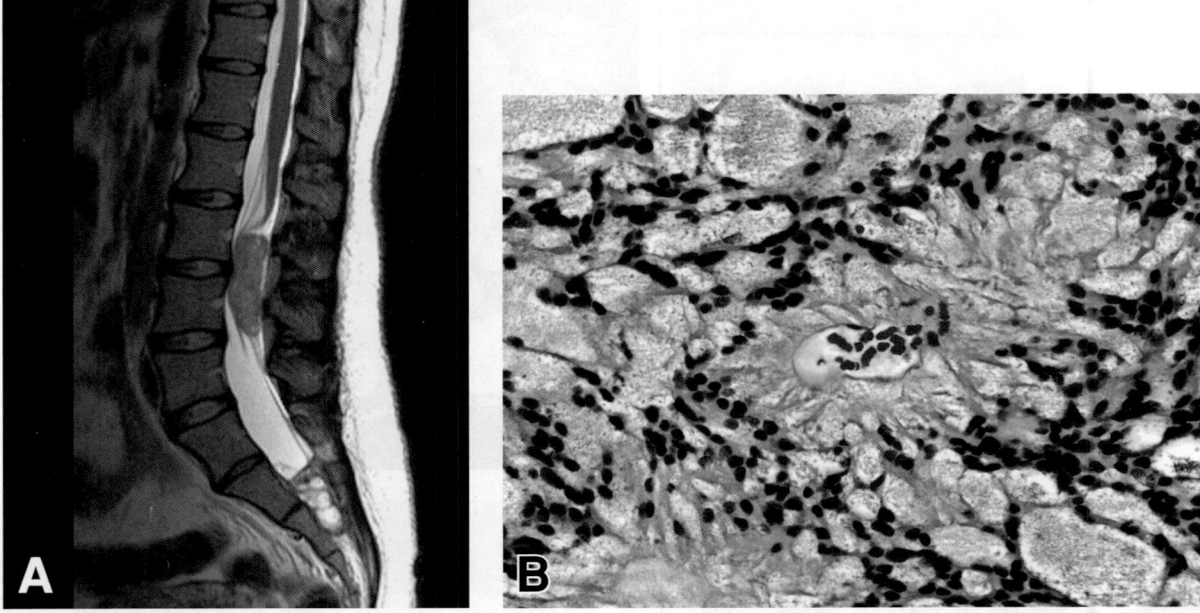

FIGURE 32-124. Myxopapillary ependymoma (MPE). A. MPEs are very low-grade (World Health Organization grade I) ependymal tumors that arise from remnants of the central canal in the spinal cord conus medullaris and filum terminale within the lumbar cistern. **B.** Histologically, nests and cords of ependymal cells are separated by prominent myxoid microcysts and perivascular myxoid cuffs.

CLINICAL FEATURES: There are four recognized MB variants: (1) classic; (2) desmoplastic/nodular; (3) medulloblastoma with extensive nodularity; and (4) large cell/anaplastic. Two of these, desmoplastic/nodular MB and MB with extensive nodularity, have better prognoses than does the classic subtype. The remaining variant, anaplastic/large cell, is the most aggressive and has a worse prognosis. CSF dissemination is common and may be a presenting feature of the tumor. MBs sometimes metastasize to regional lymph nodes, lungs or bone and may disseminate, if provided the opportunity, via ventriculoperitoneal shunts.

PATHOLOGY: MBs are composed of sheets of densely packed malignant small cells with a high nucleus:cytoplasm ratio (Fig. 32-127B). Neuroblastic (Homer Wright–type) rosettes are present in 40% of cases. Mitotic activity is high. Desmoplastic/nodular MB superficially resembles lymph node tissue, with

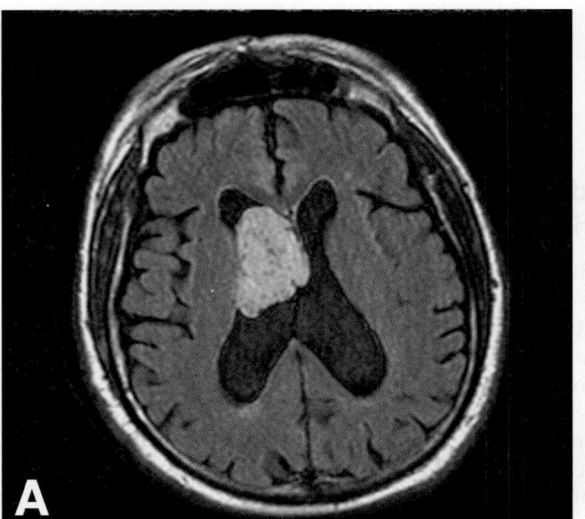
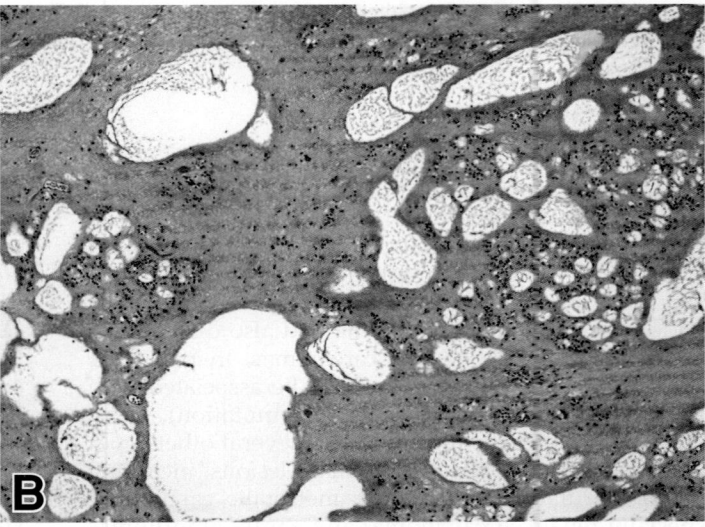

FIGURE 32-125. Subependymoma (SE). A. SE is another very low-grade (World Health Organization grade I) ependymal tumor that arises within the cerebral ventricle (shown in this magnetic resonance image) or very rarely within the spinal cord (not shown). **B.** Microscopically, SE consists of clusters of small, bland glial nuclei embedded within an abundant finely fibrillar matrix composed of tumor cell processes. Tumors located in the lateral ventricles tend to undergo microcystic degeneration as they enlarge.

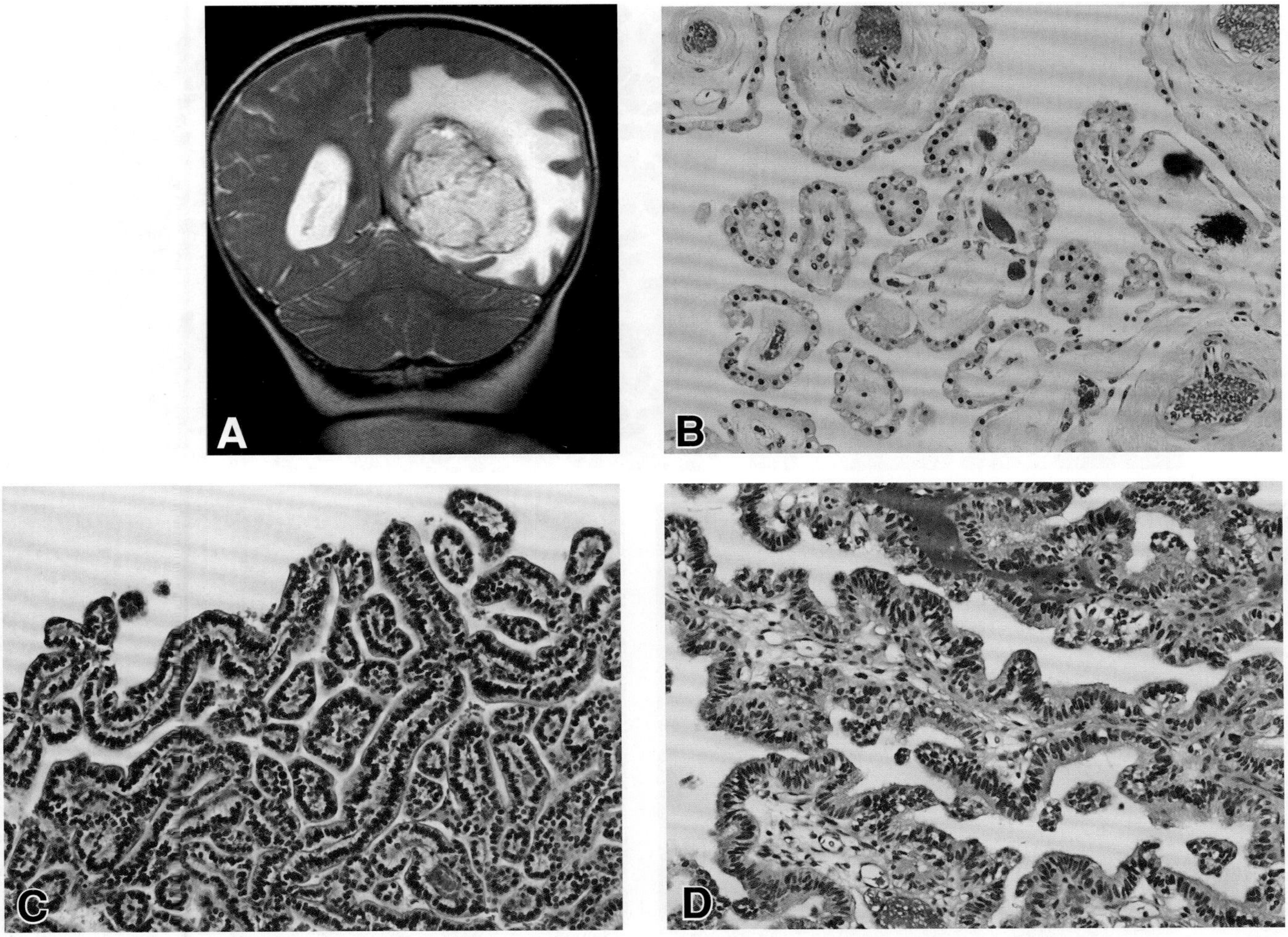

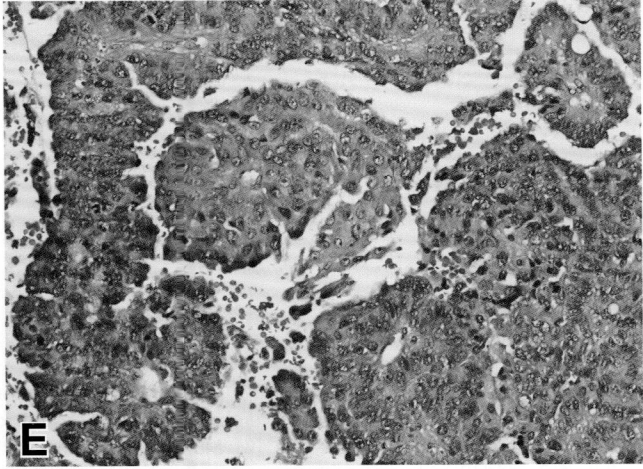

FIGURE 32-126. Choroid plexus papilloma (CPP) and carcinoma (CPC). A. CPP is a low-grade intraventricular tumor that arises from the fourth ventricular choroid plexus in adults and the lateral ventricular choroid plexus in children. **B.** Normal choroid plexus. **C.** Histologically, **CPP** retains the papillary architecture of choroid plexus, but the cells are more crowded and columnar rather than cuboidal. **D.** Atypical choroid plexus papilloma is similar to choroid plexus papilloma (C) but with increased cellular crowding and mitotic activity. **E. CPC** is a high-grade tumor that differs from CPP by showing loss of papillary architecture, marked cellular pleomorphism, increased proliferation rate and a more aggressive clinical course.

reticulin-free neurocytic islands ("pale islands") looking like germinal centers (Fig. 32-127C,D). This variant arises mainly in the cerebellar hemispheres of adults. The closely related MB with extensive nodularity is a tumor of infancy and has a distinctive multinodular appearance both on imaging and histologically.

Anaplastic MB and **large cell MB** are aggressive variants with overlapping morphologies (Fig. 32-127E). Hence,

they are combined into the large cell/anaplastic MB subtype. The former shows marked nuclear pleomorphism, nuclear molding, and cell–cell wrapping. By contrast, the large cell variant has a monomorphous population of large cells whose nuclei have prominent nucleoli. Both variants have high proliferative rates and conspicuous apoptosis. Most MBs show neuronal differentiation, in the form of immunoreactivity for synaptophysin; some

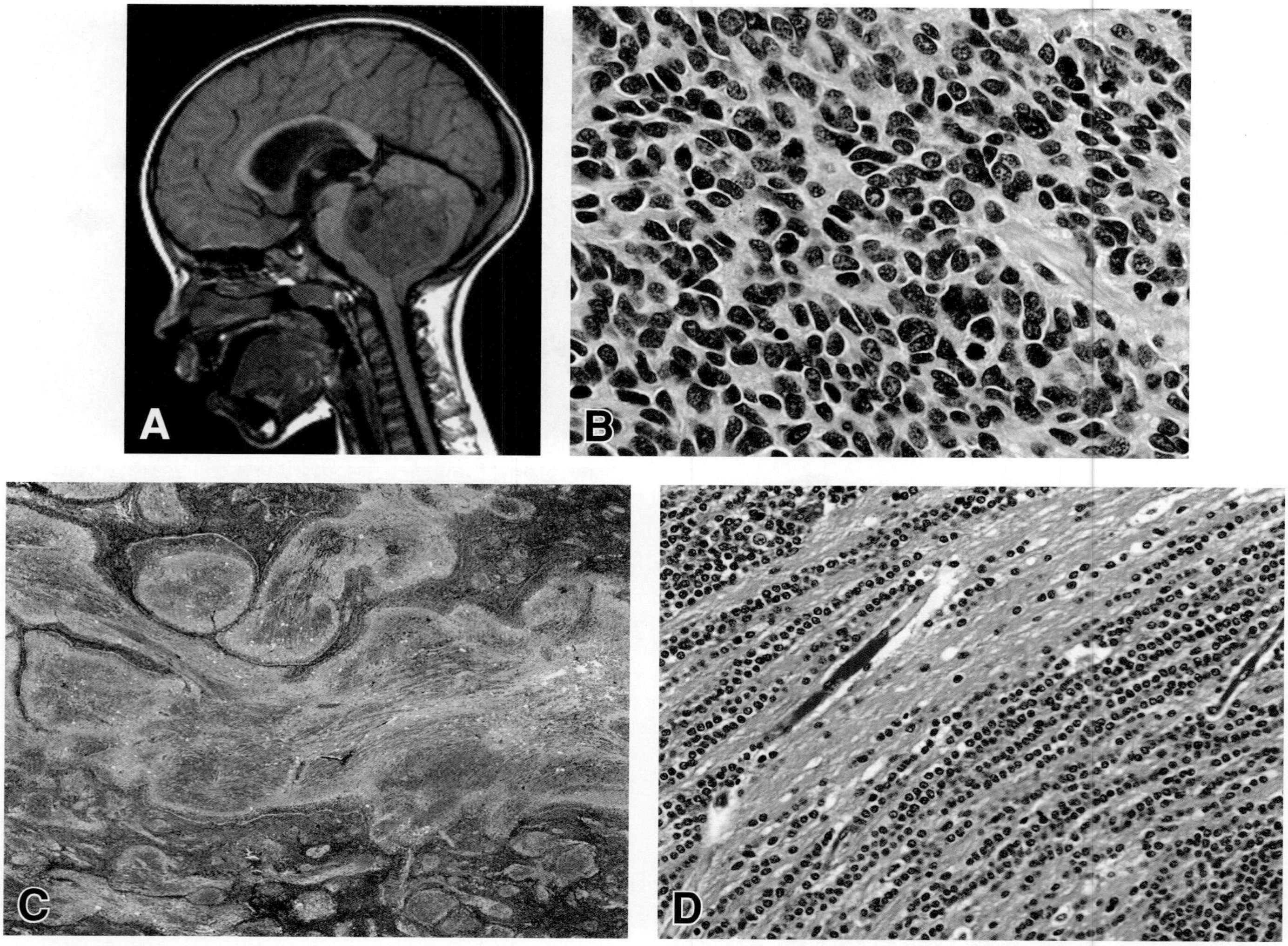

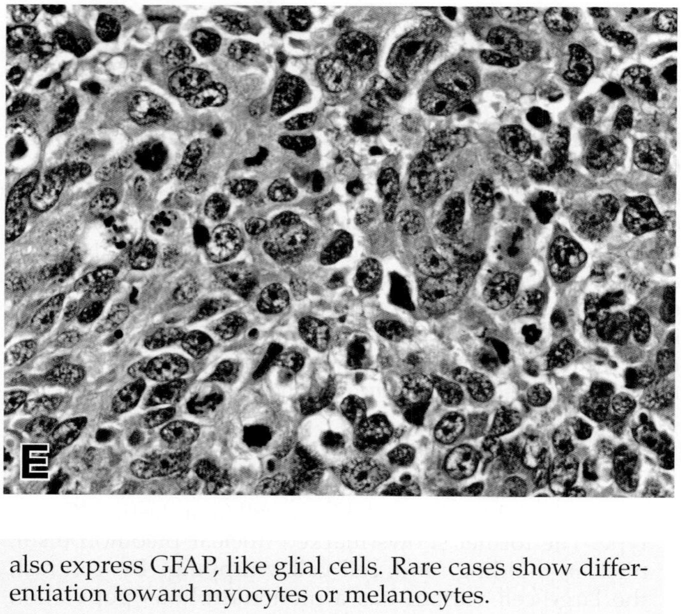

FIGURE 32-127. Medulloblastoma (MB). A. MB, the most common type of embryonal tumor, arises in the cerebellum. **B.** By light microscopy, MB is a "small blue cell" tumor. **C, D.** Two MB variants, desmoplastic/nodular MB and MB with extensive nodularity, have a better prognosis. **E.** Variants with large, anaplastic cells pursue a more aggressive clinical course.

also express GFAP, like glial cells. Rare cases show differentiation toward myocytes or melanocytes.

MOLECULAR PATHOGENESIS: MBs are thought to arise from stem cells of the fetal external granular layer and/or the periventricular germinal matrix. Molecular studies have implicated derangement in Wnt and sonic hedgehog signaling in tumor genesis. Differential activation of these pathways likely determines the MB subclass: the SHH pathway underlies desmoplastic/nodular MB and MB with extensive nodularity variants. The Wnt pathway favors the classic and anaplastic/large cell variants. In addition to the

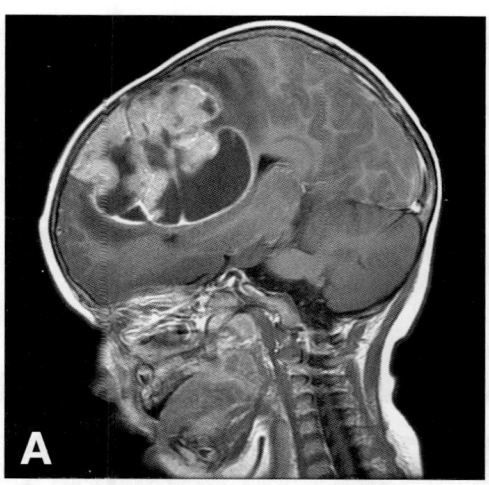
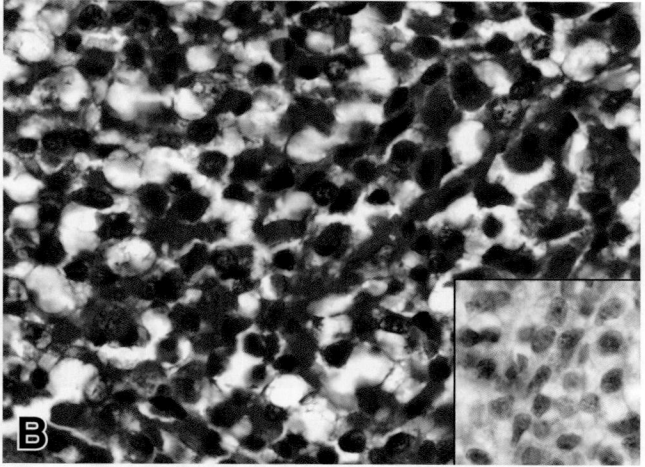

FIGURE 32-128. Atypical teratoid/rhabdoid tumor (ATRT). A. ATRT is a highly malignant neoplasm (World Health Organization grade IV) of early childhood that can arise in the cerebellum or, as illustrated here, in the cerebrum. **B.** Histologic features vary but usually include a rhabdoid cell component featuring plump hypereosinophilic cytoplasm. The molecular signature of ATRT is mutation or deletion of the *INI-1* gene, which can be detected as loss of immunostaining in tumor cell nuclei (*inset*). Normal host cells, such as vascular endothelium, serve as positive internal control in this immunostain.

four histologic subtypes mentioned above, medulloblastomas are genetically classified into three groups: (1) MB, WNT-activated; (2) MB, SHH-activated; and (3) MB, non-WNT/non-SHH. The presence of *TP53* mutations indicates worse prognosis in the MB, SHH-activated subgroup. By contrast, MB, WNT-activated, seen in 5% to 10% of all MBs, has a better prognosis. Clinical trials evaluating less aggressive therapy for this particular subtype are ongoing.

Embryonal Tumor With Multilayered Rosettes, C19MC-Altered

Embryonal tumor with multilayered rosettes (ETMRs), C19MC-altered can occur in the cerebrum, brainstem, or cerebellum, although the cerebral hemisphere is the most common location. This tumor primarily affects children and can show a wide range of histologic patterns, including multilayered rosettes, tubular structures resembling primitive neural tubes, and areas with abundant neuropil containing true rosettes (i.e., rosettes with a central lumen). ETMRs are immunoreactive for nestin and vimentin, and the neuropil areas are immunoreactive for synaptophysin. A majority of ETMRs display amplification of chromosomal region 19q13.42, which contains a cluster of microRNA genes named C19MC. C19MC amplification is restricted to embryonal tumors and serves as a specific diagnostic marker. Although not specific, these tumors also express LIN28A, an RNA-binding protein that enhances translation of insulin-like growth factor 2 (IGF-2) mRNA.

Atypical Teratoid/Rhabdoid Tumor (WHO Grade IV) Shows Multilineage Differentiation

Atypical teratoid/rhabdoid tumor (ATRT) is a malignant tumor of early childhood (although it can rarely present in adults as well) with divergent differentiation along rhabdoid, epithelial, mesenchymal, neuronal, and glial lines. The posterior fossa is most frequently affected (75%), followed by the supratentorial compartment (25%). The entire tumor may rarely be composed of rhabdoid cells, with eccentrically located nuclei and eosinophilic globular cytoplasm (referred to as "CNS rhabdoid tumor") but most often these cells are only one component of a heterogeneous malignancy (Fig. 32-128). *Inactivation of the INI-1 (hSNF5/SMARCB1) tumor suppressor gene through mutation or deletion is the molecular hallmark of ATRT* and is detected as loss of immunostaining for INI1 protein (Fig. 32-128). Renal rhabdoid tumors (see Chapter 22) share the same genetic alteration as ATRT. Germline *INI1* mutations result in **rhabdoid tumor predisposition syndrome**, with CNS and systemic rhabdoid tumors in infancy.

Craniopharyngiomas (WHO Grade I) Arise in the Sella Turcica and Suprasellar Region

Craniopharyngiomas (CPs) are circumscribed epithelial tumors, presumptively derived from Rathke cleft remnants. They arise mainly in children but also occur in adults. They typically show complex heterogeneous solid and cystic areas on imaging (Fig. 32-129A). Given the origin and expansile growth in the sellar/suprasellar region (Fig. 32-129B), CPs typically present with mixed endocrine and visual disturbances, due to compression of the pituitary below and optic chiasm above. Surgical resection is the preferred treatment. However, encroachment on the many vital structures in this area, including cranial nerves and blood vessels, often limits resectability, and residual tumor inexorably occurs.

 PATHOLOGY: CPs have two morphologic subtypes: **adamantinomatous** (by far the more common), which arises in children and adults, and the rarer **papillary**, which occurs almost exclusively in adults. The former has distinctive morphology consisting of sheets of squamous epithelium with prominent peripheral palisading, hydropic degeneration of central areas of the epithelium ("stellate reticulum"), and nodular aggregates of plump keratinocytes ("wet keratin") that tend to calcify (Fig. 32-129C). Long-standing compression of surrounding brain parenchyma may cause reactive piloid astrocytosis with prominent Rosenthal fibers. Papillary CPs contain exclusively nonkeratinizing squamous epithelium. Their

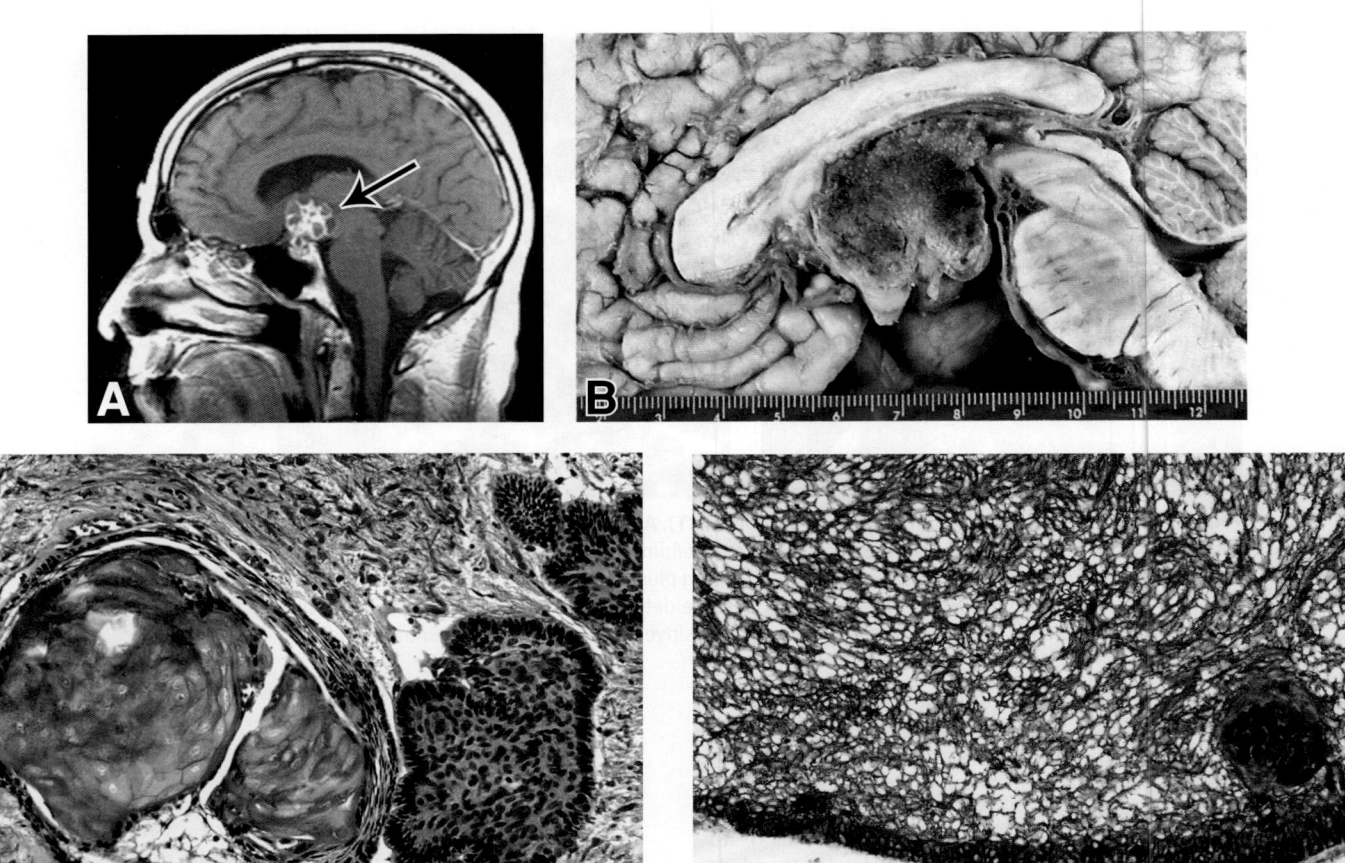

FIGURE 32-129. Craniopharyngioma. A. Craniopharyngiomas arise in the sellar/suprasellar region (*arrow*). **B.** Craniopharyngioma, gross photograph. (Courtesy of Dr. F. Stephen Vogel, Duke University.) **C.** Histologically, craniopharyngiomas are composed of squamous epithelium that displays a number of distinctive morphologic features, including peripheral palisaded nuclei and nodules of plump keratinocytes ("wet keratin") that are prone to calcify. **D.** Virtually all adamantinomatous craniopharyngiomas have mutations in *CTNNB1* resulting in nuclear localization of β-catenin in the cellular nodules.

histologic appearance is bland compared to the variegated morphology of the adamantinomatous subtype.

MOLECULAR PATHOGENESIS: Each CP morphologic subtype is associated with recurrent genetic alterations. Adamantinomatous CPs, in ~95% of cases, exhibit mutations in *CTNNB1*, which encodes β-catenin. Adamantinomatous CPs with *CTNNB1* mutations can be identified by immunohistochemistry using antibodies directed against β-catenin (Fig. 32-129D). Tumors with *CTNNB1* mutations show nuclear localization of β-catenin in nodules of squamous cells. By contrast, the vast majority of papillary CPs exhibit *BRAF* mutations, in particular, BRAF p.V600E.

Germinoma (WHO Grade III) and Other CNS Germ Cell Tumors Often Involve the Pineal Gland

Germ cell tumors (GCTs) of the CNS most often arise in midline structures, especially the pineal gland and third ventricular region (Fig. 32-130A). **Germinomas** tend to have biphasic cell composition: large malignant cells are interspersed with swarms of small reactive lymphocytes

(Fig. 32-130B). In some cases, a granulomatous response may predominate and obscure the neoplastic germ cell component. The tumors are characterized by strong immunoreactivity for OCT3/4 and c-kit, with focal positivity for placental alkaline phosphatase (PLAP) (Fig. 32-130C). In some cases, β-human chorionic gonadotropin (β-HCG) expression identifies isolated syncytiotrophoblastic cells. Pure germinomas are highly radiosensitive, and patients may receive radiation therapy, chemotherapy or a combination of the two. Other GCTs from the pineal region and at other CNS sites include **teratoma** (mature and immature), **yolk sac tumor, embryonal carcinoma,** and **choriocarcinoma**.

After germinomas, teratomas are the most common of this group to occur as pure (nonmixed) tumors. The remaining GCTs are mostly **mixed GCTs**. The prognosis for nongerminomatous GCTs is less favorable than for pure germinoma and largely depends on the extent of surgical resection.

Hemangioblastomas (WHO Grade I) Occur Most Often in the Cerebellum

Hemangioblastomas (HBs) are highly vascular tumors that arise mainly in the cerebellum but may also occur in the spinal cord and brainstem, especially in von Hippel–Lindau disease. They are among a group of low-grade circumscribed

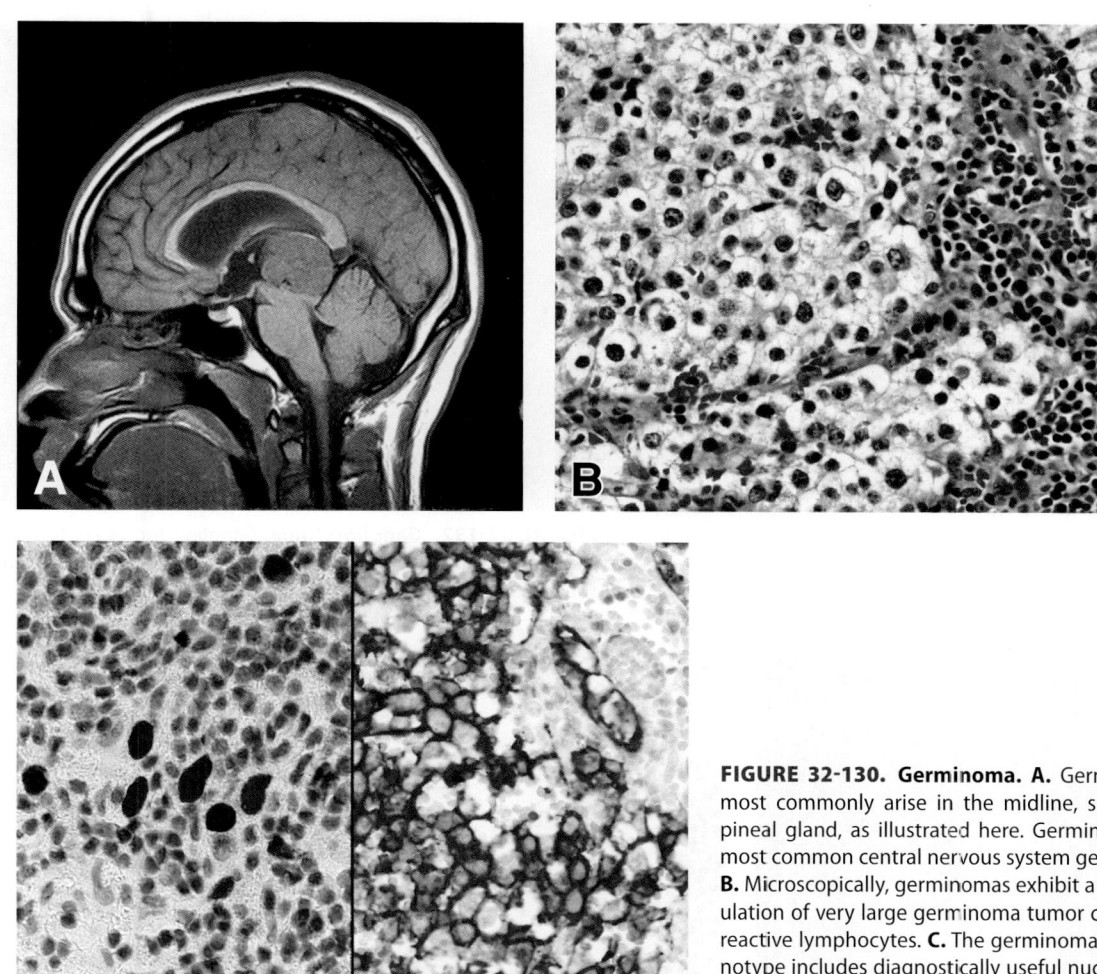

FIGURE 32-130. Germinoma. A. Germ cell tumors most commonly arise in the midline, such as in the pineal gland, as illustrated here. Germinomas are the most common central nervous system germ cell tumor. **B.** Microscopically, germinomas exhibit a biphasic population of very large germinoma tumor cells and small reactive lymphocytes. **C.** The germinoma immunophenotype includes diagnostically useful nuclear positivity for OCT3/4 (*left panel*) and cytoplasmic positivity for placental alkaline phosphatase (PLAP) (*right panel*).

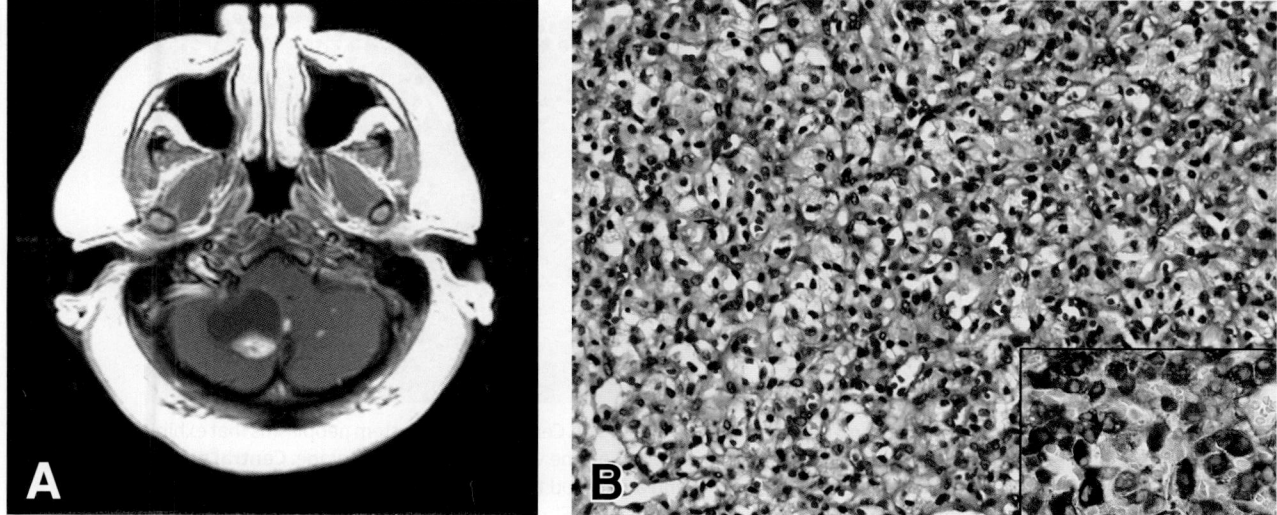

FIGURE 32-131. Hemangioblastoma (HB). A. HB most commonly arises in the cerebellum either sporadically or as part of von Hippel–Lindau disease. A common imaging presentation is as a cyst with a mural nodule. **B.** Microscopically, HB is a highly vascular tumor, with neoplastic stromal cells enmeshed in a dense capillary network. Tumor cells of HB display strong cytoplasmic positivity for inhibin-α (*inset*).

CNS tumors that appear on preoperative imaging studies as cysts with enhancing mural nodules (Fig. 32-131A). They usually present clinically as expanding masses in patients 20 to 40 years old. In 20% of cases, HBs secrete erythropoietin and induce secondary polycythemia. They can often be cured by surgical resection alone.

 PATHOLOGY: HBs consist of vacuolated stromal cells amid a dense capillary vasculature (Fig. 32-131B). The stromal cells are the neoplastic element and are immunoreactive for inhibin-α.

Tumors That Show Only Neuronal Differentiation Are Rare

All such tumors are low grade (WHO grade I or II). **Gangliocytoma (WHO grade I)** is a very well-differentiated, circumscribed tumor composed entirely of dysmorphic mature ganglion cells (Fig. 32-132). The temporal lobe is a favored

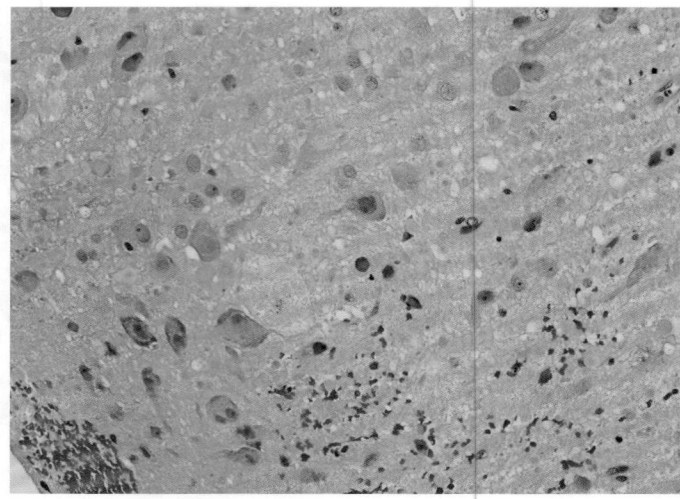

FIGURE 32-132. Gangliocytoma. Gangliocytomas are tumors formed by neoplastic ganglion cells, often with prominent nucleoli, coarse Nissl substance, and binucleation.

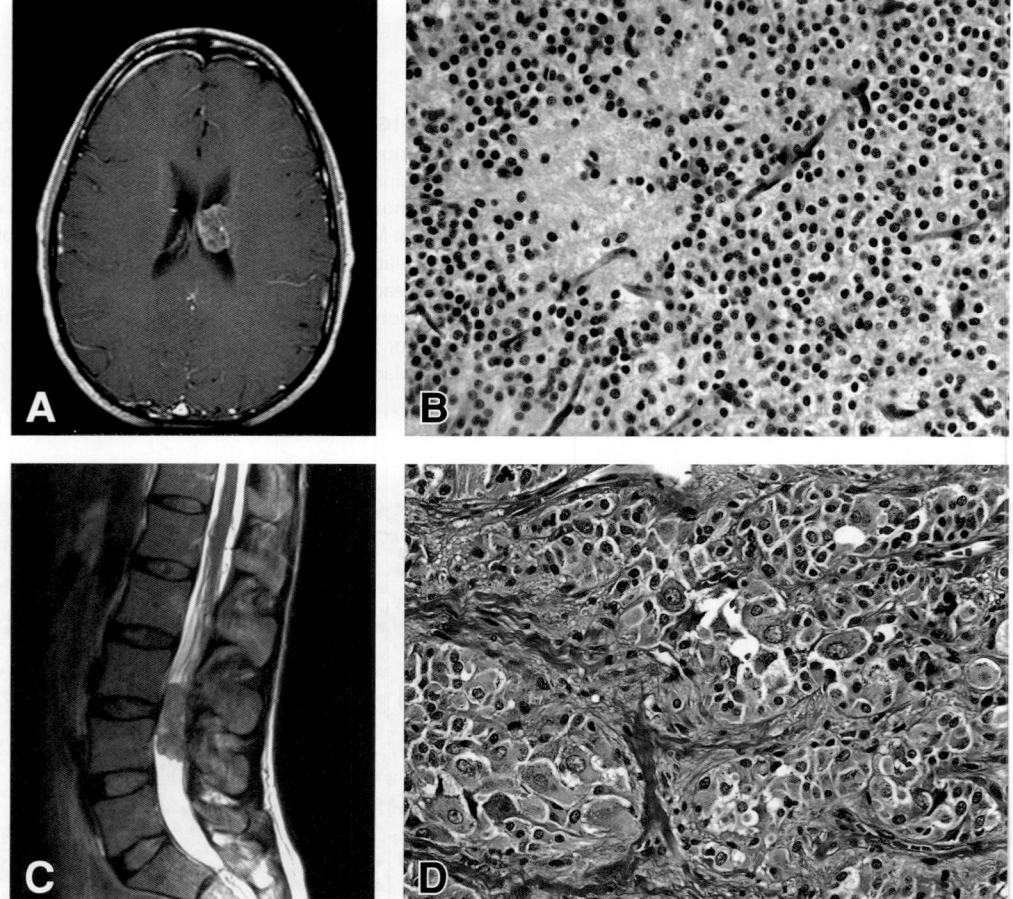

FIGURE 32-133. Neuronal and neuroendocrine tumors. A. Central nervous system neoplasms that exhibit purely neuronal/neuroendocrine differentiation are rare, and the vast majority are low grade. **Central neurocytoma** (CN) is a low-grade neuronal tumor of young adulthood that arises within the lateral ventricle. **B.** CN cells closely mimic those in oligodendrogliomas (compare to Fig. 32-122A) but exhibit a neuronal immunophenotype, including immunoreactivity for synaptophysin. **C. Paraganglioma of the filum terminale** arises, as the name implies, from the distal spinal cord terminus within the lumbar cistern. **D.** Paraganglioma tumor cells exhibit a neuroendocrine phenotype, with strong reactivity for synaptophysin and chromogranin. Frank ganglion cell differentiation is seen in about 25% of cases.

location. **Dysplastic gangliocytoma of the cerebellum (Lhermitte–Duclos disease; WHO grade I)** is a distinctive entity of the cerebellum, presenting with gross enlargement of the folia (as easily seen by MR imaging) and disorganized cerebellar cortical histology with large ganglion cells derived from granular cell neurons. A layer of myelinated axons in the outermost molecular layer just beneath the pia is another distinctive feature. Half of patients have **Cowden syndrome** (see Chapter 5). Complete surgical resection is curative.

Central neurocytoma (CN; WHO grade II) and **extraventricular neurocytoma (WHO grade II)** are low-grade tumors of young adults that arise from the septum pellucidum, grow into the lateral ventricles and often extend into the third ventricle (Fig. 32-133A). CNs contain monomorphous round cells that look like oligodendrocytes (Fig. 32-133B) but, like neurons, strongly express synaptophysin. Extraventricular neurocytomas look and behave similarly but occur in the brain parenchyma rather than the ventricles. Surgery can be curative for small tumors, but partially resected tumors may recur, and central neurocytomas also have the potential for CSF dissemination.

Paraganglioma of the filum terminale (PFT; WHO grade I) is an uncommon neuroendocrine tumor that, like MPE, arises in the lumbar cistern from the conus medullaris or filum terminale of the spinal cord (Fig. 32-133C). Like paragangliomas elsewhere in the body, PFTs show compact acinar ("zellballen") architecture (Fig. 32-133D) and express neuronal markers including synaptophysin and chromogranin. They often show ganglion cell differentiation. Most are "encapsulated" by an investing layer of leptomeninges and are cured by surgical excision.

Mixed Glioneuronal Tumors

Gangliogliomas (GGs; WHO grades I and III) are well-differentiated, circumscribed tumors of neoplastic ganglion cells, with a glioma component. The temporal lobe is its favored location. GGs are the most common tumors associated with chronic temporal lobe epilepsy (40% of tumor-associated temporal lobe epilepsy cases). Atypical ganglion cells are intermixed with the glioma element, usually astrocytoma. Although low grade (WHO grade I), GG can progress to **anaplastic ganglioglioma (WHO grade III)**. In either grade, prognosis depends on the extent of surgical resection. A majority of gangliogliomas have molecular alterations in proteins involved in MAPK pathways, and mutations in *BRAF, KRAS, NF1,* and *FGFR1/FGFR2. BRAF* p.V600E is the most common recurrent alteration, detected in ~20% to 30% of GGs.

Dysembryoplastic neuroepithelial tumors (DNETs; WHO grade I) are low-grade glioneuronal tumors arising superficially within the cerebral cortex of children (Fig. 32-134A). Their intracortical location correlates with the typical clinical history of long-standing seizures. They may also occur anteriorly in the frontal horn of the lateral ventricle, in association with the caudate nucleus and septum pellucidum. DNETs have multinodular architecture, with prominent nodular aggregates of small rounded oligodendroglial-like cells with interspersed neurons that appear to "float" within cystic spaces in the cortical parenchyma (Fig. 32-134B). They resemble low-grade oligodendrogliomas but do not express the characteristic translocation seen in the latter. Foci of cortical dysplasia may occur in adjacent peritumoral cortex. Resection is curative.

Pineal Parenchymal Tumors Encompass a Spectrum of Clinical Behavior

Pineal parenchymal tumors (PPTs) range from the very low-grade **pineocytoma (WHO grade I)** to **pineoblastoma,** a highly malignant PNET **(WHO grade IV)**. Between these two extremes are **pineal parenchymal tumors of intermediate differentiation (PPTIDs; WHO grade II or III)**. These are discussed in Chapter 27.

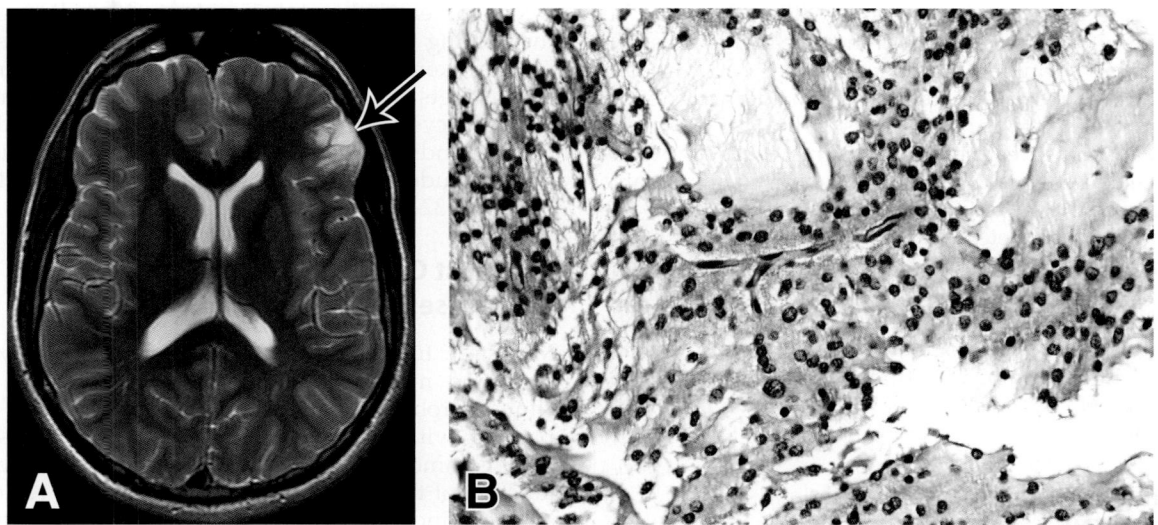

FIGURE 32-134. Dysembryoplastic neuroepithelial tumor (DNET). A. DNETs are very low-grade seizure-inducing neuronal tumors of childhood that arise superficially within the cerebral cortex (*arrow*). **B.** They are composed of monotonous round cells that resemble oligodendroglia but are not infiltrative and are potentially curable by surgical resection.

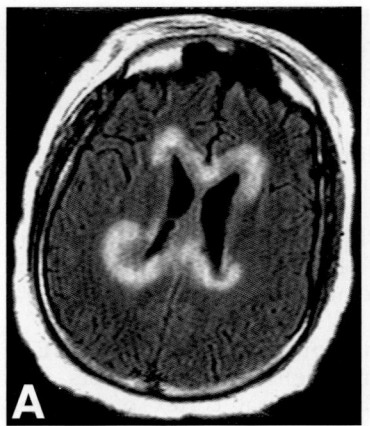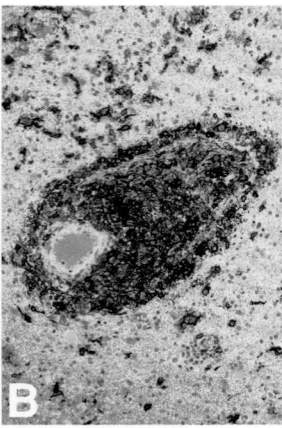

FIGURE 32-135. Primary central nervous system lymphoma (PCNSL). A. One common clinical presentation of PCNSL is as a diffuse periventricular tumor lining the lateral ventricles. **B.** The vast majority of PCNSLs are of diffuse large B-cell phenotype and thus strongly express B-cell markers such as CD20 seen here. (Courtesy of Dr. F. Stephen Vogel, Duke University.)

TABLE 32-12
CENTRAL NERVOUS SYSTEM CYSTS
Choroid plexus cyst
Pineal cyst
Epidermoid cyst
Dermoid cyst
Arachnoid cyst
Ependymal cyst
Neurenteric (enterogenous) cyst
Rathke cyst
Colloid cyst

Primary CNS Lymphomas Are Usually B-Cell Tumors

Systemic lymphomas often spread to the CNS, but lymphomas may also originate in the CNS. PCNSLs are tumors of adults and have increased in incidence in the last several decades in both immunocompromised and elderly immunocompetent patients. MR imaging reveals various patterns, including solitary or multiple tumors in superficial cortical, deep periventricular, or cerebellar locations (Fig. 32-135A).

Definitive pathologic diagnosis is usually made by stereotactic biopsy; surgical resection does not improve survival or response to treatment which involves radiation and chemotherapy. PCNSLs are composed of highly infiltrative neoplastic lymphocytes that show prominent invasion and expansion of blood vessel walls (Fig. 32-135B). The vast majority are large cell B-cell tumors that express CD20, PAX5, and other B-cell markers (Fig. 32-135B). In immunocompromised individuals, PCNSLs may be driven by EBV, which can be detected by immunohistochemistry. They are highly sensitive to steroids, often shrinking dramatically after glucocorticoid treatment, but this response is temporary. In addition, steroid therapy can make histologic diagnosis of PCNSL extremely difficult because posttreatment biopsies may show only gliosis and reactive changes. Radiation and/or chemotherapy give a median survival of 70% at 2 years and up to 45% at 5 years in immunocompetent patients. The majority (~70%) of PCNSLs have mutations in *MYD88*, whose gene product regulates immune signaling. *MYD88* p.L265P, the most common recurrent alteration in PCNSL, has not been associated with other CNS tumors. The dysregulated signaling pathway can be targeted with ibrutinib, a Brutton's tyrosine kinase (BTK) inhibitor. Thus, *MYD88* p.L265P may play both an important diagnostic and therapeutic role in PCNSL.

Many Benign (Nonneoplastic) Cysts Occur in the CNS

These are listed in Table 32-12. Some are degenerative in nature and are usually incidental findings on neuroimaging studies done for other reasons, or at autopsy. Only rarely do those such as **choroid plexus cysts** and **pineal gland cysts** cause clinical symptoms. Others, such as **arachnoid cysts** and **ependymal cysts**, are largely asymptomatic but occasionally require surgical fenestration of the cyst wall to release pressure and relieve mass effects on surrounding structures. The remaining types of cysts are primarily developmental in origin and may cause mass effects that require simple surgery as definitive treatment.

Diagnosis of specific cyst types depends on a combination of anatomic location and histology of the cyst wall lining. For example, three CNS cysts, **Rathke cyst, colloid cyst,** and **neurenteric cyst**, share virtually identical epithelial linings (i.e., ciliated pseudostratified columnar epithelium with goblet cells) but are easily and confidently diagnosed based on anatomic location: Rathke cysts arise in the sellar/suprasellar region, colloid cysts in the roof of the third ventricle near the foramen of Monro, and neurenteric cysts in the subarachnoid space anterior to the brainstem medulla or cervical spinal cord (Fig. 32-136). **Epithelial inclusion cysts** (epidermoid and dermoid cysts) are distinguished by their lining and cyst contents. Epidermoid cysts are lined only by keratinizing stratified squamous epithelium and have sheets of anucleate flattened squames for contents; dermoid cysts display dermal appendages, such as sebaceous glands and hair follicles, in their walls and their contents include not only anucleate squames but also matted hair (Fig. 32-136).

The Most Common CNS Tumors Are Metastases From Elsewhere

Metastatic tumors far surpass primary CNS tumors in numbers, and malignancies metastatic to the CNS are major clinical problems. Autopsy series show that up to 25% of patients with systemic cancers have CNS metastases. The most common site for brain metastasis is at the gray–white junction of the cerebral cortex, but any CNS region may be affected, including the choroid plexus, pineal gland, and pituitary gland.

The most common primary tumors to involve the CNS are lung (most frequent for both men and women), breast,

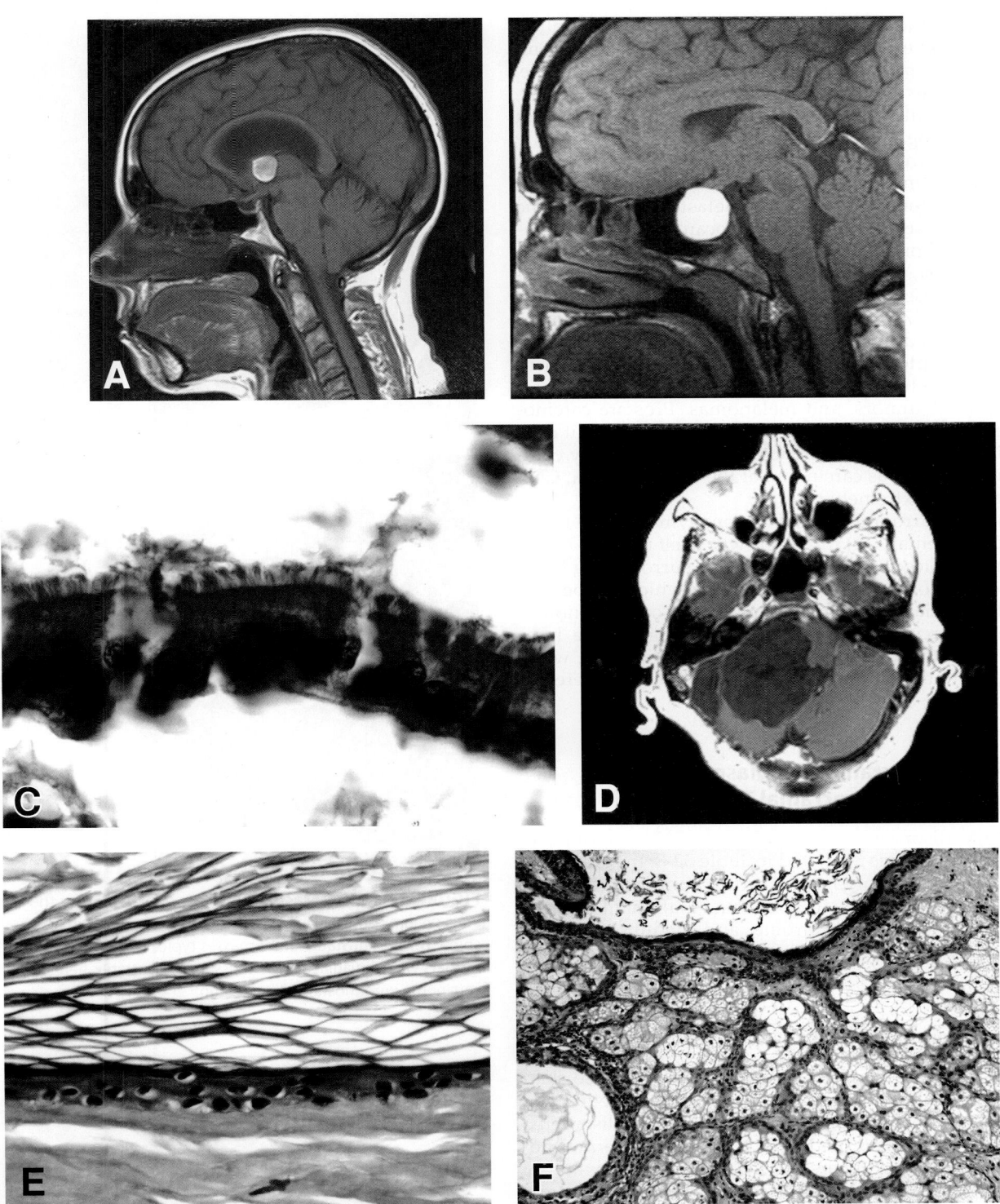

FIGURE 32-136. Cysts of the central nervous system. A. Colloid cysts arise in the rostral roof of the third ventricle. **B. Rathke cysts** are located in the sellar/suprasellar region. **C.** Both of these cysts exhibit a similar epithelial lining, consisting of ciliated pseudostratified columnar epithelium with goblet cells. **D.** A favored anatomic site for **epidermoid cysts** is the cerebellopontine angle. **E.** Epidermoid cysts differ from dermoid cysts in that the lining of epidermoids is composed of only keratinizing squamous epithelium. **F.** Dermoids also include skin adnexal appendage structures, such as sebaceous glands and hair follicles.

melanoma, kidney, and gastrointestinal tract. Over half of all cases involve multiple metastases (Fig. 32-137A), and metastatic patterns may reflect tumor type. For example, CNS metastases from cancers of gastrointestinal, breast, prostate, and uterine origin are frequently solitary, but those from lung carcinomas and melanomas are usually multiple. A rare extreme form of multiple metastasis, called miliary metastasis ("carcinomatous encephalitis"), in which innumerable minute metastases shower the brain, may be seen with lung adenocarcinomas. Metastases to cranial bones and vertebrae usually originate in the prostate, breast, kidney, thyroid, lung, or lymphoma/leukemia (giving rise to the mnemonic "Pb KTL" or "lead kettle") (Fig. 32-137B). Isolated dural metastases most often represent spread from breast cancers, and single metastases to the leptomeninges and subarachnoid space usually occur with lung, breast, and gastric adenocarcinomas; hematopoietic tumors; and melanomas. Prostate carcinomas frequently metastasize to the skull and spine but only rarely involve the brain parenchyma. For some very common cancers, such as carcinoma of the uterine cervix, CNS metastases are extremely rare.

Injury to surrounding CNS parenchyma due to metastatic tumors entails (1) tumor growth itself (Fig. 32-137C); (2) tumor-induced vasogenic edema in surrounding brain tissue; (3) hemorrhage within the tumor, which can be substantial (especially with melanomas, renal cell carcinomas and choriocarcinomas); and (4) depending on the location of metastasis, obstructive hydrocephalus (e.g., when metastases to the midbrain cause occlusion of the cerebral aqueduct).

Hereditary Intracranial Neoplasms Are Often Associated With Extracranial Tumors

Hereditary disorders associated with CNS tumors and their genetic features are listed in Table 32-8. In some, neoplasms of systemic organs are most prominent, but nervous system tumors also occur. Thus, malignant gliomas occur in Li–Fraumeni syndrome, and medulloblastomas are associated with gastrointestinal tumors in Turcot syndrome.

Tuberous Sclerosis (Bourneville Disease)

Tuberous sclerosis is an autosomal dominant disease characterized by hamartomas (tubers) of the brain, retina and viscera, as well as various neoplasms. It reflects disordered migration and arrested maturation of neuroectoderm, leading to formation of "tubers" in the cerebral cortex and of SEGAs (Fig. 32-120). The tubers are discrete cortical areas containing bizarre cells with neuronal and glial features. The SEGAs resemble "candle drippings."

In addition to intracranial lesions, tuberous sclerosis includes (1) facial angiofibromas (adenoma sebaceum), (2) cardiac rhabdomyomas, and (3) mesenchymal tumors of the kidney (angiomyolipomas). Most patients have seizures and are mentally retarded. Mutations in *TSC1* and *TSC2* are responsible: *TSC1* (9q34) encodes a protein called hamartin, and *TSC2* (16p13) encodes tuberin, which is homologous to a GTPase-activating protein. Both are tumor suppressors (see Chapter 5).

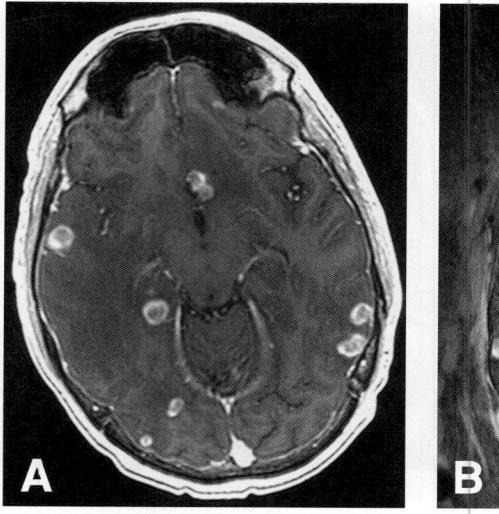
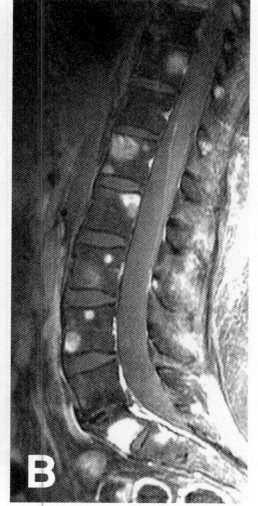
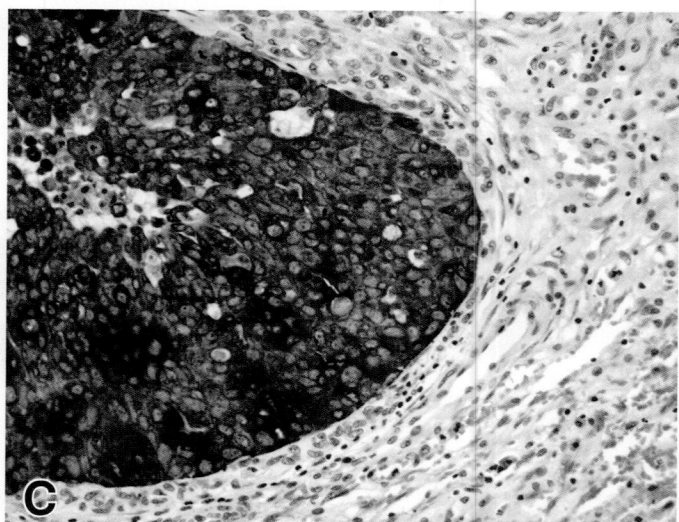

FIGURE 32-137. Metastatic disease. Metastases to the central nervous system commonly produce multiple lesions in both the brain (**A**) and spine (**B**). **C.** Metastatic tumor masses typically show very sharp "pushing" borders with the adjacent brain tissue, as illustrated here with metastatic carcinoma immunostained for keratin.

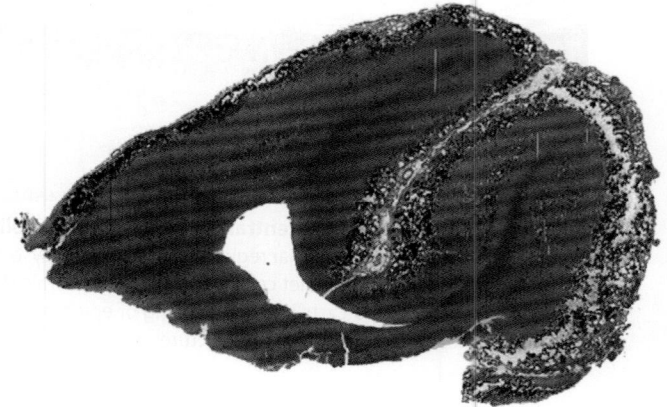

FIGURE 32-138. Sturge–Weber syndrome. A portion of cerebral cortex shows an overlying capillary angioma involving the leptomeninges and underlying cortical calcification (*purple*).

Sturge–Weber Syndrome (Encephalofacial Angiomatosis)

Sturge–Weber syndrome is a rare, nonfamilial congenital disorder characterized by angiomas of the brain and face. The facial lesion is usually unilateral and is called a **port wine stain (nevus flammeus)**. The leptomeninges contain large angiomas, which in severe cases may occupy an entire hemisphere. Cerebral calcification and atrophy often underlie the intracranial angiomas (Fig. 32-138). The link between angiomas of the face and brain may reflect the continuity of the embryologic vascular supply to the telencephalon, the eye and the overlying skin. In most instances, Sturge–Weber syndrome is associated with mental deficiency.

PHYSICAL AND CHEMICAL INJURIES

Physical trauma to the eye commonly causes ecchymosis of the highly vascular eyelids (black eye); when this occurs, other parts of the eye also may be injured. Disruption of the corneal epithelium may follow traumatic abrasion, prolonged wear of a contact lens, foreign bodies on the ocular surface, and intense exposure to ultraviolet (UV) light. The corneal epithelium has the capacity for rapid healing in most noninfectious conditions. A variety of chemicals, both household and industrial, may result in ocular surface injury (chemical burn). The nature of the injury is typically dependent on the pH of the chemical (acid vs. base).

Blunt trauma increases intraorbital pressure momentarily and may cause the bones in the floor of the orbit to fracture into the maxillary sinus (**blow-out fracture**). The inferior rectus muscle may become entrapped in such a fracture thereby causing the eye to retract into the orbit (**enophthalmos**).

An array of foreign materials can injure the eye. Whereas small particles often lodge in superficial ocular tissues, high-velocity foreign material may penetrate into (penetrating ocular trauma) or through the eye (perforating ocular injury). A foreign particle may damage the eye directly or because of secondary infection after the introduction of microorganisms into the eye. Some foreign bodies provoke a prominent acute inflammatory or granulomatous reaction. Others, such as those containing iron, cause intracellular toxicity resulting in retinal degeneration and glaucoma (**siderosis bulbi**), effects that may not be evident for several years. Other complications of ocular injuries include cataracts, retinal detachment, and optic nerve atrophy.

THE EYELIDS

Common conditions affecting the eyelids include:

- **Blepharitis** is inflammation of the eyelids. It is common and sometimes produces an acute, red, tender, inflammatory mass. Demodex mites, bacteria, and rosacea are some of the etiologies implicated in blepharitis.
- **Hordeolum (stye)** refers to an acute inflammatory, focal abscess of the eyelid. Acute inflammation involving the meibomian glands is termed an **internal hordeolum,** whereas acute folliculitis of the eyelash pilosebaceous units (glands of Zeis) is an **external hordeolum**.
- **Chalazion** is a lipogranulomatous inflammatory process centered around the meibomian glands or the glands of Zeis. It is thought to represent a reaction to extruded sebum and usually produces erythematous swelling in the eyelid.

■ **Xanthelasma** is a discrete yellow plaque consisting of aggregates of lipid-laden macrophages, usually involving the nasal aspect of the eyelids. It is often seen in adults over the age of 40 and patients with dyslipidemia.

THE ORBIT

Proptosis Is Abnormal Forward Protrusion of the Eyeball

Numerous conditions cause protrusion of the eye. The most common cause is thyroid disease. The term **exophthalmos** is typically reserved for protrusion caused by thyroid disease. Other causes of proptosis include orbital vascular malformations and hemangiomas, inflammatory lesions, and neoplasms. Proptosis also results from lesions of the paranasal sinuses and intracranial cavity that invade the orbit.

Exophthalmos of Hyperthyroidism Continues Despite Treatment

Exophthalmos caused by Graves disease may precede or follow other manifestations of thyroid dysfunction. Exophthalmos resulting from thyroid disease usually occurs in early adult life, especially in women (female to male ratio, 4:1). It may be severe and progressive, particularly in middle life, when exophthalmos no longer correlates well with the state of thyroid function. Dysthyroid exophthalmos may be associated with eyelid retraction, edema of the eyelids, red eye, dry eye, chemosis (conjunctival edema), and limitation of ocular motility. Exophthalmos is part of the constellation of ocular changes known as thyroid eye disease (TED). TED is an autoimmune process in which circulating autoantibodies are thought to bind to orbital fibroblasts resulting in increased glycosaminoglycan production in the extraocular muscles. This results in significant enlargement of the muscles that causes orbital congestion and, due to limited space in the orbit, pushes the eye forward. Fibrosis of orbital tissues may occur later in the course of TED.

CLINICAL FEATURES: Although exophthalmos of hyperthyroidism is usually bilateral, the condition may affect one eye more than the other. Other ocular manifestations of TED include upper eyelid retraction (due to increased sympathetic tone), red eye, dry eye due to increased exposure of the ocular surface, and restrictive strabismus. Compressive optic neuropathy may be vision threatening and must be treated urgently.

Nonspecific Orbital Inflammation Is a Chronic Idiopathic Inflammatory Condition

Nonspecific orbital inflammation (NSOI) is also known as *orbital pseudotumor, idiopathic orbital inflammatory syndrome, and idiopathic orbital inflammation*. It is a collection of benign inflammatory processes affecting all or part of the orbital tissues without a known systemic or local cause. It is associated with a variable degree of fibrosis. It is a common cause of proptosis and restrictive dysfunction of the extraocular muscles.

THE CONJUNCTIVA

Conjunctival Hemorrhage May Follow Blunt Trauma, Anoxia, or Severe Coughing

Conjunctival hemorrhage may occur as a result of trauma, Valsalva maneuver, or strangulation. It may also occur spontaneously, often first noted on arising after sleep. Topical steroids may result in increased vascular fragility leading to spontaneous hemorrhage. Conjunctival hemorrhage occurs in the loose collagenous connective tissue of the substantia propria and does not extend into the cornea because of the barrier imposed by the tight adherence of corneal epithelium to its underlying, avascular substantia propria.

Conjunctivitis May Be Infectious or Allergic

The most common causes of conjunctivitis are infections or allergic/atopic disease. Microorganisms infecting the surface of the eye frequently cause conjunctivitis, keratitis (corneal inflammation), or a corneal ulcer. The conjunctiva, as well as other parts of the eye, may also become infected by hematogenous spread from a focus of infection elsewhere. Adenovirus is the most common viral cause of conjunctivitis and is quite contagious. The organism may be spread by various fomites including contaminated ophthalmic instrumentation. Bacterial conjunctivitis is most common in children.

At some stage in life, virtually everyone has viral or bacterial conjunctivitis. This extremely common eye disease is characterized by hyperemic conjunctival blood vessels (pink eye). The inflammatory exudate that accumulates in the conjunctival sac commonly crusts, especially with bacterial disease, which causes the eyelids to stick together in the morning. The conjunctival discharge may be purulent, fibrinous, serous, or hemorrhagic. Participating inflammatory cells vary with the etiologic agent. As many allergens are seasonal, the allergic conjunctivitis they elicit tends to occur only at particular times of the year. Both allergic and viral conjunctivitis typically manifest with follicular lymphoid hyperplasia of the tarsal conjunctiva.

Trachoma

Trachoma is a chronic, contagious conjunctivitis caused by *Chlamydia trachomatis*. Various serotypes of *C. trachomatis* cause ocular, genital, and systemic infections (trachoma, inclusion conjunctivitis, and lymphogranuloma venereum; see Chapter 9).

EPIDEMIOLOGY: About 40 million people worldwide are afflicted by trachoma and 160 million people are at risk for infection. Trachoma is an acute, cyclic, infectious, fibrosing keratoconjunctivitis caused by *C. trachomatis* (serotypes A, B, and C). *This infection is the most common infectious cause of blindness in the world and is especially prevalent in Asia, the Middle East, and parts of Africa.* The disease has been eradicated in the United States and other developed countries. Trachoma is not particularly contagious, but overcrowding and poor hygienic conditions favor its transmission by fingers, fomites, and flies. Spontaneous healing is common in children, but in adults, the disease progresses more rapidly and rarely heals without treatment.

THE EYE

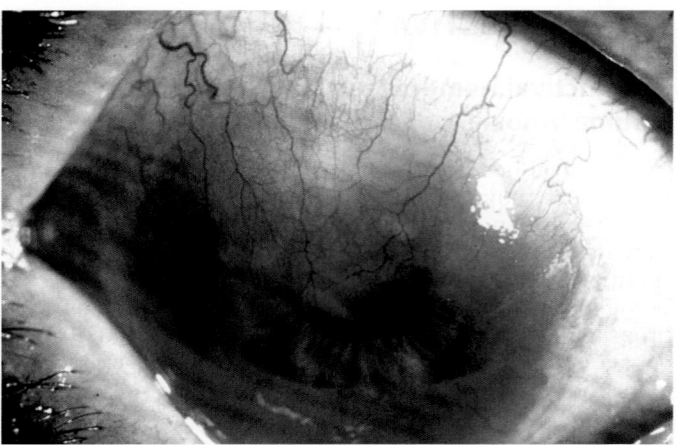

FIGURE 33-1. Trachoma. The cornea of a patient with severe trachoma shows extensive fibrovascular scarring (**pannus**) of the superior cornea.

ETIOLOGIC FACTORS: An inflammatory reaction is generated by the immune system in response to *C. trachomatis.* Serial persistent or repetitive inflammatory reactions to different strains of the pathogen are believed to cause the serious cicatricial complications.

PATHOLOGY: Trachoma is virtually always bilateral and involves the upper half of the conjunctiva more than the lower. The cellular infiltrate is predominantly lymphocytic, and conjunctival lymph follicles with necrotic germinal centers are characteristic. Eventually lymphocytes and blood vessels invade the superior portion of the cornea between the epithelium and Bowman layer (**trachomatous pannus**) (Fig. 33-1). Scarring of the conjunctiva and eyelids distorts the eyelids, resulting in misdirection of the lashes (**trichiasis**) that can rub on the cornea and cause further scarring. On microscopic examination, the desquamated conjunctival epithelium exhibits glycogen-rich intracytoplasmic inclusion bodies, and large macrophages contain nuclear fragments (Leber cells). Secondary bacterial infections occur commonly.

Other Chlamydial Infections

Chlamydia is responsible for a purulent conjunctivitis that develops in newborns who become infected during passage through the birth canal. The infection is also acquired by swimming in nonchlorinated pools (swimming pool conjunctivitis) or from contact with discharges of infected urethra or cervix.

In adults and older children, *Chlamydia* causes a chronic follicular conjunctivitis with focal lymphoid hyperplasia (**inclusion conjunctivitis**). In contrast to trachoma, the lower tarsal conjunctiva is involved. Scarring and necrosis do not develop, and keratitis is rare and mild.

Ophthalmia Neonatorum

Ophthalmia neonatorum is a severe, acute conjunctivitis with a copious purulent discharge, especially in the newborn, caused by Neisseria gonorrhoeae. The infection, which is a common early cause of blindness in some parts of the world, is complicated by corneal ulceration, perforation, scarring, and panophthalmitis. Infants usually become infected while passing through the birth canal of an infected mother. Other causative organisms for ophthalmia neonatorum include other pyogenic bacteria and *C. trachomatis.* Today, newborns are usually routinely treated with topical antimicrobials such as erythromycin, tetracycline, or povidone-iodine shortly after birth.

Pingueculum and Pterygium

Pingueculum is a yellowish conjunctival elevation adjacent to the corneoscleral limbus. It is more often located nasally but can occur temporally or on both sides of the limbus in the interpalpebral fissure. It is the most common conjunctival lesion. It consists of UV-induced elastotic degeneration of the subepithelial connective tissue similar to that seen in sun-damaged skin (actinic elastosis; see Chapter 28).

Pterygium is a band of vascularized perilimbal conjunctiva that grows horizontally onto the cornea in the shape of an insect wing (hence the name). It also consists of UV-induced elastotic stromal degeneration accompanied by neovascularization and fibrosis.

THE CORNEA

Herpes Simplex Virus Causes Corneal Infection

Herpes simplex virus (HSV) has a predilection for corneal epithelium, where it causes keratitis, but it can also involve the corneal stroma and occasionally other ocular tissues.

PRIMARY INFECTION BY HERPES SIMPLEX VIRUS TYPE 1: Subclinical or undiagnosed localized ocular lesions are caused by HSV type 1 in childhood. These infections are accompanied by regional lymphadenopathy, systemic infection, and fever. Except in newborns infected during passage through an infected mother's birth canal, HSV type 2 rarely causes ocular infection. When it does, it may produce widespread lesions of the cornea and retina. Most corneal lesions due to HSV are asymptomatic plaques of diseased epithelial cells that contain a replicating virus. These usually heal without ulceration, but an acute unilateral follicular conjunctivitis may occur. Ulcerative keratitis appears after serum antibody levels increase.

REACTIVATION OF HERPES SIMPLEX VIRUS INFECTION: Latent in the trigeminal ganglion, HSV may pass down cranial nerve V and reactivate the infection. Unlike primary HSV infection, reactivation is characterized by corneal ulceration and a more severe inflammatory reaction. Recurrence of keratitis due to HSV may be precipitated by UV light, trauma, menstruation, emotional and physical stress, exposure to light or sunlight, vaccination and other factors, similar to those causing labial recurrences.

PATHOLOGY: HSV causes multiple, minute, discrete, intraepithelial ulcerations (superficial punctate keratopathy). Although some of these lesions heal, others enlarge and eventually coalesce to form linear or branching fissures (dendritic ulcers, from the Greek *dendron,* "tree"). The epithelium between the fissures desquamates, leading to sharply demarcated, irregular geographical ulcers. Affected epithelial cells, which may become multinucleated, contain eosinophilic, intranuclear inclusion bodies (Lipschütz bodies).

The lesions of the corneal stroma vary in reactivated HSV infection. Typically, a central disc-shaped corneal opacity develops beneath the epithelium, owing to edema and minimal inflammation (**disciform keratitis**). Inflammation typically consists of lymphocytes, neutrophils, and epithelioid histiocytes. Granulomatous inflammation along Descemet membrane is highly suggestive of herpetic keratitis. The corneal stroma may become markedly thinned. Corneal perforation can also occur.

Onchocerciasis Leads to Blindness in Tropical Regions

The nematode *Onchocerca volvulus*, which is transmitted by bites of infected blackflies, is by far the most important helminthic infection of the eye (see Chapter 9). *Onchocerciasis is the second most common infectious cause of blindness worldwide, particularly in regions of Africa and Latin America where it is endemic.* Microfilariae released from fertilized adult female worms migrate into the superficial cornea, bulbar conjunctiva, aqueous humor, and other ocular tissues. The intracorneal microfilariae die and elicit an inflammatory response that leads to corneal opacification and visual impairment (**river blindness**). Less frequently, endophthalmitis, retinal lesions, and optic atrophy occur. Treatment with ivermectin is highly effective.

Corneal Arcus Is due to Lipid Deposition in the Peripheral Cornea

Also known as **arcus senilis** because of its frequency in the elderly, corneal arcus is a concentric deposition of lipid in the peripheral cornea that occurs bilaterally. If it occurs in individuals under the age of 40, clinical investigation for hyperlipidemia is indicated. Rarely, it can occur as a manifestation of a genetic corneal condition (**arcus lipoides**) or as a congenital anomaly (**arcus juvenilis**).

Common Superficial Corneal Degenerations Involve an Opaque Horizontal Band Across the Cornea

Calcium phosphate may deposit in the cornea (**calcific band keratopathy**), typically starting at 3 o'clock and 9 o'clock, at the corneoscleral limbus. It can progress centrally in a band-like fashion to occlude the visual axis. It may occur as a result of chronic intraocular inflammation, particularly in children, due to systemic hypercalcemia or hyperphosphatemia, or as a hereditary condition.

Chronic actinic keratopathy occurs worldwide but is most severe in regions in which people spend a considerable amount of time outdoors. Their unprotected eyes are exposed to excessive UV light, such as that reflected from desert, water, or snow. Actinic degeneration occurs in the subepithelial space, Bowman layer, and the superficial corneal stroma. It has a spheroidal basophilic histologic appearance.

Noninflammatory Genetic Corneal Disorders (Dystrophies) Are Diverse

Most corneal dystrophies have an autosomal dominant or recessive mode of inheritance, but rare cases are X-linked recessive. Some of these diseases affect other parts of the body (e.g., Fabry disease, cystinosis, certain types of mucopolysaccharidosis, and ichthyosis). Inherited conditions that primarily affected the cornea without clinically apparent systemic involvement were traditionally called corneal dystrophies and, before the era of molecular genetics, were classified according to the primary corneal layer that was involved: (1) the outer layer composed of epithelium, basement membrane, and Bowman layer; (2) the stroma; and (3) the endothelium and Descemet membrane, the basement membrane of the corneal endothelium. However, this classification is now considered artificial because many corneal dystrophies involve more than one layer.

EPITHELIAL DYSTROPHIES: The different epithelial dystrophies are characterized by a variety of distinct abnormalities, which include microcysts or accumulations of anomalous material within the cytoplasm of the corneal epithelium, defects in the epithelial basement membrane, and deposition of a fine fibrillar substance in the Bowman layer. In some epithelial dystrophies, faulty desmosomes may permit adjacent epithelial cells to separate, leading to accumulation of fluid-filled microcysts. Loss of hemidesmosomes between the epithelium and Bowman layer leads to painful, recurrent erosions that begin in early childhood. Although there may be a slow decrease in visual acuity, epithelial dystrophies do not ordinarily cause blindness.

 MOLECULAR PATHOGENESIS: Patients with one disorder of the corneal epithelium (*Meesmann dystrophy*) have dominant mutations in the *KRT3* or *KRT12* genes, which encode keratin 3 and keratin 12, respectively. The mutations result in aggregations of abnormal cytokeratin filaments and severely impair cytoskeletal function in the affected cells. In the rare bilateral, autosomal recessive corneal disorder *gelatinous drop-like corneal dystrophy*, the *TACSTD2* gene is mutated, and amyloid is found beneath the corneal epithelium in gelatinous drop-like deposits.

STROMAL DYSTROPHIES: The stromal corneal dystrophies are entities in which different substances (amyloid, glycosaminoglycans, proteins, or a variety of lipids) accumulate within corneal stroma because of inherited metabolic disorders. Each stromal dystrophy causes a characteristic form of corneal opacification. The age of onset and rate of progression vary with the particular disorder. Although clinical manifestations may be limited to the cornea, other tissues are involved in some of these disorders.

MOLECULAR PATHOGENESIS: Several clinically and pathologically different inherited corneal disorders, including the granular corneal dystrophies and most lattice corneal dystrophies, result from distinct mutations in the same gene, namely, *TFGBI*, which encodes transforming growth factor β-1. Another predominantly stromal corneal dystrophy (macular corneal dystrophy) results from a defect in the *CHST6* gene, which encodes a sulfotransferase that catalyzes sulfation of *N*-acetyl glucosamine and galactose in keratan sulfate. Other corneal stromal diseases are caused by mutations in *PIKFYVE* (which encodes a phosphoinositide kinase, and causes fleck corneal dystrophy), *DCN* (which encodes the extracellular matrix protein decorin, and causes congenital stromal corneal dystrophy) and *UBIAD1* (which encodes a prenyltransferase involved in cholesterol and phospholipid metabolism, and causes Schnyder corneal dystrophy).

 MOLECULAR PATHOGENESIS: *ENDOTHELIAL DYSTROPHIES:* Several different endothelial dystrophies are recognized, usually accompanied by abnormalities in Descemet membrane. In *Fuchs endothelial corneal dystrophy,* wart-like excrescences form on the posterior surface of Descemet membrane (guttae), and progressive visual loss follows endothelial cell degeneration and corneal edema. Missense mutations in *COL8A2*, the gene encoding the α_2-chain of type 8 collagen, have been identified in some patients with early-onset Fuchs dystrophy and in ***posterior polymorphous corneal dystrophy***, both of which affect the corneal endothelium and Descemet membrane.

THE LENS

Cataracts Are Opacifications in the Crystalline Lens

Cataracts are a major cause of visual impairment and blindness throughout the world and are the outcome of numerous conditions.

 ETIOLOGIC FACTORS: The most common cause of cataracts in the United States is advancing age (age-related cataract). Cataracts are also caused by diabetes, nutritional deficiencies (e.g., deficiencies in riboflavin or tryptophan), toxins (e.g., dinitrophenol, naphthalene, ergot), drugs (e.g., corticosteroids, topical phospholine iodide, phenothiazines) or physical agents (e.g., heat, ultraviolet light, trauma, intraocular surgery, ultrasound).

Cataracts may develop in ocular diseases such as uveitis, intraocular neoplasms, glaucoma, retinitis pigmentosa, and retinal detachment. Cataracts are also associated with congenital rubella virus infection, some skin diseases (e.g., atopic dermatitis, scleroderma), and various systemic diseases.

 MOLECULAR PATHOGENESIS: Cataracts may result from genetic disorders, and in some be associated with other ocular or systemic abnormalities. For example, cataracts occur with mutations in the heat shock transcription factor-4 (*HSF4*) gene and genes that encode specific lens proteins such as connexins (*GJA3*, *GJA8*), crystallins (a family of *CRY* genes), a beaded filament structural protein-2 (*BFSP2*), a putative cell-junction protein (*LIM2*), and aquaporin 0 (*MIP*). They also result from genetic mutations and chromosomal anomalies that cause numerous systemic diseases and syndromes.

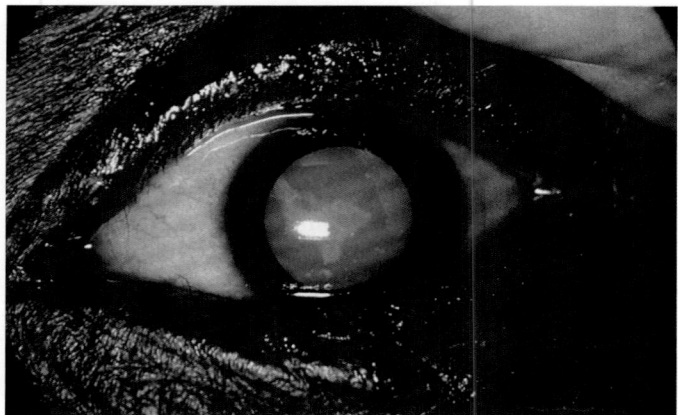

FIGURE 33-2. Cataract. The white appearance of the pupil in this eye is due to significant opacification of the lens cortex ("mature cataract").

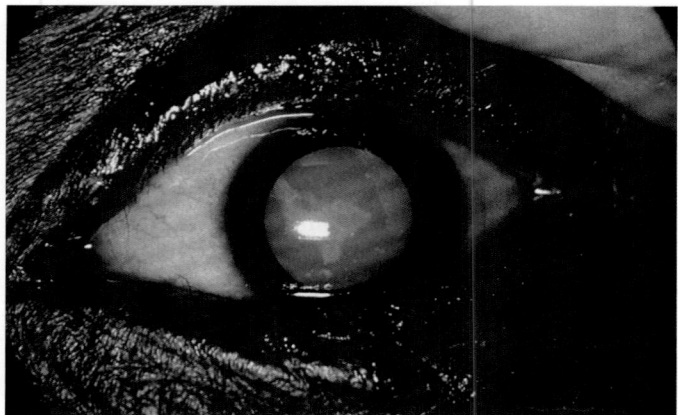 **PATHOLOGY:** In the development of cataracts, clefts appear between the lens fibers, and degenerated lens material accumulates in these spaces (morgagnian globules, incipient cataract). Degenerated lens material exerts osmotic pressure, causing the damaged lens to imbibe water. Swelling of the lens can cause anterior displacement of the iris with narrowing of the anterior chamber angle and may ultimately result in glaucoma (phacomorphic glaucoma).

In a *mature cataract* (Fig. 33-2), the entire lens degenerates and liquifies, and the lenticular debris escapes into the aqueous humor through the lens capsule, diminishing the volume of the lens (hypermature cataract). After becoming engulfed by macrophages, the extruded lenticular material may obstruct aqueous outflow and produce glaucoma (phacolytic glaucoma). The compressed lens fibers in the center of the lens normally harden with aging (simple nuclear sclerotic cataract) and may become brown or black. If the peripheral part of the lens (lens cortex) becomes liquefied (morgagnian cataract), the sclerotic nucleus may sink within the lens by gravity.

Fortunately, cataractous lenses can be surgically removed, and optical devices can be provided to permit focusing of light on the retina (typically a prosthetic intraocular lens implant).

Presbyopia Is a Failure of Accommodation as a Result of Aging

With this impairment of vision, the near point of distinct vision becomes located farther from the eye. At the equator of the crystalline lens, the cuboidal subcapsular cells normally differentiate into elongated lens fibers throughout life. Once formed, these lens fibers persist indefinitely. Older fibers become displaced into the center of the lens, causing it to thicken with age. Over the course of many years, this process reduces the elasticity of the lens. This effect interferes with the normal tendency of the lens to become spherical, and so diminishes the power of accommodation. As a result, most persons after age 40 years begin to have difficulty reading and require spectacles for near vision.

Phacoantigenic Uveitis Is an Autoimmune Granulomatous Reaction to Lens Proteins

In this disorder, an inflammatory response occurs around or within the lens (or its remains) in an eye with a traumatized or cataractous lens and sometimes after surgical removal of a cataractous lens. A similar reaction may occur spontaneously in the contralateral eye months or years later. This autoimmune reaction to unique lens proteins, which are normally sequestered from the immune system, can be provoked experimentally by immunization with autologous lens material. The inflammation has a zonal pattern surrounding lens material with neutrophils in the innermost layer, epithelioid histiocytes in the middle layer, and lymphocytes in the outer layer.

THE UVEA

A Variety of Inflammatory Conditions Affect the Uveal Tract

Inflammation of the uvea (**uveitis**) includes inflammation of the iris (**iritis**), the ciliary body (**cyclitis**), and the iris plus the ciliary body (**iridocyclitis**). Inflammation of the iris and ciliary body (**anterior uveitis**) typically causes a red eye, photophobia, moderate ocular pain, blurred vision, ciliary flush, and slight miosis. White blood cells are present in the anterior chamber. There is often a proteinaceous exudate in the aqueous humor (flare) and inflammatory deposits may be present on the posterior cornea (keratic precipitates).

Peripheral anterior synechiae are adhesions between the peripheral iris and the anterior chamber angle. **Posterior synechiae** are adhesions that develop between the iris and the lens. Both types of synechiae are complications of uveitis, and, when numerous, both can cause glaucoma.

Sympathetic Ophthalmia Can Be a Sequela of Trauma

In sympathetic ophthalmia, the posterior or entire uvea develops granulomatous inflammation after a latent period, in response to a penetrating injury in the other eye. Penetrating ocular injury and prolapse of uveal tissue through the wound likely sensitize the immune system to otherwise sequestered ocular antigens and may lead to a progressive, bilateral, diffuse, granulomatous inflammation of the uvea. This uveitis develops in the originally injured eye (exciting eye) after a latent period of 4 to 8 weeks. The latent period may, however, be as short as 10 days or as long as many years. The uninjured eye (sympathizing eye) becomes affected at the same time as the injured eye, or shortly thereafter. Vitiligo and graying of the eyelashes sometimes accompanies the uveitis. Nodules containing reactive retinal pigment epithelium, macrophages, and epithelioid histiocytes (**Dalen–Fuchs nodules**) commonly appear between Bruch membrane (**lamina vitrea**) and retinal pigment epithelium. Experimental studies suggest that the antigen(s) responsible for sympathetic ophthalmia is likely a retinal or retinal pigment epithelial protein.

Sarcoidosis Commonly Affects the Eye

Ocular involvement occurs in one-fourth to one-third of patients with sarcoidosis and is often the initial clinical manifestation. Both eyes are usually affected, most often with a granulomatous uveitis. Although any ocular and orbital tissues may be involved, this granulomatous disease has a predilection for the anterior segment of the eye. Other ocular manifestations of sarcoidosis include conjunctival micronodules, calcific band keratopathy, cataracts, retinal neovascularization, vitreous hemorrhage, and bilateral enlargement of the lacrimal and salivary glands.

THE RETINA

Retinal Hemorrhage May Occur in Both Local and Systemic Diseases

The important causes of retinal hemorrhages are hypertension, diabetes mellitus, retinal vein occlusion, bleeding diatheses, and trauma, including infantile abusive head trauma. Appearance of the hemorrhage(s) varies with cause and location. Hemorrhages in the nerve fiber layer spread between axons and causes a flame-shaped appearance on funduscopy, whereas deep retinal hemorrhages tend to be round (dot or blot hemorrhage). Hemorrhages may also occur between the vitreous face and the retina (preretinal hemorrhage) and these typically have a bright red round or boat-shaped appearance clinically. Hemorrhages may also occur between the retina and the retinal pigment epithelium or between the retinal pigment epithelium and Bruch membrane (subretinal hemorrhages). Clinically, these hemorrhages tend to appear darker red or maroon compared with those in the retina.

After accidental or surgical perforation of the globe, expulsive suprachoroidal hemorrhages may detach the choroid and displace the retina, vitreous body, and lens through the wound.

Retinal Occlusive Vascular Disease Is an Important Cause of Blindness

The retina derives its blood supply from two different sources. The inner third of the retina including the nerve fiber layer, ganglion cell layer, and inner nuclear layer is supplied by the retinal blood vessels (central retinal artery and vein). The outer two-thirds of the retina including the photoreceptors, derives its blood supply from branches of the posterior ciliary blood vessels that supply the capillary layer of the choroid (choriocapillaris). Vascular occlusion results from thrombosis (venous occlusions), embolism (arterial occlusions), stenosis (as in arteriosclerosis), vascular compression, intravascular sludging or coagulation, and vasoconstriction (e.g., in hypertensive retinopathy or migraine). Thrombosis of ocular vessels may accompany primary disease of these vessels, as in giant cell arteritis.

Certain disorders of the heart and major vessels, such as the carotid arteries, predispose to emboli that may lodge in retinal arterioles and are evident on funduscopic examination at points of vascular bifurcation. Within the optic nerve, emboli in the central retinal artery frequently lodge in the vessel in the region of the sclera (**lamina cribrosa**).

THE EYE

PATHOLOGY: The effect of vascular occlusion depends on the area of the retina supplied, the degree of resultant ischemia, and the nature of the embolus. Small emboli often do not interfere with retinal function, whereas septic emboli may cause foci of ocular infection. Retinal ischemia frequently leads to fluffy white patches that resemble cotton on ophthalmoscopic examination (**cotton-wool spots**). These spots, which are seldom wider than the optic nerve head, consist of aggregates of swollen axons in the nerve fiber layer of the retina. Affected axons contain numerous degenerated mitochondria and dense bodies related to the lysosomal system, which accumulate because of impaired axoplasmic flow. Histologically, in cross section, individual swollen axons resemble cells (cytoid bodies). Cotton-wool spots may not lead to atrophy if circulation is restored in time.

Central Retinal Artery Occlusion

Like neurons in the rest of the nervous system, those in the retina (Fig. 33-3) are extremely susceptible to hypoxia. Central retinal artery occlusion (Figs. 33-4 and 33-5) may follow thrombosis of the retinal artery, as in atherosclerosis or giant

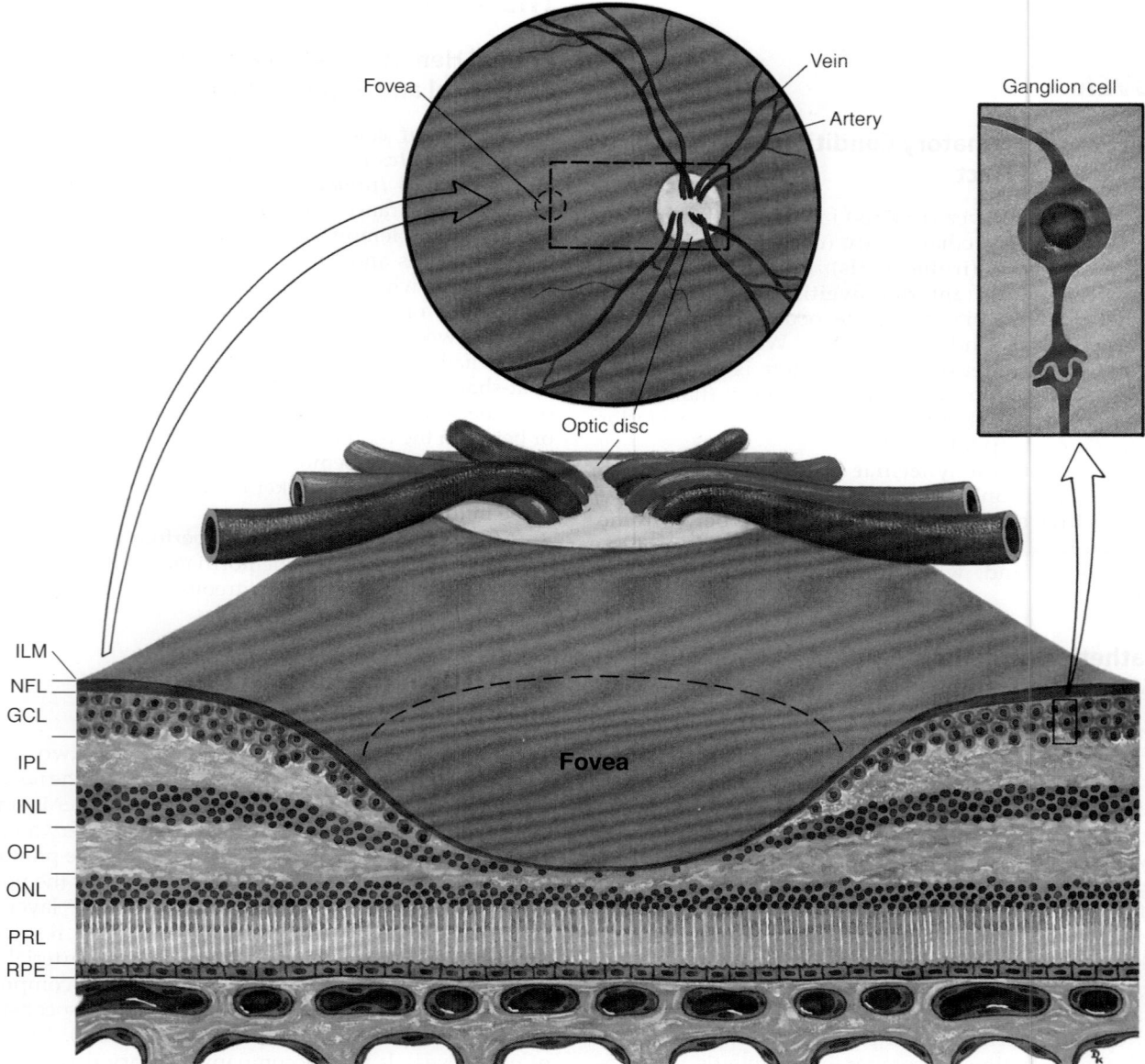

FIGURE 33-3. The normal retina. The macular region is depicted. Constituents of the normal retina are arranged in distinct layers. These include the internal limiting membrane (*ILM*), nerve fiber layer (*NFL*), ganglion cell layer (*GCL*), inner plexiform layer (*IPL*), inner nuclear layer (*INL*), outer plexiform layer (*OPL*), outer nuclear layer (*ONL*), photoreceptor layer (*PRL*) with the inner (depicted in *darker purple*) and outer segments of the photoreceptors, and the retinal pigment epithelium (*RPE*). Axons of the ganglion cells enter the nerve fiber layer and converge toward the optic nerve head. The inner retina contains arteries and veins. The retina is thinnest at the center of the macula, the fovea, where bare photoreceptors rest on the retinal pigment epithelium. Only one cell thick in most of the retina, the ganglion cell layer is multilayered at the macula.

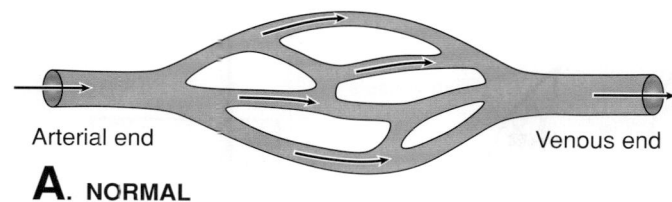

A. NORMAL

Arterial end   Venous end

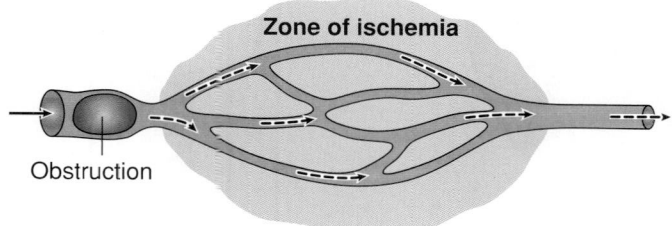

Zone of ischemia

Obstruction

Neuronal functional impairment → Visual loss
Edema → Pallor

B. RETINAL ARTERIAL OCCLUSION

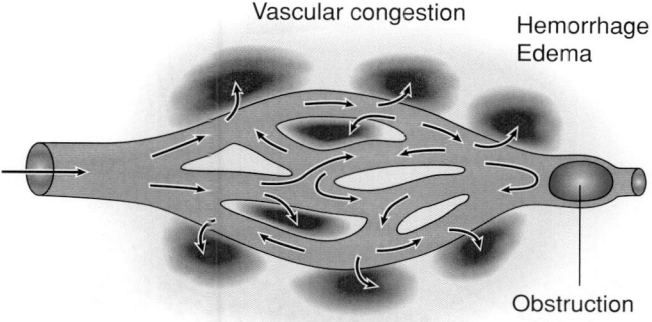

Vascular congestion   Hemorrhage
Edema

Obstruction

Mild ischemia: normal neuronal function

C. NORMAL TO MODERATELY IMPAIRED NEURONAL FUNCTION

FIGURE 33-4. Occlusion of the retinal artery and vein. A. In the retina, as in other parts of the body, blood normally flows through a capillary network. **B.** When the central retinal artery or one of its branches becomes occluded (typically by an embolus), a zone of retinal ischemia ensues. This is accompanied by impaired neuronal function and visual loss, and the ischemic retina becomes pale due to swelling of neurons. Because blood flow and intravascular pressure within the ischemic tissue are low, hemorrhage is usually not present. **C.** With occlusion of the central retinal vein or one of its branches (typically by a thrombus), there is venous stasis with vascular congestion, hemorrhage, and edema. Ischemia can be mild to severe and neuronal function may not be severely impacted.

cell arteritis, or, more commonly, embolization to that blood vessel. Intracellular edema, manifested by retinal thickening and pallor, is prominent, especially in the macula, where ganglion cells are most numerous. The fovea, the center of the macula, stands out in sharp contrast as a prominent **cherry-red spot,** because of the underlying vascularized choroid (Fig. 33-5). The lack of retinal circulation results in marked attenuation of retinal arterioles.

Permanent severe vision loss follows central retinal artery obstruction, unless the ischemia is of short duration. Unilateral loss of vision, lasting a few minutes (**amaurosis fugax**), occurs with small retinal emboli.

Central Retinal Vein Occlusion

Central retinal vein occlusion results in intraretinal hemorrhages in all four quadrants of the retina, especially around the optic nerve head. The hemorrhages reflect the high intravascular pressure that dilates and ruptures the veins and collateral vessels (Fig. 33-6). Edema of the optic nerve head and retina occurs because absorption of interstitial fluid is impaired (venous stasis).

Vision is reduced but may recover despite the severity of the funduscopic changes. An intractable, closed-angle glaucoma, with severe pain and repeated hemorrhages, commonly ensues 2 to 3 months after central retinal vein occlusion (the so-called 90-day glaucoma or neovascular glaucoma). This complication is caused by neovascularization of the iris and angle resulting in adhesions between the iris and the anterior chamber angle (**peripheral anterior synechiae**).

Hypertensive Retinopathy Correlates With the Severity of Hypertension

Increased systemic blood pressure commonly affects the retina, causing changes that can readily be seen with the ophthalmoscope (Figs. 33-7 and 33-8).

PATHOLOGY: Features of hypertensive retinopathy include:

- **Arteriolar narrowing**
- **Hemorrhages** in the retinal nerve fiber layer (flame-shaped hemorrhages)
- **Retinal exudates,** including some that radiate from the center of the macula (macular star)
- Fluffy white bodies in the superficial retina (**cotton-wool spots**)
- **Microaneurysms** of the retinal microvasculature

In the eye, arteriolosclerosis accompanies long-standing hypertension and commonly affects the retinal and choroidal vessels. Lumens of the thickened retinal arterioles become narrowed, increasingly tortuous, and of irregular caliber. At sites where arterioles cross veins, the latter appear kinked (**arteriovenous nicking**). However, the venous diameter before the site of compression is not wider than that after it. The kinked appearance of the vein reflects sclerosis within the venous walls, because retinal arteries and veins share a common adventitia at sites of arteriovenous crossings, rather than compression by a taut sclerotic artery.

By funduscopy, abnormal retinal arterioles appear as parallel white lines at sites of vascular crossings (**arterial sheathing**). Initially, the narrowed lumens of the retinal vessels decrease the visibility of the blood column and make it appear orange on ophthalmoscopic examination (**copper wiring**). However, as the blood column eventually becomes completely obscured, light reflected from the sclerotic vessels appears as threads of silver wire (**silver wiring**).

Small superficial or deep retinal hemorrhages often accompany retinal arteriolosclerosis. **Malignant hypertension** is characterized by necrotizing arteriolitis, with fibrinoid necrosis and thrombosis of precapillary retinal arterioles.

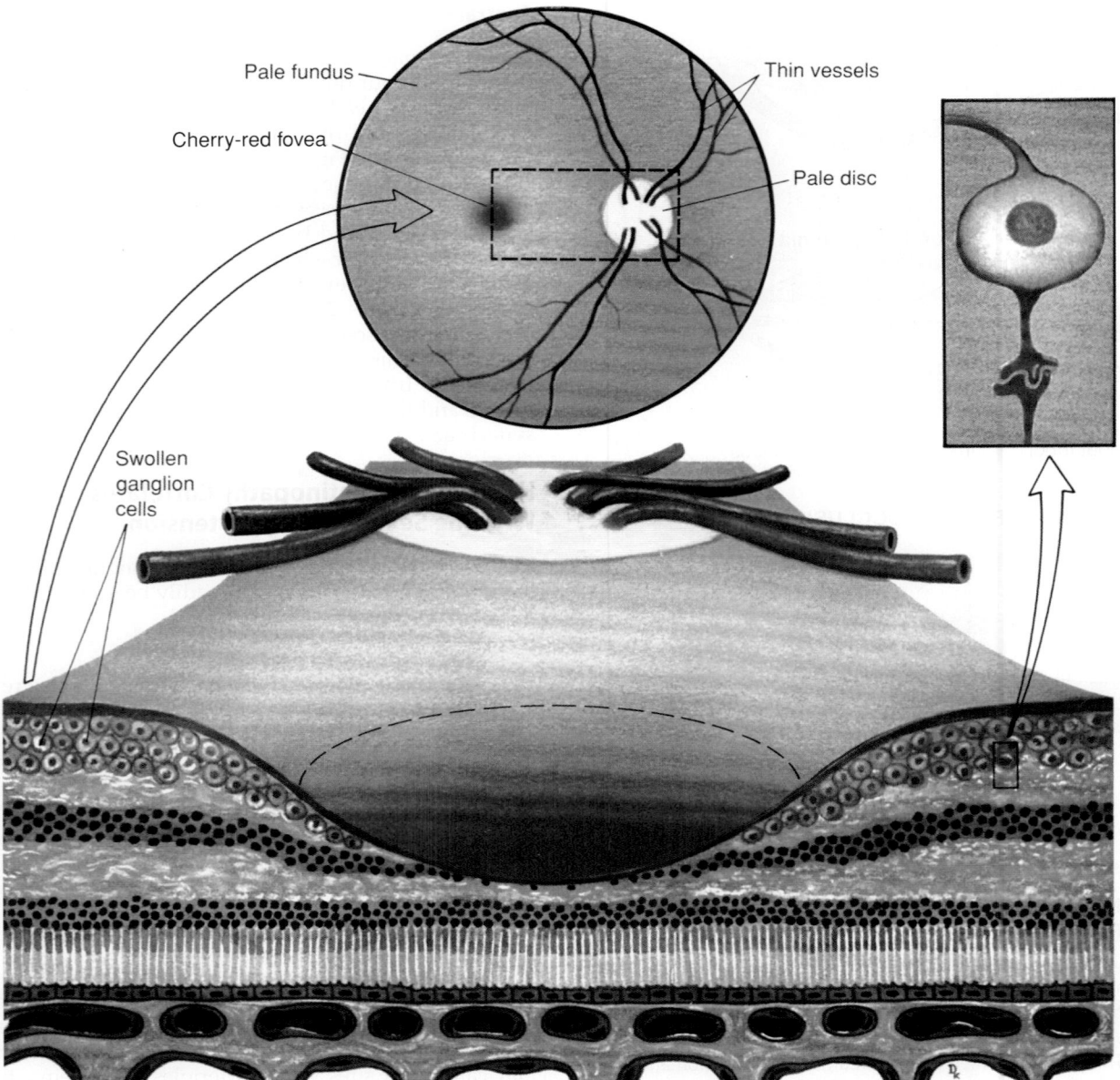

FIGURE 33-5. **Central retinal artery occlusion.** When the central retinal artery becomes occluded (e.g., with an embolus), the entire retina becomes edematous and pale. Decreased blood flow makes the retinal vessels less visible on funduscopic examination. The fovea in the center of the macula appears cherry red, owing to the normal underlying vasculature of the choroid.

Diabetic Retinopathy Is Primarily a Vascular Disease

The eye is frequently involved in diabetes mellitus. Ocular symptoms occur in 20% to 40% of diabetics and may even be evident at the time diabetes is diagnosed (in type 2 disease). Virtually all patients with type 1 (insulin-dependent) diabetes and many of those with type 2 (non–insulin-dependent) diabetes develop some background retinopathy (see below) within 5 to 15 years of the onset of diabetes (Figs. 33-9 to 33-11). The more vision-threatening **proliferative retinopathy** does not typically appear until at least 10 years after the onset of diabetes, but then its incidence increases rapidly and remains high for many years. *In type 1 diabetes, the frequency of proliferative retinopathy correlates with the degree of glycemic control; patients whose diabetes is better controlled develop retinopathy less frequently.* The relationship between retinal microvascular disease and blood glucose levels in type 2 diabetes is less clear, and other parameters (e.g., blood cholesterol levels, blood pressure) also play a role in the development of retinopathy.

Retinal ischemia can account for most features of diabetic retinopathy, including the cotton-wool spots, capillary closure, microaneurysms, and retinal neovascularization. Ischemia results from narrowing or occlusion of retinal arterioles (as from arteriolosclerosis or platelet and lipid thrombi) or from arteriovascular disease of the central retinal or ophthalmic arteries.

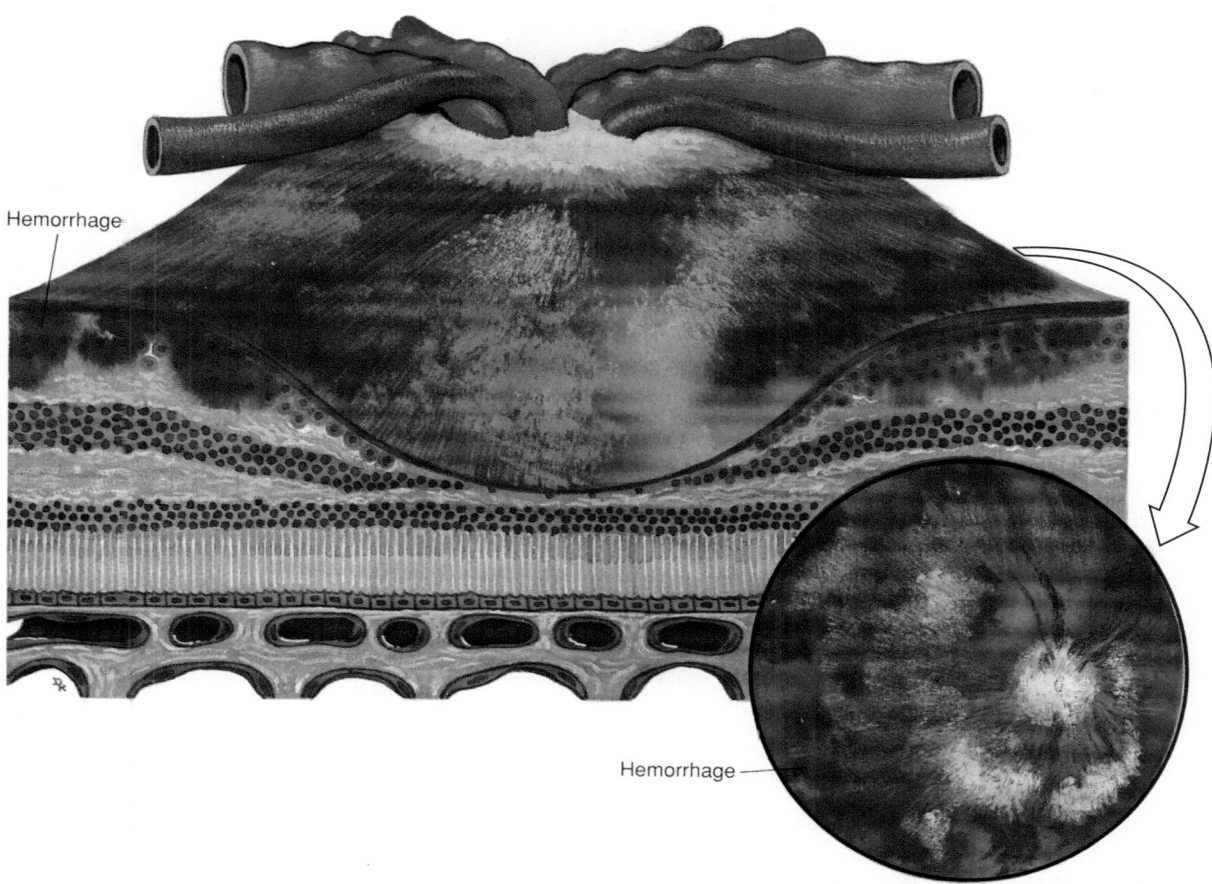

FIGURE 33-6. Central retinal vein occlusion. By contrast to central retinal artery occlusion, central retinal vein occlusion produces considerable venous engorgement and retinal hemorrhage due to increased intravascular pressure (venous stasis retinopathy).

 PATHOLOGY: The retinopathy of diabetes is characterized by background and proliferative stages.

BACKGROUND (NONPROLIFERATIVE) DIABETIC RETINOPATHY: This stage exhibits venous engorgement, small hemorrhages (dot and blot hemorrhages), cotton-wool spots, capillary microaneurysms, and exudates. These lesions usually do not impair vision unless associated with macular edema. The retinopathy typically begins at the posterior pole but eventually may involve the entire retina.

On funduscopy, the first discernible abnormality in background diabetic retinopathy is the microaneurysm. This is followed by small hemorrhages, mostly in the inner nuclear and outer plexiform layers. Engorged retinal veins, with localized sausage-shaped distentions, coils, and loops may be seen as the retinopathy advances. Yellow lipoproteinaceous exudates accumulate, chiefly in the vicinity of the microaneurysms. The retinopathy of elderly diabetic persons frequently displays numerous exudates (**exudative diabetic retinopathy**), which are not seen with type 1 diabetes.

PROLIFERATIVE RETINOPATHY: After many years, diabetic retinopathy becomes proliferative. Fragile new blood vessels grow along with fibrous and glial tissue toward the vitreous body. Retinal neovascularization is a prominent feature of diabetic retinopathy and of other conditions caused by retinal ischemia. Tortuous new vessels first appear on the surface of the retina and optic nerve head and then grow into the vitreous cavity. The newly formed friable vessels bleed easily, and resultant vitreous hemorrhages obscure vision. Neovascularization is associated with proliferation and migration of astrocytes, which grow around the new vessels to form delicate white veils (gliosis). The proliferating fibrovascular and glial tissue

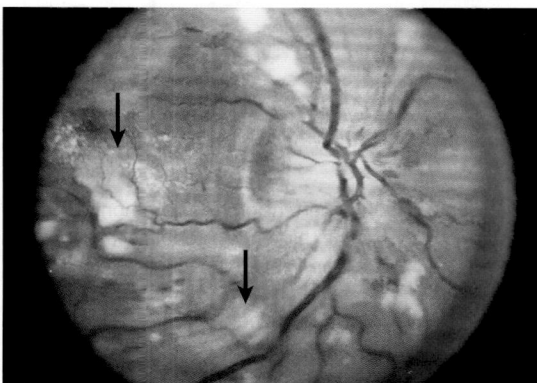

FIGURE 33-7. Hypertensive retinopathy. The ocular fundus in a patient with extensive retinopathy shows edema of the optic nerve head; the retina contains numerous "cotton-wool spots" (*arrows*) and scattered flame-shaped intraocular hemorrhages.

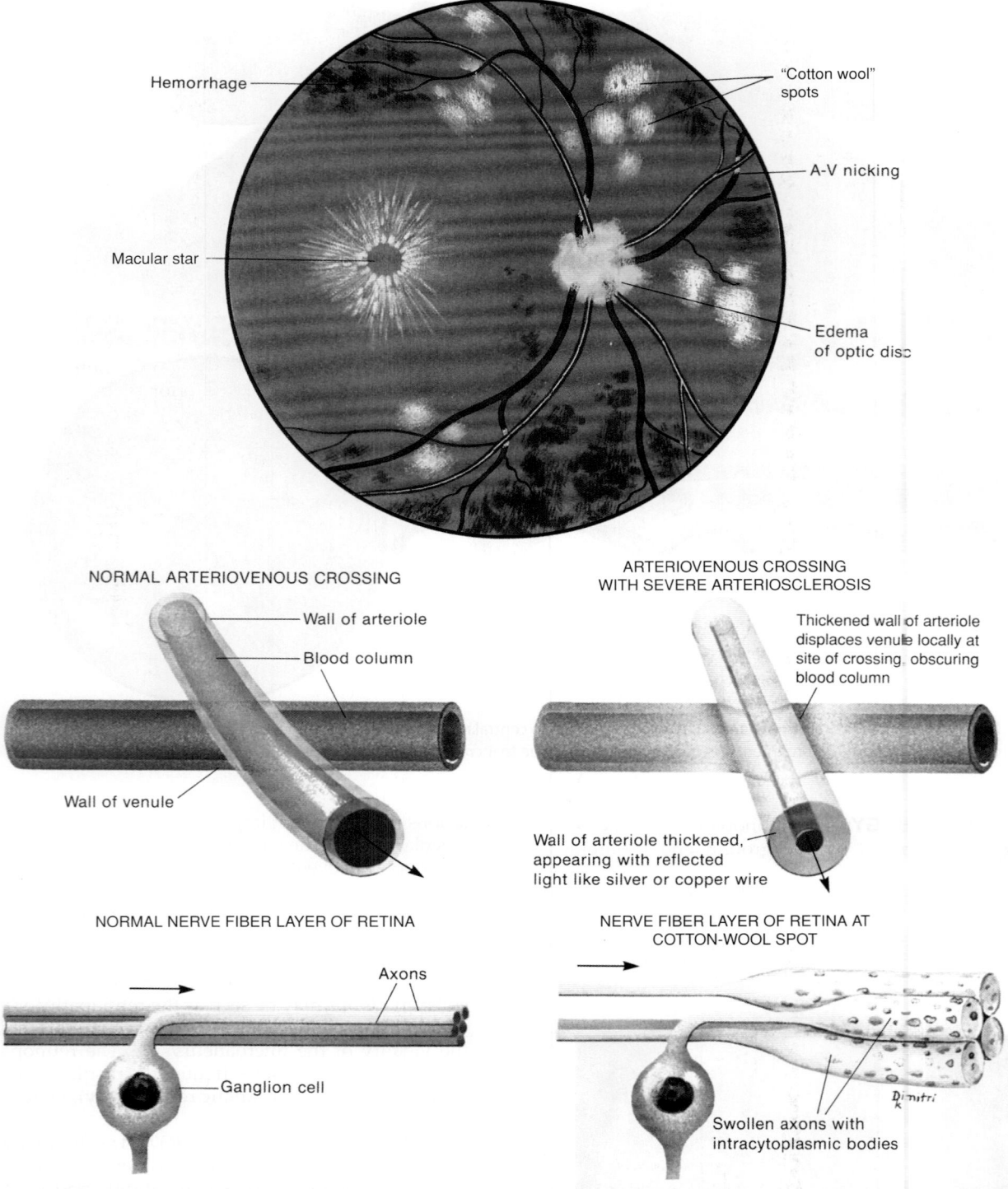

FIGURE 33-8. Hypertensive retinopathy. Various abnormalities develop within the retina in hypertension. The commonly associated arteriolosclerosis affects the appearance of the retinal microvasculature. Light reflected from the thickened arteriolar walls mimics silver or copper wire. Blood flow through the retinal venules appears pinched at the sites of arteriolar–venular crossings (A-V nicking). This effect is due to dilation of the venule rather than to an impediment to blood flow caused by compression; the column of blood proximal to the compression is not wider than the part distal to the crossing. Impaired axoplasmic flow within the nerve fiber layer, caused by focal ischemia, results in swollen axons with cytoplasmic bodies. Such structures resemble cotton on funduscopy ("cotton-wool spots"). Hemorrhages are common in the retina, and lipoproteinaceous exudates frequently form a star around the fovea.

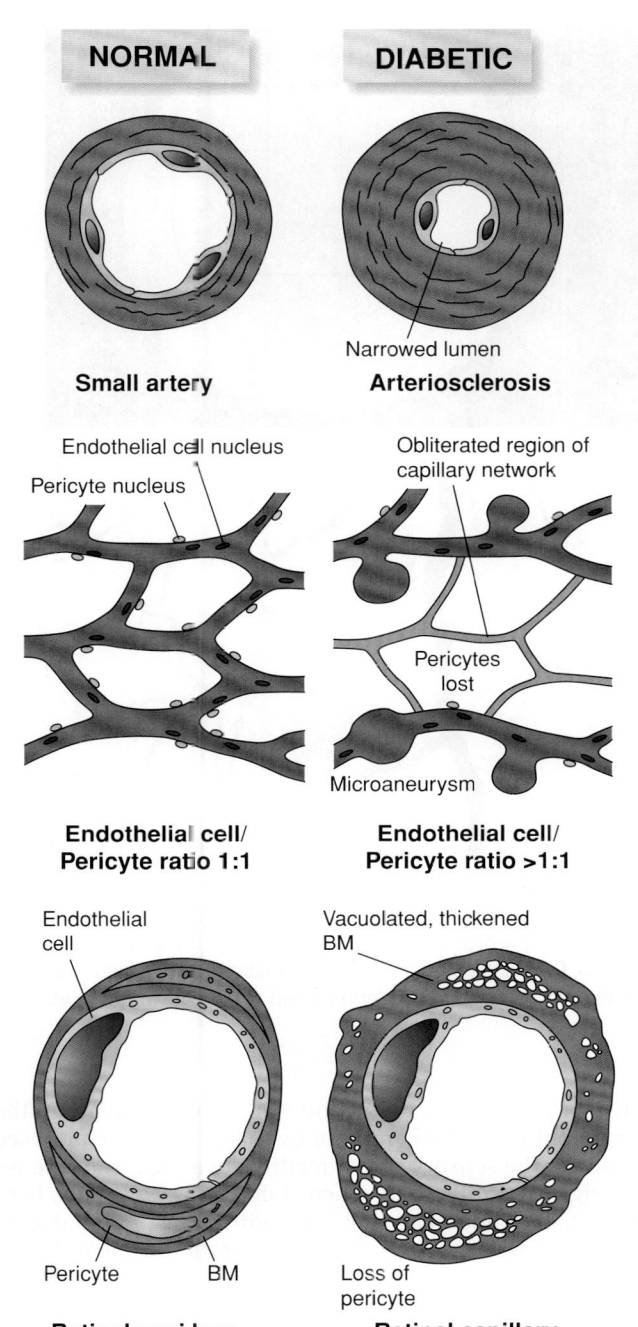

NORMAL

Small artery

Endothelial cell nucleus

Pericyte nucleus

Endothelial cell/
Pericyte ratio 1:1

Endothelial
cell

Pericyte   BM

Retinal capillary

DIABETIC

Narrowed lumen

Arteriosclerosis

Obliterated region of
capillary network

Pericytes
lost

Microaneurysm

Endothelial cell/
Pericyte ratio >1:1

Vacuolated, thickened
BM

Loss of
pericyte

Retinal capillary

FIGURE 33-9. Diabetic retinopathy. In diabetic retinopathy, the micro-vasculature is abnormal. Arteriosclerosis and thickening of the endothelial basement membrane narrow the lumens of small arteries. Pericytes are lost, and the endothelial cell to pericyte ratio is greater than 1. Capillary microaneurysms are prominent, and portions of the capillary network become acellular and lose blood flow. The basement membrane (BM) of the retinal capillaries is thickened and vacuolated.

contracts, often causing a tractional retinal detachment and blindness. Frequently, features of hypertensive and arteriolosclerotic retinopathy are associated with diabetic retinopathy.

Diabetic retinopathy, glaucoma, and age-related mac-ulopathy are the leading causes of irreversible blindness

in the United States. Blindness in diabetic retinopathy results when the macula is involved, but it also follows vitreous hemorrhage, retinal detachment, and glaucoma. Once blindness ensues, it heralds an ominous future for the patient, because death from ischemic heart disease or renal failure often follows. In fact, the mean life expectancy in such cases is less than 6 years, and only one-fifth of blind diabetics survive 10 years. Retinal laser photoco-agulation, injection of antivascular endothelial growth fac-tor agents, and strict glycemic control early in the course of proliferative retinopathy have proven effective in con-trolling the complications of this stage of retinopathy.

Diabetic Iridopathy

In diabetics with severe retinopathy, a fibrovascular layer frequently grows along the anterior surface of the iris and in the anterior chamber angle. Such iris neovascularization (**rubeosis iridis**) occurs in several conditions associated with retinal ischemia, primarily due to production of vascular endothelial growth factor (VEGF) by the ischemic retina.

PATHOLOGY: A fibrovascular membrane leads to adhesions between the iris and the peripheral cor-nea (**peripheral anterior synechiae**) and between the iris and lens (**posterior synechiae**), while traction by the fibrovascular membrane pulls the iris pigment epithe-lium anteriorly around the pupillary margin (**ectropion uveae**). The friable new vessels on the iris bleed easily and cause **hyphema** (hemorrhage within the anterior chamber of the eye). Neovascularization of the iris is clinically important because it frequently culminates in a blind, pain-ful eye, owing to secondary angle-closure glaucoma (**neo-vascular glaucoma**).

Acute hyperglycemia leads to glycogen storage in the pigmented epithelium of the iris, a phenomenon analogous to that produced in the renal tubules by glycosuria. When tissue sections of diabetic eyes are processed in the usual manner, the pigment epithelium of the iris sometimes con-tains numerous vacuoles, which imparts a lacy appearance. The vacuoles result from loss of glycogen during prepa-ration of tissue sections. Glycogen storage within the iris pigment epithelium is thought to account for the scatter-ing of iris pigment observed clinically in diabetic patients. Chronic hyperglycemia over the years results in thickening of the pigment epithelial basement membrane in the ciliary body, the structure that produces aqueous humor.

Diabetic Cataracts

Patients with type 1 diabetes often develop bilateral "snow-flake" cataracts, a blanket of white needle-shaped opacities in the lens immediately beneath the anterior and posterior lens capsule. The opacities coalesce within a few weeks in adolescents, and within days in children, until the whole lens becomes opaque. Snowflake cataracts can be produced exper-imentally in young animals and result from an osmotic effect caused by accumulation of sorbitol, the alcohol derived from glucose (see Chapter 13). The increased sorbitol content of the lens causes imbibition of water and enlargement of the lens.

Age-related cataracts occur in diabetics at an earlier age than in the general population and progress more rapidly

THE EYE

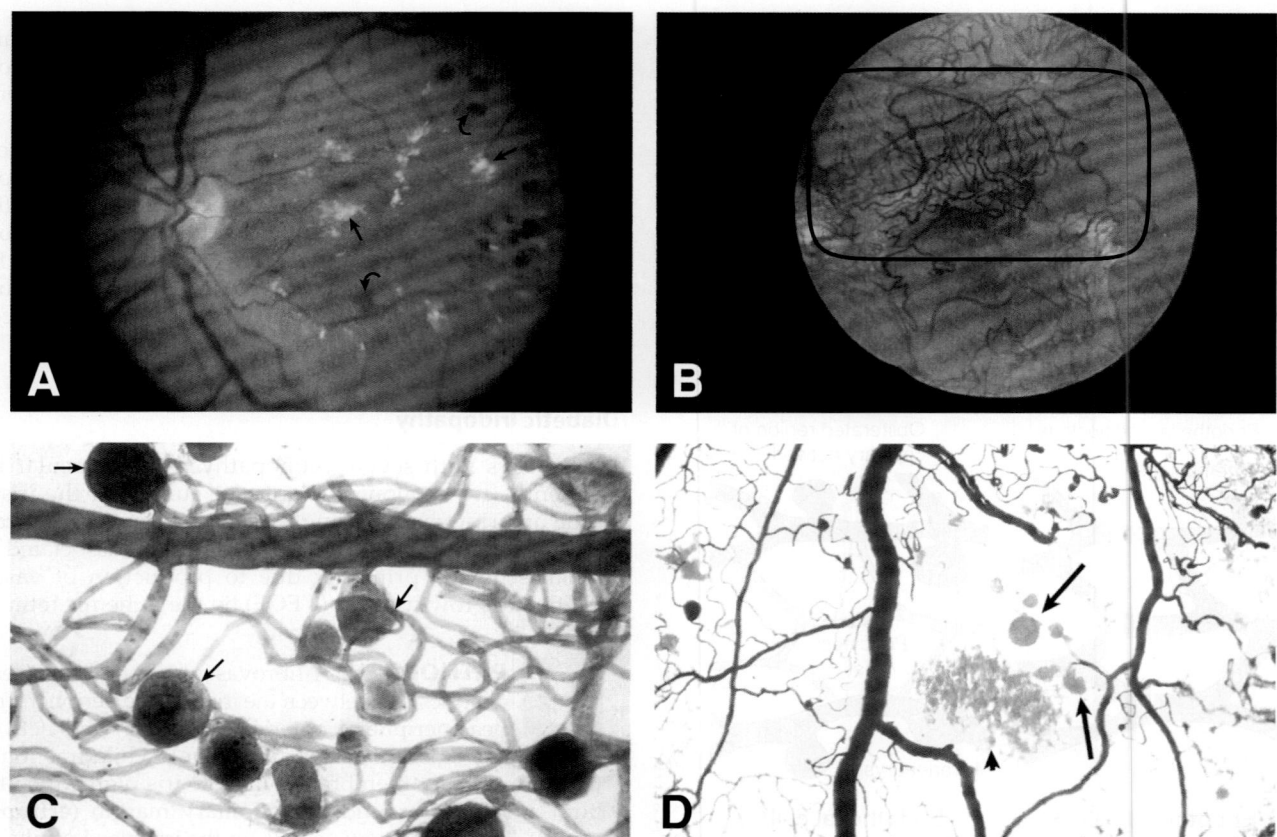

FIGURE 33-10. Diabetic retinopathy. A. The ocular fundus in a patient with background diabetic retinopathy shows several yellowish "hard" exudates (*straight arrows*), which are rich in lipids, together with several dot intraretinal hemorrhages (*curved arrows*). **B.** A neovascular frond (**circled area**) extends anteriorly from the retina into the vitreous in this example of proliferative diabetic retinopathy. **C.** Numerous microaneurysms (*arrows*) are present in this flat preparation of a diabetic retina. **D.** This flat preparation from a diabetic was stained with periodic acid–Schiff (PAS) after the retinal vessels had been perfused with India ink. Microaneurysms (*arrows*) and an exudate (*arrowhead*) are evident in a region of retinal capillary dropout.

to maturity. A sudden temporary myopia, caused by an increase in the refractive power in the lens due to thickening of the lens as described above, may be the presenting manifestation of diabetes.

Other Ophthalmic Manifestations of Diabetes

People with diabetes are at increased risk for inflammation of the anterior segment of the eye, phycomycosis (mucormycosis) of the orbit and primary open-angle glaucoma (POAG). They are also prone to the **Argyll Robertson pupil** (small pupils that react to accommodation but not to light). Cranial nerve palsies occur, especially of the oculomotor nerve (CN III). Some patients with long-standing diabetes develop recurrent corneal erosions, which are thought to be due to impaired innervation of the cornea.

The effects of diabetes mellitus on the eye are summarized in Figure 33-11.

Retinal Detachment Separates the Sensory Retina From the Pigment Epithelium

During embryogenesis, the sensory retina develops from the inner layer of the optic cup and the pigment epithelium develops from the outer layer of the optic cup. The space between the sensory retina and the retinal pigment epithelium is obliterated when these two layers become apposed. However, the sensory retina readily separates from the retinal pigment epithelium when fluid (liquid vitreous, hemorrhage, or exudate) accumulates within the potential space between these structures. Such a separation (retinal detachment) is a common cause of visual impairment and blindness. Laser therapy and surgical approaches have greatly improved the prognosis for patients with detached retina.

 ETIOLOGIC FACTORS: Retinal detachment may follow intraocular hemorrhage (e.g., after trauma) and is a potential complication of cataract extraction and several other ocular surgeries. Factors predisposing to retinal detachment include retinal defects (due to trauma or certain retinal degenerations), vitreous traction on the retinal surface, diminished pressure on the retina (e.g., after vitreous loss), and fluid leakage from the retinal or choroidal vasculature. Full-thickness holes in the retina are not complicated by retinal detachment unless liquid vitreous gains access to the potential space between the retina and the retinal pigment epithelium. Even then, some degree of vitreoretinal traction seems to be necessary for retinal detachment to occur.

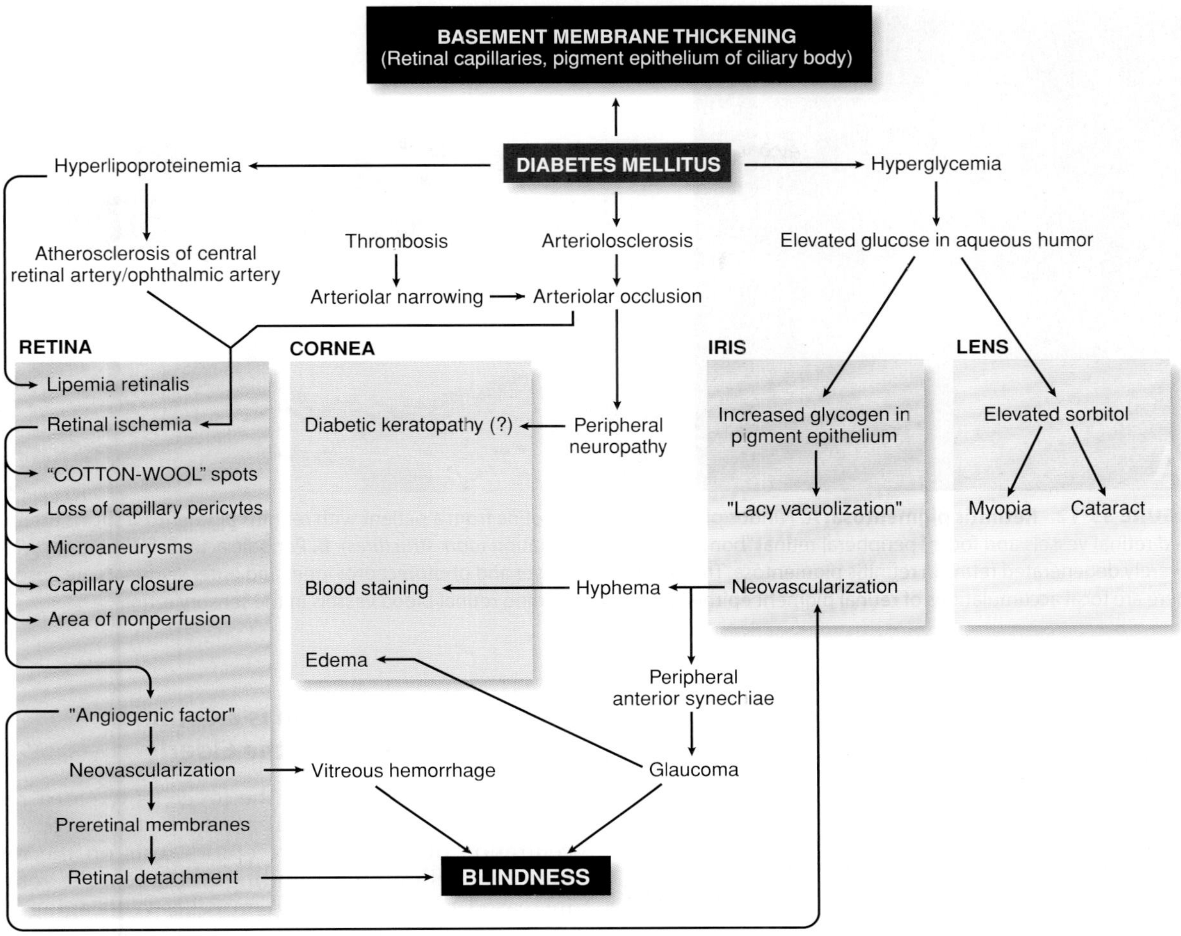

BASEMENT MEMBRANE THICKENING
(Retinal capillaries, pigment epithelium of ciliary body)

Hyperlipoproteinemia ◄——— **DIABETES MELLITUS** ———► Hyperglycemia

Atherosclerosis of central retinal artery/ophthalmic artery

Thrombosis   Arteriolosclerosis   Elevated glucose in aqueous humor

Arteriolar narrowing ——► Arteriolar occlusion

RETINA
- Lipemia retinalis
- Retinal ischemia ◄——
- "COTTON-WOOL" spots
- Loss of capillary pericytes
- Microaneurysms
- Capillary closure
- Area of nonperfusion

"Angiogenic factor"

Neovascularization ——► Vitreous hemorrhage

Preretinal membranes

Retinal detachment ———►

CORNEA

Diabetic keratopathy (?) ◄—— Peripheral neuropathy

Blood staining ◄—— Hyphema ◄—— Neovascularization

Edema ◄——

IRIS

Increased glycogen in pigment epithelium

"Lacy vacuolization"

LENS

Elevated sorbitol

Myopia   Cataract

Peripheral anterior synechiae

Glaucoma

BLINDNESS

FIGURE 33-11. Effects of diabetes on the eye.

The photoreceptors and retinal pigment epithelium normally function as a unit. Once they separate in a retinal detachment, oxygen and nutrients that normally reach the photoreceptors, cells with a high oxygen demand and metabolic rate, from the choroid must diffuse across a greater distance. This situation causes the photoreceptors to degenerate.

 PATHOLOGY: Three types of retinal detachment are recognized: rhegmatogenous, tractional, and exudative.

RHEGMATOGENOUS RETINAL DETACHMENT: This type of retinal detachment is associated with a retinal tear and also, often, with degenerative changes in the vitreous body or peripheral retina.

TRACTIONAL RETINAL DETACHMENT: In some cases of retinal detachment, the retina is pulled toward the center of the eye by adherent vitreoretinal foci or proliferations, which can occur in proliferative diabetic retinopathy, retinopathy of prematurity, and after intraocular infection.

EXUDATIVE RETINAL DETACHMENT: Accumulation of fluid in the potential space between the sensory retina and the retinal pigment epithelium causes a detached retina in disorders such as choroiditis, choroidal hemangioma, and choroidal melanoma.

Retinitis Pigmentosa Is a Heritable Bilateral Retinal Degeneration

Retinitis pigmentosa (pigmentary retinopathy) is a generic term that refers to a variety of bilateral, progressive, degenerative retinopathies characterized clinically by night blindness and constriction of peripheral visual fields, and pathologically by loss of retinal photoreceptors (rods and cones) and pigment accumulation within the retina.

The term "retinitis" is a misnomer since inflammation of the retina is not a feature of this disease.

 MOLECULAR PATHOGENESIS: A large number of retinal diseases, including retinitis pigmentosa, are caused by mutations in different genes (currently over 200; see https://www.omim.org/entry/268000). Some are isolated ocular disorders, with autosomal dominant, autosomal recessive, or X-linked recessive inheritance. Some pigmentary retinopathies are associated with neurologic and systemic disorders.

Mutations in at least 48 different genes and loci are associated with nonsyndromic retinitis pigmentosa. Some of the responsible mutated genes encode members of the rod phototransduction cascade, such as rhodopsin (*RHO*) and rod photoreceptor cyclic guanosine 3′,5′-monophosphate

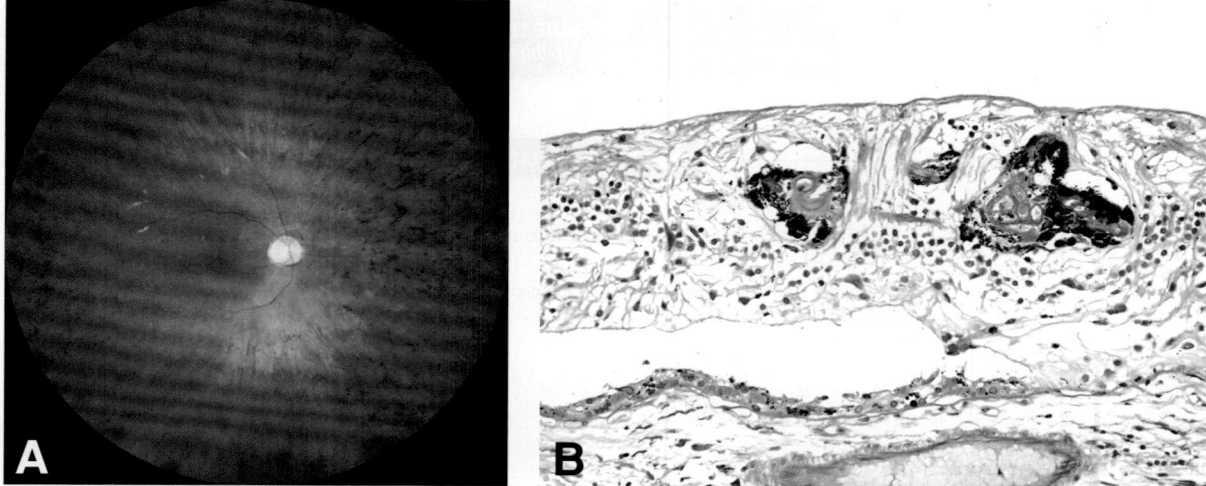

FIGURE 33-12. Retinitis pigmentosa. A. Fundus photograph of the retina from a patient with retinitis pigmentosa shows attenuated retinal vessels and foci of peripheral retinal "bone spicule" pigmentation (*dark structures*). **B.** Periodic acid–Schiff stain showing severely degenerated retina in retinitis pigmentosa. The outer nuclear layer and photoreceptor inner and outer segments are absent. There are focal accumulations of retinal pigment epithelial cells surrounding retinal blood vessels in the sensory retina.

(cGMP), phosphodiesterase α and β subunits (*PDE6A, PDE6B*), and photoreceptor structures such as peripherin (*PRPH*). How defective proteins in the rod photoreceptors lead to retinitis pigmentosa and the eventual loss of cones is not completely understood but, presumably, these disease alleles ultimately cause the death of photoreceptors due to a convergence at a final common point in key metabolic pathways.

PATHOLOGY: In retinitis pigmentosa, degeneration of rod photoreceptors, and subsequently cone photoreceptors, is followed by migration of retinal pigment epithelial cells into the sensory retina around retinal blood vessels in the more peripheral retina (Fig. 33-12). The appearance of the pigmented cells in the retina creates a "bone spicule" appearance. The retinal blood vessels then gradually attenuate, and the optic nerve head acquires a characteristic waxy pallor.

CLINICAL FEATURES: Clinical manifestations of retinitis pigmentosa, including the appearance and distribution of the retinal pigmentation, vary with the causes of the retinopathy. Half of these patients have a family history of the disease. Those with autosomal recessive and X-linked disease are more severely affected and develop night blindness and peripheral field defects in childhood. Autosomal dominant forms tend to be less severe, with symptoms beginning later in life. As the condition progresses, contraction of visual fields eventually leads to tunnel vision. Central vision is usually preserved until late in the course of the disease. In some cases, blindness follows macular involvement.

Macular Degeneration Is a Common Cause of Blindness in the Elderly

The center of the macula, the fovea, is the area responsible for the most precise visual acuity. In this area, a high concentration of cone photoreceptors rests on the retinal pigment epithelium. Surrounding the fovea, the retina has an increased density of ganglion cells. With aging, in certain drug toxicities (e.g., hydroxychloroquine) and in several inherited disorders, the macula degenerates, causing central vision to be impaired.

Age-related macular degeneration (ARMD) currently affects about 11 million people in the United States and is the most common cause of severe visual impairment among individuals of European descent older than age 50. Nonexudative (dry) and exudative (wet) forms of ARMD are recognized. The exudative variety accounts for 10% to 15% of cases and is associated with subretinal neovascularization and fibrosis and sometimes hemorrhage into the subretinal space. Repeated intraocular injections of anti-VEGF agents have become the standard of care for exudative ARMD.

ETIOLOGIC FACTORS: There is general agreement that age-related maculopathy is a multifactorial disease to which environmental and genetic factors contribute. Risk factors include advancing age, tobacco use, carotid/cardiovascular disease, and elevated serum cholesterol levels. With age, waste products accumulate in the retinal pigment epithelium and along Bruch membrane and eventually become clinically evident as **drusen** (yellow fatty deposits) in the macula. Through a complex cascade of events, local subfoveal hypoxia leads to production of VEGF, subretinal neovascularization, and fibrosis resulting in damage to the pigment epithelium and retinal photoreceptors.

MOLECULAR PATHOGENESIS: A common missense variant of the *CFH* gene that encodes complement factor H is a common risk factor for age-related macular degeneration (ARMD). Increased susceptibility to ARMD has also been associated with mutations or single-nucleotide polymorphisms in *ABCA4* (formerly called *ABCR*), *FBLN5, FBLN6, C3, CST3, LOC387715, TLR4, ERCC6, RAX2, HTRA1, CX3CR1,* and *ESR1* genes and in a mitochondrial gene (*MTTL1*). *ABCA4* encodes a rod cell protein (rim protein) thought to be a transporter involved in molecular recycling. Mutations in this gene may allow degraded material (drusen) to accumulate.

Lysosomal Storage Diseases Feature a Cherry-Red Spot at the Macula

In lysosomal storage diseases, including the gangliosidoses, myriad intracytoplasmic lysosomal inclusions within the multilayered ganglion cell layer of the macula impart a striking pallor to the affected retina due to loss of transparency of ganglion cell axons. As a result, the central fovea appears bright red because of the underlying choroidal vasculature, similar to the cherry-red spot seen in central retinal artery occlusion.

Angioid Streaks Are Vessel-Like Breaks in Bruch Membrane

Angioid streaks are seen when the fundus of the eye is examined clinically. This occurs when Bruch membrane cracks, causing characteristic irregular lines that radiate beneath the retina from the optic disc. These cracks resemble blood vessels (**angioid streaks**). This happens spontaneously in a variety of systemic disorders, most commonly pseudoxanthoma elasticum, sickle cell disease, and Paget disease of bone.

Retinopathy of Prematurity Results From Oxygen Toxicity

Retinopathy of prematurity is a bilateral, iatrogenic, retinal disorder that occurs predominantly in premature infants treated with high levels of inspired oxygen after birth. The entity was originally called **retrolental fibroplasia** because a mass of scarred tissue occurs behind the lens in advanced cases (Fig. 33-13). More than a half century ago, retinopathy of prematurity was the leading cause of blindness in infants in the United States and many other developed countries. Retinopathy of prematurity is almost always restricted to premature infants, with a birth weight of ≤1,500 g and a gestational age of ≤30 weeks, who are administered high concentrations of oxygen. In such infants, retinal vascular development is delayed, and the peripheral retina does not vascularize, leading to retinal hypoxia. Once the infant eventually returns to lower concentrations of oxygen, intense proliferation of vascular endothelium and glial cells begins at the junction of the avascular and vascularized portions of the retina. This becomes apparent by 4 to 10 weeks of postnatal age and, as in diabetic retinopathy, is thought to result from the liberation of an angiogenic factor produced by the avascular and ischemic peripheral retina. This angiogenic factor is also believed to account for the neovascularization of the iris that sometimes accompanies retinopathy of prematurity. In about 4% of US cases, the retinopathy

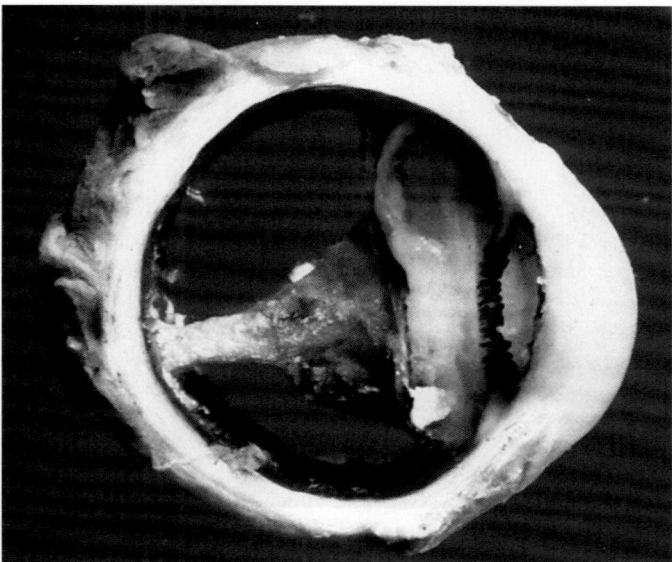

FIGURE 33-13. Retinopathy of prematurity. Anterior to posterior section through an eye with advanced retinopathy of prematurity (retrolental fibroplasia) shows a totally detached retina adherent to a fibrovascular mass behind the lens. The cornea is on the right side of the eye and the optic nerve is on the left side.

progresses to a scarring phase, characterized by traction retinal detachment and blindness. Laser photocoagulation of the avascular areas of the retina has been shown to slow or arrest progression of the condition.

THE OPTIC NERVE

Optic Nerve Head Edema Often Reflects Increased Intracranial Pressure

Optic nerve head (optic disc) edema refers to swelling of the optic nerve head (also known as papilledema). The optic disc is the location where retinal ganglion cell axons converge to form the optic nerve and exit the eye. There are many causes of optic nerve head edema, the most important of which is increased intracranial pressure. Other important causes are obstruction to venous drainage of the eye (such as may occur with compressive lesions of the orbit), infarction of the optic nerve (ischemic optic neuropathy), inflammation of the optic nerve close to the eyeball (optic neuritis), and multiple sclerosis.

Edema of the optic nerve head is characterized clinically by a swollen, congested optic nerve head that displays blurred margins and dilated vessels. Frequently, hemorrhages, exudates, and cotton-wool spots are seen (Fig. 33-14), and concentric folds of the choroid and retina may surround the nerve head. Acutely, optic nerve head edema results in few, if any, visual symptoms. As the condition becomes established, swelling of the optic nerve head enlarges the normal blind spot. After many months, atrophic changes lead to loss of visual acuity.

Optic Atrophy Is a Thinning of the Optic Nerve Caused by Loss of Axons Within Its Substance

The nerve axons within the optic nerve are lost in many conditions, including long-standing edema of the optic nerve

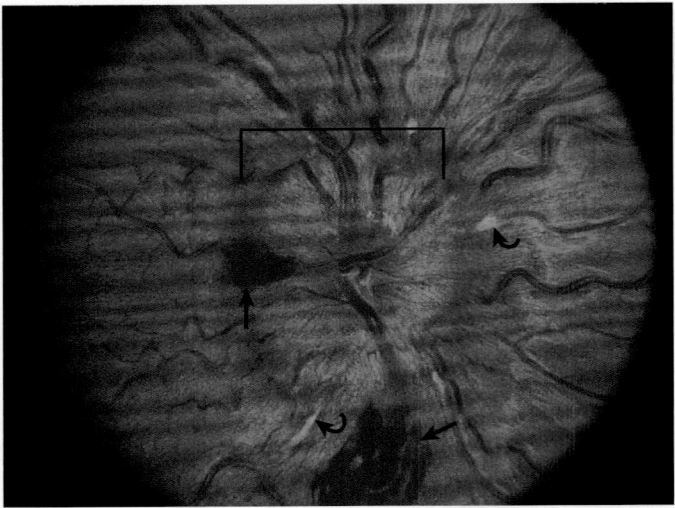

FIGURE 33-14. Papilledema. The optic nerve head (*bracket*) is markedly congested and protrudes anteriorly toward the interior of the eye. It has blurred margins, and retinal blood vessels are obscured as they cross the edge of the optic nerve head. Blood vessels are dilated and somewhat tortuous. Retinal hemorrhages are present over the optic nerve head and just peripheral to the nerve head (*straight arrows*). Several small cotton-wool spots are present within the adjacent retina (*curved arrows*).

head, optic neuritis, optic nerve compression, glaucoma, and retinal degeneration.

ETIOLOGIC FACTORS: Optic atrophy can also be caused by some drugs, such as ethambutol and isoniazid. The optic nerve head is usually flat and pale in optic atrophy, but when this disorder follows glaucoma, the optic nerve head is excavated (**glaucomatous cupping**) (Fig. 33-15).

MOLECULAR PATHOGENESIS: Optic atrophy can follow mutations in *OPA1* and *OPA3*, both of which encode mitochondrial proteins, and *WFS1*, which makes a protein involved in Ca^{2+} homeostasis.

Multiple point mutations in the mitochondrial genome are associated with **Leber hereditary optic neuropathy,** and three of them account for more than 90% of cases (*MTND1-3460, MTND4-11778,* and *MTND6-14484*).

GLAUCOMA

Glaucoma refers to a collection of disorders that feature an optic neuropathy accompanied by a characteristic progressive loss of peripheral visual field and excavation of the optic nerve head. In most cases, glaucoma is related to sustained increased intraocular pressure (**ocular hypertension**); however, increased intraocular pressure does not necessarily cause glaucoma, and not all patients with glaucoma have elevated intraocular pressure.

After being produced by the ciliary body, the aqueous humor enters the posterior chamber (the space between the iris and the zonules) before passing through the pupil to the anterior chamber (between the iris and the cornea). From that site, it drains into episcleral veins by way of the trabecular meshwork and the canal of Schlemm (Fig. 33-16). A delicate balance between production and drainage of the aqueous humor maintains physiologic intraocular pressure (10 to 21 mm Hg). In certain pathologic states, drainage of aqueous humor from the eye becomes impaired, and intraocular pressure increases. Temporary or permanent impairment of vision results from pressure-induced degenerative changes in the retina and optic nerve head (Fig. 33-15) and, when the intraocular pressure is very elevated, from edema and opacification of the cornea. Retinal ganglion cells are especially sensitive to elevated intraocular pressure and undergo selective degeneration starting in the peripheral retina and progressing centrally.

Basic Mechanisms in Glaucoma

Glaucoma, one of the most common causes of preventable blindness in the United States, almost always follows a congenital or acquired alteration in the anterior segment of the eye that mechanically obstructs aqueous drainage. The obstruction may be located between the iris and lens, or in

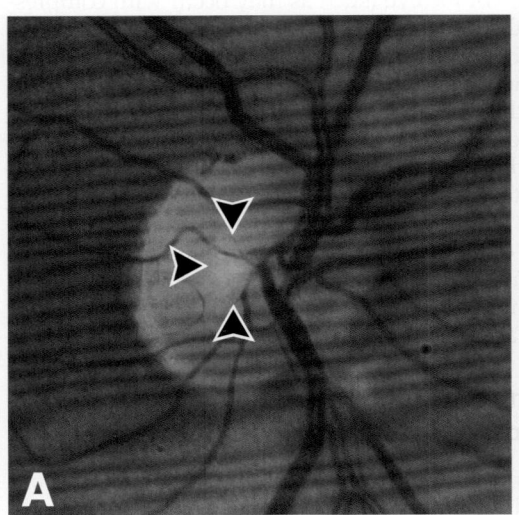

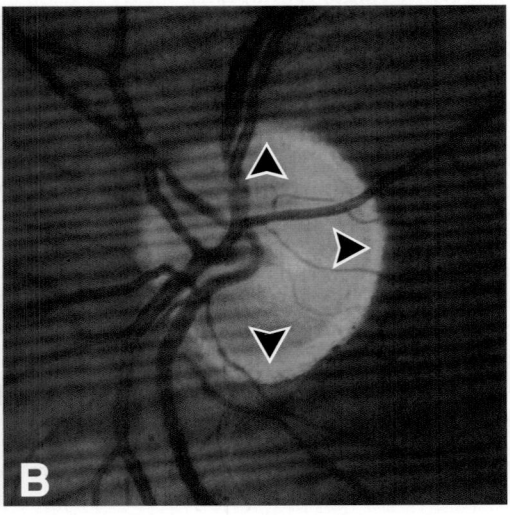

FIGURE 33-15. Glaucomatous optic atrophy. A. Normal optic nerve. The central depression in the optic nerve head (optic cup) is approximately one-third of the total optic nerve head diameter (*arrowheads*). **B.** Nerve with severe optic atrophy from glaucoma. The cup is enlarged (optic nerve cupping) (*arrowheads*) and the nerve appears pale.

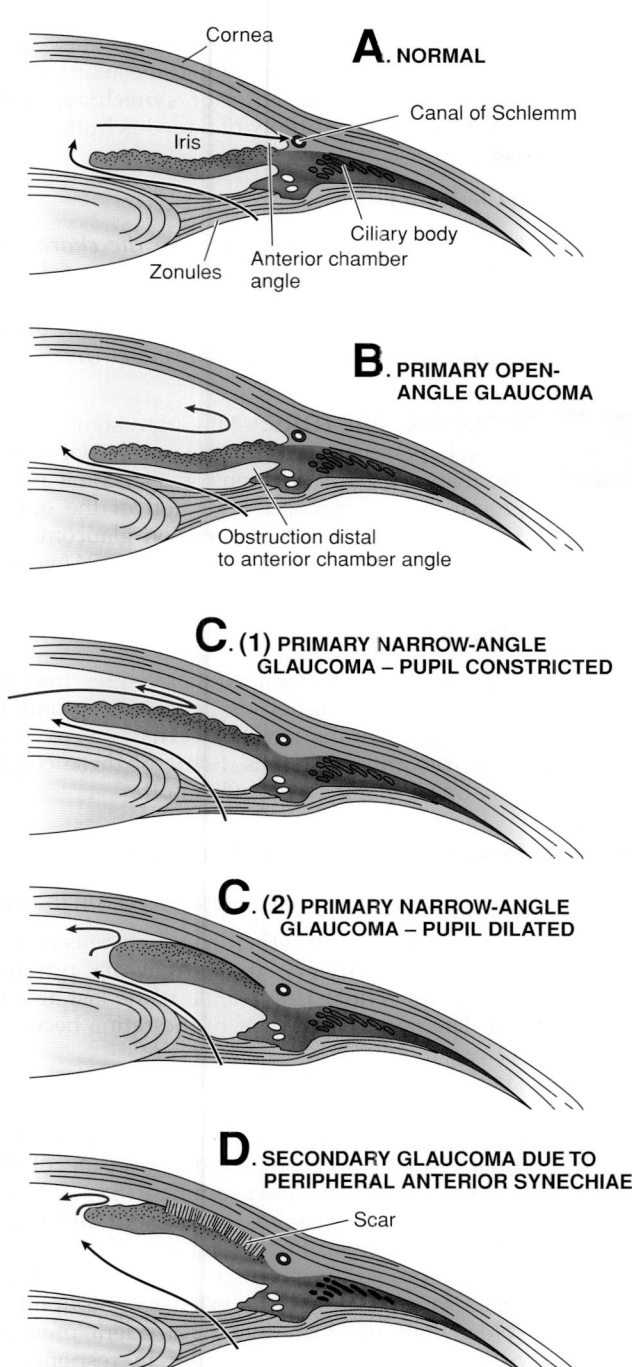

A. **NORMAL**

Cornea

Canal of Schlemm

Iris

Ciliary body

Zonules

Anterior chamber angle

B. **PRIMARY OPEN-ANGLE GLAUCOMA**

Obstruction distal to anterior chamber angle

C. (1) **PRIMARY NARROW-ANGLE GLAUCOMA – PUPIL CONSTRICTED**

C. (2) **PRIMARY NARROW-ANGLE GLAUCOMA – PUPIL DILATED**

D. **SECONDARY GLAUCOMA DUE TO PERIPHERAL ANTERIOR SYNECHIAE**

Scar

FIGURE 33-16. Pathogenesis of glaucoma. The anterior segment of the eye is affected differently in various forms of glaucoma. **A.** Anterior segment structure of the normal eye. **B.** In primary open-angle glaucoma, the obstruction to the aqueous outflow is distal to the anterior chamber angle, and the anterior segment resembles that of the normal eye. **C.** In primary narrow-angle glaucoma, the anterior chamber angle is open, but narrower than normal when the pupil is constricted (**C1**). When the pupil becomes dilated in such an eye, the thickened iris obstructs the anterior chamber angle (**C2**), causing increased intraocular pressure. **D.** The anterior chamber angle can become obstructed by a variety of pathologic processes, including an adhesion between the iris and the posterior surface of the cornea (**peripheral anterior synechiae**).

the angle of the anterior chamber, the trabecular meshwork, the canal of Schlemm, or the venous drainage of the eye.

There Are Several Types of Glaucoma

Congenital Glaucoma (Infantile Glaucoma, Buphthalmos)

Congenital glaucoma is caused by obstruction to aqueous drainage due to developmental anomalies in angle structures. This type of glaucoma develops even though intraocular pressure may not increase until early infancy or childhood. Congenital glaucoma is most often sporadic but 10% to 40% of cases have a genetic basis, most commonly with autosomal recessive inheritance. The developmental anomaly usually involves both eyes and, although often limited to the angle of the anterior chamber, it may be accompanied by other ocular malformations. Congenital glaucoma is associated with a deep anterior chamber, corneal cloudiness, sensitivity to bright lights (**photophobia**), excessive tearing, and buphthalmos. The term **buphthalmos** (from the Greek word *bous*, "ox"; *ophthalmos*, "eye") describes the enlarged eyes of patients with congenital glaucoma that result from expansion of the eye caused by increased intraocular pressure in the setting of a young, pliable sclera.

 MOLECULAR PATHOGENESIS: Several genes for primary congenital glaucoma have been identified. Homozygous mutations in the cytochrome P4501B1 gene (*CYP1B1*) and latent transforming growth factor β-binding protein 2 gene (*LTBP2*) account for some cases of autosomal recessive primary infantile glaucoma. Congenital glaucoma associated with developmental anomalies of the eye (secondary congenital glaucoma) results from mutations in the forkhead transcription factor gene (*FOXC1*), pituitary homeobox 2 gene (*PITX2*), or paired box 6 gene (*PAX6*).

Adult-Onset Primary Glaucoma

Adult-onset primary glaucoma may develop in the absence of any apparent underlying eye disease. It is subdivided into **POAG** (in which the anterior chamber angle is open and appears normal) and **primary closed-angle glaucoma** (in which the anterior chamber is shallower than normal, and the angle is abnormally narrow) (Fig. 33-16).

Primary Open-Angle Glaucoma

POAG is the most frequent type of glaucoma and a major cause of blindness in the United States. It affects 6% of Caucasian and 16% of African-American adults over the age of 40 years in the United States. The angle of the anterior chamber is open and appears normal, but there is increased resistance to the outflow of the aqueous humor in the vicinity of the canal of Schlemm. Intraocular pressure increases insidiously and asymptomatically, and although almost always bilateral, one eye may be affected more severely than the other. With time, damage to the retina and optic nerve causes irreversible loss of vision. The characteristic clinical features include elevated intraocular pressure, cupping of the optic nerve head, and progressive loss of the peripheral visual field. Flame-shaped hemorrhages may be identified occasionally on the optic nerve head.

ETIOLOGIC FACTORS: Ethnicity and age are risk factors for POAG. African-Americans and Hispanics carry a higher risk as well as age over 40 years. Other risk factors include a family history of POAG, thinner than average central corneal thickness, and diabetes mellitus and myopia.

 MOLECULAR PATHOGENESIS: POAG has been mapped to at least 13 loci on chromosomes 1, 2, 3, 5, 6, 7, 8, 9, 10, and 20, and three genes have been identified. Some cases of POAG are due to mutations in the *MYOC* gene on chromosome 1 (1q21-q31). *MYOC* encodes myocilin, a protein in the trabecular meshwork and ciliary body that functions to regulate intraocular pressure. POAG can also occur as a manifestation of the nail–patella syndrome, in association with mutations in the Lim homeobox transcription factor-1 (*LMX1B*) gene. Juvenile-onset POAG may result from mutations in *CYP1B1* (which encodes a cytochrome P450 protein involved in ocular fluid dynamics), *FKHL7* (which makes a forkhead transcription factor involved in eye development), *MYOC*, and *OPTN* (which makes optineurin, a protein that regulates apoptosis and vascular tone).

Primary Angle-Closure Glaucoma

Primary angle-closure glaucoma, differentiated from open-angle glaucoma above, is the predominant form of primary glaucoma in adults living in Asia.

 ETIOLOGIC FACTORS: The disorder afflicts people whose peripheral iris is displaced anteriorly toward the trabecular meshwork, thereby creating an abnormally narrow anterior chamber angle. When the pupil is constricted (miotic), the iris remains stretched so that the chamber angle is not occluded. However, when the pupil dilates (mydriasis), the iris obstructs drainage of aqueous humor from the eye, resulting in sudden episodes of intraocular hypertension. This is accompanied by ocular pain, and halos or rings seen around lights. In this condition, intraocular pressure may also increase if the pupil becomes blocked (e.g., by a swollen lens) and aqueous humor accumulates in the posterior chamber.

 MOLECULAR PATHOGENESIS: Primary angle-closure glaucoma has a familial predisposition, but in contrast to primary open-angle glaucoma, disease alleles have not yet been identified.

CLINICAL FEATURES: *Acute angle-closure glaucoma is an ocular emergency, and ocular hypotensive treatment or laser iridotomy must be implemented within the first 24–48 hours if vision is to be preserved.* Primary angle-closure glaucoma affects both eyes, but it may become apparent in one eye years before it is noted in the other. Intraocular pressure

is normal between attacks, but after many episodes, adhesions form between the iris and the trabecular meshwork and cornea (**peripheral anterior synechiae**) and exacerbate the block to the outflow of aqueous humor.

Low-Tension Glaucoma

In normal-tension (low-tension) glaucoma, the characteristic visual field defect and the ophthalmoscopic features of chronic open-angle glaucoma (cupping of the optic nerve head and occasional optic nerve head hemorrhages) occur, but without increased intraocular pressures over time.

 ETIOLOGIC FACTORS: Although some eyes may be hypersensitive to normal intraocular pressure, many cases of low-tension glaucoma may represent progressive microscopic infarction of the optic nerve head. Susceptibility to normal tension glaucoma is associated with an intronic polymorphism in the *OPA1* gene.

Secondary Glaucoma

In secondary glaucoma, anterior chamber angles may be open or closed. There are numerous causes of secondary glaucoma including inflammation, hemorrhage, neovascularization of the iris, and adhesions. Some of these conditions affect only one eye and others affect both.

Effects of Increased Intraocular Pressure

Prolonged ocular hypertension has several effects on the eye:

■ Selective irreversible loss of retinal ganglion cells occurs first in the retinal periphery, then involving progressively the posterior retina. The macula is the last area to be involved. The nerve fiber layer of the retina becomes thinner as a result.

■ In adults, increased intraocular pressure results in characteristic cupped excavation of the optic nerve head (glaucomatous cupping), accompanied by nasal displacement of the retinal blood vessels. In infants, cupping of the optic nerve head tends to be less prominent.

■ Optic atrophy—with loss of axons, gliosis, and thickening of the pial septa—follows retinal ganglion cell death.

■ When intraocular pressure is increased in a young child, the pliable eyeball sometimes enlarges extensively (buphthalmos). In older children, the more rigid sclera prevents the glaucomatous eyes from enlarging in response to increased pressure.

MYOPIA

Myopia (nearsightedness) is a refractive ocular abnormality in which light from the visualized object focuses at a point in front of the retina because of a longer than usual anteroposterior diameter of the eye or steeper than average corneal curvature. Myopia affects more than 120 million people in the United States and is the most common clinically significant disorder of the eye. Of the US population, 10 million individuals are classified as having high myopia (refractive error of ≥6.0 diopters). In Asia, it affects an even greater percentage of the population. Treatment requires refractive correction.

In addition to glasses and contact lenses, refractive surgery involving lasers such as laser-assisted in situ keratomileusis (LASIK) and laser epithelial keratomileusis (LASEK) is popular. Myopia usually begins in adolescents and varies in severity. A mild form (stationary or simple myopia) is generally nonprogressive after cessation of body growth, whereas a genetically determined "progressive myopia" is more severe. High myopia can be associated with vision loss due to subretinal neovascularization.

  ETIOLOGIC FACTORS AND MOLECULAR PATHOGENESIS: Strong evidence implicates excessive accommodation from reading, use of electronic devices such as phones and tablets, and other near work in childhood in the pathogenesis of myopia. In childhood, the vast majority of eyes with myopia adjust their axial length to the refraction by the anterior segment of the eye (**emmetropization**), and studies in animal models indicate that emmetropization mechanisms elongate the eye. Some nonsyndromic inherited types have been mapped to 14 different loci on various chromosomes. Myopia is also a feature of several systemic diseases, including some disorders of fibrillin (Marfan syndrome), collagen (Stickler syndrome, Knobloch syndrome), and perlecan (Schwartz–Jampel syndrome type 1).

PHTHISIS BULBI

Phthisis bulbi refers to a nonspecific, end-stage eye that is shrunken, disorganized, and atrophic. This condition (Fig. 33-17) is often the result of blindness due to previous trauma,

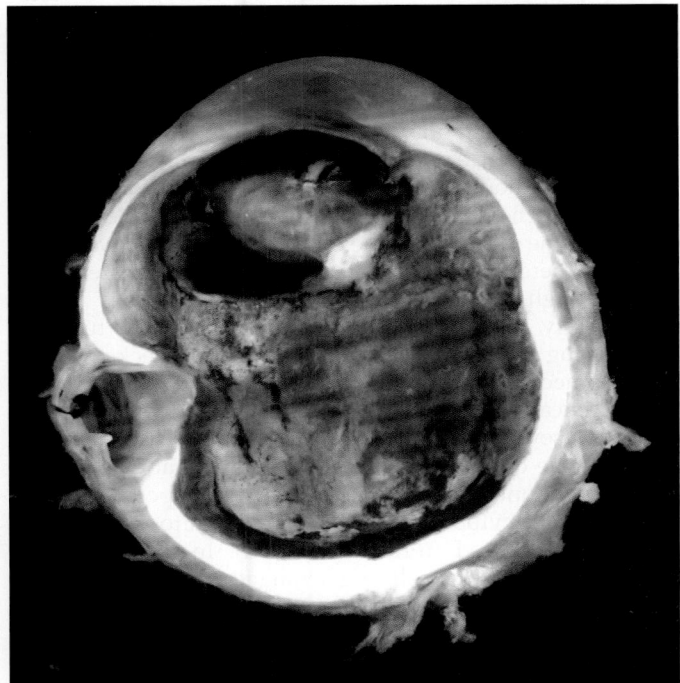

FIGURE 33-17. Phthisis bulbi. Section through an eye with phthisis bulbi shows disorganized and atrophic intraocular tissues. The globe is smaller due to overall shrinkage. Note the thickened posterior sclera due to contraction of the collagen fibers.

chronic retinal detachment, or severe inflammation. Eyes afflicted with phthisis bulbi are often enucleated (surgically removed). The eye is small and often extremely hard owing to intraocular ossification. The choroid and ciliary body are separated from the sclera, which is thickened, wrinkled, and indented owing to loss of intraocular pressure. The cornea is flattened, shrunken, and opaque. Intraocular contents are degenerated and disorganized. Retinal detachment is often present and the lens is displaced and often calcified. A typical finding in phthisis bulbi is intraocular bone formation, which may be derived from metaplasia of the pluripotent pigment epithelium.

OCULAR NEOPLASMS

The eye and adjacent structures contain a large number of cell types from which benign and malignant neoplasms may arise. Intraocular neoplasms are relatively uncommon but may be life threatening. *Intraocular neoplasms arise most commonly from immature retinal neurons (retinoblastoma) and uveal melanocytes (melanoma).* Although the retinal pigment epithelium often undergoes reactive proliferation and metaplasia, it seldom becomes neoplastic.

Intraocular Melanoma Arises From Melanocytes in the Uvea

Melanoma is the most common primary intraocular malignancy in adults. It may arise from melanocytes in any part of the eye, the choroid being the most common site.

 PATHOLOGY: Choroidal melanomas are mostly circumscribed and commonly invade Bruch membrane, causing a mushroom-shaped usually pigmented mass under the retina (Fig. 33-18). By contrast, some tumors are flat (diffuse melanoma) and cause gradual deterioration of vision over many years. Some do not become apparent until extraocular dissemination has occurred. Orange lipofuscin pigment is sometimes evident over the surface of some choroidal melanomas.

Microscopically, uveal melanomas are composed mainly of variable numbers of spindle-shaped cells without nucleoli (spindle A cells), spindle-shaped cells with prominent nucleoli (spindle B cells), polygonal cells with distinct cell borders and prominent nucleoli (epithelioid cells), or a fourth cell type that is similar to epithelioid cells but smaller with indistinct cell borders.

Prognostic factors include histologic cell type, tumor size, tumor location, extrascleral extension of tumor, and the pattern of microvasculature within the tumor. Tumors comprised entirely of spindle cells have a more favorable prognosis when compared to those comprised entirely of epithelioid cells. Most tumors are comprised of a mixture of these cell types with an intermediate survival rate. Unfavorable factors include high mitotic rate, high values for the mean diameter of the 10 largest nucleoli, monosomy of chromosome 3, mutations in the *BAP1* gene (which encodes a deubiquitinase) within the tumor, and class 2 status (high risk of metastasis) on gene expression profiling.

Melanomas of the ciliary body and iris may extend circumferentially around the globe (ring melanoma). Melanomas in the iris are usually diagnosed in younger

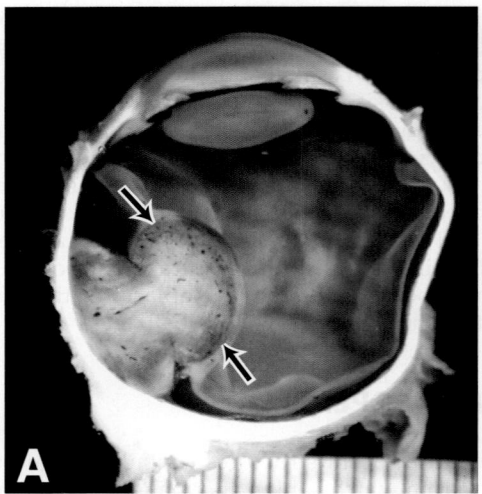
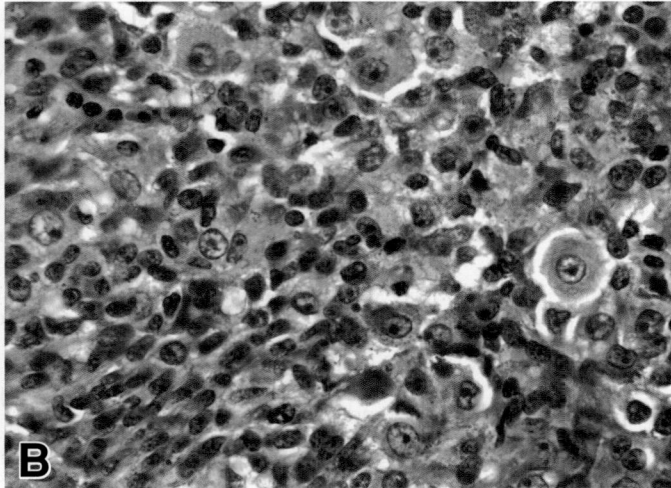

FIGURE 33-18. Choroidal melanoma. A. A lightly pigmented melanoma of the choroid with the typical mushroom shape is present in this eye (*arrows*). Choroidal melanomas commonly invade through the Bruch membrane and result in this appearance. **B.** Photomicrograph of a choroidal melanoma showing both spindle (**lower left**) and epithelioid tumor cells with prominent nucleoli. Cytoplasmic pigment is present in some cells.

adults compared with ciliary body or choroidal tumors, perhaps because they are more easily seen and are often first observed by the patient.

Spread of uveal melanomas outside of the eye occurs via direct extension through the sclera or hematogenously. Lymphatic spread does not occur because the eye has no lymphatic vessels. Uveal melanomas have a predilection for metastasizing to the liver before spreading to other sites.

CLINICAL FEATURES: Intraocular melanomas may cause cataract, glaucoma, retinal detachment, inflammation, and hemorrhage. Treatment options for uveal melanomas include enucleation of the eye, radioactive brachytherapy and, occasionally, local excision. There is an overall 20% mortality rate from ciliary body and choroidal melanomas (posterior uveal melanoma) at 5 years. Iris melanomas metastasize in less than 5% of cases and, for that reason, are categorized and staged separately from posterior melanomas.

Retinoblastomas Originate From Immature Retinal Cells

Retinoblastoma is the most common intraocular malignant neoplasm of childhood, occurring in 1 in 14,000 to 1 in 20,000 live births. It occurs most frequently within the first 2 years of life and may even be found at birth. Most retinoblastomas occur sporadically and are unilateral. Some 6% to 8% of retinoblastomas are familial and bilateral. Up to 25% of cases that arise in the absence of a family history represent new germline mutations and are also bilateral.

MOLECULAR PATHOGENESIS: Nearly all retinoblastomas are related to inherited or acquired deletions of, or mutations in, the retinoblastoma (*RB1*) tumor suppressor gene, located on the long arm of chromosome 13 (13q14) (see Chapter 6). Some patients have

homologous genomic mutations in *RB1* Others have a single genomic mutation and tumors arise when retinal cells develop a mutation in the second allele. Recently, a form of retinoblastoma without mutations in *RB1* has been described. These tumors demonstrate amplification of the *MYCN* gene, a member of the Myc family of oncogenes. Tumors due to *MYCN* amplification are typically unilateral, tend to present at an earlier age, and are more invasive.

PATHOLOGY: Some retinoblastomas grow toward the vitreous body and can be seen with an ophthalmoscope (**endophytic retinoblastoma**). Others extend between the sensory retina and the retinal pigment epithelium, thereby detaching the retina (**exophytic retinoblastoma**). Some retinoblastomas are both endophytic and exophytic. Rarely, a retinoblastoma spreads diffusely within the retina without forming an obvious mass (**diffuse retinoblastoma**). The retina often contains several distinct foci of tumor in the same eye, some of which represent multifocal origin, whereas others are tumor implants from dissemination through the vitreous body.

Grossly, retinoblastomas are cream-colored tumors containing scattered, chalky white, calcified flecks within yellow necrotic zones (Fig. 33-19), that may be detected radiologically. The tumors are intensely cellular and display several morphologic patterns. Most demonstrate some degree of necrosis. In many tumors, densely packed, round neoplastic cells with hyperchromatic nuclei, scant cytoplasm, and abundant mitoses are randomly distributed (**undifferentiated**). In differentiated retinoblastomas, the cells are arranged radially around a central tangle of neurofibrillary material (**Homer Wright rosettes**) or around a central lumen (**Flexner–Wintersteiner rosettes**), as they differentiate toward photoreceptors. In some cases, the cellular arrangement resembles a fleur-de-lis (**fleurette**). Viable tumor cells align themselves around blood vessels, and necrotic areas with calcification are seen a short distance from the vascularized regions.

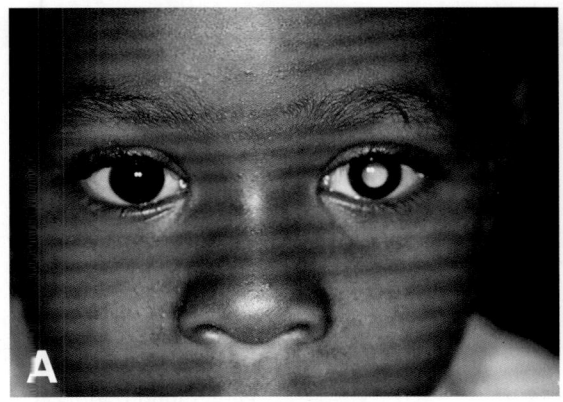

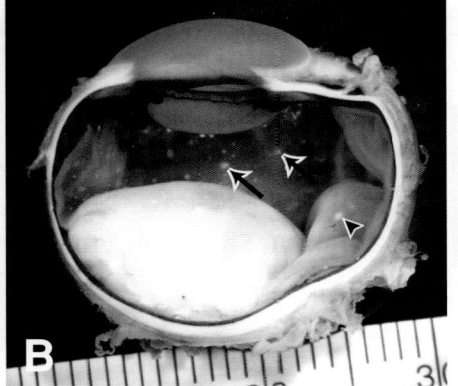

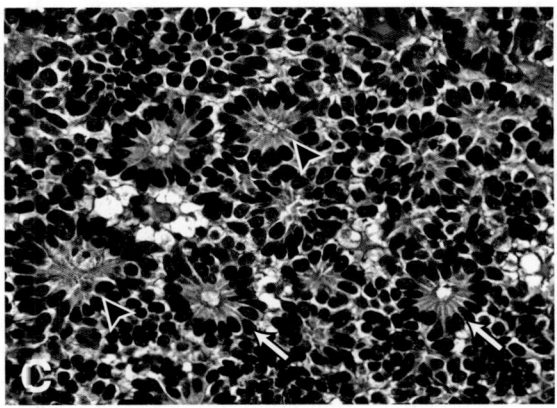

FIGURE 33-19. Retinoblastoma. A. The *white* pupil (leukocoria) in the left eye is the result of an intraocular retinoblastoma. **B.** This surgically enucleated eye demonstrates a white- to cream-colored mass with calcified flecks. Frequent vitreous seeds (*arrows*) and occasional subretinal seeds are present (*arrowhead*). **C.** Light microscopic view of a retinoblastoma showing a differentiated area with Homer Wright rosettes with a central eosinophilic fibrillary tangle (*arrowheads*) and Flexner–Wintersteiner rosettes (*arrows*) with cells arranged around a central clear lumen. Flexner–Wintersteiner rosettes demonstrate photoreceptor differentiation.

The most important histologic prognostic factors are invasion of the optic nerve and massive choroidal invasion. In an enucleation specimen for retinoblastoma, the cut end of the optic nerve is a surgical margin. If tumor is present at this surgical margin, prognosis for survival is significantly decreased. If tumor is present between the surgical margin and the lamina cribrosa, the prognosis is somewhat better. The prognosis is even more favorable if tumor is present in the optic nerve only anterior to the lamina cribrosa. The best prognosis is associated with no invasion of the optic nerve. Massive choroidal invasion refers to a tumor mass in the choroid that is at least 3 mm in greatest dimension. This is also an important factor in predicting prognosis and may dictate the therapeutic regimen for the patient. Invasion of tumor through the sclera into the orbit also portends a poor prognosis.

Retinoblastomas disseminate by several routes. They can invade the optic nerve and extend into the intracranial central nervous system. They also invade blood vessels, especially in the highly vascular choroid, before metastasizing hematogenously throughout the body. Bone marrow is a common site of blood-borne metastases, but surprisingly, the lung is rarely involved. Due to the absence of a lymphatic supply to the eye, retinoblastomas do not spread to lymph nodes of the head and neck.

 CLINICAL FEATURES: Presenting signs include a white pupil (leukocoria), strabismus, poor vision, and spontaneous hyphema or a red, painful eye.

Secondary glaucoma is a frequent complication. Light entering the eye commonly reflects a yellowish color similar to that from the tapetum of a cat (cat's eye reflex).

Retinoblastomas are almost always fatal if left untreated. However, with early diagnosis and modern therapy, survival is high (about 95%). Rarely, spontaneous regression occurs for reasons that remain unknown. Patients with bilateral retinoblastomas due to a germline mutation, presumably as a consequence of the loss of *RB1* gene function, show increased susceptibility to other malignant tumors later in life, including osteogenic sarcoma, leiomyosarcoma, and Ewing sarcoma. Approximately 5% of patients with the germline *RB1* mutation can have an ectopic focus of primitive neuroectodermal tumor of the pineal gland (the so-called trilateral retinoblastoma). These patients have a higher mortality rate compared to patients with bilateral ocular tumors but without pineal tumors.

Metastatic Tumors to the Eye Are More Common Than Primary Ocular Neoplasms

Sometimes an ocular metastasis may be the initial clinical manifestation of a cancer, but most cases are diagnosed only after death. Leukemias and cancers of the breast and lung usually metastasize to the uveal tract and account for most cases of intraocular metastases. Neuroblastoma frequently metastasizes to the orbit in infancy and childhood. The orbit may be invaded by malignant neoplasms of the eyelid, conjunctiva, paranasal sinuses, nose, nasopharynx, and intracranial cavity.

THE EYE

34 Forensic Pathology

Barbara A. Sampson, Jennifer L. Hammers

WHAT IS FORENSIC PATHOLOGY?

Forensic pathology focuses on investigations of deaths that occur from sudden, unexpected, or unnatural causes. Multiple steps are required to investigate these deaths and ensure accurate and complete determination of the cause and the manner of death. To practice as a forensic pathologist, a medical school graduate must first successfully complete training in anatomic pathology, with or without clinical pathology, or in a combined anatomic and neuropathology residency/fellowship. The resident must then successfully complete a fellowship in forensic pathology. Graduates of a forensic pathology fellowship may become certified by the American Board of Pathology.

CORONER AND MEDICAL EXAMINER SYSTEMS

Two Common Systems Investigate Deaths in the United States

The forensic pathologist serves different roles depending on the local system. Coroners and medical examiners are both responsible for investigating and determining the cause and manner of death for people who die within their jurisdiction. A coroner is an elected position. Coroners campaign, run for election, and are voted into office by local constituents. A coroner is not required to be a forensic pathologist or even a physician. Commonly, coroners have experience working in law enforcement or in the funeral industry. Because coroners are not forensic pathologists, they must hire physicians to perform autopsies. In this role, forensic pathologists serve as consultants to coroners, performing autopsies and documenting findings identified at autopsy, but the forensic pathologist is not responsible for the investigation of death or completion of the death certificate. By contrast, a

medical examiner system is led by a chief medical examiner who is responsible for death investigations and for performing autopsies and completing death certificates for people who die in their communities. The chief medical examiner is a forensic pathologist appointed by a local governmental authority to run the office and hire other medical examiners. The number of medical examiners in an office depends on the number of deaths investigated each year. Medical examiner systems are more common in large cities or states that have a single death investigation system. Coroner systems are more common in rural counties and counties with smaller populations.

Forensic Death Investigations Serve Many Purposes

These include specific medical, investigative, and lay population needs. While the ultimate product of a death investigation, the death certificate, is necessary for burial or cremation of a body, the purpose of the death certificate and forensic death investigation is to generate information to maintain and improve public health. The forensic death investigation ensures that accurate and complete information is included on the death certificate.

Public Health

Among the most important purposes of death investigation systems are to identify risks to public health and improve the health of the community. Forensic death investigations ascertain disease processes that may be rapidly transmitted to others. This helps to implement treatment plans to prevent further death and illness. Likewise, forensic death investigations document preventable injuries and prompt changes to protect others in society from suffering from the same or similar circumstances. Tracking deaths allows for identification of trends over short intervals and over many years. Using such data, federal and state agencies can target funds for preventative measures and treatment efforts to populations that will most benefit. The goal is to improve public health by preventing disease and injury and improving quality of life.

Investigation of Death

The cause and manner of death are determined only after the forensic death investigation has been completed. Such investigations involve several steps. Gathering information about the circumstances of death along with the past family, social, and medical history of the decedent is common to all forensic death investigations. This information may reveal that a decedent died of natural causes in which case the medical examiner/coroner need not be involved in determining cause of death. Rather, the decedent's treating physician is responsible for completion of the death certificate. The manner of death for such decedents is *Natural*. An autopsy is not legally required, and if one is desired by the family or the treating physician, it can only be performed with consent of the legal next of kin. Treating physicians must, therefore, know if autopsies are performed at their institutions and they must be familiar with rules regarding consent. They must also be prepared to discuss the autopsy process with a grieving family. Alternatively, the next of kin may elect to have an autopsy performed privately by a forensic pathologist, once the body has been released from the hospital.

If initial steps of the forensic death investigation reveal that the manner of death is anything other than natural, the coroner/medical examiner is responsible for determining the cause and manner of death and also has the legal responsibility to determine if an autopsy is necessary. The coroner/medical examiner takes jurisdiction over the death and proceeds with additional steps in the death investigation including examination of the body and, possibly, performing an autopsy. A visit to the location of death may be necessary, either while the body is still there or after it has been transferred to the coroner/medical examiner's office. Family members and friends may be interviewed and further investigation may be undertaken based on such interviews. The coroner/medical examiner has the authority to determine if an external examination alone is sufficient or if an autopsy is required. Factors considered in the decision to autopsy vary widely among jurisdictions. Importantly, by accepting jurisdiction over a death, the medical examiner/ coroner is not obligated to perform an autopsy. If an autopsy is performed, however, the organs are examined grossly and microscopically, and often toxicology studies are performed to help identify factors contributing to death. Other types of special studies may be performed, depending on the nature of the death, including microbiologic, genetic, and metabolic tests. Forensic death investigations and forensic autopsies require medical training, knowledge and skill, similar to taking a complete history and performing a complete physical. The forensic death investigation is equivalent to performing a thorough history and the external examination of the body and autopsy are equivalent to performing a thorough physical examination.

External Examination and Autopsy

External examination of a body may be performed without an autopsy, or it may be followed by an autopsy. As a critical part of the forensic death investigation, careful external examination is required to ensure that a death requiring autopsy is not overlooked. Just as a physician would not perform a physical examination on a fully dressed patient, external examination requires removal of clothing and obscuring objects from the decedent. External findings may be subtle. A careful and knowledgeable review is necessary to ensure that clues as to the cause and manner of death are not overlooked. External examination also aids in identifying the decedent by documenting features such as height and weight, eye and hair color, scars, and tattoos. It also documents remote and recent injuries, and evidence of previous or recent medical treatment. Analysis of changes in the skin surfaces can provide important clues to undiagnosed medical conditions or lend support to reported histories of disease processes.

Determination of Cause and Manner of Death

Cause and manner of death are statements that provide information about the reason someone died and the circumstances under which he or she died. The *cause of death statement* explains the disease process or injury that led to a person's demise. The cause of death statement begins with the immediate cause of death and ends with the underlying cause of death, with connecting statements as required. Each step in the cause of death statement can be thought of as a link in a chain, and all links must connect to one another if they are to be included in the cause of death. The *immediate cause of death* is the injury or disease process that caused someone to die at the very moment of expiration. The *underlying cause of death* is an injury or disease process that began the chain of events that ultimately led to the immediate cause of death. If these cannot be linked, then the underlying cause of death must be reconsidered. When formulating the cause of death statement, it is customary to begin with the immediate cause of death and follow with one or more statements. Thus, an example of a complete cause of death statement is: *Upper gastrointestinal bleed due to ruptured esophageal varices due to hepatic cirrhosis due to chronic alcoholism*. Occasionally the cause of death statement may be simple, for example, *hypertensive and atherosclerotic cardiovascular disease*. The specific physiologic change(s) occurring at the moment of death, known as the mechanism of death, need not be included on the death certificate. Examples of mechanisms of death include hypovolemic shock, cardiac arrhythmia, and sepsis.

The *manner of death* explains how the death occurred. In most jurisdictions, deaths are categorized as *natural* (due entirely to natural diseases processes) or, if not natural, then they are categorized as violent deaths (*homicide, suicide,* or *accident*). In some circumstances, there may be insufficient information to determine the manner of death, in which case it is *undetermined*. For example, in a patient with a fatal subdural hematoma, it might be impossible to determine if death was caused by an intentional blow to the head by another person (homicide) or by a fall (accident). Deaths caused by known complications of medical therapy, such as fatal infections or malignancies occurring in solid-organ transplant patients, are considered *natural*. However, deaths due to malfunctioning of medical devices are considered *accidental*. When a combination of natural and non-natural causes occurs, more weight is usually given to the non-natural factors. For example, a death due to heart disease in a person intoxicated by cocaine would be ruled an accident due to acute substance abuse, with heart disease as a contributing factor.

Court Testimony

Medical examiners and coroners often testify in court to the circumstances of death, autopsy findings, and cause and manner of death. Such testimony is required in criminal cases involving deaths from homicide and occasionally from accidents such as motor vehicle accidents. Some deaths investigated by the medical examiner/coroner may require civil court testimony or, more commonly, a deposition. Depositions in civil proceedings often deal with deaths occurring during or around the time of medical treatment.

NATURAL DEATH

Sudden unexpected deaths from natural causes comprise approximately half of all deaths in which the medical examiner/coroner accepts jurisdiction. The most common causes are cardiovascular diseases and processes related to obesity and diabetes.

Hypertensive and Atherosclerotic Cardiovascular Disease

Nontraumatic sudden deaths in apparently healthy adults under the age of 50 years are relatively common. They typically occur in individuals with a clinical history of coronary artery atherosclerosis but also occur in asymptomatic people with undiagnosed coronary artery disease or hypertension. Forensic pathologists commonly identify the anatomic hallmarks of atherosclerosis and hypertension in sudden death victims despite previous treatment with stents or antihypertensive medications. A negative stress test or previous medical therapy does not eliminate the risk of sudden death.

Obesity

This is an important public health concern not only because of the direct impact that excessive weight places on the body, but also because of associated disease processes, such as diabetes, hypertension, and sleep apnea. Morbidly obese decedents (BMI >40) typically show generalized organomegaly at autopsy but often, no specific immediate cause of death can be identified. It is concluded that death resulted from the long-term effects on the body, particularly the heart, from morbid obesity. Associated disease processes, both previously diagnosed and undiagnosed, that may contribute to death include diabetes mellitus and pulmonary thromboembolism from a deep vein thrombosis of the lower extremity.

Diabetes Mellitus

Diabetes is a major risk factor in various disease processes that may contribute to the cause of death. Renal changes are frequently identified and undiagnosed infectious complications are occasionally identified at autopsy. Morbidly obese decedents may die suddenly from ketoacidosis. Hyperglycemia and ketones/acetone identified in vitreous fluid and blood provide a specific determination of the immediate

cause of death or an important contributing factor to death. Evaluation of glucose levels and detection of ketones/acetone may also be helpful in investigating death in a child, teenager, or young adult when an obvious cause of death is not apparent at autopsy, as antemortem diagnosis of diabetes mellitus is occasionally not made in this population.

Other Factors in Natural Deaths

Tobacco

Tobacco use is a significant contributing factor in many deaths. It promotes coronary artery disease and hypertension and leads to respiratory compromise including chronic obstructive pulmonary disease, in addition to the known association with cancer.

Chronic Substance Abuse

Consumption of alcohol and illicit substances, and misuse of prescription medications can lead to a multitude of chronic medical problems. Complications associated with fatty liver (hepatic steatosis) and hepatic fibrosis and cirrhosis often contribute to premature death. Alcohol is cardiotoxic and dilated cardiomyopathy is commonly found at autopsy in this population. Intravenous injection of illicit substances or crushed pills may lead to cutaneous infections or infective endocarditis causing death. Infectious diseases such as hepatitis and HIV/AIDS spread by sharing of needles have long-term medical consequences and often contribute to death. Injection of crushed medications may cause respiratory complications when starch crystals in pills and tablets become trapped in the small vessels of the lungs.

Infectious Diseases

Deaths related to infections, particularly pneumonia, occur commonly in people with heart disease, diabetes, and obesity. Left untreated, infections that may be easily identified and treated can quickly become significant and difficult to treat, and may go unrecognized because symptoms can overlap with the symptoms of the underlying disease.

NON-NATURAL DEATH

Any death not solely the result of a natural cause must be categorized as a non-natural death. All of these deaths should be investigated by the medical examiner/coroner who has the legal authority and responsibility to undertake the investigation and complete the death certificate. Non-natural deaths can result from many types of injuries but they occur most commonly from a few broad categories of injury.

Blunt Force Trauma

Blunt force trauma occurs when a hard object strikes the body (or the body strikes a hard object), or when a large force is applied to the body though an acceleration or deceleration force. It results in four types of injury: abrasions, or scrapes to the skin; contusions, or bruises to the skin and internal tissues; lacerations, or tears to the skin or internal tissues; and fractures, or breaks to the bone. Such injuries occur when crushing, tearing, and/or shearing forces are applied to the body. In the clinical setting laceration is often used interchangeably with incision, but an incision results from a sharp object moving across the skin causing a clean cut, whereas a laceration produces a torn and ragged wound. Common causes of blunt force trauma include motor vehicle crashes, falls from standing or from a height, and strikes to the body with a hard object. The age of a blunt force injury can be estimated to some extent, but one must be cautious as many factors can affect healing rate and the visual appearance at different stages of healing. Microscopic examination of the wound may narrow the time frame but cannot provide definitive information. Nevertheless, careful gross and microscopic examination may support or refute a reported or suspected time frame in which an injury occurred.

Penetrating Trauma

Penetrating trauma is produced by gunshot wounds and sharp force injuries. This type of trauma often causes much more extensive internal injuries than what might be suggested by the amount of damage seen on the skin surface. Gunshot and stab wounds are the most common penetrating injuries, but any object that can pierce the skin and soft

tissues can cause injuries. A gunshot wound may penetrate or perforate the body. Penetrating gunshot wounds enter the body and then stop, or lodge without exiting. Perforating gunshot wounds enter the body, travel through the body, and exit the body. X-rays of the body are often needed to identify the path the bullet traveled, the organs injured by the bullet, and the extent of the injuries. Various features on the surface of the skin help distinguish gunshot entrance and exit wounds (Fig. 34-1 and Table 34-1). At autopsy, the path the bullet traveled must be determined and internal injuries must be documented. The caliber of a bullet cannot be determined by measuring the wound on the skin surface or by measurements from x-ray images.

A wound produced when a sharp object such as a knife penetrates the body is described as a stab wound. By contrast, a superficial wound from a sharp object is called an incised wound (a cut to the skin), and it does not penetrate the body. Stab wounds rarely enter and exit the body. The shape of the wound on the skin surface and the path of the stab wound in the body provide information about the sharp object that caused injury. Such features are shown in Figure 34-2. It is customary to describe the location of gunshot wounds and stab wounds in relation to other parts of the body, for example, indicating specific distances "below

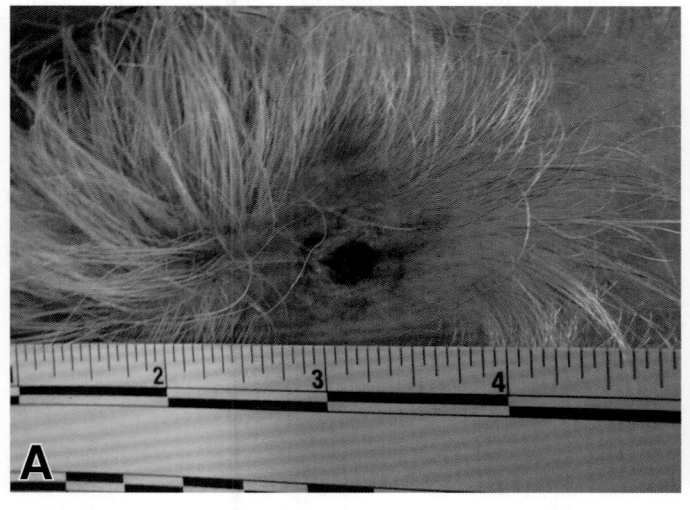
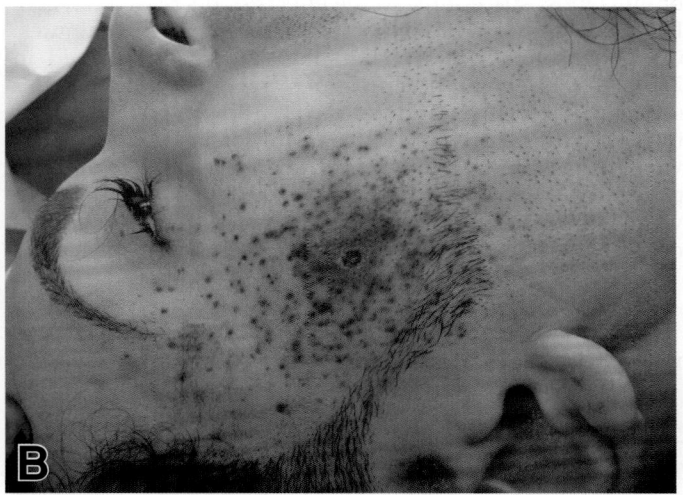
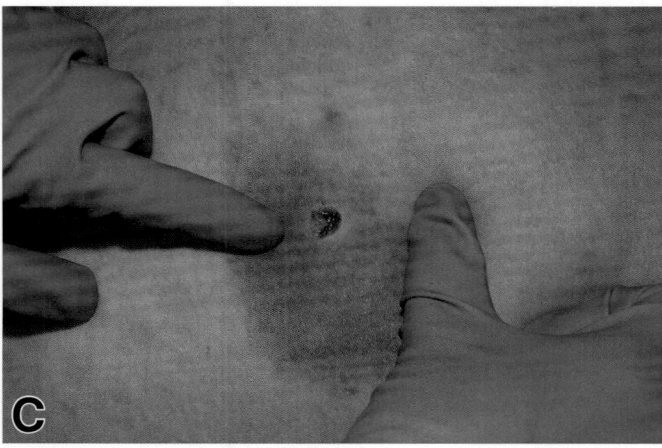
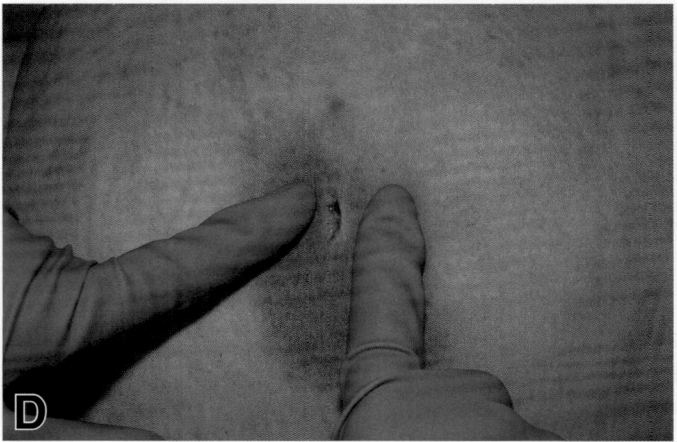

FIGURE 34-1. Gunshot wounds. A. A contact entrance wound of the scalp showing a ring of searing around the entrance due to contact of the gun with the scalp. **B.** Stippling around an entrance wound on the face from a gun fired close to the skin surface. **C,D.** An exit wound surrounded by subcutaneous hemorrhage, with reapproximation of wound edges with manipulation.

TABLE 34-1
FEATURES OF GUNSHOT ENTRANCE AND EXIT WOUNDS

Entrance	Exit
Circular to oval punched out defect	Slit-like wound
Rim of abrasion, symmetric or asymmetric	No rim of abrasion, soot or stippling around wound
Edges cannot be reapproximated	Edges can be reapproximated
Soot or stippling around wound, possible	

TABLE 34-2
CAUSES OF ASPHYXIA

Hanging
Strangulation (ligature or manual)
Smothering (covering of nose and mouth)
Environmental (e.g., carbon monoxide, hydrogen sulfide)
Compression of chest
Drowning

the top of the head," "above the heel," or "left or right of the midline," or as a measured distance from relatively fixed anatomic landmarks such as the umbilicus, nipple, or external auditory meatus.

Asphyxia

Asphyxia causes death when sufficient oxygen cannot enter the body or reach vital organs for a prolonged interval. The brain is most susceptible to the effects of decreased oxygen. Dizziness and loss of consciousness occur within minutes. Common settings in which asphyxia occurs are listed in Table 34-2. Brief temporary loss of oxygen may cause unconsciousness, but restoration of oxygen flow typically results in no long-term adverse outcomes. More prolonged intervals increase the likelihood of irreversible damage and the possibility that death will occur. Asphyxia can occur without visible injury to the body, making detailed evaluation of the death scene particularly important. Occasionally substances

in the air, such as carbon monoxide, can replace oxygen and lead to death.

Environmental Exposure

Environmental exposure to extreme temperatures, both heat and cold, may lead to death. Autopsy findings are often subtle and nonspecific, or absent entirely. A forensic death investigation focused on environmental conditions, the decedent's activities and reported symptoms before death, and the location where the decedent was found, are all critical in identifying the role of environmental exposure in causing such deaths.

Intoxication

Death from acute intoxication occurs when the level of one or more substances achieves a sufficiently toxic limit or when the drug exerts secondary effects on the body that cause death. For

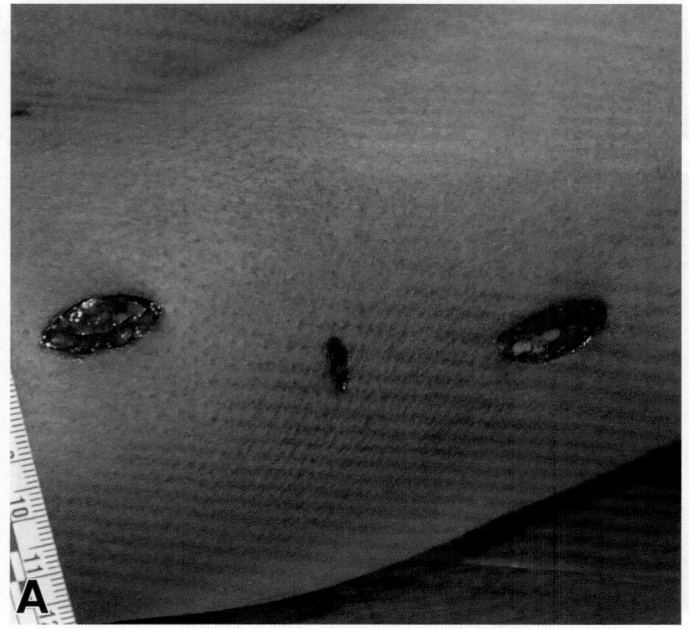

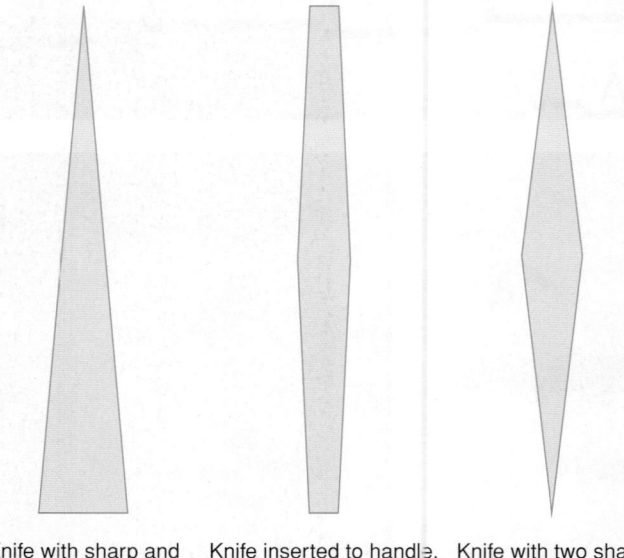

Knife with sharp and blunt edges, kitchen knife

Knife inserted to handle, cannot determine sharp and blunt edges

Knife with two sharp edges, dagger

FIGURE 34-2. Stab wounds. A. The wound features are distorted by lines of tension within the skin, masking the features of the knife. Releasing the tension aids in identification of the type of knife blade that caused the injury. **B.** Different shapes of stab wounds caused by different types of knives.

TABLE 34-3

INFORMATION REQUIRED IN REPORTING A DEATH TO THE MEDICAL EXAMINER/CORONER

Basic demographic information about the decedent:

Name

Date of birth and age

Ethnicity

Address

Date of admission (if applicable)

Date and time of death

Next of Kin Information:

Name

Relationship to decedent

Address

Contact phone numbers

Has the next of kin been notified of death?

Is the next of kin aware that decedent may come to the medical examiner/coroner?

Medical Information:

How the decedent came to the hospital

Reports from EMS or family concerning circumstances that brought decedent to hospital

Past medical, social, and family history

Findings upon physical examination

Differential diagnosis

Laboratory and radiology testing performed and results

Treatment diagnosis

Complications of treatment

Circumstances of death

Presumptive cause of death

example, the stimulant effects of cocaine can cause an abrupt surge in blood pressure which, in turn, can cause fatal aortic dissection. Deaths resulting from the direct effects of an acute intoxication or from complications resulting from the intoxication are non-natural deaths and should be investigated by the coroner/medical examiner. If blood or urine was obtained at the time of arrival to the hospital or shortly thereafter, the coroner/medical examiner can test these samples for various intoxicants. Preserving these samples is useful, particularly if the patient was maintained on life support before death, as intoxicants could be metabolized and/or eliminated from the body during this time. Discarding such samples may preclude identification of specific intoxicants responsible for death and thus directly impact public health efforts to curtail overdoses and deaths from intoxication. Drugs or paraphernalia identified on the patient at presentation should be turned over to local investigative authorities.

REPORTING A DEATH TO THE MEDICAL EXAMINER/CORONER

Treating physicians should be familiar with local statutes and requirements for reporting sudden, unexpected, or non-natural deaths, as they may vary among jurisdictions. For example, some jurisdictions require that any death occurring in the hospital within 24 hours of admission be reported. To facilitate effective and timely decisions by the medical examiner/coroner, the reporting physician should have basic demographic information about the decedent, contact information for next of kin, and information about clinical presentation, medical treatment, and circumstances of death (Table 34-3). Such information should be reported in much the same way that a physician would present a new case to a colleague or when transferring care responsibilities at the end of a shift. Reporting physicians must be prepared to address additional questions from the forensic investigator who is responsible for making a decision about accepting jurisdiction.

Note: Page numbers followed by f and t indicates figure and table respectively.